CONTENTS IN BRIEF

11TH EDITION

WONG'S Nursing Care of Infants and Children

MARILYN J. HOCKENBERRY, PhD, RN, PPCNP-BC, FAAN
Bessie Baker Professor of Nursing and Professor of Pediatrics
Associate Dean of Research Affairs, School of Nursing
Chair, Duke Institutional Review Board
Duke University
Durham, North Carolina

DAVID WILSON, MS, RNC-NIC (deceased)
Staff
Children's Hospital at Saint Francis
Tulsa, Oklahoma

CHERYL C. RODGERS, PhD, RN, CPNP, CPON (deceased)
Associate Professor
Chair, Duke Institutional Review Board
Duke University School of Nursing
Durham, North Carolina

ELSEVIER

ELSEVIER

3251 Riverport Lane
St. Louis, Missouri 63043

WONG'S NURSING CARE OF INFANTS AND CHILDREN, ELEVENTH EDITION

ISBN: 978-0-323-54939-4

Notices

Practitioners and researchers must always rely on their own experience and knowledge in evaluating and using any information, methods, compounds or experiments described herein. Because of rapid advances in the medical sciences, in particular, independent verification of diagnoses and drug dosages should be made. To the fullest extent of the law, no responsibility is assumed by Elsevier, authors, editors or contributors for any injury and/or damage to persons or property as a matter of products liability, negligence or otherwise, or from any use or operation of any methods, products, instructions, or ideas contained in the material herein.

Library of Congress Control Number: 2018941061

Senior Content Strategist: Sandra Clark
Senior Content Development Specialist: Heather Bays
Publishing Services Manager: Julie Eddy
Senior Project Manager: Tracey Schriefer
Design Direction: Renee Duenow

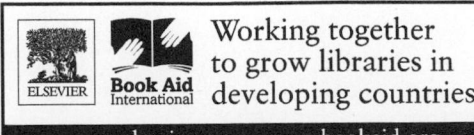

Printed in the United States of America
Last digit is the print number: 9 8 7 6 5 4

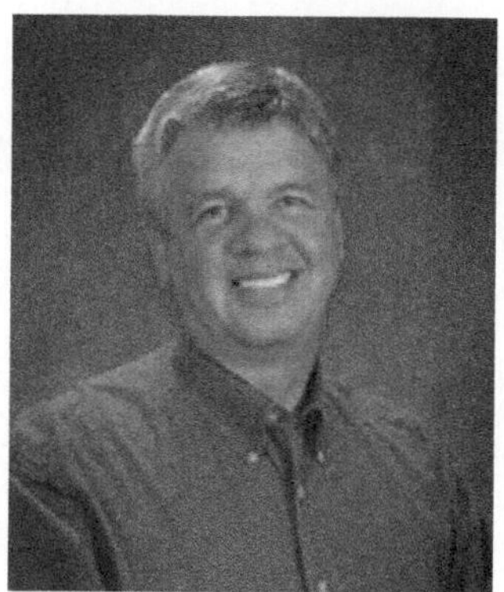

We dedicate the eleventh edition of this book to David Wilson, who passed away on March 7, 2015, after a long battle with cancer. David had been coauthor of the Wong nursing textbooks for over 15 years. He was known as an expert clinical nurse and nurse educator. His last clinical position was at St. Francis Health Services in Tulsa, Oklahoma, where he worked in the Children's Day Hospital as the coordinator for Pediatric Advanced Life Support (PALS). Students and faculty have recognized David's contributions to the Wong textbooks for many years. He was known as an outstanding educator and supporter of nursing students; his attention to clinical excellence was evident in all his work. Those who contributed to the books and had the opportunity to work with David realize the important role he played as a leader in nursing education for students and faculty. His clinical expertise provided a critical foundation for ensuring that relevant and evidence-based content was used in all the Wong textbooks. David led by example in exemplifying excellence in clinical nursing practice.

Those who knew David well will miss his humor, loyalty to friends and colleagues, and his never-ending support. He is missed greatly by those who worked closely with him on the Wong textbook over the years. Most important, we miss his friendship; he was always there to support and to encourage. We have lost an amazing nurse who worked effortlessly over the years to improve the care of children and families in need. David will not be forgotten.

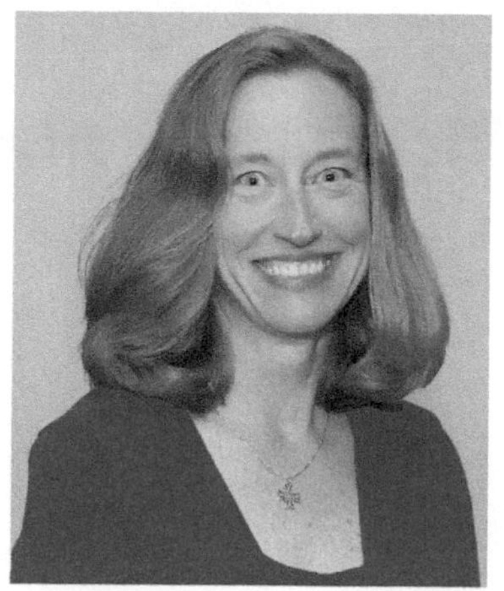

It is with great sadness that we announce the passing of Dr. Cheryl Rodgers on July 7th, 2018, following a tragic accident. Cheryl was an exemplary nurse practitioner, educator, and leader in the field of pediatric nursing. Cheryl was an Associate Professor in the Duke University School of Nursing, and she held national leadership positions in the Children's Oncology Group Nursing Discipline and the Association of Pediatric Hematology Nurses. She served on the Journal of Pediatric Oncology Nursing Editorial Board, led several funded research studies, authored numerous impactful publications, and had just been selected for induction as a Fellow in the American Academy of Nursing, the profession's highest honor. Her devotion to pediatric nursing education served her well as a Wong textbook editor and she will be greatly missed. Most importantly, Cheryl was an outstanding role model and treasured mentor to so many pediatric nurses; her loss will be felt broadly and deeply throughout the profession.

CONTRIBUTORS

Caroline E. Anderson, RN, MSN, CPHON
Clinical Practice and Advanced Education Specialist
Cook Children's Medical Center
Fort Worth, Texas

Annette L. Baker, RN, BSN, MSN, CPNP
Pediatric Nurse Practitioner
Department of Cardiology
Boston Children's Hospital
Boston, Massachusetts

Rose Ann Urdiales Baker, PhD, PMHCNS, RN
Associate Instructor
School of Nursing
College of Health Professions
University of Akron
Akron, Ohio

Raymond C. Barfield, MD, PhD
Professor of Pediatrics and Christian Philosophy; Director, Medical Humanities Pediatrics, and Trent Center for Bioethics, Humanities, and History of Medicine
Duke University
Durham, North Carolina

Amy Barry, MSN, RN, PNP-BC
Pediatric Nurse Practitioner
Children's Healthcare of Atlanta
Atlanta, Georgia

Heather Bastardi, RN, cPNP, CCTC
Pediatric Nurse Practitioner
Advanced Cardiac Therapies
Boston Children's Hospital
Boston, Massachusetts

Debra Brandon, PhD, RN, CNS, FAAN
Associate Professor
School of Nursing
Duke University
Associate Professor
Department of Pediatrics, School of Medicine
Duke University
Neonatal CNS
Duke Intensive Care Nursery
Durham, North Carolina

Rosalind Bryant, PhD, RN-CS, PNP
Clinical Instructor
Baylor College of Medicine
Houston, Texas

Cynthia J. Camille, MSN, RN, CPNP, FNP-BC
Pediatric Nurse Practitioner
Pediatric Urology
Duke University Health System
Durham, North Carolina

Brigit M. Carter, PhD, RN, CCRN
Director
Accelerated BSN Program
Duke University School of Nursing
Durham, North Carolina

Lisa M. Cleveland, PhD, RN, PNP-BC, IBCLC, NTMNC
Assistant Professor
School of Nursing
UT Health San Antonio
San Antonio, Texas

Patricia Conlon, MS, APRN, CNS, CNP
Pediatric Clinical Nurse Specialist
Assistant Professor of Nursing
Mayo Clinic Children's Center
Rochester, Minnesota

Erin Connelly, APRN, CPNP, CPON
Developmental Therapeutics Nurse Practitioner
Department of Hematology
Children's Healthcare of Atlanta
Clinical Manager of Advance Practice
Department of Oncology
Aflac Cancer and Blood Disorders Center
Atlanta, Georgia

Anne Derouin, DNP, APRN, CPNP, FAANP
Associate Professor, Faculty Lead, MSN/PNP-PC and Pediatric Behavioral Mental Health Specialty
School of Nursing
Duke University
Durham, North Carolina

Sharron L. Docherty, PhD, PNP-BC, FAAN
Associate Professor
Department of Pediatrics
Duke University
Durham, North Carolina

Angela Drummond, MS, APRN, CPNP
Pediatric Nurse Practitioner–Orthopedics
Gillette Children's Specialty Healthcare
St. Paul, Minnesota

Elizabeth A. Duffy, DNP, RN, CPNP
Clinical Assistant Professor
Health Behavior and Biological Sciences
The University of Michigan School of Nursing
Ann Arbor, Michigan

Kimberley Fisher, PhD, FNP-BC
Research Director
Neonatal Perinatal Research Unit
Division of Neonatology
Duke University
Durham, North Carolina

Jan M. Foote, DNP, CPNP, ARNP, FAANP
Pediatric Nurse Practitioner
Blank Children's Hospital
Des Moines, Iowa
Adjunct Clinical Associate Professor
University of Iowa College of Nursing
Iowa City, Iowa

Quinn Franklin, MS, CCLS
Assistant Director
Psychosocial Division
Cancer and Hematology Centers
Texas Children's Hospital
Houston, Texas

Ruth Anne Herring, MSN, RN, CPNP-AC/PC, CPHON
Pediatric Nurse Practitioner
Center for Cancer and Blood Disorders
Children's Health
Dallas, Texas

Mystii Kidd, MSN, RN, CPNP
Pediatric Nurse Practitioner
TLC Pediatrics, PA
Allen, Texas

Teri A. Huddleston Lavenbarg, MSN, APRN, PPCNP-BC, FNP-BC, CDE
Nurse Practitioner
Medical Center
University of Kansas
Kansas City, Kansas

Shirley D. Martin, PhD, RN, CPN
Outpatient Surgery
Cook Children's Medical Center
Fort Worth, Texas

Maggie Maxtin, RN, BSN, CPN
Hematology/Oncology RN
Cook Children's Medical Center
Fort Worth, Texas

Patricia Barry McElfresh, MN, RN, PNP
Clinical Program Manager - Advanced Practice Providers
Hematology Oncology-Bone Marrow Failure
Aflac Cancer & Blood Disorders Center
Atlanta, Georgia

Tara Merck, MSN, APRN, CPNP
Director of Advanced Practice Providers
Children's Specialty Group
Medical College of Wisconsin
Milwaukee, Wisconsin

Mary A. Mondozzi, MSN, BSN, WCC
Burn Center Education/Outreach Coordinator
The Paul and Carol David Foundation Burn Institute
Akron Children's Hospital
Akron, Ohio

Rebecca A. Monroe, MSN, RN, CPNP
Pediatric Nurse Practitioner
Collin County Pediatrics
Frisco, Texas

Kim Mooney-Doyle, PhD, CPNP-AC, RN
Assistant Professor
School of Nursing
University of Maryland
Baltimore, Maryland

Patricia O'Brien, CPNP-AC
Nurse Practitioner
Cardiology
Boston Children's Hospital
Boston, Massachusetts

Sue Park, APN, CPNP-PC
Pediatric Nurse Practitioner
Pediatric Anesthesia
Ann and Robert H. Lurie Children's Hospital of Chicago
Chicago, Illinois

Katherine Soss Prihoda, DNP, RN, PPCNP-BC
Assistant Professor
School of Nursing
Rutgers University, Camden
Camden, New Jersey

Cynthia A. Prows, MSN, APRN, FAAN
Clinical Nurse Specialist
Human Genetics and Patient Services
Cincinnati Children's Hospital Medical Center
Cincinnati, Ohio

Patricia A. Ring, MSN, RN, CPNP
Pediatric Nephrology
Children's Hospital of Wisconsin
Milwaukee, Wisconsin

Kathleen S. Ruccione, PhD, RN, MPH, CPON, FAAN
Associate Professor and Chair
Department of Doctoral Programs
Azusa Pacific University
Azusa, California

Margaret L. Schroeder, MSN, RN, PPCNP-BC
Pediatric Nurse Practitioner
Cardiovascular Surgery
Boston Children's Hospital
Boston, Massachusetts

Maureen Sheehan, CPNP
Child Neurology, Epilepsy, and Ketogenic Diet Nurse Practitioner
Child Neurology and Advanced Practice
Stanford Children's Health
Palo Alto, California

Katherine Smalling, RN, BSN, CPON
Nurse Case Manger
Children's Medical Center Dallas
Center for Cancer and Blood Disorders
Dallas, Texas

Anne Feierabend Stanton, APRN, PCNS, BC
Pediatric Clinical Nurse Specialist
University of Kansas Medical Center
Kansas City, Kansas

Alexandra Kathleen Superdock, MD
Pediatric Resident
University of Pittsburgh Medical Center
Pittsburgh, Pennsylvania

Barbara J. Wheeler, RN, MN, IBCLC
Neonatal Clinical Nurse Specialist
St. Boniface General Hospital
Winnipeg, Canada

Kristina D. Wilson, PhD, CCC-SLP
Senior Speech Pathologist and Clinical Research
Division of Speech, Language, and Learning
Texas Children's Hospital
Houston, Texas

CASE STUDIES AND REVIEW QUESTIONS

Stephanie Cope Evans, PhD, APRN, CPNP-PC
Assistant Professor of Nursing
Harris College of Nursing & Health Sciences
Texas Christian University
Fort Worth, Texas

KEY POINTS

Joanna Cain, BSN, BA, RN
Auctorial Pursuits, Inc.
President and Founder
Austin, Texas

POWERPOINT LECTURE SLIDES

Daryle Wane, PhD, ARNP, FNP-BC
BSN Program Director—Professor of Nursing
Department of Nursing and Health Programs
Pasco-Hernando State College
New Port Richey, Florida

TEACH FOR NURSING

Jenni Hermes
Freelance
St. Louis, Missouri

TEST BANK

Sherry Conder, BSHA, RN
Adult Career Development
Tulsa Technology Center
Tulsa, Oklahoma

REVIEWERS

Sharon Anderson, DNP, RN, APN, NNP-BC, APNG
Assistant Professor
Entry into Baccalaureate Practice
Rutgers, The State University of New Jersey
School of Nursing
Newark, New Jersey

Kristen Bagby, RN, MSN, CNL
Staff Nurse
Newborn Intensive Care Unit
Saint Louis Children's Hospital
Saint Louis, Missouri

William T. Campbell, EdD, MSN, RN
Associate Professor
Nursing
Salisbury University
Salisbury, Maryland

Rebecca E. Chatham, MSN, RN, CPN
Assistant Professor of Nursing
Jeannette C. Rudy School of Nursing
Cumberland University
Lebanon, Tennessee

Teresa M. Conte, PhD, CPNP
Associate Professor
Nursing
University of Scranton
Scranton, Pennsylvania

Claire M. Creamer, PhD, RN, CPNP-PC
Assistant Professor of Nursing
Nursing
Rhode Island College
Providence, Rhode Island

Jo Ann Cummings, PhD, RN, APN, PPCNP
Assistant Professor
Nursing
Georgian Court University
Lakewood, New Jersey

Raquel Burciaga Engolio, RN, MSN, CPN
Assistant Professor
Nursing
University of Holy Cross
New Orleans, Louisiana

Teresa Howell, DNP, RN, CNE
Professor of Nursing
Department of Nursing
Morehead State University
Morehead, Kentucky

Christine B. Kavanagh, RD, MS, PNP-BC
Instructor
Nursing Programs
School of Health Sciences
The Pennsylvania College of Technology
Williamsport, Pennsylvania

Renee C. B. Manworren, PhD, RN-BC, APRN, PCNS-BC, AP-PMN, FAAN
Posy and Fred Love Chair in Nursing Research
Director of Nursing Research and Professional Practice
Ann and Robert H. Lurie Children's Hospital of Chicago
Associate Professor of Pediatrics, Northwestern University's Feinberg School of Medicine
Chicago, Illinois

Elizabeth K. Rende, DNP, RN, CPNP-PC
Assistant Professor and Pediatric Nurse Practitioner
Duke School of Nursing and Duke Pediatric Neurology
Duke University and Duke University Medical Center
Durham, North Carolina

Deborah Spoerner, MSN, RN, CPNP, DNPc
Clinical Assistant Professor
School of Nursing
Purdue University
West Lafayette, Indiana

PREFACE

With this eleventh edition of *Wong's Nursing Care of Infants and Children*, we welcome Cheryl Rodgers, who joins Marilyn Hockenberry as coeditor. We would like to take a moment to reflect on the legacy of this textbook. The first edition, published in 1979, was the first of its kind to integrate important principles from the biologic, physical, and behavioral sciences into a pediatric nursing textbook (Whaley & Wong, 1979). With the first edition, the principles and concepts of nursing practice were conceptualized to allow both beginning students and experienced nurses an opportunity to expand and refine nursing care; this proves true with this eleventh edition.

The first edition, compared with the eleventh edition, clearly reflects 21st-century changes in pediatric nursing and demonstrates how scientific evidence has had a significant impact on the specialty. In the first edition, there is no mention of the human genome project, human immunodeficiency virus, autism disorders, respiratory syncytial virus, acute respiratory distress syndrome, acute lung injury, and cystic-fibrosis–related diabetes mellitus; they had yet to be discovered or named. The first edition of this text was perhaps the first pediatric nursing text to recognize the impact of illness and hospitalization on the child and her or his family. It was also first to introduce the concept of family-centered care in an era when the focus of care was centered on the diagnosis and treatment of the disease process.

Although the differences in content between the first *Nursing Care of Infants and Children* textbook and this eleventh edition are evident, the founding principles on which the first edition was established hold true today. This eleventh edition continues to be about families with children, and it emphasizes the philosophy of family-centered care. This book has retained the theme that Donna Wong so passionately advocated: providing atraumatic care—care that minimizes the psychologic and physical stress that health promotion and illness can inflict. The first edition's preface stated, "This books truly embodies the concept of [family-centered] care." We are proud to note that with this new edition, this foundation remains true. Features such as Family-Centered Care, Community Focus, and Atraumatic Care boxes bring these philosophies to life throughout the text. We believe strongly that children and families need consistent caregivers. Establishing therapeutic relationships with the child and family is explored as the essential foundation for providing quality nursing care.

This eleventh edition has been revised to keep pace with new innovations in pediatric nursing care. We feel a unique accountability and responsibility to continue to strive to provide students with the latest information they need to become competent critical thinkers and to attain the sensitivity necessary to become caring pediatric nurses. As editors for the Wong textbooks, we have developed an expert panel of more than 60 nurses and multidisciplinary specialists who assisted in reviewing, revising, rewriting, and authoring portions of the text on areas undergoing rapid and complex change, such as immunizations, genetics, high-risk newborn care, adolescent health issues, and numerous diseases. We have carefully preserved aspects of the book that have met with such universal acceptance—its state-of-the-art evidence-based information; strong, integrated focus on the family and community; logical and user-friendly organization; and easy reading style. We have placed additional emphasis on research with concise reviews of important evidence in Research Focus boxes. With this eleventh edition we emphasize the importance of care evaluation and have added quality indicator boxes throughout the book to demonstrate how quality of care can be assessed among the pediatric population. This format allows students to review new evidence and quality indicators on important topics in a concise way.

Throughout the chapters the reader will find quality patient outcomes that focus on serious health problems. Because nurses are the principal caregivers within health care institutions, quality patient outcomes are used as an assessment of the ability to provide excellence in patient care. Pathophysiology review figures throughout the text provide a concise evaluation of major health care diseases in children. With an understanding of the pathophysiologic process, the nurse is better prepared to develop evidence-based nursing interventions for patient care. In addition, more than 130 figures are color enhanced to focus on the importance on visual learning. This provides the visual learner with a tangible connection to the content of the text for application to clinical practice.

We have tried to meet the increasing demands of faculty and students to teach and to learn in an environment characterized by rapid change, enormous amounts of information, fewer traditional clinical facilities, and less time to teach. To help students quickly locate essential information, most of the features used in the previous edition have been retained. We continue to use Evidence-Based Practice boxes incorporating the PICOT approach and GRADE evidence quality assessment criteria. Most important, this text continues to encourage students to *think critically*.

This text serves as a reference manual for the practicing nurse. The latest recommendations have been included from authoritative organizations such as the American Academy of Pediatrics, Centers for Disease Control and Prevention, Agency for Healthcare Research and Quality, American Pain Society, American Nurses Association, and National Association of Pediatric Nurse Associates and Practitioners. To expand the universe of available information, websites and e-mail addresses have been included for hundreds of organizations and other educational resources.

ORGANIZATION OF THE BOOK

The same general approach to the presentation of content has been preserved from previous editions, although much content has been added, condensed, and rearranged within this framework to improve flow, minimize duplication, and emphasize health care trends, such as home and community care. This edition has been revised and refined to minimize content duplication, resulting in 34 chapters. The book continues to be divided into two broad parts. The first part of the book, sometimes called the "age and stage" approach, considers infancy, childhood, and adolescence from a developmental context. It emphasizes the importance of the nurse's role in health promotion and maintenance and in considering the family as the focus of care. From a developmental perspective, the care of common health problems is presented, giving readers a sense of what normal problems can be expected in otherwise healthy children and demonstrating when during childhood these problems are most likely to occur. The second part of the book presents the more serious health problems not specific to any particular age-group but that frequently require hospitalization or major medical and nursing interventions.

Unit I (Chapters 1 to 3) provides an overview of the multitude of influences on a child who is developing as a member of a family unit and maturing within a culture, community, and society. Chapter 1 includes a discussion of morbidity and mortality in infancy and childhood and examines child health care from a historical perspective. Because unintentional injury is one of the leading causes of death in children, an overview of this topic is included. The chapter presents the nursing process, with an emphasis on nursing diagnosis and outcomes and the importance of developing critical thinking skills. The critical components of evidence-based practice provide the template for exploring the latest pediatric nursing research and practice guidelines throughout the entire book. Discussion of quality patient outcomes and their importance in evaluating the quality of nursing care has been added.

Chapter 2 provides the opportunity to expand the discussion of social, cultural, religious, and family influences on child development and health promotion, including socioeconomic factors, customs, and health beliefs and practices. The content clearly describes the role of the nurse, with such content as guidelines for culturally sensitive interactions and a table discussing religious beliefs that affect nursing care. Chapter 3 has been revised by a leading genetics nursing expert, who focuses on heredity as it relates to health promotion and the influence of the Human Genome Project on future treatment strategies for inherited diseases.

Unit II (Chapters 4 to 6) is concerned with the principles of critical nursing assessment by keeping pace with the newest evaluation strategies in nursing. Chapter 4 contains guidelines for communicating with children, adolescents, and their families; telephone triage; and a detailed description of a health assessment, including an extensive discussion of family assessment and nutritional assessment. This chapter provides a comprehensive approach to physical examination and developmental assessment, using the latest literature on temperature measurement and the latest growth charts on how to assess a child's body mass index (BMI).

In this edition, an important chapter with new contributors is devoted to critical assessment and management of pain in children. Although the literature on pain assessment and management in children has grown considerably, this knowledge has not been widely applied in practice. Chapter 5 addresses this concern by presenting detailed pain assessment and management strategies, including discussion of common pain states in children. Chapter 6 is a newly developed chapter for the eleventh edition that focuses on infection control and the various infectious diseases encountered in childhood. In addition, it details hospital-acquired infections, childhood communicable diseases, and childhood immunizations.

Unit III (Chapters 7 to 9) stresses the importance of the neonatal period, the time of greatest risk to a child's survival, and discusses several health concerns encountered in the vulnerable first month of life. Chapter 7 has been updated and revised to include the latest information on the benefits of breastfeeding and dietary intake of vitamin D. Atraumatic care sections have been revised to include the latest evidence-based recommendations for pain management in newborns. This chapter also discusses the impact of prebiotics and probiotics on infant nutrition and well-being. The sections on infant safety, newborn circumcision, and circumcision analgesia have all been revised and updated. Newborn screening guidelines have also been extensively updated. Chapter 8 has been revised and updated by a new contributor who is an expert in high-risk neonatal care. The latest guidelines for the management of hyperbilirubinemia in late-preterm and term newborns and for follow-up and management of hyperbilirubinemia in the breastfeeding pair are included in this edition. The chapter includes updated sections on care of the infant with cleft lip or palate and Pierre Robin sequence. Updated management protocols for neonatal hypoglycemia are also included. Atraumatic care of the newborn remains an important concept in these chapters. Evidence-based practice and critical thinking exercises have been updated as well. Chapter 9, revised and updated by a new contributor, includes updated and revised sections on care of the preterm infant, including therapeutic positioning, preterm infant nutrition, revised guidelines for supplemental oxygen administration, noninvasive (gentle) mechanical ventilation, necrotizing enterocolitis, neonatal sepsis, discharge planning, retinopathy of prematurity, neonatal skin care guidelines, and neonatal/perinatal stroke. The most recent information regarding hypoxic ischemic reperfusion injury and therapeutic hypothermia are presented in this chapter. This chapter also contains information regarding maternal conditions that may adversely affect the fetus and newborn, including maternal viruses, maternal diabetes, fetal alcohol and tobacco exposure, and neonatal drug exposure.

Units IV through VII (Chapters 10 to 18) present the major developmental stages in childhood, expanded to provide a broader concept of the stages and the health problems most often associated with each age-group. Special emphasis is placed on the preventive aspects of care. The health promotion chapters follow a standard approach that is used consistently for each age-group.

The chapters on health problems primarily reflect typical and age-related concerns. The information on many disorders has been revised to reflect recent changes. Examples include the latest information on food sensitivity, severe acute malnutrition, colic, failure to thrive, child passenger safety, pacifier use, thumb sucking, lead poisoning, sexual abuse, attention-deficit/hyperactivity disorder, school-related violence, conduct disorders, tobacco use, contraception, teenage pregnancy, substance abuse, self-harm, and eating disorders such as anorexia nervosa and childhood obesity. This section presents the latest Dietary Reference Intake (DRI) guidelines, American Heart Association dietary guidelines for children, and U.S. Department of Agriculture dietary intake guidelines for children (MyPlate), aimed at decreasing childhood obesity and cardiovascular disease. The sections on sudden infant death syndrome (SIDS) and apparent life-threatening events (ALTEs) have been extensively updated to include the latest American Academy of Pediatrics considerations for recognized SIDS protective and risk factors. A common theme in these chapters is the recognition of the impact of accidental childhood injury on childhood morbidity and mortality and efforts for prevention of such injuries.

Childhood obesity information is now located in the school-age child chapter to emphasize the need for earlier assessment and intervention of this health problem. The chapters on adolescence include the latest information on the management of eating disorders, and also recommendations for preventive health screening in adolescents. Sections on male and female reproductive health conditions and sexual orientation have been revised and updated. The chapter includes updates on the latest screening guidelines for adolescent hypertension and hyperlipidemia.

Unit VIII (Chapters 19 and 20) deals with children who have the same developmental needs as growing children but who, because of congenital or acquired physical, cognitive, or sensory impairment, require alternative interventions to facilitate development. Chapter 19 combines discussion of chronic illness, disability, and end-of-life care for the child and family. It reflects the latest trends in the care of families and children with chronic illness or disability, such as home care, normalizing children's lives, focusing on developmental needs, enabling and empowering families, and providing early intervention. The content in Chapter 20 on cognitive, sensory, and communication impairment includes the latest information on cognitive impairment and learning disorders.

Unit IX (Chapters 21 and 22) is concerned with the impact of hospitalization on the child and the family and presents a comprehensive overview of the stressors imposed by hospitalization and nursing interventions available to prevent or eliminate these stressors. Chapter 21 discusses the care of the hospitalized child and family with consideration for increasing care in ambulatory centers. Chapter 22 explores safe implementation of procedures in children, including emphasis on the use of therapeutic holding. This chapter also includes numerous Evidence-Based Practice boxes designed to provide rationales for the interventions discussed in the chapter. Recommendations for practice are based on the evidence and are concisely presented in Evidence-Based Practice boxes throughout the chapter.

Units X through XIV (Chapters 23 to 34) consider serious health problems of infants and children primarily from a biologic system orientation, which has the practical organizational value of permitting health care problems and nursing considerations to relate to specific pathophysiologic disturbances. Important additions and revisions include discussion of hepatitis, all blood disorders, influenza management recommendations, acute respiratory distress syndrome/acute lung injury (ARDS/ALI), respiratory syncytial virus (RSV), tuberculosis, the latest classification for asthma, effects of tobacco exposure, seizures, chemotherapy, acquired immunodeficiency syndrome, diabetes mellitus, and burns. Examples of the updates and revisions for these units include the following: Chapter 27 on the child with cardiovascular dysfunction has major revisions to the latest guidelines for assessment and management of the most common heart disorders in children. Chapter 30 contains significant updates on seizures and epilepsy and cerebral abnormalities, including Chiari I and II malformations. Chapter 34 includes updates on Guillain-Barré syndrome, cerebral palsy, infant botulism, and respiratory management of neuromuscular conditions such as spinal muscular atrophy and muscular dystrophy.

UNIFYING PRINCIPLES

Several unifying principles have guided the organizational structure of this book since its inception. These principles continue to strengthen the book with each revision to maintain a consistent approach throughout each chapter.

The Family as the Unit of Care

The child is an essential member of the family unit. Nursing care is most effective when it is delivered with the belief that *the family is the patient.* This belief permeates the book. The family is seen as a myriad of structures; each has the potential to provide a caring, supportive environment in which the child can grow, mature, and maximize his or her human potential. In addition to family-centered care being integrated into every chapter, an entire chapter is devoted to understanding the family as the core focus in children's lives. Another chapter discusses the social, cultural, and religious influences on family beliefs. Separate sections in yet another chapter deal in depth with family communication and family assessment. The impact of illness, hospitalization, home care, and the death of a child are covered extensively in three additional chapters. The needs of the family are emphasized throughout the text under Nursing Care Management, with a separate section on family support. Numerous Family-Centered Care boxes are included to assist nurses in understanding and providing helpful information to families.

An Integrated Approach to Development

Children are not small adults but are special individuals with unique minds, bodies, and needs. No book on pediatric nursing is complete without extensive coverage of communication, nutrition, play, safety, dental care, sexuality, sleep, self-esteem, and, of course, parenting. Nurses promote the healthy expression of development and need to understand how this is observed in children at different ages and stages. Effective parenting depends on the parents' knowledge of development, and it is often the nurse's responsibility to provide parents with a developmental awareness of their children's needs. For these reasons, coverage of the many dimensions of childhood is integrated within each developmental-stage chapter, rather than being presented in a separate chapter. Safety concerns, for instance, are very different for a toddler than for an adolescent. Sleep needs change with age, as do nutritional needs. As a result, the units on each stage of childhood contain complete information on all these subjects as they relate to the specific age. Using the integrated approach, students gain an appreciation for the unique characteristics and needs of children at every age and stage of development.

Focus on Wellness and Illness: Child, Family, and Community

In a pediatric nursing text, a focus on illness is expected. Children become ill, and nurses typically are involved in helping children get well. However, it is not sufficient to prepare students to care primarily for sick children. First, health is more than the absence of disease. Being healthy is being whole in mind, body, and spirit; therefore the majority of the first half of the book is devoted to discussions that promote physical, psychosocial, mental, and spiritual wellness. Much emphasis is placed on anticipatory guidance of parents to prevent injury or illness in the child. Second, more than ever, health care is prevention focused. The objectives set forth in *Healthy People 2020* clearly establish a health care agenda in which solutions to medical/social problems lie in preventive strategies. Competent nursing care flows from this knowledge and is enhanced by an awareness of childhood development, family dynamics, and communication skills.

Nursing Care

Although this text incorporates information from numerous disciplines (e.g., medicine, pathophysiology, pharmacology, nutrition, psychology, sociology), its primary purpose is to provide information on the nursing care of children and families. Discussions of disorders conclude with a section on Nursing Care Management. Although many aspects of the nursing care of children and families have changed significantly over the last few decades, the focus must continue to be on the quality of care. For the quality of care to be maintained, pediatric nurses must be proactive in staying informed about the strength of evidence that supports specific nursing practices. The Nursing Care Management sections are designed to provide the latest evidence for the implementation of evidence-based nursing practice. In addition, all of the nursing care plans have been updated to current practices and include case studies to provide students with real examples to demonstrate critical thinking skills as they develop their own care plans.

Critical Role of Research and Evidence-Based Practice

This eleventh edition is the product of an extensive review of the literature published since the book was last revised. In addition, Research Focus boxes provide the student with a concise discussion of the latest research on a given topic. So that information is accurate and current, most citations are less than 5 years old, and almost every chapter has entries within 1 year of publication. Examples of current cutting-edge information include recommendations from the American Academy of Pediatrics on immunizations and media use. The chapter on pain reflects the latest guidelines from the Agency for Healthcare Research and Quality (AHRQ), formerly known as the Agency for Health Care Policy and Research (AHCPR), and the American Pain Society. The discussions on skin care reflect the AHRQ's guidelines on pressure ulcers. The American Diabetes Association's classification of diabetes mellitus is included, as are the most recent treatment guidelines for asthma.

• • •

Just as children and their families bring with them a value system and unique background that affect their role within the health care system, so too must each nurse bring to each child and family an individual set of characteristics and values that will affect their relationship. Although we have attempted to present a total picture of the child in each age-group, both in wellness and in illness, no one child, family, or nurse will be found in this book. We hope that each page, chapter, and unit builds a foundation on which the nurse can begin to construct an ideal of comprehensive, atraumatic, and individualized nursing care for infants, children, adolescents, and their families.

SPECIAL FEATURES

Much effort has been directed toward making this book easy to teach from and, more important, easy to learn from. In this edition, the following features have been included to benefit educators, students, and practitioners.

APPLYING EVIDENCE TO PRACTICE

Applying Evidence to Practice boxes are new specialty boxes throughout the text outlining up-to-date procedures to show best practice and focus on applying evidence.

ATRAUMATIC CARE

Atraumatic Care boxes emphasize the importance of providing competent care without creating undue physical and psychologic distress. Although many of the boxes provide suggestions for managing pain, atraumatic care also considers approaches to promote self-esteem and prevent embarrassment.

CONCEPTS

Concepts have been added to the beginning of each chapter to focus student attention on unique principles found in each chapter as well as aid students using concept-based curriculum, system-focused curriculum, or a hybrid approach.

COMMUNITY AND HOME HEALTH CONSIDERATIONS

Community and Home Health Considerations boxes address issues that expand to the community, such as increasing immunization rates, preventing lead poisoning, or decreasing smoking among teens.

CRITICAL THINKING CASE STUDY

Critical Thinking Case Study boxes have been revised in this edition to describe brief scenarios of the child-family-nurse interaction that depict real-life clinical situations. From the synthesis of the topical content and a critical analysis of possible options, the reader chooses the best intervention and learns to make clinical judgments. A rationale is offered for the correct answer, and explanations are given for the incorrect options at the end of the chapter.

CULTURAL CONSIDERATIONS

Cultural Considerations boxes integrate concepts of culturally sensitive care throughout the text. Their emphasis is on the clinical application of the information, whether it focuses on toilet training or on male or female circumcision.

DRUG ALERT

Drug Alert boxes highlight critical drug safety concerns for better therapeutic management.

EMERGENCY TREATMENT

Emergency Treatment boxes enable the reader to quickly learn interventions for crisis situations.

FAMILY-CENTERED CARE

Family-Centered Care boxes present issues of special significance to families who have a child with a particular disorder. This feature is another method of highlighting the needs or concerns of families that should be addressed when family-centered care is provided.

NURSING ALERT

Nursing Alert boxes call the reader's attention to considerations that if ignored could lead to a deteriorating or emergency situation. Key assessment data, risk factors, and danger signs are among the kinds of information included.

NURSING CARE GUIDELINES

Nursing Care Guidelines boxes summarize important nursing interventions for a variety of situations and conditions.

NURSING CARE PLAN

Nursing Care Plan boxes include expected patient outcomes and rationales for the included nursing interventions that may not be immediately evident to the student. The care plans include a case study that represents a "real" patient and family to demonstrate the principles of nursing care plans and how they are used to organize care.

NURSING TIP

Nursing Tip boxes present handy information of a nonemergency nature that makes patients more comfortable and the nurse's job a little easier.

PATHOPHYSIOLOGY REVIEW

Pathophysiology Review boxes have been revised in this edition to provide the student with a visual representation of the effects of the disease process on the child. These illustrations provide knowledge required for the nurse to implement appropriate evidence-based nursing interventions and provide independent care, as well as collaborative care with other health care professionals.

QUALITY PATIENT OUTCOMES

Quality Patient Outcomes boxes are added throughout the text to provide a framework for measuring nursing care performance. Nursing-sensitive outcome measures are integrated into the outcome indicators used throughout the book.

RESEARCH FOCUS

Research Focus boxes review new evidence on important topics in a concise way.

TRANSLATING EVIDENCE INTO PRACTICE

Translating Evidence into Practice boxes have been completely revised in this edition to focus the reader's attention on application of both research and critical thought processes to support and guide the outcomes of nursing care and to provide measurable outcomes that nurses can use to validate their unique role in the health care system.

Numerous pedagogic devices that enhance student learning have been retained from previous editions:

- More than 100 **COLOR PHOTOGRAPHS** are included in this edition to reflect the latest in nursing care. Anatomic drawings are easy to follow, with color appropriately used to illustrate important aspects, such as saturated and desaturated blood. New figures reflecting a **PATHOPHYSIOLOGY REVIEW** of various disorders have been added throughout the book. As an example, the full-color heart illustrations in Chapter 27 clearly depict congenital cardiac defects and associated hemodynamic changes.
- A functional and attractive **FULL-COLOR DESIGN** visually enhances the organization of each chapter, as well as the special features.
- An **INDEX,** detailed and cross-referenced, allows readers to quickly access discussions.
- **KEY TERMS** are highlighted throughout each chapter to reinforce student learning.
- **BLOOD PRESSURE LEVELS** on the inside back cover provide information nurses refer to often.
- Hundreds of **TABLES** and **BOXES** highlight key concepts and nursing interventions.

ACKNOWLEDGMENTS

This eleventh edition of *Wong's Nursing Care of Infants and Children* brings with it new contributors to the book. To continue the Wong legacy of excellence in nursing education, we have joined together numerous contributors with diverse expert nursing backgrounds to continue the commitment to providing the latest state-of-the-art information on pediatric nursing practice. We are grateful to the many nursing faculty members, practitioners, and students who have offered their comments, recommendations, and suggestions. We are grateful to the many reviewers who brought constructive criticism, suggestions, and clinical expertise to this edition. We could not have completed the enormous task of updating and adding information without the dedication of these special people.

No book is ever a reality without the dedication and perseverance of the editorial staff. Although it is impossible to list every individual at Elsevier who has made exceptional efforts to produce this text, we are especially grateful to **Heather Bays,** whose commitment to pediatric nursing education over the years is reflective of outstanding editorial staff. She is passionate about her work, and her commitment to the Wong textbooks is noted in all she does. We want to thank **Sandra Clark** for all her support, and a special thanks also to **Tracey Schriefer** for her commitment to excellence.

Finally, we thank our families and children for the unselfish love and endless patience that allows us to devote such a large portion of our lives to our careers.

Marilyn J. Hockenberry
Cheryl C. Rodgers

CONTENTS

SECTION III Family-Centered Care of the Newborn

SECTION VIII Family-Centered Care of the Child With Special Needs

SECTION IX The Child Who Is Hospitalized

SECTION X Childhood Nutrition and Elimination Problems

SECTION XI Childhood Oxygenation Problems

SECTION XII Childhood Blood Production and Circulation Problems

SECTION XIII Childhood Regulatory Problems

1

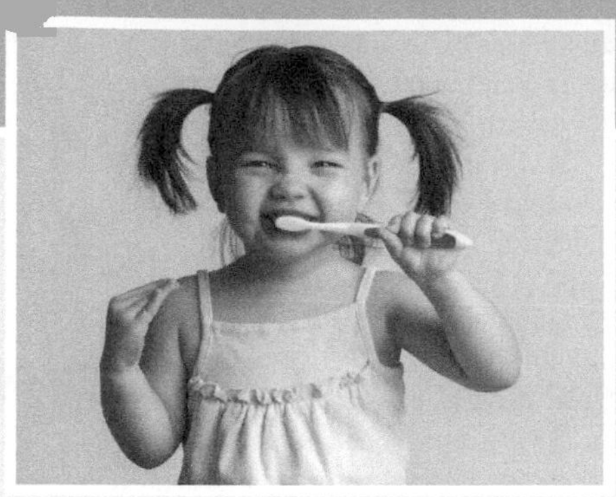

Perspectives of Pediatric Nursing

Marilyn J. Hockenberry

http://evolve.elsevier.com/wong/ncic

CONCEPTS

- Family-Centered Care
- Atraumatic Care
- Clinical Reasoning
- Nursing Process
- Research and Evidence-Based Practice
- Quality Outcome Measures

HEALTH CARE FOR CHILDREN

The major goal for pediatric nursing is to improve the quality of health care for children and their families. In 2016 almost 74 million children 0 to 17 years old lived in the United States, making up 24% of the population (Federal Interagency Forum on Child and Family Statistics, 2017). The health status of children in the United States has improved in a number of areas, including increased immunization rates for all children, decreased adolescent birth rate, and improved child health outcomes. The 2017 America's Children in Brief—Indicators of Well-Being reveals that preterm births increased slightly in 2015, after a continuous decline since 2007. Average mathematics scores for fourth- and eighth-grade students decreased, and the violent crime victimization rate among youth decreased during the last 20 years. Although the number of children living in poverty decreased slightly in 2015, overall the rate remains high at 20%. The percentage of children with at least one parent employed full time year remained steady at 75% in 2015 (see Research Focus box) (Federal Interagency Forum on Child and Family Statistics, 2017).

Millions of children and their families have no health insurance, which results in a lack of access to care and health promotion services. In addition, disparities in pediatric health care are related to race, ethnicity, socioeconomic status, and geographic factors (Flores & Lesley, 2014). Patterns of child health are shaped by medical progress and societal trends. Urgent priorities for health and health care of children in the United States are the focus for action toward new policy priorities (Box 1.1).

RESEARCH FOCUS

National Children's Study

The National Children's Study is the largest prospective, long-term study of children's health and development conducted in the United States. The study is designed to follow 100,000 children and their families from birth to 21 years old to understand the link between children's environments and their physical and emotional health and development (Duncan, Kirkendall, & Citro, 2014). Researchers hope that a study of this magnitude will provide information on innovative interventions for families, children, and health care providers to eradicate unhealthy diets, dental caries, and childhood obesity and to bring a significant reduction in violence, injury, substance abuse, and mental health disorders among the nation's children. This study supports the Healthy People 2020 primary goals to increase the quality and years of healthy life and eliminate health disparities related to race, ethnicity, and socioeconomic status (US Department of Health and Human Services, 2013).

HEALTH PROMOTION

Child health promotion provides opportunities to reduce differences in current health status among members of different groups and to ensure equal opportunities and resources to enable all children to achieve their fullest health potential. The Healthy People 2020 Leading Health Indicators (Box 1.2) provide a framework for identifying essential components for child health promotion programs designed to prevent future health

BOX 1.1 Health and Health Care Priorities for American Children

Poverty
Hunger
Lack of health insurance
Child abuse and neglect
Overweight and obesity
Firearm deaths and injuries
Mental health
Racial and ethnic disparities
Immigration

Adapted from Flores, G., & Lesley, B. (2014). Children and US federal policy on health and health care: Seen but not heard. *JAMA Pediatrics, 168*(12), 1155-1163.

BOX 1.2 Healthy People 2020

Goals

Increase quality and length of healthy life
Eliminate health disparities

Leading Health Indicators

Physical activity
Overweight and obesity
Tobacco use
Substance abuse
Responsible sexual behavior
Mental health
Injury and violence
Environmental quality
Immunization
Access to health care

From US Department of Health and Human Services, Office of Disease Prevention and Health Promotion. (2013). *Healthy People 2020.* Retrieved from http://www.healthypeople.gov/

problems in our nation's children. Bright Futures is a national health promotion initiative with a goal to improve the health of our nation's children (Bright Futures, 2016). Major themes of the Bright Futures guideline are promoting family support, child development, mental health, and healthy nutrition that leads to healthy weight, physical activity, oral health, healthy sexual development and sexuality, safety and injury prevention, and the importance of community relationships and resources.* Throughout this book, developmentally appropriate health promotion strategies are discussed. Key examples of child health promotion themes essential for all age-groups include promoting development, nutrition, and oral health. Bright Futures recommendations for preventive health care during infancy, early childhood, and adolescence are found in Chapters 7, 10, 12, 13, 15, and 17.

Development

Health promotion integrates surveillance of the physical, psychologic, and emotional changes that occur in human beings between birth and the end of adolescence. Developmental processes are unique to each stage of development, and continuous screening and assessment are essential for early intervention when problems are found. The most dramatic time of physical, motor, cognitive, emotional, and social development occurs during infancy. Interactions between the parent and infant are central to promoting optimal developmental outcomes and are a key component of infant assessment. During early childhood, early identification of developmental delays is critical for establishing early interventions. Anticipatory guidance strategies ensure that parents are aware of the specific developmental needs of each developmental stage. Ongoing surveillance during middle childhood provides opportunities to strengthen cognitive and emotional attributes, communication skills, self-esteem, and independence. Recognition that adolescents differ greatly in their physical, social, and emotional maturity is important for surveillance throughout this developmental period.

An important example for health promotion during early child development is to be aware of changing recommendations that address the fast-changing world of technology in our society. An important example is the changes in the latest American Academy of Pediatrics (2016) policy statement on screen viewing by infants and children. New guidelines for screen viewing (laptop or phone) shift the importance from what is on the screen to who is viewing the information with the young child (American Academy of Pediatrics, 2016). For infants less than 18 months of age, no screen time is recommended except for video calling with a grandparent or loved one. Parents should be advised to use technology sparingly before 5 years of age and to always participate during screen-time viewing.

Nutrition

Nutrition is an essential component for healthy growth and development. Human milk is the preferred form of nutrition for all infants. Breastfeeding provides the infant with micronutrients, immunologic properties, and several enzymes that enhance digestion and absorption of these nutrients. A recent resurgence in breastfeeding has occurred as a result of the education of mothers and fathers regarding its benefits and increased social support.

Children establish lifelong eating habits during the first 3 years of life, and the nurse is instrumental in educating parents on the importance of nutrition. Most eating preferences and attitudes related to food are established by family influences and culture. During adolescence, parental influence diminishes and the adolescent makes food choices related to peer acceptability and sociability. Occasionally these choices are detrimental to adolescents with chronic illnesses such as diabetes, obesity, chronic lung disease, hypertension, cardiovascular risk factors, and renal disease.

Families that struggle with lower incomes, homelessness, and migrant status generally lack the resources to provide their children with adequate food intake, nutritious foods such as fresh fruits and vegetables, and appropriate protein intake (Flores & Lesley, 2014). The result is nutritional deficiencies with subsequent growth and developmental delays, depression, and behavior problems.

Oral Health

Oral health is an essential component of health promotion throughout infancy, childhood, and adolescence. Preventing dental caries and developing healthy oral hygiene habits must occur early in childhood. Dental caries has been recommended for decades as a significant yet preventable health problem for children (Clark, Kent, & Jackson, 2015). Children in racial or cultural minority groups,experience disparities in oral health care and are much more likely to have dental disease. In children ages 2 to 8 years, Hispanic and non-Hispanic black children are twice as likely to experience any dental caries in primary teeth compared with non-Hispanic white children (Dye, Thornton-Evans, Li, et al., 2015).

Preschoolers of low-income families are twice as likely to develop tooth decay and only half as likely to visit the dentist as other children. Early childhood caries is a preventable disease, and nurses play an essential role in educating children and parents about practicing dental hygiene, beginning with the first tooth eruption; drinking fluoridated water,

*Bright Futures is supported by the American Academy of Pediatrics (see http://brightfutures.aap.org/about.html).

including bottled water; and instituting early dental preventive care. Oral health care practices established during the early years of development prevent destructive periodontal disease and dental decay.

CHILDHOOD HEALTH PROBLEMS

Changes in modern society, including advancing medical knowledge and technology, the proliferation of information systems, struggles with insurance disparities, economically troubled times, and various changes and disruptive influences on the family, are leading to significant medical problems that affect the health of children. Problems that can negatively affect a child's development include poverty, violence, aggression, noncompliance, school failure, and adjustment to parental separation and divorce. In addition, mental health issues cause challenges in childhood and adolescence. Recent concern has focused on groups of children who are at highest risk, such as children born preterm or with very low birth weight (VLBW) or low birth weight (LBW), children attending child care centers, children who live in poverty or are homeless, children of immigrant families, and children with chronic medical and psychiatric illness and disabilities. In addition, these children and their families face multiple barriers to adequate health, dental, and psychiatric care. A perspective of several health problems facing children and the major challenges for pediatric nurses is discussed in the following sections.

Obesity and Type 2 Diabetes

Childhood obesity, the most common nutritional problem among American children, is increasing in epidemic proportions (Martin, Saunders, Shenkin, et al., 2014). *Obesity* in children and adolescents is defined as a body mass index (BMI) at or greater than the 95th percentile for youth of the same age and gender. *Overweight* is defined as a BMI at or above the 85th percentile and below the 95th percentile for children and teens of the same age and sex. Over 30% of America's children are overweight, and 17% are obese (Flores & Lesley, 2014).

Increasing evidence associates maternal obesity as a major influence on offspring health during childhood and in adult life (Godfrey, Reynolds, Prescott, et al., 2016). An optimal nutritional and microbial environment during pregnancy may reduce the risk of infants being obese or overweight during early life (Garcia-Mantrana & Collado, 2016).

Lack of physical activity related to limited resources, unsafe environments, and inconvenient play and exercise facilities, combined with easy access to television and video games, increases the incidence of obesity among low-income, minority children. Overweight youth have increased risk for cardiometabolic changes (a cluster of cardiovascular factors that include hypertension, altered glucose metabolism, dyslipidemia, and abdominal obesity) in the future (Weiss, Bremer, & Lustig, 2013) (Fig. 1.1). The US Department of Health and Human Services (2013) suggests that nurses focus on prevention strategies to reduce the incidence of overweight children from the current 20% in all ethnic groups to less than 6%. Emphasis is on preventive strategies that start in infancy and even in the prenatal period. Lifestyle interventions show promise in preventing obesity and decreasing occurrence if targeted at children 6 to 12 years old (Martin, Saunders, Shenkin, et al., 2014).

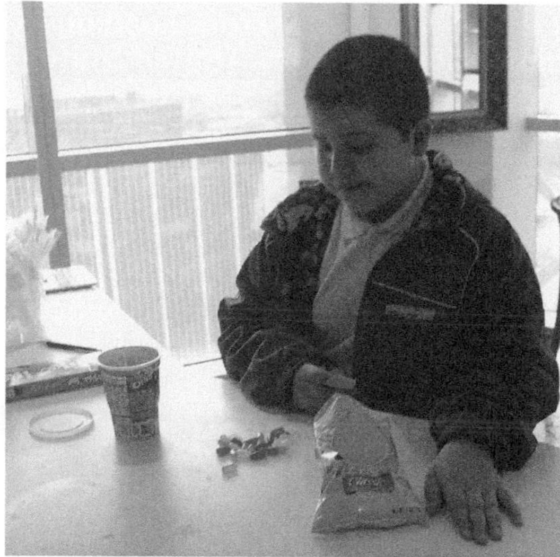

FIG. 1.1 The American culture's intake of high-caloric, fatty food contributes to obesity in children.

Childhood Injuries

Injuries are the most common cause of death and disability to children in the United States (Centers for Disease Control and Prevention, 2016) (Table 1.1). Mortality rates for suicide, poisoning, and falls rose substantially over the past decade. Other unintentional injuries (head injuries, drowning, burns, and firearm accidents) take the lives of children every day. Implementing programs of accident prevention and health promotion could prevent many childhood injuries and fatalities.

The type of injury and the circumstances surrounding it are closely related to normal growth and development (Box 1.3). As children develop, their innate curiosity compels them to investigate the environment and to mimic the behavior of others. This is essential to acquire competency as an adult, but it can also predispose children to numerous hazards.

The child's developmental stage partially determines the types of injuries that are most likely to occur at a specific age and helps provide clues to preventive measures. For example, small infants are helpless in any environment. When they begin to roll over or propel themselves, they can fall from unprotected surfaces. The crawling infant, who has a natural tendency to place objects in the mouth, is at risk for aspiration or poisoning. The mobile toddler, with the instinct to explore and investigate and the ability to run and climb, may experience falls, burns, and collisions with objects. As children grow older, their absorption with play makes them oblivious to environmental hazards such as street traffic or water. The need to conform and gain acceptance compels older children and adolescents to accept challenges and dares. Although the rate of injuries is high in children younger than 9 years old, most fatal injuries occur in later childhood and adolescence.

The pattern of deaths caused by unintentional injuries, especially from motor vehicle accidents (MVAs), drowning, and burns, is remarkably consistent in most Western societies. The leading causes of death from injuries for each age-group according to sex are presented in Table 1.1. The majority of deaths from injuries occur in boys. It is important to note that accidents continue to account for more than three times as many teen deaths as any other cause (Annie E Casey Foundation, 2016). Fortunately, prevention strategies such as the use of car restraints, bicycle helmets, and smoke detectors have significantly decreased fatalities for children. Nevertheless, the overwhelming causes of death in children are MVAs, including occupant, pedestrian, bicycle, and motorcycle deaths; these account for more than half of all injury deaths (Kidscount Data Center, 2016) (Fig. 1.2).

Pedestrian accidents involving children account for significant numbers of motor vehicle–related deaths. Most of these accidents occur at midblock, at intersections, in driveways, and in parking lots. Driveway injuries typically involve small children and large vehicles backing up.

Bicycle-associated injuries also cause a number childhood deaths. Children ages 5 to 9 years are at greatest risk of bicycling fatalities. The majority of bicycling deaths are from traumatic head injuries (Centers for Disease Control and Prevention, 2016). Helmets greatly reduce the risk of head injury, but few children wear helmets. Community-wide bicycle helmet campaigns and mandatory-use laws have resulted in significant increases in helmet use. Still, issues such as stylishness, comfort, and

TABLE 1.1 Mortality From Leading Types of Unintentional Injuries, United States*

Type of Injury	AGE (YEARS) <1	1–4	5–14	15–24
Males				
All causes	716.4	31.2	15.9	108.8
Unintentional injuries (all types)	33.3	10.5	5.8	48.1
Motor vehicle	2.8 (2)	3.0 (2)	3.0 (1)	29.5 (1)
Drowning	1.1 (4)	3.4 (1)	0.9 (2)	2.3 (3)
Fires and burns	0.5 (5)	1.1 (3)	0.5 (3)	0.4 (5)
Firearms	—	—	—	—
Choking	1.7 (3)	0.5 (5)	—	—
Falls	—	—	—	0.9 (4)
Mechanical suffocation	25.0 (1)	0.6 (4)	0.2 (4)	—
Poisoning	—	—	0.1 (5)	11.2 (2)
All other unintentional injuries	4.6	1.9	1.0	3.8
Injuries as a percent of all deaths	4.6%	33.7%	36.5%	44.2%
Females				
All causes	591.7	24.7	12.0	39.2
Unintentional injuries (all types)	28.0	6.9	3.4	16.6
Motor vehicle	2.0 (2)	2.4 (1)	2.0 (1)	11.7 (1)
Drowning	0.9 (4)	1.8 (2)	0.4 (2)	0.3 (3)
Fires and burns	0.4 (5)	0.9 (3)	0.4 (2)	0.3 (3)
Firearms	—	—	—	—
Choking	1.1 (3)	0.3 (4)	—	—
Falls	—	—	—	0.2 (5)
Mechanical suffocation	21.4 (1)	0.3 (4)	0.1 (4)	—
Poisoning	—	—	0.1 (4)	3.4 (2)
All other unintentional injuries	2.1	1.1	0.4	0.8
Injuries as a percent of all deaths	4.7%	27.9%	28.3%	42.3%

*Rate per 100,000 population in each age-group.
Adapted from National Safety Council. (2012). *Injury facts, 2012 edition.* Istaska, IL: Author.
Data from National Center for Health Statistics and US Census Bureau.

social acceptability remain important factors in noncompliance. Nurses can educate children and families about pedestrian and bicycle safety. In particular, school nurses can promote helmet wearing and encourage peer leaders to act as role models.

Drowning and burns are among the top three leading causes of deaths for males and females throughout childhood (Fig. 1.3). In addition, improper use of firearms is a major cause of death among males (Fig. 1.4). During infancy, more boys die of aspiration or suffocation than do girls (Fig. 1.5). Each year, more than 500,000 children ages 5 years and younger experience a potential poisoning related to medications (Ferguson, Osterthaler, & Kaminski, 2015). Currently, more children are brought to emergency departments (EDs) for unintentional medication overdoses. Approximately 95% of medication-related ED visits in children younger than 5 years are due to ingesting medication while unsupervised (Fig. 1.6). Intentional poisoning, associated with drug and alcohol abuse and suicide attempt, is the second leading cause of death in adolescent females and the third leading cause in adolescent males.

BOX 1.3 Childhood Injuries: Risk Factors

- *Sex*—Preponderance of males; difference mainly the result of behavioral characteristics, especially aggression
- *Temperament*—Children with difficult temperament profile, especially persistence, high activity level, and negative reactions to new situations
- *Stress*—Predisposes children to increased risk taking and self-destructive behavior; general lack of self-protection
- *Alcohol and drug use*—Associated with higher incidence of motor vehicle injuries, drownings, homicides, and suicides
- *History of previous injury*—Associated with increased likelihood of another injury, especially if initial injury required hospitalization
- *Developmental characteristics*
  - Mismatch between child's developmental level and skill required for activity (e.g., all-terrain vehicles)
  - Natural curiosity to explore environment
  - Desire to assert self and challenge rules
  - In older child, desire for peer approval and acceptance
- *Cognitive characteristics* (age specific)
  - *Infant*—Sensorimotor: explores environment through taste and touch
  - *Young child*—Object permanence: actively searches for attractive object; cause and effect: lacks awareness of consequential dangers; transductive reasoning: may fail to learn from experiences (e.g., perceives falling from a step as a different type of danger from climbing a tree); magical and egocentric thinking: is unable to comprehend danger to self or others
  - *School-age child*—Transitional cognitive processes: is unable to fully comprehend causal relationships; attempts dangerous acts without detailed planning regarding consequences
  - *Adolescent*—Formal operations: is preoccupied with abstract thinking and loses sight of reality; may lead to feeling of invulnerability
- *Anatomic characteristics* (especially in young children)
  - *Large head*—Predisposes to cranial injury
  - *Large spleen and liver with wide costal arch*—Predisposes to direct trauma to these organs
  - *Small and light body*—May be thrown easily, especially inside a moving vehicle
- *Other factors*—Poverty, family stress (e.g., maternal illness, recent environmental change), substandard alternative child care, young maternal age, low maternal education, multiple siblings

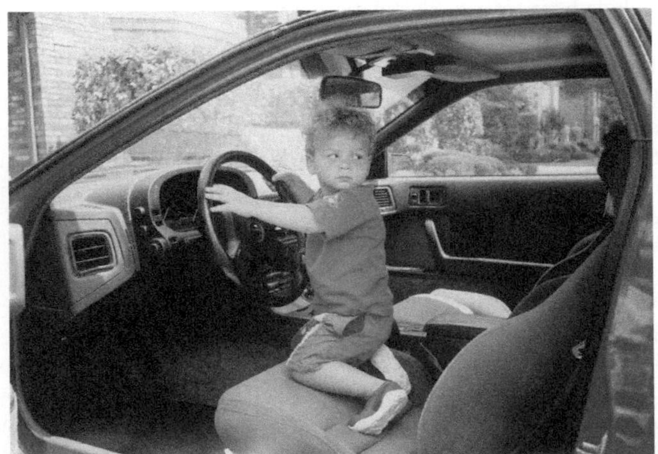

FIG. 1.2 Motor vehicle injuries are the leading cause of death in children older than 1 year of age. The majority of fatalities involve occupants who are unrestrained.

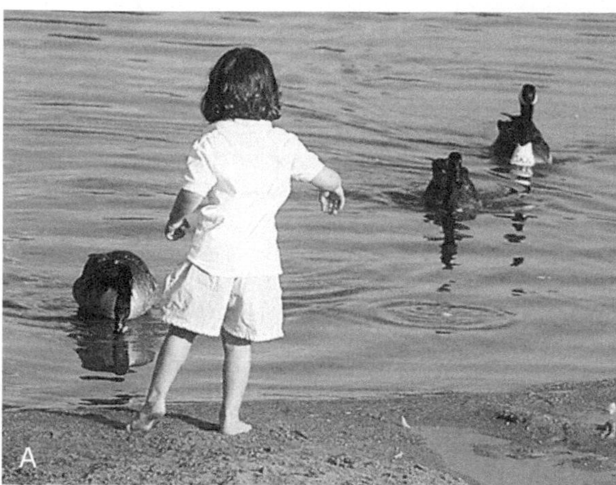

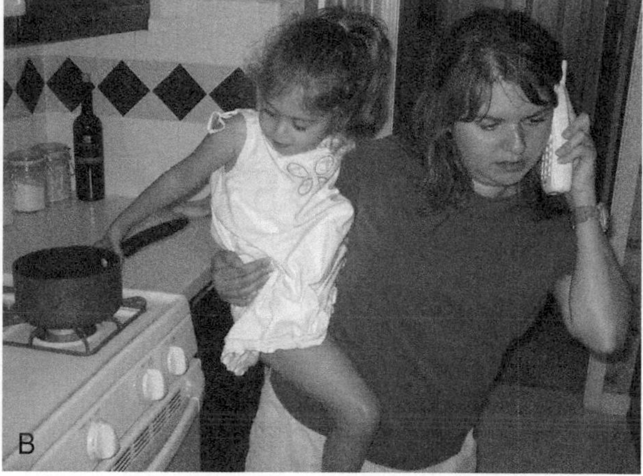

FIG. 1.3 A, Drowning is one of the leading causes of death. Children left unattended are unsafe even in shallow water. **B,** Burns are among the top three leading causes of death from injury in children 1 to 14 years old.

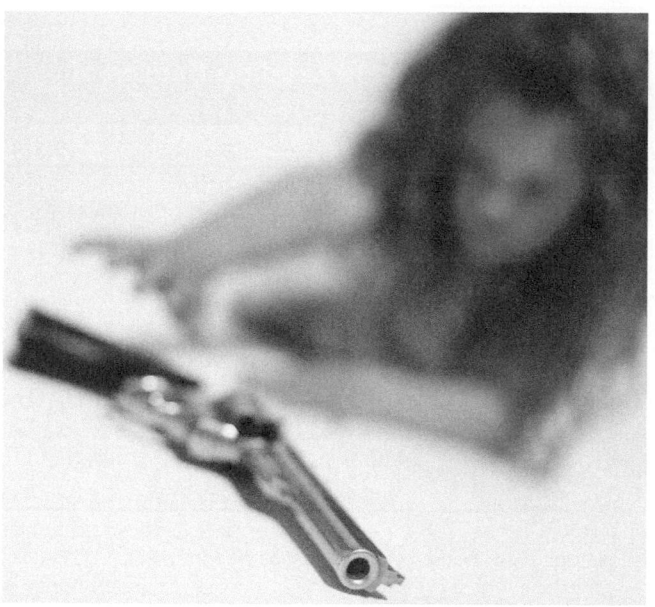

FIG. 1.4 Improper use of firearms is the fourth leading cause of death from injury in children 5 to 14 years old. (© 2012 Photos.com, a division of Getty Images. All rights reserved.)

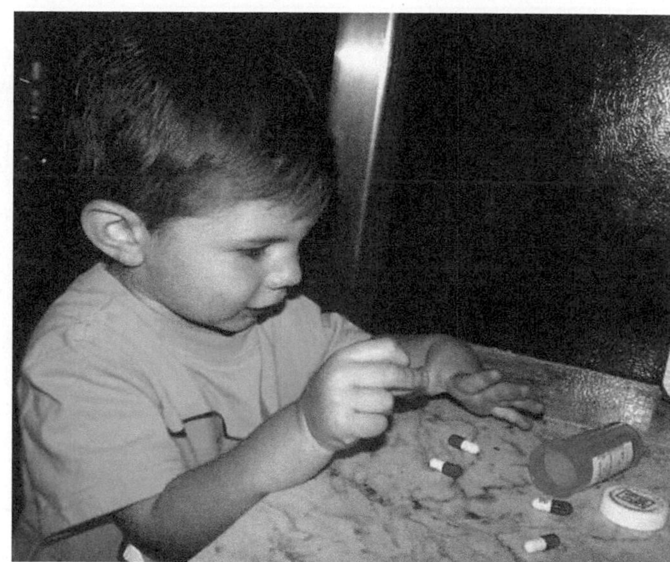

FIG. 1.6 Poisoning causes a considerable number of injuries in children younger than 4 years old. Medications should never be left where young children can reach them.

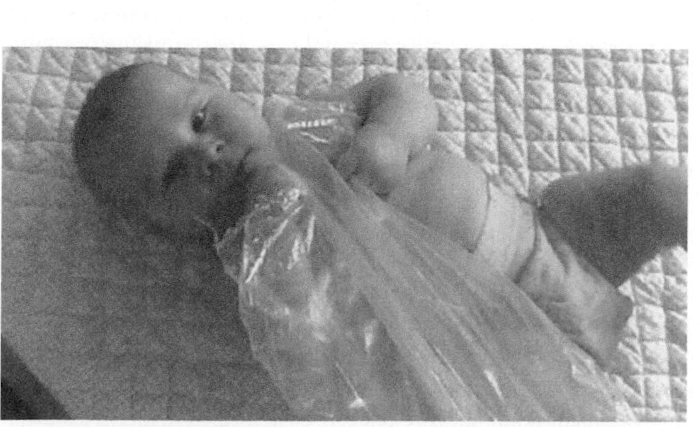

FIG. 1.5 Mechanical suffocation is the leading cause of death from injury in infants.

Violence

Youth violence is a high-visibility, high-priority concern in every sector of American society (David-Ferdon & Simon, 2014). Strikingly higher homicide rates are found among minority populations, especially African American children. The causes of violence against children and self-inflicted violence are not fully understood. Violence seems to permeate American households through television programs, commercials, video games, and movies, all of which tend to desensitize the child toward violence. Violence also permeates the schools with the availability of guns, illicit drugs, and gangs. The problem of child homicide is extremely complex and involves numerous social, economic, and other influences. Prevention lies in a better understanding of the social and psychologic factors that lead to the high rates of homicide and suicide. Nurses need to be especially aware of young people who harm animals or start fires, are depressed, are repeatedly in trouble with the criminal justice system, or are associated with groups known to be violent. Prevention requires early identification and rapid therapeutic intervention by qualified professionals.

COMMUNITY AND HOME HEALTH CONSIDERATIONS

Violence in Children

Community violence has reached epidemic proportions in the United States. The serious problem of community violence affects the lives of many children and expands throughout the family, schools, and the workplace. Nurses working with children, adolescents, and families have a critical role in reducing violence through early identification and symptom recognition of the mental-emotional stress that can result from these experiences.

Violent crimes continue to be a significant health issue for children, with homicide being the second leading cause of death in 15- to 19-year-olds (Annie E Casey Foundation, 2014). The multifaceted origins of violence include developmental factors, gang involvement, access to firearms, drugs, the media, poverty, and family conflict. Often the silent and underrecognized victims are the children who witness acts of community violence. Studies suggest that chronic exposure to violence has a negative effect on a child's cognitive, social, psychologic, and moral development. Also, multiple exposures to episodes of violence do not inoculate children against the negative effects; continued exposure can result in lasting symptoms of stress.

National concern about the increasing prevalence of violent crimes has prompted nurses to actively participate in ensuring that children grow up in safe environments. Pediatric nurses are positioned to assess children and adolescents for signs of exposure to violence and well-known risk factors; nurses also can provide nonviolent problem-solving strategies, counseling, and referrals. These activities affect community practice and expand the nurse's role in the future health environment. Professional resources include the following:

National Domestic Violence Hotline
PO Box 161810
Austin, TX 78716
800-799-SAFE
http://www.ndvh.org

Child Trends
Child Trends Databank. (2015). *Teen homicide, suicide, and firearm deaths.* Retrieved from http://www.childtrends.org/?indicators=teen-homicide-suicide-and-firearm-deaths

TABLE 1.2 Infant Mortality Rate and Percentage of Total Deaths for 10 Leading Causes of Infant Death in 2014*

Rank	Cause of Death (Based on International Classification of Diseases, 10th Revision)	Percent	Rate
	All races, all causes	100.00%	582.1
1	Congenital anomalies	20.4	119.0
2	Disorders relating to short gestation and unspecified low birth weight	18.0	104.6
3	Newborn affected by maternal complications of pregnancy	6.8	39.5
4	Sudden infant death syndrome	6.7	38.7
5	Accidents (unintentional injuries)	5.0	29.1
6	Newborn affected by complications of placenta, cord and membranes	4.2	24.2
7	Bacterial sepsis of newborn	2.3	13.6
8	Respiratory distress of newborn	2.0	11.5
9	Diseases of circulatory system	1.9	11.1
10	Neonatal hemorrhage	1.9	11.1

*Rate per 100,000 live births.
Modified from Kochanek, K.D., Murphy, S.L., Xu, J., et al. (2016). Deaths: Final data for 2014. *National Vital Statistics Report, 65*(4), 1–122.

Pediatric nurses can assess children and adolescents for risk factors related to violence. Families that own firearms must be educated about their safe use and storage. The presence of a gun in a household increases the risk of suicide by about fivefold and the risk of homicide by about threefold. Technologic changes such as childproof safety devices and loading indicators could improve the safety of firearms (see Community and Home Health Considerations box).

Mental Health Problems

One out of five children experiences mental health problems, and 1 out of 10 has a serious emotional problem that affects daily functioning (Flores & Lesley, 2014). Many adolescents with anxiety disorders and impulse control disorders (such as conduct disorder or attention-deficit/hyperactivity disorder [ADHD]) develop these during adolescence. Nurses should be alert to the symptoms of mental illness and potential suicidal ideation and be aware of potential resources for high-quality integrated mental health services.

Infant Mortality

The infant mortality rate is the number of deaths during the first year of life per 1000 live births. It may be further divided into neonatal mortality (<28 days of life) and postneonatal mortality (28 days to 11 months). In the United States the infant mortality rate was 5.82 per 1000 live births, the neonatal mortality rate was 3.94, and the postneonatal mortality rate was 1.88 in 2014 (Centers for Disease Control and Prevention, 2016).

Birth weight is considered the major determinant of neonatal death in technologically developed countries. The relatively high incidence of LBW (<2500 g [5.5 pounds]) in the United States is considered a key factor in its higher neonatal mortality rate compared with other countries. Access to and the use of high-quality prenatal care are promising preventive strategies to decrease early delivery and infant mortality.

As Table 1.2 demonstrates, many of the leading causes of death during infancy continue to occur during the perinatal period. The first four causes—congenital anomalies, disorders relating to short gestation and unspecified LBW, newborn affected by maternal complications of pregnancy, and sudden infant death syndrome—accounted for about half (53%) of all deaths of infants younger than 1 year old (Centers for Disease Control and Prevention, 2016). Many birth defects are associated with LBW, and reducing the incidence of LBW will help prevent congenital anomalies. Infant mortality resulting from human immunodeficiency virus (HIV) infection decreased significantly during the 1990s.

When infant death rates are categorized according to race, a disturbing difference is seen. Infant mortality for Caucasians is considerably lower than for all other races in the United States, with African Americans

TABLE 1.3 Five Leading Causes of Death in Children in the United States: Selected Age Intervals, 2014*

	1–4 YEARS OF AGE		5–9 YEARS OF AGE		10–14 YEARS OF AGE		15–19 YEARS OF AGE	
Rank	**Cause**	**Rate**	**Cause**	**Rate**	**Cause**	**Rate**	**Cause**	**Rate**
	All causes	24.0	All causes	11.5	All causes	14.0	All causes	45.5
1	Injuries	7.6	Injuries	3.6	Injuries	3.6	Injuries	17.7
2	Congenital anomalies	2.5	Cancer	2.1	Suicide	2.1	Suicide	8.7
3	Homicide	2.3	Congenital anomalies	0.9	Cancer	2.0	Homicide	6.7
4	Cancer	2.0	Homicide	0.6	Congenital anomalies	0.8	Cancer	2.9
5	Heart disease	0.9	Heart disease	0.3	Homicide	0.8	Heart disease	1.4

*Rate per 100,000 population.

Modified from Murphy, S. L., Mathews, T. J., Martin, J. A., et al. (2017). Annual summary of vital statistics: 2013-2014. *Pediatrics 139*(6), e20163239.

having twice the rate of Caucasians. The LBW rate is also much higher for African American infants than for any other group. One encouraging note is that the gap in mortality rates between Caucasian and non-Caucasian races (other than African Americans) has narrowed in recent years. Infant mortality rates for Hispanics and Asian–Pacific Islanders have decreased dramatically during the past two decades.

Childhood Mortality

Death rates for children older than 1 year of age have always been lower than those for infants. Children ages 5 to 14 years have the lowest rate of death. However, a sharp rise occurs during later adolescence, primarily from injuries, homicide, and suicide (Table 1.3). In 2014 accidental injuries accounted for 34.4% of all deaths. The second leading cause of death was suicide, accounting for 12.1% of all deaths. The trend in racial differences that occurs in infant mortality is also apparent in childhood deaths for all ages and for both sexes. Caucasians have fewer deaths for all ages, and male deaths outnumber female deaths.

After 1 year of age, the cause of death changes dramatically, with unintentional injuries (accidents) being the leading cause from the youngest ages to the adolescent years. Violent deaths have been steadily increasing among young people ages 10 through 25 years, especially among African Americans and males. Homicide is the third leading cause of death in the 15- to 19-year age-group (see Table 1.3). Children 12 years old and older tend to be killed by non–family members (acquaintances and gangs, typically of the same race) and most frequently by firearms. Suicide, a form of self-violence, is the third leading cause of death among children and adolescents 10 to 19 years old.

Childhood Morbidity

Acute illness is defined as an illness with symptoms severe enough to limit activity or require medical attention. Respiratory illness accounts for approximately 50% of all acute conditions, 11% are caused by infections and parasitic disease, and 15% are caused by injuries. The chief illness of childhood is the common cold.

The types of diseases that children contract during childhood vary according to age. For example, upper respiratory tract infections and diarrhea decrease in frequency with age, whereas other disorders, such as acne and headaches, increase. Children who have had a particular type of problem are more likely to have that problem again. Morbidity is not distributed randomly in children. Recent concern has focused on groups of children who have increased morbidity: homeless children, children living in poverty, LBW children, children with chronic illnesses, foreign-born adopted children, and children in day care centers. A number of factors place these groups at risk for poor health. A major cause is barriers to health care, especially for the homeless, the poverty stricken, and those with chronic health problems. Other factors include improved survival of children with chronic health problems, particularly infants of VLBW.

THE ART OF PEDIATRIC NURSING

PHILOSOPHY OF CARE

Nursing of infants, children, and adolescents is consistent with the American Nurses Association (2010) definition of nursing as the protection, promotion, and optimization of health and abilities, prevention of illness and injury, alleviation of suffering through the diagnosis and treatment of human response, and advocacy in the care of individuals, families, and populations.

Family-Centered Care

The philosophy of family-centered care recognizes the family as the constant in a child's life. Family-centered care is an approach to the planning, delivery, and evaluation of health care that is grounded in mutually beneficial partnerships among health care providers, patients, and families (Institute for Patient- and Family-Centered Care, 2014). Nurses support families in their natural caregiving and decision-making roles by building on their unique strengths and acknowledging their expertise in caring for their child both within and outside the hospital setting. The nurse considers the needs of all family members in relation to the care of the child (Box 1.4). The philosophy acknowledges diversity among family structures and backgrounds; family goals, dreams, strategies, and actions; and family support, service, and information needs.

Two basic concepts in family-centered care are enabling and empowerment. Professionals enable families by creating opportunities and means for all family members to display their current abilities and competencies and to acquire new ones to meet the needs of the child and family. *Empowerment* describes the interaction of professionals with families in such a way that families maintain or acquire a sense of control over their family lives and acknowledge positive changes that result from helping behaviors that foster their own strengths, abilities, and actions.

Although caring for the family is strongly emphasized throughout this text, it is highlighted in features such as Cultural Considerations and Family-Centered Care boxes.

Atraumatic Care

Atraumatic care is the provision of therapeutic care in settings, by personnel, and through the use of interventions that eliminate or minimize the psychologic and physical distress experienced by children and their families in the health care system. Therapeutic care encompasses the prevention, diagnosis, treatment, or palliation of acute or chronic conditions. Setting refers to the place in which that care is given—the home,

BOX 1.4 Key Elements of Family-Centered Care

- Incorporating into policy and practice the recognition that the family is the constant in a child's life, whereas the service systems and support personnel within those systems fluctuate
- Facilitating family-professional collaboration at all levels of hospital, home, and community care:
  - Care of an individual child
  - Program development, implementation, and evaluation
  - Policy formation
- Exchanging complete and unbiased information between family members and professionals in a supportive manner at all times
- Incorporating into policy and practice the recognition and honoring of cultural diversity, strengths, and individuality within and across all families, including ethnic, racial, spiritual, social, economic, educational, and geographic diversity
- Recognizing and respecting different methods of coping and implementing comprehensive policies and programs that provide developmental, educational, emotional, environmental, and financial support to meet the diverse needs of families
- Encouraging and facilitating family-to-family support and networking
- Ensuring that home, hospital, and community service and support systems for children needing specialized health and developmental care and their families are flexible, accessible, and comprehensive in responding to diverse family-identified needs
- Appreciating families as families and children as children, recognizing that they possess a wide range of strengths, concerns, emotions, and aspirations beyond their need for specialized health and developmental services and support

From Shelton, T. L., & Stepanek, J. S. (2014). *Family-centered care for children needing specialized health and developmental services.* Bethesda, MD: Association for the Care of Children's Health.

the hospital, or any other health care setting. Personnel include anyone directly involved in providing therapeutic care. Interventions range from psychologic approaches, such as preparing children for procedures, to physical interventions, such as providing space for a parent to room in with a child. Psychologic distress may include anxiety, fear, anger, disappointment, sadness, shame, or guilt. Physical distress may range from sleeplessness and immobilization to disturbances from sensory stimuli, such as pain, temperature extremes, loud noises, bright lights, or darkness. Thus atraumatic care is concerned with the where, who, why, and how of any procedure performed on a child for the purpose of preventing or minimizing psychologic and physical stress (Wong, 1989).

The overriding goal in providing atraumatic care is as follows: First, do no harm. Three principles provide the framework for achieving this goal: (1) prevent or minimize the child's separation from the family, (2) promote a sense of control, and (3) prevent or minimize bodily injury and pain. Examples of providing atraumatic care include fostering the parent-child relationship during hospitalization, preparing the child before any unfamiliar treatment or procedure, controlling pain, allowing the child privacy, providing play activities for expression of fear and aggression, providing choices to children, and respecting cultural differences.

ROLE OF THE PEDIATRIC NURSE

The pediatric nurse is responsible for promoting the health and well-being of the child and family. Nursing functions vary according to regional job structures, individual education and experience, and personal career goals. Just as patients (children and their families) have unique backgrounds, each nurse brings an individual set of variables that affect the nurse-patient relationship. No matter where pediatric nurses practice, their primary concern is the welfare of the child and family.

There are many different roles for nurses specializing in the care of children and their families. For example, a pediatric nurse can pursue an advanced degree and become a Pediatric Nurse Practitioner (PNP) or Clinical Nurse Specialist (CNS) in pediatrics. PNPs work in a variety of settings and are able to diagnose illnesses and prescribe medication. They provide a spectrum of care from children needing routine examinations and wellness care to caring for children with serious or chronic conditions. CNSs are master's-prepared nurses who function in a variety of settings in both the direct and indirect role. They model expert direct family-centered patient care.

Therapeutic Relationship

The establishment of a therapeutic relationship is the essential foundation for providing high-quality nursing care. Pediatric nurses need to have meaningful relationships with children and their families and yet remain separate enough to distinguish their own feelings and needs. In a therapeutic relationship, caring, well-defined boundaries separate the nurse from the child and family. These boundaries are positive and professional and promote the family's control over the child's health care. Both the nurse and the family are empowered and maintain open communication. In a nontherapeutic relationship, these boundaries are blurred, and many of the nurse's actions may serve personal needs, such as a need to feel wanted and involved, rather than the family's needs. Exploring whether relationships with patients are therapeutic or nontherapeutic helps nurses identify problem areas early in their interactions with children and families (see Nursing Care Guidelines box).

Family Advocacy and Caring

Although nurses are responsible to themselves, the profession, and the institution of employment, their primary responsibility is to the consumer of nursing services: the child and family. The nurse must work with family members, identify their goals and needs, and plan interventions that best address the defined problems. As an advocate, the nurse assists the child and family in making informed choices and acting in the child's best interest. Advocacy involves ensuring that families are aware of all available health services, adequately informed of treatments and procedures, involved in the child's care, and encouraged to change or support existing health care practices.

As nurses care for children and families, they must demonstrate caring, compassion, and empathy for others. Aspects of caring embody the concept of atraumatic care and the development of a therapeutic relationship with patients. Parents perceive caring as a sign of quality in nursing care, which is often focused on the nontechnical needs of the child and family. Parents describe "personable" care as actions by the nurse that include acknowledging the parent's presence, listening, making the parent feel comfortable in the hospital environment, involving the parent and child in the nursing care, showing interest in and concern for their welfare, showing affection and sensitivity to the parent and child, communicating with them, and individualizing the nursing care. Parents perceive personable nursing care as being integral to establishing a positive relationship.

Disease Prevention and Health Promotion

Every nurse involved in caring for children must understand the importance of disease prevention and health promotion. A nursing care plan must include a thorough assessment of all aspects of child growth and development, including nutrition, immunizations, safety, dental care, socialization, discipline, and education. If problems are identified, the nurse intervenes directly or refers the family to other health care providers or agencies.

NURSING CARE GUIDELINES

Exploring Your Relationships With Children and Families

To foster therapeutic relationships with children and families, you must first become aware of your caregiving style, including how effectively you take care of yourself. The following questions should help you understand the therapeutic quality of your professional relationships.

Negative Actions

- Are you overinvolved with children and their families?
- Do you work overtime to care for the family?
- Do you spend off-duty time with children's families, either in or out of the hospital?
- Do you call frequently (either the hospital or home) to see how the family is doing?
- Do you show favoritism toward certain patients?
- Do you buy clothes, toys, food, or other items for the child and family?
- Do you compete with other staff members for the affection of certain patients and families?
- Do other staff members comment to you about your closeness to the family?
- Do you attempt to influence families' decisions rather than facilitate their informed decision making?
- Are you underinvolved with children and families?
- Do you restrict parent or visitor access to children, using excuses such as the unit is too busy?
- Do you focus on the technical aspects of care and lose sight of the person who is the patient?
- Are you overinvolved with children and underinvolved with their parents?
- Do you become critical when parents do not visit their children?
- Do you compete with parents for their children's affection?

Positive Actions

- Do you strive to empower families?
- Do you explore families' strengths and needs in an effort to increase family involvement?
- Have you developed teaching skills to instruct families rather than doing everything for them?
- Do you work with families to find ways to decrease their dependence on health care providers?
- Can you separate families' needs from your own needs?
- Do you strive to empower yourself?
- Are you aware of your emotional responses to different people and situations?
- Do you seek to understand how your own family experiences influence reactions to patients and families, especially as they affect tendencies toward overinvolvement or underinvolvement?
- Do you have a calming influence, not one that will amplify emotionality?
- Have you developed interpersonal skills in addition to technical skills?
- Have you learned about ethnic and religious family patterns?
- Do you communicate directly with persons with whom you are upset or take issue?
- Are you able to "step back" and withdraw emotionally, if not physically, when emotional overload occurs, yet remain committed?
- Do you take care of yourself and your needs?
- Do you periodically interview family members to determine their current issues (e.g., feelings, attitudes, responses, wishes), communicate these findings to peers, and update records?
- Do you avoid relying on initial interview data, assumptions, or gossip regarding families?
- Do you ask questions if families are not participating in care?
- Do you assess families for feelings of anxiety, fear, intimidation, worry about making a mistake, a perceived lack of competence to care for their child, or fear of health care professionals overstepping their boundaries into family territory, or vice versa?
- Do you explore these issues with family members and provide encouragement and support to enable families to help themselves?
- Do you keep communication channels open among self, family, physicians, and other care providers?
- Do you resolve conflicts and misunderstandings directly with those who are involved?
- Do you clarify information for families or seek the appropriate person to do so?
- Do you recognize that from time to time a therapeutic relationship can change to a social relationship or an intimate friendship?
- Are you able to acknowledge the fact when it occurs and understand why it happened?
- Can you ensure that there is someone else who is more objective who can take your place in the therapeutic relationship?

The best approach to prevention is education and anticipatory guidance. In this text, each chapter on health promotion includes sections on anticipatory guidance. An appreciation of the hazards or conflicts of each developmental period enables the nurse to guide parents regarding childrearing practices aimed at preventing potential problems. One significant example is safety. Because each age-group is at risk for special types of injuries, preventive teaching can significantly reduce injuries, lowering permanent disability and mortality rates.

Prevention also involves less obvious aspects of caring for children. The nurse is responsible for providing care that promotes mental well-being (e.g., enlisting the help of a child life specialist during a painful procedure, such as an immunization).

Health Teaching

Health teaching is inseparable from family advocacy and prevention. Health teaching may be the nurse's direct goal, such as during parenting classes, or may be indirect, such as helping parents and children understand a diagnosis or medical treatment, encouraging children to ask questions about their bodies, referring families to health-related professional or lay groups, supplying patients with appropriate literature, and providing anticipatory guidance.

Health teaching is one area in which nurses often need preparation and practice with competent role models because it involves transmitting information at the child's and family's level of understanding and desire for information. As an effective educator, the nurse focuses on providing the appropriate health teaching with generous feedback and evaluation to promote learning.

Injury Prevention

Each year, injuries kill or disable more children older than 1 year old than all childhood diseases combined. The nurse plays an important role in preventing injuries by using a developmental approach to safety counseling for parents of children of all ages. Realizing that safety concerns for a young infant are completely different than injury risks of adolescents, the nurse discusses appropriate injury prevention tips to parents and children as part of routine patient care.

Support and Counseling

Attention to emotional needs requires support and, sometimes, counseling. The role of child advocate or health teacher is supportive by virtue of the individualized approach. The nurse can offer support by listening, touching, and being physically present. Touching and physical presence are most helpful with children because they facilitate nonverbal communication. Counseling involves a mutual exchange of ideas and opinions that provides the basis for mutual problem solving. It involves support, teaching, techniques to foster the expression of feelings or thoughts, and approaches to help the family cope with stress. Optimally, counseling not only helps resolve a crisis or problem but also enables the family to attain a higher level of functioning, greater self-esteem, and closer relationships. Although counseling is often the role of nurses in specialized areas, counseling techniques are discussed in various sections of this text to help students and nurses cope with immediate crises and refer families for additional professional assistance.

Coordination and Collaboration

The nurse, as a member of the health care team, collaborates and coordinates nursing care with the care activities of other professionals. A nurse working in isolation rarely serves the child's best interests. The concept of holistic care can be realized through a unified, interdisciplinary approach by being aware of individual contributions and limitations and collaborating with other specialists to provide high-quality health services. Failure to recognize limitations can be nontherapeutic at best and destructive at worst. For example, the nurse who feels competent in counseling but who is really inadequate in this area may not only prevent the child from dealing with a crisis but also impede future success with a qualified professional. Nursing should be seen as a major contributor to ensuring that the health care team focuses on high-quality, safe care.

Ethical Decision Making

Ethical dilemmas arise when competing moral considerations underlie various alternatives. Parents, nurses, physicians, and other health care team members may reach different but morally defensible decisions by assigning different weights to competing moral values. These competing moral values may include autonomy, the patient's right to be self-governing; nonmaleficence, the obligation to minimize or prevent harm; beneficence, the obligation to promote the patient's well-being; and justice, the concept of fairness. Nurses must determine the most beneficial or least harmful action within the framework of societal mores, professional practice standards, the law, institutional rules, the family's value system and religious traditions, and the nurse's personal values.

Nurses must prepare themselves systematically for collaborative ethical decision making. They can accomplish this through formal course work, continuing education, contemporary literature, and work to establish an environment conducive to ethical discourse.

The nurse also uses the professional code of ethics for guidance and as a means for professional self-regulation. Nurses may face ethical issues regarding patient care, such as the use of lifesaving measures for VLBW newborns or the terminally ill child's right to refuse treatment. They may struggle with questions regarding truthfulness, balancing their rights and responsibilities in caring for children with acquired immune deficiency syndrome (AIDS), whistle-blowing, or allocating resources. Ethical arguments are presented to help nurses clarify their value judgments when confronted with sensitive issues.

RESEARCH AND EVIDENCE-BASED PRACTICE

Nurses should contribute to research because they are the individuals observing human responses to health and illness. The current emphasis on measurable outcomes to determine the efficacy of interventions (often in relation to the cost) demands that nurses know whether clinical interventions result in positive outcomes for their patients. This demand has influenced the current trend toward evidence-based practice (EBP), which implies questioning why something is effective and whether a better approach exists. The concept of EBP also involves analyzing and translating published clinical research into the everyday practice of nursing. When nurses base their clinical practice on science and research and document their clinical outcomes, they will be able to validate their contributions to health, wellness, and cure not only to their patients, third-party payers, and institutions but also to the nursing profession. Evaluation is essential to the nursing process, and research is one of the best ways to accomplish this.

EBP is the collection, interpretation, and integration of valid, important, and applicable patient-reported, nurse-observed, and research-derived information. Using the population/patient problem, intervention, comparison, outcome, and time (PICOT) question to clearly define the problem of interest, nurses are able to obtain the best evidence to improve care. Evidence-based nursing practice combines knowledge with clinical experience and intuition. It provides a rational approach to decision making that facilitates best practice (Melnyk & Fineout-Overholt, 2014). EBP is an important tool that complements the nursing process by using critical thinking skills to make decisions based on existing knowledge. The traditional nursing process approach to patient care can be used to conceptualize the essential components of EBP in nursing. During the assessment and diagnostic phases of the nursing process, the nurse establishes important clinical questions and completes a critical review of existing knowledge. EBP also begins with identification of the problem. The nurse asks clinical questions in a concise, organized way that allows for clear answers. Once the specific questions are identified, extensive searching for the best information to answer the question begins. The nurse evaluates clinically relevant research, analyzes findings from the history and physical examination, and reviews the specific pathophysiology of the defined problem. The third step in the nursing process is to develop a care plan. In evidence-based nursing practice, the care plan is established on completion of a critical appraisal of what is known and not known about the defined problem. Next, in the traditional nursing process, the nurse implements the care plan. By integrating evidence with clinical expertise, the nurse focuses care on the patient's unique needs. The final step in EBP is consistent with the final phase of the nursing process—to evaluate the effectiveness of the care plan.

Searching for evidence in this modern era of technology can be overwhelming. For nurses to implement EBP, they must have access to appropriate, recent resources such as online search engines and journals. In many institutions, computer terminals are available on patient care units, with the Internet and online journals easily accessible. Another important resource for the implementation of EBP is time. The nursing shortage and ongoing changes in many institutions have compounded the issue of nursing time allocation for patient care, education, and training. In some institutions, nurses are given paid time away from performing patient care to participate in activities that promote EBP. This requires an organizational environment that values EBP and its potential impact on patient care. As knowledge is generated regarding the significant impact of EBP on patient care outcomes, it is hoped that the organizational culture will change to support the staff nurse's participation in EBP. As the amount of available evidence increases, so does our need to critically evaluate the evidence.

Throughout this book, Translating Evidence into Practice boxes summarize the existing evidence that promotes excellence in clinical care. The GRADE (Grading of Recommendations Assessment, Development and Evaluation) criteria are used to evaluate the quality of research articles used to develop practice guidelines (Guyatt, Oxman, Vist, et al., 2008). Table 1.4 defines how the nurse rates the quality of the evidence using the GRADE criteria and establishes a strong versus weak recommendation. Each Translating Evidence into Practice box rates the quality of existing evidence and the strength of the recommendation for practice change.

TABLE 1.4 The GRADE Criteria to Evaluate the Quality of the Evidence

Quality	Type of Evidence
High	Consistent evidence from well-performed RCTs or exceptionally strong evidence from unbiased observational studies
Moderate	Evidence from RCTs with important limitations (inconsistent results, flaws in methodology, indirect evidence, or imprecise results) or unusually strong evidence from unbiased observational studies
Low	Evidence for at least one critical outcome from observational studies, from RCTs with serious flaws, or from indirect evidence
Very low	Evidence for at least one of the critical outcomes from unsystematic clinical observations or very indirect evidence
Quality	**Recommendation**
Strong	Desirable effects clearly outweigh undesirable effects, or vice versa
Weak	Desirable effects closely balanced with undesirable effects

RCT, Randomized clinical trial.
Adapted from Guyatt, G. H., Oxman, A. D., Vist, G. E., et al. (2008). GRADE: An emerging consensus on rating quality of evidence and strength of recommendations. *British Medical Journal, 336*, 924-926.

CLINICAL REASONING AND THE PROCESS OF PROVIDING NURSING CARE TO CHILDREN AND FAMILIES

CLINICAL REASONING

A systematic thought process is essential to a profession. It assists the professional in meeting the patient's needs. Clinical reasoning is a cognitive process that uses formal and informal thinking to gather and analyze patient data, evaluate the significant of the information, and consider alternative actions (Simmons, 2010). It is based on the scientific method of inquiry, which is also the basis for the nursing process. Clinical reasoning and the nursing process are considered crucial to professional nursing in that they constitute a holistic approach to problem solving.

Clinical reasoning is a complex developmental process based on rational and deliberate thought. Clinical reasoning provides a common denominator for knowledge that exemplifies disciplined and self-directed thinking. The knowledge is acquired, assessed, and organized by thinking through the clinical situation and developing an outcome focused on optimum patient care. Clinical reasoning transforms the way in which individuals view themselves, understand the world, and make decisions. In recognition of the importance of this skill, Critical Thinking Exercises included in this text demonstrate the importance of clinical reasoning. These exercises present a nursing practice situation that challenges the student to use the skills of clinical reasoning to come to the best conclusion. A series of questions lead the student to explore the evidence, assumptions underlying the problem, nursing priorities, and support for nursing interventions that allow the nurse make a rational and deliberate response. These exercises are designed to enhance nursing performance in clinical reasoning.

NURSING PROCESS

The nursing process is a method of problem identification and problem solving that describes what the nurse actually does. The nursing process model includes assessment, diagnosis outcomes identification, planning, implementation, and evaluation.

Assessment

Assessment is a continuous process that operates at all phases of problem solving and is the foundation for decision making. Assessment involves multiple nursing skills and consists of the purposeful collection, classification, and analysis of data from a variety of sources. To provide an accurate and comprehensive assessment, the nurse must consider information about the patient's biophysical, psychologic, sociocultural, and spiritual background.

Diagnosis

The next stage of the nursing process is problem identification and nursing diagnosis. At this point, the nurse must interpret and make decisions about the data gathered. Not all children have actual health problems; some have a potential health problem, which is a risk state that requires nursing intervention to prevent the development of an actual problem. Potential health problems may be indicated by risk factors, or signs that predispose a child and family to a dysfunctional health pattern and are limited to individuals at greater risk than the population as a whole. Nursing interventions are directed toward reducing risk factors. To differentiate actual from potential health problems, the word *risk* is included in the nursing diagnosis statement (e.g., Risk for Infection).

Signs and symptoms refer to a cluster of cues and defining characteristics that are derived from patient assessment and indicate actual health problems. When a defining characteristic is essential for the diagnosis to be made, it is considered critical. These critical defining characteristics help differentiate between diagnostic categories. For example, in deciding between the diagnostic categories related to family function and coping, the nurse uses defining characteristics to choose the most appropriate nursing diagnosis.

Outcomes Identification

The goal for outcomes identification is to establish priorities and select expected patient outcomes or goals. The nurse organizes information during assessment and diagnosis and clusters these data into categories to identify significant areas and makes one of the following decisions:

- No dysfunctional health problems are evident; health promotion is emphasized.
- Risk for dysfunctional health problems exists; interventions are needed for health promotion and illness prevention.
- Actual dysfunctional health problems are evident; interventions are needed for illness management, illness prevention, and health promotion.
- Specific outcomes are formulated to address the realistic patient- and family-focused goals.

Planning

After identifying specific patient- and family-focused goals, the nurse develops a care plan specific to the identified outcomes. The outcome is the projected or expected change in a patient's health status, clinical condition, or behavior that occurs after nursing interventions have been instituted. The care plan must be established before specific nursing interventions are developed and implemented.

Implementation

The implementation phase begins when the nurse puts the selected intervention into action and accumulates feedback data regarding its effects (or the patient's response to the intervention). The feedback returns in the form of observation and communication and provides a database on which to evaluate the outcome of the nursing intervention. It is imperative that continual assessment of the patient's status occurs throughout all phases of the nursing process, thus making the process a dynamic rather than static problem-solving method. Throughout the implementation stage, the main concerns are the patient's physical safety and psychologic comfort in terms of atraumatic care.

Evaluation

Evaluation is the last step in the nursing care process. The nurse gathers, sorts, and analyzes data to determine whether (1) the established outcome has been met, (2) the nursing interventions were appropriate, (3) the plan requires modification, or (4) other alternatives should be considered. The evaluation phase either completes the nursing process (outcome is met) or serves as the basis for selecting alternative interventions to solve the specific problem.

With the current focus on patient outcomes in health care, the patient's care is evaluated not only at discharge but thereafter as well to ensure that the outcomes are met and there is adequate care for resolving existing or potential health problems. One federal agency that has developed clinical guidelines is the Agency for Healthcare Research and Quality.*

Documentation

Although documentation is not one of the steps of the nursing process, it is essential for evaluation. The nurse can assess, diagnose, and identify problems; plan; and implement without documentation. However, evaluation is best performed with written evidence of progress toward outcomes. The patient's medical record should include evidence of those elements listed in the Nursing Care Guidelines box.

NURSING CARE GUIDELINES

Documentation of Nursing Care

- Initial assessments and reassessments
- Nursing problem and/or patient care needs
- Interventions identified to meet the patient's nursing care needs
- Nursing care provided
- Patient's response to, and the outcomes of, the care provided
- Abilities of patient and/or, as appropriate, significant other(s) to manage continuing care needs after discharge

QUALITY OUTCOME MEASURES

Quality of care refers to the degree to which health services for individuals and populations increase the likelihood of desired health outcomes and are consistent with current professional knowledge (Institute of Medicine, 2000). The progress report to congress on the national strategy for quality improvement in health care focuses on six national quality priorities for health care quality improvement (National Strategy for Quality Improvement in Health Care, 2015)†:

1. Making care safer by reducing harm caused in the delivery of care.
2. Ensuring that each person and family is engaged as partners in their care.
3. Promoting effective communication and coordination of care.
4. Promoting the most effective prevention and treatment practices for the leading causes of mortality, starting with cardiovascular disease.
5. Working with communities to promote wide use of best practices to enable healthy living.
6. Making quality care more affordable for individuals, families, employers, and governments by developing and spreading new health care delivery models.

TABLE 1.5 Examples of Core Pediatric Clinical Care Quality Measures*

Clinical Care Quality Measure	How the Quality Measure Is Evaluated
Childhood Immunization Status	Percentage of children 2 years of age who had four diphtheria, tetanus, and acellular pertussis (DTaP); three polio (IPV), one measles, mumps, and rubella (MMR); three *H. influenzae* type B (HiB); three hepatitis B (Hep B); one chicken pox (VZV); four pneumococcal conjugate (PCV); one hepatitis A (Hep A); two or three rotavirus (RV); and two influenza (flu) vaccines by their second birthday.
Appropriate Treatment for Children with Upper Respiratory Infection (URI)	Percentage of children 3 months to 18 years of age who were diagnosed with upper respiratory infection (URI) and were not dispensed an antibiotic prescription on or 3 days after the episode.
ADHD: Follow-up Care for Children Prescribed Attention-Deficit/ Hyperactivity Disorder (ADHD) Medication	Percentage of children 6-12 years of age and newly dispensed a medication for ADHD who had appropriate follow-up care. Two rates are reported.
Appropriate Testing for Children with Pharyngitis	Percentage of children 2-18 years of age, who were diagnosed with pharyngitis, ordered an antibiotic, and received a group A streptococcus (strep) test for the episode.

*Endorsed by the Centers for Medicare and Medicaid Services and the National Quality Forum. 2014. https://www.cms.gov/regulations-and-guidance/legislation/ehrincentiveprograms/2014_clinicalqualitymeasures.html

The Centers for Medicare and Medicaid Services (CMS) (2017) proposed a core of pediatric clinical care quality measures that align with these high-priority health care improvement goals. These indicators are endorsed by the National Quality Forum (NQF) and designed to guide the effectiveness of pediatric health care programs. Table 1.5 presents a list of examples of quality indicators from the core set of CMS measures. Throughout the chapters, examples of quality indicators endorsed by CMS and the NQF are presented and include a description of how the indicator will be measured. In each of these boxes the measurement name is provided along with the numerator and denominator for the measure to reflect how the indicator is defined. States across the country now use these indicators, usually over a year, to determine their success in meeting the quality measure. We also have developed examples of specific patient-centered quality outcome measures for certain diseases throughout the book. These quality outcome measures

*540 Gaither Road, Suite 2000, Rockville, MD 20850; 301-427-1364; email: info@ahrq.gov; http://www.ahrq.gov.

†National Quality Strategy information can be found at http://www.ahrq.gov/workingforquality/about.htm#priorities.

promote interdisciplinary teamwork, and the boxes throughout this book exemplify measures of effective collaboration to improve care. **Pediatric Quality Indicators** and **Quality Patient Outcomes** boxes throughout this book are developed to assist nurses in identifying appropriate measures that evaluate the quality of patient care.

The Quality and Safety Education for Nurses Institute has defined quality and safety competencies for nursing. The Quality and Safety Education for Nurses Institute is now being hosted by faculty at the Case Western Reserve University and provides a comprehensive overview for the development of knowledge, skills, and attitudes related to quality and safety in health care.* In this book, each Translating Evidence into Practice box includes the Quality and Safety Education for Nurses Institute competencies related to knowledge, skills, and attitudes for evidence-based nursing practice.

*Quality and Safety Education for Nurses Institute, Frances Payne Bolton School of Nursing, Case Western Reserve University; email: qsen.institute@gmail.com.

NCLEX REVIEW QUESTIONS

1. Because injuries are the most common cause of death and disability in children in the United States, which stage of development correctly determines the type of injury that may occur? Select all that apply.
   A. A newborn may roll over and fall off an elevated surface.
   B. The need to conform and gain acceptance from his peers may make a child accept a dare.
   C. Toddlers who can run and climb may be susceptible to burns, falls, and collisions with objects.
   D. A preschooler may ride her two-wheel bike in a reckless manner.
   E. A crawling infant may aspirate due to the tendency to place objects in his mouth.
2. The National Children's Study is the largest prospective, long-term study of children's health and development in the United States. Which of these options are the goals of this study? Select all that apply.
   A. Ensure that every child is immunized at the appropriate age.
   B. Provide information for families to eradicate unhealthy diets, dental caries, and childhood obesity.
   C. Enlist the help of school lunch programs to reach the goal of vegetables and fruits as 30% of each lunch.
   D. Significantly reduce violence, substance abuse, and mental health disorders among the nation's children.
   E. Decrease tardiness and truancy and increase the high school graduation rate in each state over the next 5 years.
3. The newest nurse on the pediatric unit is concerned about maintaining a professional distance in her relationship with a patient and the patient's family. Which comment indicates that she needs more mentoring regarding her patient-nurse relationship?
   A. "I realize that caring for the child means I can visit them on my days off if they ask me."
   B. "When the mother asks if I will care for her daughter every day, I explain that the assignments change based on the needs of the unit."
   C. "When the mother asks me questions about my family, I answer politely, but I offer only pertinent information."
   D. "I engage in multidisciplinary rounds and listen to the family's concerns."
4. What is the overriding goal of atraumatic care?
   A. Prevent or minimize the child's separation from the family
   B. Do no harm
   C. Promote a sense of control
   D. Prevent or minimize bodily injury and pain
5. A family you are caring for on the pediatric unit asks you about nutrition for their baby. What facts will you want to include in this nutritional information? Select all that apply.
   A. Breastfeeding provides micronutrients and immunologic properties.
   B. Eating preferences and attitudes related to food are established by family influences and culture.
   C. Most children establish lifelong eating habits by 18 months old.
   D. During adolescence, parental influence diminishes and adolescents make food choices related to peer acceptability and sociability.
   E. Because of the stress of returning to work, most mothers use this as a time to stop breastfeeding.

Correct Answers

1. B, C, E; 2. B, D; 3. A; 4. B; 5. A, B, D

REFERENCES

American Academy of Pediatrics. (2016). *American Academy of Pediatrics announces new recommendations for children's media use*. https://www.aap.org.

American Nurses Association. (2010). *Nursing's social policy statement: The essence of the profession*. Silver Spring, MD, American Nurses Association.

Annie E Casey Foundation. (2014). *2014 Kids count data book: State profiles of child well-being*. Baltimore, MD, The Foundation.

Bright Futures. (2016). *Prevention and health promotion for infants, children, adolescents, and their families*. http://brightfutures.aap.org/index.html.

Centers for Disease Control and Prevention. (2016). *Injury and violence prevention and control*. http://www.cdc.gov/injury.

Center for Medicaid and Medicare Services. (2017). *Children's health care quality measures*. https://www.medicaid.gov/medicaid/quality-of-care/performance-measurement/child-core-set/index.html.

Clark, C. A., Kent, K. A., & Jackson, R. D. (2015). Open mouth, open mind: Expanding the role of primary care nurse practitioners. *Journal of Pediatric Health Care, 30*(5), 480–488.

David-Ferdon, C., & Simon, T. R. (2014). *Preventing youth violence: Opportunities for action*. Atlanta, GA: National Center for Injury Prevention and Control, Centers for Disease Control and Prevention.

Duncan, G. J., Kirkendall, N. J., & Citro, C. J. (Eds.). (2014). *Panel on the design of the national children's study and implications for the generalizability of results, institute of medicine*. Washington, DC: National Academies Press.

Dye, B. A., Thornton-Evans, G., Li, X., et al. (2015). Dental caries and sealant prevalence inchildren and adolescents in the United States, 2011-2012. *NCHS Data Brief, 191*, 1–7.

Federal Interagency Forum on Child and Family Statistics. (2017). *America's children: Key national indicators of well-being*. Washington, DC, U.S. Government Printing Office. http://www.childstats.gov/americaschildren/index.asp.

Ferguson, R. W., Osterthaler, K., Kaminski, S., et al. (March 2015). *Medicine safety for children: An in-depth look at poison center calls*. Washington, DC: Safe Kids Worldwide.

Flores, G., & Lesley, B. (2014). Children and US federal policy on health and health care. *JAMA Pediatrics, 168*(12), 1155–1163.

Garcia-Mantrana, I., & Collado, M. C. (2016). Obesity and overweight: Impact on maternal and milk microbiome and their role for infant health and nutrition. *Molecular Nutrition & Food Research, 60*(8), 1865–1875.

Godfrey, K. M., Reynolds, R. M., Prescott, S. L., et al. (2016). Influence of maternal obesity on the long-term health of offspring. *The Lancet. Diabetes & Endocrinology*, S2213–S8587.

Guyatt, G. H., Oxman, A. D., Vist, G. E., et al. (2008). GRADE: An emerging consensus on rating quality of evidence and strength of recommendations. *BMJ (Clinical Research Ed.), 336*(7650), 924–926.

Institute for Patient- and Family-Centered Care. (2014). *What is patient- and family-centered health care?* http://www.ipfcc.org/faq.html.

Institute of Medicine. (2000). *Crossing the quality chasm*. Washington, DC: The Institute.

Kids Count data center. (2016). *Child and teen death rate*. http://datacenter.kidscount.org.

Martin, A., Saunders, D. H., Shenkin, S. D., et al. (2014). Lifestyle intervention for improving school achievement in overweight or obese children and adolescents. *The Cochrane Database of Systematic Reviews*, (3), CD009728.

Melnyk, B. M., & Fineout-Overholt, E. (2014). *Evidence-based practice in nursing and healthcare: A guide to best practice*. Philadelphia: Lippincott Williams & Wilkins.

National Strategy for Quality Improvement in Health Care. (2015). *Annual progress report to congress*. Washington, DC: US Department of Health and Human Services.

Simmons, B. (2010). Clinical reasoning: Concept analysis. *Journal of Advanced Nursing, 66*(5), 1151–1158.

US Department of Health and Human Services. (2013). *Healthy people 2020*. http://www.healthypeople.gov/.

Weiss, R., Bremer, A. A., & Lustig, R. H. (2013). What is metabolic syndrome, and why are children getting it? *Annals of the New York Academy of Sciences, 1281*, 123–140.

Wong, D. (1989). Principles of atraumatic care. In V. Feeg (Ed.), *Pediatric nursing: forum on the future: Looking toward the 21st century*. Pitman, NJ: Anthony J Jannetti.

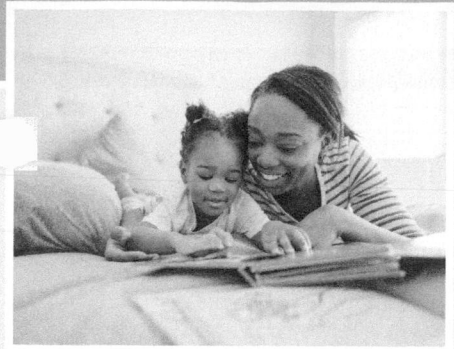

2

Social, Cultural, Religious, and Family Influences on Child Health Promotion

Quinn Franklin and Kim Mooney-Doyle

http://evolve.elsevier.com/wong/ncic

CONCEPTS

- Family Dynamics
- Culture

GENERAL CONCEPTS

DEFINITION OF FAMILY

The term *family* has been defined in many different ways according to the individual's own frame of reference, values, or discipline. There is no universal definition of family; a family is what an individual considers it to be. Biology describes the family as fulfilling the biologic function of perpetuation of the species. Psychology emphasizes the interpersonal aspects of the family and its responsibility for personality development. Economics views the family as a productive unit providing for material needs. Sociology depicts the family as a social unit interacting with the larger society, creating the context within which cultural values and identity are formed. Others define family in terms of the relationships of the persons who make up the family unit. The most common type of relationships are consanguineous (blood relationships), affinal (marital relationships), and family of origin (family unit a person is born into).

Earlier definitions of family emphasized that family members were related by legal ties or genetic relationships and lived in the same household with specific roles. Later definitions have been broadened to reflect both structural and functional changes. A family can be defined as an institution in which individuals, related through biology or enduring commitments and representing similar or different generations and genders, participate in roles involving mutual socialization, nurturance, and emotional commitment (Kaakinen & Coehlo, 2015).

Considerable controversy has surrounded the newer concepts of family, such as communal families, single-parent families, and homosexual families. To accommodate these and other varieties of family styles, the descriptive term *household* is frequently used.

! NURSING ALERT

The nurse's knowledge and the sensitivity with which he or she assesses a household will determine the types of interventions that are appropriate to support family members.

Nursing care of infants and children is intimately involved with care of the child and the family. Family structure and dynamics can have an enduring influence on a child, affecting the child's health and well-being (American Academy of Pediatrics, 2003). Consequently, nurses must be aware of the functions of the family, various types of family structures, and theories that provide a foundation for understanding the changes within a family and for directing family-oriented interventions.

FAMILY THEORIES

A family theory can be used to describe families and how the family unit responds to events both within and outside the family. Each family theory makes assumptions about the family and has inherent strengths and limitations (Kaakinen & Coehlo, 2015). Most nurses use a combination of theories in their work with children and families. Commonly used theories are family systems theory, family stress theory, and developmental theory (Table 2.1).

Family Systems Theory

Family systems theory is derived from general systems theory, a science of "wholeness" that is characterized by interaction among the components of the system and between the system and the environment (Bomar, 2004; Papero, 1990). General systems theory expanded scientific thought from a simplistic view of direct cause and effect (*A* causes *B*) to a more complex and interrelated theory (*A* influences *B*, but *B* also affects *A*). In family systems theory, the family is viewed as a system that continually interacts with its members and the environment. The emphasis is on the interaction between the members; a change in one family member creates a change in other members, which in turn results in a new change in the original member. Consequently, a problem or dysfunction does not lie in any one member but rather in the type of interactions used by the family. Because the interactions, not the individual members, are viewed as the source of the problem, the family becomes the patient and the focus of care. Examples of the application of family systems theory to clinical problems are nonorganic failure to thrive and child abuse. According to family systems theory, the problem does not rest

TABLE 2.1 **Summary of Family Theories and Application**

Assumptions	Strengths	Limitations	Applications
Family Systems Theory			
A change in any one part of a family system affects all other parts of the family system (circular causality). Family systems are characterized by periods of rapid growth and change and periods of relative stability. Both too little change and too much change are dysfunctional for the family system; therefore a balance between morphogenesis (change) and morphostasis (no change) is necessary. Family systems can initiate change, as well as react to it.	Applicable for family in normal everyday life, as well as for family dysfunction and pathology. Useful for families of varying structure and various stages of life cycle.	More difficult to determine cause-and-effect relationships because of circular causality.	Mate selection, courtship processes, family communication, boundary maintenance, power and control within family, parent-child relationships, adolescent pregnancy and parenthood.
Family Stress Theory			
Stress is an inevitable part of family life, and any event, even if positive, can be stressful for family. Family encounters both normative expected stressors and unexpected situational stressors over the life cycle. Stress has a cumulative effect on family. Families cope with and respond to stressors with a wide range of responses and effectiveness.	Potential to explain and predict family behavior in response to stressors and to develop effective interventions to promote family adaptation. Focuses on positive contribution of resources, coping, and social support to adaptive outcomes. Can be used by many disciplines in health care field.	Relationships between all variables in framework not yet adequately described. Not yet known if certain combinations of resources and coping strategies are applicable to all stressful events.	Transition to parenthood and other normative transitions, single-parent families, families experiencing work-related stressors (dual-earner family, unemployment), acute or chronic childhood illness or disability, infertility, death of a child, divorce, teenage pregnancy and parenthood.
Developmental Theory			
Families develop and change over time in similar and consistent ways. Family and its members must perform certain time-specific tasks set by themselves and by persons in the broader society. Family role performance at one stage of family life cycle influences family's behavioral options at next stage. Family tends to be in stage of disequilibrium when entering a new life cycle stage and strives toward homeostasis within stages.	Provides a dynamic, rather than static, view of family. Addresses both changes within family and changes in family as a social system over its life history. Anticipates potential stressors that normally accompany transitions to various stages and when problems may peak because of lack of resources.	Traditional model more easily applied to two-parent families with children. Use of age of oldest child and marital duration as marker of stage transition sometimes problematic (e.g., in stepfamilies, single-parent families).	Anticipatory guidance, educational strategies, and developing or strengthening family resources for management of transition to parenthood; family adjustment to children entering school, becoming adolescents, leaving home; management of "empty nest" years and retirement.

solely with the parent or child but with the type of interactions between the parent and the child and the factors that affect their relationship.

The family is viewed as a whole that is different from the sum of the individual members. For example, a household of parents and one child consists of not only three individuals but also four interactive units. These units include three dyads (the marital relationship, the mother-child relationship, and the father-child relationship) and a triangle (the mother-father-child relationship). In this ecologic model, the family system functions within a larger system, with the family dyads in the center of a circle surrounded by the extended family, the subculture, and the culture, with the larger society at the periphery.

Bowen's family systems theory (Kaakinen & Coehlo, 2015; Papero, 1990) emphasizes that the key to healthy family function is the members' ability to distinguish themselves from one another both emotionally and intellectually. The family unit has a high level of **adaptability**. When problems arise within the family, change occurs by altering the interaction or feedback messages that perpetuate disruptive behavior. **Feedback** refers to processes in the family that help identify strengths and needs and determine how well goals are accomplished. Positive feedback initiates change; negative feedback resists change (Goldenberg & Goldenberg, 2012). When the family system is disrupted, change can occur at any point in the system.

A major factor that influences a family's adaptability is its **boundary**, an imaginary line that exists between the family and its environment (Kaakinen & Coehlo, 2015). Families have varying degrees of openness and closure in these boundaries. For example, one family has the capacity to reach out for help, whereas another considers help threatening. Knowledge of boundaries is critical when teaching or counseling families. Families with open boundaries may demonstrate a greater receptivity to interventions, whereas families demonstrating closed boundaries often require increased sensitivity and skill on the part of the nurse to gain their trust and acceptance. The nurse who uses family systems theory should assess the family's ability to accept new ideas, information, resources, and opportunities and to plan strategies.

Family Stress Theory

Family stress theory explains how families react to stressful events and suggests factors that promote adaptation to stress (Kaakinen &

Coehlo, 2015). Families encounter stressors (events that cause stress and have the potential to effect a change in the family social system), including those that are predictable (e.g., parenthood) and those that are unpredictable (e.g., illness, unemployment). These stressors are cumulative, involving simultaneous demands from work, family, and community life. Too many stressful events occurring within a relatively short period (usually 1 year) can overwhelm the family's ability to cope and place it at risk for breakdown or physical and emotional health problems among its members. When the family experiences too many stressors for it to cope adequately, a state of crisis ensues. For adaptation to occur, a change in family structure or interaction is necessary.

The resiliency model of family stress, adjustment, and adaptation emphasizes that the stressful situation is not necessarily pathologic or detrimental to the family but demonstrates that the family needs to make fundamental structural or systemic changes to adapt to the situation (McCubbin & McCubbin, 1994).

Developmental Theory

Developmental theory is an outgrowth of several theories of development. Duvall (1977) described eight developmental tasks of the family throughout its life span (Box 2.1). The family is described as a small group, a semiclosed system of personalities that interacts with the larger cultural social system. As an interrelated system, the family does not have changes in one part without a series of changes in other parts.

Developmental theory addresses family change over time, using Duvall's family life cycle stages. This theory is based on the predictable changes in the family's structure, function, and roles, with the age of the oldest child as the marker for stage transition. The arrival of the first child marks the transition from stage I to stage II. As the first child grows and develops, the family enters subsequent stages. In every stage the family faces certain developmental tasks. At the same time, each family member must achieve individual developmental tasks as part of each family life cycle stage.

Developmental theory can be applied to nursing practice. For example, the nurse can assess how well new parents are accomplishing the individual and family developmental tasks associated with transition to parenthood. New applications should emerge as more is learned about developmental stages for nonnuclear and nontraditional families.

Family Nursing Interventions

In working with children, the nurse must include family members in their care plan. Research confirms parents' desire and expectation to participate in their child's care (Power & Franck, 2008). To discover family dynamics, strengths, and weaknesses, a thorough family assessment is necessary (see Chapter 4). The nurse's choice of interventions depends on the theoretic family model that is used (Box 2.2). For example, in family systems theory, the focus is on the interaction of family members within the larger environment (Goldenberg & Goldenberg, 2012). In this case using group dynamics to involve all members in the intervention process and being a skillful communicator are essential. Systems theory also presents excellent opportunities for anticipatory guidance. Because each family member reacts to every stress experienced by that system, nurses can intervene to help the family prepare for and cope with changes. In family stress theory the nurse employs crisis intervention strategies to help family members cope with the challenging event. In developmental theory the nurse provides anticipatory guidance to prepare members for transition to the next family stage. Nurses who think family involvement plays a key role in the care of a child are more likely to include families in the child's daily care (Fisher, Lindhorst, Matthews, et al., 2008).

BOX 2.1 Duvall's Developmental Stages of the Family

Stage I—Marriage and an Independent Home: The Joining of Families

Reestablish couple identity.
Realign relationships with extended family.
Make decisions regarding parenthood.

Stage II—Families With Infants

Integrate infants into the family unit.
Accommodate to new parenting and grandparenting roles.
Maintain marital bond.

Stage III—Families With Preschoolers

Socialize children.
Parents and children adjust to separation.

Stage IV—Families With Schoolchildren

Children develop peer relations.
Parents adjust to their children's peer and school influences.

Stage V—Families With Teenagers

Adolescents develop increasing autonomy.
Parents refocus on midlife marital and career issues.
Parents begin a shift toward concern for the older generation.

Stage VI—Families as Launching Centers

Parents and young adults establish independent identities.
Parents renegotiate marital relationship.

Stage VII—Middle-Aged Families

Reinvest in couple identity with concurrent development of independent interests.
Realign relationships to include in-laws and grandchildren.
Deal with disabilities and death of older generation.

Stage VIII—Aging Families

Shift from work role to leisure and semiretirement or full retirement.
Maintain couple and individual functioning while adapting to the aging process.
Prepare for own death and dealing with the loss of spouse and/or siblings and other peers.

Modified from Wright, L. M., & Leahey, M (1984). *Nurses and families: A guide to family assessment and intervention.* Philadelphia, PA: Davis.

FAMILY STRUCTURE AND FUNCTION

FAMILY STRUCTURE

The family structure, or family composition, consists of individuals, each with a socially recognized status and position, who interact with one another on a regular, recurring basis in socially sanctioned ways (Kaakinen & Coehlo, 2015). When members are gained or lost through events such as marriage, divorce, birth, death, abandonment, or incarceration, the family composition is altered and roles must be redefined or redistributed.

Traditionally, the family structure was either a nuclear or extended family. In recent years family composition has assumed new configurations, with the single-parent family and blended family becoming prominent forms. The predominant structural pattern in any society depends on the mobility of families as they pursue economic goals and

BOX 2.2 Family Nursing Intervention

- Behavior modification
- Case management and coordination
- Collaborative strategies
- Contracting
- Counseling, including support, cognitive reappraisal, and reframing
- Empowering families through active participation
- Environmental modification
- Family advocacy
- Family crisis intervention
- Networking, including use of self-help groups and social support
- Providing information and technical expertise
- Role modeling
- Role supplementation
- Teaching strategies, including stress management, lifestyle modifications, and anticipatory guidance

From Friedman, M. M., Bowden, V. R., & Jones, E. G. (2003). *Family nursing: Research theory and practice* (5th ed.). Upper Saddle River, NJ: Prentice Hall.

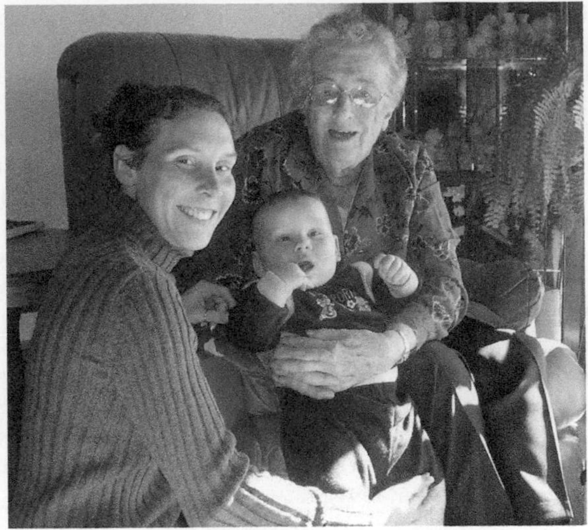

FIG. 2.1 Children benefit from interaction with grandparents, who sometimes assume the parenting role.

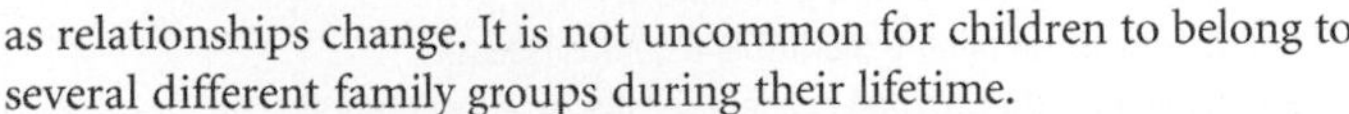

as relationships change. It is not uncommon for children to belong to several different family groups during their lifetime.

Nurses must be able to meet the needs of children from many diverse family structures and home situations. A family's structure affects the direction of nursing care. The US Census Bureau uses four definitions for families: (1) the traditional nuclear family, (2) the nuclear family, (3) the blended family or household, and (4) the extended family or household. In addition, numerous other types of families have been defined, such as single-parent; binuclear; polygamous; communal; and lesbian, gay, bisexual, and transgender (LGBT) families.

Traditional Nuclear Family

A traditional nuclear family consists of a married couple and their biologic children. Children in this type of family live with both biologic parents and, if siblings are present, only full brothers and sisters (i.e., siblings who share the same two biologic parents). No other persons are present in the household (i.e., no steprelatives, foster or adopted children, half-siblings, other relatives, or nonrelatives).

Nuclear Family

The nuclear family is composed of two parents and their children. The parent-child relationship may be biologic, step, adoptive, or foster. Sibling ties may be biologic, step, half, or adoptive. The parents are not necessarily married. No other relatives or nonrelatives are present in the household.

Blended Family

A blended family or household, also called a reconstituted family, includes at least one stepparent, stepsibling, or half-sibling. A stepparent is the spouse of a child's biologic parent but is not the child's biologic parent. Stepsiblings do not share a common biologic parent; the biologic parent of one child is the stepparent of the other. Half-siblings share only one biologic parent.

Extended Family

An extended family or household includes at least one parent, one or more children, and one or more members (related or unrelated) other than a parent or sibling. Parent-child and sibling relationships may be biologic, step, adoptive, or foster.

In many nations and among many ethnic and cultural groups, households with extended families are common. Within the extended family, grandparents often find themselves rearing their grandchildren (Fig. 2.1). Young parents are often considered too young or too inexperienced to make decisions independently. Often, the older relative holds the authority and makes decisions in consultation with the young parents. Sharing residence with relatives also assists with the management of scarce resources and provides child care for working families. A resource for extended families is the Grandparent Information Center.*

Single-Parent Family

In the United States an estimated 24.4 million or 35% of children live in single-parent families (Annie E Casey Foundation, 2017). The contemporary single-parent family has emerged partially as a consequence of the women's rights movement and also as a result of more women (and men) establishing separate households because of divorce, death, desertion, or single parenthood. In addition, a more liberal attitude in the courts has made it possible for single people, both male and female, to adopt children. Although mothers usually head single-parent families, it is becoming more common for fathers to be awarded custody of dependent children in divorce settlements. With women's increased psychologic and financial independence and the increased acceptability of single parents in society, more unmarried women are deliberately choosing mother-child families. Frequently, these mothers and children are absorbed into the extended family. The challenges of single-parent families are discussed later in the chapter.

Binuclear Family

The term *binuclear family* refers to parents continuing the parenting role while terminating the spousal unit. The degree of cooperation between households and the time the child spends with each can vary. In joint custody the court assigns divorcing parents equal rights and responsibilities concerning the minor child or children. These alternate family forms are efforts to view divorce as a process of reorganization

*For information, contact the local AARP representative or office; www.aarp.org/family/grandparenting.

and redefinition of a family rather than as a family dissolution. Joint custody and coparenting are discussed further later in this chapter.

Polygamous Family

Although it is not legally sanctioned in the United States, the conjugal unit is sometimes extended by the addition of spouses in polygamous matings. Polygamy refers to either multiple wives (polygyny) or, rarely, husbands (polyandry). Many societies practice polygyny that is further designated as sororal, in which the wives are sisters, or nonsororal, in which the wives are unrelated. Sororal polygyny is widespread throughout the world. Most often, mothers and their children share a husband and father, with each mother and her children living in the same or separate household.

Communal Family

The communal family emerged from disenchantment with most contemporary life choices. Although communal families may have divergent beliefs, practices, and organization, the basic impetus for formation is often dissatisfaction with the nuclear family structure, social systems, and goals of the larger community. Relatively uncommon today, communal groups share common ownership of property. In cooperatives, property ownership is private, but certain goods and services are shared and exchanged without monetary consideration. There is strong reliance on group members and material interdependence. Both provide collective security for nonproductive members, share homemaking and childrearing functions, and help overcome the problem of interpersonal isolation or loneliness.

Lesbian, Gay, Bisexual, and Transgender Families

A same-sex, homosexual, or lesbian/gay/bisexual/transgender (LGBT) family is one in which there is a legal or common-law tie between two persons of the same sex who have children (Blackwell, 2007). There are a growing number of families with same-sex parents in the United States, with an estimated one-fifth of all same-sex couples raising children (O'Connell & Feliz, 2011; US Census Bureau, 2011). Although some children in gay/lesbian households are biologic from a former marriage relationship, children may be present in other circumstances. They may be foster or adoptive parents, lesbian mothers may conceive through artificial fertilization, or a gay male couple may become parents through use of a surrogate mother.

When children are brought up in LGBT families, the relationships seem as natural to them as heterosexual parents do to their offspring. In other cases, however, disclosure of parental homosexuality ("coming out") to children can be a concern for families. There are a number of factors to consider before disclosing this information to children. Parents should be comfortable with their own sexual preference and should discuss this with the children as they become old enough to understand relationships. Discussions should be planned and take place in a quiet setting where interruptions are unlikely.

Nurses need to be nonjudgmental and to learn to accept differences rather than demonstrate prejudice that can have a detrimental effect on the nurse-child-family relationship (Blackwell, 2007). Moreover, the more nurses know about the child's family and lifestyle, the more they can help the parents and the child.

FAMILY STRENGTHS AND FUNCTIONING STYLE

Family function refers to the interactions of family members, especially the quality of those relationships and interactions (Bomar, 2004). Researchers are interested in family characteristics that help families function effectively. Knowledge of these factors guides the nurse throughout the nursing process and helps the nurse predict ways that families may cope and respond to a stressful event, to provide individualized support that builds on family strengths and unique functioning style, and to assist family members in obtaining resources.

Family strengths and unique functioning styles (Box 2.3) are significant resources that nurses can use to meet family needs. Building on qualities that make a family work well and strengthening family resources make the family unit even stronger. All families have strengths as well as vulnerabilities.

BOX 2.3 Qualities of Strong Families

- A belief and sense of **commitment** toward promoting the well-being and growth of individual family members, as well as the family unit
- **Appreciation** for the small and large things that individual family members do well and **encouragement** to do better
- Concentrated effort to spend **time** and do things together, no matter how formal or informal the activity or event
- A sense of **purpose** that permeates the reasons and basis for "going on" in both bad and good times
- A sense of **congruence** among family members regarding the value and importance of assigning time and energy to meet needs
- The ability to **communicate** with one another in a way that emphasizes positive interactions
- A clear set of **family rules, values,** and **beliefs** that establishes expectations about acceptable and desired behavior
- A varied repertoire of **coping strategies** that promote positive functioning in dealing with both normative and nonnormative life events
- The ability to engage in **problem-solving** activities designed to evaluate options for meeting needs and procuring resources
- The ability to be **positive** and see the positive in almost all aspects of their lives, including the ability to see crisis and problems as an opportunity to learn and grow
- **Flexibility** and **adaptability** in the roles necessary to procure resources to meet needs
- A **balance** between the use of internal and external family resources for coping and adapting to life events and planning for the future

From Dunst, C., Trivette, C., & Deal, A. (1988). *Enabling and empowering families: Principles and guidelines for practice.* Cambridge, MA: Brookline Books.

FAMILY ROLES AND RELATIONSHIPS

Each individual has a position, or status, in the family structure and plays culturally and socially defined roles in interactions within the family. Each family also has its own traditions and values and sets its own standards for interaction within and outside the group. Each determines the experiences the children should have, those they are to be shielded from, and how each of these experiences meets the needs of family members. When family ties are strong, social control is highly effective, and most members conform to their roles willingly and with commitment. Conflicts arise when people do not fulfill their roles in ways that meet other family members' expectations, either because they are unaware of the expectations or because they choose not to meet them.

PARENTAL ROLES

In all family groups, the socially recognized status of father and mother exists with socially sanctioned roles that prescribe appropriate sexual behavior and childrearing responsibilities. The guides for behavior in these roles serve to control sexual conflict in society and provide for prolonged care of children. The degree to which parents are committed and the way they play their roles are influenced by a number of variables and by the parents' unique socialization experience.

Parental role definitions have changed as a result of the changing economy and increased opportunities for women (Bomar, 2004). As the woman's role has changed, the complementary role of the man has also changed. Many fathers are more active in childrearing and household tasks. As the redefinition of sex roles continues in American families, role conflicts may arise in many families because of a cultural lag of the persisting traditional role definitions.

ROLE LEARNING

Roles are learned through the socialization process. During all stages of development, children learn and practice, through interaction with others and in their play, a set of social roles and the characteristics of other roles. They behave in patterned and more or less predictable ways because they learn roles that define mutual expectations in typical social relationships. Although role definitions are changing, the basic determinants of parenting remain the same. Several determinants of parenting infants and young children are parental personality and mental well-being, systems of support, and child characteristics. These determinants have been used as consistent measurements to determine a person's success in fulfilling the parental role.

Parents, peers, authority figures, and other socializing agents who use positive and negative sanctions to ensure conformity to their norms transmit role conceptions. Role behaviors positively reinforced by rewards such as love, affection, friendship, and honors are strengthened. Negative reinforcement takes the form of ridicule, withdrawal of love, expressions of disapproval, or banishment.

In some cultures the role behavior expected of children conflicts with desirable adult behavior. One of the family's responsibilities is to develop culturally appropriate role behavior in children. Children learn to perform in expected ways consistent with their position in the family and culture. The observed behavior of each child is a single manifestation—a combination of social influences and individual psychologic processes. In this way the uniting of the child's intrapersonal system (the self) with the interpersonal system (the family) is simultaneously understood as the child's conduct.

Role structuring initially takes place within the family unit, in which the children fulfill a set of roles and respond to the roles of their parents and other family members (Kaakinen & Coehlo, 2015). Children's roles are shaped primarily by the parents, who apply direct or indirect pressures to induce or force children into the desired patterns of behavior or direct their efforts toward modification of the role responses of the child on a mutually acceptable basis. Parents have their own techniques and determine the course that the socialization process follows.

Children respond to life situations according to behaviors learned in reciprocal transactions. As they acquire important role-taking skills, their relationships with others change. For instance, when a teenager is also the mother but lives in a household with the grandmother, the teenager may be viewed more as an adolescent than as a mother. Children become proficient at understanding others as they acquire the ability to discriminate their own perspectives from those of others. Children who get along well with others and attain status in the peer group have well-developed role-taking skills.

Family Size and Configuration

Parenting practices differ between small and large families. Small families place more emphasis on the individual development of the children. Parenting is intensive rather than extensive, and there is constant pressure to measure up to family expectations. Children's development and achievement are measured against those of other children in the neighborhood and social class. In small families, children have more democratic participation than in larger families. Adolescents in small families identify more strongly with their parents and rely more on them for advice. They have well-developed, autonomous inner controls as contrasted with adolescents from larger families, who rely more on adult authority.

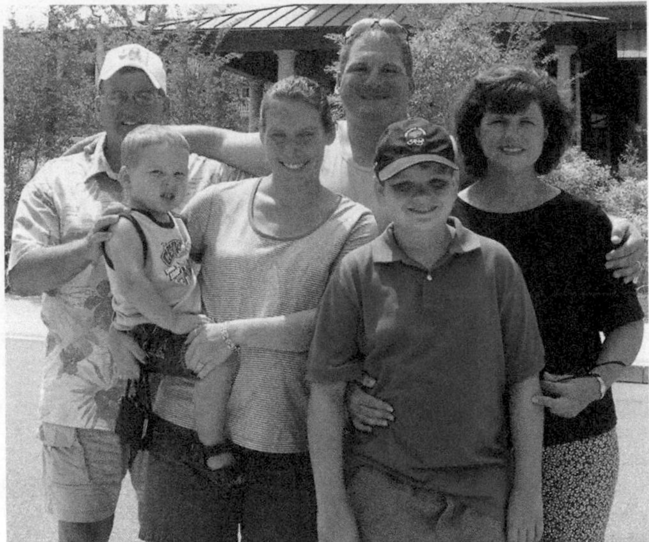

FIG. 2.2 Family structure and function promote strong relationships among its members.

Children in a large family are able to adjust to a variety of changes and crises. There is more emphasis on the group and less on the individual (Fig. 2.2). Cooperation is essential, often because of economic necessity. The large number of people sharing a limited amount of space requires a greater degree of organization, administration, and authoritarian control. A dominant family member (a parent or older child) wields control. The number of children reduces the intimate, one-to-one contact between the parent and any individual child. Consequently, children turn to each other for what they cannot get from their parents. The reduced parent-child contact encourages individual children to adopt specialized roles to gain recognition in the family.

Older siblings in large families often administer discipline (Fig. 2.3). Siblings are usually attuned to what constitutes misbehavior. Sibling disapproval or ostracism is frequently a more meaningful disciplinary measure than parental interventions. In situations such as death or illness of a parent, an older sibling often assumes responsibility for the family at considerable personal sacrifice. Large families generate a sense of security in the children that is fostered by sibling support and cooperation. However, adolescents from a large family are more peer oriented than family oriented.

PARENTING

PARENTING STYLES

Children respond to their environment in a variety of ways. A child's temperament heavily influences his or her response (see Chapter 10), but styles of parenting have also been show to affect a child and lead to particular behavioral responses. Parenting styles are often classified as authoritarian, permissive, or authoritative (Baumrind, 1971, 1996). **Authoritarian** parents try to control their children's behavior and attitudes through unquestioned mandates. They establish rules and

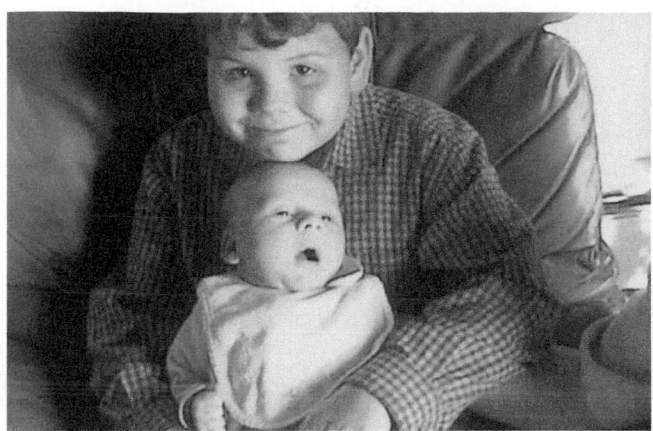

FIG. 2.3 Older school-age children often enjoy taking responsibility for the care of a younger sibling.

regulations or standards of conduct that they expect to be followed rigidly and unquestioningly. The message is: "Do it because I say so." Punishment need not be corporal but may be stern withdrawal of love and approval. Careful training often results in rigidly conforming behavior in the children, who tend to be sensitive, shy, self-conscious, retiring, and submissive. They are more likely to be courteous, loyal, honest, and dependable, but docile. These behaviors are more typically observed when close supervision and affection accompany parental authority. If not, this style of parenting may be associated with both defiant and antisocial behaviors.

Permissive parents exert little or no control over their children's actions. They avoid imposing their own standards of conduct and allow their children to regulate their own activity as much as possible. These parents consider themselves to be resources for the children, not role models. If rules do exist, the parents explain the underlying reason, elicit the children's opinions, and consult them in decision-making processes. They employ lax, inconsistent discipline; do not set sensible limits; and do not prevent the children from upsetting the home routine. These parents rarely punish the children.

Authoritative parents combine practices from both of the previously described parenting styles. They direct their children's behavior and attitudes by emphasizing the reason for rules and negatively reinforcing deviations. They respect the individuality of each child and allow the child to voice objections to family standards or regulations. Parental control is firm and consistent but tempered with encouragement, understanding, and security. Control is focused on the issue, not on withdrawal of love or the fear of punishment. These parents foster "inner-directedness," a conscience that regulates behavior based on feelings of guilt or shame for wrongdoing, not on fear of being caught or punished. Parents' realistic standards and reasonable expectations produce children with high self-esteem who are self-reliant, assertive, inquisitive, content, and highly interactive with other children.

There are differing philosophies in regard to parenting. Childrearing is a culturally bound phenomenon, and children are socialized to behave in ways that are important to their family. In the authoritative style, authority is shared and children are included in discussions, fostering an independent and assertive style of participation in family life. When working with individual families, nurses should give these differing styles equal respect.

LIMIT SETTING AND DISCIPLINE

In its broadest sense, discipline means "to teach" or refers to a set of rules governing conduct. In a narrower sense, it refers to the action taken to enforce the rules after noncompliance. Limit setting refers to establishing the rules or guidelines for behavior. For example, parents can place limits on the amount of time children spend watching television or chatting online. The clearer the limits that are set and the more consistently they are enforced, the less need there is for disciplinary action.

Nurses can help parents establish realistic and concrete "rules." Limit setting and discipline are positive, necessary components of childrearing and serve several useful functions as they help children:

- Test their limits of control
- Achieve in areas appropriate for mastery at their level
- Channel undesirable feelings into constructive activity
- Protect themselves from danger
- Learn socially acceptable behavior

Children want and need limits. Unrestricted freedom is a threat to their security and safety. By testing the limits imposed on them, children learn the extent to which they can manipulate their environment and gain reassurance from knowing that others are there to protect them from potential harm.

Minimizing Misbehavior

The reasons for misbehavior may include attention, power, defiance, and a display of inadequacy (e.g., the child misses classes because of a fear that he or she is unable to do the work). Children may also misbehave because the rules are not clear or consistently applied. Acting-out behavior, such as a temper tantrum, may represent uncontrolled frustration, anger, depression, or pain. The best approach is to structure interactions with children to prevent or minimize unacceptable behavior (see Family-Centered Care box).

General Guidelines for Implementing Discipline

Regardless of the type of discipline used, certain principles are essential to ensure the efficacy of the approach (see Family-Centered Care box). Many strategies, such as behavior modification, can only be implemented effectively when principles of consistency and timing are followed. A pattern of intermittent or occasional enforcement of limits actually prolongs the undesired behavior because children learn that if they are persistent, the behavior is permitted eventually. Delaying punishment weakens its intent, and practices such as telling the child, "Wait until your father comes home" are not only ineffectual but also convey negative messages about the other parent.

Types of Discipline

To deal with misbehavior, parents need to implement appropriate disciplinary action. Many approaches are available. Reasoning involves explaining why an act is wrong and is usually appropriate for older children, especially when moral issues are involved. However, young children cannot be expected to "see the other side" because of their egocentrism. Children in the preoperative stage of cognitive development (toddlers and preschoolers) have a limited ability to distinguish between their point of view and that of others. Sometimes children use "reasoning" as a way of gaining attention. For example, they may misbehave, thinking the parents will give them a lengthy explanation of the wrongdoing and knowing that negative attention is better than no attention. When children use this technique, parents should end the explanation by stating, "This is the rule, and this is how I expect you to behave. I won't explain it any further."

Unfortunately, reasoning is often combined with scolding, which sometimes takes the form of shame or criticism. For example, the parent may state, "You are a bad boy for hitting your brother." Children take such remarks seriously and personally, believing that they are bad.

FAMILY-CENTERED CARE

Minimizing Misbehavior

- Set realistic goals for acceptable behavior and expected achievements.
- Structure opportunities for small successes to lessen feelings of inadequacy.
- Praise children for desirable behavior with attention and verbal approval.
- Structure the environment to prevent unnecessary difficulties (e.g., place fragile objects in an inaccessible area).
- Set clear and reasonable rules; expect the same behavior regardless of the circumstances; if exceptions are made, clarify that the change is for one time only.
- Teach desirable behavior through own example, such as using a quiet, calm voice rather than screaming.
- Review expected behavior before special or unusual events, such as visiting a relative or having dinner in a restaurant.
- Phrase requests for appropriate behavior positively, such as "Put the book down," rather than "Don't touch the book."
- Call attention to unacceptable behavior as soon as it begins; use distraction to change the behavior or offer alternatives to annoying actions, such as exchanging a quiet toy for one that is too noisy.
- Give advance notice or "friendly reminders," such as "When the TV program is over, it is time for dinner" or "I'll give you to the count of three, and then we have to go."
- Be attentive to situations that increase the likelihood of misbehaving, such as overexcitement or fatigue, or decreased personal tolerance to minor infractions.
- Offer sympathetic explanations for not granting a request, such as "I am sorry I can't read you a story now, but I have to finish dinner. Then we can spend time together."
- Keep any promises made to children.
- Avoid outright conflicts; temper discussions with statements such as "Let's talk about it and see what we can decide together" or "I have to think about it first."
- Provide children with opportunities for power and control.

FAMILY-CENTERED CARE

Implementing Discipline

- **Consistency**—Implement disciplinary action exactly as agreed on and for each infraction.
- **Timing**—Initiate discipline as soon as child misbehaves; if delays are necessary, such as to avoid embarrassment, verbally disapprove of the behavior and state that disciplinary action will be implemented.
- **Commitment**—Follow through with the details of the discipline, such as timing of minutes; avoid distractions that may interfere with the plan, such as telephone calls.
- **Unity**—Make certain that all caregivers agree on the plan and are familiar with the details to prevent confusion and alliances between child and one parent.
- **Flexibility**—Choose disciplinary strategies that are appropriate to child's age and temperament and the severity of the misbehavior.
- **Planning**—Plan disciplinary strategies in advance and prepare child if feasible (e.g., explain use of time-out); for unexpected misbehavior, try to discipline when you are calm.
- **Behavior orientation**—Always disapprove of the behavior, not the child, with such statements as "That was a wrong thing to do. I am unhappy when I see behavior like that."
- **Privacy**—Administer discipline in private, especially with older children, who may feel ashamed in front of others.
- **Termination**—After the discipline is administered, consider child as having a "clean slate," and avoid bringing up the incident or lecturing.

! NURSING ALERT

When reprimanding children, focus only on the misbehavior, not on the child. Use of "I" messages rather than "you" messages expresses personal feelings without accusation or ridicule. For example, an "I" message attacks the behavior—"I am upset when Johnny is punched; I don't like to see him hurt"—not the child.

Positive and negative reinforcement is the basis of behavior modification theory—behavior that is rewarded will be repeated; behavior that is not rewarded will be extinguished. Using rewards is a positive approach. By encouraging children to behave in specified ways, the parents can decrease the tendency to misbehave. With young children, using paper stars is an effective method. For older children, the "token system" is appropriate, especially if a certain number of stars or tokens yields a special reward, such as a trip to the movies or a new book. In planning a reward system, the parents must explain expected behaviors to the child and establish rewards that are reinforcing. They should use a chart to record the stars or tokens and always give an earned reward promptly. Verbal approval should always accompany extrinsic rewards.

Consistently ignoring behavior will eventually extinguish or minimize the act. Although this approach sounds simple, it is difficult to implement consistently. Parents frequently "give in" and resort to previous patterns of discipline. Consequently, the behavior is actually reinforced because the child learns that persistence gains parental attention. For ignoring to be effective, parents should (1) understand the process, (2) record the undesired behavior before using ignoring to determine whether a problem exists and to compare results after ignoring is begun, (3) determine whether parental attention acts as a reinforcer, and (4) be aware of "response burst." Response burst is a phenomenon that occurs when the undesired behavior increases after ignoring is initiated because the child is "testing" the parents to see if they are serious about the plan.

The strategy of consequences involves allowing children to experience the results of their misbehavior. It includes three types:

1. Natural—Those that occur without any intervention, such as being late and having to clean up the dinner table
2. Logical—Those that are directly related to the rule, such as not being allowed to play with another toy until the used ones are put away
3. Unrelated—Those that are imposed deliberately, such as no playing until homework is completed or the use of time-out

Natural or logical consequences are preferred and effective if they are meaningful to children. For example, the natural consequence of living in a messy room may do little to encourage cleaning up, but allowing no friends over until the room is neat can be motivating! Withdrawing privileges is often an unrelated consequence. After the child experiences the consequence, the parent should refrain from any comment because the usual tendency is for the child to try to place blame for imposing the rule.

Time-out is a refinement of the common practice of sending the child to his or her room and is a type of unrelated consequence. It is based on the premise of removing the reinforcer (i.e., the satisfaction or attention the child is receiving from the activity). When placed in an unstimulating and isolated place, children become bored and consequently agree to behave in order to reenter the family group (Fig. 2.4). Time-out avoids many of the problems of other disciplinary approaches. No physical punishment is involved; no reasoning or scolding is given; and the parent does not need to be present for all of the time-out, thus facilitating consistent application of this type of discipline.

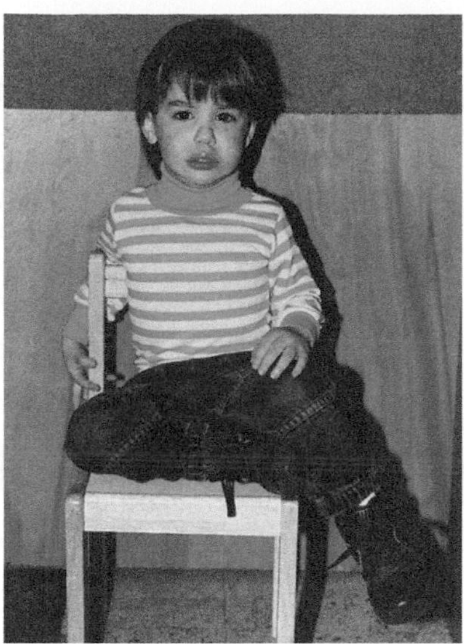

FIG. 2.4 Time-out is an excellent disciplinary strategy for young children.

Time-out offers both the child and the parent a "cooling-off" time. To be effective, however, time-out must be planned in advance (see Family-Centered Care box). Implement time-out in a public place by selecting a suitable area, or explain to children that time-out will be spent immediately on returning home.

FAMILY-CENTERED CARE

Using Time-Out

Select an area for time-out that is safe, convenient, and unstimulating, but where the child can be monitored, such as the bathroom, hallway, or laundry room.

Determine what behaviors warrant a time-out.

Make certain children understand the "rules" and how they are expected to behave.

Explain to children the process of time-out:

- When they misbehave, they will be given one warning. If they do not obey, they will be sent to the place designated for time-out.
- They are to sit there for a specified period.
- If they cry, refuse, or display any disruptive behavior, the time-out period will begin after they quiet down.
- When they are quiet for the duration of the time, they can then leave the room.

A rule for the length of time-out is 1 minute per year of age; use a kitchen timer with an audible bell to record the time rather than a watch.

Corporal or **physical punishment** most often takes the form of spanking (Zolotor & Puzia, 2010). Based on the principles of aversive therapy, inflicting pain through spanking causes a dramatic short-term decrease in the behavior. However, this approach has serious flaws: (1) it teaches children that violence is acceptable; (2) it may physically harm the child if it is the result of parental rage; and (3) children become "accustomed" to spanking, requiring more severe corporal punishment over time. Spanking can result in severe physical and psychologic injury, and it interferes with effective parent-child interaction (Gershoff, 2008). In addition, when the parents are not around, children are likely to misbehave because they have not learned to behave well for their own sake. Parental use of corporal punishment may also interfere with the child's development of moral reasoning.

SPECIAL PARENTING SITUATIONS

Parenting is a demanding task under ideal circumstances, but when parents and children face situations that deviate from "the norm," the potential for family disruption is increased. Situations that are encountered frequently are divorce, single parenthood, blended families, adoption, and dual-career families. In addition, as cultural diversity increases in our communities, many immigrants are making the transition to parenthood and a new country, culture, and language simultaneously. Other situations that create unique parenting challenges are parental alcoholism, homelessness, and incarceration. Although these topics are not addressed here, the reader may wish to investigate them further.

PARENTING THE ADOPTED CHILD

Adoption establishes a legal relationship between a child and parents who are not related by birth but who have the same rights and obligations that exist between children and their biologic parents. In the past the biologic mother alone made the decision to relinquish the rights to her child. In recent years the courts have acknowledged the legal rights of the biologic father regarding this decision. Concerned child advocates have questioned whether decisions that honor the father's rights are in the best interests of the child. As the child's rights have become recognized, older children have successfully dissolved their legal bond with their biologic parents to pursue adoption by adults of their choice. Furthermore, there is a growing interest and demand within the LGBT community to adopt.

Unlike biologic parents, who prepare for their child's birth with prenatal classes and the support of friends and relatives, adoptive parents have fewer sources of support and preparation for the new addition to their family. Nurses can provide the information, support, and reassurance needed to reduce parental anxiety regarding the adoptive process and refer adoptive parents to state parental support groups. Such sources can be contacted through a state or county welfare office.

The sooner infants enter their adoptive home, the better the chances of parent-infant attachment. However, the more caregivers the infant had before adoption, the greater the risk for attachment problems. The infant must break the bond with the previous caregiver and form a new bond with the adoptive parents. Difficulties in forming an attachment depend on the amount of time he or she has spent with caregivers early in life, as well as the number of caregivers (e.g., the birth mother, nurse, adoption agency personnel).

Siblings, adopted or biologic, who are old enough to understand should be included in decisions regarding the commitment to adopt, with reassurance that they are not being replaced. Ways that the siblings can interact with the adopted child should be stressed (Fig. 2.5).

Issues of Origin

The task of telling children that they are adopted can be a cause of deep concern and anxiety. There are no clear-cut guidelines for parents to follow in determining when and at what age children are ready for the information. Parents are naturally reluctant to present such potentially unsettling news. However, it is important that parents not withhold the adoption from the child because it is an essential component of the child's identity.

The timing arises naturally as parents become aware of the child's readiness. Most authorities believe that children should be informed at an age young enough so that, as they grow older, they do not remember a time when they did not know they were adopted. The time is highly

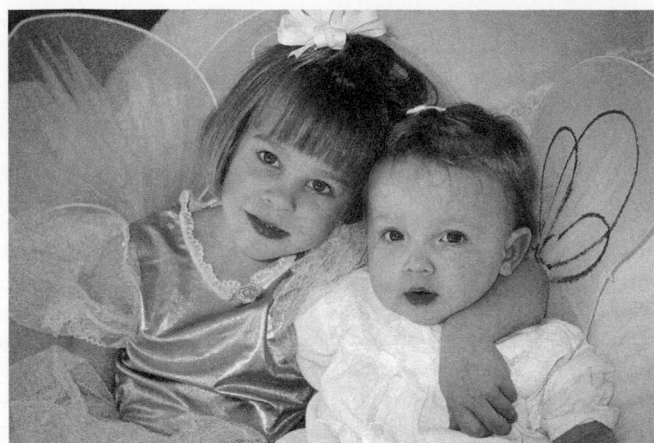

FIG. 2.5 An older sister lovingly embraces her adopted sister.

individual, but it must be right for both the parents and the child. It may be when children ask where babies come from, at which time children can also be told the facts of their adoption. If they are told in a way that conveys the idea that they were active participants in the selection process, they will be less likely to feel that they were abandoned victims in a helpless situation. For example, parents can tell children that their personal qualities drew the parents to them. It is wise for parents who have not previously discussed adoption to tell children that they are adopted before the children enter school to avoid having them learn it from third parties. Complete honesty between parents and children strengthens the relationship.

Parents should anticipate behavior changes after the disclosure, especially in older children. Children who are struggling with the revelation that they are adopted may benefit from individual and family counseling. Children may use the fact of their adoption as a weapon to manipulate and threaten parents. Statements such as "My real mother would not treat me like this" or "You don't love me as much because I'm adopted" hurt parents and increase their feelings of insecurity. Such statements may also cause parents to become overpermissive. Adopted children need the same undemanding love, combined with firm discipline and limit setting, as any other child.

Adolescence

Adolescence may be an especially trying time for parents of adopted children. The normal confrontations of adolescents and parents assume more painful aspects in adoptive families. Adolescents may use their adoption to defy parental authority or as a justification for aberrant behavior. As they attempt to master the task of identity formation, they may begin to have feelings of abandonment by their biologic parents. Gender differences in reacting to adoption may surface.

Adopted children fantasize about their biologic parents and may feel the need to discover their parents' identity to define themselves and their own identity. It is important for parents to keep the lines of communication open and to reassure their child that they understand the need to search for their identity. In some states, birth certificates are made legally available to adopted children when they come of age. Parents should be honest with questioning adolescents and tell them of this possibility (the parents themselves are unable to obtain the birth certificate; it is the children's responsibility if they desire it).

Cross-Racial and International Adoption

Adoption of children from racial backgrounds different from that of the family is commonplace. In addition to the problems faced by adopted children in general, children of a cross-racial adoption must deal with physical and sometimes cultural differences. It is advised that parents who adopt children with different ethnic background do everything to preserve the adopted children's racial heritage.

> **! NURSING ALERT**
>
> As a health care provider, it is important not to ask the wrong questions, such as "Is she yours, or is she adopted?" "What do you know about the 'real' mother?" "Do they have the same father?" or "How much did it cost to adopt him?"

Although the children are full-fledged members of an adopting family and citizens of the adopted country, if they have a strikingly different appearance from other family members or exhibit distinct racial or ethnic characteristics, challenges may be encountered outside the family. Bigotry may appear among relatives and friends. Strangers may make thoughtless comments and talk about the children as though they were not members of the family. It is vital that family members declare to others that this is their child and a cherished member of the family.

In international adoptions the medical information the parents receive may be incomplete or sketchy; weight, height, and head circumference are often the only objective information present in the child's medical record. Many internationally adopted children were born prematurely, and common health problems such as infant diarrhea and malnutrition delay growth and development. Some children have serious or multiple health problems that can be stressful for the parents.

PARENTING AND DIVORCE

Since the mid-1960s, a marked change in the stability of families has been reflected in increased rates of divorce, single parenthood, and remarriage. In 2014 the divorce rate for the United States was 3.2 per 1000 total population (Centers for Disease Control and Prevention, 2016). The divorce rate has changed little since 1987. In the decade before that, the rate increased yearly, with a peak in 1979. Although almost half of all divorcing couples are childless, it is estimated that more than 1 million children experience divorce each year.

The process of divorce begins with a period of marital conflict of varying length and intensity, followed by a separation, the actual legal divorce, and the reestablishment of different living arrangements (Box 2.4). Because a function of parenthood is to provide for the security and emotional welfare of children, disruption of the family structure often engenders strong feelings of guilt in the divorcing parents (Fig. 2.6).

During a divorce, parents' coping abilities may be compromised. The parents may be preoccupied with their own feelings, needs, and life changes and be unavailable to support their children. Newly employed parents, usually mothers, are likely to leave children with new caregivers, in strange settings, or alone after school. The parent may also spend more time away from home, searching for or establishing new relationships. Sometimes, however, the adult feels frightened and alone and begins to depend on the child as a substitute for the absent parent. This dependence places an enormous burden on the child.

Common characteristics in the custodial household after separation and divorce include disorder, coercive types of control, inflammable tempers in both parents and children, reduced parental competence, a greater sense of parental helplessness, poorly enforced discipline, and diminished regularity in household routines. Noncustodial parents are seldom prepared for the role of visitor, may assume the role of recreational and "fun" parent, and may not have a residence suitable for children's

BOX 2.4 The Divorce Process

Acute Phase

- The married couple makes the decision to separate.
- This phase includes the legal steps of filing for dissolution of the marriage and, usually, the departure of the father from the home.
- This phase lasts from several months to more than a year and is accompanied by familial stress and a chaotic atmosphere.

Transitional Phase

- The adults and children assume unfamiliar roles and relationships within a new family structure.
- This phase is often accompanied by a change of residence, a reduced standard of living and altered lifestyle, a larger share of the economic responsibility being shouldered by the mother, and radically altered parent-child relationships.

Stabilizing Phase

- The postdivorce family reestablishes a stable, functioning family unit.
- Remarriage frequently occurs, with concomitant changes in all areas of family life.

Modified from Wallerstein, J. S. (1988). Children of divorce: Stress and developmental tasks. In N. Garmezy & M. Rutter (Eds.), *Stress, coping, and development in children.* New York: McGraw-Hill.

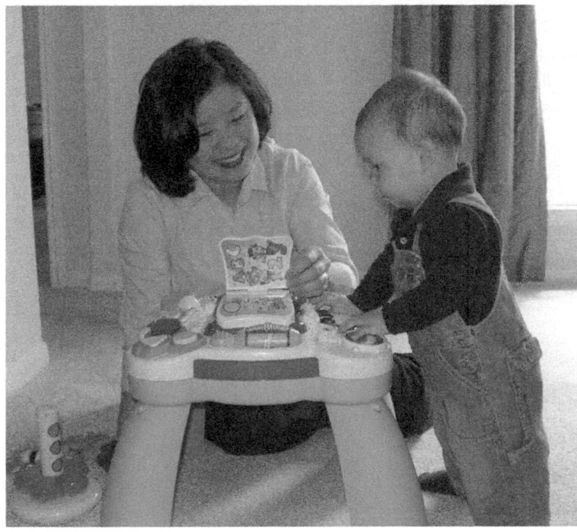

FIG. 2.6 Quality time spent with a child during a divorce is essential to a family's health and well-being.

visits. They may also be concerned about maintaining the arrangement over the years to follow.

Impact of Divorce on Children

Parental divorce is an additional childhood adversity that contributes to poor mental health outcomes, especially when combined with child abuse. Parental psychopathology may be one possible mechanism to explain the relationships between child abuse, parental divorce, and psychiatric disorders and suicide attempts (Afifi, Boman, Fleisher, et al., 2009; McLaughlin, Gadermann, Hwang, et al., 2012). Even when a divorce is amicable and open, children recall parental separation with the same emotions felt by victims of a natural disaster: loss, grief, and vulnerability to forces beyond their control.

The impact of divorce on children depends on several factors, including the age and sex of the children, the outcome of the divorce, and the quality of the parent-child relationship and parental care during the years following the divorce. Family characteristics are more crucial to the child's well-being than specific child characteristics, such as age or sex. High levels of ongoing family conflict are related to problems of social development, emotional stability, and cognitive skills for the child (see Research Focus box).

RESEARCH FOCUS

Impact of Divorce

Children who reported that their divorced parents were cooperative had better relationships with their parents, grandparents, stepparents, and siblings (Ahrons, 2007). Complications associated with divorce include efforts on the part of one parent to subvert the child's loyalties to the other, abandonment to other caregivers, and adjustment to a stepparent.

A major problem occurs when children are "caught in the middle" between the divorced parents. They become the message bearer between the parents, are often quizzed about the other parent's activities, and have to listen to one parent criticize the other. A nurse may be able to help the child get out of the middle by stating "I messages" based on the formula of "I feel (state the feeling) when you (state the source). I would like it if you …" An example of an "I message" is: "I do not feel comfortable when you ask me questions about Mom; maybe you could ask her yourself." This approach enables the child to feel in control.

Feelings of children toward divorce vary with age (Box 2.5). Previously, researchers believed that divorce had a greater impact on younger children, but recent observations indicate that divorce constitutes a major disruption for children of all ages. The feelings and behaviors of children may be different for various ages and gender, but all children suffer stress second only to the stress produced by the death of a parent. Although considerable research has looked at sex differences in children's adjustments to divorce, the findings are not conclusive.

Some children feel a sense of shame and embarrassment concerning the family situation. Sometimes children see themselves as different, inferior, or unworthy of love, especially if they feel responsible for the family dissolution. Although the social stigma attached to divorce no longer produces the emotions it did in the past, such feelings may still exist in small towns or in some cultural groups and can reinforce children's negative self-image. The lasting effects of divorce depend on the children's and the parents' adjustment to the transition from an intact family to a single-parent family and, often, to a reconstituted family.

Although most studies have concentrated on the negative effects of divorce on youngsters, some positive outcomes of divorce have been reported. A successful postdivorce family, either a single-parent or a reconstituted family, can improve the quality of life for both adults and children. If conflict is resolved, a better relationship with one or both parents may result, and some children may have less contact with a disturbed parent. Greater stability in the home setting and the removal of arguing parents can be a positive outcome for the child's long-term well-being.

Telling the Children

Parents are understandably hesitant to tell children about their decision to divorce. Most parents neglect to discuss either the divorce or its inevitable changes with their preschool child. Without preparation, even children who remain in the family home are confused by the parental separation. Frequently, children are already experiencing vague, uneasy feelings that are more difficult to cope with than being told the truth about the situation.

BOX 2.5 Feelings and Behaviors of Children Related to Divorce

Infancy
- Effects of reduced mothering or lack of mothering
- Increased irritability
- Disturbance in eating, sleeping, and elimination
- Interference with attachment process

Early Preschool Children (Ages 2 to 3 Years)
- Frightened and confused
- Blame themselves for the divorce
- Fear of abandonment
- Increased irritability, whining, tantrums
- Regressive behaviors (e.g., thumb sucking, loss of elimination control)
- Separation anxiety

Later Preschool Children (Ages 3 to 5 Years)
- Fear of abandonment
- Blame themselves for the divorce; decreased self-esteem
- Bewilderment regarding all human relationships
- Become more aggressive in relationships with others (e.g., siblings, peers)
- Engage in fantasy to seek understanding of the divorce

Early School-Age Children (Ages 5 to 6 Years)
- Depression and immature behavior
- Loss of appetite and sleep disorders
- May be able to verbalize some feelings and understand some divorce-related changes
- Increased anxiety and aggression
- Feelings of abandonment by departing parent

Middle School-Age Children (Ages 6 to 8 Years)
- Panic reactions
- Feelings of deprivation—loss of parent, attention, money, and secure future
- Profound sadness, depression, fear, and insecurity
- Feelings of abandonment and rejection
- Fear regarding the future
- Difficulty expressing anger at parents
- Intense desire for reconciliation of parents
- Impaired capacity to play and enjoy outside activities
- Decline in school performance
- Altered peer relationships—become bossy, irritable, demanding, and manipulative
- Frequent crying, loss of appetite, sleep disorders
- Disturbed routine, forgetfulness

Later School-Age Children (Ages 9 to 12 Years)
- More realistic understanding of divorce
- Intense anger directed at one or both parents
- Divided loyalties
- Ability to express feelings of anger
- Ashamed of parental behavior
- Desire for revenge; may wish to punish the parent they hold responsible
- Feelings of loneliness, rejection, and abandonment
- Altered peer relationships
- Decline in school performance
- May develop somatic complaints
- May engage in aberrant behavior such as lying, stealing
- Temper tantrums
- Dictatorial attitude

Adolescents (Ages 12 to 18 Years)
- Able to disengage themselves from parental conflict
- Feelings of a profound sense of loss—of family, childhood
- Feelings of anxiety
- Worry about themselves, parents, siblings
- Expression of anger, sadness, shame, embarrassment
- May withdraw from family and friends
- Disturbed concept of sexuality
- May engage in acting-out behaviors

If possible, the initial disclosure should include both parents and siblings, followed by individual discussions with each child. Sufficient time should be set aside for these discussions, and they should take place during a period of calm, not after an argument. Parents who physically hold or touch their children provide them with a feeling of warmth and reassurance. The discussions should include the reason for the divorce, if age appropriate, and reassurance that the divorce is not the fault of the children.

Parents should not fear crying in front of the children because their crying gives the children permission to cry also. Children need to ventilate their feelings. Children may feel guilt, a sense of failure, or that they are being punished for misbehavior. They normally feel anger and resentment and should be allowed to communicate these feelings without punishment. They also have feelings of terror and abandonment. They need consistency and order in their lives. They want to know where they will live, who will take care of them, if they will be with their siblings, and if there will be enough money to live on. Children may also wonder what will happen on special days such as birthdays and holidays, whether both parents will come to school events, and whether they will still have the same friends. Children fear that if their parents stopped loving each other, they could stop loving them. Their need for love and reassurance is tremendous at this time.

Custody and Parenting Partnerships

In the past, when parents separated, the mother was given custody of the children with visitation agreements for the father. Now both parents and the courts are seeking alternatives. Current belief is that neither fathers nor mothers should be awarded custody automatically. Custody should be awarded to the parent who is best able to provide for the children's welfare. In some cases, children experience severe stress when living or spending time with a parent. Many fathers have demonstrated both their competence and their commitment to care for their children.

Often overlooked are the changes that may occur in the children's relationships with other relatives, especially grandparents. Grandparents are increasingly involved in the care of young children (Fergusson, Maughan, & Golding, 2008). Grandparents on the noncustodial side are often kept from their grandchildren, whereas those on the custodial side may be overwhelmed by their adult child's return to the household with grandchildren.

Two other types of custody arrangements are divided custody and joint custody. **Divided custody**, or **split custody**, means that each parent is awarded custody of one or more of the children, thereby separating siblings. For example, sons might live with the father and daughters with the mother.

Joint custody takes one of two forms. In **joint physical custody**, the parents alternate the physical care and control of the children on an agreed-on basis while maintaining shared parenting responsibilities legally. This custody arrangement works well for families who live close to each other and whose occupations permit an active role in the care and rearing of the children. In **joint legal custody**, the children reside with one parent, but both parents are the children's legal guardians, and both participate in childrearing.

Coparenting offers substantial benefits for the family: children can be close to both parents and life with each parent can be more normal (as opposed to having a disciplinarian mother and a recreational father). To be successful, parents in these arrangements must be highly committed to provide normal parenting and to separate their marital conflicts from their parenting roles. No matter what type of custody arrangement is awarded, the primary consideration is the welfare of the children.

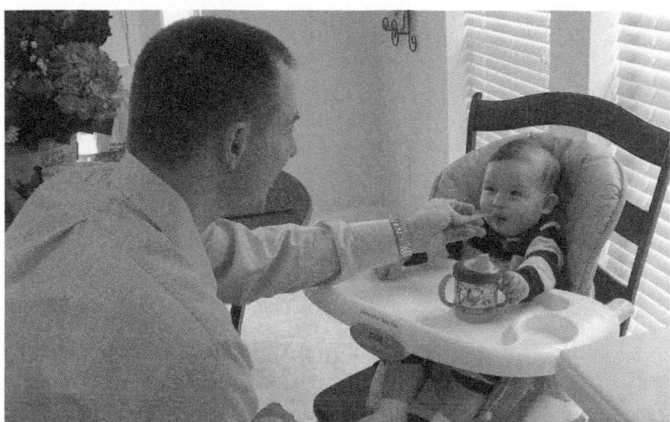

FIG. 2.7 Fathers who assume care of their children may feel more comfortable and successful in their parenting role.

SINGLE PARENTING

An individual may acquire single-parent status as a result of divorce, separation, death of a spouse, or birth or adoption of a child. Although divorce rates have stabilized, the number of single-parent households continues to rise. In 2015, 35% of single-parent families had incomes below the poverty line (Annie E Casey Foundation, 2017). In addition, 35% of children younger than 18 years of age lived in single-parent families, and the majority of single parents were women (Annie E Casey Foundation, 2017; Kreider & Elliott, 2009). Unfortunately, children raised in female-headed households are more likely to drop out of school, be a teen parent, and experience divorce in adulthood. Although some women are single parents by choice, most never planned on being single parents, and many feel pressure to marry or remarry.

Managing shortages of money, time, and energy is often a concern for single parents. Studies repeatedly confirm the financial difficulties of single-parent families, particularly single mothers. In fact, the stigma of poverty may be more keenly felt than the discrimination associated with being a single parent. These families are often forced by their financial status to live in communities with inadequate housing and personal safety concerns. Single parents often feel guilty about the time spent away from their children. Divorced mothers, from marriages in which the father assumed the role of breadwinner and the mother the household maintenance and parenting roles, have considerable difficulty adjusting to their new role of breadwinner. Many single parents have trouble arranging for adequate child care, particularly for a sick child.

Social supports and community resources needed by single-parent families include health care services that are open on evenings and weekends; high-quality child care; respite child care to relieve parental exhaustion and prevent burnout; and parent enhancement centers for advancing education and job skills, providing recreational activities, and offering parenting education. Single parents need social contacts separate from their children for their own emotional growth and that of their children. Parents Without Partners, Inc.* is an organization designed to meet the needs of single parents.

Single Fathers

Fathers who have custody of their children have many of the same problems as divorced mothers. They feel overburdened by the responsibility, depressed, and concerned about their ability to cope with the emotional needs of the children, especially girls. Some fathers lack homemaking skills. They may find it difficult at first to coordinate household tasks, school visits, and other activities associated with managing a household alone (Fig. 2.7).

PARENTING IN RECONSTITUTED FAMILIES

In the United States many of the children living in homes where parents have divorced will experience another major change in their lives, such as the addition of a stepparent or new siblings (Kaakinen & Coehlo, 2015). The entry of a stepparent into a ready-made family requires adjustments for all family members. Some obstacles to the role adjustments and family problem solving include disruption of previous lifestyles and interaction patterns, complexity in the formation of new ones, and lack of social supports. Despite these problems, most children from divorced families want to live in a two-parent home.

Cooperative parenting relationships can allow more time for each set of parents to be alone to establish their own relationship with the children. Under ideal circumstances, power conflicts between the two households can be reduced, and tension and anxiety can be lessened for all family members. In addition, the children's self-esteem can be increased, and there is a greater likelihood of continued contact with grandparents. Flexibility, mutual support, and open communication are critical in successful relationships in stepfamilies and stepparenting situations (Fig. 2.8).

PARENTING IN DUAL-EARNER FAMILIES

No change in family lifestyle has had more impact than the large numbers of women moving away from the traditional homemaker role and entering the workplace (Kaakinen & Coehlo, 2015). The trend toward increased numbers of dual-earner families is unlikely to diminish significantly. As a result, the family is subject to considerable stress as members attempt to meet often competing demands of occupational needs and those regarded as necessary for a rich family life.

Role definitions are frequently altered to arrange a more equitable division of time and labor, as well as to resolve conflict, especially conflict related to traditional cultural norms. Overload is a common source of stress in a dual-earner family, and social activities are significantly curtailed. Time demands and scheduling are major problems for all individuals who work. When the individuals are parents, the demands can be even more intense. Dual-earner couples may increase the strain on themselves to avoid creating stress for their children. Although there is no evidence to indicate that the dual-earner lifestyle is stressful to children, the stress experienced by the parents may affect the children indirectly.

*1650 South Dixie Hwy, Suite 402, Boca Raton, FL 33432; 800-637-7974; http://parentswithoutpartners.org.

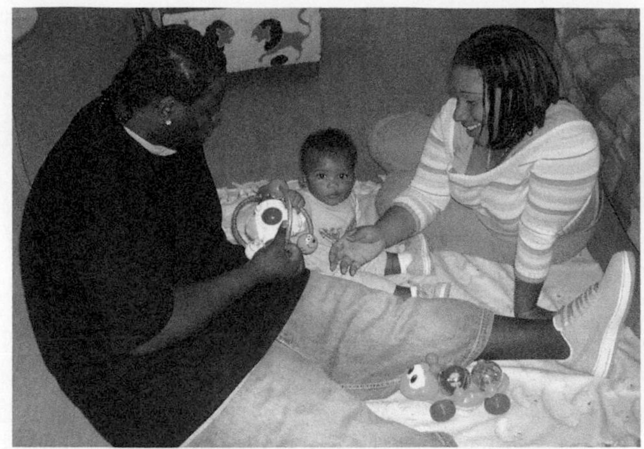

FIG. 2.8 Learning new roles in reconstituted families as a mother and father can enhance parenting relationships.

Working Mothers

Working mothers have become the norm in the United States. Maternal employment may have variable effects on preschool children's health (Goldberg, Prause, Lucas-Thompson, et al., 2008; Mindlin, Jenkins, & Law, 2009). The quality of child care is a persistent concern for all working parents. Determinants of child care quality are based on health and safety requirements, responsive and warm interaction between staff and children, developmentally appropriate activities, trained staff, limited group size, age-appropriate caregivers, adequate staff-to-child ratios, and adequate indoor and outdoor space. Nurses play an important role in helping families find suitable sources of child care and prepare children for this experience (see Alternate Child Care Arrangements, Chapter 10).

Kinship Care

Kinship care refers the the placement of a child in the care of a grandparent or other relative. According to US Census Bureau data, kinship caregivers are more likely to be poor, single, older, less educated, and unemployed than families in which at least one parent is present.

FOSTER PARENTING

The term *foster care* is the temporary placement of a child in an approved living situation away from the birth parents. The living situation may be an approved foster home, possibly with other children, or a preadoptive home. Each state provides a standard for the role of foster parent and a process by which to become one. These "parents" contract with the state to provide a home for children for a limited duration. Most states require about 27 hours of training before being on contract and at least 12 hours of continuing education a year. Foster parents may be required to attend a foster parent support group that is often separate from a state agency. Each state has guidelines regarding the relative health of the prospective foster parents and their families, background checks regarding legal issues for the adults, personal interviews, and a safety inspection of the residence and surroundings (Chamberlain, Price, Leve, et al., 2008).

Foster homes include both kinship and nonrelative placements. Since the 1980s, the proportion of children in out-of-home care placed with relatives has increased rapidly and been accompanied by a decrease in the number of foster families. As with their nonfoster counterparts, much of the child's adjustment depends on the family's stability and available resources. Even though foster homes are designed to provide short-term care, it is not unusual for children to stay for many years.

Nurses should be aware that over 400,000 children spend time living in foster care in a given year, many of them facing developmental concerns (Child Welfare Information Gateway, 2017). Children from lower-income, single-mother, and mother-partner families are considerably more likely to be living in foster care (Berger & Waldfogel, 2004). Foster children are often at risk because of their previous caretaking environment. Nurses should strive to implement strategies to improve the health care for this group of children. In particular, assessment and case management skills are required to involve other disciplines in meeting their needs.

SOCIOCULTURAL INFLUENCES ON CHILDREN AND FAMILIES

A child and his or her immediate family are nested within a local community of school, peers, and extended family and within a larger community that may be bound by common geography, background, traditions, and an even broader community that incorporates the social, political, and economic elements that influence many aspects of family life. These layers of influence are often multifactorial: parents, extended family, and community exert influence most directly when thinking about religious or ethnic background of the family. These elements do come into play when we think about children moving into the wider world, such as their interface with other children at school, or potential biases a child/adolescent might face because of religious or ethnic and racial identity. Thus the sociopolitical context, though an outer layer of a social ecologic model, can exert enormous influence on a child's daily life, opportunities, and outcomes. Equally important to child and family health outcomes, the sociopolitical context draws our attention to factors and health policies at the local, regional, state, and federal levels that can serve as barriers to health equity. This is also made evident through research on the social determinants of health. This section of the chapter will now delve into a deeper discussion of such factors.

The social ecologic model (Kazak, 2001, 2010), rooted in Bronfenbrenner's ecologic model (Bronfenbrenner, 1979, 2005), offers a perspective of viewing children and their families within the context of various circles of influence, called an ecologic framework. This framework posits that individuals adapt in response to changes in their surrounding environments, whether that be the environment of the immediate family, the school, the neighborhood in which the family lives, or the socioeconomic forces that may shape job availability in their geographic area. In addition, Kazak argues that a person's behavior results from the interaction of his or her traits and abilities with the environment. No single factor can explain the totality of a child and his or her family's health behaviors. Children possess their own factors that influence their behavior (i.e., personal history or biologic factors). In turn, they are surrounded by relationships with family, friends, and peers who influence their behavior. Children and their families are then situated within a community that establishes the context in which social relationships develop. Finally, wider sociocultural factors exist that influence whether a behavior is encouraged or prohibited (e.g., social policy on smoking, cultural norms of mothers as primary caregivers of young children, media that can influence how a teen thinks he or she should look).

Promoting the health of children requires a nurse to understand social, cultural, and religious influences on children and their families. The US population is constantly evolving. Patients experience negative health outcomes when social, cultural, and religious factors are not considered as influencing their health care (Chavez, 2012; Williams, 2012). Educating health care providers is one way to reduce disparities in health care.

INFLUENCES IN THE SURROUNDING ENVIRONMENT

SCHOOL COMMUNITIES: SCHOOL HEALTH AND SCHOOL CONNECTEDNESS

Environments differentially support learning through the kinds of opportunities and support provided. Learning and development are cumulative and synergistic; one supports the other. High-quality early childhood education is especially beneficial to set children up for success in early grades. This is especially true for children from disadvantaged backgrounds. Access to this high-quality education is key, yet also occurs along a socioeconomic gradient, with more highly resourced children attending higher-quality preschool programs.

Within communities, schools are important sites for health promotion. Initiatives, such as the Centers for Disease Control and Prevention–sponsored "Whole Child, Whole School, Whole Community," emphasize and build on this critical connection between youth academic performance and health by addressing important elements of children's and adolescents' lives that cut across domains. Examples of such elements include physical education and activity; nutritional environment; counseling; psychologic and social services; social and emotional climate; physical environment; family engagement; and community involvement (Michael, Merlo, Basch, et al., 2015). This approach acknowledges the need for multifaceted strategies to improve academic and health outcomes. It situates school not only as a place to learn but also a place to practice positive health behaviors and health promotion skills. For example, a nutritional health environment constructed in a way to promote child and adolescent health gives youth a chance to live out these skills by making healthy food choices available, by weaving nutrition education into the health curriculum, and by including supportive messaging about healthy nutrition in the school environment (Lewallen, Hunt, Potts-Datema, et al., 2015).

The Centers for Disease Control and Prevention and the World Health Organization identified place-based settings that contribute to individual, family, and population health, including educational settings. Thus schools and early childhood centers can contribute to the health of children by teaching about health and healthy behaviors and also offering ways to enact healthy behaviors (e.g., physical education, coordinated psychosocial or mental health services, healthy snacks). This position addresses potential gaps in care or assessment for children and adolescents because place-based care can improve access for many children and emphasizes coordination among services in a given neighborhood.

An important concept when considering schools as a site of health promotion is connectedness (Centers for Disease Control and Prevention, 2009). *School connectedness* is defined as students' perception that they and their learning matter to the adults at their school and their peers. It is when youth believe that their teachers, staff, and peers care about them academically and personally. The growth and implementation of this concept into educational practice stems from research indicating greater impact on youth health through bolstering protective factors that help children and adolescents avoid risky or unhealthy behaviors. This focus on strengths and promoting positive choices may also help buffer the impact of negative events on children and their health.

Feeling connected at school has important health benefits. Children and youth who feel more connected are more likely to engage in healthy behaviors and do well academically. School connectedness has been found particularly protective against substance abuse, early sexual debut, and violence in both boys and girls. In addition, school connectedness was second only to family connectedness in protection against emotional distress, disordered eating, and suicidal ideation and attempts. Finally, it also promotes academic outcomes in addition to health outcomes, including improved grades, decreased absence, and delayed dropout.

What contributes to school connectedness? Important factors include supportive teachers and school staff, membership in a positive peer group, school environment, and overall commitment to education. Teachers and staff play a pivotal role in promoting a child's sense of being part of a school community. Youth perceptions about themselves are shaped by the degree to which they believe the adults in their community care about them and are involved in their lives. Committed adults in the community create an environment in which youth flourish. When students note that teachers and staff are concerned, are invested in their learning, and care about them personally and academically, students become more engaged. Peer groups are also highly influential for positive and negative outcomes. A positive, stable peer group can protect youth against victimization, whereas a peer group composed of youth participating in negative behaviors can have a detrimental effect of health and academic outcomes. Also, the extent to which students believe their teachers, staff, and peers value education influences the overall commitment to education as a way to improve one's life and reach goals. Youth who internalize this commitment to education exhibit persistence, effort, and sustained attention to tasks. Finally, the physical and psychosocial climate of the school matters and is characterized by respectful relationships and disciplinary practices, clean and physically safe spaces for learning, and broad opportunities for student and family participation. Recommended strategies for achieving school connectedness include effective training for teachers and staff to create positive learning environments, opportunities for families to become involved in the process and associated training, and provision of important academic, emotional, and social skills to students (and addressing of barriers to achieving these skills) so that students can feel engaged and have a stake in their education (Centers for Disease Control and Prevention, 2016).

SCHOOLS

When children enter school, their radius of relationships extends to include a wider variety of peers and a new source of authority. Although parents continue to exert the major influence on children, in the school environment teachers have the most significant psychologic impact on children's development and socialization. In addition to academic and cognitive progress, teachers are concerned with the emotional and social development of the children in their care. Both parents and teachers act to model, shape, and promote positive behavior, constrain negative behavior, and enforce standards of conduct. Ideally, parents and teachers work together for the benefit of the children in their care.

Schools serve as a major source of socialization for children. Next to the family, schools exert a major force in providing continuity and passing down culture from one generation to the next. This, in turn, prepares children to carry out the social roles they are expected to assume as they develop into adults. School is the center of **cultural diffusion** wherein the cultural standards of the larger group are disseminated into the community. It governs what is taught and, to a great extent, how it is taught. School rules and regulations regarding attendance, authority relationships, and the system of rewards and penalties based on achievement transmit to children the expectations of the adult world of employment and relationships. School is an important institution in which children systematically learn about the negative consequences of behavior that departs from social expectations. School also serves as an avenue for children to participate in the larger society in rewarding ways, to promote social mobility, and to connect the family with new knowledge and services. Like parents, teachers are responsible for

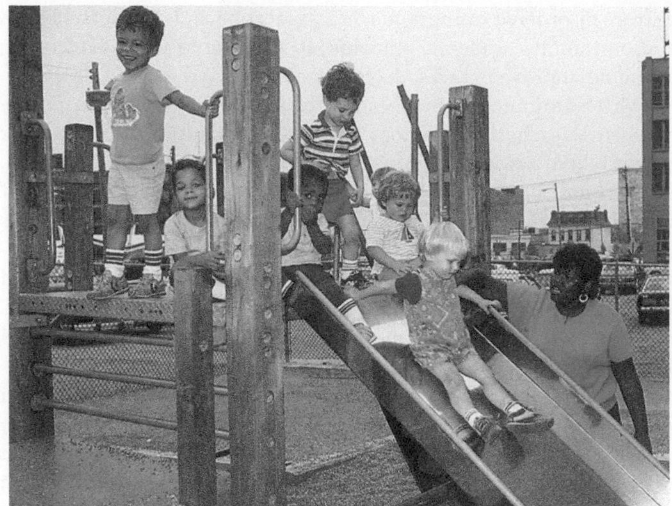

FIG. 2.9 Youngsters from different cultural backgrounds interact within the larger culture.

transmitting knowledge and culture (i.e., values on which there is a broad consensus) to the children in their care. Teachers are also expected to stimulate and guide children's intellectual development and creative problem solving.

PEER CULTURES

Peer groups also have an impact on the socialization of children (Fig. 2.9). Peer relationships become increasingly important and influential as children proceed through school. In school, children have what can be regarded as a culture of their own. This is even more apparent in unsupervised playgroups because the culture in school is partly produced by adults.

During their lives, children are subjected to many influential factors, such as family, religious community, and social class. In peer-group interactions, they confront a variety of these sets of values. The values imposed by the peer group are especially compelling because children must accept and conform to them to be accepted as members of the group. When the peer values are not too different from those of family and teachers, the mild conflict created by these small differences serves to separate children from the adults in their lives and to strengthen the feeling of belonging to the peer group.

The kind of socialization provided by the peer group depends on the subculture that develops from its members' background, interests, and capabilities. Some groups support school achievement, others focus on athletic prowess, and still others are decidedly against educative goals. Many conflicts between teachers and students and between parents and students can be attributed to fear of rejection by peers. What is expected from parents regarding academic achievement and what is expected from the peer culture often conflict, especially during adolescence.

Although the peer group has neither the traditional authority of the parents nor the legal authority of the schools for teaching information, it manages to convey a substantial amount of information to its members, especially on taboo subjects such as sex and drugs. Children's need for the friendship of their peers brings them into an increasingly complex social system. Through peer relationships, children learn to deal with dominance and hostility and to relate with persons in positions of leadership and authority. Other functions of the peer subculture are to relieve boredom and to provide recognition that individual members do not receive from teachers and other authority figures.

COMMUNITY

Families and communities are often interwoven in their impact on child health. Although both are essential to socioemotional growth and improved learning outcomes in children, their influence on children is synergistic. When families live in areas of concentrated poverty, residents experience risk at population and individual levels. Children and families living in areas of concentrated poverty are at risk for negative health outcomes and experience higher rates of crime and violence. In addition, affected neighborhoods are more likely to have poor-performing schools, limited access to high-quality preschool and diminished school readiness, and poorer overall education outcomes. If parents have grown up in the area or a similar area, they have also experienced untoward effects on their health or educational outcomes. As a result, they may not be able to secure employment that provides greater resources for them to invest in their child, or that provides economic stability for the family. Financial stressors in parents contribute to their stress and depression, which can inhibit effective parenting. Thus we see an important need for two-generation programs or strategies to both build on family and community strengths and diminish their stressors.

Community-level factors are especially important as we consider the life, safety, and causes of death in older adolescents. For example, over 70% of teen deaths are attributed to accidents, homicide, and suicide, and community-level factors, such as violence, drug use, and alcohol use, influence this number (Annie E Casey Foundation, 2017).

BROADER INFLUENCES ON CHILD HEALTH

SOCIAL MEDIA AND MASS MEDIA

Digital technologies that serve as an avenue to mass and social media are pervasive in most parts of American society. Technology has a role in the lives of children more than ever before. The American Academy of Pediatrics (2016a) found that children younger than 5 years of age, across socioeconomic levels, use digital technology daily and are frequently targeted by advertisers. This frequent use carries risks for increased rates of obesity, disrupted sleep, and delays in cognitive, social, and language development, potentially related to diminished parent-child interaction in preschoolers. Research has demonstrated that there is limited benefit of digital technology for children younger than 2 years, also likely related to diminished parent-child interaction. Benefits related to digital technology use are related to the type of content viewed and used. For example, high-quality programming, such as *Sesame Street,* can bolster cognitive and social outcomes in preschool-age children, and applications from similar organizations (e.g., PBS or Sesame Workshop) can promote literacy skills. Unfortunately, many programs and applications targeted to children and their parents or caregivers are not created under the direction of educators or developmental experts and may not prove as beneficial to child social and cognitive outcomes. In addition, less than 30% of children from lower-income homes view high-quality digital media, perpetuating potential risks posed by the technology and associated disparities. Despite technologic advances, play, social interactions with peers, and parent-child interactions remain vital to young children's development of the skills needed to succeed in school, including persistence, emotional regulation, and creative thinking (American Academy of Pediatrics, 2016a).

The digital landscape for older children and adolescents seems to change and grow on a daily basis and is woven into daily life for many youth. Indeed, recent research indicates that nearly 75% of adolescents have a smart phone or mobile technology device and approximately half report feeling addicted to their phone (American Academy of Pediatrics, 2016b). While using these mobile devices, most adolescents are engaging in social media, with nearly three-fourths engaging in multiple social media sites and cultivating a portfolio (American Academy of Pediatrics, 2016b; Reid Chassiakos, et. al, 2016). This immersion poses both benefits and risks to these youth. In terms of the benefits, youth have an unprecedented chance to learn and gather information and consider new perspectives; to connect with other youth, which is especially important for youth who may feel marginalized or isolated; and maintain connections with family and friends who live at a distance.

On the other hand, navigating this landscape includes potential risks to physical and mental health, such as obesity, disrupted sleep, addictive behavior, negative impact on academics, bullying and sexual exploitation, and normalization of maladaptive behavior (e.g., sites that promote disordered eating or self-harm). Similar to traditional forms of media (e.g., television), research has demonstrated that social media postings can influence perceptions of alcohol and drug use and younger age of initiating sexual activity as normal in the eyes of adolescents (American Academy of Pediatrics, 2016b). Traditional forms of mass media, such as television and movies, can reify gender and racial stereotypes, thus perpetuating negative mental and emotional health outcomes (American Academy of Pediatrics, 2016b; Reid Chassiakos, et. al., 2016). Finally, communication among adolescents has shifted and become more pervasive through texting, messaging through gaming systems, and messaging on social media sites. This continual access and inlet to the lives of peers can serve as both a source of support and a source of derision and stress. Thus it is essential for nurses and other health care providers to talk with older children and adolescents about the frequency, content, and nature of their digital and social media use and how they maintain their privacy and safety. Equally important, nurses can help families devise strategies and personalized plans for safe and healthy technology use (American Academy of Pediatrics, 2016b) (Box 2.6 and Table 2.2).

RACE AND ETHNICITY

Race and ethnicity are socially constructed terms used to group people who share similar characteristics, traditions, or historical experience together. **Race** is a term that groups together people by their outward, physical appearance. **Ethnicity** is a classification aimed at grouping "individuals who consider themselves, or are considered by others, to

BOX 2.6 Actions to Promote Positive Media

Parents

- Follow American Academy of Pediatrics recommendations for 2 total hours of screen time daily for children ages 2 years and older.
- Establish clear guidelines for Internet use and provide direct supervision. Have frank discussions of what youth may encounter in viewing media. Be mindful of own media use in the home.
- Encourage unstructured play in the home and plan to help children readjust to this change in family dynamic. Consider planned, deliberate use of media to experience the benefits (e.g., watching a television show together to bond or start a sensitive discussion).

Nurses/Health Care Providers

- Dedicate a few minutes of each visit to provide media screening and counseling.
- Discourage presence of electronic devices in children's rooms.
- Be sensitive to the challenges that parents face in carrying this out.

Schools

- Offer timely, accurate sexuality and drug education.
- Promote resilience.
- Develop programs to educate youth on wise use of technology.
- Develop and implement policies on dealing with cyber-bullying and sexting.

TABLE 2.2 Media Effects on Children and Adolescents

Media Effect	Potential Consequences
Violence	Government, medical, and public health data show that exposure to media violence is one factor in violent and aggressive behavior. Both adults and children become desensitized by violence witnessed through various media, including television (including children's programming), movies (including G rated), music, and video games. In addition, cyber-bullying and harassment via text messages are a growing concern among middle school and high school students.
Sex	A significant body of research shows that sexual content in the media can contribute to beliefs and attitudes about sex, sexual behavior, and initiation of intercourse. Teens access sexual content through a variety of media: television, movies, music, magazines, Internet, social media, and mobile devices. Current issues receiving attention for the role they play in teen sexual behavior include sending of sexual images via mobile devices (i.e., sexting), impact of violent media on youth views of women and forced sex/rape, cyber-bullying LGBT youth.
	Media can also serve as a positive source of sexual information (i.e., information, apps, social media about sexually transmitted infections, teen pregnancy, and promoting acceptance and support of LGBT youth).
Substance use and abuse	Although the causes of teen substance use and abuse are numerous, media play a significant role. Alcohol and tobacco are still heavily marketed to adolescents/young adults. Television and movies featuring the use of these substances can influence initiation of use. Media also show substance use to be pervasive and without consequences. Finally, content shared over social networking sites can serve as a form of peer pressure and can influence likelihood of use.
Obesity	Highly prevalent public health issue among children of all ages and increasing rates around the world. A number of studies have demonstrated a link between the amount of screen time and obesity. Advertising of unhealthy food to children is a long-standing marketing practice, which may increase snacking in the face of decreased activity. In addition, both increased screen time and unhealthy eating may also be related to unhealthy sleep.
Body image	Media may play a significant role in the development of body image awareness, expectations, and body dissatisfaction among young and older adolescent girls. Their beliefs may be influenced by images on television, movies, and magazines. New media also contribute to this through Internet images, social network sites, and websites that encourage disordered eating (Strasburger, Jordan, & Donnerstein, 2012).

share common characteristics that differentiate them from the other collectivities in a society, and from which they develop their distinctive cultural behavior" (Scott & Marshall, 2009). Ethnicities may be differentiated from one another by customs and language and may influence family structure, food preferences, and expressions of emotion. The composition and definition of ethnic groups can be fluid in response to changes in geography (i.e., moving from one country to another). Race and ethnicity influence a family's health when they are used as criteria by which a child or family is discriminated against. There is a significant body of work that describes this. In fact, 100 years of research describe racial gaps in health (Williams, 2012).

Racism remains an important social determinant of health. According to Williams (2012), for minority or other groups who experience stigmatization, "inequalities in health are created by larger inequalities in society," meaning that prevailing social conditions and obstacles to equal opportunities for all influences the health of all individuals. For example, from birth forward, African American and Native American children have a higher mortality rate than Caucasian children in general. There is also a higher death rate for babies of African American and Hispanic women versus Caucasian women. Even when controlling for maternal levels of education, the infant mortality rate for college-educated African American women is 2.5 times higher than Hispanic and Caucasian women of similar education level (Williams, 2012). These numbers demonstrate that children and families ultimately feel the effects of such health disparities.

Children and families may also experience perceived racism, which also has negative consequences. For example, in a study of more than 5000 fifth-graders, 15% of Hispanic youth and 20% of African American youth reported that they had experienced racial discrimination. Such experiences were then associated with a higher risk of mental health symptoms (Coker, Elliot, Kanouse, et al., 2009). Teens also report racial discrimination through online communities, social networking sites, and texting, which is related to increased anxiety and depression (Tynes, Giang, Williams, et al., 2008).

Ethnocentrism is the emotional attitude that one's own ethnic group is superior to others; that one's values, beliefs, and perceptions are the correct ones; and that the group's ways of living and behaving are the best (Spector, 2009). Ethnocentrism implies that all other groups are inferior. Stereotyping or labeling stems from ethnocentric beliefs. It is a common attitude among the dominant ethnic group and strongly influences a person's ability to evaluate objectively the beliefs and behaviors of others. Nurses must overcome the natural tendency to have ethnocentric attitudes when caring for people from backgrounds different from their own (Scott & Marshall, 2009).

SOCIAL CLASS

The influence of social class cannot be overlooked. This relates to the family's economic and educational levels and their ability to access resources needed to thrive in daily life. Strength of family relationships is not tied to social class. A family of lower socioeconomic status may have fewer resources, but they may be well connected to the broader family network and rely on them for support to meet physical and emotional needs. Families in higher socioeconomic groups may have access to resources that reach beyond their extended family but may be disconnected because of pressures of work and outside obligations (e.g., children's activities).

POVERTY

Our Health starts in the environment where we live, work, and playOpportunities to promote this health or risks to this health often begin in our families, schools, neighborhoods, and places of employment. Thus to fully promote child health and diminish risks to it, we need to understand how the surrounding context and environments are influential. Children are nested within layers of family, peers, school, and community; we can consider the direct impact of these outside systems interacting with the child and family. Equally important, however, is the influence of factors within the sociopolitical landscape at local/state/regional/national/and international levels. These factors affect the creation of health and social policies that may perpetuate health disparities or make health equity possible.

The circumstances into which a child is born can determine the child's exposure to factors that promote or compromise healthy development. For example, adverse events can have long-lasting impact into adulthood. Layers of the child's surrounding environment that contribute to health inequity fall into socioeconomic, political, and cultural contexts, including local, state, and federal policies; daily living conditions; and the circumstances in which people live, work, and play.

Child health disparities are discrepancies that are based in avoidable differences and are concerning because of the immense and foundational development that occurs in early childhood. Health inequities, in a similar vein, are defined as differences in health states between populations that are socially produced and systemic in unequal distribution across populations that are avoidable and unfair. Health follows a social gradient—better health outcomes with increased socioeconomic status and further improvements with movements up in socioeconomic status. Similarly, compromised health outcomes are associated with lower economic status. Inequitable access to services maintains or perpetuates health inequities in early childhood because the children most in need of services are most likely to not receive them. Multilevel, multifactorial responses to address these issues include policies that improve access to high-quality services and connect parents to secure, stable, flexible workplaces; service systems that deliver inclusive programs rooted in research and evidence; and timely assistance for parents so that they can feel successful in their parenting role.

Economy and Poverty

A major factor that affects child and family health in the United States is poverty. Nearly one fifth of all American children live in families with annual incomes below 100% of the federal poverty level (approximately $22,000) and almost one-half of children live 200% below the federal poverty limit ($44,000 for a family of four) (Fierman, Beck, Chung, et al., 2016). Poverty affects children and their families across all geographic areas, including urban, suburban, and rural. Several social factors associated with poverty that can negatively affect child health are family disruption, parental depression, substance use, other mental illnesses, unsafe homes or neighborhoods, housing instability, homelessness, decreased educational opportunities, and low parent educational levels and health literacy (Fierman, Beck, Chung, et al., 2016).

Poverty influences these social determinants of health, the circumstances and environments in which people are born, live, work, learn, and play. In turn, these social determinants shape child health in major and lasting ways. Poverty itself is a major cause of acute and chronic stress for adults and children. The daily stressors associated with poverty are overwhelming, and other circumstances, such as trauma or violence, can add to the stress experienced by parents and children. This overwhelming stress can undermine skills in dealing with challenging situations. The stressors associated with poverty can be psychologically and emotionally depleting, yet supports to deal with this depletion may not be available, such as adequate mental health services, high-quality and affordable child care, or social supports (Center on the Developing Child at Harvard University, 2016).

Considering the impact of poverty on children, an important place to look is the brain. Children's brains are dynamic and plastic and change according to what they experience. This impact is greatest in young children and adolescence because their brains go through such rapid development. Even as early as the prenatal period, children are affected by the stressors of their surrounding environments, and poverty carries multiple important stressors with it that affect health, such as housing instability, poor or compromised nutrition, unsafe living conditions, lack of insurance, or financial hardship related to insurance copayments or medications that inhibit use of prenatal care. Additionally, parents and caregivers who are overwhelmed by the stressors associated with poverty or trauma may be less able to participate in reciprocal communication with an infant or young child. Affected caregivers may not respond or infant crying or cues as needed or may become irritable, which then propels the infant toward a dysregulated state. Parent and infant are caught in a stressful cycle, and it may then be harder for the parent to prevent a harsh response in this challenging situation. Serious, early, adverse events can affect development of the prefrontal cortex, influencing later self-regulation, emotional responsiveness, and reactivity. Severe, chronic adversity early in life can trigger toxic stress responses that affect brain development and response and diminish mental health. Early exposure to stressful events is associated with challenges to working memory, attention, emotional regulation skills, and perception of new situations as potential threats that require quick action. Thus "the ways in which we have experienced the world fundamentally frame how we perceive our environment and the choices made in this environment" (Center on the Developing Child at Harvard University, 2016, p. 7).

Infants and toddlers are more likely to live in poverty than older children. Thus some of the most profound effects of poverty are demonstrated in young children, such as increased prevalence of low birth weight and infant mortality and delayed language development. These risks can perpetuate other lifetime hazards, such as diminished health status due to chronic illness or compromised academic performance.

An important element of economic status to consider is insurance status. Nearly one fifth of US children are underinsured because of the inability to pay more than one health-related cost or service in the past year. Parents' perception of their child's health is related to their state of being underinsured; in one study, approximately 60% and 90% of parents who reported that their child's health had suffered in the past several years were underinsured (Spears et al., 2013). Underinsurance imposes financial difficulties on families. This reminds us that having insurance does not automatically negate financial distress or impact on families. High out-of-pocket costs (e.g., copays, medications, supplies) and associated costs for transportation to appointments, parking at hospitals, meals while a child is hospitalized, and child care for siblings contribute to this distress (Mooney-Doyle, dos Santos, Bousso, et al., in press).

Underserved children are defined as "children who live in families who cannot afford clinician recommended health care despite having insurance coverage for children" (Spears et al., 2013). Additionally, two-thirds of families that have problems paying health care bills have health insurance. Thus for many families, especially those whose child has a significant health care need, high out-of-pocket costs are stressful and financially taxing. Underinsurance imposes financial stressors on families; having insurance does not totally eliminate financial hardship.

Parental Education

Parent level of education is another important consideration when we consider economic influences on child health. Parent educational level exerts an important influence on children and must also be considered. Child economic status is directly tied to parental earnings. Parental earnings from employment are affected by parental level of education. Income inequality is pervasive and has become worse in recent history. Although some families are catching up on what was lost in the great recession in 2008, many of the jobs that could help decrease income inequality require a college degree and only one-third of adults in the United States have such degrees. Thus many children in the United States are living in families in which parents face employment dissatisfaction and barriers, contributing to stress or negative parental or family outcomes (Annie E Casey Foundation, 2017). Although this issue affects children across races, ethnicities, and geographic settings, children of color disproportionately live in homes without sufficient finances (12% white children versus 36% African American children versus 31% Latino children). Gaps in income undermine a family's ability to access social mobility and move permanently out of poverty (American Academy of Pediatrics, 2016c).

The high incidence and pervasive nature of child poverty demands that pediatric nurses and other health care providers incorporate screening for poverty or financial hardship into everyday practice. Pediatric nurses, despite geographic context, will likely care for children and families encountering poverty. Context influences the experience of poverty and how health care providers address it. Nurses can screen in various ways and connect children and families with the right services, including Head Start, United Way, and the Nurse Family Partnership.

The American Academy of Pediatrics recommends that this screening be done at each well visit by asking about ability to meet basic needs, such as heat, shelter, and food. To address the issue, the American Academy of Pediatrics recommends that pediatric health care providers build on family strengths such as cohesion, humor, support, and spiritual beliefs, and advocate for creation of programs to address the multiple facets of childhood poverty that are rooted in research (American Academy of Pediatrics, 2016c). Barriers to screening exist, however, and derail providers with the best of intentions. Barriers include not recognizing the impact of poverty or the measurable outcomes associated with it; lack of time; limited and insufficient training in assessment, and limited familiarity with assessment tools; and limited knowledge about available community resources. Pediatric nurses and health care providers can initiate surveillance and screening to elicit and address parent concerns; identify risk and protective factors; screen for specific issues; and refer child and family to the right place with the right services. To address the social determinants of health, screening can be tailored to the most sensitive or sustained issues in the community, to parent sources of concern, and to child developmental stage.

Economic barriers impede parents' ability to provide for their children. Thus pediatric nurses and other health care providers must imbue their practice with an understanding of the challenges families face, integrate care to minimize the strain of interacting with health and social services (informed by the knowledge that emotional care of the family is within the scope of pediatrics), and minimize the effects of toxic stress through supportive care services that build on family strengths (American Academy of Pediatrics, 2013, 2016c).

In the words of Sir Michael Marmot, one of the first to recognize the impact of social determinants of health, "it is a reasonable conclusion that poverty reduction will be good for children's physical, psychological, social, and emotional development" (Marmot, 2015).

LAND OF ORIGIN AND IMMIGRATION STATUS

Cultural factors are woven into social, economic, and political influences on child health, including the misconception that children are oblivious to or not deeply affected by the world around them. This perception of children can color governments' and policymaking bodies' work on behalf of children and families. In addition, young childhood is often perceived to be in the domain of the home; thus calls for universal preschool are not heeded.

The demographics of the United States are changing, yet race and ethnicity remain important social determinants of health for many children. Children of color are disproportionately represented in impoverished communities and schools, yet they will comprise the majority of children in 13 states by 2020. This demonstrates one way in which a child's chances for thriving depend not only on child, family, and community characteristics, but also on the state in which the child lives because of variations in health and social services available. State policy choices and investments can have a tremendous impact on child health (Annie E Casey Foundation, 2014, 2017).

Considering the broader context of where children and families live, work, and play is complex when we care for children and families who are considered refugees or undocumented immigrants. For these children and families, we must consider not only where they are within the United States and in our particular site for care, but also where they been and where they have left. Nearly half of the world's displaced people are children (Murray, 2015), amounting to over 20 million children. Within this group are both children and families who have fled their home countries and those who are internally displaced within their home country. Nonetheless, these children and their families often experience mental and physical trauma; they may have experienced danger and violence in both staying in their homes and fleeing. For children and families who journey to a new destination, there are dangers along the journey, including inclement weather, discrimination in destination countries, potential loss of loved ones along the journey, further threats to safety in refugee camps, and lack of food and water. For children and adolescents who journey alone, they face heightened threats of abduction, trafficking, sexual violence and exploitation, or abuse.

For nurses caring for children who have arrived in the United States for resettlement, it is important to know that children and families will have already fled one country, arrived in a second country, and are resettled in a third country. Thus trauma and psychologic distress may come not only from extraordinary threats of violence, but also from constant disruption to family life. In fact, psychologic distress and mental illness are the major causes of disability among refugee children as they frequently experience posttraumatic stress, grief, anxiety, and depression (Murray, 2015). In terms of physical health, the greatest risks stem from infectious diseases and malnutrition. The leading causes of infectious disease related death among refugees are tuberculosis, malaria, and intestinal parasites, often due to overcrowding, poor sanitation, or inability to institute standing transmission-prevention measures in campsites. Nurses caring for these children and families must keep in mind that their assessment and treatment procedures may need to be accommodated because of trauma and stress children have already experienced. Nurses must also be aware of signs of exploitation or abuse, indicating that a child or adolescent may be a victim of trafficking, such as elevated fear or unexplained injuries. The process of disentangling the child and family's story may unfold over time after trust has been established.

Undocumented immigrants are another group of children and families that may have untoward health outcomes and for whom nurses will provide care. Undocumented immigrants are defined as "foreign-born, non-citizens residing in a country, who do not have legal documentation" (Tiedje & Plevak, 2014). Because of their own or their parents' undocumented status, children may be particularly vulnerable to limited access to health care. Negative health effects are often associated with being an undocumented immigrant and are related to poverty, poor living and working conditions, food insecurity, chronic stress, and ongoing fear of deportation and arrest. Despite the negative health effects, research demonstrates that undocumented immigrants seek health care at lower rates than other groups. Although programs such as the Migrant Health Program exist to provide access to low-cost primary care, barriers families face in accessing this care include language barriers, lack of transportation, difficulty arranging for time off from work, and limited ability to pay.

The health care system is an important layer of influence in the health of children. Although this can be a site of health promotion, health maintenance, and illness management, it may also erect barriers for families to enact the care prescribed, For example, health care system factors contribute to parents' completion of subspecialty referrals for the child (Zuckerman et al., 2013). Although child and family factors accounted for some influence (child care, transport, inadequate insurance), health care system factors had a major impact on completion of referrals. These factors included ability to get an appointment quickly, communication style of front-desk staff, and interpreter services. Thus health care system factors may be most amenable to intervention such as extended evening hours, clear directions to clinic site, and a unit navigator (Zuckerman et al., 2013).

RELIGION/SPIRITUAL IDENTITY

Religion and spirituality are powerful forces in the lives of individuals, families, and communities. Spirituality and religion are important principles around which families organize their responses to illness experiences and life transitions. Indeed, nearly 80% of people report that religion is fairly important to them. The terms, however, are often conflated. Religion and spirituality, although frequently grouped together, denote different entities. Religion is a specific set of beliefs enacted through a practice (religiosity) (Taylor, Petersen, Oyedele, et al., 2015). Spirituality is described as a unique awareness, belief, practice, and experience starting in childhood and is rooted over time. Religion and spirituality are important avenues through which children participate in meaning-making around important life events, such as illness in themselves or loved ones (Lima et al., 2013) and are shaped by the developmental stage of the child (Taylor, Petersen, Oyedele, et al., 2015). Further, spiritual assessment is necessary to provide family-centered care that is aligned with spiritual and religious needs. Finally, many regulatory bodies that guide practice call for assessment of and intervention for spiritual concerns, including the American Nurses Association, the International Council of Nurses, and The Joint Commission.

Individual, family, and community experiences of religion and spirituality are interrelated and children experience them from their own, individualized experience as someone situated within a community, and they also experience what the community as a whole experiences. For example, children whose families practice the Islamic faith experience the religion within the home and what their own relationship to Allah means. They also experience the religion from the perspective of being part of a community when attending mosque or participating in collective prayer. They also might experience being part of a faith community that may face stigma or bias or whose tenets are misunderstood. In many instances, religion and spirituality propel people toward virtuous actions and behaviors. Most of the world's religions share a common thread of "upholding humility, charity, and honesty" (Holden & Williamson, 2014).

When individuals become parents, they may connect to their religion as a guide in raising their children, to enhance their well-being, and to provide a moral and social context for their childrearing (Fig. 2.10). Although parents may employ an approach to parenting that is informed by their religion and spirituality, how this is enacted or operationalized varies dramatically because of variability in beliefs about parenting

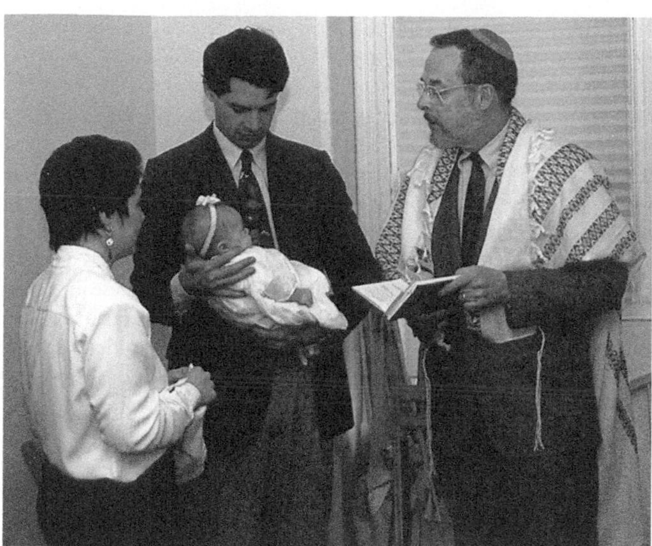

FIG. 2.10 Soon after an infant is born, many families have special religious ceremonies.

BOX 2.7 Guidelines for Integrating Spiritual Care Into Pediatric Nursing Practice

- Respect the child's and family's religious beliefs and practices.
- Consider the child's development when talking about spiritual concerns.
- Contact the institution's chaplaincy department for patients and families who have symptoms of spiritual distress or ask for specific religious rituals.
- Become knowledgeable about the religious worldviews of cultural groups found in the patients you care for.
- Encourage visitation with family members, members of the patient's spiritual community, and spiritual leaders.
- Allow children and families to teach you about the specifics of their religious beliefs.
- Develop awareness of your own spiritual perspective.
- Listen for understanding rather than agreement or disagreement.

Data from Brooks, B. (2004). Spirituality. In N. Kline (Ed.), *Essentials of pediatric oncology nursing: A core curriculum* (2nd ed.). Glenview, IL: Association of Pediatric Oncology Nurses; Barnes, L. L., Plotnikoff, G. A., Fox, K., et al. (2000). Spirituality, religion, and pediatrics: Intersecting worlds of healing. *Pediatrics 106*(4 suppl), 899-908.

goals and roles, the parent-child relationship, and child discipline and punishment (Holden & Williamson, 2014).

Additionally, parents' spirituality, religious practices, and beliefs have are a guiding force on their children. Thus considering the "family-based spirituality care," comprehensive, collaborative, spiritual care is important in addressing the spiritual needs of children who are ill and acknowledges the interrelated relationships of child, parent, and family spirituality (Box 2.7). In the context of pediatric illness, this is also important as children and families are often isolated from their faith communities and experience crises for which they have no prior experience to draw on or that cause existential questioning and meaning-seeking. Children and families receiving a new or life-threatening diagnosis often experience fear and anxiety and may benefit from health care providers helping them connect to those spiritual and religious practices that are important to them. For example, nurses can help families find a suitable place to pray and asking families which of their health care practices may be most helpful in addressing their spiritual needs.

Children who experience major life transitions, such as being diagnosed with a life-threatening illness or the death of a loved one, often experience spirituality as a source of hope and comfort that promotes their resilience and helps them discern the meaning of the life transition for them. Yet there is a paucity of research on children's spiritual development in a contemporary context (Taylor, Petersen, Oyedele, et al., 2015). Children, adolescents, and young adults have unique spiritual needs related to their developmental stage. For example, adolescents and young adults may be a greater risk for spiritual distress because of their more sophisticated understanding of the impact and risk of illness; diagnosis of a life-threatening illness can cause an internal spiritual struggle and questioning of beliefs. They may engage less with institutionalized religion, but still use spirituality as a means of finding meaning and connecting with family and loved ones (Taylor, Petersen, Oyedele, et al., 2015). By asking about and facilitating access to spiritual care, nurses can help build on child and family strengths as they deal with a critical juncture in their lives. Other key practices include avoiding assumptions about spiritual beliefs and practices; asking how the child and family understand the illness's or life event's spiritual impact on the affected individual, other family members, and the family unit; taking time to explore one's own spiritual and religious perspective so that one's values can be clarified and judgments evaluated; active listening that is compassionate and keeps the child's spiritual needs at the center, without false reassurances; and incorporating arts or storytelling into spiritual assessment and intervention. Providing space in the physical environment for children to participate in their spirituality in ways that bring them comfort and provide for meaning-making opportunities is essential as it can provide a glimpse into their spiritual distress and sources of hope. For example, the provider can elicit an adolescent's narrative of his or her illness situation or life event and invite parents or caregivers to listen and share their reaction to promote family connection and communication.

Nurses can also develop skills and access training to help them feel prepared for when children ask spiritually oriented questions. For example, Ferrell, Wittenberg, Battista, and colleagues (2016) queried children's palliative care nurses and found that children facing life-threatening illnesses most often ask questions about the time-limited nature of their illness, why this has happened to them, and why their divine would allow this to happen to them. They found that children often described the after-life without fear, sadness, or pain and with angels or predeceased loved ones caring for them in the after-life. The authors called for nurses to recognize their ideal position to facilitate spiritual care and communication between child and parents and child, family, and chaplain or some other spiritual care provider. Ill children, in particular, have spiritual care needs that must be acknowledged. Key components of spiritual care that all nurses can provide are supportive, caring presence to the child and family and taking time to reflect on one's own spirituality or beliefs in order to meet the needs of others. Nurses need not share the belief system of a child or family to sit with and support them in times of spiritual questioning or reflection. Nurses do need skills in supportive, therapeutic listening, answering children's questions about death and the afterlife, facilitating discussion between parents and children, and preserving mindfulness and family relationships (Ferrell, Wittenberg, Battista, et al., 2016). Nurses can also use these skills when engaging adolescents and young adults in spiritual assessment. Adolescents and young adults bring greater maturity, compassion, empathy, and appreciation of the difficulty of the situation and may have personal spiritual needs (loneliness) or relationship needs (discord with parents) (Taylor, Petersen, Oyedele, et al., 2015). If nurses do not take the first important steps of listening, supporting, and facilitating connection to chaplaincy or other spiritual providers, they may inadvertently contribute to health inequities because nonwhite children and families may rely more on religion and spirituality during crises of life-threatening illness (Ferrell, Wittenberg, Battista, et al., 2016).

Parents, who often experience these life transitions simultaneously with their children, have spiritual needs as well. Often their primary spiritual concern is maintaining connection to the sick child. For example, parents of children who died in the pediatric intensive care unit reported that access to clergy, prayers, and support of religious practices in caring for their child's body after death were important. Another important element of parents' spirituality that may get lost in the highly charged environment of the intensive care unit is the recognition and cultivation of the idea that the parent-child relationship transcends death and is an enduring bond (Foster & Gilmer, 2008). For parents, open, honest, clear communication from their child's health care providers can prevent moral or spiritual distress because they will believe they had all of the information needed to make the right decisions for their child.

Religion can affect children across multiple domains, including physical health, healthy behaviors, mental and emotional health, participation in risky behaviors or demonstrating externalizing problems, and academic/cognitive functioning.

Regarding physical health, religion has demonstrated mixed effects, with positive effects resulting from the emphasis on healthy behaviors and respect for others. Religiosity and spirituality have been associated with adolescent substance use and older age at sexual debut (Holden & Williamson, 2014). Conversely, deleterious effects may be associated with some religions that are more authoritarian and prohibit health care interventions, such as cases of religiously motivated medical neglect, when a child suffers injury or dies because parents did not seek treatment for a particular ailment, or when immunizations or screenings are declined. Additionally, adolescents who identified as highly religious were less likely to use contraception at sexual debut, despite being older than nonreligious adolescents, putting them at risk for unplanned pregnancy or sexually transmitted infections. Considering mental and emotional health, connection to religion or spirituality has been associated with less adolescent depression, anxiety, and suicidality, as well as lower rates of criminal or delinquent behavior. However, religion or spirituality can contribute to psychologic distress if youth are subjected to negative relationships or experiences that are imbued with demandingness and criticism. Thus the social context in which the religion is practiced may be more important than the religion itself (Holden & Williamson, 2014). Religion can be misused as a way to inflict maltreatment, in forms of physical abuse, emotional abuse, medical neglect, and sexual abuse by those in positions of authority, though this is not the norm. Parents weave religion and spirituality into their family life generally because it was an important part of their lives and because they believe it will promote their child's well-being. Religion and spirituality can help parents cope with the demands of parenting and help parents find meaning in the role.

However, conflicts can arise between religion and health care, and parental religious objections have been a major focus of literature on family spirituality versus other forms of engagement. For example, the American Academy of Pediatrics cites the intersection of religion, spirituality, and health care as potentially harmful to children based on situations in which parents refuse medical care for their children, and religious exemptions to child abuse and neglect laws. Although parents' refusal of medical care for their children falls under the scope of parental authority, the child's best interest is priority. Failure to provide essential health care is increasingly viewed as a form of neglect. Religions and spiritual traditions vary in the depth and nature of treatment they refuse, from refusal of all treatment to refusal of select interventions or therapeutics, such as blood products. Pediatric health care organizations, such as the American Academy of Pediatrics, argue that free exercise of religion should be balanced against protecting children from harm. For example, in a case where parents and health care providers differ on the proposed benefit or burden of a treatment and the primary benefit is spiritual or religious, children's future ability to decide the issue for themselves should be protected and privileged. In addition, the Supreme Court has argued that the free exercise of religion does not include the liberty to subject communities or children to disease or children, in particular, to diminished health or death. These arguments and considerations become murky when the conditions are not life threatening or when the proposed treatment has significant adverse effects, or the efficacy is limited. Negative psychologic effects must also be considered (American Academy of Pediatrics, 2013).

Complicating this debate is variation in religious exemption laws across states, creating additional uncertainty among families, health care providers, and child protection agencies about when and why to intervene and potential penalties. Thus many health care providers may perceive religion and spirituality as a negative influence in children's lives and believe such statutes should be abolished as children may be at greater risk and receive differential care across state lines. These arguments are compelling, and the welfare of children should be prioritized. However, we must walk this line carefully, as health care providers are often in positions of power and families may feel vulnerable, limit their sharing with health care providers, and ultimately withdraw from care. This hampers spiritual assessment and diminishes communication between child, parent, and health care providers. Overall, pediatric health care providers engage in a limited manner with parents around their spirituality, even if the child is engaged spiritually.

Although many health care providers support the value of religion or spirituality, there is limited discussion in clinical practice, limited assessment and inquiry into families' spiritual beliefs and needs, and limited training in nursing and medical schools on how to conduct such assessment. These limitations create an environment, then, in which limited spiritual and religious interventions that may diminish sorrow and provide comfort and solace can be provided. For example, evaluation and intervention around spiritual beliefs could be helpful for a child who has lost a sibling. Care must be taken, though, to ensure that the right person is available to conduct spiritual care interventions, such as a trained spiritual counselor or chaplain with expertise in children's spirituality and experience of religion and who can skillfully disentangle spiritual from psychologic or emotional issues or parents' spiritual perspectives from those of the child (Holden & Williamson, 2014). Indeed, assessing and addressing child and family spirituality have been incorporated into the standards of various pediatric nursing organizations (e.g., Association of Pediatric Hematology/Oncology Nurses) and other health care organizations (e.g., American Academy of Pediatrics). Spiritual care acknowledges the "transcendent dimensions of life and reflects the reality of the patient" (Taylor, Petersen, Oyedele, et al., 2015). A focused and tiered screening, as proposed by Taylor and colleagues, allows for all children to be screened for spiritual distress and identify immediate needs for support to conducting in-depth spiritual assessment or accessing someone who can (Taylor, Petersen, Oyedele, et al., 2015). The pneumonic BELIEF also allows for a guided assessment (Taylor, Petersen, Oyedele, et al., 2015):

- Belief system
- Ethics or values
- Lifestyle
- Involvement
- Education
- Future

Religion can influence community standards and norms, although context is key when we consider how religion exerts an effect on children and families. For example, the effect of religion or spirituality may be more pronounced in an isolated rural area versus a major metropolitan area with more heterogeneity in its population. The research on the influence of religion is limited in several ways: there are fewer studies about children and religion versus adults and religion; it is hard to disentangle whether other variables interact with or mediate the effect of religion on child health; whether the results are the same across levels or "doses" of religiosity; what the meaning other participation in a religious or spiritual community is for a child and how this translates into thoughts, beliefs, and behaviors ascertained through qualitative or mixed-methods research; and greater emphasis on Judeo-Christian samples.

CULTURAL HUMILITY AND HEALTH CARE PROVIDERS' CONTRIBUTION

Health care providers and the wider health care community must reassert the significance of equity, fairness, and caring as the instrumental building blocks of a strong, high-quality, and transformed health care system. One way to get to this point is through teaching and coaching trainees across health care disciplines to be more engaged in understanding the social determinants of health, their impact and roots, and how to counteract their negative effects. Betancourt, Corbett, and Bondaryk (2017) argue that, although the concept and practice have limitations, the goal of cultural competence is to "improve the ability of health care providers and health care systems to communicate effectively with and provide quality health care to patients from diverse social backgrounds" (p. 144). Effective communication with patients and families is critical to positive health outcomes, yet many trainees do not feel prepared to engage with patients and families whose backgrounds are different than their own (Betancourt, Corbett, & Bondaryk, 2017; Green, Chun, Cervantes, et al., 2017; Marshall, Cooper, Green, et al., 2017).

According to Yeager and Bauer-Wu (2013), cultural humility can be understood as the process of self-reflection to promote honest and trustworthy relationships—knowing one's self better in order to know others. Mindfulness might be an important part of this as a vehicle to understand and limit health disparities; nurses need an understanding of the context, culture, and environment of those experiencing inequities and disparities. Cultural humility is important across nursing expertise levels and functions, from student nurse, to nurse at the bedside, to advanced practice nurse, to professor and researcher. This critical consciousness leads the nurse to step back and examine his or her own beliefs, cultures, and positions in the world, as well as assumptions, biases, and values. Cultural humility cannot be collapsed into a class or education offering; rather it is viewed as an ongoing process. Tervalon and Murray-Garcia (1998) state that cultural humility is "best defined not as a discrete end point but as a commitment and active engagement in a lifelong process that individuals enter into on an ongoing basis with patients, communities, colleagues, and with themselves" (p. 118). This dynamic view acknowledges that cultures changes over time and that their influences change over time, too. For example, what is highly influential as a young child may be less so as an adolescent or young adult. Cultural competence is too limiting for this discussion because it can perpetuate stereotypes, is often limited to race/ethnicity differences, and treats those different from the white provider as "other." Humility requires courage and flexibility. Strengths and challenges of individuals and groups are explored, as well as the advantages and privileges of certain group membership. Examining and reflecting on one's own culture is an ongoing process that should prompt nurses to consider their biases, their sources of beliefs, and their own context and influences, in order to care well for people and provide the best level of care possible. An individual's culture is not a single identity, rather it is a complex intersection of various aspects of the person. Health care providers and researchers have to consider the power and privilege in their positions. Assumptions of researchers can make their way into interpretations of findings and miss heterogeneity within a group by lumping all members of one group together. Mindfulness can facilitate cultural humility by pulling nurses and health care providers out of autopilot. Cultural humility also attends to and acknowledges the systemic maltreatment of certain groups of people at the hands of health care providers/systems. Such mindful relationships can break down stereotypes. Core to any work on cultural humility is the "deliberate reflection" on their values and biases (Yeager and Bauer-Wu, 2013).

Cultural humility privileges the process of self-reflection and self-critique as an avenue to build relationships with others and to understand one's own biases, assumptions, and values. It emphasizes approaching clinical encounters with flexibility, courage, and openness versus competence or confidence. It also recognizes the dynamic nature of culture and the influence of context, place, and time. We must also recognize that "culture" is not only race and ethnicity, but also social class, age, sexual orientation, sexuality, gender, ability, and professional discipline, among other things. Thus all of us will be on the receiving and giving ends of care from and for people who do not inhabit the same space as us, yet we can connect on the desire to help and be helped and have suffering minimized. Assessing cultural impact through the lens of cultural humility also reminds us of power differentials that influence health care encounters. Humility helps us disentangle and understand the meaning of "culture" for each person—its impact, historical context, and heterogeneity within groups—and that people are often the experts in their own experiences.

Foronda and colleagues describe the attributes or characteristics of cultural humility as "openness, self-awareness, egoless, supportive interactions, self-reflection and critique" (Foronda, Baptiste, Reinholdt, et al., 2016). They found that the consequences of practicing cultural humility, as published in studies or practice guides, were "mutual empowerment, partnership, respect, optimal care, [and] lifelong learning" (Foronda, Baptiste, Reinholdt, et al., 2016) in clinical encounters. Thus transformational learning environments that can shape students' perspectives and make them aware of power imbalances and inequity in health care can promote humility in future health care encounters.

Although it is imperative to have tools to develop one's presence of mind and to assess one's own values, it is also helpful to have concrete questions and methods with which to elicit a patient's of family's health beliefs or customs. As we have seen, it is not helpful to demonstrate competence by lumping a group of people together and applying an assumed set of beliefs onto them, such as "Latinas/Latinos have strong family support," as these lump understandings can become stereotypical and not illuminate what is important for a particular patient and family in a particular context. Thus it is helpful to have a broad understanding of what health beliefs are and how to elicit them.

Religion and culture can influence the ways children, youth, and their families interact with health care providers and engage with the health care system. Various avenues for this influence include health beliefs (e.g., children should not know the severity of their illness); health customs (e.g., care of the dead); ethnic customs (e.g., gender roles and division of labor); religious beliefs (e.g., use of blood products); dietary customs (e.g., maintaining a kosher diet); and interpersonal customs (e.g., how children address parents or how touch is used in communication) (Agency for Healthcare Research and Quality, 2015). Questions to start this conversation can start with the following: "Is there anything you would like for me to know about your child or your family so that I can take the best possible care of you all?" "Can you tell me about your condition (your child's condition)?" or "Do you have any special beliefs or things you do or people you talk to when it comes to your (your child's) health?" These are example questions that are open-ended and can be adapted to anyone the nurse is caring for at any time in any given location or context. See Box 2.8 for additional questions for exploring a family's culture.

BOX 2.8 Exploring a Family's Culture, Illness, and Care

- What do you think caused your child's health problem?
- Why do you think it started when it did?
- How severe is your child's sickness? Will it have a short or long course?
- How do you think your child's sickness affects your family?
- What are the chief problems your child's sickness has caused?
- What kind of treatment do you think your child should receive?
- What are the most important results you hope to receive from your child's treatment?
- What do you fear most about your child's sickness?

NCLEX REVIEW QUESTIONS

1. Duvall's Developmental Stages of the Family include which of the following? Select all that apply.
   A. Stages an individual progresses through in his or her moral and spiritual development
   B. Stages families progress through in adulthood
   C. Stages that designate how parenting progresses as a child develops
   D. Stages that designate appropriate discipline related to developmental stages
   E. Stages that describe the journey a couple will take as their children mature
2. Family systems theory includes:
   A. Direct causality, meaning each change affects the whole family
   B. Family systems react to changes as they take place, not initiate it
   C. A balance between morphogenesis and morphostasis is necessary
   D. Theory is used primarily for family dysfunction and pathology
3. The nurse is explaining the strategy of consequences to a parent he is working with. Which response by the parent indicates that more teaching is needed when he describes the types of consequences?
   A. Natural: those that occur without any intervention
   B. Logical: those that are directly related to the rule
   C. Transforming: allowing the child to come to the conclusion on his or her own
   D. Unrelated: those that are imposed deliberately
4. Culture includes which of the following? Select all that apply.
   A. Cultural competence, which includes building skills in the health care provider, such as offering lists of common foods, health care beliefs, and important rituals
   B. Cultural humility, which requires that health care providers participate in a continual process of self-reflection and self-critique
   C. Recognizing the power of the health care provider role that views the patient and family as full members of the health care team
   D. A particular group with its values, beliefs, norms, patterns, and practices that are learned, shared, and transmitted from one generation to another
   E. A complex whole in which each part is interrelated, including beliefs, tradition, lifeways, and heritage
5. Ways to integrate spiritual practices into nursing care include:
   A. Explaining the religious practices you personally take part in
   B. Realizing that young children have little understanding regarding their spirituality
   C. Agreeing with children and their families when they explain their religious beliefs so they are not offended
   D. Becoming knowledgeable about the religious worldviews of cultural groups found in the patients you care for

Correct Answers

1. B, C, E; 2. C; 3. C; 4. B, C, D, E; 5. D

REFERENCES

Afifi, T. O., Boman, J., Fleisher, W., et al. (2009). The relationship between child abuse, parental divorce, and lifetime mental disorders and suicidality in a nationally representative adult sample. *Child Abuse and Neglect, 33*(3), 139–147.

Agency for Healthcare Research and Quality. (2015). *Consider culture, customs, and beliefs (Tool 10).* AHRQ Health Literacy Universal Precautions Toolkit (second edition). Retrieved from https://www.ahrq.gov/sites/default/files/wysiwyg/professionals/quality-patient-safety/quality-resources/tools/literacy-toolkit/healthlittoolkit2_tool10.pdf.

Ahrons, C. R. (2007). Family ties after divorce: Long-term implications for children. *Family Process, 46*(1), 53–65.

American Academy of Pediatrics Council on Communications and Media. (2016a). Media use in school-aged children and adolescents. *Pediatrics, 138*(5), e20162592.

American Academy of Pediatrics Council on Communications and Media. (2016b). Media and young minds. *Pediatrics, 138*(5), e20162591.

American Academy Council on Community Pediatrics. (2016c). Poverty and child health in the United States. *Pediatrics, 137*(4), e20160339.

American Academy of Pediatrics. (2003). Family pediatrics: Report of the task force on the family. *Pediatrics, 111*(6), 1541–1571.

American Academy of Pediatrics Section on Hospice and Palliative Medicine and Hospital Care. (2013). Pediatric palliative care commitments, guidelines, and recommendations. *Pediatrics, 132*, 966–972.

Annie E. Casey Foundation. (2014). *African American, American Indian, and Latino Children have the most barriers.* Retrieved from http://www.aecf.org/blog/african-american-american-indian-and-latino-children-have-the-most-barriers.

Annie E. Casey Foundation. (2017). *2017 kids count data book: State profiles of child well-being.* Retrieved from http://www.aecf.org/resources/2017-kids-count-data-book/.

Baumrind, D. (1971). Harmonious parents and their preschool children. *Developmental Psychology, 41*, 92–102.

Baumrind, D. (1996). The discipline controversy revisited. *Family Relations, 45*, 405–414.

Berger, L., & Waldfogel, J. (2004). Out-of-home placement of children and economic factors: An empirical analysis. *Review of Economics of the Household, 2*(4), 387–411.

Betancourt, J. R., Corbett, J., & Bondaryk, M. R. (2017). Addressing disparities and achieving equity: Cultural competence, ethics, and health-care transformation. *Chest, 145*(1), 145–148.

Blackwell, C. W. (2007). Belief in the "free choice" model of homosexuality: A correlate of homophobia in registered nurses. *Journal of LGBT Health Research, 3*(3), 31–40.

Bomar, P. J. (2004). *Promoting health in families* (3rd ed.). Philadelphia: Saunders.

Bronfenbrenner, U. (1979). *The ecology of human development: Experiments by nature and design*. Cambridge, MA: Harvard University Press.

Bronfenbrenner, U. (2005). *Making human beings human: Bioecological perspectives on human development*. Thousand Oaks, CA: Sage Publications.

Center on the Developing Child at Harvard University. (2016). *Building core capabilities for life: The science behind the skills adults need to succeed in parenting and in the workplace*. http://www.developingchild.harvard.edu.

Centers for Disease Control and Prevention. (2009). *School connectedness: Strategies for increasing protective factors among youth*. Atlanta, GA: U.S. Department of Health and Human Services.

Centers for Disease Control and Prevention. (2016). *National marriage and divorce rate trends*. Retrieved from https://www.cdc.gov/nchs/nvss/marriage_divorce_tables.htm.

Chamberlain, P., Price, J., Leve, L. D., et al. (2008). Prevention of behavior problems for children in foster care: Outcomes and mediation effects. *Prevention Science, 9*(1), 17–27.

Chavez, V. (2012). *Cultural humility: People, principles, and practices (documentary film)*. Retrieved from http://www.youtube.com/watch?v_SaSH<bslv4w).

Child Welfare Information Gateway. (2017). *Foster care statistics, 2015*. Washington DC, US Department of Health and Human Services, Children's Bureau.

Coker, T. R., Elliot, M. N., Kanouse, D. K., et al. (2009). Perceived racial/ethnic discrimination among fifth-grade students and its association with mental health. *American Journal of Public Health, 99*(5), 878–884.

Duvall, E. R. (1977). *Family development* (5th ed.). Philadelphia: Lippincott.

Fergusson, E., Maughan, B., & Golding, J. (2008). Which children receive grandparental care and what effect does it have? *Journal of Child Psychology and Psychiatry, and Allied Disciplines, 49*(2), 161–169.

Ferrell, B., Wittenberg, E., Battista, V., et al. (2016). Nurses' experiences of spiritual communication with seriously ill children. *Journal of Palliative Medicine, 19*(11), 1166–1170.

Fierman, A. H., Beck, A. F., Chung, E. K., et al. (2016). Redesigning healthcare practices to address childhood poverty. *Academic Pediatrics, 16*, S136–S146.

Fisher, C., Lindhorst, H., Matthews, T., et al. (2008). Nursing staff attitudes and behaviors regarding family presence in the hospital setting. *Journal of Advanced Nursing, 64*(6), 615–624.

Foronda, C., Baptiste, D. L., Reinholdt, M. M., et al. (2016). Cultural humility: A concept analysis. *Journal of Transcultural Nursing, 27*(3), 210–217.

Foster, T. L., & Gilmer, M. J. (2008). Continuing bonds: A human response within paediatric palliative care. *International Journal of Palliative Nursing, 14*(2), 85–91.

Gershoff, E. T. (2008). *Report on physical punishment in the United States: What research tell us about its effects on children*. Colombus, OH: Center for Effective Discipline.

Goldberg, W. A., Prause, J., Lucas-Thompson, R., et al. (2008). Maternal employment and children's achievement in context: A meta-analysis of four decades of research. *Psychological Bulletin, 134*(1), 77–108.

Goldenberg, I., & Goldenberg, H. (2012). *Family therapy: An overview* (8th ed.). Pacific Grove, CA: Brooks-Cole Cengage Learning.

Green, A. R., Chun, M. B. J., Cervantes, M., et al. (2017). Measuring medical students' preparedness and skills to provide cross-cultural care. *Health Equity, 1*(1), 15–22.

Holden, G. W., & Williamson, P. A. (2014). Religion and child well-being. In B.-A. Asher, F. Casas, I. Frones, et al. (Eds.), *Handbook of child well-being*. Dordrecht: Springer.

Kaakinen, J. R., & Coehlo, D. P. (2015). *Family health care nursing* (5th ed.). Philadelphia: Davis.

Kazak, A. E. (2001). Comprehensive care for children with cancer and their families: A social ecological framework guiding research, practice, and policy. *Children's Services: Social Policy, Research, and Practice, 4*(4), 217–233.

Kazak, A. E., Rourke, M. T., & Navasaria, N. (2010). Families and other systems in pediatric psychology. In M. C. Roberts & R. G. Steele (Eds.), *Handbook of pediatric psychology*. Guilford Press.

Kreider, R. M., & Elliott, D. B. (2009). America's families and living arrangements: 2007. In *US Census Bureau: Current population reports*. Washington, DC: The Bureau.

Lewallen, T. C., Hunt, H., Potts-Datema, W., et al. (2015). The whole school, whole community, whole child model: A new approach for improving educational attainment and healthy development for students. *The Journal of School Health, 85*, 729–739.

Lima, N. N., do Nascimento, V. B., de Carvalho, S. M., et al. (2013). Spirituality in childhood cancer care. *Neuropsychiatric Disease and Treatment, 9*, 1539–1544.

Marmot, M. (2015). *The health gap: The challenge of an unequal world*. London: Bloomsbury.

Marshall, J. K., Cooper, L. A., Green, A. R., et al. (2017). Residents' attitude, knowledge, and perceived preparedness toward caring for patients from diverse sociocultural backgrounds. *Health Equity, 1*(1), 43–49.

McCubbin, M. A., & McCubbin, H. I. (1994). Families coping with illness: The resiliency model of family stress, adjustment, and adaptation. In C. B. Danielson, B. H. Bissel, & P. Winstead-Fry (Eds.), *Families, health, and illness*. St. Louis, MO: Mosby.

McLaughlin, K. A., Gadermann, A. M., Hwang, I., et al. (2012). Parent psychopathology and offspring mental disorders: Results from the WHO World Mental Health Surveys. *The British Journal of Psychiatry: The Journal of Mental Science, 200*(4), 290–299.

Michael, S. L., Merlo, C. L., Basch, C. E., et al. (2015). Critical connections: Health and academics. *The Journal of School Health, 85*, 740–758.

Mindlin, M., Jenkins, R., & Law, C. (2009). Maternal employment and indicators of child health: A systemic review in pre-school children in OECD countries. *Journal of Epidemiology and Community Health, 63*(5), 340–350.

Mooney-Doyle, K., dos Santos, M., Bousso, R., et al. (in press). Parental expectations for support from healthcare providers: A qualitative secondary analysis. *Journal of pediatric nursing*.

Murray, J. S. (2015). Displaced and forgotten child refugees: A humanitarian crisis. *Journal for Specialists in Pediatric Nursing, 21*, 29–36.

O'Connell, M., & Feliz, S. (2011). *Same-sex couple household statistics from the 2010 Census*. SEHSD Working Paper Number 2011-26, Washington, DC, Fertility and Family Statistics Branch Social, Economic and Housing Statistics Division, US Census Bureau.

Papero, D. V. (1990). *Bowen family systems theory*. Boston, MA: Pearson.

Power, N., & Franck, L. (2008). Parent participation in the care of hospitalized children: A systematic review. *Journal of Advanced Nursing, 62*(6), 622–641.

Reid Chassiakos, Y. L., Radesky, J., Christakis, D., et al. (2016). Children and adolescents and digital media. *Pediatrics, 138*(5), e20162593.

Scott, J., & Marshall, G. (2009). *Ethnicity, oxford dictionary of sociology*. Oxford: Oxford University Press.

Spears, W., Pascoe, J., Khamis, H., et al. (2013). Parents' perspectives on their children's health insurance: Plight of the underinsured. *The Journal of Pediatrics, 162*(2), 403–408.

Spector, R. E. (2009). *Cultural diversity in health and illness* (7th ed.). Upper Saddle River, NJ: Prentice-Hall.

Strasburger, V., Jordan, A., & Donnerstein, E. (2012). Children, adolescents, and the media: Health effects. *Pediatric Clinics of North America, 59*, 533–587.

Taylor, E. J., Petersen, C., Oyedele, O., et al. (2015). Spirtualty and spiritual care of adolescents and yound adults with cancer. *Seminars in Oncology Nursing, 31*(3), 227–241.

Tervalon, M., & Murray-Garcia, J. (1998). Cultural humility versus cultural competence: A critical distinction in defining physician training outcomes in multicultural education. *Journal of Health Care for the Poor and Underserved*, *9*(2), 117–125.

Tiedje, K., & Plevak, D. J. (2014). Medical humanitarianism in the United States: Alternative healthcare, spirituality and political advocacy in the case of our Lady Guadalupe free clinic. *Social Science & Medicine*, *120*, 360–367.

Tynes, B. M., Giang, M. T., Williams, D. R., et al. (2008). Online racial discrimination and psychological adjustment among adolescents. *The Journal of Adolescent Health*, *43*(6), 565–569.

US Census Bureau. (2011). *Same sex couple households*. Washington, DC: American Community Survey Briefs.

Williams, D. R. (2012). Miles to go before we sleep: Racial inequities in health. *Journal of Health and Social Behavior*, *53*, 279–296.

Yeager, K. A., & Bauer-Wu, S. (2013). Cultural humility: Essential foundation for clinical researchers. *Applied Nursing Research*, *26*(4), 251–256.

Zolotor, A. J., & Puzia, M. E. (2010). Bans against corporal punishment: A systematic review of the laws, changes in attitudes and behaviors. *Child Abuse Review*, *19*, 229–247.

Zuckerman, K. E., Perrin, J. M., Hobrecker, K., et al. (2013). Barriers to specialty care and specialty referral completion in the community health center setting. *The Journal of Pediatrics*, *162*(2), 409–414.

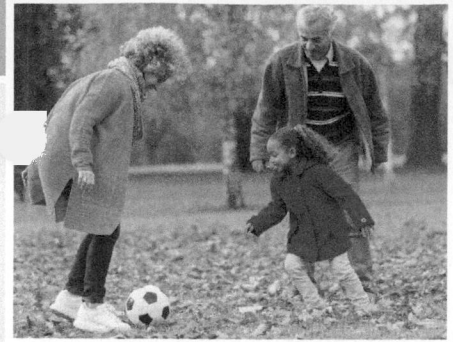

3

Hereditary Influences on Health Promotion of the Child and Family

Cynthia A. Prows

http://evolve.elsevier.com/wong/ncic

CONCEPTS

- Genetic Influences

GENETIC/GENOMIC NURSING COMPETENCIES

Nurses and other health care providers increasingly are faced with incorporating genetic-genomic information into their practice. In response to this need, the Consensus Panel on Genetic/Genomic Nursing Competencies was established in 2006. This independent panel of nurse leaders from clinical, research, and academic settings established essential minimal competencies necessary for nurses to deliver competent genetic- and genomic-focused nursing care (Consensus Panel on Genetic/Genomic Nursing Competencies, 2009). In a similar manner, genetic and genomic competencies were created and published for nurses with graduate degrees (Greco, Tinley, & Seibert, 2012). Using these documents as resources, the American Association of Colleges of Nursing published the revised *The Essentials of Baccalaureate Education for Professional Nursing Practice* (2008, http://www.aacn.nche.edu/education/pdf/BaccEssentials08.pdf), which identified genetics and genomics as strong forces influencing the role of nurses in patient care. This chapter provides foundational information to help nurses begin using genetics and genomics information and technology when caring for children and families (Box 3.1).

GENETICS AND GENOMICS

A human genome consists of 22 nuclear autosome chromosomes and a sex chromosome (either an X or a Y), as well as a single circular molecule of DNA within the mitochondria. Every cell in the human body, except the egg or the sperm, contains a maternally inherited and a paternally inherited copy of the genome in its nucleus, as well as the maternally inherited mitochondrial DNA. The ovum contains a single nuclear genome (22 autosomes and the X chromosome), as well as the circular DNA strand within the mitochondria. The sperm head contains a single nuclear genome (22 autosomes and either the X or the Y chromosome) but does not contain mitochondria. **Genes** are segments of DNA that code for structural or functional proteins. Areas of DNA that do not code for proteins still have essential regulatory functions that are beginning to be better understood. The locations of genes or noncoding regulatory elements are often referred to as *sites,* or *loci,* indicating a physical or "geographic" location on a chromosome. Each gene is made up of exons and introns. Exons are the portions of a gene that contain the code for a specific protein. Introns may have important regulatory elements or function as spacers between exons to improve the efficiency of the cellular molecules that transcribe the gene (make a copy in the form of messenger RNA [mRNA]). Although the entire gene is transcribed, the intron portions of the mRNA are removed so that only the exonic codes remain in the mature mRNA that leaves the nucleus and enters the cytoplasm where it is translated into an eventual protein. Mutations in genes may have significant qualitative and quantitative effects on the synthesis of the corresponding protein, with potential clinical consequences. Proteins can be classified as structural (or constitutive) proteins, and functional, those that affect the metabolism of other molecules or substrates (enzymes). Table 3.1 summarizes the effects of protein disorders on selected genetic diseases. Such alterations in an individual genome may have been inherited from a parent or may represent an event that is new to that person and may be the first case in that family (**new mutation**). It is therefore erroneous to consider all genetic disorders as having a positive family history.

When referring to the study of individual genes and their impact on distinct disorders we use the term *genetics.* Although often used interchangeably, the term *genomics* refers to the study of all the genes in the human genome and the multiple interactions between many genes. Whether considering single genes or the entire genome's influence on disease, environmental factors must also be considered. Most diseases are influenced by a genetic/genomic predisposition that can be activated, modified, or suppressed by environmental factors. Examples of such interactions are found in single-gene disorders, such as phenylketonuria (PKU) and sickle cell disease, and multifactorial conditions, such as cancer and neural tube defects (NTDs). PKU is a disorder resulting from the (genetically determined) absence of an enzyme that metabolizes the amino acid phenylalanine. However, the deleterious effects in the infant are expressed only after sufficient ingestion of phenylalanine-containing substances, such as milk (environmental trigger). Even in the case of a "classic" genetic condition, such as sickle cell disease, its acute signs and symptoms are precipitated by certain conditions such as lowered oxygen tension, infection, or dehydration.

BOX 3.1 Key Genetic Terms

AFP—Abbreviation of alpha-fetoprotein, a protein produced by the developing fetus. Alterations in AFP can be used as a marker suggestive of neural tube defect (increased AFP) and Down syndrome (decreased AFP).

Alleles—One version of a gene at a given location (locus) along a chromosome. The most common version of a gene in a population is called the **wild type allele**.

Amniocentesis—Prenatal diagnostic procedure that consists of transabdominally withdrawing a small sample of amniotic fluid for genetic analysis of embryonic cells. Biochemical analysis and chromosome studies can be performed in such cells. This procedure is usually performed at 14 to 20 weeks of gestation.

Aneuploidy—An abnormal chromosome pattern in which the total number of chromosomes is not a multiple of the haploid number (n = 23) (e.g., persons with 45 or 47 chromosomes, as in Turner or Down syndrome, respectively). Such monosomies and trisomies are examples of aneuploidy.

Association—Nonrandom cluster of malformations, the cause of which varies from person to person (e.g., VATER association).

Autosomes—The 22 pairs of chromosomes in somatic cells that do not greatly influence sex determination at conception. This does not include the sex chromosomes, X and Y.

Carrier—A clinically normal (asymptomatic) person who possesses a genetic alteration, either in the form of a gene or chromosome change. A carrier has the potential of transmitting that abnormality to an offspring who will then express the abnormal phenotype. Examples of carrier states include a sickle cell disease carrier ("trait") and a balanced carrier of a chromosome translocation.

Centromere—Chromosomal region that separates the chromosome arms and unites the chromatids. Centromeres attach to spindle fibers during cell division, ensuring through disjunction an equal distribution of chromosomes or chromatids.

Chromosome—Filament-like nuclear structure that consists of chromatin, stores genetic information as base sequences in DNA, and has a constant number for each species. Chromosomes are found in pairs in somatic cells (homologous chromosomes) and in single copies in germ cells. One member of a homologous pair is of paternal origin, the other of maternal origin. Homologous chromosomes have identical number and arrangement of genes.

Chromosome aberrations—Genetic disorders that result from variation in number or structure of chromosomes.

Chromosomes, acrocentric—Chromosomes in which the centromere is distally placed. Human chromosomes in groups D and G are acrocentric.

Chromosomes, metacentric—Chromosomes in which the centromere is located approximately in the midpoint of the chromosome, resulting in arms of approximately equal length. Human chromosomes A(1), A(3), and E(16) are metacentric.

Chromosomes, submetacentric—Chromosomes in which the centromere is located closer to one telomere than to the other. Human B group chromosomes are submetacentric.

Concordant—A condition in which two individuals have the same genetic trait; usually applied to monozygotic twin concordance studies.

Congenital—Present at birth. A congenital disease may or may not be genetic. Likewise, a genetic disease may or may not be congenital, although the causative genes are present at birth.

Crossing-over—The genetic event that results in exchange of genetic material between homologous chromosomes during prophase I of meiosis.

CVS—Abbreviation of chorionic villi sampling, a prenatal diagnostic procedure in which a small amount of chorionic villi material (embryonic tissue) is aspirated for genetic analysis of the developing embryo. This procedure is usually performed during the first trimester of pregnancy.

Cytogenetics—Study of chromosomes, with special focus on chromosome abnormalities.

Deformation—Fetal abnormality caused by extrinsic factors (e.g., uterine position).

Diploid—A cell that contains two copies of each chromosome. The term is often extended to include an individual carrying such cells. The diploid number (2n) in humans is 46.

Deletion—The loss of chromosomal material. An example of a terminal deletion is found in cri du chat (cat's cry) syndrome, in which there is loss of a portion of the short arm of chromosome B(5). Deleted fragments may attach to another chromosome (see Translocation).

DNA—Abbreviation of deoxyribonucleic acid, a double-helix molecule consisting of an assembly of nucleotides (phosphate–sugar [deoxyribose]–nitrogenous base). DNA bases (cytosine, guanine, thymine, adenine) encode genetic information, which is *transcribed* into messenger RNA and further *translated* into proteins.

DNA, mitochondrial (mtDNA)—DNA located in the mitochondria of cells. Inheritance of mtDNA is independent from paternal genetics.

DNA, nuclear (nDNA)—DNA located in the nucleus of cells.

Dominant—An allele that is phenotypically expressed in single copy (heterozygote) and in double copy (homozygote). Example: polydactyly.

FISH analysis—Fluorescent in situ hybridization, a process by which chromosomes or portions of chromosomes are "painted" with fluorescent molecules. This technique is useful for identifying chromosomal microdeletions.

Gamete (germ cell)—A mature reproductive cell containing the haploid number of chromosomes (n = 23); in males, the spermatozoon; in females, the ovum. The union of gametes in sexual reproduction initiates the development of a new individual.

Gametogenesis—A series of mitotic and meiotic cell divisions occurring in the gonads that lead to the production of gametes; in males, spermatogenesis; in females, oogenesis. Reduction in the number of chromosomes ($2n \rightarrow n$) during gametogenesis occurs in the first meiotic division (meiosis I).

Gene—A segment of nucleic acid that contains genetic information necessary to control a certain function, such as the synthesis of a polypeptide (structural gene). This segment is often referred to as a site, or locus, on a chromosome.

Genetic counseling—The process by which genetic information is given to patients and their families. Information about a genetic disease may include its natural history, recurrence risk, and management.

Genetics—Study of individual genes and their impact on relatively rare single-gene disorders.

Genome—Complete genetic information of an organism, usually described as total number of base pairs. The human genome contains approximately 3 billion base pairs.

Genomics—Study of all the genes in the human genome together, including their interactions with each other and the environment, and the influence of other psychosocial and cultural factors.

Genotype—Genetic constitution that determines the physical and chemical characteristics of an individual.

Haploid—The number of chromosomes present in a gamete. Also, a cell that contains one copy of each chromosome. The haploid number (n) in humans is 23. The diploid number of chromosomes (46) is reconstituted in the zygote on fertilization of two haploid gametes.

Hemizygote—A condition in which an allele is present in a single copy. Males are hemizygous for all markers (genes) located on the X chromosome.

Heterozygote—An individual who has two different alleles at a given locus on a pair of homologous chromosomes; for example, in the case of the *HexA* gene, Hh (or +/–).

Homologous—Referring to chromosomes with matching genes, or to those genes individually.

Homozygote—An individual possessing a pair of identical alleles at a given locus; for example, in the case of the *HexA* gene, above, HH (or +/+) and hh (or –/–).

Human Genome Project—International research project to map each human gene and sequence the human genome.

BOX 3.1 Key Genetic Terms—cont'd

Imprinting—Phenomenon in which an allele at a given locus is altered or inactivated, depending on whether it is inherited from mother or father; implies a functional difference in genes inherited from the two parents and explains some variation in expression.

Karyotype—The chromosome constitution of an individual represented by a laboratory-made display in which chromosomes are arranged by size and centromere position.

Locus—The chromosome location of a specific gene (or site). Plural: loci.

Malformation—A primary morphologic defect occurring as a result of abnormal morphogenesis.

Malformation, major—Structural abnormality with serious medical, surgical, or cosmetic consequences.

Malformation, minor—Structural abnormality that has no serious consequences or is a normal variation (e.g., extra nipple or umbilical hernia).

Meiosis—A reductional type of cell division, in which the chromosome number is halved. In humans, meiosis is one of the processes that lead to the formation of haploid gametes (n = 23).

Mendelian inheritance—The mode of inheritance of single-gene traits. The term is derived from Gregor Mendel, the pioneer of genetics.

Microdeletion—Chromosome deletion too small to be detected by standard cytogenetic techniques; can be detected by FISH analysis, which is a molecular cytogenetic technique.

Mitochondrion—Cellular organelle responsible for converting nutrients into energy and for many other specialized tasks. Mitochondria are the only part of the body known to have their own separate and unique DNA; mitochondrial DNA (mtDNA) is inherited exclusively from the mother. Plural: mitochondria.

Mitosis—Type of equational cell division in which the resulting daughter cells have the same number of chromosomes as each other and the mother cell.

Monosomy—The aneuploid condition of having a chromosome represented by a single copy in a somatic cell, that is, the absence of a chromosome from a given pair. Generally, monosomies are not compatible with life, except in the case of a missing X chromosome in Turner syndrome (45,XO).

Mosaicism—Condition in which an individual harbors two or more genetically distinct cell lines. Generally, one cell line is normal and one is abnormal; it results from mitotic nondisjunction, a postzygotic event.

Multifactorial—Complex interaction of both genetic and environmental factors that produces an effect on an individual. Disease processes resulting from multifactorial inheritance are referred to as *complex diseases*.

Mutation—Structural or chemical alteration in genetic material that persists and is transmitted to future generations. Mutations can occur naturally *(spontaneous)* or can be induced by a variety of physical (temperature, radiation), chemical (various substances such as nitrogen mustard), or biologic (certain viruses) mutagens.

Nondisjunction—Failure of homologous chromosomes or chromatids to separate properly during anaphase meiosis I and II, or mitosis, resulting in daughter cells with unequal chromosome numbers. Meiotic nondisjunction may result in gametes with abnormal chromosome number, which on fertilization may produce aneuploidy. Mitotic nondisjunction in a developing embryo may result in mosaicism.

Oncogene—A gene or group of genes, usually involved in cell division, whose malfunction (e.g., a mutation) will result in malignant transformation.

Pedigree chart (family tree, genogram)—A diagram that describes family relationships, gender, disease status, or other relevant information about a family, illustrating the genetic variation within a family.

Penetrance—Frequency with which a heritable trait is manifested in individuals possessing the gene.

Phenotype—Any observable or measurable expression of gene function in an individual. For instance, eye color and hemoglobin type are phenotypic expressions of specific genes. Phenotypes may result from interaction of genotype and environment.

Polygenic—Inheritance involving many genes at separate loci whose combined, additive effects produce a given phenotype.

Polyploidy—Chromosome condition in which the diploid chromosome number of a cell varies by increments of 23. For example, a triploid cell or individual would have 69 chromosomes (46 + 23); a tetraploid, 92 (46 + 23 + 23).

Proband (index case)—The clinically identified person who displays the characteristics of features of the disease in question; also referred to as propositus (feminine: proposita).

Recessive—Refers to an allele whose phenotypic expression occurs in homozygous or hemizygous conditions. In heterozygosity, a recessive allele is masked by its dominant homologous counterpart. Example: cystic fibrosis.

Recombination—The occurrence among the offspring of new combinations of alleles as a result of genetic material exchange following crossovers during parental gametogenesis.

RNA—Abbreviation of ribonucleic acid, a single-stranded molecule consisting of an assembly of nucleotides (phosphate–sugar [ribose]–nitrogenous base). RNA bases (cytosine, guanine, uracil, adenine) encode genetic information, which is *translated* into proteins.

Sex-linked—The transmission of a trait whose causative gene is located on a sex chromosome (X or Y). Most sex-linked genes in humans are located on the X chromosome (X-linked).

Somatic cell—Body tissue cells with diploid complement of 46 chromosomes.

Sporadic—A descriptor for birth defects or disorders occurring as a new case in a family and not inherited.

Syndrome—A collection of multiple primary malformations or defects all due to a single underlying cause. Examples: Down syndrome (chromosome abnormality), Marfan syndrome (single-gene disorder).

Telomere—The distal portion of a chromosome.

Teratogen—An environmental agent capable of producing a birth defect.

Transcription—The process by which genetic information is copied from DNA to RNA.

Translation—The step in protein synthesis during which an amino acid sequence is assembled according to the genetic information contained in messenger RNA (mRNA).

Translocation—Transfer of all or part of a chromosome to a different chromosome after chromosome breakage; can be balanced, producing no phenotypic effects, or unbalanced, producing severe or lethal effects.

Trisomy—An aneuploid condition caused by the presence of an extra chromosome, which is added to a given chromosome pair and results in a total number of 47 chromosomes per cell. Down syndrome is the most common human autosomal trisomy.

X inactivation (lyonization)—The process by which, in a normal female, most of genes on one of the X chromosomes are inactivated during early embryonic development, so that alleles on active chromosome are allowed full expression.

X-linked inheritance—Transmission of a trait whose causative gene is located on the X chromosome.

Zygote—Cell resulting from the fusion of male and female gametes.

TABLE 3.1 Selected Proteins Involved in Genetic Disease

Protein Involved	Altered Mechanism of Action Due to Mutations	Resulting Disorder
Constitutive Proteins		
Globins	Altered oxygen transport	Hemoglobinopathies: • Sickle cell disease • Thalassemias
Dystrophin	Muscle cell defect	Muscular dystrophies
Coagulation factors VIII and IX	Abnormal clotting activity	Hemophilia A and B
Enzymes		
Phenylalanine hydroxylase	Interrupted metabolism of phenylalanine and accumulation of toxic precursors (phenylalanine and phenylketones)	Phenylketonuria
Hexosaminidase A (HexA)	Interrupted metabolism and accumulation of precursors (GM2 ganglioside)	Tay-Sachs disease
Hypoxanthine-guanine phosphoribosyltransferase (HGPRT)	Disruption of metabolic feedback mechanism and accumulation of end product (uric acid)	Lesch-Nyhan syndrome
3-Hydroxy-3-methylglutaryl coenzyme A (HMG-CoA) reductase	Disruption of metabolic feedback mechanism and accumulation of end product (cholesterol)	Familial hypercholesterolemia

Cancer is another example of genetic-environment interplay and explains the difference between inherited conditions and somatic cell genetic disorders. A normal somatic cell (any body cell other than the ova and sperm) may become a cancer cell after acquiring a series of gene changes. This process is the typical "genetic" cause of cancer. In a small subset of families, a mutation in a gene normally involved in regulation of cell growth, DNA repair, or cell death (apoptosis) is transmitted through the germ cells (ova and sperm). Children who inherit the genetic mutation will have it in all of their somatic cells, making them more susceptible to subsequent genetic changes in one or more cells that may transform into cancer cells. Beyond the genetic component of cancer, there is little dispute that environmental insult, such as tobacco smoking, sun exposure, and radiation, can be carcinogenic. Such environmental triggers are capable of spontaneously creating noninherited mutations in genes that regulate cell growth and cell response to cell abnormalities that can eventually lead to malignant transformation.

Evidence is growing that genes play an important role in human susceptibility and resistance to infection even in cases with a clear environmental cause of the infectious disease. Evidence for this genetic element in resistance gained heightened recognition during the first decade of the acquired immunodeficiency syndrome (AIDS) epidemic. Researchers identified adults with a specific deletion in both copies of their *CCR5* genes who did not become infected with human immunodeficiency virus (HIV) despite repeated exposure. Later it was found that children exposed to HIV in utero typically had a significantly delayed onset of disease if at least one of their *CCR5* genes had the specific mutation (Romiti, Colognesi, Cancrini, et al., 2000). Understanding the mechanism of resistance associated with *CCR5* mutation led to a novel molecular therapy (Wilkin, Su, Kuritzkes, et al., 2007). This type of drug discovery or development informed by a gene is a newer aspect of pharmacogenetics.

The study of how genes influence a person's response to medication is called pharmacogenetics or pharmacogenomics. Pharmacogenetics is the study of single genes and their respective proteins that influence a medication's intended effect and the risk for adverse effects from the medication. Pharmacogenomics is the study of the portion of the genome that contributes to medication response. These terms are often used interchangeably, and a trend to simply use the term *pharmacogenomics* is becoming apparent. Genes involved in drug response may not be expressed until a medication is given. Variations in the genes predispose a person to experiencing unintended effects from normal doses of certain medications. Unintended effects include absent or reduced therapeutic effect resulting from subtherapeutic levels of the active drug or adverse drug reactions caused by toxicity from abnormally high levels of the active drug after given a normal dose. In this way, pharmacogenomics is another example of the interplay of genes and environmental factors. For more in-depth coverage of pharmacogenomics and implications for nursing practice, the reader is encouraged to consider *Mastering Pharmacogenomics: A Nurse's Handbook for Success* (Lea, Cheek, Brazeau, et al., 2015).

CONGENITAL ANOMALIES

Embryogenesis and fetal development are an intricate and precisely timed series of events in which all parts must be properly integrated to ensure a coordinated whole. Insults during development or abnormalities in differentiation or in the proper timing of organogenesis may result in a variety of congenital anomalies. Congenital anomalies, or birth defects, occur in 2% to 4% of all live-born children and are often classified as deformations, disruptions, dysplasias, or malformations. Deformations are often caused by extrinsic mechanical forces on normally developing tissue. Club foot is an example of a deformation often caused by uterine constraint. Disruptions result from the breakdown of previously normal tissue. Congenital amputations caused by amniotic bands (fibrous strands of amnion that wrap around different body parts during development) are examples of disruption anomalies (Lee, 2009). Dysplasias result from abnormal organization of cells into a particular tissue type. Congenital abnormalities of the teeth, hair, nails, or sweat glands may be manifestations of one of the more than 100 different ectodermal dysplasia syndromes (National Foundation for Ectodermal Dysplasia, 2017). Malformations are abnormal formations of organs or body parts resulting from an abnormal developmental process. Most malformations occur before 12 weeks of gestation. Cleft lip, an example of a malformation, occurs at approximately 5 weeks of gestation when the developing embryo naturally has two clefts in the area. Normally between 5 and 7 weeks, cells rapidly divide and migrate to fill in those clefts. If there is an abnormality in this developmental process, the embryo is left with either a unilateral or bilateral cleft lip that may also involve the palate.

The types of anomalies that can result from genetic or prenatal environmental agents can be major structural abnormalities with serious medical, surgical, or quality-of-life consequences, or they can be minor anomalies or normal variants with no serious consequences, such as a sacral dimple, an extra nipple, or a café-au-lait spot. Congenital anomalies can occur in isolation, such as congenital heart defect, or multiple anomalies may be present. A recognized pattern of anomalies resulting from a single specific cause is called a syndrome (e.g., Down syndrome or fetal alcohol syndrome). A nonrandom pattern of malformations for which a cause has not been determined is called an association (e.g., VACTERL [vertebral defects, anal atresia, cardiac defect, tracheoesophageal fistula, and renal and limb defects] association). When a single anomaly leads to a cascade of additional anomalies, the pattern of defects is referred to as a sequence. Pierre Robin sequence begins with the abnormal development of the mandible, resulting in abnormal placement of the tongue during development. The normal developmental process for the palate is prevented because the tongue obstructs the migration of the palatal shelves toward the midline, and a cleft palate remains. Consequently, infants born with Pierre Robin sequence have a recessed mandible and an abnormally placed tongue and are at risk for obstructive apnea. NTDs, cleft lip and palate, deafness, congenital heart defects, and cognitive impairment are examples of congenital malformations that can occur in isolation or as part of a syndrome, association, or sequence and can have different causes, such as single-gene or chromosome abnormalities, prenatal exposures, or multifactorial causes.

GENETIC DISORDERS

Genetic disorders can be caused by chromosome abnormalities as seen in Turner syndrome, Down syndrome, or velo-cardio-facial syndrome (VCFS); single-gene mutations as seen in sickle cell anemia, neurofibromatosis, or Duchenne muscular dystrophy; a combination of genetic and environmental factors as seen in NTDs or maturity-onset diabetes in the young; and mitochondrial DNA (mtDNA) mutations as seen in nonsyndromic deafness susceptibility due to aminoglycoside sensitivity. Whereas numeric or structural chromosome aberrations automatically involve large groups of genes, a small gene mutation does not alter chromosome structure and number. Alterations in single genes (single-gene disorders) or in many genes (polygenic disorders) may represent a lesion too small to cause an identifiable alteration in chromosomal structure. Human nucleated somatic cells contain approximately 25,000 genes distributed across 46 chromosomes. Because human chromosomes vary in size, the larger the chromosome, the greater the number of genes carried.

Both numeric and structural abnormalities of autosomes (all chromosomes except the X and Y chromosomes) account for a variety of syndromes usually characterized by cognitive deficiencies. A few are associated with a group of characteristics that clearly indicate the precise chromosome anomaly. Nurses often note dysmorphic facial features, behavioral characteristics such as an unusual cry and poor feeding behavior, and other neurologic manifestations such as hypotonia or abnormal reflex responses, which may alert them to these and other chromosome abnormalities.

Numeric Chromosome Abnormalities

With the exception of brief periods of gametogenesis, human beings are diploid individuals, and human somatic cells are diploid (a cell that contains two copies of each chromosome). A diploid chromosome number in humans is represented by the notation 2n = 46. A haploid chromosome constitution (n = 23) is found in germ cells, the male and female gametes (sperm and ova). Somatic cells contain 44 autosomes (the 22 pairs of chromosomes that do not greatly influence sex determination at conception) and 2 sex chromosomes: XX in females and XY in males. For the purpose of cytogenetic studies, chromosomes are usually displayed in a karyotype, the laboratory-made arrangement of specially prepared chromosomes according to their size, banding patterns, and centromere position. The location of the centromere allows the classification of human chromosomes as acrocentric, submetacentric, and metacentric chromosomes (Fig. 3.1).

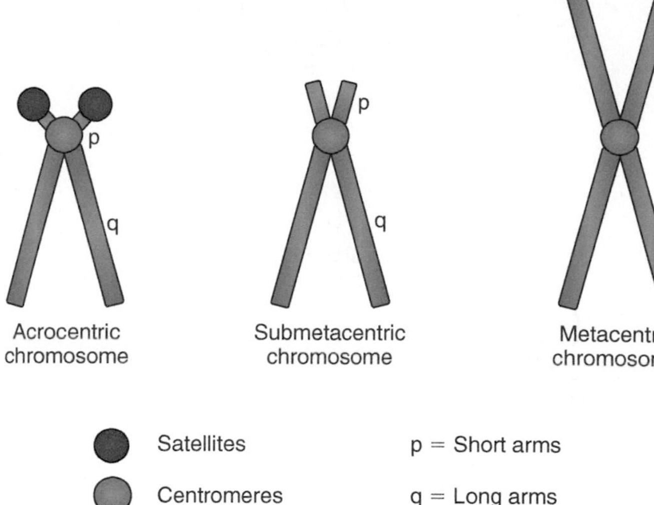

FIG. 3.1 Chromosome classification by centromere position. Positioning of centromeres results in chromosomes with extremely short arms (acrocentric chromosomes), relatively short arms (submetacentric chromosomes), or arms of equal length (metacentric chromosomes).

Numeric chromosome abnormalities occur whenever entire chromosomes are added or deleted. The addition of one or more chromosomes to each pair (increments of the haploid number, 23) will result in triploid cells with 69 chromosomes (46 + 23), or tetraploid cells with 92 chromosomes (46 + 23 + 23), and so on. The product of this uniform addition of chromosomes to all the original pairs is termed *euploidy*, a euploid cell being one whose chromosome number is a multiple of 23.

Individuals who are triploid (3n = 69) have a genetic imbalance of such magnitude that the few who are carried to term have severe multiple abnormalities that limit their life span to a few hours or days. On the other hand, one chromosome may be added to or lost from one of the pairs, creating a condition of aneuploidy. When one chromosome is added to a pair, the embryo, fetus, or child is described as having a trisomy, and the total chromosome number is 47. Most fetuses that have an autosomal trisomy are not live born. Fetuses with trisomy 21, trisomy 18, and trisomy 13 may be live born. When one chromosome is lost from the pair, the fetus is described as having a monosomy, and the total chromosome number in somatic cells is 45. The loss of a chromosome and its related complement of genes is overall more detrimental than the addition of a chromosome. The only monosomy compatible with life is monosomy X (Turner syndrome), yet most 45,X pregnancies spontaneously miscarry (Pinsker, 2012).

The most common cause of alteration in the number of chromosomes is a misdistribution of chromosomes during mitosis or meiosis. As somatic cells multiply by mitosis, each daughter cell receives the same chromosome number as the mother cell. This equitable chromosome sharing in anaphase is due to a phenomenon termed *disjunction*, by which chromatids of each chromosome separate and migrate to opposite poles of the cell. Disruption of this orderly chromosome distribution

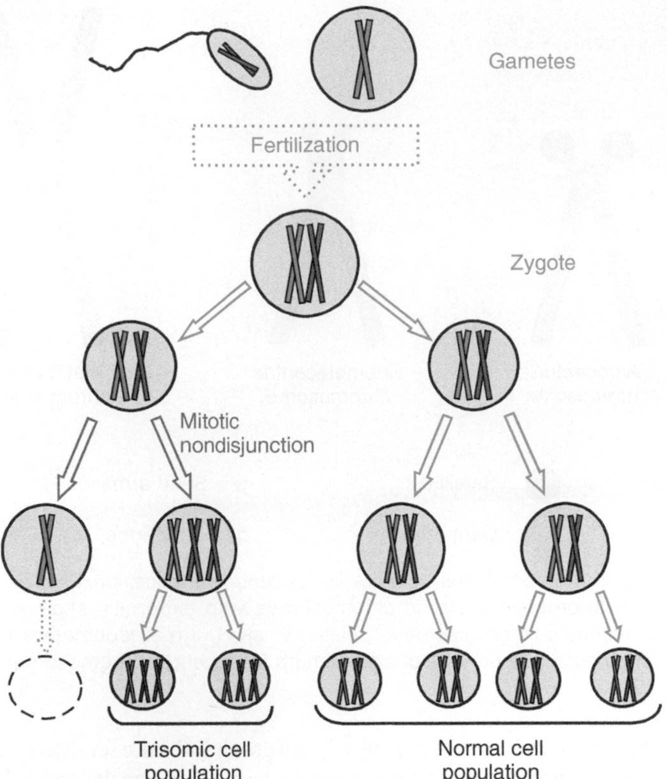

FIG. 3.2 Mitotic nondisjunction resulting in individual with different cell populations (mosaicism). This event occurs during embryonic development, after normal zygote was formed by fertilization of two normal gametes. Only one chromosome pair is represented. As represented here, mitotic nondisjunction and uneven chromosome distribution result in some cell populations with the extra chromosome, whereas other cell lines have the normal chromosome complement.

PATHOPHYSIOLOGY REVIEW

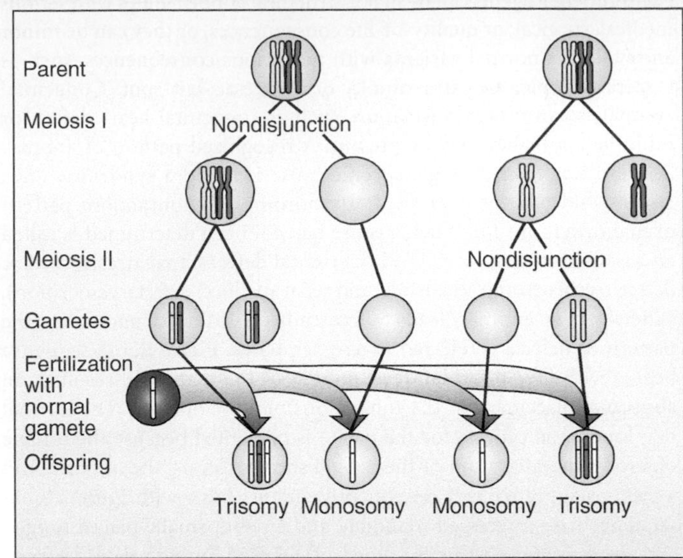

FIG. 3.3 Nondisjunction causes aneuploidy when chromosomes or sister chromatids fail to divide properly. (From Jorde, L. B., Carey, J. C., Bamshad, M. J., et al. [2003]. *Medical genetics* [3rd ed.]. St. Louis, MO: Mosby.)

occurs in ***nondisjunction***, which can occur during both mitosis and meiosis. In mitosis, failure of chromatids to separate properly during anaphase will result in daughter cells with different chromosome numbers (e.g., 45 and 47, instead of 46 and 46). Of those, the 45-chromosome monosomic cells will tend to degenerate and die, but those with the extra chromosome (trisomic) may continue to divide and generate a complete line of trisomic cells.

When **mitotic nondisjunction** occurs during embryonic development (Fig. 3.2), the trisomic cell line proliferates concomitantly with the normal cell line and results in an individual with **mosaicism** for that particular chromosome. Mosaicism therefore results in an individual (mosaic) with two or more genetically different cell populations. The chromosomal notation for a male with mosaic type of Down syndrome, for example, is 46,XY/47,XY,+21). The slash (/) indicates a dual cell population in which one has the normal chromosomal constitution (46,XY), whereas the other carries an extra chromosome 21 and has a total chromosome number of 47 (Simons, Shaffer, & Hastings, 2013). The percentage, or level, of mosaicism depends on the stage of embryonic development in which the cell division error occurs. If it occurs at the first cell division after fertilization, the level of mosaicism may be as high as 50%. If the cell division error occurs in later development, the abnormal cells may be localized to one cell type, such as the brain tissue or germ cell line (ovaries or testes). The extent of clinical manifestations is determined by the type of tissues that contain cells with abnormal chromosome numbers and the percentage of affected cells, and may vary from near normal to a fully manifested syndrome.

Meiotic nondisjunction (Fig. 3.3) is a major cause of aneuploidy, an abnormal chromosome pattern in which the total number of chromosomes is not a multiple of the haploid number, 23. Nondisjunction can occur during meiosis I and II, during both oogenesis and spermatogenesis, resulting in gametes with an aneuploid chromosome number (e.g., 22 or 24, instead of 23). As in the case of somatic cells, gametes lacking a chromosome are not likely to survive, but gametes with an extra chromosome are more often viable. Fertilization of an aneuploid gamete with a normal gamete will produce an aneuploid zygote. The most common aneuploidies in humans are trisomies.

Autosome Aneuploidies

Examples of numeric alterations affecting the autosomes include some of the most common trisomies found in humans: trisomy 21 (Down syndrome), trisomy 18 (Edwards syndrome), and trisomy 13 (Patau syndrome) (Table 3.2).

Trisomy 21

Down syndrome affects 1 in 800 to 1 in 1000 live births and is the most common aneuploidy compatible with life expectancy into adulthood. Physical and cognitive abnormalities vary (Bull & Committee on Genetics, 2011). Intelligence quotient (IQ) range is typically mild to moderate impairment. In spite of modern medical developments, life expectancy is still shortened, with 20% dying in the first decade and 50% by age 60 years. Adults with Down syndrome are also more likely to develop Alzheimer disease; more than 75% of those over age 60 are affected with the disease (Jensen & Bulova, 2014).

The chromosomal constitution of Down syndrome is variable, with three possible configurations:

1. **Trisomy**—The nomenclature for a female with trisomy is 47,XX+21 and for a male with trisomy is 47,XY,+21. Trisomy encompasses 92% of all cases of Down syndrome. The extra chromosome 21 is

TABLE 3.2 Partial List of Chromosomal Genetic Disorders

Disorder	Genetic Etiology	Possible Periods of Recognition	Major Findings	Resources*
Angelman syndrome	Chr—Deletion, uniparental disomy, or abnormal methylation of chromosome 15	Prenatal to early childhood	Significant motor, cognitive, and speech delays; microcephaly; ataxia	http://www.ncbi.nlm.nih.gov/books/NBK1144/ http://ghr.nlm.nih.gov/condition=angelmansyndrome https://www.angelman.org/
Beckwith-Wiedemann syndrome	AD or Chr—Abnormal methylation of chromosome 11, uniparental disomy of paternal chromosome 11, or structural abnormality in critical region	Prenatal to newborn	Overgrowth syndrome; often recognized in newborn period due to abnormally large tongue; abdominal wall defects; hypoglycemia in infancy	http://www.ncbi.nlm.nih.gov/books/NBK1394/ http://ghr.nlm.nih.gov/condition/beckwith-wiedemann-syndrome http://www.beckwithwiedemann.org/
Cri du chat syndrome	Chr—46,XX,del(5p) or 46,XY,del(5p)	Prenatal to newborn	Microcephaly; high-pitched, catlike cry; significant motor and cognitive delays	http://ghr.nlm.nih.gov/condition/cri-du-chat-syndrome http://www.fivepminus.org
Down syndrome (trisomy 21)	Chr—47,XX,+21 or 47,XY,+21	Prenatal to newborn	Mild to moderate cognitive impairment, characteristic facial features, hypotonia	http://ghr.nlm.nih.gov/condition/down-syndrome http://pediatrics.aappublications.org/content/128/2/393.full http://www.ndss.org http://www.nads.org
Edwards syndrome (trisomy 18)	Chr—47,XX,+18 or 47,XY,+18	Prenatal to newborn	Multiple congenital anomalies; significantly shortened life span; if survival beyond 1 year, severe cognitive impairment	http://ghr.nlm.nih.gov/condition/trisomy-18 http://www.trisomy18.org
Klinefelter syndrome	Chr—47,XXY	Prenatal; adolescence to adulthood	Gynecomastia, small testes, normal sex drive and function but infertility common	http://ghr.nlm.nih.gov/condition/klinefelter-syndrome
Patau syndrome (trisomy 13)	Chr—47,XX,+13 or 47,XY,+13	Prenatal to newborn	Multiple congenital anomalies; significantly shortened life span; if survival beyond 1 year, severe cognitive impairment	http://ghr.nlm.nih.gov/condition/trisomy-13 http://trisomy.org/
Prader-Willi syndrome	Chr—Absence of paternally derived region of chromosome 15 or abnormally methylated critical region of chromosome 15	Prenatal; infancy to early childhood	Severe hypotonia, failure to thrive in early infancy; after 1-2 years of age, excessive eating—including nonfood items; morbid obesity; cognitive impairment; distinctive behavioral problems; hypogonadism	http://www.ncbi.nlm.nih.gov/books/NBK1330/ http://ghr.nlm.nih.gov/condition/prader-willi-syndrome http://www.pwsausa.org/
Turner syndrome	Chr—45,XO	Prenatal to adolescence	Lymphedema at birth, coarctation, short stature, ovarian dysgenesis, lack of secondary sex characteristics during adolescence	http://ghr.nlm.nih.gov/condition/turner-syndrome http://jcem.endojournals.org/content/92/1/10.full http://www.turnersyndrome.org/ https://www.turnersyndromefoundation.org/

*Support groups are listed on most websites. However, before referring families to support groups, particularly for families that discovered the diagnosis prenatally, carefully review the support group and describe its focus to the couple so they can make an informed decision about whether to visit it.

AD, Autosomal dominant; *Chr,* chromosomal.

unattached and segregates freely during meiosis. The risk for this type of Down syndrome increases linearly with increasing maternal age (Allen, Freeman, Druschel, et al., 2009); however, because young women have more babies, about 75% of babies with trisomy 21 are born to younger mothers.

2. **Translocation Down syndrome**—The accepted nomenclature for a male with Down syndrome due to robertsonian translocation between acrocentric chromosomes 14 and 21 is 46,XY,t(14;21). Translocation (discussed later) accounts for approximately 4% of all male and female Down syndrome cases. The majority of cases are sporadic (without family history), but about 25% have one balanced translocation carrier parent. When one such carrier and a partner with normal chromosomes reproduce, their theoretic chances of producing a live-born child with Down syndrome are 33%, but the actual observed

risk is approximately 15% if the mother is the carrier and less than 10% if the father is the carrier. The observed chance of producing a live-born child who is a balanced translocation carrier approaches 50%. Because chromosome 21 is an acrocentric chromosome, it is possible for the translocation to be with both chromosome 21s. A carrier mother [45,XX,t(21;21)] or father [45,XY,t(21;21)] of the translocation would have a 100% chance of producing a pregnancy with Down syndrome because the other parent normally would contribute one chromosome 21. This latter situation is one of the rare examples in genetics where an abnormality is passed on to *all* living progeny.

3. **Mosaic Down syndrome**—The nomenclature for a female with mosaic Down syndrome is 46,XX/47,XX+21. This rarer type of Down syndrome can occur in males and females. It results from mitotic nondisjunction during early embryonic development of a normal zygote. Children with this type have mixed cell populations, some with the normal karyotype, others with the extra chromosome. Contrary to what one might expect, children with mosaic Down syndrome do not necessarily have a better developmental outcome than those with free trisomy type. The proportion of trisomic cells in various tissues and organs play a role in the child's developmental potential and syndrome-associated potential health problems.

Trisomy 18

Edwards syndrome is a fairly common trisomy in fetuses. Those who are live born have severe cognitive impairment and physical abnormalities that contribute to a limited life span.

Trisomy 13

Patau syndrome carries more severe malformations than the previous two trisomies discussed, consistent with the increased size of the extra chromosome and greater gene imbalance. Life span is significantly shortened.

Sex Chromosome Aneuploidies

Alterations in number may also involve the sex chromosomes (see Table 3.2). The possible mechanisms by which sex chromosome abnormalities may occur are the same as those previously described (i.e., prefertilization nondisjunction during one of the meiotic divisions of gametogenesis in either parent or in the early postfertilization divisions of the zygote). An alteration in the number of sex chromosomes usually does not produce the profound effects that are associated with the autosomal trisomies. Intelligence may be normal or low normal, or the child may have some learning disabilities, but moderate or severe cognitive impairment is less common. Some of the most common genetic disorders caused by sex chromosome aneuploidies are Klinefelter, XYY, triple-X female, and Turner syndromes.

47,XXY

Klinefelter syndrome is the most common of all sex chromosome aneuploidies. Physical abnormalities include elements of decreased masculinization, such as gynecomastia; hypogonadism (with sterility resulting from degeneration of seminiferous tubules); and increased pubis-to-sole length, reflecting elongated lower limbs (Fig. 3.4). Mental development is normal in most cases, with a mean full-scale IQ between 85 and 90. Cognitive difficulties tend to be in expressive language, auditory processing, and auditory memory. Chromosome mosaicism (46,XY/47,XXY) rarely occurs and results in individuals with milder manifestations than their trisomic counterparts. Overall, the phenotype of Klinefelter syndrome is highly variable, making it difficult, in the absence of chromosome studies, to make a prepubertal clinical diagnosis.

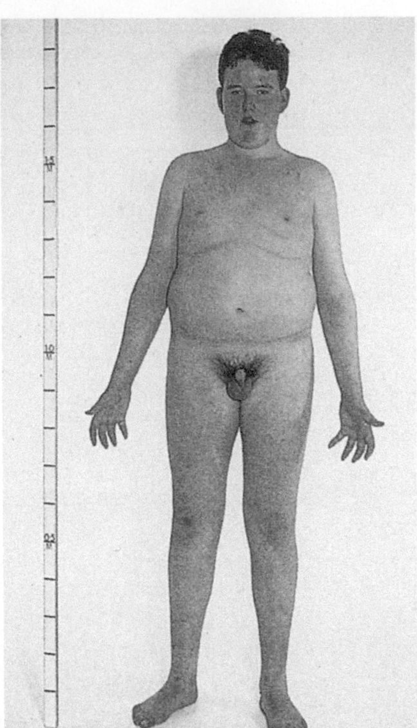

FIG. 3.4 Klinefelter syndrome. This young man exhibits many characteristics of Klinefelter syndrome: small testes, some development of the breasts, sparse body hair, and long limbs. This syndrome results from the presence of two or more X chromosomes with one Y chromosome (genotypes XXY or XXXY, for example). (From Patton, K. T. [2019]. *Anatomy and physiology* [10th ed.]. St. Louis, MO: Elsevier.)

47,XYY

This genotype was reported in the early 1960s by Patricia Jacobs, a Scottish cytogeneticist who detected an increased frequency of double-Y men among inmates of penal institutions in Great Britain. This and subsequent early studies that linked this karyotype with criminal behavior were significantly flawed by selection bias. Males with XYY may be at increased risk for autism spectrum disorder (Ross, Roeltgen, Kushner, et al., 2012). The extra Y is paternally derived. Although XYY fathers have an increased risk for offspring with abnormal Y chromosome complement, the majority of live births have a normal number of sex chromosomes.

45,XO

Turner syndrome, originally described clinically as ovarian dysgenesis (with gonads consisting of streaks of connective tissue and devoid of germ cells), is an example of a monosomy that is compatible with life. Clinical manifestations are variable in expression. Intellectually, verbal IQ exceeds performance IQ. There is no prepubertal growth spurt, and girls with Turner syndrome are generally infertile. It is common practice to administer female hormones around the time that puberty would occur to provide the girl with Turner syndrome some secondary sex characteristics; however, the female hormones may further stunt growth and must be used judiciously. The child's growth is usually normal until 3 years of age and then slows, gradually drifting away from the normal growth curve. Treatment for the decreased growth velocity includes growth hormone and anabolic steroids. Mosaicism also occurs in Turner syndrome (e.g., 46,XX/45,XO), resulting in milder expression of the phenotype. Girls with Turner syndrome may have difficulty with peer relationships and with understanding social cues. They may exhibit behavioral problems, especially immature, socially isolated behavior. Most, however, lead productive lives and function as independent adults.

47,XXX

A relatively common condition (1:1000 live female births), females with triple-X display a normal phenotype, with an increased risk of learning disabilities compared with their euploid sisters. Gynecologic complications include delayed menarche and premature menopause. As with XYY men, the offspring of XXX women is largely normal, indicative of a selective advantage of euploid gametes.

Structural Chromosome Abnormalities

Chromosomes are subject to structural alterations resulting from breakage and rearrangement. Chromosome **breakage** has long been recognized as a significant source of genetic abnormalities. Many **clastogens** (chromosome-breaking agents) have been identified, including physical (e.g., ionizing radiation), chemical (e.g., chlorpromazine), and biologic (e.g., viral infections) agents. Chromosome breakage can also result from many nonspecific causes, such as influenza. These breaks usually are restricted to somatic cells and are temporary. Chromosome breakage becomes significant when it is permanent (or long lasting) and when these permanent changes, in addition to appearing in somatic cells, are also present in germ cells and thus have the potential of being transmitted to the offspring.

A chromosome **deletion** occurs when chromosome breakage results in loss of the broken fragment at a chromosome's terminal end or within the chromosome. Chromosome deletions often have significant clinical impact, as in a chromosome 5 terminal deletion that results in cri du chat syndrome. Chromosome breakage can create unstable end points ("sticky ends"), which predispose the chromosomes to a variety of rearrangements of the fragments. A relatively rare structural abnormality that can occur as a result of chromosomal "sticky ends" is a ring chromosome. If a break occurs in the terminal end of both arms of a chromosome, the ends may fuse together, forming a circle. Like any structural alteration of a chromosome, the clinical manifestations depend on which genes are lost.

A more common rearrangement resulting from chromosome breakage is a **translocation**, which occurs when a chromosomal fragment reunites with another, nonhomologous chromosome. Two types of translocations have clinical significance: reciprocal translocations and robertsonian translocations. In a **reciprocal translocation**, breaks occur in two different chromosomes and the fragments are mutually exchanged, resulting in derivative chromosomes. **Robertsonian translocations** occur when the short arms of two acrocentric chromosomes (pairs 13 to 15 and pairs 21 and 22) break off and the remaining long arms fuse at the centromere, forming a "single chromosome" (Fig. 3.5). Both types result in individuals who have the correct amount of genetic information (although "rearranged"), and therefore no clinical manifestations are expected. These persons are termed ***balanced translocation carriers***. These asymptomatic, balanced translocation carriers (either male or female) may pass the translocation to their offspring in a balanced or unbalanced form, depending on how the chromosomes segregate to the gametes. If it is passed in the unbalanced form, the combination is often lethal, and an early spontaneous abortion occurs. The chance of having a live-born child with birth defects associated with the unbalanced translocation depends on the quantity and role of the missing or additional genetic material. Approximately 5% of cases of repeated spontaneous abortion (two or more) can be attributed to a balanced translocation carrier parent.

PATHOPHYSIOLOGY REVIEW

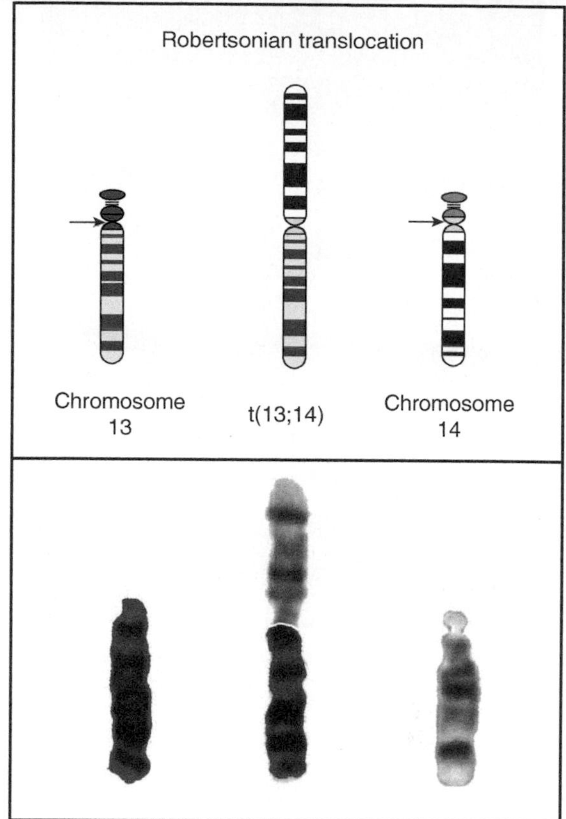

FIG. 3.5 Translocation. In a robertsonian translocation, the long arms of two acrocentric chromosomes (13 and 14) fuse, forming a single chromosome. (From Jorde, L. B., Carey, J. C., Bamshad, M. J., et al. [2003]. *Medical genetics* [3rd ed.]. St. Louis, MO: Mosby.)

Some structural chromosome abnormalities are too small to reliably visualize under a light microscope but are still clinically relevant. Fragile, or weak, sites associated with expanded triplet repeats (described later in the chapter) have been identified on both the autosomes and the X chromosome. A classic example is fragile X syndrome. **Contiguous gene syndromes** are disorders characterized by a microdeletion or microduplication of smaller chromosome segments, which may require special analysis techniques or molecular testing to detect.

46,XX,del(5p) or 46,XY,del(5p)

Cri du chat, or cat's cry, syndrome is a rare (1:50,000 live births) (Jorde, Carey, Bamshad, et al., 2016) chromosome deletion syndrome resulting from loss of the small arm of chromosome 5. In early infancy this syndrome manifests with a typical but nondistinctive facial appearance, often a "moon-shaped" face with wide-spaced eyes (hypertelorism) (Fig. 3.6). As the child grows, this feature is progressively diluted, and by age 2 years the child is indistinguishable from age-matched controls. Profound cognitive impairment persists throughout their short life; many die in infancy. Typical of this disease is a crying pattern that is abnormal and catlike. At times it sounds like an angry cat, and at others like a soft mewing sound. This is a result of a laryngeal atrophy that improves with age. By age 3 years the crying pattern is still abnormal, but it acquires a normal pitch and loses its catlike quality.

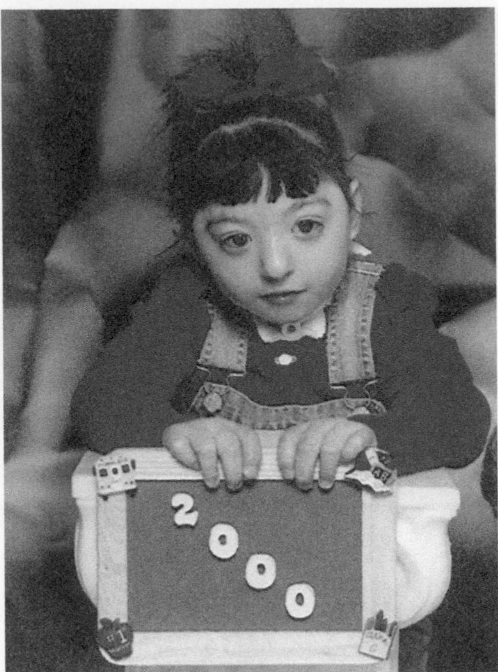

FIG. 3.6 Eight-year-old child with cri du chat (cat's cry) syndrome. Notice the wide-spaced eyes (hypertelorism) and "moon face."

Fragile X Syndrome

Fragile X syndrome acquired its name from the fact that, in special cell culture conditions, the affected X chromosome may display a gap in its terminal portion. However, it is an X-linked condition caused by an unstable expansion (described later in the chapter). Fragile X is the most common cause of inherited cognitive impairment. Common clinical features include a typical facial appearance, with an elongated face and large ears; macroorchidism in adolescent males; connective tissue dysplasia; and behavioral problems, including autism spectrum disorder (Committee on Genetics, 2011).

Velo-Cardio-Facial Syndrome

Velo-cardio-facial syndrome (VCFS), sometimes called DiGeorge syndrome or CATCH22, is a common (1:4000) microdeletion syndrome. It is caused by a specific microdeletion within the long arm of chromosome 22 (22q11.2 deletion) (McDonald-McGinn, Emanuel, & Zackai, 1999, updated 2013). Manifestations of this condition are variable, with nearly 200 different possible clinical features described. Although no one feature is found in every patient, cognitive impairment is common and can range from full-scale measured IQ in the borderline low-normal range with characteristic learning disabilities to mild cognitive impairment (Antshel, Fremont, Kates, et al., 2008). Although most patients' deletion is caused by a sporadic event, those with the condition can transmit the microdeletion in an autosomal dominant manner. Therefore their chances of producing a child with VCFS are 50% with each pregnancy.

Chromosome Instability Syndromes

Chromosome instability syndromes are a heterogeneous group of genetic disorders characterized by a high frequency of chromosome breakage observed in vitro. They include ataxia telangiectasia, Fanconi anemia, and xeroderma pigmentosum. These syndromes are associated with decreased immune function and an increased incidence of cancer.

SINGLE-GENE DISORDERS

Chromosome anomalies typically affect large numbers of genes; however, a single-gene disorder is caused by an abnormality within a gene or in a gene's regulatory region. Single-gene disorders can affect all body systems and may have mild to severe expression. These disorders display a mendelian pattern of dominant or recessive inheritance that was first delineated in the mid–nineteenth century by Gregor Mendel's experiments with plants. Single-gene disorders cannot be detected by chromosome analysis and demand specific and sophisticated molecular detection methods, such as DNA-based techniques (Table 3.3).

Mendelian inheritance laws allow for risk prediction in single-gene disorders; however, phenotypic expression may be altered by incomplete penetrance or variable expressivity of the responsible allele. An allele is said to have reduced or incomplete penetrance in a population when a proportion of persons who possess that allele do not express the phenotype. An allele is said to have variable expressivity when individuals possessing that allele display the features of the syndrome in various degrees, from mild to severe. If a person expresses even the mildest possible phenotype, the allele is penetrant in that individual.

Autosomal Inheritance Patterns

Autosomal Dominant Inheritance

General characteristics of autosomal dominant inheritance are presented in Box 3.2. A clear understanding of transmission of autosomal inheritance patterns requires the understanding of a few basic facts. First, most genetic diseases are rare. The probability that two affected persons will mate is very low for most genetic disorders (with the exception of societal selection, as in the case of achondroplasia). Second, depending on the disease, if one parent is affected, he or she is much more likely to be heterozygous (have one mutant allele) than homozygous (have two mutant alleles). Usually, an individual with two dominant mutant alleles will experience physical or cognitive abnormalities at a much more severe level.

Those assumptions being accepted, two questions remain: What are the chances of transmitting the mutant allele to the offspring? And what are the risks of the offspring being affected? If a gene has only two alleles, one normal and one mutant, three possible allele combinations exist: normal/normal, normal/mutant, and mutant/mutant. In autosomal dominant conditions, only persons with normal/normal combination will be disease free, assuming that the mutant allele is 100% penetrant. Fig. 3.7 shows the relationships between genotypes and phenotypes for an autosomal dominant trait. Considering that genetic diseases are rare and that persons who are homozygous for the mutated allele are more severely affected, it is most likely that an affected individual who is heterozygous for the mutant allele will mate with a genotypically normal partner (Fig. 3.8, *A*). The outcomes of these matings are best expressed by the use of Punnett squares. Also depicted (Fig. 3.8, *B*) is the mating of a homozygote for the mutated gene with a genotypically normal partner. The result of these matings is one of the few instances in medical genetics in which *all* progeny have a 100% chance of being affected, assuming that the mutant allele they receive is 100% penetrant. These matings, however, are extremely rare.

Many children diagnosed with an autosomal dominant disorder have a positive family history of the disease. In other instances, that child may represent the first occurrence of that condition in the family. In the latter case, the event may be due to a new mutation (de novo mutation) in that child or to the presence of the mutation only in a subset of the germ cells of a healthy parent. The birth of other affected children indicates the second possibility. The range of expression of autosomal dominant gene mutations is highly variable, from minor manifestations (e.g., polydactyly), to severe, debilitating, and life-threatening disease

TABLE 3.3 Select Techniques of DNA Analysis and Disease Detection

Technique	Purpose and Methodology	Application
Basic Techniques		
DNA extraction	Extracted DNA can be immediately analyzed or stored for future use.	DNA extracted from variety of cells (amniocytes, lymphoblasts, single cell from eight-cell stage embryo) and tissues (skin, cheek cells, hair root, chorionic villi, archived pathology specimens)
Polymerase chain reaction (PCR)	Rapid amplification of small quantities of genetic material (DNA or RNA). Short lengths of DNA (primers) bind to specific DNA regions and initiate their replication. Several repetitions of this process can amplify a desired DNA region (and only this region) several thousand fold.	Essential technique for many molecular genetic diagnostic tests, but limited to already sequenced DNA genes or regions
Post-PCR Analysis		
Sequence of all exons and intron-exon boundaries of a gene	As cost decreases, this is becoming preferred test for genes that have many possible disease-associated mutations throughout the gene.	*BRCA1, BRCA2,* familial adenomatous polyposis Picks up all mutations except large gene deletions, but may pick up a mutation not previously described and may not be able to tell if it has any pathologic significance.
Sequence-specific amplification and amplification refractory mutation system (ARMS)	Detection of already sequenced mutations by means of sequence-specific primers. ARMS detects presence or absence of specific mutation.	Cystic fibrosis Hemoglobinopathies (sickle cell disease, thalassemias)
Oligonucleotide ligation assay (OLA)	Two complementing small nucleotide probes reciprocally bind to DNA. Mutation is detected because it prevents appropriate binding of probes to DNA.	Cystic fibrosis Familial hypercholesterolemia
Restriction enzyme analysis of PCR products	Commercially available bacterial endonucleases bind to specific DNA sequences and cut molecule at that point.	Charcot-Marie-Tooth disease Duchenne and Becker muscular dystrophies
Single-stranded conformation polymorphism analysis (SSCP)	Some mutations resulting from base substitutions cause changes in secondary structure of DNA. SSCP detects such conformational changes indicative of occurring mutations.	
Heteroduplex analysis	The conformational properties of the double-stranded molecules are used to distinguish different base pairing (i.e., mutations).	
Non-PCR–Based Analysis		
Southern blotting	After cutting DNA with restriction enzymes, fragments are analyzed for mutations or repeated base sequences.	Fragile X syndrome (CGG repeats) Huntington disease (CAG repeats) Some thalassemias (e.g., Bart thalassemia)

CAG, Cytosine-adenine-guanine; *CGG,* cytosine-guanine-guanine; *DNA,* deoxyribonucleic acid; *RNA,* ribonucleic acid.

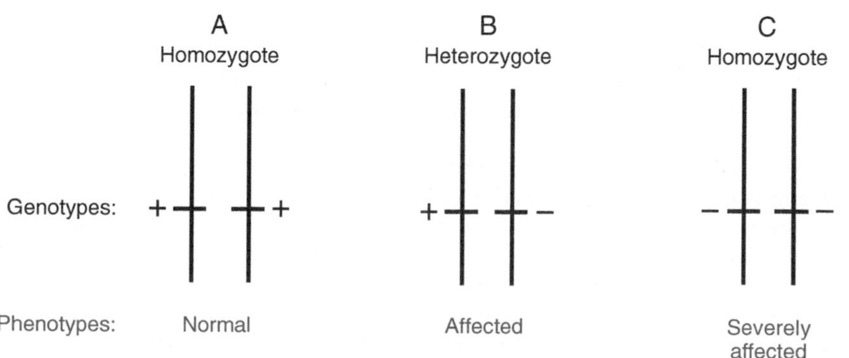

FIG. 3.7 Dominant inheritance pattern. Schematic representation of the three possible allelic arrangements of a gene with two alleles. Depicted here are genotypes and possible phenotypes for a trait transmitted by a dominant gene. The presence of a single copy of the mutant allele in heterozygous person **(B)** is sufficient to express the phenotype in question. Double dose of the mutated allele, in homozygous person **(C),** results in more severe expression of the phenotype.

BOX 3.2 Autosomal Dominant Inheritance: Characteristics*

- Males and females are equally likely to be affected.
- A single copy of the mutant allele is typically sufficient to cause the phenotype to express, and therefore a carrier state does not exist. However, if the mutant allele is not fully penetrant (some individuals in a population with the same mutant allele do not express the trait), the unaffected person with the mutant allele may be referred to as a carrier of the reduced penetrant allele.
- The homozygote for the mutant allele is usually more severely affected than the heterozygote.
- The phenotype appears in consecutive generations unless the condition was due to a new dominant mutation.
- Children of an affected parent have a 50% chance of inheriting the mutant allele and being affected.
- If the mutant allele is 100% penetrant, phenotypically normal persons in a family pedigree are free of the mutant allele and do not transmit the phenotype to their offspring. However, due to variable expressivity, careful clinical examination and laboratory studies may be necessary before concluding that a person is truly "phenotypically normal."

*All partners of affected persons here are considered genotypically normal.

A

+/− (top) / +/+ (left)	+	−
+	+/+	+/−
+	+/+	+/−

Parent 1: +/− (affected)
Parent 2: +/+ (normal)

Outcomes per pregnancy:
50% +/− (affected)
50% +/+ (normal)

B

+/+ (top) / −/− (left)	+	+
−	+/−	+/−
−	−/+	−/+

Parent 1: +/+ (normal)
Parent 2: −/− (affected)

Outcomes per pregnancy:
100% +/− (affected)

\+ Normal ("wild-type") allele
− Mutant allele

FIG. 3.8 Determination of mating outcomes in autosomal dominant inheritance obtained with Punnett squares. **A,** Possible outcomes of the mating of an affected heterozygous individual (+/–) with a normal partner (+/+). **B,** Mating of an affected homozygous individual (–/–) and a normal partner (+/+).

PATHOPHYSIOLOGY REVIEW

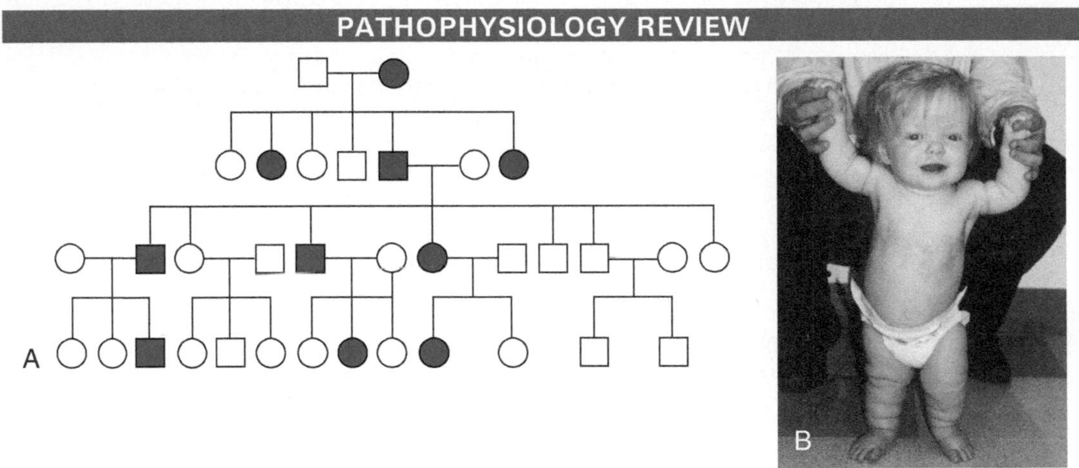

FIG. 3.9 Pedigree for achondroplasia. **A,** Pedigree showing the transmission of an autosomal dominant disease. **B,** Achondroplasia. This girl has short limbs relative to trunk length. She also has a prominent forehead, low nasal root, and redundant skin folds in the arms and legs. (*B,* From Jorde, L. B., Carey, J. C., Bamshad, M. J., et al. [2003]. *Medical genetics* [3rd ed.]. St. Louis, MO: Mosby.)

(e.g., neurofibromatosis). Depending on the degree of disability the condition imposes on the individual and the ability to procreate, the mutated gene either will be eliminated or will continue to be passed on through several generations. In addition, in diseases that have a late age of onset (e.g., Huntington disease), a person with a disease-associated mutation may be healthy and asymptomatic during childbearing years and be unaware of the risk of passing on the mutant allele to offspring. Consequently, the mutant allele continues to be passed on through several generations.

Other examples of autosomal dominant disorders include achondroplasia, neurofibromatosis, and Marfan syndrome. An idealized pedigree for autosomal dominant inheritance is found in Fig. 3.9 and discussed in the Nursing Care Guidelines box later in this chapter. The gene mutation associated with achondroplasia is considered 100% penetrant. The pedigree in the figure demonstrates that although an affected parent has a 50% chance with each pregnancy of transmitting the gene mutation associated with achondroplasia, 50% of offspring do not necessarily inherit the gene mutation. Selected examples of autosomal dominant disorders are found in Table 3.4.

Autosomal Recessive Inheritance

General characteristics of autosomal recessive inheritance are presented in Box 3.3. Children who display an autosomal recessive disorder are always homozygous for that trait (both the maternally and paternally inherited alleles contain disease-associated mutations). This is due to the fact that a recessive allele is one whose phenotypic expression occurs only when both genes have disease-associated mutations. Although this makes the alleles homozygous because both alleles are recessive, the disease-associated mutation may be different in each allele. When this is the case, the pair of alleles is more accurately referred to as compound heterozygous for the recessive trait. In the heterozygote, a recessive

Text continued on p. 56

TABLE 3.4 **Partial List of Mendelian Inherited Genetic Disorders**

Disorder	Genetic Etiology	Possible Periods of Recognition	Major Findings	Resources*
Achondroplasia	AD	Prenatal to newborn	Dwarfism with legs and arms significantly shorter than torso; characteristic facial features	http://www.ncbi.nlm.nih.gov/books/NBK1152/ http://ghr.nlm.nih.gov/condition/achondroplasia http://www.lpaonline.org/
Adenosine deaminase deficiency	AR	Prenatal[†]; infant period most common; onset can be delayed until adulthood	Enzyme deficiency that results in severe combined immunodeficiency	http://www.ncbi.nlm.nih.gov/books/NBK1483/ http://ghr.nlm.nih.gov/condition/adenosine-deaminase-deficiency http://www.primaryimmune.org
Ataxia telangiectasia	AR	Prenatal[†] to early childhood	Immunodeficiency, neurodegenerative, acute sensitivity to ionizing radiation that increases risk for cancer	https://www.ncbi.nlm.nih.gov/books/NBK26468/ http:www.cancer.gov/cancertopics/factsheet/risk/ataxia http://ghr.nlm.nih.gov/condition/ataxia-telangiectasia http://www.atcp.org
Beckwith-Wiedemann syndrome	AD or Chr—Abnormal methylation of chromosome 11, uniparental disomy of paternal chromosome 11, or structural abnormality in critical region	Prenatal to newborn	Overgrowth syndrome; often recognized in newborn period due to abnormally large tongue; abdominal wall defects; hypoglycemia in infancy	http://www.ncbi.nlm.nih.gov/books/NBK1394/ http://ghr.nlm.nih.gov/condition/beckwith-wiedemann-syndrome http://bws-support.org.uk/
Bloom syndrome	AR	Prenatal[†] to early childhood	Prenatal and postnatal growth retardation; chromosome instability leading to sun sensitivity, high cancer risk, immunodeficiency	http://www.ncbi.nlm.nih.gov/books/NBK1398/ http://ghr.nlm.nih.gov/condition/bloom-syndrome
Congenital adrenal hyperplasia	AR	Prenatal[†] to newborn	Ambiguous genitalia—virilization of female external genitalia due to elevated androgen levels; salt loss in some due to inability to reabsorb sodium	http://www.ncbi.nlm.nih.gov/books/NBK1171/ http://ghr.nlm.nih.gov/condition/21-hydroxylase-deficiency https://www.magicfoundation.org/Growth-Disorders/Congenital-Adrenal-Hyperplasia/
Cystic fibrosis	AR	Prenatal[†] to toddler	Meconium ileus at birth; pancreatic insufficiency and malabsorption; chronic pulmonary inflammation and infection	http://www.ncbi.nlm.nih.gov/books/NBK1250/ http://ghr.nlm.nih.gov/condition/cystic-fibrosis http://www.cff.org
Duchenne muscular dystrophy	XL recessive	Prenatal[†] to early childhood	Delayed milestones, progressive skeletal muscle disease, dilated cardiomyopathy	http://www.ncbi.nlm.nih.gov/books/NBK1119/ http://ghr.nlm.nih.gov/condition/duchenne-and-becker-muscular-dystrophy http://www.mda.org/disease/DMD.html
Familial adenomatous polyposis (Gardner syndrome, Turcot syndrome)	AD—Mutation in APC gene	Childhood to adulthood	Hundreds to thousands of adenomatous polyps in the distal portion of colon; colon cancer; extra colonic polyps and tumors	http://www.ncbi.nlm.nih.gov/books/NBK1345/ http://ghr.nlm.nih.gov/condition/familial-adenomatous-polyposis
Fanconi anemia	Most forms AR; at least one form XL	Prenatal[†] to childhood	Multiple malformations, progressive bone marrow failure, chromosome breakage in cell culture	http://www.ncbi.nlm.nih.gov/books/NBK1401/ https://ghr.nlm.nih.gov/condition/fanconi-anemia#

Continued

TABLE 3.4 **Partial List of Mendelian Inherited Genetic Disorders—cont'd**

Disorder	Genetic Etiology	Possible Periods of Recognition	Major Findings	Resources*
Fragile X syndrome	XL—Expanded triplet repeat	Prenatal; childhood to adolescent	Moderate cognitive impairment in males, mild cognitive impairment in females	http://www.ncbi.nlm.nih.gov/books/NBK1384/ http://ghr.nlm.nih.gov/condition/fragile-x-syndrome https://fragilex.org/
Friedreich ataxia	AR (most have expanded triplet repeat in one or both genes)	Prenatal[†] to childhood, sometimes not until adulthood	Slowly progressive ataxia, cardiomyopathy	http://www.ncbi.nlm.nih.gov/books/NBK1281/ http://ghr.nlm.nih.gov/condition/friedreich-ataxia http://www.ataxia.org/
Galactosemia	AR	Prenatal[†] to neonatal	Failure to thrive, hepatocellular damage, sepsis, bleeding, cognitive impairment, death if untreated	http://www.ncbi.nlm.nih.gov/books/NBK1518/ http://ghr.nlm.nih.gov/condition/galactosemia
Gaucher disease	AR	Prenatal[†] to adulthood	Three major types: • Type 1 most common; hepatosplenomegaly, bone disease, sometimes lung disease • Type 2 neurodegenerative, lethal by 4 years • Type 3 neurodegenerative disease, can live to adulthood	http://www.ncbi.nlm.nih.gov/books/NBK1269/ http://ghr.nlm.nih.gov/condition/gaucher-disease http://www.gaucherdisease.org/
Glucose-6-phosphate dehydrogenase (G6PD) deficiency	XL recessive	Infant to adulthood	Hemolytic anemia; expression dependent on exposure to environmental triggers (eating fava beans, certain infections, and certain drugs)	http://www.nlm.nih.gov/medlineplus/ency/article/000528.htm http://ghr.nlm.nih.gov/condition/glucose-6-phosphate-dehydrogenase-deficiency
Hemophilia A, hemophilia B	XL recessive	Prenatal[†] to adulthood depending on extent of deficient clotting activity	Hemophilia A—Factor VIII deficiency; hemophilia B—Factor IX deficiency Both diagnosed in infancy period in those with severe deficiency; brought to attention by spontaneous joint or deep muscle bleeds	http://www.ncbi.nlm.nih.gov/books/NBK1404/ http://www.ncbi.nlm.nih.gov/books/NBK1495/ http://ghr.nlm.nih.gov/condition/hemophilia
Hunter syndrome	XL recessive	Prenatal[†] to childhood	Progressive multisystem disorder due to glycosaminoglycans accumulation; CNS deterioration common in severe form but not attenuated form	http://www.ncbi.nlm.nih.gov/books/NBK1274/ http://ghr.nlm.nih.gov/condition/mucopolysaccharidosis-type-ii http://mpssociety.org/
Huntington disease	AD expanded triplet repeat	Prenatal for couples with family history; most often diagnosed in adulthood	Progressive neurodegenerative disease with mean age of onset in third to fourth decade of life; death typically within 20 years of symptom onset	http://www.ncbi.nlm.nih.gov/books/NBK1305/ http://ghr.nlm.nih.gov/condition/huntington-disease
Hurler syndrome	AR	Prenatal[†]; infant to childhood	Progressive lysosomal storage disease; death by 10 years of age in severely affected; mildly affected can live into adulthood	http://www.ncbi.nlm.nih.gov/books/NBK1162/ http://ghr.nlm.nih.gov/condition/mucopolysaccharidosis-type-i http://mpssociety.org/
Hypophosphatemic vitamin D–resistant rickets	XL dominant	Infant to adulthood	Kidney abnormality resulting in overexcretion of phosphate in urine; secondary bone defects result	http://www.ncbi.nlm.nih.gov/books/NBK83985/

TABLE 3.4 Partial List of Mendelian Inherited Genetic Disorders—cont'd

Disorder	Genetic Etiology	Possible Periods of Recognition	Major Findings	Resources*
Incontinentia pigmenti	XL dominant	Prenatal[†]; newborn to infant	Often prenatally lethal in males; those who survive should have chromosome testing; a de novo mutation is the cause in most affected individuals; blistering of skin, later linear hypopigmentation of skin; small, missing teeth; sparse, wiry hair; vascular retinal abnormalities	http://www.ncbi.nlm.nih.gov/books/NBK1472/ http://ghr.nlm.nih.gov/condition/incontinentia-pigmenti
Li-Fraumeni syndrome	AD	Prenatal[†]; 50% have first cancer by age 40	Predisposition to multiple primary cancers at various body sites	http://www.ncbi.nlm.nih.gov/books/NBK1311/ http://ghr.nlm.nih.gov/condition/li-fraumeni-syndrome
Malignant hyperthermia	AD	Prenatal[†] or before drug exposure (if family history and family mutation known)	Susceptibility to uncontrolled skeletal muscle hypermetabolism when exposed to certain anesthetics and succinylcholine; first symptoms tachycardia, tachypnea, then progressive symptoms and death if not quickly treated	http://www.ncbi.nlm.nih.gov/books/NBK1146/ http://ghr.nlm.nih.gov/condition/malignant-hyperthermia http://www.mhaus.org
Marfan syndrome	AD	Prenatal[†]; neonatal to adulthood depending on number and severity of features and presence or absence of family history	Connective tissue disorder primarily affecting cardiovascular, skeletal, and ocular systems	http://www.ncbi.nlm.nih.gov/books/NBK1335/ http://ghr.nlm.nih.gov/condition/marfan-syndrome http://www.marfan.org/
Myotonic dystrophy	AD expansion mutation; DMPK for type 1; CNBP for type 2	Prenatal if gene expansion mutation identified in affected parent Type 1—Birth in congenital form; child to adulthood for other forms Type 2—Onset typically in third decade	Variable presentation Classic type 1—Affects skeletal and smooth muscle characterized by muscle weakness, wasting, myotonia, cardiac conduction abnormalities Type 2—Muscle weakness, myotonia, posterior subcapsular cataracts, insulin insensitivity (increasingly common with age)	http://www.ncbi.nlm.nih.gov/books/NBK1165/ http://www.ncbi.nlm.nih.gov/books/NBK1466/ http://ghr.nlm.nih.gov/condition/myotonic-dystrophy
Neurofibromatosis	AD	Type 1—Childhood to adulthood Type 2— Adolescence to adulthood	Type 1—Six or more café-au-lait spots, axillary and inguinal freckling, neurofibromas, iris Lisch nodules; learning disabilities common Type 2—Vestibular schwannomas	http://www.ncbi.nlm.nih.gov/books/NBK1109/ http://ghr.nlm.nih.gov/condition/neurofibromatosis-type-1 http://www.nfnetwork.org/ http://www.ncbi.nlm.nih.gov/books/NBK1201/ http://ghr.nlm.nih.gov/condition/neurofibromatosis-type-2
Oculocutaneous albinism type 1	AR	Prenatal[†]; birth to childhood	Hypopigmentation of skin and hair due to reduced melanin production; nystagmus, iris translucency; significant vision impairment	http://www.ncbi.nlm.nih.gov/books/NBK1166/ http://ghr.nlm.nih.gov/condition/oculocutaneous-albinism
Phenylketonuria	AR	Prenatal[†]; newborn	Minimal or absent phenylalanine hydroxylase activity resulting in profound cognitive impairment if not treated early with dietary restriction of phenylalanine	http://www.ncbi.nlm.nih.gov/books/NBK1504/ http://ghr.nlm.nih.gov/condition/phenylketonuria
Pompe disease (glycogen storage disease type II)	AR	Prenatal[†]; newborn to infant	Hypotonia, cardiomegaly, and hypertrophic cardiomyopathy, failure to thrive; death within first year of life; early enzyme therapy may prevent or delay symptoms	http://www.ncbi.nlm.nih.gov/books/NBK1261/ http://ghr.nlm.nih.gov/condition/pompe-disease

Continued

TABLE 3.4 Partial List of Mendelian Inherited Genetic Disorders—cont'd

Disorder	Genetic Etiology	Possible Periods of Recognition	Major Findings	Resources*
Porphyria, acute intermittent	AD (low penetrance)	Adolescence to adulthood	Acute attacks include abdominal pain; peripheral neuropathy; neuropsychiatric symptoms	http://www.ncbi.nlm.nih.gov/books/NBK1193/ http://ghr.nlm.nih.gov/condition/porphyria
Sickle cell disorder (sickle cell anemia; sickle-hemoglobin C disease; sickle β-thalassemia)	AR	Prenatal to newborn; if missed on newborn screen, childhood	Severe pain at site of vascular occlusion leading to tissue ischemia; organ dysfunction possible at site of vascular occlusion	http://www.ncbi.nlm.nih.gov/books/NBK1377/ http://ghr.nlm.nih.gov/condition/sickle-cell-disease
Tay-Sachs disease (hexosaminidase A deficiency)	AR	Prenatal to infant	Neurodegenerative disease Acute type—Progressive weakness, loss of motor skills, seizures, blindness, spasticity, death by about 4 years Subacute type—May have onset in childhood or adulthood with variable progressive neurologic findings	http://www.ncbi.nlm.nih.gov/books/NBK1218/ http://ghr.nlm.nih.gov/condition/tay-sachs-disease
Beta-thalassemia	AR	Prenatal†; newborn screening; by 2 years of age if missed on screen	Microcytic hypochromic anemia, absent or reduced hemoglobin A; severe anemia and secondary hepatosplenomegaly	http://www.ncbi.nlm.nih.gov/books/NBK1426/ http://ghr.nlm.nih.gov/condition/beta-thalassemia
Velo-cardio-facial syndrome	AD and Chr—46,XX,del(22.11.2) or 46,XY,del(22.11.2)	Prenatal to adulthood	Extremely variable condition; nearly 200 possible features described; most common are cognitive impairment, palatal structural or functional abnormalities, conotruncal heart defects, mild immunodeficiencies	http://www.ncbi.nlm.nih.gov/books/NBK1523/ http://ghr.nlm.nih.gov/condition/22q112-deletion-syndrome
Xeroderma pigmentosum	AR (abnormalities in genes responsible for DNA repair)	Prenatal† to 2 years	Acute sun sensitivity (severe sunburns and blistering with minimal exposure) and over 1000-fold increased risk of cutaneous and ocular neoplasms; in some cases, sensitivity to x-rays	http://www.ncbi.nlm.nih.gov/books/NBK1397/ https://ghr.nlm.nih.gov/condition/xeroderma-pigmentosum

*Support groups are listed on most websites. However, before referring families to support groups, particularly for families that discovered the diagnosis prenatally, carefully review the support group and describe its focus to the couple so they can make an informed decision about whether to visit it.

†Mutation(s) in affected family member or in carrier parents need to be known before prenatal testing can be informative.

AD, Autosomal dominant; *AR*, autosomal recessive; *Chr*, chromosomal; *CNS*, central nervous system; *DNA*, deoxyribonucleic acid; *XL*, X-linked.

BOX 3.3 Autosomal Recessive Inheritance: Characteristics

- Males and females are equally likely to be affected.
- A carrier state exists. Both males and females can be carriers.
- The disease rarely appears in multiple generations unless there is consanguinity in the family or the family is part of a racial, ethnic, or cultural group in which the frequency of the mutated allele is high. Members of the generation who have affected children are usually asymptomatic (heterozygous) carriers.
- Carrier parents have a 25% chance of producing an affected child and a 50% chance of producing a carrier child in each and every pregnancy.
- Parent consanguinity may be a factor when a child is affected with a rare recessive disease.

allele is "masked" by the wild-type (normal) allele, which is dominant (Fig. 3.10). Whereas the possible pregnancy outcomes in autosomal dominant pattern (see Fig. 3.7) are children who are either affected (if the gene mutation is fully penetrant) or unaffected when completely free of the gene mutation, in autosomal recessive inheritance a third possibility arises: that of a **heterozygous carrier** (see Fig. 3.10, *B*). These are individuals who are clinically normal (or nearly normal) but who are at risk of having offspring who are affected.

Identification of such carriers is of paramount importance for genetic counseling. In the case of an unaffected couple who produce a child with a recessive disease, identification is straightforward, assuming lack of misattributed paternity; because they each must contribute a mutant allele, they are considered obligate carriers, even in the absence of specific carrier testing for that gene. Specific tests to detect heterozygous carriers of a variety of genetic diseases are available, but it would be impractical

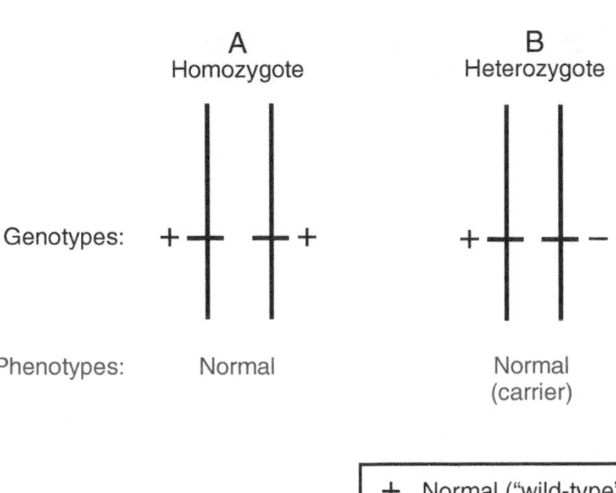

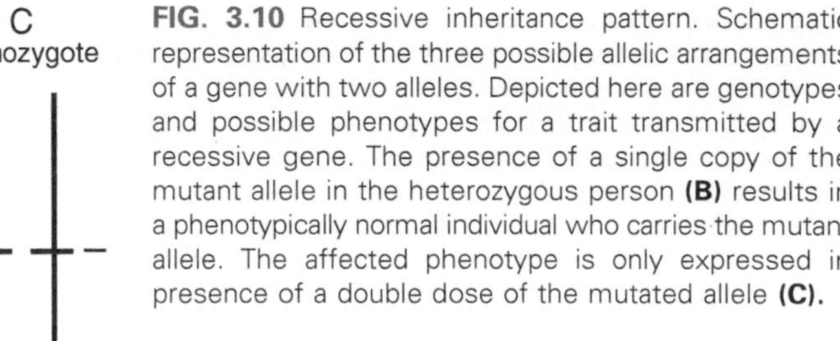

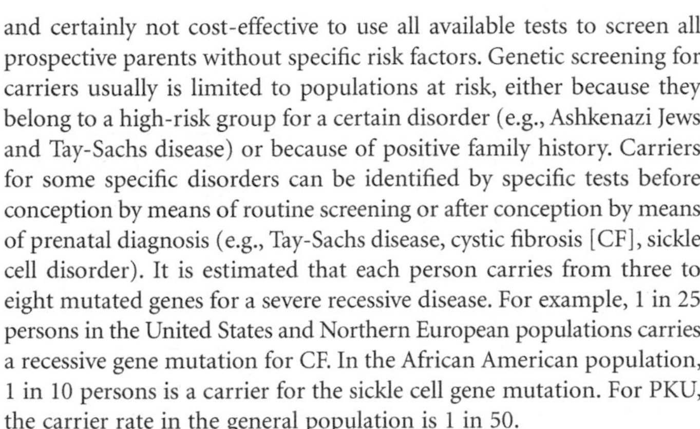

FIG. 3.10 Recessive inheritance pattern. Schematic representation of the three possible allelic arrangements of a gene with two alleles. Depicted here are genotypes and possible phenotypes for a trait transmitted by a recessive gene. The presence of a single copy of the mutant allele in the heterozygous person **(B)** results in a phenotypically normal individual who carries the mutant allele. The affected phenotype is only expressed in presence of a double dose of the mutated allele **(C)**.

and certainly not cost-effective to use all available tests to screen all prospective parents without specific risk factors. Genetic screening for carriers usually is limited to populations at risk, either because they belong to a high-risk group for a certain disorder (e.g., Ashkenazi Jews and Tay-Sachs disease) or because of positive family history. Carriers for some specific disorders can be identified by specific tests before conception by means of routine screening or after conception by means of prenatal diagnosis (e.g., Tay-Sachs disease, cystic fibrosis [CF], sickle cell disorder). It is estimated that each person carries from three to eight mutated genes for a severe recessive disease. For example, 1 in 25 persons in the United States and Northern European populations carries a recessive gene mutation for CF. In the African American population, 1 in 10 persons is a carrier for the sickle cell gene mutation. For PKU, the carrier rate in the general population is 1 in 50.

However, because genetic diseases are rare, the probability of the mating of two persons who carry the same gene in the same allelic configuration is very small. The chances are increased if mating occurs among persons who select a mate because of geographic, ethnic, or religious restrictions or blood relationship (consanguinity). For example, 1 in 30 Ashkenazi Jews is a carrier of a gene mutation associated with Tay-Sachs disease, and 1 in 3600 live births would be affected without preconception screening. For comparison, the frequency of Tay-Sachs disease outside this population is 100 times smaller (i.e., 1 in 360,000 live births).

Other examples of autosomal recessive disorders include the thalassemias, congenital adrenal hyperplasia, and galactosemia. Fig. 3.11 illustrates two situations involving autosomal recessive traits. Fig. 3.11, *A*, depicts the most common occurrence in autosomal recessive disorders: the mating of two carrier parents, with each pregnancy carrying a 25% chance of producing an affected child. Fig. 3.11, *B*, reflects the mating of an affected parent with a genotypically normal partner, in which 100% of the offspring will be carriers. An idealized pedigree representing the mating of two heterozygous (asymptomatic) carriers and its possible outcomes in each and every pregnancy is shown in Fig. 3.12. Selected examples of autosomal recessive disorders are found in Table 3.4.

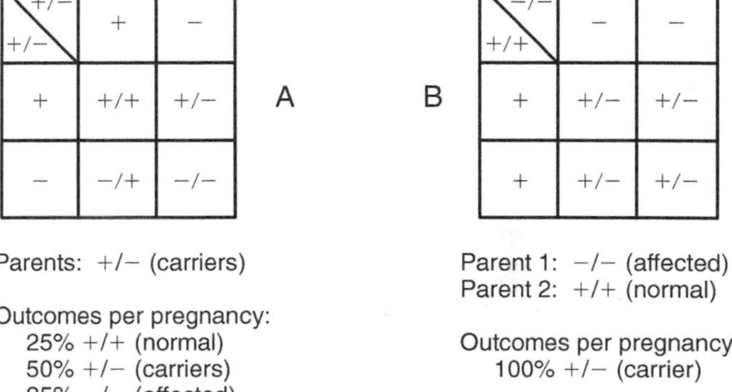

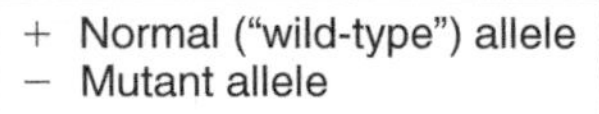

FIG. 3.11 Autosomal recessive inheritance: Punnett squares. **A,** Possible outcomes of mating of two heterozygous carriers (+/–). **B,** Mating of affected homozygous individual (–/–) and normal partner (+/+). Percentages shown refer to outcome possibilities in each pregnancy.

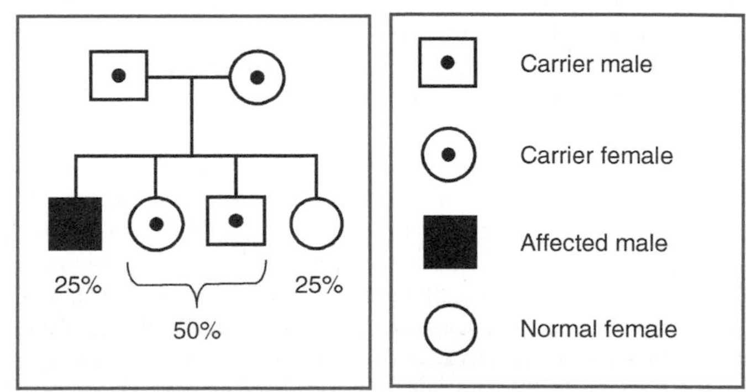

FIG. 3.12 Autosomal recessive inheritance: typical pedigree. The idealized pedigree on the left represents possible outcomes of the mating of two heterozygous carriers (+/–). Percentages express risks for each pregnancy resulting from this mating.

Sex-Linked Inheritance Patterns

The transmission of genes located on one of the sex chromosomes (either X or Y) is termed *sex-linked inheritance*. However, few genes have been found on the Y chromosome, so frequently the terms *sex-linked* and *X-linked* are interchangeably (and incorrectly) used. The testicular organizing region of the Y chromosome determines the formation of testes and the development of male sexual structures during embryonic growth. A gene for hairy ears, with high prevalence in southern Asia, has also been located on the Y chromosome. Inheritance of Y-linked genes follows a father-to-son, or male-to-male, pattern. It is important to remember that men give their X chromosomes to their daughters (and their Y to their sons), so in analyzing a family pedigree, male-to-male transmission of a gene rules out X-linked inheritance.

	A	B	C	D	E
Alleles:	Homozygote	Heterozygote	Homozygote	Hemizygote	Hemizygote
	X X	X X	X X	X	X
Genotypes:	+ +	+ −	− −	+ Y	− Y
Phenotypes:					
Dominant disease	Normal female	Affected female	Affected female	Normal male	Affected male
Recessive disease	Normal female	Carrier female	Affected female	Normal male	Affected male

\+ Normal ("wild-type") allele
− Mutant allele

FIG. 3.13 X-linked inheritance pattern. **A** to **C,** Possible allelic arrangements of an X-linked gene in females. Note that phenotypic expression of an X-linked gene in women is typically similar to that of an autosomal gene. However, unequal X inactivation could result in more active X chromosomes with the mutation and could result in symptoms. **D** and **E,** Uneven pairing of X and Y chromosomes in males, and its phenotypic expressions. Note that there are no carrier males because the phenotype is determined solely by the characteristic of X-linked allele. Hemizygous males are either normal or affected.

Sex-Linked Traits

Women have two X chromosomes; therefore inheritance of genes located on the X chromosome (X-linked inheritance) follows the same pattern as that for autosomal genes. However, in the case of males, the X and Y chromosomes have small areas of homology and therefore do not pair side-by-side during meiosis. Because of this, men are hemizygous for all genes on the X chromosome that do not have a homologous site on the Y chromosome, and their alleles are represented as single copies. Therefore, in the inheritance of an X-linked gene, the single-copy presence of its normal, or its mutant, allele will result in the expression of the normal or mutant phenotype, respectively. This is true for both dominant and recessive X-linked diseases in males (Fig. 3.13).

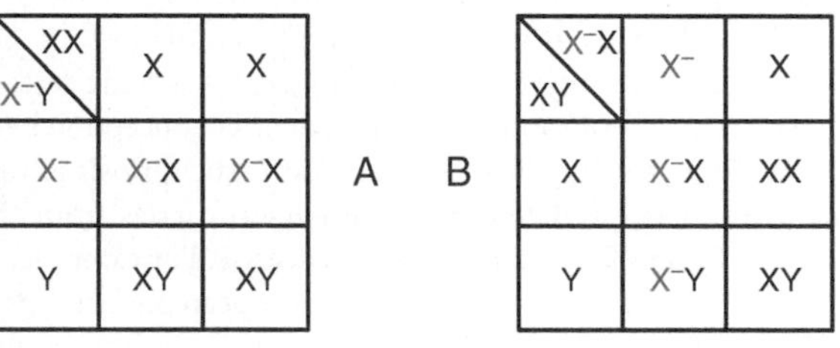

Father: X^-Y (affected)
Mother: XX (normal)

Outcomes per pregnancy:
All daughters: X^-X (carriers)
All sons: XY (normal)

Father: XY (normal)
Mother: X^-X (carrier)

Outcomes per pregnancy:
Daughters: 50% X^-X (carrier)
50% XX (normal)
Sons: 50% X^-Y (affected)
50% XY (normal)

X^- = Recessive (defective) allele on X chromosome
X = Dominant (normal) allele on X chromosome

FIG. 3.14 X-linked recessive inheritance: Punnett squares. **A,** Possible outcomes of mating of affected male with normal female. **B,** Mating of normal male and carrier female. Percentages refer to outcome possibilities in each pregnancy.

X-Linked Recessive Inheritance

In females the alleles of an X-linked recessive gene behave as the alleles of any autosomal recessive gene: the effect of the abnormal allele is "hidden" by the normal (dominant) allele. Therefore females who have a disease-associated mutation in both members of the gene pair will express the phenotype. Although it is rare for females to express the phenotype if only one member of the gene pair carries a disease-associated mutation, it is possible due to X inactivation.

Soon after fertilization, it is normal for one X chromosome in females to be inactivated through a natural process called methylation. This occurs in each cell in the early blastocyst stage, and whether the paternal or maternally inherited X is inactivated is random in each cell. At the time this occurs, the X that has been inactivated will remain so through all subsequent cell divisions. Females who express a phenotype may have a greater proportion of X chromosome with the normal allele inactivated within the tissues or organs associated with the disorder. Examples of X-linked recessive disorders include hemophilia types A and B and Duchenne muscular dystrophy. Fig. 3.14 illustrates the outcomes of each pregnancy between an affected man and a normal woman (Fig. 3.14, *A*) and between a normal man and a carrier woman (Fig. 3.14, *B*). An idealized pedigree depicting the mating between a genetically normal man and a carrier woman, and its possible outcomes per pregnancy, is shown in Fig. 3.15. The primary characteristics of X-linked recessive inheritance are listed in Box 3.4.

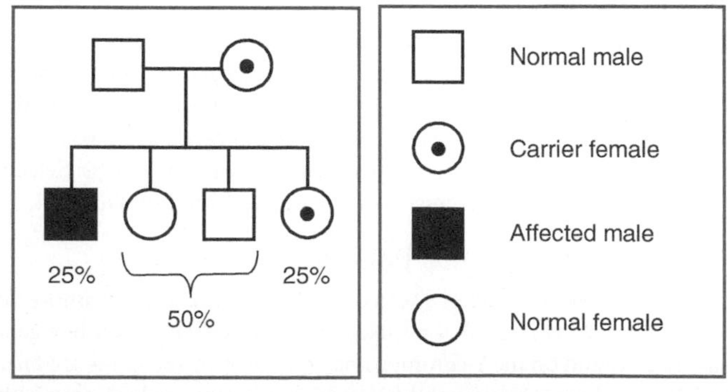

FIG. 3.15 X-linked recessive inheritance: typical pedigree. The idealized pedigree on the left represents possible outcomes of mating of normal male and carrier female. Percentages express risks for each pregnancy resulting from this mating.

X-Linked Dominant Inheritance

X-linked dominant inheritance (see Fig. 3.13) is rare. The main characteristics of X-linked dominant inheritance are (1) both males and

BOX 3.4 X-Linked Recessive Inheritance: Characteristics*

- Most affected persons are male. Affected females are extremely rare.
- Males transmit their Y chromosome to their sons; therefore father-to-son transmission of X-linked traits is not possible except in the rare instance of nondisjunction when a sperm carries both an X and Y chromosome.
- All daughters of an affected male are (heterozygous) carriers; none is affected (homozygous).
- Sons of carrier females have a 50% chance of inheriting the mutant allele and being affected (hemizygous). Daughters have a 50% risk of inheriting the mutant allele and being (heterozygous) carriers.

*Unless otherwise specified, all partners of affected or carrier persons here are genotypically normal.

A

XX \ X^-Y	X	X
X^-	X^-X	X^-X
Y	XY	XY

Father: X^-Y (affected)
Mother: XX (normal)

Outcomes per pregnancy:
All daughters: X^-X (affected)
All sons: XY (normal)

B

X^-X \ XY	X^-	X
X	X^-X	XX
Y	X^-Y	XY

Father: XY (normal)
Mother: X^-X (affected)

Outcomes per pregnancy:
Daughters: 50% X^-X (affected)
50% XX (normal)
Sons: 50% X^-Y (affected)
50% XY (normal)

X^- = Dominant (defective) allele on X chromosome
X = Recessive (normal) allele on X chromosome

FIG. 3.16 X-linked dominant inheritance: Punnett squares. **A,** Possible outcomes of mating of affected male with normal female. **B,** Mating of normal male and affected female. Percentages shown refer to outcome possibilities in each pregnancy.

females can be affected, but females, because of the random nature of X inactivation, are usually less severely affected than males; (2) affected men do not transmit the mutant allele to their sons; and (3) all daughters of an affected man are affected and have a 50% chance of passing on the mutant allele to their sons and daughters. Examples of X-linked dominant disorders are hypophosphatemic vitamin D–resistant rickets and incontinentia pigmenti. Fig. 3.16 illustrates the outcomes of each pregnancy between an affected man and an unaffected woman (Fig. 3.16, *A*) and between an unaffected man and an affected woman (Fig. 3.16, *B*). An idealized pedigree representing the mating of an affected man with a unaffected woman is shown in Fig. 3.17.

VARIABLE PATTERNS OF GENE EXPRESSION AND INHERITANCE

A number of variables have been observed that explain or modify basic inheritance patterns and the effects of chromosome abnormalities. Some of these variations have been recognized for some time; others are newly discovered phenomena that explain some apparent contradictions in the established patterns of inheritance. Also, some disorders have been reported to follow more than one inheritance pattern in different families (e.g., a classically recessive disorder occasionally may be reported to be following a dominant or X-linked pattern in other families). This phenomenon is known as locus heterogeneity (Jorde, Carey, Bamshad, et al., 2016).

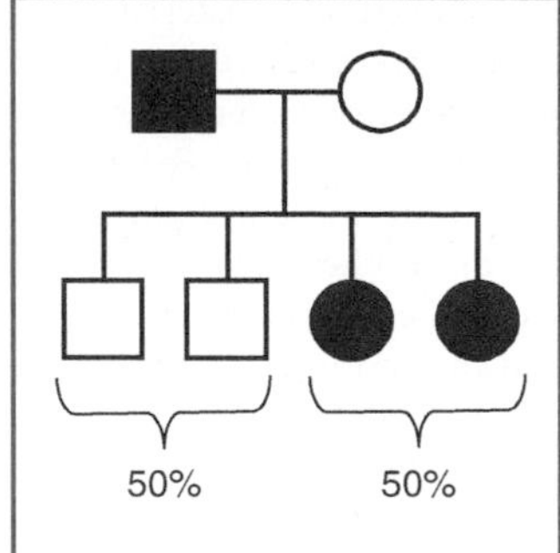

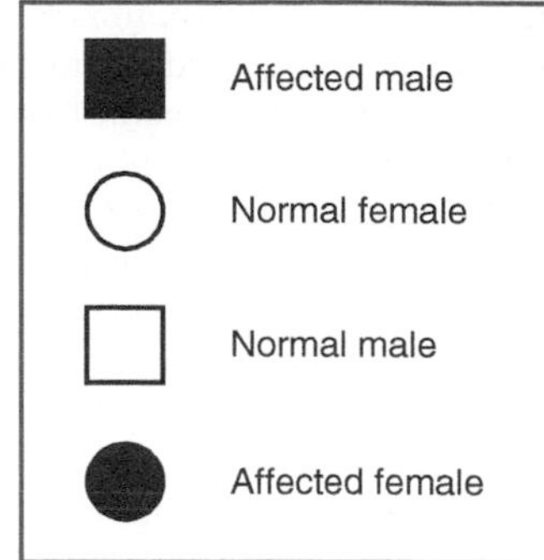

FIG. 3.17 X-linked dominant inheritance: typical pedigree. The idealized pedigree on the left represents possible outcomes of mating of affected male and normal female. Percentages depicted express risks for each pregnancy resulting from this mating. Because the mutant allele is carried in the X chromosome, an affected male will transfer it to 100% of his daughters.

The most notable of these gene variations is mutation. As discussed earlier, mutations are heritable changes in the DNA sequence of a gene. Mutations can result from a substitution of bases (point mutations) or the insertion or deletion of bases. Some genes have a high mutation rate, and various forms of the resulting disease may have varying expression. One example is the *CFTR* gene, in which more than 1000 different CF-associated mutations have been identified (the vast majority being point mutations or small deletions). Mutation rates are not constant for all genes, so some diseases may occur with much greater frequency than others.

Variable expression is an important concept that describes differences in the extent and severity and onset of phenotype. There is a continuum of expression for any affected person from very mild to severe clinical manifestations. For those with very mild manifestations, it may take an expert clinician to identify the condition. For example, a parent of a child with classic neurofibromatosis may exhibit only a few "birthmarks" that a medical geneticist, genetics advanced practice nurse, or genetic counselor would recognize as café-au-lait spots, one of the manifestations of neurofibromatosis.

Some genetic disorders are caused by an abnormal expansion of a short DNA sequence that naturally repeats. The size of an expansion mutation can influence the age of onset and severity of the disorder. For example, the *FMR1* gene on the X chromosome usually has about 5 to 40 repeats of three nucleotides: cytosine, guanine, guanine (CGG). When *FMR1* has 59 to 200 CGG repeats, that area of the gene can become unstable and gain further repeats during meiosis. Females who have this number of repeats are considered carriers of a premutation for fragile X syndrome. A person with fragile X has a full mutation allele with hundreds to thousands of repeats. Because fragile X syndrome is an X-linked disorder, females are less likely to be affected because of the presence of a normal allele on the homologous X chromosome. These expanding repeats have also been found to occur in autosomal dominant disorders such as myotonic dystrophy and in autosomal recessive disorders such as Friedreich ataxia. Expansion mutations that have a tendency to further expand when transmitted from one generation to the next can display phenotypic anticipation. Pedigrees display anticipation when individuals in successive generations develop the disorder at an earlier age and/or with more severe manifestations.

Genomic imprinting and uniparental disomy are two genetic phenomena that consider the parental origin of genetic information (i.e., maternally or paternally derived). The concept of genomic imprinting refers to modification, in some instances, of genetic material. Methyl groups are naturally added to (an in some cases removed from) certain regions of the genome to control the expression of select genes. Methylation patterns can be specific to parent of origin. For example, during sperm formation, methyl groups are removed from the father's chromosomes that were inherited from his mother and methyl groups added to areas of those chromosomes to assure that genes that should be turned on or off in paternally inherited chromosomes are transmitted to future offspring. Genomic imprinting is exhibited during pregnancy, when paternally derived chromosomes seem to positively influence placental development and maternally derived chromosomes seem to positively influence fetal development. This phenomenon also occurs in some genetic disorders, such as Prader-Willi and Angelman syndromes. In both these disorders about two-thirds of affected individuals have a deletion of the same segment of chromosome 15 that is normally methylated. However, the clinical manifestations of Prader-Willi and Angelman syndromes are markedly different. If the deletion occurs on the paternally derived chromosome 15 so only the mother's genes are expressed, the child exhibits Prader-Willi syndrome; if the deletion occurs on the maternally derived chromosome 15 so that only the father's genes are expressed, the child manifests Angelman syndrome (Jorde, Carey, Bamshad, et al., 2016). Prader-Willi syndrome is characterized by failure to thrive and central hypotonia in the newborn and infancy period with later insatiable hunger that can lead to morbid obesity during childhood. Children with Prader-Willi syndrome also have cognitive dysfunction, typical dysmorphic features, behavioral disturbances, hypothalamic hypogonadism, and short stature. In contrast, Angelman syndrome includes severe cognitive impairment, characteristic facies, abnormal (puppetlike) gait, and paroxysms of inappropriate laughter. Children with Angelman syndrome are usually nonverbal.

In some cases both copies of a chromosome pair are discovered to have come from one parent, either the mother or the father, instead of one from each; this phenomenon is called **uniparental disomy**. An example of uniparental disomy was reported with CF, in which both chromosomes, each with a mutant recessive gene, came from the carrier mother; the father was not a carrier. In cases that appear to be misattributed paternity, uniparental disomy may be a factor. One of several theories about uniparental disomy is that the chromosome pair was originally a trisomy and the father's chromosome was randomly eliminated, leaving two copies of the mother's chromosome. Because the chromosomes appear as a normal "pair," diagnosis of this situation is only possible with molecular (DNA) techniques. Uniparental disomy has also been reported with Beckwith-Wiedemann syndrome, which is characterized by overgrowth and hypoglycemia at birth (see Table 3.2).

MITOCHONDRIAL DISORDERS

Mitochondrial disorders can be caused by mutations in the nuclear genes and exhibit mendelian inheritance. However, mitochondrial disorders can also be caused by DNA found in a cytoplasmic cellular organelle, the **mitochondrion**, whose primary function in cellular metabolism is the production of energy. Mutations in mtDNA also account for nonmendelian inheritance patterns. Inheritance of traits contained in mtDNA is exclusively maternal because only the mitochondria from the ovum are transmitted to the zygote. Mitochondria are not contained within the sperm head.

An additional complexity in mitochondrial inheritance results from the fact that, during mitosis, mitochondria are randomly distributed among the daughter cells, so both normal and mutated mitochondria may be found in the same cell, a phenomenon known as **heteroplasmy**. This leads to variable dosages of mutated mtDNA between tissues and organs. This variation in mutation load leads to a highly variable spectrum of clinical manifestations, and individuals with the same mtDNA mutation may range from symptom free, to mildly affected, to severely impaired. Symptoms may include seizures, pancreatitis, and metabolic disease. Different manifestations may be seen in different members of the same family. Heteroplasmy complicates the use of prenatal diagnosis. Once the mtDNA mutation is identified in the mother, her pregnancies can be tested for the same mutation. However, the mutation load identified in sampled fetal tissue (chorionic villi or amniocytes) may not correspond to other fetal tissues, the mutational load of which will continue to change during development due to random mitotic segregation of cytoplasmic organelles. Consequently, it is not possible to predict the unborn child's phenotype based on prenatal test results.

mtDNA mutations are responsible for various childhood diseases (Table 3.5), such as Leigh syndrome (movement disorder, respiratory dyskinesia, regression, hypotonia, seizures, and failure to thrive). Because mitochondrial disorders have such variability of expression, determining the diagnosis can be confusing. However, when a child has an unexplained constellation of abnormal findings in tissue or organs that require high energy (e.g., heart, skeletal muscle, eyes), a mitochondrial disorder should be considered.

HEREDITARY CANCER PREDISPOSITION GENES

The process of carcinogenesis implies permanent changes in the DNA of the targeted cell. Early observations recognized genetic influences in cancer: (1) certain types of cancer occur more frequently within certain families (breast, colon, ovarian, some leukemias); (2) some well-defined genetic disorders show a predisposition to various malignancies (familial adenomatous polyposis and colon cancer, Bloom syndrome, and lymphomas); (3) chromosome abnormalities occur frequently with malignancies (Philadelphia chromosome in chronic myelogenous leukemia); and (4) certain chromosome aneuploidies predispose the person to cancer (Down syndrome and acute leukemias).

The discovery of **oncogenes** in the early 1970s marked the beginning of a new era in the field of cancer genetics (Box 3.5). Initially thought to be carried exclusively by retroviruses, oncogenes were later identified as natural genes that existed in all mammals. Early investigations suggested that oncogenes were found in inactive form (i.e., no correlation with cancer could be identified in this state). In reality, oncogenes are normally involved in cell growth and division. A mutation in an oncogene can disrupt this normal process and transform a normal cell into one that has uncontrolled cell growth or division, predisposing the cell to further mutations that eventually transform the cell into one that is malignant.

Since the discovery of oncogenes, two other classes of genes associated with cancer development have been identified: tumor suppressor genes and mismatch repair genes. **Tumor suppressor genes** normally inhibit cell growth and division. A mutation in these genes can interfere with this normal function and lead to uninhibited cell growth and division. Among this group is *p53* (sometimes called *TP53*), whose germ cell (or hereditary) mutations are associated with Li-Fraumeni syndrome and whose somatic cell mutations (sporadic) result in various malignancies, such as bladder cancer. Li-Fraumeni syndrome is inherited as an autosomal dominant trait that predisposes children and young adults to the development of various tumors, including osteosarcoma; soft tissue sarcomas; breast, brain, and adrenocortical carcinomas; and leukemia (Schneider, Zelley, Nichols, et al., 1999, updated 2013).

Mismatch repair genes normally function by recognizing and repairing DNA errors that occur during replication or mutations that are caused by external agents such as ultraviolet light or chemical exposure. Xeroderma pigmentosum is a classic example of inherited predisposition to cancers caused by a germline mutation in one of several possible mismatch repair genes. Infants and children with xeroderma pigmentosum are at considerable risk for skin cancers triggered by sun and ultraviolet light exposure.

TABLE 3.5 Partial List of Mitochondrial Genetic Disorders

Disorder	Genetic Etiology	Possible Periods of Recognition	Major Findings	Resources*
Kearns-Sayre syndrome	Mit—Maternal inheritance but affected women only have approximately 1 in 24 risk of having affected offspring; maternal transmission to more than one child has not been reported	Infancy; before 20 years of age	Three overlapping phenotypes that can be seen in same family and used to be distinguished as three different diseases; multisystem disease primarily affecting CNS, endocrine system, skeletal muscles, heart, retina	http://www.ncbi.nlm.nih.gov/books/NBK1203/
Leigh syndrome; NARP (neurogenic muscle weakness, ataxia, retinitis pigmentosa)	Mit—Many different mitochondrial genes implicated	Leigh—Infancy NARP—Childhood	Symptoms depend on mutation load and tissue distribution of disease causing mtDNA mutation; progressive, neurodegenerative disorder Leigh onset typically after viral infection; 75% die by 3 years of age NARP onset typically in childhood; ataxia, learning difficulties, episodic deterioration possible following viral infections	http://www.ncbi.nlm.nih.gov/books/NBK1173/
MELAS (mitochondrial encephalomyopathy, lactic acidosis, and strokelike episodes)	Mit	Early childhood	Encephalopathy, seizures, recurrent vomiting, recurrent headaches, exercise intolerance, strokelike episodes	http://www.ncbi.nlm.nih.gov/books/NBK1233/ http://ghr.nlm.nih.gov/condition/mitochondrial-encephalomyopathy-lactic-acidosis-and-stroke-like-episodes
MERRF (myoclonic epilepsy associated with ragged red fibers)	Mit	Childhood	Myoclonus, generalized epilepsy, ataxia, dementia	http://www.ncbi.nlm.nih.gov/books/NBK1520/

*Support groups are listed on most websites. However, before referring families to support groups, particularly for families that discovered the diagnosis prenatally, carefully review the support group and describe its focus to the couple so they can make an informed decision about whether to visit it.

CNS, Central nervous system; *Mit*, mitochondrial; *mtDNA*, mitochondrial deoxyribonucleic acid.

BOX 3.5 Cancer Genetics: Current Knowledge

- Genetic predispositions influence risk for malignancies.
- Environmental agents act as triggers, increasing the inherited risk factor.
- Oncogenes are normally facilitate cell growth and division. A mutation in an oncogene can disrupt this normal process and transform a normal cell into one that has uncontrolled cell growth or division, predisposing the cell to further mutations that eventually transform the cell into one that is malignant.
- Retroviruses can cause cancer by transmitting an oncogene or by insertional mutagenesis.
- Cancers may be caused by somatic mutations of genes that regulate cell growth—a localized process leading to sporadic (nonhereditary) tumors.
- Germ cell gene mutations are transmitted to the offspring—hereditary cancers.
- Tumor suppressor genes (e.g., *p53*) normally suppress cell growth. Mutations can disrupt suppression, allowing for uncontrolled cell growth that leads to cancer. Examples of other genes that suppress cell growth include *BRCA1* (female breast and ovarian cancer), *BRCA2* (male and female breast, prostate cancer), and *APC* (colon cancer).

MULTIFACTORIAL (COMPLEX) DISORDERS

A number of frequently encountered diseases and defects show an increased incidence than would be expected by chance, yet no specific mode of inheritance can be identified. In some, environmental factors, including the prenatal environment, appear to play an important role. These conditions are classified as **multifactorial disorders**, in which a genetic susceptibility and specific environmental agents interact to produce a disease state. Multifactorial disorders include NTDs, cleft lip and cleft palate, many congenital heart defects, congenital hip dislocation, and pyloric stenosis.

Recurrence risks for multifactorial conditions are empirically based on observed recurrence within a population. In general, recurrence risk is usually low (<10%). For example, NTDs occur in 1 out of 1000 births in the general population. The recurrence risk after the first affected child is 2 or 3 out of 100 births. Advances in genetics are enhancing knowledge of multifactorial inheritance and familial risks (Rimoin, Pyeritz, & Korf, 2013).

DISORDERS OF THE INTRAUTERINE ENVIRONMENT

The intrauterine environment can have a profound and permanent effect on the developing fetus, with or without chromosome or single-gene abnormalities. Intrauterine growth retardation, for example, can occur with many genetic syndromes, such as Down, Russell-Silver, Prader-Willi, and Turner syndromes (Rimoin, Pyeritz, & Korf, 2013), or it can be caused by nongenetic factors such as maternal alcohol ingestion. Placental abnormalities are increasingly being found to be the etiologic factor in neurodevelopmental disorders (such as cerebral palsy and cognitive impairment) that were previously attributed to asphyxia during delivery.

Teratogens, agents that cause birth defects when present in the prenatal environment, account for the majority of adverse intrauterine effects not attributable to genetic factors. Types of teratogens include drugs (phenytoin [Dilantin], warfarin [Coumadin], isotretinoin [Accutane]), chemicals (ethyl alcohol, cocaine, lead), infectious agents (rubella, cytomegalovirus), physical agents (maternal ionizing radiation, hyperthermia), and metabolic agents (maternal PKU). Many of these teratogenic exposures and the resulting effects are completely preventable. For example, pregnant women can avoid having a child with one of the fetal alcohol spectrum disorders by not ingesting alcohol during pregnancy.

INBORN ERRORS OF METABOLISM

Inborn errors of metabolism (IEMs) include a large number of inherited diseases caused by interruptions in the various pathways involved in the metabolism of protein, carbohydrates, or lipids. Fig. 3.18 is a conceptual model representing the multiple interactions in a metabolic pathway in health and disease. **Metabolic pathways** are series of biochemical reactions by which substrates are sequentially converted into other by-products, aiming at a final end-product that can be successfully used or eliminated by the body. Each of these transformations is mediated by an enzyme, which is under the control of a specific structural gene. Fig. 3.18, *A*, represents the normal metabolic conversion of substance **A** into end-product **K**, via by-products **B, C, D**, and so on. Enzymes **b** and **c**, whose synthesis is controlled by genes β and δ, catalyze steps **B** → **C** and **C** → **D**, respectively. A feedback loop ensures physiologic levels of **K**. A gene mutation may result in qualitative or quantitative changes in the enzyme, resulting in a different (and therefore ineffective) enzyme, or in the decreased synthesis of the enzyme, including its total absence. This ineffective (or missing) enzyme will interrupt the pathway, resulting in accumulation of the by-product that immediately precedes the blockage, as well as lack of the by-products beyond the blockage. IEMs can occur as a result of such accumulations or absences of an essential by-product.

In Fig. 3.18, *B*, a mutation in gene β prevents normal synthesis of enzyme **b**, creating an interruption of the pathway between **B** and **C**. Assuming a continuous uptake of **A**, two outcomes ensue: accumulation of **B** and depletion of all products beyond the block (**C, D, ... K**). An example of this situation is Tay-Sachs disease (or GM_2 gangliosidosis). In this disease, a mutation in the *HexA* gene (here exemplified by β) causes the lack of the enzyme hexosaminidase A (HexA), represented by **b**. Absence of **b** creates an accumulation of ganglioside GM_2 (**B**)—lipids, in nerve cells, resulting in the clinical manifestations of this progressive neurologic disorder because the lipids are not broken down by the cellular liposomes.

Fig. 3.18, *C*, depicts a mutation in gene δ, which causes depletion of enzyme **c** and interrupts the metabolic conversion of **C** into **D**. In this instance an alternative pathway **C** → **E** → **F** is opened. This event may have two outcomes: product **F** may eventually be converted into **K**, with no significant clinical consequences, or **F** may represent the endpoint to the alternative pathway. If accumulation of **F** reaches toxic levels, a disease process may occur. Such is the case with PKU, an IEM that creates an intolerance to the amino acid phenylalanine. The missing enzyme (**c**, in this case), which results from mutation in the phenylalanine hydroxylase *(PAH)* gene (δ), is phenylalanine hydroxylase. The alternative pathway leads to the formation and accumulation of phenylketones (**F**). In combination with phenylalanine deficiency, an excessive amount of phenylketones contributes to the postnatal completion of myelination of nerves, resulting in profound cognitive impairment.

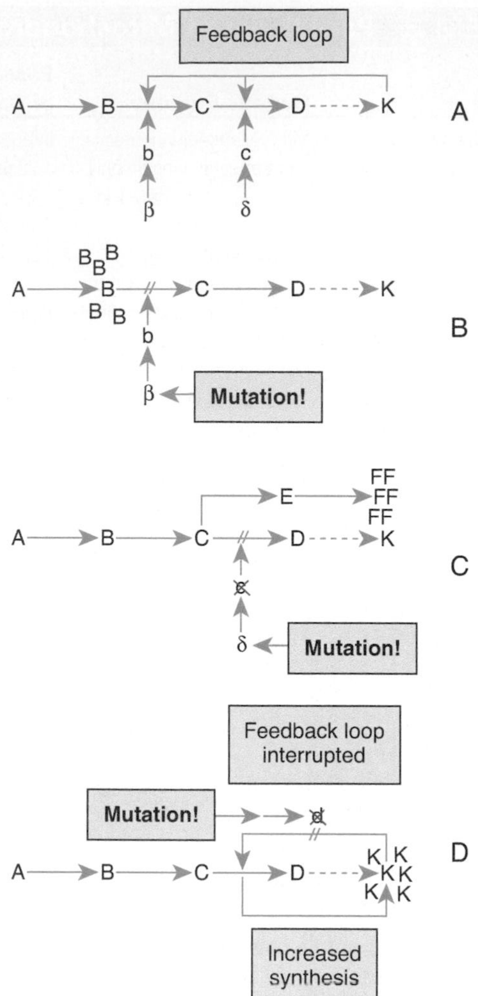

FIG. 3.18 Metabolic pathway. **A,** Normal metabolic pathway. **B,** Mutation of gene β. **C,** Mutation of gene δ. **D,** Genetic alteration of enzyme d. *A,* Substance; *B–F,* by-products; *K,* end-product; *b, c,* and, *d,* enzymes; *β* and *δ,* genes. (Adapted from da Cunha, M. F. [2000]. Genetic basis of human disease. In B. A. Bullock & R. L. Henze [Eds.], *Focus on physiology*. Philadelphia, PA: Lippincott.)

Fig. 3.18, *D*, represents a genetic alteration of the enzyme **d**, which is involved in the feedback control of synthesis of **K**. As a result, **K** may accumulate to toxic levels. The prototype genetic disease here is Lesch-Nyhan syndrome, in which **d** is the enzyme hypoxanthine-guanine phosphoribosyltransferase (HGPRT) and **K** is uric acid. A deficiency in HGPRT and accumulation of uric acid to extremely high levels will result in the development of cognitive impairment and self-mutilation tendency.

The mode of inheritance in IEMs is almost always autosomal recessive. The heterozygote has one gene with a normal effect and is still able to produce the enzyme in sufficient amounts to carry out the metabolic function under normal circumstances. Therefore the heterozygote does not exhibit symptoms of the disorder. The homozygote, who inherits a defective gene from both parents, has no functioning enzyme and thus is clinically affected.

Individually, different IEMs are rare; collectively they account for a significant proportion of health problems in children. It is becoming possible to detect and screen for an increasing number of IEMs—to detect the disease in the heterozygote, the newborn, and the fetus and to identify heterozygotes at risk for having a child with an IEM. With most IEMs, early diagnosis and prompt treatment are essential to prevent a relentless course of physical and mental deterioration. Prenatal diagnosis provides for special care of the infant immediately after birth. Neonatal screening is useful in detecting many disorders after a few days of life, but it is less helpful in detecting symptoms early in the neonatal period. Nurses caring for neonates must be certain that screening is performed, especially in infants who are discharged early, are born at home, or are in neonatal intensive care units.

A list of conditions routinely screened in each state can be found at http://genes-r-us.uthscsa.edu/sites/genes-r-us/files/nbsdisorders.pdf. Nurses also need to make certain that the neonate has a primary care provider and current home address and telephone number documented on the newborn screening blood spot card. Nurses should instruct parents to ask about newborn screening test results at their newborn's first well-child visit. Most screening tests require a heel puncture to obtain sufficient blood to completely cover circles on special blotting paper. A new screening test, tandem mass spectrometry, has the potential to identify up to 40 IEMs. With tandem mass spectrometry, earlier identification of IEMs may prevent further developmental delays and morbidities in affected children. (See Atraumatic Care box, p. 219, for measures to reduce the pain of lancing and squeezing the heel, and see Newborn Screening for Disease, Chapter 8.)

Some nonspecific manifestations—including lethargy, poor feeding, vomiting, diarrhea, hypoglycemia, metabolic acidosis, respiratory distress, apnea, hypothermia, coma, and seizures—occur in a wide variety of genetic and acquired disorders. The time of onset may be important. Most IEMs produce no symptoms during the first 24 hours of life. Other manifestations that may indicate an IEM include jaundice, hepatomegaly, unusual odor (e.g., sweat, urine, feces), abnormal eating patterns (e.g., food aversions, vomiting after eating certain foods), coarse facial features, macroglossia (enlarged tongue), abnormal hair, dysmorphic features, and abnormal eye findings (e.g., cataracts, retinal changes). A family history of neonatal deaths (within the same sibling group, or among family members) alerts the observer to the possibility of an IEM. The initial recognition of signs that might indicate an IEM is the responsibility of health professionals, including nurses.

Although there are many categories of IEMs, only three are discussed here because they can be identified in the neonatal period and because treatment has been reasonably successful. They are examples of disorders of protein metabolism (PKU), disorders of carbohydrate metabolism (galactosemia), and disorders of hormone synthesis (congenital hypothyroidism).

PHENYLKETONURIA

Phenylketonuria (PKU), a genetic disease inherited as an autosomal recessive trait, is caused by an absence of the enzyme phenylalanine hydroxylase needed to metabolize the essential amino acid phenylalanine. The prevalence of PKU varies widely in the United States because different states have different definition criteria for what constitutes hyperphenylalaninemia and PKU. The reported figures for PKU range from 1 per 10,000 to 15,000 live births (Sampson, Groshong, & Parilo, 2016). The disease has a wide variation of incidence by ethnic groups. The disease is most prevalent among individuals of Northern European ancestry, American Indians, and Alaskan Natives, whereas African American, Hispanic, Jewish, and Asian individuals account for the lowest frequencies.

Pathophysiology

In PKU the hepatic enzyme phenylalanine hydroxylase, which controls the conversion of phenylalanine to tyrosine, is absent. This results in the accumulation of phenylalanine in the bloodstream and urinary excretion of abnormal amounts of its metabolites, the phenyl acids (Fig. 3.19). One of these phenyl ketones, phenylpyruvic acid, gives urine the characteristic musty odor associated with this disease and is responsible for the term *phenylketonuria*.

Amino acids produced by the metabolism of phenylalanine are absent in PKU. One of these, tyrosine, is needed to form the pigment melanin and the hormones epinephrine and thyroxine. Decreased melanin production results in similar phenotypes of most children with PKU: blond hair, blue eyes, and fair skin that is particularly susceptible to eczema and other dermatologic problems. Children with a genetically darker skin color may be red haired or brunette.

Severe hyperphenylalaninemia (>360 to 600 mmol/L) causes progressive damage to the developing brain with severe consequences: defective myelination, cystic degeneration of the gray and white matter, and disturbances in cortical lamination. Cognitive impairment occurs before the metabolites are detected in the urine and will progress if ingested phenylalanine levels are not lowered.

Clinical Manifestations

Clinical manifestations of PKU include growth failure (failure to thrive); frequent vomiting; irritability; hyperactivity; and unpredictable, erratic behavior. Older children commonly display bizarre or schizoid behavior patterns such as fright reactions, screaming episodes, head banging, arm biting, disorientation, failure to respond to strong stimuli, and spasticity or catatonia-like positions. Many of the severely cognitively impaired children have seizures, and approximately 80% of untreated persons with PKU demonstrate abnormal electroencephalographs, regardless of whether overt seizures occur.

Diagnostic Evaluation*

The objective in diagnosing or treating the disorder is to prevent cognitive impairment. The most commonly used test for screening newborns is the Guthrie bacterial inhibition assay for phenylalanine in the blood. *Bacillus subtilis,* present in the culture medium, grows if the blood contains an excessive amount of phenylalanine. The normal range of blood phenylalanine concentration in newborns is 0.5 to 1 mg/dl. The Guthrie test detects serum phenylalanine levels greater than 4 mg/dl (normal value is 1.6 mg/dl). Only fresh heel blood, not cord blood, can be used for the test.

Newborn screening tests are mandatory in all 50 US states. The screening test is most reliable if the blood sample is taken after the infant has ingested a source of protein. Because of early discharge of newborns, recommendations for screening include (1) collecting the initial specimen as close as possible to discharge and no later than 7 days after birth, (2) obtaining a subsequent sample by 2 weeks of age if the initial specimen is collected before the newborn is 24 hours old, and (3) designating a primary care provider to all newborns before discharge for adequate newborn follow-up screening (Vockley, Andersson, Antshel, et al., 2014). In several states, a second newborn screening is performed when the infant is 1 to 2 weeks old, on the basis that a maximum number of children with genetic disorders will be identified. After a positive screen, diagnostic testing must be performed promptly (Vockley, Andersson, Antshel, et al., 2014).

*Always refer patient to a genetic metabolic specialist. For a reference list, visit the Society for Inherited Metabolic Disorders website: http://www.simd.org/.

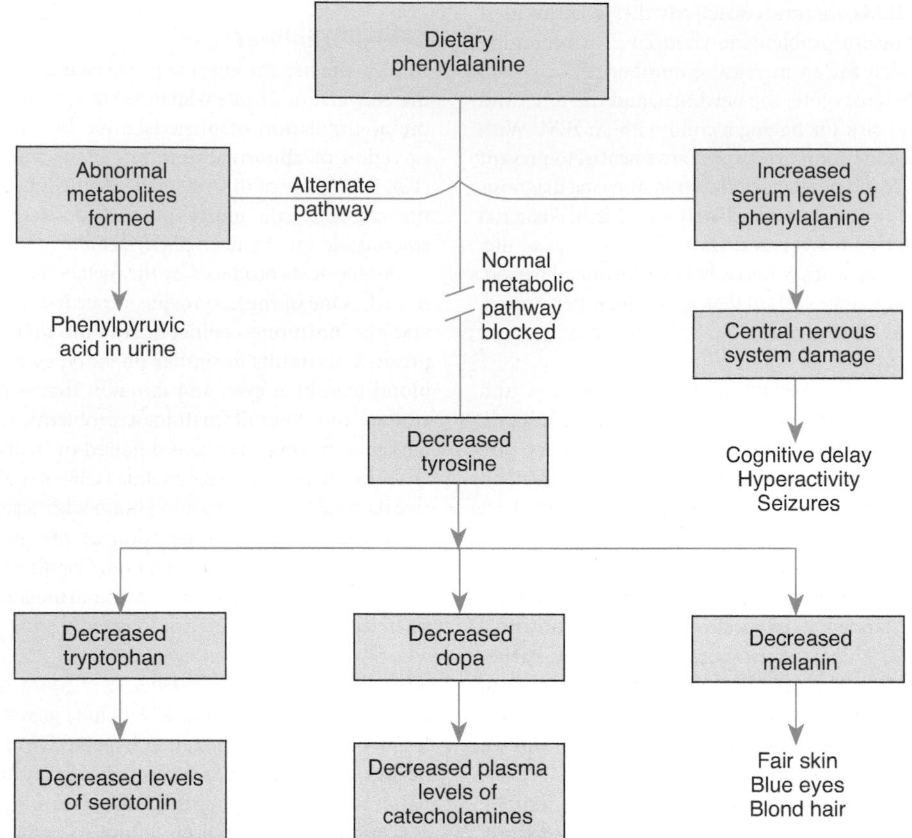

FIG. 3.19 Metabolic errors and consequences in phenylketonuria.

When collecting the specimen, avoid "layering" the blood specimen on the special Guthrie paper. Layering is placing one drop of blood on top of the other or overlapping the specimen. Best results are obtained by collecting the specimen with a pipette from the heel stick and spreading the blood uniformly over the blot paper.

A major concern is that a significant number of infants are not rescreened for PKU after early discharge and are at risk for a missed or delayed diagnosis. Give special consideration to screening infants born at home who have no hospital contact, as well as infants adopted internationally. Because of the possibility of variant forms of hyperphenylalaninemia, a natural dietary protein challenge test is recommended after approximately 3 months of dietary treatment to confirm the diagnosis of classic PKU.

Therapeutic Management*

Treatment of PKU involves the restriction of dietary protein. As with most genetic disorders, because the genetic enzyme is intracellular, systemic administration of phenylalanine hydroxylase is of no value. Phenylalanine cannot be totally eliminated because it is an essential amino acid in tissue growth. Therefore dietary management must meet two criteria: meet the child's nutritional need for optimum growth and maintain phenylalanine levels within a safe range.

Treatment for infants with sustained blood phenylalanine levels greater than 360 μmol/L is recommended. Although the threshold for adverse effects of elevated blood phenylalanine is not known, treatment of phenylalanine levels between 120 and 360 μmol/L is not recommended, but close follow-up for the first few years of life is important (Vockley, Andersson, Antshel, et al., 2014). Most clinicians now agree that, to achieve optimum metabolic control and outcome, a restricted phenylalanine diet, including medical foods and low-protein products, most likely will be medically required for virtually all individuals with classic PKU for their entire life (Vockley, Andersson, Antshel, et al., 2014). Such a lifetime reduction of phenylalanine intake is necessary to prevent neuropsychologic and cognitive deficits. To evaluate the effectiveness of dietary treatment, frequent monitoring of blood phenylalanine and tyrosine levels is necessary. The blood phenylalanine concentration in newborns is normally 0.5 to 1 mg/dl (30 to 60 μmol/L).

The diet is calculated to allow 20 to 30 mg of phenylalanine per kilogram of body weight per day, which should maintain serum phenylalanine levels between 120 and 360 μmol/L (Vockley, Andersson, Antshel, et al., 2014). For optimum growth to occur, the diet begins no later than 3 weeks of age. Phenylalanine levels should be carefully monitored throughout the first 12 years of age, and once stable, monthly assessments are still recommended.

Because all natural food proteins contain approximately 15% phenylalanine, specially prepared milk substitutes are prescribed for the infant. Some of these products are made from specially treated enzymatic casein hydrolysate, which provides only 0.4% phenylalanine (28.5 mg/8 oz). They also contain minerals and vitamins to provide a balanced nutritional formula. Tyrosine and several other amino acids are supplied in the formula. Because of the low phenylalanine content of breast milk, total or partial breastfeeding may be possible with close monitoring of phenylalanine levels (Pichler, Michel, Zlamy, et al., 2017). Diet substitutes for older children, such as Phenyl-Free 2 (Mead Johnson)

*A resource for evidence-based metabolic dietary management is the Management Guidelines Portal jointly developed by the Southeast NBS and Genetics Collaborative and the Genetic Metabolic Dieticians International: https://southeastgenetics.org/ngp/guidelines.php.

and Phenex-2 (Ross), contain no phenylalanine and allow for greater exchanges with natural low-phenylalanine foods in the diet, leading to a more normal diet.

A low-phenylalanine diet begins as soon as possible after birth and continues throughout life. Adherence to this diet can be especially challenging in adolescence and adulthood. To evaluate the effectiveness of dietary treatment, frequent monitoring of blood phenylalanine and tyrosine levels is necessary. Because phenylalanine levels greater than or equal to 20 mg/dl in mothers with PKU affect the normal embryologic development of the fetus, women with PKU who are not on a lifelong diet must resume a low-phenylalanine diet before pregnancy.

Prognosis

Although many individuals with treated PKU manifest no cognitive and behavioral deficits, many comparisons of individuals with PKU to controls show lower performance on IQ tests, with larger differences in other cognitive domains. However, their performance is still in the average range. Evidence for differences in behavioral adjustment is inconsistent despite anecdotal reports suggesting greater risk for internalizing psychopathology and attention disorders. In addition, there are insufficient data on the effects of phenylalanine restriction over many decades of life (Vockley, Andersson, Antshel, et al., 2014). Total bone mineral density is considerably lower in children who are on a low-phenylalanine diet, even though calcium, phosphorus, and magnesium intakes are higher than normal.

Currently, treatment for many genetic diseases aims at modifying the phenotypical expression of those conditions. In the case of PKU, early childhood treatment with a reduced phenylalanine diet is highly successful at removing the possibility of cognitive impairment. However, PKU-rescued adults (i.e., those treated with reduction of phenylalanine in early childhood) remain unable to metabolize the amino acid and will always exhibit phenylalaninemia. For this reason, a lifelong low-phenylalanine diet is recommended (Nardecchia, Manti, Chiarotti, et al., 2015). PKU-rescued women who do not maintain low phenylalanine levels tend to produce children with cognitive and developmental impairments. Although indirectly related to the maternal PKU genotype, this is due to the fact that embryos are developing in a uterine environment with excessive concentrations of blood phenylalanine. To avoid this possibility, PKU-rescued women contemplating motherhood need to be placed again on a low-phenylalanine diet for the duration of the pregnancy.

Nursing Care Management

The principal nursing considerations involve teaching the family regarding the dietary restrictions. Although the treatment may sound simple, the task of maintaining such a strict dietary regimen is demanding, especially for older children and adolescents. Foods with low phenylalanine levels (e.g., some vegetables [except legumes]; fruits; juices; and some cereals, breads, and starches) must be measured to provide the prescribed amount of phenylalanine. Most high-protein foods, such as meat and dairy products, are either eliminated or restricted to small amounts.

Maintaining the diet during infancy presents few problems. Parents can introduce solid foods such as cereal, fruits, and vegetables as usual to the infant. Difficulties arise as the child gets older. A decreased appetite and refusal to eat may reduce intake of the calculated phenylalanine requirement. The child's increasing independence may inhibit absolute control of what he or she eats. Either factor can result in decreased or increased phenylalanine levels. During the school years, peer pressure becomes a major force in deterring the child from eating the prescribed foods or abstaining from high-protein foods such as milkshakes or ice cream. Limitations of this diet are best illustrated by an example: a quarter-pound hamburger may provide a 2-day phenylalanine allowance for a school-age child. Illness and growth spurts increase the body's need for this essential amino acid. Adolescence is a particularly difficult period, and limiting foods containing phenylalanine in adolescents with PKU is challenging.

The assistance of a registered dietitian is essential. Parents need a basic understanding of the disorder and practical suggestions regarding food selection and preparation. A number of support groups for parents of children with PKU are available nationwide. Many Internet resources also contain valuable information regarding dietary counseling and food options. Meal planning is based on an exchange list. As soon as children are old enough, usually by early preschool, they should be involved in the daily calculation, menu planning, and formula preparation. A computer voice-activated calculator, cards, or colored beads can help children keep track of the daily allowance of phenylalanine foods. A system of goal setting, self-monitoring, contracts, and rewards can promote compliance in adolescents.

GALACTOSEMIA

Galactosemia is a rare autosomal recessive disorder that results from various gene mutations leading to three distinct enzymatic deficiencies. The most common type of galactosemia (classic galactosemia) results from a deficiency of a hepatic enzyme, galactose 1-phosphate uridyltransferase (GALT), and affects approximately 1 of 16,000 to 60,000 births (Coelho, Rubio-Gozalbo, Vicente, et al., 2017). The other two varieties of galactosemia involve deficiencies in the enzymes galactokinase (GALK) and galactose 4′-epimerase (GALE); these are extremely rare disorders. GALT, GALK, and GALE are all involved in the conversion of galactose into glucose (Fig. 3.20).

Accumulation of activated 1-phosphate metabolites of galactose (and fructose) is extremely toxic to various tissues, especially in the kidneys, liver, and nervous system. As galactose 1-phosphate accumulates in the blood, a series of abnormalities develop. Hepatic dysfunction leads to

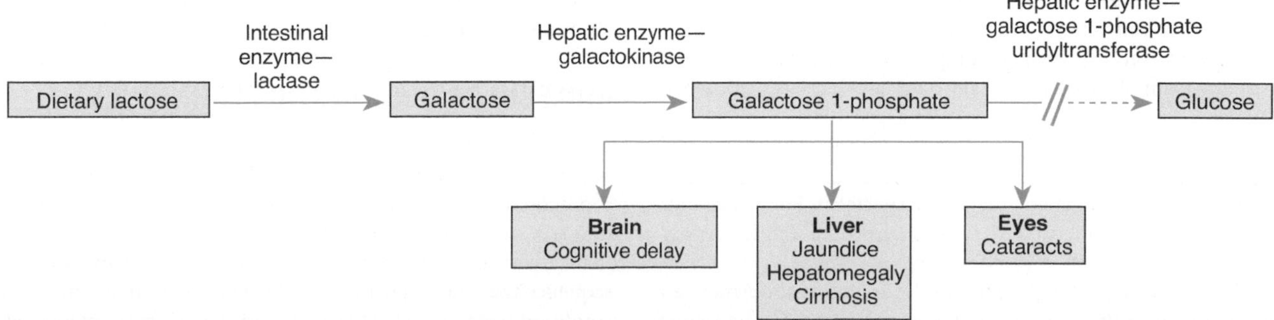

FIG. 3.20 Metabolic errors and consequences in galactosemia.

cirrhosis, resulting in jaundice in the infant by the second week of life. The spleen subsequently becomes enlarged as a result of portal hypertension. Cataracts are usually recognizable by 1 or 2 months of age; cerebral damage, manifested by the symptoms of lethargy and hypotonia, is evident soon afterward. Infants with galactosemia appear normal at birth, but on ingestion of milk (which has a high lactose content) they begin to show progressive symptoms, including vomiting, diarrhea, and weight loss. Death during the first month of life is frequent in untreated infants.

Diagnostic Evaluation*

Diagnosis is made on the basis of the infant's history, physical examination, galactosuria, increased levels of galactose in the blood, or decreased levels of uridine diphosphate–galactose transferase activity in erythrocytes. The infant may display characteristics of malnutrition and dehydration; decreased muscle mass and body fat may be evident. Newborn screening for this disease is required in all states (http://genes-r-us.uthscsa.edu/sites/genes-r-us/files/nbsdisorders.pdf). Heterozygotes can also be identified because they have significantly lower levels of the essential enzyme. Although asymptomatic, such individuals have been noted to spontaneously dislike and therefore limit the ingestion of galactose-containing foods.

Therapeutic Management

During infancy, treatment consists of eliminating all milk and lactose-containing formula, including breast milk. Traditionally, lactose-free formulas are used, with soy-protein formula being the feeding of choice. The American Academy of Pediatrics (2015) recommends the use of soy formula for infants diagnosed with galactosemia. As the infant progresses to solids, only foods low in galactose should be consumed. Certain fruits are high in galactose, and some dietitians recommend that they be avoided. Nurses should give food lists to the family to ensure appropriate foods are chosen.

If galactosemia is suspected, implement supportive treatment and care, including monitoring for hypoglycemia, liver failure, bleeding disorders, and *Escherichia coli* sepsis.

Prognosis

Follow-up studies of children treated from birth or within the first 2 months of life after symptoms appear have found long-term complications, such as ovarian dysfunction, cataracts, abnormal speech, cognitive impairment, growth restriction, and motor delay (Coelho, Rubio-Gozalbo, Vicente, et al., 2017). These findings have revealed that eliminating sources of galactose does not significantly improve the outcome. New therapeutic strategies, such as enhancing residual transferase activity, replacing depleted metabolites, or using gene replacement therapy, are needed to improve the prognosis for these children.

Nursing Care Management†

Nursing interventions are similar to those for PKU and other IEMs, except that dietary restrictions are easier to maintain because many more foods are allowed. However, reading food labels carefully for the presence of any form of lactose, especially dairy products, is mandatory. Many drugs, such as some of the penicillin preparations, contain lactose as filler and also must be avoided. Unfortunately, lactose is an unlabeled ingredient in many pharmaceuticals. Therefore instruct parents to ask their local pharmacist about galactose content of any over-the-counter or prescription medication.

CYTOGENETIC DIAGNOSTIC TECHNIQUES

Chromosomes have traditionally been studied under light microscopy. After a significant number of cells are prepared so the chromosomes can be visualized during mitotic metaphase under a light microscope and imaged through a computer, their chromosomes are displayed in a karyotype, arranged according to their size, position of their centromeres, and banding patterns. The most common human cells used for chromosomes studies are peripheral blood leukocytes obtained by venipuncture and cells obtained by biopsy from a variety of tissues, such as skin (including fetal skin cells), chorionic villi, and bone marrow. Robotic cell harvesters and computerized imaging systems have drastically cut down on manual labor; however, expert technicians and cytogeneticists are still necessary to analyze and interpret karyotypes.

Although karyotypes still have an important role in identifying large chromosomal rearrangements such as translocations, they have been replaced by chromosomal microarray testing as the preferred tool for evaluating children with congenital malformations and intellectual or global developmental delays and for whom a clinical diagnosis is uncertain (Rosenfeld & Patel, 2017). Chromosomal microarray technology is used to identify submicroscopic as well as larger segments of DNA that have more or fewer copy number than normal. Thousands to millions of DNA segments throughout the genome are examined for clinically relevant copy number variations (CNVs). Conditions caused by deletions such as velo-cardio-facial syndrome (VCFS) and cri du chat can be diagnosed, as well as very rare or previously unrecognized syndromes caused by submicroscopic deletions or duplications. Chromosomal microarrays can also identify areas where DNA is identical between one or more areas of the chromosomes inherited from the mother and father. If the identical areas are scattered throughout the genome, it is possible to estimate relatedness between the biologic parents. If the identical area is in a segment contained within a single chromosome, it may indicate uniparental disomy. An area of identical DNA between both chromosomes may offer diagnostic clues for autosomal recessive disorders.

When clinical examination, health history, and developmental history are strongly suggestive of a known condition, a less expensive targeted test can be used to identify the specific microdeletion, microduplication, or fragile site. Fluorescent in situ hybridization (FISH) uses fluorescent-labeled single-stranded DNA probes designed to attach to specific areas of chromosomes. For example, to diagnose VCFS, probes that adhere to 22q11.2 are used, as well as probes to identify chromosome 22. A positive FISH test for persons with VCFS identifies both copies of chromosome 22, but the probe specific to the q11.2 region only attaches to one of the chromosomes because the region of interest is deleted in the other chromosome 22.

MOLECULAR DIAGNOSTIC TECHNIQUES

Identification of single-gene mutations responsible for a growing number of genetic disorders is now possible with a variety of molecular tests. In some conditions, such as CF, sickle cell disease, myotonic dystrophy, and fragile X syndrome, the specific gene is known and tests are available that target many of the known disease-associated mutations or that sequence the coding portions of the gene associated with the specific condition. Gene panels for some disorders have become available as technology improves to make it easier and less expensive to analyze a

*Always refer patients to a genetic metabolic specialist. For a reference list, visit the Society for Inherited Metabolic Disorders website, http://www.simd.org/.

†Information and support for parents can be found at the American Liver Foundation, http://www.liverfoundation.org; and at Galactosemia Foundation Inc., http://www.galactosemia.org.

number of genes at one time. Finally, a new technology has made it possible to target sequencing of exons within a group of genes or the entire genome (Korf & Rehm, 2013). When exons in the entire genome are sequenced, it is called whole exome sequencing. When all accessible DNA within a genome is sequenced, it is called whole genome sequencing. Whole exome or whole genome sequencing is used to diagnose rare disorders for which specific testing is not available or when a clinically diagnosed condition can be caused by a mutation in one of many possible genes. The use of whole exome or whole genome sequencing in healthy newborns is being studied (Ceyhan-Birsoy, Machini, Lebo, et al., 2017).

PREDISPOSITION GENETIC TESTING

Molecular diagnostic techniques have enabled predisposition testing, which is the identification of gene mutations associated with genetic disorders in asymptomatic individuals. Depending on the penetrance of the allele(s), these may be considered presymptomatic or susceptibility tests.

Familial adenomatous polyposis is one of several overlapping conditions associated with mutations in the *APC* gene. These mutations are considered virtually 100% penetrant, resulting in hundreds to thousands of adenomatous polyps and eventual colon cancer. Once the *APC* mutation has been identified in an affected family member, at-risk family members can be tested for the same mutation. Because of the high penetrance, such testing in asymptomatic individuals would be considered presymptomatic testing. *APC* mutation testing in at-risk children is done to identify those who need colon screening and to identify polyp formation early so cancer-preventive surgical decisions can be made (Hegde, Ferber, Mao, et al., 2014).

Hereditary breast and ovarian cancer has primarily been associated with mutations in either *BRCA1* or *BRCA2*. Penetrance of mutations in these genes has been reported to be as high as 85% for breast cancer and lower for other associated cancers (ovarian, prostate, pancreatic, gastrointestinal, and melanoma). Once the *BRCA1* or *BRCA2* mutation has been identified in an affected family member, asymptomatic at-risk family members can be tested for the same mutation. Onset and type of cancer vary among members of a family identified with a mutation. In addition, although some members may develop one or more of the associated cancers, other mutation-carrying members may die in their eighties without ever developing cancer (Lynch, Venne, & Berse, 2015). Therefore testing for mutations in *BRCA1* and *BRCA2* in an asymptomatic family member is considered susceptibility testing.

Predisposition genetic testing for adult onset cancers is discouraged in at-risk children until they are cognitively and emotionally able to make an informed decision about testing for themselves (American Academy of Pediatrics, 2013). However, if a child has whole exome or whole genome testing to determine the cause of his or her genetic disorder, the child's parents are given the option to have their child's DNA additionally analyzed for a set of genes that include *BRCA1, BRCA2,* and other genes associated with adult-onset conditions. The set of genes were initially recommended by the American College of Medical Genetics and Genomics (ACMG) in 2013 and the organization plans to update the list on a regular basis (Kalia, Adelman, Bale, et al., 2017). Purposely analyzing the genes compromises the child's future autonomy to decide whether or not the information is desired (Prows, Tran, & Blosser, 2014).

THERAPEUTIC MANAGEMENT OF GENETIC DISEASE

Therapy for genetic disease is currently aimed at correcting the phenotypic expression of a variant gene, and therefore the major goal of therapy is modification of the internal or external environment to correct or minimize the effects of the variant gene or pair of variant genes. However, genomic advances have opened doors to genotype intervention, and clinical applications of gene manipulation techniques are currently being tested.

Phenotype Modification

Examples of currently used intervention aimed at modifying the phenotypic expression of genetic disorders follow.

Surgical Management

Surgical repair of structural defects has made it possible to prolong life in a number of multifactorial disorders, such as congenital heart disease and NTDs. Numerous facial and limb deformities can be corrected by plastic and reconstructive techniques. In the case of familial adenomatous polyposis, the colon is surgically removed to prevent colon cancer that would eventually develop in one or more of the countless polyps that line the colon. The use of splenectomy in several hereditary disorders of blood cells prevents the trapping and destruction of abnormal blood cells in that organ. Early diagnosis and enucleation in retinoblastoma have reduced the mortality rate from this malignant eye tumor. Fetal surgery may also be performed for some life-threatening anomalies such a diaphragmatic hernia. Corrective surgery for children born with ambiguous genitalia (e.g., girls with congenital adrenal hyperplasia), although widely used, has been recently the focus of controversy that involves the issue of parental versus affected individual (future) preferences.

Diet Modification

For disorders in which an enzyme deficiency causes a toxic accumulation of a substance or its by-products, restricting the intake of foods containing that substance may prevent irreversible damage from the improper metabolism of these compounds. This dietary control is lifelong and requires a high level of adherence. Examples in infants and children include the low-phenylalanine diet prescribed for PKU, elimination of dairy products containing lactose for hereditary lactase deficiency, avoidance of foods containing or producing galactose for galactosemia, and a diet low in branched-chain amino acids for maple syrup urine disease. Women with PKU who have not maintained dietary control must reinstitute a strict low-phenylalanine diet before conception and maintain it throughout pregnancy to prevent a high risk of adverse fetal effects.

Preconception and prenatal folic acid supplementation has been shown to reduce the incidence or recurrence of NTDs. Therefore in 1992 the US Public Health Service recommended that all women capable of becoming pregnant should consume 0.4 mg of folic acid per day. As of 1998 the US Food and Drug Administration mandated that folic acid be added to enriched grain products. This would add 0.1 mg folic acid to the daily diet of the average person. Women who have previously had a pregnancy affected by an NTD are advised to take 4.0 mg of folic acid per day beginning 1 month before conception and continuing throughout the first trimester of pregnancy. The risk of recurrence of an NTD in another pregnancy is reduced by 72% in women following this regimen.

Metabolic Manipulation

In some deficiency diseases, supplying the missing product that cannot be synthesized prevents undesirable effects. For example, thyroid hormone is prescribed to prevent the damaging effects of hypothyroidism, and providing the missing blood factors prevents life-threatening and debilitating hemorrhages in persons with different types of hemophilia. Other examples are insulin for diabetes mellitus, growth hormone for growth hormone deficiency, and corticosteroids for adrenogenital syndrome.

Removal of toxic substances that accumulate in vital tissues as a result of a hereditary disease can prevent disabling complications. Some of the deleterious effects of hemochromatosis, a hereditary disorder characterized by an excess accumulation of iron in the liver, heart, and pancreas, can be reduced with the removal of iron by periodic therapeutic phlebotomies or administration of chelating agents.

Diet supplements can be given when the individual is unable to synthesize or effectively utilize substances needed as cofactors in metabolism. This includes the use of vitamin B_{12} in persons with pernicious anemia, whose absorption of this vitamin is impaired. Vitamin and cofactor supplementation may be used to treat mitochondrial disease. Phenobarbitone can be used to enhance hepatic metabolism of unconjugated bilirubin in children with Crigler-Najjar syndrome type 2, thus helping prevent brain damage (kernicterus) and jaundice (Valle, Beaudet, Vogelstein, et al., 2014).

Avoidance of Drugs or Other Harmful Substances

In drug-induced disease, such as glucose-6-phosphate dehydrogenase (G6PD) deficiency and the porphyrias, avoidance of the drugs that precipitate a reaction is a simple preventive measure. These include aspirin and quinine-based antimalarial medications in the case of G6PD deficiency, and ethanol, barbiturates, anticonvulsants, sulfonamides, and oral contraceptives in the case of acute intermittent porphyria (Valle, Beaudet, Vogelstein, et al., 2014). Some anesthetic agents may precipitate symptoms of malignant hyperthermia.

Immunologic Prevention

The administration of immunoglobulin to Rh-negative mothers after the birth of an Rh-positive infant is effective in preventing Rh-antibody formation, which causes hemolytic disease of the newborn in subsequent births.

Transplantation

Better control of tissue incompatibility problems is improving the survival of children undergoing replacement of nonfunctioning organs with normal organs. Transplanted organs include the kidneys in hereditary polycystic kidneys, the heart in severe cardiac myopathy, the liver in hepatic atresia, and stem cell transplant for Fanconi anemia.

Gene Product Replacement

Recombinant DNA technology makes it possible to produce large quantities of certain gene products. Such technology avoids the infectious contamination risk that accompanied extraction of gene products from mass quantities of human blood or tissue.

The administration of gene products is especially applicable when the missing product is a circulatory peptide or protein, as in coagulation factor VIII or IX in hemophilia type A and type B, respectively (Saenko & Pipe, 2006). If the gene product is membrane bound, as is the case for enzymes deficient in various lysosomal storage diseases, the natural enzyme product may need to be purposefully altered so that it can enter the cell through a naturally occurring cell receptor. Gaucher disease was the first lysosomal disorder to be successfully treated in this manner, and lessons learned in the process have led to more recent enzyme replacement therapies for disorders such as Pompe disease and Hurler syndrome (Bailey, 2008). If the missing gene product is a substance that acts within a metabolic pathway of a specific organ protected by a barrier, such as the enzyme hexosaminidase A in Tay-Sachs disease (blood-brain barrier), injectable products become ineffective and replacement is more problematic. The introduction of a foreign gene product may eventually trigger an immune reaction, as has been observed in hemophilia when the recipient develops antibody against the clotting factor, greatly reducing the efficiency of an otherwise successful therapy.

Gene Transfer

Gene transfer is an experimental technique used to introduce a normally functioning gene into the cells of a patient with a genetic disorder. The purpose of this experimental approach is to introduce a gene that will produce a protein that can function in a patient and treat or prevent disease. Researchers are also working on strategies to turn off genes that are not functioning properly and cannot be fixed by simply adding a functioning gene into patients' cells. These approaches involve considerable risk and are focused on treatment of genetic disorders that have no other therapies. Gene transfer technology is also being studied for the treatment of cancer by targeting the tumor cells.

Environmental Modification

Inherited diseases or defects with no therapeutic modality can be modified to enhance the quality of life for the affected individual. Some examples of environmental manipulation include hearing aids for children with congenital hearing loss, glasses or vision enhancers such as books in enlarged print or Braille for the visually impaired, mobilizing devices such as braces and wheelchairs for persons with muscle and bone impairment, prosthetic devices for those with limb deficiencies, and infant stimulation programs to maximize the potential of children who are developmentally delayed. Environmental manipulation also includes protection from the damaging effects of the environment, such as exposure to sunlight, which can cause skin fragility and blistering in persons with porphyrias and increases the risk of skin cancers in patients with xeroderma pigmentosum and oculocutaneous albinism.

IMPACT OF HEREDITARY DISORDERS ON THE FAMILY

GENETIC TESTING

Genetic testing can be broadly divided into two categories: diagnostic testing and screening. Tests to detect a disease-associated gene mutation or chromosome abnormality in symptomatic individuals are rapidly assuming greater importance in management of genetic disorders as more genes and mutations are identified and techniques are developed for easy application of the tests.

With improved technology, mass screening for numerous genetic disorders will probably become routine. However, to be truly effective, screening programs depend on thorough education of both health professionals and the public regarding these programs and the limitations and implications of testing. The religious, moral, ethical, and legal issues revolving around screening and prenatal diagnosis are extensive and change over time.

Purposes of Screening

Genetic screening is presumptive identification of an unrecognized genetic predisposition for future disease in individuals or their progeny for which preventive or disease course–altering interventions exist. In general, genetic screening targets populations, whereas genetic diagnostic testing targets individuals. The first corollaries of any genetic screening intervention must be *voluntary participation, equal access to all,* and *confidentiality* (both in conducting the tests and in handling records and results). In addition, education and counseling about tests and procedures must be an integral part of any screening program. Attention must be paid to quality control of all aspects of testing and laboratory procedures.

Genetic screening has three purposes: (1) to provide for early recognition of a disease, before signs and symptoms occur, for which effective intervention and therapy exist (e.g., PKU); (2) to identify carriers of a genetic disease for the purpose of maximizing parenthood planning options (e.g., Tay-Sachs disease); and (3) to obtain population data on frequency, spectrum, and natural history of genetic variations not currently known to be associated with disease.

Screening for genetic disorders can occur during various times in a person's life: (1) preconception screening of selected populations for heterozygous carriers (e.g., Ashkenazi Jewish carrier screening panel); (2) screening of relatives of known carrier or affected individuals within a family, for the purpose of reproductive decision making; (3) postconceptional (prenatal) screening (e.g., maternal serum screen for identifying risks for NTDs and chromosome abnormalities); and (4) newborn screening.

Newborn Screening

Newborn screening began in the 1960s when Guthrie devised the blood spot test to screen for PKU. Newborn screening for PKU was begun in all states, and currently each state offers screening for a growing number of disorders such as hemoglobinopathies, galactosemia, hypothyroidism, and congenital adrenal hypoplasia. In the past, decisions about which disorder to include were based on the following criteria:

- The disease occurs with a significant frequency.
- An inexpensive and reliable method of testing exists.
- There is effective treatment and intervention.
- If untreated, the baby will die or be severely developmentally impaired.
- An affected newborn may appear normal at birth.

Because the actual disorders screened by individual states varied considerably, the American College of Medical Genetics (ACMG) was commissioned by the Maternal Child Health Bureau of the Health Resources and Services Administration to develop a uniform screening panel. The ACMG task force used the following minimum criteria when considering which disorders to include (American College of Medical Genetics Newborn Screening Expert Group, 2006):

- It can be identified at a phase (24 to 48 hours after birth) at which it would not ordinarily be clinically detected.
- A follow-up diagnostic test with appropriate sensitivity and specificity is available for it.
- There are demonstrated benefits of early detection, timely intervention, and efficacious treatment of the condition being tested.

A panel of 29 core conditions and 25 secondary conditions was recommended by ACMG in its 2006 report (Sweetman, Millington, Therrell, et al., 2006). With advancing technology the number of conditions screened by individual states can be expected to change. A regularly updated list of conditions offered in each state's newborn screening panel can be found at the National Newborn Screening and Genetics Resource Center website (http://genes-r-us.uthscsa.edu).

Because many of the conditions tested for are metabolic disorders, it is important that the first newborn screening blood sample be obtained at least 24 hours after the first protein feeding or within the first 72 hours of life. Infants found to be screen positive (thus at high risk) for a metabolic condition such as PKU or galactosemia are immediately referred to a medical center for testing to confirm the diagnosis and initiate treatment. Of course, this relies on a coordinated follow-up program that includes well-informed primary care providers and nurses who can locate newborns with abnormal screening results and facilitate the necessary follow-up visits.

Screening for Reproductive Information

Screening for heterozygotes (carriers) can detect unaffected persons with certain variant genes who, when they mate with an individual who carries a mutation in the same gene, are at high risk of producing an affected offspring. These individuals are thus provided with the information they need for making decisions about family planning. Carriers of a number of diseases can be detected by laboratory tests, but, because of the rarity of these diseases, mass screening is not feasible except in persons or populations known to be at risk. Persons at risk include close relatives of those with an inborn error of metabolism or other detectable disorder and certain ethnic populations known to have a high incidence of a specific disease, such as sickle cell anemia in African Americans, Tay-Sachs disease in Ashkenazi Jews, and thalassemia in people of Mediterranean ancestry (Holtkamp, Mathijssen, Lakeman, et al., 2016).

This type of screening is sometimes controversial. Screening for carrier status for CF is one such situation that has the potential to create ethical dilemmas. Children with CF have a disease-associated mutation in each of their *CFTR* genes. More than 1000 different *CFTR* mutations have been identified, yet carrier testing for CF typically analyzes less than 100 of the possible *CFTR* mutations. Therefore after screening, a couple may feel safe to proceed with pregnancy yet still have a child with CF. Carrier status screening has influenced marriage partner selection. Some carriers have made life choices based on inaccurate understanding of the implications of carrier status (e.g., thinking they would get the disease or that they were at high risk for having an affected child regardless of whether the partner is also a carrier). These misunderstandings and their consequences underscore the importance of careful education before decision making regarding carrier screening.

Carrier testing for children is generally not recommended because the information is for reproductive purposes (American Academy of Pediatrics, 2013). Instead, parents are counseled that the child should make a decision about carrier testing when she or he is old enough to make an informed choice. Yet newborn screening tests reveal carrier status for certain conditions such as CF and sickle cell. Careful counseling is necessary with carrier screening to ensure that individuals understand the limitations of testing and the implications of results. Even with careful counseling, there may be significant misunderstanding or misuse of information.

Screening for Epidemiologic Information

Public health officials may use screening as a method for monitoring the incidence of diseases or malformations in a population to detect environmental or other causes that might significantly influence the incidence of the disorders. For example, geographic and socioeconomic variations in the incidence of NTDs eventually led to research that determined that folic acid supplementation of 0.4 mg/day in women of childbearing age reduces NTD occurrence within the population.

Significance of Screening to Families

Mass screening programs have received mixed acceptance from health professionals and the general public. Potential benefits of carrier screening include facilitating genetic counseling and reproductive planning and providing useful information to other at-risk family members. Newborn screening provides for early detection and treatment initiation, maximizing quality of life. Yet realizing these benefits requires that couples and parents be given adequate information to make informed decisions about whether to pursue screening. For newborn screening, parent choice about testing may be limited by state regulations. Some states allow exemptions from newborn screening in certain situations, such as objections on religious grounds if there is a conflict with religious practices and beliefs of an established church. Regardless, parents need to be educated about the purpose, benefits, risks, and limitations of newborn screening and the implications of abnormal results. Parents have indicated that multiple exposures to information in different formats beginning before conception are important (Tluczek, Orland, Nick, et al., 2009).

The social stigma of being the carrier of a "defective" gene may be a side effect of screening. In some families such knowledge is embarrassing and damaging to self-esteem. Teenagers may be especially vulnerable to the effects of knowing they carry a specific disease-associated gene mutation at a time when identity formation and peer approval are extremely important. Cultural views regarding this knowledge can have profound effects on the members of some ethnic groups. In some cases, social status within the cultural group can be impaired.

Probably the most important area for nursing practice is teaching, or the ability to convey clear, precise, and unambiguous information to clients. Families need to understand why the screening is proposed, what the results mean, and how the family can interpret false-positive and false-negative results. Anxiety is greater when families have not received sufficient information about the screening or testing process and its significance for their health. Families also have a right to know who assumes the cost of additional testing or retesting—the family or the state. The nurse is a valuable resource in ensuring that families are aware of alternatives and in helping them make the best decision.

PRENATAL TESTING

Pediatric nurses may encounter couples who had prenatal testing and are preparing for the anticipated care of their unborn child. Such couples may be making primary care arrangements; meeting professionals in the newborn intensive care unit; meeting with surgeons to learn about the surgeries their newborn will need in the first few days, weeks, or months of life; and talking with other parents who have children with the same condition. Thus it is important that pediatric nurses have a general understanding of the capabilities, limitations, and risks of prenatal testing.

Advances in technology have greatly increased the spectrum of available prenatal screening and diagnostic options. Although screening options are available for all pregnant women, prenatal diagnostic testing is reserved for pregnancies considered at increased risk for less than healthy outcomes. The purposes of prenatal testing include identifying congenital anomalies and genetic disorders that may need intervention during pregnancy or soon after delivery; enabling parents to prepare for the birth of a child who will require long-term medical or developmental interventions; and enabling parents to make decisions about placing their child for adoption or terminating the pregnancy. However, even normal prenatal test results do not guarantee the birth of a healthy baby. When referring a family for prenatal testing, the nurse can benefit from general guidelines, some of which are delineated in Box 3.6.

BOX 3.6 Indications for Prenatal Testing

General Risk Factors

Maternal age of at least 35 years at time of delivery or at least 31 years if twin gestation

Elevated or low trisomy profile screen results

Specific Risk Factors

Previous child with a structural defect or chromosome abnormality

Previous stillbirth or neonatal death

Structural abnormality in mother or father

Balanced translocation in mother or father

Inherited disorders—Cystic fibrosis, metabolic disorders, sex-linked recessive disorders

Medical disease in mother—Diabetes mellitus, phenylketonuria

Exposure to a teratogen—Ionizing radiation, anticonvulsant medicines, lithium, isotretinoin, alcohol

Infection—Rubella, toxoplasmosis, cytomegalovirus

Abnormal ultrasound findings

Ethnic Risk Factors

Disorder—Ethnic or racial group

Tay-Sachs disease—Ashkenazi Jewish, French Canadian

Sickle cell anemia—Black African, Mediterranean, Arab, Indian, Pakistani

α- and β-Thalassemia—Mediterranean, Southern and Southeast Asian, Chinese

Prenatal Screening Tests

Noninvasive screening uses maternal blood or ultrasound to assess fetal risk for certain congenital malformations or chromosome abnormalities. Maternal age has been the longest-standing screening measure to detect women at increased risk for having a child with a chromosome abnormality. The most common laboratory screening method is to analyze maternal serum for abnormal levels of pregnancy-related chemical markers (such as free human chorionic gonadotropin [hCG], unconjugated estriol, and pregnancy-associated plasma protein A). Screening ultrasound can be used to measure thickness of the back of the fetal neck. Screening tests that reveal two or more abnormal markers in addition to maternal age are more likely to detect an abnormal pregnancy. Pregnancies that have a positive screen are recommended to have further evaluation with diagnostic ultrasound, amniocentesis, or fetal cord blood sampling (Dashe, 2016).

Cell free DNA screening is a first-trimester, noninvasive technique designed to detect common chromosome disorders and is increasingly being used to screen for single-gene disorders when a family mutation or pair of mutations is known. During a pregnancy, about 10% of maternal circulating DNA from broken-down cells come from the placenta or fetus. Maternal blood is analyzed for disproportionate fragments of targeted chromosomes (usually chromosomes 21, 18, and 13). Although detection of abnormally high fragments of targeted chromosomes is considered diagnostic, the absence of detection does not rule out the possibility of chromosome abnormalities. Follow-up diagnostic chorionic villi sampling or amniocentesis is recommended when noninvasive prenatal testing is normal (American College of Obstetricians and Gynecologists, 2015).

Prenatal Diagnostic Procedures

Recommendations for diagnostic testing may be triggered by preexisting risks (e.g., previous child with a genetic disorder), personal characteristics (e.g., member of subpopulation at risk for certain genetic diseases), or a newly identified risk following prenatal screening for the current pregnancy (see Box 3.6). Specific risk factors are usually identified in the family history, previous pregnancy outcomes, or the mother's medical history. Ethnic risk factors are based on a higher carrier frequency for certain genetic diseases in selected populations. Indications for prenatal diagnosis when any of these risk factors is present are based on a greater than general population risk that a congenital anomaly or genetic disorder will occur in the pregnancy. The specific risk is, of course, different for each situation.

Invasive prenatal diagnostic tests include chorionic villi sampling (CVS), amniocentesis, fetal blood sampling, and preimplantation analysis of embryonic cells (American College of Obstetricians and Gynecologists, 2016). CVS can be performed between 10 and 12 weeks of gestation. Using either a transcervical or transabdominal approach guided by ultrasound, the clinician obtains a small biopsy of the chorionic villi. Cells from the sample can be grown for chromosome and single-gene disorder studies. Contamination of the sample with maternal cells can compromise the accuracy of test results. Amniocentesis is usually performed between 14 and 18 weeks of gestation under ultrasound guidance. Fetal skin cells that have sloughed off and are present in the amniotic fluid can be isolated and cultured for chromosome or single-gene analyses. AFP can be measured in the amniotic fluid and is a much more reliable indicator of an NTD or abdominal wall defect than maternal serum AFP. An additional test for an enzyme specific to neural tissue, acetylcholinesterase, may be done; if this test is positive in the presence of an elevated AFP level, it is diagnostic of an open NTD. A diagnostic ultrasound clarifies the extent and location of the NTD or abdominal wall defect. A less frequently used test is fetal blood sampling, in which blood is drawn from the umbilical vein. This procedure can be performed after 18 weeks of gestation and is usually done for prenatal evaluation of fetal hematologic abnormalities, inborn errors of metabolism, fetal infection, and rapid chromosome analysis. **Preimplantation genetic diagnosis** first requires in vitro (test tube) fertilization followed by in vitro genetic testing of one or more cells extracted from the developing embryo or, less commonly, genetic testing of the polar bodies. Embryos without an identified genetic disorder are then candidates for implantation (Vermeesch, Voet, & Devriendt, 2016). As with all technologies, error can occur, so confirmatory testing with CVS or amniocentesis is recommended following preimplantation genetic diagnosis (American College of Obstetricians and Gynecologists, 2016).

A few additional diagnostic tests are infrequently used. Fetal biopsy is sometimes used to diagnose certain genetic skin disorders and metabolic disorders when DNA studies are unavailable or are uninformative. Fetal echocardiography may be performed for further diagnosis when a cardiac defect is noted on ultrasound or if prior prenatal procedures reveal the fetus has a genetic disorder in which cardiac malformations may occur.

GENETIC EVALUATION AND COUNSELING

The expanded recognition of genetic diseases and disorders and an increasingly well-informed public are creating a justified demand for genetic evaluation, diagnosis, information regarding risks to present and future generations, and access to available therapies. Unfortunately, however, persons who need expert genetic counseling often make uninformed decisions on their own or are the victims of well-meaning but equally uninformed relatives, acquaintances, or paraprofessionals. Nurses involved in infant and child care continually encounter families that have a risk of transmitting a disorder to an offspring, as well as children who may have an undiagnosed genetic disorder that needs expert evaluation.

Pediatric Indications for Genetic Consultation

The ACMG has produced guidelines for genetics consultation (Pletcher, Toriello, Noblin, et al., 2007). The indications can be broadly divided into preconception-prenatal, pediatric, and adult. The indications that are relevant for newborns through adolescents are as follows:

- Family history of hereditary diseases, birth defects, or developmental problems
- Family history of sudden cardiac death or early-onset cancer
- Family history of mental illness
- Abnormal newborn screen
- Abnormal genetic test result ordered by a nongenetics professional who lacks the knowledge and experience to discuss implications of results
- Progressive neurologic condition
- Major congenital anomaly (e.g., cleft lip, congenital heart defect, limb abnormality, spina bifida)
- Pattern of major or minor anomalies suggestive of genetic disorder
- Congenital or early-onset hearing loss or vision loss
- Cognitive impairment or autism
- Abnormal sexual maturation or delayed puberty
- Abnormally tall or short stature compared with other family members
- Excessive bleeding or excessive clotting
- Parental requests that child be evaluated by a genetics professional

Persons may not be affected themselves but may request genetic counseling about the heritability of a trait. A young couple contemplating childbearing may be concerned about a disorder in one of their families or may seek advice because they are related. A couple who are both members of a population at risk for certain genetic diseases may wish to determine whether they carry an associated gene mutation (e.g., African Americans and sickle cell anemia, Ashkenazi Jews and Tay-Sachs disease, or persons of Mediterranean ancestry and thalassemia). A couple planning adoption might seek genetic evaluation and counseling regarding a prospective child.

More often, persons who inquire about the possibility of recurrence of a disease or disorder have a child with a genetic disease or disorder or had a child who died of the disease. They are concerned about the likelihood of having another, similarly affected child and may want to know what reproductive choices are available. They might seek this advice before initiating another pregnancy or after the mother is already pregnant. If prenatal diagnostic testing is not done, the history of a condition in an older sibling, such as galactosemia, alerts health personnel to initiate specific and thorough testing for the condition in a newborn. In this way, early therapy can be initiated, thus minimizing or eliminating the effects of the disease or defect.

Genetic Services

Comprehensive genetic services consist of a group of specialists, which may include clinical geneticists, advanced practice nurses in genetics, genetic counselors, psychologists, biochemical geneticists, cytogeneticists, molecular geneticists, nurses, social workers, and other auxiliary personnel. Although genetic centers were typically considered a resource for genetic evaluation, diagnosis, and counseling, a growing number of centers are managing the health care needs of patients with complex, rare genetic disorders. Some centers specialize in treatment of genetic disorders (e.g., enzyme replacement therapy for lysosomal storage disorders). Most centers are associated with a large medical center, which may have extensive outreach programs with satellite clinics throughout adjacent urban and rural areas. Numerous specialty clinics also deal with specific genetic disorders (such as CF, muscular dystrophy, hemophilia, or craniofacial anomalies) and provide their own genetic counseling services. Unfortunately, these units are concentrated in and around large metropolitan areas. As a result, counseling is not always accessible to a large number of people who could benefit from the service.

As evident from the list of indicators for a genetic consultation, genetic evaluation for diagnostic purposes may occur at any point in the life span. Unlike a medical prognosis, which predicts the outcome of a disease for an individual, a genetic prognosis may have implications for members of the immediate family, other relatives, and future offspring. During a genetic evaluation or follow-up visit, a genetics professional obtains or updates the patient's family history and pedigree, developmental history, and medical history (including pregnancy, labor, and delivery information); performs a physical examination, including dysmorphic features; and orders appropriate testing such as biochemical, cytogenetic, or molecular procedures. A genetic diagnosis may or may not be made initially, and follow-up evaluations are common.

Genetic counseling is a communication process that deals with the human problems associated with the occurrence, or risk of occurrence, of a genetic disorder in a family. This process involves an attempt by one or more appropriately trained persons to help the individual or family:

- Comprehend the medical facts, including the diagnosis, the probable course of the disorder, and the available management
- Appreciate the way heredity contributes to the disorder and the risk of recurrence in specified relatives
- Understand the options for dealing with the risk of recurrence
- Choose the course of action that seems appropriate to them in view of their risk and family goals and act in accordance with that decision
- Make the best possible adjustment to the disorder in an affected family member and to the risk of recurrence of that disorder

Estimation of Risks

Risks for occurrence or recurrence of a genetic disorder are estimated from a thorough family history and any known genetic screening information. A careful, detailed family history not only provides a picture of the **proband** (the affected person, or index case) in relation to other family members, but also may identify others who are similarly affected or who might be presymptomatic or at risk of producing affected children. Analyzing the pattern of affected family members can assist in confirming a tentative diagnosis or in determining the level of risk in multifactorial inheritance.

An accurate diagnosis is essential to provide specific risk figures. There are more than 10,000 known inherited disorders, many of which have similar clinical manifestations but different modes of inheritance. For example, symptoms in the early stages of severe X-linked muscular dystrophy appear much like those of the milder autosomal recessive and autosomal dominant varieties, autosomal recessive neurogenic muscular atrophies, and nongenetic poliomyelitis. The significance of the risks related to each type of disorder is readily apparent. For disorders with an unknown or multifactorial cause, recurrence risks are termed *empiric,* meaning they are based on observations of recurrence in similar situations, rather than *theoretic,* meaning they are based on mendelian inheritance patterns.

Communicating Risks

Genetic professionals do not attempt to make recommendations or decisions for patients when discussing reproductive risks. Instead, they discuss comprehensive and current information about the nature of the disorder, the extent of risk, the probable consequences, and alternative solutions. The goal of this communication process is to enable patients to make their own decisions about whether to pursue preconception or prenatal testing and what to do in response to test results. However, genetics professionals recognize that recommendations do have a place when genetic testing is used to identify risk for diseases or disorders that have available treatments that can prevent, delay, or improve symptoms. Children who test positive for a mutation in the *APC* gene associated with familial adenomatous polyposis will eventually develop colon polyps, and eventually one or more will become cancerous. Therefore genetics professionals recommend specific screening measures for these children; when polyps are discovered, the professionals recommend a surgical consultation to discuss options. As with any health care encounter, shared decision making with parents and/or adolescents is the goal.

It is helpful to explain risks in different ways and to use examples to aid in understanding the meaning of probabilities. Most people do not have an adequate knowledge of genetics and human biology to fully comprehend these complex concepts. Words and concepts that can be used include *percentages, chance, odds,* and *likelihood.* For example, if a 40-year-old woman has a 1:112 risk of having a child with Down syndrome, other ways to explain it include "You have about a 1% chance of having a baby with Down syndrome" or "Out of 112 women your age having a baby, odds are that one of them will have a child with Down syndrome." Games of probability can also be used, such as flipping coins, baseball pools, and lotteries.

! NURSING ALERT

Families may misunderstand probability, even when it is fully explained. The nurse should impress on them that each pregnancy is an independent event. Often parents who are told that a recessive disorder carries a 1:4 risk of recurrence incorrectly reason that because they already have one affected child, the next three will be unaffected. Chance has no memory; the risk is 1:4 for each and every pregnancy.

ROLE OF NURSES

All nurses need to be prepared to use genetic and genomic information and technology when providing care. Nearly 50 nursing organizations endorsed essential minimum competencies necessary for nurses to deliver competent genetic and genomic focused nursing care (Consensus Panel on Genetic/Genomic Nursing Competencies, 2006). The professional practice domains include applying/integrating genetic knowledge into nursing assessment; identifying and referring clients who may benefit from genetic information or services; identifying genetics resources and services to meet clients' needs; and providing care and support before, during, and after providing genetic information and/or services. Often a nurse is the first one to recognize the need for genetic evaluation by identifying an inherited disorder in a family history or by noting physical, cognitive, or behavioral abnormalities when performing a nursing assessment (Box 3.7).

Nurses who specialize in genetics are guided by the Genetics/Genomics Nursing Scope and Standards of Practice (American Nurses Association and International Society of Nurses in Genetics, 2016). Genetics nurses at the basic level tend to work in clinics that focus on services for patients with specific single-gene disorders such as CF, sickle cell disease, muscular dystrophy, and hemophilia. They may also work in genetics clinics and subspecialty clinics such as cardiovascular genetics, neurogenetics, and cancer genetics clinics. Genetics nurses in advanced practice also work in a variety of specialty clinics or genetics centers. These nurses evaluate a patient's medical, developmental, prenatal, birth, and family histories; perform physical examinations, including dysmorphology examination; order tests and diagnostic procedures and evaluate their results; prescribe therapies that are within their scope of practice; and evaluate patient outcomes. Genetics nurses collaborate with teams that include medical geneticists and genetic counselors.

This chapter highlights the role of all nurses who care for children and their families. The *Essential Nursing Competencies and Curricula Guidelines for Genetics and Genomics* (Consensus Panel on Genetic/ Genomic Nursing Competencies, 2009) is used as a framework for discussion (Box 3.8).

Nursing Assessment: Applying and Integrating Genetic and Genomic Knowledge

Family health history is an important tool to identify individuals and families at increased risk for disease, risk factors for disease (such as obesity), and inheritance patterns of diseases. Because of its importance, all nurses need to be able to elicit family history information and, when feasible, document the collected information in pedigree format.

When eliciting a family health history, nurses should collect information about all family members within a minimum of three generations.

BOX 3.7 Assessment Clues to Genetic Disorders*

Major or minor birth defects (anomalies) and dysmorphic features—Cardiac defect, ear or eye abnormalities, micrognathia, forehead prominence, hairline low set on forehead or nape of neck, wide-set eyes (hypertelorism), epicanthal folds, low-set or abnormal ears.

Growth abnormalities—Short stature, overgrowth, asymmetric growth, intrauterine growth retardation

Skeletal abnormalities—Limb abnormalities, asymmetry, scoliosis, hyperextensible joints, hypotonic or hypertonic muscle tone, pectus excavatum, finger or joint abnormalities

Visual or hearing problems—Coloboma of the iris, hearing loss, congenital or early-onset cataracts

Metabolic disorders—Unusual odor of breath, urine, or stool

Sexual development abnormalities—Ambiguous genitalia, micropenis, delayed onset of puberty, primary amenorrhea, precocious sexual development, large testicles

Skin disorders—Unusual pigmentation patterns (e.g., café-au-lait spots, vitiligo), dry and scaly skin, skin tumors, hyperextensible skin

Recurrent infection or immunodeficiency—Ear infection, pneumonia, poor healing of umbilicus

Development and speech delays or loss of developmental milestones

Cognitive delays—Learning disabilities, mild to severe cognitive impairment

Behavioral disorders—Attention-deficit disorders with or without hyperactivity, autistic behavior, aggressive behavior

*Increased concern for genetic etiology if two or more findings are present.

BOX 3.8 Essential Nursing Competencies for Genetics and Genomics: Professional Practice Domain

Nursing Assessment: Applying/Integrating Genetic and Genomic Knowledge

The registered nurse:

- Demonstrates an understanding of the relationship of genetics and genomics to health, prevention, screening, diagnostics, prognostics, selection of treatment, and monitoring of treatment effectiveness
- Demonstrates ability to elicit a minimum of three-generation family health history information
- Constructs a pedigree from collected family history information using standardized symbols and terminology
- Collects personal, health, and developmental histories that consider genetic, environmental, and genomic influences and risks
- Conducts comprehensive health and physical assessments that incorporate knowledge about genetic, environmental, and genomic influences and risk factors
- Critically analyzes the history and physical assessment findings for genetic, environmental, and genomic influences and risk factors
- Assesses clients'* knowledge, perceptions, and responses to genetic and genomic information
- Develops a plan of care that incorporates genetic and genomic assessment information

Identification

The registered nurse:

- Identifies clients who may benefit from specific genetic and genomic information and/or services based on assessment data
- Identifies credible, accurate, appropriate, and current genetic and genomic information, resources, services, and/or technologies specific to given clients
- Identifies ethical, ethnic/ancestral, cultural, religious, legal, fiscal, and societal issues related to genetic and genomic information and technologies
- Defines issues that undermine the rights of all clients for autonomous, informed genetic- and genomic-related decision making and voluntary action

Referral Activities

The registered nurse:

- Facilitates referrals for specialized genetic and genomic services for clients as needed

Provision of Education, Care, and Support

The registered nurse:

- Provides clients with interpretation of selective genetic and genomic information or services
- Provides clients with credible, accurate, appropriate, and current genetic and genomic information, resources, services, and/or technologies that facilitate decision making
- Uses health promotion/disease prevention practices that (1) consider genetic and genomic influences on personal and environmental risk factors; and (2) incorporate knowledge of genetic and/or genomic risk factors (e.g., a client with a genetic predisposition for high cholesterol who can benefit from a change in lifestyle that will decrease the likelihood that the genetic risk will be expressed)
- Uses genetic- and genomic-based interventions and information to improve clients' outcomes
- Collaborates with health care providers in providing genetic and genomic health care
- Collaborates with insurance providers/payers to facilitate reimbursement for genetic and genomic health care services
- Performs interventions/treatments appropriate to clients' genetic and genomic health care needs
- Evaluates impact and effectiveness of genetic and genomic technology, information, interventions, and treatments on clients' outcome

*Clients as defined by document are recipients of health care; this may include persons, families, communities, and/or populations from any race, ethnicity or ancestry, culture, or religious background.

From Consensus Panel on Genetic/Genomic Nursing Competencies. (2009). *Essentials of genetic and genomic nursing: Competencies, curricula guidelines, and outcome indicators* (2nd ed.). Silver Spring, MD: American Nurses Association.

PATHOPHYSIOLOGY REVIEW

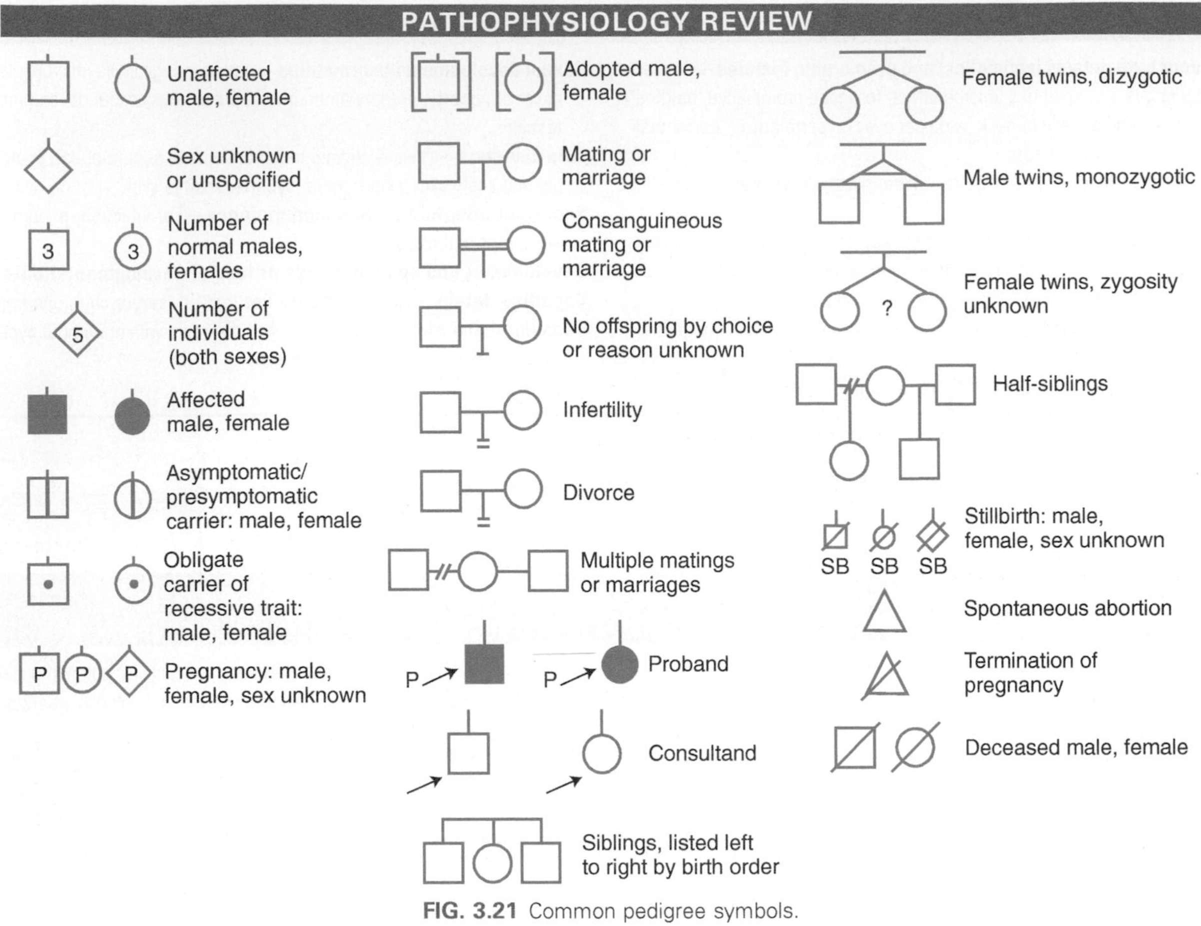

FIG. 3.21 Common pedigree symbols.

This process usually takes 20 to 30 minutes. When possible, it is best to include both parents in the interview to elicit information about relatives on both sides of the family. Medical records, birth and death records, family Bibles, and photograph albums are helpful resources, and persons being interviewed should be instructed to bring such items if they are available. It may be necessary to consult other members of the family. The level of education and the degree of understanding vary widely among informants and influence their reliability. The informants may be reticent, particularly if they view the disorder as something to be ashamed of or in some way threatening. Sometimes true relationships may be concealed, such as adoption or misattributed paternity.

Skillful interviewing is necessary to obtain essential, but often embarrassing or private, information (Prows, Hopkin, Barnoy, et al., 2013). Because the parents may not be married, they should be addressed as couples or partners and asked about other unions that may have produced a pregnancy. In eliciting a birth history from the mother and father, the nurse should specifically ask about abortions, miscarriages, and stillbirths, in addition to live births. To identify all members of the family tree, it is best to ask about pregnancies, even of young teenagers. When inquiring about family diseases, the nurse might ask the question in different ways. For example, if a person denies any cognitive impairment in the family, asking other questions, such as about learning problems, being in special education classes, and failing classes or not completing school, may uncover a family history.

The family history is recorded in the form of a **pedigree chart** or family tree (in some disciplines termed a *genogram*), using standard symbols to indicate persons, relationships, and significant details related to them (Bennett, French, Resta, et al., 2008) (Fig. 3.21). Construction of a pedigree begins with the affected child (proband, index case, or original patient) and all of the mother's pregnancies (Fig. 3.22, *A*). Next, the maternal family history is explored in a similar manner (Fig. 3.22, *B*); then information is gathered about relatives on the father's side, as well as any children or pregnancies that may have occurred through the father's previous unions (Fig. 3.22, *C*) (see Nursing Care Guidelines box). It is important at this point to determine whether the couple might be related in any way, although contrary to popular belief, this is usually a concern only for first cousins or closer relatives. The first-cousin risk for birth defects is about 5% compared with the general population risk of 2% to 3%. The primary risk increase is for autosomal recessive disorders, in which the chance that two individuals carry the same rare mutation is increased if they are related.

The nurse solicits information not only about other affected family members but also about (1) births (live birth, stillbirths, and pregnancy losses, including gestational age of pregnancy); (2) infertility problems; (3) matings (legally sanctioned, consanguineous, multiple, unwed, and other complex relationships); (4) health of family members, including any other genetic diseases or disorders or birth defects; and (5) death and causes of death, including early infant deaths. Sometimes the place of birth and ethnic background are significant. For example, the carrier frequency for Tay-Sachs disease is higher in Ashkenazi Jews from Eastern Europe than in Jews from other geographic regions. Also, when a pedigree chart is being evaluated, a sister's death in infancy

NURSING CARE GUIDELINES

Pedigree Construction

1. Begin diagram in the middle of a large sheet of paper.
2. Represent males by a square placed to the left and females by a circle placed to the right.
3. Represent the proband (index case, original patient) with an arrow (if the counselee or patient is different, place a C under that person's symbol).
4. Use a horizontal line between a square and a circle for a mating or marriage.
5. Suspend offspring vertically from the mating line and place in order of birth with oldest to the left (regardless of sex).
6. Symbolize generations by Roman numerals, with the earliest generation at the top.
7. Include three generations: grandparents, parents, offspring, siblings, aunts, uncles, and first cousins of proband.
8. Include name of each person, their age, health problems, and date and cause of death. Because of privacy concerns, include only first names of the family you are interviewing.
9. Date the pedigree and update at subsequent visits.

from a congenital heart defect might be genetically significant, whereas a healthy sibling's death in a car accident would not. Information concerning first-degree relatives is most important and should be complete.

Time is recognized as one of the biggest barriers to collecting a detailed family health history (Fuller, Myers, Webb, et al., 2010). In response to this known barrier, departments within the US Department of Health and Human Services collaborated to develop and launch the surgeon general's *My Family Health Portrait* (https://familyhistory.hhs.gov/fhh-web/home.action). Nurses can play an important role in teaching families how to access and use this web-based tool and encourage them to share the collected family history with their health care providers (Berger, Lynch, Prows, et al., 2013). The updated version of *My Family Health Portrait* allows the code to be downloaded so that patients' family histories can be imported into compatible electronic medical records. The Genetic Alliance has an online booklet about how to gather family history that is available in English and other languages (http://www.geneticalliance.org/sites/default/files/GuideToFHH/GuidetoFHH.pdf).

In addition to family history, nurses caring for children and families with, or at risk for, a genetic disorder can further facilitate a genetic

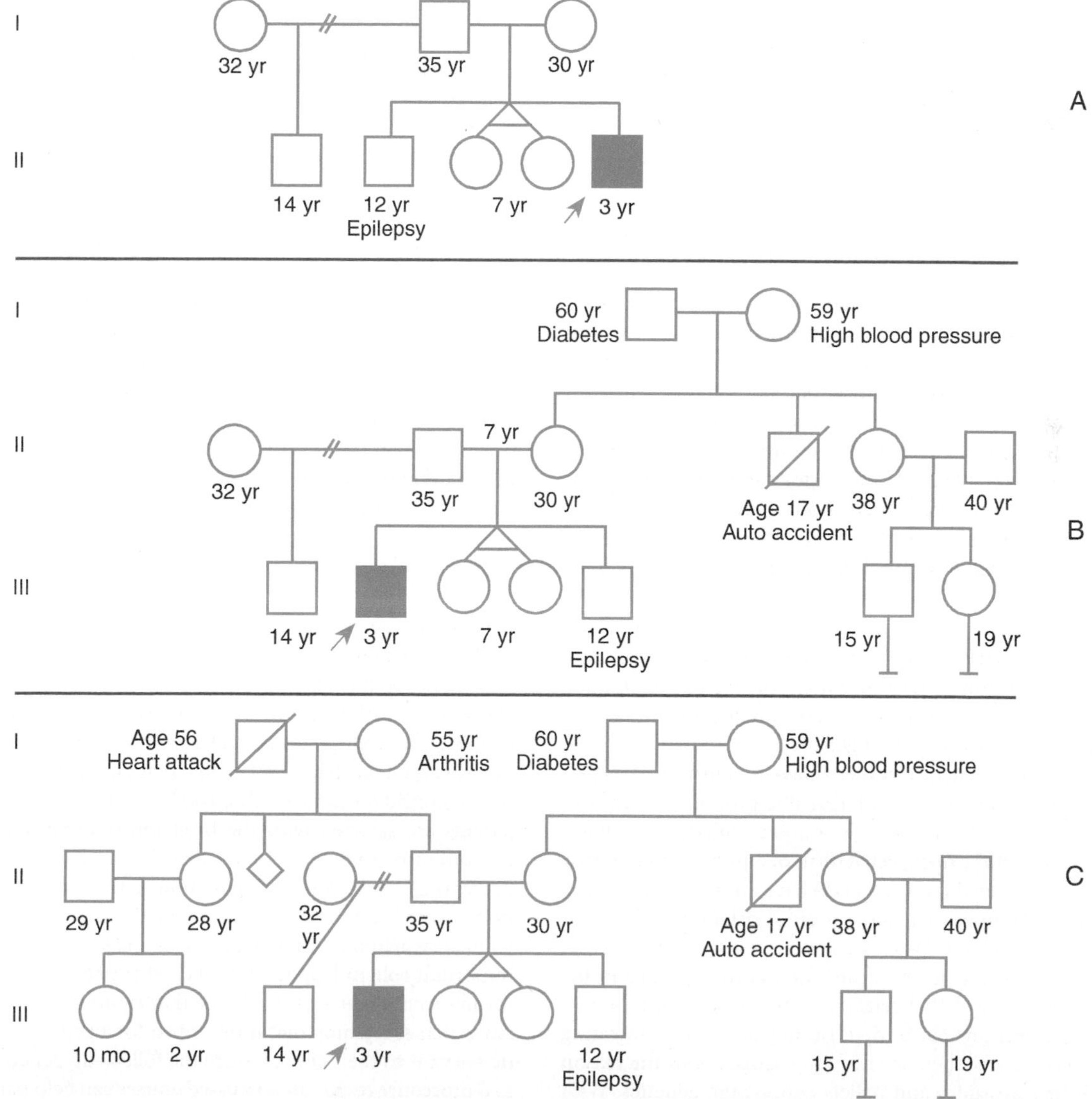

FIG. 3.22 Construction of a pedigree. **A,** Proband, siblings, and parents. **B,** Maternal relatives. **C,** Paternal relatives added.

evaluation by collecting pregnancy, labor and delivery, perinatal, medical, and developmental histories. It is recognized that time limitations of the pediatric nurse may limit the amount of assessment data that can be collected during a pediatric encounter. Electronic medical records are making it more practical to construct a comprehensive set of histories, even when many health care professionals contribute only a portion of the total history.

All nurses are taught to perform physical assessments, but they are seldom taught to recognize minor anomalies and dysmorphology that may suggest a genetic disorder. Yet nurses are keen in recognizing delays in development, behavior differences, and global appearances that raise concern that a newborn, infant, child, or adolescent needs further evaluation (Prows, Hopkin, Barnoy, et al., 2013). Although dysmorphology is beyond the scope of this chapter, readers are encouraged to review the January 2009 issue of *American Journal of Medical Genetics* (Carey, 2009). Drawings and photographs of normal and abnormal morphologic characteristics are provided for the head, face, and extremities, together with accepted dysmorphology terminology. Nurses knowledgeable in dysmorphology are able to articulate specific concerns about a child's appearance rather than relying on the outdated and offensive phrase "funny-looking kid." When a major anomaly is identified, nurses should raise suspicion that the child could have additional congenital anomalies. When three or more minor anomalies are identified, nurses should suspect the possibility of an underlying syndrome. However, it is important to consider the biologic parents' physical appearance, development, and behavior when considering the relevance of the child's combination of minor anomalies.

Identification and Referral

It is a nurse's responsibility to learn basic genetic principles, to be alert to situations in which families could benefit from genetic evaluation and counseling, to know about special services that can help manage and support affected children, and to be familiar with facilities in their areas where these services are available. In this way, nurses will be able to direct individuals and families to needed services and be active participants in the genetic evaluation and counseling process.

Nurses can contact a family before genetic consultation to assess the family's needs and attempt to reduce their anxiety. The telephone contact can also be used to obtain a family history and explain the clinic procedures. Many families are concerned about such things as whether they will be required to undress, whether blood is to be drawn, whether they can accompany the child during the visit, or whether they will be told what to do about reproduction. Families who know what to expect are able to gain more from a genetics consultation. A regularly updated resource for locating genetics clinics and professionals can be found at https://ghr.nlm.nih.gov/primer/consult/findingprofessional. In addition, state health departments either offer services or can help identify health professionals with specialty training in genetics.

Early identification of a genetic disorder allows anticipation of associated conditions and implementation of available preventive measures and therapy to avoid potential complications and to enhance the child's health. It may also prevent the unexpected birth of another affected child in the immediate or extended family. Nurses have an important role in identifying patients and families who have, or are at risk for developing or transmitting, a genetic condition. When facilitating genetics consultations, nurses should share with the genetics professional the findings in the histories the nurses collected that triggered the consultation. Nurses can also help the referral process by determining and communicating the family's initial concerns, their state of knowledge about the reason for referral, and their attitudes and beliefs concerning genetics. With so many recent advances in genetic testing, it is not unusual for a child or adult with long-standing medical problems, including cognitive impairment, to be referred for reevaluation of his or her condition as a possible genetic disorder that might not have been diagnosable a few years earlier, such as microdeletion disorders or single-gene mutations.

Providing Education, Care, and Support

Maintaining contact with the family or making a referral to a health care practice or an agency that can provide a sustained relationship is critical. It is becoming more common for genetics health care professionals to provide regular follow-up and management, particularly for children with rare genetic disorders. However, some families choose not to have follow-up visits with genetic experts.

Regardless of whether families choose to receive continued care with a genetics center, clinic, or professional, nurses can help patients and families process and clarify the information they receive during a genetics visit. Misunderstanding of this information can have many causes, including cultural differences, the disparity of knowledge between the counselor and the family, and the heightened emotion surrounding genetic counseling. Family members have difficulty absorbing all the information presented during a genetics evaluation and counseling session. Knowing this, genetics professionals write and send clinic summary letters to families. The nurse may need to help the family understand terminology in the letter, help them identify and articulate remaining questions or areas of clarification, and coach them through the process of accessing genetics health professionals to get remaining questions and concerns answered. Information often needs to be repeated several times before the family understands the content and its implications.

Nurses must assess for and address parents' feelings of guilt about carrying "bad genes" or having "made my child sick." Depending on the type of cytogenetic disorder, the nurse may be able to absolve the parents of guilt by explaining the random nature of segregation during both gamete formation and fertilization and that those errors in cell division unique to the pregnancy in question are not likely to happen again and are not inherited. If the condition is a mendelian-inherited or mitochondrial disorder, it is important to assess parents' understanding of recurrence risk, help them understand the chances that a subsequent pregnancy will not be affected, and ensure that they have been given information about their options for future children (preimplantation diagnosis, use of donor egg or sperm, prenatal diagnosis, or adoption). Families often try to reason that some unrelated event caused the abnormality (e.g., a fall, a urinary tract infection, or "one glass of wine") before the mother was aware that she was pregnant. These misconceptions need to be assessed and dispelled.

After a genetics visit, and sometimes before the visit, parents often use the Internet to find answers to their questions. During the initial genetics evaluation, a diagnosis may not be possible. Instead, findings in medical, developmental, and family histories lead the professional to order genetic tests and other diagnostic procedures. Diagnoses under consideration are discussed briefly with the parents. Some parents are satisfied with the brief information and do not care to find out more until the actual diagnosis is established. Other parents go home and seek as much information as they can about the diagnoses under consideration. The information they find can be terrifying and overwhelming and inaccurate or misleading. Nurses can play an important role in helping parents identify reliable, accurate resources for information at whatever time they desire it. It is also important to stress that everything that is described for a genetic condition may not be relevant to their child. Before the follow-up genetics visit when test and procedure results are discussed, nurses can help parents identify and write down the questions and concerns they need addressed before leaving the clinic.

Once a genetics diagnosis is made or a genetic predisposition to a delayed-onset disorder is identified, nurses need to have frequent contact with patients and families as they attempt to incorporate recommended therapies or disease-prevention strategies into their daily lives. For example, a disorder such as PKU requires conscientious diet management; therefore it is important to make certain that the family understands and follows instructions and is able to navigate the health care system to access the essential formula and low-phenylalanine food products. An infant evaluated for cleft palate and cardiac defect and subsequently found to have VCFS requires surgical intervention for the congenital malformations. Such an infant also benefits from early intervention services and eventually an individualized education plan in school because developmental delay and eventual learning problems are common.

Initial and ongoing assessment of the family's coping abilities, resources, and support systems is vital to determine their need for additional assistance and support. As with any family who has a child with chronic health care needs, nurses must teach the family to become the child's advocate. Nurses can help families locate agencies and clinics specializing in a specific disorder or its consequences that can provide services (e.g., equipment, medication, and rehabilitation), educational programs, and parent support groups. Referral to local and national support groups or contact with a local family that has a child with the same condition can be helpful for new parents. Privacy and confidentiality are imperative, and both families must give permission before their contact information is given. Nurses can also be instrumental in helping parents evaluate disease-specific social media groups and blogs or starting a local support group when none is available.

Parental attachment and adjustment to the baby can be supported and facilitated by nursing interventions. Assessing the parents' understanding of the child's disorder and providing simple and truthful explanations can help them begin to understand their child's health issues. Guiding the parents in recognizing their child's cues, responses, and strengths can be helpful even for experienced parents. A caring attitude conveys the value of their child and, by extension, their value as parents. The nurse can help the parents identify their strengths as a family and identify support that is available to them.

Giving birth to and raising a child with a genetic disorder do not necessarily result in a lifetime burden. It is important for nurses to ask parents to describe their experience raising their child with a particular genetic condition. What has been the impact on their family? Although parents may initially experience negative outcomes, such as shock, emotional distress, and grief, families can adapt and thrive. Resources for managing stress and restoring balance in the lives of families affected by a genetic condition can help. Van Riper's (2007) research has identified nursing interventions that can promote resilience and adaptation in families of children with Down syndrome. Van Riper's recommendations are useful for families of children with any type of genetic disorder:

- Recognize multiple stressors, strains, and transitions in their lives (e.g., unmet family needs).
- Discuss and implement strategies for reducing family demands (e.g., setting priorities and reducing the number of outside activities family members are involved in).
- Identify and use individual, family, and community resources (e.g., humor, family flexibility, supportive extended family, respite care, local support groups, and Internet resources).
- Expand the range and efficacy of their coping strategies (e.g., increase the use of active strategies such as reframing, mobilize their ability to acquire and accept help, and decrease the use of passive appraisal).
- Encourage the use of an affirming style of family problem-solving communication (e.g., one that conveys support and caring and exerts a calming influence).

Some families do struggle after learning their child has a genetic disorder. Families may feel ashamed of a hereditary disorder and seek to blame their partner for transmitting a faulty gene or chromosome. Intrafamilial strife, hostility, and marital or couple disharmony, sometimes to the point of family disintegration, can occur. Nurses should be alert for evidence of risk factors that indicate poor adjustment (e.g., child abuse, divorce, or other maladaptive behaviors). Referral to psychosocial professionals for crisis intervention may be necessary.

NCLEX REVIEW QUESTIONS

1. When caring for a child with a cleft lip, a parent asks the nurse, "Did I cause this defect in my child?" What is the best response by the nurse?
   A. "There are many things about embryo development we do not know; it is not you."
   B. "Cleft lip is an example of a disruption and occurs early in the pregnancy, often before you even know you are pregnant."
   C. "Is there something you took while you were pregnant?"
   D. "Early in the pregnancy there may be an abnormality in the developmental process; the reasons for this are largely still unknown."
2. The nurse may be called on to have knowledge about sex chromosome aneuploidies. In answering families' questions, the nurse can report:
   A. "Some of the most common genetic disorders caused by sex chromosome aneuploidies are Klinefelter, XXY, triple X female, and Turner syndromes."
   B. "Klinefelter syndrome is the most common of all sex chromosome aneuploidies, and mental development is normal in most cases."
   C. "Triple X females have premature menarche and delayed menopause."
   D. "Turner syndrome girls have a prepubertal growth spurt and then mostly stop growing."
3. When parents consider genetic testing, especially after having a child born with an anomaly, which information could the nurse use to further instruct the family? Select all that apply.
   A. Genetic screening can provide early recognition of a disease, before signs and symptoms occur, for which effective intervention and therapy exists.
   B. Screening can occur at different times in a person's life: preconceptual, or newborn screening, depending on the circumstances.
   C. Genetic testing can help identify carriers of a genetic disease for the purpose of maximizing parenthood planning options.
   D. A thorough family history by the nurse will include the parents' siblings, the parents, and the grandparents.
   E. Recognizing a genetic disorder can further facilitate a genetic evaluation by collecting pregnancy, labor and delivery, perinatal, medical, and developmental histories.
4. The nurse is discharging an infant diagnosed with PKU from the hospital. Which statement made by the parents indicates a further need for teaching?
   A. "I can continue breastfeeding because breast milk is low in phenylalanine."
   B. "Since my baby will begin a reduced phenylalanine diet so early, it is very likely he will have little cognitive impairment."

C. "I will bring my baby back to the doctor to obtain another blood sample by 4 weeks of age, since the first sample was drawn before he was 24 hours old."
D. "My child should remain on the special diet, which is a diet restricted in protein and close monitoring of the phenylalinenine levels."

5. The pediatric nurse may be in the unique position to talk with a family about further genetic evaluation of their child. Which assessment findings by the nurse may alert the nurse to this need? Select all that apply.
A. Digestive difficulties, especially after 6 months of age
B. Skeletal abnormalities: limb abnormalities, asymmetry, hyperextendible joints
C. Recurrent infection or immunodeficiency: ear infections, pneumonia, poor healing of the umbilicus
D. Urinary tract issues: recurrent infections, delay in toilet training
E. Development and speech delays or loss of developmental milestones

Correct Answers

1. D; 2. B; 3. A, B, C, E; 4. C; 5. B, C, E

REFERENCES

Allen, E. G., Freeman, S. B., Druschel, C., et al. (2009). Maternal age and risk for trisomy 21 assessed by the origin of chromosome nondisjunction: A report from the Atlanta and National Down Syndrome projects. *Human Genetics, 125*(1), 41–52.

American Academy of Pediatrics. *Choosing a formula, last updated 11/21/2015*, https://www.healthychildren.org/English/ages-stages/baby/feeding-nutrition/Pages/Choosing-a-Formula.aspx.

American Academy of Pediatrics. (2013). American College of Medical Genetics and Genomics: Ethical and policy issues in genetic testing and screening of children. *Pediatrics, 131*(3), 620–622.

American College of Medical Genetics Newborn Screening Expert Group. (2006). Newborn screening: Toward a uniform screening panel and system—executive summary. *Genetics in Medicine, 8*(Suppl. 5), S1–S11.

American College of Obstetricians and Gynecologists. (2016). Prenatal diagnostic testing for genetic disorders. Practice Bulleting No. 162. *Obstetrics and Gynecology, 127*, e108–e122.

American College of Obstetricians and Gynecologists. (2015). Cell-free DNA screening for fetal aneuploidy. *Obstetrics and Gynecology, 126*, e31–e37.

American Nurses Association and International Society of Nurses in Genetics (2016). *Genetics/genomics nursing: Scope and standards of practice* (2nd ed.). Silver Spring MD: Nursebooks.org.

Antshel, K. M., Fremont, W., Kates, W. R., et al. (2008). The neurocognitive phenotype in velo-cardio-facial syndrome: A developmental perspective. *Dev Disabil Res Rev, 14*(1), 43–51.

Bailey, L. (2008). An overview of enzyme replacement therapy for lysosomal storage diseases. *Online J Issues Nursing, 13*(1):Manuscript 3.

Bennett, R. L., French, K. S., Resta, R. G., et al. (2008). Standardized human pedigree nomenclature: Update and assessment of the recommendations of the National Society of Genetic Counselors. *J Genet Counsel, 17*, 424–433.

Berger, K. A., Lynch, J., Prows, C. A., et al. (2013). Mothers' perceptions of family health history and an online, parent-generated family health history tool. *Clinical Pediatrics, 52*(1), 74–81.

Bull, M. J. (2011). Committee on Genetics: Clinical report—health supervision for children with Down syndrome. *Pediatrics, 128*, 393–406.

Carey, J. C. (Ed.), (2009). Elements of morphology: Standard terminology. *American Journal of Medical Genetics. Part A, 149A*(1), 1–127.

Ceyhan-Birsoy, O., Machini, K., Lebo, M. S., et al. (2017). A curated gene list for reporting results of newborn genomic sequencing. *Genetics in Medicine*, [Epub 2017/01/12].

Coelho, A. I., Rubio-Gozalbo, M. E., Vicente, J. B., et al. (2017). Sweet and sour: An update on classic galactosemia. *Journal of Inherited Metabolic Disease*, [Epub ahead of print].

Committee on Genetics. (2011). Health supervision for children with fragile X syndrome. *Pediatrics, 127*, 994–1006.

Consensus Panel on Genetic/Genomic Nursing Competencies (2009). *Essentials of genetic and genomic nursing: Competencies, curricula guidelines, and outcome indicators* (2nd ed.). Silver Spring, MD: American Nurses Association.

Consensus Panel on Genetic/Genomic Nursing Competencies (2006). *Essential nursing competencies and curricula guidelines for genetics and genomics*. Silver Spring, MD: American Nurses Association.

Dashe, J. S. (2016). Aneuploidy screening in pregnancy. *Obstetrics and Gynecology, 128*, 181–194.

Fuller, M., Myers, M., Webb, T., et al. (2010). Primary care providers' responses to patient-generated family history. *Journal of Genetic Counseling, 19*(1), 84–96.

Greco, K. E., Tinley, S., & Seibert, D. (2012). *Essential genetic and genomic competencies for nurses with graduate degrees*. Silver Spring, MD: American Nurses Association and International Society of Nurses in Genetics.

Hegde, M., Ferber, M., Mao, R., et al. (2014). ACMG technical standards and guidelines for genetic testing for inherited colorectal cancer (Lynch syndrome, familial adenomatous polyposis, and MYH-associated polyposis). *Genetics in Medicine, 16*(1), 101–116.

Holtkamp, K. C., Mathijssen, I. B., Lakeman, P., et al. (2016). Factors for successful implementation of population-based expanded carrier screening: Learning from existing initiatives. *European Journal of Public Health*, [Epub 2016 Aug 2].

Jensen, K. M., & Bulova, P. D. (2014). Managing the care of adults with Down's syndrome. *BMJ (Clinical Research Ed.), 349*(g5596), 1–9.

Jorde, L. B., Carey, J. C., Bamshad, M. J., et al. (2016). *Medical genetics* (5th ed.). Philadelphia: Elsevier.

Kalia, S. S., Adelman, K., Bale, S. J., et al. (2017). Recommendations for reporting of secondary findings in clinical exome and genome sequencing, 2016 update (ACMG SF v2.0): A policy statement of the American College of Medical Genetics and Genomics. *Genetics in Medicine, 19*(2), 249–255.

Korf, B. R., & Rehm, H. L. (2013). New approaches to molecular diagnosis. *JAMA: The Journal of the American Medical Association, 309*(14), 1511–1521.

Lea, D. H., Cheek, D. J., Brazeau, D., et al. (2015). *Mastering pharmacogenomics: A nurse's handbook for success*. Indianapolis, IN: Sigma Theta Tau International.

Lee, K. G. *Amniotic constriction bands, 2009 (updated 11/3/2015)*. Retrieved from http://www.nlm.nih.gov/medlineplus/ency/article/001579.htm.

Lynch, J. A., Venne, V., & Berse, B. (2015). Genetic tests to identify risk for breast cancer. *Seminars in Oncology Nursing, 31*(2), 100–107.

McDonald-McGinn, D. M., Emanuel, B. S., & Zackai, E. H. (1999). 22q11.2 Deletion syndrome. In R. A. Pagon, T. D. Bird, C. R. Dolan, et al. (Eds.), *GeneReviews™ [Internet]*. Seattle, WA. Retrieved from: http://www.ncbi.nlm.nih.gov/books/NBK1523/. Updated 2013 Feb 28.

Nardecchia, F., Manti, F., Chiarotti, F., et al. (2015). Neurocognitive and neuroimaging outcome of early treated young adult PKU patients: A longitudinal study. *Molecular Genetics and Metabolism, 115*(2–3), 84–90.

National Foundation for Ectodermal Dysplasia. *Learn*. Retrieved from https://www.nfed.org/learn/.

Pichler, K., Michel, M., Zlamy, M., et al. (2017). Breast milk feeding in infants with inherited metabolic disorders other than phenylketonuria—a 10-year single-center experience. *Journal of Perinatal Medicine, 45*(3), 375–382.

Pinsker, J. E. (2012). Clinical review: Turner syndrome: Updating the paradigm of clinical care. *The Journal of Clinical Endocrinology and Metabolism, 97*(6), E994–E1003.

Pletcher, B. A., Toriello, H. V., Noblin, S. J., et al. (2007). Indications for genetic referral: A guide for healthcare providers. *Genetics in Medicine, 9*(6), 385–389.

Prows, C. A., Hopkin, R. J., Barnoy, S., et al. (2013). An update of childhood genetic disorders. *Journal of Nursing Scholarship, 45*(1), 34–42.

Prows, C. A., Tran, G., & Blosser, B. (2014). Whole exome or genome sequencing: Nurses need to prepare families for the possibilities. *Journal of Advanced Nursing, 70*(12), 2736–2745.

Rimoin, D., Pyeritz, R., & Korf, B. (2013). *Emory and Rimoin's principles and practice of medical genetics* (6th ed.). New York: Academic Press.

Romiti, M. L., Colognesi, C., Cancrini, C., et al. (2000). Prognostic value of a CCR5 defective allele in pediatric HIV-1 infection. *Molecular Medicine (Cambridge, Mass.), 6*(1), 28–36.

Rosenfeld, J. A., & Patel, A. (2017). Chromosomal microarrays: Understanding genetics of neurodevelopmental disorders and congenital anomalies. *Journal of Pediatric Genetics, 6*(1), 42–50.

Ross, J. L., Roeltgen, D. P., Kushner, H., et al. (2012). Behavioral and social phenotypes in boys with 47,XYY or 47,XXY Klinefelter syndrome. *Pediatrics, 129*, 769–778.

Saenko, E. L., & Pipe, S. W. (2006). Strategies towards a longer acting factor VIII. *Haemophilia : The Official Journal of the World Federation of Hemophilia, 12*(Suppl. 3), 42–51.

Sampson, J., Groshon, M., & Parilo, D. M. (2016). What nurses need to know about PKU. *Nursing, 46*(8), 66–67.

Schneider, K., Zelley, K., Nichols, K. E., et al. (1999). Li-Fraumeni syndrome. In R. A. Pagon, M. P. Adam, T. D. Bird, et al. (Eds.), *GeneReviews™ [Internet]*. Seattle, WA: University of Washington. http://www.ncbi.nlm.nih.gov/books/NBK1311/. [Updated 2013 Apr 11].

Simons, A., Shaffer, L. G., & Hastings, R. J. (2013). Cytogenetic nomenclature: Changes in the ISCN 2013 compared to the 2009 edition. *Cytogenetic and Genome Research, 141*, 1–6.

Sweetman, L., Millington, D. S., Therrell, B. L., et al. (2006). Naming and counting disorders (conditions) included in newborn screening panels. *Pediatrics, 117*(5 Pt. 2), S308–S314.

Tluczek, A., Orland, K. M., Nick, S. W., et al. (2009). Newborn screening: An appeal for improved parent education. *The Journal of Perinatal and Neonatal Nursing, 23*(4), 326–334.

Valle, D., Beaudet, A. L., Vogelstein, B., et al. (Eds.), (2014). *The online metabolic and molecular bases of inherited disease*. New York: McGraw-Hill. http://ommbid.mhmedical.com/content.aspx?bookid=971§ionid=62632315.

Van Riper, M. (2007). Families of children with Down syndrome: Responding to "a change in plans" with resilience. *Journal of Pediatric Nursing, 22*(2), 116–128.

Vermeesch, J. R., Voet, T., & Devriendt, K. (2016). Prenatal and pre-implantation genetic diagnosis. *Nature Reviews. Genetics, 17*(10), 643–656.

Vockley, J., Andersson, H. C., Antshel, K. M., et al. (2014). Phenylalanine hydroxylase deficiency: Diagnosis and management guideline. *Genetics in Medicine, 16*(2), 188–200.

Wilkin, J. Z., Su, Z., Kuritzkes, D. R., et al. (2007). HIV type 1 chemokine coreceptor use among antiretroviral-experienced patients screened for a clinical trial of a CCR5 inhibitor: AIDS Clinical Trial Group A5211. *Clinical Infectious Diseases: An Official Publication of the Infectious Diseases Society of America, 44*(4), 591–595.

Internet Resources

Ethical, Legal, and Social Issues (ELSI)—https://www.genome.gov/elsi/ (NIH site; program developed to study the issues surrounding the availability of genetic information).

GeneReviews—https://www.ncbi.nlm.nih.gov/books/NBK1116/ (expert-written, peer-reviewed, regularly updated resource of comprehensive descriptions of genetic conditions that include diagnosis, management, and genetic counseling for patients and their families).

GeneTests—https://www.genetests.org/ (genetic testing resource).

Genetic Alliance—http://www.geneticalliance.org/ (international nonprofit health advocacy organization).

Genetic Home Reference—http://ghr.nlm.nih.gov (consumer-friendly information about the effects of genetic variations on human health; contains handbook on basic human and clinical genetics concepts, summaries of a variety of genetic conditions and genes).

Health on the Net Code of Conduct—http://www.hon.ch/HONcode/ (describes the Health on the Net Foundation code of conduct for medical and health websites, which addresses the reliability and credibility of information).

International Society of Nurses in Genetics—http://www.isong.org/ (provides information about various education resources, conferences targeting nurses).

National Cancer Institute—https://www.cancer.gov/ (provides accurate and up-to-date cancer information).

National Human Genome Research Institute—http://www.genome.gov (information on genome research and its ethical, legal, and social implications).

National Organization for Rare Disorders—https://rarediseases.org/ (a federation of voluntary health organizations dedicated to helping people with rare "orphan" diseases).

OMIM, Online Mendelian Inheritance in Man—https://www.omim.org/ (up-to-date research summaries of human genes and genetic disorders).

United Mitochondrial Disease Foundation—http://www.umdf.org/ (provides information about mitochondrial defects, including professional and lay materials).

4

Communication, Physical, and Developmental Assessment of the Child and Family

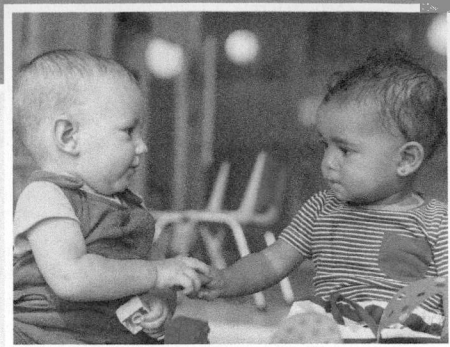

Jan M. Foote

http://evolve.elsevier.com/wong/ncic

CONCEPTS

- Communication
- Assessment

GUIDELINES FOR COMMUNICATION AND INTERVIEWING

The most widely used method of communicating with parents on a professional basis is the interview process. Unlike social conversation, interviewing is a specific form of goal-directed communication. As nurses converse with children and adults, they focus on the individuals to determine the kind of persons they are, their usual mode of handling problems, whether they need help, and the way they react to counseling. Developing interviewing skills requires time and practice, but following some guiding principles can facilitate this process. An organized approach is most effective when using interviewing skills in patient teaching.

ESTABLISHING A SETTING FOR COMMUNICATION

Appropriate Introduction

Introduce yourself and ask the name of each family member who is present. Address parents or other adults by their appropriate titles, such as "Mr." and "Mrs.," unless they specify a preferred name. Record the preferred name on the medical record. Using formal address or their preferred names, rather than using first names or "mother" or "father," conveys respect and regard for the parents or other caregivers (Ball, Dains, Flynn, et al., 2014).

At the beginning of the visit, include children in the interaction by asking them their name, preferred name, age, and other information. Nurses often direct all questions to adults even when children are old enough to speak for themselves. This only terminates one extremely valuable source of information—the patient. When including the child, follow the general rules for communicating with children given in the Nursing Care Guidelines box later in the chapter.

Assurance of Privacy and Confidentiality

The place where the nurse conducts the interview is almost as important as the interview itself. The physical environment should allow for as much privacy as possible, with distractions (such as interruptions, noise, or other visible activity) kept to a minimum. At times, it is necessary to turn off a television, radio, or cell phone. The environment should also have some play provision for young children to keep them occupied during the parent-nurse interview (Fig. 4.1). Parents who are constantly interrupted by their children are unable to concentrate fully and tend to give brief answers to finish the interview as quickly as possible.

Confidentiality is another essential component of the initial phase of the interview. Because the interview is usually shared with other members of the health care team or the teacher (in the case of students), be certain to inform the family of the limits regarding confidentiality. If confidentiality is a concern in a particular situation, such as when talking to a parent suspected of child abuse or a teenager contemplating suicide, deal with this directly and inform the person that in such instances, confidentiality cannot be ensured. However, the nurse judiciously protects information of a confidential nature.

COMPUTER PRIVACY AND APPLICATIONS IN NURSING

The use of computer technology to store and retrieve health information has become widespread; most institutions now maintain electronic health records for patients. The health care community is increasingly concerned about the privacy and security of this health information and all nurses are engaged in protecting confidentiality of health care records. Any person accessing confidential health information is charged

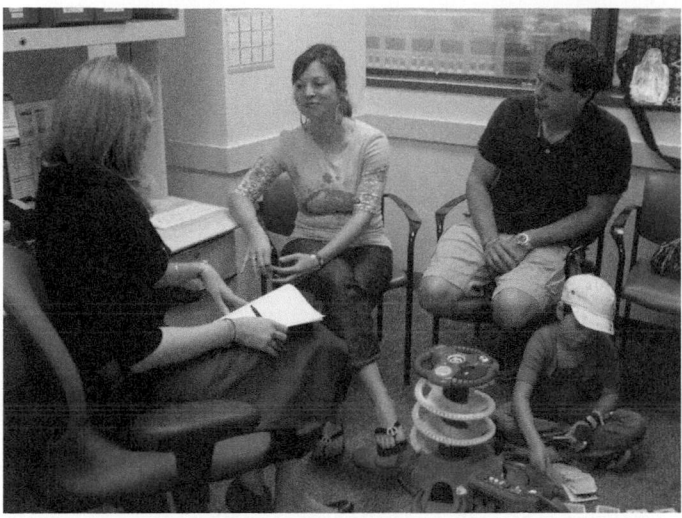

FIG. 4.1 Child plays while the nurse interviews parent.

with managing safeguards for disclosure, including password protection to prevent violation of patient privacy and confidentiality.

TELEPHONE TRIAGE AND COUNSELING

Telephone triage care management has increased access to high-quality health care services and empowered parents to participate in their child's health care. Consequently, patient satisfaction has significantly improved. Unnecessary emergency department and clinic visits have decreased, saving health care costs and time (with less absence from work) for families in need of health care.

Telephone triage is more than "just a phone call" because a child's life is a high price to pay for poorly managed or incompetent telephone assessment skills. Typically, guidelines for telephone triage include asking screening questions; determining when to immediately refer to emergency medical services (dial 911) or the emergency department; and determining when to refer to same-day appointments, appointments in 24 to 72 hours, appointments in 4 days or more, or home care (Box 4.1). Successful outcomes are based on the consistency and accuracy of the information provided. A systematic review of 49 studies where nurses triaged calls found that the appropriateness of a decision and subsequent compliance often varied (Blank, Coster, O'Cathain, et al., 2012). A meta-analysis of 13 studies provided further insight and found that patient compliance with triage recommendations were influenced by the quality of provider communication (Purc-Stephenson & Thrasher, 2012). The importance of nurse-patient communication is reinforced as an essential aspect of telephone triage training. Training of communication skills that are patient and family centered and specifically address active listening and advising skills offers the greatest opportunity for success. Assessment skills used in direct nurse-to-patient interactions are not directly transferable to the telephone and provide further support for training in decision-making skills for phone triage (Purc-Stephenson & Thrasher, 2010). Evidence-based clinical protocols for telephone triage can provide a structured method for assessment (Stacey, Macartney, Carley, et al., 2013).

BOX 4.1 Telephone Triage Guidelines

Date and time

Background

- Name, age, sex, contact information
- Chronic illness
- Allergies, current medications, treatments, or recent immunizations

Chief complaint

General symptoms

- Severity
- Duration
- Other symptoms
- Pain

Systems review

Steps taken

- Advised to call emergency medical services (911)
- Advised to go to emergency department
- Advised to see practitioner (today, tomorrow, or later appointment)
- Advised regarding home care
- Advised to call back if symptoms worsen or fail to improve

Resources for Telephone Triage Protocols

Beaulieu, R., & Jumphreys, J. (2008). Evaluation of a telephone advice nurse in a nursing faculty managed pediatric community clinic. *Journal of Pediatric Health Care, 22*(3), 175–181.

Marklund, B., Ström, M., Månsson, J., et al. (2007). Computer-supported telephone nurse triage: An evaluation of medical quality and costs. *Journal of Nursing Management, 15,* 180–187.

Schmitt, B. D. (2012). *Pediatric telephone protocols: Office version* (14th ed.). Elk Grove Village, IL: American Academy of Pediatrics.

Simonsen, S. M. (2001). *Telephone assessment: Guidelines for practice* (2nd ed.). St. Louis, MO: Mosby.

COMMUNICATING WITH FAMILIES

COMMUNICATING WITH PARENTS

Although the parent and the child are separate and distinct individuals, the nurse's relationship with the child is frequently mediated by the parent, particularly with younger children. For the most part, nurses acquire information about the child by direct observation or through communication with the parents. Usually it can be assumed that because of the close contact with the child, the parent gives reliable information. Assessing the child requires input from the child (verbal and nonverbal), information from the parent, and the nurse's own observations of the child and interpretation of the relationship between the child and the parent. When children are old enough to be active participants in their own health care, the parent becomes a collaborator.

Encouraging the Parents to Talk

Interviewing parents offers not only the opportunity to determine the child's health and developmental status but also information about factors that influence the child's life. Whatever the parent sees as a problem should be a concern of the nurse. These problems are not always easy to identify. Nurses need to be alert for clues and signals by which a parent communicates worries and anxieties. Careful phrasing with broad, open-ended questions (such as "What is Andy eating now?") provides more information than several single-answer questions (such as "Is Andy eating what the rest of the family eats?").

Sometimes the parent will take the lead without prompting. At other times, it may be necessary to direct another question on the basis of an observation, such as "Joseph seems unhappy today," or "How do you feel when Joseph cries?" If the parent appears to be tired or distraught, consider asking, "What do you do to relax?" or "What help do you have with the children?" A comment such as "You handle Jamey very well. What kind of experience have you had with babies?" to new parents who appear comfortable with their first child gives positive reinforcement and provides an opening for questions they might have on the infant's care. Often all that is required to keep parents talking is a nod or saying "yes" or "uh-huh."

Directing the Focus

Directing the focus of the interview while allowing maximum freedom of expression is one of the most difficult goals in effective communication. One approach is the use of open-ended or broad questions, followed by guiding statements. For example, if the parent proceeds to list the other children by name, say, "Tell me their ages, too." If the parent continues to describe each child in depth, which is not the purpose of the interview, redirect the focus by stating, "Let's talk about the other children later. You were beginning to tell me about Rachel's activities at school." This approach conveys interest in the other children but focuses the assessment on the patient.

Listening and Cultural Awareness

Listening is the most important component of effective communication. When the purpose of listening is to understand the person being interviewed, it is an active process that requires concentration and attention to all aspects of the conversation—verbal, nonverbal, and abstract. Major blocks to listening are environmental distraction and premature judgment.

Although it is necessary to make some preliminary judgments, listen with as much objectivity as possible by clarifying meanings and attempting to see the situation from the parent's point of view. Effective interviewers consciously control their reactions and responses and the techniques they use. (See Cultural Considerations box.)

CULTURAL CONSIDERATIONS

Interviewing Without Judgment

It is easy to inject one's own attitudes and feelings into an interview. Often nurses' own prejudices and assumptions, which may include racial, religious, and cultural stereotypes, influence their perceptions of a parent's behavior. What the nurse may interpret as a parent's passive hostility or lack of interest may be shyness or an expression of anxiety. For example, in Western cultures, eye contact and directness are signs of paying attention. However, in many non-Western cultures, including that of Native Americans, directness (e.g., looking someone in the eye) is considered rude. Children are taught to avert their gaze and to look down when being addressed by an adult, especially one with authority (Ball, Dains, Flynn, et al., 2014). Therefore nurses must make judgments about "listening," as well as verbal interactions, with an appreciation of cultural differences.

Careful listening relies on the use of clues, verbal leads, or signals from the interviewee to move the interview along. Frequent references to an area of concern, repetition of certain key words, or a special emphasis on something or someone serve as cues to the interviewer for the direction of inquiry. Concerns and anxieties are often mentioned in a casual, offhand manner. Even though they are casual, they are important and deserve scrutiny to identify problem areas. For example, a parent who is concerned about a child's habit of bed-wetting may casually mention that the child's bed was "wet this morning."

Using Silence

Silence as a response is often one of the most difficult interviewing techniques to learn. The interviewer requires a sense of confidence and comfort to allow the interviewee space in which to think without interruptions. Silence permits the interviewee to sort out thoughts and feelings and search for responses to questions. Silence can also be a cue for the interviewer to go more slowly, reexamine the approach, and not push too hard (Ball, Dains, Flynn, et al., 2014).

Sometimes it is necessary to break the silence and reopen communication. Do this in a way that encourages the person to continue talking about what is considered important. Breaking a silence by introducing a new topic or by prolonged talking essentially terminates the interviewee's opportunity to use the silence. Suggestions for breaking the silence include statements such as the following:

- "Is there anything else you wish to say?"
- "I see you find it difficult to continue; how may I help?"
- "I don't know what this silence means. Perhaps there is something you would like to put into words but find difficult to say."

Being Empathic

Empathy is the capacity to understand what another person is experiencing from within that person's frame of reference; it is often described as the ability to put oneself in another's shoes. The essence of empathic interaction is accurate understanding of another's feelings. Empathy differs from **sympathy**, which is having feelings or emotions similar to those of another person, rather than understanding those feelings.

Providing Anticipatory Guidance

The ideal way to handle a situation is to deal with it before it becomes a problem. The best preventive measure is anticipatory guidance. Traditionally, **anticipatory guidance** focused on providing families information on normal growth and development and nurturing childrearing practices. For example, one of the most significant areas in pediatrics is injury prevention. Beginning prenatally, parents need specific instructions on home safety. Because of the child's maturing developmental skills, parents must implement home safety changes early to minimize risks to the child.

Unprepared parents can be disturbed by many normal developmental changes, such as a toddler's diminished appetite, negativism, altered sleeping patterns, and anxiety toward strangers. The chapters on health promotion provide nurses with information for counseling parents. However, anticipatory guidance should extend beyond giving general information to empowering families to use the information as a means of building competence in their parenting abilities (Dosman & Andrews, 2012). To achieve this level of anticipatory guidance, the nurse should do the following:

- Base interventions on needs identified by the family, not by the professional.
- View the family as competent or as having the ability to be competent.
- Provide opportunities for the family to achieve competence.

Avoiding Blocks to Communication

A number of blocks to communication can adversely affect the quality of the helping relationship. The interviewer introduces many of these blocks, such as giving unrestricted advice or forming prejudged conclusions. Another type of block occurs primarily with the interviewees and concerns **information overload**. When individuals receive too much information or information that is overwhelming, they often demonstrate signs of increasing anxiety or decreasing attention. Such signals should alert the interviewer to give less information or to clarify what has been said. Box 4.2 lists some of the more common blocks to communication, including signs of information overload.

The nurse can correct communication blocks by careful analysis of the interview process. One of the best methods for improving interviewing skills is audiotape or videotape feedback. With supervision and guidance, the interviewer can recognize the blocks and consciously avoid them.

BOX 4.2 Blocks to Communication

Communication Barriers (Nurse)

Socializing
Giving unrestricted and sometimes unsought advice
Offering premature or inappropriate reassurance
Giving overready encouragement
Defending a situation or opinion
Using stereotyped comments or clichés
Limiting expression of emotion by asking directed, closed-ended questions
Interrupting and finishing the person's sentence
Talking more than the interviewee
Forming prejudged conclusions
Deliberately changing the focus

Signs of Information Overload (Patient)

Long periods of silence
Wide eyes and fixed facial expression
Constant fidgeting or attempting to move away
Nervous habits (e.g., tapping, playing with hair)
Sudden interruptions (e.g., asking to go to the bathroom)
Looking around
Yawning, eyes drooping
Frequently looking at a watch or clock
Attempting to change the topic of discussion

Communicating With Families Through an Interpreter

Sometimes communication is impossible because two people speak different languages. In this case it is necessary to obtain information through a third party: the interpreter. When using an interpreter, the nurse follows the same interviewing guidelines. Specific guidelines for using an adult interpreter are given in the Nursing Care Guidelines box.

Communicating with families through an interpreter requires sensitivity to cultural, legal, and ethical considerations (see Cultural Considerations box). In some cultures, class differences between the interpreter and the family may cause the family to feel intimidated and less inclined to offer information. Therefore it is important to choose the interpreter carefully and provide time for the interpreter and family to establish rapport.

In obtaining informed consent through an interpreter, the nurse should fully inform the family of all aspects of the particular procedure to which they are consenting. Issues of confidentiality may arise when family members related to another patient are asked to interpret for the family, thus revealing sensitive information that may be shared with other families on the unit. With increased sensitivity toward patient rights and confidentiality, many institutions now require consent forms translated in the patient's primary language.

NURSING CARE GUIDELINES

Using an Interpreter

- Explain to interpreter the reason for the interview and the type of questions that will be asked.
- Clarify whether a detailed or brief answer is required and whether the translated response can be general or literal.
- Introduce the interpreter to family, and allow some time before the interview for them to become acquainted.
- Communicate directly with family members when asking questions to reinforce interest in them and to observe nonverbal expressions, but do not ignore interpreter.
- Pose questions to elicit only one answer at a time, such as "Do you have pain?" rather than "Do you have any pain, tiredness, or loss of appetite?"
- Refrain from interrupting family members and the interpreter while they are conversing.
- Avoid commenting to the interpreter about family members because they may understand some English.
- Be aware that some medical words, such as *allergy,* may have no similar word in another language; avoid medical jargon whenever possible.
- Be aware that cultural differences may exist regarding views on sex, marriage, or pregnancy.
- Allow time after the interview for interpreter to share something that he or she thought could not be said earlier; ask about the interpreter's impression of nonverbal clues to communication and family members' reliability or ease in revealing information.
- Arrange for family to speak with the same interpreter on subsequent visits whenever possible.

CULTURAL CONSIDERATIONS

Using Children as Interpreters

When no one else is available to interpret, there may be temptation to use a bilingual child within the family as an interpreter. However, the use of children in health care interpreting is strongly discouraged because they are often not mature enough to understand health care questions, answers, or messages (American Academy of Pediatrics, 2017). Children may inadvertently commit interpretive errors, such as inaccuracies, omissions, or substitutions. In addition, children can be adversely affected by serious or sensitive information that may be discussed. In some cultures, using a child as an interpreter is considered an insult to an adult because children are expected to show respect by not questioning their elders. Note that some institutions prohibit the use of children as interpreters; check institutional policy for compliance. If a trained on-site or community-based interpreter is not available, a *language line* using a telephonic interpreter may be an option.

NURSING ALERT

When using translated materials, such as a health history form, be certain the informant is literate in the foreign language.

COMMUNICATING WITH CHILDREN

Although the greatest amount of verbal communication is usually carried out with the parent, do not exclude the child during the interview. Pay attention to infants and younger children through play or by occasionally directing questions or remarks to them. Include older children as active participants so that they can share their own experiences and perspectives.

In communication with children of all ages, the nonverbal components of the communication process convey the most significant messages. It is difficult to disguise feelings, attitudes, and anxiety when relating to children. They are alert to surroundings and attach meaning to every gesture and move that is made; this is particularly true of very young children.

Active attempts to make friends with children before they have had an opportunity to evaluate an unfamiliar person tend to increase their anxiety. Continue to talk to the child and parent but go about activities that do not involve the child directly, thus allowing the child to observe from a safe position. If the child has a special toy or doll, "talk" to the doll first. Ask simple questions such as "Does your teddy bear have a name?" to ease the child into conversation. Other guidelines for communicating with children are in the Nursing Care Guidelines box. Specific guidelines for preparing children for procedures are provided in Chapter 22.

NURSING CARE GUIDELINES

Communicating With Children

- Allow children time to feel comfortable.
- Avoid sudden or rapid advances, broad smiles, extended eye contact, or other gestures that may be seen as threatening.
- Talk to the parent if child is initially shy.
- Communicate through transition objects (such as dolls, puppets, and stuffed animals) before questioning a young child directly.
- Give older children the opportunity to talk without the parents present.
- Assume a position that is at the same level as the child (Fig. 4.2).
- Speak in a quiet, unhurried, and confident voice.
- Speak clearly, be specific, and use simple words and short sentences.
- State directions and suggestions positively.
- Offer a choice only when one exists.
- Be honest with children.
- Allow children to express their concerns and fears.
- Use a variety of communication techniques.

Communication Related to Development of Thought Processes

The normal development of language and thought offers a frame of reference for communicating with children. Thought processes progress from sensorimotor to perceptual to concrete and finally to abstract, formal operations. An understanding of the typical characteristics of these stages provides the nurse with a framework to facilitate social communication.

Infancy

Because they are unable to use words, infants primarily use and understand nonverbal communication. Infants communicate their needs and feelings through nonverbal behaviors and vocalizations that can be interpreted by someone who is around them for a sufficient time. Infants smile and coo when content and cry when distressed. Crying is provoked by unpleasant stimuli from inside or outside, such as hunger, pain, body restraint, or loneliness. Adults interpret this to mean that an infant needs something and consequently try to alleviate the discomfort by meeting their physical needs, speaking softly, and communicating through touch.

Infants respond to adults' nonverbal behaviors. They become quiet when they are cuddled, rocked, or receive other forms of gentle physical contact. They receive comfort from the sound of a soft voice even though they do not understand the words that are spoken. Until infants reach the age at which they experience stranger anxiety, they readily respond to any firm, gentle handling and quiet, calm speech. Loud, harsh sounds and sudden movements are frightening.

Early Childhood

Children younger than 5 years of age are egocentric. They see things only in relation to themselves and from their point of view. Therefore focus communication on them. Tell them what they can do or how they will feel. Experiences of others are of no interest to them. It is futile to use another child's experience in an attempt to gain the cooperation of small children. Allow them to touch and examine articles they will come in contact with. A stethoscope bell will feel cold; palpating a neck might tickle. Although they have not yet acquired sufficient language skills to express their feelings and wants, toddlers can effectively use their hands to communicate ideas without words. They push an unwanted object away, pull another person to show them something, point, and cover the mouth that is saying something they do not wish to hear.

Everything is direct and concrete to small children. They are unable to work with abstractions and interpret words literally. Analogies escape them because they are unable to separate reality from fantasy. For example, they attach literal meaning to such common phrases as "two-faced," "sticky fingers," or "coughing your head off." Children who are told they will get "a little stick in the arm" may not be able to envision an injection (Fig. 4.3). Therefore use simple, direct language rather than phrases that might be misinterpreted by a small child.

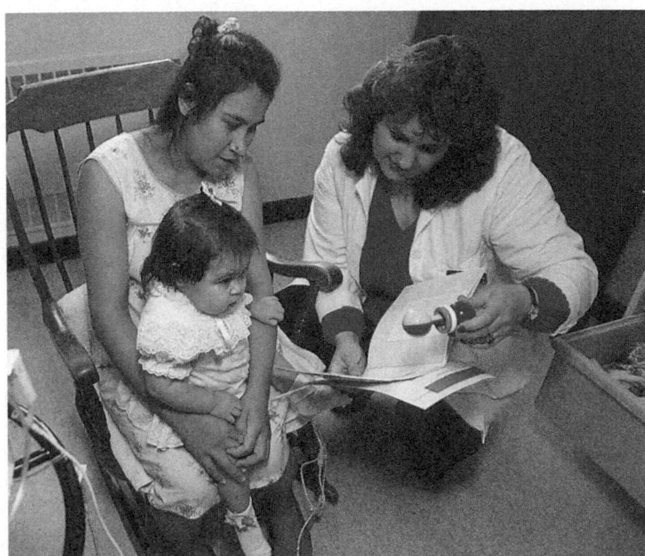

FIG. 4.2 Nurse assumes position at the child's level.

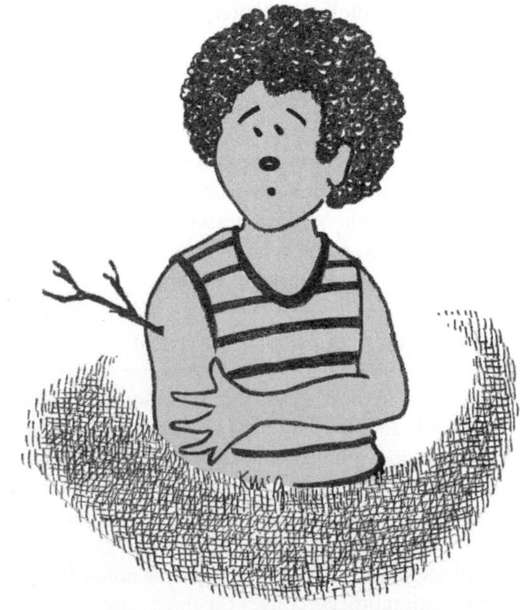

FIG. 4.3 A young child may take the expression "a little stick in the arm" literally.

School-Age Years

Younger school-age children rely less on what they see and more on what they know when faced with new problems. They want explanations and reasons for everything but require no verification beyond that. They are interested in the functional aspect of all procedures, objects, and activities. They want to know why an object exists, why it is used, how it works, and the intent and purpose of its user. They need to know what is going to take place and why it is being done to them specifically. For example, to explain a procedure such as taking blood pressure, show the child how squeezing the bulb pushes air into the cuff and makes the "arrow" move. Let the child operate the bulb. An explanation for the procedure might be as simple as, "I want to see how far the arrow moves when the cuff squeezes your arm." Consequently, the child becomes an enthusiastic participant.

School-age children have a heightened concern about body integrity. Because of the special importance they place on their body, they are sensitive to anything that constitutes a threat or suggestion of injury to it. This concern extends to their possessions, so they may appear to overreact to loss or threatened loss of treasured objects. Encouraging children to communicate their needs and voice their concerns enables the nurse to provide reassurance, to dispel myths and fears, and to implement activities that reduce their anxiety. For example, if a shy child dislikes being the center of attention, ignore that particular child by talking and relating to other children in the family or group. When children feel more comfortable, they will usually interject personal ideas, feelings, and interpretations of events.

Adolescence

As children move into adolescence, they fluctuate between child and adult thinking and behavior. They are riding a current that is moving them rapidly toward a maturity that may be beyond their coping ability. Therefore when tensions rise, they may seek the security of the more familiar and comfortable expectations of childhood. Anticipating these shifts in identity allows the nurse to adjust the course of interaction to meet the needs of the moment. No single approach can be relied on consistently, and encountering cooperation, hostility, anger, bravado, and a variety of other behaviors and attitudes is common. It is as much a mistake to regard an adolescent as an adult with an adult's wisdom and control as it is to assume that the teenager has the concerns and expectations of a child.

Interviewing the adolescent presents some special issues. The first may be whether to talk with the adolescent alone or with the adolescent and parents together. If the parents and teenager are together, talking with the adolescent first has the advantage of immediately identifying with the young person, thus fostering the interpersonal relationship. However, talking with the parents initially may provide insight into the family relationship. In either case, give both parties an opportunity to be included in the interview. If time is limited (such as during history taking), clarify this at the onset to avoid appearing to "take sides" by talking more with one person than with the other.

Privacy and confidentiality are of great importance when interviewing adolescents because it is consistent with developmental maturity and autonomy. Explain to parents and teenagers the legal and ethical protections and limits of confidentiality. Nurses need to know and understand the state and federal consent and confidentiality laws pertaining to adolescent circumstances, such as suspected abuse, alcohol or other drug use, suicidal or homicidal ideation, contraceptive care, pregnancy, sexually transmitted infections, and sexual assault (Broner, Embry, Gremminger, et al., 2013).

Another dilemma in interviewing adolescents is that two views of a problem frequently exist: the teenager's and the parents'. Clarification of the problem is a major task. However, providing both parties an opportunity to discuss their perceptions in an open and unbiased atmosphere can, by itself, be therapeutic. Demonstrating positive communication skills can help families with adolescents to communicate more effectively (see Nursing Care Guidelines box).

NURSING CARE GUIDELINES

Communicating With Adolescents

Build a Foundation
- Spend time together.
- Encourage expression of ideas and feelings.
- Respect their views.
- Tolerate differences.
- Praise good points.
- Respect their privacy.
- Set a good example.

Communicate Effectively
- Give undivided attention.
- Listen, listen, listen.
- Be courteous, calm, honest, and open minded.
- Try not to overreact. If you do, take a break.
- Avoid judging or criticizing.
- Avoid the "third degree" of continuous questioning.
- Choose important issues when taking a stand.
- After taking a stand:
  - Think through all options.
  - Make expectations clear.

COMMUNICATION TECHNIQUES

Nurses use a variety of verbal techniques to encourage communication. Some of these techniques are useful to pose questions or explore concerns in a less threatening manner. Others can be presented as word games, which are often well received by children. However, for many children and adults, talking about feelings is difficult, and verbal communication may be more stressful than supportive. In such instances, use several nonverbal techniques to encourage communication.

Box 4.3 describes both verbal and nonverbal techniques. Because of the importance of play in communicating with children, play is discussed more extensively in the section. Any of the verbal or nonverbal techniques can give rise to strong feelings that surface unexpectedly. Be prepared to handle them or to recognize when issues go beyond your ability to deal with them. At that point, consider an appropriate referral.

Play

Play is a universal language of children. It is one of the most important forms of communication and can be an effective technique in relating to them. The nurse can often pick up on clues about physical, intellectual, and social developmental progress from the form and complexity of a child's play behaviors. Play requires minimum equipment or none at all. Many providers use therapeutic play to reduce the trauma of illness and hospitalization (see Chapter 21) and to prepare children for therapeutic procedures (see Chapter 22).

Because their ability to perceive precedes their ability to transmit, infants respond to activities that register on their physical senses. Patting, stroking, and other skin play convey messages. Repetitive actions, such as stretching infants' arms out to the side while they are lying on their backs and then folding the arms across the chest or raising and revolving

BOX 4.3 Creative Communication Techniques With Children

Verbal Techniques

"I" Messages

Relate a feeling about a behavior in terms of "I."

Describe effect behavior had on the person.

Avoid use of "you."

"You" messages are judgmental and provoke defensiveness.

Example: "You" message: "You are being uncooperative about doing your treatments."

Example: "I" message: "I am concerned about how the treatments are going because I want to see you get better."

Third-Person Technique

Express a feeling in terms of a third person ("he," "she," "they"). This is less threatening than directly asking children how they feel because it gives them an opportunity to agree or disagree without being defensive.

Example: "Sometimes when a person is sick a lot, he feels angry and sad because he cannot do what others can." Either wait silently for a response or encourage a reply with a statement, such as "Did you ever feel that way?"

This approach allows children three choices: (1) to agree and, one hopes, express how they feel; (2) to disagree; or (3) to remain silent, which means they probably have such feelings but are unable to express them at this time.

Facilitative Response

Listen carefully and reflect back to patients the feelings and content of their statements.

Responses are empathic and nonjudgmental and legitimize the person's feelings.

Formula for facilitative responses: "You feel ________ because ________."

Example: If child states, "I hate coming to the hospital and getting needles," a facilitative response is, "You feel unhappy because of all the things that are done to you."

Storytelling

Use the language of children to probe into areas of their thinking while bypassing conscious inhibitions or fears.

The simplest technique is asking children to relate a story about an event, such as "being in the hospital."

Other approaches:

- Show children a picture of a particular event, such as a child in a hospital with other people in the room, and ask them to describe the scene.
- Cut out comic strips, remove words, and have child add statements for scenes.

Mutual Storytelling

Reveal the child's thinking and attempt to change his or her perceptions or fears by retelling a somewhat different story (more therapeutic approach than storytelling).

Begin by asking the child to tell a story about something; then tell another story that is similar to the child's tale but with differences that help the child in problem areas.

Example: Child's story is about going to the hospital and never seeing his or her parents again. Nurse's story is also about a child (using different names but similar circumstances) in a hospital whose parents visit every day, but in the evening after work, until the child is better and goes home with them.

Bibliotherapy

Use books in a therapeutic and supportive process.

Provide children with an opportunity to explore an event that is similar to their own but sufficiently different to allow them to distance themselves from it and remain in control.

General guidelines for using bibliotherapy:

1. Assess the child's emotional and cognitive development in terms of readiness to understand the book's message.
2. Be familiar with the book's content (intended message or purpose) and the age for which it is written.
3. Read the book to the child if child is unable to read.
4. Explore the meaning of the book with the child by having the child:
   - Retell the story.
   - Read a special section with the nurse or parent.
   - Draw a picture related to the story and discuss the drawing.
   - Talk about the characters.
   - Summarize the moral or meaning of the story.

Dreams

Dreams often reveal unconscious and repressed thoughts and feelings.

Ask the child to talk about a dream or nightmare.

Explore with the child what meaning the dream could have.

"What If" Questions

Encourage child to explore potential situations and to consider different problem-solving options.

Example: "What if you got sick and had to go the hospital?" Children's responses reveal what they know already and what they are curious about, providing an opportunity for them to learn coping skills, especially in potentially dangerous situations.

Three Wishes

Ask, "If you could have any three things in the world, what would they be?"

If the child answers, "That all my wishes come true," ask the child for specific wishes.

Rating Game

Use some type of rating scale (numbers, sad to happy faces) to have the child rate an event or feeling.

Example: Instead of asking youngsters how they feel, ask how their day has been "on a scale of 1 to 10, with 10 being the best."

Word Association Game

State key words and ask children to say the first word they think of when they hear the word.

Start with neutral words and then introduce more anxiety-producing words, such as "illness," "needles," "hospitals," and "operation."

Select key words that relate to some relevant event in the child's life.

Sentence Completion

Present a partial statement and have the child complete it. Some sample statements include the following:

- The thing I like best (least) about school is ________.
- The best (worst) age to be is ________.
- The most (least) fun thing I ever did was ________.
- The thing I like most (least) about my parents is ________.

BOX 4.3 Creative Communication Techniques With Children—cont'd

- The one thing I would change about my family is _________.
- If I could be anything I wanted, I would be _________.
- The thing I like most (least) about myself is _________.

Pros and Cons

Select a topic, such as "being in the hospital," and have the child list "five good things and five bad things" about it.

This is an exceptionally valuable technique when applied to relationships, such as things family members like and dislike about each other.

Nonverbal Techniques

Writing

Writing is an alternative communication approach for older children and adults. Specific suggestions include the following:

- Keep a journal or diary.
- Write down feelings or thoughts that are difficult to express.
- Write "letters" that are never mailed (a variation is making up a "pen pal" to write to).

Keep an account of the child's progress from both a physical and an emotional viewpoint.

Drawing

Drawing is one of the most valuable forms of communication—both nonverbal (from looking at the drawing) and verbal (from the child's story of the picture).

Children's drawings tell a great deal about them because they are projections of their inner selves.

Spontaneous drawing involves giving child a variety of art supplies and providing the opportunity to draw.

Directed drawing involves a more specific direction, such as "draw a person" or the "three themes" approach (state three things about child and ask the child to choose one and draw a picture).

Guidelines for Evaluating Drawings

Use spontaneous drawings and evaluate more than one drawing whenever possible.

Interpret the drawings in light of other available information about child and family, including the child's age and stage of development.

Interpret the drawings as a whole rather than focusing on specific details of the drawings.

Consider individual elements of the drawings that may be significant:

- Sex of figure drawn first: Usually relates to the child's perception of his or her own sex role
- Size of individual figures: Expresses importance, power, or authority
- Order in which figures are drawn: Expresses priority in terms of importance
- Child's position in relation to other family members: Expresses feelings of status or alliance
- Exclusion of a member: May denote feeling of not belonging or desire to eliminate
- Accentuated parts: Usually express concern for areas of special importance (e.g., large hands may be a sign of aggression)
- Absence of or rudimentary arms and hands: Suggest timidity, passivity, or intellectual immaturity; tiny, unstable feet may express insecurity, and hidden hands may mean guilt feelings
- Placement of drawing on the page and type of stroke: Free use of paper and firm, continuous strokes express security, whereas drawings restricted to a small area and lightly drawn in broken or wavering lines may be signs of insecurity
- Erasures, shading, or cross-hatching: Expresses ambivalence, concern, or anxiety with a particular area

Magic

Use simple magic tricks to help establish rapport with child, encourage compliance with health interventions, and provide effective distraction during painful procedures.

Although the "magician" talks, no verbal response from the child is required.

Play

Play is the universal language and "work" of children.

It tells a great deal about children because they project their inner selves through the activity.

Spontaneous play involves giving child a variety of play materials and providing the opportunity to play.

Directed play involves a more specific direction, such as providing medical equipment or a dollhouse for focused reasons, such as exploring child's fear of injections or exploring family relationships.

---

the legs in a bicycling motion, will elicit pleasurable sounds. Colorful items to catch the eye or interesting sounds, such as a ticking clock, chimes, bells, or singing, can be used to attract infants' attention.

Older infants respond to simple games. The old game of peek-a-boo is an excellent means of initiating communication with infants while maintaining a "safe," nonthreatening distance. After this intermittent eye contact, the nurse is no longer viewed as a stranger but as a friend. This can be followed by touch games. Clapping an infant's hands together for pat-a-cake or wiggling the toes for "this little piggy" delights an infant or small child. Talking to a foot or other part of the child's body is another effective tactic. Much of the nursing assessment can be carried out with the use of games and simple play equipment while the infant remains in the safety of the parent's arms or lap.

The nurse can capitalize on the natural curiosity of small children by playing games such as "Which hand do you take?" and "Guess what I have in my hand," or by manipulating items such as a flashlight or stethoscope. Finger games are useful. More elaborate materials, such as puppets and replicas of familiar or unfamiliar items, serve as excellent means of communicating with small children. The variety and extent are limited only by the nurse's imagination.

Through play, children reveal their perceptions of interpersonal relationships with their family, friends, or health care personnel. Children may also reveal the wide scope of knowledge they have acquired from listening to others around them. For example, through needle play, children may reveal how carefully they have watched each procedure by precisely duplicating the technical skills. They may also reveal how well they remember those who performed procedures. In one example, a child painstakingly reenacted every detail of a tedious medical procedure, including the role of the physician who had repeatedly shouted at her to be still for the long ordeal. Her anger at him was most evident during the play session and revealed the cause for her abrupt withdrawal and passive hostility toward the medical and nursing staff after the test.

HISTORY TAKING

PERFORMING A HEALTH HISTORY

The format used for history taking may be (1) **direct**, in which the nurse asks for information via direct interview with the informant, or (2) **indirect**, in which the informant supplies the information by

BOX 4.4 Outline of a Pediatric Health History

Identifying Information
1. Name
2. Address
3. Telephone
4. Birth date and place
5. Race or ethnic group
6. Sex
7. Religion
8. Date of interview
9. Informant

Chief complaint (CC): To establish the major specific reason for the child's and parents' seeking of health care

Present illness (PI): To obtain all details related to the chief complaint

Past history (PH): To elicit a profile of the child's previous illnesses, injuries, or surgeries
1. Birth history (pregnancy, labor and delivery, perinatal history)
2. Previous illnesses, injuries, or surgeries
3. Allergies
4. Current medications
5. Immunizations
6. Growth and development
7. Habits

Review of systems (ROS): To elicit information concerning any potential health problem
1. Constitutional
2. Integument
3. Eyes
4. Ears
5. Nose
6. Mouth
7. Throat
8. Neck
9. Chest
10. Respiratory
11. Cardiovascular
12. Gastrointestinal
13. Genitourinary
14. Gynecologic
15. Musculoskeletal
16. Neurologic
17. Endocrine
18. Hematologic/lymphatic
19. Allergic/immunologic
20. Psychiatric

Family medical history: To identify genetic traits or diseases that have familial tendencies and to assess exposure to a communicable disease in a family member and family habits that may affect the child's health, such as smoking and chemical use

Psychosocial history: To elicit information about the child's self-concept

Sexual history: To elicit information concerning the child's sexual concerns or activities and any pertinent data regarding adults' sexual activity that influences the child

Family history: To develop an understanding of the child as an individual and as a member of a family and a community
1. Family composition
2. Home and community environment
3. Occupation and education of family members
4. Cultural and religious traditions
5. Family function and relationships

Nutritional assessment: To elicit information on the adequacy of the child's nutritional intake and needs
1. Dietary intake
2. Clinical examination

completing some type of questionnaire. The direct method is superior to the indirect approach or a combination of both. However, because time is limited, the direct approach is not always practical. If the nurse cannot use the direct approach, he or she should review parents' written responses and question them regarding any unusual answers. The categories listed in Box 4.4 encompass children's current and past health status and information about their psychosocial environment.

Identifying Information

Much of the identifying information may already be available from other recorded sources. However, if the parent and child seem anxious, use this opportunity to ask about such information to help them feel more comfortable.

Informant

One of the important elements of identifying information is the **informant**, the person(s) who furnishes the information. Record (1) who the person is (child, parent, or other), (2) an impression of reliability and willingness to communicate, and (3) any special circumstances such as the use of an interpreter or conflicting answers by more than one person.

Chief Complaint

The **chief complaint** is the specific reason for the child's visit to the clinic, office, or hospital. It may be the theme, with the present illness viewed as the description of the problem. Elicit the chief complaint by asking open-ended, neutral questions (e.g., "What seems to be the matter?," "How may I help you?," or "Why did you come here today?"). Avoid labeling-type questions (e.g., "How are you sick?" or "What is the problem?"). It is possible that the reason for the visit is not an illness or problem.

Occasionally, it is difficult to isolate one symptom or problem as the chief complaint because the parent may identify many. In this situation, be as specific as possible when asking questions. For example, asking informants to state which one problem or symptom prompted them to seek help now may help them focus on the most immediate concern.

Present Illness

The history of the present illness* is a narrative of the chief complaint from its earliest onset through its progression to the present. Its four major components are the details of onset, a complete interval history, the present status, and the reason for seeking help now. The focus of the present illness is on all factors relevant to the main problem, even if they have disappeared or changed during the onset, interval, and present.

*The term *illness* is used in its broadest sense to denote any problem of a physical, emotional, or psychosocial nature. It is actually a history of the chief complaint.

Analyzing a Symptom

Because pain is often the most characteristic symptom denoting the onset of a physical problem, it is used as an example for analysis of a symptom. Assessment includes type, location, severity, duration, and influencing factors (see Nursing Care Guidelines box; see also Pain Assessment, Chapter 5).

NURSING CARE GUIDELINES

Analyzing the Symptom: Pain

Type
Be as specific as possible. With young children, asking the parents how they know the child is in pain may help describe its type, location, and severity. For example, a parent may state, "My child must have a severe earache because she pulls at her ears, rolls her head on the floor, and screams. Nothing seems to help." Help older children describe the "hurt" by asking them if it is sharp, throbbing, dull, or stabbing. Record whatever words they use in quotes.

Location
Be specific. "Stomach pains" is too general a description. Children can better localize the pain if they are asked to "point with one finger to where it hurts" or to "point to where mommy or daddy would put a Band-Aid." Determine whether the pain radiates by asking, "Does the pain stay there or move? Show me with your finger where the pain goes."

Severity
Severity is best determined by finding out how it affects the child's usual behavior. Pain that prevents a child from playing, interacting with others, sleeping, and eating is most often severe. Assess pain intensity using a rating scale, such as a numeric or Wong-Baker FACES Pain Rating Scale (see Chapter 5).

Duration
Include the duration, onset, and frequency. Describe this in terms of activity and behavior, such as "pain reported to last all night; child refused to sleep and cried intermittently."

Influencing Factors
Include anything that causes a change in the type, location, severity, or duration of the pain: (1) precipitating events (those that cause or increase the pain), (2) relieving events (those that lessen the pain, such as medications), (3) temporal events (times when the pain is relieved or increased), (4) positional events (standing, sitting, lying down), and (5) associated events (meals, stress, coughing).

History

The history contains information relating to all previous aspects of the child's health status and concentrates on several areas that are ordinarily passed over in the history of an adult, such as birth history, detailed feeding history, immunizations, and growth and development. Because this section includes a great deal of information, use a combination of open-ended and fact-finding questions. For example, begin interviewing for each section with an open-ended statement (such as "Tell me about your child's birth") to provide the informants the opportunity to relate what they think is most important. Ask fact-finding questions related to specific details whenever necessary to focus the interview on certain topics.

Birth History

The birth history includes all data concerning (1) the mother's health during pregnancy, (2) the labor and delivery, and (3) the infant's condition immediately after birth. Because prenatal influences have significant effects on a child's physical and emotional development, a thorough investigation of the birth history is essential. Because parents may question what relevance pregnancy and birth have on the child's present condition, particularly if the child is past infancy, explain why such questions are included. An appropriate statement may be "I will be asking you some questions about your pregnancy and ____'s [refer to child by name] birth. Your answers will give me a more complete picture of his [or her] overall health."

Because emotional factors also affect the outcome of pregnancy and the subsequent parent–child relationship, investigate concurrent crises during pregnancy and prenatal attitudes toward the fetus. It is best to approach the topic of parental acceptance of pregnancy through indirect questioning. Asking the parents if the pregnancy was planned is a leading statement because they may respond affirmatively for fear of criticism if the pregnancy was unexpected. Rather, encourage parents to state their true reactions by referring to specific facts relating to the pregnancy, such as the spacing between offspring, an extended or short interval between marriage and conception, or a pregnancy during adolescence. The parent can choose to explore such statements with further explanations or, for the moment, may not be able to reveal such feelings. If the parent remains silent, return to this topic later in the interview.

Dietary History

Because parental concerns are common and nursing interventions are important in ensuring optimum nutrition, the dietary history is discussed in detail under the Nutritional Assessment section of this chapter.

Previous Illnesses, Injuries, and Surgeries

When inquiring about past illnesses, begin with a general statement (e.g., "What other illnesses has your child had?"). Because parents are most likely to recall serious health problems, ask specifically about colds, earaches, and childhood diseases such as measles, rubella (German measles), chickenpox, mumps, pertussis (whooping cough), diphtheria, tuberculosis, scarlet fever, strep throat, recurrent ear infections, gastroesophageal reflux, tonsillitis, or allergic manifestations.

In addition to illnesses, ask about injuries that required medical intervention, surgeries, procedures, and hospitalizations, including the dates of each incident. Focus on injuries (e.g., accidental falls, poisoning, choking, concussion, fracture, or burns) because these may be potential areas for parental guidance.

Allergies. Ask about commonly known allergic disorders, such as hay fever and asthma; unusual reactions to drugs, food, or latex products; and reactions to other contact agents such as poisonous plants, animals, household products, or fabrics. If asked appropriate questions, most people can give reliable information about drug reactions (see Nursing Care Guidelines box).

NURSING ALERT

Information about allergic reactions to drugs or other products is essential. Failure to document a serious reaction places the child at risk if the agent is given.

Current Medications

Inquire about current medications, including vitamins, antipyretics (especially aspirin), antibiotics, antihistamines, decongestants, nutritional supplements, or herbs, essential oils, and homeopathic medications. List all medications, including name, dose, route, schedule, duration, and reasons for use. Often parents are unaware of a medication's actual name. Whenever possible, ask the parents to bring the containers with them to the next visit, or ask for the name of the pharmacy and call

NURSING CARE GUIDELINES

Taking an Allergy History

- Has your child ever taken any prescription or over-the-counter medications that have disagreed with him or her or caused an allergic reaction? If yes, can you remember the name(s) of these medication(s)?
- Can you describe the reaction?
- Was the drug taken by mouth (as a tablet or syrup), or was it an injection?
- How soon after starting the medication did the reaction happen?
- How long ago did this happen?
- Did anyone tell you it was an allergic reaction, or did you decide for yourself?
- Has your child ever taken this medication, or a similar one, again? If yes, did your child experience the same problems?
- Have you told the physicians or nurses about your child's reaction or allergy?

for a list of all the child's recent prescription medications. However, this list will not include over-the-counter medications, which are important to know.

Immunizations

A record of all immunizations is essential. As many parents are unaware of the exact name and date of each immunization, sources of information include the child's primary care provider, school record, and the state's centralized immunization registry. All immunizations and "boosters" are listed, stating (1) the name of the specific disease, (2) the number of injections, (3) the dosage (sometimes lesser amounts are given if a reaction is anticipated), (4) the date when administered, and (5) the occurrence of any reaction following the immunization. Children should be screened for contraindications and precautions before every vaccine is administered (see Immunizations, Chapter 7).

Growth and Development

Review the child's growth, including the following:

- Measurements of weight, length, and head circumference at birth
- Patterns of growth on the growth chart and any significant deviations from previous percentiles
- Concerns about growth from the family or child

Developmental milestones include the following:

- Age of holding up head steadily
- Age of sitting alone without support
- Age of walking without assistance
- Age of saying first words with meaning
- Age of achieving bladder and bowel control
- Present grade in school
- School performance
- If the child has a best friend
- Interactions with other children, peers, and adults

Use specific and detailed questions when inquiring about each developmental milestone. For example, "sitting up" can mean many different activities, such as sitting propped up, sitting in someone's lap, sitting with support, sitting up alone but in a hyperflexed position for assisted balance, or sitting up unsupported with the back slightly rounded. A clue to misunderstanding of the requested activity may be an unusually early age of achievement (see Developmental Assessment at the end of this chapter).

Habits

Habits are an important area to explore (Box 4.5). Parents frequently express concerns during this part of the history. Encourage their input by saying, "Please tell me any concerns you have about your child's habits, activities, or development." Investigate further any concerns that parents express.

BOX 4.5 Habits to Explore During a Health Interview

- Behavior patterns, such as nail biting, thumb sucking, pica (habitual ingestion of nonfood substances), rituals ("security" blanket or toy), and unusual movements (head banging, rocking, overt masturbation, walking on toes)
- Activities of daily living, such as hours of sleep and arising, duration of nighttime sleep and naps, type and duration of exercise, regularity of stools and urination, age of toilet training, and daytime or nighttime bedwetting
- Unusual disposition; response to frustration
- Use or abuse of alcohol, drugs, caffeine, or tobacco

One of the most common concerns relates to sleep. Many children develop a normal sleep pattern, and all that is required during the assessment is a general overview of nighttime sleep and nap schedules. However, a number of children develop sleep problems (see Sleep Problems, Chapters 11 and 14). When sleep problems occur, the nurse needs a more detailed sleep history to guide appropriate interventions.*

Habits related to the use of chemicals apply primarily to older children and adolescents. If a youngster admits to smoking, drinking, or using drugs, ask about the quantity and frequency. Questions such as "Many kids your age are experimenting with drugs and alcohol; have you ever had any drugs or alcohol?" may give more reliable data than questions such as "How much do you drink?" or "How often do you drink or take drugs?" Clarify that "drinking" includes all types of alcohol, including beer and wine. When quantities such as a "glass" of wine or a "can" of beer are given, ask about the size of the container.

If older children deny use of chemical substances, inquire about past experimentation. Asking "You mean you never tried to smoke or drink?" implies that the nurse expects some such activity, and the youngster may be more inclined to answer truthfully. Be aware of the confidential nature of such questioning, the adverse effect that the parents' presence may have on the adolescent's willingness to answer, and the fact that self-reporting may not be an accurate account of chemical abuse.

Sexual History

The sexual history is an essential component of adolescents' health assessment. The history uncovers areas of concern related to sexual activity, alerts the nurse to circumstances that may indicate need for screening for sexually transmitted infections or testing for pregnancy, and provides information related to the need for sexual health counseling, such as safer sex practices. Box 4.6 gives guidelines for anticipatory guidance topics for parents and adolescents.

One approach to initiating a conversation about sexual concerns is to begin with a history of peer interactions. Open-ended statements (e.g., "Tell me about your social life" or "Who are your closest friends?") generally lead into a discussion of dating and sexual issues. To probe further, include questions about the adolescent's attitudes on such topics as sex education, "going steady," "living together," and premarital sex. Phrase questions to reflect concern rather than judgment or criticism of sexual practices.

---

*A sleep history and a sleep chart for the family to record the child's daily sleep and wake activities is available in Wilson, D., & Hockenberry, M. (2012). *Wong's clinical manual of pediatric nursing* (8th ed.). St. Louis, MO: Mosby.

BOX 4.6 Anticipatory Guidance—Sexuality

Ages 12 to 14 Years

- Have the adolescent identify a supportive adult with whom to discuss sexuality issues and concerns.
- Discuss the advantages of delaying sexual activity.
- Discuss making responsible decisions regarding normal sexual feelings.
- Discuss the roles of gender, peer pressure, and the media in sexual decision making.
- Discuss contraceptive options (advantages and disadvantages).
- Provide education regarding sexually transmitted infections (STIs), including human immunodeficiency virus (HIV) infection; clarify risks and discuss condoms.
- Discuss abuse prevention, including avoiding dangerous situations, the role of drugs and alcohol, and the use of self-defense.
- Have the adolescent clarify his or her values, needs, and ability to be assertive.
- If the adolescent is sexually active, discuss limiting partners, use of condoms, and contraceptive options.
- Have a confidential interview with the adolescent (including a sexual history).
- Discuss the evolution of sexual identity and expression.
- Discuss breast examination or testicular examination.

Ages 15 to 18 Years

- Support delaying sexual activity.
- Discuss alternatives to intercourse.
- Discuss "When are you ready for sex?"
- Clarify values; encourage responsible decision making.
- Discuss consequences of unprotected sex: early pregnancy and STIs, including HIV infection.
- Discuss negotiating with partner and barriers to safer sex.
- If the adolescent is sexually active, discuss limiting partners, use of condoms, and contraceptive options.
- Emphasize that sex should be safe and pleasurable for both partners.
- Have a confidential interview with the adolescent.
- Discuss concerns about sexual expression and identity.

Data from Wright, K. (1997). Anticipatory guidance: Developing a healthy sexuality. *Pediatr Ann, 26*(2 suppl), S142-S144, C3; Fonseca, H., & Greydanus, D. (2007). Sexuality in the child, teen and young adult: Concepts for the clinician. *Prim Care Clin Office Pract, 34,* 275-292.

In any conversation regarding sexual history, be aware of the language that is used in either eliciting or conveying sexual information. For example, avoid asking whether the adolescent is "sexually active" because this term is broadly defined. "Are you having sex with anyone?" is probably the most direct and best understood question. Because same-sex experimentation may occur, refer to all sexual contacts in nongender terms, such as "partners," rather than "girlfriends" or "boyfriends."

Family Health History

The family health history is used primarily to discover any genetic or chronic diseases in the child's family members. Assess for the presence or absence of consanguinity (if anyone in the family is related to their spouse's/partner's family. Family health history is generally confined to first-degree relatives (parents, siblings, grandparents, and immediate aunts and uncles). Information includes age, marital status, health status, cause of death if deceased, and any evidence of conditions, such as early heart disease, stroke, sudden death from unknown cause, hypercholesterolemia, hypertension, cancer, diabetes mellitus, obesity, congenital anomalies, allergies, asthma, seizures, tuberculosis, abnormal bleeding, sickle cell disease, cognitive impairment, hearing or visual deficits, and psychiatric disorders (e.g., depression or psychosis, and emotional problems). Confirm the accuracy of the reported disorders by inquiring about the symptoms, course, treatment, and sequelae of each diagnosis.

Geographic Location

One of the important areas to explore when assessing the family health history is geographic location, including the birthplace and travel to different areas in or outside of the country, for identification of possible exposure to endemic diseases. Include current and past housing, whether they rent or own, reside in an urban or rural location, the age of the home and whether there are significant threats such as molds or pests within the housing structure. Although the primary interest is the child's temporary residence in various localities, also inquire about close family members' travel, especially during tours of military service or business trips. Children are especially susceptible to parasitic infestation in areas of poor sanitary conditions and to vector-borne diseases, such as those from mosquitoes or ticks in warm and humid or heavily wooded regions.

Family Structure

Assessment of the family, both its structure and function, is an important component of the history-taking process. Because the quality of the functional relationship between the child and family members is a major factor in emotional and physical health, family assessment is discussed separately and in greater detail apart from the more traditional health history.

Family assessment is the collection of data about the composition of the family and the relationships among its members. In its broadest sense, family refers to all those individuals who are considered by the family member to be significant to the nuclear unit, including relatives, friends, and social groups (e.g., the school and church). Although family assessment is not family therapy, it can and frequently is therapeutic. Involving family members in discussing family characteristics and activities can provide insight into family dynamics and relationships.

Because of the time involved in performing an in-depth family assessment as presented here, be selective in deciding when knowledge of family function may facilitate nursing care (see Nursing Care Guidelines box). During brief contacts with families, a full assessment is not appropriate, and screening with one or two questions from each category may reflect the health of the family system or the need for additional assessment.

NURSING CARE GUIDELINES

Initiating a Comprehensive Family Assessment

Perform a comprehensive assessment on the following:

- Children receiving comprehensive well-child care
- Children experiencing major stressful life events (e.g., chronic illness, disability, parental divorce, death of a family member)
- Children requiring extensive home care
- Children with developmental delays
- Children with repeated accidental injuries and those with suspected child abuse
- Children with behavioral or physical problems that could be caused by family dysfunction

The most common method of eliciting information on the family structure is to interview family members. The principal areas of concern are family composition, home and community environment, occupation and education of family members, and cultural and religious traditions (Box 4.7).

BOX 4.7 Family Assessment Interview

General Guidelines

Schedule the interview with the family at a time that is most convenient for all parties; include as many family members as possible; clearly state the purpose of the interview.

Begin the interview by asking each person's name and their relationship to one another.

Restate the purpose of the interview and the objective.

Keep the initial conversation general to put members at ease and to learn the "big picture" of the family.

Identify major concerns and reflect these back to the family to be certain that all parties receive the same message.

Terminate the interview with a summary of what was discussed and a plan for additional sessions if needed.

Structural Assessment Areas

Family Composition

Immediate members of the household (names, ages, and relationships)

Significant extended family members

Previous marriages, separations, death of spouses, or divorces

Home and Community Environment

Type of dwelling, number of rooms, occupants

Sleeping arrangements

Number of floors, accessibility of stairs and elevators

Adequacy of utilities

Safety features (fire escape, smoke and carbon monoxide detectors, guardrails on windows, use of car restraint)

Environmental hazards (e.g., chipped paint, poor sanitation, pollution, heavy street traffic)

Availability and location of health care facilities, schools, play areas

Relationship with neighbors

Recent crises or changes in home

Child's reaction and adjustment to recent stresses

Occupation and Education of Family Members

Types of employment

Work schedules

Work satisfaction

Exposure to environmental or industrial hazards

Sources of income and adequacy

Effect of illness on financial status

Highest degree or grade level attained

Cultural and Religious Traditions

Religious beliefs and practices

Cultural and ethnic beliefs and practices

Language spoken in home

Assessment questions include the following:

- Does the family identify with a particular religious or ethnic group? Are both parents from that group?
- How is religious or ethnic background part of family life?
- What special religious or cultural traditions are practiced in the home (e.g., food choices and preparation)?
- Where were family members born, and how long have they lived in this country?
- What language does the family speak most frequently?
- Do they speak and understand English?
- What do they believe causes health or illness?
- What religious or ethnic beliefs influence the family's perception of illness and its treatment?
- What methods are used to prevent or treat illness?
- How does the family know when a health problem needs medical attention?
- Whom does the family contact when a member is ill?
- Does the family rely on cultural or religious healers or remedies? If so, ask them to describe the type of healer or remedy.
- Who does the family go to for support (clergy, medical healer, relatives)?
- Does the family experience discrimination because of their race, beliefs, or practices? Ask them to describe.

Functional Assessment Areas

Family Interactions and Roles

Interactions refer to ways family members relate to each other. The chief concern is the amount of intimacy and closeness among the members, especially spouses.

Roles refer to behaviors of people as they assume a different status or position.

Observations include the following:

- Family members' responses to each other (cordial, hostile, cool, loving, patient, short tempered)
- Obvious roles of leadership versus submission
- Support and attention shown to various members

Assessment questions include the following:

- What activities does the family perform together?
- Who do family members talk to when something is bothering them?
- What are family members' household chores?
- Who usually oversees what is happening with the children, such as at school or health care?
- How easy or difficult is it for the family to change or accept new responsibilities for household tasks?

Power, Decision Making, and Problem Solving

Power refers to individual family member's control over others in family; it is manifested through family decision making and problem solving.

Chief concern is clarity of boundaries of power between parents and children.

One method of assessment involves offering a hypothetical conflict or problem, such as a child failing school, and asking family how they would handle this situation.

Assessment questions include the following:

- Who usually makes the decisions in the family?
- If one parent makes a decision, can the child appeal to the other parent to change it?
- What input do children have in making decisions or discussing rules?
- Who makes and enforces the rules?
- What happens when a rule is broken?

Communication

Communication is concerned with clarity and directness of communication patterns.

Further assessment includes periodically asking family members if they understood what was just said and to repeat the message.

Observations include the following:

- Who speaks to whom
- If one person speaks for another or interrupts
- If members appear uninterested when certain individuals speak
- If there is agreement between verbal and nonverbal messages

BOX 4.7 Family Assessment Interview—cont'd

Assessment questions include the following:

- How often do family members wait until others are through talking before "having their say"?
- Do parents or older siblings tend to lecture and preach?
- Do parents tend to "talk down" to the children?

Expression of Feelings and Individuality

Expressions are concerned with personal space and freedom to grow, with limits and structure needed for guidance.

Observing patterns of communication offers clues to how freely feelings are expressed.

Assessment questions include the following:

- Is it OK for family members to get angry or sad?
- Who gets angry most of the time? What do they do?
- If someone is upset, how do other family members try to comfort this person?
- Who comforts specific family members?
- When someone wants to do something, such as try out for a new sport or get a job, what is the family's response (offer assistance, discouragement, or no advice)?

Psychosocial History

The traditional medical history includes a personal and social section that concentrates on children's personal status, such as school adjustment and any unusual habits, and the family and home environment. Because several personal aspects are covered under development and habits, only those issues related to children's ability to cope and their self-concept are presented here.

Through observation, obtain a general idea of how children handle themselves in terms of confidence in dealing with others, answering questions, and coping with new situations. Observe the parent-child relationship for the types of messages sent to children about their coping skills and self-worth. Do the parents treat the child with respect, focusing on strengths, or is the interaction one of constant reprimands, with emphasis on weaknesses and faults? Do the parents help the child learn new coping strategies or support the ones the child uses?

Parent-child interactions also convey messages about body image. Do the parents label the child and body parts (e.g., "bad boy," "skinny legs," or "ugly scar")? Do the parents handle the child gently, using soothing touch to calm an anxious child, or do they treat the child roughly, using slaps or restraint to make the child obey? If the child touches certain parts of the body, such as the genitalia, do the parents make comments that suggest a negative connotation?

With older children, many of the communication strategies discussed earlier in this chapter are useful in eliciting more definitive information about their coping and self-concept. Children can write down five things they like and dislike about themselves. The nurse can use sentence completion statements, such as "The thing I like best (or worst) about myself is ____________;" "If I could change one thing about myself, it would be ____________;" or "When I am scared, I ____________."

Review of Systems

The review of systems is a specific review of each body system, following an order similar to that of the physical examination (see Nursing Care Guidelines box). Often the history of the present illness provides a complete review of the system involved in the chief complaint. Because asking questions about other body systems may appear irrelevant to the parents or child, precede the questioning with an explanation of why the data are necessary (similar to the explanation concerning the relevance of the birth history) and reassure the parents that the child's main problem has not been forgotten.

Begin the review of a specific system with a broad statement (e.g., "How has your child's general health been?" or "Has your child had any problems with his eyes?") If the parent states that the child has had problems with some body function, pursue this with an encouraging statement such as "Tell me more about that." If the parent denies any problems, query for specific symptoms (e.g., "No headaches, bumping into objects, or squinting?"). If the parent reconfirms the absence of such symptoms, record positive statements in the history, such as "Mother denies headaches, bumping into objects, or squinting." In this way, anyone who reviews the health history is aware of exactly what symptoms were investigated.

NUTRITIONAL ASSESSMENT

DIETARY INTAKE

Knowledge of the child's dietary intake is an essential component of a nutritional assessment. However, it is also one of the most difficult factors to assess. Individuals' recall of food consumption, especially amounts eaten, is frequently unreliable. The food intake history of children and adolescents is prone to reporting error, mostly in the form of underreporting. People from different cultures may have difficulty adequately describing the types of food they eat. Despite these obstacles, a dietary evaluation is an important component of the child's assessment. The Dietary Reference Intakes (DRIs) are a set of four evidence-based nutrient reference values that provide quantitative estimates of nutrient intake for use in assessing and planning dietary intake (US Department of Agriculture, National Agricultural Library, 2014). The specific DRIs are as follows:

Estimated Average Requirement (EAR): Estimated to meet the nutrient requirement of half of healthy individuals for a specific age and gender group

Recommended Dietary Allowance (RDA): Sufficient to meet the nutrient requirement of nearly all healthy individuals for a specific age and gender group

Adequate Intake (AI): Based on estimates of nutrient intake by healthy individuals

Tolerable Upper Intake Level (UL): Highest nutrient intake level likely to pose no risk of adverse health effects

The US Department of Agriculture has an online interactive DRI tool for health care professionals to calculate nutrient requirements based on age, gender, height, weight, and activity, although it is important to note that individual requirements may vary (available at http://fnic.nal.usda.gov/fnic/interactiveDRI/).

Fig. 4.4 illustrates Choose MyPlate for Kids, which describes the five food groups forming the foundation for a healthy diet. MyPlate Kids' Place provides resources to help families build healthy meals and be active. Specific questions used to conduct a nutritional assessment are given in Box 4.8. Every nutritional assessment should begin with a dietary history. The exact questions used to elicit a dietary history vary with the child's age. In general, the younger the child, the more specific and

NURSING CARE GUIDELINES

Review of Systems

Constitutional: Overall state of health, fatigue, recent or unexplained weight gain or loss (period of time for either), contributing factors (change of diet, illness, altered appetite), exercise tolerance, fevers (time of day), chills, night sweats (unrelated to climatic conditions), general ability to carry out activities of daily living

Integument: Pruritus, pigment or other color changes (including birthmarks), acne, eruptions, rashes (location), bruises, petechiae, excessive dryness, general texture, tattoos or piercings, disorders or deformities of nails, hair growth or loss, hair color change (for adolescents, use of hair dyes or other potentially toxic substances, such as hair straighteners)

Eyes: Visual problems (behaviors indicative of blurred vision, such as bumping into objects, clumsiness, sitting close to television, holding a book close to face, writing with head near desk, squinting, rubbing the eyes, bending head in an awkward position), crossed eyes or lazy eye (strabismus), eye infections, edema of lids, excessive tearing, use of glasses or contact lenses, date of last vision examination

Ears: Earaches, ear discharge, evidence of hearing loss (ask about behaviors, such as the need to repeat requests, loud speech, lack of response to noises, inattentive behavior), results of any previous auditory testing

Nose: Nosebleeds (epistaxis), constant or frequent runny or stuffy nose, nasal obstruction (difficulty breathing), alteration or loss of sense of smell

Mouth: Mouth breathing, gum bleeding, number of teeth and pattern of eruption/loss, toothaches, tooth brushing, use of fluoride, difficulty with teething (symptoms), last visit to dentist (especially if temporary dentition is complete)

Throat: Sore throats, difficulty swallowing, choking, hoarseness or other voice irregularities

Neck: Pain, limitation of movement, stiffness, difficulty holding head straight (torticollis), thyroid enlargement, enlarged lymph nodes or other masses

Chest: Breast enlargement, discharge, masses; for adolescent girls, ask about breast self-examination

Respiratory: Chronic cough, wheezing, shortness of breath at rest or on exertion, difficulty breathing, snoring, sputum production, infections (pneumonia, tuberculosis), skin reaction from tuberculin testing

Cardiovascular: Cyanosis or fatigue on exertion, history of heart murmur or rheumatic fever, tachycardia, syncope, edema

Gastrointestinal: Appetite, nausea, vomiting (not associated with eating; may be indicative of brain tumor or increased intracranial pressure), abdominal pain, jaundice or yellowing skin or sclera, belching, flatulence, distention, diarrhea, constipation, recent change in bowel habits, blood in stools

Genitourinary: Pain on urination, frequency, hesitancy, urgency, hematuria, nocturia, polyuria, enuresis (daytime and/or nocturnal), unpleasant odor to urine, force of stream, discharge, change in size of scrotum, date and result of last urinalysis; for adolescents, sexually transmitted infection and type of treatment; for adolescent boys, ask about testicular self-examination

Gynecologic: Menarche, date of last menstrual period, regularity or problems with menstruation, vaginal discharge, pruritus; if sexually active, type of contraception, sexually transmitted infection and type of treatment; if sexually active with weakened immune system or if 21 years old and older, date and result of last Papanicolaou (Pap) smear; obstetric history (as discussed under birth history, when applicable)

Musculoskeletal: Weakness, clumsiness, lack of coordination, unusual movements, scoliosis, back pain, joint pain or swelling, muscle pains or cramps, abnormal gait, deformity, fractures, serious sprains, activity level

Neurologic: Headaches, seizures, tremors, tics, dizziness, head injury (specific details), loss of consciousness episodes, loss of memory, developmental delays or concerns

Endocrine: Intolerance to heat or cold, excessive thirst or urination, excessive sweating, salt craving, rapid or slow growth, signs of puberty (regardless of age)

Hematologic/lymphatic: Easy bruising or bleeding, anemia, date and result of last blood count, blood transfusions, swollen or painful lymph nodes (cervical, axillary, inguinal)

Allergic/immunologic: Allergic responses, anaphylaxis, eczema, rhinitis, unusual sneezing, autoimmunity, recurrent infections, infections associated with unusual complications

Psychiatric: General affect, anxiety, depression, mood changes, hallucinations, attention span, tantrums, behavior problems, suicidal ideation, substance abuse

BOX 4.8 Assessment of Nutritional Intake

Estimated Average Requirement (EAR): Used to examine the possibility of inadequacy.

Recommended Dietary Allowance (RDA): Dietary intake at or above this level usually has a low probability of inadequacy.

Adequate Intake (AI): Dietary intake at or above this level usually has a low probability of inadequacy.

Tolerable Upper Intake Level (UL): Dietary intake above this level usually places an individual at risk of adverse effects from excessive nutrient intake.

Dietary History

What are the family's usual mealtimes?

Do family members eat together or at separate times?

Who does the family grocery shopping and meal preparation?

How much money is spent to buy food each week?

How are most foods prepared—baked, broiled, fried, other?

How often does the family or your child eat out?

- What kinds of restaurants do you go to?
- What kinds of food does your child typically eat at restaurants?

Does your child eat breakfast regularly?

Where does your child eat lunch?

What are your child's favorite foods, beverages, and snacks?

- What are the average amounts eaten per day?
- What foods are artificially sweetened?
- What are your child's snacking habits?
- When are sweet foods usually eaten?
- What are your child's tooth brushing habits?

What special cultural practices are followed? What ethnic foods are eaten?

What foods and beverages does your child dislike?

How would you describe your child's usual appetite (hearty eater, picky eater)?

What are your child's feeding habits (breast, bottle, cup, spoon, eats by self, needs assistance, any special devices)?

Does your child take vitamins or other supplements? Do they contain iron or fluoride?

Does your child have any known or suspected food allergies? Is your child on a special diet?

Has your child lost or gained weight recently?

Are there any feeding problems (excessive fussiness, spitting up, colic, difficulty sucking or swallowing)? Are there any dental problems or appliances, such as braces, that affect eating?

What types of exercise does your child do regularly?

BOX 4.8 Assessment of Nutritional Intake—cont'd

Is there a family history of cancer, diabetes, heart disease, high blood pressure, or obesity?

Additional Questions for Infants

What was the infant's birth weight? When did it double? Triple?
Was the infant premature?
Are you breastfeeding or have you breastfed your infant? For how long?
If you use a formula, what is the brand?
  How long has the infant been taking it?
  How many ounces does the infant drink a day?
Are you giving the infant cow's milk (whole, low fat, skim)?
- When did you start?
- How many ounces does the infant drink a day?

Do you give your infant extra fluids (water, juice)?
If the infant takes a bottle to bed at nap or nighttime, what is in the bottle?
At what age did the child start on cereal, vegetables, meat or other protein sources, fruit or juice, finger food, and table food?
Do you make your own baby food or use commercial foods, such as infant cereal?
Does the infant take a vitamin or mineral supplement? If so, what type?
Has the infant had an allergic reaction to any food(s)? If so, list the foods and describe the reaction.
Does the infant spit up frequently; have unusually loose stools; or have hard, dry stools? If so, how often?
How often do you feed your infant?
How would you describe your infant's appetite?

Modified from Murphy, S. P., & Poos, M. I. (2002). Dietary reference intakes: Summary of applications in dietary assessment. *Pub Health Nutr, 5*(Suppl 6A), 843-849.

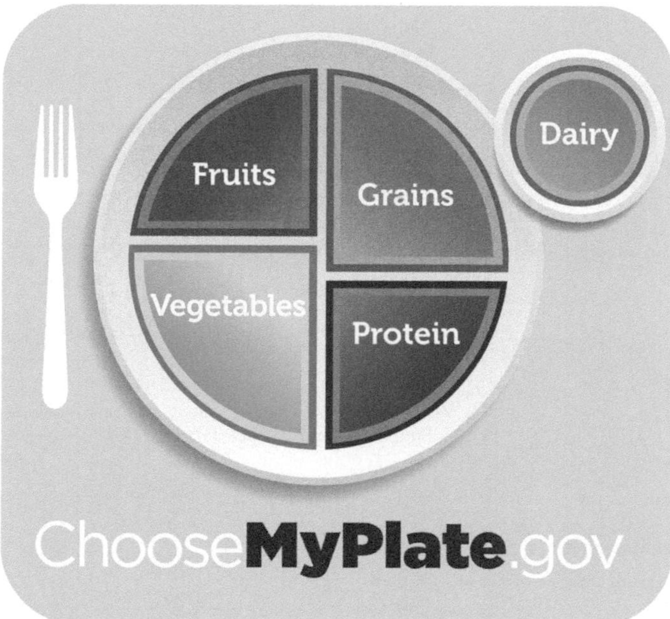

FIG. 4.4 MyPlate. MyPlate advocates building a healthy plate by making half of your plate fruits and vegetables and the other half grains and lean protein. Avoiding oversized portions, making half your grains whole grains, and drinking fat-free or low-fat (1%) milk are among the recommendations for a healthy diet. (From US Department of Agriculture, Center for Nutrition Policy and Promotion: *MyPlate,* 2015, www.ChooseMyPlate.gov.)

detailed the history should be. The overview elicited from the dietary history can be helpful in evaluating food frequency records. The history is also concerned with financial and cultural factors that influence food selection and preparation (see Cultural Considerations box).

The most common and probably easiest method of assessing daily intake is the **24-hour recall**. The child or parent recalls every item eaten and drank in the past 24 hours and the approximate amounts. The 24-hour recall is most beneficial when it represents a typical day's intake. Some of the difficulties with a daily recall are the family's inability to remember exactly what was eaten and inaccurate estimation of portion size. To increase accuracy of reporting portion sizes, the use of food models and additional questions are recommended. In general, this method is most useful in providing qualitative information about the child's diet.

CULTURAL CONSIDERATIONS

Food Practices

Because cultural practices are prevalent in food preparation, consider carefully the kinds of questions that are asked and the judgments made during counseling. For example, some cultures, such as Hispanic, African American, and Native American, include many vegetables, legumes, and starches in their diet that together provide sufficient essential amino acids, even though the actual amount of meat or dairy protein is low. (See Food Customs, Chapter 2.)

To improve the reliability of the daily recall, the family can complete a **food diary** by recording every food and liquid consumed for a certain number of days. A 3-day record consisting of 2 weekdays and 1 weekend day is representative for most people. Providing specific charts to record intake can improve compliance. The family should record items immediately after eating.

CLINICAL EXAMINATION OF NUTRITION

A significant amount of information regarding nutritional deficiencies comes from a clinical examination, especially from assessing the skin, hair, teeth, gums, lips, tongue, and eyes. Hair, skin, and mouth are vulnerable because of the rapid turnover of epithelial and mucosal tissue. Table 4.1 summarizes clinical signs of possible nutritional deficiency or excess. Few are diagnostic for a specific nutrient, and if suspicious signs are found, they must be confirmed with dietary and biochemical data. Failure to thrive is discussed in Chapter 11. Obesity and eating disorders are discussed in Chapter 18.

Anthropometry, an essential parameter of nutritional status, is the measurement of height (length), weight, head circumference, proportions, skinfold thickness, and arm circumference in children. Height and head circumference reflect past nutrition, whereas weight, skinfold thickness, and arm circumference reflect present nutritional status, especially of protein and fat reserves. Skinfold thickness is a measurement of the body's fat content because approximately half the body's total fat stores are directly beneath the skin. The upper arm muscle circumference is correlated with measurements of total muscle mass. Because muscle serves as the body's major protein reserve, this measurement is considered

TABLE 4.1 Clinical Assessment of Nutritional Status

Evidence of Adequate Nutrition	Evidence of Deficient or Excess Nutrition	Deficiency or Excess*
General Growth		
Between 5th and 95th percentiles for height, weight, and head circumference	<5th or >95th percentile for growth	Protein, calories, fats, and other essential nutrients, especially vitamin A, pyridoxine, niacin, calcium, iodine, manganese, zinc
Steady gain with expected growth spurts during infancy and adolescence	Absence of or delayed growth spurts; poor weight gain	
Sexual development appropriate for age	Delayed sexual development	Excess vitamins A, D
Skin		
Smooth, slightly dry to touch	Hardening and scaling	Vitamin A
Elastic and firm	Seborrheic dermatitis	Excess niacin
Absence of lesions	Dry, rough, petechiae	Riboflavin
Color appropriate to genetic background	Delayed wound healing	Vitamin C
	Scaly dermatitis on exposed surfaces	Riboflavin, vitamin C, zinc
	Wrinkled, flabby	Niacin
	Crusted lesions around orifices, especially nares	Protein, calories, zinc
	Pruritus	Excess vitamin A, riboflavin, niacin
	Poor turgor	Water, sodium
	Edema	Protein, thiamine
		Excess sodium
	Yellow tinge (jaundice)	Vitamin B_{12}
		Excess vitamin A, niacin
	Depigmentation	Protein, calories
	Pallor (anemia)	Pyridoxine, folic acid, vitamins B_{12}, C, E (in premature infants), iron
		Excess vitamin C, zinc
	Paresthesia	Excess riboflavin
Hair		
Lustrous, silky, strong, elastic	Stringy, friable, dull, dry, thin	Protein, calories
	Alopecia	Protein, calories, zinc
	Depigmentation	Protein, calories, copper
	Raised areas around hair follicles	Vitamin C
Head		
Even molding, occipital prominence, symmetric facial features	Softening of cranial bones, prominence of frontal bones, skull flat and depressed toward middle	Vitamin D
Fused sutures after 18 months	Delayed fusion of sutures	Vitamin D
	Hard, tender lumps in occiput	Excess vitamin A
	Headache	Excess thiamine
Neck		
Thyroid not visible, palpable in midline	Thyroid enlarged, may be grossly visible	Iodine
Eyes		
Clear, bright	Hardening and scaling of cornea and conjunctiva	Vitamin A
Good night vision	Night blindness	Vitamin A
Conjunctiva—pink, glossy	Burning, itching, photophobia, cataracts, corneal vascularization	Riboflavin
Ears		
Tympanic membrane—pliable	Calcified (hearing loss)	Excess vitamin D
Nose		
Smooth, intact nasal angle	Irritation and cracks at nasal angle	Riboflavin
		Excess vitamin A
Mouth		
Lips—smooth, moist, darker color than skin	Fissures and inflammation at corners	Riboflavin
		Excess vitamin A
Gums—firm, coral pink, stippled	Spongy, friable, swollen, bluish red or black, bleed easily	Vitamin C

TABLE 4.1 Clinical Assessment of Nutritional Status—cont'd

Evidence of Adequate Nutrition	Evidence of Deficient or Excess Nutrition	Deficiency or Excess*
Mucous membranes—bright pink, smooth, moist	Stomatitis	Niacin
Tongue—rough texture, no lesions, taste sensation	Glossitis	Niacin, riboflavin, folic acid
	Diminished taste sensation	Zinc
Teeth—uniform white color, smooth, intact	Brown mottling, pits, fissures	Excess fluoride
	Defective enamel	Vitamins A, C, D, calcium, phosphorus
	Caries	Excess carbohydrates
Chest		
In infants, shape almost circular	Depressed lower portion of rib cage	Vitamin D
In children, lateral diameter increased in proportion to anteroposterior diameter	Sharp protrusion of sternum	Vitamin D
Smooth costochondral junctions	Enlarged costochondral junctions	Vitamins C, D
Breast development—normal for age	Delayed development	See under General Growth; especially zinc
Cardiovascular System		
Pulse and blood pressure (BP) within normal limits	Palpitations	Thiamine
	Rapid pulse	Potassium
		Excess thiamine
	Arrhythmias	Magnesium, potassium
		Excess niacin, potassium
	Increased BP	Excess sodium
	Decreased BP	Thiamine
		Excess niacin
Abdomen		
In young children, cylindric and prominent	Distended, flabby, poor musculature	Protein, calories
	Prominent, large	Excess calories
In older children, flat	Potbelly, constipation	Vitamin D
Normal bowel habits	Diarrhea	Niacin
		Excess vitamin C
	Constipation	Excess calcium, potassium
Musculoskeletal System		
Muscles—firm, well-developed, equal strength bilaterally	Flabby, weak, generalized wasting	Protein, calories
	Weakness, pain, cramps	Thiamine, sodium, chloride, potassium, phosphorus, magnesium
		Excess thiamine
	Muscle twitching, tremors	Magnesium
	Muscular paralysis	Excess potassium
Spine—cervical and lumbar curves (double S curve)	Kyphosis, lordosis, scoliosis	Vitamin D
Extremities—symmetric; legs straight with minimum bowing	Bowing of extremities, knock-knees	Vitamin D, calcium, phosphorus
	Epiphyseal enlargement	Vitamins A, D
	Bleeding into joints and muscles, joint swelling, pain	Vitamin C
Joints—flexible, full range of motion, no pain or stiffness	Thickening of cortex of long bones with pain and fragility, hard tender lumps in extremities	Excess vitamin A
	Osteoporosis of long bones	Calcium
		Excess vitamin D
Neurologic System		
Behavior—alert, responsive, emotionally stable	Listless, irritable, lethargic, apathetic (sometimes apprehensive, anxious, drowsy, mentally slow, confused)	Thiamine, niacin, pyridoxine, vitamin C, potassium, magnesium, iron, protein, calories
		Excess vitamins A, D, thiamine, folic acid, calcium
Absence of tetany, convulsions	Masklike facial expression, blurred speech, involuntary laughing	Excess manganese
	Convulsions	Thiamine, pyridoxine, vitamin D, calcium, magnesium
		Excess phosphorus (in relation to calcium)
Intact peripheral nervous system	Peripheral nervous system toxicity (unsteady gait, numb feet and hands, fine motor clumsiness)	Excess pyridoxine
Intact reflexes	Diminished or absent tendon reflexes	Thiamine, vitamin E

*Nutrients listed are deficient unless specified as excess.

an index of the body's protein stores. Ideally, growth measurements are recorded over time, and comparisons are made regarding the velocity of growth based on previous and present values.

Numerous biochemical tests are available for assessing nutritional status. The most common laboratory studies to assess for undernutrition are hemoglobin, red blood cell indices, and serum albumin or prealbumin. For obese children, fasting serum glucose, lipids, and liver function studies may be performed to assess for complications.

EVALUATION OF NUTRITIONAL ASSESSMENT

After collecting the data needed for a thorough nutritional assessment, evaluate the findings to plan appropriate counseling. From the data, assess whether the child is malnourished, at risk for becoming malnourished, well nourished with adequate reserves, or overweight or obese.

Analyze the daily food diary for the variety and amounts of foods suggested in MyPlate (see Fig. 4.4). For example, if the list includes no vegetables, inquire about this rather than assuming that the child dislikes vegetables because it is possible that none were served that day. Also, evaluate the information in terms of the family's ethnic practices and financial resources. Encouraging increased protein intake with additional meat is not always feasible for families on a limited budget and may conflict with food practices that use meat sparingly, such as in Asian meal preparation.

GENERAL APPROACHES TOWARD EXAMINING THE CHILD

SEQUENCE OF THE EXAMINATION

Ordinarily, the sequence for examining patients follows a head-to-toe direction. The main function of such a systematic approach is to provide a general guideline for assessment of each body area to avoid omitting segments of the examination. The standard recording of data also facilitates exchange of information among different professionals. In examining children, this orderly sequence is frequently altered to accommodate the child's developmental needs, although the examination is recorded following the head-to-toe model. Using developmental and chronologic age as the main criteria for assessing each body system accomplishes several goals:

- Minimizes stress and anxiety associated with assessment of various body parts
- Fosters a trusting nurse-child-parent relationship
- Allows for maximum preparation of the child
- Preserves the essential security of the parent-child relationship, especially with young children
- Maximizes the accuracy and reliability of assessment findings

PREPARATION OF THE CHILD

Although the physical examination consists of painless procedures, for some children the use of a tight arm cuff, probes in the ears and mouth, pressure on the abdomen, or a cold piece of metal to listen to the chest is stressful. Therefore the nurse should use the same considerations discussed in Chapter 22 for preparing children for procedures. In addition to that discussion, general guidelines related to the examining process are given in the Nursing Care Guidelines box.

The physical examination should be as pleasant as possible, as well as educational. The paper-doll technique is a useful approach to teaching children about the body part that is being examined (Fig. 4.5). At the conclusion of the visit, the child can bring home the paper doll as a memento.

Table 4.2 summarizes guidelines for positioning, preparing, and examining children at various ages. Because the child may not fit precisely into one age category, it may be necessary to vary the approach after a preliminary assessment of the child's developmental achievements and needs. Even with the best approach, many toddlers are uncooperative and inconsolable for much of the physical examination. However, some seem intrigued by the new surroundings and unusual equipment and respond more like preschoolers than toddlers. Likewise, some early preschoolers may require more of the "security measures" employed with younger children, such as continued parent-child contact, and less of the preparatory measures used with preschoolers, such as playing with the equipment before and during the actual examination (Fig. 4.6).

PHYSICAL EXAMINATION

Although the approach to and sequence of the physical examination differ according to the child's age and development, the following discussion outlines the traditional model for physical assessment. The focus includes all pediatric age groups (see Chapter 7 for a detailed discussion of a newborn assessment). Because the physical examination is a vital part of preventive pediatric care, Fig. 4.7 gives a schedule for periodic health visits.

GROWTH MEASUREMENTS

Measurement of physical growth in children is a key element in evaluating their health status. Physical growth parameters include weight, height (length), skinfold thickness, arm circumference, and head circumference. Values for these growth parameters are plotted on percentile charts, and the child's measurements in percentiles are compared with those of the general population.

Growth Charts

Growth charts use a series of percentile curves to demonstrate the distribution of body measurements in children. The Centers for Disease Control and Prevention recommends that the World Health Organization growth standards be used to monitor growth for infants and children between the ages of 0 and 2 years old. Because breastfeeding is the recommended standard for infant feeding, the World Health Organization growth charts are used; they reflect growth patterns among children who were predominately breastfed for at least 4 months and are still breastfeeding at 12 months old. The Centers for Disease Control and Prevention growth charts (www.cdc.gov/growthcharts) are used for children 2 years old and older.

Children whose growth may be questionable include the following:

- Children whose height and weight percentiles are widely disparate (e.g., height in the 10th percentile and weight in the 90th percentile, especially with above-average skinfold thickness)
- Children who fail to follow the expected growth velocity in height and weight
- Children who show a sudden increase (except during normal puberty) or decrease in a previously steady growth pattern (i.e., crossing two major percentile lines after 3 years old)
- Children who are short in the absence of short parents

Because growth is a continuous but uneven process, the most reliable evaluation lies in comparing growth measurements over time because they reflect change. It is important to remember that same-age children (whether short, average, or tall in stature) should grow at similar rates (Fig. 4.8).

Length

The term *length* refers to measurements taken when children are supine (also referred to as recumbent length). Until children are 24 months

NURSING CARE GUIDELINES

Performing a Pediatric Physical Examination

Perform the examination in an appropriate, nonthreatening area:
- Have room well lit and decorated with neutral colors.
- Have room temperature comfortably warm.
- Place all strange and potentially frightening equipment out of sight.
- Have some toys and games available for child.
- If possible, have rooms decorated and equipped for different-age children.
- Provide privacy, especially for school-age children and adolescents.
- Provide time for play and becoming acquainted.

Observe behaviors that signal child's readiness to cooperate:
- Talking to the nurse
- Making eye contact
- Accepting the offered equipment
- Allowing physical touching
- Choosing to sit on examining table rather than parent's lap

If signs of readiness are not observed, use the following techniques:
- Talk to parent while essentially "ignoring" child; gradually focus on child or a favorite object, such as a doll.
- Make complimentary remarks about child, such as about his or her appearance, dress, or a favorite object.
- Tell a funny story or play a simple magic trick.
- Have a nonthreatening "friend" available, such as a hand puppet to "talk" to child for the nurse (see Fig. 4.26, *A*).

If child refuses to cooperate, use the following techniques:
- Assess reason for uncooperative behavior; consider that a child who is unduly afraid may have had a traumatic experience.
- Try to involve child and parent in process.
- Avoid prolonged explanations about examining procedure.
- Use a firm, direct approach regarding expected behavior.
- Perform examination as quickly as possible.
- Have attendant gently restrain child.
- Minimize any disruptions or stimulation.
- Limit number of people in room.
- Use isolated room.
- Use quiet, calm, confident voice.

Begin examination in a nonthreatening manner for young children or children who are fearful:
- Use activities that can be presented as games, such as test for cranial nerves (see Table 4.11).
- Use approaches such as Simon Says to encourage child to make a face, squeeze a hand, stand on one foot, and so on.
- Use paper-doll technique:
  1. Lay child supine on an examining table or floor that is covered with a large sheet of paper.
  2. Trace around child's body outline.
  3. Use body outline to demonstrate what will be examined, such as drawing a heart and listening with stethoscope before performing activity on child.

If several children in the family will be examined, begin with the most cooperative child to model desired behavior.

Involve child in examination process:
- Provide choices, such as sitting on table or in parent's lap.
- Allow child to handle or hold equipment.
- Encourage child to use equipment on a doll, family member, or examiner.
- Explain each step of the procedure in simple language.

Examine child in a comfortable and secure position:
- Sitting on parent's lap
- Sitting upright if in respiratory distress

Proceed to examine the body in an organized sequence (usually head to toe) with the following exceptions:
- Alter sequence to accommodate needs of different-age children (see Table 4.2).
- Examine painful areas last.
- In emergency situation, examine vital functions (airway, breathing, and circulation) and injured area first.

Reassure child throughout the examination, especially about bodily concerns that arise during puberty.

Discuss findings with family at the end of the examination.

Praise child for cooperation during the examination; give a reward such as a small toy or sticker.

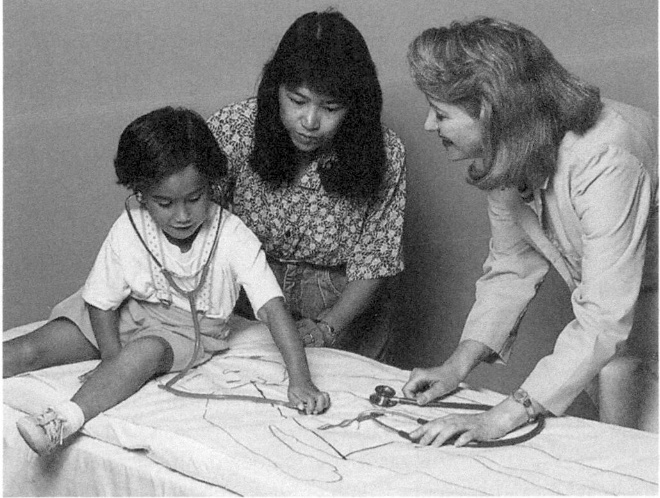

FIG. 4.5 Using the paper-doll technique to prepare a child for physical examination.

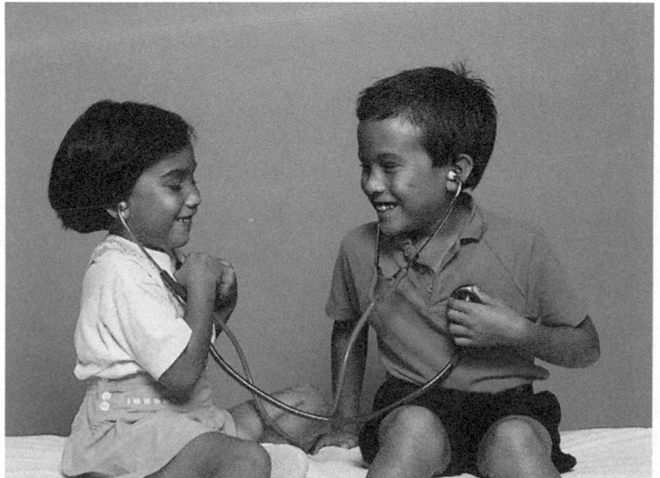

FIG. 4.6 Preparing children for physical examination.

TABLE 4.2 Age-Specific Approaches to Physical Examination During Childhood

Position	Sequence	Preparation
Infant		
Before able to sit alone—supine or prone, preferably in parent's lap; before 4-6 months, can place on examining table After able to sit alone—sitting in parent's lap whenever possible; if on table, place with parent in full view	If quiet, auscultate heart, lungs, abdomen. Record heart and respiratory rates. Palpate and percuss same areas. Proceed in usual head-to-toe direction. Perform traumatic procedures last (eyes, ears, mouth [while crying]). Elicit reflexes as body part is examined. Elicit Moro reflex last.	Completely undress if room temperature permits. Leave diaper on male infant. Gain cooperation with distraction, bright objects, rattles, talking. Smile at infant; use soft, gentle voice. Use pacifier (if used) or bottle with feeding (if bottle feeding). Enlist parent's aid for restraining to examine ears, mouth. Avoid abrupt, jerky movements.
Toddler		
Sitting or standing on or by parent Prone or supine in parent's lap	Inspect body area through play: "Count fingers," "tickle toes." Use minimum physical contact initially. Introduce equipment slowly. Auscultate, percuss, palpate whenever quiet. Perform traumatic procedures last (same as for infant).	Have parent remove outer clothing. Remove underwear as body part is examined. Allow toddler to inspect equipment; demonstrating use of equipment is usually ineffective. If uncooperative, perform procedures quickly. Use restraint when appropriate; request parent's assistance. Talk about examination if cooperative; use short phrases. Praise for cooperative behavior.
Preschool Child		
Prefer standing or sitting Usually cooperative prone or supine Prefer parent's closeness	If cooperative, proceed in head-to-toe direction. If uncooperative, proceed as with toddler.	Request self-undressing. Allow to wear underpants if shy. Offer equipment for inspection; briefly demonstrate use. Make up story about procedure (e.g., "I'm seeing how strong your muscles are" [blood pressure]). Use paper-doll technique. Give choices when possible. Expect cooperation; use positive statements (e.g., "Open your mouth").
School-Age Child		
Prefer sitting Cooperative in most positions Younger child prefers parent's presence Older child may prefer privacy	Proceed in head-to-toe direction. May examine genitalia last in older child.	Respect need for privacy. Request self-undressing. Allow to wear underpants. Give gown to wear. Explain purpose of equipment and significance of procedure, such as otoscope to see eardrum, which is necessary for hearing. Teach about body function and care.
Adolescent		
Same as for school-age child Offer option of parent's presence	Same as older school-age child. May examine genitalia last.	Allow to undress in private. Give gown. Expose only area to be examined. Respect need for privacy. Explain findings during examination (e.g., "Your muscles are firm and strong."). Matter-of-factly comment about sexual development (e.g., "Your breasts are developing as they should be."). Emphasize normalcy of development. Examine genitalia as any other body part; may leave to end.

old (or 36 months if using the chart for birth to 36 months), measure recumbent length using a length board (see Fig. 4.9, *A* and the Translating Evidence into Practice box). Because of the normally flexed position during infancy, fully extend the body by (1) holding the head in midline, (2) grasping the knees together gently, and (3) pushing down on the knees until the legs are fully extended and flat against the table. When using a length board, place the head firmly at the top of the board and the heels of the feet firmly against the footboard. A tape measure should not be used to measure the length of infants and children because the methods are inaccurate and unreliable (Foote, Brady, Burke, et al., 2009).

Clinical Preventive Services for Normal-Risk Children*

	Infancy							Early Childhood							Middle Childhood						Adolescence							
Age	Newborn	3-5 d	By1mo	2 mo	4 mo	6 mo	9 mo	12mo	15mo	18mo	24mo	30mo	3 y	4 y	5 y	6 y	7 y	8 y	9 y	10 y	11 y	12 y	13 y	14 y	15 y	16 y	17 y	18 y
History Initial/Interval	●	●	●	●	●	●	●	●	●	●	●	●	●	●	●	●	●	●	●	●	●	●	●	●	●	●	●	●
Measurements																												
Length/Height and Weight	●	●	●	●	●	●	●	●	●	●	●	●	●	●	●	●	●	●	●	●	●	●	●	●	●	●	●	●
Head Circumference	●	●	●	●	●	●	●	●	●	●	●																	
Weight for Length	●	●	●	●	●	●	●	●	●	●																		
Body Mass Index											●	●	●	●	●	●	●	●	●	●	●	●	●	●	●	●	●	●
Blood Pressure	★	★	★	★	★	★	★	★	★	★	★	★	●	●	●	●	●	●	●	●	●	●	●	●	●	●	●	●
Sensory Screening																												
Vision	★	★	★	★	★	★	★	★	★	★	★	★	●	●	●	●	★	●	★	●	★	●	★	★	●	★	★	●
Hearing	●	★	★	★	★	★	★	★	★	★	★	★	★	●	●	●	★	●	★	●	★	★	★	★	★	★	★	★
Developmental/ Behavioral Assessment																												
Developmental Screening							●			●		●																
Autism Screening										●	●																	
Developmental Surveillance	●	●	●	●	●	●		●	●		●		●	●	●	●	●	●	●	●	●	●	●	●	●	●	●	●
Psychosocial/ Behavioral Assessment	●	●	●	●	●	●	●	●	●	●	●	●	●	●	●	●	●	●	●	●	●	●	●	●	●	●	●	●
Alcohol and Drug Use Assessment																					★	★	★	★	★	★	★	★
Physical Examination	●	●	●	●	●	●	●	●	●	●	●	●	●	●	●	●	●	●	●	●	●	●	●	●	●	●	●	●
Procedures																												
Newborn Metabolic/ Hemoglobin Screening	←—	●	——	—→																								
Immunization	●	●	●	●	●	●	●	●	●	●	●	●	●	●	●	●	●	●	●	●	●	●	●	●	●	●	●	●
Hematocrit or Hemoglobin					★			●		★	★		★	★	★	★	★	★	★	★	★	★	★	★	★	★	★	★
Lead Screening						★	★	● or ★		★	● or ★		★	★	★	★												
Tuberculin Test			★			★		★		★	★		★	★	★	★	★	★	★	★	★	★	★	★	★	★	★	★
Dyslipidemia Screening											★			★		★		★		★	★	★	★	★	★	★	★	●
STI Screening																					★	★	★	★	★	★	★	★
Cervical Dysplasia Screening																					★	★	★	★	★	★	★	★
Oral Health						★	★	● or ★		● or ★	● or ★	● or ★	●			●												
Anticipatory Guidance	●	●	●	●	●	●	●	●	●	●	●	●	●	●	●	●	●	●	●	●	●	●	●	●	●	●	●	●

Key: ● = To be performed; ★ = risk assessment to be performed, with appropriate action to follow, if positive; ←●→ = range during which a service may be provided, with the symbol indicating the preferred age.

*For current immunization schedules, see Chapter 6.

FIG. 4.7 Preventive Pediatric Health Care chart. (Adapted from AAP Committee on Practice and Ambulatory Medicine and AAP Bright Futures Periodicity Schedule Workgroup. (2017). Recommendations for preventive pediatric health care. *Pediatrics. 139*(4). https://www.aap.org/en-us/Documents/periodicity_schedule.pdf.)

TRANSLATING EVIDENCE INTO PRACTICE

Linear Growth Measurement of Children

Ask the Question

PICOT Question

In children, what are the best instruments and techniques to measure linear growth (length and height)?

Search for the Evidence

Search Strategies

Search selection criteria: English language, research-based and review articles and expert opinion from databases, anthropometric and endocrinology textbooks, contact with experts in the field, and informal discovery.

Key terms: Length, height, stature, infant, children, adolescent, measurement, instrument, length board, stadiometer, calibration, technique, accuracy, reliability, diurnal variation. Exclusion criteria: Other anthropometric measurements, adults.

Databases Used

MEDLINE, CINAHL, COCHRANE, EMBASE, OCLC, ERIC, National Guideline Clearinghouse (AHRQ)

Critical Appraisal of the Evidence

An interdisciplinary team systematically and critically appraised the evidence to develop these clinical practice recommendations using an evidence-based practice rating scheme (US Preventive Services Task Force, 1996).

Measure recumbent length in children under 24 months of age and in children who cannot stand alone (Foote, 2014; Foote, Brady, Burke, et al., 2011) (see Fig. 4.9, *A*).

- Use a length board with these components: Flat, horizontal surface with stationary headboard and smoothly movable footboard, both at 90-degree angles to the horizontal surface, and attached ruler marked in millimeter and/or $\frac{1}{16}$-inch increments. Tape measures should never be used.
- Cover length board with soft, thin cloth or paper.
- Remove all clothing and shoes. Remove or loosen diaper. Remove hair ornaments on crown of head.
- Two measurers are required to accomplish correct positioning; one measurer (assistant) can be a parent or other caregiver when procedures are explained and understood.
- Place child supine on length board. Never leave unattended.

Continued

TRANSLATING EVIDENCE INTO PRACTICE—cont'd

Linear Growth Measurement of Children

- Assistant holds head in midline with crown of head against headboard, compressing the hair.
- Position head in the Frankfort vertical plane (imaginary line from the lower border of the orbit through the highest point of the auditory meatus; the line is parallel to the headboard and perpendicular to the length board).
- Lead measurer positions the body on length board with one hand placed on both legs to fully extend the body.
- Ensure that head remains against headboard, shoulders and hips are not rotated, back is not arched, and legs are not bent. Reposition as necessary.
- Using the other hand, lead measurer moves footboard against heels of both feet with toes pointing upward.
- Read measurement to the last completed millimeter or $\frac{1}{16}$ inch.
- Reposition the child and repeat procedure. Measure at least twice (ideally three times). Average the measurements for the final value. Record immediately.

Measure height in children 2 years of age and older who can stand alone well (Foote, 2014; Foote, Brady, Burke, et al., 2011) (see Fig. 4.9, *B*).

- Use a stadiometer with these components: Vertical surface to stand against, footboard or firm surface to stand on, movable horizontal headboard at 90-degree angle to the vertical surface, and attached ruler marked in millimeter and/or $\frac{1}{16}$-inch increments. Wall charts and flip-up horizontal bars (floppy-arm devices) mounted to weighing scales should never be used because these methods are inaccurate and unreliable.
- Remove shoes and heavy outer clothing. Remove hair ornaments and undo hairstyles (e.g., braids or buns) on crown of head.
- Stand child on flat surface with back against vertical surface of stadiometer.
- Weight is evenly distributed on both feet with heels together.
- Occiput, scapulae, buttocks, and heels are in contact with vertical surface.
- Encourage child to maintain fully erect position with positional lordosis minimized, knees fully extended, and heels flat. Reposition as necessary.
- Child continues normal breathing with shoulders relaxed and arms hanging down freely.
- Position head in the horizontal Frankfort plane (imaginary line from the lower border of the orbit through the highest point of the auditory meatus; the line is parallel to the headboard and perpendicular to the vertical surface).
- Move headboard down to crown of head, compressing the hair.
- Read measurement to the last completed millimeter or $\frac{1}{16}$ inch at eye level to avoid a parallax error.
- Reposition the child and repeat procedure. Measure at least twice (ideally three times). Average the measurements for the final value. Record immediately.

Quality control measures (Foote, 2014; Foote, Brady, Burke, et al., 2011).

- Personnel who measure the growth of infants, children, and adolescents need proper education. Competency should be demonstrated. Refresher sessions should occur when a lack of standardization occurs.
- Length boards and stadiometers must be assembled and installed properly and calibrated at regular intervals (ideally daily, at least monthly, and every time they are moved) due to frequent inaccuracy and the variability between different instruments. Calibration can be performed by measuring a rod of known length and adjusting the instrument accordingly.
- All children should be measured at least twice (ideally three times) during each encounter. The measurements should agree within 0.5 cm (ideally 0.3 cm). Use the mean value. If the variation exceeds the limit of agreement, measure again and use the mean of the measures in closest agreement. If none of the measures are within the limit of agreement, (1) have another measurer assist, (2) check technique, and (3) consider another education session.
- Children between 24 and 36 months of age may have length and/or height measured. Standing height is less than recumbent length due to gravity and compression of the spine. Plot length measurements on a length curve and height measurements on a height curve to avoid misinterpreting the growth pattern.

Special considerations (Foote, 2014; Foote, Brady, Burke, et al., 2011; Lohman, Roche, & Martorell, 1988).

- Some children, such as those who are obese, may not be able to place their occiput, scapulae, buttocks, and heels all in one vertical plane while maintaining their balance, so use at least two of the four contact points.
- If a child has a leg length discrepancy, place a block or wedge of suitable height under the shortest leg until the pelvis is level and both knees are fully extended before measuring height. To measure length, keep the legs together and measure to the heel of the longest leg.
- Children with special health care needs may have alternative measurements taken, such as arm span, sitting height, crown-rump length, knee height, or other segmental lengths. In general, when recumbent length is measured in a child with spasticity or contractures, measure the side of the body that is unaffected or less affected.
- Always document the presence of any condition that may interfere with an accurate and reliable measurement.

Apply the Evidence: Nursing Implications

Growth is well established as an important and sensitive indicator of health in children. Abnormal growth is a common consequence of many conditions; therefore its measurement can be a useful warning of possible pathology. In a study of 55 primary care practices within eight geographic areas in the United States, only 30% of children were measured accurately due to faulty instruments and casual techniques; an educational intervention increased measurement accuracy to 70% (Lipman, Hench, Benyi, et al., 2004). Measurement error influences growth assessment and can result in delayed evaluation and treatment of some children, as well as apparent growth deviation in others who are actually growing normally (Foote, 2014). There is good evidence with strong recommendations for using length boards and stadiometers, the described measurement techniques, and the quality control measures. There is fair evidence to recommend procedures for children with special needs (Foote, Brady, Burke, et al., 2009; Lohman, Roche, & Martorell, 1988).

Quality and Safety Competencies: Evidence-Based Practice*

Knowledge

- Differentiate clinical opinion from research and evidence-based summaries.
- Describe the appropriate instruments and techniques to obtain accurate and reliable linear growth measurements of children.

Skills

- Base individualized care plan on patient values, clinical expertise, and evidence.
- Integrate evidence into practice by using the instruments and techniques for linear growth measurement in clinical care.

Attitudes

- Value the concept of evidence-based practice as integral to determining best clinical practice.
- Appreciate strengths and weakness of evidence for measuring the linear growth of children.

References

Foote, J. M. (2014). Optimizing linear growth measurement in children. *Journal of Pediatric Health Care, 28*(5), 413–419.

Foote, J. M., Brady, L. H., Burke, A. L., et al. (2009). Evidence-based clinical practice guideline on linear growth measurement of children. Retrieved from http://www.blankchildrens.

TRANSLATING EVIDENCE INTO PRACTICE—cont'd

Linear Growth Measurement of Children

org/linear-growth-measurement.aspx (to access full-text guideline and implementation tools).

Foote, J. M., Brady, L. H., Burke, A. L., et al. (2011). Development of an evidence-based clinical practice guideline on linear growth measurement of children. *Journal of Pediatric Nursing, 26*(4), 312–324.

Lipman, T. H., Hench, K. D., Benyi, T., et al. (2004). A multicentre randomised controlled trial of an intervention to improve the accuracy of linear growth measurement. *Archives of Disease in Childhood, 89*, 342–346.

Lohman, T. J., Roche, A. F., & Martorell, R. (Eds.), (1988). *Anthropometric standardization reference manual.* Champaign, IL: Human Kinetics Books.

US Preventive Services Task Force. (1996). *Guide to clinical preventive services: Report of the US Preventive Services Task Force* (2nd ed.). Philadelphia, PA: Lippincott Williams & Wilkins.

Jan M. Foote

*Adapted from the Quality and Safety Education for Nurses (QSEN) Institute.

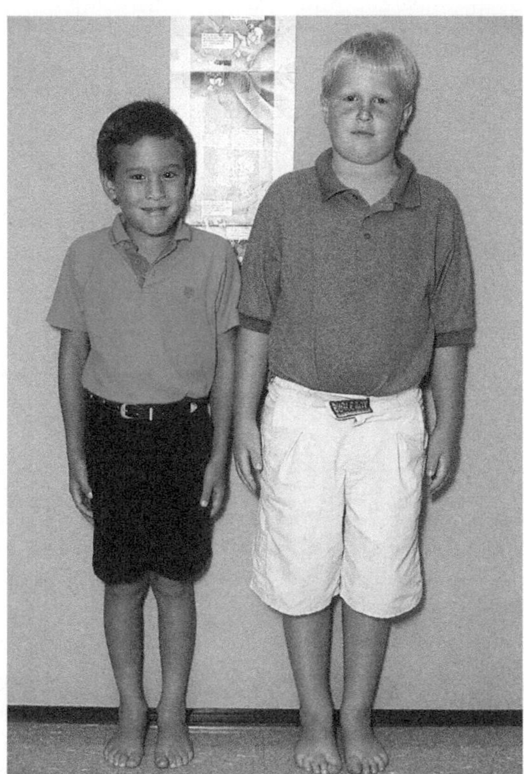

FIG. 4.8 These children of identical age (8 years) are markedly different in size. The child on the left, of Asian descent, is at the 5th percentile for height and weight. The child on the right is above the 95th percentile for height and weight. However, both children demonstrate normal growth patterns because they are growing and gaining weight at normal rates.

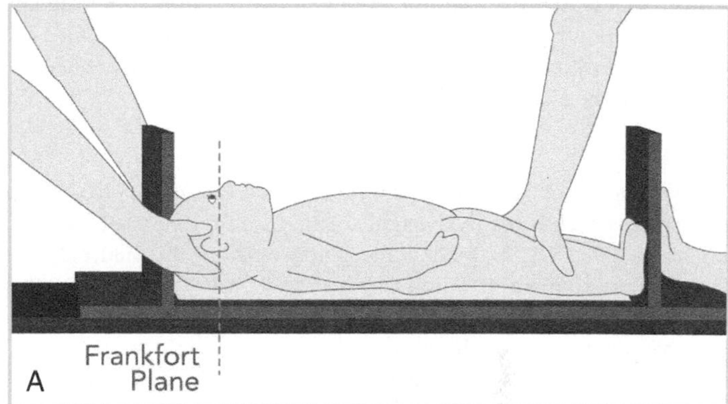

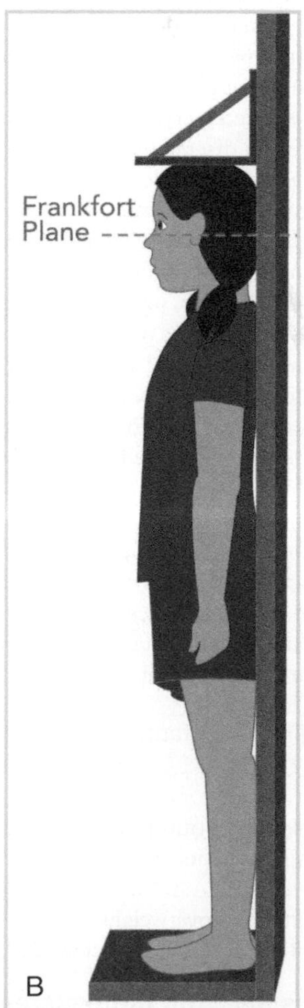

FIG. 4.9 Measurement of linear growth. **A,** Infant length. **B,** Child height. (Courtesy Jan M. Foote, Blank Children's Hospital, Des Moines, IA.)

Height

The term *height* (or *stature*) refers to the measurement taken when a child is standing upright. Wall charts and flip-up horizontal bars (floppy-arm devices) mounted to weighing scales should not be used to measure the height of children (Foote, Brady, Burke, et al., 2009). These devices are not steady and do not maintain a right angle to the vertical ruler, preventing an accurate and reliable height. Measure height by having the child, with shoes removed, stand as tall and straight as possible with the head in midline and the line of vision parallel to the ceiling and floor. Be certain the child's back is to the wall or other vertical flat surface, with the head, shoulder blades, buttocks, and heels touching the wall and the medial malleoli touching if possible (Fig. 4.9, *B*). Check for and correct slumping of the shoulders, positional lordosis, bending of the knees, or raising of the heels.

> **! NURSING ALERT**
>
> Normally height is less if measured in the afternoon than in the morning. The time of day should be recorded when measurements are taken (Foote, Brady, Burke, et al., 2009). For children in whom there are concerns about growth, serial measurements should be taken at the same time of day to establish an accurate growth velocity (see Translating Evidence into Practice box).

For the most accurate measurement, use a wall-mounted unit (**stadiometer**; see Fig. 4.9, *B*). To improvise a flat, vertical surface for measuring height, attach a paper or metal tape or yardstick to the wall, position the child adjacent to the tape, and place a three-dimensional object, such as a thick book or box, on top of the head. Rest the side of the object firmly against the wall to form a right angle. Measure height or stature to the last completed millimeter or $\frac{1}{16}$ inch.

Weight

Weight is measured with an appropriately sized electronic or balance beam scale, which measures weight to the nearest 10 g (0.35 oz) for infants and 100 g (0.22 lb) for children. Before weighing the child, balance the scale by setting it at 0 and noting if the balance registers at exactly 0 or in the middle of the mark. If the end of the balance beam rises to the top or bottom of the mark, more or less weight, respectively, is needed. Some scales are designed to self-correct, but others need to be recalibrated according to the manufacturer instructions. Scales vary in their accuracy; infant scales tend to be more accurate than adult platform scales, and newer scales tend to be more accurate than older ones, especially at the upper levels of weight measurement. When precise measurements are necessary, two nurses should take the weight independently; if there is a discrepancy, take a third reading and use the mean of the measurements in closest agreement.

Take measurements in a comfortably warm room. When birth-to-2-year or birth-to-36-month growth charts are used, children should be weighed nude. Older children are usually weighed while wearing their underpants, a gown, or light clothing, depending on the setting. However, always respect the privacy of all children. If the child must be weighed wearing some type of special device, such as a prosthesis or an armboard for an intravenous device, note this when recording the weight. Children who are measured for recumbent length are usually weighed on an infant scale and placed in a lying or sitting position. When weighing a child, place your hand slightly above the infant to prevent him or her from accidentally falling off the scale (Fig. 4.10, *A*) or stand close to the toddler, ready to prevent a fall (Fig. 4.10, *B*). For maximum asepsis, clean the scale and cover the scale with a clean sheet of paper between each child's weight measurement.

Nurses need to be familiar with determining body mass index (BMI), which requires accurate information about the child's weight and height.

$$\text{BMI} = \text{Weight in kilograms} \div [\text{Height in meters}]^2$$

or

$$\text{BMI} = [\text{Weight in pounds} \div (\text{Height in inches} \times \text{Height in inches})] \times 703$$

With the increasing number of overweight children in the United States, the BMI charts are a critical component of children's physical assessment.

Skinfold Thickness and Arm Circumference

Measures of relative weight and stature cannot distinguish between adipose (fat) tissue and muscle. One convenient measure of body fat is **skinfold thickness**, which is increasingly recommended as a routine measurement. Measure skinfold thickness with special calipers, such as the Lange calipers. The most common sites for measuring skinfold thickness are the triceps (most practical for routine clinical use), subscapular, suprailiac, abdomen, and upper thigh. For greatest reliability, follow the exact procedure for measurement and record the average of at least two measurements of one site.

Arm circumference is an indirect measure of muscle mass. Measurement of arm circumference follows the same procedure as for skinfold thickness except the midpoint is measured with a paper, nonstretchable plastic, or steel tape. Place the tape vertically along the posterior aspect of the upper arm from the acromial process to the olecranon process; half the measured length is the midpoint. World Health Organization growth curves are available for triceps skinfold and arm circumference measurements.

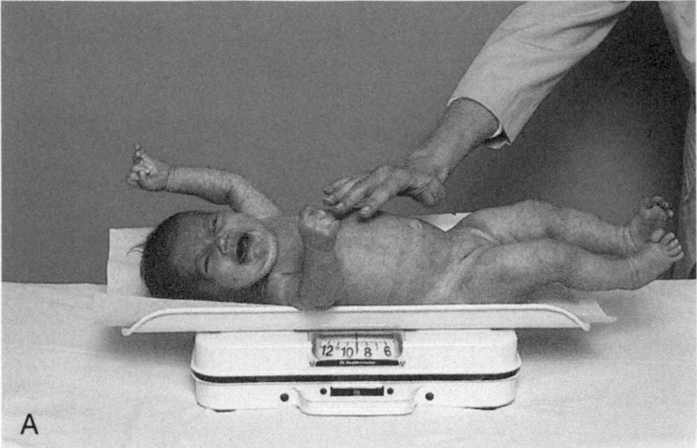

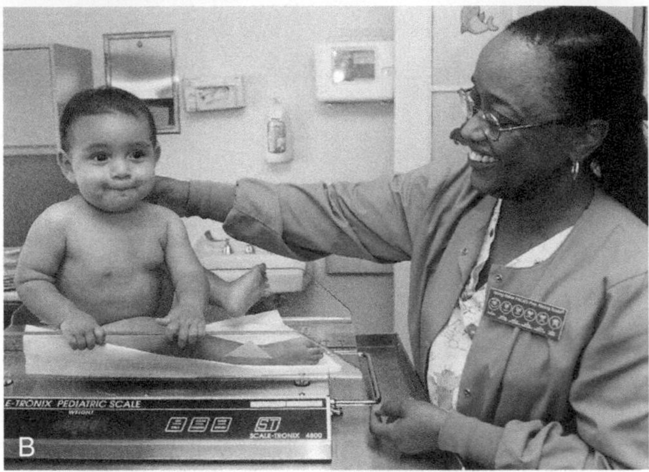

FIG. 4.10 A, Infant on scale. **B,** Toddler on scale. Note the presence of nurse to prevent falls. (*B,* Courtesy Paul Vincent Kuntz, Texas Children's Hospital, Houston, TX.)

> **! NURSING ALERT**
>
> BMI-for-age and gender is used to identify children and adolescents who are either underweight (<5th percentile), healthy weight (5th to <85th percentile), overweight (≥85th percentile and <95th percentile), or obese (≥95th percentile).

Head Circumference

Head circumference is a reflection of brain growth. Measure head circumference in children up to 36 months of age and in any child whose

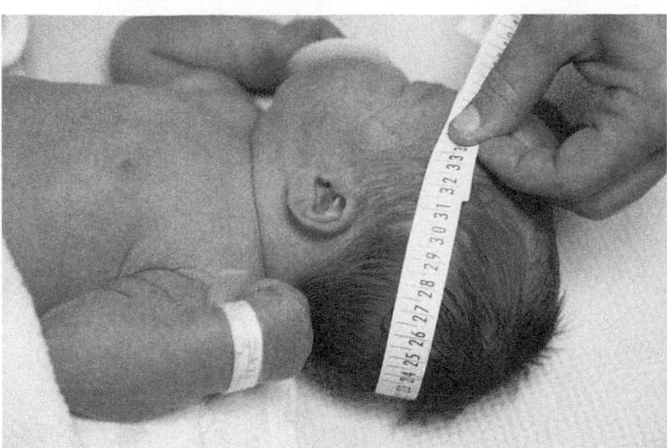

FIG. 4.11 Measurement of head circumference. (From Seidel, H. M., Ball, J. W., Dains, J. E., et al. [1999]. *Mosby's guide to physical examination* [4th ed.]. St. Louis, MO: Mosby.)

head size is questionable. Measure the head at its greatest frontooccipital circumference, usually slightly above the eyebrows and pinna of the ears and around the occipital prominence at the back of the skull (Fig. 4.11). Use a paper or nonstretchable tape, or insert-a-tape, marked in millimeter or 1/16-inch increments because a cloth tape can stretch and give a falsely small measurement. Because head shape can affect the location of the maximum circumference, more than one measurement is necessary to obtain the most accurate measure. Measure head circumference to the last completed millimeter or 1/16 inch.

Plot the head size on the appropriate growth chart for head circumference. Generally, head and chest circumferences are equal at about 1 to 2 years of age. During childhood, chest circumference exceeds head size by about 5 to 7 cm (2 to 2.75 inches). For newborns, see Chapter 7.

PHYSIOLOGIC MEASUREMENTS

Physiologic measurements, key elements in evaluating physical status of vital functions, include temperature, pulse, respiration, and blood pressure. Compare each physiologic recording with normal values for that age group. In addition, compare the values taken on preceding health visits with present recordings. For example, a falsely elevated blood pressure reading may not indicate hypertension if previous recent readings have been within normal limits. The isolated recording may indicate some stressful event in the child's life.

As in most procedures carried out with children, treat older children and adolescents much the same as adults. However, give special consideration to preschool children (see Atraumatic Care box). For best results in taking vital signs of infants, count respirations first (before the infant is disturbed), take the pulse next, and measure temperature last. If vital signs cannot be taken without disturbing the child, record the child's behavior (e.g., crying) along with the measurement.

ATRAUMATIC CARE

Reducing Young Children's Fears

Young children, especially preschoolers, fear intrusive procedures because of their poorly defined body boundaries. Therefore avoid invasive procedures, such as measuring rectal temperature, whenever possible. Also, avoid using the word "take" when measuring vital signs because young children interpret words literally and may think that their temperature or other function will be taken away. Instead, say, "I want to know how warm you are."

Temperature

Temperature is the measure of heat content within an individual's body. The core temperature most closely reflects the temperature of the blood flow through the carotid arteries to the hypothalamus. Core temperature is relatively constant despite wide fluctuations in the external environment. When a child's temperature is altered, receptors in the skin, spinal cord, and brain respond in an attempt to achieve normothermia, a normal temperature state. In pediatrics, there is a lack of consensus regarding what temperature constitutes normothermia for every child. For rectal temperatures in children, a value of 37° to 37.5° C (98.6° to 99.5° F) is an acceptable range, where heat loss and heat production are balanced. For neonates, a core body temperature between 36.5° and 37.6° C (97.7° and 99.7° F) is a desirable range. In the neonate, obtain temperature measurements for monitoring adequacy of thermoregulation, not just for fever; therefore temperature measurements in each infant should be carefully considered in the context of the purpose and the environment.

The nurse can measure temperature in healthy children at several body sites via oral, rectal, axillary, ear canal (tympanic membrane), temporal artery, or skin route. For the ill child, other sites for temperature measurement have been investigated. Skin temperature sensors are most often used for neonates and infants placed in radiant heat warmers or incubators. The pulmonary artery is the closest to the hypothalamus and best reflects the core temperature (Batra, Faridi, & Saha, 2012). Other sites used are the distal esophagus, urinary bladder, and nasopharynx. All these methods are invasive and difficult to use in clinical practice. Temperature measured by rectal thermometry is considered the closest to core temperature, but it has some drawbacks. Tympanic membrane thermometry for children older than 2 years of age and temporal artery thermometry in all age groups are taking precedence over other methods (Batra & Goyal, 2013; Batra, Faridi, & Saha, 2012). One of the most important influences on the accuracy of temperature is improper temperature-taking technique. Detailed discussion of temperature taking methods and visual examples of proper techniques are given in Table 4.3. For a critical review of the evidence on temperature taking methods, see the Translating Evidence into Practice box.

The most frequently used temperature measurement devices in infants and children include the following:

- **Electronic intermittent thermometers** measure the patient's temperature at oral, rectal, and axillary sites and are used as primary diagnostic indicators
- **Infrared thermometers** measure the patient's temperature by collecting emitted thermal radiation from a particular site (e.g., ear canal)
- **Electronic continuous thermometers** measure the patient's temperature during the administration of general anesthesia, treatment of hypothermia or hyperthermia, and other situations that require continuous monitoring

Pulse

A satisfactory pulse can be taken radially in children older than 2 years of age. However, in infants and young children, the apical impulse (heard through a stethoscope held to the chest at the apex of the heart) is more reliable (see Fig. 4.33 for location of pulses). Count the pulse for 1 full minute in infants and young children because of possible irregularities in rhythm. However, when frequent apical rates are necessary, use shorter counting times (e.g., 15- or 30-second intervals). For greater accuracy, measure the apical rate while the child is asleep; record the child's behavior along with the rate. Grade pulses according to the criteria in Table 4.4. Compare radial and femoral pulses at least once during infancy to detect the presence of circulatory impairment, such

TABLE 4.3 Temperature Measurement Locations for Infants and Children

Temperature Site

Oral

Place tip under tongue in right or left posterior sublingual pocket, not in front of tongue. Have child keep mouth closed, without biting on thermometer.

Pacifier thermometers measure intraoral or supralingual temperature and are available but lack support in the literature.

Several factors affect mouth temperature: Eating and mastication, hot or cold beverages, open-mouth breathing, and ambient temperature.

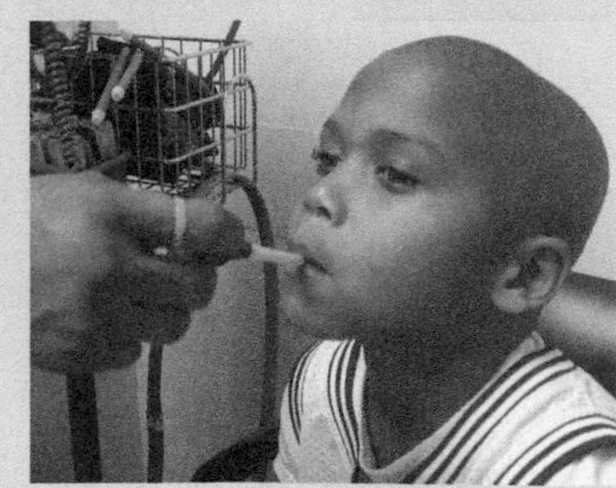

Axillary

Place tip under arm in center of axilla and keep close to skin, not clothing. Hold child's arm firmly against side. Temperature may be affected by poor peripheral perfusion (results in lower value); clothing or swaddling, use of radiant warmer, or amount of brown fat in cold-stressed neonate (results in higher value).

Advantage: Avoids intrusive procedure and eliminates risk of rectal perforation.

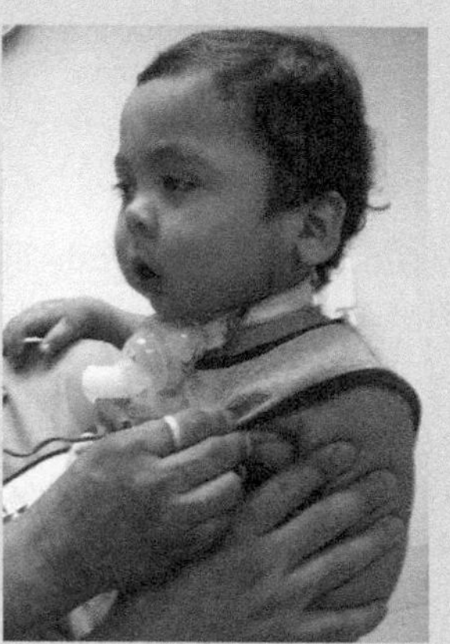

Ear Based (Aural)

Insert small infrared probe deeply into canal to allow sensor to obtain measurement from tympanic membrane.

Size of probe (most are 8 mm) may influence accuracy of result. In young children, this may be a problem because of small diameter of canal.

Proper placement of ear is controversial related to whether the pinna should be pulled in manner similar to that used during otoscopy.

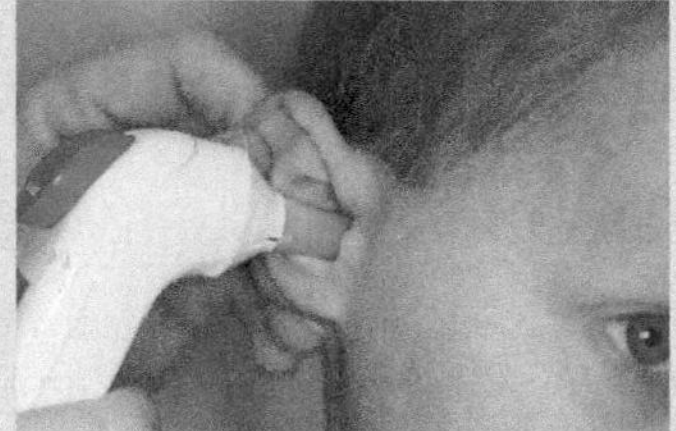

Rectal

Place well-lubricated tip at maximum 2.5 cm (1 inch) into rectum for children and 1.5 cm (0.6 inch) for infants; securely hold thermometer close to anus.

Child may be placed in side-lying, supine, or prone position (i.e., supine with knees flexed toward abdomen); cover penis because procedure may stimulate urination. A small child may be placed prone across parent's lap.

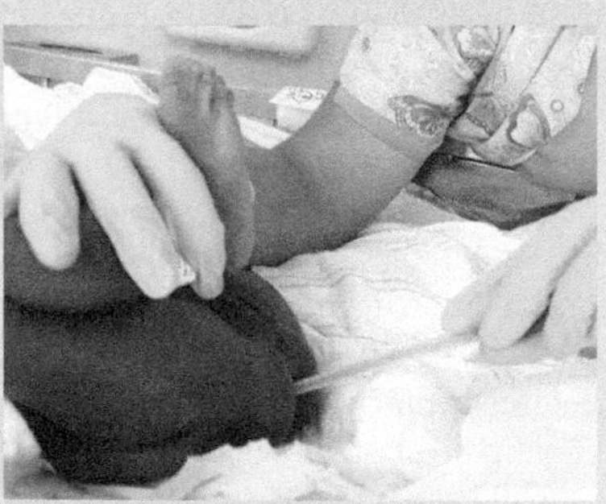

Temporal Artery

An infrared sensor probe scans across forehead, capturing heat from arterial blood flow.

Temporal artery is only artery close enough to skin's surface to provide access for accurate temperature measurement.

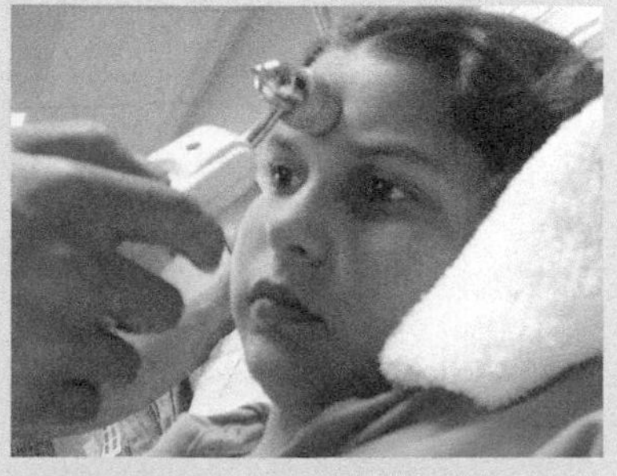

Data from Martin, S. A., & Kline, A. M. (2004). Can there be a standard for temperature measurement in the pediatric intensive care unit? *AACN Clinical Issues, 15*(2), 254-266; Falzon, A., Grech, V., Caruana, B., et al. (2003). How reliable is axillary temperature measurement? *Acta Paediatrica, 92*(3), 309-313. Oral, axillary, rectal, and temporal artery images courtesy Paul Vincent Kuntz, Texas Children's Hospital, Houston, TX.

TRANSLATING EVIDENCE INTO PRACTICE

Temperature Measurement

Ask the Question

PICOT Question

In infants and children, what is the most accurate method for measuring temperature in febrile children?

Search for the Evidence

Search Strategies

Clinical studies related to this issue were identified by searching for English publications within the past 15 years for infant and child populations; comparisons to gold standard: rectal thermometry.

Databases Used

PubMed, Cochrane Collaboration, MD Consult, Joanna Briggs Institute, National Guideline Clearinghouse (AHRQ), TRIP Database Plus, PedsCCM, BestBETs.

Critical Appraisal of the Evidence

- **Rectal temperature:** Rectal measurement remains the clinical gold standard for the precise diagnosis of fever in infants and children compared with other methods (Fortuna, Carney, Macy, et al., 2010; Holzhauer, Reith, Sawin, et al., 2009). However, this procedure is more invasive and is contraindicated for infants younger than 1 month old due to risk of rectal perforation (Batra, Faridi, & Saha, 2012). Children with recent rectal surgery, diarrhea, or anorectal lesions, or who are receiving chemotherapy (cancer treatment usually affects mucosa and causes neutropenia), should not undergo rectal thermometry.
- **Oral temperature (OT):** OT indicates rapid changes in core body temperature, but accuracy may be an issue compared with the rectal site (Batra, Faridi, & Saha, 2012). OTs are considered the standard for noninvasive temperature measurement (Gilbert, Barton, & Counsell, 2002), but they are contraindicated in children who have an altered level of consciousness, are receiving oxygen, are mouth breathing, are experiencing mucositis, had recent oral surgery or trauma, are under 5 years of age, or cannot hold the thermometer under their tongue (El-Radhi & Barry, 2006). Limitations of OTs include the effects of ambient room temperature and recent oral intake (Martin & Kline, 2004).
- **Axillary temperature:** Axillary temperature is inconsistent and insensitive in infants and children over 1 month old (Falzon, Grech, Caruana, et al., 2003; Jean-Mary, Dicanzio, Shaw, et al., 2002; Stine, Flook, & Vincze, 2012). A systematic review of 20 studies concluded that axillary thermometers showed variation in findings and are not a good method for accurate temperature assessment (Craig, Lancaster, Williamson, et al., 2005). In neonates with fever, the axillary temperature should not be used interchangeably with rectal measurement (Hissink Muller, van Berkel, & de Beaufort, 2008). It can be used as a screening tool for fever in young, clinically stable infants and children (Batra, Faridi, & Saha, 2012; Charafeddine, Tamim, Hassouna, et al., 2014).
- **Ear (aural) temperature:** This is not a precise measurement of body temperature. A meta-analysis of 101 studies comparing tympanic membrane temperatures with rectal temperatures in children concluded that the tympanic method demonstrated a wide range of variability, limiting its application in a pediatric setting (Craig, Lancaster, Taylor, et al., 2002). Other published reviews continue to find poor sensitivity using infrared ear thermometry (Devrim, Ates, Ceyhan, et al., 2007; Dodd, Lancaster, Craig, et al., 2006). Tympanic thermometry is used for screening purposes, but diagnosis of fever without a focus should not be made based on tympanic thermometry because it is not an accurate measure of core temperature (Batra, Faridi, & Saha, 2012; Devrim, Ates, Ceyhan, et al., 2007; Dodd, Lancaster, Craig, et al., 2006).
- **Temporal artery temperature (TAT):** TAT is not predictable for fever in young children. With proper use TAT can be a screening tool for detecting fever less than 38° C (100.4° F) in children 3 months to 4 years of age (Al-Mukhaizeem, Allen, Komar, et al., 2004; Callanan, 2003; Fortuna, Carney, Macy, et al., 2010; Hebbar, Fortenberry, Rogers, et al., 2005; Hoffman, Etwaru, Dreisinger, et al., 2013; Holzhauer, Reith, Sawin, et al., 2009; Reynolds, Bonham, Gueck, et al., 2014; Schuh, Komar, Stephens, et al., 2004; Siberry, Diener-West, Schappell, et al., 2002; Titus, Hulsey, Heckman, et al., 2009). However, a study by Batra and Goyal (2013) found that temporal artery temperature correlated better with rectal temperature than axillary and tympanic measures in a group of 50 febrile and 50 afebrile children between the ages of 2 and 12 years.

Apply the Evidence: Nursing Implications

- No single site used for temperature assessment provides unequivocal estimates of core body temperature.
- Studies show that the axillary and tympanic measures demonstrate poor agreement when these modes are compared with more accurate core temperature methods. The differences are more evident as temperature increases, regardless of age.
- TAT is not predictable for fever and should be only used as a screening tool in young children.
- When an accurate method for obtaining a correct reflection of core temperature is needed, the rectal temperature is recommended in younger children and the oral route in older children.
- For infants younger than 1 month of age, axillary temperatures are recommended for screening.

Quality and Safety Competencies: Evidence-Based Practice*

Knowledge

- Differentiate clinical opinion from research and evidence-based summaries.
- Demonstrate understanding of thermometry selection based on the developmental age of the child.

Skills

- Base individualized care plan on patient values, clinical expertise, and evidence.
- Integrate evidence into practice by using the correct type of thermometry to screen for fever compared with measures used for accurate determination of the degree of fever.

Attitudes

- Value the concept of evidence-based practice as integral to determining best clinical practice.
- Recognize strengths and weakness of evidence for the most accurate method for measuring temperature and fever in infants and children.

References

Al-Mukhaizeem, F., Allen, U., Komar, L., et al. (2004). Comparison of temporal artery, rectal and esophageal core temperatures in children: Results of a pilot study. *Paediatrics & Child Health, 9*(7), 461–465.

Batra, P., Faridi, M. M., & Saha, A. (2012). Thermometry in children. *Journal of Emergencies, Trauma, and Shock, 5*(3), 246–249.

Batra, P., & Goyal, S. (2013). Comparison of rectal, axillary, tympanic, and temporal artery thermometry in the pediatric emergency room. *Pediatric Emergency Care, 29*(1), 63–66.

Callanan, D. (2003). Detecting fever in young infants: Reliability of perceived, pacifier, and temporal artery temperatures in infants younger than 3 months of age. *Pediatric Emergency Care, 19*(4), 240–243.

Charafeddine, L., Tamim, H., Hassouna, H., et al. (2014). Axillary and rectal thermometry in the newborn: Do they agree? *BMC Research Notes, 7*, 584. Retrieved from http://www.biomedcentral.com/1756-0500/7/584.

Craig, J. V., Lancaster, G. A., Taylor, S., et al. (2002). Infrared ear thermometry compared with rectal thermometry in children: A systemic review. *Lancet, 360*, 603–609.

Craig, J. V., Lancaster, G. A., Williamson, P. R., et al. (2005). Temperature measured at the axilla compared with rectum in children and young people: Systematic review. *BMJ (Clinical Research Ed.), 320*(7243), 1174–1178.

Devrim, I., Ates, K., Ceyhan, M., et al. (2007). Measurement accuracy of fever by tympanic and axillary thermometry. *Pediatric Emergency Care, 23*(1), 16–19.

Continued

TRANSLATING EVIDENCE INTO PRACTICE—cont'd

Temperature Measurement

Dodd, S. R., Lancaster, G. A., Craig, J. V., et al. (2006). In a systematic review, infrared ear thermometry for fever diagnosis in children finds poor sensitivity. *Journal of Clinical Epidemiology, 59*, 354–357.

El-Radhi, A. S., & Barry, W. (2006). Thermometry in paediatric practice. *Archives of Disease in Childhood, 91*(4), 351–356.

Falzon, A., Grech, V., Caruana, B., et al. (2003). How reliable is axillary temperature measurement? *Acta Paediatrica, 92*(3), 309–313.

Fortuna, E. L., Carney, M. M., Macy, M., et al. (2010). Accuracy of non-contact infrared thermometry versus rectal thermometry in young children evaluated in the emergency department for fever. *Journal of Emergency Nursing, 36*(2), 101–104.

Gilbert, M., Barton, A. J., & Counsell, C. M. (2002). Comparison of oral and tympanic temperatures in adult surgical patients. *Applied Nursing Research, 15*(1), 42–47.

Hebbar, K., Fortenberry, J. D., Rogers, K., et al. (2005). Comparison of temporal artery thermometer to standard temperature measurement in pediatric intensive care unit patients. *Pediatric Critical Care Medicine: A Journal of the Society of Critical Care Medicine and the World Federation of Pediatric Intensive and Critical Care Societies, 6*(5), 557–561.

Hissink Muller, P. C., van Berkel, L. H., & de Beaufort, A. J. (2008). Axillary and rectal temperature measurements poorly agree in newborn infants. *Neonatology, 94*(1), 31–34.

Hoffman, R. J., Etwaru, K., Dreisinger, N., et al. (2013). Comparison of temporal artery thermometry and rectal thermometry in febrile pediatric emergency department patients. *Pediatric Emergency Care, 29*(3), 301–304.

Holzhauer, J. K., Reith, V., Sawin, K., et al. (2009). Evaluation of temporal artery thermometry in children 3-36 months old. *Journal for Specialists in Pediatric Nursing, 14*(4), 239–244.

Jean-Mary, M. B., Dicanzio, J., Shaw, J., et al. (2002). Limited accuracy and reliability of infrared axillary and aural thermometers in a pediatric outpatient population. *The Journal of Pediatrics, 141*(5), 671–676.

Martin, S. A., & Kline, A. M. (2004). Can there be a standard for temperature measurement in the pediatric intensive care unit? *AACN Clin Issues, 15*(2), 254–266.

Reynolds, M., Bonham, L., Gueck, M., et al. (2014). Are temporal artery temperatures accurate enough to replace rectal temperature measurement in pediatric ED patients? *Journal of Emergency Nursing, 40*(1), 46–50.

Schuh, S., Komar, L., Stephens, D., et al. (2004). Comparison of the temporal artery and rectal thermometry in children in the emergency department. *Pediatric Emergency Care, 20*(11), 736–741.

Siberry, G. K., Diener-West, M., Schappell, E., et al. (2002). Comparison of temple temperatures with rectal temperatures in children under 2 years of age. *Clinical Pediatrics, 41*(6), 405–414.

Stine, C. A., Flook, D. M., & Vincze, D. L. (2012). Rectal versus axillary temperatures: Is there a significant difference in infants less than 1 year of age? *Journal of Pediatric Nursing, 3*, 265–270.

Titus, M. O., Huley, T., Heckman, J., et al. (2009). Temporal artery thermometry utilization in pediatric emergency care. *Clinical Pediatrics, 48*(2), 190–193.

Jan Foote

*Based on Quality and Safety Education for Nurses (QSEN) Institute.

! NURSING ALERT

The belief that core temperature can be estimated by adding 1° F to the temperature taken in the axilla is incorrect. Do not add a degree to the finding obtained by taking a temperature by the axillary route.

TABLE 4.4 Grading of Pulses

Grade	Description
0	Not palpable
+1	Difficult to palpate, thready, weak, easily obliterated with pressure
+2	Difficult to palpate, may be obliterated with pressure
+3	Easy to palpate, not easily obliterated with pressure (normal)
+4	Strong, bounding, not obliterated with pressure

as coarctation of the aorta. (See inside back cover for normal rates for pediatric age-groups.)

Respiration

Count the respiratory rate in children in the same manner as for adult patients. However, in infants, observe abdominal movements because respirations are primarily diaphragmatic. Because the movements are irregular, count them for 1 full minute for accuracy (see also the Chest section later in this chapter). (See inside back cover for normal respiratory rates in children.)

Blood Pressure

Blood pressure (BP) should be measured annually in children 3 years of age through adolescence and in children with symptoms of hypertension, children in emergency departments and intensive care units, and high-risk infants (National High Blood Pressure Education Program Working Group on High Blood Pressure in Children and Adolescents, 2004). Auscultation remains the recommended method of BP measurement in children, under most circumstances. Use of the automated devices is preferred for BP measurement in newborns and young infants, in whom auscultation is difficult, and in the intensive care setting, where frequent BP measurement is needed.

Oscillometric devices measure mean arterial BP and then calculate systolic and diastolic values. The algorithms used by companies are proprietary and differ from company to company and device to device. These devices can yield results that vary widely when one is compared with another, and they do not always closely match BP values obtained by auscultation. An elevated BP reading obtained with an oscillometric device should be repeated using auscultation.

BP readings using oscillometry, such as Dinamap, are generally higher (10 mm Hg higher) than measurements using auscultation (Park, Menard, & Schoolfield, 2005). Differences between Dinamap and auscultatory readings prevent the interchange of the readings by the two methods.

Selection of Cuff

No matter what type of noninvasive technique is used, the most important factor in accurately measuring BP is the use of an appropriately sized cuff (**cuff size** refers only to the inner inflatable bladder, not the cloth covering). A technique to establish an appropriate cuff size is to choose a cuff with a **bladder width** that is approximately 40% of the arm circumference midway between the olecranon and the acromion (see Research Focus box). This will usually be a cuff **bladder length** that covers 80% to 100% of the circumference of the arm (Fig. 4.12). Cuffs that are either too narrow or too wide affect the accuracy of BP measurements. If the cuff size is too small, the reading on the device is falsely high. If the cuff size is too large, the reading is falsely low.

Measurement and Interpretation

Measuring and interpreting BP in infants and children requires attention to correct procedure because (1) limb sizes vary and cuff selection must accommodate the circumference; (2) excessive pressure on the antecubital fossa affects the Korotkoff sounds; (3) children easily become anxious, which can elevate BP; and (4) BP values change with age and growth. In children and adolescents, determine the normal range of BP by body size and age. BP standards that are based on gender, age, and

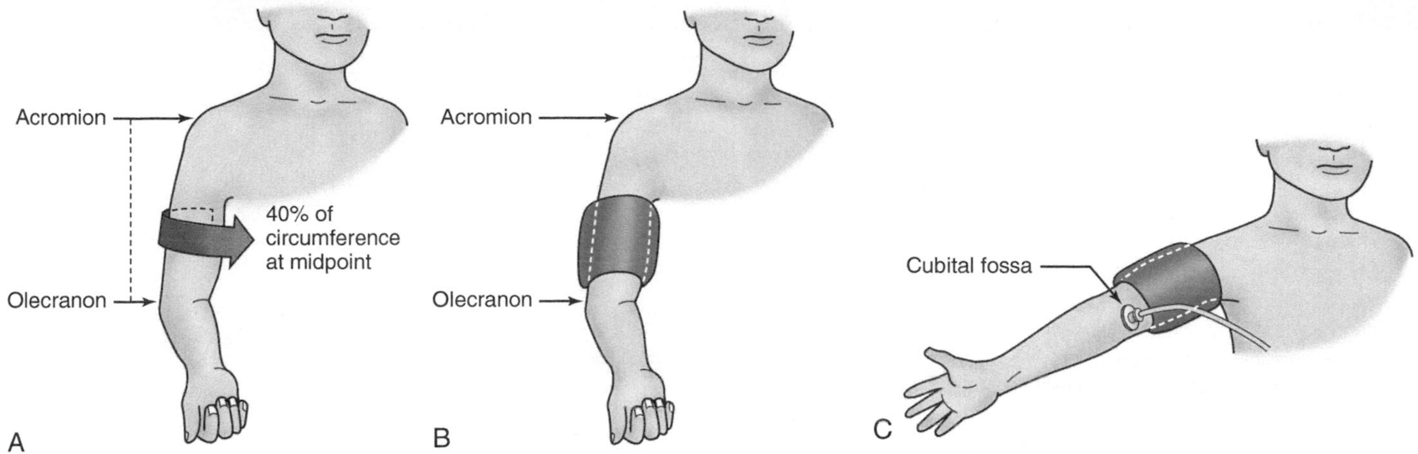

FIG. 4.12 Determination of proper cuff size. **A,** Cuff bladder width should be approximately 40% of circumference of arm measured at a point midway between olecranon and acromion. **B,** Cuff bladder length should cover 80% to 100% of circumference of arm. **C,** Blood pressure (BP) should be measured with the cubital fossa at the level of the heart. The arm should be supported. The stethoscope bell is placed over the brachial artery pulse proximal and medial to the cubital fossa and below the bottom edge of the cuff. (From National Institutes of Health, National Heart, Lung, and Blood Institute. [2005, May]. *The fourth report on the diagnosis, evaluation, and treatment of high blood pressure in children and adolescents.* NIH Pub No 05-5267 [originally printed 1996 (96-3790)]. Bethesda, MD: Author.)

! NURSING ALERT

When taking blood pressure, use an appropriately sized cuff. When the correct size is not available, use an oversized cuff rather than an undersized one or use another site that more appropriately fits the cuff size. Do not choose a cuff based on the name of the cuff (e.g., an "infant" cuff may be too small for some infants).

! NURSING ALERT

Compare blood pressure in the upper and lower extremities to detect abnormalities, such as coarctation of the aorta, in which the lower extremity pressure is less than the upper extremity pressure.

RESEARCH FOCUS

Selection of a Blood Pressure Cuff

Researchers have found that selection of a cuff with a bladder width equal to 40% of the upper arm circumference most accurately reflects directly measured radial arterial pressure (Clark, Kieh-Lai, Sarnaik, et al., 2002).

Using limb circumference for selecting cuff width more accurately reflects direct arterial blood pressure (BP) than using limb length because this method considers variations in arm thickness and the amount of pressure required to compress the artery. For measurement on sites other than the upper arms, use the limb circumference, although the shape of the limb (e.g., conical shape of the thigh) may prevent appropriate placement of the cuff and inaccurately reflect intraarterial BP (Table 4.5).

When using a site other than the arm, BP measurements using noninvasive techniques may differ. Generally, systolic BP in the lower extremities (thigh or calf) is greater than that in the upper extremities, and systolic BP in the calf is higher than that in the thigh (Schell, Briening, Lebet, et al., 2011) (Fig. 4.13).

height provide a more precise classification of BP according to body size. This approach avoids misclassifying children who are very tall or very short. The revised BP tables now include the 50th, 90th, 95th, and 99th percentiles (with standard deviations) by gender, age, and height.

To use the tables in a clinical setting, determine the height percentile by using the Centers for Disease Control and Prevention growth charts (www.cdc.gov/growthcharts). The child's measured systolic BP and diastolic BP are compared with the numbers provided in the table (boys or girls) according to the child's age and height percentile. The child is normotensive if the BP is below the 90th percentile. If the BP is at or above the 90th percentile, repeat the BP measurement to verify an elevated BP. BP measurements between the 90th and 95th percentiles indicate prehypertension and necessitate reassessment and consideration of other risk factors. In addition, if an adolescent's BP is more than 120/80 mm Hg, consider the patient prehypertensive, even if this value is below the 90th percentile. This BP level typically occurs for systolic BP at 12 years old and for diastolic BP at 16 years old. If the child's BP (systolic or diastolic) is at or above the 95th percentile, the child may be hypertensive, and the measurement must be repeated on at least two occasions to confirm diagnosis (National High Blood Pressure Education Program Working Group on High Blood Pressure in Children and Adolescents, 2004) (see Applying Evidence to Practice box).

Orthostatic Hypotension

Orthostatic hypotension (OH), also called *postural hypotension* or *orthostatic intolerance,* often manifests as syncope (fainting), vertigo (dizziness), or lightheadedness and is caused by decreased blood flow to the brain (cerebral hypoperfusion). Normally blood flow to the brain is maintained at a constant level by several compensating mechanisms that regulate systemic BP. When one assumes a sitting or standing position from a supine or recumbent position, peripheral capillary vasoconstriction occurs, and blood that was pooling in the lower vasculature is returned to the heart for redistribution to the head and remainder of the body. When this mechanism fails or is slow to respond, the person may experience vertigo or syncope. One of the most common

TABLE 4.5 Differences in Color Changes of Racial Groups

Description	Appearance in Light Skin	Appearance in Dark Skin
Cyanosis—bluish tone through skin; reflects reduced (deoxygenated) hemoglobin	Bluish tinge, especially in palpebral conjunctiva (lower eyelid), nail beds, earlobes, lips, oral membranes, soles, and palms	Ashen gray lips and tongue
Pallor—paleness; may be sign of anemia, chronic disease, edema, or shock	Loss of rosy glow in skin, especially face	Ashen gray appearance in black skin More yellowish brown color in brown skin
Erythema—redness; may be result of increased blood flow from climatic conditions, local inflammation, infection, skin irritation, allergy, or other dermatoses, or may be caused by increased numbers of red blood cells as compensatory response to chronic hypoxia	Redness easily seen anywhere on body	Much more difficult to assess; rely on palpation for warmth or edema
Ecchymosis—large, diffuse areas, usually black and blue, caused by hemorrhage of blood into skin; typically result of injuries	Purplish to yellow-green areas; may be seen anywhere on skin	Very difficult to see unless in mouth or conjunctiva
Petechiae—same as ecchymosis except for size: small, distinct, pinpoint hemorrhages ≤2 mm in size; can denote some type of blood disorder, such as leukemia	Purplish pinpoints most easily seen on buttocks, abdomen, and inner surfaces of arms or legs	Usually invisible except in oral mucosa, conjunctiva of eyelids, and conjunctiva covering eyeball
Jaundice—yellow staining of skin usually caused by bile pigments	Yellow staining seen in sclerae of eyes, skin, fingernails, soles, palms, and oral mucosa	Most reliably assessed in sclerae, hard palate, palms, and soles

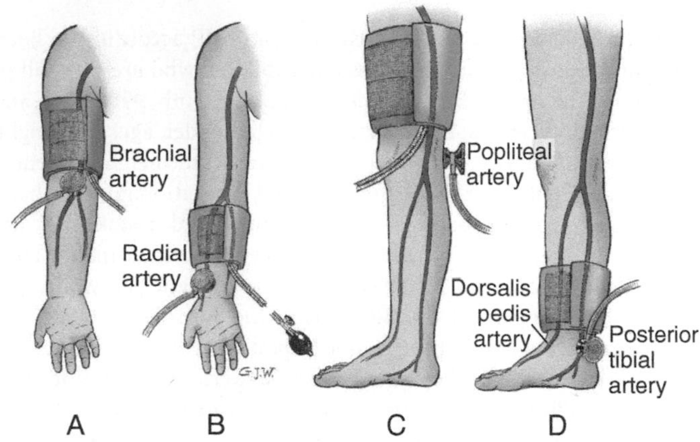

FIG. 4.13 Sites for measuring blood pressure. **A,** Upper arm. **B,** Lower arm or forearm. **C,** Thigh. **D,** Calf or ankle.

causes of OH is hypovolemia, which may be induced by medications such as diuretics, vasodilator medications, and prolonged immobility or bed rest. Other causes of OH include dehydration, diarrhea, emesis, fluid loss from sweating and exertion, alcohol intake, dysrhythmias, diabetes mellitus, sepsis, and hemorrhage.

BP measurements taken with the child first supine and then standing (at least 2 minutes in each position) may demonstrate variability and assist in the diagnosis of OH. The child with a sustained drop in systolic pressure of more than 20 mm Hg or in diastolic pressure of more than 10 mm Hg after standing for 2 minutes without an increase in heart rate of more than 15 beats/min most likely has an autonomic deficit. Nonneurogenic causes of OH have a compensatory increase in pulse of more than 15 beats/min, as well as a drop in BP, as noted previously. For children or adolescents with vertigo, lightheadedness, nausea, syncope, diaphoresis, and pallor, it is important to monitor BP and heart rate to determine the original cause. BP is an important diagnostic measurement in children and adolescents and must be a part of the routine monitoring of vital signs.

APPLYING EVIDENCE TO PRACTICE

Using the Blood Pressure Tables

1. Use the standard height charts to determine the height percentile.
2. Measure and record the child's systolic blood pressure (SBP) and diastolic blood pressure (DBP).
3. Use the correct gender table for SBP and DBP.
4. Find the child's age on the left side of the table. Follow the age row horizontally across the table to the intersection of the line for the height percentile (vertical column).
5. Then find the 50th, 90th, 95th, and 99th percentiles for SBP in the left columns and for DBP in the right columns.
   - BP less than 90th percentile is normal.
   - BP between the 90th and 95th percentiles is prehypertension. In adolescents, BP of 120/80 mm Hg or greater is prehypertension, even if this figure is less than the 90th percentile.
   - BP over the 95th percentile may be hypertension.
6. If the BP is over the 90th percentile, the BP should be repeated twice during the same patient encounter, and an average SBP and DBP should be used.
7. If the BP is over the 95th percentile, BP should be staged. If BP is stage 1 (95th to 99th percentile plus 5 mm Hg), BP measurements should be repeated on two more occasions. If hypertension is confirmed, evaluation should proceed. If BP is stage 2 (>99th percentile plus 5 mm Hg), prompt referral should be made for evaluation and therapy. If the patient is symptomatic, immediate referral and treatment are indicated.

From National High Blood Pressure Education Program Working Group on High Blood Pressure in Children and Adolescents. (2004). The fourth report on the diagnosis, evaluation, and treatment of high blood pressure in children and adolescents. *Pediatrics, 114*(2 Suppl 4th Report), 555-576.

! NURSING ALERT

Published norms for blood pressure are valid only if you use the same method of measurement (auscultation and cuff size determination) in clinical practice.

GENERAL APPEARANCE

The child's general appearance is a cumulative, subjective impression of the child's physical appearance, state of nutrition, behavior, personality, interactions with parents and nurse (also siblings if present), posture, development, and speech. Although the nurse records general appearance at the beginning of the physical examination, it encompasses all the observations of the child during the interview and physical assessment.

Note the facies, the child's facial expression and appearance. For example, the facies may give clues to children who are in pain; have difficulty breathing; feel frightened, discontented, or unhappy; are mentally delayed; or are acutely ill.

Observe the posture, position, and types of body movement. A child with hearing or vision loss may characteristically tilt the head in an awkward position to hear or see better. A child in pain may favor a body part. A child with low self-esteem or a feeling of rejection may assume a slumped, careless, and apathetic pose. Likewise, a child with confidence, a feeling of self-worth, and a sense of security usually demonstrates a tall, straight, well-balanced posture. While observing such body language, do not interpret too freely but rather record objectively.

Note the child's hygiene in terms of cleanliness; unusual body odor; the condition of the hair, neck, nails, teeth, and feet; and the condition of the clothing. Such observations are excellent clues to possible instances of neglect, inadequate financial resources, housing difficulties (e.g., no running water), or lack of knowledge concerning children's needs.

Behavior includes the child's personality, activity level, reaction to stress, requests, frustration, interactions with others (primarily the parent and nurse), degree of alertness, and response to stimuli. Some mental questions that serve as reminders for observing behavior include the following:

- What is the child's overall personality?
- Does the child have a long attention span, or is he or she easily distracted?
- Can the child follow two or three commands in succession without the need for repetition?
- What is the child's response to delayed gratification or frustration?
- Does the child use eye contact during conversation?
- What is the child's reaction to the nurse and family members?
- Is the child quick or slow to grasp explanations?

SKIN

Assess skin for color, texture, temperature, moisture, turgor, lesions, and rashes. Examination of the skin and its accessory organs primarily involves inspection and palpation. Touch allows the nurse to assess the texture, turgor, and temperature of the skin. The normal color in light-skinned children varies from a milky white and rose to a deeply hued pink. Dark-skinned children, such as those of Native American, Hispanic, or African descent, have inherited various brown, red, yellow, olive green, and bluish tones in their skin. Asian persons have skin that is normally of a yellow tone. Several variations in skin color can occur, some of which warrant further investigation. The types of color change and their appearance in children with light or dark skin are summarized in Table 4.5.

Normally the skin texture of young children is smooth, slightly dry, and not oily or clammy. Evaluate skin temperature by symmetrically feeling each part of the body and comparing upper areas with lower ones. Note any difference in temperature.

Determine tissue turgor, or elasticity in the skin, by grasping the skin on the abdomen between the thumb and index finger, pulling it taut, and quickly releasing it. Elastic tissue immediately resumes its normal position without residual marks or creases. In children with poor skin turgor, the skin remains suspended or tented for a few seconds before slowly falling back on the abdomen. Skin turgor is one of the best estimates of adequate hydration and nutrition.

Accessory Structures

Inspection of the accessory structures of the skin may be performed while examining the skin, scalp, or extremities. Inspect the hair for color, texture, quality, distribution, and elasticity. Children's scalp hair is usually lustrous, silky, strong, and elastic. Genetic factors affect the appearance of hair. For example, the hair of African American children is usually curlier and coarser than that of Caucasian children. Hair that is stringy, dull, brittle, dry, friable, and depigmented may suggest poor nutrition. Record any bald or thinning spots. Loss of hair in infants may indicate lying in the same position and may be a cue to counsel parents concerning the child's stimulation needs.

Inspect the hair and scalp for general cleanliness. Persons in some ethnic groups condition their hair with oils or lubricants that, if not thoroughly washed from the scalp, clog the sebaceous glands, causing scalp infections. Examine the scalp for lesions, scaliness, evidence of infestation (e.g., lice or ticks), and signs of trauma (e.g., ecchymosis, masses, or scars).

In children who are approaching puberty, look for growth of secondary hair as a sign of normally progressing pubertal changes. Note precocious or delayed appearance of hair growth because, although not always suggestive of hormonal dysfunction, it may be of great concern to the early-maturing child or late-maturing adolescent.

Inspect the nails for color, shape, texture, and quality. Normally the nails are pink, convex, smooth, and hard but flexible (not brittle). The edges, which are usually white, should extend over the fingers. Dark-skinned individuals may have more deeply pigmented nail beds. Short, ragged nails are typical of habitual biting. Uncut, dirty nails are a sign of poor hygiene.

The palm normally shows three flexion creases (Fig. 4.14, *A*). In some conditions, such as Down syndrome, the two distal horizontal creases may be fused to form a single horizontal crease (the single palmar crease, or transpalmar crease) (Fig. 4.14, *B*). If grossly abnormal lines or folds are observed, sketch a picture to describe them and refer the finding to a specialist for further investigation.

LYMPH NODES

Lymph nodes are usually assessed during examination of the part of the body in which they are located. The body's lymphatic drainage

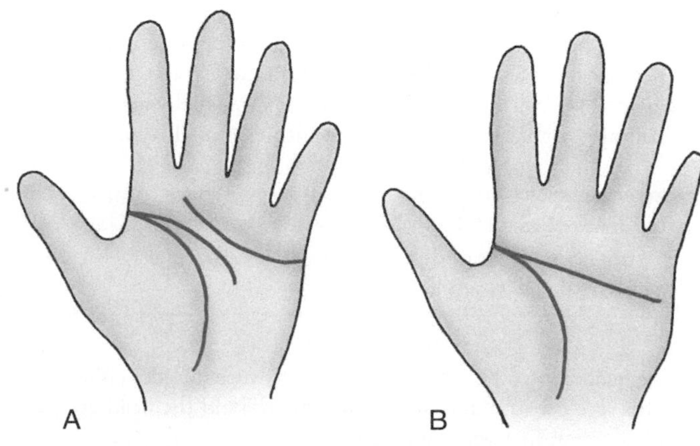

FIG. 4.14 Examples of flexion creases on palm. **A,** Normal. **B,** Single palmar crease (transpalmar crease).

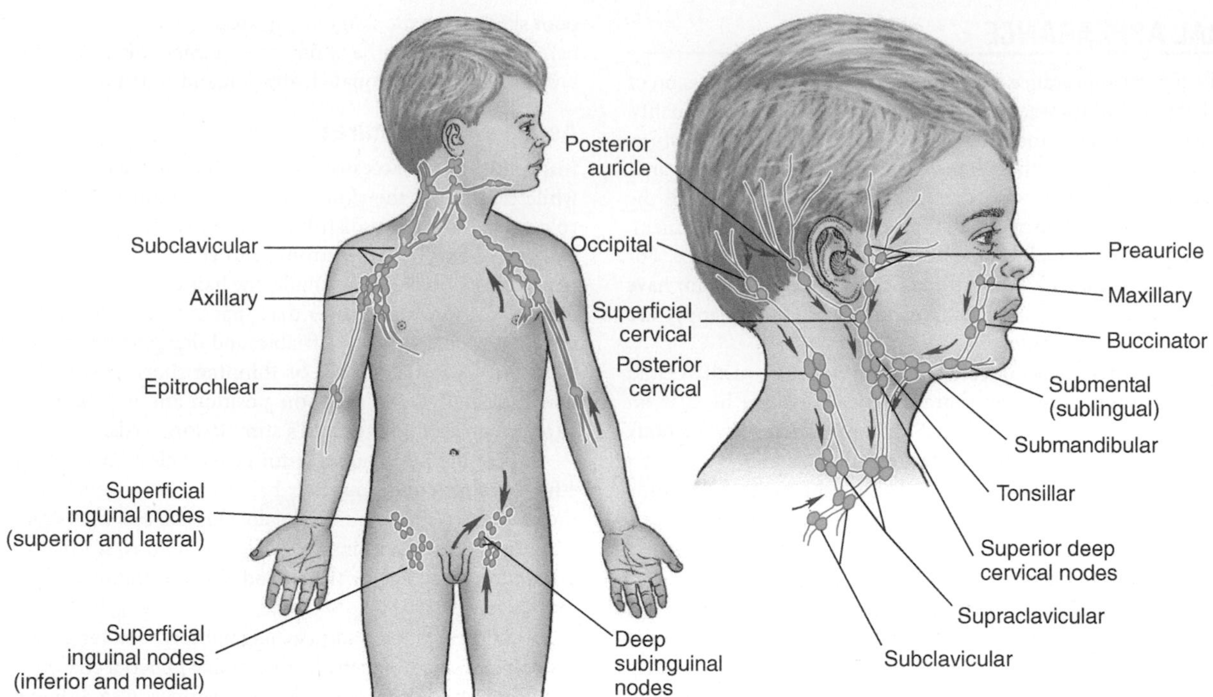

FIG. 4.15 Location of superficial lymph nodes. *Arrows* indicate directional flow of lymph.

system is extensive. Fig. 4.15 shows the usual sites for palpating accessible lymph nodes.

Palpate nodes using the distal portion of the fingers and gently but firmly pressing in a circular motion along the regions where nodes are normally present. During assessment of the nodes in the head and neck, tilt the child's head upward slightly but without tensing the sternocleidomastoid or trapezius muscles. This position facilitates palpation of the **submental**, **submandibular**, **tonsillar**, and **cervical nodes**. Palpate the **axillary nodes** with the child's arms relaxed at the sides but slightly abducted. Assess the **inguinal nodes** with the child in the supine position. Note size, mobility, temperature, and tenderness, as well as reports by the parents regarding any visible change of enlarged nodes. In children, small, nontender, movable nodes are usually normal. Tender, enlarged, warm, erythematous lymph nodes generally indicate infection or inflammation close to their location. Report such findings for further investigation.

HEAD AND NECK

Observe the head for general shape and symmetry. A flattening of one part of the head, such as the occiput, may indicate that the child continually lies in this position. Marked asymmetry is usually abnormal and may indicate premature closure of the sutures (**craniosynostosis**).

> **! NURSING ALERT**
>
> After 6 months old, significant head lag strongly indicates cerebral injury and is referred for further evaluation.

Note head control in infants and head posture in older children. By 4 months old, most infants should be able to hold the head erect and in midline when in a vertical position.

Evaluate range of motion by asking the older child to look in each direction (to either side, up, and down) or by manually putting the younger child through each position. Limited range of motion may indicate **wryneck**, or **torticollis**, in which the child holds the head to one side with the chin pointing toward the opposite side a result of injury to the sternocleidomastoid muscle.

> **! NURSING ALERT**
>
> Hyperextension of the head (opisthotonos) with pain on flexion is a serious indication of meningeal irritation and is referred for immediate evaluation.

Palpate the skull for patent sutures, fontanels, fractures, and swellings. Normally the posterior fontanel closes by 2 months old, and the anterior fontanel fuses between 12 and 18 months. Early or late closure is noted because either may be a sign of a pathologic condition.

While examining the head, observe the face for symmetry, movement, and general appearance. Ask the child to "make a face" to assess symmetric movement and disclose any degree of paralysis. Note any unusual facial proportion, such as an unusually high or low forehead; wide- or close-set eyes; or a small, receding chin.

In addition to assessment of the head and neck for movement, inspect the neck for size and palpate its associated structures. The neck is normally short, with skinfolds between the head and shoulders during infancy; however, it lengthens during the next 3 to 4 years.

> **! NURSING ALERT**
>
> If any masses are detected in the neck, report them for further investigation. Large masses can block the airway.

EYES

Inspection of External Structures

Inspect the lids for proper placement on the eye. When the eye is open, the upper lid should fall near the upper iris. When the eyes are closed, the lids should completely cover the cornea and sclera (Fig. 4.16).

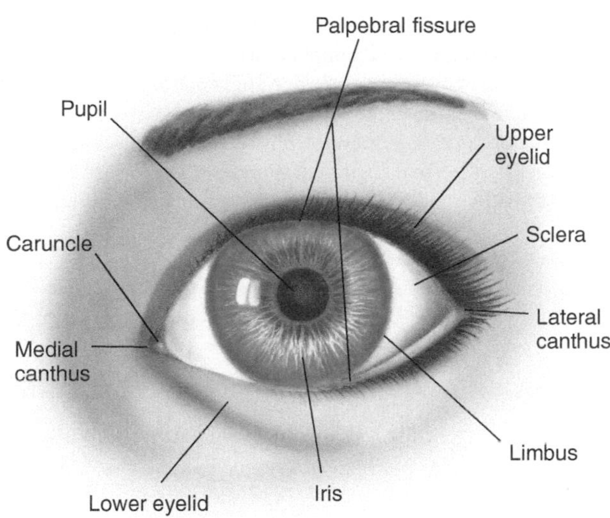

FIG. 4.16 External structures of the eye.

Determine the general slant of the palpebral fissures or lids by drawing an imaginary line through the two points of the medial canthus and across the outer orbit of the eyes and aligning each eye on the line. Usually the palpebral fissures lie horizontally. However, in Asians, the slant is normally upward.

Inspect the inside lining of the lids, the palpebral conjunctivae. To examine the lower conjunctival sac, pull the lid down while the patient looks up. To evert the upper lid, hold the upper lashes and gently pull down and forward as the child looks down. Normally the conjunctiva appears pink and glossy. Vertical yellow striations along the edge are the meibomian glands, or sebaceous glands, near the hair follicle. Located in the inner or medial canthus and situated on the inner edge of the upper and lower lids is a tiny opening, the lacrimal punctum. Note any excessive tearing, discharge, or inflammation of the lacrimal apparatus.

The bulbar conjunctiva, which covers the eye up to the limbus, or junction of the cornea and sclera, should be transparent. The sclera should be white, contrasting with the colored iris. Tiny black marks in the sclera of heavily pigmented individuals are normal.

The cornea, or covering of the iris and pupil, should be clear and transparent. Record opacities because they can be signs of scarring or ulceration, which can interfere with vision. The best way to test for opacities is to illuminate the eyeball by shining a light at an angle (obliquely) toward the cornea.

Compare the pupils for size, shape, and movement. They should be round, clear, and equal. Test their reaction to light by quickly shining a light toward the eye and removing it. As the light approaches, the pupils should constrict; as the light fades, the pupils should dilate. Test the pupil for any response of accommodation by having the child look at a bright, shiny object at a distance and quickly moving the object toward the face. The pupils should constrict as the object is brought near the eye. Record normal findings on examination of the pupils as PERRLA, which stands for "Pupils Equal, Round, React to Light, and Accommodation."

Inspect the iris and pupil for color, size, shape, and clarity. Permanent eye color is usually established by 6 to 12 months of age. While inspecting the iris and pupil, look for the lens. Normally the lens is not visible through the pupil.

Inspection of Internal Structures

The ophthalmoscope permits visualization of the interior of the eyeball with a system of lenses and a high-intensity light. The lenses permit clear visualization of eye structures at different distances from the nurse's eye and correct visual acuity differences in the examiner and child. Use of the ophthalmoscope requires practice to know which lens setting produces the clearest image.

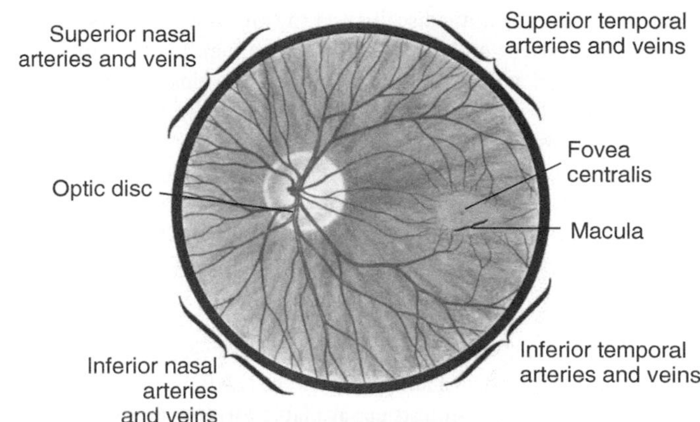

FIG. 4.17 Structures of fundus. (From Ball, J. W., Dains, J. E., Flynn, J. A., et al. [2014]. *Seidel's guide to physical examination* [8th ed.]. St. Louis, MO: Elsevier.)

The ophthalmic and otic heads may be interchangeable on one "body" or handle, which encloses the power source—either disposable or rechargeable batteries. The nurse should practice changing the heads, which snap on and are secured with a quarter turn, and replacing the batteries and light bulbs. Nurses who are not directly involved in physical assessment are often responsible for ensuring that the instrument functions properly.

Preparing the Child

The nurse can prepare the child for the ophthalmoscopic examination by showing the child the instrument, demonstrating the light source and how it shines, and explaining the reason for darkening the room. For infants and young children who do not respond to such explanations, it is best to use distraction to encourage them to keep their eyes open. Forcibly parting the eyelids results in an uncooperative, watery-eyed child and a frustrated nurse. Usually, with some practice, the nurse can elicit a red reflex almost instantly while approaching the child and may also gain a momentary inspection of the blood vessels, macula, or optic disc.

Funduscopic Examination

Fig. 4.17 shows the structures of the back of the eyeball, or the fundus. The fundus is immediately apparent as the red reflex. The intensity of the color increases in darkly pigmented individuals.

> **! NURSING ALERT**
>
> A brilliant, uniform red reflex is an important sign because it rules out many serious defects of the cornea, aqueous chamber, lens, and vitreous chamber. Any dark shadows or opacities are recorded because they indicate some abnormality in any of these structures.

As the ophthalmoscope is brought closer to the eye, the most conspicuous feature of the fundus is the optic disc, the area where the blood vessels and optic nerve fibers enter and exit the eye. The disc is orange to creamy pink with a pale center and lighter in color than the surrounding fundus. Normally, it is round or vertically oval.

After locating the optic disc, inspect the area for blood vessels. The central retinal artery and vein appear in the depths of the disc and emanate outward with visible branching. The veins are darker and about one-fourth larger than the arteries. Normally, the branches of the arteries and veins cross one another.

Other structures that are common are the macula, the area of the fundus with the greatest concentration of visual receptors, and in the center of the macula, a minute glistening spot of reflected light called the fovea centralis; this is the area of most perfect vision.

Vision Testing

The US Preventive Services Task Force (2011) recommends vision screening for the presence of amblyopia and its risk factors for all children 3 to 5 years of age. Several tests are available for assessing vision. This discussion focuses on ocular alignment, visual acuity, peripheral vision, and color vision. Chapter 20 discusses behavioral and physical signs of visual impairment. Nurses can provide accurate vision screening with appropriate training (Mathers, Keyes, & Wright, 2010).

Ocular Alignment

Normally, by the age of 3 to 4 months, children are able to fixate on one visual field with both eyes simultaneously (binocularity). In strabismus, or cross-eye, one eye deviates from the point of fixation. If the misalignment is constant, the weak eye becomes "lazy," and the brain eventually suppresses the image produced by that eye. If strabismus is not detected and corrected by 4 to 6 years old, blindness from disuse, known as amblyopia, may result.

Tests commonly used to detect misalignment are the corneal light reflex and the cover tests. To perform the corneal light reflex test, or Hirschberg test, shine a flashlight or the light of the ophthalmoscope directly into the patient's eyes from a distance of about 40.5 cm (16 inches). If the eyes are orthophoric, or normal, the light falls symmetrically within each pupil (Fig. 4.18, *A*). If the light falls off-center in one eye, the eyes are misaligned. Epicanthal folds, excess folds of skin that extend from the roof of the nose to the inner termination of the eyebrow and that partially or completely overlap the inner canthus of the eye, may give a false impression of misalignment (pseudostrabismus) (Fig. 4.18, *B*). Epicanthal folds are often found in Asian children.

In the cover test, one eye is covered, and the movement of the uncovered eye is observed while the child looks at a near (33 cm [13 inches] away) or distant (6 m [20 feet] away) object. If the uncovered eye does not move, it is aligned. If the uncovered eye moves, a misalignment is present because when the stronger eye is temporarily covered, the misaligned eye attempts to fixate on the object.

In the alternate cover test, occlusion shifts back and forth from one eye to the other, and movement of the eye that was covered is observed as soon as the occluder is removed while the child focuses on a certain point (Fig. 4.19). If normal alignment is present, shifting the cover from one eye to the other will not cause the eye to move. If misalignment is

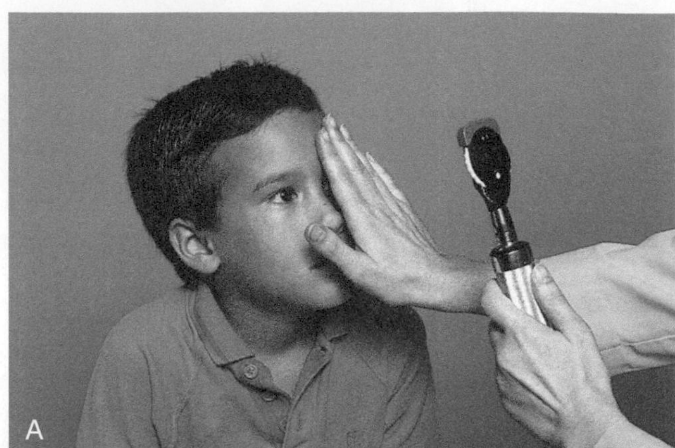

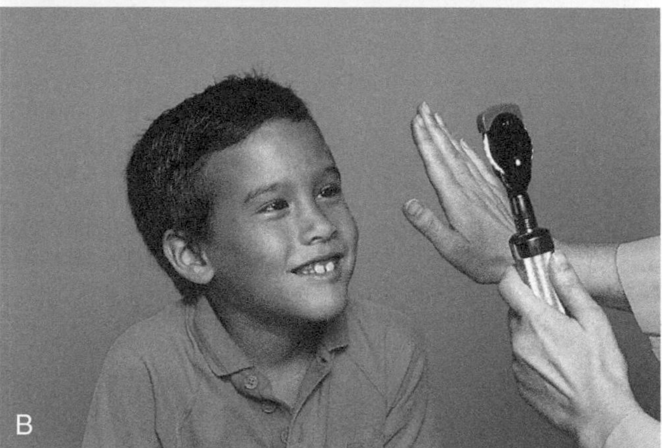

FIG. 4.19 Alternate cover test to detect amblyopia in a patient with strabismus. **A,** The eye is occluded, and the child is fixating on light source. **B,** If the eye does not move when uncovered, the eyes are aligned.

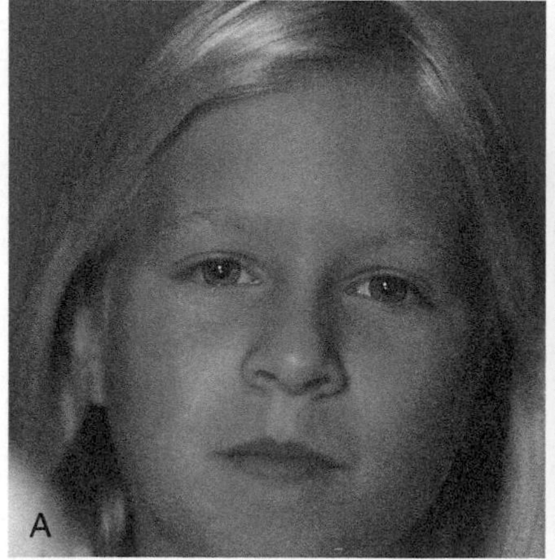

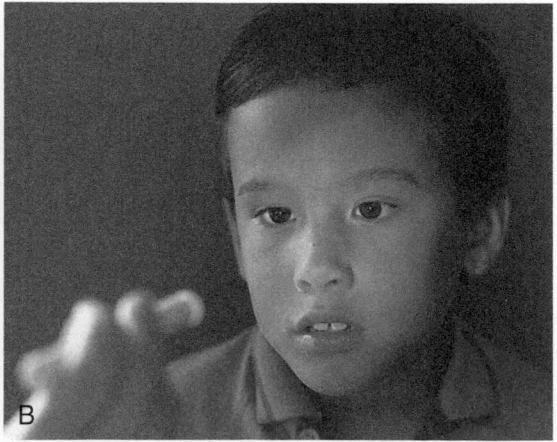

FIG. 4.18 A, Corneal light reflex test demonstrating orthophoric eyes. **B,** Pseudostrabismus. Inner epicanthal folds cause the eyes to appear misaligned; however, the corneal light reflexes fall perfectly symmetrically.

present, eye movement will occur when the cover is moved. This test takes more practice than the other cover test because the occluder must be moved back and forth quickly and accurately to see the eye move. Because deviations can occur at different ranges, it is important to perform the cover tests at both close and far distances.

! NURSING ALERT

The cover test is usually easier to perform if the examiner uses his or her hand rather than a card-type occluder (see Fig. 4.19). Attractive occluders fashioned like an ice cream cone or happy-face lollipop cut from cardboard are also well received by young children.

Visual Acuity Testing in Children

The most common test for measuring visual acuity is the Snellen letter chart, which consists of lines of letters of decreasing size. The child stands with his or her heels at a line 10 feet away from the chart. When screening for visual acuity in children, the nurse tests the child's right eye first by covering the left. Children who wear glasses should be screened with them on. Tell the child to keep both eyes open during the examination. If the child fails to read the current line, move up the chart to the next larger line. Continue up the chart until the child is able to read the line. Then begin moving down the chart again until the child fails to read the line. To pass each line, the child must correctly identify four of six symbols on the line. Repeat the procedure, covering the right eye. Table 4.6 provides a list of visual screening tests for children and guidelines for referral.

For children unable to read letters and numbers, the tumbling E or HOTV test is useful. The tumbling E test uses the capital letter **E** pointing in four different directions. The child is asked to point in the direction the **E** is facing. The HOTV test consists of a wall chart composed of the letters **H**, **O**, **T**, and **V**. The child is given a board containing a large **H**, **O**, **T**, and **V**. The examiner points to a letter on the wall chart, and the child matches the correct letter on the board held in his or her hand. The tumbling E and HOTV are excellent tests for preschool-age children.

Visual Acuity Testing in Infants and Difficult-to-Test Children

In newborns, vision is tested mainly by checking for light perception by shining a light into the eyes and noting responses, such as pupillary constriction, blinking, following the light to midline, increased alertness, or refusal to open the eyes after exposure to the light. Although the simple maneuver of checking light perception and eliciting the pupillary light reflex indicates that the anterior half of the visual apparatus is intact, it does not confirm that the infant can see. In other words, this test does not assess whether the brain receives the visual message and interprets the signals.

Another test of visual acuity is the infant's ability to fix on and follow a target. Although any brightly colored or patterned object can be used, the human face is excellent. Hold the infant upright while moving your face slowly from side to side. Signs that may indicate visual loss or other serious eye problems include fixed pupils, strabismus, constant nystagmus, the setting-sun sign, and slow lateral movements. Unfortunately, it is difficult to test each eye separately; the presence of such signs in one eye could indicate unilateral blindness.

Special tests are available for testing infants and other difficult-to-test children to assess acuity or confirm blindness. For example, in visually evoked potentials, the eyes are stimulated with a bright light or pattern, and electrical activity to the visual cortex is recorded through scalp electrodes (see Research Focus box.)

! NURSING ALERT

If visual fixation and following are not present by 3 to 4 months old, further ophthalmologic evaluation is necessary.

RESEARCH FOCUS

Instrument-Based Vision Screening

Evidence supports the use of elective instrument-based vision screening, primarily photoscreening and autorefraction, in children 6 months old to 3 years old, and as an alternative for children from 3 through 5 years old, particularly in those who are unable or unwilling to cooperate with routine vision charts (American Academy of Pediatrics Section on Ophthalmology and Committee on Practice and Ambulatory Medicine, 2012). Photoscreening uses optical images of the eye's red reflex to estimate refractive error, media opacity, ocular alignment, and other factors putting a child at risk for amblyopia. Handheld autorefraction is used to evaluate the refractive error of each eye.

Peripheral Vision

In children who are old enough to cooperate, estimate peripheral vision, or the visual field of each eye, by having the children fixate on a specific point directly in front of them while an object, such as a finger or a pencil, is moved from beyond the field of vision into the range of peripheral vision. As soon as children see the object, have them say "Stop." At that point measure the angle from the anteroposterior axis of the eye (straight line of vision) to the peripheral axis (point at which the object is first seen). Check each eye separately and for each quadrant of vision. Normally children see about 50 degrees upward, 70 degrees downward, 60 degrees nasalward, and 90 degrees temporally. Limitations in peripheral vision may indicate blindness from damage to structures within the eye or to any of the visual pathways.

Color Vision

The tests available for color vision include the Ishihara test and the Hardy-Rand-Rittler test. Each consists of a series of cards (pseudoisochromatic) containing a color field composed of spots of a certain "confusion" color. Against the field is a number or symbol similarly printed in dots but of a color likely to be confused with the field color by a person with a color vision deficit. As a result, the figure or letter is invisible to an affected individual but is clearly seen by a person with normal vision.

EARS

Inspection of External Structures

The outer portion of the ear is called the pinna, or auricle; one is located on each side of the head. Measure the height alignment of the pinna by drawing an imaginary line from the outer orbit of the eye to the occiput, or most prominent protuberance of the skull. The top of the pinna should meet or cross this line. Low-set ears are commonly associated with renal anomalies or cognitive impairment. Measure the angle of the pinna by drawing a perpendicular line from the imaginary horizontal line and aligning the pinna next to this mark. Normally the pinna lies within a 10-degree angle of the vertical line (Fig. 4.20). If it falls outside this area, record the deviation and look for other anomalies.

Normally the pinna extends slightly outward from the skull. Except in newborn infants, ears that are flat against the head or protruding away from the scalp may indicate problems. Flattened ears in an infant may suggest a frequent side-lying position and, just as with isolated

TABLE 4.6 **Eye Examination Guidelines***

Function	Recommended Tests	Referral Criteria	Comments
3-5 Years Old			
Distance visual acuity	Snellen letters Snellen numbers Tumbling E HOTV Picture test: • Allen figures • LEA symbols	1. Less than four of six correct on 20-foot (6-m) line with either eye tested at 10 feet (3 m) monocularly (i.e., <10/20 or 20/40) *or* 2. Two-line difference between eyes, even within passing range (i.e., 10/12.5 and 10/20 or 20/25 and 20/40)	1. Tests are listed in decreasing order of cognitive difficulty; highest test that child is capable of performing should be used; in general, tumbling E or HOTV test should be used for children 3-5 years old and Snellen letters or numbers for children 6 years old and older. 2. Testing distance of 10 feet (3 m) is recommended for all visual acuity tests. 3. Line of figures is preferred over single figures. 4. Nontested eye should be covered by occluder held by examiner or by adhesive occluder patch applied to eye; examiner must ensure that it is not possible to peek with nontested eye.
Ocular alignment	Cross cover test at 10 feet (3 m) Random dot E stereo test at 18 inches (40 cm) Simultaneous red reflex test (Bruckner test)	Any eye movement Less than four of six correct Any asymmetry of pupil color, size, brightness	Child must be fixing on a target while cross cover test is performed. Use direct ophthalmoscope to view both red reflexes simultaneously in a darkened room from 2-3 feet (0.6-0.9 m) away; detects asymmetric refractive errors as well.
Ocular media clarity (cataracts, tumors, and so on)	Red reflex	White pupil, dark spots, absent reflex	Use direct ophthalmoscope in a darkened room. View eyes separately at 12-18 inches (30-45 cm); white reflex indicates possible retinoblastoma.
6 Years Old and Older			
Distance visual acuity	Snellen letters Snellen numbers Tumbling E HOTV Picture test: • Allen figures • LEA symbols	1. Less than four of six correct on 15-foot (4.5-m) line with either eye tested at 10 feet (3 m) monocularly (i.e., <10/15 or 20/30) *or* 2. Two-line difference between eyes, even within the passing range (i.e., 10/10 and 10/15 or 20/20 and 20/30)	1. Tests are listed in decreasing order of cognitive difficulty; highest test that child is capable of performing should be used; in general, tumbling E or HOTV test should be used for children 3-5 years old and Snellen letters or numbers for children 6 years old and older. 2. Testing distance of 10 feet (3 m) is recommended for all visual acuity tests. 3. Line of figures is preferred over single figures. 4. Nontested eye should be covered by occluder held by examiner or by adhesive occluder patch applied to eye; examiner must ensure that it is not possible to peek with nontested eye.
Ocular alignment	Cross cover test at 10 feet (3 m) Random dot E stereo test at 18 inches (40 cm) Simultaneous red reflex test (Bruckner test)	Any eye movement Less than four of six correct Any asymmetry of pupil color, size, brightness	Child must be fixing on target while cross cover test is performed. Use direct ophthalmoscope to view both red reflexes simultaneously in a darkened room from 2-3 feet (0.6-0.9 m) away; detects asymmetric refractive errors as well.
Ocular media clarity (e.g., cataracts, tumors)	Red reflex	White pupil, dark spots, absent reflex	Use direct ophthalmoscope in a darkened room. View eyes separately at 12-18 inches (30-45 cm); white reflex indicates possible retinoblastoma.

*Assessing visual acuity (vision screening) is one of the most sensitive techniques for detection of eye abnormalities in children. The American Academy of Pediatrics Section on Ophthalmology, in cooperation with American Association for Pediatric Ophthalmology and Strabismus and American Academy of Ophthalmology, has developed these guidelines to be used by physicians, nurses, educational institutions, public health departments, and other professionals who perform vision evaluation services.

From American Academy of Pediatrics, Committee on Practice and Ambulatory Medicine, Section on Ophthalmology. (2003). Eye examination in infants, children, and young adults by pediatricians. *Pediatrics, 111*(4), 902-907.

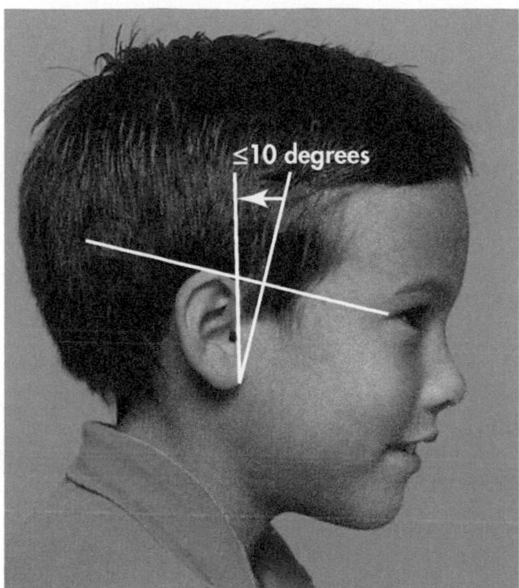

FIG. 4.20 Ear alignment.

areas of hair loss, may be a clue to investigate parents' understanding of the child's stimulation needs.

Inspect the skin surface around the ear for small openings, extra tags of skin, sinuses, or earlobe creases. If a sinus is found, note this because it may represent a fistula that drains into some area of the neck or ear. Note an earlobe crease, if found, because it may be associated with a rare syndrome. However, having one small abnormality is not uncommon and is often not associated with a serious condition. Cutaneous tags represent no pathologic process but may cause parents' concern in terms of the child's appearance.

Assess the ear for hygiene. An otoscope is not necessary for looking into the external canal to note the presence of cerumen, a waxy substance produced by the ceruminous glands in the outer portion of the canal. Cerumen is usually yellow-brown and soft. If an otoscope is used and any discharge is visible, note its color and odor. Avoid transmitting potentially infectious material to the other ear or to another child through hand washing and using disposable specula or sterilizing reusable specula between each examination.

Inspection of Internal Structures

The head of the otoscope permits visualization of the tympanic membrane by use of a bright light, a magnifying glass, and a speculum. Some otoscopes have an attachment for a pneumonic device to insert air into the canal to determine membrane compliance (movement). The speculum, which is inserted into the external canal, comes in a variety of sizes to accommodate different canal widths. The largest speculum that fits comfortably into the ear is used to achieve the greatest area of visualization. The lens, or magnifying glass, is movable, allowing the examiner to insert an object, such as a curette, into the ear canal through the speculum while still viewing the structures through the lens.

Positioning the Child

Before beginning the otoscopic examination, position the child properly and gently restrain him or her (child sits on parent's lap, and parent holds body and head) if necessary. Older children usually cooperate and do not need restraint. However, prepare them for the procedure by allowing them to play with the instrument, demonstrating how it works, and stressing the importance of remaining still. A helpful suggestion is to let them observe you examining the parent's ear. Restraint is needed for younger children because the ear examination upsets them (see Atraumatic Care box).

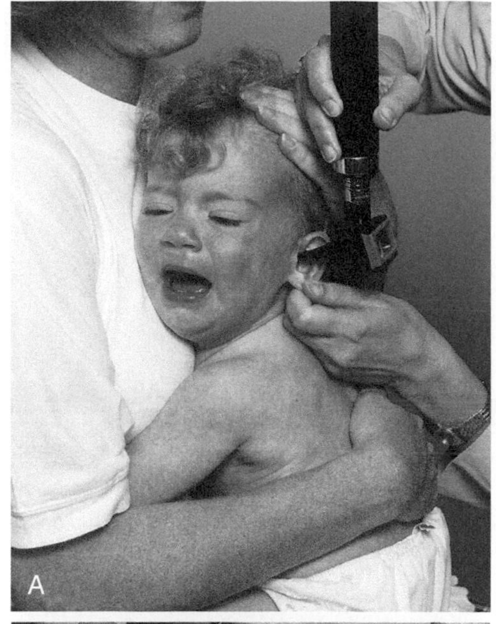

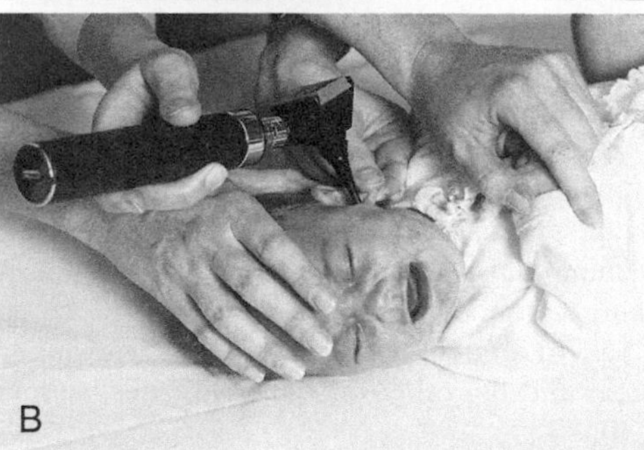

FIG. 4.21 Position for restraining a child **(A)** and an infant **(B)** during otoscopic examination.

ATRAUMATIC CARE

Reducing Distress From Otoscopy in Young Children

Make examining the ear a game by explaining that you are looking for a "big elephant" in the ear. This kind of make-believe is an absorbing distraction and usually elicits cooperation. After examining the ear, clarify that "looking for elephants" was only pretend and thank the child for letting you look in his or her ear. Another great distraction technique is asking the child to put a finger on the opposite ear to keep the light from getting out.

As you insert the speculum into the meatus, move it around the outer rim to accustom the child to the feel of something entering the ear. If examining a painful ear, examine the unaffected ear, then return to the painful ear, and touch a nonpainful part of the affected ear first. By this time, the child is usually less fearful of anything causing discomfort to the ear and will cooperate more.

For their protection and safety, restrain infants and toddlers for the otoscopic examination. There are two general positions of restraint. In one, the child is seated sideways in the parent's lap with one arm hugging the parent and the other arm at the side. The ear to be examined is toward the nurse. With one arm the parent holds the child's head firmly against his or her chest and hugs the child with the other arm, thereby securing the child's free arm (Fig. 4.21, *A*). Examine the ear using the same procedure for holding the otoscope as described later.

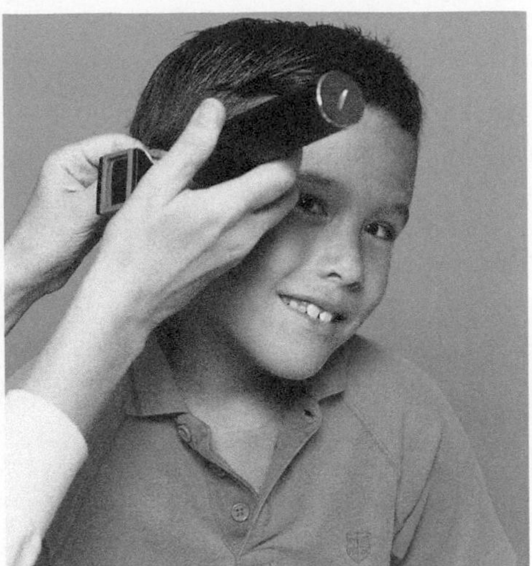

FIG. 4.22 Positioning the head by tilting it toward the opposite shoulder for full view of the tympanic membrane.

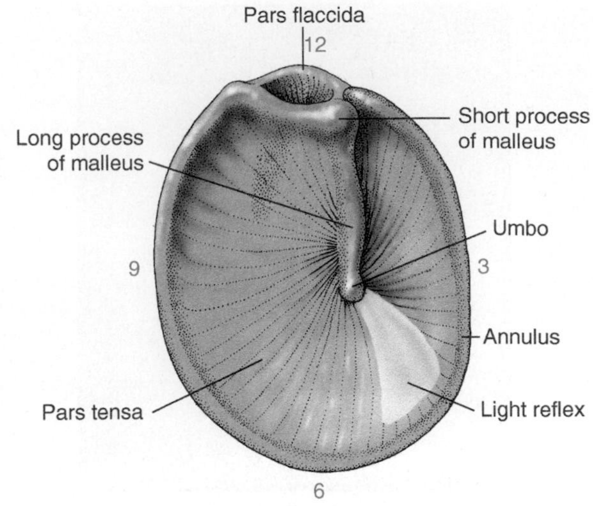

FIG. 4.23 Landmarks of the tympanic membrane. (From Ignatavicius, D. D., & Workman, M. L. [2013]. *Medical-surgical nursing: Patient-centered collaborative care* [7th ed.]. St. Louis, MO: Saunders.)

The other position involves placing the child on the side, back, or abdomen with the arms at the side and the head turned so that the ear to be examined points toward the ceiling. Lean over the child, use the upper part of the body to restrain the arms and upper trunk movements, and use the examining hand to stabilize the head. This position is practical for young infants or for older children who need minimum restraint, but it may not be feasible for other children who protest vigorously. For safety, enlist the parent's or an assistant's help in immobilizing the head by firmly placing one hand above the ear and the other on the child's side, abdomen, or back (Fig. 4.21, *B*).

With cooperative children, examine the ear with the child in a side-lying, sitting, or standing position. One disadvantage to standing is that the child may "walk away" as the otoscope enters the canal. If the child is standing or sitting, tilt the head slightly toward the child's opposite shoulder to achieve a better view of the drum (Fig. 4.22).

With the thumb and forefinger of the free hand, grasp the auricle. For the two positions of restraint, hold the otoscope upside down at the junction of its head and handle with the thumb and index finger. Place the other fingers against the skull to allow the otoscope to move with the child in case of sudden movement. In examining a cooperative child, hold the handle with the otic head upright or upside down. Use the dominant hand to examine both ears or reverse hands for each ear, whichever is more comfortable.

Before using the otoscope, visualize the external ear and the tympanic membrane as being superimposed on a clock (Fig. 4.23). The numbers are important geographic landmarks. Introduce the speculum into the meatus between the 3 and 9 o'clock positions in a downward and forward position. Because the canal is curved, the speculum does not permit a panoramic view of the tympanic membrane unless the canal is straightened. In infants, the canal curves upward. Therefore pull the pinna down and back to the 6 to 9 o'clock range to straighten the canal (Fig. 4.24, *A*). With older children, usually those older than 3 years of age, the canal curves downward and forward. Therefore pull the pinna up and back toward a 10 o'clock position (Fig. 4.24, *B*). If you have difficulty visualizing the membrane, try repositioning the head, introducing the speculum at a different angle, and pulling the pinna in a slightly different direction. Do not insert the speculum past the cartilaginous (outermost) portion of the canal, usually a distance of 0.6 to 1.25 cm (0.23 to 0.5 inch) in older children. Insertion of the speculum into the posterior or bony portion of the canal causes pain.

In neonates and young infants, the walls of the canal are pliable and floppy because of the underdeveloped cartilaginous and bony structures. Therefore the very small 2-mm speculum usually needs to be inserted deeper into the canal than in older children. Exercise great care not to damage the walls or drum. For this reason, only an experienced examiner should insert an otoscope into the ears of very young infants.

Otoscopic Examination

As you introduce the speculum into the external canal, inspect the walls of the canal, the color of the tympanic membrane, the light reflex, and the usual landmarks of the bony prominences of the middle ear. The walls of the external auditory canal are pink, although they are more pigmented in dark-skinned children. Minute hairs are evident in the outermost portion, where cerumen is produced. Note signs of irritation, foreign bodies, or infection.

Foreign bodies in the ear are common in children and range from erasers to beans. Symptoms may include pain, discharge, and affected hearing. Remove soft objects, such as paper or insects, with forceps. Remove small, hard objects, such as pebbles, with a suction tip, a hook, or irrigation. However, irrigation is contraindicated if the object is vegetative matter, such as beans or pasta, which swells when in contact with fluid.

! NURSING ALERT

If there is any doubt about the type of object in the ear and the appropriate method to remove it, refer the child to the appropriate practitioner.

The **tympanic membrane** is a translucent, light pearly pink or gray. Note marked erythema (which may indicate suppurative otitis media); a dull, nontransparent, grayish color (sometimes suggestive of serous otitis media); or ashen gray areas (signs of scarring from a previous perforation). A black area usually suggests a perforation of the membrane that has not healed.

The characteristic tenseness and slope of the tympanic membrane cause the light of the otoscope to reflect at about the 5 or 7 o'clock position. The **light reflex** is a fairly well-defined, cone-shaped reflection, which normally points away from the face.

The **bony landmarks** of the drum are formed by the **umbo**, or tip of the malleus. It appears as a small, round, opaque, concave spot near

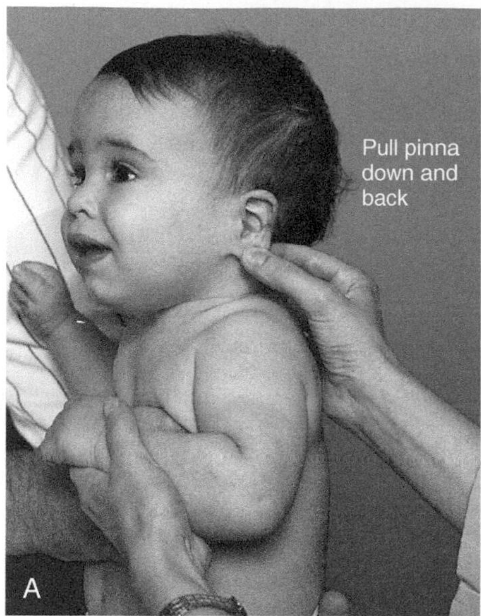

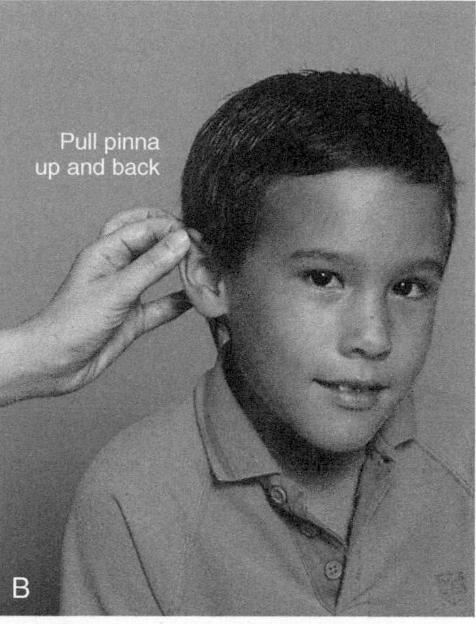

FIG. 4.24 Positioning for visualizing the eardrum in an infant **(A)** and in a child older than 3 years old **(B)**.

TABLE 4.7 Auditory Tests for Infants and Children

Age	Auditory Test	Type of Measurement	Procedure
Newborns	Auditory brainstem response (ABR)	Electrophysiologic measurement of activity in auditory nerve and brainstem pathways	Placement of electrodes on child's head detects auditory stimuli presented through earphones one ear at a time.
Infants	Behavioral audiometry	Used to observe their behavior in response to certain sounds heard through speakers or earphones	The child's responses to the sounds heard are observed.
Toddlers	Play audiometry	Uses an audiometer to transmit sounds at different volumes and pitches	The toddler is asked to do something with a toy (i.e., touch a toy, move a toy) every time the sound is heard.
Children and adolescents	Pure tone audiometry	Uses an audiometer that produces sounds at different volumes and pitches in the child's ears	The child is asked to respond in some way when the tone is heard in the earphone.
	Tympanometry (also called *impedance* or *admittance*)	Determines how the middle ear is functioning and detects any changes in pressure in the middle ear	A soft plastic tip is placed over the ear canal and the tympanometer measures eardrum movement when the pressure changes.
All ages	Evoked otoacoustic emissions (EOAE)	Physiologic test specifically measuring cochlear (outer hair cell) response to presentation of stimulus	Small probe containing sensitive microphone is placed in ear canal for stimulus delivery and response detection.

the center of the drum. The **manubrium** (long process or handle) of the malleus appears to be a whitish line extending from the umbo upward to the margin of the membrane. At the upper end of the long process near the 1 o'clock position (in the right ear) is a sharp, knoblike protuberance, representing the **short process** of the malleus. Note the absence or distortion of the light reflex or loss or abnormal prominence of any of these landmarks.

Auditory Testing

Several types of hearing tests are available and recommended for screening in infants and children (Table 4.7). The American Academy of Pediatrics recommends pure tone audiometry testing screening at 500, 1000, 2000, and 4000 Hz, with children failing if they cannot hear the tones at 20 dB (Harlor, Bower, & Committee on Practice and Ambulatory Medicine, Section on Otolaryngology Head and Neck Surgery, 2009). Universal newborn hearing screening is available in all US states (Table 4.8). The nurse must operate under a high index of suspicion for those children who may have conditions associated with hearing loss, whose parents are concerned about hearing loss, and who may have developed behaviors that indicate auditory impairment. Chapter 20 discusses types of hearing loss, causes, clinical manifestations, and appropriate treatment. (See the Research Focus box for further discussion).

TABLE 4.8 Pediatric Quality Indicator Audiologic Evaluation No Later Than 3 Months of Age*

Measure	Children who were 3 months of age or younger who received an audiological evaluation.
Numerator	Number of children who received an audiological evaluation during the measurement time.
Denominator	Number of children who were 3 months of age or younger.

*Endorsed by the National Quality Forum-0360 and 2016 Core Set of Children's Health Care Quality Measures for Medicaid and CHIP.

NOSE

Inspection of External Structures

Compare the placement and alignment of the nose by drawing an imaginary vertical line from the center point between the eyes down to the notch of the upper lip. The nose should lie in the middle of the face, with each side exactly symmetric on both sides of the imaginary line. Note its location, any deviation to one side, and asymmetry in overall size and in diameter of the nares (nostrils). The bridge of the

RESEARCH FOCUS

Hearing Loss Frequency

The prevalence of hearing loss has increased among US children, and failure to identify children even with mild high-frequency hearing loss may have long-term consequences (Sekhar, Zalewski, & Paul, 2013). Unilateral or bilateral hearing impairment within the speech frequencies is found in 3.1% of children and youth (Mehra, Eavey, & Keamy, 2009). Asking children and their parents about the presence of hearing problems is important and should be a part of every clinical visit

nose is sometimes flat in Asian and African American children. Observe the alae nasi for any sign of flaring, which indicates respiratory difficulty. Always report any flaring of the alae nasi. Fig. 4.25 illustrates the landmarks used in describing the external landmarks and internal structures of the nose.

Inspection of Internal Structures

Inspect the anterior vestibule of the nose by pushing the tip upward, tilting the head backward, and illuminating the cavity with a flashlight or otoscope without the attached ear speculum. Note the color of the mucosal lining, which is normally redder than the oral membranes, as well as any swelling, discharge, dryness, or bleeding. There should be no discharge from the nose.

On looking deeper into the nose, inspect the turbinates, or concha, plates of bone that jut into the nasal cavity and are enveloped by mucous membrane. The turbinates greatly increase the surface area of the nasal cavity as air is inhaled. The spaces or channels between the turbinates are called the meatus and correspond to each of the three turbinates. Normally the front end of the inferior and middle turbinate and the middle meatus are seen. They should be the same color as the lining of the vestibule.

Inspect the septum, which should divide the vestibules equally. Note any deviation, especially if it causes an occlusion of one side of the nose. A perforation may be evident within the septum. If this is suspected, shine the light of the otoscope into one naris and look for admittance of light to the other. Because olfaction is an important function of the nose, testing for smell may be done at this point or as part of cranial nerve assessment (see Table 4.11 later in this chapter).

MOUTH AND THROAT

With a cooperative child, the nurse can accomplish almost the entire examination of the mouth and throat without the use of a tongue blade.

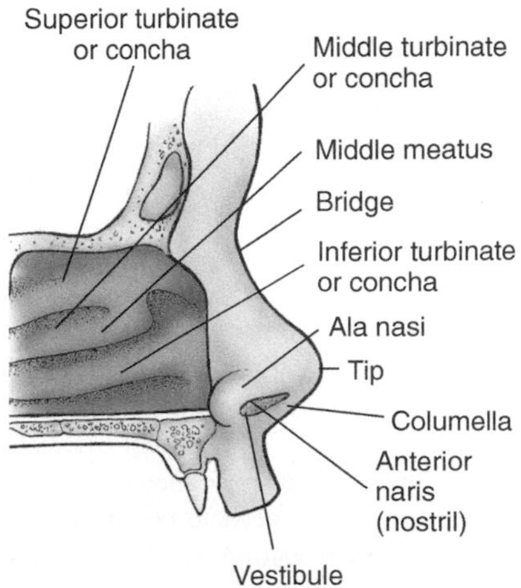

FIG. 4.25 External landmarks and internal structures of the nose.

Ask the child to open the mouth wide; to move the tongue in different directions for full visualization; and to say "ahh," which depresses the tongue for full view of the back of the mouth (tonsils, uvula, and oropharynx). For a closer look at the buccal mucosa, or lining of the cheeks, ask children to use their fingers to move the outer lip and cheek to one side (see Atraumatic Care box).

ATRAUMATIC CARE

Encouraging Opening the Mouth for Examination

- Perform the examination in front of a mirror.
- Let child first examine someone else's mouth, such as the parent, the nurse, or a puppet (Fig. 4.26, *A*), and then examine child's mouth.
- Instruct child to tilt the head back slightly, breathe deeply through the mouth, and hold the breath; this action lowers the tongue to the floor of the mouth without the use of a tongue blade.
- Lightly brushing the palate with a cotton swab also may open the mouth for assessment.

Infants and toddlers usually resist attempts to keep the mouth open. Because inspecting the mouth is upsetting, leave it for the end of the physical examination (along with examination of the ears) or do it during episodes of crying. However, the use of a tongue blade (preferably flavored) to depress the tongue may be needed. Place the tongue blade along the side of the tongue, not in the center back area where the gag reflex is elicited. Fig. 4.26, *B*, illustrates proper positioning of the child for the oral examination.

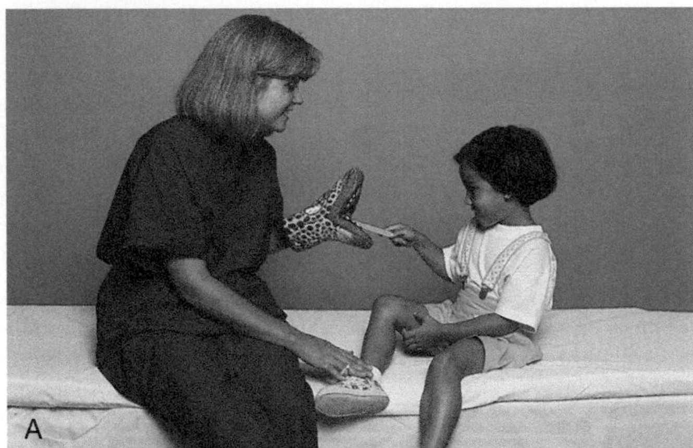

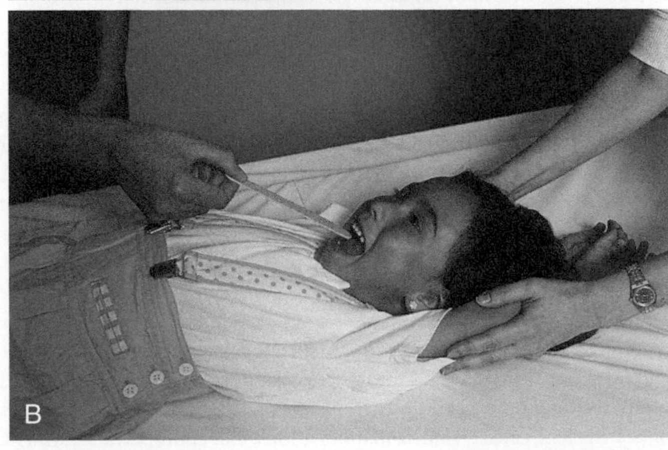

FIG. 4.26 A, Encouraging a child to cooperate. **B,** Positioning a child for examination of the mouth.

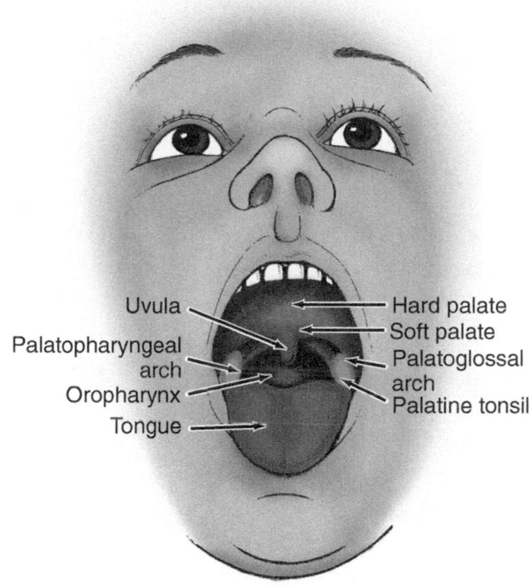

FIG. 4.27 Interior structures of the mouth.

The major structure of the exterior of the mouth is the lips. The lips should be moist, soft, smooth, and pink, or a deeper hue than the surrounding skin. The lips should be symmetric when relaxed or tensed. Assess symmetry when the child talks or cries.

Inspection of Internal Structures

The major structures that are visible within the oral cavity and oropharynx are the mucosal lining of the lips and cheeks, gums (or gingiva), teeth, tongue, palate, uvula, tonsils, and posterior oropharynx (Fig. 4.27). Inspect all areas lined with mucous membranes (inside the lips and cheeks, gingiva, underside of the tongue, palate, and back of the pharynx) for color, any areas of white patches or ulceration, petechiae, bleeding, sensitivity, and moisture. The membranes should be bright pink, smooth, glistening, uniform, and moist.

Inspect the teeth for number (deciduous, permanent, or mixed dentition) in each dental arch, for hygiene, and for occlusion or bite (see also Teething, Chapter 8). Discoloration of tooth enamel with obvious plaque (whitish coating on the surface of the teeth) is a sign of poor dental hygiene and indicates a need for counseling. Brown spots in the crevices of the crown of the tooth or between the teeth may be caries (cavities). Chalky white to yellow or brown areas on the enamel may indicate fluorosis (excessive fluoride ingestion). Teeth that appear greenish black may be stained temporarily from ingestion of supplemental iron.

Examine the gums (gingiva) surrounding the teeth. The color is normally coral pink, and the surface texture is stippled, similar to the appearance of an orange peel. In dark-skinned children, the gums are more deeply colored, and a brownish area is often observed along the gum line.

Inspect the tongue for papillae, small projections that contain taste buds and give the tongue its characteristic rough appearance. Note the size and mobility of the tongue. Normally the tip of the tongue should extend to the lips or beyond.

The roof of the mouth consists of the hard palate, which is located near the front of the oral cavity, and the soft palate, which is located toward the back of the pharynx and has a small midline protrusion called the uvula. Carefully inspect the palates to ensure they are intact. The arch of the palate should be dome shaped. A narrow, flat roof or a high, arched palate affects the placement of the tongue and can cause feeding and speech problems. Test movement of the uvula by eliciting a gag reflex. It should move upward to close off the nasopharynx from the oropharynx.

Examine the oropharynx and note the size and color of the palatine tonsils. They are normally the same color as the surrounding mucosa; glandular, rather than smooth in appearance; and barely visible over the edge of the palatoglossal arches. The size of the tonsils varies considerably during childhood. However, report any swelling, redness, or white areas on the tonsils.

CHEST

Inspect the chest for size, shape, symmetry, movement, breast development, and the bony landmarks formed by the ribs and sternum. The rib cage consists of 12 ribs on each side and the sternum, or breast bone, located in the midline of the trunk (Fig. 4.28). The sternum is composed of three main parts. The manubrium, the uppermost portion, can be felt at the base of the neck at the suprasternal notch. The largest segment of the sternum is the body, which forms the sternal angle (angle of Louis) as it articulates with the manubrium. At the end of the body is a small, movable process called the xiphoid. The angle of the costal margin as it attaches to the sternum is called the costal angle and is normally about 45 to 50 degrees. These bony structures are important landmarks in the location of ribs and intercostal spaces (ICSs), which are the spaces between the ribs. They are numbered according to the rib directly above the space. For example, the space immediately below the second rib is the second ICS.

The thoracic cavity is also divided into segments by drawing imaginary lines on the chest and back. Fig. 4.29 illustrates the anterior, lateral, and posterior divisions.

Measure the size of the chest by placing the measuring tape around the rib cage at the nipple line. For greatest accuracy, take two measurements—one during inspiration and the other during expiration—and record the average. Chest size is important mainly in relation to head circumference (see Head Circumference earlier in this chapter). Always report marked disproportions because most are caused by abnormal head growth, although some may be a result of altered chest shape, such as barrel chest (chest is round), pectus excavatum (sternum is depressed), or pectus carinatum (sternum protrudes outward).

During infancy, the chest's shape is almost circular, with the anteroposterior (front-to-back) diameter equaling the transverse, or lateral (side-to-side), diameter. As the child grows, the chest normally increases in the transverse direction, causing the anteroposterior diameter to be less than the lateral diameter. Note the angle made by the lower costal margin and the sternum, and palpate the junction of the ribs with the costal cartilage (costochondral junction) and sternum, which should be fairly smooth.

Movement of the chest wall should be symmetric bilaterally and coordinated with breathing. During inspiration, the chest rises and expands, the diaphragm descends, and the costal angle increases. During expiration, the chest falls and decreases in size, the diaphragm rises, and the costal angle narrows (Fig. 4.30). In children younger than 6 or 7 years of age, respiratory movement is principally abdominal or diaphragmatic. In older children, particularly girls, respirations are chiefly thoracic. In either case, the chest and abdomen should rise and fall together. Always report any asymmetry of movement.

While inspecting the skin surface of the chest, observe the position of the nipples and any evidence of breast development. Normally the nipples are located slightly lateral to the midclavicular line between the fourth and fifth ribs. Note symmetry of nipple placement and normal configuration of a darker pigmented areola surrounding a flat nipple in the prepubertal child.

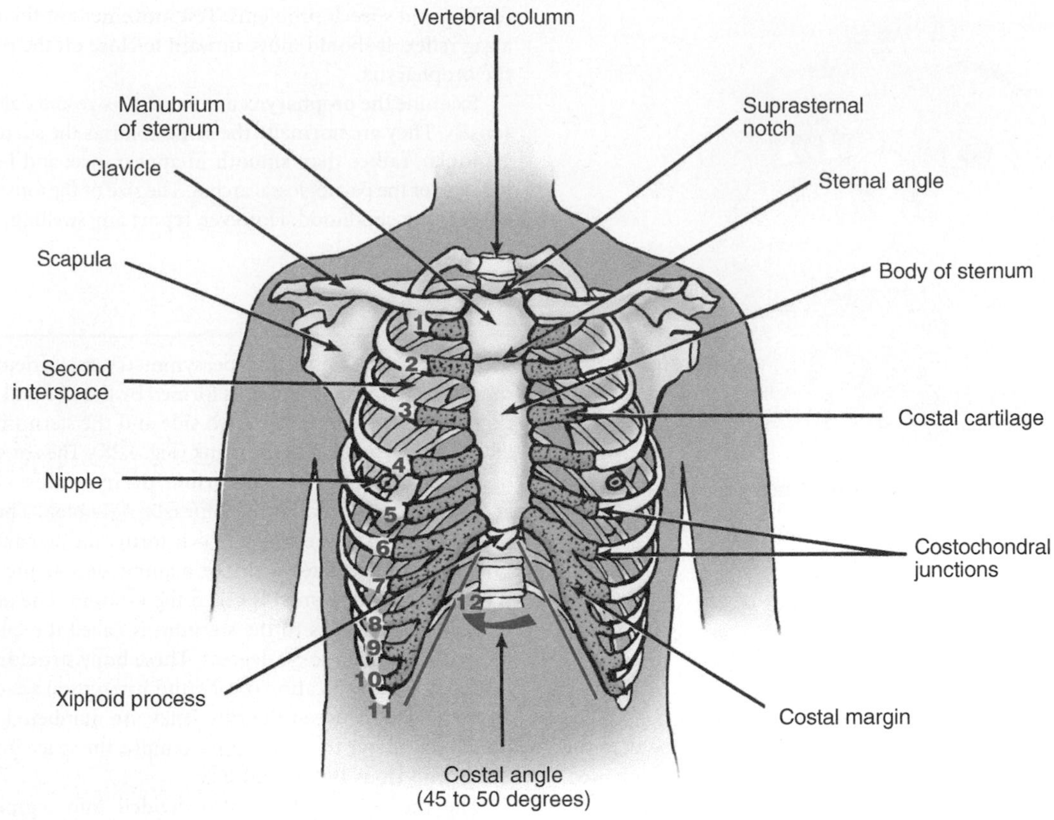

FIG. 4.28 The rib cage.

Pubertal breast development usually begins in girls between 8 and 12 years of age (see Chapter 17). Record early (precocious) or delayed breast development, as well as evidence of any other secondary sexual characteristics. In males, breast enlargement (gynecomastia) may be caused by hormonal or systemic disorders but more commonly is a result of adipose tissue from obesity or a transitory body change during early puberty. In either situation, investigate the child's feelings regarding breast enlargement.

In adolescent girls who have achieved sexual maturity, palpate the breasts for evidence of any masses or hard nodules. Use this opportunity to discuss the importance of routine breast self-examination. Emphasize that most palpable masses are benign to decrease any fear or concern that results when a mass is felt.

LUNGS

The lungs are situated inside the thoracic cavity, with one lung on each side of the sternum. Each lung is divided into an apex, which is slightly pointed and rises above the first rib; a base, which is wide and concave and rides on the dome-shaped diaphragm; and a body, which is divided into lobes. The right lung has three lobes: the right superior (upper) lobe, right middle lobe, and right inferior (lower) lobe. The left lung has only two lobes, the left superior (upper) and left inferior (lower) lobes because of the space occupied by the heart (Fig. 4.31).

Inspection of the lungs primarily involves observation of respiratory movements. Evaluate respirations for (1) rate (number per minute), (2) rhythm (regular, irregular, or periodic), (3) depth (deep or shallow), and (4) quality (effortless, automatic, difficult, or labored). Note the character of breath sounds, such as noisy, grunting, snoring, or heavy.

Evaluate respiratory movements by placing each hand flat against the back or chest with the thumbs in midline along the lower costal margin of the lungs. The child should be sitting during this procedure and, if cooperative, should take several deep breaths. During respiration, your hands will move with the chest wall. Assess the amount and speed of respiratory excursion and note any asymmetry of movement.

Experienced examiners may percuss the lungs. Percuss the anterior lung from apex to base, usually with the child in the supine or sitting position. Percuss each side of the chest in sequence to compare the sounds. When percussing the posterior lung, the procedure and sequence are the same, although the child should be sitting. Resonance is heard over all the lobes of the lungs that are not adjacent to other organs. Record and report any deviation from the expected sound.

Auscultation

Auscultation involves using the stethoscope to evaluate breath sounds (see Nursing Care Guidelines box). Breath sounds are best heard if the child inspires deeply (see Atraumatic Care box). In the lungs breath sounds are classified as vesicular, bronchovesicular, or bronchial (Box 4.9).

Absent or diminished breath sounds are always an abnormal finding warranting investigation. Fluid, air, or solid masses in the pleural space all interfere with the conduction of breath sounds. Diminished breath sounds in certain segments of the lung can alert the nurse to pulmonary areas that may benefit from chest physiotherapy. Increased breath sounds after pulmonary therapy indicates improved passage of air through the respiratory tract. Box 4.10 lists terms used to describe various respiration patterns.

Various pulmonary abnormalities produce adventitious sounds that are not normally heard over the chest. These sounds occur in addition to normal or abnormal breath sounds. They are classified into two main groups: (1) crackles, which result from the passage of air through fluid or moisture, and (2) wheezes, which are produced as air passes through narrowed passageways, regardless of the cause,

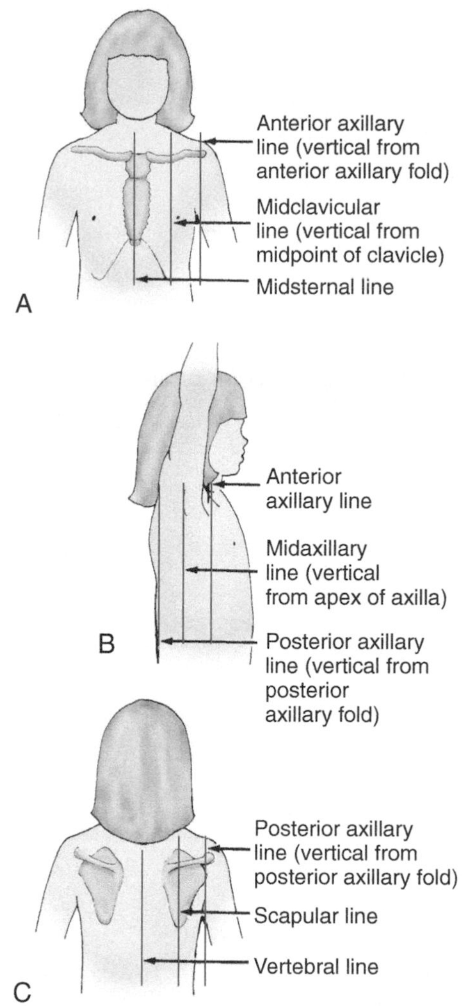

FIG. 4.29 Imaginary landmarks of the chest. **A,** Anterior. **B,** Right lateral. **C,** Posterior.

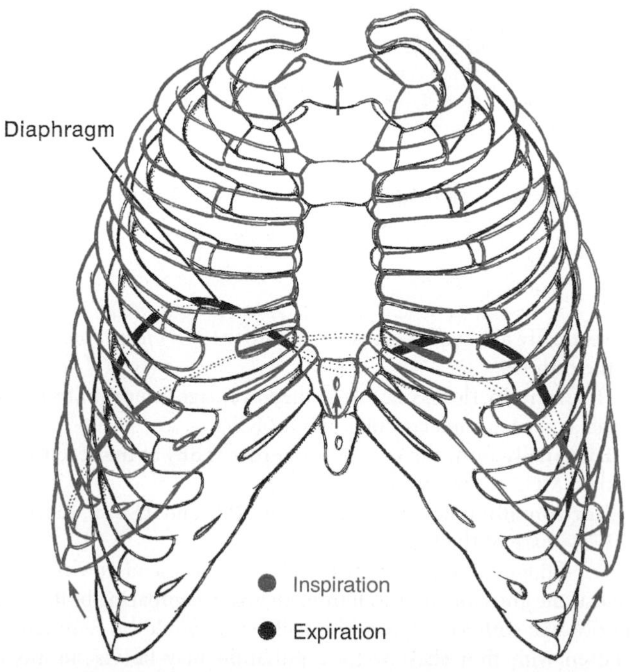

FIG. 4.30 Movement of the chest during respiration.

NURSING CARE GUIDELINES

Effective Auscultation

- Make certain child is relaxed and not crying, talking, or laughing. Record if child is crying.
- Check that room is comfortable and quiet.
- Warm stethoscope before placing it against skin.
- Apply firm pressure on chest piece but not enough to prevent vibrations and transmission of sound.
- Avoid placing stethoscope over hair or clothing, moving it against skin, breathing on tubing, or sliding fingers over chest piece, which may cause sounds that falsely resemble pathologic findings.
- Use a symmetric and orderly approach to compare sounds.

ATRAUMATIC CARE

Encouraging Deep Breaths

- Ask child to "blow out" the light on an otoscope or pocket flashlight; discreetly turn off the light on the last try so that the child feels successful.
- Place a cotton ball in child's palm; ask child to blow the ball into the air and have parent catch it.
- Hold a tissue in front of child and ask child to blow the tissue in the air.
- Have child blow a pinwheel, a party horn, or bubbles.

BOX 4.9 Classification of Normal Breath Sounds

Vesicular Breath Sounds

Heard over entire surface of the lungs, with exception of upper intrascapular area and area beneath the manubrium.

Inspiration is louder, longer, and higher pitched than expiration.

The sound is a soft, swishing noise.

Bronchovesicular Breath Sounds

Heard over the manubrium and in the upper intrascapular regions where trachea and bronchi bifurcate.

Inspiration is louder and higher pitched than in vesicular breathing.

Bronchial Breath Sounds

Heard only over trachea near the suprasternal notch.

The inspiratory phase is short, and the expiratory phase is long.

BOX 4.10 Various Patterns of Respiration

Tachypnea: Increased rate
Bradypnea: Decreased rate
Dyspnea: Distress during breathing
Apnea: Cessation of breathing
Hyperpnea: Increased depth
Hypoventilation: Decreased depth (shallow) and irregular rhythm
Hyperventilation: Increased rate and depth
Kussmaul respiration: Hyperventilation, gasping and labored respiration; usually seen in diabetic coma or other states of respiratory acidosis
Cheyne-Stokes respiration: Gradually increasing rate and depth with periods of apnea
Biot respiration: Periods of hyperpnea alternating with apnea (similar to Cheyne-Stokes except that depth remains constant)
Seesaw (paradoxic) respirations: Chest falls on inspiration and rises on expiration
Agonal: Last gasping breaths before death

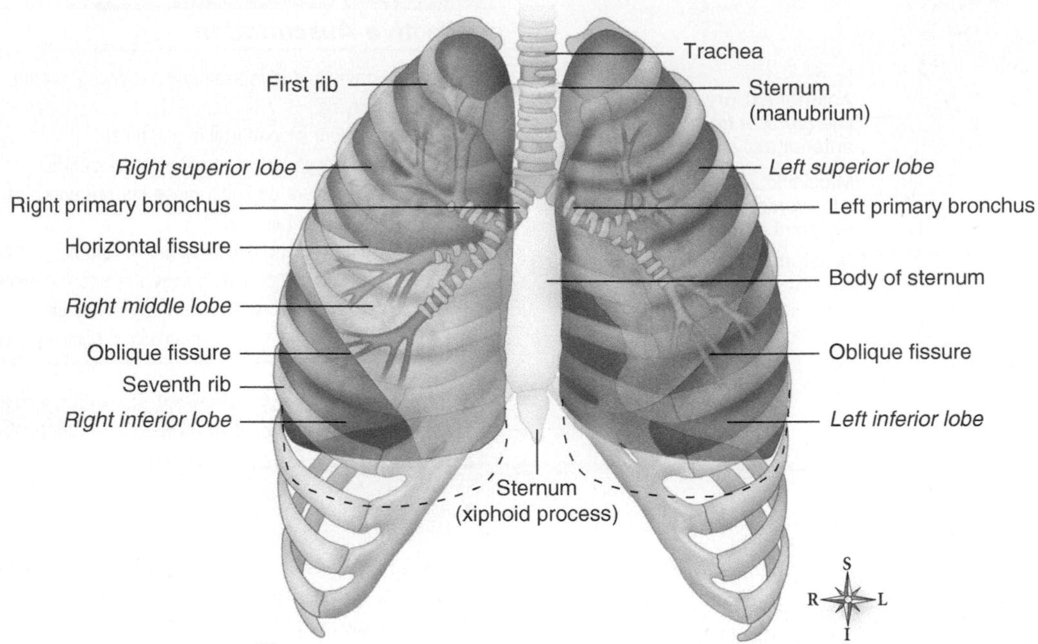

FIG. 4.31 Location of the lobes of the lungs within the thoracic cavity. (From Patton, K. T., & Thibodeau, G. A. [2013]. *Anatomy and physiology* [8th ed.]. St. Louis, MO: Mosby.)

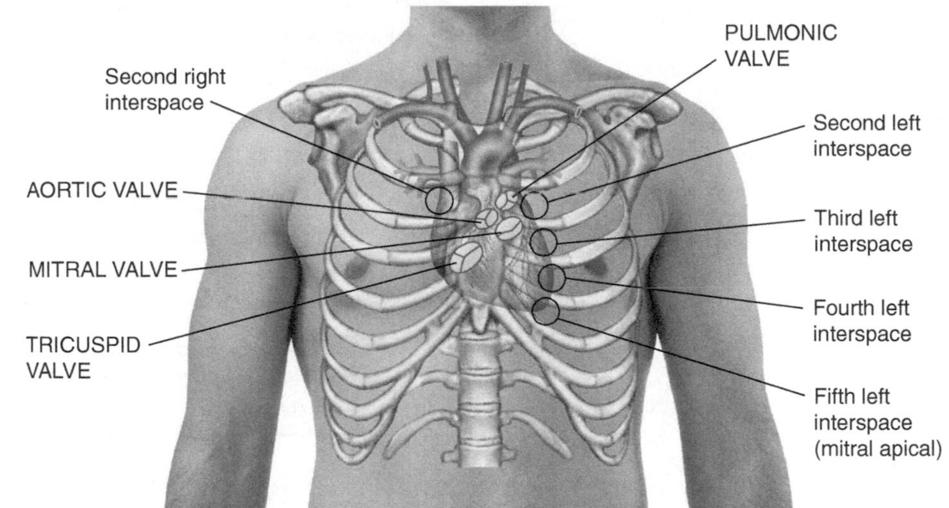

FIG. 4.32 Position of the heart within the thorax. (From Ball, J. W., Dains, J. E., Flynn, J. A., et al. [2014]. *Seidel's guide to physical examination* [8th ed.]. St. Louis, MO: Elsevier.)

such as exudate, inflammation, spasm, or tumor. Considerable practice with an experienced tutor is necessary to differentiate the various types of lung sounds. Often it is best to describe the type of sound heard in the lungs rather than trying to label it. Always report any abnormal sounds for further evaluation.

HEART

The heart is situated in the thoracic cavity between the lungs in the mediastinum and above the diaphragm (Fig. 4.32). About two-thirds of the heart lies within the left side of the rib cage, with the other third on the right side as it crosses the sternum. The heart is positioned in the thorax like a trapezoid:

- **Vertically** along the right sternal border (RSB) from the second to the fifth rib
- **Horizontally** (long side) from the lower right sternum to the fifth rib at the left midclavicular line (LMCL)
- **Diagonally** from the left sternal border (LSB) at the second rib to the LMCL at the fifth rib
- **Horizontally** (short side) from the RSB and LSB at the second ICS—base of the heart

Inspection is easiest when the child is sitting in a semi-Fowler position. Look at the anterior chest wall from an angle, comparing both sides of the rib cage with each other. Normally they should be symmetric. In children with thin chest walls, a pulsation may be visible. Because comprehensive evaluation of cardiac function is not limited to the heart,

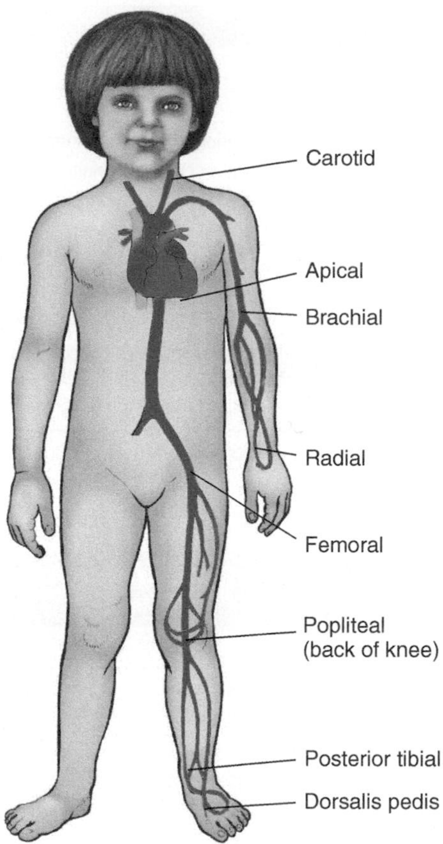

FIG. 4.33 Location of pulses.

also consider other findings such as the presence of all pulses (especially the femoral pulses) (Fig. 4.33), distended neck veins, clubbing of the fingers, peripheral cyanosis, edema, blood pressure, and respiratory status.

Use palpation to determine the location of the apical impulse (AI), the most lateral cardiac impulse that may correspond to the apex. The AI is found

- At the fifth ICS and LMCL in children older than 7 years of age
- At the fourth ICS and just lateral to the LMCL in children younger than 7 years of age

Although the AI gives a general idea of the size of the heart (with enlargement, the apex is lower and more lateral), its normal location is variable, making it an unreliable indicator of heart size.

The point of maximum intensity (PMI), as the name implies, is the area of most intense pulsation. Usually the PMI is located at the same site as the AI, but it can occur elsewhere. For this reason, the two terms should not be used synonymously.

Assess capillary refill time, an important test for circulation, by pressing the skin lightly on a central site, such as the forehead, or a peripheral site such as the nail beds, to produce a slight blanching. The time it takes for the blanched area to return to its original color is the capillary refill time.

! NURSING ALERT

Capillary refill should be brisk—less than 2 seconds. Prolonged refill may be associated with poor systemic perfusion or a cool ambient temperature.

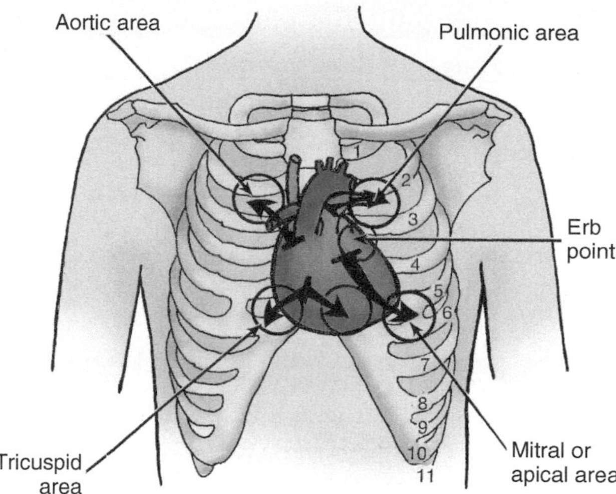

FIG. 4.34 Direction of heart sounds for anatomic valve sites and areas *(circled)* for auscultation.

Auscultation

Origin of Heart Sounds

The heart sounds are produced by the opening and closing of the valves and the vibration of blood against the walls of the heart and vessels. Normally two sounds—S_1 and S_2—are heard, which correspond, respectively, to the familiar "lub dub" often used to describe the sounds. S_1 is caused by closure of the tricuspid and mitral valves (sometimes called the atrioventricular valves). S_2 is the result of closure of the pulmonic and aortic valves (sometimes called semilunar valves). Normally the split of the two sounds in S_2 is distinguishable and widens during inspiration. Physiologic splitting is a significant normal finding.

! NURSING ALERT

Fixed splitting, in which the split in S_2 does not change during inspiration, is an important diagnostic sign of atrial septal defect.

Two other heart sounds, S_3 and S_4, may be produced. S_3 is normally heard in some children. S_4 is rarely heard as a normal heart sound; it usually indicates the need for further cardiac evaluation.

Differentiating Normal Heart Sounds

Fig. 4.34 illustrates the approximate anatomic position of the valves within the heart chambers. Note that the anatomic location of valves does not correspond to the area where the sounds are heard best. The auscultatory sites are located in the direction of the blood flow through the valves.

Normally S_1 is louder at the apex of the heart in the mitral and tricuspid area, and S_2 is louder near the base of the heart in the pulmonic and aortic area (Table 4.9). Listen to each sound by inching down the chest. Auscultate the following areas for sounds, such as murmurs, which may radiate to these sites: sternoclavicular area above the clavicles and manubrium, area along the sternal border, area along the left midaxillary line, and area below the scapulae.

Auscultate the heart with the child in at least two positions: sitting and reclining. If adventitious sounds are detected, further evaluate them with the child standing, sitting and leaning forward, and lying on the left side. For example, atrial sounds such as S_4 are heard best with the person in a recumbent position and usually fade if the person sits or stands.

TABLE 4.9 Sequence of Auscultating Heart Sounds*

Auscultatory Site	Chest Location	Characteristics of Heart Sounds
Aortic area	Second right ICS close to sternum	S_2 heard louder than S_1; aortic closure heard loudest
Pulmonic area	Second left ICS close to sternum	Splitting of S_2 heard best, normally widens on inspiration; pulmonic closure heard best
Erb's point	Third left ICS close to sternum	Frequent site of innocent murmurs and those of aortic or pulmonic origin
Tricuspid area	Fourth right and left ICSs close to sternum	S_1 heard as louder sound preceding S_2 (S_1 synchronous with carotid pulse)
Mitral or apical area	Fifth ICS, LMCL (fourth ICS and lateral to LMCL in infants)	S_1 heard loudest; splitting of S_1 may be audible because mitral closure is louder than tricuspid closure S_1 heard best at beginning of expiration with child in recumbent or left side-lying position; occurs immediately after S_2; sounds like word S_1 S_2 S_3: "Ken-tuc-ky" S_4 heard best during expiration with child in recumbent position (left side-lying position decreases sound); occurs immediately before S_1; sounds like word S_4 S_1 S_2: "Ten-nes-see"

*Use both diaphragm and bell chest pieces when auscultating heart sounds. Bell chest piece is necessary for low-pitched sounds of murmurs, S_3, and S_4.
ICS, Intercostal space; *LMCL,* left midclavicular line.

NURSING TIP

To distinguish between S_1 and S_2 heart sounds, simultaneously palpate the carotid pulse with the index and middle fingers and listen to the heart sounds; S_1 is synchronous with the carotid pulse.

Evaluate heart sounds for (1) quality (they should be clear and distinct, not muffled, diffuse, or distant); (2) intensity, especially in relation to the location or auscultatory site (they should not be weak or pounding); (3) rate (they should have the same rate as the radial pulse); and (4) rhythm (they should be regular and even). A particular arrhythmia that occurs normally in many children is **sinus arrhythmia**, in which the heart rate increases with inspiration and decreases with expiration. Differentiate this rhythm from a truly abnormal arrhythmia by having children hold their breath. In sinus arrhythmia, cessation of breathing causes the heart rate to remain steady.

Heart Murmurs

Another important category of the heart sounds is **murmurs**, which are produced by vibrations within the heart chambers or in the major arteries from the back-and-forth flow of blood. (For a more detailed discussion, see Cardiovascular Dysfunction, Chapter 27) Murmurs are classified as follows:

- **Innocent**—No anatomic or physiologic abnormality exists.
- **Functional**—No anatomic cardiac defect exists, but a physiologic abnormality (e.g., anemia) is present.
- **Organic**—A cardiac defect with or without a physiologic abnormality exists.

The description and classification of murmurs are skills that require considerable practice and training. In general, recognize murmurs as distinct swishing sounds that occur in addition to the normal heart sounds and record the (1) location, or the area of the heart in which the murmur is heard best; (2) time of the occurrence of the murmur within the S_1-S_2 cycle; (3) intensity (evaluate in relationship to the child's position); and (4) loudness. Table 4.10 lists the usual subjective method of grading the loudness or intensity of a murmur.

TABLE 4.10 Grading the Intensity of Heart Murmurs

Grade	Description
I	Very faint; often not heard if child sits up
II	Usually readily heard; slightly louder than grade I; audible in all positions
III	Loud, but not accompanied by a thrill
IV	Loud, accompanied by a thrill
V	Loud enough to be heard with a stethoscope barely touching the chest; accompanied by a thrill
VI	Loud enough to be heard with the stethoscope not touching the chest; often heard with the human ear close to the chest; accompanied by a thrill

ABDOMEN

Examination of the abdomen involves inspection, followed by auscultation and then palpation. Experienced examiners may also percuss the abdomen to assess for organomegaly, masses, fluid, and flatus. Perform palpation last because it may distort the normal abdominal sounds. Knowledge of the anatomic placement of the abdominal organs is essential to differentiate normal, expected findings from abnormal ones (Fig. 4.35).

For descriptive purposes, the abdominal cavity is divided into four quadrants by drawing a vertical line midway from the sternum to the symphysis pubis and a horizontal line across the abdomen through the umbilicus. The sections are named as follows:

- Left upper quadrant
- Left lower quadrant
- Right upper quadrant
- Right lower quadrant

Inspection

Inspect the contour of the abdomen with the child erect and supine. Normally the abdomen of infants and young children is cylindric and, in the erect position, fairly prominent because of the physiologic lordosis of the spine. In the supine position the abdomen appears flat. A midline protrusion from the xiphoid to the umbilicus or symphysis pubis is usually **diastasis recti**, or failure of the rectus abdominis muscles to join in utero. In a healthy child, a midline protrusion is usually a variation of normal muscular development.

The skin covering the abdomen should be uniformly taut, without wrinkles or creases. Sometimes silvery, whitish striae ("stretch marks") are seen, especially if the skin has been stretched as in obesity. Superficial veins are usually visible in light-skinned, thin infants, but distended veins are an abnormal finding.

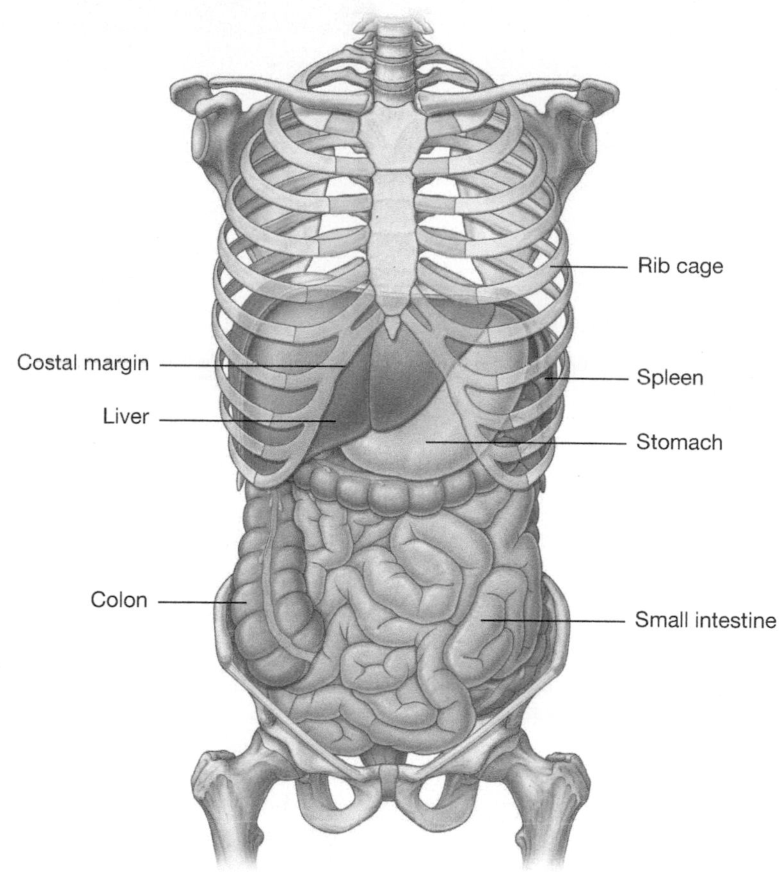

FIG. 4.35 Location of structures in the abdomen. (From Drake, R. L., Vogl, W., & Mitchell, A. W. M. [2015]. *Gray's anatomy for students* [3rd ed.]. New York: Churchill Livingstone.)

> **! NURSING ALERT**
>
> A tense, boardlike abdomen is a serious sign of paralytic ileus and intestinal obstruction.

> **NURSING TIP**
>
> If the child is too young to cough, have the child blow on a tissue or laugh to raise the intraabdominal pressure sufficiently to demonstrate the presence of an inguinal hernia.

Observe movement of the abdomen. Normally chest and abdominal movements are synchronous. In infants and thin children peristaltic waves may be visible through the abdominal wall; they are best observed by standing at eye level to and across from the abdomen. Always report this finding.

Examine the umbilicus for size, hygiene, and evidence of any abnormalities, such as hernias. The umbilicus should be flat or only slightly protruding. If a herniation is present, palpate the sac for abdominal contents and estimate the approximate size of the opening. Umbilical hernias are common in infants, especially in African American children.

Hernias may exist elsewhere on the abdominal wall (Fig. 4.36). An inguinal hernia is a protrusion of peritoneum through the abdominal wall in the inguinal canal. It occurs mostly in males, is frequently bilateral, and may be visible as a mass in the scrotum. To locate a hernia, slide the little finger into the external inguinal ring at the base of the scrotum and ask the child to cough. If a hernia is present, it will hit the tip of the finger.

A femoral hernia, which occurs more frequently in girls, is felt or seen as a small mass on the anterior surface of the thigh just below the inguinal ligament in the femoral canal (a potential space medial to the femoral artery). Feel for a hernia by placing the index finger of your right hand on the child's right femoral pulse (left hand for left pulse) and the middle finger flat against the skin toward the midline. The ring finger lies over the femoral canal, where the herniation occurs. Palpation of hernias in the pelvic region is often part of the genital examination.

Auscultation

The most important finding to listen for is peristalsis, or bowel sounds, which sound like short metallic clicks and gurgles. Record their frequency per minute (e.g., 5 sounds/min). Listen for up to 5 minutes before determining that bowel sounds are absent. Stimulate bowel sounds by stroking the abdominal surface with a fingernail. Report absence of bowel sounds or hyperperistalsis because either usually denotes an abdominal disorder.

Palpation

There are two types of palpation: superficial and deep. For superficial palpation, lightly place your hand against the skin and feel each quadrant, noting any areas of tenderness, muscle tone, and superficial lesions such as cysts. Because superficial palpation is often perceived as tickling, use several techniques to minimize this sensation and relax the child (see Atraumatic Care box). Admonishing the child to stop laughing only draws attention to the sensation and decreases cooperation.

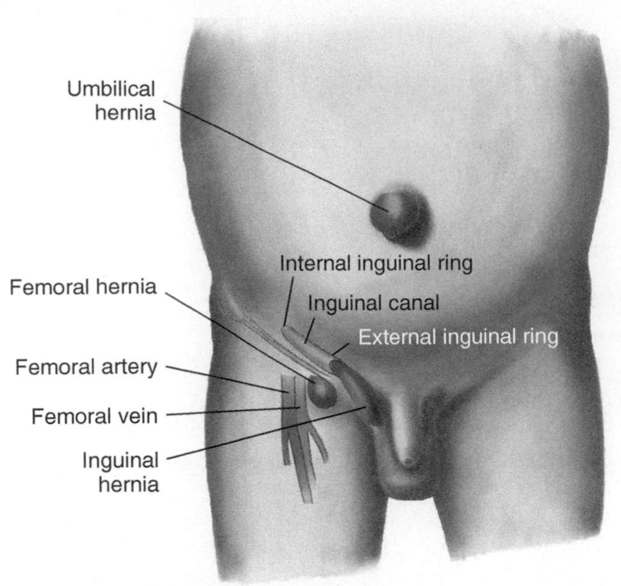

FIG. 4.36 Location of hernias.

ATRAUMATIC CARE

Promoting Relaxation During Abdominal Palpation

- Position child comfortably, such as in a semireclining position in the parent's lap, with knees flexed.
- Warm your hands before touching the skin.
- Use distraction, such as telling stories or talking to child.
- Teach child to use deep breathing and to concentrate on an object.
- Give infant a bottle or pacifier.
- Begin with light, superficial palpation and gradually progress to deeper palpation.
- Palpate any tender or painful areas last.
- Have child hold the parent's hand and squeeze it if palpation is uncomfortable.
- Use the nonpalpating hand to comfort the child, such as placing the free hand on the child's shoulder while palpating the abdomen.

To minimize sensation of tickling during palpation:

- Have children "help" with palpation by placing a hand over the palpating hand.
- Have them place a hand on the abdomen with the fingers spread wide apart, and palpate between their fingers.

Deep palpation is for palpating organs and large blood vessels and for detecting masses and tenderness that were not discovered during superficial palpation. Palpation usually begins in the lower quadrants and proceeds upward to avoid missing the edge of an enlarged liver or spleen. Except for palpating the liver, successful identification of other organs (e.g., the spleen, kidney, and part of the colon) requires considerable practice with tutored supervision. Report any questionable mass. The lower edge of the liver is sometimes felt in infants and young children as a superficial mass 1 to 2 cm (0.4 to 0.8 inch) below the right costal margin (the distance is sometimes measured in fingerbreadths). Normally the liver descends during inspiration as the diaphragm moves downward. Do not mistake this downward displacement as a sign of liver enlargement.

Palpate the **femoral pulses** by placing the tips of two or three fingers (index, middle, or ring) along the inguinal ligament about midway

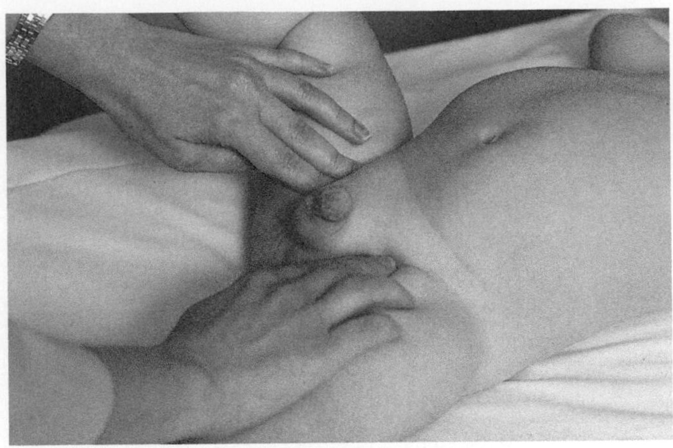

FIG. 4.37 Palpating for femoral pulses.

! NURSING ALERT

If the liver is palpable 3 cm (1.2 inch) below the right costal margin or the spleen is palpable more than 2 cm (0.8 inch) below the left costal margin, these organs are enlarged—a finding that is always reported for further investigation.

between the iliac crest and symphysis pubis. Feel both pulses simultaneously to make certain that they are equal and strong (Fig. 4.37).

! NURSING ALERT

Absence of femoral pulses is a significant sign of coarctation of the aorta and is referred for evaluation.

GENITALIA

Examination of genitalia conveniently follows assessment of the abdomen while the child is still supine. In adolescents, inspection of the genitalia may be left to the end of the examination. The best approach is to examine the genitalia matter-of-factly, placing no more emphasis on this part of the assessment than on any other segment. It helps relieve children's and parents' anxiety by telling them the results of the findings; for example, the nurse might say, "Everything looks fine here."

If it is necessary to ask questions, such as about discharge or difficulty urinating, respect the child's privacy by covering the lower abdomen with the gown or underpants. To prevent embarrassing interruptions, keep the door or curtain closed and post a "do not disturb" sign. Have a drape ready to cover the genitalia if someone enters the room.

In examining the genitalia, wear gloves when touching the child. It might be helpful for the adolescent to know that wearing gloves also prevents skin-to-skin contact.

The genital examination is an excellent time for eliciting questions or concerns about body function or sexual activity. Use this opportunity to increase or reinforce the child's knowledge of sexual anatomy by naming each body part and explaining its function. This part of the health assessment is an opportune time to teach testicular self-examination to boys.

Male Genitalia

Note the external appearance of the glans and shaft of the penis, the prepuce, the urethral meatus, and the scrotum (Fig. 4.38). The penis is generally small in infants and young boys until puberty, when it begins to increase in both length and width. In an obese child, the penis often looks abnormally small because of the folds of skin partially covering it at the base. Be familiar with normal pubertal growth of the external male genitalia to compare the findings with the expected sequence of maturation (see Chapter 17).

Examine the glans (head of the penis) and shaft (portion between the perineum and prepuce) for signs of swelling, skin lesions, inflammation, or other irregularities. Any of these signs may indicate underlying disorders, especially sexually transmitted infections.

Carefully inspect the urethral meatus for location and evidence of discharge. Normally it is centered at the tip of the glans. Note the hair distribution. Normally, before puberty, no pubic hair is present. Soft, downy hair at the base of the penis is an early sign of pubertal maturation. In older adolescents, hair distribution is diamond shaped from the umbilicus to the anus.

Note the location and size of the scrotum. The scrota hang freely from the perineum behind the penis, and the left scrotum normally hangs lower than the right. In infants, the scrota appear large in relation to the rest of the genitalia. The skin of the scrotum is loose and highly

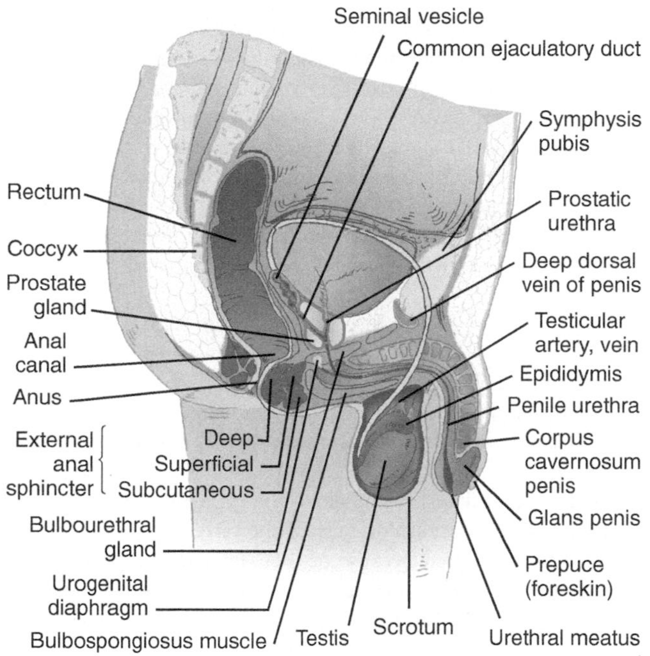

FIG. 4.38 Major structures of genitalia in an uncircumcised postpubertal male. (From Douglas, G., Nicol, F., & Robertson, C. [2013]. *Mackleod's clinical examination* [13th ed.]. Philadelphia, PA: Elsevier.)

rugated (wrinkled). During early adolescence, the skin normally becomes redder and coarser. In dark-skinned children, the scrota are usually more deeply pigmented.

Palpation of the scrotum includes identification of the testes, epididymis, and, if present, inguinal hernias. In the prepubertal child, the two testes are felt as small, ovoid bodies about 1.5 to 2 cm long (1 to 3 ml in volume)—one in each scrotal sac. They do not enlarge until puberty (see Chapter 17). Pubertal testicular development normally begins in boys between 9 and 13 years old. Record early (precocious) or delayed pubertal development, as well as evidence of any other secondary sexual characteristics.

When palpating for the presence of the testes, avoid stimulating the cremasteric reflex, which is stimulated by cold, touch, emotional excitement, or exercise. This reflex pulls the testes higher into the pelvic cavity. Several measures are useful in preventing the cremasteric reflex during palpation of the scrotum. First, warm the hands. Second, if the child is old enough, examine him in a tailor or "Indian" position, which stretches the muscle, preventing its contraction (Fig. 4.39, *A*). Third, block the normal pathway of ascent of the testes by placing the thumb and index finger over the upper part of the scrotal sac along the inguinal canal (Fig. 4.39, *B*). If there is any question concerning the existence of two testes, place the index and middle fingers in a scissors fashion to separate the right and left scrota. If, after using these techniques, you have not palpated the testes, feel along the inguinal canal and perineum to locate masses that may be undescended testes. Report any failure to palpate the testes for further evaluation.

Female Genitalia

The examination of female genitalia is limited to inspection and palpation of external structures. If a vaginal examination is required, the nurse should make an appropriate referral unless he or she is qualified to perform the procedure.

A convenient position for examination of the genitalia involves placing the young child supine on the examining table or in a semireclining position on the parent's lap with the feet supported on your knees as you sit facing the child. Divert the child's attention from the examination by instructing her to try to keep the soles of her feet pressed against each other. Separate the labia majora with the thumb and index finger and retract outward to expose the labia minora, urethral meatus, and vaginal orifice.

Examine the female genitalia for size and location of the structures of the vulva, or pudendum (Fig. 4.40). The mons pubis is a pad of adipose tissue over the symphysis pubis. At puberty, the mons is covered with hair, which extends along the labia. The usual pattern of female hair distribution is an inverted triangle. The appearance of soft, downy hair along the labia majora is an early sign of sexual maturation. Note

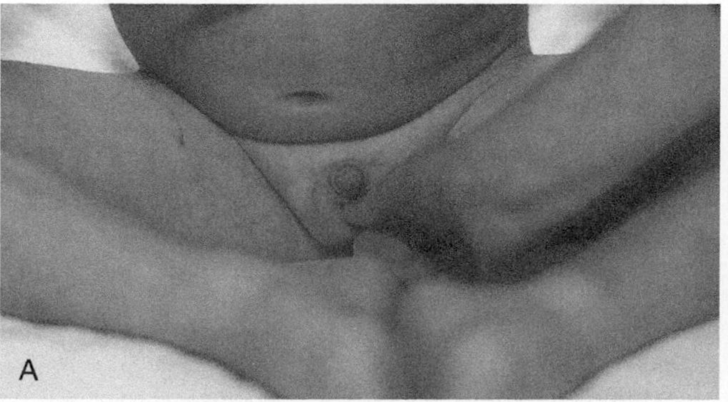

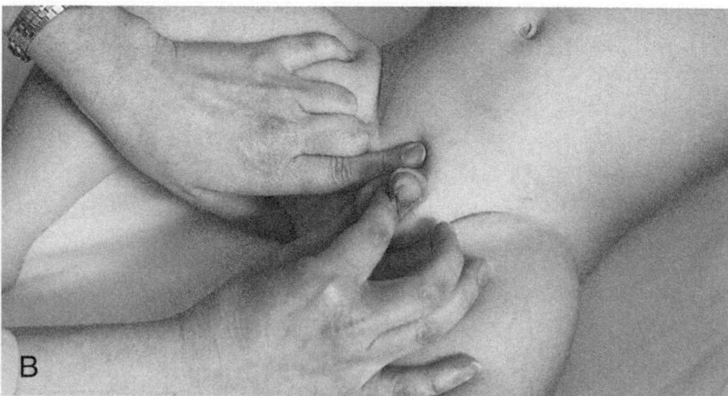

FIG. 4.39 A, Preventing the cremasteric reflex by having the child sit in the tailor position. **B,** Blocking the inguinal canal during palpation of the scrotum for descended testes.

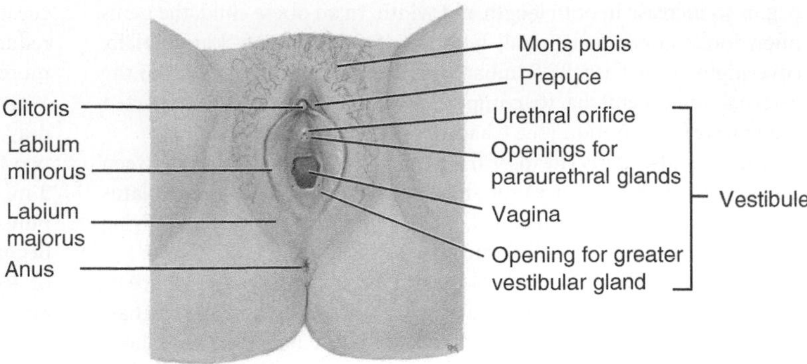

FIG. 4.40 External structures of the genitalia in a postpubertal female. The labia are spread to reveal deeper structures. (From Paulsen, F., & Waschke, J. [2013]. *Sobotta atlas of human anatomy* [2nd vol., 15th ed.]. Munich, Germany: Elsevier.)

the size and location of the clitoris, a small, erectile organ located at the anterior end of the labia minora. It is covered by a small flap of skin, the prepuce.

The labia majora are two thick folds of skin running posteriorly from the mons to the posterior commissure of the vagina. Internal to the labia majora are two folds of skin called the labia minora. Although the labia minora are usually prominent in the newborn, they gradually atrophy, which makes them almost invisible until their enlargement during puberty. The inner surface of the labia should be pink and moist. Note the size of the labia and any evidence of fusion, which may suggest male scrota. Normally, no masses are palpable within the labia.

The urethral meatus is located posterior to the clitoris and is surrounded by the Skene glands and ducts. Although not a prominent structure, the meatus appears as a small V-shaped slit. Note its location, especially if it opens from the clitoris or inside the vagina. Gently palpate the glands, which are common sites of cysts and sexually transmitted lesions.

The vaginal orifice is located posterior to the urethral meatus. Its appearance varies depending on individual anatomy and sexual activity. Ordinarily, examination of the vagina is limited to inspection. In virgins, a thin crescent-shaped or circular membrane, called the hymen, may cover part of the vaginal opening. In some instances, it completely occludes the orifice. After rupture, small rounded pieces of tissue called caruncles remain. Although an imperforate hymen denotes lack of penile intercourse, a perforate one does not necessarily indicate sexual activity (see also Sexual Abuse, Chapter 16).

! NURSING ALERT

In girls who have been circumcised, the genitalia will appear different. Do not show surprise or disgust, but note the appearance and discuss the procedure with the young woman (see also Chapter 7, Cultural Considerations: Circumcision).

Surrounding the vaginal opening are Bartholin glands, which secrete a clear, mucoid fluid into the vagina for lubrication during intercourse. Palpate the ducts for cysts. Note the discharge from the vagina, which is usually clear or white.

ANUS

After examination of the genitalia, it is easy to identify the anal area, although the child should be placed on the abdomen. Note the general firmness of the buttocks and symmetry of the gluteal folds. Assess the tone of the anal sphincter by eliciting the anal reflex (anal wink). Gently scratching the anal area results in an obvious quick contraction of the external anal sphincter.

BACK AND EXTREMITIES

Spine

Note the general curvature of the spine. Normally the back of a newborn is rounded or C shaped from the thoracic and pelvic curves. The development of the cervical and lumbar curves approximates development of various motor skills, such as cervical curvature with head control, and gives the older child the typical double S curve.

Marked curvatures in posture are abnormal. Scoliosis, lateral curvature of the spine, is an important childhood problem, especially in girls. Although scoliosis may be identified by observing and palpating the spine and noting a sideways displacement, more objective tests include the following:

- With the child standing erect, clothed only in underpants (and bra if older girl), observe from behind, noting asymmetry of the shoulders and hips.
- With the child bending forward so that the back is parallel to the floor, observe from the front and side, noting asymmetry or prominence of the rib cage.
- A slight limp, a crooked hemline, asymmetric heights of shoulders or hips, or complaints of a sore back are other signs and symptoms of scoliosis.

Inspect the back, especially along the spine, for any tufts of hair, dimples, or discoloration. Mobility of the vertebral column is easy to assess in most children because of their tendency to be in constant motion during the examination. However, you can test mobility by asking the child to sit up from a prone position or to do a modified sit-up exercise.

Movement of the cervical spine is an important diagnostic sign of neurologic problems, such as meningitis. Normally movement of the head in all directions is effortless.

! NURSING ALERT

Hyperextension of the neck and spine, or *opisthotonos,* which is accompanied by pain when the head is flexed, is always referred for immediate evaluation.

Extremities

Inspect each extremity for symmetry of length and size; refer any deviation for orthopedic evaluation. Count the fingers and toes to be certain of the normal number. This is so often taken for granted that an extra digit (polydactyly) or fusion of digits (syndactyly) may go unnoticed.

Inspect the arms and legs for temperature and color, which should be equal in each extremity, although the feet may normally be colder than the hands.

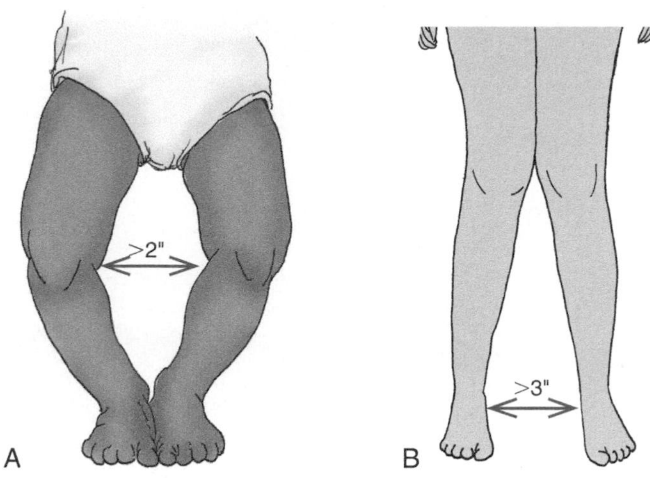

FIG. 4.41 **A,** Genu varum. **B,** Genu valgum.

Assess the shape of bones. There are several variations of bone shape in children. Although many of them cause parents concern, most are benign and require no treatment. Bowleg, or genu varum, is lateral bowing of the tibia. It is clinically present when the child stands with an outward bowing of the legs, giving the appearance of a bow. Usually there is an outward curvature of both femur and tibia (Fig. 4.41, *A*). Toddlers are usually bowlegged after beginning to walk until all their lower back and leg muscles are well developed. Unilateral or asymmetric bowlegs that are present beyond 2 to 3 years old, particularly in African American children, may represent pathologic conditions requiring further investigation.

Knock-knee, or genu valgum, appears as the opposite of bowleg, in that the knees are close together but the feet are spread apart. It is determined clinically by using the same method as for genu varum but by measuring the distance between the malleoli, which normally should be less than 7.5 cm (3 inches) (see Fig. 4.41, *B*). Knock-knee is normally present in children from about 2 to 7 years of age. Knock-knee that is excessive, asymmetric, accompanied by short stature, or evident in a child nearing puberty requires further evaluation.

Next inspect the feet. Infants' and toddlers' feet appear flat because the foot is normally wide and the arch is covered by a fat pad. Development of the arch occurs naturally from the action of walking. Normally at birth the feet are held in a valgus (outward) or varus (inward) position. To determine whether a foot deformity at birth is a result of intrauterine position or development, scratch the outer, then inner, side of the sole. If the foot position is self-correctable, it will assume a right angle to the leg. As the child begins to walk, the feet turn outward less than 30 degrees and inward less than 10 degrees.

Toddlers have a "toddling" or broad-based gait, which facilitates walking by lowering the center of gravity. As the child reaches preschool age, the legs are brought closer together. By school age, the walking posture is much more graceful and balanced.

The most common gait problem in young children is pigeon toe, or toeing in, which usually results from torsional deformities, such as internal tibial torsion (abnormal rotation or bowing of the tibia). Tests for tibial torsion include measuring the thigh-foot angle, which requires considerable practice for accuracy.

Elicit the plantar or grasp reflex by exerting firm but gentle pressure with the tip of the thumb against the lateral sole of the foot from the heel upward to the little toe and then across to the big toe. The normal response in children who are walking is flexion of the toes. Babinski sign, dorsiflexion of the big toe and fanning of the other toes, is normal during infancy but abnormal after about 1 year old or when locomotion begins (see Fig. 7.10).

Joints

Evaluate the joints for range of motion. Normally this requires no specific testing if you have observed the child's movements during the examination. However, routinely investigate the hips in infants for congenital dislocation by checking for subluxation of the hip (see Chapter 33. Report any evidence of joint immobility or hyperflexibility. Palpate the joints for heat, tenderness, and swelling. These signs, as well as redness over the joint, warrant further investigation.

Muscles

Note symmetry and quality of muscle development, tone, and strength. Observe development by looking at the shape and contour of the body in both a relaxed and a tensed state. Estimate tone by grasping the muscle and feeling its firmness when it is relaxed and contracted. A common site for testing tone is the biceps muscle of the arm. Children are usually willing to "make a muscle" by clenching their fist.

Estimate strength by having the child use an extremity to push or pull against resistance, as in the following examples:

- **Arm strength:** Child holds the arms outstretched in front of the body and tries to raise the arms while downward pressure is applied.
- **Hand strength:** Child shakes hands with nurse and squeezes one or two fingers of the nurse's hand.
- **Leg strength:** Child sits on a table or chair with the legs dangling and tries to raise the legs while downward pressure is applied.

Note symmetry of strength in the extremities, hands, and fingers, and report evidence of paresis, or weakness.

NEUROLOGIC ASSESSMENT

The assessment of the nervous system is the broadest and most diverse part of the examination process because every human function, both physical and emotional, is controlled by neurologic impulses. Much of the neurologic examination has already been discussed, such as assessment of behavior, sensory testing, and motor function. The following focuses on a general appraisal of cerebellar function, deep tendon reflexes, and the cranial nerves.

Cerebellar Function

The cerebellum controls balance and coordination. Much of the assessment of cerebellar function is included in observing the child's posture, body movements, gait, and development of fine and gross motor skills. Tests (e.g., balancing on one foot and the heel-to-toe walk) assess balance. Test coordination by asking the child to reach for a toy, button clothes, tie shoes, or draw a straight line on a piece of paper (provided the child is old enough to do these activities). Coordination can also be tested by any sequence of rapid, successive movements, such as quickly touching each finger with the thumb of the same hand.

Several tests for cerebellar function can be performed as games (Box 4.11). When a Romberg test is done, stay beside the child if there is a possibility that he or she might fall. School-age children should be able to perform these tests, although in the finger-to-nose test, preschoolers normally can only bring the finger within 5 to 7.5 cm (2 to 3 inches) of the nose. Difficulty in performing these exercises indicates a poor sense of position (especially with the eyes closed) and incoordination (especially with the eyes opened).

Reflexes

Testing reflexes is an important part of the neurologic examination. Persistence of primitive reflexes (see Chapter 7), loss of reflexes, or

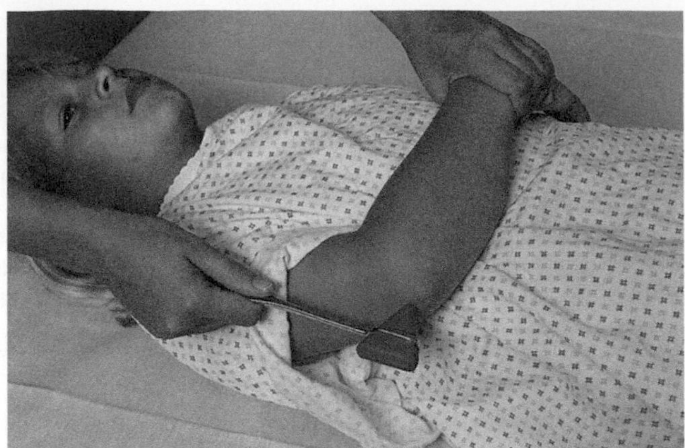

FIG. 4.42 Testing for the triceps reflex. Child is placed supine, with the forearm resting over the chest, and the triceps tendon is struck. *Alternate procedure:* The child's arm is abducted, with the upper arm supported and the forearm allowed to hang freely. The triceps tendon is struck. Normal response is partial extension of the forearm.

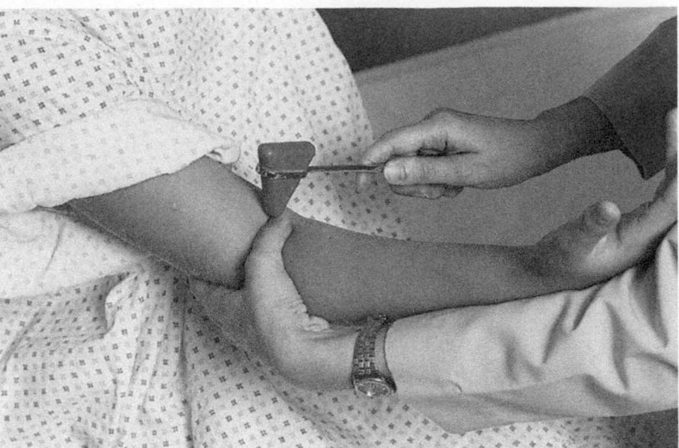

FIG. 4.43 Testing for the biceps reflex. The child's arm is held by the placing partially flexed elbow in the examiner's hand with the thumb over the antecubital space. The examiner's thumbnail is struck with a hammer. Normal response is partial flexion of the forearm.

BOX 4.11 Tests for Cerebellar Function

Finger-to-nose test: With the child's arm extended, ask the child to touch the nose with the index finger with eyes open and then closed.

Heel-to-shin test: Have the child stand and run the heel of one foot down the shin or anterior aspect of the tibia of the other leg, both with the eyes opened and then closed.

Romberg test: Have the child stand with the eyes closed and heels together; falling or leaning to one side is abnormal and is called the Romberg sign.

hyperactivity of deep tendon reflexes is usually a result of a cerebral insult.

Elicit reflexes by using the rubber head of the reflex hammer, flat of the finger, or side of the hand. If the child is easily frightened by equipment, use your hand or finger. Although testing reflexes is a simple procedure, the child may inhibit the reflex by unconsciously tensing the muscle. To avoid tensing, distract younger children with toys or talk to them. Older children can concentrate on the exercise of grasping their two hands in front of them and trying to pull them apart. This diverts their attention from the testing and causes involuntary relaxation of the muscles.

Deep tendon reflexes are stretch reflexes of a muscle. The most common deep tendon reflex is the knee jerk reflex, or patellar reflex (sometimes called the quadriceps reflex). Figs. 4.42 to 4.45 illustrate the reflexes normally elicited. Report any diminished or hyperreflexive response for further evaluation.

Cranial Nerves

Assessment of the cranial nerves is an important area of neurologic assessment (Fig. 4.46; Table 4.11). With young children, present the tests as games to foster trust and security at the beginning of the examination. Include the cranial nerve test when examining each system, such as tongue movement and strength, gag reflex, swallowing, cardinal positions of gaze (Fig. 4.47), and position of the uvula during examination of the mouth.

DEVELOPMENTAL ASSESSMENT

One of the most essential components of a complete health appraisal is assessment of developmental function. Screening procedures are designed to identify quickly and reliably children whose developmental level is below normal for their age and who therefore require further evaluation. The earlier that developmental problems are identified and treated, the more likely the child can reach his or her potential. Developmental screening also provides a means of recording objective measurements of present developmental function for future reference. Since amendments to the Individuals with Disabilities Education Act were passed by Congress in 2004, much greater emphasis is placed on the developmental assessment of infants and children, and nurses can play a vital role in providing this service. Specific timing for developmental/behavioral assessments is found in the Preventive Pediatric Health Care chart found earlier in the chapter (see Fig. 4.7). Developmental assessments can be administered in a variety of settings: home, school, day care center, hospital, practitioner's office, or clinic.

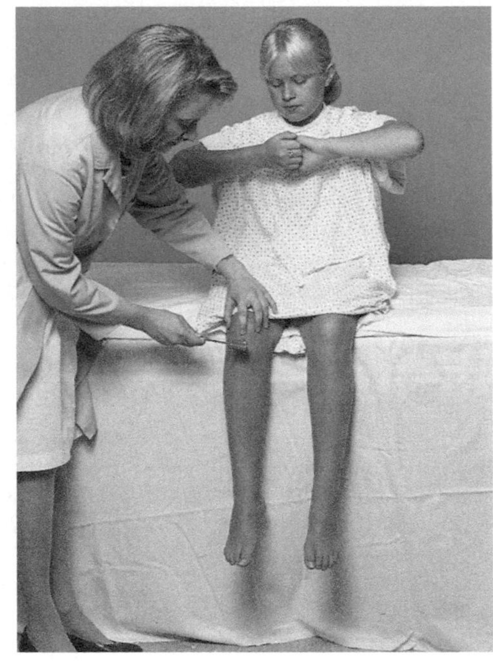

FIG. 4.44 Testing for the patellar, or knee-jerk, reflex, using distraction. The child sits on the edge of the examining table (or on the parent's lap) with the lower legs flexed at the knee and dangling freely. The patellar tendon is tapped just below the kneecap. Normal response is partial extension of the lower leg.

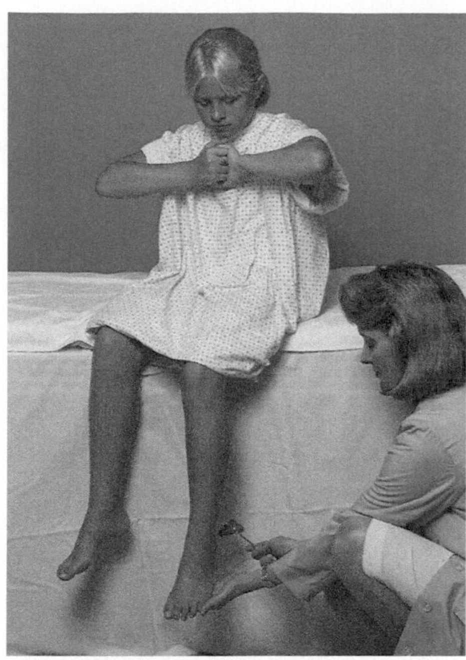

FIG. 4.45 Testing for the Achilles reflex. The child should be in the same position as for knee-jerk reflex. The foot is supported lightly in the examiner's hand, and the Achilles tendon is struck. Normal response is plantar flexion of the foot (the foot pointing downward).

The American Academy of Pediatrics (2006) does not endorse any specific developmental screening tool, but recommends a multidomain tool that addresses fine and gross motor skills, language and communication, problem solving/adaptive behavior, and personal-social skills. A comprehensive list of child development screening and assessment instruments has been developed by the National Early Childhood Technical Assistance Center as part of its cooperative agreement with the US Office of Special Education Programs (Ringwalt, 2008). The pediatric health promotion chapters in this book include detailed information on developmental assessment that is unique to the age and developmental stage of the child.

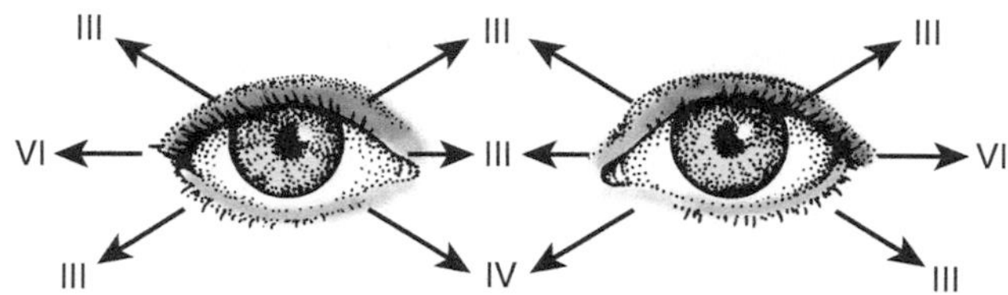

FIG. 4.47 Checking extraocular movements in the six cardinal positions indicates the functioning of cranial nerves III, IV, and VI. (From Ignatavicius, D. D., & Workman, L. M. [2016]. *Medical-surgical nursing: Patient-centered collaborative care* [8th ed.]. St. Louis, MO: Elsevier.)

PATHOPHYSIOLOGY REVIEW

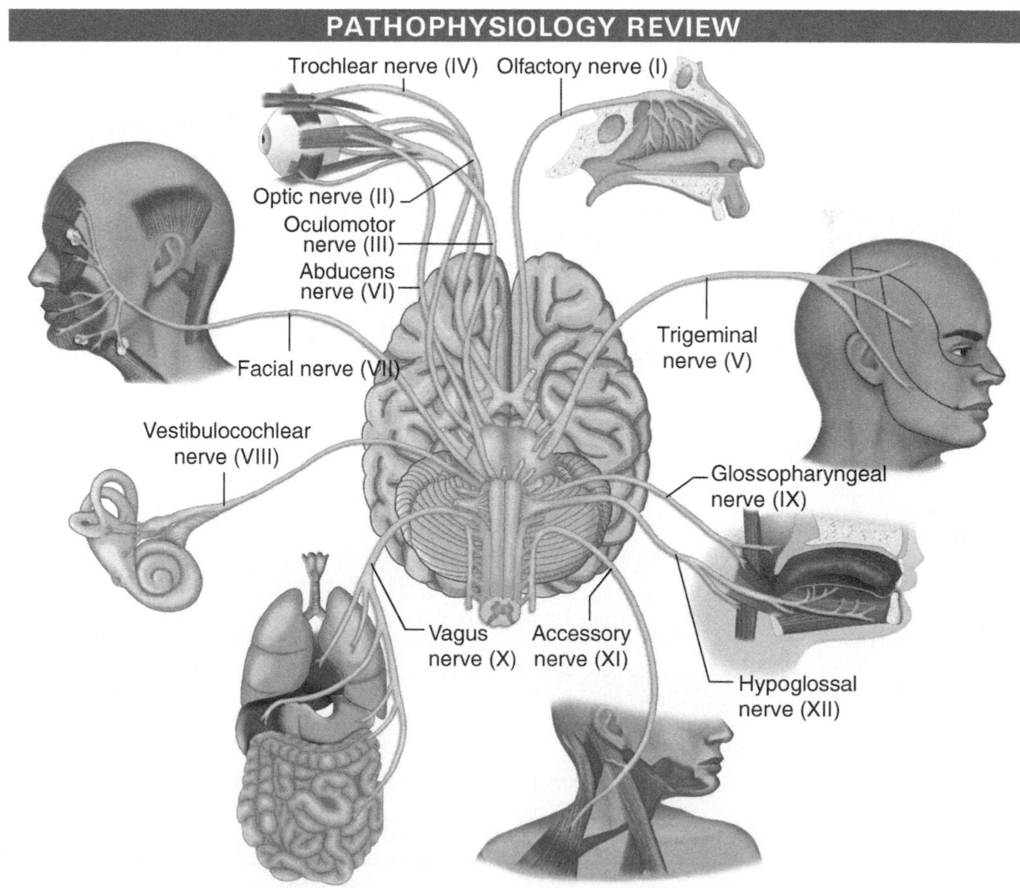

FIG. 4.46 Cranial nerves. (From Patton, K. T., & Thibodeau, G. A. [2013]. *Anatomy and physiology* [8th ed.]. St. Louis, MO: Mosby.)

TABLE 4.11 **Assessment of Cranial Nerves**

Description and Function	Tests
I—Olfactory Nerve	
Olfactory mucosa of nasal cavity Smell	With eyes closed, have child identify odors such as coffee, alcohol from a swab, or other smells; test each nostril separately.
II—Optic Nerve	
Rods and cones of retina, optic nerve Vision	Check for perception of light, visual acuity, peripheral vision, color vision, and normal optic disc.
III—Oculomotor Nerve	
Extraocular muscles of eye: • Superior rectus—moves eyeball up and in • Inferior rectus—moves eyeball down and in • Medial rectus—moves eyeball nasally • Inferior oblique—moves eyeball up and out	Have child follow an object (toy) or light in six cardinal positions of gaze (see Fig. 4.47).
Pupil constriction and accommodation	Perform PERRLA (Pupils Equal, Round, React to Light, and Accommodation).
Eyelid closing	Check for proper placement of lid.
IV—Trochlear Nerve	
Superior oblique muscle (SO)—moves eye down and out	Have child look down and in (see Fig. 4.47).
V—Trigeminal Nerve	
Muscles of mastication	Have child bite down hard and open jaw; test symmetry and strength.
Sensory—face, scalp, nasal and buccal mucosa	With child's eyes closed, see if child can detect light touch in mandibular and maxillary regions. Test corneal and blink reflex by touching cornea lightly with a whisk of cotton ball twisted into a point (approach from side so that child does not blink before cornea is touched).
VI—Abducens Nerve	
Lateral rectus (LR) muscle—moves eye temporally	Have child look toward temporal side (see Fig. 4.47).
VII—Facial Nerve	
Muscles for facial expression	Have child smile, make funny face, or show teeth to see symmetry of expression.
Anterior two-thirds of tongue (sensory)	Have child identify sweet or salty solution; place each taste on anterior section and sides of protruding tongue; if child retracts tongue, solution will dissolve toward posterior part of tongue.
VIII—Auditory, Acoustic, or Vestibulocochlear Nerve	
Internal ear Hearing and balance	Test hearing; note any loss of equilibrium or presence of vertigo.
IX—Glossopharyngeal Nerve	
Pharynx, tongue	Stimulate posterior pharynx with a tongue blade; child should gag.
Posterior third of tongue Sensory	Test sense of sour or bitter taste on posterior segment of tongue.
X—Vagus Nerve	
Muscles of larynx, pharynx, some organs of gastrointestinal system, sensory fibers of root of tongue, heart, and lung	Note hoarseness of voice, gag reflex, and ability to swallow. Check that uvula is in midline; when stimulated with tongue blade, it should deviate upward and to stimulated side.
XI—Accessory Nerve	
Sternocleidomastoid and trapezius muscles of shoulder	Have child shrug shoulders while applying mild pressure; with examiner's hands placed on shoulders, have child turn head against opposing pressure on either side; note symmetry and strength.
XII—Hypoglossal Nerve	
Muscles of tongue	Have child move tongue in all directions; have child protrude tongue as far as possible; note any midline deviation. Test strength by placing tongue blade on one side of tongue and having child move it away.

Ages and Stages

Ages and stages is a term used to broadly outline key periods in the human development timeline. During each stage, growth and development occur in the primary developmental domains, including physical, intellectual, language, and social-emotional. The Ages & Stages Questionnaires (ASQ)* are high-quality developmental screening tools that highlight a child's strengths and any areas of concern (Box 4.12). The ASQ-3 includes age-specific questionnaires about developmental skills common in daily life. Parents or other caregivers answer questions regarding their child's abilities (e.g., Does your child climb on an object such as a chair to reach something he wants? When your child wants something, does she tell you by pointing at it?). Children whose development appears to fall significantly below results of other children their age are flagged for further evaluation. The ASQ:SE2 can be used to identify children at risk for social and emotional developmental delays (Briggs, Stettler, Silver, et al., 2012).

*The ASQ can be found at www.agesandstages.com.

BOX 4.12 Ages & Stages Questionnaires*

- Type of screening: Developmental (ASQ-3) and social-emotional (ASQ:SE2)
- Age range: 1-66 months for ASQ-3, 1-72 months for ASQ:SE2
- Number of questionnaires: 21 for ASQ-3, 9 for ASQ:SE2
- Number of items: About 30 per questionnaire
- Online components: Data management and questionnaire completion
- Reading level of items: 4th to 6th grade
- Who completes it: Parents
- Time to complete: 10-15 minutes
- Who scores it: Professionals
- Time to score: 2-3 minutes
- Languages: English, Spanish (for both ASQ-3 and ASQ-SE2), and French (for ASQ-3)

*Information on the Ages & Stages Questionnaires can be found at www.agesandstages.com.

NCLEX REVIEW QUESTIONS

1. While interviewing parents who have just arrived in the health care clinic, the nurse begins the interview. Which of the following statements involve therapeutic communication techniques? Select all that apply.
   A. Allow the parents to direct the conversation so that they feel comfortable and in control.
   B. Use broad, open-ended questions so that parents can feel open to discuss issues.
   C. Redirect by asking guided questions to keep the parents on task.
   D. Use careful listening, which relies on the use of clues and verbal leads to help move the conversation along.
   E. Ask carefully worded, detailed questions to get accurate information.
2. A nurse looks over her assignment for the day, which includes an infant, a preschool-age child, a third-grader, and a sophomore in high school. Which techniques take into consideration developmental stages when working with pediatric patients?
   A. Be aware that infants will become agitated because of stranger anxiety around 4 months old.
   B. When a preschooler is having blood drawn, giving a detailed explanation will be helpful.
   C. Explain and demonstrate what the BP machine does to the third-grader before taking her blood pressure.
   D. Using a single consistent approach with the adolescent will help allay anger and hostility.
3. These general approaches can be helpful when performing a physical examination. Select all that apply.
   A. With toddlers, restraint may be necessary, and requesting a parent's assistance is appropriate.
   B. When examining a preschooler, giving a choice of which parts to examine may be helpful in gaining the child's cooperation.
   C. With a school-age child, it is always best to have the parents present when examining.
   D. Giving explanations about body systems can make adolescents nervous due to their egocentricities.
   E. An infant physical examination is done head to toe, similarly to the adult.
4. When assessing blood pressure in a child:
   A. Knowledge of normal mean is important: newborn, 65/41 mm Hg; 1 month to 2 years, 95/58 mm Hg; and 2 to 5 years, 101/57 mm Hg.
   B. Cuff size is the most important variable and should be measured using limb length.
   C. The child is considered normotensive if the BP is below the 95th percentile.
   D. Check upper- and lower-extremity BP to look for abnormalities such as aortic stenosis, which causes lower-extremity BP to be higher than upper-extremity BP.
5. Growth measurement is a key element of health status in children. One measurement is linear growth measurement. What should the nurse do to perfect this technique? Select all that apply.
   A. Understand the difference in measurement for children who can stand alone and for those who must lie recumbent.
   B. Use a length board or a tape measure to measure infant length.
   C. Two measurers are usually required for a recumbent child, although one measurer may be sufficient for a cooperative child.
   D. Reposition the child and repeat the procedure. Measure at least twice (ideally three times). Average the measurements for the final value.
   E. Demonstrate competency when measuring the growth of infants, children, and adolescents. Refresher sessions should be taken when a lack of standardization occurs.

Correct Answers

1. B, C, D; 2. C; 3. A, B; 4. A; 5. A, D, E

REFERENCES

American Academy of Pediatrics. (2017). *Culturally effective care toolkit.* https://www.aap.org/en-us/professional-resources/practice-transformation/managing-patients/Pages/effective-care.aspx.

American Academy of Pediatrics Council on Children with Disabilities, Section on Developmental Behavioral Pediatrics, Bright Futures Steering Committee, Medical Home Initiatives for Children with Special Needs Project Advisory Committee. (2006). Identifying infants and young children with developmental disorders in the medical home: An algorithm for developmental surveillance and screening. *Pediatrics, 188*(1), 405–420.

American Academy of Pediatrics Section on Ophthalmology and Committee on Practice and Ambulatory Medicine. (2012). Instrument-based pediatric vision screening policy statement. *Pediatrics, 130*(5), 983–986.

Ball, J. W., Dains, J. E., Flynn, J. A., et al. (2014). *Seidel's guide to physical examination* (8th ed.). St Louis, MO: Elsevier.

Batra, P., Faridi, M. M., & Saha, A. (2012). Thermometry in children. *Journal of Emergencies, Trauma, and Shock, 5*(3), 246–249.

Batra, P., & Goyal, S. (2013). Comparison of rectal, axillary, tympanic, and temporal artery thermometry in the pediatric emergency room. *Pediatric Emergency Care, 29*(1), 63–66.

Blank, L., Coster, J., O'Cathain, A., et al. (2012). The appropriateness of, and compliance with, telephone triage decisions: A systematic review and narrative synthesis. *Journal of Advanced Nursing, 68*(12), 2610–2621.

Briggs, R. D., Stettler, E. M., Silver, E. J., et al. (2012). Social-emotional screening for infants and toddlers in primary care. *Pediatrics, 129*, e377.

Broner, N., Embry, V. V., Gremminger, M. G., et al. (2013). *Mandatory reporting and keeping youth safe.* Washington, DC: Administration on Children, Youth and Families, Family and Youth Services Bureau.

Clark, J. A., Kieh-Lai, M. W., Sarnaik, A., et al. (2002). Discrepancies between direct and indirect blood pressure measurements using various recommendations for arm cuff selection. *Pediatrics, 110*(5), 920–923.

Dosman, C., & Andrews, D. (2012). Anticipatory guidance for cognitive and social-emotional development: Birth to five years. *Paediatrics & Child Health, 17*(2), 75–80.

Foote, J. M., Brady, L. H., Burke, A. L., et al. (2009). *Evidence-based clinical practice guideline on linear growth measurement of children.* Retrieved from http://www.blankchildrens.org/linear-growth-measurement.aspx.

Harlor, A. D., Jr., Bower, C., & Committee on Practice and Ambulatory Medicine; Section on Otolaryngology-Head and Neck Surgery. (2009). Hearing assessment in infants and children: Recommendations beyond neonatal screening. *Pediatrics, 24*(4), 1252–1263.

Mathers, M., Keyes, M., & Wright, M. (2010). A review of the evidence on the effectiveness of children's vision screening. *Child: Care, Health and Development, 36*(6), 754–780.

Mehra, S., Eavey, R. D., & Keamy, D. G. (2009). The epidemiology of hearing impairment in the United States: Newborns, children, and adolescents. *Otolaryngology–Head and Neck Surgery : Official Journal of American Academy of Otolaryngology-Head and Neck Surgery, 140*, 461–472.

National High Blood Pressure Education Program Working Group on High Blood Pressure in Children and Adolescents. (2004). The fourth report on the diagnosis, evaluation, and treatment of high blood pressure in children and adolescents. *Pediatrics, 114*(2 Suppl. 4th Report), 555–576.

Park, M. K., Menard, S. W., & Schoolfield, J. (2005). Oscillometric blood pressure standards for children. *Pediatric Cardiology, 26*(5), 601–607.

Purc-Stephenson, R. J., & Thrasher, C. (2010). Nurses' experiences with telephone triage and advice: A meta-ethnography. *Journal of Advanced Nursing, 66*(3), 482–494.

Purc-Stephenson, R. J., & Thrasher, C. (2012). Patient compliance with telephone triage recommendations: A meta-analytic review. *Patient Education and Counseling, 87*, 135–142.

Ringwalt, S. (2008). *Developmental screening and assessment instruments with an emphasis on social and emotional development for young children ages birth through five.* Chapel Hill: The University of North Carolina, FPG Child Development Institute, National Early Childhood Technical Assistance Center. http://ectacenter.org/~pdfs/pubs/screening.pdf.

Schell, K., Briening, E., Lebet, R., et al. (2011). Comparison of arm and calf automatic noninvasive blood pressures in pediatric intensive care patients. *Journal of Pediatric Nursing, 26*, 3–12.

Sekhar, D. L., Zalewski, T. R., & Paul, I. M. (2013). Variability of state school-based hearing screening protocols in the United States. *Journal of Community Health, 38*(3), 569–574.

Stacey, D., Macartney, G., Carley, M., et al. (2013). Development and evaluation of evidence-informed clinical nursing protocols for remote assessment, triage and support of cancer treatment-induced symptoms. *Nursing Research and Practice, 2013*, 171872.

US Department of Agriculture. (2014). *National Agricultural Library: Dietary reference intakes.* Retrieved from https://www.nal.usda.gov/fnic/dietary-reference-intakes.

US Preventive Services Task Force. (2011). Vision screening for children 1 to 5 years of age: US Preventive Services Task Force Recommendation statement. *Pediatrics, 127*(2), 34–346.

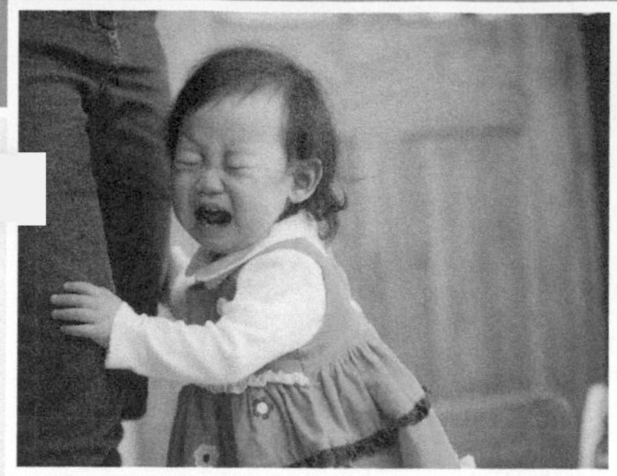

5

Pain Assessment and Management in Children

Shirley D. Martin, Maggie Maxtin, Katherine Smalling, and Sue Park

http://evolve.elsevier.com/com/wrong/ncic

CONCEPTS

- Pain
- Sensory Perception

Pain is a significant problem for children of all ages in all health care settings. Needle procedures are one of the most painful and fear-inducing procedures for children (McMurtry, Riddell, Taddio, et al., 2015). Exposure to needle procedures is highest in preterm infants in neonatal intensive care units, but neonates experience from 1 to 10 or more painful procedures during each day of hospitalization (Courtois, Droutman, Magny, et al., 2016; Johnston, Barrington, Taddio, et al., 2011). Needle pain is one cause of acute pain in hospitalized children; however, it is not the only cause. Up to 86% of hospitalized children experience acute pain (Kozlowski, Kost-Byerly, Colantuoni, et al., 2014; Solodiuk, Brighton, McHale, et al., 2014; Walther-Larsen, Pedersen, Friis, et al., 2016) from their disease or injury, treatment, and invasive procedures, including surgery; and more than 5% of children will have persistent postsurgical pain for 2 months or longer (Fortier, Chou, Maurer, et al., 2011; Kristensen, Ahlburg, Lauridsen, et al., 2012; Sieberg, Simons, Edelstein, et al., 2013). Uncontrolled acute pain has been recognized as a significant risk factor for the development of chronic pain (Chapman & Vierck, 2017). Reported prevalence rates of chronic pain in children vary from 4% to 88%, with the highest pain prevalence rates for headaches (up to 83%) and abdominal pain (up to 53%) (Craig, Hartman, Owens, et al., 2016; King, Chambers, Huguet, et al., 2011). Differences in chronic pain prevalence rates are found by gender, age, ethnicity, and geographic region.

Pediatric nurses play a pivotal role in preventing and managing children's pain. Unfortunately, evidence suggests that pediatric nurses are not translating pain prevention, assessment, and treatment knowledge into their routine care of managing children's pain (Manworren, 2017). This chapter provides an overview of pain theory, prevention, assessment, and management with a focus on pain experiences during childhood. Pain occurs in children of all ages and may manifest as acute, recurrent, chronic, or a mixture of acute and chronic pain. Examples of acute, chronic, and mixed pain and etiologies for these pain experiences are provided. Developmentally appropriate, valid, and reliable measurement tools and techniques to assess pain are discussed. Finally, pediatric pain prevention and treatment strategies are described and their mechanisms are explained. Nurses with a foundational understanding of pain, developmental differences in pain expression, and developmental implications of pain can prevent, assess, treat, and advocate for optimal pediatric pain reduction and relief.

WHAT IS PAIN AND HOW DOES IT OCCUR?

Pain is a complex biopsychosocial phenomenon with multiple components. Processes involved in the experience of pain include the peripheral and central nervous systems' reactions characteristic of acute pain. At the same time, responses and interactions within the neuronal matrix are evolving and influence both acute and chronic pain experiences (Table 5.1).

Fig. 5.1 depicts these processes and indicates areas where interventions can influence or modulate pain signaling. When a tissue injury is sustained, for example to the finger from a blood test, peripheral sensory neurons synapse onto interneurons in the spinal cord that then transmit information within a spinal segment and into ascending pathways for processing by the brain. Positron emission tomography studies confirm that painful stimulation activates somatosensory and limbic cortices of the brain. These areas have projections to the frontal cortex, an area implicated in many of our most complex human behaviors (e.g., attention, emotional regulation, mood).

A painful stimulus also activates the periaqueductal gray matter (PAG). Stimulation of the PAG with opiate administration or electrical stimulation results in significant analgesia (Mayer & Liebeskind, 1974). The PAG sends projections to the raphe nucleus magnus in the rostroventral medulla, which projects to the dorsal horn of the spinal cord. These descending projections inhibit further activation in ascending pathways, thereby modulating the amount of pain information transmitted up from the spinal cord to the brain (Basbaum & Fields, 1978, 1984; Ossipov, Morimura, & Porreca, 2014). Additionally, there are direct connections to the PAG from the frontal cortex, amygdala, and hypothalamus, and these connections are capable of eliciting analgesia (Beitz, 1982; Mantyh, 1983).

The neural network, or **brain neuromatrix** (Melzack, 2001, 2005), is a series of connected neural cells with cognitive, sensory, and affective pathways combined in a feedback loop unique to each individual. The brain neuromatrix therefore is able to assign meaning to the stimulus and modulate the perceptual experience and response through the descending pathway, which both inhibits and facilitates pain. In addition, the connections between emotional and cognitive processing areas and these descending pathways offer other paths by which pain is modulated and by which prior painful experience may affect modulatory processes.

TABLE 5.1 What Is Pain? Pain Definitions

Pain	"Pain is an unpleasant sensory and emotional experience associated with actual or potential tissue damage, or described in terms of such damage" (International Association for the Study of Pain, 2012). Pain has sensory, emotional, cognitive, and social components (Williams & Craig, 2016).
Acute pain	Pain (as described) felt acutely for a short period of time. Acute pain may occur in response to illness, stress, or injury.
Chronic pain	Persistent or recurrent pain lasting longer than 3 months.
Chronic primary pain	Pain in one or more anatomic regions that persists or recurs for longer than 3 months and is associated with significant emotional distress or significant functional disability (interference with activities of daily life and participation in social roles) and that cannot be better explained by another chronic pain condition.
Chronic cancer pain	Pain caused by the cancer itself (the primary tumor or metastases) and pain that is caused by the cancer treatment (surgical, chemotherapy, radiotherapy, and others). Cancer-related pain will be subdivided based on location into visceral, bony (or musculoskeletal), and somatosensory (neuropathic). It will be described as either continuous (background pain) or intermittent (episodic pain) if associated with physical movement or clinical procedures.
Chronic postsurgical or posttraumatic pain	Pain that develops after a surgical procedure or a tissue injury (involving any trauma, including burns) and persists at least 3 months after surgery or tissue trauma. This is a definition of exclusion, as all other causes of pain (infection, recurring malignancy) as well as pain from a preexisting pain problem need to be excluded.
Chronic neuropathic pain	Pain caused by a lesion or disease of the somatosensory nervous system.
Chronic headache or chronic orofacial pain	Pain defined as headaches or orofacial pains that occur on at least 50% of the days during at least 3 months.
Chronic visceral pain	Persistent or recurrent pain that originates from the internal organs of the head and neck region and the thoracic, abdominal, and pelvic cavities.
Chronic musculoskeletal pain	Persistent or recurrent pain that arises as part of a disease process directly affecting bone(s), joint(s), muscle(s), or related soft tissue(s).

Often the effect of descending inhibition is to increase threshold or decrease pain sensitivity during times of stress.

Prior experiences may alter the modulatory tone of this pathway, setting up circumstances where the system is perpetually sensitized and eliciting disproportionate responses to incoming painful stimuli without temporal tissue damage. Once these pain tracks are created in the brain, it is possible for pain to exist purely in the brain. This pain, however, is real and it feels the way the child says it feels—regardless of the location of origin, whether the message is coming straight from the brain or as a result of body tissue damage.

The neuromatrix is involved in both acute and chronic stress responses that contribute to pain perception. In the case of acute stress responses, each sensory, cognitive, and affective component provides input to the brain about pain. Outputs from the brain neuromatrix influence the neural web and also trigger responses in the body that are perceived as the pain experience.

WHAT DOES PAIN DO BESIDES HURT?

In addition to being uncomfortable, pain is harmful. Stress regulation includes hormonal responses and immune system activity. Pain triggers a number of physiologic stress responses in the body, and these may lead to negative consequences involving multiple systems. Long-term amplification of the sympathetic nervous system hinders healing. Unrelieved pain, whether from trauma, surgery, or disease, may prolong stress response and adversely affect a child's recovery. Box 5.1 provides a list of numerous complications of untreated pain in preterm neonates.

Poorly controlled acute pain also predisposes patients to chronic pain syndromes (Chapman & Vierck, 2017). When pain is unrelieved, sensory input from injured tissues causes recruitment of peripheral and spinal cord neurons to amplify pain responses even to nonpainful stimuli. Severe and sustained pain is more difficult to control. Nurses who care for infants and children need to consider the potential acute and long-term effects of pain on their young patients and be advocates in preventing and treating pain. The Research Focus box on the wind-up phenomenon explores this further.

RESEARCH FOCUS

What Is the Wind-Up Phenomenon?

An experience known as the wind-up phenomenon has been attributed to a decreased pain threshold and chronic pain (Chapman & Vierck, 2017). Central and peripheral mechanisms that occur in response to noxious tissue injury have been studied in an attempt to explain a prolonged neonatal response to pain characteristic of the wind-up phenomenon. After exposure to noxious stimuli, multiple levels of the spinal cord experience an altered excitability. This altered excitability may cause normal nonpainful stimuli, such as routine nursing care and handling, to be perceived as noxious stimuli. Neonates are particularly vulnerable to acute pain responses. They have more generalized spinal reflex responses and lower thresholds to stimuli than older children (Walker, 2014).

COMMON ACUTE PAIN CONDITIONS IN CHILDREN

Children experience numerous acute pain episodes during childhood, but certain children are at higher risk than others. Children may sustain acute pain from immunizations, minor injuries (e.g., knee abrasion), illnesses, or medical and surgical procedures during hospitalization. Nurses may find it easy to overlook certain painful experiences as part of normal care and perform invasive procedures without any attempts to minimize pain. Something as minor and ordinary as bandage removal, nasogastric tube placement, or urinary catheter placement is very painful to children. Premature infants are particularly vulnerable to repeated acute pain episodes from routine and frequent procedures as part of their care. Nurses need to prevent painful experiences from medical procedures and use evidence-based methods to relieve children's pain.

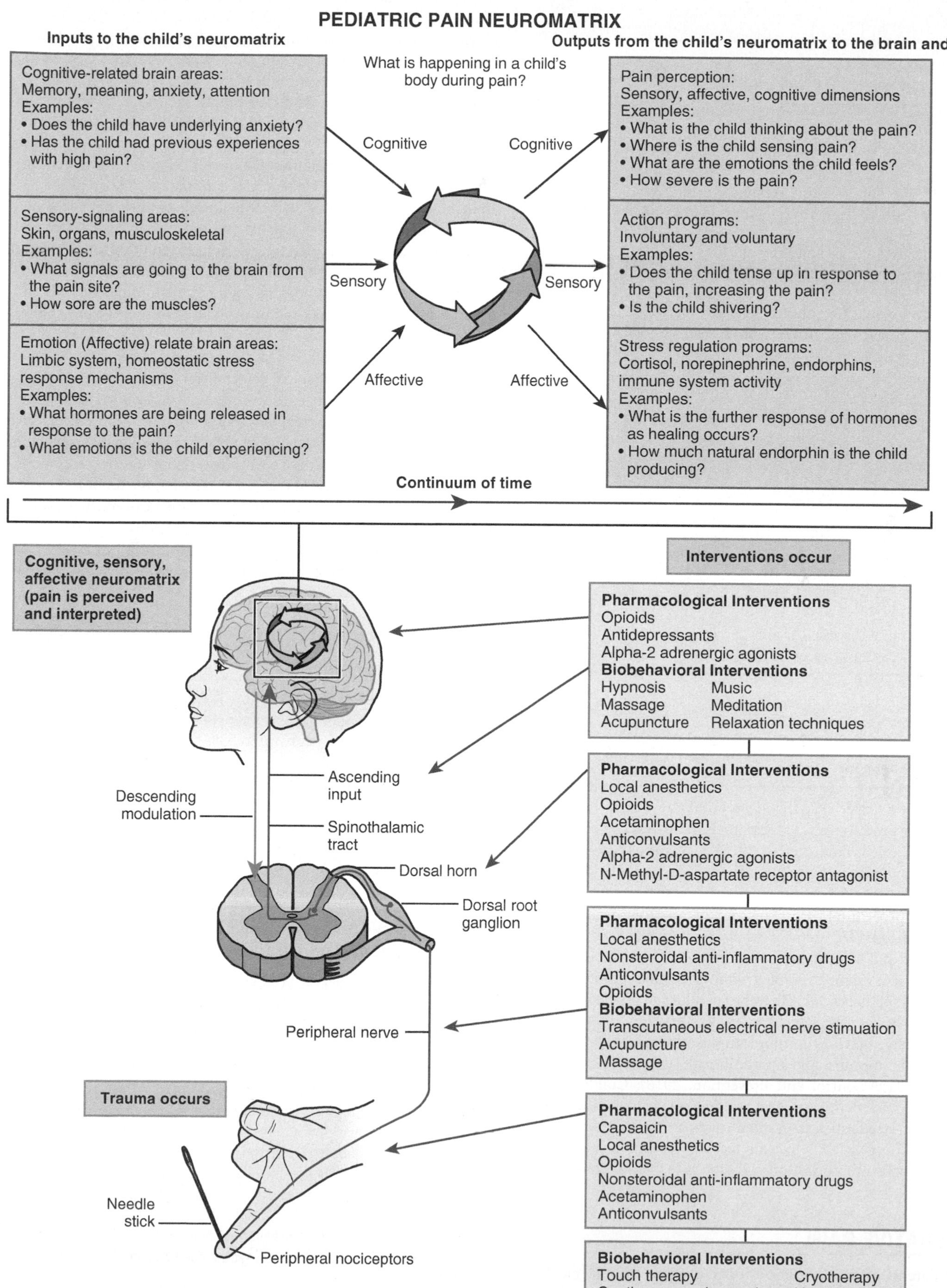
PEDIATRIC PAIN NEUROMATRIX
Inputs to the child's neuromatrix
Outputs from the child's neuromatrix to the brain and body
What is happening in a child's body during pain?
Cognitive-related brain areas: Memory, meaning, anxiety, attention Examples: • Does the child have underlying anxiety? • Has the child had previous experiences with high pain?
Sensory-signaling areas: Skin, organs, musculoskeletal Examples: • What signals are going to the brain from the pain site? • How sore are the muscles?
Emotion (Affective) relate brain areas: Limbic system, homeostatic stress response mechanisms Examples: • What hormones are being released in response to the pain? • What emotions is the child experiencing?
Cognitive
Cognitive
Sensory
Sensory
Affective
Affective
Pain perception: Sensory, affective, cognitive dimensions Examples: • What is the child thinking about the pain? • Where is the child sensing pain? • What are the emotions the child feels? • How severe is the pain?
Action programs: Involuntary and voluntary Examples: • Does the child tense up in response to the pain, increasing the pain? • Is the child shivering?
Stress regulation programs: Cortisol, norepinephrine, endorphins, immune system activity Examples: • What is the further response of hormones as healing occurs? • How much natural endorphin is the child producing?
Continuum of time
Cognitive, sensory, affective neuromatrix (pain is perceived and interpreted)
Interventions occur
Pharmacological Interventions Opioids Antidepressants Alpha-2 adrenergic agonists
Biobehavioral Interventions Hypnosis Music Massage Meditation Acupuncture Relaxation techniques
Pharmacological Interventions Local anesthetics Opioids Acetaminophen Anticonvulsants Alpha-2 adrenergic agonists N-Methyl-D-aspartate receptor antagonist
Pharmacological Interventions Local anesthetics Nonsteroidal anti-inflammatory drugs Anticonvulsants Opioids
Biobehavioral Interventions Transcutaneous electrical nerve stimuation Acupuncture Massage
Pharmacological Interventions Capsaicin Local anesthetics Opioids Nonsteroidal anti-inflammatory drugs Acetaminophen Anticonvulsants
Biobehavioral Interventions Touch therapy Cryotherapy Continous passive motion Heat therapy
Ascending input
Descending modulation
Spinothalamic tract
Dorsal horn
Dorsal root ganglion
Peripheral nerve
Trauma occurs
Needle stick
Peripheral nociceptors

FIG. 5.1 Pain model.

BOX 5.1 Consequences of Untreated Pain in Premature Neonates

Acute Consequences

Periventricular-intraventricular hemorrhage
Increased chemical and hormone release
Breakdown of fat and carbohydrate stores
Prolonged hyperglycemia
Higher morbidity
Memory of painful events
Hypersensitivity to pain
Prolonged response to pain
Inappropriate response to nonnoxious stimuli
Lower pain threshold

Potential Long-Term Consequences

Higher somatic complaints of unknown origin
Greater physiologic and behavioral responses to pain
Increased prevalence of neurologic deficits
Psychosocial problems
Neurobehavioral disorders
Cognitive deficits
Learning disorders
Poor motor performance
Behavioral problems
Attention deficits
Poor adaptive behavior
Inability to cope with novel situations
Problems with impulsivity and social control
Learning deficits
Emotional temperament changes in infancy or childhood
Accentuated hormonal stress responses in adult life

NEEDLESTICK PAIN

Children commonly experience high levels of distress and procedural fear during needle procedures, and these levels of distress correlate with age (McMurtry, Riddell, Taddio, et al., 2015). As many as two-thirds of children have needle fear related to painful injection (Taddio, Ipp, Thivakaran, et al., 2012). Procedure-related fear may be a consequence of inappropriate procedural pain management, and long-term consequences of unaddressed fear may follow. Excessive needle fear typically starts in childhood and may progress into adulthood (McMurtry, Taddio, Noel, et al., 2016). For example, fainting with vaccinations among young adults was found to be associated with fear of needles and poorly managed past needle experiences (Nir, Paz, Sabo, et al., 2003).

A child may have up to 19 immunizations by 6 months of age, an additional 5 by 12 months, and an additional 10 by 6 years of age (Centers for Disease Control and Prevention, 2016). Children also experience needlestick pain from heel and finger sticks for laboratory tests. Exposure to needlestick pain often starts on the first day of life and continues throughout life. Needle fear is a common reason for noncompliance with immunizations (Taddio, Ipp, Thivakaran, et al., 2012).

POSTOPERATIVE PAIN

Nurses and parents often consider postoperative pain an unavoidable painful consequence of surgery. About 4 million children undergo surgery each year (US Department of Health and Human Services, Centers for Disease Control and Prevention, 2006, 2015), 300,000 of whom are hospitalized for the surgical procedure in the United States (US Department of Health and Human Services, Centers for Disease Control and Prevention, 2015). At least 60% of children who undergo surgery are likely to report moderate to severe pain the first day after surgery (Kozlowski, Kost-Byerly, Colantuoni, et al., 2014).

Surgery and traumatic injuries (fractures, lacerations, burns) generate a catabolic state as a result of increased secretion of hormones (e.g., adrenalin, cortisol, glucagon). This then leads to alterations in blood flow, coagulation, fibrinolysis, substrate metabolism, and water and electrolyte balance, which increases the demands on the cardiovascular and respiratory systems. The major endocrine and metabolic changes occur during the first 48 hours after surgery or trauma. Opioids and local anesthetic nerve blocks are routinely used to alter the physiologic responses to surgical injury.

Pain associated with surgery to the chest (e.g., repair of congenital heart defects, chest wall, or spinal deformities) or abdomen (e.g., colectomy) may result in pulmonary complications. Pain leads to splinting and guarding. This decreased thoracic and abdominal muscle movement leads to decreased tidal volume, vital capacity, functional residual capacity, and alveolar ventilation. The patient is unable to cough and clear secretions, and the risk for complications (e.g., atelectasis and pneumonia) is high. Severe postoperative pain also results in sympathetic overactivity, which is manifested by increases in heart rate, peripheral resistance, blood pressure, and cardiac output. The patient eventually experiences an increase in cardiac demand and myocardial oxygen consumption and a decrease in oxygen delivery to the tissues.

COMMON CHRONIC PAIN CONDITIONS IN CHILDREN

Pain that persists for 3 months or more is defined as **chronic pain**. The three most common sites for chronic pain in pediatrics are headaches (up to 83%), abdominal pain (up to 53%), and musculoskeletal pain (up to 36%) (Friedrichsdorf, Giordano, Desai, et al., 2016). Chronic pain may also be episodic with recurrent bouts of pain at least every 3 months (see Research Focus box and Community and Home Health Considerations box).

RESEARCH FOCUS

Pain in School-Age Children

Van Dijk, McGrath, Pickett, et al. (2006) reported that 57% of school-age children have at least one recurrent pain (headaches, stomach pains, growing pains) and at least 6% have one or more chronic pain episodes (disease related, back pain).

Chronic or recurrent pain adversely affects the psychosocial and physical well-being of children. The domains for the assessment of chronic or recurrent pain are the same for acute pain (pain intensity, global judgment of satisfaction with treatment, symptoms and adverse events, physical functioning, emotional functioning, economic factors), plus two additional domains: role functioning and sleep. Because the time course of chronic or recurrent pain is different from that of acute pain, measures used to assess chronic pain often evaluate the symptom over time.

A systematic review of treatment for functional abdominal pain disorders found no evidence to support pharmacologic therapy (Korterink, Rutten, Venmans, et al., 2015).

COMMUNITY AND HOME HEALTH CONSIDERATIONS

Chronic Pain and School Absenteeism in Children

Children with chronic pain may experience a problematic cycle of school absenteeism that progresses from absences to poor performance and school refusal. Children miss school because of pain exacerbations and health care appointments. Missed days may translate into lowered academic performance and an inability to deal with the complexities of the school environment (Logan, Coakley, & Scharff, 2007). Children with various chronic pain sources have reported missing an average of 13.5 days of school in a 3-month period (Logan, Simons, & Carpino, 2012). Absence from school may require special accommodations and a modified school plan. Children with frequent or long-term absences may need a comprehensive and coordinated plan for a return to school. A team approach among health care clinicians, parents, teachers, and school administrators can help improve reintegration of children into school (Jones, King, MacLaren Chorney, et al., 2014). As part of this team approach, cognitive-behavioral therapists may provide strategies to help children work through self-esteem and peer perception issues. Nurses, physicians, and therapists can educate parents about the importance of school attendance, set boundaries for compliance with attendance policies, and teach parents to avoid reinforcement of negative behaviors.

HEADACHES

Almost every child reports having had a headache in the last 3 months. Most children with recurrent headaches have a family history of headaches. Headache prevalence also increases with age. Prevalence for boys and girls is similar before 12 years of age; after 12 years, prevalence for girls is triple that of boys.

Primary headaches, as classified by the International Headache Society, do not have an identified cause. Primary headaches common in children include migraines and tension-type headaches. Secondary headaches are associated with a cause, such as head or neck trauma, intracranial pressure, inflammatory disorders, infection, medication overuse or substance use and withdrawal, and tumor. The etiology of the headache should dictate the treatment plan. Therefore the goal of treating migraines and other headaches without known cause is pain relief or reduction to minimize associated functional disability.

Migraines are theorized to be a sensory processing disorder of dysfunctional modulation of the nociceptive system. There may be a migraine generator in the dorsal midbrain and pons. Children typically describe migraines as throbbing, unilateral or bilateral, frontotemporal, and of moderate to severe intensity. The term *migraine* is often misused to describe an intensely painful headache; however, there are specific diagnostic criteria of migraines in children. To meet these diagnostic criteria, migraine headaches must also have at least one of these characteristics: (1) aggravated by physical activity, (2) associated with nausea or vomiting, (3) photophobia, (4) phonophobia, (5) behavioral interference, or (6) lack of identified cause of recurrent headache. Children rarely report an aura with migraines.

ABDOMINAL PAIN

The Rome criteria for a diagnosis of functional abdominal pain includes episodic or continuous abdominal pain for greater than 3 months without identified pathology on physical examination and a negative stool for occult blood. Functional abdominal pain is described as nonradiating pain that lasts 1 to 3 hours and is typically located around the umbilicus. Accompanying symptoms may include altered bowel pattern, pallor, diaphoresis, nausea, vomiting, sleep disturbances, and changes in oral intake. In at least 25% of cases, patients also have some loss of daily function and other somatic symptoms, such as headache or limb pain. Other terms that have erroneously been used interchangeably with functional abdominal pain are nonorganic abdominal pain, psychogenic abdominal pain, and recurrent abdominal pain. Other common chronic abdominal pain conditions include functional dyspepsia, irritable bowel syndrome, and abdominal migraine. (See Chapter 16.)

MUSCULOSKELETAL PAIN

Chronic musculoskeletal pain can be categorized into three subtypes: injury-related, illness-related, or primary musculoskeletal pain. Pain can be localized to specific joints or muscle groups, such as ankle injuries or back pain, or may occur in multiple joints or muscle groups, as occurs with arthritis. Connective tissue disorders, such as Ehlers Danlos or other hypermobility disorders, may be associated with generalized musculoskeletal pain.

Musculoskeletal pain may also be diffuse as with fibromyalgia. Sometimes musculoskeletal pain appears as both diffuse and idiopathic in nature, making the pain difficult to characterize. Diffuse types of musculoskeletal pain have a high comorbidity with depressive symptoms (Kashikar-Zuck & Ting, 2014). Researchers believe the stress adaptation response is altered in children with fibromyalgia, possibly due to immune-mediated processes (Kashikar-Zuck & Ting, 2014).

NEUROPATHIC PAIN SYNDROMES

Neuropathic pain results from injury or dysfunction of the somatosensory system. Epidemiologic studies of adults suggest a prevalence of up to 8% (Smith & Torrance, 2012). Neuropathic pain is thought to be less common in children, but there are no current epidemiologic studies (Howard, Wiener, & Walker, 2014). Over the last 20 years, clinicians have gained increasing awareness of pediatric neuropathic conditions and are more likely to properly diagnose neuropathic pain (Walco, Dworkin, Krane, et al., 2010). Children experience neuropathic pain from nerve injury as a result of surgery or trauma (e.g., phantom limb pain or complex regional pain syndrome [CRPS]), autoimmune or degenerative neuropathies (e.g., Guillain-Barré syndrome or Charcot-Marie-Tooth disease), and neuropathies related to cancer or cancer treatment.

CRPS manifests as severe localized pain with allodynia, swelling, and color and temperature changes. CRPS typically affects a single extremity. A minor to severe injury, trauma, infection, or stressful event precipitates the syndrome. A precipitating event to any extremity can also cause CRPS to recur (Howard, Wiener, & Walker, 2014).

COMMON MIXED-PAIN CONDITIONS IN CHILDREN

BURN PAIN

Burns are the 5th most common type of nonfatal injury in children and 11th leading cause of death in children 1 to 9 years of age (World Health Organization, 2016). Burn pain is challenging to control because of multiple pain triggers, manipulations over injured sites during care, and the changing patterns of pain across time. Pain perception is mediated by the degree of the burn, sensory input, and individual child factors such as underlying anxiety (Gamst-Jensen, Vedel, Lindberg-Larsen, et al., 2014). Symptoms such as anxiety, depression, and insomnia modulate the chronicity of burn pain (McIntyre, Clifford, Maani, et al., 2016). Long-term posttraumatic stress symptoms vary inversely with early

TABLE 5.2 Cancer Pain in Children

Type	Clinical Presentation	Causes
Bone		
Skull Vertebrae Pelvis and femur	Aching to sharp, severe pain generally more pronounced with movement; point tenderness common Skull—headaches, blurred vision Spine—tenderness over spinous process Extremities—pain associated with movement or lifting Pelvis and femur—pain associated with movement; pain with weight bearing and walking	Infiltration of bone Skeletal metastases—irritation and stretching of pain receptors in periosteum and endosteum Prostaglandins released from bone destruction Aches from biologic agents and immunotherapy Bone marrow pain from immature blood cell proliferation
Neuropathic		
Peripheral Plexus Epidural Cord compression	Complaints of pain without any detectable tissue damage Abnormal or unpleasant sensations, generally described as tingling, burning, or stabbing Often a delay in onset Brief, shooting pain Increased intensity of pain with receptive stimuli	Nerve injury caused by tumor infiltration; nerve injury from treatment (e.g., vincristine toxicity) Infiltration or compression of peripheral nerves Surgical interruption of nerves (phantom pain after amputation)
Visceral		
Soft tissue Tumors of bowel Retroperitoneum	Poorly localized Varies in intensity Pressure, deep or aching	Obstruction—bowel, urinary tract, biliary tract Metabolic alteration Nociceptor activation, generally from distention or inflammation of visceral organs
Treatment Related		
Mucositis Infection typhlitis Radiation dermatitis Postsurgical Postlumbar puncture headaches	Difficulty swallowing, pain from lesions in oropharynx; may extend throughout entire gastrointestinal tract Infection may be localized pain from focused infection or generalized (i.e., tissue infection versus septicemia) Severe headache after lumbar puncture Skin inflammation causing redness and breakdown Pain related to tissue trauma secondary to surgery	Direct side effects of treatment for cancer: Chemotherapy Radiation Surgery Tumor removal Central line placement/removal Diagnostic procedures Venipuncture Lumbar puncture Bone marrow biopsy Other biopsies

opiate dosing in children recovering from serious burns (Sheridan, Stoddard, Kazis, et al., 2014).

Subtypes of burn pain have been categorized as background pain, breakthrough pain, procedural pain, and postoperative pain (Gamst-Jensen, Vedel, Lindberg-Larsen, et al., 2014). Burns often result in constant background pain that is felt at the wound sites and surrounding areas. This background pain is often described as a throbbing or burning sensation (McIntyre, Clifford, Maani, et al., 2016). Burn sites may trigger breakthrough pain during movements, such as position changes, walking, or even breathing. Procedures that cause pain include wound debridement, dressing changes, physical therapy, baths, and removal of skin graft staples (McIntyre, Clifford, Maani, et al., 2016). Postoperative pain includes both the area of the burn and the donor sites for skin grafts. Pain is commonly experienced with intense tingling or itching sensations in skin graft sites. The healing process and side effects (itch, tingling, cold sensations) may last for months to years (Van Loey, Hofland, Hendrickx, et al., 2016). Researchers have explored mechanisms of itch to develop treatments for both itch and neuropathic pain.

CANCER PAIN

Children with cancer experience pain from different causes at different points throughout their cancer experience. Pain may be a symptom of cancer and therefore children may be in pain when diagnosed with cancer (Table 5.2). Cancer treatment may also relieve cancer pain; however, treatment-related pain is also common. Survivors of childhood cancer may experience chronic pain from their cancer treatment, for example, from phantom limb pain, graft-versus-host disease, or postherpetic neuralgia.

Mucositis, inflammation of mucosal lining, is a common source of treatment-related pain. Inflammation may occur in the mouth, esophagus, stomach, intestine, rectal, and vaginal areas after patients undergo chemotherapy, radiotherapy, or bone marrow transplantation. Mucositis appears at different time intervals based on the type and duration of chemotherapy/radiology a patient receives, generally sooner after chemotherapy than after radiotherapy. Its maximum expression occurs 7 to 10 days after chemotherapy, and erythema progresses toward ulceration. Mucositis gradually subsides over a period of 2 to 3 weeks after the patient's cytotoxic treatment (Chaveli-López & Bagán-Sebastián, 2016). Mucositis after bone marrow transplantation may be prolonged and continuously intense. Mucositis pain is exacerbated by mouth care and function (swallowing, drinking, eating, and talking). There are no effective treatments to adequately relieve mucositis pain; this is an area of active research for prevention and better treatment options.

The types of treatment-related pain experienced by children with cancer vary with progression of the disease and the type of treatment protocol. Other treatment-related pain includes: (1) abdominal pain after allogeneic bone marrow transplantation, which may be associated with acute graft-versus-host disease; (2) abdominal pain associated with typhlitis (infection of the cecum), which occurs when the patient is immunocompromised; (3) phantom sensations and phantom limb pain after an amputation; (4) peripheral neuropathy after administration of vincristine; (5) medullary bone pain, which may be associated with administration of granulocyte colony–stimulating factor; and (6) pain associated with immunotherapy.

SICKLE CELL PAIN

Pain is a hallmark symptom of sickle cell disease (SCD) (see Chapter 28). The pain is severe, acute, and episodic. Vasoocclusive crisis (VOC) pain begins in infants as young as 6 months and continues throughout life. Chronic pain can also develop from repeated tissue damage or avascular joint necrosis. There are preventive treatments, but the only cure for SCD is a bone marrow transplant.

VOC pain in infants and toddlers is typically characterized by dactylitis—visible painful swelling of finger, hands, toes, or feet or extremity pain. As children get older, headaches, low back pain, and bone pain are common. Children with SCD may also have increased frequency of surgical procedures (e.g., splenectomy following splenic sequestration or cholecystectomy for gallbladder sludging). VOC, however, is the most frequent reason for emergency department visits and hospital admissions among children with SCD (Fosdal, 2015).

Sickle cell pain has been described as stronger than surgical, arthritis, and childbirth pain (Fosdal, 2015). From a very young age, children may experience this pain and changes in level of activity, guarding certain body parts, and fussiness may provide hints that the child is experiencing a pain crisis. Parents of children with SCD may notice that pain crises coincide with weather changes or acute illnesses such as respiratory viral infections or other bacterial infections.

MEASURING PAIN IN CHILDREN

Nurses may fail to recognize, treat, and prevent acute and chronic pain without a strategic plan in place to assess pain at key times during care delivery. It is important to use a pain assessment tool appropriate for the child's developmental level and condition. Pain assessment tools are available as observational pain measures, self-report rating scales, and multidimensional pain assessment tools. Pain assessment should be more thorough than merely obtaining a pain rating. Understanding the location, frequency, duration, and precipitating, aggravating, and alleviating factors of the pain experienced by the child is also essential for effective pain management. Nurses should assess other symptoms, including pain's effect on sleep, emotional function (mood, anxiety, depression), physical recovery (acute pain) or physical functioning, disability (chronic pain), role functioning (chronic pain), and satisfaction with pain treatment (Eccleston, Pelermo, Williams, et al., 2014; Eccleston, Walco, Turk, et al., 2008).

Consistent use of the same measurement tools is necessary to standardize communication related to pain and evaluate the effectiveness of pain management strategies. Clinical practice councils may select pain assessment tools appropriate for the scope of pediatric care and pain conditions treated at a hospital or organization. These decisions have become increasingly difficult because the number of pediatric pain measures available for use continues to increase in specificity.

The current trend is to choose pain assessment tools with a common metric for measurement of pain. A common metric would make pain scores easier to read, interpret, and integrate into research and practice (von Baeyer, 2009). Most instruments consist of 0 for no pain to a range of 4 to 160 for the top anchors in pain measures. A pain score of 5 may mean a lot of pain (if a 0 to 5 scale is used) or very little (if a 0 to 100 scale is used), and it may not be clearly specified which score corresponds to which scale. Tools based on a 0 to 10 scale have been reported as the metric most commonly preferred by health care professionals, but not by patients (von Baeyer, 2009). The goal of interpreting all pain scores based on a common metric is flawed because pain assessment tools measure different pain expressions; for example, self-report measures patients' perceived pain intensity, whereas observational pain measures are used to quantify patients' behavioral and physiologic responses to pain.

OBSERVATIONAL PAIN MEASURES

Observational measures of pain are generally used for children from infancy until they are able to provide a self-report of pain and distinguish increments of pain intensity, typically around 3 to 4 years of age (Table 5.3). Observational pain measurement tools require a trained observer to watch and record children's behaviors, such as vocalization, facial expression, and body movements, that are associated with painful stimulus. Facial expression is the most consistent and specific indicator of pain in infants. Scales are available to systematically evaluate facial features, such as eye squeeze, brow bulge, open mouth, and taut tongue (Figs. 5.2 and 5.3). Understanding which behaviors are associated with pain helps nurses assess pain in infants and small children who are unable to provide self-report. However, discriminating between pain

TABLE 5.3 Examples of Commonly Used Behavioral Observational Pain Assessment Scales for Children

	FLACC (Malviya, Voepel-Lewis, Burke, et al., 2006; Merkel, Voepel-Lewis, Shayevitz, et al., 1997; Voepel-Lewis, Zanotti, Dammeyer, et al., 2010)	COMFORT-B (Harris, Ramelet, van Dijk, et al., 2016; Ista, van Dijk, Tibboel, et al., 2005; van Dijk, de Boer, & Koot, 2000)
Age range	0-3 *2 months to 7 years in PACU *0-19 years in ICU *0-19 years with cognitive impairment (use revised descriptors)	0-18 years
Type of pain	Acute pain including postoperative pain, pain in children with cognitive impairment (revised descriptors), and critically ill	Acute pain in critically ill, ventilated children
Variables assessed	Face (0-2) Legs (0-2) Activity (0-2) Cry (0-2) Consolability (0-2)	Alertness Calmness/agitation Respiratory response or crying Physical movement Muscle tone Facial tension
Score range	0-10	6-30 Consider pain >17

*Crellin, Harrison, Santamaria, et al. (2015).
ICU, Intensive care unit; *PACU*, postanesthesia care unit.

behaviors and reactions to other sources of distress, such as hunger, anxiety, or other types of discomfort, is not always easy. Observational pain measures are most reliable when used to measure short, sharp procedural pain, such as pain due to heel lance or injections. They are less reliable when measuring acute pain and not reliable or valid for assessing chronic pain or pain in older children. Pain scores on observational measures do not correlate with children's own reports of pain intensity (see Cultural Considerations box).

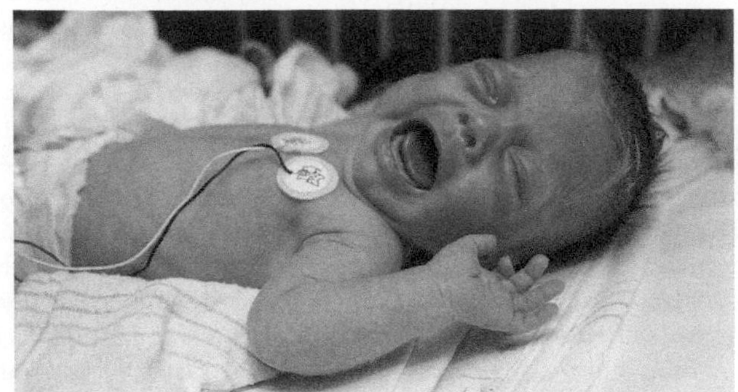

FIG. 5.2 Full, robust crying of preterm infant after heel stick. (Courtesy Halbouty Premature Nursery, Texas Children's Hospital, Houston, TX; photo by Paul Vincent Kuntz.)

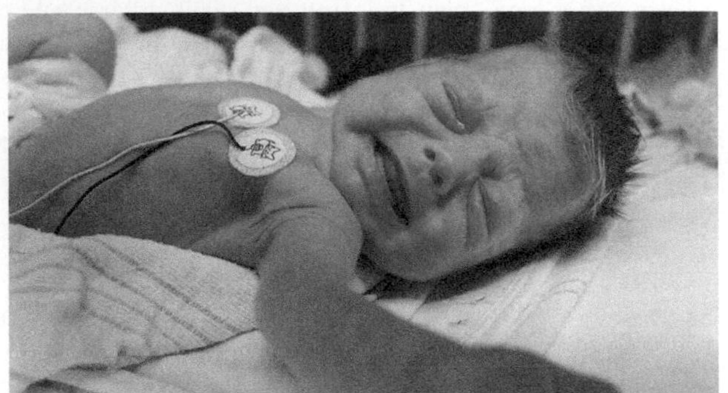

FIG. 5.3 The face of pain after heel stick. Note eye squeeze, brow bulge, nasolabial furrow, and wide-spread mouth. (Courtesy Halbouty Premature Nursery, Texas Children's Hospital, Houston, TX; photo by Paul Vincent Kuntz.)

CULTURAL CONSIDERATIONS

Pain Reporting in Non–English-Speaking Children

Jacob, McCarthy, Sambuco, et al. (2008) examined the pain experience of Spanish-speaking children with cancer who were asked about their pain during the week before a scheduled oncology clinic appointment. They found that 41% of the patients were experiencing pain. Some were experiencing moderate to severe pain and did not receive medications because they did not report their pain.

One commonly used clinical observational tool is the FLACC Pain Assessment Tool. It is an interval scale that includes the five categories of behavior: **F**acial expression, **L**eg movement, **A**ctivity, **C**ry, and **C**onsolability (Babl, Crellin, Cheng, et al., 2012; Howard, Carter, Curry, et al., 2012; Manworren & Hynan, 2003; Merkel, Voepel-Lewis, Shayevitz, et al., 1997). Observers rate each category of behavior on a 0 to 2 scale, for total scores ranging from 0 (no pain behaviors) to 10. This procedure of rating each category and then summing them for a score is common to the observational pain assessment tools (see Table 5.3).

SPECIAL POPULATIONS

Preterm Infants

Early pain experiences greatly influence the developing nervous system with persistent long-term effects. Nurses must consider the infant's maturity, behavioral state, energy resources available to respond to pain, and risk factors for pain. Evaluation of pain in preterm infants is complex and based on gestational age, state, condition, previous response to pain, physiologic changes, and validated observational tools (Hatfield & Ely, 2015). Several pain assessment tools for neonates have been validated in preterm infants (Table 5.4).

Preterm infants in awake or alert states demonstrate a more robust reaction to painful stimuli than infants in sleep states. Preterm infants' responses to pain may be behaviorally blunted or absent. Also, an infant receiving a muscle-paralyzing agent (vecuronium) is incapable of a behavioral or visible pain response; however, there is ample evidence that such infants are neurologically capable of feeling pain. In preterm infants with diminished ability to respond robustly to pain, it is imperative

TABLE 5.4 Summary of Pain Assessment Scales for Infants

	PIPP-revised (Stevens, Gibbins, Yamada, et al., 2014)	**NIPS** (Lawrence, Alcock, McGrath, et al., 1993)	**N-PASS** (Hummel, Puchalski, Creech, et al., 2008)	**COMFORT-neo** (van Dijk, Roofthooft, Anand, et al., 2009)	**CRIES** (Krechel & Bildner, 1995)
Age range	25-40 weeks	26-40 weeks	23-40 weeks	24-42 weeks	32-40 weeks
Type of pain	Procedural and postoperative		Procedural and prolonged	Prolonged pain	Postoperative pain
Variables assessed	Scored at (0-3) each	Breathing (0-1)	Scored at (0-2) each	Scored at (1-5) each	Scored at (0-2) each
	Heart rate	Face (0-1)	Vital signs	Alertness	Crying
	Oxygen saturation	Arms (0-1)	Crying/ irritability	Calmness/agitation	Oxygen requirement
	Brow bulge	Legs (0-1)	Facial expressions	Respiratory response or crying	Changes to vital signs
	Eye squeeze	Cry (0-2)	Behavioral state	Body movement	Facial expressions
	Nasolabial furrow	Arousal (0-1)	Extremities/tone	Muscle tone	Sleeplessness
	Behavioral state			Facial tension	
Score range	0-21	0-7	Pain: 0-10	6-30	0-10
Adjusted for gestational age	Yes Scored at (0-3)	No	Yes	No	No

Table 5.4 depicts various neonatal assessment scales with variables assessed and score ranges.

Adapted from Harris, J., Ramelet, A., van Dijk, M., et al. (2016). Clinical recommendations for pain, sedation, withdrawal and delirium assessment in critically ill infants and children: An ESPNIC position statement for healthcare professionals. *Intensive Care Medicine, 42,* 972-986.

to presume that pain exists in all situations that are usually considered painful for adults and children, even in the absence of behavioral or physiologic signs.

Cognitively Impaired Children

Cognitively impaired children may not be able to express pain through behaviors or self-report methods validated for developmentally similar peers. Parents of children with cognitive impairment reported their children experienced pain or severe discomfort that was not effectively managed (Crosta, Ward, Walker, et al., 2014; Malviya, Voepel-Lewis, Burke, et al., 2006). The most frequent pain behaviors reported by parents of children with cognitive impairment were crying; being less active; seeking comfort; moaning; not cooperating; being irritable; being stiff, spastic, tense, or rigid; sleeping less; being difficult to satisfy or pacify; flinching or moving body part away; and being agitated or fidgety. Parents also reported that some daily living activities were painful, such as assisted stretching and walking, independent standing, toileting, putting on splints, occupational therapy, range of motion, and physical therapy. There are three tools that have been found reliable and valid for this population: Revised Faces Legs Activity Cry Consolability Scale (rFLACC), Non-communicating Children's Pain Checklist–Revised (NCCPC-r), and Paediatric Pain Profile (PPP) (Chen-Lim, Zarnowsky, Green, et al., 2012; Hunt, Goldman, Seers, et al., 2003; Malviya, Voepel-Lewis, Burke, et al., 2006; Quinn, Seibold, & Hayman, 2015). When using the rFLACC, nurses must include parent-reported pain behaviors to customize the tool to use with individual children.

Children Postanesthesia

Pain assessment can be challenging in children recovering from anesthesia. For this reason, nurses often use observational pain assessment tools and then transition to self-report tools when the child is more alert. The only tool found reliable and valid for pain assessment of children 2 months to 7 years of age recovering in the postanesthesia care unit is the FLACC tool (Merkel, Voepel-Lewis, Shayevitz, et al., 1997).

Children in the Pediatric Intensive Care Unit

It is challenging to differentiate a child's pain from distress, anxiety, and agitation due to physiologic compromise when a child is in the pediatric intensive care unit. Sedating pain medications (opioids) and other sedatives are used to treat these complex patients. One of the most commonly used pain scales to assess critically ill ventilated children who are nonverbal due to sedation or their condition is the COMFORT behavior scale (COMFORT-B). There are six COMFORT scales: COMFORT, COMFORT plus crying, COMFORT-behavior, COMFORT-modified, COMFORT-adapted, and COMFORT-neo. Each scale has been developed and studied as measures of several different comfort concepts (pain, stress, distress and sedation) with different patient populations. See Tables 5.3 and 5.4 for examples of COMFORT-B and COMFORT-neo compared with other scales. The COMFORT-B scale is able to detect specific changes in pain or distress intensity in critically ill children (Boerlage, Ista, Duivenvoorden, et al., 2015; de Jong, Tuinebreijer, Bremer, et al., 2012; van Dijk, de Boer, Koot, et al., 2000) and is particularly helpful in children who are mechanically ventilated.

SELF-REPORT PAIN RATING SCALES

Self-report is the single most reliable indicator of pain and must be accepted and respected by nurses as the most important pain assessment data available. Self-report measures are most often used for children older than 3 to 4 years, but even 2-year-olds can report pain. Several cognitive skills, such as measurement, classification, and seriation (the ability to accurately place items in rank order), become apparent between 7 and 10 years of age. Therefore most school-age children have the cognitive ability required to use a numeric rating scale. Many self-report pain rating scales exist, but not all have well-established psychometric properties. It is necessary to have multiple tools available because validity and reliability of each tool varies across age-groups and types of pain (Manworren & Stinson, 2016).

There are many different "faces" scales for the measurement of pain intensity. Although children at 3 or 4 years of age are able to self-report pain, they do not have the cognitive ability to understand rank order. Self-report measures with "faces" provide a pictorial representation of pain intensity. The ability to discriminate degrees of pain in facial expressions appears to be reasonably established by 3 years old. However, cognitive characteristics of the preoperational stage influence their ability to separate feelings of pain and mood. It has been suggested that smiling faces on pain assessment scales may lead younger children to rate the affective domain of pain; or, in other words, rate their feelings about having pain rather than report the intensity of their physical pain (Quinn, Sheldon, & Cooley, 2014). Simple, concrete anchor words, such as the script originally used to validate the tool, should be used (Table 5.5). The faces are appealing and valid for use with children of all ages (even adults); patients can simply point to the face that represents their pain intensity to report pain.

For children 8 years old and older, there are a number of numeric rating scales. The numeric rating scales (NRSs), such as the 0 to 10 scale, are the most widely used in clinical practice because they are easy to use. The NRS is also called the verbal numeric scale (VNS) (Bailey, Daoust, Doyon-Trottier, et al., 2010). In contrast, the visual analog scale (VAS) is classically a 10-centimeter line with or without anchors from 0 to 10 or 0 to 100, sometimes anchored with the words *no pain* and *worst pain*. Word graphic scales use descriptors along a line that provides a highly subjective evaluation of a pain or other symptom. All have established reliability and validity.

Pain assessment in the patient who can provide self-report should not be limited to pain intensity. Other dimensions (such as, pain quality, location, and spatial distribution) may change without a change in pain intensity. Valid pain charts, diagrams, or drawings may be used to help children over 8 years of age describe the location of their pain (von Baeyer, Lin, Seidman, et al., 2011). The Adolescent Pediatric Pain Tool (APPT), modeled after the McGill Pain Questionnaire (Melzack, 1975), is a multidimensional pain measurement instrument used with children and adolescents to assess pain location, intensity, and quality (Fernandes, DeCampos, Batalha, et al., 2014) (Fig. 5.4). The APPT is an instrument with an anterior and posterior body outline on one side and a 100-mm word-graphing rating scale with a pain descriptor on the other side (Savedra, Holzemer, Tesler, et al., 1993; Savedra, Tesler, Holzemer, et al., 1989; Tesler, Savedra, Holzemer, et al., 1991). Each of the three components of the APPT is scored separately. The scorer may obtain a pain measurement by placing a clear plastic template overlay with 43 body areas on top of the body outline diagram. The number of body areas marked is counted to estimate the pervasiveness of the pain. A ruler or micrometer is used to score the word-graphic rating scale. The number of millimeters from the left side of the scale to the point marked by the child is measured, and the numeric value provides an overall evaluation of the amount of pain the child is experiencing. The total number of words on the descriptor list is counted, and scores range from 0 to 56. The clinician then counts the number of words selected in each of three categories—evaluative (0 to 8), sensory (0 to 37), and affective (0 to 11)—and calculates a percentage score for each one (Savedra, Holzemer, Tesler, et al., 1993). A systematic review of the APPT concluded that this tool can be helpful for customizing pain management interventions for adolescents (Fernandes, DeCampos, Batalha, et al., 2014).

TABLE 5.5 Pain Rating Scales for Children

Pain Scale, Description	Instructions	Recommended Age, Comments
Wong-Baker FACES Pain Rating Scale*		
Consists of six cartoon faces ranging from smiling face for "no pain" to tearful face for "worst pain"	*Original instructions:* Explain to child that each face is for a person who feels happy because there is no pain (hurt) or sad because there is some or a lot of pain. FACE 0 is very happy because there is no hurt. FACE 1 hurts just a little bit. FACE 2 hurts a little more. FACE 3 hurts even more. FACE 4 hurts a whole lot, but FACE 5 hurts as much as you can imagine, although you don't have to be crying to feel this bad. Ask child to choose face that best describes own pain. Record number under chosen face on pain assessment record. *Brief word instructions:* Point to each face using the words to describe the pain intensity. Ask child to choose face that best describes own pain, and record appropriate number.	For children as young as 3 years old. Using original instructions without affect words, such as happy or sad, or brief words resulted in same range of pain rating, probably reflecting child's rating of pain intensity. For coding purposes, numbers 0, 2, 4, 6, 8, and 10 can be substituted for 0-5 system to accommodate 0-10 system. The Wong-Baker FACES Pain Rating Scale provides three scales in one: facial expressions, numbers, and words. Research supports cultural sensitivity of FACES for Caucasian, African American, Hispanic, Thai, Chinese, and Japanese children.

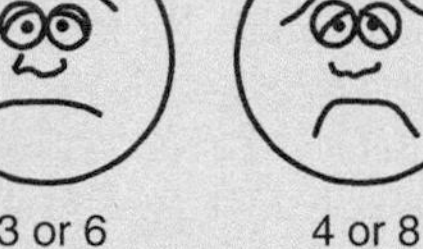

Pain Scale, Description	Instructions	Recommended Age, Comments
Faces Pain Scale–Revised (FPS-R) (Hicks, von Baeyer, Spafford, et al., 2001)		
Consists of six cartoon faces ranging from neutral face for "no pain" to grimacing face "worst possible pain" The child is asked to select the picture of a face that best represents their pain intensity For children 5-17		
Word-Graphic Rating Scale† (Tesler, Savedra, Holzemer, et al., 1991)		
Uses descriptive words (may vary in other scales) to denote varying intensities of pain	Explain to child, "This is a line with words to describe how much pain you may have. This side of the line means no pain, and over here the line means worst possible pain." (Point with your finger where "no pain" is, and run your finger along the line to "worst possible pain," as you say it.) "If you have no pain, you would mark like this." (Show example.) "If you have some pain, you would mark somewhere along the line, depending on how much pain you have." (Show example.) "The more pain you have, the closer to worst pain you would mark. The worst pain possible is marked like this." (Show example.) "Show me how much pain you have right now by marking with a straight, up-and-down line anywhere along the line to show how much pain you have right now." With millimeter rule, measure from the "no pain" end to mark and record this measurement as pain score.	For children 8-17 years old.

No pain — Little pain — Medium pain — Large pain — Worst possible pain

Cultural Considerations

Expression of pain can be greatly affected by communication barriers (Azize, Humphreys, & Cattani, 2011). Culture also exerts a profound influence on pain expression. Some cultures train children to withhold pain expression whereas others encourage pain expression (Bisogni, Calzolai, Olvini, et al., 2014). In addition, underlying genetic and biologic factors contribute to ethnic and gender differences in pain expression and pain perceptions (Kozlowski, Kost-Byerly, Colantuoni, et al., 2014).

Special Populations

Children with autism spectrum disorder. Children with autism may be unable to engage in the social interactions required to both verbally and nonverbally communicate pain. Because there is a wide range of cognitive abilities among individuals with autism spectrum disorder (ASD), self-report measures should be used whenever possible. Ask the verbal child with ASD where the pain is located and to describe how it feels (Ely, Chen-Lim, Carpenter, et al., 2016). Individuals with ASD

TABLE 5.5 Pain Rating Scales for Children—cont'd

Pain Scale, Description	Instructions	Recommended Age, Comments
Oucher (Villarruel & Denyes, 1991)		
Consists of six photographs of a white child's face representing "no hurt" to "biggest hurt you could ever have;" also includes vertical scale with numbers from 0-100; scales for African American and Hispanic children have been developed	*Numeric scale:* Point to each section of scale to explain variations in pain intensity: "0 means no hurt." "This means little hurts" (pointing to lower part of scale, 1-29). "This means middle hurts" (pointing to middle part of scale, 30-69). "This means big hurts" (pointing to upper part of scale, 70-99). "100 means the biggest hurt you could ever have." Score is actual number stated by child. *Photographic scale:* Point to each photograph and explain variations in pain intensity using following language: First picture from the bottom is "no hurt," second is "a little hurt," third is "a little more hurt," fourth is "even more hurt than that," fifth is "pretty much or a lot of hurt," and sixth is "biggest hurt you could ever have." Score pictures from 0-5, with bottom picture scored as 0. *General:* Practice using Oucher by recalling and rating previous pain experiences (e.g., falling off bike). Child points to number or photograph that describes pain intensity associated with experience. Obtain current pain score from child by asking, "How much hurt do you have right now?"	For children 3-13 years old. Use numeric scale if child can count off any two numbers or by 10s Determine whether child has cognitive ability to use photographic scale; child should be able to rate six geometric shapes from largest to smallest. Determine which ethnic version of Oucher to use; allow child to select version of Oucher or use version that most closely matches physical characteristics of child. *Note:* Ethnically similar scale may not be preferred by child when given choice of ethnically neutral cartoon scale (Luffy & Grove, 2003).
Numeric Rating Scale		
Verbal scale or may have a line If a line is used, it may be oriented horizontally or vertically.	Explain to child that is 0 is no pain (hurt), and 5 or 10, is the worst pain. Ask child to choose number that best describes own pain.	For children as young as 8 years old, as long as they can count and have some concept of numbers and their values in relation to other numbers.
No pain — 0 1 2 3 4 5 6 7 8 9 10 — Worst pain		
Visual Analog Scale (VAS) (Cline, Herman, Shaw, Et Al., 1992)		
Defined as vertical or horizontal line that is drawn to certain length, such as 10 cm (4 inches), and anchored by items that represent extremes of the subjective phenomenon being measured, such as pain	Ask child to place mark on line that best describes amount of own pain. With centimeter ruler, measure from "no pain" end to the mark, and record this measurement as the pain score.	For children as young as 8 years old. Vertical or horizontal scale may be used. Research shows that children ages 3-18 years old least prefer VAS compared with other scales (Luffy & Grove, 2003; Wong & Baker, 1988).
No pain — Worst pain		

†Word-Graphic Rating Scale is part of the Adolescent Pediatric Pain Tool and is available from Pediatric Pain Study, University of California, School of Nursing, Department of Family Health Care Nursing, San Francisco, CA 94143-0606; 415-476-4040.

who are nonverbal may have an escalation of repeated self-stimulating activities (i.e., rocking or hand flapping) when in pain.

CHRONIC AND RECURRENT PAIN ASSESSMENT

Tools that measure acute pain intensity may not be sensitive to the subtle changes and slow resolution characteristic of chronic and recurrent pain because pain expression becomes more complex. Specialized assessment tools are used to assess the domains of pain experienced by children with chronic or recurrent pain and the accompanying functional disability.

MULTIDIMENSIONAL MEASURES

The Pediatric Pain Questionnaire (PPQ), like the APPT, is a multidimensional pain instrument to assess patients' perceptions of their pain

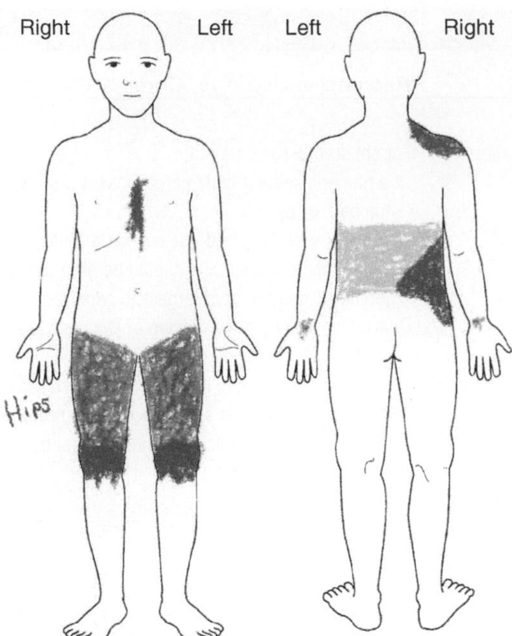

FIG. 5.4 Adolescent Pediatric Pain Tool (APPT): Body outlines for pain assessment. Instructions: "Color in the areas on these drawings to show where you have pain. Make the marks as big or as small as the place where the pain is." Tool has been completed by a child with sickle cell disease. (From Savedra, M. C., Tesler, M. D., Holzemer, W. L., Ward, J. A., School of Nursing, University of California–San Francisco; copyright 1989, 1992.)

experience in a manner appropriate for the cognitive-developmental level of the child (Lootens & Rapoff, 2011). The PPQ consists of eight areas of inquiry: pain history, pain language, the colors the child associates with pain, emotions the child experiences, the worst pain experiences, the way the child copes with pain, the positive aspects of pain, and the location of the current pain. The three components of the PPQ are (1) VASs; (2) color-coded rating scales; and (3) verbal descriptors to provide information about the sensory, affective, and evaluative dimensions of chronic pain. There is also information about the child's and family's pain history, symptoms, pain relief interventions, and socioenvironmental situations that may influence pain. The child, parent, and physician each complete the form separately to report their individual perceptions of the child's pain experiences.

For the child with chronic pain, a measure such as the Functional Disability Inventory (FDI) (Walker & Greene, 1991) provides a more comprehensive evaluation of the influence of pain on physical functioning. The FDI assesses the child's ability to perform everyday physical activities and has established psychometric properties with different populations (Claar & Walker, 2006; Kashikar-Zuck, Flowers, Claar, et al., 2011). For the child younger than 7 years old, the Pediatric Quality of Life Scale (PedsQL) is a multidimensional scale with both parent and child versions. It is recommended for assessing physical, emotional, social, and academic functioning as they relate to the child's pain (Varni, Seid, & Rode, 1999). The PedsQL and the PedMIDAS (Gold, Mahrer, Yee, et al., 2009; Hershey, Powers, Vockell, et al., 2001, 2004) have been validated for measurement of role functioning in the child with chronic or recurrent pain. The PedMIDAS is specifically designed to evaluate pain caused by migraines.

Pain diaries are commonly used to assess pain symptoms and response to treatment in children and adolescents with recurrent or chronic pain (Fortier, Wahi, Bruce, et al., 2014; Stinson, Stevens, Feldman, et al., 2008). Diary studies have included children as young as 6 years old. Conventional paper-and-pencil measures have been associated with several limitations, such as poor compliance, missing data, hoarding of responses, and back and forward filling. Electronic diaries to assess pediatric chronic pain have been developed to address these limitations. Refinement continues and holds promise for efficient clinical translation.

Chronic and recurrent types of pain often occur with some level of depression and anxiety in children (Fisher, Law, Palermo, et al., 2015). Among the many validated tools to measure anxiety and depression in children are the Children's Depression Inventory (CDI) (Kovacs, 1981) and the Revised Child Anxiety and Depression Scale (Chorpita, Yim, Moffit, et al., 2000). These two validated scales may be used together to better measure negative affect (Manworren & Stinson, 2016).

Sleep disruption is also common in children with chronic or recurrent pain (Valrie, Bromberg, Palermo, et al., 2013). A sleep diary can be useful in keeping a record of activities surrounding sleep, including bedtime, time to fall asleep, number of night awakenings, waking in the morning, and especially any pain or other circumstance that interfered with sleeping. Sleep diaries have been validated using actigraphy in healthy adolescents (Gaina, Sekine, Chen, et al., 2004). The Sleep Habits Questionnaire, which is useful for assessing sleep behaviors in school-age children with chronic or recurrent pain, has also been evaluated for use in preschool and toddlers using parent proxy (Sneddon, Peacock, & Crowly, 2013).

PREVENTION AND TREATMENT OF PAIN IN CHILDREN

Nurses' knowledge, unfortunately, does not always translate into improved pain outcomes for children. Nurses and other clinicians may hold onto outdated or incorrect beliefs and attitudes about pain or may work in a culture that does not support good pain management practices. Improving pain prevention and management requires a multifaceted approach of education, institutional support, attitude shifts, and change leadership. Pain management outcomes for children improve when several organizational strategies are used simultaneously (Twycross, Dowden, & Stinson, 2013). A national curriculum is available as a free download to facilitate pediatric nurses' efforts to improve knowledge and change organizational culture to be more sensitive to children's pain (http://www.childkindinternational.org). See Nursing Care Guidelines: Goals of a Pain Treatment Program.

NURSING CARE GUIDELINES

Goals of a Pain Treatment Program

A multidisciplinary approach helps provide the most comprehensive treatment of acute, chronic, and mixed types of pain. The primary care provider must first rule out and/or treat any systemic disease. When children experience chronic pain, intensive physical therapy, occupational therapy, and psychologic support for parents and children can be especially helpful. The ultimate goal in the experience of any pain is to improve function, quality of life, and a return to daily activities. Clinicians may emphasize the importance of participation in normal activities, including daily school attendance, sports or physical activities, social life, and adequate sleep (see Community and Home Health Considerations: Chronic Pain and School Absenteeism in Children).

Biobehavioral interventions and adequate analgesics are essential for effective pain prevention and treatment. Biobehavioral interventions are also known as nonpharmacologic interventions. The term *biobehavioral intervention* is preferred over *nonpharmacologic* because it is a term that reflects the mechanism of action. The term *nonpharmacologic* reflects the lack of pharmaceutical treatment as though medications are the gold standard of treatment. Sometimes biobehavioral interventions are as effective as, or even more effective than, pharmacologic interventions. The type of intervention(s) needed to prevent and treat a child's pain depends on the situation and specific needs of the child. Multimodal, also known as combinations of analgesic and biobehavioral therapies, is the preferred pain treatment plan. By targeting different mechanism of pain, medications combined with biobehavioral interventions are more effective at relieving pain.

BIOBEHAVIORAL INTERVENTIONS

Pain is often associated with fear, anxiety, and stress. Most biobehavioral interventions prevent and treat pain by interrupting the pain, fear, anxiety, and stress cycle. A number of biobehavioral techniques such as distraction, relaxation, guided imagery, hypnosis, cognitive-behavioral therapy, massage, heat, cold, and transcutaneous nerve stimulation (TENS) can help with pain control. Some techniques have combined targets of action. For example, music therapy is used for both distraction and relaxation. Coping strategies can help reduce pain perception, make pain more tolerable, decrease anxiety, and enhance the effectiveness of analgesics or reduce the dosage required. Biobehavioral interventions are accompanied by few if any side effects and at the same time may have crossover benefits in unintended areas. For example, use of regular relaxation and deep breathing practice to reduce chronic headaches could also improve a child's sleep.

It is helpful to think of biobehavioral pain prevention and treatment strategies as a box of available tools for acute, chronic, or recurrent pain (Figs. 5.5 and 5.6 and Table 5.6). Nurses may consider the individual child's needs when deciding on a strategy or series of strategies to use in prevention and treatment of pain. What helps one child may not be as effective for another. The child's developmental age and cognitive abilities are important considerations when choosing biobehavioral strategies.

If the child cannot identify a familiar coping technique, the nurse can describe several strategies (e.g., distraction, breathing, guided imagery) and let the child select the most appealing one (see Research Focus box). Experimentation with several strategies that are suitable to the child's developmental abilities is often necessary to determine the most effective approach. Parents should be involved in the selection process; they may be familiar with the child's usual coping style and can help identify potentially successful strategies. Involving parents also encourages their participation in learning the skill with the child and acting as coach. If the parent cannot assist the child, other appropriate persons may include a grandparent, older sibling, nurse, or child-life specialist.

RESEARCH FOCUS

Biobehavioral Methods of Pain Management—Preterm and Newborn Infants

Sucrose is safe and effective in reducing pain during needlesticks in neonates (Pillai Riddell, Racine, Gennis, et al., 2015; Stevens, Yamada, Ohlsson, et al., 2004). In a randomized controlled trial of 71 infants comparing oral sucrose, facilitated tucking, and a combination of both interventions, sucrose with and without facilitated tucking had pain-relieving effects (Cignacco, Sellam, Stoffel, et al., 2012) (see Fig. 5.9). Significant differences were found in pain responses during heel lancing between infants who were held skin-to-skin and those who were not. Infant responses to pain during heel-lance procedures were studied using skin-to-skin care (see Fig. 5.10), with the neonate held upright at a 60-degree angle between the mother's breasts for maximal skin-to-skin contact (Johnston, Stevens, Pinelli, et al., 2003). A blanket was placed over the neonate's back, and the mother's clothes were wrapped around the neonate for 30 minutes before the lancing procedure, during, and at least 30 minutes after the heel stick. Another group remained in the isolette in a prone position, swaddled with a blanket and the heel accessible, for 30 minutes before the heel-lancing procedure. Pain scores were significantly lower in skin-to-skin–held infants.

Although there is lack of evidence on the effectiveness of sweet-tasting solutions in reducing injection pain in infants and children 1 to 12 months old, the data are promising (Kassab, Foster, Fourerur, et al., 2012). A recent randomized controlled trial found that sucrose reduced 16- to 19-month-old infant distress during immunizations (Yilmaz, Caylan, Oguz, et al., 2014). Breastfeeding, but not breast milk, is as effective as sucrose and skin-to-skin care (Johnston, Campbell-Yeo, Disher, et al., 2017).

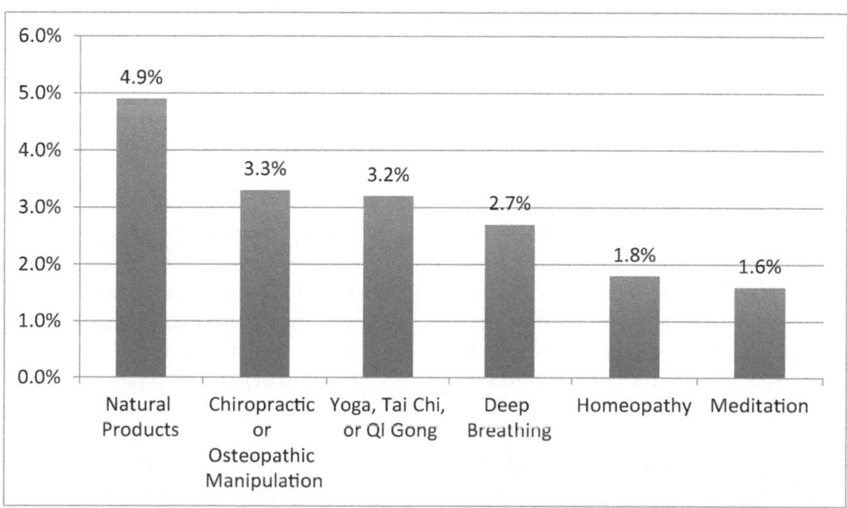

FIG. 5.5 Six most common complementary health approaches among children in the United States—2012. (Adapted from Black, L., Clarke, T., Stussman, B., et al. [2015]. Use of complementary health approaches among children aged 4-17 years in the United States: National Health Interview Survey 2007-2012. National health statistics reports no. 78. Hyattsville, MD: National Center for Health Statistics. Retrieved from https://nccih.nih.gov/health/children.)

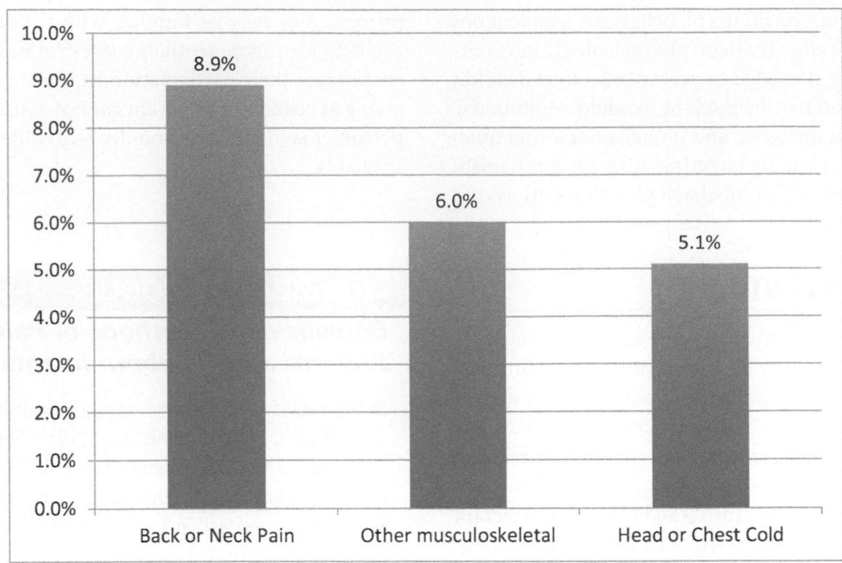

FIG. 5.6 Three most common painful conditions for which complementary health approaches are frequently used among children in the United States—2012. (Adapted from Black, L., Clarke, T., Stussman, B., et al. [2015]. Use of complementary health approaches among children aged 4-17 years in the United States: National Health Interview Survey 2007-2012. National health statistics reports no. 78. Hyattsville, MD: National Center for Health Statistics. Retrieved from https://nccih.nih.gov/health/children.)

TABLE 5.6 Classification of Biobehavioral Approaches

Biobehavioral Therapies Are Grouped Into Five Classes:	
Biologically based	Foods, special diets, herbal or plant preparations, vitamins, other supplements
Manipulative treatments	Physical therapy, chiropractic, osteopathy, massage
Energy based	TENS, Reiki, bioelectric or magnetic treatments, pulsed fields, alternating and direct currents
Mind-body techniques	Distraction, guided imagery, hypnosis, relaxation, biofeedback, yoga, spiritual healing/prayer
Alternative medical systems	Homeopathy; naturopathy; ayurvedic; traditional Chinese medicine, including acupuncture and moxibustion
Physical treatments	Heat, ice

TENS, Transcutaneous electrical nerve stimulation.

Children should learn to use a specific strategy before pain occurs or before it becomes severe. Instructions for a strategy, such as distraction or relaxation, can be audiotaped and played during a period of comfort. However, even after they have learned an intervention, children often need help using it during a painful procedure. The intervention can also be used after the procedure. This gives the child a chance to recover, feel mastery, and cope more effectively.

Biobehavioral interventions used to treat certain disease-specific pain syndromes may be helpful in prevention and treatment of other types of pain. Researchers have found good effect sizes and significant results using virtual reality, various mind-body techniques, creative arts therapy, listening to music, massage, and hypnosis in treatment of pain and anxiety in children with cancer (Thrane, 2013). Creative arts therapy incorporates any of the following into a program to reduce pain and anxiety: dance, movement, music, art, theater, yoga, and/or poetry (Poder & Lemieux, 2014).

An outdated term for biobehavioral therapies is complementary and alternative therapies (CAMs). There are some important distinctions to consider in the name of these types of therapies. Alternative refers to use of a nonmainstream practice to replace standard medical care. Complementary care is used together with standard medical care. Integrative medicine refers to the integration of conventional and biobehavioral approaches.

About 10% of infants are given teas or botanical supplements by their parents, usually for fussiness or stomach problems (National Institutes of Health, June 2016). For safety, nurses must ask about nonprescribed pain treatments and facilitate integration into the child's pain treatment plan. Dietary supplements must be used with caution in children. About 23,000 visits to the emergency department each year are associated with supplement use, either accidental or nonaccidental (National Institutes of Health, July 2016). Some biobehavioral treatments are well researched and low risk, including biofeedback, guided imagery, hypnosis, mindfulness, and yoga. Other alternative treatments may have higher risks; for example, spinal manipulation is associated with rare but serious complications (National Institutes of Health, June 2016).

PHARMACOLOGIC MANAGEMENT OF PAIN

The World Health Organization (2012) states that the principles for pharmacologic pain management should include the following:

- Using a two-step strategy
- Dosing at regular intervals
- Using the appropriate route of administration
- Adapting treatment to the individual child

The traditional World Health Organization stepladder has been replaced with a two-step approach for use with children. For children older than 3 months of age the first step is to administer a nonopioid analgesic. Opioids are started when pain is severe or unrelieved by nonopioids. Morphine is the medicine of choice for the second step, although other opioids may be considered (World Health Organization, 2012). The following sections discuss the most common pain medications used in children in the nonopioid and opioid categories.

Nonopioids

Nonopioids include medications such as acetaminophen (Table 5.7) and nonsteroidal antiinflammatory drugs (NSAIDs) (Table 5.8). NSAIDs are known for their antipyretic, antiinflammatory, and analgesic actions. Acetaminophen has antipyretic and analgesic actions, but no antiinflammatory action. Nonopioids are usually the first analgesics for pain related to tissue injury, also known as *nociceptive pain.* Nonopioid analgesics can provide safe and effective pain relief when dosed at appropriate levels with adequate frequency.

TABLE 5.7 Acetaminophen Dosing for Children

Drug	Dosage	Comments
Acetaminophen (Tylenol)	10-15 mg/kg/dose q 4-6 h PO not to exceed five doses in 24 h or 75 mg/kg/day, or 3-4000 mg/day	Available in numerous preparations Nonprescription

TABLE 5.8 Nonsteroidal Antiinflammatory Drugs for Children

Drug	Dosage	Comments
Choline magnesium trisalicylate (Trilisate)	25 mg/kg every 12 hours PO Maximum dose 3000 mg/day	Available in suspension, 500 mg/5 ml Prescription
Ibuprofen (children's Motrin, children's Advil)	Children >6 months old: 5-10 mg/kg/dose every 6-8 hours Maximum dose 40 mg/kg/day or 3200 mg/day	Available in numerous preparations Available in suspension, 100 mg/5 ml, and drops, 100 mg/2.5 ml Nonprescription
Naproxen (Naprosyn)	Children >2 years old: 5-10 mg/kg/dose every 12 hours Maximum 20 mg/kg/day or 1250 mg/day	Available in suspension, 125 mg/5 ml, and several different dosages for tablets Prescription
Indomethacin	1 mg/kg every 8 hours Maximum 3 mg/kg/day or 200 mg/day	Available in 25 mg and 50 mg capsules and suspension 25 mg/5 ml Prescription
Diclofenac	1-2 mg/kg every 8 hours PO Maximum 3 mg/kg day or 150 mg/day	Available in 50 mg tablet and extended release 100 mg tablets Prescription
Celecoxib	>2 years: >10 kg and <25 kg: 50 mg every 12 hours PO >25 kg:100 mg every 12 hours PO	Prescription
Ketorolac	1 mg/kg IV up to 60 mg as initial dose then 0.5 mg/kg IV every 6 hours (initial dose may be 0.5 mg/kg)	Prescription

PO, By mouth.
Data from American Pain Society. (2016). *Principles of analgesic use* (7th ed.). Chicago, IL.

Opioids

Opioids are indicated for nociceptive pain that is severe or unrelieved by nonopioids (Table 5.9). Morphine remains the standard agent used for comparison to other opioids. Opioids are titrated to safely achieve optimal analgesia.

Genetic Variants of Drug Metabolism

Genetic background influences how children and adults metabolize medications, placing certain children at particular risk. Codeine was

TABLE 5.9 Starting Dosages for Opioid Analgesics in Opioid-Naive Children (for Infants Start at 25%-33% of Dose and Titrate Analgesia and Sedation)

Medicine	Route of Administration	Starting Dosage
Morphine	Oral (immediate release)	0.3 mg/kg every 3-4 hours PO
	Oral (prolonged release)	0.3-0.9 mg/kg every 8-12 hours PO
	IV injection* SC injection	0.1 mg/kg every 1-2 hours IV or SC
	IV Infusion SC infusion	0.02 mg/kg/h
Fentanyl	IV injection	0.5-1 mCg/kg,† repeated every 30-60 min
	IV infusion	0.5-1 mCg/kg†
Hydromorphone‡	Oral (immediate release)	60 mCg/kg every 3-4 hours (maximum: 2-4 mg/dose)
	IV injection* or SC injection	15 mCg/kg every 2-3 hours
Methadone	Oral (immediate release) IV injection† or SC injection	0.1 mg/kg Every 4 h for the first two to three doses, then as analgesia duration increases, wean to every 6-8 hour intervals analgesia beyond 8 hours is rare, but may be dosed every 12-24 hours to treat withdrawal¶
Oxycodone	Oral (immediate release)	0.2 mg/kg every 3-4 hours (maximum: 10 mg/dose)
	Oral (prolonged release)	0.2-0.6 mg/dose or 10 mg every 12 hours

*Administer IV opioids over 3 to 5 minutes.
†Due to the complex nature and wide interindividual variation in the pharmacokinetics of methadone, methadone should only be commenced by practitioners experienced with its use.
‡Hydromorphone is a potent opioid and significant differences exist between oral and IV dosing. Use extreme caution when converting from one route to another.
¶Methadone should initially be titrated like other strong opioids. The dosage may need to be reduced by 50% 2 to 3 days after the effective dose has been found to prevent adverse effects due to methadone accumulation. From then on, dosage increases should be performed at intervals of 1 week or over and with a maximum increase of 50%.
IV, Intravenous; *SC,* subcutaneous.
Data from American Pain Society. (2016). *Principles of analgesic use* (7th ed.). Chicago, IL.

once a commonly used opioid in children. Children with CYP2D6 allele combinations associated with poor metabolism of codeine may get no analgesia, whereas children with combinations associated with ultrarapid metabolism are at risk of morphine toxicity and death (Isaacson, 2014; Manworren, Jeffries, Pantaleao, et al., 2016). Over 400 variations of the CYP2D6 gene are known (Baugh, Archer, Mitchell, et al., 2011; Isaacson, 2013; Khetani, Madadi, Sommer, et al., 2012; Lauder & Emmott, 2014). In 2017, the US Food and Drug Administration (FDA) issued a black box warning on the use of codeine in children because of reported deaths. Genetic differences in metabolism, however, may explain differences in opioid analgesic effectiveness and adverse reactions to an estimated 50% of currently available medications, including opioids, NSAIDs, and coanalgesics (Trescot, 2014).

Coanalgesic Drugs

Several drugs, known as coanalgesics or adjuvants (Table 5.10), may be used alone or with nonopioids and opioids to control pain and associated symptoms, including opioid side effects (Table 5.11). Benzodiazepines are frequently used to treat anxiety; however, these drugs do not provide analgesia and should not be used as a substitute for analgesics. The concomitant use of opioids and sedatives, such as diazepam, is associated with increased risk of death. Tricyclic antidepressants (e.g., amitriptyline, imipramine), antiepileptics (e.g., gabapentin, pregabalin), steroids, α_2-agonists, ketamine, and intravenous (IV) lidocaine are being used to treat chronic pain; these coanalgesics are also being used with increased frequency to treat acute pain (American Pain Society, 2016). Other medications commonly prescribed to address opioid-related side effects include peristaltics for constipation, antiemetics for nausea and vomiting, opioid antagonists for itching, and stimulants for sedation (see Table 5.11).

Choosing the Pain Medication Dose

Children's dosages are usually calculated according to body weight, with two exceptions. First, children achieve adult capabilities of cytochrome P450 metabolism (CYP2D6) by 1 year of age and over 50% by 6 months of age. Therefore doses of opioids for infants less than 6 months of age should be one-fourth to one-third of the starting dose recommended for children over 6 months of age. The infant receiving opioid analgesics should be monitored closely for signs of pain relief and respiratory depression (see Nursing Care Guidelines). Doses of other analgesics are also adjusted to account for this age difference in drug metabolism. Second, most adult analgesic doses are based on a weight of 50 to 60 kg. Children with a weight greater than 50 kg (110 lb) should be prescribed the average adult dose (see Pain Management in Obese and Overweight Children later in this chapter).

A major difference between opioids and nonopioids is that nonopioids have a ceiling effect. This means that doses higher than the recommended dose will not produce greater pain relief. Opioids do not have a ceiling effect other than that imposed by side effects. Therefore recommended initial opioid dosages are titrated to effect. If the patient experiences pain relief and opioid side effects, the dosage should be titrated downward. However, if pain relief is inadequate, the dosage is increased to provide greater analgesic effect. Decreasing the interval between doses may also provide more continuous pain relief. Because tolerance to opioids can develop, large doses may be needed for continued or increasing pain.

Parenteral and oral dosages of opioids are not the same. Because of the first-pass effect, an oral opioid is absorbed from the gastrointestinal tract and is partially metabolized in the liver before reaching the central circulation. Therefore oral dosages must be larger to compensate for the partial loss of analgesic potency to achieve an equal analgesic effect. Conversion factors (Table 5.12) for selected opioids should be used when a change is made from the IV to the oral route.

NURSING CARE GUIDELINES

Managing Opioid-Induced Respiratory Depression

Assess sedation level.
If sedated, stimulate patient (shake shoulder gently, call by name, ask to breathe).
Stop or reduce opioid.
Monitor closely for pain and progressive sedation and respiratory depression.
If patient cannot be aroused and respirations are depressed or patient is apneic:
Stop or reduce opioid.
Administer oxygen.
Support respirations.
Initiate resuscitation efforts as appropriate.
Administer naloxone (Narcan):

- For children weighing less than 40 kg (88 lb), dilute 0.1 mg naloxone in 10 ml sterile saline to make 10 mcg/ml solution and give up to 0.5 mcg/kg.
- For children weighing more than 40 kg (88 lb), dilute 0.4-mg ampule in 10 ml sterile saline (usually only 40 to 50 mcg are needed except with unwitnessed acute intoxication such as in emergency department).

Administer bolus by slow intravenous push until effect is obtained.
Closely monitor patient. Naloxone's duration of antagonist action may be shorter than that of the opioid, requiring repeated doses of naloxone.

Note: Respiratory depression caused by benzodiazepines (e.g., diazepam [Valium] or midazolam [Versed]) can be reversed with flumazenil (Romazicon). Pediatric dosing experience suggests 0.01 mg/kg (0.1 ml/kg); if no (or inadequate) response after 1 to 2 minutes, administer same dose and repeat as needed at 60-second intervals for maximum dose of 1 mg (10 ml).

NURSING ALERT

The optimum dosage of an opioid analgesic is one that controls pain without causing undesirable side effects. This usually requires titration, the gradual adjustment of drug dosage (usually by increasing the dose) until optimum pain relief without excessive sedation is achieved. Dosage recommendations are considered safe initial dosages (see Tables 5.10 to 5.13), not optimum dosages or maximum dosages. Monitoring is required to determine safe and optimal dose for each patient.

Choosing the Timing of Analgesia

The right timing for administering analgesics depends on the type of pain and the drug-specific duration of analgesia. For continuous pain control, such as for postoperative or VOC pain, medications should be administered around the clock (ATC). The ATC schedule achieves steady-state analgesia. If analgesics are administered only when the patient has pain or requests pain medications (a typical use of the prn, or "as needed," order), the child is then being required to endure pain to demonstrate a need for pain treatment. Pain then is not controlled. Uncontrolled pain is less responsive to pain medications and thus requires more and higher doses of medications. This places the child at greater risk for adverse analgesic effects. This cycle of erratic pain control also promotes "clock watching," which may be erroneously equated with addiction. Nurses can effectively use prn orders by giving the drug at regular intervals because "as needed" should be interpreted "as needed to prevent and treat pain," not "as little as possible."

Choosing the Method of Administration

Several routes of analgesic administration can be used (Box 5.2), and the most effective and least traumatic route of administration should be selected. The intramuscular route is never appropriate. Continuous

TABLE 5.10 Coanalgesic Adjuvant Drugs

Drug	Dosage	Indications	Comments
Antidepressants			
Amitriptyline	0.05-1 mg/kg/day PO hs Titrate upward by 0.25 mg/kg every 5-7 days prn Available in 10- and 25-mg tablets Usual starting dose: 10-25 mg	Chronic pain Continuous neuropathic pain with burning, aching, dysesthesia with insomnia	Provides analgesia by blocking reuptake of serotonin and norepinephrine, possibly slowing transmission of pain signals Helps with pain related to insomnia and depression (use nortriptyline if patient is oversedated) Analgesic effects seen earlier than antidepressant effects
Nortriptyline	0.05-1 mg/kg/day PO am or bid Titrate up by 0.5 mg every 5-7 days Maximum: 25 mg/dose	Chronic pain Neuropathic pain as above without insomnia	Side effects include dry mouth, constipation, urinary retention
Anticonvulsants			
Gabapentin	Initially 2 mg/kg/day, titrate to 5-30 mg/kg/day orally in 3 divided doses Maximum: 300 mg/day	Chronic pain Neuropathic pain	Mechanism of action unknown Side effects include sedation, ataxia, nystagmus, dizziness
Pregablin	Safety and efficacy in pediatric patients have not been established Dose may be approximately one-sixth of gabapentin dose	Chronic pain Neuropathic pain	Mechanism of action unknown Side effects include sedation, ataxia, nystagmus, dizziness
Carbamazepine	Initially, 10 mg/kg/day orally in 2 or 3 divided doses May increase dose by 100 mg/day at weekly intervals as needed Do not exceed 30 mg/kg/day	Sharp, lancinating neuropathic pain Peripheral neuropathies Phantom limb pain	Similar analgesic effect to amitriptyline Monitor blood levels for toxicity only Side effects include decreased blood counts, ataxia, gastrointestinal irritation
Anxiolytics			
Lorazepam	0.02-0.09 mg/kg tid Maximum: 2 mg/dose	Muscle spasm Anxiety	May increase sedation in combination with opioids Can cause depression with prolonged use
Diazepam	For skeletal muscle spasm: Adjunct: 6 months or older, initial, 1-2.5 mg orally 3-4 times daily, may increase gradually as needed Maximum: 10 mg/dose		
Corticosteroids			
Dexamethasone	Dose dependent on clinical situation; higher bolus doses in cord compression, then lower daily dose 0.02-0.3 mg/kg/day in 3 or 4 divided doses	Pain from increased intracranial pressure Bony metastasis Spinal or nerve compression	Side effects include edema, gastrointestinal irritation, increased weight, acne Use gastro protectants such as H_2-blockers (ranitidine) or proton pump inhibitors, such as omeprazole for long-term administration of steroids or NSAIDs in end-stage cancer with bony pain
Others			
Clonidine	2-5 mcg/kg orally in 4 divided doses May also use a 100 mcg transdermal patch every 7 days for patients >40 kg (88 lb)	Chronic pain Neuropathic pain Lancinating, sharp, electrical, shooting pain Phantom limb pain	α_2-Adenoreceptor agonist modulates ascending pain sensations Routes of administration: oral, transdermal, and spinal Management of withdrawal symptoms Monitor for orthostatic hypertension, decreased heart rate Sedation common
Mexiletine	Initially, 150 mg at hs; titrate to 10-15 mg/kg Maximum: 300 mg/dose	Neuropathic pain Lancinating, sharp, electrical, shooting pain Phantom limb pain	Similar to lidocaine, longer acting Stabilizes sodium conduction in nerve cells, reduces neuronal firing Can enhance action of opioids, antidepressants, anticonvulsants Side effects include dizziness, ataxia, nausea, vomiting May measure blood levels for toxicity

bid, Twice a day; *hs,* at bedtime; *IV,* intravenous; *NSAID,* nonsteroidal antiinflammatory drug; *PO,* by mouth; *prn,* as needed; *q,* every; *tid,* three times a day.

Data from American Pain Society. (2016). *Principles of analgesic use* (7th ed.). Chicago, IL.

TABLE 5.11 Management of Opioid Side Effects

Side Effect	Adjuvant Drugs	Nondrug Techniques
Constipation	Senna and docusate sodium *Tablet:* 2-6 years old: Start with ½ tablet once a day; maximum: 1 tablet twice a day 6-12 years old: Start with 1 tablet once a day; maximum: 2 tablets twice a day >12 years old: Start with 2 tablets once a day; maximum: 4 tablets twice a day *Liquid:* 1 month old to 1 year old: 1.25-5 ml q hs 1-5 years old: 2.5-5 ml q hs 5-15 years old: 5-10 ml q hs >15 years old: 10-25 ml q hs Casanthranol and docusate sodium *Liquid:* 5-15 ml q hs *Capsules:* 1 cap PO q hs Bisacodyl: PO or PR 3-12 years old: 5 mg/dose/day >12 years old: 10-15 mg/dose/day Magnesium citrate <6 years old: 2-4 ml/kg PO once 6-12 years old: 100-150 ml PO once >12 years old: 150-300 ml PO once Milk of magnesia <2 years old: 0.5 ml/kg/dose PO once 2-5 years old: 5-15 ml/day PO 6-12 years old: 15-30 ml PO once >12 years old: 30-60 ml PO once	Increase water intake Chewing gum Exercise
Sedation	Caffeine: Single dose of 1-1.5 mg PO Dextroamphetamine: 2.5-5 mg PO in AM and early afternoon Methylphenidate: 2.5-5 mg PO in AM and early afternoon Consider opioid switch if sedation persists	Caffeinated drinks (e.g., Mountain Dew, cola drinks)
Nausea, vomiting	Ondansetron: 0.1-0.15 mg/kg IV or PO q 4 h; maximum: 8 mg/dose Granisetron: 10-40 mCg/kg q 2-4 h; maximum: 1 mg/dose Droperidol: 0.05-0.06 mg/kg IV q 4-6 h; can be very sedating	Acupressure Imagery, hypnosis, relaxation Deep, slow breathing
Pruritus	Naloxone: 1-2 mCg/kg q/hr IV infusion Nalbuphine mixed agonist-antagonist 0.1-0.2 mg/kg every 4 hours	Exclude other causes of itching Change opioids
Respiratory depression—mild to moderate	Hold dose of opioid Reduce subsequent doses by 25%	Arouse gently, give oxygen, encourage to deep breathe
Respiratory depression—severe	Naloxone During disease pain management: 0.5 mcg/kg in 2 min increments until breathing improves (Pasero & McCaffrey, 2011) Reduce opioid dose if possible Consider opioid switch During sedation for procedures: 5-10 mcg/kg until breathing improves Reduce opioid dose if possible Consider opioid switch	Oxygen, bag and mask if indicated
Dysphoria, confusion, hallucinations	Evaluate medications, eliminate adjuvant medications with central nervous system effects as symptoms allow Consider opioid switch if possible Haloperidol (Haldol): 0.05-0.15 mg/kg/day divided in two to three doses; maximum: 2-4 mg/day	Rule out other physiologic causes
Urinary retention	Evaluate medications, eliminate adjuvant medications with anticholinergic effects (e.g., antihistamines, tricyclic antidepressants) Occurs more frequently with spinal analgesia than with systemic opioid use Oxybutynin 1 year old: 1 mg tid 1-2 years old: 2 mg tid 2-3 years old: 3 mg tid 4-5 years old: 4 mg tid >5 years old: 5 mg tid	Rule out other physiologic causes In/out or indwelling urinary catheter

hs, At bedtime; *IV,* intravenous; *PO,* by mouth; *PR,* by rectum; *prn,* as needed; *q,* every; *tid,* three times a day.

TABLE 5.12 Approximate Equianalgesia Ratios for Switching Between Parenteral and Oral Dosage Forms

Medicine	Dosage Ratio Parenteral	Dosage Ratio Oral
Morphine	1	3
Hydromorphone	0.15	0.6
Fentanyl	0.01	—
Hydrocodone	—	3
Oxycodone	—	2

Data from American Pain Society. (2016). *Principles of analgesic use* (7th ed.). Chicago, IL.

analgesia is not always appropriate because not all pain is continuous. Frequently, temporary pain control or sedation is needed to provide analgesia for medical procedures. When pain can be predicted, the drug's peak effect should be timed to coincide with the painful event. For example, with opioids the onset of effect is usually 5 to 10 minutes after administration and peak effect is approximately 30 minutes for the IV route. Analgesics given by the oral route typically have onset of action by 30 minutes and the peak effect occurs about 60 minutes after administration. Time of onset and peak effect is dependent on drug metabolism and therefore varies by drug, route, and patient. For extended pain control with fewer administration times, drugs that provide longer duration of action (e.g., some NSAIDs, time-released morphine or oxycodone, methadone) can be used.

BOX 5.2 Routes and Methods of Analgesic Drug Administration

Oral

Oral route preferred because of convenience, cost, and relatively steady blood levels

Higher dosages of oral form of opioids required for equivalent parenteral analgesia

Peak drug effect occurring after 1 hour for most analgesics

Delay in onset a disadvantage when rapid control of severe or fluctuating pain is desired

Sublingual, Buccal, or Transmucosal

Tablet or liquid placed between cheek and gum (buccal) or under tongue (sublingual)

Highly desirable because more rapid onset than oral route

- Produces less first-pass effect through liver than oral route, which normally reduces analgesia from oral opioids (unless sublingual or buccal form is swallowed, which occurs often in children)

Few drugs commercially available in this form

Many drugs can be compounded into sublingual troche or lozenge.*

- Actiq: Oral **transmucosal** fentanyl citrate in hard confection base on a plastic holder; indicated only for management of breakthrough cancer pain in patients with malignancies who are already receiving and are tolerant to opioid therapy

Intravenous (Bolus)

Preferred for rapid control of severe pain

First-choice alternative when oral route not available

Provides most rapid onset of effect, usually in about 5 minutes

Advantage for acute pain, procedural pain, and breakthrough pain

Needs to be repeated for continuous pain control

Intravenous (Continuous)

Preferred for sedation

Easy to titrate dosage

Need to provide boluses for analgesia

Subcutaneous (Continuous)

Used when oral and intravenous (IV) routes not available

Provides equivalent blood levels to continuous IV infusion

Total 24-hour dose usually requires concentrated opioid solution to minimize infused volume; use smallest gauge needle that accommodates infusion rate

Patient-Controlled Analgesia

Generally refers to self-administration of drugs, regardless of route

Typically uses programmable infusion pump (IV, epidural, subcutaneous [SC]) that permits self-administration of boluses of medication at preset dose and time interval (lockout interval is time between doses)

Patient-controlled analgesia (PCA) bolus administration often combined with initial bolus may be combined with continuous (basal or background) infusion of opioid, but not recommended in opioid-naïve patients or unless sedation is desired

Optimum lockout interval not known but must be at least as long as time needed for onset of drug

- Should effectively control pain during movement or procedures

Family-Controlled Analgesia

One family member (usually a parent) or other caregiver designated as child's primary pain manager with responsibility for pressing PCA button

Guidelines for selecting a primary pain manager for family-controlled analgesia:

- Spends a significant amount of time with the patient
- Is willing to assume responsibility of being primary pain manager
- Is willing to accept and respect patient's reports of pain (if able to provide) as best indicator of how much pain the patient is experiencing; knows how to use and interpret a pain rating scale
- Understands the purpose and goals of patient's pain management plan
- Recognizes signs of pain and side effects and adverse reactions to opioid
- Agrees to not activate device when patient is sleeping

Nurse-Activated Analgesia

Child's primary nurse designated as primary pain manager and is only person who presses PCA button during that nurse's shift

Guidelines for selecting primary pain manager for family-controlled analgesia also applicable to nurse-activated analgesia

Because nurse is not with patient at all times, dose is typically higher than PCA but lower than traditional boluses and lockout is longer

May be used in addition to basal rate to treat breakthrough pain with bolus doses; patient assessed every 30 minutes for need for bolus dose

May be used without a basal rate as a means of maintaining analgesia with around-the-clock bolus doses

Intramuscular

Note: Not recommended for pain control; not current standard of care

Painful administration (hated by children)

Tissue and nerve damage caused by some drugs

Wide fluctuation in absorption of drug from muscle

Time consuming for staff and unnecessary delay for child

Intranasal

Available commercially as butorphanol (Stadol NS) and approved for those older than 18 years old

Should not be used in patients receiving morphine-like drugs because butorphanol is partial antagonist that will reduce analgesia and may cause withdrawal

Continued

BOX 5.2 Routes and Methods of Analgesic Drug Administration—cont'd

Intradermal

Used primarily for skin anesthesia (e.g., before lumbar puncture, bone marrow aspiration, arterial puncture, skin biopsy)

Local anesthetics (e.g., lidocaine) cause stinging, burning sensation

- Duration of stinging dependent on type of "caine" used
- To avoid stinging sensation associated with lidocaine:
  - Buffer the solution by adding 1 part sodium bicarbonate (1 mEq/ml) to 9 to 10 parts 1% or 2% lidocaine with or without epinephrine

Normal saline with preservative, benzyl alcohol, anesthetizes venipuncture site

Same dose used as for buffered lidocaine

Topical or Transdermal (Zempsky, 2014)

EMLA (eutectic mixture of local anesthetics [lidocaine and prilocaine]) cream

- Eliminates or reduces pain from most procedures involving skin puncture
- Must be placed on intact skin over puncture site and covered by occlusive dressing for 1 hour or more before procedure

Lidocaine-tetracaine (Synera, S-Caine)

- Apply for 20 to 30 minutes
- Do not apply to broken skin

LAT (lidocaine-adrenaline-tetracaine), tetracaine-phenylephrine (tetraphen)

- Provides skin anesthesia about 15 minutes after application on nonintact skin
- Gel (preferable) or liquid placed on wounds for suturing
- Adrenaline not for use on end arterioles (fingers, toes, tip of nose, penis, earlobes) because of vasoconstriction

Transdermal fentanyl (Duragesic)

- Available as patch for continuous pain control
- Safety and efficacy not established in children younger than 12 years old
- Not appropriate for initial relief of acute pain because of long interval to peak effect (24-72 hours); for rapid onset of pain relief, give an immediate-release opioid
- Orders for "rescue doses" of an immediate-release opioid recommended for breakthrough pain, a flare of severe pain that breaks through the medication being administered at regular intervals for persistent pain
- Has duration of up to 72 hours for prolonged pain relief
- If respiratory depression occurs, possible need for several doses of naloxone

Regional Nerve Block

Use of long-acting local anesthetic (bupivacaine or ropivacaine) injected to block nerve transmission of pain

Provides up to 8 hours of analgesia postoperatively, such as after inguinal herniorrhaphy

May be used to provide local anesthesia for surgery, such as dorsal penile nerve block for circumcision, or for reduction of fractures

Inhalation

Use of anesthetics, such as nitrous oxide, to produce partial or complete analgesia for painful procedures

Side effects (e.g., headache) possible from occupational exposure to high levels of nitrous oxide

Epidural or Intrathecal

Involves catheter placed into epidural, caudal, or intrathecal space for continuous infusion or single or intermittent administration of opioid with or without a long-acting local anesthetic (e.g., bupivacaine, ropivacaine)

Analgesia primarily from drug's direct effect on opioid receptors in spinal cord

Respiratory depression rare but may have slow and delayed onset; can be prevented by checking level of sedation and respiratory rate and depth hourly for initial 24 hours and decreasing dose when excessive sedation is detected

Nausea, pruritis, and urinary retention common dose-related side effects from the epidural opioid

Hypotension, urinary retention, pruritis and temporary motor or sensory deficits common unwanted effects of epidural local anesthetic

Catheter for urinary retention inserted during surgery to decrease trauma to child; if inserted when child is awake, anesthetize urethra with lidocaine

*For further information about compounding drugs in troche or suppository form, contact Professional Compounding Centers of America (PCCA), 9901 S. Wilcrest Drive, Houston, TX 77009; 800-331-2498; http://www.pccarx.com.

Data from Pasero, C., & McCaffrey, M. (2011). *Pain assessment and pharmacologic management.* St Louis, MO: Elsevier.

American Pain Society. (2016). *Principles of analgesic use* (7th ed.). Chicago, IL.

Patient-Controlled Analgesia

A significant advance in the administration of IV or epidural analgesics is the use of patient-controlled analgesia (PCA). As the name implies, the patient controls the frequency of analgesic administration, which is typically delivered through a special infusion device. Children who are physically able to activate the device and who can understand the concept of cause and effect (usually by 7 to 8 years of age) can use PCA. Nurses can also efficiently use the infusion device to administer analgesics. The pump is typically locked, programmed, and verified to deliver a specific dose, making the infusion device an efficient alternative to witnessing and preparing each dose every time it is needed. Specific education and safety assessment are required when parents act as a proxy and control the infusion pump doses because this practice negates the inherent safety of PCA (Cooney, Czarnecki, Dunwoody, et al., 2013; Oakes, 2011) (Fig. 5.7).

PCA infusion devices typically allow for three modes of drug administration:

1. Patient-administered boluses that can be infused at a preset dose and lockout interval (time between doses). More frequent attempts at self-administration may mean the patient needs the dose and time adjusted for better pain control.
2. Nurse-administered boluses are typically used to give an initial loading dose to increase analgesia rapidly and to relieve breakthrough pain (pain not relieved with the usual programmed dose).
3. Continuous infusion that delivers a constant analgesic amount. This mode has been shown to increase sedation from opioids without providing improved analgesia, but may be appropriate in critical care settings.

PCA is typically used for controlling pain from surgery, sickle cell crisis, trauma, and cancer. If more than one dose of an IV opioid is needed, it is more cost effective to administer intermittent doses by infusion pump or PCA. Table 5.13 provides initial PCA settings for opioid-naive children. As with any type of analgesic management plan, continued assessment of the child is essential for the greatest benefit from PCA.

Epidural Analgesia

Epidural analgesia is recommended to manage postoperative pain in children hospitalized for pain control from surgeries below the neck

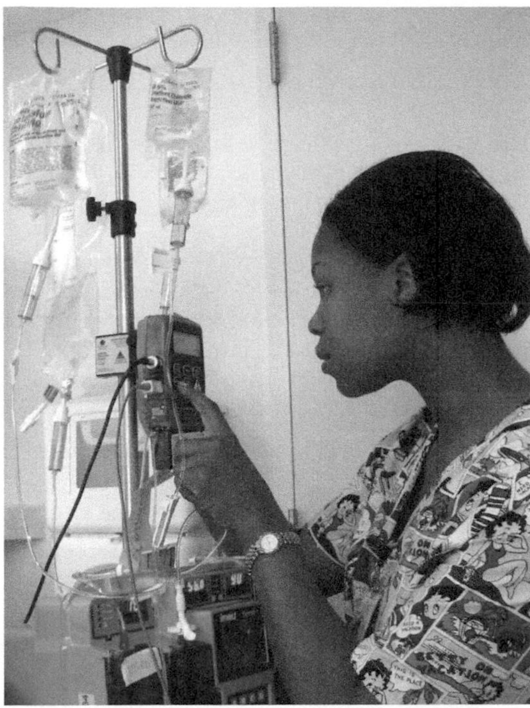

FIG. 5.7 Nurse programming a patient-controlled analgesia (PCA) pump to administer analgesia.

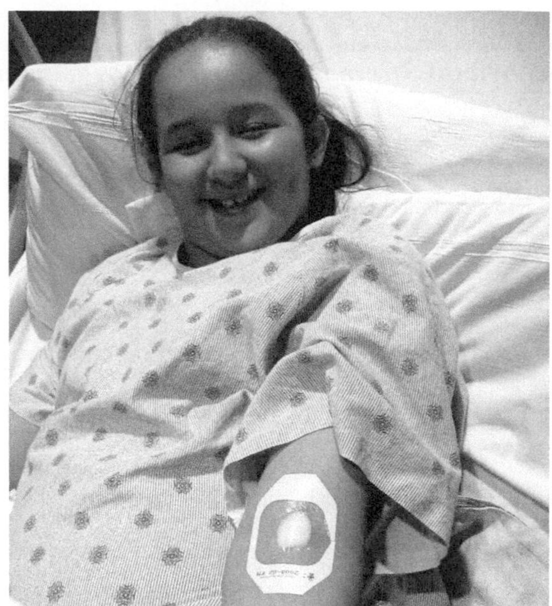

FIG. 5.8 Topical anesthetics are effective before intravenous (IV) insertion or blood draw.

TABLE 5.13 Initial Patient-Controlled Analgesia Settings for Opioid-Naive Children

Drug	Continuous Infusion Dosage	Bolus Dosage/ Frequency
Morphine	0-0.02 mg/kg/h	0.02 mg/kg q 6-10 min
Hydromorphone	0-0.004 mg/kg/h	0.004 mg/kg q 6-10 min
Fentanyl	0-0.5-1 mcg/kg/h	0.2-0.5 mcg/kg q 6-10 min

Data from American Pain Society. (2016). *Principles of analgesic use* (7th ed.). Chicago, IL.

(Chou, Gordon, de Leon-Casasola, et al., 2016). Although an epidural catheter can be inserted at any vertebral level, it is usually placed into the epidural space at the lumbar or caudal level (Suresh, Birmingham, & Kozlowski, 2012). The thoracic level is usually reserved for older children or adolescents who have had an upper abdominal or thoracic procedure, such as a cardiac or chest surgery. A local anesthetic (which is often combined with a preservative-free opioid such as fentanyl, hydromorphone, or morphine) is instilled by continuous infusion, with or without patient-controlled epidural analgesia. Careful monitoring of sedation level and respiratory status is critical to prevent opioid-induced respiratory depression. Assessments of pain and motor function are also critical to promptly identify epidural hematoma and avoid paralysis.

Transmucosal and Transdermal Analgesia

One of the most significant improvements in the ability to provide atraumatic care to children undergoing procedures is the development of anesthetic creams. EMLA (a eutectic mixture of local anesthetics: lidocaine 2.5% and prilocaine 2.5%) is one well-studied topical anesthetic found to be effective in children when applied to intact skin, but must be administered at least an hour before the painful intervention (Olsen & Weinberg, 2017). EMLA and other topical anesthetic creams should be used with caution in neonates (Watterberg, Cummings, Benitz, et al., 2016) (Fig. 5.8). Topical anesthetics can reduce pain of immunization when allowed sufficient time for action (Shah, Taddio, McMurtry, et al., 2015).

The intradermal route is sometimes used to inject a local anesthetic, typically lidocaine, into the skin to reduce the pain from a lumbar puncture, bone marrow aspiration, or venous or arterial access. One problem with the use of lidocaine is the stinging and burning that initially occurs. However, the use of buffered lidocaine with sodium bicarbonate reduces the stinging sensation. Needleless injection systems (i.e., J-tip) can be used to numb the skin for needle procedures.

Local anesthetics are lipophilic and have been successfully manipulated to penetrate intact skin. Fentanyl is also lipophilic. Fentanyl is available as a transdermal patch for continuous administration through intact skin for 72 hours per patch. The transdermal fentanyl patch is contraindicated for acute pain management but is FDA approved for use in opioid-tolerant children over 12 years of age who require chronic continuous opioid treatment (US Food and Drug Administration, 2015).

Monitoring Side Effects

All analgesics have side effects and risk of adverse effects. Respiratory depression is rare, but is the most serious adverse effect from analgesics. Respiratory depression from opioids progresses in a predictable pattern. The patient first becomes sedated and unarousable. Then depth of respirations decreases and rate of respirations increases. End-tidal CO_2 increases, oxygen saturation decreases, and respiratory rate decreases and then ceases. Sedation from opioids is to be avoided and nurses must increase their monitoring vigilance while patients sleep. Early recognition of respiratory compromise and prompt intervention is critical. See Nursing Care Guidelines box and Box 5.3 for further discussion of opioid side effects.

Although respiratory depression is the most dangerous side effect, nausea is the most common side effect of analgesics. Nonsedating

NURSING CARE GUIDELINES

Biobehavioral Strategies for Pain Management

General Strategies

Form a trusting relationship with child and family.

Express concern regarding their reports of pain and intervene appropriately.

Take an active role in seeking effective pain management strategies.

If available, consult a child-life specialist.

Use biobehavioral interventions to supplement, not replace, pharmacologic interventions.

Use general guidelines to prepare child for procedure.

Prepare child before potentially painful procedures. Honestly describe procedure.

- For example, instead of saying, "This doesn't hurt," say, "Sometimes this feels like pushing, sticking, or pinching, and sometimes it hurts and sometimes it doesn't bother people. Tell me what it feels like to you."
- Use descriptors when possible (e.g., "It feels like heat" rather than "It's a burning pain"). This allows for variation in sensory perception and gives the child control in describing reactions.
- Avoid evaluative statements or descriptions (e.g., "This is a terrible procedure" or "It really will hurt a lot").

Stay with child during a painful procedure.

Allow parents to stay with child if child and parent desire; encourage parent to talk softly to child and to remain near child's head.

Involve parents in learning specific biobehavioral strategies and in coaching child in their use.

Educate child about the pain, especially when explanation may lessen anxiety (e.g., that pain may occur after surgery and does not indicate something is wrong); reassure the child that he or she is not responsible for the pain.

Educate the child in a developmentally appropriate manner, for example, offer the child a doll, which represents "the patient," and allow child to do everything to the doll that is done to the child; emphasize pain control through the doll by stating, "Dolly feels better after the medicine."

Teach procedures to child and family for later use.

Specific Strategies

Distraction

Involve parent and child in identifying strong distractors.

Involve child in play; use radio, CD player, or computer game, smart phone; have child sing or use rhythmic breathing.

Have child take a deep breath and blow it out until told to stop.

Have child blow bubbles to "blow the hurt away."

Have child concentrate on yelling or saying "ouch," with instructions to "yell as loud or soft as you feel it hurt; that way I know what's happening."

Have child look through kaleidoscope (type with glitter suspended in fluid-filled tube) and encourage him or her to concentrate by asking, "Do you see the different designs?"

Use humor, such as watching cartoons, telling jokes or funny stories, or acting silly with child.

Have child read, play games, or visit with friends.

Relaxation

With an infant or young child:

- Hold in a comfortable, well-supported position, such as vertically against the chest and shoulder.
- Rock in a wide, rhythmic arc in a rocking chair or sway back and forth, rather than bouncing child.
- Repeat one or two words softly, such as "Mommy's here."

With a slightly older child:

- Ask child to take a deep breath and "go limp as a rag doll" while exhaling slowly; then ask child to yawn (demonstrate if needed).
- Help child assume a comfortable position (e.g., pillow under neck and knees).
- Begin progressive relaxation: starting with the toes, systematically instruct child to let each body part "go limp" or "feel heavy." If child has difficulty relaxing, instruct child to tense or tighten each body part and then relax it.
- Allow child to keep eyes open because children may respond better if eyes are open rather than closed during relaxation.

Guided Imagery

Have child identify some highly pleasurable real or imaginary experience.

Have child describe details of the event, including as many senses as possible (e.g., "feel the cool breezes," "see the beautiful colors," "hear the pleasant music").

Have child write down or tape record script.

Encourage child to concentrate only on the pleasurable event during the painful time; enhance the image by recalling specific details by reading the script or playing the tape.

Combine with relaxation and rhythmic breathing.

Positive Self-Talk

Teach child positive statements to say when in pain (e.g., "I will be feeling better soon," or "When I go home, I will feel better, and we will eat ice cream").

Thought Stopping

Identify positive facts about the painful event (e.g., "It does not last long").

Identify reassuring information (e.g., "If I think about something else, it does not hurt as much").

Condense positive and reassuring facts into a set of brief statements and have child memorize them (e.g., "Short procedure, good veins, little hurt, nice nurse, go home").

Have child repeat the memorized statements whenever thinking about or experiencing the painful event.

Behavioral Contracting

Informal: May be used with children as young as 4 or 5 years old:

- Use stars, tokens, or cartoon character stickers as rewards.
- Give a child who is uncooperative or procrastinating during a procedure a limited time (measured by a visible timer) to complete the procedure.
- Proceed as needed if child is unable to comply.
- Reinforce cooperation with a reward if the procedure is accomplished within specified time.

Formal: Use written contract, which includes the following:

- Realistic (seems possible) goal or desired behavior
- Measurable behavior (e.g., agrees not to hit anyone during procedures)
- Contract written, dated, and signed by all persons involved in any of the agreements
- Identified rewards or consequences that are reinforcing
- Goals that can be evaluated
- Commitment and compromise requirements for both parties (e.g., while timer is used, nurse will not nag or prod child to complete procedure)

BOX 5.3 Side Effects of Opioids

General
Nausea and vomiting
Miosis (may be sign of toxicity)
Constipation (possibly severe)
Sedation
Euphoria
Agitation
Mental clouding
Hallucinations
Pruritus
Orthostatic hypotension
Respiratory depression
Anaphylaxis (rare)

Signs of Tolerance
Decreasing pain relief
Decreasing duration of pain relief

Signs of Withdrawal Syndrome in Patients With Physical Dependence
Initial Signs of Withdrawal
Lacrimation
Rhinorrhea
Yawning
Sweating
Restlessness

Later Signs of Withdrawal
Irritability
Tremors
Anorexia
Dilated pupils
Piloerection
Nausea, vomiting
Abdominal cramping, diarrhea
Seizure

antiemetics should be given to prevent nausea. Sedating antiemetics such as lorazepam may be tried in the vomiting child, but the patient must be monitored for sedation. Constipation is also a common side effect of opioids due to a decrease in gastric peristalsis. Prevention of constipation with peristaltic agents and laxatives is more effective than treatment once constipation occurs. Dietary treatment, such as increased fiber and the use of stool softeners, is usually not sufficient to promote regular bowel evacuation. However, increased fluid intake and physical activity, such as rocking and walking, should be encouraged. Gum chewing has also been used to effectively increase peristalsis. Pruritus from epidural or IV opioid infusions is treated with low-dose opioid agonists such as naloxone or nalbuphine. Diphenhydramine is often erroneously used to treat opioid-related pruritus; however, appreciable relief is the result of sedation rather than the antihistamine effect. Ondansetron has also been effective for opioid and epidural pruritus. Nausea, vomiting, pruritus, and sedation usually subside after 2 days of regular opioid administration.

Both tolerance and physical dependence can occur with prolonged use of opioids. Tolerance occurs when the dose of an opioid needs to be increased to achieve the same analgesic effects that was previously achieved at a lower dose. Treatment of tolerance involves increasing the dose or decreasing the duration between doses.

Physical dependence to opioids is a normal, natural, physiologic state of "neuroadaptation." When opioids are abruptly discontinued in physically dependent patients without weaning, withdrawal symptoms occur. Symptoms of withdrawal include signs of neurologic excitability (irritability, tremors, increased motor tone, insomnia, seizures), gastrointestinal dysfunction (nausea, vomiting, diarrhea, abdominal cramps), and autonomic dysfunction (sweating, fever, chills, tachypnea, nasal congestion, rhinitis). Withdrawal symptoms can be anticipated and prevented by weaning patients from opioids that were administered for more than 5 days. In children (7 months to 10 years old) the Withdrawal Assessment Tool–1 may be use to assess and monitor withdrawal symptoms in pediatric critically ill children who are exposed to opioids and benzodiazepines for prolonged periods (Franck, Harris, Soetenga, et al., 2008).

Opioids are rarely indicated for long-term management of chronic pain in children (Palermo, Eccleston, Goldschneider, et al., 2013) but may be indicated for short-term treatment. Parents and older children may fear addiction when opioids are prescribed. The nurse should address these concerns (see Community and Home Health Considerations box). Infants may be at risk for physical tolerance and physical dependence but not psychologic dependence or addiction when using opioids for short-term pain management. The use of opioid analgesics early in life has not been demonstrated to increase the risk for addiction later in life. However, there is new evidence of increased risk of prescription opioid misuse in young adults who were treated with opioids as adolescents (Miech, Johnston, O'Malley, et al., 2015). Nurses need to explain to parents the differences between tolerance, physical dependence, and addiction and allow patients and parents to express concerns about the use and duration of opioid use. Nurses must counsel parents to secure opioids used to treat pain and promptly dispose of opioids that are no longer needed for pain treatment (Manworren & Gilson, 2015).

Specific Strategies for Special Populations

Pain Prevention for Needlestick

A number of interventions have been studied for prevention of needlestick pain in children. The most effective biobehavioral intervention to reduce needlestick pain in infants is breastfeeding (Benoit, Martin-Misener, & Newman, 2017). Other effective methods to reduce needlestick distress include the use of 24% sucrose or glucose and skin-to-skin care in infants; comfort holds for toddlers and small children; and deep breathing, distraction, hypnosis, and virtual reality for children and adolescents (Stevens & Marvicsin, 2016). There is strong evidence that these strategies are effective interventions to manage distress and help children and adolescents cope with needle pain, but there is no evidence these interventions prevent, reduce, or relieve needle pain (Birnie, Noel, Parker, et al., 2014; Jones, Moore, & Choo, 2016). Local anesthetics are the most effective pharmacologic agents for preventing and reducing needlestick pain (Box 5.4, Figs. 5.9 and 5.10, and Table 5.14). Best practice to manage needlestick pain requires a team approach with clinicians and families. Resources on the Internet are available (Box 5.5).

Care During Painful and Invasive Procedures

Combining pharmacologic and biobehavioral interventions provides the best approach for reducing pain from invasive procedures (see Research Focus box). Severe pain associated with invasive procedures and anxiety associated with diagnostic imaging may require sedation and analgesia.

Procedural sedation and analgesia. Sedation involves a wide range of levels of consciousness (Box 5.6). A thorough patient assessment including the child's history is essential before procedural sedation.

BOX 5.4 Evidence-Based Strategies to Reduce Needlestick Pain

Vaccination Specific

Injection technique	Avoid aspiration, use rapid injection technique
Vaccination order and sequencing	• Administer the least painful vaccine first when administering multiple vaccines in one visit (e.g., Priorix before MMR-II) • Consider simultaneous vaccine administration if possible

General Needlestick Pain Prevention Strategies

Positioning	Avoid supine position if possible Use position of comfort in all ages; use breastfeeding for small infants or at least skin-to-skin care
Type of soothing	Caregivers and nurses should *avoid* verbal reassurance, empathy, and apology Caregivers can be encouraged to use physical soothing and coaching
Topical agents/numbing agents/sucrose. See Table 5.14 and Figs. 5.9 and 5.10	Topical numbing recommended in appropriate age groups Sucrose recommended in children under 6 months of age
Other	Consider use of hypnosis or age-appropriate distraction

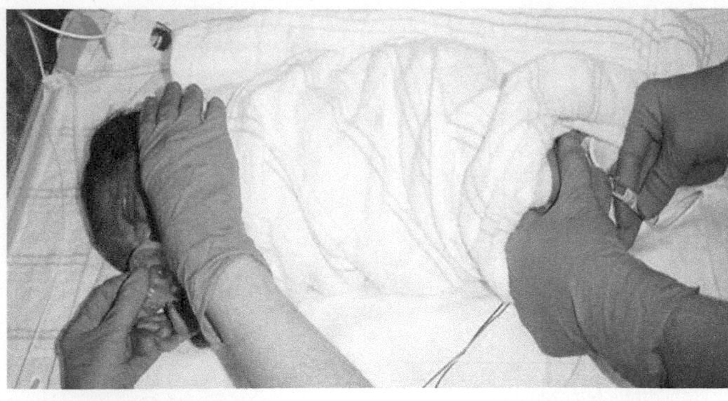

FIG. 5.9 Sucking following oral sucrose can enhance analgesia before a heel stick in a preterm infant.

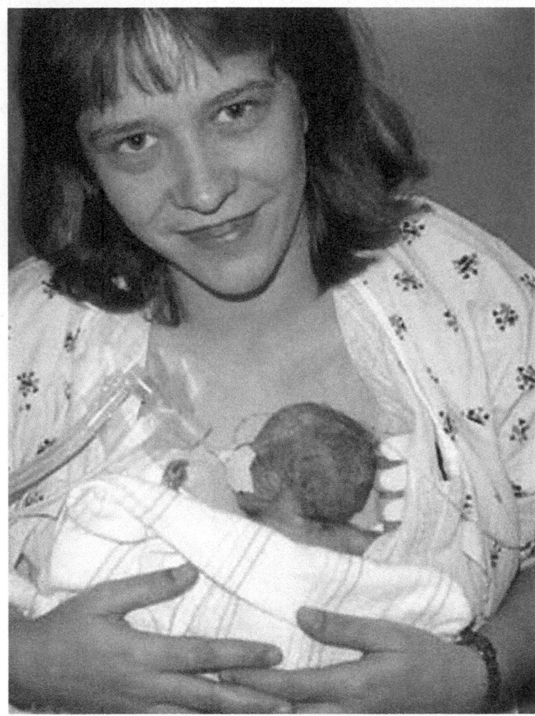

FIG. 5.10 Mother using skin-to-skin hold with her newborn infant. Note placement of the infant directly on the mother's skin.

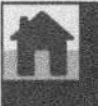

COMMUNITY AND HOME HEALTH CONSIDERATIONS

*Prescription Drug Abuse**

Prescription opioid diversion, misuse, and addiction are at epidemic levels. Deaths from opioid misuse now outnumber deaths from motor vehicle crashes (Centers for Disease Control and Prevention, National Center for Injury Prevention and Control, 2013; Manchikanti, Helm, Fellows, et al., 2012; Paulozzi, Jones, Mack, et al., 2011). Prescription drug misuse is defined as use other than prescribed, including use of another person's prescription or use only for the feeling the drug causes (Hasin, O'Brien, Auriacombe, et al., 2013). From 2011 to 2014, trend data reveal that prevalence of prescription opioid misuse increases from 1% to 2% of 8th graders, to 3% to 6% of 10th graders, and to 4% to 8% of 12th graders (Johnston, O'Malley, Miech, et al., 2015). Over 20% of young adults report misuse of opioid during their lifetime (Centers for Disease Control and Prevention, National Center for Injury Prevention and Control, 2013).

Opioids are appropriate for treating severe acute pain. Opioids are prescribed at greater than 5% of adolescents' primary care and emergency department visits (Fortuna, Robbins, Caiola, et al., 2010). Previous prescriptions for acute pain are a commonly identified source of opioids for misuse (Boyd, Young, Grey, et al., 2009). Legitimately prescribed opioid use by the 12th grade is independently associated with increased risk of future opioid misuse as a young adult (before 23 years of age) (Miech, Johnston, & O'Malley, 2015). This association is strongest among young adults who reported little to no previous history of drug use and disapproval of illegal drug use as adolescents.

Nurses should counsel families to monitor home opioid use and to secure opioids in locked medication safes or other locked cabinets to protect their children and children who visit (Manworren & Gilson, 2015). Nurses should also inform families of methods to dispose of opioids when they are no longer needed for the reason they are prescribed. Nurses must model this behavior in their use and control of medications.

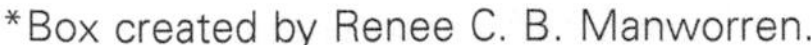

*Box created by Renee C. B. Manworren.

Key components of the patient's history include the following:

- Past medical history: Major illnesses, such as asthma, psychiatric disorders, cardiac disease, hepatic or renal impairment; previous hospitalizations or surgeries; history of previous anesthesia or sedation
- Allergies: Opiates, benzodiazepines, barbiturates, local anesthetics, or other drug allergies and side effects
- Current medications: Cardiovascular medications, central nervous system depressants; use caution with chronic benzodiazepine and opiate users; administration of reversal agents may induce withdrawal or seizures
- Drug use: Opiates, benzodiazepines, barbiturates, cocaine, tobacco, marijuana, and alcohol
- Last oral intake: For nonemergent cases, some guidelines recommend more than 6 hours for solid food and more than 2 hours for clear liquid
- Volume status: Vomiting, diarrhea, fluid restriction, urinary output, making tears

TABLE 5.14 Use of Needlestick Pain Prevention Products

Product	Onset	Duration	Appropriate Age/Weight	Potential Adverse Effects; Contraindications
EMLA	1 hour	4 hours	Approved by FDA for use in neonates over 27 weeks of gestation Has been used in preterm infants <37 weeks; safety of repeated dosages in preterm infants not established (Biran, Gourrier, Cimerman, et al., 2011)	Blanching, erythema Methemoglobinemia
Needle-free jet injection with buffered lidocaine	10-30 seconds	1-4 hours	Theoretic safety for ≥37 weeks of gestation but no published research Safety established for use in children ≥1 year of age (Lunoe, Drendel, Levas, et al., 2015)	Blanching, erythema, bleeding with improper placement; do not use in children with bleeding disorders or especially fragile skin
Sucrose pacifier	2 minutes	10 minutes	Newborn to 6 months	
Cold vibration device	15 seconds	Limit use to 3 minutes	≥1 year of age; assess cold tolerance before use	Blanching, erythema

BOX 5.5 Needlestick Pain Prevention Resources

Found online at the Centers for Disease Control and Prevention website at https://www.cdc.gov/vaccines/pubs/pinkbook/vac-admin.html and https://www.cdc.gov/vaccines/parents/downloads/parent-ver-sch-0-6yrs.pdf.

In addition, handouts with tips for clinical staff and parents are available in an article by Stevens and Marviscin (2016) at https://www.pediatricnursing.net/ce/2018/article4206267274.pdf.

Clinical practice guidelines for reducing pain during immunization by Taddio, McMurtry, Shah, et al. (2015) found online at http://www.apsoc.org.au/PDF/SIG-Pain_in_Childhood/20150824_CMAJ_Reducing_pain_during_vaccine_injections_full.pdf

RESEARCH FOCUS

Deep Intraoperative Anesthesia: Landmark Study

In the landmark study by Anand and Hickey (1992), 30 neonates received deep intraoperative anesthesia with high doses of the opioid sufentanil, followed postoperatively by an infusion of opioids for 24 hours; and 15 neonates received lighter anesthesia with halothane and morphine, followed postoperatively by intermittent morphine and diazepam. The 15 neonates who received the lighter anesthesia and intermittent postoperative opioids had more severe hyperglycemia and lactic acidemia, and four postoperative deaths occurred in the group. The 30 neonates who received deep anesthesia had a lower incidence of complications (sepsis, metabolic acidosis, disseminated intravascular coagulation) and no deaths.

A physical status evaluation using the American Society of Anesthesiologists Physical Status Classification (Meredith, O'Keefe, & Galwankar, 2008) is documented before administering analgesia and sedation:

- Class I: A normally health patient
- Class II: A patient with mild systemic disease
- Class III: A patient with severe systemic disease
- Class IV: A patient with severe systemic disease that is a constant threat to life
- Class V: A moribund patient who is not expected to survive without the operation

To provide a safe environment for procedural sedation and analgesia, equipment should be readily available to prevent or manage adverse events and complications (Box 5.7). If nitrous oxide alone is not appropriate, the patient should have IV access for titration of sedatives and analgesics and for administration of antagonists and fluids, if needed. A trained health care provider whose sole responsibility is to monitor the patient (rather than performing or assisting with the procedure) should be present to monitor for level of pain, sedation, and adverse events and complications.

BOX 5.6 Levels of Sedation

Minimal Sedation (Anxiolysis)

Patient responds to verbal commands.

Cognitive function may be impaired.

Respiratory and cardiovascular systems are unaffected.

Moderate Sedation

Patient responds to verbal commands but may not respond to light tactile stimulation.

Cognitive function is impaired.

Respiratory function is adequate; cardiovascular system is unaffected.

Deep Sedation

Patient cannot be easily aroused except with repeated or painful stimuli.

Ability to maintain airway may be impaired.

Spontaneous ventilation may be impaired; cardiovascular function is maintained.

General Anesthesia

Loss of consciousness, patient cannot be aroused with painful stimuli.

Airway cannot be maintained adequately and ventilation is impaired.

Cardiovascular function may be impaired.

From Meredith, J. R., O'Keefe, K. P., & Galwankar, S. (2008). Pediatric procedural sedation and analgesia. *Journal of Emergencies, Trauma, and Shock, 1*(2), 88-96.

Biobehavioral Interventions With Postsurgical Pain

A number of biobehavioral interventions have been studied to manage children's postoperative pain. Parental presence has been associated with significantly lower pain scores after surgery (Scalford, Flynn-Roth, Howard, et al., 2013). Therapeutic suggestion under anesthesia, a script of positively worded suggestions (no mention of pain or nausea) for promoting a sense of calm and healing delivered to a child while emerging

BOX 5.7 Procedural Sedation and Analgesia Equipment Needs

- High-flow oxygen and delivery method
- Airway management materials: endotracheal tubes, bag valve masks, and laryngoscopes
- Pulse oximetry, blood pressure monitor, electrocardiography,* capnography*
- Suction and large-bore catheters
- Vascular access supplies
- Resuscitation drugs, intravenous fluids
- Reversal agents, including flumazenil and naloxone

*May be optional devices.

from anesthesia, significantly lowered pain in children after tonsillectomy (Martin, Smith, Newcomb, et al., 2014) (see Research Focus Box). Music therapy (Van der Heijden, Oliai Araghi, van Dijk, et al., 2015) has also been successfully used to reduce postoperative pain in conjunction with pharmacologic management. However, there is limited and conflicting research support for these interventions. An expert panel from the American Pain Society and American Society of Anesthesia reviewed the evidence for postoperative pain interventions and the only recommended biobehavioral strategy with clear evidence of effectiveness was TENS (Chou, Gordon, Leon-Casasola, et al., 2016). Additional research is requested on other nondrug therapies.

RESEARCH FOCUS

Therapeutic Suggestions

Therapeutic suggestions (TS) delivered to children while emerging from anesthesia may be a potential tool to lower pain and reduce opioid use in children after painful surgery. TS are positively worded statements with suggestions for feeling comfortable. TS do not include references to pain or nausea. Martin, Smith, Newcomb, et al. (2014) found that children ages 4 to 8 who had TS in the postanesthesia care unit (PACU) after tonsillectomy had significantly lowered pain scores 30 minutes after extubation compared with children who heard PACU noises only ($p = .04$, Mann Whitney U for independent samples). The children who received TS also had 70% lower risk of receiving higher opioid doses. Further research is necessary to determine generalizability to other age-groups.

Pain Management in Obese and Overweight Children

Little evidence exists on proper dosing of pharmaceuticals in children, including obese and overweight (OB/OW) children. Pediatric medication doses are calculated based on measures of height and weight. Children with excess body fat may have altered metabolism of medications compared with normal-weight peers (Ross, Heizer, Mixon, et al., 2015). There is some evidence that OB/OW children may be at risk for prolonged episodes of acute pain after painful surgery (Martin, 2016). There are no current practice guidelines across all settings for OB/OW children requiring dosing of analgesics. Ross and colleagues (2015) produced a support tool to guide medication use in critically ill OB children. This tool includes some of the commonly used analgesic medications and contains instructions to adjust medications based on calculations of ideal body weight (IBW) and adjusted body weight (ABW). When medications are calculated using the ABW calculation, the ABW has been multiplied by a medication-specific cofactor. Controlled trials of this support tool, use of adult dose limits, IBW, and ABW are needed to provide evidence for safety and effectiveness.

Adjusted weight calculations for obese and overweight children

Calculate IBW:

$$(50\%\ \text{BMI for age})/[\text{height (in meters)}]^2$$

Calculate ABW doses:

$$\text{IBW} + (\text{total body weight} - \text{IBW}) \times \text{specific cofactor}$$

Treatment for Chronic Pain

Management of chronic pain is highly individualized to reflect the causes of the pain and the psychosocial needs of the child and family. A clear understanding of the child's characteristics (anxiety, physical health, temperament, coping skills, experience, learned response, depression), child's disability (school attendance, activities with family, social interactions, pain behaviors), environmental factors (family attitudes and behavioral patterns, school environment, community, friendships), and the pain stimulus (disease, injury, stress) is important in planning management strategies (Oakes, 2011).

Before any workup of chronic pain, the nurse informs the family that chronic pain is common in children and only 10% of children with chronic pain have an identifiable and treatable organic cause for their pain symptom. Medical workup is dictated by the child's symptoms in combination with knowledge about common organic causes of chronic pain. Even if no organic cause is found, the nurse needs to communicate to the child and family acceptance of the pain and the belief that the pain is real.

The management plan includes regular follow-up at 3- to 4-month intervals, a list of symptoms that call for earlier contact, and biobehavioral pain management techniques. Cognitive-behavioral therapy (CBT) may be required. The goal is to minimize the impact of the pain on the child's activities and the family's quality of life.

The use of CBT has been documented to reduce or eliminate pain in children with chronic pain. Parent involvement is a necessary supportive component. Case reports have demonstrated the effectiveness of implementing a time-out procedure, token systems, and positive reinforcement based on operant theory treatment modalities. Parent training in how to avoid positive reinforcement of sick behaviors and focus on rewarding healthy behaviors is important. Stress management strategies may be taught as part of the training. Over the course of several sessions, parents are educated about the chronic pain syndrome, how to distinguish between sick and well behaviors, how to implement a reward system for well behaviors, and how to reinforce relaxation and coping skills taught to children for pain management. Treatment may consist of a varying number of sessions over 1 to 6 months and may include various components, such as monitoring symptoms, limiting parent attention, relaxation training, and requiring school attendance. No negative side effects of symptom substitution occurred with the interventions (see the Research Focus box).

RESEARCH FOCUS

What Is Cognitive-Behavioral Therapy?

Cognitive-behavioral therapy (CBT) is an evidence-based psychologic approach for managing pediatric pain. Environmental and psychologic factors exert a powerful influence on children's pain perceptions. CBT uses strategies that focus on thoughts and behaviors to modify negative beliefs and enhance the child's ability to solve pain-related problems that result in better pain management.

Pain With Pediatric Cancer

Sedation or general anesthesia may be required to prevent the significant pain of procedures performed to diagnose and treat cancer. The pain related to bone marrow aspiration is due to the insertion of a large needle into the posterior iliac space and the unpleasant sensation experienced at the time of marrow aspiration. Lumbar puncture (LP) for administration of chemotherapy (e.g., cytarabine, methotrexate) and collection of cerebrospinal fluid may lead to a leak at the puncture site and low intracranial pressure. Some children may experience post–dural puncture headache after LP, which may be treated by administering nonopioid analgesics and placing the patient in the supine position. Rarely, post–dural puncture pain that persists may require a blood patch. Adequate pain control during immunotherapy infusions may minimize other side effects such as bronchospasm (Parsons, Bernhardt, & Strickland, 2013).

The most common clinical syndrome of cancer-related neuropathic pain is painful peripheral neuropathy caused by chemotherapeutic agents, particularly vincristine and cisplatin, and rarely cytarabine (Hickman, Varadarajan, & Weisman, 2014). After withdrawal of the chemotherapy, the neuropathy may resolve over weeks to months, or it may persist. Neuropathic pain is associated with at least one of the following: (1) pain that is described as a tingling, pins-and-needles, electric or shock-like, stabbing, allodynia, burning or numbness; (2) signs of neurologic involvement (paralysis, neuralgia) other than those associated with the progression of the tumor; or (3) the location of the solid organ cancer consistent with neurologic damage that could give rise to neuropathic pain. Tricyclic antidepressants (amitriptyline, desipramine) and anticonvulsants (gabapentin, pregabalin) have demonstrated effectiveness in neuropathic cancer pain (Rastogi & Campbell, 2014) (see Research Focus box).

RESEARCH FOCUS

Tricyclic Antidepressants to Treat Neuropathic Pain

Although there is limited evidence for the use of antidepressants for the management of pain in children, there is clinical use of amitriptyline for pain management in children (World Health Organization, 2012). A study of 90 children with irritable bowel syndrome, functional abdominal pain, or functional dyspepsia randomized participants to 4 weeks of placebo or amitriptyline (Saps, Youssef, Miranda, et al., 2009). Both amitriptyline and placebo were associated with excellent therapeutic response. There was no significant difference between amitriptyline and placebo after 4 weeks of treatment. Patients with mild to moderate intensity of pain responded better to treatment.

If the patient has neutropenia (absolute neutrophil count less than $500/mm^3$), the antipyretic action of acetaminophen may mask a fever. Therefore acetaminophen should only be administered as needed and with timed temperature monitoring. NSAIDs are contraindicated in patients with thrombocytopenia (platelet count less than $50{,}000/mm^3$) who may be at risk for bleeding. Trilisate and Cox-2 inhibitors do not affect platelet function and may be used to treat pain in patients with thrombocytopenia.

Pain Prevention and Treatment for Children With Sickle Cell Disease

A multidisciplinary approach combining pharmacologic and biobehavioral modalities is useful in treating the pain of SCD (Williams & Tanabe, 2016). The main treatment goal of the acute episode is to make the pain tolerable because complete pain relief is usually impossible even with the use of high-dose opioids. Other goals include patient participation in activities of daily living and a return to baseline physical function (Oakes, 2011).

SCD pain has both acute and chronic pain components; clinicians should not rely on typical physiologic response (outward distress, guarding) during assessment to determine level of pain. There is evidence that clinicians have undervalued patient-reported pain due to mismatch of observed and expected behaviors in relation to the severity of self-reported pain intensity (Schiavenato & Alvarez, 2013). Nurses should ask patients to rate their pain, and believe the patient's response, even if the patient's appearance does not match the nurses' expectations. The nurse should expect and not promote functional disability with reports of severe pain.

At home, most patients with SCD have treatment protocols that include escalation of opioids to prevent hospitalization. For example, patients may be given a regimen where they attempt to control pain and prevent hospitalization. Therefore patients coming to an emergency department for acute painful episodes usually have exhausted all home management options or outpatient therapy. Nurses should be aware that patients may be on long-term opioid therapy at home and may have developed some degree of tolerance (Han, Saraf, Zhang, et al., 2016). It is important to collect accurate information on the patient's current doses and home treatment for pain control so that hospital dosing may be adequate during times of crisis.

Patients may require inpatient management of severe pain if adequate relief is not achieved in the emergency department. For severe pain, IV administration with bolus dosing and continuous infusion using a PCA device may be necessary. Rapid treatment is needed to prevent chest syndrome and further patient deterioration. VOC lasts an average 7 to 10 days, but hospitalization is typically less than half this time. The goal while inpatient is to provide adequate pain control and transition from IV pain medication to oral so that the patient may be discharged home. Rehospitalization is common after a rapid return to home. Dehydration can trigger and prolong the sickle cell pain crisis. Close attention should be given to the patient's fluid status to ensure adequate hydration. IV fluids may be necessary to achieve optimal intake. In addition to opioids (oral or IV), the patient may also be on oral or IV NSAIDs such as Motrin or ketorolac. Patients with localized pain can benefit from heat applied to the affected area. Use of cold therapy should be avoided because cold is known to precipitate VOC. Other treatments that may be effective for pain from SCD include massage therapy, physical therapy, distraction, music therapy, art therapy, and CBT.

Pain Treatment During End-of-Life Care

Many patients at the end of life require doses of opioids to treat the pain of their disease as their disease progresses (e.g., cancer, human immunodeficiency virus, cystic fibrosis, neurodegenerative diseases). Patients achieve comfort with a combination of opioids and adjuvant analgesics in most situations. Parents need reassurance that the opioids are treating pain but not causing the child's death and that the child's advancing disease is the cause of death.

A small group of patients have intolerable side effects or inadequate analgesia despite extremely aggressive use of medications to relieve pain and side effects. Continuous sedation may be a means of relieving suffering when there is no feasible or acceptable means of providing analgesia that preserves alertness. A continuing high-dose infusion of opioids along with sedation is prescribed to reduce the possibility that a child might experience unrelieved pain but be too sedated to report it. Sedation in these situations is widely regarded as providing comfort, not euthanasia. Clinicians and ethicists have a range of views regarding assisted suicide and euthanasia, but they all agree that no child or parent should choose death because of inadequate efforts to relieve pain and suffering.

NCLEX REVIEW QUESTIONS

1. When caring for their infant, a parent asks you, "Is Emily in a lot of pain? How would you know since she can't really tell you?" The best answer to this question is:
   A. "Infants don't feel pain as we do because their pain receptors are not fully developed yet."
   B. "The nurses give pain medication before she really feels the pain."
   C. "We assess her pain using an infant pain assessment tool and give the medicine as needed."
   D. "Although we try to give her medicine before she feels pain, we watch her very closely and use different techniques to help relieve the pain."
2. Pain scales for infants and their uses include but are not limited to:
   A. CRIES: Crying, Requiring increased oxygen, Inability to console, Expression, and Sleeplessness
   B. FLACC: child's face, legs, activity, cry, and consolability
   C. NCCPC: parent and health caregiver questionnaire assessing acute and chronic pain
   D. NPASS: neonatal pain, agitation, and sedation scale for infants from 3 to 6 months
3. As the nurse is getting Nathan ready for surgery, his doctor asked you to explain preemptive analgesic to Nathan's mother. Which response leads you to believe his mother needs more teaching?
   A. "I understand that preemptive analgesia is giving Nathan pain medication before he has pain and could be given before surgery."
   B. "This medication will control Nathan's pain so he doesn't feel anything."
   C. "Giving this medicine early may help prevent complications after surgery."
   D. "By controlling Nathan's pain, he will be more comfortable and may be able to go home sooner."
4. When teaching a 6-year-old child with sickle cell disease and his family about pain management, which of the following should the nurse discuss? Select all that apply.
   A. When pain medications are used, all pain will be eliminated.
   B. Nonpharmacologic methods of pain relief, including heat, massage, physical therapy, humor, and distraction.
   C. It is helpful to use a "passport card" that includes information about the diagnosis, any previous complications, and the pain regimen.
   D. Only the physician can decide the best course of treatment, and the other health care providers follow that plan.
   E. Long-term medication use considers many factors.
5. How can the nurse prepare a child for a painful procedure? Select all that apply.
   A. Be honest and use correct terms so that the child trusts the nurse.
   B. Involve the child in the use of distraction, such as using bubbles, music, or playing a game.
   C. Kindly ask parents to leave the room so they don't have to watch the painful procedure.
   D. Use positive self-talk such as "When I go home, I will feel better and be able to see my friends."
   E. Use guided imagery that involves recalling a previous pleasurable event.

Correct Answers

1. D; 2. B; 3. B; 4. B, C, D; 5. B, D, E

REFERENCES

American Pain Society. (2016). *Principles of Analgesic Use, 7th Ed.* Chicago, IL: APS.

Anand, K. J., & Hickey, P. R. (1992). Halothane-morphine compared with high-dose sufentanil for anesthesia and postoperative analgesia in neonatal cardiac surgery. *The New England Journal of Medicine, 326*(1), 1–9.

Azize, P. M., Humphreys, A., & Cattani, A. (2011). The impact of language on the expression and assessment of pain in children. *Intensive & Critical Care Nursing, 27*(5), 235–243.

Babl, F. E., Crellin, D., Cheng, J., et al. (2012). The use of faces, legs, activity, cry, and consolability scale to assess procedural pain and distress in young children. *Pediatric Emergency Care, 28*(12), 1281–1296.

Bailey, B., Daoust, R., Doyon-Trottier, S., et al. (2010). Validation and properties of the verbal numeric scale in children with acute pain. *Pain, 149*, 216–221.

Basbaum, A. I., & Fields, H. L. (1978). Endogenous pain control mechanisms: Review and hypothesis. *Annals of Neurology, 4*(5), 451–462.

Basbaum, A. I., & Fields, H. L. (1984). Endogenous pain control systems: Brainstem spinal pathways and endorphin circuitry. *Annual Review of Neuroscience, 7*(1), 309–338.

Baugh, R. F., Archer, S. M., Mitchell, R. B., et al. (2011). Clinical practice guideline. *Otolaryngology–Head and Neck Surgery: Official Journal of American Academy of Otolaryngology–Head and Neck Surgery, 144*(1 Suppl.), S1–S30.

Beitz, A. J. (1982). The organization of afferent projections to the midbrain periaqueductal gray of the rat. *Neuroscience, 7*(1), 133–159.

Benoit, B., Martin-Misener, R., Newman, A., et al. (2017). Neurophysiological assessment of acute pain in infants: A scoping review of research methods. *Acta Paediatrica, 106*(7), 1053–1066.

Biran, V., Gourrier, E., Cimerman, P., et al. (2011). Analgesic effects of EMLA cream and oral sucrose during venipuncture in preterm infants. *Pediatrics, 128*(1), e63–e70.

Birnie, K. A., Noel, M., Parker, J. A., et al. (2014). Systematic review and meta-analysis of distraction and hypnosis for needle-related pain and distress in children and adolescents. *Journal of Pediatric Psychology, 39*(8), 783–808.

Bisogni, S., Calzolai, M., Olivini, N., et al. (2014). Cross-sectional study on differences in pain perception and behavioral distress during venipuncture between Italian and Chinese children. *Pediatric Reports, 6*(3), 5660.

Black, L. I., Clarke, T. C., Barnes, P. M., et al. (2015). *Use of complementary health approaches among children aged 4–17 years in the United States: National Health Interview Survey, 2007–2012.* National health statistics reports, 78, Hyattsville, MD: National Center for Health Statistics.

Boerlage, A. A., Ista, E., Duivenvoorden, H. J., et al. (2015). The COMFORT behavior scale detects clinically meaningful effects of analgesic and sedative treatment. *European Journal of Pain, 19*(4), 473–479.

Boyd, C. J., Young, A., Grey, M., et al. (2009). Teens' nonmedical use of prescription medications and other problem behaviors. *The Journal of Adolescent Health, 45*(6), 543–550.

Centers for Disease Control and Prevention (CDC). (2016 Dec).*2017 Recommended Immunizations for Children from Birth Through 6 Years Old.* https://www.cdc.gov/vaccines/parents/downloads/parent-ver-sch-0-6yrs.pdf.

Centers for Disease Control and Prevention, National Center for Injury Prevention and Control. (2013). *Division of Unintentional Injury Prevention: Policy Impact. Prescription Painkiller Overdoses.* http://www.cdc.gov/homeandrecreationalsafety/rxbrief/.

Chapman, C. R., & Vierck, C. J. (2017). The transition of acute postoperative pain to chronic pain: An integrative overview of research on mechanisms. *The Journal of Pain, 18*(4), 359.e1–359.e38.

Chaveli-López, B., & Bagán-Sebastián, J. V. (2016). Treatment of oral mucositis due to chemotherapy. *Journal of Clinical and Experimental Dentistry, 8*(2), e201.

Chen-Lim, M. L., Zarnowsky, C., Green, R., et al. (2012). Optimizing the assessment of pain in children who are cognitively impaired through the quality improvement process. *Journal of Pediatric Nursing, 27*(6), 750–759.

Chorpita, B. F., Yim, L., Moffitt, C., et al. (2000). Assessment of symptoms of DSM-IV anxiety and depression in children: A revised child anxiety and depression scale. *Behaviour Research and Therapy, 38*(8), 835–855.

Chou, R., Gordon, D. B., de Leon-Casasola, O. A., et al. (2016). Management of postoperative pain: A clinical practice guideline from the American pain society, the American Society of Regional Anesthesia and Pain Medicine, and the American Society of Anesthesiologists' committee on regional anesthesia, executive committee, and administrative council. *The Journal of Pain, 17*(2), 131–157.

Cignacco, E. L., Sellam, G., Stoffel, L., et al. (2012). Oral sucrose and "facilitated tucking" for repeated pain relief in preterms: A randomized controlled trial. *Pediatrics, 129*(2), 299–308.

Claar, R. L., & Walker, L. S. (2006). Functional assessment of pediatric pain patients: Psychometric properties of the functional disability inventory. *Pain, 121*(1–2), 77–84.

Cline, M. E., Herman, J., Shaw, E. R., et al. (1992). Standardization of the visual analogue scale. *Nursing Research, 41*(6), 378–380.

Cooney, M. F., Czarnecki, M., Dunwoody, C., et al. (2013). American Society for Pain Management Nursing position statement with clinical practice guidelines: Authorized agent controlled analgesia. *Pain Management Nursing, 14*(3), 176–181.

Courtois, E., Droutman, S., Magny, J. F., et al. (2016). Epidemiology and neonatal pain management of heelsticks in intensive care units: EPIPPAIN 2, a prospective observational study. *International Journal of Nursing Studies, 59*, 79–88.

Craig, B. M., Hartman, J. D., Owens, M. A., et al. (2016). Prevalence and losses in quality-adjusted life years of child health conditions: A burden of disease analysis. *Maternal and Child Health Journal, 20*(4), 862–869.

Crellin, D. J., Harrison, D., Santamaria, N., et al. (2015). Systematic review of the Face, Legs, Activity, Cry and Consolability scale for assessing pain in infants and children. *Pain, 156*(11), 2132–2151.

Crosta, Q. R., Ward, T. M., Walker, A. J., et al. (2014). A review of pain measures for hospitalized children with cognitive impairment. *Journal for Specialists in Pediatric Nursing, 19*(2), 109–118.

De Jong, A. E., Tuinebreijer, W. E., Bremer, M., et al. (2012). Construct validity of two pain behavior observation measurement instruments for yound children with burns by Rasch analysis. *Pain, 153*(11), 2260–2266.

Eccleston, C., Palermo, T. M., Williams, A. C. D., et al. (2014). Psychological therapies for the management of chronic and recurrent pain in children and adolescents. *The Cochrane Library*.

Ely, E., Chen-Lim, M. L., Carpenter, K. M., et al. (2016). Pain assessment of children with autism spectrum disorders. *Journal of Developmental and Behavioral Pediatrics : JDBP, 37*(1), 53–61.

Fernandes, A. M., De Campos, C., Batalha, L., et al. (2014). Pain assessment using the adolescent pediatric pain tool: A systematic review. *Pain Research & Management, 19*(4), 212–218.

Fisher, E., Law, E., Palermo, T. M., et al. (2015). Psychological therapies (remotely delivered) for the management of chronic and recurrent pain in children and adolescents. *The Cochrane Database of Systematic Reviews*, (3), CD011118.

Fortier, M. A., Chou, J., Maurer, E. L., et al. (2011). Acute to chronic postoperative pain in children: Preliminary findings. *Journal of Pediatric Surgery, 46*, 1700–1705.

Fortier, M. A., Wahi, A., Bruce, C., et al. (2014). Pain management at home in children with cancer: A daily diary study. *Pediatric Blood & Cancer, 61*(6), 1029–1033.

Fortuna, R. J., Robbins, B. W., Caiola, E., et al. (2010). Prescribing of controlled medications to teens and young adults in the United States. *Pediatrics, 126*(6), 1108–1116.

Fosdal, M. B. (2015). Perception of pain among pediatric patients with sickle cell pain crisis. *Journal of Pediatric Oncology Nursing, 32*(1), 5–20.

Franck, L. S., Harris, S. K., Soetenga, D. J., et al. (2008). The Withdrawal Assessment Tool–1 (WAT-1): An assessment instrument for monitoring opioid and benzodiazepine withdrawal symptoms in pediatric patients. *Pediatric Critical Care Medicine: A Journal of the Society of Critical Care Medicine and the World Federation of Pediatric Intensive and Critical Care Societies, 9*(6), 573–580.

Friedrichsdorf, S. J., Giordano, J., Desai Dakoji, K., et al. (2016). Chronic pain in children and adolescents: Diagnosis and treatment of primary pain disorders in head, abdomen, muscles and joints. *Children, 3*(4), 42.

Gaina, A., Sekine, M., Chen, X., et al. (2004). Validity of child sleep diary questionnaire among junior high school children. *Journal of Epidemiology, 14*(1), 1–4.

Gamst-Jensen, H., Vedel, P. N., Lindberg-Larsen, V. O., et al. (2014). Acute pain management in burn patients: Appraisal and thematic analysis of four clinical guidelines. *Burns: Journal of the International Society for Burn Injuries, 40*(8), 1463.

Gold, J. I., Mahrer, N. E., Yee, J., et al. (2009). Pain, fatigue and health-related quality of life in children and adolescents with chronic pain. *The Clinical Journal of Pain, 25*(5), 407.

Han, J., Saraf, S. L., Zhang, X., et al. (2016). Patterns of opioid use in sickle cell disease. *American Journal of Hematology, 91*(11), 1102–1106.

Harris, J., Ramelet, A. S., van Dijk, M., et al. (2016). Clinical recommendations for pain, sedation, withdrawal and delirium assessment in critically ill infants and children: An ESPNIC position statement for healthcare professionals. *Intensive Care Medicine, 42*(6), 972–986.

Hasin, D. S., O'Brien, C. P., Auriacombe, M., et al. (2013). DSM-5 criteria for substance use disorders: Recommendations and rationale. *The American Journal of Psychiatry, 170*(8), 834–851.

Hatfield, L. A., & Ely, E. A. (2015). Measurement of acute pain in infants: A review of behavioural and physiological variables. *Biological Research for Nursing, 17*(1), 100–111.

Hershey, A. D., Powers, S. W., Vockell, A. L., et al. (2001). PedMIDAS development of a questionnaire to assess disability of migraines in children. *Neurology, 57*(11), 2034–2039.

Hershey, A. D., Powers, S. W., Vockell, A. L., et al. (2004). Development of a patient-based grading scale for PedMIDAS. *Cephalalgia: An International Journal of Headache, 24*(10), 844–849.

Hickman, J., Varadarajan, J., Weisman, S. J., et al. (2014). Paediatric cancer pain. In P. C. McGrath, B. J. Stevens, & S. M. Walker (Eds.), *Oxford textbook of paediatric pain*. Oxford: Oxford University Press.

Hicks, C. L., von Baeyer, C. L., Spafford, P. A., et al. (2001). The faces pain scale–revised: Toward a common metric in pediatric pain measurement. *Pain, 93*(2), 173–183.

Howard, R., Carter, B., Curry, J., et al. (2012). Good practice in postoperative and procedural pain management. *Paediatric Anaesthesia, 22*(July Suppl. 1), 1–79.

Howard, R. F., Wiener, S., & Walker, S. M. (2014). Neuropathic pain in children. *Archives of Disease in Childhood, 99*(1), 84–89.

Hummel, P., Puchalski, M., Creech, S. D., Weiss, M. G., et al. (2008). Clinical reliability and validity of the N-PASS: Neonatal pain, agitation and sedation scale with prolonged pain. *Journal of Perinatology, 28*(1), 55–60.

Hunt, A., Goldman, A., Seers, K., et al. (2003). Clinical validation of the Paediatric Pain Profile. *Developmental Medicine and Child Neurology, 46*(01).

International Association for the Study of Pain (IASP). (2012 May). *Pain Terms, IASP Taxonomy*. http://www.iasp-pain.org/Taxonomy?navItemNumber=576#Pain.

Isaacson, G. (2013). Further concerns regarding opioids after tonsillectomy in children. *Otolaryngology–Head and Neck Surgery : Official Journal of American Academy of Otolaryngology-Head and Neck Surgery, 148*, 892.

Isaacson, G. (2014). Pediatric tonsillectomy: An evidence-based approach. *Otolaryngologic Clinics of North America, 47*, 673–690.

Ista, E., van Dijk, M., Tibboel, D., et al. (2005). Assessment of sedation levels in pediatric intensive care patients can be improved by using the COMFORT "behavior" scale. *Pediatric Critical Care Medicine: A Journal of the Society of Critical Care Medicine and the World Federation of Pediatric Intensive and Critical Care Societies, 6*(1), 58–63.

Jacob, E., McCarthy, K. S., Sambuco, G., et al. (2008). Intensity, location, and quality of pain in Spanish-speaking children with cancer. *Pediatric Nursing, 34*(1), 45.

Johnston, C., Barrington, K. J., Taddio, A., et al. (2011). Pain in Canadian NICUs: Have we improved over the past 12 years? *The Clinical Journal of Pain, 27*(3), 225–232.

Johnston, C., Campbell-Yeo, M., Disher, T., et al. (2017). Skin-to-skin care for procedural pain in neonates. *The Cochrane Database of Systematic Reviews.*

Johnston, C. C., Stevens, B., Pinelli, J., et al. (2003). Kangaroo care is effective in diminishing pain response in preterm neonates. *Archives of Pediatrics and Adolescent Medicine, 157*(11), 1084–1088.

Johnston, L. D., O'Malley, P. M., Miech, R. A., et al. (2015). *Monitoring the Future Study: Trends in Prevalence of various drugs for 8th graders, 10th graders, and 12th graders, 2011-2014 from Monitoring the Future national results on adolescent drug use: overview of key findings, 2014, Ann Arbor, Mich: Institute for Social Research, University of Michigan.* http://www.drugabuse.gov/trends-statistics/monitoring-future/.

Jones, K. M., King, S., & MacLaren Chorney, J. E. (2014). Supporting children with chronic pain in their return to school. *Pediatric Pain Letter, 16*(1–2), 8–14. http://www.childpain.org/ppl.

Jones, T., Moore, T., & Choo, J. (2016). The impact of virtual reality on chronic pain. *PLoS ONE, 11*(12), e0167523.

Kashikar-Zuck, S., Flowers, S. R., Claar, R. L., et al. (2011). Clinical utility and validity of the Functional Disability Inventory among a multicenter sample of youth with chronic pain. *Pain, 152*(7), 1600–1607.

Kashikar-Zuck, S., & Ting, T. V. (2014). Juvenile fibromyalgia: Current status of research and future developments. *Nature Reviews. Rheumatology, 10*(2), 89–96.

Kassab, M., Foster, J. P., Foureur, M., et al. (2012). Sweet-tasting solutions for needle-related procedural pain in infants one month to one year of age. *The Cochrane Database of Systematic Reviews,* (12), CD008411.

Khetani, J. D., Madadi, P., Sommer, D. D., et al. (2012). Apnea and oxygen desaturations in children treated with opioids after adenotonsillectomy for obstructive sleep apnea syndrome. *Paediatric Drugs, 14,* 411–415.

King, S., Chambers, C. T., Huguet, A., et al. (2011). The epidemiology of chronic pain in children and adolescents revisited: A systematic review. *Pain, 152,* 2729–2738.

Korterink, J. J., Rutten, J. M., Venmans, L., et al. (2015). Pharmacologic treatment in pediatric functional abdominal pain disorders: A systematic review. *The Journal of Pediatrics, 166*(2), 424–431.

Kovacs, M. (1981). Rating scales to assess depression in school-aged children. *Acta Paedopsychiatrica, 46*(5–6), 305–315.

Kozlowski, L. J., Kost-Byerly, S., Colantuoni, E., et al. (2014). Pain prevalence, intensity, assessment and management in a hospitalized pediatric population. *Pain Management Nursing, 15,* 22–35.

Krechel, S. W., & Bildner, J. (1995). CRIES: A new neonatal postoperative pain measurement score. Initial testing of validity and reliability. *Paediatric Anaesthesia, 5,* 53–61.

Kristensen, A. D., Ahlburg, P., Lauridsen, M. C., et al. (2012). Chronic pain after inguinal hernia repair in children. *British Journal of Anaesthesia, 109*(4), 603–608.

Lauder, G., & Emmott, A. (2014). Confronting the challenges of effective pain management in children following tonsillectomy. *International Journal of Pediatric Otorhinolaryngology, 78,* 1813–1827.

Lawrence, J., Alcock, D., McGrath, P., et al. (1993). The development of a tool to assess neonatal pain. *Neonatal Network: NN, 12*(6), 59–66.

Logan, D. E., Coakley, R. M., & Scharff, L. (2007). Teachers' perceptions of and responses to adolescents with chronic pain syndromes. *Journal of Pediatric Psychology, 32*(2), 139–149.

Logan, D. E., Simons, L. E., & Carpino, E. (2012). Too sick for school? Parent influences on school functioning among children with chronic pain. *Pain, 153*(2), 437–443.

Lootens, C. C., & Rapoff, M. A. (2011). Measures of pediatric pain: 21-numbered circle visual analog scale (VAS), E-Ouch electronic pain diary, Oucher, pain behavior observation method, pediatric pain assessment tool (PPAT), and pediatric pain questionnaire (PPQ). *Arthritis Care and Research, 63*(Suppl. 11), S253–S262.

Luffy, R., & Grove, S. K. (2003). Examining the validity, reliability, and preference of three pediatric pain measurement tools in African-American children. *Pediatric Nursing, 29*(1), 54–60.

Lunoe, M. M., Drendel, A. L., Levas, M. N., et al. (2015). A randomized clinical trial of jet-injected lidocaine to reduce venipuncture pain for young children. *Annals of Emergency Medicine, 66*(5), 466–474.

Malviya, S., Voepel-Lewis, T., Burke, C., et al. (2006). The revised FLACC observational pain tool: Improved reliability and validity for pain assessment in children with cognitive impairment. *Paediatric Anesthesia, 16*(3), 258–265.

Manchikanti, L., Helm, S., Fellows, B., et al. (2012). Opioid epidemic in the United States. *Pain Physician, 15*(3 Suppl.), ES9–ES38.

Mantyh, P. W. (1983). Connections of midbrain periaqueductal gray in the monkey. I. Ascending efferent projections. *Journal of Neurophysiology, 49*(3), 567–581.

Manworren, R. C. B. (2017). We do still hurt babies. *Journal of Perinatal & Neonatal Nursing,* NIHMS855388, Publ.ID: JPNN-D-17-00014, (in press).

Manworren, R. C. B., & Gilson, A. M. (2015). Nurses' role in preventing prescription opioid diversion. *The American Journal of Nursing, 115*(8), 34–40. http://journals.lww.com/ajnonline/Abstract/2015/08000/CE___Nurses__Role_in_Preventing_Prescription.21.aspx.

Manworren, R. C. B., & Hynan, L. S. (2003). Clinical validation of FLACC: Preverbal patient pain scale. *Pediatric Nursing, 29*(2), 140. http://www.pediatricnursing.org.

Manworren, R. C. B., Jeffries, L., Pantaleao, A., et al. (2016). Pharmacogenetic testing for analgesic adverse effects: Pediatric case series. *The Clinical Journal of Pain, 32*(2), 109–115.

Manworren, R. C. B., & Stinson, J. (2016). Pediatric pain measurement, assessment, and evaluation. *Seminars in Pediatric Neurology, 23*(3), 189–200.

Martin, S. (2016). *Associations between weight status and post-tonsillectomy pain experiences in children: A retrospective study* (Order No. 10585181), available from Dissertations & Theses @ University of Texas–Arlington; ProQuest Dissertations & Theses Global.

Martin, S., Smith, A. B., Newcomb, P., et al. (2014). Effects of therapeutic suggestion under anesthesia on outcomes in children post tonsillectomy. *Journal of Perianesthesia Nursing, 29*(2), 94–106.

Mayer, D. J., & Liebeskind, J. C. (1974). Pain reduction by focal electrical stimulation of the brain: An anatomical and behavioral analysis. *Brain Research, 68*(1), 73–93.

McGrath, P. J., Walco, G. A., Turk, D. C., et al. (2008). Core outcome domains and measures for pediatric acute and chronic/recurrent pain clinical trials: PedIMMPACT recommendations. *The Journal of Pain, 9*(9), 771–783.

McIntyre, M. K., Clifford, J. L., Maani, C. V., et al. (2016). Progress of clinical practice on the management of burn-associated pain: Lessons from animal models. *Burns: Journal of the International Society for Burn Injuries, 42*(6), 1161–1172.

McMurtry, C. M., Riddell, R. P., Taddio, A., et al. (2015). Far from "Just a Poke": Common painful needle procedures and the development of needle fear. *The Clinical Journal of Pain, 31,* S3–S11.

McMurtry, C. M., Taddio, A., Noel, M., et al. (2016). Exposure-based interventions for the management of individuals with high levels of needle fear across the lifespan: A clinical practice guideline and call for further research. *Cognitive Behaviour Therapy, 45*(3), 217–235.

Melzack, R. (1975). The McGill pain questionnaire: Major properties and scoring methods. *Pain, 1*(3), 277–299.

Melzack, R. (2001). Pain and the neuromatrix in the brain. *Journal of Dental Education, 65*(12), 1378–1382.

Melzack, R. (2005). Evolution of the neuromatrix theory of pain: The Prithvi Raj lecture: Presented at the third world congress of world institute of pain, Barcelona 2004. *Pain Practice, 5*(2), 85–94.

Meredith, J. R., O'Keefe, K. P., & Galwankar, S. (2008). Pediatric procedural sedation and analgesia. *Journal of Emergencies, Trauma, and Shock, 1*(2), 88–96.

Merkel, S. I., Voepel-Lewis, T., Shayevitz, J. R., et al. (1997). The FLACC: A behavioral scale for scoring postoperative pain in young children. *Pediatric Nursing, 23*(3), 293–297.

Miech, R., Johnston, L., O'Malley, P. M., et al. (2015). Prescription opioids in adolescence and future opioid misuse. *Pediatrics, 136*(5), e1169–e1177.

National Institutes of Health. (2016 June). *Complimentary, alternative, or integrative health: What's in a name?* National Center for Complementary and Integrative Health, https://nccih.nih.gov/health/integrative-health#cvsa.

National Institutes of Health. (2016 July). *Children and the use of complimentary health approaches*. National Center for Complementary and Integrative Health. https://nccih.nih.gov/health/children#hed1.

Nir, Y., Paz, A., Sabo, E., et al. (2003). Fear of injections in your adults: Prevalence and associations. *The American Journal of Tropical Medicine and Hygiene, 68*(3), 341–344.

Oakes, L. L. (2011). *Infant and child pain management*. New York: Springer Publishing.

Olsen, K., & Weinberg, E. (2017). Pain-less practice: Techniques to reduce procedural pain and anxiety in pediatric acute care. *Clinical Pediatric Emergency Medicine, 18*(1), 32–41.

Ossipov, M. H., Morimura, K., & Porreca, F. (2014). Descending pain modulation and chronification of pain. *Current Opinion in Supportive and Palliative Care, 8*(2), 143–151.

Palermo, T., Eccleston, C., Goldschneider, K., et al. (2013). *Assessment and management of children with chronic pain: A position statement from the American Pain Society*. http://americanpainsociety.org/uploads/get-involved/pediatric-chronic-pain-statement.pdf.

Parsons, K., Bernhardt, B., & Strickland, B. (2013). Targeted immunotherapy for high-risk Neuroblastoma—The role of monoclonal antibodies. *The Annals of Pharmacotherapy, 47*(2), 210–218.

Pasero, C., & McCaffrey, M. (2011). *Pain assessment and pharmacologic management*. St. Louis, MO: Elsevier.

Paulozzi, L. J., Jones, C. M., Mack, K. A., et al. (2011). Vital signs: Overdoses of prescription opioid pain relievers—United States, 1999-2008. *Morbidity and Mortality Weekly Report, 60*(43), 1487–1492.

Pillai Riddell, R. R., Racine, N. M., Gennis, H. G., et al. (2015). Non-pharmacological management of infant and young child procedural pain. *The Cochrane Database of Systematic Reviews*.

Poder, T. G., & Lemieux, R. (2014). How effective are spiritual care and body manipulation therapies in pediatric oncology? A systematic review of the literature. *Global Journal of Health Science, 6*(2), 112.

Quinn, B. L., Seibold, E., & Hayman, L. (2015). Pain assessment in children with special needs: A review of the literature. *Exceptional Children, 82*(1), 44–57.

Quinn, B. L., Sheldon, L. K., & Cooley, M. E. (2014). Pediatric pain assessment by drawn faces scales: A review. *Pain Management Nursing, 15*(4), 909–918.

Rastogi, S., & Campbell, F. (2014). Drugs for neuropathic pain. In P. C. McGrath, B. J. Stevens, S. M. Walker, et al. (Eds.), *Oxford textbook of paediatric pain*. Oxford: Oxford University Press.

Ross, E. L., Heizer, J., Mixon, M. A., et al. (2015). Development of recommendations for dosing of commonly prescribed medications in critically ill obese children. *American Journal of Health-System Pharmacy, 72*(7), 542–556.

Saps, M., Youssef, N., Miranda, A., et al. (2009). Multicenter, randomized, placebo-controlled trial of amitriptyline in children with functional gastrointestinal disorders. *Gastroenterology, 137*(4), 1261–1269.

Savedra, M. C., Holzemer, W. L., Tesler, M. D., et al. (1993). Assessment of postoperation pain in children and adolescents using the adolescent pediatric pain tool. *Nursing Research, 42*(1), 5–9.

Savedra, M. C., Tesler, M. D., Holzemer, W. L., et al. (1989). Pain location: Validity and reliability of body outline markings by hospitalized children and adolescents. *Research in Nursing and Health, 12*(5), 307–314.

Scalford, D., Flynn-Roth, R., Howard, D., et al. (2013). Pain management of children aged 5 to 10 years after adenotonsillectomy. *Journal of Perianesthesia Nursing, 28*(6), 353–360.

Schiavenato, M., & Alvarez, O. (2013). Pain assessment during a vaso-occlusive crisis in the pediatric and adolescent patient: Rethinking practice. *Journal of Pediatric Oncology Nursing, 30*(5), 242–248.

Shah, V., Taddio, A., McMurtry, C. M., et al. (2015). Pharmacological and combined interventions to reduce vaccine injection pain in children and adults: Systematic review and meta-analysis. *The Clinical Journal of Pain, 31*(Suppl. 10), S38–S63.

Sheridan, R. L., Stoddard, F. J., Kazis, L. E., et al. (2014). Long-term posttraumatic stress symptoms vary inversely with early opiate dosing in children recovering from serious burns. *The Journal of Trauma and Acute Care Surgery, 76*(3), 828–832.

Sieberg, C. B., Simons, L. E., Edelstein, M. R., et al. (2013). Pain prevalence and trajectories following pediatric spinal fusion surgery. *The Journal of Pain, 14*(12), 1694–1702.

Smith, B. H., & Torrance, N. (2012). Epidemiology of neuropathic pain and its impact on quality of life. *Current Pain and Headache Reports, 16*(3), 191–198.

Sneddon, P., Peacock, G. G., & Crowley, S. L. (2013). Assessment of sleep problems in preschool aged children: An adaptation of the children's sleep habits questionnaire. *Behavioral Sleep Medicine, 11*(4), 283–296.

Solodiuk, J. C., Brighton, H., McHale, J., et al. (2014). Documented electronic medical record-based pain intensity scores at a tertiary pediatric medical center: A cohort analysis. *Journal of Pain and Symptom Management, 48*(5), 924–933.

Stevens, B. J., Gibbins, S., Yamada, J., et al. (2014). The premature infant pain profile-revised (PIPP-R): Initial validation and feasibility. *The Clinical Journal of Pain, 30*, 238–243.

Stevens, K. E., & Marvicsin, D.J. (2016). Evidence-based recommendations for reducing pediatric distress during vaccination. *Pediatric Nursing, 42*(6), 267.

Stevens, B., Yamada, J., & Ohlsson, A. (2004). Sucrose for analgesia in newborn infants undergoing painful procedures. *The Cochrane Library*.

Stinson, J. N., Stevens, B. J., Feldman, B. M., et al. (2008). Construct validity of a multidimensional electronic pain diary for adolescents with arthritis. *Pain, 136*(3), 281–292.

Suresh, S., Birmingham, P. K., & Kozlowski, R. J. (2012). Pediatric pain management. *Anesthesiology Clinics, 30*(1), 101–117.

Taddio, A., Ipp, M., Thivakaran, S., et al. (2012). Survey of the prevalence of immunization non-compliance due to needle fears in children and adults. *Vaccine, 30*(32), 4807–4812.

Taddio, A., McMurtry, C. M., Shah, V., et al. (2015). Reducing pain during vaccine injections: Clinical practice guideline. *Canadian Medical Association Journal, 187*(13), 975–982.

Tesler, M. D., Savedra, M. C., Holzemer, W. L., et al. (1991). The word-graphic rating scale as a measure of children's and adolescents' pain intensity. *Research in Nursing and Health, 14*(5), 361–371.

Thrane, S. (2013). Effectiveness of integrative modalities for pain and anxiety in children and adolescents with cancer. *Journal of Pediatric Oncology Nursing, 30*(6), 320–332.

Trescot, A. M. (2014). Genetics and implications in perioperative analgesia. *Best Practice & Research Clinical Anaesthesiology, 28*(2), 153–166.

Twycross, A., Dowden, S., & Stinson, J. (2013). *Where to from here?* In Managing Pain in Children: A Clinical Guide for Nurses and Healthcare Professionals, 2013. http://www.eblib.com.

U.S. Department of Health and Human Services, Centers for Disease Control and Prevention. (2006). *National Health Statistics Reports. Ambulatory Surgery in the United States*. http://www.cdc.gov/nchs/data/nhsr/nhsr011.pdf.

U.S. Department of Health and Human Services, Centers for Disease Control and Prevention. (2015). *National Health Statistics Reports*. Health, United States, DHHS Publication No. 2016-1232. http://www.cdc.gov/nchs/hus.htm.

U.S. Food and Drug Administration. (2015 June). *FDA blueprint for prescriber education for extended-release and long-acting opioid analgesics*. Silver Spring, MD; http://www.fda.gov/downloads/Drugs/DrugSafety/InformationbyDrugClass/UCM277916.pdf.

Valrie, C. R., Bromberg, M. H., Palermo, T., et al. (2013). A systematic review of sleep in pediatric pain populations. *Journal of Developmental and Behavioral Pediatrics : JDBP, 34*(2), 120–128.

Van der Heijden, M. J. E., Oliai Araghi, S., van Dijk, M., et al. (2015). The effects of perioperative music interventions in pediatric surgery: A systematic review and meta-analysis of randomized controlled trials. *PLoS ONE, 10*(8).

van Dijk, M., de Boer, J., & Koot, H. (2000). The reliability and validity of the COMFORT scale as a postoperative pain instrument in 0 to 3-year-old infants. *Pain, 84*(2–3), 367–377.

van Dijk, A., McGrath, P. A., Pickett, W., et al. (2006). Pain prevalence in nine-to 13-year-old school children. *Pain Research and Management, 11*(4), 234–240.

van Dijk, M., Roofthooft, D. W. E., Anand, K. J. S., et al. (2009). Taking up the challenge of measuring prolonged pain in (premature) neonates: The COMFORTneo scale seems promising. *The Clinical Journal of Pain, 25*(7), 607–616.

Van Loey, N. E., Hofland, H. W., Hendrickx, H., et al. (2016). Validation of the burns itch questionnaire. *Burns: Journal of the International Society for Burn Injuries, 42*(3), 526–534.

Varni, J. W., Seid, M., & Rode, C. A. (1999). The PedsQL: Measurement model for the pediatric quality of life inventory. *Medical Care, 37*(2), 126–139.

Villarruel, A. M., & Denyes, M. J. (1991). Pain assessment in children: Theoretical and empirical validity. *Advances in Nursing Science, 14*(2), 32–41.

Voepel-Lewis, T., Zanotti, J., Dammeyer, J. A., et al. (2010). Reliability and validity of the face, legs, activity, cry, consolability behavioral tool in assessing acute pain in critically ill patients. *American Journal of Critical Care, 19*(1), 55–61.

von Baeyer, C. L. (2009). Children's self-report of pain intensity: What we know, where we are headed. *Pain Research & Management, 14*(1), 39–45.

von Baeyer, C. L., Lin, V., Seidman, L. C., et al. (2011). Pain charts (body maps or manikins) in assessment of the location of pediatric pain. *Pain Management, 1*(1), 61–68.

Walco, G. A., Dworkin, R. N., Krane, E. J., et al. (2010). Neuropathic pain in children: Special considerations. *Mayo Clinic Proceedings, 85*(3), S33–S41.

Walker, L. S., & Greene, J. W. (1991). The functional disability inventory: Measuring a neglected dimension of child health status. *Journal of Pediatric Psychology, 16*(1), 39–58.

Walker, S. M. (2014). Neonatal pain. *Pediatric Anesthesia, 24*(1), 39–48.

Walther-Larsen, S., Pedersen, M. T., Friis, S. M., et al. (2016). Pain prevalence in hospitalized children. *Acta Anaesthesiologica Scandinavica, 61*(3).

Watterberg, K. L., Cummings, J. J., Benitz, W. E., et al. (2016). Prevention and management of procedural pain in the neonate. *Pediatrics, 137*(2).

Williams, A. C. C., & Craig, K. D. (2016). Updating the definition of pain. *Pain, 157*(11), 2420–2423.

Williams, H., & Tanabe, P. (2016). Sickle cell disease: A review of nonpharmacological approaches for pain. *Journal of Pain and Symptom Management, 51*(2), 163–177.

Wong, D. L., & Baker, C. M. (1988). Pain in children: Comparison of assessment scales. *Pediatric Nursing, 14*(1), 9–17.

World Health Organization. (2012). *WHO guidelines on the pharmacological treatment of persisting pain in children with medical illnesses*. Geneva: World Health Organization.

World Health Organization. (2016, Sept). *Burns. Media center*. http://www.who.int/mediacentre/factsheets/fs365/en/.

Yilmaz, G., Cavlan, N., Oguz, M., et al. (2014). Oral sucrose administration to reduce pain response during immunization in 16-19-month infants: A randomized, placebo-controlled trial. *European Journal of Pediatrics, 173*(11), 1527–1532.

Zempsky, W. T. (2014). Topical anesthetics and analgesics. In P. C. McGrath, B. J. Stevens, S. M. Walker, et al. (Eds.), *Oxford textbook of paediatric pain*. Oxford: Oxford University Press.

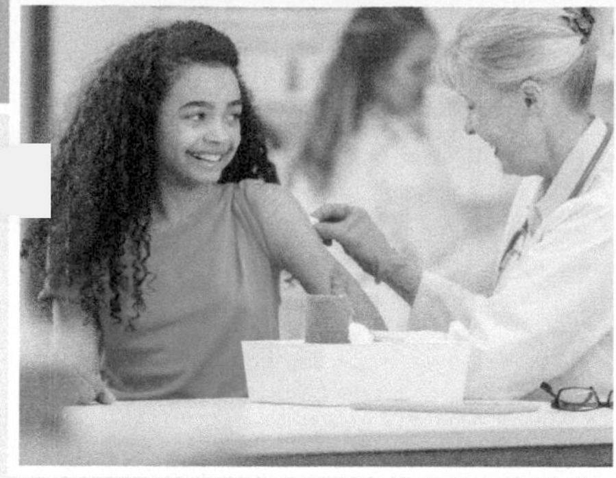

6

Childhood Communicable and Infectious Diseases

Cheryl C. Rodgers

http://evolve.elsevier.com/wong/ncic

CONCEPTS

- Immunity
- Infection
- Safety

INFECTION CONTROL

According to the Centers for Disease Control and Prevention (CDC), approximately 2 million patients each year develop hospital-acquired infections (HAIs). The overall cost of HAIs to US hospitals is $96 billion to $147 billion annually (Marchetti & Rossiter, 2013). These infections occur when there is interaction among patients, health care personnel, equipment, and bacteria. HAIs are preventable if caregivers practice meticulous hand washing, cleaning, and disposal techniques.

Standard Precautions synthesize the major features of universal (i.e., blood and body fluid) precautions (designed to reduce the risk of transmission of blood-borne pathogens) and body substance isolation (designed to reduce the risk of transmission of pathogens from moist body substances). Standard Precautions involve the use of barrier protection (personal protective equipment [PPE]), such as gloves, goggles, gowns, and masks, to prevent contamination from blood; all body fluids, secretions, and excretions, except sweat, regardless of whether they contain visible blood; nonintact skin; and mucous membranes. Standard Precautions are designed for the care of all patients to reduce the risk of transmission of microorganisms from both recognized and unrecognized sources of infection.

In 2007 the Centers for Disease Control and Prevention recommended adding Respiratory Hygiene/Cough Etiquette and safe injection practices to Standard Precautions. Respiratory Hygiene/Cough Etiquette stresses the importance of source control measures to contain respiratory secretions to prevent droplet and fomite transmission of viral respiratory tract infections such as respiratory syncytial virus, influenza, and adenovirus. Safe injection practices involve the use of safety-engineered sharp devices to prevent sharps injury as a component of Standard Precautions.

Hand hygiene continues to be the single most important practice to reduce the transmission of infectious diseases in health care settings (Bolon, 2016). Hand hygiene includes hand washing with soap and water, as well as the use of alcohol-based products for hand disinfection.

Transmission-Based Precautions are designed for patients with documented or suspected infection or colonization (i.e., presence of microorganisms in or on patient but without clinical signs and symptoms of infection) with highly transmissible or epidemiologically important pathogens for which additional precautions beyond Standard Precautions are needed to interrupt transmission in hospitals. The three types of Transmission-Based Precautions are (1) Airborne Precautions, (2) Droplet Precautions, and (3) Contact Precautions. They may be combined for diseases that have multiple routes of transmission (Box 6.1). They are to be used in addition to Standard Precautions.

Airborne Precautions reduce the risk of airborne transmission of infectious agents. Airborne transmission occurs by dissemination of either airborne droplet nuclei (i.e., small-particle residue [≤5 mm] of evaporated droplets that may remain suspended in the air for long periods) or dust particles containing the infectious agent. Microorganisms carried in this manner can be dispersed widely by air currents and may become inhaled by or deposited on a susceptible host within the same room or over a longer distance from the source patient, depending on environmental factors. Special air handling and ventilation are required to prevent airborne transmission. The term *airborne infection isolation room* (AIIR) has replaced *negative pressure isolation room;* this room is used to isolate persons with a suspected or confirmed airborne infectious disease transmitted by the airborne route such as measles, varicella, and tuberculosis.

Droplet Precautions reduce the risk of droplet transmission of infectious agents. Droplet transmission involves contact of the conjunctivae or the mucous membranes of the nose or mouth of a susceptible person with large-particle droplets (>5 mm) containing microorganisms generated from a person who has a clinical disease or who is a carrier of the microorganism. Droplets are generated from the source person primarily during coughing, sneezing, or talking and during procedures such as suctioning and bronchoscopy. Transmission requires close contact between source and recipient persons because droplets do not remain suspended in the air and generally travel only short distances, usually 3 feet or less, through the air. Because droplets do not remain suspended in the air, special air handling and ventilation are not required to prevent droplet transmission. Droplet Precautions apply to any patient with known or suspected infection with pathogens that can be transmitted by infectious droplets (see Box 6.1).

Contact Precautions reduce the risk of transmission of microorganisms by direct or indirect contact. Direct-contact transmission involves skin-to-skin contact and physical transfer of microorganisms to a susceptible host from an infected or colonized person, such as occurs when turning or bathing patients. Direct-contact transmission also can occur between two patients (e.g., by hand contact). Indirect contact

BOX 6.1 Types of Precautions and Patients Requiring Them

Standard Precautions for Prevention of Transmission of Pathogens

Use Standard Precautions for the care of all patients. Hand hygiene should be emphasized as part of Standard Precautions.

Respiratory Hygiene/Cough Etiquette

In addition to Standard Precautions, the CDC suggests a combination of measures designed to minimize the transmission of respiratory pathogens via droplet or airborne routes in the health care environment. Measures include covering the mouth and nose during coughing and sneezing; offering a surgical mask to persons who are coughing; using tissues to contain respiratory secretions; turning the head away from others and keeping a space of 3 feet or more when coughing. These measures should be used on entry to the health care institution for patients and visitors or family members who have symptoms of respiratory infection.

Airborne Precautions

In addition to Standard Precautions, use Airborne Precautions and an airborne infection isolation room (AIIR) for patients known or suspected to have serious illnesses transmitted by airborne droplet nuclei. Examples of such illnesses include measles, varicella (including disseminated zoster), and tuberculosis.

Droplet Precautions

In addition to Standard Precautions, use Droplet Precautions for patients known or suspected to have serious illnesses transmitted by large particle droplets. Examples of such illnesses include the following:

- Invasive *Haemophilus influenzae* type b disease, including meningitis, pneumonia, epiglottitis, and sepsis
- Invasive *Neisseria meningitidis* disease, including meningitis, pneumonia, and sepsis
- Other serious bacterial respiratory tract infections spread by droplet transmission, including diphtheria (pharyngeal), mycoplasmal pneumonia, pertussis, pneumonic plague, streptococcal pharyngitis, pneumonia, or scarlet fever in infants and young children
- Serious viral infections spread by droplet transmission, including adenovirus, influenza, mumps, human parvovirus B19, and rubella

Contact Precautions

In addition to Standard Precautions, use Contact Precautions for patients known or suspected to have serious illnesses easily transmitted by direct patient contact or by contact with items in the patient's environment. Examples of such illnesses include the following:

- Gastrointestinal, respiratory, skin, or wound infections or colonization with multidrug-resistant bacteria judged by the infection control program, based on current state, regional, or national recommendations, to be of special clinical and epidemiologic significance
- Enteric infections with a low infectious dose or prolonged environmental survival, including *Clostridium difficile;* for diapered or incontinent patients: enterohemorrhagic *Escherichia coli* 0157:H7, *Shigella* organisms, hepatitis A, or rotavirus
- Respiratory syncytial virus, parainfluenza virus, or enteroviral infections in infants and young children
- Skin infections that are highly contagious or that may occur on dry skin, including diphtheria (cutaneous), herpes simplex virus (neonatal or mucocutaneous), impetigo, major (noncontained) abscesses, cellulitis or decubitus, pediculosis, scabies, staphylococcal furunculosis in infants and young children, zoster (disseminated or in the immunocompromised host)
- Viral or hemorrhagic conjunctivitis
- Viral hemorrhagic infections (Ebola, Lassa, or Marburg)

Modified from Siegel, J. D., Rhinehart, E., Jackson, M., et al. (2007). *2007 Guideline for isolation precautions: Preventing transmission of infectious agents in healthcare settings.* Retrieved from https://www.cdc.gov/hicpac/pdf/isolation/Isolation2007.pdf.

transmission involves contact of a susceptible host with a contaminated intermediate object, usually inanimate, in the patient's environment. Contact Precautions apply to specified patients known or suspected to be infected or colonized with microorganisms that can be transmitted by direct or indirect contact.

! NURSING ALERT

The most common piece of medical equipment, the stethoscope, can be a potent source of harmful microorganisms and nosocomial infections. Consider also the keyboard and desktop as potential sources.

Nurses caring for young children are frequently in contact with body substances, especially urine, feces, and vomitus. Nurses need to exercise judgment concerning those situations when gloves, gowns, or masks are necessary. For example, wear gloves and possibly gowns for changing diapers when there are loose or explosive stools. Otherwise, the plastic lining of disposable diapers provides a sufficient barrier between the hands and body substances and gloves are adequate.

Antimicrobial-resistant organisms are causing increasing numbers of HAIs. In hospitals, patients are the most significant sources of methicillin-resistant *Staphylococcus aureus* (MRSA), and the main mode of transmission is patient-to-patient transmission via the hands of a health care provider. Hand washing is the most critical infection control practice.

During feedings, wear gowns if the child is likely to vomit or spit up, which often occurs during burping. When wearing gloves, wash the hands thoroughly after removing the gloves because gloves fail to provide complete protection. The absence of visible leaks does not indicate that gloves are intact.

Another essential practice of infection control is that all needles (uncapped and unbroken) are disposed of in a rigid, puncture-resistant container located near the site of use. Consequently, these containers are installed in each patient's room. Because children are naturally curious, extra attention is needed in selecting a suitable type of container and a location that prevents access to the discarded needles (Fig. 6.1). The use of needleless systems allows secure syringe or intravenous (IV) tubing attachment to vascular access devices without the risk of needle stick injury to the child or nurse.

IMMUNIZATIONS*

One of the most dramatic advances in pediatrics has been the decline of infectious diseases during the twentieth century because of the widespread use of immunization for preventable diseases. This trend has continued

*Additional information on immunizations and recommendations for specific conditions can be found in the *2015 Red Book: Report of the Committee on Infectious Diseases* (American Academy of Pediatrics, 2015), and from the Centers for Disease Control and Prevention website: https://www.cdc.gov/vaccines/.

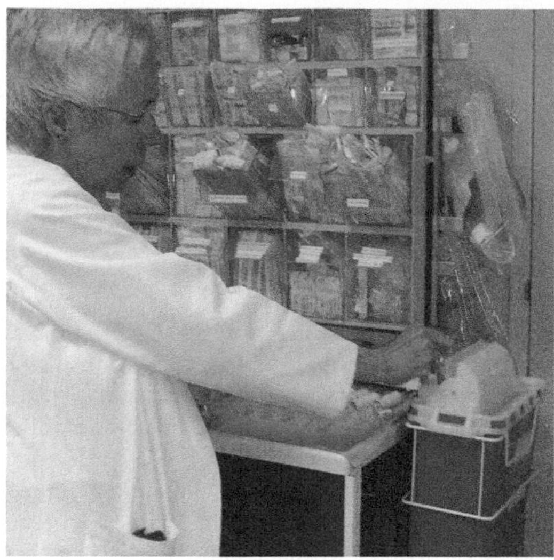

FIG. 6.1 To prevent needlestick injuries, used needles (and other sharp instruments) are not capped or broken and are disposed of in a rigid, puncture-resistant container located near site of use. Note placement of container to prevent children's access to contents.

into the twenty-first century with the development of newer vaccines. Although many of the immunizations can be given to individuals of any age, the recommended primary schedule begins during infancy and, with the exception of boosters, is completed during early childhood. This section includes a discussion of childhood immunizations for diphtheria, tetanus, and acellular pertussis (DTaP); poliovirus; measles, mumps, and rubella (MMR); *Haemophilus influenzae* type b (Hib); hepatitis B virus (HBV); hepatitis A virus (HAV); meningococcal; pneumococcal conjugate vaccine (PCV); influenza (and H1N1); varicella-zoster virus (VZV; chickenpox); rotavirus; and human papillomaviruses. Selected vaccines generally reserved for children considered at high risk for the disease are discussed here and as appropriate throughout the text.

To facilitate an understanding of immunizations, key terms are listed in Box 6.2. Although in this discussion the terms *vaccination* and *immunization* are used interchangeably in reference to active immunization, they are not synonymous because the administration of an immunobiologic such as a vaccine cannot automatically be equated with the development of adequate immunity.

Schedule for Immunizations

In the United States, two organizations, the Advisory Committee on Immunization Practices (ACIP) of the Centers for Disease Control and

BOX 6.2 Key Immunization Terms

Immunization—Inclusive term denoting the process of inducing or providing active or passive immunity artificially by administering an immunobiologic

Immunity—An inherited or acquired state in which an individual is resistant to the occurrence or the effects of a specific disease, particularly an infectious agent

Natural immunity—Innate immunity or resistance to infection or toxicity

Acquired immunity—Immunity from exposure to the invading agent, either bacteria, virus, or toxin

Active immunity—A state where immune bodies are actively formed against specific antigens, either naturally by having had the disease clinically or subclinically or artificially by introducing the antigen into the individual

Passive immunity—Temporary immunity obtained by transfusing immunoglobulins or antitoxins either artificially from another human or an animal that has been actively immunized against an antigen or naturally from the mother to the fetus via the placenta

Antibody—A protein, found mostly in serum, that is formed in response to exposure to a specific antigen

Antigen—A variety of foreign substances, including bacteria, viruses, toxins, and foreign proteins, that stimulate the formation of antibodies

Attenuate—Reduce the virulence (infectiousness) of a pathogenic microorganism by such measures as treating it with heat or chemicals or cultivating it on a certain medium

Immunobiologic—Antigenic substances (e.g., vaccines and toxoids) or antibody-containing preparations (e.g., globulins and antitoxins) from human or animal donors, used for active or passive immunization or therapy

Vaccine—A suspension of live (usually attenuated) or inactivated microorganisms (e.g., bacteria, viruses, or rickettsiae) or fractions of the microorganism administered to induce immunity and prevent infectious disease or its sequelae

Toxoid—A modified bacterial toxin that has been made nontoxic but retains the ability to stimulate the formation of antitoxin

Antitoxin—A solution of antibodies (e.g., diphtheria antitoxin, botulinum antitoxin) derived from the serum of animals immunized with specific antigens and used to confer passive immunity and for treatment

Immunoglobulin (Ig) or intravenous immunoglobulin (IVIG)—A sterile solution containing antibodies from large pools of human blood plasma; primarily indicated for routine maintenance of immunity of certain immunodeficient persons and for passive immunization against measles and hepatitis A

Specific immunoglobulins—Special preparations obtained from blood plasma from donor pools preselected for a high antibody content against a specific antigen (e.g., hepatitis B immunoglobulin, varicella zoster immunoglobulin, rabies immunoglobulin, tetanus immunoglobulin, and cytomegalovirus immunoglobulin); as with Ig and IVIG, do not transmit hepatitis B virus, human immunodeficiency virus, or other infectious diseases

Vaccination—Originally referred to inoculation with vaccinia smallpox virus to make a person immune to smallpox; currently denotes physical act of administering any vaccine or toxoid

Herd immunity—A condition in which the majority of the population community is vaccinated and the spread of certain diseases is stopped because the population that has been vaccinated protects those in the same population who are unvaccinated

Monovalent vaccine—Vaccine designed to vaccinate against a single antigen or organism

Conjugate vaccine—A carrier protein with proven immunologic potential combined with a less antigenic polysaccharide antigen to enhance the type and magnitude of the immune response (e.g., *Haemophilus influenzae* type b [Hib])

Combination vaccine—Combination of multiple vaccines into one parenteral form

Polyvalent vaccine—Vaccine designed to vaccinate against two or more antigens or organisms (e.g., inactivated poliovirus vaccine [IPV])

Cocooning—strategy of protecting infants from pertussis by vaccinating all persons who come in close contact with the infant, including the mother, grandparents, and health care workers.

Prevention and the Committee on Infectious Diseases of the American Academy of Pediatrics, govern the recommendations for immunization policies and procedures. In Canada, recommendations are from the National Advisory Committee on Immunization under the authority of the Minister of Health and Public Health Agency of Canada. The policies of each committee are recommendations, not rules, and they change as a result of advances in the field of immunology. Nurses need to be knowledgeable about the purpose of each organization, view immunization practices in light of the needs of each individual child and the community, and keep informed of the latest advances and changes in policy.

The recommended age for beginning primary immunizations of infants is at birth or within 2 weeks of birth. Children born preterm should receive the full dose of each vaccine at the appropriate chronologic age. A recommended catch-up schedule for children not immunized during infancy is available at the Centers for Disease Control and Prevention website (http://www.cdc.gov/vaccines/schedules/downloads/child/catchup-schedule-pr.pdf). Immunization recommendation schedules for Canadian children are available at http://www.phac-aspc.gc.ca/im/is-cv/index-eng.php.

Children who began primary immunization at the recommended age but fail to receive all the doses do not need to begin the series again but instead receive only the missed doses. For situations in which there is doubt that the child will return for immunization according to the optimum schedule, HBV vaccine (HepB), DTaP, IPV (poliovirus vaccine), MMR, varicella, and Hib vaccines can be administered simultaneously at separate injection sites. Parenteral vaccines are given in separate syringes in different injection sites (American Academy of Pediatrics, 2015).

Recommendations for Routine Immunizations*

Hepatitis B Virus

HBV is a significant pediatric disease because HBV infections that occur during childhood and adolescence can lead to fatal consequences from cirrhosis or liver cancer during adulthood. Up to 90% of infants infected perinatally and 25% to 50% of children infected before age 5 years become chronically infected (American Academy of Pediatrics, 2015). It is recommended that newborns receive HepB before hospital discharge if the mother is hepatitis B surface antigen (HBsAg) negative. Monovalent HepB should be given as the birth dose, whereas combination vaccine containing HepB may be given for subsequent doses in the series. Both full-term and preterm infants born to mothers whose HBsAg status is positive or unknown should receive HepB and hepatitis B immune globulin (HBIG), 0.5 ml, within 12 hours of birth at two different injection sites. Because the immune response to HepB is not optimum in newborns weighing less than 2000 grams (4.4 pounds), the first HepB dose should be given to such infants at a chronologic age of 1 month, as long as the mother's HBsAg status is negative (American Academy of Pediatrics, 2015). In the event that the preterm infant is given a dose at birth, the current recommendation is that the infant be given the full series (three additional doses) at 1, 2, and 6 months of age. The American Academy of Pediatrics (2015) also encourages immunization of all children by age 11 years.

*Because of constant changes in the pharmaceutical industry, trade names of single and combination vaccines in this section may differ from those currently available. The reader is encouraged to access the vaccine page of the Center for Biologics Evaluation and Research (CBER) of the Food and Drug Administration (FDA) for the latest licensed vaccine trade names: http://www.fda.gov/BiologicsBloodVaccines/Vaccines/ApprovedProducts/ucm093833.htm.

The vaccine is given intramuscularly in the vastus lateralis in newborns or in the deltoid for older infants and children. Regardless of age, avoid the dorsogluteal site because it has been associated with low antibody seroconversion rates, indicating a reduced immune response. No data exist regarding the seroconversion when the ventrogluteal site is used. The vaccine can be safely administered simultaneously at a separate site with DTaP, MMR, and Hib vaccines.

Hepatitis A Virus

Hepatitis A has been recognized as a significant child health problem, particularly in communities with unusually high infection rates. HAV is spread by the fecal-oral route and from person-to-person contact, by ingestion of contaminated food or water, and, rarely, by blood transfusion. The illness has an abrupt onset, with fever, malaise, anorexia, nausea, abdominal discomfort, dark urine, and jaundice being the most common clinical signs of infection. In children under 6 years of age, who represent approximately one-third of all cases of hepatitis A, the disease may be asymptomatic, and jaundice is rarely evident.

HepA vaccine is now recommended for all children beginning at age 1 year (i.e., 12 months to 23 months). The second dose in the two-dose series may be administered no sooner than 6 months after the first dose. Since the implementation of widespread childhood HepA vaccination, infection rates among children ages 5 to 14 years have declined significantly.

Diphtheria

Although cases of diphtheria are rare in the United States, the disease can result in significant morbidity. Respiratory manifestations include respiratory nasopharyngitis or obstructive laryngotracheitis with upper airway obstruction. The cutaneous manifestations of the disease include vaginal, otic, conjunctival, or cutaneous lesions, which are primarily seen in urban homeless persons and in the tropics (American Academy of Pediatrics, 2015). Administer a single dose of equine antitoxin intravenously to the child with clinical symptoms because of the often fulminant progression of the disease (American Academy of Pediatrics, 2015). Diphtheria vaccine is commonly administered (1) in combination with tetanus and pertussis vaccines (DTaP) or DTaP and Hib vaccines for children younger than 7 years of age, (2) in combination with a conjugate *H. influenzae* type B vaccine, (3) in a combined vaccine with tetanus (DT) for children younger than 7 years of age who have some contraindication to receiving pertussis vaccine, (4) in combination with tetanus and acellular pertussis (Tdap) for children 11 years and older, or (5) as a single antigen when combined antigen preparations are not indicated. Although the diphtheria vaccine does not produce absolute immunity, protective antitoxin persists for 10 years or more when given according to the recommended schedule, and boosters are given every 10 years for life (see following discussion for adolescent diphtheria and acellular pertussis and tetanus toxoid recommendation). Several vaccines contain diphtheria toxoid (e.g., Hib, meningococcal, pneumococcal), but this does not confer immunity to the disease.

Tetanus

Three forms of tetanus vaccine—tetanus toxoid, tetanus immunoglobulin (TIG) (human), and tetanus antitoxin (equine antitoxin)—are available; however, tetanus antitoxin is no longer available in the United States. Tetanus toxoid is used for routine primary immunization, usually in one of the combinations listed for diphtheria, and provides protective antitoxin levels for approximately 10 years.

Tetanus and diphtheria toxoids along with acellular pertussis vaccine (Tdap) are now recommended for persons ages 11 to 12 years who have completed the recommended DTaP/DTP vaccine series but have not received the tetanus (Td) booster dose. Adolescents 13 to 18 years of age who have not received the Td/Tdap booster should receive a single Tdap booster, provided the routine DTaP/DTP childhood immunization series has been previously received. In addition, children ages 7 to 10 years who are not fully vaccinated for pertussis (i.e., did not receive 5 doses of DTaP or 4 doses of DTaP with the fourth dose being administered on or after the fourth birthday) should receive a dose of Tdap (American Academy of Pediatrics, 2015). It is recommended that children receive subsequent Td boosters every 10 years (American Academy of Pediatrics, 2015). Boostrix (Tdap) is currently licensed for persons 10 years of age (including those ≥65 years of age) and older, whereas Adacel (Tdap) is licensed for individuals 10 to 64 years of age.

For wound management, passive immunity is available with TIG. Persons with a history of two previous doses of tetanus toxoid can receive a booster dose of the toxoid. Separate syringes and different sites are used when tetanus toxoid and TIG are given concurrently.

For children over 7 years who require wound prophylaxis, tetanus immunization may be accomplished by administering Td (adult-type diphtheria and tetanus toxoids). If TIG is not available, the equine antitoxin (not available in the United States) may be administered after appropriate testing for sensitivity. The antitoxin is administered in a separate syringe and at a separate intramuscular site if given concurrently with tetanus toxoid.

Pertussis

Pertussis vaccine is recommended for all children 6 weeks through 6 years of age (up to the seventh birthday) who have no neurologic contraindications to its use. Concerns over outbreaks of the disease in the past decade have prompted discussion about vaccinating infants and adults. Many cases of pertussis have occurred in children less than 6 months or persons over 7 years, both groups falling in the category for which pertussis immunization previously was not recommended. The tetanus and diphtheria toxoids and acellular pertussis vaccine (Tdap) is now recommended at ages 11 to 12 years for persons who have completed the DTaP/DTP childhood series. The Tdap is also recommended for adolescents 13 to 18 years old who have not received a tetanus booster (Td) or Tdap dose and have completed the childhood DTaP/DTP series. When the Tdap is used as a booster dose, it may be administered regardless of the interval from the previous tetanus, diphtheria, and pertussis-containing vaccine. Children ages 7 through 10 years who are not fully vaccinated for pertussis (i.e., did not receive 5 doses of DTaP or 4 doses of DTaP with the fourth dose being administered on or after the fourth birthday) should receive a dose of Tdap (American Academy of Pediatrics, 2015) (see discussion in Tetanus).

The Advisory Committee on Immunization Practices and the American College of Obstetricians and Gynecologists have recommended that pregnant adolescents and women who are not protected against pertussis receive the Tdap vaccine optimally between 27 and 36 weeks of gestation or postpartum before discharge from the hospital; breastfeeding is not a contraindication to Tdap vaccination (Centers for Disease Control and Prevention, 2013a). The concept of cocooning has been promoted since 2006 to reduce the spread of pertussis to vulnerable infants. Cocooning involves the strategy of vaccinating pregnant women during or after pregnancy, as well as all persons who will have close contact with the infants (including health care workers, fathers, and adults [especially those ages 65 years and older]) (Blain, Lewis, Banerjee, et al., 2016). Cocooning can prevent pertussis in vulnerable infants; however, actual implantation of the cocooning strategy among all family members is difficult (Blain, Lewis, Banerjee, et al., 2016).

Currently, two forms of pertussis vaccine are available in the United States. The whole-cell pertussis vaccine is prepared from inactivated cells of *Bordetella pertussis* and contains multiple antigens. In contrast, the acellular pertussis vaccine contains one or more immunogens derived from the *B. pertussis* organism. The highly purified acellular vaccine is associated with fewer local and systemic reactions than those occurring with the whole-cell vaccine in children of similar age. The acellular pertussis vaccine is recommended by the American Academy of Pediatrics (2015) for the first three immunizations and is usually given at 2, 4, and 6 months of age with diphtheria and tetanus (DTaP). Several forms of acellular pertussis vaccine are currently licensed for use in infants: Daptacel, Pediatrix, Kinrix (DTaP and IPV), and Infanrix (diphtheria, tetanus toxoid, and acellular pertussis conjugate). Pentacel is licensed for use in infants 4 weeks old and older; in addition to acellular pertussis, diphtheria, and tetanus, this vaccine also contains inactivated poliovirus (IPV) and Hib conjugate. Either the acellular or whole-cell vaccine may be given for the fourth and fifth doses, but the acellular is preferred. It is also recommended that the first three DTaP vaccinations be from the same manufacturer. The fourth dose may be from a different manufacturer. The child who has received one or more whole-cell vaccines may complete the series of five with the acellular vaccine.

Health care workers who may be susceptible to pertussis as a result of waning immunity and who have potential exposure to children or adults with pertussis should receive a single dose of Tdap (if not previously vaccinated with same) and take the necessary protective precautions against droplet contamination (i.e., wear procedural or surgical masks and practice hand washing). The diagnosis of pertussis may be missed or delayed in unvaccinated infants, who often are seen with respiratory distress and apnea without the typical cough.

Additional guidelines for prevention and treatment of pertussis among health care workers and close contacts can be found on the Centers for Disease Control and Prevention website: http://www.cdc.gov/vaccines/.

Polio

An all-IPV (inactivated poliovirus vaccine) schedule for routine childhood polio vaccination is now recommended for children in the United States. All children should receive four doses of IPV at 2 months, 4 months, 6 to 18 months, and 4 to 6 years of age (American Academy of Pediatrics, 2015).

The change from the exclusive use of oral polio vaccine (OPV) to the exclusive use of IPV is related to the rare risk of vaccine-associated polio paralysis (VAPP) from OPV. The exclusive use of IPV eliminates the risk of VAPP but is associated with an increased number of injections and increased cost. Since IPV usage was instituted in the United States in 2000, no new indigenously acquired cases of VAPP have occurred. Pediarix is a **combination vaccine** containing DTaP, hepatitis B, and IPV; this may be used as the primary immunization beginning at 2 months of age (American Academy of Pediatrics, 2015). Kinrix contains DTaP and IPV, and it may be used as the fifth dose in the DTaP series and the fourth dose in the IPV series in children ages 4 to 6 years whose previous vaccine doses have been with Infanrix and/or Pediarix for the first three doses and Infanrix for the fourth dose. As noted earlier, Pentacel is also licensed for use in infants 4 weeks old and older and contains DTaP, Hib, and inactivated poliovirus. Pediarix has been licensed for use in children as young as 6 weeks and contains DTaP, Hep B, and inactivated poliovirus.

Measles

The measles (rubeola) vaccine is given at 12 to 15 months of age. During the course of measles outbreaks, the vaccine can be given at 6 to 11 months of age, followed by a second inoculation after age 12 months. The second measles immunization is recommended at 4 to 6 years of age (at school entry) but may be given earlier provided that 4 weeks have elapsed since the administration of the previous dose. Revaccination should occur by 11 to 12 years of age if the measles vaccine was not administered at school entry (4 to 6 years). Any child who is vaccinated before 12 months of age should receive two additional doses beginning at 12 to 15 months and separated by at least 4 weeks (American Academy of Pediatrics, 2015). Revaccination should include all individuals born after 1956 who have not received two doses of measles vaccine after 12 months of age. Individuals born before this date are thought to be immune from exposure to natural measles virus. Because of the continuing occurrence of measles in older children and young adults, identify potentially susceptible adolescents and young adults and immunize them if two doses of measles vaccine have not been administered previously or the person had a confirmed case of the illness. For postexposure prophylaxis, one dose of MMR may be administered within 72 hours of exposure in vaccine-eligible individuals ≥12 months of age and is preferable to immunoglobulin (Centers for Disease Control and Prevention, 2013b).

The measles, mumps, rubella, and varicella (MMRV) vaccine is an attenuated live virus vaccine and may be given to children 12 months to 15 months of age or at 4 through 6 years of age concurrent with other vaccines. Children with HIV should not receive the MMRV vaccine because of a lack of evidence of its safety in this population. The risks and benefits of administering the MMRV vaccine should be fully explained to the parent or caregiver; the risk for a febrile seizure at 5 to 12 days in children 12 to 23 months old remains relatively low and should be weighed with the benefit of one fewer intramuscular injection (American Academy of Pediatrics, 2015). The American Academy of Pediatrics (2015) recommends that either the MMR or MMRV vaccine be given as the first dose of measles, mumps, rubella, and varicella vaccine at ages 12 through 47 months; for children 48 months and older, the first dose with MMRV is recommended to decrease the number of injections; for the second dose at any age (15 months through 12 years), MMRV is also recommended for the same reason.

Vitamin A supplementation has been effective in decreasing the morbidity and mortality risks associated with measles in developing countries.

Mumps

Mumps virus vaccine is recommended for children at 12 to 15 months of age and is typically given in combination with measles and rubella. It should not be administered to infants younger than 12 months because persisting maternal antibodies can interfere with the immune response. Because of continued occurrence of the disease, especially in children 10 to 19 years of age, mumps immunization is recommended for all individuals born after 1957 who may be susceptible to mumps (i.e., those who have no history of having had the disease or vaccine and who have no laboratory evidence of immunity).

Rubella

Rubella is a relatively mild infection in children, but in a pregnant woman the actual infection presents serious risks to the developing fetus. Therefore the aim of rubella immunization is actually protection of the unborn child rather than the recipient of the immunization.

Rubella immunization is recommended for all children at 12 to 15 months of age and at age of school entry or 4 to 6 years of age or sooner, according to the routine recommendations for the MMRV vaccine (American Academy of Pediatrics, 2015). Increased emphasis should also be placed on vaccinating all unimmunized prepubertal children and susceptible adolescents and adult women in the childbearing age-group. Postpubertal females without evidence of rubella immunity should be immunized unless they are pregnant; they should be counseled not to become pregnant for 28 days after receiving the rubella-containing vaccine (American Academy of Pediatrics, 2015). Because the live attenuated virus may cross the placenta and theoretically present a risk to the developing fetus, rubella vaccine is currently not given to any pregnant woman. Although this is standard practice, current evidence from women who received the vaccine while pregnant and delivered unaffected offspring indicates that the risk to the fetus is negligible (de Martino, 2016). In addition, there is no reported danger of administering rubella vaccine to a child if the mother is pregnant.

Haemophilus influenzae Type b

Hib conjugate vaccines protect against a number of serious infections caused by *H. influenzae* type b, especially bacterial meningitis, epiglottitis, bacterial pneumonia, septic arthritis, and sepsis (Hib is not associated with the viruses that cause influenza, or "flu"). Hib vaccines that are currently available include PedvaxHIB, Pentacel, and Comvax, which are combination vaccines, and Hiberix and ActHib. Pentacel is described in the previous section on Pertussis. MenHibrix has been licensed for administration to children ages 6 weeks to 18 months and provides protection against meningococcal (groups A, C, Y, and W-135), as well as Hib. MenHibrix is administered in a four-dose series at 2, 4, 6, and 12 to 15 months of age. These conjugate vaccines connect Hib to a nontoxic form of another organism, such as meningococcal protein, tetanus toxoid, or diphtheria protein. There is no antibody response to these nontoxic proteins, but they significantly improve the antibody response to Hib, especially in infants. The use of combination vaccines provides equivalent immunogenicity and decreases the number of injections an infant receives. However, it is important that they be given to the appropriate-age child. Hiberix is a conjugate vaccine licensed for use as the booster (final) dose of the Hib vaccine series for children ages 15 months to 4 years (American Academy of Pediatrics, 2013). In 2013 the American Academy of Pediatrics clarified that only one dose of Hib should be given to children 15 months old or older who have not been previously vaccinated (American Academy of Pediatrics, 2013).

When possible, the Hib conjugate vaccine used at the first vaccination should be used for all subsequent vaccinations in the primary series. All Hib vaccines are administered by intramuscular injection using a separate syringe and at a site separate from any concurrent vaccinations.

! NURSING ALERT

The use of meningococcal and diphtheria proteins in combination vaccines does not mean the child has received adequate immunization for meningococcal or diphtheria illnesses; the child must be given the appropriate vaccine for that specific disease.

Varicella

Administration of the cell-free live-attenuated varicella vaccine is recommended for any susceptible child (i.e., one who lacks proof of varicella vaccination or has a reliable history of varicella infection). A single dose of 0.5 ml should be given by subcutaneous injection. The first dose of varicella vaccine is recommended for children ages 12 to 15 months, and to ensure adequate protection, a second varicella vaccine is recommended for children at 4 to 6 years of age. The second varicella vaccine may be administered before 4 years of age as long as a period of 3 months occurs between the first and second doses. Children 13 years of age or older who are susceptible should receive two doses administered at least 4 weeks apart. Children in the same age-group (13 to 18 years) who have received only one previous varicella vaccine should receive a second varicella vaccine. The two-dose regimen was adopted to protect children who did not have adequate protection with one dose, not because of waning immunity to the vaccine (American Academy of Pediatrics, 2015). The combination vaccine MMRV (ProQuad) is licensed for use in children ages 12 months to 12 years (see discussion under Measles.)

According to the American Academy of Pediatrics (2015), children who have received two doses of the varicella vaccine are one-third less likely to have breakthrough illness in the first 10 years of immunization in comparison with those who have received one dose. Children who do contract varicella after immunization reportedly have milder cases with fewer vesicles, lower degree of fever, and faster recovery. Antibodies persist for at least 8 years.

Keep the vaccine frozen in the lyophilic form (i.e., stable particles that readily go into solution), and use it within 30 minutes of being reconstituted to ensure viral potency.

Varicella vaccine may be administered simultaneously with MMR. However, separate syringes and injection sites should be used. If they are not administered simultaneously, the interval between administration of varicella vaccine and MMR should be at least 1 month. Varicella vaccine may also be given simultaneously with DTaP, IPV, HepB, or Hib (American Academy of Pediatrics, 2015). The vaccine is administered subcutaneously.

Pneumococcal Disease

Streptococcal pneumococci are responsible for a number of bacterial infections in children under 2 years, which may cause serious morbidity and mortality. Among these are generalized infections, such as septicemia and meningitis, or localized infections, such as otitis media, sinusitis, and pneumonia. These illnesses are particularly problematic in children who attend day care facilities (the incidence in day care children is two or three times higher than in children not attending out-of-home day care) and in those who are immunocompromised. A 13-valent pneumococcal vaccine (PCV13 [Prevnar13]) has been licensed for use and is currently recommended as the standard pneumococcal vaccine for children ages 6 weeks to 24 months old. Children who have started the PCV series with PCV7 may complete the vaccine series with PCV13 (American Academy of Pediatrics, 2015).

The PCV13 vaccine is administered at 2, 4, and 6 months of age, with a fourth dose at 12 to 15 months of age. A single supplemental dose of PCV13 is recommended for children ages 14 through 59 months who have received an age-appropriate series of PCV7. PCV13 is also recommended for all children younger than 24 months old and for children 24 to 71 months of age with sickle cell disease; functional or anatomic asplenia; nephrotic syndrome or chronic renal failure; conditions associated with immunosuppression, such as solid organ transplantation, drug therapy, or cytoreduction therapy (including long-term systemic corticosteroid therapy); diabetes mellitus; cochlear implants; congenital immunodeficiency; human immunodeficiency virus (HIV) infection; cerebrospinal fluid leaks; chronic cardiovascular disease (e.g., congestive heart failure or cardiomyopathy); chronic pulmonary disease (e.g., emphysema or cystic fibrosis, but not asthma); chronic liver disease (e.g., cirrhosis); or exposure to living environments or social settings in which the risk of invasive pneumococcal disease or its complications is very high (e.g., Alaskan Native, African American, and certain Native American populations). The PCV13 vaccine may be administered in conjunction with all other immunizations in a separate syringe and at a separate intramuscular site.

The PPSV23 (pneumococcal polysaccharide [23-valent] vaccine) is not recommended for children younger than 24 months who do not have one of the high-risk conditions described previously. One dose of PPSV23 is recommended in children older than 23 months who have one of the high-risk conditions after primary immunization with PCV13.

Influenza

The influenza vaccine is recommended annually for children ages 6 months to 18 years. Influenza vaccine (inactivated influenza vaccine [IIV]) may be given to any healthy children 6 months old and older. The trivalent inactivated influenza vaccine (TAIV) was changed to inactivated influenza vaccine (IIV) (American Academy of Pediatrics, 2013). The vaccine is administered in early fall before the flu season begins and is repeated yearly for ongoing protection. The intramuscular vaccine is administered as two separate doses 4 weeks apart in first-time recipients younger than 9 years old. The dose is 0.25 ml for children 6 to 35 months old and 0.5 ml for children 3 years old and older. An intradermal form of IIV has been licensed for persons 18 to 64 years of age. The vaccine may be given simultaneously with other vaccines but in a separate syringe and at a separate site. The vaccine is administered yearly because different strains of influenza are used each year in the manufacture of the vaccine. The American Academy of Pediatrics (2015) recommends an assessment of the egg allergenic reaction—mild (such as hives alone) versus severe (such as an anaphylactic reaction)—before making a decision about the vaccine administration to children who have a history of egg allergy. Several options for administering the influenza vaccine are described in the literature, and individuals should discuss the risks and benefits with a knowledgeable health care practitioner.

During the 2016–2017 influenza season, the live attenuated influenza vaccine (LAIV) was determined not to be an acceptable alternative for the influenza vaccine due to concerns about its effectiveness (Belongia, Karron, Reingold, et al., 2017). The US Advisory Committee on Immunization Practices is monitoring ongoing research to determine recommendations for future influenza seasons.

The H1N1 virus (swine flu) is a subtype of influenza type A. Previous outbreaks of H1N1 influenza occurred in 1918, and the mortality rates were significant both in the United States and worldwide (American Academy of Pediatrics, 2015). The pandemic of H1N1 in 2009–2010 caused significant morbidity and mortality worldwide, but particularly in Mexico and the United States. Antigenic shift occurs when influenza viruses undergo significant changes that result in new infection subtypes; such is the case in the 2009 pandemic. The signs and symptoms of H1N1 flu are the same as those mentioned for influenza. The most updated information on the status of this disease may be found at the websites for the Centers for Disease Control and Prevention (http://www.cdc.gov/flu/about/season/index.htm).

Meningococcal Disease

Invasive meningococcal disease continues to be the cause of high morbidity in children in the United States. Infants younger than 1 year of age are particularly susceptible, yet the highest fatalities occur in adolescents and young adults with 50 to 60 cases and 5 to 10 deaths reported annually (Centers for Disease Control and Prevention, 2015). There is also evidence that the risk of meningococcal infections is high in college freshmen living in dormitories. Meningococcal infections are also responsible for significant morbidities, including limb or digit amputation, skin scarring, hearing loss, and neurologic disabilities.

Neisseria meningitidis is the leading cause of bacterial meningitis in the United States. It is not recommended that children 9 months to 10 years old routinely receive the meningococcal conjugate vaccines because the infection rate is low in this age-group. Children at increased risk for meningococcal infection should receive a two-dose series of either MenACY-D (Menactra) or MenACY-CRM (Menveo), both of which are MCV4 vaccines, or the infant series of MenHibrix (Hib-MenCY) given at least 2 months apart. These include children with terminal complement component deficiency, anatomic or functional asplenia, or HIV. Children ages 2 to 18 years who travel to or reside in countries where *N. meningitidis* is hyperendemic or epidemic or who are at risk during a community outbreak should receive one dose of MCV4 (either Menveo or Menactra). Menactra is licensed for administration in children as young as 9 months of age, whereas Menveo is only licensed for children 2 years of age and older.

Children and adolescents 11 to 12 years of age should receive a single immunization of MCV4 (either Menactra or Menveo) and a booster of the same at age 16 to 18 years. Others at high risk who should receive MCV4 include college freshmen living in dormitories and military recruits. MenHibrix has been licensed for administration to children ages 6 weeks to 18 months and provides protection against meningococcal (groups A, C, Y, and W-135), as well as Hib. MenHibrix is administered in a four-dose series at 2, 4, 6, and 12 to 15 months of age. Persons who are at high risk for the disease and previously received meningococcal polysaccharide vaccine (MPSV4) 3 or more years previously should be reimmunized with MCV4. MCV4 (Menveo or Menactra) is administered as an intramuscular injection (0.5 ml) and may be administered in conjunction with other vaccines in a separate syringe and at a separate site. Immunization with MCV4 is contraindicated in persons with hypersensitivity to any components of the vaccine, including diphtheria toxoid, and to rubber latex (part of vial stopper).

Rotavirus

Rotavirus is one of the leading causes of severe diarrhea in infants and young children and is transmitted by the fecal-oral route. The incidence of rotavirus has decreased dramatically since rotavirus vaccines became available in 2006. Two rotavirus vaccines, RotaTeq (RV5) and Rotarix (RV1), have received a license from the US Food and Drug Administration (FDA) for distribution in the United States. Infants in the United States are routinely immunized with three doses of RotaTeq at 2, 4, and 6 months of age or two doses of Rotarix at 2 and 4 months of age. RotaTeq is licensed for administration to infants at 6 to 14 weeks of age, with two additional doses administered at 4- to 10-week intervals but not after 32 weeks of age (American Academy of Pediatrics, 2015). Rotarix (1 ml) may be administered beginning at 6 weeks of age, with a second dose at least 4 weeks after the first dose but before 32 weeks of age (American Academy of Pediatrics, 2015). Both vaccines are administered orally. Infants who contract rotavirus infection before completing the vaccine series should complete the vaccinations following the standard intervals (American Academy of Pediatrics, 2015).

Human Papillomavirus

Human papillomaviruses (HPVs) are a large family of viruses that consist of cutaneous (i.e., skin warts) and genital (i.e., mucosal) types. Genital HPVs can be classified as low risk and high risk according to their association with cancers. Three human papillomavirus (HPV) vaccines have been licensed for use in adolescents but Gardasil 9 is the only available HPV vaccine in the United States (Centers for Disease Control and Prevention, 2016). The vaccine is administered intramuscularly, preferably in the deltoid muscle, in three separate doses; the first dose in the series is commonly administered at 11 to 12 years of age, and the second dose is given 1 to 2 months after the first, with the third dose given 6 months after the first dose (American Academy of Pediatrics, 2015). The vaccine is recommended for both boys and girls at a minimum age of 9 years and a maximum age of 26 years (Centers for Disease Control and Prevention, 2016). Women who receive the HPV vaccines must continue to have regular Papanicolaou (Pap) tests (American Academy of Pediatrics, 2015).

Reactions

Vaccines for routine immunizations are among the safest and most reliable drugs available. However, minor side effects do occur after many of the immunizations and, rarely, a serious reaction may result from the vaccine. A number of inactive components are incorporated in vaccines to enhance their effectiveness and safety. Some of these components include preservatives, stabilizers, adjuvants, antibiotics (e.g., neomycin), and purified culture medium proteins (e.g., egg) to enhance effectiveness. A child may react to the preservative in the vaccine rather than the vaccine component; an example of this is the hepatitis B vaccine, which is prepared from yeast cultures. Yeast hypersensitivity therefore would preclude one from receiving that particular vaccine without consulting an allergist. Trace amounts of neomycin are used to decrease bacterial growth within certain vaccine preparations, and persons with documented anaphylactic reactions to neomycin should avoid those vaccines.

Most vaccine preparations now contain vial stoppers with a synthetic rubber to prevent latex allergy reactions, but health care personnel administering vaccines should make sure that the package insert specifies there is no latex in the stopper. In the event that an individual has a severe reaction to a vaccine and subsequent immunizations are required, an allergist should be consulted to determine the best course of action. Although influenza vaccines contain small amounts of egg protein, recent evidence shows no risk of an anaphylactic reaction with the inactivated influenza vaccine among children with an egg allergy and these children should receive the influenza vaccine (American Academy of Pediatrics, Committee on Infectious Diseases, 2016). Some vaccines contain a preservative, thimerosal, which contains ethyl mercury. Concerns regarding possible mercury poisoning in the 1990s prompted many to put off vaccination of infants and small children for fear of childhood developmental problems, such as autism. A number of manufacturers have since stopped producing vaccines containing thimerosal. No local hypersensitivity reactions to thimerosal have been recorded, and studies on thimerosal and the potential link to autism or any other pervasive developmental disorder failed to establish a causal relationship between the two (DeStefano, Price, & Weintraub, 2013; Yoshimasu, Kiyohara, Takemura, et al., 2014). The Institute of Medicine (2004), following an in-depth 3-year study, concluded that there was no link between autism and the MMR vaccine or vaccines containing the preservative thimerosal.

With inactivated antigens, such as DTaP, side effects are most likely to occur within a few hours or days of administration and are usually limited to local tenderness, erythema, and swelling at the injection site; low-grade fever; and behavioral changes (e.g., drowsiness, eating less, prolonged or unusual cry). Local reactions tend to be less severe when a needle of sufficient length to deposit the vaccine in the muscle is used (see Atraumatic Care box). Rarely, more severe reactions may occur. If epinephrine is administered, observe for adverse reactions such as tachycardia, hypertension, irritability, headaches, nausea, and tremors.

Contraindications and Precautions

Nurses need to be aware of the reasons for withholding immunizations—both for the child's safety in terms of avoiding reactions and for the child's maximum benefit from receiving the vaccine. Unfounded fears and lack of knowledge regarding contraindications can needlessly prevent a child from having protection from life-threatening diseases. Issues that have surfaced regarding vaccines include the misconception that administering combination vaccines may overload the child's immune system; the combined vaccines have undergone rigorous study in relation to side effects and immunogenicity rates following administration. Others may express concern that vaccines are not a part of the individual's natural immunity and that administering too many vaccines may decrease the child's immunity to such diseases. A recent evaluation of parents' vaccination concerns identified through posts on social media found that parents were concerned about adverse reactions, such as autism, pain, compromised immunity, and death associated with vaccinations (Tangherlini, Roychowdhury, Glenn, et al., 2016).

ATRAUMATIC CARE

Immunizations

Needle length and injection techniques are important factors and must be considered for each individual child. Fewer reactions to immunizations are observed when the vaccine is given deep into the muscle rather than into subcutaneous tissue. The dorsogluteal site is not recommended as an injection site for children because of the potential for sciatic nerve damage (Rishovd, 2014). In addition, aspiration for blood is no longer recommended for an intramuscular injection because large blood vessels are not present at recommended injection sites and slow aspiration causes more pain than injection without aspiration (Rishovd, 2014).

To ensure appropriate needle size for vaccine administration (Rishovd, 2014):

- Newborns (0-28 days old): recommended needle size is ⅝ inch, 22 to 25 gauge, recommended injection site: vastus lateralis.
- Infant/Toddler (1 month to 2 years): recommended needle size/site is 1 inch, 22 to 25 gauge for vastus lateralis or ⅝ to 1 inch, 22 to 25 gauge in the deltoid only if muscle mass is adequately developed.
- Child/Adolescent (3 to 18 years): less than 60 kg: ⅝ to 1 inch, 22 to 25 gauge in deltoid, and greater than 60 kg: 1 to 1.5 inch, 22 to 25 gauge in deltoid.

Use one or more of the following techniques to minimize pain (Rishovd, 2014; World Health Organization, 2015):

- Apply the topical anesthetic EMLA (lidocaine-prilocaine) to the injection site and cover with an occlusive dressing for at least 1 hour* or apply the topical anesthetic LMX4 (4% lidocaine) to the injection site and cover with an occlusive dressing for 30 minutes before the injection.
- Apply a vapocoolant spray (e.g., ethyl chloride or FluoriMethane) directly to the skin; however, some children may report pain associated with the cooling sensation.
- Ensure beneficial positioning of the patient: being held by a parent or caregiver for infants and young children, and sitting upright for older children and adolescents.
- Encourage breastfeeding during or before the immunizations.
- For children less than 6 years old, use distraction, such as asking the child to blow bubbles or telling the child to "take a deep breath and blow and blow and blow until I tell you to stop." Evidence does not show any benefit in using distraction during injections with adolescents.
- Nurses administering the injections should remain calm and use neutral words such as "here I go" instead of "here comes the sting."
- Do not manually stimulate (i.e., rubbing or applying pressure) the injection site.

*The use of the EMLA patch before administration of diphtheria-tetanus–acellular pertussis–inactivated poliovirus–*Haemophilus influenzae* type b (DTaP-IPV-Hib) and hepatitis B vaccines did not decrease antibody titers in immunized infants and was effective in reducing pain in 6-month-old children (Halperin, Halperin, McGrath, et al., 2002).

DRUG ALERT

*Emergency Management of Anaphylaxis**

EpiPen Jr (0.15 mg; 0.3 ml of 1 : 2000) intramuscularly (IM) for child weighing 15 to 30 kg (33 to 66 lb)

EpiPen (0.3 mg; 0.3 ml of 1 : 1000) IM for child weighing 30 kg (66 lb) or more

*Lieberman, P., Nicklas, R. A., Randolph, C., et al. (2015). Anaphylaxis—a practice parameter update 2015. *Ann Allergy Asthma Immunol, 115,* 341-384.

A *contraindication* is considered as a condition in an individual that increases the risk for a serious adverse reaction (e.g., not administering a live virus vaccine to a severely immune-compromised child). Thus one would not administer a vaccine when a contraindication is present. A *precaution* is a condition in a recipient that might increase the risk for a serious adverse reaction or that might compromise the ability of the vaccine to produce immunity. If conditions are such that the benefit of receiving the vaccine would outweigh the risk of an adverse event or incomplete response, a precaution would not prevent vaccine administration (American Academy of Pediatrics, 2015).

The general contraindication for all immunizations is a severe febrile illness. This precaution avoids adding the risk of adverse side effects from the vaccine to an already ill child or mistakenly identifying a symptom of the disease as having been caused by the vaccine. The presence of minor illnesses, such as the common cold, is not a contraindication. Live virus vaccines are generally not administered to anyone with an altered immune system because multiplication of the virus may be enhanced, causing a severe vaccine-induced illness.

In general, live virus vaccines should not be administered to persons who are severely immunocompromised or among persons whose immune function is not known (American Academy of Pediatrics, 2015). Another contraindication to live virus vaccines (e.g., MMR, varicella, and rotavirus) is the presence of recently acquired passive immunity through blood transfusions, immunoglobulin, or maternal antibodies. Administration of MMR and varicella should be postponed for a minimum of 3 months after passive immunization with immunoglobulins and blood transfusions (except washed red blood cells, which do not interfere with the immune response). Suggested intervals between administration of immunoglobulin preparations and MMR and varicella depend on the type of immune product and dosage. If the vaccine and immunoglobulin are given simultaneously because of imminent exposure to disease, the two preparations are injected at sites far from each other. Vaccination should be repeated after the suggested intervals unless there is serologic evidence of antibody production.

A final contraindication is a known allergic response to a previously administered vaccine or a substance in the vaccine. An anaphylactic reaction to a vaccine or its component is a true contraindication. MMR vaccines contain minute amounts of neomycin; measles and mumps vaccines, which are grown on chick embryo tissue cultures, are not believed to contain significant amounts of egg cross-reacting proteins. Therefore only a history of anaphylactic reaction to neomycin, gelatin, or the vaccine itself is considered a contraindication to their use.

Pregnancy is a contraindication to MMR vaccines, although the risk of fetal damage is primarily theoretic. Breastfeeding is not a contraindication for any vaccine. The only vaccine virus that has been isolated in human milk is rubella, and there is no indication that this is harmful to infants; rubella infection in an infant as a result of exposure to rubella virus in human milk would likely be well tolerated because the vaccine is attenuated (American Academy of Pediatrics, 2015).

To identify the rare child who may not be able to receive the vaccines, take a careful allergy history. If the child has a history of anaphylaxis, report this to the practitioner before administering the vaccine. Contact dermatitis in reaction to neomycin is not considered a contraindication to immunization. Evidence indicates that children who are egg sensitive are not at increased risk for untoward reactions to MMR vaccine. Furthermore, skin testing of egg-allergic children with vaccine has failed to predict immediate hypersensitivity reactions (American Academy of Pediatrics, 2015). A family history of seizures, or adverse event following vaccination, penicillin allergy, allergies to duck meat or duck feathers, and a family history of sudden infant death syndrome (SIDS) are not considered contraindications to receiving childhood vaccines (American Academy of Pediatrics, 2015).

Nurses are at the forefront in providing parents with appropriate information regarding childhood immunization benefits, contraindications, and side effects and the effects of nonvaccination on the child's health. Some suggestions for communicating with parents about the benefits of immunizations in childhood include the following (portions adapted from Coyer, 2002; Fredrickson, Davis, Arnold, et al., 2004; Rosenthal, 2004):

- Provide accurate and user-friendly information on vaccines (the necessity for each one, the disease each prevents, potential adverse effects).
- Realize that the parent is expressing concern for the child's health.
- Acknowledge the parent's concerns in a genuine, empathetic manner.
- Tailor the discussion to the needs of the parent; avoid judgmental or threatening language.
- Be knowledgeable about the benefits of individual vaccines, the common adverse effects, and how to minimize those effects.
- Give the parent the vaccine information statement (VIS) beforehand, and be prepared to answer any questions that may arise.
- Help the parent make an informed decision regarding the administration of each vaccine.
- Be flexible and provide parents options regarding the administration of multiple vaccines, especially in infants, who must receive multiple injections at 2, 4, and 6 months (i.e., allow parents to space the vaccinations at different visits to decrease the total number of injections at each visit; make provisions for office visits for immunization purposes only [does not incur a practitioner fee except for administration of vaccine], provided the child is healthy).
- Involve the parent in minimizing the potential adverse effects of the vaccine (e.g., administering an appropriate dose of acetaminophen 45 minutes before administering the vaccine [as warranted]; applying eutectic mixture of local anesthetics [EMLA; lidocaine-prilocaine] or 4% lidocaine [LMX4] to the injection sites before administration [see Atraumatic Care box in this chapter]; following up to check on the child if untoward reactions have occurred in the past or parent is especially anxious about the child's well-being).
- Respect the parent's ultimate wishes.

Administration

The principal precautions in administering immunizations include proper storage of the vaccine to protect its potency and institution of recommended procedures for injection. The nurse must be familiar with the manufacturer's directions for storage and reconstitution of the vaccine. For example, if the vaccine is to be refrigerated, it should be stored on a center shelf, not in the door, where frequent temperature increases from opening the refrigerator can alter the vaccine's potency. For protection against light, the vial can be wrapped in aluminum foil. Periodic checks are established to ensure that no vaccine is used after its expiration date.

The DTP (or DTaP) vaccines contain an adjuvant to retain the antigen at the injection site and prolong the stimulatory effect. Because subcutaneous or intracutaneous injection of the adjuvant can cause local irritation, inflammation, or abscess formation, excellent intramuscular injection technique must be used (see Atraumatic Care box in this chapter).

The total series requires several injections, and every attempt is made to rotate the sites and administer the injections as painlessly as possible. (See discussion on intramuscular injections, Chapter 22.) When two or more injections are given at separate sites, the order of injections is arbitrary. Some practitioners suggest injecting the less painful one first. Some believe this is DTP (or DTaP), whereas others suggest the MMR or Hib vaccine. Still others advocate injecting at two sites simultaneously (requires two operators) (see Research Focus box).

Nurses often administer vaccines, and thus they may have the responsibility for adequately informing parents of the nature, prevalence, and risks of the disease; the type of immunization product to be used; the expected benefits and risks of side effects of the vaccine; and the need for accurate immunization records. Referring to immunizations as "baby shots" and limiting the discussion to vague statements about the vaccines are unacceptable practices.

Although immunization rates have increased significantly, health professionals should use every opportunity to encourage complete immunization of all children (see Community and Home Health Considerations box). Table 6.1 reports the quality indicator for childhood immunization status.

Another important nursing responsibility is accurate documentation. Each child should have an immunization record for parents to keep, especially for families who move frequently. Blank immunization records may be downloaded from a number of websites, including the

RESEARCH FOCUS

Order of Injections

Ipp, Parkin, Lear, and colleagues (2009) evaluated the administration order of the vaccines diphtheria-tetanus–acellular pertussis–*Haemophilus influenzae* type b (DTaP-Hib) and pneumococcal conjugate vaccine (PCV) and pain perception in 120 infants 2 to 6 months of age. The infants who were given the primary DTaP-Hib vaccine before the PCV vaccine had significantly lower pain scores than those who received the PCV vaccine first. Fallah, Gholami, Ferdosian, and colleagues (2016) evaluated the best order for immunizations: intramuscular injection (diphtheria, pertussis, and tetanus) versus subcutaneous injection (measles, mumps, and rubella) among 70 children. Pain was significantly lower when the subcutaneous injection was administered before the intramuscular injection.

One of the most important features of injecting vaccines is adequate penetration of the muscle for deposition of the drug intramuscularly and not subcutaneously (depending on the manufacturer's recommendation for administration). The use of appropriate needle length is an essential component of administering vaccines. A recent systematic review reported the appropriate needle size to be $\frac{5}{8}$ inch for infants less than 28 days old; 1 inch for infants 1 month to 2 years; and $\frac{5}{8}$ inch for the skin is stretched tightly and not bunched to 1 inch for children 3 to 18 years (Beirne, Hennessy, Cadogan, et al., 2015). In two studies, the use of longer needles significantly decreased the incidence of localized edema and tenderness when vaccines were administered to a group of infants (Diggle & Deeks, 2000; Diggle, Deeks, & Pollard, 2006). Similar findings have been recorded for children 4 to 6 years of age receiving the fifth DTaP vaccine (Jackson, Yu, Nelson, et al., 2011).

TABLE 6.1 Pediatric Quality Indicator*

CHILDHOOD IMMUNIZATION STATUS	
Measure	Children 2 years of age who had four diphtheria, tetanus and acellular pertussis (DTaP); three polio (IPV); one measles, mumps, and rubella (MMR); three *H. influenzae* type B (HiB); three hepatitis B (HepB); one chickenpox (VZV); four pneumococcal conjugate (PCV); two hepatitis A (HepA); two or three rotavirus (RV); and two influenza (flu) vaccines by their second birthday.
Numerator	Number of children who have evidence showing they received recommended vaccines during the measurement time.
Denominator	Number of children who turn 2 years of age during the measurement year are eligible for inclusion.

*Endorsed by the National Quality Forum–0038 and Center for Medicare and Medicaid Services–146v1.

COMMUNITY AND HOME HEALTH CONSIDERATIONS

Keeping Current on Vaccine Recommendations

It is much easier to keep current if you know where to look for the official recommendations of the American Academy of Pediatrics and the Centers for Disease Control and Prevention's Advisory Committee on Immunization Practices (ACIP). The primary sources are publications and the Internet. You can also contact each organization to request information:

American Academy of Pediatrics
141 Northwest Point Blvd.
Elk Grove Village, IL 60007
847-434-4000
Fax: 847-434-8000
http://www.aap.org

Centers for Disease Control and Prevention
1600 Clifton Road
Atlanta, GA 30333
404-639-3311
Information: 800-232-4636
https://www.cdc.gov
Vaccine and immunization information: https://www.cdc.gov/vaccines

Immunization Action Coalition (http://www.immunize.org), which has vaccine information and records in a number of languages.

Document the following information on the medical record: day, month, and year of administration; manufacturer and lot number of vaccine; and name, address, and title of the person administering the vaccine. Additional data to record are the site and route of administration and evidence that the parent or legal guardian gave informed consent before the immunization was administered. Report any adverse reactions after the administration of a vaccine to the Vaccine Adverse Event Reporting System (http://www.vaers.hhs.gov; 1-800-822-7967).

Many states and territories participate in the Immunization Information System (IIS), which provides immunization information for parents and health professionals, as well as a local or regional registry of immunizations children have received. In addition the IIS can provide parents with information about missed scheduled immunizations. This information is also useful for schools and health clinics.

An additional source of vaccine information that must be given to parents (as required by the National Childhood Vaccine Injury Act, 1986) before the administration of vaccines is the VIS for the particular vaccine being administered. Practitioners are required by law to fully inform families of the risks and benefits of the vaccines. VISs are designed to provide updated information to the adult vaccinee or parents or legal guardians of children being vaccinated regarding the risks and benefits of each vaccine. The practitioner should answer questions regarding the information in the VISs. VISs are available for the following vaccines: adenovirus, anthrax, tetanus, diphtheria, pertussis, MMR, MMRV, IPV, HPV, varicella, Hib, influenza, meningococcal, pneumococcal (13 and 23), rabies, rotavirus, shingles, smallpox, yellow fever, Japanese encephalitis, typhoid, and hepatitis A and B. An updated VIS should be provided, and documentation in the patient's chart should state that the VIS was given and include the publication date of the VIS; this represents **informed consent** once the parent or caregiver gives permission to administer the vaccines. VISs are available from state or local health departments or from the Immunization Action Coalition* and Centers for Disease Control and Prevention.†

*http://www.immunize.org/vis.
†http://www.cdc.gov/vaccines/pubs/vis/default.htm.

In response to the concerns of manufacturers, practitioners, and parents of children with serious vaccine-associated injuries, the National Childhood Vaccine Injury Act of 1986 and the Vaccine Compensation Amendments of 1987 were passed. These laws are designed to provide fair compensation for children who are inadvertently injured and provide greater protection from liability for vaccine manufacturers and providers. (See *2015 Red Book: Report of the Committee on Infectious Diseases* [American Academy of Pediatrics, 2015] for further details of this program.)

The American Academy of Pediatrics' Report of the Committee on Infectious Diseases, known as the *Red Book,* is an authoritative source of information on vaccines and other important pediatric infectious diseases. However, it lacks an in-depth review and reference list of controversial issues. The recommendations in the *Red Book* first appear in the journal *Pediatrics* and/or the *AAP News.* Typically, the most recent immunization schedule appears in the January issue of the journal.

The Centers for Disease Control and Prevention now offers a valuable online resource tool for parents and clinicians. The tool prints out an individualized vaccination schedule with dates associated with each vaccination based on the child's date of birth. Clinicians can use this tool for children under 5 years of age to serve as a reminder for parents. Nurses should note that the personalized tool is based on the current immunization schedule and may need to be adjusted with the yearly updates from the American Academy of Pediatrics and the ACIP. The tool is available at www2a.cdc.gov/nip/kidstuff/newscheduler_le.

A publication of the Centers for Disease Control and Prevention (CDC), *Morbidity and Mortality Weekly Report* (MMWR), contains comprehensive reviews of the literature and important background data regarding vaccine efficacy and side effects. To receive an electronic copy, send an e-mail message to listserv@listserv.cdc.gov. The body content should read: SUBscribe mmwr-toc. An electronic copy also is available from the CDC's website at https://www.cdc.gov.

Vaccine information statements (VISs) are available by calling your state or local health department. They can also be downloaded from the Immunization Action Coalition's website at http://www.immunize.org/vis or Centers for Disease Control and Prevention's website at https://www.cdc.gov/vaccines/hcp/vis/index.html. Some translations are available.

Another resource to keep up to date on the vaccines that are licensed and commercially available is the US Food and Drug Administration's Center for Biologics Evaluation and Research report for each year, http://www.fda.gov/BiologicsBloodVaccines/Vaccines/default.htm.

COMMUNICABLE DISEASES

The incidence of childhood communicable diseases has declined significantly since the advent of immunizations. The use of antibiotics and antitoxins has further reduced serious complications resulting from such infections. However, infectious diseases do occur, and nurses must be familiar with the infectious agent to recognize the disease and to institute appropriate preventive and supportive interventions (Table 6.2 and Figs. 6.2 to 6.7).

NURSING CARE MANAGEMENT

Table 6.2 describes the more common communicable diseases of childhood, their therapeutic management, and specific nursing care. The following is a general discussion of nursing care management for communicable diseases.

Identification of the infectious agent is of primary importance to prevent exposure to susceptible individuals. Nurses in ambulatory care

Text continued on p. 186

TABLE 6.2 Communicable Diseases of Childhood

Disease	Clinical Manifestations	Therapeutic Management and Complications	Nursing Care Management
Chickenpox (Varicella) (Fig. 6.2)			
Agents—Varicella-zoster virus (VZV) **Source**—Primary secretions of respiratory tract of infected persons; to a lesser degree, skin lesions (scabs not infectious) **Transmissions**—Direct contact, droplet (airborne) spread, and contaminated objects **Incubation period**—2-3 weeks, usually 14-16 days **Period of communicability**—Probably 1 day before eruption of lesions (prodromal period) to 6 days after first crop of vesicles when crusts have formed	**Prodromal stage**—Slight fever, malaise, and anorexia for first 24 hours; rash highly pruritic; begins as macule, rapidly progresses to papule and then vesicle (surrounded by erythematous base; becomes umbilicated and cloudy; breaks easily and forms crusts); all three stages (papule, vesicle, crust) present in varying degrees at one time **Distribution**—Centripetal, spreading to face and proximal extremities but sparse on distal limbs and less on areas not exposed to heat (i.e., from clothing or sun) **Constitutional signs and symptoms**—Elevated temperature from lymphadenopathy, irritability from pruritus	**Specific**—Antiviral agent acyclovir (Zovirax); varicella-zoster immune globulin or intravenous immune globulin (IVIG) after exposure in high-risk children **Supportive**—Diphenhydramine hydrochloride or antihistamines to relieve itching; skin care to prevent secondary bacterial infection **Complications**—Secondary bacterial infections (abscesses, cellulitis, necrotizing fasciitis, pneumonia, sepsis) Encephalitis Varicella pneumonia (rare in healthy children) Hemorrhagic varicella (tiny hemorrhages in vesicles and numerous petechiae in skin) Chronic or transient thrombocytopenia **Preventive**—Childhood immunization	Maintain Standard, Airborne, and Contact Precautions if hospitalized until all lesions are crusted; for immunized child with mild breakthrough varicella, isolate until no new lesions are seen. Keep child in home away from susceptible individuals until vesicles have dried (usually 1 week after onset of disease), and isolate high-risk children from infected children. Administer skin care: give bath and change clothes and linens daily; administer topical calamine lotion; keep child's fingernails short and clean; apply mittens if child scratches. Keep child cool (may decrease number of lesions). Lessen pruritus; keep child occupied. Remove loose crusts that rub and irritate skin. Teach child to apply pressure to pruritic area rather than scratching it. Avoid use of aspirin (possible association with Reye syndrome).
Diphtheria			
Agent—*Corynebacterium diphtheriae* **Source**—Discharges from mucous membranes of nose and nasopharynx, skin, and other lesions of infected person **Transmission**—Direct contact with infected person, a carrier, or contaminated articles **Incubation period**—Usually 2-5 days, possibly longer **Period of communicability**—Variable; until virulent bacilli are no longer present (identified by three negative cultures); usually 2 weeks but as long as 4 weeks	Vary according to anatomic location of pseudomembrane **Nasal**—Resembles common cold, serosanguineous mucopurulent nasal discharge without constitutional symptoms; may have frank epistaxis **Tonsillar-pharyngeal**—Malaise; anorexia; sore throat; low-grade fever; pulse increased above expected for temperature within 24 hours; smooth, adherent, white or gray membrane; lymphadenitis possibly pronounced ("bull's neck"); in severe cases, toxemia, septic shock, and death within 6-10 days **Laryngeal**—Fever, hoarseness, cough, with or without previous signs listed; potential airway obstruction; apprehensive; dyspneic retractions; cyanosis	Equine antitoxin (usually intravenously); preceded by skin or conjunctival test to rule out sensitivity to horse serum Antibiotics (penicillin G procaine or erythromycin) in addition to equine antitoxin Complete bed rest (prevention of myocarditis) Tracheostomy for airway obstruction Treatment of infected contacts and carriers **Complications**—Toxic cardiomyopathy (2nd to 3rd week) Toxic neuropathy **Preventive**—Childhood immunization	Follow Standard and Droplet Precautions until two cultures are negative for *C. diphtheriae;* use Contact Precautions with cutaneous manifestations. Administer antibiotics in timely manner. Participate in sensitivity testing; have epinephrine available. Administer complete care to maintain bed rest. Use suctioning as needed. Observe respiration for signs of obstruction. Administer humidified oxygen as prescribed.

TABLE 6.2 Communicable Diseases of Childhood—cont'd

Disease	Clinical Manifestations	Therapeutic Management and Complications	Nursing Care Management
Erythema Infectiosum (Fifth Disease) (Fig. 6.3)			
Agent—Human parvovirus B19 **Source**—Infected persons, mainly school-age children **Transmission**—Respiratory secretions and blood, blood products **Incubation period**—4-14 days; may be as long as 21 days **Period of communicability**—Uncertain but before onset of symptoms in children with aplastic crisis	Rash appears in three stages: **I**—Erythema on face, chiefly on cheeks ("slapped face" appearance); disappears by 1-4 days **II**—About 1 day after rash appears on face, maculopapular red spots appear, symmetrically distributed on upper and lower extremities; rash progresses from proximal to distal surfaces and may last ≥1 week **III**—Rash subsides but reappears if skin is irritated or traumatized (sun, heat, cold, friction) In children with aplastic crisis, rash usually absent and prodromal illness includes fever, myalgia, lethargy, nausea, vomiting, and abdominal pain Child with sickle cell disease may have concurrent vaso-occlusive crisis	**Symptomatic and supportive**—Antipyretics, analgesics, antiinflammatory drugs Possible blood transfusion for transient aplastic anemia **Complications**—Self-limited arthritis and arthralgia (arthritis may become chronic); more common in adult women May result in serious complications (anemia, hydrops) or fetal death if mother infected during pregnancy (primarily second trimester) Aplastic crisis in children with hemolytic disease or immunodeficiency Myocarditis (rare)	Isolation of child is not necessary, except hospitalized child (immunosuppressed or with aplastic crises) suspected of parvovirus infection is placed on Droplet Precautions and Standard Precautions. Pregnant women need not be excluded from workplace where parvovirus infection is present; they should not care for patients with aplastic crises. Explain low risk of fetal death to those in contact with affected children; assist with routine fetal ultrasound for detection of fetal hydrops.
Exanthem Subitum (Roseola Infantum) (Fig. 6.4)			
Agent—Human herpesvirus type 6 (HHV-6; rarely HHV-7) **Source**—Possibly acquired from saliva of healthy adult person; entry via nasal, buccal, or conjunctival mucosa **Transmission**—Year round; no reported contact with infected individual in most cases (virtually limited to children <3 years but peak age is 6-15 months old) **Incubation period**—Usually 5-15 days **Period of communicability**—Unknown	Persistent high fever >39.5°C (103°F) for 3-7 days in child who appears well Precipitous drop in fever to normal with appearance of rash Bulging fontanel Rash—Discrete rose-pink macules or maculopapules appearing first on trunk, then spreading to neck, face, and extremities; nonpruritic; fades on pressure; lasts 1-2 days **Associated signs and symptoms**—Cervical and postauricular lymphadenopathy, inflamed pharynx, cough, coryza	Nonspecific Antipyretics to control fever **Complications**—Recurrent febrile seizures (possibly from latent infection of central nervous system that is reactivated by fever) Encephalitis Hepatitis (rare)	Use Standard Precautions. Teach parents measures for lowering temperature (antipyretic drugs); ensure adequate parental understanding of specific antipyretic dosage to prevent accidental overdose. If child is prone to seizures, discuss appropriate precautions and possibility of recurrent febrile seizures.
Mumps			
Agent—Paramyxovirus **Source**—Saliva of infected persons **Transmission**—Direct contact with or droplet spread from an infected person **Incubation period**—14-21 days **Period of communicability**—Most communicable immediately before and after swelling begins	**Prodromal stage**—Fever, headache, malaise, and anorexia for 24 hours, followed by "earache" that is aggravated by chewing **Parotitis**—By third day, parotid gland(s) (either unilateral or bilateral) enlarges and reaches maximum size in 1-3 days; accompanied by pain and tenderness; other exocrine glands (submandibular) may also be swollen	**Preventive**—Childhood immunization **Symptomatic and supportive**—Analgesics for pain and antipyretics for fever Intravenous fluid if needed for child who refuses to drink or vomits because of meningoencephalitis **Complications**—Sensorineural deafness Postinfectious encephalitis Myocarditis Arthritis Hepatitis Epididymo-orchitis Oophoritis Pancreatitis Sterility (extremely rare in adult men) Meningitis	Maintain isolation during period of communicability; institute Droplet and Contact Precautions during hospitalization. Encourage rest and decreased activity during prodromal phase until swelling subsides. Give analgesics for pain; if child is unwilling to swallow pills or tablets medication, use elixir form. Encourage fluids and soft, bland foods; avoid foods requiring chewing. Apply hot or cold compresses to neck, whichever is more comforting. To relieve orchitis, provide hot or cold packs for analgesia and scrotal elevation.

Continued

TABLE 6.2 Communicable Diseases of Childhood—cont'd

Disease	Clinical Manifestations	Therapeutic Management and Complications	Nursing Care Management
Measles (Rubeola) (Fig. 6.5)			
Agent—Virus **Source**—Respiratory tract secretions, blood, and urine of infected person **Transmission**—Usually by direct contact with droplets of infected person; primarily in the winter **Incubation period**—10-20 days **Period of communicability**—From 4 days before to 5 days after rash appears, but mainly during prodromal (catarrhal) stage	**Prodromal (catarrhal) stage**—Fever and malaise, followed in 24 hours by coryza, cough, conjunctivitis, Koplik spots (small, irregular red spots with a minute, bluish-white center first seen on buccal mucosa opposite molars 2 days before rash); symptoms gradually increasing in severity until second day after rash appears, when they begin to subside Rash—Appears 3-4 days after onset of prodromal stage; begins as erythematous maculopapular eruption on face and gradually spreads downward; more severe in earlier sites (appears confluent) and less intense in later sites (appears discrete); after 3-4 days assumes brownish appearance, and fine desquamation occurs over area of extensive involvement **Constitutional signs and symptoms**—Anorexia, abdominal pain, malaise, generalized lymphadenopathy	**Preventive**—Childhood immunization **Supportive**—Bed rest during febrile period; antipyretics Antibiotics to prevent secondary bacterial infection in high-risk children **Complications**—Otitis media Pneumonia (bacterial) Obstructive laryngitis and laryngotracheitis Encephalitis (rare but has high mortality) **Treatment**—Administer vitamin A (World Health Organization recommendation) for children with acute illness: 200,000 international units for children 12 months and older; 100,000 international units for children 6 through 11 months old; 50,000 international units for infants younger than 6 months (American Academy of Pediatrics, 2015)	Maintain isolation until fifth day of rash; if child is hospitalized, institute Airborne Precautions. Encourage rest during prodromal stage; provide quiet activity. Fever—Instruct parents to administer antipyretics; avoid chilling; if child is prone to seizures, institute appropriate precautions. Eye care—Dim lights if photophobia present; clean eyelids with warm saline solution to remove secretions or crusts; keep child from rubbing eyes. Coryza, cough—Use cool-mist vaporizer; protect skin around nares with layer of petrolatum; encourage fluids and soft, bland foods. Skin care—Keep skin clean; use tepid baths as necessary.
Pertussis (Whooping Cough)			
Agent—Bordetella pertussis **Source**—Discharge from respiratory tract of infected persons **Transmission**—Direct contact or droplet spread from infected person; indirect contact with freshly contaminated articles **Incubation period**—6-20 days; usually 7-10 days **Period of communicability**—Greatest during catarrhal stage before onset of paroxysms	**Catarrhal stage**—Begins with symptoms of upper respiratory tract infection, such as coryza, sneezing, lacrimation, cough, and low-grade fever; symptoms continue for 1-2 weeks, when dry, hacking cough becomes more severe **Paroxysmal stage**—Cough most common at night, consists of short, rapid coughs followed by sudden inspiration associated with a high-pitched crowing sound or "whoop"; during paroxysms, cheeks become flushed or cyanotic, eyes bulge, and tongue protrudes; paroxysm may continue until thick mucus plug is dislodged; vomiting frequently follows attack; stage generally lasts 4-6 weeks, followed by convalescent stage Infants <6 months old may not have characteristic whoop cough, but have difficulty maintaining adequate oxygenation with amount of secretions, frequent vomiting of mucus and formula or breast milk Pertussis may occur in adolescents and adults with varying manifestations; cough and whoop may be absent, however, as many as 50% of adolescents may have a cough for up to 10 weeks (American Academy of Pediatrics, 2015) Additional symptoms in adolescents include difficulty breathing and posttussive vomiting (See also Immunizations, for discussion of pertussis immunization schedule.)	**Preventive**—Immunization; current belief is that childhood immunizations for pertussis do not confer lifelong immunity to adolescents and adults, so a pertussis booster is recommended for adolescents (see Immunizations section in this chapter) Antimicrobial therapy (e.g., erythromycin, clarithromycin, azithromycin) **Supportive**—Hospitalization sometimes required for infants, children who are dehydrated, or those who have complications Increased oxygen intake and humidity Adequate fluids Intensive care and mechanical ventilation if needed for infants <6 months old **Complications**—Pneumonia (usual cause of death in younger children) Atelectasis Otitis media Seizures Hemorrhage (scleral, conjunctival, epistaxis; pulmonary hemorrhage in neonate) Weight loss and dehydration Hernias (umbilical and inguinal) Prolapsed rectum Complications reported among adolescents include syncope, sleep disturbance, rib fractures, incontinence, and pneumonia (American Academy of Pediatrics, 2015)	Maintain isolation during catarrhal stage; if child is hospitalized, institute Standard and Droplet Precautions. Obtain nasopharyngeal culture for diagnosis. Encourage oral fluids; offer small amount of fluids frequently. Ensure adequate oxygenation during paroxysms; position infant on side to decrease chance of aspiration with vomiting. Provide humidified oxygen; suction as needed to prevent choking on secretions. Observe for signs of airway obstruction (e.g., increased restlessness, apprehension, retractions, cyanosis). Encourage compliance with antibiotic therapy for household contacts. Encourage adolescents to obtain pertussis booster (Tdap) (see Immunizations section in this chapter). Use Standard Precautions and Droplet in health care workers exposed to children with persistent cough and high suspicion of pertussis.

TABLE 6.2 Communicable Diseases of Childhood—cont'd

Disease	Clinical Manifestations	Therapeutic Management and Complications	Nursing Care Management
Poliomyelitis			
Agent—Enteroviruses, three types: type 1, most frequent cause of paralysis, both epidemic and endemic; type 2, least frequently associated with paralysis; type 3, second most frequently associated with paralysis **Source**—Feces and oropharyngeal secretions of infected persons, especially young children **Transmission**—Direct contact with persons with apparent or inapparent active infection; spread via fecal-oral and pharyngeal-oropharyngeal routes; vaccine-acquired paralytic polio may occur as a result of the live oral polio vaccination (no longer available in the United States) **Incubation period**—Usually 7-14 days, with range of 5-35 days **Period of communicability**—Not exactly known; virus present in throat and feces shortly after infection and persists for about 1 week in throat and 4-6 weeks in feces	May be manifested in three different forms: **Abortive or inapparent**—Fever, uneasiness, sore throat, headache, anorexia, vomiting, abdominal pain; lasts a few hours to a few days **Nonparalytic**—Same manifestations as abortive but more severe, with pain and stiffness in neck, back, and legs **Paralytic**—Initial course similar to nonparalytic type, followed by recovery and then signs of central nervous system paralysis	**Preventive**—Childhood immunization **Supportive**—Complete bed rest during acute phase Mechanical or assisted ventilation in case of respiratory paralysis Physical therapy for muscles after acute stage **Complications**—Permanent paralysis Respiratory arrest Hypertension Kidney stones from demineralization of bone during prolonged immobility	Institute Contact Precautions. Administer mild sedatives as necessary to relieve anxiety and promote rest. Participate in physical therapy procedures (use of moist hot packs and range-of-motion exercises). Position child to maintain body alignment and prevent contractures or skin breakdown; use footboard or appropriate orthoses to prevent footdrop; use pressure mattress for prolonged immobility. Encourage child to perform activities of daily living to capability; promote early ambulation with assistive devices; administer analgesics for maximum comfort during physical activity; give high-protein diet and bowel management for prolonged immobility. Observe for respiratory paralysis (e.g., difficulty talking, ineffective cough, inability to hold breath, shallow and rapid respirations); report such signs and symptoms to practitioner.

Continued

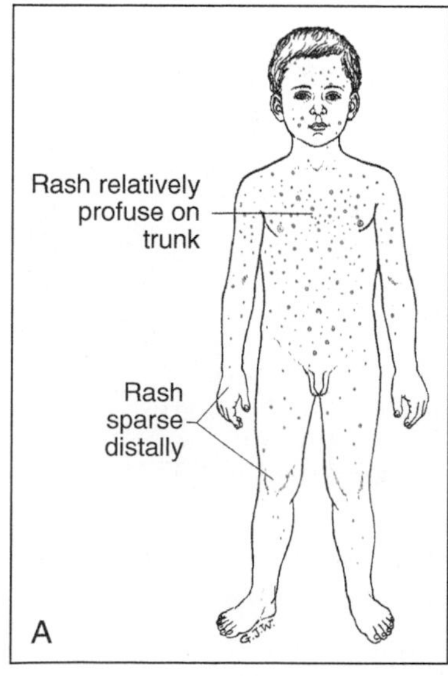

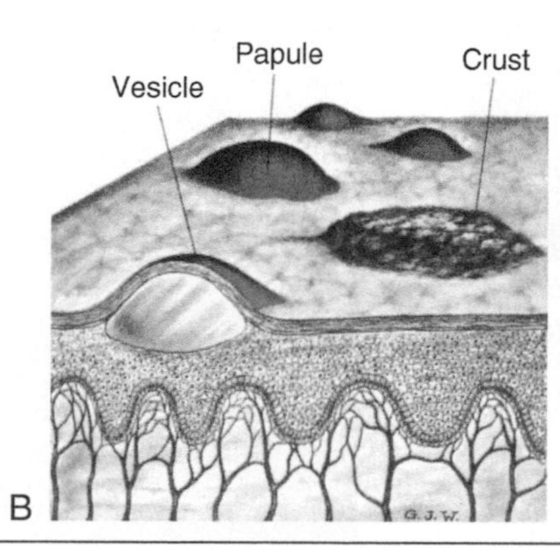

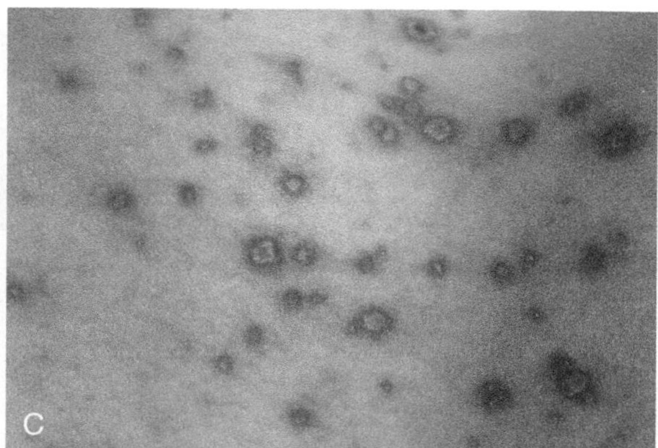

FIG. 6.2 Chickenpox (varicella). **A,** Progression of disease. **B,** Simultaneous stages of lesions. **C,** Clinical view. (*C,* From Habif, T. P. [2016]. *Clinical dermatology: A color guide to diagnosis and therapy* [6th ed.]. St. Louis, MO: Mosby.)

TABLE 6.2 Communicable Diseases of Childhood—cont'd

Disease	Clinical Manifestations	Therapeutic Management and Complications	Nursing Care Management
Rubella (German Measles) (Fig. 6.6)			
Agent—Rubella virus **Source**—Primarily nasopharyngeal secretions of person with apparent or inapparent infection; virus also present in blood, stool, and urine **Incubation period**—14-21 days **Period of communicability**—7 days before to about 5 days after appearance of rash **Constitutional signs and symptoms**—Occasionally low-grade fever, headache, malaise, and lymphadenopathy	**Prodromal stage**—Absent in children, present in adults and adolescents; consists of low-grade fever, headache, malaise, anorexia, mild conjunctivitis, coryza, sore throat, cough, and lymphadenopathy; lasts 1-5 days, subsides 1 day after appearance of rash Rash—First appears on face and rapidly spreads downward to neck, arms, trunk, and legs; by end of first day, body is covered with discrete, pinkish-red maculopapular exanthema; disappears in same order as it began and is usually gone by third day	**Preventive**—Childhood immunization No treatment necessary other than antipyretics for low-grade fever and analgesics for discomfort **Complications**—Rare (arthritis, encephalitis, or purpura); most benign of all childhood communicable diseases; greatest danger is teratogenic effect on fetus	Institute Droplet Precautions. Reassure parents of benign nature of illness in affected child. Use comfort measures as necessary. Avoid contact with pregnant woman. Monitor rubella titer in pregnant adolescent.

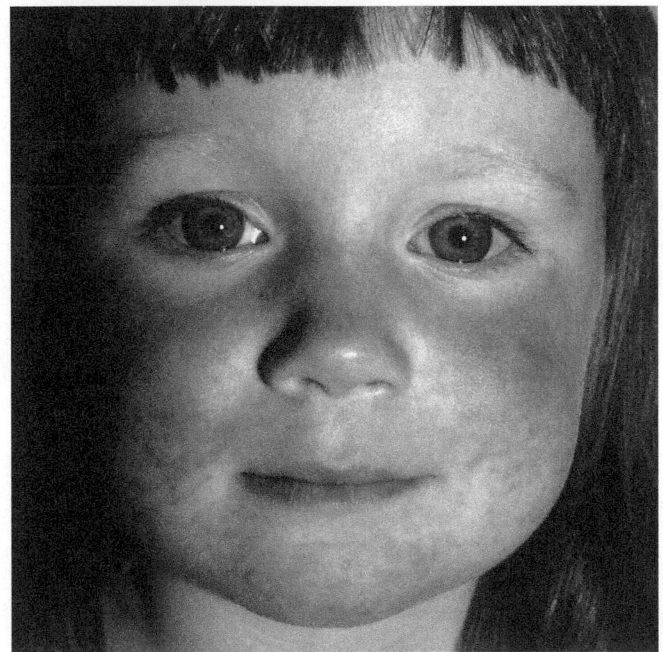

FIG. 6.3 Erythema infectiosum (fifth disease). (From Habif, T. P. [2016]. *Clinical dermatology: A color guide to diagnosis and therapy* [6th ed.]. St. Louis, MO: Mosby.)

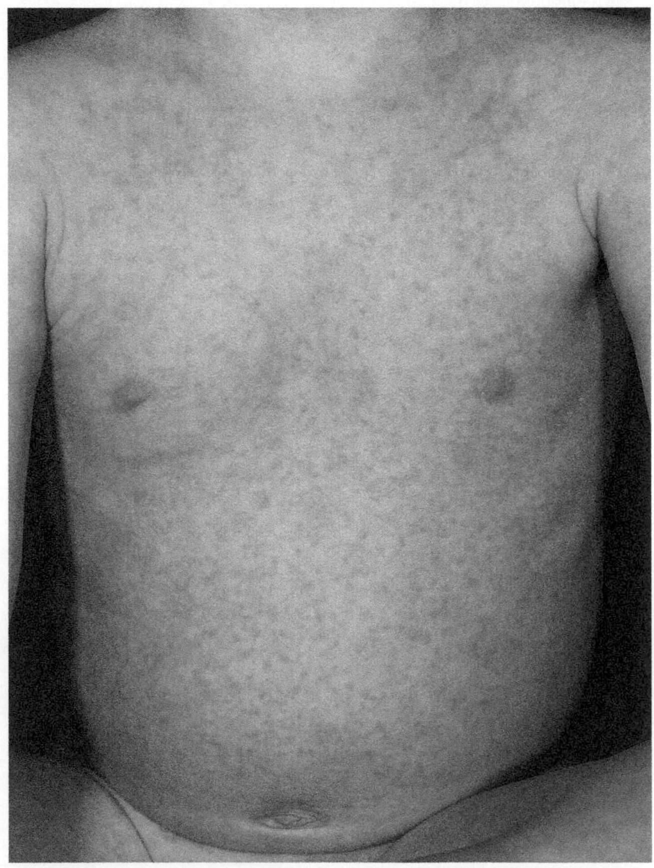

FIG. 6.4 Exanthem subitum (roseola infantum). (From Habif, T. P. [2016]. *Clinical dermatology: A color guide to diagnosis and therapy* [6th ed.]. St. Louis, MO: Mosby.)

TABLE 6.2 Communicable Diseases of Childhood—cont'd			
Disease	**Clinical Manifestations**	**Therapeutic Management and Complications**	**Nursing Care Management**
Scarlet Fever (Fig. 6.7)			
Agent—Group A β-hemolytic streptococci **Source**—Usually from nasopharyngeal secretions of infected persons and carriers **Transmission**—Direct contact with infected person or droplet spread; indirectly by contact with contaminated articles or ingestion of contaminated milk or other food **Incubation period**—2-5 days, with range of 1-7 days **Period of communicability**—During incubation period and clinical illness, approximately 10 days; during first 2 weeks of carrier phase, although may persist for months	**Prodromal stage**—Abrupt high fever, pulse increased out of proportion to fever, vomiting, headache, chills, malaise, abdominal pain, halitosis Enanthema—Tonsils enlarged, edematous, reddened, and covered with patches of exudates; in severe cases appearance resembles membrane seen in diphtheria; pharynx is edematous and beefy red; during first 1-2 days tongue is coated and papillae become red and swollen (white strawberry tongue); by fourth or fifth day white coat sloughs off, leaving prominent papillae (red strawberry tongue); palate is covered with erythematous punctate lesions Exanthema—Rash appears within 12 hours after prodromal signs; red pinhead-sized punctate lesions rapidly become generalized but are absent on face, which becomes flushed with striking circumoral pallor; rash more intense in folds of joints; by end of first week desquamation begins (fine, sandpaper-like on torso; sheetlike sloughing on palms and soles), which may be complete by 3 weeks or longer	Full course of penicillin (or erythromycin in penicillin-sensitive children) or oral cephalosporin Antibiotic therapy for newly diagnosed carriers (nose or throat cultures positive for streptococci) **Supportive**—Rest during febrile phase, analgesics for sore throat; antipruritics for rash if bothersome **Complications**—Peritonsillar and retropharyngeal abscess Sinusitis Otitis media Acute glomerulonephritis Acute rheumatic fever Polyarthritis (uncommon)	Institute Standard and Droplet Precautions until 24 hours after initiation of treatment. Ensure compliance with oral antibiotic therapy; intramuscular benzathine penicillin G [Bicillin] may be given. Encourage rest during febrile phase; provide quiet activity during convalescent period. Relieve discomfort of sore throat with analgesics, gargles, lozenges, antiseptic throat sprays, and inhalation of cool mist. Encourage fluids during febrile phase; avoid irritating liquids (e.g., citrus juices) or rough foods (e.g., chips); when child is able to eat, begin with soft diet. Advise parents to consult practitioner if fever persists after beginning therapy. Discuss procedures for preventing spread of infection—discard toothbrush; avoid sharing drinking and eating utensils.

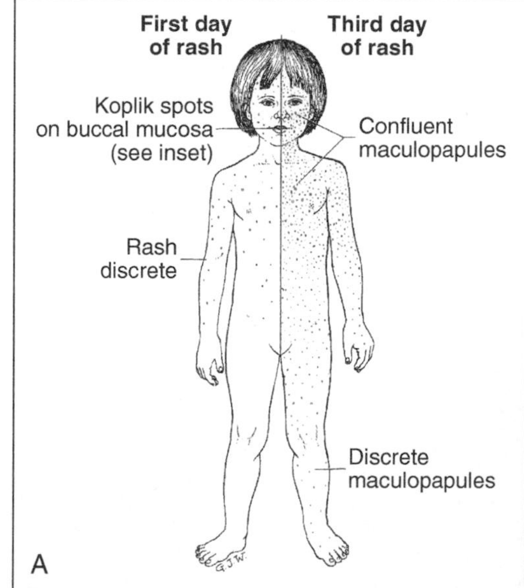

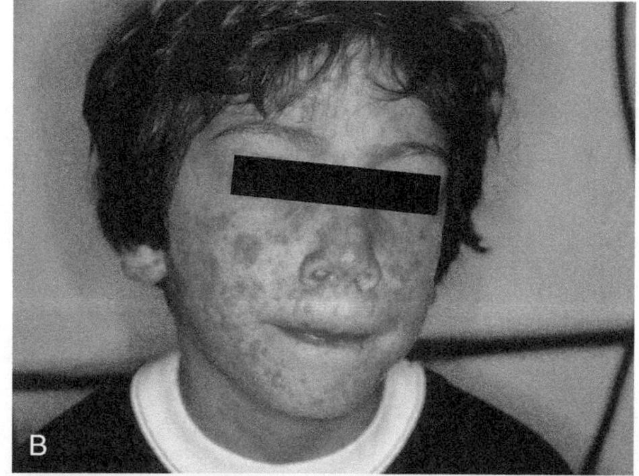

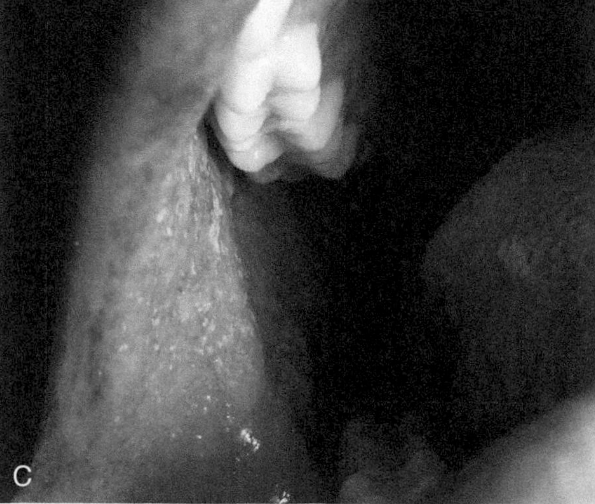

FIG. 6.5 Measles (rubeola). **A,** Progression of disease. **B,** Clinical view. **C,** Koplik spots. (*B,* From Paller, S. A., & Mancini, A. J. [2011]. *Hurwitz clinical pediatric dermatology* [4th ed.]. St. Louis, MO: Saunders; *C,* From Habif, T. P. [2016]. *Clinical dermatology: A color guide to diagnosis and therapy* [6th ed.]. St. Louis, MO: Mosby.)

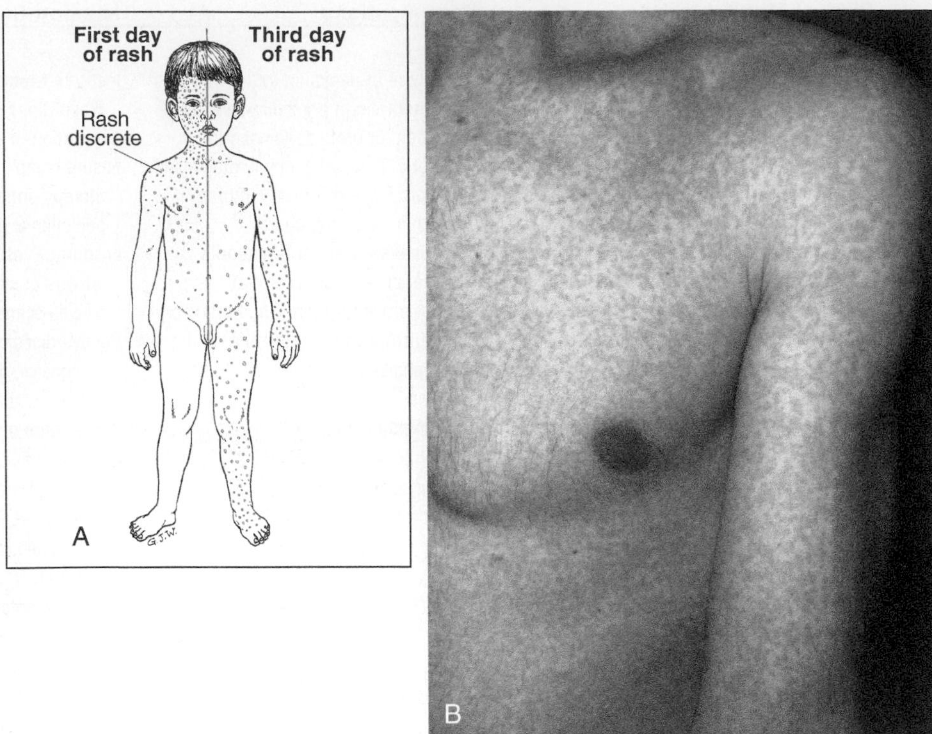

FIG. 6.6 Rubella (German measles). **A,** Progression of rash. **B,** Clinical view. (*B,* From Zitelli, B. J., & Davis, H. W. [2007]. *Atlas of pediatric physical diagnosis* [5th ed.]. St. Louis, MO: Mosby; courtesy Dr. Michael Sherlock, Lutherville, Md.)

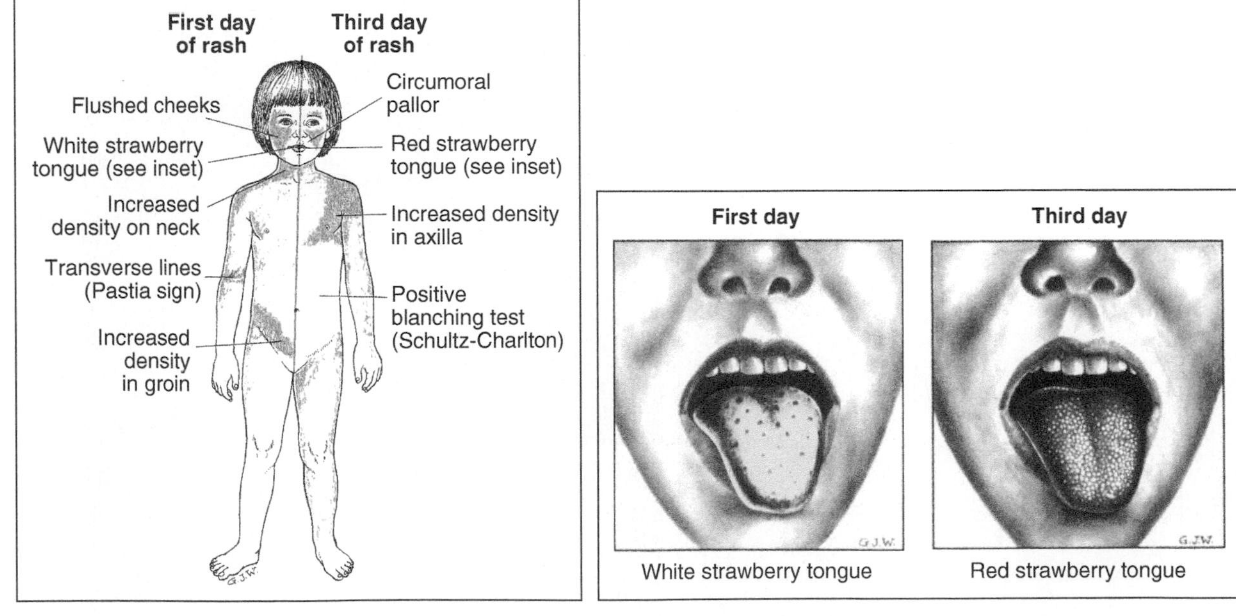

FIG. 6.7 Scarlet fever.

settings, child care centers, and schools are often the first persons to see signs of a communicable disease, such as a rash or sore throat. The nurse must operate under a high index of suspicion for common childhood diseases to identify potentially infectious cases and to recognize diseases that require medical intervention. An example is the common complaint of sore throat. Although most often a symptom of a minor viral infection, it can signal diphtheria or a streptococcal infection, such as scarlet fever. Each of these bacterial conditions requires appropriate medical treatment to prevent serious complications.

When the nurse suspects a communicable disease, it is important to assess the following:

- Recent exposure to a known case
- Prodromal symptoms (symptoms that occur between early manifestations of the disease and its overt clinical syndrome) or evidence of constitutional symptoms, such as a fever or rash (see Table 6.2)
- Immunization history
- History of having the disease

Immunizations are available for many diseases, and infection usually confers lifelong immunity; therefore the possibility of many infectious agents can be eliminated based on these two criteria.

Prevent Spread

Prevention consists of two components: prevention of the disease and control of its spread to others. Primary prevention rests almost exclusively on immunization.

Control measures to prevent spread of disease should include techniques to reduce risk of cross-transmission of infectious organisms between patients and to protect health care workers from organisms harbored by patients. If the child is hospitalized, follow the facility's policies for infection control. The most important procedure is hand washing. Persons directly caring for the child or handling contaminated articles must wash their hands and practice effective Standard Precautions in care of their patients.

Instruct the child to practice good hand-washing technique after toileting and before eating. For those diseases spread by droplets, instruct the parents in measures to reduce airborne transmission. The child who is old enough should use a tissue to cover the face during coughing or sneezing; otherwise the parent should cover the child's mouth with a tissue and then discard it (see Respiratory Hygiene/Cough Etiquette). Stress the usual hygiene measures of not sharing eating and drinking utensils to the family.

> **! NURSING ALERT**
>
> If a child is admitted to the hospital with an undiagnosed exanthema, institute strict Transmission-Based Precautions (contact, airborne, and droplet) and Standard Precautions until a diagnosis is confirmed. Childhood communicable diseases requiring these precautions include diphtheria, varicella-zoster virus (VZV; chickenpox), measles, tuberculosis, adenovirus, *Haemophilus influenzae* type b (Hib), influenza, mumps, *Neisseria meningitides, Mycoplasma pneumoniae* infection, pertussis, plague, rhinovirus, group A streptococcal pharyngitis, severe acute respiratory syndrome, pneumonia, or scarlet fever (American Academy of Pediatrics, 2015).

Prevent Complications

Although most children recover without difficulty, certain groups are at risk for serious, even fatal, complications from communicable diseases, especially the viral diseases chickenpox and erythema infectiosum (fifth disease) caused by human parvovirus B19.

Children with immunodeficiency—those receiving steroid or other immunosuppressive therapy, those with a generalized malignancy such as leukemia or lymphoma, or those with an immunologic disorder—are at risk for viremia from replication of the varicella-zoster virus (VZV)* in the blood. VZV is so named because it causes two distinct diseases: varicella (chickenpox) and zoster (herpes zoster or shingles). Varicella occurs primarily in children younger than 15 years of age. However, it leaves the threat of herpes zoster, an intensely painful varicella that is localized to a single dermatome (body area innervated by a particular segment of the spinal cord). Immunocompromised patients and healthy infants younger than 1 year of age (who also have reduced immunity) are at a higher risk for reactivation of VZV causing herpes zoster, probably as a result of a deficiency in cellular immunity (American Academy of Pediatrics, 2015). Complications of herpes zoster virus in children include secondary bacterial infection, depigmentation, and scarring. Postherpetic neuralgia in children is uncommon (American Academy of Pediatrics, 2015).

The use of varicella-zoster immune globulin (VariZIG) or intravenous immune globulin (IVIG) is recommended for children who are immunocompromised, who have no previous history of varicella, and who are likely to contract the disease and have complications as a result (American Academy of Pediatrics, 2015). The antiviral agent acyclovir (Zovirax) or valacyclovir may be used to treat varicella infections in susceptible immunocompromised persons. It is effective in decreasing the number of lesions; shortening the duration of fever; and decreasing itching, lethargy, and anorexia. Consider oral valacyclovir for immunocompromised children without a history of varicella disease, newborns whose mother had varicella within 5 days before delivery or within 48 hours after delivery, and hospitalized preterm infants with significant varicella exposure (American Academy of Pediatrics, 2015).

Children with hemolytic disease, such as sickle cell disease, are at risk for aplastic anemia from erythema infectiosum. Human parvovirus B19 infects and lyses red blood cell precursors, thus interrupting the production of red blood cells. Therefore the virus may precipitate a severe aplastic crisis in patients who need increased red blood cell production to maintain normal red blood cell volumes. Thrombocytopenia and neutropenia may also occur as a result of human parvovirus B19 infection. The fetus has a relatively high rate of red blood cell production and an immature immune system; it may develop severe anemia and hydrops as a result of maternal human parvovirus infection. Fetal death rates as a result of human parvovirus B19 have been estimated to be between 2% and 6%, with the greatest risk appearing to be in the first 20 weeks (American Academy of Pediatrics, 2015; Koch, 2016).

> **! NURSING ALERT**
>
> Refer children at risk for contracting these communicable diseases to the practitioner immediately in case of known exposure or outbreaks.

In the past decade the incidence of pertussis has increased, particularly in infants less than 6 months old and in children 10 to 14 years of age. Early clinical manifestations of pertussis in infants may include gagging and gasping, followed by posttussive emesis, apnea, and cyanosis; the typical "whoop" associated with the disease is absent (Long, 2016). In older children the disease may manifest as a common cold, but a prolonged cough (at least 21 days) is common in adolescents (Long, 2016) (see Table 6.2). There is now a recommendation that children ages 11 to 12 receive a booster pertussis vaccine (Tdap) to prevent the disease. Because pertussis is contagious, especially among close household members, identify pertussis early and initiate treatment for the child and those who have been exposed. Azithromycin (for infants younger than 1 month old) and erythromycin, clarithromycin, or azithromycin are administered to infants and children with pertussis (American Academy of Pediatrics, 2015).

Prevention of complications from diseases such as diphtheria, pertussis, and scarlet fever requires compliance with antibiotic therapy. With

*Educational materials may be obtained from the National Shingles Foundation, 590 Madison Ave., 21st Floor, New York, NY 10022; 212-222-3390; http://www.vzvfoundation.org.

oral preparations, educate the importance to complete the entire course of therapy. (See Compliance, Chapter 22.)

Evidence suggests that vitamin A supplementation reduces both morbidity and mortality in measles and that all children with severe measles should receive vitamin A supplements. A single oral dose of 200,000 international units for children at least 1 year old is recommended (use half that dose for children 6 to 12 months of age) (see Table 6.2). The higher dose may be associated with vomiting and headache for a few hours. The dose should be repeated the next day and at 4 weeks for children with ophthalmologic evidence of vitamin A deficiency (American Academy of Pediatrics, 2015).

> **! NURSING ALERT**
>
> Although the risk of vitamin A toxicity from these doses (they are 100 to 200 times the recommended dietary allowance) is relatively low, nurses should instruct parents on safe storage of the drug. Ideally, vitamin A should be dispensed in the age-appropriate unit dose to prevent excessive administration and possible toxicity.

Provide Comfort

Many communicable diseases cause skin manifestations that are bothersome to the child. The chief discomfort from most rashes is itching, and measures such as cool baths (usually without soap) and lotions (e.g., calamine) are helpful. Cooling the lotion in the refrigerator beforehand often makes it more soothing on the skin than at room temperature.

> **! NURSING ALERT**
>
> When lotions with active ingredients such as diphenhydramine in Caladryl are used, they are applied sparingly, especially over open lesions, where excessive absorption can lead to drug toxicity. Use these lotions with caution in children who are simultaneously receiving an oral antihistamine.

To avoid overheating, which increases itching, children should wear lightweight, loose, nonirritating clothing and keep out of the sun. If the child persists in scratching, keep the nails short and smooth or use mittens and clothes with long sleeves or legs. For severe itching, antipruritic medication, such as diphenhydramine (Benadryl) or hydroxyzine (Atarax), may be required, especially when the child has trouble sleeping because of itching. Loratadine, cetirizine, and fexofenadine do not cause drowsiness and may be preferred for urticaria during the day.

An elevated temperature is common, and both antipyretic medicine (acetaminophen or ibuprofen) and environmental manipulation are implemented. (See Controlling Elevated Temperatures, Chapter 22.) Acetaminophen is effective in lowering the fever but does not significantly reduce the symptoms of itching, anorexia, abdominal pain, fussiness, or vomiting.

A sore throat, another frequent symptom, is managed with lozenges, saline rinses (if the child is old enough to cooperate), and analgesics. Because most children are anorectic during an illness, bland foods and increased liquids are usually preferred. During the early stages of the disease, children voluntarily curtail their activity, and although bed rest is beneficial, it should not be imposed unless specifically indicated. During periods of irritability, quiet activity (e.g., reading, music, television, video games, puzzles, coloring) helps distract children from the discomfort.

Support Child and Family

Most communicable diseases are benign but may produce considerable concern and anxiety for parents. Often the occurrence of a disease, such as chickenpox, is the first time the child is acutely uncomfortable. Parents need assistance to cope with manifestations of the illness, such as intense itching. The family and child need reassurance that recovery is generally rapid. However, visible signs of the dermatosis may be present for some time after the child is well enough to resume usual activities.

> **! NURSING ALERT**
>
> The occurrence of a communicable disease provides the opportunity to ask parents about the child's immunization status and reinforce the benefits of vaccines for children.

CONJUNCTIVITIS

Acute **conjunctivitis** (inflammation of the conjunctiva) occurs from a variety of causes that are typically age related. In newborns conjunctivitis can occur from infection during birth, most often from *Chlamydia trachomatis* (inclusion conjunctivitis) or *Neisseria gonorrhoeae.* Conjunctivitis in a neonate is a serious condition and can potentially lead to blindness; all signs of conjunctivitis require prompt reporting and a comprehensive evaluation (Olitsky, Hug, Plummer, et al., 2016). The clinical signs of conjunctivitis are similar regardless of the cause: redness and swelling of the conjunctiva, eyelid edema, and discharge (Olitsky, Hug, Plummer, et al., 2016). In infants recurrent conjunctivitis may be a sign of nasolacrimal (tear) duct obstruction or dacryocystitis, an infection of the lacrimal sac. Timing of the infection may provide signs of the cause. A chemical conjunctivitis may occur within 24 hours of instillation of neonatal ophthalmic prophylaxis; *N. gonorrhoeae* usually occurs within 2 to 5 days after birth, and *C. trachomatis* occurs 5 to 14 days after birth (Olitsky, Hug, Plummer, et al., 2016). In children the usual causes of conjunctivitis are viral, bacterial, allergic, or related to a foreign body. Bacterial infection accounts for most instances of acute conjunctivitis in children. Diagnosis is made primarily from the clinical manifestations (Box 6.3), although cultures of purulent drainage may be needed to identify the specific cause.

Therapeutic Management

Treatment of conjunctivitis depends on the cause. Viral conjunctivitis is self-limiting, and treatment is limited to removal of the accumulated secretions. Bacterial conjunctivitis has traditionally been treated with topical antibacterial agents such as polymyxin and bacitracin (Polysporin), sodium sulfacetamide (Sulamyd), or trimethoprim and polymyxin (Polytrim). Infants with bacterial conjunctivitis may require systemic antibiotics (Olitsky, Hug, Plummer, et al., 2016). For children 1 year and older, fluoroquinolones and aminoglycosides are commonly used ophthalmic antimicrobial agents. Fourth-generation fluoroquinolones such as moxifloxacin, gatifloxacin, and besifloxacin provide broad-spectrum coverage, are bactericidal, and are generally well tolerated (Alter, Vidwan, Sobande, et al., 2011). Drops may be used during the day and an ointment at bedtime because the ointment preparation remains in the eye longer but blurs the vision. Corticosteroids are avoided because they reduce ocular resistance to bacteria.

Nursing Care Management

Nursing care includes keeping the eye clean and properly administering ophthalmic medication. Remove accumulated secretions by wiping from

BOX 6.3 Clinical Manifestations of Conjunctivitis

Bacterial Conjunctivitis ("Pink Eye")
Purulent drainage
Crusting of eyelids, especially on awakening
Inflamed conjunctiva
Swollen eyelids

Viral Conjunctivitis
Usually occurs with upper respiratory tract infection
Serous (watery) drainage
Inflamed conjunctiva
Swollen eyelids

Allergic Conjunctivitis
Itching
Watery to thick, stringy discharge
Inflamed conjunctiva
Swollen eyelids

Conjunctivitis Caused by Foreign Body
Tearing
Pain
Inflamed conjunctiva
Usually only one eye affected

the inner canthus downward and outward, away from the opposite eye. Warm, moist compresses, such as a clean washcloth wrung out with hot tap water, are helpful in removing the crusts. Compresses are *not* kept on the eye because an occlusive covering promotes bacterial growth. Instill medication immediately after the eyes have been cleaned and according to correct procedure. (See Chapter 22.)

Prevention of infection in other family members is an important consideration with bacterial conjunctivitis. Keep the child's washcloth and towel separate from those used by others. Discard tissues used to clean the eye. Instruct the child to refrain from rubbing the eye and to use good hand-washing technique.

! NURSING ALERT

Signs of serious conjunctivitis include reduction or loss of vision, ocular pain, photophobia, exophthalmos (bulging eyeball), decreased ocular mobility, corneal ulceration, and unusual patterns of inflammation (e.g., the perilimbal flush associated with iritis or localized inflammation associated with scleritis). If a patient has any of these signs, refer him or her immediately to an ophthalmologist.

STOMATITIS

Stomatitis is inflammation of the oral mucosa, which may include the buccal (cheek) and labial (lip) mucosa, tongue, gingiva, palate, and floor of the mouth. It may be infectious or noninfectious and may be caused by local or systemic factors. In children, aphthous stomatitis and herpetic stomatitis are typically seen. Children with immunosuppression and those receiving chemotherapy or head and neck radiotherapy are at high risk for developing mucosal ulceration and herpetic stomatitis.

Aphthous stomatitis (aphthous ulcer, canker sore) is a benign but painful condition whose cause is unknown. Its onset is usually associated with mild traumatic injury (e.g., biting the cheek, hitting the mucosa with a toothbrush, or a mouth appliance rubbing on the mucosa), allergy, or emotional stress. The lesions are painful, small, whitish ulcerations surrounded by a red border. They are distinguished from other types of stomatitis by healthy adjacent tissues, absence of vesicles, and no systemic illness. The ulcers persist for 4 to 12 days and heal uneventfully.

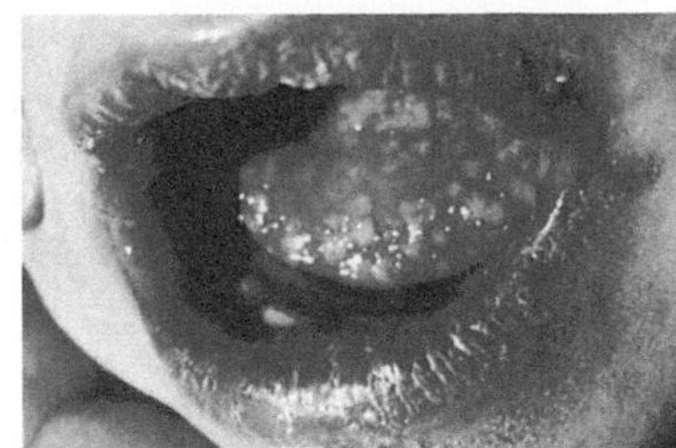

FIG. 6.8 Primary gingivostomatitis. (From Thompson, J. M., McFarland, G. M., Hirsch, J. E., et al. [2002]. *Mosby's clinical nursing* [5th ed.]. St. Louis, MO: Mosby.)

Herpetic gingivostomatitis (HGS) is caused by HSV, most often type 1, and may occur as a primary infection or recur in a less severe form known as recurrent herpes labialis (commonly called *cold sores* or *fever blisters*). The primary infection usually begins with a fever; the pharynx becomes edematous and erythematous; and vesicles erupt on the mucosa, causing severe pain (Fig. 6.8). Cervical lymphadenitis often occurs, and the breath has a distinctly foul odor. In the recurrent form, the vesicles appear on the lips, usually singly or in groups. The precipitating factors for the cold sores include emotional stress, trauma (often related to dental procedures), immunosuppression, or exposure to excessive sunlight. The disease can last 5 to 14 days, with varying degrees of severity.

Stomatitis may occur as a manifestation of hand-foot-and-mouth disease (HFMD) and herpangina; both manifest with scattered vesicles on the buccal mucosa and are commonly caused by the nonpolio enteroviruses (primarily coxsackieviruses). Children with either HFMD or herpangina often have poor intake as a result of the mouth sores; infants may refuse to nurse or take a bottle or may pull away and cry after a few seconds of nursing.

Therapeutic Management

Treatment for all types of stomatitis is aimed at relief of symptoms, primarily pain. Acetaminophen and ibuprofen are usually sufficient for mild cases, but with more severe HGS, stronger analgesics such as codeine may be needed. Topical anesthetics are helpful and include over-the-counter preparations such as Orabase, Anbesol, and Kank-A. Lidocaine (Xylocaine Viscous) can be prescribed for the child who can keep 1 tsp of the solution in the mouth for 2 to 3 minutes and then expectorate the drug. A mixture of equal parts of diphenhydramine elixir and Maalox (aluminum and magnesium hydroxide) provides mild analgesia, antiinflammatory properties, and a protective coating for the lesions. Sucralfate can also be used as a coating agent for oral mucous membranes. Treatment for children with severe cases of HGS includes the use of antiviral agents such as acyclovir (Tinanoff, 2016).

Nursing Care Management

The chief nursing goals for children with stomatitis are relief of pain and prevention of spread of the herpes virus. Analgesics and topical anesthetics are used as needed to provide relief, especially before meals to encourage food and fluid intake. For younger infants and toddlers who cannot swish and swallow, apply the diphenhydramine and Maalox solution with a cotton-tipped applicator before feedings to minimize pain. Educating parents regarding the use of these medications is important to maintain adequate hydration in the child whose mouth is too sore to take liquids. Drinking bland fluids through a straw is helpful in avoiding the painful lesions. Encourage mouth care; the use of a very soft bristle toothbrush or disposable foam-tipped toothbrush provides gentle cleaning near ulcerated areas.

Careful hand washing is essential when caring for children with HGS. Because the infection is autoinoculable, children should keep their fingers out of the mouth; contaminated hands can infect other body parts. Very young children may require elbow restraints to ensure compliance. Articles placed in the mouth are cleaned thoroughly. Newborns and individuals with immunosuppression should not be exposed to infected children.

> **! NURSING ALERT**
>
> When examining herpetic lesions, wear gloves. The virus easily enters breaks in the skin and can cause herpetic whitlow of the fingers.

Because herpes infection is often associated with sexual transmission, explain to parents and older children that HGS is usually caused by type 1 HSV, the type not associated with sexual activity.

ZIKA VIRUS

The Zika virus (ZIKV) was initially discovered almost 70 years ago in the Zika Forrest in Uganda with sporadic outbreaks, but in 2013 occurrences of the virus in Polynesia then spread to various areas of South America leading to a major epidemic by 2016. ZIKV is transmitted to humans primarily via an infected *Aedes* species mosquito bite; however, the virus can also be transferred from mother to child during pregnancy (transplacental) and to others by contact with urine, blood, semen, or vaginal fluid (Centers for Disease Control and Prevention, 2016). There is no current evidence that the Zika virus is in breastmilk, and mothers are encouraged to continue breastfeeding (Centers for Disease Control and Prevention, 2016).

Most infected individuals are asymptomatic but approximately 18% will develop fever, arthralgia, maculopapular rash, or conjunctivitis 3 to 12 days after being infected, with symptoms lasting up to 7 days (Murray, 2016). The most serious manifestations of the ZIKV are fetal brain defects, including microcephaly, that occur in the developing fetus when a pregnant woman contracts the virus (Murray, 2016). Preliminary diagnosis is based on the patient's symptoms and recent travel (Centers for Disease Control and Prevention, 2016). Confirmation of the diagnosis can be made through molecular diagnostic techniques of blood or urine from the individual.

Therapeutic Management

There is no current therapy available to treat ZIKV (Murray, 2016). Provide the patient with supportive care measures including rest, adequate hydration, analgesics, and antipyretics as needed. As with any other viral illness, aspirin and other salicylates should not be administered to children to avoid Reye syndrome (Murray, 2016). Avoiding mosquito bites is the best method to prevent the disease.

Nursing Care Management

Nurses must remain informed about emerging ZIKV developments and educate patients, parents, and caretakers with accurate information. The Centers for Disease Control and Prevention provides thorough and updated information on the virus on its website (https://www.cdc.gov/zika). Resources such as fact sheets, posters, and communication toolkits in several different languages are also available on the website.

Preventing mosquito bites is one of the most effective ways to prevent ZIKV infection. When traveling to areas known to have ZIKV, preventive measures include wearing appropriate clothing to have as little skin exposed as possible, using insect repellent, and using screens on windows and doors or insecticide-treated nets if windows and doors are not available (Murray, 2016). (See insect repellent discussion later in this chapter.)

INTESTINAL PARASITIC DISEASES

Intestinal parasitic diseases, including helminths (worms) and protozoa, constitute the most frequent infections in the world. In the United States the incidence of intestinal parasitic disease, especially giardiasis, has increased among young children who attend day care centers. Young children are especially at risk because of typical hand-to-mouth activity and uncontrolled fecal activity.

Various infecting organisms cause intestinal parasitic diseases in humans. This discussion is limited to the two most common parasitic infections among children in the United States: giardiasis and pinworms. Table 6.3 describes the outstanding features of selected helminths that belong to the family of nematodes.

GENERAL NURSING CARE MANAGEMENT

Nursing responsibilities related to intestinal parasitic infections involve assistance with identification of the parasite, treatment of the infection, and prevention of initial infection or reinfection. Laboratory examination of substances containing the worm, its larvae, or ova can identify the organism. Most are identified by examining fecal smears from the stools of persons suspected of harboring the parasite. Fresh specimens are best for revealing parasites or larvae; therefore take collected specimens directly to the laboratory for examination. If this is not possible, place the specimen in a container with a preservative. Parents need clear instructions on obtaining an adequate sample and the number of samples required (see Stool Specimens, Chapter 22). In most parasitic infections, other family members, especially children, may be examined to identify those who are similarly affected.

After the diagnosis is confirmed and appropriate treatment is planned, parents need further explanation and reinforcement. Compliance in terms of drug therapy and other measures, such as thorough hand washing, is essential for eradication of the parasite. The family needs to understand the nature of transmission and that in some cases the medication must be repeated in 2 weeks to 1 month to kill organisms hatched since initial treatment.

The nurse's most important function is preventive education of children and families regarding hygiene and health habits. Thorough hand washing before eating or handling food and after using the toilet is the most important precautionary method. The Family-Centered Care box lists other preventive practices.

GIARDIASIS

Giardiasis is caused by the protozoan *Giardia intestinalis* (formerly called *Giardia lamblia* and *Giardia duodenalis*). It is the most common intestinal parasitic pathogen in the United States, with an estimated 1.2 million people affected annually (Painter, Gargano, Collier, et al., 2015). Child care centers and institutions providing care for persons with developmental disabilities are common sites for urban giardiasis, and the children may pass cysts for months. Also consider giardiasis in those with a history of recent travel to an endemic area or drinking untreated water.

TABLE 6.3 Selected Intestinal Parasites

Clinical Manifestations	Comments
Ascariasis—*Ascaris lumbricoides* (Common Roundworm)	
Light infections/asymptomatic: Parent may find roundworm in child's diaper with/without stool or see roundworms in the toilet Heavy infections: Anorexia, irritability, nervousness, enlarged abdomen, weight loss, fever, intestinal colic Severe infections: Intestinal obstruction, appendicitis, perforation of intestine with peritonitis, obstructive jaundice, lung involvement (pneumonitis)	Transferred to mouth by way of contaminated food, fingers, or toys (ascaris lays eggs in soil, which children play in) No person-to-person transmission Largest of the intestinal helminths Affects principally young children 1-4 years of age Prevalent in warm climates Treatment with albendazole (single dose); OR mebendazole for 3 days; OR oral ivermectin (children >15 kg) as a single dose; OR nitazoxanide for 3 days Reexamine stool specimen in 2 weeks to establish need for further pharmacologic therapy (American Academy of Pediatrics, 2015).
Hookworm—Necator Americanus and Ancylostoma Americanalis	
Light infections in well-nourished individuals: No problems Heavier infections: Mild to severe hypochromic, microcytic anemia, malnutrition, hypoproteinemia and edema May be itching and burning followed by erythema and a papular eruption in areas to which the organism migrates	Transmitted by discharging eggs on the soil, which are picked up by human host, commonly in the feet, causing infection from direct skin contact with contaminated soil Recommend wearing shoes, although children playing in contaminated soil expose many skin surfaces Diagnosis established by presence of hookworm eggs in stool (humans are the only host of hookworms) Treat with albendazole, mebendazole, and pyrantel pamoate
Strongyloidiasis—*Strongyloides Stercoralis* (Threadworm)	
Light infection: Asymptomatic Heavy infection: Respiratory signs and symptoms; abdominal pain, distention; nausea and vomiting; diarrhea (large, pale stools, often with mucus) Larva migration manifests as pruritic skin lesions in the perianal area, buttocks, and upper thighs, creating serpiginous, erythematous tracks called *larva currens* (American Academy of Pediatrics, 2015) Life threatening in children with weakened immunologic defenses	Transmission is same as for hookworm except autoinfection common; humans are hosts, but cats, dogs, and other animals may also be hosts for the threadworm Older children and adults affected more often than young children Severe infections may lead to severe nutritional deficiency Diagnosis: often difficult; several stool specimens may be required Treat with oral ivermectin (preferred); OR thiabendazole and albendazole (both less effective than oral ivermectin)
Visceral Larva Migrans—*Toxocara Canis* (Dogs) (Roundworm)	
Intestinal Toxocariasis—*Toxocara Cati* (Cats) (Roundworm)	
Depends on reactivity of infected individual May be asymptomatic except for eosinophilia or pulmonary wheezing Specific diagnosis difficult Visceral toxocariasis: Fever, leukocytosis, eosinophilia, hepatomegaly, and hypogammaglobulinemia, malaise, anemia, cough (American Academy of Pediatrics, 2015) Ocular invasion may occur Rarely pneumonia, myocarditis, encephalitis	Transmitted by direct contamination of hands from contact with soil or contaminated objects; less commonly by direct contact with dog or cat More common in children or adults with pica Keep dogs and cats away from areas where children play; sandboxes especially important transmission areas; more common in hot, humid regions Hand washing is imperative in children playing in soil or around domestic animals such as cats and dogs Periodic deworming of diagnosed dogs and cats Control of dog and cat population Diagnosis: hypergammaglobulinemia and hypereosinophilia; increased titers of anti-A or anti-B blood group antigens; liver biopsy in some cases Treatment: albendazole; specific symptoms may require additional treatment
Trichuriasis—*Trichuris Trichiura* (Whipworm or Human Whipworm)	
Light infections: Asymptomatic Heavy infections: Abdominal pain and distention, diarrhea; failure to thrive, impaired cognitive development; stools may have mucus, water, and blood	Transmitted from contaminated soil, fruit, vegetables, toys, and other objects Most frequent in warm, moist climates Occurs most often in undernourished children living in unsanitary conditions where human feces is not disposed of properly. Diagnosis by microscopic examination of stool specimen Treat with albendazole, mebendazole, or oral ivermectin

FAMILY-CENTERED CARE

Preventing Intestinal Parasitic Disease

- Always wash hands and fingernails with soap and water before eating and handling food and after toileting.
- Avoid placing fingers in mouth and biting nails.
- Discourage children from scratching bare anal area.
- Use superabsorbent disposable diapers to prevent leakage.
- Change diapers as soon as soiled and dispose of diapers in closed receptacle out of children's reach.
- Do not rinse cloth or disposable diapers in toilet.
- Disinfect toilet seats and diaper-changing areas; use dilute household bleach (10% solution) or ammonia (Lysol) and wipe clean with paper towels.
- Drink only treated water or bottled water, especially if camping.
- Wash all raw fruits and vegetables and food that have fallen on the floor.
- Avoid growing foods in soil fertilized with human or untreated animal excreta.
- Teach children to defecate only in a toilet, not on the ground.
- Keep dogs and cats away from playgrounds and sandboxes.
- Avoid swimming in pools frequented by diapered children.
- Wear shoes outside.

The potential for transmission is great because the cysts—the nonmotile stage of the protozoa—can survive in the environment for months. Chief modes of transmission are person to person, food, and animals. Contaminated water, especially in lakes and streams, and swimming or wading pools frequented by diapered infants are common sources of transmission (Painter, Gargano, Collier, et al., 2015). In children, person-to-person transmission is the most likely cause. Although individuals infected with giardiasis may be asymptomatic, common symptoms include abdominal cramps, bloating, and diarrhea (Box 6.4).

Diagnosis of giardiasis may be made by microscopic examination of stool specimens or duodenal fluid or by identification of *G. intestinalis* antigens in these specimens by techniques such as enzyme immunoassay (EIA) and direct fluorescence antibody (DFA) assays. Because the *Giardia* organisms live in the upper intestine and are excreted in a highly variable pattern, repeated microscopic examination of stool specimens may be required to identify trophozoites (active parasites) or cysts. Duodenal specimens are obtained by direct aspiration, biopsy, or the string test. In the string test, the child swallows a gelatin capsule with a nylon string attached. Several hours later, the string is withdrawn, and the contents are sent for laboratory analysis. With the availability of EIA techniques to identify *Giardia* antigens in stool specimens, other tests are being used less often.

BOX 6.4 Clinical Manifestations of Giardiasis

Infants and young children:
- Diarrhea
- Vomiting
- Anorexia
- Failure to thrive—if chronic exposure

Children older than 5 years of age:
- Abdominal cramps
- Intermittent loose stools
- Constipation
- Stools that are malodorous, watery, pale, and greasy
- Spontaneous resolution of most infections in 4 to 6 weeks

Rare, chronic form:
- Intermittent loose, foul-smelling stools
- Possibility of abdominal bloating, flatulence, sulfur-tasting belches, epigastric pain, vomiting, headache, and weight loss

Therapeutic Management

The drugs of choice for treatment of giardiasis are metronidazole (Flagyl), tinidazole (Tindamax), and nitazoxanide (Alinia). Tinidazole is said to have an 80% to 100% cure rate after a single dose (American Academy of Pediatrics, 2015). Metronidazole and tinidazole have a metallic taste and gastrointestinal side effects, including nausea and vomiting. Nitazoxanide does not have a bitter taste and should be taken with food to avoid gastrointestinal symptoms; it reportedly has very few adverse effects and is available in suspension form. Alternative drug therapy includes albendazole, furazolidone, and quinacrine (John, 2016). Quinacrine is only available from a compounding pharmacy.

The most important nursing consideration is prevention of giardiasis and education of parents, child care center staff, and others who assume the daily care of small children. Attention to meticulous sanitary practices, especially during diaper changes, is essential (see Family-Centered Care box and Fig. 6.9). Nurses can play an important role in educating parents of small children and day care staff regarding appropriate sanitation practices. In addition, discourage young children who are infected or who have diarrhea from swimming in community or private pools until they have been infection free for 2 weeks (American Academy of Pediatrics, 2015). Lakes and streams may contain high numbers of *Giardia* spore cysts, which can be swallowed in the water. Discourage children from swimming in stagnant bodies of water and in water where there are known infected children swimming when there is a high chance of swallowing water. *Giardia* organisms are resistant to chlorine (Painter, Gargano, Collier, et al., 2015). Encourage parents to take small children to the restroom frequently when swimming, avoid letting children in diapers in swimming areas, and change diapers away from the water source. (See also Centers for Disease Control and Prevention information on recreational water illnesses, http://www.cdc.gov/

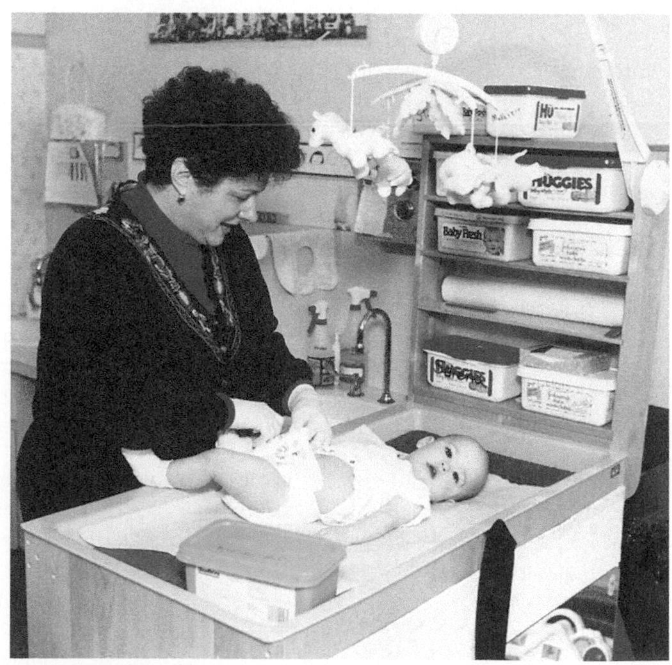

FIG. 6.9 Prevention of giardiasis, especially in day care centers, requires sanitary practices during diaper changes, such as discarding paper diapers in a covered receptacle, changing paper covers on the diaper-changing surface, and having facilities for hand washing nearby. Note: Soiled cloth diapers and clothing should be stored in a plastic bag for transport home.

BOX 6.5 Clinical Manifestations of Pinworms

Intense perianal itching is the principal symptom. Evidence of itching in young children includes the following:

- General irritability
- Restlessness
- Poor sleep
- Bed-wetting
- Distractibility
- Short attention span
- Perianal dermatitis and excoriation secondary to itching
- If worms migrate, possible vaginal (vulvovaginitis) and urethral infection

healthywater/swimming.) After children are infected, family education regarding drug administration is essential.

ENTEROBIASIS (PINWORMS)

Enterobiasis, or pinworms, caused by the nematode *Enterobius vermicularis,* is the most common helminthic infection in the United States. It is universally present in temperate climatic zones and may infect more than 30% of all children at any one time. Transmission is favored in crowded conditions, such as in classrooms and day care centers. Infection begins when the eggs are ingested or inhaled (the eggs float in the air). The eggs hatch in the upper intestine and then mature and migrate through the intestine. After mating, adult females migrate out the anus and lay eggs (American Academy of Pediatrics, 2015). The movement of the worms on skin and mucous membrane surfaces causes intense itching. As the child scratches, eggs are deposited on the hands and underneath the fingernails. The typical hand-to-mouth activity of young children makes them especially prone to reinfection. Pinworm eggs persist in the indoor environment for 2 to 3 weeks, contaminating anything they contact, such as toilet seats, doorknobs, bed linen, underwear, and food. Except for the intense rectal itching associated with pinworms, the clinical manifestations are nonspecific (Box 6.5).

Diagnostic Evaluation

Diagnosis is most commonly made from the tape test (see Nursing Care Management). Repeated tests to collect eggs may be necessary (3 consecutive days in the early morning before the child washes are recommended for testing [American Academy of Pediatrics, 2015]), and if there is a possibility that other family members may be infected, a tape test should be performed on them.

Therapeutic Management

The drugs available for treatment of pinworms include pyrantel pamoate (Pin-Rid, Antiminth) and albendazole. Mebendazole is not recommended for children younger than 2 years of age. Because pinworms are easily transmitted, all household members should be treated. The dose of antiparasitic medication should be repeated in 2 weeks to completely eradicate the parasite and prevent reinfection.

Nursing Care Management

Direct nursing care at identifying the parasite, eradicating the organism, and preventing reinfection. Parents need clear, detailed instructions for the tape test. A loop of transparent (not "frosted" or "magic") tape, sticky side out, is placed around the end of a tongue depressor, which is then firmly pressed against the child's perianal area. A convenient, commercially prepared tape is also available for this purpose. Pinworm specimens are collected in the morning as soon as the child awakens and *before* the child has a bowel movement or bathes. The procedure may need to be performed on 3 or more consecutive days before eggs are collected. Parents are instructed to place the tongue blade in a glass jar or loosely in a plastic bag so it can be brought in for microscopic examination. For specimens collected in the hospital, practitioner's office, or clinic, place the tape smoothly on a glass slide, sticky side down, for examination.

Adherence to the drug regimen is usually excellent because only one or two doses are needed. The family should be reminded of the need to take a second dose in 2 weeks to ensure eradication of the eggs.

To prevent reinfection, washing all clothes and bed linens in hot water and vacuuming the house may be recommended. However, there is little documentation on the effectiveness of these measures because pinworms survive on many surfaces. Helpful suggestions include hand washing after toileting and before eating, keeping the child's fingernails short to minimize the chance of ova collecting under the nails, dressing children in one-piece sleeping outfits, and daily showering rather than tub bathing. Inform families that recurrence is common. Treat repeated infections in the same manner as the first one.

BEDBUGS

Bedbugs are classified as insects, and the most common types seen are *Cimex lectularis* (common bedbug) and *Cimex hemipterus* (tropical bedbug). Although once considered to be practically nonexistent in the United States, these parasites have reemerged and are increasing by 100% to 500% annually (Lai, Ho, Glick, et al., 2016). Bedbugs are troublesome because they are difficult to diagnose and among the most challenging pests to eradicate. Mention is made herein primarily because of the secondary health problems that may occur as a result of their bites: infection, cellulitis, folliculitis, intense urticaria, impetigo, anaphylactic reaction, and sleep loss. However, in some cases the person may be asymptomatic (McMenaman & Gausche-Hill, 2016).

Bedbugs undergo various life stages, but the small ones are approximately 5 mm in length and are light yellow; once the bedbugs "feed" on blood, they enlarge and become reddish-brown. They tend to inhabit warm, dark areas such as bed mattresses, sofas, and other furniture and emerge at night to feed. Although there is speculation of bedbugs being vectors to transmit other dieases, there is currently no evidence that bedbugs are associated with disease transmission (Lai, Ho, Glick, et al., 2016).

The clinical manifestations of bedbug bites are outlined in Box 6.6. The cutaneous manifestations of bedbug bites tend to be primarily on arms, legs, and trunk areas.

The treatment of bedbugs should focus on proper identification, treatment of the symptoms, and eradication. Bedbugs can be identified on bedding at night because of their nighttime activity. They tend to hide in dark crevices (e.g., floor, walls, furniture) during the daytime and do not stay on the human host. Contrary to several myths, bedbugs do not fly or jump. It is not uncommon for bedbug bites to be misdiagnosed as scabies, chickenpox, spider or mosquito bites, and even food anaphylaxis in some cases. There is no specific treatment for bedbugs; topical steroids and systemic antihistamines may be used to treat the urticaria. Secondary skin infections are treated with antibiotics as described previously in this chapter. Eradication of bedbugs is complex and must be handled by professional exterminators; multiple chemical applications are often required to completely eradicate the insects. Suggestions for minimizing exposure when traveling include inspecting the mattresses for signs of infestation; encasing mattress covers may be helpful. Thorough washing of all clothing and bed linens may also help minimize exposure. The use of pesticides and various other control measures is discussed in Bennett, Gondhalekar, Wang, et al. (2016).

BOX 6.6 Clinical Manifestations of Bedbugs

Cutaneous Reactions
- Erythematous papule
- Linear papules
- Red macular lesion
- Rash
- Wheal
- Vesicles
- Bullae
- Urticaria

Secondary
- Impetiginous lesions with scratching
- Folliculitis
- Cellulitis
- Eczematoid dermatitis

Systemic Reactions
- Asthma exacerbation
- Anaphylaxis
- Fever and malaise (chronic exposure)

Data from Doggett, S. L., Dwyer, D., Peñas, P. F., et al. (2012). Bed bugs: Clinical relevance and control options. *Clin Microbiol Rev, 25*(1), 164-192; Haisley-Royster, C. (2011). Cutaneous infestations and infections. *Adolesc Med State Art Rev, 22*(1), 129-145.

NCLEX REVIEW QUESTIONS

1. Which of the following should be used in the care of all pediatric patients to reduce the risk of transmission of microorganisms from both recognized and unrecognized sources of infection?
   A. Transmission-Based Precautions
   B. Airborne Precautions
   C. Standard Precautions
   D. Droplet Precautions
2. Which childhood vaccine provides some protection against bacterial meningitis, epiglottitis, and bacterial pneumonia?
   A. Hib vaccine
   B. Hepatitis B vaccine
   C. Varicella vaccine
   D. Influenza vaccine
3. Which vaccine do the Centers for Disease Control and Prevention (CDC) and American College of Obstetricians and Gynecologists recommend that pregnant adolescents and women who are not protected against pertussis receive optimally between 27 and 36 weeks of gestation or postpartum before discharge from the hospital?
   A. DTaP
   B. Td
   C. IPV
   D. Tdap
4. Which childhood vaccine provides protection against streptococcal infections such as otitis media, sinusitis, and pneumonia?
   A. Rotavirus
   B. Hib
   C. Pneumococcal
   D. MMR
5. One of the most common intestinal parasitic pathogens in the United States acquired from a contaminated water source such as a lake or swimming pool is:
   A. Tinea capitis
   B. *Giardia intestinalis*
   C. Pediculosis capitis
   D. Enterobiasis

Correct Answers

1. C; 2. A; 3. D; 4. C; 5. B

REFERENCES

Alter, S. J., Vidwan, N. K., Sobande, P. O., et al. (2011). Common childhood bacterial infections. *Current Problems in Pediatric and Adolescent Health Care, 41*(10), 256–283.

American Academy of Pediatrics. (2013). Recommended childhood and adolescent immunization schedule—United States, 2013. *Pediatrics, 131*(2), 397–398.

American Academy of Pediatrics, Committee on Infectious Diseases (2015). L. Pickering (Ed.), *2015 red book: Report of the committee on infectious diseases* (30th ed.). Elk Grove Village, Ill: The Academy.

American Academy of Pediatrics, Committee on Infectious Diseases. (2016). Recommendations for prevention and control of influenza in children, 2016-2017. *Pediatrics, 138*, 1–20.

Beirne, P. V., Hennessy, S., Cadogan, S. L., et al. (2015). Needle size for vaccination procedures in children and adolescents. *Cochrane Database of Systematic Reviews*, (6), CD010720.

Belongia, E. A., Karron, R. A., Reingold, A., et al. (2017). The Advisory Committee on Immunization Practices recommendation regarding the use of live influenza vaccine: A rejoinder. *Vaccine*, epub ahead of print.

Bennett, G. W., Gondhalekar, A. D., Wang, C., et al. (2016). Using research and education to implement practical bed bug control programs in multifamily housing. *Pest Management Science, 72*, 8–14.

Blain, A. E., Lewis, M., Banerjee, E., et al. (2016). An assessment of the cocooning strategy for preventing infant pertussis – United States, 2011. *Clinical Infectious Diseases, 63*(suppl. 4), S221–S226.

Bolon, M. K. (2016). Hand hygiene: An update. *Infectious Disease Clinics of North America, 30*, 591–607.

Centers for Disease Control and Prevention. (2013a). Updated recommendations for use of tetanus toxoid, reduced diphtheria toxoid and acellular pertussis vaccine (Tdap) in pregnant women—Advisory Committee on Immunization Practices (ACIP), 2012. *MMWR. Morbidity and Mortality Weekly Report, 62*(7), 131–135.

Centers for Disease Control and Prevention. (2013b). Prevention of measles, rubella, congenital rubella syndrome, and mumps, 2013: Summary recommendations of the Advisory Committee on Immunization Practices (ACIP). *MMWR. Recommendations and Reports: Morbidity and Mortality Weekly Report. Recommendations and Reports, 62*(4), 1–25.

Centers for Disease Control and Prevention. (2015). Use of serogroup B meningococcal vaccines in adolescents and young adults: Recommendations of the Advisory Committee on Immunization Practices, 2015. *MMWR. Morbidity and Mortality Weekly Report, 64*(41), 1171–1176.

Centers for Disease Control and Prevention. (2016). *Human papillomavirus (HPV)*. Obtained from https://www.cdc.gov/hpv/.

Centers for Disease Control and Prevention. (2016). *Zika virus*. Retrieved from https://www.cdc.gov/zika/.

Coyer, S. M. (2002). Understanding parental concerns about immunizations. *Journal of Pediatric Health Care, 16*(4), 193–196.

de Martino, M. (2016). Dismantling the taboo against vaccines in pregnancy. *International Journal of Molecular Sciences, 17*, 1–8.

DeStefano, F., Price, C. S., & Weintraub, E. S. (2013). Increasing exposure to antibody-stimulating proteins and polysaccharides in vaccines is not associated with risk of autism. *The Journal of Pediatrics, 163*(2), 561–567.

Diggle, L., & Deeks, J. (2000). Effect of needle length on incidence of local reactions to routine immunizations in infants aged 4 months: Randomized controlled trial. *BMJ (Clinical Research Ed.), 321*(7266), 931–993.

Diggle, L., Deeks, J. J., & Pollard, A. J. (2006). Effect of needle size and immunogenecity and reactogenecity of vaccines in infants: A randomized controlled trial. *BMJ (Clinical Research Ed.), 333*(7568), 571.

Fallah, R., Gholami, H., Ferdosian, F., et al. (2016). Evaluation of vaccines injection order on pain score of intramuscular injection of diphtheria, whole cell pertussis and tetanus vaccine. *Indian Journal of Pediatrics, 83*, 1405–1409.

Fredrickson, D. D., Davis, T. C., Arnold, C. L., et al. (2004). Childhood immunization refusal: Provider and parent perceptions. *Family Medicine, 36*(6), 431–438.

Halperin, B. A., Halperin, S. A., McGrath, P., et al. (2002). Use of lidocaine-prilocaine patch decrease intramuscular injection pain does not adversely affect the antibody response to diptheria-tetanus-acellular pertussis-inactivated poliovirus-Haemophilus influenzae type B conjugate and hepatitis B vaccines in infants form birth to 6 months of age. *Pediatric Infectious Disease, 21*(5), 399–405.

Institute of Medicine (2004). *Immunization safety review: Vaccines and autism*. Washington, DC: National Academies Press.

Ipp, M., Parkin, P. C., Lear, N., et al. (2009). Order of vaccine injection and infant pain response. *Archives of Pediatrics and Adolescent Medicine, 163*(5), 469–472.

Jackson, L. A., Yu, O., Nelson, J. C., et al. (2011). Injection site and risk of medically attended local reactions to acellular pertussis vaccine. *Pediatrics, 127*(3), e681–e687.

John, C. C. (2016). Giardia lamblia. In R. M. Kliegman, B. F. Stanton, J. W. St. Geme, et al. (Eds.), *Nelson textbook of pediatrics* (20th ed.). Philadelphia: Saunders/Elsevier.

Koch, W. C. (2016). Parvoviruses. In R. M. Kliegman, B. F. Stanton, J. W. St Geme, et al. (Eds.), *Nelson textbook of pediatrics* (20th ed.). Philadelphia: Saunders/Elsevier.

Lai, O., Ho, D., Glick, S., et al. (2016). Bed bugs and possible transmission of human pathogens: A systematic review. *Archives of Dermatological Research, 308*, 531–538.

Long, S. S. (2016). Pertussis. In R. M. Kliegman, B. F. Stanton, J. W. St. Geme, et al. (Eds.), *Nelson textbook of pediatrics* (20th ed.). Philadelphia: Saunders.

Marchetti, A., & Rossiter, R. (2013). Economic burden of healthcare-associated infection in US acute care hospitals: Societal perspective. *Journal of Medical Economics, 16*, 1399–1404.

McMenaman, K. S., & Gausche-Hill, M. (2016). Cimex lectularius ("Bed Bugs") recognition, management, and eradication. *Pediatric Emergency Care, 32*, 801–806.

Murray, J. S. (2016). Understanding zika virus. *Journal for Specialists in Pediatric Nursing, 109*, 2016.

National Childhood Vaccine Injury Act: 42 U.S.C. Sec 300aa-1 to 300aa-34, Rockville, Md, 1986, Public Health Service.

Olitsky, S. E., Hug, D., Plummer, L. S., et al. (2016). Disorders of the conjunctiva. In R. M. Kliegman, B. F. Stanton, J. W. St. Geme, et al. (Eds.), *Nelson textbook of pediatrics* (20th ed.). Philadelphia: Saunders.

Painter, J. E., Gargano, J. W., Collier, S. A., et al. (2015). Giardiasis surveillance – United States, 2011-2012. *MMWR Supplements, 64*(3), 15–25.

Rishovd, A. (2014). Pediatric intramuscular injections: Guidelines for best practice. *MCN. The American Journal of Maternal Child Nursing, 39*, 107–112.

Rosenthal, M. (2004). Bacterial colonization, hyperresponsive immune systems conspire in eczema: Diagnosing dermatological disorders. *Infectious Diseases in Children, 17*(3), 47–48.

Tangherlini, T. R., Roychowdhury, V., Glenn, B., et al. (2016). "Mommy blogs" and the vaccination exemption narrative: Results from a machine-learning approach for story aggregation on parenting social media sites. *JMIR Public Health and Surveillance, 2*, 1–15.

Tinanoff, N. (2016). Common lesions of the oral soft tissues. In R. M. Kliegman, B. F. Stanton, J. W. St. Geme, et al. (Eds.), *Nelson textbook of pediatrics* (20th ed.). Philadelphia: Saunders.

World Health Organization. (2015). Reducing pain at the time of vaccination: WHO position paper – September 2015. *World Health Organization Weekly Epidemiological Record, 39*, 505–516.

Yoshimasu, K., Kiyohara, C., Takemura, S., et al. (2014). A meta-analysis of the evidence on the impact of prenatal and early infancy exposures to mercury on autism and attention deficit/hyperactivity disorder in the childhood. *Neurotoxicology, 44*, 121–131.

7 Health Promotion of the Newborn and Family

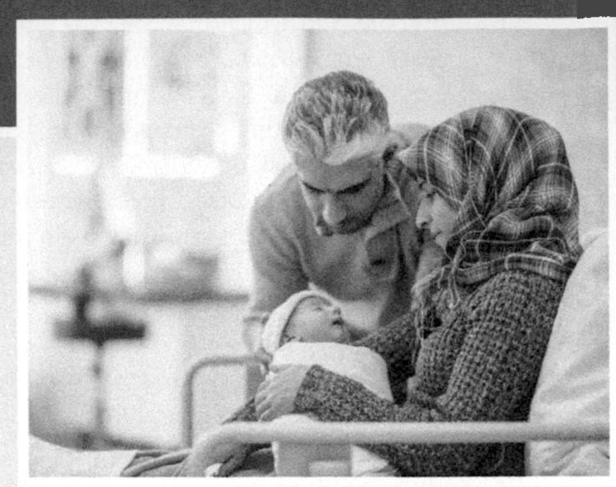

Barbara J. Wheeler

http://evolve.elsevier.com/wong/ncic

CONCEPTS

- Perfusion
- Thermoregulation

ADJUSTMENT TO EXTRAUTERINE LIFE

The most profound physiologic change required of the newborn is transition from fetal or placental circulation to independent respiration. The loss of the placental connection means the loss of complete metabolic support, particularly the supply of oxygen and the removal of carbon dioxide. The normal stresses of labor and delivery cause alterations in placental gas exchange patterns, acid-base balance in the blood, and cardiovascular activity in the neonate. Factors that interfere with normal transition or that interfere with fetal oxygenation (including conditions such as hypoxemia, hypercapnia, and acidosis) will affect the fetus's adjustment to extrauterine life.

IMMEDIATE ADJUSTMENTS

Respiratory System

The most critical and immediate physiologic change required of the newborn is the onset of breathing. The stimuli that help initiate respiration are primarily chemical and thermal. Chemical factors in the blood (low oxygen, high carbon dioxide, and low pH) initiate impulses that excite the respiratory center in the medulla. The primary thermal stimulus is the sudden chilling of the infant, who leaves a warm environment and enters a relatively cooler atmosphere. This abrupt change in temperature excites sensory impulses in the skin that are transmitted to the respiratory center. Tactile stimulation may assist in initiating respiration. Descent through the birth canal and normal handling during delivery, such as drying the skin, help stimulate respiration in uncompromised infants. Acceptable methods of tactile stimulation include slapping or flicking the soles of the feet or gently rubbing the newborn's back, trunk, or extremities (American Academy of Pediatrics, 2016a). Slapping the newborn's buttocks or back is a harmful technique and should not be done. Prolonged tactile stimulation, beyond one or two slaps or flicks to the soles of the feet or rubbing the back once or twice, can waste precious time in the event of respiratory difficulty and can cause additional damage in infants who have become hypoxemic before or during the birth process.

The initial entry of air into the lungs is opposed by the surface tension of the fluid that filled the fetal lungs and alveoli. Some fetal lung fluid is removed during the normal forces of labor and delivery. As the chest emerges from the birth canal, fluid is squeezed from the lungs through the nose and mouth. After complete emergence of the neonate's chest, a brisk recoil of the thorax occurs. Air enters the upper airway to replace the lost fluid. In cesarean birth the chest is not compressed, and the newborn may need additional respiratory support or monitoring until remaining fetal lung fluid is absorbed by the pulmonary capillaries and lymphatic vessels.

In the alveoli the fluid's surface tension is reduced by **surfactant**, a substance produced by the alveolar epithelium that coats the alveolar surface. Chapter 9 discusses the effect of surfactant in facilitating breathing in relation to respiratory distress syndrome.

Circulatory System

As important as the initiation of respiration are the circulatory changes that allow blood to flow through the lungs. These changes occur more gradually and are the result of pressure changes in the lungs, heart, and major vessels. The transition from fetal circulation to postnatal circulation involves the functional closure of the **fetal shunts**: the foramen ovale, the ductus arteriosus, and eventually the ductus venosus. (For a brief review of fetal circulation, see Chapter 27)

Once the lungs are expanded, the inspired oxygen dilates the pulmonary vessels, which decreases pulmonary vascular resistance and consequently increases pulmonary blood flow. As the lungs receive blood, the pressure in the right atrium, right ventricle, and pulmonary arteries decreases. At the same time, there is a progressive rise in systemic vascular resistance and an increased volume of blood as a result of cord clamping. This increases the pressure in the left side of the heart. Because blood flows from an area of high pressure to one of low pressure, the circulation of blood through the fetal shunts is reversed (see Fig. 27.2).

The most important factor controlling ductal closure is the increased oxygen concentration of the blood. Secondary factors are the fall in endogenous prostaglandins and acidosis. The foramen ovale closes functionally at or soon after birth from compression of the two portions of the atrial septum. The ductus arteriosus is closed functionally by the fourth day in well neonates, but closure may be delayed in ill or preterm infants. Anatomic closure from deposition of fibrin and cell products takes considerably longer. Because of the reversible flow of blood through the ductus arteriosus during the early neonatal period, a functional murmur is occasionally heard.

PHYSIOLOGIC STATUS OF OTHER SYSTEMS

Thermoregulation

Next to establishing respiration, heat regulation is most critical to the newborn's survival. Although the newborn's capacity for heat production is adequate, several factors predispose the newborn to excessive heat loss. First, the newborn's large surface area relative to his or her weight facilitates heat loss to the environment. The newborn's large body surface is partially compensated for by a usual position of flexion, which decreases the amount of surface area exposed to the environment.

The second factor that contributes to loss of body heat is the newborn's thin layer of subcutaneous fat. Because core body temperature is approximately 1°F (~0.5°C) higher than surface body temperature, this temperature gradient (difference) causes a heat transfer from a higher to lower temperature.

A third factor is the newborn's mechanism for producing heat. Unlike the child or adult, who can increase heat production through shivering, the chilled neonate cannot shiver but produces heat through nonshivering thermogenesis (NST). NST (or chemical thermogenesis) is produced by stimulating cellular respiration, resulting in increased need for oxygen and glucose (see Thermoregulation, Chapter 9). A thermogenic source, once believed to be unique to the full-term newborn, is brown adipose tissue (BAT), or brown fat, which owes its name to its larger content of mitochondrial cytochromes. BAT has a greater capacity for heat production through intensified metabolic activity than does ordinary adipose tissue. Heat generated in the brown fat is distributed to other parts of the body by the blood, which is warmed as it flows through the layers of this tissue. Superficial deposits of brown fat are located between the scapulae, around the neck, in the axillae, and behind the sternum. Deeper layers surround the kidneys, trachea, esophagus, some major arteries, and adrenals. The location of the brown fat may explain why the nape of the neck often feels warmer than the rest of the body.

Because of these factors predisposing infants to loss of body heat, it is essential that newly born infants are quickly dried and either placed skin-to-skin with their mothers after delivery and covered with a blanket, or, if that is not possible, wrapped with warm, dry blankets.

Although concern is usually for newborns' ability to conserve heat, they may also have difficulty dissipating heat in an overheated environment, increasing the risk of hyperthermia.

Hematopoietic System

The blood volume of the newborn depends largely on the amount of blood transferred via the placenta before clamping of the cord. The blood volume of the full-term infant is about 80 to 85 ml/kg of body weight. Immediately after birth, the total blood volume averages 300 ml, but, depending on how long cord clamping is delayed, or if cord is milked, as much as 100 ml may be added to the blood volume (Rabe, Jewison, Alvarez, et al., 2011).

Fluid and Electrolyte Balance

Changes occur in the total body water volume, extracellular fluid volume, and intracellular fluid volume during the transition from fetal to postnatal life. The fetus is composed almost entirely of water early in gestation and at term is 73% fluid, compared with 58% in the adult. The fetus has more extracellular fluid than intracellular fluid, but this shifts progressively throughout postnatal life, probably because of the growth of cells at the expense of extracellular fluid.

An important aspect of fluid balance is its relationship to other systems. The infant's rate of metabolism is twice that of an adult in relation to body weight. As a result, more acid is formed, leading to more rapid development of acidemia. In addition, the immature kidneys cannot sufficiently concentrate urine to conserve body water. These three factors make the infant more prone to dehydration, acidosis, and overhydration.

Gastrointestinal System

The newborn's ability to digest, absorb, and metabolize food is adequate but limited in certain functions. Enzymes are available to catalyze proteins and simple carbohydrates (monosaccharides and disaccharides), but deficient production of pancreatic amylase impairs utilization of complex carbohydrates (polysaccharides). A deficiency of pancreatic lipase limits the absorption of fats, especially with ingestion of foods that have high saturated fatty acid content, such as cow's milk. Human milk, despite its high fat content, is easy to digest and absorb because it contains enzymes such as lipase, which assist in digestion.

The liver is the most immature of the gastrointestinal organs. The activity of the enzyme glucuronyl transferase is reduced, affecting the conjugation of bilirubin with glucuronic acid, which contributes to physiologic jaundice of the newborn. The liver is also deficient in forming plasma proteins, which likely plays a role in the edema usually seen at birth. Prothrombin and other coagulation factors are also low. The liver stores less glycogen at birth than later in life. Consequently, the newborn is prone to hypoglycemia, which may be prevented by early and effective feeding, ideally breastfeeding.

Some salivary glands are functioning at birth, but the majority do not begin to secrete saliva until about age 2 to 3 months, when drooling is common. Newborn stomach capacity is difficult to determine; however, Bergman (2013) reviewed six published studies exploring this, concluding that stomach capacity is about 20 ml at birth, thus the infant requires frequent small feedings. Newborns who breastfeed usually have more frequent feedings and more frequent stools than infants who receive formula.

The infant's intestine is longer in relation to body size than that in the adult. Therefore it has a proportionately larger number of secretory glands and a larger surface area for absorption compared with the adult's intestine. Rapid peristaltic waves and simultaneous nonperistaltic waves occur along the entire intestine. These waves, called the migrating motor complex (MMC), propel nutrients forward. The relative immaturity of the MMC, combined with decreased lower esophageal sphincter (LES) pressure, inappropriate relaxation of the LES, and delayed gastric emptying, makes regurgitation a common occurrence. Progressive changes in the stooling pattern indicate a properly functioning gastrointestinal tract (Box 7.1).

Renal System

All structural components are present in the renal system, but the kidney has a functional deficiency in its ability to concentrate urine and to cope with fluid and electrolyte fluctuations, such as dehydration or a concentrated solute load.

BOX 7.1 Change in Stooling Patterns of Newborns

Meconium

This is the infant's first stool, composed of amniotic fluid and its constituents, intestinal secretions, shed mucosal cells, and possibly blood (ingested maternal blood or minor bleeding of alimentary tract vessels).

Passage of meconium occurs within the first 24 hours for the vast majority of newborns, although it is delayed in premature infants.

Transitional Stools

These usually appear by the third day after initiation of feeding.

They are greenish brown to yellowish-brown, thin, and less sticky than meconium and may contain some milk curds.

Milk Stools

These usually appear by the fourth day.

In breastfed infants stools are yellow to golden, are pasty in consistency, and have an odor similar to that of sour milk.

In formula-fed infants stools are pale yellow to light brown, are firmer in consistency, and have a more offensive odor.

Total volume of urinary output per 24 hours is about 200 to 300 ml by the end of the first week. The bladder involuntarily empties when stretched by a volume of 15 ml, resulting in as many as 20 voidings per day. The first voiding should occur within 24 hours. The urine is colorless and odorless and has a specific gravity of approximately 1.020.

Integumentary System

At birth all the structures within the skin are present, but many of the functions of the integument are immature. The two layers of the skin, the epidermis and dermis, are loosely bound to each other and are very thin. Rete pegs, which later in life anchor the epidermis to the dermis, are not developed. Slight friction across the epidermis, such as from rapid removal of tape, can cause separation of these layers and blister formation or loss of the epidermis. In full-term infants the transitional zone between the cornified and living layers of the epidermis is effective in preventing fluid from reaching the skin surface.

The sebaceous glands are active late in fetal life and in early infancy because of high levels of maternal androgens. They are most densely located on the scalp, face, and genitalia and produce the grayish-white, greasy **vernix caseosa** that covers the infant at birth. Plugging of the sebaceous glands causes **milia**.

The eccrine glands, which produce sweat in response to heat or emotional stimuli, are functional at birth, and by 3 weeks of age palmar sweating on crying reaches levels equivalent to those of anxious adults. The eccrine glands produce sweat in response to higher temperatures than those required in adults, and the retention of sweat may result in milia. The apocrine glands, sweat glands that develop as attachments to hair follicles, remain small and nonfunctional until puberty.

The growth phases of hair follicles usually occur simultaneously at birth. During the first few months, the synchrony between hair loss and regrowth is disrupted, and there may be overgrowth of hair or temporary alopecia.

Because the amount of melanin is low at birth, newborns are lighter skinned than they will be as children. Consequently, infants are more susceptible to the harmful effects of ultraviolet light such as the sun.

Musculoskeletal System

At birth the skeletal system contains more cartilage than ossified bone, although the process of ossification is fairly rapid during the first year. The nose, for example, is predominantly cartilage at birth and is frequently flattened by the force of delivery. The six skull bones are relatively soft and not yet joined. The sinuses are incompletely formed as well.

Unlike the skeletal system, the muscular system is almost completely formed at birth. Hypertrophy, rather than hyperplasia, of cells causes the growth in the size of muscular tissue.

Defenses Against Infection

The infant is born with several defenses against infection. The first line of defense is the skin and mucous membranes, which protect the body from invading organisms. The second line of defense is the cellular elements of the immunologic system, which produces several types of cells capable of attacking a pathogen. The neutrophils and monocytes are **phagocytes**, cells that engulf, ingest, and destroy foreign agents. Eosinophils also probably have a phagocytic property because in the presence of foreign protein they increase in number. The **lymphocytes** (T and B cells) are capable of being converted to other cell types, such as monocytes and antibodies. Although the phagocytic properties of the blood are present in the infant, the tissues' inflammatory response to localize an infection is immature.

The third line of defense is the formation of specific antibodies to an antigen. This process requires exposure to various foreign agents for antibody production to occur. Infants are generally not capable of producing their own immunoglobulins until the beginning of the second month of life, but they receive considerable passive immunity in the form of immunoglobulin G (IgG) from the maternal circulation and from human milk (see p. 224). They are protected against most major childhood diseases, including diphtheria, measles, poliomyelitis, and rubella, for about 3 months, provided that the mother has developed antibodies to these illnesses.

Endocrine System

Ordinarily, the newborn's endocrine system is adequately developed, but its functions are immature. For example, the posterior lobe of the pituitary gland produces limited quantities of antidiuretic hormone, or vasopressin, thus risk of diuresis is increased. This renders the newborn highly susceptible to dehydration.

The effect of maternal sex hormones is particularly evident in the newborn. The labia are hypertrophied, and the breasts in both sexes may be engorged and secrete milk during the first few days of life to as long as 2 months of age. Female newborns may have pseudomenstruation (more often seen as a milky secretion rather than actual blood) from a sudden drop in progesterone and estrogen levels.

Neurologic System

At birth the nervous system is incompletely integrated but sufficiently developed to sustain extrauterine life. Most neurologic functions are primitive reflexes. The autonomic nervous system is crucial during transition because it stimulates initial respirations, helps maintain acid-base balance, and partially regulates temperature control.

Myelination of the nervous system follows the **cephalocaudal-proximodistal** (head-to-toe–center-to-periphery) laws of development and is closely related to the observed mastery of fine and gross motor skills. Myelin is necessary for rapid and efficient transmission of some, but not all, nerve impulses along the neural pathway. Tracts that develop myelin earliest are the sensory, cerebellar, and extrapyramidal. This accounts for the acute senses of taste, smell, and hearing and the perception of pain in the newborn. All cranial nerves are myelinated except the optic and olfactory nerves.

Sensory Functions

The newborn's sensory functions are remarkably well developed and have a significant effect on growth and development, including the attachment process.

Vision

At birth the eye is structurally incomplete. The fovea centralis is not yet completely differentiated from the macula. The ciliary muscles are also immature, limiting the eyes' ability to accommodate and fixate on an object for any length of time. The pupils react to light, the blink reflex is responsive to minimum stimulus, and the corneal reflex is activated by a light touch. Tear glands usually do not begin to function until 2 to 4 weeks of age.

The newborn has the ability to momentarily fixate on a bright or moving object that is within 20 cm (8 inches) and in the midline of the visual field. The infant's ability to fixate or coordinate movement is greater during the first hour of life than during the succeeding several days. Visual acuity is reported to be between 20/100 and 20/400, depending on the vision measurement techniques (see Chapter 4).

The infant also demonstrates visual preferences: medium colors (yellow, green, pink) over dim or bright colors (red, orange, blue); black-and-white contrasting patterns, especially geometric shapes and checkerboards; large objects with medium complexity rather than small, complex objects; and reflecting objects over dull ones.

Hearing

Once the amniotic fluid has drained from the ears, the infant probably has auditory acuity similar to that of an adult. The newborn is able to detect a loud sound of about 90 dB and reacts with a startle (Moro) reflex. The newborn's response to sounds of low frequency and high frequency differs; the former, such as a heartbeat, metronome, or lullaby, tends to decrease an infant's motor activity and crying, whereas the latter elicits an alerting reaction.

Infants have an early sensitivity to the sound of human voices and to specific speech sounds. For example, infants younger than 3 days of age can distinguish their mother's voice from that of other females. As early as 5 days, newborns can differentiate between stories read by their mother's voice (in utero) versus stories read by another woman's voice after birth.

The internal and middle ear structures are large at birth, but the external canal is small. The mastoid process and the bony part of the external canal have not yet developed. Consequently, the tympanic membrane and facial nerve are close to the surface and can be easily damaged.

Smell

Newborns react to strong odors such as alcohol or vinegar by turning their heads away. Breastfed infants are able to smell breast milk and will cry for their mothers when the breasts are leaking. Infants are also able to differentiate their mother's breast milk from that of other women by scent alone. Many believe maternal odors influence the attachment process and successful breastfeeding. Unnecessary routine washing of the breasts may interfere with establishment of early breastfeeding.

Taste

The newborn can distinguish between tastes, and various types of solutions elicit differing facial reflexes. A tasteless solution elicits no facial expression; a sweet solution elicits an eager suck and a look of satisfaction; a sour solution causes the usual puckering of the lips; and a bitter liquid produces an angry, upset expression.

Touch

The newborn perceives tactile sensation in any part of the body, although the face (especially the mouth), hands, and soles of the feet seem to be most sensitive. Sufficient evidence now shows that touch and motion are essential components in the attachment process and in normal growth and development. Gentle patting of the back or rubbing of the abdomen usually elicits a calming response from the infant. However, painful stimuli, such as a pinprick, elicit an upset response.

NURSING CARE OF THE NEWBORN AND FAMILY

ASSESSMENT

The newborn requires thorough, skilled observation to ensure a satisfactory adjustment to extrauterine life. Physical assessment after delivery is divided into four phases: (1) the initial assessment, which includes the Apgar scoring system; (2) transitional assessment during periods of reactivity; (3) assessment of gestational age; and (4) a comprehensive, systematic physical examination. In addition, the nurse must be aware of those behaviors that signal successful attachment between the infant and parents. Awareness of the expected normal findings during each assessment process helps the nurse recognize any deviation that may prevent the infant from progressing uneventfully through the early postnatal period. With shorter hospital stays, accomplishing a thorough newborn assessment and comprehensive parent teaching requires focused nursing observations and interventions with every parent and newborn encounter.

Initial Assessment: Apgar Scoring

The most frequently used method to assess the newborn's immediate adjustment to extrauterine life is the Apgar scoring system. The score is based on observation of heart rate, respiratory effort, muscle tone, reflex irritability, and color (Table 7.1). Each item is given a score of 0, 1, or 2. Evaluations of all five categories are made 1 and 5 minutes after birth and are repeated every 5 minutes until the infant's condition stabilizes. Total scores of 0 to 3 represent severe distress, scores of 4 to 6 signify moderate difficulty, and scores of 7 to 10 indicate absence of difficulty in adjusting to extrauterine life. Many healthy newborns do not achieve a score of 10 because the body is not completely pink. The degree of physiologic immaturity affects the Apgar score. For example, a healthy preterm infant may receive a low score due to low tone and reduced reflex irritability. Infection, congenital anomalies, maternal sedation or analgesia, hypovolemia, and neuromuscular disorders also affect the Apgar score.

TABLE 7.1 Infant Evaluation at Birth: Apgar Scoring System

Sign	0	1	2
Heart rate	Absent	Slow, <100 beats/min	>100 beats/min
Respiratory effort	Absent	Irregular, slow, weak cry	Good, strong cry
Muscle tone	Limp	Some flexion of extremities	Well flexed
Reflex irritability	No response	Grimace	Cry, sneeze
Color	Blue, pale	Body pink, extremities blue	Completely pink

The Apgar score reflects the infant's general condition at 1 and 5 minutes based on the five parameters described previously. The Apgar score is not a tool, however, that stands on its own to interpret past events, determine need for newborn resuscitation, or predict future events linked to the infant's neurologic or physical status (American Academy of Pediatrics & American College of Obstetricians and Gynecologists, 2015a).

Transitional Assessment: Periods of Reactivity

The newborn exhibits behavioral and physiologic characteristics that can at first appear to be signs of stress. During a newborn's initial 24 hours, changes in heart rate, respiration, motor activity, color, mucus production, and bowel activity occur in an orderly, predictable sequence, which is normal and indicates lack of stress. Distressed infants also progress through these stages but at a slower rate.

For 6 to 8 hours after birth the newborn is in the first period of reactivity. During the first 30 minutes the infant is alert, cries vigorously, may suck his or her fingers or fist, and appears interested in the environment. At this time the neonate's eyes are usually open; thus this is an excellent opportunity for mother, father, and child to see one another. Because the healthy, full-term newborn has a vigorous suck reflex, this is an opportune time to begin breastfeeding. The newborn usually grasps the nipple quickly, satisfying both mother and child. This is important to remember because it is likely that after this initial highly active state, the infant may be sleepy and uninterested in sucking. Physiologically the respiratory rate can be as high as 80 breaths/min, crackles may be heard, heart rate may reach 180 beats/min, bowel sounds are active, mucus secretions are increased, and temperature may decrease slightly. Maintaining appropriate temperature for the newborn is best accomplished by practicing skin-to-skin care, whereby only a diaper is worn, to allow the majority of the skin surface to be in contact with the mother's skin. A light blanket is used to cover the mother and newborn. Research has shown that skin-to-skin care is effective in ensuring the newborn remains normothermic (Moore, Bergman, Anderson, et al., 2016).

After this initial stage of alertness and activity, the infant enters the second stage of the first reactive period, which generally lasts 2 to 4 hours. Heart and respiratory rates decrease, temperature continues to fall, mucus production decreases, and urine or stool is usually not passed. The infant is in a state of sleep and relative calm. Any attempt at stimulation usually elicits a minimal response. Because of the decrease in body temperature, avoid undressing or bathing the infant during this time.

The second period of reactivity begins when the infant wakes from this deep sleep; it lasts about 2 to 5 hours and provides another excellent opportunity for child and parents to interact. The infant is again alert and responsive, heart and respiratory rates increase, the gag reflex is active, gastric and respiratory secretions are increased, and passage of meconium commonly occurs. This period is usually over when the amount of respiratory mucus has decreased. After this stage is a period of stabilization of physiologic systems and a vacillating pattern of sleep and activity.

Behavioral Assessment

An important area of assessment is observation of behavior. Infants' behavior helps shape their environment, and their ability to react to various stimuli affects how others relate to them. The principal areas of behavior for newborns are sleep, wakefulness, and activity such as crying.

One method of systematically assessing the infant's behavior is use of the Brazelton Neonatal Behavioral Assessment Scale (BNBAS) (Brazelton & Nugent, 1996). The BNBAS is an interactive examination that assesses the infant's response to 28 items organized in clusters (Box 7.2). It is generally used as a research or diagnostic tool and requires special training.

BOX 7.2 Clusters of Neonatal Behaviors in Brazelton Neonatal Behavioral Assessment Scale

Habituation—Ability to respond to and then inhibit response to discrete stimulus (light, rattle, bell, pinprick) while asleep
Orientation—Quality of alert states and ability to attend to visual and auditory stimuli while alert
Motor performance—Quality of movement and tone
Range of state—Measure of general arousal level or arousability of infant
Regulation of state—How infant responds when aroused
Autonomic stability—Signs of stress (tremors, startles, skin color) related to homeostatic (self-regulating) adjustment of the nervous system
Reflexes—Assessment of several neonatal reflexes

Data from Brazelton, T. B., & Nugent, J. K. (1996) *Neonatal behavioural assessment scale.* London: MacKeith Press.

The scale may be used to assess and support parent-child relationships guiding parents to focus on their infant's individuality and develop a deeper attachment. Studies have demonstrated that exposure to the NBAS results in increased maternal confidence, and improved parent-infant interaction and developmental outcome (Nugent, 2013).

The Newborn Behavioral Observations (NBO) system, inspired by the NBAS, is an interactive relationship-building instrument that highlights the baby's capacities and individuality (Nugent, Keefer, Minear, et al., 2007). It is much shorter than the NBAS, consisting of 18 neurobehavioral observation, which are easily integrated into routine care (Sanders & Buckner, 2006). There has been renewed interest in the NBO recently, and it is being used by nurses, doctors, home visitors, and others to optimize parent-infant relationships (Holland & Watkins, 2015).

Patterns of Sleep and Activity

Newborns begin life with a systematic schedule of sleep and activity that is initially evident during the periods of reactivity. For the next 2 or 3 days most infants sleep almost constantly to recover from the exhausting birth process.

Infants have six distinct sleep-wake states, which represent a particular form of neural control (Table 7.2). As gestational and postconceptional maturity increases, each state becomes more precisely defined according to the behaviors observed. State is defined as a "group of characteristics that regularly occur together" (Blackburn, 2013); these include body activity, eye and facial movements, respiratory pattern, and response to internal and external stimuli. The six sleep-wake states are quiet (deep) sleep, active (light) sleep, drowsy, awake (quiet), active alert, and crying. Infants respond to internal and external environmental factors by controlling sensory input and regulating the sleep-wake states; the ability to make smooth transitions between states is called state modulation. The ability to regulate sleep-wake states is essential in the infant's neurobehavioral development. The more immature the infant, the less he or she is able to cope with factors, external or internal, that affect the sleep-wake patterns.

Recognition and knowledge of sleep-wake states are important in planning nursing care. It is also important for nurses to help parents and caregivers understand the significance of the infant's behavioral responses to daily caregiving and how these states can be altered. A classic example is the newborn who feeds vigorously in the active alert

TABLE 7.2 States of Sleep and Activity

State and Behavior	Implications for Parents
Deep Sleep (Quiet)	
Closed eyes Regular breathing No movement except for occasional sudden bodily twitch No eye movement	Continue usual household noises because external stimuli do not arouse infant. Leave infant alone if sudden loud noise awakens infant and child cries. Do not attempt to feed.
Light Sleep (Active)	
Closed eyes Irregular breathing Slight muscular twitching of body Rapid eye movements under closed eyelids May smile	External stimuli that did not arouse infant during regular sleep may minimally arouse child. Periodic groaning or crying is usual; do not interpret as indication of pain or discomfort.
Drowsy	
Eyes may be open Irregular breathing Active body movement variable, with occasional mild startles	Most stimuli arouse infant, but infant may return to sleep state. Pick infant up during this time rather than leaving in crib. Provide mild stimulus to awaken. Infant may enjoy nonnutritive sucking.
Quiet Alert	
Eyes wide open and bright Responds to environment by active body movement and staring at close-range objects Minimum body activity Regular breathing Focuses attention on stimuli	Satisfy infant's needs such as hunger or nonnutritive sucking. Place infant in area of home where activity is continuous. Place toys in crib or playpen. Place objects within 17.5-20 cm (7-8 inches) of infant's view. Intervene to console.
Active Alert	
May begin with whimpering and slight body movement Eyes open Irregular breathing	Remove intense internal or external stimuli because of increased sensitivity to stimuli.
Crying	
Progresses to strong, angry crying and uncoordinated thrashing of extremities Eyes open or tightly closed Grimaces Irregular breathing	Comforting measures that were effective during alert state are usually ineffective. Rock and swaddle to decrease crying. Intervene to reduce fatigue, hunger, or discomfort.

Portions adapted from Blackburn, S., & Loper, D. L. (2007). *Maternal, fetal, and neonatal physiology: A clinical perspective.* Philadelphia, PA: Saunders.

state but poorly once he or she progresses to the crying state. The neurologic assessment of a newborn in the active alert state will differ significantly from the deep sleep state.

Newborns typically spend as much as 16 to 18 hours a day sleeping and do not necessarily follow a pattern of light-dark diurnal rhythm. With increasing age, sleep-wake states change, with increasing amounts of time spent in awake alert states and decreasing amounts in sleep time. Approximately 50% of total sleep time is spent in irregular or rapid eye movement sleep.

Cry

The newborn should begin extrauterine life with a strong, lusty cry. The duration of crying in each infant varies as much as the duration of sleep. Some newborns may cry for as little as 5 minutes or as much as 2 hours or more per day. Holding the infant skin-to-skin or swaddling or wrapping an infant snugly in a blanket (while ensuring the hands are free to allow self-calming and avoid overheating) calms infants, promotes sleep, and maintains body temperature. Rocking the infant may reduce crying and induce quiet alertness or sleep.

Variations in the initial cry can indicate underlying abnormalities. A weak, groaning cry or grunting during expiration usually indicates a respiratory disturbance. Absent, weak, or constant crying requires further investigation for possible drug withdrawal or a neurologic problem. Crying status alone, however, is not a diagnostic tool.

Assessment of Attachment Behaviors

One of the most important areas of assessment is careful observation of those behaviors thought to indicate the formation of emotional bonds between the newborn and family, especially the mother. Although **bonding** and **attachment** are sometimes referred to as separate phenomena, with bonding representing the development of emotional ties from parent to infant and attachment representing the emotional ties from infant to parent, in this discussion and the one on p. 230, the terms are used interchangeably to denote both processes.

Unlike physical assessment of the neonate, which follows concrete guidelines, assessment of parent-child attachment requires much more skill in terms of observation and interviewing. The assessment process is even more challenging with short hospital stays for mothers and their newborn infants. Rooming-in of mother and infant and visits by partner, siblings, and grandparents facilitate recognition of behaviors that demonstrate positive or negative attachment. Guidelines for assessment of bonding behaviors are in the Nursing Care Guidelines box.

NURSING CARE GUIDELINES

Assessing Attachment Behavior

- When you bring the infant to the parents, do they reach out for the child and call the child by name?
- Do the parents speak about the child in terms of identification (e.g., whom the infant looks like; what appears special about their child compared with other infants)?
- When parents are holding the infant, what kind of body contact is there? Do parents feel at ease in changing the infant's position; are fingertips or whole hands used; are there parts of the body they avoid touching or parts of the body they investigate and scrutinize?
- When the infant is awake, what kinds of stimulation do the parents provide? Do they talk to the infant, to each other, or to no one? How do they look at the infant—direct visual contact, avoidance of eye contact, or looking at other people or objects?
- How comfortable do the parents appear in terms of caring for the infant? Do they express any concern regarding their ability or disgust for certain activities, such as changing diapers?
- What type of affection do they demonstrate to the newborn, such as smiling, stroking, kissing, or rocking?
- If the infant is fussy, what kinds of comforting techniques do the parents use, such as rocking, swaddling, talking, or stroking?

Talking to the parents uncovers many variables that can affect the development of attachment and parenting. (See also Child Maltreatment, Chapter 14.) What expectations do they have for this child? In other words, how similar are their predictions of the fantasy child and their realizations about the real child? Encourage them to talk about their relationship with their own parents because the type of parenting that parents received as children influences their childrearing practices.

The labor process significantly affects the immediate attachment of mothers to their newborn children. Factors such as a long labor, feeling tired or "drugged" after delivery, and problems with breastfeeding may delay the development of initial positive feelings toward the newborn.

During pregnancy, and often even before conception, parents develop an image of the "ideal or fantasy infant." The unborn child has an imagined appearance, pattern of behavior, expected accomplishments, and predetermined effect on the family's lifestyle. At birth the fantasy infant becomes the real infant. How closely the dream child resembles the real child influences the bonding process. Assessing such expectations during pregnancy and at the time of the infant's birth allows identification of discrepancies in the parents' fantasy versus the real child.

Clinical Assessment of Gestational Age

Assessment of gestational age is important because perinatal morbidity and mortality are related to gestational age and birth weight. A frequently used method is the New Ballard Scale (NBS) by Ballard, Khoury, Wedig, and colleagues (1991) (Fig. 7.1, *A*). The NBS, an abbreviated version of the Dubowitz scale (Dubowitz & Dubowitz, 1977), assesses six external physical and six neuromuscular signs. Each sign has a number score, and the cumulative score correlates with a maturity rating of 20 to 44 weeks of gestation.

The New Ballard Scale can be used with newborns as young as 20 weeks of gestation, as it includes scores that reflect signs of extremely

ESTIMATION OF GESTATIONAL AGE BY MATURITY RATING

NEUROMUSCULAR MATURITY

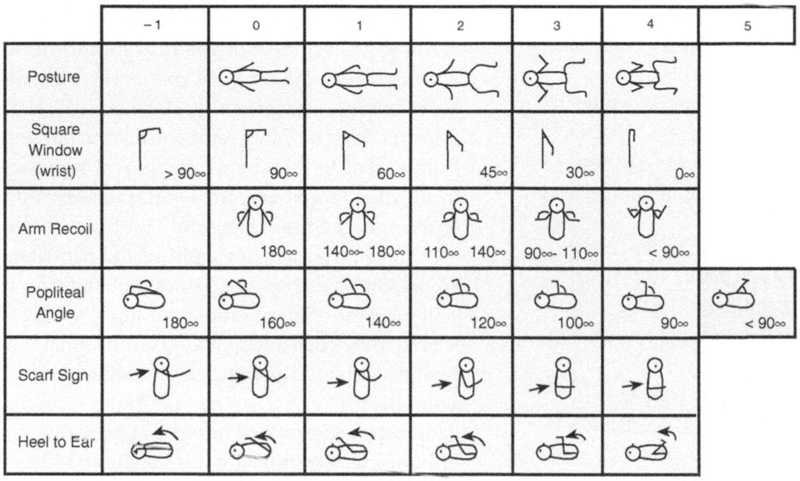

	-1	0	1	2	3	4	5
Posture							
Square Window (wrist)	> 90°	90°	60°	45°	30°	0°	
Arm Recoil		180°	140°- 180°	110° 140°	90°- 110°	< 90°	
Popliteal Angle	180°	160°	140°	120°	100°	90°	< 90°
Scarf Sign							
Heel to Ear							

PHYSICAL MATURITY

Skin	sticky friable transparent	gelatinous red, translucent	smooth pink, visible veins	superficial peeling &/or rash, few veins	cracking pale areas rare veins	parchment deep cracking no vessels	leathery cracked wrinkled
Lanugo	none	sparse	abundant	thinning	bald areas	mostly bald	
Plantar Surface	heel-toe 40-50 mm: -1 <40 mm: -2	>50 mm no crease	faint red marks	anterior transverse crease only	creases ant. 2/3	creases over entire sole	
Breast	imperceptible	barely perceptible	flat areola no bud	stippled areola 1-2 mm bud	raised areola 3-4 mm bud	full areola 5-10 mm bud	
Eye/Ear	lids fused loosely: -1 tightly: -2	lids open pinna flat stays folded	slightly curved pinna; soft; slow recoil	well-curved pinna; soft but ready recoil	formed & firm instant recoil	thick cartilage ear stiff	
Genitals (male)	scrotum flat, smooth	scrotum empty faint rugae	testes in upper canal rare rugae	testes descending few rugae	testes down good rugae	testes pendulous deep rugae	
Genitals (female)	clitoris prominent labia flat	prominent clitoris small labia minora	prominent clitoris enlarging minora	majora & minora equally prominent	majora large minora small	majora cover clitoris & minora	

MATURITY RATING

score	weeks
-10	20
-5	22
0	24
5	26
10	28
15	30
20	32
25	34
30	36
35	38
40	40
45	42
50	44

A

FIG. 7.1 A, Ballard scale for newborn maturity rating. Expanded scale includes extremely premature infants and has been refined to improve accuracy in more mature infants. (*A*, From Ballard, J. L., Khoury, J. C., Wedig, K., et al. [1991]. New Ballard score expanded to include extremely premature infants. *J Pediatr, 119,* 417.)

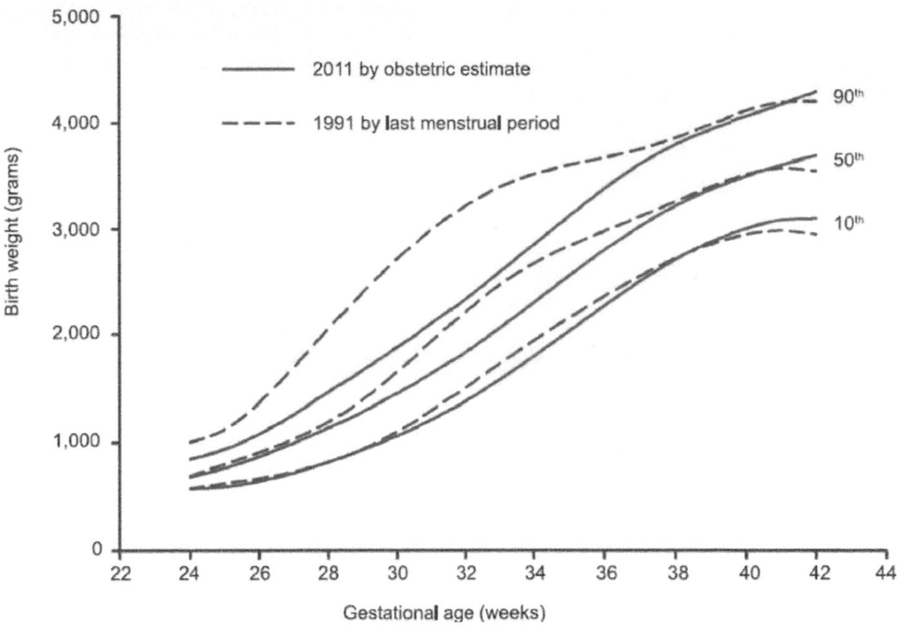

FIG. 7.1,cont'd B, Intrauterine growth: Birth weight curves for 1991 neonates dated by last menstrual period compared with 2011 neonates dated by obstetrics estimate. (*B,* From Duryea, E. L., Hawkins, J. S., McIntire, D. D., et al. [2014]. A revised birth weight reference for the United States. *Obstet Gynecol, 124*[1], 16-22.)

BOX 7.3 Tests Used in Assessing Gestational Age

See Fig. 7.1, *A,* for score categories and maneuvers.

Posture—With infant quiet and in a supine position, observe degree of flexion in arms and legs. Muscle tone and degree of flexion increase with maturity. *Score:* Full flexion of the arms and legs = 4.

Square window—With thumb supporting back of arm below wrist, apply gentle pressure with index and third fingers on dorsum of hand without rotating infant's wrist. Measure angle between base of thumb and forearm. *Score:* Full flexion (hand lies flat on ventral surface of forearm) = 4.

Arm recoil—With infant supine, fully flex both forearms on upper arms, hold for 5 seconds; pull down on hands to fully extend and rapidly release arms. Observe rapidity and intensity of recoil to a state of flexion. *Score:* A brisk return to full flexion = 4.

Popliteal angle—With infant supine and pelvis flat on a firm surface, flex lower leg on thigh and then flex thigh on abdomen. While holding knee with thumb and index finger, extend lower leg with index finger of other hand. Measure degree of angle behind knee (popliteal angle). *Score:* An angle of less than 90 degrees = 5.

Scarf sign—With infant supine, support head in midline with one hand; use other hand to pull infant's arm across the shoulder so that infant's hand touches shoulder. Determine location of elbow in relation to midline. *Score:* Elbow does not reach midline = 4.

Heel to ear—With infant supine and pelvis flat on a firm surface, pull foot as far as possible up toward ear on same side. Measure distance of foot from ear and degree of knee flexion (same as popliteal angle). *Score:* Knees flexed with a popliteal angle of less than 10 degrees = 4.

premature infants such as fused eyelids; imperceptible breast tissue; sticky, friable, transparent skin; no lanugo; and square-window (flexion of wrist) angle of greater than 90 degrees (see Fig. 7.1, *A,* and a description of the tests in Box 7.3). For infants with a gestational age of at least 26 weeks, the examination may be performed up to 96 hours after birth, but it is recommended that the initial examination be performed within the first 48 hours of life. In a study of preterm infants ranging from 29 to 35 weeks at birth, Ballard scores completed 7 days after birth were found to either overestimate or underestimate gestational age by up to 2 weeks (Sasidharan, Dutta, & Narang, 2009).

Weight Related to Gestational Age

The infant's weight at birth also correlates with the incidence of perinatal morbidity and mortality. Birth weight alone, however, is a poor indicator of gestational age and fetal maturity. Maturity implies functional capacity—the degree to which the neonate's organ systems are able to adapt to the requirements of extrauterine life. Therefore gestational age is more closely related to fetal maturity than is birth weight. Because heredity influences size at birth, it is important to note the sizes of other family members as part of the assessment process.

Many intrauterine growth charts have been published, generally reflecting data for a particular geographic region. Duryea, Hawkins, McIntire, and colleagues (2014) have published national reference charts which are representative of more than 3.2 million live births in the United States, using data from births in 2011. Compared with national reference data reflecting 3.2 million US births in 1991 (Alexander, Himes, Kaufman, et al., 1996) the Duryea group found that birth weights for preterm newborns were overestimated in the 1991 reference curves, compared with the 2011 reference (Fig. 7.1, *B*). This difference was attributed to the different methods used to establish gestational age (GA) in the two references. Alexander, Himes, Kaufman and colleagues (1996) used the last menstrual period to establish GA; Duryea, Hawkins, McIntire, and colleagues (2014) used the obstetric estimate, which often included ultrasound, to determine GA. For many women, menstrual dating may be inaccurate as a result of impaired recall, or cycles which do not occur regularly every 28 days. Thus determining GA based on menses alone is believed to be less precise than using this information in combination with obstetric estimates. Intrauterine growth curses

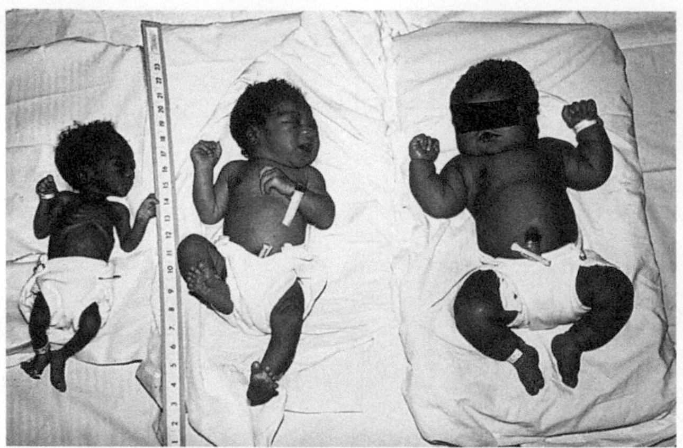

FIG. 7.2 Three infants, same gestational age, weighing 600, 1400, and 2750 g (1.3, 3, and 6 lb), respectively, from left to right. (From *Perinatal assessment of maturation,* National Audiovisual Center, Washington, DC.)

are important, as newborns labeled large for gestational age are often placed on hospital care protocols requiring glucose monitoring and prescribed feedings—measures that are not necessary if these infants are actually appropriate for gestational age.

Thomas, Peabody, Turnier, and colleagues (2000) suggested that intrauterine growth measured by head circumference, birth weight, and length varies according to race and gender. These researchers also found that altitude did not seem to significantly affect birth weight as other authors have suggested. It is recommended that the reader access and use the most current intrauterine growth chart specific to the population being evaluated.

Classification of infants at birth by both birth weight and gestational age provides a more satisfactory method for predicting mortality risks and providing guidelines for management of the neonate than estimating gestational age or birth weight alone. The infant's birth weight, length, and head circumference are plotted on standardized graphs that identify normal values for gestational age. The infant whose weight is appropriate for gestational age (AGA) (between the 10th and 90th percentiles) can be presumed to have grown at a normal rate regardless of the length of gestation—preterm, term, or postterm. The infant who is large for gestational age (LGA) (>90th percentile) can be presumed to have grown at an accelerated rate during fetal life; the small-for-gestational-age (SGA) infant (<10th percentile) can be presumed to have grown at a restricted rate during intrauterine life. When gestational age is determined according to the NBS, the newborn will fall into one of the following nine possible categories for birth weight and gestational age: AGA—term, preterm, postterm; SGA—term, preterm, postterm; or LGA—term, preterm, postterm. Fig. 7.2 illustrates the disparity between birth weights of three preterm infants of the same gestational age. Birth weight influences mortality rate: the lower the birth weight, the higher the mortality rate. The same is true for gestational age: the lower the gestational age, the higher the mortality rate.

Physical Assessment

The discussion of physical examination focuses on normal findings, variations from the norm that require little or no intervention, and specific potential danger signs that require more careful observation. General guidelines for conducting a physical examination are in the Nursing Care Guidelines box. Table 7.3 summarizes the physical examination of the newborn. (See Chapter 4 for further discussion of examination techniques.)

NURSING CARE GUIDELINES

Physical Examination of the Newborn

Provide a normothermic and nonstimulating examination area.
Check that equipment and supplies are working properly and are accessible.
Proceed quickly to avoid stressing infant.
Undress only body area examined to prevent heat loss.
Proceed in an orderly sequence (usually head to toe) with the following exceptions:

- Perform all procedures that require quiet first, such as auscultating the lungs, heart, and abdomen.
- Perform disturbing procedures, such as testing reflexes, last.
- Measure head, crown-to-rump, and head-to-heel length at same time to compare results.

Comfort infant during and after examination; involve parent in the following:

- Talking softly
- Holding the infant's hands against the chest
- Swaddling and holding
- Giving a pacifier or gloved finger to suck

General Measurements

Several measurements of the newborn are significant compared with each other, as well as when recorded over time on a graph. For the full-term infant, average head circumference is between 33 and 35 cm (13 and 14 inches). Head circumference may be somewhat less than that immediately after birth because of the molding process that occurs during vaginal delivery. Usually by the second or third day the normal size and contour of the skull have replaced the molded one. Head circumference may be compared with crown-to-rump length, or sitting height, to provide a means for identifying infants at risk, as head circumference is generally equal to or up to 2 cm (0.8 inches) more than crown-to-rump length in a majority of the infants determined to be normocephalic. Crown-to-rump measurements are usually 31 to 35 cm (12.5 to 14 inches).

However, if the head is significantly smaller than the crown-to-rump length, microcephaly or premature closure of the sutures (craniosynostosis) is a possibility. If the head is more than 4 cm (1.6 inches) larger than the crown-to-rump length and this relationship remains constant or increases over several days, then hydrocephalus must be considered. Other causes of increased head circumference are caput succedaneum, cephalhematoma, subgaleal hemorrhage, and subdural hematoma. Prematurity and intrauterine malnutrition also may disrupt the relationship between head circumference and crown-to-rump length.

Head-to-heel length is also measured. It is important to extend the legs completely when measuring total body length (Fig. 7.3). The average length of the newborn is 48 to 53 cm (19 to 21 inches).

Abdominal circumference need not be routinely measured in the newborn but should be done in the event of abdominal distention to determine changes in girth over time. Abdominal circumference is measured just above the level of the umbilicus. Because the umbilical cord is still attached, measurements across the umbilicus are too variable in newborns. Measuring the abdominal circumference below the umbilical region is also unsuitable because bladder status may affect the reading.

Measure body weight soon after birth because weight loss occurs fairly rapidly. Normally the newborn loses up to 10% of the birth weight by 3 to 4 days of age because of loss of excessive extracellular fluid and meconium, as well as limited food intake, especially in

TABLE 7.3 Summary of Physical Assessment of the Newborn

Usual Findings	Common Variations, Minor Abnormalities	Potential Signs of Distress, Major Abnormalities
General Measurements		
Head circumference—33-35 cm (13-14 inches); equal or up to 2 cm (0.8 inches) larger than crown-to-rump length	Molding after birth altering head circumference	Head circumference <10th or >90th percentile
Crown-to-rump length—31-35 cm (12.2-14 inches); approximately equal to head circumference		
Head-to-heel length—48-53 cm (19-21 inches)		
Birth weight—2700-4000 g (6-9 lb)	Loss of 10% of birth weight in first week; regained in 10-14 days, depending on feeding method	Birth weight <10th or >90th percentile Loss of >10% of birth weight in first week
Vital Signs		
Temperature, axillary—36.5°-37°C (97.7°-98°F)	Crying increasing body temperature slightly Radiant warmer falsely increasing axillary temperature	Hypothermia Hyperthermia
Heart rate, apical—120-140 beats/min	Crying increasing heart rate; sleep decreasing heart rate During 1st period of reactivity (6-8 hr), rate ≤180 beats/min	Bradycardia—Resting rate <80-100 beats/min Tachycardia—Rate >160-180 beats/min Irregular rhythm
Respirations—30-60 breaths/min	Crying increasing respiratory rate; sleep decreasing respiratory rate During 1st period of reactivity (6-8 hours), rate up to 80 breaths/min	Tachypnea—Rate >60 breaths/min Apnea—cessation of respirations for 20 seconds or more
Blood pressure (BP), oscillometric: 65/41 mm Hg in arm and calf	Crying and activity increasing BP	Oscillometric systolic pressure in calf 6-9 mm Hg less than in upper extremity (possible sign of coarctation of aorta) Systolic pressure >90 mm Hg is considered hypertension
General Appearance		
Posture—Flexion of head and extremities, which rest on chest and abdomen	Frank breech—Extended legs, abducted and fully rotated thighs, flattened occiput, extended neck	Limp posture—Extension of extremities
Skin		
At birth, bright red, puffy, smooth 2nd-3rd day, pink, flaky, dry Vernix caseosa Lanugo Edema around eyes, face, legs, dorsa of hands, feet, and scrotum or labia Acrocyanosis—Cyanosis of hands and feet Cutis marmorata—Transient mottling when infant is exposed to decreased temperature	Neonatal jaundice after first 24 hours Ecchymoses or petechiae caused by birth trauma Milia—Distended sebaceous glands that appear as tiny white papules on cheeks, chin, and nose Miliaria or sudamina—Distended sweat (eccrine) glands that appear as minute vesicles, especially on face Erythema toxicum—Pink papular rash with vesicles superimposed on thorax, back, buttocks, and abdomen; may appear in 24-48 hours and resolve after several days Harlequin color change—Clearly outlined color change as infant lies on side; lower half of body becomes pink, and upper half is pale	Progressive jaundice, especially in first 24 hours after birth Generalized cyanosis Pallor Mottling Grayness Plethora Hemorrhage, ecchymoses, or petechiae that persist Sclerema—Hard and stiff skin Poor skin turgor (tenting) Rashes, pustules, or blisters Café-au-lait spots—Light brown spots Nevus flammeus—Port-wine stain Herpetic blister(s) (see also Chapter 8) Capillary hemangiomas—Bright red, raised, soft, lobulated tumor occurring on the head, neck, trunk, or extremities; does not blanch with pressure (see also Birthmarks, Chapter 8)

Continued

TABLE 7.3 Summary of Physical Assessment of the Newborn—cont'd

Usual Findings	Common Variations, Minor Abnormalities	Potential Signs of Distress, Major Abnormalities
	Mongolian spots—Irregular areas of deep blue pigmentation, usually in sacral and gluteal regions; seen predominantly in newborns of African, Native American, Asian, or Hispanic descent (see figure at right)	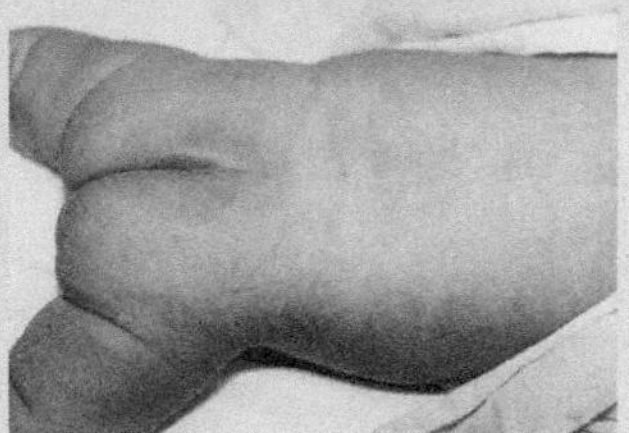
	Nevus simplex (stork bite or salmon patch)—Flat, deep pink, localized areas usually seen on nape of neck, upper eyelid, glabella, or on the upper lip; blanches with pressure and frequently becomes more prominent with crying	
Head		
Anterior fontanel—Diamond shaped; size varies from barely palpable to 4-5 cm (0.5-2 inches) (see Fig. 7.7) Posterior fontanel—Triangular, 0.5-1 cm (0.2-0.4 inches) Fontanels flat, soft, and firm Widest part of fontanel measured from bone to bone, not suture to suture	Molding after vaginal delivery Third sagittal (parietal) fontanel Bulging fontanel because of crying or coughing Caput succedaneum—Edema of soft scalp tissue Cephalhematoma (uncomplicated)—Hematoma between periosteum and skull bone	Fused sutures Bulging or depressed fontanels when quiet Widened sutures and fontanels Craniotabes—Snapping sensation along lambdoid suture that resembles indentation of Ping-Pong ball
Eyes		
Lids usually edematous Color—Slate gray, dark blue, brown Absence of tears Red reflex Corneal reflex in response to touch Pupillary reflex in response to light Blink reflex in response to light or touch Rudimentary fixation on objects and ability to follow to midline	Epicanthal folds in Asian infants Searching nystagmus or strabismus Subconjunctival (scleral) hemorrhages—Ruptured capillaries, usually at limbus	Pink color of iris Purulent discharge Upward slant in non-Asians Hypertelorism (≥3 cm [1.8 inches]) Hypotelorism Congenital cataracts Constricted or dilated fixed pupil Absence of red reflex Absence of pupillary or corneal reflex Inability to follow object or bright light to midline Yellow sclera Leukocoria (white pupil)—Possible retinoblastoma
Ears		
Position—Top of pinna on horizontal line with outer canthus of eye Startle (Moro) reflex elicited by loud, sudden noise or stimulus Pinna flexible, cartilage present	Inability to visualize tympanic membrane because of filled aural canals Pinna flat against head Irregular shape or size Pits or skin tags	Low placement of ears Absence of startle (Moro) reflex in response to loud noise or stimulus Minor abnormalities possible signs of various syndromes, especially renal
Nose		
Nasal patency Nasal discharge—Thin white mucus Sneezing	Flattened and bruised	Nonpatent canals Thick, bloody nasal discharge Flaring of nares (alae nasi) Single nasal canal Copious nasal secretions or stuffiness (may be minor)

TABLE 7.3 Summary of Physical Assessment of the Newborn—cont'd

Usual Findings	Common Variations, Minor Abnormalities	Potential Signs of Distress, Major Abnormalities
Mouth and Throat		
Intact, high-arched palate Uvula in midline Frenulum of tongue Frenulum of upper lip Sucking reflex—Strong and coordinated Rooting reflex Gag reflex Extrusion reflex Absent or minimum salivation Vigorous cry	Natal teeth—Teeth present at birth; benign but may be associated with congenital defects Epstein pearls—Small, white epithelial cysts along midline of hard palate	Cleft lip Cleft palate Large, protruding tongue or posterior displacement of tongue Profuse salivation or drooling Candidiasis (thrush)—White, adherent patches on tongue, palate, and buccal surfaces Inability to pass nasogastric tube to stomach Hoarse, high-pitched, weak, absent, or other abnormal cry Stridor Micrognathia—Small lower jaw seen in Pierre-Robin sequence (see Chapter 8)
Neck		
Short, thick, usually surrounded by skinfolds Tonic neck reflex	Torticollis (wry neck)—Head held to one side with chin pointing to opposite side	Excessive skinfolds or webbing Resistance to flexion Absence of tonic neck reflex Fractured clavicle; crepitus
Chest		
Anteroposterior and lateral diameters equal Slight sternal retractions evident during inspiration Xiphoid process evident Breast enlargement	Funnel chest (pectus excavatum) Pigeon chest (pectus carinatum) Supernumerary nipples Secretion of milky substance from breasts ("witch's milk")	Depressed sternum Marked retractions of chest and intercostal spaces during respiration Asymmetric chest expansion Redness and firmness around nipples Wide-spaced nipples
Lungs		
Respirations chiefly abdominal Cough reflex absent at birth, present by 1-2 days Bilateral equal bronchial breath sounds	Rate and depth of respirations may be irregular; periodic breathing Crackles shortly after birth	Inspiratory stridor Expiratory grunting Retractions Persistent irregular breathing Periodic breathing with repeated apneic spells Seesaw respirations (paradoxic) Apnea Unequal breath sounds Persistent fine, medium, or coarse crackles Wheezing Diminished breath sounds Peristaltic bowel sounds on one side, with diminished breath sounds on same side
Heart		
Apex—4th-5th intercostal space, lateral to left sternal border S_2 slightly sharper and higher in pitch than S_1	Sinus arrhythmia—Heart rate increasing with inspiration and decreasing with expiration Transient cyanosis on crying or straining	Dextrocardia—Heart on right side Displacement of apex, muffled heart sound Cardiomegaly Abdominal shunts Murmur Thrill Persistent central cyanosis Hyperactive precordium

Continued

TABLE 7.3 **Summary of Physical Assessment of the Newborn—cont'd**

Usual Findings	Common Variations, Minor Abnormalities	Potential Signs of Distress, Major Abnormalities
Abdomen		
Cylindric in shape Liver—Palpable 2-3 cm (0.8-1.8 inches) below right costal margin Spleen—Tip palpable at end of 1st week of age Kidneys—Palpable 1-2 cm (0.4-0.8 inches) above umbilicus Umbilical cord—Bluish white at birth with 2 arteries and 1 vein Femoral pulses—Equal bilaterally	Umbilical hernia Diastasis recti—Midline gap between recti muscles Wharton jelly—Unusually thick umbilical cord	Abdominal distention Localized bulging Distended veins Absent bowel sounds Enlarged liver and spleen Ascites Visible peristaltic waves Scaphoid or concave abdomen (possible congenital diaphragmatic hernia) Moist umbilical cord Presence of only 1 artery in cord Urine, stool, or pus leaking from cord or cord insertion site Periumbilical erythema Palpable bladder distention after scant voiding Absent femoral pulses Cord bleeding or hematoma Omphalocele or gastroschisis—Protrusion of abdominal contents through umbilical cord or abdominal wall Bladder exstrophy (exteriorized bladder; also associated with epispadias or cloaca)
Female Genitalia		
Labia and clitoris usually edematous Urethral meatus behind clitoris Vernix caseosa between labia Urination within 24 hours	Pseudomenstruation—Blood-tinged or mucoid discharge Hymenal tag	Enlarged clitoris with urethral meatus at tip Fused labia Absence of vaginal opening Meconium from vaginal opening No urination within 24 hours Masses in labia Ambiguous genitalia Bladder exstrophy
Male Genitalia		
Urethral opening at tip of glans penis Testes palpable in each scrotum Scrotum usually large, edematous, pendulous, and covered with rugae; usually deeply pigmented in dark-skinned ethnic groups Smegma Urination within 24 hours	Urethral opening covered by prepuce Inability to retract foreskin Epithelial pearls—Small, firm, white lesions at tip of prepuce Erection or priapism Testes palpable in inguinal canal Scrotum small	Hypospadias—Urethral opening on ventral surface of penis Epispadias—Urethral opening on dorsal surface of penis Chordee—Ventral curvature of penis Testes not palpable in scrotum or inguinal canal No urination within 24 hours Inguinal hernia Hypoplastic scrotum Hydrocele—Fluid in scrotum Masses in scrotum Meconium from scrotum Discoloration of testes Ambiguous genitalia Bladder exstrophy
Back and Rectum		
Spine intact; no openings, masses, or prominent curves Trunk incurvation reflex Anal reflex Patent anal opening Passage of meconium within 48 hours	Green liquid stools in infant under phototherapy Delayed passage of meconium in very-low-birth-weight neonates	Anal fissures or fistulas Imperforate anus Absence of anal reflex No meconium within 36-48 hours Pilonidal cyst or sinus Tuft of hair along spine Spina bifida (any degree)

TABLE 7.3 **Summary of Physical Assessment of the Newborn—cont'd**

Usual Findings	Common Variations, Minor Abnormalities	Potential Signs of Distress, Major Abnormalities
Extremities		
10 fingers and toes Full range of motion Nail beds pink, with transient cyanosis immediately after birth Creases on anterior ⅔ of sole Sole usually flat Symmetry of extremities Equal muscle tone bilaterally, especially resistance to opposing flexion Equal bilateral brachial pulses	Partial syndactyly between 2nd and 3rd toes 2nd toe overlapping 3rd toe Wide gap between 1st (hallux) and 2nd toes Deep crease on plantar surface of foot between 1st and 2nd toes Asymmetric length of toes Dorsiflexion and shortness of hallux	Polydactyly—Extra digits Syndactyly—Fused or webbed digits Phocomelia—Hands or feet attached close to trunk Hemimelia—Absence of distal part of extremity Hyperflexibility of joints Persistent cyanosis of nail beds Yellowing of nail beds Sole covered with creases Transverse palmar (simian) crease Fractures Decreased or absent range of motion Dislocated or subluxated hip Limitation in hip abduction Unequal gluteal or leg folds Unequal knee height (Allis or Galeazzi sign) Audible clunk on abduction (Ortolani sign) Asymmetry of extremities Unequal muscle tone or range of motion
Neuromuscular System		
Extremities usually in some degree of flexion Extension of extremity followed by previous position of flexion Head lag while sitting, but momentary ability to hold head erect Ability to turn head from side to side when prone Ability to hold head in horizontal line with back when held prone	Quivering or momentary tremors	Hypotonia—Floppy, poor head control, extremities limp Hypertonia—Jittery, arms and hands tightly flexed, legs stiffly extended, startles easily Asymmetric posturing (except tonic neck reflex) Opisthotonic posturing—Arched back Signs of paralysis Tremors, twitches, and myoclonic jerks Marked head lag in all positions

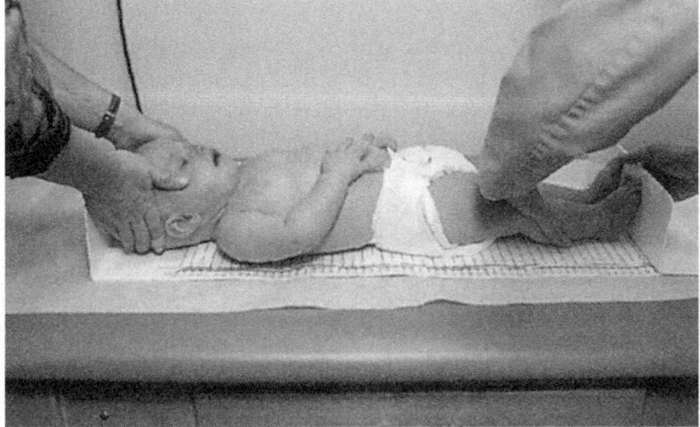

FIG. 7.3 Measurement of infant length.

breastfed infants. The birth weight is usually regained by the tenth to fourteenth day of life, depending on the method of feeding. Most newborns weigh 2700 to 4000 g (6 to 9 lb), with the average weight being about 3400 g (7.5 lb). Accurate birth weights and lengths are important because they provide a baseline for assessment of risk status and future growth.

Vital Signs

Another category of measurements is vital signs. Although rectal temperature measurement has traditionally been considered the gold standard for temperature-taking because it reflects core body temp, this route has largely been abandoned for newborns due to the risk of perforation of the rectal mucosa. The axilla route is safer and has demonstrated significant correlation with rectal temperature. Friedrichs, Staffileno, Fogg, and colleagues (2013) found a mean difference of 0.23°C when comparing rectal temperature with temperature taken in the left axilla of full-term infants (Fig. 7.4; see Table 4.3). Core (internal) body temperature varies according to the period of reactivity but is normally 36.5° to 37.6°C (97.7° to 99.7°F).

In addition to axilla temperature measurements, several other techniques may be used for newborns; however, the single best and most accurate method for determining the newborn infant's temperature is unclear when considering published research.

Despite their usefulness in older children and adults, the accuracy of tympanic membrane thermometers has been problematic in infants. A comprehensive review of the literature exploring methods and devices for temperature measurement in the newborn resulted in the authors concluding that the accuracy of the tympanic route in the neonate is controversial (Smith 2014; Smith, Alcock, & Usher, 2013). The Canadian Paediatric Society (2015a) has outlined concerns regarding safety and

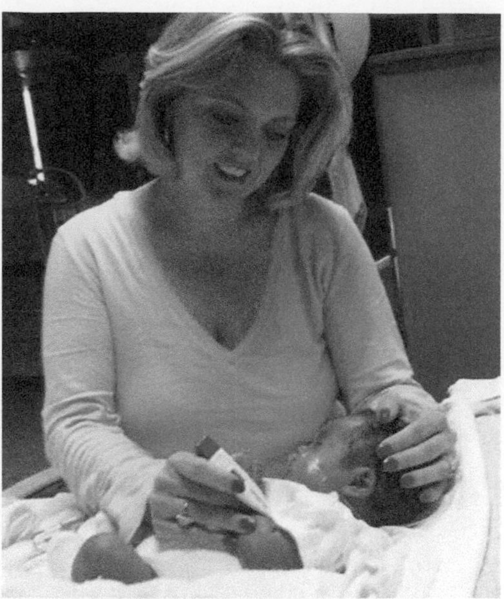

FIG. 7.4 Mother taking axillary temperature with digital thermometer. (Courtesy E. Jacob, Texas Children's Hospital, Houston.)

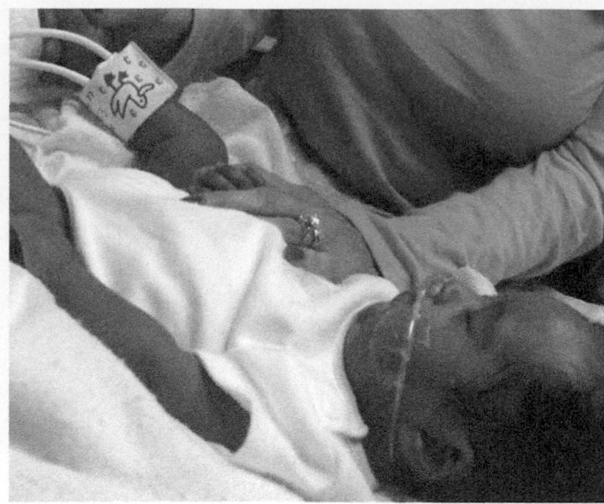

FIG. 7.5 Measurement of blood pressure using oscillometry. (Courtesy E. Jacob, Texas Children's Hospital, Houston.)

accuracy of tympanic temperature measurement in newborns because of the size of a newborn's external ear canal relative to the size of the thermometer probe. To ensure accuracy, the probe, which may be up to 8 mm (0.3 inch) in diameter, must be deeply inserted into the ear canal to allow orientation of the sensor near or against the tympanic membrane. At birth, the average diameter of the canal is just 4 mm (0.16 inch); at 2 years of age it is just 5 mm (0.2 inch). The CPS concludes that current infrared tympanic thermometry lacks sufficient safety and precision to meet clinical needs for use in newborn infants and children under 2 years of age.

Temporal artery thermometers (TATs), in which a battery-powered instrument is gently slid across the newborn's forehead, are available for use in the general pediatric population, and parents often report ease of use and increased comfort with such methods. Beginning research in the neonatal population suggests that TAT may be a reasonable method for newborn temperature measurement in healthy full-term newborns. Haddad, Smith, Phillips, and colleagues (2012), in a study of healthy newborns in a mother-baby unit, compared TAT with auxiliary temperature measurement. Although a slightly statistically significant difference was found between TAT and axillary temperatures, the difference was deemed clinically insignificant, and the unit has adopted TAT as their standard of care for healthy newborns. Similarly, Sim, Leow, Hao, and colleagues (2016) report, after a prospective comparative study, that TAT and axillary temperatures did not differ significantly for newborns nursed in room air. They recommend that TAT measurements are a reasonable alternative to axillary temperatures for stable, afebrile infants nursed in room air. The use of TAT for infants under phototherapy or those in incubators or under radiant warmers was deemed inappropriate in this study, as there was poor correlation between TAT and axillary temperatures in those newborns.

Infrared axillary and digital thermometers are used in many neonatal units because they give rapid readings and are easy to clean. Smith, Alcock, and Usher's (2013) extensive review of the literature on temperature measurement in term and preterm infants reported that the axillary route is the most common one used in newborns.

Nurses must be cognizant of the many variables involved in measuring temperature, and be able to make clear clinical decisions based on accurate and objective data. Variables include the following:

- **Site**—Axillary, temporal arterial, skin
- **Environment**—Open crib, radiant warmer, incubator, clothing, or blankets
- **Purpose**—Fever, possible sepsis (in which case the temperature may be lower than normal in newborns), and thermoregulation in the transition phase
- **Instrument**—Electronic, digital, or infrared

Nurses must also consider cost-effectiveness (i.e., nursing care time and instrument operation cost) and potential cross-contamination risks when evaluating neonatal temperature measurement. Ease of use and infant comfort are important factors to consider when teaching parents about taking the newborn's temperature at home.

Pulse and respirations vary according to the periods of reactivity and to the infant's behavior but are usually 120 to 140 beats/min and 30 to 60 breaths/min. Both are counted for a full 60 seconds to detect irregularities in rate, rhythm, and quality. The heart rate is taken apically with a stethoscope, and the brachial and femoral arteries are palpated for equality of strength or fullness. A suggested schedule for monitoring heart and respiratory rates and temperature for healthy full-term newborns is within the first hour of life, once every 30 minutes until the newborn has been stable for 2 hours, and then once every 8 hours until discharge. This schedule may vary according to institutional policy. Any change in the infant's color, breathing, muscle tone, or behavior necessitates more frequent monitoring.

Measurement of blood pressure (BP) provides baseline data and may indicate cardiovascular problems. BP is affected by gestational age and birth weight. For infants with murmurs, suspicion of congenital heart disease, or any concerns regarding tissue perfusion or fluid volume, BP is most easily and accurately assessed using oscillometry (Dinamap) (Fig. 7.5). Oscillometric BP is more accurate when the newborn is in a quiet or sleep state and an appropriate cuff width–to–arm or calf ratio of 0.45 to 0.70 is used. It is recommended that two or three BP measurements be taken in sick infants and that the mean BP be used because there is less error than when using systolic and diastolic readings. For healthy full-term infants, the average oscillometric systolic/diastolic BP is 65/45 mm Hg on day 1 of life, changing to 69.5/44.5 by day 3 (Kent, Kecskes, Shadbolt, et al., 2007). Compare BP in the upper and lower extremities, which should be equal.

Although uncommon, neonatal hypertension may be a sign of a significant underlying problem such as a renal, cardiac, or thromboembolic pathologic condition, or it may be associated with a medication treatment regimen. The nurse should bring neonatal hypertension to the primary practitioner's attention for further evaluation.

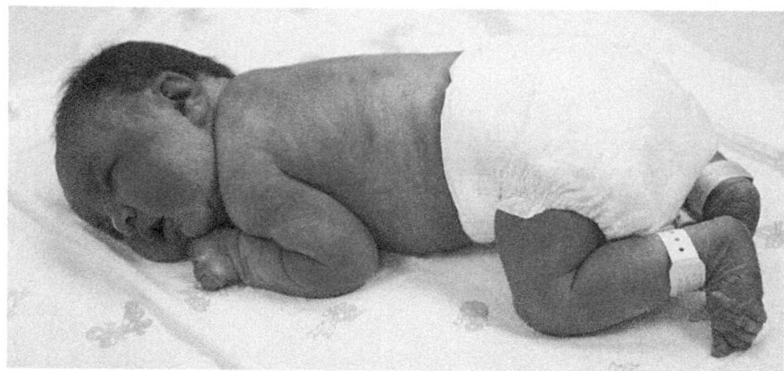

FIG. 7.6 Flexion position of neonate. *Note:* Prone position is avoided for infant sleeping.

The American Academy of Pediatrics (2012a) recommends routine pulse oximetry screening for critical congenital heart disease (CCHD) for all newborns. Universal screening for CCHD with pulse oximetry has been adopted in many states (see also http://www.cchdscreeningmap.org). Delayed diagnosis of CCHD can result in morbidity or mortality to infants. Research has demonstrated that adding pulse oximetry, a noninvasive, painless technology, to newborn assessment can detect CCHD. Practitioners are directed to use motion-tolerant pulse oximeters and to screen infants after 24 hours of age to reduce false-positive results. Because the ductus arteriosus may not be fully closed at 24 hours of age, oxygen saturation must be measured in the right hand (preductal circulation) and in one foot. A reading of 95% or greater in either extremity with a 3% or less difference between the upper and lower extremities (preductal and postductal circulation) is considered to be a "pass." Infants with saturation of less than 90% need immediate evaluation.

General Appearance

In the full-term newborn the posture is one of flexion, a result of in utero position (Fig. 7.6). Most infants are born in a vertex (head first) presentation and keep the head flexed, with the chin resting on the upper chest. The arms are flexed at the elbows and rest, folded, on the chest with hands clenched or fisted. The legs are flexed at the knees, the hips are flexed with thighs resting on the abdomen, and the feet are dorsiflexed against the anterior aspect of the legs. The vertebral column is also flexed.

Note any deviation from this characteristic fetal position. For example, preterm and hypoxic infants do not assume an attitude of total flexion but rather one of limp or hypotonic extension. Nonvertex presentations also result in variations in posture. In breech presentations the posture depends on the presenting part; a frank breech presentation results in extended legs, abducted and fully rotated thighs, a flattened head on top, and a neck that appears elongated.

Observe the infant's behavior, especially the degree of alertness, drowsiness, and irritability, which are common signs of neurologic problems. Ask the following questions when assessing behavior:

- Is the infant easily awakened by a loud noise?
- Is the infant comforted by rocking, sucking, or cuddling?
- Does the infant seem to have periods of deep and light sleep?
- When awake, does the infant seem satisfied after a feeding?
- What stimuli elicit responses from the infant?

Skin

The texture of the newborn's skin is velvety smooth and puffy, especially about the eyes, the legs, the dorsal aspect of the hands and feet, and the scrotum or labia.

Skin color depends on racial and familial background and varies greatly among newborns. In general, the Caucasian infant is usually pink to red; the African American newborn may appear a pinkish- or yellowish-brown; infants of Hispanic descent may have an olive tint or a slight yellow cast to the skin; infants of Asian descent may be a rosy- or yellowish-tan; and the color of Native American newborns varies from light pink to dark reddish-brown. By the second or third day the skin tone may change, and skin is drier and flakier.

Observe the color of the skin in relation to activity, position, and temperature changes. In general, the infant becomes redder when crying and may demonstrate transient periods of cyanosis during the first few hours of life (not associated with apnea or bradycardia). Table 7.3 describes several other color changes and minor skin blemishes.

At birth the skin may be covered with a grayish-white, cheeselike substance called vernix caseosa, a mixture of sebum and desquamating cells. If it is not removed during the bath, it will be absorbed by about 24 to 48 hours. A fine, downy hair called lanugo may be present on the skin, especially on the forehead, cheeks, shoulders, and back.

Head

General observation of the head's contour is important because molding occurs in almost all vaginal deliveries. In a vertex delivery the head is usually flattened at the forehead, with the apex rising and forming a point at the end of the parietal bones, and the posterior skull or occiput dropping abruptly. The usual, more oval contour of the head is apparent by 1 or 2 days after birth. The change in shape occurs because the bones of the cranium are not fused, allowing for overlapping of the edges of these bones to accommodate to the size of the birth canal during delivery. Such molding does not occur in infants born by cesarean section unless there has been prolonged labor or the head has been engaged in the pelvis.

Six bones—the frontal, occipital, two parietals, and two temporals—constitute the cranium. Between the junctions of these bones are bands of connective tissue called sutures. At the junction of the suture are wider spaces of unossified membranous tissue called fontanels. The two most prominent fontanels are the anterior fontanel, formed by the junction of the sagittal, coronal, and frontal sutures, and the posterior fontanel, formed by the junction of the sagittal and lambdoid sutures (Fig. 7.7, *A*).

NURSING TIP

The location of the sutures is easily remembered because the coronal suture "crowns" the head, and the sagittal suture "separates" the head.

Palpate the skull for all sutures and fontanels by using the tip of the index finger and running it along the ends of the bones (Fig. 7.7, *B*). Sutures feel like cracks between the skull bones; fontanels feel like wider "soft spots" at the junction of sutures. Note their size, shape, molding, and any abnormal closure.

The anterior fontanel is diamond shaped and measures 4 to 5 cm (about 2 inches) at its widest point (from bone to bone, rather than from suture to suture). The posterior fontanel is triangular, measuring between 0.5 and 1 cm (0.5 inch) at its widest part. It is easily located by following the sagittal suture toward the occiput. The posterior fontanel may not be palpable after birth because of edema (caput) or other cranial molding.

The fontanels should feel flat, firm, and well demarcated against the bony edges of the skull. Frequently pulsations are visible at the anterior fontanel. Coughing, crying, or lying down may temporarily cause the fontanels to bulge and become more taut.

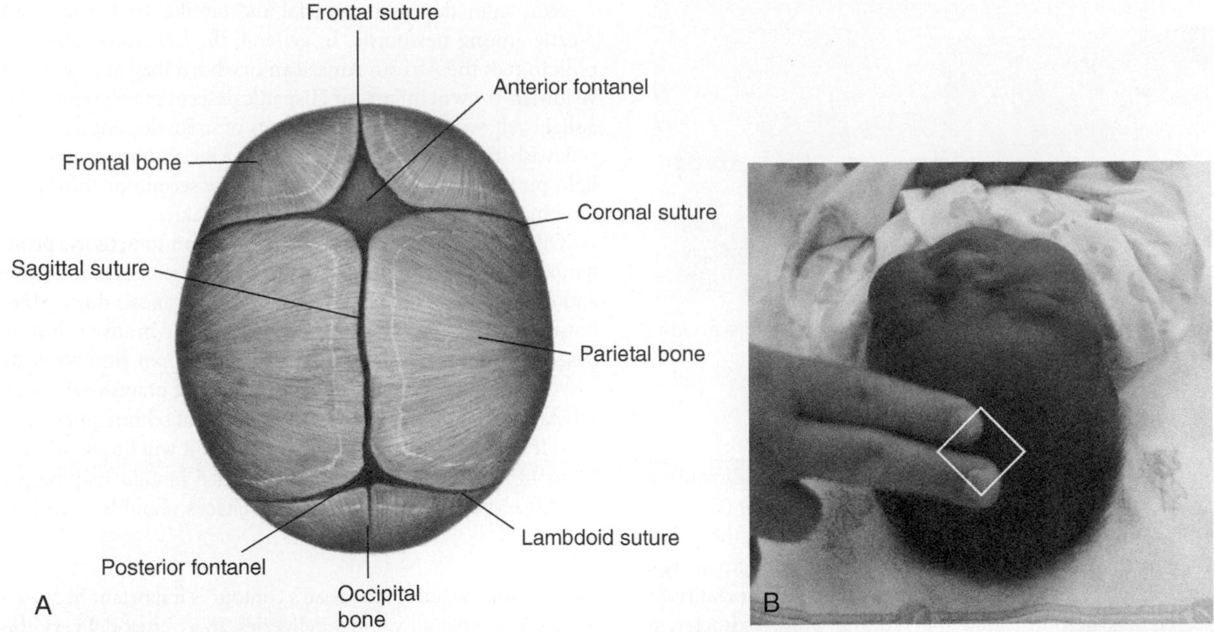

FIG. 7.7 **A,** Location of sutures and fontanels. **B,** Palpating anterior fontanel.

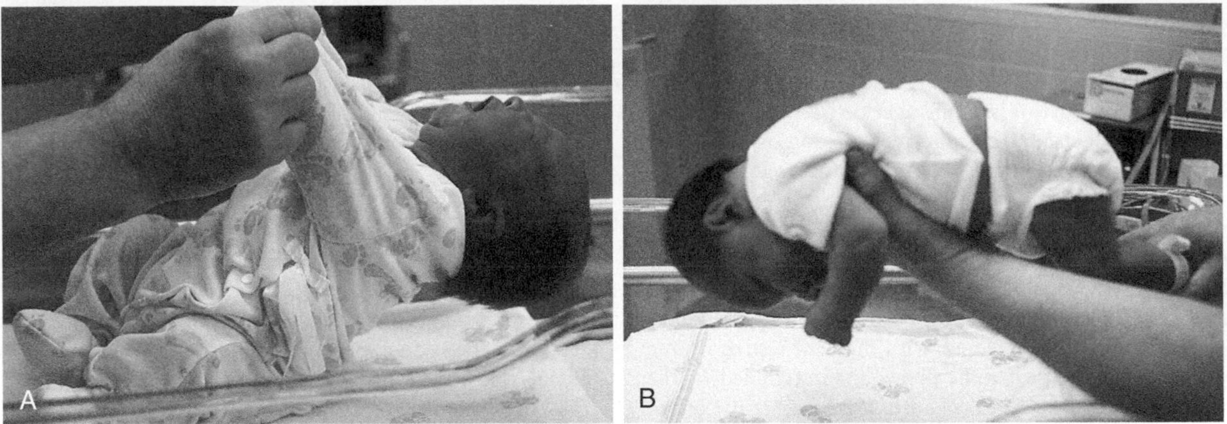

FIG. 7.8 Head control in infant. **A,** Inability to hold head erect when pulled to sitting position. **B,** Ability to hold head erect when placed in ventral suspension.

Palpate the skull for any unusual masses or prominences, particularly those resulting from birth trauma, such as caput succedaneum or cephalhematoma (see Chapter 8). Because of the pliability of the skull, exerting pressure at the margin of the parietal and occipital bones along the lambdoid suture may produce a snapping sensation similar to the indentation of a Ping-Pong ball. This phenomenon, known as physiologic **craniotabes**, may be found normally, especially in newborns of breech birth, but also may be associated with hydrocephalus, congenital syphilis, or rickets.

Assess the degree of head control. Although head lag is normal, the full-term newborn has some ability to control the head in certain positions. If the supine infant is pulled by the arms into a semi-Fowler position, head lag and hyperextension occur (Fig. 7.8, *A*). However, as infants are brought forward into a sitting position, they attempt to control their heads in an upright position. As the head falls forward onto the chest, many infants attempt to right it into the erect position. If they are held in ventral suspension (i.e., held prone above and parallel to the examining surface), the head is held in a straight line with the spinal column (Fig. 7.8, *B*). When lying on the abdomen, newborns have the ability to lift the head slightly, turning it from side to side. Marked head lag is seen in neonates with Down syndrome, prematurity, hypoxia, and metabolic and neurologic disorders.

Eyes

Because newborns tend to keep their eyes tightly closed, begin the examination of the eyes by observing the lids for edema, which is normally present for 2 days after delivery. Observe the eyes for symmetry and for hypertelorism (wide spacing between the eyes), but do not measure the distance between the inner canthi unless there is cause for further investigation. Tears may be present at birth, but purulent discharge from the eyes shortly after birth is abnormal.

To visualize the surface structures of the eye, hold the infant supine and gently lower the head. The eyes will usually open, similar to the mechanism of a doll's eyes. The sclera should be white and clear.

Examine the cornea for any opacities or haziness. The corneal reflex is present at birth but is generally not elicited unless cerebral or eye damage is suspected. The pupil usually responds to light by constricting. Absence of the pupillary reflex, particularly by 3 weeks of age, suggests blindness. A fixed, dilated, or constricted pupil may indicate central nervous system damage. A searching nystagmus is common after birth. Strabismus is a normal finding because of the lack of binocularity.

Note the color of the iris. Most light-skinned newborns have slate gray or dark blue eyes, whereas dark-skinned infants have brown eyes. Absence of color is characteristic of albinism.

Although it is difficult to perform a complete funduscopic examination of the retina, the nurse should elicit a red reflex.

NURSING TIP

To elicit a red reflex, place the infant in a dark room. In an alert state many newborns will open the eyes in a supported sitting position.

! NURSING ALERT

Always record and report absence of the red reflex. It may indicate the presence of glaucoma, retinal abnormality, retinoblastoma, cataracts, or a systemic disease (American Academy of Pediatrics, 2016b).

Ears

Examine the ears for position, structure, and auditory function. The pinna is often flattened against the side of the head from pressure in utero. An otoscopic examination may not always be performed because the canals are filled with vernix caseosa and amniotic fluid, making visualization of the tympanic membrane difficult. Periauricular skin tags, sinuses, and misshapen or low-set ears may be familial or associated with other congenital defects such as trisomy 18 and renal defects.

One way to assess auditory ability is by making a sharp, loud noise close to the infant's head and noting the presence of the startle reflex (Table 7.4 and Fig. 7.9) or twitching of the eyelids. However, the absence of a response to a loud noise in the newborn is not diagnostic for hearing deficit. Full-term newborns have the ability to habituate to noxious stimuli such as noise and may not react every time. Also, be aware of newborns considered at risk for hearing loss so that early testing can be performed (see Universal Newborn Hearing Screening, p. 220). (See Auditory Testing, Chapter 4, and Hearing Impairment, Chapter 20.)

Nose

Assess patency of the nasal canals by holding your hand over the infant's mouth and one canal and noting the passage of air through the unobstructed opening. If nasal patency is questionable, report it because most newborns are obligatory nose breathers and are unable to breathe orally in response to nasal occlusion.

The nose is usually flattened after birth, and bruises are common, especially if forceps were used. Thin, white mucus is common in the newborn, but a thick, bloody nasal discharge should be evaluated. Sneezing is common.

Mouth and Throat

Inspect the mouth's existing structures. The palate is normally high arched and somewhat narrow. Inspect the hard and soft palates for any clefts, which warrant further investigation. A common finding is **Epstein pearls**—small, white, epithelial cysts along both sides of the midline of the hard palate. They are insignificant and disappear in several weeks.

The **frenulum** of the upper lip is a band of thick, pink tissue that lies under the inner surface of the upper lip and extends to the maxillary alveolar ridge. It usually disappears as the maxilla grows. It is particularly evident when the infant yawns or smiles.

The **lingual frenulum** attaches the underside of the tongue midway between the ventral surface of the tongue and the tip to the lower palate. It is estimated that 4% to 16% of newborns have a tight lingual frenulum, sometimes referred to as tongue-tie, which may restrict adequate sucking (Brookes & Bowley, 2014). Further evaluation may be required to ascertain sucking ability, particularly in breastfed infants. Some practitioners recommend frenotomy as a safe and effective surgical procedure that improves comfort, effectiveness, and ease of breastfeeding for mother and infant. A recent Cochrane review of five published studies concluded, however, that although a reduction in maternal pain was generally reported, breastfeeding was not consistently improved postprocedure (O'Shea, Foster, O'Donnell, et al., 2017). Research continues in an effort to determine how best to select which infants may benefit from the procedure and when to perform it (Emond, Ingram, Johnson, et al.; 2014; Power & Murphy, 2015).

Elicit the **sucking reflex** by placing a nipple or nonlatex gloved finger in the infant's mouth. The infant should exhibit a strong, vigorous suck. To stimulate the **rooting reflex**, stroke the cheek and note the infant's response of turning toward the stimulated side and sucking. Assess the **gag reflex** when using a tongue blade to visualize the oropharynx.

Inspect the uvula while the infant is crying and the chin is depressed. However, the uvula may be retracted upward and backward during crying. Tonsillar tissue is generally not seen in the newborn. Natal teeth (i.e., teeth present at birth as opposed to neonatal teeth—teeth that erupt during the first month of life) are seen infrequently and erupt chiefly at the position of the lower central incisors. They are reported because they are sometimes found in infants with developmental abnormalities and syndromes, including cleft lip and palate. Most natal teeth are loosely attached. However, current research suggests preserving them until they exfoliate naturally (Maheswari, Kumar, Karunakaran, et al., 2012), unless breastfeeding is impaired by the neonate biting the breast or the teeth are very loose.

Neck

Because the newborn's neck is short and covered with folds of tissue, for adequate assessment allow the head to fall gently backward in slight hyperextension while supporting the back in a slightly raised position. Observe for range of motion, shape, and any abnormal masses, and palpate each clavicle for possible fractures. (See Fractures, Chapter 8.)

Chest

The shape of the newborn's chest is almost circular, with equal anteroposterior and lateral diameters. The ribs are flexible, and slight **intercostal retractions** are normal on inspiration. The xiphoid process is commonly visible as a small protrusion at the end of the sternum. The sternum is raised and slightly curved.

Inspect the breasts for size; shape; and nipple formation, location, and number. Maternal hormones cause breast enlargement that appears in many newborns of either gender by the second or third day. Occasionally the infant's breasts will secrete a milky substance. Infrequently, more than two nipples are present; if these are found, evaluate the kidneys because of the association of extra nipples with renal anomalies.

Lungs

The newborn's normal respirations are irregular and abdominal, and the rate is between 30 and 60 breaths/min. Periods of **apnea** lasting more than 20 seconds are abnormal and may be accompanied by **bradycardia**. After the first forceful breaths required to initiate respiration, subsequent breaths should be easy and fairly regular in rhythm. Occasional irregularities occur in relation to crying, sleeping, and feeding.

TABLE 7.4 Assessment of Reflexes in the Newborn

Reflexes	Expected Behavioral Responses
Localized	
Eyes	
Blinking or corneal reflex	Infant blinks at sudden appearance of bright light or at approach of object toward cornea; persists throughout life.
Pupillary	Pupil constricts when bright light shines toward it; persists throughout life.
Doll's eye	As head is moved slowly to right or left, eyes lag behind and do not immediately adjust to new position of head; disappears as fixation develops; if persists, indicates neurologic damage.
Nose	
Sneeze	Nasal passages respond spontaneously to irritation or obstruction; persists throughout life.
Glabellar	Tapping briskly on glabella (bridge of nose) causes eyes to close tightly; usually disappears in infancy.
Mouth and Throat	
Sucking	Infant begins strong sucking movements of circumoral area in response to stimulation; persists throughout infancy, even without stimulation, such as during sleep.
Gag	Stimulation of posterior pharynx by food, suction, or passage of tube causes infant to gag; persists throughout life.
Rooting	Touching or stroking cheek along side of mouth causes infant to turn head toward that side and begin to suck; should disappear at about age 3-4 months but may persist for up to 12 months.
Extrusion	When tongue is touched or depressed, infant responds by forcing it outward; disappears by age 4 months.
Yawn	Infant has spontaneous response to decreased oxygen by increasing amount of inspired air; persists throughout life.
Cough	Irritation of mucous membranes of larynx or tracheobronchial tree causes coughing; persists throughout life; usually present after 1st day of birth.
Extremities	
Grasp	Touching palms or soles near base of digits causes flexion of hands and toes (see Fig. 7.10, *A*); palmar grasp lessens after age 3 months, to be replaced by voluntary movement; plantar grasp lessens by 8 months of age.
Babinski	Stroking outer sole of foot upward from heel and across ball of foot causes toes to hyperextend and hallux to dorsiflex (see Fig. 7.10, *B*); disappears after age 1 year.
Ankle clonus	Briskly dorsiflexing foot while supporting knee in partially flexed position results in 1-2 oscillating movements ("beats"); eventually no beats should be felt.
Mass	
Moro	Sudden jarring or change in equilibrium causes sudden extension and abduction of extremities and fanning of fingers, with index finger and thumb forming a C shape, followed by flexion and adduction of extremities; legs may weakly flex; infant may cry (Fig. 7.9, *A*); disappears after age 3-4 months, usually strongest during first 2 months.
Startle	Sudden loud noise causes abduction of arms with flexion of elbows; hands remain clenched; disappears by age 4 months.
Perez	While infant is prone on firm surface, thumb is pressed along spine from sacrum to neck; infant responds by crying, flexing extremities, and elevating pelvis and head; lordosis of spine, defecation, and urination may occur; disappears by age 4-6 months.
Asymmetric tonic neck	When infant's head is turned to one side, arm and leg extend on that side, and opposite arm and leg flex (Fig. 7.9, *B*); disappears by age 3-4 months, to be replaced by symmetric positioning of both sides of body.
Trunk incurvation (Galant) reflex	Stroking infant's back alongside spine causes hips to move toward stimulated side; disappears by age 4 weeks.
Dance or step	If infant is held so that sole of foot touches hard surface, there is reciprocal flexion and extension of leg, simulating walking (Fig. 7.9, *C*); disappears after age 3-4 weeks, to be replaced by deliberate movement.
Crawl	When placed on abdomen, infant makes crawling movements with arms and legs; disappears at about age 6 weeks (Fig. 7.9, *D*).
Placing	When infant is held upright under arms and dorsal side of foot is briskly placed against hard object, such as table, leg lifts as if foot is stepping on table; age of disappearance varies.

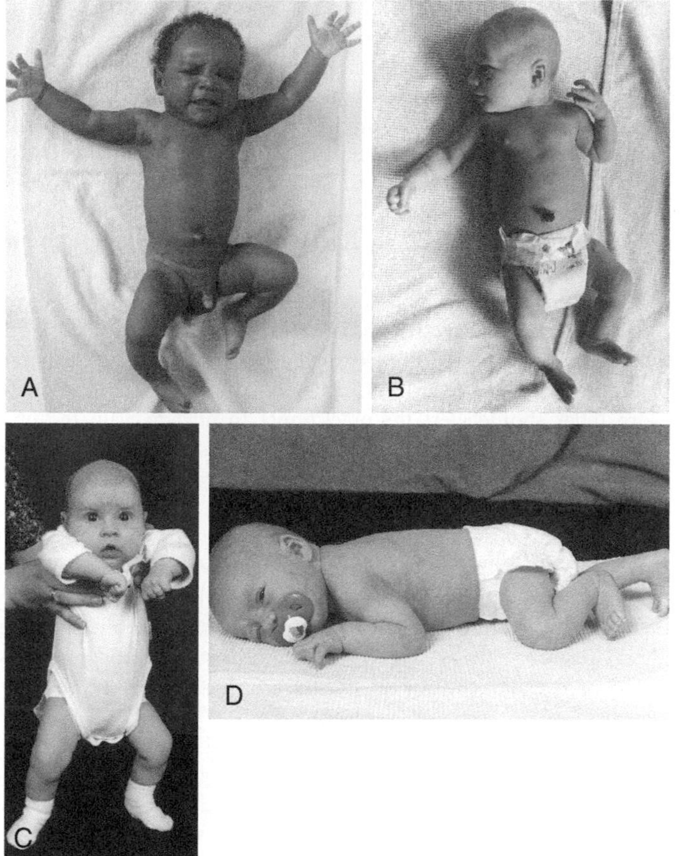

FIG. 7.9 **A,** Moro reflex. **B,** Tonic neck reflex. **C,** Dance reflex. **D,** Crawl reflex. (Courtesy Paul Vincent Kuntz, Texas Children's Hospital, Houston.)

Periodic breathing is common in full-term newborns and consists of rapid nonlabored respirations followed by pauses of less than 20 seconds; periodic breathing may be more prominent during sleep and is not accompanied by status changes such as cyanosis or bradycardia.

Perform auscultation when the infant is quiet. Bronchial breath sounds should be equal bilaterally. Report any differences in auscultatory findings between symmetric sites. Crackles soon after birth may indicate areas of atelectasis or the presence of fluid, which represents the normal transition of the lungs to extrauterine life. However, wheezes, persistence of crackles, and stridor should be reported.

! NURSING ALERT

Signs of respiratory distress include tachypnea, grunting, nasal flaring, intercostal retractions, stridor, abnormal breath sounds, cyanosis, and pallor.

Heart

Heart rate may range from 100 to 180 beats/min shortly after birth and, when the infant's condition has stabilized, from 120 to 140 beats/min. Palpate to find the point of maximum intensity (PMI), which is usually in the fourth to fifth intercostal space, medial to the left midclavicular line. The PMI gives some indication of the location of the heart, which may be displaced in conditions such as congenital diaphragmatic hernia or pneumothorax. Dextrocardia, an anomaly wherein the heart is on the right side of the body, should be reported (the abdominal organs may also be reversed), along with associated circulatory abnormalities.

NURSING TIP

Because auscultation of neonatal breath sounds and heart tones is often difficult for the untrained ear, practice auscultating one parameter at a time. Close your eyes and mentally block out the extraneous sounds heard, such as room noise or neonatal movement; offer the newborn a pacifier or gloved finger. Auscultation of a murmur and decreased air movement in specific lung fields requires patience and practice; it may require auscultating the heart tones or breath sounds for 1 to 3 minutes each.

Auscultation of the specific components of the heart sounds is difficult because of the rapid rate and effective transmission of respiratory sounds. However, the first (S_1) and second (S_2) sounds should be clear and well defined; the second sound is somewhat higher in pitch and sharper than the first. Murmurs are frequently heard in the newborn as a whooshing, blowing, or rasping sound, especially over the base of the heart or at the left sternal border in the third or fourth interspace. Ordinarily they are not associated with specific cardiac defects but frequently represent the incomplete functional closure of fetal shunts. (Chapter 4 discusses grading of heart murmurs.) However, always record and report any murmur or other unusual sounds.

Abdomen

The normal contour of the abdomen is cylindric and prominent with visible veins. Bowel sounds are audible within the first 15 to 20 minutes after birth. Visible peristaltic waves may be observed in thin newborns but should not be seen in well-nourished infants.

Inspect the umbilical cord to determine the presence of two arteries, which look like papular structures, and one vein, which has a larger lumen than the arteries and a thinner vessel wall. At birth the cord appears bluish-white and moist. After clamping, it begins to dry and appears a dull, yellowish-brown. It progressively shrivels and turns greenish-black. If the umbilical cord appears unusually large in diameter at the base, inspect for the presence of a hematoma or small omphalocele. The cord must not be clamped over an omphalocele because part of the intestine will be clamped, causing tissue necrosis. One practical rule of thumb is to cut the cord distally 10 to 12 cm (4 to 5 inches) from a questionable enlargement until further examination is carried out by a practitioner. The extra length can be cut once normal anatomy has been identified.

A cord that is draining and erythematous at the base should be investigated by the primary practitioner. The cord undergoes a process of dry gangrene decay, which has an odor; therefore odor alone may not be a reliable index of suspicion for omphalitis.

Palpate after inspecting the abdomen. The liver is normally palpable 1 to 3 cm (about 0.5 to 1 inch) below the right costal margin. The tip of the spleen can sometimes be felt, but a palpable spleen more than 1 cm below the left costal margin suggests enlargement and warrants further investigation. Although the nurse should palpate both kidneys, this maneuver requires considerable practice. When felt, the lower half of the right kidney and the tip of the left kidney are 1 to 2 cm (about 0.5 to 1 inch) above the level of the umbilicus. During examination of the lower abdomen, palpate for femoral pulses, which should be strong and equal bilaterally.

Female Genitalia

Normally the labia majora and minora (the minora may be more prominent) and clitoris are edematous, especially after a breech delivery. However, carefully inspect the labia and clitoris to identify any evidence of ambiguous genitalia or other abnormalities. Normally in a girl the urethral opening is located behind the clitoris. Any deviation from this may mistakenly suggest that the clitoris is a small penis, which can occur in conditions such as congenital adrenal hyperplasia.

A hymenal tag is occasionally visible from the posterior opening of the vagina. It is composed of tissue from the hymen and the labia minora and usually disappears in several weeks. Generally, the vaginal vault is not inspected.

Vaginal discharge may be noted during the first week of life. This pseudomenstruation is a manifestation of the abrupt decrease in maternal hormones and usually disappears by 2 to 4 weeks of age. Fecal discharge from the vaginal opening indicates a rectovaginal fistula and must be reported. Vernix caseosa may be present in large amounts between the labia. Vigorous attempts to remove all the vernix through bathing are avoided to prevent tissue damage. With routine bathing and care, vernix will disappear after several days.

Male Genitalia

Inspect the penis for the urethral opening, which is located at the tip. However, the opening may be totally covered by the prepuce, or foreskin, which covers the glans penis. A tight prepuce is a common finding in newborns and does not indicate phimosis. It should not be forcefully retracted; locating the urinary meatus is usually possible without retracting the foreskin. Smegma, a white, cheesy substance, is commonly found around the glans penis, under the foreskin. An erection is common in the newborn. Small, white, firm lesions called epithelial pearls may be seen at the tip of the prepuce.

The scrotum may be large, edematous, and pendulous in the full-term neonate, especially in the infant born in breech position. It is more deeply pigmented in dark-skinned infants. A noncommunicating hydrocele commonly occurs unilaterally and disappears within a few months. Palpate the scrotum for the presence of testes. (See Chapter 4.)

In small newborns, particularly premature infants, the undescended testes may be palpable within the inguinal canal. Absence of the testes may also be a sign of ambiguous genitalia, especially when accompanied by a small scrotum and penis. Inguinal hernias may or may not be manifested immediately after birth. A hernia is easier to detect when the infant is crying. Palpable lymph nodes are most commonly found in the inguinal area. Report a discolored or dusky scrotum, scrotal edema, or palpation of a small mass to the practitioner because these may be a sign of testicular torsion.

Back and Anus

Inspect the spine with the infant prone. The shape of the spine is gently rounded, with none of the characteristic S-shaped curves seen later in life. Any abnormal openings or sinuses, masses, dimples, or soft areas are noted. A protruding sac anywhere along the spine, but most commonly in the sacral area, indicates some type of spina bifida. A small sinus, which may or may not be communicating with the spine, is a pilonidal sinus; the sinus is usually located on the lower spine at the coccyx. It is frequently covered with a tuft of hair. Although it may have no pathologic significance, a pilonidal cyst may indicate the existence of spina bifida occulta or be a portal of entry into the spinal column. With the infant still prone, note symmetry of the gluteal folds. Report any evidence of asymmetry. Skilled examiners test for developmental dysplasia of the hip. (See Chapter 33)

The presence of an anal orifice and passage of meconium through the orifice during the first 24 to 48 hours of life indicates anal patency. If the nurse suspects an imperforate anus, report this to the practitioner for further evaluation. The presence of meconium or stool on the perineum is not an indication of rectal patency; a fistula may exist wherein stool is evacuated via the vagina, scrotum, or raphe. Therefore further investigations to ascertain anal patency may be done should any doubt regarding patency exist.

Extremities

Examine the extremities for symmetry, range of motion, and signs of malformation or trauma. Count the fingers and toes, and note supernumerary digits (polydactyly) or fusion of digits (syndactyly). A partial syndactyly between the second and third toes is a common variation seen in otherwise normal infants. More extensive fusion is abnormal, and the nurse should report this to the practitioner.

Observe range of motion of the extremities throughout the entire examination. The newborn will demonstrate full range of motion in the elbow, hip, shoulder, and knee joints. Movements should be symmetric, smooth, and unrestricted. The absence of arm movement signals a potential birth injury paralysis such as Klumpke or Erb-Duchenne paralysis. (See Birth Injuries, Chapter 8.) An asymmetric or partial Moro reflex should alert the practitioner to further evaluate upper extremity mobility. Examine the lower extremities for limb length, symmetry, and hip abduction and flexion.

Examine the nails; the nail beds should be pink, although slight blueness is evident in acrocyanosis. Persistent cyanosis of the nail beds may indicate hypoxia or vasoconstriction. Yellowing of the nail beds may indicate intrauterine distress (as nails may be stained after intrauterine expulsion of meconium), postterm birth, or hemolytic disease. Short or absent nails are seen in preterm infants, whereas long nails, extending over the ends of the fingers, are characteristic of postterm newborns.

The palms of the hands should have the usual creases (see Fig. 4.14). A transverse palmar crease (simian crease) suggests Down syndrome but may also be a normal finding. The full-term newborn usually has creases covering the entire sole of the foot. In postterm infants the sole is covered with deep creases, and in preterm infants the creases may partially cover the sole or may be absent. The soles are flat with prominent fat pads. Note any foot abnormalities.

Two reflexes are elicited. The first is the grasp reflex. Touching the palms or soles near the base of the digits causes flexion or grasping (Fig. 7.10, *A*). The other is the Babinski reflex. Stroking the outer sole of the foot upward from the heel across the ball of the foot causes the big toe to dorsiflex and the other toes to hyperextend (Fig. 7.10, *B*, and Table 7.4).

Inspect the extremities for evidence of fractures from birth trauma. The clavicle, humerus, and femur are most commonly involved. Limitation of movement, crepitus, visible deformity, asymmetry of reflexes, and malposition of the site suggest a fracture.

It is important to assess neonatal muscle tone. By attempting to extend a flexed extremity, determine whether tone is equal bilaterally. Extension of any extremity is usually met with resistance, and when released, the extremity returns to its previous flexed position. Hypotonia suggests some degree of hypoxia, neurologic or muscular disorder, or condition such as Down syndrome. Asymmetry of muscle tone may indicate a degree of paralysis from damage to the central nervous system. Failure to move the lower limbs suggests a spinal cord lesion or injury. Sustained rhythmic tremors, twitches, and myoclonic jerks characterize neonatal seizures or may indicate neonatal abstinence syndrome. (See Neonatal Seizures and Drug-Exposed Infants, Chapter 9.) Sudden asynchronous jerking movements, quivering, or momentary tremors are usually normal.

Neurologic System

Assessing neurologic status is a critical part of the physical examination of the newborn. Much of the neurologic testing takes place during evaluation of body systems, such as eliciting localized reflexes and observing posture, muscle tone, head control, and movement. However, several important mass (total body) reflexes also need to be elicited.

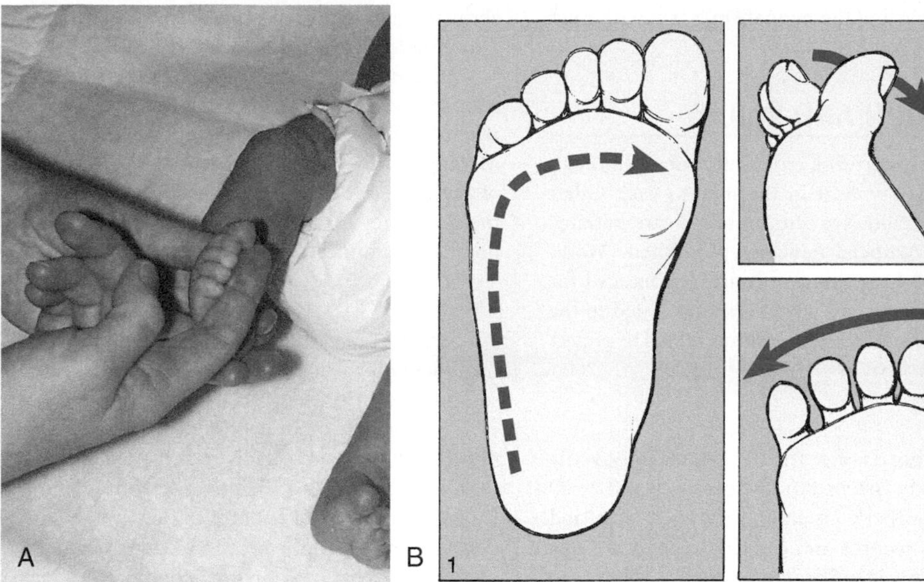

FIG. 7.10 A, Plantar or grasp reflex. **B,** Babinski reflex. **1,** Direction of stroke. **2,** Dorsiflexion of big toe. **3,** Fanning of toes. (*A,* From Zitelli, B. J., & Davis, H. W. [2002]. *Atlas of pediatric physical diagnosis* [4th ed.]. St. Louis, MO: Mosby.)

Test these at the end of the examination because they may disturb the infant and interfere with auscultation. Table 7.4 describes these reflexes and several local reflexes. Record and report the absence, asymmetry, persistence, or weakness of a reflex.

MAINTAIN A PATENT AIRWAY

Establishing a patent airway is the primary objective in the delivery room. When the newborn is supine, a neutral neck position (i.e., avoiding neck flexion or hyperextension) is critical to achieving and maintaining a patent airway. After feeding, position the infant to facilitate drainage of secretions.

The American Academy of Pediatrics (2016c) recommends the supine position during sleep for all newborns. This recommendation is based on the association between sleeping prone and sudden infant death syndrome. (See Chapter 11.) Since the initial recommendation in 1992 that all infants be placed in the supine position to sleep, there has been no evidence of an increased number of complications, such as choking or vomiting, when infants are placed in a supine sleep position. There has, however, been an increase in the number of infants with cranial asymmetry, particularly unilateral flattening of the occiput, and the American Academy of Pediatrics (2016d) has endorsed guidelines for the management of positional plagiocephaly. Health care professionals must educate parents on prevention of deformational plagiocephaly by encouraging alternate positions when baby is awake. (See also Positional Plagiocephaly, Chapter 11.)

Suctioning of secretions, if needed, may be done with a bulb syringe. Compress the bulb syringe before insertion to avoid forcing secretions into the bronchi. If more forceful removal of secretions is required, mechanical suction is used. Use of the proper-sized catheter and correct suctioning technique are essential to prevent mucosal damage and edema. Gentle suctioning is necessary to prevent laryngospasm, reflex bradycardia, and other cardiac arrhythmias from vagal stimulation. Oropharyngeal suctioning is performed for up to 5 seconds with sufficient time between each attempt to allow the infant to reoxygenate. If nasal suctioning is necessary, it must be done *after* oral suctioning to minimize the possibility of aspiration of oropharyngeal contents (American Academy of Pediatrics, 2016a). Closely monitor vital signs, and report immediately any indication of respiratory distress.

MAINTAIN A STABLE BODY TEMPERATURE

Conserving the newborn's body heat is an essential nursing goal. At birth a major cause of heat loss is **evaporation**, the loss of heat through moisture. The amniotic fluid that bathes the infant's skin favors evaporation, especially when combined with the cool atmosphere of the delivery room. Rapidly drying the skin and hair with a warmed towel and placing the infant in skin-to-skin contact with his mother, covered by a blanket, will minimize heat loss through evaporation.

Another source of heat loss is **radiation**, the loss of heat to cooler solid objects in the environment that are not in direct contact with the infant. Loss of heat through radiation increases as these solid objects become colder and closer to the infant. The temperature of ambient (surrounding) air has no effect on loss of heat through radiation. This is a critical point to remember when attempting to maintain a constant temperature for the infant because even when the temperature of the ambient air is optimum, the infant can become hypothermic. Radiant heat loss may occur if the crib or incubator is placed close to a cold window or air conditioning unit. The cold from either source will cool the crib or incubator walls and subsequently the neonate's body. To prevent this, place cribs or incubators as far away as possible from cool walls, windows, or ventilating units.

Heat loss can also occur through conduction and convection. **Conduction** involves loss of body heat from direct skin contact with a cooler solid object. The nurse can minimize this by placing the infant on a padded, covered surface rather than directly on a cool hard table and by providing insulation with clothes and blankets. Placing the newborn nestled close to the mother, such as in her arms or on her abdomen or chest immediately after delivery in **skin-to-skin** (kangaroo care) contact, is beneficial in terms of conserving newborn heat and fostering maternal attachment and breastfeeding.

Convection is similar to conduction, except that heat loss is aided by surrounding air currents. For example, placing the infant in the direct flow of air from a fan or air conditioner vent causes rapid heat loss through convection. Transporting the neonate in a crib with solid sides reduces airflow around the infant.

PROTECT FROM INFECTION AND INJURY

The most important practice for preventing cross-infection is thorough hand washing by all individuals involved in the infant's care. Other procedures to prevent infection include eye care, umbilical care, bathing, and care of the circumcision. Artificial nails are prohibited (World Health Organization, 2009) and long fingernails are discouraged for health care providers because the former have been implicated in the transmission of harmful pathogens. Vitamin K is administered to protect against hemorrhage.

Identification

Proper identification of the newborn is essential. The nurse must verify that identifying bands are securely fastened on the newborn and verify the information (name, sex, mother's admission number, date, and time of birth) against the birth records and the child's gender. Some institutions use methods of infant identification such as a color photograph kept in the medical record, storage of blood for DNA genotyping, and electronic surveillance systems for infant security. The National Center for Missing and Exploited Children (NCMEC) recommends the use of footprints as a form of identification in addition to a cord blood sample, which is stored until the day after discharge (National Center for Missing and Exploited Children, 2015). Electronic tags that give off a radio frequency are also being used to prevent newborn abductions. A tag is placed on the newborn and removed at the time of discharge by hospital personnel. Another measure to decrease infant abduction is to discontinue the publication of birth announcements in the local newspaper.

A proactive hospital emergency plan should be implemented to prevent infant abduction and to respond promptly and effectively if one occurs (National Center for Missing and Exploited Children, 2015). A mock newborn abduction drill is an effective method to evaluate staff competence and response to the incident (National Center for Missing and Exploited Children, 2015). *All* hospital personnel should be educated regarding newborn abduction, preventive strategies, and methods to identify the potential risk of such an occurrence.

The nurse needs to discuss safety issues with the mother before and after delivery of the newborn to ensure adequate understanding of safety measures to prevent newborn abduction. A written copy of safety instructions should also be given to the parent. Instruct parents to look at identification badges of nurses and any hospital personnel who come in contact with the infant and not to relinquish their infants to anyone without proper identification. Mothers are also advised not to leave the infant alone in the crib while they shower or use the bathroom; rather, they should ask a health care worker to watch the infant if a family member is not present in the room. Encourage parents and staff to use a password system when the newborn is taken from the room as a routine security measure. The nurse should document in the chart that these instructions were given and that appropriate identification band checks are routinely made throughout each shift.

Nursing staff are also educated regarding the "typical" abductor profile and to be constantly aware of visitors with unusual behavior. The typical abductor is a female between the ages of 15 and 44 who often has a large build and low self-esteem. She may be emotionally disturbed because of the loss of her own child or inability to conceive and may have a strained relationship with her husband or partner. The typical abductor may also be seen visiting the newborn nursery or neonatal intensive care unit (NICU) before the abduction and may ask questions about the care of or the health of a specific newborn. The abductor may familiarize herself with the hospital routine and may also impersonate a health care worker.

The nurse should advise parents that infant safety measures must be implemented after discharge from the hospital as well because the majority of infant abductions are from the home (National Center for Missing and Exploited Children, 2015). Instruct parents to be cautious of anyone they do not know well, particularly persons they met during the pregnancy who show excessive interest or who show up at their home unannounced.

Eye Care

Prophylactic eye treatment against **ophthalmia neonatorum**, infectious conjunctivitis of the newborn, includes the use of silver nitrate (1%) solution, erythromycin (0.5%) ophthalmic ointment, or tetracycline (1%) ophthalmic ointment or drops (preferably in single-dose ampules or tub). All three are effective against gonococcal conjunctivitis. *Chlamydia trachomatis* is a major cause of ophthalmia neonatorum in the United States; topical antibiotics (tetracycline and erythromycin) and silver nitrate have not proved to be effective in the prevention and treatment of chlamydial conjunctivitis. A 14-day course of oral erythromycin or a 3-day course of azithromycin may be given for chlamydial conjunctivitis (American Academy of Pediatrics, 2015b). The administration of oral erythromycin to infants less than 6 weeks old has been associated with the development of infantile hypertrophic pyloric stenosis; therefore parents should be informed of the potential risks and signs of the illness (American Academy of Pediatrics, 2015b).

Although eye prophylaxis is mandatory in the United States, health care facilities are free to choose specific drugs. Effective prophylaxis may be better directed at treating maternal chlamydial infection in areas where that organism is prevalent.

> **NURSING TIP**
>
> A chemical conjunctivitis may occur within 24 hours of instillation of ophthalmic prophylaxis. The clinical features include mild lid edema and a sterile, nonpurulent eye discharge. Report any purulent eye discharge to the primary practitioner for further investigation.

Studies on maternal attachment suggest that in the first hour of life, a newborn has a greater ability to focus on coordinated movement than at any other time during the next several days. Because eye contact is important in the development of maternal-infant bonding, routine administration of silver nitrate or antibiotics may be postponed for up to 1 hour after birth. However, practitioners must ensure that the drug is given by 1 hour of age.

Vitamin K Administration

Shortly after birth, vitamin K is administered to prevent hemorrhagic disease of the newborn. (See Chapter 8.) The intestinal flora synthesizes vitamin K, however, because the infant's intestine is sterile at birth, vitamin K levels are insufficient in newborns. A dose of vitamin K provides protection until the newborn's intestinal flora is established, which usually occurs by 3 to 4 days of age. The major function of vitamin K is to catalyze the synthesis of prothrombin in the liver, which is needed for blood clotting. The vastus lateralis muscle is the traditionally recommended injection site, but the ventrogluteal (not dorsogluteal) muscle may also be used.

Several countries have noted a resurgence in later onset of vitamin K deficiency bleeding (VKDB) after practicing orally administered prophylaxis (American Academy of Pediatrics, 2014a). Current recommendations are that vitamin K be given to all newborns as a single intramuscular dose of 0.5 to 1.0 mg (American Academy of Pediatrics, 2014a; Canadian Paediatric Society, 2016b). Additional study is needed on the efficacy, safety, and bioavailability of oral preparations and on the most effective dosing regimens to prevent VKDB.

Hepatitis B Vaccine Administration

To decrease the incidence of hepatitis B virus (HBV) in children and its serious consequences (cirrhosis and liver cancer) in adulthood, the first of three doses of HBV vaccine is recommended after birth and before hospital discharge for all newborns born to hepatitis B surface antigen (HBsAg)–negative mothers. The injection is given in the vastus lateralis muscle because this site is associated with a better immune response than the dorsogluteal area (American Academy of Pediatrics, 2015b). (See Immunizations, Chapter 6.) Giving the infant concentrated oral sucrose can reduce the pain of the injection (Stevens, Yamada, Ohlsson, et al., 2016). Infants born to HBsAg-negative mothers with a birth weight of less than 2000 g (4.4 lb) should receive the first dose of the Hep B vaccine at 1 month of chronologic age or at hospital discharge if before 1 month of chronologic age. Infants born to HBsAg-positive mothers should be immunized within 12 hours after birth with HBV vaccine and hepatitis B immune globulin at separate sites, regardless of gestational age or birth weight (American Academy of Pediatrics, 2015b).

Newborn Screening

Blood sampling can detect a large number of congenital disorders in the newborn period so that early intervention can take place to decrease the long-term effects and cost of not treating such conditions. Currently no national policy regulates newborn screening; therefore the extent of screening has been largely determined by state laws and individual practice. All states now mandate screening tests for phenylketonuria (PKU) and congenital hypothyroidism (see Chapters 3 and 8); many states also have programs that include screening for sickle cell disease and galactosemia. Because of concern regarding the inconsistency among states in screening for such conditions based on cost, population demographics, resource availability, and political environment, the American Academy of Pediatrics and other federal health care agencies have developed a number of recommendations to better address the issue of newborn screening (American Academy of Pediatrics, 2016e).

The nurse's responsibility is to educate parents regarding the importance of screening and to collect appropriate specimens at the recommended time (after 24 hours of age or after the introduction of feedings; hospitalized infants must be screened before 7 days of age). With early newborn discharge before 24 hours, some authorities recommend a repeat screening for PKU within 2 weeks. Accurate screening depends on high-quality blood spots on approved filter paper forms. The blood should completely saturate the filter paper spot on one side only. The paper should not be handled, placed on wet surfaces, or contaminated with any substance (see Atraumatic Care box). The American Academy of Pediatrics (2015b) recommends routine prenatal and perinatal human immunodeficiency virus (HIV) counseling and testing for all pregnant women. Benefits of early identification of HIV-infected infants include the following:

- Early antiretroviral therapy and aggressive nutritional supplementation
- Appropriate changes in their immunization schedule
- Monitoring and evaluation of immunologic, neurologic, and neuropsychologic functions for possible changes caused by antiretroviral therapy
- Initiation of special educational services
- Evaluation of the need for other therapies, such as immunoglobulin for the prevention of bacterial infections
- Tuberculosis screening and treatment
- Management of communicable disease exposures

ATRAUMATIC CARE

Heel Punctures

Heel lancing is necessary to obtain blood for newborn tests, including newborn metabolic screening. Heel lancing is recognized as a painful procedure, and numerous nonpharmacologic strategies have demonstrated pain relief potential.

The American Academy of Pediatrics (2016f) has written a comprehensive policy statement on prevention and management of pain in the neonate. It outlines the importance of preventing and minimizing pain with interventions such as nonnutritive sucking, skin-to-skin holding, swaddling/facilitated tucking, and providing breastfeeding or sucrose. These strategies can significantly manage pain behaviors associated with painful procedures in neonates.

Oral sucrose and nonnutritive sucking have proved effective in decreasing the pain associated with heel punctures and other painful procedures in preterm and full-term infants; however, the exact dosage range that provides optimal effectiveness varies among studies. Evidence indicates that as little as 0.05 to 0.5 ml of a 24% oral sucrose solution is effective in decreasing pain in full-term and preterm infants (Stevens, Yamada, Ohlsson, et al., 2016). The best analgesic effect is achieved when sucrose is administered 2 minutes before the painful procedure with a pacifier or syringe and is repeatedly administered in small amounts (i.e., 0.05 to 0.5 ml) at 2-minute intervals throughout the painful procedure. The effect appears to begin at 2 minutes and lasts about 4 minutes, thus analgesic effect may wane if procedures are prolonged (Stevens, Yamada, Ohlsson, et al., 2016).

A number of commercially available oral sucrose solutions now exist. When these are not available, the pharmacy may mix an oral sucrose solution to ensure a clean product. Strict attention must be paid to aseptic technique with this method to prevent contamination of the solution and subsequent problems.

Breastfeeding is correlated with pain relief for full-term newborns undergoing painful procedures, as demonstrated by reduction in infants' crying time and reduction in pain scores, but breast milk given by syringe has not shown the same efficacy as breastfeeding itself (Shah, Herbozo, Aliwalas, et al., 2012). Comparison of sucrose with breastfeeding has produced mixed results, thus it is difficult to determine optimal pain prevention treatment when comparing breastfeeding with sucrose, and more research is needed (Shah, Herbozo, Aliwalas, et al., 2012).

A review of eight randomized controlled studies explored the use of topical anesthetics such as the eutectic mixture of local anesthetic (EMLA) cream before venipuncture in term and preterm infants. The authors concluded that analgesic effects were of uncertain clinical significance, and concerns regarding the risk of methemaglobinemia need to be further evaluated in future studies (Foster, Taylor, & Spence, 2017).

Having the mother hold the infant in skin-to-skin contact has been shown to significantly reduce the child's distress during painful procedures, as measured by physiologic indices such as heart rate and behaviors such as crying. Studies published are diverse with respect to outcomes measured, and it is impossible to have observers be blinded to pain prevention treatments. The authors of a comprehensive review of 25 studies concluded that more research is needed to better understand optimal strategies for, and effects of, skin-to-skin holding for pain prevention and relief (Johnston, Campbell-Yeo, Disher, et al., 2017).

There are many effective ways to decrease the pain associated with heel puncture in newborns. It is essential that nurses use all available resources to advocate for the prevention and management of neonatal pain during such procedures as heel puncture. (See also Atraumatic Care box later in this chapter.)

The American Academy of Pediatrics (2015b) provides comprehensive direction for care of mothers affected with HIV and their newborns. Cesarean section performed before the rupture of membranes or the onset of labor may prevent mother-to-child transmission of HIV in optimally treated women, and is associated with a reduction in the risk of mother-to-child transmission among HIV-infected women who are either not receiving antiretroviral therapy or are receiving minimal therapy. For infants whose mother's HIV status is unknown, rapid HIV antibody testing provides information within 12 hours of the infant's birth. Antiretroviral prophylaxis is started as soon as possible, pending completion of confirmatory HIV testing. Breastfeeding is delayed until confirmatory testing is done. If the test is negative, prophylaxis is stopped and breastfeeding may start. If the test is positive, infants should be treated with antiretroviral prophylaxis for 6 weeks, and the mother should not breastfeed (American Academy of Pediatrics, 2015b).

Universal Newborn Hearing Screening

It is estimated that screening children for hearing loss by risk factors alone fails to identify approximately 50% of all newborns with a congenital hearing loss. Auditory deprivation in early infancy results in structural and functional reorganization at a cortical level, leading to lifelong deficits (Canadian Paediatric Society, 2016c). Thus without early diagnosis and intervention, hearing loss leads to irreversible deficits in communication and psychosocial skills, cognition, and literacy (Canadian Paediatric Society, 2016c). For these reasons the American Academy of Pediatrics (2007, 2017) and the Canadian Paediatric Society (2016c) recommend universal hearing screening of all newborns before discharge from the birthing hospital.

Infants may be screened for hearing loss by auditory brainstem response or evoked otoacoustic emissions. For infants born by cesarean delivery, it is preferable to delay otoacoustic emission (OAE) testing until after 48 hours of age, as testing earlier than this is associated with significantly higher rates of failure, possibly as a result of retained fluid in the middle ear (Smolkin, Mick, Dabbah, et al., 2012). Newborns who fail the initial screening require referral for outpatient retesting and intervention by 1 month of age; newborns who do not receive initial screening before discharge should also be tested by 1 month (American Academy of Pediatrics, 2007).

Bathing

Bath time is an opportunity for the nurse to accomplish much more than general hygiene. It is an excellent time for observing the infant's behavior, state of arousal, alertness, and muscular activity. With the possibility of transmission of organisms such as HBV and HIV via maternal blood and blood-stained amniotic fluid, as part of Standard Precautions nurses should wear gloves when handling the newborn until blood and amniotic fluid are removed by bathing.

Early bathing (within the first hour of life) interferes with skin-to-skin holding and breastfeeding, thus compromising basic protection against neonatal infection. In a large study of more than 800 late preterm infants, researchers concluded that early bathing may interfere with transition to extrauterine life and optimal adaption of body processes, possibly contributing to problems such as hypothermia and hypoglycemia (Medoff Cooper, Holditch-Davis, Verklan, et al., 2012). Time of initial bathing should be based on individualized assessment, and the initial newborn bath is best delayed for at least 2 hours, until thermal and cardiorespiratory stabilization has been achieved and initial skin-to-skin holding and breastfeeding is complete (Association of Women's Health, Obstetric and Neonatal Nurses, 2013).

The bath time provides an opportunity for the nurse to involve the parents in the care of their child, to teach correct hygiene procedures, and to help them learn about their infant's individual characteristics (Fig. 7.11). The bath may also be used to help parents learn and better understand their newborn's behavioral characteristics. The nurse stresses appropriate bathing supplies and the need for safety in terms of water temperature and supervision of the infant at all times during the bath.

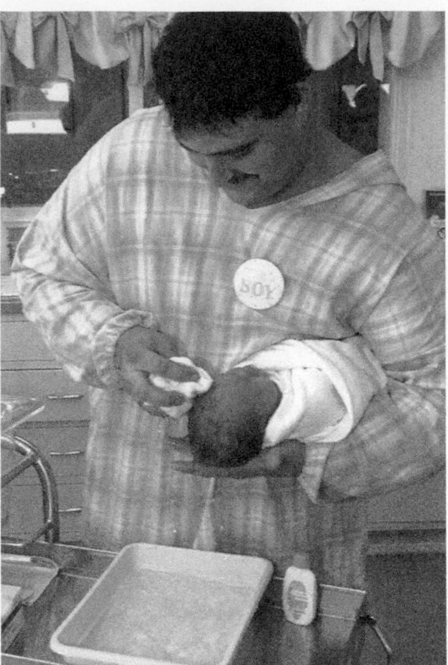

FIG. 7.11 Bath time is an excellent opportunity for parents to learn about their newborn.

The infant's skin surface has a pH of about 5 soon after birth, and the bacteriostatic effects of this pH are significant. In addition, newborn skin is covered with vernix caseosa, a chemical and mechanical skin barrier for newborns. Vernix protects newborns from infection, and assists in the development of the skin's acid mantle. Vernix should not be removed with bathing; allow it to absorb or wear off with normal care and handling (Lund, 2016). Consequently, plain warm water is appropriate for routine bathing. If a cleanser is needed, it should be mild and have a neutral pH. Alkaline soaps, oils, powder, and lotions are not used because they alter the acid mantle, thus providing a medium for bacterial growth. Talcum or cornstarch powders have the added risk of aspiration if they are applied close to the infant's face. (See Diaper Dermatitis, Chapter 11.)

Parents should be involved in a discussion regarding the newborn's bath at home. It is recommended that for the first 2 to 4 weeks the infant be bathed no more than two or three times per week with a plain warm sponge bath. This practice will help maintain the integrity of the newborn's skin and allow time for the umbilical cord to dry completely. Routine daily bathing for newborns is no longer recommended.

Cleansing should proceed in the cephalocaudal (head-to-toe) direction. Remind parents not to vigorously rub infant's skin to remove vernix. A diaper is applied after the bath, and the infant is clothed appropriately to prevent heat loss.

Care of the Umbilicus

Because the umbilical stump is an excellent medium for bacterial growth, various methods of cord care have been practiced to prevent infection. Some methods popular in the past include the use of an antimicrobial agent such as bacitracin or triple dye, or agents such as alcohol or povidone. A Cochrane Review of 21 studies (most of which were conducted in developed countries) found no significant difference between cords treated with antiseptics compared with dry cord care or placebo; there were no reported systemic infections or deaths, and a trend toward reduced colonization was found in cords treated with antibiotics (Zupan, Garner, & Omari, 2013). Current recommendations for cord care for infants in the developed world includes cleaning the cord initially with sterile water or a neutral pH cleanser, then subsequently cleaning the cord with water (American Academy of Pediatrics, 2016g; Association of Women's Health, Obstetric and Neonatal Nurses, 2013).

Nurses working in neonatal care must carefully evaluate the available studies and compare the risks and benefits regarding the method of cord care within their own population of newborns and families. Particularly in the developing world, infants may encounter increased risk of potentially life-threatening sepsis, thus antimicrobial treatment may be appropriate in such settings (American Academy of Pediatrics, 2016g; Association of Women's Health, Obstetric and Neonatal Nurses, 2013).

Regardless of the method used, nurses must teach parents about the importance of observation and monitoring of the cord, in addition to cord care methods, in discharge planning. The diaper is placed below the cord to avoid irritation and wetness on the site. Parents are instructed regarding stump deterioration and proper umbilical care. The stump deteriorates through the process of dry gangrene, with an average separation time of 5 to 15 days. Cord separation time is influenced by a number of factors, including type of cord care, type of delivery, and other perinatal events. It takes a few more weeks for the cord base to heal completely after cord separation. During this time, care consists of keeping the base clean and dry and observing for any signs of infection.

Circumcision

Circumcision, the surgical removal of the foreskin on the glans penis, is not a common practice in most countries. In the United States, however, between 40% and 70% of newborn males are circumcised, depending on the region (Owings, Uddin, Williams, et al., 2013). The Centers for Disease Control and Prevention reports that the overall rate of newborn circumcision in the United States has fallen from 64.5% in 1979 to 58.3% in 2010 (Owings, Uddin, Williams, et al., 2013). Despite the frequency of the procedure in the United States, there is some controversy regarding the benefits and risks (Box 7.4).

BOX 7.4 Risks and Benefits of Neonatal Circumcision

Risks (Complications)

Hemorrhage
Infection
Dehiscence (separation of approximated edges of skin)
Meatitis (from loss of protective foreskin)
Adhesions
Concealed penis
Urethral fistula
Meatal stenosis
Pain in unanesthetized infants (long-term consequences unknown, but short-term stresses include increased heart rate, behavior changes, prolonged crying, increased cortisol levels, and decreased blood oxygenation)

Benefits

Prevention of penile cancer and posthitis (inflammation of prepuce)
Decreased incidence of balanitis (inflammation of glans) and possibly urinary tract infection in infants
Reduction or prevention of acquisition and transmission of sexually transmitted infections (see text)
Prevention of complications associated with later circumcision

Research has explored the possible link between circumcision and reduced transmission of communicable illnesses such as human papillomavirus (HPV) and HIV in later life. Current evidence suggests circumcision reduces incidence of urinary tract infections, penile and vaginal cancer, and the acquisition of sexually transmitted infections; however, benefits are most significant for high-risk populations in the developing world (Canadian Paediatric Society, 2015b). The American Academy of Pediatrics (2012b) states that current evidence indicates the health benefits of newborn male circumcision outweigh the risks, and that the procedure should be made available to families who choose it (American Academy of Pediatrics, 2012b). Despite encouraging outcome data, the health benefits are not yet great enough to recommend *routine* circumcision for all male newborns (American Academy of Pediatrics, 2012b; Canadian Paediatric Society, 2015b; Jagannath, Fedorowicz, Sud, et al., 2012).

The American Academy of Pediatrics statement emphasizes parental autonomy to determine what is in the best interest of their newborn. The policy encourages the primary care practitioner to ensure that parents have been given accurate and unbiased information about the risks, benefits, and alternatives before making an informed choice and that they understand that circumcision is an elective procedure. In addition to examining the medical benefits of newborn circumcision, the Academy recommends that if parents decide to have their male infant circumcised, procedural analgesia should be provided.

Nurses are in a unique position to educate parents regarding the care of their newborns, and they must ensure that parents have accurate and unbiased information with which to make an informed decision. Parents should discuss the options for pain control, and the possibility of observing the procedure, with the primary practitioner.*

The nurse should use nonpharmacologic interventions as an adjunct to reduce the pain of this operative procedure (see Atraumatic Care box). Despite adequate scientific evidence that newborns feel and respond to pain, circumcisions may still be performed with either insufficient analgesia or no analgesia at all. Nurses can use the Academy's policy statement to advocate for the use of optimum pain relief during circumcision.

Circumcision is usually performed in the nursery. It should not be performed immediately after delivery because of the neonate's unstable physiologic status and increased susceptibility to stress. Preoperative nursing care includes allowing the infant nothing by mouth before the procedure to prevent aspiration of vomitus (about 1 to 2 hours); however, the necessity of this practice has been challenged. Additional measures include the surgical time-out, checking for a signed consent form, and adequately restraining the infant, usually on a special board (Fig. 7.12)

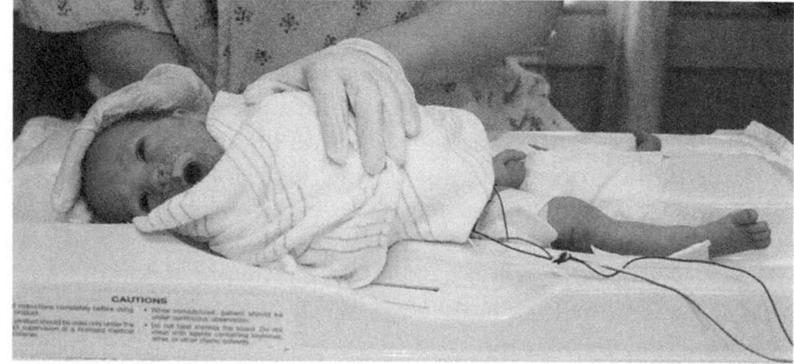

FIG. 7.12 Proper positioning of infant in Circumstraint. (Courtesy Paul Vincent Kuntz, Texas Children's Hospital, Houston.)

**Should the baby be circumcised?* is available from the American Academy of Pediatrics, 141 Northwest Point Blvd., Elk Grove Village, IL 60009-1098; 847-434-4000; fax: 847-434-8000; http://www.aap.org.

ATRAUMATIC CARE

*Guidelines for Pain Management During Neonatal Circumcision**

Pharmacologic Interventions

The primary practitioner is responsible for ordering analgesics, which may include preprocedure and postprocedure acetaminophen, topical creams such as EMLA to numb the operative site, and lidocaine, which is administered by injection to perform a nerve block.

Nonpharmacologic Interventions

Comfort measures such as music, sucking on a pacifier, and soothing voices are helpful; however, these strategies have *not* proved to be sufficient in reducing the pain of circumcision when used alone. In addition to the practitioner-ordered pharmacologic interventions:

- If using a circumcision board, pad as needed with blankets or other thick, soft material. A more comfortable, padded, and physiologic restraint that places the infant semireclining may also decrease distress.
- Provide the parents with the option to be present during the circumcision, after ascertaining that this is an option by discussing with primary practitioner.
- Swaddle the upper body and legs to provide warmth and containment and to reduce movement.
- If the newborn is not swaddled and is unclothed, use a radiant warmer to prevent hypothermia. Shield newborn's eyes from overhead lights.
- Prewarm any topical solutions to be used in sterile preparation of the surgical site by placing in a warm blanket or towel.
- Play infant relaxation music before, during, and after procedure; allow parents or other caregiver the option of choosing the music.
- After the procedure, remove restraints and swaddle. Immediately have the parent, other caregiver, or nursing staff hold the infant. Continue to have the infant suck on pacifier or offer feeding.

*There is sufficient evidence and support for use of a combination of pharmacologic and nonpharmacologic interventions to holistically manage neonatal pain. Combined analgesia, including pharmaceuticals and nonpharmacologic interventions (such as swaddling, sucking, and sucrose), are recommended during the procedure to provide holistic pain management (American Academy of Pediatrics, 2012b).

or physiologic circumcision restraint chair. The circumcision chair is padded and allows free movement of the newborn's extremities without compromising the surgical field. In addition, the chair allows the infant to sit at a 30- to 45-degree angle, and it is adjustable to accommodate smaller newborns. All the equipment used for the procedure, such as gloves, instruments, dressings, and draping towels, must be sterile.

The procedure involves freeing the foreskin from the glans penis by using a scalpel, Gomco or Mogen clamp (see Cultural Considerations box), or Plastibell. In the Gomco technique the foreskin is clamped, cut with a scalpel, and removed; the clamp crushes the nerve endings and blood vessels, promoting hemostasis. In the Plastibell procedure the foreskin is removed using a plastic ring and a string tied around the foreskin like a tourniquet. The excess foreskin is trimmed. In about 5 to 8 days the plastic ring separates and falls off.

Once the procedure is completed, the infant is released from the restraints and comforted. If the parents were not present during the procedure, they are informed of the infant's status and reunited with their son.

Care of the circumcision depends on the type of procedure. If a clamp was used, a petrolatum gauze dressing may be applied loosely to prevent adherence to the diaper. If the Plastibell was applied, no special dressing is required; however, a petrolatum jelly gauze dressing may be used to prevent adherence of the glans to the diaper. Because the area is tender, the diaper is applied loosely to prevent friction against the penis. The circumcision is evaluated for excessive bleeding in the first few hours after the procedure, and the first void is recorded. A recommended standard is to evaluate the site every 30 minutes for at least 2 hours and then at least every 2 hours thereafter.

Normally, on the second day a yellowish white exudate forms as part of the granulation process. This is not a sign of infection and is not forcibly removed. As healing progresses, the exudate disappears. Parents are educated to report any evidence of bleeding, unusual swelling, or absence of voiding to the practitioner.

PROVIDE OPTIMUM NUTRITION

Selection of a feeding method is one of the major decisions parents face. It is best to explore feeding options before the infant is born when parents are better able to understand the importance of infant nutrition

CULTURAL CONSIDERATIONS

Circumcision

In the Jewish culture circumcision is performed during a ceremony called a berith, or bris, which takes place on the eighth day of life. A specially trained professional known as a mohel stretches the prepuce over the glans, pulling it through a slit in a shield (usually a Mogen clamp) and cutting it with a knife. The traditional technique is not sterile, and bleeding is controlled by tight bandaging around the penis. The infant may be given some sweet wine before the procedure. Blankets instead of straps are usually used to restrain the infant to a board, and the parents are present. Although the risk of injury as a result of neonatal circumcision is low, risk is increased when circumcision is done outside of the hospital by nonprofessional practitioners. Suggested techniques for avoiding injury, and for repair of injury, are available (Banihani, Fox, Gander, et al., 2014; Pippi Salle, Jesus, Lorenzo, et al., 2013).

Female circumcision (mutilation) is practiced in some parts of Africa, the Middle East, Southeast Asia, and South America—and in some immigrants from these areas. In the most extensive operations, the vaginal orifice is narrowed with creation of a covering seal by cutting and appositioning the labia minora and/or the labia majora, with or without excision of the clitoris (Bazi, 2017). Sharp objects such as glass, razors, scissors or sharpened rocks are typically used, often without anesthesia of any type. Hemorrhage, trauma, and sepsis are potential complications. Female genital mutilation may be done on infants, or may be delayed until puberty. In some cultures, female circumcision is used to prove virginity and to reduce sexual pleasure, thus promoting fidelity.

The World Health Organization (2017) condemns all forms of female genital mutilation. It is associated with an increased risk for adverse obstetric outcomes and numerous physical problems, which often may not receive adequate medical care.

NURSING TIP

To check for the first void in disposable diapers made of absorbent gelling material, pinch the crotch of the diaper for a "clumpy, doughy" feeling because these diapers will feel dry despite voiding.

BOX 7.5 Advantages of Human Milk Compared With Formula

- Contains adequate (not excessive) protein; has greater quantities of certain amino acids, including cystine and taurine
- Contains more lactalbumin (produces easily digested curds) than casein (produces large, hard curds)
- Contains more lactose, which in the gut stimulates growth of microorganisms, which synthesize some B vitamins and produce organic acids that may restrict or prevent the growth of harmful bacteria
- Contains more monounsaturated fatty acids, which enhance absorption of fat and calcium
- Contains adequate (not excessive) minerals, with exception of fluoride (low)
- Contains low amounts of iron and zinc, but these are more readily absorbed
- Contains less calcium and phosphorus but a more favorable ratio of the minerals, which prevents excessive calcium excretion
- Contains adequate amounts of vitamins A, B complex, and E; vitamin C content depends on maternal intake; vitamin D is low but more readily absorbed (see text)
- Contains growth modulators that modify growth or maturation
- Offers several immunologic benefits: contains various immunoglobulins, especially immunoglobulin A; macrophages, granulocytes, T- and B-cell lymphocytes; and other factors that inhibit bacterial growth
- Has laxative effect
- Is economical, readily available, and sanitary
- Has psychologic benefits of a close bond between infant and mother during feeding

and the choices available. Nurses should be at the forefront in providing parent(s) with accurate and unbiased information needed to make a conscientious, informed decision regarding feeding method. In general, there are two choices: human milk and commercially prepared cow's milk–based formula. These two methods have significant nutritional, economic, and psychologic differences (Box 7.5).

Cultural Influences on Infant Feeding

Cultural beliefs and practices may significantly influence infant feeding methods. Many cultures typically do not give colostrum to newborns and only begin breastfeeding after the milk has "come in" (i.e., milk is produced in larger volumes than those seen with initial colostrum production). These groups include mothers in Asia, Latin America, and sub-Saharan Africa, and often mothers who have emigrated from these areas (Agho, Ogeleka, Ogbo, et al., 2016). When breastfeeding is delayed until the mother's milk is available in larger volumes (generally a few days after delivery), babies are given prelacteal liquids such as tea, juice, water, or water sweetened with sugar or honey before the initiation of breastfeeding (Agho, Ogeleka, Ogbo, et al., 2016). Some rationales for this practice include a concern that because colostrum volume is small, the baby may be at risk for dehydration, or that nonmilk feeds are needed to "cleanse" the gastrointestinal tract for digestion. Although perhaps intuitively logical, neither of these rationales is based in evidence. The use of prelacteal feedings significantly increases the risk of infection, particularly in developing countries where sanitation may be poor. In addition, failure to empty the breasts regularly in the early hours and days after delivery contributes to suboptimal milk supply.

A recent study of Chinese immigrant women in Australia reported that Chinese women were more likely to combine breastfeeding with formula and to introduce solids earlier than the general Australian population (Kuswara, Laws, Kremer, et al., 2016). Chinese mothers shared that although they supported exclusive breastfeeding, grandparents frequently pressured them to use formula, believing that "a fat baby is a healthy baby." Wandel, Terragni, Nguyen, and colleagues (2016) report similar findings after studying a small group of Somali women who immigrated to Norway. Although family support for breastfeeding is generally reported as strong, early formula supplementation is common, as is the belief in the need to introduce water feedings early. Somali culture apparently favors "chubby" babies, and formula is seen as the best way ensure this weight gain.

Waldrop (2013) describes the practice of *los dos* (which means *the two* or *both*) among Hispanic women living in the United States, which involves supplementing breastfeeding with infant formula. Women in this study stated that reasons for choosing *los dos* were based on previous experience with infant feeding; not wanting the baby to cry from hunger; to improve the infant's health; and to prevent the baby from suffering when the mother had to return to work. Many mothers believed that breast milk alone was inadequate for the infant's nutrition and that the mother did not have an adequate supply of breast milk to keep the infant satisfied. Breastfeeding was also perceived as being somewhat laborious and at times painful and embarrassing in comparison to bottle-feeding. Family and cultural beliefs were also cited as reasons for not exclusively breastfeeding and practicing *los dos*.

In a recent small study of Mexican American women from a midwestern US city, the authors reported that 43% of women exclusively breastfed, and only a minority of these mothers used formula in the early days of breastfeeding (Wambach, Domain, Page-Goertz, et al., 2016). This finding illustrates the danger of making assumptions about any cultural group, as education and exposure to different practices may influence change in breastfeeding practice. Traditional cultural ideas and practices may evolve over time, thus cultural background does not always predict behavior—individual assessment is necessary.

Sociocultural values may preclude the mother receiving adequate information regarding breastfeeding. If the family is strongly patriarchal and the father is the only English-speaking person in the family, the necessary information being conveyed to the family by the health care provider may not be correctly translated, thus the need to continually assess mothers' beliefs and practices. Variation in dialect may also contribute to confusion. For example, among Hispanic Spanish-speaking people, terminology used in one country for the act of breastfeeding or describing the breasts may be offensive in another Spanish-speaking country. Cultural attitudes regarding modesty and breastfeeding are sometimes important considerations. (See Cultural Considerations box.)

CULTURAL CONSIDERATIONS

Acculturation

Acculturation is a process whereby members of one cultural group adopt the beliefs and behaviors of another group. There may be language or literacy issues that interfere with acquisition of up-to-date breastfeeding information. There may be limited family support for immigrant women, and cultural norms may be at odds with information presented by care providers in their new country.

Jones, Power, Queenan, and colleagues (2015) report that although there are potential barriers to breastfeeding common to all women, such as pain, embarrassment, employment, or inconvenience, immigrant women often have additional concerns. Strategies to increase the likelihood of breastfeeding success include prenatal breastfeeding education, enhanced breastfeeding support programs in hospitals, and linking mothers with nonprofessional peer supporters (Jones, Power, Queenan, et al., 2015).

With the increasing numbers of immigrants in the United States, it is incumbent on nurses to discuss cultural values related to breastfeeding and the benefits of breastfeeding so the mother can make an informed decision. Nurses must clarify with the mother what her expectations are regarding infant feeding and assist her in meeting those goals.

Human Milk

Human milk is the best option for infant nutrition. Breast milk consists of a number of micronutrients that are bioavailable, meaning these nutrients are available in quantities and qualities that make them easily digestible by the newborn and absorbed for energy and growth. A variety of immunologic properties are found exclusively in human milk.

Lysozyme is found in large quantities in human milk with bacteriostatic functions against gram-positive bacteria and *Enterobacteriaceae* organisms. Human milk also contains numerous other host defense factors such as macrophages, granulocytes, and T and B lymphocytes. Casein in human milk greatly enhances the absorption of iron, thus preventing iron-dependent bacteria from proliferating in the gastrointestinal tract. Secretory immunoglobulin A (IgA) is found in high levels in colostrum, but levels gradually decrease over the first 14 days of life. Secretory IgA is an immunoglobulin that prevents viruses and bacteria from invading the intestinal mucosa in breastfed newborns, thus protecting them from infection. This whey protein is also believed to play an important role in preventing the development of allergies.

The fat content of human milk is composed of lipids, triglycerides, and cholesterol; cholesterol is an essential element for brain growth. The function of these lipids is to allow optimum intestinal absorption of fatty acids and provide essential fatty acids and polyunsaturated fatty acids. Furthermore, lipids contribute approximately 50% of the total calories in human milk. Although the overall fat content in human milk is higher than that of cow's milk–based formula, it is used more efficiently by the infant.

The primary source of carbohydrate in human milk is lactose, which is present in higher concentrations (6.8 g/dl) than in cow's milk–based formula (4.9 g/dl). Other carbohydrates found in human milk include glucose, galactose, and glucosamine. The carbohydrates serve not only as a large percentage of the total calories in human milk but also have a protective function; the oligosaccharides (**prebiotic**) in human milk stimulate the growth of *Lactobacillus bifidus* (a **probiotic**) and prevent bacteria from adhering to epithelial surfaces.

Human milk contains the two proteins whey (lactalbumin) and casein (curd) in a whey-dominant ratio of 70 to 80:20 to 30 in early lactation, decreasing to 50:50 in late lactation. Cow's milk is casein-dominant, with a ratio of approximately 20:80 whey to casein ratio. Cow's milk–based formulas vary in their whey-casein ratios, as some have added whey to alter their formulation to more closely resemble human milk (Martin, Ling, & Blackburn, 2016). This ratio of whey dominance in human milk makes it more digestible and produces the soft stools seen in breastfed infants. Thus human milk has a laxative effect, and constipation is uncommon. The whey protein lactoferrin in human milk has iron-binding characteristics with bacteriostatic capabilities, particularly against gram-positive and gram-negative aerobes, anaerobes, and yeasts.

Several digestive enzymes are present in human milk, such as amylases, lipases, proteases, and ribonucleases, which enhance digestion and absorption of various nutrients. The amounts of lipid- and water-soluble vitamins, as well as electrolytes, minerals, and trace elements, in human milk are sufficient for infant growth, development, and energy needs during the first 6 months of life. The one possible exception is vitamin D, which is found in varying amounts depending on the mother's intake of vitamin D–fortified food and exposure to ultraviolet light. Therefore to prevent vitamin D–deficiency rickets, the American Academy of Pediatrics (2014b) recommends that unless the lactating mother is taking supplements of approximately 6000 IU per day, breastfed and partially breastfed infants should be supplemented with 400 IU of vitamin D (oral) per day, beginning in the first few days of life. Supplementation should continue until the infant is consuming at least 1 L/day of vitamin D–fortified infant formula or cow's milk (American Academy of Pediatrics, 2014b). The Canadian Paediatric Society (2017) suggests that for infants and children living in its northernmost climates, it may be reasonable to supplement with 800 IU per day, to compensate for extremely limited exposure to sunlight.

Breastfeeding is associated with a decrease in the incidence of type 2 diabetes and obesity, fewer hospital admissions for respiratory tract illnesses in generally healthy infants, and higher intelligence scores compared with formula-fed infants (Horta, Loret de Mola, & Victora, 2015; Wang, Collins, Ratliff, et al., 2017). Breastfeeding has an analgesic effect on newborns during painful procedures such as heel puncture (Shah, Herbozo, Aliwalas, et al., 2012), and it has also been found to decrease pain scores in full-term and older infants receiving routine childhood immunizations (Modarres, Jazayeri, Rahnama, et al., 2013).

Additional beneficial components of human milk include stem cells, prostaglandins, epidermal growth factor, docosahexaenoic acid (DHA), arachidonic acid (AA), taurine, carnitine, cytokine, interleukins, and natural hormones such as thyroid-releasing hormone, gonadotropin-releasing hormone, and prolactin.

Human milk changes over the course of the lactation cycle. **Colostrum**, for example, is rich in immunoglobulins and vitamin K and has a higher protein content than mature milk; however, it has a lower fat content. Transitional milk replaces colostrum when the mother's milk supply starts increasing, and eventually mature milk becomes the primary milk source. There is also diurnal variation in the biochemistry of mature human milk. Human milk also varies with respect to gestational age; preterm human milk differs from mature milk in its biochemical composition. Nonphysiologic advantages of human milk are discussed in the next section.

Breastfeeding

Human milk is the preferred form of nutrition for the full-term infant. *Healthy People 2020* has a goal to increase breastfeeding rates in the United States to 81.9% in early postpartum and to 60.6% for mothers who continue to breastfeed for at least 6 months (US Department of Health and Human Services, 2013). Data from the US Department of Health and Human Services (2013) indicate that in 2011 the overall rate of breastfeeding was 79.2%; breastfeeding at 6 months of age was reported to be 49.4%. Among infants born in 2011, 40.7% and 18.8% were exclusively breastfeeding at 3 and 6 months, respectively (US Department of Health and Human Services, 2013). Rates of breastfeeding varied among different demographic groups, with lower breastfeeding rates at 6 months reported in African American women and higher rates in women of Asian descent. Interestingly, enrollment in the Women, Infants, and Children (WIC) program is consistently found to have a negative impact on breastfeeding rates in the United States (Houghtaling, Byker Shanks, & Jenkins, 2017). Several strategies have been identified to mitigate the negative influences, including environmental, social, and individual WIC participant strategies (Houghtaling, Byker Shanks, & Jenkins, 2017).

Studies exploring mothers' reasons for early cessation of breastfeeding suggest several factors may contribute to this decision, such as the perception of insufficient milk, difficulties with lactation such as nipple trauma, and concerns with maternal or newborn health (Newby & Davies, 2016; Odom, Li, Scanlon, et al., 2013). Modifiable factors associated with decreased risk of early cessation of breastfeeding include professional and social support (Newby & Davies, 2016; Odom, Li, Scanlon, et al., 2013). These findings have important implications for nurses in education and discussion regarding breastfeeding before, during, and after the pregnancy. Teaching families about the importance of breastfeeding and supporting mothers learning this skill will contribute to mothers' success.

The American Academy of Pediatrics (2012c) has reaffirmed its position recommending exclusive breastfeeding until 6 months of age, with continued breastfeeding to at least 1 year of age and beyond as long as is mutually desirable by mother and infant. The Academy also supports programs that enable women to continue breastfeeding after returning to work. In its support of breastfeeding practices, the Academy further discourages the advertisement of infant formula to breastfeeding mothers and distribution of formula discharge packs without the advice of a health care provider.

The Baby-Friendly Initiative (BFI) is a joint effort of the World Health Organization and UNICEF to encourage, promote, and support breastfeeding as the model for optimum infant nutrition. BFI developed 10 research-supported practices as guidelines for caregivers worldwide to promote breastfeeding (World Health Organization, UNICEF, & Wellstart International, 2009) (Table 7.5). Research indicates that BFI designation is sometimes associated with higher rates of breastfeeding initiation; however, the designation does not appear to affect breastfeeding rates among women with higher educational levels in US populations (Hawkins, Stern, Baum, et al., 2014, 2015). Howe-Heyman and Lutenbacher (2016), after reviewing 25 studies published over 23 years, concluded that although there are more studies that support the BFI as an intervention to increase breastfeeding rates than there are studies than demonstrate no effect, many of the studies are methodologically weak. These authors suggest that peer support, formal prenatal breastfeeding education, and needs-based informal postpartum support may be more effective than the BFI for increasing breastfeeding rates (Howe-Heyman & Lutenbacher, 2016).

In addition to the physiologic qualities of human milk, the most outstanding psychologic benefit of breastfeeding is the close maternal-child relationship. The infant is nestled close to the mother's skin, can hear the rhythm of her heartbeat, can feel the warmth of her body, and has a sense of peaceful security. The mother has a close feeling of union with her child and feels a sense of accomplishment and satisfaction as the infant suckles milk from her.

Human milk is the most economical form of feeding. It is always available, ready to serve at room temperature, and free of contamination. Although human milk is not sterile, healthy full-term infants can tolerate, and in fact benefit from, varying amounts of nonpathogenic and pathogenic organisms. The protection against infection can provide additional cost savings in terms of fewer medical visits and less time lost from work for the employed mother. Breastfed infants, especially beyond 2 to 3 months of age, tend to grow at a satisfactory but slower rate than bottle-fed infants.

Contraindications to breastfeeding include the following (American Academy of Pediatrics, 2012c):

- Maternal chemotherapy—antimetabolites and certain antineoplastic drugs
- Active tuberculosis not under treatment in mother

TABLE 7.5 Ten Steps to Successful Breastfeeding

Every facility providing maternity services and care for newborn infants should:

WHO 10 Steps	BCC Interpretation
1. Have a written breastfeeding policy that is routinely communicated to all health care staff.	Have a written breastfeeding policy that is routinely communicated to all health care providers and volunteers.
2. Train all health care staff in skills necessary to implement this policy.	Ensure all health care providers have the knowledge and skills necessary to implement the breastfeeding policy.
3. Inform all pregnant women about the benefits and management of breastfeeding.	Inform all pregnant women and their families about the importance and process of breastfeeding.
4. Help mothers initiate breastfeeding within a half hour of birth (WHO, 2009). Place babies in skin-to-skin contact with their mothers immediately following birth for at least an hour. Encourage mothers to recognize when their babies are ready to breastfeed and offer help if needed.	Place babies in uninterrupted skin-to-skin contact with their mothers immediately following birth for at least an hour or until completion of the first feeding or as long as the mother wishes; encourage mothers to recognize when their babies are ready to feed, offering help as needed.
5. Show mothers how to breastfeed and how to maintain lactation even if they are separated from their infants	Assist mothers to breastfeed and maintain lactation should they face challenges including separation from their infants.
6. Give newborn infants no food or drink other than breast milk, unless medically indicated.	Support mothers to exclusively breastfeed for the first 6 months, unless supplements are *medically* indicated.
7. Practice rooming-in—allow mothers and infants to remain together—24 hours a day.	Facilitate 24 hour rooming-in for all mother-infant dyads: mothers and infants remain together.
8. Encourage breastfeeding on demand.	Encourage baby-led or cue-based breastfeeding. Encourage sustained breastfeeding beyond 6 months with appropriate introduction of complementary foods.
9. Give no artificial teats or pacifiers (also called dummies or soothers) to breastfeeding infants.	Support mothers to feed and care for their breastfeeding babies without the use of artificial teats or pacifiers (dummies or soothers).
10. Foster the establishment of breastfeeding support groups and refer mothers to them on discharge from the hospital or clinic.	Provide a seamless transition between the services provided by the hospital, community health services, and peer support programs. Apply principles of Primary Health Care and Population Health to support the continuum of care and implement strategies that affect the broad determinants that will improve breastfeeding outcomes.

From The WHO 10 Steps to Successful Breastfeeding (1989) and The Interpretation for Canadian Practice (2011).
From The Breastfeeding Committee for Canada (BCC). Retrieved from http://www.breastfeedingcanada.ca/documents/2012-05-14_BCC_BFI_Ten_Steps_Integrated_Indicators_Summary.pdf.

- HIV in mothers *in the industrialized world* (In the developing world, risks to nonbreastfeeding infants from malnutrition and infectious disease are significant, so the benefits of breastfeeding may outweigh the risk of acquiring HIV from human milk [American Academy of Pediatrics, 2015b])
- Galactosemia in infant
- Maternal herpes simplex lesion on a breast
- Cytomegalovirus (CMV): may be a risk to extremely low birth weight preterm infants (<1500 g); not a risk for full-term infants whose mother is seropositive for CMV
- Maternal substance abuse with street drugs (e.g., phencyclidine [PCP], cocaine, and cannibis) (Note: Adequately nourished narcotic-dependent mothers may be encouraged to breastfeed if they are enrolled in a supervised methadone maintenance program and have negative screening for HIV and illicit drugs.)
- Human T-cell leukemia virus type I or II
- Mothers receiving diagnostic or radioactive isotopes or who have had exposure to radioactive materials (for as long as there is radioactivity in the milk)

A small number of medications are contraindicated for breastfeeding mothers. Consult a reference such as LactMed, an online source published by the National Library of Medicine/National Institutes of Health (National Institutes of Health, 2017). Mastitis is usually not a contraindication if the discomfort is tolerable; however, each case should be treated on an individual basis.

Some herbal products are marketed as safe and effective alternatives to prescription medications, and claims may be made about efficacy for which there is no evidence. Certain agents, called galactogogues, are reported to increase breast milk production. Data are insufficient to confirm or deny the assertion of increased milk production using herbal galactogogues, and nurses should caution mothers to seek advice from a practitioner to ensure that the herbal preparations do not have the potential for harm (Bazzano, Hofer, Thibeau, et al., 2016).

Breastfeeding with twins and other multiples requires specialized professional support. If the infants are full term, they can begin feedings immediately after birth (Fig. 7.13); late preterm infants should be evaluated individually but may be put to breast if stable. Simultaneous feeding promotes the rapid production of milk needed for both infants and makes the milk that would normally be lost in the let-down reflex available to one of the twins. When only one infant is hungry, the mother should feed singly. She should also alternate breasts when feeding each infant and avoid favoring one breast for one infant. The sucking patterns of infants vary, and each infant needs the visual stimulation and exercise that alternating breasts provides.

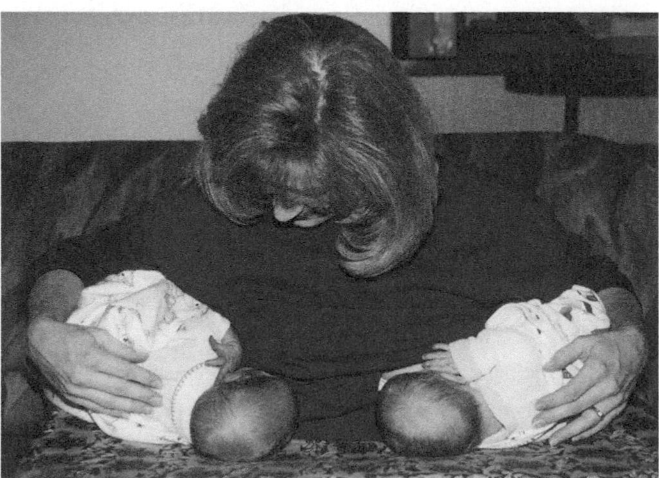

FIG. 7.13 Simultaneous breastfeeding of twins.

! NURSING ALERT

Do not use microwaves to defrost or warm human milk. High-temperature microwaving (72° to 98°C [162° to 208°F]) significantly destroys antiinfective factors and vitamin C and may cause hot spots that could burn the baby's mouth (American Dietetic Association, 2011). Human milk may be thawed or warmed in warm tap water (be sure the milk is not contaminated by the water bath) or by placing in a commercial bottle warmer. Test the temperature of the milk before feeding.

A concern many mothers have is the perceived inconvenience of loss of freedom and independence. Being committed to feeding the infant every 2 to 3 hours can seem overwhelming, especially to women with multiple responsibilities. Many women resume their careers shortly after delivery and prefer to bottle-feed. Combining breastfeeding and employment is possible, and many employers provide space for mothers to pump and store their milk. This is an acknowledgment of the demonstrated health benefits of breastfeeding, as a breastfed infant is far less likely to have infection of any sort; thus the infant's mother is far less likely to need time away from work to care for an ill infant. Although breastfeeding is the preferred form of infant feeding, mothers' decisions regarding their preferences must be respected and supported.

Mothers need encouragement and assistance during their postpartum hospital stay and at home to enhance their opportunities for success and satisfaction. Successful breastfeeding is facilitated by the mother's desire to breastfeed, satisfaction with breastfeeding, and available support systems, both personal and professional. The following interventions promote breastfeeding:

- Frequent and early breastfeeding, especially during the first hour of life; immediate skin-to-skin contact; rooming-in; and feeding on demand
- Correct positioning of the infant at the breast to achieve a deep alveolar latch, that is, a wide-open mouth, tongue under the areola, and expression of milk by effective alveolar compressions (Fig. 7.14)

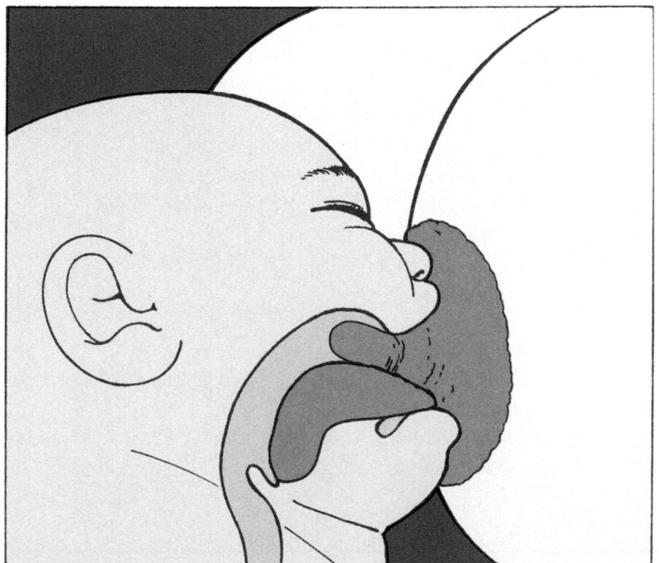

FIG. 7.14 The tongue is under the areola, with tip of the nipple at back of the wide-open mouth.

- Direct modeling of the importance of breastfeeding by health care providers, such as encouraging demand nursing with no formula supplementation and decreased emphasis on infant formula products
- Increased information and support to mothers after discharge, especially follow-up telephone calls
- Early breast pumping every 2 to 3 hours for 20 minutes bilaterally if the newborn is unable to nurse immediately (increases oxytocin production and thus milk production)

Nurses play a significant role in the breastfeeding decision and must make themselves available to families for guidance and support. Several excellent books and organizations, such as La Leche League International,* are available as resources for professionals and breastfeeding mothers.

Breastfeeding Problems

Mothers may have concerns regarding breastfeeding, and, with earlier discharge from hospital or birth centers, problems may develop after the mother is home. New mothers are often concerned about their milk supply, and excessive anxiety can affect successful lactation (see Family-Centered Care box).

FAMILY-CENTERED CARE

Breastfeeding and Infant Weight Gain

Breastfed infants are leaner and have less body fat than formula-fed infants, but growth in head circumference is greater in the breastfed group. There is evidence that breastfed infants regulate their energy intake, thus decreasing the propensity toward obesity in later life.

An important factor in the development of the Dietary Reference Intakes by the Institute of Medicine (see Chapter 12) that affects children, particularly infants 0 to 6 months, is that the Adequate Intakes are based on the nutrient intake of full-term, healthy, breastfed infants (by well-nourished mothers), which now represents the gold standard for infant nutrition in this age-group.

Table 7.6 summarizes some common breastfeeding problems and suggested interventions to correct them. Most of these problems are easily prevented or easily remedied, provided the mother receives education and guidance. Assessment should include a detailed history, examination of the breasts, and observation of the breastfeeding (see Nursing Care Guidelines box).

Encourage frequent feedings to increase milk production; use of supplemental formula, water, glucose water, or solid foods will result in decreased breast milk intake and ultimately decreased production.

Many breastfeeding problems respond rapidly to simple interventions, such as correcting the infant's feeding position. However, the mother needs continual reassurance of success and the support that allows her the needed rest and relaxation to breastfeed her infant. Referral to a peer supporter or to supportive agencies, such as local groups of La Leche League International, or to a lactation specialist, may be beneficial.

Bottle-Feeding

Bottle-feeding generally refers to the use of bottles for feeding commercial or evaporated milk formula rather than using the breast, although in some instances human milk may be expressed and fed with a bottle.

NURSING CARE GUIDELINES

Observing the Breastfeeding Pair

- Position of mother, her body language, and any possible tension.
- Position of infant. Infant's ventral (front) surface is next to mother's ventral surface with the face directly in front of the breast ("tummy to tummy"). The infant cannot swallow if the head has to turn to the breast.
- Position of mother's hand on the breast. Using the thumb on top and fingers supporting the breast encircling the areola (the C-hold) facilitates infant's ability to grasp the areola properly.
- Flanged position of infant's lips on the areola. The lips should gently grasp most of the areola, with the lower lip covering more of the areola than the upper lip.
- Baby's chin, not the nose, touching mother's breast
- Use of alternate breasts and feeding time on each breast.
- Technique to break suction. The mother should release suction using fingers between the areola and lips, not pulling infant from the breast abruptly.

Bottle-feeding is an acceptable method of feeding. Nurses should not assume, however, that new parents automatically know how to bottle-feed their infant. Parents who choose bottle-feeding also need support and assistance in meeting their infant's needs.

Providing newborns with nutrition is only one aspect of the feeding. Holding them close to the body while rocking or cuddling them helps ensure the emotional component of feeding. Like breastfed infants, bottle-fed infants need to be held on alternate sides of the lap to expose them to different stimuli. The feeding should not be hurried. Even though they may suck vigorously for the first 5 minutes and seem to be satisfied, they should be allowed to continue sucking. Infants need at least 2 hours of sucking a day. If there are six feedings per day, about 20 minutes of sucking at each feeding provides for oral gratification.

Propping the bottle is discouraged for the following reasons:

- It denies the infant the important component of close human contact.
- The infant may aspirate formula into the trachea and lungs.
- It may facilitate the development of middle ear infections. As the infant lies flat and sucks, milk that has pooled in the pharynx becomes a suitable medium for bacterial growth. Bacteria may then enter the eustachian tube, which leads to the middle ear, causing acute otitis media.
- It encourages continuous pooling of formula in the mouth, which can lead to caries when the teeth erupt. (See Chapter 12.)

NURSING ALERT

Warming bottles in the microwave oven is not recommended because of the risk of burns from excessively hot temperatures of the milk or bottles exploding. When milk is warmed in the microwave, it is not warmed evenly and may be too hot in places, causing mouth burns (American Dietetic Association, 2011). Milk may be warmed in warm tap water (be sure the milk is not contaminated by the water bath) or in a commercial bottle warmer. Test the temperature of the milk before feeding.

Preparation of Formula

The two traditional ways of preparing formula are the terminal heat method (all the utensils and formula are boiled together for 25 minutes) and the aseptic method (the equipment is boiled separately, after which the formula is poured into the bottles). Because of improved sanitary conditions in developed countries, neither of these methods is considered essential. The clean technique is generally satisfactory, including using

*110 Horizon Drive, Suite 210, Raleigh, NC 27615; 800-LA-LECHE or 877-452-5324; http://www.llli.org. In Canada: PO Box 307, Silton SK, S0G 4L0; 306-992-2125 or 800-665-4324; http://www.lllc.ca.

TABLE 7.6 Breastfeeding Problems*

Problem	Comments	Interventions
Engorgement	Best intervention is *prevention* with deep areolar latch-on and frequent nursing on both breasts for complete emptying of ducts. If engorgement occurs, infant may be unable to properly grasp distended areola.	Manually express small amount of milk; electric pump may be beneficial for some. Use warm compresses or a warm shower *before feeding;* for severely engorged breasts, cold compresses may be helpful to reduce vascularity *after feeding.* Compress areola with fingers before attempting to latch. This may reduce superficial edema and facilitate infant's grasp. This is known as *reverse pressure softening.* Use well-fitting nursing brassiere and wear 24 hours a day. For excessive discomfort, take ibuprofen or acetaminophen 30 minutes before feeding. Massage breasts; vary position of infant's mouth on nipple and areola.
Painful nipples	Most common causes are shallow latch, improper care of breasts, bacterial or fungal infection, or infant tongue-tie (tight lingual frenulum). If left untreated, discomfort may cause mother to terminate breastfeeding.	Care of breasts: Avoid soaps, oils, or self-prescribed treatments. Gently massage a small amount of expressed breast milk onto sore nipples after feeding. Expose nipples to air as much as possible. Change breast pads frequently; avoid plastic-backed pads (may trap moisture). Feeding: Start let-down reflex by manual expression before putting infant to breast. Begin nursing with less affected breast, then nurse on affected side. Position infant properly at breast to achieve deep areolar grasp. Vary infant's position during feeding Take analgesics 30 min before feeding; apply cool compresses to nipples after feeding.
Delayed let-down reflex	Reflex essential to optimal delivery of milk from alveoli and smaller milk ducts into larger lactiferous ducts; controlled primarily by release of oxytocin. Pain, stress, and anxiety can interfere with reflex.	Provide quiet, relaxing atmosphere for breastfeeding (e.g., soothing music, privacy, pillows for positioning, decreased distractions). Stroke breast gently. Apply warmth to breast. May need to use oxytocin nasal spray (compounded prescription) to induce reflex (use only in newborn period).
Inadequate milk supply	Production of milk depends primarily on supply and demand. Inadequate supply rarely is related to organic causes, such as decreased glandular tissue, but may occur after breast augmentation or reduction surgery, or as a result of a hormonal imbalance such as polycystic ovarian syndrome.	Continue breastfeeding every 2-3 hours. Massage breasts before feeding. Apply warm compresses before pumping or feeding. Avoid use of supplemental formula before breastfeeding is well established to prevent nipple preference and satiation (infant will not be hungry enough to breastfeed). Reassure mother that her milk supply will likely be adequate and it depends on frequent nursing. Encourage more frequent nursing (at least 8-10 times daily, initially at both breasts). Encourage adequate rest, nutrition, and fluids. Monitor infant's growth; in some cases formula supplementation may be indicated. An alternative to bottle-feeding is use of a supplemental feeding device consisting of a plastic bag or syringe for formula and a thin feeding tube placed next to mother's nipple during nursing.
Plugged ducts	This may occur at any time, especially during first 6 weeks.	Continue breastfeeding every 2-3 hours. Massage breasts before feeding. Apply warm compresses before pumping or feeding. Alternate feeding positions, positioning infant's chin toward obstructed area.
Mastitis	Inflammation or infection in mammary gland or tissue, most often by *Staphylococcus aureus;* results from inadequate emptying of ducts or from cracks in nipple skin; may be associated with fever and flulike symptoms. Prevention: see Interventions for Plugged ducts, above. If mastitis occurs, current treatment is 10 days of antibiotics (usually amoxicillin or cephalexin, started with onset of symptoms). If symptoms of intense "burning" in breasts with erythema of nipples, consider *Candida* infection of ducts (oral fluconazole [Diflucan] is treatment).	Continue breastfeeding during this time to keep breast well drained (unless contraindicated for medical reasons such as systemic illness).
Unsuccessful latch-on	Improper positioning of infant at breast, inability to achieve deep areolar grasp, sleepiness, or improper suckling technique may cause this common problem; flat, large, or inverted nipples may also be a factor.	Mother and newborn must be positioned so that infant's mouth is in full contact with breast; mother should use C-hold; newborn's mouth is opened wide, and most of areola is grasped (see Fig. 7.14), especially with lower lip; frequent swallowing should be heard as evidence of spontaneous and successful suckling. Anatomic problems such as flat or inverted nipples may be managed by mother wearing nipple shields to elongate or make nipples more accessible. Additional pumping may be necessary after nursing when shield is used.

*Consult a Lactation Consultant as needed to resolve problems.

a dishwasher. Persons preparing the formula wash their hands well and then wash all the equipment used to prepare the formula, including the cans of formula or evaporated milk.

When reconstituting formula, care providers should be aware that powdered infant formula is not sterile, and it has occasionally been associated with severe illness attributed to *Cronobacter* species (formerly known as *Enterobacter sakazakii*) and *Salmonella enterica* (American Academy of Pediatrics, 2015b). Careful preparation and handling of formula decrease risk. Reconstitution with water brought to a rolling boil, and mixed when it is at or above 70°C is helpful because this is hot enough to deactivate *Cronobacter* and other pathogens (American Academy of Pediatrics, 2015b). Bottled water is not considered sterile, and it may also be boiled before use to reduce risk.

The formula is prepared and bottled and refrigerated if not used for feeding immediately. Warming the formula is optional. Discard any milk remaining in the bottle after the feeding is completed because it is an excellent medium for bacterial growth. Cover opened cans of formula and refrigerate until the next feeding.

Stress to families that the proportions must not be altered—neither diluted to extend the amount of formula nor concentrated to provide more calories, unless directed by the practitioner to increase caloric content. Recommendations for labeling infant formulas require that the directions for preparation and use of the formula include pictures and symbols for nonreading individuals. In addition, manufacturers are translating the directions into foreign languages, such as Spanish and Vietnamese, to prevent misunderstanding and errors in formula preparation.

Feeding Schedules

Ideally, feeding times should be determined by the infant's hunger. Demand feedings are given when the infant signals readiness; scheduled feedings are arranged at predetermined intervals. Although schedules may be satisfactory for bottle-fed infants, they hinder the breastfeeding process. Because of the easy digestibility of human milk, breastfed infants should be fed on demand. At times, breastfed infants will *cluster-feed,* that is, have several short feedings within an hour or two, and then sleep for several hours. It is important for mothers to understand that cluster-feeding is a normal, expected pattern for breastfed infants, especially during a growth spurt, to prevent them worrying that their milk is of insufficient quality or quantity. Cluster-feeding is recognized as a mechanism that facilitates increased milk production to meet the infant's increasing metabolic needs, thus it is imperative that mothers understand and facilitate cluster-feeding.

Supplemental feedings should not be offered to breastfed infants before lactation is well established because they may satiate the infant and may contribute to nipple preference. Supplemental water is not needed by breastfed or bottle-fed infants, even in hot climates (Kleinman & Greer, 2014). Satiated infants suck less vigorously at the breast, and optimal milk production depends on the breast being emptied at each feeding. If milk is allowed to accumulate in the breast, engorgement and ischemia follow, which suppresses the activity of the acini, or milk-secreting cells. Consequently, milk production is reduced. In addition, the process of sucking from a bottle is different from breast nipple compression. The relatively inflexible rubber nipple prevents the tongue from its usual rhythmic action. Infants learn to put the tongue against the nipple holes to slow down the more rapid flow of fluid. When infants use these same tongue movements during breastfeeding, they may push the human nipple out of the mouth and may not grasp the areola properly.

Usually by 3 weeks of age, lactation is well established, and breastfed infants may feed as frequently as 10 to 12 times per day. Bottle-fed infants feed about six times per day, consuming about 2 to 3 oz of formula at each feeding.

Feeding Behavior

Five behavioral stages occur during successful feeding. Recognizing these steps can assist nurses in identifying potential feeding problems caused by improper feeding techniques. Prefeeding behavior, such as crying or fussing, demonstrates the infant's level of arousal and degree of hunger. To encourage the infant to grasp the breast or bottle properly, it is preferable to begin feeding during the quiet alert state, before the infant becomes upset. Approach behavior is indicated by sucking movements or the rooting reflex.

Attachment behavior includes those activities that occur from the time the infant receives the nipple and sucks (sometimes more pronounced during initial attempts at breastfeeding). Consummatory behavior consists of coordinated sucking and swallowing. Persistent gagging might indicate unsuccessful consummatory behavior. Satiety behavior is observed when infants let the parent know that they are satisfied, usually by falling asleep.

Commercially Prepared Formulas

The analysis of human and whole cow's milk indicates that the latter is unsuitable for infant nutrition. Whole cow's milk has a high protein content and low fat content, and may cause intestinal bleeding and lead to iron deficiency anemia in infants. There has also been some question regarding the unmodified protein content of whole cow's milk, which may trigger an undesired immune response and thus increase the incidence of allergies in children exposed at an early age.

Commercially prepared formulas are cow's milk–based formulas that have been modified to more closely resemble the nutritional content of human milk. These formulas are altered from cow's milk by removing butterfat, decreasing the protein content, and adding vegetable oil and carbohydrate. Some cow's milk–based formulas have demineralized whey added to yield a whey/casein ratio of 60:40. Standard cow's milk–based formulas, regardless of the commercial brand, have similar compositions of vitamins, minerals, protein, carbohydrates, and essential amino acids, with possible variations such as the source of carbohydrate, nucleotides to enhance immune function, and long-chain polyunsaturated fatty acids (LCPUFAs) DHA and AA, which are believed to improve brain function. DHA and AA are both found in large quantities in human milk but until recently were not present in most infant formulas.

A meta-analysis of 15 randomized controlled studies (RCTs) explored outcomes such as physical growth, visual acuity, and neurodevelopmental outcomes among term infants fed formula milk fortified with LCPUFAs, compared with infants fed formula that was not enriched with LCPUFAs. The authors concluded that most studies reported no beneficial effects or harms of LCPUFA supplementation on neurodevelopmental outcomes of formula-fed infants, and no consistent beneficial effects on visual acuity (Jasani, Simmer, Patole, et al., 2017). Thus routine supplementation of term infant formula with LCPUFAs is not recommended at this time (Jasani, Simmer, Patole, et al., 2017).

The presence of the probiotics *Lactobacillus rhamnosus GG* and *Bifidobacterium lactis* in breast milk has led to the addition of prebiotic components to some cow's milk–based formula. Prebiotic oligosaccharides are food ingredients that promote the growth and activity of bacteria such as *Lactobacillus* and *Bifidobacterium,* which benefit the host. Although some studies report increasing bifidobacterial counts with prebiotic-supplemented formula, others report that although stool frequency is increased, prebiotic infant formula failed to increase bifidobacteria or lactobacillus levels, or to decrease the level of pathogens such as *E. coli* (Bertelsen, Jensen, & Ringel-Kulka, 2016). To date, there is insufficient evidence that changes in gastrointestinal microbiota resulting from fortified formula induce a significant clinical benefit for the immune system (Bertelsen, Jensen, & Ringel-Kulka, 2016). Further, long-term health effects of prebiotic formula supplementation are unknown.

Commercially prepared infant formulas fall into four main categories: (1) cow's milk–based formulas, available in 20 kcal/fl oz as liquid (ready to feed), as powder (requires dilution with water), or as a concentrated liquid (requires dilution with water); (2) soy-based formulas, available commercially in ready-to-feed 20 kcal/fl oz powder and concentrated liquid forms, commonly used for children who are lactose or cow's milk protein intolerant; (3) casein- or whey-hydrolysate formulas, commercially available in ready-to-feed and powder forms and used primarily for children who cannot tolerate or digest cow's milk or soy-based formulas; and (4) amino acid formulas.

The American Academy of Pediatrics Committee on Nutrition (Kleinman & Greer, 2014) recommends the use of soy protein–based formulas for infants with galactosemia and primary (very rare) and secondary lactose intolerance, and in situations where a vegetarian diet is preferred. For infants with documented allergies caused by cow's milk, extensively hydrolyzed protein formula should be considered because up to 14% of these infants will also have a soy protein allergy. The casein- or whey-hydrolysate formulas are considered to be less antigenic than either cow's milk or soy-based formulas. The protein hydrolysate formulas (casein and whey) are derived from cow's milk–based formula by a process of heat, filtration, and enzyme treatment designed to break the peptide chains into more digestible proteins. There are also amino acid formulas, designed for infants who are extremely sensitive to cow's milk–based, soy-based, and partially or extensively hydrolyzed casein- and whey-based formulas. A variety of formulas are manufactured for infants and children with special needs. A formula company representative can provide product books that describe the purpose and content of each formula.

Follow-up formulas are marketed as a transitional formula for infants older than 6 months who are also eating solid foods. These generally contain a higher percentage of calories from protein and carbohydrate sources, a higher amount of iron and vitamins, and a lower amount of fat than standard cow's milk–based formulas. Many nutrition experts and the American Academy of Pediatrics Committee on Nutrition (Kleinman & Greer, 2014), however, discount the necessity of follow-up formulas if the infant is receiving an adequate amount of solid food containing sufficient iron, vitamins, and minerals.

Alternate Milk Products

In the United States few infants are fed evaporated milk formula, and its use is not recommended by the American Academy of Pediatrics Committee on Nutrition (Kleinman & Greer, 2014). However, it has some advantages over whole milk. It is readily available in cans, needs no refrigeration if unopened, is less expensive than commercial formula, provides a softer, more digestible curd, and contains more lactalbumin and a higher calcium/phosphorus ratio. Disadvantages of evaporated milk for infant nutrition include low iron and vitamin C concentrations, excessive sodium and phosphorus, decreased vitamin A and D (except in fortified forms), and poorly digested fat. A common method for preparing evaporated milk formula is diluting the 13-oz can of milk with 19½ oz of water and adding 3 tbsp of sugar or commercially processed corn syrup.

Evaporated milk must not be confused with condensed milk, which is a form of evaporated milk with 45% more sugar. Because of its high carbohydrate concentration and disproportionately low fat and protein content, condensed milk is not used for infant feeding. Likewise, skim milk and low-fat milk must not be used because they are deficient in caloric concentration, significantly increase the renal solute load and water demands, and deprive the body of essential fatty acids.

Goat's milk is a poor source of iron and folic acid. It has an excessively high renal solute load as a result of its high protein content and can cause metabolic acidosis, making it unsuitable for infant nutrition (Kleinman & Greer, 2014). Some caretakers believe that goat's milk is less allergenic than other available milk sources and may feed it to their infants to reduce allergic milk reactions. However, infants allergic to cow's milk have experienced anaphylaxis with their first exposure to goat's milk (Pessler & Nejat, 2004). Raw, unpasteurized milk from any animal source is unacceptable for infant nutrition.

PROMOTE PARENT-INFANT BONDING (ATTACHMENT)

The process of parenting is based on a relationship between parent and infant. As more is learned of the complexity of neonates and their potential for influencing and shaping their environments, particularly their interaction with significant others, it is apparent that promoting positive parent-child relationships necessitates an understanding of behavioral steps in attachment, including variables that enhance or hinder this process. Nurses also must be skilled in methods of teaching parents to develop a stronger relationship with their children, especially by recognizing potential problems (see Assessment of Attachment Behaviors, p. 201).

Infant Behavior

Nurses must appreciate the individuality and uniqueness of each infant. According to the individual temperament, the infant will change and shape the environment, which will undoubtedly influence future development. An infant who sleeps 20 hours a day will be exposed to fewer stimuli than one who sleeps 16 hours a day. In turn, each infant will likely elicit a different response from parents. The infant who is quiet, undemanding, and passive may receive much less attention than the infant who is responsive, alert, and active. Behavioral characteristics such as irritability and consolability can influence the ease of transition to parenthood and the parent's perception of the infant.

Nurses can positively influence the attachment of parent and child. The first step is recognizing individual differences and explaining to parents that such characteristics are normal. For example, some people believe that infants sleep throughout the day, except for feedings. For some newborns this may be true, but for many it is not. Understanding that the infant's wakefulness is part of biologic rhythm and not a reflection of inadequate parenting can be crucial in promoting healthy parent-child relationships. Another aspect of helping parents involves supplying guidelines on how to enhance the infant's development during awake periods. Placing the child in a crib to stare at the same mobile every day is not exciting, but carrying the infant into each room as one does daily chores can be fascinating.

Maternal Attachment

Mothers often demonstrate a predictable and orderly pattern of behavior during the attachment process. When mothers are presented with their nude infants, they begin to examine the infant with their fingertips, concentrating on touching the extremities, and then proceed to massage and encompass the trunk with their entire hands. Assuming the **en face** position, in which the mother's and infant's eyes meet in visual contact in the same vertical plane, is significant in the formation of affectional ties (Fig. 7.15). Some authors have reported that mothers experiencing depression, as well as adolescent mothers, may have lower rates of secure attachment with their infants (Behrendt, Konrad, Goecke, et al., 2016; Flaherty & Sadler, 2011), necessitating the need for caregivers to monitor such mothers closely and to model attachment behaviors.

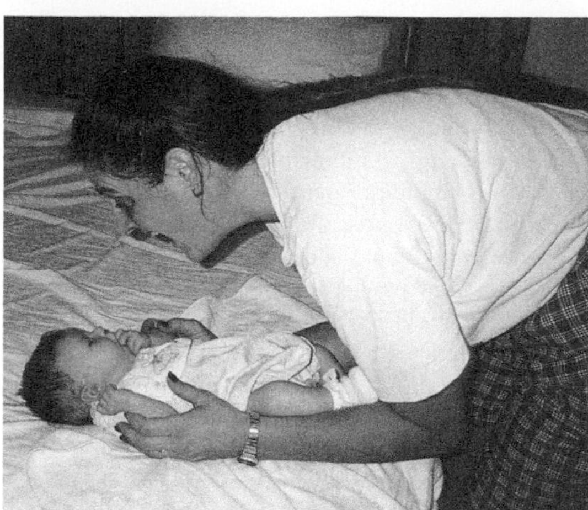

FIG. 7.15 En face position between parent and infant can be significant in the attachment process.

Nurses must observe for maternal attachment behaviors and exercise caution in interpreting such behaviors.

The long-term benefits of providing parents with opportunities to bond with their infant during the initial postpartum period are unclear; however, skin-to-skin contact with the mother immediately after delivery enhances the likelihood of success in breastfeeding. The nurse should stress to parents that, although early bonding may be valuable, it does not represent an "all or none" phenomenon. Throughout the child's life there will be multiple opportunities for the development of parent-child attachment. Bonding is a complex process that develops gradually and is influenced by numerous factors, only one of which is the type of initial contact between the newborn and parent.

One component of successful maternal attachment is reciprocity (Brazelton, 1974). As the mother responds to the infant, the infant must respond to the mother by some signal, such as sucking, cooing, eye contact, grasping, or molding (conforming to other's body during close physical contact). The first step in this complex process is *initiation,* in which interaction between infant and parent begins. Next is *orientation,* which establishes the partners' expectations of each other during the interaction. Following orientation is *acceleration* of the attention cycle to a peak of excitement. The infant reaches out and coos, both arms jerk forward, the head moves backward, the eyes dilate, and the face brightens. After a short time, *deceleration* of the excitement and *turning away* occur, in which the infant's eyes shift away from the mother's and the child may grasp his or her own shirt. During this cycle of nonattention, repeated verbal or visual attempts to reinitiate the infant's attention are ineffective. This deceleration and turning away probably prevent the infant from being overwhelmed by excessive stimuli. In a good-quality interaction, both participants have synchronized their attention-nonattention cycles. Parents or other caregivers who do not allow the infant to turn away and who continually attempt to maintain visual contact may encourage the infant to turn off the attention cycle and thus prolong the nonattention phase.

Although this description of reciprocal interacting behavior is usually observed in the infant by 2 to 3 weeks of age, nurses can use this information to teach parents how to interact with their newborn infant. Recognizing the attention versus nonattention cycles and understanding that the latter is not a rejection of the parent helps parents develop competence in parenting.

Paternal Engrossment

Fathers also show specific attachment behaviors to the newborn. This process of paternal engrossment, forming a sense of absorption, preoccupation, and interest in the infant, includes (1) visual awareness of the newborn, especially focusing on the child's beauty; (2) tactile awareness, often expressed in a desire to hold the infant; (3) awareness of distinct characteristics with emphasis on those features of the infant that resemble the father; (4) perception of the infant as perfect; (5) development of a strong feeling of attraction to the child that leads to intense focusing of attention on the infant; (6) extreme elation; and (7) a sense of deep self-esteem and satisfaction. These responses are greatest during the early contacts with the infant and are intensified by the neonate's normal reflex activity, especially the grasp reflex and visual alertness. In addition to behavioral reactions, fathers also demonstrate physiologic responses such as increased heart rate and blood pressure during interactions with their newborns.

The process of engrossment has significant implications for nurses. It is imperative to recognize the importance of early father-infant contact in this process. Fathers need to be encouraged to express their positive feelings, especially if such emotions are contrary to any belief that fathers should remain stoic. If this is not clarified, fathers may feel confused and attempt to suppress the natural sensations of absorption, preoccupation, and interest to conform to societal expectations.

Mothers also need to be aware of the responses of the father toward the newborn because one of the consequences of paternal preoccupation with the infant is less overt attention toward the mother. If both parents are able to share their feelings, each can appreciate the process of attachment toward their child and will avoid the unfortunate conflict of being insensitive and unaware of the other's needs. In addition, a father who is encouraged to form a relationship with his newborn is less likely to feel excluded and abandoned once the family returns home and the mother directs her attention toward caring for the infant.

Ideally, the process of engrossment should be discussed with parents before the delivery, such as in prenatal classes, to reinforce the father's awareness of his natural feelings toward the expected child. Focusing on the future experience of seeing, touching, and holding one's newborn may also help expectant fathers become more comfortable in accepting their paternal feelings. This in turn can assist them in being more supportive toward the mother, especially as labor and delivery draw near.

At the infant's birth the nurse can play a vital role in helping the father express engrossment by assessing the neonate in front of the couple; pointing out normal characteristics; encouraging identification through consistent referral to the child by name; encouraging the father to cuddle, hold, and talk to the infant; and demonstrating whenever necessary the soothing powers of caressing, stroking, and rocking the child (Fig. 7.16).

The father's role in supporting the mother during this period cannot be overemphasized. Once the mother has held the newborn skin-to-skin, the father may also be encouraged to hold the newborn skin-to-skin while the mother rests. Fathers are encouraged to be with the mother during labor and delivery, to spend time alone with the mother and newborn after delivery, and to "room-in" with the mother and infant. Education programs should be made available to new fathers and include information on holding the newborn, bathing, assisting the mother with breastfeeding, problems associated with breastfeeding and potential solutions, and care of the newborn at home (including safety). The integration of the father into the existing dyad of mother-newborn to form a new family—a triad—will help solidify his role as parent and partner in the care and support of his family.

The indications of affection from the father are the same as those expected in the mother, such as visual contact in the en face position and embracing the infant close to the body. When present, such behaviors

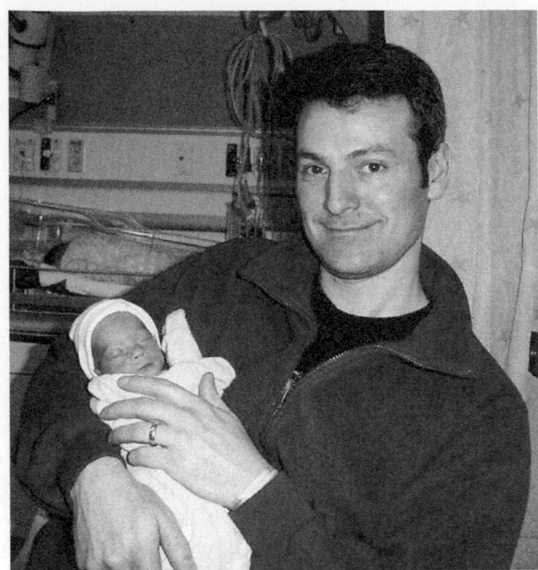

FIG. 7.16 A desire to hold the infant and participate in caregiving activities is an important step in the paternal attachment process.

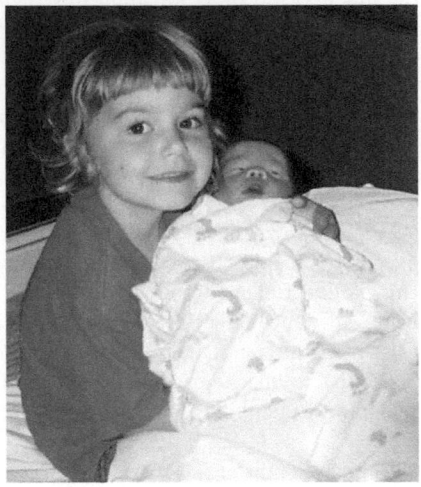

FIG. 7.17 Sibling visitation shortly after birth can be significant in the attachment process.

should be reinforced. If such responses are not obvious, the nurse needs to assess the father's feelings regarding this birth, cultural beliefs that may prevent his expression of emotions, and other factors to facilitate his positive attachment during the newborn period.

Siblings

Although the attachment process has been discussed almost exclusively in terms of the parents and infants, it is essential that nurses be aware of other family members, such as siblings, grandparents, and members of the extended family, who need preparation for the acceptance of this new child. Young children in particular need sensitive preparation for the birth to minimize sibling jealousy.

In support of family-centered care, there is an increasing trend to encourage siblings to visit the mother on the postpartum unit and to hold the newborn (Fig. 7.17). Another trend has been the presence of siblings at childbirth. Unlike sibling visitation, this practice has been controversial, yet family-centered care encompasses siblings, grandparents, and other significant persons from the extended family unit. Children exhibit different degrees of involvement in the birth process. Some reported benefits include children's increased knowledge of the birth process, less regressive behavior after the birth, and more mothering and caregiving behavior toward the infant. Some practitioners add facilitated family bonding and assimilation of the newborn into the family as positive outcomes. Parents whose children attended the birth have echoed these same benefits and have expressed their desire to repeat the experience should another pregnancy occur. Despite these positive findings, some practitioners believe that allowing children to observe a delivery could lead to emotional difficulties, although no research supports this contention. Birthing centers that allow siblings at the birth are developing more definitive guidelines, such as an age requirement of at least 4 to 5 years, the presence of a supportive person for the sibling only, and an adequate sequence of preparation in which parents explore all options for preparing their other children.

From observations during sibling visitation, there is evidence that sibling attachment occurs. However, the en face position is assumed much less often among the newborn and siblings than between mother and newborn, and when this position is used, it is brief. Siblings focus more on the head or face than on touching or talking to the infant. The siblings' verbalizations are focused less on attracting the infant's attention and more on addressing the mother about the newborn. Children who have established a prenatal relationship with the fetus have demonstrated more attachment behaviors, supporting the suggestion of encouraging prenatal acquaintance. Additional research is needed to establish theories on sibling bonding like those that have been constructed for parental bonding.

Multiple Births and Subsequent Children

A component of attachment that has special meaning for families with multiple births, *monotropy* refers to the principle that a person can become optimally attached to only one individual at a time. If a parent can form only one attachment at a time, how can all the siblings of a multiple birth receive optimum emotional care? In regard to maternal-twin bonding, the conclusions of different authors vary. Some report that mothers bond equally to each twin at the time of birth, even if one twin is ill. Others suggest that mothers of twins may take months or even years to form individual attachments and even longer if the twins are identical.

Nurses can be instrumental in promoting bonding at multiple births. The most important principle is to assist the parents in recognizing the individuality of the children, especially monozygotic (identical) twins. The mother should visit with each newborn, including a sick infant, as much as possible after birth. Rooming-in and breastfeeding are encouraged. The nurse emphasizes any characteristics that are unique to each child and calls each infant by name, rather than calling them "the twins." Asking the family questions such as "How do you tell Ashley and Amy apart?" and "In what ways are Ashley and Amy different and similar?" helps point out their individual characteristics. Behaviors on the BNBAS can be used to illustrate these differences and to stress effective strategies for dealing with multiple personalities at the same time. Co-bedding of twins or other multiples in the hospital has at times been suggested to maintain the bond between siblings that was formed in utero. A review of five studies exploring the safety and benefits of the practice of co-bedding stable preterm twins concluded that available evidence is insufficient to recommend this practice (Lai, Foong, Foong, et al., 2016). (See also Sudden Infant Death Syndrome, Chapter 11.) The American Academy of Pediatrics (2016c) has also recommended against parents or other family members sleeping in the same bed with infants at home. Because neither the safety nor the benefits of co-bedding for newborns has been documented in the literature, the

Academy recommends that families be counseled to follow safe sleeping practices, which currently dictate that infants sleep alone for optimal safety.

Another area of attachment that has received minimal attention is maternal bonding of multiparous mothers. Research suggests that "taking on" a second or third child has several additional tasks:

- Promoting acceptance and approval of the second child
- Grieving and resolving the loss of an exclusive dyadic relationship with the first child
- Planning and coordinating family life to include a second child
- Reformulating a relationship with the first child
- Identifying with the second child by comparing this child with the first child in terms of physical and psychologic characteristics
- Assessing one's affective capabilities in providing sufficient emotional support and nurturance simultaneously to two children

PREPARE FOR DISCHARGE AND HOME CARE

With shorter postpartum stays, as well as a trend toward mother-infant care (also called dyad or couplet care), discharge planning and postdischarge follow-up have become important components of comprehensive newborn care. First-time, as well as experienced, parents benefit from guidance and assistance with the infant's care, such as breastfeeding or bottle-feeding, and with the family's integration of a new member, particularly sibling adjustment.

To assess and meet these needs, teaching must begin early, ideally before the birth. Not only is the postpartum stay sometimes very short (as little as 12 to 24 hours), but mothers are also in the taking-in phase, where they may demonstrate passive and dependent behaviors. On the first postpartum day, because of fatigue and excitement about the newborn, mothers may not be able to absorb large amounts of information. This time may need to be spent highlighting essential aspects of care, such as infant safety and feeding. Parents may also be given a list of mother and infant care topics so they can choose issues they wish to review before going home. Teaching before discharge should focus on newborn feeding patterns, monitoring diapers for stools and voiding, jaundice, and infant crying (see Family-Centered Care box).

Although legislation has been enacted guaranteeing most mothers a minimum of 48 hours' hospitalization, some mothers leave the hospital as early as 8 to 12 hours after vaginal delivery. The American Academy of Pediatrics (2015c) has established guidelines for discharge criteria for healthy-term newborns. The Academy emphasizes that the primary care practitioner, in consultation with the mother, the midwife or obstetrician, and other health care providers, should make the determination of appropriate discharge time.

Follow-up home care within days (or even hours after discharge when minor problems are anticipated) is important to provide adequate maternal-newborn care with minimal complications. Despite the changing spectrum of well-newborn health care, the nurse's role continues to be that of providing ongoing assessments of each mother-newborn dyad to ensure a safe transition to home and a successful adaptation into the family unit. The ultimate safety and success of early newborn discharge from the hospital are contingent on using clear discharge criteria and having a high-quality early follow-up program (see Community and Home Health Considerations box).

With family structures changing, it is essential that nurses identify the primary caregiver, which may not always be the mother but may be a partner, spouse, grandparent, or babysitter. The primary caregiver should be present, along with the mother, for teaching sessions, to ensure that they understand how to safely care for the newborn. Nurses should avoid using terminology that may be unfamiliar to families when teaching about newborn care. Mothers with other children do not necessarily understand more words, and young maternal age and less education may contribute to confusion or decreased comprehension. Ensure that parents understand pertinent areas of newborn care by having them demonstrate skills such as diaper changing or by repeating back to the nurse critical knowledge such as when to seek assistance.

An essential area of discharge counseling is the safe transport of the newborn home from the hospital. Ideally this information should be provided *before* delivery to allow parents to purchase a federally approved infant car safety seat restraint. When purchasing a car safety

FAMILY-CENTERED CARE

*Healthy Term Newborn Discharge Criteria**

- Infant born between 37 and 41 completed weeks of gestation.
- Clinical course and physical examination at discharge have not revealed abnormalities that require continued hospitalization.
- Vital signs are within normal range and stable for the 12 hours preceding discharge.
- Infant has urinated regularly and passed at least one stool spontaneously.
- Infant has completed at least two successful feedings. For breastfed infants: A caregiver knowledgeable in breastfeeding must observe a feeding and assess latch, swallow, and infant satiety. For bottle-fed infants: Assess ability to coordinate sucking, swallowing, and breathing while feeding. These assessments must be documented in the health record.
- There is no significant bleeding at the circumcision site.
- Clinical risk of development of hyperbilirubinemia has been assessed, and follow-up plans per American Academy of Pediatrics clinical practice guidelines are in place.
- Infant has been adequately evaluated and monitored for sepsis based on maternal risk factors, including group B streptococcal disease.
- Maternal blood test and screening results are available and have been reviewed, including syphilis, hepatitis B, and HIV as per state regulations.
- Infant blood tests are available and have been reviewed, including cord or infant blood type and direct Coombs test results, as clinically indicated.
- Initial hepatitis B vaccine has been administered.
- If a mother has not previously been vaccinated, she should receive tetanus toxoid, reduced diphtheria toxoid, and acellular pertussis (Tdap) vaccine immediately after delivery.
- If a mother who delivers during the flu season has not been previously immunized, she should receive flu vaccine.
- Newborn metabolic, hearing, and congenital heart disease screening has been completed per hospital protocol and state regulations.
- Family, environmental, and social risk factors have been assessed and proactive management is in place.
- Mother's knowledge, ability, and confidence to provide adequate infant care have been assessed for competency.
- An appropriate car seat is available before hospital discharge, and mother has demonstrated competence in its use.
- Continuing medical care is planned; infants discharged sooner than 48 hours should be examined within 48 hours of discharge from the hospital.
- Barriers to adequate follow-up care (e.g., lack of telephone or transportation) have been assessed, and a plan is in place to manage issues.

*See American Academy of Pediatrics (AAP) Policy Statement: "Hospital Stay for Healthy Term Newborn Infants" (2015) for comprehensive discussion of each criterion.

Data from American Academy of Pediatrics. (2015). Policy statement: Hospital stay for healthy term newborn infants. *Pediatrics, 135*(5), 948-953.

COMMUNITY AND HOME HEALTH CONSIDERATIONS

*Newborn Home Care After Early Discharge**

- **Wet diapers**—Minimum of one for each day of life (day 2 = 2 wets; day 3 = 3 wets) until fifth or sixth day, at which time 5 or 6 per day to 14 days, then 6 to 10 or more per day.
- **Breastfeeding**—Successful latch-on and feeding every 2 to 3 hours daily. Swallowing should be audible.
- **Formula feeding**—Successfully taking at least 1 to 2 oz every 3 to 4 hours. Should be easily aroused for feeding.
- **Circumcision**—Wash with warm water only; yellow exudate forming, nonbleeding, Plastibell intact for 48 hours.
- **Stools**—At least one soft stool every 48 to 72 hours (bottle-feeding), or two or three per day (breastfeeding).
- **Color**—Pink to ruddy when crying; pink centrally when at rest or asleep.
- **Activity**—Four or five wakeful periods per day; alerts to environmental sounds and voices.
- **Jaundice**—Physiologic jaundice (not appearing in first 24 hours), feeding, voiding, and stooling as noted above. Notify practitioner of suspicion of pathologic jaundice (if it appears within 24 hours of birth, ABO or Rh problems are suspected), decreased activity, poor feeding, dark orange skin color persisting after the fifth day in light-skinned newborn. Obtain transcutaneous bilirubin before discharge and identify risk per hour-specific risk nomogram; follow up with practitioner within 48 hours after discharge if discharged home before 24 hours old (see Hyperbilirubinemia, Chapter 8).
- **Cord**—Kept above diaper line; drying, no drainage; periumbilical area nonerythematous.
- **Vital signs**—Heart rate 120 to 140 beats/min at rest; respiratory rate 30 to 55 breath/min at rest without evidence of sternal retractions, grunting, or nasal flaring; temperature 36.3° to 37°C (97.3° to 98.6°F) axillary.
- **Position of sleep**—On back.

*Any deviation from the above or suspicion of poor newborn adaptation should be reported to the practitioner at once.

seat restraint, parents should consider cost and convenience. The convertible-type seats are more expensive initially but cost less than two separate car restraint systems (infant-only model or infant-toddler convertible model). (See Chapter 10.) Convenience is a major factor because a cumbersome restraint may be used less and improperly. Before buying a car safety seat restraint, it is best to try out different models. For example, some types are too large for subcompact cars. Asking friends about the advantages and disadvantages of their restraints is helpful, but borrowing their car seat or purchasing a used one can be dangerous. Parents should use only a restraint that has directions for use and a certification label stating that it complies with federal motor vehicle safety standards (both should be on the seat). They should not use a restraint that has been involved in a crash. Some service clubs and hospitals have loan programs for vehicle safety restraints. Information about approved models and other aspects of car safety seat restrains is available from several sources.*

Parents should not place an infant in the front seat of a car with a passenger-side air bag. Infants and toddlers should ride in a rear-facing child safety seat in the back seat of the car until age 2 years or until they reach the highest weight or height recommended by the car seat manufacturer (American Academy of Pediatrics, 2014c).

! NURSING ALERT

In the United States and Canada, all states and provinces have mandated the use of child restraints. Therefore hospitals and birthing centers should have policies regarding the safe discharge of a newborn in a car safety seat and provisions for parents to learn to use the device correctly. In addition, hospital personnel should ensure that infants born before 37 weeks of gestation have a period of observation in the selected car seat to monitor for possible apnea, bradycardia, and oxygen desaturation (American Academy of Pediatrics, 2014c). Parents are more likely to use a restraint correctly and consistently if the proper use of one is demonstrated and its necessity is stressed.

Although federal safety standards do not specify the minimum weight of an infant and the appropriate type of restraint, newborns weighing 2000 g (4.4 lb) receive relatively good support in convertible seats with a seat back–to–crotch strap height of 14 cm (5.5 inches) or less. Rolled blankets and towels may be needed between the crotch and legs to prevent slouching and can be placed along the sides to minimize lateral movements. Placing the infant in a safety seat at a 45-degree angle will prevent slumping and airway obstruction (American Academy of Pediatrics, 2014c). Seats with shields (large padded surfaces in front of the child) and armrests (found on some older models) are unacceptable because of their proximity to the infant's face and neck. (For a discussion of appropriate car restraints for preterm infants, see Discharge Planning and Home Care in Chapter 9, and for infants, see Motor Vehicle Injuries in Chapters 10 and 12.) Padding is never placed underneath or behind the infant because it creates slack in the harness, leading to the possibility of the child's ejection from the seat in the event of a crash.

The use of an appropriate car safety seat restraint is also encouraged to prevent injuries to children riding in airplanes.

*American Academy of Pediatrics, 141 Northwest Point Blvd., Elk Grove Village, IL 60007-1098; phone: 847-434-4000 or (toll-free) 800-433-9016. Car seats: Information for families for 2017 is available at http://www.healthychildren.org/English/safety-prevention/on-the-go/Pages/Car-Safety-Seats-Information-for-Families.aspx. National Highway Traffic Safety Administration Auto Safety Hotline, 888-327-4236; http://www.nhtsa.gov. For children with special needs, contact the National Easter Seal Society, 800-221-6827, and ask about Special KARS (Kids Are Riding Safe); http://www.easterseals.com. The National Center for the Safe Transportation of Children with Special Healthcare Needs, 800-755-0912; http://www.preventinjury.org.

NCLEX REVIEW QUESTIONS

1. Identify the anatomic changes that occur shortly after birth that affect the newborn's adaptation to extrauterine existence. Select all that apply.
   A. Closure of the foramen ovale
   B. Closure of the ductus arteriosus
   C. Increase in pulmonary vascular resistance
   D. Closure of the ductus venosus
   E. Decrease in pulmonary vascular resistance
2. In the newly born infant thermogenesis is achieved by:
   A. Shivering
   B. Brown fat metabolism
   C. Overhead warming unit
   D. Skin-to-skin contact with mother
3. What does the Apgar scoring system assess? Select all that apply.
   A. Respiratory effort
   B. Heart rate
   C. Core temperature
   D. Reflex irritability
   E. Muscle tone
   F. Color
4. A newborn whose mother is positive for *Chlamydia trachomitis* should be optimally treated with which of these to prevent ophthalmia?
   A. Silver nitrate solution (1%)
   B. Tetracycline ophthalmic ointment (1%)
   C. Oral erythromycin
   D. Erythromycin ophthalmic solution (0.5%)
5. A healthy infant is born to a mother with known high-risk behaviors whose HIV status is undetermined. The mother states that she wishes to breastfeed her infant. The nurse's response to the mother's request should be based on which of the following information?
   A. HIV is rarely transmitted to the newborn through maternal milk.
   B. Breastfeeding should be withheld until HIV status (maternal) is determined.
   C. Breastfeeding should be avoided completely in mothers with high-risk behaviors.
   D. In such infants antiretroviral medication should be started within 12 hours of birth.

Correct Answers

1. A, B, D, E; 2. B; 3. A, B, D, E, F; 4. C; 5. B

REFERENCES

Agho, K. E., Ogeleka, P., Ogbo, F. A., et al. (2016). Trends and predictors of prelacteal feeding practices in Nigeria (2003–2013). *Nutrients, 8*(8), E462.

Alexander, G. R., Himes, J. H., Kaufman, R. B., et al. (1996). A United States national reference for fetal growth. *Obstetrics and Gynecology, 87*(2), 163–168.

American Academy of Pediatrics, Joint Committee on Infant Hearing. (2007). Year 2007 position statement: Principles and guidelines for early hearing detection and intervention programs. *Pediatrics, 120*, 898–921.

American Academy of Pediatrics, Section on Cardiology and Cardiac Surgery Executive Committee. (2012a). Endorsement of Health and Human Services recommendation for pulse oximetry screening for critical congenital heart disease. *Pediatrics, 129*(1), 190–192.

American Academy of Pediatrics, Task Force on Circumcision. (2012b). Circumcision policy statement. *Pediatrics, 130*(3), 585–586.

American Academy of Pediatrics. (2012c). Policy statement: Breastfeeding and the use of human milk. *Pediatrics, 129*(3), e827–e841.

American Academy of Pediatrics. (2003; reaffirmed 2014a). Policy statement: Controversies concerning vitamin K and the newborn. *Pediatrics, 112*(1), 191–192.

American Academy of Pediatrics Committee on Nutrition Clinical Report. (2014b). Optimizing bone health in children and adolescents. *Pediatrics, 134*(4), e1229–e1243.

American Academy of Pediatrics, Council on Injury, Violence and Poison Prevention. (2011; reaffirmed 2014c). Child passenger safety. *Pediatrics, 127*(4), 788–793.

American Academy of Pediatrics Committee on Fetus and Newborn, American College of Obstetricians and Gynecologists Committee on obstetric practice. (2015a). The Apgar score. *Pediatrics, 136*(4), 819–822.

American Academy of Pediatrics, Committee on Infectious Diseases. (2015b). *Red book: 2015 Report of the Committee on Infectious Diseases* (30th ed.). Elk Grove Village, IL: The Academy.

American Academy of Pediatrics, Committee on Fetus & Newborn, Policy statement. (2015c). Hospital stay for healthy term newborn infants. *Pediatrics, 135*(5), 948–953.

American Academy of Pediatrics. (2016a). *Neonatal resuscitation textbook* (7th ed.). Elk Grove Village, IL: American Academy of Pediatrics & American Heart Association.

American Academy of Pediatrics, Committee on Practice and Ambulatory Medicine, Section on Ophthalmology, American Association of Certified Orthoptists, American Association for Pediatric Ophthalmology and Strabismus, and American Academy of Ophthalmology. (2016b). Visual system assessment in infants, children, and young adults by pediatricians. *Pediatrics, 137*(1), 28–30.

American Academy of Pediatrics, Task Force on Sudden Infant Death Syndrome Policy Statement. (2016c). SIDS and other sleep-related infants deaths: Updated 2016 recommendations for a safe infant sleeping environment. *Pediatrics, 138*(5), e20162938.

American Academy of Pediatrics, Statement of Endorsement. (2016d). Systematic review and evidence-based guidelines for the management of patients with positional plagiocephaly. *Pediatrics, 138*(5), e20162802.

American Academy of Pediatrics, Clinical Report. (2008; reaffirmed 2016e). Newborn screening expands: Recommendations for pediatricians and medical homes – implications for the system. *Pediatrics, 121*(1), 192–217.

American Academy of Pediatrics, Committee on Fetus and Newborn, and Section on Anesthesiology and Pain Medicine, Policy Statement. (2016f). Prevention and management of procedural pain in the neonate: An update. *Pediatrics, 137*(2), e20154217.

American Academy of Pediatrics, Committee on fetus and newborn. (2016g). Umbilical cord care in the newborn infant. *Pediatrics, 138*(3), e201622149.

American Academy of Pediatrics, Committee on Practice and Ambulatory Medicine, Policy Statement. (2017). 2017 Recommendations for preventive pediatric health care. *Pediatrics, 139*(4), e20170254.

American Dietetic Association, Pediatric Nutrition Practice Group. (2011). *Guidelines for preparation of human milk and formula in health care facilities* (2nd ed.). Washington, DC: American Dietetic Association.

Association of Women's Health, Obstetric and Neonatal Nurses. (2013). *Neonatal skin care evidence-based clinical practice guideline* (3rd ed.). Washington, DC: The Association.

Ballard, J. L., Khoury, J. C., Wedig, K., et al. (1991). New Ballard score expanded to include extremely premature infants. *The Journal of Pediatrics, 119*, 417–423.

Banihani, O. I., Fox, J. A., Gander, B. H., et al. (2014). Complete penile amputation during ritual neonatal circumcision and successful replantation using postoperative leech therapy. *Urology, 84*(2), 472–474.

Bazzano, A. N., Hofer, R., Thibeau, S., et al. (2016). A review of herbal and pharmaceutical galactogogues for breast-feeding. *The Ochsner Journal, 16*(4), 511–514.

Bazi, T. (2017). Female genital mutilation: The role of medical professional organizations. *International Urogynecology Journal, 28*(4), 537–541.

Behrendt, H. R., Konrad, K., Goecke, T. W., et al. (2016). Post-natal mother-to-infant attachment in sub-clinically depressed mothers: Dyads at risk? *Psychopathology, 49*(4), 269–276.

Bergman, N. J. (2013). Neonatal stomach volume and physiology suggest feeding at 1 hour intervals. *Acta Paediatrica, 102*(8), 773–777.

Bertelsen, R. J., Jensen, E. T., & Ringel-Kulka, T. (2016). Use of probiotics and prebiotics in infant feeding. *Best Practice & Research. Clinical Gastroenterology, 30*(1), 39–48.

Blackburn, S. T. (2013). *Maternal, fetal, and neonatal physiology: A clinical perspective* (4th ed.). St. Louis, MO: Saunders.

Brazelton, T. B. (1974). Mother-infant reciprocity. In M. H. Klaus, T. Leger, & M. A. Trause (Eds.), *Maternal attachment and mothering disorders: A round table*. Sausalito, CA: Johnson & Johnson Baby Products.

Brazelton, T. B., & Nugent, J. K. (1996). *Neonatal behavioral assessment scale*. London: MacKeith Press.

Brookes, A., & Bowley, D. M. (2014). Tongue tie: The evidence for frenotomy. *Early Human Development, 90*(11), 765–768.

Canadian Paediatric Society, First Nations, Inuit and Métis Health Committee. (reaffirmed 2017). Vitamin D supplementation: Recommendations for Canadian mothers and infants. *Paediatrics & Child Health, 12*(7), 583–589.

Canadian Paediatric Society, Fetus and Newborn Committee. (reaffirmed January 2016b). *Routine administration of vitamin K to newborns*. Retrieved from http://www.cps.ca/en/documents/position.

Canadian Paediatric Society, Community Paediatrics Committee. (2011, reaffirmed 2016c). Universal newborn hearing screening. *Paediatrics & Child Health, 16*(5), 301–305.

Canadian Paediatric Society, Community Paediatrics Committee. (updated 2015a). *Temperature measurement in paediatrics*. Retrieved from http://www.cps.ca/en/documents/position.

Canadian Paediatric Society, Position Statement. (2015b). Newborn male circumcision. *Paediatrics & Child Health, 20*(6), 311–315.

Dubowitz, L. M. S., & Dubowitz, V. (1977). *Gestational age of the newborn*. Menlo Park, CA: Addison Wesley.

Duryea, E. L., Hawkins, J. S., McIntire, D. O., et al. (2014). A revised birthweight reference for the United States. *Obstetrics & Gynecology, 124*(1), 16–22.

Emond, A., Ingram, J., Johnson, D., et al. (2014). Randomized controlled trial of early frenotomy in breastfed infants with mild-moderate tongue-tie. *Archives of Disease in Childhood. Fetal and Neonatal Edition, 99*(3), F189–F195.

Flaherty, S. C., & Sadler, L. S. (2011). A review of attachment theory in the context of adolescent parenting. *Journal of Pediatric Health Care, 25*(2), 114–121.

Foster, J. P., Taylor, C., & Spence, K. (2017). Topical anaesthesia for needle-related pain in newborn infants. *The Cochrane Database of Systematic Reviews*, (2), CD010331.

Friedrichs, J., Staffileno, B. A., Fogg, L., et al. (2013). Axillary temperatures in full-term newborn infants: Using evidence to guide safe and effective practice. *Advances in Neonatal Care, 13*(5), 361–368.

Haddad, L., Smith, S., Phillips, K. D., et al. (2012). Comparison of temporal artery and axillary temperatures in healthy newborns. *Journal of Obstetric, Gynecologic, and Neonatal Nursing, 41*, 383–388.

Hawkins, S. S., Stern, A. D., Baum, C. F., et al. (2014). Compliance with the Baby-Friendly Hospital Initiative and impact on breastfeeding rates. *Archives of Disease in Childhood. Fetal and Neonatal Edition, 99*(2), F138–F143.

Hawkins, S. S., Stern, A. D., Baum, C. F., et al. (2015). Evaluating the impact of the Baby-Friendly Hospital Initiative on breast-feeding rates: A multi-state analysis. *Public Health Nutrition, 18*(2), 179–187.

Holland, A., & Watkins, D. (2015). Flying Start health visitors' views of implementing the Newborn Behavioural Observation: Barriers and facilitating factors. *Community Practitioner, 88*(6), 33–36.

Horta, B. L., Loret de Mola, C., & Victora, C. G. (2015). Breastfeeding and intelligence: A systematic review and meta-analysis. *Acta Paediatrica, 104*(467), 14–19.

Houghtaling, B., Byker Shanks, C., & Jenkins, M. (2017). Likelihood of breastfeeding within the USDA's Food and Nutrition Service Special Supplementation Nutrition Program for women, infants, and children population. *Journal of Human Lactation, 33*(1), 83–97.

Howe-Heyman, A., & Lutenbacher, M. (2016). The Baby-Friendly Hospital Initiative as an intervention to improve breastfeeding rates: A review of the literature. *Journal of Midwifery & Women's Health, 61*(1), 77–102.

Jagannath, V. A., Fedorowicz, Z., Sud, V., et al. (2012). Routine neonatal circumcision for the prevention of urinary tract infections in infancy. *The Cochrane Database of Systematic Reviews*, (11), CD009129.

Jasani, B., Simmer, K., Patole, S. K., et al. (2017). Long chain polyunsaturated fatty acid supplementation in infants born at term. *The Cochrane Database of Systematic Reviews*, (3), CD000376.

Johnston, C., Campbell-Yeo, M., Disher, T., et al. (2017). Skin-to-skin care for procedural pain in neonates. *The Cochrane Database of Systematic Reviews*, (2), CD008435.

Jones, K. M., Power, M. L., Queenan, J. T., et al. (2015). Racial and ethnic disparities in breastfeeding. *Breastfeeding Medicine: The Official Journal of the Academy of Breastfeeding Medicine, 10*(4), 186–196.

Kent, A. L., Kecskes, Z., Shadbolt, B., et al. (2007). Blood pressure in the first year of life in healthy infants born at term. *Pediatric Nephrology (Berlin, Germany), 22*(10), 1743–1749.

Kleinman, R. E., & Greer, F. R. (Eds.), (2014). *Pediatric nutrition* (7th ed.). Elk Grove Village, IL: American Academy of Pediatrics.

Kuswara, K., Laws, R., Kremer, P., et al. (2016). The infant feeding practices of Chinese immigrant mothers in Australia: A qualitative exploration. *Appetite, 105*, 375–384.

Lai, N. M., Foong, S. C., Foong, W. C., et al. (2016). Co-bedding in neonatal nursery for promoting growth and neurodevelopment in stable preterm twins. *The Cochrane Database of Systematic Reviews*, (4), CD008313.

Lund, C. (2016). Bathing and beyond: Current bathing controversies for newborn infants. *Advances in Neonatal Care, 16*(5S), S13–S20.

Maheswari, N. U., Kumar, B. P., Karunakaran, A., et al. (2012). "Early baby teeth": Folklore and facts. *Journal of Pharmacy & Bioallied Sciences, 4*(Suppl. 2), S329–S333.

Martin, C. R., Ling, P.-R., & Blackburn, G. L. (2016). Review of infant feeding: Key features of breast milk and infant formula. *Nutrients, 8*(5), 279–290.

Medoff Cooper, B., Holditch-Davis, D., Verklan, M. T., et al. (2012). Newborn clinical outcomes of the AWHONN Late Preterm Infant Research-Based Practice Project. *Journal of Obstetric, Gynecologic, and Neonatal Nursing, 41*(6), 774–785.

Modarres, M., Jazayeri, Q., Rahnama, P., et al. (2013). Breastfeeding and pain relief in full-term neonates during immunization injections: A clinical randomized trial. *BMC Anesthesiology, 13*(1), 22–28.

Moore, E. R., Bergman, N., Anderson, G. C., et al. (2016). Early skin-to-skin contact for mothers and their healthy newborn infants. *The Cochrane Database of Systematic Reviews*, (11), CD003519.

National Center for Missing and Exploited Children (NCMEC). (2015). *Child safety and prevention*. http://www.missingkids.com/Safety. NEMEC.

National Institutes of Health, US National Library of Medicine, Toxicology Data Network, Drugs and Lactation Database. *LactMed*. http://toxnet.nlm.nih.gov/newtoxnet/lactmed.htm.

Newby, R. M., & Davies, P. S. (2016). Why do women stop breast-feeding? Results from a contemporary prospective study in a cohort of Australian women. *European Journal of Clinical Nutrition, 70*(12), 1428–1432.

Nugent, J. K. (2013). The competent newborn and the Neonatal Behavioral Assessment State: T. Berry Brazelton's legacy. *Journal of Child and Adolescent Psychiatric Nursing, 26*, 173–179.

Nugent, J. K., Keefer, C. H., Minear, S., et al. (2007). *Understanding newborn behavior and early relationships: The Newborn Behavioral Observations (NBO) system handbook*. Baltimore, MD: Paul H. Brookes Publishing Company.

Odom, E. C., Li, R., Scanlon, K. S., et al. (2013). Reasons for earlier than desired cessation of breastfeeding. *Pediatrics, 131*(3), e726–e732.

O'Shea, J. E., Foster, J. P., O'Donnell, C. P. F., et al. (2017). Frenotomy for tongue-tie in newborn infants. *The Cochrane Database of Systematic Reviews*, (3), CD011065.

Owings, M., Uddin, S., Williams, S., et al. (2013). *Trends in circumcision for male newborns in US hospitals: 1979-2010.* http://www.cdc.gov/nchs/data/hestat/circumcision_2013/circumcision_2013.pdf.

Pessler, R. F., & Nejat, M. (2004). Anaphylactic reactions to goat's milk in a cow's milk allergic infant. *Pediatric Allergy and Immunology, 15*(2), 183–185.

Pippi Salle, J. L., Jesus, L. E., Lorenzo, A. J., et al. (2013). Glans amputation during routine neonatal circumcision: Mechanism of injury and strategy for prevention. *Journal of Pediatric Urology, 9*(6 Pt. A), 763–768.

Power, R. F., & Murphy, J. F. (2015). Tongue-tie and frenotomy in infants with breastfeeding difficulties: Achieving a balance. *Archives of Disease in Childhood, 100*(5), 489–494.

Rabe, H., Jewison, A., Alvarez, R. F., et al. (2011). Milking compared with delayed cord clamping to increase placental transfusion in preterm neonates, a randomized controlled trial. *Obstetrics and Gynecology, 117*(2 Pt. 1), 205–211.

Sanders, L., & Buckner, E. B. (2006). The Newborn Behavioral Observations (NBO) system as a nursing intervention to enhance engagement in first-time mothers: Feasibility and desirability. *Pediatric Nursing, 32*(5), 455–459.

Sasidharan, K., Dutta, S., & Narang, A. (2009). Validity of New Ballard score until 7th day of postnatal life in moderately preterm neonates. *Archives of Disease in Childhood. Fetal and Neonatal Edition, 94*, F39–F44.

Shah, P. S., Herbozo, C., Aliwalas, L. L., et al. (2012). Breastfeeding or breast milk for procedural pain in neonates. *The Cochrane Database of Systematic Reviews*, (12), CD004950.

Sim, M. A., Leow, S. Y., Hao, Y., et al. (2016). A practical comparison of temporal artery thermometry and axillary thermometry in neonates under different environments. *Journal of Paediatrics and Child Health, 52*(4), 391–396.

Smith, J. (2014). Methods and devices of temperature measurement in the neonate: A narrative review of practice recommendations. *Newborn and Infant Nursing Reviews, 14*(2), 64–71.

Smith, J., Alcock, G., & Usher, K. (2013). Temperature measurement in the preterm and term neonate: A review of the literature. *Neonatal Network, 32*(1), 16–25.

Smolkin, T., Mick, O., Dabbah, M., et al. (2012). Birth by cesarean delivery and failure of first otoacoustic emissions hearing test. *Pediatrics, 130*(1), e95–e100.

Stevens, B., Yamada, J., Ohlsson, A., et al. (2016). Sucrose for analgesia in newborn infants undergoing painful procedures. *The Cochrane Database of Systematic Reviews*, (7), CD001069.

Thomas, P., Peabody, J., Turnier, V., et al. (2000). A new look at intrauterine growth and the impact of race, altitude, and gender. *Pediatrics, 106*(2), e21.

US Department of Health and Human Services. (2013). *Healthy people 2020*, Washington, DC, The Department. Retrieved from http://www.healthypeople.gov/2020/topics-objectives.

Waldrop, J. (2013). Exploration of reasons for feeding choices of Hispanic mothers. *MCN. The American Journal of Maternal Child Nursing, 38*(5), 282–288.

Wambach, K., Domain, E. W., Page-Goertz, S., et al. (2016). Exclusive breastfeeding experiences among Mexican-American women. *Journal of Human Lactation, 32*(1), 103–111.

Wandel, M., Terragni, L., Nguyen, C., et al. (2016). Breastfeeding among Somali mothers living in Norway: Attitudes, practices and challenges. *Women and Birth, 29*(6), 487–493.

Wang, L., Collins, C., Ratliff, M., et al. (Feb 2017). Breastfeeding reduces childhood obesity risks. *Childhood Obesity epub.*

World Health Organization. (2009). *WHO guidelines on hand hygiene in health care, 2009,* World Health Organization. http://whqlibdoc.who.int/publications/2009/9789241597906_eng.pdf.

World Health Organization. (2017). *Female genital mutilation, Fact Sheet 241.* Retrieved from http://www.who.int/mediacentre/factsheets/fs241/en.

World Health Organization, UNICEF, Wellstart International. (2009). *Baby-friendly hospital initiative: revised, updated and expanded for integrated care*, World Health Organization.

Zupan, J., Garner, P., & Omari, A. A. (2013). Topical umbilical cord care at birth. *The Cochrane Database of Systematic Reviews*, (3), CD001057, 2004; edited, no change to conclusions.

8

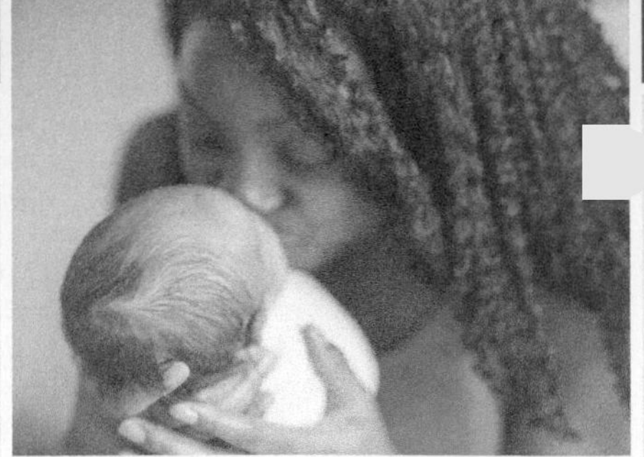

Health Problems of the Newborn

Kimberley Fisher and Kristina D. Wilson

http://evolve.elsevier.com/wong/ncic

CONCEPTS

- Birth Injuries
- Congenital Abnormalities
- Thermoregulation
- Glucose Regulation

BIRTH INJURIES

Several factors predispose an infant to birth injuries. Maternal factors include uterine dysfunction that leads to prolonged or precipitous labor, preterm or postterm labor, and cephalopelvic disproportion. Injury may result from dystocia caused by fetal macrosomia, multifetal gestation, abnormal or difficult presentation (not caused by maternal uterine or pelvic conditions), and congenital anomalies. Intrapartum events that can result in scalp injury include the use of intrapartum monitoring of fetal heart rate and collection of fetal scalp blood for acid-base assessment. Obstetric birth techniques can cause injury. Forceps birth, vacuum extraction, version and extraction, and cesarean birth are potential contributory factors. Often more than one factor is present, and multiple predisposing factors may be related to a single maternal condition.

Many injuries are minor and resolve spontaneously in a few days; others, although minor, require some degree of intervention. Still others can be serious or even fatal. Part of the nurse's responsibility is to identify such injuries so that appropriate interventions can be initiated as soon as possible. Birth injuries are classified according to the type of body structure involved (Box 8.1).

SOFT TISSUE INJURY

Infants may sustain various types of soft tissue injury during birth, primarily in the form of bruises and abrasions secondary to dystocia. Soft tissue injury usually occurs when there is some degree of disproportion between the presenting part and the maternal pelvis (cephalopelvic disproportion). Box 8.2 lists common types of soft tissue injury. The use of forceps to facilitate a difficult vertex delivery may produce discoloration or abrasions with the same configuration as the forceps on the sides of the neonate's face. Petechiae or ecchymoses may be observed on the presenting part after a breech or brow delivery. After a difficult or precipitous delivery, the sudden release of pressure on the head can produce scleral hemorrhages or generalized petechiae over the face and head. Petechiae and ecchymoses may also appear on the head, neck, and face of an infant born with a nuchal cord, giving the infant's face a cyanotic appearance. A well-defined circle of petechiae and ecchymoses may also appear on the occipital region of the newborn's head when a vacuum suction cup is applied during delivery. Metal suction cups are associated with more scalp injuries than silastic; alopecia has been reported in association with vacuum-associated scalp trauma (Doumouchtsis & Arulkumaran, 2008). Rarely, lacerations occur during cesarean section.

These traumatic lesions generally fade spontaneously and without treatment within a few days. However, petechiae may be a manifestation of an underlying bleeding disorder and require further evaluation.

Nursing Care Management

Nursing care is directed primarily toward assessing the injury, maintaining asepsis of the area to prevent additional skin breakdown and infection, and providing an explanation and reassurance to the parents. The nurse should record an accurate description of the injury in writing (e.g., the location, color, size, and shape) and via photographs, when possible, to facilitate subsequent comparative nursing evaluations.

Regardless of how benign the injury, parents may be concerned and mourn the loss of the expected "perfect" infant. Explanations of the cause and treatment, if any, need to be thorough and repeated frequently. If the injury is temporarily disfiguring, such as extensive facial bruising, nurses can demonstrate acceptance of the child through their example of sensitive, personal care.

HEAD INJURY

Head injury that occurs during the birth process is usually benign but occasionally results in more serious injury. The injuries that produce serious trauma, such as intracranial hemorrhage and subdural hematoma, are discussed in relation to neurologic disorders in the newborn (See Chapters 9 and 32). Skull fractures are discussed with other fractures sustained during the birth process. The three most common types of extracranial hemorrhagic injury are caput succedaneum, subgaleal hemorrhage, and cephalhematoma.

Caput Succedaneum

The most commonly observed scalp lesion is caput succedaneum, a vaguely outlined area of edematous tissue situated over the portion of

BOX 8.1 Types of Neonatal Physical Injuries at Birth*

Soft Tissue Injury
Erythema
Abrasion
Petechiae
Ecchymoses
Subcutaneous fat necrosis
Retinal hemorrhage
Scalp laceration

Head Injury
Caput succedaneum
Subgaleal hemorrhage
Cephalhematoma
Fracture (depressed or linear)
Intracranial hemorrhage
Subdural or epidural hematoma

Nerve Injury
Facial paralysis
Brachial palsy (Erb-Duchenne paralysis, Klumpke palsy)
Phrenic nerve palsy (diaphragmatic paralysis)
Spinal cord injury
Vocal cord paralysis

Other
Fracture-clavicle, femur
Torticollis
Scalp abscess
Subconjunctival (scleral) hemorrhage
Liver, spleen rupture
Hemorrhage into abdominal organ(s)

*Partial adaptation from Rozance, P. J., & Rosenberg, A. A. (2012). The neonate. In S. G. Gabbe, J. R. Niebyl, J. L. Simpson, et al. (Eds.), *Obstetrics: Normal and problem pregnancies* (6th ed.). Philadelphia, PA: Elsevier/Saunders.

BOX 8.2 Common Types of Soft Tissue Injury

Erythema and abrasions—Usually the result of the application of forceps; discoloration the same configuration as the instrument

Petechiae—Nonraised, pinpoint hemorrhages caused by a sudden increase and then release of pressure during passage through the birth canal; may be seen on the chest, face, and head

Ecchymoses—Small hemorrhagic areas (larger than petechiae) that may occur after traumatic, precipitous, or breech delivery

Subcutaneous fat necrosis—Clearly outlined masses located in the subcutaneous tissues that are firm to the overlying skin but movable over the underlying tissue; most likely caused by traumatic manipulation during delivery

Subconjunctival (scleral) hemorrhages—The result of rupture of capillaries in the sclera from pressure on the fetal head during delivery; most commonly located in the limbus of the iris

Retinal hemorrhages—Flame-shaped, irregular, or round areas of bleeding in the retina from excessive pressure on the fetal head during delivery; extensive areas possibly indicative of subdural hematoma or brain trauma

the scalp that presents in a vertex delivery (Fig. 8.1, *A*). The swelling consists of serum and/or blood that has accumulated in the tissues above the bone. Typically the swelling extends beyond the bone margins (or sutures) and may be associated with overlying petechiae or ecchymosis. It is present at or shortly after birth. No specific treatment is necessary, and the swelling subsides within a few days.

Subgaleal Hemorrhage

Subgaleal hemorrhage is bleeding into the subgaleal compartment (Fig. 8.1, *B*). The subgaleal compartment is a potential space that contains loosely arranged connective tissue. It is located beneath the galea aponeurosis, the tendinous sheath that connects the frontal and occipital muscles and forms the inner surface of the scalp. The injury occurs as a result of forces that compress and then drag the head through the pelvic outlet (Parsons, Seay, & Jacobson, 2016; Shah & Wusthoff, 2016). Instrumented delivery, particularly vacuum extraction and forceps delivery, increases the risk of subgaleal hemorrhage. Additional risk factors include prolonged second stage of labor, fetal distress, macrosomia, failed vacuum extraction, and maternal primiparity. The bleeding extends beyond bone, often posterior into the neck, and continues after birth, with the potential for serious complications and morbidity.

Early detection of the hemorrhage is vital; serial head circumference measurements and inspection of the back of the neck for increasing edema and a firm mass are essential. A boggy fluctuant mass over the scalp that crosses the suture line and moves as the baby is repositioned is an early sign of subgaleal hemorrhage (Smith, Kandamany, Okafor, et al., 2016). Other signs include pallor, tachycardia, a forward and lateral positioning of the newborn's ears as the hematoma extends posteriorly, and increasing head circumference. Computed tomography (CT) or magnetic resonance imaging (MRI) is useful in confirming the diagnosis. Replacement of lost blood and clotting factors is required in acute cases of hemorrhage. Monitoring the infant for changes in level of consciousness and a decrease in the hematocrit is also vital to early recognition and management. An increase in serum bilirubin levels may occur as a result of the degrading red blood cells within the hematoma.

Cephalhematoma

A cephalhematoma forms when blood vessels rupture during labor or delivery and produce bleeding into the area between the bone and its periosteum. The injury occurs most often with primiparous women and is often associated with forceps delivery and vacuum extraction. Unlike caput succedaneum, the boundaries of the cephalhematoma are distinguishable and do not extend beyond the limits of the bone (Fig. 8.1, *C*). The cephalhematoma may involve one or both parietal bones but rarely affects the occipital and frontal bones. The swelling is usually minimal or absent at birth and increases in size on the second or third day. Blood loss is usually not significant.

No treatment is indicated for uncomplicated cephalhematoma. Most lesions are absorbed within 2 weeks to 3 months. Lesions that result in severe blood loss to the area or that involve an underlying fracture require further evaluation. Hyperbilirubinemia may result during resolution of the hematoma. A local infection can develop and is suspected when swelling suddenly increases.

Nursing Care Management

Nursing care is directed toward assessment, observation, and accurate documentation of the common scalp injuries. Vigilance in observing for possible associated complications, such as infection or, as in the case of subgaleal hemorrhage, acute blood loss and hypovolemia, is important. Nursing care of a newborn with a subgaleal hemorrhage includes careful monitoring for signs of hemodynamic instability and shock (Modanlou, Hutson, & Merritt, 2016). Because caput succedaneum

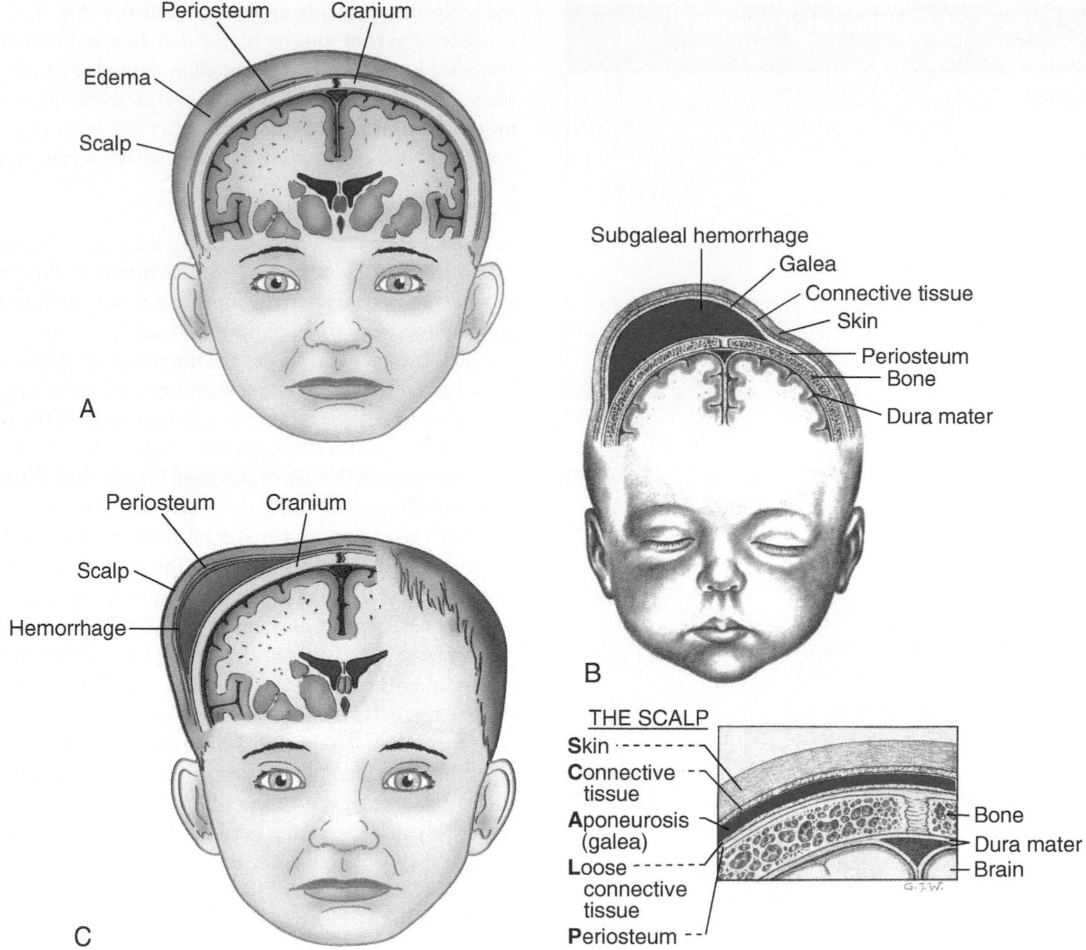

FIG. 8.1 A, Caput succedaneum. **B,** Subgaleal hemorrhage. **C,** Cephalhematoma. (*A* and *C*, From Seidel, H. M., Ball, J. W., Dains, J. E., et al. [2006]. *Mosby's guide to physical examination* [6th ed.]. St. Louis, MO: Mosby.)

and cephalhematoma usually resolve spontaneously, parents need reassurance of their usually benign nature.

FRACTURES

Fracture of the clavicle, or collarbone, is the most common birth injury. It is often associated with difficult vertex or breech deliveries of infants of greater-than-average size. Further examination usually reveals **crepitus** (i.e., the coarse, crackling sensation produced by the rubbing together of fractured bone fragments), and radiographs usually reveal a complete fracture with overriding of the fragments. A palpable spongy mass, representing localized edema and hematoma, is also a sign of a fractured clavicle.

The newborn with a fractured clavicle may have no symptoms, but the nurse should suspect a fracture if an infant has limited use of the affected arm, malpositioning of the arm, an asymmetric Moro reflex, or focal swelling or tenderness or cries when the arm is moved. Eliciting the scarf sign (i.e., extending arm across chest toward opposite shoulder) for assessment of gestational age is contraindicated if a fractured clavicle is suspected.

In neonates, fractures of long bones, such as the femur or the humerus, are often difficult to detect by radiographic examination. Although osteogenesis imperfecta is a rare finding, assess a newborn infant with a fracture for other evidence of this congenital disorder.

Fractures of the neonatal skull are uncommon. The bones, which are less mineralized and more compressible than bones in older infants and children, are separated by membranous seams that allow the head contour to adjust to the birth canal during delivery. Skull fractures usually follow a prolonged, difficult delivery or forceps extraction. Most fractures are linear, but some may be visible as depressed indentations that compress or decompress like a Ping-Pong ball. Management of depressed skull fractures is controversial; many resolve without intervention. Nonsurgical elevation of the indentation using a hand breast pump or vacuum extractor has been reported (Mangurten & Puppala, 2015). Surgery may be required in the presence of bone fragments or signs of neurologic changes and increased intracranial pressure (ICP). A similar finding in neonates is *craniotabes,* which is usually benign or may be associated with prematurity or hydrocephalus (Johnson, 2016). In this condition the cranial bone(s) moves freely on palpation and may be easily compressed.

Nursing Care Management

Often no intervention is prescribed other than proper body alignment, careful dressing and undressing of the infant, and handling and carrying techniques that support the affected bone. If the infant has a fractured clavicle, it is important to support the upper and lower back rather than pull the infant up from under the arms. Occasionally, for immobilization and relief of pain, the arm on the side of the fractured clavicle may be abducted at more than 60 degrees with the elbow flexed at more than 90 degrees for 7 to 10 days.

Linear skull fractures usually require no treatment. A Ping-Pong–type fracture may require decompression by surgical intervention. The infant is carefully observed for signs of neurologic complications. The parents of an infant with a fracture of any bone should be involved in caring for the infant during hospitalization as part of discharge planning for care at home. Evaluate any newborn large for gestational age and delivered vaginally for a fractured clavicle. The newborn with a fractured clavicle may have no symptoms, but suspect a fracture if the infant has limited use of the affected arm, malpositioning of the arm, an asymmetric Moro reflex, or focal swelling or tenderness or cries in pain when the arm is moved.

! NURSING ALERT

Any newborn who is large for gestational age or weighs more than 4000 g (8 lb, 8 oz) and is delivered vaginally should be evaluated for a fractured clavicle.

NERVE INJURIES

Facial Paralysis

Pressure on the facial nerve (the seventh cranial nerve) during delivery may result in injury to the nerve. The primary clinical manifestations are loss of movement on the affected side, such as an inability to completely close the eye, drooping of the corner of the mouth, and absence of wrinkling of the forehead and nasolabial fold (Fig. 8.2). The paralysis is most noticeable when the infant cries. The mouth is drawn to the unaffected side, the wrinkles are deeper on the normal side, and the eye on the involved side remains open.

No medical intervention is necessary. The paralysis usually disappears spontaneously in a few days but may take as long as several months.

Brachial Palsy

Brachial plexus injury results from forces that alter the normal position and relationship of the arm, shoulder, and neck. Erb palsy (Erb-Duchenne paralysis) is caused by damage to the upper plexus and usually results from stretching or pulling away of the shoulder from the head, as might occur with shoulder dystocia or with a difficult vertex or breech delivery. Other identified clinical situations that are considered to place the baby at risk for brachial palsy include a significantly larger than normal baby with a fetal weight exceeding 5000 g in women without diabetes or 4500 g in women with diabetes, prior recognized shoulder dystocia, or a midpelvic operative vaginal delivery with a fetal birth weight in excess of 4000 g (American College of Obstetricians and Gynecologists' Task Force on Neonatal Brachial Plexus Palsy, 2014). The less common lower plexus palsy, or Klumpke palsy, results from severe stretching of the upper extremity while the trunk is relatively less mobile.

The clinical manifestations of Erb palsy are related to the paralysis of the affected upper extremity and muscles. The arm hangs limp alongside the body. The shoulder and arm are adducted and internally rotated. The elbow is extended and the forearm is pronated, with the wrist and fingers flexed; a grasp reflex may be present because finger and wrist movement remain normal, but the Moro reflex is absent (Tappero, 2016) (Fig. 8.3). In lower plexus palsy the muscles of the hand are paralyzed, with consequent wrist drop and relaxed fingers. In a third and more severe form of brachial palsy, total plexus injury, the entire arm and hand are paralyzed and hang limp and motionless at the side. The Moro reflex is absent on the affected side for all forms of brachial palsy.

Treatment of the affected arm is aimed at preventing contractures of the paralyzed muscles and maintaining correct placement of the humeral head within the glenoid fossa of the scapula. Complete recovery from stretched nerves usually takes 3 to 6 months. Full recovery is expected in the majority of infants (Parsons, Seay, & Jacobson, 2016), but there are specific peripartum and neonatal factors associated with persistent neonatal brachial plexus palsy at 1 year (Wilson, Chang, Chauhan, et al., 2016). Cephalic presentation, induction of labor, birth weight greater than 9 pounds, and the presence of Horner syndome significantly increase the odds of persistence of brachial palsy. Cesarean delivery and Narakas grade I to II injury (Narakas grading defines the severity of nerve damage) significantly reduced the chance of brachial palsy continuing after 1 year. For those injuries that do not improve spontaneously by 3 months, surgical intervention may be needed to relieve pressure on the nerves or to repair the nerves with grafting (Carlo & Ambalavanan, 2016b). In some cases injection of botulinum toxin A into the pectoralis major muscle may be effective in reducing muscle contractures after birth-related brachial plexus injuries (Dahan-Oliel, Kasaai, Montpetit, et al., 2012).

A condition that may occur in association with brachial plexus injury is *torticollis*. This symptom, as it is called by many, is observed as a

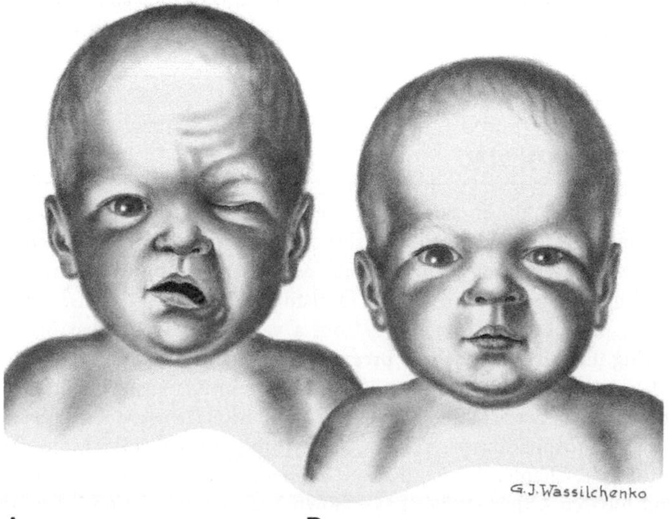

FIG. 8.2 A, Paralysis of right side of face 15 minutes after forceps delivery. Absence of movement on affected side is especially noticeable when infant cries. **B,** Same infant 24 hours later.

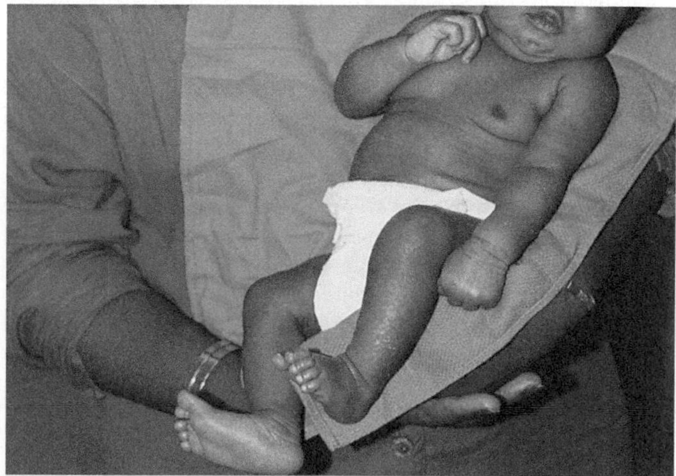

FIG. 8.3 Left-sided brachial plexus (Erb-Duchenne) palsy. Note extended, internally rotated arm and pronated wrist on affected side.

tilting of the head to one side in combination with rotation of the head to the opposite side due to the unilateral contracture of the sternocleidomastoid muscle; it has been reported to occur in as many as 43% of infants with brachial plexus injury (Hervey-Jumper, Justice, & Vanaman, 2011; O'Toole & Spiegel, 2016). Torticollis may also occur in older infants with positional plagiocephaly (see Chapter 11) and in association with other conditions such as spinal cord tumors, clavicle fracture, congenital scoliosis, Klippel-Feil anomalies, and cervical spine subluxation (Hervey-Jumper, Justice, & Vanaman, 2011). The treatment of torticollis involves massage, stimulation, and stretching programs under the supervision of a physical therapist (Hervey-Jumper, Justice, & Vanaman, 2011; O'Toole & Spiegel, 2016). Additional pathology associated with torticollis may occur, but it is not within the scope of this section to discuss the range of possibilities.

Phrenic Nerve Paralysis

Phrenic nerve paralysis results in diaphragmatic paralysis as demonstrated by ultrasonography, which shows paradoxic chest movement and an elevated diaphragm. Initially, chest radiography may not demonstrate an elevated diaphragm if the neonate is receiving positive pressure ventilation. The injury sometimes occurs in conjunction with brachial palsy. Respiratory distress is the most common and important sign of injury. Because injury to the phrenic nerve is usually unilateral, the lung on the affected side does not expand, and respiratory efforts are ineffectual. Breathing is primarily thoracic, and cyanosis, tachypnea, or complete respiratory failure may be seen. Pneumonia and atelectasis on the affected side may also occur.

Nursing Care Management

Nursing care of the infant with facial nerve paralysis involves aiding the infant in suckling and helping the mother with feeding techniques. A comprehensive evaluation of the infant's oral motor skills by both an infant feeding specialist and a Lactation Consultant are recommended to develop an effective multidisciplinary feeding regimen. The infant may require partial gavage feeding and supplemental oral stimulation with a minimum amount of expressed breast milk to prevent aspiration. Breastfeeding is recommended and the mother will need assistance in helping the infant grasp and compress the areolar area to ensure effective milk transfer from the mother to the infant.

If the lid of the eye on the affected side does not close completely, instill artificial tears as needed to prevent drying of the conjunctiva, sclera, and cornea. The lid is often taped shut to prevent injury. If the infant requires eye care at home, teach the parents the procedure for administering eye drops before the infant is discharged from the nursery. (See Chapter 23.)

Nursing care of the newborn with brachial palsy is concerned primarily with proper positioning of the affected arm. The affected arm should be gently immobilized on the upper abdomen; passive range-of-motion exercises of the shoulder, wrist, elbow, and fingers are initiated at 7 to 10 days of age (Carlo & Ambalavanan, 2016b; Roland & Hill, 2016). Wrist flexion contractures may be prevented with the use of supportive splints or braces. In dressing the infant, give preference to the affected arm. Undressing begins with the unaffected arm, and redressing begins with the affected arm to prevent unnecessary manipulation and stress on the paralyzed muscles. Teach parents to use the "football" position when holding the infant and to avoid picking the child up from under the axillae or by pulling on the arms.*

*United Brachial Plexus Network, 1610 Kent St., Kent, OH 44240; 866-877-7004; email: info@ubpn.org; http://www.ubpn.org/.

The infant with phrenic nerve paralysis requires the same nursing care as any infant with respiratory distress. The family's emotional needs are also an important part of nursing care; the family needs reassurance regarding the neonate's progress toward an optimal outcome. Follow-up care is also essential because of the extended length of recovery.

CRANIAL DEFORMITIES

In the normal newborn the cranial sutures are separated by membranous seams several millimeters wide. For the first few hours to 1 to 2 days after birth, the cranial bones are highly mobile, which allows the bones to mold and overlap one another, adjusting the circumference of the head to accommodate to the changing shape and character of the birth canal. The principal sutures in the infant's skull are the sagittal, coronal, and lambdoid sutures, and the major soft areas at the juncture of these sutures are the anterior and posterior fontanels. (See Fig. 7.7.)

After birth, growth of the skull bones occurs in a direction perpendicular (at right angles) to the line of the suture, and normal closure occurs in a regular and predictable order. Although the age at which closure takes place varies widely in individual children, solid union of all sutures is not completed until late childhood. Normally, sutures and fontanels are ossified by the following ages:

- Eight weeks—Posterior fontanel closed
- Six months—Fibrous union of suture lines and interlocking of serrated edges
- Eighteen months—Anterior fontanel closed
- Twelve years and older—Sutures not separable by ICP

Closure of a suture before the expected time inhibits the perpendicular growth. Because normal increase in brain volume requires expansion, the skull is forced to grow in a direction parallel to the fused suture. This alteration in skull growth always distorts the head shape when the underlying brain growth is normal. The small head with closed sutures and a normal shape is a result of deficient brain growth; the suture closure is secondary to this brain growth failure. Failure of brain growth is not secondary to suture closure.

Various types of cranial deformities are encountered in early infancy. These include the enlarged head with frontal protrusion, or bossing (characteristic of hydrocephalus); the parietal bossing that is seen in chronic subdural hematoma; the small head; and a variety of skull deformities (Fig. 8.4). Some occur during prenatal development. In others, head circumference is usually within normal limits at birth, and the deviation from normal development becomes apparent with advancing age.

MICROCEPHALY

Primary (genetic) microcephaly refers to a small head size that may be caused by an autosomal recessive or autosomal dominant disorder or a chromosomal abnormality such as Down syndrome or Cornelia de Lange syndrome (Kinsman & Johnston, 2016). Secondary (nongenetic) microcephaly can result from a variety of insults that occur during the third trimester of pregnancy, the perinatal period, or early infancy (Kinsman & Johnston, 2016). These stimuli may be irradiation (especially between 4 and 20 weeks of gestation), maternal infection (notably toxoplasmosis, rubella, or cytomegalovirus [see Maternal Infections, Chapter 9]), irradiation, or chemical agents such as alcohol and tobacco. Other studies have shown a strong association between maternal alcohol ingestion and microcephaly and low birth weight and length (Feldman, Jones, Lindsay, et al., 2012). Infection, trauma, metabolic disorders, and anoxia are all capable of causing decreased brain growth. Microcephaly is defined as an occipitofrontal circumference greater

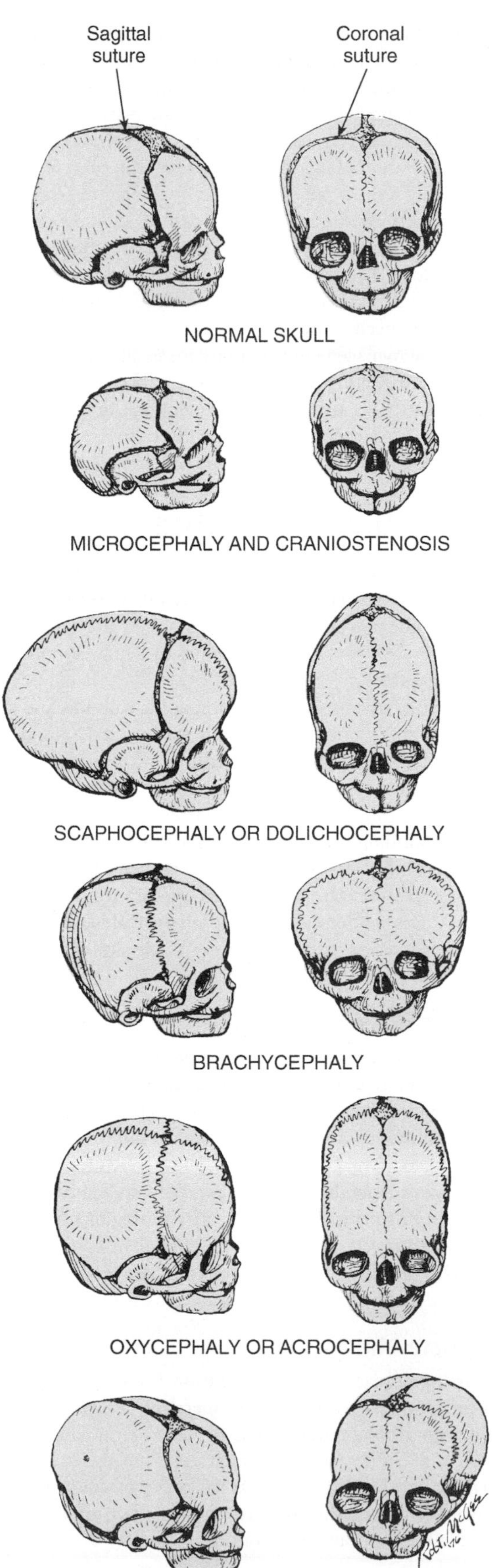

FIG. 8.4 Abnormal skull configurations.

than 3 standard deviations below the mean for age and sex (Kinsman & Johnston, 2016).

The Zika virus (ZIKV), transmitted by the Aedes mosquito, is identified as a causal contributor to microcephaly in infancy (Cauchemez, Besnard, Bompard, et al., 2016; Chibueze, Tirado, Lopes, et al., 2017). In 2016 ZIKV infection was declared a Public Health Emergency of International Concern. Although it causes simple flulike symptoms in the pregnant mother, ZIKV can lead to serious complications (including microcephaly) in the newborn (Passi, Sharma, Dutta, et al., 2017).

Secondary microcephaly may also occur as a result of maternal diabetes and maternal hyperphenylalanemia. Fetal exposure to alcohol and tobacco use was shown to result in a 2.6-fold increase in the risk of isolated secondary microcephaly compared with other causes, including syndromes (Feldman, Jones, Lindsay, et al., 2012). Kuban, Allred, O'Shea, and colleagues (2009) found that 71% of extremely low-birth-weight (ELBW) infants born with microcephaly had a normal head circumference at age 2 years; however, their study concluded that ELBW infants with microcephaly at 2 years of age had a poor neurodevelopmental outcome.

In both types the neurologic manifestations range from decerebration, complete unresponsiveness, and autistic behavior to mild motor impairment, educable neurocognitive impairment, and mild hyperkinesis. There appears to be a decided relationship between microcephaly and cognitive delays of varying degrees; however, not all children with microcephaly have cognitive delays.

Nursing Care Management

There is no specific treatment. Nursing care is supportive and may be directed toward helping parents adjust to rearing a child with cognitive impairment when this condition is present. (See Chapter 20.)

CRANIOSTENOSIS

Craniostenosis is defined as the premature closure at birth of one or more cranial sutures (Kinsman & Johnston, 2016). The clinical picture depends on which sutures close, the duration of the closure process, and the success or failure of the other sutures to compensate by expansion (see Fig. 8.4). The condition may be divided according to the number of sutures involved; primary craniostenosis involves one or more sutures as a result of abnormalities of skull development, whereas secondary craniostenosis involves the failure of brain growth and expansion (Kinsman & Johnston, 2016). Focal hydrodynamic mechanisms are involved in the compensatory skull changes seen in craniostenosis. Brain atrophy and an underlying motor delay account for the position-induced skull changes. Craniostenosis is also a common feature of children with genetic syndromes such as Crouzon, Apert (Box 8.3), Pfeiffer, Chotzen, Carpenter, and Jackson-Weiss syndromes (Kinsman & Johnston, 2016). Potential risk factors for craniostenosis include maternal Caucasian race, advanced maternal age, male infant, use of nitrosatable drugs, fertility treatments, and certain paternal occupations (e.g., agriculture, repairmen, mechanics, forestry). Diagnosis is established with CT scan, and MRI is useful in identifying accompanying brain abnormalities. Ultrasound is also shown to be a reliable screening tool to rule out craniostenosis in newborns with abnormal head shape (Hall, Beasachio, Moore, et al., 2017). Increased ICP is more frequent in children with more than one prematurely fused suture.

The most common form of craniostenosis is premature closure of the sagittal suture (scaphocephaly) with resulting elongation of the skull in the anteroposterior direction. This occurs more commonly in males and does not result in increased ICP or hydrocephalus. A similar head shape (dolicocephaly) occurs as a result of postnatal position

BOX 8.3 Cranial Abnormalities Associated With Abnormal Bone Growth

Crouzon syndrome—Craniofacial dysostosis (abnormal ossification of fetal cartilages) with shallow orbits and underdevelopment of the middle third of the face

Apert syndrome—Craniostenosis resulting in a prominent forehead; may be extracranial abnormalities, such as syndactyly (webbing) of fingers and toes and cardiac defects

Treacher Collins syndrome—Asymmetric facial deformity, including absent cheekbones, underslung jaw, and small chin; also downward slant of the eyes and other minor defects

Pierre Robin sequence—Displacement of the chin as a result of micrognathia (mandibular hypoplasia) or retrognathia (normal-sized mandible positioned posteriorly); also glossoptosis with obstruction of the airway and sometimes a cleft palate

maintenance in some preterm infants (McCarty, Peat, Malcolm, et al., 2016); however, in this case there is no premature closure of sutures. In some types of craniostenosis an increase in ICP may occur, which may or may not cause cognitive delays but can result in progressive papilledema, optic atrophy, and eventual blindness. Other complications include facial asymmetry and malocclusion.

Trigonocephaly, or metopic craniostenosis, represents a premature closure of the metopic suture in utero, a congenital problem that is familial and often requires surgical treatment to prevent forebrain abnormalities. The metopic suture occurs where the right and left frontal bones meet on the forehead. Craniostenosis of the metopic suture may be an autosomal dominantly inherited disorder not associated with functional brain or other abnormalities. Other types of craniostenosis include frontal plagiocephaly (fusion of coronal and sphenofrontal sutures), occipital plagiocephaly (fusion of lambdoid suture or positional), turricephaly (fusion of coronal and frontoethmoidal sutures), and kleebattschädel deformity (skull resembles a cloverleaf and hydrocephalus is common) (Kinsman & Johnston, 2016).

Therapeutic Management

Treatment involves surgical excision of long bars of bone (strip craniectomy) along or parallel to the fused suture. Various surgical procedures are employed in an effort to release the fused suture and direct growth. Surgery is performed to achieve the best possible cosmetic effect and, in severe cases, to relieve cerebral pressure symptoms and complications. The advised timing of suture release is before 6 months of age for best cosmetic and neurodevelopmental results. For optimal outcomes, it is imperative that a multidisciplinary craniofacial team is involved in the care of the child with craniostenosis.

Nursing Care Management

Nursing care primarily involves the early identification of persistent cranial molding weeks after regular birth molding would have resolved and referral for follow-up evaluation. In the postoperative period, nursing care includes observation for changes in neurologic status, hemorrhage, or infection.

Because of the type of bone surgery involved with craniostenosis, blood loss can be significant. Therefore the nurse should carefully monitor hematocrit and hemoglobin after surgery. Parents may also wish to provide a compatible blood donor for their infant. Nurses should inform and guide parents through this blood bank procedure. With endoscopic surgery, blood loss is minimized, but the child must wear a cranial molding helmet for 3 to 4 months. The helmet should be worn 23 hours each day and a second helmet may be fitted as a result of rapid head growth; erythematous areas should be examined closely by the orthotist and adjustments made accordingly. Instructions regarding compliance with the helmet and skin care are essential.

Most children have substantial swelling of the eyelids postoperatively; careful handling and talking to the child may help calm fears while the eyelids are swollen shut. Eye care should be limited to gentle cleansing with a moist cloth. Pain management measures should be instituted in infants experiencing postoperative pain as they would be for older children or adults. Fluids and adequate hydration are essential. Oral feedings resume as soon as possible for hydration and for the infant's nutritive sucking needs.

Early surgical management of craniostenosis allows proper expansion of the brain and the creation of an acceptable appearance. Parents require special support and education during this time, especially from other parents whose infants have undergone similar operations. The nurse can serve as a liaison for this type of parental support.

CRANIOFACIAL ABNORMALITIES

Craniofacial abnormalities are those deformities involving the skull and facial bones. They have a low incidence rate in the population, but their effects can be psychologically devastating to affected children and their families. Box 8.3 lists some deformities caused by abnormal growth of cranial bone(s).

Most craniofacial anomalies are compatible with life, and all efforts are made to help the child and family live as normal a life as possible. Advances in microscopic, endoscopic, orthopedic, neurologic, and plastic reconstructive surgery techniques have made it possible for children with craniofacial anomalies not only to survive beyond childhood but also to live a fulfilling life without the social stigmas of past decades. These children, however, may continue to face erroneous assumptions of cognitive impairment because of their appearance. Multidisciplinary craniofacial teams are dedicated to helping the child and family achieve optimum potential for intellectual growth, physical competence, and social acceptance.

Therapeutic Management

Craniofacial surgical correction involves peeling the patient's face away from the skull and remolding the understructures. Parts can be brought together, the skull reshaped and remodeled, and bone fragments removed or reshaped. Bone segments from the child's hip or ribs may be used to reshape the skull or facial features. The procedures are performed at various ages, depending on the anomaly, in craniofacial centers specializing in this pediatric problem. The timing of surgery is before school entry and is determined on an individual basis to ensure normal growth and development. Depending on the abnormality, other surgeries are performed, such as mandibular and digit correction.

Nursing Care Management

Direct nursing efforts involve preparation for surgery (often several surgical procedures over time), postoperative care similar to care of any child with cranial surgery, and support of the child and family. Frequently this child and family must adjust to the unfamiliar body image, which may be as traumatic as the previous deformity. A helmet may be worn to protect the operative site and bone grafts for 6 months to 2 years. Follow-up care is important.

PIERRE ROBIN SEQUENCE

Pierre Robin sequence (PRS) is a defect characterized by retroposition of the tongue and mandible, which often results in neonatal respiratory and feeding problems. The condition has an incidence of 1 in 8500 to 14,000 live births, and about one-half of those with PRS have other congenital anomalies (Breugem, Evans, Poets, et al., 2016). The tongue may be large (glossoptosis) and frequently falls over the neonate's airway, causing occlusion and respiratory distress. In severe upper airway obstruction a tracheotomy may be required; however, an alternative is to place a modified nasopharyngeal tube and bypass the upper airway obstruction (Gangopadhyay, Mendonca, Woo, et al., 2012). From a lateral view the infant's lower jaw can be seen to be positioned posterior (micrognathia) to the upper jaw. PRS may be observed in the newborn nursery when the infant has apnea and cyanosis in the supine position, due primarily to upper airway obstruction. The neonate is positioned to facilitate an open airway. A tongue-lip adhesion is a common surgical procedure that repositions the tongue anteriorly. Surgical mandibular distraction osteogenesis is another technique used to correct the condition (Cicchetti, Cascone, Caresta, et al., 2012; Scott, Tibesar, Lander, et al., 2011). There are usually no associated neurocognitive defects in isolated (nonsyndromic) PRS.

CLEFT LIP AND CLEFT PALATE

Cleft lip (CL) with or without cleft palate (CP) is the most common birth defect in the United States and occurs with a frequency of 1 in 600 live births (Cleft Palate Foundation, 2013). Isolated CL with or without CP is more common in males, and CP alone is more common in females. See Table 8.1 for a comparison of the two defects.

Etiology

Most cases of CL and/or CP result from a combination of genetic and environmental factors. The gene(s) responsible for clefting in individuals without syndromes is not yet known. However, some genetic syndromes are known to be associated with clefting in approximately 15% of individuals with clefts (such as 22q11.2 deletion). Exposure to environmental factors or teratogens may be responsible for clefts at a critical point in embryonic development. Alcohol use, cigarette smoking, and prescription drugs, including anticonvulsants, steroids, and retinoids, are associated with higher rates of oral clefting. Conversely, folic acid supplements may protect against clefting.

Pathophysiology

Development of the primary and secondary palates takes place at different times and involves different developmental processes, which is why clefts can vary significantly. The primary palate includes the medial portion of the upper lip and the portion of the alveolar ridge that contains the central and lateral incisors. The secondary palate contains the remaining portion of the hard palate and all of the soft palate. A cleft lip can occur unilaterally or bilaterally, and it may present as a simple notch in the upper lip or extend completely to the base of the nose. CL occurs from failure of the maxillary processes to fuse with the nasal elevations on the frontal prominence to form the primary palate, which normally occurs during the sixth week of gestation (Fig. 8.5, *A*). A cleft palate is a midline defect and may vary from a bifid uvula (the mildest form of a cleft palate with essentially no functional impact on speech or feeding), to a complete cleft palate that extends from the soft palate into the hard palate. CP occurs from a failed fusion of the secondary palate (hard and soft palates), which takes place later in development, between the seventh and twelfth weeks of gestation (Fig. 8.5, *B–D*).

Diagnostic Evaluation

A cleft that involves the lip and/or CP is readily apparent at birth. The cleft palate is detected through visual inspection of the oral cavity or

TABLE 8.1 Comparison of Cleft Lip and Cleft Palate

	Cleft Lip	Cleft Palate
Incidence	1:600	1:2500
Inheritance	Multifactorial inheritance, environmental factors, familial occurrence Male predominance	Associated with syndromes (chromosomal), familial occurrence; environmental factors such as maternal alcohol ingestion, smoking, or teratogens Female predominance
Anatomy	Unilateral or bilateral May involve external nose, nasal cartilages, nasal septum, maxillary alveolar ridges, and dental anomalies	Soft palate and/or hard palate Midline of posterior palate May involve nostril and absence of nasal septal development (communication with oral and nasal cavity)
Management	Surgical repair at approximately 2-3 months Early use of orthodontics Nasal alveolar molding	Surgical repair for isolated CP between 6 and 12 months; infants with CL/CP between 9 and 15 months
Short-term problems (before surgical repair)	Feeding and weight gain	Feeding efficiency; growth failure
Special postoperative care	Suture line protection and care Position on right side or upright in infant seat; avoid prone positioning to protect suture line Special feeding—slow-flow nipple, plastic squeezable bottle, syringe feeding—until suture line heals Care of suture line in postoperative period with massage (after 2-3 weeks) and tape	Feeding cup, syringe feeding, Special Needs Feeder, Pigeon bottle, Cleft Palate Nurser; avoid spoon, fork (also tongue blade and other objects that could damage palatal suture line)
Long-term problems	Social acceptance (depends on success of repair) Dental or orthodontic if associated with cleft palate	Speech, otitis media, middle ear effusion, possible hearing loss, upper respiratory tract infections Orthodontic or dental Feeding Social acceptance (voice changes, facial appearance if with cleft lip)

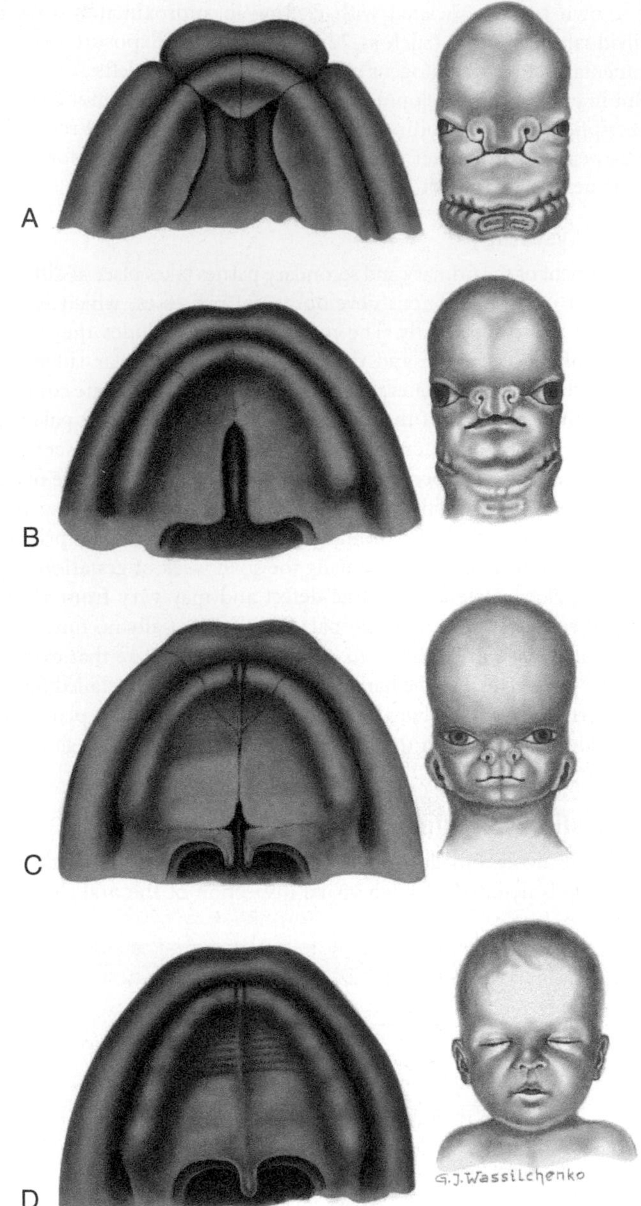

FIG. 8.5 **A–D,** Stages in palatine development. (See text for discussion.)

by palpating the hard palate and soft palate with a gloved finger. The degree of malformation of the CL or CP can then be evaluated (Figs. 8.6 and 8.7). The presence of a cleft palate likely affects feeding even though in most cases the infant's ability to swallow is normal. Poor feeding skills may be an indicator to further evaluate the palate in case a minor palatal defect was not readily detected at birth.

Therapeutic Management

Individuals with clefts should always be treated by a cleft/craniofacial multidisciplinary team, including plastic surgery, otolaryngology, orthodontics, speech-language pathology, pediatrics, nursing, audiology, social work, and psychology. Although the initial cleft lip and cleft palate are both repaired within the first year of life, treatment to repair the deformity may continue into early adulthood. Management of both defects is directed toward surgical closure of the cleft, prevention of complications, and facilitation of normal growth and development of the child.

Surgical Correction: Cleft Lip

Cleft lip repair typically occurs when the baby is between 2 and 3 months of age. Surgical correction is performed when the infant is free of any oral, respiratory, or systemic infection. There are numerous techniques to repair the cleft lip defect, including Millard, Tennison-Randall, and Fisher techniques. Some surgeons work closely with orthodontists and use nasal alveolar molding (NAM) or taping of the upper lip before surgical repair in order to bring the segments of the lip and alveolus into better alignment before the surgical repair, resulting in less tension on the lip repair following surgery and an improved esthetic outcome.

Improved surgical techniques have minimized deformity related to scar retraction, but optimum cosmetic results are difficult to obtain in severe defects. Lip, nose, and scar revisions may be required at a later age.

Surgical Correction: Cleft Palate

CP repair is typically completed between 6 and 12 months. Although early repair of the cleft palate may restrict skeletal growth of the midface, delaying palate repair after first words emerge may result in significant speech disorders. Children who are younger and less advanced in terms of speech development exhibit better articulation and resonance than those who have their palates repaired when they are older and exhibit more speech and language development. Common techniques used to repair the cleft palate include Veau-Wardill-Kilner V-Y pushback and Furlow double-opposing Z-plasty. Approximately 20% to 30% of patients with repaired cleft palate will exhibit features of velopharyngeal dysfunction such as audible nasal air emission and hypernasality; these features require additional surgery such as levator repositioning, Furlow palatoplasty, pharyngeal flap, sphincter pharyngoplasty, or posterior pharyngeal wall augmentation to improve velopharyngeal closure. Nasopharyngoscopy and/or videofluoroscopy should be used to determine which surgery is needed to enhance the function of the velopharynx. Speech pathologists work closely with the team's surgeon to ensure that speech therapy services are provided when the child exhibits speech production errors, and surgery is provided when the child exhibits ongoing velopharyngeal dysfunction that will not respond to therapy.

Long-Term Problems

The care of children with CL and CP often involves a team of specialists who meet periodically to examine the child and consult with one another and with the parents. Although the CL and CP are repaired within the first year of life, some children will require additional surgeries to refine the repairs. Many children with CP and/or CL have some degree of speech impairment that requires speech therapy or even further surgery to improve speech if the errors arise from a faulty mechanism. Rotated, missing, or malformed teeth, as well as differences in facial skeletal development, may require orthodontic and orthognathic intervention. Varying degrees of hearing loss throughout early childhood also place children with clefts at higher risk for speech and language delays.

Children with CL and CP may require additional surgeries to the lip, nose, and palate throughout childhood. Cleft lip and nose revisions may be needed to modify scars or improve symmetry. Additionally, the surgeon will likely perform an alveolar bone graft to repair the cleft defect in the alveolar ridge. If the child with CP exhibits velopharyngeal dysfunction following the initial repair, a secondary surgery for speech will need to be performed. Sometimes an appliance is fabricated to help obturate the velopharyngeal port. Finally, once the child has reached skeletal maturity, orthognathic surgery may be necessary to achieve appropriate alignment of the bony structures of the face and an optimal esthetic outcome.

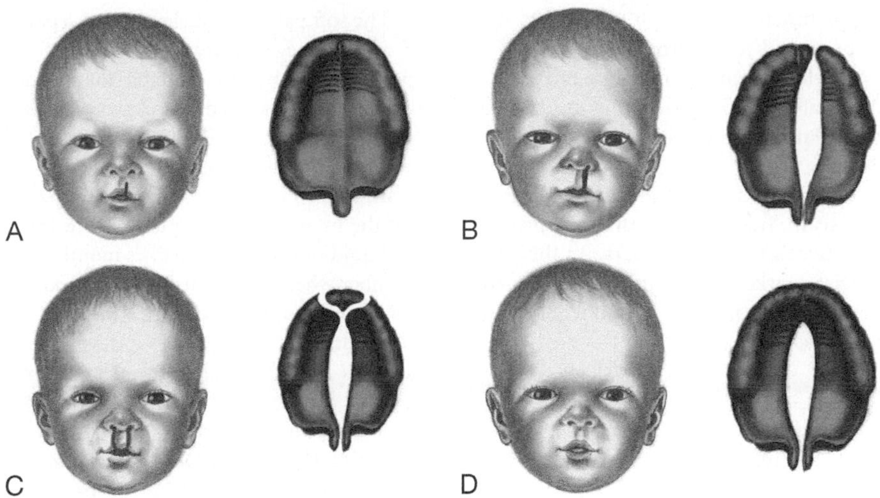

FIG. 8.6 Variations in clefts of lip and palate at birth. **A,** Notch in vermilion border. **B,** Unilateral cleft lip and cleft palate. **C,** Bilateral cleft lip and cleft palate. **D,** Cleft palate.

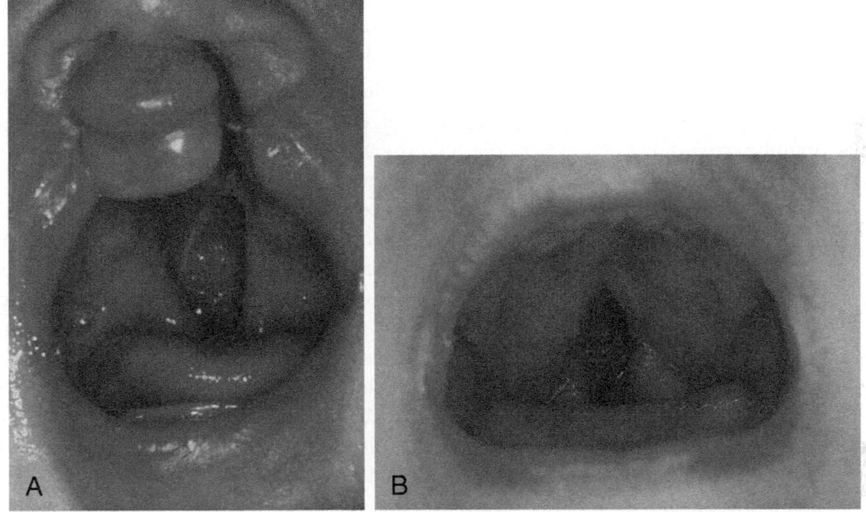

FIG. 8.7 A, Bilateral cleft lip with complete cleft palate. Cleft extends from soft to hard palate, exposing nasal cavity. **B,** Midline cleft of soft palate. (From Zitelli, B. J., & Davis, H. W. [2007]. *Atlas of pediatric physical diagnosis* [5th ed.]. St. Louis, MO: Mosby. *B,* Courtesy Barbara Elster, Cleft Palate Center, Pittsburgh.)

Improper drainage of the middle ear, as a result of inefficient function of the eustachian tube secondary to the CP, causes increased pressure in the middle ear and contributes to recurrent middle ear effusion or otitis media, which can lead to hearing impairment in some children with CP. The insertion of pressure-equalizing (PE) tubes by an otolaryngologist has become standard procedure in the child with CL/CP and is often performed at the same time as other surgical procedures (such as CP repair) to facilitate fluid drainage from the middle ear and prevent middle ear effusion and recurrent otitis media. Audiologists evaluate the child's hearing throughout early childhood and work closely with otolaryngologists to determine whether PE tubes are needed.

A child with a cleft will go through multiple phases of orthodontic intervention to align teeth and the maxillary arches. At some centers, NAM is fabricated by the orthodontist and used before surgical repair of the cleft lip. Children with clefts may then go through a period of active orthodontic treatment before the alveolar bone graft, at which time they may have maxillary expansion and limited orthodontics. Comprehensive orthodontic treatment of the permanent teeth is then accomplished in much the same manner as for children without clefts, except that children with clefts often have more dental anomalies such as missing teeth, extra teeth, malformed teeth, and more teeth out of alignment. Finally, orthognathic surgery to improve alignment of the mandible and maxilla may be completed once the child has reached skeletal maturity (often in the late teen years).

With isolated CL, minimal speech problems are anticipated. The child with CP usually requires the services of a speech-language pathologist at some point throughout childhood. A major problem for a child with CP may be "cleft palate" speech patterns. Features such as audible nasal air emission and hypernasality are addressed surgically. However, children with repaired CP and/or CL may exhibit active errors relating to velopharyngeal dysfunction or malocclusion. If the child exhibits velopharyngeal dysfunction while developing speech, the child may actively shift the place of articulation to a place lower in the vocal tract that allows him or her to produce a similar sound as the intended speech sound. These errors are often referred to as "compensatory" speech errors, and the errors will often require speech therapy even after the velopharyngeal mechanism has been surgically corrected. Early intervention that involves the education of parents and the child is critical to ensuring appropriate speech development. In addition to errors relating to velopharyngeal function, children with clefts may exhibit distortions on sounds produced in the front of the mouth if teeth are misaligned or absent, as well as when the mandible and maxilla are not in proper alignment. Finally, hearing loss from middle ear infection or middle ear effusion is an additional impediment because of difficulty in interpreting sounds.

Psychosocial development of the child with CP and/or CL is an important consideration for the team. Initially, the team may provide assistance and support to the patient's family members. As the child grows, the psychologist or social worker monitors the emotional, behavioral, and educational development of the child and will provide intervention to the child or family as needed.

Nursing Care Management

The immediate nursing problems in the care of an infant with CL and CP deformities are related to feeding the infant and dealing with the parental reaction to the defect. Facial deformities are particularly disturbing to parents. CL, especially, is a disfiguring, visible defect that may generate a strong negative response in parents. During the initial phase after birth of an infant with CL or CP, it is important for the nurse to address not only the infant's physical needs but also the parents' emotional needs.

The nurse should encourage expression of parental grief and fears. Such expression may promote attachment in the preoperative period. It is especially important to emphasize the positive aspects of the infant's physical appearance and to express optimism regarding surgical correction while acknowledging the parents' concern.

Feeding

Feeding the newborn with CL/CP can be a challenge, and teaching the parent to successfully feed the child is perhaps one of the most significant and challenging nursing roles. Growth failure in these infants has been attributed to feeding difficulties; however, with appropriate modifications to positioning, infants with nonsyndromic CP and/or CL should be able to feed successfully by mouth. Mothers should be encouraged to provide the protective benefits of breastmilk. These infants may require lactation and nutritional counseling and evaluation. Weekly weight checks at the practitioner's office assist in monitoring the infant's weight preoperatively.

Infants with an isolated cleft lip may have difficulty achieving an adequate anterior lip seal (Gailey, 2016). The infant with an isolated CL can often breastfeed without difficulty, as the breast tissue is able to conform to the cleft. If bottle-fed, systems that have a wider base, such as a NUK (orthodontic) nipple or a Playtex nurser, may allow the baby with a CL to feed more successfully. Finally, cheek support (i.e., squeezing the cheeks together to decrease the width of the cleft) may also help the infant achieve an adequate anterior lip seal during feeding.

Although infants with isolated CL are typically able to breastfeed without difficulty, breastfeeding can be a more difficult process for infants with an unrepaired CP. Infant feeding requires compression and suction. An infant with CP has difficulty creating adequate suction to extract breast milk directly from the breast or a standard bottle. Modified bottles or specialized feeding systems are needed. Accepting that she may not be able to breastfeed can be difficult for a new mother. However, La Leche League International and the Cleft Palate Foundation recommend that a mother of a child with a cleft should be encouraged to try the following strategies:

- She should pump her breast milk and provide the milk with an adapted bottle made for children with clefts.
- Skin-to-skin contact should be encouraged.
- After bottle-feeding, the infant may be put to the mother's breast for nonnutritive sucking.

The soft palate must elevate and separate the oral and nasal cavities to achieve negative intraoral pressure and achieve suction. Several specialized bottles are available that do not require suction, including the Special Needs Feeder (formerly Haberman bottle), Pigeon, and the Mead-Johnson Cleft Palate Nurser (Gailey, 2016). The Special Needs Feeder and the Pigeon bottles use a one-way flow valve that allows the infant to feed by compressing the nipple chamber between the tongue and the intact palatal segments. With the one-way flow valve in place, the liquid flows into the baby's mouth rather than back into the bottle chamber when the nipple is compressed. The Special Needs Feeder also has a long nipple chamber that can be compressed by the feeder for additional support. It comes in regular and mini nipple sizes, and also has a slit-cut tip, which the feeder can rotate within the baby's mouth to allow for increased or decreased flow of liquid. The Pigeon bottle has a wide, bulbous nipple and Y-cut tip, which allows for a faster flow of liquid. The Special Needs Feeder and the Pigeon bottle allow the infant to develop relatively independent feeding skills using these bottles. The third modified bottle, the Mead-Johnson Cleft Palate Nurser, is a squeezable bottle with a long, thin X-cut nipple; this bottle requires the feeder to compress the bottle in coordination with the infant's suck-swallow-breathe pattern throughout the feeding.

Regardless of the type of nipple used, the person doing the feeding should resist the temptation to remove the nipple because of the noise the infant makes or because of fear that the infant will choke. Infants with clefts do tend to be "noisy feeders" because they swallow excessive amounts of air throughout the feeding due to their inability to separate the nose and mouth. These infants should be burped following every ounce of liquid, or two to three times during a feeding. Additionally, they often have some degree of liquid that enters the nasal cavity during the feed, which may alarm the feeder who is not used to feeding babies with clefts. An indication that the infant needs to stop feeding momentarily is the facial signal, which involves elevated eyebrows, a wrinkled forehead, or watery eyes; the nipple may be gently removed to allow the infant to swallow milk in the mouth without getting upset.

Mothers will need immediate access to a lactation specialist before discharge from the hospital to assist with positioning and management of milk supply (Reilly, Reid, Skeat, et al., 2013). Regardless of the feeding method used, the mother will need ongoing support from the health care team before and after discharge from the hospital.

Preoperative Care

In preparation for the surgical repair, instruct the parents to accustom the infant to some of the needs of the early postoperative period. Some craniofacial surgery teams encourage the transition to cup-feeding before CP surgery, and this feeding method is used postoperatively as well. Alternative methods, such as syringe-feeding, should be introduced several days before surgery. Preoperative preparation, including medication, is determined by the surgeon and anesthesiologist.

Postoperative Care: Cleft Lip

The major efforts in the postoperative period are directed toward protecting the operative site. Avoid the prone position to prevent suture damage. After CL repair (cheiloplasty), some surgeons allow the infant to return to breastfeeding or bottle-feeding, whereas others require syringe-feeding once the child is awake and alert. CL repair may be performed on an outpatient basis, or the child may stay in the hospital overnight for monitoring.

Careful supervision of the child is recommended to ensure that the suture line is not damaged by an object or fingers entering the mouth. Pain management should continue in the home setting, and parents are taught how to administer the appropriate dosage of analgesic. A thin layer of antibiotic ointment may be prescribed for application to the suture line for 3 days, followed by application of petroleum jelly for several weeks. Parents should be taught how to properly clean the sutures by using water or diluted hydrogen peroxide. Inflammation or infection interferes with optimum healing and the ultimate cosmetic effect of the surgical repair.

! NURSING ALERT

Avoid the use of suction or objects in the mouth such as tongue depressors, thermometers, spoons, or straws.

The infant should be positioned to prevent airway obstruction by secretions, blood, or the tongue. Gentle aspiration of mouth and nasopharyngeal secretions may be necessary to prevent aspiration and respiratory complications. Because of vascularity of the lip and palate, postoperative care involves monitoring operative sites for bleeding. Excessive swallowing may be a sign of bleeding and swallowing blood.

Postoperative Care: Cleft Palate

Postoperative care varies according to surgeon's preference. The child should be closely observed postoperatively for signs of airway obstruction, hemorrhage, and laryngeal spasm. A face mask is often used to deliver oxygen. A tongue stitch may be used to prevent the tongue from obstructing the airway; it is taped to the cheek and may be removed per surgeon's preference. Observe the child's vital signs and oxygen saturation for potential airway compromise. Signs of stridor, croup, or difficulty breathing and/or swallowing should be carefully evaluated. The child with a CP repair may be placed on clear liquids for 24 hours followed by a liquid diet for 2 weeks. A soft diet may be encouraged for a full 6 weeks following palate repair. Acceptable feeding devices include open cup for liquids, but rigid utensils such as spoons, straws, or hard-tipped sippy cups should not be used to avoid accidental injury to the repair.

Elbow restraints can keep the hands away from the mouth, and the parents should maintain this precaution at home until the palate is healed. However, studies have demonstrated no statistically significant benefit to the use of arm restraints in children having cleft lip and palate surgery (Huth, Petersen, Lehman, et al., 2013). Evidence-based information should be provided to parents so that they can make informed decisions related to the care of their child.

Assess the infant for pain postoperatively. Opiates may be prescribed for the first 24 to 48 hours, or longer if needed, and acetaminophen may be given thereafter.

Preparation for Discharge and Home Care

Parents should participate in the infant's care as soon as possible after surgery. They should learn the feeding method recommended by the team's surgeon. Parents should also know how to cleanse the suture line to free any crust that might form and to replace elbow restraints (if used). Carefully evaluate and discuss car seat restraint appropriate to the infant's condition with the parents before discharge. Also discuss the infant sleep position based on the infant's condition and the American Academy of Pediatrics recommendation for supine sleeping in infants. (See Chapter 10.)

Long-Term Family Guidance

Individuals with clefts are followed well into their teenage years by the cleft/craniofacial team. Team members work together to ensure that care is delivered in a coordinated manner between surgeons, orthodontic/dental intervention, and therapy services. Agencies that provide services and information for children with CL/CP and their families include the American Cleft Palate-Craniofacial Association,* the Cleft Palate Foundation,† the March of Dimes‡ (http://www.marchforbabies.org), and various state and local agencies.

DERMATOLOGIC PROBLEMS IN THE NEWBORN

ERYTHEMA TOXICUM NEONATORUM

Erythema toxicum neonatorum, also known as *flea bite dermatitis* or *newborn rash,* is a benign, self-limiting eruption that usually appears within the first 2 days of life. The 1- to 3-mm lesions are firm, pale yellow or white papules or pustules on an erythematous base that resemble flea bites. Erythema toxicum may appear as one or two isolated lesions or as multiple lesions; the rash commonly disappears from one location and reappears elsewhere hours later. The rash appears most commonly on the face, proximal extremities, trunk, and buttocks, but it may be located anywhere on the body except the palms and soles. The rash may be more obvious during crying episodes. There are no systemic manifestations, and successive crops of lesions heal without pigmentation changes. The rash usually lasts approximately 5 to 7 days.

The cause is unknown. However, a smear of the pustule shows numerous eosinophils and a relative absence of neutrophils. Obtain bacterial, fungal, or viral cultures when the diagnosis is questionable. Although no treatment is necessary, parents are usually concerned about the rash and need to be reassured of the benign and transient nature.

CANDIDIASIS

Candidiasis, also known as moniliasis, is not uncommon in the newborn. *Candida albicans,* the organism usually responsible, may cause disease in any organ system. It is a yeast-like fungus (produces yeast cells and spores) that can be acquired from a maternal vaginal infection during delivery; by person-to-person transmission (especially from poor hand-washing technique); or from contaminated hands, bottles, nipples, or other articles. Mucocutaneous, cutaneous, and disseminated candidiasis are observed in this age-group. It is usually a benign disorder in the neonate and is often confined to the oral and diaper regions. (See Diaper Dermatitis, Chapter 11.)

ORAL CANDIDIASIS

Oral candidiasis (thrush) is characterized by white adherent patches on the tongue, palate, and inner aspects of the cheeks (Fig. 8.8). Oral candidiasis can be distinguished from coagulated milk when attempts to remove the patches with a tongue blade are unsuccessful. The infant may refuse to suck or may feed poorly because of pain in the mouth. This condition tends to be acute in the newborn and chronic in older infants and young children. Thrush appears when the oral flora is altered as a result of antibiotic therapy or poor hand washing by the infant's caregiver. Although the condition is usually self-limiting, spontaneous resolution may take as long as 2 months, during which time lesions may spread to the larynx, trachea, bronchi, and lungs and along the gastrointestinal tract.

---

*1504 E. Franklin St., Suite 102, Chapel Hill, NC 27514-2820; 919-933-9044; email: info@acpa-cpf.org; http://www.acpa-cpf.org.

†1504 E. Franklin St., Suite 102, Chapel Hill, NC 27514-2820; 800-242-5338; http://www.cleftline.org.

‡1275 Mamaroneck Ave., White Plains, NY 10605; 914-997-4488, http://www.marchofdimes.com. In Canada, http://www.marchofdimes.ca.

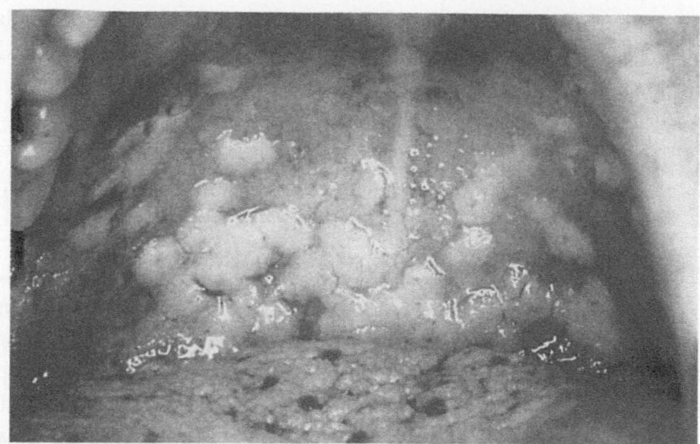

FIG. 8.8 Oral candidiasis (thrush). (Courtesy of J.A. Innes. In Goering, R. A., Dockrell, H. A., Zuckerman, M. Chiodini, P. L., Roitt, I. M. [2013]. Mims' medical microbiology [5th ed.]. Philadelphia: Saunders.)

Oral candidiasis in the newborn is treated with good hygiene and application of a fungicide. The source of infection, usually the mother, should be treated to prevent reinfection. Topical application of 1 ml of nystatin (Mycostatin) over the surfaces of the oral cavity four times a day or every 6 hours is usually sufficient to prevent spread of the disease or prolongation of its course. Oral fluconazole is an alternative for the infant with esophageal and gastrointestinal candidiasis and for the breastfeeding mother. To prevent relapse, therapy should be continued for at least 2 weeks after the lesions disappear (Lawrence & Lawrence, 2015). Gentian violet solution may be used in addition to one of the antifungal drugs in chronic cases of oral thrush; however, gentian violet does not treat gastrointestinal *Candida* organisms and may irritate the oral mucosa. Preterm infants are at risk for developing a systemic infection, which can be fatal; treatment is described elsewhere in this text.

Nursing Care Management

Direct nursing care toward preventing spread of the infection and correct application of the prescribed topical medication. For candidiasis in the diaper area, teach the caregiver to keep the diaper area clean and dry. Medication should be applied to the affected areas as prescribed. (See Diaper Dermatitis, Chapter 11.) Older infants can introduce *Candida* organisms into their mouths with hands contaminated by contact with diaper dermatitis.

In cases of oral thrush, administer nystatin after feedings. Distribute the medication over the surface of the oral mucosa and tongue with an applicator or syringe; the remainder of the dose is deposited in the mouth to be swallowed by the infant to treat any gastrointestinal lesions. In addition to good hygienic care, other measures to control thrush include rinsing the infant's mouth with plain water after each feeding before applying the medication and boiling reusable nipples and bottles for at least 20 minutes after a thorough washing (spores are heat resistant). Boil pacifiers for at least 20 minutes once daily, and treat the nipples of breastfeeding mothers to prevent reinfection. If the mother is breastfeeding, simultaneous treatment of the infant and mother is recommended if either is infected (Lawrence & Lawrence, 2015).

HERPES SIMPLEX VIRUS

Neonatal herpes is one of the most serious viral infections in the newborn, with a mortality rate of up to 60% in infants with disseminated disease. The disease may be classified according to the following types: (1) skin, eye, and mouth; (2) localized central nervous system (CNS) disease; or (3) disseminated infection involving multiple sites such as the lungs, liver, adrenal glands, CNS, skin, eyes, and mouth. Approximately 86% to 90% of herpes simplex virus (HSV) transmission occurs during delivery. The rash appears as vesicles or pustules on an erythematous base. Clusters of lesions are common. The lesions ulcerate and crust over rapidly. Fetal scalp monitoring sites are commonly the primary site of infection. The risk of infection during vaginal birth in the presence of genital herpes is estimated to be 25% to 60% with active primary infection at term (American Academy of Pediatrics, 2015). Infants born to mothers with a recurrent case of HSV are less likely to contract the virus (Kimberlin, Baley, & American Academy of Pediatrics, 2013).

Most infants with neonatal herpes eventually develop this characteristic rash, but many neonates with disseminated disease do not develop a skin rash (Wang, Wohrley, & Rosebush, 2017). Because signs and symptoms resemble those of bacterial sepsis, close assessment is extremely important. Ophthalmologic clinical findings include chorioretinitis and microphthalmia; neurologic involvement such as microcephaly and encephalomalacia may also develop (Wang, Wohrley, & Rosebush, 2017). Disseminated infections may involve virtually every organ system, but the liver, adrenal glands, and lungs are most commonly affected. In HSV meningitis infants develop multiple lesions of cortical hemorrhagic necrosis. It can occur alone or with oral, eye, or skin lesions. The presenting symptoms, which may occur in the second to fourth week of life, include lethargy, poor feeding, irritability, and local or generalized seizures.

Infants with CNS and disseminated disease have a much higher mortality rate than those initially seen with skin, eye, or mouth disease. Neonatal HSV may be difficult to detect in the early newborn period, and nonspecific signs such as irritability, fever, poor feeding, or lethargy may be seen. When the diagnosis is delayed, mortality rates may be high even with antiviral therapy, and long-term irreversible complications such as seizures, blindness, and psychomotor and learning delays are not uncommon.

Nursing Care Management

Neonates with herpes virus or suspected infection (as a result of exposure) should be carefully evaluated for clinical manifestations. The absence of skin lesions in the neonate exposed to maternal herpes virus does not indicate absence of disease. Implement Contact Precautions (in addition to Standard Precautions) according to American Academy of Pediatrics and American College of Obstetricians and Gynecologists (2012) guidelines or hospital protocol. It is recommended that swabs of the mouth, nasopharynx, conjunctivae, rectum, and any skin vesicles be obtained from the exposed neonate. In addition, obtain urine, stool, blood, and cerebrospinal fluid specimens for culture. Antiviral therapy with acyclovir is initiated if the cultures are positive or if there is strong suspicion of herpes infection (American Academy of Pediatrics, 2015). An algorithm for the evaluation and treatment of asymptomatic infants born to women with active genital herpes lesions has been published (Kimberlin, Baley, & American Academy of Pediatrics, 2013).

Early recognition and treatment with antiviral therapy are essential elements to the prevention of serious and often fatal complications. Closely evaluate infants who are seen in the first 5 or 6 weeks of life with the nonspecific signs of poor feeding, lethargy, fever, and irritability, with or without the characteristic rash.

BULLOUS IMPETIGO

Bullous impetigo is an infectious superficial skin condition most often caused by various strains of *Staphylococcus aureus.* Bullous vesicular lesions erupt on previously untraumatized or intact skin. The lesions may appear on any surface of the body and sometimes become widespread, but the usual distribution involves the buttocks, perineum, trunk, face, and extremities. The neonatal form may appear first in the diaper region

(Shulman, 2016). They vary in size from a few millimeters to several centimeters, contain turbid fluid, and are easily ruptured (Shulman, 2016). The bullae normally rupture in 1 or 2 days, leaving a superficial red, moist, denuded area with little crusting. In some cases the condition may be mistaken for thermal injury or *staphylococcal scalded skin syndrome* (SSSS). Bullous impetigo lesions develop on intact skin, whereas lesions of SSSS spread systemically from an original infection site. There is no cutaneous sensitivity with bullous impetigo, and the Gram stain and blister cultures are positive for staphylococci.

Treatment usually involves the administration of oral antibiotics and topical application of mupirocin (Bactroban). Systemic treatment with erythromycin may be required if the lesions are near the mouth or in the event of abscess formation. Recovery is usually rapid and uneventful.

Nursing Care Management

Once the diagnosis is suspected, the infant is isolated until therapy is instituted to prevent spread of the infection to other infants. Persons who have come in contact with the infant are investigated to determine a possible source of the infecting organism. Scrutinize other infants who have mutual contacts for early detection of any infection. Instruct parents and other visitors regarding precautions for the prevention of infection, especially through hand washing and Standard Precautions. (See Infection Control, Chapter 6.)

To prevent older infants from scratching the lesions, the arms may need to be confined by using elbow restraints, by pulling the undershirt sleeves over the hands and securing the openings with tape, or by applying mittens. If restraints of any kind are used, the infant is allowed freedom of movement at supervised times. Rocking, cuddling, and holding during feeding are essential components of care.

BIRTHMARKS

Discolorations of the skin are common findings in the newborn infant. (See discussion on skin assessment under Physical Assessment, Chapter 4.) Most, such as mongolian spots or nevus simplex, involve no therapy other than reassuring parents of the benign nature of these discolorations. However, some can be the manifestation of a disease that suggests further examination of the child and other family members (e.g., multiple flat, light-brown café-au-lait spots often characterize the autosomal dominant hereditary disorder neurofibromatosis and are common findings in Albright syndrome).

Darker or more extensive lesions demand further inspection. Excision of the lesion may be recommended for biopsy. Such lesions include the reddish-brown solitary nodule that appears on the face or upper arm and usually represents a spindle and epithelioid cell nevus (juvenile melanoma); a giant pigmented nevus (bathing trunk nevus), a dark-brown to black irregular plaque that is at risk of transformation to malignant melanoma; and the dark-brown or black macules that become more numerous with age (junctional or compound nevi).

Vascular birthmarks may be divided into vascular malformations and vascular tumors (hemangiomas). Experts now recommend labeling vascular tumors as **hemangiomas of infancy** or **infantile hemangiomas** to differentiate them from other vascular tumors and malformations. A vascular tumor often mislabeled as a hemangioma is a congenital hemangioma; this differs from an infantile hemangioma in that the former is fully formed at birth and may or may not involute over time, whereas the infantile hemangioma typically grows after birth. Hemangiomas may be further classified as localized (sometimes labeled focal), segmental, or multifocal (sometimes labeled indeterminate) (Chen, Eichenfield, & Friedlander, 2013; Labreze, Harper, & Hoeger, 2017). Localized superficial infantile hemangiomas tend to appear early in infancy and spontaneously resolve without therapy within several years, whereas the segmental variety is more likely to cause complications such as ulceration and vital organ compromise and to involve developmental defects. Multifocal hemangiomas are less likely to be associated with the complications seen with the segmental variety (Chen, Eichenfield, & Friedlander, 2013).

Vascular stains (malformations) are permanent lesions that are present at birth and are initially flat and erythematous. Any vascular structure—capillary, vein, artery, or lymphatic—may be involved. The two most common vascular stains are port-wine stains (nevus flammeus) and transient macular stains (nevus simplex) such as the stork bite or salmon patch, usually located on the glabella or nape of the neck. Port-wine lesions are pink, red, or, rarely, purple stains of the skin that thicken, darken, and proportionately enlarge as the child grows (Fig. 8.9, *A*).

Port-wine stains may also be associated with structural malformations, such as glaucoma or leptomeningeal angiomatosis (i.e., tumor of blood or lymph vessels in the pia arachnoid, or Sturge-Weber syndrome) or bony or muscular overgrowth (Klippel-Trénaunay-Weber syndrome). Monitor children with port-wine stains on the eyelids, forehead, cheeks, or extremities for these syndromes with periodic ophthalmologic examination, neurologic imaging, and measurement of extremities.

The treatment of choice for port-wine stains is the pulsed-dye laser. A series of treatments is usually needed (see Atraumatic Care box). The treatments can significantly lighten or completely clear the lesions with almost no scarring or pigment change. Other treatments for port-wine stains include the use of intense pulsed light, epidermal cooling, and combination treatments (Chen, Ghasri, & Aguilar, 2012).

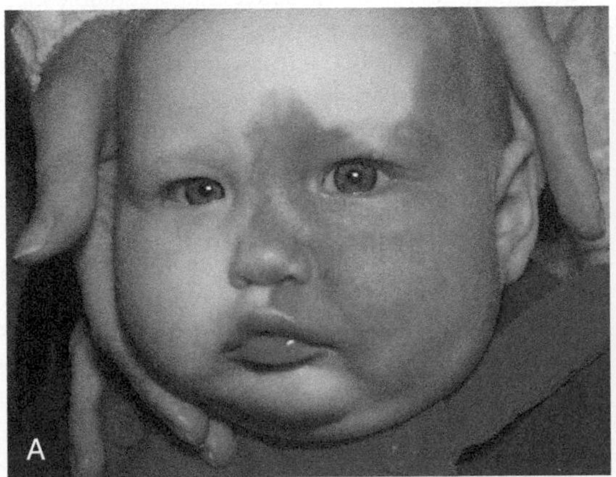

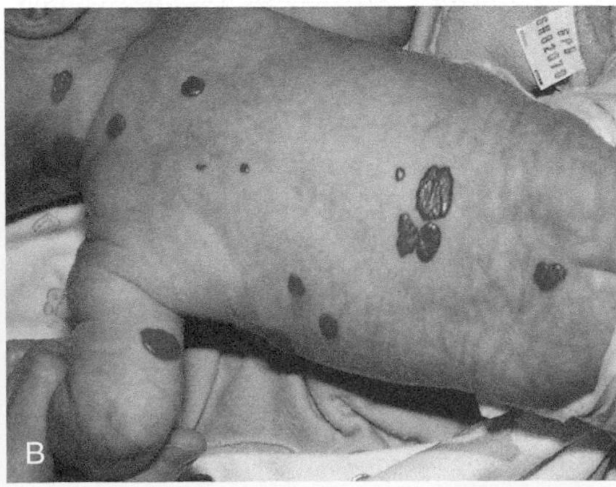

FIG. 8.9 A, Port-wine stain. **B,** Strawberry hemangioma. (From Zitelli, B. J., & Davis, H. W. [2002]. *Atlas of pediatric physical diagnosis* [4th ed.]. St. Louis, MO: Mosby.)

ATRAUMATIC CARE

Laser Therapy

The laser pulse feels like the sharp snap of a rubber band on the skin, and each treatment may involve from 15 to 100 pulses. Therefore children should be given a general anesthetic, sedation, or a topical anesthetic.

Infantile hemangiomas, also sometimes referred to as strawberry or capillary hemangiomas, are benign cutaneous tumors that involve only capillaries. These are often not apparent at birth but may appear within a few weeks as an erythematous patch, enlarge considerably during the first year of life, and then begin to involute spontaneously. It may take 5 to 9 years for complete resolution. Many patients may be left with residual findings such as telangiectasia, redundant fatty tissue, or skin atrophy (Martin, 2016). These hemangiomas are bright red, rubbery nodules with a rough surface and a well-defined margin (Fig. 8.9, *B*).

Cavernous venous hemangiomas involve deeper vessels in the dermis and have a bluish-red color and poorly defined margins. These latter forms may be associated with the trapping of platelets (Kasabach-Merritt syndrome) and subsequent thrombocytopenia.

Hemangiomas may also occur as part of the PHACE syndrome:

P—Posterior fossa brain malformation
H—Hemangiomas (segmental cervicofacial)
A—Arterial anomalies
C—Cardiac defects, including coarctation of the aorta
E—Eye anomalies

PHACE syndrome hemangiomas occur predominantly in females, term infants, singleton births, and infants of normal birth weight; in addition, PHACE syndrome hemangiomas are primarily large, segmental facial hemangiomas (Labreze, Harper, & Hoeger, 2017).

This neurocutaneous syndrome is diagnosed by the presence of a facial hemangioma in addition to either one or several of the other associated conditions; clinical outcomes vary according to the organs involved.

Although many localized superficial hemangiomas require no treatment because of their high rate of spontaneous involution, some vision and airway obstruction may necessitate therapy. Infants with a beard-distribution hemangioma often have airway involvement and must be closely evaluated for airway compromise (Hartzell & Buckmiller, 2012). Ulceration is a common complication, especially when the hemangioma is perineal or perioral. This may result in pain, bleeding, infection, and scarring. The pulsed-dye laser can effectively reduce some hemangiomas; systemic prednisone administered for 2 to 3 weeks or longer may also deter further growth. Optional treatments may include interferon alfa, imiquimod, propanolol, vincristine, bleomycin, cyclophosphamide, becaplermin, debulking surgery, and no treatment but simple observation (Hartzell & Buckmiller, 2012; Martin, 2016). Propanolol is reported to be the first-line treatment for hemangiomas, but the U.S. Food and Drug Administration has not approved it for the treatment of hemangiomas, so it is considered an experimental treatment (Drolet, Frommelt, Chamlin, et al., 2013; Hartzell & Buckmiller, 2012).

Nursing Care Management

Birthmarks, especially those on the face, are upsetting to parents. Families need an explanation of the type of lesion, its significance, and possible treatment.*

*Information is available from Birthmarks and Hemangiomas InterNETwork Support Group, http://members.tripod.com/~Michelle_G/SPTGP.html; and Vascular Birthmarks Foundation, 877-VBF-4646; http://www.birthmark.org.

Parents can benefit from seeing photographs of other infants before and after treatment for port-wine stains or after the passage of time for hemangiomas. Pictures taken to follow the involution process may further help parents gain confidence that progress is taking place.

If laser therapy is performed, the lesion will have a purplish-black appearance for 7 to 10 days, after which the blackness will fade and give way to redness with an eventual lightening of the treated area. During the treatment phase, caution parents to avoid any trauma to the lesion or picking at the scab. Trim the infant's fingernails as an added precaution. Washing the area gently with water and dabbing it dry are adequate, although in some cases a topical antibiotic ointment may be used. Do not give any salicylates during the treatment phase because they decrease the effects of the therapy. Keep the infant out of the sun for several weeks and then protected with a sunscreen of at least sun protection factor 15. Complications associated with laser treatment include possible secondary infection, keloid or pyogenic granuloma formation, localized dermatitis, and hyperpigmentation or hypopigmentation.

PROBLEMS RELATED TO PHYSIOLOGIC FACTORS

HYPERBILIRUBINEMIA

The term **hyperbilirubinemia** refers to an excessive level of accumulated bilirubin in the blood and is characterized by **jaundice**, or **icterus**, a yellowish discoloration of the skin and other organs. Hyperbilirubinemia is a common finding in the newborn and in most instances is relatively benign. However, in extreme cases, it can indicate a pathologic state.

Hyperbilirubinemia may result from increased unconjugated or conjugated bilirubin. The unconjugated form (Table 8.2) is the type most commonly seen in newborns. The following discussion of hyperbilirubinemia is limited to unconjugated hyperbilirubinemia.

Pathophysiology

Bilirubin is one of the breakdown products of hemoglobin that results from red blood cell (RBC) destruction. When RBCs are destroyed, the breakdown products are released into the circulation, where the hemoglobin splits into two fractions: heme and globin. The globin (protein) portion is used by the body, and the heme portion is converted to unconjugated bilirubin, an insoluble substance bound to albumin.

In the liver the bilirubin is detached from the albumin molecule and, in the presence of the enzyme glucuronyl transferase, is conjugated with glucuronic acid to produce a highly soluble substance, conjugated bilirubin glucuronide, which is then excreted into the bile. In the intestine, bacterial action reduces the conjugated bilirubin to urobilinogen, the pigment that gives stool its characteristic color. Most of the reduced bilirubin is excreted through the feces; a small amount is eliminated in the urine (Fig. 8.10).

Normally the body is able to maintain a balance between the destruction of RBCs and the use or excretion of by-products. However, when developmental limitations or a pathologic process interferes with this balance, bilirubin accumulates in the tissues to produce jaundice. Possible causes of hyperbilirubinemia in the newborn include the following:

- Physiologic (developmental) factors (e.g., prematurity)
- An association with breastfeeding or inadequate breast milk, especially unsuccessful breastfeeding and/or weight loss of 8% to 10% (Muchowski, 2014).
- Excess production of bilirubin (e.g., hemolytic disease, biochemical defects, bruises)

TABLE 8.2 **Comparison of Major Types of Unconjugated Hyperbilirubinemia***

Physiologic Jaundice	Breastfeeding-Associated Jaundice (Early Onset)	Breast Milk Jaundice (Late Onset)	Hemolytic Disease
Cause			
Immature hepatic function plus increased bilirubin load from red blood cell (RBC) hemolysis; enterohepatic shunting	Decreased milk intake related to fewer calories consumed by infant before mother's milk is well established; enterohepatic shunting; less frequent stooling	Possible factors in breast milk that prevent bilirubin conjugation Less frequent stooling	Blood antigen incompatibility causing hemolysis of large numbers of RBCs Functional inability of liver to conjugate and excrete excess bilirubin from hemolysis
Onset			
After 24 hours (preterm infants, prolonged)	3rd-4th day	4th day	During first 24 hours (levels increase ≥5 mg/dl/day)
Peak			
2nd-5th day, depending on ethnic origin, method of feeding	3rd-5th day	10th-15th day	Variable
Duration			
Declines on 5th-7th day	Variable	May remain jaundiced for 3-12 weeks or more	Depends on severity and treatment
Therapy			
Increase frequency of feedings and avoid supplements. Evaluate stooling pattern. Monitor transcutaneous bilirubin (TcB) or total serum bilirubin (TSB) level. Perform risk assessment (see Fig. 8.11). Use phototherapy if bilirubin levels increase significantly or significant hemolysis is present.	Breastfeed frequently (10-12 times/day); avoid supplements such as water, dextrose water, or formula. Evaluate stooling pattern; stimulate as needed. Perform risk assessment (see Fig. 8.11). Use phototherapy if bilirubin levels increase significantly or significant hemolysis is present. If phototherapy is instituted, evaluate benefits and harm of temporarily discontinuing breastfeeding; additional assessments may be required. Assist mother with maintaining milk supply; feed expressed milk as appropriate. After discharge, follow up according to age of infant at discharge and hour-specific nomogram bilirubin level at discharge (see p. 256).	Increase frequency of breastfeeding; use no supplementation such as glucose water; cessation of breastfeeding is not recommended. Perform risk assessment (see Fig. 8.11). Consider performing additional evaluations: glucose-6-phosphate dehydrogenase, direct and indirect serum bilirubin, family history, and others as necessary. May include home phototherapy with a temporary (10-12 hours) discontinuation of breastfeeding; a subsequent TSB may be drawn to evaluate a drop in serum levels (see text). Assist mother with maintenance of milk supply and reassurance regarding her milk supply and therapy. Use formula supplements only at practitioner's discretion.	Monitor TcB or TSB level. Perform risk assessment (see Fig. 8.11). Postnatal—Use phototherapy; administer tin-mesoporphyrin, administer intravenous immunoglobulin per protocol; if severe, perform exchange transfusion. Prenatal—Perform intrauterine transfusion (fetus). Prevent sensitization (Rh incompatibility) of Rh-negative mother with Rh immune globulin (RhIg) administration. If mother is breastfeeding, assist with maintenance and storage of milk; may bottle-feed expressed milk as appropriate to therapy. Minimize maternal-infant separation, and encourage contact as appropriate.

*Table depicts patterns of jaundice in term infants; patterns in preterm infants will vary according to factors such as gestational age, birth weight, and illness.

- Disturbed capacity of the liver to secrete conjugated bilirubin (e.g., enzyme deficiency, bile duct obstruction)
- Combined overproduction and underexcretion (increased hemolytic process)
- Some conditions or disease states (e.g., glucose-6-phosphate dehydrogenase [G6PD] deficiency, hypothyroidism, galactosemia, infant of a diabetic mother)
- Genetic predisposition to increased production (e.g., Native Americans, Asians)

The first two causes, physiologic factors and an association with breastfeeding, are discussed in the following sections; the third major cause, hemolytic disease, is presented on p. 259.

Complications

Unconjugated bilirubin is highly toxic to neurons; therefore an infant with severe hyperbilirubinemia is at risk of developing **bilirubin encephalopathy**, a term that describes early varying degrees of acute symptoms of bilirubin toxicity resulting from the deposition of unconjugated bilirubin in brain cells (Blackburn, 2013). **Kernicterus**, or **bilirubin-induced neurologic dysfunction**, describes the yellow staining of the brain cells and brain cell necrosis that results in chronic, permanent changes to the brain secondary to bilirubin deposition in the brain (Ambalavanan & Carlo, 2016; Blackburn, 2013). The damage occurs when the serum concentration reaches toxic levels, regardless of cause.

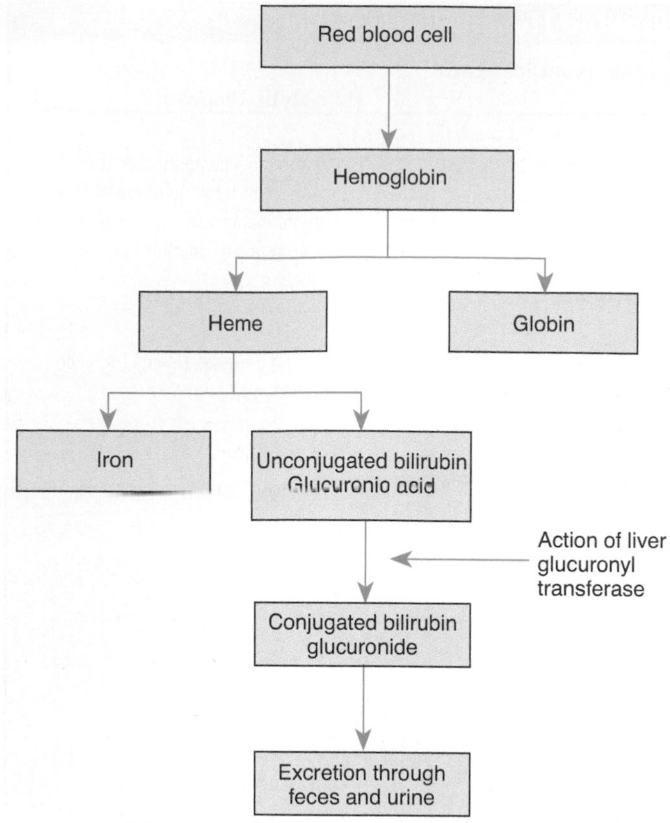

FIG. 8.10 Formation and excretion of bilirubin.

There is evidence that a fraction of unconjugated bilirubin crosses the blood-brain barrier in neonates with physiologic hyperbilirubinemia. When certain pathologic conditions exist in addition to elevated bilirubin levels, the infant has an increased permeability of the blood-brain barrier to unconjugated bilirubin and thus potential irreversible damage. The exact level of serum bilirubin required to cause damage is not yet known.

Multiple factors contribute to bilirubin neurotoxicity; therefore serum bilirubin levels alone do not predict the risk of CNS injury. Factors that enhance the development of bilirubin encephalopathy include acidosis, lowered serum albumin levels, intracranial infections such as meningitis, and abrupt fluctuations in blood pressure. In addition, any condition that increases the metabolic demands for oxygen or glucose (e.g., fetal distress, hypoxia, hypothermia, or hypoglycemia) also increases the risk of CNS damage despite lower serum levels of bilirubin. The administration of hypertonic solutions such as glucose and sodium bicarbonate in acutely ill infants, which causes a sudden rise in serum osmolality, has also been a contributing factor in the development of bilirubin encephalopathy.

The risk is increased in late-preterm infants, infants born preterm, male infants, inadequately breastfeeding infants, and those who are discharged early from the birth hospital without adequate follow-up (Blackburn, 2013). Late-preterm infants, especially those who are breastfed, may be at increased risk for hyperbilirubinemia and should be followed closely. Because of their immaturity, late-preterm infants are less alert, have less stamina, and have greater difficulty with latch, suck, and swallow than full-term infants (Boies & Vaucher, 2016). Proactive lactation management, strategies, support, and follow-up for late-preterm infants and some early term infants are important components that affect breastfeeding success (Boies & Vaucher, 2016).

The signs of bilirubin encephalopathy are those of CNS depression or excitation. Prodromal symptoms consist of decreased activity, increasing lethargy, irritability, poor feeding, hypotonia, high-pitched cry, and temperature instability, although some infants, particularly very low-birth-weight infants, may be asymptomatic. Later these subtle findings are followed by development of athetoid cerebral palsy, extrapyramidal symptoms, opisthotonos, dental enamel hyperplasia of the primary teeth, motor delay, seizures, and sensorineural hearing deficits (Blackburn, 2013). Long-term effects include evidence of neurologic damage, such as cognitive impairment, attention-deficit/hyperactivity disorder, delayed or abnormal motor movement (especially ataxia or athetosis), behavior disorders, perceptual problems, or sensorineural hearing loss.

Physiologic Jaundice

The most common evidence of hyperbilirubinemia is the relatively mild and self-limited physiologic jaundice, or icterus neonatorum. Unlike hemolytic disease of the newborn (HDN) (see p. 259), physiologic jaundice is not associated with any pathologic process. Although almost all newborns experience elevated serum bilirubin levels, only about half demonstrate observable signs of jaundice.

Two phases of physiologic jaundice have been identified in full-term infants. In the first phase, bilirubin levels of formula-fed Caucasian and African American infants gradually increase to approximately 5 to 6 mg/dl by 2 to 5 days of life, then decrease to a plateau of less than 3 mg/dl by the fifth day (Blackburn, 2013). Bilirubin levels maintain a steady plateau state in the second phase without increasing or decreasing until approximately 12 to 14 days, at which time levels decrease to the normal value of 1 mg/dl (Blackburn, 2013). In Asian American infants serum bilirubin levels peak by the fourth or fifth day of life at 10 to 14 mg/dl and gradually decrease to less than 3 mg/dl by 7 to 10 days of life (Blackburn, 2013). This pattern varies according to racial group, method of feeding (breast versus bottle), and gestational age. Breastfed term infants tend to have higher peak levels of serum bilirubin (7 to 14 mg/dl), and the plateau phase is reached later. In preterm formula-fed infants, serum bilirubin levels may peak as high as 10 to 12 mg/dl at approximately 5 days of life and decrease slowly over a period of 2 to 4 weeks (Blackburn, 2013) (see also Table 8.2).

As noted, infants of Asian descent (as well as Native Americans) have mean bilirubin levels almost twice those seen in Caucasians or African Americans. An increased incidence of hyperbilirubinemia occurs in newborns from certain geographic areas, particularly areas around Greece. These populations may have G6PD deficiency, which can cause acute hemolytic anemia. Hyperbilirubinemia also develops in a small number of newborns with Crigler-Najjar syndrome, an inherited disorder in which there is an absence of glucuronyl transferase. Infants with metabolic disorders such as galactosemia or hypothyroidism may also develop hyperbilirubinemia.

Mechanisms Involved in Physiologic Jaundice

On average, newborns produce twice as much bilirubin as do adults because of higher concentrations of circulating erythrocytes and a shorter life span of RBCs (only 70 to 90 days, in contrast to 120 days in older children and adults). In addition, the liver's ability to conjugate bilirubin is reduced because of limited production of glucuronyl transferase. Newborns also have a lower plasma-binding capacity for bilirubin because of lower albumin concentrations than older children. Normal changes in hepatic circulation following birth may contribute to excessive demands on liver function.

Normally, conjugated bilirubin is reduced to urobilinogen by the intestinal flora and excreted in feces. However, the relatively sterile and less motile newborn bowel is initially less effective in excreting urobilinogen. In the newborn intestine the enzyme β-glucuronidase is able to convert conjugated bilirubin into the unconjugated form, which is subsequently reabsorbed by the intestinal mucosa and transported to the liver. This process, known as enterohepatic circulation or enterohepatic shunting, is accentuated in the newborn and is believed to be a significant factor in physiologic jaundice (Blackburn, 2013). Feeding stimulates peristalsis and produces more rapid passage of meconium, thus diminishing the amount of reabsorption of unconjugated bilirubin, and introduces bacteria to aid in the reduction of bilirubin to urobilinogen. Colostrum, a natural cathartic, facilitates meconium evacuation.

Jaundice in Breastfeeding Infants

The American Academy of Pediatrics recommends exclusive breastfeeding for the first 6 months of life. Because breastfeeding can be associated with an increased incidence of jaundice, carefully monitoring of the infant while supporting and establishing successful breastfeeding is important (Chantry, Eglash, Labbok, et al., 2015). Two types of jaundice have been identified. Breastfeeding-associated jaundice (early-onset jaundice) may begin as early as 2 to 4 days of age. The jaundice is related to the process of breastfeeding and probably results from decreased caloric and fluid intake by breastfed infants before the milk supply is well established, because fasting is associated with decreased hepatic clearance of bilirubin. A decrease in milk (fluid) intake may result in decreased stooling, increased weight loss, and increased fatty acid formation, which may interfere indirectly with hepatic uptake of bilirubin and conjugation. Blackburn (2013) asserts, however, that breastfeeding-associated jaundice is most likely a result of enterohepatic shunting rather than an increase in new bilirubin formation or abnormal bilirubin conjugation. Supplemental fluids such as glucose water or water do not enhance bilirubin excretion and may delay the excretion process. The current philosophy is to encourage more frequent effective breastfeeding, and thus increase stooling, while monitoring the infant's bilirubin levels with transcutaneous monitoring or serum levels.

Breast milk jaundice (late-onset jaundice) begins around the fourth day. Rising levels of bilirubin peak during the second week and gradually diminish. Despite high levels of bilirubin that may persist for 3 to 12 weeks, these infants are well. The jaundice may be caused by factors in the breast milk (pregnanediol, fatty acids, and β-glucuronidase) that either inhibit the conjugation or decrease the excretion of bilirubin (see also Table 8.2).

Clinical Manifestations

The most obvious sign of hyperbilirubinemia is jaundice, the yellowish discoloration primarily of the sclera, nails, or skin. As a rule, jaundice that appears within the first 24 hours is caused by HDN, sepsis, or one of the maternally derived diseases such as diabetes mellitus or infections. Jaundice that appears on the second or third day, peaks on the third to fifth day, and declines on the fifth to seventh day is usually the result of physiologic jaundice; as noted earlier, this pattern may vary according to ethnic origin. The intensity of the jaundice is not always related to the degree of hyperbilirubinemia; therefore transcutaneous screening or serum bilirubin levels are necessary.

Diagnostic Evaluation

Total serum bilirubin is measured to determine the degree of hyperbilirubinemia. Normal values of unconjugated bilirubin are 0.2 to 1.4 mg/dl. In the newborn, levels must exceed 5 mg/dl before jaundice (icterus) is observable. However, evaluation of jaundice is not based solely on serum bilirubin levels, but also on the timing of the appearance of clinical jaundice; gestational age at birth; age in days since birth; family history, including maternal Rh factor; evidence of hemolysis; feeding method; infant's physiologic status; and progression of serial serum bilirubin levels. The following risk factors are associated with pathologic hyperbilirubinemia in term and late-preterm infants; further investigation is warranted as to the cause, although the exact cause may remain undetermined (Ambalavanan & Carlo, 2016; Blackburn, 2013):

- Appearance of clinical jaundice within 24 hours of birth
- Serum bilirubin level or transcutaneous bilirubin in the high-risk zone of the hour-specific nomogram (Fig. 8.11)

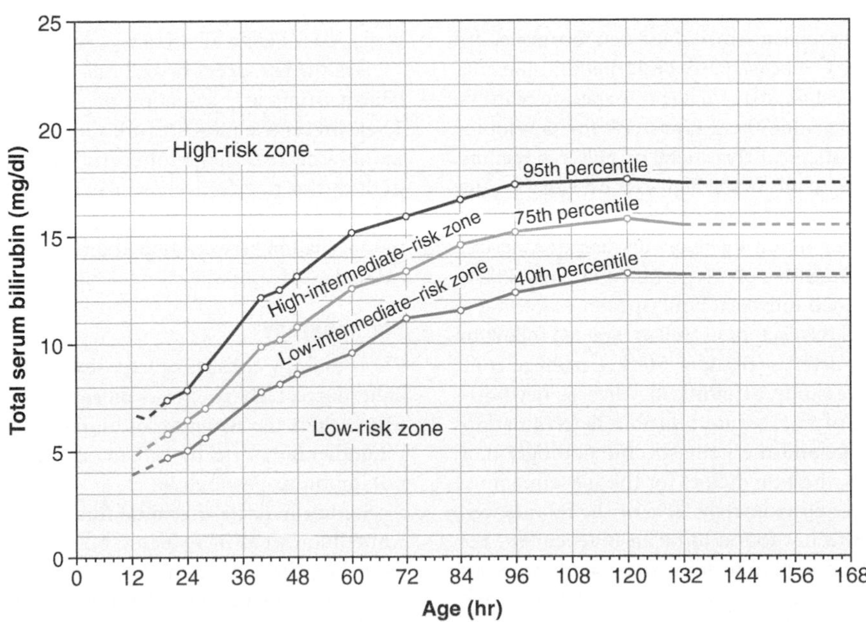

FIG. 8.11 A, Nomogram for designation of risk in 2840 well newborns at 36 or more weeks of gestational age with birth weight of 2000 g (4.4 lb) or more, or 35 or more weeks of gestational age and birth weight of 2500 g (5.5 lb) or more, based on the hour-specific serum bilirubin values. (This nomogram should not be used to represent the natural history of neonatal hyperbilirubinemia.) (*A,* From Bhutani, V. K., Johnson, L., & Sivieri, E. M. [1999]. Predictive ability of a predischarge hour-specific serum bilirubin for subsequent significant hyperbilirubinemia in healthy term and near-term newborns. *Pediatrics, 103*(1), 6-14.)

- Blood group incompatibility with a positive direct Coombs test
- Hereditary hemolytic disease such as G6PD deficiency
- Gestational age 35 to 36 weeks
- East Asian or Asian American race
- Cephalhematoma or significant bruising
- Exclusive breastfeeding, especially infants experiencing difficulty breastfeeding or significant weight loss
- History of sibling with hyperbilirubinemia

Noninvasive monitoring of bilirubin via cutaneous reflectance measurements (transcutaneous bilirubinometry [TcB]) allows for repetitive estimations of total serum bilirubin and, when used correctly, may decrease the need for invasive monitoring. With shorter maternity stays, the value of transcutaneous bilirubin measurements as a screening tool for evaluating the need for obtaining serum bilirubin levels or closely monitoring the infant has received considerable attention. Some TcB monitors provide accurate measurements within 2 to 3 mg/dl in most neonatal populations at serum levels below 15 mg/dl (American Academy of Pediatrics, Subcommittee on Hyperbilirubinemia, 2004). Regardless of the screening instrument chosen or the decision method used to treat, it is important to note that, to date, no transcutaneous bilirubin meter measures the total serum bilirubin level, and they must be used according to published guidelines as screening tools, not as predictors of need for therapy (Taylor, Burgos, Flaherman, et al., 2016). Multiple readings over time at a consistent site (e.g., sternum, forehead) are more valuable than a single reading. Once phototherapy has been initiated, TcB is no longer useful as a screening tool.

The use of hour-specific serum bilirubin levels to predict newborns at risk for rapidly rising levels is now considered the gold standard for monitoring healthy neonates more than 35 weeks of gestation before discharge from the hospital (American Academy of Pediatrics, Subcommittee on Hyperbilirubinemia, 2004). Using a nomogram (see Fig. 8.11, *A*) with three designated risk levels (high, intermediate, or low risk) of hour-specific total serum bilirubin values assists in determining which newborns might need further evaluation before and after discharge. Universal bilirubin screening based on hour-specific total serum bilirubin, performed possibly at the same time as other routine newborn metabolic screening (e.g., phenylketonuria, galactosemia), has been recommended (American Academy of Pediatrics, Subcommittee on Hyperbilirubinemia, 2004; Bhutani, Stark, Lazzeroni, et al., 2013). The hour-specific bilirubin risk nomogram is used to determine the infant's risk for developing hyperbilirubinemia requiring medical treatment or closer screening. Risk factors recognized to place infants in the high-risk category include gestational age of less than 38 weeks, breastfeeding, a sibling who had significant jaundice, and jaundice appearing before discharge (American Academy of Pediatrics, Subcommittee on Hyperbilirubinemia, 2004). Some experts have recommended universal hour-specific screening in combination with these clinical risk factors, as well as targeted follow-up to prevent further cases of kernicterus (Bhutani, Stark, Lazzeroni et al., 2013). A prospective multisite study of ethnically diverse newborns found that the combined use of total serum bilirubin determinations at 24 to 48 hours postnatal age and the hour-specific nomogram, as well as gestational age, were the best predictors for the subsequent use of phototherapy. In this study approximately 90% of the infants were breastfed, but breastfeeding was not found to be an independent risk factor for the development of hyperbilirubinemia (Bhutani, Stark, Lazzeroni et al., 2013).

It is also recommended that healthy late-preterm and term infants (≥35 weeks of gestation) receive follow-up care and assessment of bilirubin within 3 days of discharge, if discharged at less than 24 hours, and a risk assessment with the hour-specific nomogram; likewise, newborns discharged at 24 to 47.9 hours should receive follow-up evaluation within 4 days, and those discharged between 48 and 72 hours should receive follow up within 5 days (American Academy of Pediatrics, Subcommittee on Hyperbilirubinemia, 2004). The guidelines for monitoring and treating neonatal hyperbilirubinemia are published extensively elsewhere, and the reader is referred to the American Academy of Pediatrics, Subcommittee on Hyperbilirubinemia (2004) reference for an in-depth overview of management guidelines. Guidelines have also been published for the management of hyperbilirubinemia in preterm infants less than 35 weeks of gestation (Maisels, Watchko, Bhutani, et al., 2012).

Therapeutic Management

The primary goals in the treatment of hyperbilirubinemia are to prevent bilirubin encephalopathy and kernicterus, and, as in any blood group incompatibility, to reverse the hemolytic process (see p. 254). The main form of treatment involves the use of phototherapy. Exchange transfusion is generally used for reducing dangerously high bilirubin levels that occur with hemolytic disease.

The pharmacologic management of hyperbilirubinemia with phenobarbital has centered primarily on the infant with hemolytic disease and is most effective when given to the mother several days before delivery. Phenobarbital promotes hepatic glucuronyl transferase synthesis, which increases bilirubin conjugation and hepatic clearance of the pigment in bile, and protein synthesis, which may increase albumin for more bilirubin binding sites. However, the use of phenobarbital in either the antenatal or the postnatal period has not proved to be as effective as other treatments in reducing bilirubin. Bilirubin production in the newborn can be decreased by inhibiting heme oxygenase—an enzyme needed for heme breakdown (to biliverdin)—with metalloporphyrins, especially tin protoporphyrin and tin mesoporphyrin.

Intravenous immunoglobulin (IVIG) is effective in reducing bilirubin levels in infants with Rh isoimmunization and ABO incompatibility (Bratlid, Nakstad, & Hansen, 2011; Schwartz, Haberman, & Ruddy, 2011). Studies have shown a decrease in hospital stay and duration of phototherapy when IVIG is administered either as single-dose or two-dose regimens in neonates with hemolytic disease (Demirel, Akar, Celik, et al., 2011; Elalfy, Elbarbary, & Abaza, 2011).

Healthy late-preterm and full-term infants with jaundice may also benefit from early initiation of feedings and frequent breastfeeding. These preventive measures are aimed at promoting increased intestinal motility, decreased enterohepatic shunting, and normal bacterial flora in the bowel to effectively enhance the excretion of unconjugated bilirubin. Ensuring that breastfeeding is successful is the best way to mitigate the association between hyperbilirubinemia and exclusive breastfeeding (Maisels, 2015).

Phototherapy

Phototherapy consists of exposing the infant's skin to an appropriate light source. Light promotes bilirubin excretion by photoisomerization, which alters the structure of bilirubin to a soluble form (lumirubin). Phototherapy works by enhancing the excretion of bilirubin but does not inhibit its production.

Studies indicate that blue fluorescent light is more effective than white fluorescent in reducing bilirubin levels. However, because blue light alters the infant's coloration, the normal light of fluorescent bulbs in the spectrum of 420 to 460 nm is often preferred so the infant's skin can be better observed for color (e.g., jaundice, pallor, cyanosis) or other conditions. Increasing irradiance to the 460- to 490-nm band provides best results (Bhutani & American Academy of Pediatrics Committee on Fetus and Newborn, 2011). For phototherapy to be effective, the infant's skin must be fully exposed to an adequate amount of the light source. A diaper and boundary materials for postural support may be left in place; periodically turning the neonate under phototherapy has not been shown to accelerate bilirubin clearance (Stokowski, 2011). When serum bilirubin levels are rapidly increasing or approximating critical levels, intensive phototherapy is recommended. Intensive phototherapy with a higher irradiance is considered to be more effective than standard phototherapy for rapid reduction of serum bilirubin levels. The color of the infant's skin does not influence the efficacy of phototherapy. Best results occur within the first 4 to 6 hours of treatment (Bhutani & American Academy of Pediatrics Committee on Fetus and Newborn, 2011; Stokowski, 2011). Phototherapy alone is not effective in the management of hyperbilirubinemia when levels are at a critical level or are rising rapidly; it is designed primarily for the treatment of moderate hyperbilirubinemia. Available commercial phototherapy delivery systems are numerous and include halogen spotlights, light-emitting diodes, fluorescent tubes or bank lights, and fiberoptic mattresses (Stokowski, 2011).

The American Academy of Pediatrics, Subcommittee on Hyperbilirubinemia (2004) practice parameter guidelines provide suggestions for initiating phototherapy and for implementing exchange transfusion in infants 35 weeks of gestation or more. The initiation of phototherapy should always be based on individual clinical judgment rather than serum bilirubin levels alone.

Preterm infants are thought to have a higher risk of developing pathologic jaundice at lower serum bilirubin levels than healthy term infants because of associated illness factors that may increase the entry of bilirubin into the brain; however, research has failed to confirm this belief (Maisels, Watchko, & Bhutani, 2012). Prophylactic phototherapy is often used in preterm infants to prevent a significant increase in serum bilirubin levels (Maisels, Watchko, & Bhutani, 2012). A Cochrane study found that prophylactic phototherapy in such infants lowered serum bilirubin levels and reduced the rate of exchange transfusions, but the authors also concluded that further data are needed to determine the efficacy and safety of prophylactic phototherapy in preterm infants less than 37 weeks of gestation and weighing less than 2500 g (Okwundu, Okoramah, & Shah, 2012).

Phototherapy has not been found to cause long-term adverse effects. However, American Academy of Pediatrics guidelines noted that the following gaps in knowledge still remain: standardization of irradiance meters, improvements in device design, and lower-upper limits of light intensity for phototherapy units (Bhutani & American Academy of Pediatrics Committee on Fetus and Newborn, 2011). The effectiveness of treatment is determined by a decrease in total serum bilirubin levels. Concurrently, the infant's total physical status is assessed continually because the suppression of jaundice by phototherapy may mask signs of sepsis, hemolytic disease, or hepatitis.

Management of Breastfeeding Jaundice

Recommendations for prevention and management of early-onset jaundice in breastfed infants include encouraging frequent effective breastfeeding, preferably every 1.5 to 2 hours; avoiding glucose water, formula, and water supplementation; and monitoring for early stooling. The infant's weight, voiding, and stooling should be evaluated along with the breastfeeding pattern and the transfer of milk from the mother to the infant (Lawrence & Lawrence, 2015). Parents are taught to evaluate the number of voids and evidence of adequate breastfeeding after the infant is home. Notification of the primary care practitioner if there are indications the infant is not feeding well, is difficult to arouse for feedings, or is not voiding and stooling adequately is paramount to breastfeeding success.

Bilirubin levels are monitored in late-onset jaundice, and treatment options vary. It is not within the scope of this text to discuss the full spectrum of treatment possibilities; therefore consult other sources to ensure that breastfeeding is supported. Home phototherapy and continued breastfeeding are options for the family of a newborn with mild to moderate hyperbilirubinemia.

Prognosis

Early recognition and treatment of neonatal jaundice prevent unnecessary medical therapies, parent-infant separation, breastfeeding disruption and possibly failure, and bilirubin-induced neurologic dysfunction. Close follow-up after discharge home in infants with certain risk factors (e.g., exclusive breastfeeding, Asian ethnicity, gestational age less than 38 weeks, and increased hemolysis) for hyperbilirubinemia can minimize risks for a poor outcome. Phototherapy is a safe and effective method of decreasing serum bilirubin levels in newborns with mild to moderate hyperbilirubinemia.

Nursing Care Management

Part of the routine physical assessment includes observing for evidence of jaundice at regular intervals. Jaundice is most reliably assessed by observing the infant's skin color from head to toe and the color of the sclerae and mucous membranes. Applying direct pressure to the skin, especially over bony prominences such as the tip of the nose or the sternum, causes blanching and allows the yellow stain to be more pronounced. Also, bilirubin (especially at high levels) is not uniformly distributed in skin. The nurse should observe the infant in natural daylight for a true assessment of color.

The transcutaneous bilirubin meter is a useful screening device to detect neonatal jaundice in full-term infants. Because phototherapy reduces the accuracy of the instrument, its value is limited to assessments made before the initiation of phototherapy.

In many cases, jaundice may appear after discharge in the term and late-preterm infant. A careful history from the parents may reveal significant familial patterns of hyperbilirubinemia (e.g., older siblings of the infant). Other considerations in assessment include the family's ethnic origin (e.g., higher incidence in Asian infants), type of delivery (e.g., induction of labor), and infant characteristics such as significant weight loss after birth, gestational age, sex, and bruising. Assess the method and frequency of feeding, as well as the infant's apparent hydration status. In general, healthy term newborns under 1 week of age will have a number of voidings roughly equal to the number of days in age up to the fifth or sixth day, at which time adequate voiding is considered to be 6 to 10 times per day (e.g., day 2 = 2 voids, day 3 = 3 voids, etc.). Encourage parents to keep a log of number of feedings, wet diapers, and stools, especially if the mother is breastfeeding and this is her first newborn. Parents may indicate they cannot tell if the baby has voided because there is also stool in the diaper crotch; show the parents how to remove the diaper's outer plastic layer and observe the absorbent gel material granules for yellowish-green moisture that is an indication of urine. Another method is to place several cotton balls in the crotch of the diaper (inside) to verify voiding. The number of voids per day coincidentally increases when the mother transitions to mature milk.

Prevention of physiologic and breastfeeding jaundice may be possible with early introduction of feedings and frequent nursing without water supplementation. Make every effort to provide an optimum thermal environment to reduce metabolic needs.

QUALITY PATIENT OUTCOMES

Neonatal Hyperbilirubinemia

Total serum bilirubin level will be maintained below high-risk zone on the hour-specific bilirubin nomogram.

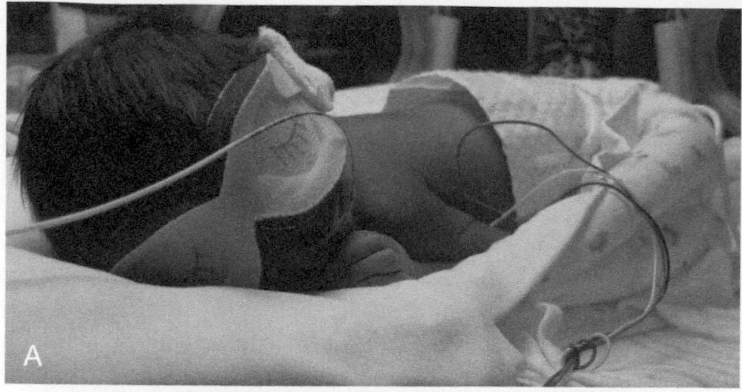

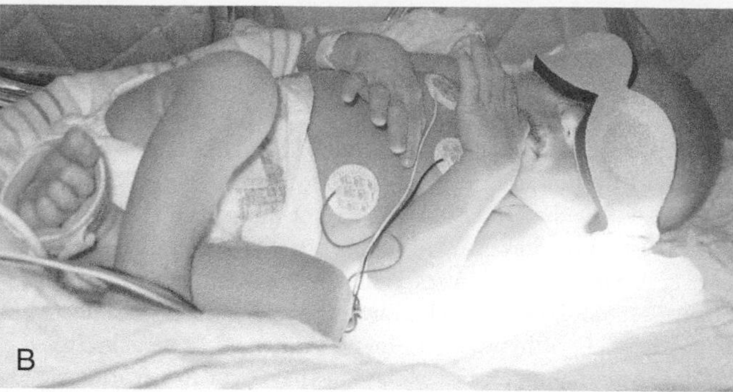

FIG. 8.12 A, Infant receiving phototherapy; note eye protection and nested boundaries for comfort. **B,** Newborn lying on phototherapy light source, which may be used with overhead lights to provide intensive phototherapy. (Courtesy E. Jacobs, Texas Children's Hospital, Houston.)

Phototherapy

The infant who receives phototherapy is placed under the light source, exposing as much skin surface as possible, and repositioned frequently to expose all body surface areas to the light. Once phototherapy has been initiated, frequent (every 6 to 12 hours) serum bilirubin levels are necessary because visual and transcutaneous assessments of jaundice are no longer considered valid.

The nurse should implement several precautions to protect the infant during phototherapy. An opaque mask shields the infant's eyes to prevent exposure to the light (Fig. 8.12). The eye shield should be properly sized and positioned to cover the eyes completely but prevent any occlusion of the nares. The infant's eyelids are closed before the mask is applied because the corneas may become excoriated if they come in contact with the dressing. The nurse checks the newborn's eyes at least every 4 to 6 hours for evidence of discharge, excessive pressure on the lids, or corneal irritation. Remove eye shields during feedings, which provide the opportunity for visual and sensory stimulation.

Monitor infants who are in an open crib receiving phototherapy for temperature instability because phototherapy may cause an increase in the body temperature. The distance between the phototherapy light source and the infant must be maintained as outlined by the manufacturer's guidelines; halogen lights placed too close to the infant's skin may cause burns (Stokowski, 2011). Maintaining the infant in a flexed position with rolled blankets along the sides of the body helps maintain heat and provides comfort.

Accurate charting is another important nursing responsibility and includes (1) times that phototherapy is started and stopped, (2) proper shielding of the eyes, (3) type of phototherapy unit (by manufacturer), (4) number of lamps, (5) distance between surface of lamps and infant, (6) use of phototherapy in combination with an incubator or open bassinet, (7) photometer measurement of light intensity (microwatts), and (8) observed side effects.

Side Effects of Phototherapy

Minor side effects for which the nurse should be alert include loose, greenish stools, transient skin rashes, mild hyperthermia, and increased metabolic rate. Dehydration and electrolyte disturbances, such as hypocalcemia, are uncommon, yet may occur. To prevent or minimize these effects, the nurse monitors the temperature to detect early signs of hypothermia or hyperthermia and observes the skin for evidence of dehydration and drying, which can lead to excoriation and breakdown. Oily lubricants or lotions are not used on the skin to prevent increased tanning. Full-term and late-preterm infants receiving phototherapy may require additional fluid volume or feedings to compensate for insensible and intestinal fluid loss. Because phototherapy enhances the excretion of unconjugated bilirubin through the bowel, loose stools may indicate accelerated bilirubin excretion. Frequent stooling can cause perianal irritation; therefore meticulous skin care, especially keeping the skin clean and dry, is essential.

Once phototherapy is permanently discontinued, there is often a subsequent increase in the serum bilirubin level, often called the "rebound effect." This is usually transient and resolves without resuming therapy.

Another reaction to phototherapy is the **bronze-baby syndrome**, in which the serum, urine, and skin turn grayish-brown several hours after the infant is placed under the light. This reaction is probably caused by retention of a bilirubin breakdown product of phototherapy, possibly copper porphyrin. The syndrome almost always occurs in infants who have elevated conjugated hyperbilirubinemia and some degree of cholestasis. The browning generally resolves after discontinuation of phototherapy.

Family Support

Parents need reassurance concerning their infant's progress. The nurse explains all the procedures to familiarize them with the benefits and risks. Reassure parents that the infant under the bilirubin light is warm and comfortable. Remove eye shields and turn off phototherapy when the parents are visiting to facilitate the attachment process. Also reassure parents that the neonate is accustomed to darkness after months of intrauterine existence and benefits a great deal from auditory and tactile stimulation (see Family-Centered Care box).

FAMILY-CENTERED CARE

Phototherapy and Parent-Infant Interaction

The traditional use of phototherapy has evoked concerns regarding a number of psychobehavioral issues, including parent-infant separation, potential social isolation, decreased sensorineural stimulation, altered biologic rhythms, altered feeding patterns, and activity changes. Parental anxiety is greatly increased, particularly at the sight of the newborn blindfolded and under special lights. The interruption of breastfeeding for phototherapy is a potential deterrent to successful maternal-infant attachment and interaction.

Because research has demonstrated that bilirubin catabolism occurs primarily within the first few hours of the initiation of phototherapy, there is increased support for the removal of the infant from treatment for feeding and holding. The benefits of stopping phototherapy for parental feeding and holding outweigh concerns related to the clearance of bilirubin in the healthy full-term newborn with mild to moderate hyperbilirubinemia. Home phototherapy offers an additional opportunity to foster parent-infant attachment.

The initiation of any treatment requires informed consent by the parents; however, in the case of phototherapy, parents may feel considerable anxiety when nurses use such words as "kernicterus" and "possible harm to the brain" to describe possible effects of hyperbilirubinemia. It is imperative that nurses remain sensitive to parents' feelings and information needs during this process. An important nursing intervention is the assessment of the parents' understanding of the treatment involved and clarification of the nature of the therapy.

One of the most important nursing interventions is recognition of breastfeeding jaundice. Historically, lack of familiarity among health professionals has caused many newborns prolonged hospitalization, termination of breastfeeding, and unnecessary phototherapy. Parents often receive contradictory information about jaundice. Care of the new mother includes supporting successful and frequent breastfeeding. Parents also need reassurance of the benign nature of the jaundice and encouragement to resume breastfeeding if temporary cessation is prescribed. Unfortunately, jaundice increases the risk of breastfeeding being discontinued and development of the vulnerable child syndrome—the parents' belief that their child has suffered a "close call" and is vulnerable to serious injury.

Discharge Planning and Home Care

With short hospital stays, mothers and infants may be discharged before evidence of jaundice is present. It is imperative that the nurse discuss signs of jaundice with the mother because any clinical symptoms will probably appear at home. Helping parents recognize risk factors and providing suggestions for further surveillance are important aspects of discharge planning. Teach parents to evaluate the number of voids and evidence of adequate breastfeeding once the infant is home, and encourage them to bring the newborn to the hospital, clinic, or primary care practitioner if there are problems related to elimination and feeding. Breastfeeding mother-infant dyads must receive appropriate guidance and assistance with breastfeeding to ensure the infant is receiving an adequate amount of breast milk and that stooling is occurring. A follow-up visit to the health care practitioner within 2 or 3 days after discharge to evaluate feeding and elimination patterns and jaundice is important in the posthospital care of the full-term newborn (see Diagnostic Evaluation, p. 255, for follow-up recommendations). Some infants may require follow up for serum bilirubin determination within 24 to 48 hours of discharge.

If home phototherapy is instituted, the hospital, durable medical equipment company representative, or home health care nurse is usually responsible for teaching family members and assessing their abilities to implement the treatment safely and in a timely manner. General guidelines for home care preparation and education are discussed in Chapters 7 and 22. Written instructions and supervision of care—especially the application of eye shields, if needed—are essential. The minor side effects of phototherapy are reviewed, and parents may need instruction in taking axillary temperatures and recording times and amounts of feedings and the number of wet diapers and stools. Infants on home phototherapy will often have serum levels drawn every 24 hours or more depending on individual risk factors, the serum bilirubin level on the hour-specific nomogram, and rising bilirubin levels.

Regardless of how benign the disorder or the therapy, parents need support and understanding. In jaundice associated with breastfeeding, follow-up blood studies are usually required to assess the progress of the jaundice. Nurses should take measures to help the mother achieve successful breastfeeding, including consultation with a lactation specialist on an outpatient basis. According to the American Academy of Pediatrics Subcommittee on Hyperbilirubinemia, for every newborn born at 35 or more weeks of gestation, health care providers should promote and support successful breastfeeding: nurses should advise mothers to nurse their infants at least 8 to 12 times per day for the first several days; the nurse should recommend against routine supplementation of nondehydrated breastfed infants with water or dextrose (sugar) water (Centers for Disease Control and Prevention, 2015).

HEMOLYTIC DISEASE OF THE NEWBORN

Hyperbilirubinemia in the first 24 hours of life is most often the result of hemolytic disease of the newborn (HDN), an abnormally rapid rate of RBC destruction. Anemia caused by this destruction stimulates the production of RBCs, which in turn provides increasing numbers of cells for hemolysis. Major causes of increased erythrocyte destruction are isoimmunization (primarily RhD) and ABO incompatibility.

Blood Incompatibility

The membranes of human blood cells contain a variety of antigens, also known as agglutinogens, substances capable of producing an immune response if recognized by the body as foreign. The reciprocal relationship between antigens on RBCs and antibodies in the plasma causes agglutination (clumping). In other words, antibodies in the plasma of one blood group (except the AB group, which contains no antibodies) produce agglutination when mixed with antigens of a different blood group. In the ABO blood group system the antibodies occur naturally. In the Rh system the person must be exposed to the Rh antigen before significant antibody formation takes place and causes a sensitivity response known as isoimmunization.

Rh Incompatibility (Isoimmunization)

The Rh blood group consists of several antigens (with D being the most prevalent). For simplicity, only the terms Rh positive (presence of antigen) and Rh negative (absence of antigen) are used in this discussion. (See Autosomal Inheritance Patterns, Chapter 3.) The presence or absence of the naturally occurring Rh factor determines the blood type.

Ordinarily, no problems are anticipated when the Rh blood types are the same in both mother and fetus or when the mother is Rh positive and the infant is Rh negative. Difficulty may arise when the mother is Rh negative and the infant is Rh positive. Although the maternal and fetal circulations are separate, there is evidence of a bidirectional trafficking of fetal RBCs and cell-free DNA to the maternal circulation (Moise, 2012). More commonly, however, fetal RBCs enter into the maternal circulation at the time of delivery. The mother's natural defense mechanism responds to these alien cells by producing anti-Rh antibodies.

Under normal circumstances, this process of isoimmunization has no effect on the fetus during the first pregnancy with an Rh-positive fetus because the initial sensitization to Rh antigens rarely occurs before the onset of labor. However, with the increased risk of fetal blood being transferred to the maternal circulation during placental separation, maternal antibody production is stimulated. During a subsequent pregnancy with an Rh-positive fetus, these previously formed maternal antibodies to Rh-positive blood cells enter the fetal circulation, where they attach to and destroy fetal erythrocytes (Fig. 8.13). Multiple gestations, abruptio placentae, placenta previa, manual removal of the placenta, and cesarean delivery increase the incidence of transplacental hemorrhage and subsequent isoimmunization.

Because the condition begins in utero, the fetus attempts to compensate for the progressive hemolysis by accelerating the rate of erythropoiesis. As a result, immature RBCs (erythroblasts) appear in the fetal circulation—hence the term erythroblastosis fetalis.

The development of maternal sensitization to Rh-positive antigens exhibits wide variability. Sensitization may occur during the first pregnancy if the woman previously received an Rh-positive blood

PATHOPHYSIOLOGY REVIEW

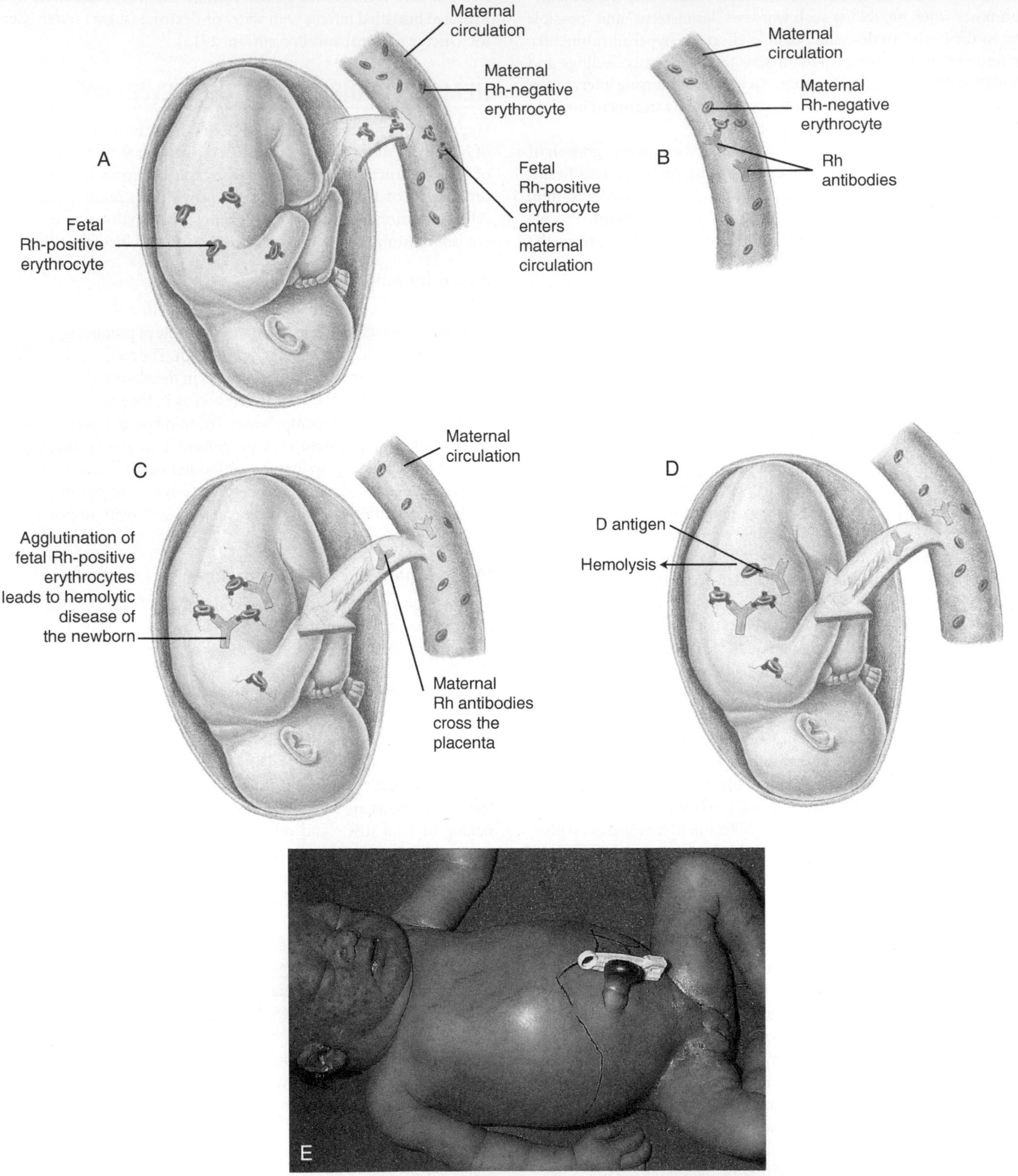

FIG. 8.13 Hemolytic disease of the newborn (HDN). **A,** Before or during delivery, Rh-positive erythrocytes from the fetus enter the blood of an Rh-negative woman through a tear in the placenta. **B,** The mother is sensitized to the Rh antigen and produces Rh antibodies. Because this usually happens after delivery, there is no effect on the fetus in the first pregnancy. **C,** During a subsequent pregnancy with an Rh-positive fetus, Rh-positive erythrocytes cross the placenta, enter the maternal circulation, and **(D)** stimulate the mother to produce antibodies against the Rh antigen. **E,** The Rh antibodies from the mother cross the placenta, causing agglutination and hemolysis of fetal erythrocytes, and HDN develops. (From McCance, K., & Huether, S. [2010]. *Pathophysiology: The biological basis for disease in adults and children* [6th ed.]. St. Louis, MO: Mosby.)

transfusion. No sensitization may occur in situations in which a strong placental barrier prevents transfer of fetal blood into the maternal circulation. Approximately 10% to 15% of sensitized mothers have no hemolytic reaction and no adverse effects on the fetus. In addition, some Rh-negative women, even though exposed to Rh-positive fetal blood, are immunologically unable to produce antibodies to the foreign antigen.

In the most severe form of erythroblastosis fetalis (**hydrops fetalis**), the progressive hemolysis causes fetal hypoxia; cardiac failure; generalized edema (anasarca); and fluid effusions into the pericardial, pleural, and peritoneal spaces (hydrops). The fetus may be delivered stillborn or in severe respiratory distress. Maternal Rh immunoglobulin (RhIg) administration, early intrauterine detection of fetal anemia by ultrasonography (i.e., serial Doppler assessment of the peak velocity in the fetal middle cerebral artery), and subsequent treatment by fetal blood transfusions or high-dose IVIG have dramatically improved the outcome of affected fetuses.

ABO Incompatibility

Hemolytic disease can also occur when the major blood group antigens of the fetus are different from those of the mother. The major blood groups are A, B, AB, and O. The incidence of these blood groups varies according to race and geographic location. In the North American Caucasian population, 46% have type O blood, 42% have type A blood, 9% have type B blood, and 3% have type AB blood.

The presence or absence of antibodies and antigens determines whether agglutination will occur. Antibodies in the plasma of one blood group (except the AB group, which contains no antibodies) will produce agglutination (clumping) when mixed with antigens of a different blood group. Naturally occurring antibodies in the recipient's blood cause agglutination of a donor's RBCs. The agglutinated donor cells become trapped in peripheral blood vessels, where they hemolyze releasing large amounts of bilirubin into the circulation.

The most common blood group incompatibility in the neonate is between a mother with O blood group and an infant with A or B blood group. Hemolysis due to anti-A is more common than for anti-B (see Table 8.3 for possible ABO incompatibilities). Naturally occurring anti-A or anti-B antibodies already present in the maternal circulation cross the placenta and attach to fetal RBCs, causing hemolysis. Unlike the Rh reaction, ABO incompatibility may occur in the first pregnancy. The risk of significant hemolysis in subsequent pregnancies is higher when the first pregnancy is complicated by ABO incompatibility.

Clinical Manifestations

Jaundice usually appears during the first 24 hours after birth, and serum levels of unconjugated bilirubin rise rapidly (see Table 8.2). Anemia results from the hemolysis of large numbers of erythrocytes, and hyperbilirubinemia and jaundice result from the liver's inability to conjugate and excrete the excess bilirubin. Most newborns with HDN are not jaundiced at birth. However, hepatosplenomegaly and varying degrees of hydrops may be evident. If the infant is severely affected, hydrops, anemia, and hypovolemic shock are apparent. Hypoglycemia may occur as a result of pancreatic cell hyperplasia.

TABLE 8.3 Potential Maternal-Fetal ABO Incompatibilities

Maternal Blood Group	Incompatible Fetal Blood Group
O	A or B
B	A or AB
A	B or AB

Diagnostic Evaluation

Early identification and diagnosis of Rh sensitization is important in the management and prevention of fetal complications. A maternal antibody titer (indirect Coombs test) should be drawn at the first prenatal visit. Genetic testing allows early identification of paternal zygosity at the Rh gene locus, thus allowing earlier detection of the potential for isoimmunization and avoiding further maternal or fetal testing (Hendrickson & Delaney, 2016).

Amniocentesis can be used to test the fetal blood type of a woman whose antibody screen is positive; the use of polymerase chain reaction may determine the fetal blood type, hemoglobin, hematocrit, and presence of maternal antibodies. Chorionic villus sampling has drawbacks that preclude its use, including possible spontaneous abortion of the fetus and fetomaternal hemorrhage. With either method the determination of an Rh-negative fetus requires no further treatment. The detection of cell-free fetal DNA in the maternal plasma of Rh-negative women to detect an Rh-positive fetus has been used successfully (Hendrickson & Delaney, 2016). Such testing usually negates the necessity for amniocentesis for fetal blood type (Moise & Argoti, 2012).

Ultrasonography is an important adjunct in the detection of isoimmunization. Alterations in the placenta, umbilical cord, and amniotic fluid volume, as well as the presence of fetal hydrops, can be detected with high-resolution ultrasonography, allowing early, noninvasive treatment before the development of erythroblastosis. Serial Doppler ultrasonography of fetal middle cerebral artery peak velocity is now the gold standard to detect and measure fetal hemoglobin and, subsequently, fetal anemia (Moise & Argoti, 2012). Erythroblastosis fetalis caused by Rh incompatibility can also be assessed by evaluating rising anti-Rh antibody titers in the maternal circulation (indirect Coombs test), or by testing the optical density of amniotic fluid (delta OD 450 test) because bilirubin discolors the fluid. The condition in the newborn is suspected on the basis of the timing and appearance of jaundice (see Table 8.2) and can be confirmed postnatally by detecting antibodies attached to the circulating erythrocytes of affected infants (direct Coombs test or direct antiglobulin test). The Coombs test may be performed on umbilical cord blood samples from infants born to Rh-negative mothers if there is a history of incompatibility or if further investigation is warranted.

Therapeutic Management

The primary aim of therapeutic management of isoimmunization is prevention. Postnatal therapy usually entails phototherapy for mild cases and exchange transfusion for more severe forms. In severe cases of hydrops, aggressive interventions such as pericardial and pleural fluid aspiration, mechanical ventilatory support, and inotrope therapy may be required for stabilization. Although phototherapy may control bilirubin levels in mild cases, the hemolytic process may continue, causing severe anemia (if untreated) between 7 and 21 days of life.

Prevention of Rh Isoimmunization

The administration of RhIg, a human gamma-globulin concentrate of anti-D, to all unsensitized Rh-negative mothers after delivery or abortion of an Rh-positive infant or fetus prevents the development of maternal sensitization to the Rh factor. The injected anti-Rh antibodies destroy (by subsequent phagocytosis and agglutination) fetal RBCs passing into the maternal circulation before the mother's immune system can recognize them. Because the immune response is blocked, anti-D antibodies and memory cells (which produce the primary and secondary immune responses, respectively) are not formed. The inhibition of memory cell formation is especially important because memory cells provide long-term immunity by initiating a rapid immune response once the antigen is reintroduced (McCance & Huether, 2014).

To be effective, RhIg (such as RhoGAM) must be administered to unsensitized mothers within 72 hours (but possibly as long as 3 to 4 weeks) after the first delivery, miscarriage, or abortion, and repeated after subsequent pregnancies. The administration of RhIg at 26 to 28 weeks of gestation further reduces the risk of Rh isoimmunization. RhIg is not effective against existing Rh-positive antibodies in the maternal circulation. RhIg is administered intramuscularly, not intravenously, and only to Rh-negative women with a negative Coombs test—never to the infant.

Studies have demonstrated the effectiveness of neonatal IVIG therapy at decreasing the severity of RBC destruction (hemolysis) in HDN and subsequent development of neonatal jaundice (Elalfy, Elbarbary, & Abaza, 2011). IVIG is believed to attack the maternal cells that destroy neonatal RBCs, slowing the progression of bilirubin production (Hendrickson & Delaney, 2016). This therapy, often used in conjunction with phototherapy, may decrease the necessity for exchange transfusion. Maternal administration of high-dose IVIG, alone or in combination with plasmapheresis, decreases the fetal effects of Rh isoimmunization (Hendrickson & Delaney, 2016). The use of a heme-oxygenase inhibitor such as tin mesoporphyrin (administered intramuscularly to the newborn) has proved effective in treating hyperbilirubinemia in newborns with hemolytic disease (Maisels & Yang, 2012).

Intrauterine Transfusion

Infants of mothers already sensitized may be treated by intrauterine transfusion, which consists of infusing blood into the umbilical vein of the fetus. The need for therapy is based on the antenatal diagnosis of fetal anemia by serial Doppler assessments of middle cerebral artery peak systolic velocity (Moise & Argoti, 2012). With the advance of ultrasound technology, fetal transfusion may be accomplished directly via the umbilical vein, infusing type O Rh-negative packed RBCs to raise the fetal hematocrit to 40% to 50%; fetal movement and transfusion risks are minimized by administering a drug such as vecuronium bromide for temporary fetal paralysis. The frequency of intrauterine transfusions may vary according to institution and fetal hydropic status, but one recommendation is in intervals of 10 days, 2 weeks, and then 3 weeks for subsequent procedures until the fetus reaches pulmonary maturity at approximately 37 to 38 weeks of gestation (Moise & Argoti, 2012). Intraperitoneal blood transfusions are used less commonly for isoimmunization because of higher associated fetal risks; however, they may be used when intravascular access is impossible.

Exchange Transfusion

Exchange transfusion, in which the infant's blood is removed in small amounts (usually 5 to 10 ml at a time) and replaced with compatible blood (Rh-negative blood), is a standard mode of therapy for treatment of severe hyperbilirubinemia that is unresponsive to phototherapy or other therapies such as tin-mesoporphyrin. However, there are reports that this procedure is less common with closer monitoring of rising bilirubin levels, maternal administration of RhIg, intensive phototherapy, and the use of prophylactic phototherapy in preterm infants (Maisels, Watchko, Bhutani, et al., 2012). Exchange transfusion removes the sensitized erythrocytes, lowers the serum bilirubin level to prevent bilirubin encephalopathy, corrects the anemia, and prevents cardiac failure. Indications for exchange transfusion include rapidly increasing serum bilirubin levels and hemolysis despite aggressive phototherapy. The criteria for exchange transfusion in preterm infants vary according to associated illness factors. The American Academy of Pediatrics, Subcommittee on Hyperbilirubinemia (2004) practice parameter guidelines provide suggestions for initiating phototherapy and exchange transfusion in infants 35 weeks of gestation or more. An infant born with hydrops fetalis or signs of cardiac failure is a candidate for immediate exchange transfusion with fresh whole blood.

For exchange transfusion, fresh whole blood is typed and cross-matched to the mother's serum. The amount of donor blood used is usually double the infant's blood volume, which is approximately 85 ml/kg body weight. The double-volume exchange transfusion replaces approximately 85% of the neonate's blood.

An exchange transfusion is a sterile surgical procedure. A catheter is inserted into the umbilical vein and threaded into the inferior vena cava. Depending on the infant's weight, 5 to 10 ml of blood is withdrawn within 15 to 20 seconds, and the same volume of donor blood is infused until the targeted volume (double the estimated blood volume) is reached.

ABO Incompatibility

The treatment for ABO hemolytic disease is early detection and implementation of phototherapy for the reduction of hyperbilirubinemia. The initial diagnosis is often more difficult because the direct Coombs test may be negative or weakly reactive. The presence of jaundice within the first 24 hours, elevated serum bilirubin levels, RBC spherocytosis, and increased erythrocyte production is diagnostic of ABO incompatibility. In some centers IVIG transfusions are used in combination with phototherapy to treat ABO incompatibility. Exchange transfusion is not commonly required for ABO incompatibility except when phototherapy fails to decrease bilirubin concentrations. As stated previously the neonatal administration of tin-mesoporphyrin may also serve to decrease the effects of hemolysis associated with ABO incompatibility.

Prognosis

The severe anemia of isoimmunization may result in stillbirth, shock, congestive heart failure, poor feeding, or poor weight gain. Complications from exchange transfusion are uncommon; however, close monitoring during the procedure is imperative.

Nursing Care Management

The initial nursing responsibility is recognizing the early onset of neonatal jaundice. The possibility of hemolytic disease can be anticipated from the prenatal and perinatal history. Prenatal evidence of incompatibility, maternal blood type O, and a positive Coombs test are cause for increased vigilance for early signs of jaundice in an infant.

The nursing care of the infant undergoing phototherapy has been described in detail earlier and is no different for infants with hyperbilirubinemia from hemolytic disease. If an exchange transfusion is required, the nurse prepares the infant and the family and assists the practitioner with the procedure. The infant must remain NPO ("nothing by mouth") during the procedure; therefore a peripheral infusion of dextrose and electrolytes is established. The nurse documents blood volumes exchanged, including the amount of blood withdrawn and infused; the time of each procedure; and the cumulative record of the total volume exchanged. The nurse also evaluates vital signs frequently (monitored electronically during the procedure) and correlates them with the removal and infusion of blood. If signs of cardiac or respiratory problems occur, the procedure is stopped temporarily and resumed once the infant's cardiorespiratory function stabilizes. The nurse also observes for signs of transfusion reaction (e.g., temperature instability, hypotension, tachycardia, bradycardia, rash) and maintains adequate neonatal thermoregulation, blood glucose levels, and fluid balance.

Family Support

Parents often feel guilty because they think they have caused the blood incompatibility. Parents should never be made to feel responsible or negligent. The nurse encourages them to express their thoughts. The nurse should praise parents for actions they took to prevent any problems, such as frequent antepartum examinations and blood tests.

HYPOGLYCEMIA

Neonatal hypoglycemia has many recognized causes; the following discussion primarily focuses on transient neonatal hypoglycemia.

Hypoglycemia is present when the newborn's blood glucose concentration is lower than the body's requirement for cellular energy and metabolism. However, the precise definition of hypoglycemia for every newborn in regard to gestational age, birth weight, metabolic needs, and illness or wellness state remains unknown. Because some infants experience metabolic complications at higher levels than previously thought, some researchers recommend that serum glucose levels be maintained above 45 mg/dl in infants with abnormal clinical symptoms (Gregory, 2016). Other researchers state the goal of the "golden hour," the first hour of the preterm newborn after birth, is to maintain a glucose value between 50 and 110 mg/dl (Sharma, 2016). Newborns most at risk for hypoglycemeia include those who are large or small for gestational age, infants of diabetic mothers, and those with intrauterine growth restriction (Sharma, Sharma, & Shastri, 2017).

Pathophysiology

After birth the infant must supply nutrients to meet energy requirements for maintaining body temperature, respiration, muscular activity, and regulation of blood glucose. Glucose comes primarily from glycogen stores deposited in the liver, heart, and skeletal muscles during the last trimester of pregnancy.

The brain is especially dependent on adequate glucose supply for appropriate function. Studies demonstrate that a majority of fetal and neonatal glucose produced is used by neuronal cells; a decreased availability of glucose predisposes both the fetal and neonatal brain to potential permanent damage (Tam, Haeusslein, Bonifacio, et al., 2012). There is evidence of a major shift in energy metabolism from glucose to carbohydrate in newborns during the first several hours of life—hence the importance of providing adequate energy substrate. Although newborns demonstrate the ability to use ketones and amino acids as energy substrate, there are certain limitations. Infants with severe hyperinsulinism are unable to compensate metabolically and require more glucose than normal. Conditions that decrease the availability of substrate or prevent appropriate metabolism of available substrate place the infant at risk for pathologic hypoglycemia. These include intrauterine growth restriction; preterm birth; gestational diabetes mellitus; maternal use of hypoglycemic drugs; maternal administration of tocolytics such as terbutaline and ritodrine; intrapartum administration of glucose; perinatal hypoxia; infection; hypothermia; polycythemia; fetal hydrops; inborn errors of metabolism (IEMs), such as galactosemia; certain congenital malformations; endocrine disorders; abnormal extrauterine transition; and failure to receive adequate perinatal nutrition.

Both transient neonatal hypoglycemia and recurrent hypoglycemia are based on conditions with decreased hepatic glucose production. Transient neonatal hypoglycemia is associated with intrapartum glucose administration, terbutaline administration, gestational diabetes mellitus, intrauterine growth restriction, perinatal stress or asphyxia, prematurity, cold stress, polycythemia, and large for gestational age. Recurrent hypoglycemia is observed in neonates with excessive insulin production or hyperinsulinism and includes infants with IEMs, Beckwith-Wiedmann syndrome, nesidioblastosis, Rh isoimmunization, and certain rare endocrine disorders (Sperling, 2016).

Clinical Manifestations

The signs of hypoglycemia are usually vague and often indistinguishable from those observed in other newborn conditions, such as hypocalcemia, septicemia, CNS disorders, or cardiorespiratory problems. Many newborns with hypoglycemia, however, are asymptomatic. Because the brain depends on glucose for energy, cerebral signs such as jitteriness, tremors, twitching, weak or high-pitched cry, lethargy, hypotonia, seizures, and coma are prominent. Other clinical manifestations are cyanosis, apnea, rapid and irregular respirations, sweating, eye rolling, and refusal to feed. The symptoms often are transient but recurrent.

Diagnostic Evaluation

Diagnosis is confirmed by direct analysis of blood glucose concentration. Two consecutive specimens of blood should be analyzed because of the many factors that can affect readings.

Bedside point-of-care blood glucose monitors in neonatal care must be accurate, rapid, and inexpensive; must demonstrate reliability with neonatal hematocrit ranges; must accept small blood volumes; and must provide reliable data for diagnosing neonatal hypoglycemia and hyperglycemia (Raizman, Shea, Daly, et al., 2016). Strict quality monitoring, regular calibration, and adherence to strict protocols are necessary to ensure accuracy.

The most accurate method is the laboratory analysis of serum glucose. Blood specimens may be obtained from heel, arterial, or venous punctures. (See Atraumatic Care box, p. 219 [Chapter 7].)

Proper handling of the specimen is essential because storage at room temperature increases glycolysis. Accurate readings can be facilitated by storing the blood sample on ice to slow cellular metabolism or by removing the RBCs through centrifugation.

Continuous glucose monitoring to measure interstitial glucose levels has been used in preterm and late-preterm infants (McKinlay, Alsweiler, Ansell, et al., 2015).

Therapeutic Management

Self-limiting or transient hypoglycemia is common in the first few hours following delivery. In healthy full-term infants who are borderline hypoglycemic and clinically asymptomatic, the early initiation of feeding (breast or formula) may reestablish normoglycemia. Most newborns compensate for this low blood glucose with "counterregulation" of endogenous fuel production through gluconeogenesis, glycogenolysis, and ketogenesis, collectively (Wight & Marinelli, 2014). Infants at risk for hypoglycemia should be monitored within the first 2 hours of life and monitoring should continue until acceptable, prefeed levels are obtained. Acceptable levels are defined as an infant with at least two consecutive satisfactory glucose measurements (Hawdon, 2014).

Oral glucose feedings have been used as a treatment for hypoglycemia in healthy newborns. However, formula and breast milk are probably more effective because of the carbohydrate content. Hypoglycemia is preventable in most instances by the initiation of early feeding in healthy, asymptomatic, term and late-preterm newborns. Breastfed infants should be put to breast as soon as possible after delivery. (See Infants of Diabetic Mothers, Chapter 9, for management of hypoglycemia related to transient hyperinsulinemia.)

The American Academy of Pediatrics (Adamkin, 2011) recommends that newborns be fed within an hour after birth and the blood glucose level checked 30 minutes after feeding. If the blood glucose level is less than 25 mg/dl, the newborn should be fed and checked again within the hour. If the blood glucose level remains under 25 mg/dl, the infant should receive intravenous glucose to maintain a glucose level from 25 to 40 mg/dl (Gregory, 2016). During the first 24 hours of life the newborn should be fed every 2 to 3 hours, with a blood glucose checked before each feeding, and the glucose level should be maintained at 45 to 50 mg/dl or above. The decision of when to treat the hypoglycemic newborn is not based on a single plasma glucose value, but on a number of clinical factors.

In 2015 the Pediatric Endocrine Society published new recommendations regarding the management of the hypoglycemic newborn (Thornton, Stanley, De Leon, et al., 2015). The main goals for the recommendations from this group were to help guide clinicians toward the target threshold plasma glucose concentration for treatment set at 50 mg/dl. This study also cited that neurogenic symptoms occur in newborns below the same glucose concentrations found in adults (55 to 54 mg/dl) and recommended that in certain patients an even higher glucose target threshold of 60 mg/dl should be implemented (Thornton, Stanley, De Leon, et al., 2015). The inconsistencies among these recommendations reflect the need for further research to help establish guidelines for therapeutic management of hypoglycemia of the newborn.

QUALITY PATIENT OUTCOMES

Neonatal Hypoglycemia

- No clinical evidence of hypoglycemia
- Receives adequate carbohydrate (milk) intake

Nursing Care Management

Although management strategies for infants with hypoglycemia remain unclear, the nursing responsibility involves identification of the problem through careful observation of physical status. Another concern is to reduce environmental factors, such as cold stress and respiratory distress, which predispose the infant to the development of a decreased blood glucose level. Infants who are at risk for hypoglycemia (late-preterm, infants of diabetic mothers/large for gestational age, term small for gestational age) should be carefully screened and observed for symptoms of hypoglycemia and other comorbidities often observed (e.g., respiratory distress syndrome, feeding intolerance) within the first several hours of life when glucose levels are known to fluctuate. An important nursing intervention is to assist the mother and infant in establishing successful breastfeeding.

An intravenous glucose infusion is required for infants with symptomatic hypoglycemia who are unable to tolerate oral feedings, infants who are unable to maintain adequate glucose levels with oral feedings, and infants with profound hypoglycemia. Major nursing objectives include preventing, anticipating, and recognizing potential dangers of concentrated dextrose infusion. Too-rapid infusion of the hypertonic solution can cause circulatory overload, hyperglycemia, glycosuria, and intracellular dehydration. Maintaining the ordered flow rate with an intravenous pump and checking and charting hourly intake decrease the chance of such problems.

Because hypoglycemia may be a symptom of some other underlying pathophysiologic process, parents are usually concerned about their infant's progress, particularly because these infants do not feed well or demonstrate behaviors that are typical of healthy infants. Nurses need to be aware of parents' thoughts, allow them to express their feelings, and update them on the infant's progress.

HYPERGLYCEMIA (TRANSIENT)

Hyperglycemia in the newborn is usually defined as a blood glucose concentration greater than 125 mg/dl in the full-term infant or greater than 150 mg/dl in the preterm infant. The condition in preterm infants is associated with increased morbidity and mortality, but the best treatment method to maintain euglycemia in preterm infants has not been defined (Alsweiler, Harding, & Bloomfield, 2013). Those affected are usually low-birth-weight infants, particularly those with weights less than 1000 g who are unable to tolerate intravenous glucose infusions at the usual rate. The glucose intolerance is probably related to general immaturity of the usual regulatory mechanisms. Increased blood glucose levels may also occur in infants with sepsis or decreased insulin sensitivity (such as infants with transient diabetes mellitus), infants receiving methylxanthines, and infants who are stressed (e.g., infants with respiratory distress syndrome, infants undergoing surgical procedures).

Hyperglycemia is usually asymptomatic but detected on routine screening. Most often, hyperglycemia is treated by reducing the infant's glucose intake. Untreated hyperglycemia may result in an osmotic diuresis with subsequent fluid volume loss and dehydration; if severe, it may result in an intraventricular hemorrhage as a result of fluid shifts in the CNS (Blackburn, 2013). Insulin infusion is sometimes administered to very low-birth-weight infants who require but are unable to tolerate intravenous dextrose.

Nursing Care Management

Monitor blood glucose frequently, especially in the infant receiving insulin. This requires numerous heel sticks, and sites should be rotated to minimize tissue damage. (See Blood Specimens, Chapter 22, and the Atraumatic Care box titled "Heel Punctures" in Chapter 7.) Closely monitor and measure the infant's urinary output to detect any evidence of glycosuria and possible osmotic diuresis.

Continuous glucose monitoring has the potential to decrease multiple heel sticks, to observe glycemic trends, and to promptly detect episodes of both hypoglycemia and hyperglycemia. The utilization of this technology in very low-birth-weight infants has been described in the literature and found to be safe and reliable (Tiberi, Cota, Barone, et al., 2016). However, studies with a larger population of preterm infants are needed to better establish safety, reliability, and the therapeutic application of continuous glucose monitoring.

As in the care of all infants, give parents a careful explanation of the therapy, provide frequent progress reports, and support them to reduce anxiety. (See Chapter 9.)

HYPOCALCEMIA

As with many conditions in the neonate, transient hypocalcemia is difficult to differentiate from other disorders (e.g., sepsis, meningitis, narcotic withdrawal, hypoglycemia), and the etiology may not be clear. The incidence is highest at two times during the neonatal period. *Early-onset hypocalcemia,* which appears within the first 24 to 48 hours, is the more common form and typically affects the preterm or small-for-gestational-age infant and any infant who has experienced perinatal asphyxia. Preterm infants may have hypocalcemia as a result of inadequate calcium intake, increased calcitonin levels, possibly resistance to parathyroid hormone activation preventing calcium removal from bones, acidosis, and decreased vitamin D intake and absorption (Blackburn, 2013). An infant born to a diabetic mother may also experience early hypocalcemia, possibly as a result of relative maternal hyperparathyroidism and transient neonatal hypoparathyroidism. Symptoms include jitteriness, prolonged QT interval, apnea, cyanotic episodes, a high-pitched cry, and abdominal distention.

Late-onset hypocalcemia, which is not apparent until after the first 3 or 4 days of life, is referred to as cow's milk–induced hypocalcemia or neonatal tetany. Although uncommon in developed countries, it may be observed in well-nourished infants who are fed modified cow's milk, such as evaporated milk formula. Cow's milk, which has a high phosphorus content, produces hyperphosphatemia and a resultant hypocalcemia by increasing calcium deposition in the bone and soft tissues. Late hypocalcemia may also be seen in infants with intestinal malabsorption, hyperinsulinemia, hypoparathyroidism, or hypomagnesemia. Maternal hyperparathyroidism and elevated maternal serum calcium levels may suppress fetal parathyroid gland function, resulting in a transient neonatal hypocalcemia that may not be apparent (tetany) until 3 or 4 weeks after birth, especially if the newborn is breastfeeding; the mother is usually asymptomatic (Doyle, 2016).

The manifestations of neonatal tetany reflect neuromuscular irritation: twitching; tremors; irritability; high-pitched cry; tachycardia; and, rarely, seizures (Blackburn, 2013). The preterm neonate with hypocalcemia may be asymptomatic. Neonatal tetany is rarely seen in industrialized countries because of the prevalent use of commercial formula or human milk as the newborn's primary source of nutrition.

In some preterm neonates, rickets and osteopenia may occur as a result of calcium or phosphorus deficiency in association with vitamin D deficiency, which prevents adequate intestinal absorption of minerals (Blackburn, 2013). Very low-birth-weight infants, infants with chronic conditions such as chronic lung disease (bronchopulmonary dysplasia), and infants on prolonged diuretic management are at particular risk for developing rickets and osteopenia (Blackburn, 2013). There have been reported cases of vitamin D deficiency in healthy breastfed infants who received minimal ultraviolet light exposure or whose breastfeeding mother had a diet deficient in vitamin D—hence the American Academy of Pediatrics' (2008) recommendation for vitamin D supplementation (400 IU/day, oral) in all newborns exclusively breastfed.

Diagnostic Evaluation

Diagnosis of hypocalcemia is confirmed with serum electrolyte determinations. Normal infant serum calcium values are usually in the range of 7.0 to 8.0 mg/dl (1.75 to 2.0 mmol/L) (Blackburn, 2013).

In full-term infants hypocalcemia is present at total serum calcium levels below 7.8 to 8 mg/dl (1.95 to 2.0 mmol/L) or ionized calcium levels (the biologically important fraction of calcium) below 3.0 to 4.4 mg/dl (1.1 mmol/L). In preterm infants a lower limit of 7.0 mg/dl (1.8 mmol/L) is considered hypocalcemic (Blackburn, 2013). Most clinicians consider the serum ionized calcium to be the best standard for monitoring blood calcium activity.

Therapeutic Management

In most instances early-onset hypocalcemia is transient and resolves in 1 to 3 days. Restoration of a normal calcium level is facilitated by early feedings, physiologic correction of hypoparathyroidism, and, sometimes, administration of calcium supplements.

Treatment of hypocalcemia involves intravenous administration of 10% calcium gluconate. The drug is administered slowly over 10 to 30 minutes or as a continuous infusion; intravenous administration should not exceed 100 mg/min (Tschudy & Arcara, 2012). Rapid intravenous calcium administration may cause cardiac dysrhythmias and circulatory collapse. The heart rate and blood pressure should be electronically monitored. Take care to ascertain that the infusion device is positioned within the vein because extravasation into surrounding tissue causes local necrosis, calcification, and sloughing. Intramuscular administration of calcium gluconate is contraindicated because it precipitates in the tissue, causing necrosis. If the infant can tolerate oral fluids, oral doses of calcium are given with formula. Adequate intake of vitamin D and phosphorus is imperative, especially in low-birth-weight infants. Exercise caution in the use of oral calcium salts because of their hypertonicity and subsequent effects on the bowel of at-risk infants.

Nursing Care Management

Nursing care of the infant with hypocalcemia is directed toward identifying infants at risk for early hypocalcemia, observing for clinical manifestations in such infants, and administering supplemental calcium, vitamin D, and phosphorus. Monitor the infant continuously during intravenous infusions. Calcium gluconate can cause tissue necrosis and scar formation; therefore it is recommended that superficial veins such as those on the scalp be avoided. To prevent tissue necrosis, carefully observe the infusion site and change it as needed. Calcium gluconate is also incompatible with a number of drugs, most notably sodium bicarbonate.

The nurse also observes for signs of acute hypercalcemia (e.g., vomiting, bradycardia). If such symptoms occur, discontinue the injection or infusion and notify the practitioner. Seizure precautions must be initiated immediately because seizures are common with acute hypercalcemia.

To prevent late-onset hypocalcemia, the nurse provides preventive care and anticipatory guidance regarding the correct use of an infant formula containing the appropriate balance of calcium and phosphorus and assists the parent in planning for meeting the growing infant's nutritional needs through an affordable commercial infant formula. If powder formula is used, ensure that the recommended amount of water is used to avoid inappropriate amounts of calcium and phosphorous ingestion.

If the infant is discharged on formula feedings supplemented with calcium, teach the parents the correct procedure for diluting the mineral in the formula and advise them to use only the prescribed formula. Also teach parents to observe for any signs of hypocalcemia or hypercalcemia in the infant receiving supplemental calcium.

HEMORRHAGIC DISEASE OF THE NEWBORN

Hemorrhagic disease of the newborn, or vitamin K–deficiency bleeding, is a bleeding disorder that occurs as a result of a vitamin K deficiency. Hemorrhagic disease may be classified according to appearance as early, classic, or late onset. Newborns' vitamin K stores are virtually absent, and prothrombin activity is moderately deficient, decreases until approximately 72 hours after birth, and then begins to increase. Consequently, vitamin K–dependent coagulation factors (e.g., II, VII, IX, X) are significantly reduced. In addition, the newborn's relatively sterile intestinal tract is unable to synthesize the vitamin until feedings have begun.

Signs and symptoms of early hemorrhagic disease typically appear within 1 to 2 days and can include oozing from the umbilicus or circumcision site, bloody or black stools, hematuria, ecchymoses on the skin and scalp, epistaxis, or bleeding from punctures. Early hemorrhagic disease may occur as late as 14 days after birth. Diagnosis is confirmed by findings of prolonged prothrombin time and partial thromboplastin time accompanied by normal platelet count and fibrinogen level. Factor VII levels may be low in early disease, and levels of undercarboxylated proteins (i.e., proteins induced by vitamin K absence, or PIVKA-II) are elevated with mild disease (Greenbaum, 2016).

Another form of hemorrhagic disease occurs in infants born to mothers who are taking the antiepileptic drugs phenytoin and phenobarbital, or warfarin drugs that cross the placenta and interfere with vitamin K function. The newborn may have a severe form of hemorrhagic disease and should be carefully evaluated and treated accordingly. The bleeding is most severe within the first 24 hours of life and may require treatment with intravenous vitamin K and fresh frozen plasma (Greenbaum, 2016).

A late form of hemorrhagic disease (late onset) appears at approximately 2 to 12 weeks of age. This form occurs in totally or predominantly breastfed infants who did not receive adequate vitamin K prophylaxis at birth. Although vitamin K levels in breast milk appear to be lower than in cow's milk–based formulas, previous studies indicate that hemorrhagic disease occurred in infants who were exclusively breastfed and who did not receive the standard prophylaxis at birth or were given a single dose of oral vitamin K (Lawrence & Lawrence, 2015). Manifestations of late-onset disease include evidence of intracranial hemorrhage; jaundice; failure to thrive; deep ecchymoses; and bleeding from the gastrointestinal tract, mucous membranes, skin punctures, or surgical incisions. Both the American Academy of Pediatrics and the World Health Organization recommend that vitamin K should be given to all newborns as a single, intramuscular dose (American Academy of Pediatrics, 2014; Tiberi, Cota, Barone, et al., 2016).

Therapeutic Management

The goal of management is prevention of hemorrhagic disease of the newborn with prophylactic administration of vitamin K. In the United States intramuscular administration of vitamin K (phytonadione [AquaMEPHYTON, Mephyton]) in a dose of 0.5 to 1 mg once during the first few hours after birth is standard practice. The current recommendation to prevent hemorrhagic disease in infants who are breastfed is to provide intramuscular vitamin K at birth and for the mother to have a well-balanced diet (American Academy of Pediatrics, 2014). The administration of oral vitamin K is currently not recommended to prevent neonatal hemorrhagic disease (Greenbaum, 2016).

In newborns with hemorrhagic disease, treatment is the same as the preventive measures except that the vitamin may be given intravenously to prevent a hematoma at an intramuscular site. Bleeding usually ceases within 2 to 4 hours of vitamin K administration.

Nursing Care Management

Nursing care primarily involves prevention through careful administration of the vitamin into the vastus lateralis or ventrogluteal (not dorsogluteal) muscle. In instances in which this procedure is not routinely carried out (e.g., home births or emergency deliveries), the nurse observes for signs of the bleeding disorder and notifies the practitioner for appropriate diagnosis and treatment. Mothers should be encouraged to consume a healthy, well-balanced diet. However, maternal dietary intake of vitamin K–enriched foods has very little impact on the vitamin K content of breast milk due to varying bioavaibility of the food source (Phillippi, Holley, Morad, et al., 2016).

PROBLEMS CAUSED BY PERINATAL ENVIRONMENTAL FACTORS

CHEMICAL AGENTS

Prenatal environmental effects from chemicals such as alcohol, medications, or drugs; infectious disease; or radiation or other environmental factors may be regarded as nongenetic causes of congenital anomalies because these substances can produce congenital structural, functional, or growth defects. An agent that produces congenital malformations or increases their incidence is called a teratogen.

The relationship of the fetal and maternal circulations allows for the interchange of chemical substances across the placental membrane. Many drugs have been suspected of producing congenital malformations, and some have been definitely implicated. Some of the most recognized teratogenic drugs include alcohol, tobacco, antiepileptic medications (valproic acid, phenytoin), isotretinoin (Accutane), lithium, methotrexate, cocaine, and diethylstilbestrol. (See Chapter 9, Drug-Exposed Infants and Fetal Alcohol Syndrome or Alcohol-Related Birth Defects.) The limited metabolic capabilities of the fetal liver and its immature enzyme and transport systems render the unborn child ill equipped for maintaining homeostasis when chemical disturbances are imposed by the mother or the environment. This includes both substances produced by the mother in response to a disease state (such as gestational diabetes mellitus) and exogenous substances ingested or inhaled by the mother. Neural tube defects (e.g., anencephaly, myelomeningocele) may be caused in part by folic acid deficiency, so appropriate supplementation before conception is imperative.

The teratogenic effect of drugs is not believed to affect developing tissue until day 15 of gestation, when tissue differentiation begins to take place. Before that time, drugs usually have little effect because they are believed to have an insignificant affinity for undifferentiated tissue. Also, until implantation takes place, at approximately 7 days after conception, the embryo is not exposed to maternal blood that contains the drug. However, some drugs may affect the uterine lining, making it unsuitable for implantation. Drugs administered between days 15 and 90 may produce an effect if the tissue for which the drug has an affinity is in the process of differentiation at that time. After 90 days, when differentiation is complete, most fetal tissues are relatively resistant to teratogenic effects of drugs. However, the impact on ongoing neurologic development is not known.

Nursing Care Management

Caution expectant mothers against ingesting any medication without first consulting a practitioner. To help ensure that fewer women will inadvertently take some chemical that might harm the fetus, medication labels are now required to include information regarding the possible teratogenic effects. Excessive use of some commonplace drugs, such as alcohol, valproic acid, and isotretinoin, produces characteristic malformations in the fetus. Nurses should also caution mothers-to-be about appropriate dietary intake and necessary supplements should it be impossible to consume a well-balanced diet. One of the goals of preventing birth defects in diabetic mothers is maintenance of strict glycemic control and avoidance of excessive weight gain.

Nurses should be aware of Birth Defect Research for Children, Inc.,* which offers help and information to families with children with defects caused by maternal exposure to drugs, chemicals, radiation, or other environmental agents.

RADIATION

Ionizing radiation in large doses has been shown to be both mutagenic and teratogenic in humans. Pelvic irradiation of pregnant women—from natural background radiation that is present everywhere in varying degrees, from occupational exposure, or from diagnostic or therapeutic procedures—is believed to be hazardous to the embryo, although the extent of teratogenicity and the exact dosage required to induce somatic change are not yet known. There is a theoretic risk of carcinogenesis when the fetus is exposed to diagnostic radiation; however, with the radiation levels currently used, there are no known risks for congenital malformations or cognitive impairment. These authors present an extensive review of diagnostic radiation methods used for pregnant and lactating mothers. Carlo and Ambalavanan (2016a) indicate that single diagnostic radiation doses are not adequate to cause harm in the fetus. Diagnostic CT and MRI radiation can be modified to decrease the amount of radiation to the fetus. Radiation may damage the conceptus at any time during its prenatal existence, and it is known that rapidly

*800 Celebration Ave., Suite 225, Celebration, FL 34747; 407-466-8304; http://www.birthdefects.org.

dividing and differentiating cells, such as those of the embryo, have increased radiosensitivity. As with other teratogens, the type of effect produced is closely correlated with the stage of development at which the radiation exposure occurs.

To help prevent the possibility of radiation damage, it is advisable (1) to avoid unnecessary radiation exposure, such as elective radiographs to the pelvis and abdomen, in women of childbearing age except during the 2 weeks immediately after menstruation; (2) to ascertain whether pregnancy is a possibility; and (3) to advise both men and women who have lower abdominal or pelvic radiographs to avoid conception for several months. Pregnant women should avoid radioactive iodine exposure because iodine has an affinity for fetal thyroid tissue and can lead to developmental problems such as fetal goiter, microcephaly, intrauterine growth restriction, malignancy, and death. Women should also avoid the use of nonradioactive iodides in vaginal douche solutions, vaginal suppositories containing povidone-iodine (Betadine), and iodinized drugs for asthmatics during pregnancy (Blackburn, 2013).

The occurrence of childhood cancer as a result of prenatal or preconceptual radiation exposure has been debated for more than 50 years. Epidemiology studies have demonstrated that high dose rates to the embryo or fetus increase the risk of cancer (Slovis & Frush, 2016). The risk of cancer in offspring exposed in utero at low dose remains controversial and has not yet been determined (Brent, 2014). Brent (2009) cites studies that support the concept that the carcinogenic risk for the fetus being exposed to radiation during diagnostic tests is negligible. Maternal treatment for cancer has also received considerable attention, and it has been determined that many diagnostic and treatment methods pose no additional risk to the growing fetus (Backes, Moorehead, Nelin, et al., 2011).

NCLEX REVIEW QUESTIONS

1. Nursing care of a 9-month-old who has recently undergone cleft palate repair can be expected to include feeding with a(n):
   A. Plastic spoon
   B. Open cup
   C. Pigeon bottle
   D. Special Needs feeder
2. Nursing care of a healthy term newborn aimed at preventing significant hyperbilirubinemia includes:
   A. Encourage mother to breastfeed the infant frequently
   B. If the mother cannot breastfeed at night, give the infant feedings of water and dextrose
   C. Observe the number of voids and stools, especially in the first 72 hours
   D. Promote newborn rooming-in with the mother
   E. Observe infant for appearance of jaundice and obtain transcutaneous bilirubin reading
   F. Feed the infant formula on a schedule of every 4 to 5 hours
3. Nursing care of a 2-day-old infant undergoing phototherapy in the mother's hospital room should include:
   A. Ensure proper fit of eye covering (patches)
   B. Monitor bilirubin levels with transcutaneous monitor every 8 hours
   C. Record number of infant voidings and stools
   D. Examine infant's eyes for presence of drainage every 8 hours or as warranted
   E. Avoid removing the infant from phototherapy except for brief periods of feeding and cuddling
4. An infant born at term and weighing 3.0 kg (6 lb, 6 oz) has Apgar scores of 8 and 9 at 1 and 5 minutes, respectively, and is in the nursery until the mother's blood pressure is stabilized. The infant has some tremors of the extremities but is otherwise alert and active at 4 hours of age with vital signs within normal limits for age. Prenatal history and delivery are uneventful, and the infant is appropriate for gestational age. A priority nursing intervention should include:
   A. Obtain vital signs every hour until stable
   B. Consider transferring the infant to a transitional unit for closer observation
   C. Obtain bedside serum glucose per standing orders
   D. Feed infant 20 ml of infant formula
5. The nurse notes that a healthy term infant appears jaundiced at 12 hours of age. The nurse understands that there is probably an ABO incompatibility based on the following information:
   A. The direct Coombs test is weakly positive.
   B. The infant's hemoglobin is 11.3 mg/dl.
   C. The mother's blood type is O positive.
   D. This is the mother's first pregnancy.
   E. The infant's serum bilirubin (indirect) is 2.6 mg/dl.

Correct Answers

1. B; 2. A, C, D, E; 3. A, C, D; 4. C; 5. A, C, D, E

REFERENCES

Adamkin, D. H., & American Academy of Pediatrics: Committee on Fetus and Newborn. (2011). Postnatal glucose homeostasis in late-preterm and term infants. *Pediatrics, 127*(3), 575–579.

Alsweiler, J. M., Harding, J. E., & Bloomfield, F. H. (2013). Neonatal hyperglycaemia increases mortality and mordbidity in pretem lambs. *Neonatology, 103*(2), 83–90.

Ambalavanan, N., & Carlo, W. (2016). Jaundice and hyperbilirubinemia in the newborn. In R. M. Kliegman, B. F. Stanton, J. W. St. Geme, et al. (Eds.), *Nelson textbook of pediatrics* (20th ed.). Philadelphia: Elsevier.

American Academy of Pediatrics. (2008). Prevention of rickets and vitamin D deficiency in infants, children, and adolescents. *Pediatrics, 122*(5), 1142–1148.

American Academy of Pediatrics. (2014). *Pediatric nutrition handbook* (7th ed.). Elk Grove Village, IL: The Academy.

American Academy of Pediatrics, American College of Obstetricians and Gynecologists. (2012). *Guidelines for perinatal care* (7th ed.). Elk Grove Village, IL: The Academy.

American Academy of Pediatrics, Committee on Infectious Diseases, Pickering L., (Eds.). (2015). *2015 Red book: report of the Committee on Infectious Diseases*, ed 30, Elk Grove Village, IL: The Academy.

American Academy of Pediatrics, Subcommittee on Hyperbilirubinemia. (2004). Clinical practice guideline: Management of hyperbilirubinemia in the newborn infant 35 or more weeks of gestation. *Pediatrics, 114*(1), 297–316.

American College of Obstetricians and Gynecologists' Task Force on Neonatal Brachial Plexus Palsy. (2014). Neonatal brachial plexus palsy. *Obstetrics and Gynecology, 123*(4), 902–904.

Backes, C. H., Moorehead, P. A., & Nelin, L. D. (2011). Cancer in pregnancy: Fetal and neonatal outcomes. *Clinical Obstetrics and Gynecology, 54*(4), 574–590.

Bhutani, V. K., & American Academy of Pediatrics Committee on Fetus and Newborn. (2011). Phototherapy to prevent severe neonatal hyperbilirubinemia in the newborn infant 35 or more weeks of gestation. *Pediatrics, 128*(4), e1046–e1052.

Bhutani, V. K., Stark, A. R., Lazzeroni, L. C., et al. (2013). Predischarge screening for severe neonatal hyperbilirubinemia identifies infants who need phototherapy. *The Journal of Pediatrics, 162*(3), 477–482.

Blackburn, S. (2013). *Maternal, fetal, and neonatal physiology: A clinical perspective* (4th ed.). St. Louis, MO: Saunders.

Boies, E. G., Vaucher, Y. E., & the Academy of Breastfeeding Medicine. (2016). ABM Clinical Protocol #10: Breastfeeding the Late Preterm (34–36 6/7 Weeks of Gestation) and Early Term Infants (37–38 6/7 Weeks of Gestation), Second Revision 2016. *Breastfeeding Medicine, 11*(10), 494–500.

Bratlid, D., Nakstad, B., & Hansen, T. W. (2011). National guidelines for treatment of jaundice in the newborn. *Acta Paediatrica, 100*(4), 499–505.

Brent, R. L. (2009). Saving lives and changing family histories: Appropriate counseling of pregnant women and men and women of reproductive age, concerning the risk of diagnostic radiation exposures during and before pregnancy. *American Journal of Obstetrics and Gynecology, 200*(1), 4–24.

Brent, R. L. (2014). Carcinogenic risks of prenatal ionizing radiation. *Seminars in Fetal & Neonatal Medicine, 19*(3), 203–213.

Breugem, C. C., Evans, K. N., Poets, C. F., et al. (2016). Best practices for the diagnosis and evaluation of infants with Robin Sequence. *JAMA Pediatrics, 9*, 894–902.

Carlo, W. A., & Ambalavanan, N. (2016a). Radiation. In R. M. Kliegman, B. F. Stanton, J. W. St. Geme, et al. (Eds.), *Nelson textbook of pediatrics* (20th ed.). Philadelphia: Elsevier.

Carlo, W. A., & Ambalavanan, N. (2016b). Peripheral nerve injuries. In R. M. Kliegman, B. F. Stanton, J. W. St. Geme, et al. (Eds.), *Nelson textbook of pediatrics* (20th ed.). Philadelphia: Elsevier.

Cauchemez, S., Besnard, M., Bompard, P., et al. (2016). Association between Zika virus and microcephaly in French Polynesia, 2013–15: A retrospective study. *Lancet (London, England), 387*(10033), 2125–2132.

Center for Disease Control and Prevention. (2015). *Should a mother continue breastfeeding if her child has jaundice?* Update from CDC. https://www.cdc.gov/breastfeeding/disease/jaundice.htm.

Chantry, C. J., Eglash, A., Labbok, M., et al. (2015). ABM Position on Breastfeeding – Revised 2015. *Breastfeeding Medicine, 10*(9), 407–411.

Chen, T. S., Eichenfield, L. F., & Friedlander, S. F. (2013). Infantile hemangiomas: An update on pathogenesis and therapy. *Pediatrics, 131* (1), 99–108.

Chen, J. K., Ghasri, P., Aguilar, G., et al. (2012). An overview of clinical and experimental treatment modalities for port wine stains. *Journal of the American Academy of Dermatology, 67*(2), 289–304.

Cicchetti, R., Cascone, P., Caresta, E., et al. (2012). Mandibular distraction osteogenesis for neonates with Pierre Robin sequence and airway obstruction. *The Journal of Maternal-fetal and Neonatal Medicine, 25*(Suppl. 4), 141–143.

Chibueze, E. C., Tirado, V., Lopes, K., et al. (2017). Zika virus infection in pregnancy: A systematic review of disease course and complications. *Reproductive Health, 14*(28), 1–14.

Cleft Palate Foundation. Retrieved from http://www.cleftline.org/parents-individuals/.

Dahan-Oliel, N., Kasaai, B., Montpetit, K., et al. (2012). Effectiveness and safety of botulinum toxin type a in children withmusculoskeletal conditions: What is the current state of evidence? *International Journal of Pediatrics*, 1–16.

Demirel, G., Akar, M., Celik, I. H., et al. (2011). Single versus multiple dose intravenous immunoglobulin in combination with LED phototherapy in the treatment of ABO hemolytic disease in neonates. *International Journal of Hematology, 93*(6), 700–703.

Doumouchtsis, S. K., & Arulkumaran, S. (2008). Head trauma after instrumental births. *Clinics in Perinatology, 35*(1), 69–83.

Doyle, D. A. (2016). Hypoparathyroidism. In R. M. Kliegman, B. F. Stanton, J. W. St. Geme, et al. (Eds.), *Nelson textbook of pediatrics* (20th ed.). Philadelphia: Elsevier.

Drolet, B. A., Frommelt, P. C., Chamlin, S. L., et al. (2013). Initiation and use of propanolol for infantile hemangioma: Report of a consensus conference. *Pediatrics, 131*(1), 131–140.

Elalfy, M. S., Elbarbary, N. S., & Abaza, H. W. (2011). Early intravenous immunoglobulin (two-dose regimen) in the management of severe Rh hemolytic disease of newborn—a prospective randomized controlled trial. *European Journal of Pediatrics, 170*(4), 461–467.

Feldman, H. S., Jones, K. L., Lindsay, S., et al. (2012). Prenatal alcohol exposure patterns and alcohol-related birth defects and growth deficiencies: A prospective study. *Alcoholism, Clinical and Experimental Research, 36*(4), 670–676.

Gailey, D. G. (2016). Feeding infants with cleft and the postoperative cleft management. *Oral and Maxillofacial Surgery Clinics of North America, 28*, 153–159.

Gangopadhyay, N., Mendonca, D. A., & Woo, A. S. (2012). Pierre Robin sequence. *Seminars in Plastic Surgery, 26*(2), 76–82.

Gregory, K. A. (2016). New approaches to care of the infant with hypoglycemia. *The Journal of Perinatal & Neonatal Nursing, 34*(4), 284–286.

Greenbaum, L. A. (2016). Vitamin K deficiency. In R. M. Kliegman, B. F. Stanton, J. W. St. Geme, et al. (Eds.), *Nelson textboobrachial plexyk of pediatrics* (20th ed.). Philadelphia: Elsevier.

Hall, K. M., Besachio, D. A., Moore, M. D., et al. (2017). Effectiveness of screening for craniosynostosis with ultrasound: A retrospective review. *Pediatric Radiology, 47*(5), 606–612.

Hartzell, L. D., & Buckmiller, L. M. (2012). Current management of infantile hemangiomas and their common associated conditions. *Otolaryngologic Clinics of North America, 45*(3), 545–556.

Hawdon, J. (2014). Neonatal hypoglycemia: Are evidence-based clinical guidelines available? *Neoreviews, 15*, 91–98.

Hendrickson, J. E., & Delaney, M. (2016). Hemolytic disease of the fetus and newborn: Modern practice and future investigations. *Transfusion Medicine Reviews, 30*, 159–164.

Hervey-Jumper, S. L., Justice, D., & Vanaman, M. M. (2011). Torticollis associated with neonatal brachial plexus palsy. *Pediatric Neurology, 45*(5), 305–310.

Huth, J., Petersen, J., & Lehman, J. The use of postoperative restraints in children after cleft lip or cleft palate repair: A preliminary report. *Plastic Surgery*, 1–3, 2013.

Johnson, P. J. (2016). Head, eyes, ears, nose, mouth and neck assessment. In E. P. Tappero & M. E. Honeyfield (Eds.), *Physical assessment of the newborn: a comprehensive approach to the art of physical assessment* (5th ed.). New York: Springer Publishing Company.

Kimberlin, D. W., Baley, J., & American Academy of Pediatrics. (2013). Guidance on management of asymptomatic neonates born to women with active genital herpes lesions. *Pediatrics, 131*(2), e635–e648.

Kinsman, S. L., & Johnston, M. V. (2016). Congenital anomalies of the central nervous system. In R. M. Kleigman, B. F. Stanton, J. W. St. Geme, et al. (Eds.), *Nelson textbook of pediatrics* (20th ed.). Philadelphia: Elsevier.

Kuban, K. C., Allred, E. N., O'Shea, T. M., et al. (2009). Developmental correlates of head circumference at birth and two years in a cohort of extremely low gestational age newborns. *The Journal of Pediatrics, 155*(3), e1–e3.

Labreze, C. L., Harper, H. I., & Hoeger, P. H. (Jan 12, 2017). Infantile haemangioma. *Lancet.*

Lawrence, R. A., & Lawrence, R. M. (2015). *Breastfeeding: a guide for the medical profession* (8th ed.). Philadelphia: Elsevier.

Maisels, M. J. (2015). Managing the jaundiced newborn: A persistent challenge. *Canadian Medical Association Journal, 187*(5), 335–343.

Maisels, M. J., Watchko, J. F., Bhutani, V. K., et al. (2012). An approach to the management of hyperbilirubinemia in the preterm infant less than 35 weeks of gestation. *Journal of Perinatology, 32*(9), 660–664.

Maisels, M. J., & Yang, H. (2012). Tin-mesoporphyrin in the treatment of refractory hyperbilirubinemia due to Rh incompatibility. *Journal of Perinatology, 32*(11), 899–900.

Mangurten, H. H., & Puppala, B. L. (2015). Birth injuries. In R. J. Martin, A. A. Fanaroff, & M. C. Walsh (Eds.), *Fanaroff and Martin's neonatal-perinatal medicine: diseases of the fetus and infant* (10th ed.). Philadelphia, PA: Saunders, an imprint of Elsevier Inc.

Martin, K. L. (2016). Vascular disorders. In R. M. Kliegman, B. F. Stanton, J. W. St. Geme, et al. (Eds.), *Nelson textbook of pediatrics* (20th ed.). Philadelphia: Elsevier.

McCance, K., & Huether, S. (2014). *Pathophysiology: The biological basis for disease in adults and children* (7th ed.). St. Louis, MO: Mosby.

McCarty, D., Peat, J., Malcolm, W., et al. (2016). Dolichocephaly in preterm infants: Prevalence, risk factors, and early motor outcomes. *American Journal of Perinatology*, 1–7.

McKinlay, C., Alsweiler, J. M., Ansell, J. M., et al., for the Children with Hypoglycemia and their Later Development. (2015). Neonatal glycemia and neurodevelopmental outcomes at 2 years. *The New England Journal of Medicine, 373*(16), 1507–1518.

Modanlou, H., Hutson, S., & Merritt, A. T. (2016). Early blood transfusion and resolution of disseminated intravascular coagulation associated with massive subgaleal hemorrhage. *Neonatal Network, 35*(1), 37–41.

Moise, K. J. (2012). Red cell alloimmunization. In S. G. Gabbe, J. R. Niebyl, K. L. Simpson, et al. (Eds.), *Obstetrics: Normal and problem pregnancies* (6th ed.). London: Churchill Livingstone.

Moise, K. J., & Argoti, P. S. (2012). Management and prevention of red cell alloimmunization in pregnancy: A systematic review. *Obstetrics and Gynecology, 120*(5), 1132–1139.

Muchowski, K. E. (2014). Evaluation and treatment of neonatal hyperbilirubinemia. *American Family Physician, 89*(11), 873–878.

Okwundu, C. I., Okoramah, C. A., & Shah, P. S. (2012). Prophylactic phototherapy for preventing jaundice in preterm or low birth weight infants. *Cochrane Database of Systematic Review*, (1), CD0007966.

O'Toole, P., & Spiegel, D. A. (2016). The neck: Torticollis. In R. M. Kliegman, B. F. Stanton, J. W. St. Geme, et al. (Eds.), *Nelson textbook of pediatrics* (20th ed.). Philadelphia: Elsevier.

Parsons, J. A., Seay, A. R., & Jacobson, M. (2016). Neurologic disorders. In S. L. Gardner, B. S. Carter, M. Enzman-Hines, et al. (Eds.), *Merenstein and Gardner's handbook of neonatal intensive care* (8th ed.). St. Louis, MO: Mosby Elsevier.

Passi, D., Sharma, S., Dutta, S. R., et al. (2017). Zika virus diseases: The new face of an ancient enemy as global public health emergency (2016): Brief review and recent updates. *International Journal of Preventive Medicine, 8*(6).

Phillippi, J. C., Holley, S. L., Morad, A., et al. (2016). Prevention of vitamin k deficiency bleeding. See comment in PubMed Commons below *Journal of Midwifery and Women's Health, 4*, 632–636..

Raizman, J. E., Shea, J., Daly, C. H., et al. (2016). Clinical impact of improved point-of-care glucose monitoring in neonatal intensive care using Nova StatStrip: Evidence for improved accuracy, better sensitivity, and reduced test utilization. *Clinical Biochemistry, 49*, 879–884.

Reilly, S., Reid, J., Skeat, J., et al. (2013). ABM Clinical Protocol #18: Guidelines for Breastfeeding Infants with Cleft Lip, Cleft Palate, or Cleft Lip and Palate, Revised 2013. *Breastfeeding Medicine, 8*(4), 349–353.

Roland, E., & Hill, A. (2016). Neurological problems of the newborn. In R. D. Daruff, J. Jankovic, J. C. Mazziotta, et al. (Eds.), *Bradley's neurology in clinical practice* (7th ed.). Philadelphia: Elsevier.

Schwartz, H. P., Haberman, B. E., & Ruddy, R. M. (2011). Hyperbilirubinemia: Current guidelines and emerging therapies. *Pediatric Emergency Care, 27*(9), 884–889.

Scott, A. R., Tibesar, R. J., Lander, T. A., et al. (2011). Mandibular distraction osteogenesis in infants younger than 3 months. *Archives of Facial Plastic Surgery, 13*(3), 173–179.

Shah, N. A., & Wusthoff, C. J. (2016). Intracranial hemorrhage in the neonate. *Neonatal Network, 35*(2), 67–72.

Sharma, D. (2016). Golden 60 minutes of newborn's life: Part 1: Preterm neonate. *The Journal of Maternal-Fetal & Neonatal Medicine: The Official Journal of the European Association of Perinatal Medicine, the Federation of Asia and Oceania Perinatal Societies, the International Society of Perinatal Obstetricians*, 1–12.

Sharma, D., Sharma, P., & Shastri, S. (2017). Golden 60 minutes of newborn's life: Part 2: Term neonate. *The Journal of Maternal-Fetal & Neonatal Medicine: The Official Journal of the European Association of Perinatal Medicine, the Federation of Asia and Oceania Perinatal Societies, the International Society of Perinatal Obstetricians, 30*(22), 2728–2733.

Shulman, S. T. (2016). Group A Streptococcus. In R. M. Kliegman, B. F. Stanton, J. W. St. Geme, et al. (Eds.), *Nelson textbook of pediatrics* (20th ed.). Philadelphia: Elsevier.

Slovis, T. L., & Frush, D. P. (2016). Environmental health hazards: Biological effects of radiation in children. In R. M. Kliegman, B. F. Stanton, J. W. St Geme, et al. (Eds.), *Nelson textbook of pediatrics* (20th ed.). Philadelphia: Elsevier.

Smith, A., Kandamany, H., Okafor, I., et al. (2016). Delayed infant subaponeurotic (subgaleal) fluid collections: A case series of 11 infants. *The Journal of Emergency Medicine, 50*(6), 881–886.

Sperling, M. A. (2016). Hypoglycemia. In R. M. Kliegman, B. F. Stanton, J. W. St. Geme, et al. (Eds.), *Nelson textbook of pediatrics* (20th ed.). Philadelphia: Elsevier.

Stokowski, L. A. (2011). Fundamentals of phototherapy for neonatal jaundice. *Advances in Neonatal Care: Official Journal of the National Association of Neonatal Nurses, 11*(5S), S10–S21.

Tam, E. W., Haeusslein, L. A., Bonifacio, S. L., et al. (2012). Hypoglycemia associated with increased risk for brain injury and adverse neurodevelopmental outcome in neonates at risk for encephalopathy. *The Journal of Pediatrics, 161*(1), 88–93.

Tappero, E. (2016). Musculoskeletal system assessment. In E. Tappero & M. A. Honeyfield (Eds.), *Physical assessment of the newborn: a comprehensive approach to the art of physical examination* (5th ed.). New York: Springer Publishing Company.

Taylor, J. A., Burgos, A. E., Flaherman, V., et al., on behalf of the BORN Investigators. (2016). Utility of decision rules for transcutaneous bilirubin measurements. *Pediatrics, 137*(5), 1–8.

Tiberi, E., Cota, F., Barone, G., et al. (2016). Continuous glucose monitoring in preterm infants: Evaluation by a modified Clarke error grid. *Italian Journal of Pediatrics, 42*, 29, 1–7.

Thornton, P. S., Stanley, C. A., De Leon, D. D., et al. (2015). Recommendations from the Pediatric Endocrine Society for Evaluation and Management of Persistent Hypoglycemia in Neonates, Infants, and Children. *The Journal of Pediatrics, 167*, 238–245.

Tschudy, M. M., & Arcara, K. M. (Eds.), (2012). *Harriet Lane handbook* (19th ed.). Philadelphia: Mosby.

Wang, A., Wohrley, J., & Rosebush, J. (2017). Herpes simplex virus in the neonate. *Pediatric Annals, 46*(2), e42–e46.

Wight, N., Marinelli, K., & Academy of Breastfeeding Medicine. (2014). Guidelines for blood glucose monitoring and treatment of hypoglycemia in term and late-preterm neonates. *Breastfeeding Medicine, 9*(4), 173–179.

Wilson, T. J., Chang, K. W. C., Chauhan, S. P., et al. (2016). Peripartum and neonatal factors associated with the persistence of neonatal brachial plexus palsy at 1 year: A review of 382 cases. *Journal of Neurosurgery. Pediatrics, 17*, 618–624.

9

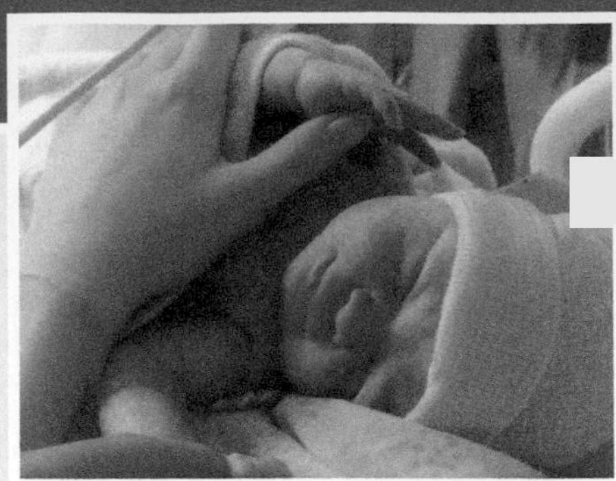

The High-Risk Newborn and Family

Kimberly Fisher

CONCEPTS

- Thermoregulation
- Perfusion
- Infection

GENERAL MANAGEMENT OF HIGH-RISK NEWBORNS

IDENTIFICATION OF HIGH-RISK NEWBORNS

The **high-risk neonate** is a newborn, regardless of gestational age or birth weight, with a greater-than-average chance of morbidity or mortality, usually because of conditions beyond the normal events related to birth and subsequent adjustment to extrauterine life. The high-risk period begins at the time of viability (i.e., the gestational age at which survival outside the uterus is thought possible, or as early as 23 weeks of gestation) up to 28 days after birth and includes threats to life and health that occur during the prenatal, perinatal, and postnatal periods.

In the past, the late-preterm infants of 34 to 36$\frac{6}{7}$ weeks of gestation often received the same treatment as term infants. Late-preterm infants actually experience morbidities that are similar to those of preterm infants: respiratory distress, hypoglycemia requiring treatment, jaundice, feeding difficulties, and adverse neurodevelopmental outcomes (Gill & Boyle, 2017; Natarajan & Shankaran, 2016). Assessment and prompt intervention in life-threatening perinatal emergencies often make the difference between a favorable outcome and a lifetime of disability. The nurse in the intensive care nursery knows the characteristics of neonates and recognizes the significance of serious deviations from expected observations. The probability of a successful outcome increases when the care team anticipates the need for specialized care and plans for it.

Late-Preterm Infant

Within the past two decades, several significant changes have occurred in neonatal care. Early postpartum discharge for term and preterm infants gained popularity as health care institutions attempted to cut health care costs. Infants who appeared to be "near" term began to be treated much like term infants, avoiding the costs of neonatal intensive care for infants who appeared to be healthy. Experts have recommended that infants born between 34 and 36$\frac{6}{7}$ weeks of gestation be referred to as **late-preterm infants** rather than *near-term infants* (Natarajan & Shankaran, 2016). Late-preterm infants may transition effectively to extrauterine life. However, because of their limited gestation, they remain at risk for problems related to feeding, breathing, neurodevelopment, thermoregulation, hypoglycemia, hyperbilirubinemia, and sepsis (Gill & Boyle, 2017; Natarajan & Shankaran, 2016). Studies have shown an increase risk for children born at 34 to 36 weeks to be diagnosed with cerebral palsy (CP) (Gill & Boyle, 2017; Natarajan & Shankaran, 2016). Late- and moderate-preterm infants represent an estimated 70% of the total preterm infant population. The mortality rate for this group is up to five times higher than that of term infants (Bulut, Gursoy, & Ovali, 2016; De Carolis, Pinna, Cocca, et al., 2016; Natarajan & Shankaran, 2016). Because late-preterm infants' birth weights often range from 2000 to 2500 g (4.4 to 5.5 lb) and they appear relatively mature in comparison to smaller preterm infants, they may be cared for in the same way as healthy term infants and their risk factors may be overlooked. Late-preterm infants are often discharged early and have a threefold higher rate of rehospitalization than term infants (Natarajan & Shankaran, 2016). Discussions regarding high-risk infants in this chapter also refer to late-preterm infants who are experiencing a delayed transition to extrauterine life.

The Association of Women's Health, Obstetric and Neonatal Nurses has published the *Assessment and Care of the Late Preterm Infant* guide (2010) to teach perinatal nurses about the late-preterm infant's risk factors and appropriate care and follow-up (Table 9.1).

Classification of High-Risk Newborns

High-risk infants are most often classified according to birth weight, gestational age, and main pathophysiologic problems. The more common problems related to physiologic status involve the infant's maturity and usually chemical disturbances (e.g., hypoglycemia, hypocalcemia) and consequences of immature organs and systems (e.g., hyperbilirubinemia, respiratory distress, hypothermia). Box 9.1 outlines terms describing the developmental status of the newborn.

Weight at birth formerly reflected a reasonably accurate estimation of gestational age; that is, if an infant's birth weight exceeded 2500 g (5.5 lb), the infant was considered mature. However, accumulated data have shown that intrauterine growth rates are not the same for all infants and that other factors (e.g., heredity, placental insufficiency, and maternal disease) affect intrauterine growth and the infant's birth weight.

TABLE 9.1 Late-Preterm Infant Assessment and Interventions

Risk Factors	Assessment	Interventions*
Respiratory distress	Assess for cardinal signs of respiratory distress (nasal flaring, grunting, tachypnea, central cyanosis, retractions) and presence of apnea, especially during feedings. Assess for hypothermia, hypoglycemia.	Perform gestational age assessment. Observe for signs of respiratory distress; monitor oxygenation by pulse oximetry; provide supplemental oxygen judiciously.
Thermal instability	Monitor axillary temperature every 30 minutes immediately postpartum until stable; thereafter every 1-4 hours, depending on gestational age and ability to maintain thermal stability.	Provide skin-to-skin care in immediate postpartum period for stable infant. Implement measures to avoid excess heat loss (adjust environmental temperature, avoid drafts). Bathe only after thermal stability has been maintained for 1 hour.
Hypoglycemia	Monitor for signs and symptoms of hypoglycemia. Assess feeding ability (latch-on, nipple-feeding). Assess thermal stability and signs and symptoms of respiratory distress. Monitor bedside glucose in infants with additional risk factors (IDM, prolonged labor, respiratory distress, poor feeding).	Initiate early feedings of human milk or formula. Avoid dextrose water or water feedings. Provide IV dextrose as necessary for hypoglycemia.
Jaundice	Observe for appearance of jaundice in first 24 hours. Evaluate maternal-fetal history for additional risk factors that may cause increased hemolysis and circulating levels of unconjugated bilirubin (Rh, ABO, spherocytosis, bruising). Assess feeding method, voiding and stooling patterns.	Monitor transcutaneous or serum bilirubin and note risk zone on hour-specific nomogram (see Fig. 8.11).
Feeding problems	Assess suck-swallow and breathing. Assess for respiratory distress, hypoglycemia, thermal stability. Assess latch-on, maternal comfort with feeding method. Determine weight loss (should be ≤10% of birth weight).	Initiate early feedings (human milk or formula). Ensure maternal knowledge of feeding method and signs of inadequate feeding (sleepiness, lethargy, color changes during feeding, apnea during feeding, decreased or absent urine output).
Neurodevelopmental problems	Assess for respiratory distress, neonatal jaundice, hypoglycemia, and thermal instability. Assess neurodevelopmental status. Assess for seizure activity.	Perform newborn screening, including hearing test. Implement individualized developmental care. Encourage parents to keep follow-up appointments with primary care provider for evaluation of growth and development (including cognitive function and achievement of appropriate milestones).
Infection	Evaluate maternal-fetal history for risk factors that may contribute to neonatal septicemia. Assess for signs and symptoms of neonatal infection.	Use Standard Precautions, especially hand washing between infants and contact with surfaces that may harbor bacteria (e.g., keyboards, telephones). Maintain thermal stability. Administer hepatitis B vaccine. Encourage breastfeeding and assist mother-baby pair with breastfeeding. Encourage parents to decrease infant exposure to respiratory viruses postdischarge and obtain vaccines as appropriate to prevent development of respiratory viruses (e.g., influenza).

*This is not an exhaustive list of nursing interventions; additional interventions include those discussed under the care of the high-risk infant in this chapter.

IDM, Infant of diabetic mother; *IV,* intravenous.

Portions adapted from Askin, D. F., Bakewell-Sachs, S., Medoff-Cooper, B., et al. (2010). *Late preterm infant assessment guide.* Washington, DC: Association of Women's Health, Obstetric and Neonatal Nurses.

From these data a more meaningful classification system that encompasses birth weight, gestational age, and neonatal outcome has been developed. It has also been found that the lowest perinatal mortality rate occurs in the infant who weighs between 3000 and 4000 g (6.4 and 8.8 lb) and whose gestational age is between 36 and 42 weeks (Walsh & Fanaroff, 2015). (See Fig. 7.2 for size comparison of newborn infants.)

Many perinatal problems can be anticipated before delivery. Prenatal testing and labor monitoring have reduced perinatal mortality rate, and specialized care of the distressed newborn is improving the survival rate. If the infant is likely to require special therapy at or soon after birth, plans can be made for the delivery to take place at a hospital with the appropriate level of care. This eliminates delay in starting care and avoids some of the dangers associated with transporting the sick newborn. Prenatal evaluation of fetal well-being along with advanced surgical and anesthetic techniques have made intrauterine treatment of certain pathologic conditions possible, while enhancing the neonate's chances for survival.

INTENSIVE CARE FACILITIES

Intensive care of the ill and immature newborn requires specialized knowledge and skill in a number of areas. Much of the equipment used in the care of the critically ill adult is unsuited to the needs of the very small infant, so equipment has been modified to meet these needs.

BOX 9.1 Classification of High-Risk Infants

Classification According to Size

Low-birth-weight (LBW) infant—An infant whose birth weight is less than 2500 g (5.5 lb), regardless of gestational age

Very-low-birth-weight (VLBW) infant—An infant whose birth weight is less than 1500 g (3.3 lb)

Extremely low-birth-weight (ELBW) infant—An infant whose birth weight is less than 1000 g (2.2 lb)

Appropriate-for-gestational-age (AGA) infant—An infant whose weight falls between the 10th and 90th percentiles on intrauterine growth curves

Small-for-date (SFD) or small-for-gestational-age (SGA) infant—An infant whose rate of intrauterine growth was slowed and whose birth weight falls below the 10th percentile on intrauterine growth curves

Intrauterine growth restriction (IUGR)—Found in infants whose intrauterine growth is restricted (sometimes used as a more descriptive term for the SGA infant)

Large-for-gestational-age (LGA) infant—An infant whose birth weight falls above the 90th percentile on intrauterine growth charts

Classification According to Gestational Age

Preterm (premature) infant—An infant born before completion of 37 weeks of gestation, regardless of birth weight

Full-term infant—An infant born between the beginning of 38 weeks and the completion of 42 weeks of gestation, regardless of birth weight

Postterm (postmature) infant—An infant born after 42 weeks of gestational age, regardless of birth weight

Late-preterm infant—An infant born between 34 $^{0}/_{7}$ and 36 $^{6}/_{7}$ weeks of gestation, regardless of birth weight

Classification According to Mortality

Live birth—Birth in which the neonate manifests any heartbeat, breathes, or displays voluntary movement, regardless of gestational age

Fetal death—Death of the fetus after 20 weeks of gestation and before delivery, with absence of any signs of life after birth

Neonatal death—Death that occurs in the first 27 days of life; early neonatal death occurs in the first week of life; late neonatal death occurs at 7 to 27 days

Perinatal mortality—Describes the total number of fetal and early neonatal deaths per 1000 live births

Postnatal death—Death that occurs at 28 days to 1 year after birth

Examples of modifications include ventilators that deliver small volumes of oxygen in the proper concentration and pressure, infusion pumps that accurately deliver very small volumes, and radiant heat warmers that provide a constant source of warmth and allow maximum access to the infant. Most important, advances in intensive care have created a need for highly skilled personnel trained in neonatal intensive care.

The diversity of special care needs requires that the unit be arranged for graduated care of the infant population. There should be adequate facilities and skilled personnel to provide one-to-one nursing care for each seriously ill infant, as well as a means for graduation to one-to-three or one-to-four nursing care in a quieter area where infants require less intensive care until they are ready to be discharged. Family-centered care and a quieter environment are often difficult to provide in a busy neonatal intensive care unit (NICU), so some units have developed step-down and single-room units where staff can observe high-risk infants. Such areas are designed for family-centered care alongside appropriate neurodevelopmental care.

Organization of Services

The most efficient organization of services is a regionalized system. Neonatal intensive care facilities may provide four prescribed levels of care with special equipment, skilled personnel, and ancillary services concentrated in a centralized institution (American Academy of Pediatrics, Committee on Fetus and Newborn, 2012):

- **Level I facility**—Provides management of normal maternal and newborn care inclusive of the following:
  - Provide neonatal resuscitation at every delivery
  - Evaluate and provide postnatal care to stable term newborn infants
  - Stabilize and provide care for infants born 35 to 37 weeks of gestation who remain physiologically stable
  - Stabilize newborn infants who are ill and those born at <35 weeks of gestation until transfer to a higher level of care
- **Level II facility**—Provides Level I capabilities plus the following:
  - Provide care for infants born ≥32 weeks gestation and weighing ≥1500 g who have physiologic immaturity or who are moderately ill with problems that are expected to resolve rapidly and are not anticipated to need subspecialty services
  - Provide care for infants convalescing after intensive care
  - Provide mechanical ventilation for brief duration (<24 hours) or continuous positive airway pressure or both
  - Stabilize infants born before 32 weeks of gestation and weighing less than 1500 g until transfer to a neonatal intensive care facility
- **Level III facility**—Level II capabilities plus the following:
  - Provide sustained life support
  - Provide comprehensive care for infants born <32 weeks of gestation and weighing <1500 g and infants born at all gestational ages and birth weights with critical illness
  - Provide prompt and readily available access to a full range of pediatric medical subspecialists, pediatric surgical specialists, pediatric anesthesiologists, and pediatric ophthalmologists
  - Provide a full range of respiratory support that may include conventional and/or high-frequency ventilation and inhaled nitric oxide
  - Perform advanced imaging, with interpretation on an urgent basis, including computed tomography (CT), magnetic resonance imaging (MRI), and echocardiography
- **Level IV**—Level III capabilities plus the following:
  - Located within an institution with the capability to provide surgical repair of complex congenital or acquired conditions
  - Maintain a full range of pediatric medical subspecialists, pediatric surgical subspecialists, and pediatric anesthesiologists at the site
  - Facilitate transport and provide outreach education

Transporting High-Risk Newborns

When an at-risk infant is identified or anticipated, arrangements are made for care in the intensive care facility. The uterus is the ideal transport unit for the infant with anticipated difficulties: whenever possible, transport the mother where special care is available for her delivery.

Some infants develop difficulties after a seemingly normal pregnancy and uncomplicated labor. Because it is impossible to always predict when infants will require intensive care, a coordinated system ensures the best chance for survival. Each hospital that delivers infants should be able to provide for appropriate neonatal stabilization and transportation to a tertiary care facility. The infant must be kept warm, be adequately oxygenated (including intubation if indicated), have vital signs and oxygen saturation monitored, and, when indicated, receive an intravenous (IV) infusion. The infant is transported in a specially designed incubator unit that contains a complete life-support system and other emergency equipment that can be carried by ambulance, van, plane, or helicopter.

The transport team may consist of one or more of the highly trained persons from the NICU: a neonatologist (or a fellow in neonatology), a neonatal nurse practitioner, a respiratory therapist, and one or more nurses. The accompanying professional must be constantly alert to every change in the infant's condition and able to intervene appropriately. The neonate who must be moved from one place to another within the hospital (e.g., to surgery, or from delivery room to nursery) is transported in an incubator or radiant warmer and accompanied by the necessary personnel and equipment.

NURSING CARE OF HIGH-RISK NEWBORNS

Because the majority of infants admitted to intensive care facilities are born before the estimated date of delivery, this chapter focuses primarily on the preterm infant. (See p. 296 for the characteristics of preterm infants.) The rate of neonatal complications (e.g., respiratory distress and hypoglycemia) is highest in this group, and often other high-risk factors (e.g., sepsis and congenital malformations) are associated with prematurity. This chapter discusses nursing problems encountered in the intensive care nursery and considers common complications. Nursing care of high-risk infants with more serious disorders is examined in relation to specific high-risk conditions.

ASSESSMENT

At birth the newborn is given a cursory yet thorough assessment to determine any apparent problems and identify those that demand immediate attention. This examination is most concerned with the evaluation of cardiopulmonary and neurologic functions. The assessment includes the assignment of an Apgar score (see Chapter 7) and an evaluation for any obvious congenital anomalies or evidence of neonatal distress. The infant is stabilized and evaluated before being transported to the NICU for therapy and more extensive assessment. (See Clinical Assessment of Gestational Age, Chapter 7.)

A thorough, systematic physical assessment is an essential component in the care of the high-risk infant (see Nursing Care Guidelines box). Subtle changes in feeding behavior, activity, color, oxygen saturation (Spo_2), or vital signs often indicate an underlying problem. The preterm infant, especially the extremely low-birth-weight (ELBW) infant, is not able to withstand prolonged physiologic stress and may die within minutes of exhibiting abnormal symptoms if the underlying pathologic process is not corrected. Through ongoing observations of the infant, the alert nurse recognizes subtle changes and reacts promptly to implement interventions that promote optimum function in the high-risk neonate.

Observational assessments of the high-risk infant are made according to the infant's acuity (seriousness of condition). The critically ill infant requires close observation and assessment of respiratory function, including continuous pulse oximetry, electrolytes, and blood gases. Accurate documentation of the infant's status is a key part of nursing care. With the aid of continuous, sophisticated cardiopulmonary monitoring, nursing assessments and daily care can be coordinated to allow for minimum handling of the infant (especially the very-low-birth-weight [VLBW] or ELBW infant) to decrease the effects of environmental stress.

MONITORING PHYSIOLOGIC DATA

Most neonates under intensive observation are placed in a controlled thermal environment and monitored for heart rate, respiratory activity, and temperature. The monitoring devices are equipped with an alarm system that indicates when the vital signs are above or below preset limits. However, a "hands-on" assessment, including auscultation of heart tones and breath sounds, is essential.

The placement of electrodes may be challenging because of the lack of flat areas on the neonate's chest, the limited space for alternating sites, the size of the electrodes, and irritation from the adhesive. Hydrogel electrodes are gentler on the skin and are easily removed by lifting an edge from the skin and moistening it with plain water to release the adhesive (Association of Women's Health, Obstetric and Neonatal Nurses, 2013). If the same electrode is reapplied to the skin, rinse the hydrogel with plain water to remove accumulated sodium, which can eventually irritate the skin. It is important to follow the manufacturer's directions for care and handling of electrodes to avoid malfunction or burns to sensitive skin.

Monitor blood pressure routinely in the sick neonate by either internal or external means. Direct recording with arterial catheters is often used but carries inherent risks, as with any arterial catheterization. Oscillometry (Dinamap) or Doppler transcutaneous apparatus is a simple, effective means for detecting changes in systemic blood pressure (hypotension or hypertension). Table 9.2 lists normal blood pressure ranges for healthy preterm infants. Infants who have birth asphyxia, have low Apgar scores, or are mechanically ventilated have lower systolic and diastolic pressures.

In the NICU frequent laboratory examinations and their interpretation are integral parts of the ongoing assessment of infants' progress. The nurse keeps accurate intake and output records on all acutely ill infants. An accurate output can be obtained by collecting urine in a plastic urine collection bag specifically made for preterm infants (see Urine Specimens, Chapter 22) or by weighing the diapers, which is the simplest and least traumatic means of measuring urinary output. The preweighed wet diaper is weighed on a gram scale, and the gram weight of the urine is converted directly to milliliters (e.g., 25 g = 25 ml).

Urine obtained from cloth diapers and disposable diapers containing absorbent gel material may yield inaccurate results for urine specific gravity, pH, and protein. Urine samples obtained from cotton balls made from 100% cotton strategically placed in the diaper proved to be the most accurate.

TABLE 9.2 Blood Pressure Ranges in Different Weight Groups of Healthy Preterm Infants*

Birth Weight	Systolic Pressure (mm Hg)	Diastolic Pressure (mm Hg)
501-750 g (1.1-1.6 lb)	50-62	26-36
751-1000 g (1.6-2.2 lb)	48-59	23-36
1001-1250 g (2.2-2.7 lb)	49-61	26-35
1251-1500 g (2.7-3.3 lb)	46-56	23-33
1501-1750 g (3.3-3.8 lb)	46-58	23-33
1751-2000 g (3.8-4.4 lb)	48-61	24-35

*Defined as infants without a history of maternal hypertension, Apgar scores of <3 at 1 min and <6 at 5 min, pneumothorax, hematocrit 0.32, serum pH 7.1, use of dopamine, infusion of erythrocytes or colloid, mechanical ventilation, or cardiopulmonary resuscitation.
Modified from Hegyi, T., Carbone, M. T., Anwar, M., et al. (1994). Blood pressure ranges in premature infants, part I: The first hours of life. *Journal of Pediatrics, 124*(4), 630.

NURSING CARE GUIDELINES

Physical Assessment

General Assessment

Using electronic scale, weigh daily or as the baby's condition dictates.
Measure length and head circumference periodically.
Describe general body shape and size, posture at rest, ease of breathing, presence and location of edema.
Describe any apparent deformities.
Describe any signs of distress (e.g., poor color, mottling, hypotonia).

Respiratory Assessment

Describe shape of chest (e.g., concave, barrel shaped), symmetry, chest tubes, or other deviations.
Describe use of accessory muscles: nasal flaring or substernal, intercostal, or suprasternal retractions.
Determine respiratory rate and regularity.
Auscultate and describe breath sounds: stridor, crackles, wheezing, areas of absence of sound, grunting, diminished air entry, equality of breath sounds.
Determine whether suctioning is needed.
Describe ambient oxygen and method of delivery; if intubated, describe size of tube, type of ventilator and settings, and method of securing tube.
Determine oxygen saturation by pulse oximetry.

Cardiovascular Assessment

Determine heart rate and rhythm.
Describe heart sounds, including any murmurs.
Determine the point of maximum intensity (PMI), the point at which the heartbeat sounds and palpates loudest (a change in the PMI may indicate a mediastinal shift).
Describe infant's color (abnormalities may be of cardiac, respiratory, or hematopoietic origin): cyanosis, pallor, plethora, jaundice, mottling.
Assess color of mucous membranes and lips.
Determine blood pressure. Indicate extremity used and cuff size.
Describe peripheral pulses, capillary refill (<2 to 3 seconds), peripheral perfusion (mottling).
Describe monitors, their parameters, and whether alarms are in "on" position.

Gastrointestinal Assessment

Determine presence of abdominal distention: increase in circumference, shiny skin, evidence of abdominal wall erythema, visible peristalsis, visible loops of bowel, status of umbilicus.
Determine any signs of regurgitation and time related to feeding; character and amount of residual if gavage fed; if nasogastric tube in place, describe type of suction, drainage (e.g., color, consistency).
Describe amount, color, and consistency of any emesis.
Palpate liver margin.
Describe amount, color, and consistency of stools.
Describe bowel sounds: presence or absence.

Genitourinary Assessment

Describe any abnormalities of genitalia.
Describe urine amount (as determined by weight), color, pH, and specific gravity (to screen for adequacy of hydration).

Neurologic-Musculoskeletal Assessment

Describe infant's movements (e.g., random, purposeful, jittery, twitching, spontaneous, elicited); level of activity with stimulation; evaluate based on gestational age.
Describe infant's position or attitude: flexed, extended.
Describe reflexes observed: Moro, sucking, Babinski, plantar, and other age-appropriate reflexes.
Determine level of response and consolability.
Determine changes in head circumference (if indicated); size and tension of fontanels, suture lines.

Temperature

Determine axillary temperature.
Determine relationship to environmental temperature.

Skin Assessment

Describe any discoloration, reddened area, signs of irritation, blisters, abrasions, or denuded areas, especially where monitoring equipment, infusions, or other apparatus come in contact with skin; also check and note any skin preparation used (e.g., povidone-iodine).
Determine texture and turgor of skin: dry, smooth, flaky, peeling, etc.
Describe any rash, skin lesion, or birthmarks.
Determine whether intravenous infusion catheter is in place, and observe for signs of infiltration.
Describe parenteral infusion lines: location, type (e.g., arterial, venous, peripheral, umbilical, central, peripherally inserted central catheter); type of infusion (e.g., medication, saline, dextrose, electrolytes, lipids, total parenteral nutrition); type of infusion pump and rate of flow; type of catheter; and appearance of insertion site.

NURSING TIP

When small volumes of urine are measured, superabsorbent disposable diapers, especially when kept closed, give more accurate volume measurements than cloth diapers because they are less affected by evaporative losses.

Laboratory examinations are a necessary part of the ongoing assessment and monitoring of the sick newborn's progress. The tests most often performed are blood glucose, bilirubin, electrolytes, calcium, hematocrit, and blood gases. Samples may be obtained by heel stick, venipuncture, arterial puncture, or an indwelling catheter in an umbilical vein, umbilical artery, or peripheral artery. (See Atraumatic Care box, Heel Punctures, in Chapter 7.) When collecting blood samples from the heel, studies have shown that the use of alternative therapies (e.g., nonnutritive sucking, oral sucrose, mechanical vibration, skin-to-skin contact) results in less pain and trauma for infants in the NICU (McGinnis, Murray, Cherven, et al., 2016; Yin, Yang, Lee, et al., 2015). When skilled phlebotomists are available, venipuncture for blood collections may be preferred.

When infants require close monitoring of oxygenation, **pulse oximetry**, a noninvasive measurement of the saturation or percent of oxygen in hemoglobin, is typically used. The nurse notes changes in oxygenation (or other aspects being monitored) associated with handling and adjusts the infant's care accordingly. The frequency of taking vital signs depends on the infant's acuity level and response to handling.

Safety Measures

The increased sophistication of supportive technology, including delivery systems, monitors, ventilator devices, and warmers, creates technology dependence for nurses providing care to high-risk infants. Although built-in safety systems and better engineering have made these devices more reliable and easier to use, our increasing reliance on them carries with it the additional risks of electrical biohazards and inaccurate function. Additionally, untrained or inexperienced operators confer an extra element of risk. Parents need instruction regarding safety precautions and observations. They are usually uncomfortable around the equipment and atmosphere of an intensive care unit and therefore appreciate an explanation of the devices and pertinent safety aspects. Although most NICUs are closed units, parents must also learn about specific safety measures designed to prevent infant abduction. Most institutions have their own protocols for preventing such an occurrence. (See Protect from Infection and Injury, Chapter 7.)

Respiratory Support

The primary objective in the care of high-risk infants is to establish and maintain respiration. Many infants require supplemental oxygen and assisted ventilation. All infants require appropriate positioning to ensure an open airway and to maximize oxygenation and ventilation. Oxygen therapy is provided on the basis of the infant's requirements and illness (see Respiratory Distress Syndrome, p. 299, and Oxygen Therapy, p. 303).

Thermoregulation

Along with the establishment of respiration, the most crucial need of the low-birth-weight (LBW) infant is external warmth. Prevention of heat loss in the distressed infant is essential for survival, and maintaining a neutral thermal environment is a challenging aspect of neonatal intensive nursing care. Heat production is a complicated process that involves the cardiovascular, neurologic, and metabolic systems, and the immature neonate has all the problems related to heat production that are faced by the full-term infant. (See Thermoregulation, Chapter 7.) However, LBW infants are placed at further disadvantage by a number of additional problems. They have an even smaller muscle mass and fewer deposits of brown fat for producing heat, lack insulating subcutaneous fat, and have poor reflex control of skin capillaries.

Pathophysiology

The immature neonate, who cannot increase activity and lacks a shivering response, produces heat mainly through increasing metabolic rate. Some heat is generated by liver, heart, brain, and skeletal muscles, but the major source of increased heat production during cold stress is **nonshivering thermogenesis**. Norepinephrine, secreted by the sympathetic nerve endings in response to chilling, stimulates fat metabolism in the richly vascularized brown adipose tissue to produce internal heat, which is then conducted through the blood to surface tissues. A significant increase in metabolism requires increased oxygen consumption.

Cold stress poses hazards to the neonate through hypoxia, metabolic acidosis, and hypoglycemia. Increased metabolism in response to chilling creates a compensatory increase in oxygen and calorie consumption.

Norepinephrine released in response to cold stress causes pulmonary vasoconstriction, which further reduces the effectiveness of pulmonary ventilation. Decreased oxygen intake reduces the supply available for glucose metabolism. As a result, glucose is broken down by an alternate, hypoxic pathway (anaerobic glycolysis) that generates increased lactic acid. This, together with acid end-products of brown fat metabolism, contributes to the acidotic state. Anaerobic metabolism consumes glycogen at a faster rate compared with aerobic metabolism, causing hypoglycemia. This condition is especially marked when glycogen stores are diminished at birth and caloric intake is inadequate after birth.

Maintaining Thermoneutrality

To delay or prevent the effects of cold stress, at-risk newborns are placed in a heated environment immediately after birth, where they remain until they are able to independently maintain **thermal stability**—a balance of heat production and conservation and heat dissipation. Because overheating produces an increase in oxygen and calorie consumption, the infant is also compromised in a hyperthermic environment. A **neutral thermal environment** is one that permits the infant to maintain a normal core temperature with minimum oxygen consumption and calorie expenditure. Studies indicate that optimum environmental temperature cannot be predicted for every high-risk infant's needs (Blackburn, 2012; Gardner, Goldson, & Hernandez, 2016).

VLBW and ELBW infants, with thin skin and almost no subcutaneous fat, can control body heat loss or gain only within a limited range of environmental temperatures. In these infants heat loss from radiation, evaporation, and **transepidermal water loss** is three to five times greater than in larger infants. A decrease in body temperature is associated with increased mortality rate.

The three main methods for maintaining a neutral thermal environment are the use of an incubator, a radiant warming panel, and an open bassinet with cotton blankets. The healthy, full-term infant dressed and under blankets can maintain a stable temperature within a wider range of environmental temperatures. However, the infant requiring close observation or treatments such as phototherapy may need to be cared for in an incubator or under radiant heat (Fig. 9.1). The incubator should always be prewarmed before placing an infant in it. Double-walled incubators significantly improve the infant's ability to maintain a desirable temperature and reduce energy expenditure related to heat regulation. The infant is clothed and warmly wrapped in blankets when removed from the warm environment of the incubator for feeding or cuddling. Inside or outside the incubator, head coverings prevent heat loss. A fabric-insulated cap is more effective than one fashioned from stockinette (Blackburn, 2012).

An automatically controlled (servocontrolled) incubator is an effective means for maintaining the desired range of temperature in the infant. The mechanism adjusts automatically in response to preset limits and signals from a thermal sensor attached to the abdomen. If the infant's temperature drops, the warming device is triggered to increase heat

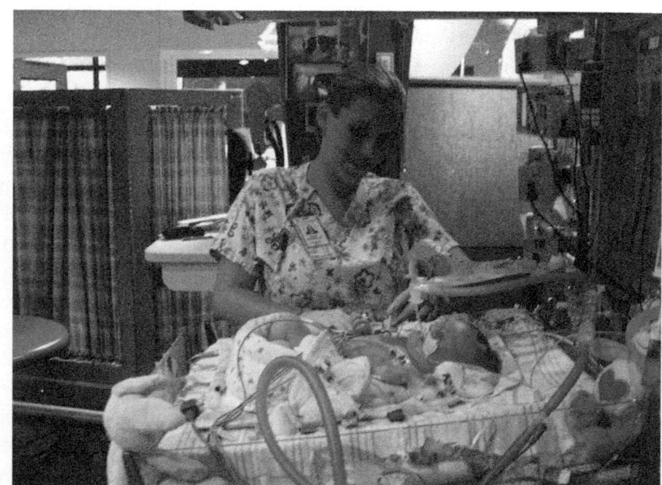

FIG. 9.1 Nurse caring for infant in radiant warmer. (Courtesy E. Jacobs, Texas Children's Hospital, Houston.)

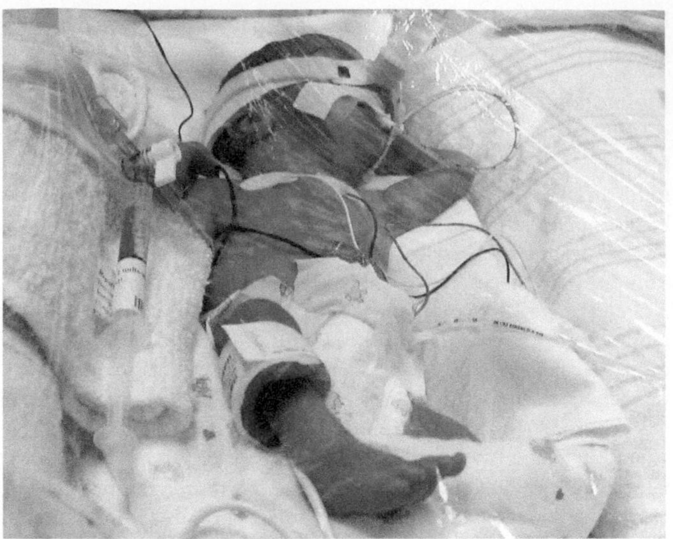

FIG. 9.2 Infant under plastic wrap, which produces a draft-free environment. (Courtesy E. Jacobs, Texas Children's Hospital, Houston.)

output. The servocontrol is usually set to a desired skin temperature between 36° and 36.5°C (96.8° and 97.7°F) (Gardner & Hernandez, 2016).

Convective heat loss occurs when infants are exposed to increased air flow velocity and turbulence (e.g., drafts from doors, ventilation system, opening and closing incubator portholes and side panels). The infant in a radiant warmer also experiences convective heat losses in response to ventilation drafts and traffic flow around the bed. These losses may be partially countered with plastic wrap placed directly on the infant's body or stretched over the side guards of the warmer unit (Fig. 9.2). A plastic bag or wrap that encloses the infant's trunk and lower extremities is also effective in decreasing heat loss in ELBW and VLBW infants. Oxygen or any source of air, such as an oxygen mask or tube, should not blow directly on the infant's face. Oxygen concentrated around the head, such as that supplied to a hood (if used) or nasal cannula, must be warmed and humidified.

Radiant heat loss is one of the greatest threats to temperature regulation in the incubator because the temperature of circulating air within has no influence on heat loss to windows, walls, or a lower nursery temperature. Such losses can be effectively reduced with the use of double-walled incubators; the infant radiates heat to the inner wall, which is surrounded by the warmed incubator air.

A high-humidity atmosphere reduces evaporative heat loss. Humidity is provided in some incubators by circulating air over a heated water reservoir, which has the additional advantage of decreasing heat loss by convection as the air flows over the infant. The water reservoir in older incubators was often a source of water-borne bacteria, requiring frequent water changes. Newer technologies such as ultrasonic nebulizers may reduce the risk of such infections. Follow manufacturer's recommendations in determining the frequency of water changes. The recommended humidity is 50% to 65%; higher humidity and a warmer environment are recommended for VLBW and ELBW infants.

A number of "microenvironments" may be used with the VLBW and ELBW infant to minimize evaporative and insensible water losses (IWLs). These include items such as bubble wrap blankets, humidified reservoirs for incubators, humidified tents, humidified Plexiglas boxes with plastic wrap coverings, polyethylene bags, and plastic wrap blankets. In cold-stressed infants, heat shields may be inappropriate because they may block heat from reaching the infant. Emollient cream has been used to prevent transepidermal water loss; however, this therapy has increased the risk of infection with coagulase-negative staphylococcus. In preterm infants weighing 750 g or less, it should be used with caution (Association of Women's Health, Obstetric and Neonatal Nurses, 2013).

The nurse can reduce conductive heat loss by warming all items that come in direct contact with the infant, such as scales, radiographic film, blankets, mattress, and the hands of caregivers. For example, the nurse can store blankets in a warming unit ready for use and place a freestanding warming unit or a heat lamp over a scale before weighing an infant.

Although the open radiant warmer unit allows easier access to the infant, there is an inherent rise in evaporative water and heat loss from the skin, especially in ELBW and VLBW infants. Transepidermal water losses, a form of IWL, may be increased by as much as 50% to 200%, thus predisposing the infant to dehydration; daily fluid requirements are generally increased to compensate for such losses. The use of plastic wrap over the ELBW or VLBW infant in a radiant warmer will help reduce IWL and convective losses.

The infant being cared for in a radiant warmer is kept warm using the servocontrol method. Air temperature manual control should not be used because of the danger of overheating the infant. A reflective aluminum temperature probe cover is used to allow proper function of the servocontrol heating unit. The temperature probe should be placed over a nonbony, well-perfused tissue area such as the abdomen or flank. In general, the probe site is changed when the infant's position is changed to prevent the probe from coming in contact with the bed surface and potentially trapping heat at the probe site, causing an abnormal ambient temperature. Chaseling, Molgat-Seon, Daboval, and colleagues (2016) found that the levels of temperature agreement between the skin (taken at different anatomic sites) and the core body temperature of neonates under a radiant warmer were poorly correlated. The researchers raised two points of concern. First, the feedback provided from a single skin temperature is unlikely to be a reliable representation of true deep core temperature. Second, skin temperature values across the body are nonuniform and the differences between the feet and the forehead/torso have up to a 6°C observed difference (Chaseling, Molgat-Seon, Daboval, et al., 2016). Minimizing thermal instability is important for infants being cared for in the NICU environment.

Sterile cloth or disposable drapes also block radiant heat waves in a radiant warmer. During such procedures, a warmed blanket or heating pad under the infant is appropriate.

Prolonged exposure to cold stress in the sick or preterm infant, particularly the ELBW or VLBW infant, may have detrimental results. Thermoregulation measures in the labor and delivery area and during transport to the NICU are essential. The use of a plastic bag or plastic wrap; careful drying; prewarming of equipment such as scales, stethoscopes, and incubators; and prompt placement of the VLBW or ELBW newborn in a proper heat source are key to the prevention of further morbidity.

High-risk infants typically have a limited ability to perspire, thus decreasing heat dissipation and increasing risk of hyperthermia. In high-risk neonates hyperthermia is usually a result of overheating rather than increased metabolism. Therefore knowledge of proper care and use of external heating devices, such as radiant warmers or incubators, is as important as knowing the conditions for which they are being used.

Protection From Infection

Protection from infection is an integral part of all newborn care, but preterm and sick neonates are particularly susceptible. Thorough and frequent hand washing is the foundation of a preventive program. This includes all persons who come in contact with infants and their equipment. After handling another infant or equipment, no one should ever touch an infant without first washing hands.

Personnel with infectious disorders are either barred from the unit until they are no longer infectious or are required to wear suitable shields, such as masks or gloves, to reduce the likelihood of contamination. Standard Precautions as a method of infection control are instituted in all nursery areas to protect the infants and staff. (See Chapter 6.)

Readmission of infants from home or admission of infants delivered in unsterile conditions or suspected of having communicable illnesses is handled per institutional protocol. Such infants should at least be initially physically isolated from other high-risk infants. (See American Academy of Pediatrics, American College of Obstetricians and Gynecologists [2012] for further infection control recommendations, including nursery care of infants with specific communicable diseases.)

Hydration

High-risk infants often receive supplemental parenteral fluids to supply additional calories, electrolytes, and/or water. Adequate hydration is particularly important in preterm infants because their extracellular water content is higher (70% in full-term infants and up to 90% in preterm infants), their body surface area is larger in comparison to their weight, and ability to concentrate urine is limited in their underdeveloped kidneys. Therefore these infants are highly vulnerable to water retention and fluid overload.

Parenteral fluids may be given to the high-risk neonate via several routes depending on the nature of the illness, the duration and type of fluid therapy, and unit preference. Common routes of fluid infusion include peripheral, peripherally inserted central venous (or percutaneous central venous), surgically inserted central venous or arterial, and, at times, umbilical venous or umbilical arterial catheterization. Special precautions and frequent observations (at least once every hour) must accompany the use of peripheral lines with hypertonic solutions (dextrose 10% to 12%) and parenteral hyperalimentation solutions. In many neonatal centers the percutaneous central venous catheter, also called the peripherally inserted central venous catheter, is used for IV hydration therapy and medication administration because of less expense and decreased neonatal trauma and because of the ease of insertion (Bradshaw & Tanaka, 2016).

In most facilities NICU nurses insert peripheral IV catheters and maintain the infusions. IV fluids must always be delivered by continuous infusion pumps that deliver minute volumes at a preset flow rate. Secure the catheter to the skin with transparent tape or a specialized IV dressing, taking care not to cause undue pressure from the needle hub and tubing. Because ELBW and VLBW infants are highly vulnerable to any fluid shifts, infusion rates are carefully regulated and checked hourly to prevent tissue damage from extravasation, fluid overload, or dehydration (Nyp, Brunkhorst, Reavey, et al., 2016). Pulmonary edema, congestive heart failure, patent ductus arteriosus (PDA), and intraventricular hemorrhage (IVH) may occur with fluid overload. Dehydration may cause electrolyte disturbances (particularly sodium), with potentially serious central nervous system (CNS) effects.

> **! NURSING ALERT**
>
> Nurses should be constantly alert for signs of infiltration (e.g., redness, edema, or color change of tissue; blanching at site) and for signs of overhydration (e.g., weight gain of >30 g/24 hr [0.07 lb], periorbital edema, tachypnea, tachycardia, and crackles on lung auscultation).

Small, fragile peripheral blood vessels are subject to rupture and subsequent infiltration. This problem is compounded by the use of infusion pumps that may continue to infuse fluid into surrounding tissues. Observations are especially important when using hypertonic solutions (e.g., calcium, sodium bicarbonate, parenteral hyperalimentation) and IV drugs (e.g., antibiotics and vasoactive drugs such as dopamine and dobutamine), which can cause serious tissue damage. With flexible catheters and small IV catheter shields, arm boards and limb restraints are usually unnecessary. If used, restraints should be checked frequently to ensure that no harm to the patient's extremity occurs and that peripheral circulation is adequate.

Infants who are ELBW, tachypneic, receiving phototherapy, or under a radiant warmer have increased IWL and require appropriate fluid adjustments. Nurses must monitor fluid status by taking daily (or more frequent) weights; accurately monitoring intake and output of all fluids, including medications and blood products; and evaluating serum electrolyte levels. ELBW infants require more frequent monitoring of these parameters because of their excessive transepidermal fluid loss, immature renal function, and tendency to become dehydrated or overhydrated. Intolerance of even dextrose 5% is not uncommon in the ELBW infant, with subsequent glycosuria and osmotic diuresis. Alterations in behavior, alertness, or activity level in infants receiving IV fluids may signal an electrolyte imbalance, hypoglycemia, or hyperglycemia. The nurse is also alert for tremors or seizures in the VLBW or ELBW infant because these may be a sign of hyponatremia or hypernatremia.

A common problem observed in infants who have an umbilical arterial catheter in place is vasoconstriction of peripheral vessels, which can seriously impair circulation. The response is triggered by arterial vasospasm caused by the presence of the catheter, the infusion of fluids, or injection of medication. Blanching of the buttocks, genitalia, or legs or feet is an indication of vasospasm. The problem must be recognized and reported promptly. The nurse must also observe for signs of thrombi in infants with umbilical venous or arterial lines. The precipitation of microthrombi in the vascular bed with the use of such catheters is commonly manifested by a sudden bluish discoloration seen in the toes, called "cath toes." Failure to alleviate the pathologic condition may result in permanent injury to the toes, foot, or leg.

Circulatory effects are observed first in the toes but may extend to include the legs and buttocks. The toes first flush and then turn a mulberry color; if the condition is not corrected, there may be serious complications involving the loss of a limb. The infant with an umbilical venous or arterial catheter should also be observed closely for catheter dislodgment and subsequent bleeding or hemorrhage; urinary output, renal function, and gastrointestinal (GI) function are also evaluated in these infants. Although the intent of such catheters is to effectively deliver IV fluids (and sometimes medications) and to obtain arterial blood gas samples, they are not without inherent complications.

Nutrition

Optimum nutrition is critical in the management of preterm infants, but difficulties arise in providing for their nutritional needs. The various mechanisms for ingestion and digestion of foods are not fully developed. The problem of providing optimal nutrition to the infant is greatest in the more immature infant.

Physiologic Characteristics

The preterm infant's need for rapid growth and daily maintenance must be met in the presence of several anatomic and physiologic challenges. Although infants demonstrate some sucking and swallowing activities before birth, coordination of these mechanisms does not occur until approximately 32 to 34 weeks of gestation, and they are not fully synchronized until 36 to 37 weeks. Initial sucking is not accompanied by swallowing, and esophageal contractions are uncoordinated. As infants mature, the suck-swallow pattern develops but is slow and ineffectual, and these reflexes may easily become exhausted.

As with most full-term infants, preterm infants have poor muscle tone in the area of the lower esophageal (cardiac) sphincter. This causes milk in the stomach to be easily regurgitated into the esophagus, where it can trigger the chemoreceptors and cause apnea (vagal stimulation) and bradycardia and increase the risk of aspiration. The stomach has a limited capacity in preterm infants and is easily overdistended, further compromising respiration.

Physiologically, late-preterm infants have approximately the same capacity to digest and absorb protein as full-term infants. However, carbohydrates and fats are less well tolerated. The secretion of lactase, a late-developing enzyme, is low in infants born before 34 weeks of gestation; formulas containing lactose may not be well tolerated. Although amylase is deficient in preterm infants, an alternative enzyme (glucoamylase) is able to compensate in most neonates so that they can tolerate moderate amounts of starch. Preterm infants are inefficient in digesting and absorbing lipids, especially the saturated triglycerides of cow's milk, because they have low levels of pancreatic lipase and low bile acid.

Nutritional Needs

The demand for nutrients in LBW infants is much higher than that in larger infants. Individual infants vary in activity level, ease of achieving basal energy expenditure, thermoneutrality, physical condition, and efficacy of nutrient absorption. The American Academy of Pediatrics, Committee on Nutrition (Kleinman & Greer, 2014) recommends an energy intake of 105 to 130 kcal/kg/day (taken enterally) for most preterm infants to achieve a satisfactory growth rate. It is estimated that for a daily weight gain of 15 g/kg, a caloric expenditure of 45 to 67 kcal/kg above the maintenance expenditure of 50 kcal/kg (Table 9.3) would be required (Kleinman & Greer, 2014). Thus the number of calories required for optimum growth in sick and VLBW infants is significantly higher than in their healthy full-term counterparts. Providing adequate calories for growth in the preterm infant with limited capability to ingest and absorb nutrients is an important part of nursing care for this population.

TABLE 9.3 Estimated Energy Requirement in Low-Birth-Weight Infants

Energy Expenditure	Average Estimation (kcal/kg/day)
Total energy used	40-60
• Resting metabolic rate	40-50*
• Activity	0-5*
Thermoregulation	0-5*
Energy synthesis	15†
Stored energy	20-30†
Stool loss (energy)	15
Energy intake	110-135†

*Energy required for maintenance.
†Energy expenditure for growth.
Adapted from Kleinman, R. E., & Greer, F. R. (Eds.). (2014). *Pediatric nutrition* (7th ed.). Elk Grove Village, IL: The Academy; and Committee on Nutrition, Enteral Nutrient Supply for Preterm Infants. (2010). Commentary from the European Society for Paediatric Gastroenterology, Hepatology, and Nutrition Committee on Nutrition. *Journal of Pediatric Gastroenterology and Nutrition, 50*(1), 85-91.

Table 9.3 shows the caloric requirements of healthy, growing preterm infants at 3 to 4 weeks of age. The energy requirements for sick and VLBW infants remain unknown; estimates are an intake of up to 105 to 115 kcal/kg/day, including a protein intake of 3.5 to 4.0 g/kg/day, for the ELBW infant (Kleinman & Greer, 2014). Because most of the nutritional stores are accumulated in the final months of gestation, preterm infants also have low stores of calcium, iron, phosphorus, proteins, and vitamins A and C.

The infant's size and condition determine the amount and method of feeding. Nutrition can be provided by either the parenteral or enteral route, or both. Total parenteral nutritional support of acutely ill infants may be accomplished with commercially available IV solutions specifically designed to meet the infant's nutritional needs, including protein, amino acids, trace minerals, vitamins, carbohydrates (dextrose), and fat (lipid emulsion). Experts recommend a protein intake of at least 2 to 3 g/kg/day started within the first few hours of life in VLBW infants to preserve body protein stores and increase plasma concentrations (Kleinman & Greer, 2014; Su, 2014). Daily monitoring of weight, electrolytes, renal function, calcium, and hydration status is carried out to ensure adequate therapy. The maintenance of adequate serum glucose homeostasis in sick preterm infants, who may depend on exogenous glucose sources for several days or weeks, is also important. Rozance, McGowan, Price-Douglas, and colleagues (2016) recommend that in sick preterm infants an operational threshold blood glucose value of 40 to 45 mg/dl (2.4 to 2.6 mmol/L) be maintained.

Studies have revealed benefits to the early introduction of small amounts of oral colostrum priming (OCP) in preterm infants (Civardi, Garofoli, Mazzucchelli, et al., 2014; Romano-Keeler, Azcarate-Peril, Weitkamp, et al., 2017). These OCP feedings have been shown to stimulate the infant's GI tract, preventing mucosal atrophy and subsequent enteral feeding difficulties. They have also been shown to reduce the risk of sepsis and shorten hospitalization (Civardi, Garofoli, Mazzucchelli, et al., 2014; Romano-Keeler, Azcarate-Peril, Weitkamp, et al., 2017).

A Cochrane review (2013) showed that infants receiving trophic feedings versus no feedings had an overall reduction in the number of days to full feedings and a shorter length of stay (Tyson & Kennedy, 2013). However, the researchers suggested that there was insufficient evidence to conclude that trophic feedings would prevent necrotizing enterocolitis (NEC).

Human milk is considered to be the ideal form of infant nutrition, and is both nationally and internationally endorsed by health organizations (American Academy of Pediatrics, 2012). There exists in the literature an abundance of evidence linking the association of human milk and improved medical outcomes for preterm infants. Overall, the evidence supports that the immune components present in human milk play a role in reducing the incidence of a variety of immune-related conditions in the preterm infant, such as NEC, retinopathy of prematurity, bronchopulmonary disease, and allergies (Abrams, Schanler, Lee, et al., 2014; Cacho, Parker, & Neu, 2016; Lechner & Vohr, 2017; Lewis, Richard, Larsen, et al., 2016).

In the preterm newborn, the mother's own milk is the first choice; when it is unavailable, donor milk is considered as the next best choice (Martin, Ling, & Blackburn, 2016). Alternatively, if breast milk is not available, commercial formulas designed specifically to meet the needs of small preterm infants that provide for adequate growth and metabolic stability can be used. Prepared formulas have the advantage of allowing more concentrated feedings.

Studies regarding the effects of long-chain polyunsaturated fatty acids (LCPUFAs) on cognitive development, visual acuity, and physical growth in full-term and preterm infants have prompted formula companies to add docosahexaenoic acid (DHA) and arachidonic acid

(AA) to their infant formulas. AA and DHA are in human milk, and their presence has been assumed to increase cognitive development in human milk–fed infants compared with infants fed a formula without these fatty acids (Tai, Wang, & Chen, 2013). A Cochrane review (2016) of 17 trials involving 2260 preterm infants concluded that no clear long-term benefit or harm was demonstrated for preterm infants receiving LCPUFA-supplemented formula (Moon, Rao, Schulzke, et al., 2016).

Milk from mothers whose infants are born before term contains more protein, sodium, chloride, and immunoglobulin A (IgA). Thus mothers are the preferred source of milk for their preterm infants. Growth factors, hormones, prolactin, calcitonin, thyroxine, steroids, and taurine (an essential amino acid) are also found in human milk. The milk produced by mothers for their infants changes in content over the first 30 days postnatally, at which time it is similar to full-term human milk. Preterm infants who received human milk during their hospitalization demonstrated better intellectual performance scores at 7½ to 8 years of age compared with children who received formula (Colaizy, Bell, Carlo, et al., 2012). Improved psychomotor development at 18 months has also been observed in preterm infants fed donor human milk compared with formula-fed preterm infants. Despite its benefits, LBW infants (<1500 g [3.3 lb]) who are exclusively fed unfortified human milk demonstrate decreased growth rates and nutritional deficiencies even beyond the hospitalization period. These infants often have inadequate calcium, phosphorus, protein, sodium, vitamins, and energy intake (Colaizy, Bell, Carlo, et al., 2012). Specially designed supplements for human milk have been developed to address these deficits. Preterm infants fed fortified human milk (FHM) have shorter hospital stays and less infection and NEC than infants given preterm formulas. Fortifiers are commercially available, usually as a liquid or powder containing protein, carbohydrate, calcium, phosphorus, magnesium, sodium, and varied amounts of zinc, copper, and vitamins. Because fortifiers do not contain sufficient iron, an exogenous source must be administered after enteral feeding. Fortifiers should be added to milk as close as possible to feeding time, and FHM should be refrigerated until it is used.

The anti-infection attributes of human milk provide more benefits for preterm infants. Secretory IgA concentration is higher in milk from mothers of preterm infants than in milk from mothers of full-term infants. IgA is important in the control of bacteria in the intestinal tract, where it inhibits adherence and proliferation of bacteria on epithelial surfaces. Additional protection from infection is provided by leukocytes, lactoferrin, and lysozyme, all of which are in human milk. Research suggests that administration of **probiotics**, live microbial supplements, decreases the incidence of NEC by normalizing intestinal flora, reducing intestinal permeability, and reducing gut inflammation (Dermyshi, Wang, Yan, et al., 2017; Sawh, Deshpande, Jansen, et al., 2016).

NEC has been shown to occur more often in formula-fed infants than in preterm infants fed human milk (Caplan, 2015). Research also suggests that NEC is less severe and the prevalence of intestinal perforation lowered when preterm infants are fed human milk (Colaizy, Bell, Carlo, et al., 2012).

Preterm infants exclusively fed human milk have demonstrated significantly decreased NEC, fewer positive blood cultures, and decreased need for antibiotics (Meier, Johnson, Patel, et al., 2017). In one study infants fed human milk also received more skin-to-skin (STS) contact with their mothers and shorter hospital stays. Neu and Sullivan (2012) suggest that STS contact might potentially stimulate the enteromammary immune system to produce specific antibodies against nosocomial pathogens in the nursery. Gastric emptying is improved with human milk feedings for preterm infants, primarily because of increased intestinal lactase and possibly decreased intestinal permeability. Finally, the psychologic advantages the mother gets from using her own milk cannot be overlooked.

For VLBW infants who cannot be breastfed, banked donor milk may be an option. Because of the anti-infective and growth-promoting properties of human milk, as well as its superior nutrition, donor milk is used in many NICUs for preterm or sick infants when the mother's own milk is not available (American Academy of Pediatrics, 2012; O'Hare, Wood, & Fiske, 2013). Unprocessed human milk from unscreened donors is not recommended because of the risk of transmission of infectious agents (American Academy of Pediatrics, 2012).

The Human Milk Banking Association of North America (HMBANA; http://www.hmbana.org) has established guidelines for donor human milk banks (Human Milk Banking Association, 2013). Donor milk banks collect, screen, process (pasteurize), and distribute milk donated by breastfeeding mothers who are feeding their own infants and pumping a few extra ounces each day for the milk bank. All donors are screened both by interview and serologically for communicable diseases. Donor milk is stored frozen until it is heat processed to kill potential pathogens (bacteria and viruses), and then it is refrozen for storage until it is dispensed for use. Heat processing adds a level of protection for the recipient that is not possible with any other donor tissue or organ. Milk is dispensed only by prescription. A per-ounce fee is charged by the bank for processing, but the HMBANA guidelines prohibit payment to donors.

Early feeding (provided that the infant is medically stable) reduces the incidence of complicating factors such as hypoglycemia and dehydration and reduces the degree of hyperbilirubinemia. The feeding regimen used varies in different units. One strategy for the prevention of NEC that has been supported by research is the use of standardized feeding protocols. A review of the literature found evidence of a significant reduction in NEC in infants fed by a standard protocol (Gephart & Hanson, 2013).

Feeding tolerance and feeding success are not entirely the same concept. **Feeding tolerance** is evaluated by (1) a soft abdomen; (2) an absence of abdominal distention or visible bowel loops on the skin surface; (3) minimum or no aspirated gastric residual; (4) presence of bowel sounds; (5) usual frequency, color, and consistency of stools; (6) minimum to no spitting up or vomiting; (7) infant's continued interest in feeding; and (8) consistent behavior pattern. Successful oral feeding should be safe, functional, and pleasurable. **Feeding success** can be measured by an infant's ability to (1) participate in feeding with energy, (2) coordinate sucking and swallowing with adequate pauses for breathing, (3) maintain vital signs and oxygenation within normal limits, (4) maintain normal muscle tone in face and body, (5) complete feeding in about 20 to 25 minutes, (6) manage a liquid bolus with minimum or no loss of liquid from mouth, (7) sustain alertness for feeding, (8) maintain strength and endurance for entire feeding, and (9) measure appropriate-for-age on standard growth curve. A preterm infant's success with feeding is first measured in terms of safety and functionality. Nurturing by holding close, but not socializing, during a feeding creates a warm and pleasurable experience. Later, after the infant is a competent feeder, socialization will enrich both parents' and infant's mealtime enjoyment.

Gavage Feeding

Gavage feeding is a safe means of meeting the nutritional requirements of infants who are not yet ready to feed orally. These infants are usually too weak to suck effectively, are unable to coordinate swallowing, or lack a gag reflex. Studies have demonstrated that both bolus and continuous feeding are equally suitable feeding strategies for preterm neonates (Bozzetti, Paterlini, De Lorenzo, et al., 2016; Rovekamp-Abels,

Hogewind-Schoonenboom, de Wijs-Meijler, et al., 2015). Intermittent gavage feeding is used as an energy-conserving technique for infants learning to nipple-feed who become excessively tired, listless, or cyanotic. Some evidence exists that preterm infants fed in response to feeding and satiation cures achieve full oral feeding earlier than infants fed prescribed volumes at scheduled intervals (Shaker, 2013; Whetten, 2016). However, a Cochrane review (2015) found that feeding preterm infants in response to their hunger and satiation cues compared with feedings done at scheduled intervals was not supported by the data as affecting important outcomes for these infants (Watson & McGuire, 2016). Optimizing enteral nutrition is very important for improving the health outcomes of preterm infants. However, further research is needed to explore how different feeding strategies affect optimal nutrition.

A size 3.5-, 5-, 6-, or 8-French feeding tube is usually used to instill the feeding, and the usual methods for determining correct placement are used. (See Chapter 22 for technique.) Although the more relaxed cardiac sphincter makes passage of the tube easier, the heart rate and blood pressure may change in response to vagal stimulation. The procedure is best accomplished when an infant is in a prone or a right side-lying position with the head slightly elevated. Small flexible nasogastric (NG) tubes (3.5 and 5 French) may be maintained as an indwelling feeding tube and used for prolonged periods without complications of intermittent removal and insertion.

The stomach is aspirated, the contents measured, and the aspirate returned as part of the feeding. However, this practice may vary, depending on circumstances and individual unit protocol.

! NURSING ALERT

An increase in gastric residuals, abdominal distention, bilious vomiting, temperature instability, apneic episodes, and bradycardia may indicate early NEC and should be called to the attention of the practitioner.

The feeding is allowed to flow by gravity, and the length of time varies. This procedure is not used as a time-saving method for the nurse. Complications of indwelling tubes include obstructed nares, mucous plugs, purulent rhinitis, epistaxis, infection, and possible stomach perforation.

Current best practice dictates a radiograph as the only certain way to determine NG tube placement in the stomach. Methods such as auscultation of an air bubble, neck-ear-xiphoid measurements for insertion depth, or pH measurements are considered imprecise when used as the only method for determination of placement of feeding tubes in infants (Taylor, Allan, McWilliam, et al., 2014). Ellett, Cohen, Perkins, and colleagues (2012) developed an age-related, height-based regression equation for determining adequate gastric tube insertion length for use in neonates less than 1 month old (corrected age). Others have developed guidelines for correct NG tube insertion and placement in LBW and term infants based on the infant's weight (Freeman, Saxton, & Holberton, 2012). Future research focusing on MRI-guided NG feeding tube placement for neonates has demonstrated feasibility and benefits (Daniels, Ireland, Kraus, et al., 2016). Further research is needed to determine optimal verification of feeding tube placement in high-risk infants.

The infant may be held during gavage feedings by the caregiver or parent. Nonnutritive sucking (NNS) on a pacifier helps infants associate sucking with satiety. A Cochrane review (2016) of NNS demonstrated a significant reduction in length of stay in preterm infants receiving an NNS intervention. Other positive outcomes of NNS included enhanced transition from tube- to bottle-feeding and better bottle-feeding performance (Foster, Psaila, & Patterson, 2016).

Oral Feeding

Vigorous infants can be fed orally with little difficulty, but compromised preterm infants require alternative methods. The amount to be fed is determined largely by the infant's weight gain and tolerance of previous feeding and is increased by small increments until a satisfactory caloric intake is ensured.

The rate of tolerated increase varies from one infant to another, and determining this rate is often a nursing responsibility. Preterm infants require more time and patience to feed than full-term infants, and the oropharyngeal mechanism may be stressed by an attempt to feed too rapidly. It is important not to tire the infants or overtax their capacity to retain the feedings. When infants require a prolonged time (25 to >30 minutes) to complete a feeding, gavage feeding may be considered.

The decision regarding when to start breastfeeding or bottle-feeding is somewhat controversial. In many cases it is based on the infant's developmental maturity, weight, activity level, respiratory status (absence of apnea and adequate oxygen saturation levels), and sucking capabilities. Infant behavioral organizational skills, such as the ability to maintain a quiet alert state and display engagement cues, also influence the preterm infant's successful transition to oral feedings (Lau, 2012; Lubbe, 2017). When infants are unable to tolerate breastfeedings or bottle-feedings, intermittent feedings by gavage begin until they gain enough strength and coordination to use the nipple.

! NURSING ALERT

Poor feeding behaviors such as apnea, bradycardia, cyanosis, pallor, and decreased oxygen saturation in any infant who has previously fed well may indicate an underlying illness in the preterm infant.

Although the nurse's role in relation to feeding depends on the institution, some suggested nursing responsibilities are: (1) recognize feeding readiness cues; (2) identify feeding behaviors typical of preterm infants; (3) understand the infant's history and current medical condition; (4) consider environment, behavioral state, time of day, nipple type, and positioning; (5) understand rationale for different facilitation techniques and use appropriately; (6) evaluate feeding ability and tolerance; (7) identify infants with poor progress, structural defects, or abnormal feeding patterns who would benefit from specific therapy; and (8) support mothers who choose to breastfeed.

A developmental approach to feeding considers the individual infant's readiness rather than initiating feedings based on weight and age. Feeding readiness is determined by each infant's medical status, energy level, ability to sustain a brief quiet alert state, gag reflex (demonstrated with gavage tube insertion), spontaneous rooting and sucking behaviors, and functional sucking reflex (Jones, 2012; Newland, L'huillier, & Petrey, 2013).

Oral feeding guidelines for preterm infants remain unclear. Feeding preterm infants in response to their hunger and satiation cues (responsive, cue-based, or infant-led feeding) rather than at scheduled intervals might enhance infants' and parents' experience and satisfaction, help in the establishment of independent oral feeding, increase nutrient intake and growth rates, and allow earlier hospital discharge. However, a Cochrane review (2016) found that the data did not provide strong or consistent evidence that responsive feeding (initiating feeds based on the readiness cures of the infant) affected important outcomes for preterm infants (Watson & McGuire, 2016). Nurse responsibilities for assessing, monitoring, and assisting with oral feedings are paramount to preterm infants' ability to master oral feedings. The nurse must first assess the following:

BOX 9.2 Feeding Stress Cues

Color Change
Pallor, dusky, gray, central cyanosis—perioral/periorbital

Changes in State of Alertness
Increasing drowsiness, falling asleep
Restlessness

Breathing
Respiratory fatigue
Tachypnea
Nasal flaring, retractions (increased work of breathing)
Chin tugging/head bobbing

Swallowing
Drooling
Gulping
Gurgling sounds
Coughing, choking, spitting up

Modified from Gardner, S. L., Goldson, E., & Hernandez, J. A. (2016). The neonate and the environment: Impact on development. In S. L. Gardner, B. S. Carter, M. Enzman-Hines, et al. (Eds.), *Merenstein and Gardner's handbook of neonatal intensive care* (8th ed.). St. Louis, MO: Mosby.

BOX 9.3 Feeding Facilitation Techniques for Preterm Infants

Environment
Prepare calm, quiet area with dim lighting and no distractions.
Ensure restful environment between feedings.

Direct Care
Avoid trial oral feedings after stressful procedures.
Choose slightly firm nipple with slower flow.
Gently arouse to alert state.
Swaddle in gentle flexion with infant's hands midline and toward face.
Support positioning with infant cradled close to body in semiupright or upright position, with neck in neutral to slightly flexed position.
Continuously observe physiologic, behavioral, and oral-motor functioning.
Provide adequate breathing and rest periods for infants who cannot pace themselves by gently removing nipple or, if that is too stressful, tipping bottle gently downward to drain milk from nipple.
Provide firm but gentle jaw and cheek support for problems with latching onto nipple (e.g., weak seal, loss of milk bolus).
Institute "developmental burping" on shoulder with postural support and gentle back rubbing in an upward motion to stimulate burp.
Recognize infant's limits and when to stop feeding.
Use gavage for the rest of the feeding as needed.
Schedule plenty of undisturbed rest between feedings.

Family Support and Education
Model appropriate feeding techniques.
Provide opportunity for feeding.
Educate on infant cues and how to measure feeding success.

Modified from Hunter, J. (2010). The neonatal intensive care unit. In J. Case-Smith (Ed.), *Occupational therapy for children* (6th ed.). St. Louis, MO: Mosby.

1. Assessing individual physiologic, motor, and state behaviors during feeding
2. Individualizing the feeding plan based on specific infant cues at each feeding opportunity
3. Fostering parental skill and confidence with feeding

The nurse's support of feeding, skill development, and protection from behavioral and physiologic stress during the feeding may have significant implications for the both the infant and the mother as both build confidence (Park, Thoyre, Estrem, et al., 2016; Thoyre, Hubbard, Park, et al., 2016).

The goal of feeding must be well understood. A key concept is recognizing the difference between a successful feeding (volume and time) and a successful feeder (infant ability and enjoyment). This is the difference between task and developmental feeding techniques. Planning the progression and nature of feedings requires close monitoring and careful documentation. Baseline assessment data are collected before each feeding and observed during and after the feeding to make a comparative evaluation of feeding success. Assessment is ongoing throughout the feeding. Facilitation techniques are chosen based on the individual infant's responses to improve the chance for feeding success and tolerance (Thoyre, Hubbard, Park, et al., 2016). Feeding stress and performance (Box 9.2) are evaluated and documented. Planning is done in collaboration with the health care team and family before the next feeding to determine appropriate strategies for the infant. Box 9.3 gives examples of ways to facilitate feeding.

Breastfeeding

The American Academy of Pediatrics (2012) recommends human milk for all infants, including sick newborns and preterm infants (with rare exceptions). The Academy recognizes that the choice of what to feed is the parents' prerogative but advises that providers give parents complete and accurate information on the benefits and the risks of not providing breast milk to ensure that an informed decision is made. Barriers to initiation and continuation of breastfeeding include physician indifference, misinformation, lack of prenatal education about breastfeeding, distracting hospital policies, lack of follow-up, maternal employment, lack of support from family or society, hospital discharge packs with formula or coupons for formula, and media portrayal of bottle-feeding.

Studies indicate that even small preterm infants are able to breastfeed if they have adequate sucking and swallowing reflexes and no other contraindications, such as respiratory complications or concurrent illness (Meier, Johnson, Patel, et al., 2017). Mothers who wish to breastfeed their preterm infants should pump their breasts until their infants are stable enough to tolerate breastfeeding. Protecting maternal human milk volumes in breast pump–dependent mothers of preterm infants is paramount to breastfeeding success. Appropriate guidelines for the storage of expressed mother's milk should be followed to decrease the risk of milk contamination and destruction of its beneficial properties. (See Chapter 7.)

Preterm infants may be able to successfully breastfeed earlier than previously believed (28 to 36 weeks). In addition, preterm infants who are breastfed rather than bottle-fed demonstrate fewer oxygen desaturation episodes, an absence of bradycardia, warmer skin temperature, and better coordination of breathing, sucking, and swallowing (Gardner & Lawrence, 2016). The nurse should carefully evaluate the preterm infant for readiness to breastfeed, including assessment of behavioral state, ability to maintain body temperature outside an artificial heat source, respiratory status, and readiness to suckle at the mother's breast. The latter may be accomplished with NNS at the breast during STS (or kangaroo) contact so the mother and newborn can become accustomed to each other (Gardner & Lawrence, 2016; Meier, Johnson, Patel, et al.,

2017). Nasal cannula oxygen may also be provided during breastfeeding if required by the infant.

Time, patience, and dedication on the part of the mother and the nursing staff are necessary to ensure breastfeeding success. The process starts slowly, beginning with one oral feeding daily and gradually increasing the feedings as the infant tolerates them. Human milk provides both short-term and long-term advantages in a dose-dependent relationship in that the more breast milk the preterm receives, the more benefits are gained (Gardner & Lawrence, 2016; Meier, Johnson, Patel, et al., 2017). Supplementary bottle-feeding is inefficient because the infant expends energy and calories to feed twice. Feeding more often and/or supplementing with gavage feeding are more energy and calorie efficient. Breastfeeding the preterm infant often requires additional guidance by a lactation consultant and continued support and encouragement by the nursing staff. In addition, postdischarge breastfeeding often requires further guidance, counseling, and support.

Social support for the mother is a major influence on the decision to breastfeed. To be effective advocates for mothers of all ethnicities, nurses must understand the cultural aspects that influence, whether positively or negatively, breastfeeding choices (Fabiyi, Peacock, Hebert-Beirne, et al., 2016). African American women, for example, identify prenatal health care providers and friends as influential in decisions regarding breastfeeding. They tend to breastfeed less than women from other cultures and should be provided with appropriate information on breastfeeding by health care providers. Breastfeeding materials are available from organizations such as La Leche League International.*

Nipple-Feeding

The infant is positioned in the feeder's arms or placed semiupright in the lap and is held with the back curved slightly to simulate the position assumed naturally by most full-term newborns. Oral sensitivity can be promoted by the stroking of the infant's lips, cheeks, and tongue before feeding.

Brown, Hendrickson, Evans, and colleagues (2016) used the semi–elevated side-lying (ESL) position when introducing bottle feedings to preterm infants between 32 and 36 weeks of age. The ESL position better mimics the breastfeeding position and allows for better coordination of breathing with swallowing (Fig. 9.3). Supported infants had fewer and shorter pauses during feeding and had higher postfeeding oxygen saturations than infants not receiving oral support (Brown, Hendrickson, Evans, et al., 2016). As infants mature, they can be transitioned to the semi–elevated recumbent position. Bottle-feedings continue if infants are able to tolerate the feedings. The infant is best fed when fully alert. Drowsy infants feed more slowly, and liquid is more likely to fill the relaxed pharynx before the infant swallows, causing choking. Many digestive processes are believed to require signal stimulation to respond. Some preterm infants respond more slowly than full-term infants, so the feeding interval and amount are individualized. Preterm infants are often slow feeders and require patience, frequent rest periods, and burping (or bubbling). Provider pacing is important until the infant learns to self-pace during a feeding (Brown, Hendrickson, Evans, et al., 2016).

Choosing an appropriate nipple is important. The nipple used should be relatively firm and stable. Although a high-flow, pliable nipple requires less energy to use, it may provide a flow rate that is too rapid for some preterm infants to manage without risk of aspiration. A firmer nipple facilitates a more "cupped" tongue configuration and allows for a more controlled, manageable flow rate.

*PO Box 4079, Schaumburg, IL 60618; 847-519-9585 (order department); http://www.llli.org. In Canada, La Leche League Canada, PO Box 700, Winchester, ON KOC 2KO; 613-774-4900; http://www.lalecheleaguecanada.ca.

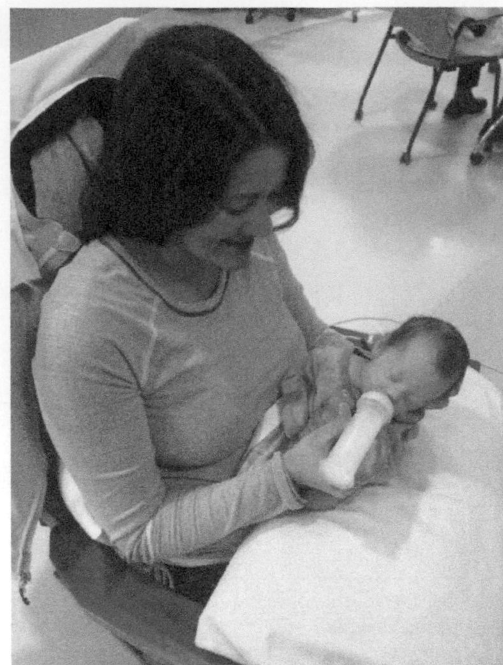

FIG. 9.3 Nipple-feeding the preterm infant using ESL technique.

Prodding techniques to encourage sucking can increase the risk of aspiration, especially if adequate breathing opportunities are not provided. The preterm infant has difficulty managing rapid or continuous milk flow with suck, swallow, and breathing coordination when the nipple is manipulated frequently by twisting or turning; the bottle is moved up and down or in and out of the mouth; or the infant's jaw is moved up and down (not the same as cheek and jaw support). The infant will try to continue to suck or swallow at the risk of physiologic and behavioral consequences.

Garber (2013) has demonstrated that a paced bottle-feeding protocol structured to limit the length of sucking bursts and lengthen the duration of swallowing and breathing resulted in earlier emergence of organized sucking patterns than traditional approaches to feeding. Lau (2012) found that a systematic protocol of oral motor stimulation enhanced tongue and jaw muscle strength and coordination.

Feeding Resistance

Any feeding technique that bypasses the mouth prevents the infant from practicing sucking and swallowing or experiencing normal hunger and satiation cycles. Infants may demonstrate aversion to oral feedings by averting the head from the nipple, extruding the nipple by tongue thrust, gagging, or even vomiting.

Developmental delays have occurred in perceptual-motor performance among infants with feeding refusal as measured by standard tests, although intellectual function remains within normal limits. Other observations include disinterest in or active resistance to oral play, diminished spontaneity and motivation, and shallow interpersonal relationships, probably related to the absence of some early incorporative patterns of normal oral experiences. The longer the period of nonoral feeding, the more severe the feeding problems, especially if this period occurs during a time when the infant progresses from reflexive to learned and voluntary feeding actions. During infancy the mouth is the primary instrument for reception of stimulation and pleasure.

Infants identified as being at risk for feeding resistance should receive regular oral stimulation based on the child's developmental level. Those who exhibit feeding aversion should begin a stimulation program to overcome resistance and acquire the ability to take nourishment by mouth. Because management requires long-term commitment, successful implementation of a plan for oral stimulation depends on maximum parental involvement and promotion of primary nursing. Key strategies and interventions are in Box 9.4.

BOX 9.4 Strategies to Prevent or Overcome Feeding Resistance

Minimize noxious stimuli to the mouth
- Suction only as needed (not routinely)
- Consider indwelling gastric tube rather than intermittent gavage
- Use perioral and intraoral stimulation techniques

Enhance pleasant stimuli to mouth
- Have infant smell or taste breastmilk
- Provide nonnutritive suckling while tube feeding
- Use nipple with proper flow
- Use perioral and intraoral stimulation

Use proper position to facilitate swallow and improve suction
- Hold with feedings
- Swaddle
- Facilitate swallowing (e.g. position with chin tucked)
- Improve formation of suction (e.g. cupping both cheeks for support)

Timing
- Do not allow infant to cry before feeding
- Keep external stimuli to a minimum
- Feed for short periods at first

Modified from Gardner, S. L., Goldson, E., & Hernandez, J. A. (2016). The neonate and the environment: Impact on development. In S. L. Gardner, B. S. Carter, M. Enzman-Hines, et al. (Eds.), *Merenstein and Gardner's handbook of neonatal intensive care* (8th ed.). St. Louis, MO: Mosby.

Skin Care

Preterm infants have immature skin with increased sensitivity and fragility. Alkaline-based soap that might destroy the "acid mantle" of the skin should be avoided. The increased permeability of the skin facilitates absorption of ingredients. All skin products (e.g., alcohol or povidone-iodine) are used with caution. The skin is rinsed with water afterward because these substances may cause severe irritation and chemical burns in LBW infants.

The skin is easily excoriated and denuded; therefore take care to avoid damage to the delicate structure. The total skin is thinner than that of full-term infants and lacks rete pegs, appendages that anchor the epidermis to the dermis. Therefore there is less cohesion between the thinner skin layers. Adhesives used after heel sticks or to secure monitoring equipment or IV infusions may excoriate the skin or adhere to the skin surface so well that the epidermis can be separated from the dermis and pulled away with the tape. The use of a zinc oxide–based tape is encouraged to minimize epidermal stripping: the tape is flexible, waterproof, and washable. Skin barriers protect healthy skin and help excoriated skin heal.

Use scissors very carefully to remove dressings or tape from the extremities of very small and immature infants because it is easy to snip off tiny extremities or nick loosely attached skin. Avoid solvents because they tend to dry and burn delicate skin. Guidelines for skin care are given in the Applying Evidence to Practice box.

Although no studies comparing the effectiveness of different commercially available neonatal bedding have been done, a number of products are useful in minimizing skin problems. The Applying Evidence to Practice box gives general information about bedding. Particularly vulnerable areas of the skin, such as bony prominences, can be protected with clear dressings. Gel pads or mattresses can also be used to prevent pressure ulcers (Association of Women's Health, Obstetric and Neonatal Nurses, 2013).

APPLYING EVIDENCE TO PRACTICE

Neonatal Skin Care

General Skin Care*

Assessment

Assess skin once each shift for redness, dryness, flaking, scaling, rashes, lesions, excoriation, or breakdown.

Consider using a validated skin assessment tool such as the Neonatal Skin Condition Score (Lund & Osborne, 2004) or the Delphi Skin Assessment Tool (Vance, Demel, Kirksey, et al., 2015).

Identify those infants at increased risk for skin breakdown.

Evaluate and report abnormal skin findings and analyze for possible causation.

Intervene according to interpretation of findings or physician order.

Bathing

Initial Bath

Assess for stable temperature a minimum of 2 to 4 hours before first bath.

Use cleansing agents with neutral pH or minimum dyes or perfume, in water.

Do not completely remove vernix caseosa.

Bathe preterm infant (<32 weeks of gestation) in sterile water alone.

Routine

Decrease frequency of baths to every second or third day by daily cleansing of eye, oral, and diaper areas, and pressure points.

Use cleanser or soaps no more than two or three times a week.

Avoid rubbing skin during bathing or drying.

Immerse stable infants fully (except head) in an appropriate-sized tub.

Use swaddled immersion bathing technique: slow unwrapping after gently lowering into water for sensitive, but stable, infants needing assistance with motor system reactivity.

Emollients

Follow hospital protocol or consider the following:
- Apply emollient as needed for dry, flaking skin.
- Use only emollients without perfumes, preservatives, or dyes.

Adhesives

Decrease use as much as possible.

Use transparent semipermeable adhesive dressings to secure intravenous lines, catheters, and central lines.

Use hydrogel electrodes.

Consider using pectin or hydrocolloid barriers beneath adhesives to protect skin.

Secure pulse oximeter probe or electrodes with elasticized dressing material (carefully avoid restricting blood flow).

Do not use adhesive remover, solvents, and bonding agents.

Avoid removing adhesives for at least 24 hours after application.

Use water, mineral oil, or petrolatum to facilitate adhesive removal.

Remove adhesives or skin barriers slowly, supporting the skin underneath with one hand and gently peeling away from the skin with the other hand.†

Continued

APPLYING EVIDENCE TO PRACTICE—cont'd

Neonatal Skin Care

Antiseptic Agents

Apply before invasive procedures.

Evaluate the risks and benefits of any antiseptic agent. Chlorhexidine gluconate and 10% povidone-iodine have both been shown to reduce skin bacterial counts in newborns. Povidone-iodine may be absorbed systemically. Chlorhexidine 2% may cause burns in VLBW infants; the US Food and Drug Administration (2012) recommends that it be used with care in premature infants or those under 2 months of age. Avoid use of alcohol.

Transepidermal Water Loss

Minimize transepidermal water loss and heat loss in small preterm infants (<30 weeks of gestation) by measuring ambient humidity during first weeks of life and considering an increase in humidity to 70% for the first week of life by using one or more of the following options or hospital guidelines:

- Transparent dressings
- Servocontrolled humidifying incubator
- Supplemental conductive heat sources such as heated mattresses
- Polyethylene coverings (but avoid having plastic wraps in contact with skin surfaces for long periods)

Skin Breakdown*

Prevention

Decrease pressure from externally applied forces using water, air, or gel mattresses; sheepskin; or cotton bedding.

Provide adequate nutrition, including protein, fat, and zinc.

Apply transparent adhesive dressings to protect arms, elbows, and knees from friction injury.

Use tracheostomy and gastrostomy dressings for drainage and relief of pressure from tracheostomy or gastrostomy tube (Hydrasorb or Lyofoam).

Use emollient in the diaper area (groin and thighs) to reduce urine irritation.

Treating Skin Breakdown

Irrigate wound every 4 to 6 hours with warm half-strength normal saline using a 30-ml or larger syringe and 20-gauge Teflon catheter.

Culture wound and treat if signs of infection are present (e.g., excessive redness, swelling, pain on touch, heat, or resistance to healing).

Use petrolatum-based ointments for uninfected wounds.

Apply hydrogel with or without antibacterial or antifungal ointments (as ordered) for infected wounds (may need to moisten before removal).

Use hydrocolloid for deep, uninfected wounds (leave in place for 5 to 7 days) or as an ostomy barrier and to improve appliance adhesion; warm barrier in hand for several minutes to soften before applying to skin.

Avoid use of antiseptic solutions for wound cleansing (used for intact skin only).

Treating Diaper Dermatitis

Maintain clean, dry skin; use absorbent diapers and change often.

If mild irritation occurs, use petrolatum barrier.

For developing dermatitis, apply a generous quantity of zinc-oxide barrier.

For severe dermatitis, identify cause and treat (e.g., frequent stooling from spina bifida, severe opiate withdrawal, or malabsorption syndrome).

Treat *Candida albicans* with antifungal ointment or cream.

Avoid talcum powders and antibiotic ointments. (See Care of the Umbilicus and Circumcision, Chapter 7.)

Other Skin Care Concerns‡

Use of Substances on Skin

Evaluate all substances that come in contact with infant's skin.

Before using any topical agent, analyze components of preparation and:

- Use sparingly and only when necessary.
- Confine use to smallest possible area.
- Whenever possible and appropriate, wash off with water.
- Monitor infant carefully for signs of toxicity and systemic effects.

Use of Fluid Therapy and Hemodynamic Monitoring

Be certain fingers or toes are visible whenever extremity is used for intravenous or arterial line.

Secure catheter with transparent dressing or tape to promote easy visualization of site.

Assess site hourly for signs of ischemia, infiltration, and inadequate perfusion (check capillary refill).

Avoid use of restraints (e.g., arm boards); if used, check that they are secured safely and not restricting circulation or movement (check for pressure areas).

Use commercial intravenous protector (e.g., I.V. House) with minimum tape.

*From Association of Women's Health, Obstetric and Neonatal Nurses. (2013). *Evidence-based clinical practice guideline: Neonatal skin care* (3rd ed.). Washington, DC: The Association.

†CAUTION: Scissors are not to be used for tape or dressing removal because of hazard of cutting skin or tiny digits.

‡Data from Ness, M. J., Davis, D. M., & Carey, W. A. (2013). Neonatal skin care: A concise review. *International Journal of Dermatology, 52*(1), 14-22; Fox, M. D. (2011). Wound care in the neonatal intensive care unit. *Neonatal Network, 30*(5), 291-303.

Skin injuries have been reported with phototherapy blankets. Caution is needed in using these products with extremely preterm infants or infants with birth trauma, poorly perfused skin, or hypotension. Manufacturers of phototherapy blankets recommend that practitioners monitor skin color, observe for rashes or excoriation, keep skin clean with warm water, promptly clean perineum after stooling, reposition every 2 hours, carefully monitor cleanliness and skin integrity, and avoid direct contact of blanket with infant's skin.

Administration of Medications

Administration of therapeutic agents, such as drugs, ointments, IV infusions, and oxygen, requires careful attention to detail. The computation, preparation, and administration of drugs in minute amounts require collaboration among nurses, physicians, and pharmacists to reduce the chance for error. The immaturity of an infant's detoxification mechanisms and inability to demonstrate symptoms of toxicity (e.g., signs of auditory nerve involvement from ototoxic drugs such as gentamycin) complicate drug therapy and require that nurses be particularly alert for signs of adverse reaction. (See Administration of Medication, Chapter 22.)

Nurses should be aware of the hazards of administering bacteriostatic and hyperosmolar solutions to infants. Benzyl alcohol, a common preservative in bacteriostatic water, heparin sodium, and some saline flushes, is toxic to newborns and should not be used to flush IV catheters or to dilute or reconstitute medications. It is recommended that medications with preservatives such as benzyl alcohol be avoided. Nurses must read labels carefully to detect the presence of preservatives in any medication administered to an infant.

Hyperosmolar solutions present a potential danger to preterm infants. Hyperosmolar solutions given orally to infants can produce clinical, physiologic, and morphologic alterations, the most serious of which is NEC. Oral or parenteral medications should be sufficiently diluted to prevent complications related to hyperosmolality.

Take caution to reduce adverse effects of medication administration in preterm infants. Strategies to heighten awareness and decrease unnecessary morbidity in such infants include having two registered nurses double-check the dosages of potentially lethal medications (high-risk medications) and providing calculators in neonatal units to perform dosage calculations, double-check unit dose medications, and have the hospital pharmacy reconstitute medications. Another strategy is to develop computerized guidelines for managing dose ranges based on the neonate's most recent weight so medications ordered outside the appropriate dose range are reevaluated by the pharmacist and practitioner. Information technology (e.g., computerized practitioner order entry and clinical participation by a clinical pharmacist) is available to reduce medication errors, yet this technology does not provide the entire solution (Campino, Santesteban, Pascual, et al., 2016). Medication errors are rarely the result of one, single individual action; more often, multiple mistakes during the medication use process occur resulting in an error. Nurses, physicians, and pharmacists are at times affected by internal and external environmental factors that lead to a medication error: excessive workload; distractions such as a monitor alarm or questions asked during medication administration; boredom; work hours (nighttime or daytime); lack of updated or consistent drug information; ambiguous drug labeling; and dosage calculation errors (Sorrentino & Alegiani, 2012). The variables involved are numerous and multifaceted, yet can be decreased by simple cautionary measures, extensive education, and verification of medication orders written. Evidence-based interventions implemented in collaboration with pharmacist can be an effective way of reducing medication errors (Santesteban, Arenas, & Campino, 2015).

Developmental Outcome

Neonatal intensive care and rapid improvements in technology are associated with improved survival of critically ill newborn and preterm infants. Survival rates have increased to 94% for VLBW infants (1001 to 1500 g [2.2 to 3.3 lb]), 88% for ELBW infants (751 to 1000 g [1.6 to 2.2 lb]), and 63% for infants weighing 501 to 750 g [1.1 to 1.6 lb] (Horbar, Carpenter, Badger, et al., 2012). With decreasing mortality rates, morbidity rates have remained stable. At highest risk for unfavorable outcomes are preterm infants compromised during the neonatal period by respiratory distress syndrome (RDS), bronchopulmonary dysplasia (BPD, or chronic lung disease), NEC, sepsis, anemia, IVH, hydrocephalus, meningitis, or seizures (Rogers & Hintz, 2016). These serious sequelae of prematurity correlate with the degree of immaturity, demonstrating the relationship of increasing morbidity associated with decreasing gestational age. A greater incidence of CP, attention-deficit/hyperactivity disorder, visual-motor deficits, mild to severe cognitive disabilities, hearing loss, speech and language impairment, and neuromotor problems has been reported in outcome studies of preterm infants (Church, Luther, & Asztalos, 2012; Rogers & Hintz, 2016). Moderate and late-preterm infants also exhibit developmental delay compared with their term-born peers, most often noted in the language domain (Cheong, Doyle, Burnett, et al., 2017).

An increased need for special school services, especially in reading and math, has been reported in former LBW infants at 8 years of age (Litt, Glymour, Hauser-Cram, et al., 2015). A study of 576 preterm infants found that, when evaluated at 8 and 18 years of age, 80% of the cohort had special health care needs (SHCN) and those with SHCN had lower mean achievement scores in both math and reading (Litt & McCormick, 2016). The researchers concluded that SHCN are associated with poor academic achievement and recommended targeted interventions for improving the burden of chronic health problems through prevention strategies for LBW infants (Litt & McCormick, 2016). Neurodevelopmental impairment also occurs in preterm infants without the complications of IVH, sepsis, and hypoxemia. Conversely, some preterm infants do well and function at age level without evidence of neurobehavioral limitations. Improved developmental outcomes are more likely for these infants with the finest medical and nursing care within a developmentally supportive framework. This philosophy requires caregivers to evaluate their own knowledge, skills, and attitudes and expand their thinking beyond the traditional medical and nursing models of care.

The rates of survival have increased among infants born at the borderline of viability (22 to 24 weeks of gestation). Younge, Goldstein, Bann, and colleagues (2017) reported on survival outcomes for periviable infants born at 11 centers across the United States and concluded that the rate of survival without neurodevelopmental impairment increased between 2000 and 2011. Despite these improvements for periviable infants, the incidence of death, neurodevelopmental impairment, and other adverse outcomes remains high in this population (Younge, Goldstein, Bann, et al., 2017). The researchers cautioned that despite improvements over time in this periviable population, the incidence of death, neurodevelopmental impairment, and other adverse outcomes remains high.

Developmental Assessment

One approach to NICU care is based on Als's (1982) **synactive theory of infant development**, which provides a framework for understanding the preterm infant's development. The model proposes a systematic method for observing NICU infants to collect information concerning each infant's competencies, vulnerabilities, and thresholds. This information forms the basis for planning individualized care appropriate for a particular infant (Table 9.4). The major assumption of this model is that infants, even ELBW infants, can communicate through physical and behavioral responses that provide us with the best information for planning their care. Communication by the infant is seen through three subsystems of function (autonomic, motor, and state) that can be readily observed in the clinical setting during rest, care, or procedures and during recovery from care or procedures. Responses by an infant's autonomic (physiologic), motor, and state systems to the environment, physical care, or procedures help the nurse make necessary adjustments to optimize the infant's stability and function.

Individualized developmental care has had positive effects on medical and neurobehavioral outcomes in high-risk newborn infants. A study of developmental care for preterm infants found earlier oral feeding; reduced need for mechanical ventilation or supplemental oxygen; decreased time in the hospital; improved weight gain; enhanced autonomic, motor, state, attention, and self-regulatory function; and lowered family stress (Als, 2009; Macho, 2017). In contrast, a systematic review done by Ohlsson and Jacobs (2013) noted that the evidence did not demonstrate that individualized developmental care improved long-term neurodevelopmental or short-term medical outcomes for preterm infants.

Because each infant is unique, supportive developmental care requires ongoing data collection of moment-by-moment responses and flexible care to address the infant's cues. For example, an infant who demonstrates altered vital signs and even apnea after being weighed might benefit from swaddled weighing to support the infant's competence and organization during a stressful procedure.

Knowledge of behavioral assessment and infant development assists the nurse in providing care that supports each infant's ongoing function in a manner consistent with current evidence. Nurses have the greatest impact on the daily routine experienced by their patients. The CNS is undergoing rapid and significant change during the preterm infant's

TABLE 9.4 **Synactive Theory of Development: Neurobehavioral Subsystems**

Subsystem	Signs of Stress	Signs of Stability
Autonomic	Physiologic instability	Physiologic stability
Respiratory	Tachypnea, pauses, gasping, sighing	Smooth, stable respirations; regular rate and pattern
Color	Mottled, flushed, dusky, pale or gray	Pink, stable color
Visceral	Hiccups, gagging, choking, spitting up, grunting and straining as if having a bowel movement; coughing, sneezing, yawning	Absence of hiccups, gagging, spitting up, etc.
Autonomic	Tremors, startles, twitches	Absence of tremors, startles, twitches
Motor	Fluctuating tone; lack of control over movement, activity, and posture	Consistent tone; controlled or improved movement, activity, and posture
Flaccidity	Low tone in trunk; limp, floppy upper and lower extremities; limp, drooping jaw (gape face)	Tone consistent and appropriate for postmenstrual age Well-maintained posture
Hypertonicity	Arm or leg extensions, arm(s) outstretched with fingers splayed in salute gesture, fingers stiffly outstretched, trunk arching, neck hyperextended	Smooth, controlled movements
Hyperflexion activity	Trunk hyperflexion, hyperflexion of extremities, fisting; squirming; frantic diffuse activity or little or no activity or responsiveness	Successful motor strategies for self-regulation (see Self-Regulation below)
State	Disorganized quality to state behaviors, including range of available states, maintenance of state control, and transition from one state to another	Easy-to-read state behaviors that are maintained; calm, focused alertness, well-modulated sleep
Sleep	Whimpering sounds, facial twitching, irregular respirations, fussing, grimacing, restless appearance	Clear, well-defined sleep states; periods of quiet, restful sleep
Awake	Glazed unfocused look, staring, worried or pained expression, hyperalert or panicked appearance, eye roving, crying, "cry-face," actively averting gaze or closing eyes, irritability, prolonged awake periods, inconsolability, frenzy Abrupt or rapid state changes	Alert with bright, shiny eyes; focused attention on object or person; animated expression (e.g., cheek softening, frowning, "ooh-face," cooing, smiling) Robust crying Good calming, consolability Smooth changes between states, full range of sleep-wake states
Other state-related behaviors and attention-interaction	Efforts to attend to and interact with environmental stimulation eliciting signs of stress and disorganized subsystem functioning	Responsive to auditory, visual, and social stimuli
Autonomic	Physiologic instability of varying degrees with autonomic, respiratory, color, and visceral responses	Responsiveness to stimuli well maintained and prolonged
Motor	Fluctuating tone, increased motor activity, progressively frantic diffuse activity if stimulation continues	Actively seeking auditory stimulus, minimum motor activity
State	Roving eyes, gaze averted, glazed-unfocused look or worried, panicked expression; weak cry; cry-face; irritability Closed eyes and sleeplike withdrawal Abrupt state changes Signs of stress when presented with more than one type of stimulus at a time	Bright, shiny-eyed, alert, and attentive expression Sustained awake and alert state Shifting attention smoothly to more than one type of stimulation

Self-regulation—Infant's efforts to achieve, maintain, or regain a balanced, stable, and relaxed stated of subsystem functioning and integration. Success of these efforts will vary among infants depending on maturity, available self-regulatory skills, and overall subsystem organization. Examples of self-regulatory strategies include the following:

Motor—Foot bracing against a boundary or blanket nest, hand holding, clasping hands together, hand to mouth or face, grasping blanket, tubing, tucking trunk, sucking, position changes

State—Lowering state from high arousal to quiet alert or sleep state; releasing energy by rhythmic, robust crying; focused attention and orientation

Facilitation by caregivers—Environmental modifications or developmental care techniques to aid infant's own self-regulatory abilities when environmental challenges exceed infant's capabilities.

Modified from Als, H. (1982). Toward a synactive theory of development: Promise for the assessment and support of infant individuality. *Infant Mental Health Journal, 3*(4), 229-243; Als, H. (1986). A synactive model of neonatal behavior organization: Framework for the assessment of neurobehavioral development in the premature infant and for support of infants and parents in the neonatal intensive care environment. *Physical & Occupational Therapy in Pediatrics, 6,* 3-55; and Hunter, J. (2010). The neonatal intensive care unit. In J. Case-Smith (Ed.), *Occupational therapy for children* (6th ed.). St. Louis, MO: Mosby.

stay in the NICU. This vulnerable period of brain growth, differentiation, and organization is combined with the challenge of developing in environmental conditions that are not typical for the fetus and newborn (Blackburn, 2012). Brain organization peaks from about 20 weeks of gestation to several years after birth. The product of this complex process is establishment of an elaborate circuitry unique to the human brain.

Behavioral State Organization

Traditional nursing placed emphasis on interpreting physiologic data as the basis of caregiving. Developmentally supportive care uses both physiologic and behavioral information to better understand the needs of infants in the NICU setting. Behavioral states are highly individualized

TABLE 9.5 **Arousal States**

State	Description
Deep sleep	Regular breathing; eyes closed with no movement of eyes under lid; relaxed face; little or no movement or activity except for possible startle response
Active sleep	Sometimes called light sleep; may see rapid eye movements under closed lids, low activity level, breathing regular or irregular, occasional sighing or smiling
Drowsy	Eyes open or closed, unfocused expression; activity level varied
Quiet awake	Different qualities of alerting
• Robust	Bright, shiny appearance to eyes; focused attention; minimum motor activity
• Low level	Dull or unfocused eyes; little energy; appears to look through object or caregiver
• Hyperalert	Wide eyes, panicked expression; may fixate on object or caregiver intensely and have trouble breaking away
Active awake	Active; eyes open or closed; fussy but not crying robustly
Crying	Highest level of arousal; agitated, rhythmic, and robust crying

Modified from Als, H. (1995). *Manual for the naturalistic observation of newborn behavior, Newborn Individualized Developmental Care and Assessment Program (NIDCAP).* Boston, MA: Harvard Medical School.

and formed by experience, maturation, circadian rhythms, and genetic inheritance. The emerging availability and regulation of arousal states mark a balancing of CNS inhibitory and excitatory processes that affect attention states and also mark executive functions (prefrontal cortex) that influence information processing, learning, and socialization. **State organization** has been described as a gating mechanism that protects the cortex from overstimulation and promotes coordination among attentional, executive, and sensory cortical systems.

Infant responsiveness to environmental stimuli depends on the quality, amount, and availability of particular states of arousal. States can be organized into five levels of arousal (Table 9.5). Transitional states such as drowsiness are not considered true states, but are in-between levels of arousal in which the infant either moves toward wakefulness or back into sleep.

Distinct sleep and awake states are observable in infants between 25 and 27 weeks (Buenoa & Menna-Barretob, 2016; Guyer, Huber, Fontijn, et al., 2015). Young preterm infants spend 70% or more of their time in active sleep. Developmental maturation for the young preterm infant is seen by a decrease in the amount of active sleep with an increase in quiet sleep, awake periods, and crying. Around 30 to 32 weeks, quiet alert states with some focused attention can occur. Before 32 to 34 weeks, attempts to attend to stimuli may have physiologic consequences for the immature infant (Raoof & Ohlsson, 2013). Responsiveness to sound and touch is greater during active or light (**rapid eye movement** [REM]) sleep, resulting in longer periods of vulnerability to sleep disturbance (Gardner, Goldson, & Hernandez, 2016). Maturation continues throughout the first year of life. By 6 months, the amount of quiet sleep is greater than that of active sleep. By 1 year, infants usually sleep 10 to 12 hours at night and take one or two naps during the day. Preterm infants generally sleep for shorter periods at night and awaken more frequently than full-term infants. Other maturational changes include organization of the standard sleep cycle and electroencephalogram sleep patterns comparable to those of adults. Neurologic insults, severity of illness, hyperbilirubinemia, and prenatal exposure to drugs can alter behavioral state patterns.

Physiologic parameters vary depending on level of arousal. Heart rate is higher during waking periods but more variable during active sleep. Blood pressure is higher during wakefulness. Cerebral blood flow is greater during active sleep (greater during quiet sleep in full-term infants). Respiratory rates vary more and are higher in active sleep. Arterial oxygen and carbon dioxide levels are lower in active sleep than in quiet sleep or awake states. Hypoventilation and poorly coordinated chest wall and abdominal movements are reported during active sleep. Apneic pauses of less than 20 seconds are more frequent in active than quiet sleep in preterm infants.

Nursing care should be timed to the responsiveness of the infant as much as possible to optimize the development of sleep organization and enhance alerting as it emerges. Sensory stimulation can influence behavioral state as seen by either increased or decreased infant arousal when presented with a stimulus and its removal; the type of stimulus (e.g., loud bell or soft lullaby) also is a factor. The quality of each state, its duration, and the movement between states provide information about how well organized the state is and how much state control the infant has. Protection of sleep is an important goal for both the preterm and full-term infant. Environmental modifications and timing of care to provide longer episodes of undisturbed sleep should be planned into care.

Nurses can also support transitions between states. Gentle arousal to wakefulness by soft speech or gentle touch before caregiving is preferable to the traditional model in which care is begun without warning and with abrupt disruption of sleep. Slow movements and gentle handling support quiet alerting or return to sleep without periods of arousal after care is over. Nurses should facilitate return to sleep or interact with a quietly alert infant after care events.

An infant's state of arousal allows for communication of responses that are valuable for individualized caregiving. By observing state patterns and individual responses of infants, nurses can better know their patients and support behavioral state organization. The nurse can also share this knowledge with parents to foster intimacy with the child.

Sensory System

Atypical sensory experiences, whether overstimulating or depriving, can modify the developing brain (Gardner, Goldson, & Hernandez, 2016). In fact, much of the cerebral cortex is associated with the sensory system. Most sensory systems develop prenatally and are capable of functioning before birth. The onset of sensory function proceeds in the same order for each individual (i.e., tactile, vestibular, gustatory-olfactory, auditory, and visual). The visual system becomes functional after birth. Sensory input provided before the stimulation would typically occur has been shown to interfere with perceptual and behavioral development (Gardner, Goldson, & Hernandez, 2016).

The normal experience for the preterm infant is within the womb and for the full-term infant is the home environment with a few primary caregivers. These environments are vastly different from the NICU. The NICU experience for the high-risk infant is made up of external conditions and interactions with caregivers. Often that experience is overstimulating to later-developing sensory systems (i.e., auditory and visual) and understimulating to earlier ones (i.e., tactile, vestibular, gustatory-olfactory). Alterations in the sensory environment may have developmental consequences. The nurse should consider (1) timing of stimulation in relation to the infant's current developmental stage, (2) amount of stimulation provided or denied, (3) type of stimulation, and (4) the infant's response to the stimulation (Gardner, Goldson, & Hernandez, 2016).

By the age of viability, infants in the NICU have sophisticated perioral sensation and perceive pressure, pain, and temperature (Gardner, Goldson, & Hernandez, 2016). Touch in the NICU frequently involves routine, sometimes impersonal, caregiving and procedures that are either intrusive or painful. Even nonpainful care has been associated with adverse responses in preterm infants.

Preterm infants demonstrate cry expression, grimacing, and knee and leg flexion during major reposition changes. Hypoxemia has been reported with nonpainful or routine caregiving activities such as suctioning, repositioning, taking vital signs, and changing diapers. Other physiologic changes involve blood pressure, heart rate, and respiratory rhythm (Gardner, Goldson, & Hernandez, 2016). Nursing activities that are painful or especially intrusive, such as needle puncture, have negative physiologic repercussions such as acute decreases in Sao_2 and behavioral state changes in preterm infants (Gardner, Enzman-Hines, & Nyp, 2016). Increased motor activity, agitation, crying, and startle reflex have also been described as negative behavioral responses to touch (Gardner, Goldson, & Hernandez, 2016).

Touch is the first sensory system to develop and forms the basis for early communication between infants and caregivers. In particular, touch is a powerful means of emotional exchange for parents and infants. Positioning and handling techniques promote comfort and minimize stress while creating a balance between nurturing care and necessary interventions.

Therapeutic Handling

Using the developmental model of supportive care, the nurse closely monitors physiologic and behavioral signs to promote organization and well-being of high-risk infants during handling (Box 9.5). The type, timing, and amount of handling are carefully considered in terms of the infant's current age, condition, vulnerabilities, thresholds for stress, and capabilities. Because touch can be disruptive to maturing sleep-wake states, avoid waking an infant for care or nurturing. Sleep deprivation may affect secretion of growth hormone and interfere with growth and development (Gardner, Goldson, & Hernandez, 2016).

Respectful approach before touching an infant allows more time for transition and adaptation from being alone to being handled. The nurse can use the infant's own cues to determine optimum times for caregiving rather than following a rigid schedule. The best time for care is when an infant is awake. If the care or procedure cannot be postponed, softly calling an infant by name and then gently placing a hand on the body signals care is beginning and avoids the abrupt interruption that frequently precedes caregiving. Abrupt transitions can disrupt even organized functioning of an infant's autonomic, motor, and state subsystems.

Infants who are unable to maintain a gently flexed position during repositioning or care procedures may benefit from containment. Gently holding the infant's arms and legs in a tucked, flexed position close to the body can be accomplished with hands or blanket swaddling. **Facilitated tucking** was shown to decrease physiologic and behavioral distress in preterm infants during painful procedures (Hartley, Miller, & Gephart, 2015; Lavoie, Stritzke, Ting, et al, 2015). Blanket swaddling and nesting or containment decreased physiologic and behavioral stress during routine care procedures such as bathing and heel lance (Hartley, Miller, & Gephart, 2015; Quraishy, Bowles, & Moore, 2013).

Because repositioning has been associated with significant physiologic distress in immature infants, avoid sudden postural changes. Slow turning while containing the infant's extremities in a gently tucked, midline position may reduce the impact of this procedure.

Stroking preterm infants who are not physiologically stable has been reported to result in signs of distress such as gasping, grunting, gaze aversion, and decreased $tcPO_2$ levels (Gardner, Enzman-Hines, & Nyp, 2016). Some infants experience apnea and bradycardia during massage or tactile-kinesthetic stimulation (Gardner, Enzman-Hines, & Nyp, 2016). Other researchers report positive benefits of gentle human touch, including heart rate and oxygen saturation stability (Herrington & Chiodo, 2013). Individual infants show varied responses to tactile intervention, further supporting the need for close monitoring of behavioral and physiologic parameters.

Investigators have reported positive results of massage on stable, growing preterm infants. A systematic review by Alvarez, Fernandez, Gomez-Salgado, and colleagues (2017) found that when infant massage therapy is properly applied to stable preterm infants, they respond with increased weight gain and shortened hospital stays. Parents of the preterm infant also benefit because infant massage enhances bonding with their child and increases confidence in their parenting skills (Lai, D'Acunto, Guzzetta, et al., 2016). Wang, He, and Zhang (2013) conducted a meta-analysis of studies relevant to infant massage and concluded that available studies showed benefits of massage on weight gain and length of stay, but no conclusive benefits were shown for the outcome of neurobehavioral outcome.

Kangaroo care, or STS holding, has been advocated for fostering neurobehavioral development and supporting parent-infant intimacy and attachment. STS contact is maintained with the diaper-clad infant resting prone and semiupright on the bare chest of either parent, who encloses the infant in his or her own clothing to maintain temperature stability. Kangaroo care is reported to reduce the incidence of severe illness and nosocomial infection, support breastfeeding duration until discharge, improve maternal satisfaction and parental interaction, and quicken neurologic maturation (Gardner, Goldson, & Hernandez, 2016). Others have reported maintenance of skin temperature, reduction of apnea and bradycardia, stable $tcPO_2$ level, increased frequency and duration of quiet sleep, and less time crying during kangaroo care (Kommers, Joshi, van Pul, et al., 2017). A Cochrane reviewed (2017) examined the effect of kangaroo care on pain from medical and nursing procedures in neonates and determined it to be an effective intervention (Johnston, Campbell-Yeo, Disher, et al., 2017).

BOX 9.5 Considerations for Tactile Interventions in the Neonatal Intensive Care Unit

- Modify all handling and touch so that it is supportive and calming.
- Consider sleep-wake states and behavioral cues to determine optimum times for handling and touch.
- Adjust handling and touch based on continual observation of the infant's autonomic and behavioral responses.
- Ensure appropriate touch opportunities for parents aside from routine caregiving.
- Encourage parents to be primary providers of social touch.
- Avoid using massage with vulnerable high-risk infants (e.g., medically unstable, low-birth-weight infants less than 32 weeks of gestation; easily disorganized, low-threshold infants; chronically ill infants with chronic lung disease or cardiac disorders known to display physiologic and behavioral disorganization).
- Assist parents in identifying the most appropriate type of touch and handling for their infant.
- Teach infant cues to parents for monitoring responses to handling and touch.
- Weigh the risks and benefits for any tactile intervention.

Therapeutic Positioning

The American Academy of Pediatrics, Task Force on Sudden Infant Death Syndrome (2011) recommends the supine sleeping position for healthy infants in the first year of life as a preventive measure for sudden infant death syndrome (SIDS). Prone sleeping has decreased from more than 70% to about 13% in the United States since the guidelines were published in 1992. SIDS is the third highest cause of infant death after the neonatal period (28 days); the rate has decreased by more than 50% with the advent of supine sleeping. (See Sudden Infant Death Syndrome, Chapter 8.) However, after an initial decrease in the 1990s, the overall death rate attributable to sleep-related infant deaths has not declined in more recent years (American Academy of Pediatrics Task Force on SIDS and Other Sleep-Related Infant Deaths, 2016).

Parents of infants in the NICU should be educated on the safe sleeping position at home as part of discharge instructions. Supportive positioning in the NICU for acutely ill or recovering infants may look different from the Academy's recommendations, depending on each infant's changing clinical condition, maturation, and readiness for the supine sleeping position and minimum bedding. Routine care practices in the NICU may serve as a model for parents who, without proper instruction, may reproduce the environment and care techniques at home. Position and bedding choices in the unit, such as prone positioning, nests, and sheepskin, may be lethal for infants who have been discharged home.

Infants in the NICU are at increased risk for acquiring position-related deformities for a variety of reasons. Weakness, low tone, immature motor control, the effects of gravity, and treatments such as sedation are a few of the factors associated with prolonged immobility or decreased spontaneous movement (Byrne & Garber, 2013). Common position-related deformities include the following:

- Hyperabduction and flexion of the arms, causing upper extremity external rotation, resulting in a persistent "W" positioning of the arms, can interfere with later midline skills that form the foundation for feeding, crawling, reaching, and midline play with objects (Vaivre-Douret, Ennouri, Jrad, et al., 2004)
- Lower extremity external rotation deformities occurring when the trunk and pelvis are flat on the mattress, causing extreme hip abduction and outward rotation of the lower limbs, or the frog-leg appearance (Gardner, Goldson, & Hernandez, 2016)
- Neck extension and arching posture often observed in infants pulling away from endotracheal (ET) tubes or nasal prongs during mechanical ventilation or nasal continuous positive airway pressure (CPAP)
- Motor asymmetries reported in preterm infants at 32 weeks of gestation or who are small for gestational age, occurring more often than in full-term infants even after 4 months corrected age (Samsom & de Groot, 2000, 2001)

Therapeutic positioning reduces the potential for acquired positional deformities that can affect motor development, play skills, and social attachment (Altimier & Phillips, 2013). Positioning can affect stability and comfort, and each infant must be observed for the effects of any position or repositioning. A position may also need to be adapted to accommodate necessary medical equipment or particular conditions, such as myelomeningocele, where the supine position is contraindicated before surgical repair of the defect. Deciding on which position and supportive aids to use requires the caregiver to consider the medical and developmental risks and benefits unique to a specific infant and situation (see Nursing Care Guidelines box).

The goal of therapeutic positioning for preterm and high-risk infants is to provide adequate support and containment as indicated to sustain flexed and midline postures in an attempt to minimize positional deformities and assist infants in remaining calm and organized (Altimier & Phillips, 2013).

The supine position requires support for the weak or immature infant. Because this position can create the most disorganization, make the position comfortable using positioning aids or blanket boundaries that support the head, trunk, and extremities according to the general positioning principles.

Although the prone position may appear to be the easiest to maintain, mistakes are often made with infants who are unable to sustain rounded shoulders, trunk, and pelvis without assistance. Use of a postural support roll has been shown to prevent shoulder retraction (Figs. 9.4 and 9.5) (Versaw-Barnes & Wood, 2015).

NURSING CARE GUIDELINES

General Considerations for Positioning

- Neutral or slightly flexed neck
- Gently rounded shoulders (no flattened posture against bed as in supine or prone positions)
- Elbows flexed
- Hands to face or midline as position allows
- Trunk slightly rounded with pelvic tilt
- Hips partially flexed and adducted to near midline (not medial or neutral alignment) and knee flexion (no frog leg or externally rotated hips flat against bed)
- Lower boundary secured for foot bracing

Modified from Biber, P. (1995). When to seek consultation. In P. J. Creger & J. V. Browne, *Developmental interventions for preterm and high-risk infants: Self-study modules for professionals.* Tucson, AZ: Therapy Skill Builders.

Auditory Environment

The auditory system of the human fetus is mature enough for sound to produce physiologic effects as early as 22 to 24 weeks of gestation (Gardner, Goldson, & Hernanez, 2016). Physical and behavioral responses to sudden, loud NICU noise have been observed in preterm and full-term infants (Hassanein, Raggal, & Shalaby, 2013). Physiologic changes include apnea and bradycardia; fluctuations in heart and respiratory rates, blood pressure, and oxygen saturation; and changes in sleep-wake states (Kuhn, Zores, Langlet, et al., 2013; Pineda, Durant, Mathur, et al., 2017). These data demonstrate that infants in the NICU are capable of perceiving and responding to sounds around them.

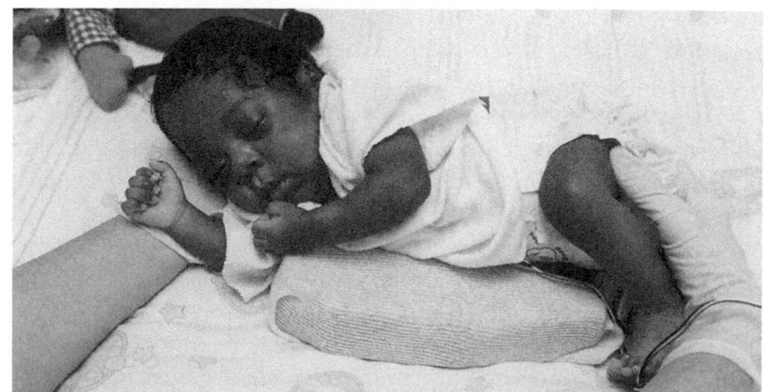

FIG. 9.4 Preterm infant slowly and gently transitioned to prone position on prone roll designed with stockinette-covered foam cut to individual specifications to prevent flattening of shoulders and pelvis against mattress and to support stable breathing base for the infant. (Courtesy Paul Vincent Kuntz, Halbouty Premature Nursery, Texas Children's Hospital, Houston.)

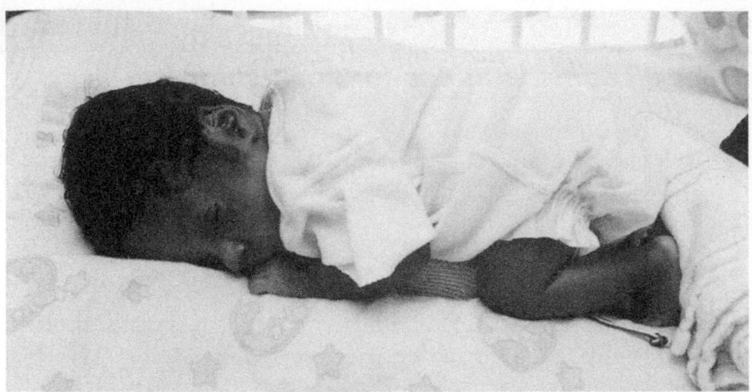

FIG. 9.5 Preterm infant positioned on prone roll. (Courtesy Paul Vincent Kuntz, Halbouty Premature Nursery, Texas Children's Hospital, Houston.)

The primary auditory environment in fetal life is made up of the maternal voice, respirations, heartbeat, and intestinal sounds. Soon after birth, newborn infants demonstrate preference for their own mother's voice and the language heard in utero (Gardner, Goldson, & Hernandez, 2016). The acoustic environment of most NICUs is vastly different from that of the uterus or home. Currently no data are available on the effects of long-term exposure to NICU noise levels. Of serious concern is the increased risk of language delays in infants born prematurely (Kuhn, Zores, Langlet, et al., 2013; Pineda, Durant, Mathur, et al., 2017). NICU noise may interfere with developing auditory pathways and mask socially relevant sounds of the human voice necessary for language development.

Maintaining recommended sound levels (<45 dB) in the NICU may provide (1) increased physiologic stability, (2) improved growth, (3) more natural and consistent neurosensory maturation, (4) enhanced parent-infant interaction and subsequent attachment, and (5) fewer speech and language difficulties (Byrne & Garber, 2013; Gardner, Goldson, & Hernandez, 2016).

Visual Environment

Sight is the least mature of the newborn's senses. The preterm infant's eyes undergo significant maturation and differentiation of the retina and its connections to the visual cortex that typically occur in utero during the last trimester of pregnancy (Atkinson & Braddick, 2012). Early intense visual stimulation for preterm infants could adversely affect visual pathways and alter the developmental course for other sensory systems.

Visual function in preterm infants is more limited than that in full-term infants, who, although restricted in ability to focus (accommodation to near and far distances) and discriminate (acuity), will actively explore the environment. Preterm infants are less responsive to visual stimulation and have less acuity and accommodation than full-term infants. The ability to visually attend emerges around 30 to 32 weeks, and the infant may become stressed if the visual stimulus is intense and prolonged. Strong visual stimulation such as high-contrast black-and-white patterns can evoke an obligatory staring response by the immature infant who is unable to break away from it. This behavior is neither appropriate nor desired.

A variety of lighting conditions exist for NICUs: continuous 24-hour illumination, continuous dim lighting, day-night cycled lighting, or unpredictable periods of light-dark, depending on staff or situations. Cycled lighting is done to follow the natural day and night light rhythm, levels, and colors or light. Preterm infants have shown a faster weight increase and further development and an earlier day/activity and night/rest pattern (Engwall, Fridh, Bergbom, et al., 2014; Guyer, Huber, Fontijn, et al., 2012). A Cochrane Systematic Review (2016) showed the benefit of cycled light compared with continuous bright light for preterm infants and low-weight infants investigated in an NICU (Morag & Ohlsson, 2016).

BOX 9.6 Visual Stimulation: Considerations for Infants

- Decrease ambient light levels by dimming lights or using incubator covers for lower-birth-weight and lower-gestational-age infants.
- Facilitate eye opening and visual attention in older preterm and term infants by dimming overhead lights.
- Direct procedure lights toward the necessary visual field and away from infants' eyes when performing tasks that require visual acuity such as intravenous catheter insertion.
- Shield infants' eyes from bright procedure lights or full ambient lighting as needed during examinations, treatments, or procedures.
- Avoid placing a cloth over the face or using eye patches that provide tactile irritation unless necessary for phototherapy or special circumstances.
- Ensure eye patches are securely in place during phototherapy.
- Introduce day-night cycling of lighting in the neonatal intensive care unit and intermediate nursery before discharge.
- Consider the human face the most appropriate visual stimulation in early infancy.
- Avoid leaving visual stimuli in the beds of infants who cannot escape from it.
- Provide appropriate visual stimuli or toys for recovering full-term or older infants.

Staff needs to carefully consider the impact of visual stimuli on the NICU infant. For preterm infants whose visual system is undergoing maturation, it is probably wiser to provide stimulation to the earlier-developing senses first and minimize the impact of the NICU visual milieu. As attention and alerting emerge, the most appropriate visual stimulus is likely to be the human face, especially that of the parent. Box 9.6 provides some suggested approaches to visual stimulation in the NICU (Guyer, Huber, Fontijn, et al., 2012; Hunter, 2010).

Facilitating Parent-Infant Relationships

Because of their physiologic instability, preterm infants are immediately separated from their mothers and surrounded by a complex barrier of glass windows, mechanical equipment, and special caregivers. Increasing evidence indicates that the emotional separation that accompanies the physical separation of mothers and infants interferes with the normal maternal-infant attachment process, discussed in Chapter 7. Maternal attachment is a cumulative process that begins before conception, strengthens by significant events during pregnancy, and matures through maternal-infant contact during the neonatal period.

When an infant is sick, the necessary physical separation appears to be accompanied by an emotional estrangement in the parents, which may seriously damage their capacity for parenting their infant. This detachment is further hampered by the tenuous nature of the infant's condition. When survival is in doubt, parents may be reluctant to establish a relationship with their infant, unconsciously preparing themselves for the infant's death. This **anticipatory grief** (see Chapter 19) and hesitancy to embark on a relationship are evidenced by behaviors such as delay in giving the infant a name, reluctance to visit the nursery (or focusing on equipment and treatments rather than on their infant when they do visit), and hesitancy to touch or handle the infant when given the opportunity.

Comprehensive management of high-risk newborns includes encouraging and facilitating parental involvement rather than isolating

BOX 9.7 Psychologic Tasks of Parents of a High-Risk Infant

- Work through the events surrounding labor and delivery.
- Acknowledge that the infant's life is endangered and begin the anticipatory grieving process.
- Recognize and confront feelings of inadequacy and guilt in not delivering a healthy child.
- Adapt to the neonatal intensive care environment.
- Resume parental relationships with the sick infant and initiate the caregiving role.
- Prepare to take the infant home.

Modified from Gardner, S. L., Voos, K., & Hills, P. (2016). Families in crisis: Theoretical and practical considerations. In S. L. Gardner, B. S. Carter, M. Enzman-Hines, et al. (Eds.), *Merenstein and Gardner's handbook of neonatal intensive care* (8th ed.). St. Louis, MO: Mosby.

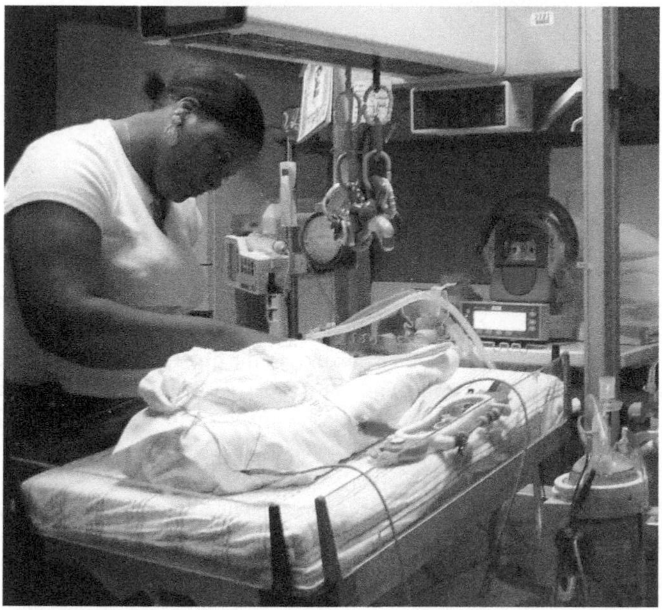

FIG. 9.6 Encouraging interaction of mother and her preterm infant in intensive care unit facilitates the mother-infant attachment process. (Courtesy E. Jacobs, Texas Children's Hospital, Houston.)

parents from their infant and associated care (Box 9.7). This is particularly important for mothers; to reduce the effects of physical separation, mothers are united with their newborns at the earliest opportunity (Fig. 9.6). Preparing the parents to see their infant for the first time is a nursing responsibility.

Before the first visit, the nurse prepares parents for their infant's appearance, the equipment attached to the child, and the general atmosphere of the unit. The initial encounter with the intensive care unit is stressful, and the frightening array of people, equipment, and activity is likely to be overwhelming. A book of photographs or pamphlets describing the NICU environment (e.g., infants in incubators or under radiant warmers, monitors, mechanical ventilators, and IV equipment) provides a useful and nonthreatening introduction to the NICU.

Encourage parents to visit their infant as soon as possible. Even if they saw the infant at the time of transport or shortly after birth, the infant may have changed considerably, especially if there are a number of medical and equipment requirements associated with the infant's hospitalization. At the bedside the nurse should explain the function of each piece of equipment and the role it plays in facilitating recovery. Explanations may need to be patiently repeated because parents' anxiety over the infant's condition and the surroundings may prevent them from really "hearing" what is said. When possible, some items related to therapy can be removed; for example, phototherapy can be temporarily discontinued and eye patches removed to permit eye-to-eye contact.

Parents appreciate the support of a nurse during the initial visit with their infant, but they may also want some time alone with the infant. It is important during the early visits to emphasize the positive aspects of their infant's behavior and development so that parents can focus on their infant as an individual rather than on the equipment that surrounds the child. For example, the nurse may describe the infant's spontaneous behaviors during care, such as grasp, sucking, and movement, or make comments about the infant's biologic functions. Most institutions promote family-centered care and have open visiting policies so that parents and siblings can visit as often as they wish. Although pediatric health care providers are embracing family-centered care, successful implementation of initiative to support this model is challenging. Uhl, Fisher, Docherty, and colleagues (2013) demonstrated from parent focus groups evidence of parental stress throughout hospitalization. Parents reported that uncertainty, fear, and lack of control were the predominant factors in this distress (Uhl, Fisher, Docherty, et al., 2013). In the NICU environment, the focus has shifted from parents being participants in performing limited care tasks to being active contributors to the health care and management of their infant.

Parents vary greatly in the degree to which they are able to interact with their infant. Some may wish to touch or hold their infant during the first visit, whereas others may not feel comfortable enough to even enter the nursery. Parents may not be receptive to early and extended infant contact because they need time to adjust to having an infant with birth problems and must be helped to grieve before they can accept their infant. Parents have noted that the most important aspect of care participation was simply having the opportunity to be engaged in the activity whether they chose to participate or not (Uhl, Fisher, Docherty, et al., 2013).

The parents' inability to focus on their infant is a clue for the nurse to assist the parents in expressing feelings of guilt, anxiety, helplessness, inadequacy, anger, and ambivalence. Nurses can help parents deal with these distressing feelings and recognize that they are normal responses shared by other parents. It is important to point out and reinforce the positive aspects of parents' behavior and interactions with their infant.

To meet parental needs in the NICU, nurses must provide accurate information regarding treatment plan and procedures; answer parents' questions honestly; actively listen to parents' fears and expectations; and help parents understand infant responses to hospitalization (Gardner, Goldson, Hernandez, & 2016).

Most parents feel shaky and insecure about initiating interaction with their infant. Nurses can sense parents' level of readiness and offer encouragement in these initial efforts. Parents of preterm infants follow the same acquaintance process as do parents of full-term infants. They may quickly proceed through the process or may require several days, or even weeks, to complete it. Parents begin by touching their infant's extremities with their fingertips and poking the infant tenderly, and then proceed to caresses and fondling (Fig. 9.7). Touching is the first act of communication between parents and child. Parents need to be prepared for their infant's exaggerated and generalized startle responses to touch so that they will not interpret these as negative reactions to their overtures. It may be necessary to limit tactile stimuli when the infant is critically ill and labile, but the nurse can offer other options, such as speaking softly or sitting at the bedside.

Parents of acutely ill preterm infants may express feelings of helplessness and lack of control. Involving the parent in some type of caregiving activity, no matter how minor it may seem to the nurse, enables the parent to take on a more active role. Examples of such caregiving for

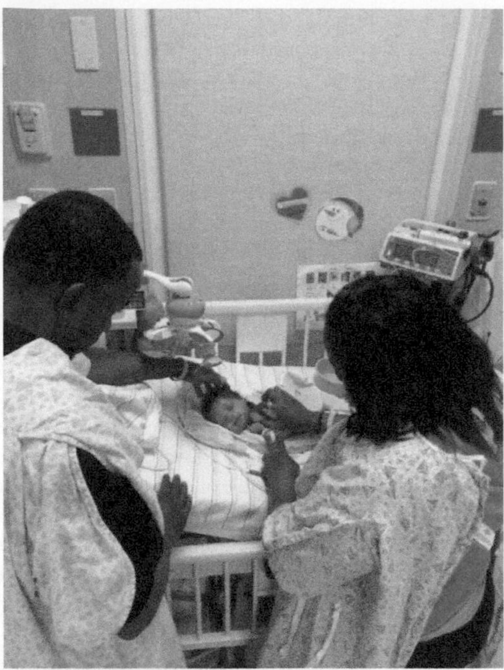

FIG. 9.7 Mother and father interact with their preterm infant. (Courtesy K. Fisher, Duke University.)

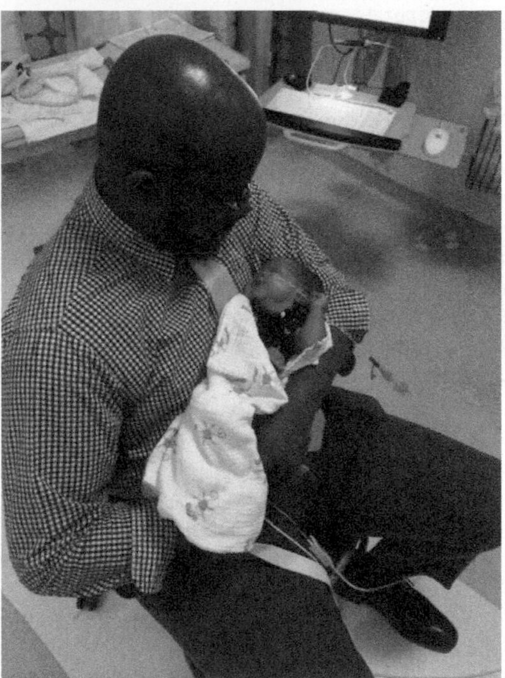

FIG. 9.8 Father holding preterm infant. (Courtesy K. Fisher, Duke University.)

the acutely ill infant who cannot be held and is seemingly not responding positively include moistening the infant's lips with a small amount of sterile water on a cotton-tipped swab or slipping the diaper from under the infant when it is wet or soiled.

The nurse encourages parents to bring in clothes, a toy, a stuffed animal, or a family snapshot for their infant. The nurse can also help parents set goals for themselves and for the infant. Parents may become involved by reading a children's storybook or nursery rhymes in a soft, soothing voice. The nurse encourages parents to visit at times when they can become involved in their infant's care (Figs. 9.8 and 9.9).

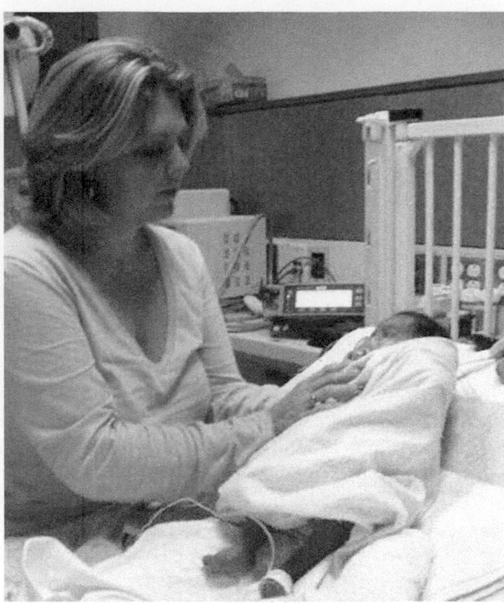

FIG. 9.9 Mother consoling preterm infant. (Courtesy E. Jacobs, Texas Children's Hospital, Houston.)

Throughout the parent-infant acquaintance process, the nurse listens carefully to what the parents say to assess their concerns and their progress toward incorporating their infant into their lives. The manner in which parents refer to their infant and the questions they ask reveal their worries and feelings and can serve as valuable clues to future relationships with the infant. The alert nurse is attuned to these subtle indications of parents' needs, which provide guidelines for nursing intervention. Often all that the parents need is reassurance that they will have the nurse's support during caregiving activities and that the behaviors about which they are concerned are normal reactions and will disappear as the infant matures (e.g., an exaggerated Moro reflex or inability to coordinate swallowing).

Parents need guidance in their relationships with their infant and assistance in their efforts to meet their infant's physical and developmental needs. The nursing staff must help parents understand that their preterm infant offers few behavioral rewards and show them how to accept small rewards from their infant. They need reassurance that avoidance behaviors are not a reflection on their parenting skills. Teach parents to recognize their infant's cues regarding stimulation, handling, and other interaction, especially aversive behaviors that indicate a need for rest. Nurses need to include parents in planning their infant's care.

Above all, nurses must encourage parents during their caregiving activities and interactions with their infant to promote healthy parent-child relationships. It is also helpful for the parents to have contact and communication with the infant's primary nurse and associate primary nurse (according to unit model of nursing care). This decreases the amount of different information given to parents and often instills confidence that, although the parents cannot be at their infant's bedside 24 hours a day, they can call competent and caring nurses to inquire about the infant's status. Periodic parent conferences involving the primary practitioner, primary nurse, and associate primary nurse serve to clarify misunderstandings or problems related to the infant's condition. Other members of the NICU team, such as the perinatal social worker, lactation consultant, discharge coordinator, or surgeon, may become involved as necessary.

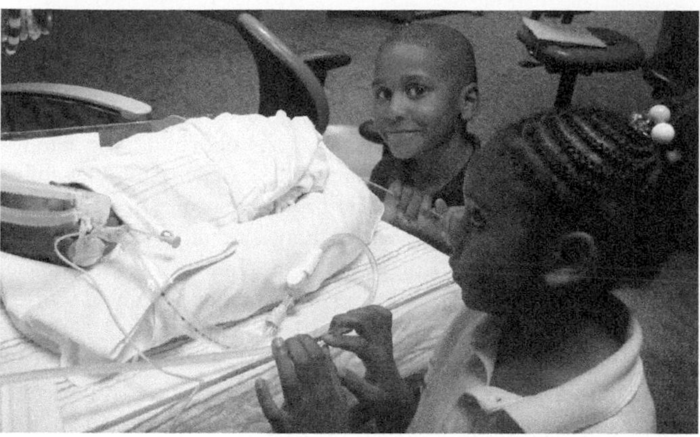

FIG. 9.10 Siblings visiting in the neonatal intensive care unit. (Courtesy E. Jacobs, Texas Children's Hospital, Houston.)

Siblings

In the past, concerns about sibling visitation in the NICU focused on fears of infection and disruption of nursing routines. These fears have not been substantiated, and sibling visits should be a part of the normal operation of NICUs (Fig. 9.10).

The birth of a preterm infant is a difficult time for siblings, who rely on the support of understanding parents. When the happy anticipation changes to sadness, worry, and altered routines, siblings are bewildered and deprived of their parents' attention. They know something is wrong, but they do not completely understand what it is. Concern about the negative effects on visiting siblings of seeing the ill newborn has not been confirmed. Children have not hesitated to approach or touch the infant, and children less than 5 years of age have been less reluctant than older children. In addition, no measurable differences were found between previsit and postvisit behaviors.

The potential benefits of sibling visits must be weighed against the negatives of exposing the child to the NICU environment. Children must be prepared for the unfamiliar NICU atmosphere, but contact with the infant appears to have a positive effect on siblings by helping them deal with the reality rather than the fantasies that are characteristic of young children. Such visits also help bond the family as a unit.

Support Groups

Parents need to feel they are not alone. Parent support groups have been of great value to families of infants in the NICU. Some groups consist of parents who have infants in the hospital and share the same anxieties and concerns. Other groups include parents who have had infants in the NICU and who have dealt with the crisis effectively. The groups are usually under the leadership of a staff person and may involve physicians, nurses, and social workers, but it is the parents who can offer other parents something that no one else can provide.

Family Support America* (formerly Family Resource Coalition) is a North American network of family support programs designed to help families of preterm infants. An excellent resource for parents of preterm infants is the book by J. Zaichkin, *Understanding the NICU: What Parents of Preemies and Other Hospitalized Newborns Need to Know* (2017). This resource has technical and anecdotal information regarding different problems facing preterm infants, common treatments and therapies, preparation for home discharge, and home care for the preterm infant.

Discharge Planning and Home Care

Parents become apprehensive and excited as the time for discharge approaches. They have many concerns and insecurities regarding the care of their infant. They fear that the child may still be in danger, that they will be unable to recognize signs of distress or illness, and that the infant may not be ready for discharge. Nurses need to begin early to assist parents in acquiring or increasing their skills in the care of their infant. Appropriate instruction must be provided and sufficient time allowed for the family to take in the information and learn special care requirements. Where rooming-in or other live-in arrangements are available, parents can stay for a few days and nights and assume the care of their infant under the supervision and support of the nursery staff.

There should be appropriate medical and nursing follow-up care, including developmental follow-up, and referrals to services that can benefit the family. Parents of preterm infants should also receive information about immunizations, including respiratory syncytial virus (RSV) prophylaxis, as well as other discharge planning information. Home health agencies provide nursing supervision, counseling, and referrals for nursing visits. With early discharge, many hospital-based home health care agencies become involved in the follow-up monitoring and care of the NICU "graduate" in the home. For an infant being discharged with equipment such as an oxygen tank, apnea monitor, or even a ventilator, discharge planning requires multidisciplinary, collaborative practice to ensure that the family has not only the appropriate resources but also assistance for dealing with the infant's needs. Many communities have organized support groups, including those discussed previously, those designed for parents of infants who require special care because of specific defects or disabilities, and those for parents of multiple births.

Car seat safety is an essential aspect of discharge planning. It is recommended that infants less than 37 weeks of gestation have an infant car seat challenge (ICSC) for a period of observation to monitor for possible apnea, bradycardia, and decreased Sao_2 (Bull, Engle, & American Academy of Pediatrics, 2009; Davis, Zenchenko, Lever, et al., 2013). Davis (2015) found an overall failure rate of 4.8%, which is similar to that in published reports on the failure rates in large cohorts of preterm infants. The only significant difference in clinical and demographic characteristics between those who passed the ICSC and those who failed was maternal urine toxicology positive for opiates (Davis, 2015). Davis, Condon, and Rhein (2013) used the American Academy of Pediatrics (2009) guidelines for ICSC and determined that there were major barriers to the standardization of testing infants across many NICUs and recommended universal testing parameters to help improve generalizability of the ICSC between nurseries. (See Family-Centered Care box.)

Several car seat models can be adapted for small infants with the placement of blanket rolls on each side of the infant, but never behind, to support the head and trunk. For adequate support without slumping, the seat back–to–crotch strap distance must be 14 cm (5.5 inches) or less. A small rolled blanket may be placed between the crotch strap and the infant to reduce slouching. If the child's head drops forward because the position of the seat is upright, a roll cloth or blanket may be placed in the vehicle seat crease and under the safety base so the infant reclines at no more than a 45-degree angle. A car seat restraint without a shield is recommended; if the infant needs to be supine, a crash-tested car bed may be used (Bull, Engle, & American Academy of Pediatrics, 2009).

The rear-facing position provides support for the head, neck, and back, thereby reducing the stress to the neck and spinal cord in a vehicle crash. It is recommended that, before discharge from the hospital, the

*307 W. 200 S., Suite 2004, Salt Lake City, 84101; http://www.familysupportamerica.org.

FAMILY-CENTERED CARE

Preterm and Late-Preterm Infant Car Seat Evaluation

The American Academy of Pediatrics recommends that infants born before 37 weeks of gestation be evaluated for apnea, bradycardia, and oxygen desaturation episodes before hospital discharge. The Academy suggests that facilities develop policies for implementing an evaluation program; however, few evidence-based practice recommendations have been published to date delineating specific requirements for such a program. Based on the available literature, suggestions for providing a car seat evaluation of infants born before 37 weeks of gestation include the following:

- Use the parents' car seat for the evaluation.
- Perform the evaluation 1 to 7 days before the infant's anticipated discharge.
- Secure infant in car seat per guidelines using blanket rolls on side.
- Set pulse oximeter low alarm at 88% (arbitrary).
- Set heart rate low alarm limit at 80 beats/min and apnea alarm at 20 seconds (cardiorespiratory monitor).
- Leave the infant undisturbed in car seat for 90 to 120 minutes or for the time parents state it takes to arrive at their home (if >90 minutes).
- Document infant's tolerance to car seat evaluation.
- An episode of desaturation, bradycardia, or apnea (≥20 seconds) constitutes a failure, and evaluation by the practitioner must occur before discharge.
- Repeat the test after 24 hours once modifications are made to the car seat, car bed, or infant's position in either restraint system.
- It is recommended that a certified car seat technician place the infant in the car seat (or bed) if a failure occurs (see National Highway Traffic Safety Administration website [http://www.nhtsa.dot.gov] for car seat inspection station). The technician will demonstrate appropriate positioning of the infant in the restraint device to the parents and have the parents do a return demonstration.
- Document the interventions, the infant's tolerance, and the parents' return demonstration.

Modified from Bull, M. J., Engle, W. A., & American Academy of Pediatrics. (2009). Safe transportation of preterm and low birth weight infants at hospital discharge. *Pediatrics, 123*(5), 1424-1429.

preterm infant have an evaluation in the designated car seat restraint by a staff member who is knowledgeable in car seat restraint positioning. Parents should learn how to properly restrain the child in the car seat for safe transportation (Bull, Engle, & American Academy of Pediatrics, 2009).

Additional guidelines are available from the American Academy of Pediatrics, including a videotape for the safe transportation of preterm infants. (See Chapter 10 for a discussion of infant car restraints and American Academy of Pediatrics website [http://www.aap.org] for a list of appropriate car seats for infants.)

An important part of discharge planning and care of the preterm infant is nutrition for continued growth; thus choice of feeding must be carefully addressed. Human milk is the preferred form of infant nutrition. An enriched postdischarge formula has been used for preterm infants born at less than 36 weeks to meet appropriate growth standards (Gardner, Goldson, & Hernandez, 2016). However, a Cochrane reviews of studies examining growth in preterm infants fed an enriched post-discharge formula did not find strong evidence of enhanced growth and development compared with infants fed standard formula (Young, Embleton, & McGuire, 2016; Young, Morgan, McCormick, et al., 2012).

The term **vulnerable child syndrome** is applied to physically healthy children who are perceived by their parents to be at high risk for medical or developmental problems. The syndrome has been observed in parents of children who had an illness or injury from which they had not been expected to recover. The family continues to perceive the child as fragile, vulnerable, and "different" and as having needs that warrant special status in the family, which adversely affects the child's and family's behavior. The parents may lack confidence in their parenting ability that persists beyond the illness. The parents may also become overly indulgent and have difficulty setting limits, resulting in interference with normal development. Consequently, the child becomes dependent, demanding, and out of control. Overprotection and frequent visits to the health care provider are characteristic.

Problems that may arise in the high-risk newborn include overfeeding, underfeeding, feeding resistance, aversion to human touch or interaction, and difficulty separating the child from the parent. To help parents deal with the stress of home care for the infant, nurses can discuss the family's fears and anxieties, which are exaggerated in parents of preterm infants, and encourage them to create a normal routine in caring for the infant. Parents need to learn the normal developmental delays expected of formerly preterm infants and the importance of setting disciplinary limits and schedules. Continued explanations and clarification of the infant's true health status and ongoing support of the parents' efforts are important aspects of follow-up care.

Neonatal Loss

The precarious nature of many high-risk infants makes death a real and ever-present possibility. Although infant mortality has been reduced sharply with improved technology, the mortality rate is still greatest during the neonatal period. Nurses in the NICU must prepare the parents for an inevitable death and facilitate a family's grieving process after an expected or unexpected death.

The loss of an infant has special meaning for the grieving parents. It represents a loss of a part of themselves; a loss of the potential for immortality that offspring represent; and a loss of the dream child that has been fantasized throughout the pregnancy. The parents have a sense of emptiness and failure. In addition, when an infant has lived for such a short time, they may have few, if any, pleasant memories to serve as a basis for the identification and idealization that are part of the resolution of a loss.

To help parents understand that the death is a reality, it is important that they be given the opportunity to hold their infant before death and, if possible, be present at the time of death so their infant can die in their arms if they choose.

Parents should have the opportunity to actually "parent" the infant in any manner they wish or are able to before and after the death. This may include seeing, touching, holding, caressing, and talking to their infant privately. The parents may also wish to bathe and dress the infant. If parents are hesitant to see their deceased infant, it is advisable to keep the body in the unit for a few hours because many parents change their minds after the initial shock of the death.

Parents may need to see and hold the infant more than once—the first time to say "hello" and the last time to say "good-bye." If parents wish to see the infant after the body has been taken to the morgue, the infant should be retrieved, wrapped in a blanket, rewarmed in a radiant warmer, and taken to the mother's room or other private place. The nurse should plan to stay with the parents but also provide them an opportunity for private time alone with their dead infant if they wish. Individual grief responses of the mother and father should be recognized and handled appropriately. Gender differences and cultural and religious beliefs will affect the parents' grief responses (Koopmans, Wilson, Cacciatore, et al., 2013).

Some units have implemented a hospice approach for families with infants for whom the decision has been made not to prolong life and who are receiving only palliative care. A special "family" room is set aside and contains all supportive equipment needed for the care of the infant. It also provides a homelike atmosphere for the family. All hospice services are available to the family, and the infant remains under the care and supervision of a primary nurse on the NICU staff. (See Chapter 19, End-of-Life Care, for further discussion of hospice care.)

When available, providers trained in palliative care bring additional expertise in effective acute and chronic pain management for infants and their families (Marc-Aurele & English, 2016). The 2014 Institute of Medicine report recommends that all health care providers who care for people with advanced serious illness should be competent in basic palliative care (*Dying in America,* Institute of Medicine of the National Academies Report, 2014). Early integration of palliative care permits involvement of decision support for both the family and the clinicians. A fundamental focus of palliative care is on maximizing quality of life for both the patient and the family throughout the process of illness (Lemmon, Bidegain, & Boss, 2016). Integrating this focus early may help families begin to formulate their goals related to quality of life and thus lessen the burden of decision making on the family.

A photograph of the infant taken before or after death is highly desirable. Parents may wish to have a special family portrait taken with the infant and other family members. This often helps personalize the experience and make it more tangible. The parents may not wish to see the photograph at the time of death, but the chance to refer to it later will help make their infant seem more real, which is a part of the normal grieving process. A photograph of their infant being held by the hand or touched by an adult offers a more positive image than a morgue photograph. The photographs and other personal effects of the deceased infant were perceived as critically important in the grieving process by one group of parents in a survey. Photographs are helpful in remembering the infant's actual appearance during this stressful period (Michelson, Blehart, Hochberg, et al., 2013; Swaney, English, & Carter, 2016). Naming the deceased infant is an important step in the grieving process. Some parents may hesitate to give the newborn a name that had been chosen during the pregnancy for their special "baby." However, it helps to have a tangible person for whom to grieve. In supporting parental responses to the loss of a child, care providers must understand and respect the cultural and religious practices.

A primary nurse who is familiar to the family should be present during the discussion about the dead or dying infant. A *Resolve Through Sharing* or bereavement counselor is often involved in helping the family through this difficult period. The nurse should talk with parents openly and honestly about funeral arrangements because few of them have had experience with this aspect of death. Someone from the NICU should take responsibility for acquiring this information. It is often helpful to parents for the NICU to have a list of local funeral homes, services offered, and prices. Families need to be informed of the options available, but a funeral is preferable because the ritual provides an opportunity for parents to feel the support of friends and relatives. A clergyman of the appropriate faith may be notified if the parents wish. Issues regarding an autopsy or organ donation (when appropriate) are approached in a multidisciplinary fashion (primary practitioner and primary nurse) with respect, tact, and consideration of the family's wishes. (See also "Grief and Perinatal Loss" in Gardner & Carter, 2016.)

Before the parents leave the hospital, the nurse should provide them with the telephone number of the unit (if they do not have it) and invite them to call any time they have any further questions. Many intensive care units make it a point to contact the parents after a neonatal death to assess the parents' coping mechanisms, evaluate the grieving process, and provide support as needed. Several organizations are available to offer support and understanding to families who have lost a newborn, including the Compassionate Friends* and Aiding Mothers and Fathers Experiencing Neonatal Death (AMEND).† (See Chapter 19 for further discussion of the family and the grieving process.)

Nurses who care for critically ill infants also experience grief. NICU nurses may feel helpless and sorrowful. It is important that such grief be allowed and that nurses attend the funeral or memorial service as a part of working through the grieving process. Nurses may fear that showing emotion is unprofessional and that the expression of grief demonstrates "loss of control"; these fears are unfounded. Studies have demonstrated that to continue to be effective providers of care, nurses must be allowed to grieve and support one another through the process (Jonas-Simpson, Pilkington, MacDonald, et al., 2013).

Education regarding bereavement, end-of-life care, and culturally sensitive care of families and their dying infants may help nurses comfort families during this stressful period (Mancini, Kelly, & Bluebond-Langner, 2013).

Baptism

Many Christian parents wish to have their child baptized if death is anticipated or likely. Whenever possible, a representative of the parents' faith (e.g., a Roman Catholic priest or a Protestant minister) should perform such a ritual. When death is imminent, a nurse or a physician can perform the baptism by simply pouring a few drops of water on the infant's forehead (a medicine dropper is a convenient means) while repeating the words, "I baptize you in the name of the Father and of the Son and of the Holy Spirit." This includes an infant of any gestational age, particularly when the parents are Roman Catholic.

When the faith of the parents is uncertain, a conditional baptism can be carried out by saying, "If you are capable of receiving baptism, I baptize you in the name of the Father and of the Son and of the Holy Spirit." The fact of the baptism is recorded in the infant's chart. Parents are informed at the first opportunity.

HIGH-RISK CONDITIONS RELATED TO DYSMATURITY

PRETERM INFANTS

Prematurity of infants accounts for the largest number of admissions to the NICU. Immaturity not only places infants at risk for neonatal complications (e.g., hyperbilirubinemia and RDS, which has the highest incidence in preterm infants), but it may also predispose the infant to problems that persist into adulthood (e.g., learning disabilities, growth deficiencies, asthma).

Etiology

A variety of maternal and pregnancy-related complications increase the risk of preterm delivery; however, the actual cause of prematurity is not known in most instances. The incidence of prematurity is lowest in the middle to high socioeconomic classes, in which pregnant women are generally in good health, are well nourished, and receive prompt and comprehensive prenatal care. The incidence is highest in the lower socioeconomic classes, in which a combination of negative circumstances is present. Other factors, such as multiple pregnancies,

*PO Box 3696, Oak Brook, IL 60522-3696; 630-990-0010, 877-969-0010; http://www.compassionatefriends.org.

†Contact Maureen Connelly, 4324 Berrywick Terr., St. Louis, MO 63128; 314-487-7582; e-mail: martha@amendgroup.com; http://www.amendgroup.com.

gestational hypertension, and placental problems that interrupt the normal course of gestation, are responsible for a large number of preterm births.

The outlook for preterm infants is largely, but not entirely, related to the state of physiologic and anatomic immaturity of the various organs and systems at the time of birth. Infants at term have advanced to a state of maturity sufficient to allow a successful transition to the extrauterine environment. Infants born prematurely must make the same adjustments but with functional immaturity proportional to the stage of development reached at the time of birth. The degree to which infants are prepared for extrauterine life can be predicted to some extent by estimated gestational age. (See Clinical Assessment of Gestational Age, Chapter 7.) An understanding of prenatal development provides some concept of the status of the developing systems that must cope with functional changes that occur with birth.

Characteristics

Preterm infants have distinct characteristics at various stages of development. Identification of these characteristics provides valuable clues to the gestational age and hence to the infant's physiologic capabilities. Physical appearance changes as the fetus progresses to maturity. Skin, posture and tone, distribution of hair, and amount of subcutaneous fat provide clues to a newborn's physical development. Observation of spontaneous, active movements and response to stimulation and passive movement contributes to the assessment of neurologic status. The appraisal is made as soon as possible after admission to the nursery because much of the observation and management of infants depend on this information.

On inspection, preterm infants are very small and appear scrawny because they have little to no subcutaneous fat deposits. They also have a proportionately large head in relation to the body, which reflects the cephalocaudal direction of growth. The skin is bright pink (often translucent, depending on the degree of immaturity), smooth, and shiny (may be edematous), with small blood vessels clearly visible. The fine lanugo is abundant over the body (depending on gestational age) but is sparse, fine, and fuzzy on the head. The ear cartilage is soft and pliable, and the soles and palms have minimum creases, resulting in a smooth appearance. The bones of the skull and the ribs feel soft, and before 26 weeks the eyes may be fused. Male infants have few scrotal rugae, and the testes are undescended; the labia minora and clitoris are prominent in females. Fig. 9.11 compares the features of full-term and preterm infants.

In contrast to full-term infants' overall attitude of flexion and continuous activity, preterm infants are inactive and listless. The extremities maintain an attitude of extension and remain in any position in which they are placed. Physiologically immature, many preterm infants are unable to maintain body temperature, have limited ability to excrete solutes in the urine, and have increased susceptibility to infection. A pliable thorax, immature lung tissue, and an immature regulatory center lead to periodic breathing, hypoventilation, and frequent periods of apnea. These infants are more susceptible to biochemical alterations such as hyperbilirubinemia and hypoglycemia (see Chapter 8), and they have a higher extracellular water content that renders them more vulnerable to fluid and electrolyte imbalance. Preterm infants exchange fully half their extracellular fluid volume every 24 hours, compared with one-seventh of the volume turnover in adults.

The soft cranium is subject to characteristic unintentional deformation (**dolichocephaly**) caused by positioning from one side to the other on a mattress (McCarty, Peat, & Malcolm, 2016). The head looks disproportionately long from front to back, is flattened on both sides, and lacks the usual convexity seen at the temporal and parietal areas. This positional molding is often a concern to parents and may influence their perception of the infant's attractiveness and their responsiveness to the infant. Frequent repositioning of the infant and positioning on a gel mattress can reduce or minimize cranial molding.

Late-preterm infants may not have the immature appearance characteristic of infants born at a lower gestational age (<34 weeks of gestation). However, late-preterm infants are at risk for the development of some of the same physiologic adaptation problems: respiratory distress syndrome, hyperbilirubinemia, thermoregulation difficulties, hypoglycemia, and feeding problems. Late-preterm infants are at greater risk for a number of transitional and feeding-related morbidities (Boies & Vaucher, 2016).

Therapeutic Management

When delivery of a preterm infant is anticipated, the intensive care nursery is alerted and a team approach implemented. Ideally, a neonatologist or a neonatal nurse practitioner, a staff nurse, and a respiratory therapist are present for the delivery. Infants who do not require resuscitation are immediately transferred in a heated incubator to the NICU, where they are weighed and where IV access, oxygen therapy, and other therapeutic interventions are initiated as needed. Resuscitation is conducted in the delivery area until infants can be safely transported to the NICU. Ongoing care is described elsewhere in the chapter.

Nursing Care Management

As with therapeutic management, individualize nursing care for each infant. See appropriate discussions under Nursing Care of High-Risk Newborns for details of care.

POSTTERM INFANTS

Infants born after 42 weeks as calculated from the mother's last menstrual period (or by gestational age assessment) are **postterm**, or postmature, regardless of birth weight. This constitutes 3.5% to 15% of all pregnancies. The cause of delayed birth is unknown. Postterm infants display the characteristics of infants who are 1 to 3 weeks of age, such as absence of lanugo, little if any vernix caseosa, abundant scalp hair, and long fingernails. The skin is often cracked, parchmentlike, and peeling. A common finding in postterm infants is a wasted physical appearance that reflects intrauterine nutritional deprivation. Depletion of subcutaneous fat gives them a thin, elongated appearance. The little vernix caseosa that remains in the skin folds may be stained a deep yellow or green, which is usually an indication of meconium in the amniotic fluid.

Fetal and neonatal mortality rates increase significantly in postterm infants compared with those born at term. They are especially prone to fetal distress associated with the decreasing efficiency of the placenta, **macrosomia**, and meconium aspiration syndrome (MAS). The greatest risk occurs during labor and delivery, particularly in infants of primigravidas, or women delivering their first child. Induction of labor is usually recommended when infants are significantly overdue.

HIGH RISK RELATED TO DISTURBED RESPIRATORY FUNCTION

APNEA OF PREMATURITY

Preterm infants are characteristically periodic breathers. They have periods of rapid respiration separated by periods of very slow breathing, and often short periods with no visible or audible respirations. **Apnea** is primarily an extension of this periodic breathing and can be defined as a lapse of spontaneous breathing for 20 or more seconds, or shorter pauses accompanied by bradycardia or oxygen desaturation (Gardner, Enzman-Hines, & Nyp, 2016).

CLINICAL EVALUATION

PRETERM | TERM

Posture—The preterm infant lies in a "relaxed attitude," limbs more extended; the body size is small, and the head may appear somewhat larger in proportion to the body size. The term infant has more subcutaneous fat tissue and rests in a more flexed attitude.

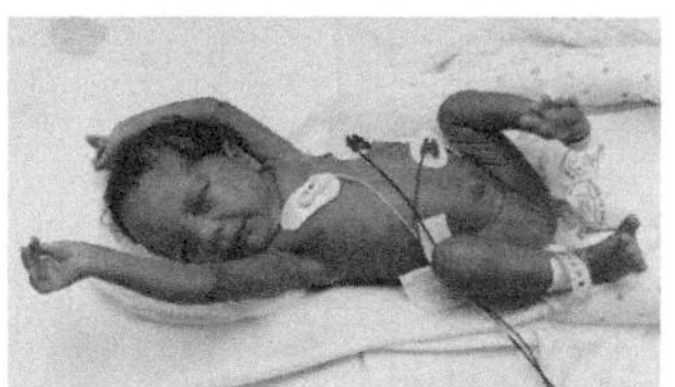

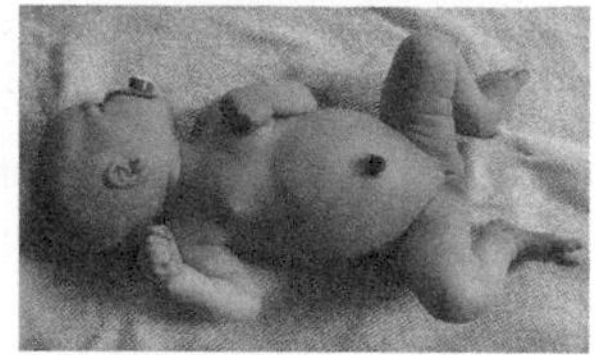

Ear—The preterm infant's ear cartilages are poorly developed, and the ear may fold easily; the hair is fine and feathery, and lanugo may cover the back and face. The mature infant's ear cartilages are well formed, and the hair is more likely to form firm, separate strands.

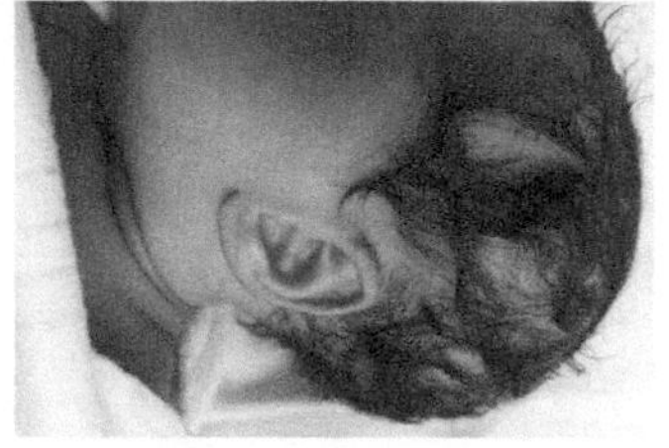

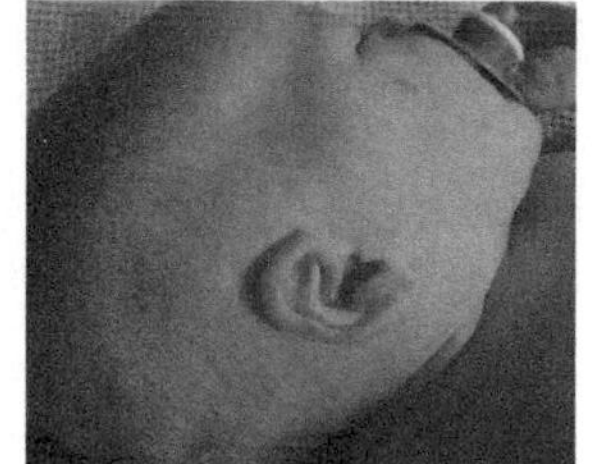

Sole—The sole of the foot of the preterm infant appears more turgid and may have only fine wrinkles. The mature infant's sole (foot) is well and deeply creased.

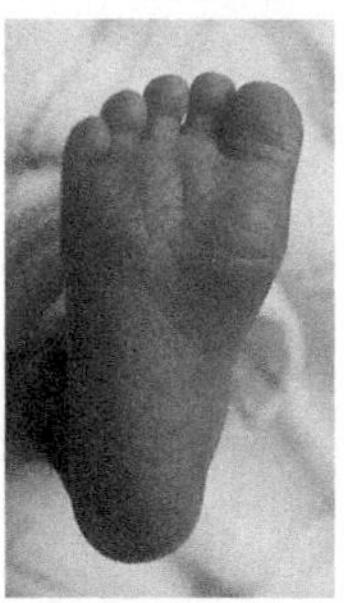

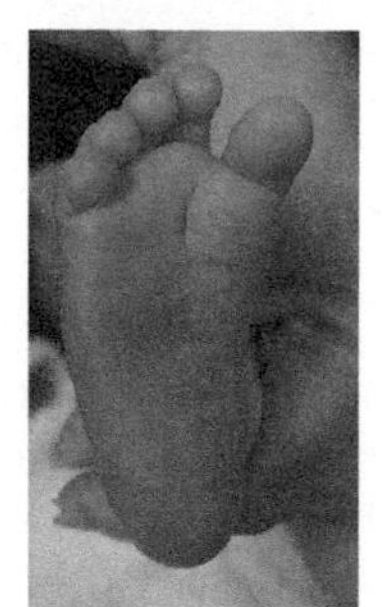

Female genitalia—The preterm female infant's clitoris is prominent, and labia majora are poorly developed and gaping. The mature female infant's labia majora are fully developed, and the clitoris is not as prominent.

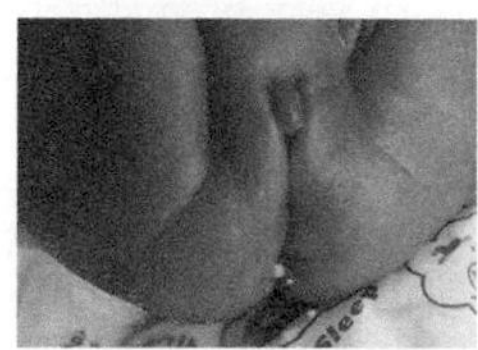

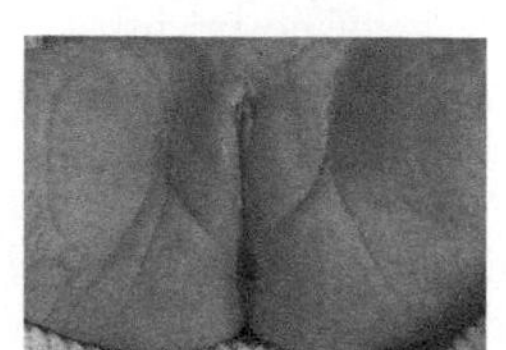

Male genitalia—The preterm male infant's scrotum is undeveloped and not pendulous; minimal rugae are present, and the testes may be in the inguinal canals or in the abdominal cavity. The term male infant's scrotum is well developed, pendulous, and rugated, and the testes are well down in the scrotal sac.

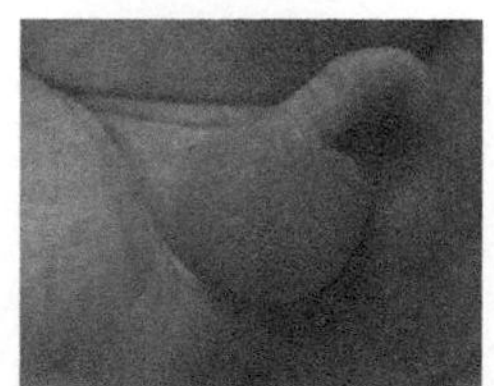

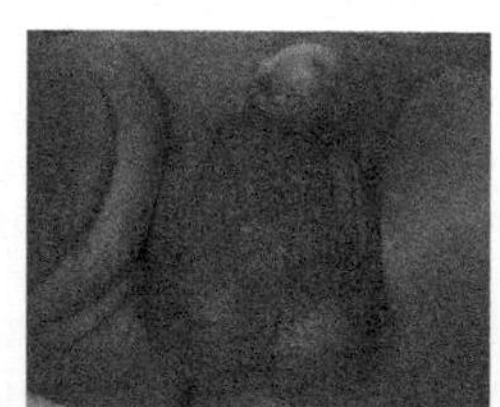

Scarf sign—The preterm infant's elbow may be easily brought across the chest with little or no resistance. The mature infant's elbow may be brought to the midline of the chest, resisting attempts to bring the elbow past the midline.

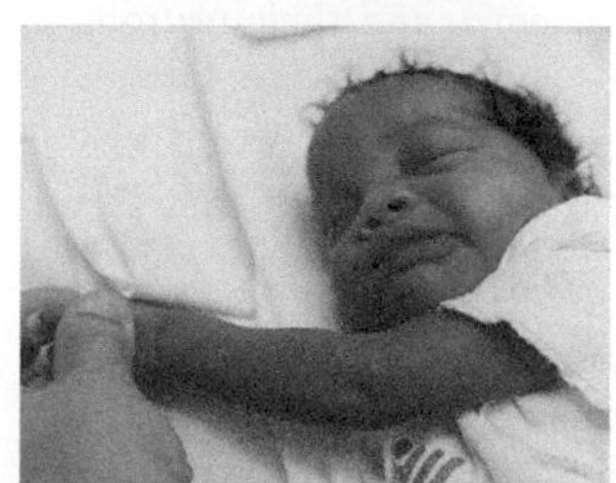

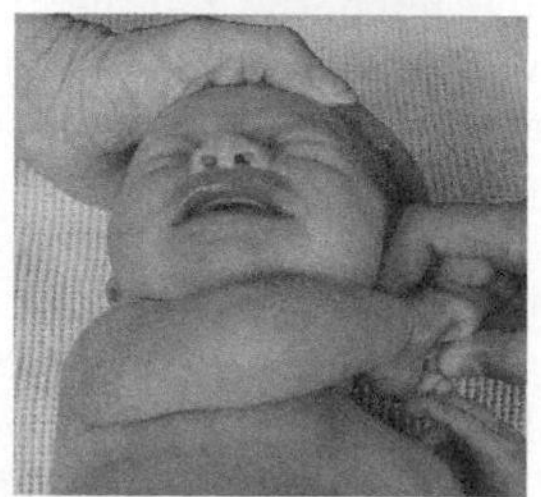

FIG. 9.11 Clinical and neurologic examinations comparing preterm and full-term infants. (Data from Pierog, S. H., & Ferrara, A. [1976]. *Medical care of the sick newborn* [2nd ed.]. St. Louis, MO: Mosby; photos courtesy Paul Vincent Kuntz, Texas Children's Hospital, Houston.)

NEUROLOGIC EVALUATION

PRETERM | TERM

Grasp reflex—The preterm infant's grasp is weak; the term infant's grasp is strong, allowing the infant to be lifted up from the mattress.

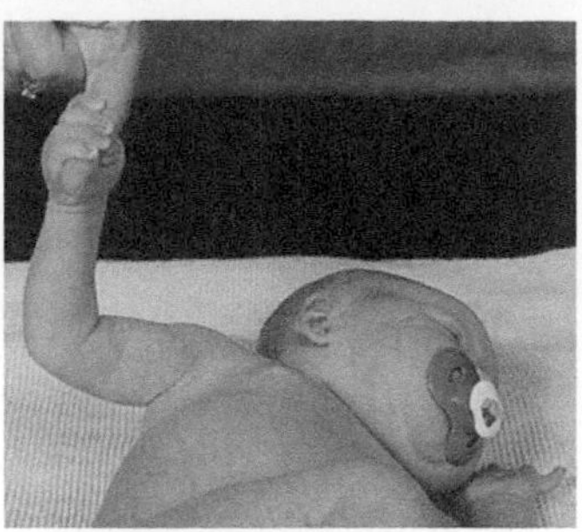

Heel-to-ear maneuver—The preterm infant's heel is easily brought to the ear, meeting with no resistance. This maneuver is not possible in the term infant, since there is considerable resistance at the knee.

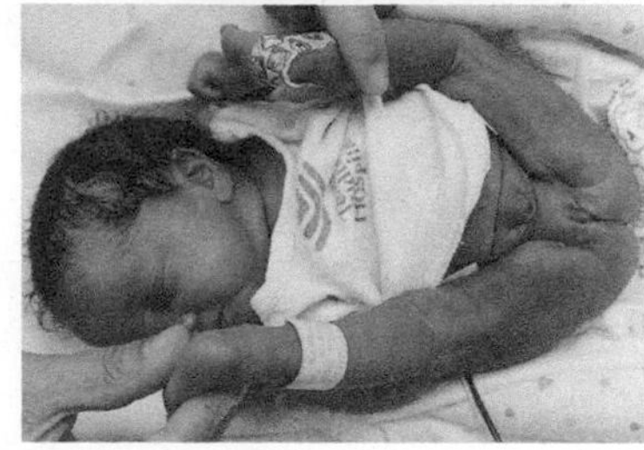

FIG. 9.11, cont'd

Apnea of prematurity (AOP) is a common phenomenon in the preterm infant. Rarely observed in full-term infants, apneic spells increase in prevalence the younger the gestational age. Most infants less than 32 weeks of gestation and nearly all apparently healthy infants less than 30 weeks of gestation have apneic spells (Gardner, Enzman-Hines, & Nyp, 2016). Apnea usually resolves as the infant approaches 37 weeks of postmenstrual age, but in those born very prematurely, apnea can persist up to 43 weeks of postmenstrual age (Alvaro, 2012).

AOP may be further classified according to origin. The three recognized types are (1) central apnea, an absence of diaphragmatic and other respiratory muscle function that causes a lack of respiratory effort and occurs when the CNS does not transmit signals to the respiratory muscles; (2) obstructive apnea, when air flow stops because of upper airway obstruction, yet chest or abdominal wall movement is present; and (3) mixed apnea, a combination of central and obstructive apnea and the most common form of apnea seen in preterm infants (Gardner, Enzman-Hines, & Nyp, 2016).

Pathophysiology

AOP reflects the immature and poorly refined neurologic and chemical respiratory control mechanisms in preterm infants. These infants are not as responsive to hypercarbia and hypoxemia, and their neurons have fewer dendritic associations than those of more mature infants. The respiratory reflexes of these infants are significantly less mature, which may be a contributing factor in the etiology. Overall weakness of the muscles of the thorax, diaphragm, and upper airway may also contribute to apneic episodes in the preterm infant. In addition, apnea is characteristically observed during periods of REM sleep. A variety of factors, including infection, intracranial hemorrhage (ICH), or PDA, can make apnea worse. Secondary causes of apnea should be investigated in infants with new-onset apnea or when there is a significant change in the frequency or severity of apneic episodes. Apnea in full-term infants should always be considered secondary and the cause investigated.

Clinical Manifestations

Factors that contribute to apnea in preterm neonates should be investigated and treated. Apnea can be anticipated in infants with a variety of conditions (Box 9.8); conversely, one of these disorders may be suspected in infants with persistent apneic spells. Although apnea is an expected event in preterm neonates, it should not be designated benign until all other causes have been ruled out. Apnea is a reason to screen for any of the causes listed in Box 9.8.

Therapeutic Management

Caffeine is often effective in reducing the frequency of primary apnea-bradycardia spells in newborns. Caffeine acts as a CNS stimulant to breathing. Neonates receiving caffeine must be closely observed for symptoms of toxicity. Caffeine has come to the forefront of pharmacologic therapy for AOP because it has fewer side effects than previously used aminophylline or theophylline, requires dosing once daily, has more predictable plasma concentrations, has slower elimination, and has a wider therapeutic range (trough, 5 to 20 mcg/ml) (Carlo, 2016). Caffeine citrate (Cafcit) has been approved for use in preterm infants with AOP. It can be injected or administered orally. Weight and urinary output should be closely monitored because caffeine acts as a mild diuretic.

DRUG ALERT

Caffeine Toxicity

Signs of caffeine toxicity are tachycardia (>180 to 190 beats/min) at rest, vomiting, irritability, restlessness, diuresis, dysrhythmias, jitteriness, and gastritis (hemorrhagic).

BOX 9.8 Possible Causes of Apnea of Prematurity

- Prematurity
- Airway obstruction with mucus or milk, or poor positioning
- Anemia, polycythemia
- Dehydration
- Cooling or overheating
- Hypoxemia
- Hypercapnia or hypocapnia
- Hypoglycemia
- Hypocalcemia
- Hyponatremia
- Sepsis, meningitis
- Seizures
- Increased vagal tone (in response to suctioning nasopharynx, gavage tube insertion, reflux of gastric contents, endotracheal intubation)
- Central nervous system depression from pharmacologic agents
- Intraventricular hemorrhage
- Patent ductus arteriosus, congestive heart failure
- Depression following maternal obstetric sedation
- Respiratory distress as a result of pneumonia, inborn errors of metabolism such as hyperammonemia, congenital defects of the upper airways

Nasal CPAP and, more recently, nasal intermittent positive pressure ventilation has been used as an adjunct treatment for AOP. CPAP acts to stabilize the airway and improve lung volumes; hence it is most effective for obstructive or mixed apnea.

Nursing Care Management

Management of apnea consists of monitoring respiration and heart rate routinely in all preterm infants and preventing contributing conditions. Cardiorespiratory monitors alert the staff to cessation of breathing according to a preset delay time—usually 15 to 20 seconds. Effective monitoring devices do not eliminate the need for alert nursing observation. Nursing observation combined with monitoring is the most effective means of identifying neonatal apnea.

If begun early, gentle tactile stimulation (e.g., rubbing the back or chest gently, repositioning the infant) will stop most apneic spells. If tactile stimulation fails to reinstitute respiration, flow-by oxygen and suctioning of the nose and mouth may be required. If breathing does not begin, the chin is raised gently to open the airway, and sufficient positive pressure is applied with a resuscitation mask and bag to lift the rib cage. The infant is never shaken. After breathing is restored, the infant is assessed for possible precipitating factors, such as unstable temperature, abdominal distention (if not observed earlier), or malpositioning of the airway. The use of pulse oximetry has helped detect the onset of an apneic episode.

! NURSING ALERT

When the alarm sounds, infants are first assessed for color and for presence of respiration. If they display the usual color and respirations, the nurse should investigate possible causes of a false alarm, such as faulty lead placement, detached or disconnected leads, improper alarm setting, or mechanical failure.

Nurses should maintain a careful record of episodes of apnea, including the number of apneic spells, the infant's appearance during and after the episode, and whether the infant self-recovers or if tactile stimulation, supplemental oxygen, or other measures are needed to restore breathing. Subsequent investigation into the possible cause of the apneic episode is vital to the care of the preterm infant because it may signal an underlying condition such as sepsis or NEC.

RESPIRATORY DISTRESS SYNDROME

RDS refers to a condition of surfactant deficiency and physiologic immaturity of the thorax. The terms *respiratory distress syndrome* and *hyaline membrane disease* are most often applied to this severe lung disorder. It is seen almost exclusively in preterm infants but may also be associated with multifetal pregnancies, infants of diabetic mothers, cesarean section delivery, cold stress, asphyxia, and a family history of RDS (Carlo & Ambalavanan, 2016c). The disorder is rarely observed in drug-exposed infants or infants who have been subjected to chronic intrauterine stress (e.g., maternal preeclampsia or hypertension). Respiratory distress of a nonpulmonary origin in neonates may also be caused by sepsis, cardiac defects (structural or functional), exposure to cold, airway obstruction (atresia), IVH, hypoglycemia, metabolic acidosis, acute blood loss, and drugs. Pneumonia in the neonatal period is respiratory distress caused by bacterial or viral agents and may occur alone or as a complication of RDS.

Pathophysiology

Preterm infants are born before the lungs are fully prepared to serve as efficient organs for gas exchange. This appears to be a critical factor in the development of RDS. RDS results from a combination of structural and functional immaturity of the lungs.

Because the final unfolding of the alveolar septa, which increases the surface area of the lungs, occurs during the last trimester of pregnancy, preterm infants are born with numerous underdeveloped and many uninflatable alveoli. In addition, the fetal chest wall is highly compliant because of the predominance of cartilage rather than bone, and the diaphragm, the dominant respiratory muscle, is prone to fatigue.

Functionally, the fetal lungs are deficient in **surfactant**, a surface-active phospholipid secreted by type II cells in the alveolar epithelium. Surfactant is first produced at about 24 weeks of gestational age, but the type II cells in the lung do not fully mature until about 36 weeks of gestation (Fig. 9.12). Acting much like a detergent, this substance reduces the surface tension of fluids that line the alveoli and respiratory passages, resulting in uniform expansion and maintenance of lung expansion at low intraalveolar pressure. Immature development of these functions seriously compromises respiratory efficiency. Deficient surfactant production causes unequal inflation of alveoli on inspiration and the collapse of alveoli on end expiration. Without surfactant, infants are unable to keep their lungs inflated and therefore exert a great deal of effort to reexpand the alveoli with each breath. It has been estimated that each breath requires as much negative pressure (60 to 75 cm H_2O) as the initial lung expansion at birth. With increasing exhaustion they are able to open fewer and fewer alveoli. This inability to maintain lung expansion produces widespread atelectasis.

In the absence of alveolar stability (i.e., normal functional residual capacity) and with progressive atelectasis, pulmonary vascular resistance (PVR) increases, whereas with normal lung expansion it would decrease. Consequently, there is hypoperfusion to the lung tissue, with a decrease in effective pulmonary blood flow. The increase in PVR causes partial reversion to the fetal circulation, with a right-to-left shunting of blood through the persisting fetal communications—the ductus arteriosus and foramen ovale.

Inadequate pulmonary perfusion and ventilation produce hypoxemia and hypercapnia. Pulmonary arterioles, with their thick muscular layer, are markedly reactive to diminished oxygen concentration. Thus a decrease in oxygen tension causes vasospasm in the pulmonary arterioles

PATHOPHYSIOLOGY REVIEW

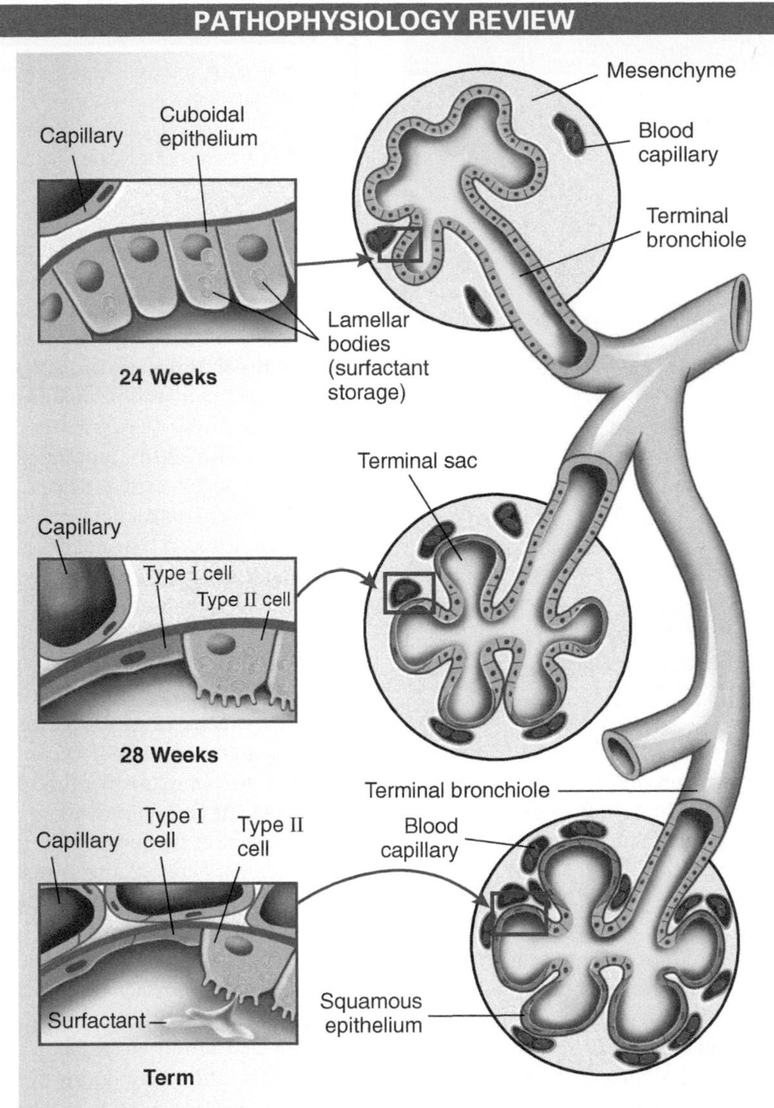

FIG. 9.12 Prenatal development of the alveolar unit. (From McCance, K., & Huether, S. [2010]. *Pathophysiology: The biological basis for disease in adults and children* [6th ed.]. St. Louis, MO: Mosby.)

that is worsened by a decrease in blood pH. This vasoconstriction contributes to a marked increase in PVR. In normal ventilation with increased oxygen concentration, the ductus arteriosus constricts and the pulmonary vessels dilate to decrease PVR (Fig. 9.13).

Prolonged hypoxemia activates anaerobic glycolysis, which produces increased amounts of lactic acid. An increase in lactic acid causes metabolic acidosis. Inability of the atelectatic lungs to blow off excess carbon dioxide produces respiratory acidosis. Lowered pH causes further vasoconstriction. With deficient pulmonary circulation and alveolar perfusion, Pao_2 continues to fall, pH falls, and the materials needed for surfactant production are not circulated to the alveoli.

Pulmonary edema observed in the early stages of RDS also contributes to impaired gas exchange. Factors believed to facilitate this fluid accumulation in the lungs include renal immaturity or insufficiency resulting from hypoxemia, high fluid intake and PDA, left ventricular dysfunction associated with papillary muscle necrosis, low serum protein concentration and low colloid osmotic pressure, increased alveolar surface tension that enhances the shift of interstitial fluid to alveolar spaces, oxygen toxicity, and high plasma vasopressin.

Pulmonary interstitial emphysema (PIE) may develop in preterm infants with RDS and immature lungs as a result of overdistention of distal airways. This condition further complicates adequate oxygenation in the immature airways (see Air Leak Syndromes, p. 307).

Deficiencies in other systems contribute to respiratory distress. For example, a high threshold of the respiratory center to afferent stimuli and weak or absent gag and cough reflexes reflect the immaturity of the nervous system. In addition, the persistence of fetal hemoglobin may place the infant at a disadvantage during respiratory distress. Although the binding power of fetal hemoglobin for oxygen is much greater than that of adult hemoglobin, this increased affinity also causes less oxygen to be released to the tissues at normal oxygen tension. In the newborn the arterial oxygen concentration must fall to a lower level for bound oxygen to be released from fetal hemoglobin.

A hyaline membrane is formed as hypoxemia and the increased pulmonary vascular pressure cause transudation of fluid into the alveoli. Necrotic cells from damaged alveoli plus the fibrin in the transudate form a membranous layer that lines the alveoli and inhibits gas exchange. The hyaline membrane contributes to respiratory problems by greatly

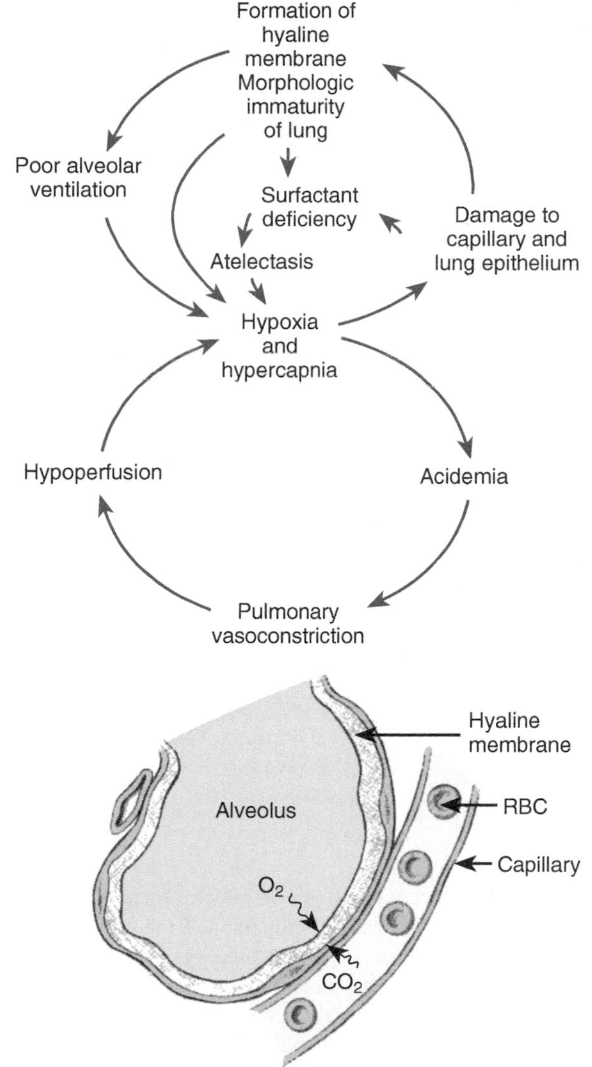

FIG. 9.13 Interdependent relationship of factors involved in pathology of respiratory distress syndrome. *CO_2,* Carbon dioxide; *O_2,* oxygen; *RBC,* red blood cell. (From Pierog, S. H., & Ferrara, A. [1976]. *Medical care of the sick newborn* [2nd ed.]. St. Louis, MO: Mosby.)

reducing lung distensibility, or compliance, the elastic quality of lung tissue that permits expansion in response to a given amount of applied pressure during inspiration. Affected lungs are stiffer and require far more pressure than do normal lungs to achieve an equal amount of expansion. Table 9.6 summarizes the major factors that produce RDS in immature infants.

Clinical Manifestations

Infants with RDS can develop respiratory distress either acutely or over a period of hours, depending on the acuity of pulmonary immaturity, associated illness factors, and gestational maturity. The observable signs produced by the pulmonary changes usually begin to appear in infants who apparently achieve normal breathing and color soon after birth. In a matter of a few hours, breathing gradually becomes more rapid (>60 breaths/min). Infants may display retractions—suprasternal or substernal, and supracostal, subcostal, or intercostal—which result from a compliant chest wall. Weak chest wall muscles and the highly cartilaginous rib structure produce an abnormally elastic rib cage, resulting in indrawing, or retraction, of the skin between the ribs. During this period the infant's color may remain good, and auscultation reveals air entry. Some of the criteria for evaluating respiratory distress in infants are illustrated in Fig. 9.14.

TABLE 9.6 Major Factors in Respiratory Distress Syndrome

Cause	Effect
Increased pulmonary vascular resistance	Alveolar collapse; atelectasis; increased difficulty breathing
Impaired gas exchange	Hypoxemia and hypercapnia with respiratory acidosis
Increased transudation of fluid into lungs	Hypoperfusion of pulmonary circulation
Hypoperfusion (with hypoxemia)	Tissue hypoxia and metabolic acidosis
Hyaline membrane formation; impaired gas exchange	Increased surface tension of alveoli (surfactant deficiency)

Within a few hours, respiratory distress becomes more obvious. The respiratory rate continues to increase (to 80 to 120 breaths/min), and breathing becomes more labored. Infants increase the rate rather than the depth of respiration when in distress. Substernal retractions become more pronounced as the diaphragm works hard in an attempt to fill collapsed air sacs. Fine inspiratory crackles can be heard over both lungs, and there is an audible expiratory grunt. This grunting, a useful mechanism observed in the earlier stages of RDS, serves to increase end-expiratory pressure in the lungs, thus maintaining alveolar expansion and allowing gas exchange for an additional brief period. Flaring of the nares is also a sign that accompanies tachypnea, grunting, and retractions in respiratory distress. Central cyanosis (i.e., a bluish discoloration of oral mucous membranes and generalized body cyanosis) is a late and serious sign of respiratory distress. Initially supplemental oxygen may eliminate cyanosis. The use of pulse oximetry and arterial blood gas sampling prevents dependence on color to determine oxygen requirements.

Severe RDS is often associated with a shocklike state, with diminished cardiac inflow and low arterial blood pressure. As a result of extreme pulmonary immaturity, decreased glycogen stores, and lack of accessory muscles, the ELBW and VLBW infant may have severe RDS at birth, bypassing the aforementioned steps in the development of RDS.

Infants with RDS who are treated with exogenous surfactant have a good chance for recovery. Complications of RDS include those described as complications of positive pressure ventilation (see p. 305). Associated complications (of prematurity and RDS) include PDA and congestive heart failure, retinopathy of prematurity, IVH, BPD, NEC, and neurologic sequelae.

Diagnostic Evaluation

Laboratory data are nonspecific, and the abnormalities observed are identical to those observed in numerous biochemical abnormalities of the newborn (i.e., the findings of hypoxemia, hypercapnia, and acidosis). Specific tests are used to determine complicating factors, such as blood glucose (to test for hypoglycemia), blood gas measurements for serum pH (to test for acidosis), and Pao_2 (to test for hypoxia). Pulse oximetry is an important component for determining hypoxia. Other special examinations may be used to diagnose or rule out complications.

Radiographic findings characteristic of RDS include (1) a diffuse granular pattern over both lung fields that resembles ground glass and represents alveolar atelectasis and (2) dark streaks, or air bronchograms, within the ground glass areas that represent dilated, air-filled bronchioles.

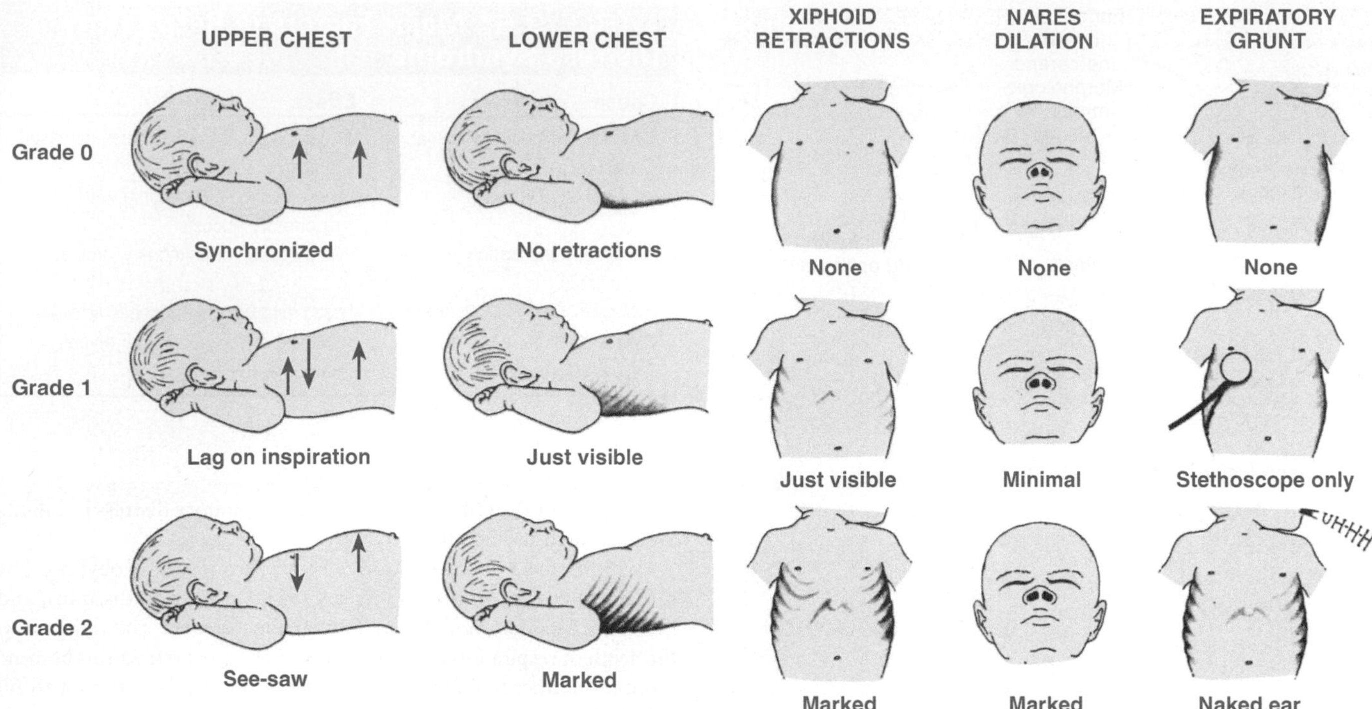

FIG. 9.14 Criteria for evaluating respiratory distress. (Modified from Silvermann, W. A., & Anderson, D. H. [1956]. A controlled clinical trial of effects of water mist on obstructive respiratory signs, death rate, and necropsy findings among premature infants. *Pediatrics, 17,* 1.)

It is important to distinguish between RDS and pneumonia in infants with respiratory distress.

Prenatal Diagnosis

Fetal lung maturity depends on gestational age and maternal illnesses. Problems such as maternal diabetes delay fetal lung maturation, whereas fetuses exposed to chronic stress (intrauterine growth restriction [IUGR], drug exposure) often have more mature lungs. Antenatal administration of glucocorticoids enhances fetal lung maturity, especially when combined with postnatal surfactant administration (Gardner, Enzman-Hines, & Nyp, 2016; Surbek, Drack, Irion, et al., 2012).

Functional maturity of the fetal lung is indicated by surfactant phospholipids in amniotic fluid. The most commonly tested is the lecithin/sphingomyelin (L/S) ratio, which represents the relationship between these two lipids during gestation. Phospholipids are synthesized by fetal alveolar cells, and the concentrations in amniotic fluid change during gestation. Initially there is more sphingomyelin, but at approximately 32 to 33 weeks the concentrations become equal; sphingomyelin then diminishes and lecithin increases significantly until the fetus has developed sufficient surfactant to maintain alveolar stability at approximately 35 weeks. An L/S ratio of 2 : 1 in nondiabetic mothers indicates virtually no risk of RDS.

Other key surfactant compounds (also phospholipids) that are needed to stabilize surfactant are phosphatidylcholine (PC) and phosphatidylglycerol (PG). Without these compounds, lecithin is not functional as a surfactant. Concentrations of PC parallel those of lecithin, peaking at 35 weeks and then gradually decreasing. At 36 weeks PG appears in amniotic fluid and increases until term. By measuring these phospholipids—L/S ratio, PC, and PG—the clinician can estimate the maturity of the lungs with a high degree of accuracy. Other, less commonly used methods have been devised to provide rapid, inexpensive, and accurate measures of lung maturity. These include the "shake" or "bubble" test, in which stable foam or bubbles form when amniotic fluid is shaken in the presence of ethanol, and the tap test, in which abundant bubbles appear in a test tube of amniotic fluid with 6*N*-hydrochloric acid and diethyl ether.

Another test that may be used to evaluate fetal lung maturity is the TDx Fetal Lung Maturity (FLM) assay, which determines PG levels in amniotic fluid or neonatal tracheal aspirates. The FLM test compared with the L/S ratios was a better predictor of long maturity with the utilization of the L/S ratios as a reflex test to confirm lung maturity associated with a high risk of respiratory morbidity (Tennant, Friedman, Pare, et al., 2012). The researchers hypothesized that the poor performance of L/S ratios may be due to increased disease prevalence in the population undergoing testing (Tennant, Friedman, Pare, et al., 2012).

Lamellar bodies, representing the storage form of surfactant, are found in amniotic fluid in increasing quantities with the advancement of gestational age and lung maturity. A quantitative count of lamellar bodies has been reported to be as accurate as the L/S ratio in determining fetal lung maturity. The count can be obtained faster than the L/S ratio, thus making it clinically appealing (Welch, Shaw, & Welch, 2016).

Therapeutic Management

The treatment of RDS includes all the general measures required for any preterm infant, as well as those instituted to correct imbalances. The supportive measures most crucial to a favorable outcome are: (1) maintain adequate ventilation and oxygenation with CPAP, high-flow nasal cannula, or mechanical ventilation; (2) maintain acid-base balance; (3) maintain a neutral thermal environment; (4) maintain adequate tissue perfusion and oxygenation; (5) prevent hypotension; and (6) maintain adequate hydration and electrolyte status. Nipple and gavage feedings are avoided in any situation that creates a marked increase in respiratory rate because of the greater hazards of aspiration.

QUALITY PATIENT OUTCOMES

Neonatal RDS

- Room air or oxygen saturation ≥88%
- Respiratory rate <60 breaths/min
- Blood pH ≥7.30

Surfactant

The administration of exogenous surfactant to preterm neonates with RDS has become an accepted and common therapy in most neonatal centers worldwide. Numerous clinical trials involving the administration of exogenous surfactant to infants with or at high risk for RDS demonstrate improvements in blood gas values and ventilator settings, decreased incidence of pulmonary air leaks, decreased deaths from RDS, and a lower infant mortality rate (Gardner, Enzman-Hines, & Nyp, 2016; Polin, Carlo, & Committee on Fetus and Newborn, 2014). Exogenous surfactant comes from a natural source (e.g., porcine or bovine) or from the production of artificial surfactant. Commercially available surfactant products include beractant (Survanta), poractant alfa (Curosurf), and calfactant (Infasurf).

Studies have been done comparing one surfactant product with another. Jordan and Donn (2013) found that an investigational synthetic surfactant—lucinactant—mimics the action of human surfactant protein-B (SP-B), and it was more effective than beractant and colfosceril palmitate at reducing the RDS-related mortality by 14 days of life. BPD was significantly less common in infants at 36 weeks of postmenstrual age who had received lucinactant.

Additional benefits of surfactant replacement therapy include decreased oxygen requirements and mean airway pressure (MAP) within hours of administration and an overall decrease in the incidence of pulmonary air leaks. To date, long-term improvement in the decrease of BPD and IVH has not been evidenced in all surfactant clinical trials.

Complications seen with surfactant administration include pulmonary hemorrhage and mucous plugging. Use of surfactant in infants with meconium aspiration resulted in a reduction in the severity of respiratory illness and subsequent need for extracorporeal membrane oxygenation (ECMO) support (Gardner, Enzman-Hines, & Nyp, 2016). Other studies continue to investigate the potential benefits of exogenous surfactant for the treatment of infectious pneumonia and lung hypoplasia associated with congenital diaphragmatic hernia (Zani, Eaton, Puri, et al., 2016). Acute RDS/acute lung injury may also respond favorably to surfactant administration (see Acute Respiratory Distress Syndrome/Acute Lung Injury, Chapter 26. Surfactant may be administered at birth as a prophylactic treatment of RDS or later in the course of RDS as a rescue treatment. Studies found improved clinical outcomes and fewer adverse effects when surfactant is administered prophylactically to infants at risk for developing RDS; early rescue (within 2 hours of birth) surfactant administration in ELBW with RDS resulted in lower rates of BPD, mortality, and air leaks (Bahadue & Soll, 2012; Polin, Carlo, & Committee on Fetus and Newborn, 2014). Surfactant is administered via the ET tube directly into the infant's trachea (Fig. 9.15); the exact number of doses (single versus multiple) that are most effective has yet to be determined.

Nursing responsibilities with surfactant administration include assistance in the delivery of the product, collection and monitoring of arterial blood gases, scrupulous monitoring of oxygenation, and assessment of the infant's tolerance of the procedure. Once surfactant is absorbed, there is usually an increase in respiratory compliance that requires adjustment of ventilator settings to decrease MAP and prevent overinflation or hyperoxemia. Suctioning is usually delayed for an hour or so (depending on the type of surfactant, delivery system, and unit protocol) to allow maximum effects to occur. Current research is investigating the possibility of delivering an aerosolized surfactant. This method would decrease the problems associated with current delivery systems (e.g., contamination of the airway, interruption of mechanical ventilation, and loss of the drug in the ET tubing from reflux) (see Fig. 9.16 of an infant in an oxyhood).

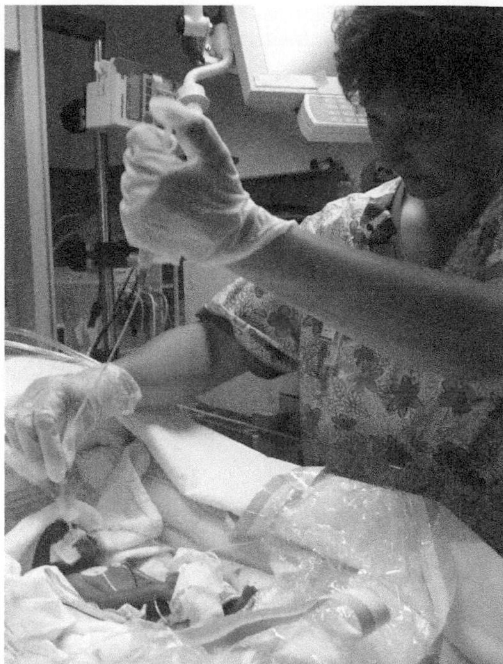

FIG. 9.15 Exogenous surfactant administration to infant on mechanical ventilation. (Courtesy E. Jacobs, Texas Children's Hospital, Houston.)

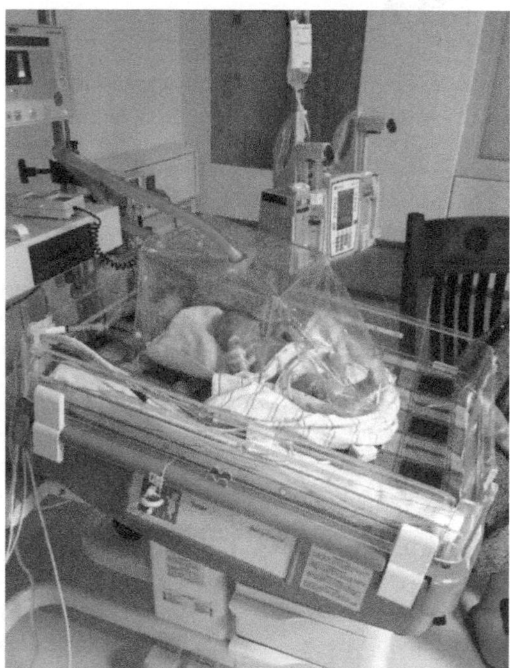

FIG. 9.16. Infant in an Oxyhood. (Courtesy K. Fisher, Duke University.)

Oxygen Therapy

The goals of oxygen therapy are to provide adequate oxygen to the tissues, prevent lactic acid accumulation resulting from hypoxia, and

TABLE 9.7 Common Methods for Assisted Ventilation in Neonatal Respiratory Distress

Method	Description	How Provided
Conventional Methods		
Continuous positive airway pressure (CPAP)	Provides constant distending pressure to airway in spontaneously breathing infant	Nasal prongs Endotracheal tube Face mask
Positive end-expiratory pressure (PEEP)*	Provides increased end-expiratory pressure during expiration and between mandatory breaths, which prevents alveolar collapse; maintains residual airway pressure	Endotracheal intubation and either volume-limited or pressure-limited ventilator
Intermittent mandatory ventilation (IMV)*	Allows infant to breathe spontaneously at own rate but provides mechanical cycled respirations and pressure at regular preset intervals	Endotracheal intubation and ventilator
Synchronized intermittent mandatory ventilation (SIMV)	Mechanically delivers breaths synchronized to onset of spontaneous patient breaths; uses assist/control mode to facilitate full inspiratory synchrony; involves signal detection of onset of spontaneous respiration from abdominal movement, thoracic impedance, and airway pressure or flow changes	Patient-triggered infant ventilator with signal detector and assist/control mode; endotracheal tube
Volume guarantee ventilation	Delivers predetermined volume of gas using inspiratory pressure that varies according to infant's lung compliance (often used in conjunction with SIMV)	Volume guarantee ventilator with flow sensor; endotracheal tube
Alternative Methods		
High-frequency oscillatory ventilation (HFOV)	Application of high-frequency, low-volume, sine-wave flow oscillations to airway at rates between 480 and 1200 breaths/min	Variable-speed piston pump (or loudspeaker, fluidic oscillator); endotracheal tube
High-frequency jet ventilation (HFJV)	Uses separate, parallel, low-compliant circuit and injector port to deliver small pulses or jets of fresh gas deep into airway at rates between 250 and 900 breaths/min	May be used alone or with low-rate IMV; endotracheal tube

*Also referred to as conventional ventilation (versus HFOV).

avoid the potentially negative effects of oxygen toxicity. Numerous methods have been devised to improve oxygenation (Table 9.7). All require that the gas be warmed and humidified before entering the respiratory tract. If the infant does not require ventilatory assistance, oxygen can be given via nasal prongs to supply variable concentrations of humidified oxygen. (See Oxygen Therapy, Chapter 26.) If oxygen saturation cannot be maintained at a satisfactory level and the carbon dioxide level ($Paco_2$) rises, infants will need ventilatory assistance.

Oxygen should be administered judiciously to preterm infants being stabilized in labor and delivery and for oxygenation maintenance in the NICU. Much attention has been focused recently on high oxygen concentration and the effect of free oxygen radicals on the development of conditions such as NEC, BPD, and retinopathy of prematurity (ROP). The current Neonatal Resuscitation Program guidelines recommend the use of oxygen concentrations between 21% and 100% to achieve an oxygen saturation appropriate to the infant's age in minutes (American Academy of Pediatrics & American Heart Association, 2011). Research indicates that optimal target ranges for maintaining adequate oxygenation while preventing ROP and BPD or other conditions is not clearly defined, but avoiding saturation levels lower than 88% or higher than 94% is prudent (Vain & Garcia, 2013) (see also Retinopathy of Prematurity later in this chapter).

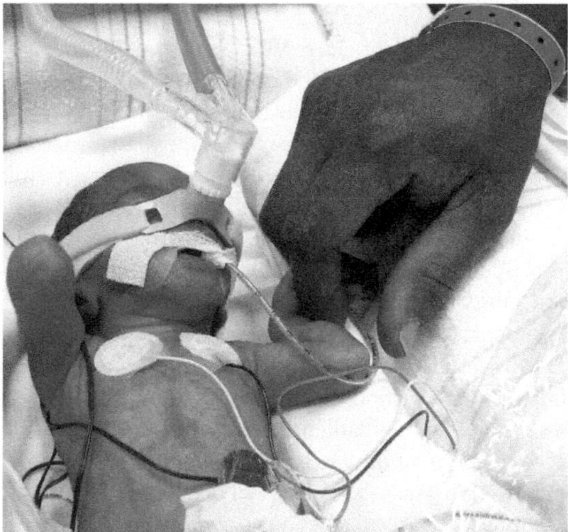

FIG. 9.17 Infant on nasal continuous positive airway pressure with father's finger in hand. (Courtesy E. Jacobs, Texas Children's Hospital, Houston.)

CPAP, the application of 3 to 8 cm H_2O (positive) pressure to the airway, uses the infant's spontaneous respiration to improve oxygenation by helping prevent alveolar collapse and increasing diffusion time. CPAP may be delivered via fitted face mask or nasal prongs (Fig. 9.17). Ventilation with CPAP is done entirely by the infant. The use of high-flow nasal cannulae (HFNC) at flow rates greater than or equal to 2 liters per minute is an alternative to nasal cannula for infants with RDS; the infant may be given surfactant shortly after birth then placed on either nasal CPAP or HFNC.

If oxygenation is not improved and the infant requires assisted ventilation, intermittent mandatory ventilation (IMV) is used with positive end-expiratory pressure (PEEP). This allows infants to breathe at their own rate but provides positive pressure breaths with end-expiratory pressure to prevent alveolar collapse and overcome airway resistance. IMV also involves peak inspiratory pressure (PIP) and rate (number of breaths per minute). The PIP is the maximum amount of positive pressure applied to the infant on inspiration. The total amount of pressure transmitted to the airway throughout an entire respiratory cycle is called the *mean airway pressure* (MAP or P_{aw}). Increasing MAP in infants with severe RDS correlates positively with improved oxygenation by maintaining functional residual capacity and overcoming the resistive forces of the atelectatic lung. The MAP is affected by changes in the PEEP, PIP, and inspiratory/expiratory ratio. Although MAP is now recognized as the major determinant of oxygenation, this does not imply that simply increasing MAP will automatically improve oxygenation (Keszler & Abubakar, 2017).

Improved technology has provided to preterm or sick neonates a form of mechanical ventilatory assistance previously used in adults: synchronized intermittent mandatory ventilation (SIMV). With this method breaths delivered by the ventilator are synchronized to the onset of spontaneous infant breaths. The net effect is to produce full respiratory synchrony rather than asynchronous respiratory efforts (commonly called "fighting the ventilator") that are believed to significantly impede the ability to adequately oxygenate infants without sedation or muscle paralysis. With SIMV, the operator sets the number of breaths per minute delivered by the ventilator, and the patient may breathe spontaneously between mechanical breaths. In the "assist-control" mode a mechanical breath is delivered each time a spontaneous respiration is detected; the "control" mode includes the delivery of a mechanical breath at a regular rate if the patient fails to initiate a spontaneous respiration. Additional benefits of SIMV are improved oxygenation, decreased incidence of BPD, and decreased time on mechanical ventilation.

If adequate oxygenation cannot be maintained and hypercarbia persists, infants may benefit from one of the two high-frequency ventilation (HFV) modalities. HFV delivers gas at very rapid rates to provide adequate minute volumes using lower proximal airway pressures by way of high-frequency oscillatory ventilation (HFOV) or high-frequency jet ventilation (HFJV). HFV was initially recommended for intractable respiratory failure, especially for infants with pulmonary air leaks and PIE. Many clinicians have now begun recommending earlier use of HFOV to prevent volutrauma to the lungs of very preterm infants (Clark, 2017).

Volutrauma is believed to be a key factor in the development of BPD. Sun, Cheng, Kang, and colleagues (2013) reported that HFOV was associated with improved survival and a decreased incidence of neurologic disability. HFJV is most often used in the treatment of full-term infants with meconium aspiration, persistent pulmonary hypertension, or air leak syndromes.

Complications of Positive Pressure Ventilation

Mechanical ventilation is not without hazards. Positive pressure introduced by mechanical apparatus increases complications such as PIE, pneumothorax, and pneumomediastinum (see p. 307). The avoidance of intubation and mechanical ventilation reduces the incidence of BPD (Gardner, Enzman-Hines, & Nyp, 2016). Other complications directly related to positive pressure include various problems associated with intubation, such as nasal, tracheal, or pharyngeal perforation; stenosis; inflammation; palatal grooves; subglottic stenosis; tube obstruction; and infection.

Nitric Oxide

Inhaled nitric oxide (NO) has emerged as a significant treatment modality for neonates with conditions that cause persistent pulmonary hypertension, pulmonary vasoconstriction, and subsequent acidosis and severe hypoxia. Infants with conditions such as MAS, pneumonia, sepsis, and congenital diaphragmatic hernia with pulmonary hypoplasia often require intervention in an attempt to reverse pulmonary hypertension. NO is a colorless, highly diffusible gas that causes smooth muscle relaxation and reduces pulmonary vasoconstriction and subsequent pulmonary hypertension when inhaled. NO may be administered through the ventilator circuit and blended with oxygen. It attaches readily to hemoglobin and is thus deactivated so that systemic vasculature is not affected. NO is toxic in large quantities, but the amount required to induce pulmonary vasculature relaxation (6 to 20 ppm) is well below toxic levels.

Studies of term and near-term infants being treated with NO for respiratory failure have been positive (Barrington, Finer, Pennaforte, et al., 2017; Peliowski & Canadian Paediatric Society, 2012). One exception is the study of newborns with congenital diaphragmatic hernia (CDH), whose morbidity and mortality rates were not significantly improved with NO (Putnam, Tsao, Morini, et al., 2016). Surfactant replacement therapy may be performed in combination with NO therapy in infants with inadequate pulmonary maturity. Nursing care of the infant receiving NO is the same as for the newborn with PPHN: continuous assessment of respiratory status and response to treatment is essential. A Cochrane Review (2017) concluded that NO was effective at an initial concentration of 20 ppm for term and near-term infants with hypoxic respiratory failure who do not have CDH (Barrington, Finer, Pennaforte, et al., 2017).

The use of NO for preterm infants remains controversial. A Cochrane Review (2017) concluded that NO for the treatment of very ill preterm infants as a rescue therapy does not appear to be effective (Barrington, Finer, & Pennaforte, 2017). Some studies have proposed a role for NO in the treatment of RDS and respiratory failure in these infants, whereas others suggest no benefit (Barrington, Finer, Pennaforte, et al., 2017; Kumar & Committee on Fetus and Newborn, 2014; Love & Bradshaw, 2012).

Medical Therapies

The treatment of the infant with RDS requires one or more IV lines to maintain hydration and nutrition, monitor arterial blood gases, and administer medications. Systemic antibiotics may be administered during the acute phase if sepsis is suspected (see Sepsis, p. 311). Caffeine may be used to treat apnea and to prepare for weaning VLBW and ELBW infants from mechanical ventilation. Inotropes such as dopamine and dobutamine may be required to support the infant's systemic blood pressure and maintain effective cardiac output during the acute phase of illness.

Prevention

The most successful approach to prevention of RDS is prevention of preterm delivery, especially elective early delivery and cesarean section. Improved methods for assessing the maturity of the fetal lung by amniocentesis, although not a routine procedure, allow a reasonable prediction of adequate surfactant formation (see Diagnostic Evaluation, p. 301). Because estimation of a delivery date can be miscalculated by as much as 1 month, such tests are particularly valuable when scheduling an elective cesarean section. Studies indicate that the combination of maternal glucocorticoid administration before delivery and surfactant administration postnatally has a synergistic effect on neonatal lungs, with the net result being a decrease in infant mortality, and incidence of IVH or infection (Gardner, Enzman-Hines, & Nyp, 2016; Hallman & Saarela, 2012).

Nursing Care Management

Care of infants with RDS involves all the observations and interventions previously described for high-risk infants. In addition, the nurse is concerned with the complex problems related to respiratory therapy and the constant threat of hypoxemia and acidosis that complicates the care of patients in respiratory difficulty.

The respiratory therapist is often responsible for the maintenance and regulation of respiratory equipment. Nevertheless, nurses should understand the equipment and be able to recognize when it is not functioning correctly. The most essential nursing function is to observe and assess the infant's response to therapy. Continuous monitoring and close observation are key because an infant's status can change rapidly and because oxygen concentration and ventilation parameters are prescribed according to the infant's blood gas measurements and pulse oximetry readings. Changes in oxygen concentration are based on these observations.

The nurse determines the amount of oxygen administered, expressed as the fraction of inspired air (Fio_2), on an individual basis according to pulse oximetry and/or arterial oxygen concentration. Capillary samples collected from the heel (see Chapter 22 for procedure) are useful for pH and $Paco_2$ determinations but not for oxygenation status. Continuous pulse oximetry readings are recorded hourly or more often as required in critically ill infants. Blood sampling is performed after ventilator changes for the acutely ill infant and thereafter when clinically indicated.

In infants with RDS who are acutely ill or extremely preterm, an umbilical arterial catheter (UAC) may be used to draw arterial blood for monitoring oxygenation. The catheter is inserted under sterile conditions via one of the umbilical arteries to the premeasured desired position (either at the level of the diaphragm, T6–T10, or between L3 and L4) and rests in the descending aorta. Continuous arterial pressure monitoring may be carried out with an "in-line" transducer. Practices vary regarding medication administration via a UAC. The nurse is aware of the potential hazards associated with these catheters (e.g., infection, hemorrhage, thrombus formation and subsequent vessel occlusion, arterial vasospasm) and implements monitoring and observation strategies to promptly intervene should complications occur (see Hydration, p. 277). An umbilical venous catheter (UVC) may be used separately or in conjunction with the UAC, depending on the severity of the infant's illness, the fluid requirements, and preferred medical practice.

Mucus may collect in the respiratory tract as a result of the infant's pulmonary condition. Secretions interfere with gas flow and may obstruct the passages, including the ET tube. Suctioning should occur only when necessary and should be based on individual infant assessment, which includes auscultation of the chest, evidence of decreased oxygenation, excess moisture in the ET tube, or increased infant irritability. It is recommended that, where possible, an in-line suction device be used on infants who are acutely ill and who do not tolerate any procedure without profound decreases in oxygen saturation, blood pressure, and heart rate. The purpose of suctioning an artificial airway is to maintain patency of that airway, not the bronchi. Suction applied beyond the ET tube can cause traumatic lesions of the trachea.

Research indicates that suctioning to a point where the catheter meets resistance and is then withdrawn causes trauma to the tracheobronchial wall. To remove secretions without damage to the tracheobronchial mucosa, the suction catheter is premeasured and inserted to a predetermined depth to avoid extension beyond the ET tube. The practice of suctioning patients on mechanical ventilation has undergone close scrutiny in recent years. Further studies are needed to validate this practice and to determine the best methods for maintaining a patent airway without compromising the patient's well-being. All efforts are made to prevent *ventilator-associated pneumonia* in mechanically ventilated high-risk infants. (see also Mechanical Ventilation, Chapter 26).

! NURSING ALERT

Suctioning is not an innocuous procedure; it may cause bronchospasm, bradycardia because of vagal nerve stimulation, hypoxia, and increased intracranial pressure, predisposing the infant to IVH. It should never be carried out on a routine basis. Improper suctioning technique can also cause infection, airway damage, or even pneumothorax.

Inspection of the skin is part of routine infant assessment. Position changes and the use of gel mattresses are helpful in guarding against skin breakdown.

Mouth care is especially important when infants are receiving nothing by mouth. The problem is often aggravated by the drying effect of oxygen therapy. The nurse can prevent drying and cracking by good oral hygiene using sterile water. Irritation to the nares or mouth that occurs from appliances used to administer oxygen may be reduced with a water-soluble ointment (see Skin Care section, p. 283).

Nursing care of an infant with RDS is demanding. Pay meticulous attention to subtle changes in the infant's oxygenation status. The importance of attention to detail cannot be overemphasized, particularly in regard to medication administration.

MECONIUM ASPIRATION SYNDROME

Meconium aspiration occurs when a fetus has been subjected to asphyxia or other intrauterine stress that causes relaxation of the anal sphincter and passage of meconium into the amniotic fluid. Most meconium aspiration occurs with the first breath. However, a severely compromised fetus may aspirate in utero. At delivery of the chest and initiation of the first breath, infants inhale fluid and meconium into the nasooropharynx (Fig. 9.18).

Pathophysiology

MAS involve the passage of meconium in utero as a result of hypoxic stress. It occurs primarily in full-term and postterm infants but has been reported in infants at less than 37 weeks of gestation. Once the fetus ingests meconium, any gasping activity occurring as a result of intrauterine stress may cause the sticky and tenacious substance to be aspirated into the lower airways. The net results are partial airway obstruction, air trapping, hyperinflation distal to the obstruction, and atelectasis caused by surfactant deactivation. A "ball-valve" situation exists wherein gas flows into the lungs on inspiration but is trapped there on exhalation as a result of the small airway diameter. As the infant struggles to take in more air (air hunger), even more meconium may be aspirated. Hyperinflation, hypoxemia, and acidemia result in increased PVR.

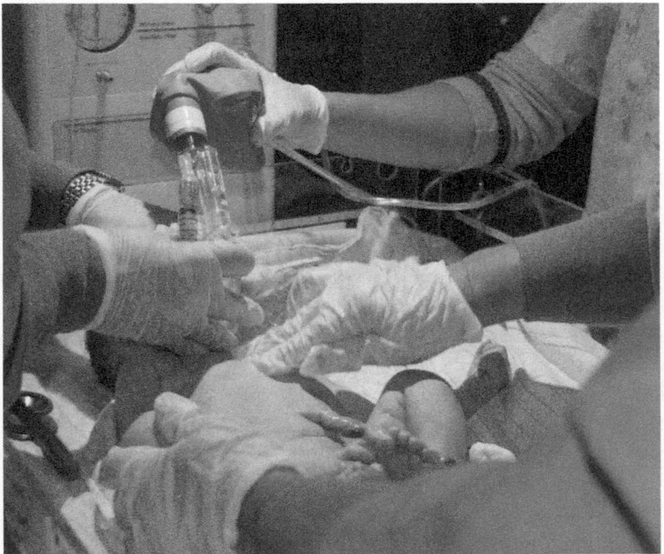

FIG. 9.18 Infant being resuscitated at birth. Note presence of meconium on abdomen and umbilical cord. (Courtesy Shannon Perry, Phoenix.)

In turn, shunting of blood through the ductus arteriosus (right to left) occurs because of increased resistance to blood flow through the pulmonary arteries (and to the lungs), leading to further hypoxemia and acidosis. Ductal shunting increases with hypoxia; some blood may enter the left atrium (LA) from the right atrium (RA) via the foramen ovale because there is a net decrease in blood returning to the LA via the pulmonary venous system, preventing closure of the foramen ovale. This pathologic process is essentially persistence of the fetal circulation, or PPHN, which is discussed later in this chapter. The air trapping of MAS causes overdistention of the alveoli and often air leaks. There is evidence that meconium contributes to the destruction of surfactant, increasing surface tension and further predisposing the alveoli to decreased functional capacity.

Clinical Manifestations

Infants who have released meconium in utero for some time before birth are stained from green meconium stools (those with more recent meconium passage may not be stained), tachypneic, hypoxic, and often depressed at birth. They develop expiratory grunting, nasal flaring, and retractions similar to those of infants with RDS. They may initially be cyanotic or pale, as well as tachypneic, and they may demonstrate the classic barrel chest from hyperinflation. The infants are often stressed, hypothermic, hypoglycemic, and hypocalcemic. Severe meconium aspiration progresses rapidly to respiratory failure if untreated. These infants exhibit profound respiratory distress with gasping, ineffective ventilations, marked cyanosis and pallor, and hypotonia.

Diagnostic Evaluation

At birth, meconium can often be visualized via laryngoscopy in the respiratory passages and vocal cords. Chest radiographs show uneven distribution of patchy infiltrates, air trapping, hyperexpansion, and atelectasis. Air leaks may occur as the illness progresses. Oxygenation will be poor, as evidenced by pulse oximetry and arterial blood gases. These infants may quickly develop metabolic and respiratory acidosis. Echocardiography assists in the diagnosis of right-to-left shunting of blood away from the pulmonary system.

Therapeutic Management

After delivery, the need for tracheal suctioning is based on infant assessment. Infants who are vigorous with strong, stable respiratory effort, good muscle tone, and heart rate greater than 100 beats/min should not undergo tracheal suctioning but should be closely monitored (Weiner, 2016). On the other hand, infants with poor respiratory effort, low heart rate, and poor tone should be rapidly intubated, suctioned, and resuscitated according to clinical status after suctioning.

Infants with respiratory distress are admitted to the NICU. Management of MAS consists of ventilatory support, exogenous surfactant administration, IV fluids, systemic antibiotics, and in some cases inotropes. Because these infants are prone to development of persistent pulmonary hypertension, they should be supported to maintain normal pH, carbon dioxide, and oxygen levels; they may be candidates for ECMO therapy, HFV, or NO (see Nitric Oxide, p. 305, and Persistent Pulmonary Hypertension of the Newborn, p. 308). Complications are managed symptomatically or as described under the specific disorder.

Nursing Care Management

Nursing care management is the same as for any high-risk neonate (see nursing care in sections on oxygen therapy, persistent pulmonary hypertension, and other complications).

QUALITY PATIENT OUTCOMES

MAS

- Room air oxygen saturation ≥90%
- Maintains arterial/venous pH ≥7.35

AIR LEAK SYNDROMES

Air leaks result from alveolar rupture and subsequent escape of air to tissues in which air is not normally present. Air leaks (1) may occur spontaneously in normal neonates, (2) can result from congenital renal or pulmonary malformations, and (3) often complicate underlying respiratory disease and its therapy (e.g., positive pressure ventilation, especially when high distending pressures are required).

After alveolar rupture, air often vents directly into the pleural space to create a pneumothorax. Air may vent into the perivascular interstitium, a condition termed *pulmonary interstitial emphysema (PIE)*. PIE may be seen on radiographs as early as 2 to 3 hours after birth in ELBW and VLBW infants with severe RDS. Localized PIE may resolve by itself or may lead to pneumothorax. HFV has been reported to improve the outcome in infants with PIE (Squires, De Paoli, Williams, et al., 2013). Air can dissect along the perivascular sheaths to eventually enter the mediastinum and cause pneumomediastinum. More extensive leaks involve the pericardium (manifested as pneumopericardium) or emphysema in the cervical, subcutaneous, or retroperitoneal soft tissues.

Clinical Manifestations

Spontaneous pneumothorax usually occurs during the first few breaths after birth, primarily in full-term or postterm infants, and is evident by the gradual onset of symptoms of respiratory distress after arrival in the nursery. Use of positive pressure ventilation in resuscitation may cause air leaks. In some cases, such as in extreme prematurity and meconium aspiration, air leaks may not be altogether preventable. The nurse suspects an air leak on the basis of respiratory manifestations, a decrease in oxygen saturation, and a shift in location of maximum intensity of heart sounds and absent or diminished breath sounds (although breath sounds may not be altered because of the small diameter of the chest and auscultation of referred breath sounds).

A tension pneumothorax occurs more frequently in infants requiring ventilatory assistance but may also occur in term infants at birth. In preterm infants being mechanically ventilated, an air leak may be demonstrated by hypotension, bradycardia, decreased or absent breath sounds unilaterally, decreased oxygenation (by pulse oximetry), and cyanosis, none of which responds to efforts for oxygenation (a resuscitation bag connected to the ET tube and manual ventilations). There may also be chest asymmetry, altered cardiac sounds (diminished, shifted, or muffled), a palpable liver and spleen, and subcutaneous emphysema. Infants on HFV may demonstrate an air leak by a sudden decrease in systemic blood pressure or an absence of chest movement (because of difficulty in auscultation of the chest with such modalities). The otherwise healthy full-term infant may exhibit only mild to moderate signs of respiratory distress. Air leaks contribute to the risk of an adverse developmental outcome in preterm infants (Pishva, Parsa, Saki, et al., 2012).

Therapeutic Management

Diagnosis is confirmed by transillumination of the chest with a fiberoptic light and/or radiographic examination. In symptomatic infants, treatment is urgent. Trapped air is evacuated by chest tube insertion into the pleural space through a small chest incision. The chest tube is then attached to continuous water-seal or dry suction

! NURSING ALERT

Early manifestations of pneumothorax include tachypnea, restlessness and irritability, lethargy, grunting, nasal flaring, and retractions. Pneumothorax during ventilatory assistance is evident from abrupt and profound duskiness or cyanosis; significant declines in heart rate, arterial blood pressure, and pulse pressure; and poor peripheral perfusion.

control drainage. In situations requiring infant transport, a pocket-sized Heimlich valve may be used until an appropriate drainage system can be established. The valve is not effective when fluid drainage is required. Needle aspiration serves as an emergency measure until a chest tube can be inserted. Pneumomediastinum seldom requires treatment, but pneumopericardium is managed by needle aspiration or pericardial tube drainage. The full-term newborn with a small tension pneumothorax may require oxygen therapy and parenteral fluids for a brief period if respiratory distress is not severe.

Nursing Care Management

The most important nursing function is close observation for the possibility of an air leak in susceptible infants. Nurses have a high level of suspicion in (1) infants with RDS with or without positive pressure ventilation, (2) infants with meconium-stained amniotic fluid or MAS, (3) infants with radiographic evidence of interstitial or lobar emphysema, (4) infants who required resuscitation at birth, or (5) infants receiving CPAP or positive pressure ventilation. For infants at risk, needle aspiration equipment (e.g., 30-ml syringe, three-way stopcock, and 23- to 25-gauge needles) should be available for emergency use.

The general nursing care of the infant with an extraneous air syndrome is the same as that for all high-risk neonates. Respiratory management is similar to that for infants with RDS. Assessing breath sounds frequently, monitoring the efficacy of gas exchange, and regulating oxygen therapy according to the infant's needs are vital nursing functions. Pain management is vital in these preverbal and significantly stressed infants.

PERSISTENT PULMONARY HYPERTENSION OF THE NEWBORN

PPHN results from elevated pulmonary artery pressure with levels equal to or greater than systemic pressure, and large right-to-left shunts through both the foramen ovale and the ductus arteriosus (Parker & Kinsella, 2012). Because full development of pulmonary arterial musculature occurs late in gestation, PPHN is primarily a condition of late-preterm, full-term, or postterm infants, many of whom were products of complicated pregnancies or deliveries. The condition is often associated with meconium aspiration, congenital diaphragmatic hernia with severe respiratory distress, cold stress, respiratory distress (e.g., RDS or pneumonia), and septicemia (group B streptococci [GBS]). PPHN is believed to be precipitated by perinatal factors, such as perinatal asphyxia, that cause or contribute to constriction of the pulmonary vasculature.

PPHN can be either primary or secondary. Primary PPHN occurs when the pulmonary vessels fail to relax and open with the initial respiration at birth. Secondary PPHN results from hypoxic stress that increases PVR and causes a return to fetal cardiopulmonary circulation. PPHN is most commonly observed in infants at 35 to 44 weeks of gestation who have a history of perinatal asphyxia, metabolic acidosis, or sepsis and respiratory distress within the first 24 hours. The infants become hypoxic and display marked cyanosis, tachypnea with grunting and retractions, and decreased peripheral perfusion. A loud pulmonary component of the second heart sound and, sometimes, a systolic ejection murmur are present. Diagnosis is established from clinical signs and diagnostic tests, including chest radiography, electrocardiogram, and echocardiography.

Therapeutic Management

Early recognition and management of conditions that contribute to or cause hypoxia and pulmonary vascular vasoconstriction are the primary goals in the prevention of PPHN. Additional treatment includes careful fluid regulation and evaluation of intravascular fluid volume. Supplemental oxygen reduces hypoxia and decreases pulmonary vasoconstriction. Assisted ventilation, often by HFV, is required if hypoxia is severe. Vasodilators, such as sildenafil (a phosphodiesterase [PDE5] inhibitor) or epoprostenol (prostacyclin), are sometimes prescribed to decrease PVR, thereby avoiding ECMO and NO. Sildenafil administered in intravenous or oral form has been shown to reduce PVR (hypertension) in neonates and improve oxygenation, but further controlled clinical trials are needed (Lakshminrusimha, Konduri, & Steinhorn, 2016; Sayed & Bisheer, 2015).

Additional drug therapy used in the management of PPHN includes the vasopressors dopamine, dobutamine, epinephrine, and nitroprusside to increase systemic vascular resistance. Inhaled NO has been successfully used to reverse pulmonary vascular vasoconstriction and is usually tried before other therapies such as ECMO (see Nitric Oxide, p. 305).

Another approach to management of infants with pulmonary complications is the use of ECMO with a modified heart-lung machine. Blood is shunted from a catheter in the right atrium or right internal jugular vein by gravity to a servoregulated roller pump; pumped through a membrane lung and a small heat exchanger; and returned to the systemic circulation via a major artery, such as the carotid artery, to the aortic arch. A venovenous approach (femoral vein) may be used, avoiding the need to ligate the carotid artery. ECMO provides oxygen to the circulation and allows the lungs to rest. The goal of ECMO is to "buy time" for the severely injured lung to heal while effectively oxygenating major organ systems, including the brain, heart, kidneys, and lungs (Fig. 9.19).

ECMO is labor intensive and expensive. Technical malfunctions may occur, requiring frequent monitoring of the equipment and the patient's response to treatment. Typically, two nurses, or a nurse and a perfusionist, are minimum staffing for the ECMO patient; more staff, including a respiratory therapist, are required in the acute phase. ECMO requires heparinization of the blood and blood circuit. For this reason it is not used in infants at less than 35 weeks of gestation, who are prone to intraventricular hemorrhage. Bleeding is one of the major complications associated with ECMO. The need for ECMO has decreased with increased

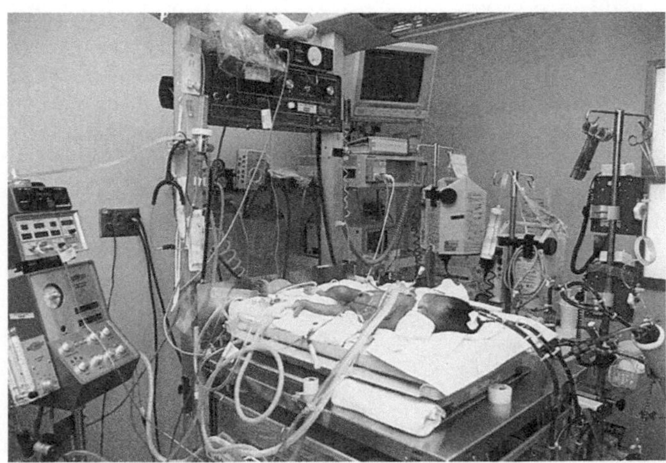

FIG. 9.19 Infant on extracorporeal membrane oxygenation (ECMO).

use of exogenous surfactant, inhaled NO, and HFV for neonatal hypoxemic respiratory failure (Sharma, Berkelhamer, & Lakshminrusimha, 2015).

Nursing Care Management

Nursing care for PPHN is the same as for infants with severe respiratory difficulties and those given mechanical ventilation and cardiovascular support. The infant with PPHN is often the sickest on the unit, depending on the causative factors and reaction to treatment. Because handling for any reason causes a decrease in arterial oxygen concentration, the nurse must weigh the stresses imposed by routine care against the risk of iatrogenic hypoxia. It is important to decrease noxious stimuli that cause hypoxia and to use clustered nursing interventions that keep nonsedated infants calm. Continuous monitoring of oxygenation, temperature, central venous pressure, vital signs, blood pressure, and acid-base balance decreases the need for physical manipulation and disturbance. Infants are further assessed for response to treatments, including IV therapy, fluids, electrolytes, and exogenous glucose.

BRONCHOPULMONARY DYSPLASIA

BPD, sometimes referred to as chronic lung disease, is a pathologic process that develops primarily in ELBW and VLBW infants with RDS. BPD may also develop in infants with MAS, persistent pulmonary hypertension, pneumonia, and cyanotic heart disease. Infants who develop BPD are at risk for frequent hospitalization because of their borderline respiratory reserve, hyperactive airway, and increased susceptibility to respiratory infection.

Mild BPD is operationally defined by the need for supplemental oxygen for 28 days or more but room air by 36 weeks corrected gestational age or at discharge. Moderate BPD is defined by the need for oxygen for 28 days or more and less than 30% oxygen at 36 weeks corrected gestational age. With severe BPD infants require more than 30% oxygen at 36 weeks corrected gestational age (Botet, Figueras-Aloy, Miracle-Echegoyen, et al., 2012). An inverse relationship between incidence of BPD and birth weight is emphasized in the Vermont-Oxford Network report, which found a 60% incidence for ELBW infants (501 to 750 g [1.1 to 1.6 lb]) versus 21% for infants weighing 1001 to 1250 g (2.2 to 2.7 lb). Risk factors for BPD include assisted ventilation, oxygen administration, prenatal and postnatal (nosocomial) infections, PDA, and fluid imbalance (Fraser, 2012; Gardner, Enzman-Hines, & Nyp, 2016).

The more severe form of BPD usually begins with severe respiratory failure secondary to RDS or with pneumonia requiring mechanical ventilation with high airway pressure and oxygen supplementation during the first few days of life (Gardner, Enzman-Hines, & Nyp, 2016). Since the advent of antenatal glucocorticoid therapy, surfactant replacement, and new ventilator strategies, a "new" BPD is emerging (Philip, 2012). These infants experience a milder initial respiratory course but continue to require ventilatory support or oxygen supplementation and show radiographic pulmonary changes characteristic of BPD.

Pathophysiology

The pathogenesis of BPD is complex and multifactorial. BPD begins when the immature lung undergoes an initial injury, leading to a chronic inflammatory process which results in recurrent injury and abnormal healing (Fraser, 2012). A variety of mechanisms have been related to the initial injury, including (1) prenatal infection (inflammatory process before birth), (2) mechanical ventilation (volutrauma, intubation), (3) supplemental oxygen (oxygen-derived free radicals), (4) increased pulmonary blood flow from PDA, or (5) postnatal infection.

The pulmonary changes are characterized by interstitial edema and epithelial swelling, followed by thickening and fibrotic proliferation of the alveolar walls and squamous metaplasia of the bronchiolar epithelium. Areas of atelectasis and cystlike foci of hyperaeration are visible on radiographs between 10 and 20 days of life and persist for weeks; however, some infants may not demonstrate cystic foci. Ciliary activity is paralyzed by high oxygen concentrations that interfere with the ability to clear the lung of mucus, thus aggravating airway obstruction and atelectasis. As the infant's lungs begin healing, the process is altered, possibly by continuous high oxygenation, inadequate nutrition, or vitamin E deficiency, resulting in decreased surface for oxygen and carbon dioxide exchange. The overall results of this process are hypercarbia, hypoxemia, and subsequent inability to wean successfully from oxygen.

As survival of immature preterm infants (<28 weeks of gestation) increases, the occurrence of BPD also increases.

In addition to BPD, other diseases associated with similar radiographic findings include congenital heart disease and viral pneumonia caused by cytomegalovirus. There are no laboratory alterations that confirm a diagnosis. Diagnosis is made on the basis of radiographic findings, oxygen therapy or positive pressure ventilation after 28 days, signs of respiratory distress, and a history of requiring mechanical ventilation in the first week of life for more than 3 days.

Therapeutic Management

The first approach to management is prevention of the disorder in susceptible infants. A meta-analysis demonstrated that early administration of surfactant (within 2 hours of birth) in ELBW infants with RDS resulted in lower rates of air leak, mortality, and BPD (Polin, Carlo, & Committee on Fetus and Newborn, 2014). To reduce the risk of volutrauma with positive pressure ventilation, maintain the lowest PIP necessary to obtain adequate ventilation, and use the lowest level of inspired oxygen to maintain adequate oxygenation. HFOV has been beneficial in reducing the risk of BPD, as has the administration of vitamin A (Guimaraes, Guedes, Rocha, et al., 2012). Fluid administration is carefully controlled and restricted. Drug or surgical intervention is indicated when there is significant shunting of blood through the PDA.

No specific treatment exists for BPD except to maintain adequate arterial blood gases with the administration of oxygen and to avoid progression of the disease. Corticosteroid therapy has been shown to benefit infants with BPD by decreasing the pulmonary inflammatory response and improving oxygenation and gas exchange, resulting in earlier weaning from mechanical assistance. However, with complications such as sepsis, hypertension, and hyperglycemia and an overall lack of decreased mortality in such infants, this therapy remains controversial. Other adverse effects of this long-acting, potent glucocorticoid have been reported, including growth restriction, GI hemorrhage, and cardiomyopathy. In light of studies that show an increased incidence of periventricular leukomalacia, neuromotor abnormalities, CP, decreased cerebral cortical gray matter volume, and adverse long-term neurologic outcome, the benefits of this treatment may not outweigh the risks (Shah, Ohlsson, Halliday, et al., 2017). It is possible that inhaling the steroids, so that the drug directly reaches the lung, may reduce the observed adverse events (Shah, Ohlsson, Halliday, et al., 2017). Research examining whether an alternative dosing regimen of postnatal steroids can reduce the incidence of BPD without associated neurodevelopmental side effects showed an increased risk of BPD and adverse neurodevelopmental outcomes for infants receiving a lower cumulative dose (Onland, De Jaegere, Offringa, et al., 2017).

Weaning infants from oxygen is difficult and must be accomplished gradually. These infants do not tolerate excessive or even normal amounts of fluid well and have a tendency to accumulate interstitial fluid in the lungs, which aggravates the condition. Oral diuretics may be used to control interstitial fluid.

Growth and development are often delayed in infants with BPD, which is related in part to the difficulties in providing adequate nutrition and in part to the lack of normal sensory stimulation because of prolonged hospitalization. Infants with BPD have far greater metabolic needs. This can create a problem for the caregiver, who must ensure adequate nutrition while avoiding overhydration, especially if the infant is ill, eats poorly, or has cardiopulmonary instability. The infant may be further compromised by gastroesophageal reflux, a frequent complication in preterm infants. Adequate intake of protein is particularly important in preventing postnatal growth failure in LBW infants. Protein supplements may be necessary to ensure adequate intake.

Osteopenia may occur in infants with BPD and in preterm infants, with higher incidence among the infants with BPD, presumably because of low calcium and vitamin D intake secondary to the calciuric effects of diuretic therapy. Dietary supplementation with human milk fortifier, calcium and phosphorus, and vitamin D has reduced the incidence of osteopenia in preterm infants.

RSV prophylaxis with the monoclonal antibody palivizumab (Synagis) is effective in diminishing the complications of RSV. RSV is a common cause of hospitalization and death in growing preterm neonates, including those with BPD. Palivizumab is given intramuscularly to high-risk infants, does not interfere with immunizations, and has few side effects. Palivizumab is administered in a dose of 15 mg/kg once a month, usually beginning in October and ending in May. (See Respiratory Syncytial Virus, Chapter 26.)

Despite the efficacy and excellent safety record of palivizumab, the majority of infants at risk for severe RSV do not receive palivizumab (Hall, Weinberg, Blumkin, et al., 2013). Although palivizumab is indicated for the broader population of high-risk children for the prevention of serious RSV lower respiratory tract disease, the American Academy of Pediatrics (AAP) and other pediatric society position statements recommend restricting its use to only infants at the highest-risk category due to the high cost of palivizumab (Hall, Weinberg, Blumkin, et al., 2013).

Prognosis

Reports vary regarding the mortality rate for BPD. The hospital stay is often long because of the infant's need for supplemental oxygen, although home oxygen therapy provides some infants the opportunity for discharge. A nasal cannula is an acceptable way to administer oxygen for the dependent infant to promote development of motor and social skills. Long-term problems seen in older children who had BPD as infants include growth failure, airway hyperreactivity, hyperexpansion, increased incidence of respiratory infections, and airway obstruction.

A diagnosis of BPD can have a long-term impact on a child. Lodha, Ediger, Ravil, and colleagues (2015) concluded that at 36 months children diagnosed with BPD with chronic oxygen dependency at NICU discharge were more likely to need respiratory medications and supplemental oxygen in the previous 12 months compared with the no-BPD group. These children were also more likely to require more frequent physician visits than the no-BPD group (Lodha, Ediger, Ravil, et al., 2015). An 8-year follow-up study comparing the outcomes of preterm infants with BPD and preterm infants without BPD found that children with a history of BPD are significantly more likely to have lung function abnormalities, such as airway obstruction and respiratory symptoms, at school age compared with preterm-born children without BPD (vom Hove, Prenzel, Uhlig, et al., 2014). BPD was also associated with reductions in both diffusion capacity and spirometry when lung function was measured at school age for children born preterm with BPD (Ronkainen, Dunder, Peltoniemi, et al., 2015).

Nursing Care Management

Infants with BPD expend considerable energy in their efforts to breathe, so they must receive plenty of opportunities for rest and additional calories. Growth records provide clues to the need for change in their diets. Some infants require nutritional supplements. Because these infants tire easily and because large quantities of milk might compromise respiration, small, frequent feedings are better tolerated. Reducing environmental stimuli and subsequent hypoxia is an important aspect in the care of these infants. The older infant's behavioral cues may signal carbon dioxide retention.

Adequate hydration is extremely important because a large amount of fluid is lost through respiration, and secretions must be thinned sufficiently to facilitate removal by suctioning. However, because BPD increases lung permeability, many infants are subject to pulmonary edema and require fluid restriction. Nurses must be alert to signs of both overhydration and underhydration, such as changes in weight, electrolytes, output measurements, and urine specific gravity and signs of edema.

Because the growing infant with BPD has a restricted fluid intake, has higher than average caloric requirements, and often requires many oral medications, the nurse is challenged by the complexity of care involved. Infants with BPD may become difficult or maladaptive feeders if they are aware of hunger yet compromised by not being able to eat fast enough to satiate that hunger because of the increased labor of breathing. Individualized nursing efforts to monitor oxygenation requirements during feedings, decrease environmental stimuli, fortify feedings, and provide more contact with a primary caregiver may facilitate the infant's care. Feeding schedules should be individualized as much as possible. Oral medications that taste bad to the infant may be given at times separate from feedings to ensure that feeding time is pleasant. Adjustments to overall fluid administration requirements are made, taking into account that the oral medications are also fluids. Regurgitated medications and feedings need to be dealt with in regard to fluid and caloric needs and the amount of absorption of medication that occurs before emesis.

Parents are extremely anxious regarding the prognosis when their infant has BPD. The lengthy hospitalization interferes with parent-child relationships and deprives the infant of appropriate parental contact and stimulation. Nurses should encourage the parents to visit the infant and become involved in the routine care. The parents need to be informed regarding medical care, equipment, and procedures related to their infant and taught procedures such as suctioning.

The older infant with BPD should have normal nurturing and developmental opportunities appropriate to the infant's condition and abilities. Careful monitoring of physiologic and behavioral systems during any activity is necessary so that activity can be stopped before the infant becomes irritable or tired. Opportunities out of bed in an infant seat or on a floor mat with a nurse or physical or play therapist provide one-on-one interaction that can enhance the infant's experience of the world and people.

Irritability has been associated with infants who have BPD, making their care often challenging and frustrating (see Developmental Outcome, p. 285). Some strategies to facilitate infant coping during prolonged hospitalization include (1) decreased number of unfamiliar caregivers, (2) increased access to parents, (3) predictability in schedule and caregivers, (4) consistency of care routines and practices, (5) pleasurable opportunities for play and socialization within physical tolerance, (6) adequate nutrition, and (7) uninterrupted rest cycles with diurnal variation to facilitate biologic rhythms. Parental involvement is critical because they are the one constant for the infant.

Home Care

Because the availability of home cardiac and apnea monitors and home oxygen therapy has increased, many infants with BPD can be discharged when they are gaining weight and their oxygen need is low. Home care promotes parent-infant bonding, minimizes health care costs, and prevents nosocomial infections. Preparation for home care requires education and considerable reassurance. Management of home monitoring equipment and home oxygen therapy provokes stress, but most families become comfortable with the machinery while their infant is still in the hospital. Families need reminders about their infant's increased risk of infection and about limiting contact with persons who have respiratory tract infections. Because of their minimum respiratory reserve, even a minor illness can threaten these infants.

Some infants are discharged with a tracheostomy on oxygen supplementation or home ventilators. Discharge teaching and home care nursing (minimum of 2 weeks to several months) is crucial to these infants' safe and successful transition into the community and home setting. Parents need to learn how to advocate for appropriate home care and supplies in anticipation of future needs.

Because of the high mortality rate in the first year, parents should learn cardiopulmonary resuscitation and how to manage any other emergency that might be anticipated for their infant. Helping families cope with their anxieties and reassuring them of their ability to manage the care of their infant are important nursing functions. Parents need follow-up visits in the home and the comfort of knowing that help is only a phone call away.

HIGH RISK RELATED TO INFECTIOUS PROCESSES

SEPSIS

Sepsis, or septicemia, refers to a generalized bacterial infection in the bloodstream. Neonates are highly susceptible to infection because of diminished nonspecific (inflammatory) and specific (humoral) immunity, such as impaired phagocytosis, delayed chemotactic response, minimum or absent IgA and immunoglobulin M (IgM), and decreased complement levels. Because of the infant's poor response to pathogenic agents, there is usually no local inflammatory reaction at the portal of entry to signal an infection, and the resulting symptoms tend to be vague and nonspecific. Consequently, diagnosis and treatment may be delayed.

Although the mortality rate from sepsis has decreased, the incidence has not. Nursery epidemics are not infrequent, and the high-risk infant has a four-times greater chance of developing septicemia than does the normal neonate. The frequency of infection is almost twice as great in male infants as in females and also carries a higher mortality for males. Other risk factors are prematurity, congenital anomalies or acquired injuries that disrupt the skin or mucous membranes, invasive procedures such as placement of IV lines and ET tubes, administration of total parenteral nutrition, and nosocomial exposure to pathogens in the NICU. Thorough hand washing is the single most important infection control measure in the NICU. Proper handling of formula and supplies such as syringes and gavage tubes is also vital to prevent infection.

Breastfeeding has a protective effect against infection and should be promoted for all newborns. It is of particular benefit to the high-risk neonate (Lewis, Richard, Larsen, et al., 2016). Colostrum contains agglutinins that are effective against gram-negative bacteria. Human milk contains large quantities of IgA and iron-binding protein that exert a bacteriostatic effect on *Escherichia coli.* Human milk also contains macrophages and lymphocytes that promote a local inflammatory reaction.

Pathophysiology

The premature withdrawal of the placental barrier leaves infants vulnerable to most common viral, bacterial, fungal, and parasitic infections. Immune substances, primarily immunoglobulin G (IgG), are normally acquired from the maternal system and stored in fetal tissues during the final weeks of gestation to provide newborns with passive immunity to a variety of infectious agents. Early birth interrupts this transplacental transmission; thus preterm infants have a low level of circulating IgG. The concentrations of immune substances directly relate to the length of gestation. IgA, which plays a role in defense against viral infections, and IgM, with properties that are most efficient in dealing with gram-negative organisms, are not transferred to the fetus, leaving the infant highly vulnerable to invasion by these organisms.

Defense mechanisms of neonates are further hampered by a low level of complement, diminished opsonization ability, monocyte dysfunction, and a reduced number and inefficient function of circulating leukocytes. Furthermore, leukocytes with diminished motility and phagocytic capacity are unable to concentrate their limited numbers selectively at the site of infection. In addition, a hypofunctioning adrenal gland contributes only a meager antiinflammatory response. These deficiencies permit rapid invasion, spread, and multiplication of organisms. An immature gut mucosal barrier further predisposes the preterm infant to bacteria, which may easily cross the mucosa into the bloodstream.

Sources of Infection

Sepsis in the neonatal period can be acquired prenatally across the placenta from the maternal bloodstream or during labor from ingestion or aspiration of infected amniotic fluid. Prolonged rupture of the membranes always presents a risk for maternal-fetal transfer of pathogenic organisms. In utero transplacental transfer can occur with a variety of organisms and viruses such as cytomegalovirus, toxoplasmosis, and *Treponema pallidum* (syphilis), which cross the placental barrier during the latter half of pregnancy.

Early-onset sepsis (EOS) (<3 days after birth) is acquired in the perinatal period. EOS is defined as a positive blood culture in an infant who is less than 72 hours of age. EOS remains an important cause of serious illness and death among neonates of all birth weights and gestational ages. Despite the widespread use of intrapartum chemoprophylaxis for prevention of EOS due to GBS, 1 out of every 1000 newborns develops EOS and 16% of these infants die, most commonly with infection due to *Escherichia coli* (Camacho-Gonzalez, Spearman, & Stoll, 2013; Simonsen, Anderson-Berry, Delair, et al., 2014).

Infection can occur from direct contact with organisms from the maternal GI and genitourinary tracts. Organisms associated with early-onset infection include GBS, *E. coli,* and other gram-negative enteric organisms. Despite the development of maternal screening and prophylaxis, infection rates for early-onset GBS infection remain at approximately 0.3 per 1000 live births (Centers for Disease Control and Prevention, 2016). GBS is an extremely virulent organism in neonates, with a high death rate in affected infants (Cortese, Scicchitano, Gesualdo, et al., 2015). Gestational age is tightly related to death in GBS EOS, with a mortality rate of 20% to 30% among infants with gestational ages less than 33 weeks, and this was noted to be 2% to 3% in full-term newborns (Le Doare & Heath, 2013). Other bacteria noted to cause early-onset infection include *E. coli, Haemophilus influenzae, Enterobacter* organisms, and coagulase-negative staphylococci (Pammi, Brand, & Weisman, 2016; Resch, Renoldner, & Hofer, 2016). Other pathogens that are harbored in the vagina and may infect the infant include gonococci, *Candida albicans,* herpes simplex virus (type II), and chlamydia.

Late-onset sepsis (1 to 3 weeks after birth) is primarily nosocomial (**health care–associated infection**), and the offending organisms are usually staphylococci, *Klebsiella* organisms, enterococci, *E. coli,* and *Candida* species (Pammi, Brand, & Weisman, 2016). Coagulase-negative staphylococci, considered to be primarily a contaminant in older children and adults, is commonly found to be the cause of septicemia in ELBW and VLBW infants. Bacterial invasion can occur through the umbilical stump; the skin; mucous membranes of the eye, nose, pharynx, and ear; and internal systems such as the respiratory, nervous, urinary, and GI systems.

Postnatal infection is acquired by cross-contamination from other infants, personnel, or objects in the environment. Bacteria, such as *Klebsiella* and *Pseudomonas* organisms, commonly called "water bugs" (because they are able to grow in water), are found in water supplies; humidifying apparatus; sink drains; suction machines; most respiratory equipment; and indwelling venous and arterial catheters used for infusions, blood sampling, and monitoring vital signs. These organisms are often transmitted from person to person or object to person by poor hand washing and inadequate housecleaning.

Neonatal sepsis is most common in the "at risk" infant, particularly the preterm infant or the infant born after a difficult or traumatic labor and delivery, who is least capable of resisting such bacterial invasion.

Clinical Manifestations

A few neonatal infections (e.g., pyoderma, conjunctivitis, omphalitis, and mastitis) are easy to recognize. However, systemic infections are characterized by subtle, vague, nonspecific, and almost imperceptible physical signs. Often the only complaint concerns an infant's "failure to do well," not looking "right," or nonspecific respiratory distress. Rarely is there any indication of a local inflammatory response, which would suggest the portal of entry into the bloodstream. The presence of bacteria is indicated by a specific characteristic. For example, group B β-hemolytic streptococci usually results in severe respiratory distress, periods of apnea, and a chest radiograph similar to that of RDS.

All body systems tend to show some indication of sepsis, although often little correlation exists between the manifestations and the etiologic factors involved. For example, seizures and fever, a universal feature of infection in older children, may be absent in neonates. It is usually the nursing observation of subtle changes in appearance and behavior that leads to the detection of infection. The nonspecific, early signs are hypothermia and changes in color, tone, activity, and feeding behavior. In addition, sudden episodes of apnea and unexplained oxygen desaturation (hypoxia) may signal an infection. Significantly, similar signs may be manifestations of a number of clinical conditions unrelated to sepsis, such as hypoglycemia, hypocalcemia, opioid withdrawal, or a CNS disorder.

Preterm infants, particularly ELBW and VLBW infants, are highly susceptible to early sepsis and pneumonia occurring concurrently with RDS. Preterm delivery has been increasingly shown to be associated with a maternal bacterial pathogen. ELBW and VLBW infants are also highly susceptible to fungal and viral infections. Investigation for such agents should begin when sepsis is suspected in this population. Because meningitis is a common sequela of sepsis, the neonate is evaluated for bacterial growth in cerebrospinal fluid (CSF). Clinical signs of neonatal meningitis, particularly in VLBW infants, may not have typical features of older infants. Clinical signs that may indicate possible neonatal sepsis are listed in Box 9.9.

BOX 9.9 Manifestations of Neonatal Sepsis

General Signs

Infant generally "not doing well"
Poor temperature control—hypothermia (common), hyperthermia (rare)

Circulatory System

Pallor, cyanosis, or mottling
Cold, clammy skin
Hypotension
Edema
Irregular heartbeat—bradycardia, tachycardia

Respiratory System

Irregular respirations, apnea, or tachypnea
Cyanosis
Grunting
Dyspnea
Retractions

Central Nervous System

Diminished activity—lethargy, hyporeflexia, coma
Increased activity—irritability, tremors, seizures
Full fontanel
Increased or decreased tone
Abnormal eye movements

Gastrointestinal System

Poor feeding
Vomiting
Diarrhea or decreased stooling
Abdominal distention
Hepatomegaly
Hemoccult-positive stools

Hematopoietic System

Jaundice
Pallor
Petechiae, ecchymosis
Splenomegaly

Diagnostic Evaluation

Because sepsis is easy to confuse with other neonatal disorders, the definitive diagnosis is established by laboratory and radiographic examination. Isolation of the specific organism is always attempted through cultures of blood, urine, and CSF. Blood studies may show signs of leukocytosis or leukopenia. Leukopenia is usually an ominous sign because of its frequent association with high mortality rates. An elevated number of immature neutrophils (**left-shift**), decreased or increased total neutrophils, and changes in neutrophil morphologic characteristics also suggest an infectious process in the neonate. Other diagnostic data that are helpful in the determination of neonatal sepsis include C-reactive protein and interleukins, specifically interleukin-6 (Pammi, Brand, & Weisman, 2016).

Therapeutic Management

In addition to the institution of rigorous preventive measures such as good hand washing, early recognition and diagnosis are essential to increase the infant's chance for survival and reduce the likelihood of permanent neurologic damage. Diagnosis of sepsis is often based on suspicion of initial clinical signs and symptoms. Antibiotic therapy is initiated before laboratory results are available for confirmation and identification of the exact organism. Treatment consists of circulatory support, respiratory support, and aggressive administration of antibiotics.

Supportive therapy usually involves administration of oxygen (if respiratory distress or hypoxia is evident), careful regulation of fluids, correction of electrolyte or acid-base imbalance, and temporary discontinuation of oral feedings. Blood transfusion may be needed to correct anemia. IV fluids for shock, electronic monitoring of vital signs, and regulation of the thermal environment are mandatory.

Antibiotic therapy is continued for 7 to 10 days if cultures are positive, discontinued in 36 to 48 hours if cultures are negative and the infant is asymptomatic, and most often administered via IV infusion. Antifungal and antiviral therapies are implemented as appropriate, depending on causative agents.

Prognosis

The prognosis for neonatal sepsis is variable. Severe neurologic and respiratory sequelae may occur in ELBW and VLBW infants with early-onset sepsis. Late-onset sepsis and meningitis may also result in poor outcomes for immunocompromised neonates.

The introduction of new markers for neonatal sepsis such as acute phase proteins, cytokines, cell surface antigens, and bacterial genomes may prove to be particularly helpful in early differentiation of true sepsis from RDS and in guidance for antibiotic therapy (Camacho-Gonzalez, Spearman, & Stoll, 2013; Gilfillan & Bhandari, 2017). Future experimental methods being explored to combat infection in neonates include monoclonal antibody therapy, fibronectin infusion, and lymphokine enhancement.

Nursing Care Management

Nursing care of the infant with sepsis involves observation and assessment as outlined for any high-risk infant. Recognition of the problem is of paramount importance. It is usually the nurse who observes and assesses infants and identifies that "something is wrong" with the infant. Awareness of the potential modes of infection transmission also helps the nurse identify those at risk for developing sepsis. Much of the care of infants with sepsis involves the medical treatment of the illness. Knowledge of the side effects of the specific antibiotic and proper regulation and administration of the drug are vital. Antibiotics are usually administered via a special injection port near the infusion site. The appropriately diluted medication is administered slowly by mechanical pump.

Prolonged antibiotic therapy poses additional hazards for affected infants. Oral antibiotics, if administered, destroy intestinal flora responsible for the synthesis of vitamin K, which can reduce blood coagulability. In addition, antibiotics predispose the infant to growth of resistant organisms and superinfection from fungal or mycotic agents, such as *C. albicans.* Nurses must be alert for evidence of such complications. Nystatin oral suspension may be administered for prophylaxis against oral candidiasis.

Part of the total care of infants with sepsis is to decrease any additional physiologic or environmental stress. This includes providing an optimum thermoregulated environment and anticipating potential problems such as dehydration or hypoxia. Precautions are implemented to prevent the spread of infection to other newborns, but to be effective, activities must be carried out by all caregivers. Proper hand washing, the use of disposable equipment (e.g., linens, catheters, feeding supplies, and IV equipment), disposal of secretions (e.g., vomit and stool), and adequate housekeeping of the environment and equipment are essential. Because nurses are the most consistent caregivers involved with sick infants, it is usually their responsibility to ensure that everyone maintains all phases of contact isolation or Standard Precautions (see also Infection Control, Chapter 6).

Another aspect of caring for infants with sepsis involves observation for signs of complications, including meningitis and septic shock, a severe complication caused by toxins in the bloodstream.

A number of viral agents—namely, cytomegalovirus, herpes, hepatitis, and human immunodeficiency virus (HIV)—may also be transmitted to the fetus from the mother. When acquired prenatally (congenital), these viruses represent a serious threat to the infant's life. (See Table 9.10 for viral infections.)

NECROTIZING ENTEROCOLITIS

NEC is an acute inflammatory disease of the bowel with increased incidence in preterm and other high-risk infants; it is most common in preterm infants. Because the signs are similar to those observed in many other disorders of the newborn, nurses must constantly be aware of the possibility of this disease.

Pathophysiology

The precise cause of NEC is still uncertain, but it appears to occur in infants whose GI tract has suffered vascular compromise. Contributory factors for NEC include the following: intestional immaturity, such as gastrointestional dysmotility; impaired digestive capacity; altered regulation of intestinal blood blow; barrier dysfunction; altered antiinflammatory control; and impaired host defense (Chang, Chen, Chang, et al., 2017). Frequent use of antibiotic therapy and antiacid medications, followed by enteral feeding, are believed to increase the risk of NEC (Chang, Chen, Chang, et al., 2017). Prematurity remains the greatest risk factor in this disease (Sharma & Hudak, 2013).

The damage to mucosal cells lining the bowel wall is great. Diminished blood supply to these cells causes their death in large numbers. They stop secreting protective, lubricating mucus, and the thin, unprotected bowel wall is attacked by proteolytic enzymes. It is unable to synthesize protective IgM, and the mucosa is permeable to macromolecules (e.g., exotoxins), which further hamper intestinal defenses. Gas-forming bacteria invade the damaged areas to produce intestinal **pneumatosis**, air in the submucosal or subserosal surfaces of the bowel.

Clinical Manifestations

The prominent clinical signs of NEC are a distended abdomen, gastric residuals, and blood in the stools. Because NEC closely resembles septicemia, the infant may "not look well." Nonspecific signs include lethargy, poor feeding, hypotension, apnea, vomiting (often bile-stained), decreased urinary output, and hypothermia. The onset is usually between 4 and 10 days after the initiation of feedings, but signs may be evident as early as 4 hours of age and as late as 30 days. NEC in full-term infants almost always occurs in the first 10 days of life. The early clinical signs of NEC are subtle and nonspecific and may often be overlooked for other conditions; the earliest clinical signs include lethargy, abdominal distention, and high gastric residuals (Bucher, Pacetti, Lovvorn, et al., 2016; Kastenberg & Sylvester, 2013). Late-onset NEC is confined primarily to preterm infants and coincides with the onset of feedings after they have passed through the acute phase of an illness such as RDS.

Diagnostic Evaluation

Radiographic studies show a sausage-shaped dilation of the intestine that progresses to marked distention and the characteristic intestinal pneumatosis—"soapsuds," or the bubbly appearance of thickened bowel wall and ultralumina. Air may be present in the portal circulation or free air observed in the abdomen, indicating perforation. Laboratory findings may include anemia, leukopenia, leukocytosis, metabolic acidosis, and electrolyte imbalance. In severe cases, coagulopathy (disseminated intravascular coagulation) or thrombocytopenia may be evident. Organisms may be cultured from blood, although bacteremia or septicemia may not be prominent early in the course of the disease.

Therapeutic Management

Treatment of NEC begins with prevention. Oral feedings may be withheld for 24 to 48 hours from infants who are believed to have suffered birth asphyxia. Breast milk is the preferred enteral nutrient because it confers some passive immunity (IgA), macrophages, and lysozymes. There is evidence that human milk may have a protective effect against the development of NEC (Cacho, Parker, & Neu, 2016; Ramani & Ambalavanan, 2013).

Minimal enteral feedings (trophic feeding, GI priming) in VLBW infants have gained acceptance. Some studies have shown that such feedings may be protective against NEC in nonasphyxiated preterm infants (Bingham, 2012; Ramani & Ambalavanan, 2013). The administration of maternal antenatal steroids may prevent NEC in some infants by promoting early gut closure and maturation of the gut barrier mucosa (Wapner, Gyamfi-Bannerman, Thom, et al., 2016).

Many meta-analyses of randomized controlled trials have confirmed that oral probiotics effectively prevent NEC when given within the first 7 days and continued for 14 days in preterm infants (≤34 weeks of gestation) and/or those of a birth weight ≤1500 g (Aceti, Gori, & Barone, 2015; Alfaleh, Anabrees, Bassler, et al., 2014; Athalye-Jape, Rao, & Patole, 2016; Lau & Chamberlain, 2015; Wang, Dong, & Zhu, 2012). Lactoferrin, the major whey protein in human milk, in combination with lysozyme, which is also found in human milk, may have a significant role in the prevention of NEC and neonatal sepsis in high-risk preterm infants; both act in the intestine to kill harmful bacteria and enhance intestinal immune properties (Chang, Chen, Chang, et al., 2017; Sherman, 2013).

Medical treatment of confirmed NEC consists of discontinuation of all oral feedings; institution of abdominal decompression via nasogastric suction; administration of IV antibiotics; and correction of extravascular volume depletion, electrolyte abnormalities, acid-base imbalances, and hypoxia. Replacing oral feedings with parenteral fluids decreases the need for oxygen and circulation to the bowel. Serial abdominal radiograph films (every 4 to 6 hours in the acute phase) are taken to monitor for possible progression of the disease to intestinal perforation.

With early recognition and treatment, medical management is increasingly successful. If there is progressive deterioration under medical management or evidence of perforation, surgical resection and anastomosis are performed. Extensive involvement may necessitate surgical intervention and establishment of an ileostomy, jejunostomy, or colostomy. Sequelae in surviving infants include short-bowel syndrome, colonic stricture with obstruction, fat malabsorption, and failure to thrive secondary to intestinal dysfunction. Various surgical interventions for NEC are available and depend on the extent of bowel necrosis, associated illness factors, and infant stability. Intestinal transplantation has been successful in some former preterm infants with NEC-associated short-bowel syndrome who had already developed life-threatening complications related to total parenteral nutrition. More than 50% of these patients survived with improved quality of life. Bowel lengthening procedures and intestinal transplantation may be lifesaving options for infants who previously faced high morbidity and mortality rates (Höllwarth, 2017; Javid, Sanchez, Horslen, et al., 2013).

Nursing Care Management

Astute nursing care is a key factor in the prompt recognition of the early warning signs of NEC. When the disease is suspected, the nurse assists with diagnostic procedures and implements the therapeutic regimen. Vital signs, including blood pressure, are monitored for changes that might indicate bowel perforation, septicemia, or cardiovascular shock. Measures are instituted to prevent possible transmission to other infants. It is especially important to avoid rectal temperatures because of the increased danger of perforation. To avoid pressure on the distended abdomen and to facilitate continuous observation, infants are often left undiapered and positioned supine or on the side.

> **! NURSING ALERT**
>
> Observe for indications of early development of NEC by checking the abdomen frequently for distention (measuring abdominal girth, measuring residual gastric contents before feedings, and listening for the presence of bowel sounds) and performing all routine assessments for high-risk neonates.

Conscientious attention to nutrition and hydration needs is essential, and antibiotics are administered as prescribed. The time at which oral feedings are reinstituted varies considerably but is usually at least 7 to 10 days after diagnosis and treatment.

Because NEC is an infectious disease, one of the most important nursing functions is control of infection. Strict hand washing is the primary barrier to spread, and confirmed multiple cases are isolated. Persons with symptoms of a GI infection should not care for these or any other infants.

The infant undergoing surgery requires the same careful attention and observation as any infant with abdominal surgery, including ostomy care (as applicable). This disorder is one of the most common reasons for performing ileostomies on newborns. Throughout the medical and surgical management of infants with NEC, the nurse is continually alert for signs of complications, such as septicemia, disseminated intravascular coagulation, hypoglycemia, and other metabolic derangements.

HIGH RISK RELATED TO CARDIOVASCULAR AND HEMATOLOGIC COMPLICATIONS

PATENT DUCTUS ARTERIOSUS

PDA is a common complication of severe respiratory disease in preterm infants. It occurs in the majority of preterm infants under 1200 g (2.6 lb), and the incidence diminishes in direct relationship to increasing birth weight. During fetal life the ductus remains patent through the vasodilatory action of prostaglandin, which is produced by the placenta and circulated to the fetus. Postnatally the increase in oxygen tension has a constricting effect on the ductus, but it may reopen in preterm infants in response to the lowered oxygen tension associated with respiratory impairment.

Lack of ductal smooth muscle in preterm infants also prolongs patency of the ductus arteriosus. Functional closure occurs usually within 3 to 4 days, but complete anatomic closure with fibrosis and permanent sealing of the lumen may take up to 2 to 3 weeks.

Clinical Manifestations

Signs of PDA may appear within the first week of life. Early signs are increased Pa_{CO_2}, decreased Pa_{O_2}, increased Fi_{O_2}, increased work of breathing, and recurrent apnea. Other signs include bounding peripheral pulses; wide pulse pressure with decreased diastolic blood pressure; pericardial hyperactivity; cardiomegaly; and a systolic or continuous murmur usually referred to as a "machinery-type" murmur, heard loudest in systole. If the PDA is wide open, a murmur may not be heard. Spontaneous closure usually occurs within 12 weeks, but in infants with severe lung involvement, the left-to-right shunting of blood leads to pulmonary edema and may prevent timely weaning from mechanical ventilation. The diagnosis is confirmed by echocardiography.

Therapeutic Management

Therapy consists of careful fluid regulation; respiratory support; and administration of indomethacin or ibuprofen, which inhibits prostaglandin synthetase. However, indomethacin inhibits platelet function and affects renal function in neonates, so close monitoring for bleeding and renal dysfunction is necessary if this drug is used. If a ductus reopens after cessation of therapy, readministration of the medication may produce a favorable response. As many as six doses may be used to accomplish ductal closure. Surgical ligation may be necessary if medical therapy is unsuccessful because ductal shunting is perceived as an important contributor to respiratory distress and BPD.

Nursing Care Management

Nursing observations are important in the recognition and management of PDA. Assisting in early detection, carefully assessing cardiovascular status, and monitoring for complications after implementation of therapy are nursing responsibilities. Activities related to therapy include collection of specimens for laboratory examination, continued assessment of renal function (e.g., adequate urinary output, any abnormal laboratory findings such as blood urea nitrogen and creatinine levels), and observation for any bleeding tendencies (e.g., Hematest-positive stools or gastric aspirate, oozing from heel sticks or venipuncture sites, and laboratory evidence of clotting abnormalities).

Postoperative care includes monitoring for pneumothorax or atelectasis on the affected side, assessment for bleeding and signs or symptoms of infection, supportive respiratory care, and pain management. Other nursing observations and management are the same as for the high-risk infant and the infant with congenital heart disease. (See Chapter 27.)

ANEMIA

Preterm infants tend to develop anemia that is more severe and appears earlier than in more mature infants. It may be a result of hemorrhage during pregnancy or labor and delivery (e.g., loss of placental integrity, anomalies of the umbilical cord, fetomaternal hemorrhage), hemorrhage during the neonatal period (e.g., ICH, visceral trauma), or blood disorders (e.g., hemolytic disease, thrombocytopenia). Anemia may also be iatrogenic from blood withdrawn in the NICU for laboratory tests. Physiologic characteristics of prematurity tend to contribute to the development of anemia (i.e., a decreased red blood cell mass at birth, a drop in the production of hemoglobin, and shortened survival time of red blood cells). This lag in hematopoiesis during continued growth results in physiologic anemia, probably as a consequence of diminished erythropoietin values.

Fortunately, even VLBW infants are able to accommodate the GI absorption of iron required for their high needs. Iron is supplied in iron-fortified formulas or iron supplements as both a preventive and therapeutic measure. Transfusions with packed red blood cells are often required for severe anemia, usually for replacement of blood loss from iatrogenic measures. At 4 to 12 weeks of age, "physiologic anemia" reaches a peak, at which time infants sometimes display signs that suggest true anemia (e.g., poor feeding, decreased oxygen saturation, pallor).

Nursing Care Management

One of the most common causes of anemia in acutely ill preterm infants is blood loss associated with frequent sampling for blood gas and metabolic analyses. Repeated blood sampling depletes the small total blood volume of preterm infants quickly. In light of hepatitis and HIV transmission and the potential for other blood-borne pathogens, measures to reduce iatrogenic blood loss and to minimize the need for transfusions of blood products are important considerations.

The nurse observes for signs of anemia in the preterm infant: poor feeding, decreased oxygen saturation, systolic murmur, dyspnea, tachycardia, tachypnea, diminished activity, and pallor. However, some infants may not display all these signs. Poor weight gain may be an indication of a lowered hemoglobin level. (Chapter 28 discusses nursing precautions and observations during blood transfusion.)

POLYCYTHEMIA

The current definition of polycythemia is a venous hematocrit of 65% or more (Maheshwari & Carlo, 2016). With a hematocrit above 65%, blood flow becomes increasingly sluggish and hyperviscous, resulting in hypoperfusion of organs. Polycythemia may result from in utero twin-to-twin transfusion and maternal-fetal transfusion, delayed cord clamping or stripping of the umbilical cord, maternal diabetes mellitus, or intrapartum asphyxia. The small-for-gestational-age infant is the most at risk for polycythemia. Increased red blood cell consumption of glucose further predisposes the infant to hypoglycemia. Infants with polycythemia have a high incidence of cardiopulmonary distress symptoms (e.g., PPHN, cyanosis, and apnea), seizures, hyperbilirubinemia, and GI abnormalities.

Appropriate therapy for correcting metabolic disturbances (e.g., hypoxia, hypoglycemia, and hyperbilirubinemia) is implemented. Lowering blood viscosity by partial plasma exchange transfusion may be considered in symptomatic cases.

Nursing Care Management

Nursing care involves watching for signs of polycythemia (e.g., plethora, peripheral cyanosis, respiratory distress, lethargy, jitteriness or seizure activity, hypoglycemia, hyperbilirubinemia) and assisting with diagnostic tests and therapeutic procedures. (Care of the infant with hyperbilirubinemia is discussed in Chapter 8.)

RETINOPATHY OF PREMATURITY

Although often discussed in relation to respiratory dysfunction, retinopathy of prematurity (ROP) is a disorder involving immature retinal vasculature. Formerly known as retrolental fibroplasia, ROP is a term used to describe retinal changes observed in preterm infants. The incidence and severity of the disease correlate with the degree of the infant's maturity, the younger the gestational age, the greater the likelihood of ROP, with extremely preterm infants being most at risk. However, cases have been documented of ROP in full-term infants who received no oxygen therapy (Carter, Gratny, & Carter, 2016; Chen, He, & Huang, 2012).

In addition to immaturity, contributory factors for ROP include oxygenation, respiratory distress, apnea, bradycardia, heart disease, infections, hypercarbia, acidosis, anemia, and the need for transfusions (Olitsky, Hug, Plummer, et al., 2016). Previously considered an iatrogenic disease related to hyperoxia, ROP is now believed to be a complex disease of prematurity with multiple causes and therefore difficult to completely prevent. A study done by Owen, Morrison, Hoffman, and colleagues (2017) conducted a comprehensive risk assessment for prediction of ROP and found that severe ROP was best predicted by estimated gestational age (week), the need for any surgery and increased probability of death or moderate/severe BPD at 7 days. The most predictive model for type 1 ROP included estimated gestational age (week) and the presence of severe chronic lung disease (Owen, Morrison, Hoffman, et al., 2017).

BOX 9.10 Stages of Retinopathy of Prematurity

1. A demarcation line (separates the avascular retina anteriorly from the vascularized retina posteriorly)
2. A ridge (formed from the demarcation line with the height and width, occupies volume, and extends beyond the plane of the retina)
3. A ridge with extraretinal fibrovascular proliferation
4. Partial retinal detachment
5. Total retinal detachment

"Plus" disease—increased dilation and tortuosity of peripheral retinal vessels (e.g., stage 2 plus ROP)

Data from International Committee for the Classification of Retinopathy of Prematurity. (2005). The international classification of retinopathy of prematurity revisited. *Arch Ophthalmol, 123*(7), 991-999.

Pathophysiology

Severe vascular constriction in the immature retinal vasculature, followed by hypoxia in those areas, is characteristic of ROP. This appears to stimulate vascular proliferation of retinal capillaries into the hypoxic areas, where veins become numerous and dilate. As new vessels multiply toward the lens, the aqueous humor and vitreous humor become turbid. The retina becomes edematous, and hemorrhages and scarring occur, which separate the retina from its attachment. This process results in irreversible blindness.

Diagnostic Evaluation

The International Committee for the Classification of Retinopathy of Prematurity (2005) established a system of classification to describe the location and extent of the developing vasculature involved. Normal vascular growth proceeds in an orderly fashion from the optic disc toward the ora serrata, the irregular anterior margin of the retina. Box 9.10 outlines the stages of ROP. ROP is further classified by location of damage in the retina and by the extent of abnormally developing vascularization. Current US guidelines recommend that all infants with a birth weight of less than 1500 g (3.3 lb) or a gestational age of less than 30 weeks, and selected infants who are believed to be at high risk, undergo ROP screening (American Academy of Pediatrics, American Association for Pediatric Ophthalmology and Strabismus, & American Academy of Ophthalmology, 2013). The frequency of follow-up examination is determined by the ophthalmologist and is outlined in the 2013 recommendations. With increased survival of extremely preterm infants, most authorities agree that the incidence of ROP is not likely to decrease until definitive causative factors are identified.

Therapeutic Management

Studies have shown an association between the development of ROP and high or fluctuating arterial oxygen saturations in ELBW and VLBW infants. Although there is no consensus on the ideal arterial oxygen saturation in preterm infants—to prevent either hypoxemia or hyperoxemia—evidence is mounting that oxygen saturations of over 94% are undesirable and may have a significant role in the development of ROP (Darlow, Lui, Kusuda, et al., 2017; Owen, Morrison, Hoffman, et al., 2017). Recent clinical trials that evaluated two sets of desired oxygenation ranges, low (85% to 89%) and high (91% to 95%), found that the rate of severe ROP was lower in the low-range group of infants; however, the low-range group had a higher overall mortality rate than the high-range group (Fleck & Stenson, 2013). Management and treatment of ROP is primarily aimed at preventing fluctuations in arterial concentrations of oxygen in preterm neonates.

The early recognition of ROP, treatment, and follow-up care are essential components of disease management. Although prevention is the primary goal of therapeutic management, treatment of retinal pathologic conditions is directed toward arresting the proliferation process. Early treatment of high-risk prethreshold ROP significantly reduced unfavorable outcomes (Olitsky, Hug, Plummer, et al., 2016). Laser photocoagulation therapy is the most common treatment for ROP.

Clinical trials using systemic propranolol or intravitreal VEGF antagonists are currently ongoing and being evaluated for efficacy and risk for ROP (Olitsky, Hug, Plummer, et al., 2016).

Nursing Care Management

The nursing care of extremely preterm infants and those at risk for development of ROP should focus on decreasing or avoiding events known to cause fluctuations in systemic blood pressure and oxygenation. The infant's oxygenation status should be carefully monitored and targeted SpO_2 ranges maintained. Individualized care of the preterm infant is essential to aid in further decreasing the incidence of ROP. For infants undergoing ophthalmic examination for ROP, concentrated sucrose has proved effective in decreasing pain responses (Stevens, Yamada, Lee, et al., 2013).

Intraoperative nursing care for the infant undergoing laser surgery involves proper infant identification, stabilization and monitoring of vital signs as required, monitoring of IV therapy, and administration of the necessary medications. Postoperative nursing care also includes monitoring the infant for signs of pain and appropriate pain management as needed. After surgery the infant's eyelids will be edematous and closed; the nurse informs the parents of this preoperatively. Eye medications are administered as ordered, and the infant's tolerance of these medications is monitored. Most infants are able to feed once awake and alert in the postoperative period. When the infant suffers partial or complete visual impairment, the parents need a considerable amount of support and assistance in meeting his or her special developmental needs. (See Chapter 20.)

HIGH RISK RELATED TO NEUROLOGIC DISTURBANCE

Neurologic complications are observed with increased frequency in preterm infants and in infants born after a difficult labor and delivery. A disproportionately high incidence of perinatal encephalopathy and psychomotor delay occurs in the high-risk infant population, especially ELBW and VLBW infants. Preterm infants are also more vulnerable to cerebral insults (e.g., hypoxia) and chemical alterations (e.g., decreased blood glucose). Fragility and increased permeability of capillaries and prolonged prothrombin time predispose the preterm infant's brain to trauma when subjected to increased pressure, such as the forces of labor, high ventilatory pressures, fluid and electrolyte imbalances, sepsis, acidosis, and seizure activity. All these factors contribute to intracranial insults, including traumatic bleeding in the newborn, which consists of four major types: intraventricular, subdural, primary subarachnoid, and intracerebellar.

PERINATAL HYPOXIC-ISCHEMIC BRAIN INJURY

Hypoxic-ischemic brain injury, or hypoxic-ischemic reperfusion injury, is the most common cause of neurologic impairment in term and preterm infants. The brain damage usually results from asphyxia before, during, or after delivery. Ischemia and hypoxemia may occur simultaneously, or one may precede the other. The fetal brain is somewhat protected against mild hypoxic events but may be damaged when there is a decrease in cerebral blood flow, systemic blood pressure, and oxygen and nutrients such as glucose. Subsequent reperfusion after the event may further result in bleeding of the fragile capillaries and tissue ischemia.

Hypoxic-ischemic encephalopathy (HIE) is the resultant cellular damage from hypoxic-ischemic injury that causes the clinical manifestations observed in each case. Such clinical manifestations are variable and may be mild, moderate, or severe. In some infants little or no residual damage may be observed. In general, hypoxia that is severe enough to cause HIE will also damage other organs such as the liver, kidneys, myocardium, and GI tract (Carlo & Ambalavanan, 2016a; Parsons, Seay, & Jacobson, 2016). In the preterm infant HIE may occur in conjunction with IVH. Prematurity and general organ and system immaturity may result in hypoxic-ischemic brain damage in the neonatal period due to altered cerebral blood flow, systemic hypotension, and decreased cellular nutrients (blood glucose and oxygen).

The site of the hypoxic-ischemic injury varies according to the infant's gestational age. In the full-term infant the primary ischemic damage is parasagittal cerebral injury with cortical necrosis (deeper region of the brain). In the preterm infant the primary ischemic lesion is in the white matter near the ventricles, or periventricular, with resultant periventricular leukomalacia (Volpe, 2008).

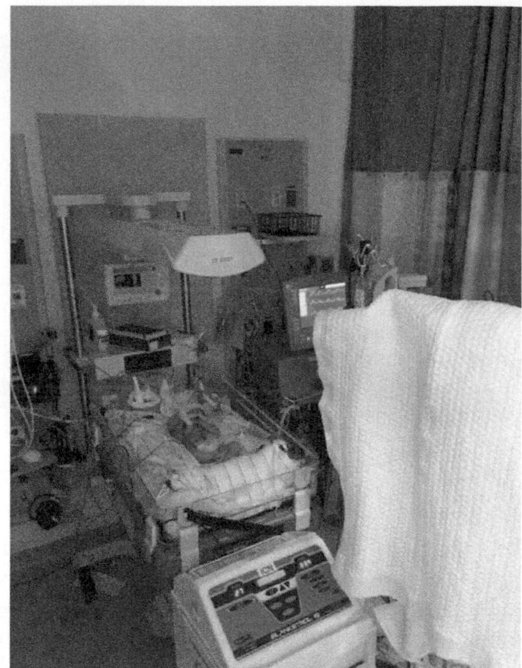

FIG. 9.20 Whole body cooling for HIE.

Clinical Manifestations

The neurologic signs of encephalopathy appear within the first hours after the hypoxic episode, with manifestations of bilateral cerebral dysfunction. The infant may be stuporous or comatose. Seizures begin after 6 to 12 hours in approximately 50% of the infants, and they become more frequent and severe by 12 to 24 hours. Between 24 and 72 hours the level of consciousness may deteriorate, and after 72 hours persistent stupor, abnormal tone (usually hypotonia), and evidence of disturbances of sucking and swallowing may occur. Muscular weakness of the hips and shoulders occurs in full-term infants, and lower limb weakness occurs in preterm infants. Apneic episodes happen in approximately 50% of the affected infants.

Improvement in neurologic deficiencies is highly variable and difficult to predict. Infants who demonstrate the most rapid initial improvement appear to have the best prognosis. Myocardial failure and acute tubular necrosis are frequent complications. The major long-term sequelae of hypoxic-ischemic injury are cognitive impairment, seizures, and CP.

Therapeutic Management

Treatment involves aggressive resuscitation at birth, supportive care to provide adequate ventilation and avoid aggravating the existing hypoxia, and measures to maintain adequate cerebral perfusion and prevent cerebral edema.

Therapeutic hypothermia provided by either cooling the infant's head or the whole body has been shown to reduce the severity of the neurologic damage when it is applied in the early stages of injury (first 6 hours after delivery) (Carlo & Ambalavanan, 2016a; Jacobs, Berg, Hunt, et al., 2013; Parsons, Seay, & Jacobson, 2016). Currently this therapy is being used only in infants who are 36 weeks gestation or more. Clinical trials are currently ongoing to evaluate the efficacy and safety of using whole body cooling for infants with HIE born at 33 to 35 weeks of gestational age (Fig. 9.20). Seizures are managed as described on p. 321. However, prevention is the most important therapy, and every effort should be made to recognize high-risk pregnancies, monitor the fetus, and initiate appropriate therapy early.

Another potential treatment for infants born with HIE is the therapeutic use of autologous cord blood. A pilot study assessing the safety and feasibility of providing autologous umbilical cord blood (UCB) cells to neonates with HIE has demonstrated feasibility (Cotten, Murtha, Goldberg, et al., 2014). The study hypothesized that early infusion of autologous volume- and red blood cell (RBC)–reduced UCB cells in infants with HIE would improve outcomes (Cotten, Murtha, Goldberg, et al., 2014). These promising results dictate the need for a randomized double-blind study to prove efficacy (Cotten, Murtha, Goldberg, et al., 2014).

Nursing Care Management

Nursing care is primarily the same as for any high-risk infant: careful assessment and observation for signs that might indicate cerebral hypoxia or ischemia; monitoring of ventilatory and IV therapy; observation and management of seizures; and general supportive care to infants and parents, including guidelines for management in the event of cognitive impairment. During therapeutic hypothermia, the nurse carefully regulates the infant's body temperature according to the parameters in the cooling protocol being used. The protocol also directs the frequency of blood work, vital signs, and other parameters to be monitored such as a continuous brain wave recording.

INTRAVENTRICULAR HEMORRHAGE

Germinal matrix–intraventricular hemorrhage is known by a variety of terms according to the locus of bleeding: intraventricular hemorrhage, periventricular hemorrhage, and subependymal-intraventricular hemorrhage. Most authorities use the term intraventricular hemorrhage (IVH) to describe this disorder, which is responsible for a significant percentage of seriously ill infants and neonatal mortality. IVH is said to occur in approximately 30% of preterm infants weighing less than 1500 g; the incidence is inversely related to gestational age, with a higher incidence seen in those weighing less than 750 g (Carlo & Ambalavanan, 2016a). IVH is extremely common in preterm infants, especially ELBW and VLBW infants less than 32 weeks of gestation. The degree of neonatal immaturity correlates with the incidence of hemorrhage, and subsequent neurologic handicap is not uncommon.

TABLE 9.8 Severity of Germinal Matrix—Intraventricular Hemorrhage

Grade	Extent of Hemorrhage
I	Germinal matrix hemorrhage with minimum to no IVH; <10% of the ventricle
II	IVH in roughly 10%-50% of ventricle
III	IVH with lateral ventricular distention; >50% of ventricle
III+*	IVH and periventricular hemorrhage

*Another classification system considers this a grade IV involving parenchymal hemorrhage (Carlo & Ambalavanan, 2016a).
IVH, Intraventricular hemorrhage.
Data modified from Volpe, J. J. (2008). *Neurology of the newborn* (5th ed.). Philadelphia, PA: Saunders.

Pathophysiology

During the early months of prenatal development an extensive but fragile vascular network in the region of the ventricles receives a disproportionately large amount of cerebral blood flow. Blood is directed to the germinal matrix located in the periventricular region near the caudate nuclei of the cerebrum. Preterm infants are subject to bleeding in this heavily vascularized region, especially during events that are likely to cause fluctuations in cerebral blood flow, such as hypoxic episodes and the associated increased venous pressure. In IVH the bleeding originates in these capillaries. The blood may rupture through the ependymal lining of the ventricles and fill all or part of the ventricular system. In severe cases the hemorrhage extends into the cerebral parenchyma. Bleeding in the cerebral parenchyma may lead to the development of cystic lesions referred to as periventricular leukomalacia, which is a significant risk factor for CP. Table 9.8 lists the classification of degrees of IVH.

Following bleeding in the ventricle, clots and other debris can obstruct the passages between the ventricles, causing the ventricles to dilate and resulting in the development of hydrocephalus (posthemorrhagic hydrocephalus).

Several clinical features are associated with IVH: birth asphyxia, early gestational age, LBW, respiratory distress, asynchronous breathing on ventilatory therapy, pneumothorax, low blood glucose, noxious stimuli, hypercarbia, coagulation and platelet disorders, and hypotension. Posthemorrhagic hydrocephalus and damage to the periventricular white matter of the brain (such as in grade III+) are major determinants of associated chronic problems and prognosis.

Clinical Manifestations

Volpe (2008) classifies clinical manifestations of IVH into three categories:

1. **Catastrophic deterioration**—Begins within minutes to hours of the insult with a coma or deep stupor, respiratory abnormalities such as apnea and hypoventilation, fixed pupils, decerebrate posturing, generalized tonic seizures, flaccid quadriparesis, and cardiac arrhythmias
2. **Saltatory deterioration**—More subtle; signs appear over several hours; may stop altogether, then reappear; signs consist of altered level of consciousness, hypotonia, subtle abnormal eye position and movements, decreased spontaneous or abnormal movements and an abnormally tight popliteal angle; respiratory abnormalities observed in some cases
3. **Clinically silent deterioration**—Often overlooked clinically; a sudden unexplained decrease in hematocrit may be the only clinical sign of IVH

Approximately 50% of all IVHs occur on the first postnatal day of life, 25% on the second, 15% on the third, and 10% on or after the fourth day of life (Volpe, 2008).

Diagnostic Evaluation

When IVH is suspected or the infant is at risk, studies of intracranial structures are performed by ultrasonography, CT, or MRI. In many NICUs screening with cranial ultrasonography is performed at the bedside (via the anterior fontanel) within hours of birth if there is suspicion of IVH or within 4 to 7 days for high-risk infants (<32 weeks of gestation). A positron emission tomography (PET) scan may also be helpful in identifying cerebral blood flow in and around the site of the hemorrhage.

Therapeutic Management

Management of IVH is aimed at prevention, particularly of prematurity and any events that may lead to IVH. The maintenance of adequate oxygenation by decreasing iatrogenic events is the key to keeping ELBW and VLBW infants neurologically intact. Factors associated with prematurity and RDS may predispose the preterm infant to IVH: acidosis, electrolyte imbalances and rapid fluid shifts (extracellular to intracellular), administration of hyperosmolar solutions (such as sodium bicarbonate), and hypotension followed by rapid volume expansion. Medical treatments aimed at preventing IVH with vitamin E, maternal vitamin K, pancuronium (to decrease blood pressure fluctuations), ibuprofen, phenobarbital, ethamsylate, magnesium sulfate, indomethacin, and surfactant (for RDS) have met with varying degrees of success. Antenatal betamethasone administration has played a significant role in the reduction of IVH in preterm infants (Ballabh, 2014; Volpe, 2008).

In the event of IVH, treatment is both preventive and supportive. Prompt detection by clinical signs or periodic ultrasonography is a key element in implementing strategies to prevent further damage. Posthemorrhagic hydrocephalus is a common occurrence within 1 month of the event. Serial lumbar punctures may be used to decrease the amount of CSF and thus decrease ventricular size. A closed reservoir may be attached to an intraventricular shunt, with the reservoir tapped or drained intermittently to relieve pressure on the ventricles. Ventricular dilation (grade III to grade III+) may be managed with shunting (ventriculoperitoneal or subgaleal) or a temporary external ventricular drainage.

The long-term outcome of IVH is unpredictable and is influenced by the size of the hemorrhage and the extent of parenchymal involvement. Infants with small lesions have an excellent prognosis for neurologic outcome (Parsons, Seay, & Jacobson, 2016).

Nursing Care Management

In addition to routine observations and management, the nurse directs care toward prevention of fluctuations in cerebral blood flow. Some nursing procedures increase intracranial pressure. For example, blood pressure increases significantly during ET suctioning in preterm infants, and head positioning produces measurable changes in intracranial pressure. Researchers have found that intracranial pressure is highest when infants are in the dependent position and decreases when the head is in a midline position and elevated 30 degrees.

Cerebral pressure is lower when infants are in a midline position as opposed to a side-lying position. When the head is turned to the side without body alignment, the resulting venous congestion creates hydrostatic pressure fluctuations that increase intracranial pressure. Infants encumbered with tubes and monitoring equipment are more difficult to turn while maintaining head-body alignment.

Other interventions that may reduce the risk of increased intracranial pressure include avoiding interventions that cause crying (such as painful procedures). Crying (which essentially creates a Valsalva effect) can impede venous return, increase cerebral blood volume, and compromise cerebral oxygenation in LBW infants. Avoid rapid volume expansion following hypotension (primarily in preterms) and administration of hyperosmolar solutions such as sodium bicarbonate. Because air leaks such as pneumothorax produce variable cerebral blood flow, rapid detection and intervention are key components of nursing care of the high-risk infant. Monitoring serum blood glucose levels and preventing hypoglycemia are also important factors in keeping the infant neurologically intact. Many units practice minimum handling of infants at high risk to avoid fluctuations in cerebral blood flow. In addition, research has suggested that noxious external stimuli (e.g., pain and noise) have a potential role in stimulation that may lead to IVH. Care includes evaluating manipulations and handling and administering analgesics to reduce discomfort.

INTRACRANIAL HEMORRHAGE

ICH in neonates, although manifested in the same ways as in older children, occurs with different frequencies and degrees of severity.

Subdural Hemorrhage

A subdural hematoma is a life-threatening collection of blood in the subdural space. The stretching and tearing of the large veins in the tentorium cerebelli, the dural membrane that separates the cerebrum from the cerebellum, is the most common cause. With improved obstetric care this condition has become relatively uncommon; however, it is especially serious because of the inaccessibility of the hematoma to aspiration by subdural tap. Less commonly, hemorrhage occurs when veins in the subdural space over the surface of the brain are torn. (See Head Injury, Chapter 30.)

Subarachnoid Hemorrhage

Subarachnoid hemorrhage, the most common type of ICH, occurs in full-term infants as a result of trauma and in preterm infants as a result of the same types of events that cause IVH. Small hemorrhages are the most common. Bleeding is of venous origin, and underlying contusion may also occur.

Intracerebellar Hemorrhage

Intracerebellar hemorrhage is a common finding on postmortem examination of the preterm infant and can be a primary hemorrhage in the cerebellum associated with skull compression during abrupt, precipitous delivery. It may occur secondary to extravasation of blood into the cerebellum from a ventricular hemorrhage. In the full-term infant the bleeding may follow a difficult delivery.

Nursing Care Management

Nursing care is the same as care of the infant with IVH or with perinatal hypoxic-ischemic brain injury.

NEONATAL/PERINATAL STROKE

Neonatal stroke is reported to occur in 1 in 6000 live term births (Cole, Dewey, Letourneau, et al., 2017). Inconsistent terminology and classification of neonatal hemorrhagic stroke (NHS) continues to complicate studies examining NHS (Cole, Dewey, Letourneau, et al., 2017). Perinatal intracerebral hemorrhage is defined with the National Institutes of Health Common Data Elements as a term neonate with encephalopathy, seizures, altered mental status, and/or neurologic deficit within the first 28 days of life with a focal collection of blood within the brain parenchyma confirmed by neuroimaging or autopsy (Saver, Warach, Janis, et al., 2012).

Neonatal stroke is the second leading cause of seizures in term neonates and may be caused by arterial, thrombotic, or ischemic events that result in altered brain blood flow and infarction. Neonatal stroke is more predominant in males, and there is an increased tendency toward left-sided involvement. Known risk factors for neonatal and perinatal stroke are not clearly defined or described. However, even without clear evidence for risk factors and etiology, perinatal stroke is a leading cause of cerebral palsy and lifelong neurologic morbidity (Cole, Dewey, Letourneau, et al., 2017). Diagnosis with MRI is most accurate because head ultrasonography may be negative with an ischemic event (Cole, Dewey, Letourneau, et al., 2017).

Because neonatal stroke can only be diagnosed retrospectively, it is important for the nurse to be vigilant for apnea or seizure activity in the first year of life, the time when clinical manifestations will appear.

NEONATAL SEIZURES

Seizures in the neonatal period are usually the clinical manifestation of a serious underlying disease. The most common cause of seizures in the neonatal period (for term and preterm infants) is HIE secondary to perinatal asphyxia (Mikati & Hani, 2016; Volpe, 2008). Although not life threatening as an isolated entity, seizures constitute a medical emergency because they signal a disease process that may produce irreversible brain damage. Consequently, it is imperative to recognize a seizure and its significance so that the cause, as well as the seizure, can be treated (Box 9.11).

Pathophysiology

The features of neonatal seizures are different from those observed in the older infant or child. For example, the well-organized, generalized tonic-clonic seizures seen in older children are rare in infants, especially preterm infants. The newborn brain, with its immature anatomic and physiologic status and reduced cortical organization, is developmentally insufficient to allow ready development and maintenance of a generalized seizure. The advanced degree of development of limbic structures with connections to the diencephalon and brainstem probably accounts for the higher frequency of seizure manifestations (such as oral movements, oculomotor deviations, and apnea) that originate in these structures.

Clinical Manifestations

Seizures in newborns may be subtle and barely discernible or grossly apparent. Because most neonatal seizures are subcortical, they do not have the etiologic and prognostic significance of seizures in children. The type of seizure is seldom important because one may produce a variety of manifestations. Neonatal seizures can be divided into four major types: clonic, tonic, myoclonic, and subtle seizures. Table 9.9 lists these classifications in order of frequency (Volpe, 2008). Clonic, multifocal clonic, and migratory clonic seizures are more common in full-term infants.

Jitteriness or tremulousness in the newborn is a repetitive shaking of an extremity or extremities that may be observed with crying, may occur with changes in sleeping state, or may be elicited with stimulation. Jitteriness is relatively common in newborns, and to a mild degree may be considered normal during the first 4 days of life. Jitteriness can be distinguished from seizures by several characteristics: jitteriness is not accompanied by abnormal ocular movement as are seizures; the dominant movement in jitteriness is tremor, whereas seizure movement is clonic jerking that cannot be stopped by flexion of the affected limb; and jitteriness is highly sensitive to stimulation, whereas seizures are not.

BOX 9.11 Causes of Neonatal Seizures

Metabolic
Hypoglycemia, hyperglycemia
Hypernatremia, hyponatremia
Hypocalcemia
Hypomagnesemia
Pyridoxine deficiency
Aminoacidurias (e.g., phenylketonuria, maple syrup urine disease)
Hyperammonemia

Toxic
Uremia
Bilirubin encephalopathy (kernicterus)

Prenatal Infections
Toxoplasmosis
Syphilis
Cytomegalovirus
Herpes simplex
Hepatitis

Postnatal Infections
Bacterial meningitis
Viral meningoencephalitis
Sepsis
Brain abscess

Trauma at Birth
Hypoxic brain injury
Intracranial hemorrhage
Subarachnoid, subdural hemorrhage
Intraventricular hemorrhage

Malformations
Central nervous system agenesis
Hydranencephaly
Panencephaly
Tuberous sclerosis

Miscellaneous
Degenerative disease
Benign familial neonatal seizures
Narcotic withdrawal
Stroke (fetal, perinatal, or neonatal)

TABLE 9.9 Classifications of Neonatal Seizures

Type	Characteristics
Clonic	Slow, rhythmic jerking movements Approximately 1-3/second
Focal	Involves face, upper or lower extremities on one side of body May involve neck or trunk Infant is conscious during event
Multifocal	May migrate randomly from one part of the body to another Movements may start at different times
Tonic	Extension, stiffening movements
Generalized	Extension of all four limbs (similar to decerebrate rigidity) Upper limbs maintained in a stiffly flexed position (resembles decorticate rigidity)
Focal	Sustained posturing of a limb Asymmetric posturing of trunk or neck
Subtle	May develop in either full-term or preterm infants but more common in preterm Often overlooked by inexperienced observers Signs: • Horizontal eye deviation • Repetitive blinking or fluttering of the eyelids, staring • Sucking or other oral-buccal-lingual movements • Arm movements that resemble rowing or swimming • Leg movements described as pedaling or bicycling • Apnea (common) Signs may appear alone or in combination
Myoclonic	Rapid jerks that involve flexor muscle groups
Focal	Involves upper extremity flexor muscle group No electroencephalogram (EEG) discharges observed
Multifocal	Asynchronous twitching of several parts of the body No associated EEG discharges observed
Generalized	Bilateral jerks of upper and lower limbs Associated with EEG discharges

Adapted from Volpe, J. (2008). Neonatal seizures. In J. Volpe, *Neurology of the newborn* (5th ed.). Philadelphia, PA: Saunders.

Further evaluation is indicated if jittery movements persist beyond the fourth day, if the movements are persistent and prolonged after a stimulus, or if they are easily elicited with minimum stimulus.

Spasms are sudden generalized jerks lasting briefly (1 to 2 seconds) that are distinguished from generalized tonic spells by their short duration and by the fact that spasms are most often associated with a single, brief generalized discharge (Mikati & Hani, 2016). A **tremor** is repetitive movements of both hands (with or without movement of legs or jaws) at a frequency of two to five per second and lasting more than 10 minutes. It is common in newborn infants and has a variety of causes, including neurologic damage, hypoglycemia, and hypocalcemia. Tremors are usually of no pathologic significance.

Diagnostic Evaluation

Early evaluation and diagnosis of seizures are urgent. In addition to a careful physical examination, the pregnancy and family histories are investigated for familial and prenatal causes. Blood is drawn for glucose and electrolyte examination, and CSF is obtained for examination for gross blood, cell count, protein, glucose, and culture. Electroencephalography (EEG) may help identify subtle seizures but is less helpful in establishing a diagnosis; continuous video EEG is the gold standard for monitoring neonatal seizures (Glass, 2014; Mikati & Hani, 2016). Other diagnostic procedures, such as CT, ultrasonography, and echoencephalography, may be indicated. Inborn errors of metabolism should also be evaluated on an individual basis.

Therapeutic Management

Treatment is directed toward the prevention of cerebral damage, correction of metabolic abnormalities, respiratory and cardiovascular support, and suppression of the seizure activity. The underlying cause is treated (e.g., glucose infusion for hypoglycemia, calcium for hypocalcemia, and antibiotics for infection). If needed, respiratory support is provided for hypoxia. Anticonvulsants may be administered, especially when the other measures fail to control the seizures. Lorazepam is the initial drug of choice used to control acute seizures because it is distributed to the brain quickly and exerts its anticonvulsant effect in less than 5 minutes (Mikati & Hani, 2016). Phenobarbital is the first drug of choice for a long-acting drug. It is given intravenously or orally if seizures are severe and persistent. Other drugs that may be used are diazepam, midazolam, phenytoin, and fosphenytoin. If EEG done at the time of discharge does not show evidence of epileptiform activity, medications are usually tapered at that time.

Nursing Care Management

The major nursing responsibilities in the care of infants with seizures are to recognize when the infant is having a seizure so that therapy can be instituted, to carry out the therapeutic regimen, and to observe the response to the therapy and any further evidence of seizures or other symptoms. Assessment and other aspects of care are the same as for all high-risk infants. Parents need to be informed of their infant's status, and the nurse should reinforce and clarify the practitioner's explanations. The infant's behaviors need to be interpreted for the parents, and the infant's responses to the pharmacologic treatment must be anticipated and their significance explained. Encourage parents to visit their infant and perform parenting activities. Parents are also educated regarding the administration of prescribed anticonvulsant drugs and common adverse effects. Seizures generate a great deal of anxiety and fear, and the staff's concern, which is justifiable, can heighten that anxiety. Providing support and guidance is an important nursing function.

HIGH RISK RELATED TO MATERNAL CONDITIONS

INFANTS OF DIABETIC MOTHERS

The morbidity and mortality rates of infants of diabetic mothers (IDMs) have been significantly reduced as a result of effective control of maternal diabetes mellitus and an increased understanding of fetal disorders. However, the offspring of diabetic mothers (type 1, type 2, and gestational) are at risk for a greater number of adverse outcomes. The incidence of congenital anomalies is increased threefold in infants of diabetic mothers (Carlo, 2016). CNS anomalies such as anencephaly and spina bifida occur at rates 16 times higher than in nondiabetic mothers (Hay, 2012). Cardiac anomalies such as ventriculoseptal defects occur in 30% of IDMs (Carlo, 2016; Hay, 2012). Because infants born to women with gestational diabetes mellitus are at risk for many of the same complications as IDMs, the following discussion includes both types of infants. Hypoglycemia associated with congenital hyperinsulinism and hypoglycemia due to inborn metabolic defects is beyond the scope of this discussion.

The severity of the maternal diabetes affects infant survival. Several factors determine the severity: duration of the disease before pregnancy; age of onset; extent of vascular complications; and abnormalities of the current pregnancy such as pyelonephritis, diabetic ketoacidosis, gestational hypertension, and noncompliance. *The single most important factor influencing fetal well-being is the mother's normoglycemic status.* Reasonable metabolic control that begins before conception and continues during the first weeks of pregnancy can prevent malformation in an IDM.

Effects of Diabetes on the Fetus

Hypoglycemia may appear a short time after birth and in IDMs is associated with increased insulin activity in the blood. A standardized definition for neonatal hypoglycemia remains elusive and controversial. At best, authorities agree that reliance on a single numeric value for every clinical situation is inadequate (see Therapeutic Management section). Hypoglycemia in the IDM is related to hypertrophy and hyperplasia of the pancreatic islet cells, causing transient hyperinsulinism.

High maternal blood glucose levels during fetal life provide a continuous stimulus to the fetal islet cells for insulin production. This sustained hyperglycemia promotes fetal insulin secretion that ultimately leads to excessive growth and deposition of fat, which probably accounts for the infants who are large for gestational age, or macrosomic. Hay (2012) suggests that maternal hyperlipidemia and increased lipid transfer to the fetus are responsible for the excessive weight gain and fat deposition seen in such infants. When the neonate's glucose supply is removed abruptly at the time of birth, the continued production of insulin soon depletes the blood of circulating glucose, creating a state of hyperinsulinism and hypoglycemia within 1.5 to 4 hours, especially in infants of mothers with poorly controlled diabetes. Precipitous drops in blood glucose levels can cause serious neurologic damage or death. The birth defects observed in IDMs are thought to occur as a result of multifactorial teratogenic factors rather than hyperglycemia alone (Carlo, 2016; Hay, 2012).

Clinical Manifestations

IDMs have a characteristic appearance (Fig. 9.21). They are usually macrosomic for their gestational age, very plump and full faced, liberally coated with vernix caseosa, and plethoric. The placenta and umbilical cord are also larger than average. However, infants of mothers with advanced diabetes may be small for gestational age, have IUGR, or be appropriate for gestational age because of maternal vascular (placental) involvement. IDMs have an increased incidence of hypoglycemia, hypocalcemia, hyperbilirubinemia, hypomagnesemia, and RDS. Hyperglycemia in the diabetic mother and subsequent fetal hyperinsulinism may be a factor in reducing fetal surfactant synthesis, contributing to the development of RDS. Morbidities in IDMs are the result of exposure to elevated glucose and ketone levels, placental insufficiency, and prematurity. Although large, these infants may be delivered before term because of maternal complications or increased fetal size.

Therapeutic Management

The management of IDMs includes careful monitoring of serum glucose levels and observation for accompanying complications such as RDS. Examine these infants for any anomalies or birth injuries, and regularly

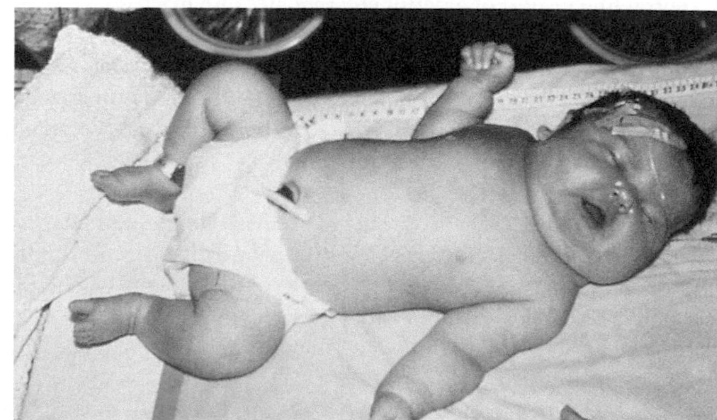

FIG. 9.21 Large-for-gestational-age infant. This infant of a diabetic mother weighed 5 kg (11 lb) at birth and exhibits the typical round facies. (From Zitelli, B. J., & Davis, H. W. [2007]. *Atlas of pediatric physical diagnosis* [5th ed.]. Philadelphia, PA: Mosby.)

obtain blood studies for determinations of glucose, calcium, hematocrit, and bilirubin. A common definition of hypoglycemia has not been established. Several authors have suggested the use of operational thresholds at which hypoglycemia should be closely monitored and treated. Close observation in infants with known risk factors such as maternal diabetes mellitus or with plasma glucose values below 45 mg/dl (2.5 mmol/L) is recommended (Carlo, 2016). If two feeding attempts fail to increase the glucose levels or if symptoms of hypoglycemia develop, IV glucose should be administered to maintain glucose levels above 45 mg/dl (2.5 mmol/L). A newborn less than 4 hours of age with levels at or below 25 mg/dl, or less than 35 mg/dl if greater than 4 hours of age, should receive IV glucose (Adamkin & American Academy of Pediatrics, Committee on Fetus and Newborn, 2011). Rozance, McGowan, Price-Douglas, and colleagues (2016) further recommend that therapeutic glucose levels be kept at or above 50 mg/dl in neonates with profound, recurrent, or persistent hyperinsulinemic hypoglycemia. Studies confirm the importance of maintaining serum glucose levels above 45 mg/dl (2.6 mmol/L) in hyperinsulinemic infants with hypoglycemia to prevent serious neurologic sequelae (Rozance, McGowan, Price-Douglas, et al., 2016).

Because the hypertrophied pancreas is so sensitive to blood glucose concentrations, the administration of oral glucose may trigger a massive insulin release, resulting in rebound hypoglycemia. Therefore feedings should begin within the first hour after birth provided that the infant's cardiorespiratory condition is stable. Approximately half of IDMs do well and adjust without complications. Infants born to mothers with uncontrolled diabetes may require IV infusion of dextrose. Oral and IV intake may be titrated to maintain adequate blood glucose levels. Frequent blood glucose determinations are needed for the first 2 days of life to assess the degree of hypoglycemia present at any given time. Testing blood taken from the heel with point-of-care portable reflectance meters (e.g., glucometer) is a simple and effective screening evaluation that can then be confirmed by laboratory examination.

Nursing Care Management

The nursing care of IDMs involves early examination for congenital anomalies and signs of possible respiratory or cardiac problems, maintenance of adequate thermoregulation, early introduction of carbohydrate feedings as appropriate, and monitoring of serum blood glucose levels. The latter is of particular importance because many hypoglycemic infants may remain asymptomatic. IV glucose infusion requires careful monitoring of the site and the neonate's reaction to therapy. High glucose concentrations (>12.5%) should be infused via a central line instead of a peripheral one. Because macrosomic infants are at risk for problems associated with a difficult delivery, they are monitored for birth injuries such as brachial plexus injury and palsy, fractured clavicle, and phrenic nerve palsy. Additional monitoring of the infant for associated problems (e.g., RDS, polycythemia, hypocalcemia, poor feeding, and hyperbilirubinemia) is also a vital nursing function.

Continuous glucose monitoring has been used to monitor interstitial glucose levels in infants at high risk for neonatal hypoglycemia; although there was good agreement between intermittent blood glucose and continuous interstitial glucose results, there was greater variability among measurements obtained on the first day of life (Wackernagel, Dube, Blennow, et al., 2016).

There is evidence that IDMs have an increased risk of acquiring metabolic syndrome (i.e., obesity, hypertension, dyslipidemia, and glucose intolerance) in childhood or early adulthood (Carlo, 2016). Nursing care of IDMs should also focus on healthy lifestyle and prevention later in life.

DRUG-EXPOSED INFANTS*

Overview

In the 2012 to 2013 National Survey on Drug Use and Health, 5.4% of pregnant women ages 15 to 44 years reported illicit drug use within the past month (Substance Abuse and Mental Health Services Administration, 2012). Given the self-reporting nature of the data, it is likely that there are considerably more substance-using pregnant women. Determining the effects of intrauterine drug and alcohol exposure is difficult for a variety of reasons. Many substance-using women ingest multiple drugs or a combination of drugs and alcohol, and some women who use drugs or alcohol may be undernourished or suffer from chronic medical conditions. Some may not seek prenatal care. For others, the drugs used may be cut with a variety of materials, and the strength, dose, and duration of exposure are likely unknown (Hudak, Tan, Committee on Drugs, et al., 2012).

Clinical Manifestations

Most infants of drug-dependent mothers appear normal at birth but may begin to exhibit signs of drug withdrawal within 12 to 24 hours, depending on the substance and the mother's pattern of use. If mothers have been taking methadone, the signs appear somewhat later—anywhere from 1 or 2 days to 2 to 3 weeks or more after birth. The clinical manifestations of withdrawal may fall into one or all of the following categories: CNS, GI, respiratory, and autonomic nervous system signs (Weiner & Finnegan, 2016). The manifestations become most pronounced between 48 and 72 hours of age and may last from 6 days to 8 weeks (Box 9.12).

BOX 9.12 Signs of Withdrawal in the Neonate

- Irritability
- Tachypnea (>60 beats/min)
- Tremors
- Excoriations (knees, face)
- Shrill cry
- Mottling (skin)
- Hypertonicity of muscles
- Sneezing
- Frantic sucking of hands
- Yawning
- Poor feeding
- Vomiting, often projectile
- Hyperactivity
- Temperature instability
- Perspiring
- Loose diarrheal stools
- Fever
- Seizures
- Nasal stuffiness
- Sleep disturbances

*The term *addiction* is often associated with drug-seeking to experience a high or euphoria, escape from reality, or satisfy a personal need. Newborns are not addicted in a behavioral sense, yet they may experience mild to strong physiologic signs as a result of the mother's drug use. Therefore saying that an infant born to a mother who uses substances is addicted is incorrect; *drug-exposed newborn* is a better term, which implies intrauterine drug exposure.

Signs of withdrawal include increased tone, irritability, increased respiratory rate, disturbed sleep, fever, excessive sucking, and loose, watery stools. Other signs observed include projectile vomiting, mottling, crying, nasal stuffiness, hyperactive Moro reflex, and tremors (Malcolm, 2015). Although these infants suck avidly on fists and display an exaggerated rooting reflex, they are poor feeders with uncoordinated and ineffectual sucking and swallowing reflexes.

One observation in a large percentage of these infants is generalized perspiring, which is unusual in newborn infants. It is significant that although drug-exposed infants may have some tachypnea, cyanosis, or apnea, they rarely develop RDS when born near term. Narcotics or stress factors in the intrauterine environment apparently accelerate lung maturation even with a high incidence of prematurity.

Not all infants of narcotic-addicted mothers show signs of withdrawal. Because of irregular and varying degrees of drug use, quality of drug, and mixed drug usage by the mother, some infants display mild or variable manifestations. Most manifestations are the vague, nonspecific signs characteristic of infants in general; therefore it is important to differentiate between drug withdrawal and other disorders before instituting specific therapy. Other states (e.g., hypocalcemia, hypoglycemia, or sepsis) often coexist with the drug withdrawal.

Many of the mothers often use several drugs, such as tranquilizers, nicotine, sedatives, narcotics, amphetamines, phencyclidine (PCP), marijuana, and other psychotropic agents. Of increasing concern in the United States is the number of newborns who are exposed to methamphetamines and selective serotonin reuptake inhibitors in utero.

Therapeutic Management

The treatment of the drug-exposed infant initially consists of modulating the environment to decrease external stimuli. Drug therapies to decrease withdrawal side effects are implemented once neonatal abstinence syndrome (NAS) is identified. This term is used to describe the behaviors exhibited by the infant exposed to drugs in utero.

Nursing Care Management

When possible, nursery personnel should be alerted to the likelihood of a drug-exposed infant requiring admittance. If the mother has had good prenatal care, the practitioner is aware of the problem and substance abuse treatment may have been instituted before delivery. However, a number of mothers deliver their infants without the benefit of adequate care, and the addiction is unknown to health care personnel at the time of delivery. The degree of narcosis or withdrawal is closely related to the amount of drug the mother has habitually taken, the length of time she has been taking the drug, and her drug level at the time of delivery. The most severe symptoms occur in the infants of mothers who have taken large amounts of drugs over a long period. In addition, the nearer to the time of delivery that the mother takes the drug, the longer it takes the infant to develop withdrawal, and the more severe the manifestations. The infant may not exhibit withdrawal symptoms until 7 to 10 days after delivery.

Once the presence of NAS is identified in an infant, direct nursing care is provided toward reducing external stimuli that might trigger hyperactivity and irritability (e.g., dimming the lights and decreasing noise levels), providing adequate nutrition and hydration, and promoting positive maternal-infant relationships. Providing care on demand rather than on a fixed schedule may help reduce irritability for infants. Appropriate individualized developmental care is implemented, such as facilitating self-consoling and self-regulating behaviors (see Table 9.5). Some irritable and hyperactive infants respond to comforting, movement, containment, and close contact. Wrapping infants snugly and rocking and holding them tightly limit their ability to self-stimulate. The infant's arms should remain flexed with hands close to the mouth for sucking as appropriate; sucking on fingers or hands is a form of self-control and comfort. Arranging nursing activities to reduce disturbances helps decrease exogenous stimulation.

The Neonatal Abstinence Scoring System has been developed to monitor infants in an objective manner and evaluate the infant's response to clinical and pharmacologic interventions (Finnegan, 1985). This system also assists nurses and other health care workers in evaluating the severity of the infant's withdrawal symptoms.

Another scoring tool has been developed specifically aimed at measuring neurologic behavior and resultant effects on the neonate when substances are used during pregnancy. The NICU Network Neurobehavioral Scale (NNNS), developed by the National Institutes of Health, provides an assessment of neurologic, behavioral, and stress-abstinence function in the neonate. The NNNS was designed to provide a comprehensive assessment of both neurologic integrity and behavioral function (Lester, Tronick, & Brazelton, 2004).

Loose stools and poor intake and regurgitation after feeding predispose the infants to malnutrition, dehydration, and electrolyte imbalance. An oral opioid such as morphine may be administered to control loose, watery stools (Weiner & Finnegan, 2016). It takes considerable time and patience to ensure that these infants receive sufficient caloric and fluid intake.

Monitoring and recording activity level and its relationship to other activities, such as feeding and preventing complications, are important nursing functions.

A valuable aid to anticipating problems in the newborn is recognizing drug abuse in the mother. Unless the mother is enrolled in a methadone rehabilitation program, she seldom risks calling attention to her habit by seeking prenatal care. Consequently, infants and mothers are exposed to the additional hazards of obstetric and medical complications resulting from the lack of adequate prenatal care. Moreover, the nature of heroin addiction makes the user susceptible to disorders such as infection (hepatitis B and HIV related to IV needle use), foreign body reaction, and inadequate nutrition and preterm birth. Methadone treatment does not prevent withdrawal reaction in neonates, but the clinical course may be modified. Intensive psychologic support of mothers is a factor in the treatment and reduction of perinatal mortality. Mothers are usually anxious and depressed, lack confidence, have poor self-image, and have difficulty with interpersonal relationships. They may have a psychologic need for the pregnancy and an infant.

Initial symptoms or the recurrence of withdrawal symptoms may develop after discharge from the hospital. Therefore it is important to establish rapport and maintain contact with the family so that they return for treatment if this occurs. The demands of the drug-exposed infant on the caregiver are enormous and unrewarding in terms of positive feedback. The infants are difficult to comfort, and they cry for long periods, which can be especially trying for the caregiver after the infant's discharge. Long-term follow-up to evaluate the status of the infant and family is important.

An important aspect of nursing care is identification of an infant who was exposed to drugs in utero. Observation of signs mentioned previously may warrant further investigation so prompt treatment can be implemented. Newborn urine, rarely hair, or meconium sampling may be required to identify drug exposure and implement appropriate early interventional therapies aimed at minimizing the consequences of intrauterine drug exposure. Meconium sampling for fetal drug exposure provides more screening accuracy than urine because drug metabolites accumulate in meconium (Weiner & Finnegan, 2016). Urine toxicology screening has less accuracy because it only reflects recent substance intake by the mother (Soni & Singh, 2012). Meconium testing for drug metabolites has the advantages of being easy to collect, noninvasive, and more accurate.

Pharmacologic treatment is usually based on the severity of withdrawal symptoms, as determined by an assessment tool. Drug therapies to decrease withdrawal side effects include administration of phenobarbital, morphine, diluted tincture of opium methadone buprenorphine, or clonidine (Carlo & Ambalavanan, 2016b; Weiner & Finnegan, 2016). A combination of these drugs may be necessary to treat infants exposed to multiple drugs in utero, careful attention should be given to possible adverse effects (Weiner & Finnegan, 2016).

Many problems relate to the disposition of infants of drug-dependent mothers. Those who advocate separation of mothers and children argue that the mothers are not capable of assuming responsibility for their infant's care, that child care is frustrating to them, and that their existence is too disorganized and chaotic. Others encourage the maternal-infant bond and recommend a protected environment such as a therapeutic community; a halfway house; or ongoing supportive services in the home after discharge. Careful evaluation and the cooperative efforts of a variety of health professionals are required, whether the choice is foster home placement or supportive follow-up care of mothers who keep their infants.

Opiate Exposure

Narcotics have a low molecular weight, allowing them to readily cross the placental membrane and enter the fetal system. When the mother is a habitual user of narcotics, especially heroin or methadone, the unborn child may also become passively physiologically addicted to the drug, which places the infant at risk during the early neonatal period.

Prescription opioids such as oxycodone (OxyContin) have been identified as increasingly popular drugs of abuse, which may cause withdrawal symptoms in neonates (Carlo & Ambalavanan, 2016b). Other chemical substances that may cause neonatal withdrawal include methadone, caffeine, and PCP.

Methadone Exposure

Methadone, a synthetic opiate, has been the therapy of choice for heroin addiction since 1965. Methadone crosses the placenta. An increasing number of infants have been born to methadone-maintained mothers who seem to have better prenatal care and a somewhat better lifestyle than those taking heroin.

Some question exists concerning the benefits of methadone therapy during pregnancy because of its effect on the fetus. Methadone withdrawal resembles heroin withdrawal but tends to be more severe and prolonged. Signs of methadone withdrawal include tremors, irritability, fever, hypertonicity, hyperactive Moro reflex, vomiting, and sleep disturbances (Gaalema, Scott, Heil, et al., 2012; Kraft, Stover, & Davis, 2016). These infants exhibit a disturbed sleep pattern similar to that seen in heroin withdrawal. They have a higher birth weight than those infants in heroin withdrawal, usually appropriate for gestational age. No increased incidence of congenital anomalies is seen. The American Academy of Pediatrics (2012) has suggested that mothers in a methadone treatment program can be encouraged to breastfeed if they are adequately nourished and negative for HIV or illicit drug use.

Late-onset withdrawal occurs at age 2 to 4 weeks and may continue for weeks or months. A higher incidence of SIDS has been reported in these infants (Weiner & Finnegan, 2016). This factor is important for perinatal nurses who coordinate follow-up care for the infant and education for the mother or caregiver. Community health nurses must know about the potential for withdrawal symptoms.

Therapy for methadone withdrawal is similar to that for heroin withdrawal. The few available follow-up studies of these infants reveal a high incidence of hyperactivity, learning and behavior disorders, and poor social adjustment.

Cocaine Exposure

Cocaine, a common illicit drug in the United States, has multiple forms. Prenatal cocaine exposure is commonly associated with a number of adverse consequences throughout development (Ross, Graham, Money, et al., 2015). Use of the relatively inexpensive and easily administered "crack" form increased significantly among pregnant women and women of childbearing age in the 1980s and 1990s (Ryder & Brisgone, 2013). Because crack vaporizes at relatively low temperatures, it is smoked and absorbed in large quantities through the pulmonary vasculature. The drug readily enters the placenta, placing the fetus at risk (Cain, Bornick, & Whiteman, 2013).

Cocaine is a CNS stimulant and peripheral sympathomimetic, and the effects on the fetus may be direct or indirect. Indirect effects include fetal hypoxemia secondary to impaired uterine blood flow. Cocaine also appears to affect fetal cardiac function and suppresses the fetal immune system (Weiner & Finnegan, 2016). Exposure to cocaine is typified by abnormal arousal and attention regulation. One study demonstrated functional connectivity and behavioral disruptions in the thalamus of neonates exposed to cocaine prenatally (Salzwedel, Grewen, Goldman, et al., 2016). The difficulties encountered by cocaine-exposed infants are compounded when the mother takes the drug in conjunction with other illicit drugs (Cain, Bornick, & Whiteman, 2013).

Adolescence follow-up of 218 children exposed prenatally to cocaine demonstrated poorer perceptual organization IQ, visual-spatial information processing, attention, language, executive function, and behavior regulation through age 14 (Singer, Minnes, Min, et al., 2015). Another compounding factor for prenatal drug exposure and later substance abuse risk is that cocaine-exposed adolescents self-reported that they were more likely to use alcohol, tobacco, and/or marijuana by age 15 compared with non–cocaine-exposed adolescents (Minnes, Singer, Min, et al., 2014).

Clinical Manifestations

Infants who are exposed to cocaine in utero may demonstrate no immediate untoward effects. Previous reports of catastrophic neurologic effects have been published, yet the findings have considerable variability because of poor reliability of maternal history, maternal polydrug use, prematurity, poor social environment, and poor specificity in detecting cocaine exposure. It may be, however, that habitual cocaine use in pregnancy has negative effects that are too subtle to notice in the newborn and infancy period (Lambert & Bauer, 2012).

Clinical manifestations of intrauterine cocaine exposure include IUGR; decreased head circumference; and association with preterm delivery, NEC, cerebral infarcts, respiratory disturbances such as apnea, tachycardia, transient EEG abnormalities, and tremors (Weiner & Finnegan, 2016). Other findings related to neurobehavioral effects include sleep disturbances, increased tone, jitteriness, delayed language acquisition, behavior problems in school, poor impulse control, hypertonia, abnormal reflexes, motor asymmetry, significant cognitive delays, and poor responses to stimuli (Kim & Koren, 2012; Salzwedel, Grewen, Goldman, et al., 2016). Environmental and sociodemographic factors likely play an important role in the outcome of children exposed to cocaine in utero.

Therapeutic Management

Infants exposed to cocaine alone are less likely than other drug-exposed infants to demonstrate signs of withdrawal. Regardless of the type of drug or substance to which the newborn was exposed, treatment begins with prompt identification of a potential problem by obtaining a comprehensive maternal history, identifying potential risks associated with exposure, and maintaining a safe environment. Newborn urine, hair (rarely), or meconium sampling may be required to identify intrauterine drug exposure and implement appropriate early interventional therapies aimed at minimizing the consequences.

Nursing Care Management

Nursing care of cocaine-exposed infants is similar to that of infants exposed to other drugs. Individualized assessment helps determine appropriate intervention strategies. If the nurse identifies hypertonicity and sleep disturbance, the environment is modified accordingly to decrease noxious stimuli. The use of swaddling, containment, gentle rocking, NNS, and undisturbed periods of rest may help promote self-containment and state regulation. As previously noted, tissue samples may be required for identification of drug exposure. Because cocaine is easily passed in breast milk, mothers should be counseled to avoid breastfeeding (D'Apolito, 2013; Jones, 2015). A fussy newborn may be thought by caretakers to be consistently hungry, and thus overfeeding and vomiting may be problematic. Provision of a safe environment in which the mother and newborn may interact is imperative. Opportunities for appropriate family bonding and attachment should be provided as with any other newborn. Because a large percentage of women who use cocaine during pregnancy have sexually transmitted infections, consider screening for the newborn (Cain, Bornick, & Whiteman, 2013).

Referral to early intervention programs, including child health care, parental drug treatment, individualized developmental care, and parenting education, is essential in promoting optimum outcomes for these children. Children exposed to maternal cocaine use often live in impoverished conditions and are at high risk for cognitive delays, poor child health care, and abuse or neglect; they would benefit from an early intervention program (Solis, Shadur, Burns, et al., 2012). It is essential that nurses caring for these infants and their mothers understand the depth of the problem of prenatal drug exposure, have a positive attitude toward cocaine-using mothers and their children, be aware of community resources, and encourage positive parenting (Hill, 2012).

Methamphetamine Exposure

The fetal and neonatal effects of maternal use of methamphetamines in pregnancy are not well known but appear to be dose related (Soto & Bahado-Singh, 2013). Continuous methamphetamine use during pregnancy is associated with preterm delivery and low birth weight, both of which contribute to neonatal morbidity and mortality (Wright, Schuetter, Tellei, et al., 2015). Stopping methamphetamine use at any time during pregnancy improves birth outcomes (Wright, Schuetter, Tellei, et al., 2015).

Methamphetamine use continues to be prevalent in the United States, especially in young adults of childbearing age, and has increased significantly among women and girls 12 years of age and older. In the Infant Development, Environment, and Lifestyle (IDEAL) study (Della Grotta, LaGasse, Arria, et al., 2010), 42% of pregnant women using methamphetamines reported using the drug throughout the pregnancy. A higher incidence of preterm delivery and placental abruption was associated with methamphetamine use. The IDEAL study follow-up at ages 3 and 5 years demonstrated increased scores for emotional reactivity, anxious/depressed problems, and attention-deficit/hyperactivity disorder (LaGasse, Derauf, Smith, et al., 2012). School-age outcomes (7.5 years of age) of the IDEAL subjects concluded that methamphetamine use continued to be associated with behavioral problems, but noted that early adversity may be a strong determinant of behavioral outcomes for these children (Eze, Smith, LaGasse, et al., 2016).

Infants exposed to methamphetamine in utero have significantly smaller head circumferences and birth weights than those not exposed (Shah, Diaz, Arria, et al., 2012). In addition, exposed infants may exhibit agitation, vomiting, and tachypnea (Davis, Roberds, Hannaford, et al., 2012). After birth, infants may experience bradycardia or tachycardia that resolves as the drug is cleared from the system. Lethargy may continue for several months, along with frequent infections and poor weight gain. Emotional disturbances and delays in gross and fine motor coordination may occur during early childhood.

The long-term effects of methamphetamine exposure on children living in households where the product is manufactured are not known, but there are early reports of burns in exposed children and concerns regarding the effects of the toxic by-products on small children. Skin rashes and respiratory tract illnesses are common problems seen in methamphetamine-exposed children. Physical neglect and speech and language developmental delays are of significant concern as well (Messina & Jeter, 2012).

Marijuana Exposure

Marijuana is the most common illicit drug used by women ages 18 to 44 years (nonpregnant and pregnant) in the United States (McCabe & Arndt, 2012). Marijuana crosses the placenta. Some studies have shown that use during pregnancy resulted in decreased birth weight and a need for placement in an NICU (Conner, Carter, & Tuuli, 2015; Gunn, Rosales, Center, et al., 2016). Warshak, Regan, Moore, and colleagues (2015) concluded that marijuana use, as an independent factor, had no poor neonatal outcomes in term pregnancies. A review of studies examining the effects of marijuana during pregnancy found inconsistent results regarding the drug's effect on birth weight and gestational age (Soto & Bahado-Singh, 2013). Compounding the issue of the effects of marijuana is multidrug use, which combines the harmful effects of marijuana, tobacco, alcohol, opiates, and cocaine (Gunn, Rosales, Center, et al., 2016). Long-term follow-up studies on exposed infants are needed.

Fetal Alcohol Spectrum Disorder

Infants and children exposed to alcohol in utero were previously reported to have characteristic facial features, prenatal and postnatal growth failure, and neurodevelopmental deficits. This triad of findings, termed fetal alcohol syndrome (FAS), was attributed to excessive ingestion of alcohol by the mother during pregnancy. It has since been shown that infants may not initially display the dysmorphic facial features. These are believed to become more defined with increasing age during childhood. A number of terms (including *alcohol-related neurodevelopmental birth defects* and *fetal alcohol spectrum disorders*) have been proposed to describe the combination of findings. The umbrella term fetal alcohol spectrum disorder (FASD) is now recommended to describe the continuum of defects seen in children affected by maternal alcohol intake, including classic FAS at the most severe end of the spectrum.

Three categories described by the Centers for Disease Control and Prevention (2016) for diagnosis of FAS are growth restriction, both prenatal and postnatal; midfacial dysmorphic facial features; and CNS involvement (i.e., structural, neurologic, or functional abnormality). Any single or combination of these may be present in addition to a history of maternal alcohol consumption. The diagnosis of FASD is complicated by the absence of a specific single biologic marker and by manifestations that are often seen in other childhood conditions.

When possible, long-term disabilities are prevented by early evaluation and implementation of therapy. The family should learn any special handling techniques needed for the care of their infant and signs of complications or possible sequelae. When sequelae are inevitable, the family needs assistance in determining how to best cope with the problems, such as with home care assistance, referral to appropriate agencies, or placement in an institution for care.

The major goal of nursing care is prevention of these disorders through provision of adequate prenatal care for the expectant mother and precautions regarding exposure to potentially harmful infections.

FASD is recognized as the leading preventable cause of cognitive impairment (Tai, Piskorski, Kao, et al., 2017). The incidence of FASD is on the rise in the United States despite public warnings, including the US Surgeon General's warning that consumption of alcohol during pregnancy may cause cognitive impairment and other defects. The incidence of FASD in the United States is about 2 to 7 per 1000 live births (May, Baete, Russo, et al., 2014). The reported incidence of maternal alcohol consumption during pregnancy did not change substantially from 1991 to 2005 despite widespread education and information regarding periconceptional and gestational effects of drinking (Centers for Disease Control and Prevention, 2016). Among pregnant women ages 18 to 44, the average annual rates were 12.2% for alcohol use and 1.9% for binge drinking. Among nonpregnant women, 53.7% reported alcohol consumption and 12.1% binge drinking. The Centers for Disease Control and Prevention (2016) found that pregnant women who were older, unmarried, more educated, and employed were more likely to use alcohol.

Alcohol (ethanol and ethyl alcohol) interferes with normal fetal development. The effects on the fetal brain are permanent, and even moderate use of alcohol during pregnancy may cause long-term postnatal difficulties, including impaired maternal-infant attachment. Because there is no known safe level of alcohol consumption in pregnancy, the current recommendation is that women stop consuming alcohol at least 3 months before they plan to conceive.

Fetal abnormalities are not related to the amount of the mother's alcohol intake, but to the amount consumed in excess of the liver's ability to detoxify it. The liver's capacity to detoxify alcohol is limited and inflexible; when the liver receives more alcohol than it is able to handle, the excess is continually recirculated until the organ is able to reduce it to carbon dioxide and water. This circulating alcohol has a special affinity for brain tissue. There is no specific critical period at which alcohol toxicity may occur, although early gestation is considered the most vulnerable period. Exposure at any period may cause subtle damage to the developing fetus (Tai, Piskorski, Kao, et al., 2017). Other factors that contribute to the teratogenic effects include toxic acetyl aldehyde (a degradation by-product of ethanol) and other substances that may be added to the alcohol. Poor nutritional state, smoking, polydrug intake, and infrequent or lack of prenatal care may compound the problem of alcohol abuse (Paintner, Williams, & Burd, 2012a).

The effects on the fetal brain are reflected in CNS manifestations of FASD (Box 9.13). Cognitive and motor delays, hearing disorders, and a variety of defects in craniofacial development are prominent features (Fig. 9.22). MRI studies of children with diagnosed FASD revealed a high incidence of midbrain anomalies, including displacements in the corpus callosum and changes in symmetry in the temporal lobes. Alcohol-exposed infants also demonstrate narrowing in the temporal region and reduced brain growth in portions of the frontal lobe (Wilhoit, Scott, & Simecka, 2017). Some affected infants display physical features of the syndrome; behaviors, however, are nonspecific in newborns and may therefore pass undetected. These include difficulty in establishing respiration, irritability, lethargy, poor suck reflex, and abdominal distention.

Nursing Care Management

Nursing care of affected infants involves the same assessment and observations that are employed for any high-risk infant. Poor feeding is characteristic of infants with FASD and is a significant problem throughout infancy. Strategies to provide individualized developmental care are aimed at reducing noxious environmental stimuli and helping the infant achieve self-regulation (see Developmental Outcome, p. 285). Monitoring weight gain, analyzing feeding behaviors, and devising strategies to promote nutritional intake are especially important.

BOX 9.13 Major Features of Fetal Alcohol Syndrome*

Facial Features

Short palpebral fissures
Hypoplastic or smooth philtrum (vertical ridge in upper lip)
Thinned upper lip (vermilion)
Short, upturned nose
Hypoplastic maxilla
Micrognathia or prognathia in adolescence
Retrognathia in infancy

Neurologic

Cognitive impairment
Motor delays
Microcephaly (head circumference below 10th percentile)
Poor coordination
Hypotonia
Hearing disorders

Behavior

Irritability (infancy)
Hyperactivity (child)

Growth

Disproportionately low weight to height
Prenatal growth restriction
Persistent postnatal growth lag

*For a comprehensive list of fetal alcohol–related birth defects, see Fig. 1 in American Academy of Pediatrics, Committee on Substance Abuse and Committee on Children with Disabilities. (2000). Fetal alcohol syndrome and alcohol-related neurodevelopmental disorders. *Pediatrics, 106*(2), 358-361.

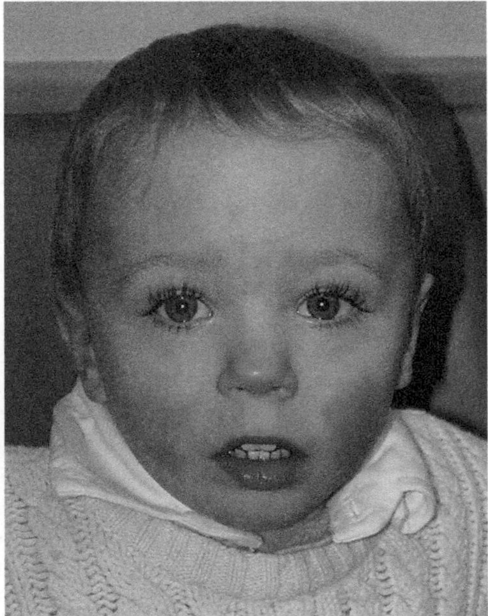

FIG. 9.22 Child with fetal alcohol syndrome.

The effects of FASD have been identified in adolescents and young adults, primarily in relation to growth deficiencies, delayed motor development, and cognitive impairment. Children exposed to alcohol prenatally showed more aggressiveness, delinquent behavior, and attention problems (Wilhoit, Scott, & Simecka, 2017). Facial characteristics in adults tend to be more subtle than in infants and children.

Early diagnosis and intervention are reported to be beneficial for reducing the effects of alcohol exposure on the growing child (Paintner, Williams, & Burd, 2012b; Popova, Lange, Probst, et al., 2017; Wilhoit, Scott, & Simecka, 2017). Nurses should be actively involved in identifying and referring children exposed to alcohol prenatally.

The dangers of heavy drinking are known, and *all* women should be counseled regarding the risks to the fetus. The nurse should emphasize to women of all ages that there is no known "safe" amount of alcohol intake during pregnancy that will prevent FASD. Furthermore, FASD is a totally preventable birth defect. A change in drinking habits even as late as the third trimester (when brain growth in the fetus is greatest) is associated with improved fetal outcome.*

Infants of Mothers Who Smoke

Cigarette smoking during pregnancy is clearly associated with significant birth weight deficits, and there is a definitive dose-response relationship between the number of cigarettes smoked by the mother and these deficits (Abraham, Alramadhan, Iniguez, et al., 2017; Himes, Stroud, Scheidweiler, et al., 2013). This dose-related response also affects the Apgar scores. Nearly four times more infants whose mothers smoked three packs per day had low Apgar scores compared with infants whose mothers did not smoke or smoked only one pack per day. Studies indicate that almost 30% of women smoke and the majority of this population are in their childbearing period (Sabra, Gratocos, & Gomez Roig, 2017)

The rate of preterm births is increased in mothers who smoke, but the infants are smaller at all stages of gestation. They show fetal growth restriction in length, weight, and chest and head circumference; these deficits are not related to maternal appetite or weight gain. The concentration of a pharmacologically active substance found in tobacco—nicotine—has been found to be higher in newborns of mothers who smoke than in the mothers themselves. Nicotine is metabolized to cotinine and secreted in breast milk and has a half-life of 70 to 80 minutes. In addition, it is now recognized that neonates may experience withdrawal symptoms after exposure to nicotine, whether smoked or chewed. It has also been shown that cigarette smoking has detrimental effects beyond the neonatal period, with deficits in growth, intellectual and emotional development, and behavior. Maternal smoking and passive smoking by household members has been correlated with higher rates of SIDS (Sabra, Gratocos, & Gomez Roig, 2017), spontaneous abortion, premature rupture of membranes, preterm delivery, and learning and behavior deficits (Sabra, Gratocos, & Gomez Roig, 2017).

The popularity of electronic cigarettes has increased significantly within the last few years, especially among middle school– and high school–age children (Centers for Disease Control and Prevention, 2013). There is currently no evidence that "vaping," or smoking e-cigarettes, is less harmful than regular cigarettes; nicotine is a product found in e-cigarettes and maternal use can pass nicotine to the unborn child just as easily as regular cigarette smoking.

Nursing Care Management

Nurses are prime candidates for disseminating information to expectant mothers regarding smoking-related risks. Mothers who stop or substantially reduce smoking during pregnancy improve the quality of life for their unborn infants. In one study, infants of expectant mothers who were given information, support, encouragement, practical guidance, and behavior modification during pregnancy delivered infants with significantly higher birth weights than did controls. If mothers continue to smoke while breastfeeding, encourage them to do so immediately after breastfeeding to reduce the amount of nicotine and cotinine in the breast milk. Smoking decreases milk production in the breastfeeding mother (Napierala, Mazela, Merritt, et al., 2016). Parents should make all efforts to avoid secondhand smoke around all infants, but especially around those born with respiratory or cardiac problems and those born prematurely.

MATERNAL INFECTIONS

The range of pathologic conditions produced by infectious agents is large, and the difference between the maternal and fetal effects caused by any one agent is also great. Some maternal infections, especially during early gestation, can result in fetal loss or malformations because the fetus's ability to handle infectious organisms is limited and the fetal immunologic system is unable to prevent the dissemination of infectious organisms to the various tissues.

Not all prenatal infections produce teratogenic effects. Furthermore, disorders caused by transplacental transfer of infectious agents are not always well defined clinically. Some microbial agents can cause remarkably similar manifestations, and it is not uncommon to test for all when a prenatal infection is suspected. This is the so-called TORCHS complex:

T—Toxoplasmosis
O—Other (e.g., hepatitis B, parvovirus, HIV)
R—Rubella
C—Cytomegalovirus infection
H—Herpes simplex
S—Syphilis

To determine the causative agent in a symptomatic infant, perform tests to rule out each of these infections. The *O* category may involve testing for several viral infections (e.g., hepatitis B, varicella-zoster, measles, mumps, HIV, human papillomavirus, and human parvovirus). Bacterial infections are not included in the TORCHS workup because they are usually identified by clinical manifestations and readily available laboratory tests. Gonococcal conjunctivitis (ophthalmia neonatorum) and chlamydial conjunctivitis have been significantly reduced by prophylactic measures at birth. (See Chapter 7.) HIV infection is discussed in Chapter 28. The major maternal infections, their possible effects, and specific nursing considerations are outlined in Table 9.10.

The Zika virus (ZIKV), transmitted by the Aedes mosquito, is identified as a causal contributor to microcephaly in infancy (Cauchemez, Besnard, Bompard, et al., 2016; Chibueze, Tirado, Lopes, et al., 2017). In 2016 ZIKV infection was declared a Public Health Emergency of International Concern. Although it may cause only simple flulike symptoms in the pregnant mother, ZIKV can lead to serious complications (including microcephaly) in the newborn (Passi, Sharma, Dutta, et al., 2017).

Nursing Care Management

One of the major goals in care of infants suspected of having an infectious disease is identification of the causative agent. Until the diagnosis is

*Further information is available from National Organization on Fetal Alcohol Syndrome, 900 17th St. NW, Washington, DC 20006; 202-785-4585; http://www.nofas.org; and Fetal Alcohol Syndrome Branch, National Center on Birth Defects and Developmental Disabilities, Centers for Disease Control and Prevention, Atlanta, GA; http://www.cdc.gov/ncbddd/fas.

TABLE 9.10 Infections Acquired From Mother Before, During, or After Birth*

Fetal or Newborn Effect	Transmission	Nursing Considerations†
Human Immunodeficiency Virus (HIV)		
No significant difference between infected and uninfected infants at birth in some instances Embryopathy reported by some observers: • Depressed nasal bridge • Mild upward or downward obliquity of eyes • Long palpebral fissures with blue sclerae • Patulous lips • Ocular hypertelorism • Prominent upper vermilion border	Transplacental; during vaginal labor and delivery; breast milk; feeding infant blood-tinged premasticated food	Administer combination antiretroviral prophylaxis to human immunodeficiency (HIV)–positive mother; prophylaxis to prevent perinatal transmission may begin after first trimester. Choice of regimens is determined by examining a number of factors, including mother's current treatment. Detailed recommendations can be obtained from Panel on Treatment of HIV-Infected Pregnant Women and Prevention of Perinatal Transmission (2012). During labor ZDV is recommended for all HIV-infected pregnant women who have HIV RNA ≥400 copies ml, regardless of antepartum regimen; those with less than 400 copies/ml and receiving combination antiretroviral regimen may not be required to receive ZDV during labor. HIV-exposed neonates (regardless of maternal antiretroviral dosing) should receive a 6-wk course of ZDV starting as soon after birth as possible but preferably within 6-12 hours; nevirapine may also be given in 3 doses during the first week of life. ZDV dosing varies according to infant gestational age and route of administration (see Panel on Treatment, Table 9, 2012 for dosage regimen). Discuss avoidance of premasticated foods given to infant from HIV-infected mother. Cesarean section at 38 weeks of gestation in HIV-positive mothers is recommended to reduce transmission. Avoid breastfeeding in HIV-positive mother. For chemoprophylaxis against *Pneumocystis carinii* pneumonia in HIV-exposed infants, drug of choice is trimethoprim-sulfamethoxazole (Bactrim, Septra). ZDV and nevirapine are the only ART drugs recommended for preterm infants (see Table 9, Panel on Treatment, 2012)
Chickenpox (Varicella-Zoster Virus [VZV])		
Intrauterine exposure—congenital varicella syndrome: limb dysplasia, microcephaly, cortical atrophy, chorioretinitis, cataracts, cutaneous scars, other anomalies, auditory nerve palsy, motor and cognitive delays Severe symptoms (rash, fever) and higher mortality in infant whose mother develops varicella 5 days before to 2 days after delivery	First trimester (fetal varicella syndrome); perinatal period (infection)	Use varicella zoster immune globulin or IVIG to treat infants born to mothers with onset of disease within 5 days before or 2 days after birth. Healthy term infants exposed postnatally to varicella (especially if mother's rash does not appear until after 48 hours of birth) should not receive varicella zoster immune globulin (American Academy of Pediatrics, Committee on Infectious Diseases, 2015). (See also Immunizations, Chapter 6, for administration recommendations for preterm infants.) Institute Isolation Precautions in newborn born to mother with varicella up to 21-28 days (latter time if newborn received varicella zoster immune globulin or IVIG after birth (if hospitalized).† Prevention—Immunize all children with varicella vaccine.
Chlamydia Infection *(Chlamydia trachomatis)*		
Conjunctivitis, pneumonia	Last trimester or perinatal period	Standard ophthalmic prophylaxis for gonococcal ophthalmia neonatorum (topical antibiotics, silver nitrate, or povidone-iodine) is not effective in treatment or prevention of chlamydial ophthalmia. Treat with oral erythromycin for 14 days.
Coxsackievirus (Group B Enterovirus–Nonpolio)		
Poor feeding, vomiting, diarrhea, fever; cardiac enlargement, arrhythmias, congestive heart failure; lethargy, seizures, meningeal involvement Mimics bacterial sepsis	Peripartum	Treatment is supportive. Provide IVIG in neonatal infections.

TABLE 9.10 Infections Acquired From Mother Before, During, or After Birth*—cont'd

Fetal or Newborn Effect	Transmission	Nursing Considerations†
Cytomegalovirus (CMV)		
Variable manifestation from asymptomatic to severe Microcephaly, cerebral calcifications, chorioretinitis Jaundice, hepatosplenomegaly Petechial or purpuric rash Neurologic sequelae—seizure disorders, sensorimotor deafness, cognitive impairment	Throughout pregnancy	Infection acquired at birth, shortly thereafter, or via human milk is not associated with clinical illness. Affected individuals excrete virus in saliva and other oropharyngeal secretions. Virus is detected in urine or tissue by electron microscopy. Pregnant women should avoid close contact with known cases. To treat infection, administer IV antivirals such as ganciclovir to newborn.
Erythema Infectiosum (Parvovirus B19)		
Fetal hydrops and death from anemia and heart failure with early exposure Anemia with later exposure No teratogenic effects established Ordinarily, low risk of ill effect to fetus	Transplacental	First trimester infection has most serious effects. Pregnant health care workers should not care for patients who might be highly contagious (e.g., child with aplastic crisis). Aggressive cardiovascular and respiratory support is required in newborn with hydrops. Routine exclusion of pregnant women from workplace where disease is occurring is not recommended.
Gonococcal Disease *(Neisseria gonorrhoeae)*		
Ophthalmitis Neonatal gonococcal arthritis, septicemia, meningitis	Last trimester or perinatal period	Preventive: Apply prophylactic medication to eyes at time of birth. Infant with confirmed ophthalmia, scalp abscess, or disseminated infection should be hospitalized, and cultures obtained to determine antimicrobial treatment. Consider testing infant for *Chlamydia*, HIV, and syphilis. Irrigate infant's eyes with saline until discharge is eliminated. Obtain smears for culture. To treat ophthalmia and nondisseminated infection, administer IV or IM ceftriaxone, once. Disseminated disease requires cefotaxime treatment for 1 week.
Hepatitis B Virus (HBV)		
May be asymptomatic at birth Acute hepatitis, changes in liver function	Transplacental; contaminated maternal fluids or secretions during delivery	Administer HBIG to all infants of HBsAG-positive mothers within 12 hours of birth; in addition, administer HepB vaccine at separate site. Prevention—Immunize all infants with HepB vaccine. Infants born to HBsAG-positive mothers and weighing <2000 g should receive 3-dose vaccine series in addition to birth dose (See Immunizations, Chapter 6.)
Herpes, Neonatal (Herpes Simplex Virus)		
Cutaneous lesions—vesicles at 6-10 days of age; may be no lesions Disseminated disease resembling sepsis—encephalitis in 60%-70% Visceral involvement—granulomas Early nonspecific signs—fever, lethargy, poor feeding, irritability, vomiting May include hyperbilirubinemia, seizures, flaccid or spastic paralysis, apneic episodes, respiratory distress, lethargy, or coma	History of genital infection in mother or partner in 50% of cases Transmitted intrapartum, either by ascending infection or direct contact, especially primary infection	Absence of skin lesions in neonate exposed to maternal herpesvirus does not indicate absence of disease. Contact Precautions (in addition to Standard Precautions) should be instituted. It is recommended that swabs of mouth, nasopharynx, conjunctivae, rectum, and any skin vesicles be obtained from exposed neonate; in addition, urine, stool, blood, and CSF specimens should be obtained for culture. Therapy with IV acyclovir is initiated if culture results are positive or if there is strong suspicion of herpesvirus infection; ophthalmic treatment (e.g., 1% trifluridine or 3% vidarabine) is required for ocular involvement in addition to acyclovir. Therapy with oral acyclovir for 6 months is recommended for neonates with HSV CNS disease (American Academy of Pediatrics, Committee on Infectious Diseases, 2015).
Listeriosis *(Listeria monocytogenes)*		
Maternal infection associated with abortion, preterm delivery, and fetal death Preterm birth, sepsis, and pneumonia seen in early-onset disease; late-onset disease usually manifests as meningitis	Transplacental, by ascending infection or exposure at delivery	Hand washing is essential to prevent nosocomial spread. Treat infected newborn with antibiotics—ampicillin and gentamicin.

Continued

TABLE 9.10 Infections Acquired From Mother Before, During, or After Birth*—cont'd

Fetal or Newborn Effect	Transmission	Nursing Considerations†
Rubella, Congenital (Rubella Virus)		
Eye defects—cataracts (unilateral or bilateral), microphthalmos, retinitis, glaucoma CNS signs—microcephaly, seizures, severe cognitive impairment Congenital heart defects—patent ductus arteriosus Auditory—high incidence of delayed hearing loss Intrauterine growth restriction Hyperbilirubinemia, meningitis, thrombocytopenia, hepatomegaly	First trimester; early second trimester	Pregnant women should avoid contact with all affected persons, including infants with rubella syndrome. Emphasize vaccination of all unimmunized prepubertal children, susceptible adolescents, and women of childbearing age (nonpregnant). Caution women against pregnancy for at least 3 months after vaccination.
Syphilis, Congenital *(Treponema pallidum)*		
Stillbirth, prematurity, hydrops fetalis May be asymptomatic at birth and in 1st few weeks of life or may have multisystem manifestations: hepatosplenomegaly, lymphadenopathy, hemolytic anemia, and thrombocytopenia Copper-colored maculopapular cutaneous lesions (usually after 1st few weeks of life), mucous membrane patches, hair loss, nail exfoliation, snuffles (syphilitic rhinitis), profound anemia, poor feeding, pseudoparalysis of one or more limbs, dysmorphic teeth (older child)	Transplacental; can be anytime during pregnancy or at birth	This is most severe form of syphilis. Treatment consists of IV penicillin. Diagnostic evaluation depends on maternal serology testing and infant symptoms (American Academy of Pediatrics, Committee on Infectious Diseases, 2015).
Toxoplasmosis *(Toxoplasma gondii)*		
May be asymptomatic at birth (70%-90% of cases) or have maculopapular rash, lymphadenopathy, hepatosplenomegaly, jaundice, thrombocytopenia Hydrocephaly, cerebral calcifications, chorioretinitis (classic triad) Microcephaly, seizures, cognitive impairment, deafness Encephalitis, myocarditis, hepatosplenomegaly, anemia, jaundice, diarrhea, vomiting, purpura	Throughout pregnancy Predominant host for organism is cats May be transmitted through cat feces or poorly cooked or raw infected meats	Caution pregnant women to avoid contact with cat feces (e.g., emptying cat litter boxes). Administer sulfadiazine (with folinic acid) and pyrimethamine (Daraprim). Spiramycin may be administered to infected pregnant female to reduce transmission to fetus but has no effect if fetal infection has occurred.

*This table is not an exhaustive representation of all perinatally transmitted infections. For further information regarding specific diseases or treatment not listed here, refer to American Academy of Pediatrics, Committee on Infectious Diseases, Kimberlin, D. W. (Ed.). (2015). *2015 Red Book: Report of the Committee on Infectious Diseases* (30th ed.). Elk Grove Village, IL: The Academy.

†Isolation Precautions depend on institutional policy. (See Infection Control.)

CNS, Central nervous system; *HBsAg,* hepatitis B surface antigen; *IV,* intravenous.

established, implement Standard Precautions according to institutional policy. In suspected cytomegalovirus and rubella infections, pregnant personnel are cautioned to avoid contact with the infant. Herpes simplex is easily transmitted from one infant to another; therefore risk of cross-contamination is reduced or eliminated by wearing gloves for patient contact. The American Academy of Pediatrics, Committee on Infectious Diseases' *2015 Red Book: Report of the Committee on Infectious Diseases* (2015) provides guidelines for the types and durations of precautions for most bacterial and viral exposures. Careful hand washing is the most important nursing intervention in reducing the spread of any infection.

Specimens need to be obtained for laboratory examinations, and the infant and parents need to be prepared for diagnostic procedures. When possible, long-term disabilities are prevented by early evaluation and implementation of therapy. Teach the family any special handling techniques needed for the care of their infant and signs of complications or possible sequelae. If sequelae are inevitable, the family will need assistance in determining how they can best cope with the problems, such as assistance with home care, referral to appropriate agencies, or placement in an institution for care. The major goal of nursing care is prevention of these disorders with provision of adequate prenatal care for the expectant mother and precautions regarding exposure to teratogenic infections.

NCLEX REVIEW QUESTIONS

1. Lung maturity may be enhanced by which of the following? Select all that apply.
   A. Antenatal (maternal) glucocorticoid administration
   B. Maternal chorioamnionitis
   C. Neonatal administration of exogenous surfactant
   D. Maternal diabetes mellitus
   E. Maternal tobacco smoking
2. A late-preterm infant (estimated 35 weeks of gestation) is admitted to the neonatal intensive care nursery at 2 hours of age with the following: respiratory rate 68; heart rate 132; bilateral nasal flaring; audible grunting on expiration; intercostal retractions; systolic blood pressure 35; hypotonia; and acrocyanosis and pulse oximetry reading of 89% on 30% inspired oxygen. The radiograph shows a diffuse ground glass appearance. The nurse recognizes these as signs of:
   A. Hypoglycemia
   B. Respiratory distress syndrome
   C. Meconium aspiration
   D. Apnea of prematurity

The following information relates to questions 3 and 4.

An infant born at 27 weeks of gestation is now 3 weeks old and on supplemental oxygen by nasal cannula. Feedings are being administered by gavage: 12 ml of expressed breast milk and human milk fortifier every 2 hours. On assessment the nurse notes that the infant's abdomen appears slightly distended, the infant's activity is decreased from previous assessment, and there is a prefeeding gastric residual of 6 ml. The infant's core temperature is 35.8°C (it was 36.4°C 2 hours before).

3. Based on these findings, what are the nurse's priority interventions? Select all that apply.
   A. Obtain a full set of vital signs, including BP and pulse oximetry
   B. Withhold the next feeding (now due)
   C. Discuss findings with the primary practitioner
   D. Observe the infant closely and administer the current feeding
   E. Measure the infant's abdominal girth
4. The nurse recognizes that these symptoms are most likely associated with:
   A. Transient feeding intolerance
   B. Respiratory distress syndrome
   C. Necrotizing enterocolitis
   D. Bronchopulmonary dysplasia
5. In addition to hypoglycemia, the infant of a diabetic mother should be observed for:
   A. Hydrocephalus
   B. Hyperglycemia
   C. Respiratory distress
   D. Sepsis

Correct Answers

1. A, C; 2. B; 3. A, B, C, E; 4. C; 5. C

REFERENCES

Abraham, M., Alramadhan, S., Iniguez, C., et al. (2017). A systematic review of maternal smoking during pregnancy and fetal measurements with meta-analysis. *PLoS ONE*, 1–13.

Abrams, S. A., Schanler, R. J., Lee, M. L., et al. (2014). Greater mortality and morbidity in extremely preterm infants fed a diet containing cow milk protein products. *Breastfeed Medicine*, *9*, 281–285.

Aceti, A., Gori, D., Barone, G., et al. (2015). Probiotics for prevention of necrotizing enterocolitis in preterm infants: systematic review and meta-analysis. *Italian Journal of Pediatrics*, *41*, 1–20.

Adamkin, D. H., & American Academy of Pediatrics, Committee on Fetus and Newborn. (2011). Clinical report—postnatal glucose homeostasis in late-preterm and term infants. *Pediatrics*, *127*(3), 575–579.

Alfaleh, K., Anabrees, J., Bassler, D., et al. (2014). Probiotics for prevention of necrotizing enterocolitis in preterm infants. *Cochrane Database of Systematic Review*, (4), CD005496.

Als, H. (1982). Toward a synactive theory of development: promise for the assessment and support of infant individuality. *Infant Mental Health Journal*, *3*(4), 229–243.

Als, H. (2009). Newborn Individualized Developmental Care and Assessment Program (NIDCAP): new frontier for neonatal and perinatal medicine. *The Journal of Neonatal-Perinatal Medicine*, *2*(3), 135–147.

Altimier, L., & Phillips, R. M. (2013). The neonatal integrative developmental care model: seven neuroprotective core measures for family-centered developmental care. *Newborn and Infant Nursing Reviews*, *13*(1), 9–22.

Alvarez, M. J., Fernandez, D., Gomez-Salgado, J., et al. (2017). The effects of massage therapy in hospitalized preterm neonates: A systematic review. *International Journal of Nursing Studies*, *69*, 119–136.

Alvaro, R. E. (2012). Neonatal Apnea. In D. Fraser (Ed.), *Acute respiratory care of the neonate* (3rd ed., pp. 51–64). Santa Rosa, CA: NICU Ink Books.

American Academy of Pediatrics. (2016). SIDS and Other Sleep-Related Infant Deaths: Updated 2016 Recommendations for a Safe Infant Sleeping Environment: Task Force on Sudden Infant Death Syndrome (SIDS). *Journal of Pediatrics*, *138*(5), 1–12.

American Academy of Pediatrics. (2009). Safe transportation of preterm and low birth weight infants at hospital discharge. *Pediatrics*, *123*(5), 1424–1429.

American Academy of Pediatrics. (2012). Breastfeeding and the use of human milk. *Pediatrics*, *129*(3), e827–e884.

American Academy of Pediatrics, American Association for Pediatric Ophthalmology and Strabismus, American Academy of Ophthalmology. (2013). Screening examination of premature infants for retinopathy of prematurity. *Pediatrics*, *131*(1), 189–195.

American Academy of Pediatrics, American College of Obstetricians and Gynecologists (2012). *Guidelines for perinatal care* (ed. 7). Elk Grove Village, Ill: The Academy and The College.

American Academy of Pediatrics, American Heart Association (2011). *Neonatal resuscitation textbook* (ed. 6). Elk Grove Village, IL: The Academy and The Association.

American Academy of Pediatrics, Committee on Fetus and Newborn. (2012). Levels of neonatal care. *Pediatrics*, *130*(3), 587–597.

American Academy of Pediatrics, Committee on Infectious Diseases, & Kimberlin, D. W. (Eds.), (2015). *2015 Red book: report of the Committee on Infectious Diseases* (30th ed.). Elk Grove Village, IL: The Academy.

American Academy of Pediatrics, Task Force on Sudden Infant Death Syndrome. (2011). SIDS and other sleep-related infant deaths: expansion of recommendations for a safe infant sleeping environment. *Pediatrics*, *128*(5), e1341–e1367.

Association of Women's Health, Obstetric and Neonatal Nurses (2010). *Assessment and care of the late preterm infant.* Washington, DC: The Association.

Association of Women's Health, Obstetric and Neonatal Nurses (AWHONN) (2013). *Evidence-based clinical practice guideline: neonatal skin care* (3rd ed.). Washington, DC: The Association.

Athalye-Jape, G., Rao, S., & Patole, S. (2016). Lactobacillus reuteri DSM 17938 as a probiotic for preterm neonates: A strain-specific systematic review. *The Journal of Parenteral and Enteral Nutrition, 40*, 783–794.

Atkinson, J., & Braddick, O. (2012). Visual and visuocognitive development of children born very prematurely. In V. R. Preedy (Ed.), *Handbook of growth and growth monitoring in health and disease* (Vol. 1). New York: Springer.

Bahadue, F. L., & Soll, R. (2012). Early versus delayed selective surfactant treatment for neonatal respiratory distress syndrome. *Cochrane Database of Systematic Reviews*, (11), CD001456.

Ballabh, P. (2014). Pathogenesis and prevention of intraventricular hemorrhage. *Clinics in Perinatology, 41*(1), 47–67.

Barrington, K. J., Finer, N., Pennaforte, T., et al. (2017). Nitric oxide for respiratory failure in infants born at or near term. *Cochrane Database of Systematic Reviews*, (1), CD000399.

Barrington, K. J., Finer, N., & Pennaforte, T. (2017). Inhaled nitric oxide for respiratory failure in preterm infants. *Cochrane Database of Systematic Reviews*, (1), CD000509.

Bingham, E. M. (2012). Optimizing nutrition in the neonatal intensive care unit: a look at enteral nutrition and the prevention of necrotizing enterocolitis. *Topics in Clinical Nutrition, 27*(3), 250–259.

Blackburn, S. T. (2012). *Maternal, fetal, and neonatal physiology: a clinical perspective* (4th ed.). St. Louis: Elsevier.

Boies, E. G., Vaucher, Y. E., & the Academy of Breastfeeding Medicine. (2016). ABM Clinical Protocol #10: Breastfeeding the Late Preterm (34–36 6/7 Weeks of Gestation) and Early Term Infants (37–38 6/7 Weeks of Gestation), Second Revision 2016. *Breastfeeding Medicine, 11*(10), 494–500.

Botet, F., Figueras-Aloy, J., Miracle-Echegoyen, X., et al. (2012). Trends in survival among extremely-low-birth-weight infants (less than 1000 g) without significant bronchopulmonary dysplasia. *BMC Pediatrics, 63*, 63–74.

Bozzetti, V., Paterlini, G., De Lorenzo, P., et al. (2016). Impact of continuous vs bolus feeding on splanchnic perfusion in very low birth weight infants: a randomized trial. *Journal of Pediatrics, 176*, 86–92.

Bradshaw, W. T., & Tanaka, D. T. (2016). Physiologic monitoring. In S. L. Gardner, B. S. Carter, M. Enzman-Hines, et al. (Eds.), *Merenstein & Gardner's handbook of neonatal intensive care* (8th ed.). St. Louis: Mosby.

Brown, L. D., Hendrickson, K., Evans, R., et al. (2016). Enteral nutrition. In S. L. Gardner, B. S. Carter, M. Enzman-Hines, et al. (Eds.), *Merenstein & Gardner's handbook of neonatal intensive care* (8th ed.). St. Louis: Mosby.

Bucher, B. T., Pacetti, A. S., Lovvorn, H. N., et al. (2016). Neonatal surgery. In S. L. Gardner, B. S. Carter, M. Enzman-Hines, et al. (Eds.), *Merenstein & Gardner's handbook of neonatal intensive care* (8th ed.). St. Louis: Mosby.

Buenoa, C., & Menna-Barretob, L. (2016). Development of sleep/wake, activity and temperature rhythms in newborns maintained in a neonatal intensive care unit and the impact of feeding schedules. *Infant Behavior & Development, 44*, 21–28.

Bull, M. J., Engle, W. A., & American Academy of Pediatrics. (2009). Safe transportation of preterm and low birth weight infants at hospital discharge. *Pediatrics, 123*(5), 1424–1429.

Bulut, C., Gursoy, T., & Ovali, F. (2016). Short-term outcomes and mortality of late preterm infants. *Balkan Medical Journal, 33*(2), 198–203.

Byrne, E., & Garber, J. (2013). Physical therapy intervention in the neonatal intensive care unit. *Physical and Occupational Therapy in Pediatrics, 33*(1), 75–110.

Cacho, N. T., Parker, L. A., & Neu, J. (2016). Necrotizing enterocolitis and human milk feeding: a systematic review. *Clinics in Perinatology, 3*(1), 49–67.

Cain, M. A., Bornick, P., & Whiteman, V. (2013). The maternal, fetal, and neonatal effects of cocaine exposure in pregnancy. *Clinical Obstetrics and Gynecology, 56*(1), 124–132.

Camacho-Gonzalez, A., Spearman, P. W., & Stoll, B. J. (2013). Neonatal infectious diseases: evaluation of neonatal sepsis. *Pediatric Clinics of North America, 60*(2), 367–389.

Campino, A., Santesteban, E., Pascual, P., et al. (2016). Strategies implementation to reduce medicine preparation error rate in neonatal intensive care units. *European Journal of Pediatrics, 175*, 755–765.

Caplan, M. S. (2015). Neonatal necrotizing enterocolitis: clinical observations, pathophysiology and prevention. In R. J. Martin, A. A. Fanaroff, & M. C. Walsh (Eds.), *Fanaroff and Martin's neonatal-perinatal medicine: diseases of the fetus and newborn*. St. Louis: Elsevier Mosby.

Carlo, W. A. (2016). Apnea. In R. M. Kliegman, B. F. Stanton, J. W. St. Geme, et al. (Eds.), *Nelson textbook of pediatrics*. Philadelphia: Saunders.

Carlo, W. A., & Ambalavanan, N. (2016a). Intracranial-intraventricular hemorrhage and periventricular leukomalacia. In R. M. Kliegman, B. F. Stanton, J. W. St. Geme, et al. (Eds.), *Nelson textbook of pediatrics*. Philadelphia: Saunders.

Carlo, W. A., & Ambalavanan, N. (2016b). Metabolic disturbances. In R. M. Kliegman, B. F. Stanton, J. W. St. Geme, et al. (Eds.), *Nelson textbook of pediatrics*. Philadelphia: Saunders.

Carlo, W. A., & Ambalavanan, N. (2016c). Respiratory distress syndrome. In R. M. Kliegman, B. F. Stanton, J. W. St. Geme, et al. (Eds.), *Nelson textbook of pediatrics*. Philadelphia: Saunders.

Carlo, W. A. (2016). Infants of Diabetic Mothers. In R. M. Kliegman, B. F. Stanton, J. W. St. Geme, et al. (Eds.), *Nelson textbook of pediatrics*. Philadelphia: Saunders.

Carter, A., Gratny, L., & Carter, B. S. (2016). Discharge planning and follow-up of the neonatal intensive care unit infant. In S. L. Gardner, B. S. Carter, M. Enzman-Hines, et al. (Eds.), *Merenstein & Gardner's handbook of neonatal intensive care* (8th ed.). St. Louis: Mosby.

Cauchemez, S., Besnard, M., Bompard, P., et al. (2016). Association between Zika virus and microcephaly in French Polynesia, 2013–15: a retrospective study. *The Lancet, 10033*, 2125–2132.

Centers for Disease Control and Prevention: *Guidelines for identifying and referring persons with fetal alcohol syndrome*. https://www.cdc.gov/ncbddd/fasd/. (Updated 14 October 2016).

Centers for Disease Control and Prevention: *Group B Strep (GBS): Clinical Overview*. 2010. Retrieved from: https://www.cdc.gov/groupbstrep/. (Updated 27 October 2016).

Centers for Disease Control and Prevention. (2013). Tobacco product use among middle and high school students—United States, 2011 and 2012. *MMWR Weekly Report, 62*(45), 893–897.

Chang, H., Chen, J., Chang, J., et al. (2017). Multiple strains probiotics appear to be the most effective probiotics in the prevention of necrotizing enterocolitis and mortality: An updated meta-analysis. *PLoS ONE, 12*(2), 1–14.

Chaseling, G. K., Molgat-Seon, Y., Daboval, T., et al. (2016). Body temperature mapping in critically ill newborn infants nursed under radiant warmers during intensive care. *Journal of Perinatology, 36*, 540–543.

Chen, L.-N., He, X.-P., & Huang, L.-P. (2012). A survey of high risk factors affecting retinopathy in full-term infants in China. *International Journal of Ophthalmology, 5*(2), 117–180.

Cheong, J. L., Doyle, L. W., Burnett, A. C., et al. (2017). Association between moderate and late preterm birth and neurodevelopment and social-emotional development at age 2 years. *JAMA Pediatrics*, 1–7.

Chibueze, E. C., Tirado, V., Lopes, K., et al. (2017). Zika virus infection in pregnancy: A systematic review of disease course and complications. *Reproductive Health, 14*(28), 1–14.

Church, P. T., Luther, M., & Asztalos, E. (2012). The perfect storm: the high prevalence low severity outcomes of the preterm survivors. *Current Pediatric Reviews, 8*(2), 142–151.

Civardi, E., Garofoli, F., Mazzucchelli, I., et al. (2014). Enteral nutrition and infections: the role of human milk. *Early Human Development, 3*(90), 1–3.

Clark, R. H. (2017). High-frequency oscillatory ventilation. In S. M. Donn & S. K. Sinha (Eds.), *Manual of neonatal respiratory care* (4th ed.). New York: Springer.

Colaizy, T., Bell, E., Carlo, W., et al.: *Neurodevelopmental effects of donor human milk vs preterm formula in ELBW infants: the MILK trial*, 2012, National Institute of Child Health and Human Development. Retrieved from: http://www.nichd.nih.gov/about/Documents/Milk_Protocol.pdf.

Cole, L., Dewey, D., Letourneau, N., et al. (2017). Clinical characteristics, risk factors, and outcomes associated with neonatal hemorrhagic stroke: a population-based case-control study. *JAMA Pediatrics, 1*, 1–9.

Conner, S. N., Carter, E. B., Tuuli, M. G., et al. (2015). Maternal marijuana use and neonatal morbidity. *American Journal of Obstetrics and Gynecology, 213*(3), 422–425.

Cortese, F., Scicchitano, P., Gesualdo, M., et al. (2015). Early and late infections in newborns: where do we stand? A Review. *Pediatrics and Neonatology, 57*, 265–273.

Cotten, M., Murtha, A., Goldberg, R., et al. (2014). Feasibility of autologous cord blood cells for infants with hypoxic-ischemic encelphalopathy. *Journal of Pediatrics, 164*, 973–979.

Daniels, B., Ireland, C., Kraus, S., et al. (2016). Magnetic resonance–guided nasogastric feeding tube placement for neonates: a preclinical study. *Journal of Parenteral and Enteral Nutrition*, 1–7.

D'Apolito, K. (2013). Breastfeeding and substance abuse. *Clinics in Obstetrics and Gynaecology, 56*(1), 202–211.

Darlow, B. A., Lui, K., Kusuda, S., et al. on behalf of the International Network for Evaluating Outcomes of Neonates. (2017). International variations and trends in the treatment for retinopathy of prematurity. *British Journal of Ophthalmology, 0*, 1–6.

Davis, A. S., Roberds, E. L., Hannaford, M., et al. (2012). Early childhood cognitive disorders: perinatal complications. In A. S. Davis (Ed.), *Psychopathology of childhood and adolescence: a neurophysical approach*. New York: Springer.

Davis, N. L. (2015). Car seat screening for low birth weight term neonates. *Pediatrics, 136*(1), 89–96.

Davis, N. L., Condon, F., & Rhein, L. M. (2013). Epidemiology and predictors of failure of the infant car seat challenge. *Pediatrics, 131*(5), 951–957.

Davis, N. L., Zenchenko, Y., Lever, A., et al. (2013). Car seat safety for preterm neonates: implementation and testing parameters of the infant car seat challenge. *Academic Pediatrics, 13*(3), 272–277.

De Carolis, M. P., Pinna, G., Cocca, C., et al. (2016). The transition from intra to extra-uterine life in late preterm infant: a single-center study. *Italian Journal of Pediatrics, 42*(1), 1–7.

Della Grotta, S. H., LaGasse, L. L., Arria, A. M., et al. (2010). Patterns of methamphetamine use during pregnancy from the Infant Development, Environment, and Lifestyle (IDEAL) study. *Maternal and Child Health Journal, 14*(4), 519–527.

Dermyshi, E., Wang, Y., Yan, C., et al. (2017). The "golden age" of probiotics: a systematic review and meta-analysis of randomized and observational studies in preterm infants. *Neonatology, 112*(1), 9–23.

Dying in America: improving quality and honoring individual preferences near the end of life. Institute of Medicine of the National Academies Report, September 17, 2014.

Ellett, M. L., Cohen, M. D., Perkins, S. M., et al. (2012). Comparing methods of determining insertion length for placing gastric tubes in children 1 month to 17 years of age. *Journal for Specialists in Pediatric Nursing, 17*(1), 19–32.

Engwall, M., Fridh, I., Bergbom, I., et al. (2014). Let there be light and darkness: findings from a prestudy concerning cycled light in the intensive care unit environment. *Critical Care Nursing Quarterly, 37*(3), 273–298.

Eze, N., Smith, L. M., LaGasse, L. L., et al. (2016). School-aged outcomes following prenatal methamphetamine exposure: 7.5-year follow-up from the infant development, environment, and lifestyle study. *The Journal of Pediatrics, 170*, 34–38.

Fabiyi, C., Peacock, N., Hebert-Beirne, J., et al. (2016). A qualitative study to understand nativity differences in breastfeeding behaviors among middle-class African American and African-Born women. *Maternal and Child Health Journal, 20*(10), 2100–2111.

Finnegan, L. P. (1985). Neonatal abstinence. In N. Nelson (Ed.), *Current therapy in neonatal perinatal medicine* (pp. 1985–1986). Toronto: BC Decker.

Fleck, B. W., & Stenson, B. J. (2013). Retinopathy of prematurity and the oxygen conundrum: Lessons learned from recent randomized trials. *Clinics in Perinatology, 40*(2), 229–240.

Foster, J. P., Psaila, K., & Patterson, T. (2016). Non-nutritive sucking for increasing physiologic stability and nutrition in preterm infants. *Cochrane Database Syst Review*, (10), CD001071.

Fraser, D. (2012). Complications of positive pressure ventilation. In D. Fraser (Ed.), *Acute respiratory care of the neonate* (3rd ed.). Santa Rosa, CA: NICU Ink Books.

Freeman, D., Saxton, V., & Holberton, J. (2012). A weight-based formula for the estimation of gastric tube insertion length in newborns. *Advances in Neonatal Care, 12*(3), 179–182.

Gaalema, D. E., Scott, T. L., Heil, S. H., et al. (2012). Differences in the profile of neonatal abstinence syndrome signs in methadone-versus buprenorphine-exposed neonates. *Addiction (Abingdon, England), 107*(S1), 53–62.

Garber, J. (2013). Oral-motor function and feeding intervention. *Physical and Occupational Therapy in Pediatrics, 33*(1), 111–138.

Gardner, S. L., Enzman-Hines, M., & Nyp, M. (2016). Respiratory diseases. In S. L. Gardner, B. S. Carter, M. Enzman-Hines, et al. (Eds.), *Merenstein & Gardner's handbook of neonatal intensive care* (8th ed.). St. Louis: Mosby.

Gardner, S. L., Goldson, E., & Hernandez, J. A. (2016). The neonate and the environment: impact on development. In S. L. Gardner, B. S. Carter, M. Enzman-Hines, et al. (Eds.), *Merenstein & Gardner's handbook of neonatal intensive care* (8th ed.). St. Louis: Mosby.

Gardner, S. L., & Hernandez, J. A. (2016). Heat balance. In S. L. Gardner, B. S. Carter, M. Enzman-Hines, et al. (Eds.), *Merenstein & Gardner's handbook of neonatal intensive care* (ed. 8). St. Louis: Mosby.

Gardner, S. L., & Lawrence, R. A. (2016). Breast-feeding the neonate with special needs. In S. L. Gardner, B. S. Carter, M. Enzman-Hines, et al. (Eds.), *Merenstein & Gardner's handbook of neonatal intensive care* (ed. 8). St. Louis: Mosby.

Gephart, S. M., & Hanson, C. K. (2013). Preventing necrotizing enterocolitis with standard feeding protocols: not only possible, but imperative. *Advances in Neonatal Care, 13*(1), 48–54.

Gilfillan, M., & Bhandari, V. (2017). Biomarkers for the diagnosis of neonatal sepsis and necrotizing enterocolitis: Clinical practice guidelines. *Early Human Development, 105*, 25–33.

Gill, J. V., & Boyle, E. M. (2017). Outcomes of infants born near term. *Archives of Disease in Childhood, 102*, 194–198.

Glass, H. C. (2014). Neonatal seizures: advances in mechanisms and management. *Clinics in Perinatology, 41*(1), 177–190.

Guimaraes, H., Guedes, M., Rocha, G., et al. (2012). Vitamin A in prevention of bronchopulmonary dysplasia. *Current Pharmaceutical Design, 18*(21), 3101–3113.

Gunn, J. K., Rosales, C. B., Center, K. E., et al. (2016). Prenatal exposure to cannabis and maternal and child health outcomes: a systematic review and meta-analysis. *BMJ (Clinical Research Ed.), 6*(4), 1–8.

Guyer, C., Huber, R., Fontijn, J., et al. (2015). Very preterm infants show earlier emergence of 24-hour sleep–wake rhythms compared to term infants. *Early Human Development, 91*, 37–42.

Guyer, C., Huber, R., Fontijn, J., et al. (2012). Cycled light exposure reduces fussing and crying in very preterm infants. *Pediatrics, 130*(1), E145–E151.

Hall, C. B., Weinberg, G. A., Blumkin, A. K., et al. (2013). Respiratory syncytial virus-associated hospitalizations among children less than 24 months of age. *Pediatrics, 132*(2), e341–e348.

Hallman, M., & Saarela, T. (2012). Respiratory distress syndrome: predisposing factors, pathophysiology, and diagnosis. In G. Buonocore, R. Bracci, & M. Weindling (Eds.), *Neonatology: a practical approach to neonatal diseases*. New York: Springer.

Hartley, K. A., Miller, C. S., & Gephart, S. M. (2015). Facilitated tucking to reduce pain in neonates: evidence for best practice. *Advances in Neonatal Care, 15*(3), 201–208.

Hassanein, S., Raggal, N., & Shalaby, A. (2013). Neonatal nursery noise: practice-based learning and improvement. *The Journal of Maternal-fetal and Neonatal Medicine, 26*(4), 392–395.

Hay, W. W. (2012). Care of the infant of the diabetic mother. *Current Diabetes Reports, 12*(1), 4–15.

Herrington, C. J., & Chiodo, L. M. (2013). Human touch effectively and safely reduces pain in the newborn intensive care unit. *Pain Management Nursing*. Retrieved from: http://www.painmanagementnursing.org/article/S1524-9042%2812%2900086-0/abstract.

Hill, P. (2012). Perinatal addiction: providing compassionate and competent care. *Clinics in Obstetrics and Gynaecology*, *56*(1), 178–185.

Himes, S. K., Stroud, L. R., Scheidweiler, K. B., et al. (2013). Prenatal tobacco exposure, biomarkers for tobacco in meconium, and neonatal growth outcomes. *The Journal of Pediatrics*, *162*(5), 970–975.

Höllwarth, M. E. (2017). Surgical strategies in short bowel syndrome. *Pediatric Surgery International*, *33*(4), 413–419.

Horbar, J. D., Carpenter, J. H., Badger, G. J., et al. (2012). Mortality and neonatal morbidity among infants 501 to 1500 grams from 2000 to 2009. *Pediatrics*, *129*(6), 1019–1026.

Hudak, M. L., Tan, R. C., & The Committee On Drugs, The Committee On Fetus And Newborn. (2012). Neonatal drug withdrawal: clinical report. *Journal of Pediatrics*, *129*(2), 1–25.

Human Milk Banking Association: *2008 Guidelines for the establishment and operation of a donor human milk bank*, 2013. Retrieved from: http://www.hmbana.org.

Hunter, J. (2010). The neonatal intensive care unit. In J. Case-Smith (Ed.), *Occupational therapy for children* (ed. 6). St. Louis: Mosby.

International Committee for the Classification of Retinopathy of Prematurity. (2005). The International Classification of Retinopathy of Prematurity revisited. *Archives of Ophthalmology*, *123*(7), 991–999.

Jacobs, S. E., Berg, M., Hunt, R., et al. (2013). Cooling for newborns with hypoxic ischaemic encephalopathy. *Cochrane Database of Systematic Review*, (1), CD003311.

Javid, P. J., Sanchez, S. E., Horslen, S. P., et al. (2013). Intestinal lengthening and nutritional outcomes in children with short bowel syndrome. *American Journal of Surgery*, *205*(5), 576–580.

Johnston, C., Campbell-Yeo, M., Disher, T., et al. (2017). Skin-to-skin care for procedural pain in neonates. *Cochrane Database of Systematic Review*, (2), CD008435.

Jonas-Simpson, C., Pilkington, F. B., MacDonald, C., et al. (2013). Nurses' experiences of grieving when there is a perinatal death. *SAGE Open*, *3*(2). Retrieved from: http://sgo.sagepub.com/content/3/2/2158244013486116.short.

Jones, L. R. (2012). Oral feeding readiness in the neonatal intensive care unit. *Neonatal Network*, *31*(3), 148–155.

Jones, W. (2015). Cocaine use and the breastfeeding mother. *The Practising Midwife*, *18*(1), 19–22.

Jordan, B. K., & Donn, S. M. (2013). Lucinactant for the prevention of respiratory distress syndrome in premature infants. *Expert Review of Clinical Pharmacology*, *6*(2), 115–121.

Kastenberg, Z. J., & Sylvester, K. G. (2013). The surgical management of necrotizing enterocolitis. *Clinics in Perinatology*, *40*(1), 135–148.

Keszler, M., & Abubakar, K. (2017). Physiologic principles. In J. P. Goldsmith & E. H. Karotkin (Eds.), *Assisted ventilation of the neonate* (6th ed.). Philadelphia: Elsevier.

Kim, E., & Koren, G. (2012). Infants of drug-addicted mothers. In G. Buonocore, R. Bracci, & M. Weindling (Eds.), *Neonatology: a practical approach to neonatal diseases*. New York: Springer.

Kleinman, R. E., & Greer, F. R. (Eds.), (2014). *Pediatric nutrition* (7th ed.). Elk Grove Village, IL: The Academy.

Kommers, D. R., Joshi, R., van Pul, C., et al. (2017). Features of heart rate variability capture regulatory changes during kangaroo care in preterm infants. *Journal of Pediatrics*, *182*, 92–98.

Koopmans, L., Wilson, T., Cacciatore, J., et al. (2013). Support for mothers, fathers and families after perinatal death. *Cochrane Database of Systematic Review*, (6), CD000452.

Kraft, W. K., Stover, M. W., & Davis, J. M. (2016). Neonatal abstinence syndrome: Pharmacologic strategies for the mother and infant. *Seminars in Perinatology*, *40*, 203–212.

Kuhn, P., Zores, C., Langlet, C., et al. (2013). Moderate acoustic changes can disrupt the sleep of very preterm infants in their incubators. *Acta Paediatrics*, *102*(10), 949–954.

Kumar, P., & Committee on Fetus and Newborn. (2014). Use of inhaled nitric oxide in premature infants. *Pediatrics*, *133*(1), 164–170.

LaGasse, L. L., Derauf, C., Smith, L. M., et al. (2012). Prenatal methamphetamine exposure and childhood behavior problems at 3 and 5 years of age. *Pediatrics*, *129*, 681–688.

Lai, M. M., D'Acunto, G., Guzzetta, A., et al. (2016). PREMM: preterm early massage by the mother: protocol of a randomised controlled trial of massage therapy in very preterm infants. *BMC Pediatrics*, *16*, 1–12.

Lakshminrusimha, S., Konduri, G. G., & Steinhorn, R. H. (2016). Considerations in the management of hypoxemic respiratory failure and persistent pulmonary hypertension in term and late preterm neonates. *Journal of Perinatology*, *36*, 12–19.

Lambert, B. L., & Bauer, C. R. (2012). Development and behavioral consequences of prenatal cocaine exposure: a review. *Journal of Perinatology*, *32*, 819–828.

Lau, C. (2012). Development of oral feeding skills in the preterm infant. In V. R. Preedy (Ed.), *Handbook of growth and growth monitoring in health and disease* (Vol. 1). New York: Springer.

Lau, C. S., & Chamberlain, R. S. (2015). Probiotic administration can prevent necrotizing enterocolitis in preterm infants: A meta-analysis. *Journal of Pediatric Surgery*, *50*, 1405–1412.

Lavoie, P. M., Stritzke, A., Ting, J., et al. (2015). A randomized controlled trial of the use of oral glucose with or without gentle facilitated tucking of infants during neonatal echocardiography. *PLoS ONE*, 1–11.

Lechner, B. E., & Vohr, B. R. (2017). Neurodevelopmental outcomes of preterm infants fed human milk: a systematic review. *Clinics in Perinatology*, *3*(1), 69–83.

Le Doare, K., & Heath, P. T. (2013). An overview of global GBS epidemiology. *Vaccine*, *31*, 7–12.

Lemmon, M. E., Bidegain, M., & Boss, R. D. (2016). Palliative care in neonatal neurology: robust support for infants, families and clinicians. *Journal of Perinatology*, *36*, 331–337.

Lester, B. M., Tronick, E. Z., & Brazelton, T. B. (2004). The Neonatal Intensive Care Unit Network Neurobehavioral Scale Procedures. *Pediatrics*, *113*(3), 641–667.

Lewis, E. D., Richard, C., Larsen, B. M., et al. (2016). The importance of human milk for immunity in preterm infants. *Clinics in Perinatology*, *3*(1), 23–47.

Litt, J. S., Glymour, M., Hauser-Cram, P., et al. (2015). The effect of the Infant Health and Development Program on special education use at school age. *Journal of Pediatrics*, *166*(2), 457–462.

Litt, J. S., & McCormick, M. C. (2016). The impact of special health care needs on academic achievement in children born prematurely. *Academic Pediatrics*, *16*(4), 350–357.

Lodha, A., Ediger, K., Rabil, Y., et al. (2015). Does chronic oxygen dependency in preterm infants with bronchopulmonary dysplasia at NICU discharge predict respiratory outcomes at 3 years of age? *Journal of Perinatology*, *35*, 530–536.

Love, L. E., & Bradshaw, W. T. (2012). Efficacy of inhaled nitric oxide in preterm neonates. *Advances in Neonatal Care*, *12*(1), 15–20.

Lubbe, W. W. (2017). Clinicians guide for cue-based transition to oral feeding in preterm infants: An easy-to-use clinical guide. *Journal of Evaluation in Clinical Practice*, 1–9.

Lund, C. H., & Osborne, C. W. (2004). Validity and reliability of the neonatal skin condition score. *Journal of Obstetric, Gynecologic, and Neonatal Nursing*, *33*(3), 320–327.

Macho, P. (2017). Individualized developmental care in the NICU: a concept analysis. *Advances in Neonatal Care*, 1–13.

Maheshwari, A., & Carlo, W. A. (2016). Plethora in the newborn infant (polycythemia). In R. M. Kliegman, B. F. Stanton, J. W. St. Geme, et al. (Eds.), *Nelson textbook of pediatrics*. Philadelphia: Saunders.

Malcolm, W. (2015). *Beyond the NICU: comprehensive care of the high-risk infant*. New York: McGraw Hill.

Mancini, A., Kelly, P., & Bluebond-Langner, M. (2013). Training neonatal staff for the future in neonatal palliative care. *Seminars in Fetal and Neonatal Medicine*, *18*(2), 111–115.

Marc-Aurele, K. L., & English, N. K. (2016). Primary palliative care in neonatal intensive care. *Seminars in Perinatology*, 1–7.

Martin, C. R., Ling, P., & Blackburn, G. L. (2016). Review of infant feedings: key features of breast milk and infant formula. *Nutrients*, *8*(279), 1–11.

May, P. A., Baete, A., Russo, J., et al. (2014). Prevalence and characteristics of fetal alcohol spectrum disorders. *Pediatrics*, *134*, 855–866.

McCabe, J. E., & Arndt, S. (2012). Demographic and substance abuse trends among pregnant and non-pregnant women: eleven years of treatment admission data. *Maternal and Child Health Journal, 16*(8), 1696–1702.

McCarty, D., Peat, J., & Malcolm, W. (2016). Dolichocephaly in preterm infants: prevalence, risk factors, and early motor outcomes. *American Journal of Perinatology*, 1–7.

McGinnis, K., Murray, E., Cherven, B., et al. (2016). Effect of vibration on pain response to heel lance: a pilot randomized control trial. *Advances in Neonatal Care, 16*(6), 439–448.

Meier, P. P., Johnson, T. J., Patel, A. L., et al. (2017). Evidence-based methods that promote human milk feeding of preterm infants: an expert review. *Clinics in Perinatology, 44*(1), 1–22.

Messina, N., & Jeter, K. (2012). Parental methamphetamine use and manufacture: child and familial outcomes. *Journal of Public Child Welfare, 6*(3), 296–312.

Michelson, K., Blehart, K., Hochberg, T., et al. (2013). Bereavement photography for children: program development and health care professionals' response. *Death Studies, 37*(6), 513–528.

Mikati, M. A., & Hani, A. J. (2016). Neonatal seizures. In R. M. Kliegman, B. F. Stanton, J. W. St. Geme, et al. (Eds.), *Nelson textbook of pediatrics* (20th ed.). Philadelphia: ELSEVIER.

Minnes, S., Singer, L., Min, M. O., et al. (2014). Effects of prenatal cocaine/polydrug exposure on substance use by ate 15. *Drugs Alcohol Dependence, 134*, 201–210.

Moon, K., Rao, S. C., Schulzke, S. M., et al. (2016). Longchain polyunsaturated fatty acid supplementation in preterm infants. *Cochrane Database of Systematic Review*, (12), CD000375.

Morag, I., & Ohlsson, A. (2016). Cycled light in the intensive care unit for preterm and low birth weight infants. *Cochrane Database of Systematic Reviews*, (8), CD006982.

Napierala, M., Mazela, J., Merritt, T. A., et al. (2016). Tobacco smoking and breastfeeding: Effect on the lactation process, breast milk composition and infant development. A critical review. *Environmental Research, 151*, 321–338.

Natarajan, G., & Shankaran, S. (2016). Short- and long-term outcomes of moderate and late preterm infants. *American Journal of Perinatology, 33*, 305–317.

Neu, J., & Sullivan, S. (2012). Baby and breast: a dynamic interaction. *Pediatric Research, 71*, 135.

Newland, L., L'huillier, M. W., & Petrey, B. (2013). Implementation of cue-based feeding in a level III NICU. *Neonatal Network, 32*(2), 132–137.

Nyp, M., Brunkhorst, J. L., Reavey, D., et al. (2016). Fluid and electrolyte management. In S. L. Gardner, B. S. Carter, M. Enzman-Hines, et al. (Eds.), *Merenstein & Gardner's handbook of neonatal intensive care* (8th ed.). St. Louis: Elsevier.

O'Hare, E. M., Wood, A., & Fiske, E. (2013). Human milk banking. *Neonatal Network, 32*(3), 175–183.

Ohlsson, A., & Jacobs, S. E. (2013). NIDCAP: a systematic review and meta-analyses of randomized controlled trials. *Pediatrics, 131*(3), 881–893.

Olitsky, S., Hug, D., Plummer, L. S., et al. (2016). Disorders of the retina and vitreous. In R. M. Kliegman, B. F. Stanton, J. W. St. Geme, et al. (Eds.), *Nelson textbook of pediatrics* (20th ed.). Philadelphia: Elsevier.

Onland, W., De Jaegere, A. P. M. C., Offringa, M., et al. (2017). Systemic corticosteroid regimens for prevention of bronchopulmonary dysplasia in preterm infants. *Cochrane Database of Systematic Reviews*, (1), CD010941.

Owen, L. A., Morrison, M. A., Hoffman, R. O., et al. (2017). Retinopathy of prematurity: A comprehensive risk analysis for prevention and prediction of disease. *PLoS ONE, 12*(2), 1–14.

Paintner, A., Williams, A. D., & Burd, L. (2012a). Fetal alcohol spectrum disorders—implications for child neurology, part 1: prenatal exposure and dosimetry. *Journal of Child Neurology, 27*(2), 258–263.

Paintner, A., Williams, A. D., & Burd, L. (2012b). Fetal alcohol spectrum disorders—implications for child neurology, part 2: diagnosis and management. *Journal of Child Neurology, 27*(3), 355–362.

Pammi, M., Brand, M. C., & Weisman, L. E. (2016). Infection in the neonate. In S. L. Gardner, B. S. Carter, M. Enzman-Hines, et al. (Eds.), *Merenstein & Gardner's handbook of neonatal intensive care* (8th ed.). St. Louis: Mosby.

Panel on Treatment of HIV-Infected Pregnant Women and Prevention of Perinatal Transmission (2012). *Recommendations for use of antiretroviral drugs in pregnant HIV-infected women for maternal health and interventions to reduce perinatal HIV transmission in the United States* (pp. 1–235). Washington, DC: National Institutes of Health. aidsinfo.nih.gov/contentfiles/lvguidelines/perinatalgl.pdf.

Park, J., Thoyre, S., Estrem, H., et al. (2016). Mothers' psychological distress and feeding of their preterm infants. *MCN. The American Journal of Maternal Child Nursing, 41*(4), 221–229.

Parker, T. A., & Kinsella, J. P. (2012). Respiratory failure in the term newborn. In C. A. Gleason & S. U. Devaskar (Eds.), *Avery's diseases of the newborn*. Philadelphia: Elsevier Saunders.

Parsons, J. A., Seay, A. R., & Jacobson, M. (2016). Neurologic disorders. In S. L. Gardner, B. S. Carter, M. Enzman-Hines, et al. (Eds.), *Merenstein & Gardner's handbook of neonatal intensive care* (8th ed.). St. Louis: Mosby.

Passi, D., Sharma, S., Dutta, S. R., et al. (2017). Zika virus diseases—The new face of an ancient enemy as global public health emergency (2016): Brief review and recent updates. *International Journal of Preventive Medicine, 8*(6).

Peliowski, A., & Canadian Paediatric Society. (2012). Inhaled nitric oxide use in newborns. *Paediatrics and Child Health, 17*(2), 95–97.

Philip, A. G. S. (2012). Bronchopulmonary dysplasia: then and now. *Neonatology, 102*, 1–8.

Pineda, R., Durant, P., Mathur, A., et al. (2017). Auditory exposure in the neonatal intensive care unit: room type and other predictors. *Journal of Pediatrics*, 1–11.

Pishva, N., Parsa, G., Saki, F., et al. (2012). Intraventricular hemorrhage in premature infants and its association with pneumothorax. *Acta Medica Iranica, 50*(7), 473–476.

Polin, R. A., Carlo, W. A., & Committee on Fetus and Newborn. (2014). Surfactant replacement therapy for preterm and term neonates with respiratory distress. *Pediatrics, 133*(1), 158–163.

Popova, S., Lange, S., Probst, C., et al. (2017). Estimation of national, regional, and global prevalence of alcohol use during pregnancy and fetal alcohol syndrome: a systematic review and meta-analysis. *The Lancet Global Health, 5*(3), 290–299.

Putnam, L. R., Tsao, K., Morini, G., et al. for the Congenital Diaphragmatic Hernia Study Group. (2016). Evaluation of variability in inhaled nitric oxide use and pulmonary hypertension in patients with congenital diaphragmatic hernia. *JAMA Pediatrics, 170*(12), 1188–1194.

Quraishy, K., Bowles, S., & Moore, J. (2013). A protocol for swaddled bathing in the neonatal intensive care unit. *Neonatal Therapists, 13*(1), 48–50.

Ramani, M., & Ambalavanan, N. (2013). Feeding practices and necrotizing enterocolitis. *Clinics in Perinatology, 40*(1), 1–10.

Raoof, A., & Ohlsson, A. (2013). Noise reduction management in the neonatal intensive care unit for preterm or very low birthweight infants. *Cochrane Database of Systematic Review*, (1), CD010333.

Resch, B., Renoldner, B., & Hofer, N. (2016). Comparison between pathogen associated laboratory and clinical parameters in early-onset sepsis of the newborn. *The Open Microbiology Journal, 10*, 133–139.

Rogers, E. E., & Hintz, S. R. (2016). Early neurodevelopmental outcomes of extremely preterm infants. *Seminars in Perinatology, 40*, 497–509.

Romano-Keeler, J., Azcarate-Peril, M. A., Weitkamp, J. H., et al. (2017). Oral colostrum priming shortens hospitalization without changing the immunomicrobial milieu. *Journal of Perinatology, 37*, 36–41.

Ronkainen, E., Dunder, T., Peltoniemi, O., et al. (2015). New BPD predicts lung function at school age: follow-up study and meta-analysis. *Pediatric Pulmonology, 50*, 1090–1098.

Ross, E. J., Graham, D. L., Money, K. M., et al. (2015). Developmental consequences of fetal exposure to drugs: what we know and what we still must learn. *Neuropsychopharmacology, 40*, 61–87.

Rovekamp-Abels, L. W., Hogewind-Schoonenboom, J. E., de Wijs-Meijler, D. P., et al. (2015). Intermittent bolus or semicontinuous feeding for preterm infants? *Journal of Pediatric Gastroenterol Nutrition, 61*(6), 659–664.

Rozance, P. J., McGowan, J. E., Price-Douglas, W., et al. (2016). Glucose homeostasis. In S. L. Gardner, B. S. Carter, M. Enzman-Hines, et al. (Eds.), *Merenstein & Gardner's handbook of neonatal intensive care* (8th ed.). St. Louis: ELSEVIER.

Ryder, J. A., & Brisgone, R. E. (2013). Cracked perspectives: reflections of women and girls in the aftermath of the crack cocaine era. *Fem Crim, 8*(1), 40–62.

Sabra, S., Gratocos, E., & Gomez Roig, M. D. (2017). Smoking-induced changes in the maternal immune, endocrine, and metabolic pathways and their impact on fetal growth: a topical review. *Fetal Diagnosis and Therapy*, 1–10.

Salzwedel, A. P., Grewen, K. M., Goldman, B. D., et al. (2016). Thalamocortical functional connectivity and behavioral disruptions in neonates with prenatal cocaine exposure. *Neurotoxicology and Teratology, 56*, 16–25.

Samsom, J. F., & de Groot, L. (2000). The influence of postural control on motility and hand function in a group of "high risk" preterm infants at 1 year of age. *Early Human Development, 60*(2), 101–113.

Samsom, J. F., & de Groot, L. (2001). Study of a group of extremely preterm infants (25-27 weeks): how do they function at 1 year of age? *Journal of Child Neurology, 16*(11), 832–837.

Santesteban, E., Arenas, S., & Campino, A. (2015). Medication errors in neonatal care: A systematic review of types of errors and effectiveness of preventive strategies. *Journal of Neonatal Nursing, 12*, 200–208.

Saver, J. L., Warach, S., Janis, S., National Institute of Neurological Disorders and Stroke (NINDS) Stroke Common Data Element Working Group, et al. (2012). Standardizing the structure of stroke clinical and epidemiologic research data: the National Institute of Neurological Disorders and Stroke (NINDS) Stroke Common Data Element (CDE) project. *Stroke; a Journal of Cerebral Circulation, 43*(4), 967–973.

Sawh, S. C., Deshpande, S., Jansen, S., et al. (2016). Prevention of necrotizing enterocolitis with probiotics: a systematic review and meta-analysis. *PeerJ, 10*(4), 1–29.

Sayed, A., & Bisheer, N. (2015). Outcome of oral sildenafil in neonatal persistent pulmonary hypertension of non-cardiac causes. *Journal of neonatal-perinatal medicine, 8*(3), 215–220.

Shah, R., Diaz, S. D., Arria, A., et al. (2012). Prenatal methamphetamine exposure and short-term maternal and infant medical outcomes. *American Journal of Perinatology, 29*, 391–400.

Shah, V. S., Ohlsson, A., Halliday, H. L., et al. (2017). Early administration of inhaled corticosteroids for preventing chronic lung disease in very low birth weight preterm neonates. *Cochrane Database of Systematic Reviews*, (1), CD001969.

Shaker, C. S. (2013). Cue-based feeding in the NICU: using the infant's communication as a guide. *Neonatal Network, 32*(6), 404–408.

Sharma, R., & Hudak, M. L. (2013). A clinical perspective of necrotizing enterocolitis: Past, present, and future. *Clinics in Perinatology, 40*(1), 27–51.

Sharma, V., Berkelhamer, S., & Lakshminrusimha, S. (2015). Persistent pulmonary hypertension of the newborn. *Maternal Health Neonatology Perinatology, 3*, 1–18.

Sherman, M. P. (2013). Lactoferrin and necrotizing enterocolitis. *Clinics in Perinatology, 40*(1), 79–91.

Simonsen, K. A., Anderson-Berry, A. L., Delair, S. F., et al. (2014). Early-onset neonatal sepsis. *Clinical, Microbiology Review, 27*(1), 21–47.

Singer, L. T., Minnes, S., Min, M. O., et al. (2015). Prenatal cocaine exposure and child outcomes: a conference report based on a prospective study from Cleveland. *Human Psychopharmacology, 30*, 285–289.

Solis, J. M., Shadur, J. M., Burns, A. R., et al. (2012). Understanding the diverse needs of children whose parents abuse substances. *Current Drug Abuse Reviews, 5*(2), 135–147.

Soni, A., & Singh, S. (2012). Neonatal abstinence syndrome. In A. Sachdeva, A. K. Dutta, M. P. Jain, et al. (Eds.), *Advances in pediatrics* (2nd ed.). London: JP Medical.

Sorrentino, E., & Alegiani, C. (2012). Medication errors in the neonate. *The Journal of Maternal-Fetal & Neonatal Medicine, 25*(S4), 83–85.

Soto, E., & Bahado-Singh, R. (2013). Fetal abnormal growth associated with substance abuse. *Clinical Obstetrics and Gynecology, 56*(1), 142–153.

Squires, K. A. G., De Paoli, A. G., Williams, C., et al. (2013). High-frequency oscillatory ventilation with low oscillatory frequency in pulmonary interstitial emphysema. *Neonatology, 104*(4), 243–249.

Stevens, B., Yamada, J., Lee, G. Y., et al. (2013). Sucrose for analgesia in newborn infants undergoing painful procedures. *Cochrane Database of Systematic Review*, (1), CD001069.

Su, B. (2014). Optimizing nutrition in preterm infants. *Pediatrics and Neonatology, 55*(1), 5–13.

Substance Abuse and Mental Health Services Administration (2012). *Results from the 2011 National Survey on Drug Use and Health: summary of national findings* NSDUH Series H-44, HHS Publication No. 12-4713. Rockville, Md: The Administration.

Sun, H., Cheng, R., Kang, W., et al. (2013). High-frequency oscillatory ventilation versus synchronized intermittent mandatory ventilation plus pressure support in preterm infants with severe respiratory distress syndrome. *Respiratory Care*. Retrieved from: http://rc.rcjournal.com/content/early/2013/06/13/respcare.02382.abstract.

Surbek, D., Drack, G., Irion, O., et al. (2012). Antenatal corticosteroids for fetal lung maturation in threatened preterm delivery: indications and administration. *Archives of Gynecology and Obstetrics, 286*(2), 277–281.

Swaney, J. R., English, N., & Carter, B. S. (2016). Ethics, values, and palliative care in neonatal intensive care. In S. L. Gardner, B. S. Carter, M. Enzman-Hines, et al. (Eds.), *Merenstein & Gardner's handbook of neonatal intensive care* (8th ed.). St. Louis: Mosby.

Tai, E., Wang, X., & Chen, Z. (2013). An update on adding docosahexaenoic acid (DHA) and arachidonic acid (AA) to baby formula. *Food Function, 4*, 1767–1775.

Tai, M., Piskorski, A., Kao, J. C., et al. (2017). Placental morphology in fetal alcohol spectrum disorders. *Alcohol and alcoholism, 52*(2), 138–144.

Taylor, S. J., Allan, K., McWilliam, H., et al. (2014). Nasogastric tube depth: the 'NEX' guideline is incorrect. *British Journal of Nursing, 23*(12), 641–644.

Tennant, C., Friedman, A. M., Pare, E., et al. (2012). Performance of lecithin-sphingomyelin ratio as a reflex test for documenting fetal lung maturity in late preterm and term fetuses. *The Journal of Maternal-Fetal & Neonatal Medicine, 25*(8), 1460–1462.

Thoyre, S. M., Hubbard, C., Park, J., et al. (2016). Implementing co-regulated feeding with mothers of preterm infants. *MCN. The American Journal of Maternal Child Nursing, 41*(4), 204–211.

Tyson, J. E., & Kennedy, K. A. (2013). Trophic feedings for parenterally fed infants. *Cochrane Database of Systematic Review*, (3), CD000504.

Uhl, T., Fisher, K., Docherty, S. L., et al. (2013). Insights into patient and family-centered care through the hospital experiences of parents. *Journal of Obstetric, Gynecologic & Neonatal Nursing, 42*(1), 121–131.

U.S. Food and Drug Administration (2012). *Drug Safety Labeling changes: 2% Chlorhexidine Gluconate (CHG) Cloth*. Silver Spring, MD: U.S. Food and Drug Administration. Retrieved from: http://www.fda.gov/Safety/MedWatch/SafetyInformation/SafetyRelatedDrugLabelingChanges/ucm307387.htm.

Vain, N., & Garcia, C. (2013). "Safe" oxygen saturation levels in extremely preterm infants: have we found a definite answer? *Arch Argent Pediatrics, 111*(5), 372–376.

Vaivre-Douret, L., Ennouri, K., Jrad, I., et al. (2004). Effect of positioning on the incidence of abnormalities of muscle tone in low-risk, preterm infants. *European Journal of Paediatric Neurology, 8*(1), 21–34.

Vance, D. A., Demel, S., Kirksey, K., et al. (2015). A Delphi Study for the Development of an Infant Skin Breakdown Risk Assessment Tool. *Advances in Neonatal Care, 15*(2), 150–157.

Versaw-Barnes, D., & Wood, A. (2015). The infant at high risk for developmental delay. In J. S. Tecklin (Ed.), *Pediatric physical therapy* (5th ed.). Philadelphia: Lippincott Williams & Wilkins.

Volpe, J. J. (2008). *Neurology of the newborn* (5th ed.). Philadelphia: Saunders.

vom Hove, M., Prenzel, F., Uhlig, H., et al. (2014). Pulmonary outcome in former preterm, very low birth weight children with bronchopulmonary dysplasia: a case-control follow-up at school age. *The Journal of Pediatrics, 164*(1), 40–45.

Wackernagel, D., Dube, M., Blennow, M., et al. (2016). Continuous subcutaneous glucose monitoring is accurate in term and near-term infants at risk of hypoglycaemia. *Acta Paediatrics, 105*(8), 917–923.

Walsh, M. C., & Fanaroff, A. A. (2015). Epidemiology for neonatologists. In R. M. Martin, A. A. Fanaroff, & M. C. Walsh (Eds.), *Neonatal-perinatal medicine: diseases of the fetus and infant* (10th ed.). Philadephia: Saunders.

Wang, L., He, J. L., & Zhang, X. H. (2013). The efficacy of massage on preterm infants: a meta-analysis. *American Journal of Perinatology, 30*(9), 731–738.

Wang, Q., Dong, J., & Zhu, Y. (2012). Probiotic supplement reduces risk of necrotizing enterocolitis and mortality in preterm very low-birth-weight infants: an updated meta-analysis of 20 randomized, controlled trials. *Journal of Pediatric Surgery, 47*, 241–248.

Wapner, R. J., Gyamfi-Bannerman, C., & Thom, E., for the Eunice Kennedy Shriver National Institute of Child Health and Human Development Maternal-Fetal Medicine Units Network. (2016). What we have learned about antenatal corticosteroid regimens. *Seminars in Perinatology, 40*, 291–297.

Warshak, C. R., Regan, J., Moore, B., et al. (2015). Association between marijuana use and adverse obstetrical and neonatal outcomes. *Journal of Perinatology, 35*, 991–995.

Watson, J., & McGuire, W. (2016). Responsive versus scheduled feeding for preterm infants. *Cochrane Database of Systematic Review*, (8), CD005255.

Weiner, G. M. (Ed.), (2016). *Textbook of neonatal resuscitation* (7th ed.). Elk Grove Village, IL: American Academy of Pediatrics and American Heart Association.

Weiner, S. M., & Finnegan, L. P. (2016). Drug withdrawal in the neonate. In S. L. Gardner, B. S. Carter, M. Enzman-Hines, et al. (Eds.), *Merenstein & Gardner's handbook of neonatal intensive care* (8th ed.). St. Louis: Mosby.

Welch, R. A., Shaw, M. K., & Welch, K. C. (2016). Amniotic fluid LPCAT1 mRNA correlates with the lamellar body count. *Journal of Perinatal Medicine, 44*(5), 531–555.

Whetten, C. H. (2016). Cue-based feeding in the NICU. *Nursing for Women's Health, 20*(5), 507–510.

Wilhoit, L. F., Scott, D. A., & Simecka, B. A. (2017). Fetal alcohol spectrum disorders: characteristics, complications, and treatment. *Community Mental Health*, 1–8.

Wright, T. E., Schuetter, R., Tellei, J., et al. (2015). Methamphetamines and pregnancy outcomes. *Journal Addict Medicine, 9*(2), 111–117.

Yin, T., Yang, L., Lee, T., et al. (2015). Development of atraumatic heel-stick procedures by combined treatment with non-nutritive sucking, oral sucrose, and facilitated tucking: a randomized, controlled trial. *International Journal of Nursing Studies, 52*(8), 1288–1299.

Young, L., Morgan, J., McCormick, F., et al. (2012). Nutrient-enriched formula versus standard term formula for preterm infants following hospital discharge. *Cochrane Database of Systematic Review*, (3), CD004696.

Young, L., Embleton, N. D., & McGuire, W. (2016). Nutrient-enriched formula versus standard formula for preterm infants following hospital discharge. *Cochrane Database of Systematic Review*, (12), CD004696.

Younge, N., Goldstein, R., Bann, C. M., et al. for the Eunice Kennedy Shriver National Institute of Child Health and Human Development Neonatal Research Network. (2017). Survival and neurodevelopmental outcomes among periviable infants. *The New England Journal of Medicine, 376*(7), 617–628.

Zaichkin, J. (2017). *Understanding the NICU: what parents of preemies and other hospitalized newborns need to know*. Elk Grove Village, IL: American Academy of Pediatrics.

Zani, A., Eaton, S., Puri, P., EUPSA Network Office, et al. (2016). International Survey on the Management of Congenital Diaphragmatic Hernia. *European Journal of Pediatric Surgery, 25*(1), 38–46.

10

Health Promotion of the Infant and Family

Mystii Kidd and Cheryl C. Rodgers

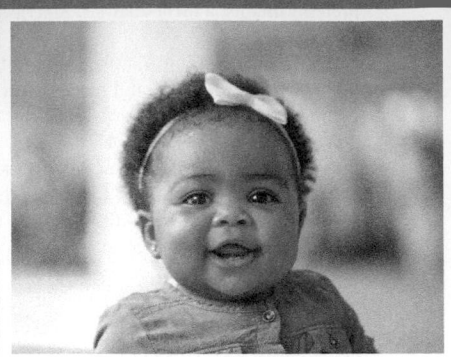

http://evolve.elsevier.com/wong/ncic

CONCEPTS

- Development
- Functional Ability
- Nutrition
- Safety

PROMOTING OPTIMUM GROWTH AND DEVELOPMENT

BIOLOGIC DEVELOPMENT

At no other time in life are physical changes and developmental achievements so dramatic as during infancy. All body systems undergo progressive maturation. Concurrent development of skills allows infants to increasingly respond to the environment. Acquisition of these fine and gross motor skills occurs in an orderly head-to-toe and center-to-periphery (cephalocaudal-proximodistal) sequence.

Proportional Changes

Growth is rapid during the first year, especially during the initial 6 months. Infants gain 680 g (1.5 lb) per month until age 5 months, when the birth weight has at least doubled. An average weight for a 6-month-old child is 7.26 kg (16 lb). Weight gain decreases by half that amount during the second 6 months. By 1 year of age the infant's birth weight has tripled, to an average of 9.75 kg (21.5 lb). Infants who are breastfed beyond 4 to 6 months of age typically gain less weight than those who are bottle-fed, yet head circumference is more than adequate.

Height increases by 2.5 cm (1 inch) per month during the first 6 months and by half that amount per month during the second 6 months. Increases in length occur in sudden spurts rather than in a slow, gradual pattern. Average height is 65 cm (25.5 inches) at 6 months and 74 cm (29 inches) at 12 months. By 1 year birth length has increased by almost 50%. This increase occurs mainly in the trunk rather than the legs and contributes to the characteristic physique of the older infant (see Fig. 10.8, *A*, later in this chapter).

Head growth is also rapid and an important determinant of brain growth. Head circumference increases approximately 2 cm (0.75 inch) per month from birth to 3 months, 1 cm (0.4 inch) per month from 4 to 6 months, and 0.5 cm (0.2 inch) per month during the second 6 months. The average head size is 43 cm (17 inches) at 6 months and 46 cm (18 inches) at 12 months. By 1 year of age head size has increased by almost 33%. Closure of the cranial sutures occurs, with the posterior fontanel fusing by 6 to 8 weeks of age and the anterior fontanel closing by 12 to 18 months of age (the average age being 14 months).

It is important to note that genetic, metabolic, environmental, and nutritional factors strongly influence infant growth; thus the previous statements are general guidelines only. Use the appropriate growth charts reflecting weight for length and head circumference in each case to determine appropriate growth parameters. The World Health Organization growth charts released in 2006 are now recommended as reference growth charts in children 0 to 24 months of age because they represent growth parameters in healthy breastfed infants worldwide (Turck, Michaelson, Shanir, et al., 2013).

Expanding head size reflects the growth and differentiation of the nervous system. By the end of the first year the brain has increased in weight approximately 2.5 times. Maturation of the brain is exhibited in the dramatic developmental achievements of infancy. The primitive reflexes (see Table 7.4) are replaced by voluntary, purposeful movement, and new reflexes that influence motor development appear (Box 10.1 and Fig. 10.1).

The chest assumes a more adult contour, with the lateral diameter becoming larger than the anteroposterior diameter. The chest circumference approximately equals head circumference by the end of the first year. The heart grows less rapidly than does the rest of the body. Its weight is usually doubled by 1 year of age, whereas body weight triples over the same period. The size of the heart is still large in relation to the chest cavity; its width is approximately 55% of the chest width.

Sensory Changes

During infancy, visual acuity gradually improves and binocular fixation is established. Box 10.2 lists the major developmental characteristics of vision during infancy. Binocularity, or the fixation of two ocular images

BOX 10.1 Neurologic Reflexes That Appear During Infancy

Labyrinth righting—Infant in prone or supine position is able to raise head; appears at 2 months, strongest at 10 months

Neck righting—While infant is supine, head is turned to one side; shoulder, trunk, and finally pelvis will turn toward that side; appears at 3 months, until 24 to 36 months

Body righting—A modification of the neck-righting reflex in which turning hips and shoulders to one side causes all other body parts to follow; appears at 6 months, until 24 to 36 months

Otolith righting—When body of an erect infant is tilted, head is returned to upright, erect position; appears at 7 to 12 months, persists indefinitely

Landau—When infant is suspended in a horizontal prone position, the head is raised and legs and spine are extended; appears at 6 to 8 months, lasts until 12 to 24 months

Parachute—When infant is suspended in a horizontal prone position and suddenly thrust downward, hands and fingers extend forward as if to protect against falling (see Fig. 10.1); appears at 7 to 9 months, persists indefinitely

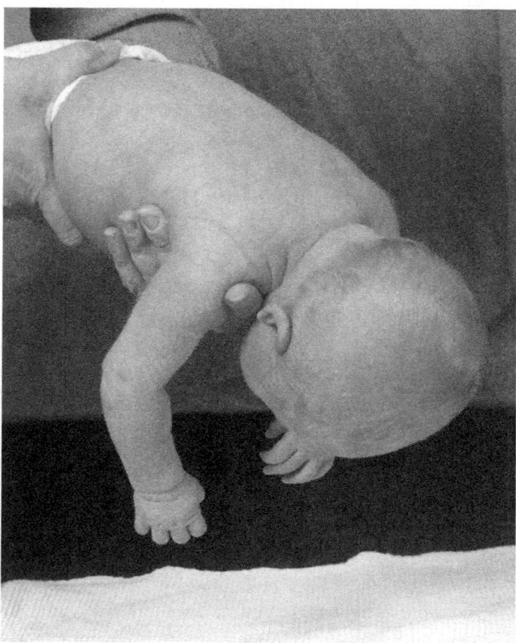

FIG. 10.1 Parachute reflex. (Courtesy Paul Vincent Kuntz, Texas Children's Hospital, Houston.)

into one cerebral picture (fusion), begins to develop by 6 weeks of age and should be well established by age 4 months (Fig. 10.2). Lack of binocular vision results in strabismus and must be detected early to prevent permanent blindness.

Depth perception (stereopsis) begins to develop by age 7 to 9 months but may exist earlier as an innate safety mechanism. At approximately 7 months the parachute reflex appears and may be a protective response during a fall (see Fig. 10.1 and Box 10.1).

Infants have a visual preference for looking at the human face; this preference also has a developmental sequence. At age 6 weeks infants show more interest in a picture of a face with eyes than in one without eyes. By 10 weeks of age a picture with both eyes and eyebrows elicits more response, and by 20 weeks of age the mouth is also necessary. By age 6 months infants respond to facial expressions and can distinguish between familiar and strange faces. This is about the time that separation anxiety begins to occur (see information later in this chapter).

BOX 10.2 Major Developmental Characteristics of Vision

Birth

Visual acuity: 20/100 to 20/400*

Pupillary and corneal (blink) reflexes present

Able to fixate on moving object in range of 45 degrees when held 20 to 25 cm (8 to 10 inches) away

Cannot integrate head and eye movements well (doll's eye reflex—eyes lag behind if head is rotated to one side; note that the presence of this reflex at any other time in childhood is abnormal and may indicate a neurologic problem)

4 Weeks

Can follow in range of 90 degrees

Can watch parent intently as he or she speaks to infant

Tear glands beginning to function

Visual acuity hyperoptic because of less spheric eyeball than in adult

6 to 12 Weeks

Has peripheral vision to 180 degrees

Has binocular vision beginning at age 6 weeks, well established by age 4 months

Convergence on near objects beginning by age 6 weeks, developed by age 3 months

Disappearance of doll's eye reflex

12 to 20 Weeks

Recognizes feeding bottle

Able to fixate on a 1.25-cm (0.5-inch) block

Looks at hand while sitting or lying on back

Able to accommodate to near objects

20 to 28 Weeks

Adjusts posture to see an object

Able to rescue a dropped toy

Develops color preference for yellow and red

Able to discriminate between simple geometric forms

Prefers more complex visual stimuli

Develops hand-eye coordination

28 to 44 Weeks

Can fixate on very small objects

Depth perception beginning to develop

Lack of binocular vision indicative of strabismus

44 to 52 Weeks

Visual acuity: 20/40 to 20/60

Visual loss developing if strabismus is present

Can follow rapidly moving objects

*Measurement of visual acuity differs according to testing procedures. (See Chapter 4.)

With progressive myelination of the auditory pathway, the specific responses of locating sound replace the generalized response of the neonate. Box 10.3 lists the major developmental characteristics of hearing. (See Chapter 7 for further discussion of hearing and the senses of smell, taste, and touch.)

Maturation of Systems

Other organ systems also change and grow during infancy. The respiratory rate slows somewhat (see inside back cover) and is relatively stable.

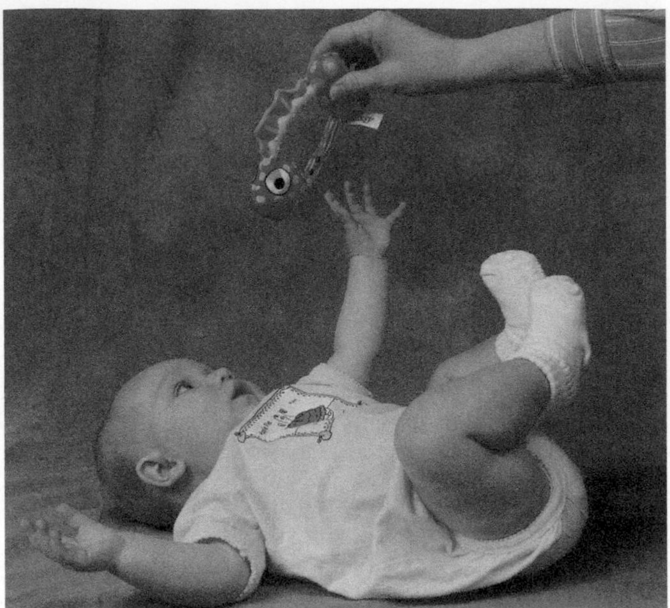

FIG. 10.2 Three-month-old infant focuses on visual object and reaches toward it. (Courtesy Paul Vincent Kuntz, Texas Children's Hospital, Houston.)

BOX 10.3 Major Developmental Characteristics of Hearing

Birth

Responds to loud noise by startle, or Moro reflex

Responds to sound of human voice more readily than to any other sound

Quieting effect from low-pitched sounds, such as lullaby, metronome, or heartbeat

8 to 12 Weeks

Turns head to side when sound is made at level of ear

12 to 16 Weeks

Locates sound by turning head to side and looking in same direction

16 to 24 Weeks

Locates sound by turning head to side and then looking up or down

24 to 32 Weeks

Locates sounds by turning head in a curving arc

Responds to own name

32 to 40 Weeks

Localizes sounds by turning head diagonally and directly toward sound

40 to 52 Weeks

Knows several words and their meaning, such as "no," and names of family members

Learns to control and adjust own response to sound, such as listening for the sound to occur again

Respiratory movements continue to be abdominal. Several factors predispose the infant to severe and acute respiratory problems. Given the proximity of the trachea to the bronchi and its branching structures, an infectious agent is rapidly transmitted to the respiratory system and ears. The short, straight eustachian tube closely communicates with the ear, allowing infection to ascend from the pharynx to the middle ear. In addition, the immune system's inability to produce immunoglobulin A (IgA) in the mucosal lining provides less protection against infection in infancy than in later childhood. The entire respiratory tract's ability to produce mucus is diminished, decreasing the humidification of the large volume of inspired air.

Although the lumen of the trachea and bronchi enlarges during infancy, it remains small in comparison with the total size of the lung, maintaining high resistance to the volume of air inspired. The small airways are easily blocked by edema, mucus, or a foreign body. The pliant (flexible) rib cage has less elastic recoil, and during respiratory distress, the work of breathing is increased. In addition, the volume of dead space (i.e., that amount of air needed to fill the respiratory passages with each breath) is large, requiring the infant to breathe approximately twice as fast as the adult to provide the body with the needed amount of oxygen.

As the infant grows, the heart rate slows (see inside back cover), and the rhythm is often **sinus arrhythmia** (rate increases with inspiration and decreases with expiration). Blood pressure also changes during infancy (see inside back cover). Systolic pressure rises during the first 2 months as a result of the left ventricle's increasing ability to pump blood into the systemic circulation. Diastolic pressure decreases during the first 3 months, then gradually rises to values close to those at birth. Fluctuations in blood pressure occur during varying states of activity and emotion.

Significant hematopoietic changes occur during the first year. Fetal hemoglobin (HgbF) is present up to the first 5 months, with adult hemoglobin steadily increasing through the first half of infancy. HgbF results in a shortened survival of red blood cells (RBCs) and thus a decreased number of RBCs. A common result at 3 to 6 months of age is *physiologic anemia.* High levels of HgbF depress the production of **erythropoietin**, a hormone released by the kidney that stimulates RBC production.

Maternally derived iron stores are present for the first 5 to 6 months and gradually diminish, which also accounts for lowered hemoglobin levels toward the end of the first 6 months. The occurrence of physiologic anemia is not affected by an adequate iron supply. However, when erythropoiesis is stimulated, iron stores are necessary for the formation of adequate amounts of hemoglobin.

The digestive processes are relatively immature at birth. Although full-term newborn infants have some limitations in digestive function, human milk has properties that partially compensate for decreased digestive enzymatic activity, thus enabling the infant to receive optimum nutrition during the first several months of life (Lawrence & Lawrence, 2016). The enzyme amylase is present in small amounts but usually has little effect on the foodstuffs because of the small amount of time the food stays in the mouth. Gastric digestion in the stomach relies primarily on the action of hydrochloric acid and rennin, an enzyme that acts specifically on the casein in milk to cause the formation of curds (coagulated semisolid particles of milk). The curds cause the milk to be retained in the stomach long enough for digestion to occur.

Digestion also takes place in the duodenum, where pancreatic enzymes and bile begin to break down protein and fat. Secretion of the pancreatic enzyme amylase, which is needed for digestion of complex carbohydrates, is limited until about the fourth to sixth months of life. Lipase is also limited, and infants do not achieve adult levels of fat absorption until 4 to 5 months of age. Trypsin is secreted in sufficient quantities to catabolize protein into polypeptides and some amino acids.

The immaturity of the digestive processes is evident in the appearance of stools. During infancy, solid foods (e.g., peas, carrots, corn, raisins) are passed incompletely broken down in the feces. An excessive quantity of fiber easily disposes the child to loose, bulky stools. During infancy the stomach enlarges to accommodate a greater volume of food. By the end of the first year the infant is able to tolerate three meals a day and an evening bottle and may have one or two bowel movements daily.

However, with any type of gastric irritation, the infant is vulnerable to diarrhea, vomiting, and dehydration.

The liver is the most immature of all the gastrointestinal organs throughout infancy. The ability to conjugate bilirubin and secrete bile is achieved after the first couple of weeks of life. However, the capacities for gluconeogenesis, formation of plasma protein and ketones, storage of vitamins, and deaminization of amino acids remain relatively immature for the first year of life.

Maturation of the sucking, swallowing, and breathing reflexes and the later eruption of teeth parallel the changes in the gastrointestinal tract and prepare the infant for the introduction of solid foods.

Sucking activity can occur in utero as early as 15 to 18 weeks of gestation. Weak, disorganized mouthing movements may be noted at 27 to 28 weeks of gestation. Complete maturation of sucking, swallowing, and breathing patterns are usually synchronized by 34 to 36 weeks, although some sucking and swallowing synchrony skills are seen by 30 to 33 weeks (Lau, 2015). Sucking is further divided into nutritive and nonnutritive; the latter is observed in infants of all ages and is reported to be primarily for the purpose of satisfying the basic sucking urge. On the other hand, nutritive sucking has as its primary purpose the intake of food. *Suckling* is a term often used for breastfeeding (Lawrence & Lawrence, 2016), yet use of the term varies among different sources.

Swallowing (deglutition) is the ability to collect the food (bolus) and propel it into the esophagus. During the infantile (visceral) swallow reflex food lies in a shallow groove on the top (dorsum) of the tongue. As the tongue is pressed upward toward the palate, the milk flows by gravity down the sloping tongue and along the sides of the mouth in lateral furrows between the tongue, cheek, and gum pads. As the bolus moves downward, the posterior wall of the pharynx comes forward to displace the soft palate. This swallowing process is efficient for fluids but not for solids.

As the infant grows, the tongue becomes smaller in proportion to the oral cavity and attains greater motility, the orofacial muscles develop, and teeth erupt. Consequently, the mature (somatic) swallow reflex is significantly different. The tongue remains behind the central incisors, and the mandible no longer thrusts forward. The dorsum of the tongue is less concave and remains higher and parallel, not inclined, against the palate. The lateral furrows are absent because of tooth eruption. Tongue pressure and movement against the hard palate push the bolus back into the pharynx.

Healthy infants also exhibit a special reflex called the *Santmyer swallow.* When a puff of air is directed at the face, the infant will exhibit a reflexive swallow (Khan & Orenstein, 2016). This reflex may be useful in the administration of small amounts of fluids or medications, but caution is recommended to prevent aspiration.

The immunologic system undergoes numerous changes during the first year. Full-term newborns receive significant amounts of maternal immunoglobulin G (IgG), which for approximately 3 months confers immunity against many antigens to which the mother was exposed. During this time, IgG levels gradually fall as maternal IgG is catabolized, and the newborn produces limited IgG. Infants reach approximately 40% of adult levels by 1 year of age; therefore during the first 6 to 12 months of life, the infant is at higher risk for infections. Significant amounts of immunoglobulin M (IgM) are produced at birth, yet specificity is decreased, thus limiting recognition of certain pathogens. Adult levels of IgM are reached by 9 to 12 months of age. The production of immunoglobulins A, D, and E (IgA, IgD, and IgE) is much more gradual, and maximum levels are not attained until early childhood.

Prebiotic oligosaccharides found in breast milk produce probiotic bacteria such as bifidobacteria and lactobacilli, which in turn stimulate synthesis and secretion of secretory IgA (sIgA). Secretory IgA is present in large amounts in colostrum; IgA confers protection to the mucous membranes of the gastrointestinal tract (Durand, Ochoa, Bellomo, et al., 2013) against many bacteria, such as *Escherichia coli,* and viruses, such as rubella, poliovirus, and the enteroviruses. The development of the mucosa-associated lymphoid tissue occurs during infancy; in part, this system is believed to prevent colonization and passage of bacteria across the infant's mucosal barrier. The function and quantity of T-lymphocytes, lymphokines, interferon-γ, interleukins, tumor necrosis factor–α, and complement are reduced in early infancy, thus preventing optimal response to certain bacteria and viruses. The production of IgA, IgD, and IgE is much more gradual, and maximum levels are not attained until early childhood. Probiotics may have a significant role in helping the gastrointestinal tract establish a "good" bacterial colonization in the gut to prevent many illnesses, including antibiotic-induced diarrhea and possibly *Helicobacter pylori* gastritis (Vitetta, Briskey, Alford, et al., 2014).

There is evidence that vernix caseosa, a white, oily substance that coats the term infant's body and is often found in abundance in the creases of the axillae and groin, has innate immunologic properties that serve to protect the newborn from infection (Visscher & Narendran, 2014). Vernix also appears to have a role in maintaining the integrity of the stratum corneum and facilitating acid mantle development (Visscher & Narendran, 2014). The epidermis of the full-term infant undergoes maturation during the first month of life; the newborn's skin acts as a barrier to infection, assists in thermal regulation, and prevents transepidermal water loss in term infants.

During infancy thermoregulation becomes more efficient; the skin's ability to contract and of muscles to shiver in response to cold increases. The peripheral capillaries respond to changes in ambient temperature to regulate heat loss. The capillaries constrict in response to cold, conserving core body temperature and decreasing potential evaporative heat loss from the skin surface. The capillaries dilate in response to heat, decreasing internal body temperature through evaporation, conduction, and convection. Shivering (thermogenesis) causes the muscles and muscle fibers to contract, generating metabolic heat, which is distributed throughout the body. Increased adipose tissue during the first 6 months insulates the body against heat loss.

A shift in total body fluid occurs. At birth 75% of the infant's body weight is water, and a significant amount of that is extracellular fluid (ECF). As the percentage of body water decreases, so does the amount of ECF—from 40% at term to 20% in adulthood. The high proportion of ECF, which is composed of blood plasma, interstitial fluid, and lymph, predisposes the infant to more rapid loss of total body fluid and, consequently, dehydration. The loss of 5% to 10% of the term newborn's initial birth weight in the first 5 days of life is attributed to ECF compartment contraction, enhanced renal tubular function, and rapidly increasing glomerular filtration rate (O'Brien & Walker, 2014).

The immaturity of the renal structures also predisposes the infant to dehydration. Complete maturity of the kidney occurs during the latter half of the second year, when the cuboidal epithelium of the glomeruli becomes flattened. Before this time the filtration capacity of the glomeruli is reduced. Infants void urine frequently, and it has a low specific gravity (1.008 to 1.012). At term most infants produce and excrete approximately 45 to 50 ml/kg/24 hr and the volume increases to 60 to 80 ml/kg/24 hr as the infant grows (O'Brien & Walker, 2014). Insensible water loss caused from radiant warmers, increased body temperature, and some types of phototherapy may cause the newborn to have little or no urine output in the first 24 hours; however, infants should have at least 1 ml/kg/hr by the second day of life (O'Brien & Walker, 2014).

The endocrine system is adequately developed at birth, but its functions are immature. The interrelatedness of all the endocrine organs has a major effect on the function of any one gland. The lack of homeostatic control because of various functional deficiencies renders the infant especially vulnerable to imbalances in fluid and electrolytes,

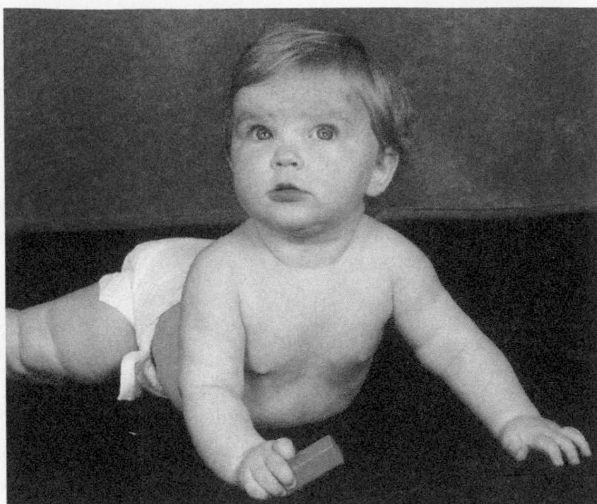

FIG. 10.3 Crude pincer grasp at 8 to 10 months of age. (Courtesy Paul Vincent Kuntz, Texas Children's Hospital, Houston.)

glucose levels, and amino acid metabolism. For example, corticotropin (adrenocorticotropic hormone [ACTH]) is produced in limited quantities during infancy. ACTH acts on the adrenal cortices to produce their hormones, particularly the glucocorticoids and aldosterone. Because the feedback mechanism between ACTH and the adrenal cortex is immature during infancy, there is much less tolerance for stressful conditions, which affect fluid and electrolytes and the metabolism of fats, proteins, and carbohydrates. In addition, although the islets of Langerhans produce insulin and glucagon during fetal life and early infancy, blood glucose levels tend to remain labile, particularly under conditions of stress.

Fine Motor Development

Fine motor behavior includes the use of the hands and fingers in the **prehension** (grasp) of an object. Grasping occurs during the first 2 to 3 months as a reflex and gradually becomes voluntary. At 1 month of age the hands are predominantly closed, and by 3 months they are mostly open. By this time infants demonstrate a desire to grasp an object, but they "grasp" it more with the eyes than with the hands. If a rattle is placed in the hand, the infant will actively hold onto it. By 4 months of age the infant regards both a small pellet and the hands and then looks from the object to the hands and back again. By 5 months the infant is able to voluntarily grasp an object.

Gradually the palmar grasp (using the whole hand) is replaced with a **pincer grasp** (using the thumb and index finger). By 8 to 9 months of age the infant uses a crude pincer grasp (Fig. 10.3), and by 10 months of age the pincer grasp is sufficiently established to enable infants to pick up a raisin and other finger foods. By 11 months the infant has progressed to a neat pincer grasp (Fig. 10.4).

By 6 months of age infants have increased manipulative skill. They hold their bottle, grasp their feet and pull them to their mouth, and feed themselves a cracker. By 7 months they transfer objects from one hand to the other, use one hand for grasping, and hold a cube in each hand simultaneously. They enjoy banging objects and will explore the movable parts of a toy. By 10 months of age infants can deliberately let go of an object and will offer it to someone. By 11 months they put objects into a container and like to remove them. By age 1 year infants try to build a tower of two blocks but fail.

Gross Motor Development

Gross motor behavior includes developmental maturation in posture, head balance, sitting, creeping, standing, and walking. The full-term neonate is born with some ability to hold the head erect and reflexively assumes the postural tonic neck position when supine. Several of the primitive reflexes have significance in terms of development of later gross motor skills. The righting reflexes elicit certain postural responses, particularly of flexion or extension. They are responsible for certain motor activities, such as rolling over, assuming the crawl position, and maintaining normal head-trunk-limb alignment during all activities. The neck-righting reflex, which turns the body to the same side as the head, enables the child to roll over from supine to prone. Other reflexes, such as the otolith-righting and labyrinth-righting reflexes, enable the infant to raise the head (see Box 10.1).

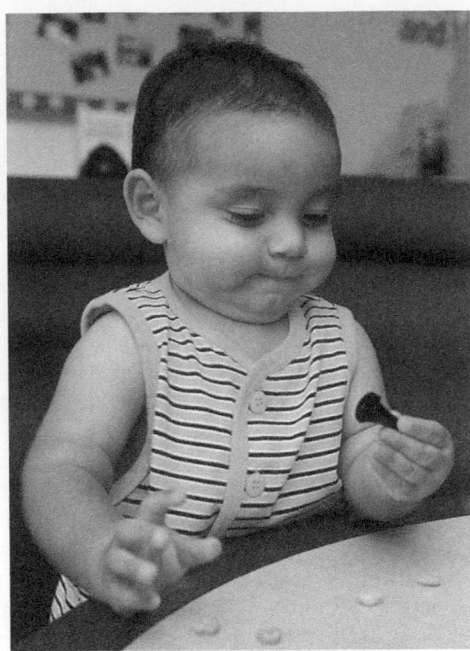

FIG. 10.4 Neat pincer grasp at 11 months of age. (Courtesy Paul Vincent Kuntz, Texas Children's Hospital, Houston.)

The asymmetric tonic neck reflex, which persists from birth to 3 months, prevents the infant from rolling over. The symmetric tonic neck reflex, which is evoked by flexing or extending the neck, helps the infant assume the crawl position. When the head and neck are extended, the extensor tone of the upper extremities and the flexor tone of the lower extremities increase. The child extends the arms and bends the knees. Because of the strong flexor tone of the lower extremities, the infant may initially crawl backward before crawling forward. This reflex disappears when neurologic maturity allows actual crawling to occur because independent limb movement is required.

Head Control. The full-term newborn can momentarily hold the head in midline and parallel when the body is suspended ventrally and can lift and turn the head from side to side when prone (see Fig. 7.8). This is not the case when the infant is lying prone on a pillow or soft surface; infants do not have the head control to lift their head out of the depression of the object and therefore risk possible suffocation. (See Sudden Infant Death Syndrome, Chapter 11.) Marked head lag is evident when the infant is pulled from a lying to a sitting position. By 3 months of age infants can hold their head well beyond the plane of the body. By 4 months of age infants can lift the head and front portion of the chest approximately 90 degrees above the table, bearing their weight on the forearms. Only slight head lag is evident when the infant is pulled from a lying to a sitting position, and by 4 to 6 months head control is well established (Figs. 10.5 and 10.6).

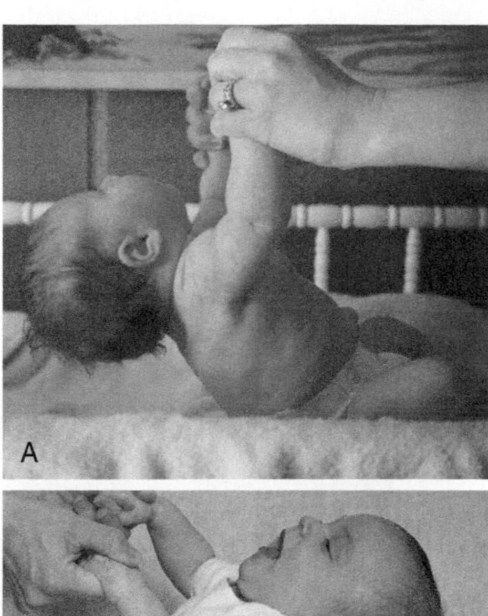

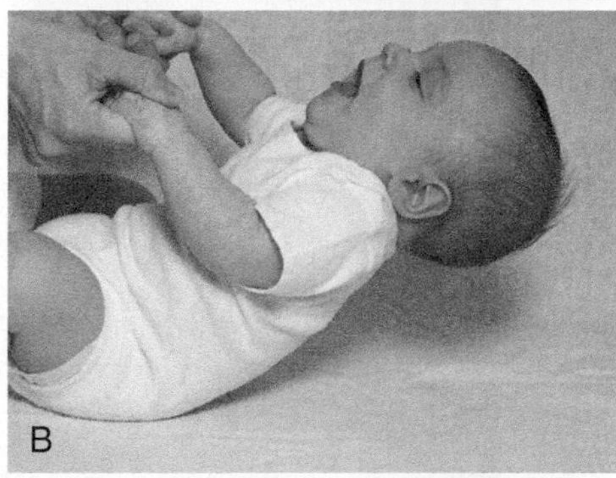

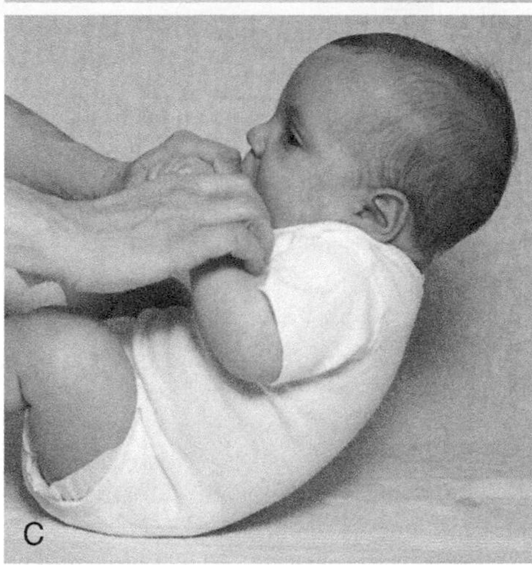

FIG. 10.5 Head control while pulled to sitting position. **A,** Complete head lag at 1 month. **B,** Partial head lag at 2 months. **C,** Almost no head lag at 4 months.

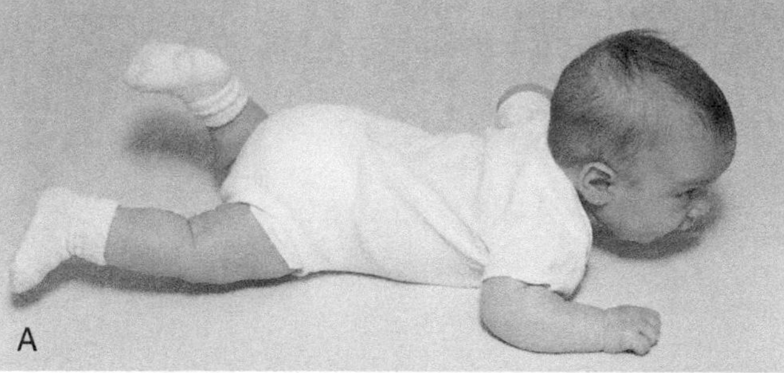

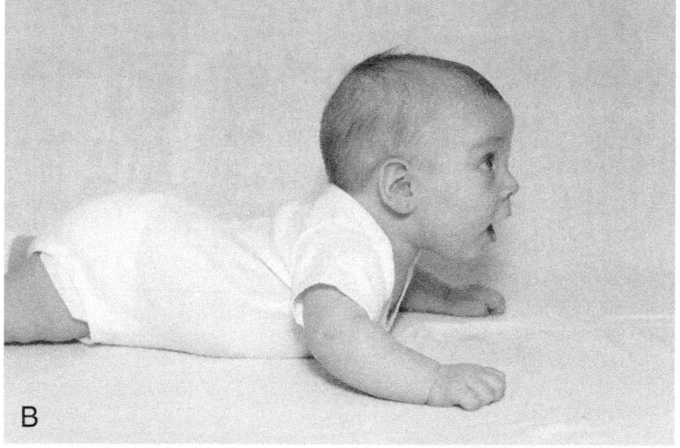

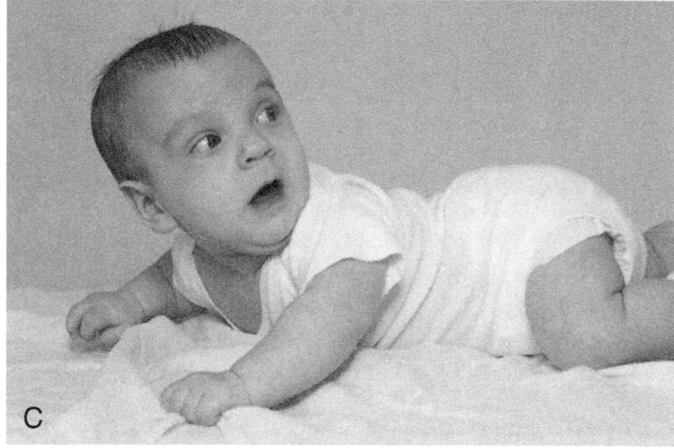

FIG. 10.6 Head control while prone. **A,** Infant momentarily lifts head at 1 month. **B,** Infant lifts head and chest 90 degrees and bears weight on forearms at 4 months. **C,** Infant lifts head, chest, and upper abdomen and can bear weight on hands at 6 months. Note how this position facilitates turning from abdomen to back.

Rolling Over. Newborns may roll over accidentally because of their rounded back. The ability to willfully turn from the abdomen to the back occurs at 5 months, and the ability to turn from the back to the abdomen occurs at 6 months. It is noteworthy that the parachute reflex (see Fig. 10.1), which elicits a protective response to falling, appears at 7 months.

Sitting. The ability to sit follows progressive head control and straightening of the back (Fig. 10.7). For the first 2 to 3 months the back is uniformly rounded. The convex cervical curve forms at approximately 3 to 4 months of age, when head control is established. The convex lumbar curve appears when the child begins to sit, at about age 4 months. As the spinal column straightens, the infant can be propped in a sitting position. By age 7 months infants can sit alone, leaning forward on their hands for support. By age 8 months they can sit well while unsupported and begin to explore their surroundings in this position rather than in a lying position. By 10 months they can maneuver from a prone to a sitting position.

An infant who does not pull to a standing position by 11 to 12 months of age should be further evaluated for possible developmental dysplasia of the hip. (See Chapter 33.) Although infants vary considerably in regard to the achievement of these milestones, they provide guidelines for early intervention.

Locomotion. Locomotion involves acquiring the ability to bear weight, propel forward on all four extremities, stand upright with support, and, finally, walk alone (Fig. 10.8). After a cephalocaudal pattern, infants 4 to 6 months old have increasing coordination in their arms. Initial locomotion results in infants propelling themselves backward by pushing with the arms. By 6 to 7 months of age they are able to bear all their

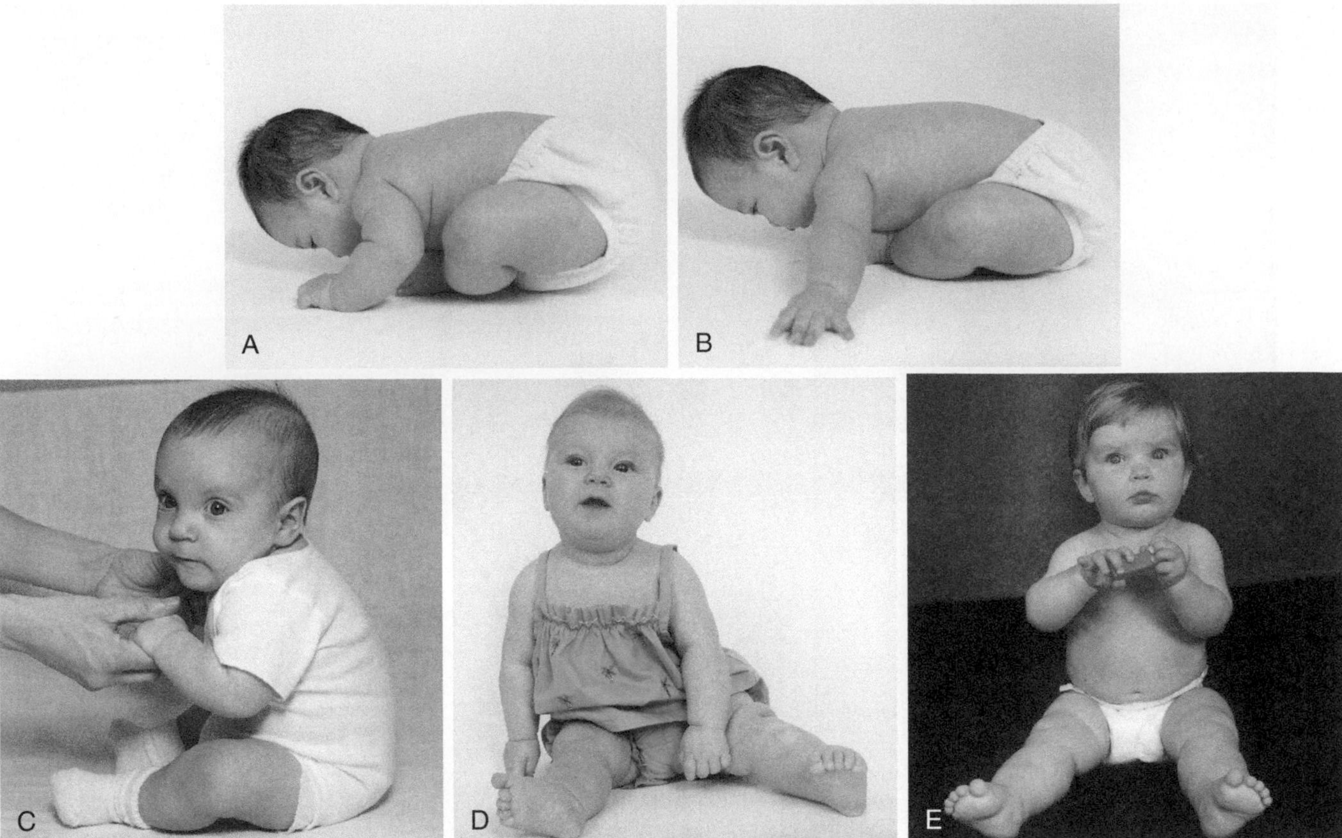

FIG. 10.7 Development of sitting. **A,** Back is completely rounded; infant has no ability to sit upright at 1 month. **B,** At 2 months, infant exhibits more control; back is still rounded, but infant can try to pull up with some head control. **C,** Back is rounded only in lumbar area; infant is able to sit erect with good head control at 4 months. **D,** Infant can sit alone, leaning on hands for support, at 7 months. **E,** Infant sits without support at 8 months. Note the transferring of objects that occurs at 7 months. (Courtesy Paul Vincent Kuntz, Texas Children's Hospital, Houston.)

weight on their legs with assistance. Crawling (propelling forward with belly on floor) progresses to creeping on hands and knees (with belly off floor) by 9 months. At this time they stand while holding onto furniture and can pull themselves to the standing position, but they are unable to maneuver back down except by falling. By 11 months they walk while holding onto furniture or with both hands held, and by age 1 year they may be able to walk with one hand held. A number of infants attempt their first independent steps by their first birthday.

PSYCHOSOCIAL DEVELOPMENT

Developing a Sense of Trust (Erikson)

Erik Erikson's (1963) phase I (birth to 1 year) is concerned with acquiring a sense of trust while overcoming a sense of mistrust. The trust that develops is a trust of self, of others, and of the world. Infants "trust" that their feeding, comfort, stimulation, and caring needs will be met. The crucial element for the achievement of this task is the quality of both the relationship between the parent (or caregiver) and child and the care the infant receives. The provision of food, warmth, and shelter by itself is inadequate for the development of a strong sense of self. The infant and parent must jointly learn to satisfactorily meet their needs for mutual regulation of frustration to occur. When this synchrony fails to develop, mistrust is the eventual outcome. Frustration is heightened in situations in which the parent is emotionally immature and does not understand the infant's behavioral cues because of his or her own self-centered phase of development.

Failure to learn delayed gratification leads to mistrust. Mistrust can result from either too much or too little frustration. If parents always meet their children's needs before the children signal their readiness, infants will never learn to test their ability to control the environment. If the delay is prolonged, infants will experience constant frustration and eventually mistrust others in their efforts to satisfy them. Therefore consistency of care is essential.

The trust acquired in infancy provides the foundation for all succeeding phases. Trust allows infants a feeling of physical comfort and security, which assists them in experiencing unfamiliar, unknown situations with a minimum of fear. Erikson has divided the first year of life into two oral-social stages. During the first 3 to 4 months, food intake is the most important social activity in which the infant engages. The newborn can tolerate little frustration or delay of gratification. Primary narcissism (total concern for oneself) is at its height. However, as bodily processes such as vision, motor movements, and vocalization become better controlled, infants use more advanced behaviors to interact with others. For example, rather than cry, infants may put their arms up to signify a desire to be held.

The next social modality involves a mode of reaching out to others through grasping. Grasping is initially reflexive, but even as a reflex it has a powerful social meaning for the parents. The reciprocal response to the infant's grasping is the parents' holding on and touching. There is pleasurable tactile stimulation for both the child and the parents.

Tactile stimulation is extremely important in the total process of acquiring trust. The degree of mothering skill, the quantity of food, or

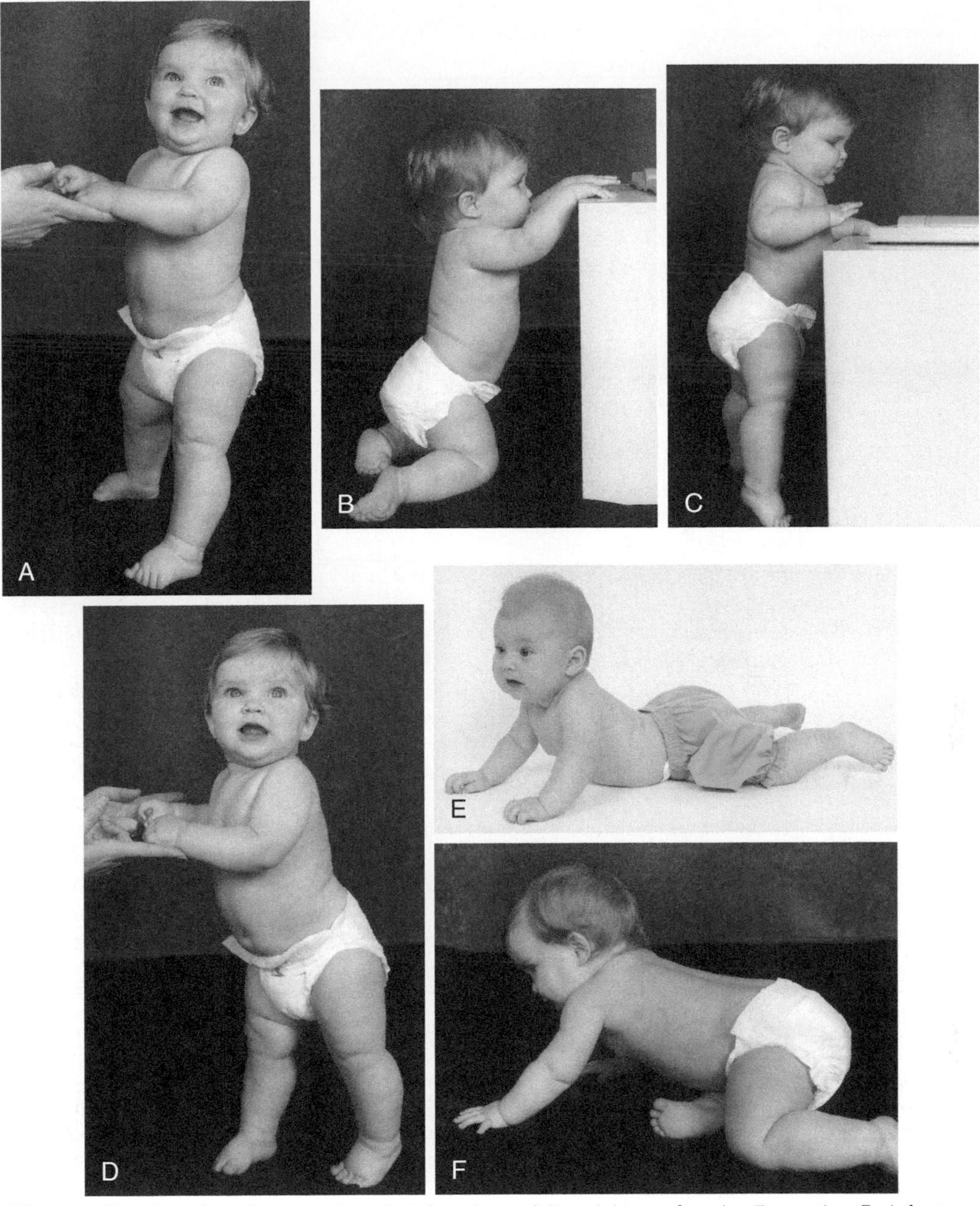

FIG. 10.8 Development of locomotion. **A,** Infant bears full weight on feet by 7 months. **B,** Infant can maneuver from sitting to kneeling position by 8 months. **C,** Infant can stand holding onto furniture at 8 to 9 months. **D,** While standing, infant takes deliberate step at 9 to 10 months. **E,** Infant crawls with abdomen on floor and pulls self forward and then, **F,** creeps on hands and knees at 9 months. (Courtesy Paul Vincent Kuntz, Texas Children's Hospital, Houston.)

the length of sucking does not determine the quality of the experience. Rather, it is the total quality of the interpersonal relationship that influences the infant's formulation of trust.

During the second stage, the more active and aggressive modality of biting occurs. Infants learn that they can hold onto what is their own and can more fully control their environment. During this stage infants may be confronted with one of their first conflicts. If they are breastfeeding, they quickly learn that biting causes the mother to become upset and withdraw the breast. Yet biting also brings internal relief from teething discomfort and a sense of power or control.

This conflict has a variety of solutions. The mother may wean the infant from the breast and begin bottle-feeding, or the infant may learn to bite substitute "nipples," such as a pacifier, and retain pleasurable breastfeeding. The successful resolution of this conflict strengthens the mother-child relationship because it occurs at a time when infants are recognizing the mother as the most significant person in their life.

COGNITIVE DEVELOPMENT

Sensorimotor Phase (Piaget)

The theory most commonly used to explain *cognition,* or the ability to know, is that of Piaget (1952). The period from birth to 24 months is termed the sensorimotor phase and is composed of six stages. However,

TABLE 10.1 Sensorimotor Phase During Infancy*

Stage and Age	Cognitive Development	Behavior
I. Use of reflexes (birth–1 month)	Repetitious use of reflexes establishing pattern of experiences Totally narcissistic (self-centered) being	Mostly reflective (e.g., sucking, swallowing, rooting, grasping, crying) Little or no tolerance for frustration of delayed gratification
II. Primary circular reactions (1-4 months)	Use of reflexes gradually replaced by voluntary activity Recognition of causality occurring when repetition of events causes one stimulus to produce consistent response Beginning notion of temporal space of time as infant realizes progression of orderly sequence of events Beginning separation of self from others Learns from type of interaction between objects or individual rather than from object itself Engages in activity for pleasure of the activity more than for its results	Recognizes familiar faces and objects (e.g., bottle) Shows anticipation before feeding Shows awareness of strange surroundings, indicating memory Discovers parts of own body—plays with hands, fingers, feet Becomes bored when left alone Shows no separation anxiety unless caregiver's skill differs from usual routine
III. Secondary circular reactions (4-8 months)	Intentional activity replaces repetitious activity that did not produce desired result Beginning of object permanence when object is beyond perceptual range Progressive idea of time; awareness of before and after in sequence of events Able to imitate selective activity from several events Further separation of self from environment Idea of quality and quantity Beginning recognition of symbols as type of communication	Secures objects by pulling on string Searches for objects that have fallen Shows separation anxiety Able to tolerate some frustration and delayed gratification Imitates sounds and simple gestures Shows interest in mirror image (see Fig. 10.10) Beginning independence in self-feeding Shows displeasure if activity is inhibited Language development; attracts attention by methods other than crying Realizes that parents are present even if not in visual field
IV. Coordination of secondary schemas and their application to new situations (9-12 months)	Concept of object permanence advancing; beginning of intellectual reasoning Associates symbols with events, but classification is based on own experience Distinguishes objects from related activity and perceives them as objects Distinguishes end products from their means; attempts to remove barriers to achieve the end	Actively searches for hidden object (see Fig. 10.9) Comprehends meanings of words and simple commands Know that gestures (e.g., bye-bye, kiss) have certain meanings Is able to put objects in container Works to get toy that is out of reach Ventures away from parent to explore surroundings

*For phases during toddlerhood, see Table 12.1.

because this discussion centers on ages birth to 12 months, only the first four stages are discussed (Table 10.1; see Table 12.1 for the stages from 13 to 24 months).

During the sensorimotor phase, infants progress from reflexive behaviors to simple repetitive acts to imitative activity. Three crucial events take place during this phase. The first event involves separation, in which infants learn to separate themselves from other objects in the environment. They realize that others besides themselves control the environment and that certain adjustments must take place for mutual satisfaction to occur. This coincides with Erikson's concept of the formation of trust and mutual regulation of frustration.

The second major accomplishment is achieving the concept of object permanence, or the realization that objects that leave the visual field still exist. A typical example of the development of object permanence is when infants are able to pursue objects they observe being hidden under a pillow or behind a chair (Fig. 10.9). This skill develops at approximately 9 to 10 months of age, which corresponds to the time of increased locomotion skills.

The last major intellectual achievement of this period is the ability to use symbols, or mental representation. The use of symbols allows the infant to think of an object or situation without actually experiencing it. The recognition of symbols is the beginning of the understanding of time and space.

The first stage, from birth to 1 month, is identified by the infant's use of reflexes. At birth the infant expresses individuality and temperament through the physiologic reflexes of sucking, rooting, grasping, and crying. The repetitious nature of the reflexes is the beginning of associations between an act and a sequential response. When infants cry because they are hungry, a nipple is put in the mouth, and they suck, feel satisfaction, and sleep. They are assimilating this experience while perceiving auditory, tactile, and visual cues. This experience of perceiving certain patterns, or ordering, provides a foundation for the subsequent stages.

The second stage, primary circular reactions, marks the beginning of the replacement of reflexive behavior with voluntary acts. During the period from 1 to 4 months, activities such as sucking or grasping become deliberate acts that elicit certain responses. The beginning of accommodation is evident. Infants incorporate and adapt their reactions to the environment and recognize the stimulus that produced a response. Previously they would cry until the nipple was brought to the mouth. Now they associate the nipple with the sound of the parent's voice. They accommodate this new piece of information and adapt by ceasing to cry when they hear the voice—before receiving the nipple. What is taking place is a realization of causality and recognition of an orderly sequence of events. The infant takes in the environment with all the senses and with whatever motor ability is present.

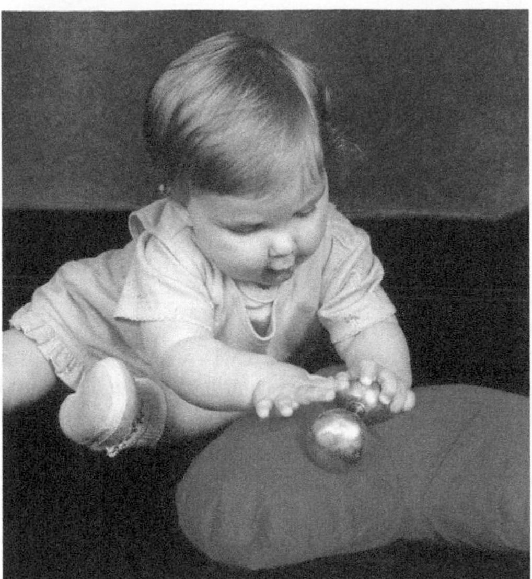

FIG. 10.9 Nine-month-old is able to find hidden object under pillow. (Courtesy Paul Vincent Kuntz, Texas Children's Hospital, Houston.)

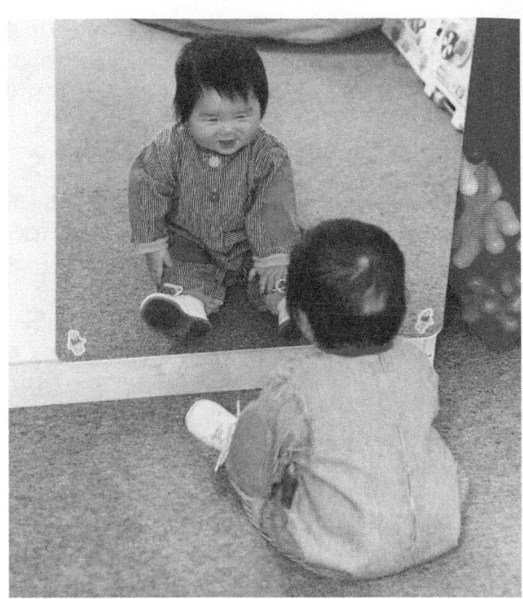

FIG. 10.10 Nine-month-old infant enjoying own image in mirror.

The secondary circular reactions stage is a continuation of primary circular reactions and lasts until 8 months of age. In this stage the primary circular reactions are repeated and prolonged for the response that results. Grasping and holding now become shaking, banging, and pulling. Infants shake objects to hear a noise, not solely for the pleasure of shaking. Quality and quantity of an act become evident. "More" or "less" shaking produces different responses. Causality, time, deliberate intention, and separateness from the environment begin to develop.

Three new processes of human behavior occur. Imitation requires the differentiation of selected acts from several events. By the second half of the first year infants can imitate sounds and simple gestures. Play becomes evident as they take pleasure in performing an act after they have mastered it. Much of infants' waking hours are absorbed in sensorimotor play. Affect (outward manifestation of emotion and feeling) is evident as infants begin to develop a sense of permanency. During the first 6 months infants believe that an object exists only for as long as they can visually perceive it; in other words, out of sight, out of mind. A reaction to external objects is evident when the object continues to be remembered even though it is beyond the range of perception. Object permanence is a critical component of parent-child attachment and is seen in the development of separation anxiety at 6 to 8 months of age (see discussion later in this chapter).

During the fourth sensorimotor stage, coordination of secondary schemas and their application to new situations, infants use previous behavioral achievements primarily as the foundation for adding new intellectual skills to their expanding repertoire. This stage is largely transitional. Increasing motor skills allow for greater exploration of the environment. They begin to discover that hiding an object does not mean that it is gone but that removing an obstacle will reveal the object. This marks the beginning of intellectual reasoning. Furthermore, they can experience an event by observing it, and they begin to associate symbols with events (e.g., "bye-bye" with "Mommy goes to work"), but the classification is purely their own. In this stage they learn from the object itself. This is in contrast to the second stage, in which infants learn from the type of interaction between objects or individuals. Intentionality is further developed in that infants now actively attempt to remove a barrier to the desired (or undesired) action (see Fig. 10.9). If something is in their way, they attempt to climb over it or push it away, whereas previously they would have given up any attempt to achieve the desired goal.

DEVELOPMENT OF BODY IMAGE

The development of body image parallels sensorimotor development. Infants' kinesthetic and tactile experiences are the first perceptions of their body, and the mouth is the principal area of pleasurable sensations. Other parts of the body are primarily objects of pleasure—the hands and fingers to suck and the feet to play with. As physical needs are met, they feel comfort and satisfaction with their body. Messages conveyed by the caregivers reinforce these feelings. For example, when infants smile, they receive emotional satisfaction from others who smile back.

Achieving the concept of object permanence is basic to the development of self-image. By the end of the first year infants recognize that they are distinct from their parents. At the same time they have increasing interest in their image, especially in the mirror (Fig. 10.10). As motor skills develop, they learn that parts of the body are useful; for example, the hands bring objects to the mouth, and the legs help them move to different locations. All these achievements transmit messages to them about themselves. Therefore it is important to transmit positive messages to infants about their bodies.

DEVELOPMENT OF GENDER IDENTITY

Gender identity is reported to begin in utero because of hormonal influences that are not entirely understood. Such hormones are also thought to influence sexual differentiation of the brain. One's gender identity as being male or female is established by 2 to 3 years of life (Bockting, 2016). The final determination of gender identity is influenced by environmental, biologic, and sociocultural factors. At birth the child is named, and significant others, especially the parents, act certain ways toward the infant because of its gender. Touch is crucial to infant development and plays a primary role in gender development. Infants have great oral sensitivity, which is manifested through sucking and mouthing. They enjoy skin-to-skin contact and explore their own body for pleasure. Infants are capable of genital self-stimulation to orgasm;

erections in male infants are common. Parents' responses to these early manifestations of sexuality influence children's evolving attitudes. Therefore a healthy, accepting response by parents is important.

SOCIAL DEVELOPMENT

Infants' social development is initially influenced by their reflexive behavior, such as the grasp, and eventually depends primarily on the interaction between them and the principal caregivers. Attachment to the parent is increasingly evident during the second half of the first year. In addition, infants make tremendous strides in communication and personal-social behavior. Play is a major socializing agent and provides the stimulation needed to learn from interactions with the environment.

Attachment

Human physical contact is extremely important. Parenting is not an instinctual ability but a learned, acquired process. The attachment of parent and child, which begins before birth and assumes even more importance at birth (see Chapter 7), continues during the first year. In the following discussion of attachment, the word *mother* is used in the broad context of the consistent caregiver with whom the child relates more than anyone else. However, in a society with a changing social climate and dissolving sex-role stereotypes, this person may well be the father, grandmother, or other family member.

Studies on father-child attachment demonstrate that stages similar to maternal attachment occur and that fathers are more involved in child care when mothers are employed. Additional research has shown that inexperienced first-time fathers are as capable as experienced fathers of developing a close attachment with their infants. Studies of fathers of high-risk infants demonstrate that fathers experience feelings of love and affection toward their offspring during the newborn period; fathers in one study verbalized more positive feelings of love and affection toward the newborn when they were able to have close physical contact such as holding the child (Feeley, Sherrard, Waitzer, et al., 2013). The father has also been reported to have a significant role in supporting the mother in the perinatal period; fathers of high-risk infants reported concern about their mates' well-being in addition to the status of the ill infant (Feeley, Sherrard, Waitzer, et al., 2013). Research demonstrates that fathers develop feelings of attachment with their offspring and that their relationship with the infant is an important factor in the mother's emotional well-being.

With many single-parent families in existence, a grandmother (or other significant caretaker) may become the primary caretaker. It is important for nurses to recognize that infant-parent attachments may be present or absent in situations where caretaker roles are less well defined by those involved.

When the infant is not provided a safe haven and consistent and loving care, an insecure attachment develops; such infants do not feel they can trust the world in which they live. This insecure attachment may result in psychosocial difficulties as the child grows and may persist even into adulthood. Perinatal maternal depression has been postulated to alter fetal and neonatal neuroendocrine development, which negatively affects the infant's growth and development (Miklush & Connelly, 2013).

Attachment progresses during infancy, with the child assuming an increasingly significant role in the family. Two components of cognitive development are required for attachment: (1) the ability to discriminate the mother from other individuals and (2) the achievement of object permanence. Both these processes prepare the infant for an equally important aspect of attachment: separation from the parent. Separation-individuation should occur as a harmonious, parallel process with emotional attachment.

During the formation of attachment to the parent, the infant progresses through four distinct but overlapping stages. For the first few weeks infants respond indiscriminately to anyone. Beginning at approximately 8 to 12 weeks of age, they cry, smile, and vocalize more to the mother than to anyone else but continue to respond to others, whether familiar or not. At approximately 6 months of age, infants show a distinct preference for the mother. They follow her more, cry when she leaves, enjoy playing with her more, and feel most secure in her arms. About 1 month after showing attachment to the mother, many infants begin attaching to other members of the family, most often the father.

Infants acquire other developmental behaviors that influence the attachment process. These include (1) differential crying, smiling, and vocalization (more to mother than to anyone else); (2) visual-motor orientation (looking more at mother, even if she is not close); (3) crying when the mother leaves the room; (4) approaching through locomotion (crawling, creeping, or walking); (5) clinging (especially in the presence of a stranger); and (6) exploring away from mother while using her as a secure base.

Effects of Prolonged Separation. Attachment is considered so critical to optimum child development that many researchers have documented the effects of prolonged and early separation on infants in the absence of high-quality parent substitutes. Some of the most famous research on emotional deprivation has been done by John Bowlby, John Robertson, and René Spitz. Bowlby (1969) studied the effects of the infant's separation from the mother and noted severe cognitive and physical impairment, particularly if emotional deprivation occurred during the first 3 years of life. He observed that progressive impairment could be arrested or reversed if no further emotional deprivation occurred after the first 2 years, whereas prolonged, severe deprivation beginning early in the first year and lasting for 3 years led to severe, permanent effects. Among these were the inabilities to form trusting, intimate interpersonal relationships; language impairment; and deficiency in abstract thinking. Robertson (1953) and Bowlby (1969) found typical behavioral reactions of infants who were hospitalized and separated from their mothers. (See Separation Anxiety, Chapter 22.)

Spitz (1945) studied the effects of emotional deprivation on children raised in foundling homes or institutions. The infants were cared for by one nurse who had responsibility for eight children. Although the caregiver might be a loving, motherly person, she lacked the time to devote individual attention and stimulation to each child. As a result, the children were delayed in physical growth, were more susceptible to disease, and demonstrated decreasing developmental quotients over a 2-year period. Spitz found that children developed normally if given one-to-one attention by a mother substitute.

Although these studies represent extreme examples of young children reared in environments essentially devoid of high-quality mothering, rather than temporary separation such as day care, the question remains regarding the long-term effects of separation and other stresses on children.

Severe attachment disorders are psychologic and developmental problems that stem from maladaptive or absent attachment between the infant and parent and may persist into childhood and even adulthood (Zeanah & Gleason, 2015). Infants at risk for severe attachment disorders include those who have been victims of physical or sexual abuse or neglect; infants exposed to parental alcoholism, mental illness, or substance abuse; and infants who have experienced the absence of a consistent primary caregiver as a result of foster care, institutionalization, parental abandonment, or parental incarceration (Zeanah & Gleason, 2015). Historically, two different patterns of attachment disorders were described: the emotionally withdrawn–inhibited pattern and an indiscriminate-disinhibited pattern (Zeanah & Gleason, 2015). These patterns have been classified into separate disorders: disinhibited social engagement disorder (DSED) and reactive attachment disorder (RAD) of infancy or early childhood. Children with RAD may manifest behaviors such as not being cuddly with parents, failing to seek and respond to comfort when distressed, minimal social and emotional reciprocity, and emotional deregulation such unexplained fearfulness or irritability (Zeanah & Gleason, 2015). Children with DSED may exhibit behaviors such as inappropriate approach to unfamiliar adults, lack of suspicion of strangers, and poor impulse control (Zeanah & Gleason, 2015). Either or both of these complex disorders are diagnosed with maltreated and orphaned children. Without early intervention, some of these children fail to develop a conscience and suffer from an antisocial personality disorder that may lead to criminal acts. Children with autism or other pervasive developmental disorders have behaviors that are categorically different from those with RAD (Zeanah & Gleason, 2015).

Based on such findings, nurses need to assess each family with the understanding that stress may or may not be necessarily harmful and that children can adapt even under adverse conditions. The nurse evaluates individual risk factors that influence a child's coping ability, using tools such as the Revised Infant Temperament Questionnaire (see later in this chapter) to assess "goodness of fit." When prolonged parental separation occurs, make every effort to help the family provide suitable caregiver substitutes for the child. Individuals who are warm, responsive, and interactive with the infant during separation can significantly minimize the physiologic and behavioral effects. The nurse should emphasize the child's plasticity and resiliency in coping to minimize the family's feelings of responsibility and guilt.

Separation Anxiety. Between the ages of 4 and 8 months the infant progresses through the first stage of separation-individuation and begins to have some awareness of self and mother as separate beings. At the same time, object permanence is developing, and the infant is aware that the parent can be absent. Therefore separation anxiety develops and is manifested through a predictable sequence of behaviors.

During the early second half of the first year, infants protest when placed in their crib, and a short time later they object when the mother leaves the room. Infants may not notice the mother's absence if they are absorbed in an activity. However, when they realize her absence, they protest. From this point on they become very alert to her activities and whereabouts. By 11 to 12 months they are able to anticipate her imminent departure by watching her behaviors, and they begin to protest before she leaves. At this point many parents learn to postpone alerting the child to their departure until just before leaving.

Stranger Fear. As infants demonstrate attachment to one person, they correspondingly exhibit less friendliness to others. Between ages 6 and 8 months fear of strangers and stranger anxiety become prominent and are related to infants' ability to discriminate between familiar and unfamiliar people. Behaviors such as clinging to the parent, crying, and turning away from strangers are common (Fig. 10.11). Suggestions for coping with stranger fear and separation anxiety are listed later in this chapter.

Language Development

The infant's first means of verbal communication is crying. Crying as a biologic sign conveys a message of urgency and signals displeasure, such as hunger. However, crying is also a social event that affects the development of the parent-infant relationship—either by its absence, which usually has a positive effect on parents, or its presence, which may evoke a negative response or persuade parents to minister to the child's physical or emotional needs.

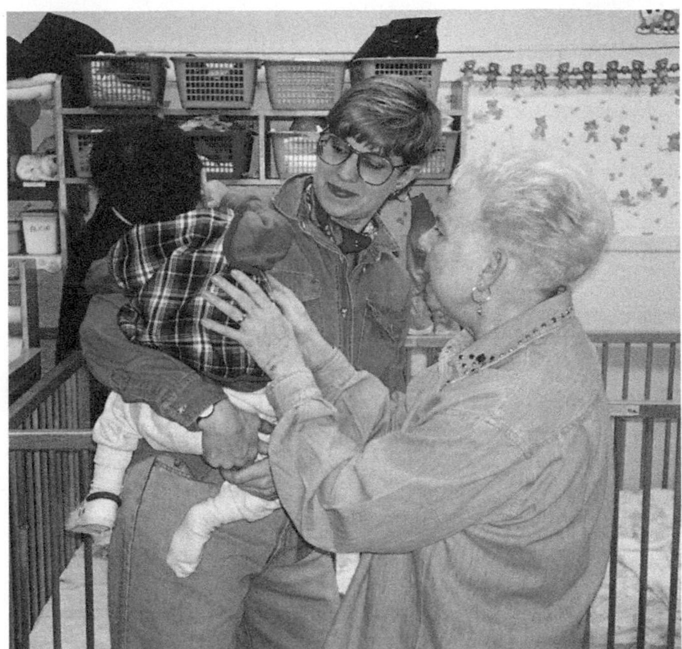

FIG. 10.11 Stranger fear behaviors include clinging to the parent and turning away from a stranger.

In the first few weeks of life, crying has a reflexive quality and is mostly related to physiologic needs. Infants cry for 1 to 1½ hours per day up to 3 weeks of age and then build up to 2 hours and even 4 hours by 6 weeks. Crying tends to decrease by 12 weeks. It is thought that the increase in crying for no apparent reason during the first few months may be related to the discharge of energy and the maturational changes in the central nervous system. By the end of the first year infants cry for attention; from fear (especially stranger fear); and from frustration, usually in response to their developing but inadequate motor skills.

Many parents state that they can distinguish between different types of crying and from these messages are able to interpret the infant's needs. However, crying can be a source of acute distress for parents, especially the inconsolable crying of colic. (See Chapter 11.) Parents benefit from an explanation of the variability of crying among infants and an assurance that periods of "unexplained fussiness" are normal. Some parents may need guidance in consoling techniques, such as holding, swaddling, massaging, caressing, rocking, walking, or stimulating sucking.

Vocalizations heard during crying eventually become syllables and words (e.g., the "mama" heard during vigorous crying). Infants vocalize as early as 5 to 6 weeks of age by making small throaty sounds. By 2 months they make single vowel sounds such as *ah, eh,* and *uh.* By 3 to 4 months the consonants *n, k, g, p,* and *b* are added, and the infants coo, gurgle, and laugh aloud. By 6 months they imitate sounds; add the consonants *t, d,* and *w;* and combine syllables (e.g., "dada"), but they do not ascribe meaning to the word until 10 to 11 months of age. By 9 to 10 months they comprehend the meaning of the word "no" and obey simple commands accompanied by gestures. By age 1 year they can say 3 to 5 words with meaning and may understand as many as 100 words. Because language development is based on expressive (i.e., ability to make thoughts, ideas, and desires known to others) and receptive skills (i.e., ability to understand the words being spoken), it is important that infants are exposed to expressive speech and that delays in achieving milestones are carefully evaluated for potential hearing loss. (See Universal Newborn Hearing Screening, Chapter 7.)

Personal-Social Behavior

Personal-social behavior includes the child's personal responses to the environment. It is the area most influenced by external stimuli, but, as in the other fields of behavior, it follows certain developmental laws. Personal-social behavior implies communication with one's self and with others. It provides the foundation for the successful mastery of skills such as feeding, control of bodily functions, independence, and cooperativeness in play.

Infants have the ability to shape their environment and to elicit certain responses. Newborns show visual preference for the human face and, as early as 1 week of age, begin to watch the parent intently as he or she speaks to them. As they regard the parent's face, activity diminishes, their head bobs up and down, and their mouth moves, almost as if they were trying to say something.

By 6 to 8 weeks a social smile in response to pleasurable stimuli is present. This has a profound effect on family members and evokes continued responses from others. By 3 months infants show considerable interest in the environment—excitement when a toy is presented, refusal to be left alone, recognition of parent, and demonstration of pleasure by squealing. By 4 months they laugh aloud and enjoy strange, novel stimuli.

By 6 months infants are very personable. They play games such as peek-a-boo when their head is hidden in a towel, signal their desire to be picked up by extending their arms, and show displeasure when a toy is removed or their face is washed. They increasingly demonstrate their ability to control the environment. The acquisition of fine and gross motor skills allows much more independence in movement.

By the second half of the first year infants understand simple discipline, such as the meaning of the word "no" or a scolding remark. They comprehend different facial expressions and are sensitive to emotional changes in others. Imitation is developing during this time. They imitate actions and noises by 7 months, sounds by 8 months, and games such as pat-a-cake and peek-a-boo by 10 months.

From 11 months onward they are increasingly independent. They are learning to feed themselves; are using their fingers, spoon, and cup (with much spilling); and can help with dressing by putting the foot out for a shoe or pushing the arm through the sleeve. They not only comprehend the meaning of "no" but also shake their head to indicate "no." They can follow simple directions and gladly perform for others to attract and prolong attention.

Play

Play during infancy represents the various social modalities observed during cognitive development. Infants' activity is primarily narcissistic and revolves around their own body. As discussed under Development of Body Image, body parts are primarily objects of play and pleasure.

During the first year, play becomes more sophisticated and interdependent. From birth to 3 months, infants' responses to the environment are global and largely undifferentiated. Play is dependent; pleasure is demonstrated by a quieting attitude (1 month), a smile (2 months), and a squeal (3 months). From 3 to 6 months infants show more discriminate interest in stimuli and begin to play alone with a rattle or soft stuffed toy or with someone else. They interact much more during play. By 4 months of age they laugh aloud, show preference for certain toys, and become excited when food or a favorite object is brought to them. They recognize an image in a mirror, smile at it, and vocalize to it.

By 6 months to 1 year, play involves sensorimotor skills. Infants play actual games such as peek-a-boo and pat-a-cake. They demonstrate verbal repetition and imitation of simple gestures. Play is much more selective, not only in terms of specific toys but also in terms of "playmates." Although play is solitary or one sided, infants choose with whom they will interact. At 6 to 8 months they usually refuse to play with strangers. Parents are definite favorites, and infants know how to attract their attention. At 6 months they extend the arms to be picked up, at 7 months cough to make their presence known, at 10 months pull the parent's clothing, and at 12 months call them by name. This represents a tremendous advance from the newborn who signaled biologic needs by crying to express displeasure.

Stimulation is as important for psychosocial growth as food is for physical growth. Knowledge of developmental milestones allows nurses to guide parents regarding proper play for infants. It is not sufficient to place a mobile over a crib and toys in a play yard for a child's optimum social, emotional, and intellectual development. Media, other than video-chatting, should be discouraged in all children under the age of 18 months because it does not provide infants with appropriate sensory stimulation and does not increase language skills (American Academy of Pediatrics, Council on Communications and Media, 2016). Play must provide interpersonal contact and recreational and educational stimulation. Infants need to be played with, not merely be allowed to play. Although the type of play infants engage in is called solitary, this is only a figurative, not literal, term to denote one-sided play. The types of toys given to the child are much less important than the quality of personal interaction that occurs.

Table 10.2 lists play activities appropriate for the infant's developmental level in terms of motor, language, and personal-social achievements. Although the activities are grouped according to the major mode of stimulation provided, many examples overlap. In addition, play activities suggested for one age-group may be appropriate for older infants but inappropriate for younger ones.

TEMPERAMENT

The infant's temperament or behavioral style influences the type of interaction that occurs between the child and parents and other family members. In assessing a child's temperament, it is the parents' perception of the child and the degree of fit between their expectations and the child's actual temperament that are important. The more dissonance (or lack of harmony) between the child's temperament and the parent's ability to accept and deal with the behavior, the greater the risk for subsequent parent-child conflicts.

Although many behavioral researchers agree that temperament has a strong biologic component, researchers also suggest that the environment, particularly the family, may modify temperament (Gallitto, 2015). Family interaction with the infant is perceived as a circular process wherein each family member affects one another and the family as a unit. With these concepts in mind, the nurse has an important role in helping the family understand the infant's temperament as it relates to family dynamics and the eventual well-being of the child and family unit (Gallitto, 2015).

Some researchers speculate that maternal depression is linked to infant temperament. Postpartum depression is associated with a difficult infant temperament that negatively affects the maternal-infant relationship (Behrendt, Konrad, Goecke, et al., 2016; Rode & Kiel, 2016). In other studies, infant sleep problems along with temperament affected maternal-infant bonding (Hairston, Solnik-Menilo, Deviri, et al., 2016). Indeed, when there is a lack of reciprocity between the infant and mother, there is increased risk for discord. Fathers also experience postnatal depression when infants have a difficult temperament; other factors influencing fathers' affect included previous loss of a pregnancy, parenting distress, decreased marital adjustment, and perceived low parenting efficacy (Demontigny, Girard, Lacharité, et al., 2013).

TABLE 10.2 Play During Infancy

Age (Months)	Visual Stimulation	Auditory Stimulation	Tactile Stimulation	Kinetic Stimulation
Suggested Activities				
Birth-1	Look at infant at close range. Hang bright, shiny object within 20-25 cm (8-10 inches) of infant's face and in midline. Hang mobiles with black-and-white designs.	Talk to infant; sing in soft voice. Play music box, tape, or compact disc. Have ticking clock or heartbeat doll nearby.	Hold, caress, cuddle. Keep infant warm. Swaddle infant with hands to face.	Rock infant; place in cradle. Use stroller for walks.
2-3	Provide bright objects. Make room bright with pictures or mirrors. Take infant to various rooms while doing chores. Place in infant seat for vertical view of environment (use a safe surface).	Talk to infant. Include infant in family gatherings. Expose to various environmental noises other than those of home. Use rattles, wind chimes.	Caress infant while bathing or changing diaper. Comb hair with a soft brush. Give massage.	Use infant swing. Take in car for rides. Exercise body by moving extremities in swimming motion. Use cradle gym.
4-6	Place infant in front of unbreakable mirror. Give brightly colored toys to hold (small enough to grasp).	Talk to infant; repeat sounds infant makes. Laugh when infant laughs. Call infant by name. Place rattle or bell in hand.	Give infant soft squeeze toys of various textures. Allow to splash in bath. Place nude on soft, furry rug and move extremities.	Use swing or stroller. Bounce infant in lap while holding in standing position. Support infant in sitting position; let infant lean forward to balance self. Place infant on floor to crawl, roll over, sit.
7-9	Give infant large toys with bright colors, movable parts, and noisemakers. Play peek-a-boo, especially hiding face in towel. Make funny faces to encourage imitation. Give ball of yarn or string to pull apart.	Call infant by name. Repeat simple words such as "dada," "mama," "bye-bye." Speak clearly. Name parts of body, people, and foods. Tell infant what you are doing. Use "no" only when necessary. Give simple commands. Show how to clap hands, bang a drum.	Let infant play with fabrics of various textures. Have bowl with foods of different sizes and textures to feel. Let infant "catch" running water. Encourage supervised "swimming" in large bathtub or shallow pool. Give wad of sticky tape to manipulate.	Hold upright to bear weight and bounce. Pick up, say "up." Put down, say "down." Place toys out of reach; encourage infant to get them. Play pat-a-cake.
10-12	Show infant large pictures in books. Play ball by rolling it to child, demonstrate "throwing" it back. Demonstrate building a two-block tower.	Read infant simple nursery rhymes. Point to body parts and name each one. Imitate sounds of animals.	Give infant finger foods of different textures. Let infant mess and squash food. Let infant feel cold (ice cube) or warm objects; say what temperature each is. Let infant feel a breeze (fan blowing).	Give large push-pull toys. Turn in different positions.
Suggested Toys				
Birth-6	Nursery mobiles Unbreakable mirrors	Music boxes Musical mobiles Crib dangle bells Small-handled clear rattle	Stuffed animals Soft clothes* Soft or furry quilt* Soft mobiles	Rocking crib or cradle Weighted or suction toy Infant swing
7-12	Colored blocks Nested boxes or cups Books with rhymes and bright pictures Strings of big beads Simple take-apart toys Large ball Cup and spoon Large-piece wood puzzles Jack-in-the-box	Rattles of different sizes, shapes, tones, and bright colors Squeaky animals and dolls Records with light, rhythmic music	Soft, different-texture animals and dolls Sponge toys, floating toys Squeeze toys Teething toys Books with textures and objects, such as fur and zipper	Activity box for crib Push-pull toys Wind-up swing

*Remove from crib when child is put to sleep to avoid possible suffocation (see suffocation later in this chapter).

TABLE 10.3 Pediatric Quality Indicator*

Developmental Screening in the First 3 Years of Life

Measure	Developmental screen performed during the first 3 years of life
Numerator	Number of children who turn 1, 2, 3 years of age who received developmental screening during the measurement time
Denominator	Number of children who turn 1, 2, 3 years of age who were eligible for developmental screening

*Endorsed by the National Quality Forum-1448 and 2016 Core Set of Children's Health Care Quality Measures for Medicaid and CHIP.

Several instruments can measure infant temperament. These instruments include the Revised Infant Temperament Questionnaire (Carey & McDevitt, 1978), the Infant Behavior Questionnaire (Gartstein & Rothbart, 2003), and the Early Infancy Temperament Questionnaire (Medoff-Cooper, Carey, & McDevitt, 1993). In discussing test results to parents, it is best to avoid descriptors (e.g., "difficult"); instead, infants can be described in terms of characteristics (e.g., "intense" or "less predictable"). With knowledge of the infant's temperament, nurses are better able to (1) provide parents with background information that will help them see their child in a better perspective, (2) offer a more organized picture of their child's behavior and possibly reveal distortions in their perceptions of the behavior, and (3) guide parents regarding appropriate childrearing techniques.

Appropriate guidance based on awareness of the child's temperament can greatly enhance the quality of interaction between parents and infant. Even just letting parents know that "difficult" traits are innate can relieve feelings of guilt and incompetence.

Knowledge of the developmental sequence allows the nurse to assess normal growth and minor or abnormal deviations. It also helps parents gain realistic expectations of their child's ability and provides guidelines for suitable play and stimulation. Parents who lack knowledge of child growth and development may set inappropriate behavioral expectations for their child. Emphasizing the child's developmental rather than chronologic age strengthens the parent-child relationship by fostering trust and lessening frustration. Therefore thorough understanding and appreciation of children's growth and development are essential.

Because of the complexity of the developmental process during the first 12 months, Table 10.4 is presented to help organize and clarify the data already discussed. Although all milestones are important, some represent essential integrative aspects of development that lay the foundation for achievement of more advanced skills. These essential milestones are designated by an asterisk (*) in the table. The table represents the average monthly age at which various skills are attained. It must be remembered that although the sequence is the same, the rate will vary among children. Because of this variation, it is important for nurses to conduct developmental screening with all children. Table 10.3 lists the pediatric quality indicator for developmental screening in early childhood.

COPING WITH CONCERNS RELATED TO NORMAL GROWTH AND DEVELOPMENT

Separation Anxiety and Stranger Fear

A number of fears can appear during infancy. However, the fear that causes many parents concern is related to strangers and separation. Although some erroneously interpret this as a sign of undesirable, antisocial behavior, stranger fear and separation anxiety are important components of a strong, healthy parent-child attachment. Nevertheless, this period can present difficulties for the parent and child. Parents may be more confined to the home because the infant violently protests to being left at day care or having a babysitter. To accustom the infant to new people, encourage parents to have close friends or relatives visit often. This provides other persons with whom the child is comfortable and who can give parents time for themselves.

Infants also need opportunities to safely experience strangers. Usually toward the end of the first year infants begin to venture away from the parent and demonstrate curiosity about strangers. If allowed to explore at their own rate, many infants eventually "warm up." If parents hold the child away from their face, the infant can observe while maintaining close physical contact.

A number of factors influence the intensity of a child's stranger fears:

Gender, age, and size of the stranger—Female, younger age, and smaller size (including kneeling or sitting rather than standing) are less stressful.

Approach—Loud, sudden, intrusive approach causes more distress.

Child's proximity to parent—Being closer to parent (on parent's lap rather than in infant seat) is less stressful.

Consequently, the best approach for the stranger (including the nurse) is to talk softly; meet the child at eye level (to appear smaller); maintain a safe distance from the infant; and avoid sudden, intrusive gestures, such as holding the arms out and smiling broadly.

Parents also may wonder whether they should encourage the child's clinging, dependent behavior, especially if there is pressure from others who view this as spoiling the child (see following discussion). Parents need reassurance that such behavior is healthy, desirable, and necessary for the child's optimum emotional development. If parents can reassure the infant of their presence, the infant will learn to realize that they are still there even if not physically present. Techniques to reassure infants of the parent's continued presence include talking to infants when leaving the room, allowing them to hear one's voice on the telephone, and using transitional objects (e.g., a favorite blanket or toy).

This is no less trying, but a necessary time for infants because parents cannot always be with them. An excellent example of necessary separation is bedtime. Fear of going to bed or being left alone in the dark commonly occurs during the second half of the first year. Fear at bedtime is only one of the many bedtime problems that can occur in young children (see Chapter 11).

Limit Setting and Discipline

As infants' motor skills advance and mobility increases, parents are faced with the need to set safe limits (see Safety Promotion and Injury Prevention later in this chapter). Although numerous disciplinary techniques exist, some are more appropriate for this age than others. Parents can begin discipline using a negative voice and stern eye contact. When parents need to use more definitive measures, one of the most effective approaches is time-out. The basic principles are the same as those discussed in Chapter 2, except that the place for time-out needs to correspond with the child's abilities. For example, the play yard is better for most infants than a chair. Although parents may be concerned with instituting discipline during infancy, it is important to stress that the earlier effective disciplinary methods are employed, the easier it is to continue these approaches.

Parents must recognize the infant's cognitive and behavioral limitations and implement adequate protection from hazards because infants and toddlers do not understand a cause-and-effect relationship between dangerous objects and physical harm. Additionally, parents may need

Text continued on p. 358

TABLE 10.4 **Growth and Development During Infancy**

Age (Months)	Physical	Gross Motor	Fine Motor	Sensory	Vocalization	Socialization/Cognition
1	Weight gain of 150-210 g (5-7 oz) weekly for first 6 months Height gain of 2.5 cm (1 inch) monthly for first 6 months Head circumference increases by 1.5 cm (0.6 inch) monthly for first 6 months Primitive reflexes present and strong Doll's eye reflex and dance reflex fading Obligatory nose breathing (most infants)	■ Assumes flexed position with pelvis high but knees not under abdomen when prone (at birth, knees flexed under abdomen) ■ Can turn head from side to side when prone; lifts head momentarily from bed (see Fig. 10.6, *A*) Has marked head lag, especially when pulled from lying to sitting position (see Fig. 10.5, *A*) Holds head momentarily parallel and in midline when suspended in prone position Assumes asymmetric tonic neck reflex position when supine When held in standing position, is limp at knees and hips In sitting position, has uniformly rounded back, absence of head control	Hands predominantly closed Grasp reflex strong Clenches hand on contact with rattle	■ Able to fixate on moving object in range of 45 degrees when held at distance of 20-25 cm (8-10 inches) Visual acuity approaches 20/100* Follows light to midline Quiets when hears a voice	Cries to express displeasure Makes small, throaty sounds Makes comfort sounds during feeding	Is in sensorimotor phase, stage I, use of reflexes (birth–1 month); and stage II, primary circular reactions (1-4 months) Watches parent's face intently as she or he talks to infant
2	Posterior fontanel closed Crawling reflex disappears	■ Assumes less flexed position when prone—hips flat, legs extended, arms flexed, head to side Less head lag when pulled to sitting position (see Fig. 10.5, *B*) Can maintain head in same plane as rest of body when held in ventral suspension When prone, can lift head almost 45 degrees off table When held in sitting position, can hold head up, but bends forward (see Fig. 10.7, *B*) Assumes asymmetric tonic neck reflex position intermittently	Hands often open Grasp reflex fading	Binocular fixation and convergence to near objects beginning When supine, follows dangling toy from side to point beyond midline Visually searches to locate sounds Turns head to side when sound is made at level of ear	■ Vocalizes, distinct from crying Crying becomes differentiated Coos Vocalizes to familiar voice	■ Demonstrates social smile in response to various stimuli

Continued

TABLE 10.4 **Growth and Development During Infancy—cont'd**

Age (Months)	Physical	Gross Motor	Fine Motor	Sensory	Vocalization	Socialization/Cognition
3	Primitive reflexes fading	Able to hold head more erect when sitting, but still bobs forward Has only slight head lag when pulled to sitting position Assumes symmetric body positioning Able to raise head and shoulders from prone position to 45- to 90-degree angle from table; bears weight on forearms When held in standing position, able to bear slight fraction of weight on legs Regards own hand	■ Actively holds rattle but will not reach for it Grasp reflex absent Hands kept loosely open Clutches own hand; pulls at blankets and clothes	■ Follows objects to periphery (180 degrees) ■ Locates sound by turning head to side and looking in same direction Begins to have ability to coordinate stimuli from various sense organs	■ Squeals aloud to show pleasure Coos, babbles, chuckles Vocalizes when smiling "Talks" a great deal when spoken to Less crying during periods of wakefulness	Displays considerable interest in surroundings Ceases crying when parent enters room Can recognize familiar faces and objects, such as feeding bottle Shows awareness of strange situations
4	Drooling begins ■ Moro, tonic neck, and rooting reflexes disappear	■ Has almost no head lag when pulled to sitting position (see Fig. 10.5, *C*) ■ Balances head well in sitting position (see Fig. 10.7, *C*) Back less rounded, curved only in lumbar area Able to sit erect if propped up Able to raise head and chest off surface to angle of 90 degrees (see Fig. 10.6, *B*) Assumes predominant symmetric position ■ Rolls from back to side	■ Inspects and plays with hands; pulls clothing or blanket over face in play Tries to reach objects with hand but overshoots Grasps object with both hands Plays with rattle placed in hand, shakes it, but cannot pick it up if dropped Can carry objects to mouth	Able to accommodate to near objects Binocular vision fairly well established Can focus on a 1.25-cm (0.5-inch) block Beginning eye-hand coordination	Makes consonant sounds *n, k, g, p, b* ■ Laughs aloud Vocalization changes according to mood	Is in stage III, secondary circular reactions Demands attention by fussing; becomes bored if left alone Enjoys social interaction Anticipates feeding when sees bottle or mother if breastfeeding Shows excitement with whole body, squeals, breathes heavily Shows interest in strange stimuli Begins to show memory
5	Beginning signs of tooth eruption Birth weight doubles	No head lag when pulled to sitting position When sitting, able to hold head erect and steady Able to sit for longer periods when back is well supported Back straight When prone, assumes symmetric positioning with arms extended ■ Can turn over from abdomen to back When supine, puts feet to mouth	■ Able to grasp objects voluntarily Uses palmar grasp, bidextrous approach Plays with toes Takes objects directly to mouth Holds one cube while regarding a second one	Visually pursues dropped object Is able to sustain visual inspection of object Can localize sounds made below ear	Squeals Makes cooing vowel sounds interspersed with consonant sounds (e.g., *ah-goo*)	Smiles at mirror image Pats bottle or breast with both hands More enthusiastically playful, but may have rapid mood swings Is able to discriminate strangers from family Vocalizes displeasure when object is taken away Discovers parts of body

6	Growth rate may begin to decline Weight gain of 90-150 g (3-5 oz) weekly for next 6 months Height gain of 1.25 cm (0.5 inch) monthly for next 6 months ■ May begin teething with eruption of two lower central incisors ■ May chew and bite	When prone, can lift chest and upper abdomen off surface, bearing weight on hands (see Fig. 10.6, *C*) When about to be pulled to sitting position, lifts head Sits in highchair with back straight ■ Rolls from back to abdomen When held in standing position, bears almost all of weight Hand regard absent	Resecures a dropped object Drops one cube when another is given Grasps and manipulates small objects Holds bottle Grasps feet and pulls to mouth	Adjusts posture to see object Prefers more complex visual stimuli Can localize sounds made above ear Will turn head to side, then look up or down	■ Begins to imitate sounds ■ Babbling resembles one-syllable utterances—*ma, mu, da, di, hi* Vocalizes to toys, mirror image Takes pleasure in hearing own sounds (self-reinforcement)	Recognizes parents; begins to fear strangers Holds arms out to be picked up Has definite likes and dislikes Begins to imitate (cough, protrusion of tongue) Excites on hearing footsteps Laughs when head is hidden in towel ■ Briefly searches for dropped object (object permanence beginning) Frequent mood swings from crying to laughing with little or no provocation
7	Eruption of upper central incisors Parachute reflex appears (see Fig. 10.1)	When supine, spontaneously lifts head off surface ■ Sits, leaning forward on both hands (see Fig. 10.7, *D*) When prone, bears weight on one hand Sits erect momentarily Bears full weight on feet (see Fig. 10.8, *A*) When held in standing position, bounces actively	■ Transfers objects from one hand to other (see Fig. 10.7, *E*) Has unidextrous approach and grasp Holds two cubes more than momentarily Bangs cubes on table Rakes at small object	■ Can fixate on very small objects Responds to own name Localizes sound by turning head in curving arch Beginning awareness of depth and space Has taste preferences	■ Produces vowel sounds and chained syllables—*baba, dada, kaka* Vocalizes four distinct vowel sounds "Talks" when others are talking	■ Increasing fear of strangers; shows signs of fretfulness when parent disappears Imitates simple acts and noises Tries to attract attention by coughing or snorting Plays peek-a-boo Demonstrates dislike of food by keeping lips closed Exhibits oral aggressiveness in biting and mouthing Demonstrates expectation in response to repetition of stimuli
8	Begins to show regular patterns in bladder and bowel elimination	■ Sits steadily unsupported (see Fig. 10.7, *E*) Readily bears weight on legs when supported; may stand holding onto furniture Adjusts posture to reach object	Has beginning pincer grasp using index, fourth, and fifth fingers against lower part of thumb Releases objects at will Rings bell purposely Retains two cubes while regarding third cube Secures object by pulling on string Reaches persistently for toys out of reach		Makes consonant sounds *t, d, w* Listens selectively to familiar words Utterances signal emphasis and emotion Combines syllables, such as *dada*, but does not ascribe meaning to them	Exhibits increasing anxiety over loss of parent, particularly mother, and fear of strangers Responds to word "no" Dislikes dressing, diaper change

Continued

TABLE 10.4 **Growth and Development During Infancy—cont'd**

Age (Months)	Physical	Gross Motor	Fine Motor	Sensory	Vocalization	Socialization/Cognition
9	Eruption of upper lateral incisor may begin	Creeps on hands and knees Sits steadily on floor for prolonged time (10 min) Recovers balance when leaning forward but cannot do so when leaning sideways ■ Pulls self to standing position and stands holding onto furniture (see Fig. 10.8, *B* and *C*)	■ Uses thumb and index finger in crude pincer grasp (see Fig. 10.3) Grasps third cube Compares two cubes by bringing them together	Localizes sounds by turning head diagonally and directly toward sound Depth perception increasing	Responds to simple verbal commands Comprehends "no-no"	Parent (mother) is increasingly important for own sake Shows increasing interest in pleasing parent Begins to show fears of going to bed and being left alone Puts arms in front of face to avoid having it washed
10	Labyrinth-righting reflex strongest when infant in prone or supine position; is able to raise head	Can change from prone to sitting position Stands while holding onto furniture, sits by falling down Recovers balance easily while sitting While standing, lifts one foot to take step (see Fig. 10.8, *D*)	Crude release of an object beginning Grasps bell by handle		■ Says "dada," "mama" with meaning Comprehends "bye-bye" May say one word (e.g., "hi," "bye," "no")	Inhibits behavior to verbal command of "no-no" or own name Imitates facial expressions; waves bye-bye Extends toy to another person but will not release it ■ Develops object permanence Repeats actions that attract attention and cause laughter Pulls clothes of another to attract attention Plays interactive games such as pat-a-cake Reacts to adult anger; cries when scolded Demonstrates independence in dressing, feeding, locomotive skills, and testing of parents Looks at and follows picture in book

11	Eruption of lower lateral incisor may begin	When sitting, pivots to reach toward back to pick up an object ■ Cruises or walks holding onto furniture or with both hands held	Explores objects more thoroughly (e.g., clapper inside bell) Has neat pincer grasp Drops object deliberately for it to be picked up Puts one object after another into container (sequential play) Able to manipulate object to remove it from tight-fitting enclosure		Imitates definite speech sounds	Experiences joy and satisfaction when task is mastered Reacts to restrictions with frustration Rolls ball to another on request Anticipates body gestures when familiar nursery rhyme or story is being told (e.g., holds toes and feet in response to "This little piggy went to market") Plays games up-down, "so big," or peek-a-boo Shakes head for "no"
12	■ Birth weight tripled ■ Birth length increased by 50% Head and chest circumference equal (head circumference 46 cm [18 inches]) Has six to eight deciduous teeth Anterior fontanel almost closed Landau reflex fading Babinski reflex disappears Lumbar curve develops; lordosis evident during walking	■ Walks with one hand held Cruises well ■ May attempt to stand alone momentarily; may attempt first step alone Can sit down from standing position without help	Releases cube in cup Attempts to build two-block tower but fails Tries to insert pellet into narrow-necked bottle but fails Can turn pages in book, many at a time	Discriminates simple geometric forms (e.g., circle) Amblyopia may develop with lack of binocularity Can follow rapidly moving object Controls and adjusts response to sound; listens for sound to recur	■ Says three to five words besides "dada," "mama" Comprehends meaning of several words (comprehension always precedes verbalization) Recognizes objects by name Imitates animal sounds Understands simple verbal commands (e.g., "Give it to me," "Show me your eyes")	Shows emotions such as jealousy, affection (may give hug or kiss on request), anger, fear Enjoys familiar surroundings and explores away from parent Is fearful in strange situation; clings to parent May develop habit of "security blanket" or favorite toy Has increasing determination to practice locomotor skills ■ Searches for object even if it has not been hidden, but searches only where object was last seen

■Milestones that represent essential integrative aspects of development that lay the foundation for the achievement of more advanced skills.
*Degree of visual acuity varies according to vision measurement procedure used.

reassurance that their infant's behavior is exploratory, not oppositional (at this age) and primarily centered on needs for warmth, love, food, security, and comfort. Parents may verbalize that comforting the infant too much or meeting his or her needs will result in a spoiled child; there is no substantial evidence that meeting the infant's basic needs will result in such behaviors later in life. Children will innately test limits and explore during the exploratory phase of growth; instead of discouraging exploration, parents should provide safe alternatives, put away dangerous household items, and give children consistent discipline and nurturing. Effective teaching for injury prevention optimally begins in infancy by helping parents understand their child's normal development. It must be reiterated continually that infants cry because a need is not being met, not to intentionally irritate an adult. The fussy or irritable infant is a potential victim of traumatic brain injury or shaken baby syndrome* (or other bodily harm) because adults and caretakers may not understand the nature of the infant's crying (see also Chapter 11, Colic).

A common concern of parents is that too much attention can spoil a child. Many of the recommendations for promoting attachment, such as attending to the infant's needs to establish trust, accepting fear of strangers and separation from parent, and holding and rocking the crying child, are described by parents as methods of spoiling. However, research on parents' response to crying during early infancy does not support the contention that picking up a crying baby leads to spoiling. Ainsworth (1982) found that the amount an infant cried during the first 3 months had no correlation with the frequency of crying during the rest of the first year. However, the degree of maternal responsiveness to crying did. Parents who were less responsive, such as not picking up the infant immediately on crying, had infants who cried more than those of parents who responded promptly to crying. Parents of colicky infants less than 3 months old who responded to the crying with increased attention successfully decreased the overall crying time.

If too much attention does not cause spoiling in early infancy, parents need to understand what "spoiling" really is and how it differs from normal behavior that may mimic aspects of spoiling. The spoiled child syndrome has been defined as "excessive self-centered and immature behavior, resulting from the failure of parents to enforce consistent, age-appropriate limits" (McIntosh, 1989). Spoiled children demand to have their own way; are inconsiderate of others; and have intrusive, obstructive, and manipulative behavior. Indulging children, when combined with clear expectations and limits, does not cause spoiling. However, indulgence with failure to provide guidelines for acceptable behavior can result in a child who expects to get her or his way all the time. Such expectations are unrealistic and do not help the child in the transition to older childhood, adolescence, and adulthood.

Several age-related normal behaviors and child characteristics can be mistaken for evidence of spoiling:

- Crying during early infancy that may or may not be associated with colic
- Crying associated with unmet basic physical need (e.g., soiled diaper, hunger, physical contact)
- Toddler behaviors such as negativism, persistent exploration, and temper tantrums
- Children experiencing extreme stress from marital discord; physical, emotional, or sexual abuse; substance abuse; or mental illness in a parent

*One resource for parents and health care professionals is the National Center on Shaken Baby Syndrome and the Period of Purple Crying Program, 1433 North 1075 W, Suite 110, Farmington, UT, 84025; 801-447-9360; http://www.dontshake.org.

With anticipatory guidance regarding expected but challenging behaviors and situations that may produce extreme stress in children, parents should feel comfortable in loving their infant without fear of spoiling. However, as the infant gets older, parents may need assistance in providing limits that prevent normal, disruptive behaviors, such as temper tantrums, from becoming problems.

Alternative Child Care Arrangements

For many parents, especially working mothers, locating safe and competent child care facilities for the infant is a challenge—one that is compounded by the number of mothers working outside the home. Over the past 40 years a marked shift has occurred in child care arrangements, with fewer children cared for at home and more children cared for in group centers or other settings.

Types of Child Care. The basic types of care are in-home care, either in the parents' or caregivers' home (family day care); and center-based care, usually in a day care center. In-home care may consist of a full-time babysitter who lives in the home, a full-time babysitter who comes to the home, cooperative arrangements such as exchange babysitting, and family day care. A licensed small family child day care home typically provides care and protection for up to six children for part of a day and does not include informal arrangements such as exchange babysitting or caregivers in the child's own home. The six children include the family day care provider's own children younger than 5 years of age living in the home. Large family child care homes may provide care for 8 to 12 children.

Child center–based care usually refers to a licensed day care facility that provides care for six or more children for 6 or more hours a day. Work-based group care is another option that is becoming increasingly popular as employers recognize the benefit of providing high-quality and convenient child care to their employees. Sick-child care may also be available for times when the child is ill. Such programs are often located in community hospitals or in work settings.

Guiding Parents in Selecting Child Care. An important nursing responsibility is guiding parents in locating suitable facilities that have a well-qualified staff. State licensing agencies can help parents identify day care centers that accept children of specific age-groups and are convenient to home and work. Their records are available to the public and provide reports from the health, safety, and fire departments; periodic evaluations from the licensing agency; complaints filed against the center; and qualification of the center's employees. State-licensed programs are supposed to follow established standards, which represent the minimum requirements and safeguards. However, enforcement of the standards is sometimes inadequate. Early childhood programs may also belong to a voluntary accreditation system, the National Academy of Early Childhood Programs/NAEYC,* which serves as a model for

*Information about accreditation criteria and procedures of the National Academy for Early Childhood Program Accreditation/NAEYC is available from the National Association for the Education of Young Children, 1313 L St. NW, Suite 500, Washington, DC 20005; 800-424-2460 or 202-232-8777; http://www.naeyc.org. These criteria are excellent guidelines for evaluating child care facilities. Other resources are (1) Choosing Quality Childcare: What's Best for Your Family? and a number of other child care articles and pamphlets from American Academy of Pediatrics, 141 Northwest Point Blvd., Elk Grove Village, IL 60007; 800-433-9016 or 847-434-4000; http://aap.org; and (2) Child Care Aware, 800-424-2246; http://www.childcareaware.org.

optimum care. References from other parents are also helpful, provided they have investigated the center carefully and have remained involved with the agency's activities.

Other areas for parents to evaluate are the center's daily program, teacher qualifications, nurturing qualities of caregivers, student-to-staff ratio, discipline policy, emergency protocols (e.g., fire, tornado), environmental safety precautions, provision of meals, sanitary conditions, adequate indoor and outdoor space per child, and fee schedule. Although fees vary considerably, a program that charges a minimum fee may also be providing minimum services. In terms of an overall evaluation, there is no substitute for personal observation of the facility. Parents should arrange to meet the director and some of the employees, especially those who would be caring for the child. Resources to familiarize parents with characteristics of quality child care and checklists to systematically evaluate the center and compare it with other facilities can help parents make successful choices. At all times the parent should have the right to visit the child, and regular conferences should occur to review the child's progress.

Parents should apply the same conscientious attention to locating competent babysitters. References from other employers are essential, and there is no substitute for observing the interaction between the individual and the child. Although very young infants need little if any preparation for the introduction of a new caregiver, older infants may benefit from a gradual placement to reduce stranger fear. (See Preschool and Kindergarten Experience, Chapter 13.)

One of the areas that is increasingly important in selecting child care is the center's health practices; however, parents often do not check the center for health and safety features. Children in day care centers, especially children under age 3 years, have more illnesses—including diarrhea, otitis media, respiratory tract infections (especially if the caregiver smokes), hepatitis A, meningitis, and cytomegalovirus—than children cared for in their home. The strongest predictor of risk of illness is the number of unrelated children in the room. Proactive infection control measures and education of staff are effective in reducing the incidence of upper respiratory tract infections, diarrhea, and rotavirus. Parents should inquire about the center's policy regarding the attendance and care of sick children. Parents with children in day care or even with in-home care need to discuss safe sleep positions and environments for infants in order to prevent SIDS; a number of SIDS cases have occurred in day care centers (Matthews & Moore, 2013).

Nurses play an important role in infection control and injury prevention. Not only can they advise parents on evaluating a center's sanitary and safety practices, but they can also take an active part in educating staff in measures to minimize the transmission of infection and injury. Guidelines for diapering and toileting recommended by the American Academy of Pediatrics, Committee on Infectious Diseases (2015) include the following:

- Washing hands by children and personnel after diaper changing and toileting
- Using disposable paper diapers, single-unit reusable cloth diapers with an inner cotton lining attached to an outer waterproof cover, or single-unit reusable systems with an inner cotton lining attached to an outer waterproof covering that are changed as a unit
- Changing diapers as soon as they are soiled
- Never rinsing reusable diapers, although fecal contents can be flushed down the toilet
- Sending soiled reusable diapers or clothing home in a sealed plastic bag
- Cleaning the diaper-changing surface properly after each use and using it only for this purpose
- Using child-sized toilets or access to steps and modified toilet seats that provide easier maintenance
- Sanitizing toilets, seats, potty chairs, and diaper-changing areas with a fresh solution of 1:64 dilution of household bleach (one-quarter cup of bleach diluted in 1 gallon of water), applied for 2 minutes and rinsed

The American Academy of Pediatrics' *2015 Red Book: Report of the Committee on Infectious Diseases* (2015) contains additional infection control guidelines regarding day care hand hygiene; cleaning sleep equipment and toys; food handling, preparation, and disposal; handling, storage, and feeding of human milk; care of pets; and conditions or illnesses for which children should be kept out of day care to prevent the spread of illness. In addition, such centers should share information about nationally notifiable infectious diseases that could be communicated to the child or immediate family member (American Academy of Pediatrics, Committee on Infectious Diseases, 2015).

Thumb Sucking and Use of Pacifier

Sucking is the infant's chief pleasure and may not be satisfied by breastfeeding or bottle-feeding. It is such a strong need that infants who are deprived of sucking, such as those with a cleft lip repair, will suck on their tongues. Some newborns are born with sucking blisters on their hands from in utero sucking activity.

Problems arise when parents are overly concerned about the sucking of the fingers, thumb, or pacifier and attempt to restrain this natural tendency. Before giving advice, nurses should investigate the parents' feelings and base guidance on this information.

Pacifier use, particularly in the early days after birth and in the birth hospital, has gained considerable attention in the scientific literature. In the past, experts on breastfeeding recommended that health care workers not introduce pacifiers to breastfed infants unless the parent requested it; however, recent research has shown no effects on pacifier use and breastfeeding (see Research Focus box). Researchers and experts have proposed that the pacifier itself may not be the cause of premature cessation of breastfeeding, but rather signal a decision by the mother to stop breastfeeding (Goldman, 2013). Still, pacifier use should not replace actual feeding or suckling, and there should be an emphasis on allowing the infant to control the pace, frequency, and termination of feeding rather than allowing the pacifier (or anything else) to become the focus of the interaction.

RESEARCH FOCUS

Pacifier Use and Breastfeeding

Jaafar, Ho, Jahanafar, and colleagues (2016) performed a meta-analysis on the effects of pacifier use on healthy full-term newborns whose mothers initiated breastfeeding and concluded that pacifier use did not adversely affect breastfeeding duration or exclusivity. Others found that restricting pacifier distribution at the birth hospital did not increase exclusive breastfeeding; instead, they noted a significant increase in the use of supplemental formula feedings in breastfed newborns and a concomitant decrease in the incidence of exclusive breastfeeding (Kair, Kenron, Etheredge, et al., 2013).

Pacifier use has been associated with an increased risk of otitis media in several studies (Ilia & Galanakis, 2013; Salah, Abdel-Aziz, Al-Farok, et al., 2013). The American Academy of Pediatrics and American Academy of Family Physicians recommend using a pacifier during the first 6 months because of the benefit with regard to pain management during painful procedures and prevention of sudden infant death syndrome (SIDS), but they recommend that the child be weaned from the pacifier during the second 6 months of life (American Academy of Pediatrics, Task Force on Sudden Infant Death Syndrome, 2016). However, non-nutritive sucking such as a pacifier during painful procedures in neonates has been shown to produce an analgesic effect. (See Atraumatic Care box, Chapter 7.)

The American Academy of Pediatrics, Task Force on Sudden Infant Death Syndrome (2016) cites strong evidence for pacifier use and its protective effect in SIDS reduction and recommends pacifier use as soon as desired in infants who are not directly breastfed and as soon as breastfeeding is established in infant who are breastfed. The exact mechanism involved in the protection for SIDS is not known.

If the child uses a pacifier, stress safety considerations in purchasing one. Caution parents against altering a pacifier, thus making it more dangerous (see Aspiration and Suffocation, Chapter 12). Pacifiers with added decorative gems or "bling" may be dangerous because the infant or child may remove the decorative object and swallow it or aspirate it into the airway.

During infancy and early childhood there is no need to restrain nonnutritive sucking of the fingers. Malocclusion may occur if thumb sucking persists past approximately 4 years of age, or when the permanent teeth erupt. Some parents may perceive pacifiers as less damaging because they are discarded by 2 to 3 years of age, whereas thumb sucking may persist well into school-age years. Both pacifier use and thumb sucking may also have significant cultural variations. Thumb sucking reaches its peak at age 18 to 20 months and is most prevalent when the child is hungry, tired, or feeling insecure. Persistent thumb sucking in a listless, apathetic child always warrants investigation. It may be a sign of an emotional problem between parent and child or of boredom, isolation, and lack of stimulation.

There is recent evidence that pacifier use may improve nonnutritive sucking in preterm infants. A randomized control trial with 70 preterm infants found that infants who received a pacifier had significantly better sucking skills and shorter time to transition to full breastfeeding compared with a control group of preterm infants without pacifiers (Kaya & Aytekin, 2016). Nonnutritive sucking should not be withheld from preterm infants.

Teething

One of the more difficult periods in the infant's (and parents') life is the eruption of the deciduous (primary) teeth, often referred to as teething. The age of tooth eruption shows considerable variation among children, but the order of their appearance is fairly regular and predictable (Fig. 10.12). The first primary teeth to erupt are the lower central incisors, which appear at approximately 6 to 10 months of age (average 8 months). These are followed closely by the upper central incisors. The following is a quick guide to assessment of deciduous teeth during the first 2 years: Age of the child in months − 6 = Number of teeth. For example, 8 months of age − 6 = 2 teeth at this time.

Teething is a physiologic process. Some discomfort is common as the crown of the tooth breaks through the periodontal membrane. Some children show minimum evidence of teething, such as drooling, increased finger sucking, or biting on hard objects. Others are irritable and have difficulty sleeping, mild temperature elevation, ear rubbing, and decreased appetite for solid foods. Generally, signs of illness such as fever (>39°C [102°F]), vomiting, or diarrhea are not symptoms of teething but of illness and may warrant further investigation.

Because teething pain is a result of inflammation, cold is soothing. Giving the child a frozen teething ring or an ice cube wrapped in a washcloth helps relieve the inflammation. Several nonprescription topical anesthetic ointments are available, although the active ingredient in most of them is benzocaine, which if ingested may cause a rare but serious disorder called *methemoglobinemia.* Therefore anesthetic ointments should only be used under the direct advice and supervision of a health care provider (US Food and Drug Administration, 2017). If persistent irritability affects sleeping and feeding, systemic analgesics such as acetaminophen or ibuprofen (if *age appropriate*) can be given for no more than 3 days. However, parents should know that this is a temporary measure and should contact the practitioner if symptoms persist or if the child's condition changes. Discourage the use of teething powders or procedures such as cutting or rubbing the gums with aspirin or liquor because ingestion of the powder, infection or irritation of the tissue, or aspiration of the aspirin can occur. Hard candy may cause accidental choking or aspiration and should be avoided at this age. Amber teething necklaces should not be worn by infants and small children because of the danger of choking and suffocation, as well as the danger that beads may become dislodged and ingested by the infant.

PROMOTING OPTIMUM HEALTH DURING INFANCY

NUTRITION

Ideally, discussion of optimum nutrition should begin prenatally with the decision to breastfeed or bottle-feed the newborn. The choice for either is highly individual and is discussed in Chapter 7. This section is primarily concerned with infant nutrition during the next 12 months, when growth needs and developmental milestones ready the child for the introduction of solid foods.

Despite adequate availability of optimum nutrient sources, experts are concerned that infants are not fed appropriately (Moss & Yeatin, 2014). Infants may be given solid foods when their digestive system is not ready to completely absorb such foods. In addition, drinks that are inappropriate for growing infants may be given in place of enriched

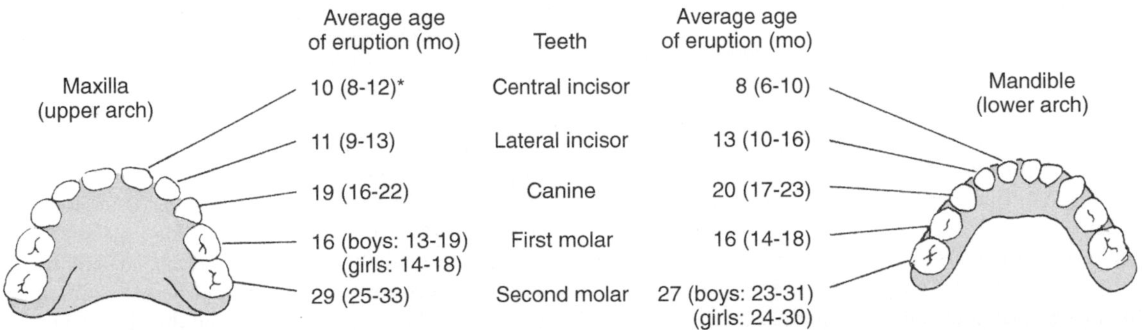

FIG. 10.12 Sequence of eruption of primary teeth. *Range represents 1 standard deviation, or 67% of subjects studied. (Data from American Dental Association. Retrieved from: http://www.mouthhealthy.org/en/az-topics/e/eruption-charts.)

infant milk and may only provide "empty" calories and contribute to childhood and adult cardiovascular disease or obesity and place the infant at risk for iron deficiency anemia, vitamin D deficiency, and rickets. A survey of infant feeding practices found that about 24% of infants had consumed infant cereal, fruit, or vegetables by 4 months of age, despite recommendations that such foods not be introduced until 4 to 6 months (Moss & Yeatin, 2014). There is evidence that early introduction of solid food before 4 months of life is correlated with obesity later in life (Barrera, Perrine, Li, et al., 2016; Moss & Yeatin, 2014); however, there is no correlation between length of breastfeeding duration and obesity later in life (Barrera, Perrine, Li, et al., 2016; Redsell, Edmonds, Swift, et al., 2016).

Infant nutrition has a far-reaching, long-term impact on the child's life. Growth and development could be negatively affected, as could the risk of acquiring certain chronic health conditions. Nurses must be proactive in teaching parents what constitutes appropriate infant nutrition and nutritional habits, which provide the child with an optimum opportunity to grow and develop into a healthy child and adult.

Health Canada, in concert with the Canadian Paediatric Society, Dietitians of Canada, and Breastfeeding Committee for Canada, has published and recently updated nutrition guidelines for healthy term infants from birth to 6 months of age. Most of the previous discussions reflect these guidelines, as well as those promoted by the American Academy of Pediatrics. The Canadian guidelines are available in English online at http://www.hc-sc.gc.ca/fn-an/nutrition/infant-nourisson/recom/index-eng.php.

The First 6 Months*

Human milk is the most desirable complete diet for the infant during the first 6 months. Breastfeeding is rarely contraindicated; the main contraindications to breastfeeding include mothers who are HIV-positive; mothers taking illicit drugs such as heroin, cocaine, methamphetamines, or PCP (angel dust); mothers taking antimetabolites or radioactive medications; and maternal illnesses such as T-cell leukemia/lymphoma (Lawrence & Lawrence, 2016). Although very few routinely prescribed drugs are hazardous to breastfeeding infants, experts recommend consulting with the health care provider to determine the benefits and hazards of certain maternal medications (Lawrence & Lawrence, 2016).

The healthy term infant receiving breast milk from a well-nourished mother usually requires no specific vitamin and mineral supplements, with a few exceptions. Daily supplements of vitamin D and vitamin B_{12} may be indicated if the mother's intake of these vitamins is inadequate. The American Academy of Pediatrics (Kleinman & Greer, 2014) recommends that all infants (including those exclusively breastfed) receive a daily supplement of 400 international units (IU) of vitamin D beginning in the first few days of life to prevent rickets and vitamin D deficiency. Vitamin D supplementation should occur until the infant is consuming at least 1 L/day (or 1 quart/day) of vitamin D–fortified formula. Nonbreastfed infants who are taking less than 1 L/day of vitamin D–fortified formula should also receive a daily vitamin D supplement of 400 IU. If the infant is exclusively breastfed after 4 months (when fetal iron stores are depleted), iron supplementation (1 mg/kg/day) is recommended until appropriate iron-containing complementary foods such as iron-fortified cereal are introduced (Kleinman & Greer, 2014) (see Community and Home Health Considerations). Infants, whether breastfed or bottle-fed, do not require additional fluids, especially water or juice, during the first 4 months of life. Excessive intake of water in infants may result in water intoxication and hyponatremia.

*A comprehensive list of infant feeding resources is available from the US Department of Agriculture website at https://wicworks.fns.usda.gov/infants/complementary-foods.

COMMUNITY AND HOME HEALTH CONSIDERATIONS

Safety Alert

There are reports of accidental overdoses of liquid vitamin D in infants because of packaging errors; the syringe for liquid administration may not be labeled clearly for 400 IU. Nurses should educate parents to read the syringe and to avoid administering more than 400 IU of vitamin D.

Substituting skim or low-fat milk is unacceptable because the essential fatty acids are inadequate and the solute concentration of protein and electrolytes, such as sodium, is too high.

Fluoride supplementation in exclusively breastfed children is not required for the first 6 months because of the risk of dental fluorosis. However, fluoride supplementation may be necessary if the breastfeeding mother's water supply does not contain the required amount of fluoridation (see information later in this chapter).

An acceptable alternative to breastfeeding is commercial iron-fortified formula. Like human milk, it supplies all nutrients needed by the infant for the first 6 months. Unmodified whole cow's milk, low-fat cow's milk, skim milk, other animal milks, and imitation milk drinks are not acceptable as a major source of nutrition for infants because of their limited digestibility, increased risk of contamination, and lack of components needed for appropriate growth. Whole milk can cause iron deficiency anemia in infants, possibly as a result of occult gastrointestinal blood loss. Pasteurized whole cow's milk is deficient in iron, zinc, and vitamin C and has a high renal solute load, which makes it undesirable for infants less than 12 months of age (Kleinman & Greer, 2014). Dietary fat should not be restricted in infancy unless under medical supervision. Substituting skim or low-fat milk is unacceptable because the essential fatty acids are inadequate and the solute concentration of protein and electrolytes, such as sodium, is too high.

Honey should be avoided in the first 12 months because of the risk of infant botulism (see Chapter 34); pacifiers should not be coated with honey to encourage the infant to take it. Socializing the infant to food flavors of the family's culture is common in addition to continuing breastfeeding for 2 to 4 years (see Cultural Considerations box). The amount of formula per feeding and the number of feedings per day vary among infants.

CULTURAL CONSIDERATIONS

Multicultural Feeding Practices

Cultural beliefs and values often influence infant feeding practices. Health care professionals may benefit from understanding the multicultural feeding practices that parents choose for their infant. Traditional feeding practices include offering a variety of liquids or foods, such as sugared wine, water, or honey, during the first few days of life and thereafter.

Employed mothers can continue breastfeeding with guidance and encouragement.* Encourage mothers to set realistic goals for employment and breastfeeding, with accurate information regarding the costs, risks, and benefits of available feeding options. Barriers encountered by working breastfeeding mothers include lack of employer or co-worker support,

*See also *The CDC Guide to Strategies to Support Breastfeeding Mothers and Babies,* which includes information for breastfeeding in the workplace. This guide can be downloaded at http://www.cdc.gov/breastfeeding/pdf/BF-Guide-508.PDF.

unavailable or inadequate facilities for pumping and storing milk, and insufficient time allowed during work time to pump. Many mothers may find that a program of breast-pumping when away from home and bottle-feeding the infant the expressed milk with or without formula supplementation is successful. Expressed breast milk may be stored in the refrigerator (4°C [39°F]) but should be used within 48 hours (Parks, Shaikhkhalil, Groleau, et al., 2016). Breast milk should never be thawed or rewarmed in a microwave oven (Parks, Shaikhkhalil, Groleau, et al., 2016). To thaw the frozen milk, either place container under a lukewarm water bath (40.5°C [105°F]), use a commercial breast milk warmer, or place in a refrigerator overnight.

Although at home the infant may be fed on a demand basis, pumping milk away from home may be needed every 3 to 4 hours to maintain an adequate supply. Breast milk may be expressed by hand or pump (manual or electric) and stored in an appropriate airtight glass or plastic container. Expressed breast milk may be frozen (−18°C [0°F] or lower) for up to 6 months (depending on the type of freezer used), but take care to prevent freezer burn (see Lawrence & Lawrence, 2016, for further guidelines on storing and freezing human milk).

One recent survey of breastfeeding mothers found that mothers stopped breastfeeding before 6 months because they were concerned about infant weight gain and adequate milk supply, difficulties with lactation, illness or need to take medications, and the effort associated with pumping milk to maintain milk supply (Odom, Li, Scanlon, et al., 2013).

> **! NURSING ALERT**
>
> Neither infant formula nor breast milk should be warmed in a microwave oven because this may cause oral burns as a result of uneven heating in the container; the bottle or container may remain cool while hot spots develop in the formula.

The addition of solid foods before 4 to 6 months of age is not recommended. During the early months solid foods are not yet compatible with the ability of the gastrointestinal tract and the infant's nutritional needs. Despite the recommendations not to introduce food into the infant's diet until after 4 to 6 months, studies have found that many parents continue to introduce solid foods sometimes as early as 2 weeks of life (Clayton, Li, Perrine, et al., 2013; Heinrich, Koletzko, & Koletzko, 2014). Developmentally, infants are not ready for solid food. The extrusion (protrusion) reflex is strong and often causes food to be pushed out of the mouth. Infants instinctively suck when given food. Because of their limited motor abilities, infants are unable to deliberately push food away or avoid feeding.

Early introduction of solid food may also reduce the frequency of breastfeeding or cause eventual cessation of breastfeeding before 6 months of age (Clayton, Li, Perrine, et al., 2013). Caution parents concerning the excessive use of juices and nonnutritive drinks such as fruit-flavored drinks or carbonated beverages (soda or pop) during this period. Many juices and nonnutritive drinks, although readily available to consumers, do not provide sufficient and appropriate caloric intake for infants less than 12 months of age. Such drinks may replace the nutrients in milk (formula) and lead to growth or health problems. Fruit juices are not required in the first 6 months; there are no studies demonstrating benefits of giving fruit juice to infants.

Bottled water for mixing powdered or concentrated formula is a relatively safe alternative to tap water if available tap water has a high content of contaminants such as lead. Do not assume, however, that bottled water is sterile unless specifically stated on the container. Fluoridated bottled water is not necessary for mixing powdered formula unless the local water source is low in fluoride, in which case fluoride supplementation is recommended after age 6 months (see Dental Health later in this chapter).

The Second 6 Months

During the second half of the first year, human milk or formula continues to be the primary source of nutrition. Fluoride supplementation begins depending on the infant's intake of fluoridated tap water when mixing commercial formula. Breast milk remains the best source of nutrition well into the second half of the first year; however, if it is discontinued, a commercial iron-fortified formula should be substituted. Formulas specially marketed for older infants, or follow-up formulas, offer no advantages over other infant formulas and provide excessive protein (Kleinman & Greer, 2014).

The major change in feeding habits is the addition of solid foods to the infant's diet. Physiologically and developmentally, the infant 4 to 6 months of age is in a transition period. By this time the gastrointestinal tract has matured sufficiently to handle more complex nutrients and is less sensitive to potentially allergenic foods. Tooth eruption is beginning and facilitates biting and chewing. The extrusion reflex has disappeared, and swallowing is more coordinated to allow the infant to accept solids easily. Head control is well developed, which permits infants to sit with support and purposely turn the head away to communicate a lack of interest in food. Voluntary grasping and improved eye-hand coordination gradually allow infants to pick up finger foods and feed themselves. Their increasing independence is evident in their desire to hold the bottle and try to "help" during feeding. The major developmental milestones associated with feeding are listed in Box 10.4.

BOX 10.4 Developmental Milestones Associated With Feeding

Birth

Sucking, rooting, and swallowing reflexes

Feels hunger and indicates desire for food by crying; expresses satiety by falling asleep

Strong extrusion reflex

3 to 4 Months

Extrusion reflex fading

Beginning eye-hand coordination

4 to 5 Months

Can approximate lips to the rim of a cup but may spill contents

5 to 6 Months

Can use fingers to feed self a cracker

6 to 7 Months

Chews and bites

May hold own bottle, but may not drink from it (prefers for it to be held)

7 to 9 Months

Refuses food by keeping lips closed; has preferences

Holds a spoon and plays with it during feeding

May drink from a straw

Drinks from a cup with assistance

9 to 12 Months

Picks up small morsels of food (finger foods) and feeds self

Holds own bottle and drinks from it

Drinks from a cup but spills some of the contents

Uses a spoon with much spilling

Previous recommendations for preventing food allergies and atopy in children have been to avoid introducing potentially allergenic foods after 6 to 8 months of life, but there is now some debate about whether avoidance of such foods is preventive (Heinrich, Koletzko, & Koletzko 2014; Kleinman & Greer, 2014) (see also Chapter 11, Food Sensitivity).

Selection and Introduction of Solid Foods

The choice of solid foods to introduce first is variable but should meet the reasons for feeding solids, such as supplying nutrients not found in formula or breast milk. Iron-fortified infant cereal is generally introduced first because of its high iron content (7 mg/3 tbsp of prepared dry cereal). Commercially prepared ready-to-serve dry cereals for infants include rice, barley, oatmeal, and high-protein cereals. Rice is usually suggested as an initial food because of its easy digestibility and low allergenic potential. Some of the commercial baby cereals are combined with fruit. These preparations have little nutritional benefit and are more expensive. Parents should add new foods one at a time; therefore parents should avoid cereal combinations when beginning a new grain.

Infant cereal may be mixed with formula in a bowl until whole milk is given. If the infant is breastfed, the cereal is mixed with expressed breast milk or water. After 6 months of age, fruit juices can be mixed with the dry cereal. The vitamin C content of the juice enhances the absorption of iron in the cereal. Because of their benefit as a source of iron, continue iron-fortified infant cereals until the child is 18 months of age.

Parents can offer fruit juice from a cup as a rich source of vitamin C and as a substitute for milk for one feeding a day. Avoid certain juices (e.g., apple, pear, prune, sweet cherry, peach, grape) because they contain high amounts of fructose and sorbitol and may cause abdominal pain, diarrhea, or bloating in some children. The American Academy of Pediatrics (Kleinman & Greer, 2014) recommends that fruit juice intake not exceed 4 to 6 oz/day in children 1 to 6 years of age and that juices not be given to infants less than 4 to 6 months old; only 100% fruit juice should be offered. Because heat destroys vitamin C, juice is not warmed. Juice containers are always kept covered and refrigerated to prevent further vitamin loss. In addition, fruit juice may be offered from a cup, rather than a bottle, to prevent the development of dental caries. (See Dietary Factors, Chapter 12.)

The order of introduction of other foods is arbitrary. A common sequence is strained fruits, followed by vegetables, and, finally, meats. Some clinicians recommend adding vegetables before fruit. Only one solid is introduced every 5 to 7 days so that a reaction to a particular food can be distinguished. At 6 months foods such as a cracker or zwieback can be offered as finger and teething food. By 8 to 9 months junior foods and nutritious finger foods such as a firmly cooked vegetable, raw pieces of fruit (except grapes), or cheese can be given. By 1 year well-cooked table foods may be served.

The introduction of solid foods into the infant's diet at this age is primarily for taste and chewing experience. The majority of the infant's caloric needs come from the primary milk source (human or formula); therefore solids should not be perceived as a substitute for milk until the child is older than 12 months. Portion sizes may vary according to the infant's taste. In general, 1 tbsp per year of age (i.e., ½ to ¾ tbsp for most infants under 12 months) is adequate for most infants. In most cases 2 tbsp may be served, but because of the infant's focus on the texture and feel of the food, smaller amounts than those served will be consumed. Another consideration for smaller portions is the concern over feeding habits in early childhood and obesity; early feeding of smaller portions may help prevent the "clean your plate" or "eat all your food or you can't get down from the table" concepts, which are known to contribute to overeating in later life. The addition of solids to the diet of exclusively breastfed infants has not been found to significantly increase overall caloric intake or weight gain.

In general, low-calorie milk and foods should be avoided in infants and toddlers unless a strict medically prescribed diet is required. The infant's growth during this phase is crucial to future development, and dietary fat should be curtailed with great caution. At the same time it is important to recognize that certain types of dietary fat are unacceptable for infants; fried potatoes, candy, ice cream, cake, soda pop and other sweetened drinks, and other such items do not constitute an appropriate amount of fat intake and may contribute to childhood obesity. One suggestion is to limit the *amount* (serving size) of dietary fat in foods provided rather than eliminate them altogether, especially during infancy.

Commercially prepared baby foods are the most common types of food served to infants in the United States. They are convenient and usually contain no added salt or sugar, but they are relatively expensive. An alternative is preparing baby foods at home, which is simple and inexpensive.

When solid foods are introduced, the safety and digestibility of the selections must be considered. Raw fruits with seeds, vegetables, and nuts are hazardous for infants and young children because of the danger of aspiration. Beans, grain cereals, and vegetables should be served well cooked and mashed during infancy (to prevent choking).

Preferably, home-prepared infant foods should be fresh or frozen because canned foods, except for those prepared for infants, may contain excessive sodium or sugar. If sweetening is needed, refined sugar can be used, but avoid honey and corn syrup because of the risk of infant botulism. Parents are cautioned to avoid reliance on food supplements marketed as iron- or vitamin-fortified as primary sources of minerals. Instead, encourage parents to offer the child a variety of fruits, vegetables, and whole grains, including those known to be naturally rich in iron.

Weaning

Defined as the process of giving up one method of feeding for another, **weaning** usually refers to relinquishing the breast or bottle for a cup. In Western societies this is generally regarded as a major task for infants and is often seen as a potentially traumatic experience. It is psychologically significant because the infant is required to give up a major source of oral pleasure and gratification.

Other cultural groups define weaning in relation to significant life events (e.g., teething) or reaching a specific age. No one time for weaning is best for every child, but generally most infants show signs of readiness during the second half of the first year. It is recommended that weaning occur with the infant's needs as a guide (Lawrence & Lawrence, 2016). Infants learn that good things come from a spoon. Their increasing desire for freedom of movement may lessen their desire to be held close for feedings. They are acquiring more control over their actions and can easily manipulate a cup to their lips. Imitation becomes a powerful motivator by age 8 or 9 months, and they enjoy using a cup or glass like others do.

Weaning should be gradual by replacing one bottle-feeding or breastfeeding at a time. The nighttime feeding is usually the last feeding to be discontinued. If breastfeeding ends before 5 or 6 months of age, weaning should be to a bottle (not in bed) to provide for the infant's continued sucking needs. If discontinued later, weaning can be directly to a cup, especially by age 12 to 14 months. Any liquid containing sucrose or other sugars, such as fruit juice, should be given in a cup.

SLEEP AND ACTIVITY

Sleep patterns vary among infants, with active infants typically sleeping less than milder children. Generally by 3 months of age, most infants sleep is 15 total hours with a nocturnal pattern of sleep that lasts from

9 to 11 hours and approximately three 1- to 2-hour naps during the day (Feigelman, 2016). Consolidation of nocturnal sleep hours occurs during the first 12 months, with decreasing daytime sleep and increasing nighttime sleep (approximately 11.7 hours) by 1 year of age. The number of naps per day varies, but infants may take one or two naps by the end of the first year. Daytime naps usually decline during the toddler years to no daytime naps by preschool age. Breastfed infants usually sleep for shorter periods, with more frequent waking, especially during the night, than do bottle-fed infants (Middlemiss, Yaure, & Huey, 2015). Average total sleep for 4-week-old infants in this study was 14 hours. (For a discussion of sleep position and sleep problems, see Chapter 11.) Others have correlated frequent nighttime awakenings in infants to boys, breastfeeding, having a difficult temperament, and maternal depression; notably this review found an overall pattern of less frequent wakings by 6 months of age (Middlemiss, Yaure, & Huey, 2015).

Most infants are naturally active and need no encouragement to be mobile. Problems can arise when devices such as play yards, strollers, commercial swings, and walkers are used excessively to limit the infant's naturally curious exploratory nature and activity or to be a "sitter" while the parent is otherwise occupied. These items restrict movement and prevent infants from exploring and developing necessary gross motor skills. Contrary to popular belief, walkers do not enhance walking and coordination, and they are dangerous if tipped over or placed near the top of stairs, porches, decks, in-ground pools, floor furnaces, and other hazardous surfaces.

DENTAL HEALTH

Good dental hygiene begins with appropriate maternal dental health and counseling during early infancy regarding dietary intake for the promotion of optimal oral hygiene. Counsel parents early regarding feeding practices that increase the risk of poor dental health. Some of these, as previously mentioned, include avoiding propping the milk bottle or giving the milk bottle in the bed, and avoiding fruit juices in a bottle, especially before 6 months of age. These contribute to enamel erosion and early childhood caries (previously called *baby bottle tooth decay*).

Once the primary teeth erupt, cleaning should begin. Parents should clean the teeth and gums initially by wiping with a damp cloth; toothbrushing is too harsh for the tender gingiva. The caregiver can stabilize the infant by cradling him or her with one arm and using the free hand to cleanse the teeth. Oral hygiene can be made pleasant by singing or talking to the infant. It is recommended that the infant have a brief oral health examination by 6 months of age from a qualified pediatric health practitioner; infants at high risk for caries are identified and oral health counseling is implemented. It is also recommended that the infant have an established dental home by 1 year of age (American Academy of Pediatric Dentistry, 2014). It is generally recommended that a small, soft-bristled toothbrush be used as more teeth erupt and the infant adjusts to the routine of cleaning. Water is preferred to toothpaste, which the infant will swallow (and if the toothpaste is fluoridated, the infant may ingest excessive amounts of fluoride). The American Academy of Pediatric Dentistry (2014) recommends a "smear" of fluoridated toothpaste for children younger than 2 years and a pea-size amount for those 2 to 5 years old.

Fluoride, an essential mineral for building caries-resistant teeth, is needed beginning at 6 months of age if the infant does not receive water with adequate fluoride content. The American Academy of Pediatric Dentistry (2014) recommends that children 6 months to 3 years of age take 0.25 mg fluoride daily if water fluoride content is less than 0.3 ppm. The fluoride dosage has been decreased from earlier recommendations because of an increased occurrence of dental fluorosis from excessive fluoride ingestion. If bottled water is used to reconstitute powdered or concentrated formula, it should either be fluoride free or contain low levels of fluoride.

Dietary considerations are also important because habits begun during infancy tend to continue into later years. Avoid foods with concentrated sugar (sucrose) in the infant's diet. Parents need to be counseled regarding the detrimental effects of frequent and prolonged bottle-feeding or breastfeeding during sleep, when the milk or other fluid, such as juice, bathes the teeth, producing nursing caries. The practice of coating pacifiers with honey or using commercially available hard-candy pacifiers is discouraged. Besides being cariogenic, honey also may cause infant botulism, and parts of the candy pacifier can be aspirated. (See Chapter 12 for a more extensive discussion of dental care, including early child caries and fluoride.)

SAFETY PROMOTION AND INJURY PREVENTION

Injuries are a major cause of death during infancy. In 2011 unintentional injuries (accidents) were the leading cause of death in children ages 1 to 4 years, and accidents were the fifth leading cause of death in infants ages birth to 12 months (Hamilton, Hoyert, Martin, et al., 2013). The three leading cause of accidental death injury in infants were suffocation, motor vehicle–related injuries, and drowning (Kochanek, Murphy, Xu, et al., 2016).

Falls are the leading cause of nonfatal injuries among infants (Centers for Disease Control and Prevention, 2015) and account for approximately half of hospitalizations in this age-group (Vallmuur & Barker, 2016). Furniture, such as cribs, highchairs, baby walkers, changing tables, and bouncers, are commonly associated with infant falls (Vallmuur & Barker, 2016). Constant vigilance, awareness, and supervision are essential as children gain increased locomotor and manipulative skills that are coupled with an insatiable curiosity about the environment. Box 10.5 lists the major developmental achievements of each period during infancy and the appropriate injury prevention plan. Table 10.5 lists common types of injuries and associated objects that predispose to such injuries. Suggestions for promoting safety in the home environment are given for specific types of injuries. The acronym SAFE PAD, described in Table 10.5, may be used to identify common types of injuries to infants and older children.

Motor Vehicle Injuries

The use of infant and child safety seats in cars has dramatically reduced motor vehicle–related fatalities, up to 71% in infants younger than 1 year of age (Lee, Farrell, & Mannix, 2015). However, a significant number of infants are injured or die from improper restraint within vehicles, either inappropriate restraint or incorrect use of restraint. An analysis of fatality reports from the National Highway Transportation Safety Administration noted that only 53% of children ages 0 to 9 years were using any child restraint system and 20% were sitting in the front seat (Lee, Farrell, & Mannix, 2015). Lack of proper child restraint continues to be a major factor in fatal accidents involving children. One observational report of newborns being placed in a car seat restraint by their family and transported home found that there was an 86% incidence of newborn infants placed incorrectly in car seat restraints and a 77% incidence of errors in the placement of infant car seat restraints in a vehicle (Hoffman, Gallardo, & Carlson, 2016). All infants must be secured in federally approved restraints rather than held or placed on the seat of the car. There is no safe alternative.

Infant restraints are designed either as an infant-only model or as a convertible infant-toddler model. Either restraint is a semireclined seat that faces the rear of the car. A rear-facing car seat provides the best protection for the disproportionately heavy head and weak neck

BOX 10.5 Injury Prevention During Infancy

Birth to 4 Months

Major Developmental Accomplishments

Involuntary reflexes, such as the crawling reflex, may propel infant forward or backward; the startle reflex may cause the body to jerk.

May roll over

Has increased eye-hand coordination and voluntary grasp reflex

Injury Prevention

Aspiration

This is not as great a danger to this age-group, but parents should begin practicing safeguarding early (see under 4 to 7 Months).

Hold infant for feeding; do not prop bottle.

Know emergency procedures to relieve choking.

Use pacifier with one-piece construction and loop handle.

Suffocation and Drowning

Keep all plastic bags stored out of infant's reach; discard large plastic garment bags after tying in a knot.

Do not cover mattress with plastic.

Use firm mattress and loose blankets; no pillows.

Make certain crib design follows federal regulations and mattress fits snugly—crib slats 6 cm (2.375 inches) apart.*

Do not use drop-side crib. Obtain hardware to permanently secure older dropside cribs to avoid suffocation.

Position crib away from other furniture and away from radiators.

Do not tie pacifier on a string around infant's neck.

Remove bibs at bedtime.

Never leave infant alone in bath.

Do not leave infant under 12 months alone on adult or youth mattress or "beanbag" type pillows.

Do not leave infant in a car.

Falls

Use crib with fixed, raised rails.

Never leave infant on a raised, unguarded surface.

When in doubt as to where to place infant, use floor.

Restrain infant in infant seat and never leave infant unattended while the seat is resting on a raised surface.

Avoid using a highchair until infant can sit well with support.

Accidental Poisoning

This is not as great a danger to this age-group, but begin practicing safeguards early (see under 4 to 7 Months).

Burns

Install smoke detectors in home.

Avoid warming formula in microwave oven; always check temperature of liquid before feeding.

Check bath water temperature.

Do not pour hot liquids when infant is close by, such as sitting on lap.

Beware of cigarette ashes that may fall on infant.

Do not leave infant in sun for more than a few minutes; keep exposed areas covered.

Wash flame-retardant clothes according to label directions.

Use cool-mist vaporizers.

Do not leave infant in parked car.

Check surface heat of car restraint before placing infant in seat.

Motor Vehicles

Transport infant in federally approved, rear-facing car seat, preferably in back seat.

Do not place infant on seat of car or in lap.

Do not place infant in a carriage or stroller behind a parked car.

Do not place infant or child (in car seat) in front passenger seat with an air bag unless air bag is deactivated.

Bodily Damage

Keep sharp, jagged objects out of infant's reach.

Keep diaper pins closed and away from infant.

4 to 7 Months

Major Developmental Accomplishments

Rolls over

Sits momentarily

Grasps and manipulates small objects

Resecures a dropped object

Has well-developed eye-hand coordination

Can focus on and locate small objects

Can push up on hands and knees

Crawls backward

Places objects in mouth (hand-to-mouth)

Injury Prevention

Aspiration

Keep buttons, beads, syringe caps, and other small objects out of infant's reach.

Keep floor free of any small objects.

Do not feed infant hard candy, nuts, food with pits or seeds, or whole or circular pieces of hot dog.

Exercise caution when giving teething biscuits because large chunks may be broken off and aspirated.

Do not feed infant while he or she is lying down.

Inspect toys for removable parts.

Suffocation

Keep all latex balloons out of reach.

Remove all crib toys that are strung across crib or play yard when infant begins to push up on hands or knees or is 5 months old.

Use only cribs with well secured crib sides; avoid use of drop-side cribs.

Falls

Restrain in a highchair.

Accidental Poisoning

Make sure that paint for furniture or toys does not contain lead.

Place toxic substances on a high shelf or in locked cabinet.

Keep medication vials and bottles locked in a secure place.

Hang plants or place on high surface rather than on floor.

Avoid storing large quantities of cleaning fluid, paints, pesticides, and other toxic substances.

Discard used containers of poisonous substances.

Do not store toxic substances in food containers.

Keep cosmetic and personal products out of infant's reach.

Discard used button-size batteries; store new batteries in safe area.

Know telephone number of local poison control center.

*Information on many items such as cribs or walkers available from US Consumer Product Safety Commission, 800-638-2772; http://www.cpsc.gov.

Continued

BOX 10.5 Injury Prevention During Infancy—cont'd

Burns

Keep faucets out of reach.
Place hot objects (e.g., cigarettes, candles, incense) on high surface.
Limit exposure to sun; apply sunscreen.

Motor Vehicles

See under Birth to 4 Months

Bodily Damage

Give toys that are smooth and rounded, preferably made of wood or plastic.
Avoid long, pointed objects as toys.
Avoid toys that are excessively loud.
Keep sharp objects out of infant's reach.

8 to 12 Months

Major Developmental Accomplishments

Crawls, creeps
Stands holding onto furniture
Stands alone
Cruises around furniture
Walks
Climbs
Pulls on objects
Throws objects
Picks up small objects; has pincer grasp
Explores by putting objects in mouth
Dislikes being restrained
Explores away from parent
Has increasing understanding of simple commands and phrases

Injury Prevention

Aspiration

Keep lint and small objects off floor, off furniture, and out of reach of infants.
Take care in feeding solid table food to give very small pieces.
Do not use beanbag toys or allow infant to play with small objects.
See also under 4 to 7 Months.

Suffocation and Drowning

Keep doors of ovens, dishwashers, refrigerators, coolers, and front-loading clothes washers and dryers closed at all times.
If storing an unused appliance, such as a refrigerator, remove the door.
Supervise contact with inflated balloons, immediately discard popped balloons, and keep uninflated balloons out of reach.
Fence area around swimming pools.
Always supervise when near any source of water, such as cleaning buckets, drainage areas, toilets, ponds, or other bodies of water within infant's access.
Keep bathroom doors closed.
Eliminate unnecessary pools of water.
Keep one hand on infant at all times when in tub.
When swimming keep infant within arm's reach at all times.

Falls

Avoid walkers, especially near stairs.
Ensure that furniture is sturdy enough for infant to pull self to standing position and cruise.
Fence stairways at top and bottom if infant has access to either end.

Accidental Poisoning

Administer medications as a drug, not as a candy.
Avoid use of over-the-counter cough and cold preparations for infants.
Replace medications and poisons immediately after use; replace caps properly if a child-protector cap is used.
Keep phone number for poison control center readily available.

Burns

Place guards in front of or around any heating appliance, fireplace, or furnace.
Keep electrical wires hidden or out of reach.
Place plastic guards over electrical outlets; place furniture in front of outlets.
Keep hanging tablecloths out of reach (infant may pull down hot liquids or heavy or sharp objects).

of an infant (Fig. 10.13). This position minimizes the stress on the neck by spreading the forces of a frontal crash over the entire back, neck, and head; the spine is supported by the back of the car seat. If the seat were faced forward, the head would whip forward because of the force of the crash, creating enormous stress on the neck. It is now recommended that all infants and toddlers ride in rear-facing car safety seats until they reach age 2 years or the weight recommended by the car seat manufacturer (Rivara & Grossman, 2016).* Some infant-only rear-facing infant car safety seats can accommodate children weighing up to a maximum of 35 pounds. Studies indicate that toddlers up to 24 months of age are safer riding in convertible seats in the rear-facing position (Truong, Hill, & Cole, 2013).

The restraint is anchored to the vehicle with the vehicle's seat belt, and the restraint has a harness system for securing the infant. Some

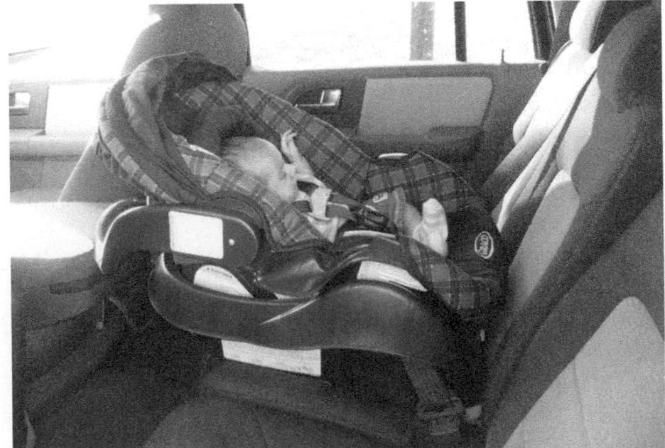

FIG. 10.13 Rear-facing infant seat in rear seat of car. (Courtesy Brian and Mayannyn Sallee, Las Vegas.)

harness systems require a clip to keep the shoulder straps correctly positioned. Vehicles manufactured after 1999 have tether straps that attach to anchors in the car seat to better secure the seat and minimize forward movement of the forward-facing convertible seats in the event of an accident. The LATCH (lower anchor and tether for children)

*Car seat information is available from the American Academy of Pediatrics at https://healthychildren.org/English/safety-prevention/on-the-go/; and from the Insurance Institute for Highway Safety, 1005 N. Glebe Road, Suite 800, Arlington, VA 22201; 703-247-1500; http://www.iihs.org. The National Highway Traffic Safety Administration, http://www.nhtsa.gov, also provides child passenger safety and air bag safety information for parents.

system provides car seat anchors between the front cushion and backrest so that the seat belt does not have to be used. Some automobiles have tether straps for rear-facing infant-only seats as well (see Fig. 12.12). Although many infant restraints can be recliners, they are used in the car only in the position specified by the manufacturer. The National Highway Transportation Safety Administration changed the rule about the use of the LATCH system if the combined weight of the child and the car seat is more than 65 pounds; since 2014, parents are instructed to use the shoulder–lap belt restraint to restrain the child in the car seat instead of relying on the LATCH system for maximum protection if the combined weight of the child and car seat is more than 29.5 kg (65 lb).

TABLE 10.5 Common Infant Injuries, Associated Risk Factors, and Safety Promotion

Safe Pad	Risk Factors	Suggested Safety Interventions
S—Suffocation, Sleep position	Latex balloons	Avoid latex balloons except with close adult supervision.
	Plastic bags	Tie unused plastic bags in a knot and dispose of in a safe container.
	Bed surface (noninfant) such as sofa or adult bed	Avoid placing infants to sleep on sofas, soft bedding, or adult bed.
	Pillows	Avoid use of pillows for sleep.
	Soft cushions and blankets	Clear bedding of soft cushions and blankets.
	Prone sleeping	Place infant to sleep on back at all times.
A—Asphyxia, animal bites	Food items: cylindrical items such as hot dogs, hard candy, peanuts, almonds	Cut hot dogs lengthwise; avoid hard candy in infants and toddlers. Infants should completely chew up each food item in mouth; do not feed more until item is swallowed.
	Toys: small toys such as Legos	As a general rule of thumb, if the toy fits into a toilet paper cardboard roll, it can be swallowed by a small child.
	Small objects: batteries, buttons, beads, dried beans, syringe caps, safety pins	Keep out of reach of infants, who are naturally inquisitive.
	Pacifiers	Pacifiers should be one piece.
	Baby (talc) powder	Avoid shaking powder over infant; if used, place on adult's hand and then place on infant's skin.
	Domestic dogs, cats	Supervise child around domestic animals; teach not to approach dog that is eating, has puppies, or is not feeling well. Animals that are "tame" can be unpredictable. Small children are the right size for most domesticated animals to come face to face. Closely supervise child around visiting pets. (See Pet Bites, Chapter 32.)
F—Falls	Stairs	Infants like to climb; place childproof gate at top and bottom of stairs.
	Diaper changing table	Infants do not have depth perception and cannot perceive a dangerous height from one that is safe. Never leave infants unattended on a flat surface even if not rolling over.
	Crib, bed-crib sides can fall when infant leans on them	In 2011 a mandate was made to stop selling drop-side infant cribs because of safety problems with infants being trapped against a wall or mattress and asphyxiation or falling out of bed when the latches do not hold.*
	Infant carriers	Never leave infant unattended in a carrier on top of a surface such as a shopping cart, clothes dryer, washer, kitchen cabinet; place carrier on floor.
	Car seat restraints	Secure infant in car seat restraint securely and never leave unattended.
	Highchair	Restrain infant in highchair; avoid using highchair except for feeding and only if adult supervision is adequate; even restrained infants can squirm out of some restraints and fall.
	Infant walkers	Use only stationary walkers. There is no evidence that walkers help infants "walk" any sooner. Wheeled walkers can easily be propelled off stairs and other platforms such as porches or decks, causing significant injury.
	Windows, screens	Avoid placing furniture next to a window. Infants learn to climb and can fall out of open windows, even with screens.
	Television, stereos, sound systems	These must be secured to the stand; infants can pull the stand over, causing the TV or sound system to land on their heads, causing significant injury.
E—Electrical burns or burns	Electrical outlets	Place safety cap over electrical outlets; infants may be burned by placing conductive object into outlet.
	Irons, curlers	Keep out of reach of infant and keep turned off when not in use.
	Water	Infants may turn on tap or faucet in bathtub and burn self. Lower the water heater to a safe temperature of 49°C (120°F). Before placing infant in tub, check temperature of water and completely turn off faucet so child cannot alter temperature of water. NEVER leave infant unattended in tub or sink of water.
	Fireplace	Place a childproof screen in front of fireplace.
	Stove, hot liquids	Keep top front burners off and keep pot handles turned toward back to avoid infant pulling hot pot onto self and causing burn injuries.
	Cigarettes	Avoid smoking and holding infant on lap while smoking cigar or cigarette.

Continued

TABLE 10.5 Common Infant Injuries, Associated Risk Factors, and Safety Promotion—cont'd

Safe Pad	Risk Factors	Suggested Safety Interventions
P—Poisoning, ingestions	Medication, ointments, cream, lotions	Medications left in purses or handbags or on a table top can often be ingested by the curious infant. Keep Poison Control Center number readily available (800-222-1222).
	Plants: household plants may be a source of accidental poisoning	Keep plants out of child's reach.
	Cleaning solutions and laundry pods	Store in locked cabinet or in top cabinet where there are no drawers or shelves for infant to climb on. Avoid storing cleaning and caustic solutions in containers such as a soda bottle or jar—infants and toddlers cannot differentiate a soda from a caustic drain cleaner.
	Inhalation or oral or nasal ingestion of poisonous or harmful chemicals such as methamphetamine, gasoline, turpentine	Keep gasoline and turpentine stored in a locked cabinet or closet out of child's reach. Avoid storing in containers that are also used to keep drinks or food.
A—Automobile safety	Car or truck and hot weather	An automobile-related hazard for infants is overheating (hyperthermia) and subsequent death when left in a vehicle in hot weather (>26.4°C [80°F]). Infants dissipate heat poorly, and an increase in body temperature may cause death in a few hours. Caution parents against leaving infants in a vehicle alone for *any reason.*
	Air bags	Avoid placing infant in a car restraint behind an air bag. Deactivate the air bag (available in certain models) or place the infant in the back seat in a proper car seat restraint.
	Car seat restraint	See discussion later in this chapter.
D—Drowning	Bathtub	NEVER leave infant unattended in tub, sink, or pool of water.
	Swimming pools, birdbaths, decorative ponds of water, splash pads	Place fence around pools with gate lock that is out of child's reach. Supervise infants in water at ALL times; an infant may drown in as little as 2 inches of water. Swimming lessons are encouraged but are not foolproof for drowning; use touch supervision—keep child within arm's reach at all times while swimming.
	5-gal or larger buckets	Keep buckets empty of water or elevated out of child's reach.

*A number of parent education pamphlets—such as *Crib Safety Tips* and *Is Your Used Crib Safe?*—are available in English and Spanish from the US Consumer Product Safety Commission, 4330 East-West Highway, Bethesda, MD 20814; 301-504-7923 or 800-638-2772; http://www.cpsc.gov.

Severe injuries and deaths in children have occurred from air bags deploying on impact in the front passenger seat. The back seat is the safest area of the car for children. For restraints to be effective, they must be used properly. Dressing the infant in an outfit with sleeves and legs allows the harness to hold the child securely in the seat. A small blanket or towel rolled tightly can be placed on either side of the head to minimize movement and keep the infant's hips against the back of the seat. Padding between the infant's legs and crotch is added to prevent slouching. Thick, soft padding is not placed under the infant or behind the back because during the impact, the padding will compress, leaving the harness straps loose. Preterm infants being discharged home from the hospital should be placed in appropriate car seat restraints as they would be placed in the car, and their heart rate and oxygen saturation should be monitored to detect any potential problems with airway occlusion. (For further discussion of car seat restraints, see Chapter 12.)

! NURSING ALERT

Rear-facing infant safety seats must not be placed in the front seats of cars equipped with an air bag on the passenger side. If an infant safety seat is placed in the passenger seat with an air bag, the child could be seriously injured if the air bag is released because rear-facing infant seats extend closer to the dashboard.

Nurse's Role in Injury Prevention

The task of injury prevention begins to be appreciated only when the potential environmental dangers to which infants are vulnerable are considered. Injury prevention and parent education should be handled on a growth and developmental basis. It is simply impossible to completely protect infants and small children from all potential dangers without placing them in a sterile, impractical environment. However, a large percentage of childhood deaths continue to occur as a result of preventable injuries (Kochanek, Murphy, Xu, et al., 2016). Nurses must be aware of the possible causes of injury in each age-group to provide anticipatory, preventive teaching. For example, the nurse should discuss guidelines for injury prevention during infancy (see Box 10.5) before the child reaches the susceptible age-group. Preventive teaching ideally begins during pregnancy.

One-third of all injuries to children occur in the home, and therefore the importance of safety cannot be overemphasized. The Family-Centered Care box summarizes a home safety checklist that can be presented to parents to increase their awareness of danger areas in the home and assist them in implementing safety devices and practices *before* their absence can inflict injury on infants. Hands-on displays such as cabinet latches or toilet seat locks can familiarize parents with inexpensive, commercial devices that can be used in the home to prevent injuries.

ANTICIPATORY GUIDANCE—CARE OF FAMILIES

Childrearing is no easy task; it presents challenges to both new and seasoned parents. With society's changing roles and mores, combined with a highly mobile population, traditional role models and time-honored methods of raising children are declining. As a result, parents look to professionals for guidance. Nurses are in an advantageous position to render assistance and offer suggestions. Every phase of a child's life has its particular traumas—toilet training for toddlers, unexplained fears for preschoolers, and identity crises for adolescents. For parents of an infant some challenges center around dependency, discipline, increased mobility, and safety. Major areas for parental guidance during the first year are listed in the Family-Centered Care box.

FAMILY-CENTERED CARE

Child Safety Home Checklist

Safety: Fire, Electrical, Burns

- ☐ Guards in front of or around any heating appliance, fireplace, or furnace (including floor furnace)*
- ☐ Electrical wires hidden or out of reach*
- ☐ No frayed or broken wires; no overloaded sockets
- ☐ Plastic guards or caps over electrical outlets; furniture in front of outlets*
- ☐ Hanging tablecloths out of reach, away from open fires*
- ☐ Smoke detectors tested and operating properly
- ☐ Kitchen matches stored out of child's reach*
- ☐ Large, deep ashtrays throughout house (if used)
- ☐ Small stoves, heaters, and other hot objects (e.g., cigarettes, candles, coffee pots, slow cookers) placed where they cannot be tipped over or reached by children
  - Hot water heater set at 49°C (120°F) or lower
  - Pot handles turned toward back of stove, center of table
  - No loose clothing worn near stove
  - No cooking or eating hot foods or liquids with child standing nearby or sitting in lap
- ☐ All small appliances, such as iron, turned off, disconnected, and placed out of reach when not in use
- ☐ Cool, not hot, mist vaporizer used
- ☐ Fire extinguisher available on each floor and checked periodically
- ☐ Electrical fuse box and gas shutoff accessible
- ☐ Family escape plan in case of a fire practiced periodically; fire escape ladder available on upper-level floors
- ☐ Telephone number of fire or rescue squad and address of home with nearest cross street posted near phone

Safety: Suffocation and Aspiration

- ☐ Small objects stored out of reach*
- ☐ Toys inspected for small removable parts or long strings*
- ☐ Hanging crib toys and mobiles placed out of reach
- ☐ Plastic bags stored away from young child's reach; large plastic garment bags discarded after tying in knots*
- ☐ Mattress or pillow not covered with plastic or in manner accessible to child*
- ☐ Crib design according to federal regulations (crib slats <6 cm [2.375 inches] apart) with snug-fitting mattress*
- ☐ Avoid use of drop-side cribs; for older models crib sides are permanently secured with approved hardware
- ☐ Crib positioned away from other furniture or windows*
- ☐ Portable play yard gates up at all times while in use*
- ☐ Accordion-style gates not used*
- ☐ Bathroom doors kept closed and toilet seats down*
- ☐ Faucets turned off firmly*
- ☐ Pool fenced with locked gate
- ☐ Proper safety equipment at poolside
- ☐ Electric garage door openers stored safely and garage door adjusted to rise when door strikes object
- ☐ Doors of ovens, trunks, dishwashers, refrigerators, and front-loading clothes washers and dryers kept closed*
- ☐ Unused appliance, such as a refrigerator, securely closed with lock or doors removed*
- ☐ Food served in small, noncylindric pieces*
- ☐ Toy chests without lids or with lids that securely lock in open position*
- ☐ Buckets and wading pools kept empty when not in use*
- ☐ Clothesline above head level
- ☐ At least one member of household trained in basic life support (cardiopulmonary resuscitation), including first aid for choking

Safety: Accidental Poisoning

- ☐ Toxic substances, including batteries, placed on a high shelf, preferably in locked cabinet
- ☐ Toxic plants hung or placed out of reach*
- ☐ Excess quantities of cleaning fluid, paints, pesticides, drugs, and other toxic substances not stored in home
- ☐ Used containers of poisonous substances discarded where child cannot obtain access
- ☐ Telephone number of local poison control center and address of home with nearest cross street posted near each phone
- ☐ Medicines clearly labeled in childproof containers and stored out of reach
- ☐ Household cleaners, disinfectants, and insecticides kept in their original containers, separate from food and out of reach
- ☐ Cosmetics and personal use items kept out of child's reach.

Safety: Falls

- ☐ Nonskid mats, strips, or surfaces in tubs and showers
- ☐ Exits, halls, and passageways in rooms kept clear of toys, furniture, boxes, or other items that could be obstructive
- ☐ Stairs and halls well lighted, with switches at both top and bottom of stairs
- ☐ Sturdy handrails for all steps and stairways
- ☐ Nothing stored on stairways
- ☐ Treads, risers, and carpeting in good repair
- ☐ Glass doors and walls marked with decals
- ☐ Safety glass used in doors, windows, and walls
- ☐ Gates on top and bottom of staircases and elevated areas, such as porch, fire escape*
- ☐ Guardrails on upstairs windows with locks that limit height of window opening and access to areas such as fire escape*
- ☐ Crib side rails raised to full height; mattress lowered as child grows*
- ☐ Restraints used in high chairs, walkers, or other baby furniture; preferably walkers not used*
- ☐ Scatter rugs secured in place or used with nonskid backing
- ☐ Walks, patios, and driveways in good repair

Safety: Bodily Injury

- ☐ Knives, power tools, and unloaded firearms stored safely or placed in locked cabinet
- ☐ Garden tools returned to storage racks after use
- ☐ Pets properly restrained and immunized for rabies
- ☐ Swings, slides, and other outdoor play equipment kept in safe condition
- ☐ Yard free of broken glass, nail-studded boards, other litter
- ☐ Cement birdbaths placed where young child cannot tip them over*

*Safety measures are specific for homes with young children. All safety measures should be implemented in homes where children reside and visit frequently, such as those of grandparents or babysitters.

FAMILY-CENTERED CARE

Guidance During Infant's First Year

Birth to 6 Months

Teach parents about car safety with use of federally approved restraint, facing rearward, in the middle of the back seat—not in a seat with an air bag.

Understand each parent's adjustment to newborn, especially mother's postpartum emotional needs.

Teach care of infant and help parents understand the infant's individual needs and temperament and that the infant expresses wants through crying.

Reassure parents that infant cannot be spoiled by too much attention during the first 4 to 6 months.

Encourage parents to establish a schedule that meets needs of infant and themselves.

Help parents understand infant's need for stimulation in environment.

Support parents' pleasure in seeing infant's growing friendliness and social response, especially smiling.

Plan anticipatory guidance for safety.

Stress need for immunization.

Prepare for introduction of solid foods.

6 to 12 Months

Prepare parents for infant's "stranger anxiety."

Encourage parents to allow infant to cling to them and avoid long separation from either parent.

Guide parents concerning discipline because of infant's increasing mobility.

Encourage use of negative voice and eye contact rather than physical punishment as a means of discipline.

Encourage showing most attention when infant is behaving well, rather than when infant is crying.

Teach injury prevention because of infant's advancing motor skills and curiosity.

Encourage parents to leave infant with suitable caregiver to allow some free time.

Discuss readiness for weaning.

Explore parents' feelings regarding infant's sleep patterns.

NCLEX REVIEW QUESTIONS

1. In relation to developmental milestones, the infant can be expected to roll over from back to abdomen at approximately:
   A. 2 months
   B. 4 months
   C. 6 months
   D. 8 months
2. An important milestone in the infant's life is the development of object permanence. This milestone is represented by which of these statements?
   A. The infant smiles at the mother when she talks to him.
   B. The infant repeatedly flexes and extends his arms and legs when the mother picks him up.
   C. The infant turns and looks for the mother when she walks out of his view.
   D. The infant cries when the mother hands him to a babysitter.
3. An important nutritional supplement recommended to prevent rickets in infants who are exclusively breastfeeding is:
   A. Vitamin A
   B. Fluoride
   C. Vitamin D
   D. Folic acid
4. A 4-month-old infant is brought to the well-child clinic for immunizations. The mother indicates that the infant often strains to have a bowel movement, so she has been giving him honey and has stopped feeding him iron-fortified formula, based on her sister's recommendations. The nurse recognizes that the infant is at risk for the development of which of the following? Select all that apply.
   A. Obesity
   B. Iron-deficiency anemia
   C. Rickets
   D. Infant botulism
   E. Cow's milk allergy
5. The type of play in which infants engage is called:
   A. Solitary
   B. Parallel
   C. Associative
   D. Cooperative

Correct Answers

1. C; 2. C; 3. C; 4. B, D; 5. A

REFERENCES

Ainsworth, M. (1982). Early caregiving and later patterns of attachment. In M. Klaus & M. Robertson (Eds.), *Birth, interaction, and attachment.* Skillman, NJ: Johnson & Johnson Baby Products.

American Academy of Pediatric Dentistry. (2014). Guideline on infant oral health care. *Clinical Guidelines Reference Manual, 35*(6), 137–141. Retrieved from: http://www.aapd.org/media/Policies_Guidelines/G_InfantOralHealthCare.pdf.

American Academy of Pediatrics, Committee on Infectious Diseases, & Pickering, L. (Eds.), (2015). *2015 Red Book: report of the Committee on Infectious Diseases* (30th ed.). Elk Grove Village, IL: The Academy.

American Academy of Pediatrics, Council on Communications and Media. (2016). Media and young minds. *Pediatrics, 138*(5), 1–7.

American Academy of Pediatrics, Task Force on Sudden Infant Death Syndrome. (2016). SIDS and other sleep-related infant deaths: Updated 2016 recommendations for a safe infant sleeping environment. *Pediatrics, 138*(5), e20162938.

Barrera, C. M., Perrine, C. G., Li, R., et al. (2016). Age at introduction to solid foods and child obesity at 6 years. *Childhood Obesity (Print), 12*(3), 188–192.

Behrendt, H. F., Konrad, K., Goecke, T. W., et al. (2016). Postnatal mother-to-infant attachment in subclinically depressed mothers: Dyads at risk? *Psychopathology, 49*(4), 269–276.

Bockting, W. (2016). Sexual identity development. In R. M. Kliegman, B. F. Stanton, J. W. St. Geme, et al. (Eds.), *Nelson textbook of pediatrics* (20th ed.). Philadelphia: Elsevier/Saunders.

Bowlby, J. (1969). *Attachment and loss* (Vol. 1). New York: Basic Books.

Carey, W. B., & McDevitt, S. C. (1978). Revision of the infant temperament questionnaire. *Pediatrics, 61*(5), 735–739.

Centers for Disease Control and Prevention. (2015). *CDC childhood injury report.* Retrieved from: https://www.cdc.gov/safechild/child_injury_data.html.

Clayton, H. B., Li, R., Perrine, C. G., et al. (2013). Prevalence and reasons for introducing infants early to solid foods: Variations by milk feeding type. *Pediatrics, 131*(4), e1108–e1114.

Demontigny, F., Girard, M. E., Lecharite, C., et al. (2013). Psychosocial factors associated with paternal postnatal depression. *Journal of Affective Disorders*, SO165-0327(13)00173-0.

Durand, D., Ochoa, T. J., Bellomo, S. M. E., et al. (2013). Detection of secretory immunoglobulin A in human colostrum as mucosal immune response against proteins of the type III secretion system of Salmonella, Shigella and enteropathogenic *Escherichia coli. The Pediatric Infectious Disease Journal, 32*(10), 1122–1126.

Erikson, E. (1963). *Childhood and society*. New York: WW Norton.

Feeley, N., Sherrard, K., Waitzer, E., et al. (2013). The father at the bedside: Patterns of involvement in the NICU. *The Journal of Perinatal & Neonatal Nursing, 27*(1), 72–80.

Feigelman, S. (2016). The first year. In R. M. Kliegman, B. F. Stanton, J. W. St. Geme, et al. (Eds.), *Nelson textbook of pediatrics* (20th ed.). Philadelphia: Elsevier/Saunders.

Gallitto, E. (2015). Temperment as a moderator of the effects of parenting on children's behavior. *Development and Psychopathology, 27*(3), 757–773.

Gartstein, M. A., & Rothbart, M. K. (2003). Studying infant temperament via the Revised Infant Behavior Questionnaire. *Infant Behavior and Development, 26*(1), 64–86.

Goldman, R. D. (2013). Pacifier use in the first month of life. *Canadian Family Physician, 59*(5), 499–500.

Hairston, I. S., Solnik-Menilo, T., Deviri, D., et al. (2016). Maternal depressed mood moderates the impact of infant sleep on mother-infant bonding. *Archives of Women's Mental Health, 19*(6), 1029–1039.

Hamilton, B. E., Hoyert, D. L., Martin, J. A., et al. (2013). Annual summary of vital statistics: 2010-2011. *Pediatrics, 131*(3), 548–558.

Heinrich, J., Koletzko, B., & Koletzko, S. (2014). Timing and diversity of complementary food introduction for prevention of allergic diseases. How early and how much? *Expert Review of Clinical Jmmunology, 10*(6), 701–704.

Hoffman, B. D., Gallardo, A. R., & Carlson, K. F. (2016). Unsafe from the start: Serious misuse of car safety seats at newborn discharge. *The Journal of Pediatrics, 171*, 48–54.

Ilia, S., & Galanakis, E. (2013). Clinical features and outcomes of acute otitis media in early infancy. *International Journal of Infectious Diseases, 17*(5), e317–e320.

Jaafar, S. H., Ho, J. J., Jahanafar, S., et al. (2016). Effect of restricted pacifier use in breastfeeding term infants for increasing duration of breastfeeding. *Cochrane Database of Systematic Review*, (8), CD007202.

Kair, L. R., Kenron, D., Etheredge, K., et al. (2013). Pacifier restriction and exclusive breastfeeding. *Pediatrics, 131*(4), e1101–e1107.

Kaya, V., & Aytekin, A. (2016). Effects of pacifier use on transition to full breastfeeding and sucking skills in preterm infants: A randomised controlled trial. *Journal of Clinical Nursing*, epub ahead of print.

Khan, S., & Orenstein, S. R. (2016). The esophagus. In R. M. Kliegman, B. F. Stanton, J. W. St. Geme, et al. (Eds.), *Nelson textbook of pediatrics* (20th ed.). Philadelphia: Elsevier/Saunders.

Kleinman, R. E., & Greer, F. R. (Eds.), (2014). *Pediatric nutrition* (7th ed.). Elk Grove Village, IL: American Academy of Pediatrics.

Kochanek, K. D., Murphy, S. L., Xu, J., et al. (2016). Deaths: Final data for 2014. *National Vital Statistics Reports: From the Centers for Disease Control and Prevention, National Center for Health Statistics, National Vital Statistics System, 64*(4), 1–122.

Lau, C. (2015). Development of suck and swallow mechanisms in infants. *Annals of Nutrition and Metabolism, 66*(suppl5), 7–14.

Lawrence, R. A., & Lawrence, R. M. (2016). *Breastfeeding: a guide for the medical profession* (ed. 8). Philadelphia: Elsevier.

Lee, L. K., Farrell, C. A., & Mannix, R. (2015). Restraint use in motor vehicle crash fatalities in children 0 year to 9 years old. *The Journal of Trauma and Acute Care Surgery, 79*, S55–S60.

Matthews, R., & Moore, A. (2013). Babies are still dying of SIDS. *The American Journal of Nursing, 113*(2), 59–64.

McIntosh, B. (1989). Spoiled child syndrome. *Pediatrics, 83*(1), 108–114.

Medoff-Cooper, B., Carey, W. B., & McDevitt, S. C. (1993). The Early Infancy Temperament Questionnaire. *Journal of Developmental and Behavioral Pediatrics : JDBP, 14*(4), 230–231.

Middlemiss, S., Yaure, R., & Huey, E. (2015). Translating research-based knowledge about infant sleep into practice. *Journal of the American Association of Nurse Practitioners, 27*(6), 328–337.

Miklush, L., & Connelly, C. D. (2013). Maternal depression and infant development: Theory and current evidence. *MCN. The American Journal of Maternal Child Nursing, 38*(6), 369–374.

Moss, B. G., & Yeaton, W. H. (2014). Early childhood healthy and obese weight status: Potentially protective benefits of breastfeeding and delaying solid foods. *Maternal and Child Health Journal, 18*(5), 1224–1232.

O'Brien, F., & Walker, I. A. (2014). Fluid homeostasis in the neonate. *Pediatric Anesthesia, 24*, 49–59.

Odom, E. C., Li, R., Scanlon, K. S., et al. (2013). Reasons for earlier than desired cessation of breastfeeding. *Pediatrics, 131*(3), e726–e732.

Parks, E. P., Shaikhkhalil, A., Groleau, V., et al. (2016). Feeding healthy infants, children, and adolescents. In R. M. Kliegman, B. F. Stanton, J. W. St. Geme, et al. (Eds.), *Nelson textbook of pediatrics* (20th ed.). Philadelphia: Elsevier/Saunders.

Piaget, J. (1952). *The origins of intelligence in children*. New York: International University Press.

Redsell, S. A., Edmonds, B., Swift, J. A., et al. (2016). Systematic review of randomised controlled trials of interventions that aim to reduce the risk, either directly or indirectly, of overweight and obesity in infancy and early childhood. *Maternal and Child Nutrition, 12*(1), 24–38.

Rivara, F. P., & Grossman, D. C. (2016). Injury control. In R. M. Kliegman, B. F. Stanton, J. W. St. Geme, et al. (Eds.), *Nelson textbook of pediatrics* (20th ed.). Philadelphia: Elsevier/Saunders.

Robertson, J. (1953). Some responsesof young children to loss of maternal care. *Nursing Care, 49*, 382–386.

Rode, J. L., & Kiel, E. J. (2016). The mediated effects of maternal depression and infant temperament on maternal role. *Archives of Women's Mental Health, 19*, 133–140.

Salah, M., Abdel-Aziz, M., Al-Farok, A., et al. (2013). Recurrent acute otitis media in infants: Analysis of risk factors. *International Journal of Pediatric Otorhinolaryngology, 77*(10), 1665–1669.

Spitz, R. A. (1945). Hospitalism: an inquiry into the genesis of psychiatric conditioning in early childhood. In O. Fenichel, P. Greenacre, & H. Hartmann (Eds.), *Psychoanalytic studies of the child* (Vol. 1). New York: International University Press.

Truong, W. H., Hill, B. W., & Cole, P. A. (2013). Automobile safety in children: A review of North American evidence and recommendations. *The Journal of the American Academy of Orthopaedic Surgeons, 21*(6), 323–331.

Turck, D., Michaelsen, K. F., Shamir, R., et al. (2013). World Health Organization 2006 child growth standards and 2007 growth reference charts: A discussion paper by the committee on nutrition of the European Society for Pediatric Gastroenterology, Hepatology, and Nutrition. *Journal of Pediatric Gastroenterology and Nutrition, 57*(2), 258–264.

US Food and Drug Administration. *Do teething babies need medicine on their gums?* No, 2017. Retrieved from: http://www.fda.gov/ForConsumers/ConsumerUpdates/ucm385817.htm.

Vallmuur, K., & Barker, R. (2016). Infant product-related injuries: Comparing specialized injury surveillance and routine emergency department data. *Australian and New Zealand Journal of Public Health, 40*, 37–42.

Visscher, M., & Narendran, V. (2014). The ontogeny of skin. *Adv Wound Care, 3*(4), 291–303.

Vitetta, L., Briskey, D., Alford, H., et al. (2014). Probiotics, prebiotics and the gastrointestinal tract in health and disease. *Inflammopharmacology, 22*(3), 135–154.

Zeanah, C. H., & Gleason, M. M. (2015). Attachment disorders in early childhood—clinical presentation, causes, correlates, and treatment. *Journal of Child Psychology and Psychiatry, and Allied Disciplines, 56*(3), 207–222.

11

Health Problems of the Infant

Lisa M. Cleveland

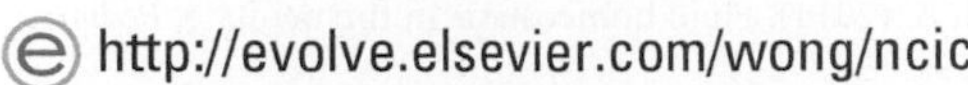

CONCEPTS

- Development
- Nutrition
- Cellular Regulation
- Safety

NUTRITIONAL IMBALANCES

Severe nutritional disorders are uncommon in children who live in developed countries, yet a small number of children may experience a nutritional deficiency of some kind. Children in the United States who are less than 2 years old have an adequate intake of most nutrients (Ahluwalia, Herrick, Rossen, et al., 2016). However, 10% of these children had an iron intake below the Estimated Average Requirement (EAR), and only 21% had a vitamin D intake that met or exceeded the recommended Adequate Intake (AI). More nutrient deficiencies were noted among toddlers; one in four had a lower-than-recommended fat intake, and most had intakes that were below the EAR for vitamins E (82%) and D (74%). Few toddlers (1%) met or exceeded the AI for fiber and potassium. In contrast, one in two toddlers had sodium intakes that exceeded the Tolerable Upper Intake Level; 16% had excessive intake of vitamin A and 41% had an excess intake of zinc. The findings of this study and other similar reports are important for nurses who care for infants and children. Nurses must strive to promote healthy nutritional habits early in childhood through proper education of families and children about healthy lifestyle practices. This includes diet and exercise for health promotion and prevention of morbidities associated with poor micronutrient intake and sedentary lifestyle.

VITAMIN IMBALANCES

Although true vitamin deficiencies are considered rare in the United States, subclinical deficiencies are commonly seen in certain maternal-child populations in which dietary intake is imbalanced and contains inadequate amounts of vitamins. Vitamin D–deficiency rickets, once rarely seen because of the widespread commercial availability of vitamin D–fortified milk, increased before the turn of the century. Populations at risk include the following:

- Children who are exclusively breastfed by mothers with an inadequate intake of vitamin D or are exclusively breastfed longer than 6 months without adequate maternal vitamin D intake or supplementation
- Children with dark skin pigmentation who (1) are exposed to minimal sunlight because of socioeconomic, religious, or cultural beliefs; (2) live in urban areas with high levels of pollution; or (3) live above or below a latitude of 33 degrees north and south where sunlight does not produce vitamin D (Wacker & Holick, 2013)
- Children whose diets that are low in sources of vitamin D and calcium
- Children who receive milk products not supplemented with vitamin D (e.g., yogurt,* raw cow's milk) as their primary dairy source
- Children who are overweight or obese (Turer, Lin, & Flores, 2013)

The findings of population-based studies in the United States show that childhood rates of vitamin D deficiency are 21% to 23.7% for normal-weight children but can be as high as 49% for obese children (Turer, Lin, & Flores, 2013). Clinical manifestations of vitamin D deficiency include abdominal pain, seizures, limb pain, and weakness. Further, a correlation has been found between the incidence of childhood upper respiratory infections and vitamin D deficiency, but the implications of these research findings have yet to be completely understood (Esposito & Lelii, 2015).

Exclusively breastfed infants may also be at risk for vitamin D deficiency. Therefore the American Academy of Pediatrics recommends that infants who are exclusively breastfed receive 400 IU of vitamin D beginning shortly after birth to prevent vitamin D deficiency and rickets (Kleinman & Greer, 2014). Vitamin D supplementation of infants should continue until they are consuming at least 1 L/day (or 1 quart/day) of vitamin D–fortified infant formula. Despite these recommendations, national studies conducted before and after their publication indicate that only one in five breastfed US infants receive this recommended vitamin D supplementation (Furman, 2015). Parent adherence to the recommendations may be a contributing factor. To address this issue, a clinical trial was conducted to determine the feasibility and efficacy of supplementing maternal diets with vitamin D as a means for ensuring adequate intake in exclusively breastfed infants. Researchers learned that 6400 IU of daily maternal vitamin D_3 supplementation for 6 months successfully supported maternal vitamin D status that was effective in producing sufficient vitamin D levels in their breastfeeding infants. This approach has the added benefit of improving maternal as well as infant health (Furman, 2015).

*Yogurt does not contain adequate amounts of vitamins A and D, but it is an acceptable source of calcium and phosphorus.

Nonbreastfed infants who are taking less than 1 L/day of vitamin D–fortified infant formula should also receive a daily vitamin D supplement of 400 IU. The National Institutes of Health Office of Dietary Supplements (2016) recommends a daily intake of 400 IU for infants (with an upper limit of 1000 to 1500 IU/day) and 600 IU for children older than 1 year (with an upper limit of 2500 to 3000 IU). Food sources that are high in vitamin D are salmon, sardines, tuna, and cod liver oil. Vitamin D–fortified foods include orange juice, oatmeal, whole milk, yogurt, and certain breakfast cereals (Wacker & Holick, 2013).

Children may also be at risk for vitamin deficiencies secondary to special diets, disorders, or medical treatment. For example, children on vegetarian diets, especially vegan diets, are at risk for vitamin B_{12} deficiency so it must be ensured that an adequate source of this vitamin is consumed (Pawlak, Parrott, Raj, et al., 2013). Although scurvy (caused by a deficiency of vitamin C) is rare in developed countries, cases have been reported in children who have low intake of vitamin C due to poor oral intake, oral motor dysfunction, or feeding problems (Agarwal, Shaharyar, Kumar, et al., 2014). Vitamin deficiencies of the fat-soluble vitamins A and D may occur in malabsorptive disorders such as cystic fibrosis and short bowel syndrome. Preterm infants may develop rickets in the second month of life as a result of inadequate intake of vitamin D, calcium, and phosphorus. Children receiving high doses of salicylates may have impaired vitamin C storage. Therefore children with chronic illnesses resulting in anorexia, decreased food intake, or possible nutrient malabsorption as a result of multiple medications should be carefully evaluated for adequate vitamin and mineral intake in some form (parenteral or enteral).

Children with sickle cell disease (SCD) may have suboptimal intakes of calcium, iron, and vitamins B_1 and C. This is problematic because low intake of calcium and vitamin B_1 has been correlated with more severe SCD symptoms (Mandese, Marotti, Bedetti, et al., 2016). Further, significant vitamin D deficiencies have been found in children with intestinal failure who received parenteral nutrition at home; therefore routine screening and consideration of vitamin D supplementation are recommended (Wozniak, Bechtold, Reyen, et al., 2015).

Vitamin A deficiency can occur in children as a result of diarrhea or infection. Vitamin A deficiency has been associated with an increased risk for blindness in children with measles. However, in a recent Cochrane review of studies assessing the efficacy of vitamin A in preventing blindness in children with measles, researchers found no evidence specifically related to ocular morbidities (Bello, Meremikwu, Ejemot-Nwadiaro, et al., 2016). Despite this lack of evidence, vitamin A supplementation has minimal side effects and should be administered to children with measles (Bello, Meremikwu, Ejemot-Nwadiaro, et al., 2014).

Excessive doses of vitamins can be concerning as well. In general, an excessive dose is defined as 10 or more times the Recommended Dietary Allowance (RDA). Although the water-soluble vitamins, primarily niacin, B_6, and C, can cause toxicity, the fat-soluble vitamins, especially vitamins A and D, tend to cause toxic reactions at lower doses. With the addition of vitamins to commercially prepared foods, the potential for **hypervitaminosis** has increased, especially when combined with excessive use of vitamin supplements. Hypervitaminosis of A and D presents the greatest problems because these fat-soluble vitamins are stored in the body and severe anemia and thrombocytopenia have resulted from megadoses of vitamin A. Hypercalcemia has been reported in children receiving therapeutic doses of vitamin D for the prevention of rickets (Talarico, Barreca, Galiano, et al., 2016) and in children on high doses of vitamin A for the treatment of autism (Boyd & Moodambail, 2016). Vitamin D is the most likely of all vitamins to cause toxic reactions in relatively small overdoses.

Inadequate maternal ingestion of cobalamin (vitamin B_{12}) may contribute to infant neurologic impairment when exclusive breastfeeding (past 6 months) is the only source of the infant's nutrition. One vitamin supplementation that is recommended for all women of childbearing age is a daily dose of 0.4 mg of folic acid, the usual RDA. Folic acid taken before conception and during early pregnancy can reduce the risk of neural tube defects such as spina bifida by as much as 70%. Drugs such as oral contraceptives and antidepressants may decrease folic acid absorption; thus adolescent girls taking these medications should consider supplementation. (See Spina Bifida, Chapter 34.)

MINERAL IMBALANCES

A number of minerals are essential nutrients. The **macrominerals** refer to those with daily requirements greater than 100 mg and include calcium, phosphorus, magnesium, sodium, potassium, chloride, and sulfur. **Microminerals**, or **trace elements**, have daily requirements of less than 100 mg and include several essential minerals that have an unclear role in nutrition. The greatest concern with minerals is deficiency, especially iron-deficiency anemia (see Chapter 28). However, other minerals that may be inadequate in children's diets, even with supplementation, include calcium, phosphorus, magnesium, and zinc. Low levels of zinc can cause nutritional failure to thrive (FTT). Some of the macrominerals may be inadvertently overlooked when a child with intestinal failure or recent surgery is making the transition from total parenteral nutrition to enteral feedings.

An imbalance in the intake of calcium and phosphorous may occur in infants less than 1 year old who are given whole cow's milk instead of infant formula, and neonatal tetany may be observed in these cases (see also Chapter 8). Whole cow's milk is a poor source of iron, and inadequate intake of iron from other food sources such as iron-fortified cereal may cause iron-deficiency anemia.

The regulation of mineral balance in the body is a complex process. Dietary extremes of mineral intake can cause a number of mineral interactions that could result in unexpected deficiencies or excesses. Poor outcomes in infants (e.g., fatal hypermagnesemia) have been associated with megavitamin therapy with high doses of magnesium oxide. Further, excessive amounts of one mineral, such as zinc, can result in a deficiency of another mineral, such as copper, even if sufficient amounts of copper are ingested. Thus megadose intake of one mineral may cause an inadvertent deficiency of another essential mineral by blocking its absorption in the blood or intestinal wall or by competing with binding sites on protein carriers needed for metabolism.

Deficiencies can also occur when various substances in the diet interact with minerals. For instance, iron, zinc, and calcium can form insoluble complexes with **phytates** or **oxalates** (substances found in plant proteins), which impair the bioavailability of the mineral. This type of interaction is important in vegetarian diets because plant foods such as soy are high in phytates. Further, contrary to popular opinion, spinach is not an ideal source of iron or calcium because of its high oxalate content (see also Box 12.2).

Children with certain illnesses are at greater risk for growth failure, especially in relation to bone mineral deficiency resulting from medical treatments, decreased nutrient intake, or decreased absorption of necessary minerals. Those at risk for these deficiencies include children who are have (1) human immunodeficiency virus (HIV), (2) sickle cell disease, (3) cystic fibrosis, (4) gastrointestinal (GI) malabsorption, or (5) nephrosis. Extremely low-birth-weight (ELBW) and very-low-birth-weight (VLBW) preterm infants and children who are receiving or have received radiation and/or chemotherapy for cancer are also at risk.

Nursing Care Management

A primary goal of pediatric nursing is to ensure adequate nutrition in children. This requires a nutritional assessment based on a thorough dietary history and physical examination for signs of deficiency or excess (see Nutrition, Chapter 12, and Nutritional Assessment, Chapter 4). After assessment data are collected, this information is compared with standardized intakes to identify areas of potential concern. One source of standardized nutrient intakes is the Dietary Reference Intakes.

Standardized growth reference charts are used in infants, children, and adolescents to compare and assess growth parameters such as height and head circumference with the percentile distribution of other children at the same ages. The World Health Organization's growth charts represent standardized growth references now recommended for infants and toddlers up to age 24 months. These growth charts include head circumference, height, and weight references that were derived from healthy children in six different countries around the world. These growth standards are based on the growth of healthy infants who were predominantly breastfed for at least 4 months and still breastfeeding to some extent at 12 months (World Health Organization, 2017a). The Centers for Disease Control and Prevention also offers a set of growth charts for children; however, these charts are only recommended for children 2 to 19 years of age (Kleinman & Greer, 2014).

Current recommendations for infant feeding include exclusive breastfeeding for the first 6 months with continued breastfeeding for at least 1 year or longer, if desired, with the addition of age-appropriate complementary foods (Academy of Breastfeeding Medicine, 2015). The introduction of some solid complementary foods may begin around 4 to 6 months and should include iron-fortified cereal for at least 18 months (see Chapter 10). The introduction of complementary foods in vegetarian infants may occur using the same guidelines used for other children (see Nutrition, Chapter 10). A variety of foods should be introduced during the early years to ensure a well-balanced nutritional intake. Infants who have a particular nutritional deficiency should be identified. A multidisciplinary approach should be taken to identify the deficiency, determine its etiology, and establish a plan with the caregiver to promote adequate growth and development.

HEALTH PROBLEMS RELATED TO NUTRITION

SEVERE ACUTE MALNUTRITION (PROTEIN-ENERGY MALNUTRITION)

Malnutrition continues to be a major health problem in the world today, particularly in children younger than 5 years of age. However, lack of food is not always the primary cause of malnutrition. In many developing and underdeveloped nations, diarrhea (gastroenteritis) is a major factor. Additional contributors are (1) bottle-feeding (in poor sanitary conditions), (2) inadequate knowledge of proper child care practices, (3) parental illiteracy, (4) economic and political factors, (5) climate conditions, (6) cultural and religious food preferences, and (7) a lack of adequate food. Poverty and food insecurity, which is the lack of a consistent and reliable food source, play an important role in worldwide malnutrition (US Department of Agriculture, 2016). The most extreme forms of malnutrition, or **protein-energy malnutrition**, are **kwashiorkor** and **marasmus**. Some authorities believe that severe malnutrition encompasses more than protein-energy deficits and thus prefer the term *severe childhood undernutrition* (SCU). However, entities such as the World Health Organization (2017b) now use the term *severe acute malnutrition* (SAM). SAM may be subdivided into edematous (kwashiorkor) and nonedematous with severe wasting (marasmus) types. A third type, marasmic kwashiorkor, has features of both marasmus and kwashiorkor (Ashworth, 2016).

In the United States milder forms of SAM are seen as a result of primary malnutrition, although classic cases of marasmus and kwashiorkor may occur but are rare. Unlike in developing countries, where the main reason for SAM is inadequate food, in the United States SAM may occur despite ample food supplies (see Failure to Thrive, later in this chapter). SAM may also be seen in children with chronic health problems, such as (1) cystic fibrosis, (2) renal disease, (3) cancer, (4) bone marrow transplantation, (5) HIV, (6) inborn errors of metabolism, (7) GI malabsorption, and (8) prolonged, untreated anorexia nervosa. Kwashiorkor has been reported in the United States in children fed only a rice beverage diet (Rice Dream) and few solid foods (Ashworth, 2016). This rice drink contains only 0.13 g of protein per ounce (compared with the 0.5 g found in human milk and infant formulas) and is an inadequate source of nutrition for children. Thus it is important for nurses to recognize that SAM can occur in developed countries; therefore a comprehensive dietary history is essential for any child with clinical features resembling SAM.

Kwashiorkor

Taken from the Ga language (Ghana), the word ***kwashiorkor*** means "the sickness the older child gets when the next baby is born." It clearly describes the syndrome that develops in the first child, usually between 1 and 4 years of age, when weaned from the breast after the second child is born. Kwashiorkor has been defined as primarily a deficiency of protein with an adequate supply of calories. A diet consisting mainly of starchy grains or tubers provides adequate calories in the form of carbohydrates but an inadequate amount of high-quality proteins. Some evidence supports a multifactorial etiology, including cultural, psychologic, and infectious factors that may interact to place the child at risk for kwashiorkor. Further, kwashiorkor may result from the interplay of nutrient deprivation and infectious or environmental stresses that produce an imbalanced response to these insults (Trehan & Manary, 2015). For example, kwashiorkor often occurs subsequent to an infectious outbreak of measles and dysentery.

The child with kwashiorkor has thin, wasted extremities and a prominent abdomen from edema (ascites) (Fig. 11.1). The edema often masks severe muscular atrophy making the child appear less debilitated than he or she actually is. The skin is scaly and dry and has areas of

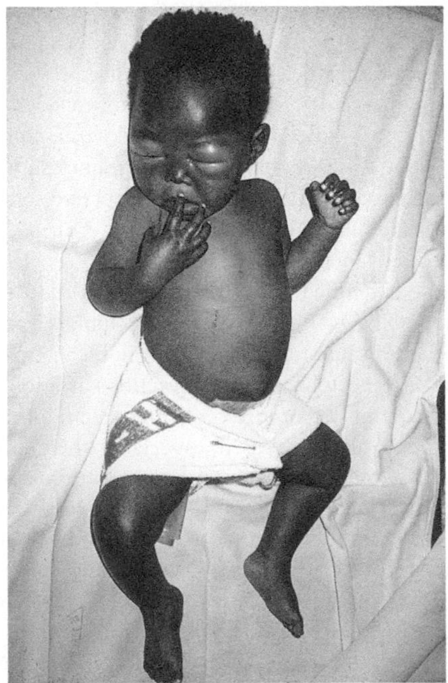

FIG. 11.1 Kwashiorkor. The infant shows generalized edema, seen in the puffiness of the face, arms, and legs. (From Kumar, V., Abbas, A., Fausto, N., et al. [2007]. *Robbins basic pathology* [8th ed.]. Philadelphia, PA: Saunders.)

depigmentation. Several dermatoses may be evident partly resulting from vitamin deficiencies. Permanent blindness often results from a severe lack of vitamin A. Mineral deficiencies are also common, especially iron, calcium, and zinc. Acute zinc deficiency is a common complication of severe SAM and results in (1) skin rashes, (2) loss of hair, (3) impaired immune response and susceptibility to infections, (4) digestive problems, (5) night blindness, (6) changes in affective behavior, (7) ineffective wound healing, and (8) impaired growth. Its depressant effect on appetite further impedes food intake.

Diarrhea (persistent diarrhea malnutrition syndrome) commonly occurs from a lowered resistance to infection and further complicates the often-concurrent electrolyte imbalance observed with kwashiorkor, leading to fatal deterioration and circulatory collapse. Low levels of cytokines (i.e., protein cells involved in the primary response to infection) have been reported in children with kwashiorkor, suggesting that these children have a blunted immune response to infection. Protein deficiency increases the child's susceptibility to infection, which eventually results in death. Many deaths also occur in children with kwashiorkor who develop HIV infection. GI disturbances such as fatty infiltration of the liver and atrophy of the acini cells of the pancreas are additional complications of kwashiorkor. Anemia is also common in these children.

Marasmus

Marasmus results from general malnutrition of both calories and protein. It is common in underdeveloped countries during times of drought, especially in cultures where adults eat first. The remaining food is often insufficient in quality or quantity for children. Marasmus is typically a syndrome of physical and emotional deprivation and is not confined to geographic areas where food supplies are inadequate. It may be seen in children with growth failure for whom the cause is not solely nutritional but primarily emotional. Marasmus may be seen in infants as young as 3 months of age if breastfeeding is unsuccessful and there are no suitable alternatives.

Marasmic kwashiorkor is a form of SAM where clinical findings of both kwashiorkor and marasmus are evident; the child has edema, severe wasting, and stunted growth. In marasmic kwashiorkor the child has inadequate nutrient intake and superimposed infection. Co-occurring fluid and electrolyte disturbances, hypothermia, and hypoglycemia are associated with a poor prognosis.

Marasmus is characterized by gradual wasting and atrophy of body tissues, especially of subcutaneous fat. The child has an aged appearance with loose and wrinkled skin, unlike the child with kwashiorkor, who appears more rounded by edema. Fat metabolism is less impaired than in kwashiorkor; thus deficiency of fat-soluble vitamins is usually minimal or absent. In general, the clinical manifestations of marasmus are similar to those seen in kwashiorkor. However, with marasmus there is no edema from hypoalbuminemia or sodium retention, which contributes to a severely emaciated appearance. There are also no dermatoses caused by vitamin deficiencies, little or no depigmentation of hair or skin, moderately normal fat metabolism and lipid absorption, a smaller head size, and a delayed recovery after treatment. The child is fretful, apathetic, withdrawn, and so lethargic that collapse frequently occurs. Concurrent infection with debilitating diseases such as tuberculosis, parasitosis, HIV, and dysentery is common.

Therapeutic Management

The treatment of SAM includes providing a diet with high-quality proteins, carbohydrates, vitamins, and minerals. When SAM occurs as a result of persistent diarrhea, there are three management goals:

1. Rehydration with an oral rehydration solution that also replaces electrolytes
2. Administration of antibiotics to prevent concurrent infections
3. Provision of adequate nutrition by either breastfeeding or a proper weaning diet

Local protocols are used in developing countries to treat SAM, but experts recommend a three-phase management protocol. The first phase is the acute or initial phase, which occurs in the first 2 to 10 days. During this phase, management involves initiation of oral rehydration and treatment of diarrhea and intestinal parasites. A focus is also placed on prevention of hypoglycemia and hypothermia and subsequent dietary management. Phase two, recovery or rehabilitation, occurs during the next 2 to 6 weeks, and treatment is focused on increasing dietary intake and weight gain. Management in phase 3, the follow-up phase, is focused on care after discharge in an outpatient setting to prevent relapse and promote weight gain, provide developmental stimulation, and evaluate cognitive and motor development.

In the acute phase of SAM, extreme care must be taken to prevent fluid overload. The child is observed closely for signs of food or fluid intolerance. Refeeding syndrome may occur if caloric intake progresses too rapidly. The resulting cardiac failure may cause sudden death in a child who has been malnourished and is fed too rapidly (Ashworth, 2016). Because severely malnourished children cannot tolerate a high-protein, high-energy diet, a modest-energy food source is given initially. These children are then slowly progressed to high-protein and high-energy foods as tolerated. A variety of food sources may be used to treat SAM, including oral rehydration solutions (ReSoMal), therapeutic milks (F75 and F100), and ready-to-use therapeutic foods (RUTF) that do not require the addition of water, thus preventing exposure to contaminated water sources (see Cultural Considerations box). In addition, parenteral and oral antibiotics are often part of the standard treatment for SAM (Jones & Berkley, 2014).

CULTURAL CONSIDERATIONS

World Health Organization Child Growth Standards

The World Health Organization has published growth standards for children that are based on the growth of healthy breastfed infants throughout the first year of life. The World Health Organization growth standards are designed to evaluate the growth of children ages birth to 5 years. The growth charts were compiled from a multicenter project conducted in Brazil, Ghana, India, Norway, Oman, and the United States and included 8440 children raised in environments that promoted healthy growth habits, including being breastfed and born to nonsmoking mothers. The growth standards are representative of an international standard of growth designed to promote healthy eating and living habits in all countries. These growth charts and additional information may be accessed at http://www.who.int/childgrowth/standards/en.

Vitamin and mineral supplementations are also required in most cases of SAM with vitamin A, zinc, and copper recommended. In contrast, iron supplementation is not recommended until the child can tolerate a steady food source. During recovery, the child is observed for signs of skin breakdown, which should be treated to prevent infection. Breastfeeding is encouraged if the mother and child are able to do so effectively; however, in some cases partial supplementation with a modified cow's milk–based infant formula may be necessary.

The World Health Organization has issued a statement recognizing the importance of breastfeeding for the first 6 months in developing countries where HIV is prevalent among childbearing women and children (Lawrence, 2013). Further, the World Health Organization recognizes that safe sources of food and water may not be available or adequate for infants after the first 6 months of life and that the risk of malnutrition in these children is greater than their theoretic risk of contracting HIV. Thus the organization recommends that breastfeeding continue after 6 months with the introduction of complementary foods provided there are safe sources of food available.

Nursing Care Management

Because SAM appears early in childhood, primarily in children 6 months to 2 years of age, and is associated with early weaning, maternal illiteracy, poverty, large family size, and incomplete vaccinations (Mishra, Kumar, Basu, et al., 2014), it is essential that nursing care focus on the *prevention* of SAM through parent education about feeding practices and infant care during this critical period. Prevention should also focus on the nutritional health of pregnant women because this will directly affect the health of their unborn children. Breastfeeding is the optimal method of infant feeding for the first 6 months. The immune properties naturally found in breast milk not only nourish infants but also help prevent opportunistic infections that may contribute to SAM. It is essential to ensure that infants' physiologic needs are met, including adequate nutrition and hydration, protection from infection, and appropriate skin care. Additional nursing care should be focused on educating parents about the importance of (1) childhood vaccinations to prevent illness, (2) nutrition and well-being for lactating mothers, (3) attending well-child visits for infants and toddlers, (4) appropriate food sources for children being weaned from breastfeeding, and (5) sanitation practices to prevent childhood GI illnesses.

Nursing care of young infants should also include appropriate skin care because poor skin integrity contributes to infection, hypothermia, water loss, and skin breakdown. If an infant is not well enough to effectively breastfeed or bottle-feed, tube feedings may be required to ensure adequate nutrition. Oral rehydration with an approved oral rehydration solution is commonly used in cases of SAM in which diarrhea and infection are not immediately life threatening.

Further, infants may be treated with higher-calorie (24 to 27 kcal per ounce) commercial infant formulas when appropriate. One potential drawback of using therapeutic milks (F75 and F100 formulas) is that they require water and may become contaminated during mixing, whereas RUTF, a peanut-based paste containing dried skim milk, vitamins, and minerals, has little water content (UNICEF, 2013). Therefore the home-based use of RUTF has gained acceptance for treating childhood malnutrition in developing countries. The packaged RUTF can be stored without refrigeration, has a long shelf-life, and improves survival rates in malnourished children (UNICEF, 2013). Further, RUTF can be administered by community health workers and offers the added advantage of home-based treatment of SAM, which can prevent exposure to hospital-acquired infections in already vulnerable children. Finally, by mobilizing communities and providing access to RUTF, 80% of children with SAM can be successfully treated at home. Rapid and appropriate care management can lower case-fatality rates to as low as 5% in both the community and health care setting (UNICEF, 2013).

It is imperative that nurses be at the forefront of educating and reinforcing healthy nutrition habits with parents of small children to prevent malnutrition. Because children with marasmus may experience emotional as well as nutritional deprivation, care should be consistent with the typical, age-appropriate, developmentally supportive care provided for children with failure to thrive.

The World Health Organization has published guidelines for the dietary treatment and management of children with SAM (available at http://www.who.int/elena/titles/full_recommendations/sam_management/en/). These guidelines include 11 recommendations for the management of SAM in infants 6 to 59 months of age, as well as hospital admission and discharge criteria for these infants (World Health Organization, 2017b).

FOOD SENSITIVITY

In 2010 the National Institute of Allergy and Infectious Diseases, working with 34 other professional organizations, published new evidence-based guidelines for the diagnosis and management of food allergy. **Food allergies** are adverse immunologic reactions to foods (Nowak-Węgrzyn, Sampson, & Sicherer, 2016). They are defined as specific components of a food or ingredients in a food, such as a protein, that are recognized by allergen-specific immune cells eliciting an immune reaction that results in the characteristic symptoms of an allergic response. A **food intolerance** exists when a food or food component elicits a reproducible adverse reaction but does not have an established or likely immunologic mechanism (Nowak-Węgrzyn, Sampson, & Sicherer, 2016). For example, a person with a milk allergy may have an immune-mediated response to cow's milk protein; however, a person who is unable to digest the lactose in cow's milk is intolerant to cow's milk, not allergic to it. True food allergies may involve anaphylaxis, GI food allergies, and cutaneous reactions to foods (Nowak-Węgrzyn, Sampson, & Sicherer, 2016). Further, food allergies may manifest in specific syndromes, such as Heiner syndrome, which is a rare but reversible non–immunoglobulin E (IgE)–mediated hypersensitivity to cow's milk resulting in atypical pulmonary disease in infants and young children (Sigua & Zacharisen, 2013). The exact prevalence of food allergies in children is believed to be much lower than what parents report. Approximately 6% of children may experience an allergic reaction to foods in the first 2 to 3 years of life. Food allergy symptoms are most common in infants and young children but can occur at any age. Clinical manifestations of food allergies are described as follows (Nowak-Węgrzyn, Sampson, & Sicherer, 2016):

Systemic—Anaphylaxis, growth failure
GI—Abdominal pain, vomiting, cramping, diarrhea
Respiratory—Cough, wheezing, rhinitis, infiltrates
Cutaneous—Urticaria, rash, atopic dermatitis

Approximately 90% of adverse reactions to foods are associated with eight specific types of foods: eggs, milk, peanuts, tree nuts, fish, shellfish, wheat, and soy (American College of Allergy, Asthma and Immunology, 2014). In food-allergic children, peanuts are the most prevalent allergen followed by milk and then shellfish (American Academy of Allergy, Asthma and Immunology, 2017). The National Institute of Allergy and Infectious Diseases further points out that most children will eventually be able to tolerate milk, eggs, soy, and wheat, but far fewer will ever tolerate tree nuts and peanuts (Nowak-Węgrzyn, Sampson, & Sicherer, 2016).

Children (50%) will typically outgrow milk and egg allergies by the time they are school age; however, 80% to 90% of children with peanut, nut, or seafood allergies will retain them for life. Further, it is important to note that peanut allergy prevalence has tripled over the past decade (Nowak-Węgrzyn, Sampson, & Sicherer, 2016). As many as 6% of children will experience a food-caused allergic reaction within the first 3 years of life—2.5% with cow's milk allergy, 1.5% with egg allergy, and 1% with peanut allergy. Recommendations for the prevention of food allergies in young children include the following:

- Exclusive breastfeeding for the first 4 to 6 months of life.
- Soy-based infant formulas will not prevent the development of food allergy.
- Introduce complementary solid foods only after 4 to 6 months of exclusive breastfeeding.
- Introduce high allergy-causing foods (eggs, nut products, fish, milk and wheat) soon after low allergy-causing foods. Delaying the introduction of these foods will not prevent food allergies. Further, avoiding allergy-causing foods during pregnancy or lactation will not prevent food allergy.

- Children, even with an egg allergy, should be vaccinated with the measles, mumps, and rubella (MMR) or measles, mumps, rubella, and varicella (MMRV) vaccines.
- Patients with severe egg allergy reactions should be referred to an allergist before considering receiving the influenza vaccine (Nowak-Węgrzyn, Sampson, & Sicherer, 2016) (see also Chapter 6, Immunizations).

Food allergies usually occur either as IgE-mediated or non–IgE-mediated immune responses. Some toxic reactions may occur because of a toxin found within the food. Food allergy is caused by exposure to allergens, usually proteins (but not the smaller amino acids), that are capable of inducing IgE antibody formation (sensitization) when ingested. Sensitization refers to the initial exposure of an individual to an allergen resulting in an immune response. Subsequent exposure induces a much stronger response that is clinically apparent. Consequently, food allergy typically occurs after the food has been ingested one or more times. Sensitization alone is not sufficient to be classified as a food allergy. Rather, an immune-mediated response *and* manifestation of specific signs and symptoms are necessary to categorize an individual as having a food allergy. The most common food allergens are listed in Box 11.1.

Oral allergy syndrome occurs when a food allergen (commonly fruits and vegetables) is ingested and there is subsequent edema and pruritus involving the lips, tongue, palate, and throat. Recovery from these symptoms is usually rapid. Immediate GI hypersensitivity is an IgE-mediated reaction to a food allergen that can result in nausea, abdominal pain, cramping, diarrhea, vomiting, anaphylaxis, or all of these. Additional food allergies seen in young children can cause allergic eosinophilic esophagitis, allergic eosinophilic gastroenteritis, food protein–induced proctocolitis, and food protein–induced enterocolitis.

BOX 11.1 Hyperallergenic Foods and Sources

Milk*—Ice cream, butter, margarine (if it contains dairy products), yogurt, cheese, pudding, baked goods, wieners, bologna, canned creamed soups, instant breakfast drinks, powdered milk drinks, milk chocolate
Eggs*—Mayonnaise, creamy salad dressing, baked goods, egg noodles, some cake icing, meringue, custard, pancakes, French toast, root beer
Wheat*—Almost all baked goods, wieners, bologna, pressed or chopped cold cuts, gravy, pasta, some canned soups
Legumes—Peanuts,* peanut butter or oil, beans, peas, lentils
Nuts*—Some chocolates, candy, baked goods, cherry soda (may be flavored with a nut extract), walnut oil
Fish or shellfish*—Cod liver oil, pizza with anchovies, Caesar salad dressing, any food fried in same oil as fish
Soy*—Soy sauce, teriyaki or Worcestershire sauce, tofu, baked goods using soy flour or oil, soy nuts, soy infant formulas or milk, soybean paste, tuna packed in vegetable oil, many margarines
Chocolate—Cola beverages, cocoa, chocolate-flavored drinks
Buckwheat—Some cereals, pancakes
Pork, chicken—Bacon, wieners, sausage, pork fat, chicken broth
Strawberries, melon, pineapple—Gelatin, syrups
Corn—Popcorn, cereal, muffins, cornstarch, cornmeal, corn bread, corn tortilla; many processed foods also contain corn syrup
Citrus fruits—Orange, lemon, lime, grapefruit; any of these in drinks, gelatin, juice, or medicines
Tomatoes—Juice, some vegetable soups, spaghetti, pizza sauce, catsup
Spices—Chili, pepper, vinegar, cinnamon

*Most common allergens.

Food allergy or hypersensitivity may also be classified by the interval between ingestion and the manifestation of symptoms: immediate (within minutes to hours) or delayed (2 to 48 hours).

Further, food allergies may occur at any time throughout the life span but are most common during infancy because the immature intestinal tract is more permeable to proteins than the mature intestinal tract thus increasing the likelihood of an immune response. Allergies in general have a genetic component. For example, children who have one parent with allergy have a 50% or greater risk of developing allergy. Children who have both parents with allergy have up to a 100% risk of developing allergy. Allergy with a hereditary tendency is referred to as atopy. Some infants with atopy can be identified at birth from elevated levels of IgE in umbilical cord blood.

Deaths have been reported in children who experienced an anaphylactic reaction to food. Onset of the reactions occurred shortly after ingestion (5 to 30 minutes). In most of these children, the reactions did not begin with skin signs, such as hives, red rash, and flushing, but rather mimicked an acute asthma attack (e.g., wheezing, decreased air movement in airways, dyspnea). Watch children with food anaphylaxis closely because a biphasic reaction has been reported in as many as 35% of children. This may manifest as an immediate response to treatment, apparent recovery, and then acute recurrence of symptoms (Keet & Wang, 2014). Children with extremely sensitive food allergies should wear a medical identification bracelet and have an injectable epinephrine cartridge (EpiPen) readily available. (See Anaphylaxis, Chapter 6.) Any child with a history of food allergy or previous severe reaction to food should have a written emergency treatment plan, as well as an EpiPen. Note that diphenhydramine (Benadryl) and cetirizine (Zyrtec) are effect for cutaneous and nasal symptoms but not for airway symptoms (Keet & Wang, 2014).

Because there is a tendency for children to lose their hypersensitivity, allergenic foods should be reintroduced into the diet after a period of abstinence to evaluate whether the food can be safely added back to the diet. There is evidence that children may tolerate foods to which they were previously allergic when these foods are extensively heated as in muffins or breads. The prolonged or complete avoidance of foods to prevent food allergy is not recommended, and there is some evidence that lack of exposure to antigens may be detrimental (Kleinman & Greer, 2014; Longo, Berti, Burks, et al., 2013).

! NURSING ALERT

The administration of **intramuscular** epinephrine in a child with a life-threatening anaphylactic reaction or one who is experiencing severe symptoms is indicated when the child has any one of the following symptoms (Keet & Wang, 2014):

- Itching sensation or tightness in throat, hoarseness, difficulty swallowing
- "Barky" cough, wheezing, dyspnea, cyanosis, respiratory arrest
- Mild cardiac dysrhythmia or mild hypotension
- Severe bradycardia, hypotension, cardiac arrest, or loss of consciousness

Diagnosis and Therapeutic Management

The diagnosis of food allergy is made based on several factors, including the occurrence of anaphylaxis or any combination of 37 symptoms listed in the National Institute of Allergy and Infectious Diseases guidelines within minutes to hours of ingesting food or if such symptoms have occurred after the ingestion of a specific food on one or more occasions. The gold standard is the double-blind, placebo-controlled food challenge. The skin prick test and serum IgE measurements may be used as an adjunct to diagnosing food allergy but singly should not be used for diagnosis (Nowak-Węgrzyn, Sampson, & Sicherer, 2016).

The atopy patch test, intradermal test, and serum IgE test are not recommended for establishing a diagnosis. A single oral food challenge may be used in certain circumstances (Bock & Sampson, 2016). Recently several trials of oral immunotherapy (OIT) and sublingual immunotherapy (SLIT) for cow's milk allergy, egg allergy, and peanut allergy in children have yielded mixed results. OIT consists of administering small amounts of an offending food to the child (which is then swallowed) over a lengthy period to induce tolerance to the food. SLIT consists of administering a small portion of food (e.g., 8 g of peanut powder) that is held under the tongue. The results of a few trials have shown that OIT results were better than SLIT but study participants experienced more systemic reactions with OIT. With both methods, avoidance of the food over time resulted in loss of sensitization (Fleischer, Burks, Vickery, et al., 2013); however, researchers suggest that further clinical trials are needed before peanut allergy OIT can be fully endorsed as being safe and effective (Sampson, 2013).

The traditional management of food allergy consists of avoiding the specific food or ingredient that causes the reaction. Because children with food allergies (usually two or more) are at risk for inadequate nutrient intake and growth failure, it is recommended that they have an annual nutritional assessment to prevent these problems. Dietary restrictions of milk may lead to calcium, vitamin D, calorie, and protein deficiencies in young children. Further, elimination of wheat may result in inadequate intake of the B vitamins, iron, and calories.

Nursing Care Management

A primary prevention strategy for avoiding food atopy in children includes parent education about the importance of exclusive breastfeeding for at least 4 to 6 months. There is no evidence that maternal avoidance (during pregnancy or lactation) of common food allergens (eggs, peanuts) prevents food allergies in children (Kleinman & Greer, 2014). Moreover, researchers have found that delaying the introduction of highly allergenic foods past 4 to 6 months of age may not be as protective against food allergy as previously believed (Nowak-Węgrzyn & Sicherer, 2016). Further, there is no evidence that soy formulas prevent allergic disease in infants and children (Kleinman & Greer, 2014).

Nursing care of children with potential food allergy consists of collecting vital health assessment data for the establishment of a diagnosis and assisting with diagnostic testing. It is important for nurses to be informed about food allergy and provide parents and caregivers, as well as older children, with accurate information regarding food allergy. This includes the education of parents, teachers, and day care workers regarding signs and symptoms of food allergy and reactions (see Critical Thinking Case Study box). Children with diagnosed food allergy should avoid unfamiliar foods and restaurants that do not disclose food ingredients. New labeling guidelines require that food additives such as spices and flavoring be clearly labeled on commercially sold, store-bought foods. Hidden ingredients in prepared foods are also potential sources of food allergy. In children with diagnosed allergies to certain foods, a nutritional consultation is imperative for the development of a dietary plan that includes sufficient nutrients for growth and development while avoiding the offending food.

Children with a history of food allergy may spend a considerable amount of time in day care; therefore persons working in day care centers and other children's settings need to be properly educated regarding recognition and management of severe anaphylactic reactions. Further, it is important for schools to ensure that children who have potentially life-threatening food allergies are recognized so plans can be implemented to prevent contact with allergy-producing foods. A written emergency action or food-allergy plan should be kept for the child and a self-injectable epinephrine device should be readily available for these children (Keet & Wang, 2014). Families of children with life-threatening food allergies are at risk for increased psychosocial distress, so health care workers should be prepared to meet the families' psychosocial as well as physical needs regarding their child.

? CRITICAL THINKING CASE STUDY

Food Allergy Anaphylaxis

A group of nursing students is holding a health promotion fair at a local elementary school for first-, second-, and third-graders. The nursing students have several booths set up in the school cafeteria. Three second-grade boys are playing around in front of one of the booths when one of the boys, Jason, an 8-year-old, suddenly starts coughing and clutching his throat. The nursing students also observe that he is developing red splotches on his face, neck, and throat and that he is scratching. Jason says, "I'm having trouble breathing!" The school nurse is nearby and comes over to see what the commotion is about. One of the boys with Jason says, "We didn't mean any harm—we were just goofing around when we put peanuts in his trail mix." One of the student nurses says, "He's in obvious distress—what should we do?"

1. Evidence—Is there sufficient evidence to draw any conclusions at this time about Jason's condition?
2. Assumptions—Describe some underlying assumptions about the following:
   a. Clinical manifestations of food allergy
   b. The emergency treatment of a food allergy "reaction," or anaphylaxis
   c. Which one of the following interventions would have highest immediate priority?
      1. Call Jason's parents and ask them to come pick him up from school.
      2. Call Jason's family practitioner to obtain orders for medication.
      3. Promptly administer an intramuscular dose of epinephrine.
      4. Call 911 and wait for the emergency response personnel to arrive.
   d. Based on your answer to item 2c, identify the appropriate medication dosage for this child (his weight is 56 lb).
3. What implications for nursing care exist in this situation after an intervention in item 2c has been chosen and implemented?
4. Describe the potential results of taking a "Let's observe Jason for a few minutes before we do anything" stance in this scenario.
5. Is there evidence to support your immediate and secondary nursing interventions?

Provide objective evidence to support your decisions for action.

Answers are available at http://evolve.elsevier.com/wong/ncic.

Cow's Milk Allergy

Cow's milk allergy (CMA) is a multifaceted disorder representing adverse systemic and local GI reactions to cow's milk protein. Approximately 2.5% of infants develop cow's milk hypersensitivity with 60% of those being IgE mediated. It is estimated that 50% of those children may outgrow the hypersensitivity by 3 to 4 years of age (Groetch & Sampson, 2016). (This discussion relates to cow's milk protein contained in commercial infant formulas. Whole milk is not recommended for infants younger than 12 months of age.) The allergy may be manifested within the first 4 months of life through a variety of signs and symptoms that may appear within 45 minutes of milk ingestion or after several days (Box 11.2). The diagnosis may initially be made from the history, although the history alone is not diagnostic. The timing and diversity of clinical symptoms vary greatly. For example, CMA may be manifested as colic (see information later in the chapter), diarrhea, vomiting, GI bleeding, gastroesophageal reflux, chronic constipation, or sleeplessness in an otherwise healthy infant.

Diagnostic Evaluation

Several diagnostic tests may be performed, including stool analysis for blood (both frank and occult bleeding can occur from colitis), eosinophils,

BOX 11.2 Common Clinical Manifestations of Cow's Milk Sensitivity

Gastrointestinal
Diarrhea
Vomiting
Colic
Wheezing
Gastroesophageal reflux
Bloody stools
Rectal bleeding

Respiratory
Rhinitis
Bronchitis
Asthma
Sneezing
Coughing
Chronic nasal discharge

Other Signs and Symptoms
Eczema
Excessive crying
Pallor (from anemia secondary to chronic blood loss in gastrointestinal tract)
Fussiness, irritability

leukocytes, serum IgE levels, and skin-prick testing. Skin testing may help identity the offending food, but the results are not always conclusive. No single diagnostic test is considered definitive for the diagnosis (Kleinman & Greer, 2014).

The most definitive diagnostic strategy is elimination of cow's milk in the diet followed by challenge testing after improvement of symptoms. Challenge testing involves reintroducing small quantities of milk in the diet to detect resurgence of symptoms. It may also involve the use of a placebo so that the parent is unaware of (or "blind" to) the timing of allergen ingestion. A double-blind, placebo-controlled food challenge is the gold standard for diagnosing food allergies such as CMA. Careful observation of the child is required during a challenge test because of the possibility of anaphylactic reaction. A clinical diagnosis is made when symptoms improve after removal of milk from the diet and two or more challenge tests produce symptoms (Groetch & Sampson, 2016).

Therapeutic Management

Treatment of CMA is elimination of cow's milk–based formula and all other dairy products. For infants fed commercial cow's milk infant formula, this primarily involves changing the formula to a casein hydrolysate milk formula (Pregestimil, Nutramigen, or Alimentum) in which the protein has been broken down into its amino acids through enzymatic hydrolysis. Although the American Academy of Pediatrics (Kleinman & Greer, 2014) recommends the use of extensively hydrolyzed formulas for CMA, many practitioners may start a soy-based infant formula instead because of the expense of the hydrolyzed formulas. Unfortunately, approximately 50% of infants who are sensitive to cow's milk protein will also demonstrate a sensitivity to soy-based formulas. Other choices for children who are intolerant to cow's milk–based formulas include the amino acid–based formulas, Neocate or EleCare, but their cost is a major consideration. Infants with CMA usually remain on a cow's milk–free diet for 12 months after which time small quantities of milk are reintroduced.

Nursing Care Management

The principal nursing objectives are identification of potential CMA and appropriate counseling of parents regarding substitute infant formulas. Parents often interpret GI symptoms such as spitting up, loose stools, or fussiness as CMA and switch the infant to a variety of formulas in an attempt to resolve the problem. Parents need reassurance regarding the needs of nonverbal infants who have an array of symptoms. Endless nights of lost sleep and a crying infant may promote feelings of parenting inadequacy and role conflict, thus aggravating the situation. Nurses can reassure parents that many of these symptoms are common and the reasons are often never discovered, yet the child does achieve appropriate growth and development. Parents should be advised to report acute symptoms to the practitioner for further evaluation. They should be reassured that the infant will receive complete nutrition from the new formula and will have no ill effects from the absence of cow's milk–based formula.

When solid foods are introduced, parents need guidance in avoiding cow's milk products. Carefully reading all food labels helps avoid exposure to prepared foods containing milk products. Although labeled as nondairy, cream and butter substitutes may contain cow's milk protein.

Lactose Intolerance

The term *lactose intolerance* encompasses at least four different conditions that involve a deficiency of the enzyme lactase, which is needed for the hydrolysis or digestion of lactose in the small intestine. Lactose is hydrolyzed into glucose and galactose. Congenital lactase deficiency occurs soon after birth when the newborn has consumed lactose-containing milk (human milk or commercial infant formula). This inborn error of metabolism involves the complete absence or severely reduced presence of lactase, is extremely rare, and requires a lifelong lactose-free or extremely reduced lactose diet.

Primary lactase deficiency, sometimes referred to as late-onset lactase deficiency, is the most common type of lactose intolerance and is manifested usually after 4 or 5 years of age, although the time of onset is variable. Ethnic groups with a high incidence of lactase deficiency include Asians, southern Europeans, Arabs, Israelis, and African Americans. Scandinavians tend to have the lowest incidence. Lactose malabsorption manifests as lactose intolerance and is characterized by an imbalance between the ability for lactase to hydrolyze the ingested lactose and the amount of lactose ingested (Högenauer & Hammer, 2016).

Secondary lactase deficiency may occur secondary to damage that has occurred in the intestinal lumen which decreases or destroys the enzyme lactase. For example, diseases such as cystic fibrosis, sprue, celiac disease, or kwashiorkor and infections such as giardiasis, HIV, or rotavirus may cause a temporary or permanent lactose intolerance.

Developmental lactase deficiency refers to the relative lactase deficiency observed in preterm infants of less than 34 weeks of gestation (Albenberg, Evans, & Piccoli, 2016). The primary symptoms include abdominal pain, bloating, flatulence, and diarrhea after the ingestion of lactose. The onset of symptoms occurs within 30 minutes to several hours of lactose consumption.

Lactose intolerance can be diagnosed based on the history and improvement of symptoms with a lactose-reduced diet. The breath hydrogen test can be used to diagnose lactase deficiency. However, it is more common to try dietary elimination of lactose and subsequent challenge. The testing of stool pH and glucose content can also be used (Kleinman & Greer, 2014). Specific to infants, lactose malabsorption may be diagnosed by evaluating fecal pH and reducing substances. Fecal pH in infants is usually lower than in older children, but an acidic pH may indicate malabsorption (Högenauer & Hammer, 2016).

Treatment of lactose intolerance is elimination of offending dairy products; however, some advocate decreasing amounts of dairy products rather than total elimination, especially in small children. Over-the-counter lactase enzyme supplements may be helpful in these cases (Högenauer & Hammer, 2016). In infants, lactose-free or low-lactose formula may be used until diarrhea has resolved (Kleinman & Greer, 2014).

One dietary concern is that dairy avoidance in children and adolescents with lactose intolerance will contribute to reduced bone mineral density and osteoporosis later in life (Kleinman & Greer, 2014). Evidence shows that dietary lactose enhances calcium absorption and that lactose-free diets may negatively affect bone mineralization (Porto, 2016). Therefore it is recommended that individuals with lactose maldigestion but no lactose intolerance symptoms continue to consume small amounts of dairy products with meals to prevent reduced bone mass density and subsequent osteoporosis. Some evidence shows that probiotics (i.e., food preparations containing microorganisms such as *Lactobacillus,* which alter the gastrointestinal microflora and thus are beneficial to the host) improve lactose intolerance when live cultures are fermented in dairy products (Canani, Sangwan, & Stefka, 2016). The positive attributes of probiotics for those with lactose maldigestion include delayed gastrointestinal transit (slower than with milk), positive effects on intestinal and colonic microflora, and a reduction of maldigestion symptoms.

Most people can tolerate small amounts of lactose (approximately 1 cup of milk per day [12 g]) even in the presence of deficient lactase activity and should be encouraged to continue their intake of dairy products in small amounts to obtain much-needed nutrients (Porto, 2016). Milk taken at meals may be better tolerated than when taken alone. Pretreated milk (with microbial-derived lactase) is reported to be effective in improving lactose absorption. Because dairy products are a major source of calcium and vitamin D, supplementation of these nutrients is needed to prevent deficiency. Yogurt contains inactive lactase enzyme which is activated by the temperature and pH of the duodenum. This lactase activity substitutes for the lack of endogenous lactase. Fresh, plain yogurt may be tolerated better than frozen or flavored yogurt. Hard cheeses, lactase-treated dairy products, and lactase tablets taken with dairy products are also viable options. An important distinction between lactose intolerance and food allergy is that lactose intolerance will not manifest as an anaphylactic-type reaction.

Nursing Care Management

Nursing care is similar to that discussed for CMA and includes (1) explaining the dietary restrictions to the family; (2) reviewing sources of lactose, including hidden sources; (3) identifying alternate sources of calcium, such as yogurt; (4) discussing the importance of calcium supplementation; and (5) reviewing strategies for controlling symptoms.

FAILURE TO THRIVE

Failure to thrive (FTT) is inadequate growth resulting from an inability to obtain or use calories required for growth. FTT has no universal definition; however, the objective parameter is usually the deceleration of growth—both height and weight. If FTT is severe, poor brain growth may occur as evidenced by a smaller than normal head circumference. The diagnosis is based on growth parameters that (1) drop more than 2 percentiles from baseline, (2) are persistently below the third to fifth percentiles, or (3) are less than the 80th percentile of median weight for height measurement. The term *growth failure* is now generally considered to be overly simplistic and obsolete (Sirotnak & Chiesna, 2016). Weight for length is reported to be a more accurate indicator of undernutrition (Becker, Carney, Corkins, et al., 2015).

Growth measurements alone are not used to diagnose children with FTT. Rather, the finding of a pattern of persistent deviation from established growth parameters is cause for concern. In addition to the lack of consensus on the exact definition of FTT, some advocate for a change in terminology; thus terms such as *growth faltering* and *pediatric undernutrition* are used in the literature for FTT. Further, some experts suggest that the previously used classifications of *organic FTT* and *nonorganic FTT* are too simplistic because in most cases growth failures have mixed causes. Therefore experts suggest that FTT be classified by pathophysiology in the following categories (McLean & Price, 2016; Sirotnak & Chiesna, 2016):

Inadequate caloric intake—Incorrect formula preparation, neglect, food fads, excessive juice consumption, poverty, breastfeeding problems, behavioral problems affecting eating, parental restriction of caloric intake, or central nervous system problems affecting intake

Inadequate absorption—Cystic fibrosis, celiac disease, Crohn's disease, vitamin or mineral deficiencies, cow's milk allergy, biliary atresia, or hepatic disease

Increased metabolism—Hyperthyroidism, congenital heart disease, or chronic immunodeficiency

Defective utilization—Genetic anomaly such as trisomy 21 or 18, congenital infection, or metabolic storage diseases

Rates of true FTT in US children are not clearly known. However, poverty is believed to be the greatest risk factor for FTT in developed and developing countries (Sirotnak & Chiesna, 2016). Nearly 20% of children younger than 4 years live in poverty and are unable to obtain adequate food on a regular basis (Sirotnak & Chiesna, 2016). The cause of FTT is often multifactorial and involves a combination of infant organic disease, dysfunctional parenting behaviors, subtle neurologic or behavioral problems, and disturbed parent-child interactions (Sirotnak & Chiesna, 2016). However, the primary etiology of FTT is inadequate caloric intake regardless of the cause.

Infants who are born preterm with very low birth weight (VLBW), extremely low birth weight (ELBW), and those with intrauterine growth restriction (IUGR) are often referred for FTT within the first 2 years of life. This is because they typically do not grow physically at the same rate as term cohorts even after discharge from the hospital. Catch-up growth is more difficult to achieve in VLBW and ELBW infants. As children, former VLBW and ELBW infants are more likely to have small stature and demonstrate lower cognitive and academic achievement scores than term cohorts (Darlow, Horwood, Pere-Bracken, et al., 2013). Children with congenital heart disease are also more likely to develop FTT in infancy due to inadequate caloric intake, malabsorption, increased energy expenditure that supersedes caloric intake, and pulmonary hypertension (McLean & Price, 2016).

Other factors that can lead to inadequate caloric intake in infancy include (1) health or childrearing beliefs such as fad diets, (2) child neglect, (3) child abuse, (4) inadequate nutritional knowledge, (5) financial difficulties, (6) family stress, (7) feeding resistance, and (8) insufficient breast milk intake. In infants younger than 8 weeks of age, breastfeeding problems as a result of inadequate latch or uncoordinated sucking and swallowing may occur (Sirotnak & Chiesna, 2016).

Diagnostic Evaluation

Diagnosis of FTT is initially made clinically through identification of signs and symptoms. If FTT is acute, the weight, but not the length/height, is below accepted standards (usually the 5th percentile). If FTT is chronic, both weight and length/height are low, indicating ongoing malnutrition. The use of weight velocities (according to the World Health Organization growth charts at http://www.who.int/childgrowth/

standards/height_for_age/en/) may be a better indicator of acute growth failure while considering age-dependent changes in growth. Perhaps as important as anthropometric measurements is a complete health and dietary history (including perinatal history), physical examination for evidence of organic causes, developmental assessment, and family assessment. A dietary intake history, either in the form of a 24-hour dietary recall or a history of food consumed over a 3- to 5-day period, is also essential. In addition, explore the child's activity level, parental stature, perceived food allergies, and dietary restrictions.

An assessment of household organization and mealtime behaviors and rituals is an important component in the collection of pertinent data. It is often helpful to obtain the growth patterns of the affected child's parents and siblings because these can be compared with norm-referenced standards to evaluate the child's growth (McLean & Price, 2016). An assessment of the home environment and parent-child interaction may be helpful as well. Other tests (e.g., lead toxicity, anemia, stool-reducing substances, occult blood, ova and parasites, alkaline phosphatase, and zinc levels) are selected only as indicated to rule out organic problems. To prevent the overuse of diagnostic procedures, consider FTT early in the differential diagnosis. To avoid the social stigma of FTT during the early investigative phase, some health care workers use the term *growth delay* (or *growth failure*) until the actual cause is established.

Therapeutic Management

The primary management of FTT is focused on reversing the cause of the growth failure. If malnutrition is severe, the initial treatment is directed at reversing the malnutrition while avoiding refeeding syndrome (see information earlier in this chapter). The goal is to provide sufficient calories to support "catch-up" growth, which is a rate of growth greater than the expected rate for age. A suggested goal for catch-up growth is 2 to 3 times the average rate of weight gain for the child's corrected age (Kleinman & Greer, 2014). In addition to adding caloric density to feedings, the child may require multivitamin supplementation. Further, any coexisting medical problems must be addressed.

An interprofessional team, consisting of physicians, nurses, dietitians, child life specialists, occupational therapists, pediatric feeding specialists, and social workers or mental health professionals, is important for managing complex cases of FTT. Care providers should make efforts to relieve any additional stresses on the family by offering referrals for public assistance or supplemental food programs. In some cases, family therapy may be helpful. Behavior modification focused on mealtime rituals (or lack thereof) and family social time may also be helpful. Hospitalization is indicated for (1) evidence (anthropometric) of SAM, (2) child abuse or neglect, (3) significant dehydration, (4) caretaker substance abuse or psychosis, (5) serious concurrent infection, or (6) if outpatient management fails to result in weight gain (McLean & Price, 2016; Sirotnak & Chiesna, 2016). Depending on the cause of the growth failure and the child's response to nutritional intervention, many children can be treated on an outpatient basis.

Prognosis

The prognosis for children with FTT is related to the cause. If parents lack knowledge of the infant's needs, teaching may remedy the child's limited caloric intake and permanently reverse the growth failure. Inadequate or infrequent feedings by the infant's primary caretaker, in conjunction with family disorganization, are often the underlying cause of FTT.

There are few long-term studies to provide data on the prognosis of children with FTT; however, some researchers have found that children who had FTT as infants had shorter statures, lower weights, and lower scores on measures of psychomotor development than their peers (Nangia & Tiwari, 2013). Factors that are related to poor prognosis include (1) severe feeding resistance, (2) lack of awareness in parents, (3) poor parental cooperation, (4) low family income, (5) low maternal educational level, (6) adolescent mothers, (7) preterm birth, (8) IUGR, and (9) early age of onset of FTT. Because later cognitive and motor function is affected by malnourishment in infancy, many of these children are below normal in intellectual development resulting in childhood IQ scores that are significantly lower than their peers who have no history of malnourishment (Romano, Hartman, Privitera., et al, 2015). In addition, there is a higher likelihood of eating and behavioral issues among children with a history of malnutrition compared with their peers (Romano, Hartman, Privitera., et al, 2015). These findings indicate that a long-term plan and follow-up care are needed for the optimum development of these children.

Nursing Care Management

Nurses play a critical role as part of the interprofessional team in the diagnosis of FTT through their assessment of the child, parents, and family interactions. Knowledge of the characteristics of children with FTT and their families is essential in the identification of these children and the rapid confirmation of a diagnosis (Box 11.3). The accurate assessment of initial weight, head circumference, length/height, and daily weight is an essential component of nursing care for children with FTT. Further, keeping a record of all food intake is imperative. The nurse documents the child's feeding behaviors, as well as the parent-child interaction during feedings, and assesses other caregiving activities, including play.

Children with FTT may have a history of difficult feeding, vomiting, sleep disturbance, and excessive irritability. Patterns such as crying during feedings, vomiting, hoarding food in the mouth, ruminating after feeding, refusing to switch from liquids to solids, and displaying aversion behavior, such as turning from food or spitting food, can become attention-seeking behaviors to prolong interaction with caregivers at mealtime. Besides showing signs of malnutrition and delayed social development, children with FTT may exhibit altered behavioral interactions with others. In some cases, the child may use feeding as a control mechanism in a poorly organized or chaotic family situation. Parents may allow the child to dictate the norms for behavior and feeding because of inexperience with parenting or poor parenting role models. Thus refusing to eat or only eating sweets and snacks with nonnutritive value may be the child's norm based on food availability and family tradition. In these cases, family therapy is indicated to address this trend and improve the parent-child relationship.

Some of the relationship strain that may occur between parent and child may be the result of dissatisfaction and frustration; therefore the

BOX 11.3 Clinical Manifestations of Failure to Thrive

- Growth failure
- Developmental delays—social, motor, adaptive, language
- Undernutrition
- Apathy
- Withdrawn behavior
- Feeding or eating disorders, such as vomiting, feeding resistance, anorexia, pica, rumination
- No fear of strangers (at age when stranger anxiety is normal)
- Avoidance of eye contact
- Wide-eyed gaze and continual scan of the environment ("radar gaze")
- Stiff and unyielding or flaccid and unresponsive
- Minimal smiling

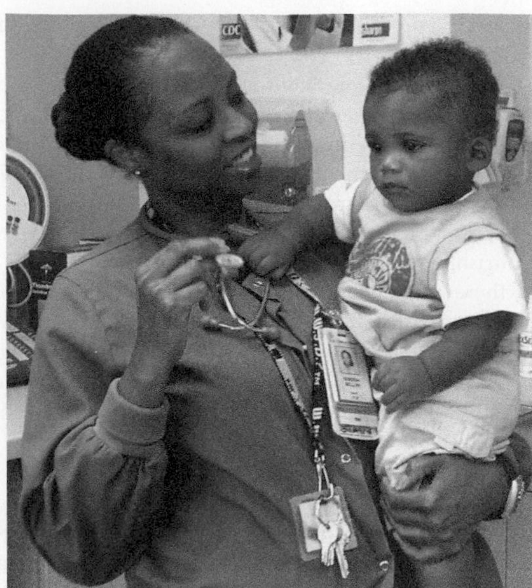

FIG. 11.2 A consistent nurse is important in developing trust with infants who have failure to thrive.

child should have a consistent core team of primary nurses (Fig. 11.2). These nurses caring for the child can learn to perceive his or her cues and address the cycle of dissatisfaction, especially around feeding.

Because many children with FTT are responding to stimuli that have led to the negative feeding patterns, an important primary intervention is to structure the feeding environment to encourage healthful eating. Initially, staff members and a feeding specialist may need to feed these children to thoroughly assess the difficulties encountered during the feeding process and to devise strategies that eliminate or minimize these problems.

There are four primary goals in the nutritional management of children with FTT: (1) correcting nutritional deficiencies and achieving ideal weight for height, (2) providing adequate calories for catch-up growth, (3) restoring optimum body composition, and (4) educating the parents or primary caregivers about the child's nutritional requirements and age-appropriate feeding methods. For infants, higher-calorie formulas (24 kcal/oz) may be provided to increase caloric intake. Older children (1 to 6 years) may benefit from 30-kcal/oz milk formulas (Kleinman & Greer, 2014). For example, toddlers may be given a high-calorie milk drink such as PediaSure to increase caloric intake. The nurse should carefully monitor for signs of intolerance to the formula. Usually only in extreme cases of malnourishment are tube feedings or intravenous therapy required. Finally, carbohydrate additives including fortified cereals and vegetable oil may be indicated. Because vitamin and mineral deficiencies may occur, multivitamin supplementation, including zinc and iron, is recommended.

Maladaptive feeding practices often contribute to growth failure; therefore parents should be given specific, step-by-step directions for formula preparation, as well as a written schedule of feeding times. Fruit juice is restricted in children with FTT until adequate weight gain has been achieved using appropriate milk sources. At that time, juice may be reintroduced but limited to no more than 4 oz/day.

Behavior modification techniques may be used with older infants and toddlers to interrupt maladaptive feeding patterns. Feeding times can become a "war of wills" resulting in food refusal and eventually FTT. These behaviors are different from the occasional toddler behavior of food refusal, which is primarily developmental, not pathologic.

In addition to attending to the child's physical needs, the interdisciplinary team must plan care for appropriate developmental stimulation. After an approximate developmental age is established, a planned program of play should be initiated. Ideally, a child life specialist is involved in this plan to implement and supervise the child's play activities. Every effort should be made to educate parents about how to play and interact with their child at a developmentally appropriate level. A pediatric nutrition specialist should also be involved in planning and implementing a diet specifically tailored for the child's growth needs.

Nursing care of children with FTT involves a "family systems" approach. Therefore if the goal is for the entire family to become healthy, all members should be engaged in the change process. Nursing care of the child's parents is focused on improving their self-esteem and supporting them as they acquire positive, successful parenting skills. Initially, this necessitates providing an environment in which they feel welcomed and accepted.

SPECIAL HEALTH PROBLEMS

COLIC (PAROXYSMAL ABDOMINAL PAIN)

Colic is believed to occur in 15% to 20% of all infants (Milidou, Sondergaard, Jensen, et al., 2014; Savino, Ceratto, Poggi, et al., 2015). Yet an organic cause may be identified in less than 5% of infants seen by practitioners for excessive crying (Akhnikh, Engelberts, van Sleuwen, et al., 2014). The condition is generally described as abdominal pain or cramping that is manifested by loud crying and drawing the legs up to the abdomen. Parents typically express dissatisfaction with the amount of time the infant spends crying each day. Colic can be characterized by crying (1) greater than 3 hours a day, (2) for more than 3 days per week, and (3) for more than 3 weeks. Symptoms may increase in the late afternoon or evening (Deshpande, 2015); however, in some infants the onset of symptoms occurs at varying times. Colic is more common in younger infants under the age of 3 months than in older infants. Further, infants with difficult temperaments are more likely to be colicky.

Despite the obvious behavioral indications of pain, the infant with colic gains weight and usually thrives. There is no evidence of a residual effect of colic on older children, except perhaps a strained parent-child relationship in some cases. Typically, colicky infants grow up to be normal children and adults. Colic is self-limiting and usually resolves as the infant matures, generally around 12 to 16 weeks of age (Akhnikh, Engelberts, van Sleuwen, et al., 2014).

Etiology

The potential causes of colic include (1) feeding too rapidly, (2) overfeeding, (3) swallowing excessive air, (4) improper feeding technique (especially positioning and burping), and (5) emotional stress or tension between parent and infant. Although all of these may occur, there is no evidence that one factor is consistently present. Infants with CMA symptoms have a high rate of colic (44%), and eliminating cow's milk products from these infants' diets can reduce the symptoms.

Although the exact cause of colic is not fully understood, some experts believe maternal smoking, inadequate parent-infant interaction, firstborn status, lactase deficiency, difficult infant temperament, difficulty self-regulating, and abnormal GI motility are potential causes (Drug and Therapeutics Bulletin, 2013). Some experts have suggested that inadequate amounts of lactobacilli in the GI tract influences gut motor functioning and gas production (Drug and Therapeutics Bulletin, 2013). The consensus of many experts who study colic is that colic is multifactorial and that no single treatment will effectively alleviate the symptoms for every infant.

Therapeutic Management

Management of colic should begin with an investigation of possible organic causes such as CMA, intussusception, or other GI problems. If a sensitivity to cow's milk is strongly suspected, a trial substitution with another formula such as an extensively hydrolyzed (Nutramigen, Alimentum, Pregestimil) whey hydrolysate or amino acid (Neocate, EleCare) formula is warranted. Soy formulas are frequently prescribed for infants who do not tolerate cow's milk–based formulas although 10% to 14% of those infants will develop a sensitivity to soy protein as well (Kleinman & Greer, 2014). The addition of lactase to infant formula has produced mixed results as far as reduction of overall symptoms. Oral administration of *Lactobacillus reuteri* to colicky breastfed infants has been found to decrease crying symptoms within 21 days of initiation (Szajewska, Gyrczuk, & Horvath, 2013); however, the widespread use of probiotics for the treatment of infantile colic is not currently recommended (Anabrees, Indrio, Paes, et al., 2013). When no specific cause can be found, the supportive measures discussed in the Nursing Care Management section are used.

The use of medications such as antispasmodics, antihistamines, and antiflatulents are sometimes recommended. Simethicone (Mylicon) may help relieve the symptoms of colic; however, in most controlled studies no medications completely resolved the symptoms of colic. Behavioral interventions have not proven effective at reducing symptoms of colic either but have helped parents deal with the crying infant in a more positive manner.

> **! NURSING ALERT**
>
> To date, there is no evidence to support one remedy that will relieve symptoms in every infant. Dietary changes including the elimination of cow's milk protein in the infant's diet may be effective in reducing the infant's crying, yet these interventions have been found to be only moderately effective (Drug and Therapeutics Bulletin, 2013).
>
> If cow's milk sensitivity is suspected, breastfeeding mothers should follow a milk-free diet for a minimum of 3 to 5 days to see if this is effective in reducing the infant's symptoms. Caution mothers that some nondairy creamers may contain calcium caseinate, a cow's milk protein. If a milk-free diet is helpful, lactating mothers may need calcium supplements to meet requirements. Formula-fed infants may improve with the same dietary modifications as for infants with CMA.

Nursing Care Management

The initial step in managing colic is to take a thorough, detailed history of the usual daily events. Areas that should be stressed include (1) the infant's diet; (2) diet of the breastfeeding mother; (3) timing of the crying; (4) relationship of crying to feedings; (5) presence of a specific family member during crying; (6) habits of family members, such as smoking; (7) activity of the mother or usual caregiver before, during, and after crying; (8) characteristics of the cry (e.g., duration, intensity); (9) measures used to relieve crying and their effectiveness; and (10) the infant's stooling, voiding, and sleeping patterns. Of particular importance is a careful assessment of the feeding process via demonstration by the parent.

One important nursing intervention is to reassure parents they are not to blame for their infant's discomfort. Parents, especially mothers, may become frustrated with their infant's crying and perceive this as a sign that something is horribly wrong. Caregivers express feelings of helplessness and frustration at being unable to console the crying infant. Additionally, colicky infants may be at increased risk for being shaken by their caregivers and experiencing traumatic brain injury. An empathetic, gentle, and reassuring attitude, in addition to suggestions for treatment, will help allay parents' anxieties, which are usually exacerbated by lack of sleep and preoccupation over their infant's welfare. Colic disappears spontaneously, usually by 3 to 4 months of age, although guarantees should never be made because it may continue for longer.

Helping caregivers understand the nature of the infant's crying and methods to effectively cope may be more important than finding a specific cause or treatment for colic. Because excessive infant crying increases the risk for abusive head trauma, disrupted caregiver-infant relationships, strained marital relationships, and maternal and paternal depression, the nurse should provide understanding and encourage parents to seek support from family members and friends.*

Sleep Problems

Sleep problems can be common in young children. The two major categories are the dyssomnias and parasomnias. With dyssomnias, the child has trouble either falling or staying asleep at night or has difficulty staying awake during the day. Parasomnias consist of confusional arousals, sleepwalking, sleep terrors, nightmares, and rhythmic movement disorders. These typically occur in children 3 to 8 years old (Carter, Hathaway, & Lettieri, 2014). This discussion focuses on minor sleep issues in infants such as refusal to go to sleep or frequent waking during the night. Later in this text, other sleep disturbances will be discussed such as obstructive sleep-disordered breathing and sleep terrors.

Concerns regarding sleep are common during infancy. Sometimes these concerns are as basic as parents' questions about whether the infant needs additional sleep. In this case it is best to investigate the reason for their concern, stressing the individual needs of each child. Infants who are active during wakeful periods and growing normally are typically receiving adequate sleep.

However, several more serious concerns require intervention. Sleep disturbances of physiologic origin are less common in infants with the exception of colic. The more common sleep disturbances are a learned pattern or developmental characteristic of some infants (Table 11.1). Although many families may report sleep problems typical of these patterns, interventions are offered only when the pattern is disruptive to the family. Sleep problems in early infancy have been positively correlated with higher maternal depression scores (Muscat, Obst, Cockshaw, et al., 2014); therefore nurses should discuss infant sleep problems with the mother (and family) in addition to other developmental aspects of newborn care.

When a sleeping problem is presented, a careful assessment is essential. Charting sleep habits both before and after interventions is an important strategy. Questions regarding the frequency and duration of waking, the usual bedtime routine, the number of nighttime feedings, the perceived problem (e.g., how much disruption the behavior generates), and the attempted interventions are important in planning effective approaches for the specific sleep problem. The common suggestion given to parents for any type of sleep problem, "Let the child cry until falling asleep," is difficult to implement and inappropriate for certain conditions.

The best way to prevent sleep problems is to encourage parents to establish bedtime routines that do not foster problematic patterns (Owens, 2016). One of the most constructive routines consists of placing infants in their crib while still awake. When infants become accustomed to falling asleep somewhere else, such as in their parent's arms, and then being transferred to their crib, they awaken in unfamiliar surroundings

---

*Parents may find this resource helpful: The Period of Purple Crying, at http://purplecrying.info/.

TABLE 11.1 Selected Sleep Disturbances During Infancy and Early Childhood

Disorder and Description	Management
Nighttime Feeding	
Child has a prolonged need for middle-of-night bottle-feeding or breastfeeding. Child goes to sleep at breast or with bottle. Awakenings are frequent (may be hourly). Child returns to sleep after feeding; other comfort measures (e.g., rocking or holding) are usually ineffective.	Increase daytime feeding intervals to >4 hr (may need to be done gradually). Offer last feeding as late as possible at night; may need to gradually reduce amount of formula or length of breastfeeding. Offer no bottles in bed. Put to bed awake. When child is crying, check at progressively longer intervals each night; reassure child but do not hold, rock, take to parents' bed, or give bottle or pacifier.
Developmental Night Crying	
Child ages 6-12 months with undisturbed nighttime sleep now awakens abruptly; may be accompanied by nightmares.	Reassure parents that this phase is temporary. Enter room immediately to check on child but keep reassurances brief. Avoid feeding, rocking, taking to parents' bed, or any other routine that may initiate trained night crying.
Refusal to Go to Sleep	
Child resists bedtime and comes out of room repeatedly. Nighttime sleep may be continuous, but frequent awakenings and refusal to return to sleep may occur and become a problem if parent allows child to deviate from usual sleep pattern.	Evaluate whether hour of sleep is too early (child may resist sleep if not tired). Assist parents in establishing consistent before-bedtime routine and enforcing consistent limits regarding child's bedtime behavior. If child persists in leaving bedroom, close door for progressively longer periods. Use reward system with child to provide motivation.
Trained Night Crying (Inappropriate Sleep Associations)	
Child typically falls asleep in place other than own bed (e.g., rocking chair or parents' bed) and is brought to own bed while asleep; on awakening, cries until usual routine is instituted (e.g., rocking).	Put child in own bed when awake. If possible, arrange sleeping area separate from other family members. When child is crying, check at progressively longer intervals each night; reassure child but do not resume usual routine.
Nighttime Fears	
Child resists going to bed or wakes during night because of fears. Child seeks parent's physical presence and falls asleep easily with parent nearby, unless fear is overwhelming.	Evaluate whether hour of sleep is too early (child may fantasize when nothing to do but think in dark room). Calmly reassure frightened child; keeping night-light on may be helpful. Use reward system with child to provide motivation to deal with fears. Avoid patterns that can lead to additional problems (e.g., sleeping with child or taking child to parents' room). If child's fear is overwhelming, consider desensitization (e.g., progressively spending longer time alone; consult professional help for protracted fears). Distinguish between nightmares and sleep terrors (confused partial arousals).

Modified from Ferber, R. (1987). Behavioral "insomnia" in the child. *Psychiatric Clinics of North America, 10*(4), 641-653.

and may be unable to fall back to sleep until the routine is repeated. Also, the bed should be used for sleeping only, not for play. Although the interventions that have been described and those listed in Table 11.1 are usually successful, it is much easier to prevent the problem with appropriate counseling during the early months of the infant's life.*

SUDDEN INFANT DEATH SYNDROME

Sudden infant death syndrome (SIDS) is defined as the sudden death of an infant younger than 1 year of age that remains unexplained after a complete postmortem examination (autopsy), including an investigation of the death scene and a review of the case history. An autopsy is essential to identify possible natural explanations for sudden unexpected death such as congenital anomalies or infection and to identify a death that was the result of child abuse. The autopsy typically cannot distinguish between SIDS and intentional suffocation, but the scene investigation and medical history may be of help if inconsistencies are discovered.

There has been much debate over the term *SIDS*, yet the definition noted earlier remains for the time being. Other terms have been developed to explain sudden deaths in infants. Sudden unexpected early neonatal death (SUEND) and sudden unexpected infant death (SUID) share similar features but differ in regard to the timing of death: whereas SUID is considered a death in the postneonatal period, SUEND occurs in the first week of life. The American Academy of Pediatrics Task Force on Sudden Infant Death Syndrome considers SIDS to be a component of SUID.

SIDS is the third leading cause of infant mortality in the United States, accounting for approximately 8% of all infant deaths and claiming the lives of 3500 US infants each year (Centers for Disease Control and Prevention, 2016). It is the most common cause of postneonatal infant

*A resource for parents is Ferber, R. (2006). *Solve your child's sleep problems.* New York, NY: Simon & Schuster (800-223-2336; http://www.simonandschuster.com). Also available in Spanish.

TABLE 11.2 Epidemiology of Sudden Infant Death Syndrome

Factor	Occurrence
Incidence	3500 US infants each year (Centers for Disease Control and Prevention, 2016)
Peak age	2-3 months; 95% occur by 6 months; preterm infants die of sudden infant death syndrome (SIDS) at mean age of 6 weeks later than mean age of death from SIDS for term infants
Sex	Higher percentage of boys affected
Time of death	During sleep
Time of year	Increased incidence in winter
Racial	Greater incidence in African American, American Indian, and Alaskan Native infants
Socioeconomic	Increased occurrence in lower socioeconomic class
Birth	Higher incidence in:
	Preterm infants, especially infants of extremely and very low birth weight
	Multiple births*
	Neonates with low Apgar scores
	Infants with central nervous system disturbances and respiratory disorders such as bronchopulmonary dysplasia
	Increasing birth order (subsequent siblings as opposed to firstborn child)
Health status	Infants with a recent history of illness; lower incidence in immunized infants
Sleep habits	Highest risk associated with prone position; use of soft bedding; overheating (thermal stress); cosleeping with adult, especially on sofa or noninfant bed; higher incidence in cosleeping with adult smoker
	Infants cosleeping with adult at higher risk if younger than 11 weeks
Feeding habits	Lower incidence in breastfed infants
Pacifier	Lower incidence in infants put to sleep with pacifier
Siblings	May have greater incidence in siblings of SIDS victims
Maternal	Young age; cigarette smoking, especially during pregnancy; poor prenatal care; substance abuse (heroin, methadone, cocaine). A few studies have shown an increased risk in infants exposed to secondhand environmental tobacco smoke.

*Although a rare event, simultaneous death of twins from SIDS can occur.

Data from American Academy of Pediatrics Task Force on Sudden Infant Death Syndrome. (2005). The changing concept of sudden infant death syndrome: Diagnostic coding shifts, controversies regarding the sleeping environment, and new variables to consider in reducing risk. *Pediatrics, 116*(5), 1245-1255; American Academy of Pediatrics Task Force on Sudden Infant Death Syndrome. (2011). SIDS and other sleep-related infant deaths: Expansion of recommendations for a safe infant sleeping environment. *Pediatrics, 128*(5), 1030-1038.

mortality, accounting for 40% to 50% of all deaths between 1 month and 1 year of age (Hunt & Hauck, 2016). Since 1994, the incidence of SIDS in the United States has steadily decreased due to the Back to Sleep campaign.* Despite dramatic decreases in SIDS rates, African American, American Indian, and Alaskan Native infants are disproportionately affected by higher rates than the rest of the population. Between 2010 and 2013, SIDS rates for infants in these groups were more than twice those of non-Hispanic white infants (Centers for Disease Control and Prevention, 2016). See Table 11.2.

Etiology

There are numerous theories regarding the etiology of SIDS, but the cause remains unknown. One hypothesis is that SIDS is related to brainstem abnormalities in the neurologic regulation of cardiorespiratory control. This maldevelopment affects arousal and physiologic responses to a life-threatening challenge during sleep (Bejjani, Machaalani, & Waters, 2013). Abnormalities include prolonged sleep apnea, increased frequency of brief inspiratory pauses, excessive periodic breathing, and impaired arousal responsiveness to increased carbon dioxide or decreased oxygen. However, *sleep apnea is not the cause of SIDS.* The majority of infants with apnea do not die and only a minority of SIDS victims have documented apparent life-threatening events (ALTEs) (see Apparent Life-Threatening Event later in this chapter). Further, the findings of numerous studies indicate that no association exists between SIDS and any childhood vaccine.

A genetic predisposition to SIDS has been suspected as a potential cause. In particular, differences in genes pertinent to immune system functioning and the development of the autonomic nervous system have been discovered in infants who died of SIDS compared with typical infants (Hunt & Hauck, 2016). Several "triple-risk factor" hypotheses have been proposed to explain the etiology of SIDS. The proposed risk factors include an underlying infant vulnerability such as a brain abnormality, a critical incident in the fetal developmental period or in early neonatal life, and an environmental stressor such as prone sleep positioning (Matthews & Moore, 2013).

Risk Factors for Sudden Infant Death Syndrome

Maternal smoking during pregnancy is a major modifiable risk factor for SIDS. The incidence of SIDS is approximately 3 times greater among infants whose mothers smoked during pregnancy, and risk of death is progressively greater as daily cigarette use increases (Hunt & Hauck, 2016). The effects of smoking by the father and other household members are more difficult to interpret because they are highly correlated with maternal smoking. There appears to be a small independent effect of paternal smoking but data on other household members have been inconsistent. Thus it is difficult to assess the independent effect of infant exposure to environmental tobacco smoke because parental smoking behaviors during and after pregnancy are also highly correlated. However, an increased risk for SIDS has been found in infants exposed only to postnatal maternal environmental tobacco smoke (Hunt & Hauck, 2016).

*Back to Sleep materials may be ordered by contacting the National Institute of Child Health and Human Development Information Resource Center, Back to Sleep, PO Box 3006, Rockville, MD 20847; 800-505-CRIB (2742); http://www.nichd.nih.gov/sids.

Further, a meta-analysis showed that exposure to tobacco smoke significantly increases an infant's risk for SIDS with an odds ratio of 2.25 for prenatal maternal smoking and 1.97 for postnatal maternal smoking (Zhang & Wang, 2013).

Co-sleeping, or an infant sharing a bed with an adult or older child in a noninfant bed, is associated with SIDS. In two studies, researchers found a significant increase in the risk of SIDS among infants who bed-shared compared with infants who slept alone (Carpenter, McGarvey, Mitchell, et al., 2013; Das, Sankar, Agarwal, et al., 2014). The findings of a retrospective analysis of infant deaths showed a twofold increase in accidental suffocation or strangulation when infants were sleeping on a sofa compared with other locations. This is likely due to sharing the sleeping area with another person (Rechtman, Colvin, Blair, et al., 2014).

Prone sleeping may cause oropharyngeal obstruction or affect thermal balance or arousal state. Rebreathing of carbon dioxide by infants due to sleeping in the prone position is also a possible cause of SIDS. Infants sleeping prone and on soft bedding may be unable to move their heads to the side, thus increasing the risk of suffocation and lethal rebreathing. Therefore the side-lying position is no longer recommended for infants sleeping at home, day care, or hospitals (unless medically indicated). Further, most preterm infants being discharged from the hospital should be placed in a supine sleeping position unless special factors predispose them to airway obstruction.

Another potential cause of SIDS may be a prolonged Q-T interval or other cardiac arrhythmias (Hunt & Hauck, 2016). Recently cardiac ion channelopathies, which occur as a result of gene mutations and may result in lethal arrhythmias, have been proposed as a possible risk factor for SIDS (Hunt & Hauck, 2016).

Soft bedding (waterbeds, sheepskins, beanbags, pillows, and quilts) should be avoided for infant sleeping surfaces. Bedding items, such as stuffed animals and toys, should be removed from the crib while the infant is asleep. Head covering by a blanket has also been found to be a risk factor for SIDS, thus supporting the recommendation to avoid extra bed linens and other items (Hunt & Hauck, 2016). Further, crib bumper pads should not be used (American Academy of Pediatrics, 2016).

Protective Factors for Sudden Infant Death Syndrome

The findings of a meta-analysis indicate that SIDS rates may be reduced by 45% for infants who are breastfed and this protective effect increases with exclusive breastfeeding (Hunt & Hauck, 2016). Pacifier use has also been associated with a lower risk of SIDS. Although it is uncertain if this is a direct effect of the pacifier itself or from associated infant or parental behavior, there is increasing evidence that pacifier use even with dislodgment can increase the arousability of infants during sleep. There has been some concern about recommending pacifiers for reducing the risk of SIDS out of fear this may interfere with breastfeeding. The findings of rigorous studies have failed to show an association between pacifier use and breastfeeding duration (Hunt & Hauck, 2016).

The American Academy of Pediatrics, Task Force on Sudden Infant Death Syndrome (2016) recommends that *all infants* be placed to sleep in the supine (on the back) position. They also recommend that medically stable preterm infants and infants diagnosed with gastroesophageal reflux (GER) be placed in a supine sleep position unless they have a specific upper airway disorder that places them at greater risk of death than the risk of death from SIDS. Further, in their new Safe Sleep recommendations, the American Academy of Pediatrics recommends that infants share a bedroom with parents, but not the same sleeping surface, preferably until the infant is a year old but at least for the first 6 months. Room-sharing decreases the risk of SIDS by as much as 50% (American Academy of Pediatrics, Task Force on Sudden Infant Death Syndrome, 2016).

Since the 1994 Back to Sleep campaign began advocating for nonprone sleeping for infants, an increased incidence of positional plagiocephaly has been observed (see later in the chapter). Therefore it is recommended that an infant's head position be alternated during sleep time to prevent plagiocephaly. Infants should also be placed prone in "tummy time" during awake periods for 10 to 15 minutes three times a day to prevent positional plagiocephaly and to encourage development of upper shoulder girdle strength (Hunt & Hauch, 2016). Updated childhood immunization status has also been shown to be protective against SIDS.

Although the cause of SIDS is unknown, autopsies reveal consistent pathologic findings, such as pulmonary edema and intrathoracic hemorrhages that confirm the diagnosis. Consequently, autopsies should be performed on all infants suspected of dying of SIDS, and findings should be shared with the parents as soon as possible after the death. Postmortem findings in SIDS and accidental suffocation or intentional suffocation, such as in Munchausen syndrome by proxy (see Child Maltreatment, Chapter 14), are practically the same. Individuals with less experience and training in performing autopsies, such as coroners instead of medical examiners, may not correctly identify some deaths as SIDS. Therefore mortality statistics can vary in different regions.

Infant Risk Factors

Certain groups of infants are at increased risk for SIDS:

- Low birth weight or preterm birth (<37 weeks gestation)
- Low Apgar scores
- Recent viral illness
- Siblings of two or more SIDS victims
- Male gender
- Infants of Native American or African American ethnicity

No diagnostic tests exist to predict which infants, including those in the above-listed groups, will die of SIDS. The next-born siblings of first-born infants who died of any noninfectious natural cause are at significantly increased risk for infant death from the same cause, including SIDS. This increased risk for recurrent SIDS in families is consistent with genetic risk factors interacting with environmental risk factors (Hunt & Hauck, 2016). Home monitoring is not recommended for this group of children, but it is often used by practitioners and may even be requested by parents. There is no evidence that home apnea monitoring prevents SIDS (Hunt & Hauck, 2016).

Nursing Care Management

Nurses have a vital role in preventing SIDS by educating families about the risk of prone sleeping in infants from birth to 6 months of age. This education should include the use of appropriate bedding surfaces, the association between SIDS and maternal smoking, and the dangers of co-sleeping on noninfant surfaces with adults or other children. Additionally, nurses have an important role in modeling behaviors for parents that decrease SIDS risk such as placing infants in a supine sleeping position while in the hospital. Unfortunately, research shows that some nurses are still placing healthy infants in a side-lying position due to their safety concerns about placing infants supine to sleep (Mason, Ahlers-Schmidt, & Schunn, 2013). However, research shows that education can change practice. After an educational session and laminated reminder cards on safe sleep recommendations, neonatal intensive care unit nurses had a significant increase in their patients' supine sleeping rates (39% before and 83% after), firm sleeping surfaces (5% before and 96% after), and soft, object-free beds (45% before and 75% after) (Gelfer, Cameron, Masters, et al., 2013).

Role modeling safe sleep practices and providing education to parents is imperative before hospital discharge because limited opportunities exist for parents to receive information about caring for their infant after discharge (Ateah, 2013). Nurses must be proactive in further decreasing the incidence of SIDS through providing education during postpartum discharge planning, newborn discharge teaching, follow-up home visits, well-baby clinic visits, and immunization visits. Further, nurses must continue to take every opportunity to advocate for infants by providing information for parents and caretakers about the modifiable risk factors for SIDS that can be implemented to prevent its occurrence across all sectors of the population.

Caring for the Family After Sudden Infant Death Syndrome

Loss of a child from SIDS presents several crises for the infant's parents. In addition to grief and mourning the death of their child, the parents must face a tragedy that was sudden, unexpected, and unexplained. This discussion focuses primarily on the objectives of care for families experiencing SIDS rather than on the process of grief and mourning, which is explored in Chapter 19.

The first persons to arrive at the scene may be the police and emergency medical service personnel. They should handle the situation by (1) asking few questions; (2) giving no indication of wrongdoing, abuse, or neglect; (3) making sensitive judgments concerning any resuscitation efforts for the child; and (4) comforting the family members as much as possible. A compassionate, sensitive approach to the family may help minimize some of the overwhelming guilt and anguish that commonly follow this type of loss.

The medical examiner or coroner may go to the home or place of death and make the death pronouncement. Until then, the sleep environment should remain as it was when the infant was initially found. If the infant is not pronounced dead at the scene, he or she may be transported to the emergency department to be pronounced dead by a physician. Usually there is no attempt at resuscitation in the emergency department. While in the emergency department, the parents should only be asked factual questions such as when they found the infant, how he or she looked, and whom they called for help. The nurse should avoid any remarks that may suggest responsibility, such as "Why didn't you go in earlier?" or "Didn't you hear the infant cry out?" It is the coroner's responsibility to document these findings at the scene rather than have parents recount the painful experience in the emergency department. Parents may also express feelings of guilt about administering cardiopulmonary resuscitation (CPR) correctly or the timing of CPR in relation to finding the infant.

The physician should initiate the discussion of an autopsy often with the nurse being present to support the family. The physician or medical examiner, depending on the circumstances, should emphasize that a diagnosis cannot be confirmed until the postmortem examination is completed. Instructions about the autopsy and funeral arrangements may need to be repeated or put in writing. If the mother was breastfeeding, she will need information about abrupt discontinuation of lactation. The nurse or physician should contact the primary care practitioner for the infant and the mother to avoid any miscommunications or telephone calls later inquiring about the child's health status.

Parents experiencing perinatal death perceive health care workers' responses as having a significant impact on their grieving process. A family-centered approach that involves the sociocultural context and unique needs of the family is essential for perinatal bereavement care (Flenady, Boyle, Koopmans, et al., 2014). Health care workers require adequate training and support to deliver appropriate care and prevent burnout (Flenady, Boyle, Koopmans, et al., 2014).

An important aspect of compassionate care for parents is allowing them to say good-bye to their child. These are the parents' last moments with their child, and they should be as quiet, meaningful, peaceful, and undisturbed as possible. Encourage parents to hold their infant before leaving the emergency department. Because the parents will be leaving the hospital without their infant, it may be helpful to accompany them to the car or arrange for someone else to take them home. A debriefing session may help health care workers who cared for the family cope with troubling emotions.

When the parents return home, a competent, qualified professional should visit them as soon after the death as possible. They should receive printed material that contains accurate information about SIDS (available from the national organizations*). During the initial visit, the nurse should help the parents gain an intellectual understanding of the condition. The nursing objectives are to assess what the parents have been told about SIDS, what they think happened, and how they explained the death to the other siblings, family members, and friends. One question that the nurse will not be able to answer and therefore should never attempt is, "Why did this happen to our baby?" or "Who is responsible for this tragedy?" These and other questions may linger in the parents' minds for months or even years.

When the unexpected death of a child occurs, it is common for one parent to blame the other. Parents may also experience guilt over the child's death. For example, they may feel that if they had checked on their child earlier, he or she might still be alive. It is important that the nurse assist parents in working through these feelings to prevent marital disruption in addition to the loss of the loved child.

Some parents are able to discuss their feelings openly and the nurse should support this coping skill. However, others may be reluctant to express their grief and the nurse can encourage the expression of emotions by asking about crying and feeling sad, angry, or guilty. During their interaction, the nurse can help the parents explore their typical coping strategies and, if these are ineffectual, to investigate new approaches. For example, one parent may refrain from discussing the death for fear of upsetting the other parent but each may need to hear how the other is feeling.

Ideally, the number of visits and plans for subsequent intervention needs to be flexible. Parents facing the question of having a subsequent child will need support. Both the birth of a subsequent child and the survival of that child, especially past the age of death of the previous child, are important transitional stages for parents.

POSITIONAL PLAGIOCEPHALY

Since the Back to Sleep campaign began in 1994 that advocated nonprone sleeping for infants to prevent SIDS, an increase in the incidence of positional plagiocephaly has been reported (Myers, Duncan, & Girotto, 2016). Approximately 20% of infants have this type of skull deformity that is most prevalent between 2 and 4 months of age (van Wijk, van Vlimmeren, Groothuis-Oudshoorn, et al., 2014). The term **plagiocephaly** connotes an oblique or asymmetric head. Positional plagiocephaly, deformational plagiocephaly, or nonsynostotic plagiocephaly implies an acquired skull deformity that occurs as a result of cranial molding during infancy usually as a result of lying in the supine position (van Wijk, van Vlimmeren, Groothuis-Oudshoorn, et al., 2014). Because infants' sutures are not yet fused, the skull is pliable so when infants are placed on their backs to sleep, the posterior occiput flattens over time (Fig. 11.3). A typical bald spot develops over the area, which is

*American SIDS Institute, 528 Ravens Way, Naples, FL 34110, 239-431-5425, http://www.sids.org; First Candle, 1314 Bedford Ave., Suite 210, Baltimore, MD 21208, 800-221-7437, http://www.firstcandle.org; National Sudden and Unexpected Infant/Child Death and Pregnancy Loss Resource Center, Georgetown University, Box 571272, Washington, DC 20057-1272, 866-866-7437, 202-687-7466, http://www.sidscenter.org.

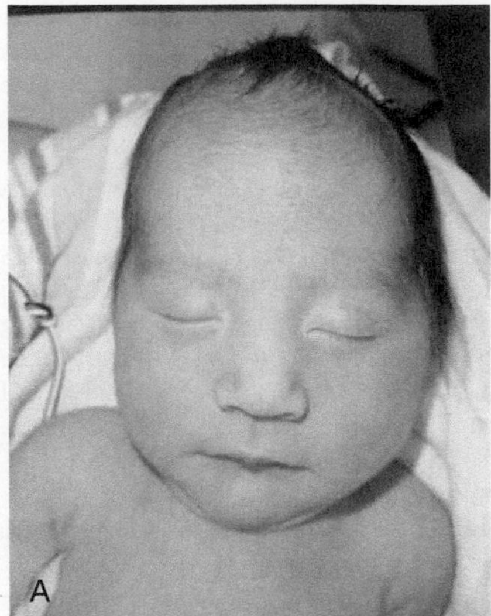

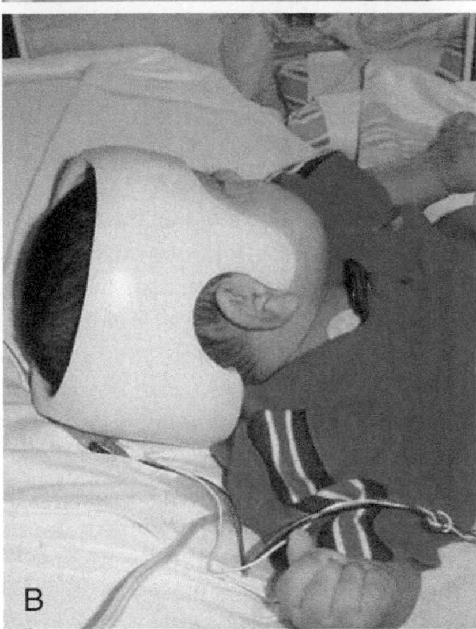

FIG. 11.3 A, Plagiocephaly. **B,** Helmet used to correct plagiocephaly. (Courtesy Dr. Gerardo Cabrera-Meza, Department of Neonatology, Baylor College of Medicine, Houston, TX.)

usually transient. Prolonged pressure on one side of the skull can result in that side becoming misshapen. Mild facial asymmetry may also develop. The sternocleidomastoid muscle may tighten on the preferential side resulting in a condition called *torticollis.* Congenital or acquired torticollis may also cause plagiocephaly. Other causes of deformational plagiocephaly include certain craniofacial syndromes. The following discussion is focused only on positional plagiocephaly (PP) caused by supine sleeping position.

Diagnostic Evaluation

The diagnosis of PP may be made on physical examination of the infant's head, which is viewed frontally and from above. The typical infant's head shape will resemble a parallelogram with unilateral flattening of the occiput, frontal and parietal bossing, a prominent cheekbone, and an anterior ear displacement. An evaluation of neck movement and range of motion is also made to determine the presence of torticollis. In most cases skull films and further radiologic studies (computed tomography scan) are used only to rule out craniosynostosis or other cranial deformities that may affect brain growth.

Therapeutic Management

Prevention of PP should begin shortly after birth by placing the infant to sleep supine and alternating the infant's head position nightly, avoiding prolonged placement in car safety seats and swings, and using prone positioning or "tummy time" for approximately 10 to 15 minutes three times per day while the infant is awake (Myers, Duncan, & Girotto, 2016).

The watch and wait method of treatment for torticollis and PP is not recommended (Myers, Duncan, & Girotto, 2016). Repositioning and physical therapy (RPPT), which includes providing counseling and teaching for parents as to positional changes and tummy time for their child, is recommended. A referral to physical therapy may be needed in the case of congenital torticollis. RPPT is the optimal treatment choice for patients younger than 4 months of age who have mild to moderately severe PP. The earliest types of behavioral modifications can be as simple as increasing tummy time or repositioning the infant's crib such that everything interesting in the room is on the side opposite the plagiocephaly (Myers, Duncan, & Girotto, 2016).

Molding therapy (helmet therapy) is the use of an orthotic helmet to promote the resolution of cranial asymmetry while the infant's head is still rapidly growing (Myers, Duncan, & Girotto, 2016). Orthotic helmets do not actively mold the skull; instead, they protect the areas that are flattened and allow the child to "grow into" the flat spots. Studies have shown helmet therapy to achieve correction 3 times faster and better than repositioning alone. This therapy is still debated, however, due to its expense, time requirements, and side effects (irritation, rashes, and pressure sores). The findings of recent studies suggest that combined treatment with helmet therapy and physical therapy is the most beneficial for the management of infants older than 4 months who are severely affected or with worsening of mild/moderate plagiocephaly who have been trialed on physical therapy. Infants with severe plagiocephaly should be considered for helmet therapy at any age (Myers, Duncan, & Girotto, 2016).

Nursing Care Management

Minor skull deformation is not considered significant, but parents should learn to prevent plagiocephaly by altering the infant's head position during sleep. Infants should be placed prone on a firm surface during awake time (tummy time) for at least 10 to 15 minutes three times a day (Myers, Duncan, & Girotto, 2016), which prevents plagiocephaly and facilitates development of upper shoulder girdle strength. The latter helps in the progressive development of movements such as rolling over and starting to rise on all fours that are precursors to crawling and eventually walking. Despite the perceived increase in incidence of positional plagiocephaly, the supine sleeping position is still recommended because it has led to a significant decrease in loss of infant lives from SIDS. When a nurse or parent notices plagiocephaly, a consultation with the primary practitioner is recommended to evaluate the head shape and ascertain the need for early intervention.

Nurses are in a unique position in well-child care settings to assess parents' ability to follow guidelines for preventing plagiocephaly by observing them alternating head placement for sleeping, demonstrating sternocleidomastoid muscle exercises (as appropriate to the condition), and implementing tummy time for infants during awake periods. Most important, nurses should continue to encourage parents to place the infant in a supine sleep position despite the development of plagiocephaly. Nurses can also assist parents in the proper use of a skull-molding helmet and reassure them of the high rate of success with the helmet. Allowing parents to verbalize concerns and feelings related to the health status of their child, as well as the provision of current best practice, is an important nursing function.

APPARENT LIFE-THREATENING EVENT

An apparent life-threatening event (ALTE), formerly referred to as an *aborted SIDS death* or a *near-miss SIDS,* generally refers to an event that is sudden and frightening to the observer in which the infant exhibits a combination of apnea, change in color (e.g., pallor, cyanosis, redness), change in muscle tone (usually hypotonia), and choking, gagging, or coughing that usually involves a significant intervention such as CPR provided by the caregiver who witnesses the event (Carolan, 2016). The definition of ALTE may include apnea, but ALTE may occur without apnea (Carolan, 2016). In 2016 the American Academy of Pediatrics released a new clinical practice guideline that recommended the replacement of the term *ALTE* with a new term, *brief resolved unexplained event (BRUE).* The American Academy of Pediatrics defines BRUE as an event observed in infants younger than 1 year of age during which an observer reports a sudden, brief (less than 1 minute), but then resolved episode including at least one of the following: (1) cyanosis or pallor; (2) absent, decreased, or irregular breathing; (3) marked change in muscle tone (hypertonia or hypotonia); or (4) altered responsiveness. The guidelines also state that a BRUE is diagnosed only when there is no explanation for a qualifying event after completion of a thorough history and physical examination (Carolan, 2016).

It is erroneous to characterize ALTE as a near-miss SIDS incident. A history of an unexplained ALTE occurs in 5% to 9% of SIDS victims and the risk of SIDS appears to be higher with two or more unexplained events, but no definitive incidence rates are available. Compared with healthy control infants, the risk for SIDS may be as much as 3 to 5 times greater in infants having experienced an ALTE.

Results from the Collaborative Home Infant Monitoring Evaluation (CHIME) study showed that apnea and bradycardia occurred at conventional and extreme alarm thresholds in all groups of infants studied: siblings of SIDS infants, infants with ALTEs, symptomatic (of apnea and bradycardia) and asymptomatic preterm infants weighing less than 1750 g (3 lb, 13 oz) at birth, and healthy term infants. Many infants experience apnea and bradycardia in each of these groups, yet do not die (Hunt & Hauck, 2016).

Diagnostic Evaluation

An essential component of the diagnostic process includes a detailed description of the event, including who witnessed the event, where the infant was during the event, and what, if any, activities were involved (e.g., during or after a feeding, riding in a car seat restraint, presence of siblings or any minor children, what clothing the infant was wearing). In addition, a prenatal and postnatal history must be obtained. A short period of observation in the emergency department may be appropriate to observe the infant's respiratory pattern and response to feeding. Further, a careful evaluation of late-preterm and preterm infants in their car seat restraint is essential. Upper airway occlusion and subsequent apnea and cyanosis may occur if the infant is not positioned properly. Reported diagnoses in infants with ALTE include (1) neurologic events such as a seizures (10% to 20% of cases seen); (2) GI problems, including GER (48%); (3) respiratory conditions (20% to 30%); (4) cardiac conditions (10% to 20%); (5) ear, nose, and throat abnormalities; (6) ingestions; and (7) Munchausen syndrome by proxy or child abuse (each less than 5%) (Chu & Hageman, 2013).

If an underlying diagnosis cannot be established, home monitoring may be recommended. The most common monitoring used is continuous recording of cardiorespiratory patterns (cardiopneumogram or pneumocardiogram). Four-channel pneumocardiograms (or multichannel pneumogram) monitor heart rate, respirations (chest impedance), nasal airflow, and oxygen saturation. A more sophisticated test, polysomnography (sleep study), also records brain waves, eye and body movements, esophageal manometry, and end-tidal carbon dioxide measurements. However, none of these tests can predict risk. Some children with normal results may still have subsequent apneic episodes.

Therapeutic Management

The treatment of an infant with an ALTE depends on the underlying condition. Several diagnostic tests may be carried out to determine the cause of the ALTE; however, a cause may not be determined in up to 50% of the cases. Further, testing for seizures, GER, or sepsis is not recommended unless signs were present on the physical examination and history. However, testing for a urinary tract infection is recommended (Tieder, Altman, Bonkowski, et al., 2013).

Nursing Care Management

The diagnosis of an ALTE causes great anxiety and concern in parents, and the initiation of home monitoring presents additional physical and emotional burdens. Parents of infants on home apnea monitors report experiencing emotional distress, especially depression and hostility, during the first few weeks after hospital discharge. For parents of a SIDS victim who have a new infant on home apnea monitoring, the anxiety is compounded by the uncertainty of the future of the living child and grief for the lost child. Home apnea monitoring may offer some predictability and control over the current child's survival through the period of uncertainty.

If home monitoring is required, the nurse can be a major source of support to the family in terms of education about the equipment, education regarding observation of the infant's status, and instructions on immediate intervention during apneic episodes, including CPR. To help the family cope with the numerous procedures they must learn, adequate preparation before discharge and written instructions are essential. In the first few weeks after discharge, parents may benefit by having a practitioner readily available to answer questions regarding false alarms and for other technical assistance.

Several types of home monitors are available and are set up by either a home monitor equipment company or home health staff. Nurses, especially those involved in the care at home, must become familiar with the equipment, including its advantages and disadvantages. Safety is a major concern because monitors can cause electrical burns and electrocution. The following precautions are recommended:

- Remove leads from infant when not attached to the monitor.
- Unplug the power cord from the electrical outlet when the cord is not plugged into the monitor.
- Use safety covers on electrical outlets to discourage children from inserting objects into sockets.

Additional home use instructions should focus on troubleshooting the monitor alarms. Encourage the parents to look first at the infant if an alarm goes off and ensure that the infant is breathing, and then determine the cause of the alarm. Parents also need information about traveling or running necessary errands with an infant on an apnea monitor, what to do in case of power failure, and whom to contact if the monitor alarm goes off continuously but the infant appears well. Siblings should be supervised when near the infant and taught that the monitor is not a toy. Other safety practices include informing local utility and rescue squads (fire and/or emergency services) of the home monitoring in case of an emergency, especially if the family lives in a remote rural area. Telephone numbers for these services should be posted in the home or set up as speed dial on certain phones if a universal 911 system is not available. Post instructions for infant CPR in a central location of the house and encourage parents to tell visitors and other family members about the location of these instructions. If a cellular phone is the main house phone, make sure it stays in a central location for all family members to access in an emergency.

> **! NURSING ALERT**
>
> If the infant is apneic, gently stimulate the trunk by patting or rubbing it. Call loudly for help even if alone. If the infant is prone, turn to the supine position and flick the heels of the feet. If there is still no response, immediately begin CPR starting with chest compressions. After approximately 2 minutes of CPR, activate the emergency medical service—"Call 911!" and then resume CPR until emergency responders arrive or the infant starts breathing. Never vigorously shake the child. No more than 10 to 15 seconds are spent on stimulation before implementing CPR (American Heart Association, 2015).

Caregivers need detailed information regarding proper attachment of the electrodes to the infant's chest with impedance monitors that detect chest movement. The electrodes are placed in the midaxillary line at a space one or two fingerbreadths below the nipple. For home use, electrodes attached to a belt that is placed around the child's trunk are preferred (Fig. 11.4). The belt is positioned so that the electrodes contact the skin in the same area. Monitors may have memory chips that allow for event recording, which can be an effective tool in evaluating the use of the monitor, events immediately before and after the ALTE, and reported frequency of alarms. Monitors are effective only if they are used. They do not prevent death but alert the caregiver to the ALTE in time to intervene. The need to use the monitor and to respond appropriately to alarms must be stressed. Noncompliance can result in the infant's death.

Many of the stresses observed during the home monitoring period are characteristic of families with chronically ill children. The child with an apnea or cardiorespiratory monitor may have additional health care needs such as a gastrostomy, tracheostomy, and multiple medications or treatments that exacerbate the parents' stress. Parents report increased stress, including concern for the child's survival, fear of incompetence in assuming home responsibility, inadequate respite care, lack of time for other children and spouse, social isolation from friends and extended family, constant work, and fatigue. To deal with these potential stressors, nurses need to use the same interventions as those discussed for children with chronic illnesses and be aware of the need for referral when difficulties are suspected.

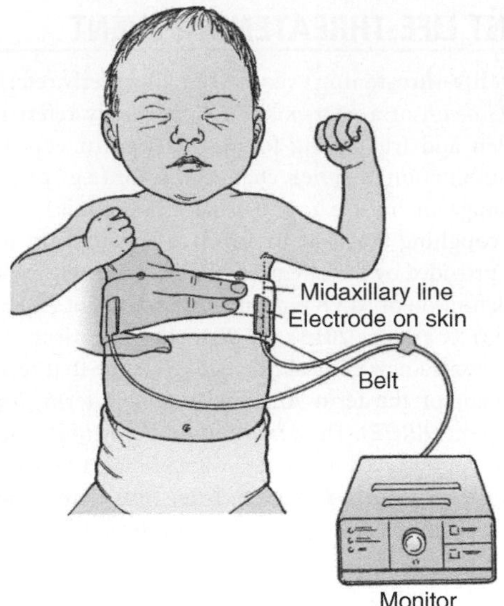

FIG. 11.4 Electrode placement for apnea monitoring. In small infants, one fingerbreadth may be used.

To lessen the continuous responsibility of monitoring, other family members, such as grandparents and other immediate family members, should be taught how to assess the infant for responsiveness, manipulate the equipment, read and interpret the signals, and administer CPR (if needed). They are encouraged to stay with the infant for regular periods to allow the parents respite. Support groups of other families who have successfully completed monitoring can also be of benefit. Because reliable babysitters can be difficult to locate, support group members and nursing students may be potential sources of qualified caregivers.

NCLEX REVIEW QUESTIONS

1. Vitamin A may be administered in significant amounts to children with this childhood communicable illness to decrease morbidity and mortality:
   A. Pertussis
   B. Varicella
   C. Rubella
   D. Measles
2. A 10-year-old child with a peanut allergy would be expected to have which of these as an early manifestation of his allergy? Select all that apply.
   A. Wheezing
   B. Nausea
   C. Headache
   D. Trouble breathing
   E. Urticaria
3. The recommended treatment for cow's milk protein allergy is the substitution of cow's milk–based formula for:
   A. Goat's milk
   B. Soy milk or a hydrolyzed formula
   C. Whole milk
   D. Evaporated milk
4. Which factors are considered protective factors for sudden infant death syndrome (SIDS)?
   A. Side sleeping position, breastfeeding, updated childhood immunization status
   B. Supine sleeping position, breastfeeding, soft bedding
   C. Prone sleeping position, exposure to maternal tobacco use, updated childhood immunization status
   D. Supine sleeping position, breastfeeding, updated childhood immunization status
5. A 3-month-old is being seen in the well-child clinic for positional plagiocephaly. The nurse knows that the initial interventions for this condition involve which of the following? Select all that apply.
   A. Place the infant to sleep in the prone position.
   B. Place the infant in a prone position when awake (approximately 15 min).
   C. Alternate the infant's head position (side of head) when asleep.
   D. Have the infant wear a soft helmet for 23 to 24 hours a day.
   E. Place the infant to sleep in an infant seat twice a day.

Correct Answers

1. D; 2. A, D, E; 3. B, C; 4. D; 5. B, C

REFERENCES

Academy of Breastfeeding Medicine. (2015). Position on breastfeeding—Revised 2015. *Breastfeeding Medicine: The Official Journal of the Academy of Breastfeeding Medicine, 10*(9).

Agarwal, A., Shaharyar, A., Kumar, A., et al. (2014). Scurvy in pediatric age group—A disease often forgotten. *Journal of Orthopaedic Trauma, 6,* 101–107.

Ahluwalia, N., Herrick, K. A., Rossen, L. M., et al. (2016). Usual nutrient intakes of US infants and toddlers generally meet or exceed Dietary Reference Intakes: findings from NHANES 2009–2010. *The American Journal of Clinical Nutrition, 104,* 1167–1174.

Akhnikh, S., Engelberts, A. C., van Sleuwen, B. E., et al. (2014). The excessively crying infant: etiology and treatment. *Pediatric Annals, 43*(4), e69–e75.

Albenberg, L., Evans, J., & Piccoli, D. A. (2016). Protracted diarrhea. In R. Wyllie, J. S. Hyams, & M. Kay (Eds.), *Pediatric gastrointestinal and liver disease* (5th ed.). Pennsylvania: Elsevier.

American Academy of Allergy, Asthma and Immunology. (2017) *Allergy statistics.* Retrieved from: http://www.aaaai.org/about-aaaai/newsroom/allergy-statistics.

American Academy of Pediatrics. (2016). *American academy of pediatrics announces new safe sleep recommendations to protect against SIDS, sleep-related infant deaths.* Retrieved from: https://www.aap.org/en-us/about-the-aap/aap-press-room/pages/american-academy-of-pediatrics-announces-new-safe-sleep-recommendations-to-protect-against-sids.aspx.

American Academy of Pediatrics. (2016). Task Force on Sudden Infant Death Syndrome: SIDS and other sleep-related infant deaths: Updated 2016 recommendations for a safe infant sleeping environment. *Pediatrics, 138*(5), 1–14.

American College of Allergy, Asthma and Immunology. (2014). *Types of allergies, food allergies.* Retrieved from: http://acaai.org/allergies/types/food-allergy.

American Heart Association. (2015). *Highlight of the 2015 American Heart Association guidelines update for CPR and ECC.* Retrieved from: http://eccguidelines.heart.org/wp-content/uploads/2015/10/2015-AHA-Guidelines-Highlights-English.pdf.

Anabrees, J., Indrio, F., Paes, B., et al. (2013). Probiotics for infantile colic: a systematic review. *BMC Pediatrics, 13*(1), 186.

Ashworth, A. (2016). Nutrition, food security, and health. In R. M. Kliegman, B. F. Stanton, J. W. St. Geme, et al. (Eds.), *Nelson textbook of pediatrics* (20th ed.). Philadelphia: Elsevier/Saunders.

Ateah, C. A. (2013). Prenatal parent education for first-time expectant parents: "Making it through labor is just the beginning…". *Journal of Pediatric Health Care, 27*(2), 91–97.

Becker, P., Carney, L. N., Corkins, M. R., et al. (2015). Consensus statement of the Academy of Nutrition and Dietetics/American Society for Parenteral and Enteral Nutrition: indicators recommended for the identification and documentation of pediatric malnutrition (undernutrition). *Nutrition in Clinical Practice, 30*(1), 147–161.

Bejjani, C., Machaalani, R., & Waters, K. A. (2013). The dorsal motor nucleus of the vagus (DMNV) in sudden infant death syndrome (SIDS): pathways leading to apoptosis. *Respiratory Physiology & Neurobiology, 185*(2), 203–210.

Bello, S., Meremikwu, M. M., Ejemot-Nwadiaro, R. I., et al. (2014). Routine vitamin A supplementation for the prevention of blindness due to measles infection in children. *The Cochrane Database of Systematic Reviews,* Retrieved from: http://onlinelibrary.wiley.com/doi/10.1002/14651858.CD007719.pub3/full.

Bello, S., Meremikwu, M. M., Ejemot-Nwadiaro, R. I., et al. (2016). Vitamin A for preventing blindness in children with measles. *The Cochrane Database of Systematic Reviews,* Retrieved from: http://www.cochrane.org/CD007719/ARI_vitamin-preventing-blindness-children-measles.

Bock, A. S., & Sampson, H. A. (2016). Evaluation of food allergy. In D. Y. Leung, S. J. Szefler, F. A. Bonilla, et al. (Eds.), *Pediatric allergy: principles and practice* (3rd ed.). New York: Elsevier.

Boyd, C., & Moodambail, A. (2016 October 6). Severe hypercalcaemia in a child secondary to use of alternative therapies. *BMJ Case Reports, 2016.*

Canani, R. B., Sangwan, N., & Stefka, A. T. (2016). Lactobacillus rhamnosus GG-supplemented formula expands butyrate-producing bacterial strains in food allergic infants. *The ISME Journal, 10,* 742–750.

Carpenter, R., McGarvey, C., Mitchell, E. A., et al. (2013). Bed-sharing when parents do not smoke: is there a risk of SIDS? An individual level analysis of five major case-control studies. *BMJ Open, 2013*(3), 1–12.

Carolan, P. L. (2016). Brief resolved unexplained events (apparent life-threatening events). In M. L. Windle & G. D. Sharma (Eds.), *Pediatric, general medicine.* Retrieved from: http://emedicine.medscape.com/article/1418765-overview.

Carter, K. A., Hathaway, N. E., & Lettieri, C. F. (2014). Common sleep disorders in children. *American Family Physician, 89*(5), 368–377.

Centers for Disease Control and Prevention. (2016). *Sudden unexpected infant death and sudden infant death syndrome, data and statistics.* Retrieved from: https://www.cdc.gov/sids/data.htm.

Chu, A., & Hageman, J. R. (2013). Apparent life-threatening events in infancy. *Pediatric Annals, 42*(2), 78–83.

Das, R. R., Sankar, M. J., Agarwal, R., et al. (2014). Is "bed sharing" beneficial and safe during infancy? A systematic review. *International Journal of Pediatrics, 1-16,* 2014.

Darlow, B. A., Horwood, J., Pere-Bracken, H. M., et al. (2013). Psychosocial outcomes of young adults born very low birth weight. *Pediatrics, 132*(6), e1521–e1528.

Deshpande, P. G. (2015). Colic. In M. L. Windle, S. Guandalini, & C. Cuffari (Eds.), *Pediatrics: general medicine.* Retrieved from: http://emedicine.medscape.com/article/927760-overview.

Drug and Therapeutics Bulletin. (2013). Management of infantile colic. *BMJ (Clinical Research Ed.), 347,* f4102.

Esposito, S., & Lelii, M. (2015). Vitamin D and respiratory tract infections in childhood. *BMC Infectious Diseases, 16,* 487.

Fleischer, D. M., Burks, A. W., Vickery, B. P., et al. (2013). Sublingual immunotherapy for peanut allergy: a randomized, double-blind, placebo-controlled multicenter trial. *Journal of Allergy and Clinical Immunology, 131*(1), 119–127.

Flenady, V., Boyle, F., Koopmans, L., et al. (2014). Meeting the needs of parents after a stillbirth or neonatal death. *BJOG: An International Journal of Obstetrics and Gynaecology, 121*(Suppl. 4), 137–140.

Furman, L. (2015). Maternal vitamin D supplementation for breastfeeding infants: will it work? *Pediatrics, 136*(4), 763–764.

Gelfer, P., Cameron, R., Masters, K., et al. (2013). Integrating "back to sleep" recommendations into neonatal ICU practice. *Pediatrics, 131*(4), e1264–e1270.

Groetch, M., & Sampson, H. A. (2016). Management of food allergy. In D. Y. Lueng, S. J. Szefler, F. A. Bonilla, et al. (Eds.), *Pediatric allergy principles and practice* (3rd ed.). Pennsylvania: Elsevier.

Högenauer, C., & Hammer, H. F. (2016). Maldigestion and malabsorption. In M. Feldman, L. S. Friedman, & L. J. Brandt (Eds.), *Sleisenger and fordtran's gastrointestinal and liver disease* (10th ed.). New York: Elsevier.

Hunt, C. E., & Hauck, F. R. (2016). Sudden infant death syndrome. In R. M. Kliegman, B. F. Stanton, J. W. St Geme, et al. (Eds.), *Nelson textbook of pediatrics* (20th ed.). Pennsylvania: Elsevier.

Jones, K. D., & Berkley, J. A. (2014). Severe acute malnutrition and infection. *Paediatrics and International Child Health, 34*(Suppl. 1), S1–S29.

Keet, C., & Wang, J. (2014). Acute reactions and anaphylaxis. In S. H. Sicherer (Ed.), *Food allergy practical diagnosis and management* (1st ed.). Florida: CRC Press.

Kleinman, R. E., & Greer, R. F. (Eds.), (2014). *Pediatric nutrition* (7th ed.). Elk Grove Village, IL: American Academy of Pediatrics.

Lawrence, R. M. (2013). Circumstances when breastfeeding is contraindicated. *Pediatric Clinics of North America, 60*(1), 295–318.

Longo, G., Berti, I., Burks, A. W., et al. (2013). IgE-mediated food allergy in children. *Lancet, 382*(9905), 1656–1664.

Mandese, V., Marotti, F., Bedetti, L., et al. (2016). Effects of nutritional intake on disease severity in children with sickle cell disease. *Nutrition Journal, 15*(1).

Mason, B., Ahlers-Schmidt, C. R., & Schunn, C. (2013). Improving safe sleep environments for well newborns in the hospital setting. *Clinical Pediatrics, 52*(10), 969–975.

Matthews, R., & Moore, A. (2013). Babies are still dying of SIDS. *The American Journal of Nursing, 113*(2), 59–64.

McLean, H. S., & Price, D. T. (2016). Failure to thrive. In R. M. Kliegman, B. F. Stanton, J. W. St Geme, et al. (Eds.), *Nelson textbook of pediatrics* (20th ed.). Pennsylvania: Elsevier.

Milidou, I., Sondergaard, C., Jensen, M. S., et al. (2014). Gestational age, small for gestational age, and infantile colic. *Paediatric and Perinatal Epidemiology, 28*(2), 138–145.

Mishra, K., Kumar, P., Basu, S., et al. (2014). Risk factors for severe acute malnutrition in children below 5 y of age in India: a case-control study. *Indian Journal of Pediatrics, 81*(8), 762–765.

Muscat, T., Obst, P., Cockshaw, W., et al. (2014). Beliefs about infant regulation, early infant behaviors and maternal postnatal depressive symptoms. *Birth (Berkeley, Calif.), 41*(2), 206–213.

Myers, R. P., Duncan, A. N., & Girotto, J. A. (2016). Deformational plagiocephaly. In R. M. Kliegman, B. F. Stanton, J. W. St Geme, et al. (Eds.), *Nelson textbook of pediatrics* (20th ed.). Pennsylvania: Elsevier.

Nangia, S., & Tiwari, S. (2013). Failure to thrive. *Indian Journal of Pediatrics, 80*(7), 585–589.

National Institutes of Health Office of Dietary Supplement. (2016). *strengthening knowledge and understanding of dietary supplements.* Retrieved from: https://ods.od.nih.gov/factsheets/VitaminD-Consumer/.

Nowak-Węgrzyn, A., Sampson, H. A., & Sicherer, S. H. (2016). Food allergy and adverse reactions to foods. In R. M. Kliegman, B. F. Stanton, J. W. St Geme, et al. (Eds.), *Nelson textbook of pediatrics* (20th ed.). Pennsylvania: Elsevier.

Nowak-Węgrzyn, A., & Sicherer, S. H. (2016). Serum sickness. In R. M. Kliegman, B. F. Stanton, J. W. St Geme, et al. (Eds.), *Nelson textbook of pediatrics* (20th ed.). Pennsylvania: Elsevier.

Owens, J. A. (2016). Sleep medicine. In R. M. Kliegman, B. F. Stanton, J. W. St Geme, et al. (Eds.), *Nelson textbook of pediatrics* (20th ed.). Pennsylvania: Elsevier.

Pawlak, R., Parrott, S. J., Raj, S., et al. (2013). How prevalent is vitamin B (12) deficiency among vegetarians? *Nutrition Reviews, 71*(2), 110–117.

Porto, A. (2016). Lactose intolerance in infants & children: Parent FAQs. Retrieved from: https://www.healthychildren.org/English/healthy-living/nutrition/Pages/Lactose-Intolerance-in-Children.aspx.

Rechtman, L. R., Colvin, J. D., Blair, P. S., et al. (2014). Sofas and infant mortality. *Pediatrics, 134*(5), e1293–e1300.

Romano, C., Hartman, C., Privitera, C., et al. (2015). Current topics in the diagnosis and management of the pediatric non organic feeding disorders (NOFEDs). *Clinical Nutrition: Official Journal of the European Society of Parenteral and Enteral Nutrition, 34*(2), 195–200.

Sampson, H. A. (2013). Peanut oral immunotherapy: is it ready for clinical practice? *The Joural of Allergy and Clinical Immunology. in Practice, 1*(1), 15–21.

Savino, F., Ceratto, S., Poggi, E., et al. (2015). Preventive effects of oral probiotic on infantile colic: a prospective, randomized blinded, controlled trial using Lactobacillus reuteri DSM 17938. *Beneficial Microbes, 6*(3), 245–251.

Sigua, J. A., & Zacharisen, M. (2013). Heiner syndrome mimicking an immune deficiency. *Official Publication of the State Medical Society of Wisconsin, 112*(5), 215–217.

Sirotnak, A. P., & Chiesa, A. (2016). Failure to thrive. In M. L. Windle & C. Pataki (Eds.), *Pediatrics: developmental and behavioral articles.* Retrieved from: http://emedicine.medscape.com/article/915575-overview.

Szajewska, H., Gyrczuk, E., & Horvath, A. (2013). Lactobacillus reuteri DSM 17938 for the management of infantile colic in breastfed infants: a randomized, double-blind, placebo-controlled trial. *The Journal of Pediatrics, 162*(2), 257–262.

Talarico, V., Barreca, M., Galiano, R., et al. (2016). Vitamin D and risk for vitamin A intoxication in an 18-month-old boy. *Case Reports in Pediatrics, 2016* (article id 1395718), 1–3.

Tieder, J. S., Altman, R. L., Bonkowsky, J. L., et al. (2013). Management of apparent life-threatening events in infants: A systematic review. *The Journal of Pediatrics, 163*(1), 94–99.

Trehan, I., & Manary, M. J. (2015). Management of severe acute malnutrition in low-income and middle-income countries. *Archives of Disease in Childhood, 100*(3), 283–287.

Turer, C. B., Lin, H., & Flores, G. (2013). Prevalence of vitamin D deficiency among overweight and obese US children. *Pediatrics, 131*(1), e152–e161.

UNICEF. (2013). *Position paper, ready-to-use therapeutic food for children with severe acute malnutrition.* Retrieved from: https://www.unicef.org/media/files/Position_Paper_Ready-to-use_therapeutic_food_for_children_with_severe_acute_malnutrition__June_2013.pdf.

US Department of Agriculture. (2016). *Economic Research Service: Definitions of food security.* Retrieved from: https://www.ers.usda.gov/topics/food-nutrition-assistance/food-security-in-the-us/definitions-of-food-security.aspx.

van Wijk, R. M., van Vlimmeren, L. A., Groothuis-Oudshoorn, C. G., et al. (2014). Helmet therapy in infants with positional skull deformation: randomized controlled trial. *BMJ (Clinical Research Ed.), 348*, g2741.

Wacker, M., & Holick, M. F. (2013). Vitamin D—Effects on skeletal and extraskeletal health and the need for supplementation. *Nutrients, 5*(1), 111–148.

WHO Child Growth Standards. (2017a). *Length/height-for-age, weight-for-age, weight-for-length, weight-for-height and body mass index-for-age methods and development.* Retrieved from: http://www.who.int/childgrowth/standards/technical_report/en/.

World Health Organization. (2017b). *Management of severe acute malnutrition in infants and children.* Retrieved from: http://www.who.int/elena/titles/full_recommendations/sam_management/en/.

Wozniak, L. J., Bechtold, H. M., Reyen, L. E., et al. (2015). Vitamin D deficiency in children with intestinal failure receiving home parenteral nutrition. *Journal of Parenteral Enteral Nutr, 39*(4), 471–475.

Zhang, K., & Wang, X. (2013). Maternal smoking and increased risk of sudden infant death syndrome: a meta-analysis. *Legal Medicine, 15*(3), 115–121.

12

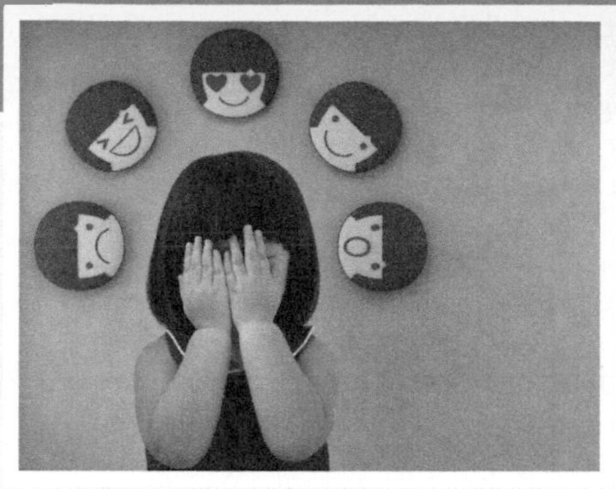

Health Promotion of the Toddler and Family

Elizabeth A. Duffy

http://evolve.elsevier.com/wong/ncic

CONCEPTS

- Development
- Functional Ability
- Communication
- Nutrition
- Safety

PROMOTING OPTIMUM GROWTH AND DEVELOPMENT

The term *terrible twos* has often been used to describe the toddler years, the period from 12 to 36 months of age. It is a time of intense exploration of the environment as children attempt to find out how things work; what the word "no" means; and the power of temper tantrums, negativism, and obstinacy. "Getting into things" is their way of learning about their world, especially relationships. Successful mastery of the tasks of this age requires a strong foundation of trust during infancy and frequently necessitates guidance from others when parent and toddler face the struggles of toilet training, limit setting, and sibling rivalry. Nurses who understand the dynamics of growth and development of the toddler can help families deal effectively with the tasks of this age.

BIOLOGIC DEVELOPMENT

Proportional Changes

Physical growth slows considerably during toddlerhood. The average weight at 2 years is 12 kg (26.5 lb). The average weight gain is 1.8 to 2.7 kg (4 to 6 lb) per year. The birth weight is quadrupled by 2½ years old. The rate of increase in height also slows. The usual increment is an addition of 7.5 cm (3 inches) per year and occurs mainly in elongation of the legs rather than the trunk. The average height of a 2-year-old is 86.6 cm (34 inches). In general, adult height is about twice the child's height at 2 years of age. Accurate measurement of height and weight during the toddler years should reveal a steady growth curve that is *steplike* rather than linear (straight), which is characteristic of the growth spurts during the early childhood years.

The rate of increase in head circumference slows somewhat by the end of infancy, and head circumference is usually equal to chest circumference by 1 to 2 years of age. The usual total increase in head circumference during the second year is 2.5 cm (1 inch). Then the rate of increase slows until age 5 years, when the increase is less than 1.25 cm (0.5 inch) per year. The anterior fontanel closes between 12 and 18 months of age.

Chest circumference continues to increase and exceeds head circumference during the toddler years. The chest's shape also changes as the transverse (or lateral) diameter exceeds the anteroposterior diameter. After the second year the chest circumference exceeds the abdominal measurement, which, in addition to the growth of the lower extremities, gives the child a taller, leaner appearance. However, the toddler retains a squat, "potbellied" appearance because of the less well-developed abdominal musculature and short legs (Fig. 12.1). The legs retain a slightly bowed or curved appearance during the second year from the weight of the relatively large trunk.

Sensory Changes

Visual acuity of 20/40 is considered acceptable during the toddler years. Full binocular vision is well developed, and any evidence of persistent strabismus should receive professional attention as early as possible to prevent amblyopia. Depth perception continues to develop, but because of the child's lack of motor coordination, falls from heights remain a persistent danger.

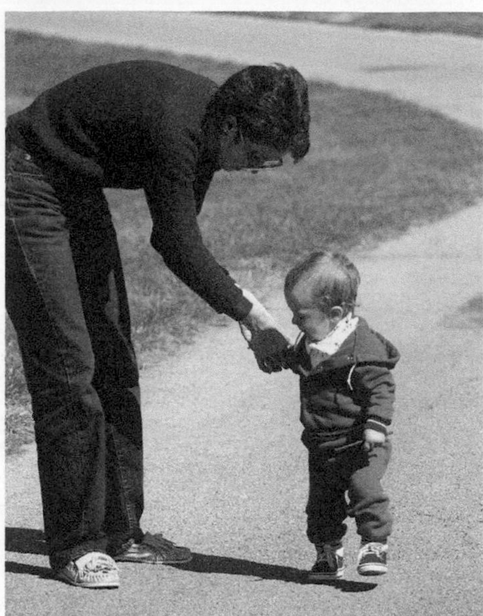
FIG. 12.1 Typical toddling gait.

The senses of hearing, smell, taste, and touch become increasingly well developed, coordinated with one another, and associated with other experiences. All of the senses are used to explore the environment. Toddlers visually inspect an object by turning it over; they may taste it, smell it, and touch it several times before they are satisfied with their investigation. They will shake it to see if it makes noise and vigorously test its durability.

Another example of the integrated function of the senses is the toddlers' development of specific taste and texture preferences. Toddlers are much less likely than infants to try a new food because of its appearance or smell, not just its taste. Likewise, a toddler is likely to reject a new food because of its texture. Nonsensory associations with objects also take on significance. For example, if parents refuse a particular food because of their dislike, they will transfer this negative connotation to the child before the child has had an opportunity to taste it. Awareness of these factors is important in several areas of childrearing, such as feeding, teaching socially acceptable habits, and reinforcing appropriate behavioral responses to various situations.

Touch continues to be important to the toddler. Descending development of the spinal tract is evidenced by increased sensation in the lower extremities, such as ticklish feet. Pleasant tactile sensations soothe and comfort the toddler, especially in times of stress or fatigue.

Maturation of Systems

Most of the physiologic systems are relatively mature by the end of toddlerhood. By the end of the first year, all the brain cells are present but continue to increase in size. Myelination of the spinal cord is almost complete by 2 years old, which parallels the completion of most of the gross motor skills associated with locomotion. Brain growth is 75% completed by the end of 2 years.

Development of various areas of the brain seems to correspond with the child's progressive intellectual capacity. As development progresses, specific changes take place in various areas of the cerebral cortex, such as the Broca area for speech and cortical areas for control of the legs, hands, feet, and sphincters. Because this neuromotor organization is so inclusive, complex, and intricate, the child is limited in the ability to attend to any one aspect of behavior for more than a few minutes.

Between 2 and 3 years old, coordination and consolidation of these voluntary functions allow the toddler to listen better, look longer, and have an extended attention span. Although postural control is increasingly developed as myelination of the spinal cord advances, the immaturity of this control, combined with the child's limited experiences and lack of visual perception, makes it difficult to do simple acts such as seating oneself in a chair or climbing down stairs.

Volume of the respiratory tract and growth of associated structures continue to increase during early childhood, lessening some of the factors that predisposed the child to frequent and serious infections during infancy. The internal structures of the ear and throat continue to be short and straight, and the lymphoid tissue of the tonsils and adenoids continues to be large. As a result, otitis media, tonsillitis, and upper respiratory tract infections are common. The respiratory and heart rates slow, and the blood pressure increases (see inside back cover). Respirations continue to be abdominal.

The digestive processes are fairly complete by the beginning of toddlerhood. The acidity of the gastric contents continues to increase and has a protective function because it destroys many types of bacteria. Stomach capacity increases to allow for the usual schedule of three small meals a day.

One of the more prominent changes of the gastrointestinal system is the voluntary control of elimination. With complete myelination of the spinal cord, control of anal and urethral sphincters is gradually achieved. The physiologic ability to control the sphincters occurs somewhere between ages 18 and 24 months old. Bladder capacity also increases considerably. By 14 to 18 months old the child is able to retain urine for up to 2 hours or longer.

The skin functionally matures during early childhood. The epidermis and dermis are more tightly bound together, increasing their resistance to infection and irritation and creating a more effective barrier against fluid loss. Production of sebum is minimal, which contributes to the development of dry skin. The eccrine glands are functional during early childhood and react to changes in temperature, but they produce minimum amounts of sweat. Hair grows thicker and coarser and usually darkens and loses some curliness. Fine hair is evident on the lower arms and legs. Production of adipose tissue declines as hyperplasia of muscle cells increases. With the concurrent growth of the lower extremities, the child assumes more adultlike proportions.

Under conditions of moderate variation in temperature, the toddler rarely has the difficulties of the young infant in maintaining body temperature. The capillaries are able to conserve core body temperature by constricting in response to cold and dilating in response to heat. Shivering, an involuntary act that results in rhythmic muscle contraction, which increases cellular metabolism and produces heat, is much more effective as a source of thermogenesis. The child also learns mechanisms to control body temperature—putting on clothing when cold or removing it when warm.

The defense mechanisms of the tissues and blood, particularly phagocytosis and chemotaxis, are much more efficient in the toddler than in the infant. The production of antibodies is well established. Immunoglobulin G, which neutralizes microbial toxins, reaches adult levels by the end of the second year of life. Passive immunity from maternal transfer during fetal life disappears by the beginning of toddlerhood. Immunoglobulin M, which responds to artificial immunizing techniques and combats serious infection, attains adult levels during late infancy. Immunoglobulins A, D, and E increase gradually, not reaching eventual adult levels until later childhood. However, many young children demonstrate a sudden increase in colds and minor infections when entering day care or preschool because of exposure to new antigens.

Gross and Fine Motor Development

The major gross motor skill during the toddler years is the development of locomotion. By 12 to 13 months old, toddlers walk alone, using a wide stance for extra balance; by age 18 months old, they try to run but fall easily. Between 2 and 3 years of age, refinement of the upright, biped position is evident in improved coordination and equilibrium. At 2 years old toddlers can walk up and down stairs, and by age 2½ years they jump using both feet, stand on one foot for a second or two, and manage a few steps on tiptoe. By the end of the second year they stand on one foot, walk on tiptoe, and climb stairs with alternate footing.

Fine motor development is demonstrated in increasingly skillful manual dexterity. Once toddlers achieve pincer grasp, usually at 9 to 10 months old, they combine this skill with other developing sensory and cognitive abilities. For example, by age 12 months old they are able to grasp a very small object. By age 15 months they can drop a pellet into a narrow-necked bottle. Casting or throwing objects and retrieving them become an almost obsessive activity at about 15 months old. By 18 months old, toddlers can throw a ball overhand without losing their balance.

Visual perception of geometric shapes is also evident at this time. At 12 months old children selectively look at a round hole in a special form board but are unable to insert a round object. By age 15 months they promptly place the round object in the hole, even if the board is revised or turned upside down. Spatial relations also are evident in their ability to build a tower with blocks: by age 18 months, a tower of three or four blocks; by age 24 months, a tower of six or seven blocks; and by age 30 months, a tower of eight blocks or more.

Fine motor skill and visual ability are demonstrated in toddlers' progressive adeptness in manipulating a pencil or crayon. By age 15 months they scribble spontaneously, and by age 24 months they imitate a circular stroke and a vertical line. By the end of the toddler period, the child can copy a circle and imitate a cross.

Mastery of gross and fine motor skills is evident in all phases of the child's activity, such as play, dressing, language comprehension, response to discipline, social interaction, and propensity for injuries. Activities occur less in isolation and more in conjunction with other physical and mental abilities to produce a purposeful result. For example, the toddler walks to reach a new location, releases a toy and picks it up again or chooses a new one, and scribbles to look at the image produced. The possibilities of the exploration, investigation, and manipulation mastery of the environment—and its hazards—are endless.

Psychosocial Development

Toddlers are faced with the mastery of several important tasks. If the need for basic trust has been satisfied, they are ready to give up dependence for control, independence, and autonomy. Some of the specific tasks include the following:

- Differentiation of self from others, particularly the mother or primary caregiver
- Toleration of separation from parents
- Ability to withstand delayed gratification
- Control over bodily functions
- Acquisition of socially acceptable behavior
- Verbal means of communication
- Ability to interact with others in a less egocentric manner

Mastery of these goals is only begun during late infancy and the toddler years, and such tasks as developing interpersonal relationships with others may not be completed until adolescence. However, crucial foundations for successful completion of such developmental tasks are laid during these early formative years.

Developing a Sense of Autonomy (Erikson)

According to Erikson (1963), the developmental task of toddlerhood is acquiring a sense of **autonomy** while overcoming a sense of doubt and shame. As infants gain trust in the predictability and reliability of their parents, environment, and interaction with others, they begin to discover that their behavior is their own and that it has a predictable, reliable effect on others. Although they are aware of their will and control over others, they are confronted with the conflict of exerting autonomy and relinquishing the much enjoyed dependence on others. Exerting their will has definite negative consequences, whereas retaining dependent, submissive behavior is generally rewarded with affection and approval. On the other hand, continued dependency creates a sense of doubt regarding their potential capacity to control their actions. This doubt is compounded by a sense of *shame* for feeling this urge to revolt against others' will and a fear that they will exceed their own capacity for manipulating the environment. The latter fear is a basis for instituting limit setting and consistent discipline at this age. Without appropriate limits on what is acceptable versus unacceptable behavior, children have no guidelines for establishing the end-points of their ability to control.

Just as the infant has the social modalities of grasping and biting, the toddler has the newly gained modality of holding on and letting go. Holding on and letting go are evident in how the toddler uses the hands, mouth, eyes, and, eventually, sphincters when toilet training is begun. Children constantly express these social modalities in play activities such as casting or throwing objects; taking objects out of boxes, drawers, or cabinets; holding on tighter when someone says, "No, don't touch"; and refusing to eat certain foods as taste preferences become strong.

Several characteristics, especially **negativism** and **ritualism**, are typical of toddlers in their quest for autonomy. As toddlers attempt to express their will, they often act with negativism, giving a negative response to requests. The words "no" or "me do" can be the sole vocabulary. Emotions become strongly expressed, usually in rapid mood swings. One minute toddlers can be engrossed in an activity, and the next minute they might be violently angry because they were unable to manipulate a toy or open a door. If scolded for doing something wrong, they can have a temper tantrum and almost instantaneously pull at the parent's legs to be picked up and comforted. Understanding and coping with these swift changes is often difficult for parents. Many parents find the negativism exasperating and, instead of dealing constructively with it, give in to it, which further threatens the child's search for acceptable methods of interacting with others.

In contrast to negativism, which frequently disrupts the environment, ritualism, the need to maintain sameness and reliability, provides a sense of comfort. Toddlers can venture out with security when they know that familiar people, places, and routines still exist. One can easily understand why change, such as hospitalization, represents such a threat to these children. Without the comfortable rituals, they have little opportunity to exert autonomy. Consequently, dependency and regression occur (see Regression, later in this chapter).

Erikson focuses on the development of the ego, which may be thought of as reason or common sense, during this phase of psychosocial development. The child struggles to deal with the impulses of the id, tolerate frustration, and learn socially acceptable ways of interacting with the environment. The ego becomes evident as the child is able to delay gratification.

Toddlers also have a rudimentary beginning of the superego, or conscience, which is the incorporation of the morals of society and the process of acculturation. With the development of the ego, children further differentiate themselves from others and expand their sense of trust in self. But as they begin to develop awareness of their own will and capacity to achieve, they also become aware of their ability to fail.

This ever-present awareness of potential failure creates doubt and shame. Successful mastery of the task of autonomy necessitates opportunities for self-mastery while withstanding the frustration of necessary limit setting and delayed gratification. Opportunities for self-mastery are present in appropriate play activities, toilet training, the crisis of sibling rivalry, and successful interactions with significant others.

COGNITIVE DEVELOPMENT

Sensorimotor Phase (Piaget)

The period from 12 to 24 months old is a continuation of the final two stages of the sensorimotor phase (Table 12.1). During this time the cognitive processes develop rapidly and at times seem similar to mature thinking. However, reasoning skills are still primitive and need to be understood to effectively deal with the typical behaviors of this age child. The main cognitive achievement of early childhood is the acquisition of language, which represents mental symbolism.

In the fifth stage, **tertiary circular reactions** (from 13 to 18 months old), the child uses active experimentation to achieve previously unattainable goals. Newly acquired physical skills are increasingly important for the function they serve rather than for the acts themselves. The child incorporates the old learning of secondary circular reactions and applies the combined knowledge to new situations, with emphasis on the results of the experimentation. In this way there is the beginning of rational judgment and intellectual reasoning. During this stage the child further differentiates self from objects. This is evident in the child's increasing ability to venture away from the parent and to tolerate longer periods of separation.

Awareness of a **causal relationship** between two events is apparent. After flipping a light switch, toddlers are aware that a response occurs. However, they are not able to transfer that knowledge to new situations. Therefore every time they see what appears to be a light switch, they must reinvestigate its function. Such behavior demonstrates the beginning of categorizing data into distinct classes, subclasses, and so

TABLE 12.1 Sensorimotor and Preoperational Phases During Toddlerhood*

Stage and Age	Cognitive Development	Behavior
Sensorimotor		
V. Tertiary circular reactions (13-18 months)	Active experimentation to achieve previously unattainable goals Increased concept of object permanence Differentiation of oneself from objects Early traces of memory Beginning awareness of spatial, causal, and temporal relationships Able to enter into an action at any point without reproducing entire sequence	Insatiable curiosity about environment Uses all sensory cues for exploration Ventures away from parent for longer periods Uses physical skills to achieve particular goal Can find hidden objects, but only in first location Able to insert round object into hole Fits smaller objects into each other (nesting) Gestures "up" and "down" Puts objects into container and takes them out Realizes that "out of sight" is not out of reach; opens doors and drawers to find objects Gains comfort from parent's voice even if parent is not visible
VI. Invention of new means through mental combinations (19-24 months)	Awareness of object permanence regardless of number of invisible displacements Can infer a cause only while experiencing the effect Imitation increasingly symbolic Beginning sense of time in terms of anticipation, memory, and ability to wait Egocentrism in thought and behavior Global organization of thought	Searches for object through several hiding places Will infer cause by associating two or more experiences (such as candy missing, sister smiling) Imitates words and sounds of animals Imitates adult behavior (domestic mimicry) Follows directions and understands requests Uses words "up," "down," "come," and "go" with meaning May sit and wait for meals at table for short period Has some sense of time; waits in response to "just a minute"; may use word "now" Refers to self by name Engages in parallel play; demonstrates awareness of ownership Concerned with ritualistic, routinized schedule
Preoperational		
2-4 year	Increased use of language as mental symbolization Egocentrism still present in thought, play, and behavior Increased sense of time, space, causality See Box 12.1	Uses two- or three-word phrases Increased vocabulary Refers to self by pronoun Possessive of own toys; uses word "mine" Begins to use past tense of verbs Uses phrases "going to," "in a minute," "today," "all done" Uses many future-oriented words, such as "tomorrow," "next day," "afternoon," but has poor concept of passage of time Follows directions using prepositions, such as "up," "behind," "under," "in back of"

*For the previous four stages during early infancy, see Table 10.1.

on. Innumerable examples of this type of behavior occur as toddlers repeatedly explore the same object each time it appears in a new place. A classic example is their curiosity about electrical outlets. Even if they receive a shock from one of them, they will adamantly poke and inspect every other outlet. This inability to transfer information leaves toddlers particularly vulnerable to injuries. However, traces of memory are evident because they usually avoid the outlet where the shock occurred.

Because classification of objects is still basic, the appearance of an object indicates its function. For example, if the child's toys are stored in a paper bag or large container, the toddler does not perceive a difference between that toy receptacle and the garbage pail or laundry basket. If allowed to turn over the toy receptacle, the child will just as quickly do the same to other similar objects because, in the child's mind, there is no difference. Expecting toddlers to judge which receptacles are permissible to explore and which are not is inappropriate for this age-group. Instead, the forbidden object, such as the garbage pail, should be placed out of reach. This has significant implications for prevention of accidents and accidental ingestion of injurious agents.

The discovery of objects as objects leads to an awareness of their spatial relationships. Children are able to recognize different shapes and their relationship to one another. For example, they can fit slightly smaller boxes into each other (nesting) and can place a round object into a hole, even if the board is turned around, upside down, or reversed. However, they cannot do the same thing with a square until 2 years of age. Children are also aware of space and the relationship of their body to dimensions such as height. They will stretch, stand on a low stair or stool, and pull a string to reach an object.

Object permanence has also advanced. Although they still cannot find an object that has been displaced and is no longer visible or has been moved from under one pillow to another without their seeing the change, toddlers are increasingly aware of the existence of objects behind closed doors, in drawers, and under tables. Parents are usually acutely aware of this developmental achievement because they find high places and locked cabinets to be the only areas inaccessible to toddlers. Parents also experience toddlers' protest behaviors when the parents leave because toddlers are aware that their parents are absent when they cannot see them.

During ages 19 to 24 months the child is in the final sensorimotor stage, invention of new means through mental combinations. This stage completes the more primitive, autistic thought processes of infancy and prepares the way for more complex mental operations during the phase of preoperational thought. One of the most dramatic achievements of this stage is in the area of object permanence. Toddlers will now actively search for an object in several potential hiding places. In addition, they can infer a cause when only experiencing the effect. They can infer that an object was hidden in any number of places even if they only saw the original hiding place.

Imitation displays deeper meaning and understanding. Earlier, imitation was concrete and action oriented. For example, "bye-bye" was a behavioral response more than a conceptual gesture of departure. Now it has a broader meaning, such as Mommy is going to work, it is time for a walk, or something is no longer present. There is greater symbolization to imitation.

One type of symbolic imitation is domestic mimicry, the imitation of household activity. Toddlers are acutely aware of others' actions and attempt to copy them in gestures and in words. They can imitate the parents' performance of a household task both physically and verbally (Fig. 12.2). Parents often remark how accurately they see themselves when the toddler engages in domestic mimicry. Such activity is part of the toddler's learning sex-role behavior. Identification with the parent of the same sex becomes apparent by the second year and represents the toddler's intellectual ability to differentiate models of behavior and to imitate them appropriately.

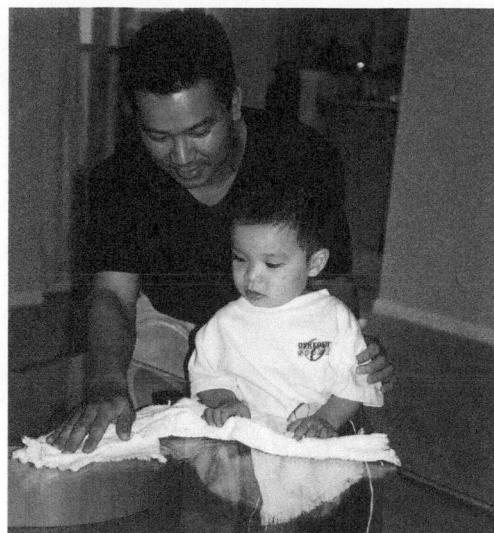

FIG. 12.2 Domestic mimicry is common during toddlerhood.

The concept of time is still embryonic, but toddlers have some sense of timing in terms of anticipation, memory, and the limited ability to wait. They may listen to the command "Just a minute" and behave appropriately. However, their sense of timing is exaggerated—1 minute can last an hour. Toddlers' limited attention spans also indicate their sense of immediacy and concern for the present.

Egocentrism, or the inability to envision situations from perspectives other than one's own, is evident in all aspects of toddlers' behavior. They see, experience, and live every event in reference to themselves. A common example of egocentric behavior is the toddler who takes a toy away from another child. The toddler is concerned only with playing with the toy and is unable to conceptualize that taking the toy away will make the other child unhappy.

Preoperational Phase (Piaget)

At approximately 2 years of age the child enters the preconceptual phase of cognitive development, which lasts until about age 4 years. The preconceptual phase is a subdivision of the preoperational phase, which spans ages 2 to 7 years. The preconceptual phase is primarily one of transition that bridges the purely self-satisfying behavior of infancy and the undeveloped socialized behavior of latency. Preoperational thinking implies that children cannot think in terms of operations—the ability to manipulate objects in relation to each other in a logical fashion. Rather, toddlers think primarily on the basis of their perception of an event. Problem solving is based on what the toddler sees or hears directly rather than on what the toddler recalls about objects or events. The principal characteristics of this stage are egocentric use of language and dependence on perception in problem solving.

From ages 2 to 4 years old children learn a variety of words and increasingly use language. In fact, toddlers talk a lot. Speech is primarily of two types: egocentric or socialized. Egocentric speech consists of repeating words and sounds for the pleasure of hearing oneself and is not intended to communicate. This collective monologue reflects the child's lingering self-centeredness.

Socialized speech is for communication; however, it is still egocentric in that children communicate about themselves to others. Before age 3 most speech is directed at self-fulfillment or self-reference, such as "Want drink" or "I do," and it is directed mostly toward adults. Because children think that everyone else's world is the same as theirs, they expect others to understand their verbal messages even when limited information is conveyed.

Preoperational thinking implies that children cannot think in terms of operations—the ability to manipulate objects in relation to one another in a logical fashion. Rather, toddlers think primarily based on their perception of an event. Problem solving is based on what they see or hear directly rather than on what they recall about objects and events (Box 12.1).

Within the second year the child increasingly uses language symbolically and is concerned with the "why" and "how" of things. For example, a pencil is "something to write with" and food is "something to eat." However, such **mental symbolization** is closely associated with prelogical reasoning. For instance, a needle is "something that hurts." Such painful experiences take on new significance because memory is associated with the specific event, and fears are likely to develop, such as resistance to people who wear uniform scrubs or rooms that look like the practitioner's office. Sometimes parents and health care personnel underestimate the child's ability to recall events and give little thought to preparation for visits to a practitioner's office or other health facility, resulting in fears that can last a lifetime. Because of the vulnerability of these early years, it is essential to prepare children for new experiences, whether it is a new babysitter, a primary practitioner, or a visit to the dentist.

BOX 12.1 Characteristics of Preoperational Thought

Egocentrism—Inability to envision situations from perspectives other than one's own

- Example—If a person is positioned between the toddler and another child, the toddler, who is facing the person, will explain that both children can see the middle person's face. The toddler is unable to realize that the other child views the middle person from a different perspective, the back.

Transductive—Reasoning from the particular to the particular

- Example—Child refuses to eat a food because something previously eaten did not taste good.

Global organization—Belief that a change in any one part of the whole changes the entire whole

- Example—Child refuses to sleep in room because location of bed is changed.

Centration—Focusing on one aspect rather than considering all possible alternatives

- Example—Child refuses to eat a food because of its color, even though its taste and smell are acceptable.

Animism—Attributing lifelike qualities to inanimate objects

- Example—Child scolds stairs for making child fall down.

Irreversibility—Inability to undo or reverse the actions initiated physically

- Example—When told to stop doing something, such as talking, child is unable to think of opposite activity.

Magical—Believing that thoughts are all-powerful and can cause events

- Example—Child wishes someone dead; then if the person dies, child feels at fault because of the "bad" thought that made the death happen.
- Example—Calling children "bad" because they did something wrong makes children feel as though they are bad.

Inability to conserve—Inability to understand the idea that a mass can be changed in size, shape, volume, or length without losing or adding to the original mass (instead, children judge what they see by the immediate perceptual clues given to them)

- Example—If two lines of equal length are presented in such a way that one appears longer than the other, the child will state that one line is longer even if he or she measures both lines with a ruler and finds that they are the same length.

MORAL DEVELOPMENT: PRECONVENTIONAL OR PREMORAL LEVEL

Toddlers' development of moral judgment is at the most basic level. They have little, if any, concern for why something is wrong. Kohlberg's theory of moral development is influenced by Piaget's theory of moral thought; the first phase of Kohlberg's theory is called the preconventional phase, and it involves punishment and obedience. Young children behave in accordance with the freedom or restriction that is placed on actions. In the punishment and obedience orientation, whether an action is good or bad depends on whether it results in reward or punishment. If children are punished for it, the action is bad. If they are not punished, the action is good, regardless of the meaning of the act. For example, if parents allow hitting, the child will perceive that hitting is good because it is not associated with punishment. By age 36 months, developmental aspects of conscience may be present.

The type of discipline also affects children's moral development. When parents use power to control behavior, such as physical punishment or withholding privileges, children receive a negative view of morals, especially toward authority figures, such as law enforcement officials. When parents withdraw love or attention, children behave primarily because of guilt, rather than from an internalization of morals. However, when parents give explanations for the misbehavior and try to help children change through positive approaches, such as consequences or rewards, children feel less hostility and are more likely to base their actions on an analysis of why an act may be wrong. Of course, the effect of discipline is not limited to the toddler years, and the sole use of explanation is inappropriate during this period. Because parents usually establish disciplinary techniques at this time, the use of constructive approaches should begin early. (See Limit Setting and Discipline, Chapter 2.)

SPIRITUAL DEVELOPMENT

Spiritual development in children is often discussed in terms of the child's developmental level because the evolution of spirituality often parallels cognitive development (Lima, do Nascimento, de Carvalho et al., 2013). The child's family and environment strongly influence his or her perception of the world around him or her, and this often includes spirituality. Furthermore, family values, beliefs, customs, and expressions of these influence the child's perception of his or her spiritual self (Lima, do Nascimento, de Carvalho et al., 2013). Neuman (2011) proposes that Fowler's stages of faith (Fowler, 1981) be used to better understand children and spirituality; she provides an excellent overview of the stages of faith in childhood. The relationship among spirituality, illness in childhood, and nursing has been studied in the context of suffering, terminal illness such as cancer, and end-of-life care. In the past decade there has been an increased interest in and focus on spiritual care in adults and children as further understanding of the influence of one's spirituality on health, illness, and well-being has progressed.

Toddlers learn about God through the words and actions of those closest to them. They have only a vague idea of God and religious teachings because of their immature cognitive processes; however, if God is spoken about with reverence, young children associate God with something special. During this period the assignment of powerful religious symbols and images is strongly influenced by the manner in which it is presented; therein lies the potential for the development of guilt and fear, or conversely, love and companionship with religious symbols (Lima, do Nascimento, de Carvalho, et al., 2013). Toddlers are said to be in the intuitive-projective phase of Fowler's faith construct (Fowler, 1981) wherein thinking is largely based on fantasy and rather fluid in relation to reality and fantasy. God may be described as being around like air by the toddler because of the fluidity in dividing fantasy and reality (Neuman, 2011).

Toddlers begin to assimilate behaviors associated with the divine (e.g., folding hands in prayer). Routines such as saying prayers before meals or at bedtime can be important and comforting. Because toddlers tend to find solace in ritualistic behavior and routines, they incorporate routines associated with religious practices into their behavioral patterns without understanding all of the implications of the rituals until later. Near the end of toddlerhood, when children use preoperational thought, there is some advancement of their understanding of God. Religious teachings such as reward or fear of punishment (heaven or hell) and moral development may influence their behavior (see Chapter 13).

DEVELOPMENT OF BODY IMAGE

As in infancy, the development of body image closely parallels cognitive development. With increasing motor ability, toddlers recognize the usefulness of body parts and gradually learn their respective names. They also learn that certain body parts have various meanings; for example, during toilet training, the genitalia become significant and cleanliness is emphasized. By 2 years old toddlers recognize gender differences and refer to self by name and then by pronoun. Gender identity is developed by age 3 years old. Also by this time, children begin to remember events with reference to their personal significance, forming an autobiographic memory that helps establish a continuous identity throughout life's events.

Once they begin preoperational thought, toddlers can use symbols to represent objects, but their thinking may lead to inaccuracies. For example, if someone who is pregnant is called "fat," they will describe all "fat" women as having babies. They have a beginning recognition of words used to describe physical appearance, such as "pretty," "handsome," or "big boy." Such expressions eventually influence how children view their own bodies, and such labeling (negative or positive) becomes part of their body image.

It is evident that body integrity is poorly understood in young children and that intrusive experiences are threatening. For example, toddlers forcefully resist procedures such as examining the ear or mouth and taking an axillary temperature. The procedure itself (e.g., taking vital signs) does not hurt the child, but it represents an intrusion into the child's personal space, which elicits a strong protest. Toddlers also have unclear body boundaries and may associate nonviable parts, such as feces, with essential body parts. This can be seen in a toddler who is upset by flushing the toilet and watching the stool disappear.

Researchers have found that children possess a rudimentary topographic (i.e., children's awareness of their body's shape and spatial configuration) representation of their own body's shape, structure, and size by 30 months of age (Waugh & Brownell, 2015). Research has also shown that toddlers are beginning to develop body self-awareness as a dimension of reflective self-awareness (Waugh & Brownell, 2015). There is evidence that one's awareness and perception of self may be partially developed by the end of the toddler period, but further development takes place as one grows (Waugh & Brownell, 2015). Nurses can help parents foster a positive body image in their child by encouraging them to avoid negative labels, such as "skinny arms" or "chubby legs"; such self-perceptions are internalized and can last a lifetime. Body parts, especially those related to elimination and reproduction, should be called by their correct names. Respect for the body should be practiced.

DEVELOPMENT OF GENDER IDENTITY

Just as toddlers explore their environment, they also explore their bodies and find that touching certain body parts is pleasurable; this process actually begins in infancy as infants become aware of pleasurable effects of human touch. Genital fondling (masturbation) can occur and involves manual stimulation and posturing movements (especially in young girls) such as tightening the thighs or applying mechanical pressure to the pubic or suprapubic area. Other demonstrations of pleasurable activities include rocking, swinging, and hugging people and toys. Parental reactions to toddlers' behavior influence the children's own attitudes and should be accepting rather than critical. If such acts are performed in public, parents should not condone or bring attention to the behavior but should teach the child that it is more acceptable to perform the behavior in private.

Children in this age-group are learning vocabulary associated with anatomy, elimination, and reproduction. Certain associations between words and functions become significant and can influence future attitudes about sexual matters. For example, if parents refer to the genitalia as dirty, especially in the context of elimination, this association between "genitalia" and "dirty" may be transferred to sexual functions later in life. Sex-role differences become obvious to children and are evident in much of toddlers' imitative play. Although current research indicates that prenatal exposure to testosterone strongly influences the individual's gender identity, researchers also indicate that there are sensitive periods (e.g., puberty) that may influence the development of gender identity (Hines, Constantinescu, & Spencer, 2015; Stortelder, 2014). A sense of maleness or femaleness, or gender identity, is formed by age 24 months old when children are able to label their own and other's gender (Steensma, Kreukels, deVries, et al., 2013). Early attitudes are formed about affectionate behaviors between adults from observing parental and other adult intimate activities. (See also Sex Education, Chapter 13.) The quality of relationships with parents is important to the child's capacity for sexual and emotional relationships later in life.

SOCIAL DEVELOPMENT

Separation and Individuation

A major task of the toddler period is differentiation of self from significant others, usually the mother. The differentiation process consists of two phases: separation, the children's emergence from a symbiotic fusion with the mother, and individuation, those achievements that mark children's assumption of their individual characteristics in the environment. Although the process begins during the latter half of infancy, the major achievements occur during the toddler years.

Toddlers have an increased understanding and awareness of object permanence and some ability to withstand delayed gratification and tolerate moderate frustration. They begin to lose some of their resistance to separation, yet appear even more concerned about the parent's whereabouts. They have learned from experience that parents exist when physically absent. Repetition of events such as going to bed without the parents but waking to find them again reinforces the reliability of such brief separations. Consequently, toddlers are able to venture away from their parents for brief periods because of the security of knowing that the parents will be there when they return. Verbal and visual reassurance from the parent gradually replaces some of the previous need to be physically close for comfort.

Toddlers react differently to strangers than do infants. The appearance of unfamiliar people does not represent such a significant threat to their attachment to their mothers. In addition, toddlers show less fear of strangers, but only when their parents are present. When left alone with a stranger, they are fearful and acutely anxious; manifest depressive behavior, such as crying and withdrawal; and may become restless, hyperactive, or passive, reverting to regressive behaviors. Such reactions may be evident when a child is left with a babysitter; is beginning kindergarten, preschool, or day care; or is hospitalized. (See Chapter 22.)

These behaviors are not pathologic or harmful if parents realize how desperately their children need them. Indiscriminate friendliness toward strangers and lack of anxiety during separation from parents may be reasons for concern. Sensitive, perceptive parents will be aware of the child's need for increased love, affection, and attention when they are together. An attitude such as "They will get used to the babysitter" will not help young children positively tolerate separation.

The separation-individuation phase encompasses the phenomenon of rapprochement; as the toddler separates from the mother and begins to make sense of experiences in the environment, the child is drawn back to the mother for assistance in verbally articulating the meaning of the experiences (Zimmer-Gembeck, Webb, Thomas, et al., 2015). Developmentally the term **rapprochement** means the child moves away and returns for reassurance. If the mother's response to the toddler is inappropriate, the toddler may experience insecurity and confusion.

Parents often need help in realizing the necessity of preparing children for an inevitable separation. Particularly with the firstborn, parents tend to overprotect children, shield them from any anxiety-producing experience, and insulate them from less than immediate gratification. Although this is not necessarily harmful, especially if opportunities for independence are allowed later, it does not prepare children for unexpected events. A typical example is the birth of a sibling. The child is faced with the crisis of sibling rivalry and separation from the parent. Allowing children to experience brief periods of separation during early infancy prepares them for such experiences later. Indeed, they may still manifest the typical behaviors of protest, but they will also have learned that their mother or father always returns. Therefore it is important to appreciate the tremendous loss that the death of a parent represents for young children; unlike their other experiences with separation, this time the parent will not return.

Transitional objects, such as a favorite blanket or toy, provide security for young children, especially when they are separated from parents, are dealing with a new stress, or are just fatigued (Fig. 12.3). Security objects often become so important to toddlers that they refuse to let them be taken away. Such behavior is normal; there is no need to discourage this tendency. During separations, such as day care, hospitalization, or even overnight stays with a relative, transitional objects should be provided to minimize any feelings of fear or loneliness.

Learning to tolerate and mastering brief periods of separation are important developmental tasks of children in this age-group. In addition, it is a necessary component of parenting because brief periods of separation from their children allow parents to recoup their energy and patience and to avoid directing their irritations and frustrations at the children.

Language Development

The most striking characteristic of language development during early childhood is the increasing level of comprehension. Although the number of words acquired—from about 4 at 1 year of age to approximately 300 at age 2 years—is notable, the ability to understand speech is much greater than the number of words the child can say. Bilingual children can also achieve their early linguistic milestones in each of the languages at the same time and produce a substantial number of semantically corresponding words in each of their two languages from the very first words or signs (Estes & Hay, 2015).

At age 1 year the child uses one-word sentences, or holophrases. The word "up" can mean "pick me up" or "look up there." For the child

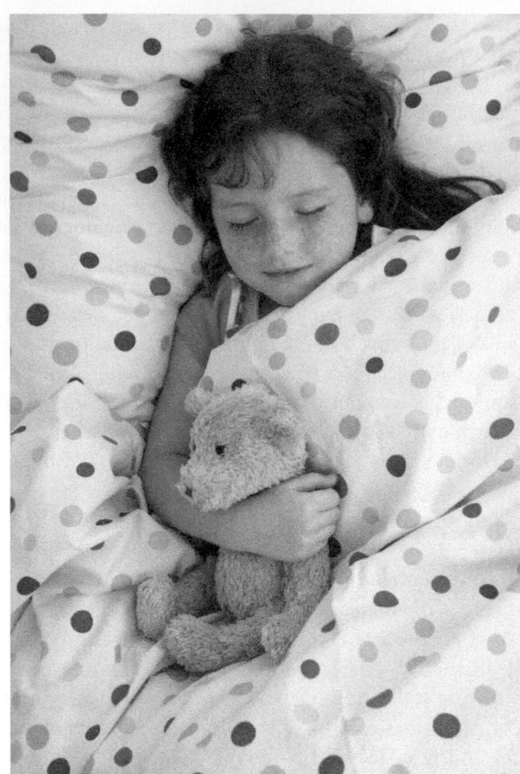

FIG. 12.3 Transitional objects, such as a warm and fuzzy stuffed animal, are sources of security to a toddler.

the one word conveys the meaning of a sentence, but to others it may mean many things or nothing. At this age about 25% of the vocalizations are intelligible. By the age of 2 years the child uses multiword sentences by stringing together two or three words, such as the phrases, "Mama go bye-bye" or "all gone," and approximately 65% of the speech is understandable. At 30 months the toddler knows her or his full name. By 3 years the child puts words together into simple sentences, begins to master grammatical rules, acquires five or six new words daily, knows his or her age and gender, and can count three objects correctly (Feigelman, 2016). Reading books together during this period provides an ideal setting for further language development. Language development among infants and toddlers is positively affected by adult-child conversations including reading, storytelling, and interactive adult-child communication. Because of their immature symbolic, memory, and attentional skills, infants and toddlers cannot learn from traditional digital media as they do from interactions with caregivers and they have difficulty transferring that knowledge to their three-dimensional experience (Barr, 2013). Emerging evidence shows that at 24 months of age, children can learn words from live video-chatting with a responsive adult or from an interactive touchscreen interface that scaffolds the child to choose the relevant answers (Kirkorian, Choi, & Pempek, 2016; Roseberry, Hirsh-Pasek, & Golinkoff, 2014). The American Academy of Pediatrics, Council on Communications and Media (2016) discourage the use of screen media other than video-chatting for children younger than 18 months. However, children 18 to 24 months of age can be introduced to digital media consisting of high-quality programming/apps but should be viewed together with parents and children. Allowing children to use media alone should be avoided.

Gestures (such as putting phone to ear or pointing) precede or accompany each of the language milestones up to 30 months of age. Once language is sufficiently mastered, gestures phase out and the pace of word learning increases.

Personal-Social Behavior

One of the most dramatic aspects of development in the toddler is personal-social interaction. Parents frequently wonder why their manageable, docile, lovable infant has turned into a determined, strong-willed, volatile-tempered little "tyrant." In addition, the tyrant can swiftly and unpredictably revert back to the adorable infant. All this is part of growing up as toddlers acquire an awareness that others' feelings and desires can be different than their own. Through interactions with caregivers, children are able to explore these differences and their consequences which are evident in such areas as dressing, feeding, playing, and establishing self-control.

Toddlers are developing skills of independence, which are evident in all areas of behavior. By 15 months of age children feed themselves, drink well from a covered cup, and manage a spoon, with considerable spilling. By 2 years old they use a spoon well, and by 3 years old they may be using a fork. Between ages 2 and 3 years old they eat with the family and like to help with chores such as setting the table or removing dishes from the dishwasher, but they lack table manners and may find it difficult to sit through the family's entire meal.

In dressing, toddlers also demonstrate strides in independence. The 15-month-old child helps by putting the arm or foot out for dressing and pulls shoes and socks off. The 18-month-old child removes gloves, helps with pullover shirts, and may be able to unzip. By 2 years old toddlers remove most articles of clothing and puts on socks, shoes, and pants without regard for right or left and back or front. Toddlers still need help to fasten clothes.

Toddlers also begin to develop concern for the feelings of others and develop an understanding of how adult expectations for behavior apply to specific situations (e.g., causing a sibling to cry while playing rough). As their understanding increases, they develop control. Age-appropriate discipline contributes to healthy social and emotional development. Positive reinforcement, redirection, and time-out are appropriate for most toddlers. It is recognized that social and emotional problems can develop in the youngest children. Early screening and intervention promote more positive outcomes as the young child grows and develops.

Play

Play magnifies toddlers' physical and psychosocial development. Interaction with people becomes increasingly important. The solitary play of infancy progresses to parallel play: the toddler plays alongside, not with, other children. Although sensorimotor play is still prominent, there is much less emphasis on the exclusive use of one sensory modality. The toddler inspects the toy, talks to the toy, tests its strength and durability, and invents several uses for it.

Play assumes many forms and serves several functions. Toddlers benefit from a wide variety of play interactions (e.g., alone, with other children, with adults), environments (e.g., own home, other children's homes, park, playgrounds), and activities (e.g., active, quiet, organized, unstructured).

Imitation is one of the most distinguishing characteristics of play and enriches children's opportunity to engage in fantasy. With less emphasis on sex-stereotyped toys, play objects such as dolls, dollhouses, dishes, cooking utensils, child-sized furniture, trucks, and dress-up clothes are used by both sexes; however, boys may be more interested than girls in activities related to trucks, trailers, cars, plastic soldiers or superheroes, and building blocks, whereas girls may prefer doll-related activities (Fig. 12.4).

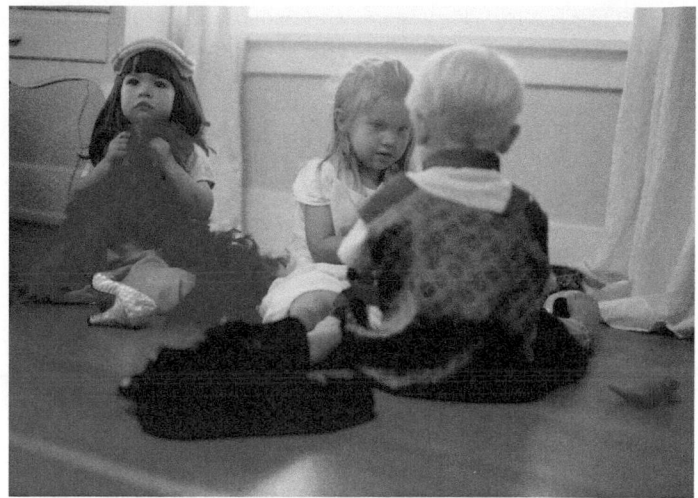

FIG. 12.4 Young children enjoy dressing up.

Increased locomotive skills make push-pull toys; stick horses; straddle trucks or cycles; a small gym and slide; balls of various sizes, and riding toys appropriate for the energetic toddler. Finger paints, thick crayons, chalk, blackboard, paper, and puzzles with large, simple pieces use the toddlers' developing fine motor skills. Interlocking blocks in varied sizes (but large enough to avoid aspiration) and shapes provide hours of fun and, during later years, are useful objects for creative and imaginative play. The most educational toy is the one that fosters the interaction of an adult with a child in supportive, unconditional play. Parents and other providers are encouraged to allow children to play with a variety of simple toys that foster creative thinking (such as blocks, dolls, and clay), rather than passive toys that the child observes (battery-operated or mechanical). Active play time should also be encouraged over the use of computer or video games, which are more passive (American Academy of Pediatrics, Council on Communications and Media, 2016). Toys are never substitutes for the attention of devoted caregivers, but toys can enhance these interactions.

Certain aspects of play are related to emerging linguistic abilities. Talking is a form of play for toddlers, who enjoy musical toys such as "talking" dolls and animals and toy telephones. Children's television programs are appropriate for some children over 2 years of age who learn to associate words with visual images. However, total media time should be limited to 1 hour or less of quality programming per day. Parents are encouraged to allow the child to engage in unstructured playtime, which is considered much more beneficial than any electronic media exposure (American Academy of Pediatrics, Council on Communications and Media, 2016). Toddlers also enjoy "reading" stories from a picture book and imitating the sounds of animals.

Tactile play is also important for the exploring toddler. Water toys, a sandbox with pail and shovel, finger paints, soap bubbles, and clay provide excellent opportunities for creative and manipulative recreation. Adults sometimes forget the fascination of feeling slippery textures such as slippery cream, mud, or pudding; catching air bubbles; squeezing and reshaping clay, or smearing paints. These types of unstructured activities are as important as educational play to allow children freedom of expression.

Selection of appropriate toys must involve safety factors, especially in relation to size and sturdiness. The oral activity of toddlers puts them at risk for aspirating small objects and ingesting toxic substances. Parents need to be especially vigilant of toys played with in other children's homes and those of older siblings. Toys are a potential source of serious bodily damage to toddlers, who may have the physical strength to manipulate them but not the knowledge to appreciate their danger.

Ride-on toys (i.e. tricycles, wagons, scooters) and early exploratory toys (i.e. blocks, stacking toys, building sets) were the most common type of toy causing injury to children younger than 5 years old (Abraham, Gaw, Chounthirath, et al., 2015). Government agencies do not inspect and police all toys on the market. Therefore adults who purchase play equipment, supervise purchases, or allow children to use play equipment need to evaluate its safety, including toys that are gifts or those that are purchased by the children themselves. Adults should also be alert to notices of toys determined to be defective and recalled by the manufacturers. Parents and health care workers can obtain information on a variety of recalled products and report potentially dangerous toys and child products to the US Consumer Product Safety Commission* or in Canada, the Canadian Toy Testing Council.† Printable tips on toy safety are also available from Safe Kids Worldwide (http://www.safekids.org).

TEMPERAMENT

Temperamental characteristics of children during infancy tend to predominate during toddlerhood. Most difficult infants remain difficult during early childhood, but the easy infants also become less easy. Parents often perceive toddlers as more challenging, especially considering the typical negativistic traits of this age-group. Parents of easy infants may be particularly distressed by the behavior change, whereas parents of difficult children may be more prepared because of a previously troublesome year, or be overwhelmed by the additional behaviors. For practitioners in a busy setting, asking parents about their impression of the child's temperament can help professionals understand the parent-child interactional process.

Guyer, Jarcho, Perez-Edgar, and colleagues (2015) emphasize that parenting style influences children's social and emotional development. Parents are often concerned that their child with an adverse temperament will develop a behavioral dysfunction that persists for a lifetime. The lack of fit between the child's temperament and the parents' expectations is often a source of conflict that may escalate if providers do not intervene. The authors point out that behavioral problems in children can be managed appropriately, but the child's temperament cannot be changed (Guyer, Jarcho, Perez-Edgar, et al., 2015).

Eisenberg, Taylor, Widaman, and colleagues (2015) found evidence of bidirectional and interactive effects between parenting and children's characteristics of fear, self-regulation, frustration, and impulsivity. Children with high frustration levels, impulsivity, and low effortful control were more vulnerable to negative parenting behaviors. Such parental behaviors served to predict an increase in children's fearfulness, frustration, and effortful control. The authors present information that can be used to evaluate the goodness of fit between the toddler's parents and the toddler's behavior and make adjustments in parenting style accordingly.

Although temper tantrums are common in toddlers, certain temperament characteristics make some children more prone to such outbursts. Active, intensely responding children are apt to yell, scream, and fling items during tantrums. Discipline is also influenced by temperament. Easy children generally respond well to mild forms of discipline, including a stern voice and sustained eye contact. However, difficult children often need more structured types of discipline, such as time-out, physical containment, or rewards, and the effectiveness of one approach may be short lived. Efforts at preventing misbehavior are especially important with children who have persistent natures. (See Limit Setting and Discipline, Chapter 2.) Without "friendly warnings" such children often have difficulty terminating an activity. These children may be punished for behavior that is merely typical of their temperament, and if the unwarranted punishment continues, the pattern can develop into a behavior problem. Slow-to-warm-up children may also present challenges, especially when this characteristic is combined with the toddler's usual fear of strangers. These children require gradual introduction to new situations, such as day care and babysitters.

COPING WITH CONCERNS RELATED TO NORMAL GROWTH AND DEVELOPMENT

Table 12.2 summarizes the major features of growth and development for the age-groups of 15, 18, 24, and 30 months. The key developmental ages are 18 and 24 months, although the chronologic ages of 15 and 30 months are also significant. Fifteen months of age is a particularly integrative period of developmental achievement because it represents the completion or fruition of many skills that were unperfected at 1 year of age.

TOILET TRAINING

One of the major tasks of toddlerhood is toilet training. Anticipatory guidance and clinical intervention for families surrounding toilet training should begin during routine well-child visits before the child's developmental readiness to toilet train. Preparation and education reveal and allay misconceptions; lead to the development of appropriate expectations; and provide information, guidance, and support to parents for managing this potentially frustrating process.

Voluntary control of the anal and urethral sphincters is achieved sometime after the child is walking, probably between ages 18 and 24 months. However, complex psychophysiologic factors are required for readiness. The child must be able to recognize the urge to let go and hold on and be able to communicate this sensation to the parent. In addition, some motivation is probably involved in the desire to please the parent by holding on rather than pleasing oneself by letting go. Cultural beliefs may also affect the age at which children demonstrate readiness (Feigelman, 2016).

Trends in toilet training have changed, likely due to the availability of disposable diapers. In the 1920s toilet training began at around 12 months old, which changed to at least 18 months old in the 1960s, and now is initiated at around 21 months old with approximately 26% of children toilet trained by 24 months old and 88% of children toilet trained by 30 months (Kimball, 2016).

Three markers signal a child's readiness to toilet train: (1) being aware of the urge to void or stool, (2) interest in and/or motivation to use the toilet, and (3) being dry for at least 2 hours during the day (Kimball, 2016). According to some experts, physiologic and psychologic readiness is not complete until ages 24 to 30 months (Rogers, 2013); however, parents should begin preparing their children for toilet training earlier than 30 months. By this time the child has mastered the majority of essential gross motor skills, can communicate intelligibly, is in less conflict with parents in terms of self-assertion and negativism, and is aware of the ability to control the body and please the parent. Some studies have linked starting toilet training at a later age with urinary incontinence, but as Kiddoo (2012) suggests, there are no strong evidence-based studies demonstrating the best toilet training time. Furthermore, dysfunctional voiding has not been linked to any specific method of toilet training (Colaco, Johnson, Schneider, et al., 2013).

*800-638-2772; https://www.cpsc.gov/safety-education/toy-recall-statistics (assistance is also available in Spanish).

†1973 Baseline Road, Ottawa, Ontario K2C 0C7 Canada; 613-228-3155; http://www.toy-testing.org.

TABLE 12.2 Growth and Development During the Toddler Years

Physical	Gross Motor	Fine Motor	Sensory	Language	Socialization/ Cognition
Age 15 Month					
Steady growth in height and weight Head circumference 48 cm (19 inches) Weight 11 kg (24 lb) Height 78.7 cm (31 inches)	Walks without help (usually since age 13 months) Creeps up stairs Kneels without support Cannot walk around corners or stop suddenly without losing balance Assumes standing position without support Cannot throw ball without falling	Constantly casting objects to floor Builds tower of two cubes Holds two cubes in one hand Releases pellet into narrow-necked bottle Scribbles spontaneously Uses cup well but often rotates spoon	Able to identify geometric forms; places round object into appropriate hole Binocular vision well developed Displays intense and prolonged interest in pictures	Uses expressive jargon Says four to six words, including names Asks for objects by pointing Understands simple commands May shake head to denote "no" Uses "no" even while agreeing to the request Uses common gestures such as putting cup to mouth when empty	Tolerates some separation from parent Less likely to fear strangers Beginning to imitate parents, such as cleaning house (sweeping, dusting), folding clothes May discard bottle Manages spoon but rotates it near mouth Kisses and hugs parents; may kiss pictures in book Expresses emotions; has temper tantrums
Age 18 Month					
Physiologic anorexia from decreased growth needs Anterior fontanel closed Physiologically able to control sphincters	Runs clumsily; falls often Walks up stairs with one hand held Pulls and pushes toys Jumps in place with both feet Seats self on chair Throws ball overhand without falling	Builds tower of three or four cubes Release, prehension, and reach well developed Turns two or three pages in book at a time In drawing, makes stroke imitatively Manages spoon without rotation		Says 10 or more words Points to common object, such as shoe or ball, and to two or three body parts Forms word combinations Forms gesture-word combinations (points while naming) Forms gesture-gesture combinations	Great imitator (domestic mimicry) Takes off gloves, socks, and shoes, and unzips zippers Temper tantrums may be more evident Beginning awareness of ownership ("my toy") May develop dependency on transitional objects, such as security blanket
Age 24 Month					
Head circumference 49-50 cm (19.5-20 inches) Chest circumference exceeds head circumference Lateral diameter of chest exceeds anteroposterior diameter Usual weight gain of 1.8-2.7 kg (4-6 lb) Usual gain in height of 10-12.5 cm (4-5 inches) Adult height approximately double height at 2 years May be ready to begin daytime control of bowel and bladder Primary dentition of 16 teeth	Goes up and down stairs alone with two feet on each step Runs fairly well, with wide stance Picks up object without falling Kicks ball forward without overbalancing	Builds tower of six to seven cubes Aligns two or more cubes like a train Turns pages of book one at a time In drawing, imitates vertical and circular strokes Turns doorknob, unscrews lid	Accommodation well developed in geometric discrimination; able to insert square block into oblong space	Has vocabulary of approximately 300 words Uses two- or three-word phrases Uses pronouns "I," "me," "you" Understands directional commands Gives first name; refers to self by name Verbalizes need for toileting, food, or drink Talks incessantly Able to remember and imitate arbitrary sequences of manual actions and gestures	Stage of parallel play Has sustained attention span Temper tantrums decreasing Pulls people to show them something Increased independence from parent Dresses self in simple clothing Develops visual recognition and verbal self-reference ("me big") Develops awareness that feelings and desires of others may be different and begins to explore implications and consequences

Continued

TABLE 12.2 Growth and Development During the Toddler Years—cont'd

Physical	Gross Motor	Fine Motor	Sensory	Language	Socialization/ Cognition
Age 30 Month					
Birth weight quadrupled Primary dentition (20 teeth) completed May have daytime bowel and bladder control	Jumps with both feet Jumps from chair or step Stands on one foot momentarily Takes a few steps on tiptoe	Builds tower of eight cubes Adds chimney to train of cubes Good hand-finger coordination; holds crayon with fingers rather than fist In drawing, imitates vertical and horizontal strokes; makes two or more strokes for cross; draws circles		Gives first and last name Refers to self by appropriate pronoun Uses plurals Names one color	Separates more easily from parent In play, helps put things away; can carry breakable objects; pushes with good steering Begins to notice gender differences; knows own gender May attend to toilet needs without help except for wiping Emotions expand to include pride, shame, guilt, embarrassment

One of the nurse's most important responsibilities is to help parents identify the readiness signs in their child (see Nursing Care Guidelines box).* On average, girls are developmentally ready to begin toilet training 2 to 3 months before boys (Kimball, 2016).

NURSING CARE GUIDELINES

Assessing Toilet Training Readiness

Physical Readiness

Voluntary control of anal and urethral sphincters, usually by ages 24 to 30 months
Ability to stay dry for 2 hours; decreased number of wet diapers; waking dry from nap
Regular bowel movements
Gross motor skills of sitting, walking, and squatting
Fine motor skills to remove clothing

Mental Readiness

Recognition of urge to defecate or urinate
Verbal or nonverbal communication skills to indicate when wet or has urge to defecate or urinate
Cognitive skills to imitate appropriate behavior and follow directions

Psychologic Readiness

Expressing willingness to please parent
Ability to sit on toilet for 5 to 8 minutes without fussing or getting off
Curiosity about adults' or older sibling's toilet habits
Impatience with soiled or wet diapers; desire to be changed immediately

Parental Readiness

Recognition of child's level of readiness
Willingness to invest the time required for toilet training
Absence of family stress or change, such as a divorce, moving, new sibling, or imminent vacation

*Helpful books to guide toilet training are available from the American Academy of Pediatrics, 847-434-4000; https://shop.aap.org/toilet-training/.

Nighttime bladder control normally takes several months to years after daytime training begins. This is because the sleep cycle needs to mature so the child can awake in time to urinate. Feigelman (2016) indicates that bedwetting is normal in girls up to age 4 years old and in boys up to age 5 years. Few children have night wetting episodes after daytime dryness is totally achieved; however, children who do not have nighttime dryness by the age of 6 years old are likely to require intervention.

Bowel training is usually accomplished before bladder training because of its greater regularity and predictability. The sensation for defecation is stronger than that for urination and easier for children to recognize. A well-balanced diet that includes dietary fiber helps keep stool soft and supports the development and maintenance of regular bowel movements.

A number of techniques are helpful when initiating training, and cultural differences should be considered (see Cultural Considerations box). In the United States some of the options recommended by practitioners include the Brazelton child-oriented approach, the American Academy of Pediatrics guidelines (which are similar to the Brazelton method), Dr. Spock's training method, and the intensive "toilet-training-in-a-day" (operant conditioning) approach by Azrin and Foxx. A systematic review by the by the Agency for Healthcare Research and Quality concluded that the child-oriented method and the Azrin and Foxx methods were effective at toilet training healthy children (Kiddoo, 2012). The following discussion of toilet training methods includes suggestions from the child-oriented approach.

Parents should begin the readiness phase of toilet training by teaching the child about how the body functions in relation to voiding and having a stool. Parents can talk about how adults and animals perform such functions on a routine basis. Toilet training should be made as easy and simple as possible. Important considerations are the selection of the child's clothing and the potty chair or use of the toilet. A freestanding potty chair allows children a feeling of security (Fig. 12.5, *A*). Planting the feet firmly on the floor also facilitates defecation. Another option is a portable seat attached to the regular toilet, which may ease the transition from potty chair to regular toilet. Placing a small bench under the feet helps stabilize the child's position. It is probably best to keep the potty in the bathroom and to let the child observe the excreta being

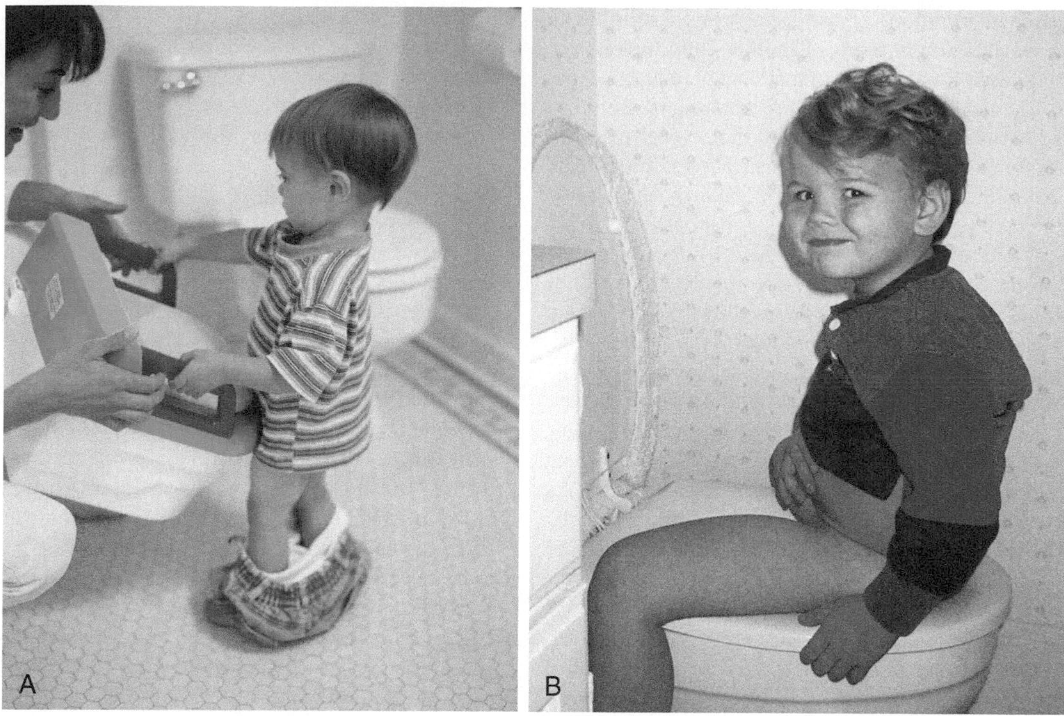

FIG. 12.5 **A,** Children may begin toilet training sitting on a small toilet. **B,** Sitting in reverse fashion on a regular toilet provides additional security to a young child.

CULTURAL CONSIDERATIONS

Toilet Training

Cultural practices influence the timing, method, and significance of toilet training. For many families in China, the timing is liberal, the method is distinct, and the significance is low. Children are diapered during infancy. Once they are walking, they wear loose pants with a long slit between the legs, and they eliminate on the ground. This practice may continue until the child is 5 years of age. In cold weather, a piece of cloth, like a "curtain," may be inserted. However, the Chinese have a concept that the buttocks are not susceptible to cold, so this is not a common practice.

flushed down the toilet to associate these activities with usual practices. If a potty chair is not available, having the child sit facing the toilet tank provides added support (Fig. 12.5, *B*). Practice sessions should be limited to 5 to 8 minutes, and a parent should stay with the child, practicing sanitary habits after every session. Children should be praised for cooperative behavior and successful evacuation. Dressing children in easily removed clothing; using training pants, "pull-on" diapers, or underwear; and encouraging imitation by watching others are other helpful suggestions.

When the child begins to experience regular daytime dryness, parents may experiment with underwear during the day. Daytime accidents are common, particularly during periods of intense activity. Young children become so engrossed in play activity that, if they are not reminded, they will wait until it is too late to reach the bathroom. Therefore frequent reminders and trips to the toilet are necessary. Parents may forget to plan ahead when their toddlers are being toilet trained; before trips outside the house, it is important to remind children to at least try to urinate to decrease the chance of needing to use the toilet while the car is stuck in traffic.

As the child masters each step of toileting (discussion, undressing, going, wiping, dressing, flushing, and hand washing), he or she gains a sense of accomplishment that parents should reinforce. If the parent-child relationship becomes strained, both may need a break to focus on enjoyable activities together. Regression may coincide with a stressful family situation or the child being pushed too hard and too fast. Regression is a normal part of toilet training and does not mean failure but should be viewed as a temporary setback to a more comfortable place for the child.

Day care providers also play a role in the support and education of parents regarding toilet training practices. It is important for parents to inform all caregivers of their individual family values and the child's specific needs when planning for training away from home. Ensuring consistency in care of toddlers and ensuring healthy practices in a sanitary environment allow for safe and effective toilet practices in all settings.

SIBLING RIVALRY

The term **sibling rivalry** refers to the natural jealousy and resentment of children to a new child in the family. It typically involves the arrival of a new infant but may be associated with anyone who joins the family. A common example is the merging of stepfamilies (**blended families**). However, the following discussion focuses on the sibling's response to the birth of a newborn.

The arrival of a new infant represents a crisis for even the best-prepared toddlers. They do not hate or resent the infant; rather they hate the changes that this additional sibling brings, especially the separation from the mother during the birth. The parents now share their love and attention with someone else, the usual routine is disrupted, and toddlers may lose their crib or room—all at a time when they thought they were in control of their world. Sibling rivalry tends to be most pronounced in the firstborn, who experiences "dethronement" (i.e., loss of sole parental attention). It also seems to be most difficult for young children, particularly in terms of mother-child interaction.

Preparation of children for the birth of a sibling is individual, but age dictates some important considerations. For toddlers, time is a vague concept. A good time to start talking about the new baby is when toddlers become aware of the pregnancy and the changes occurring in the home in anticipation of the new member. Jealousy can develop from feeling left out; because fantasy dictates reality, fear of the unknown can lead to fear of abandonment, separation anxiety, and insecurity.

Toddlers need to have a realistic idea of what the newborn will be like. Telling them that a new playmate will come home soon sets up unrealistic expectations. Rather, parents should stress the activities that will take place when the baby arrives home, such as diapering, bottle-feeding or breastfeeding, bathing, and dressing. At the same time, parents should emphasize which routines will stay the same, such as reading stories or going to the park. If toddlers have had no contact with an infant, it is a good idea to introduce them to one, if feasible. Providing a doll on which toddlers can imitate parental behaviors is another excellent strategy. They can tend to the doll's needs (diapering, feeding) at the same time the parent is performing similar activities for the infant, then progress to helping with the sibling (Fig. 12.6).

Regardless of how well adjusted and accepting toddlers or preschoolers appear, infants must be protected by supervising the interaction between siblings. Other safety considerations are "baby-proofing" the house and instructing children regarding the dangers to infants of small, sharp, or pointed objects.

The first few weeks at home with a newborn and toddler can be challenging for parents. Assuring them that this period will pass, that the toddler will learn to accept the changes in lifestyle, and that the newborn will sleep through the night is part of the intervention. Allowing parents to talk about their feelings of ambivalence and frustration and suggesting ways of dealing with the sibling jealousy help all members of the family with this experience. Indeed, sibling rivalry is so common, regardless of the children's ages, that it is a part of family life. Suggestions such as spending time with each child, letting children settle their arguments, and accepting angry feelings while teaching children appropriate ways to express hostility are general guidelines for dealing with the eventual conflicts between brothers and sisters.

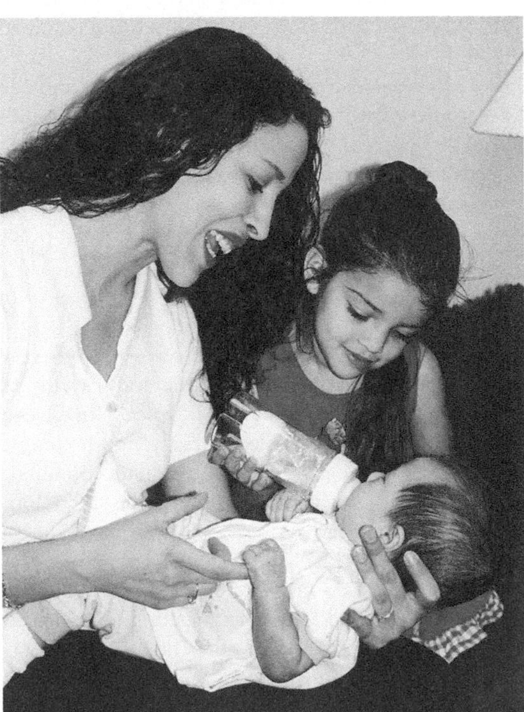

FIG. 12.6 To minimize sibling rivalry, parents should include the toddler during caregiving activities.

TEMPER TANTRUMS

Toddlers may assert their independence by violently objecting to discipline. They may lie down on the floor, kick their feet, and scream as loud as possible. Some have learned the effectiveness of holding their breath until the parent relents. Although holding one's breath may cause fainting from lack of oxygen, the accumulation of carbon dioxide will stimulate the respiratory control center, resulting in no physical harm. Tantrums are an indication of the child's inability to control emotions; toddlers are particularly prone to tantrums because their strong drive for mastery and autonomy is frustrated by adult figures or lack of motor and cognitive skills. Temper tantrums commonly occur when the child is ill, hungry, frustrated, or tired; some children may use temper tantrums to get parental attention, get something they want, or avoid having to do something they do not want to do (El-Radhi, 2015). **Temper tantrums** have been linked to two emotional and behavioral processes: anger and distress (Eisbach, Cluxton-Keller, Harrison, et al., 2014). Anger increases rapidly and peaks near the beginning of the tantrum; components of distress, such as crying and comfort seeking, increase as anger subsides. The majority of temper tantrums (75%) last 5 minutes or less (Eisbach, Cluxton-Keller, Harrison, et al., 2014).

The best approach toward tapering temper tantrums requires consistency and developmentally appropriate expectations and rewards. Ensuring consistency among all caregivers in expectations, prioritizing what rules are important, and developing consequences that are reasonable for the child's level of development help manage the behavior. For example, a popular time for a tantrum is before bedtime. Active toddlers often have trouble slowing down and, when placed in bed, resist staying there. Parents can reinforce consistency and expectations by stating, "After this story it is bedtime." Starting at 18 months, time-outs work well for managing temper tantrums.

During tantrums ignore the behavior, provided the behavior is not injurious to the child, such as violently banging the head on the floor. Continue to be present to provide a feeling of control and security to the child once the tantrum has subsided. If the tantrum occurs on an outing such as a visit to the store, the child may need to be removed from the public place until the tantrum has subsided. Provide realistic expectations on such outings; if the child goes into the store expecting to receive a toy or candy and does not, a tantrum is likely. Remember that toddlers like routines, so try to adhere to the child's routine for naps, playtime, and meals to decrease the child's frustration. During periods of no tantrums, practice developmentally appropriate positive reinforcement.

Other suggestions for handling tantrums include the following (El-Radhi, 2015):

- Offering the child options instead of an "all or none" position
- Ensuring a consistent response to child's behavior by all caregivers
- Praising the child for positive behavior when he or she is not having a tantrum or providing a reward system (e.g., sticker chart)

Temper tantrums are common during the toddler years and essentially represent normal developmental behaviors. However, temper tantrums can be signs of serious problems. Temper tantrums that occur past 5 years of age, last longer than 15 minutes, or occur more than five times a day are considered abnormal and may indicate a serious problem

(El-Radhi, 2015). Nurses should be alert to situations that require further evaluation.

NEGATIVISM

One of the more difficult aspects of rearing toddlers is related to their persistent negative response to every request. The negativism is not an expression of being stubborn or disrespectful, but a necessary assertion of control. One method of dealing with **negativism** is by reducing the opportunities for a "no" answer. Asking the child, "Do you want to go to sleep now?" is almost certain to be met with an emphatic "no." A more appropriate approach is to tell the child when it will be time to go to sleep (preferably within a specific time frame, such as "after reading a story") and proceed accordingly.

In an attempt to exert control, toddles like to make choices. When confronted with appropriate choices, such as "You can have a peanut butter–and–jelly sandwich or chicken noodle soup for lunch," they are more likely to choose one than to automatically say no. However, if their response is negative, parents should make the choice for the child. This behavior is frustrating for both the child and the parent. Parents need to respond in a calm, reassuring manner. Many of the suggestions for preventing misbehavior in Chapter 2 also help minimize negativism.

STRESS

Adults rarely think of young children as being exposed to stress or suffering its consequences. However, the normal demands of growing up coupled with the usual pressures most families experience mean that few, if any, young children grow up stress free. Small amounts of stress are beneficial during the early years to help children develop effective coping skills. However, excessive stress is destructive, and young children are especially vulnerable because of their limited ability to cope.

To deal with stress in their children's lives, parents must be aware of the signs of stress and be able to identify the source. Any number of other stresses may be imposed on children, such as alternative caregiving arrangements, birth of a sibling, separation and divorce, relocation, or illness. Watching children at play can help identify stressors. Other signs of increased stress in a toddler's life may include increased thumb sucking, aggressive behavior, and biting.

The best approach to dealing with stress is prevention—monitoring the amount of stress in children's lives so that levels do not exceed their coping ability. In many instances this is as simple as increasing the child's rest periods to allow for quiet recovery time. Often it involves adequately preparing the child for change, such as day care or a new sibling. It also requires helping the child cope with stress. Unsupervised play is an excellent vehicle for releasing anger or frustration, and toys such as drums, play nails and hammer, clay, and play dough provide alternative methods of dissipating anxiety. They also begin to teach socially acceptable ways of dealing with such feelings. Another approach is the use of relaxation and imagery.

REGRESSION

Regression involves a retreat from one's present pattern of functioning to past levels of behavior. It usually occurs in instances of stress, when one attempts to cope by reverting to patterns of behavior that were successful in earlier stages of development. Regression is common in toddlers because almost any additional stress lessens their ability to master present developmental tasks. Any threat to their autonomy, such as illness, hospitalization, separation, or adjustment to a sibling, represents a need to revert to earlier forms of behavior, such as increased dependency. This can include refusal to use the potty chair; temper tantrums; demand for the bottle or crib; and loss of newly learned motor, language, social, and cognitive skills.

At first, such regression appears acceptable and comfortable for children, but on closer inspection it becomes evident that the loss of newly acquired achievements is frightening and threatening because children are aware of their total helplessness in the recent past. Parents, too, become concerned about regressive behavior and may force the child to cope with an additional source of stress: the pressure of living up to expected standards. Brazelton (1999) suggests that these predictable times of regression, or **touchpoints**, are an opportunity to prepare parents for the next step in their child's development.

When regression does occur, the best approach is to ignore it while praising existing patterns of appropriate behavior. The child is saying, "I can't cope with this present stress and accomplish this new skill as well, but I will eventually if given patience and understanding." For this reason, it is advisable not to introduce new areas of learning when an additional crisis is present or expected, such as beginning toilet training shortly before a sibling is born or during a brief hospitalization.

Fears are common during this age and include fear of annihilation, going to sleep, animals, and engines, with the greatest fear continuing to be fear of strangers and separation from parents or other caregivers. Because fear of strangers and separation begins in infancy, it is discussed in Chapter 10. The other fears often escalate in the preschool period and consequently are discussed in Chapter 13.

PROMOTING OPTIMUM HEALTH DURING TODDLERHOOD

NUTRITION

During the period from 12 to 18 months of age the growth rate slows, decreasing the child's need for calories, protein, and fluid. However, the protein (13 g/day) and energy requirements are still relatively high to meet the demands for muscle tissue growth and high activity level. The need for minerals such as iron, calcium, and phosphorus may be difficult to meet, considering the characteristic food habits of children in this age-group. Parents may be tempted to rely on vitamin supplementation rather than a well-balanced diet to meet these requirements. Toddlers usually require three meals and two snacks per day; however, the portions consumed are generally much smaller compared with those of older children.

The Feeding Infants and Toddlers Study (FITS) (Saavedra, Denning, Dattilo, et al., 2013) found that in general toddlers met or exceeded the requirements for daily energy and protein requirements. However, intake of a variety of foods was seen with advancing age in toddlers as their food preferences changed. There was an increase in the intake of sweets, snacks, and soda; french fried potatoes were the most commonly consumed vegetable by toddlers, and sweetened beverages were often substituted for 100% fruit juices. Researchers voiced concern that parents administering multivitamin preparations to toddlers failed to understand that such vitamins, although appropriate in most cases, failed to address the problem of excessive sodium, saturated fats, sugars, and overall energy intake (Saavedra, Denning, Dattilo, et al., 2013). The FITS recommended that toddlers be fed a more balanced diet of vegetables, fruits, and whole grains.

At approximately 18 months of age most toddlers manifest this decreased nutritional need with a decreased appetite, a phenomenon known as **physiologic anorexia**. They become picky, fussy eaters with strong taste preferences. They may eat large amounts one day and almost nothing the next. They are increasingly aware of the nonnutritive function

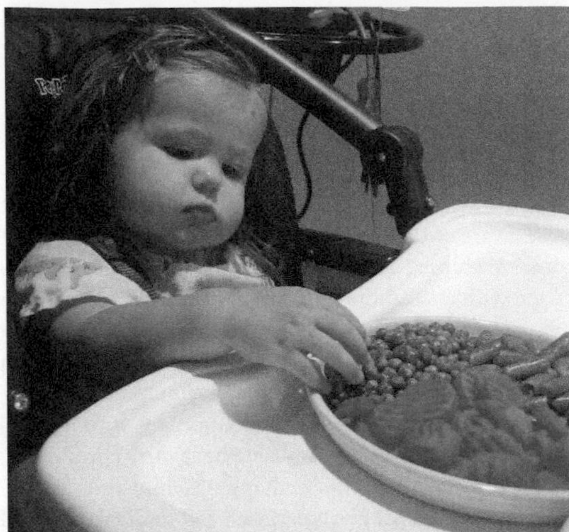

FIG. 12.7 Toddlers enjoy finger foods such as green peas. (Courtesy E. Jacobs, Texas Children's Hospital, Houston.)

TABLE 12.3 Developmental Milestones Associated With Feeding

Age (Month)	Development
12-18	Drools less Drinks well from cup with lid but may drop it when finished Holds cup with both hands Begins to use spoon but turns it before reaching mouth
24	Can use straw and cup Chews food with mouth closed, and shifts food in mouth Distinguishes between finger and spoon foods Uses spoon correctly but with some spilling
36	Spills small amount from spoon Begins to use fork; holds it in fist Uses adult pattern of chewing, which involves rotary action of jaw

of food (i.e., the pleasure of eating, the social aspect of mealtime, and the control of refusing food). They are influenced by factors other than taste when choosing food. If a family member refuses to eat something, toddlers are likely to imitate that response. If the plate is overfilled, they are likely to push it away, overwhelmed by its size. If food does not appear or smell appetizing, they will probably not agree to try it. In essence mealtime is more closely associated with psychologic rather than nutritional components. Toddlers like to eat with their fingers and enjoy foods of different colors and shapes (Fig. 12.7).

The ritualism of this age also dictates certain principles in feeding practices. Toddlers like to have the same dish, cup, or spoon every time they eat. They may reject a favorite food simply because it is served in a different dish. If one food touches another, they often refuse to eat it. Mixed foods such as stews or casseroles are rarely favorites. Because toddlers have unpredictable table manners, it is best to use plastic dishes and cups for both economic and safety reasons. For some children a regular mealtime schedule also contributes to their desire and need for predictability and ritualism.

Developmentally by 12 months of age most children eat many of the same foods prepared for the rest of the family. Some may have mastered using a cup with occasional spilling, although most cannot use a spoon adeptly until 18 months of age or later and generally prefer using their fingers (Table 12.3).

Nutritional Counseling

The emphasis on preventing childhood obesity and subsequent cardiovascular disease in the United States has prompted a number of changes in dietary recommendations for children and adults alike. It is now recognized that lifetime eating habits are established in early childhood, possibly by the end of the toddler period; health care workers are increasingly emphasizing the role of food selection choices, exercise, stress reduction, and other lifestyle choices (e.g., tobacco and alcohol use) on the quality of adult life and survival. Conditions such as obesity and cardiovascular disease can be prevented by encouraging healthy eating habits in toddlers and their families.

If food is used as a reward or sign of approval, a child may overeat for nonnutritive reasons. If food is forced and mealtime is consistently unpleasant, the usual pleasure associated with eating may not develop. Mealtimes should be enjoyable rather than times for discipline or family arguments. The social aspect of mealtime may be distracting for young children; therefore an earlier feeding hour may be appropriate. Young children are unable to sit through a long meal and become restless and disruptive. This is particularly common when children are brought to the table just after active play. Calling them in from play 15 minutes before mealtime allows them ample opportunity to get ready for eating while settling down their active minds and bodies.

The method of serving food also takes on more importance during this period. Toddlers need to have a sense of control and achievement in their abilities. Giving them large, adult-size portions can overwhelm them. In general, what is eaten is much more significant than how much is consumed. Toddlers usually restrict their food preference to four or five main foods and rarely try new foods; in some cases, a toddler may insist on one food such as mashed potatoes for lunch and dinner. Small amounts of meat and vegetables supply greater food value than a large consumption of bread or potato. Serving sizes need to be appropriate for age. Young children tend to like less spicy, bland food, although this is a culturally determined preference. Substitutions can be provided for foods that they do not enjoy, although parents need not cater to all of their desires. Frequent, small nutritious snacks can replace a meal.

To determine serving size for young children, use the following guidelines:

- A general guide to the serving size of food is 1 tablespoon of solid food per year of age, or one-fourth to one-third of the adult portion size.
- Use the tablespoon guide for easily measured foods such as vegetables or rice.
- Use the fraction guide for bread or milk.

Mastication skills continue to mature, putting children at risk for choking; therefore large round foods (e.g., hot dogs, grapes, peas, carrots, popcorn, fruit gel snacks) should be avoided until the child is able to chew them effectively. Active play while eating should be discouraged to prevent choking. Appetite and food preferences are sporadic. Often the interest in food parallels a growth spurt; thus periods of good eating are interspersed with phases of poor eating. If exposed to the same food every day, a young toddler does not learn how to manage the complex sensory information needed to eat new, more difficult foods (e.g., vegetables with a different texture versus pureed, slippery fruits). To help prevent "food jags" it is recommended that parents present food in various physical forms. The child may need to progress to eating new foods in a stepwise fashion such as visually tolerating the food, interacting with it, smelling it, touching it, tasting it, and then eating it.

This period of picky eating can be trying for both parents and child. Many authorities consider it to be a developmental phase and stress that most toddlers will consume the necessary amount of food required for growth (Saavedra, Denning, Dattilo, et al., 2013). Parents are encouraged to plan a nutritionally balanced week instead of day because of the way toddlers restrict food intake in their effort to exert control over their environment (Schwartz & Benuck, 2013).

Dietary Guidelines

Dietary guidelines are necessary to promote adequate energy and nutrient intake to support physical, emotional, psychologic, and cognitive development. A number of new dietary guidelines have been developed to address the issues of childhood obesity, sedentary lifestyles, and increase in cardiovascular disease mortality in the United States.

The National Academy of Medicine (2017) has guidelines for nutritional intake that encompass the Recommended Daily Allowances (RDAs), yet extend their scope to include additional parameters related to nutritional intake. The Dietary Reference Intakes (DRIs)* are composed of four categories: Estimated Average Requirements (EARs) for age and gender categories, tolerable upper-limit nutrient intakes that are associated with a low risk of adverse effects, Adequate Intakes (AIs) of nutrients, and new standard RDAs. The guidelines present information about lifestyle factors that may affect nutrient function such as caffeine intake and exercise and about how the nutrient may be related to chronic disease. An important factor in the development of the DRIs that affects children, particularly infants from birth to age 6 months, is that the AIs are based on the nutrient intake of full-term, healthy, breastfed infants (by well-nourished mothers), which now represents the gold standard for infant nutrition in this age-group.

The 2015-2020 Dietary Guidelines for Americans may also be used to encourage healthy dietary intakes and regular exercise designed to decrease obesity, cardiovascular risk factors, and subsequent cardiovascular disease, which is now known to occur in both young children and adults. The 2015-2020 Dietary Guidelines recommend a caloric intake for a moderately active boy, ages 2 to 3 years, of 1000 to 1400 calories per day. The emphasis in the Dietary Guidelines is in decreasing overall fat and sodium intakes and increasing the amount of daily exercise to reduce the incidence of obesity and cardiovascular disease. The 2015-2020 Dietary Guidelines† are for children ages 2 years and older. They encourage a variety of fruits, vegetables, whole grains, and low-fat and nonfat dairy products in addition to fish, beans, and lean meat.

Additional resources for dietary counseling include MyPlate,‡ developed by the US Department of Agriculture to replace MyPyramid. This colorful plate shows the five main food groups (i.e., fruits, grains, vegetable, protein, and dairy) with the intended purpose to involve children and their families in making appropriate food choices for meals and decrease the incidence of overweight and obesity in the United States. MyPlate provides an online interactive feature that allows the individual to select (click on) an individual food group and see choices for foods in that group. Approximate serving sizes are suggested, and vegetarian substitutions are also provided.

Nutrition during toddlerhood involves a transition as a young toddler is weaned off milk- or formula-based diets. Milk intake, the chief source of calcium and phosphorus, should average two or three servings (24 to 30 oz) a day. Consuming more than a quart of milk daily considerably limits the intake of solid foods, resulting in a deficiency of dietary iron and other nutrients. After 2 years of age children can be given low-fat milk to reduce daily total fat to less than 30% of calories, saturated fatty acids to less than 10% of calories, and cholesterol to less than 300 mg. Other measures to reduce dietary fat include using lean meats, fat-modified products (e.g., low-fat cheese), and low-fat cooking. Because less fat in children's diets can also mean fewer calories and nutrients, caregivers must know what kinds of food to choose. However, *trans* fatty acids and saturated fats should be avoided.

Iron-fortified cereals and iron-rich foods are recommended for all children older than 6 months of age. Parents should be encouraged to provide an iron-rich diet that includes heme and nonheme iron sources (e.g., red meats, poultry, fish, green leafy vegetables, dried fruit, beans) and limits whole-milk consumption. Iron supplementation may be necessary in some cases; the EAR for iron in a child age 1 to 3 years is 7.0 mg/day (US Department of Health and Human Services, 2016).

Calcium and vitamin D are essential for healthy bone development. Adequate intake of calcium for children 1 to 3 years of age is 500 mg per day. Whole milk, cheese, yogurt, legumes (beans), and vegetables (e.g., broccoli, collard greens, kale) are good sources for calcium. Popular calcium-fortified foods include waffles, cereals and cereal bars, orange juice, and some white breads. Vitamin D is essential if exposure to sunlight is inadequate (≅5 to 15 min/day on the hands, arms, and face of light-skinned persons; slightly more in darker-pigmented individuals) or in people who are dark skinned or who live in northern latitudes or cloudy or smoky areas. Adequate vitamin D intake is essential to prevent rickets; it is now recommended that children and adolescents have an intake of at least 600 IU of vitamin D daily (US Department of Health and Human Services, 2016). Multivitamin preparations containing 600 IU of vitamin D (by tablet or liquid) are adequate if food intake is poor or exposure to sunlight is minimal; vitamin D–only preparations containing 600 IU are also available commercially. Sources of vitamin D include fish, fish oils, and egg yolks. Fortified cereals, dairy products, and meat are also good sources of zinc and vitamin E.

It is also recommended that toddlers have 1 cup of fruit each day. Vitamin C enhances iron absorption. Children ages 2 years and older may consume approximately 4 to 6 ounces of juice per day. It tastes good to toddlers and is readily available. A 6-ounce glass of fruit juice equals one fruit serving; however, juices lack the fiber of whole fruit and should not be a substitution for whole fruit. High intake of juice can contribute to diarrhea, overnutrition or undernutrition, and the development of caries; thus only 4 to 6 ounces of 100% fruit juice per day is recommended for toddlers (American Academy of Pediatrics, Committee on Nutrition, 2014). Fruit-flavored drinks advertised as juices may not actually contain 100% juice and should be avoided. Dietary fiber intake in children and adults in the United States has been documented to be deficient. The recommended average intake for fiber in toddlers is 14 g/1000 kcal (US Department of Health and Human Services, 2016). The benefits of adequate fiber consumption include a reduced body weight in adults, prevention of type 2 diabetes, and reduction in childhood constipation (Kranz, Brauchla, Slavin, et al., 2012).

VEGETARIAN DIETS

Vegetarian diets have become increasingly popular in the United States because people are concerned about hypertension; cholesterol; obesity; cardiovascular disease; cancer of the stomach, intestine, and colon; and the influence of the animal rights movement. The Academy of Nutrition and Dietetics and the American Academy of Pediatrics endorse vegetarian diets for adults and children (Schurmann, Kersting, & Alexy, 2017): well-planned vegetarian diets are adequate for all stages of the life cycle promote normal growth, and have been shown to have lower intakes

*http://www.nationalacademies.org/hmd/Home/Global/News%20 Announcements/DRI

†https://health.gov/dietaryguidelines/2015/guidelines/

‡http://www.choosemyplate.gov/

of cholesterol, saturated fat, and total fat and higher intakes of fruits, fiber, and vegetables than nonvegetarians. However, vegetarian diets may vary considerably, and assessment of dietary adequacy is essential to ensure that children are receiving adequate nutrients (Schurmann, Kersting, & Alexy, 2017).

The major types of vegetarianism are as follows:

- *Lacto-ovo vegetarians,* who exclude meat from their diet but consume dairy products and rarely fish
- *Lacto-vegetarians,* who exclude meat and egg products
- *Ovo-vegetarian,* who exclude meat and milk products
- *Vegans,* who eliminate all foods of animal origin, including milk and eggs

Other types of vegetarian diets include fruitarian, sproutarian, nutritarian, raw food eaters, and anthroposophic (Kleinman & Greer, 2014). Many individuals who are concerned about healthy diets subscribe to vegetarian diets that may not be typified by the previous categories. Therefore during nutritional assessment it is necessary to clearly list exactly what the diet includes and excludes.*

The major deficiencies that may occur in the stricter vegan diets are inadequate protein for growth; inadequate calories for energy and growth; poor digestibility of many of the bulky natural, unprocessed foods, especially for infants; and deficiencies of vitamin B_6, niacin, riboflavin, vitamin D, iron, calcium, and zinc. Many of these deficiencies can be avoided with the use of some dietary supplements such as calcium for bone health or a multivitamin supplement, which are not considered to be complementary and alternative medicine (National Center for Complementary and Integrative Health, 2016).

Evaluate for iron-deficiency anemia and rickets in children on strict vegetarian and macrobiotic diets; this may occur as a result of consuming plant foods such as unrefined cereals, which impair the absorption of iron, calcium, and zinc. The American Academy of Pediatrics, Committee on Nutrition (2014) recommends iron supplementation of 1 mg/kg/day in infants exclusively breastfed after 4 to 6 months of age by vegetarian mothers and no dietary fat restrictions in vegetarian children younger than age 2 years. Other factors that affect iron absorption are listed in Box 12.2.

Achieving a nutritionally adequate vegetarian diet is not difficult (except with the strictest diets), but it requires careful planning and knowledge of nutrient sources (American Academy of Pediatrics, Committee on Nutrition, 2014). For children the lacto-ovo vegetarian diet is nutritionally adequate; however, the vegan diet requires supplementation with vitamins D and B_{12} for children ages 2 to 12 years. Breastfeeding mothers on a strict vegan diet should supplement their infants with vitamin B_{12} because their milk will be low in vitamin B_{12}. In addition, breastfeeding infants of strict vegans should receive foods fortified with zinc after 7 months of age (Canadian Paediatric Society, 2016).

To ensure sufficient protein in the diet, foods with incomplete proteins (i.e., those that do not have all the essential amino acids) must be eaten at the same meal with other foods that supply the missing amino acids. Three basic combinations of foods consumed by vegetarians generally provide the appropriate amounts of essential amino acids:

- Grains (cereal, rice, pasta) and legumes (beans, peas, lentils, peanuts)
- Grains and milk products (milk, cheese, yogurt)
- Seeds (sesame, sunflower) and legumes

*Additional information regarding vegetarian diets may be found at the Vegetarian Resource Group; 410-366-8343; http://www.vrg.org. Another helpful resource for adolescents and parents is the KidsHealth website: http://kidshealth.org/parent/nutrition_center/dietary_needs/vegetarianism.html.

BOX 12.2 Factors That Affect Iron Absorption

Increase

- Acidity (low pH)—Administer iron between meals (gastric hydrochloric acid)
- Ascorbic acid (vitamin C)—Administer iron with juice, fruit, or multivitamin preparation
- Vitamin A
- Tissue (cellular) need
- Meat, fish, poultry
- Cooking in cast iron pots

Decrease

- Alkalinity (high pH)—Avoid any antacid preparation
- Phosphates—Milk is unfavorable vehicle for iron administration
- Phytates—Found in cereals
- Oxalates—Found in many fruits and vegetables (plums, currants, green beans, spinach, sweet potatoes, tomatoes)
- Tannins—Found in tea, coffee
- Tissue (cellular) saturation
- Malabsorptive disorders
- Disturbances that cause diarrhea or steatorrhea
- Infection
- Calcium

COMPLEMENTARY AND ALTERNATIVE MEDICINE

There are four complementary and alternative medicine (CAM) domains according to the National Center for Complementary and Integrative Health; this discussion centers on only one of those biologically based practices that include herbs, vitamins, and foods. The National Center for Complementary and Integrative Health (2016) classifies probiotics as a type of natural product and CAM. Many CAM products are sold over the counter as dietary supplements, but the use of some dietary supplements, such as calcium for bone health or a multivitamin supplement, is not considered to be CAM (National Center for Complementary and Integrative Health, 2016). The National Center for Complementary and Integrative Health(2016) reports that natural products are the most commonly used CAM products in children. CAM is often used for children's chronic remedies for which traditional therapy is not effective (National Center for Complementary and Integrative Health, 2016).

The misuse of CAM has the potential for placing some children at risk for health problems. Although 55% of children have used CAM at least once, only 4.4% of CAM use was reported to emergency department physicians primarily because the parent or child did not think it was important to inform the physician and/or the physician did not ask about use (Taylor, Dhir, Craig, et al., 2015). The most common CAM remedies used in children seen in the emergency department were homeopathy (77%), herbs (64%), and traditional Chinese medicine (13%) (Zuzak, Zuzak-Siegrist, Rist, et al., 2010). A survey of four pediatric emergency departments found that child herbal use was common, especially among children 6 years of age and older (Taylor, Dhir, Craig, et al., 2015). Some of the herbs used by the children in the survey included chamomile, cranberry, parsley, ginger, celery, amino acids, and green tea, and herbal therapies with known toxicity included garlic, licorice, bella donna, and ginko biloba.

There is concern that terms often used to market supplements such as megavitamins may mislead parents regarding the actual benefits (or harms) of such therapies. The intention herein is not to discredit the use of CAM such as vitamin supplements but rather to ensure safety and efficacy in children who may experience inadvertent harm. The use of various herbal therapies, or intake of herbs, is also popular; many of these have been a part of medicine since the early days and are beneficial in some cases. Growing evidence from clinical samples suggest that CAM therapies are desired by families and may benefit some children with pain conditions (Groenewald, Beals-Erickson, Ralston-Wilson, et al., 2017).

Herbs known to have adverse effects in children include ephedra, comfrey, and pennyroyal; some herbs may not be harmful taken alone but may counteract or potentiate prescription medications when taken together. Parents should be fully informed of the use of herbs to ensure that there is more benefit than potential harm in the ingredients being used. Health care workers also need to be knowledgeable of the benefits or potential harm in herbs to counsel parents and address their concerns appropriately. Little research has been performed in children on many over-the-counter (OTC) herbal medicines, yet some herbs are known to cause harm. Parents should be cautioned not to exceed the upper limits of vitamin intake according to the new DRIs (see dietary guideline section earlier in this chapter).*

Nursing Care Management

Evaluation of adequacy of nutrient intake is the initial nursing goal and requires assessment based on a dietary history and physical examination for signs of deficiency or excess. Once assessment data are collected, this information is evaluated against standard intakes to identify areas of concern. (See Nutritional Assessment, Chapter 4.)

The American Heart Association Dietary Guidelines, patterned after the Dietary Guidelines for Americans, may also be used to encourage healthy dietary intakes designed to decrease obesity and cardiovascular risk factors and subsequent cardiovascular disease, which is now known to occur in both young children and adults (Steinberger, Daniels, Hagberg, et al., 2016). The American Heart Association guidelines have been endorsed by the American Academy of Pediatrics, but it is important to note that these guidelines are for children ages 2 years and older. The guidelines encourage a variety of fruits, vegetables, whole grains, and low-fat dairy and nonfat dairy products, in addition to fish, beans, and lean meat.

The nurse has an important role in evaluating the food intake of infants, children, and adolescents and may serve as a resource for parents; the overall nutritional goal should be to provide the best sources of vitamin and mineral intake through food intake rather than rely on supplemental vitamins, which may not always be as well absorbed as food products. In addition, parents are encouraged to read labels of food products and CAM products to ensure that their child is receiving an adequate portion of recommended nutrients for proper growth and development.

SLEEP AND ACTIVITY

Total sleep time decreases only slightly during the second year and averages about 11 to 12 hours. Most toddlers take one nap a day, and by the end of the second or third year, many relinquish this habit.

Toddlers are more prone to having bedtime resistance (refusal to go to bed) and frequent night waking. Fears can be provoked by a child's daily stressors, such as pressure to toilet train, moves, sibling birth, experiences of loss, or separation from parents. Consistent nightly bedtime is associated with better sleep patterns, such as shorter sleep onset latency, decreased waking, longer total sleep, and decreased daytime behavior problems (Mindell, Li, Sadeh, et al., 2015). In addition, providing transitional objects, such as a favorite stuffed animal or blanket, can ease the child's insecurity at bedtime. Children may need a light snack before bedtime; a heavy meal immediately before bedtime may interfere with sleep. Other suggestions to help small children sleep better include keeping the television out of the child's room, making the hour before bedtime a quiet time of reading stories, and avoiding stimulating activities such as computer games and roughhousing (Owens, 2016). Toddlers who are no longer sleeping in a crib may come out of their rooms after being put to bed. Limit prolonged bedtime rituals by defining a length of time and set of activities ("one more story, one more drink"). Toddlers who are too immature to respond to the measures identified may need their doorways gated. For problems that persist, parents should consider the interventions outlined in Table 11.1.

Toddler's activity level is high, and rarely is there a problem with too little physical exercise, provided that inappropriate restrictions are not instituted. Recently, however, there has been concern that decreased time spent in actual physical play and more time involved with computers and television watching have increased the tendency toward being overweight. This is especially true in large urban centers during the winter months where there may not be adequate "safe" play and physical exercise space. With increasing numbers of young children being cared for outside the home, attention to the kinds of activity provided is important. For example, children with high activity levels may benefit from an environment that encourages vigorous play whether outside or in a large indoor play area.

DENTAL HEALTH

Regular Dental Examinations

The American Academy of Pediatric Dentistry (2016a) recommends that every child have an oral health examination by a practitioner by 6 months of age; if the child is in a high-risk category for caries, it is recommended that an initial visit to a dentist or pedodontist (pediatric dentist) occur by age 6 months or within 6 months of the eruption of the first tooth. Every child should have an established dental home by age 12 months (American Academy of Pediatric Dentistry, 2016a). Initial visits to the dentist should be nontraumatizing. Because toddlers react negatively to new and potentially frightening experiences, the initial visit can center around meeting the dentist, seeing the equipment, and sitting in the chair. If the child is cooperative, the dentist may just look at the teeth but reserve a more thorough examination for another visit. Modeling, in which the child observes procedures performed on the parent or a cooperative sibling, can also be effective but may not work on all toddlers.

Removal of Plaque

Oral hygiene measures should be implemented in toddlers to remove plaque (i.e, soft bacterial deposits that adhere to the teeth and cause dental caries [decay or cavities] and periodontal [gum] disease). Poor oral hygiene and dietary habits are associated with the development of caries in children. Table 12.4 lists the pediatric quality indicator for children with cavities.

The most effective methods for plaque removal are brushing and flossing. Several brushing techniques exist, although there is no universal agreement regarding the best method. One that is suitable for cleaning the primary teeth is the scrub method. The tips of the bristles are placed firmly at a 45-degree angle against the teeth and gums and moved back and forth in a vibratory motion. The ends of the bristles should be wiggling but not moving forcefully back and forth, which can damage the gums and enamel. All the surfaces of the teeth are cleaned in this

*Helpful websites for health care and consumer information concerning herbs are NCCAM, http://www.nccam.nih.gov; American Botanical Council, http://abc.herbalgram.org; and Herb Research Foundation, http://www.herbs.org.

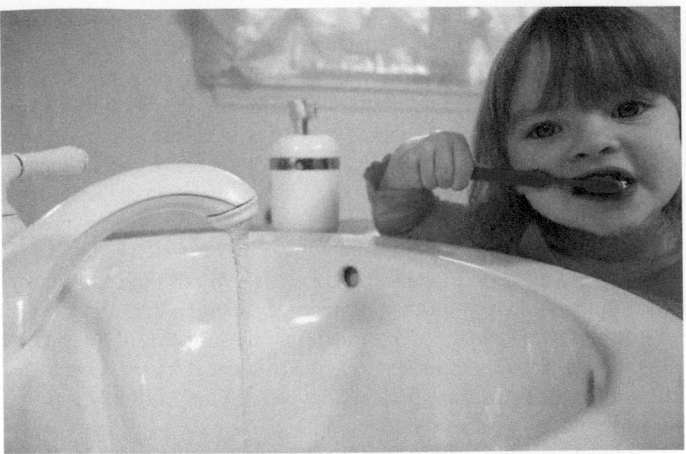

FIG. 12.8 Young children can participate in tooth brushing.

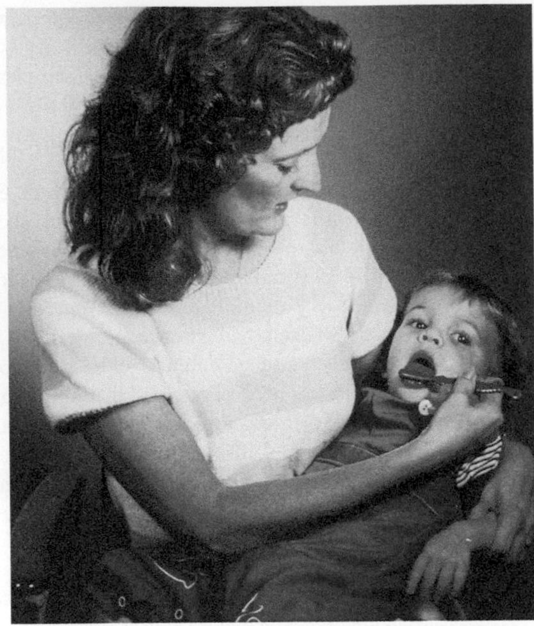

FIG. 12.9 The most effective cleaning of the teeth is done by parents.

TABLE 12.4 Pediatric Quality Indicator*

Dental Decay or Cavities

Children who have dental decay or cavities	
Measure	Children ages 0-20 years, who have had tooth decay or cavities during the measurement period
Numerator	Number of children who had cavities or decayed teeth during the measurement time
Denominator	Number of children, age 0-20 years, with at least one outpatient visit

*Endorsed by the Center for Medicare and Medicaid Services-75v1.

manner except the lingual (inner) surfaces of the anterior teeth. To clean these surfaces, the toothbrush is placed vertical to the teeth and moved up and down. Only a few teeth are brushed at one time, using six to eight strokes for each section. A systematic approach is used so all surfaces are thoroughly cleaned (Fig. 12.8).

For young children the most effective cleaning is done by parents (Fig. 12.9). Several positions can be used that facilitate access to the mouth and help stabilize the head for comfort:

- Stand with the child's back toward the adult. (When done in front of a bathroom mirror, both the child and adult can see what is being done in the mirror.)
- Sit on a couch or bed with the child's head resting in the adult's lap.
- Sit on the floor or a stool with the child's head resting between the adult's thighs.

Use one hand to cup the chin and one to brush the teeth. For easier access to back teeth, hold the mouth partially open. After brushing with an appropriate amount of fluoridated paste or gel, avoid rinsing the mouth to maximize the beneficial effects of the fluoride.

For effective cleaning a small toothbrush with soft, rounded, multitufted nylon bristles that are short and uniform in length is recommended. Nylon bristles dry more rapidly after use and retain their shape better than natural bristles. Toothbrushes are replaced as soon as the bristles are frayed or bent. With young children, brushing may be more easily accomplished using only water because many children dislike the foam from toothpaste, and the foam interferes with visibility. Use a "smear" or "rice-like" amount of toothpaste for children younger than 3 years old (apply across the narrow width of the toothbrush, rather than along its length, to decrease the chance of applying an excessive amount) and a pea-size amount of toothpaste for children 3 to 6 years old (American Academy of Pediatric Dentistry, 2016b).

After the teeth have been cleaned, the teeth are flossed to remove plaque and debris from between the teeth and below the gum margin, where brushing is ineffective. Because young children do not have the dexterity to manipulate dental floss, parents must perform the procedure.

Ideally the teeth should be cleaned after each meal and especially before bedtime, and the child should be given nothing to eat or drink after the night brushing except water. At times when brushing is impractical, the "swish-and-swallow" method of cleaning the mouth is taught; with a mouthful of water, the child rinses the mouth and swallows, repeating the procedure three or four times.*

Fluoride

Fluoride supplementation should be considered for any child. Fluoride, a mineral, is found in water, foods, or drinks in which fluoridated water was used as part of the processing system. Because the water fluoridation process and manufacturing of fluoride toothpaste are almost impossible to standardize in the United States, the dosage of fluoride should be determined in consultation with a medical professional (American Academy of Pediatric Dentistry, 2016b) (Table 12.5). Increased fluoride ingestion leads to fluorosis, which consists of enamel protein retention, hypomineralization of the enamel and dentin, and disturbance of crystal formation. The effects caused by this change range from barely discernible white fiberlike lines or spots to gray-brown stains or pitted areas. Parents should be cautioned against regular use of fluoridated water or beverages such as bottled water containing fluoride if the community water supply already has an adequate amount of fluoride (see Community and Home Health Considerations box).

Topical fluoride treatments (e.g., fluoride varnish) performed in the dental home are also effective in decreasing caries (American Academy of Pediatric Dentistry, 2014).

*More detailed information can be obtained from the American Academy of Pediatric Dentistry, http://www.aapd.org.

TABLE 12.5 Dietary Fluoride Supplementation

	WATER FLUORIDE CONTENT (ppm)		
Age	**<0.3**	**0.3-0.6**	**>0.6**
Birth–6 months	0	0	0
6 months–3 years	0.25 mg	0	0
3-6 years	0.5 mg	0.25 mg	0
6-16 years	1.00 mg	0.50 mg	0

From American Academy of Pediatric Dentistry. (2014). *Reference manual, 2013-2014: Guideline on fluoride therapy*. Available at http://www.aapd.org/media/Policies_Guidelines/G_FluorideTherapy.pdf.

COMMUNITY AND HOME HEALTH CONSIDERATIONS

An Optimum Fluoride Regimen in Young Children

Base recommendations on the fluoride concentration in child's drinking water, including bottled water, filtered water, and well water.

If the water is fluoridated, encourage use of tap water for drinking and for preparation of formula (except soy formula, which has twice the fluoride of regular formula), frozen-concentrated juices, powdered mixes, soups, ice, and gelatin.

If the water is nonfluoridated or contains less than 0.3 ppm (ages 6 months to 3 years) or less than 0.6 ppm (ages 3 to 6 years) fluoride, or if child refuses to drink tap water or refuses drinks or foods made with tap water, consider fluoride supplements (see Table 12.5).

If the water, such as water from some wells or springs, has a concentration of fluoride above the recommended level, encourage use of bottled non-fluoridated water for drinking.

Encourage supervision of toddler when brushing teeth or using a fluoridated mouth rinse to prevent overingestion of fluoridated topical supplement.

Use fluoridated toothpaste only in children 2 years old and older.

Consider other sources of fluoride from diet, such as tea.

If fluoride supplements are needed, give special instructions to family, including the following:

- Give supplements on an empty stomach without calcium-rich products, such as milk or cheese.
- Do not give food or drink for at least 30 minutes after taking the supplement.
- Place drops on tongue; it should be mixed with saliva and swished around in the mouth so that fluoride comes in contact with the teeth.
- Chewable tablets should be chewed and then mixed with saliva and swished in mouth for 30 seconds so that fluoride comes in contact with the teeth.
- Store fluoride products away from toddlers to avoid overingestion.
- Keep only a 4-month supply.
- Administer supplement at same time daily; post reminders if necessary.

Stress that dental appointments should be scheduled every 6 months for professional topical fluoride treatment.

Fluoride rinses are usually only suggested for children at high cariogenic risk or over the age of 6 years.

Modified from American Academy of Pediatric Dentistry. (2014). *Reference manual, 2014: Guideline on fluoride therapy, 35*(6), 167-170. Available at http://www.aapd.org/media/Policies_Guidelines/G_FluorideTherapy.pdf.

Dietary Factors

Diet is critical to developing good teeth because the carious process depends primarily on fermentable sugars, especially sucrose, and other carbohydrates. Refined table sugar, honey, molasses, corn syrup, and dried fruits such as raisins are highly cariogenic. Complex carbohydrates such as breads, potatoes, and pasta also contribute to caries because they lower the plaque pH. Sugary beverages that are commonly consumed by children and adolescents and sugar-containing medications are also highly cariogenic (Llena, Leyda, Forner, et al., 2015).

Ideally, highly cariogenic foods, especially those containing complex sugars, should be eliminated. However, because this is impractical, some suggestions can be helpful. First, *the frequency with which sugar is consumed is more important than the total amount eaten.* Therefore when sweets are eaten, they are less damaging if consumed immediately after a meal rather than as a snack between meals. When they are served as the dessert, the teeth can be cleaned afterward, decreasing the amount of time the sugar is in the mouth.

Second, the form of sugar (sucrose) is important. The more cariogenic foods are those that are sticky or hard because they remain in the mouth longer. Consequently, sucking on lollipops is more cariogenic than eating a chocolate bar. Sometimes the source of the sugar is "hidden," as in numerous prescription and nonprescription drugs and many popular cereals, including the "all-natural" variety. Reading food labels is essential in eliminating sources of sucrose.

Some snacks do not contribute to tooth decay. Aged cheeses such as cheddar may alter the pH and delay bacterial growth. Sugarless gum chewed after eating may actually protect against cavities by stimulating saliva that neutralizes acid.

A special form of tooth decay in children between 18 months and 3 years of age is early childhood caries (ECC) (historically called *nursing caries* or *baby bottle tooth decay*) (Fig. 12.10). This often occurs when a child is routinely given a bottle of milk or juice at naptime or bedtime or uses the bottle as a pacifier while awake. Frequent nocturnal breastfeeding for prolonged periods also leads to extensive destruction of the teeth. The practice of coating pacifiers in honey can also contribute to caries and may be a potential source of botulism poisoning. As the sweet liquid pools in the mouth, the teeth are bathed for several hours in this cariogenic environment. Prolonged bottle-feeding, fruit-juice consumption, lack of periodic dental examination, and nocturnal feeding contribute to significant ECC (Ozen, Van Strijp, Ozer, et al., 2016). The maxillary (upper) incisors and molars are affected most because the mandibular (lower) incisors are protected by the lower lip, tongue, and saliva. Severely decayed teeth may require the application of stainless-steel bands to preserve the spacing until the permanent teeth erupt.

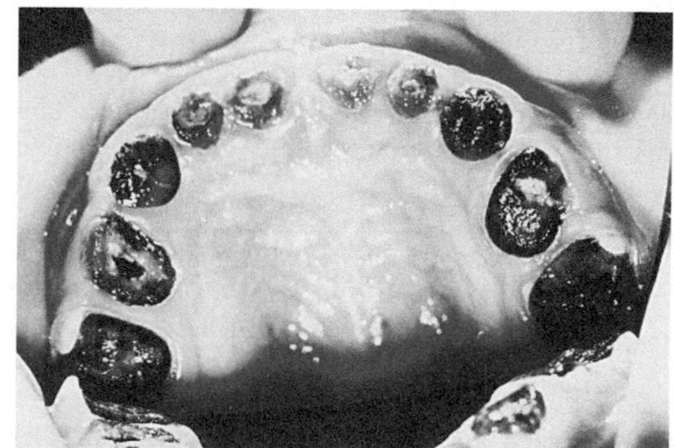

FIG. 12.10 Early childhood caries. Note extensive carious involvement of maxillary primary incisors. (Courtesy Bruce Carter, DDS, Texas Children's Hospital, Houston.)

ECC is now considered to be an infectious disease of childhood. There is evidence that *Streptococcus mutans* is a highly cariogenic bacteria (American Academy of Pediatric Dentistry, 2016b). One of the early origins of *S. mutans* is the mother's saliva; infants of mothers with high counts of the bacteria have a greater incidence of ECC. Therefore it is important to discuss oral hygiene with pregnant women because of its impact on their children's tooth development.

Prevention involves eliminating the bedtime bottle completely, feeding the last bottle before bedtime, not using the bottle as a pacifier, and never coating pacifiers in sweet substances. Juice in bottles, especially commercially available ready-to-use bottles, is discouraged; these beverages are especially damaging because the sugar is more readily converted to acid. Juice should always be offered in a cup to avoid prolonging the bottle-feeding habit. Toddlers should be encouraged to drink from a cup at the first birthday and weaned from a bottle by 14 months of age. Nurses are in an excellent position to counsel parents regarding the dangers of this habit and other aspects of dental care.*

SAFETY PROMOTION AND INJURY PREVENTION

Unintentional childhood injury was the leading cause of death among children ages 1 to 4 years in 2013, accounting for 32% of all deaths in this age-group (Centers for Disease Control and Prevention, 2016). Males have a higher rate of death (36%) than females (28%). Leading causes of accidental death include suffocation for children less than 1 year of age and drowning for children 1 to 4 years of age (Centers for Disease Control and Prevention, 2016). Falls are the leading cause of nonfatal injuries among children. These deaths and injuries are preventable, and they highlight the need for public health action and education. There is evidence that one-on-one and face-to-face education in the home, safety interventions, and safety equipment are effective in reducing the number of unintentional childhood injuries that can have catastrophic results (Folger, Bowers, Dexheimer, et al., 2017).

A major factor in the critical increase of injuries during early childhood compared with the number in preschoolers and school-age children is the unrestricted freedom achieved through locomotion combined with an unawareness of danger within the environment. Toddlers are very curious about how things work and exploration of previously unknown or unseen objects and places is common. Toddlers also have not fully developed or understand the cause-and-effect principles and often are unable to gauge danger; poorly developed depth perception may also contribute to falls and tumbles, as does the general bodily structure of toddlers. Specific categories of injuries and appropriate prevention are best understood by associating them with the major developmental achievements of young children. The discussions of injuries in Chapters 2, 10, and 13 are also relevant to safety concerns at this age.

Motor Vehicle Injuries

Motor vehicle injuries cause more accidental deaths in children ages 5 to 19 years than any other type of injury and are responsible for a significant number of all accidental deaths among children ages 1 to 4 years (Centers for Disease Control and Prevention, 2016). Many of the deaths are caused by injuries within the car when restraints have not been used or age-related guidelines have not been properly followed. Unrestrained children riding in the vehicle's front seat are at the highest risk for injury. Approved restraints properly installed and applied can reduce the majority of fatalities and injuries.

Car Restraints

Nurses are responsible for educating parents regarding the importance of car restraints and their proper use. Five types of restraints are available: infant-only devices, convertible models for both infants and toddlers, booster seats, safety belts, and devices for children with special needs (see Chapter 22). Chapter 10 discusses the infant-type restraints; convertible restraints and boosters are included here. The convertible restraint is suitable for infants in the rearward-facing position (see Fig. 10.13). It is now recommended that children up to the age of 2 years ride in a rear-facing safety seat until the child has outgrown the car seat manufacturer's height and weight recommendations; then transition the child to a forward-facing safety seat with a harness in the backseat of the vehicle (Rivara & Grossman, 2016). Many rear-facing car safety seats can accommodate children weighing up to a maximum of 35 pounds (according to manufacturer specifications). Studies indicate that toddlers up to 24 months of age are safer riding in convertible seats in the rear-facing position (American Academy of Pediatrics, 2015). Another study confirmed that children 0 to 3 years of age riding properly restrained in the rear seat had significantly less risk of death than passengers in the front seats (Durbin, Jermakian, Kallan, et al., 2015).

Convertible restraints use different types of harness systems: a five-point harness that consists of a strap over each shoulder, one on each side of the pelvis, and one between the legs (all five come together at a common buckle) and a padded overhead shield that uses shoulder straps attached to a shield that is held in place by a crotch strap. The overhead shield convertible seats are no longer manufactured but if in one's possession may be used until the manufacturer's weight limit is reached. With both the infant and toddler restraints it is important not to add extra blankets, head cushions, or padding between the child and the restraint straps that did not come as original equipment because these "add-ons" create spaces of air between the child and the restraint and decrease support for the back, head, and neck. A 3-in-1 convertible seat is also available that can be used rear-facing, forward-facing, and as a belt-positioning seat for toddlers; this seat is larger than other convertible seats, so it is important to verify that the seat fits in the car in the rear-facing position.

Cars with free-sliding latch plates on the lap or shoulder belt require the use of a metal locking clip to keep the belt in a tight-holding position. The locking clip is threaded onto the belt above the latch plate (Fig. 12.11, *A*). If parents have cars with automatic lap and shoulder belts, they need to have additional lap belts installed to properly secure the restraint.

Booster seats are not restraint systems like the convertible devices because they depend on the vehicle safety belts to hold the child and booster seat in place. Three booster models have been approved by the National Highway Traffic Safety Administration: the high-back belt-positioning seat (Fig. 12.11, *B*), which provides head and neck support for the child riding in a vehicle seat without a headrest; the no-back belt-positioning seat, which should be used only if the vehicle seat has a headrest; and a combination seat, which converts from a forward-facing toddler seat to a booster seat. This last model is equipped with a harness for use by toddlers; the harness may be removed, and a lap shoulder belt can be used when the child outgrows the harness. The belt-positioning booster seats are used for children who are less than 145 cm (4 feet, 9

*Sources of information about nursing caries and other aspects of child dental health include the National Institute of Dental and Craniofacial Research, National Institutes of Health, Bethesda, MD 20892-2190, 301-496-4261, http://www.nidcr.nih.gov; American Academy of Pediatric Dentistry, 211 E. Chicago Ave., Suite 1700, Chicago, IL 60611, 312-337-2169, http://www.aapd.org; American Dental Association, 211 E. Chicago Ave., Chicago, IL 60611, 312-440-2500, http://www.ada.org/; and Canadian Dental Association, 1815 Alta Vista Drive, Ottawa, Ontario K1G 3Y6, 613-523-1770, http://www.cda-adc.ca.

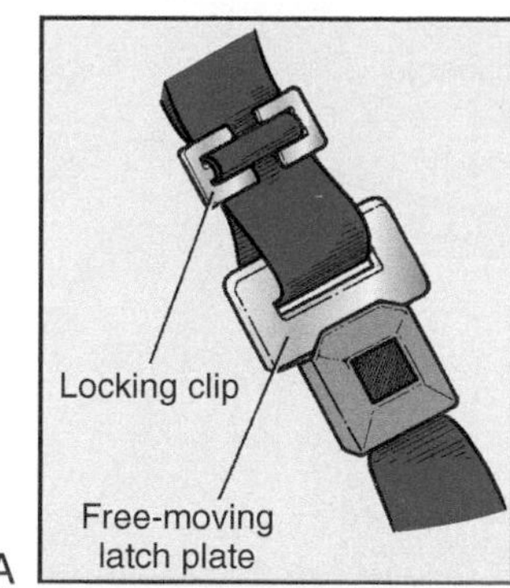

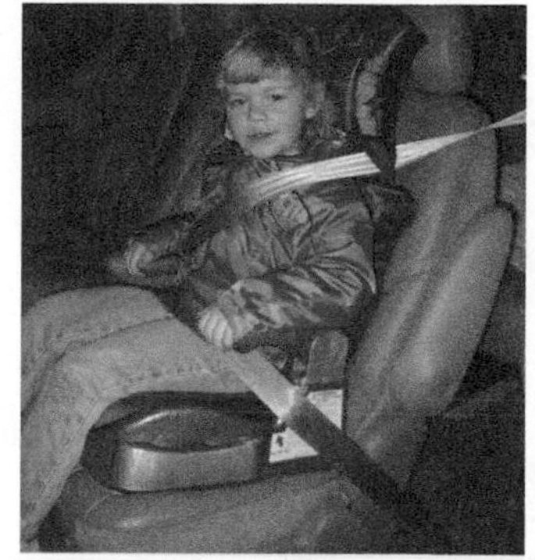

FIG. 12.11 **A,** Locking clip used with free-sliding lap-shoulder belt to keep the belt in a tight-holding position. **B,** Automobile booster seat. Note placement of shoulder strap (away from neck and face).

inches) tall and weigh 15.9 kg to 36.3 kg (35 to 80 lb, depending on the type of booster seat). In general school-age children should ride in a belt-positioning seat booster until approximately 7 to 8 years of age. However, note that because children's sizes vary considerably, manufacturer recommendations should be followed regarding height and weight limitations. A booster seat should be used until the child is able to sit against the back of the seat with feet hanging down and legs bent at the knees. The belt-positioning booster model raises a child higher in the seat, moving the shoulder part of the belt off the neck and the lap portion off the abdomen onto the pelvis. Children who outgrow the convertible restraint may still be able to ride safely in a booster seat until the midpoint of the head is higher than the vehicle seat back.

Children should use a specially designed car restraint (such as those discussed previously) until they are 145 cm (4 feet, 9 inches) in height or 8 to 12 years old (American Academy of Pediatrics, 2015). Shoulder-lap safety belts should be worn low on the hips, snug, and not on the abdominal area. Children should be taught to sit up straight to allow for proper fit. The shoulder belt is used only if it does not cross the child's neck or face.

Shoulder-only automatic belts are designed to protect adults. Children should use the manual shoulder belts in the rear seat. Air bags do not take the place of child safety seats or seat belts and can be lethal to young children. The safest area of the car for children is the backseat.

For any restraint to be effective, it must be used consistently and properly. Examples of misuse include misrouting the vehicle seat belt through the restraint; failing to use the vehicle seat belt to secure the restraint; failing to use a tether strap; failing to use the restraint harness system; and incorrectly positioning the child, especially by facing infants forward instead of rearward. To address these issues nurses must stress correct use of car restraints and rules that ensure compliance (see Family-Centered Care box). Additional information about child safety restraints is available from various sources.*

The LATCH (lower anchors and tethers for children) universal child safety seat system was implemented as a requirement starting in 2002 for all new automobiles and child safety seats. This system provides uniform anchorage consisting of two lower anchorages and one upper anchorage in the rear seat of the vehicle (Fig. 12.12). When used appropriately, the top anchor (tether) strap prevents the child from pitching forward in a crash. If the tether strap is not used, up to 90% of the protection of the restraint is lost. Instructions for proper installation of the tether strap and permanent bracket are included with the car restraint. New child safety seats have a hook, buckle, strap, or other connector that attaches to the anchorage. Concerns about the increased weight of children in the United States has led some to question the safety of the LATCH system with child restraints (car seats) and the child whose combined weight is more than 29.5 kg (65 lb). The National Highway Traffic Safety Administration recommends the shoulder–lap belt restraint to restrain the child in the car seat instead of relying on the LATCH system for maximum protection if the combined weight of the child and car seat is more than 29.5 kg (65 lb).

Children with disabilities may require a restraint system that secures them appropriately in the event of a crash. Examples of such devices include car-bed restraints for infants who cannot tolerate a semireclining position and specially adapted molded-plastic chairs for children who have spica casts. The E-Z-On vest is a special safety harness for larger children with poor trunk control. A HIPPO (Spica Cast) Car Seat is available for transporting children with spica casts; these are sold only in the United States. Additional safety restraints and a list of distributors are available at the SafetyBeltSafe US website (http://www.carseat.org). See also Chapter 9 for a discussion of preterm infants being discharged home and car seat evaluation.

Children should never ride in the open back of a truck. The danger of falls can be compounded by another vehicle striking the child or by the truck rolling over. In addition, leaving children unsupervised in a

FAMILY-CENTERED CARE

Using Car Safety Seats

- Read manufacturer's directions and follow them exactly.
- Anchor safety seat securely to car's seat and apply harness (depending on model) snugly to child.
- Do not start car until everyone is properly restrained.
- Always use the car seat restraint, even for short trips.
- If child begins to climb out or undo harness, firmly say, "no." It may be necessary to stop the car to reinforce the expected behavior. Use rewards, such as stars or stickers, to encourage cooperative behavior.
- Allow child to hold favorite toy, blanket, or stuffed animal in car seat.
- Encourage child to help attach buckles, straps, and shields.
- Decrease boredom on long trips. Keep special toys in car for quiet play; talk to child; point out objects and teach child about them. Stop periodically. If child wishes to sleep, make certain child stays in restraint seat.
- Insist that others who transport children also follow these safety rules.

*American Academy of Pediatrics, 141 Northwest Point Blvd., Elk Grove Village, IL 60007, 847-434-4000, http://www.aap.org; and local division of traffic safety or National Highway Traffic Safety Administration, 1200 New Jersey Ave. SE, West Building, Washington, DC 20590, 888-327-4236, http://www.nhtsa.dot.gov.

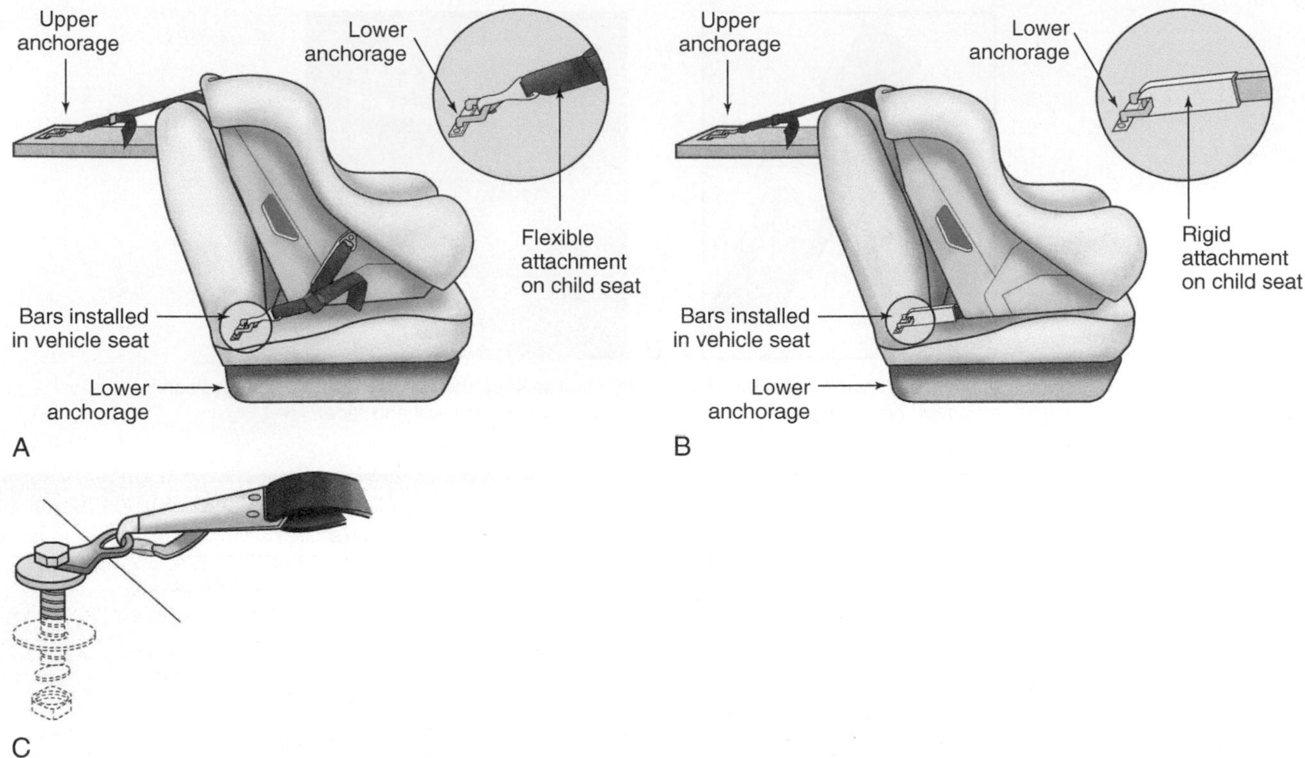

FIG. 12.12 Lower anchors and tethers for children (LATCH). **A,** Flexible two-point attachment with top tether. **B,** Rigid two-point attachment with top tether. **C,** Top tether. (Courtesy U.S. Department of Transportation, National Highway Traffic Safety Administration.)

parked vehicle, especially in a private driveway, provides an opportunity for a child to release the brake or put the car in gear. The child also can be injured from a collision with or a fall from a bicycle-towed trailer or bicycle-mounted child seat.

Toddlers are often involved in pedestrian traffic injuries. Because of their gross motor skills of walking, running, and climbing and their fine motor skills of opening doors and fence gates, they are likely to be in hazardous areas unsupervised. Unaware of danger and unable to estimate the speed of a car, children may be hit by moving vehicles. Running after a ball, playing in a pile of leaves or snow or inside a cardboard box, riding a tricycle, and playing behind a parked car or near the curb are common activities that may result in a vehicular tragedy.

One type of injury that has become more common occurs when children crawl into an open trunk and pull it closed. Asphyxia may occur in such cases; therefore car trunks should not be left open when children are unsupervised. Some cars are equipped with a safety switch that can be activated from inside the trunk to open a closed trunk door.

Another automobile-related hazard for toddlers is overheating (hyperthermia) and subsequent death when left in a vehicle in hot weather (>27° C [80° F]). Small children dissipate heat poorly, and an increase in body temperature can cause death in a few hours. Since 1998, a total of 661 children died from hyperthermia when left alone in parked cars; in 2014, the total number of child deaths was 41, and it is estimated that an average of 37 children die each year from overheating in cars (Null, 2015). It is estimated that, with the ambient temperature at 22° to 35.5° C (72° to 96° F), the vehicle interior temperature rises by 10.5° to 11° C (19° to 20° F) for each 10 minutes, even with a window cracked (Duzinski, Barczyk, Wheeler, et al., 2014). Approximately 50% of adults who left a child in a car either forgot or were unaware that the child was still in the car (Duzinski, Barczyk, Wheeler, et al., 2014). Parents are cautioned against leaving infants alone in a vehicle for *any reason.*

Preventing vehicular injuries involves protecting and educating children about the danger of moving and parked vehicles. Although toddlers are too young to be trusted to always obey, parents should emphasize looking for moving vehicles before crossing the street and recognizing the stop and go colors of traffic lights. Physical barriers limiting children from playing near vehicles help prevent these injuries. Most important, what is preached must be practiced. Children learn through imitation, and consistency reinforces learning.

Drowning

The highest rates of drowning occur in children ages 1 to 4 years; one-third of these children died from drowning (Centers for Disease Control and Prevention, 2016). Drowning deaths in infants occur most commonly in the bathtub and large buckets. With well-developed skills of locomotion, toddlers are able to reach potentially dangerous areas such as bathtubs, toilets, buckets, swimming pools, hot tubs, and ponds or lakes. Toddlers' intense drive for exploration and investigation, combined with an unawareness of the danger of water and their helplessness in water, makes drowning always a viable threat. It is also one category of injury that results in death within minutes, diminishing the chance for rescue and survival. Close adult supervision of children when near any source of water is essential; many drownings in this age-group occur when a supervising adult becomes distracted. The American Academy of Pediatrics recommends "touch" supervision for small children; the adult can reach out and touch or grab the child having difficulty. Teaching swimming and water safety can be helpful but cannot be regarded as sufficient protection. Pool fencing, although critical, does not always deter fast-moving children.

Burns

Toddlers' ability to climb, stretch, and reach objects above their heads makes any hot surface a potential source of danger. Children pulling pots with hot liquids, especially oil and grease, on top of themselves are a major source of burns. As a precaution, turn pot handles toward the back of the stove, and electric pots (e.g., coffee maker, frying pan, slow cooker), including cords, should be placed out of reach. Ideally, the knobs for controlling the range burners should be out of reach, not on the front panel where nimble fingers can turn them on and accidentally touch the hot burner.

Other sources of heat, such as radiators, fireplaces, accessible furnaces, kerosene heaters, or wood-burning stoves, should have guards placed in front of them. The tops of some of these heaters are designed to become hot enough to boil water to provide humidity. They are hazardous if touched or if the pan of water is spilled. Portable electric heaters must be placed in a high area, well out of reach of climbing young children.

Hot objects such as candles, incense, hot embers and ashes, cigarettes, pots of tea or coffee, or irons must be placed away from children. Hair curling irons and hot curlers may also be easily reached and can burn the hands of curious toddlers. Ashtrays with a center well are preferred to prevent the cigarette from falling off the rim, and adults should try not to smoke, cook, or drink hot liquids when children are nearby. Flame burns represent one of the most fatal types of burns and commonly occur when children play with matches or lighters and accidentally set themselves (and the home) on fire (Fig. 12.13). To prevent flame burns, all matches must be stored safely away from children, and parents need to teach children the dangers of playing with matches and lighters. In addition, all homes should have smoke detectors installed to alert the occupants of a fire. A safety plan for immediate escape is also essential.

Electrical burns represent an immediate danger to children. With the ability to manipulate small, thin objects, they are able to insert hairpins or other conductive articles into electrical sockets. Young toddlers may explore outlets and wires by mouthing them. Because saliva is an excellent conductor, the chance for a severe circumoral electrical burn is great. Electrical outlets should have protective guards plugged into them when not in use or be made inaccessible by placing furniture in front of them when feasible (Fig. 12.14). Children should not be allowed to play with electrical cords, appliances, or batteries.

Scald burns are the most common type of thermal injury in children, especially 1- and 2-year-olds. Scalding often occurs because the child is reaching toward a stove or other surface and pulling hot water onto herself or because the child has spilled a hot liquid container (such as a parent's coffee or tea) onto himself. A scalding burn is often caused by high-temperature tap water, which children come in contact with as a result of turning on the hot-water faucet, falling into a bathtub of hot water, or suffering deliberate abuse. Besides the obvious prevention of always supervising children when they are near tap water and checking bathwater temperatures, household water temperatures should be limited to less than 49° C (120° F). At this temperature it takes 10 minutes for exposure to the water to cause a full-thickness burn. Conversely, water temperatures of 54° C (130° F), the usual setting of most water heaters, expose household members to the risk of full-thickness burns within 30 seconds.

Nurses can help prevent such burns by advising parents of this common household danger and recommending that they adjust the water heater to a safe temperature. An easy-to-read hot-water gauge that changes color to show water temperatures between 49° C and 65.5° C (120° F and 150° F) is available; it shows "hot," "cool," or "OK" water temperature. A special device can also be added to the faucet that reduces the water flow if the set temperature is reached. (See also Burns, Chapter 23.)

Sunburns are a special concern for this age-group. Children spend a large amount of time outdoors, and their increased mobility makes it difficult to prevent sun exposure. Sunburn can be prevented by applying a sunscreen with a sun protection factor (SPF) of 15 or greater, dressing in protective clothing (e.g., wide-brimmed hat, protective cotton clothing with a tight weave), and avoiding sun exposure between 10 AM and 2 PM.

FIG. 12.13 Matches are a potentially deadly hazard for young children.

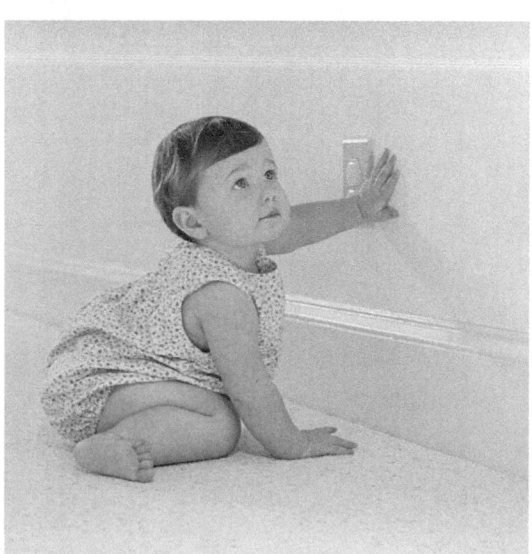

FIG. 12.14 Special plastic caps in electrical sockets prevent young fingers from exploring dangerous areas.

Accidental Poisoning

Toddlers are at the highest risk for accidental poisoning because of their innate curiosity and ability to open "childproof" containers. Because mouthing activity continues to be prevalent after 1 year of age and exploring objects by tasting them is part of children's curious investigation, ingestion is the most common form of exposure (Kostic, 2016). Toddlers' curiosity and inability to understand logical consequences further place them at risk for ingesting harmful substances. About 50% of accidental exposures in children involve cosmetics and personal care products, cleaning solutions, plants, and foreign bodies, including toys (Kostic, 2016). Pharmaceutical agents, such as analgesics, topical preparations, cough and cold products, and vitamins, account for most of the other types of ingested agents (Kostic, 2016). Although in many instances poisoning does not result in death, it may cause significant morbidity such as esophageal erosion and stricture from lye ingestion. Toddlers are able to climb most heights, open most drawers or closets, and unscrew most lids. By trial and error younger children also manage to undo tops of bottles, plastic containers, aerosol cans, and jars, including those with child-resistant lids. Newer forms of drugs such as transdermal patches and cough-suppressant lozenges have created additional dangers because they are not packaged with safety caps and the lozenges look like candy.

The major reason for poisoning is improper storage (Fig. 12.15). The guidelines suggested in Chapter 14 apply to children in this age-group as well. However, unlike infants, who are confined to certain heights and unable to unlatch inventive locks, young children manage to find access to many high-level, tight-security places. For this age-group only a locked cabinet is safe.

Recent attention has focused on OTC medications used for cough and colds as a common cause of accidental poisonous ingestion in toddlers. Ingestion of acetaminophen is also a common cause of morbidity because it is found in many combination OTC products; caregivers may unknowingly administer a dose of acetaminophen in addition to an OTC drug containing the product without knowing the danger.

A recent study by the Centers for Disease Control and Prevention (2014) noted that the number of calls to poison control centers involving e-cigarette liquids containing nicotine rose from one per month in September 2010 to 215 per month in February 2014. More than half (51.1%) of the calls to poison centers due to e-cigarettes involved children under 5 years of age.

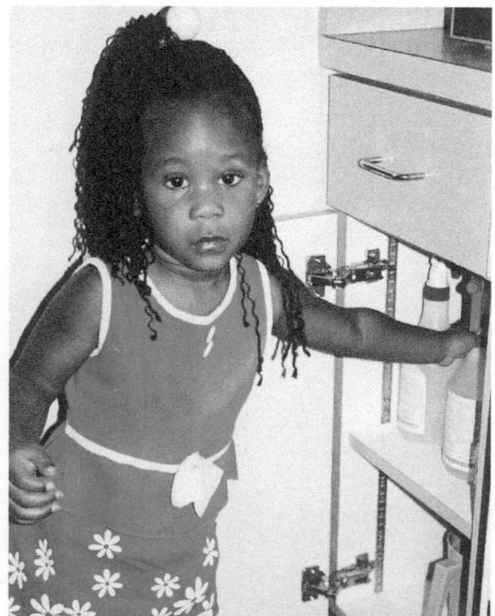

FIG. 12.15 Children are most likely to ingest substances that are on their level, such as cleaning agents stored under sinks, rat poison, plants, or diaper pail deodorants.

Poison prevention for toddlers is critical. The Centers for Disease Control and Prevention developed a comprehensive program to educate parents on preventive measures for medications.* Parents should have ready access to the telephone number for the poison control center (National Poison Control, 800-222-1222) and be prepared to act on the advice of the center. Emergency and preventive measures for accidental poisoning are further discussed in Chapter 14.

Falls

Falls are still a hazard to children in this age-group, although by the later part of early childhood, gross and fine motor skills are well developed, decreasing the incidence of falls down stairs or from chairs. However, playground injuries are common. Children need to learn safety at play areas, such as no horseplay on high slides or jungle gyms, sitting on swings, and staying away from moving swings. Prevention includes placement of grass, sand, or wood chips under play equipment. Swing seats should be made of plastic, canvas, or rubber and have smooth or rounded edges. Slides should have inclines of no more than 30 degrees and have evenly spaced rungs for climbing.

The climbing and running activity of the typical toddler is complicated by total neglect for and lack of appreciation of danger, immature coordination, and a high center of gravity. Falling from furniture is a major cause of injury, with more children in this age-group sustaining head injuries than older children. Gates must be placed at both ends of stairs. Accessible windows that are left open during warm weather must be guarded with a rail. Falling from open windows is a major cause of accidental death in urban lower socioeconomic groups; screens are not designed to prevent falls. Doors leading to stairwells or porches must be locked. A convenient type of lock is a sliding bar or hook that can be attached to the door and frame at a level higher than the child can reach, provided that inventive youngsters do not pull a chair over to unlatch the device.

Cribs are other sources of falls. Ideally the floor under the crib should be carpeted or have a throw rug. The manufacture and sale of drop-side cribs have been banned by the Consumer Product Safety Commission. When children reach a height of 89 cm (35 inches), they should sleep in a bed rather than a crib. If a bunk bed is selected, parents should be aware of possible dangers, including falls from the top bed and the ladder and head entrapment between the mattress and guardrail or between the supporting mattress slats.

Children can fall from high chairs, shopping carts, carriages, car seats, and strollers if not properly restrained or if balance changes when the place where they are sitting is weighed down with heavy objects. Therefore proper restraint and adequate supervision are essential. Children, especially older infants who are mobile, should not be placed in an infant seat on top of a shopping cart because the infant seat may fall off the cart. The safest place for an infant seat is inside the cart's bed.

Windows, stairs, and playgrounds are additional sites that have been associated with a large number of accidental falls in children (Centers for Disease Control and Prevention, 2016). Falls in hospitalized children have received little attention in the scientific literature but are known to occur.

*Up and Away Project information can be retrieved from http://www.upandaway.org/.

Aspiration and Suffocation

Suffocation death rates are the leading cause of accidental death among infants less than 1 year of age (Centers for Disease Control and Prevention, 2016). Some link the high prevalence to the inability to differentiate between sudden infant death syndrome and accidental suffocation in such infants. Suffocation deaths usually occur in this age-group by choking on food items; other causes include choking on undersized infant pacifiers, small balls, and latex balloons (Rivara & Grossman, 2016). As noted earlier, the Consumer Public Safety Commission issued a ban on the manufacture of drop-side cribs in 2010 because of deaths attributed to infants becoming trapped between the crib mattress and side rail and suffocating.

Usually by 1 year of age children chew well, but they may have difficulty with large pieces of food, such as meat or whole hot dogs, and with hard foods, such as nuts or dried beans. Small items such as colored beads, green peas, pellets, or beans are often placed into the nose by toddlers and may present a danger if aspirated into the airway. Young children cannot discard pits from fruit or bones from fish as older children can. Gel snacks that are sealed in plastic wrappers can be difficult to manage, and the plastic wrapper can be aspirated. Therefore implement the same precautions as discussed for infants regarding food selection. (See Chapter 10.)

Play objects for toddlers must still be chosen with an awareness of the danger of small parts. Large, sturdy toys without sharp edges or removable parts are safest. Coins, paper clips, pull tabs on cans, thumbtacks, nails, screws, jewelry (especially pierced earrings), and all types of pins are common household objects that can cause significant harm if swallowed or aspirated. Because of the danger of aspiration, parents should know emergency procedures for choking.

Suffocation is less frequent from causes seen during infancy but old refrigerators, car trunks, ovens, and other large appliances are an ever-present threat. Toddlers can climb inside these appliances and, if they close the door behind them, can become trapped inside. Discarding old appliances and removing all doors during storage can prevent such tragic injuries. Toddlers may also suffocate when toy boxes with heavy, hinged lids accidentally close on their head or neck. Advise parents of this danger and encourage them to buy storage chests with lightweight, removable covers.

Bodily Harm

Toddlers are still clumsy in many of their skills and can seriously harm themselves when walking while holding a sharp or pointed object or having food or objects such as spoons in their mouths. Preventing such occurrences is the best approach with toddlers. Teach the child that when walking with a pointed object, such as a fork, knife, or scissors, the pointed end is held away from the face. Dangerous garden or workshop equipment and all firearms should be stored in a locked cabinet. Power lawn mowers are especially dangerous, and young children should not be allowed in an area where a mower is being used, nor should they be taken for a ride on a mower or allowed to operate the device.

Toddlers are often unable to understand that all pets are not as safe as their own; because of toddlers' height, they are often at the eye level of some dogs and may be bitten on the face. It is imperative to teach pet safety to toddlers and keep animals at a safe distance because even the most loving pet may perceive a threat and react accordingly.

Although accidental firearm injuries and deaths among children have declined significantly since the 1990s, such injuries and deaths continue to be a concern. Safety education should include respect for firearms and their proper and appropriate use, including nonpowder guns, such as air guns, rifles (BB and pellet), and paintball guns, which can cause serious penetrating injuries. Firearm safety devices such as trigger locks, gun safes, and personalized locks are necessary to prevent unintentional firing of guns and subsequent injuries or fatalities.

Toys can be a source of danger, and safety must be a prime consideration when selecting toys. Most toys have age ranges written on them to designate their safety, but parents should also consider the specific child's readiness.

Strategies for ensuring safety in households with toddlers include the usual precautions recommended for any age-group (see Family-Centered Care box). An additional safeguard for young children is the use of safety glass in doors, windows, and tabletops and the application

FAMILY-CENTERED CARE

Guidance During Toddler Years

12 to 18 Months

Prepare parents for expected behavioral changes of toddler, especially negativism and ritualism.

Assess present feeding habits and encourage gradual weaning from bottle and increased intake of solid foods.

Stress expected feeding changes of physiologic anorexia, presence of food fads and strong taste preferences, need for scheduled routine at mealtimes, inability to sit through an entire meal, and lack of table manners.

Assess sleep patterns at night, particularly habit of a bedtime bottle, which is a major cause of dental caries, and procrastination behaviors that delay hour of sleep.

Prepare parents for potential dangers, particularly motor vehicle, poisoning, and falling injuries; give appropriate suggestions for childproofing the home.

Discuss need for firm but gentle discipline and ways to deal with negativism and temper tantrums; stress positive benefits of appropriate discipline.

Emphasize importance for both child and parents of brief, periodic separations.

Discuss toys that use developing gross and fine motor, language, cognitive, and social skills.

Emphasize need for dental supervision, types of basic dental hygiene at home, and food habits that predispose the child to caries; stress importance of supplemental fluoride.

18 to 24 Months

Stress importance of peer companionship in play.

Explore need for preparation for additional sibling; stress importance of preparing child for new experiences.

Discuss present discipline methods, their effectiveness, and parents' feelings about child's negativism; stress that negativism is important aspect of developing self-assertion and independence and is not a sign of spoiling.

Discuss signs of readiness for toilet training; emphasize importance of waiting for physical and psychologic readiness.

Discuss development of fears, such as fear of darkness or loud noises, and of habits, such as security blanket or thumb sucking; stress normalcy of these transient behaviors.

Continued

FAMILY-CENTERED CARE—cont'd

Guidance During Toddler Years—cont'd

Prepare parents for signs of regression in time of stress.

Assess child's ability to separate easily from parents for brief periods under familiar circumstances.

Allow parents opportunity to express their feelings of weariness, frustration, and exasperation; be aware that it is often difficult to love toddlers at times when they are not asleep!

Point out some of the expected changes of the next year, such as longer attention span, somewhat less negativism, and increased concern for pleasing others.

24 to 36 Months

Discuss importance of imitation and domestic mimicry and need to include child in activities.

Discuss approaches toward toilet training, particularly realistic expectations and attitude toward accidents.

Stress uniqueness of toddlers' thought processes, especially through their use of language, poor understanding of time, causal relationships in terms of proximity of events, and inability to see events from another's perspective.

Stress that discipline still must be structured and concrete and that relying solely on verbal reasoning and explanation leads to confusion, misunderstanding, and even injuries.

Discuss investigation of preschool or day care center toward completion of second year.

of decals on glassed areas to lessen the likelihood of running through glass. Also, children should not be allowed to run, jump, wrestle, or play ball in areas where glass litter may be a hazard. (See Injury Prevention, Chapter 13; Pet and Human Bites, Chapter 32.)

ANTICIPATORY GUIDANCE—CARE OF FAMILIES

Understanding toddlers is fundamental to successful childrearing. Nurses, particularly those in ambulatory or child health centers, are in a most favorable position to assist parents in meeting the tasks and needs of children in this age-group. Anticipatory guidance in each of the areas presented in the Family-Centered Care box can prevent future problems. Advice is sometimes not the sole answer. Actual assistance, such as being available for telephone consulting, should be a part of the nurse's flexible repertoire of interventions. Whether parents are experiencing the challenges of rearing a first or a subsequent child, they benefit from sharing their feelings, frustrations, and satisfactions. They need adult companionship, shared childrearing responsibilities, and periodic separation from their children. For single parents such goals can be especially difficult to achieve. Part of a nurse's responsibility is to provide opportunities for parents to express their feelings and to meet their emotional and physical needs.

NCLEX REVIEW QUESTIONS

1. The typical play activity in which toddlers engage is called:
   A. Solitary
   B. Parallel
   C. Associative
   D. Cooperative
2. One indication that the toddler is ready to begin toilet training is:
   A. Child recognizes urge to void and is able to communicate this sensation to the parent
   B. Child is able to stay dry all night
   C. Child demonstrates mastery of dressing and undresssing self
   D. Child asks parent to have wet or soiled diaper changed
3. A mother brings her 3-year-old daughter to the well-child clinic and expresses concern that the child's behavior is worrisome and possibly requires therapy or medication at minimum. The mother further explains that the child constantly responds to the mother's simple requests with a "no" answer even though the activity has been a favorite in the recent past. Furthermore, the child has had an increase in the number of temper tantrums at bedtime and refuses to go to bed. The mother is afraid her daughter will hurt herself during a temper tantrum because she holds her breath until the mother picks her up and gives in to her request. The nurse's best response to the mother is that:
   A. The child probably would benefit from some counseling with a trained therapist.
   B. The mother and father should evaluate their childrearing practices.
   C. The child's behavior is normal for a toddler and may represent frustration with control of her emotions; further exploration of events surrounding temper tantrums and possible interventions should be explored.
   D. The child's behavior is typical of toddlers, and the parents should just wait for the child to finish this phase because this will end soon.
4. Toddlers are often known to be finicky eaters and may exhibit abnormal eating patterns that may concern parents. Which of the following actions for feeding toddlers should be suggested so adequate amounts of nutrients for growth and development are consumed? Select all that apply.
   A. Avoid placing large food portions on the toddler's plate
   B. Allow the child to graze on nutritious (not "junk" food) snacks during the day
   C. Insist that the child sit at the table until all persons have completed their meals
   D. Allow the child to make certain food choices (within reasonable limits)—for example, "Would you like a half peanut butter or ham sandwich?"
   E. Provide meals at the same time of day as much as possible so the toddler has a sense of consistency
   F. Make the child eat all of the food provided, and provide disciplinary actions such as a "time-out" if the plate is not cleaned
5. A common cause of accidental death in children ages 1 to 19 years involves motor vehicle crashes. Evidence from test crashes indicates that the safest action to prevent accidental deaths in toddlers includes:
   A. Placing the child in a rear-facing weight-appropriate car restraint seat until the child has outgrown the car seat manufacturer's height and weight recommendations
   B. Allowing the child to ride in the front seat with a lap-shoulder seat restraint to avoid emotional outbursts

C. Allowing the child to ride in a forward-facing booster restraint seat after 12 months of age
D. Placing the child in the regular seat using the lap-shoulder belt as long as the child weighs at least 45 pounds

6. One of the primary reasons for monitoring the toddler's activities and intervening to prevent accidental injury is that:
A. Toddlers have oppositional defiant behavior and negativism
B. Toddlers do not understand the concept of "cause and effect," so explaining that certain actions will result in serious injury is useless
C. Toddlers will often listen to reasoning about why an activity should be avoided
D. Toddlers enjoy making their parents worry about their safety and like to see the parents' reactions to the behavior

Correct Answers

1. B; 2. A; 3. C; 4. A, B, D, E; 5. A; 6. B

REFERENCES

Abraham, V. M., Gaw, C. E., Chounthirath, T., et al. (2015). Toy-related injuries among children treated in US emergency departments, 1990-2011. *Clinical Pediatrics, 54*(2), 127–137.

American Academy of Pediatric Dentistry. (2016a). *Guideline on perinatal and infant oral health care.* http://www.aapd.org/assets/1/7/G_PerinatalOralHealthCare1.PDF.

American Academy of Pediatric Dentistry. (2016b). *Policy on early childhood caries (ECC): classifications, consequences, and preventive strategies.* http://www.aapd.org/assets/1/7/P_ECCClassifications1.PDF.

American Academy of Pediatric Dentistry. (2014). *Policy on use of fluoride.* http://www.aapd.org/media/Policies_Guidelines/P_FluorideUse.pdf.

American Academy of Pediatrics. (2015). *Car seats: a guide for families 2015.* http://www.healthychildren.org/English/safety-prevention/on-the-go/Pages/Car-Safety-Seats-Information-for-Families.aspx.

American Academy of Pediatrics, Committee on Nutrition. (2014). *Pediatric nutrition handbook* (7th ed.). Elk Grove Village, IL: American Academy of Pediatrics.

American Academy of Pediatrics, Council on Communications and Media. (2016). Media use by young minds. *Pediatrics, 138*(5).

Barr, R. (2013). Memory constraints on infant learning from picture books, television, and touchscreens. *Child Developmental Perspective, 7*(4), 205–210.

Brazelton, T. B. (1999). How to help parents of young children: The touchpoints model. *Journal of Perinatology, 19*(6 Pt. 2), S6–S7.

Canadian Paediatric Society. (2016). *Position Statement: Vegetarian diets in children and adolescents.* Available at: http://www.cps.ca/en/documents/position/vegetarian-diets.

Centers for Disease Control and Prevention. (2014). *New CDC study finds dramatic increase in e-cigarette-related calls to poison centers, MMWR Weekly Report.* Available at https://www.cdc.gov/media/releases/2014/p0403-e-cigarette-poison.html.

Centers for Disease Control and Prevention. (2016). Deaths: Leading causes for 2013. *National Vital Statistics Reports, 65*(2), 1–95.

Colaco, M., Johnson, K., Schneider, D., et al. (2013). Toilet training method is not related to dysfunctional voiding. *Clinical Pediatrics, 52*(1), 49–53.

Durbin, D. R., Jermakian, J. S., Kallan, M. J., et al. (2015). rear seat safety: Variation in protection by occupant, crash and vehicle characteristics. *Accident Analysis and Prevention, 80*, 185–192.

Duzinski, S. V., Barczyk, A. N., Wheeler, T. C., et al. (2014). Threat of paediatric hyperthermia in an enclosed vehicle: A year-round study. *Injury Prevention: Journal of the International Society for Child and Adolescent Injury Prevention, 20*(4), 220–225.

Eisbach, S. S., Cluxton-Keller, F., Harrison, J., et al. (2014). Characteristics of temper tantrums in preschoolers with disruptive behavior in a clinical setting. *Journal of Psychosocial Nursing and Mental Health Services, 52*(5), 32–40.

Eisenberg, N., Taylor, Z. E., Widaman, et al. (2015). Externalizing symptom, effortful control, and intrusive parenting: A test of bidirectional longitudinal relations during early childhood. *Development and Psychology, 27*(4), 953–968.

El-Radhi, A. S. (2015). Management of common behavior and mental health problems. *British Journal of Nursing, 24*(11), 586–590.

Erikson, E. H. (1963). *Childhood and society* (2nd ed.). New York: Norton.

Estes, K. G., & Hay, J. F. (2015). Flexibility in bilingual infants' word learning. *Child Development, 86*(5), 1371–1385.

Feigelman, S. (2016). The second year. In R. M. Kliegman, B. F. Stanton, J. W. St. Geme, et al. (Eds.), *Nelson textbook of pediatrics* (20th ed.). Philadelphia: Saunders/Elsevier.

Folger, A., Bowers, K. A., Dexheimer, J. W., et al. (2017). Education of early childhood home visiting to prevent medically attended unintentional injury. *Annals of Emergency Medicine*, epub ahead of print.

Fowler, J. W. (1981). *Stages of faith: the psychology of human development and the quest for meaning.* San Francisco: Harper & Row.

Groenewald, C. B., Beals-Erickson, S. E., Ralston-Wilson, J., et al. (2017). Complementary and alternative medicine use by children with pain in the united states. *Academic Pediatrics*, epub ahead of print.

Guyer, A. E., Jarcho, J. M., Perez-Edgar, K., et al. (2015). Temperament and parenting styles in early childhood differentially influence neural response to peer evaluation in adolescence. *Journal of Abnormal Child Psychology, 43*(5), 863–875.

Hines, M., Constantinescu, M., & Spencer, D. (2015). Early androgen exposure and human gender development. *Biology of Sex Differences, 6*(3).

Kiddoo, D. A. (2012). Toilet training children: When to start and how to train. *CMAJ: Canadian Medical Association Journal = Journal de l'Association Medicale Canadienne, 184*(5), 511–512.

Kimball, V. (2016). The perils and pitfalls of potty training. *Pediatric Annals, 45*(6), e199–e201.

Kirkorian, H. L., Choi, K., & Pempek, T. A. (2016). Toddlers' word learning from contingent and noncontingent video on touch screens. *Child Development, 87*(2), 405–413.

Kleinman, R. E., & Greer, F. R. (Eds.), (2014). *Pediatric nutrition* (7th ed.). Elk Grove Village, IL: American Academy of Pediatrics.

Kostic, M. A. (2016). Poisoning. In R. M. Kliegman, B. F. Stanton, J. W. St. Geme, et al. (Eds.), *Nelson textbook of pediatrics* (20th ed.). Philadelphia: Elsevier/Saunders.

Kranz, S., Brauchla, M., Slavin, J. L., et al. (2012). What do we know about dietary fiber intake in children and health? The effects of fiber intake on constipation, obesity, and diabetes in children. *Advances in Nutrition, 3*(1), 47–53.

Lima, N. N. R., do Nascimento, V. B., de Carvalho, S. M. F., et al. (2013). Spirituality in childhood cancer care. *Neuropsychiatic Disease and Treatment, 9*, 1539–1544.

Llena, C., Leyda, A., Forner, L., et al. (2015). Association between the number of early carious lesions and diet in children with a high prevalence of caries. *European Journal of Paediatric Dentistry, 16*(1), 7–12.

Mindell, J. A., Li, A. M., Sadeh, A., et al. (2015). Bedtime routines for young children: A dose-dependent association with sleep outcomes. *Sleep, 38*(5), 717–722.

National Academies of Medicine. (2017). *Dietary reference intakes tables and application*, Washington DC. http://www.nationalacademies.org/hmd/Activities/Nutrition/SummaryDRIs/DRI-Tables.aspx.

National Center for Complementary and Integrative Health. (2016). *Complementary, Alternative, or Integrative Health: What's in a name?* Bethesda, MD, National Institutes of Health, National Center for Complementary and Integrative Health. https://nccih.nih.gov/health/integrative-health.

Neuman, M. E. (2011). Addressing children's beliefs through Fowler's stages of faith. *Journal of Pediatric Nursing*, *26*(1), 44–50.

Null, J. (2015). *Heatstroke deaths of children in vehicles*. Available at: http://noheatstroke.org/.

Owens, J. A. (2016). Sleep medicine. In R. M. Kliegman, B. F. Stanton, J. W. St. Geme, et al. (Eds.), *Nelson textbook of pediatrics* (20th ed.). Philadelphia: Saunders/Elsevier.

Ozen, B., Van Strijp, A. J., Ozer, L., et al. (2016). Evaluation of possible associated factors for early childhood caries and severe early childhood caries: A multicenter cross-sectional survey. *The Journal of Clinical Pediatric Dentistry*, *40*(2), 118–123.

Rivara, F. P., & Grossman, D. C. (2016). Injury control. In R. M. Kliegman, B. F. Stanton, J. W. St. Geme, et al. (Eds.), *Nelson textbook of pediatrics* (20th ed.). Philadelphia: Elsevier/Saunders.

Rogers, J. (2013). Daytime wetting in children and acquisition of bladder control. *Nursing Children and Young People*, *25*(6), 26–33.

Roseberry, S., Hirsh-Pasek, K., & Golinkoff, R. M. (2014). Skype me: Socially contingent interactions to help toddlers learn. *Child Development*, *85*(3), 956–970.

Saavedra, J. M., Deming, D., Dattilo, A., et al. (2013). Lessons from the feeding infants and toddlers study in North America: What children eat, and implications for obesity prevention. *Annals of Nutrition and Metabolism*, *62*(supp3), 27–36.

Schurmann, S., Kersting, M., & Alexy, U. (2017). Vegetarian diets in children: A systematic review. *European Journal of Nutrition*, epub ahead of print.

Schwartz, S., & Benuck, I. (2013). Strategies and suggestions for a healthy toddler diet. *Pediatric Annals*, *42*(9), 181–183.

Steensma, T. D., Kreukels, B. P., de Vries, A. L., et al. (2013). Gender identity development in adolescence. *Hormones and Behavior*, *64*(2), 288–297.

Steinberger, J., Daniels, S. R., Hagberg, N., et al. (2016). American Heart Association: *Cardiovascular health promotion in children: challenges and opportunities for 2020 and beyond: a scientific statement from the American heart association.*

Stortelder, F. (2014). Varieties of male-sexual identity development in clinical practice: A neuropsychoanalytic model. *Frontiers in Psychology*, *5*(1512).

Taylor, D. M., Dhir, R., Craig, S. S., et al. (2015). Complementary and alternative medicine use among paediatric emergency department patients. *Journal of Paediatrics and Child Health*, *51*(9), 895–900.

US Department of Health and Human Services. (2016). *2015-2020 Dietary Guidelines for America*. Available at https://health.gov/dietaryguidelines/2015/guidelines/.

Waugh, W. E., & Brownell, C. E. (2015). Development of body part vocabulary in toddlers in relation to self understanding. *Early Child Development and Care*, *185*(7).

Zimmer-Gembeck, M. J., Webb, H. J., Thomas, R., et al. (2015). A new measure of toddler-parenting practices and associations with attachment and mothers' sensitivity, competence, and enjoyment of parenting. *Early Child Development and Care*, *185*(9).

Zuzak, T. J., Zuzak-Siegrist, I., Rist, L., et al. (2010). Medicinal systems of complementary and alternative medicine: A cross-sectional survey at a pediatric emergency department. *Journal of Alternative and Complementary Medicine (New York, N.Y.)*, *16*(4), 473–479.

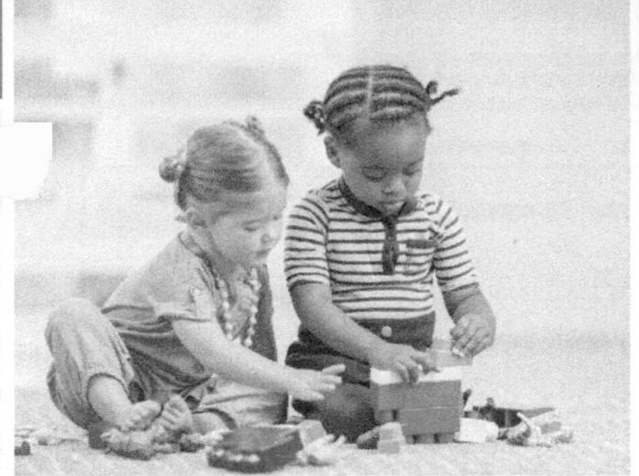

13

Health Promotion of the Preschooler and Family

Rebecca A. Monroe

http://evolve.elsevier.com/wong/ncic

CONCEPTS

- Development
- Behavior
- Temperament

PROMOTING OPTIMUM GROWTH AND DEVELOPMENT

The combined biologic, psychosocial, cognitive, spiritual, and social achievements during the preschool period (3 to 5 years of age) prepare preschoolers for their most significant change in lifestyle: entrance into school. Their control of bodily systems, experience of brief and prolonged periods of separation, ability to interact cooperatively with other children and adults, use of language for mental symbolization, and increased attention span and memory prepare them for the next major period: the school years. Successful achievement of previous levels of growth and development is essential for preschoolers to refine many of the tasks that were mastered during the toddler years.

BIOLOGIC DEVELOPMENT

The rate of physical growth slows and stabilizes during the preschool years. The average weight is 14.5 kg (32 lb) at 3 years, 16.5 kg (36.5 lb) at 4 years, and 18.5 kg (41 lb) at 5 years. The average weight gain remains approximately 2 to 3 kg (4.5 to 6.5 lb) per year.

Growth in height also remains steady at a yearly increase of 6.5 to 9 cm (2.5 to 3.5 inches). The legs of a preschooler, rather than the trunk, increase in length. The average height is 95 cm (37.5 inches) at 3 years, 103 cm (40.5 inches) at 4 years, and 110 cm (43.5 inches) at 5 years.

Physical proportions no longer resemble those of the squat, pot-bellied toddler. The preschooler is slender but sturdy, graceful, agile, and posturally erect. There is little difference in physical characteristics according to sex, except in factors such as dress and hairstyle.

Most organ systems can adjust to moderate stress and change. During this period, most children are toilet trained. For the most part, motor development consists of increases in strength and refinement of previously learned skills, such as walking, running, and jumping. However, muscle development and bone growth are still far from mature. Excessive activity and overexertion can injure delicate tissues. Good posture, appropriate exercise, and adequate nutrition and rest are essential for optimum development of the musculoskeletal system.

Gross and Fine Motor Behavior

By 36 months, preschoolers are walking, running, climbing, and jumping well. Refinement in eye-hand and muscle coordination is evident in several areas. At age 3 years, the preschooler rides a tricycle, walks on tiptoe, balances on one foot for a few seconds, and broad jumps. By age 4 years, the child skips and hops proficiently on one foot (Fig. 13.1) and catches a ball reliably. By age 5 years, the child skips on alternate feet, jumps rope, and begins to skate and swim.

Achievement in fine motor development is evident in the child's increasingly skillful manipulation. Drawing shows several advancements in the perception of shape and the development of fine muscle coordination. The 3-year-old child copies a circle and imitates a cross and vertical and horizontal lines. He or she holds the writing instrument with the fingers rather than the fist. The child scribbles or scrawls drawings but can name what has been drawn. The 3-year-old is not able to draw a complete stick figure but draws a circle, later adds facial features, and by age 5 or 6 years can draw several parts (head, arms, legs, body, and facial features). Between 4 and 5 years of age, the child can trace a cross and copy a square. The triangle and diamond are usually the last geometric figures to be mastered, sometime between ages 5 and 6 years.

As children progress from scribbling to picture making, they advance through four distinguishable stages (Kellogg, 1969). In the placement stage, 15-month-old children place their earliest spontaneous scribbling on the paper in a specific placement pattern, such as in the center, all over, across the lower half, or across the page in a diagonal direction (Fig. 13.2). Approximately 17 different placement patterns appear by age 2 years and, once developed, are never lost.

By 3 years of age, children are in the shape stage. They draw single-line outline forms such as rectangles, circles, ovals, crosses, and other odd shapes. As soon as they draw diagrams, they almost immediately progress to the design stage, in which simple forms are drawn together to make structured designs. When two diagrams are united, the resulting design is called a combine. Three or more united diagrams produce an aggregate. Between ages 4 and 5 years, most children enter the pictorial stage, in which their designs are recognizable as familiar objects. Early pictorial drawings are suggestive of human figures, houses, animals, and trees.

Later pictorial drawings are more clearly defined and recognizable; they are not representations of the actual object but esthetically satisfying structures that resemble familiar objects. For example, the initial human figure drawing is a circle with arms attached to the head. It is more an aggregate drawing than any attempt to copy a human figure. Drawings of animals follow the human figure drawing but are only a slight modification, such as attaching ears to the top of the head.

Kellogg (1969) suggests that uninhibited scribbling and drawing are necessary for children to learn to read and that children who have been free to experiment and produce abstract forms have developed the mental set required for learning symbolic language. Scribbling and drawing also help develop the fine muscle skills and eye-hand coordination eventually required for making precise letters and numbers.

Drawing is also a tool used for assessing intelligence, personality development, and psychosocial adjustment. The precise value of using drawing to measure such concepts is still a nebulous science. However, children (especially school-age children) do reveal thoughts about themselves in their drawings. It is not necessary to have in-depth knowledge of children's drawings to make assumptions about their significance. Being receptive to all the clues, both verbal and nonverbal, is essential to understanding how and what children are communicating to others (see Cultural Considerations box).

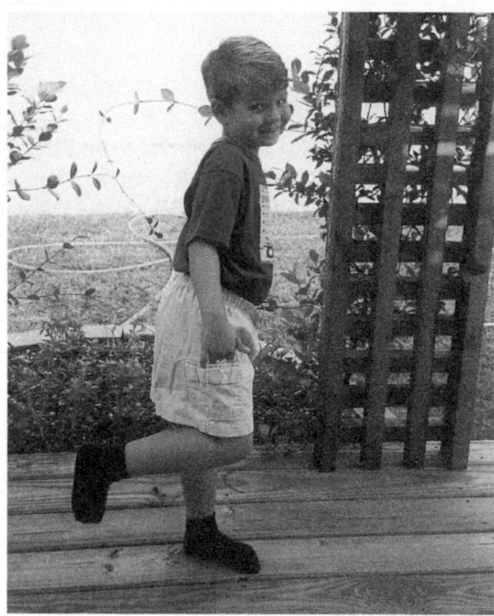

FIG. 13.1 A 4-year-old child has sufficient balance to hop on one foot.

CULTURAL CONSIDERATIONS

Drawings

Children's drawings before age 6 years are strikingly similar universally, suggesting that some inherent neurologic mechanisms influence the type of self-taught art forms. After age 6 years, cultural and environmental influences, particularly from parents and teachers, shape much of what children draw. For example, drawings of physical characteristics (skin color, hair type, and facial features), style of dress, type of housing, and scenery may reflect ethnic or geographic variations. Therefore nurses need to consider children's backgrounds when interpreting drawings.

PSYCHOSOCIAL DEVELOPMENT

Developing a Sense of Initiative (Erikson)

If preschoolers have mastered the tasks of the toddler period, they are ready to face the developmental challenges of the preschool period. Erikson maintained that the chief psychosocial task of this period is acquiring a sense of initiative. Children are in a stage of energetic learning. They play, work, and live to the fullest and feel a real sense of accomplishment and satisfaction in their activities. Conflict arises when children overstep the limits of their ability and inquiry and experience guilt for not having behaved appropriately. Feelings of guilt, anxiety, and fear may also result from thoughts that differ from expected behavior.

A particularly stressful thought is wishing one's parent dead. As a sense of rivalry or competition develops between the child and the same-sex parent, the child may think of ways to get rid of the interfering parent. In most situations, this contest is resolved when the child strongly identifies with the same-sex parent and peers during the school years. However, if that parent dies before the identification process is completed, the preschooler can be overwhelmed with guilt for having wished and therefore "caused" the death. Clarifying for children that wishes cannot make events occur is essential in helping them overcome their guilt and anxiety.

Development of the **superego**, or conscience, starts toward the end of the toddler years and is a major task for preschoolers. Learning right from wrong and good from bad is the beginning of morality (see Cultural Considerations box). Children in this age-group are generally unable to understand why something is acceptable or unacceptable. They are aware of appropriate behavior primarily through punishment or reward and rely almost completely on parental principles for developing their own moral judgment. Verbal enforcement of limits is much more effective

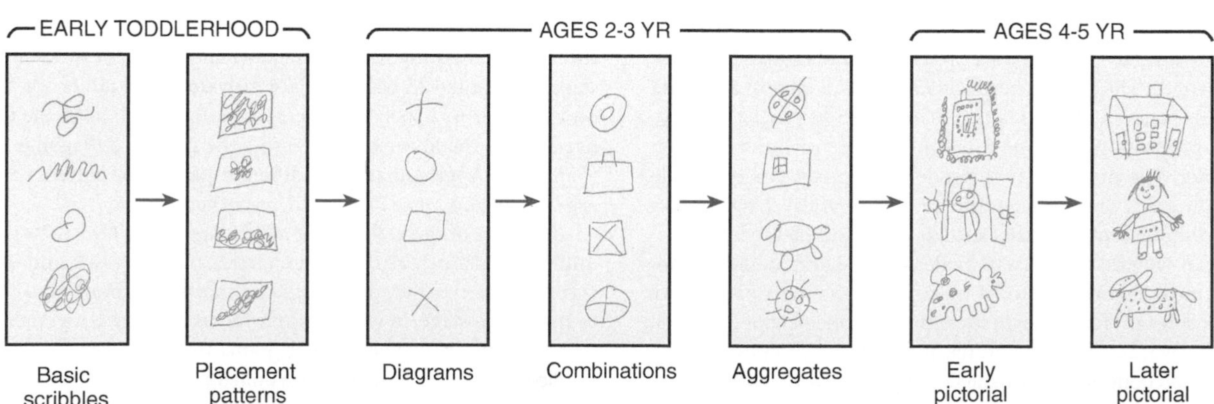

FIG. 13.2 Sequential development in self-taught art. (From Kellogg, R. [1969]. Understanding children's art. In *Readings in psychology today.* Del Mar, CA: Communications/Research/Machines.)

in this age-group than with toddlers. For example, to prevent injuries, parents need to supervise toddlers, keep them contained within protected areas, and tell them not to run into the street. The preschooler still needs close supervision but is much more aware of danger and can listen and obey in most instances. If allowed to disagree and question, they will develop socially acceptable behavior and independence in thought and action.

CULTURAL CONSIDERATIONS

Learning Sociocultural Mores

Developing a conscience implies learning the sociocultural mores of the family's heritage. Depending on the type of attitudes conveyed, children will learn not only appropriate behaviors but also tolerant, biased, or prejudicial values concerning their ethnic, religious, and social background and those of other groups. Much of this influence may remain dormant until they associate with children or adults of a different heritage. Then, depending on the particular group, they may be accepted or excluded for their attitudes.

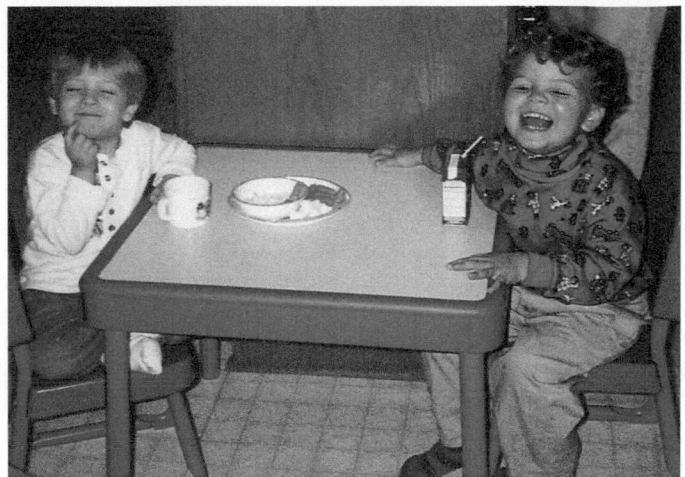

FIG. 13.3 Preschool children enjoy friends and often use nonverbal messages to communicate.

Oedipal Stage (Freud)

As soon as children comprehend their separateness as persons, they begin to realize that there are categories of objects, such as things, people, males, females, children, and adults. One of the principal goals in further differentiation of oneself from others is learning sex differences and sexually appropriate behavior.

Freud described this goal in psychosexual terms and labeled the period the oedipal, or phallic, stage. He believed that conflict arises when a boy realizes that his father is much stronger and more powerful than he. Subconsciously, he wishes that his father were dead so he could marry his mother (Oedipus complex). Concurrently, he notices physical sexual differences, specifically that boys have a penis and girls do not. In his mind, he supposes that girls have lost their penis for some wrongdoing. His guilt regarding his feelings toward his father makes him fear the same punishment of mutilation, resulting in the castration complex. Girls have similar wishes to marry their father and kill their mother (the Electra complex). However, girls do not fear castration; rather they experience penis envy (desire to have a penis). The resolution of the Oedipus or Electra complex is identification with the same-sex parent.

COGNITIVE DEVELOPMENT

One of the tasks related to the preschool period is readiness for school and scholastic learning. Many of the thought processes of this period are crucial for achieving such readiness, and it is intentional that the child begins school between ages 5 and 6 years, rather than earlier.

Preoperational Phase (Piaget)

Piaget's cognitive theory does not include a period specifically for children 3 to 5 years old. The preoperational phase covers the age span from 2 to 7 years and is divided into two stages: the preconceptual phase, ages 2 to 4 years, and the phase of intuitive thought, ages 4 to 7 years. One of the main transitions during these two phases is the shift from totally egocentric thought to social awareness and the ability to consider other viewpoints (Fig. 13.3). Egocentricity, however, is still evident. Children are able to think and verbalize their mental processes without having to act out their thinking. They can think of only one idea at a time and are unable to think of all parts in terms of the whole.

Language continues to develop during the preschool period. Speech remains primarily a vehicle of egocentric communication. Preschoolers assume that everyone thinks as they do and that a brief explanation of their thinking makes them understood by others. Because of this self-referenced, egocentric verbal communication, it is often necessary to explore and understand young children's thinking through other, nonverbal approaches. For children in this age-group, the most enlightening and effective method is play, which becomes the child's way of understanding, adjusting to, and working out life's experiences. Because of a child's rich imagination and unlimited ability to invent and imitate, all types of play hold therapeutic and communicative value.

Preschoolers increasingly use language without comprehending the meaning of words, particularly concepts of right and left, causality, and time. Children may use the concepts correctly but only in the circumstances in which they have learned them. For example, they may know how to put on shoes by remembering that the buckle is always on the outside of the foot. However, if different shoes have no buckles, they cannot reason which shoe fits which foot. They do not understand the concept of right and left.

Superficially, causality resembles logical thought. Preschoolers explain a concept as they have heard it described by others, but their understanding is limited. For example, because preschoolers do not completely understand time, they interpret it according to their own frame of reference, such as "A long time means until Christmas." Consequently, time is best explained in relation to an event, such as "Your mother will visit you after you finish your lunch." Avoiding words such as "yesterday," "tomorrow," "next week," or "Tuesday" to express when an event is expected to occur and associating time with usual expected daily occurrences help children learn about temporal relationships while increasing their trust in others' predictions.

Preschoolers' thinking is often described as magical thinking. Because of their egocentrism and transductive reasoning, they believe that thoughts are all powerful. Such thinking places them in the vulnerable position of feeling guilty and responsible for bad thoughts that may coincide with the occurrence of a wished event. A typical example is wishing a new sibling dead. If that sibling does die, young children think their wish caused the death. Their inability to reason the cause and effect of illness or injury makes it especially difficult for them to understand such events.

Preschoolers believe in the power of words and accept their meaning literally. A significant example of this type of thinking is calling children "bad" because they did something wrong. In their minds, telling children that they are bad means that they are bad. For this reason, it is better to relate such words to the act by saying, for example, "That was a bad thing to do."

MORAL DEVELOPMENT (KOHLBERG)

Moral development theory is based on cognitive development theory and consists of three major levels: preconventional, conventional, and postconventional (Kohlberg, 1968). Young children's development of moral judgment is at the most basic level. They have little, if any, concern for why something is wrong. They behave because of the freedoms or restrictions placed on actions. In the punishment and obedience orientation, children (approximately ages 2 to 4 years) judge whether an action is good or bad according to whether it results in reward or punishment. If children are punished for it, the action is bad. If they are not punished, the action is good, regardless of its meaning. For example, if parents allow hitting, the child will perceive that hitting is good because it is not associated with punishment.

From approximately 4 to 7 years of age, children are in the stage of naive **instrumental orientation**, in which actions are directed toward satisfying their needs and, less commonly, the needs of others. They have a concrete sense of justice and fairness during this period of development.

SPIRITUAL DEVELOPMENT

Children learn about faith and religion from significant others in their environment, usually from parents and their religious beliefs and practices. However, cognitive level influences young children's understanding of spirituality. Preschoolers have a concrete conception of a god with physical characteristics, often like an imaginary friend. They understand simple stories and memorize short prayers, but have limited understanding of the meaning of these rituals. They benefit from concrete representations of religious practices, such as picture books and small statues.

Development of the conscience is strongly linked to spiritual development. At this age, children are learning right from wrong and behave correctly to avoid punishment. Wrongdoing provokes guilt, and preschoolers often misinterpret illness as punishment for real or imagined transgressions. It is important that children view God as one who bestows unconditional love, rather than as a judge of good or bad behavior. Spirituality and participation in religious traditions often help children cope during illness and hospitalization (Drutchas & Anandarajah, 2014). Therefore it is important to address children's spiritual needs to provide the most comprehensive care, especially during times of distress.

DEVELOPMENT OF BODY IMAGE

The preschool years play a significant role in the development of body image. With increasing comprehension of language, preschoolers recognize that individuals have undesirable and desirable appearances. They recognize differences in skin color and racial identity and are vulnerable to learning prejudices and biases. They are aware of the meaning of words such as "pretty" or "ugly," and they reflect the opinions of others regarding their own appearance. By 5 years of age, children compare their size with that of their peers and can become conscious of being large or short, especially if others refer to them as "so big" or "so little" for their age. Research indicates that children as young as preschool age experience body dissatisfaction (Tatangelo, McCabe, Mellor, et al., 2016). Because these are formative years, parents should make efforts to instill positive principles regarding body image.

Despite the advances in body image development, preschoolers have poorly defined body boundaries and little knowledge of their internal anatomy. Intrusive experiences are frightening, especially those that disrupt the integrity of the skin (e.g., injections and surgery). They fear that all their blood and "insides" can leak out if the skin is "broken." Therefore preschoolers may believe it is critical to use bandages after an injury.

DEVELOPMENT OF SEXUALITY

Sexual development during the preschool years is important to a person's overall sexual identity and beliefs. Preschoolers form strong attachments to the opposite-sex parent, while identifying with the same-sex parent. **Sex typing**, or the process by which an individual develops the behavior, personality, attitudes, and beliefs appropriate for his or her culture and sex, occurs through several mechanisms during this period. Probably the most powerful mechanisms are childrearing practices and imitation. The ways in which parents dress, hold, cuddle, caress, discipline, and talk to their child express some aspect of gender-oriented behavior. Gender identification is a result of complex prenatal and postnatal psychologic factors, as well as biologic, social, and genetic influences. It is believed that most children are aware of their sex and the expected set of related behaviors by 1½ to 2½ years of age. Although toddlers might be aware of their particular sex, they do not possess the language and cognitive skills to investigate sexual identity as fully as preschoolers do.

As sexual identity develops beyond gender recognition, modesty and fears of mutilation may become a concern. Sex-role imitation and "dressing up" like Mommy or Daddy are important activities. Attitudes and responses of others to role-playing can condition the child to adopt particular views of self or others. For example, comments such as "Boys shouldn't play with dolls" can influence a boy's masculine self-concept.

Sexual exploration may be more pronounced now, particularly in terms of exploring and manipulating the genitalia. Preschoolers may have questions about sexual reproduction as they search for understanding. (See Sex Education, p. 432, and also Chapters 15 and 17.)

SOCIAL DEVELOPMENT

During the preschool period, the separation-individuation process is completed. Preschoolers have overcome much of their anxiety associated with strangers and the fear of separation of earlier years. They relate to unfamiliar people easily and tolerate brief separations from parents with little or no protest. However, they still need parental security, reassurance, guidance, and approval, especially when entering preschool or elementary school. Prolonged separation, such as that imposed by illness and hospitalization, is difficult; however, preschoolers respond well to anticipatory preparation and concrete explanation. They can cope with changes in daily routine much better than toddlers but may develop more imaginary fears. They gain security and comfort from familiar objects such as toys, dolls, or photographs of family members. They are able to work through many of their unresolved fears, fantasies, and anxieties through play, especially if guided with appropriate play objects (e.g., dolls or puppets) that represent family members, health professionals, and other children.

Language

Language becomes more sophisticated and complex during the preschool years. Both cognitive ability and environment, particularly consistent role models, influence vocabulary, speech, and comprehension. Language becomes a major mode of communication and social interaction. Vocabulary increases dramatically, from 300 words at age 2 years to more than 2100 words at the end of age 5 years. Sentence structure, grammatical usage, and intelligibility also advance to a more adult level. Preschool children may even become bilingual (see Cultural Considerations box).

CULTURAL CONSIDERATIONS

Bilingual Children

Many children in the United States are bilingual. Children who learn two languages simultaneously or develop bilingualism in early childhood reach language milestones at similar stages to monolinguals (McCabe, Tamis-LeMonda, Bornstein, et al., 2013). The type, quantity, and quality of language input determines successful acquisition of each language (McCabe, Tamis-LeMonda, Bornstein, et al., 2013). If a child has a language disability, it will manifest in both languages (American Speech-Language-Hearing Association, 2017a). Nurses should inquire about each child's language repertoire and identify the child's primary language, especially when assessing a child's development.

Children between ages 3 and 4 years form sentences of approximately three or four words and include only the words most essential to convey meaning. Such speech is often termed *telegraphic* because of its brevity. Three-year-old children ask many questions and use plurals, correct pronouns, and the past tenses of verbs. They name familiar objects (such as animals and parts of the body), relatives, and friends. They can give and follow simple commands. They talk incessantly, regardless of whether anyone is listening to or answering them. They enjoy musical or talking toys or dolls and imitate new words proficiently.

From ages 4 to 5 years, preschoolers use longer sentences of four or five words and use more words to convey a message, such as prepositions, adjectives, and a variety of verbs. They follow simple directional commands, such as "Put the ball on the chair," but can carry out only one request at a time. They answer questions such as "What do you do when you are hungry?" by describing the appropriate action. The pattern of asking questions is at its peak, and children usually repeat the question until they receive an answer.

By age 6 years, children can use all parts of speech correctly, except for deviations from the rule. They can define simple objects and actions by describing their use, shape, or general category of classification, rather than simply describing their outward appearance. For example, they can define a ball as "round, something you bounce, or a toy," rather than only describing its color. They can give some examples of opposites, such as "If Mommy is a woman, Daddy is a man." They can also describe an object according to its composition, such as "A spoon is made of metal."

Personal-Social Behavior

The pervasive ritualism and negativism of toddlerhood gradually diminish during the preschool years. Although self-assertion is still a major theme, preschoolers demonstrate their sense of autonomy differently. They are able to verbalize their request for independence and perform independently because of their much-refined physical and cognitive development. By 4 or 5 years of age, they need little if any assistance with dressing, eating, or toileting (Fig. 13.4). They can also be trusted to obey warnings of danger, although 3- or 4-year-old children may exceed their boundaries at times.

Preschoolers are much more sociable and willing to please than toddlers. They have internalized many of the standards and values of the family and culture. However, by the end of early childhood, they begin to question parental values and compare them with those of their peer group and other authority figures. As a result, they may be less willing to abide by the family's code of conduct. Preschoolers become

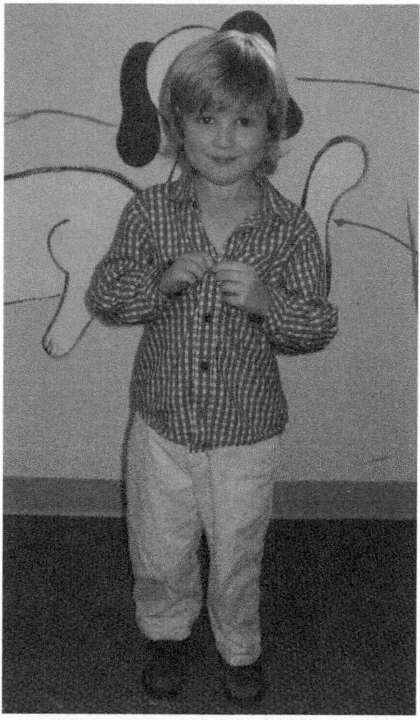

FIG. 13.4 Most preschoolers are able to dress themselves but need help with more difficult items of clothing.

increasingly aware of their position and role within the family. Although this is a more secure age for experiencing the addition of another sibling, relinquishing the position of first or youngest is still difficult and requires appropriate preparation. (See Sibling Rivalry, Chapter 15.)

Play

Various types of play are typical of this period, but preschoolers especially enjoy associative play, group play in similar or identical activities but without rigid organization or rules. Play should provide for physical, social, and mental development (Table 13.1).

Play activities for physical growth and the refinement of motor skills include jumping, running, and climbing. Tricycles, wagons, gym and sports equipment, sandboxes, wading pools, and winter sleds can help develop muscles and coordination. Activities such as swimming, skating, and skiing teach safety and can also help develop muscles and coordination.

Manipulative, constructive, creative, and educational toys provide for quiet activities, fine motor development, and self-expression. Easy construction sets, large blocks of various sizes and shapes, a counting frame, alphabet or number flash cards, paints, crayons, simple carpentry tools, musical toys, illustrated books, simple sewing or handicraft sets, large puzzles, and clay are suitable toys (Fig. 13.5). Electronic games and computer programs can also be valuable in helping children learn basic skills, such as letters and simple words. Although their attention span is still short, preschoolers are beginning to enjoy crafts, especially with the guidance and assistance of adults. A helpful rule in planning creative activities is one simple project per year of age. For example, a 3-year-old child usually has the patience to decorate three eggs but will become bored and restless with more.

Probably the most characteristic and pervasive preschooler activity is imitative, imaginative, and dramatic play. Dress-up clothes, dolls, housekeeping toys, dollhouses, telephones, farm animals and equipment, village sets, trains, trucks, cars, planes, hand puppets, and medical kits provide hours of self-expression (Fig. 13.6). Probably more than

TABLE 13.1 **Growth and Development During Preschool Years**

Physical	Gross Motor	Fine Motor	Language	Socialization	Cognition	Family Relationships
Age 3 Years						
Usual weight gain of 1.8-2.7 kg (4-6 lb) Average weight of 14.5 kg (32 lb) Usual gain in height of 7.5 cm (3 inches) per year Average height of 95 cm (3 feet, 1½ inches) May have achieved nighttime control of bowel and bladder	Rides tricycle Jumps off bottom step Stands on one foot for few seconds Goes up stairs using alternate feet; may still come down using both feet on step Broad jumps May try to dance, but balance may not be adequate	Builds tower of 9-10 cubes Builds bridge with three cubes Adeptly places small pellets in narrow-necked bottle In drawing, copies circle, imitates cross, names what has been drawn; cannot draw stick figure but may make circle with facial features	Has vocabulary of about 900 words Uses primarily "telegraphic" speech Uses complete sentences of three or four words Talks incessantly regardless of whether anyone is paying attention Repeats sentence of six syllables Asks many questions	Dresses self almost completely if helped with back buttons and told which shoe is right or left Pulls on shoes Has increased attention span Feeds self completely Can prepare simple meals, such as cold cereal and milk Can help set table; can dry dishes without breaking any May have fears, especially of dark and going to bed Knows own gender and gender of others Play is parallel and associative; begins to learn simple games, but often follows own rules; begins to share	Is in preconceptual phase Is egocentric in thought and behavior Has beginning understanding of time; uses many time-oriented expressions, talks about past and future as much as about present, pretends to tell time Has improved concept of space, as demonstrated by understanding of prepositions and ability to follow directional command Has beginning ability to view concepts from another perspective	Attempts to please parents and conform to their expectations Is less jealous of younger sibling; may be opportune time for birth of additional sibling Is aware of family relationships and sex-role functions Boys tend to identify more with father or other male figure Has increased ability to separate easily and comfortably from parents for short periods
Age 4 Years						
Pulse and respiration rates decrease slightly Growth rate is similar to that of previous year Average weight of 16.5 kg (36.5 lb) Average height of 103 cm (3 feet, 4½ inches) Length at birth is doubled Maximum potential for development of amblyopia	Skips and hops on one foot Catches ball reliably Throws ball overhead Walks downstairs using alternate footing	Uses scissors successfully to cut out picture following outline Can lace shoes but may not be able to tie bow In drawing, copies square, traces cross and diamond, adds three parts to stick figure	Has vocabulary of 1500 words or more Uses sentences of four or five words Questioning is at peak Tells exaggerated stories Knows simple songs May be mildly profane if associates with older children Obeys prepositional phrases, such as "under," "on top of," "beside," "in back of," or "in front of" Names one or more colors Comprehends analogies, such as "If ice is cold, fire is ___"	Very independent Tends to be selfish and impatient Aggressive physically as well as verbally Takes pride in accomplishments Has mood swings Shows off dramatically, enjoys entertaining others Tells family tales to others with no restraint Still has many fears Play is associative Imaginary playmates common Uses dramatic, imaginative, and imitative devices Sexual exploration and curiosity demonstrated through play, such as being "doctor" or "nurse"	Is in phase of intuitive thought Causality is still related to proximity of events Understands time better, especially in terms of sequence of daily events Unable to conserve matter Judges everything according to one dimension, such as height, width, or order Immediate perceptual clues dominate judgment Is beginning to develop less egocentrism and more social awareness May count correctly but has poor mathematic concept of numbers Obeys because parents have set limits, not because of understanding of right or wrong	Rebels if parents expect too much, such as impeccable table manners Takes aggression and frustration out on parents or siblings Do's and don'ts become important May have rivalry with older or younger siblings; may resent older sibling's privileges and younger sibling's invasion of privacy and possessions May "run away" from home Identifies strongly with parent of opposite sex Is able to run simple errands outside the home

Age 5 Years						
Pulse and respiration rates decrease slightly Average weight of 18.5 kg (41 lb) Average height of 110 cm (3 feet, 7½ inches) Eruption of permanent dentition may begin Handedness is established (about 90% are right-handed)	Skips and hops on alternate feet Throws and catches ball well Jumps rope Skates with good balance Walks backward with heel to toe Jumps from height of 12 inches and lands on toes Balances on alternate feet with eyes closed	Ties shoelaces Uses scissors, simple tools, or pencil well In drawing, copies diamond and triangle; adds seven to nine parts to stick figure; prints a few letters, numbers, or words, such as first name	Has vocabulary of about 2100 words Uses sentences of six to eight words, with all parts of speech Names coins (e.g., nickel, dime) Names four or more colors Describes drawing or pictures with much comment and enumeration Knows names of days of week, months, and other time-associated words Knows composition of articles, such as "A shoe is made of ____" Can follow three commands in succession	Less rebellious and quarrelsome than at age 4 yr More settled and eager to get down to business Not as open and accessible in thoughts and behavior as in earlier years Independent but trustworthy, not fool-hardy; more responsible Has fewer fears; relies on outer authority to control world Eager to do things right and to please; tries to "live by the rules" Has better manners Cares for self totally, occasionally needing supervision in dress or hygiene Not ready for concentrated close work or small print because of slight farsightedness and still unrefined eye-hand coordination Play is associative; tries to follow rules but may cheat to avoid losing	Begins to question what parents think by comparing them with age-mates and other adults May notice prejudice and bias in outside world Is more able to view other's perspective, but tolerates differences rather than understanding them May begin to show understanding of conservation of numbers through counting objects regardless of arrangement Uses time-oriented words with increased understanding Cautious about factual information regarding world	Gets along well with parents May seek out parent more often than at age 4 yr for reassurance and security, especially when entering school Begins to question parents' thinking and principles Strongly identifies with parent of same sex, especially boys with their fathers Enjoys activities such as sports, cooking, and shopping with parent of same sex

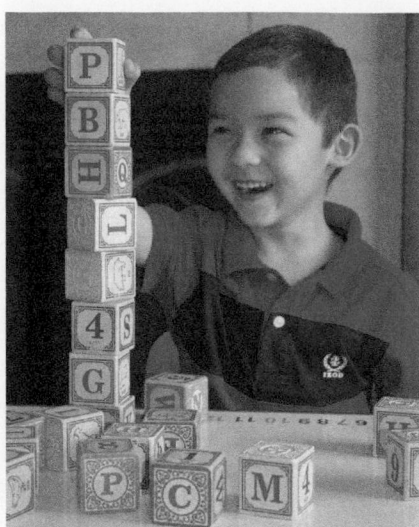

FIG. 13.5 Preschoolers enjoy a sense of accomplishment from activities such as stacking blocks.

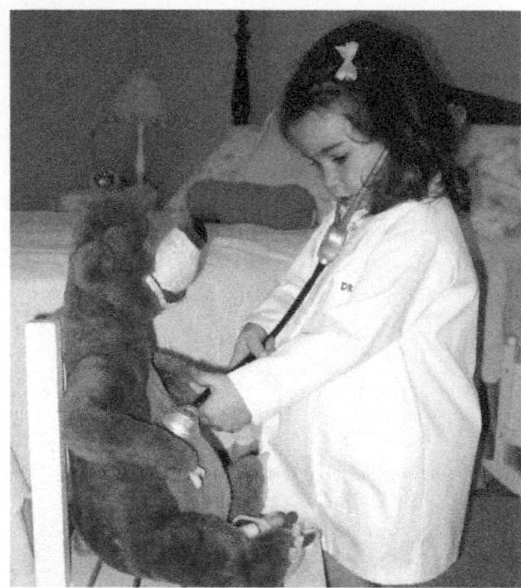

FIG. 13.6 Imaginative and imitative play is typical of preschoolers.

any other age-group, 4- and 5-year-old children are absorbed in the reproduction of the behavior of significant adults. Toward the end of the preschool period, children are less satisfied with make-believe or pretend objects and enjoy actually doing the activity, such as cooking and carpentry.

Television programs and other forms of electronic media also have their place in children's play, although each should be only one part of the total repertoire of social and recreational activities. Parents and other caregivers should supervise the selection of programs and applications, co-view and discuss programs with their children, co-play games and applications, limit media exposure, and set a good example of media use (American Academy of Pediatrics Council on Communications and Media, 2016). Children enjoy and learn from educational programs and applications; however, television viewing and other media exposure limit time spent in other meaningful activities such as reading, physical activity, and socialization (American Academy of Pediatrics Council on Communications and Media, 2016). Television viewing and digital play can become an interactive activity when adults participate in these activities with children and discuss the content.

Play is so much a part of the young child's life that reality and fantasy become blurred. The make-believe is reality during play and becomes fantasy only when toys are put away or dress-up clothes are removed. It is no wonder that imaginary playmates are so much a part of this age period. Imaginary companions usually appear between ages 2½ and 3 years and, for the most part, last until the child enters school.

Imaginary companions serve many purposes; they become friends in times of loneliness, they accomplish what the child is still attempting, and they experience what the child wants to forget or remember. It is not unusual for the "friend" to have a myriad of vices and to be blamed for wrongdoing. Sometimes the child hopes to escape punishment by saying, "My friend Brian broke the glass." At other times the preschooler may fantasize that the "companion" misbehaved and play the role of parent. This becomes a way of assuming control and authority in a safe situation.

Parents often worry about their child having imaginary playmates, not realizing how normal and useful they are. Parents should be reassured that the child's fantasy is a sign of health that helps differentiate between make-believe and reality. Parents can acknowledge the presence of the imaginary companion by calling him or her by name and even agreeing to simple requests such as setting an extra place at the table, but they should not allow the child to use the playmate to avoid punishment or responsibility. For example, if the child blames the companion for messing up a room, the parents need to clearly state that the child is the only person they see, and therefore the child is responsible for cleaning up (see Critical Thinking Case Study box).

CRITICAL THINKING CASE STUDY

Imaginary Playmates

Mrs. Preston tells you, the nurse, that her 3-year-old daughter, Libby, has an imaginary playmate named Allison. She was not concerned about this until Libby started asking her to put a plate on the table for Allison at mealtimes. What is your response?

1. What evidence should you consider regarding this situation?
2. What additional information is required at this time?
3. Describe the nursing intervention(s) that have the highest priority.
4. Identify important patient-centered outcomes with reference to your nursing interventions.

Answers are available at http://evolve.elsevier.com/wong/ncic.

Children also benefit from play that occurs between them and a parent. Mutual play fosters development from birth through the school years and provides enriched opportunities for learning. Through mutual play, parents can provide tactile and kinesthetic experiences, can maximize verbal and language abilities, and can offer praise and encouragement for exploration of the world. Additionally, mutual play encourages positive interactions between the parent and child, strengthening their relationship. Recommendations for mutual play should reflect the child's developmental level and can incorporate readily available items found in the home or community (e.g., musical CDs, puppets, games, and puzzles).

TEMPERAMENT

Temperament influences children's social development and interactions. Chapters 12 and 13 discuss the importance of temperament during early childhood. Because temperamental characteristics tend to remain stable, the same considerations in terms of childrearing apply during the preschool years.

One major concern in the preschool age-group is the effect of temperament on adjustment in group situations, especially school, and the long-term consequences of temperamental characteristics. In particular, the degree of adaptability to new situations, intensity of response, distractibility, amount of persistence, mood, and activity level influence a child's chances for success in school. Consequently, parents can benefit from suggestions that can promote preschoolers' adjustment. For example, children who are slow to warm up need gradual introduction to new situations and may benefit from the parent's presence until they have settled in. Children with high activity levels tend to adjust better to environments that allow freedom of movement, rather than a structured or regimented classroom. The more aware parents are of their children's unique behaviors, the better they are able to inform teachers or other caregivers of the children's needs and successful approaches to handling the youngsters.

The Behavioral Style Questionnaire helps identify temperamental characteristics in children from 3 to 7 years old (McDevitt & Carey, 1978). Simply asking parents to rate their child as being much easier than, easier than, as easy as, more difficult than, or much more difficult than the average child may also be a valuable screening method. Table 13.1 summarizes the major developmental achievements for children 3, 4, and 5 years old.

COPING WITH CONCERNS RELATED TO NORMAL GROWTH AND DEVELOPMENT

Preschool and Kindergarten Experience

Many children attend some type of early childhood program, usually preschool or a day care center. Group care has become commonplace with the large number of parents currently employed outside the home. The effects of early education and stimulation on children have increasingly gained recognition. Because social development widens to include age-mates and other significant adults, preschool provides an excellent vehicle for expanding children's experiences with others. It is also excellent preparation for entrance into elementary school.

In preschool or day care centers, children have opportunities to learn about group cooperation; adjustment to sociocultural differences; and coping with frustration, dissatisfaction, and anger. Preschool center activities often provide for mastery and achievement, which allow children to gain increased feelings of success, self-confidence, and personal competence. Whether structured learning is imposed is less important than the social climate, type of guidance, and attitude that the teacher or leader displays toward the children. With a teacher who is aware of preschoolers' developmental abilities and needs, children will learn from the activity provided. Most programs incorporate a daily schedule of quiet play, outdoor activity, group activities such as games and projects, creative or free play, and snack and rest periods.

Preschool is particularly beneficial for children who lack a peer-group experience, such as an only child, and for children from impoverished homes. It provides extensive stimulation for language, physical, and social development. It is also excellent preparation for kindergarten. For a child from an underprivileged home, elementary school can be so overwhelming that the sensory overload impedes all learning. Regular school places many more demands on children for prolonged attention, self-disciplined behavior, and demonstrated progress in performance and achievement than does the less-structured atmosphere of preschool.

One of the issues that parents face is the child's readiness for preschool or kindergarten. School readiness is influenced by a myriad of elements, including a child's social, emotional, and physical development; health status; ability and desire to learn; life experiences; family environment; and parental support. There are no absolute indicators for school readiness. The child's social maturation, especially attention span, is as important as academic readiness.

The use of developmental screening tools and readiness testing varies by state and local district. Developmental screening differs from readiness testing, and there is controversy over the most beneficial form of evaluation in determining a child's readiness to enter school. Readiness testing focuses on evaluation of skill acquisition, whereas developmental screening focuses on the potential to learn. Developmental screening tools address cognitive (especially language), social, and physical milestones and can identify children who may benefit from further diagnostic testing.

Schools and parents play integral roles in a child's school readiness. Schools must be able to assist children with varying learning and physical abilities and should be able to provide diverse learning situations that serve as a foundation for continued growth and maturation. Parents should promote a positive attitude toward learning, participate in their child's learning, read to their child, provide opportunities for social and emotional growth, and choose programs or schools that will partner with the family to foster learning (National Center on Parent, Family, and Community Engagement, 2014).

Nurses can help parents assess a child's readiness in terms of age, physical ability, and cognitive and social development (see Table 13.1). For example, a group experience may be difficult for young children with short attention spans. These children may require a different type of experience with more individualized attention.

Nurses can also help guide parents in selecting enriched social and educational early intervention programs, schools, and child care centers. Careful selection of early childhood education is fundamental to future learning and development. Licensed and regulated programs must follow established standards, which represent minimum requirements and safeguards. Regulation is important to protect children from harm and to promote the conditions essential for a child's healthy development and learning. The National Association for the Education of Young Children supports early childhood regulation on all levels.*

Other areas to evaluate are the facility's daily program, teacher qualifications, staff/student ratio, discipline policy, environmental safety precautions, provision of meals, sanitary conditions, amount of indoor and outdoor space per child, and fee schedule. Evaluation of the facility's health practices is extremely important. When children are in group settings such as child care centers, preschool, and kindergarten, they are exposed to more illnesses. Nurses can advise parents regarding the evaluation of a facility's sanitary practices and can actively participate in educating staff in measures to minimize infection.

References from other parents help evaluate a facility, but personal observation of the facility is recommended. Encourage parents to meet the director and some of the employees at a few facilities to make an informed choice.

Preparing the Child

Children need preparation for the preschool and kindergarten experience.† For young children, these programs represent a change from their usual home environment and prolonged separation from their parents. Even if children have been cared for by a babysitter or in a group setting, preschool and kindergarten differ because there is less individualized attention, programs are more structured, and learning is expected.

Before children begin school, parents should present the idea as exciting and pleasurable. Talking to them about activities such as painting, building with blocks, or enjoying swings and other outdoor equipment

*Young Children, 1313 L St. NW, Suite 500, Washington, DC 20005; 800-424-2460 or 202-232-8777; www.naeyc.org.

†Resources for developmental and learning activities can be found at Teacher Created Resources, 12621 Western Ave., Garden Grove, CA 92841; 800-662-4321; www.teachercreated.com.

allows children to fantasize about the forthcoming event in a positive manner. When the first day of school arrives, parents should behave confidently. Such behavior requires parents to have resolved their own feelings regarding the experience.

Parents should introduce their child to the teacher and the facility. In some instances, it is helpful for parents to remain for at least part of the first day until the child is comfortable. If parents stay, they should be available to the child but inconspicuous. A full-day routine is often too overwhelming for a child and could be shortened to a morning or afternoon session if possible. To decrease separation anxiety, parents can provide the school with detailed information about the child's home environment, such as familiar routines, favorite activities, food preferences, names of siblings or pets, and personal habits. Such information helps the child feel at ease in the strange surroundings. A school that automatically requests this information demonstrates the staff's awareness of each child's needs, and the parent has a valuable clue to evaluating the quality of the program. Transitional objects, such as a favorite toy, may also help the child bridge the gap from home to school.

Sex Education

Preschoolers have assimilated a tremendous amount of information during their short lifetimes. Although their thinking may not be mature, they search constantly for explanations and reasons that are logical and reasonable to them. The word "why" seems to supplant the word "no," which was common in toddlerhood. It is only natural that as they learn about "me," they will also want to know "why me" and "how me." Questions such as "Where do babies come from?" are as casual as "Why is the sky blue?," "What makes it rain?," or "Who is that?" It is the way in which adults answer questions about procreation that conditions children, even the youngest, to separate these questions from others about their world. If adults answer these questions honestly and as matter-of-factly as any other inquiry, children will feel comfortable asking questions as they explore their bodies and world. If they are answered with a "tall tale" or an anxious "You are too young to know about that," children will learn to keep such questions to themselves. Unfortunately, as they harbor these silent mysteries, they formulate their own theories to explain birth. Because magical thinking need not be based on logic or fact, any fantastic and often terrifying explanation can substitute for the truth.

Two rules govern answering sensitive questions about topics such as sex. The first is to find out what children know and think. While investigating the theories children have produced as reasonable explanations, parents can give correct information and also help children understand why their explanations are inaccurate. Another reason for ascertaining what the child thinks before offering any information is to avoid giving an "unasked for" answer. For example, 4-year-old Lauren asked her father, "Where did I come from?" Both parents quickly took this inquiry as a clue for offering sex education. After the explanation, Lauren exclaimed, "I don't know about all that! All I know is Mary came from New York, and I want to know where I came from."

The second rule for giving information is to be honest. True, the preschooler will forget or misunderstand much of the correct information, but the correct information can be restated until the child absorbs and comprehends the facts. Even though the correct anatomic words may be hard to pronounce or difficult to remember, they become important for explaining other concepts later on. Nurses have the opportunity to contribute to early sex education by conveying accurate information regarding genital terms during physical examinations.

Honesty does not imply imparting every fact of life or allowing excessive permissiveness in sexual curiosity. A child who asks one question is looking for one answer. When they are ready, children will ask about the other "unfinished" parts of the story. Sooner or later they will wonder how the "sperm meets the egg" and "how the baby gets out," but it is best to wait until they ask.

If parents offer too much information, the child will simply become bored or end the conversation with an irrelevant question. Parents worry a great deal about whether they can "harm" their children with "too much" information or tell them things they will not understand. In general, knowledge is not harmful when delivered in a developmentally appropriate manner. It is likely that children will not comprehend everything parents explain initially; they will process information at their own pace. What matters is that parents are approachable and do not dismiss their child's inquiries. It is also important for parents to recognize that children's sex education is affected not only by the information they receive verbally but also by the relationship and sexual behavior they see their parents modeling and by the sexual content they are exposed to in their everyday environment (e.g., television, magazines, movies).

When a child does not ask questions, parents and health professionals should take advantage of natural opportunities to discuss reproduction, such as talking about someone who is pregnant or discussing a television program or movie about biologic aspects. Many excellent books on sex education are available for preschool children at public libraries. In addition, the Sexuality Information and Education Council of the United States* and the American Academy of Pediatrics† have bibliographies of suggested reading material. Parents should read the material before giving or reading it to a child.

Regardless of whether children are given sex education, they will engage in games of sexual curiosity and exploration. At approximately 3 years of age, children are aware of the anatomic differences between the sexes and are concerned with how the other "works." This is not really "sexual" curiosity because many children are still unaware of the reproductive function of the genitalia. They are curious about the eliminative function of the anatomy. Little boys wonder how girls can urinate without a penis, so they watch girls go to the bathroom. Because they cannot see anything but the stream of urine coming out, they want to observe further. "Doctor play" is often a game invented for such investigation. Little girls are no less curious about boys' anatomy. They find it intriguing to inspect this "thing" that girls do not have.

Parents often wonder how to handle such sexual curiosity. A positive approach is to neither condone nor condemn the behavior, but to tell the children that, if they have questions, they should ask the parents; the parents should then encourage the children to engage in some other activity. In this way, children understand that they can satisfy their sexual curiosity in ways other than playing investigative games. This in no way condemns the act but stresses alternative methods by which to seek solutions and answers. Allowing children unrestricted permissiveness only intensifies their anxiety and concern because exploring and searching usually yield little evidence to satisfy their curiosity.

Occasionally, parents are faced with special dilemmas (e.g., when a child accidentally witnesses sexual intercourse). When such an event occurs, parents must remember that sex education is much more than textbook facts. It is part of a broader concept called sexuality; two people unite intimately because of the special relationship they have together. Intercourse is not a physical act apart from feeling or emotion, but a private act that two people share for pleasure and to

*1012 14th St., NW, Suite 1108, Washington, DC 20005; 202-265-2405; fax: 202-462-2340; www.siecus.org.

†American Academy of Pediatrics, 141 Northwest Point Blvd., Elk Grove Village, IL 60007; 847-434-4000 or 800-433-9016; fax: 847-434-8000; www.aap.org.

express caring for each other. Offering such an explanation teaches appropriate social behavior and, in particular, stresses the meaningful, intimate relationship between two adults. When children witness sexual acts, parents should use the opportunity to communicate that sex is part of a healthy and natural adult relationship. However, to prevent subsequent interruptions, children are cautioned to always knock first; if they are too young to understand or comply, a lock on the door is appropriate.

Another concern for some parents is masturbation, or self-stimulation of the genitalia. This occurs at any age for a variety of reasons and, if not excessive, is normal and healthy. For preschoolers, it is part of sexual curiosity and exploration. If parents are concerned about their child masturbating, it is essential for nurses to investigate the circumstances associated with the activity. Masturbation can be an expression of anxiety, boredom, or stress. In the case of excessive masturbation, it may be associated with emotional or behavioral problems and physical or sexual abuse (Strachan & Staples, 2012). Management of normal childhood masturbation includes parent education and reassurance, redirection of the child to other activities, and discussion with the child regarding appropriate boundaries (Strachan & Staples, 2012). In addition, parents should emphasize that masturbation is a private act, thus teaching children socially acceptable behavior.

Gifted Children

The importance of identifying gifted children and their needs is increasingly being acknowledged. Although the definition of gifted varies, **giftedness** is commonly recognized as a minimum intelligence quotient (IQ) of 130 (Vaivre-Douret, 2011). A broader view, reflected in the term *gifted-talented,* considers signs of giftedness to include specific academic aptitudes, advanced memory skills, creative thinking, ability in the visual or performing arts, and psychomotor ability, either individually or in combination. Children may be identified as gifted when they enter school or are referred by parents or teachers and receive IQ or achievement tests. However, parents and caregivers should be aware that giftedness may be present in both academic and nonacademic areas. Therefore not all gifted children are identified when IQ tests or achievement tests alone are used to determine giftedness. Identification of giftedness based solely on test scores may result in the tragic loss of the opportunity to develop a child's full potential. It is also important to recognize that giftedness can exist in children who have learning disabilities, students who are often referred to as "twice-exceptional" (McCallum, Bell, Coles, et al., 2013).

Gifted children can present unique challenges to parents. They often demand increased stimulation as infants and continue to seek a great deal of attention from their parents. Their high energy level and persistence can lead to discipline problems similar to those seen in children with difficult temperaments. Parents may be intimidated by having a child smarter than themselves and be hesitant to set limits. However, gifted children are children first and have the same needs for love, security, and consistent boundaries as other youngsters. Children's advanced skills in one area may also cause adults to exaggerate their abilities in all areas and thus expect excessively mature behavior. Parents may mislabel slower achievement in a particular skill as lack of trying, when really it represents children's natural progression of abilities.

Gifted children benefit from academic settings that provide enrichment and accelerated learning commensurate with their capabilities. Early identification of a gifted child and nurturance of the child's potential and abilities are vital to the child's optimum development (Coleman, 2016). Nurses who are aware of the behavioral and developmental characteristics of giftedness can assess children's mental and physical capabilities and assist in early identification (Box 13.1).

BOX 13.1 Understanding Gifted Children

- Interests similar to those of older individuals
- Language development advanced for age
- Inquisitive, always asking questions
- Especially curious about facts
- Developmental tasks varied across domains
- Memory skills are pronounced, especially long-term memory
- Intuitive in questions and thought processes
- Easily able to connect two concepts
- Eager to learn about connections
- Interest in configurations and interactions
- Exceptional sense of humor
- Always eager to try new pathways of thinking
- Takes pride in solving and posing new problems
- Capacity for independent, self-directed activities
- Often demonstrates talent in one area: drawing, music, games, math, reading
- Perfectionism is a focus
- Displays intense feelings and emotion

Information on parenting gifted and talented children is available from the National Association for Gifted Children,* the Council for Exceptional Children,† and local associations.

Aggression

The term **aggression** refers to behavior that attempts to hurt a person or destroy property. Aggression differs from anger, which is a temporary emotional state, but anger may be expressed through aggression. Hyperaggressive behavior in preschoolers is characterized by unprovoked physical attacks on other children and adults, destruction of others' property, frequent intense temper tantrums, extreme impulsivity, disrespect, and noncompliance.

A complex set of biologic, sociocultural, and familial variables influence aggression. Research indicates that types of aggression differ between genders. Boys exhibit more physical aggression than girls during preschool years (Lussier, Corrado, & Tzoumakis, 2012). Relational aggression is exhibited at similar rates in boys and girls of this age-group; however, differences in the frequency of relational aggression among genders can vary depending on peer interactions in various situations and settings (McEachern & Snyder, 2012). Sociocultural factors that are associated with childhood aggression include exposure to community violence (Fleckman, Drury, Taylor, et al., 2016) and violence in the media (Fitzpatrick, Barnett, & Pagani, 2012). Familial variables such as maternal depression, low level of maternal education, and low socioeconomic status contribute to childhood aggression (Provencal, Booij, & Tremblay, 2015). Family conflict, hostile parenting, low levels of positive interactions and parental warmth, physical and verbal abuse, and punitive interactions also contribute to childhood aggression (Jia, Wang, Shi, et al., 2016). Other factors that tend to increase aggressive behavior are frustration, modeling, and reinforcement.

Frustration, or the continual thwarting of self-satisfaction by parental disapproval, humiliation, punishment, and insults, can lead children to act out against others as a means of release. These children displace their anger on others, particularly peers and other authority figures,

*1331 H St. NW, Suite 1001, Washington, DC 20005; 202-785-4268, fax: 202-785-4248; www.nagc.org.

†2900 Crystal Drive, Suite 1000, Arlington, VA 22202; 888-232-7733; fax: 703-264-9494; www.cec.sped.org.

especially if they fear their parents. This type of aggression often applies to the child who is well behaved at home but a discipline problem at school or a bully among playmates.

Modeling, or imitating the behavior of significant others, is a powerful influencing force in preschoolers. Children who are exposed to family violence are observing behavior that they perceive as acceptable and therefore may exhibit aggressive behavior with others (Liu, Lewis, & Evans, 2013). Also, early harsh discipline may lead to aggressive behavior (Jia, Wang, Shi, et al., 2016). Another aspect of modeling is establishing a double-standard for acceptable conduct. For example, in some families aggression is synonymous with masculinity, and boys are encouraged to defend themselves. Although defending one's rights is to be encouraged for both sexes, at times the principle of "being tough" or "standing up for yourself" is not tempered with judgment, fairness, or equality but becomes an excuse for ruling and dominating others. Such permissive aggression can produce extreme anxiety in children because it makes them feel out of control, even though outwardly they may appear to be the "boss" or "bully."

Another significant source for modeling is media exposure. Numerous studies have found a positive correlation between viewing violent programs and developing aggression; therefore parents need encouragement to supervise programming, especially for children with aggressive tendencies (Fitzpatrick, Barnett, & Pagani, 2012). The American Academy of Pediatrics Council on Communications and Media (2016) offers recommendations for healthy media exposure.

Reinforcement can also shape aggressive behavior and is closely associated with modeling "masculine" behavior. Sometimes the reward for aggressive behavior is negative (e.g., punishment or disapproval) yet reinforcing because it brings attention. For example, children who are ignored by their parents until they hit a sibling learn that this act attracts attention. Additionally, parents who permit aggressive behavior by not interfering communicate silent, implicit approval of such acts.

One of the tasks of preschoolers is learning socially acceptable behavior and the ability to control aggression and redirect their anger. Parents can help children by modeling the appropriate behavior and encouraging children to express themselves verbally. For example, rather than condoning the hitting of another child for taking a toy, parents can suggest that the child state how he or she feels, such as "I get angry when you take my ball. Please give it back."

Children should not be made to feel guilty or ashamed for being angry or frustrated. When children recognize these feelings, they are better able to channel them into constructive, not destructive, outlets. One of the earliest demonstrations of aggression is temper tantrums. (See Chapter 14.) Parents can handle them constructively by not attending to or reinforcing them and by helping children find control through appropriate play situations. In this way, young children learn to acknowledge such feelings and express them in alternate ways, such as pounding on clay or hitting a punching bag. When children are out of control, they may need to be physically restrained or removed from the scene to prevent them from hurting themselves or others.

Sometimes the type of discipline used to extinguish other forms of unacceptable behavior actually promotes aggressive behavior. For example, if a child is spanked for an aggressive act, aggression is being used to "teach" a lesson against aggression. In addition to physically aggressive discipline, inconsistency in disciplinary practices may also foster behavior problems in children (Duncombe, Havighurst, Holland, et al., 2012). The use of time-out and solitary play are effective disciplinary measures in the preschool years. Additionally, minimizing anger and frustration can lead to fewer opportunities for acting out.

When a child exhibits extreme behaviors, such as aggression, parents are often concerned about the need for professional help. Generally, the difference between normal and problematic behavior is not the behavior itself but its quantity (number of occurrences), severity (interference with social or cognitive functioning), distribution (different manifestations), onset (when the behavior started), and duration (at least 4 weeks). When aggressive tendencies are evaluated, these factors are assessed to distinguish between behaviors typically seen at various ages and those that may represent an underlying problem. Extreme aggression requires professional treatment and is often difficult to change.*

Speech Problems

The most critical period for speech development occurs between 2 and 4 years of age. During this period, children are using their rapidly growing vocabulary faster than they can produce the words. A failure to master sensorimotor integration results in stuttering or stammering as children try to say the word they are already thinking about. This disfluency in speech pattern is called developmental stuttering and is common during language development in children ages 2 to 5 years (Nelson, 2013). Stuttering affects boys more frequently than girls, has been shown to have a genetic link, and usually resolves during childhood (American Speech-Language-Hearing Association, 2017b). The National Institute on Deafness and Other Communication Disorders (2016) encourages parents and caregivers of children who stutter to speak slowly and relaxed, refrain from interrupting the child's speech, resist completing the child's sentences, and take time to listen attentively. When parents or other significant caregivers place undue emphasis on a child's stuttering, they may exacerbate the problem. A speech evaluation is indicated if stuttering persists for 3 to 6 months, there is a family history of stuttering, or there is evidence of struggling or distress related to stuttering (National Institute on Deafness and Other Communication Disorders, 2016).

The best therapy for speech problems is prevention and early detection. Common causes of speech problems are hearing deficits, developmental delay, and physical conditions that impede normal speech production. Referral for evaluation and treatment may be necessary to prevent a problem from interfering with learning. Anticipatory preparation of parents for expected developmental norms may calm caregiver anxiety.

Children pressured into producing sounds ahead of their developmental level may develop dyslalia (articulation problems) or revert to using infantile speech. Prevention involves educating parents regarding the usual achievement of speech production during childhood.

Stress

Although for parents the preschool years generally are less troublesome than toddlerhood, this period presents children with many unique stresses. Some are innate and stem from preschoolers' unique understanding of the world, such as fears. Others are imposed, such as beginning school. Although minimal amounts of stress are beneficial during the early years to help children develop effective coping skills, excessive stress is harmful. Young children are especially vulnerable because of their limited capacity to cope.

To help parents deal with stress in their child's life, they must be aware of signs of stress and be helped to identify the source (Box 13.2). Any number of stresses may be present, such as the birth of a sibling, marital discord, relocation, or illness. The best approach to dealing with stress is prevention. It is important to monitor the amount of stress

---

*Information on child development and behavior can be obtained through the American Academy of Pediatrics Section on Developmental and Behavioral Pediatrics, www.aap.org/en-us/about-the-aap/Committees-Councils-Sections/sodbp/Pages/default.aspx.

BOX 13.2 Sources of Stress in Preschoolers

Age 3 Years

Stubbornness—Despite developing interest in social relationships and a concept of "we," may lapse into uncooperative behavior
Belongings—Guards possessions
Jealousy—Particularly when it comes to parents' love
Separation anxiety—Difficulty leaving the parent
Stranger anxiety—Expresses fear being around someone unknown
Confusion—Cannot always discriminate between fantasy and reality
Fears—May be precipitated by imagination; may also fear dogs or other animals
Speech—May stutter or stumble over words
Activity level—Seems to be in perpetual motion; may exhaust himself or herself
Mealtime—May forget to eat or lose interest in food
Nap or bedtime—May fear bad dreams, the dark, or missing out on some fun while asleep
Destructiveness—May damage or destroy objects
Questions—Continually asks "Why?" and is upset if trusted adults do not respond or do not know the answer

Age 4 Years

Insecurity—May develop nervous habits such as nail biting, facial tics, thumb sucking, genital manipulation, eye blinking, or nose picking; may insist on bringing a familiar item from home to preschool
Companionship—Enjoys interacting with friends, although they may quarrel
Belongings—Protects possessions
Sex—Interested in the human body; may engage in exhibitionism
Activity level—Enjoys running, jumping, and slamming doors; may be punished for disruptive behavior
Fears—Picks up fears from adults; may fear dark room or anything perceived as "creepy"
Attention—Likes to talk and is frustrated if ignored or put off

Age 5 Years

Approval—Parents' love and acceptance are vital; seeks praise
School—May have difficulty adjusting to kindergarten
Separation anxiety—Particularly fears loss of mother
Worrying—May develop irrational fears; take information out of context; or fret over a misinterpreted, overheard conversation
Belongings—Protects possessions
Procrastination—Delays completing chores or activities
Name calling—Insults others to boost self-image but is upset when he or she is the victim of mockery

Modified from Kuczen, B. (1982). *Childhood stress: Don't let your child be a victim.* New York: Delacorte.

in the child's life so that levels do not exceed ability to cope. In many instances, structuring the child's schedule to allow rest and preparing the child for change, such as entering school, are sufficient measures.

Because stress is a constant aspect of daily living, it is not too early to help preschool children learn to cope with it. They can learn the meaning of the word *stress* and recognize physical signs of a stress reaction, such as a rapid pulse, a pounding heart, or fatigue. Teaching children relaxation and imagery is effective. Young children can learn to "let their bodies go limp like a rag doll." Parents can use stories to help their child imagine pleasurable events. As language skills improve, parents can encourage preschoolers to talk about their feelings and explore other ways of expressing emotions. Play is an excellent vehicle for venting anger or frustration, and toys such as drums, clay, and punching bags provide alternative methods of dissipating anxiety and teach socially acceptable ways of dealing with such feelings.

Fears

The greatest number and variety of real and imagined fears are present during the preschool years. Preschoolers may fear the dark, being left alone (especially at bedtime), animals (particularly large dogs and snakes), ghosts, sexual matters (castration), and objects or persons associated with pain. The exact cause of children's fears is unknown. Freudians believe that the upsurge of fears during the preschool years results from the anxiety of being injured and mutilated (castration complex). Piaget views fears as a product of the type of thinking in this age-group; preschoolers are caught between the egocentric thinking of infants, which protects them from imagined fears, and the more logical thought processes of school-age children, which help explain and dispel potential fears. Children in the preconceptual stage still engage in egocentric thought but are now able to imagine an event without actually experiencing it. For example, seeing someone hurt is sufficient for realizing what the hurt must be like and for consequently fearing that hurt. This is commonly observed in medical practice. When watching another child get an injection, the preschooler may become upset, almost as if he or she received the injection.

The concept of animism (i.e., ascribing lifelike qualities to inanimate objects) helps explain why children fear objects. For example, a child may refuse to use the toilet after watching a television commercial in which the toilet bowl is portrayed as turning into a monster.

One fear peculiar to this age is fear of annihilation. Because of poorly defined body boundaries and improved cognitive abilities, young children develop concerns related to loss of body parts, such as their body going down the drain. Because preschool children cannot understand concepts of size, they cannot understand that their body is too large to disappear down the drain.

Preschoolers are also likely to develop parent-induced fears. When parents demonstrate their fears, these concerns are communicated to the children. Such fears tend to be long-lasting and difficult to dispel.

The best way to help children overcome their fears is by actively involving them in finding practical methods to deal with frightening experiences. This may be as simple as keeping a dim night-light in the child's bedroom for reassurance or letting the child bathe a doll so that the child can observe that large objects cannot go down the drain. In this way, the experience that created the fear in the child can be reconstructed without involving the child directly as the victim. The child is allowed alternative methods by which to feel in control while overcoming fear.

Exposing children to the feared object in a safe situation provides a type of conditioning, or desensitization. For instance, children who are afraid of dogs should never be forced to approach or touch one, but they may be gradually introduced to the experience by watching other children play with the animal. This type of modeling, having others demonstrate fearlessness, can be effective if children are allowed to progress at their own rate.

Usually by 5 or 6 years of age, children relinquish many of their fears. Explaining the developmental sequence of fears and their gradual disappearance may help parents feel more secure in handling preschoolers' fears. However, sometimes fears do not subside with simple measures or developmental maturation. When children experience severe fears that disrupt family life, professional help is required. Successful training programs may include (1) muscle relaxation; (2) guided imagery; (3) positive self-talk or recitation of brave statements; or (4) thought stopping, or repetition of reassuring statements that block fearful thoughts. Rewards or "tokens" may be given for "bravery" and not being afraid. Nurses can apply such interventions in clinical settings to reduce fears (e.g., of being alone or of painful procedures).

PROMOTING OPTIMUM HEALTH DURING THE PRESCHOOL YEARS

NUTRITION

Healthy nutrition during childhood should include eating a variety of nutrient-dense foods, ensuring sufficient energy to promote growth and development, and balancing energy intake with energy expenditure to maintain a healthy weight (American Academy of Pediatrics Committee on Nutrition, 2014b). For moderately active preschoolers, the estimated daily caloric requirement ranges from 1200 to 1400 calories (US Department of Health and Human Services and US Department of Agriculture, 2015). Fluid requirements depend on activity level, climatic conditions, and state of health. The recommended daily allowance of protein increases with age; the recommended intake for preschoolers is 13 to 19 g/day (US Department of Health and Human Services & US Department of Agriculture, 2015). The recommended daily intake of fiber is 19 g for children 3 years of age and 25 g for children 4 and 5 years of age (American Academy of Pediatrics Committee on Nutrition, 2014a).

The American Academy of Pediatrics Committee on Nutrition (2014b) recommends that the total fat intake, averaged over several days, be reduced to 30% of total caloric intake for children 2 years and older. These efforts are important in the prevention of childhood obesity, cardiovascular disease, diabetes, and metabolic syndrome. While limiting fat consumption, it is also important to ensure that the diet contains adequate nutrients. This can be done simultaneously, as in the following example regarding calcium. The recommended daily allowance for calcium for children 1 to 3 years old is 700 mg, and the recommendation for children 4 to 8 years old is 1000 mg (US Department of Health and Human Services & US Department of Agriculture, 2015). Milk and dairy products provide a major source of calcium. Consuming less fat does not necessarily require drinking less milk or eating fewer dairy products but instead replacing higher-fat milk, cheese, and yogurt with lower-fat or nonfat choices.

Excessive consumption of fruit juices and other sugar-sweetened beverages has been associated with dental caries (Marshall, 2013) and adverse cardiometabolic effects (Kosova, Auinger, & Bremer, 2013). The American Academy of Pediatrics recommends limiting the intake of fruit juice to 4 to 6 oz/day for children 1 to 6 years of age (American Academy of Pediatrics, 2016). Nurses should counsel moderation in the consumption of fruit juice and sugar-sweetened beverages and provide suggestions for more appropriate sources of nutrients with fewer empty calories.

In 2011 the US Department of Agriculture released a new food guide system called MyPlate, with customizable daily food plans created specifically for children ages 2 to 5 years (US Department of Agriculture, 2015). This new system is comprehensive and provides information for developing a healthy lifestyle at an early age. Parents and providers can develop food plans and access information on growth during the preschool years, healthy eating habits, physical activity, and food safety at www.ChooseMyPlate.gov. Parents can use this information to assist their children in making healthy lifestyle choices and to help prevent adverse health conditions secondary to poor nutrition.

Some preschoolers still have food habits typical of toddlers, such as food fads and strong taste preferences. When children reach 4 years of age, they seem to enter another period of finicky eating, which is generally characteristic of the more rebellious behavior of children in this age-group. By age 5 years, children are more agreeable to trying new foods, especially if encouraged by an adult who allows the child to help with food preparation or to experiment with a new taste or different dish (Fig. 13.7). Mealtime can become a battle if parents expect excellent table manners. A 5-year-old child is usually ready for the "social" side of eating, but the younger child still has difficulty sitting quietly through a long family meal.

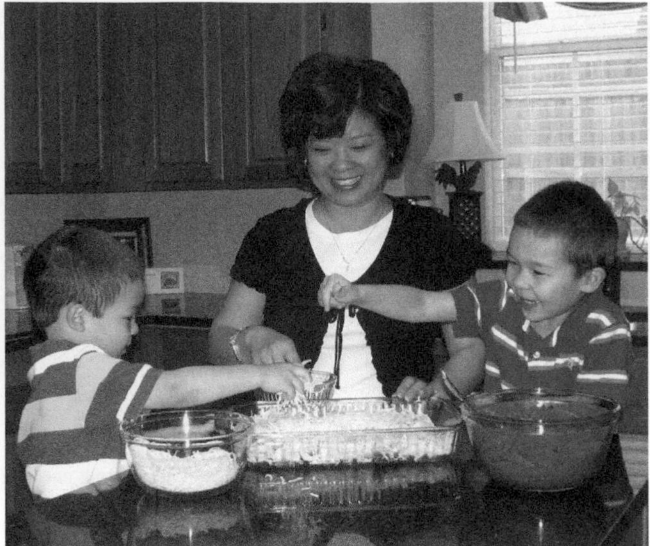

FIG. 13.7 Preschool children enjoy helping adults and are more likely to try new foods if they are included in the preparation.

> **! NURSING ALERT**
>
> Obesity in young children has dramatically increased over the past two decades, and efforts to provide a healthy diet and to encourage physical activity should begin early to help children achieve optimum health (Ford, Slining, & Popkin, 2013). The 5-2-1-0 framework recommended by the American Academy of Pediatrics provides a foundation for patient education regarding healthy lifestyle choices. This framework refers to 5 servings of fruits and vegetables per day, 2 hours or less of screen time per day, 1 hour of physical activity per day, and 0 (or limited) servings of sugar-sweetened beverages (American Academy of Pediatrics, 2015).

The amount and variety of foods young children eat vary greatly from day to day. Consequently, parents sometimes worry about the quantity and quality of food consumed by preschoolers. In general, the quality is much more important than the quantity, which nurses should stress during nutritional counseling. There is some evidence that children self-regulate their caloric intake. If they eat less at one meal, they compensate at another meal or snack.

One approach toward lessening parental concern is advising parents to keep a weekly record of everything the child eats. In particular, stress the need to measure the amount of food, such as setting aside ½ cup of vegetables and serving the child from this premeasured amount, to provide a more accurate estimate of food intake at each meal. When parents look at the food chart at the end of the week, they are usually amazed at how much the child consumed. In general, preschoolers eat only slightly more than toddlers, or approximately half of an adult's portion. Resources are available for the health care provider and the caregiver to help build healthy eating habits for children* (see Critical Thinking Case Study box).

*A nutritional resource for the health care provider is American Academy of Pediatrics Committee on Nutrition. (2014). *Pediatric nutrition.* Elk Grove, IL: American Academy of Pediatrics. A nutritional resource for parents and caregivers is Food Fights. To order, contact the American Academy of Pediatrics, 800-433-9016; www.aap.org.

CRITICAL THINKING CASE STUDY

Nutrition

Mrs. Pierce reports that she thinks her 3-year-old daughter, Hannah, is not eating enough, and she is concerned about her overall nutrition. Mealtimes are difficult, and sometimes it takes an hour to get Hannah to eat what is on her plate. She seems to only want to eat chicken nuggets. Mrs. Pierce feels discouraged that mealtimes are such a battle but knows it is important for Hannah to get the nutrients she needs for growth. Many times she uses activities to entice Hannah to eat, such as allowing her to watch her favorite video while eating or allowing her to bring her doll to the table. Today, Hannah weighed 14.2 kg (31.3 lb), and her height was 94.1 cm (3 feet, 1 inch). She has been growing along the 50th percentile on growth curves for both height and weight for the past 1½ years. Her assessment reveals a healthy, well-nourished, well-developed preschooler.

1. What evidence should you consider regarding this situation?
2. What additional information is required at this time?
3. Describe the nursing interventions that have the highest priority.

Answers are available at http://evolve.elsevier.com/wong/ncic.

SLEEP AND ACTIVITY

Sleep patterns vary widely, but the average preschooler sleeps approximately 12 hours a night and infrequently takes daytime naps. Waking during the night is common throughout early childhood. An appropriate and consistent bedtime, nap schedule (as needed), and bedtime routine can help prevent and treat common sleep problems and night wakings experienced by young children (Honaker & Meltzer, 2014). (See Chapter 14 for discussion of sleep problems in preschoolers.)

Motor activity levels continue to be high and allow preschoolers to explore their environment, begin learning physical games and sports, and interact with others. Motor activity is therefore encouraged. Quiet activities, such as television and video games, are increasingly appealing and can become an unhealthy substitute for active play.

Preschoolers' increased gross motor abilities and coordination allow them to engage in many physical activities, if only at a novice level. At this age, children benefit from free play and exposure to a variety of physical activities (Stricker, 2015). Whether young children should begin formalized training in an activity at this early age is controversial. Training programs must consider the child's physical and psychologic immaturity, and readiness must be determined individually. The most important aspect of organized play for preschoolers is that the activity is developmentally appropriate and occurs in a nonthreatening, fun, and safe environment.

DENTAL HEALTH

By the beginning of the preschool period, the eruption of the deciduous (primary) teeth is complete. Dental care is essential to preserve these temporary teeth and to teach good dental habits. (See Chapter 14.) Although preschoolers' fine motor control is improved, they still require assistance and supervision with brushing, and parents should perform flossing. Professional care and routine prophylaxis, especially fluoride supplements, should continue. The frequency of professional dental care should be based on a child's individual needs and risk assessment, including family oral health habits, dental development, presence or absence of dental disease, special health care needs, and dietary habits (American Academy of Pediatric Dentistry, 2016). Primary care providers are in an ideal position to perform dental screenings and risk assessments and refer children to a dental home (American Academy of Pediatrics Section on Oral Health, 2014). The American Academy of Pediatric Dentistry offers a Caries-Risk Assessment Tool for health care providers (www.aapd.org/media/Policies_Guidelines/G_CariesRiskAssessment.pdf), and the American Academy of Pediatrics provides practice tools for pediatric health care professionals that include information on dental screenings, risk assessments, and patient education (www2.aap.org/oralhealth/PracticeTools.html).

Trauma to teeth during this period is not uncommon, and prompt evaluation by a dentist is necessary if oral trauma occurs. Preservation of the space previously occupied by an avulsed tooth is necessary for proper eruption of the secondary tooth.

INJURY PREVENTION

Because of improved gross and fine motor skills, coordination, and balance, preschoolers are less prone to falls than toddlers. They tend to be less reckless; listen more to parental rules; and are aware of potential dangers, such as hot objects, sharp instruments, and dangerous heights. Putting objects in the mouth as part of exploration has all but ceased, but poisoning is still a danger. Cognitive ability may play a role in injury avoidance, especially in girls, who are less daring and risk-taking. Inform parents that children as young as 4½ years old have been shown to engage in risk-taking behaviors. Intervention strategies targeted at high-risk populations need to be part of safety education. Pedestrian motor vehicle injuries increase because of activities such as playing in the street, riding tricycles, running after balls, or forgetting safety regulations when crossing streets.

In general, the guidelines suggested for injury prevention for toddlers may be applied to children in this age-group as well. However, injury prevention measures can now include education regarding safety and potential hazards. Because preschoolers are great imitators, it is essential that parents set a good example by "practicing what they preach." Children quickly observe discrepancies between what they are told to do and what they observe. Establishing habits at this time, such as wearing bicycle helmets, can create long-term safety behaviors.

ANTICIPATORY GUIDANCE—CARE OF FAMILIES

The preschool years present fewer childrearing difficulties than the earlier years, and this stage of development is facilitated by appropriate anticipatory guidance in the areas already discussed (see Family-Centered Care box). Injury prevention also shifts from protection to education. For example, at this age the use of electrical outlet caps may be discontinued, with verbal explanations given of why danger exists and how to avoid it.

During this period, an emotional transition between parent and child occurs. Although children are still attached to their parents and accept all their values and beliefs, they are nearing the period of life when they will question previous teachings and prefer the companionship of peers. Entry into school marks a separation for both parents and children. Parents may need help in adjusting to this change, particularly if one parent has focused his or her daily activities on home responsibilities. As a child begins preschool or elementary school, parents may need to seek activities outside the home, such as community involvement or a career. In this way, all family members are adjusting to change, which is part of the process of growth and development.

FAMILY-CENTERED CARE

Guidance During Preschool Years

Age 3 Years

Prepare parents for the child's increasing interest in widening personal relationships.
Encourage enrollment in preschool or other socialization activities.
Emphasize importance of setting limits.
Prepare parents to expect exaggerated tension-reduction behaviors, such as need for "security blanket."
Encourage parents to offer the child choices.
Prepare parents to expect marked changes at 3½ years, when the child becomes insecure and exhibits emotional extremes.
Prepare parents for normal dysfluency in speech and advise them to avoid focusing on the pattern.
Prepare parents to expect extra demands on their attention as a reflection of the child's emotional insecurity and fear of loss of love.
Warn parents that the equilibrium of a 3-year-old will change to the aggressive, out-of-bounds behavior of a 4-year-old.
Prepare parents to handle anger appropriately and constructively.
Inform parents to anticipate a more stable appetite with more food selections.
Stress the need for protection and education of the child to prevent injury. (See Injury Prevention, Chapter 14.)

Age 4 Years

Prepare parents for more aggressive behavior, including motor activity and offensive language.
Prepare parents to expect resistance to parental authority.
Explore parental feelings regarding the child's behavior.
Suggest some type of respite for primary caregivers, such as placing the child in preschool for part of the day.
Prepare parents for the child's increasing sexual curiosity.
Emphasize the importance of realistic limit setting on behavior and appropriate disciplinary techniques.
Prepare parents for the highly imaginative 4-year-old who indulges in "tall tales" (to be differentiated from lies) and develops imaginary playmates.
Prepare parents to expect nightmares or an increase in them.
Provide reassurance that a period of calm begins at 5 years of age.

Age 5 Years

Inform parents to expect a tranquil period at 5 years.
Help parents prepare the child for entrance into the school environment.
Make certain immunizations are up to date before entering school.
Encourage parents to establish safety rules regarding interaction with strangers.
Suggest that unemployed mothers or fathers consider own activities when child begins school.
Suggest swimming lessons for child.
Encourage parents to limit television viewing and to preview shows and movies for inappropriate content.

NCLEX REVIEW QUESTIONS

1. The nurse caring for a preschool child understands which of the following developmental concepts? Select all that apply.
   A. Preschoolers have egocentric thought and believe that everyone thinks as they do.
   B. Play can be therapeutic and enlightening into a child's level of understanding.
   C. Explanations are helpful when using detail to allay the preschooler's stress.
   D. Preschoolers understand inferences and can relate to others' feelings with empathy.
   E. Preschoolers have magical thinking and believe their thoughts have power.
2. When her preschool son is in the hospital, the parent tells the nurse, "I think there is something wrong with him because he is so skinny." The most appropriate answer by the nurse is:
   A. Most preschoolers weigh between 10 and 14 kilograms.
   B. The legs of a preschooler, rather than the trunk, increase in length, which may make him look slimmer.
   C. Preschoolers usually keep that pot-bellied appearance until about 4 years old.
   D. Most preschoolers gain 2 to 3 pounds per year.
3. At the clinic appointment, a 4-year-old's mother wants to discuss several concerns. Which statements require more teaching by the nurse? Select all that apply.
   A. My husband feels that TV is okay as long as it is educational.
   B. I think it is okay for my son to play dress-up along with the girls.
   C. I told my son that his imaginary playmate moved away because it did not seem normal.
   D. My mother-in-law thinks I should be working around the house all the time, but I believe playing with my son is very important.
   E. My neighbor gave me some flash cards with letters and numbers for my son to use, but I said, "What's the rush? He's only 4."
4. One of the concerns of the preschool period is adequate nutrition. What can the nurse say to give anticipatory guidance to parents?
   A. Preschoolers are growing during this period and need to increase their caloric intake to 110 kcal/kg, for an average daily intake of 2200 calories.
   B. There is some evidence that children self-regulate their caloric intake. If they eat less at one meal, they compensate at another meal or snack.
   C. To monitor fat intake, dairy and meat should be limited to twice a day.
   D. For children who do not like milk, consumption of fruit juices is a healthy alternative.
5. At an appointment at the pediatrician's office, a patient's mother states, "My son gets rough with some of the neighborhood kids. I am worried that he is becoming a bully." Which statements by the mother need more teaching? Select all that apply.
   A. When my son becomes aggressive, I feel he needs to be punished.
   B. I think it is good for him to bond with his dad, so they often watch TV together.
   C. I am trying to get him to learn to say what he is upset about in words.
   D. Boys will be boys, so I think this can be considered a normal stage in development.
   E. I am thinking that a time-out would be a better strategy than spanking when my son shows this behavior.

Correct Answers

1. A, B, E; 2. B; 3. A, C, E; 4. B; 5. C, E

REFERENCES

American Academy of Pediatric Dentistry. (2016). Guideline on periodicity of examination, preventive dental services, anticipatory guidance/counseling, and oral treatment for infants, children, and adolescents. *Pediatric Dentistry, 38*(6), 133–141.

American Academy of Pediatrics. (2015). *Healthy active living for families*, American Academy of Pediatrics. https://www.healthychildren.org/English/healthy-living/nutrition/Pages/Healthy-Active-Living-fo r-Families.aspx.

American Academy of Pediatrics. (2016). *Fruit juice and your child's diet*, American Academy of Pediatrics. https://www.healthychildren.org/English/healthy-living/nutrition/Pages/Fruit-Juice-and-Your-Childs-Diet.aspx.

American Academy of Pediatrics Committee on Nutrition (2014a). Carbohydrate and dietary fiber. In R. E. Kleinman & F. R. Greer (Eds.), *Pediatric nutrition* (7th ed.). Elk Grove Village, IL: American Academy of Pediatrics.

American Academy of Pediatrics Committee on Nutrition (2014b). Feeding the child. In R. E. Kleinman & F. R. Greer (Eds.), *Pediatric nutrition* (7th ed.). Elk Grove Village, IL: American Academy of Pediatrics.

American Academy of Pediatrics Council on Communications and Media. (2016). Media and young minds. *Pediatrics, 138*(5), e20162591.

American Academy of Pediatrics Section on Oral Health. (2014). Maintaining and improving the oral health of young children. *Pediatrics, 134*(6), 1224–1229.

American Speech-Language-Hearing Association. (2017a). *The advantages of being bilingual*, American Speech-Language-Hearing Association. http://www.asha.org/public/speech/development/The-Advantages-of-Bein g-Bilingual/.

American Speech-Language-Hearing Association. (2017b). *Stuttering*, American Speech-Language-Hearing Association. http://www.asha.org/public/speech/disorders/stuttering/.

Coleman, M. R. (2016). Recognizing young children with high potential: U-STARS~PLUS. *Annals of the New York Academy of Sciences, 1377*(1), 32–43.

Drutchas, A., & Anandarajah, G. (2014). Spirituality and coping with chronic disease in pediatrics. *Rhode Island Medical Journal, 97*(3), 26–30.

Duncombe, M. E., Havighurst, S. S., Holland, K. A., et al. (2012). The contribution of parenting practices and parent emotion factors in children at risk for disruptive behavior disorders. *Child Psychiatry and Human Development, 43*(5), 715–733.

Fitzpatrick, C., Barnett, T., & Pagani, L. S. (2012). Early exposure to media violence and later child adjustment. *Journal of Developmental and Behavioral Pediatrics : JDBP, 33*(4), 291–297.

Fleckman, J. M., Drury, S. S., Taylor, C. A., et al. (2016). Role of direct and indirect violence exposure on externalizing behavior in children. *Journal of Urban Health, 93*(3), 479–492.

Ford, C. N., Slining, M. M., & Popkin, B. M. (2013). Trends in dietary intake among US 2- to 6-year-old children, 1989-2008. *Journal of Nutrition and Dietetics, 113*(1), 35–42.

Honaker, S. M., & Meltzer, L. J. (2014). Bedtime problems and night wakings in young children: an update of the evidence. *Paediatric Respiratory Reviews, 15*(4), 333–339.

Jia, S., Wang, L., Shi, Y., et al. (2016). Family risk factors associated with aggressive behavior in Chinese preschool children. *Journal of Pediatric Nursing, 31*(6), e367–e374.

Kellogg, R. (1969). Understanding children's art. In *Readings in psychology today*. Del Mar, CA: Communications/Research/Machines.

Kohlberg, L. (1968). Moral development. In D. L. Sills (Ed.), *International encyclopedia of the social sciences*. New York: MacMillan.

Kosova, E. C., Auinger, P., & Bremer, A. A. (2013). The relationships between sugar-sweetened beverage intake and cardiometabolic markers in young children. *Journal of the Academy of Nutrition & Dietetics, 113*(2), 219–227.

Liu, J., Lewis, G., & Evans, L. (2013). Understanding aggressive behaviour across the lifespan. *Journal of Psychiatric and Mental Health Nursing, 20*(2), 156–168.

Lussier, P., Corrado, R., & Tzoumakis, S. (2012). Gender differences in physical aggression and associated developmental correlates in a sample of Canadian preschoolers. *Behavioral Sciences and the Law, 30*(5), 643–671.

Marshall, T. A. (2013). Preventing dental caries associated with sugar-sweetened beverages. *J Am Dental Assoc, 144*(10), 1148–1152.

McCabe, A., Tamis-LeMonda, C. S., Bornstein, M. H., et al. (2013). Multilingual Children: beyond myths and toward best practices. *Social Policy Report, 27*(4), 1–36.

McCallum, R. S., Bell, S. M., Coles, J. T., et al. (2013). A model for screening twice-exceptional students (gifted with learning disabilities) within a response to intervention paradigm. *Gifted Child Quarterly, 57*(4), 209–222.

McDevitt, S., & Carey, W. (1978). The measurement of temperament in 3-7 year old children. *Journal of Child Psychology and Psychiatry, and Allied Disciplines, 19*(3), 245–253.

McEachern, A. D., & Snyder, J. (2012). Gender differences in predicting antisocial behaviors: developmental consequences of physical and relational aggression. *Journal of Abnormal Child Psychology, 40*(4), 501–512.

National Center on Parent, Family, and Community Engagement. (2014). *Family engagement and school readiness*. http://eclkc.ohs.acf.hhs.gov/hslc/tta-system/family/docs/schoolreadiness-pfce-rtp.pdf.

National Institute on Deafness and Other Communication Disorders, National Institutes of Health. (2016). *Stuttering*. https://www.nidcd.nih.gov/health/stuttering.

Nelson, A. (2013). *Stuttering*, KidsHealth. http://kidshealth.org/en/parents/stutter.html.

Provencal, N., Booij, L., & Tremblay, R. E. (2015). The developmental origins of chronic physical aggression: biological pathways triggered by early life adversity. *Journal of Experimental Biology, 218*(Pt. 1), 123–133.

Strachan, E., & Staples, B. (2012). Masturbation. *Pediatrics in Review, 33*(4), 190–191.

Stricker, P. R. (2015). *Sports goals and applications—preschoolers*. American Academy of Pediatrics, https://www.healthychildren.org/English/ages-stages/preschool/nutrition-fitness/Pages/Sports-Goals-an d-Applications-Preschoolers.aspx.

Tatangelo, G., McCabe, M., Mellor, D., et al. (2016). A systematic review of body dissatisfaction and sociocultural messages related to the body among preschool children. *Body Image, 18*, 86–95.

US Department of Agriculture (2015). *Preschoolers: health and nutrition information*. US Department of Agriculture. https://www.choosemyplate.gov/health-and-nutrition-information.

US Department of Health and Human Services and US Department of Agriculture (2015). *2015–2020 Dietary guidelines for Americans* (8th ed.). US Department of Health and Human Services and US Department of Agriculture. http://health.gov/dietaryguidelines/2015/guidelines/.

Vaivre-Douret, L. (2011). Developmental and cognitive characteristics of "high-level potentialities" (highly gifted) children. *Int J Pediatr, 2011*, 420297.

14

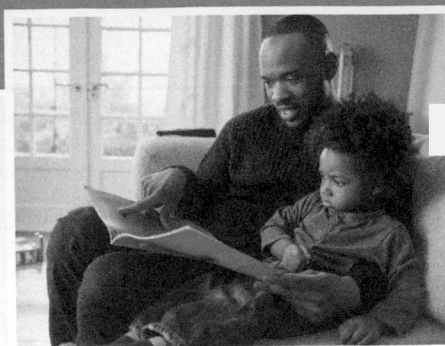

Health Problems of Early Childhood

Brigit M. Carter

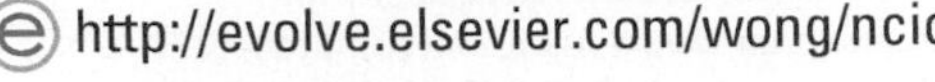

CONCEPTS

- Sleep
- Ingestion of Injurious Agents
- Abuse

SLEEP PROBLEMS

The preschool years are a prime time for sleep disturbances. Children may have trouble going to sleep, wake during the night, have difficulty resuming sleep after waking during the night, have nightmares or sleep terrors, or prolong the inevitable bedtime through elaborate rituals. Such sleep disturbances are typically related to increasing autonomy, negative sleep associations, nighttime fears, inconsistent bedtime routines, and lack of limit setting (Babcock, 2011).

Media use can also contribute to sleep disturbances. Research has revealed a direct correlation between sleep problems in preschool children and evening media use, as well as daytime exposure to violent media content (Garrison, Liekweg, & Christakis, 2011). Specific sleep problems associated with media use include delayed sleep onset, nightmares, night wakings, daytime tiredness, and difficulty waking in the morning (Garrison, Liekweg, & Christakis, 2011). In addition to limiting the duration of television viewing and other media exposure, parents should ensure that all types of media are age appropriate and are not too frightening or overstimulating.

Consequences of inadequate sleep include daytime tiredness, behavior changes, hyperactivity, difficulty concentrating, impaired learning ability, poor control of emotions and impulses, and strain on family relationships (Bhargava, 2011). Nurses should incorporate assessment of sleep patterns and education about the development of healthy sleep behaviors into every well-child visit. Recommendations for handling a sleep disturbance are offered only after a thorough assessment. Cultural traditions may dictate sleep practices contrary to certain well-accepted professional recommendations. Thus parents may not perceive particular sleep habits as problematic (see Cultural Considerations box).

Interventions differ greatly; for example, nightmares and sleep terrors require different approaches (Table 14.1). For children who delay going to bed, a recommended approach involves counseling consistent bedtime ritual and emphasizing the normalcy of this type of behavior in young children. Parents should ignore attention-seeking behavior, and the child should not be taken into the parents' bed or allowed to stay up past a reasonable hour. Other measures that may be helpful include keeping a light on in the room, providing transitional objects such as a favorite toy, or leaving a drink of water by the bed.

CULTURAL CONSIDERATIONS

Co-Sleeping

Many experts recommend that infants and children be trained to always sleep in their own crib or bed. However, co-sleeping, or the "family bed" (in which parents allow the children to sleep with them), is an accepted cultural practice among many African American and Asian families (Mindell, Sadeh, Kohyama, et al., 2010; Ward & Doering, 2014). Others who have adopted co-sleeping include parents who believe that co-sleeping promotes parent-child bonding, parents who think that co-sleeping diminishes their child's nighttime fears or other sleep disturbances, and mothers who are breastfeeding. Co-sleeping may be a practical solution to limited numbers of bedrooms or beds in lower-socioeconomic families. Controversy exists regarding the medical, developmental, and social advantages and disadvantages of co-sleeping. Studies have indicated that co-sleeping is associated with sleep problems, such as frequent night wakings, poor sleep quality, and decreased length of sleep (Mindell, Sadeh, Kohyama, et al., 2010). Parents who are considering co-sleeping should fully investigate the potential risks and benefits. Health care providers should be proactive in discussing sleeping arrangements with families at each visit to ensure children's safety and healthy sleep habits.

Helping children slow down before bedtime also reduces resistance to going to bed. One approach is to establish soothing, limited rituals that signal readiness for bed, such as a bath or story. Parents can reinforce the pattern by stating, "After this story, it is bedtime," and consistently carrying through the routine. If anticipated extra stimulation (e.g., having visitors arrive at the children's bedtime) disrupts this routine, it is advisable to settle children in bed beforehand.

INGESTION OF INJURIOUS AGENTS

Since the passage of the Poison Prevention Packaging Act of 1970, which requires that certain potentially hazardous drugs and household products be sold in child-resistant containers, the incidence of poisonings in children has decreased dramatically. However, despite these advances, poisoning remains a significant health concern, with most cases (49%

TABLE 14.1 **Comparison of Nightmares to Sleep Terrors**

Characteristics	Nightmares	Sleep Terrors
Description	A scary dream; takes place during REM sleep and is followed by full waking	A partial arousal from very deep sleep (stage IV, non-REM) sleep
Time of distress	After dream is over, child wakes and cries or calls; not during nightmare itself	During terror itself, as child screams and thrashes; afterward is calm
Time of occurrence	In second half of night, when dreams are most intense	Usually 1-4 hours after falling asleep, when non-REM sleep is deepest
Child's behavior	Crying in younger children, fright in all; behaviors persistent even though child is awake	Initially may sit up, thrash, or run in bizarre manner, with eyes bulging, heart racing, and profuse perspiring; may cry, scream, talk, or moan; shows apparent fright, anger, or obvious confusion, which disappears when child is fully awake
Responsiveness to others	Is aware of and reassured by another's presence	Is not very aware of another's presence, is not comforted, and may push person away and scream and thrash more if held or restrained
Return to sleep	May be considerably delayed because of persistent fear	Usually rapid; often difficult to keep child awake
Description of dream	Yes (if old enough)	No memory of dream or of yelling or thrashing
interventions	Accept dream as real fear Sit with child; offer comfort, assurance, and sense of protection Avoid forcing child back to his or her own bed Consider professional counseling for recurrent nightmares unresponsive to above approaches	Observe child for a few minutes, without interfering, until child becomes calm or wakes fully Intervene only if necessary to protect child from injury Guide child back to bed if needed Stress to parents that sleep terrors are a normal, common phenomenon in preschoolers that requires relatively little intervention

REM, Rapid eye movement.
Modified from Haupt, M., Sheldon, S. H., & Loghmanee, D. (2013). Just a scary dream? A brief review of sleep terrors, nightmares, and rapid eye movement sleep behavior disorder. *Pediatric Annals, 42*(10), 211-216.

in 2011) occurring in children younger than 6 years old (Bronstein, Spyker, Cantilena, et al., 2012). Although pharmaceuticals (e.g., analgesics, cough and cold preparations, topical preparations, antibiotics, vitamins, gastrointestinal preparations, hormones, and antihistamines) are frequently the agents of poisonings, a variety of other substances can also poison children. The most frequently ingested poisons reported in the American Association of Poison Control Centers' 2015 annual report for children under age 6 include the following:*

- Cosmetics and personal care products (deodorants, makeup, perfume, cologne, mouthwash)
- Household cleaning products (bleaches, laundry pods, disinfectants)
- Medications (acetaminophen, acetylsalicylic acid, ibuprofen, opioids)
- Foreign bodies, toys, and miscellaneous substances (desiccants, thermometers, bubble-blowing solutions)
- Topical preparations
- Vitamins
- Antihistamines
- Pesticides
- Dietary supplements, herbals, homeopathic plants

The American Association of Poison Control Centers also reported recent concerns related to the exposure of e-cigarettes and liquid nicotine. Many poisonings reflect the ready accessibility of the products in the home, which is where more than 90% of poisonings occur (Bronstein, Spyker, Cantilena, et al., 2012). In a review of the American Association of Poison Control Centers, more than 60% of exposures to plants occurred in children 5 years old and younger (Bronstein, Spyker, Cantilena, et al., 2012; Petersen, 2011). Box 14.1 lists common poisonous and nonpoisonous plants.

The developmental characteristics of young children predispose them to poisoning by ingestion. Infants and toddlers explore their environment through oral experimentation. Because their sense of taste is not discriminating at this age, they ingest many unpalatable substances. In addition, toddlers and preschoolers are developing autonomy and initiative, which increases their curiosity and noncompliant behavior. Imitation is also a powerful motivator, especially when combined with a lack of awareness of danger.

This section is primarily concerned with the immediate emergency treatment of ingestion of injurious agents. Box 14.2 summarizes specific management of corrosive, hydrocarbon, acetaminophen, salicylate, iron, and plant poisoning. Because of the importance of lead poisoning among young children, ingestion of lead is discussed separately. Appropriate suggestions for poison prevention are discussed on p. 445.

PRINCIPLES OF EMERGENCY TREATMENT

A poisoning may or may not require emergency intervention, but in every instance medical evaluation is necessary to initiate appropriate action. Advise parents to call the poison control center (PCC) *before* initiating any intervention. Parents should post the local PCC telephone number (usually listed in the front of the telephone directory) near each phone in the house* (see Emergency Treatment box).

Based on the initial telephone assessment, the PCC counsels the parents to begin treatment at home or to take the child to an emergency facility. When a call is taken, the name and telephone number of the caller are recorded to reestablish contact if the connection is interrupted. Because most poisonings are managed in the home, expert advice is essential in minimizing adverse effects. When the exact quantity or type

*The most common substances in each category are in parentheses. Substances ingested are not necessarily the most toxic but often are readily available.

*Also available by calling 800-222-1222 or online at American Association of Poison Control Centers, http://www.aapcc.org.

BOX 14.1 Poisonous and Nonpoisonous Plants

Poisonous Plants (Toxic Parts)

Apple (leaves, seeds)
Apricot (leaves, stem, seed pits)
Azalea (all parts)
Buttercup (all parts)
Castor oil plant (bean or seeds—extremely toxic)
Cherry (wild or cultivated) (twigs, seeds, foliage)
Daffodil (bulbs)
Dumb cane (dieffenbachia) (all parts)
Elephant ear (all parts)
Foxglove (leaves, seeds, flowers)
Holly (berries)
Hyacinth (bulbs)
Ivy (leaves)
Mistletoe* (berries, leaves)
Oak tree (acorn, foliage)
Philodendron (all parts)
Plum (pit)
Poinsettia† (leaves)
Poison ivy, poison oak (leaves, stems, sap, fruit, smoke from burning plants)
Pokeweed, pokeberry (roots, berries, leaves [when eaten raw])
Pothos (all parts)
Rhubarb (leaves)
Tulip (bulbs)
Wisteria (seeds, pods)
Yew (all parts)

Nonpoisonous Plants

African violet
Aluminum plant
Asparagus fern
Begonia
Boston fern
Christmas cactus
Coleus
Gardenia
Grape ivy
Jade plant
Piggyback plant
Poinsettia†
Prayer plant
Rose
Rubber tree
Snake plant
Spider plant
Swedish ivy
Wax plant
Weeping fig
Zebra plant

*Eating one or two berries or leaves is probably nontoxic.
†Mildly toxic if ingested in massive quantities.

BOX 14.2 Selected Poisonings in Children

Corrosives (Strong Acids or Alkalis)

Drain, toilet, and oven cleaners
Electric dishwasher detergent (liquid because of higher pH, is more hazardous than granular)
Mildew remover
Batteries
Clinitest tablets
Denture cleaners
Bleach

Clinical Manifestations

Severe burning pain in the mouth, throat, and stomach
White, swollen mucous membranes; edema of the lips, tongue, and pharynx (respiratory obstruction)
Coughing, hemoptysis
Drooling and inability to clear secretions
Signs of shock
Anxiety and agitation

Comments

Household bleach is a frequently ingested corrosive but rarely causes serious damage.
Liquid corrosives are easily ingested and cause more damage than granular/solid preparations. Liquids may also be aspirated, causing upper airway injury.
Solid products tend to stick to and burn tissues, causing localized damage.

Treatment

Inducing emesis is contraindicated (vomiting further damages the mucosa).
Contact the PCC immediately. If the PCC or medical advice and treatment not immediately available, it may be appropriate to dilute corrosive with water or milk (usually ≤120 ml [4 oz]).
Do not neutralize. Neutralization can cause an exothermic reaction (which produces heat and causes increased symptoms or produces a thermal burn in addition to a chemical burn).
Maintain patent airway as needed.
Administer analgesics.
Give oral fluids when tolerated.
Esophageal stricture may require repeated dilations or surgery.

Hydrocarbons

Gasoline
Kerosene
Lamp oil
Mineral seal oil (found in furniture polish)
Lighter fluid
Turpentine
Paint thinner and remover (some types)

Clinical Manifestations

Gagging, choking, and coughing
Burning throat and stomach
Nausea

BOX 14.2 Selected Poisonings in Children—cont'd

Vomiting
Alterations in sensorium, such as lethargy
Weakness
Respiratory symptoms of pulmonary involvement
- Tachypnea
- Cyanosis
- Retractions
- Grunting

Comments

Immediate danger is aspiration (even small amounts can cause bronchitis and chemical pneumonia).

Gasoline, kerosene, lighter fluid, mineral seal oil, and turpentine cause severe pneumonia.

Treatment

Inducing emesis is generally contraindicated.

Gastric decontamination and emptying are questionable even when the hydrocarbon contains a heavy metal or pesticide; if gastric lavage must be performed, a cuffed endotracheal tube should be in place before lavage because of a high risk of aspiration.

Symptomatic treatment of chemical pneumonia includes high humidity, oxygen, hydration, and acetaminophen.

Acetaminophen

Clinical Manifestations

Occurs in four stages after ingestion:

1. 0 to 24 hours
   - Nausea
   - Vomiting
   - Sweating
   - Pallor
2. 24 to 72 hours
   - Patient improves
   - May have right upper quadrant abdominal pain
3. 72 to 96 hours
   - Pain in right upper quadrant
   - Jaundice
   - Vomiting
   - Confusion
   - Stupor
   - Coagulation abnormalities
   - Sometimes renal failure, pancreatitis
4. More than 5 days
   - Resolution of hepatoxicity or progress to multiple organ failure
   - May be fatal

Comments

This is the most common accidental drug poisoning in children.

Toxicity occurs from acute ingestion. Toxic dose is 150 mg/kg or greater in children.

Treatment

Antidote *N*-acetylcysteine (Mucomyst) is equally effective given intravenously or orally. When given orally may first be diluted in fruit juice or soda because of the antidote's offensive odor. An antiemetic may be given if vomiting occurs.

Given as 1 loading dose followed by 17 additional doses in different dosages. IV administration is given as a continuous infusion.

Aspirin (Acetylsalicylic Acid)

Clinical Manifestations

Acute poisoning (early symptoms):
- Nausea
- Hyperventilation
- Vomiting
- Tinnitus

Acute poisoning (later symptoms):
- Hyperactivity
- Fever
- Confusion
- Seizures
- Renal failure
- Respiratory failure

Chronic poisoning:
- Same as listed above but subtle onset and nonspecific symptoms (often mistaken for viral illness)
- Bleeding tendencies

Comments

May be caused by acute ingestion (severe toxicity occurs with 300 to 500 mg/kg).

May be caused by chronic ingestion (i.e., >100 mg/kg/day for ≥2 days); can be more serious than acute ingestion.

Time to peak serum salicylate level can vary with enteric aspirin or the presence of concretions (bezoars).

Treatment

Hospitalization is necessary for severe toxicity.

Activated charcoal is given as soon as possible (unless contraindicated by altered mental status). If bowel sounds are present, may be repeated every 4 hours until charcoal appears in the stool.

Lavage will not remove concretions of ASA.

Sodium bicarbonate transfusions are used to correct metabolic acidosis, and urinary alkalinization may be effective in enhancing elimination; hypokalemia may interfere with achieving urinary alkalinization.

Be aware of the risk for fluid overload and pulmonary edema.

Use external cooling for hyperpyrexia.

Administer anticonvulsants if seizures present.

Provide oxygen and ventilation for respiratory depression.

Administer vitamin K for bleeding.

In severe cases, hemodialysis (not peritoneal dialysis) is used.

Iron

Mineral supplement or vitamin containing iron

Clinical Manifestations

Occurs in five stages (may have significant variation in symptoms and their progression):

1. Within 6 hours (if child does not develop gastrointestinal symptoms in 6 hours, toxicity is unlikely)
   - Vomiting
   - Hematemesis
   - Diarrhea
   - Hematochezia (bloody stools)
   - Abdominal pain
   - Severe toxicity may have tachypnea, tachycardia, hypotension, coma

Continued

BOX 14.2 Selected Poisonings in Children—cont'd

2. Latency period—up to 24 hours of apparent improvement
3. 12 to 24 hours
    - Metabolic acidosis
    - Fever
    - Hyperglycemia
    - Bleeding
    - Seizures
    - Shock
    - Death (may occur)
4. 2 to 5 days
    - Jaundice
    - Liver failure
    - Hypoglycemia
    - Coma
5. 2 to 5 weeks
    - Pyloric stenosis or duodenal obstruction may occur secondary to scarring.

Comments

Factors related to frequency of iron poisoning include the following:

- Widespread availability
- Packaging of large quantities in individual containers
- Lack of parental awareness of iron toxicity
- Resemblance of iron tablets to candy (e.g., M&Ms)

Toxic dose is based on the amount of elemental iron ingested. Common preparations include ferrous sulfate (20% elemental iron), ferrous gluconate (12%), and ferrous fumarate (33%). Ingestions of 20 to 60 mg/kg are considered mildly to moderately toxic, and >60 mg/kg is severely toxic and may be fatal.

Treatment

Hospitalization is required when more than mild gastroenteritis is present.

Use whole bowel irrigation if radiopaque tablets are visible on abdominal x-ray; may need to be given via nasogastric tube.

Emesis empties the stomach more effectively than lavage.

Activated charcoal does not absorb iron.

Chelation therapy with deferoxamine should be used in severe intoxication (may turn urine red to orange).

If IV deferoxamine is given too rapidly, hypotension, facial flushing, rash, urticaria, tachycardia, and shock may occur; stop the infusion, maintain the IV line with normal saline, and notify the practitioner immediately.

Plants

Poisonous plants listed in Box 14.1

Clinical Manifestations

Depends on type of plant ingested.

May cause local irritation of oropharynx and entire gastrointestinal tract.

May cause respiratory, renal, and central nervous system symptoms.

Topical contact with plants can cause dermatitis.

Comments

Plants are some of the most frequently ingested substances.

They rarely cause serious problems, although some plant ingestions can be fatal.

Plants can also cause choking and allergic reactions.

Treatment

Wash from skin or eyes.

Provide supportive care as needed.

ASA, Acetylsalicylic acid; *IV*, intravenous; *PCC*, poison control center.

EMERGENCY TREATMENT

Poisoning

1. Assess the victim:
    - Initiate cardiorespiratory support if needed (circulation, airway, breathing).
    - Assess mental status; reevaluate routinely.
    - Take vital signs; reevaluate routinely.
    - Evaluate for possibility of concomitant trauma or illness; treat before initiation of gastric decontamination.
2. Terminate exposure:
    - Empty mouth of pills, plant parts, or other material.
    - Flush any body surface (including the eyes) exposed to a toxin with large amounts of moderately warm water or saline.
    - Remove contaminated clothes, including socks and shoes, and jewelry. Ensure protection of rescuers and health care workers from exposure.
    - Bring victim of an inhalation poisoning into fresh air.
3. Identify the poison:
    - Question the victim and witnesses.
    - Observe the circumstances surrounding the poisoning (e.g., location, activity before ingestion).
    - Look for environmental clues (empty container, nearby spill, odor on breath) and save all evidence of poison (container, vomitus, urine).
    - Be alert to signs and symptoms of potential poisoning in the absence of other evidence, including symptoms of ocular or dermal exposure.
    - Call the poison control center or other competent emergency facility for immediate advice regarding treatment.
4. Prevent poison absorption:
    - Place the child in a side-lying, sitting, or kneeling position with the head below the chest to prevent aspiration.

of ingested toxin is not known, admission to a health care facility with pediatric emergency treatment services for laboratory evaluation and surveillance during the time after ingestion is critical.

Assessment

The first and most important principle in dealing with a poisoning is to treat the child first, not the poison. This requires an immediate concern for life support. Vital signs are taken, mental status assessed, and respiratory or circulatory support is instituted as needed. The child's condition is routinely reevaluated. Because shock is a complication of several types of household poisons, particularly corrosives, measures to reduce the effects of shock are important, beginning with circulation, airway, and breathing support measures—the CABs of resuscitation. Establishing and maintaining vascular access for rapid intravascular volume expansion is vital in the treatment of pediatric shock.

The emergency department nurse's responsibility is to be prepared for immediate intervention with all of the necessary equipment. Because time and speed are critical factors in recovery from serious poisonings, anticipation of potential problems and complications may mean the difference between life and death.

Gastric Decontamination

Although pediatric poison ingestions are common, they rarely result in significant morbidity or mortality (Bronstein, Spyker, Cantilena, et al., 2012). Consider using gastrointestinal decontamination (GID) only after careful evaluation of the potential toxicity of the poison and the risks versus benefits. GID (e.g., ipecac, activated charcoal, and gastric lavage) is not routinely recommended for most childhood poisonings. Because of continuing controversy regarding the use of these methods, treat each toxic ingestion individually (Albertson, Owen, Sutter, et al., 2011). Specific antidotes may be administered for certain poisonings.

! NURSING ALERT

Syrup of ipecac is not recommended for routine poison treatment intervention in the home (Albertson, Owen, Sutter, et al., 2011; Theurer & Bhavsar, 2013). Syrup of ipecac is an emetic that exerts its action through irritation of the gastric mucosa and by stimulation of the vomiting center; however, the American Academy of Pediatrics no longer recommends its use for routine treatment of poison ingestion and suggests disposal of bottles of syrup of ipecac from the home.

One method of GID is the use of activated charcoal, an odorless, tasteless, fine black powder that absorbs many compounds, creating a stable complex (Frithsen & Simpson, 2010). The use of activated charcoal has become less common, and it was used in only 1.1% of pediatric toxic exposures in 2015 (Mowry, Spyker, Brooks, et al., 2016). Activated charcoal may be considered in the following situations:

- Child may have ingested large amounts of carbamazepine, dapsone, phenobarbital, quinine, or theophylline.
- Time to activated charcoal administration is within 1 hour after the poison ingestion.
- Child has an intact or protected airway.

Activated charcoal is mixed with water or a saline cathartic to form a slurry. Slurries are neither gritty nor distasteful but resemble black mud. To increase the child's acceptance of activated charcoal, the nurse should mix it with small amounts of chocolate milk, fruit syrup, or cola drinks and serve it through a straw in an opaque container with a cover (e.g., a disposable coffee cup and lid) or an ordinary cup covered with aluminum foil or placed inside a small paper bag. Superactivated charcoal has three to four times the surface area and can absorb greater quantities of poison (Olson, 2010). For small children, a nasogastric tube may be required to administer activated charcoal. Potential complications from the use of activated charcoal include vomiting and potential aspiration, constipation, and intestinal obstruction (in multiple doses) (Albertson, Owen, Sutter, et al., 2011).

If the child is admitted to an emergency facility, gastric lavage may be performed to empty the stomach of the toxic agent; however, this procedure can be associated with serious complications (gastrointestinal perforation, hypoxia, aspiration). There is no conclusive evidence that gastric lavage decreases morbidity, and it is no longer recommended to be performed routinely, if at all (Albertson, Owen, Sutter, et al., 2011; Benson, Hoppu, Troutman, et al., 2013). In addition, gastric lavage may be of little benefit if used later than 1 hour after ingestion (Albertson, Owen, Sutter, et al., 2011; McGregor, Parkar, & Rao, 2009). Conditions that may be appropriate for the use of gastric lavage include presentation within 1 hour of ingestion of a toxin, ingestion in patient who has decreased gastrointestinal motility, the ingestion of a toxic amount of sustained-release medication, and a large or life-threatening amount of poison (Albertson, Owen, Sutter, et al., 2011). When gastric lavage is used, the patient requires a protected airway, possible sedation, and the largest diameter tube that can be inserted to facilitate passage of gastric contents. Gastric lavage should only be performed by medical personnel with proper training and expertise (Benson, Hoppu, Troutman, et al., 2013).

In a minority of poisonings, specific antidotes are available to counteract the poison. They are highly effective and should be available in all emergency facilities. The supply of antidotes should be checked routinely and replaced as used or according to expiration dates. Antidotes available to treat toxin ingestion include *N*-acetylcysteine for acetaminophen poisoning, oxygen for carbon monoxide inhalation, naloxone for opioid overdose, flumazenil (Romazicon) for benzodiazepine (diazepam [Valium], midazolam [Versed]) overdose, digoxin immune fab (Digibind) for digoxin toxicity, amyl nitrate for cyanide, and antivenin for certain poisonous bites.

Prevention of Recurrence

The ultimate objective is to prevent poisonings from occurring or recurring. Home safety education improves poison prevention practices (Kendrick, Young, Mason-Jones, et al., 2012). Research supports the effectiveness of parent education on preventing unintentional injuries (Kendrick, Mulvaney, Ye, et al., 2013). One effective counseling method is first to discuss the difficulties of constantly watching and safeguarding young children (see Family-Centered Care box). In this way, the challenging task of raising children can lead to a discussion of injury prevention as part of the parental role. This approach also incorporates contributory causes for the incident, such as inadequate support systems; marital discord; discipline techniques (especially use of physical punishment); and any disruption in the family or family activities, such as vacations, moves, visitors, illnesses, or births. A visit to the home, especially after repeat poisonings, is recommended as part of the follow-up care to assess hazards, including family factors, and to evaluate appropriate injury-proofing measures. One method of identifying risk areas is to ask specific questions or to have the parent complete a questionnaire designed to isolate factors that predispose children to poisoning. Another approach is to encourage parents to bend down to the child's eye level and survey the home environment for potential hazards. Have the parents try to open cabinets and reach shelves to access poisons.

FAMILY-CENTERED CARE

Poisoning

A poisoning is more than a physical emergency for the child; it also usually represents an emotional crisis for the parents, particularly in terms of guilt, self-reproach, and insecurity in the parenting role. The emergency department is no place to admonish the family for negligence, lack of appropriate supervision, or failure to injury-proof the home. Rather, it is a time to calm and support the child and parents while unaccusingly exploring the circumstances of the injury. If the nurse prematurely attempts to discuss ways of preventing such an incident from recurring, the parents' anxiety will block out any suggestions or offered guidance. Therefore it is preferable for the nurse to delay the discussion until the child's condition is stabilized or, if the child is discharged immediately after emergency treatment, to make a public health referral or send a packet of information.

Passive measures (those that do not require active participation) have been the most successful in preventing poisoning and include using child-resistant closures and limiting the number of tablets in one container. However, these measures alone are not sufficient to prevent poisoning because most toxic agents in the home do not have safety closures. Therefore active measures (those that require participation) are essential. The Nursing Care Guidelines box lists the guidelines for preventing the occurrence or recurrence of a poisoning.

HEAVY METAL POISONING

Heavy metal poisoning can occur from the ingestion of a variety of substances, the most common being lead. Other sources that are important in terms of children are iron and mercury. Mercury toxicity, a rare form of heavy metal poisoning, has occurred in children from a

NURSING CARE GUIDELINES

Poison Prevention

- Assess possible contributing factors in occurrence of injury, such as discipline, parent-child relationship, developmental ability, environmental factors, and behavior problems.
- Institute anticipatory guidance for possible future injuries based on child's age and developmental level.
- Initiate referral to appropriate agency to evaluate home environment and need for injury-proofing measures.
- Provide assistance with environmental manipulation, such as lead removal, when necessary.
- Educate parents regarding safe storage of toxic substances.
- Advise parents to take drugs out of sight of children.
- Teach children the hazards of ingesting nonfood items.
- Advise parents against using plants for teas or medicine.
- Discuss problems of discipline and children's noncompliance and offer strategies for effective discipline.
- Instruct parents regarding correct administration of drugs for therapeutic purposes and to discontinue drug if there is evidence of mild toxicity.
- Advise parents to contact the PCC (800-222-1222) or practitioner immediately when a poisoning occurs.
- Tell them to post the number of the regional PCC with an emergency phone list by the telephone.
- Include by the telephone the home address with nearest cross street in case an ambulance is needed. (In an emergency, family members may not remember the house address, and babysitters may not be aware of the information.)

PCC, Poison control center.

variety of sources, such as predator fish (king mackerel, shark, swordfish, tilefish), broken thermometers or thermostats, broken fluorescent light bulbs, disk batteries, topical medications, gas regulators, cathartics, and interior latex house paint (Bose-O'Reilly, McCarthy, Steckling, et al., 2010). Elemental mercury (also called *metallic mercury* or *quicksilver*) is nontoxic if ingested and if the gastrointestinal tract is healthy (e.g., has no fistulas). However, mercury is volatile at room temperature and enters the bloodstream after it is inhaled. Chronic exposure produces symptoms ranging from nonspecific (e.g., anorexia, weight loss, memory loss, insomnia, gingivitis, diarrhea) to severe (e.g., tremors, extreme behavior changes, delirium). The classic form of mercury poisoning is called acrodynia (or "painful extremities").

NURSING ALERT

Mercury thermometers are no longer recommended because if they are broken, the inhaled vapors can cause toxicity. To prevent inhalation, clean up spilled mercury quickly, using disposable towels and rubber gloves and washing the hands well afterward.

Heavy metals have an affinity for certain essential tissue chemicals, which must remain free for adequate cell functioning. When metals are bound to these substances, cellular enzyme systems are inactivated. Treatment involves chelation, use of a chemical compound that combines with the metal for rapid and safe excretion.

LEAD POISONING

Poisoning from lead has been a problem throughout history and throughout the world. In the United States the problem became apparent in the early 1900s when white lead was added to paints and when tetraethyl lead was added to gasoline as an antiknock compound. Lead content in paint was decreased in 1950, and in 1978 the use of lead in household paint was banned. The use of lead in paint and leaded gasoline has been banned in the United States. After this change in policy, the average blood lead level (BLL) in the United States for people 1 to 74 years old dropped from 12.8 mcg/dl in 1980 to 1.3 mcg/dl in 2010 (Centers for Disease Control and Prevention, 2012; 2017). However, children continue to be exposed to lead; an estimated 0.8% of children in the United States 1 to 5 years old had BLLs of more than 10 mcg/dl in 2010, and more than 5% had BLLs of 5 mcg/dl or higher (Centers for Disease Control and Prevention, 2017).

Causes of Lead Poisoning

Although there are numerous sources of lead (Box 14.3), in most instances of acute childhood lead poisoning, the source is nonintact lead-based paint in an older home or lead-contaminated bare soil in the yard. Microparticles of lead gain entrance into a child's body through ingestion or inhalation and, in the case of an exposed pregnant woman, by placental transfer. When measured, a mother's lead level is nearly the same as

BOX 14.3 Sources of Lead*

Lead-based paint in deteriorating condition
Lead solder
Lead crystal
Battery casings
Lead fishing sinkers
Lead curtain weights
Lead bullets
Some of these may contain lead:

- Ceramic ware
- Water
- Pottery
- Pewter
- Dyes
- Industrial factories
- Vinyl miniblinds
- Playground equipment
- Collectible toys
- Some imported toys or children's metal jewelry
- Artists' paints
- Pool cue chalk

Occupations and hobbies involving lead:

- Battery and aircraft manufacturing
- Lead smelting
- Brass foundry work
- Radiator repair
- Construction work
- Furniture refinishing
- Bridge repair work
- Painting contracting
- Mining
- Ceramics work
- Stained-glass making
- Jewelry making

*The US Consumer Product Safety Commission issues alerts and recalls for products that contain lead and may unexpectedly pose a hazard to young children. Additional information is available from Alliance for Healthy Homes, http://www.cehn.org/alliance_healthy_homes.

that of her unborn child. Although the level of lead may not be harmful to adult women, it can be harmful to the fetuses.

Whereas inhalation exposure usually occurs during renovation and remodeling activities in the home, ingestion happens during normal day-to-day play and mouthing activities. Sometimes a child will actually swallow loose chips of lead-based paint because it has a sweet taste. Water and food may also be contaminated with lead. A child does not need to eat loose paint chips to be exposed to the toxin; normal hand-to-mouth behavior, coupled with the presence of lead dust in the environment that has settled over decades, is the usual method of poisoning (Bose-O'Reilly, McCarthy, Steckling, et al., 2010; Campbell, Gracely, Tran, et al., 2012).

Because of family, cultural, or ethnic traditions, a source of lead may be a routine part of life for a child. Nurses must educate themselves about the practices of their patients and identify when such products may be a source of lead. The use of pottery or dishes containing lead may be an issue, as may the use of folk remedies for stomachaches or the use of some cosmetics (see Cultural Considerations box). Children of immigrants and internationally adopted children may have been exposed to sources of lead before arrival in the United States and should be carefully evaluated for lead exposure (Raymond, Kennedy, & Brown, 2013). Other risk factors for having an elevated BLL include living in poverty, being younger than 6 years old, dwelling in urban areas, and living in older rental homes where lead decontamination may not be a priority. Nurses are often in a position to observe or elicit information about these practices and educate families about their potential harm.

CULTURAL CONSIDERATIONS

Sources of Lead

In some cultures, the use of traditional ethnic remedies that contain lead may increase children's risk of lead poisoning. These remedies include the following:

Azarcon (Mexico): For digestive problems; a bright orange powder; usual dose is 0.25 to 1 tsp, often mixed with oil, milk, or sugar or sometimes given as a tea; sometimes a pinch is added to a baby bottle or tortilla dough for preventive purposes

Greta (Mexico): A yellow-orange powder used in the same way as azarcon

Paylooah (Southeast Asia): Used for rash or fever; an orange-red powder given as 0.5 tsp straight or in a tea

Surma (India and Pakistan): Black powder used as a cosmetic and as teething powder

Unknown ayurvedic (Tibet): Small, gray-brown balls used to improve slow development; two balls are given orally three times a day

Tamarind jellied, fruit candy (Mexico): Fruit candy packaged in paper wrappers that contain high lead levels

Lozeena (Iraq): A bright orange powder used to color meat and rice

Litargirio (Dominican Republic): Yellow or peach-colored powder used as a folk remedy and as an antiperspirant/deodorant

Ba-Baw-San (China): Herbal medicine used to treat colic pain

Modified from Centers for Disease Control and Prevention. (1993). Lead poisoning associated with use of traditional ethnic remedies—California, 1991-1992. *MMWR Morbidity and Mortality Weekly Report, 42*(27), 521-524; Centers for Disease Control and Prevention. (1998). Lead poisoning associated with imported candy and powdered food coloring—California and Michigan. *MMWR Morbidity and Mortality Weekly Report, 47*(48), 1041-1043; Centers for Disease Control and Prevention. (2002). Childhood lead poisoning associated with tamarind candy and folk remedies—California, 1992-2000. *MMWR Morbidity and Mortality Weekly Report, 51*(31), 684-686; Centers for Disease Control and Prevention. (2005). Lead poisoning associated with use of litargirio—Rhode Island. *MMWR Morbidity and Mortality Weekly Report, 54*(09), 227-229.

Pathophysiology and Clinical Manifestation

Lead can affect any part of the body, including the renal, hematologic, and neurologic systems (Fig. 14.1). Of most concern for young children is the developing brain and nervous system, which are more vulnerable than those of older children and adults. Lead in the body moves via an equilibration process between the blood, the soft tissues and organs, and the bones and teeth. Lead ultimately settles in the bones and teeth, where it remains inert and in storage. This makes up the largest portion of the body burden, approximately 75% to 90%. At the cellular level, it competes with molecules of calcium, interfering with the regulating action of calcium. In the brain, lead disrupts the biochemical processes and may have a direct effect on the release of neurotransmitters, may cause alterations in the blood-brain barrier, and may interfere with the regulation of synaptic activity (Cunningham, 2012; Jones, 2009).

There is a relationship between anemia and lead poisoning. Children who are iron deficient absorb lead more readily than those with sufficient iron stores. Lead can interfere with the binding of iron onto the heme molecule. This sometimes creates a picture of anemia even though the child is not iron deficient. Lead toxicity to the erythrocytes leads to the release of the enzyme erythrocyte protoporphyrin (EP). Because EP is not sensitive to BLLs of less than about 16 to 25 mcg/dl, it is no longer used as a screening test. Therefore the BLL test is currently used for screening and diagnosis. However, elevation of the EP level (>35 mcg/dl of whole blood) is a good indicator of toxicity from lead and reflects the length of exposure and body burden of lead in an individual child.

Although adults have been shown to experience adverse renal effects from occupational lead exposure, few studies document renal effects in children except at extremely high lead levels. One can hypothesize that lead can affect the renal integrity of children as well as adults. Therefore the renal system of a child is still considered a potential target for the harmful effects of lead.

The lead levels identified in children have declined since the initiation of screening for children at risk for lead poisoning. With earlier intervention, the most prevalent effects have changed. Since the late 1960s, children have rarely died of lead poisoning, and seizures and cognitive impairment have become less likely. However, even mild and moderate lead poisoning can cause a number of cognitive and behavioral problems in young children, including aggression, hyperactivity, impulsivity, delinquency, disinterest, and withdrawal. Long-term neurocognitive signs of lead poisoning include developmental delays, lowered intelligence quotient (IQ), reading skill deficits, visual-spatial problems, visual-motor problems, learning disabilities, and lower academic success. Chronic lead toxicity may also affect physical growth and reproductive efficiency (Jones, 2009).

Diagnostic Evaluation

Children with lead poisoning rarely have symptoms even at levels requiring chelation therapy. A diagnosis of lead poisoning is based only on the lead testing of a venous blood specimen from a venipuncture. The collection process is important. Blood must be collected carefully to avoid contamination by lead on the skin. The acceptable BLL has dropped from 40 mcg/dl in 1970 to 10 mcg/dl today (Chandran & Cataldo, 2010).

Anticipatory Guidance

The most effective prevention of lead exposure is ensuring that environmental exposures are reduced before children are exposed. The following information should be made available to families beginning during prenatal and postnatal care (Centers for Disease Control and Prevention Advisory Committee on Childhood Lead Poisoning Prevention, 2012):

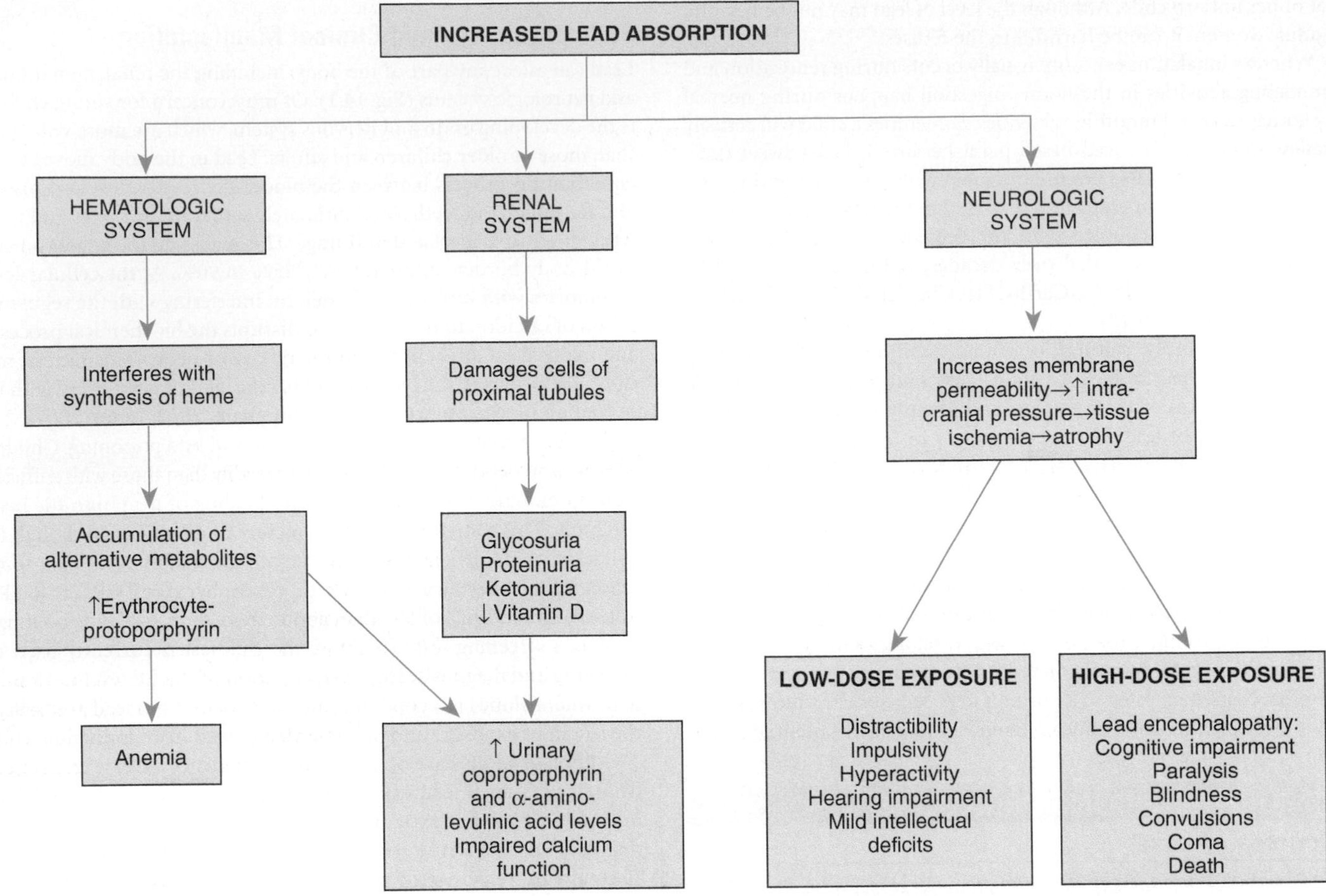

FIG. 14.1 Main effects of lead on body systems.

- Hazards of lead-based paint in older housing
- Ways to control lead hazards safely
- How to choose safe toys
- Hazards accompanying repainting and renovation of homes built before 1978
- Other exposure sources, such as traditional remedies, that might be relevant for a family

There has been recent concern regarding toys and other imported items children play with that were found to contain lead. Parents should carefully evaluate the source of the toy (manufacturer) or item the child may play with and not assume it is safe because it is sold in a US market. The US Consumer Product Safety Commission (http://www.cpsc.gov) is an excellent resource for parents and caregivers concerned about the safety of a given toy or product that may be harmful.

Screening for Lead Poisoning

When primary prevention fails, secondary prevention screening efforts for elevated BLLs can identify children much earlier than in the past. This need is established using BLL surveillance and other risk factor data collected over time to establish the status and risk of children throughout the state. Universal screening should be done at 1 and 2 years old. Any child between 3 and 6 years old who has not been previously screened should also be tested. All children with risk factors should be screened more often.

Targeted screening is acceptable when an area has been determined by existing data to have less risk. Children should be screened when they live in a high-risk geographic area or are members of a group determined to be at risk (e.g., Medicaid recipients) or if their family cannot answer "no" to the following personal risk questions:

- Does your child live in or regularly visit a house that was built before 1950?
- Does your child live in or regularly visit a house built before 1978 with recent or ongoing renovations or remodeling within the past 6 months?
- Does your child have a sibling or playmate who has or had lead poisoning?

Therapeutic Management

The degree of concern, urgency, and need for medical intervention change as the lead level increases. Education is one of the most important elements of the treatment process. Areas that the nurse needs to discuss with the family of every child who has an elevated BLL (≥5 mcg/dl) include the following (Centers for Disease Control and Prevention Advisory Committee on Childhood Lead Poisoning Prevention, 2012):

- The child's BLL and what it means
- Potential adverse health effects of an elevated BLL
- Sources of lead exposure and suggestions on how to reduce exposure, such as the importance of wet cleaning to remove lead dust on floors, windowsills, and other surfaces
- Importance of good nutrition in reducing the absorption and effects of lead; for persons with poor nutritional patterns, adequate intake of calcium and iron and importance of regular meals
- Need for follow-up testing to monitor the child's BLL
- Results of an environmental investigation if applicable

TABLE 14.2 Centers for Disease Control and Prevention's Blood Lead Level Test

Blood Lead Level (mcg/dl)	Action
<5	Provide family with lead education. Reassess or rescreen in 1 year. If exposure status changes, do this sooner.
5-14	Provide family with lead education, regular developmental/behavioral surveillance, and social service referral if necessary. Provide follow-up testing within 1 month, and then every 3-4 months.
15-19	Provide family with lead education, regular developmental/behavioral surveillance, and social service referral if necessary. Provide follow-up testing within 1 month, and then every 3-4 months. Initiate professional environmental cleanup. Follow guidelines for BLL of 20-44 mcg/dl if BLL remains 15 mcg/dl or higher on two samples obtained at least 3 months apart.
20-44	Provide family with lead education, regular developmental/behavioral surveillance, and social service referral if necessary. Refer to clinical center specializing in lead poisoning. Provide both clinical and environmental management. Consider treating with appropriate chelation therapy.
45-69	Provide lead education. Refer to clinical center specializing in lead poisoning; provide coordination of care. Provide diagnostic testing within 24-48 hours. Perform clinical evaluation and management within 48 hours. Provide appropriate chelation therapy. Ensure aggressive environmental intervention. Follow up testing at least once per month.
70 or over	*Immediately* provide diagnostic testing and initiate chelation therapy. Begin other activities (listed above).

- Hazards of improper removal of lead paint (dry sanding, scraping, or open-flame burning)

Treatment actions vary depending on the child's BLL. Based on a diagnosis from a venous BLL test, the Centers for Disease Control and Prevention (2002) recommends the actions found in Table 14.2.

Chelation Therapy

Chelation is the term used for removing lead from circulating blood and, theoretically, some lead from organs and tissues. It is unclear whether chelation affects lead stores in bones. Although not an antidote in the truest sense, it does serve a similar purpose in that the toxic substance or poison is removed from the body. However, chelation does not counteract any effects of the lead.

Historically, three chelating agents have been used consistently: calcium disodium edetate ($CaNa_2EDTA$, or calcium EDTA), British antilewisite (BAL; dimercaprol, dimercaptopropanol), and meso-2,3-dimercaptosuccinic acid (DMSA, Chemet, Succimer). BAL (dimercaprol, dimercaptopropanol) is used in conjunction with EDTA with high lead levels or the presence of lead encephalopathy. All of the agents have potential toxic side effects and contraindications. Renal, hepatic, and hematologic parameters should be monitored.

Because of the equilibration process between blood, soft tissues, and other sites in the body, there is often a rebound of the BLL after chelation. After the body burden of lead is reduced enough to stabilize the BLL, rebound will cease. Multiple chelation treatments may be necessary. Adequate hydration is essential during therapy because the chelates are excreted via the kidneys.

Severe lead toxicity (lead level ≥70 mcg/dl) requires immediate inpatient treatment, whether symptoms are present or not. BAL is contraindicated in children with peanut allergies or hepatic insufficiency, nor should it be given in conjunction with iron. Also, use with caution in children with renal impairment or hypertension; monitor for hemolysis with presence of glucose 6-phosphate dehydrogenase deficiency. It must be given only at a deep intramuscular site, in repeated doses over several days. Calcium EDTA should be given intravenously or intramuscularly (in a different site from BAL). The intravenous route should not be used in children with cerebral edema.

For lead levels of 45 to 69 mcg/dl and an absence of symptoms, DMSA can be used. The capsule is opened and sprinkled on a small amount of food or may be swallowed whole. DMSA can be used in conjunction with iron. Adverse effects include nausea, vomiting, diarrhea, loss of appetite, rash, elevated liver function tests, and neutropenia. Because the chelates are excreted via the kidneys, adequate hydration is essential.

A less used oral chelating agent, d-penicillamine, is sometimes used to treat lead poisoning, but the medication is not approved by the US Food and Drug Administration for use in the United States (Dapul & Laraque, 2014).

Prognosis

Although most of the pathophysiologic effects of lead are reversible, the most serious consequences of both high and low lead exposure are the effects on the central nervous system. In children with lead encephalopathy, permanent brain damage can result in cognitive impairment, behavior changes, possible paralysis, and seizures. However, low-dose exposure may also cause permanent neurologic deficits. Increased distractibility, short attention span, impulsivity, reading disabilities, and school failure have been associated with lead exposure (Centers for Disease Control and Prevention Advisory Committee on Childhood Lead Poisoning Prevention, 2012).

Nursing Care Management

The primary nursing goal in lead poisoning is to prevent the child's initial or further exposure to lead. For children with low-level exposure, this requires identifying the sources of lead in the environment. Careful history taking is the most useful and most valuable tool and should concentrate on the personal risk questions. Suggestions for reducing lead in the child's environment are listed in the Community and Home Health Considerations box.

For children who undergo chelation therapy, the nurse prepares them for the injections and makes all efforts to reduce injection pain. Chelating agents are administered deeply into a large muscle mass (see Atraumatic Care box). To lessen the pain from calcium EDTA, the local anesthetic procaine is injected with the drug. Rotation of sites is essential to prevent the formation of painful areas of fibrotic tissue. Because calcium EDTA and lead are toxic to the kidneys, keep records of intake and output, and assess the results of urinalysis to monitor renal functioning.

Discharge planning for children with lead poisoning must include thorough education of families regarding safety from lead hazards, clear instructions regarding medication administration and follow-up, and confirmation that the child will be discharged to a home without lead

COMMUNITY AND HOME HEALTH CONSIDERATIONS

Reducing Blood Lead Levels

- Make certain children do not have access to peeling paint or chewable surfaces painted with lead-based paint, especially windowsills and wells.
- If a house was built before 1978 and has hard-surface floors, wet mop them at least once per week. Wipe other hard surfaces (e.g., windowsills, baseboards). If there are loose paint chips in an area, such as a window well, use a wet disposable cloth to pick up and discard them. Do not vacuum hard-surfaced floors or windowsills or wells because this spreads dust. Use vacuum cleaners with agitators to remove dust from rugs rather than vacuum cleaners with suction only. If a rug is known to contain lead dust and cannot be washed, it should be discarded.
- Wash and dry children's hands and faces frequently, especially before eating.
- Wash toys and pacifiers frequently.
- Wipe your feet on mats before entering the home, especially if you work in occupations where lead is used. Removing your shoes when you are entering the home is a good practice to control lead.
- If soil around home is or is likely to be contaminated with lead (e.g., if the home was built before 1978 or is near a major highway), plant grass or other ground cover; plant bushes around outside of the house so that children cannot play there.
- During remodeling of older homes, follow correct procedures. Be certain children and pregnant women are not in the home, day or night, until the process is completed. After deleading, thoroughly clean the house using cleaning solution to a damp mop and dust before inhabitants return.
- In areas where lead content of water exceeds the drinking water standard and a particular faucet has not been used for 6 hours or more, "flush" the cold-water pipes by running the water until it becomes as cold as it will get (30 seconds to 2 minutes). The more time water has been sitting in pipes, the more lead it may contain.
- *Use only cold water* for consumption (drinking, cooking, and especially for reconstituting powder infant formula). Hot water dissolves lead more quickly than cold water and thus contains higher levels of lead. It is acceptable to use first-flush water for nonconsumption uses (e.g., bathing).
- Have water tested by a competent laboratory. This action is especially important for apartment dwellers; flushing may not be effective in high-rise buildings and in other buildings with lead-soldered central piping.
- Do not store food in open cans, particularly if cans are imported.
- Do not use pottery or ceramic ware that was inadequately fired or is meant for decorative use for food storage or service. Do not store drinks or food in lead crystal.
- Avoid folk remedies or cosmetics that contain lead.
- Avoid candy imported from Mexico (e.g., tamarind hard candy).
- Avoid imported toys and toy jewelry that may contain lead.
- Make certain that home exposure is not occurring from parental occupations or hobbies. Household members employed in occupations such as lead smelting should shower and change into clean clothing before leaving work. Construction and lead abatement workers may also bring home lead contaminants.
- Ensure that children eat regular meals because more lead is absorbed on an empty stomach.
- Ensure that children's diets contain sufficient iron and calcium and not excessive fat.
- Consider iron supplementation if child does not regularly consume foods rich in iron.

Modified from Centers for Disease Control and Prevention. (2017). *Lead home.* Retrieved from http://www.cdc.gov/nceh/lead/

ATRAUMATIC CARE

Lead Chelation Therapy

To lessen the pain from intramuscular injection of calcium disodium edetate ($CaNa_2EDTA$ or calcium EDTA), the local anesthetic procaine is injected with the drug. Apply topical anesthetic cream such as eutectic mixture of local anesthetic (e.g., lidocaine-prilocaine [EMLA]) or LMX4 (4% lidocaine) over the puncture site before the injection of EDTA and British antilewisite (BAL) (time per manufacturer's guidelines).

! NURSING ALERT

Use extreme caution with chelating agents. Incidences of child death from hypocalcemia have been recorded when Na_2EDTA was substituted for $CaNa_2EDTA$ and used as a chelating agent (Fountain & Reith, 2014).

! NURSING ALERT

Adequate urinary output must be ensured with administration of calcium EDTA. Children receiving the drug intramuscularly must be able to maintain adequate oral intake of fluids.

hazards. Although the nurse must use caution to avoid alarming parents unnecessarily, it is important that they know the risk implications for their child's behavior and cognitive functions. Nurses should observe the development and behavior of children who are hospitalized. Thoroughly evaluate any concerns that are identified. Referral to a child development or speech and language specialist may be necessary.

As in any situational crisis, parents need support and understanding if their child is treated for lead poisoning. Many families at the highest risk for lead poisoning have the fewest resources to comply with measures such as relocation or removal of lead from the environment where the child experiences exposure.

CHILD MALTREATMENT

The broad term child maltreatment includes intentional physical abuse or neglect, emotional abuse or neglect, and sexual abuse of children, usually by adults. It is one of the most significant social problems affecting children. In 2015 Child Protective Service agencies in the United States confirmed that an estimated 683,000 children were victims of one or more types of child maltreatment. Of the confirmed cases, about 17.2% suffered physical abuse, 8.4% sexual abuse, 75.3% neglect, and 6.9% psychologic maltreatment or emotional abuse. In 2015 there were an estimated 1585 child fatalities as a result of child abuse and neglect (US Department of Health and Human Services, 2015). Reported statistics only partially represent the actual incidence of child maltreatment because many cases are believed to go unreported.*

CHILD NEGLECT

Child neglect is the most common form of maltreatment, and 74.8% of reported neglect cases involve children 3 years old or younger (US

*Additional information is available from the Children's Bureau, Administration for Children and Families, 370 L'Enfant Promenade SW, Washington, DC 20447; https://www.acf.hhs.gov/cb.

Department of Health and Human Services, 2015). Of the children who died, 72.9% suffered from neglect either exclusively or in combination with another type of maltreatment (US Department of Health and Human Services, 2015). Neglect is generally defined as the failure of a parent or other person legally responsible for the child's welfare to provide for the child's basic needs and an adequate level of care.

Important contributing factors for child neglect are lack of knowledge of child's needs, lack of resources, and caregiver substance abuse. For example, neglectful parents often demonstrate poor parenting skills. They may be unaware that an infant needs to be fed every 3 to 4 hours, may not know what to feed the child, and may have insufficient funds to buy food. The most serious lack of knowledge is failure to recognize emotional nurturing as an essential need of children. (See also Failure to Thrive, Chapter 8.)

Types of Neglect

Neglect takes many forms and can be classified broadly as physical or emotional maltreatment. Physical neglect involves the deprivation of necessities, such as food, clothing, shelter, supervision, medical care, and education. Emotional neglect generally refers to failure to meet the child's needs for affection, attention, and emotional nurturance.

Neglect may also include lack of intervention for or fostering of maladaptive behavior, such as delinquency or substance abuse. Emotional abuse or psychologic maltreatment, an even more difficult aspect of maltreatment to define, refers to the deliberate attempt to destroy or significantly impair a child's self-esteem or competence. Emotional abuse may take the form of rejecting, isolating, terrorizing, ignoring, corrupting, verbally assaulting, or over pressuring the child (Hibbard, Barlow, MacMillan, et al., 2012).

PHYSICAL ABUSE

The deliberate infliction of physical injury on a child, usually by the child's caregiver, is termed *physical abuse.* Physical abuse can include anything from bruises and fractures to brain damage. Minor physical injury is responsible for more reported cases of maltreatment than major physical injury, but major physical abuse causes more deaths. In 2015, 43.9% of fatalities from abuse suffered physical abuse alone or in combination with other types of maltreatment (US Department of Health and Human Services, 2015). Despite the importance of the problem, a universally accepted definition of what constitutes minor and major physical abuse does not exist. Rather, each state in the United States defines abuse according to its individual reporting laws.

Abusive Head Trauma

Abusive head trauma (AHT) is a serious form of physical abuse caused by violent shaking of infants and young children. Other commonly used terms include *shaken baby syndrome, inflicted head injury,* and *neuroinflicted brain injury.* This violent shaking would be easily recognized by others as dangerous (American Academy of Pediatrics Committee on Child Abuse and Neglect, 2009; Kemp, 2011) and is most often a result of the caregiver's frustration with crying, maternal stress, or depression (Kemp, 2011). Every year in the United States, an estimated 1200 to 1400 children are shaken, and of these victims, 25% to 30% die as a result of their injuries. The rest have lifelong complications (National Center on Shaken Baby Syndrome, n.d.).

It is important to understand what happens in AHT. Infants have a large head-to-body ratio, weak neck muscles, and a large amount of water in the brain. Violent shaking causes the brain to rotate within the skull, resulting in shearing forces that tear blood vessels and neurons. The characteristic injuries that occur are intracranial bleeding (subdural and subarachnoid hematomas) and, in approximately 80% of cases, bilateral retinal hemorrhages, which are classic results of repetitive acceleration-deceleration head trauma (Maguire, Watts, Shaw, et al., 2013). Injuries may also include fractures of the ribs and long bones. Most often, there are no signs of external injury, making diagnosis difficult. Clinicians base an abusive diagnosis on patterns of injuries to the infant, but this can be subjective. PredAHT, a prediction tool, assists clinicians with an AHT diagnosis by listing six key clinical features of AHT obtained from high-quality publications (Cowley, Morris, Maguire, et al., 2015). The PredAHT has high sensitivity and specificity in estimating the probability of AHT when three or more of the six features are present in the patient (Cowley, Morris, Maguire, et al., 2015).

Traumatic brain injury is often not an isolated event, with a large number of children showing evidence of a previous injury (Kemp, 2011). Victims of AHT can be seen with a variety of symptoms, from generalized flulike symptoms to unresponsiveness with impending death (Altimier, 2008). Many of the presenting symptoms, such as vomiting, irritability, poor feeding, and listlessness, are often mistaken for common infant and childhood ailments. In more severe forms, presenting symptoms may include seizures, posturing, alterations in level of consciousness, apnea, bradycardia, or death. The long-term outcomes of AHT include seizure disorders; visual impairments, including blindness; developmental delays; hearing loss; cerebral palsy; and mild to profound mental, cognitive, or motor impairments (Altimier, 2008). Nurses can take an active role in prevention of AHT by teaching caregivers about care for infants and techniques to cope with inconsolable crying (Barr, 2012).

> **! NURSING ALERT**
>
> Stress to parents the danger of shaking infants (shaking can cause AHT). Education must include coping mechanisms on caring for children with inconsolable crying.

Munchausen Syndrome by Proxy

Munchausen syndrome by proxy (MSBP), also known as *medical child abuse* or *factitious disorder by proxy,* is a rare but serious form of child abuse in which caregivers deliberately exaggerate or fabricate histories and symptoms or induce symptoms. It is a form of child maltreatment that may include physical, emotional, and psychologic abuse for the gratification of the caregiver. In most cases, the perpetrator is the biologic mother with some degree of health care knowledge and training. Health care providers can become easily misled and unknowingly enable the perpetrator (Squires & Squires, 2013). Because of the history of symptoms provided by the caregiver, the child endures painful and unnecessary medical testing and procedures. Common symptoms presented are seizures, nausea and vomiting, diarrhea, and altered mental status; they are usually witnessed only by the perpetrator.

Considerations when determining whether a child is a victim of MSBP include the following:

- Is the child's condition consistent with the reported history?
- Does diagnostic evidence support the reported history?
- Has anyone other than the caregiver witnessed the symptoms?
- Is treatment being provided primarily because of the caregiver's demands?

The resolution of symptoms after separation from the perpetrator confirms the diagnosis.

Factors Predisposing to Physical Abuse

The causes of child abuse are multifaceted. Child maltreatment occurs across all socioeconomic, religious, cultural, racial, and ethnic groups (US Department of Health and Human Services, 2015). Three risk factors are commonly identified in child abuse: (1) parental characteristics, (2) characteristics of the child, and (3) environmental characteristics. However, no single factor or group of factors is predictive of abuse. Rather, the interaction of these factors is thought to increase the risk of abuse occurring in a particular family.

Parental Characteristics

Some identified characteristics occur more frequently in parents who abuse their children and are therefore considered risk factors. Younger parents more often are abusers of their children. Single-parent families are at higher risk for abuse; and in single-parent families that include an unrelated partner, the partner is sometimes the abuser, although a biologic parent is most commonly the perpetrator (US Department of Health and Human Services, 2015).

Abusive families are often socially isolated and have few supportive relationships. They often have additional stressors, such as low-income circumstances with little education. Parents with substance abuse problems pose a greater risk for abuse and neglect because of a variety of factors. The additional stressors of substance abuse with the demands of normal care of children create situations in which abuse and neglect can occur because these parents have impaired judgment and may react with violence while under the influence of drugs or alcohol (Lyden, 2011). With little or no available support system and concurrent stressors imposed by the child or environment, these parents are vulnerable to additional crises of any nature and may strike out at the child as a method of releasing their frustration and anxiety.

Other factors identified in abusive parents include low self-esteem and little knowledge of appropriate parenting skills. Parenting skills are learned behaviors, and parents who grew up with poor parental role models may have difficulty parenting their own children. Often, child abusers were abused themselves or observed some type of abuse in their home (Lyden, 2011).

Characteristics of the Child

The onus for child abuse is always on the abuser. However, children who are abused do have some common characteristics. Children from birth to 1 year old are at highest risk for being abused (US Department of Health and Human Services, 2012). Infants and small children require constant attention and must have all their needs met by others. This can result in parental or caregiver fatigue that results in striking out at the child with physical force, shaking the child, or ignoring the child's needs.

The physical and emotional demands placed on the parents or caregiver of an unwanted, brain-damaged, hyperactive, or physically disabled child may overwhelm them, resulting in abuse. Children with disabilities may not understand that abusive behaviors are not appropriate, so they may not tell others or defend themselves. Premature infants may be at risk for maltreatment because of failure of parent-child bonding during early infancy, increased physical needs, or irritability. One child may be singled out in an abusive family. Removing that child from the home often places the other siblings at risk for abuse. Therefore no child is safe if left in the abusive environment unless the parents can be helped to learn new parenting skills, to meet the children's needs, and to release their frustration through alternatives other than attacking their children.

Environmental Characteristics

The environment is a significant part of the potentially abusive situation. A typical environment is one of chronic stress, including problems of divorce, poverty, unemployment, poor housing, frequent relocation, alcoholism, and drug addiction. Increased exposure between children and parents, such as that which occurs in crowded living conditions, also increases the likelihood of abuse.

Although most reporting of abuse has been from lower socioeconomic populations, as stated earlier, child abuse is not a problem of any one societal group. Stresses imposed by poverty predispose lower socioeconomic families to abusive situations, and abuse in these groups is more likely to be reported. However, concealed crises may also be present in upper-class families. Families who have substitute caregivers (e.g., daycare providers and babysitters) may also be at risk for child abuse, especially if the family has not fully evaluated the caregiver. Nurses need to be aware of all these factors to identify the less obvious examples of child abuse and neglect.

SEXUAL ABUSE

Sexual abuse is one of the most devastating types of child maltreatment, and estimates indicate that it has increased significantly during the past decade (US Department of Health and Human Services, 2015). Some of the apparent increase is due to increased awareness and increased reporting (Evans, 2011).

As with all forms of child maltreatment, no universal definition for sexual abuse exists. The Child Abuse Prevention and Treatment Act (CAPTA), amended by the CAPTA Reauthorization Act of 2010, defines **sexual abuse** as "the employment, use, persuasion, inducement, enticement, or coercion of any child to engage in, or assist any other person to engage in, sexually explicit conduct or any simulation of such conduct; or the rape, molestation, prostitution, or other form of sexual exploitation of children, or incest with children" (US Department of Health and Human Services, 2015).

Sexual abuse includes the following types of sexual maltreatment (see also Sexual Assault [Rape], Chapter 18):

Incest: Any physical sexual activity between family members; blood relationship is not required (abusers can include stepparents, unrelated siblings, grandparents, uncles, and aunts); does not include sexual relations between legally sanctioned partners, such as spouses

Molestation: A vague term that includes "indecent liberties," such as touching, fondling, kissing, single or mutual masturbation, or oral-genital contact

Exhibitionism: Indecent exposure, usually exposure of the genitalia by an adult man to children or women

Child pornography: Arranging and photographing, in any media, sexual acts involving children, alone or with adults or animals, regardless of consent by the child's legal guardian; also may denote distribution of such material in any form with or without profit

Child prostitution: Involving children in sex acts for profit and usually with changing partners

Pedophilia: Literally means "love of child" and does not denote a type of sexual activity but rather the preference of an adult for prepubertal children as the means of achieving sexual excitement

Characteristics of Abusers and Victims

Anyone, including siblings and mothers, can be sexual abusers, but a typical abuser is a man whom the victim knows. Offenders come from all levels of society; however, a higher risk of child abuse has been noted among families with incomes below the poverty level (Breyer & MacPhee, 2015). In addition, parents with a high school education are more likely than parents with a college education to be abusers (Breyer & MacPhee, 2015). Many offenders hold full-time jobs, are active in community affairs, and may not have prior criminal records. Offenders often are employed (or volunteers) in positions such as teaching or coaching that bring them into contact with young girls and boys. Offenders may commit many assaults before being caught.

Incestuous relationships between father or stepfather and daughter are generally prolonged, and the victims are usually reluctant to report the situation because of fear of retaliation and fear that they will not be believed. Typically, incestuous relationships begin later than other forms of child abuse. The eldest daughter is usually abused, but in her absence, another sister may be substituted. Sibling incest may also occur. Sexual abuse by relatives with a strong emotional bond with the victim, such as a parent, is often the most devastating to the child.

Boys are also victims of both intrafamilial and extrafamilial abuse. Compared with female victims, male victims are much less likely to report abuse, and they may suffer much greater emotional harm from incestuous relationships. Boys are likely to be subjected to anal penetration and oral-genital contact. They often have subtle physical findings and are abused by a father, stepfather, or mother's boyfriend.

Significant risk factors for child sexual abuse include parental unavailability, lack of emotional closeness and flexibility, social isolation, emotional deprivation, and communication difficulties. Most sexual abuse is committed by men and by persons known to the child, such as family members (Forsdike, Tarzia, Hindmarsh, et al., 2014). Around 20% to 25% of child sexual abuse cases involve penetration or oral-genital contact. In 2011 more than 26% of sexual abuse victims were between 12 and 14 years old, and nearly 22% were between 15 and 17 years old (US Department of Health and Human Services, 2012).

Initiation and Perpetuation of Sexual Abuse

The cycle of sexual abuse often starts insidiously unless it involves an isolated attack, such as rape. Often offenders spend time with the victims to gain their trust before initiating any sexual contact. Most victims are then pressured into being an accessory to the sexual activity through various means (Box 14.4) and may be unaware that sexual activity is part of the offer. Children may not reveal the truth for fear that their parents would not believe them if they told, especially if the offender is a trusted member of the family. Some fear that they will be blamed for the situation, and many young children with limited vocabulary have difficulty describing the activity when they do have the courage or opportunity to reveal the abuse.

Incest most frequently occurs between siblings, but it may also be between fathers or stepfathers and daughters, or grandfather and granddaughter. Sibling incest has been found to have adverse outcomes during childhood that extend into adulthood and are just as damaging as father-daughter abuse (Krienert & Walsh, 2011). Victims may take years to disclose this abuse. However, not all incestuous relationships follow this pattern of silence. Reports of father-daughter incest during child custody conflicts have become more common and have raised serious concerns regarding the possibility of false accusation. Rather than tolerating or denying the child's sexual abuse, the other parent (usually the mother) is typically the chief accuser.

BOX 14.4 Methods Used to Pressure Children Into Sexual Activity

- The child is offered gifts or privileges or has privileges withheld.
- The adult misrepresents moral standards by telling the child that it is "okay to do."
- Isolated and emotionally and socially impoverished children are enticed by adults who meet their needs for warmth and human contact.
- The successful sex offender pressures the victim into secrecy by describing it as a "secret between us" that other people would take away if they found out.
- The offender plays on the child's fears, including fear of punishment by the offender, fear of repercussions if the child tells, and fear of abandonment or rejection by the family.

NURSING CARE OF THE MALTREATED CHILD

A critical responsibility of health professionals is identifying abusive situations as early as possible. Nurses who increase their knowledge of the different types of abuse and neglect and underlying causes will enhance their ability to identify, intervene, and prevent children from maltreatment and neglect (Lyden, 2011). The characteristics that may predispose members of some families to commit abuse can serve as a framework for assessing vulnerability but are never predictive of actual abuse. A careful, detailed history and interview combined with a thorough physical examination are the diagnostic tools needed to identify abuse. Nurses have a special role because they may be the first person to see the child and parent and are the consistent caregivers if the child is hospitalized (see Nursing Care Guidelines box).

NURSING CARE GUIDELINES

Talking With Children Who Reveal Abuse

- Provide a private time and place to talk.
- Do not promise not to tell; tell them that you are required by law to report the abuse.
- Do not express shock or criticize their family.
- Use their vocabulary to discuss body parts.
- Avoid using any leading statements that can distort their report.
- Reassure them that they have done the right thing by telling.
- Tell them that the abuse is not their fault and that they are not bad or to blame.
- Determine their immediate need for safety.
- Let the child know what will happen when you report.

In interviewing the child and family, the nurse must be careful to avoid biasing the child's retelling of the events. Some experts suggest that health professionals limit the interview to the child's physical and mental health concerns and leave topics of the family's social, legal, or other problems to the police or the Child Protective Services (Mollen, Goyal, & Frioux, 2012). If this is not possible, make an effort to coordinate the interview process so that all pertinent health care professionals can be present for the interview.

Recognition of abuse or neglect necessitates a familiarity with both physical and behavioral signs that suggest maltreatment (Box 14.5). No one indicator can be used to diagnose maltreatment. It is a pattern or combination of indicators that should arouse suspicion and lead to further investigation. It is important to note that some situations (e.g., bleeding disorders, osteogenesis imperfecta, or sudden infant death syndrome) may be misinterpreted as abuse. Also, some cultural practices, such as cupping or coin rubbing (see Health Practices, Chapter 2), may mimic physical abuse. Unintentional injuries, such as burns from metal buckles on car seats, bruising from seat belts, or spiral fractures from a twist-and-fall injury, may also be wrongly diagnosed as abuse. Normal variants, such as mongolian spots and congenital anomalies of genitalia, can be mistaken for abuse.

Caregiver-Child Interaction

The nurse can use the initial contact with the family to assess the interaction between the caregiver and the child. Observations of the caregivers should include emotional support for the child, attentiveness to the child's needs, and concern for the child's injury. Although caregivers and children may vary in responses to a stressful event, note an unusual caregiver-child relationship and factor this into the overall evaluation of the child.

BOX 14.5 Warning Signs of Abuse

- Child has physical evidence of abuse or neglect, including previous injuries.
- History is incompatible with the pattern or degree of injury, such as bilateral skull fractures after being dropped.
- Explanation of how injury occurred is vague or the parent or guardian is reluctant to provide information.
- The patient is brought in with a minor, unrelated complaint, and significant trauma is found.
- Histories are contradictory among caregivers.
- The mechanism of injury provided is not possible given age or developmental level of the patient, such as 6-month-old turning on hot water.
- Bruising or other injury is present in a nonmobile patient.
- The patient's affect is inappropriate in relation to the extent of injury.
- Evidence of abusive or neglectful parent-child interaction is present.
- The parent, guardian, or custodian disappears after bringing in the patient for trauma or a patient with suspicious injury is brought in by an unrelated adult.
- The patient has multiple fractures of differing ages.
- There was a delay in seeking care.
- The parent or caregiver discloses that abuse has or may have occurred.
- The patient makes an outcry of abuse or neglect.

Certain behavioral responses of the parents to their child and to the interviewer should alert the nurse to the possibility of maltreatment. Abusive parents may have difficulty showing concern toward their child. They may be unable or unwilling to comfort the child. Abusers may blame the child for the injuries or belittle him or her for being clumsy or stupid. When interacting with health care workers, the parent may become hostile or uncooperative. During the child's hospitalization, they may not participate in the child's care and may show little concern for his or her progress, eventual discharge, or need for follow-up care.

Abused children's responses to their parents or the injury may also support the suspicion of abuse. Although no one pattern is typical, extremes of behavior may be observed. Children may be unresponsive to the parent or excessively clinging and intolerant of separation. They may be overly attached to the abusive parent, possibly in the hope of preventing any upset that may precipitate anger and another attack. During care of the injury, children may be passive and accepting of the discomfort or uncooperative and fearful of any physical contact. They may avoid eye contact. Some children maintain a wary watchfulness of all strangers; some shy away from strangers as if frightened; others are unusually affectionate and outgoing.

History and Interview

Child Physical Abuse

It is often difficult to distinguish child maltreatment from accidental injuries. Caregivers whose history of events may be deceptive or incomplete and children who are nonverbal may make the assessment more complex. A purposeful, skilled history and appropriate interview questions help the nurse ensure the right course of action. Knowledge of mechanism of injury and child development is essential. Cases of abuse are often detected when the child or caregiver history of events does not match with physical findings. Children who are verbal can often give a history of the injury. Separating the child from the caregiver may provide a more reliable history. It is important to ask nonleading, open-ended questions. The history should include a narrative of the injury from both caregiver and child (if verbal). Date, time, and location where the injury took place, along with who was present at the time of the injury, are essential questions. Family history for bleeding and bone disorders is important. Box 14.5 outlines areas of history that are concerning for abuse.

Neglect and Emotional Abuse

Each child may manifest different responses to neglect, depending on the situation and developmental age of the child. The goal of the interview is to determine whether the child is in a safe environment and whether the caregiver has the skills and resources to care for the child. It is often difficult to determine whether the circumstances constitute poor parenting skills or true neglect. Box 14.6 lists flags for behaviors to look for in neglected and abused children.

Sexual Abuse

An essential component to identifying sexual abuse is the interview. Several dynamics may impede the child's revelation of sexual abuse. Child sexual abuse is often perpetrated by someone known to the child, including family members. In some cases, the child may have been sworn to secrecy. The child may have been told that no one will believe the story or that his or her family would be harmed if he or she told someone about the abuse. Small children may imitate behaviors they have had perpetrated on themselves or have seen others do. The nurse must be able to recognize normal, age-related sexual curiosity and self-stimulating behaviors. Typically, children do not act out specific details of the sexual act or perform intrusive acts on others unless they have sexual knowledge beyond their normal age-related development (Dubowitz & Lane, 2016).

Children's reports of sexual abuse may vary from contradictory stories to unwavering versions of the experience. Stories that sound contradictory may reflect the child's experiences in several instances of abuse. Also, children who repeatedly tell identical facts may have been prompted to do so.

Increasing evidence suggests that the types of interrogation children are exposed to after reports of sexual abuse shape their thinking. To avoid biasing the interaction, nurses must be skillful interviewers when questioning children who may be victims of abuse. Medical records should include verbatim statements made by the child and interviewer that reflect appropriate nonleading questions and statements (Lyden, 2011). The child may not be emotionally ready to discuss the abuse. Establishing rapport with the child is essential to gaining his or her trust. Interviews should not be rushed. Engaging the child in play activities while encouraging conversation may help the child discuss the abuse. It may take several interviews or psychologic counseling for the child to be forthcoming about the abuse. Information regarding the last sexual contact is important because it determines the need for a forensic evaluation. Children who have been sexually abused within the past 72 to 96 hours should be considered for forensic testing.

Unfortunately, there is no typical profile of the victim, and the nurse must have a high index of suspicion to identify these children. Physical signs vary and may include any of those listed for sexual abuse. The victim may exhibit various behavioral manifestations, but none of these behaviors is diagnostic. When abused children exhibit these behaviors, the signs may be incorrectly attributed to the normal stresses of childhood, especially in older school-age children or adolescents. Even signs considered most predictive of sexual abuse (e.g., certain genital findings, sexually inappropriate behavior for age, enactment of adult sexual activity, and intense focus on sexual activity [e.g., masturbation]) do not always indicate that sexual abuse has occurred. Conversely, abused children may not demonstrate more knowledge of sexual activity than nonabused children. However, one difference in the abused children's explanation of sexual activity may be unusual affective responses. For example, abused children have an increased risk for conduct disorders, aggressive behavior, and poor academic performance (Dubowitz & Lane, 2016).

BOX 14.6 Clinical Manifestations of Potential Child Maltreatment

Physical Neglect

Suggestive Physical Findings

Growth failure

Signs of malnutrition, such as thin extremities, abdominal distention, lack of subcutaneous fat

Poor personal hygiene

Unclean or inappropriate dress

Evidence of poor health care, such as delayed immunization, untreated infections, frequent colds

Frequent injuries from lack of supervision

Suggestive Behaviors

Dull and inactive affect; excessively passive or sleepy

Self-stimulatory behaviors, such as finger sucking or rocking

Begging or stealing food

Absenteeism from school

Substance abuse

Vandalism or shoplifting

Emotional Abuse and Neglect

Suggestive Physical Findings

Growth failure (failure to thrive)

Eating or feeding disorder

Enuresis

Sleep disorder

Suggestive Behaviors

Self-stimulatory behaviors, such as biting, rocking, or sucking

During infancy, lack of social smile and stranger anxiety

Withdrawal from environment and people

Unusual fearfulness

Antisocial behavior, such as destructiveness, stealing, cruelty to animals or people

Extremes of behavior, such as overcompliant and passive or aggressive and demanding

Lags in emotional and intellectual development, especially language

Suicide attempts

Physical Abuse

Suggestive Physical Findings

Bruises and welts (may be in various stages of healing)

- On face, lips, mouth, back, buttocks, thighs, or areas of torso
- Regular patterns descriptive of object used, such as belt buckle, hand, wire hanger, chain, wooden spoon, squeeze or pinch marks
- May be present in various stages of healing

Burns

- On soles, palms, back, or buttocks
- Patterns descriptive of object used, such as round cigar or cigarette burns; sharply demarcated areas from immersion in scalding water; rope burns on wrists or ankles from being bound; burns in the shape of an iron, radiator, or electric stove burner
- Absence of "splash" marks and presence of symmetric burns
- Stun gun injury: Lesions circular, fairly uniform (≤0.5 cm), and paired about 5 cm apart

Fractures and dislocations

- Skull, nose, or facial structures
- Injury denoting type of abuse, such as spiral fracture or dislocation from twisting of an extremity or whiplash from shaking the child
- Multiple new or old fractures in various stages of healing

Lacerations and abrasions

- On backs of arms, legs, torso, face, or external genitalia
- Unusual symptoms, such as abdominal swelling, pain, and vomiting from punching
- Descriptive marks, such as from human bites or pulling out of hair

Chemical

- Unexplained repeated poisoning, especially drug overdose
- Unexplained sudden illness, such as hypoglycemia from insulin administration

Suggestive Behaviors

Wary of physical contact with adults

Apparent fear of parents or going home

Lying very still while surveying environment

Inappropriate reaction to injury, such as failure to cry from pain

Lack of reaction to frightening events

Apprehensive when hearing other children cry

Indiscriminate friendliness and displays of affection

Superficial relationships

Acting-out behavior, such as aggression, to seek attention

Withdrawal behavior

Sexual Abuse

Suggestive Physical Findings

Bruises, bleeding, lacerations, or irritation of external genitalia, anus, mouth, or throat

Torn, stained, or bloody underclothing

Pain on urination or pain, swelling, and itching of genital area

Penile discharge

Sexually transmitted disease, nonspecific vaginitis

Difficulty in walking or sitting

Unusual odor in the genital area

Recurrent urinary tract infections

Presence of sperm

Pregnancy in young adolescent

Suggestive Behaviors

Sudden emergence of sexually related problems, including excessive or public masturbation, age-inappropriate sexual play, promiscuity, or overtly seductive behavior

Withdrawn behavior, excessive daydreaming

Preoccupation with fantasies, especially in play

Poor relationships with peers

Sudden changes, such as anxiety, loss or gain of weight, clinging behavior

In incestuous relationships, excessive anger at mother for not protecting daughter

Regressive behavior, such as bedwetting or thumb sucking

Sudden onset of phobias or fears, particularly fears of the dark, men, strangers, or particular settings or situations (e.g., undue fear of leaving the house or staying at the daycare center or the babysitter's house)

Running away from home

Substance abuse, particularly of alcohol or mood-elevating drugs

Profound and rapid personality changes, especially extreme depression, hostility, and aggression (often accompanied by social withdrawal)

Rapidly declining school performance

> **! NURSING ALERT**
>
> When children report potentially sexually abusive experiences, take their reports seriously but also cautiously to avoid alarming the child or falsely accusing someone.

Physical Assessment

Child Physical Abuse

The goal of the physical assessment for child physical abuse is identification of all injuries. A system approach ensures that the whole body is evaluated. In instances of severe abuse and injuries, the assessment should begin with a rapid assessment of airway, breathing, circulation, and neurologic systems. A systematic head-to-toe examination follows. Attention to areas often overlooked, such as the scalp, behind the ears, and the frenulum, is essential. The child's exterior genital area and posterior surface should be completely examined.

Record the location and a detailed description of all injuries. Note the color, size, and location of all bruising. Burn documentation should include the location, pattern, demarcation lines, and presence of eschar or blisters. Diagrams of the injuries using a body diagram form are helpful. If possible, obtain photographs of the injuries using a measurement tool.

Not all forms of physical abuse have obvious signs. Intraabdominal organ injury from blunt trauma to the abdomen can occur without signs of external abdominal bruising. Nurses should consider intraabdominal injury in infants and children who have any other signs of abuse.

> **! NURSING ALERT**
>
> Incompatibility between the history and the injury is probably the most important criterion on which to base the decision to report suspected abuse.

All evidence collected must adhere to strict guidelines for legal purposes; the chain of custody must be appropriately maintained with local law enforcement personnel. Documentation on the chain of custody form should include the names of persons collecting and receiving evidence (e.g., photographs and DNA samples), types of evidence collected and received, and date of receipt (Lyden, 2011).

Neglect and Emotional Abuse

Neglect from deprivation of necessities is easier to identify than emotional neglect or psychologic maltreatment because physical signs are usually evident. Assessment of the child's height, weight, nutritional status, hygiene, and age-appropriate interactions is important for the overall picture of potential neglect. Emotional maltreatment may be readily suspected, but it is difficult to substantiate. Physical signs are often nonspecific, and nurses must rely on behavioral indicators, which range from depression to acting-out behavior, to help identify a possibly abusive situation. Any persistent and unexplained change in the child's behavior is an important clue to possible emotional abuse.

Sexual Abuse

Identifying instances of sexual abuse is particularly difficult because, often, few if any obvious physical indications of the activity exist. Physical signs vary and may include any of those listed in Box 14.6 for sexual abuse. The goal of the physical examination is to document genital findings. In most cases, the genital examination findings are normal, which does not mean that sexual abuse did not occur. Fondling or genital-to-genital contact without penetration may leave no physical findings. Forensic evidence obtained directly from a prepubertal victim's body diminishes greatly after 24 hours, with the best chance for evidence collection coming from bed linens or the child's underwear (Girardet, Bolton, Lohoti, et al., 2011). The female genital examination should include a description of the vulva, hymen, and surrounding tissue. Abnormal findings of concern are injuries to the posterior vulva or the lower half of the hymeneal ring or abrasions, bruising, or bleeding of the genital or anal tissue. It is often helpful to use a magnifying instrument (colposcope) to detect subtle injuries. There are many variants of normal findings for female genital anatomy, so it is recommended that the examination be done by a practitioner experienced with these types of cases. Contrary to popular myth, the size of the hymeneal opening is not predictive of the likelihood of sexual abuse (Adams, 2011). For male victims, swelling, abrasions, or bruising of the genital tissue raises concerns for abuse. Examine the anal area for symmetry, tone, fissures, or scars. Genital tissue heals very quickly and most often without scars. Therefore unless the child is seen within a few days of injury, the genital tissue may appear normal. In addition, the vaginal and anal mucosa is elastic; therefore penetration without disruption of tissue is possible. This defies another myth that there is always evidence of female virginity. Consider the collection of specimens for determining the presence of sexually transmitted infections, which may have been contracted during the sexual contact.

Nursing Care Management

Protect the Child From Further Abuse

Initially, identification of instances of suspected abuse or neglect is essential. The nurse may come in contact with abused children in an emergency department, practitioner's office, home, daycare center, or school.

> **! NURSING ALERT**
>
> The priority is to remove the child from the abusive situation to prevent further injury.

All states and provinces in North America have laws for mandatory reporting of child maltreatment. Suspected child abuse is reported to the local authorities.* Referrals usually come to the state child welfare department and are assigned to a caseworker in an agency, such as Child Protective Services. After a referral has been made, a caseworker is assigned to investigate the report. Based on the findings, the child is left in the home or temporarily removed.

A court proceeding may be necessary before the child can be placed outside the home or when parental rights are to be terminated. When the courts are involved, they usually require firsthand testimony by the referring parties. Nurses may be subpoenaed to appear in court, or their notes may be introduced as evidence in court hearings. Accurate and factual documentation is essential. Behaviors are described, not interpreted, and are recorded daily to establish a progress record (see Nursing Care Guidelines box). Conversations among the nurse, child, and parent are recorded verbatim as much as possible.

Support the Child

Children suspected of being abused are often hospitalized for medical management of their injuries and to allow further assessment of their safety needs. The needs of these children are the same as those of any hospitalized child. The child should be treated as a child with the usual physical needs, developmental tasks, and play interests—not as a victim of abuse. The goal of the nurse-child relationship is to provide a role model for the parents in helping them relate positively and constructively

---

*Telephone numbers are usually listed under "Child Abuse" in the business white pages of the local directory, or you can call the emergency child abuse hotline: 800-422-4453 (800-4-A-CHILD).

NURSING CARE GUIDELINES

Recording Assessment Data in Suspected Abuse

History of Injury

Date, time, and place of occurrence
Sequence of events with recorded times
Presence of witnesses, especially person caring for child at time of incident
Time lapse between occurrence of injury and initiation of treatment
Interview with child when appropriate, including verbal quotations and information from drawing or other play activities
Interview with parent, witnesses, and other significant persons, including verbal quotations
Description of parent-child interactions (verbal interactions, eye contact, touching, parental concern)
Name, age, and condition of other children in home (if possible)

Physical Examination

Location, size, shape, and color of bruises; approximate location, size, and shape on drawing of body outline
Distinguishing characteristics, such as a bruise in the shape of a hand or a round burn (possibly caused by cigarette)
Symmetry or asymmetry of injury; presence of other injuries
Degree of pain; any bone tenderness
Evidence of past injuries; general state of health and hygiene
Developmental level of child; screening test

to their child and to foster a therapeutic environment for the child in his or her reprieve from the abusing situation.

Support the Family

The nurse also encourages the child's relationship with nonoffending parents. The nurse does not become a substitute parent but rather acts as a role model for parents in helping them relate positively and constructively to their child. When parental ignorance of childrearing practices has played a part in the abuse, the nurse can educate the parent regarding children's physical and emotional needs. Because of the parents' own childrearing, they may not be aware of nonviolent methods of discipline, such as time-outs. They may also need help in dealing with their frustration so that they do not vent anger on the child. Because these parents may be sensitive to criticism or resistant to authority figures, teaching is implemented through demonstration and example rather than through lecturing. Praise any competent parenting abilities they demonstrate to promote their sense of parental adequacy.

Advise family members to encourage the child to resume normal activities and observe the child for signs of distress (see Posttraumatic Stress Disorder, Chapter 16). Children express their feelings primarily through behavior. Parents should be alert for changes in behavior that indicate distress resulting from the incident, such as remaining in the house, refusal to go to school, changes in sleeping patterns, and frequency of dreams and nightmares.

Referral to appropriate social service agencies is also essential. Many abusive parents live in poverty, and the daily stresses imposed by their circumstances are overwhelming. Seek resources for financial aid, improved housing, and child care. Self-help groups also provide important services. Groups such as Parents Anonymous* (a group for parents who have abused or fear that they may abuse their child but only in terms of physical abuse, not sexual abuse) are accepting and nonjudgmental.

*250 West First Street, Suite 250, Claremont, CA 91711; 909-621-6184; http://www.parentsanonymous.org.

Plan for Discharge

Discharge planning should begin as soon as the legal disposition for placement has been decided, which may be temporary foster home placement, return to the parents, or permanent termination of parental rights. The latter is the most drastic solution, but it is necessary in situations of life-threatening abuse. Whenever children are sent to a foster home or juvenile institution, they must be allowed an opportunity to express their feelings. No matter how severe the abuse, they usually mourn the loss of their parents. They need help to understand why they must not return home and that this new home is in no way a punishment. Whenever possible, foster parents are encouraged to visit in the hospital, and the nurse should take an active role in helping the new parents understand the child, as well as the child's health care needs, because studies have shown that the health care needs of children in foster care often go unmet (Schneiderman, Smith, & Palinkas, 2012).

Prevent Abuse

Prevention of child maltreatment has been an extremely difficult goal. However, nurses have played an important role in such programs. For example, home visits based on identified risk factors (e.g., mothers who are teenagers, unmarried, or of low socioeconomic status) were noted to be an effective preventive measure (Selph, Bougatsos, Blazina, et al., 2013). The nurses provided information on normal child growth and development and routine health care needs, served as informal support persons, and referred families to appropriate services when a need for assistance was identified. The Nurse-Family Partnership is one program that has demonstrated evidence-based interventions resulting in the prevention of child maltreatment (Lane, 2014).

Nurses in a variety of settings can implement similar activities. For example, nurses in prenatal clinics can prepare expectant families for adjustment to parenthood. Nursery and postpartum nurses can foster the attachment process by encouraging parents to hold and look at their infant, as well as teach coping mechanisms for prolonged crying. Nurses in neonatal intensive care units can minimize the effects of separation by encouraging parents to visit and can help parents become comfortable caring for their child. Nurses in ambulatory settings can teach parents appropriate methods of bathing, feeding, toileting, disciplining, and preventing injuries while stressing the normal needs and developmental characteristics of children. Nurses must be sensitive to parental needs for attention, reassurance, and reinforcement and should refer parents to community services and self-help groups.

Unlike preventive efforts for neglect and physical abuse, which have been aimed at the potential offender, prevention of child sexual abuse has centered on education of children to protect themselves. Materials are available for parents that describe sexual abuse and its prevention.* Helpful games such as "What if the babysitter wants to wrestle and hug but tells you to keep it a secret?" can be used to explore dangerous situations in advance and help children learn the importance of saying "no." They need reassurance that no matter what the other person says or does, the parents want to know about it and will not punish them. Even if children participate in the activity before telling their parents, they must be reassured that it was not their fault. It is equally important to teach children safety in terms of potential risk situations. Several suggestions for parents regarding protecting and educating children against possible molestation are presented in the Family-Centered Care

*Sources of information are Prevent Child Abuse America, 228 S. Wabash Ave., 10th Floor, Chicago, IL 60604; 312-663-3520 or 800-Children (800-244-5373); http://www.preventchildabuse.org; and American Humane Association, 1400 16th Street NW, Suite 360, Washington DC 20036; 800-227-4645; http://www.americanhumane.org.

box. The nurse is frequently in a position to discuss the topic of abuse with parents and to provide guidelines. In addition, parents need to be made aware that "nice" people, including friends and relatives, can be offenders; parents should carefully observe how others act toward the child. A sudden change in the child's behavior and a response such as "I don't like Uncle Bob anymore" are clues to investigate the relationship. In the event of any doubt, prevent further solitary encounters with this person and the child. It is sometimes to the child's great misfortune that parents do not take certain comments seriously, such as "He hugs me too tight" or "I don't want to go with him." Casual parental statements such as "He just loves you" or "You do whatever adults tell you to do" can place children in jeopardy. Health professionals must alert parents to such dangers and guide them toward an appreciation of the problem, providing concrete guidelines toward child education and protection.

FAMILY-CENTERED CARE

Preventing and Dealing With Sexual Abuse of Children

Sexual assault of children is much more common than most people realize. It may be preventable if children have good preparation. *To provide protection and preparation:*

- Pay careful attention to who is around children. (Unwanted touch may come from someone liked and trusted.)
- Back up a child's right to say no.
- Encourage communication by taking seriously what children say.
- Take a second look at signals of potential danger.
- Refuse to leave children in the company of those who are not trusted.
- Include information about sexual assault when teaching about safety.
- Provide specific definitions and examples of sexual assault.
- Remind children that even "nice" people sometimes do mean things.
- Urge children to tell about *anybody* who causes them to be uncomfortable.
- Prepare children to deal with bribes, threats, and possible physical force.
- Virtually eliminate secrets between children and parents.
- Teach children how to say no, ask for help, and control who touches them and how.
- Model self-protective and limit-setting behavior for children.

If it ever becomes necessary to help a child recover from a sexual assault:

- Listen carefully to understand the child.
- Support the child for telling through praise, belief, sympathy, and lack of blame.
- Know local resources and choose help carefully.
- Provide opportunities to talk about the assault.
- Provide opportunities for the entire family to go through a recovery process.

Sexual assault affects everyone. To help deal with this social problem:

- Provide care and support to those who have been victimized.
- Recognize that offenders may not change behavior even with intervention.
- Organize neighborhood programs to support each other's efforts to protect children.
- Encourage schools to provide information about sexual assault as a problem of health and safety.
- Organize community groups to support educational treatment and law enforcement programs.

Modified from Adams, C., & Fay, J. (1981). *No more secrets: Protecting your child from sexual assault.* San Luis Obispo, CA: Impact.

NCLEX REVIEW QUESTIONS

1. The mother of a 4-year-old health clinic patient asks the nurse about night terrors. Which statement by the mother reveals a need for further teaching? Select all that apply.
   A. He will grow out of this stage when he is a little older.
   B. Getting into a specific routine is helpful and can be calming to my son.
   C. Watching TV with an adult is helpful so that he understands what is real.
   D. I can help my child with sleep by giving him his favorite stuffed animal or using a night-light.
   E. Our family often sleeps together, and this seems to help.
2. A child is brought to the emergency department by his parents after noted to be "acting funny" a few hours ago while he was being cared for by his grandmother. When she went to take her evening medication, the grandmother noted that her pill container had been opened and some pills were missing. The parents state that the grandmother has a heart condition. Anticipating the emergency care this child will receive, you know:
   A. The majority of medications have a specific antidote.
   B. In this case gastric lavage may be used.
   C. Activated charcoal will most likely be used, and it can be mixed with another drink (milk or juice) to make it more palatable.
   D. The main concerns are for vital sign assessment, assessment of mental status, and giving cardiac and respiratory support as needed.
3. You are working with the family of a 4-year-old patient and have concerns about possible exposure to lead poisoning. Which information will determine whether follow-up is needed? Select all that apply.
   A. The child goes daily to the older home of a babysitter.
   B. One of the child's playmates in the neighborhood has lead poisoning.
   C. Although living in a newer neighborhood, one of the child's playmates' homes is being renovated.
   D. The child is out of the danger age range for screening (1 to 2 years old), so screening is not needed.
   E. Past BLL was 12, so no follow-up is needed at this time.
4. When assessing a child's injury in the emergency department, a nurse suspects physical abuse. Based on this suspicion, the nurse's primary legal responsibility is to
   A. Assist the family in identifying resources for support
   B. Report the case in which the abuse is suspected to the local authorities
   C. Document the child's physical assessment findings accurately and thoroughly
   D. Refer the family to the hospital support group
5. Nursing care of a child in the hospital with suspected abuse should include which of the following actions?
   A. Assign a variety of nurses to the child so that he can get to know and trust the whole staff.
   B. Praise the child's ability to minimize feelings of shame and guilt.
   C. Treat the child as someone with a specific problem, not as an "abuse" victim, to promote self-esteem and minimize feelings of guilt.
   D. Talk with and ask questions as often as possible to show interest and get to know the child better.

Correct Answers

1. A, C, E; 2. D; 3. A, B; 4. B; 5. C

REFERENCES

Adams, J. A. (2011). Medical evaluation of suspected child sexual abuse: 2011 update. *Journal of Child Sexual Abuse, 20*(5), 588–605.

Albertson, T. E., Owen, K. P., Sutter, M. E., et al. (2011). Gastrointestinal decontamination in the acutely poisoned patient. *International Journal of Emergency Medicine, 4*, 65.

Altimier, L. (2008). Shaken baby syndrome. *J Perinat Neonat Nurs, 22*(1), 68–76.

American Academy of Pediatrics Committee on Child Abuse and Neglect. (2009). Abusive head trauma in infants and children. *Pediatrics, 123*(5), 1409–1411.

Babcock, D. A. (2011). Evaluating sleep and sleep disorders in the pediatric primary care setting. *Pediatric Clinics of North America, 58*(3), 543–554.

Barr, R. G. (2012). Preventing abusive head trauma resulting from a failure of normal interaction between infants and their caregivers. *Proc Natl Acad Sci, 109*(Suppl. 2), 17294–17301.

Benson, B. E., Hoppu, K., Troutman, W. G., et al. (2013). Position paper update: gastric lavage for gastrointestinal decontamination. *Clinical Toxicology (Philadelphia, Pa.), 51*(3), 140–146.

Bhargava, S. (2011). Diagnosis and management of common sleep problems in children. *Pediatrics in Review, 32*(3), 91–98.

Bose-O'Reilly, S., McCarthy, K. M., Steckling, N., et al. (2010). Mercury exposure and children's health. *Current Problems in Pediatric and Adolescent Health Care, 40*(8), 186–215.

Breyer, R. J., & MacPhee, D. (2015). Community characteristics, conservative ideology, and child abuse rates. *Child Abuse Neglect, 41*, 126–135.

Bronstein, A. C., Spyker, D. A., Cantilena, L. R., Jr., et al. (2012). 2011 Annual report of the American Association of Poison Control Centers' National Poison Data System (NPDS): 29th annual report. *Clinical Toxicology (Philadelphia, PA), 50*(10), 911–1164.

Campbell, C., Gracely, E., Tran, M., et al. (2012). Primary prevention of lead exposure—blood lead levels at age two years. *International Journal of Environmental Research and Public Health, 9*(4), 1216–1226.

Centers for Disease Control and Prevention (2002). *Managing elevated blood lead levels among young children: Recommendations from the Advisory Committee on Childhood Lead Poisoning Prevention*. Atlanta, GA: Author.

Centers for Disease Control and Prevention: *Lead*. https://www.cdc.gov/nceh/lead/ Updated 9 February 2017.

Centers for Disease Control and Prevention Advisory Committee on Childhood Lead Poisoning Prevention: *CDC response to Advisory Committee on Childhood Lead Poisoning Prevention recommendations in "low level lead exposure harms children: a renewed call of primary prevention,"* 2012, http://www.cdc.gov/nceh/lead/acclpp/final_document_030712.pdf.

Chandran, L., & Cataldo, R. (2010). Lead poisoning: basics and new developments. *Pediatrics in Review, 31*(10), 399–406.

Cowley, L. E., Morris, C. B., Maguire, S. A., et al. (2015). Validation of a prediction tool for abusive head trauma. *Pediatrics, 136*(2), 290–298.

Cunningham, E. (2012). What role does nutrition play in the prevention or treatment of childhood lead poisoning? *Journal of the Academy of Nutrition & Dietetics, 112*(11), 1916.

Dapul, H., & Laraque, D. (2014). Lead poisoning in children. *Advances in Pediatrics, 61*(1), 313–333.

Dubowitz, H., & Lane, W. (2016). Abused and neglected children. In R. M. Kliegman, B. F. Stanton, J. W. St Geme, et al. (Eds.), *Nelson textbook of pediatrics* (20th ed.). Philadelphia: Saunders/Elsevier.

Evans, H. (2011). Pediatrics tackles child sexual abuse. *Archives of Pediatrics and Adolescent Medicine, 165*(9), 783–784.

Forsdike, K., Tarzia, L., Hindmarsh, E., et al. (2014). Family violence across the life cycle. *Australian Family Physician, 43*(11), 768–774.

Fountain, J. S., & Reith, D. M. (2014). Dangers of "EDTA. *The New Zealand Medical Journal, 127*(1398), 126–127.

Frithsen, I., & Simpson, W. (2010). Recognition and management of acute medication poisoning. *American Family Physician, 81*(3), 316–323.

Garrison, M. M., Liekweg, K., & Christakis, D. A. (2011). Media use and child sleep: the impact of content, timing and environment. *Pediatrics, 128*(1), 29–35.

Girardet, R., Bolton, K., Lohoti, S., et al. (2011). Collection of forensic evidence from pediatric victims of sexual assault. *Pediatrics, 128*(2), 233–238.

Hibbard, R., Barlow, J., MacMillan, H., et al. (2012). Psychological maltreatment. *Pediatrics, 130*(2), 372–378.

Jones, A. L. (2009). Emerging aspects of assessing lead poisoning in childhood. *Emerg Health Threats J, 2*, e3.

Kemp, A. M. (2011). Abusive head trauma: recognition and the essential investigation. *Arch Dis Child Educ Pract Ed, 96*(6), 202–208.

Kendrick, D., Mulvaney, C. A., Ye, L., et al. (2013). Parenting interventions for the prevention of unintentional injuries in childhood. *Cochrane Database of Systematic Review*, (3), CD006020.

Kendrick, D., Young, B., Mason-Jones, A. J., et al. (2012). Home safety education and provision of safety equipment for injury prevention. *Cochrane Database of Systematic Review*, (9), CD005014.

Krienert, J. L., & Walsh, J. A. (2011). Sibling sexual abuse: an empirical analysis of offender, victim, and event characteristics in National Incident-based Reporting System (NBRS) data, 2000-2007. *Journal of Child Sexual Abuse, 20*(4), 353–372.

Lane, W. G. (2014). Prevention of child maltreatment. *Pediatric Clinics of North America, 61*(5), 873–888.

Lyden, C. (2011). Uncovering child abuse. *Nursing Management, 42*(Suppl.), 1–5.

Maguire, S. A., Watts, P. O., Shaw, A. D., et al. (2013). Retinal hemorrhages and related findings in abusive and non-abusive head trauma: a systematic review. *Eye, 27*(1), 28–36.

McGregor, T., Parkar, M., & Rao, S. (2009). Evaluation and management of common childhood poisonings. *American Family Physician, 79*(5), 397–403.

Mindell, J. A., Sadeh, A., Kohyama, J., et al. (2010). Parental behaviors and sleep outcomes in infants and toddlers: a cross-cultural comparison. *Sleep Medicine, 11*(4), 393–399.

Mollen, C. J., Goyal, M. K., & Frioux, S. M. (2012). Acute sexual abuse. *Pediatric Emergency Care, 28*(6), 584–590.

Mowry, J. B., Spyker, D. A., Brooks, D. E., et al. (2016). 2015 Annual report of the American Association of Poison Control Centers' National poison data system (NPDS): 33rd annual report. *Clinical Toxicology, 54*(10), 924–1109.

National Center on Shaken Baby Syndrome: *All about SBS/AHT*, n.d., http://www.dontshake.org/sbs.php?topNavID=3&subNavID=317.

Olson, K. R. (2010). Activated charcoal for acute poisoning: one toxicologist's journey. *J Med Toxicol, 6*(2), 190–198.

Petersen, D. D. (2011). Common plant toxicology: a comparison of national and southwest Ohio data trends in plant poisonings in the 21st century. *Toxicology and Applied Pharmacology, 254*(2), 148–153.

Raymond, J. S., Kennedy, C., & Brown, M. J. (2013). Blood lead level analysis among refugee children resettled in New Hampshire and Rhode Island. *Public Health Nursing, 30*(1), 70–79.

Schneiderman, J. U., Smith, C., & Palinkas, L. A. (2012). The caregiver as gatekeeper for accessing health care for children in foster care: a qualitative study of kinship and unrelated caregivers. *Children and Youth Services Review, 34*(10), 2123–2130.

Selph, S. S., Bougatsos, C., Blazina, I., et al. (2013). Behavioral interventions and counseling to prevent child abuse and neglect: a systematic review to update the US Preventative Services Task Force recommendations. *Annals of Internal Medicine, 158*(3), 179–190.

Squires, J. E., & Squires, R. H. (2013). A review of Munchausen syndrome by proxy. *Pediatric Annals, 42*(4), 67–71.

Theurer, W. M., & Bhavsar, A. K. (2013). Prevention of unintentional childhood injury. *American Family Physician, 87*(7), 502–509.

US Department of Health and Human Services (2012). *Child maltreatment 2011*. Washington, DC: US Government Printing Office.

US Department of Health and Human Services (2015). *The Child Abuse Prevention and Treatment Act (CAPTA) 2010*. Washington, DC: US Government Printing Office.

Ward, T. C., & Doering, J. J. (2014). Application of a socio-ecological model to mother-infant bed-sharing. *Health Education & Behavior, 41*(6), 577–589.

15

Health Promotion of the School-Age Child and Family

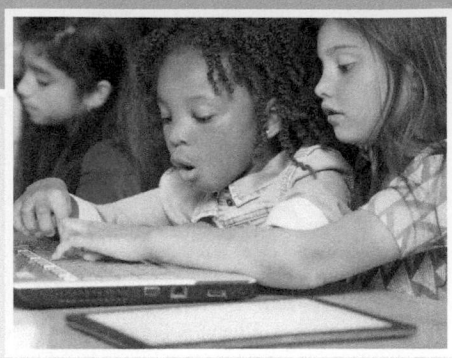

Cheryl C. Rodgers

http://evolve.elsevier.com/wong/ncic

CONCEPTS

- Development
- Functional Ability
- Culture
- Family Dynamics
- Sexuality
- Stress
- Safety

PROMOTING OPTIMUM GROWTH AND DEVELOPMENT

The segment of the life span that extends from age 6 years to approximately age 12 years has a variety of labels, each of which describes an important characteristic of the period. The middle years are most often referred to as school-age or the school years. This period begins with entrance into the wider sphere of influence represented by the school environment, which has a significant impact on development and relationships.

Physiologically the middle years begin with the shedding of the first deciduous tooth and end at puberty with the acquisition of the final permanent teeth (with the exception of the wisdom teeth). In the 5 to 6 years before the school-age period, children progressed from helpless infants to sturdy, complicated individuals with the capacity to communicate, conceptualize in a limited way, and become involved in complex social and motor behaviors. Physical growth has been equally rapid. In contrast, the period of middle childhood—between the rapid growth of early childhood and the prepubescent growth spurt—is a time of gradual growth and development, with even more progress in both physical and emotional aspects.

BIOLOGIC DEVELOPMENT

During middle childhood, growth in height and weight assumes a slower but steady pace compared with the earlier years. Between ages 6 and 12 years, children grow an average of 5 cm (2 inches) per year to gain 30 to 60 cm (1 to 2 feet) in height and will almost double in weight, increasing 2 to 3 kg (4.4 to 6.6 lb) per year. The average 6-year-old child is about 116 cm (46 inches) tall and weighs about 21 kg (46 lb); the average 12-year-old child stands about 150 cm (59 inches) tall and weighs approximately 40 kg (88 lb). During this age period girls and boys differ little in size, although boys tend to be slightly taller and somewhat heavier than girls. Toward the end of the school-age years both boys and girls begin to increase in size, although most girls begin to surpass boys in both height and weight, to the acute discomfort of both girls and boys.

Physical Changes

School-age children are more graceful than they were as preschoolers, and they are steadier on their feet. Their bodies take on a slimmer look, with longer legs, varying body proportions, and a lower center of gravity. Posture improves over that of the preschool period to facilitate locomotion and efficiency in using the arms and trunk. These proportions make climbing, bicycle riding, and other activities much easier. Fat gradually diminishes, and its distribution patterns change, contributing to the thinner appearance of children during the middle years.

Accompanying the skeletal lengthening and fat diminution is an increase in the percentage of body weight represented by muscle tissue. By the end of this age period, both boys and girls double their strength and physical capabilities, and their steady and relatively consistent acquisition of refined coordination increases their poise and skill. However, this increased strength is often misleading. Although strength increases, muscles are still functionally immature compared with those of the adolescent, and they are more readily injured by overuse.

The most pronounced changes that seem best to indicate increasing maturity in children are a decrease in head circumference in relation to standing height, a decrease in waist circumference in relation to height, and an increase in leg length related to height. These indicators

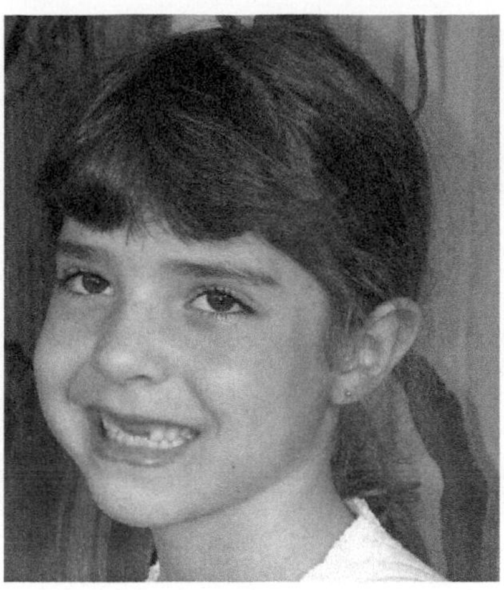

FIG. 15.1 Middle childhood is the stage of development when deciduous teeth are shed.

often provide a clue to a child's degree of maturity. Certain physiologic and anatomic characteristics are typical of school-age children. Facial proportions change as the face grows faster in relation to the remainder of the cranium. The skull and brain grow very slowly during this period and increase little in size thereafter. Because all of the primary (deciduous) teeth are lost during this age span, middle childhood is sometimes known as the age of the loose tooth (Fig. 15.1). The early years of middle childhood are known as the ugly duckling stage, when the new secondary (permanent) teeth appear to be much too large for the face.

Maturation of Systems

As the gastrointestinal system matures, the child has fewer stomach upsets; better maintenance of blood glucose levels; and an increased stomach capacity, which permits retention of food for longer periods. The school-age child does not need to be fed as carefully, as promptly, or as frequently as before. Caloric needs are lower than they were in the preschool years and lower than they will be during the coming adolescent growth spurt.

Physical maturation occurs in other body tissues and organs. Bladder capacity, although differing widely among individual children, is generally greater in girls than in boys. There are individual variations in frequency of urination and differences in the same child according to circumstances such as temperature, humidity, time of day, amount of fluids ingested, and emotional state.

The heart grows more slowly during the middle years and is smaller in relation to the rest of the body than at any other period of life. Heart and respiratory rates steadily decrease and blood pressure increases between ages 6 and 12 years (see inside back cover).

The immune system becomes more competent in its ability to localize infections and produce an antibody-antigen response. Because of increased exposure to others in school classes, children can have several infections in the first 1 to 2 years of school while immunity develops.

Bones continue to ossify throughout childhood, but because mineralization is not completed until maturity, children's bones resist pressure, and muscles pull less than with mature bones. Consequently, parents must be careful to prevent alterations in bone structure and provide children with well-fitted shoes and with chairs and desks that allow correct sitting posture with the feet able to reach the floor and the hips able to fit well back in the seat. Children should have ample opportunity to move around and be cautious about carrying heavy loads. For example, they should shift books and/or tote bags from one arm to the other. Back packs, when worn correctly, distribute weight more evenly.

Wider differences between children are seen at the end of middle childhood than at the beginning. These differences become increasingly apparent and, if extreme or unique, may create emotional problems. The nurse explains the associated characteristics of height and weight relationships, rapid or slow growth, and other important features of development to children and their families. Physical maturity is not necessarily correlated with emotional and social maturity. Seven-year-old children who look like 10-year-old children will think and act like 7-year-olds. Expecting behavior appropriate for 10-year-old children from them is unrealistic and can be detrimental to their development of competence and self-esteem. Conversely, treating 10-year-old children as though they were 7 years old is an equal disservice to them.

Prepubescence

Preadolescence is the period that begins toward the end of middle childhood and ends with the thirteenth birthday. Puberty signals the beginning of the development of secondary sex characteristics, and prepubescence, the 2-year period that precedes puberty, typically occurs during preadolescence.

Toward the end of middle childhood the discrepancies in growth and maturation between boys and girls become apparent. On average, there is a difference of approximately 2 years between girls and boys in the age of onset of pubescence. For many, especially for girls, preadolescence is a period of rapid growth. For others, mostly boys, it is generally a period of continued steady growth in height and weight.

There is no universal age at which children assume the characteristics of preadolescence. The first physiologic signs appear at about 9 years (particularly in girls) and are usually clearly evident in 11- to 12-year-old children. Although preadolescent children do not want to be different, variability in physical growth and physiologic changes among children of the same sex, and between the two sexes, is often striking at this time. This variability, especially in relation to the onset of secondary sex characteristics, is of utmost concern to the preadolescent. Either early or late appearance of these characteristics is a source of embarrassment and uneasiness to both sexes. Early appearance of secondary sex characteristics in girls is often associated with dissatisfaction with physical appearance, greater general unhappiness, and lower self-esteem. Late-developing boys often have a negative self-concept. Both early appearance of physical characteristics in girls and late appearance in boys have been linked to participation in risk-taking behaviors (e.g., early sexual activity, substance use, and reckless vehicle use).

Preadolescence is a time when considerable overlapping of developmental characteristics occurs, with elements of both middle childhood and early adolescence apparent. However, there are sufficient unique characteristics to set this period apart as an age category. Generally, puberty begins at 10 years in girls and 12 years in boys, but its onset in either sex after age 8 years is considered normal. The average age of puberty is 12 years in girls and 14 years in boys. Boys experience little sexual maturation during preadolescence.

Psychosocial Development

Middle childhood is the period of psychosexual development that Freud described as the latency period, a time of tranquility between the oedipal phase of early childhood and the eroticism of adolescence. During this time children experience relationships with same-sex peers following the indifference of earlier years and preceding the heterosexual fascination that occurs for most boys and girls in puberty.

Developing a Sense of Industry (Erikson)

Successful mastery of Erikson's first three stages of psychosocial development is probably the most important accomplishment in terms of development of a healthy personality (Erikson, 1963).

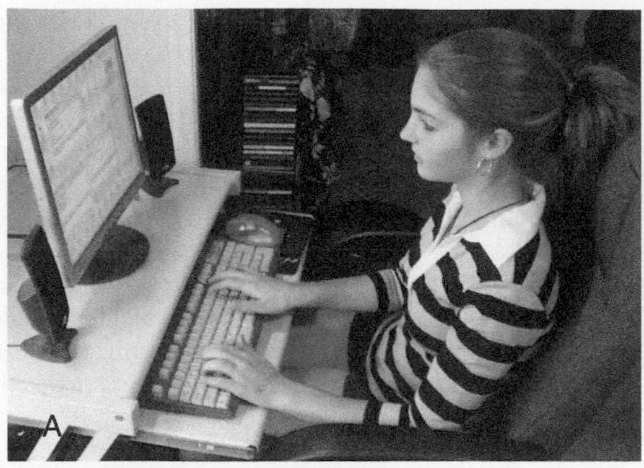
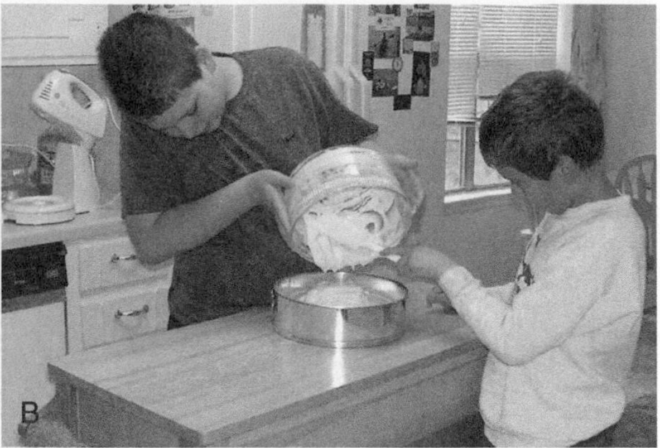

FIG. 15.2 School-age children are motivated to complete tasks. **A,** Working alone. **B,** Working with others.

Successful completion of these stages requires a loving environment within a stable family unit that has prepared the child to engage in experiences and relationships beyond this intimate group. During childhood, children affiliate with age-mates, receive the systematic instruction prescribed by their individual cultures, and develop the skills needed to become useful, contributing members of their social communities.

A sense of industry, or a stage of accomplishment, occurs somewhere between age 6 years and adolescence. The goal of this stage of development is to achieve a sense of personal and interpersonal competence through the acquisition of technologic and social skills. School-age children are eager to build skills and participate in meaningful and socially useful work. Interests expand, and, with a growing sense of independence, children want to engage in tasks that they can complete (Fig. 15.2). Failure to develop a sense of accomplishment may result in a sense of inferiority.

Many aspects of industry contribute to the child's sense of competence and mastery. Intrinsic motivation is associated with increased competence in mastering new skills and assuming new responsibilities. Children gain a great deal of satisfaction from independent behavior in exploring and manipulating their environment and from interaction with peers. Extrinsic sources of reinforcement in the form of grades, material rewards, additional privileges, and recognition provide encouragement and stimulation. Often the acquisition of skills is a means for achieving success in special activities such as athletics or social organizations. Peer approval is a strong motivating factor.

The danger inherent in this period of personality development is the occurrence of situations that might result in a sense of inadequacy or inferiority. This may happen if the previous stages have not been successfully mastered or if a child is incapable of assuming or unprepared to assume the responsibilities associated with developing a sense of accomplishment. Feelings of inferiority or lack of worth come from children themselves or from the social environment. Children with physical or mental limitations are sometimes at a disadvantage for acquisition of certain skills. When the reward structure is based on evidence of mastery, children who are incapable of developing these skills are at risk for feeling inadequate and inferior.

Even children without chronic disabilities show such a wide range of individual differences in capabilities and preferences that they experience feelings of inadequacy in some areas. No child is able to do well in everything, and children must learn that they will not be able to master each skill that they attempt. All children, even children who usually have positive attitudes toward work and their own capabilities, feel some degree of inferiority in regard to a specific skill that they cannot master.

For some children, success or aptitude in one area may compensate for failure or ineptitude in another. However, the differences in reinforcement provided for success in various areas have significant effects on feelings of adequacy. For example, society places a higher value on success in team sports than on success in repairing a bicycle. Compensating for the inability to excel in more socially valued skills through mastery of other, less valued skills is difficult for children. If the social environment places a negative value on any failure, feelings of inferiority may be increased in the less capable child. Repeated failures can generate such strong feelings that eventually the child is reluctant to attempt any new task or is fearful of not being able to perform as well as his or her peers. Thus intrinsic motivation toward engaging in a task for the pleasure of the challenge conflicts with the external forces that cause feelings of doubt and inferiority. Consequently, the child may no longer try.

A child's concept of success or failure is important. Children who aspire to more than they are capable of usually experience failure. In contrast, children who set their aspirations lower than their level of achievement are likely to experience success. Most accomplishments during the school years are very public. Family, teachers, and peers are all aware of success or failure in school. In school and sometimes at home, feelings of inferiority may be produced through comparisons with others that suggest the child is not as good as a peer, sibling, or member of another group. This inadequacy becomes a source of embarrassment. The child may even be shamed for the failure. Earlier conflicts of doubt and guilt are closely associated with feelings of inferiority.

A sense of accomplishment also involves the ability to cooperate, to compete with others, and to cope effectively with people. Middle childhood is the time when children learn the value of doing things with others and the benefits derived from division of labor in the accomplishment of goals. Children need and want real achievement. When they can accomplish tasks that need to be done and perform well despite individual differences in capacities and emotional development, and when they are suitably rewarded, children develop a sense of industry and accomplishment that prepares them for establishing a stable identity later in life.

Temperament

The reactivity patterns or temperamental traits identified in infancy may continue to influence behavior in middle childhood. Analyzing behavioral patterns observed in past situations can provide clues to the way that a child may react to new situations, although long-range projections are not always successful. Through interaction with the environment, experiences, motives, and abilities, many children change. In some children, major temperamental characteristics persist into adolescence; in others they do not.

Many children tend to be identified with one of three broad temperament categories: easy, slow to warm up, and difficult. Parents and teachers are in an excellent position to assess a child's behavioral style and to try to make their demands and expectations consonant with the individual child's temperamental characteristics. With easy children this rarely poses a problem. They adapt readily to many childrearing programs and new situations. School entry and other changes usually go smoothly and are accomplished with minimal stress. Difficulties arise with children who are slow to warm up or are difficult or easily distracted.

Slow-to-warm-up children usually exhibit discomfort when introduced to new situations and need time to become accustomed to a new environment, authority figures, and expectations. These children may respond with tears, somatic complaints, or other maneuvers to avoid the event. The nurse should encourage them to try new experiences but allow them to adapt to their surroundings at their own speed. Pressure to move quickly into new situations only strengthens the tendency to withdraw. After-school activities can be a cause for reaction, but attending with a friend or contracting for permission to withdraw after a trial of a specified number of times may provide them with sufficient incentive to try (see Critical Thinking Case Study box).

CRITICAL THINKING CASE STUDY

Temperament in the School-Age Child

Mary's teacher asks the school nurse for guidance. Mary is 8 years old and has just entered the third grade. In the classroom Mary is quiet and passive, and she frequently cries when the teacher talks with her. Mary's mother describes her daughter as a healthy child who has always required more time and effort to adapt to changes in her routine. In counseling Mary's teacher, what should the nurse encourage the teacher to do?

1. Evidence—Is there sufficient evidence to draw any conclusions about Mary's behavior?
2. Assumptions—Describe the underlying assumptions about each of the following:
   a. Factors and timing related to establishment of a child's temperament
   b. Ease or difficulty of adapting to new situations in relation to temperament
   c. Helping the slow-to-warm-up child adjust to new situations
3. What priorities for nursing care can be drawn from this situation?
4. Does the evidence support your conclusion?

Answers are available at http://evolve.elsevier.com/wong/ncic.

Difficult or easily distracted children may benefit from "practice" sessions in which they are prepared for a given event by role playing, visiting the site, or reading or listening to stories, or use of other methods to acquaint them with what to expect. Children who are persistent need to know when to stop what they are doing so that the signal to stop will not come as a surprise or trigger a reaction. Nurses need to handle children with difficult temperaments with exceptional patience, firmness, and understanding so that they can learn appropriate behavior in their interactions with others. If possible, teachers' styles and characteristics should match the temperament of children to ensure a good fit.

COGNITIVE DEVELOPMENT (PIAGET)

When children enter the school years, they begin to acquire the ability to relate a series of events and actions to mental representations that they can express both verbally and symbolically. This is the stage that Piaget describes as **concrete operations**, when children are able to use their thought processes to experience events and actions. The term *operation* implies an action that is performed on an object or set of objects; thus a mental operation is an alteration or transformation that an individual carries out in thought rather than in action. Toddlers or preschool children can perform acts that involve ordering, such as correctly arranging a graduated set of circles from largest to smallest on a stick, and can find their way to a friend's house, but they are unable to verbalize the actions involved in the process. School-age children are able to articulate the process and perform the actions mentally without the need to carry out the behaviors.

As children move from the preschool years into the school years, their conceptual abilities become increasingly flexible. During the concrete operational period, they acquire the ability to perform cognitive operations and apply these new skills when thinking about objects, situations, and events. Their rigid, egocentric outlook is replaced by thought processes that allow them to see things from another's point of view. They become aware of a variety of perspectives and become more sensitive to the fact that others do not always perceive events exactly as they do. They are able to delay an action until they have evaluated alternative responses to situations. Their steady reduction in egocentricity helps form the basis for logical thought and the development and maturation of morality.

The concrete operational stage occurs between ages 7 and 11 years. During this stage children develop an understanding of relationships between things and ideas. They progress from making judgments based on what they see (perceptual thinking) to making judgments based on what they reason (conceptual thinking). They are increasingly able to master symbols and to use their memories of past experiences to evaluate and interpret the present.

One of the major cognitive tasks of school-age children is mastering the concept of **conservation**—that physical matter does not appear and disappear by magic. They learn that certain properties of the environment are not changed simply by altering their disposition in space. They are able to resist perceptual cues that suggest alterations in the physical state of an object. The nurse can use commonplace items to demonstrate the conservation of liquid, mass, number, length, area, and volume (Fig. 15.3). To explain the observation that the mass of the clay in the figure has not been altered, children use one of three concepts:

1. Identity—Because nothing has been added and nothing has been taken away, the pancake is still the same clay. Nothing has changed but the shape.
2. Reversibility—The clay can be reshaped into its original form (a ball).
3. Reciprocity—Although the pancake appears larger in circumference, the ball is much thicker. In this instance the child demonstrates the ability to deal with two dimensions at the same time and to comprehend that a change in one dimension compensates for a change in another.

When children are able to use the concepts of identity, reversibility, and reciprocity, they can conserve along any physical dimension. They perceive the concept of volume in relation to container size and shape, recognize that size is not necessarily related to weight or volume, and are able to manipulate or "see" in a concrete manner. They recognize that logical operations move in two directions (such as addition and subtraction or multiplication and division) and that certain properties are invariant (e.g., 7 remains 7 whether it is represented by 3 + 4, 2 + 5, seven buttons, seven stars, or seven boys).

There appears to be a developmental sequence in children's capacity to conserve matter. Children usually grasp conservation of numbers (ages 5 to 6 years) before conservation of substance. Conservation of liquids, mass, and length usually is accomplished at about ages 6 to 7, conservation of weight sometime later (ages 9 to 10 years), and conservation of volume or displacement last (ages 9 to 12 years).

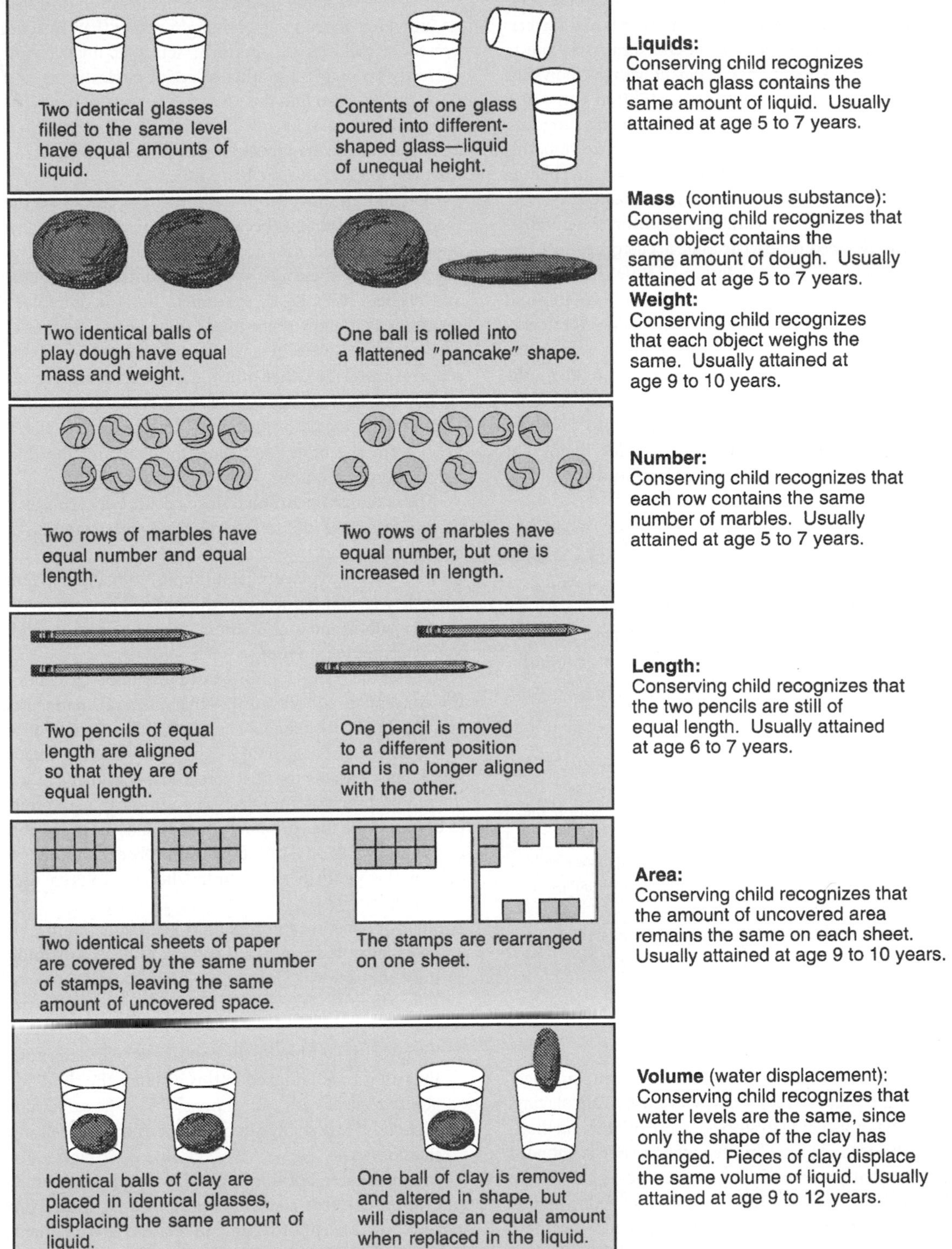
Two identical glasses filled to the same level have equal amounts of liquid.
Contents of one glass poured into different-shaped glass—liquid of unequal height.
Liquids:
Conserving child recognizes that each glass contains the same amount of liquid. Usually attained at age 5 to 7 years.
Two identical balls of play dough have equal mass and weight.
One ball is rolled into a flattened "pancake" shape.
Mass (continuous substance):
Conserving child recognizes that each object contains the same amount of dough. Usually attained at age 5 to 7 years.
Weight:
Conserving child recognizes that each object weighs the same. Usually attained at age 9 to 10 years.
Two rows of marbles have equal number and equal length.
Two rows of marbles have equal number, but one is increased in length.
Number:
Conserving child recognizes that each row contains the same number of marbles. Usually attained at age 5 to 7 years.
Two pencils of equal length are aligned so that they are of equal length.
One pencil is moved to a different position and is no longer aligned with the other.
Length:
Conserving child recognizes that the two pencils are still of equal length. Usually attained at age 6 to 7 years.
Two identical sheets of paper are covered by the same number of stamps, leaving the same amount of uncovered space.
The stamps are rearranged on one sheet.
Area:
Conserving child recognizes that the amount of uncovered area remains the same on each sheet. Usually attained at age 9 to 10 years.
Identical balls of clay are placed in identical glasses, displacing the same amount of liquid.
One ball of clay is removed and altered in shape, but will displace an equal amount when replaced in the liquid.
Volume (water displacement):
Conserving child recognizes that water levels are the same, since only the shape of the clay has changed. Pieces of clay displace the same volume of liquid. Usually attained at age 9 to 12 years.

FIG. 15.3 Common examples that demonstrate the child's ability to conserve (ages are approximate).

Children use reversibility in selecting a course of action, which thus provides greater control over themselves and their environment. They have the ability to think through an action sequence, anticipate the consequences, and, if needed, return to the beginning and rethink the action in a different direction. They no longer need to experience an action before they can anticipate the results. Reversibility allows mental action and enables children to disassemble and reassemble certain kinds of things in their thoughts.

Classification skills involve the ability to group objects according to the attributes that they have in common. School-age children can place things in a sensible and logical order, group and sort, and hold a concept in their minds while they make decisions based on that concept. In middle childhood children get a great deal of enjoyment from classifying and ordering their environment. They become occupied with numerous and varied collections of objects, such as shells, dolls, cars, stones, cards, stuffed animals, and anything that is classifiable

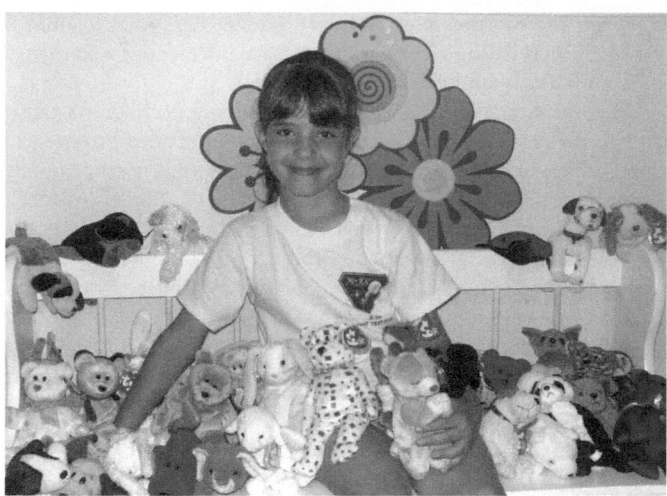

FIG. 15.4 School-age children are often avid collectors.

(Fig. 15.4). They even begin to order friends and relationships (e.g., first best friend, second best friend).

As children mature, they progress from collecting simply for the sake of collecting and become more selective and discriminating. Their classification systems become more complex and are based on abstract ideas rather than on perception and experience. Much of the pleasure of collections is in the appraising, ordering, and reordering of the parts.

School-age children are able to serialize, or to arrange objects according to some ordinal scale or quantified dimension such as size, weight, or color. They develop the ability to understand relational terms and concepts, such as bigger and smaller; darker and paler; heavier and lighter; to the right of and to the left of; first, last, and intermediate (e.g., fourth, second); and more than and less than. They can see family relationships in terms of reciprocal roles—for example, to be a brother, one must have a sibling.

During the school-age years children develop combinatorial skills—the ability to manipulate numbers and to learn the skills of addition, subtraction, multiplication, and division. They learn to apply the basic operations to any object or quantity. They learn the alphabet and the world of symbols called words that can be arranged in terms of structure and their relationship to the alphabet. They learn to tell time, to see the relationship of events in time (history) and places in space (geography), and to combine time and space relationships (geology and astronomy).

The most significant skill, the ability to read, is acquired during the school years and becomes the most valuable tool for independent inquiry. Children's capacity for exploration, imagination, and expansion of knowledge is enhanced by the ability to read as they progress from the repetition and confusion of early efforts to increasing facility and comprehension. Formal academic learning begins at ages 5 to 6 years, when children's intellectual capabilities and cognitive processes allow them to attain intellectual achievements.

MORAL DEVELOPMENT (KOHLBERG)

As children move from egocentrism to more logical patterns of thought, they also move through stages in the development of conscience and moral standards. Young children do not believe that standards of behavior come from within themselves but that others establish and enforce these rules. During preschool years, children perceive rules as definite and require no reason or explanation. Children learn the standards for acceptable behavior, act according to these standards, and feel guilty when they violate the standards. Although children 6 or 7 years old know the rules and behaviors expected of them, they do not understand the reasons behind them. Young children usually judge an act by its consequences. Rewards and punishment guide their judgment; a "bad" act is one that breaks a rule or causes harm. When a child and an adult differ in judging an act, the adult is right. Children may believe that what other people tell them to do is right and that what they themselves think is wrong. Consequently, children 6 or 7 years old are more likely to interpret accidents and misfortunes as punishment for misdeeds or "bad" acts.

Older school-age children are able to judge an act by the intentions that prompted it rather than just by the consequences. Rules and judgments become less absolute and authoritarian and begin to be founded more on the needs and desires of others. Rules of conduct are more readily considered in terms of mutual agreement and are based on cooperation and respect for others. Older children will likely view a rule violation in relation to the total context in which it appears; reactions are influenced by the situation as well as by the morality of the rule itself. However, it is not until adolescence or beyond that children are able to view morality on an abstract basis with sound reasoning and principled thinking. Although younger children can judge an act only according to whether it is right or wrong, older children take into account a different point of view to make a judgment. They are able to understand and accept the concept of treating others as they would like to be treated.

SPIRITUAL DEVELOPMENT

Children at this age think in very concrete terms but are avid learners and have a great desire to learn about their God or deity. They picture God as human and use adjectives such as "loving" and "helping" to describe their deity. They are fascinated by heaven and hell and, with a developing conscience and concern about rules, they fear going to hell for misbehavior. School-age children want and expect to be punished for misbehavior and, if given the option, tend to choose a punishment that "fits the crime." Often they view illness or injury as a punishment for a real or imagined misdeed. The beliefs and ideals of family and religious personages are more influential than those of their peers in matters of faith.

School-age children begin to learn the difference between the natural and the supernatural but have difficulty understanding symbols. Consequently, religious concepts must be presented to them in concrete terms. They try to relate phenomena in the world in a logical, systematic manner, which is both satisfying and occasionally disheartening. Religion is a means whereby children can relate to their deity in a direct and personal way.

Prayer and other religious rituals are often a comfort to children, and if these activities are a part of children's daily lives, they can help children cope with threatening situations (Fig. 15.5). Their petitions to their God in prayers tend to be for tangible rewards. Although younger children expect their prayers to be answered, as children get older they begin to recognize that this does not always occur and become less concerned when prayers are not answered. They are able to discuss their feelings about their faith and how it relates to their lives (see Cultural Considerations box).

LANGUAGE DEVELOPMENT

Children enter middle childhood with remarkably efficient language skills, but they make many important linguistic achievements during the school-age years. During the elementary school years they learn to correct previous syntactic errors and begin to use more complex

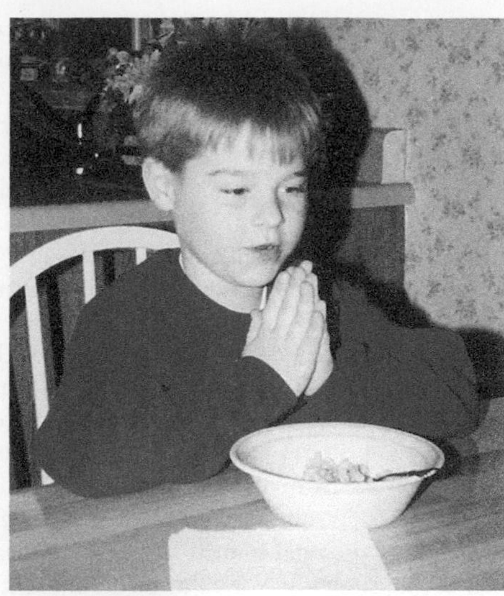

FIG. 15.5 Children are comforted by prayer or other religious rituals.

CULTURAL CONSIDERATIONS

Religious Orientation

Many schools and communities have a Judeo-Christian orientation toward prayer, holidays, and values. This may result in conflict and discomfort for children of other religious and ethnic groups. Sensitivity must be exercised so as not to offend and confuse children from other religious backgrounds, such as the Buddhist, Hindu, and Muslim faiths, and those with no religious backgrounds.

grammatical forms, such as correct past tenses for irregular verbs, correct plurals for irregular nouns, and correct personal pronouns.

Word usage and the ability to find and retrieve words quickly when called on to produce what they know in a relatively short time grow considerably during the school years. Children learn to apply the minimum-distance principle—the rule that the subject of a verb in an active sentence is the noun or pronoun that immediately precedes it. For example, a 6-year-old child will understand the sentence "Ask Mary her last name" but until age 9 or 10 years will be confused by the sentence "Ask Mary what to bring to the party."

Narrative skills improve markedly. School-age children are increasingly able to provide directives that others can correctly interpret without visual data (e.g., explain directions over the telephone). By ages 10 to 12 years the child should be able to use factitive words (such as *know, think,* and *believe*), as well as complex pronouns and conjunctions, and be able to form grammatically correct sentences. School-age children gradually become more proficient at making inferences about meanings and learn the subtle exceptions to grammatical rules. This makes them less likely to engage in literal interpretation of messages.

They rapidly develop *metalinguistic awareness*—an ability to think about language and to comment on its properties. This enables them to appreciate jokes, riddles, and puns that involve play on words, sounds, or double meanings. They are beginning to understand metaphors and figurative statements, such as "A stitch in time saves nine." The acquisition of cognitive skills enables them to think about the quality of their own and others' speech and to evaluate and clarify messages.

SOCIAL DEVELOPMENT

At the beginning of middle childhood, children enter a period of less intense emotions, secure in their dependency on their parents and family and with self-confidence tempered by a more realistic perspective. They have the energy to explore the environment beyond the family, to gradually increase the scope of interpersonal interactions, and to invest their curiosity in understanding the world.

Identification with peers is a strong influence in children's gaining independence from parents. The aid and support of peers provides children with enough security to risk the moderate parental rejection brought about by each small victory in their development of independence.

Questions of masculinity and femininity take on importance as sex-role learning assumes more prominence. Boys associate with boys, and girls with girls, each group pursuing its own interests, with communication between the sexes confined to that which is necessary. Much of the child's concept of the appropriate sex role is acquired through relationships with peers. During the early school years there is little difference relative to sex in the play experiences of children. Both girls and boys share games and other activities. However, in the later school years the differences become marked.

Social Relationships and Cooperation

Daily relationships with peers provide the most important social interactions for school-age children. For the first time, children are able to join in group activities with unrestrained enthusiasm and steady participation. Previously, interactions were limited to short periods under considerable adult supervision. With increased skills and wider opportunities, children become involved with one or several peer groups in which they can gain status as respected members.

Valuable lessons are learned from daily interaction with age-mates. First, children learn to appreciate the numerous and varied points of view that are represented in the peer group. As they play together, children discover that there are many occupations for fathers and mothers, more than one version of the same song, different rules for the same game, and different customs for celebrating the same holiday. As children interact with peers who see the world in ways that are different from their own, they become aware of the limits of their own point of view. Because age-mates are peers and are not forced to accept one another's ideas as they are expected to accept those of adults, other children have a significant influence on decreasing the egocentric outlook of the individual child. Consequently, children learn to argue, persuade, bargain, cooperate, and compromise to maintain friendships.

Second, children become increasingly sensitive to the social norms and pressures of their peer group. The peer group establishes standards for acceptance and rejection, and children may be willing to modify their behavior to be accepted by the group. They are judged by the physical impression they convey, the skills they possess, and other abilities they can demonstrate. The need for peer approval becomes a powerful influence toward conformity. Children learn to dress, talk, and otherwise behave in a manner acceptable to the group. A variety of roles, such as class joker or class hero, may be assumed by the individual child to gain approval from the group. However, no child can adapt perfectly to all the requirements of the peer group. If some children find differences between the values of the peer group and the values of their families to be too great, they may relinquish the pleasure of interaction with the group to abide by the regulations established in the home. Thus to diminish conflict within the family, some children may be forced into a position outside the peer group.

Third, the interaction among peers leads to the formation of intimate friendships between same-sex peers (Fig. 15.6). School age is the time when children have "best friends" with whom they share secrets, private jokes, and adventures; they come to one another's aid in times of trouble. In the course of these friendships, children also fight, threaten, break up, and reunite. These dyadic relationships, in which children experience love for and closeness with a peer, seem to be important as a foundation for relationships in adulthood. The conflicts encountered

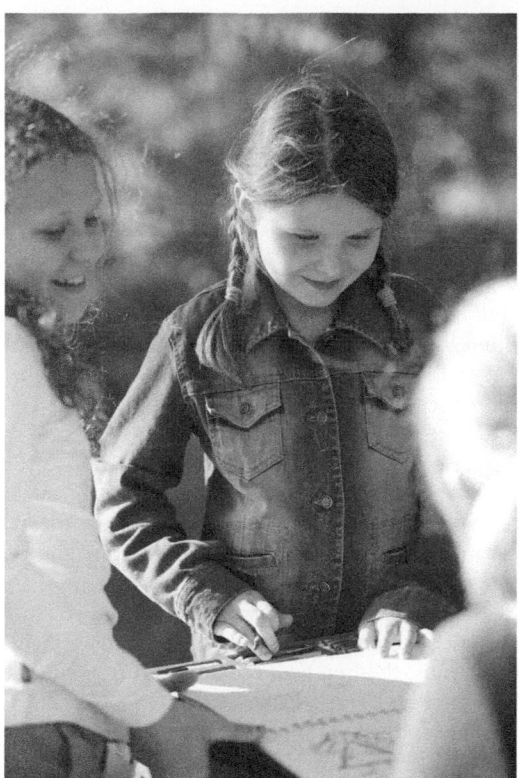

FIG. 15.6 School-age children enjoy engaging in activities with a "best friend."

in the relationship are usually resolved in terms that children are able to control. Because neither child has authority over the other, as in an adult-child relationship, children must work through their differences within the framework of their commitment to each other.

Clubs and Peer Groups

One of the outstanding characteristics of middle childhood is the formation of formalized groups or clubs. Initially, children in the early middle years merely hang around the periphery of the formalized group, watching, learning, practicing various skills, and participating in group activities whenever the members of the group allow them to do so. As they age, children eventually take their places as full-fledged participating group members.

A prominent feature of middle childhood groups is the code of rigid rules imposed on the members. Exclusiveness is evident in the selection of persons given the privilege of joining. Acceptance in the group often depends on a pass-fail basis according to social or behavioral criteria. Conformity is the core of the group structure. There are often secret codes, shared interests, special styles of dress, and special words that signify membership in the group. Each child must follow a standard of behavior established by the group. Conforming to the rules provides children with feelings of security and relieves them of the responsibility of making decisions.

Membership in the group provides children with a comfortable place in society. Many of the qualities valued by the group, such as physical strength, daring, ingenuity, and comradeship, have not been stressed in the family. However, these are values that contribute to an individual child's total personality. By merging their identity with the identities of their peers, children move from the family group to an outside group as a step toward further independence. They substitute conformity to a peer-group pattern for conformity to a family pattern while they are still too insecure to function independently.

During the early school years, groups are small and loosely organized, with changing membership and no formal structure. They do not demonstrate the elements of cooperation and order that are seen in groups of older children. As a rule, girls' groups are less formalized than boys' groups, and although there may be a mixture of both sexes in groups in the earlier school years, those of later school years are composed predominantly of children of the same sex. Common interests are frequently the central element around which a group is structured.

Children's strong desire not to be different creates problems for those who are, for various reasons, unable to meet the accepted standards of the peer group. Children with disabilities or those who are in some way unable to compete have a difficult time. Children become self-conscious when they are unable to dress like other children, do not have spending money like other children, or appear different from other children.

Children who have physical characteristics that are obviously different (such as birthmarks, ears that "stick out," or physical defects) may be set apart from the peer group and become a target for the criticism and ridicule. Peer-group identification and association are essential to socialization.

Poor relationships with peers and a lack of group identification can also contribute to bullying behavior. **Bullying** is any recurring activity that intends to cause harm, distress, or control toward another individual where there is a perceived imbalance of power between the aggressor(s) and the victim (Rettew & Pawlowski, 2016). Bullying can occur in varying degrees of severity in a physical, social, or emotional context. Although bullying can occur in any setting, it usually takes place in school hallways or on the playground where supervision is minimal but peers are present to witness the attack (Shetgiri, 2013). Cyberbullying involves an electronic medium to harm or bother another individual and can be more harmful than traditional bullying because the attack can instantly reach a wider audience, while allowing the bully to remain anonymous (Sticca & Perren, 2013). Up to 30% of school-age children engage in bullying (Rettew & Pawlowski, 2016) and approximately 11% to 42% engage in cyberbullying as the bully or the victim (Hamm, Newton, Chisholm, et al., 2015). The risk for bullying is greater in elementary and middle school than high school, but cyberbullying occurs more frequently in high school (Simon & Olson, 2014). Children who are targeted for bullying often have internalizing characteristics such as anxiety, depression, low self-esteem, and reduced assertiveness that may make them an easy target for bullying (Flannery, Todres, Bradshaw, et al., 2016). Bullies are generally defiant toward adults, manipulative, and likely to break school rules. They have aggressive attitudes, have a positive view of violence, and may experience or witness violence or abuse at home (Simon & Olson, 2014). Boys who bully tend to use physical force, referred to as *direct bullying,* but girls usually use bullying methods, such as exclusion, gossip, or rumors, which is referred to as *indirect bullying* (Simon & Olson, 2014).

The long-term consequences of bullying are significant. Future problems of bullies include a higher risk for antisocial behavior and participation in criminal behavior (Simon & Olson, 2014). Victims of bullying are at increased risk for low self-esteem; anxiety; depression, feelings of insecurity, and loneliness; poor academic performance; and self-harm behaviors (Flannery, Todres, Bradshaw, et al., 2016). Bullying can be reduced or prevented through supportive relationships with family, intervention of school personnel, and involvement with positive peer groups.* Many school districts have developed bullying prevention programs. The most effective aspects of bullying prevention programs

*For information on bullying, go to https://www.stopbullying.gov, a federal government website managed by the US Department of Health and Human Services.

include high levels of playground supervision, schoolwide rules related to bullying, teacher training, and parent training activities and meetings (Simon & Olson, 2014). Ineffective antibullying policies include grouping students who bully together and brief (e.g., 1-day) awareness campaigns (Simon & Olson, 2014).

Although peer-group identification and association are essential to a child's emergence into the world, dangers are inherent in strong peer-group attachment. Peer pressure may force children into taking risks or engage in behaviors that are against their better judgment. The frequency of gang membership increases during the preteen years and peaks at 14 years of age (Pyrooz & Sweeten, 2015). A child's membership in a gang is associated with marked increases in delinquent behavior, substance abuse, unsafe sexual activity, illicit drug use, nonfatal intentional injury, homicide, and educational and economic hardship (Pyrooz & Sweeten, 2015). An integration of family-centered and school-based programs is needed to reduce the influences for children to become affiliated with gangs (see Community and Home Health Considerations box).

COMMUNITY AND HOME HEALTH CONSIDERATIONS

Providing Guidance About Gangs

Parents of school-age children often worry about the informal and unstructured social groups that their children are attracted to and wish to join. Parents of boys seem particularly concerned about "boys only" groups and the possibility that such groups could become gangs and participate in violent activities.

To help parents cope with these fears, nurses can encourage parents to become aware of any gang-related activities in their community. Typically, activities of organized gangs are illegal, and children involved in gang activities may experience frequent accidents or trips to the emergency department or police station. In addition, gang members frequently have characteristics that parents can identify, such as graffiti, a particular clothing style, unique tattoos, hand signals, or violent illegal initiation rituals. Nurses can also encourage parents to become acquainted with their child's friends and to become involved in providing positive recreational activities for their children.

The community's awareness of gangs that promote violence is essential to stop the spread of gang membership among youth. The media can inform the community of gang influx, identification, and activities to raise parents' awareness of the potential dangers to their children. Community services that promote a sense of belonging among children and offer structured recreational and social events can help youth find alternatives to being a gang member.

Relationships With Families

Although the peer group is highly influential and necessary to normal child development, parents are the primary influence in shaping children's personalities, setting standards for behavior, and establishing value systems. Family values usually predominate when parental and peer value systems come into conflict. Although children may appear to reject parental values while testing the new values of the peer group, ultimately they retain and incorporate many parental values into their own value systems.

As children move into a wider world of peer-group relationships, parents are faced with the task of letting go of control. Parents may find it difficult to face the rejection that children demonstrate as they become more involved with their peer groups. Children may want to spend more time in the company of their peers, may seem eager to leave the house, and often prefer activities of the peer group to family activities. During this time, children discover that parents can be wrong, and they begin to question the knowledge and authority of the parents who previously were considered to be all-knowing and all-powerful. Parents can best serve the interests of their children through tolerant understanding and support.

Although increased independence is the goal of middle childhood, children are not yet prepared to abandon parental control. Children need and want restrictions placed on their behavior; they are not yet prepared to cope with all of the problems of their expanding environment. They feel more secure knowing that there is an authority greater than themselves to implement controls and restrictions. Children may complain loudly about the restrictions and try to break down parental barriers, but they are uneasy if they succeed in doing so. Children feel secure with reasonable, consistent controls. They respect the adults on whom they can rely to prevent them from acting on each and every urge. Children see this behavior as an expression of love and concern for their welfare.

Children also need their parents as adults, not as "pals." Sometimes parents, hurt by their children's rejection, attempt to maintain their children's love and gratitude by assuming the role as a friend. Children need the stable, secure strength provided by mature adults to whom they can turn during troubled relationships with peers or stressful changes in their world. During a disruption in their lives, such as times of failure, periods of illness, or a move that separates them from the security of friends, children need the firm, secure anchor of parental interest and concern. With a secure base in a loving family, children are able to develop the self-confidence and maturity needed to stand independently.

Children's relationships with siblings change during the middle years. Children view siblings as equal in power and status. In earlier years, older siblings were influential in the younger siblings' learning. In the middle years the relationship becomes one of companionship. Positive emotional tone increases, but sibling conflict also increases as the siblings get older. Middle childhood is a period of transition for sibling relationships, a juncture between the open bickering of early childhood and the supportive relationships observed in adult siblings.

PLAY

As children enter the school years, their play takes on new dimensions that reflect a new stage of development. Not only does play involve increased physical skill, intellectual ability, and fantasy, but as children form groups and cliques, they begin to evolve a sense of belonging to a team or club. Belonging to a group is of vital importance. Clubs, societies, and organizations are important parts of the culture of childhood.

Rules and Rituals

The need for conformity in middle childhood is strongly manifested in the activities and games of school-age children. Up to this point, they have either played games they have invented themselves or have played in the company of a friend or an adult, and rules more or less evolved with the game. Now they begin to see the need for rules, and the games they play have fixed and unvarying rules that may be bizarre and extraordinarily rigid (especially those made up by the group). But part of the enjoyment of the game is knowing the rules because knowing means belonging. Once the rules are established and agreed on, the demand for conformity is strong (Fig. 15.7).

Conformity and ritual characterize the play of school-age children, not only in games, but also in behavior and language. Childhood is full of chants and taunts, such as "Eeny, meeny, miney, mo," "Last one is a rotten egg," and "Step on a crack, break your mother's back." Children receive a great deal of pleasure and power from such sayings, which have been handed down with few changes through generations.

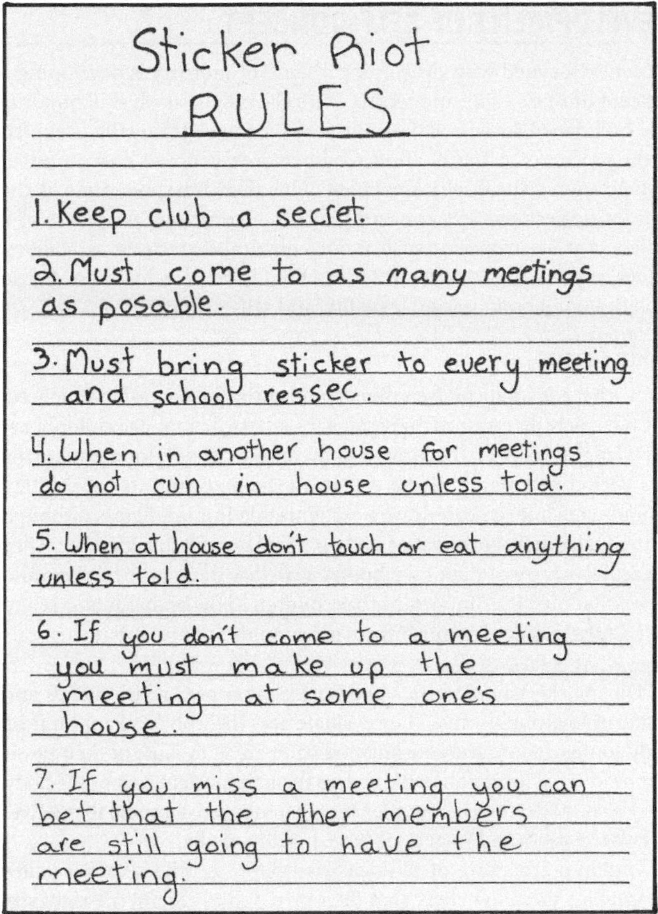

Sticker Riot
RULES

1. Keep club a secret.

2. Must come to as many meetings as posable.

3. Must bring sticker to every meeting and school ressec.

4. When in another house for meetings do not run in house unless told.

5. When at house don't touch or eat anything unless told.

6. If you don't come to a meeting you must make up the meeting at some one's house.

7. If you miss a meeting you can bet that the other members are still going to have the meeting.

FIG. 15.7 A list of club rules compiled by a group of 9-year-old children.

Team Play

A more complex form of group play that develops from the need for peer interaction involves the team games and sports that are part of the school years. Such games may require a referee, umpire, or person of authority so the rules can be followed more accurately. Team membership has several characteristics that promote child development during the middle years.

Children learn to subordinate personal goals to group goals. Team membership means that each child is accountable to the other team members and that acts may affect the success or failure of the entire group. Each member's behavior is open to public evaluation, and children risk ostracism, ridicule, or scapegoating if they contribute to a team loss. Although individual skills are recognized, team successes and failures are shared by all members. Children learn the concept of interdependence and the reliance of all players on one another.

Children learn that division of labor is an effective strategy for the attainment of a goal. Each person on a team has a specific function, which increases the team's chances of winning. Once children learn that certain goals are best accomplished by dividing tasks among several individuals, they can transfer this knowledge to other social situations. Children also learn that some children are best equipped to perform one part of the task and other children are best suited to another aspect of the task.

Team play helps children learn about the nature of competition. In all team play there is a winning side and a losing side. Because losing is often interpreted as failure, children go to great lengths to avoid the public embarrassment and personal shame that accompany failure. The more a child identifies with the team and values membership in the group, the more distasteful losing becomes. Fear of losing and the failure it implies are strong incentives for group commitment; however, winning is not universally given high value. Some cultures and subcultures emphasize the game and consideration for one's companions rather than the outcome.

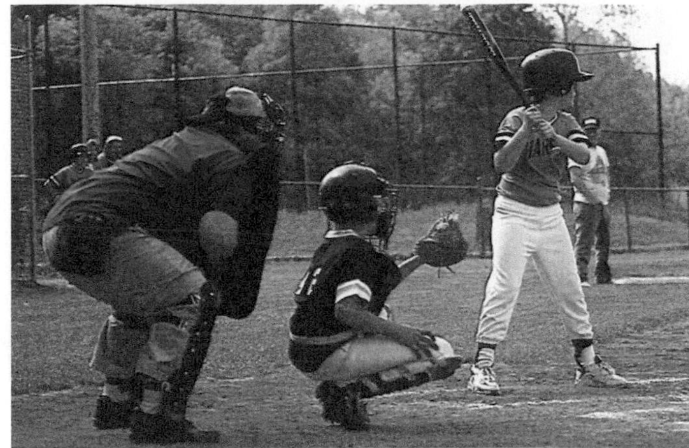

FIG. 15.8 Activities engaged in by school-age children, such as Little League baseball, vary according to each child's interest and opportunity.

Team play also contributes to children's social, intellectual, and skill growth (Eime, Young, Harvey, et al., 2013). Children work hard to develop the skills needed to become members of a team, to improve their contribution to the group, and to anticipate the consequences of their behavior for the group. Team play helps stimulate cognitive growth because children are called on to learn many complex rules, make judgments about those rules, plan strategies, and assess the strengths and weaknesses of members of their own and the opposing teams (Fig. 15.8).

Quiet Games and Activities

Although the play of school-age children can be highly active, they also enjoy many quiet and solitary activities. The middle childhood years are the time for collections, and young school-age children's collections are an odd assortment of unrelated objects in messy, disorganized piles. Collections of later years are more orderly and selective and often are organized neatly in scrapbooks, on shelves, or in boxes.

School-age children become fascinated with complex board, card, computer, and electronic games. Children play these games alone or in groups. As in all games, the adherence to rules is fanatic. Disagreements over the rules can cause much discussion and argument, but are easily resolved reading the rules of the game.

The newly acquired skill of reading becomes increasingly satisfying as school-age children begin to expand their knowledge of the world through books (Fig. 15.9). School-age children never tire of stories, and, like preschool children, they love to have stories read aloud. They also enjoy sewing, cooking, carpentry, gardening, and creative endeavors, such as painting. Many creative skills, such as those involving music and art, and athletic skills, such as swimming, hiking, dancing, and karate, are acquired during childhood and continue to be enjoyed into adolescence and adulthood (Fig. 15.10).

Hero worship is another characteristic of children and adolescents. The object of the adoration can be a friend, relative, teacher, or national sports or entertainment figure. However, problems can arise when the idol proves to be an inappropriate role model.

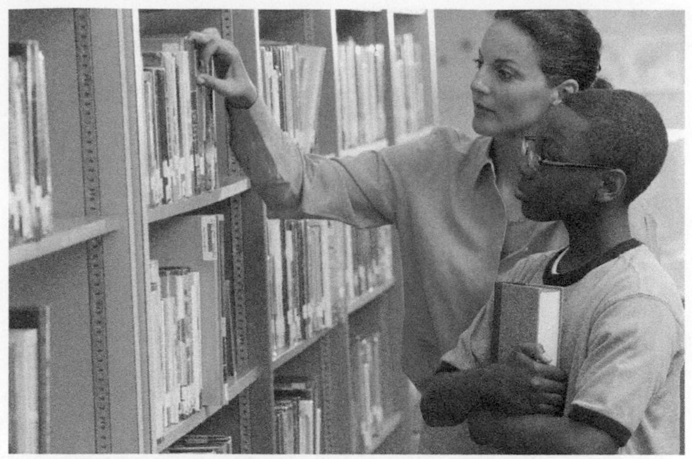

FIG. 15.9 Selecting a book with the assistance of an adult.

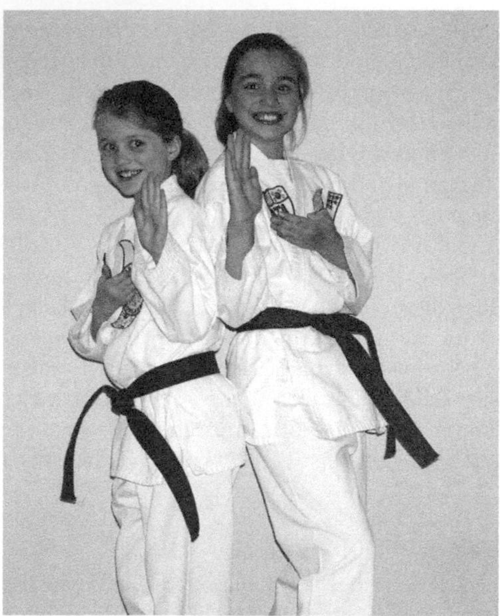

FIG. 15.10 School-age children take pride in learning new skills.

Ego Mastery

Play affords children the means to acquire representational mastery over themselves, their environment, and others. Through play, children can feel as big, as powerful, and as skillful as their imaginations will allow, and they can attain vicarious mastery and power over whomever and whatever they choose. They need to feel in control in their play. School-age children still need the opportunity to use large muscles in exuberant outdoor play and the freedom to exert their newfound autonomy and initiative. They need space in which to exercise and to work off tensions, frustrations, and hostility. Physical skills practiced and mastered in play help develop a feeling of personal competence, which contributes to a sense of accomplishment and helps provide a place of status in the peer group.

Table 15.1 presents a summary of growth and development in middle childhood. Because each child has a unique developmental pattern, any descriptions of the typical child of any age-group can represent only an average and should not be considered as absolute criteria for any given child.

DEVELOPMENT OF SELF-CONCEPT

Closely associated with developing a sense of industry is developing a concept of one's value and worth. With the emphasis on skill building and broadened social relationships, children are continually occupied in the process of self-evaluation. Children's self-concepts are composed of their own critical self-assessments plus their interpretations of the opinions of others. Self-concept refers to a conscious awareness of a variety of self-perceptions, such as one's physical characteristics, abilities, values, and self-ideals, and one's idea of self in relation to others. It also includes one's body image, sexuality, and self-esteem.

Body Image

Body image is what children think about their bodies and is influenced, but not solely determined, by significant others. School-age children are knowledgeable about the human body, and social development during this period focuses to a large extent on the body and its capabilities. School-age children can draw a recognizable human figure, although individually their portrayal of body parts may vary considerably. They are acutely aware of their own bodies as well as those of their peers and those of adults. It is important that children know body functions and that adults correct any misinformation children have about the body (e.g., what is fat).

During the school years, children focus on peer relationships and conform to group norms. They evaluate how their physical appearance, body configuration, and coordination compare with those of their peers. The head is the most noticeable and, to them, important part of the body. They also model themselves after their parents and compare themselves to favored peers and images observed in the media.

Children are aware of physical disabilities in others, and it is not unusual for them to believe that their own bodies are not the right size or the right shape or are in some way defective. They respond to such concerns in a variety of ways. For example, they will conceal perceived shortcomings of body or performance, as in the obese child who refrains from going swimming, the child who conveniently forgets a gym suit, the child who conceals an imagined defect, or the child with enuresis who declines invitations to slumber parties. Children seldom express these concerns to families. However, they need reassurance about both the uniqueness and the sameness of their bodies, while their privacy is respected, and they are allowed appropriate protective strategies. Children who are different become aware of the differences and may find themselves excluded from the group. When children are teased or criticized about being different, the effect can last even into adulthood.

Self-Esteem

Self-esteem is children's pictures of their individual worth and consists of both positive and negative qualities. Children actively strive to achieve internalized goals. At the same time, they continually receive feedback on the quality of their performance from individuals they consider to be authorities. By the time they reach school age, children have received messages regarding the extent to which they are able to accomplish tasks that have been delegated to them. For example, one child may have been given prestigious responsibilities at home or at school or received special commendation for an achievement. On the other hand, another child may have been sent to a special class for slow learners or may have been the last person selected when children chose sides for a game. These and other signs serve as clues to social worth that children incorporate as part of their self-evaluation.

Children approach the process of self-evaluation from a framework of either self-confidence or self-doubt. Children who have mastered the maturational crises of autonomy and initiative are able to face the world with feelings of pride rather than shame. At first, children's

TABLE 15.1 Growth and Development During School-Age Years

Physical and Motor	Mental	Adaptive	Personal-Social
Age 6 Years			
Height and weight gain continues slowly Weight—16-26.3 kg (35.5-58 lb); height—106.7-123.5 cm (42-49 inches) Central mandibular incisors erupt Loses first tooth Demonstrates gradual increase in dexterity Active age; constant activity Often returns to finger feeding More aware of hand as a tool Likes to draw, print, color Vision reaches maturity	Develops concept of numbers Can count 13 pennies Knows whether it is morning or afternoon Defines common objects (such as fork and chair) in terms of their use Obeys triple commands in succession Knows right and left hands Says which is pretty and which is ugly of a series of drawings of faces Describes the objects in a picture rather than simply enumerating them Attends first grade	At table, uses knife to spread butter or jam on bread At play, cuts, folds, pastes paper; sews crudely if needle is threaded Takes bath without supervision; performs bedtime activities alone Reads from memory; enjoys oral spelling game Likes table games, checkers, simple card games Giggles a lot Sometimes steals money or attractive items Has difficulty owning up to misdeeds Tries out own abilities	Can share and cooperate better Has great need for children of own age Will cheat to win Often engages in rough play Often jealous of younger brother or sister Does what adults are seen doing May have occasional temper tantrums Is a boaster Is more independent, probably influence of school Has own way of doing things Increases socialization
Age 7 Years			
Begins to grow at least 5 cm (2 inches) in height per year Weight—17.7-30 kg (39-66 lb); height—111.8-129.5 cm (44-51 inches) Maxillary central incisors and lateral mandibular incisors erupt More cautious in approaches to new performances Repeats performances to master them Jaw begins to expand to accommodate permanent teeth	Notices that certain items are missing from pictures Can copy a diamond Repeats three numbers backward Develops concept of time; reads ordinary clock or watch correctly to nearest quarter-hour; uses clock for practical purposes Attends second grade More mechanical in reading; often does not stop at the end of a sentence, skips words such as *it, the,* and *he*	Uses table knife for cutting meat; may need help with tough or difficult pieces Brushes and combs hair acceptably without help May steal Likes to help and have a choice Is less resistant and stubborn	Is becoming a real member of the family group Takes part in group play Boys prefer playing with boys; girls prefer playing with girls Spends a lot of time alone; does not require a lot of companionship
Ages 8-9 Years			
Continues to gain 5 cm (2 inches) in height per year Weight—19.6-39.6 kg (43-87 lb); height—116.8-141.8 cm (46-56 inches) Lateral incisors (maxillary) and mandibular cuspids erupt Movement fluid; often graceful and poised Always on the go; jumps, chases, skips Increased smoothness and speed in fine motor control; uses cursive writing Dresses self completely Likely to overdo; hard to quiet down after recess More limber; bones grow faster than ligaments	Gives similarities and differences between two things from memory Counts backward from 20-1; understands concept of reversibility Repeats days of the week and months in order; knows the date Describes common objects in detail, not merely their use Makes change out of a quarter Attends third and fourth grades Reads more; may plan to wake up early just to read Reads classic books, but also enjoys comics More aware of time; can be relied on to get to school on time Can grasp concepts of parts and whole (fractions) Understands concepts of space, cause and effect, nesting (puzzles), conservation (permanence of mass and volume) Classifies objects by more than one quality; has collections Produces simple paintings or drawings	Makes use of common tools such as hammer, saw, screwdriver Uses household and sewing utensils Helps with routine household tasks such as dusting, sweeping Assumes responsibility for share of household chores Looks after all of own needs at table Buys useful articles; exercises some choice in making purchases Runs useful errands Likes pictorial magazines Likes school; wants to answer all the questions Is afraid of failing a grade; is ashamed of bad grades Is more critical of self Takes music and sports lessons	Is easy to get along with at home Likes the reward system Dramatizes Is more sociable Is better behaved Is interested in boy-girl relationships but will not admit it Goes about home and community freely, alone or with friends Likes to compete and play games Shows preference in friends and groups Plays mostly with groups of own sex but is beginning to mix Develops modesty Compares self with others Enjoys organizations, clubs, and group sports

Continued

TABLE 15.1 Growth and Development During School-Age Years—cont'd

Physical and Motor	Mental	Adaptive	Personal-Social
Ages 10-12 Years			
Weight—24.3-58 kg (54-128 lb); height—127-162.6 cm (50-64 inches) Remainder of teeth erupt and tend toward full development (except wisdom teeth) *Boys*—Slow growth in height and rapid weight gain; may become obese in this period *Girls*—Pubescent changes may begin to appear; body lines soften and round out	Writes brief stories Attends fifth to seventh grades Writes occasional short letters to friends or relatives on own initiative Uses telephone for practical purposes Responds to magazine, radio, or other advertising Reads for practical information or own enjoyment—stories or library books of adventure or romance, animal stories	Makes useful tools or does easy repair work Cooks or sews in small ways Raises pets Washes and dries own hair, but may need reminding to do so Is sometimes left alone at home for an hour or so Is successful in looking after own needs or those of other children left in his or her care	Loves friends; talks about them constantly Chooses friends more selectively; may have a "best friend" Enjoys conversation Develops beginning interest in opposite sex Is more diplomatic Likes family; family really has meaning Likes mother and wants to please her in many ways Demonstrates affection Likes father, who is admired and may be idolized Respects parents

self-concepts are formed exclusively from their perceptions of their parents' evaluation of them. During middle childhood the opinions of peers and teachers are important. Criticisms and peer approval are additional sources of data for evaluation. Parents and other adults are no longer the only persons who respond to their skills, talents, and abilities; peers also identify skills and capabilities. Each child soon begins to internalize these outside opinions. If children regard themselves as worthwhile or satisfactory persons, they have high self-esteem, self-confidence, and a positive self-concept. If they view themselves as worthless, they have low self-esteem.

For adults, owning a pet has been linked to better physical and mental health, but little evidence exists for children and adolescents about the benefits of pets. Owning a dog has been shown to reduce anxiety among children (Gadomski, Scribani, Krupa, et al., 2015) and loneliness among adolescents (Black, 2012), but no differences in weight or fitness level has been noted among children with and without pets (Westgarth, Boddy, Stratton, et al., 2016).

Children encounter difficulties assessing their own abilities because they rely on their own expectations or on the expectations expressed by others regarding their performance. They depend almost entirely on external evidence of worth, such as school grades, teachers' comments, and parental and peer approval. Children do not yet have the capacity to develop their own independent criteria to evaluate their own accomplishments. It is especially difficult for them to assess their achievement in abstract skills.

Nothing succeeds like success. Significant adults in children's lives can often manage to manipulate the environment so that children meet with success. Each small success can improve a child's self-image. The more positive children feel about themselves, the more confident they feel in trying again for success. All children profit from feeling that they are special to significant adults. A positive self-image makes them feel likable, worthwhile, and capable of valuable contributions. Such feelings lead to self-respect, self-confidence, and a general feeling of happiness. Parents can help their school-age children develop self-esteem by being honest, by providing opportunities for creativity, by helping them succeed in activities, and by providing positive reinforcement. Nurses can enhance self-esteem by fostering supportive relationships between children and members of their families and by emphasizing children's strengths and positive aspects of their behavior (see Community and Home Health Considerations box).

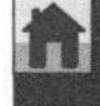

COMMUNITY AND HOME HEALTH CONSIDERATIONS

Socialization of Boys and Girls

Health professionals have long been aware that boys and girls are socialized differently by parents and teachers. Girls are encouraged to express their emotions and to be sensitive and responsive to others. Boys, on the other hand, are often told to hide their feelings and are criticized if they are "too sensitive." In school, boys are encouraged to take the most challenging courses, to do well in math and science, and to participate in athletic endeavors. Girls may be discouraged from taking math and science and ostracized socially if they take typically "male" courses. These differences in socialization may contribute to stereotypic behavior and the way that boys and girls relate to each other. Boys may feel entitled to life's opportunities and benefits, and girls may think that they need to be submissive and deferential to succeed. Such beliefs may ultimately influence participation in risk-taking behaviors in adolescence.

To prevent the development of a sense of entitlement in boys and to foster self-reliance in girls, parents can children to be socially and interpersonally sensitive and responsive to others. Teachers can encourage girls, as well as boys, to take the challenging courses in math and science, foster cooperation between boys and girls on school projects, and facilitate the development of athletic endeavors for not only boys but also girls. Some schools are providing same-sex courses to provide a more neutral and nurturing environment for students.

DEVELOPMENT OF SEXUALITY

Evidence indicates that many children experience some form of sex play during or before preadolescence as a response to normal curiosity, not as a result of love or sexual urge. Children are experimentalists by nature, and this play is incidental and transitory. Any adverse emotional consequences or guilt feelings depend on how the parents manage the behavior and whether children view their actions as wrong in the eyes of significant persons, particularly their parents.

Children's attitudes toward sex are acquired indirectly at an early age and affect the way they respond to sexual information. Many parents discourage sexual exploration, either through subtle substitution of activities that divert their children's attention from the genitalia or by expressions of anger or disgust at their children's behavior. These tactics clearly communicate to children that they should not engage in such activities, discourage questions about sex, and limit the sources of information.

Sex Education

Parents may not teach young children the correct terminology for sexual organs or sexual feelings. Often the only vocabulary available to children is one that identifies sexual organs with excretory functions. If children learn that excretory organs and functions are dirty, they may associate "dirtiness" with the reproductive organs and functions. If children learn the correct terminology for the organs and their functions, this will eliminate or reduce this association.

Because parents often either repress or avoid their children's sexual curiosity, sexual information received in childhood is often acquired almost entirely from peers. One study found the majority of parents of preadolescent and adolescent children believed they were open with sex education discussions; however, only a few parents communicated direct information about safe sex practices (Hyde, Drennan, Butler, et al., 2013). When peers are the primary source of sexual information, it is often transmitted and exchanged in secret conversation and contains misinformation. These communications can also create anxiety in children and inhibit spontaneous expressions or questioning of their parents.

Although middle childhood is an ideal time for formal sex education, this subject has created considerable controversy. Many parents and groups are unconditionally opposed to the inclusion of sex education in the schools. Others believe that information relating to sexual maturation and the process of reproduction should be presented as naturally as information about other natural phenomena, such as the growth of plants, the changing seasons, and the migratory habits of birds. When sex education is presented from a life span perspective and treated as a normal part of growth and development, the information is less likely to contain overtones of uncertainty, guilt, or embarrassment that could in turn produce anxiety in children.

Sex education programs have been successfully incorporated into a number of elementary school curricula. In many of these programs, sexuality is presented in the context of its central role as a biologic mechanism for the survival of the culture. Children learn that sexual maturation and reproduction represent each individual's contribution to the natural order of things. This approach provides a natural entry into discussion of sexuality as a basis for family units, marriage, and attitudes toward children, as well as an entry into a presentation of the biologic facts of sexuality. Many sex education programs also emphasize that sexual intimacy is part of a close, personal relationship and a means of conveying love, as well as a means for ensuring the survival of the species.

Nurse's Role in Sex Education

No matter where nurses practice, they can provide information on human sexuality to both parents and children. To discuss the topic adequately, nurses must understand the physiologic aspects of sexuality; know the common myths and misconceptions associated with sex and the reproductive process; understand cultural and societal values; and be aware of their own attitudes, feelings, and biases.

When nurses present sexual information to children, they should treat sex as a normal part of growth and development. Nurses should answer questions honestly, matter-of-factly, and at the child's level of understanding. School-age children may be more comfortable when boys and girls are segregated for discussions; however, each group needs information about both sexes.

Children need help to differentiate sex and sexuality. Exercises focused on clarifying values, identifying role models, solving problems, and practicing responsibility are important to prepare school-age children for early adolescence and puberty. In addition, children need explanations of sexual information that is discussed via the media or jokes. A comprehensive sex education program including information about anatomy, pregnancy, contraceptives, and sexually transmitted diseases should be presented in simple, accurate terms. Teaching a child to be sexually responsible is an essential component of sex education. Preadolescents need precise and concrete information that will allow them to answer questions such as "What if I start my period in the middle of class?" or "How can I keep people from telling I have an erection?" It is important to tell them what they want to know and what they can expect to happen as they mature sexually.

During encounters with parents, nurses can be open and available for questions and discussion. They can set an example by the language they use in discussing body parts and their function and by the way in which they deal with problems that have emotional overtones, such as exploratory sex play and masturbation. Parents need help to understand normal behaviors and to view sexual curiosity in their children as a part of the developmental process. Assessing the parents' level of knowledge and understanding of sexuality provides cues to their need for supplemental information that will prepare them for increasingly complex explanations as their children grow older.

Children with developmental disabilities need emotional and sexual relationships. Parents of children with developmental disabilities may need special assistance and help with sex education. In 1996 the American Academy of Pediatrics developed specific guidelines that discuss ways to teach these children about human anatomy, pubertal changes, expression of physical affection, protection from sexual abuse or exploitation, and independence in personal hygiene and self-care. A clinical report was released in 2016 provided updated evidence on sexual and reproductive health education, including intimate relationships, sexually transmitted infections, sexual orientation, gender identity, and reproductive rights and responsibilities (Breuner, Mattson, Committee on Adolescence, et al., 2016). Sex education for children with chronic health conditions and disabilities requires individualized techniques, depending on the health issues and disabilities (Breuner, Mattson, Committee on Adolescence, et al., 2016). Nurses must take an active role in broaching the issue of sexuality and promoting the idea that sexuality is a part of every individual's identity in order to address educational needs.

Sometimes participation in short classes or group discussions can help parents address disturbing behaviors and anticipate their children's questions and learning needs. It is wise to include both parents in such activities when possible. Both parents should assume responsibility for sex education in the home so that the children will not acquire a distorted view of either the male or the female role that may alter relationships with the opposite sex in later life.

COPING WITH CONCERNS RELATED TO NORMAL GROWTH AND DEVELOPMENT

SCHOOL EXPERIENCE

School serves as an agent for transmitting societal values to each succeeding generation of children and as a setting for many peer relationships. As a socializing agent second only to the family, school exerts a profound influence on the social development of children.

School entrance causes a sharp break in the structure of a child's world. For some children it is their first experience in conforming to a group pattern imposed by an adult who is not a parent and who has responsibility for too many children to be constantly aware of each child as an individual. Children want to go to school and usually adapt to the new environment with little difficulty. Successful adjustment is directly related to the child's physical and emotional maturity and the parents' readiness to accept the separation associated with school entrance. Cooperation among parents and support for the child are successful ways of coping with school entry stress. Unfortunately, some parents express their unconscious attempts to delay their child's maturity by clinging behavior, particularly with their youngest child.

Anticipatory Socialization

By the time they enter school, most children have a fairly realistic concept of what school involves. They receive information regarding the role of pupil from parents, playmates, and the media. In addition, most children have had experience with day care or preschool and kindergarten.

Children's attitudes toward school and the extent of their adjustment are influenced by their parents, siblings, and playmates. Middle-class children have fewer adjustments to make and less to learn about expected behavior because the school tends to reflect dominant middle-class customs and values, although this may be tempered by the school's location and predominant teachers and student body. Parents who view school as a place that they have helped create and support and that is directed toward the same objectives for socialization as their own usually prepare their children with useful anticipatory socialization and furnish them with confidence to meet the challenge. Parents who view the school as an alien culture and one that they have little, if any, power to affect may unknowingly teach their children to be fearful and resentful toward school, even though the parents agree with its purposes and objectives.

Television influences the acquisition of information and attitudes and provides anticipatory socialization. Television viewing has the potential to increase a child's vocabulary, extend the child's horizons, and enrich the school experience. However, television relies heavily on images to convey information. Consequently, it is difficult to explore complex issues by this medium. Extensive television viewing may also encourage children to seek simple answers to tough problems and to believe that violence is the most effective and quick solution to conflict.

Although most children have had some experience with schooling before they enter the first grade, the extent to which early childhood education prepares children for primary school varies. Some preschool programs provide custodial care; others also emphasize emotional, social, and intellectual development. Early childhood programming that stresses cognitive more than social aspects appears to be more effective in facilitating later academic achievement.

Role of the Teacher

To facilitate the transition from home to school, teachers should have personality characteristics that allow them to deal with the needs of young children. Because they react to the teacher on the basis of past experience, children respond best to teachers with attributes that they would find in a warm, loving parent. As a parental surrogate, teachers in the early grades perform many of the activities formerly assumed by the parents, such as recognizing the children's personal needs (e.g., a need to go to the bathroom or for assistance with clothing) and helping develop their social behavior (e.g., manners).

Teachers, like parents, are concerned about the psychologic and emotional welfare of children. Although the functions of teachers and parents differ, both place constraints on behavior, and both are in a position to enforce standards of conduct. However, the teacher's primary responsibility is stimulating and guiding children's intellectual development as opposed to providing for their physical welfare beyond the school setting.

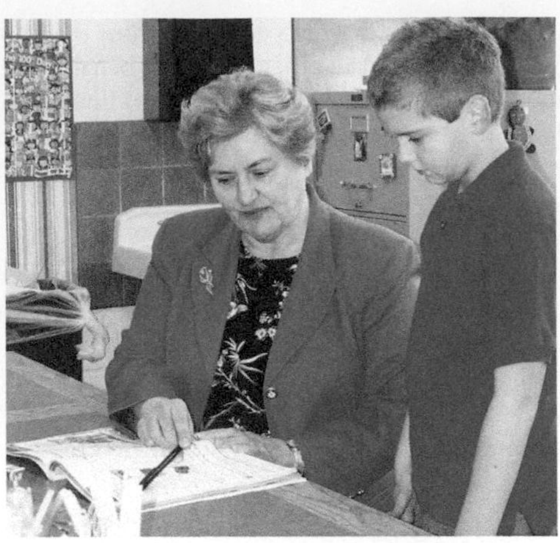

FIG. 15.11 School represents an important change in a child's life, and teachers exert a significant influence on the child.

Teachers share the parental influence in shaping a child's attitudes and values. They serve as models with whom children can identify and whom they try to emulate. Children seek a teacher's approval and avoid a teacher's disapproval. The teacher is a significant person in the life of the early school-age child, and hero worship of a teacher may extend into late childhood and preadolescence. It is not uncommon for the first or second grader to be heartbroken and tearful at leaving a familiar teacher at the end of the school term or to be upset when faced with a substitute teacher for even a short period.

Children's interest in school and learning and much of their social interaction and self-concept are related to interactions with the teacher (Fig. 15.11). The differential systems of reward and punishment administered by teachers affect the emotional adjustment and self-concept of children and how they respond to school in general.

The interaction between the teacher and an individual pupil affects the pupil's acceptance by other children, which in turn affects the child's self-concept. Behaviors praised by the teacher usually acquire a positive value, whereas those viewed negatively by the teacher are devalued by the children. In this way the teacher exerts considerable influence in a number of areas, such as attitudes toward minority groups, the disabled, or less favorably endowed children. Teacher approval of children and their self-acceptance are closely related.

The teacher sets the emotional tone of the classroom. Those who are able to establish a positive social climate are usually concerned about the mental health and social dynamics of children. Feeling a responsibility for personality development in their pupils, they are alert and sensitive to a child's anxieties, peer-group relationships, self-concepts, and general attitudes toward school. Learner-centered behaviors, such as supportive statements that reassure or commend children, accepting and clarifying statements that help them refine ideas and feelings to provide a sense of being understood, and constructive assistance that aids them with their own problem solving, contribute to the expansion and development of a positive self-concept.

Role of the Parents

Parents share responsibility with the schools for helping children achieve their maximum potential. Parents can supplement the school program in numerous ways (see Family-Centered Care box). Cultivating responsibility is the goal of parental assistance. Being responsible for schoolwork helps children learn to keep promises, meet deadlines, and succeed at their jobs as adults. Responsible children may occasionally ask for help (e.g., with a spelling list), but usually they like to think through their work by themselves. Excessive pressure or lack of encouragement from parents may inhibit the development of these desirable traits.

FAMILY-CENTERED CARE

Helping Children in School

General Guidelines

Be supportive; provide companionship; share ideas and thoughts.
Be positive; every child should experience some success each day.
Share an interest in reading; use the library, and discuss books they are reading.
Support and encourage activity rather than passivity.
Encourage originality; help children make their own projects from discarded articles or other available materials.
Foster the development of hobbies and collections.
Encourage children to wonder and reflect during free time.
Encourage family experiences and trips to places of interest.
Encourage questions; help children discover sources for information or places to explore and investigate.
Stimulate creative thinking and problem solving; help children try out new solutions to problems without fear of making mistakes.
Use rewards rather than punishment.

Specific Guidelines

Meet the teacher at the beginning of school and plan to visit the school to see what is taught and expected.
Send the child to school every day. Teachers are concerned when parents make other plans for their children; it conveys the impression that school is unimportant.
Demonstrate an interest in what the child is learning.
Demonstrate an interest in content and growth more than in grades.
Make it clear to the child that schoolwork is between the child and the teacher; teacher and child should set goals for better school performance to allow the child to feel responsible for school successes and failures.
Take advantage of situations that support and reinforce school learning.
Share information with teachers that will help them understand the child better.
Communicate with the teacher if there appears to be a problem; avoid waiting for a scheduled conference.
Provide a quiet, well-lit area for study that is safe from interruption; do not allow television or music.
Avoid dictating a study time, but do enforce rules, such as no video games until homework is done; accept the child's word that work is complete.
Help with homework should focus on explaining the question, not giving the answer.
Teach the child to break large tasks (such as a report) into smaller, manageable tasks spread over the allotted time rather than to attempt the entire project the night before it is due.
Request special help for children with learning problems.
Support the school staff by showing respect for both the school system and the teacher, at least in the child's presence.

DISCIPLINE

Numerous factors influence the amount and manner of discipline imposed on school-age children: the parents' psychosocial maturity, their own childrearing experiences during childhood, the children's temperament, the context of the children's misconduct, and the children's response to rewards and punishments. Discipline serves many purposes: (1) to help the child interrupt or inhibit a forbidden action; (2) to point out a more acceptable form of behavior so that the child knows what is right in a future situation; (3) to provide some reason, understandable to the child, that explains why one action is inappropriate and another action is more desirable; and (4) to stimulate the child's ability to empathize with the victim of a misdeed.

As children are increasingly able to see a situation from the point of view of another, they are able to understand the effects of their reactions on others and themselves. Disciplinary techniques should help children control their own behavior.

To be effective, discipline should take place in an environment characterized by positive, supportive parent-child relationships and should involve strategies that educate and guide desired behaviors and eliminate undesired or ineffective behaviors. The American Academy of Pediatric developed a comprehensive program to educate healthcare providers and parents on preventing violence that includes information on how to discipline.*

Parents should not use punitive actions or corporal punishment because these methods are of limited value and are associated with multiple negative consequences. In particular, physically aggressive parenting practices that involve spanking are linked to children with poor internalizing behaviors such as depression, anxiety, and hopelessness; poor externalizing behaviors such as aggression and violence; slower cognitive development; and increased risk for physical abuse (Hornor, Bretl, Chapman, et al., 2015). Reasoning, on the other hand, is an effective disciplinary technique for school-age children; however, use of a time-out may be necessary to stop the behavior acutely.

As their cognitive skills advance, school-age children are able to benefit from more complex disciplinary strategies. For example, withholding privileges, requiring recompense, imposing penalties, and contracting can be used with great success. Problem solving is the best approach to limit setting, and children themselves can be included in the process of determining appropriate disciplinary measures.

Dishonest Behavior

During middle childhood, children may engage in what is considered to be antisocial behavior. Lying, stealing, and cheating may become manifest in previously well-behaved children. This is especially disturbing to parents, who may have difficulty coping with such behavior.

Lying can occur for a number of reasons. Preschool children often have difficulty distinguishing between fact and fantasy. They do not have the cognitive capacity to deliberately mislead. Sometimes they misperceive or fail to remember an event. By the time they reach school age, they still tell stories but can distinguish between what is real and what is make-believe. If not, they need to learn to distinguish between fantasy and reality. Often children will exaggerate a story or situation as a means to impress their family or friends.

Young children lie to escape punishment or get out of some difficulty, even when the evidence of their misbehavior is evident. Lying is more common in families in which punishment is severe. When parents model honesty and veracity, the children will often behave in the same way. If parents lie, the children will emulate their behavior. Older children may lie to meet expectations set by others to which they have been unable to measure up. They may also lie because of low self-esteem or as a means of getting ahead or acquiring something with little effort. However, most children are concerned with the wrongfulness of lying and cheating—especially in their friends. They are quick to tell on others when they detect cheating.

*Connected Kids: Safe, Strong, Secure. Website: https://www2.aap.org/connectedkids/.

Parents need to be reassured that all children lie sometimes and that they often have difficulty separating fantasy from reality. Providers should help parents understand the importance of their own behavior as role models and of being truthful in their relationships with children. Parents can discuss the issue with the children directly to impress on them how much of their own security and respect is lost when they are not believed.

Cheating is most common in young children, ages 5 to 6 years. They find it difficult to lose at a game or contest, and they cheat to win. They have not yet acquired the full realization of the wrongfulness of this behavior and do it almost automatically. It usually disappears as they mature. However, when children observe parental behaviors such as boasting about cheating on income taxes, they assume this to be appropriate behavior. Parents need to be aware of the types of behaviors they model for their children. When they set examples of honesty, children are more likely to conform to these standards.

As with other ethically related behavior, stealing is not an unexpected event in the younger child. Between ages 5 and 8 years, children's sense of property rights is limited; they tend to take something simply because they are attracted to it, or they take money for what it will buy. They are equally likely to give away something valuable that belongs to them. When young children are caught and punished, they are penitent—they "didn't mean to" and promise "never to do it again," but they may well repeat the performance the following day. Often they not only steal but lie about it as well or attempt to justify the act with excuses. It is seldom helpful to trap children into admission by asking directly if they did the offensive thing. Children do not take on such responsibility until nearer the end of middle childhood.

Children steal for several reasons: lack of a sense of property rights, an attempt to acquire the means with which to bribe other children for favors, a strong desire to own the coveted item, or a wish for revenge to "get back at someone" (usually a parent) for what they consider to be unfair treatment. Older children may steal to supplement an inadequate income from other sources. Sometimes stealing is an indication that something is seriously wrong or lacking in the child's life. Children may steal to make up for a perceived lack of love or another satisfaction.

In some settings in which living arrangements are crowded, children have little privacy, and much of the family property is communal, children may fail to develop a sense of property rights. Sometimes parents unintentionally confuse children with seemingly conflicting values. In an attempt to teach unselfishness, they may force children to share belongings with others, with the result that the children fail to understand property rights.

If children are told not to take money from their mother's purse or their father's pocket but observe the parents doing the same thing, they receive conflicting messages. Parents may go through a child's pockets or other private areas at night and even discard, without explanation, items of which they do not approve. Children should have a place that is private to them alone that other family members respect. If children's personal rights are respected, they are more likely to respect the rights of others.

It is difficult for many parents to cope with stealing by their children. In most situations it is best not to attempt to find a hidden or deep meaning to the stealing. A reprimand, together with an appropriate and reasonable punishment, such as having the older child pay back the money or return the stolen items, will ordinarily take care of most cases. Most children can learn to respect the property rights of others with little difficulty despite temptations and opportunities. Some children simply need more time to learn the importance of the culture's rules regarding private property.

COPING WITH STRESS

Children today experience significant amounts of stress. This stress comes from a variety of sources. Other sections in this book discuss dealing with specific types of stresses, especially those in which nurses assume a major role, such as hospitalization, illness, abuse, disabling injuries, and death or the threat of death.

In the normal course of growing up, children are pressured by their peers to identify with their friends; to eat, dress, and look like their friends; to talk about the same things that their friends talk about; to engage in the same activities as their friends; and yet to compete with them. They are pressured by parents to excel in school, in athletics, and in social situations at ever-younger ages. Children in the middle school years can be overcommitted with activities such as dance lessons, music lessons, athletics, and other activities until the cumulative effect is overwhelming.

Although children receive better treatment than in earlier times, when beatings and child labor were common, their physical and emotional well-being is threatened by different stresses. The high divorce rate and the number of single-parent families result in altered relationships and increasing responsibilities for children. Children are stressed by various conflicts within the home.

Children's exposure to household activities such as alcohol or drug abuse, domestic violence, or criminal activity is a significant problem in the United States. At least 700,000 children who are exposed to one of these negative household influences will experience some form of maltreatment (Hunt, Slack, & Berger, 2016). Parents of violent households may be unable to meet their children's needs and may have ineffective relationships with their children. These children are at risk for physical consequences such as obesity, chronic obstructive pulmonary disease, or heart disease; psychologic consequences, including aggression or depression; and social consequences such as teen pregnancy (Hunt, Slack, & Berger, 2016). In addition, longitudinal studies have shown that children exposed to domestic violence are more likely to display antisocial behavior and potentially become abusive parents (Jaffe, Campbell, Hamilton, et al., 2012).

Exposure to violence in the family, school, or community affects children's ability to concentrate and function. Children may be traumatized by witnessing violence and develop fear, insecurity, and a sense of helplessness, which can result in social withdrawal and behavioral regression (Levendosky, Bogat, & Martinez-Torteya, 2013). Children exposed to repeated violence can display hyperarousal symptoms leading to posttraumatic stress disorder and symptoms such as nightmares, flashbacks, a fatalistic orientation to the future, depression, and anxiety (Levendosky, Bogat, & Martinez-Torteya, 2013).

School itself is stressful for many children, and school has become a more violent environment. A recent national survey found that 4.1% of students brought a weapon such as a gun, knife, or club to school in the last 30 days and 6.0% of students were threatened or injured with a weapon on school property in the last 12 months (Kann, McManus, Harris, et al., 2016). In addition, 7.8% of students were involved in a physical fight on school property and 2.9% of students in a physical fight required medical attention (Kann, McManus, Harris, et al., 2016).

The school environment may also pose a threat to the middle schooler's self-image. School-age children have a high fear of failure and criticism (Muris, Ollendick, Roelofs, et al., 2014). Competing with classmates for grades and teacher recognition, failing an examination, being teased or made fun of in school, or being labeled as "stupid" or "learning disabled" all result in emotional distress. Teachers or parents may not always recognize or appreciate the worries or sources of stress for school-age children.

Students' relationships with their teachers are an important component of children's social and cognitive development and can affect students' motivation to learn (Spilt, Leflot, Onghena, et al., 2016). Children become distressed when teachers raise their voices, yell or scream, or use fear of physical punishment in the classroom. Students exposed to such behavior may show symptoms of stress, express excessive worry about school, demonstrate negative self-perceptions, and verbalize fear of physical harm by the teacher. Although parents and nurses should be cautious in interpreting such behaviors (they are in many ways similar to school phobia; see Chapter 16), a high degree of suspicion might be justified if the symptoms are not explained by other factors or if they represent a marked change from previous patterns.

Some children are encouraged to feel, think, and behave at a level of maturity far beyond what could reasonably be expected of individuals their age. They are expected to take on many adult-type responsibilities, to make decisions they may not be able to make, and to achieve more. An emphasis on high test score achievement can increase stress. Children have little time for being young and enjoying the spontaneous activities of childhood.

When asked to describe sources of worry, school-age children identified concerns such as social threats (e.g., conflicts with friends), medical procedures, danger and death, and the unknown (Muris, Ollendick, Roelofs, et al., 2014). These worries were more prominent in girls versus boys and tend to decrease as children became older (Muris, Ollendick, Roelofs, et al., 2014). Other potential sources of stress are listed in Box 15.1.

Children respond to stress by using various adaptive and maladaptive coping mechanisms (Skinner, Pitzer, & Steele, 2016). Adaptive coping consists of problem solving, emotional regulation such as mediation or talking with friends, and cognitive reappraisal such as reshaping one's thoughts about a situation. Maladaptive coping techniques include internalizing symptoms such as withdrawal and helplessness along with externalizing symptoms such as aggression and blaming others (Skinner, Pitzer, & Steele, 2016). Variables that contribute to children's ability to use adaptive coping include socioeconomic status, family relationships, social support, gender, and previous life experiences.

To help children cope with the stresses in their lives, the parent, teacher, or health care worker must recognize signs that indicate that

BOX 15.1 Potential Sources of Stress in Middle Childhood*

Sources of Stress for the 6-Year-Old

Expectations—Parents, teachers, and other adults beginning to demand more

School—First grade introduces the child to the more formal, academic setting; may be the child's first experience away from home all day

Activity level—May find it difficult to sit still for long periods or control impulses

Competition—Wants to be "first" or best

Shyness—May initially be shy in a new situation but usually recovers quickly

Aggression—May become hostile or aggressive; temper tantrums peak

Sensitivity—Begins to read body language or facial expressions and becomes upset when sensing disapproval

Teasing—Engages in teasing but becomes upset when on the receiving end

Decisions—Has difficulty coping with increasing independence

Jealousy—Sibling rivalry is common

Fears—Usually center around newly found independence and might include fear of getting lost or fear of making an embarrassing social blunder

Sources of Stress for the 7-Year-Old

Moodiness—Is often moody, unhappy, or pensive

Approval—Continues to need praise and approval from peer group and parents

Modesty—Demands privacy when in the bathroom or dressing

Organization—Is comfortable with rules, regulations, routines, and order; becomes upset when they are disrupted

Interruptions—Hates to be disturbed when intensely involved in an activity

Idols—Has a desire to be more like an admired idol

Friendship—Becomes more selective about playmates

Sources of Stress for the 8-Year-Old

Self-criticism—Is very critical of personal ability and performance

Parental authority—Is beginning to resent parental authority

Loneliness—Likes frequent interaction with friends; may hate to miss school

Praise—Continues to seek approval but can identify when praise is not genuine

Independence—May begin to stay alone for brief periods while parents run errands, with resulting feelings of uneasiness

Sources of Stress for the 9-Year-Old

Rebelliousness—Occasionally tests independence by rebelling

Opposite sex—Engages in sex-segregated play; expresses an aversion to the opposite sex

Fair play—Has a keen sense of what is fair and is vehement in demanding personal rights when a situation is perceived as unfair

Interruptions—Continues to dislike interruptions but will usually resume an activity after an interruption

Propriety—Has a sense of propriety and will often be upset if siblings or parents offend the child's notion of decorum or dignity

Sources of Stress for the 10- to 12-Year-Old

Sexual maturation—Girls, in particular, may become self-conscious regarding obvious signs of puberty

Social issues—A new level of awareness can generate concern regarding pressing societal problems

Stature—Both boys and girls may be upset by the fact that the girls are taller; the extremely small or extremely large child may be concerned about his or her size

Shyness—If the child already has a problem in this area, it is likely to become more pronounced at this stage

Opposite sex—May become interested, yet shy, around members of the opposite sex

Confusion—Too much freedom can cause the child to flounder or make bad decisions

Health—May become a hypochondriac during this period of development

Money—Is anxious to earn and handle money but often uses poor judgment

Competition—Continues to be highly competitive and looks to peer group for prestige

Burnout—May become vigorously involved in so many activities that he or she finally becomes exhausted

Self-concept—May engage in teasing, scapegoating, or vicious attacks to temporarily boost his or her self-image; guilt often ensues; may be self-conscious about attempting a new skill

Parents—Often becomes highly critical or intolerant of parents

Idols—Continues hero worshipping

Fair play—Continues to have a highly developed sense of fair play

Drugs and sex—May be tempted to experiment with drugs or sex because "everyone" is doing it

Peer pressure—Becomes a powerful motivating force

Self-criticism—May be highly critical of personal performance

*Violence is a universal stress at all ages (see text).

From Kuczen, B. (1982). *Childhood stress: Don't let your child be a victim.* New York: Delacorte Press.

! NURSING ALERT

The nurse who observes the following signs of stress in a child should explore the situation further:

- Stomach pains or headache
- Sleep problems
- Bedwetting
- Changes in eating habits
- Aggressive or stubborn behavior
- Withdrawal or reluctance to participate
- Regression to earlier behaviors (e.g., thumb sucking)
- Trouble concentrating or changes in academic performance

a child is undergoing stress (see Box 15.1) and identify the source promptly. Children need to learn how to recognize signs of stress in themselves, such as a pounding heart, rapid breathing, or "butterflies" in the stomach. Once they are able to recognize that they are stressed, they can employ techniques for managing their stress. Children can learn relaxation techniques such as deep-breathing exercises, progressive relaxation of muscle groups, and positive imagery to reduce stress. Encouraging them to "blow off steam" through physical activity reduces tension and anxiety. Children need to learn to identify their stress reactions and strategies to reduce stress. Children should list all possibilities to reduce or minimize stress, including those they know will not work. They need to examine what might happen as a consequence of each alternative. The final step is to select what they perceive to be the best option. It is sometimes helpful to have children model their behavior after that of someone they know who has successfully coped with a similar problem. When children work through this process a few times, they are able to apply problem solving automatically.

Fears

Several anxiety symptoms, including fear of the dark, excessive worry about past behavior, self-consciousness, social withdrawal, and an excessive need for reassurance, are considered normal developmental events for children. School-age children are less fearful of body safety than they were as preschoolers, although they still fear being hurt, kidnapped, or having to undergo surgery. They also fear death and are fascinated by all aspects of death and dying. They have less fear of noises, darkness, storms, and dogs. Most new fears that trouble school-age children are related to school and family (e.g., fear of failing, fear of teachers and bullies, or fear of something bad happening to their parents).

Parents and other persons involved with children should discuss children's fears with them individually or through group activities. Their viewpoints must be respected, and their need to communicate their concerns should be recognized. Sometimes school-age children are inclined to hide their fears to avoid being ridiculed or labeled as a "baby" or "chicken." Hiding fears does not end them, and children who are afraid to communicate their fears may develop displaced fears or phobias. Children need to know that their concerns are heard and understood. Parents who convey this to their children without becoming overprotective help their children feel less lonely and less frightened.

Latchkey Children

The term latchkey children is used to describe children in elementary school who are left to care for themselves before or after school without supervision of an adult (Fig. 15.12). Due to an increased availability of after school programs, the number of school-age children spending time alone has decreased to about 15% (Rajalakshmi & Thanasekaran, 2015). The number of single-parent families and working parents,

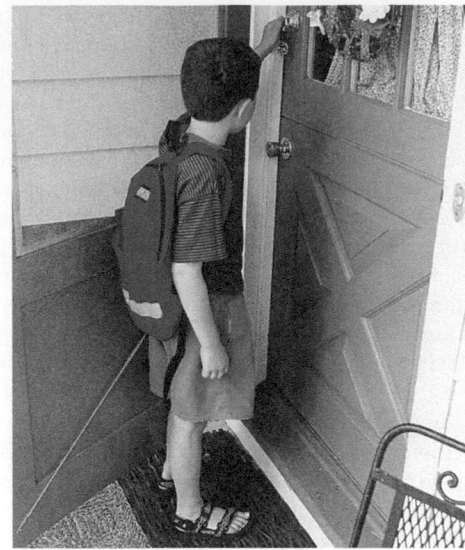

FIG. 15.12 A child unlocks the door to let himself into his home after school.

together with a lack of child care, has created a situation for many school-age children to be home alone.

Inadequate adult supervision after school leaves children at greater risk for injury and delinquent behavior. Latchkey children can feel more lonely, isolated, and fearful than children who have someone to care for them. To cope with their fears and anxieties while alone, these children may devise strategies such as hiding (in a bathroom, closet, or shower or under a bed), playing the television loudly to drown out noises, and using pets as a comfort.

Many communities and persons concerned about such children's welfare are trying to help children and their parents deal with this potentially serious problem. School-age child care programs have been implemented by some communities and employers. Some guidelines appropriate for presentation to parents and/or children to help alleviate their stress and increase the children's safety are listed in the Family-Centered Care box. Other types of programs include those designed to teach self-help skills to children, hotlines that provide telephone check-in and reassurance programs for children, and programs that link latchkey children with reassuring older persons in their community.

Nurses should be aware of services in their communities designed to meet the needs of latchkey children and include this information in anticipatory guidance of school-age children and their families. It is vital that children have adequate supervision and companionship.

PROMOTING OPTIMUM HEALTH DURING THE SCHOOL YEARS

HEALTH BEHAVIORS

During the middle childhood years, children acquire increased cognitive skills that allow them to make decisions about health behaviors they will select and pursue. In addition to personal traits, children establish health behaviors through social and environmental variables. By the end of middle childhood, children should be able to assume personal responsibility for self-care in the areas of hygiene, nutrition, exercise, recreation, sleep, and safety. In general, school-age boys and girls view themselves as healthy and can manage their own care in the areas of seat belt use, exercise, emergency situations, and dental health.

FAMILY-CENTERED CARE

Latchkey Children

Safety

Teach the child not to display keys and to always lock doors.
Tell the child not to enter the house after school if the door is ajar, a window is open, or anything appears unusual.
Talk through the after-school routine with the child.
Consult with public safety officials about burglar-proofing and fireproofing the home.
Teach the child first-aid procedures.
Teach safety rules to the child who is expected to cook (microwave ovens are safest).
Emphasize fire safety rules and conduct practice fire drills.
Teach and reinforce traffic and bicycle safety.
Teach the child weather-related safety (e.g., stay inside during an electrical storm; go to a storm cellar during a tornado warning).
Teach and reinforce water safety practices (e.g., warn the child not to go swimming alone; caution about safe bathing methods and keeping the toilet lid down when infants or toddlers are in their care).
Keep firearms securely locked away and teach the child that they are for adult use only.
Teach the child not to open the door to anyone.

Telephone Use

Teach the child his or her home telephone number, address, and parents' names.
Teach the child to tell callers that parents are "busy" and cannot come to the phone right now; instruct the child not to tell a caller that parents are not at home.
Teach the child not to tell casual callers the home address.
Keep a list of emergency numbers by the telephone. Make certain that the child knows how to report emergencies.
Have a list of telephone numbers of friends or neighbors who are available for help with emergencies.
Ask public safety officials to offer classes about when and how to call them.
If a telephone hotline for latchkey children exists, teach the child how to use it.

After-School Activities

Arrange for the child to spend some afternoons with friends.
Provide structured activities for the child.
Have the child attend a public library–sponsored activity rather than being home alone.
Discuss with the child things to do after school.
Emphasize positive aspects of independence and resourcefulness, but do not demand too much from the child.
Help the child feel successful in self-care.
Consider the potential problems of letting an older child assume care of younger ones before the child is developmentally ready.

Loneliness

Help the child talk about experiences and feelings about being alone after school.
Consider getting a pet to help provide company for the child.
Be punctual in arriving home. A child's anxiety level accelerates when parents are not home when expected.
Call the child if there is a delay in arriving home.
Leave a tape-recorded message for the child to play on arrival home from school.
Form a group of parents with flex-time so that children can be cared for by one of the group after school.

Health education is a primary component of comprehensive health care, and health education programs should promote desired health behavior through guided learning and modeling. An optimum program helps children learn about their bodies and about the effect of their behavior on their health.

Health promotion projects teach school-age children that social decision making to promote health is important. Children who engage in healthy behaviors, attain skills in self-control and problem solving, and know others care about them engage in fewer health risk behaviors (Horner, Rew, & Brown, 2012).

Children can also learn to take a more active role in relationships with health care providers. If asked what they would like to ask the health practitioner, most children are able to formulate several questions related to the reason for their visit. Providers can also teach children how to ask these questions so they can learn about their health during well-child visits to the pediatrician, nurse practitioner, and school nurse.

NUTRITION

Although caloric needs are diminished in relation to body size during middle childhood, resources are being laid down for the increased growth needs of the adolescent period. It is important to impress on children and their parents the value of a balanced diet to promote growth (Box 15.2). When children enter school, they develop an eating style that is increasingly independent from parental influence and scrutiny. Parents do not know what their children eat when they are away from home. A parent may pack a lunch to be eaten at school but be unaware of how much is eaten, traded, sold, or thrown away.

Likes and dislikes established at an early age continue in middle childhood, although the inclination for single-food preferences begins to end and children acquire a taste for an increasing variety of foods. Because children usually eat as the family does, the quality of their diet depends to a large extent on their family's pattern of eating. Other interests and participation in outside activities often compete with mealtime.

Outside Influences

With the influence of the mass media and the temptation of an immense variety of "junk food," it is all too easy for children to fill up on empty calories—foods that do not promote growth, such as sugars, starches, and excess fats. They have more freedom to move without parental supervision and often have small amounts of money to spend on candy, soft drinks, and other easily accessible treats. Midafternoon snacks are common, and it is wise to encourage consumption of fruit, nuts, and other wholesome finger foods to meet this need. Nutrition is a joint responsibility of both the child and the family.

The popularity of fast-food restaurants has aroused the attention of nutritionists and other health care professionals concerned with children's nutrition. The restaurants provide fast service, they are relatively inexpensive and appealing to children, and their convenience makes them attractive to busy parents as an alternative to eating at home. Because the nutritional content of fast foods is usually available, it is easier for nutrition-conscious parents to help children select appropriate items from the available menu. Nurses can support consumer advocate groups to encourage restaurants to offer items higher in nutritional value (such as skim milk, broiled meats, and fresh fruits and vegetables)

BOX 15.2 School-Based Interventions to Promote Nutrition Education

- Have young children collect pictures of healthy foods and make a poster for display at school.
- Ensure healthy foods (fruits, vegetables, whole grains, low-fat snacks) are available in school vending machines and at school sporting events.
- Discourage the use of high-fat foods (candy bars) as part of school fund-raising projects.
- Avoid the use of food as rewards for behavior; use verbal praise and token gifts to reinforce healthy eating and physical activity.
- Have teachers and school personnel model healthy eating habits.
- Ask children to select foods from a fast-food restaurant menu and to identify those foods high in fat, cholesterol, and sodium.
- Ask each child to keep a diary of foods eaten in 1 day, using MyPlate to evaluate these foods.
- Incorporate nutrition education into other classes (such as using a computer to analyze the nutritional content of foods).
- Have students keep a diary to identify cues for their eating behavior (e.g., hunger, stress, other people, social situations).
- Teach students how to read and discuss the nutrition labels on foods.
- Ask students to examine television commercials, magazine advertisements, and billboards to identify social influences on eating and physical activities.
- Use role playing to help students learn to cope with social and peer pressures to eat specific foods.
- Have students identify environmental barriers to healthy eating.
- Have students prepare nutritious foods, plan menus, and develop a recipe book of healthy foods.
- Involve parents in nutrition education through homework assignments or by inviting parents to attend student-led nutrition fairs.

Modified from Center for Communicable Diseases. (1996). Guidelines for school programs to promote lifelong healthy eating. *Journal of School Health, 67,* 9-26.

and to list ingredients and nutritional content on the menu as required for packaged foods.

Childhood obesity is a common health problem in school-age children. Obesity prevalence among school-age children in the United States has remained relatively stable over the past 3 years at 17% with higher prevalence among non-Hispanic blacks (19.5%) and Hispanics (21.9%) (Ogden, Carroll, Lawman, et al., 2016). The availability of inexpensive high-calorie foods, the tendency toward sedentary activities (such as watching television and playing electronic games), and the trend toward transportation by automobile instead of walking or cycling have reduced caloric expenditure. The consumption of a high-fat diet also contributes to obesity. The problem of childhood obesity is discussed further in Chapter 16. Given the threat of obesity and a diet-conscious society, many school-age children start to diet in an effort to prevent obesity or lose weight or to conform to peer behaviors and pressures. Children need education about food selection and the importance of body-building nutrients as opposed to empty caloric intake.

School Programs

Working parents assume that their children are sufficiently mature and frequently leave the responsibility of meal preparation to them. Although most older school-age children are capable of preparing simple meals, all too often breakfast and lunch may be inadequate, makeshift, or nonexistent. In recognition of this problem, the federal government has established the National School Lunch Program and the School Breakfast Program to provide low-cost or free meals to children at

BOX 15.3 Sample Menu for School-Age Children Based on MyPlate

Breakfast

Cold cereal (1 cup bran flakes, ½ cup fat-free milk, 1 medium banana)
1 slice whole-wheat toast with 1 tsp tub margarine
1 cup prune juice

Lunch

Tuna fish sandwich (2 slices rye bread, 2 oz tuna [packed in water, drained], 1 Tbsp mayonnaise, 1 Tbsp diced celery, ½ cup shredded lettuce)
1 medium peach
1 cup fat-free milk

Dinner

3 oz cooked chicken breast
1 large baked sweet potato, roasted
½ cup succotash (limas and corn) with 1 tsp tub margarine
1 oz whole-wheat dinner roll with 1 tsp tub margarine
1 cup water

Snack

¼ cup dried apricots
1 cup flavored yogurt

Obtained from US Department of Agriculture. (n.d.). *Sample menus for a 2000-calorie food pattern.* Retrieved from https://www.choosemyplate.gov/sites/default/files/misc/tools/Sample_Menus-2000Cals-DG2010.pdf

school or in afterschool programs, and the Healthy, Hunger Free Kids Act of 2010 to ensure availability of fruits, vegetables, and whole grains in the school menu. These meals must meet specified nutritional requirements and furnish one-third of the daily recommended dietary allowance for children in the United States. Most schools subscribe to the programs, and although the results are difficult to measure directly, it is believed that these school meal programs positively influence the behavior and learning capacity of children. However, the average school lunch may also exceed the recommended dietary guidelines for saturated and total fat. In addition, children who purchase school lunches often select only the items they want. In general, food choices of American children do not meet recommended intakes outlined in the US Department of Agriculture's MyPlate. Many Americans consume too many foods and drinks high in fat and carbohydrates and too little nutrient-dense foods and drinks such as fruits, vegetables, and low-fat milk (Keast, Fulgoni, Nicklas, et al., 2013).

Nutrition Education

Nutrition education should be integrated throughout the school years into classroom learning. In school, children can learn daily food choices, serving sizes, portion control, and the elements of a wholesome diet using ChooseMyPlate (Box 15.3). Guidelines from the US Department of Agriculture (2016) include the following:

- Follow a healthy eating pattern across the life span.
- Focus on variety, nutrient density, and amount.
- Limit calories from added sugars and saturated fats and reduce sodium intake.
- Shift to healthier food and beverage choices.
- Support healthy eating patterns for all—including home, school, work, and communities.

The school nurse should take an active role in nutrition education and work with teachers to implement nutrition instruction that is relevant and interesting to children (see Box 15.2 and Critical Thinking

Case Study box). The US Department of Agriculture maintains a website called Team Nutrition that provides nutrition education information and resources for schools, students, parents, and communities.*

CRITICAL THINKING CASE STUDY

Physical Growth in the School-Age Child

Janie, an 8-year-old girl, has just received her annual school physical examination. Janie weighs 30 kg (66 lb) and is 127 cm (50 inches) tall. Janie has gained 4.5 kg (10 lb) since last year and is otherwise reported as in good health with no acute illnesses.

1. Evidence—Is there sufficient evidence to draw conclusions about this situation?
2. Assumptions—Describe the underlying assumption about each of the following:
   a. Changing eating patterns among children
   b. Genetic, environmental, and societal risk factors associated with becoming overweight and obese
   c. Comorbidities associated with overweight and obesity in children
   d. Healthy food choice education for the school-age child
3. What implications for nursing care can be drawn from this situation?
4. Does the evidence support your conclusion?

Answers are available at http://evolve.elsevier.com/wong/ncic.

SLEEP AND REST

The amount of sleep and rest required during middle childhood is highly individualized. The specific amount of needed sleep depends on the child's age, activity level, and other factors such as health status. The growth rate slows in the school-age years; therefore less energy is expended in growth than during the preceding periods.

Sleep requirements decrease during school-age years; 5-year-olds generally require 10 to 13 hours of sleep, whereas 11-year-olds require approximately 9 to 11 hours of sleep (Allen, Howlett, Coulombe, et al., 2016). School-age children usually do not require a nap. Fewer bedtime problems occur during these years, but occasional difficulties are still associated with the necessary bedtime ritual. Usually children 6 and 7 years old have few problems, and encouraging quiet activity before bedtime, such as coloring and reading, can facilitate the task of going to bed. Although most children in middle childhood must be reminded to go to bed, 8- to 9-year-old children and 11-year-old children are particularly resistant. Often children are unaware that they are tired; if they are allowed to remain up later than usual, they are fatigued the following day. Sometimes parents can resolve bedtime resistance by allowing a later bedtime in deference to their advancing age. Twelve-year-old children usually offer no difficulty in relation to bedtime. Some even retire early to enjoy slow preparations for bed, to read, or to listen to music.

A firm approach to bedtime is usually the most successful. Parents can help children by giving them a little advance warning, but children should realize that when the final bedtime is announced, the parents mean it.

Sleep Problems

During middle childhood, nighttime sleep is usually continuous, and the child has developed a repertoire of tactics (such as reading or playing quietly without involving the parents) to deal with occasional difficulties in falling asleep. If a child has a sleep problem, a thorough assessment may be necessary to plan appropriate interventions.

The cause of bedtime resistance is not always clear. For some children it is related to normal fears of their age, such as fear of the dark, strange noises, intruders, or other imagined phenomena. Children who are subject to frightening dreams are hesitant to retire, and their sleep is more likely to be disturbed after emotional stimulation before bedtime. Sometimes children are unwilling to give up an exciting or interesting activity, or they are reluctant to leave the protective social circle of the family. Another factor associated with reluctance to go to bed is related to status. For example, older children are given the privilege of a later bedtime than younger children. Promotion to a later bedtime is highly prestigious, and age-mates compare their bedtimes. This may explain why children who believe that playmates enjoy a more privileged position strongly oppose parental decisions. In some situations going to bed is used as a method of control. When going to bed early is imposed as a punishment or when staying up late is a reward, children may view bedtime as punitive or status degrading.

Some children resort to multiple "curtain calls," such as wanting a drink of water, asking for one more story, needing to go to the bathroom, or wanting to watch television. Some children persist in coming out of their rooms repeatedly after being put back to bed. Some voice fears, such as "there is someone outside the window." Parents may have difficulty determining whether the fear is legitimate or whether the behavior is a bid for attention. Consistent reassurance and limit setting usually resolve the problem. Children feel tense and insecure when limits are applied inconsistently, such as when parents grant permission one night and punish the next for the same behavior.

The night terrors of preschool children may be replaced by sleepwalking and sleep talking. Like night terrors, sleepwalking is associated with the transition from stage 4 to stage 1 of non–rapid eye movement sleep. When children arouse from stage 4 sleep, it is often difficult for them to reach a fully alert, wakeful state rapidly. Sleepwalking occurs in the first 3 to 4 hours of sleep. Children often have no memory of sleepwalking in the morning. The episode begins when the child sits up abruptly and walks, usually with open eyes. During sleepwalking, movements are clumsy and repetitive; parents often observe finger and hand movements. Most commonly, children move about restlessly, then lie down and return to sleep. Children rarely perform purposeful acts during sleepwalking. Any attempts to communicate with the child elicit only mumbled and slurred responses. Sleep talking, like sleepwalking, is not purposeful, and speech is usually incomprehensible and monosyllabic.

The best approach is to leave sleepwalking children alone unless they are in danger or may endanger others. However, clumsiness and stereotyped movements can make sleepwalking very dangerous. If the environment is not safe, children can get hurt. Instruct parents to gently redirect children back to bed without waking them, if possible. If children must be wakened, it is best to call them by name slowly and softly, orient them to where they are, explain that they were walking in their sleep, and assure them that it will not happen when they are more relaxed. Preventive measures include avoiding overfatigue in children, making certain they get adequate rest, employing relaxation techniques, and relieving any stress the children may be experiencing.

Sleepwalking is usually self-limiting and resolves spontaneously. About 17% of children sleepwalk once during childhood, with a peak onset of 8 to 12 years of age (Carter, Hathaway, & Lettieri, 2014). Persistent sleepwalking occurs in children and adolescents who tend to repress strong emotions, such as anger. They may benefit from learning to express their feelings and from doing self-relaxation before bedtime.

Nightmares are a part of the normal developmental process; up to 50% of children experience nightmares during childhood (Carter,

*US Department of Agriculture's Team Nutrition, 3101 Park Center Drive, Room 632, Alexandria, VA 22302; 703-305-1624; www.fns.usda.gov/tn/.

Hathaway, & Lettieri, 2014). Nightmares can begin in children 3 to 6 years of age and peak at 6 to 10 years of age (Carter, Hathaway, & Lettieri, 2014). Repetitive nightmares or increased nightmare frequency may indicate a specific underlying conflict or stressor that is strongly influencing the child's behavior and thought. Resolving worries or stress will often reduce nightmares. If nightmares become chronic, parents should consider professional counseling (Carter, Hathaway, & Lettieri, 2014).

A traumatic event often produces posttraumatic nightmares, which are anxiety provoking and literal in their depiction of the trauma. As time goes on, the dreams of affected children may consist of "modified repetitions" that may add more current material to the recurrent dreams (e.g., involving others who were not a part of the traumatic event). Current external stresses, movies, or stories may also precipitate a nightmare by reactivating old traumas. (For a comparison of nightmares and sleep terrors, see Table 14.1.)

PHYSICAL ACTIVITY

Exercise is essential for muscle development and tone, refinement of balance and coordination, gaining of strength and endurance, and stimulation of body functions and metabolic processes. Throughout middle childhood, children's increasing capabilities and adaptability permit greater speed and effort in motor activities. Larger, stronger muscles with greater efficiency and skill permit longer and increasingly strenuous play without exhaustion. During this period, children acquire the coordination, timing, and concentration that are required to participate in adult-type activities, even though they may lack the strength, stamina, and control of the adolescent and adult. Consequently, parents should expect and encourage a larger amount of physical activity during the school years.

Children should have opportunities that provide satisfying experiences to meet individual likes and dislikes. Children need space to run, jump, skip, and climb, as well as safe facilities and equipment to use both inside and outside. Appropriate activities that promote coordination and development include running, jumping rope, swimming, skating, dancing, and bicycle riding. Positive reinforcement achieved by experiencing increasingly smooth, rhythmic, and efficient use of the body conditions the child toward regular physical activity. However, one must keep in mind that although school-age children are large and appear to be strong, they may not be prepared for strenuous competitive athletics.

Most children need little encouragement to engage in physical activity. They have so much energy that they seldom know when to stop. However, children with disabilities or those who hesitate to become involved in active play, such as obese children, require special assessment and help in determining activities that appeal to them, are compatible with their limitations, and meet their developmental needs.

Physical Fitness

The development of physical fitness is a goal for all children. This goal was easy to accomplish in the past when school-age children spent a considerable amount of time each day playing on playgrounds, walking to school, and participating in games or sports at school or in their communities. With the advent of technology and the information age, many children are less active physically and spend large portions of their day in front of electronic devises (see Research Focus box).

Counseling should include developing goals, identifying fun and safe physical activities, addressing potential barriers, and encouraging support from family and friends. Nurses can further promote efforts to include physical fitness in school programs and encourage children to engage in aerobic physical activities during their free time. Such activities provide cardiopulmonary benefits, maintain normal weight, and have the potential to contribute to lifelong fitness. *Exergaming,* the use of active video games to promote physical activity, is a new method that can be used to increase physical activity. Children perceive exergaming as fun and motivating, but its effectiveness has not yet been established (Gao, Chen, & Stodden, 2015).

> **RESEARCH FOCUS**
>
> ***Strategies to Increase Physical Activity in Children***
>
> Strategies focusing on increasing physical activity and reducing sedentary behavior have become a priority; however, only 30% of students participate in daily physical education classes (Kann, McManus, Harris, et al., 2016). In addition, children spend less than 50% of their time in moderate or vigorous physical activity during recess (Gao, Chen, & Stodden, 2015). Furthermore, safety concerns (e.g., traffic and stranger danger) along with the appeal of sedentary activities (e.g., video games) have contributed to a significant decline in children's outdoor play time, resulting in a decrease in physical activity (Ergler, Kearns, & Witten, 2013).

Sports

Much controversy has surrounded the trend toward earlier participation in competitive athletics and the amount and type of competitive sports that are appropriate for children in the elementary grades. The current view is that virtually every child is suited for some type of sport, and authorities do not discourage participation if children are matched to the type of sport appropriate to their abilities and to their physical and emotional constitutions. School-age children enjoy competition, and when teachers, parents, and coaches understand children's physical limitations and teach them the proper techniques and safety measures to avoid injury to developing bones and muscles, a safe and appropriate sport can be found for even the most unskilled and uncompetitive child.

During middle childhood, girls have the same basic structure as boys and thus have a similar response to systematic exercise training. At puberty, when boys become larger and have more muscle mass, it is usually recommended that girls compete only against other girls. Before puberty there is no essential difference in strength and size between girls and boys, which makes these precautions unnecessary.

Well-organized extracurricular sports programs based in the community or school encourage enjoyment of sports and fitness in childhood (Box 15.4). Preadolescence is a time to teach fundamental motor skills; develop fitness in a practical, safe, and gradual manner; and promote desired attitudes and values. Activities should include practice sessions

> **BOX 15.4 Goals of Organized Athletics for Preadolescent Children**
>
> Organized extracurricular athletic programs for preadolescent children should focus on helping children develop the following:
>
> - Enjoyment of sports and fitness that will be sustained through adulthood
> - Physical fitness
> - Basic motor skills
> - A positive self-image
> - A balanced perspective on sports in relation to the child's school and community life
> - A commitment to the values of teamwork, fair play, and sportsmanship

Modified from American Academy of Pediatrics, Committee on Sports Medicine and Committee on School Health. (2001). Organized athletics for preadolescent children. *Pediatrics, 107*(6), 1459-1462.

BOX 15.5 Safeguards for Athletic Programs

Every athletic program should require the following:

- Participation physical examinations at least every 2 years
- Warm-up and cool-down stretching exercises
- The availability of a medically trained person who is competent in recognizing significant injuries during practices and games of contact sports
- The establishment of policies for first aid, referral of injured participants, treatment, rehabilitation, and certification for return to participation
- Suitable and well-maintained sports facilities
- Appropriate protective and safety equipment
- Strict enforcement of rules concerning safety
- A formal surveillance method to ensure that goals are met

Modified from American Academy of Pediatrics, Committee on Sports Medicine and Committee on School Health. (2001). Organized athletics for preadolescent children. *Pediatrics, 107*(6), 1459-1462; and Veigel, J. D., & Pleacher, M. D. (2008). Injury prevention in youth sports. *Current Sport Medicine Reports, 7*(6), 348-352.

and unstructured play. The actual game or event should be managed in a manner that stresses mastery of the sport and enhancement of self-image rather than winning or pleasing others. All children should have an opportunity to participate, and special ceremonies should recognize all participants rather than individuals.

In addition to ensuring the interest, suitability, and safety (Box 15.5) of the sport, parents must make certain that coaches (if involved in the sport) are skillful in managing children and do not engage in abusive behavior. Coaches, parents, and others involved in children's sports play critical roles in shaping children's self-esteem. Any sport for children should emphasize the pleasure of the activity. It is wise to expose children to a variety of individual sports. The overall emphasis of both team and individual sports should be on playing and learning. Parents who pressure their children to perform beyond their capabilities run the risk of the child's being injured, developing a dislike for the activity, and developing a lowered self-image (see Family-Centered Care box).

FAMILY-CENTERED CARE

Athletic Stress in School-Age Children

Participating in a competitive sport should be an enjoyable experience for school-age children. For some children, however, this activity is associated with considerable stress and anxiety. Their parents' reaction to their performance serves as the source of this stress. Children state that they feel awful when they strike out or are unable to catch a fly ball or when their team loses a game. These children report that their parents often yell at them and are more upset over a lost game than their coach is. Children notice that their mothers and fathers consider themselves a failure if their child is not a star player.

Parents of children who participate in competitive sports need to praise and support their children regardless of whether games are won or lost. Parents need to avoid the temptation to identify with their child. Parents' success and self-worth should not depend on whether their child wins. At the very minimum, parents should monitor their behavior at games and avoid criticizing their child, other players, the officials, or the coaches.

The same principles described in the preceding paragraphs apply to children with chronic illnesses, such as diabetes, epilepsy, asthma, or allergies, if the disorder is mild and can be controlled with medication. Children with cognitive impairment do not need to be excluded from sports competition if they are matched evenly against other children of equal abilities and provided with skilled supervision and coaching.

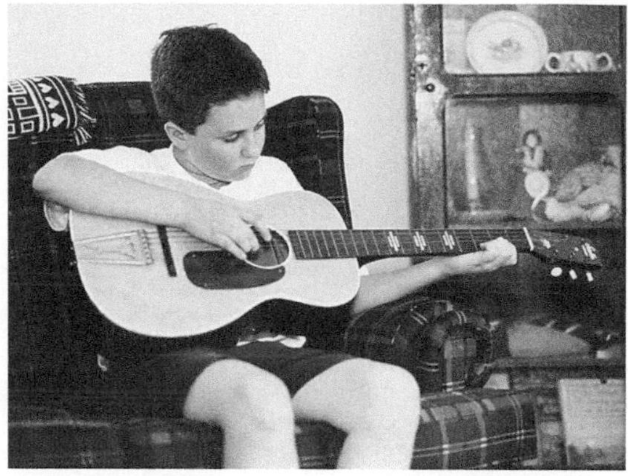

FIG. 15.13 Music is a favorite form of expression for school-age children.

Some activities need to be modified to accommodate the skills of these children.

Acquisition of Skills

School-age children demonstrate increasing capacity in fine muscle facility and complex artistic skills. Handedness is well established by the beginning of the school years, and children make great strides in writing and drawing during this age period. It is a time of energetic and vibrant creative productivity. With the tools of language and reading, children can create poems, stories, and plays. With more advanced fine motor skills, they are able to master an unlimited variety of handicrafts, such as ceramics, needlework, wood carving, and beadwork. They avidly pursue these skills in solitude, with a friend, or in programs offered through organizations such as boys' or girls' clubs or special interest groups that use crafts as a means to occupy, entertain, and educate children.

Music is a favorite form of expression in middle childhood (Fig. 15.13). Music stimulates and invigorates school-age children. They can sing in harmony, play instruments in orchestras and bands, and manage music at a more complex level. They can compose original songs, learn lyrics almost effortlessly, and turn any empty moment into an occasion for singing.

School-age children are capable of assuming responsibility for their own needs, although their distaste for soap and water and "dress" clothes is legendary. School-age children can and want to assume their share of household tasks, which usually are related to the male and female roles that have been defined by their culture (Fig. 15.14). Many also assume responsibility for tasks outside the home, such as babysitting, yard work, or paper routes.

Television, Video Games, and the Internet

For some time, child development specialists and parents have been concerned about the effect of media on child development and behavior. Children spend a significant amount of time each day involved in media-related activities, including the use of television, the Internet, electronic games, and cell phones. Children ages 8 to 12 years spend at least 6 hours every day with various forms of media for entertainment, not including time spent for schoolwork, and children ages 13 to 18 years spend an average of 9 hours every day (Rideout, 2016). Because of the long periods of exposure, the media have more time to develop children's attitudes than do parents and teachers.

There is no doubt that children learn from various forms of media, but the values and attitudes depicted on these forums are not always realistic and may conflict with values that children were previously

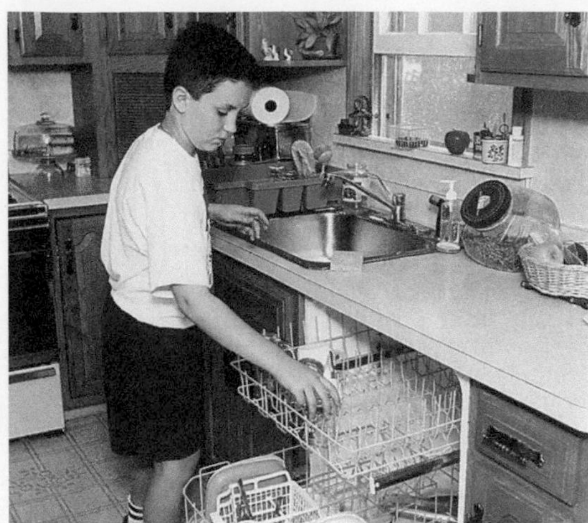

FIG. 15.14 Children can assume responsibility for a variety of household tasks.

taught. School-age children can distinguish fantasy from reality, and some have had sufficient life experience to view information from media with skepticism. However, violence is common in various forms of media, and significant exposure to media violence increases aggressive behavior, aggressive thoughts, and angry feelings in some children (American Academy of Pediatrics, Council on Communications and Media, 2016). In addition, repeated exposure to violence can desensitize children to violence, convey a message that violence is acceptable, and teach children that initiating violent behavior is a way to protect themselves (Brockmyer, 2015).

Violence in the media can also increase fear and anxiety in children. Events such as terrorist attacks and mass shootings have infiltrated television and the Internet, frequently exposing children to real-life violence. Viewing violence in the news can cause immediate effects such as fear, worry, and attention difficulty, and can also cause long-term effects such as emotional problems and poor school performance (Leiner, Peinado, Villanos, et al., 2016). Parents should make the ultimate decisions about which programs their child will watch and which sites their child can use on the Internet. To reduce exposure to violence and maximize the beneficial effects of television, parents are advised to monitor program selection, view programs with their children, and discuss program content when the programs are finished (Leiner, Peinado, Villanos, et al., 2016). (See Chapter 2 for a more in-depth discussion of children and mass media.)

Electronic and Internet games have been both criticized and supported in relation to their effect on children and adolescents. Critics maintain that games keep children from schoolwork and can cause tension, sleeplessness, and violence. Others support the activity as a means for improving hand-eye coordination and as a substitute for the inactivity of passive television viewing. Benefits may also include development of inductive reasoning (i.e., drawing generalizations from specific observations), improving spatial perception, and learning to handle multiple variables that interact simultaneously.

Research suggests that electronic games may affect physical and psychologic functioning. Physical effects, including flickering of lights produced by video games, may trigger a reflex seizure (Koepp, Caciagli, Pressler, et al., 2016). (See seizure discussion, Chapter 30.) However, research has noted some positive applications of electronic games with dyslexic children (Franceschini, Gori, Ruffino, et al., 2013).

The Internet is a popular means for obtaining educational and recreational information. Approximately 83% of children have Internet access at home and spend varying amounts of time with reading

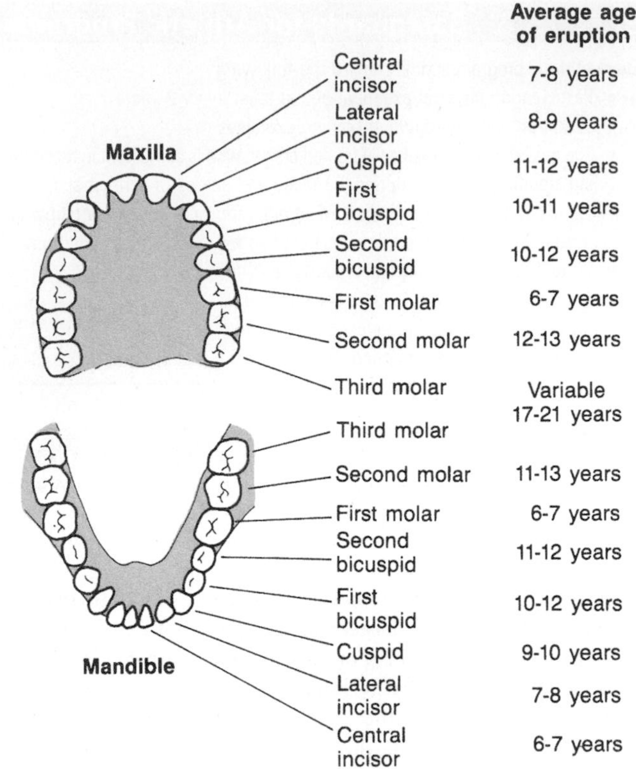

FIG. 15.15 Sequence of eruption of secondary teeth. (Data from Dean, J. A. [2016]. *McDonald and Avery's dentistry for the child and adolescent* [10th ed.]. St. Louis, MO: Mosby.)

information, gaming, and social networking (Rideout, 2016). Although these opportunities provide valuable educational opportunities for children, there are also many risks that parents must acknowledge before children access the Internet. Major risks include exposure to inappropriate, dangerous, or illegal material; sexual solicitation; exposure to harassment; revelation of financial information that leads to negative consequences; and safety issues relating to sharing personal information or meeting strangers. The best way to eliminate potential risks is to educate parents and children about the Internet and to provide adult supervision when children use the Internet.

Parent and teacher education relating to television, electronic games, and the Internet (including social networking) should include recommendations to limit media time, monitor content, and increase access to games and information that are educational.

DENTAL HEALTH

The first permanent (secondary) teeth erupt at about 6 years of age. Before their appearance they have been developing in the jaw beneath the deciduous (primary) teeth. The roots of the latter are gradually absorbed, so when a deciduous tooth is shed, only the crown remains. At 6 years of age, all of the primary teeth are present, and those of the secondary dentition are relatively well formed. Eruption of the permanent teeth begins with the 6-year molar, which erupts posterior to the deciduous molars. The others appear in approximately the same order as in eruption of the primary teeth and follow shedding of the deciduous teeth (Fig. 15.15).

The pattern of shedding of primary teeth and eruption of secondary teeth is subject to wide variation among children. To allow the larger permanent teeth to occupy the limited space left by shed primary teeth, a series of complicated changes must take place in the jaws. At this time many of the difficulties created by crowding of teeth become apparent. With the appearance of the second permanent (12-year) molars, most of the permanent teeth are present. The third permanent molars, or wisdom teeth, may erupt from 18 to 25 years of age or later. Permanent dentition is somewhat more advanced in girls than in boys.

Because permanent teeth erupt during the school-age years, good dental hygiene and regular attention to dental caries are vital parts of health supervision during this period. Caries is a common problem, and 42% of children ages 2 to 11 years have caries in their primary teeth (Moyer, 2014). Children of this age tend to become careless about oral hygiene unless they are carefully supervised. Although children are assuming more responsibility for their own care, they are not as motivated by improved appearance and odor as they will be during adolescence. School nurses should be alert for opportunities to teach correct brushing and flossing techniques; to reinforce avoidance of fermentable carbohydrates and sticky sweets; and to be alert for problems of malocclusion, toothache, and mouth infections.

Comprehensive dental supervision should be an integral part of the health maintenance program. Regular dental prophylaxis (teeth cleaning) by a dentist or dental hygienist and continued fluoride supplementation are essential to decrease the susceptibility of the tooth enamel to acid breakdown. (See Chapter 12 for a discussion of fluoride and other aspects of dental care.)

Brushing

The most effective means of preventing dental caries is a regimen of proper oral hygiene. Children should learn to carry out their own dental care with the supervision and guidance of parents. Parents should learn proper brushing technique along with their children and should inspect their children's efforts until the children can assume full responsibility for their own care.

Most practitioners believe that the majority of children do not possess the fine motor skills needed to brush their teeth properly until approximately second grade. Ideally, children should brush teeth after meals, after snacks, and at bedtime. The bedtime brushing is especially important because there is more time overnight for interaction between oral bacteria and unremoved substrate on the tooth substance. Children who brush their teeth frequently and become accustomed to the feel of a clean mouth at an early age usually maintain the habit throughout life.

The thoroughness of plaque removal (cleaning) can be checked using a plaque-disclosing agent that stains any remaining plaque red. The child should inspect the teeth closely with the aid of a mirror and under adequate light. The teeth then are again cleansed with a fluoridated dentifrice to remove the remaining plaque and provide further protection. This procedure may be carried out regularly or occasionally, according to instructions from the child's dentist. Toothpaste recommended by the American Dental Association Council on Dental Therapeutics carries a seal of approval, which is easily identified on the package. They have been submitted to testing and demonstrate the ability to reduce the incidence of dental caries when used correctly.

For school-age children with mixed and permanent dentition, the best toothbrush is one with soft nylon bristles and an overall length of about 21 cm (8 inches). There are numerous methods of brushing the teeth for children, but no conclusive evidence indicates that one method is superior to another. The thoroughness of the cleaning is more important than the specific technique used. The dentist will assess all factors, such as the child's manipulative skills and special needs, and suggest the most appropriate brushing technique and regimen. Flossing follows brushing. Parents usually floss until children acquire the manual dexterity needed. Most children are not able to floss properly until about 8 or 9 years of age.

SCHOOL HEALTH

Child health maintenance is ultimately the responsibility of parents; however, public schools and health departments in the United States have contributed to the improvement of child health by providing a healthful school environment, health services, and health education functions that emphasize sound health practices. These functions constitute major components of community health services and involve large amounts of public funds and many health professionals, including nurses.

A school health program is involved in ongoing health maintenance through assessment, screening, and referral activities. Routine health services provided by most schools include health appraisal, emergency care, safety education, communicable disease control, counseling, and follow-up care. One model that has been used to provide information about the essential components of school health is the Coordinated School Health Program (Centers for Disease Control and Prevention, 2015). The 10 basic components of this program are health education; physical education and physical activity; nutrition environment and services; health services; counseling, psychologic, and social services; social and emotional climate; physical environment; employee wellness; family engagement; and community involvement (Centers for Disease Control and Prevention, 2015). See Boxes 15.6 and 15.7 for factors that contribute to a healthful school setting and for characteristics of school health programs.

Health Education

Health education of school-age children focuses on providing knowledge of health and influencing habits, attitudes, and conduct in relation to health (Box 15.8). A viable health education program is based on sound health concepts but should be adjusted to meet specific local needs, objectives, and legal requirements. Parents must understand and approve the health education curriculum so that its teaching will be reinforced at home. A comprehensive approach to health education is more successful in developing positive health practices than one in which the subjects are taught in isolation. Many topics presented in health education classes are associated with differing social and cultural attitudes and should be presented accurately and with sensitivity to these attitudes.

Health education concerning AIDS is a specific example. Most authorities agree that AIDS education should begin in the elementary grades to prevent high-risk behaviors. However, educational programs concerning AIDS must be developmentally appropriate and, to be effective, must be implemented with parental and community support. Young children need information on how HIV is transmitted in simple, accurate terms without elaborate, unnecessary discussions of sex. Misconceptions that increase children's anxiety about contracting the virus should be corrected. Although many children have heard that sex and drugs cause AIDS, some children also have misconceptions about AIDS. Children need information that HIV is transmitted through infected blood on shared drug needles and that the virus is not spread through common forms of expressing affection such as hugging and holding hands.

School Nursing Services

School nurses assume a major role in the school health program and can affect the lives of school-age children significantly. Working in collaboration with others in the school and community, school nurses provide health supervision, health counseling, and health education. The responsibilities of the school nurse can include providing education and interventions for acute and chronic illness, safety, health promotion, normal development, nutrition, mental health, dental disease, and sexually transmitted infections (American Academy of Pediatrics, Council

BOX 15.6 Components of a Coordinated School Health Program: The Whole School, Whole Community, Whole Child (WSCC) Model

Health Services—Services provided to students to protect and promote health through health appraisals, prevention and control of communicable diseases, emergency care, and educational counseling

Health Education—A planned, sequential, prekindergarten to grade 12 curriculum and instructions that addresses physical, mental, emotional, and social dimensions of health

Nutrition Environment and Services—Food service that conforms to federal nutrition standards and ensures balanced diets and, when needed, special diets

Counseling, Psychologic, and Social Services—Services provided to students to improve mental, behavioral, and social-emotional health through psychologic, psychoeducational, and psychosocial assessments, direct and indirect intervention, and referral to such support services as needed

Employee Wellness—Services to promote health and wellness (e.g., blood pressure screening, stress reduction programs, fitness activities) among school staff to improve the health of staff and serve as role models for students

Physical Education and Physical Activity—Physical activity for students in kindergarten to grade 12 that provides cognitive learning and physical fitness experiences with a variety of activities

Community Involvement—Dynamic partnerships with community groups, organizations, and local businesses to enhance the health and well-being of students

Family Engagement—Families working with school staff to support and improve learning, development, and the health of students

Social and Emotional Climate—A positive social and emotional school climate is conducive to effective teaching and learning by promoting health, growth, and development in a safe and supportive learning environment

Physical Environment—The physical environment encompasses the school building and its content and the land and area surrounding the school; a healthy physical environment protects students from physical threats and biologic and chemical agents, and maintains normal operations during renovations

From Centers for Disease Control and Prevention. (2015). *Whole school, whole community, whole child (WSCC)*. Retrieved from www.cdc.gov/healthyschools/wscc/index.htm.

BOX 15.7 Content of School Health Services

Health appraisal—Screening tests (vision, hearing); measurements (height, weight); and medical, dental, and psychologic examinations

Health promotion—Teaching healthy lifestyles and encouraging avoidance of health risks through promotion and awareness programs

Emergency care and safety—Emergency treatment (first aid), notification of parents, and transportation of the ill or injured child to home or hospital

Communicable disease control—Detection and exclusion of affected children and policies for readmission and attendance at school (immunizations required in most states before school entry)

Counseling and guidance—Health guidance, referral, and follow-up for parents and children with special health needs

Adjustment to individual student needs

BOX 15.8 Recommendations for School Health Programs

- Health and safety education should be taught as part of basic education and deserves the same priority in the curriculum as traditional subjects.
- Planned integrated programs of comprehensive health and safety education should be a requirement for students from kindergarten through grade 12 and should be taught by specially qualified teachers or those certified to teach health education.
- Health and safety education should include the active participation of students for the most effective learning of sound health concepts.
- Financial support for health and safety education programs must be ensured. Proper funding is critical to the development of effective programs, and the agencies responsible must be convinced to continue or increase funding.
- Comprehensive health and safety education programs should be directed by qualified health educators who function in consultation and cooperation with school personnel and administrators.
- The programs should be monitored by a well-organized school health committee composed of representative parents, students, pediatricians, and health agency personnel (e.g., public health nurses) in the community.
- Health and safety education should be a part of every elementary school and secondary school teacher's training program.
- School districts, other public agencies, the medical community, and private agencies should intensify their health and safety education program for adults as part of a coordinated community health and safety education effort, and pediatricians should make health and safety education a regular component of child health supervision and routine illness visits.
- Research studies to evaluate the impact of such programs on students must be carried out at local and national levels.

Data from American Academy of Pediatrics. (2013). *Health, mental health and safety guidelines for schools.* Retrieved from http://www.nationalguidelines.org

on School Health, 2016). These functions are not necessarily limited to the confines of the school environment but extend into the community in which the students live. As a health care practitioner, the school nurse is in a position to promote and evaluate health services throughout the community as they affect children and to collaborate with agencies in planning for health and safety. For some children, especially those in poverty, the school nurse may be the only contact with illness prevention and health promotion. For children with chronic health conditions, the school nurse provides leadership within the school health team and assesses the student's health status, develops an individualized health care plan by interpreting medical recommendations into the school environment, and provides feedback regarding the student's response to treatment plans (American Academy of Pediatrics, Council on School Health, 2016).

Traditionally, school nurses have been viewed from a limited perspective that placed them in the role of disease detector, applier of bandages, and official caregiver in cases of illness and injury. Although these are still important functions, this traditional role has acquired much broader dimensions. School nurses develop, implement, and evaluate health care plans and programs. In some settings a school-based health center is near or within a school to provide additional health services. In these centers, school nurse practitioners provide primary health care, including treatment of acute illnesses, screening for vision and hearing, administration of immunizations, nutrition counseling, and anticipatory guidance, including substance abuse assessments (American Academy of Pediatrics, Council on School Health, 2016).

Unlicensed assistive personnel (UAP) may be a part of the school health care team. These paraprofessionals have a state certification and are trained to assist a professional but must be trained, evaluated for competency, and monitored by the school nurse (Rose, Disney, Andresen, et al., 2016). The school nurse must have awareness of state regulation and use professional judgment in deciding which procedures may be delegated to UAP.

! NURSING ALERT

In the delegation or transfer of responsibility for the performance of an activity to an assistant, the nurse remains accountable for the outcome.

The passage of Public Law 94-142, now known as the Individuals with Disabilities Education Act (IDEA), requires equal access to education in the least restrictive environment for children with chronic illness or disability. School nurses are responsible for the medical and nursing needs of these children in the school setting. School nurses assess and monitor all health problems in children who come into the school and compile a health care list of all of these problems and their associated therapies. The nurse may call the parents of the child and arrange a visit to the home, made by either the school nurse or a public health nurse. After gathering information, the nurse can develop a nursing care plan for use in the school. The nurse collaborates with the family and includes their suggestions in the care plan. The nurse then discusses the plan with the child's teachers and provides any needed education. School nurses are the only ones in the school system qualified to deal with medical problems. However, in many instances school nurses can collaborate with teachers to provide atraumatic care (see Community and Home Health Considerations box).

COMMUNITY AND HOME HEALTH CONSIDERATIONS

Collaboration Between School Nurse and Teachers

- All students should have health cards completed by their parents.
- All teachers should receive a list of students who have health problems.
- Teachers should schedule students who miss physical education into an adaptive physical education class if possible.
- All students with asthma should have their metered-dose inhalers available to them for emergency use in physical education and all other classes.
- In physical education, evaluation of a skill or activity should be repeated several times if some students score extremely high and others extremely low because every child has good and bad days.
- Teachers should never question a child's ability in front of other students.
- Nurses should maintain privacy for height and weight checks and for vision and hearing tests. (Students should be taken into the nurse's office individually so other students do not hear the test results.)

Sometimes all that is required is conducting an assessment and making the teacher aware that the child has a health problem. In other cases more complex teaching is needed, such as how to observe for certain signs (e.g., insulin reaction); how to perform certain techniques (e.g., tracheostomy suctioning, gastrostomy or nasogastric tube feedings); and how to manage emergencies (e.g., care of a child during a seizure). School nurses instruct teachers in the necessary procedures and review their performance.

The American Academy of Pediatrics, Council on School Health (2008) established guidelines for emergency medical care of children in schools in 2008 and reaffirmed the guidelines in 2012. These guidelines include developing emergency policies and procedures, clarifying school staff roles, collecting emergency data on all schoolchildren, making emergency equipment and medication easily accessible, and adequately training staff. It is recommended that at least one staff member, in addition to the school nurse, have cardiopulmonary resuscitation, first aid, and automated external defibrillator training.

A child who must take medication at school needs written authorization from his or her health care provider and/or written permission from the parents allowing the nurse to administer or supervise the administration of the medication. The medication must be brought to the school in a container appropriately labeled by the pharmacist or prescribing provider. Medications are kept locked up in the nurse's office; usually the child is not allowed to carry medications at school. The policy may vary in some school districts or situations. For example, some children may be allowed to carry metered-dose inhalers that contain their asthma medication, provided that their health care provider and a parent provide the required authorization. Guidelines for administration of medications in schools are also available from the National Association of School Nurses.*

INJURY PREVENTION

Because school-age children have developed more refined muscular coordination and control and can apply their cognitive capacities to select a more judicious course of action, the incidence of unintentional injury is diminished in middle childhood compared with the incidence in early childhood. School-age children have exposure to more environments in which they need protection, they acquire skills and interests that expose them to new perils, they have less supervision, and they take more responsibility as they begin to participate in the adult world.

Injuries most prevalent in school-age children reflect their developmental stage. Table 15.2 outlines the developmental characteristics and accomplishments of middle childhood that predispose children to physical injury and offers guidelines for injury prevention.

The incidence of injury during middle childhood is significantly higher in school-age boys than in school-age girls, and their death rate is twice that of girls (see Chapter 1). Most injuries occur in or near the home or school. The prevalence of injury depends on the dangers present in the environment, the protection offered by adults, and the behavior patterns of the children. Safety helmets, protective eye and mouth shields, and protective padding are strongly recommended for children engaging in active sports, even though they may not be required equipment. Although school age children are conscious of rules and frequently impose them in relationships with peers, they also tend to challenge established rules. It is often difficult to maintain a balance between the level of supervision and restriction needed by children and their need for freedom and independence.

The incidence of transportation-related injuries is higher in school-age children than in younger children, and the incidence of bicycle injury not involving a motor vehicle is higher than that in teenagers and preschool children. Injuries from burns and poisonings are lowest in school-age children. However, physically active school-age children are susceptible to cuts and abrasions, and the incidence of childhood fractures, strains, and sprains is high.

Risk-Taking Behavior

Achieving social acceptance is a primary objective for school-age children. They often attempt dangerous acts (sometimes extreme behaviors) to

*1100 Wayne Avenue, Suite 925, Silver Springs, MD 20910; 240-821-1130; e-mail: nasn@nasn.org; www.nasn.org.

TABLE 15.2 Injury Prevention During School-Age Years

Developmental Abilities Related to Risk of Injury	Injury Prevention
Motor Vehicle Accidents	
Is increasingly involved in activities away from home Is excited by speed and motion Is easily distracted by environment Can be reasoned with	Educate child regarding proper use of seat belts while a passenger in a vehicle. Maintain discipline while the child is a passenger in a vehicle (e.g., ensure that child keeps arms inside, does not lean against doors or interfere with driver). Remind parents and children that no one should ride in the bed of a pickup truck. Emphasize safe pedestrian behavior. Insist that child wear safety apparel (e.g., helmet) when applicable, such as riding bicycle (see Family-Centered Care box).
Drowning	
Is apt to overdo May work hard to perfect a skill Has cautious, but not fearful, gross motor actions Likes swimming	Teach child to swim. Teach basic rules of water safety. Select safe and supervised places to swim. Check sufficient water depth for diving. Caution child to swim with a companion. Ensure that child uses an approved flotation device in water or boat. Advocate for legislation requiring fencing around pools. Learn cardiopulmonary resuscitation.
Burns	
Has increasing independence Is adventurous Enjoys trying new things	Make sure smoke detectors are in homes. Set water heaters to 48.9°C (120°F) to avoid scald burns. Instruct child regarding behavior in areas involving contact with potential burn hazards (e.g., gasoline, matches, bonfires or barbecues, lighter fluid, firecrackers, cigarette lighters, cooking utensils, chemistry sets). Instruct child to avoid climbing or flying kite around high-tension wires. Instruct child in proper behavior in the event of fire (e.g., fire drills at home and school). Teach child safe cooking (e.g., use low heat; avoid any frying; be careful of steam burns, scalds, or exploding foods, especially from microwaving).
Poisoning	
Adheres to group rules May be easily influenced by peers Has strong allegiance to friends	Educate child regarding hazards of taking nonprescription drugs and chemicals, including aspirin and alcohol. Teach child to say "no" if offered illegal or dangerous drugs or alcohol. Keep potentially dangerous products in properly labeled receptacles, preferably out of reach.
Bodily Damage	
Has increased physical skills Needs strenuous physical activity Is interested in acquiring new skills and perfecting attained skills Is daring and adventurous, especially with peers May play in hazardous places Confidence often exceeds physical capacity Desires group loyalty and has strong need for friends' approval Attempts hazardous feats Accompanies friends to potentially hazardous facilities Delights in physical activity Is likely to overdo Growth in height exceeds muscular growth and coordination	Help provide facilities for supervised activities. Encourage playing in safe places. Keep firearms safely locked up except with adult supervision. Teach proper care of, use of, and respect for potentially dangerous devices (e.g., power tools, firecrackers). Teach children not to tease or surprise dogs, invade their territory, take dogs' toys, or interfere with dogs' feeding. Stress use of eye, ear, or mouth protection when using potentially hazardous objects or devices or when engaged in potentially hazardous sports. Do not permit use of trampolines except as part of supervised training. Teach safety regarding use of corrective devices (glasses); if child wears contact lenses, monitor duration of wear to prevent corneal damage. Stress careful selection, use, and maintenance of sports and recreation equipment, such as skateboards and in-line skates (see Family-Centered Care box, Skateboard, Skates, and Scooter Safety). Emphasize proper conditioning, safe practices, and use of safety equipment for sports or recreational activities. Caution against engaging in hazardous sports, such as those involving trampolines. Use safety glass and decals on large glassed areas, such as sliding glass doors. Use window guards to prevent falls. Teach name, address, and phone number and emphasize that child should ask for help from appropriate people (e.g., cashier, security guard, police) if lost; have identification on child (e.g., sewn in clothes, inside shoe). Teach safety and stranger awareness: • Avoid personalized clothing in public places. • Never go with a stranger. • Have child tell parents if anyone makes child feel uncomfortable in any way. • Teach child to say "no" when confronted with uncomfortable situations. • Always listen to child's concerns regarding others' behavior.

prove themselves worthy of acceptance and improve their status in the peer group. Peer pressure is a normal part of psychologic development, but it is also a major contributor to risk-taking behaviors. Peer challenges often encourage problem behaviors that place children at risk for injury or hazardous habits. School-age children are in the process of moving from preoperational to concrete operational thinking and are only beginning to understand causal relationships. Therefore they may attempt certain activities without planning or evaluating the consequences.

Children who are risk takers may have inadequate self-regulatory behavior. These children need to learn the motivation or the incentives for such behavior and to visualize the possible consequences if the risk-taking behavior ends in a tragic outcome.

Motor Vehicle Injury

As in all other age-groups, the most common cause of severe accidental injury and death in school-age children is involvement in motor vehicle accidents—either as a pedestrian or as a passenger. In 2014 approximately 19% of traffic-related fatalities involved pedestrians under the age of 14 years (National Highway Traffic Safety Administration, 2016a). Most of the injuries occur when children misinterpret traffic signs or disobey common traffic safety regulations, cross the street against a red light, cross at places other than designated crosswalks, dart into the street, or walk in the same direction as the traffic. Parents consistently overestimate the street-crossing skills of young children ages 5 to 6 years and need education about their children's developmental abilities and competence as pedestrians. Nurses can help parents develop more realistic expectations of their children's behavior and teach them to model safe street-crossing behaviors through pedestrian skills training programs.

Use of restraint systems, door-lock mechanisms, and appropriate passenger seating and behavior are simple but effective measures for eliminating noncrash injuries and reducing the severity of crash injuries. The correct use of seat restraints is essential.

In 2014, 602 children ages 0 to 12 years died in motor vehicle accidents, and 121,350 received injuries (Centers for Disease Control and Prevention, 2016a). Investigations of motor vehicle accidents showed that 34% of those who died were not using a seat belt (Centers for Disease Control and Prevention, 2016a). When in the car, school-age children should always be buckled properly in a weight-, height-, and age-appropriate seat. Booster seats should be used until the child is 57 inches tall (Centers for Disease Control and Prevention, 2016b). The rear vehicle seat is the safest place for children younger than 13 years old (Centers for Disease Control and Prevention, 2016b).

Injuries to children ages 5 to 9 years restrained in adult-type seat belts are related to anatomic differences between adults and children. The child's sitting height is less than the adult's, and the child's center of gravity is located above the level of the lap belt. Consequently, the greater proportion of body mass above the belt may cause more forward motion and jackknifing over the belt, which increases the risk of head injury from impact with interior vehicle parts. The child's smaller and less developed iliac crests are not suited to serve as an anchor for belts designed to restrain adults, and their intraabdominal organs are less protected by the bony pelvis. The natural behavior of children, such as readjusting the seating position, moving about, and otherwise altering the fit of the restraint, also influences its effectiveness.

When children use adult-type seat belts, parents should make certain that the restraints are fitted to their children and fastened correctly. To reduce their risk of sliding beneath the standard seat belt during a collision, children should sit up straight and well back in the seat, and the seat should be moved forward until the feet fit firmly against the toe board. Caution children against assuming alternate seating positions, such as tailor fashion, while riding in the car. (See Chapter 12 for a comprehensive discussion of car restraints.)

Each year 23 million children are transported to and from school on school buses. The majority of school travel–related injuries and deaths occur from passenger vehicles, whereas only an average of 11 school-age children die in school bus–related crashes annually (National Highway Traffic Safety Administration, 2016b). However, the National Highway Traffic Safety Administration and the American Academy of Pediatrics have developed minimum standards to enhance school bus safety. These standards state that all children should travel to and from school in an age-appropriate, properly secured child-restraint system; all school buses should be equipped with lap and lap-shoulder restraint systems that can accommodate safety seats, booster seats, and harness systems; and school districts should encourage appropriate education on safety devices (National Highway Traffic Safety Administration, 2016b).

All-terrain vehicles (ATVs), designed for off-road use by children and adolescents, are popular with children under 16 years of age but are responsible for a significant number of childhood injuries. These vehicles have a short wheelbase and low profile, which make them relatively unstable and unable to be seen easily. The vehicles can also achieve substantial speed. Most injuries occur when the driver loses control of the vehicle, is thrown from the vehicle, or collides with fixed objects or other vehicles. Immature judgment and poorly developed motor skills also contribute to injury. The American Academy of Pediatrics views ATVs as a major hazard to the health of children and recommends that children younger than 16 years of age should not ride in or operate ATVs (Denning, Harland, & Jennissen, 2014).

Bicycle Injury

The majority of school-age children have bicycles and love riding them, but this increases their risk of injury on streets and byways. In 2014 bicycle injuries in children age 14 years and younger accounted for approximately 6000 nonfatal injuries and 50 fatal injuries (National Highway Traffic Safety Administration, 2016a).

Many injuries are related to violations of traffic laws by the bicyclist, including wrong-way riding (facing traffic), failure to yield the right of way, and turning violations. Others are related to road conditions described as hazardous: bumps, potholes, and gravel. Bicycle-related injuries occur in young children playing in their own neighborhoods and in older children using their bicycles for transportation on streets with heavy traffic.

In addition to major injuries, cuts and bruises from falls and collisions account for a large number of injuries. Other injuries include trauma to internal organs. These injuries initially seem trivial, but injured children can develop serious symptoms (e.g., pain, vomiting, or collapse) hours later.

Many of the injuries to school-age children on bicycles occur because of children's developmentally limited range of vision and their inability to process perceptions of road situations sufficiently well and quickly enough to ride safely in traffic. Other important factors are lack of instruction in use of the equipment, lack of safety equipment, and unfamiliarity with the bicycle (e.g., having ridden the bicycle for less than a month).

To prevent bicycle injuries, both parents and children should learn and periodically review bicycle safety. Children need bicycles that are suited to their size and age; they should be able to stand with the balls of both feet on the ground when seated on the bicycle, be able to place both feet flat on the ground when straddling the center bar, and be able to grasp the brake lever comfortably and easily enough to apply sufficient pressure to brake the bicycle. Discourage parents from buying their child a bicycle that the child can "grow into."

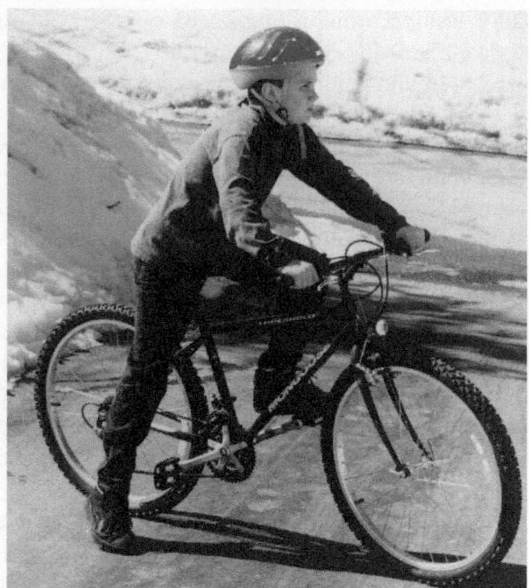

FIG. 15.16 The right-size bike is important; the child should be able to sit on the bike and place the balls of both feet on the ground. The foot should comfortably reach and manipulate the pedal in the down position. Wearing a protective helmet is mandatory for safe cycling. The helmet should sit on top of the head in a level position and should not rock back and forth or from side to side. The strap should always be fastened securely under the chin.

Because head injury is the major cause of bicycle-related fatalities, the single most important aspect of bicycle safety is to encourage the rider to wear a protective helmet (Fig. 15.16). Helmet use has caused a 51% reduction in head injury, 69% reduction in serious head injury, 33% reduction in facial injury, and 65% reduction in fatal head injury (Olivier & Creighton, 2016). Hard-shelled helmets lined with expanded polystyrene (Styrofoam) provide the best head protection. The helmet should be one that can be adjusted to the individual child's head, fits securely, and does not limit the child's vision or hearing. A brightly colored helmet improves visibility. The helmet should carry a seal indicating that it is approved by the US Consumer Product Safety Commission. All helmets should be replaced after any damage or crash.

Legislative interventions in the United States significantly increase children's usage of bicycle helmets, with 51% of children always wearing a helmet in states that have helmet laws and only 40% of children always wearing a helmet in states that do not have helmet laws (Jewett, Beck, Taylor, et al., 2016). Although most young riders acknowledge that wearing a helmet is important for safety, reasons for not wearing them include discomfort (especially heat), presumed lack of importance for casual riding, lack of style, and peer pressure.

Parental attitudes and behaviors also influence children's use of bicycle helmets. Ninety percent of children reported they were likely to wear a helmet if their parent used a helmet, compared with only 38% of children reporting a likelihood to wear a helmet if their parent did not use a helmet (Jewett, Beck, Taylor, et al., 2016). Parents, as well as children, need to be educated on safety. The American Academy of Pediatrics recommends that (1) parents be informed of the dangers of riding without a helmet, (2) only helmets that meet the standards of the Consumer Product Safety Commission (CPSC) be purchased, (3) state and local governments continue to enact legislation requiring helmet use by all bicyclists, (4) parents and community-based programs promote bicycle safety and helmet use, and (5) the media depict helmet use in all programs and promotional materials.

Schools, hospital emergency departments, and communities have developed numerous bicycle helmet promotion programs. Programs that are most successful are those that address the cost of helmets and peer pressure and combine multimedia public education announcements with the support of community organizations. The Family-Centered Care box lists guidelines for bicycle safety, and the Critical Thinking Case Study box discusses bicycle helmets.

FAMILY-CENTERED CARE

Bicycle Safety

- Always wear a properly fitted helmet that is approved by the US Consumer Product Safety Commission; replace a damaged helmet.
- Ride bicycles with traffic and away from parked cars.
- Ride single file.
- Walk bicycles through busy intersections and at crosswalks.
- Give hand signals well in advance of turning or stopping.
- Keep as close to the curb as practical.
- Watch for drain grates, potholes, soft shoulders, and loose dirt or gravel.
- Keep both hands on handlebars except when signaling.
- Never ride double on a bicycle.
- Do not carry packages that interfere with vision or control; do not drag objects behind bike.
- Watch for and yield to pedestrians.
- Watch for cars backing up or pulling out of driveways; be especially careful at intersections.
- Look left, right, then left before turning into traffic or roadway.
- Never hitch a ride on a truck or other vehicle.
- Learn rules of the road and respect for traffic officers.
- Obey all local ordinances.
- Wear shoes that fit securely while riding.
- Wear light colors at night, and attach fluorescent material to clothing and bicycle.
- Be certain the bicycle is the correct size.
- Equip the bicycle with proper lights and reflectors.
- Have the bicycle inspected to ensure good mechanical condition.
- When riding as a passenger, wear appropriate-size helmet and sit in a specially designed protective seat.

Modified from American Academy of Pediatrics, Committee on Injury and Poison Prevention. (2001). Bicycle helmets. *Pediatrics, 108*(4), 1030-1032.

CRITICAL THINKING CASE STUDY

Bicycle Helmets

During the past month in your school district, one child died and another sustained a serious head injury from bicycle-vehicle collisions. Neither child wore a bicycle helmet. As a school nurse, you are considering effective approaches to increase the students' use of bicycle helmets.

1. Evidence—Is there sufficient evidence to draw any conclusions?
2. Assumptions—Describe the underlying assumption about each of the following:
   a. Potential hazards to children associated with bicycling
   b. Intrinsic and extrinsic risk factors for bicycle injuries
   c. Factors associated with deciding whether to wear a bicycle helmet
   d. Strategies for pediatricians and nurses to help decrease bicycle-related injuries
3. What implications for nursing care can be drawn from this situation?
4. Does the evidence support your conclusion?

Answers are available at http://evolve.elsevier.com/wong/ncic.

Other Vehicle-Related Injuries

Ride-on toys allow a child to move forward either by his or her own power or through the use of a motor. These toys are very popular among children and can assist in the development of balance, coordination, and physical fitness; however, the toys can be dangerous. Among all toy-related injuries from 1990 to 2011, ride-on toys accounted for 35% of the injuries and 43% of hospital admissions in children less than 18 years of age (Abraham, Gaw, Chounthirath, et al., 2015). Ride-on toys were three times more likely to cause a fracture or dislocation compared with other toys (Abraham, Gaw, Chounthirath, et al., 2015). Although the majority of injuries involve the upper extremities, severe injuries of the head and neck can occur. School-age children often use ride-on toys on streets and highways, which increases the likelihood of collisions with objects or vehicles. Parents should carefully evaluate the skill level of the child before allowing the child to use any ride-on toy. Recommendations for wheeled toys are in the Family-Centered Care boxes.

FAMILY-CENTERED CARE

Ride-On Toys

- Children under 1 year old cannot use any ride-on toys because of their inability to balance themselves.
- Children 1 to 2 years old can use ride-on toys that are propelled by their feet only after they learn to walk.
- Children 2 to 3 years old are beginning to learn to pedal and to coordinate with a steering wheel but lack control to avoid hazards.
- Children 4 to 5 years old are interested in battery-operative vehicles but are at high risk of falling or colliding with objects and must have adult supervision.
- Children 6 to 8 years old have developed coordination for steering and can operate slow-moving vehicles; they are very interested in scooters and skateboards.
- Children 9 to 12 years old are usually capable of operating a motorized vehicle that does not exceed 10 miles per hour, scooters, and skateboards but may engage in high-risk behaviors such as stunt riding.

Modified from US Consumer Product Safety Commission. (2016). *CPSC guidelines for age-related activities.* Retrieved from http://www.helmets.org/ageguide.htm

FAMILY-CENTERED CARE

Skateboard, Skates, and Scooter Safety

- Children younger than 5 years should not ride skateboards because they are not developmentally prepared to protect themselves from injury. Children ages 6 to 10 years should use skateboards only with close adult supervision.
- The age when children are ready to use skates safely is not known because of differences in the ability to acquire the skills needed to participate in the sport. Novice skaters should learn indoors on a flat, smooth surface.
- Children who use skateboards, skates, and scooters should wear helmets and other protective padding, especially on wrists, knees, and elbows, to prevent injury.
- Skateboards, skates, and scooters should never be ridden near traffic. Their use should be prohibited on streets and highways. Activities that bring these items and cars together (e.g., "catching a ride") are especially dangerous.
- Some types of use, such as riding homemade ramps on hard surfaces, may be particularly hazardous.

Modified from American Academy of Pediatrics, Committee on Injury and Poison Prevention. (2009). In-line skating injuries in children and adolescents. *Pediatrics, 123,* 1421-2422.

Ride-on mower and other power mower injuries also occur among school-age children. Approximately 12,000 children under age 18 years experienced lawn mower–related injuries in the United States in 2015 (American Academy of Orthopaedic Surgeons, 2016). These injuries occur when children are allowed to operate a mower, when they are run over or backed over by another driver, or when they fall from a mower or from a trailer pulled by a mower. Although there are no age-specific criteria for the use of lawn mowers, children should not operate lawn mowers until they have appropriate levels of judgment, strength, coordination, and maturity, which is usually over age 12 years for walk-behind mowers and over age 16 years for riding mowers (American Academy of Orthopaedic Surgeons, 2016).

Similar injuries occur with snowmobiles. Most deaths and injuries involving snowmobiles occur when the vehicle collides with a stationary object or when riders fall or are ejected from the vehicle. Because children lack the strength and skill that is necessary to safely operate or travel on a snowmobile, the American Academy of Pediatrics (2016) recommends that persons under 16 years of age be prohibited from operating snowmobiles and children under 6 years of age should never ride on snowmobiles.

Injuries at School

The risk of injury at school is relatively low, despite the amount of time children spend in that environment. Some injuries occur in gyms, shops, and laboratories, as well as on playgrounds and playing fields. Most injuries occur on the way to and from school. Many are related to sports activities (see Chapter 33). Persons concerned with child safety should be alert to hazards in the school environment and should become involved in efforts to make the environment safe in every aspect—physical facilities, equipment, training practices, and supervision.

Trampolines and indoor trampoline parks are popular with young children and can cause significant injuries, including fractures, sprains, and head injuries. Trampoline injuries result in approximately 100,000 visits to the emergency department every year (Kasmire, Rogers, & Sturm, 2016). The most common mechanisms of injury occur during landing (33%), collision with another jumper (8%), performing flips (8%), or coming in contact with the trampoline structure (7%) (Kasmire, Rogers, & Sturm, 2016). Warnings with trampoline equipment should include avoiding flips, restricting multiple jumpers, and improving padding around the structure (Kasmire, Rogers, & Sturm, 2016).

Other Injuries

Falls are still a source of injury in school age children but less so than in preschool children and toddlers. "Flipping," a popular activity in which children jump from an elevated surface and perform an aerial flip with the idea of landing upright, has resulted in serious injuries to the face and head and places children at risk for back and spinal cord injury. Seasonal injuries such as sledding accidents are common and more likely to occur when children ride sleds without adult supervision and in streets, as opposed to parks. Horseback riding injuries are another source of concern for parents of school-age children. The most common cause of death from horseback riding activities is head injury, followed by injuries to the chest and abdomen. Before enrolling children for riding lessons, parents should determine the instructor's safety record with students, verify that safety helmets will be used, and confirm that the instructor is certified by a recognized organization. Injuries at public playgrounds and amusement parks (especially water slides) and around the home (e.g., power tools, ladders, fireworks) are ongoing concerns of parents and health care providers.

Injuries to eyes and teeth are a constant threat to school-age children involved in rough play. (See Chapter 20 [eyes] and Chapter 16 [teeth].) The normally shallow bony orbit of children in this age-group makes them particularly vulnerable to eye trauma, especially during contact sports or activities such as basketball, baseball, or softball. Wearing protective eye and mouth gear is essential (Pollard, Xiang, & Smith, 2012).

Injuries have been reported from a variety of toys (e.g., slingshots, water balloons, lawn darts, chemistry sets) and household equipment (e.g., mowers, lawn trimmers). Gunshot wounds have become a significant problem during past years. The overall rate of firearm-related homicides in the United States is nearly seven times greater than rates found in other high-income countries (Grinshteyn & Hemenway, 2016). So-called toy firearms (air guns and air rifles) also cause frequent firearm injuries to children. Most of these injuries involve the face or eyes.

Nurse's Role in Injury Prevention

Nurses are primary advocates for preventive care and guidance. Safety education and anticipatory guidance for both parents and school-age children can be incorporated in all nursing interventions. The most effective means of prevention is education of the child and family regarding the hazards of risk-taking behavior and improper use of equipment. No piece of equipment is safe unless a child is physically and mentally equipped to use it. A careful history and knowledge of normal growth and development serve as guidelines for both planned and impromptu education.

Parents are often unaware of hazards to their children at various ages, especially those related to normal developmental progress. Susceptibility to injuries and understanding of safety issues are influenced by children's developmental level. Nurses who understand the growth and development of school-age children can provide effective safety education to parents and children and can correct misconceptions before injuries occur.

School nurses should be alert to hazards in the school and instrumental in evaluating safety risks and implementing safety programs. Characteristics of the school-age child and preventive measures are outlined in Table 15.2.

ANTICIPATORY GUIDANCE—CARE OF FAMILIES

The parents of the school-age child find themselves in the position of sharing their child's time and interests with the increasingly important peer group. As a child feels the need to fit into a peer group and gain a sense of industry through individual and cooperative production and performance, he or she moves away from the close, familiar relationships of the family group. It is through these early peer relationships that children prepare for moving from narrow, sheltered family relationships to a broader world of relationships and increased independence. Parents must learn to provide support as unobtrusively as possible without feeling rejected, hurt, or angry. The nurse can help parents of the school-age child by providing anticipatory guidance and reassurance throughout this period of child development and maturation (see Family-Centered Care box).

FAMILY-CENTERED CARE

Guidance During School Years

Age 6 Years

Prepare parents to expect strong food preferences and frequent refusal of specific food items.
Prepare parents to expect increasingly ravenous appetite.
Prepare parents for emotional reactions as child experiences erratic mood changes.
Help parents anticipate continued susceptibility to illness.
Teach injury prevention and safety, especially bicycle safety.
Encourage parents to respect child's need for privacy and to provide a separate bedroom for child, if possible.
Prepare parents for child's increasing interests outside the home.
Help parents understand the need to encourage child's interactions with peers.

Ages 7 to 10 Years

Prepare parents to expect improvement in health with fewer illnesses, but warn them that allergies may increase or become apparent.
Prepare parents to expect an increase in minor injuries.
Emphasize caution in selecting and maintaining sports equipment and reemphasize safety.
Prepare parents to expect increased involvement with peers and interest in activities outside the home.
Emphasize the need to encourage independence while maintaining limit setting and discipline.
Prepare parents to expect more demands at 8 years.
Prepare fathers to expect increasing admiration at 10 years; encourage father-child activities.
Prepare parents for prepubescent changes in girls.

Ages 11 to 12 Years

Help parents prepare child for body changes of pubescence.
Prepare parents to expect a growth spurt in girls.
Make certain child's sex education is adequate with accurate information.
Prepare parents to expect energetic but stormy behavior at 11 years, with child becoming more even tempered at 12 years.
Encourage parents to support child's desire to "grow up" but to allow regressive behavior when needed.
Prepare parents to expect an increase in masturbation.
Instruct parents that the child may need more rest.
Help parents educate child regarding experimentation with potentially harmful activities.

Health Guidance

Help parents understand the importance of regular health and dental care for child.
Encourage parents to teach and model sound health practices, including diet, rest, activity, and exercise.
Stress the need to encourage children to engage in appropriate physical activities.
Emphasize providing a safe physical and emotional environment.
Encourage parents to teach and model safety practices.

NCLEX REVIEW QUESTIONS

1. A hallmark of cognitive development in the school-age child is in what Piaget describes as concrete operations. In this stage the child:
   A. Uses thought processes to experience events and actions
   B. Is unable to see things from another's point of view
   C. Has a limited perspective of how others' interpretations of a given event differ
   D. Makes judgments based on what he or she sees
2. In terms of social development, the school-age child does which of the following? Select all that apply.
   A. Begins to explore the environment beyond the family
   B. Has an increased interest in persons of the opposite sex (gender)
   C. May actively participate in same-sex groups or clubs
   D. Strives to be different from those in the peer group
   E. Begins to form strong relationships with persons of the same sex (gender)
3. Characteristics of bullying include:
   A. Unintentional harm inflicted on another person that is part of the socialization process in childhood
   B. The infliction of repetitive physical, verbal, or emotional abuse on another person with intent to harm
   C. An attempt to gain acceptance and be liked by same-sex peers
   D. An early sign of a severely disturbed personality disorder that escalates in adulthood
4. A school nurse in middle school (grades 6, 7, and 8) is preparing an outline for a sex education class. Which of these statements represent important concepts to be covered in discussing this topic with this age-group? Select all that apply.
   A. Consider separating the boys and girls into same-sex groups with a leader of the same sex.
   B. Answer questions matter-of-factly and honestly and appropriate to the children's level of understanding.
   C. Use vernacular or slang terms to describe human physiologic functions.
   D. Avoid discussing sexually transmitted diseases in this age-group.
   E. Discuss common myths and misconceptions associated with sex and the reproductive process.
   F. Avoid controversial topics such as birth control.
5. School-age children are prone to accidental injury primarily because of:
   A. Peer pressure and risk-taking behaviors
   B. Physical awkwardness and clumsiness
   C. Parents' lack of supervision
   D. Attempts to impress members of the opposite sex

Correct Answers

1. A; 2. A, C, E; 3. B; 4. A, B, E; 5. A

REFERENCES

Abraham, V. M., Gaw, C. E., Chounthirath, T., et al. (2015). Toy-related injuries among children treated in US emergency departments 1990-2011. *Clinical Pediatrics*, *54*, 127–137.

Allen, S. L., Howlett, M. D., Coulombe, J. A., et al. (2016). ABCs of SLEEPING: A review of the evidence behind pediatric sleep practice recommendations. *Sleep Medicine Reviews*, *29*, 1–14.

American Academy of Orthopaedic Surgeons. (2016). *Lawn mower injuries in children*. Available at http://orthoinfo.aaos.org/topic.cfm?topic=A00611.

American Academy of Pediatrics. (2016).*Winter safety tips*. Available at https://www.aap.org/en-us/about-the-aap/aap-press-room/news-features-and-safety-tips/Pages/Winter-Safety-Tips.aspx.

American Academy of Pediatrics, Council on Communications and Media. (2016). Virtual violence. *Pediatrics*, *138*, 1–7.

American Academy of Pediatrics, Council on School Health. (2008). Medical emergencies occurring at school. *Pediatrics*, *122*(4), 887–894.

American Academy of Pediatrics, Council on School Health. (2016). Role of the school nurse in providing school health services. *Pediatrics*, *137*, 1–8.

Black, K. (2012). The relationship between companion animals and loneliness among rural adolescents. *Journal of Pediatric Nursing*, *27*(2), 103–112.

Breuner, C. C., Mattson, G., Committee on Adolescence, et al. (2016). Sexuality education for children and adolescents. *Pediatrics*, *138*, e1–e13.

Brockmyer, J. F. (2015). Playing violent video games and desensitization to violence. *Child Adolescent Psychiatric Clinics of North Ammerica*, *24*, 65–77.

Carter, K. A., Hathaway, N. E., & Lettieri, C. F. (2014). Common sleep disorders in children. *American Family Physician*, *89*, 368–377.

Centers for Disease Control and Prevention. (2015). *Whole School, Whole Community, Whole Child*. Available at www.cdc.gov/healthyschools/wscc/index.htm.

Centers for Disease Control and Prevention. (2016a). *Child passenger safety: Get the facts*. Available at www.cdc.gov/MotorVehicleSafety/Child_Passenger_Safety/cps-factsheet.html.

Centers for Disease Control and Prevention.(2016b). *Use the correct car seat*. Available at https://www.cdc.gov/features/passengersafety/ingofraphic.html.

Denning, G. M., Harland, K. K., & Jennissen, C. A. (2014). Age-based risk factors for pediatric ATV-related fatalities. *Pediatrics*, *134*, 1094–1102.

Eime, R. M., Young, J. A., Harvey, J. T., et al. (2013). A systematic review of the psychological and social benefits of participation in sport for children and adolescents: Informing development of a conceptual model of health through sport. *The International Journal of Behavioral Nutrition and Physical Activity*, *10*, 98.

Ergler, C. R., Kearns, R. A., & Witten, K. (2013). Seasonal and locational variations in children's play: Implications for wellbeing. *Social Science and Medicine*, *91*, 178–185.

Erikson, E. H. (1963). *Childhood and society* (2nd ed.). New York: Norton.

Flannery, D. J., Todres, J., Bradshaw, C. P., et al. (2016). Bullying prevention: A summary of the report of the national academies of sciences, engineering, and medicine. *Prevention Science*, *17*, 1044–1053.

Franceschini, S., Gori, S., Ruffino, M., et al. (2013). Action video games make dyslexic children read better. *Current Biology*, *23*, 462–466.

Gadomski, A. M., Scribani, M. B., Krupa, N., et al. (2015). Pet dogs and children's health: Opportunities for chronic disease prevention? *Preventing Chronic Disease*, *12*, E205.

Gao, Z., Chen, S., & Stodden, D. F. (2015). A comparison of children's physical activity levels in physical education, recess, and exergaming. *Journal of Physical Activity and Health*, *12*, 349–354.

Grinshteyn, E., & Hemenway, D. (2016). Violent death rates: The US compared with other high-income OECD countries, 2010. *The American Journal of Medicine*, *129*, 266–273.

Hamm, M. P., Newton, A. S., Chisholm, A., et al. (2015). Prevalence and effect of cyberbullying on children and young people, a scoping review of social media studies. *JAMA Pediatrics*, *169*, 770–777.

Horner, S. D., Rew, L., & Brown, A. (2012). Risk-taking behaviors engaged in by early adolescents while on school property. *Issues in Comprehensive Pediatric Nursing*, *35*, 90–110.

Hornor, G., Bretl, D., Chapman, E., et al. (2015). Corporal punishment: Evaluation of an intervention by PNPs. *Journal of Pediatric Health Care*, *29*, 526–535.

Hunt, T., Slack, K. S., & Berger, L. M. (2016). Adverse childhood experiences and behavioral problems in middle childhood. *Child Abuse & Neglect*, epub ahead of print.

Hyde, A., Drennan, J., Butler, M., et al. (2013). Parents' constructions of communication with their children about safer sex. *Journal of Clinical Nursing*, *22*(23–24), 3438–3446.

Jaffe, P. G., Campbell, M., Hamilton, L., et al. (2012). Children in danger of domestic homicide. *Child Abuse and Neglect*, *36*, 71–74.

Jewett, A., Beck, L. F., Taylor, C., et al. (2016). Bicycle helmet use among persons 5 years and older in the United States, 2012. *Journal of Safety Research*, *59*, 1–7.

Kann, L., McManus, T., Harris, W. A., et al. (2016). Youth risk behavior surveillance—United States, 2015. *MMWR. Surveillance Summaries*, *65*, 1–177.

Kasmire, K. E., Rogers, S. C., & Sturm, J. J. (2016). Trampoline park and home trampoline injuries. *Pediatrics*, *138*, 1–10.

Keast, D. R., Fulgoni, V. L., Nicklas, T. A., et al. (2013). Food sources of energy and nutrients among children in the United States: National health and nutrition examination survey 2003-2006. *Nutrients*, *5*, 283–301.

Koepp, M. J., Caciagli, L., Pressler, R. M., et al. (2016). Reflex seizures, traits, and epilepsies: From physiology to pathology. *The Lancet. Neurology*, *15*, 92–105.

Leiner, M., Peinado, J., Villanos, M. T. M., et al. (2016). Mental and emotional health of children exposed to news media of threats and acts of terrorism: The cumulative and pervasive effects. *Frontiers in Pediatrics*, *4*, 1–4.

Levendosky, A. A., Bogat, G. A., & Martinez-Torteya, C. (2013). PTSD symptoms in young children exposed to intimate partner violence. *Violence Against Women*, *19*, 187–201.

Moyer, V. A. (2014). Prevention of dental caries in children from birth through age 5 years: US preventive services task force recommendation statement. *Pediatrics*, *133*, 1102–1111.

Muris, P., Ollendick, T. H., Roelofs, J., et al. (2014). The short form of the fear survey schedule for children-revised (PSSC-R-SF): An efficient, reliable, and valid scale for measuring fear in children and adolescents. *Journal of Anxiety Disorders*, *28*, 957–965.

National Highway Traffic Safety Administration. (2016a). *Traffic safety facts, 2014 data* (DOT HS 812 270), Washington DC, U.S. Department of Transportation.

National Highway Traffic Safety Administration. (2016b). *School-transportation-related crashes* (DOT HS 812 272), Washington, DC, U.S. Department of Transportation.

Ogden, C. L., Carroll, M. D., Lawman, H. G., et al. (2016). Trends in obesity prevalence among children and adolescents in the United States, 1988-1994 through 2013-2014. *JAMA: The Journal of the American Medical Association*, *315*, 2292–2299.

Olivier, J., & Creighton, P. (2016). Bicycle injuries and helmet use: A systematic review and meta-analysis. *International Journal of Epidemiology*, *1-7*, 2016.

Pollard, K. A., Xiang, H., & Smith, G. A. (2012). Pediatric eye injuries treated in US emergency departments, 1990-2009. *Clinical Pediatrics*, *51*(4), 374–381.

Pyrooz, D. C., & Sweeten, G. (2015). Gang membership between ages 5 and 17 years in the United States. *The Journal of Adolescent Health*, *56*, 414–419.

Rajalaksmhi, J., & Thanasekaran, P. (2015). The effects and behaviours of home alone situation by latchkey children. *The American Journal of Nursing Science*, *4*(4), 207–211.

Rettew, D. C., & Pawlowski, S. (2016). Bullying. *Child Adolescent Psychiatric Clinics of North America*, *25*, 235–242.

Rideout, V. J..(2016). *The common sense census: Media use by tweens and teens.* Common Sense Media. Available at https://www.commonsensemedia.org/sites/default/files/uploads/research/census_executivesummary.pdf.

Rose, K. C., Disney, J., Andresen, K., et al. (2016). Unlicensed assistive personnel, their role on the school health service team: Position statement. *NASN School Nurse*, *2016*, 299–301.

Shetgiri, R. (2013). Bullying and victimization among children. *Advances in Pediatrics*, *60*(1), 33–51.

Simon, P., & Olson, S. (2014). *Building capacity to reduce bullying, workshop summary*. Washington, DC: The National Academies Press.

Skinner, E. A., Pitzer, J. R., & Steele, J. S. (2016). Can student engagement serve as a motivational resource for academic coping, persistence, and learning during late elementary and early middle school? *Developmental Psychology*, *52*, 2099–2117.

Spilt, J. L., Leflot, G., Onghena, P., et al. (2016). Use of praise and reprimands as critical ingredients of teacher behavior management: Effects on children's development in the context of a teacher-mediated classroom intervention. *Prevention Science*, *17*, 732–742.

Sticca, F., & Perren, S. (2013). Is cyberbullying worse than traditional bullying? Examining the differential roles of medium, publicity, and anonymity for the perceived severity of bullying. *Journal of Youth and Adolescence*, *42*, 739–750.

US Department of Agriculture.(2016). *Dietary Guidelines 2015-2020.* Available at https://health.gov/dietaryguidelines/2015/guidelines/executive-summary/.

Westgarth, C., Boddy, L. M., Stratton, G., et al. (2016). The association between dog ownership or dog walking and fitness or weight status in childhood. *Pediatric Obesity*, epub ahead of print.

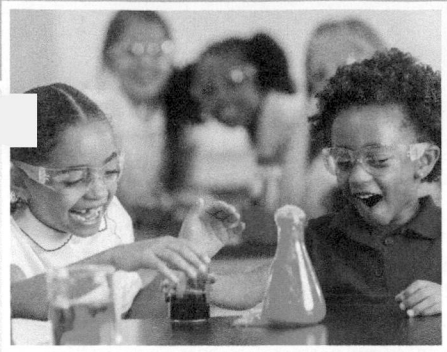

16

Health Problems of the School-Age Child

Katherine Soss Prihoda and Cheryl C. Rodgers

http://evolve.elsevier.com/wong/ncic

CONCEPTS

- Nutrition
- Elimination
- Cognition
- Mood and Affect
- Stress
- Anxiety
- Psychosis

The vast majority (more than 80%) of school-age children in the United States are considered to be in very good or excellent health. The most common acute health concerns of children ages 5 to 11 years are obesity, enuresis, attention-deficit/hyperactivity disorder, and learning disorders. This chapter discusses common health problems experienced by school-age children.

OBESITY: COMPLICATIONS, TREATMENT, AND PREVENTION

OBESITY

Few problems in childhood and adolescence are so obvious to others, are so difficult to treat, and have such long-term effects on health as obesity. **Overweight** refers to the state of weighing more than average for height and body build. **Obesity** is defined as an increase in body weight resulting from an excessive accumulation of body fat relative to lean body mass. The **body mass index (BMI)** measurement is recommended as the most accurate method for screening children and adolescents for obesity (Gahagan, 2016). Overweight status is described as an age- and gender-specific BMI between the 85th and 94th percentiles based on the Centers for Disease Control and Prevention Growth Charts for the United States. Obesity is classified as an age- and gender-specific BMI at or above the 95th percentile for children of the same age and sex. Pediatric growth charts for age and gender are available from the Centers for Disease Control and Prevention (http://www.cdc.gov/growthcharts). BMI measurements are strongly associated with subcutaneous and total body fat and also with skinfold thickness measurements. However, a subset of adolescents (e.g., athletes) may have a high BMI because of increased muscle mass rather than fat mass. Clinical judgment is needed to understand if the youth is at risk for overweight or obesity.

The number of overweight and obese children in the United States is significant. Approximately one in three children and adolescents (32%) in the United States are overweight or obese (Gahagan, 2016). Numerous studies referred to as the National Health and Nutrition Examination Surveys (NHANES) dating back to the early 1960s have documented childhood overweight through comprehensive evaluations of dietary intake, physical activity, and anthropometric measures. The NHANES studies are sponsored by the Centers for Disease Control and Prevention and provide valuable data on trends in overweight and obesity. Over the past 10 years, obesity rates have reached a plateau among children and adolescents; however, extreme obesity has increased (Ogden, Carroll, Lawman, et al., 2016). The prevalence of obesity is disproportionately high among non-Hispanic black and Hispanic youth (19.5% and 21.9%, respectively) compared with non-Hispanic white children and adolescents (14.7%) (Ogden, Carroll, Lawman, et al., 2016). Parent education also has a significant influence on the prevalence of obesity among youth. A recent survey found that 21% of youth were obese in households headed by individuals with less than a high school degree and a 22% prevalence in which the household head had a high school degree compared with 14% in households headed by someone with greater than a high school degree (Ogden, Carroll, Lawman, et al., 2016). Furthermore, parental obesity increases the risk of overweight by twofold to threefold (Altman & Wilfley, 2015).

In the United States it is estimated that childhood obesity costs $14 billion in direct medical care costs alone (Finkelstein, Graham, & Malhotra, 2014). The direct health costs of childhood overweight can only be estimated; however, obese children are more likely to become obese adults and experience health and social consequences of obesity much earlier than children and adolescents of normal weight (Olson, Aldrich, Callahan, et al., 2015). Because of the health-related problems related to obesity, reports indicate that for the first time in US history, the current generation of children will have a shorter life expectancy than their parents (American Heart Association, 2017).

Obesity contributes to some of the most prevalent, costly, debilitating, and potentially fatal conditions in the United States. Obesity in childhood and adolescence has been related to elevated blood cholesterol, high blood pressure, respiratory disorders, orthopedic conditions, cholelithiasis,

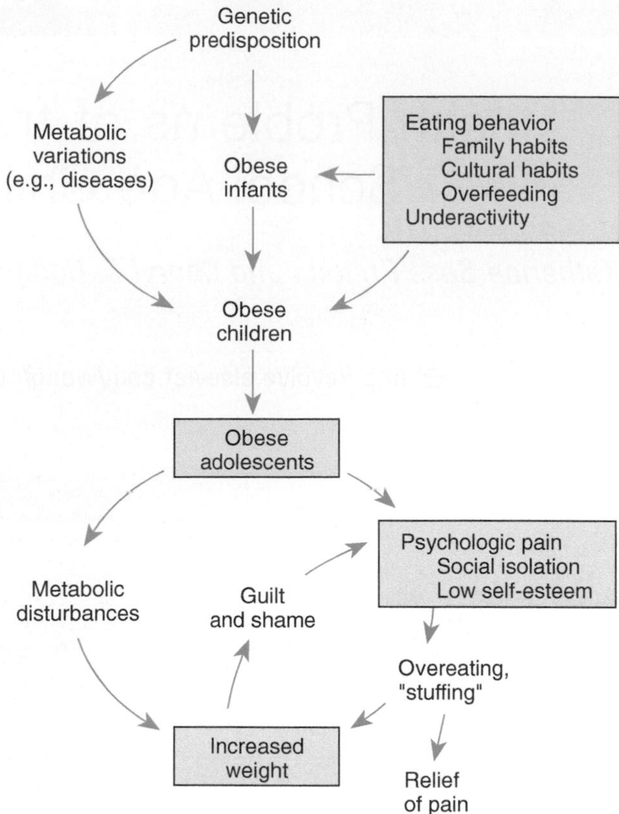

FIG. 16.1 Complex relationships in adolescent obesity.

some types of adult-onset cancer, nonalcoholic fatty liver disease, and type 2 diabetes mellitus. The incidence of metabolic syndrome was 30% in obese children (Kiess, Kratzsch, Sergeyev, et al., 2014). Common emotional consequences of obesity include low self-esteem, social isolation, anxiety, depression, and an increased risk for the development of eating disorders (Altman & Wilfley, 2015).

Etiology and Pathophysiology

Obesity results from a caloric intake that consistently exceeds caloric requirements and expenditure and may involve a variety of interrelated influences, including metabolic, hypothalamic, hereditary, social, cultural, and psychologic factors. Because the etiology of obesity is multifactorial, the treatment requires multilevel interventions. Fig. 16.1 illustrates an ecologic approach to understanding the multitude of risk factors associated with childhood and adolescent obesity. This framework suggests that the dominant factors, such as the availability of fast-food restaurants, may influence food choices of the children and adolescents who live there. An ecologic approach helps promote a better understanding of the roles that institutional, community, and societal factors play in the development of children's eating practices and activity levels, thereby taking some of the blame off children for their overweight.

Energy Balance

A balance between energy intake and energy expenditure is a critical factor in regulating body weight. Factors that raise energy intake or decrease energy expenditure by even small amounts can have a long-term impact on the development of overweight and obesity. For example, eating one small chocolate chip cookie (50 calories) is equivalent to walking briskly for 10 minutes. Factors that raise energy intake or decrease energy expenditure by even small amounts can have a long-term impact on the development of overweight and obesity.

Genetic Factors

Genetic influence is an epidemiologic consideration in regard to children's weight. Genetic mutations, such as FTO (fat mass and obesity), are rare but can predispose individuals to becoming overweight or obese (Gahagan, 2016). Studies have also suggested a tendency for a combination of genetic and environmental factors. Parental BMI is a potent predictor of obesity than genetics, suggesting that behaviors and environment play a greater role in obesity (Morandi, Meyre, Lobbens, et al., 2012). The increasing rates of obesity within genetically stable populations suggest that environmental and some perinatal factors (e.g., bottle feeding) and possible intrauterine factors (e.g., maternal gestational weight gain and stress) are contributors to the current increases in childhood obesity (Li, Magadia, Fein, et al., 2012). More research is needed to better understand the influences of family behavior and adolescent overweight.

Diseases

Fewer than 5% of the cases of childhood obesity can be attributed to an underlying disease. Such diseases include hypothyroidism; adrenal hypercorticoidism; hyperinsulinism; and dysfunction or damage to the central nervous system as a result of tumor, injury, infection, or vascular accident. Obesity is a frequent complication of muscular dystrophy, paraplegia, Down syndrome, spina bifida, and other chronic illnesses that limit mobility.

Several congenital syndromes have obesity as a feature, including Laurence-Moon-Biedl, Prader-Willi, and Alström syndromes and pseudohypoparathyroidism. The most common of these is Prader-Willi syndrome, a disorder characterized by hypogonadism; slow intellectual development; short stature; and dysmorphic facial features, including a narrowed bifrontal diameter, almond-shaped eyes, and triangular mouth. These children are hypotonic and hyperphagic. They lack the internal mechanism that regulates satiety and as a result go to great lengths to obtain food.

Molecular, Metabolic, and Endocrine Factors: Regulators of Appetite

A major focus of obesity research has been appetite regulation. The expression of appetite is chemically coded in the hypothalamus by distinctive circuitry involved in drive and motivation. Orexigenic substances produce signals that increase appetite, and anorexigenic substances promote the cessation of appetite. Feedback loops between signals have been identified where one signal peptide is able to alter the secretion of another signal peptide. No one signal has been identified as the gatekeeper of appetite. It is apparent that an entire network of signals, including their frequency and amplitude, is responsible for triggering eating behaviors.

This network of appetite signals explains the behavioral observations that appetite and food consumption patterns are dynamic and influenced by biologic, environmental, and psychologic events. Internal cues such as habitual intake, memories of food-related activities, and anticipation of consumption easily modify human eating behaviors. External cues that modify the perception of appetite include plate/utensil size, portion sizes served, food aroma, anticipation, and the number food choices (Berthoud, 2012; Lee, Carter, Owen, et al., 2012).

Researchers have identified a number of hormones and proteins that regulate appetite and weight in animal models. It is likely that these same mechanisms apply to humans. However, the role of hormones and neurotransmitters in determining overweight in humans remains unknown. There is little evidence to support a relationship between obesity and *low metabolism.* There may be small differences in regulation of dietary intake or metabolic rate between obese and nonobese children that could lead to an energy imbalance and inappropriate weight gain, but these small differences are difficult to accurately quantify. Obese children tend to be less active than lean children, but it is uncertain whether inactivity creates the obesity or obesity is responsible for the inactivity. Obesity in adolescents and children can be caused by overeating, low activity levels, or both.

Caloric Equilibrium: Sociocultural Factors

The tendency toward obesity occurs whenever environmental conditions are favorable toward excessive caloric intake, such as an abundance of high-calorie/low-nutrient foods, limited access to nutrient-dense foods, reduced or minimum physical activity, and snacking combined with excessive screen (e.g., computer, television, video games, cell phone) time. Family and cultural eating patterns, as well as psychologic factors, play an important role. Some families and cultures consider plumpness to be an indication of good health, a status symbol, or an indication of affluence. It is not uncommon for obese children to have families that emphasize large portion sizes, admonish children for leaving food on their plates, or use food as a reward or punishment. Parents may not have a concept of the amount of food children require and expect them to eat more than they need.

Disparities in obesity rates exist among racial/ethnic minorities, immigrant communities, and refugee communities, as well as across socioeconomic status, with differences often becoming apparent before 6 years of age. Lower-socioeconomic groups have a greater prevalence of obesity. Youth immigrating to the United States tend to have lower initial weight statuses, but on a population level, immigrant youth have higher BMIs than their native-born counterparts after one generation of living in the United States. This is particularly true for Hispanic immigrants (Xi, Takyi, & Lamptey, 2015). Sociocultural factors also influence physical activity. Studies have shown that activity and inactivity patterns differ by ethnicity, and minority adolescents (e.g., non-Hispanic black, Hispanics) engage in less physical activity and more inactivity than their non-Hispanic white counterparts (Kann, McManus, Harris, et al., 2016).

Community and Institutional Contributors

Some community factors that influence eating and activity patterns include a lack of a built environment (e.g., food deserts, community gardens, farmers markets, sidewalks, parks, bike paths) or affordable and accessible facilities for low-income youth to be active, thus limiting their opportunities to participate in physical activities or eat healthfully. Social policies also contribute to obesity. The increased availability of energy-dense foods, pricing strategies that promote unhealthy food choices, and overzealous food advertising that targets children and adolescents with high-fat and high-sugar foods are some examples.

Schools have made efforts to limit their influence on patterns of obesity, especially with regards to available foods. In 2010 the Healthy Hunger-Free Kids Act was passed, which resulted in healthier foods offered in school meals and during the school day (including in vending machines and a la carte lines). However, some school policies allow students to leave school for lunch, and fast-food restaurants are often allowed to advertise to children in schools. Although well-balanced, nutritious school lunches may be available, students will often opt for no lunch or one that is of less nutritious choices such as high-fat and high-sugar snacks.

Physical inactivity has also been identified as an important contributing factor in the development and maintenance of childhood overweight. There is little doubt that physical activity has decreased in elementary and secondary schools in the United States. The percentage of high school students who attended physical education classes daily was 25% in 1995, increased to 29.3% in 2013, and remained stable at 29.8% in 2015 (Kann, McManus, Harris, et al., 2016). By 2010, 42% of ninth-grade students but only 22% of twelfth-grade students attended physical education class daily (Kann, McManus, Harris, et al., 2016). Consequently, most of a child's physical activity must occur within the family or outside of school, which is also often limited due to community factors (e.g., unsafe neighborhoods). Decreased physical activity within the family and community is a powerful influence on children because children imitate their parents and other adults.

The attraction and availability of many sedentary activities, including television, video games, computers, and the Internet, have greatly influenced the amount of exercise that children get. Studies have shown the association between screen time and obesity among children (Berlin, Kamody, Thurston, et al., 2017; Zhang, Wu, Zhou, et al., 2016). The American Academy of Pediatrics (2016a) issued a policy statement encouraging parents to limit media viewing in children to 2 hours or less per day.

Personal and Interpersonal Factors

Psychologic factors also affect eating patterns. Infants experience relief from discomfort through feeding and learn to associate eating with a sense of well-being, security, and the comforting presence of a nurturing person. Eating is soon associated with the feeling of being loved. In addition, the pleasurable oral sensation of sucking provides a connection between emotions and early eating behavior. Many parents use food as a positive reward for desired behaviors. This practice may become a habit, and the child may continue to use food as a reward, a comfort, and a means of dealing with feelings of depression or hostility. Many individuals eat when they are not hungry or in response to stress, boredom, loneliness, sadness, depression, or tiredness. Difficulty in determining feelings of satiety can lead to weight problems and may compound the factor of eating in response to emotional rather than physical hunger cues.

Skipping breakfast is associated with a higher BMI. In addition, the frequency of family meals has consistently been shown to be a protective factor for obesity (Gahagan, 2016). Family meals tend to provide access to a variety of nutrient-rich foods, particularly fruits and vegetables. Family meals also create a forum for increased family communication and connectedness, both of which promote healthy weight behaviors. This is also a time when parents can model healthy behaviors (Tandon, Zhou, Sallis, et al., 2012).

Friends have also been shown to be associated with adolescents' eating, physical activity, and weight (Bruening, Eisenberg, MacLehose, et al., 2012; Sirard, Bruening, Wall, et al., 2013). Friends have been shown to have similar weights and to share both healthy and unhealthy weight-related behaviors. However, research is still needed to determine the causality of these relationships and their relative contribution to obesity risk.

Cultural impact of childhood obesity. Child overweight and obesity are not confined to affluent countries such as the United States and Europe. The World Health Organization (2017) estimates that in 2015, 42 million children under the age of 5 years were overweight. More than two-thirds of these children live in urban settings in low- and middle-income countries. In 2007 the World Health Organization made available new childhood growth standards that were compiled from a Multicentre Growth reference study of 8500 children in countries around the world. These growth standards include body mass index reference standards for children ages 5 to 19 years, as well as weight and height for age growth charts. These growth charts may be downloaded from www.who.int/growthref/en.

Diagnostic Evaluation

A careful history is obtained regarding the development of obesity, and a physical examination is performed to differentiate simple obesity from increased fat that results from organic causes. A family history of obesity, diabetes, coronary heart disease, and dyslipidemia should be obtained for all children who are overweight or at risk for overweight. Specific information from the patient and family about the effects of obesity on daily functioning—for example, problems with nighttime breathing and sleep, daytime sleepiness, joint pain, ability to keep up with family activities and peers at school—is helpful. The physical examination should focus on identifying comorbid conditions and identifiable causes of obesity. For some, psychologic assessment, by interviews and standardized personality tests, may provide insight into the personality and emotional problems that contribute to obesity and that might interfere with therapy.

It is useful to estimate the degree of obesity to determine the component of body weight that can be modified. All the following methods have been used to assess obesity: BMI, body weight, weight-height ratios, weight-age ratios, hydrostatic weight, dual-energy x-ray absorptiometry, skinfold measurements, bioelectrical analysis, computed tomography (CT), magnetic resonance imaging (MRI), and neutron activation. Each of these methods has advantages and disadvantages. Hydrostatic weighing provides the most accurate measurement of lean body weight. In hydrostatic weighing, total body density is determined by total submersion in a water-filled tank. However, this method is not practical in clinical settings. Skinfold thickness uses special calipers to measure the subcutaneous fat deposits. Human error is a problem with this method; results can vary greatly for health care professionals who do not perform these measurements frequently. The bioelectrical impedance method determines body fat from measures of impedance of electrical current by way of electrodes attached to the arm and leg. CT is used to estimate subcutaneous and intraabdominal fat deposition. MRI provides clear images of fat deposits compared with tissues containing water and other components. Total-body neutron activation provides an estimation of water and fat, as well as calcium, protein, and other components. These techniques are expensive and are typically used in specialized clinical settings.

BMI is currently considered the best method to assess weight in children and adolescents (Gahagan, 2016). The calculation is based on the individual's height and weight. In adults, BMI definitions are fixed measures without regard for sex and age. The BMI in children and adolescents varies to accommodate age- and gender-specific changes in growth. The formula for BMI calculation is weight in kilograms divided by height in meters squared (weight (kg)/[height $(m)^2$]). BMI measures in children and adolescents are plotted on growth charts that enable heath care professionals to determine BMI-for-age for the patient. The initial assessment of obese children and adolescents should include screening to evaluate for comorbidities. The history is an important guide to determine the workup. A complete physical examination is important. Some areas to focus on include (1) skin for stretch markings and discolorations (e.g., acanthosis nigricans), (2) joints for swelling and evidence of pain, and (3) airway for evidence of obstruction and enlarged tonsils. Basic laboratory studies include a fasting lipid panel; fasting insulin level; fasting glucose hepatic enzymes, including gamma-glutamyl transferase (GGT); and, in some institutions, hemoglobin A1c. Other studies, such as a polysomnogram (sleep study), metabolic studies, and radiographic evaluations, may be added based on the history and physical examination. These assessments may determine whether the patient needs a referral to specialty services for more focused evaluation and treatment, such as endocrinology (insulin resistance, diabetes), hepatology (elevated liver enzymes, nonalcoholic fatty liver disease), orthopedics (Blount disease), or pulmonary medicine (sleep-disordered breathing).

Complications of Obesity

Adults with longstanding obesity are at risk for medical complications that include hypertension, diabetes, coronary heart disease, stroke, fatty liver disease, and colorectal cancer. Although obesity-related complications occur frequently in adults, children and adolescents are experiencing significant health consequences as well. Health care providers, researchers, and government agencies discovered that children and adolescents are developing these complications sooner rather than later in adult life. Childhood obesity has become an increasingly important medical problem, resulting in hypertension, type 2 diabetes, pulmonary complications (e.g., asthma, sleep apnea), growth acceleration, dyslipidemia, musculoskeletal problems, fatty liver disease, and a potential for psychosocial problems. Diagnostic evaluations of children and adolescents who are overweight or obese have expanded to screen for these complications.

Physical Complications of Obesity

Insulin resistance and type 2 diabetes. Along with obesity, type 2 diabetes mellitus is reaching epidemic proportions in children and adolescents. Up to 45% of all new cases of type 2 diabetes consist of children or adolescents (Temneanu, Trandafir, & Purcarea, 2016). Inactivity and obesity influence insulin resistance. Insulin resistance syndrome, also known as metabolic syndrome, is characterized by hyperinsulinemia, obesity, hypertension, and dyslipidemia and develops before any of these conditions develops.

Insulin is necessary for the metabolism of fats, proteins, and carbohydrates and must be present for glucose to enter the fat and muscle cells. Insulin facilitates the storage of glucose in the form of glycogen in the liver and muscle cells and further prevents the mobilization of fat from fat cells. The cell membrane has special receptor sites for insulin. Once the receptor site has been established, a chemical reaction results and glucose enters the cell. If the amount of insulin is inadequate, glucose cannot enter the cell. In response to elevated levels of glucose in the body, the pancreas increases the production of insulin, resulting in hyperinsulinemia. Type 2 diabetes develops when the pancreas is no longer able to lower the blood glucose level by hypersecretion of insulin.

Children and adolescents with type 2 diabetes often have decreased high-density lipoprotein cholesterol levels, increased triglyceride levels, and increased blood pressure causing them to be at risk for cardiovascular disease (Berquist, 2015).

Fatty liver disease. Recently a growing number of children and adolescents have been diagnosed with nonalcoholic fatty liver disease (NAFLD), which has been recognized as one of the leading causes of chronic liver disease in the general population. Between 10% and 25% of obese children and adolescents are diagnosed with NAFLD, which is the most common liver disease in children (Gahagan, 2016). The increased prevalence of NAFLD in the pediatric population appears to coincide with the increasing prevalence of obesity.

NAFLD is generally a benign condition in which a buildup of fat infiltrates the liver. Liver blood tests, including alanine aminotransferase (ALT) and aspartate aminotransferase (AST), are either normal or slightly elevated. Nonalcoholic steatohepatitis (NASH) is a stage within the spectrum of NAFLD where the fatty infiltration causes liver inflammation (steatohepatitis) and may cause scarring. Approximately 25% of pediatric patients with NAFLD will progress to NASH (Temple, Cordero, Li, et al., 2016). Although the disease process is not completely understood, some factors contribute to the development of NASH including insulin resistance; diabetes; and obesity. People with NASH may feel healthy and show no outward signs of liver disease. NASH and NAFLD are diagnosed by imaging tests such as an ultrasound, CT scan, or liver biopsy. NASH can be treated with weight loss for most people; however, for some it will progress leading to cirrhosis and end-stage liver disease, which may require liver transplantation (Temple, Cordero, Li, et al., 2016).

Pulmonary complications. Childhood obesity is related to pulmonary complication, including sleep apnea, exercise intolerance, and asthma.

Asthma and exercise intolerance can in turn worsen obesity by limiting physical activity and causing further weight gain. A recent study of 472 children (49% were overweight/obese) with asthma found that compared with normal-weight children, overweight/obese children had more days with asthma symptoms (3.42 versus 4.25, $p = 0.035$), more days with activity limitation (2.55 versus 3.34, $p = 0.013$), and more acute asthma medical visits (1.31 versus 1.68, $p = 0.09$) (Wiesenthal, Fagnano, Cook, et al., 2016). This difference in obesity between asthmatics and non-asthmatics was controlled for race, ethnicity, and caregiver age. The mechanisms for the relationship between asthma and obesity are still unknown.

Sleep-disordered breathing is another significant problem with obese adults and children. Obstructive sleep apnea (OSA) is reported in 20% to 30% of obese children and adolescents (Thompson, Mansfield, Stringer, et al., 2016). Evaluating OSA includes assessing for snoring, daytime drowsiness, poor quality of sleep, and presence of apneic episodes (Thompson, Mansfield, Stringer, et al., 2016). Any suspected cases should be referred to an otolaryngologist. Airway obstructions such as enlarged tonsils and adenoids may require assessment and intervention. Continuous positive airway pressure (CPAP) and bilevel positive airway pressure (BiPAP) are used for obese children requiring additional nighttime respiratory support.

Musculoskeletal and abnormal growth acceleration. Obesity has been associated with musculoskeletal problems resulting from increased body weight on the supporting structures of the hips, knees, and feet. Slipped capital femoral epiphysis is the most common hip disorder among young teenagers and occurs when the cartilage plate (epiphysis) at the top of the femur slips out of place. Blount disease, another orthopedic problem, is the overgrowth of the medial aspect of the proximal tibial metaphysis that causes the lower leg to angle inward (tibia vara). The inner part of the tibia, just below the knee, fails to develop normally, resulting in angulation of the bone. The cause is unknown, but it is thought to be due to the effects of weight on the growth plate (Sabharwal, 2015). Studies have shown a dose-response relationship between BMI and Blount disease (Sabharwal, 2015).

Psychologic and Social Complications of Obesity

Childhood obesity has been associated not only with metabolic health risk but also with problems in social interactions and relationships. Obese children become targets of early and systematic discrimination. Early studies reported that children at a young age are sensitized to obesity and have begun to incorporate the culture's preference for thinness.

Obesity status is inversely related to several self-perception factors. Many appear to develop a negative self-image and low body satisfaction that persists into adulthood (Rankin, Matthews, Cobley, et al., 2016). Obese children may develop anxiety, depression, and a decreased quality of life (Kumar & Kelly, 2017). In fact, youth who are obese are more likely to practice unhealthy weight control behaviors (e.g., using diet pills, induced vomiting) that may lead to eating disorders (see Chapter 18) (Rankin, Matthews, Cobley, et al., 2016).

Studies have examined the association between overweight and obesity and bullying in adolescents. They found that overweight children are more frequently the victims of bullying compared with children of normal weight (Puhl & King, 2013; Rankin, Matthews, Cobley, et al., 2016). Bullying behaviors included name calling, teasing, threats, physical harm, rejection, rumors, and sexual harassment. Because adolescents are extremely reliant on their peers for social support, identity, and self-esteem, they are particularly at risk for the negative consequences of bullying and victimization. More studies are needed to better understand the effects of overweight and obesity on the psychologic and social functioning of children and adolescents.

TABLE 16.1 Pediatric Quality Indicator: Weight Assessment and Counseling*

Weight Assessment and Counseling for Nutrition and Physical Activity	
Measure	Children/adolescents 3-17 years of age who had an outpatient visit and had evidence of the following during the measurement period: height, weight, and body mass index (BMI) percentile documentation counseling on nutrition and physical activity.
Numerator	Number of children with BMI percentile documentation, counseling for nutrition, and counseling for physical activity during the measurement time.
Denominator	Number of children 3-17 years of age with at least one outpatient visit.

*Endorsed by the National Quality Forum-0024 and Center for Medicare and Medicaid Services-155v1.

Therapeutic Management

The best approach to the management of obesity is a preventive one. Early recognition and control measures are essential before the child or adolescent reaches an obese state. A pediatric quality indicator for weight assessment and nutrition and physical activity counseling is listed in Table 16.1. Health care providers need to educate families about the medical complications of obesity.

Treatments recommended for obese children include diet, exercise, behavior modification, and in some situations pharmacologic agents such as orlistat. The treatment of obesity is difficult. Many approaches do not achieve long-term success. The average individual only loses about 5% to 10% of his or her weight with available therapies. Losing weight can have a significant positive effect on many comorbidities, but unfortunately the lost weight is frequently regained in a year or two. A number of multidisciplinary programs offer interventions combining medical, dietary, exercise, and psychologic support. This therapy is labor intensive and fairly costly.

Diet

Diet modification is an essential part of weight reduction programs. Dietary counseling focuses on improving the nutritional quality of the diet rather than on dietary restriction. Children should avoid fad diets. Most dietitians and nutrition experts recommend a diet with no trans fats, low saturated fat, moderate total fat (≤30%), low sodium, and at least nine servings of fruits and vegetables, consistent with the MyPlate food guide for children (www.choosemyplate.gov). Also, promoting high-fiber foods and avoiding highly refined starches and sugars will decrease caloric intake. Many programs recommend using a food diary as a helpful tool to increase awareness of food choices and eating behaviors. The goal is to encourage the individual to make healthier choices in food selection and discourage using food by habit or to appease boredom. Box 16.1 contains helpful suggestions.

Many dietitians recommend encouraging parents to take charge of family meals and the home food environment to improve their nutritional quality. Getting families to sit down together at the table, away from distractions such as television, makes dinner time more than just eating. Dinnertime becomes a time to share the events of the day and build relationships. Being able to create an environment in the home where healthy choices are readily available for adolescents is also important. For example, having cut fruit and vegetables in the refrigerator and limiting unhealthy snack foods at home can help adolescents make better choices.

BOX 16.1 Recommended Behaviors for Preventing Obesity

In counseling adolescents whose body mass index is between the 5th and 84th percentiles, physicians and health care providers should recommend the following steps to prevent obesity:

- Limit consumption of sugar-sweetened beverages.
- Consume recommended quantities of fruits and vegetables.
- Limit television and other screen time to no more than 2 hours per day.
- Remove television and computer screens from primary sleeping areas.
- Eat breakfast daily.
- Limit eating at restaurants.
- Have frequent family meals in which parents and youth eat together.
- Limit portion sizes.

Adapted from Davis, D. M., Gance-Cleveland, B., Hassink, S., et al. (2007). Recommendations for prevention of childhood obesity. *Pediatrics, 120,* S229-S253.

BOX 16.2 Strategies to Increase Physical Activities Among Adolescents

- Start by identifying how much time is spent in sedentary activities and screen time (e.g., television, computer, video games).
- Decrease television and sedentary activities to 1 to 2 hours per day or less.
- Put more physical activities into daily routines. Small changes can result in healthful outcomes.
- Take the stairs.
- Walk with friend instead of talking or texting on the phone.
- Walk to school.
- Walk the dog.
- Get off the bus or train one stop earlier.
- In parking lots, select spaces farther from the door.
- Consider purchasing a pedometer ($10 to $15) and aim for 10,000 to 15,000 steps daily.
- Take classes—dance, yoga, spinning, swimming, soccer.
- Take aerobic classes or use videos. YouTube has free exercise videos to get you started.
- Participate in team sports.
- Ride bicycles for fun and to get to places.
- Consider an hour of activity after school before sitting down for homework.
- Buy active toys rather than computer games and videotapes.
- Involve the whole family in activities together.

Special Diets

In patients with severe obesity, strict diets have been used, such as the protein-sparing modified fast, hypocaloric diet, or ketogenic diet (Castaldo, Palmieri, Galdo, et al., 2016; Sukkar, Signori, Borrini, et al., 2013). These diets are designed to provide enough protein to minimize loss of lean body mass during weight loss. Such diets need to be closely monitored and should be used only with multidisciplinary teams that include a physician, nutritionist, and behavior therapist. Generally, the diet consists of 1.5 to 2.5 g of protein per kilogram. The intake of carbohydrates is low enough to induce ketosis. The benefits of the diet are relatively rapid weight loss and anorexia induced by ketosis. Potential complications include protein losses, electrolyte imbalances, hypoglycemia, inadequate calcium intake, orthostatic hypotension, and increased risk for osteoporosis. Low-carbohydrate supplements containing vitamins, minerals, and trace minerals, along with therapeutic doses of vitamin D is recommended (Luat, Coyle, & Kamat, 2016). It is difficult to sustain these diets over the long term, and the long-term outcomes of using these diets have not been established.

Physical Activity

Regular physical activity is incorporated into all weight reduction programs. Recommendations for physical activity need to consider the patient's current health status and developmental level. Current recommendations encourage children to be physically active for 60 minutes or more a day (Centers for Disease Control and Prevention, 2017). The best choice for exercise is any form that is enjoyable and likely to be sustainable. Aerobic and endurance exercises help oxidize body fats. Light exercises such as walking may provide an opportunity for the family to increase time together and increase caloric expenditure. Weight training can increase basal metabolic rate and replace fat mass with muscle mass. However, weight training is not generally recommended for prepubertal children until they have reached physical and skeletal maturity. In prepubertal children increasing outdoor playtime is likely to be beneficial. Many children find exercise videos and treadmills boring and may not continue these activities. Children and adolescents are more likely to exercise when they have a choice. Individuals can choose from a large variety of physical activities, including team sports and individual sports such as yoga, dance, bike riding, and swimming.

Limiting sedentary screen time behaviors, such as viewing television, social media sites, and video games, is the most effective way to encourage physical activity. The American Academy of Pediatrics (2016a) recommends limiting sedentary screen time to less than 2 hours a day. Box 16.2 shows more strategies to increase physical activities.

Behavior Modification

Behavior modification approaches to weight loss are based on the observation that obese individuals have abnormal eating practices that can be altered. Attention is focused not on food but on the social and behavioral aspects surrounding food consumption. Successful behavior modification weight programs help children identify and eliminate inappropriate eating habits and include a problem-solving component that enables children to identify problems and determine solutions. Combining behavioral modifications with pharmacologic therapy in children 12 years and older has produced mixed results with regard to total weight loss maintained over a significant period of time (Wright & Wales, 2016). Programs including family-based behavioral modification, dietary modification, and exercise have been shown to be successful in reducing obesity in some children (Altman & Wilfley, 2015). Behavior modification is an important part of multidisciplinary intervention programs.

Drugs

A number of medications have been used in adults with varying results. Currently, multicenter clinical trials are being conducted to evaluate the effects of medications on weight loss in children. To date the only drug approved for use in children 12 years of age and older is orlistat, a lipase inhibitor. Currently no long-term data are available regarding the benefits of such drugs for obesity management in children and adolescents (Mead, Atkinson, Richter, et al., 2016). Some drugs have been used to promote weight loss in children with certain conditions such as metformin in obese adolescents with insulin resistance and hyperinsulinemia, octreotide for hypothalamic obesity caused by intracranial tumors, growth hormone in children with Prader-Willi syndrome, and metreleptin for congenital leptin deficiency (Meehan, Cochran, Kassai, et al., 2016; Stagi, Ricci, Bianconi, et al., 2017; Xu & Xue, 2016); however, given the risks involved, drug trials are limited in children and adolescents.

Surgical Techniques

Surgical techniques (bariatric surgery) that bypass portions of the intestine or occlude a segment of the stomach to produce a marked diet restriction and weight loss are hazardous and cause many metabolic complications. These complications include severe water and electrolyte depletion, persistent diarrhea, vitamin deficiency, internal herniation, and fatty infiltration and degeneration of the liver. In the past, these procedures were considered contraindicated for pediatric patients. Surgical intervention for children and adolescents is being reevaluated in the context of the significant increase in the prevalence of obesity and concomitant comorbidities within this population. The most common surgical methods used in youth include the Roux-en-Y gastric bypass, adjustable gastric banding, and sleeve gastrectomy (Rajjo, Mohammed, Alsawas, et al., 2017). Minimally invasive surgical techniques are being used with increased frequency.

Bariatric surgery may be the only practical alternative for increasing numbers of severely overweight adolescents who have failed organized attempts to lose or maintain weight loss through conventional nonoperative approaches and who have serious life-threatening conditions. There are few studies in adults and no information for adolescents that suggest surgical weight loss improves the early mortality rates of patients with severe obesity. Therefore in general, bariatric surgery should be reserved for severely obese adolescents with comorbidities after careful consideration. Physicians must define clear, realistic, and restrictive guidelines to apply with younger patients when surgery is considered. Candidates for surgery should be referred to centers that offer a multidisciplinary team experienced in the management of childhood and adolescent obesity. The surgery should be performed by surgeons who have participated in subspecialty training in bariatric medical and surgical care as detailed by the American College of Surgeons and the American Society for Metabolic and Bariatric Surgery.

It is recommended that a pediatric review process be in place to carefully screen patients. Candidates should undergo complete medical assessments and psychologic evaluations that include the patient and parents. The most important ethical considerations for bariatric surgery in an adolescent are whether (1) the patient's health is severely compromised by severe obesity, (2) the patient has failed more conservative treatment options, and (3) the patient (adolescent) has the ability to make this decision. Current criteria for bariatric surgery include (1) attainment of physical maturity (Tanner stage 4 or 95% of linear growth based on bone age); (2) BMI greater than or equal to 35 kg/m^2 with a severe comorbidity; (3) BMI of at least 40 kg/m^2 with less severe comorbidities; (4) understanding of the importance of behavioral change, and role of diet and physical activity necessary for long-term success after surgery; (5) agreement to avoid pregnancy for at least 18 months postoperatively; and (6) ability to understand the risks and benefits of weight loss surgery (Desai, Wulkan, & Inge, 2016).

Surgical treatment options for adolescents should be chosen carefully and with the support of the multidisciplinary team, the patient, and the family (Black, White, Viner, et al., 2013). It is strongly recommended that all patients who have bariatric surgery be monitored throughout their lives (Beamish & Reinehr, 2017). Knowledge about appropriate timing and better surgical and postoperative management of adolescent surgical patients depends on the rigorous collection of high-quality outcome data (Black, White, Viner, et al., 2013).

Nursing Care Management

Nurses play a key role in the adherence and maintenance phases of many weight reduction programs. Nurse practitioners assess, manage, and evaluate the progress of many overweight adolescents. They also play an important role in recognizing potential weight problems and assisting parents and adolescents in preventing obesity.

The presence of obesity may not be obvious from appearance alone. Regular assessment of height and weight and computation of the BMI facilitate early recognition of risk. Guidelines for childhood obesity prevention and treatment are available (Styne, Arslanian, Connor, et al., 2017). Evaluation includes a height and weight history of the adolescent and family members, eating habits, appetite and hunger patterns, and physical activities. A psychosocial history is also helpful in understanding the impact of obesity on the child's life. Steps to approaching behavior change with youth are described in Box 16.3.

Before initiating a treatment plan, it is important to be certain that the family is ready for change. Lack of readiness may result in failure, frustration, and reluctance to address the problem in the future. It may be wiser to defer treatment until the family is ready (Box 16.4). Children need to take a personal responsibility for dietary habits and physical activity. Youth who are forced by their parents to seek help are seldom motivated, become rebellious, and are unwilling to control their dietary intake.

BOX 16.3 Pediatric Obesity Prevention Protocol for Primary Care

Step 1: Assess

Explain and conduct assessments of:
- Weight, height, and body mass index percentile
- Dietary intake (fruit, vegetables, sweetened beverages, and fast food)
- Activity (screen time, moderate-to-vigorous activity)
- Eating behaviors (breakfast, portion sizes, family meals)

Provide and elicit feedback on body mass index and behaviors found to be inside and outside the optimal range.

Step 2: Set Agenda

Explore interest in changing behaviors not in the optimal range.

Agree on target behaviors with the patient and caregiver.

Step 3: Assess Motivation and Confidence

With regard to interest in changing weight status or behaviors, assess:
- Willingness/ability to make change
- Perceived importance
- Confidence in having success

Probe the patient regarding ratings of willingness, perceived importance, and confidence to explore the advantages and disadvantages of changing.

Step 4: Summarize and Explore Possible Changes

Summarize the advantages and disadvantages of change.

Query possible next steps. Allow the adolescent to suggest ideas.

Provide guidance for getting started in making a change as needed. Encourage achievable goals.

Summarize the change plan.

Provide positive feedback.

Step 5: Schedule Follow-Up Visit

If a change plan is made, agree on a follow-up appointment within a specified number of weeks or months.

If no change plan is made, agree to revisit the topic within a specific number of weeks or months.

Data from Davis, D. M., Gance-Cleveland, B., Hassink, S., et al. (2007). Recommendations for prevention of childhood obesity. *Pediatrics, 120*, S229-S253.

BOX 16.4 Stages of Change Model

Precontemplation—Not yet acknowledging that there is a problem behavior that needs to be changed
Contemplation—Acknowledging there is a problem but not yet ready or sure of wanting change
Preparation/determination—Getting ready to change
Action/willpower—Changing behavior
Maintenance—Maintaining the behavior change
Relapse—Returning to older behaviors and abandoning the new changes

Data from Prochaska, J. O., & DiClemente, C. C. (1984). *The transtheoretical approach: Crossing traditional boundaries of change.* Homewood, IL: Dorsey Press.

! NURSING ALERT

The nurse should explore with children and adolescents the reasons behind the desire to lose weight because motivation to lose weight is the key to success.

Nutritional Counseling

Preventing an increase in body fat during growth is a realistic approach. This is often accomplished by adjusting four aspects of eating: (1) reducing the quantity eaten by purchasing, preparing, and serving smaller portions; (2) altering the quality consumed by substituting low-calorie, low-fat foods for high-calorie foods (especially for snacks); (3) eating regular meals and snacks, particularly breakfast; and (4) altering situations by severing associations between eating and other stimuli, such as eating while watching television. Nutrition counseling incorporates health behavior theories to help motivate and maintain behavior change. The most successful changes are those that are attainable, reasonable, and sustainable.

The nurse teaches children and parents how to incorporate favorite foods into their diet and to select satisfying substitutes. To maintain a healthy diet, it is necessary to encourage the consumption of nutrient-dense foods such as fruits, vegetables, whole grains, and low-fat dairy protein products. Keep calories and fat to a healthy level without being significantly restricted. To be successful, a dietary program should be nutritionally sound with sufficient satiety value, produce the desired weight loss, and be accompanied by nutrition education and continued support.

Behavior Therapy

Altering eating behavior and eliminating inappropriate eating habits are essential to weight reduction, especially in maintaining long-term weight control. Most behavior modification programs include the following concepts:

- A description of the behavior to be controlled, such as eating habits
- Attempts to modify and control the stimuli that govern eating
- Development of eating techniques designed to control speed of eating
- Positive reinforcement for these modifications through a suitable reward system that does not include food
- Create environments where the healthy choice is the easy choice

Group Involvement

Commercial groups (e.g., Weight Watchers) or diet workshops are usually directed to adults; a group of other peers is often more effective for children and adolescents. Groups include summer camps designed for obese young people and conducted by health professionals, school groups organized and led by a school nurse or health professional, and groups associated with special clinics.

These groups are concerned not only with weight loss but also with the development of a positive self-image and the encouragement of physical activity. Nutrition education, diet planning, and the improvement of social skills are essential components of these groups. Improvement is determined by positive changes in all aspects of behavior.

Family Involvement

There is a definite connection between family environment, interaction, and obesity. The nurse needs to educate parents in the purposes of the therapeutic measures and their role in management. The family needs nutrition education and counseling regarding the reinforcement plan, alterations in the food environment, and ways to maintain proper attitudes. They can support their child in efforts to change eating behaviors, food intake, and physical activity.

Prognosis

Lifelong eating habits and psychologic problems make weight reduction difficult. Compared with normal-weight peers, adolescents with severe obesity are 70% more likely to be obese adults and overweight adolescents are 8% more likely to be obese adults (Kumar & Kelly, 2017). Obesity is consistently linked to poorer health outcomes. Obese children have a higher incidence of diabetes and coronary heart disease as adults (Llewellyn, Simmonds, Owen, et al., 2016). Overweight or obese children are almost twice as likely to develop metabolic syndrome as their normal-weight peers (Kim, Lee, & Lim, 2017). Weight loss in obese children can improve health outcomes. Obese adolescents who had an 8% reduction in weight experienced a reduction in blood glucose and liver fat, resulting in a lower incidence of diabetes and nonalcoholic fatty liver disease (Gow, Baur, Johnson, et al., 2017). Lifestyle modification approaches to promote energy balance through healthy eating and adequate physical activity have shown modest improvements in risk for obesity; however, interventions that include components about the built environment (e.g., sidewalks, fewer fast-food restaurants in the neighborhood) have had the greatest impact on obesity (Schmiege, Gance-Cleveland, Gilbert, et al., 2016; Slawson, Fitzgerald, & Morgan, 2013).

Prevention

Reducing adolescent obesity has been identified as a national public health priority by the Institute of Medicine and numerous other expert groups. Prevention of obesity should begin in early childhood with the development of healthy eating habits, regular exercise patterns, and a positive relationship between parents and children. Prevention of adolescent obesity is best accomplished by early identification of obesity in the preschool, school-age, and preadolescent periods. Health care professionals should encourage frequent health care visits for children who are overweight or obese and incorporate a dietary history and counseling into each well-infant, well-child, and well-adolescent visit.

DENTAL DISORDERS

DENTAL CARIES

Dental caries (cavities) is one of the most common chronic diseases that affect individuals at all ages, and it is the principal oral problem in children and adolescents. Although the overall incidence of dental caries in children has decreased since the introduction of fluoridation, more than half of the children in the United States have dental caries (Tinanoff, 2016). Reducing the incidence and consequences of the disorder remains important. Dental caries, if untreated, results in total destruction of the involved teeth and can lead to significant health risks like endocarditis and sinus and neurologic infections.

Pathophysiology

Dental caries is a multifactorial disease. It involves a number of elements: the host, microorganisms, substrate, and time.

Host

The prevalence of caries is directly related to the tooth size and morphologic characteristics and to the consistency, composition, and amount of saliva. The incidence of caries is higher in teeth that are improperly developed, crowded, or deeply fissured. The areas most subject to attack by bacteria are grooves and fissures, interdermal areas, gum margins, and other smooth surfaces. Newly erupted teeth that have not yet acquired sufficient surface minerals are more susceptible to decay than those that have been erupted for 2 years or longer. Hereditary factors influence resistance and susceptibility, and similar patterns and anatomic characteristics often appear in successive generations. Salivary flow can mechanically clean away bacteria and food debris. It also contains buffering systems, lysozymes, peroxidases, and immunoglobulins that influence the development of caries.

Microorganisms

Certain types of microflora contribute to the formation of dental caries. Acidogenic bacteria act on fermentable carbohydrates in dental plaque to produce organic acids that decalcify hard surface tooth enamel. With the inner organic matrix exposed, proteolytic organisms and acids digest and destroy the inner tooth structure. These destructive organisms are harbored and protected in a gelatinous plaque formed on the tooth surface by another group of bacteria that are thought to play no primary role in production of decay.

Substrate

Caries formation is strongly influenced by the two concurrent processes that continually operate on enamel surfaces: acid production and acid neutralization by saliva. The material on which the acid-forming bacteria act consists essentially of carbohydrates. Among the fermentable carbohydrates, sucrose has been consistently implicated as the most cariogenic. Sucrose-containing substances, especially in acidic forms that cling (such as sour chewy candy) or that promote prolonged contact with the teeth (such as hard candy and lollipops), when ingested between meals, contribute markedly to the development of dental caries. Saliva, some foods, and chewing gum after a meal tend to help neutralize much of the acid formed from sucrose.

Time and Other Factors

Bacterial enzymes act on salivary glycoproteins to produce a tenacious protein matrix on the tooth surface. This substance, along with the microorganisms, forms dental plaque. If plaque removal (brushing with a fluorinated toothpaste) is inadequate or nonexistent for a significant length of time (a few days), the plaque is metabolized by the bacteria to form acid, which initiates the demineralization of enamel.

Other factors that contribute to caries formation are heredity, diet, the amount of fluoride in drinking water, and acute illnesses. Hereditary factors influence both resistance and susceptibility to dental caries. For example, structural defects, such as deep fissures or crowding of teeth on occlusive surfaces, may be genetically passed from parents to children. The effectiveness of the buffering action of saliva is also highly variable among individuals.

The susceptibility to dental decay is also influenced by the child's general health. Children with special health care needs show increased caries activity, likely due to the sugar content of their drug therapy and lower salivary flow (Solanki, Kumar, Awasthi, et al., 2016). Children with developmental delays also have an increase incidence of decayed teeth compared with children of similar age without developmental delays (Chi, Rossitch, & Beeles, 2013). Poor oral hygiene that permits the accumulation of food debris on tooth surfaces allows acid-forming bacteria to thrive and proliferate. Removal of food particles and bacteria-laden plaque inhibits destructive acid formation. The American Dental Association recommends careful brushing and flossing of teeth after every meal.

Diagnostic Evaluation

Children are more susceptible for the development of dental caries during middle childhood, when permanent teeth erupt. Carious activity is slower and more irregular at later ages but remains a significant health risk to older children and adolescents. Large or extensive caries are usually accompanied by the child's complaint of oral pain and will be apparent on examination to the untrained eye, especially if on visible tooth surfaces. Smaller lesions or cracks in the dentation are best identified by trained dental professionals. Caries between the teeth may not be located without x-ray examination. A common site of decay is the fissures of the molars.

Therapeutic Management

Nurses and other health care professionals can provide dental hygiene information and assist families in making periodic dental assessments. However, dentists are the only health professionals qualified to treat caries and most other dental problems. Prevention, including routine daily hygiene and biannual fluoride treatment, is the major thrust of dental therapy. Plasticized sealant, applied to the deep fissures and grooves of healthy teeth, is effective in blocking cavity formation. Treatment of dental caries involves removal of all carious portions of the tooth as soon as decay is detected, preparation of a retentive cavity, and replacement of the lost portion of the tooth with a material that is durable in the mouth environment. This restoration of involved teeth not only prevents progression of established caries but also reduces the number of harmful bacteria in the oral cavity, reducing the risk of caries to uninvolved teeth.

Nursing Care Management

Oral inspection is an integral part of the nursing assessment of the child. If there is evidence of dental caries or another unhealthy state, the child is referred for dental services. Many families have a family dentist or a pedodontist who can provide needed care. However, an alarming number of children do not receive regular preventative dental services; a significant number reach adulthood without being examined or treated by a dentist. Pediatric nurses working in schools and community health centers are instrumental in preventing severe caries through routine assessments and the application of fluoride dental varnish to children during annual health visits. The varnish, topically applied to primary and permanent teeth of children and adolescents on an annual basis, is an effective measure to reduce childhood caries (Sievers & Silk, 2016).

Nurses can also serve as participants in preventive educational programs, as counselors to families regarding the importance of oral hygiene, and as dietary managers and advocates for regular dental care. School nurses, in particular, have an excellent opportunity to not only participate in the detection of dental needs but to make referrals and educate and motivate children to comply with prophylaxis and treatment. Children should brush their teeth and use dental floss according to the method recommended by their dentists. Regular administration of fluoride is also important. (See Chapter 12.) Families should be aware of the fluoride content of their drinking water, including bottled water if it is used. School-age children can usually manage the chewable fluoride tablets, which have both topical and systemic effects.

Restriction of cariogenic foods is important to prevent dental caries, but this should be viewed as an activity in which all family members are involved and not simply a directive for the child to obey. Routinely choosing "healthy food" rather than sweets should be communicated during health visits so the child interprets caring for his teeth (and smile) as a benefit rather than thinking that limiting sweets is a punishment. Children should be prepared for dental services in such a way that visits to the dentist are a positive experience. Keeping appointments and following through on recommended treatments and practices are habits that extend beyond childhood.

There is a significant concern about the sugar content of children's pharmaceutical products, especially because children with chronic conditions such as seizure disorders, asthma, depression, and recurrent urinary tract infections take medications over a period of years. These children are cautioned to brush their teeth after taking the medication just as they would after eating any meal or snack to reduce their risk for caries.

PERIODONTAL DISEASE

Periodontal disease, an inflammatory and degenerative condition involving the gums and tissues supporting the teeth, often begins in childhood and accounts for a significant amount of tooth loss in adulthood. The more common periodontal problems are **gingivitis** (simple inflammation of the gums) and **periodontitis** (inflammation of the gums and loss of connective tissue and bone in the supporting structures of the teeth). An uncommon condition is acute necrotizing ulcerative gingivitis ("trench mouth"). Children with these conditions will complain of oral pain, especially when eating or chewing, and have gingival tissues that are erythematous, edematous, and subject to bleeding at slight irritation.

Management is directed toward prevention by conscientious daily oral care: brushing and flossing after meals to deprive the bacteria of the substrates required to produce the disease. The implementation and maintenance of preventive dental practices, including the use of fluoride, are effective in preventing both caries and periodontal disease.

Nursing Care Management

Nursing care of the child with periodontal disease is primarily supportive; it includes education regarding dental hygiene and regular inspection of the gingival tissues for signs of early inflammation. Advise the child to see the dentist at any sign of oral pain, inflammation, or irritation.

MALOCCLUSION

When teeth of the upper and lower dental arches do not approximate in the proper relationships, the physiologic function of mastication is less effective, and the cosmetic effect is less pleasing. Teeth that are uneven, crowded, or overlapping or are otherwise unable to meet their opponents in the opposite jaw in the appropriate relationships may be predisposed to dental disease. More than half of children 12 to 17 years of age suffer from malocclusions that could be corrected with professional dental care.

The most common cause of malocclusion is hereditary factors, but abnormal growth and habits such as thumb sucking and tongue thrusting also contribute to the disordered alignment and occlusion of the teeth. Treatment of malocclusion includes eliminating habits that aggravate the deformity and initiating corrective therapy at the optimum time. Orthodontic treatment is usually most successful when it is started in the later school-age years or the early adolescent years, after the last primary teeth have been shed and before growth ceases. However, because some deformities can be corrected at an earlier age, referral should be made as soon as malocclusion is evident. Rather than waiting until later in childhood, early removal of "extra" or impacted teeth or provision of a prosthetic tooth or retainer by a dentist or orthodontist can often prevent problems from developing.

Nursing Care Management

Malocclusions and missing teeth can have adverse effects on a child's self-esteem and body image. Many children with severe malocclusion are teased by their peers or siblings, causing both psychologic and physical stress to affected children. The nurse who detects malocclusion is obligated to recommend that the teeth be examined by a dentist. The sooner the child is evaluated, the sooner treatment can begin. Orthodontic treatment averages 16 to 30 months, with frequent visits, usually scheduled every 3 to 6 weeks, to the orthodontist who monitors the progress. When fixed appliances or orthodontic braces are applied or adjusted during the treatment of malocclusion, the child should be advised that there will be discomfort for a few days. Use of mild analgesia medications and a soft diet are usually recommended during this period. Although the bands or brackets protect the teeth they cover, plaque can collect on the unprotected surfaces or under loose-fitting bands, so proper oral hygiene is vital. Some orthodontists recommend using an oral irrigating device to remove food from between the teeth and around the braces. However, the device does not remove plaque and is not a substitute for thorough brushing. Forbidden foods during orthodontic treatment typically include chewing gum, ice, nuts, hard candy, corn on the cob, uncut apples, hard taco shells, nachos, and popcorn because they may damage braces or dental appliances or be difficult to remove from the teeth during cleaning.

Occasionally, tooth movement or poking at the braces with a pencil or other object may cause an arch wire to break or protrude. If this happens, cover the broken wire with dental wax (provided by the dentist) and schedule an appointment with the orthodontist as soon as possible. After the braces are taken off, a removable or permanent retainer is used to maintain the desired position of the teeth. Placement of a permanent wire behind the front teeth may also be used to prevent recurrence of malocclusion until the child is fully matured.

Sometimes children need considerable reinforcement for compliance with orthodontic treatment. It may be difficult for some to value the long-term result of the treatment compared with the present-day discomfort, inconvenience, and embarrassment of wearing braces or a fixed dental appliance. Early adolescents with a heightened awareness of body image and physical attractiveness are especially at risk for noncompliance in maintaining their routine appointments and abiding by the recommendations for bands and hygienic practices while wearing orthodontics.

TRAUMA

Dental injury is common in childhood. Most injuries occur after bicycle accidents, playground mishaps, or sports and athletic activities and include fractures of varying degrees of severity, including chipping, dislocation, or avulsion. Trauma usually involves the maxillary incisors. Children with protruding teeth, craniofacial abnormalities, or neuromuscular disorders are more likely to sustain dental injuries. All tooth injuries require prompt treatment by a dentist to prevent permanent displacement or loss of the tooth or infection.

Nursing Care Management: Tooth Avulsion

A permanent tooth that is avulsed (exarticulated, or "knocked out") should be reimplanted by the child, adult caregiver, or nurse and stabilized as soon as possible so that the blood supply to the tooth can be reestablished and the tooth kept alive (see Emergency Treatment box). If the avulsed tooth is replaced within 1 hour of the injury, there is a better chance of full recovery (Tinanoff, 2016). Avulsed primary teeth are usually not reimplanted.

EMERGENCY TREATMENT

Avulsed Tooth

1. Recover tooth.
2. Hold tooth by crown; avoid touching root area.
3. If tooth is dirty, rinse it gently under running water or saline; be sure to insert stopper in sink or basin (to avoid losing the tooth) and do not scrub the tooth.
4. Insert tooth into gingiva socket.
5. Have child hold tooth in place with tongue or clean finger.
6. Transport child to dentist immediately.
7. Avoid sudden stops or sharp turns to prevent dislodging tooth.

After reimplantation, the tooth usually becomes firmly attached, although endodontic therapy may be required. If permanent reimplantation is not successful, the tooth may be retained anywhere from 6 months to 12 years, which facilitates normal dental growth, development, and occlusion.

All mouth trauma, including tooth avulsion, causes a large amount of bleeding due to the vascularity of the tissues. The bleeding can be frightening to children and their families. The nurse should be prepared to effectively manage the emotionality that accompanies tooth avulsion, while also controlling bleeding, pain, and reimplantation of a tooth. Using a calm, confident, and reassuring approach toward the child and caregivers is often successful in reducing anxiety and ensuring an injury to a tooth or mouth is effectively managed.

DISORDERS OF CONTINENCE

ENURESIS

Enuresis (bed-wetting) is a common and troublesome disorder that is defined as intentional or involuntary passage of urine in children who are beyond the age when voluntary bladder control should normally have been acquired. Medical evaluation is recommended when inappropriate voiding of urine occurs at least twice a week for a minimum of 3 consecutive months in a child with the chronologic or developmental age of at least 5 years (Sinha & Raut, 2016). In addition, the urinary incontinence must not be related to the direct physiologic effects of a medication (e.g., diuretics) or a general medical condition (e.g., diabetes mellitus or diabetes insipidus, spina bifida, or seizure disorder). Enuresis is more common in boys (Sinha & Raut, 2016). Enuresis occurs in approximately 20% of children 5 years of age, 10% of children 8 years of age, and 3% of children 12 years of age (Caldwell, Sureshkumar, & Wong, 2016; Sinha & Raut, 2016). If untreated, enuresis can persist into adulthood.

Enuresis can also be defined as **primary** (bed-wetting in children who have never been dry for extended periods) or **secondary** (the onset of wetting after a period of established urinary continence). The passage of urine may occur only during nighttime sleep, with the child remaining dry during the day (monosymptomatic), or it may be nonmonosymptomatic, where the child has daytime urinary urgency and an occasional daytime incontinence in conjunction with other conditions such as emotional stressors (Elder, 2016). Although most children with enuresis do not have coexisting psychopathology, medical evaluation is recommended. Spontaneous recovery occurs in 14% of children (Arda, Cakiroglu, & Thomas, 2016).

Enuresis can cause serious psychologic problems in affected children. The degree of psychologic effect may be related to the impact of enuresis on the child's social life—for example, not being able to attend overnight camps, school field trips, or "sleep-over" parties with peers. Adolescents with enuresis have described themselves as being anxious or tense, having difficulty sleeping, and having bad dreams; many delay or avoid treatment, believing they will eventually "grow out of it." Children with enuresis may have significant stress and anxiety in the home environment if parental response to the disorder is harsh or punitive and often demonstrate low self-esteem. In some instances, enuresis may serve as a trigger for child abuse. Although behavior problems can be associated with these psychologic effects, adults who were successfully treated for enuresis as children have normal psychologic, social, and academic profiles.

Etiology and Pathophysiology

No clear etiology for enuresis has been determined. However, several factors and theories are associated with enuresis. There is a high concordance rate of enuresis in monozygotic (identical) twins and an even higher one in dizygotic (nonidentical) twins. Additionally, up to 77% of children develop enuresis if both parents were enuretic (Sinha & Raut, 2016). Emotional factors may influence enuresis. Some children exhibit temporary regressive behavior resulting in enuresis after family events such as the birth of a sibling or divorce of parents. Other children, such as those with attention-deficit/hyperactivity disorder (ADHD), may have occasional "accidents" when they become so involved in play that they are unaware of a full bladder or "forget" to empty the bladder. In other children enuresis may be related to attempts to toilet train before they are developmentally mature enough to maintain bladder control, the emotional atmosphere surrounding the training situation, or an excessive amount of emotional dependence on the caregiver.

Several additional theories have been proposed to explain enuresis. The *sleep theory* stems from parental reports that these children sleep more soundly and are difficult to arouse from sleep. The *functional bladder capacity theory* suggests that the volume of urine voided after maximum delay of micturition. Another theory suggests that the kidneys of these children fail to concentrate urine during sleep because of insufficient secretion of antidiuretic hormone (ADH). The ADH circadian rhythm may thus be a significant biologic marker in enuresis (Arda, Cakiroglu, & Thomas, 2016). The *dysfunctional detrusor activity theory* suggests that an unstable bladder detrusor muscle spontaneously contracts to produce bed-wetting, either because of abnormal innervation or as a result of other, unknown reasons (Arda, Cakiroglu, & Thomas, 2016). Emotional factors may influence the symptom. Some children exhibit temporary regressive behavior resulting in enuresis after the birth of a sibling or other trauma. Occasionally enuresis can be a behavioral manifestation of a personality disorder.

Clinical Manifestations

The predominant symptom of enuresis is immediate urgency that is accompanied by acute discomfort, restlessness, and sometimes urinary frequency. With nocturnal enuresis, the child may or may not feel urgency. If awareness of the urgency is present, the child often reports difficulty awakening to urinate. Spontaneous voiding during sleep occurs, which usually results in multiple nightly incidents. Spontaneous remission of nocturnal enuresis occurs in approximately 15% of cases. However, in some cases nocturnal enuresis continues into adolescence and adulthood.

Diagnostic Evaluation

During the initial phases of evaluation, a routine physical examination is performed to rule out physical causes. These include urinary tract infection, structural disorders of the urinary tract, neurologic deficits, disorders that increase the normal output of urine (e.g., diabetes mellitus and diabetes insipidus), and disorders that impair the concentrating ability of the kidneys (e.g., chronic renal failure). If psychologic difficulties are evident or a personality disorder is suspected, a routine psychiatric evaluation is warranted.

A detailed history of voiding and bowel habits is obtained, including information about the toilet training process. Assess parental attitudes by listening and asking parents how they have attempted to cope with the bed-wetting. An important feature of assessment is a baseline count of enuretic incidents and the time of day when each occurs. This is necessary not only to establish diagnostic reliability but also to confirm outcome success after treatment. It usually consists of a chart or calendar given to the family on which they indicate the date of the incident, the time of the incident, and the approximate volume of the urinary output.

The physical examination may be followed by diagnostic evaluation of functional bladder capacity. Functional bladder capacity is determined by having the child hold off voiding until the strongest urgency is felt, at which time the child voids into a measurement container. Normal bladder capacity (in ounces) is the child's age plus 2 (up to 14 years of age); therefore normal bladder capacity for a 6-year-old is 8 ounces (237 ml). A bladder volume of 10 to 12 ounces (300 to 350 ml) is sufficient for retention of a night's urine.

Therapeutic Management

Enuresis has been treated in several ways. No single method has achieved universal endorsement, and more than one technique is often employed by families coping with enuresis. Therapeutic techniques used to manage nocturnal enuresis include medications, complementary and alternative medicine techniques, such as hypnotherapy, restriction or elimination of fluids after the evening meal, avoidance of caffeinated and sugar-containing beverages after 4 PM, purposeful interruption of sleep to void, and motivational therapy. In approximately 14% to 16% of cases, a spontaneous decrease in bed-wetting occurs irrespective of the treatments used (Sinha & Raut, 2016). Successful treatment is defined as a specified period of dry nights, varying from 7 to 28 consecutive nights.

Initial treatment consists of behavioral therapy such as a reward system, retention control training, and a waking schedule treatment. A star chart for every dry night with a reward after a preset number of stars have been earned is an example of a reward system, providing rewards to the child for the desired behavior. Retention control training was developed after the observation of reduced functional bladder capacity in children who were bed-wetters. The child drinks fluids while awake and alert, then delays urination as long as can be tolerated to stretch the bladder to accommodate increasingly larger volumes of urine. The use of Kegel or pelvic muscle exercises may be helpful in children with daytime enuresis. In the waking schedule treatment, the child is awakened during the night at intervals to void. This method has been successful in reducing, but not eliminating, bed-wetting incidents.

Conditioning therapy involves training the child to awaken to urinate after a stimulus is given, such as an urine alarm. The device contains a moisture-sensitive wire pad that is placed inside the underpants and is attached to a bell or buzzer. When the system detects moisture, the bell or buzzer sounds, which fully awakens the child. The child is thus conditioned to awaken at the initiation of micturition or to the stimulus of the bell or buzzer and eventually learns to continue voiding in the toilet. The urine alarm can be very effective after a period of at least 6 to 8 weeks, but children may relapse once they stop using it (Arda, Cakiroglu, & Thomas, 2016). Relapse is addressed by reinstituting the alarm during sleep. This method is inexpensive compared with drug therapy and has no side effects.

Drug therapy is increasingly being prescribed to treat enuresis; however, drugs are considered second-line management for enuresis. Parents should be cautioned not to think that these agents will cure the condition and should also be advised of the drug's side effects (Elder, 2016). Desmopressin, anticholinergic therapy, and imipramine are common medications used in the treatment of enuresis. The selection depends on the interpretation of the cause.

Desmopressin acetate is a synthetic analog of antidiuretic hormone, which reduces nighttime urinary output. Desmopressin acetate is available in tablet form and is the preferred method of delivery. In the past, the medication was delivered in a nasal spray but this formulation caused hyponatremia and seizures and is no longer recommended (Elder, 2016). Response to therapy has been noted to be as high as 70% but the medication must tapered off because sudden discontinuation has a high relapse rate (Arda, Cakiroglu, & Thomas, 2016).

Anticholinergic drugs are indicated for children with an overactive bladder or a poor response to desmopressin. These medications reduce uninhibited bladder contractions and may be helpful for children with daytime urinary frequency. Oxybutynin is a commonly prescribed anticholinergic medication.

A third-line medication is imipramine, a tricyclic antidepressant that exerts an anticholinergic action in the bladder to inhibit urination. The dosage and time of administration are individualized, and the drug is given in amounts sufficient to lighten sleep but not to cause wakefulness. The medication is cardiotoxic at high doses causing death from cardiotoxicity; therefore this medication is not used for front-line treatment and parents are cautioned about safe use and keeping the medication out of reach of other children (Arda, Cakiroglu, & Thomas, 2016). The suggested length of treatment is delivered over 4 to 6 months, followed by a gradual withdrawal over at least 4 weeks to prevent relapse.

Other therapies and treatment options include stream interruption training, overlearning, fluid restriction, and self-monitoring (motivation therapy). Frequently these therapies are coupled with other treatment modalities. Counseling may be beneficial in helping the child, and sometimes the family, adjust to the bed-wetting.

It is imperative that punishment not be used to correct enuresis. Supportive therapy such as teaching the child to change soiled pajamas and bed linens and restriction of fluid intake (especially those containing caffeine) before bedtime should be used instead. Social reinforcement can also be used to enhance the rewards for success. Positive reinforcement in the form of keeping diaries to record dry nights has also been effective in fostering motivation in children.

Nursing Care Management

No matter what therapeutic methods are used, the nurse can support both children and parents who are coping with the problem of enuresis, the treatment plan, and the difficulties they may encounter in the process. Both need encouragement and patience. The problem is discussed with both the parent and the child because any treatment involves and requires the child's active participation. In some treatment interventions the child is in charge of the intervention; therefore parents must learn to support the child rather than intervene themselves. Parents should also be taught to observe for side effects of any medications used. Parents should encourage the child to maintain a regular bowel evacuation regimen; constipation can contribute to nocturnal enuresis (Elder, 2016). A calendar with wet and dry nights may be helpful to motivate the child to stay dry and maintain a positive perspective on the problem.

Many parents believe that enuresis is caused by a fear that they have somehow produced the situation by improper childrearing practices. They need reassurance that the bed-wetting does not represent willful misbehavior. Parents need to understand that punishment such as scolding, shaming, and threatening is contraindicated because of their negative emotional impact and limited success in reducing the behavior. Encourage parents to be patient and understanding and to communicate love and support to the child.

Communication with children is directed toward eliminating the emotional impact of the problem; relieving feelings of shame, guilt, and the burden of parental disapproval; building self-confidence; and motivating them toward independent control. More important, the nurse can provide consistent support and encouragement to help children through the inconsistent and unpredictable treatment process. Children need to believe that they are helping themselves and to maintain feelings of confidence and hope.

ENCOPRESIS

Encopresis is repeated voluntary or involuntary passage of feces of normal or near-normal consistency in places not appropriate for that purpose according to the individual's own sociocultural setting. The event must occur at least once a month for a minimum of 3 months, and the child's chronologic or developmental age must be at least 4 years (Fiorino & Liacouras, 2016). The fecal incontinence must not be caused by physiologic effects of a substance (e.g., laxatives) or a general medical condition except through a mechanism involving constipation. The consistency of the stool may vary from normal to liquid, with a more liquid stool seen especially in individuals who have overflow incontinence secondary to fecal retention.

A child 4 years of age or older who has never achieved fecal continence is said to have primary encopresis. This type is more frequently observed as a result of neglect, lax training methods, mental subnormalities, and familial causes. Secondary encopresis is fecal incontinence occurring in a child over 4 years of age after a period of established fecal continence. The disorder is more common in males than in females.

Etiology

One of the most common causes of encopresis is constipation, which may be precipitated by environmental change, such as having a new sibling, moving to a new house, changing schools, or even having to use new or unfamiliar toilet facilities. Chronic, severe constipation has a tendency to impair the usual movement and contractions of the colon, which can lead to fecal obstruction. Abnormalities in the digestive tract (e.g., Hirschsprung disease, anorectal lesions, malformations, rectal prolapse) and medical conditions (e.g., hypothyroidism, hypokalemia, hypercalcemia, lead intoxication, myelomeningocele, cerebral palsy, muscular dystrophy, irritable bowel syndrome) are also associated with constipation, which can lead to encopresis. Voluntary retention of stool may also follow an incident of painful defecation (e.g., in a child with anal fissures). Involuntary retention may be produced by emotional problems caused by the encopresis, which sets up a fear-pain cycle and results in learned abnormal defecation patterns. Psychogenic encopresis includes soiling caused by emotional problems.

Normally, children and adolescents have one or two soft-formed stools per day. Children with soiling problems tend to form large-bore stools, which are painful to excrete. Therefore they tend to avoid defecation and withhold stooling. Stool held in the rectum and sigmoid colon loses water and progressively hardens, which causes successively more painful bowel movements and a stretched rectal vault. Over time the child will lose the urge to defecate on his or her own (Colombo, Wassom, & Rosen, 2015). A pain-retention-pain cycle is established. Many children have diarrhea or loose leakage in their clothing and pass small amounts of hard stool, which suggests leakage around an impaction.

Children may experience exacerbations with transitions in the school setting. Some reasons for developing retentive tendencies at this time are fear of using school bathrooms, a busy schedule, and the interruption of an established time schedule for bowel evacuation. Children may also react to stress with bowel dysfunction.

Clinical Manifestations

The manifestation of simple constipation is painful expulsion of hard, pellet-like stools. Voluntary retention is usually temporary, with a history of a painful precipitating episode and blood-streaked stools. Involuntary retention is associated with a history of abdominal pain, distention, moodiness, poor appetite, and accumulation of stools with periodic passage of voluminous stools. Children display a characteristic posturing during suppression of colonic signals to defecate—stiffening, standing in a corner with straight legs and a bright red face, "doing a little dance," "crawling," or hiding behind furniture or behind a tree when playing outdoors. They typically hide soiled underwear. It is not unusual for soiling to take place after bathing because of reflex stimulation.

The child with encopresis often feels ashamed and may wish to avoid social situations (e.g., camp or school) that might lead to embarrassment. School performance and attendance are affected as the child's offensive odor becomes a target for scorn and derision by classmates. The child is not well liked by peers and may be severely rejected by the parents as a result of the symptom. Rejection by peers and parents causes further withdrawal and other behavioral manifestations.

Therapeutic Management

Treatment is aimed toward alleviating the cause of the soiling. To determine the cause, a detailed medical history including risk factors (e.g., negative toilet training, child abuse or neglect, fear of bathrooms), comorbid conditions (e.g., attention deficit disorder, cognitive delays, oppositional disorders), and associated symptoms of bowel movements (e.g., retention, overflow soiling, incontinence) are obtained (Mosca & Schatz, 2013). Next, a thorough physical examination, including a rectal examination, is completed. An abdominal x-ray film may be obtained to determine the severity of impaction.

Many children require an extensive and invasive bowel cleansing, to remove the bowel impaction before starting treatment (Colombo, Wassom, & Rosen, 2015). Fecal impaction is relieved by lubricants such as mineral oil; osmotic laxatives such as lactulose or polyethylene glycol (PEG or MiraLax); and magnesium hydroxide. Customary dosages are usually insufficient to produce a therapeutic response. Mineral oil should be avoided in children who have dysphagia or vomiting to prevent risk of aspiration.

Dietary changes are helpful: elimination of milk and dairy products and consumption of increased amounts of high-fiber foods, such as fruits, vegetables, and cereals, as well as increased hydration with water. Behavior therapy is a vital part of the treatment plan and is indicated to eliminate any fear that has developed as a result of painful defecation. Psychotherapeutic intervention with the child and the family may become necessary.

Nursing Care Management

Education regarding the physiology of normal defecation, toilet training as a developmental process, and the treatment outlined for the particular family is a prerequisite to a successful outcome. The regimen prescribed for stimulating elimination is explained to parents. Bowel retraining with mineral oil, a high-fiber diet, and a regular toileting routine is essential in treating encopresis.

The child is typically encouraged to sit on the toilet 10 to 15 minutes after meals for intervals of 10 minutes. Placing a footstool below the feet may relax the abdomen and make the child more comfortable. Enemas may be needed for impactions, but long-term use prevents the child from assuming responsibility for defecation. Initially lubricants are given liberally, but stimulant cathartics often cause abdominal cramps that can frighten the child. Positive reinforcement such as giving stickers, praising the child, and awarding special activities may encourage the child to participate in the bowel regimen.

> **! NURSING ALERT**
>
> A thorough history of the soiling is essential: when soiling began, how often it occurs and under what circumstances, and whether the child uses the toilet successfully at all. Because the parents and child are reluctant to volunteer information, direct questioning about the soiling is more successful.

Family counseling is directed toward reassurance that most problems resolve successfully, although the child may have relapses during periods of stress, such as vacations or illness. If encopresis persists beyond occasional relapses, the condition needs to be reevaluated. Behavior modification techniques are explained, and the family is assisted with a plan suited to the particular situation.

DISORDERS WITH BEHAVIORAL COMPONENTS

Attention-Deficit/Hyperactivity Disorder

Attention-deficit/hyperactivity disorder (ADHD) refers to developmentally inappropriate degrees of inattention, impulsiveness, and hyperactivity (American Psychiatric Association, 2013). It is a common neurobehavioral disorder of childhood, affecting 11% of school-age children, and often persists into adulthood (Children and Adults with Attention-Deficit/Hyperactivity Disorder, 2017). Prevalence rates for ADHD vary depending on whether they are based on school samples or community samples. Parent-reported data have been used to monitor the number of children with ADHD; however, there is limited evidence about the validity of these reports as an indicator of a medical diagnosis (Centers for Disease Control and Prevention, 2016). ADHD is seen more frequently in boys than in girls. The symptoms of ADHD were first recognized in the early 1900s. Several different names have been applied to the disorder. According to the *Diagnostic and Statistical Manual of Mental Disorders, Fifth Edition* (DSM-5), there are two acknowledged dimensions of ADHD: hyperactivity/impulsivity (HI), represented by symptoms of poor impulse control, difficulty sitting still, and fidgeting or squirming; and inattention (IA), represented by symptoms including difficulty sustaining attention, carelessness, and disorganization.

Individuals with ADHD can be very successful in life. However, without identification and proper treatment, ADHD may have serious consequences, including school failure, family stress and disruption, depression, problems with relationships, substance abuse, delinquency, accidental injuries, and job failure (Children and Adults with Attention-Deficit/Hyperactivity Disorder, 2017). Difficulties associated with ADHD are most often school related or academic. Children with ADHD are at greater risk for conduct disorders, oppositional defiant disorders, depression, anxiety disorders, and developmental disorders such as speech and language delays and learning disabilities than are children without ADHD (American Academy of Pediatrics, 2016b).

Early identification of affected children is important because the characteristics of ADHD significantly interfere with the normal course of emotional and psychologic development. Some researchers suggest that poor academic, social, and behavioral outcomes are directly related to ADHD; others propose poor outcomes are predicted by co-occurring psychiatric disorders. Therefore in the evaluation of a child for ADHD, the health care provider should assess for coexisting conditions such as emotional or behavioral (e.g., anxiety, depressive, oppositional defiant, and conduct disorders), developmental (e.g., learning and language disorders or other neurodevelopmental disorders), and physical (e.g., tics, sleep apnea) conditions.

Etiology

The exact cause of ADHD is unknown. A combination of organic, genetic, and environmental factors is probably involved. A variety of factors put a child at risk for symptoms of ADHD, including a family history of ADHD. Parents with ADHD have more than 50% chance of having a child with ADHD (American Academy of Pediatrics, 2016b). Other risk factors include exposure to toxins or medications, perinatal complications, infectious diseases, such as Lyme disease and pediatric autoimmune neuropsychiatric disorder associated with streptococcus (PANDAS), and head trauma.

Some children may have an absence or insufficiency of norepinephrine, dopamine, or serotonin. These neurotransmitters normally occur in high concentrations in the brain and affect activity level, mood, and awareness. It is hypothesized that children who lack these neurotransmitters experience learning difficulties in reading, math, and language and are prone to impulsivity. The dopamine system is exquisitely sensitive to hypoxia, particularly in the fetus or infant. Thus any prenatal or postnatal disruption of the flow of blood or oxygen to the brain might set the stage for later ADHD behaviors. Support for a neurochemical etiology is suggested by the fact that many children with ADHD respond to medications that affect the central nervous system. Many of these children respond to psychostimulants such as methylphenidate hydrochloride, which increases dopamine and norepinephrine levels (American Academy of Pediatrics, 2016b).

Another *neurochemical theory* suggests that symptoms result from an excess of norepinephrine and/or an alteration in the reticular activating system of the midbrain, an area that controls consciousness and attention. This excess or abnormality interferes with the function of filtering out extraneous stimuli. Consequently, children are unable to focus on one stimulus and are compelled to respond to every stimulus in the environment. They demonstrate hyperactive behaviors that result from cognitive "flooding" and exaggerated arousal that overwhelms the attention filters and overrides inhibitory processes. Other theories maintain that symptoms of ADHD result from dysfunction in the brain circuits of the behavioral inhibition system; structural abnormalities in the prefrontal cortex, caudate, and thalamus; and a gene variant known to code for a receptor for dopamine.

Interest in *diet as a factor* in hyperactivity continues to generate controversy. For years, healthcare providers have speculated that certain foods may correlate with ADHD. However this theory has not been validated by empirical studies. Nevertheless, some children do have worse ADHD symptoms when certain foods are consumed. Some believe that the observed behavior patterns are related to an innate sensitivity to food items such as sucrose or food additives such as aspartame.

The role that environmental factors play in ADHD should not be minimized. Early psychosocial deprivation, such as children who are raised in institutions, can result in ADHD symptoms in later childhood, including increased rates of attention deficit and hyperactivity (Kennedy, Kreppner, Knights, et al., 2016).

Clinical Manifestations

The behaviors exhibited by the child with ADHD are not unusual aspects of child behavior. The difference lies in the quality of motor activity and the developmentally inappropriate inattention, impulsivity, and hyperactivity that the child displays; the degree of severity is highly variable (Parker & Corkum, 2016). The manifestations may be numerous or few, mild or severe, and vary with the child's developmental level. Mild manifestations of the symptoms are apparent in at least two settings, usually educational and family environments. Every child with ADHD is different from all other children with ADHD (American Psychiatric Association, 2013).

BOX 16.5 Clinical Characteristics of Attention-Deficit/Hyperactivity Disorder

Inattentive type—six or more symptoms (or five for people over 17 years) must be present for at least 6 months:

- Does not pay close attention to details or makes careless mistakes in school or job tasks.
- Has problems staying focused on tasks or activities, such as lectures, conversations, or long reading.
- Does not appear to listen when spoken to (i.e., seems to be elsewhere).
- Does not follow through on instructions and does not complete schoolwork, chores, or job duties (may start tasks but quickly loses focus).
- Has problems organizing tasks and work (i.e., does not manage time well; has messy, disorganized work; misses deadlines).
- Avoids or dislikes tasks that require sustained mental effort (i.e., preparing reports, completing forms).
- Often loses things needed for tasks or daily life (i.e., school papers, books, keys, wallet, cell phone, eyeglasses).
- Is easily distracted.
- Forgets daily tasks, such as doing chores and running errands. Older teens and adults may forget to return phone calls, pay bills, and keep appointments.

Hyperactive/impulsive type—six symptoms (or five for people over 17 years) must be present for at least the past 6 months:

- Fidgets with or taps hands or feet, or squirms in seat.
- Not able to stay seated (in classroom, workplace).
- Runs about or climbs where it is inappropriate.
- Unable to play or do leisure activities quietly.
- Always "on the go," as if driven by a motor.
- Talks too much.
- Blurts out an answer before a question has been finished (i.e., finishes people's sentences, can't wait to speak in conversations).
- Has difficulty waiting his or her turn while waiting in a line.
- Interrupts or intrudes on others (i.e., cuts into conversations, games or activities, starts using other people's things without permission). Older teens and adults may take over what others are doing.

Children diagnosed with ADHD demonstrate a persistent pattern of inattention and/or hyperactivity-impulsivity that interferes with functioning or development. Box 16.5 lists the clinical characteristics of individuals with inattention and hyperactivity and impulsivity. The diagnosis is made when six or more of the symptoms (five symptoms required for individuals 17 years of age and older) are present to a degree that is inconsistent with developmental level for a minimum of 6 months; occur before 12 years of age; are present in two or more settings; and negatively affect social and academic/occupational activities (American Psychiatric Association, 2013). The symptoms are not solely a manifestation of oppositional behavior, defiance, hostility, or failure to understand tasks or instructions. In addition, symptoms do not occur during the course of schizophrenia or another psychotic disorder and are not better explained by another mental disorder (e.g., mood disorder, anxiety disorder, dissociative disorder, personality disorder, substance intoxication or withdrawal).

Most behavioral manifestations are apparent at an early age, but the learning disabilities may not become evident until the child enters school. A major clinical manifestation is distractibility. The stimuli may come from external sources or internal sources. Children frequently demonstrate immaturity relative to chronologic age. Selective attention is often seen, in which the child has difficulty attending to "nonpreferred" tasks, such as completing chores or finishing homework. The child may not consider the consequences of behavior, may take excessive physical risks (often beginning early in life), and may demonstrate inappropriate social skills.

There is also an increased incidence of comorbid disorders, such as oppositional defiant disorder, mood and anxiety disorders, and learning disabilities, in children diagnosed with ADHD (Parker & Corkum, 2016). Furthermore, substance abuse and antisocial personality disorders are common in families of children with ADHD.

Course of ADHD

ADHD is relatively stable throughout early adolescence for most children. Some children experience decreased symptoms during adolescence and adulthood, but a significant number of these children carry symptoms into adulthood. The goal for children with ADHD who have any learning disabilities is to help them identify areas of weakness and learn to compensate for them.

Diagnostic Evaluation

There is no single diagnostic test for ADHD. It is important to emphasize the need for a complete and thorough multidisciplinary evaluation of the child, incorporating the efforts of the primary pediatric health care provider and the family, as well as possible support from a psychologist, developmental pediatrician, neurologist, pediatric nurses, classroom teachers, and administrators. Health care providers must first determine whether the child's behavior is age appropriate or related to a psychiatric disorder.

Before diagnosis, a complete medical and developmental history is obtained. Detailed descriptions of the child's behavior in the home, in school, and in social situations are also obtained from as many observers of the child as possible, particularly from the parents and teachers involved in the child's care.

A physical examination, including vision and hearing screening and a detailed neurologic evaluation, is completed. Psychologic testing, especially projective tests, is used to identify visual-perceptual difficulties, problems with spatial organization, and other phenomena that suggest cortical or diencephalic involvement, and it helps identify the child's intelligence and achievement levels.

Behavioral checklists and adaptive scales should be completed by the child's caregivers and educators and scored by the primary care provider. Samples of these tools can be found at the Children and Adults with ADHD website: http://www.chadd.org/Understanding-ADHD/For-Professionals/For-Healthcare-Professionals/Clinical-Practice-Tools/Evaluation-and-Assessment-Tools.aspx. The assessment tools are also helpful in measuring social adaptive functioning and behavioral concerns in children with ADHD, as well as providing benchmarks for evaluation of improved or worsening behavioral changes once therapy has begun. Psychiatric disorders, medical problems, and traumatic experiences are ruled out, including lead poisoning, seizures, partial hearing loss, psychosis, and witnessing of sexual activity and/or violence.

Therapeutic Management

Treatment of ADHD depends on the child's age and severity of symptoms. Evidence supports behavioral therapy as the first-line treatment, but other approaches include family education and counseling, medications, environmental manipulation, and psychotherapy for the child. The most effective treatment approach is multimodal (Antai-Otong & Zimmerman, 2016).

Behavior Therapy and Psychotherapy

Behavior therapy focuses on the prevention of undesired behaviors. Families are helped to identify new appropriate contingencies and reward systems to meet the child's developing needs. They may also receive instruction in parenting skills, such as delivering positive reinforcement, rewarding small increments of desired behaviors, and providing age-appropriate consequences (e.g., time-out, response cost). Through collaborative teamwork, parents learn techniques to help the child become more successful at home and in school.

Pharmacologic Therapy

The most effective and most frequently used medications are stimulants: methylphenidate and dextroamphetamine (Weyandt, Marraccini, Gudmundsdottir, et al., 2014). Nonstimulant medications, including norepinephrine reuptake inhibitors and adrenergic agonists, have also shown to be effective with fewer side effects in school-age and adolescent children (American Academy of Pediatrics, 2016b; Weyandt, Marraccini, Gudmundsdottir, et al., 2014). Children are given a small dosage initially, and the dosage is gradually increased until the desired response is achieved. Children who receive stimulants should be monitored carefully for side effects of medication: appetite loss, abdominal pain, headaches, sleep disturbances, and growth velocity. Stimulants are avoided in children who have a history of tic-like behaviors, a family history of Tourette syndrome (TS), or ADHD combined with TS because these medications may exaggerate tics. Other medications, including tricyclic antidepressants and extended-release clonidine, may be used as adjunct therapy for ADHD, primarily for children with coexisting conditions such as sleep disturbances (American Academy of Pediatrics, 2011).

For preschool-age children (4 to 5 years of age), behavior therapy is the first line of treatment. Methylphenidate may be prescribed if behavior interventions do not provide significant improvement and there is moderate to severe continuing disturbance in the child's function. In areas where evidence-based behavioral treatments are not available, the health care provider weighs the risks of starting medication at an early age with the harm of delaying treatment (American Academy of Pediatrics, 2011).

Elementary school–age children (6 to 11 years of age) receive a US Food and Drug Administration–approved medication and/or evidence-based parent and teacher-administered behavior therapy as treatment for ADHD, preferably both. The evidence is particularly strong for stimulant medications and less strong but sufficient for atomoxetine, extended-release guanfacine, and extended-release clonidine (in that order). Assistance in the school environment is a part of all treatment plans (American Academy of Pediatrics, 2011).

For adolescents (12 to 18 years of age), a US Food and Drug Administration–approved medications is prescribed with the assent of the adolescent and/or behavior therapy as treatment for ADHD, preferably both (American Academy of Pediatrics, 2011).

Regularly scheduled reevaluation of the child is essential with all of these medications to determine medication effectiveness, detect and evaluate any side effects, monitor development and health status (especially growth and blood pressure), and assess family and social status. The pediatric quality indicator for follow up care for children prescribed with ADHD medication is listed in Table 16.2.

TABLE 16.2 Pediatric Quality Indicator: Children on ADHD Medications*

Follow-Up Care for Children Prescribed ADHD Medications	
Measure	Children 6-12 years of age who were given a prescription of ADHD medication had at least two follow-up visits within 270 days including one visit within 30 days after starting the medication.
Numerator	Number of children who had at least one face-to-face visit with a practitioner with prescribing authority within 30 days after starting the medication during the measurement time.
Denominator	Number of children who were dispensed an ADHD medication during the intake period and who had a visit during the measurement period.

*Endorsed by the National Quality Forum-0108 and Center for Medicare and Medicaid Services-146v1.
ADHD, Attention-deficit/hyperactivity disorder.

Nursing Care Management

It has long been recognized that appropriately educated nurses can assist in the management of ADHD. Nurses, especially school nurses, are active participants in all aspects of management of the child with ADHD. Nurses in the community setting work with families in the home on a long-term basis to help plan and implement therapeutic regimens and to evaluate the effectiveness of therapy. They coordinate services and serve as a liaison between health and education professionals directly involved in the child's therapy program. School nurses understand the child's special needs and work with teachers. Nurses in any setting (e.g., community, school, hospital, practitioner's office) provide support and guidance to children and families during the difficult experience of growing up with a disabling condition and assist in providing education and supportive resources.

To some parents, a diagnosis of ADHD is confirmation of the fear that their child has some irreversible, serious disease; to others it is a relief. All need the opportunity to vent their feelings and suspicions. It is important that they understand that the therapy is not necessarily a panacea and that it will extend over a long period. This has particular significance for changes they need to make in environmental management. Reading material to help the child and family is available from a variety of sources. Resources the nurse may suggest are the National Resource Center for ADHD (http://www.help4adhd.org) and the Centers for Disease Control and Prevention ADHD resource guide available at http://www.cdc.gov/features/adhdresources/.

> **! NURSING ALERT**
>
> Parents need information about the prognosis and an understanding of the treatment plan. The greater their understanding of the disorder and its effects, the more likely they will be to carry out the recommended program of therapy.

Paidipati and Deatrick (2015) describe family phenomena across multiple disciplines in ADHD research. The findings of this review highlight the importance of the intersection between family phenomena and ADHD youth. The four major themes that emerged are related to family stress and strain, parenting practices and caregiver health, family relationships, and family processes related to ADHD management. Priorities in the management of a family with ADHD include addressing issues of parental knowledge, decision making, treatment plans, neurobiologic views of ADHD, behavioral management, advocacy, and sibling and marital relationships. Positive family relationships may facilitate or enhance clinical outcomes whereas tenuous relationships may impede or inhibit the effectiveness of ADHD treatment (Paidipati & Deatrick, 2015).

Medication

Two forms of stimulant medications are available: (1) short-acting medications that are immediate release and require administration throughout the day; and (2) intermediate-acting or long-acting medications that are extended release and are administered once a day, usually in the morning. Because the symptoms of ADHD do not disappear on weekends or during vacations, continuous medication may provide therapy that allows them not only to succeed in school but also to function successfully in other social situations and to develop a positive self-image.

Many school-age children take their short-acting medication at home in the morning before going to school and at lunchtime in the school health suite. Both parents and school nurses should be sensitive to the issue of peer stigma and children's feelings about taking these medications at school.

Parents need to be informed of the possible side effects of medications. The use of caffeine decreases the efficacy of these drugs, and insulin requirements for children with diabetes may also be altered. If decreased appetite is a concern, giving the psychostimulants with or after meals rather than before, encouraging consumption of nutritious snacks in the evening when the effects of the medication are decreasing, and serving frequent small meals with healthy "on-the-go" snacks are helpful interventions. Sleeplessness is reduced by administering medication early in the day and using the minimal effective dosages.

The issue of stimulants and their relationship to growth suppression is another area of concern for parents. Long-term use of dextroamphetamine may result in suppression of growth. Nurses monitor growth closely and provide information on the child's growth, as well as discuss options for diet and nutrition to the child and caregivers.

Parents often express concern that their child will become addicted to the psychostimulants or the antidepressant drugs. Both types of drugs have the potential for abuse, and all children taking these drugs should be monitored closely for psychologic dependence, tolerance, depression, and other adverse behavior changes or idiosyncratic effects. A potential exists for misuse and dependence with stimulant medications due to the pharmacologic action on neurotransmission. The level of misuse of prescribed stimulants is increasing. Adolescents with ADHD may misuse their medication to augment cognitive function for academic purposes. Nurses must explore this potential with their patients and caution parents to keep these drugs safely stored.

Environmental Manipulation

Encourage families to learn how to modify the environment to allow the child to be more successful. Consistency is especially important for children with ADHD. Consistency between families and teachers in terms of reinforcing the same goals is essential. Fostering improved organizational skills requires a more highly structured environment than most children need. The child should be encouraged to make more appropriate choices and to take responsibility for his or her actions.

Other helpful interventions include teaching parents how to make organizational charts (e.g., listing all activities that must be performed before leaving for school), suggesting how to decrease distractions in the environment while the child is completing homework (e.g., turning off the TV, having a consistent study area equipped with needed supplies), and helping parents understand ways to model positive behaviors and problem solving. The focus is on strategies to help the child succeed and cope with deficits while emphasizing strengths.

Appropriate Classroom Placement

Children with ADHD need an orderly, predictable, and consistent classroom environment with clear and consistent rules. Homework and classroom assignments may need to be reduced, and more time may need to be allotted to allow the child to complete tests. Verbal instructions should be accompanied by visual references such as written instructions on the chalkboard. Schedules may need to be arranged so that academic subjects are taught in the morning when the child is experiencing the effects of the morning dose of medication. Low-interest and high-interest classroom activities should be intermingled to maintain the child's attention. Regular and frequent breaks in activity are helpful because sitting in one place for an extended period of time may be difficult. Computers are helpful for children who have difficulty with written assignments and fine motor skills.

If learning disabilities exist, special training activities may be accomplished in self-contained classes limited to six to eight children, in special resource rooms with equipment and teaching teams, by mobile consultants who move from room to room to provide assistance to teachers and children, and in special first-grade programs in which high-risk children receive special attention to prevent or reduce the need for services as they progress. The purpose of programs for children with special learning disabilities is to assist them toward more successful achievement, personal adjustment, and retention in the regular classroom. Under the law students are provided with these services under the designation of an Individualized Educational Plan (IEP) or a 504 Plan. The IEP is a program to ensure that children with disabilities receive specialized instruction and related services while attending an elementary or secondary educational institution. The 504 Plan assures accommodations to children with disabilities to promote their academic success and access to the learning environment while attending an elementary or secondary educational institution. According to Public Law 94-142, the Education for All Handicapped Children Act, children with learning disorders must receive free public education in the least-restrictive environment possible.

Psychiatric, Psychologic, and Social Therapies

Counseling or therapy can be helpful for children who demonstrate signs of anxiety or depression. Therapy can help the child develop a healthier self-esteem and practice problem-solving strategies. The adolescent may benefit from group work focusing on social skill development. Parents of children with ADHD can face a lot of stress, and therapy may be indicated for parents and other family members.

LEARNING DISABILITY

Learning disabilities consist of three characteristics: (1) lower intellectual ability; (2) childhood onset; and (3) significant impairment of social functioning or adaptation (Blows, Teoh, & Paul, 2016). The disabilities are related to communication, reading, writing, and/or learning new things requiring individualized support and resources (Blows, Teoh, & Paul, 2016). The types of disabilities include dyslexia (difficulty with reading, letter reversal), dysgraphia (difficulty with writing), dyscalculia (difficulty with calculation), right-left confusion, and short attention span. Not included are learning problems that result primarily from visual, hearing, or motor disabilities; cognitive impairment; emotional disturbances; or environmental disadvantage.

A comprehensive battery of tests is needed to confirm a learning disability. These include intelligence tests (these children tend to have normal or above-average intelligence); hand-eye coordination tests; and measurements of auditory and visual perception, comprehension, and memory. Often a wide gap exists between verbal and performance scores on intelligence tests.

Therapeutic Management

Nurses must understand which type of learning disability a child has to best provide direction for the child, parents, and teachers. Children with an auditory perceptual deficit appear unable to follow directions or to comprehend large amounts of verbal teaching. These children need to learn with diagrams, pictures, demonstrations, and written lists. Children with a visual perceptual deficit may have difficulty reading, lining up numbers for mathematical operations, or judging distance. These children may have dyslexia and may do better with demonstration and a verbal approach. Children with an integrative deficit may have difficulty sequencing data or storing and retrieving sensory data. Multisensory techniques should be used, and comprehension should be checked frequently throughout instruction. Children with motor deficits may need to use computers in the classroom because their handwriting will not improve. They may need to find alternatives to physical competition that requires coordination of movement. The Learning Disabilities Association of America provides information and support to families who have a child with a learning disability. An online interactive website (www.ldonline.org) is also available for parents, teachers, and children with learning disabilities. Children with learning disorders grow up to be adults with learning disorders. The goal is to help them identify their area of weakness and to compensate for it.

TIC DISORDERS

A **tic** is an involuntary, recurrent, random, rapid, highly stereotyped movement or vocalization (Table 16.3). Approximately 6 cases per 1000, or 300,000 school-age children in the United States, have a tic disorder (Scahill, Specht, & Page, 2014). Boys are affected three times more often than girls (Scahill, Specht, & Page, 2014).

Tics can be simple or complex and can involve eye movements, other motor movements, or vocalizations (Box 16.6). Tics decrease during concentration, are markedly diminished during sleep, and become more exaggerated when the affected children are experiencing stress or excitement. Obsessive-compulsive behaviors in the form of ritualistic activities may also be present and can occur in individuals free of tics. A number of medications can precipitate or exacerbate tics.

Almost all mild, transient tic disorders of childhood are self-limiting and disappear within a few months, usually less than a year. The most common tics involve the eyes, head, and face, and treatment does not affect recovery. Tic disorders can begin at any time during childhood.

TABLE 16.3 Spectrum of Tic Disorders

	Mild (Provisional)	↔	Chronic (Persistent)
Duration	Acute	Subacute	Chronic, persists for more than 1 year since first tic onset
Motor tics	Simple Few	Complex	Obscene gestures Multiple
Vocal tics	None	Noises	Coprolalia
Suppressible	Yes		No

BOX 16.6 Types of Tics

Simple motor—Eye blinking, grimacing, neck jerking, shoulder jerking
Complex motor—Jumping, squatting, stamping the foot, thrusting out the arm, hitting or biting self, ritualistic movements (smelling an object, touching own or another's body, obsessive or compulsive patterns of behavior), grooming behaviors
Simple vocal—Throat clearing, sniffing, grunting, coughing, snorting, lip noises
Complex vocal—Echolalia (repeating last-heard sound, word, or phrase of another), palilalia (repeating own sounds or words), coprolalia (use of socially unacceptable words, often obscene), shouting of words out of context

PANDAS is the abbreviation for *pediatric autoimmune neuropsychiatric disorders associated with streptococcal infections* (National Institute of Mental Health, 2016). The term is used to describe a subset of children and adolescents who have obsessive-compulsive disorder and/or tic disorders and in whom symptoms worsen after strep. The disorder results from postinfectious autoimmunity after a streptococcal infection. Diagnostic criteria for PANDAS are as follows (National Institute of Mental Health, 2016):

- Presence of obsessive-compulsive disorder and/or a tic disorder
- Pediatric onset of symptoms (age 3 years to puberty)
- Episodic course of symptom severity
- Association with group A β-hemolytic streptococcal infection (a positive throat culture for strep or history of scarlet fever)
- Association with neurologic abnormalities (motoric hyperactivity or adventitious movements, such as choreiform movements)

Motor or vocal tics are considered chronic if they persist for longer than 1 year. The most severe of the chronic tic disorders is Gilles de la Tourette syndrome, more commonly referred to as Tourette syndrome (American Psychiatric Association, 2013). Diagnosis of a tic disorder is based on clinical observations.

Therapeutic Management

Most tic disorders resolve by late childhood or adolescence without treatment and cause no physical harm to the child. Therapeutic management consists primarily of support to the child and family, reassurance about the prognosis, and education regarding expectations (of the child) for control. Although the child is able to suppress the manifestations to some degree, persistent pressure for control constitutes an additional stress to an affected child. Medications may provide some relief of symptoms of chronic tics. Therapeutic plasma apheresis to remove the offending autoantibodies is under investigation for children with PANDA (see Research Focus box). Genetic counseling is advisable for families of children with chronic tics.

RESEARCH FOCUS

Therapeutic Plasma Apheresis for PANDAS

The efficacy of three treatments of therapeutic plasma apheresis was evaluated in 35 children with pediatric autoimmune neuropsychiatric disorder associated with streptococcus (PANDAS) (Latimer, L'Etoile, Seidlitz, et al., 2015). All children in the study experienced some benefit from the treatment, including a decrease in obsessive-compulsive disorder, anxiety, tics, and/or somatic symptoms. The researchers conclude that therapeutic plasma apheresis is beneficial, but it is an invasive intervention with potential for complications and should be reserved only for children and adolescents with severe PANDAS.

GILLES DE LA TOURETTE SYNDROME

Tics are the defining feature of Gilles de la Tourette syndrome (GTS). GTS is the most complex and severe of the tic disorders (American Psychiatric Association, 2013). According to DSM-5 criteria, the presence of motor and vocal (or phonic) tics manifesting before 18 years of age for more than 12 months in the absence of secondary causes warrants diagnosis of GTS (American Psychiatric Association 2013). It begins between ages 2 and 16 years, is more common in boys than girls, persists throughout life, and is characterized by rapidly repetitive multiple motor and vocal movements. The prevalence of GTS is approximately 0.8% between the ages of 6 and 18 years. GTS is complicated by psychiatric comorbidities (ADHD, obsessive-compulsive disorder, anxiety/depressive disorders, and autism spectrum disorders) in about 90% of cases.

Secondary tic disorders are less frequent than primary tic disorders and should be suspected in older onset (>20 years) and associated neurologic abnormalities. Various conditions may present with secondary tics, including neurodevelopmental disorders, acute brain lesions, neurodegenerative illnesses, immune-mediated conditions, and drugs or toxins. A later age at onset (e.g., late adolescence or adulthood), abrupt onset, and association with other neurologic manifestations represent red flags that should prompt the exclusion of secondary causes of tics (Ganos, 2016).

The cause of GTS is uncertain; most theories implicate abnormalities of various neurotransmitters or a dysregulation in brain circuits that connect the basal ganglia to the motor cortex. Family research illustrates a genetic influence for GTS (Ong, Mordekar, & Seal, 2016).

The manifestations of GTS wax and wane in intensity and exhibit a continuing pattern of change in which old tics disappear and new tics develop. The onset is usually mild, and the initial tic is of brief duration. The minor tics then come and go, becoming more intense and lasting longer. Some tics may be severe from the onset, often with no symptom-free periods. A high percentage of children with GTS have associated obsessive-compulsive symptoms (e.g., recurring thoughts or the need to arrange and rearrange objects, repeatedly turn the light switch off and on, tie and retie their shoes, and so on). Other problems associated with GTS include ADHD, disruptive behavior, and learning disabilities. For some children, these associated symptoms may be more disturbing than the tics. Diagnosis is based on clinical observations, especially if other family members are affected. The tics do not lead to physical deterioration or affect the child's life expectancy.

Therapeutic Management

Treatment of GTS is primarily symptomatic and consists of child and family education and support. Children with more severe tics sometimes obtain symptomatic relief from medications. Various α_2-agonists (clonidine and guanfacine) are first-line medications for the treatment of tics in the United States and Canada and may be more effective in patients with GTS and ADHD compared with GTS alone. Antipsychotic medications (mostly risperidone, haloperidol, pimozide, fluphenazine, aripiprazole) are also effective, but with a less favorable side-effect profile. The goal is to use the lowest dose of medication that reduces symptoms to an acceptable level while enhancing the child's development. Genetic counseling is also advised for families of children affected by GTS (Ganos, 2016).

Nursing Care Management

Education of children, families, teachers, and others involved in the affected child's everyday life is a major aspect of therapy. Affected children are often quick to become angry or easily frustrated. They may also have temper tantrums. These children need to be guided toward acceptable substitute behaviors to develop normally, both socially and emotionally. Punishment for the behaviors is inappropriate because these actions are involuntary.

Children with GTS are in a constant, ongoing battle to control their impulses and need positive relationships with their parents, peers, health care providers, and educators to become well adjusted. A child's self-concept can be damaged if parents react to the disability with controlling behaviors, guilt, anger, or hostility.

School nurses can help children with GTS cope with their condition by advocating positive support from peers, ensuring the child has access to extracurricular activities and academic support or classroom accommodations, and educating teachers, administrators, and classmates about GTS.

Nurses can assist families in long-term monitoring of symptoms and determining whether symptoms interfere with the child's development or require more intensive therapy. Families of children taking medication need to be alert to possible side effects, including lethargy, personality change, increased appetite and weight gain, depression or parkinsonian symptoms (e.g., tremor; muscle rigidity; shuffling gait; hypokinesia; and difficulty chewing, swallowing, and speaking), and anticholinergic symptoms (e.g., confusion, excitement, dilated pupils, blurred vision, dry mouth, and dysphagia).

The nurse may advocate for additional family support by referral to health agencies such as the local health departments, social services, and parent groups. The Tourette Syndrome Association is active in research and education and provides services to affected children and their families. Resources may be found at http://www.tsa-usa.org.

POSTTRAUMATIC STRESS DISORDER

Posttraumatic stress disorder (PTSD) refers to the development of characteristic symptoms after exposure to an extremely traumatic experience or catastrophic event. The traumatic experience or catastrophic event is typically life threatening to self or a significant other and may involve witnessing mutilation or death, experiencing or witnessing a serious injury, or physical coercion. The disturbance causes clinically significant distress or impairment in social, occupational, or other important areas of functioning and is not attributable to the physiologic effects of a medication or illicit substance or another medical condition (Connor, Ford, Arnsten, et al., 2014). It is important to note that PTSD is not limited to children who have lived in war-torn countries. Events such as automobile, school, and recreational accidents and bullying have been identified as causes of PTSD.

After a horrific event, the child's response involves intense fear, helplessness, or horror, resulting in behavior that is disorganized, depressed, or agitated. The characteristic symptoms include persistent reexperiencing of the traumatic event, persistent avoidance of stimuli associated with the trauma, numbing of general responsiveness, and persistent symptoms of increased arousal. The response to the event occurs in three stages. The initial response to the stressor is intense arousal, which usually lasts from a few minutes to 1 or 2 hours, depending on the stressor and the individual. The stress hormones are at the maximum as the individual prepares for "fight or flight." A prolonged arousal phase may indicate psychosis.

The second phase, which lasts approximately 2 weeks, is one in which defense mechanisms are mobilized. It is a period of calm in which the event appears to have produced no impression. The victim feels numb, and stress hormone secretion is absent. The reaction is outside the individual's awareness, is not well controlled, and involves some type of behavior pattern. Defense mechanisms are less adaptive to specific situations and may not be what the situation demands. Denial that anything is wrong is a frequently observed defense mechanism. Without professional support, the child may develop severe depression, aggression, or psychosis (Gerson & Rappaport, 2013).

The third phase is one of coping, which normally extends over 2 to 3 months. This is a phase of consciously directed inquiry. The victim wants to know what happened and appears to be getting worse, when actually he or she is getting better. Numerous psychologic symptoms such as depression, repetitive phenomena, phobic symptoms, anxiety symptoms, and conversion reactions may be apparent. Children frequently display repetitive actions. They play out the situation over and over again in an attempt to come to terms with their fear. Flashbacks are common. This phase can be self-perpetuating, and a prolonged reaction can develop into an obsession with the traumatic event. Some traumatic effects remain indefinitely.

Nursing Care Management

Health care providers are often the first to identify and treat traumatized children. Appropriate interventions early can decrease the sequelae of the traumatic event such as PTSD. There are various brief systematic tools that providers can use to screen children after a traumatic event for symptoms of PTSD (Connor, Ford, Arnsten, et al., 2014). Children need to deal with any traumatic event; much hinges on the intensity of the event and their reactions to it. Children's reactions depend heavily on their social environment and the way in which their caretaking adults react to the event. Children usually react in the same manner as their caregivers (contagious pathology); therefore it is important to be aware of these reactions. In the second, or defense, phase of PTSD, the appropriateness of the defense mechanism must be assessed, and children must be assisted in coping with their emotions.

Coping is a learned response, and children in the third phase can be helped to use their coping strategies to deal with their fears. Children usually are willing to accept reasoning. Those who are assisted in their catharsis and allowed expression will survive without serious lasting effects. Encourage them to play out the stress and/or discuss their feelings about the event.

Children need professional help if any of the phases of PTSD are prolonged. Boys are more likely to have a prolonged defense phase than girls. Occasionally the precipitating event will go unrecognized (bullying and psychologic abuse are most common in school-age children), and the affected child will engage in what is considered to be unusual behavior. Children exhibiting any sudden change in behavior need to be assessed for exposure to a traumatic event. When the change in behavior is determined to be caused by a traumatic event, treatment should be implemented immediately to prevent or reduce the long-term emotional and psychologic effects of PTSD (Gerson & Rappaport, 2013).

SCHOOL PHOBIA

Children other than beginning students who resist going to school or who demonstrate extreme reluctance to attend school for a sustained period as a result of severe anxiety or a fear of school-related experiences are said to have school phobia. The terms *school refusal* and *school avoidance* are also used to describe this behavior. School phobia occurs in children of all ages, but it is more common in children 10 years of age and older. School avoidance behaviors occur in both boys and girls and in children from all socioeconomic levels.

Anxiety that verges on panic is a constant manifestation, and children can develop symptoms as a protective mechanism to keep them from facing the situation that distresses them. Physical symptoms are prominent and may affect any part of the body; headache, nausea, vomiting, diarrhea, dizziness, anorexia, leg pains, or abdominal pains are most common. The children may even develop a low-grade fever. A striking feature of school phobia is the prompt subsiding of symptoms when it is evident that the child can remain at home. Another significant observation is absence of symptoms on weekends and holidays, unless they are related to other places such as Sunday school or parties. Occasional mild reluctance to attend school is not uncommon among schoolchildren, but if the fear continues for longer than a few days, it must be considered a serious problem.

The onset is usually sudden and precipitated by a school-related incident. By taking a careful history, nurses find out whether a poor attendance record is due to trivial reasons.

Etiology

A number of factors can cause school phobia. Sometimes the complaints are related to a transient, specific cause, such as fear of a mismatched or overcritical teacher; fear of failing an examination or giving an oral presentation for a painfully shy child; or discrimination based on race, dress, or physical appearance. School avoidance may also be related to a safety concern, such as a bully, cyberbullying, or a threatening gang. An insecure home situation in which children fear that they may be deserted by a parent may be the basis of anxiety, especially if the parent has previously threatened to leave.

A frequent source of fear is separation anxiety growing out of a strong, dependent relationship between the mother and child in which the child is reluctant to leave the mother and she is equally reluctant to have the child leave her (although this feeling may be unconscious on the mother's part). The intense need for closeness between mother and child is normal in infancy, but the persistence of this type of relationship into childhood is inappropriate.

Characteristically, these children are not afraid to go to school; rather, they are afraid to leave home. They fear that something dreadful might happen while they are separated from their families. These symptoms may be precipitated by a situation that intensifies the mutual dependency between the mother and the child, such as illness, arrival of a new baby, a move to a new neighborhood or school, or parental discord.

In some instances children have an unrealistic, exaggerated view of their abilities and achievements. When they feel threatened by incidents that challenge their estimates of themselves, such as a minor episode that leads to embarrassment, return to school after an absence, transfer to another class, or even imagined social or academic failure, they become anxious and withdraw, frequently seeking proximity to the mother. Sometimes the step-up in expectations at school or a change in important personnel at school (e.g., teacher or principal) is a contributing factor. Occasionally the child may be suffering from an undiagnosed learning disability.

Therapeutic Management

The treatment for school phobia depends on the cause. If the reason for the problem is an examination, a relationship with a bully, or a mismatch between teacher and child, it can be dealt with accordingly. When the child is helped to understand and cope with the fear, the symptoms usually disappear. In severe cases when returning to school is unsuccessful, professional psychiatric consultation is usually desirable to help identify possible distorted family relationships or a personality disturbance in the child and to help both the child and the family understand the sources of the problem.

Some children with a moderately severe separation anxiety disorder and school refusal may be treated with an antidepressant. However, medical and psychiatric evaluation is always required before anxiolytic agents are prescribed.

Nursing Care Management

School nurses play a vital role in the identification and management of school phobia as many of these students will visit the school nurse. Treatment of school phobia depends on the cause but all students should be treated with support and reassurance. Parents must be convinced gently but firmly that immediate return to school is essential and that it is their responsibility to insist on school attendance.

! NURSING ALERT

The primary goal of school phobia is school attendance. The longer the child is permitted to stay out of school, the more difficult it is to reenter.

A school reentry protocol may be necessary for a child with severe symptoms. In reentry programs, the child role-plays routines that are involved in getting ready for school and that occur at school. Relaxation techniques are also useful. The child usually goes to school for a half-day initially and then progresses to a full day. Children may be rewarded with points for each period during the day that they are able to remain in school. These points are then redeemed for rewards (e.g., playing with favorite toys or social rewards). Often the school nurse can provide both the teacher and the parents with support in carrying out this plan.

Prevention

School phobia and other dependency problems can be avoided by encouraging independence at appropriate times during infancy and early childhood. For example, by 6 months of age children can be left with a babysitter during a parents' night out. Two-year-olds can be left at home (while awake) with a sitter. By 3 years of age children should experience being left somewhere other than their home (e.g., grandparents' home). As soon as they are able, they should be able to feed, dress, and wash themselves. By 3 to 4 years of age children can be allowed to play in the yard by themselves, and later they should be allowed to play in the neighborhood by themselves.

For most first-time school fears, simple reassurances and a little advance preparation are all that is necessary. Direct contact with the school and teachers is an excellent way to allay anticipatory anxiety. Parents can take the child to visit the school about a month before school starts, introduce the child to the teacher, and let the child experience the classroom firsthand.

Bedtime is also an excellent time to help children resolve first-day jitters. Bedtime stories and books suited to the occasion are available from bookstores and libraries. Several videotapes and tape recordings are also available to help children cope with a variety of common fears (e.g., dark, nightmares, babysitters, doctors, dentists, monsters).

Parents who suspect that their child may be especially frightened may want to accompany the child to school and wait outside the classroom the first day. A gradual breakaway over succeeding days should relieve their child's and their own anxiety. If the distress extends over a long period, professional help may be necessary.

FUNCTIONAL ABDOMINAL PAIN

Functional abdominal pain (FAP) is a complaint of childhood that is often attributed to psychogenic causes, although it can be a symptom of either psychosomatic or organic disease. The disorder commonly affects school-age children and is more common in children over 8 years of age and in girls more often than in boys (Sood & Matta, 2016). FAP is traditionally defined as three or more separate episodes of abdominal pain at least 3 months before diagnosis that interferes with functioning. FAP can be diagnosed by a primary care provider in children 4 to 18 years of age with chronic abdominal pain when there are no warning symptoms or signs, the physical examination is normal, and the stool sample tests are negative for occult blood. Warning symptoms and signs include involuntary weight loss, deceleration of linear growth, gastrointestinal blood loss, persistent vomiting, chronic severe diarrhea, persistent right upper or right lower quadrant pain, unexplained fever, family history of inflammatory bowel disease, or abnormal or unexplained physical findings (Korterink, Devanarayana, Rajindrajith, et al., 2015). Any of these symptoms or signs is indication to pursue diagnostic testing for specific anatomic, infectious, inflammatory, or metabolic etiologies on the basis of specific symptoms in an individual case. Significant vomiting includes bilious emesis, protracted vomiting, cyclic vomiting, or a pattern worrisome to the health care provider. Alarm signs on abdominal examination include localized tenderness in the right upper or right lower quadrants, a localized fullness or mass effect, hepatomegaly, splenomegaly, abdominal distention, and perianal abnormalities (e.g., tags, fissures, or fistulas) (Almadhoun, 2012).

Etiology and Pathophysiology

Only a minority of youngsters with FAP have an organic basis for their pain. Organic causes include inflammatory bowel disease, peptic ulcer disease, lactose intolerance, pelvic inflammatory disease, urinary bladder infection, and pancreatitis. Psychogenic causes of abdominal pain, such as school phobia, depression, acute reactive anxiety, and conversion reaction, account for a small number of cases.

In cases in which no organic disorder is identifiable, the abdominal pain of FAP has been attributed to dysfunction. Dysfunctional conditions causing FAP include constipation, chronic stool retention, overeating, irritable colon, and intestinal gas, with heightened awareness of intestinal motility or dysmotility. Normally, intestinal contents arrive at the distal portion of the intestine with a relatively high fluid content, and fluid is extracted in the distal colon and rectum. If the normally relaxed distal intestine fails to relax and prevents the flow of its contents toward the rectum, the resulting excessive distention and spasms of the distal intestinal musculature produce pressure on nerve endings, causing pain.

The symptoms of FAP may result from multiple causes, and it is important to assess a number of factors that could place a child at risk for this condition, including somatic predisposition, dysfunction, or disorder; lifestyle and habit, including routines, diet, and life tempo; temperament and learned response patterns, such as the child's behavior style, personality, and learned coping skills; and milieu and critical events (i.e., the child's intimate surroundings [familial, social, and cultural norms] and unexpected sources of stress or gratification).

Children at risk for FAP tend to be high achievers who have extensive personal goals or whose parents have unusually high expectations. They are described as being more mature and sensitive than others or as worriers. At risk are children who are overly concerned about what others think about them but have difficulty meeting the expectations of parents, teachers, and others. They are uncomfortable with expressions of anger or argument, especially directed at those persons who are significant in their lives. School attendance is adversely affected, and these children generally exhibit poor learning performance. It is not uncommon for symptoms to be aggravated during school days.

Clinical Manifestations

Children with FAP have real pain that is usually located in the periumbilical and/or epigastric area. On palpation the pain is more likely to be experienced in the epigastric area or in the lower right or left quadrant and is accompanied by vague tenderness without muscle guarding. The pain is irregular in time, duration, and intensity and is associated with either loose or pellet-formed stools. Other symptoms that may accompany the abdominal pain are headache, flushing, pallor, dizziness, and fatigue. Nausea, vomiting, diarrhea, and dysuria are sometimes part of the syndrome. The symptoms reflect the heightened intensity of response to stimulation of the autonomic bowel sites. Loose stools are a result of the exaggerated propulsive motility, and the pain is caused by the sharply increased mechanical tension in the gut.

Pain on morning wakening, which improves in the afternoon and becomes severe again before bedtime, suggests FAP. A hallmark of FAP is school absenteeism whereas children with organic diseases attend school regularly. Children with FAP rarely remain in bed, instead lying on the couch watching television. At night, pain may delay the onset of sleep but seldom wakes the child (Brett, Rowland, & Drumm, 2012).

Diagnostic Evaluation

Diagnosis is based on a complete family history, the child's health history, physical examination, and laboratory tests. The family history may provide evidence of a hereditary disorder or mimicry of adult symptoms. The child is evaluated for evidence of an organic basis for symptoms, such as pain that radiates to the back, pain that awakens the child from sleep, persistent right upper or right lower quadrant pain, unexplained or recurrent fever, weight loss, gastrointestinal blood loss, significant vomiting, chronic severe diarrhea, or family history of inflammatory bowel disease (Korterink, Devanarayana, Rajindrajith, et al., 2015). Pain is assessed for location, quality, frequency, duration, any associated symptoms, alleviating factors, and exacerbating factors. Pain diaries can assist in clarifying details of abdominal pain and triggering factors. An organic cause is found in less than 10% of children diagnosed with FAP.

Therapeutic Management

Treatment involves providing reassurance and reducing or eliminating symptoms. Hospitalization may be necessary, and the child frequently shows improvement in the hospital environment. Initial efforts are directed toward ruling out organic causes of the pain, relieving discomfort, and attempting to determine the situations that precipitate attacks.

Emphasize a high-fiber diet, psyllium bulk agents, lubricants such as mineral oil, and bowel training for pain associated with bowel patterns. Treatment may also include acid-reduction therapy for pain associated with dyspepsia, antispasmodic agents, smooth muscle relaxants, or low doses of psychotropic agents for pain. Dietary modifications may include removal of dairy products, fructose, and gluten for 2 to 3 weeks to rule out lactose intolerance, sensitivity to high sugar content, and celiac disease. Other treatments include cognitive-behavioral therapy and biofeedback.

Nursing Care Management

The nurse is instrumental in assessment and management of FAP in children. Many techniques used in a routine assessment elicit information that might help identify factors that contribute to the child's symptoms. Evaluate the child's social and psychologic adjustment, and obtain the details of the pain directly from the child. Questions that provide clues to parent-child relationships and the way the family deals with angry feelings provide information for diagnosis and management. Relationships with peers, school problems, and other concerns of the child need to be explored. Note any evidence of depression.

Once the diagnosis has been established, the parents and the child need an explanation of the pain, which can be compared with a skeletal muscle cramp, "charley horse," or headache for easier comprehension. Reassurance that the symptoms are not unique to their child and that the pain is rarely associated with a severe disease can help relieve parental fears and anxieties.

Discuss a high-fiber diet with the child and family, and emphasize bowel training. The child is encouraged to establish a pattern of sitting on the toilet for 10 to 15 minutes immediately after breakfast to take advantage of the increased colonic activity after meals. If necessary, have the child use stimulatory suppositories to induce early-morning defecation.

Once parents are reassured that there is no organic cause for the pain, they need guidance on what to do during a pain episode. Often they feel helpless and anxious, which tends to compound the child's distress. The simple measure of having the child rest in a peaceful, quiet environment and providing comfort will often relieve the symptoms in a short time. Application of a heating pad may also ease the discomfort. (See Nonpharmacologic [Pain] Management, Chapter 5.) If pain is not relieved by these simple measures, teach parents how to administer antispasmodics, if prescribed. For example, if pain is precipitated by meals, having the child take the medication 20 to 30 minutes before mealtime may prevent an episode.

The most valuable assistance that the nurse can provide is support and reassurance to the family. When open communication is established and families are able to see a relationship between stress-provoking situations and the child's symptoms, the chance for remedial action is enhanced.

> **! NURSING ALERT**
>
> Follow-up care and continued support of FAP are essential because the symptoms tend to remit and exacerbate. The availability of a supportive health professional can be a source of comfort to the child and family.

CONVERSION REACTION

Conversion reaction, also known as hysteria, hysterical conversion reaction, and childhood hysteria, is a psychophysiologic disorder with a sudden onset that can usually be traced to a precipitating environmental event. The disorder is observed with equal frequency in both sexes in childhood, but affected girls outnumber affected boys during adolescence. The manifestations involve primarily the voluntary musculature and special senses and include abdominal pain, fainting, pseudoseizures, paralysis, headaches, and visual field restriction. Once considered rare in childhood, the disorder occurs more frequently than has generally been acknowledged. The most commonly observed symptom is seizure activity, which can be differentiated from symptoms of neurogenic origin by formal tests, the most useful of which is the finding of a normal electroencephalogram.

Many children with conversion reaction have experienced a major family crisis before the onset of symptoms, such as loss of a parent or other significant person through death, divorce, or moving. The families of children with conversion reaction characteristically display problems in communication and depression or hypochondriasis in a parent.

Educating the child and family regarding the cause of emotional stresses or feelings and alternative approaches to coping with stress may alleviate the child's symptoms. If deep personality problems are evident, psychiatric consultation is indicated. Nursing care is similar to that for the child with FAP.

CHILDHOOD DEPRESSION

Depression in childhood is often difficult to detect because many children may be unable to adequately express their feelings and tend to act out their problems and concerns rather than identify them verbally. Adult caregivers, health care professionals, and educators may not recognize early warning signs of depression in children or may delay referral and treatment, believing symptoms of depression in children are "just a stage of development" and will resolve with maturation. Childhood depression does exist, but the manifestations often differ from those in depressed adults. The characteristics of depression are largely determined by parallel developments in symbolism, language, and cognitive development. Younger children demonstrate a more cause-and-effect relationship between the stressors and the depressive manifestations. In older children the relationships between stressful events and depression are less clear. Their reactions are less physiologic and more cognitively complex, and the observed behaviors tend to be age specific. Depressed children often exhibit a distinctive style of thinking characterized by low self-esteem, hopelessness, poor social engagement with peers, and a tendency to explain negative events in terms of personal shortcomings.

Some states of depression are temporary (e.g., acute depression precipitated by a traumatic event). The causative event might be a period of hospitalization, loss of a parent through death or divorce, or loss of a significant relationship with something (a pet), someone (a friend or family member), or a place (move from a familiar home, neighborhood, or city). The easily identified manifestations include a sad, downcast face; tearfulness; irritability; and withdrawal from previously enjoyed activities and relationships. The child tends to spend more time in solitary activities, especially television viewing. Schoolwork is impaired. Some children become more dependent and clinging, whereas others become more aggressive and disruptive. Sleeplessness or hypersomnia, changes in appetite or weight (either increased or decreased), constipation, tiredness, and nonspecific complaints of not feeling well are common reactions. Responses are not sustained and can be modified with social and family support.

More serious and less common are depressive responses to more chronic stress and loss. These are frequently observed in children with chronic illness or disability. There is no apparent precipitating event, but a history of frequent disruptions in important relationships often occurs. A history of depressive illness in one or both parents during the child's lifetime is also common. The manifestations are similar to those seen in acute reactions. Major depressive disorders in childhood have a number of similarities with several other psychologic disorders. Some forms of depression develop under unique circumstances, such as the following:

1. **Persistent depressive disorder** (also called *dysthymia*) is a depressed mood that lasts for at least 2 years. A person diagnosed with persistent depressive disorder may have episodes of major depression along with periods of less severe symptoms, but symptoms must last for 2 years (National Institute of Mental Health, 2016).
2. **Psychotic depression** occurs when a person has severe depression plus some form of psychosis, such as having disturbing false fixed beliefs (delusions) or hearing or seeing upsetting things that others cannot hear or see (hallucinations). The psychotic symptoms typically have a depressive "theme," such as delusions of guilt, poverty, or illness (National Institute of Mental Health, 2016).
3. **Seasonal affective disorder** is characterized by the onset of depression during the winter months, when there is less natural sunlight. This depression generally lifts during spring and summer; however, the depression predictably returns every winter. Winter depression is typically accompanied by social withdrawal, increased sleep, and weight gain (National Institute of Mental Health, 2016)
4. **Bipolar disorder** is different from depression, but it is included here because individuals experience episodes of extremely low moods that meet the criteria for major depression (called *bipolar depression*). A person with bipolar disorder also experiences extreme high—euphoric or irritable—moods called *mania* or a less severe form called *hypomania* (National Institute of Mental Health, 2016).

Examples of other types of depressive disorders added to the diagnostic classification of DSM-5 include disruptive mood dysregulation disorder (diagnosed in children and adolescents) and premenstrual dysphoric disorder (American Psychiatric Association, 2013).

Therapeutic Management

Depressed children are managed by a health team specially trained in the care of children with mental disorders. Treatment is highly individualized and should be undertaken in the least constrictive environment, usually an outpatient setting. Suicidal children are admitted to the hospital for protection if the family is unable to provide constant monitoring (see Suicide section in Chapter 18). Hospitalization may also be advised for children with associated disruptive behavior, such as fighting with peers or family. Most therapeutic regimens focus on various combinations of counseling, psychotherapy, family therapy, cognitive therapy, education (teaching social and life skills that facilitate coping), environmental improvement, and pharmacotherapy.

Pharmacotherapy may involve tricyclic antidepressants or selective serotonin reuptake inhibitors such as sertraline (Zoloft), paroxetine (Paxil), bupropion (Wellbutrin), or venlafaxine (Effexor). There have been reports that antidepressant medications may cause increased suicidal thinking and behaviors in pediatric patients. This prompted the US Food and Drug Administration to require black box drug labeling detailing potential suicide-related risks for pediatric patients.

Nursing Care Management

Nurses should be aware that depression is a problem that can easily be overlooked in the school-age child and one that can interrupt normal growth and development. Recognizing depression (Box 16.7) and making appropriate referrals are important nursing functions. Identification of the depressed child requires a careful history taking (e.g., health, growth and development, social family health); interviews with the child; and observations by the nurse, parents, and teachers. If antidepressants are prescribed, the child and family need to know that antidepressants must be at a therapeutic level for 2 to 4 weeks to achieve a beneficial effect. The child and family also need to monitor the child for side effects of the specific drug prescribed and any interactions with other drugs.

CHILDHOOD SCHIZOPHRENIA

Childhood schizophrenia refers to severe deviations in ego functioning and is generally reserved for psychotic disorders that appear in children younger than 15 years of age. Childhood schizophrenia is a very rare illness among children in the general population; only about 2 in every 1000 children with mental illness have childhood schizophrenia.

The cause of schizophrenia is unknown, but three risk factors have been identified: genetic characteristics, gestational and birth complications, and winter birth. Biologic relatives of affected individuals have an increased chance of developing the disorder. For example, the risk for the children if both parents have schizophrenia is 40%. The rate of concordance is 10% for dizygotic (nonidentical) twins and 40% to 50% for monozygotic (identical) twins.

Altered development of the central nervous system is an etiologic factor. Psychosocial theories, especially those focusing on the parent-child relationship, have not been supported, but certain social and

BOX 16.7 Characteristics of Children With Depression

Behavior

- Predominantly sad facial expression with absent or diminished range of affective response
- Solitary play or work; tendency to be alone; disinterest in play
- Withdrawal from previously enjoyed activities and relationships
- Lowered grades in school; lack of interest in doing homework or achieving in school
- Diminished motor activity; tiredness
- Tearfulness or crying
- Dependent and clinging or aggressive and disruptive behavior

Internal States

- Utterance of statements reflecting lowered self-esteem, sense of hopelessness, or guilt
- Suicidal ideations

Physiologic Manifestations

- Constipation
- Nonspecific complaints of not feeling well
- Change in appetite resulting in weight loss or gain
- Alterations in sleeping pattern, sleeplessness, or hypersomnia

BOX 16.8 Characteristics of Childhood Schizophrenia

- Bizarre behavior patterns and stereotyped movements such as robotlike walking, whirling, or graceful gyrations
- Periods of hypoactivity alternating with periods of hyperactivity
- Inappropriate affect that ranges from flatness to explosiveness
- Common occurrence of temper tantrums
- Language disturbances such as speaking in fragmented sentences, parrotlike repetition of words, development of a private language, and altered tone of voice; for some schizophrenic children, muteness or uttering only a single word on rare occasions
- Distorted time orientation with a blending of past, present, and future
- Distorted sense of and use of the body
- Apparent denial of the human quality in people, such as attempting to use a person as a step stool to reach an object
- Conveying of a nonhuman identity by action, sounds, or posture, such as barking or calling self a vacuum cleaner
- Frequent occurrence of compulsive behavior and phobias

environmental factors may play a role in a child's vulnerability to developing schizophrenia.

Childhood schizophrenia is characterized by symptoms that last at least 6 months and that seriously interfere with the child's functioning at school, at home, or in other social situations. However, the basic core disturbance is the child's lack of contact with reality and the subsequent development of a world of his or her own.

The most common manifestations are language disturbances, impaired interpersonal relationships, and inappropriate affect (outward expression of emotion) (Box 16.8). Treatment involves management of symptoms, prevention of relapse, and social and occupational rehabilitation of the young person. In some individuals drug therapy produces dramatic improvement in symptoms and social adjustment. Antipsychotic drugs that may be used include haloperidol, clozapine, chlorpromazine, and risperidone. Family interventions and family therapy often result in improvements in psychotic symptoms, thought disorders, and social functioning among children with schizophrenia.

Nursing Care Management

Nursing of psychotic children is a highly specialized area, but because such problems are occurring with increasing frequency, nurses should recognize children who consistently demonstrate abnormal behavior and refer them for evaluation.

Nurses should also instruct family members of children taking antipsychotic drugs to observe for possible side effects. Common side effects of these drugs include dizziness, drowsiness, tachycardia, hypotension, and extrapyramidal effects such as abnormal movements and seizures. Agranulocytosis occurs in 1% of patients who take clozapine in the first few months of treatment. Therefore a mandatory monitoring program requires that patients taking clozapine have a white blood cell (WBC) count performed every week during the first 6 months of therapy and every other week for the second 6 months of therapy. Pharmacies and clinicians report the weekly WBC count and cannot dispense clozapine to the patient without evidence of a safe WBC count.

ANXIETY DISORDERS

Anxiety disorders include a range of conditions characterized by excessive fear and anxiety (Ege & Reinholdt-Dunne, 2016). They are the most common type of mental health disorder in childhood, affecting up to 31% of all children and adolescents (Ege & Reinholdt-Dunne, 2016).

BOX 16.9 Symptoms of Anxiety Disorders

- Recurring fears and worries about routine parts of everyday life
- Physical complaints, like stomachache or headache
- Trouble concentrating
- Trouble sleeping
- Fear of social situations
- Fear of leaving home
- Fear of separation from a loved one
- Refusing to go to school

Reused with permission from American Academy of Pediatrics. (2017). *Anxiety fact sheet.* Retrieved from https://www.aap.org/en-us/advocacy-and-policy/aap-health-initiatives/resilience/Pages/Anxiety-Fact-Sheet.aspx

There are many types of anxiety disorders that affect youth, the most common being generalized anxiety disorder, panic disorder, separation anxiety disorder, social anxiety disorder, and phobic disorders. Comorbid disorders, in particular ADHD and depression, commonly occur with anxiety disorders.

Symptoms of anxiety disorders are listed in Box 16.9. Evaluation for an anxiety disorder often begins with a visit to a primary care provider. Some physical health conditions (i.e., thyroid dysfunction or hypoglycemia) and some medications can imitate or worsen an anxiety disorder. A thorough mental health evaluation is also helpful because anxiety disorders often coexist with other related conditions, such as depression or obsessive-compulsive disorder (National Institute of Mental Health, 2016).

Therapeutic Management

Anxiety disorders are treated with psychotherapy, medication, or both (Dillon-Naftolin, 2016). Cognitive-behavioral therapy (CBT) is an effective psychotherapy for people with anxiety disorders by teaching individuals different ways of thinking, behaving, and reacting to anxiety-producing and fearful situations. CBT also teaches social skills, which is vital for treating social anxiety disorder (National Institute of Mental Health, 2016). Two specific components of CBT used to treat social anxiety disorder are cognitive therapy and exposure therapy. Cognitive therapy focuses on identifying, challenging, and then neutralizing unhelpful thoughts underlying anxiety disorders. Exposure therapy focuses on confronting the fears underlying an anxiety disorder to help people engage in activities they have been avoiding. Exposure therapy is used along with relaxation exercises and/or imagery (National Institute of Mental Health, 2016).

Medications are sometimes used as the initial treatment of an anxiety disorder, or for an insufficient response to psychotherapy. The most common classes of medications are antidepressants, antianxiety drugs, and β-blockers. Antidepressants may be risky for children, adolescents, and young adults. Therefore a black box warning for suicide and suicide ideation is added to the labels of antidepressants. Any child, adolescent, or young adult taking an antidepressant should be monitored closely, especially during the initial phase of the medication (National Institute of Mental Health, 2016).

CONDUCT DISORDERS

Conduct disorder is categorized under the broad heading of disruptive behavior disorders and is defined as repetitive behaviors through which the rights of others are violated and societal rules are broken (American Psychiatric Association, 2013). The disruptive behavior causes clinically significant impairment in social, academic, or occupational functioning.

TABLE 16.4 Criteria for Conduct Disorder Diagnosis

Diagnostic Criteria	Examples
A. A repetitive and persistent pattern of behavior in which the basic rights of others or other age-appropriate societal norms or rules are violated, as manifested by the presence of at least three of the following 15 criteria in the past 12 months from any of the categories below, with at least one criterion present in the past 6 months.	
Aggression to People and Animals	1. Often bullies, threatens, or intimidates others. 2. Often initiates physical fights. 3. Has used a weapon that can cause serious physical harm to others (e.g., a bat, brick, broken bottle, knife, and gun). 4. Has been physically cruel to people. 5. Has been physically cruel to animals. 6. Has stolen while confronting a victim (e.g., mugging, purse snatching, extortion, armed robbery). 7. Has forced someone into sexual activity.
Destruction of Property	8. Has deliberately engaged in fire setting with the intention of causing serious damage. 9. Has deliberately destroyed others' property (other than by fire setting).
Deceitfulness or Theft	10. Has broken into someone else's house, building, or car. 11. Often lies to obtain goods or favors or to avoid obligations (i.e., "cons" others). 12. Has stolen items of nontrivial value without confronting a victim (e.g., shoplifting without breaking and entering; forgery).
Serious Violations of Rules	13. Often stays out at night despite parental prohibitions, beginning before age 13 years. 14. Has run away from home overnight at least twice while living in the parental or parental surrogate home, or once without returning for a lengthy period. 15. Is often truant from school, beginning before age 13 years.
B. The disturbance in behavior causes clinically significant impairment in social, academic, or occupational funding.	
C. If the individual is age 18 years or older, criteria are not met for antisocial personality disorder.	

From American Psychiatric Association. (2013). *Diagnostic and statistical manual of mental disorders: DSM* (5th ed.). Washington, DC: American Psychiatric Publishing.

A pattern of three or more specific criteria must be present for at least 12 months and one criterion for 6 months to make the diagnosis. Table 16.4 lists the criteria and examples.

Children who exhibit these behaviors should receive a comprehensive evaluation by an experienced mental health professional. Children with a conduct disorder may have coexisting conditions such as mood disorders, anxiety, PTSD, substance abuse, ADHD, learning problems, or thought disorders. Without treatment, many children with conduct disorder are unable to adapt to the demands of adulthood and continue to have problems with relationships and holding a job. They often break laws or behave in an antisocial manner (American Academy of Adolescent and Child Psychiatry, 2013).

Therapeutic Management

Children with conduct disorder are likely to have ongoing problems if they and their families do not receive early and comprehensive treatment. Treatment of children with conduct disorder can be complex and challenging depending on the severity of the behaviors. Adding to the challenge of treatment may include the child's uncooperative attitude, fear, and distrust of adults. The pediatric psychiatrist uses information from the child, family, teachers, community (including the legal system), and other health care providers to identify the causes of the disorder (American Academy of Adolescent and Child Psychiatry, 2013).

Treatment options include psychotherapy, behavioral therapy, family therapy, and pharmacotherapy. Although there is no medication approved for the treatment of conduct disorder, medications may relieve specific symptoms. Stimulant medications including methylphenidate and risperidone have a large effect on childhood aggression, whereas antipsychotics have clinical efficacy on conduct disorders (Balia, Carucci, Coghill, et al., 2017).

! NURSING ALERT

When working with children with conduct disorder, nurses assess for comorbid mood and anxiety disorders. Management of the child's aggression is the main focus of interventions for conduct disorders.

NCLEX REVIEW QUESTIONS

1. Which of the following conditions may lead to the development of obesity in children? Select all that apply.
   A. Physical inactivity
   B. Low socioeconomic status
   C. Use of food as a positive reinforcement of desired behaviors
   D. Consumption of energy-dense foods and drinks
   E. Positive self-esteem
2. Which child should receive further diagnostic testing for chronic abdominal pain? Select all that apply.
   A. An 11-year-old boy with a 1-month history of generalized periumbilical pain
   B. An 8-year-old girl with a 1-week history of right lower quadrant pain
   C. A 12-year-old girl with a 6-week history of constipation
   D. A 6-year-old boy with a 1-month of diarrhea and a rectal fistula

3. You are working with a family whose 7-year-old has just been diagnosed with attention-deficit/hyperactivity disorder. Which statements by the mother indicate a need for further teaching? Select all that apply.
   A. "My child will respond best to verbal instructions, since that will help him learn to pay attention and listen intently."
   B. "A consistent schedule for homework and activities will help him be organized."
   C. "I need to bring him for routine checkups while he is taking his medication because the medication can affect his appetite and growth."
   D. "I am going to ask the principal if my son can change classrooms because his current teacher has too many rules and he seems to get in trouble."
   E. "We might consider counseling because this has been stressful for the whole family."
4. A good understanding of enuresis will help the nurse work with children and their families. Which of the following teaching points should be included? Select all that apply.
   A. Enuresis is primarily an alteration of neuromuscular bladder functioning and as such is benign and self-limiting.
   B. Spontaneous remission of nocturnal enuresis occurs in approximately 35% of cases.
   C. Normal bladder capacity (in ounces) is the child's age plus 4; therefore normal bladder capacity for a 6-year-old is 10 ounces (600 ml).
   D. Success has also been achieved with desmopressin acetate nasal spray, which reduces nighttime urinary output to a volume less than functional bladder capacity.
   E. Parents need reassurance that bed-wetting is not a manifestation of emotional disturbance but just represents willful misbehavior.
5. As a nurse caring for children, an understanding of childhood depression is essential. Some important information about depression includes which of the following statements? Select all that apply.
   A. Authorities agree that childhood depression exists, and the manifestations are often similar to adult depression.
   B. Identification of the depressed child requires a careful history taking (e.g., health, growth and development, social and family health); interviews with the child; and observations by the nurse, parents, and teachers.
   C. If antidepressants are prescribed, the child and family need to know that antidepressants must be at a therapeutic level for 4 to 6 weeks to achieve a beneficial effect.
   D. Depressed children often exhibit a distinctive style of thinking characterized by low self-esteem, hopelessness, poor social engagement with peers, and a tendency to explain negative events in terms of personal shortcomings.
   E. Nurses should be aware that depression is a problem that can be easily overlooked in the school-age child and one that can interrupt normal growth and development.

Correct Answers

1. A, B, C, D; 2. B, D; 3. A, D; 4. A, D; 5. B, D, E

REFERENCES

Almadhoun, O. (2012). Managing chronic abdominal pain in children. *Contemporary Pediatrics, 29*(3), 18–20.

Altman, M., & Wilfley, D. E. (2015). Evidence update on the treatment of overweight and obesity in children and adolescents. *Journal of Clinical Child and Adolescent Psychology, 44*(4), 521–537.

American Academy of Adolescent and Child Psychiatry. (2013). *Conduct Disorder*. https://www.aacap.org/AACAP/Families_and_Youth/Facts_for_Families/FFF-Guide/Conduct-Disorder-033.aspx.

American Academy of Pediatrics, Council on Communications and Media. (2016a). Media use in school-aged children and adolescents. *Pediatrics, 138*(5), e20162592.

American Academy of Pediatrics. (2016b). *Causes of ADHD: what we know today*. https://www.healthychildren.org/English/health-issues/conditions/adhd/pages/Causes-of-ADHD.aspx.

American Academy of Pediatrics. (2011). ADHD: Clinical practice guideline for the diagnosis, evaluation and treatment of the school-aged child with attention-deficit/hyperactivity disorder in children and adolescents. *Pediatrics, 128*(5), 1007–1022.

American Heart Association. (2017). *Overweight in children*. http://www.heart.org/HEARTORG/HealthyLiving/HealthyKids/ChildhoodObesity/OverweigOv-in-Children_UCM_304054_Article.jsp#.WSDBBca1vlU.

American Psychiatric Association. (2013). *Diagnostic and statistical manual of mental disorders* (5th ed.). Arlington, VA: American Psychiatric Association.

Antai-Otong, D., & Zimmerman, M. L. (2016). Treatment approaches to attention deficit hyperactivity disorder. *The Nursing Clinics of North America, 51*, 199–211.

Arda, E., Cakiroglu, B., & Thomas, D. T. (2016). Primary nocturnal enuresis: A review. *Nephro-Urology Monthly, 8*(4), e35809.

Balia, C., Carucci, S., Coghill, D., et al. (2017). The pharmacological treatment of aggression in children and adolescents with conduct disorder; do callous-unemotional traits modulate the efficacy of medication? *Neuroscience and Biobehavioral Reviews*, epub ahead of print.

Beamish, A. J., & Reinehr, T. (2017). Should bariatric surgery be performed in adolescents? *European Journal of Endocrinology, 176*, D1–D15.

Berlin, K. D., Kamody, R. C., Thurston, I. B., et al. (2017). Physical activity, sedentary behaviors, and nutritional risk profiles and relations to body mass index, obesity, and overweight in eighth grade. *Behavioral Medicine (Washington, D.C.), 43*(1), 31–39.

Berquist, M. J. (2015). Understanding type 2 diabetes in students with obesity and the role of the school nurse. *NASN School Nurse, 30*(2), 81–84.

Berthoud, H.-R. (2012). The neurobiology of food intake in an obesogenic environment. *The Proceedings of the Nutrition Society, 1*(1), 1–10.

Black, J., White, B., Viner, R., et al. (2013). Bariatric surgery for obese children and adolescents: A systematic review and meta-analysis. *Obesity Reviews : An Official Journal of the International Association for the Study of Obesity, 14*(8), 634–644.

Blows, E. S., Teoh, L., & Paul, S. P. (2016). Recognition and management of learning disabilities in early childhood by community practitioners. *Community Practitioner, 89*(5), 32–35.

Brett, T., Rowland, M., & Drumm, B. (2012). An approach to functional abdominal pain in children and adolescents. *The British Journal of General Practice, 62*(600), 386–387.

Bruening, M., Eisenberg, M., MacLehose, R., et al. (2012). Relationship between adolescents' and their friends' eating behaviors: Breakfast, fruit, vegetable, whole-grain, and dairy intake. *Journal of the Academy of Nutrition & Dietetics, 112*(10), 1608–1613.

Caldwell, P. H. Y., Sureshkumar, P., & Wong, W. C. F. (2016). Tricyclic and related drugs for nocturnal enuresis in children. *Cochrane Database of Systematic Reviews*, CD02117.

Castaldo, G., Palmieri, V., Galdo, G., et al. (2016). Aggressive nutritional strategy in morbid obesity in clinical practice: Safety, feasibility, and effects on metabolic and haemodynamic risk factors. *Obesity Research & Clinical Practice, 10*(2), 169–177.

Centers for Disease Control and Prevention. (2016). *Attention deficit/ hyperactivity disorder (ADHD)*. From https://www.cdc.gov/ncbddd/adhd/features/adhd-keyfindings-parents-jama.html.

Centers for Disease Control and Prevention. (2017). *Youth physical activity guidelines toolkit*. From https://www.cdc.gov/healthyschools/physicalactivity/guidelines.htm.

Chi, D. L., Rossitch, K. C., & Beeles, E. M. (2013). Developmental delays and dental cares in low-income preschoolers in the USA: A pilot cross-sectional study and preliminary explanatory model. *BMC Oral Health, 13*, 53.

Children and Adults with Attention-Deficit/Hyperactivity Disorder. (2017). *About ADHD*. http://www.chadd.org/Understanding-ADHD/About-ADHD.aspx.

Colombo, J. M., Wassom, M. C., & Rosen, J. M. (2015). Constipation and encopresis in childhood. *Pediatrics in Review, 36*(9), 393–402.

Connor, D. F., Ford, J. D., Arnsten, A. F. T., et al. (2014). An update on posttraumatic stress disorder in children and adolescents. *Clinical Pediatrics, 54*(6), 517–528.

Desai, N. K., Wulkan, M. L., & Inge, T. H. (2016). Update on adolescent bariatric surgery. *Endocrinology and Metabolism Clinics of North America, 45*(3), 667–676.

Dillon-Naftolin, E. (2016). Identification and treatment of generalized anxiety disorder in children in primary care. *Pediatric Annals, 45*(10), e349–e355.

Ege, S., & Reinholdt-Dunne, M. L. (2016). Improving treatment response for paediatric anxiety disorders: An information-processing perspective. *Clinical Child and Family Psychology Review, 19*, 392–402.

Elder, J. S. (2016). Enuresis and voiding dysfunction. In R. M. Kliegman, B. F. Stanton, J. W. St. Geme, et al. (Eds.), *Nelson textbook of pediatrics* (20th ed.). Philadelphia: Saunders/Elsevier.

Finkelstein, E. A., Graham, W. C. K., & Malhotra, R. (2014). Lifetime direct medical costs of childhood obesity. *Pediatrics, 133*(5), 854–862.

Fiorino, K. N., & Liacouras, C. A. (2016). Encopresis and functional constipation. In R. M. Kliegman, B. F. Stanton, J. W. St. Geme, et al. (Eds.), *Nelson textbook of pediatrics* (20th ed.). Philadelphia: Saunders/Elsevier.

Gahagan, S. (2016). Overweight and obesity. In R. M. Kliegman, B. F. Stanton, J. W. St. Geme, et al. (Eds.), *Nelson textbook of pediatrics* (20th ed.). Philadelphia: Saunders/Elsevier.

Ganos, C. (2016). Tics and tourette's: Update on pathophysiology and tic control. *Current Opinion in Neurology, 29*(4), 513–518.

Gerson, R., & Rappaport, N. (2013). Traumatic stress and posttraumatic stress disorder in youth: Recent research findings on clinical impact, assessment and treatment. *The Journal of Adolescent Health, 52*(2), 137–143.

Gow, M. L., Baur, L. A., Johnson, N. A., et al. (2017). Reversal of type 2 diabetes in youth who adhere to a very-low-energy diet: A pilot study. *Diabetologia, 60*(3), 406–415.

Kann, L., McManus, T., Harris, W. A., et al. (2016). Youth risk behavior surveillance – United States, 2015. *MMWR. Surveillance Summaries, 65*(6), 1–180.

Kennedy, M., Kreppner, J., Knights, N., et al. (2016). Early severe institutional deprivation is associated with a persistent variant of adult attention-deficit/hyperactivity disorder: Clinical presentation, developmental continuities and life circumstances in the English and Romanian adoptees study. *Journal of Child Psychology and Psychiatry, and Allied Disciplines, 57*(10), 1113–1125.

Kiess, W., Kratzsch, J., Sergeyev, E., et al. (2014). Metabolic syndrome in childhood and adolescence. *Clinical Biochemistry, 47*(9), 695.

Kim, J., Lee, I., & Lim, S. (2017). Overweight or obesity in children aged 0 to 6 and the risk of adult metabolic syndrome: A systematic review and meta-analysis. *Journal of Clinical Nursing*, epub ahead of print.

Korterink, J., Devanarayana, N. M., Rajindrajith, S., et al. (2015). Childhood functional abdominal pain: Mechanisms and management. *Nature Reviews. Gastroenterology & Hepatology, 12*, 159–171.

Kumar, S., & Kelly, A. S. (2017). Review of childhood obesity: From epidemiology, etiology, and comorbidities to clinical assessment and treatment. *Mayo Clinic Proceedings. Mayo Clinic, 92*(2), 251–265.

Latimer, M. E., L'Etoile, N., Seidlitz, J., et al. (2015). Therapeutic plasma apheresis as a treatment for 35 severely ill children and adolescent with pediatric autoimmune neuropsychiatric disorders associated with streptococcal infections. *Journal of Child and Adolescent Psychopharmacology, 25*(1), 70–75.

Lee, N. M., Carter, A., Owen, N., et al. (2012). The neurobiology of overeating. *EMBO Reports, 13*(9), 785–790.

Li, R., Magadia, J., Fein, S. B., et al. (2012). Risk of bottle-feeding for rapid weight gain during the first year of life. *Archives of Pediatrics and Adolescent Medicine, 166*(5), 431–436.

Llewellyn, A., Simmonds, M., Owen, C. G., et al. (2016). Childhood obesity as a predictor of morbidity in adulthood: A systematic review and meta-analysis. *Obesity Reviews : An Official Journal of the International Association for the Study of Obesity, 17*(1), 56–67.

Luat, A. F., Coyle, L., & Kamat, D. (2016). The ketogenic diet: A practice guide for pediatricians. *Pediatric Annals, 45*(12), e446–e450.

Mead, E., Atkinson, G., Richter, B., et al. (2016). Drug interventions for the treatment of obesity in children and adolescents. *Cochrane Database of Systematic Review*, (11), CD012436.

Meehan, C. A., Cochran, E., Kassai, A., et al. (2016). Metreleptin for injection to treat the complications of leptin deficiency in patients with congenital or acquired generalized lipodystrophy. *Expert Review of Clinical Pharmacology, 9*(1), 59–68.

Morandi, A., Meyre, D., Lobbens, S., et al. (2012). Estimation of newborn risk for child or adolescent obesity: Lessons from longitudinal birth cohorts. *PLoS ONE, 7*(11), e49919.

Mosca, N. W., & Schatz, M. L. (2013). Encopresis, not just an accident. *NASN School Nurse, 28*(5), 218–221.

National Institute of Mental Health. (2016). *PANDAS – question and answers*. https://www.nimh.nih.gov/health/publications/pandas/index.shtml.

Ogden, C. L., Carroll, M. D., Lawman, H. G., et al. (2016). Trends in obesity prevalence among children and adolescents in the United States, 1988-1994 through 2013-2014. *JAMA: The Journal of the American Medical Association, 315*(21), 2292–2299.

Olson, J., Aldrich, H., Callahan, T. J., et al. (2015). Characterization of childhood obesity and behavioral factors. *Journal of Pediatric Health Care, 30*(5), 444–452.

Ong, M. T., Mordekar, S. R., & Seal, A. (2016). Fifteen minute consultation: Tics and tourette syndrome. *Archives of Disease in Childhood. Education and Practice Edition 101*, 87–94.

Paidipati, C. P., & Deatrick, J. A. (2015). The role of family phenomena in children and adolescents with attention deficit hyperactivity disorder. *Journal of Child and Adolescent Psychiatric Nursing, 28*(1), 3–13.

Parker, A., & Corkum, P. (2016). ADHD diagnosis: As simple as administering a questionnaire or a complex diagnostic process? *Journal of Attention Disorders, 20*(6), 478–486.

Puhl, R. M., & King, K. M. (2013). Weight discrimination and bullying. *Best Practice & Research. Clinical Endocrinology & Metabolism, 27*(2), 117–127.

Rajjo, T., Mohammed, K., Alsawas, M., et al. (2017). Treatment of pediatric obesity: An umbrella systematic review. *Journal of Clinical Endocrinology and Metabolism, 102*(3), 763–775.

Rankin, J., Matthews, L., Cobley, S., et al. (2016). Psychological consequences of childhood obesity: Psychiatric comorbidity and prevention. *Adolescent Health, Medicine and Therapeutics, 7*, 125–146.

Sabharwal, S. (2015). Blount disease: An update. *The Orthopedic Clinics of North America, 46*(1), 37–47.

Scahill, L., Specht, M., & Page, C. (2014). The prevalence of tic disorders and clinical characteristics in children. *Journal of Obsessive-Compulsive and Related Disorders, 3*(4), 394–400.

Schmiege, S. J., Gance-Cleveland, B., Gilbert, L., et al. (2016). Identifying patterns of obesity risk behavior to improve pediatric primary care. *Journal for Specialists in Pediatric Nursing, 21*, 18–28.

Sievers, K., & Silk, H. (2016). Fluoride varnish for preventing dental cares in children and adolescents. *American Family Physician, 93*(9), 743–744.

Sinha, R., & Raut, S. (2016). Management of nocturnal enuresis – myths and facts. *World Journal of Nephrology, 5*(4), 328–338.

Sirard, J. R., Bruening, M., Wall, M. M., et al. (2013). Physical activity and screen time in adolescents and their friends. *American Journal of Preventive Medicine, 44*(1), 48–55.

Slawson, D. L., Fitzgerald, N., & Morgan, K. T. (2013). Position of the academy of nutrition and dietetics: The role of nutrition in health promotion and chronic disease prevention. *Journal of the Academy of Nutrition & Dietetics, 113*(7), 972–979.

Solanki, N., Kumar, A., Awasthi, N., et al. (2016). Assessment of oral status in pediatric patients with special health care needs receiving dental rehabilitation procedures under general anesthesia: A retrospective analysis. *The Journal of Contemporary Dental Practice, 17*(6), 476–479.

Sood, M. R., & Matta, S. R. (2016). Approach to a child with functional abdominal pain. *Indian Journal of Pediatrics, 83*(12), 1452–1458.

Stagi, S., Ricci, F., Bianconi, M., et al. (2017). Retrospective evaluation of metformin and/or metformin plus a new polysaccharide complex in treating severe hyperinsulinism and insulin resistance in obese children and adolescents with metabolic syndrome. *Nutrients, 9*(5), E524.

Styne, D. M., Arslanian, S. A., Connor, E. L., et al. (2017). Pediatric obesity-assessment, treatment, and prevention: An endocrine society clinical practice guideline. *Journal of Clinical Endocrinology and Metabolism, 102*(3), 709–757.

Sukkar, S. G., Signori, A., Borrini, C., et al. (2013). Feasibility of protein-sparing modified fast by tube (ProMoFasT) in obesity treatment: A phase II pilot trial on clinical safety and efficacy (appetite control, body composition, muscular strength, metabolic pattern, pulmonary function test). *Mediterranean Journal of Nutrition and Metabolism, 6*, 165–176.

Tandon, P. S., Zhou, C., Sallis, J. F., et al. (2012). Home environment relationships with children's physical activity, sedentary time, and screen time by socioeconomic status. *The International Journal of Behavioral Nutrition and Physical Activity, 9*, 88.

Temneanu, O. R., Trandafir, L. M., & Purcarea, M. R. (2016). Type 2 diabetes mellitus in children and adolescents: A relatively new clinical problem within pediatric practice. *Journal of Medicine and Life, 9*(3), 235–239.

Temple, J. L., Cordero, P., Li, J., et al. (2016). A guide to non-alcoholic fatty liver disease in childhood and adolescence. *International Journal of Molecular Sciences, 17*(6), 947.

Thompson, N., Mansfield, B., Stringer, M., et al. (2016). An evidence-based resource for the management of comorbidities associated with childhood overweight and obesity. *Journal of the American Association of Nurse Practitioners, 28*(10), 559–570.

Tinanoff, N. (2016). Dental caries. In R. M. Kliegman, B. F. Stanton, J. W. St. Geme, et al. (Eds.), *Nelson textbook of pediatrics* (20th ed.). Philadelphia: Saunders/Elsevier.

Weyandt, L. L., Marraccini, M. E., Gudmundsdottir, B. G., et al. (2014). Pharmacological interventions for adolescents and adults with ADHD: Stimulant and nonstimulant medications and misuse of prescription stimulants. *Psychology Research and Behavior Management, 9*(7), 223–249.

Wiesenthal, E. N., Fagnano, M., Cook, S., et al. (2016). Asthma and overweight/obese: Double trouble for urban children. *The Journal of Asthma, 53*(5), 485–491.

World Health Organization. (2017). *Childhood overweight and obesity*. http://www.who.int/dietphysicalactivity/childhood/en/.

Wright, N., & Wales, J. (2016). Assessment and management of severely obese children and adolescents. *Archives of Disease in Childhood, 101*(12), 1161–1167.

Xi, J., Takyi, B., & Lamptey, E. (2015). Are recent immigrants larger than earlier ones at their arrival? Cohort variation in initial BMI among US immigrants, 1989-2011. *Journal of Immigrant and Minority Health, 17*, 1854–1862.

Xu, S., & Xue, Y. (2016). Pediatric obesity: Causes, symptoms, prevention and treatment. *Experimental and Therapeutic Medicine, 11*(1), 15–20.

Zhang, G., Wu, L., Zhou, L., et al. (2016). Television watching and risk of childhood obesity: A meta-analysis. *European Journal of Public Health, 26*(1), 13–18.

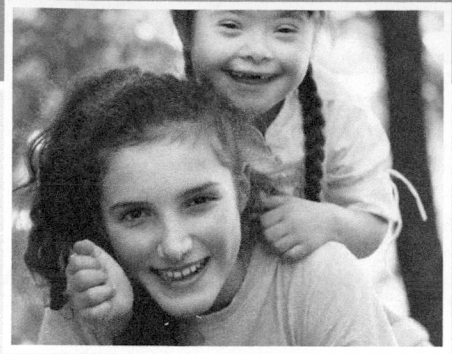

17

Health Promotion of the Adolescent and Family

Anne Derouin

http://evolve.elsevier.com/wong/ncic

CONCEPTS

- Development
- Functional Ability
- Family Dynamics
- Reproduction
- Sexuality
- Mood and Affect
- Safety
- Health Promotion

PROMOTING OPTIMUM GROWTH AND DEVELOPMENT

Adolescence is a dynamic period of transition from childhood to adult maturity; a time of profound biologic, intellectual, psychosocial, and economic change—this phase of rapid growth and development is second only to the first of life. During this period individuals progress through phases of physical and sexual maturity, gradually develop more sophisticated intellectual and reasoning capabilities, and make critical social, emotional, educational, and occupational decisions that will ultimately shape their adult careers and health outcomes. The changes that occur during adolescence have important health risk implications. Young people are exposed to a wide variety of opportunities and behaviors that could have long-term health consequences, underlining the key role nurses have in promoting safety and health practices among this population.

When examining widely accepted theories of adolescent development, researchers have challenged many popular notions. For example, a common belief is that teenagers' behaviors are overwhelmingly negative, controlled by "raging hormones," and that adolescence is a period when rebellious and risky behavior is the norm causing struggles with adult caregivers. Although these notions are mistaken, the foundational ideal is not benign; choices and behaviors that some adolescents make during this period have detrimental effects on their long-term health outcomes, so health care provider attitudes, interactions with adolescents, and the application of consistent, safety-first policies and program development are vital. Current research supports a positive view of this developmental period, confirming that adolescence involves a complex interplay of biologic, cognitive, psychologic, and social change. These changes occur at predicable but highly variable individual timeframes that is interdependent on multiple variables, including the social determinates of health. On the individual level, changes include biologic maturation, cognitive development, and psychologic development. Change also occurs in the social contexts of adolescents' families, peer groups, schools, faith communities, and workplaces.

Adolescence progresses for each child in three distinct phases: (1) early adolescence, also termed *pubescent,* typically ages 11 to 14 years; (2) middle adolescence, typically ages 15 to 17 years; and (3) late adolescence, also termed *young adulthood,* typically ages 18 to 22 years. Many researchers feel that neurodevelopment is not complete until 25 years old, so consideration has been given to young adulthood extending later into the second decade of life (Arain, Haque, Johal, et al., 2013). The physical, emotional, and psychologic changes, opportunities, challenges, social pressures, and resources available to young people differ during these three unique phases. Early adolescence is characterized primarily by the physical changes of puberty and the emotional responses to those changes. Middle adolescence is characterized by transition from adult-caregiver to peer-dominant orientation, often with intense self-focus preoccupations and experimentation with of music, technology, dress, and physical appearance. Wide variations of cognitive development, gender, peer, and future-career exploration, as well as experimental social behaviors, including sexuality and recreational drug use, typically occur at this time. Late adolescence features full physical maturation and the transition toward adult behaviors, sustainable emotional and

TABLE 17.1 Growth and Development During Adolescence

Early Adolescence (11-14 years)	Middle Adolescence (15-17 years)	Late Adolescence (18-20 years)
Growth		
Rapidly accelerating growth Reaches peak velocity Secondary sexual characteristics appear	Growth decelerating in girls Stature reaches 95% of adult height Secondary sexual characteristics well advanced	Physically mature Structure and reproductive growth almost complete
Cognition		
Explores newfound ability for limited abstract thought Clumsy groping for new values and energies Comparison of "normality" with peers of same sex	Developing capacity for abstract thinking Enjoys intellectual powers, often in idealistic terms Concern with philosophic, political, and social problems	Established abstract thought Can perceive and act on long-range options Able to view problems comprehensively Intellectual and functional identity established
Identity		
Preoccupied with rapid body changes Trying out of various roles Measurement of attractiveness by acceptance or rejection by peers Conformity to group norms Decline in self-esteem	Modified body image Self-centered; increased narcissism Tendency toward inner experience and self-discovery Rich fantasy life Idealistic Able to perceive future implications of current behavior and decisions; variable application	Body image and gender-role definition nearly secured Mature sexual identity Phase of consolidation of identity Increase in self-esteem Comfortable with physical growth Social roles defined and articulated
Relationships With Parents		
Defining independence-dependence boundaries Strong desire to remain dependent on parents while trying to detach No major conflicts over parental control	Major conflicts over independence and control Low point in parent-child relationship Greatest push for emancipation; disengagement Final and irreversible emotional detachment from parents	Emotional and physical separation from parents completed Independence from family with less conflict Emancipation nearly secured
Relationships With Peers		
Seeks peer affiliations to counter instability generated by rapid change Upsurge of close, idealized friendships with members of same sex Struggle for mastery within peer group	Strong need for identity to affirm self-image Behavioral standards set by peer group Acceptance by peers extremely important—fear of rejection Exploration of ability to attract opposite sex	Peer group recedes in importance in favor of individual friendship Testing of romantic relationships against possibility of permanent alliance Relationships characterized by giving and sharing
Sexuality		
Self-exploration and evaluation Limited dating, usually group Limited intimacy	Multiple plural relationships Internal identification of heterosexual, homosexual, or bisexual attractions Exploration of "self-appeal" Feeling of "being in love" Tentative establishment of relationships	Forms stable relationships and attachment to another Growing capacity for mutuality and reciprocity Dating as a romantic pair May publicly identify as gay, lesbian, or bisexual Intimacy involves commitment rather than exploration and romanticism
Psychologic Health		
Wide mood swings Intense daydreaming Anger outwardly expressed with moodiness, temper outbursts, and verbal insults and name calling	Tendency toward inner experiences; more introspective Tendency to withdraw when upset or feelings are hurt Vacillation of emotions in time and range Feelings of inadequacy common; difficulty asking for help	More constancy of emotion Anger more likely to be concealed

intimate relationships, and critical thinking skills to independently manage health care, career, and responsibilities (Table 17.1).

BIOLOGIC DEVELOPMENT

Neuroendocrine Events of Puberty

The fundamental biologic changes of adolescence are collectively referred to as puberty. Puberty involves a predictable sequence of physical changes that occur sequentially during adolescence that results in sexual and physical maturation. The events of puberty are triggered by hormonal influences and are controlled by the anterior pituitary gland in response to stimulus from the hypothalamus.

Puberty begins as the hypothalamus produces increased levels of gonadotropin-releasing hormone (GnRH). GnRH travels through a network of capillaries to the anterior pituitary gland, where it stimulates the production and secretion of follicle-stimulating hormone (FSH)

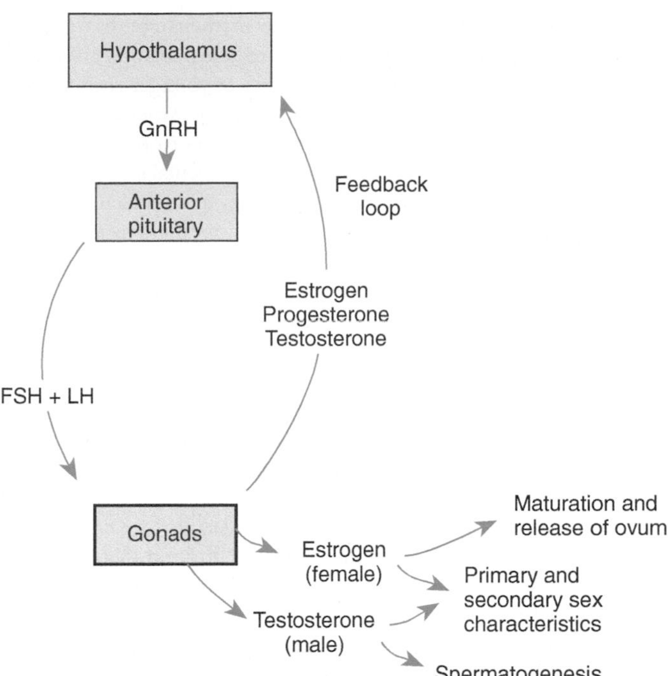

FIG. 17.1 Hormonal interaction among hypothalamus, pituitary, and gonads. *GnRH,* Gonadotropin-releasing hormone; *FSH,* follicle-stimulating hormone; *LH,* luteinizing hormone.

and luteinizing hormone (LH) (Fig. 17.1). Increasing levels of FSH and LH in the blood stimulate gonadal response. The sequential response varies for the two genders: for females, FSH stimulates growth of ovarian follicles and production of estrogen. LH initiates ovulation, the formation of the corpus luteum, and progesterone production. For males, LH acts on testicular Leydig cells, prompting maturation of the testicles and testosterone production. FSH, acting with LH, stimulates sperm production. Sex steroids—estrogen, progesterone, and testosterone and other androgens—are released from the gonads and effect biologic changes in various organs, including muscles, bones, skin, and hair follicles. Increasing serum levels of sex steroids also provide feedback to the hypothalamus, causing decreases in GnRH secretion. When serum sex hormone levels decrease, the hypothalamus is stimulated to increase GnRH secretion, again initiating the sequence that produces the appropriate gonadal responses.

Initiation of Puberty

The precise mechanism that institutes the changes at puberty is not completely understood. Although the pituitary gland and gonads are capable of mature function and can respond to stimuli at any age, the hypothalamic-pituitary-gonadal system is kept in a dormant state throughout childhood by some central nervous system inhibitory mechanism in the region of the hypothalamus. It is believed that the receptor sites in the hypothalamus are so sensitive that minute quantities of circulating sex hormones are sufficient to inhibit the secretion of GnRH during childhood. The hypothalamus loses this negative sensitivity at puberty, which allows the hypothalamic-pituitary-gonadal mechanism to attain full secretory function. As puberty progresses, the pituitary and gonads become increasingly sensitive to positive hormonal stimulation.

Changes in Reproductive Hormones

Females

The primary sexual characteristic in girls is the development and release of an egg, or ovum, from the ovaries approximately every 28 days. Beginning in early puberty, FSH stimulates estrogen production by the ovaries. However, concentrations of estrogen do not reach levels high enough to cause ovulation. By the time girls reach midpuberty, the body produces estrogen in larger amounts. This quantity of estrogen production results in the building of an endometrial lining of the uterus and first menstruation, or menarche. At menarche, ova still do not generally mature enough to be released. However, as puberty progresses, usually one ovarian follicle becomes dominant during each menstrual cycle and produces increasing amounts of estrogen during the early-cycle, follicular phase. This follicle then releases an ovum, a process termed *ovulation,* around day 14 of the menstrual cycle. After ovulation the follicle involutes and its estrogen production decreases. This leads to a drop in serum estrogen and progesterone. The pituitary gland responds to the drop in these hormone levels with increased production of FSH, initiating the start of a new menstrual cycle.

By direct action, estrogens cause growth and development of the vagina, uterus, and fallopian tubes. The skin of the labia majora, as well as that of the breast areola and nipples, grows and darkens under the influence of estrogen. Estrogen is responsible for breast enlargement. Estrogen also promotes the growth of pubic and axillary hair, and widening of the hips. At low levels estrogen tends to stimulate skeletal growth in both boys and girls, but at higher levels it inhibits growth.

Males

The primary male sexual characteristic is the development of viable sperm. During puberty, FSH acts on testicular cells, stimulating the production of viable sperm. FSH and LH also act on a different group of testicular cells, resulting in increased production and secretion of testosterone. In this process of sexual development, boys do not experience a discrete event analogous to menstruation or ovulation in girls. However, just as the production of a mature ovum tends to occur 1 year or more after menarche in girls, the production of viable sperm tends to follow boys' first ejaculations. The capacity to ejaculate appears relatively early in boys' sexual development, approximately 1 year after initial testicular enlargement and the appearance of pubic hair. From a clinical perspective, however, an adolescent should be considered potentially fertile with a first menstrual period or a first ejaculation.

Testosterone and other androgens have a direct impact on growth of the penis, scrotum, prostate, and seminal vesicles of the testicles. The tremendous growth-promoting properties of these hormones also result in rapid increases in muscle mass, skeletal growth, bone age, and bone density. In both sexes androgens are responsible for the development of pubic, axillary, facial, and body hair. Clinically, increased activity of androgens is associated with pubertal conditions such as acne, body odor, deepening of the voice, a spurt in height, and an increase in red blood cell levels.

Pubertal Sexual Maturation

Increases in reproductive hormones are responsible for dramatic changes in secondary sexual characteristics that occur during puberty. As with general growth, development of secondary sexual characteristics occurs in a predictable sequence. This sequence has been divided into a series of five phases termed the Tanner stages (Box 17.1 and Figs. 17.2 to 17.6). Although the sequence of sexual development is predictable, the age at which these changes occur and the rate of developmental progression vary considerably among individuals. Over the course of pubescence, many young people have questions about the timing, rate, and normalcy of their body changes. These concerns provide nurses with excellent opportunities to discuss health-related topics such as puberty, sexuality, contraception options, and prevention of sexually transmitted infections (STIs), as well as promotion of nutrition, exercise, and safe methods for weight control.

Sexual Maturation in Girls

The earliest, most easily visible changes of puberty in girls are changes in the nipple and areola and development of a small bud of breast tissue (thelarche). The average age of thelarche varies among ethnic groups: African American girls have an average age of 8.8 years, Caucasian girls average is 9.7 years, and Hispanic girls average 9.3 (Herman-Giddens, 2013).

The appearance of pubic hair (pubarche) typically follows initial breast development though many have strands of underarm and/or pubic hair before breast development. Early in puberty there is often an increase in clear, white or yellowish vaginal discharge (physiologic leukorrhea), associated with hormonal changes and uterine development. Girls or their parents may be concerned that this vaginal discharge is a sign of infection. The nurse can reassure them that the discharge is normal and a sign that their body is maturing; the uterus is preparing for menstruation. Throughout puberty, there is continued breast enlargement and pubic hair progresses to adult-type sexual hair covering the mons pubis and labia majora.

The hallmark of late puberty is the first menstrual period, or *menarche.* Initial menstrual cycles are usually scanty and irregular (unpredictable) and are not always accompanied by ovulation. Gradually ovulation and regular, predicable menstrual periods occur about a year after menarche. The maturation cycle is typically a 2-year period from the appearance of breast buds to regular menstrual cycles but can range from 1 to 6 years. The mean age of menarche in the United States is 10½ to 15½ years, with an average age being 12.2 years for African American girls and 12.8 years for non-Hispanic Caucasian girls (Cabrera, Bright, Frane, et al., 2014). Girls may be considered to have pubertal delay if breast development has not occurred by age 13 years or if menarche has not occurred within 2 to 2½ years of the onset of breast development (Villanueva & Argente, 2014).

BOX 17.1 Tanner Stages

The Tanner stages were developed by Dr. J. M. Tanner and colleagues. Tanner stages describe the stages of pubertal growth and are numbered from stage 1 (immature) to stage 5 (mature) for both males and females. In females the Tanner stages describe pubertal development based on breast size and the shape and distribution of pubic hair. In males the Tanner stages describe pubertal development based on the size and shape of the penis and scrotum and the shape and distribution of pubic hair.

Data from Tanner, J. M. (1962). *Growth of adolescents.* Oxford: Blackwell Scientific Publications.

There is evidence that the mean age of menarche has gradually decreased over the past century in the United States and other developing countries. Females are experiences puberty at younger ages, with differences noted between Caucasian and African American girls. The explanation for this is not yet clear but appears to be influenced by complex physiologic, psychological, and environmental interrelationships and the reduced rates of disease as technology and medicine advances. This decline in the average age of menarche appears to have leveled off in recent years but continues to be studied (Papadimitriou, 2016). Internationally, a decline in the average age at first menses has not been seen in countries where children are more likely to be malnourished and suffer from chronic illness.

Sexual maturation influences young people's satisfaction with their appearance, but the effects differ for girls and boys. For girls, physical maturation can lead to greater dissatisfaction with their appearance. For example, adolescent girls are more dissatisfied with their appearance and significantly likely to identify themselves as being overweight, even when they are at a normal weight for height (Fan, Jin, & Khubchandani, 2014). Normal increases in weight and fat deposition that accompany puberty among girls conflict with cultural norms that emphasize a slender look. Early-maturing girls suffer most because they begin to develop at a time when their peers still exemplify prepubertal slimness. Unfortunately, one response to changes in body shape among teenagers is to engage in extensive dieting at a time when nutritional requirements are at a peak. For some, the focus on slimness and dieting may trigger the development of eating disorders (see Chapter 18). Consequently, nurses play a key role in providing health promotion and educating teens about pubertal growth, eating behaviors, and body image, especially for early-maturing girls.

Sexual Maturation in Boys

The first pubescent changes in boys are testicular enlargement accompanied by thinning, reddening, and increasing looseness of the scrotum. These events usually occur between 9½ and 14 years of age. Early puberty is also characterized by the initial appearance of scant pubic hair, which continues throughout puberty. Penile enlargement begins, and testicular enlargement and pubic hair growth continue throughout midpuberty. During this period boys also undergo increasing muscularity, early voice changes, and development of early facial hair. Gynecomastia (breast enlargement and tenderness) is common during midpuberty, occurring in up to 70% of boys (Ali & Donohoue, 2016). Gynecomastia disappears within 2 years of development; however, it may persist in obese individuals. By midpuberty there is a definite increase in the length and width of the penis, testicular enlargement continues, and first ejaculation

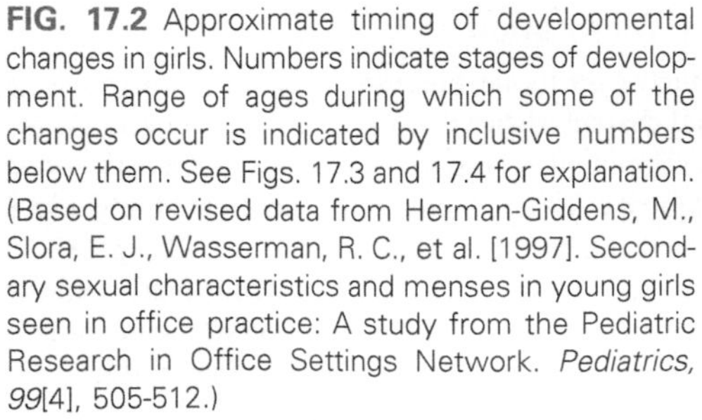

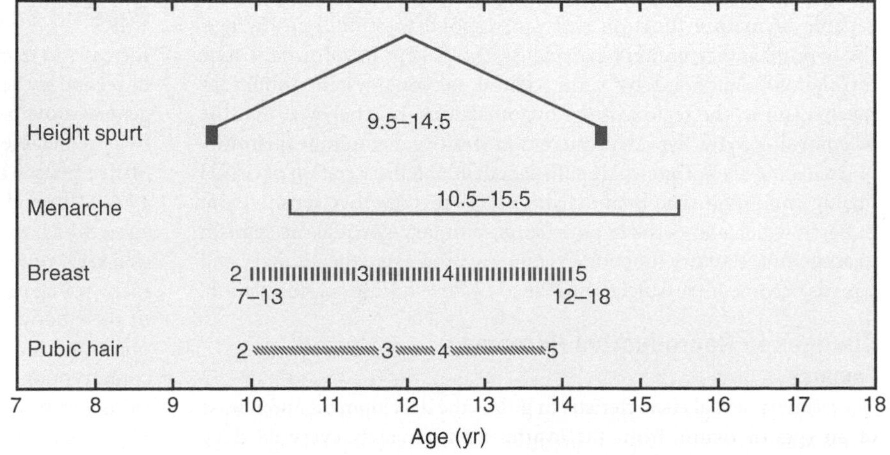

FIG. 17.2 Approximate timing of developmental changes in girls. Numbers indicate stages of development. Range of ages during which some of the changes occur is indicated by inclusive numbers below them. See Figs. 17.3 and 17.4 for explanation. (Based on revised data from Herman-Giddens, M., Slora, E. J., Wasserman, R. C., et al. [1997]. Secondary sexual characteristics and menses in young girls seen in office practice: A study from the Pediatric Research in Office Settings Network. *Pediatrics, 99*[4], 505-512.)

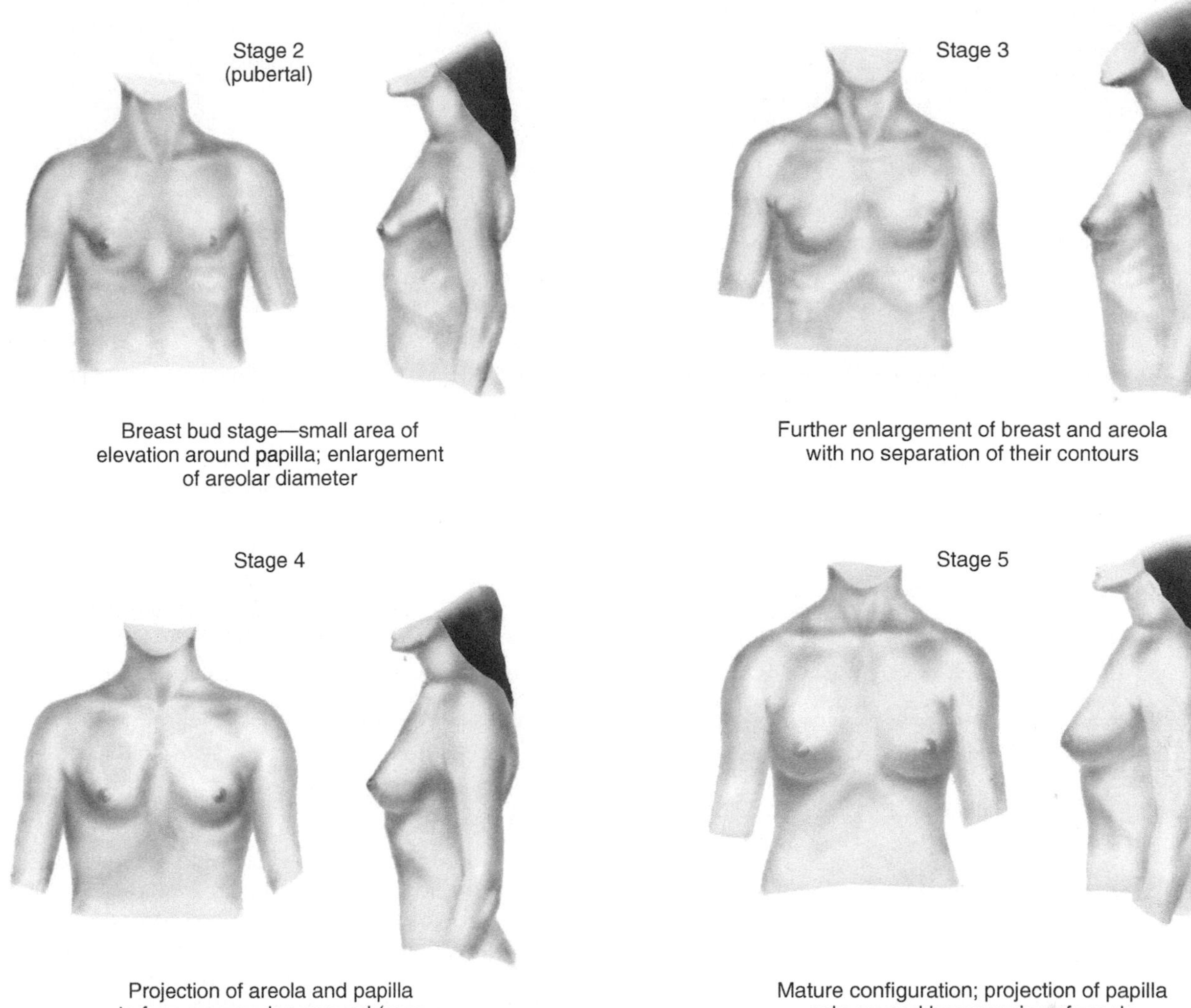
Stage 2
(pubertal)
Breast bud stage—small area of elevation around papilla; enlargement of areolar diameter
Stage 3
Further enlargement of breast and areola with no separation of their contours
Stage 4
Projection of areola and papilla to form a secondary mound (may not occur in all girls)
Stage 5
Mature configuration; projection of papilla only caused by recession of areola into general contour

FIG. 17.3 Development of breasts in girls. Average age span is 8 to 12¾ years. Stage 1 (prepubertal—elevation of papilla only) is not shown. (Modified from Marshall, W. A., & Tanner, J. M. [1969]. Variations in pattern of pubertal changes in girls. *Archives of Disease in Childhood, 44*[235], 291-303; and Daniel, W. A., & Paulshock, B. Z. [1979]. A physician's guide to sexual maturity. *Patient Care, 13,* 122-124.)

occurs. Axillary hair develops, and facial hair extends to cover the anterior neck. Final voice changes occur secondary to the growth of the larynx.

Herman-Giddens, Steffes, Harris, and colleagues (2012) found that secondary sexual characteristics occurred earlier in US adolescents than those described in Tanner's studies in England in 1969. Mean ages for onset of Tanner 2 stage of genital development in African American males was 9.14 years, in Hispanic males the average onset was 10.04 years, and among non-Hispanic white males it was 10.14 years. The authors suggest that genetic factors, environmental factors, and lifestyle changes may be the cause for the earlier appearance of secondary sexual characteristics but note that further studies are needed to clarify these findings.

Changes in the size and shape of the penis and testicles and changes in genital functioning can be areas of great concern for adolescent boys. Although the ability for penile erection is present at birth, only with pubertal maturation do boys have seminal emissions. Ejaculation may occur spontaneously as a nocturnal emission, or "wet dream"; as a result of self-stimulation (masturbation); or during sexual activity with others. Unless they are prepared, boys may find spontaneous ejaculations puzzling, troublesome, and embarrassing. Pubertal changes and related concerns create important opportunities for health promotion among young teenage boys. Nurses are valuable resources of accurate information and anticipatory guidance around issues related to sexual maturation.

Precocious (early) puberty in both females and males may be a concern if secondary sexual characteristics occur before 8 years old. Concerns about pubertal delay should be considered for girls who do not exhibit menarche by age 15 years and among boys who exhibit no enlargement of the testes or scrotal changes by 14 years old (Villanueva & Argente, 2014).

Physical Growth During Puberty

Along with increases in reproductive hormones and sexual maturation, major changes in skeletal and lean body mass occur during puberty. The final 20% to 25% of linear growth is achieved during puberty, and up to 50% of ideal adult body weight is gained during this time as well. The **pubertal growth spurt** refers to the general increase in growth of

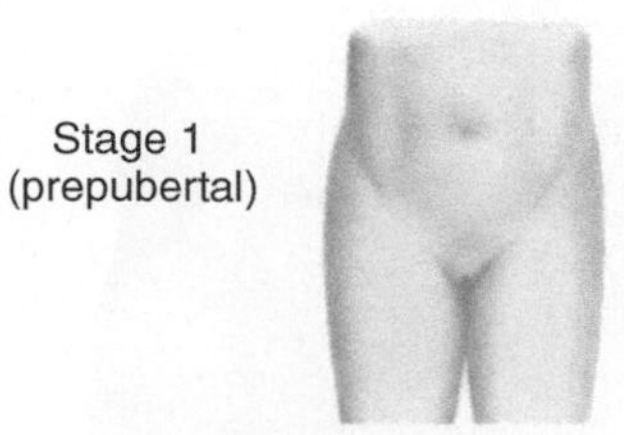
Stage 1
(prepubertal)
No pubic hair; essentially the same as during childhood; no distinction between hair on pubis and over the abdomen

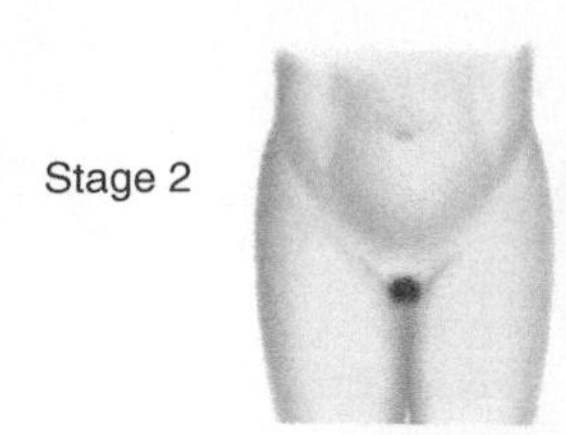
Stage 2
Sparse growth of long, straight, downy, and slightly pigmented hair extending along labia; between stages 2 and 3 begins to appear on pubis

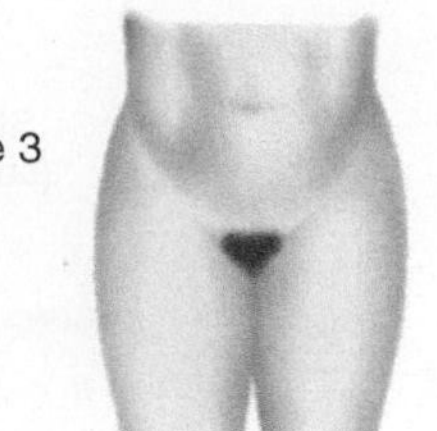
Stage 3
Hair darker, coarser, and curly and spread sparsely over entire pubis in the typical female triangle

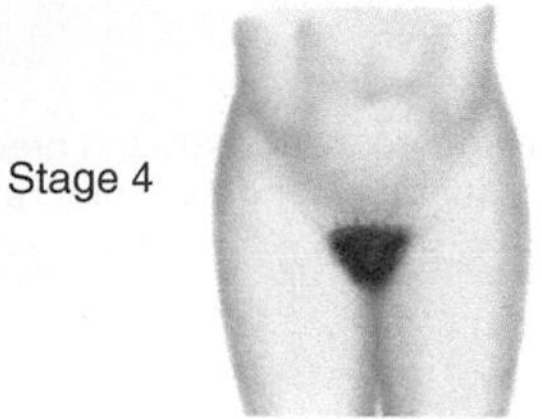
Stage 4
Pubic hair denser, curled, and adult in distribution but less abundant and restricted to the pubic area

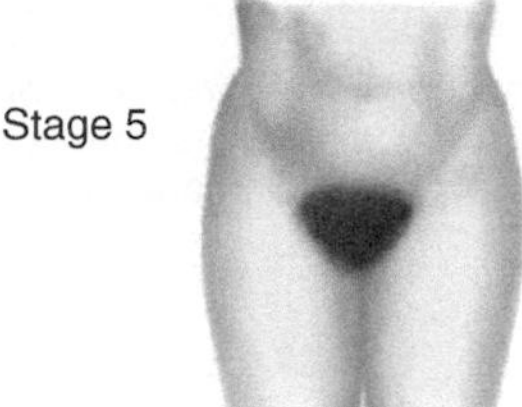
Stage 5
Hair adult in quantity, type, and pattern with spread to inner aspect of thighs

FIG. 17.4 Growth in pubic hair in girls. Average age span for stages 2 through 5 is 11 to 14 years. (Modified from Marshall, W. A., & Tanner, J. M. [1969]. Variations in pattern of pubertal changes in girls. *Archives of Disease in Childhood, 44*[235], 291-303; and Daniel, W. A., & Paulshock, B. Z. [1979]. A physician's guide to sexual maturity. *Patient Care, 13,* 122-124.)

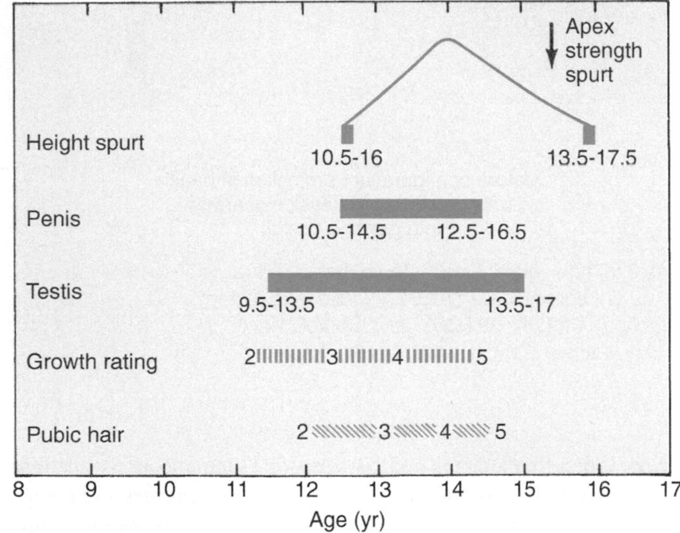
Apex strength spurt
Height spurt
10.5-16
13.5-17.5
Penis
10.5-14.5
12.5-16.5
Testis
9.5-13.5
13.5-17
Growth rating
2 3 4 5
Pubic hair
2 3 4 5
8 9 10 11 12 13 14 15 16 17
Age (yr)

FIG. 17.5 Approximate timing of developmental changes in boys. Numbers indicate stages of development. Range of ages during which some of the changes occur is indicated by inclusive numbers below them. See Fig. 17.6 for explanation. (From Marshall, W. A., & Tanner, J. M. [1970]. Variations in the pattern of pubertal changes in boys. *Archives of Disease in Childhood, 45*[239], 13-23.)

the skeleton, muscles, and internal organs, which reaches a peak rate at about 12 years of age in girls and about 14 years of age in boys. Although accelerated growth occurs in all adolescents, the age of onset, duration, and extent vary among individuals. Genetic endowment is the most important determinant of the onset, rate, and duration of pubertal growth, although adequate nutrition, environment, and health status also play important roles.

Normal Patterns of Growth

Once the process of growth begins, the sequence of changes is progressive and usually predictable. Awareness of this sequence is not only important for reassuring concerned adolescents and parents but also useful in diagnosing conditions associated with abnormal growth. In general, girls begin puberty and reach maturity about 2 years earlier than boys. The pubertal growth spurt begins as early as 9½ years or as late as 14½ years in girls, and as early as 10½ years and as late as 16 years in boys.

General growth includes accumulation of body mass, along with increases in height and weight. Lean body mass, primarily muscle mass, increases in both girls and boys during early puberty. For girls, the rate of muscle mass growth peaks at menarche and then slows. For boys, muscle mass continues to increase throughout puberty, resulting in the attainment of significantly higher lean body mass in boys than in girls. In girls, gain in fat mass increases markedly early in puberty and continues to increase after menarche. In boys there is a peak deceleration in the rate of fat mass accumulation at the time of their growth spurt, and thereafter a slower and much less dramatic increase than in girls.

The rate of linear growth (height) (Fig. 17.7) begins to increase in girls during early puberty, whereas in boys the rate does not increase until midpuberty. Peak height velocity (PHV) occurs at about 12 years of age in girls, around 6 to 12 months before menarche. PHV is used as a predictor of menarche; height at menarche is a predictor of ultimate adult height. Few girls grow more than 5 cm (2 inches) in height after menarche. Growth in girls' height usually ceases 2 to 2½ years after menarche. Boys typically reach PHV at about 14 years of age, after growth of the testicles and penis and the appearance of axillary and mature pubic hair. Among most boys, growth in height ceases at 18 or 20 years of age. Increases in leg length tend to precede growth of the trunk by about 6 to 9 months and that of the shoulders and chest by about 1 year. In short, teenagers tend to follow a linear growth pattern, in which they outgrow their shoes first, then their pants, and finally their shirts. Peak weight velocity occurs about 6 months after PHV in

Stage 1 (prepubertal)

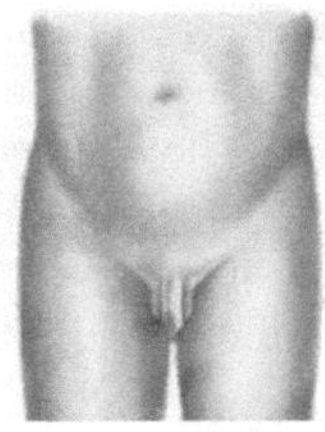

No pubic hair; essentially the same as during childhood; no distinction between hair on pubis and over the abdomen

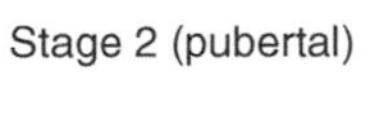

Stage 2 (pubertal)

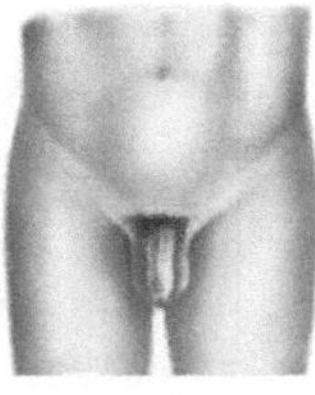

Initial enlargement of scrotum and testes; reddening and textural changes of scrotal skin; sparse growth of long, straight, downy, and slightly pigmented hair at base of penis

Stage 3

Initial enlargement of penis, mainly in length; testes and scrotum further enlarged; hair darker, coarser, and curly and spread sparsely over entire pubis

Stage 4

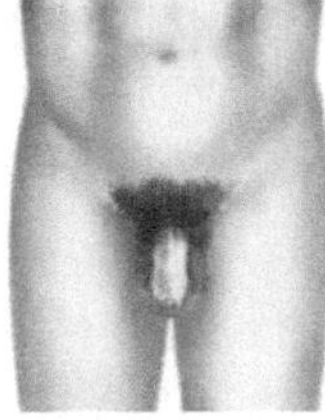

Increased size of penis with growth in diameter and development of glans; glans larger and broader; scrotum darker; pubic hair more abundant with curling but restricted to pubic area

Stage 5

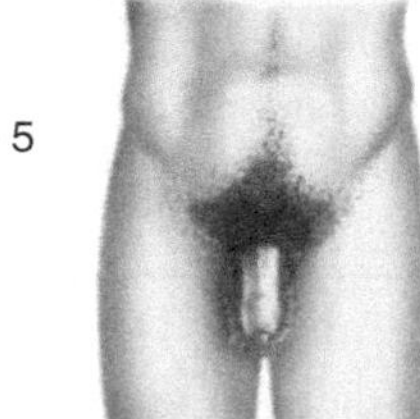

Testes, scrotum, and penis adult in size and shape; hair adult in quantity and type with spread to inner surface of thighs

FIG. 17.6 Developmental stages of secondary sexual characteristics and genital development in boys. Average age span is $12\frac{1}{2}$ to 16 years. (Modified from Marshall, W. A., & Tanner, J. M. [1970]. Variations in the pattern of pubertal changes in boys. *Archives of Disease in Childhood, 45*[239], 13-23; and Daniel, W. A., & Paulshock, B. Z. [1979]. A physician's guide to sexual maturity. *Patient Care, 13,* 122-124.)

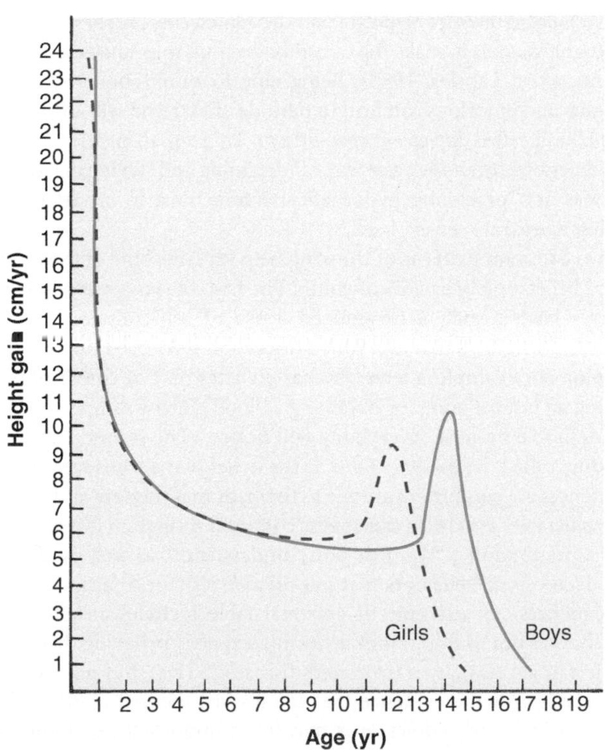

FIG. 17.7 Linear growth in centimeters per year. (From Tanner, J. M., Whitehouse, R. H., & Takaishi, M. [1966]. Standards from birth to maturity for height, weight, height velocity and weight velocity: British children, 1965. *Archives of Disease in Childhood, 41,* 454-471.)

girls. In contrast, weight and height spurts occur simultaneously for boys. On average, girls gain 5 to 20 cm (2 to 8 inches) in height and 7 to 25 kg (15.5 to 55 lb) in weight during adolescence, and boys gain 10 to 30 cm (4 to 12 inches) in height and 7 to 30 kg (15.5 to 66 lb) in weight during adolescence.

Other Physiologic Changes

In addition to the sexual development changes of puberty, numerous body systems mature as well. The size and strength of the heart, blood volume, and systolic blood pressure increase, and the heart rate decreases. Consistent with the general developmental timetable, these changes appear earlier in girls, who establish a slightly higher pulse rate and a slightly lower systolic blood pressure than boys. Blood volume and values in blood components steadily increase during childhood to reach adult levels in adolescence. There is an increase in serum iron, the number of red blood cells, hemoglobin, and hematocrit levels more so in boys compared with girls, which is likely related to the increased muscle mass in pubertal boys.

The lungs increase in both diameter and length during puberty. The respiratory rate, decreasing steadily throughout childhood, reaches the adult rate in adolescence. Respiratory volume, vital capacity, and other physiologic properties related to respiratory function are increased, and to a greater extent in boys than in girls. The differences between the sexes are a result of the greater lung growth associated with boys' increased shoulder and chest size.

The rate of steady decline in basal metabolic rate from birth to adulthood slows during puberty, coinciding with the growth spurt in both sexes, reflecting the increase in physiologic activities. A slightly higher metabolic rate in boys than in girls is probably a function of differences in androgenic hormones. Basal body temperature gradually decreases with age in both sexes, reaching adult values by 12 years of age in girls and somewhat later in boys.

Adolescence is also a time of continued brain growth. Although the number of neurons does not increase, there is a proliferation of the support cells that brace and nourish the neurons, and an increase in the number of neural connections. Development of these connections within the cortex of the brain continues during adolescence and may not reach adult levels until 26 years old. In addition, the growth of the myelin sheath around the nerve cells continues through and beyond puberty, enabling faster neural processing. This "fine-tuning" of the neurosystem, also called neuroplasticity, coincides with development of the more advanced cognitive capacities of youth and continues into early adulthood. Recent studies have shown that the frontal cortex areas of the brain, associated with executive functions, continue myelinization throughout adolescence and may not be complete until as late as age 26 years (Fuhrmann, Knoll, & Blakemore, 2015).

COGNITIVE DEVELOPMENT

Emergence of Formal Operational Thought (Piaget)

Jean Piaget (1972) described the shift from childhood to adolescence as a movement from concrete to formal operational thought. Children's thinking is oriented to things and events that they can observe directly. Unable to think in terms of abstract possibilities, they process information based on what is directly observable. For most young people, emergence of formal operational thinking occurs between the ages of 11 and 14 years. **Formal operational thought** includes being able to think in abstract terms, consider consequences to actions, and hypothesize possibilities. Adolescents gradually become able to symbolically associate behaviors with abstract concepts such as attractiveness, adult status, responsibilities or happiness. They also become capable of conceptualizing a future time perspective rather than being tied to the concrete thinking of "here-and-now" that is common during the latency period. They are able to imagine a sequence of future events that might occur including college or occupational opportunities, or how current situations, such as relationships with parents or friends, could change to meet an imagined ideal.

The nurse's ability to assess an adolescent's level of cognitive development has important implications for health promotion. Younger teens need concrete communication strategies, support of a parent, and frequent reminders (verbal, written, and electronic), whereas older adolescents, who have developed abstract thinking, may well be able to manage responsibilities of self-care and independently consider long-term implications of their behaviors. Younger adolescents require health promotion efforts that emphasize immediate risks or benefits of the behavior. Older adolescents may respond to health promotion efforts that focus on concrete health benefits of the future or acknowledge ability to make conscious decisions which result in health consequences or rewards.

Along with cognitive development, decision-making abilities increase over the adolescent period. Young people gradually develop their ability to consider risks and benefits of behaviors, along with potential consequences of such behaviors. Most teens evolve from relying on parents and adult caregivers to consulting peers and adults outside of the home, mentors, and role models outside of the home as they mature, as well as resources found on the Internet and through social media. If teens routinely attend health care visits, their nurse is often considered a reliable source of information. By middle adolescence, most healthy teens are able to reason as well as adults and will seek information independently as well as from their peers. Health promotion efforts, especially those aimed at younger adolescents, should offer learning strategies that promote and enhance decision-making skills including peer-led initiatives, mentoring, instruction or workshops offered at school, vocational settings and shared evidence-based resources available on the Internet or via social media. During health care visits, nurses can screen for risk behaviors, offer resources that emphasize health-promotion norms for young people, and discuss alternatives to unhealthy behaviors along with opportunities to practice skills necessary to resist unhealthy behaviors.

Even with the best framework for health promotion, persons who are capable of formal operational thought and reasoned decision making do not always choose safe, healthy options of behavior. This is especially true for developing adolescents; when faced with time constraints, personal stress from home, community and school settings, sleep deprivation, social media influences, or overwhelming peer pressure, young people are more likely to abandon their rational thought processes. Unfortunately, many of the health-related decisions adolescents confront, such as those related to illicit substance use, safety practices, or sexual behavior, involve issues that are personally stressful, emotionally overwhelming, or new and novel/interesting to adolescents. Under such conditions, young people tend to diminish their capacities for abstract formal reasoning even if they typically use advanced decision-making skills.

Adolescent Conceptions of Self

With development of formal operational thought, adolescents begin thinking in more abstract capacities and are able to verbalize personal and interpersonal characteristics, beliefs, and emotional states. Compared with children, they develop a more differentiated self-concept, recognizing that their behavior and performance vary from setting to setting and that they are separate with varied thoughts and ideals from their parents. Over time, adolescents integrate these disparate observations of their selves into abstract personal characterizations (e.g., "I am a sensitive person").

Psychologic theories help explain how adolescents use these powerful new cognitive tools to make the transition to adult roles and relationships (Elkind, 1978; Lapsley, 1993). Being able to think about one's own thoughts and emotions can lead to periods of extreme self-absorption, what Elkind called *adolescent egocentrism.* This self-absorption has also been described by Lapsley as a way of imagining and "trying on" various personas and practicing hypothetical interactions in an attempt to develop a separate sense of self.

Two common patterns of thinking help explain some of the health-related beliefs and behaviors of youth. The first, the *imaginary audience,* involves having such a heightened sense of self-consciousness; an adolescent imagines that everyone notices and is focused on his or her behavior. For example, a teen who has diabetes may be convinced that wearing an insulin pump or obtaining a blood glucose sample at school is undesirable because "everybody will notice." The second pattern of thinking, called the *personal fable,* is the belief that a teens feelings and experiences are completely unique to them, or that they are all-knowing or invulnerable. This helps explain the common accusation from younger teens toward adults, "You just don't understand!" as well as some of their decisions or behaviors that put them at risk for significant health consequences. An example of personal fable includes an adolescent who chooses not to use condoms during sex, truly believing that "other people can get sexually transmitted diseases (STDs), but not me."

There is growing evidence that the inward-focused or narcissistic egocentrism of early adolescence may be an important developmental mechanism that leads to positive mental health among mature adults, but adolescents with a strong sense of invulnerability to danger in their personal fable are more likely to engage in risky behaviors that can lead to significant morbidity and mortality. Teens who feel invincible to danger have more delinquent behaviors and drug use, whereas teens with psychological invulnerability have better mastery and coping skills (Hill, Duggan, & Lapsley, 2012).

Changes in Social Cognition

Gains in cognitive abilities also have an impact on perspective-taking capacities of young people. As adolescents mature, they are increasingly able to "step into the shoes" of others. Preadolescents develop limited perspective-taking skills, first learning to step into the shoes of their closest friends, and then, during adolescence, the skills develop toward considering the experiences of other peers and family members, and finally people outside their social circle. Perspective-taking capacities develop further as adolescents engage in mutual role-taking. As they mature, teens are able to discuss various issues highlighting points of importance to people in various social roles (e.g., "From a parent's perspective, having a curfew is important because it means I'm safely home"). Older adolescents also realize that the perspectives people hold are influenced by a range of intrapersonal, interpersonal, and sociocultural factors and can be acceptable but varied from their own. They are typically able to consider the choices, behaviors, and outcomes experienced by other people while making their own health-related choices. The ability to consider alternative choices that may or may not apply to the teen significantly expands the opportunities to develop health-promoting behaviors or adapt new strategies of self-care.

DEVELOPMENT OF VALUE AUTONOMY

With advances in cognitive development, adolescents' beliefs become more abstract and increasingly rooted in general ideological principles with gradual independence from their parents' beliefs and values. Adolescents progress toward greater behavioral independence as they encounter new social situations and make independent decisions. They face a variety of cognitive conflicts as they compare past experiences and the advice of their parents to the views and influence of peers and deal with competing pressures to behave in given ways. Earlier in life most teens accept the decisions or points of view of their parents while maturing adolescents begin to "test," substitute, or adopt a set of values distinct from those significant adults in their lives. This struggle to clarify values, created in part by an expanded behavioral independence, is a large part of the process of developing what has been termed **value autonomy** (Steinberg, 1990). The development of a personal value system is a gradual process, with evidence that value autonomy occurs relatively late in adolescence, between the ages of 18 and 20 years (Steinberg, 1990).

Moral Development

Moral development parallels advances in reasoning and social cognition. With the attainment of abstract thought and the realization that people's perspectives and opinions may differ, the ways adolescents approach moral issues change. According to one theory of moral development (Kohlberg & Gilligan, 1972), older children and young adolescents function at a conventional level of moral reasoning in which absolute moral guidelines are seen to emanate from authorities such as parents or teachers. Thus judgments of right and wrong are made according to a set of concrete rules. A major concern is to act or behave in ways that will gain or maintain the approval of others.

Elements of **principled moral reasoning** emerge during adolescence. With this level of reasoning, adolescents question absolutes and rules and view moral standards as subjective and based on points of view that are subject to disagreement. One may have a moral duty to abide by social standards for behavior, but only insofar as those standards support and serve human ends. Thus occasions arise in which social conventions should be questioned and when principles such as justice, caring, or quality of life take precedence over established social norms. Empirical research on Kohlberg's theory has demonstrated that aspects of both conventional and principled reasoning are present during adolescence, and different levels of reasoning are used at different times and in different situations.

Kohlberg's scheme of moral development focuses on an orientation to justice. This orientation holds as its ideal a morality based on reciprocity and equal respect. From this orientation the most important consideration in making moral decisions would be whether the individuals involved were treated "fairly" by the ultimate decision. Gilligan (1982) proposes that an equally valid alternative to the justice orientation is one that emphasizes caring. From this perspective, the ideal is a morality of attention to others and responses to human need. As opposed to the justice orientation, which assumes that moral decisions are best made from a detached position of objectivity, the caring orientation is rooted in the belief that moral decisions should be shaped by attachments and responsiveness to others. Studies have found that although both men and women are capable of approaching moral problems from the perspectives of justice and caring, women may be more likely to give caring-oriented responses before justice-oriented ones, whereas men are more likely to follow the opposite pattern (Gilligan, 1986; Walker, de Vries, & Trevethan, 1987).

Spiritual Development

Religious beliefs also become more abstract and principled during the adolescent years. Specifically, adolescents' beliefs become more oriented toward spiritual and ideological matters and less oriented toward rituals, practice, and the strict observance of religious customs. Compared with children, adolescents place more emphasis on the internal aspects of religious commitment, such as what a person believes, and less on the external manifestations, such as whether an individual attends religious worship (Elkind, 1978).

Generally, the stated importance of participation in organized religion declines somewhat during the adolescent years. More high school students than young adults attend religious services regularly, and, not surprisingly, the younger the adolescents, the more likely they are to view religion as being important to them. Among older adolescents, the importance of organized religion declines more among college students than among those not in college. Late adolescence appears to be a time when individuals reexamine and reevaluate many of the beliefs and values of their childhood. Consistent with developmental changes in value autonomy, the religious beliefs of young people are likely to become more personalized and less bound to the traditional religious practices they may have been exposed to when they were younger. As adolescents mature and form an identity, they may either reject or conform to their family's traditional beliefs (Neuman, 2011).

Nurses play an important role for teens by providing an opportunity to discuss issues viewpoints and practices regarding morality and spirituality. These aspects are especially important to younger and middle-age adolescents who may be contemplating or participating in risky behaviors because greater levels of religiosity and spirituality are associated with protective, health-promoting behaviors, especially for youth living in environments lacking positive influences (Horton, 2015).

PSYCHOSOCIAL DEVELOPMENT

Identity Development

The task of **identity** formation is to develop a stable, coherent picture of oneself that includes integrating one's past and present experiences with a sense of where one is headed in the future. Erik Erikson (1968) describes identity achievement as one of the main psychosocial tasks of the adolescent years; "From among all possible and imaginable relations [the adolescent] must make a series of ever-narrowing selections of personal, occupational, gender-related, and ideological commitments."

The cognitive development and social environment that occur during adolescence push individuals to reflect on their place in society, the way others view them, their own sense of self-worth, and their options regarding career, service, and contributions in the future. For most individuals, the formation of a coherent self-identity occurs sometime during late adolescence and early adulthood.

Erikson (1968) suggests that the key to identity achievement lies in adolescents' interactions with others—role model adults, caregivers, and, most significantly, peers. Cultural influences, the environmental surroundings, and the society norms in which an adolescent lives play important roles in determining the range of available alternatives for identity formation. Optimally, adolescents have the opportunity to explore a range of possible options related to ideological, occupational, and interpersonal roles before making an identity commitment.

Experiences and opportunities within one's social environment influence both the content of identity and progression toward identity achievement. Among ethnic minority adolescents, those from a majority culture may experience restricted opportunities to explore alternative roles due to pressure from the community leaders who aim to preserve the contextual norm within the emerging generation. However, as the "melting pot" of America becomes more diverse with an increasing number of mixed-race families, and as political pressures and social media influences pervade all aspects of our culture, there are multiple forces among minority youth attempting to attain cultural identity. Possible barriers to identity formation among minority youth may include conflicting values between their minority ethnic group and the broader society, lack of adult role models who exemplify positive ethnic identity, and inadequate preparation or coping strategies for adolescents to manage stereotyping and prejudice that are frequently experienced among youth who derive from various cultures. However, many ethnic minority adolescents develop unique cultural norms within their community or adapt bicultural identities with the ability to navigate the cultural expectations of home, community, and society, creating positive connections to cultural identities that ultimately foster healthy adolescent development.

It is critical for the nurse to be sensitive to variations in family systems and cultural variations among their adolescent patients, as well as in general within the community where they serve. Asking the adolescent about the home and school environment as well as cultural beliefs helps establish therapeutic communication.

Development of Autonomy

Becoming an autonomous, self-governing person is another fundamental psychosocial task of adolescence. Autonomy includes emotional, cognitive, and behavioral components. Emotional autonomy is that aspect of independence related to changes in an individual's close relationships, and behavioral autonomy is the capacity to make independent decisions and follow through with them. Individuals generally begin the process of emotional autonomy during early adolescence by becoming more emotionally independent from their parents but remain cohesive with their friends. In the process of separating from their parents, younger adolescents often shift a portion of their emotional ties to other adults, often developing "crushes" on teachers, coaches, celebrities, or the parent/caregiver of a trusted friend while gradually becoming less emotionally dependent.

This emotional autonomy typically progresses in phases. First, adolescents no longer rush to their parents for advice or comfort when they are worried or upset. Second, conformity to parents' opinions declines and peer influence increases. Young and middle adolescents no longer see their parents/caregivers as all-knowing or all-powerful. Third, teenagers invest more emotional energy in relationships outside their families.

Decision-making abilities improve over the adolescent years; older adolescents become more aware than younger adolescents of risks and benefits involved with decisions, consider future consequences, turn to "experts" for advice rather than impulsively acting, and realize when vested interests may influence the advice of others. During middle and late adolescence, conformity to both parent and peer opinions declines, allowing for genuine behavioral autonomy. Subjective feelings of self-reliance increase steadily over the adolescent years until finally, older adolescents begin interacting with their parents as people and confidants, recognizing that both peers and parents have value.

In contrast to popular stereotypes, the development of autonomy during adolescence does not always involve rebellion nor is it always accompanied by strained or tense family relationships, especially among families in which there is mutual respect, consistent communication, and support. In households where guidelines for adolescent behavior are clear and consistently enforced; where changes in guidelines are open to discussion; and where an atmosphere of interpersonal warmth, concern, and fairness exists, a gradual and smooth maturational process occurs over the course of the adolescent years. Problems in the development of autonomy are often understandable reactions to excessively controlling circumstances, lack of nurturing environment or consistency in caregiving, or growing up in the absence of clear expectations. In addition to dispelling the myths that major parent-child conflicts and adolescent rebellion are essential to the development of autonomy, research has shown that parent and peer influences are not necessarily opposing forces but can play complementary roles in the development of a healthy degree of individual independence. Experts emphasize that adolescents still need monitoring and input by parents during their search for an identity; abandonment of the adolescent during this phase is undesirable and may leave the adolescent feeling fragmented, alone, and adrift, resulting in the development of psychopathology (Meeus, 2016).

Sexuality

Adolescence represents a critical time in the development of sexuality. Hormonal, physical, cognitive, and social changes that occur during adolescence all have an impact on sexual development and ultimately gender identity. Of all the developmental changes that affect adolescent sexuality, none is more obvious than the impact of puberty. Adolescents must come to terms with hormonal influences, physiologic manifestations such as menstruation and ejaculation, and physical changes such as breast and genital development. All these changes have a profound impact on the way teenagers perceive their bodies (i.e., body image). In addition to transitions in body image, increasing levels of pubertal hormones contribute to emotional liability and increased levels of sexual motivation among both boys and girls. The degree to which adolescents feel comfortable with their bodies may affect sexual behaviors and varies widely among teens.

Changes in sexual motivations and feelings, happening at the same time as shifts in cognitive skills, contribute to painful conjectures ("Is what I'm feeling normal?"), self-conscious concerns ("Am I good looking enough?"), and hypothetical thinking ("What if he/she wants to have sex?"). The emergence of formal operational thinking also increases adolescents' decision-making capabilities concerning sexual issues. The important task of successfully incorporating sexuality into a developing or establishing intimate relationship is made possible by the advanced cognitive abilities that emerge over the course of adolescence.

Part of adolescent identity formation involves the development of gender identity. For young adolescents, the process of gender identity development usually involves forming close friendships with same-gender peers with whom they may discuss various sexual topics or experiment sexually, often to satisfy curiosity. Sexual activity among young teenagers varies by gender. Masturbation provides an opportunity for sexual self-exploration; participation in this behavior is influenced by learned cultural attitudes and sex-role expectations. Boys typically begin masturbating during early adolescence; the age of first masturbation varies greatly for girls. Although some girls begin masturbating during early adolescence, many do not masturbate until after they have had intercourse. Once sexual exploration begins, approximately 33% of teens engage in oral sex and sexual intercourse in the same year (Haydon, Herring, Prinstein, et al., 2012). National reports show that 24% of teens have had vaginal intercourse by ninth grade; nearly 58% of teens graduating from high school report at least one sexual encounter (Kann, McManus, Harris, et al., 2016). Among teens who choose to delay sexual debut, the top three reasons reported are religious or moral beliefs, desire to postpone becoming a parent, and "haven't found the right person yet" (Reese, Choukas-Bradley, Herring, et al., 2014).

Many teens choose to experiment or intentionally shift from typical intimate relationships with opposite-gender partners to same-gender experiences during middle adolescence. Opposite-gender romantic relationships typically begin after peer activities involving both boys and girls. The type and degree of seriousness of partner relationships vary; pairing off as couples becomes more common as middle adolescence progresses (Fig. 17.8). Initial relationships are usually noncommittal, extremely mobile, and seldom characterized by any deep romantic attachments. Sexual activity (whether with same- or opposite-gender or both-gender partners) becomes more common during middle to late adolescence. The relationship between romance and expressions of love and sexual expression is brought into focus during middle adolescence. Most young people oppose exploitation, or being pressured into participating in a sexual act, and typically do not consider sex solely for the sake of physical enjoyment without a personal relationship. Many adolescents find it hard to believe that sex can exist without love; therefore they view each relationship as "real love." However, some teen social groups have embraced "friends with benefits" norms that includes sexual activity among friends who are not considered exclusive or committed romantic partners.

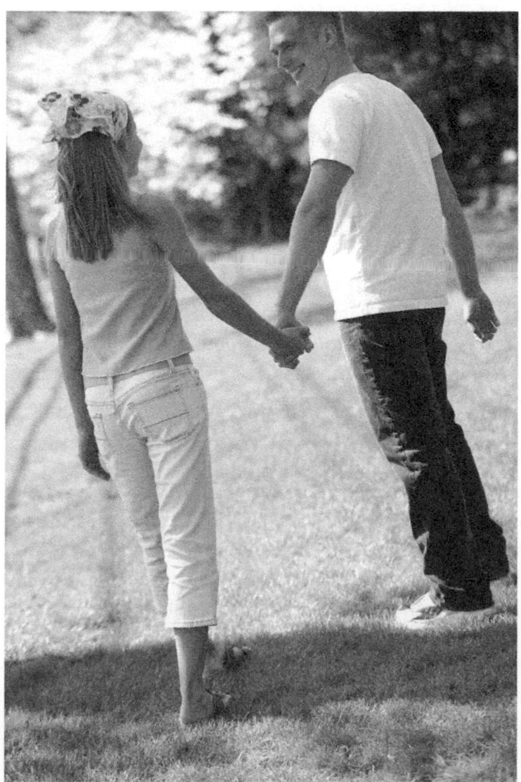

FIG. 17.8 Romantic relationships are an important part of adolescence.

The meaning and implication of sexual activity as it affects psychosocial development may be quite different for adolescent boys and girls; that is, sexual socialization differs for males and females in our society. Typically, adolescent boys' first sexual experiences are in early adolescence through masturbation. Before dating or interest in romance, most boys have already experienced orgasm and know how to arouse themselves sexually. For boys, the development of sexuality during adolescence revolves around efforts to integrate the formation of close relationships into an already existing sense of sexual capability. Girls' first sexual experiences are likely to have a different meaning. The adolescent girl is more likely to experience sexual intercourse for the first time in a perceived intimate or meaningful relationship and may not experience organism. For girls, the development of sexuality involves the integration of sexual activity into an existing capacity for emotional involvement.

An integrated sexual identity often emerges during late adolescence as individuals incorporate sexual experiences, feelings, and knowledge. For most, this identity is consistent with their own physical and mental capacities and with societal limits and expectations. Whatever their gender orientation, most older teenagers possess the capacity to have intimate relationships that satisfy the emotional and sexual needs of both partners.

Sexual orientation is an important aspect of sexual identity. **Sexual orientation** is defined as a pattern of sexual arousal or romantic attraction toward persons of the opposite gender (heterosexual); of the same gender (homosexual, often called gay, lesbian, or queer); of both genders (bisexual); or may be in the process of gender transition (transgender) or asexual (not sexually aroused by either gender). Sexual orientation encompasses several dimensions: (1) sexual orientation identity that consists of how an individual defines his or her sexual orientation; (2) sexual attraction that includes the gender to which the individual is romantically and physically attracted; and (3) sexual behavior that consists of whom an individual has sexual relationships with (O'Neill & Wakefield, 2017). In individuals the direction and intensity of each dimension are not necessarily consistent with any of the others. For example, individuals may be attracted most strongly to their same gender, have sexual activity only with the opposite gender, and identify as gay or lesbian. As with all aspects of sexual identity, cultural meaning and expectation, gender, peer groups, opportunities for intimacy, and other environmental contexts all influence sexual orientation. Nurses who ask teens what gender term they prefer as identification in health care settings demonstrate support and understanding of emerging gender issues. The information is also important as the provider considers clinical management and screening for risks.

Adolescence is the period during which individuals commonly begin to identify their sexual orientation as part of their developing sexual identity. However, cultural beliefs and values, societal and family pressures, or a lack of similar peers can influence this identification process. Among adolescents whose orientation encompasses any same-gender dimensions, the identity process during adolescence can be complicated, especially when community norms disapprove of orientations other than heterosexual. Adolescents who have witnessed harassment or violence directed at gay, lesbian, bisexual, and transgender people may be reluctant to self-identify their sexual orientation, even when their attractions and behaviors are exclusively same-gender or bisexual.

The development of sexual orientation as part of sexual identity includes several developmental milestones during late childhood and throughout adolescence. These milestones do not necessarily occur in the same order for everyone, nor are they completed in the same amount of time. They include (1) the realization of romantic or erotic attraction to people of one (or both) genders; (2) erotic daydreaming about one or both genders; (3) romantic partners or dates without sexual activity; (4) sexual activity with people of the preferred gender or genders (also, for some teens, sexual activity with a nonpreferred gender, due to curiosity or social pressure); (5) self-identification of the orientation that best fits one's current circumstances and understanding; (6) publicly self-identifying that orientation, usually to intimate friends and family first, then the wider social group; and (7) an intimate, committed sexual relationship with a person of the gender appropriate to one's orientation.

The order of these milestones varies greatly among adolescents, but adolescents who identify as gay, lesbian, bisexual, transgender, or queer (LGBTQ) tend to publicly self-identify later than their heterosexual peers. Without positive LGBTQ role models or a supportive family member or peer group, sexual minority teens can feel isolated, confused, and depressed, and they may delay or avoid sharing their gender orientation with anyone for fear of rejection or violence (see Critical Thinking Case Study box). When adolescents who would otherwise identify as bisexual can only find a peer group of gay and lesbian teens, they may focus on their same-gender dimensions of orientation and adopt the label of lesbian or gay; later, they may self-label as bisexual. Likewise, some gay and lesbian adolescents may first identify as heterosexual, then bisexual, before identifying as gay or lesbian.

CRITICAL THINKING CASE STUDY

Discussing Sexual Orientation With Adolescents

John, a 17-year-old adolescent, comes into the school-based clinic and tells the nurse practitioner that he thinks he is gay. What is the most appropriate response for the nurse practitioner?

1. What evidence should you consider regarding this condition?
2. What additional information is required at this time?
3. List the nursing intervention(s) that have the highest priority.
4. Identify important patient-centered outcomes with reference to your nursing intervention.

Answers are available at http://evolve.elsevier.com/wong/ncic.

There is no evidence that gay, lesbian, or bisexual adults are more or less likely to create long-term, stable relationships than are heterosexual couples. It should be noted that bisexual adolescents and adults do not generally engage in sexual relationships with both genders concurrently; self-identification as bisexual usually refers to the ability to be attracted to either gender but does not imply that such a person requires partners of both genders or that one must be equally attracted to and have sexual experience with both genders in order to be bisexual.

Intimacy

Intimate relationships are emotional attachments between two people characterized by concern for each other's well-being; a willingness to disclose private, possibly sensitive topics; and a sharing of common interests and activities. Intimate relationships are distinct from sexual relationships; it is possible for individuals to have close intimate relationships without becoming sexually involved. At the same time, people can be involved in sexual relationships that are not particularly intimate.

Intimate relationships first emerge during adolescence. Adolescents' close friendships are likely to include a strong emotional foundation in which individuals understand and care about one another. Puberty and its resultant changes in sexual impulses often raise new issues and concerns requiring serious, intimate discussions. Over the course of the adolescent years, individuals become more capable of and interested in emotional closeness with other people. The greater degree of behavioral independence often accompanying the transition into adolescence provides more opportunities for teenagers to be alone with friends and to come into meaningful contact with adults outside their families. Although research on intimacy during adolescence has focused on peer friendships, intimate relationships are by no means limited to peers. Teenagers may also develop intimate relationships with parents, siblings, and adults who are not part of their immediate families.

Harry Stack Sullivan (1953) was among the first to describe the developmental course of intimacy. Usually adolescents develop the capacity for intimacy through preadolescent and early adolescent relationships with same-gender peers. Intimate relationships with opposite-sex peers develop relatively late during adolescence. Opposite-gender friendships may play a more important role in the development of intimacy among boys than among girls, who may develop and experience intimacy with other girls earlier in adolescence.

Although teenagers may begin dating during early adolescence, these early dating relationships are not usually psychosocially intimate. Early dating relationships typically follow highly ritualized "scripts," in which adolescents are more likely to play stereotypic roles than to really be themselves. Participating in mixed-gender group activities, such as going to parties or other events, may have a positive impact on young teenagers' well-being. One-on-one dating during early adolescence, however, with a lot of time spent alone, may lead to sexual intimacy before a teen is ready. A moderate degree of dating, with serious relationships delayed until late adolescence, may be the ideal pattern of interpersonal involvement.

SOCIAL ENVIRONMENTS

Although all adolescents experience similar biologic and cognitive changes and face similar psychosocial tasks, the health-related effects of these changes are not the same for all people. Why are individuals not affected in the same ways by puberty, by changes in thinking patterns, and by changes in social and legal status? The answer lies in the fact that biologic, cognitive, and social changes of adolescence are shaped by the social environment in which the changes take place. The social environment provides the opportunities, barriers, role models, and support for individuals' development and health. Systems within the social environment, including family, peers, schools, community, social determinates of health, social media community, and the larger society, all contribute uniquely to an adolescent's development and health.

Families

Over the past several decades, changes have taken place within the family microsystem that have important implications for adolescent health. Higher rates of divorce and remarriage, increasing numbers of single parents, same-gender parents, older parents (including grandparents), and blended families have affected youth. There is also an increasing percentage of dual-parents or working mothers among contemporary US society. Higher rates of divorce and the decisions of single women to have children have increased the number of US children spending at least part of their childhood in a single-parent family. Correspondingly, many young people find themselves in blended families, thus developing relationships with stepparents during their adolescent years. A growing number of same-gender couples are raising their own or adopted children as well; in 2015 an estimated 859,000 households, or 17% of American households, were headed by same-gender partners (Lofquist & Lewis, 2015). Changes in family structure have been accompanied by changes in parent employment patterns and a dramatic increase in the percentage of mothers who work outside the home. (See Family Structure, Chapter 2.)

These changes in family structure and parent employment have resulted in young people having more time unsupervised by adults and increased time alone or with peers. Although for mature adolescents little risk may be involved with minimum supervision, for younger, less competent teenagers, decreased adult supervision may result in more risk-taking behaviors, such as poor diet, increased screen time and reduced exercise, substance use, and sexual intercourse. Poorly monitored teenagers may also socialize with peers who engage in risky behaviors. Lack of consistent adult supervision in the home also decreases adolescents' opportunities for communication and intimacy with parents. Although quantity of time does not guarantee quality, sufficient quantity is necessary for communication and the development of intimate relationships. The National Center on Abuse and Addiction (2010) reports that families who eat meals together at least five to seven times per week benefit by feeling more connected and the teens perform better academically, and participate in fewer risky behaviors.

Consistently, adolescents with a sense of family belonging along with connectedness with school and community show less susceptibility to negative peer pressure, and lower tendencies to be involved in risk-taking behaviors (Brooks, Magnusson, Spencer, et al., 2012). In many situations lack of direct adult supervision may be counterbalanced by parent monitoring and communication about adolescents' activities during parental absence. On the other hand, in dysfunctional or abusive families, spending greater amounts of time with parents may compromise the health of teenagers. In these situations the type and content of communication may be the most important factors to address.

In addition to adult supervision, the overall parenting style affects adolescent development. Both effective conflict resolution within families and family cohesion create environments conducive to healthy adolescent development. These two characteristics, along with parent expectations for mature behavior on the part of the adolescent and the practice of setting and enforcing reasonable limits for behavior, form the basis of effective parenting. This parenting style, termed **authoritative parenting**, is related to greater psychosocial maturity and school performance and less substance abuse among young people.

Adolescents from low-income households are more likely to have less supervised time with adults, to have parents who work at more than one job, to drop out of high school, and to experience violence in their homes and communities. Additionally, low-income teens typically experience less quality time with trusted adults besides their parents and often experience fewer health-enhancing supervision or mentoring activities. Nurses should avoid attributing differences in adolescent risk behaviors to racial or ethnic group membership, socioeconomic status, or family structure.

Peer Groups

One hallmark of adolescence is the increasing value young people place on friendships and relationships with peers (Fig. 17.9). Adolescents spend more time with their peers than do children. Compared with younger children, adolescent peer groups are more autonomous and more likely to include members of the opposite gender. Because of the changes that have taken place within family systems in contemporary society, peer groups play a significant role in the socialization of adolescents.

Peers serve as credible sources of information, serve as role models of social behaviors, and provide sources of social reinforcement or a bridge to alternative lifestyles. Close and supportive peer friendships have beneficial effects for young people (Fig. 17.10); however, adolescents with greater peer identification than parental identification, especially when the peers model or promote risky behaviors, are more prone to negative and health-compromising behaviors. Thus the transition to greater peer involvement, like other developmental transitions of adolescence, is a process requiring guidance and skill and, optimally, a prolonged time to complete the transition. At a time when they are developing interpersonal skills to deal with peer pressure, young adolescents who lack adult supervision and opportunities for communication with adults may be more susceptible to peer influences and at a higher risk for poor peer-group selection than teenagers who have close relationships with caring adults.

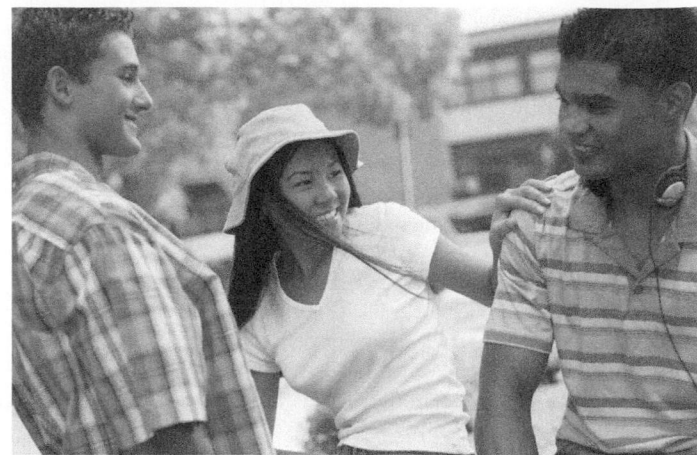

FIG. 17.9 The peer group is a major influence in adolescent development.

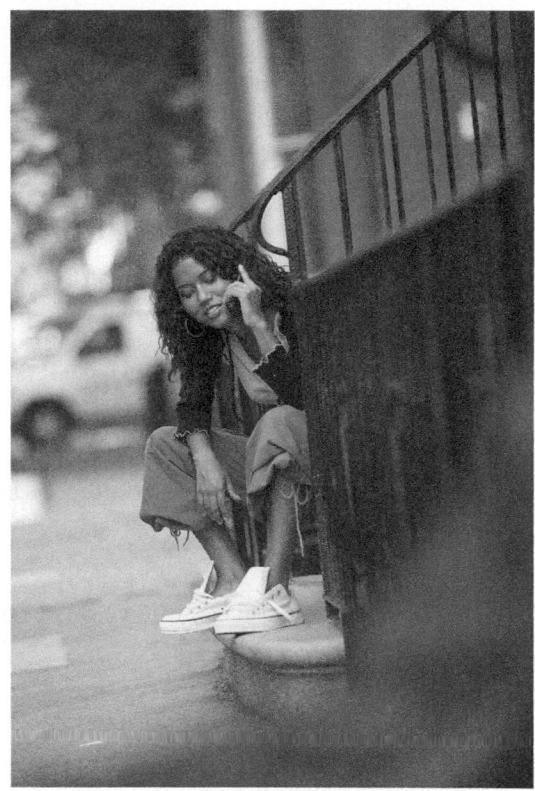

FIG. 17.10 The cell phone allows adolescents to talk or text message for hours with peers.

The heightened value placed on adolescent peer relationships leads to questions about the quality and nature of peer influence. Rather than thinking of all peer influence as either good or bad, it is important to recognize that the influence of peers varies from one adolescent to another, from one peer group to another, and across different societies and cultures. Adolescents' selection of peer groups seems to be most strongly influenced by sociodemographic factors and the common patterns of behavior, including school achievement, religious participation, and social interactions such as sports, clubs, and employment. Peers can have either positive or negative effects on adolescent behavior. Negative effects include alcohol or illicit substance use, gang membership, and violent or reckless behaviors. Positive effects include an orientation supporting academic achievement, volunteer efforts or community engagement, or a commitment to religious, athletic, scholastic, philanthropic, or social youth groups.

Peers can also be a positive force in health promotion. Same-age and older adolescents can encourage healthy behavior by serving as positive role models and promoting positive health norms in the peer group. Nurses can often gain insight on health behaviors and potential risks to adolescents by inquiring about peers during conversation and health histories. Examples of this include asking "Do any of your friends drink?" or "Are any of your friends driving yet?" Questions such as these give the nurse valuable information that typically reflects similar behaviors of the teen.

Schools

In contemporary society, schools play an increasingly important role in preparing young people for adulthood. Schooling is essential for a successful future for both boys and girls. Failure to complete high school reduces employment opportunities and the probability of earning an adequate income. Yet many schools in the United States do not meet the developmental needs of all young people. Because of a variety of reasons, including safety, academic performance, and access issues, many families choose to homeschool their teens.

Another important problem is the lack of parental involvement in schools. Parental involvement increases the effectiveness of schools at all levels. However, with a large number of single-parent and two–working-parent families, parents have less time for involvement in schools.

The timing of school transition may be important, especially if the school environment is not appropriate to the adolescent's developmental needs. In particular, the transition into a middle or junior high school at age 12 or 13 years typically occurs at the same time as the rapid physical changes of puberty.

Another characteristic of school that may have negative effects is a system of grading that acknowledges few young people for their academic successes. Teenagers whose grades fall below average may spend much of their time in environments in which they perceive negative evaluations by adult authorities. As a result, they may feel alienated from school. Students who repeat one or more academic years of school exhibit greater emotional distress than those who do not. Students with below-average grades are more likely to be engaged in health-compromising behaviors such as tobacco and alcohol use, unprotected sexual intercourse, and self-harm behaviors, including suicide attempts.

The social environment of schools has an impact on student outcomes. Small classroom size and small school size are both related to higher-quality social environments within schools. Safety and respect for all students are critical issues because students have difficulty learning in unsafe environments. In many schools, violence toward and harassment of students on the basis of race, gender, or sexual orientation are common, affecting more than half of all students. Students targeted for repeated teasing and harassment are more likely to skip school, to report symptoms of depression, and to attempt suicide (Troop-Gordon, 2017). Equally troubling, teens who are regularly harassed or bullied are also more likely to bring weapons to school to feel safe. In 2015, 16.2% of high school students nationwide reported carrying a weapon one or more days in the past month, which is a decline since 1991, when 26.1% of youth reported carrying a weapon (Kann, McManus, Harris, et al., 2016). School practices and conditions that lead to better student outcomes stress the importance of supportive environments that foster positive peer group relationships, promote health and fitness, encourage family involvement in school, and strengthen connections between schools and communities.

Work

For many young people in the United States, the workplace becomes a fourth microsystem that affects their development, behavior, and health. Most teenagers are employed in a relatively restricted array of jobs as restaurant workers, cashiers, sales clerks, clerical assistants, and laborers. The jobs tend to be monotonous, require little initiative or decision making, and rarely use skills learned in school. Furthermore, some are highly stressful, requiring work under extreme time pressure. Greater involvement as an employee can also lead to fatigue, decreased sleep, declining interest in academics and poorer grades, reduced extracurricular involvement, and limited social time with family and peers. Detrimental effects are more likely for adolescents who work more than 20 hours a week.

Although some teen employment may not contribute to healthy maturation, jobs that allow young people to develop intellectual and social skills, have some autonomy, or offer teens the sense that their contributions matter can be positive experiences and promote healthy development. Jobs that provide adolescents with experiences relevant to future employment or that link them to adults who serve as vocational mentors may be especially valuable.

Technology as a Social Environment

The role of social media and advanced technology are prominent in the lives of most adolescents. Studies show increasingly universal access to the Internet; a national survey in 2015 found that 87% own or have access to a computer, 88% own or have access to a mobile phone, and 73% have smartphones (Lenhart, 2015).

The widespread availability of the Internet and access to social networking sites such as Facebook, Twitter, Instagram, email, blogs, and countless others that are rapidly evolving have created virtual communities and multiple opportunities for young people to interact with one another; web cameras even allow those interactions to include real-time video communication. Cellular telephones offer mobile opportunities to talk on the phone or send text messages, photos, or videos.

Social networking sites have created a more public arena for trying out identities, having multiple identities, and developing interpersonal skills with a wider network of people, occasionally with anonymity. These virtual opportunities provide a source for socialization for young people who have a limited access to friends (because of rural location, shyness, or chronic conditions) to interact with people like themselves. However, many adolescents use online social environment to interact with the same peers they spend their day with at school.

Text messaging via cell phones is also a common activity and can be disruptive during school. Both the online and text environment can create opportunities for **cyberbullying**, in which teens engage in insults, harassment, and publicly humiliating statements online or on cell phones. There is a recognized danger of adolescents coming in contact and sharing personal information with sexual predators who pose as adolescents in an attempt to make personal contact with underage victims or engage them in "sexting" (i.e., sending sexually explicit or suggestive pictures or messages online). Adolescent sexting, rather than being an innocent anonymous activity, has been linked to risky sexual behaviors (Morelli, Bianchi, Baiocco, et al., 2016).

Studies note that teens are not only enthusiastic technology users but also frequently use multiple types of technology at the same time. They may be listening to music on their digital music player and using the Internet to complete a homework assignment while texting friends on their cell phone. It is unclear at present how this multitasking and multiple media exposure will affect development of the brain and attention, though frequent media use has been associated with late nights and sleep deprivation. In addition, there are some demonstrated affective and behavioral effects among adolescents who are exposed to high levels of violence or sexual content in the technology sources they use, which can become a cause of concern for health promotion (Jacobson, Bailin, Milanaik, et al., 2016).

There is increased concern focusing on adolescent vehicle driving and distractions such as texting or concurrent handheld cellular phone usage. More than 80% of US teens own cell phones and more than 60% reported having texted or emailed while driving (Kann, McManus, Harris, et al., 2016). Studies have shown that drivers using handheld devices are considerably more distracted and spend less time looking at the road or paying attention to driving conditions (McKeever, Schultheis, Padmanaban, et al., 2013). Many states have outlawed the use of handheld mobile devices while actively operating a vehicle (Chase, 2014).

PROMOTING OPTIMUM HEALTH DURING ADOLESCENCE

Health promotion involves empowering individuals, families, and communities to take developmentally and contextually appropriate actions toward realizing their potential. It includes physical, cognitive, emotional, and social dimensions. Health promotion involves helping youth acquire the power (including knowledge, attitudes, and skills), authority (permission to use their power), and opportunities to make choices that increase the likelihood of creating positive expressions of health for themselves in their contexts.

A comprehensive approach to health promotion combines activities aimed at individuals with interventions focused on changing norms, attitudes, and behaviors of peer groups, families, communities, and society at large. For example, prevention of tobacco use involves more than a teacher's lecture on the consequences of cigarette and smokeless tobacco use, a ban on tobacco use in schools, a parent's admonition not to smoke, or a nurse's question to an adolescent about smoking history. In reality, it requires all these components and more; the support of the community leaders, policies, and institutions that affect the lives of adolescents.

The rationale for focusing on these health issues becomes obvious when one examines the major sources of mortality and morbidity during adolescence. The four leading causes of mortality during adolescence in the United States are motor vehicle crashes, other accidental injuries, homicide, and suicide; together these causes are responsible for more than 70% of all adolescent deaths (Kann, McManus, Harris, et al., 2016). Major causes of adolescent morbidity include the use of motor and recreational vehicles, sexual and physical abuse, sexual activity such as unwanted pregnancy and STIs, and substance use. Mental disorders, chronic illness, eating disorders, and oral health problems are other important sources of morbidity (Kann, McManus, Harris, et al., 2016). Chapter 18 provides further information about threats to adolescent health and well-being.

A number of inequities exist in relation to health status among subsets of the US population. Adolescents are one subgroup that experiences health inequities. For example, a substantial gap in life expectancy exists between African American and Caucasian adolescents. African American and Native American males have a higher risk of premature death than any other racial or ethnic group. Adolescent males die at a rate more than twice that of girls. Mortality rates increase by more than 200% between early and late adolescence. There are also age differences in the causes of death, with a shift toward more violent deaths occurring in late adolescence. Among Caucasian adolescents a dramatic increase in suicide occurs during later adolescence, making it the second leading cause of death in this group. For older African American adolescents, homicide ranks as the most likely cause of death. Similar to mortality, patterns of morbidity vary within the adolescent population. For example, rates of vehicular injury are high among males, whereas for females morbidities associated with "quietly disturbed" behaviors such as eating disorders and emotional distress are common (Kann, McManus, Harris, et al., 2016).

ADOLESCENTS' PERSPECTIVES ON HEALTH

To be most effective, adolescent health promotion efforts must incorporate adolescents' perspectives on what health means. Such efforts also must focus on adolescents' concerns and priorities related to health and health care services. From a positive perspective, adolescents' developmentally based sense of curiosity and movement toward autonomy provide opportunities for health promotion that should not be wasted.

Adolescents define health as being able to live up to one's potential; being able to function physically, mentally, and socially; and experiencing positive emotional states. The content of their definitions often goes beyond an "absence of illness" and includes what can be done to maintain and enhance health.

Adolescents' health-related interests and concerns include stress and anxiety, sleep hygiene, relationships with adults and peers, weight, acne, and feelings of sadness or depression. Health concerns are often consistent with the immediate developmental tasks that teenagers face. For example, younger adolescents—in the midst of the physical changes of puberty—have a particular interest in issues related to hygiene, growth and development, and social relationships. In the process of making transitions from middle or junior high school to senior high school, middle adolescents have questions and concerns related to peer-group acceptance, relationships with friends, and physical appearance. Older adolescents focus increasingly on intimacy issues, academic performance, future career and employment plans, and emotional health issues.

Among the behaviors that adolescents view as risky are substance use, sexual activity, and the use of recreational and motor vehicles. Adolescents also identify health threats that primarily involve psychologic issues, such as anxiety, depression, and body image problems. Other perceived health threats include violence and pollution and threats within the more immediate social environment, including school problems and conflicts with parents, teachers, and friends. When adolescents are asked about general threats to youth, they respond differently than if asked about how their own personal behaviors produce certain risks. Like adults, adolescents tend to underestimate the potentially negative consequences of their own behaviors.

Although young people identify health risks and concerns that are primarily social and psychologic, many are reluctant to seek health services for problems they do not consider to be organic, despite the fact that they indicate they would like help with these problems. A variety of factors influence an adolescent's ability to seek health care, including access to services, characteristics of health care providers (often their "baby doctor" is the only known provider), perceived availability of confidential services, geographic access, and financial limitations.

The availability of confidential services is particularly important to adolescents, especially when they have concerns related to sensitive issues such as sexual/gender issues, mental health concerns, or substance use behaviors. Many teenagers are unwilling to seek health care related to sensitive topics if their parents/caregivers will know about the visit. Although most states have provisions for confidential care for adolescents 16 years or older and for problems related to substance abuse, mental health, and sexual health, adolescents often are unaware of their ability to receive confidential health care. Laws vary by state, and since 2001 a number of states have either enacted or are considering laws requiring parental notification for a variety of health care services for adolescents, including reproductive health care. Adolescents may be more likely to participate in health care services when such services are delivered by caring, respectful providers.

FACTORS THAT PROMOTE ADOLESCENT HEALTH AND WELL-BEING

Even when they are exposed to risk factors such as poverty, violence, parental abuse or neglect, or divorce of parents, most adolescents become competent, healthy adults. It is important to understand how this group of young people succeeds despite odds against them. Health promotion efforts with adolescents should focus on nurturing such protective factors in addition to reducing risk factors. Indeed, a large body of research has shown that fostering protective factors can reduce a wide range of health risk behaviors, so it may be more effective than health promotion efforts solely focused on reducing the problem behavior.

Adolescents who cope successfully in the midst of adverse circumstances are often supported by caring, cohesive families. Protective factors within the community include connections with adults outside the family, with the school, or with a church group. Health care providers who are able to connect with adolescents support successful coping. Schools that are safe and intellectually engaging can make a difference in the health and well-being of young people. Involvement with healthy peer groups, guided by caring adults who are good role models, also prevents poor outcomes. Community engagement where young people think their involvement is meaningful, and they are listened to, is associated with better adjustment during adolescence.

The potential positive impact of social interactions suggests guidelines for making changes in adolescent environments that support overall health and well-being. Nurses involved with adolescents can develop interventions that shift the balance for young people from vulnerability to resilience by decreasing exposures to health risks or stressful life events (e.g., the impact of parental alcoholism or threats of violence) and by increasing the number of protective factors (e.g., communication and problem-solving skills or sources of emotional support).

Contexts for Adolescent Health Promotion

A consensus is growing that the most effective adolescent health promotion efforts involve multiple systems and address multiple issues. Interventions integrating programs and expertise from health care, school, and community-based settings can effectively increase adolescents' prevention skills, improve their access to health care services, build adult motivation and support for adolescent prevention practices, and change physical environments and social norms to support healthy behavior. Such a comprehensive approach to health promotion requires a great deal of cooperation and coordination on the part of complex institutions. On the other hand, by not limiting the responsibility for adolescent health to one person or one setting, multiple opportunities for health promotion arise. Individual efforts reinforce important themes and become an integral part of an overall health promotion strategy. For example, a plan for smoking cessation devised by a teenager with the help of a nurse is most likely to be successful if the teenager is encouraged by peers and family members to abstain and if use of and access to tobacco products are discouraged through policy interventions such as smoke-free schools and bans on cigarette vending machines.

Schools

Schools are a primary site for adolescent health promotion and disease prevention. Large numbers of young people can be affected by school-based health promotion efforts because virtually all teenagers attend school at least through the early adolescent years. Group interventions offer adolescents a sense of anonymity, which they prefer when obtaining information about sensitive topics. School personnel often have special expertise and experience with health education. Through daily contact, school staff can develop supportive relationships with a limited number of students. Parent-teacher associations and school boards also link schools with the larger community in ways that can be used to expand the scope of adolescent health promotion efforts.

School-based health promotion interventions include classroom health education, school-level policies, and environmental changes. School systems often offer classroom program which include components that focus on building students' knowledge and skills and establish peer support for health-enhancing behaviors. Some programs effectively use classroom peer leaders as positive role models and social support for healthy behaviors. Out-of-class assignments often involve parents or other admired adults, emphasizing the roles that adults play as resources regarding health issues. Classroom programs have been designed to address health-related issues, including healthy eating and exercise habits (Fig. 17.11), nonviolent conflict resolution, substance use and abuse prevention, and responsible sexual behavior.

Other school-level interventions involve changing the school environment itself, including improving or enhancing physical education options, adding clubs or after-school programming, enhancing the food service

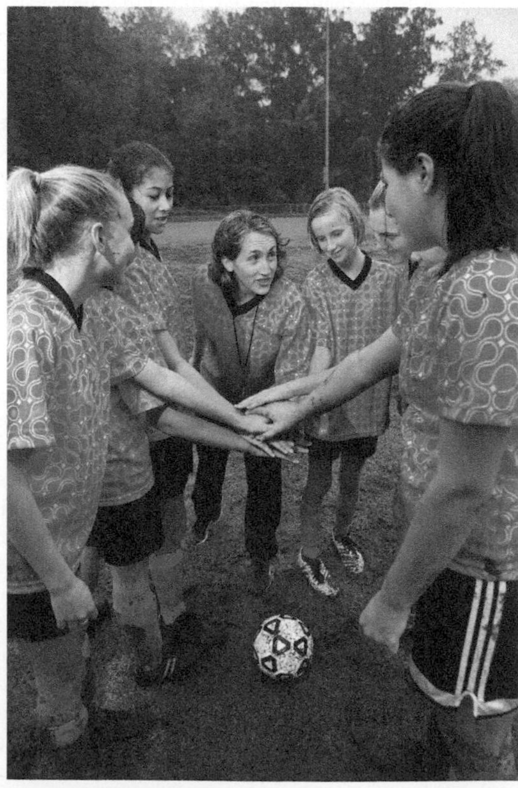

FIG. 17.11 Adolescents should be encouraged to participate in activities that contribute to lifelong physical fitness.

programs with gardening programs and limited sugar-sweetened beverages, and enforcing tobacco-free school policies.

School-Based and School-Linked Health Services

Another avenue for health promotion is school-based and school-linked clinics. School-based health clinics (SBHCs) are located on school grounds and serve adolescents within a specific school, in which a primary care provider and health care team are collated within a school community to enhance access to health care services to the teens (see http://www.sbh4all.org for listings). School-linked clinics (SLCs) may be located off school grounds or on school campuses but serve more than one school. Originally designed to address issues related to adolescent pregnancy, SBHCs and SLCs have expanded to address a broad range of health problems and psychosocial issues. In combination, school-linked health services and traditional school-based health promotion efforts provide a comprehensive approach to health promotion that integrates health care, education, and environmental support.

Several private foundations, as well as state and local governments, have provided considerable resources to initiate school-linked health services that offer adolescents confidential services at minimum cost. Parental consent for services is usually obtained on a blanket basis before adolescents seek services. These services increase adolescents' access to preventive and primary care services through highly visible locations, convenient hours, affordability, and confidential care. SLCs have made a concerted effort to provide the services of a multidisciplinary team of health professionals—which may include nurses, nurse practitioners, health educators, medical assistants, physicians, psychologists, nutritionists, and social workers—skilled in meeting both the mental and physical health needs of adolescents. Adolescents are receptive to services offered by SLCs, especially when they address emotionally charged issues such as depression.

Communities

Community-level approaches to adolescent health promotion, involving both media campaigns and initiatives on the part of community groups, offer the advantage of reaching a broad audience. Specifically, community-based approaches can reach adolescents who do not attend school or have no source of preventive health care. This type of approach directly addresses changing social environments where high-risk behaviors occur. For example, violence prevention may be more effectively addressed by changing community-wide standards related to issues such as conflict resolution than by focusing on the individual. Community-based approaches have the potential to be most effective when they involve various sectors of the community (including adolescents) and include persons representing a variety of youth-serving agencies. With the involvement of multiple sectors, adolescents have the opportunity to hear consistent health messages across a variety of social contexts.

Media campaigns can be an effective but somewhat costly way to reach adolescents in community-level health promotion efforts. Adolescents receive considerable information from sources such as television, the Internet, radio, and magazines. Messages can also be targeted to appeal to parents and other adults who have an impact on the health-related behavior of youth. Media campaigns use brief images and provide short, superficial coverage of specific issues. Podcasts and youth-created videos uploaded to public websites such as YouTube are other ways of using media for health promotion efforts (see The Internet and Other Technologies, later in this chapter).

Coalitions and task forces are another setting in which nurses can raise awareness about health issues or influence the larger environments for health promotion. This is an opportunity to partner with parents, community agencies, and concerned community groups. The goal of initiatives launched by parent and community groups is often to build climates within communities that support health-enhancing behaviors. Such initiatives create social contexts in which teenagers encounter more health-promoting messages and norms.

Health Care Settings

Consistent, supportive, one-on-one interactions over time between adolescents and members of the health care team provide significant opportunities for health promotion. These relationships can create "safe environments" in which adolescents can disclose sensitive information related to health risk. In turn, this information should be incorporated into preventive interventions specific to individual adolescent needs.

Health care settings offer the advantage of being able to provide confidential services, which are especially important in sensitive situations such as those involving substance use and sexual behavior. Interventions provided through health care settings can include parents and help create social environments that support adolescents' health-enhancing behaviors. Another advantage is that health care settings have resources available to address various components of health, including physical, emotional, and social needs.

Health promotion interventions provided in health care settings do have limitations. Individual care is time-consuming, limiting the number of adolescents who can be reached in one-on-one encounters. Although one-on-one interventions can foster health-enhancing attitudes and behaviors of individual adolescents, they do not address changes in social environments, such as peer groups and communities, that may be necessary to support these attitudes and behaviors.

To be effective, health care services for adolescents must be accessible and appropriate. To be accessible, services must be available, affordable, and approachable. Services must include outreach to adolescents and their parents, informing them of the availability of services. Mechanisms for low- or no-cost services must be developed because cost is a major barrier to adolescents receiving appropriate care. Locating health care services in places such as schools, youth services centers, shopping malls, and detention facilities and offering convenient clinical hours are two strategies that increase accessibility for teenagers who may not use traditional services.

The Internet and Other Technologies

A growing number of health promotion activities use the communication technologies that adolescents surround themselves with. Health-related websites designed to appeal to youth (often designed with youth) offer extensive information on nearly every topic that can affect adolescent health, although the accuracy and quality of such websites varies greatly. Programs for helping youth manage their chronic conditions can include a web-based or electronic "health passport," with information about their condition, their medications, and their health regimen. Social networking sites have been created to help youth with specific health issues. Some youth clinics offer text message reminders of appointments and cell phone calls to return for STI testing results. Other programs even offer text message or email encouragements for youth who are trying to quit smoking; reminders about safer sex practices; or tips to improve nutrition, exercise, and weight management. Although clinicians need to consider carefully the levels of privacy and confidentiality in the use of different forms of technology, there is growing evidence of effectiveness in engaging youth through the technology they use to communicate.

Adolescent Health Screening

One strategy for health promotion by nurses and other professionals in health care settings is one-on-one health screening. Through information gained during a health screening interview, the health professional can identify both assets and threats to an adolescent's health and well-being. The health screening interview also offers an opportunity for health professionals to build trusting relationships with adolescents. This sense of trust may be critical for adolescents to act on information, attitudes, and skills that are shared to help them successfully negotiate particular stressors.

In addition, the health screening interview provides an opportunity for teaching adolescents self-advocacy skills. Nurses in schools and clinic settings can use several specific strategies to promote self-advocacy skills. These strategies include (1) maintaining an up-to-date file of handouts, pamphlets, and websites to show adolescents during "teachable moments"; (2) directing adolescents to resources in their community and to appropriate, accurate sources of health information on the Internet; and (3) teaching adolescents how the health care system works, how to schedule their health care appointments, and how to keep their own personal health records of immunizations, allergies, and health care encounters.

HEALTH CONCERNS OF ADOLESCENCE

Effective health education for adolescents should incorporate a developmentally appropriate, multifaceted approach. Motivational interviewing improves adherence to health care advice by using a collaborative approach. In this process, the adolescent is encouraged to introspectively explore ambivalence and develop solutions for effecting change. Education alone is not enough to change behavior. Effective programs for adolescents must include opportunities to improve communication and empowerment skills (Hoying, Melnyk, & Arcoleo, 2016).

As adolescents progress through adolescence, they are able to assume additional responsibility for their own health, including maintaining health practices, taking prescribed medications, keeping appointments, and performing procedures when necessary. Health care professionals who work with adolescents should consider the adolescent's developmental age and promote increased independence and responsibility, while maintaining privacy and ensuring confidentiality (see Nursing Care Guidelines box). Parents should also respect their teenager's independence and move toward the role of consultant about health issues, while also maintaining some level of parental involvement throughout adolescence.

NURSING CARE GUIDELINES

Interviewing Adolescents

- Ensure confidentiality and privacy; interview adolescent without parents.
- Explain the limits of confidentiality (e.g., legal duty to report physical or sexual abuse, or to get others involved if patient is suicidal).
- Show concern for the adolescent's perspective: "First, I'd like to talk about your main concerns" and "I'd like to know what you think is happening."
- Offer a nonthreatening explanation for the questions you ask and assure teens it is normal and routine: "I'm going to ask a number of questions to help me better understand your health. These are questions we ask all teens in effort to provide the best possible care."
- Maintain objectivity; avoid assumptions, judgments, and lectures.
- Ask open-ended questions when possible; move to more directive questions if necessary.
- Begin with less sensitive issues and proceed to more sensitive ones.
- Use language that both the adolescent and you understand.
- Restate: Reflect back to the adolescent what he or she has said, along with feelings that may be associated with the descriptions.

Several professional organizations have published guidelines aimed at improving and maintaining health care for adolescents and young adults. The American Academy of Pediatrics, American Academy of Family Physicians, American Medical Association, and US Preventive Services Task Force have similar guidelines for health supervision of adolescents. These guidelines emphasize the need to provide health services to adolescents that meet their physical and emotional needs. They place great import on provision of health care by health care providers who are trained in meeting adolescents' needs. Bright Futures (American Academy of Pediatrics, 2017) emphasizes that the following issues should be addressed with adolescents at each health visit:

- Physical growth and development (physical and dental health, body image, healthy nutrition, physical activity)
- Social and academic competence (relationships with peers and family, school performance, interpersonal relationships)
- Emotional well-being (mental health, sexuality)
- Risk reduction (tobacco, alcohol, other drugs, pregnancy, STIs)
- Violence and injury prevention

Some practical suggestions for addressing the adolescent's individual health care needs are found in the following mnemonic:

H—Home environment ("Where do you stay? Who else lives with you?")
E—Education/employment (congruent with age/developmental stage?)
E—Eating/nutrition/elimination
A—Activities, physical activities ("What do you do for fun? Who do you do this with?")
D—Drugs (tobacco, alcohol, illicit substance use, caffeine)
S—Sexuality (gender orientation, sexual debut, use of contraception)
S—Suicide/depression
S—Safety (seat belt, texting, sports equipment, gun in the home)

The following discussion of adolescent health focuses on some of the topics from this mnemonic, as well as the Bright Futures topics listed earlier; other adolescent health issues are discussed later in this chapter.

Parenting and Family Adjustment

Having family members who are emotionally available and appropriately involved in their lives has proved to be a key factor in adolescents' well-being. A wide variety of family disorders, including parental discord, alcohol or drug abuse, mental illness, and sexual and physical abuse, can lead to additional stresses in teenagers coping with the tasks of adolescence.

Screening questions such as "Who is your primary caregiver? Tell me about your family," "How are things going at home?" and "Who in your family could you talk with about problems you are having?" help give a general sense of family relationships. More directed questions that give insight into family functioning include "How does your family generally solve disagreements?" "What are some of the rules in your family related to issues such as underage drinking, curfew, and friends?" "Who sets these rules?" and "Are you currently having conflicts with your family?"

Many parents are interested in and involved in the lives of their adolescent. Parents who are appropriately involved serve as an important protective influence, and efforts to exclude parents from adolescent health services are both unrealistic and unwise. While providing health care, a balance must be sought between the individual adolescent's growing autonomy and the parents' diminishing control over, and responsibility for, the adolescent.

Offer parents the opportunity to share concerns and provide them with an overview of health guidance information offered at least once during their child's early adolescence, once during middle adolescence, and once during late adolescence. Such guidance can include information about normative adolescent development, along with signs and symptoms of troubled adolescents. Engage parents in discussion of parenting behaviors that promote healthy adolescent adjustment, including maintaining open communication, setting age-appropriate limits, monitoring their child's social and recreational activities, and acting as role models for health-enhancing behaviors. Encourage parents to discuss health-related behaviors with their adolescents (see Family-Centered Care box later in this chapter).

Psychosocial Adjustment

As adolescents experience the many changes of adolescence, they redefine who they are and what they want out of life. Most individuals progress through the changes of their adolescent years with minimum emotional upheaval, countering the belief that this period in life is one of "storm and stress." Some adolescents, however, do have difficulty coping and exhibit emotional distress, especially when multiple normative events happen simultaneously and are combined with nonnormative life events.

Adolescence is characterized by change within multiple domains. Changes associated with pubertal development typically take place during the early adolescent years. Early- and late-maturing adolescents who feel they are "out of sync" with their age-mates' growth patterns may have a more difficult time emotionally than those who develop "on time" with their peers. Another normative change, typically occurring during middle adolescence, is the transition from middle or junior high school to high school. With this transition, adolescents often are increasingly concerned about peer relationships. During older adolescence, psychosocial concerns focus on school achievement and future career plans.

Questions such as "Do you think that your development is going too fast, too slow, or at about the right speed?" may allow young adolescents to discuss issues related to physical development. Questions about feeling cared for and connected to teachers, counselors, students, and others at school, along with questions about their involvement in school-related activities, give teenagers an opportunity to talk about strengths and deficits they experience within their school environments. Questions about the quality of peer relationships may help identify teenagers who feel socially isolated. Finally, questions about future plans related to education and employment or career choices may give older youth the chance to talk through significant sources of stress.

As sources of credible information, support, and encouragement, nurses can help adolescents cope with the changes and challenges they face. To promote both emotional health and psychosocial adjustment, nurses and other health care professionals can encourage adolescents to develop (1) skills to cope with stress and change and (2) skills to become involved in personally meaningful activities.

Intentional and Unintentional Injury

The rationale for focusing on health issues becomes obvious when one examines the major sources of mortality and morbidity during adolescence. The leading causes of mortality during adolescence in the United States are motor vehicle crashes, other accidental injuries, homicide, and suicide, which together are responsible for approximately 71% of all adolescent deaths (Kann, McManus, Harris, et al., 2016). (See Childhood Mortality, Chapter 1.) Motor vehicle crashes are the single greatest source of unintentional injury and death in young people. Many factors contribute to the higher rate of crashes among teen drivers, including lacking driving experience and maturity, driving too fast, having other teen passengers in the car, texting, and using alcohol. Homicide, a form of intentional injury, is the third leading cause of death among all US adolescents. In the United States homicides among teenagers are most likely to involve firearms and to occur among friends or gangs.

In addition to being the leading cause of death, injuries also account for substantial morbidity among youth. Certain behaviors increase the risk of injury. For example, 6% of high school students nationwide report rarely or never using seat belts, 20% of high school students reported riding with a driver who had been drinking alcohol, and 7.8% of students had driven a vehicle after drinking alcohol (Kann, McManus, Harris, et al., 2016). In 2015, 16.2% of high school students reported carrying a weapon (e.g., a gun, knife, or club) at some point during the previous month, with 4.1% noting that they carried a weapon on school property during that same time period (Kann, McManus, Harris, et al., 2016). Nationwide, 22.6% of students reported being in a physical fight during the 12 months before the survey (Kann, McManus, Harris, et al., 2016). Many adolescents have easy access to a gun in their home, and such accessibility is significantly associated with involvement in violent behavior and with fatal suicide attempts.

During an interview, the segment addressing injury prevention should include screening and counseling related to motor vehicle crashes, firearm use, and suicide. In relation to prevention of motor vehicle injury, one might initially ask how the adolescent "gets around town." Further questions and health education might focus on seat belt or helmet use and the practice of drinking and driving or riding with drivers who have been drinking. Ask adolescents whether they have access, at home or elsewhere, to firearms or a weapon; whether they carry a gun for safety or protection; and whether they ever use alcohol or other substances in combination with handling guns.

Health education related to firearm injury prevention should include advising parents to limit their children's household access to firearms, counseling on nonviolent ways to resolve conflicts, and discouraging use of weapons. Family members and acquaintances are a common source of guns for young people. Having a gun in the home increases the risk of adolescent suicide and homicide. Assess all families for the presence of a gun in the home and inform them of the increased risk for suicide and homicide. When guns are present in the home, families must take preventive action to be certain that the guns are never loaded, that they are locked up in a safe place, and that ammunition is locked up in a separate location accessible only to appropriate adults.

Dietary Habits and Eating Disorders

Puberty marks the beginning of accelerated physical growth, which can as much as double adolescents' nutritional requirements for iron, calcium, zinc, and protein. At the same time, growing independence, the need for peer acceptance, concern with physical appearance, and an active lifestyle may affect eating habits, food choices, nutrient intake, and thus nutritional status. Iron-deficiency anemia and obesity are increasingly common among adolescents; they are found in all income and racial/ethnic groups and both genders (Fig. 17.12). Inadequate intake of certain vitamins (e.g., folic acid, vitamin B_6, vitamin A) and minerals (e.g., iron, calcium, zinc) is also evident, particularly among girls and teenagers of low socioeconomic status. In combination with other factors, these dietary patterns could result in increased risk for chronic diseases such as heart disease, osteoporosis, and some types of cancer later in life. Girls, in particular, are susceptible to iron deficiency at menarche. Maximum bone mass is also acquired during adolescence; therefore the calcium deposited during these years determines the risk of osteoporosis.

Routine nutrition screening for all adolescents should include questions about meal patterns, dieting behaviors, consumption of high-fat and high-salt foods, and recent changes in weight. In terms of weight control, the number of adolescents who are overweight has increased significantly over the past decade, with more than 18% of 12- to 19-year-olds qualifying as overweight (Child Trends, 2014a). (See Obesity, Chapter 16.) In 2016 one-third of adolescents reported drinking sweetened soda daily, and only 15% ate the recommended

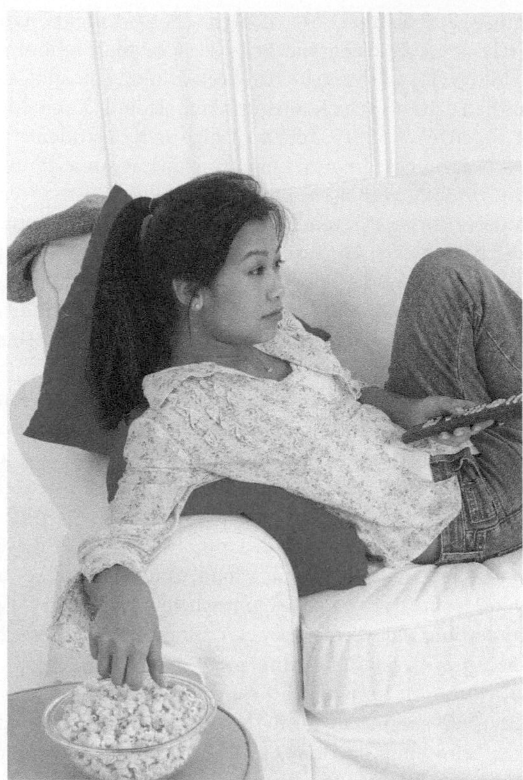

FIG. 17.12 Snacking on empty calories is common among adolescents, especially during inactivity.

five or more servings of fruits and vegetables. Discuss healthy dietary habits with all adolescents, including the benefits of a healthy diet; ways to consume foods rich in calcium, iron, and other vitamins and minerals; and safe weight management.

Female adolescents who are normal weight are also more likely to be currently attempting to lose weight, whereas male adolescents are more often trying to gain weight (Kann, McManus, Harris, et al., 2016). Although most teens trying to lose weight exercise or diet, a small percent of students engage in risky weight-loss practices such as vomiting after meals or taking laxatives. Anorexia nervosa and bulimia nervosa also commonly occur during the adolescent and young adult years. If left untreated, these disorders can lead to considerable morbidity and mortality. (See Eating Disorders, Chapter 18.)

A screening hemoglobin or hematocrit is recommended at the first encounter with an adolescent, at the end of puberty, or at both screening visits and at the end of pubertal development. The American Academy of Pediatrics (2017) recommends annual measures of weight and height and calculation of body mass index. Along with height and weight measurements, an appropriate screening or interview question related to obesity and eating disorders might be "Do you feel that you are too heavy, too thin, or about the right weight?"

Physical Fitness

Nationwide, in 2015 nearly one-half (49.6%) of all high school students reported that they had participated in activities that made them "sweat and breathe hard for at least 20 minutes" (i.e., vigorous physical activity) five or more times in the past week. Male students were more likely than female students to engage in vigorous physical activity (Kann, McManus, Harris, et al., 2016). Participation in school physical education classes declines with age because schools often do not have mandatory requirements past grade 9 or 10.

High levels of physical activity and fitness may reduce cardiovascular disease risk factors during adolescence, including obesity, high blood pressure, and hyperlipidemia. In addition, routine exercise may reduce adolescents' risk for depression and emotional distress. Although some evidence supports a positive relationship between a person's level of physical activity and fitness during adolescence and this level as an adult, the association between exercise and physical fitness and reduced risk for cardiovascular disease during adulthood is well documented.

Routine screening related to exercise should include questions about frequency, intensity, and type of physical activity. Health care organizations such as the American Academy of Pediatrics (2017) recommend discussing the emotional, social, and physical benefits of exercise with all adolescents. Furthermore, encourage all adolescents to engage in physical activity on a daily regular basis. Nurses should encourage adolescents to be physically active daily, or nearly every day, as part of play, games, sports, work, transportation, recreation, physical education, or other planned exercise. However, adolescents should not be encouraged to engage in physical activities that are beyond their physical or emotional capacity.

Sedentary activities, such as watching television, playing video games, and using a computer, can also contribute to obesity and cardiovascular health problems in later life. Youth should limit their "sedentary screen time" to 2 hours or less per day to get enough exercise. Some new forms of video games include equipment for more active involvement, such as dance or musical performance video games or "virtual" sports. A meta-analysis evaluating health outcomes of children and adolescents noted a large effect when comparing active video games to sedentary behaviors but no effect when comparing active video games to field-based physical activity (Gao, Chen, Pasco, et al., 2015). It is unclear if active video games will offer levels of aerobic activity equivalent to those of more traditional forms of sports and exercise.

Sexual Behavior, Sexually Transmitted Infections, and Unintended Pregnancy

Sexual activity significantly decreased among US youth in the 1990s through 2015 with 61.8 live births per 1000 teens in 1991, 39.1 live births per 1000 teens in 2009, and 22.3 live births per 1000 teens in 2015 (Centers for Disease Control and Prevention, 2017). Despite this decline, less than 5% of teens use the most effective types of birth control (long-acting reversible contraceptives) and instead rely on condoms or birth control pills, which require consist and correct use (Centers for Disease Control and Prevention, 2017). Furthermore, rates of STIs among teens, including human papillomavirus (HPV), chlamydia, and human immunodeficiency virus (HIV), have increased, although this may be partly due to increased testing and better sensitivity of testing.

Many sexually active young people engage in behaviors that put them at risk for STIs or pregnancy, such as having sex with multiple partners and having sex without using condoms or other forms of contraception. Approximately 11.5% of US high school students reported having had four or more sexual partners during their lifetime (Kann, McManus, Harris, et al., 2016). Among the sexually active students, nearly 57% reported using a condom during their most recent experience of intercourse, 18% reported using birth control pills, and 3% reported using an intrauterine device (IUD) or implant at the time of their most recent experience of intercourse (Kann, McManus, Harris, et al, 2016). Since 2013 rates of condom or oral contraceptive use have remained stable, and rates of IUD or implant use have increased 1.7% (Kann, McManus, Harris, et al., 2016).

Obtaining a confidential sexual history can be an important step in promoting sexual health and preventing STIs and unintended pregnancies among young people. Given their sensitive nature, questions about sexuality should be prefaced by an explanation of their purpose and the limits of confidentiality. Initial questions can cover less sensitive topics, such as milestones in pubertal development and, for girls, the menstrual history (including the age at menarche, timing of menstrual cycles, duration of menstrual flow, and symptoms of dysmenorrhea). Questions should also address dating behavior, same- and opposite-gender attractions, and same- and opposite-gender sexual behavior (e.g., "There are many ways people can be sexual with others, such as kissing; touching; and having oral, vaginal, and anal sex. In what ways have you been sexual with others?"). Adolescents should be asked about a history of uninvited or nonconsensual sexual contact (e.g., "Has anyone ever touched you in a sexual way that felt uncomfortable or when you did not want them to? Has anyone ever forced you to have sex?").

Sexually active youth should be asked about their consistency and motivation to use condoms or other barrier methods for preventing STIs; the number of sexual partners they have had over the past 6 months; and the use of alcohol or other substances in connection with sexual activity. The use of birth control pills or other forms of hormonal contraception is not protective against STIs. Sexually active adolescents should also be asked about any history of pregnancies or STIs. Adolescents who reveal a history of physical or sexual abuse, who admit to heavy use of alcohol or other drugs, or who have unstable social or economic support systems should also be asked whether they have ever exchanged sex for money, shelter, or drugs.

Sexually active adolescents should be screened for STIs. A Papanicolaou (Pap) smear is recommended for detection of cervical dysplasia at age 21 years unless the family history reveals high risk. Both males and females should be evaluated for HPV by visual inspection, and the HPV vaccine series should be promoted. Sexually active teenagers should have a serologic test for syphilis if they have lived in an area endemic for syphilis, have had other STIs, have had more than one sexual partner within the past 6 months, have exchanged sex for drugs or money, or are males who have had sex with other males.

One of the goals for *Healthy People 2020* is to test all adolescents for HIV at least once before adulthood (US Department of Health and Human Services, 2017). Adolescents at risk for HIV infection should be offered confidential HIV screening tests. HIV risk status includes having a history of injecting drug use (including anabolic steroid injections), having sexual intercourse in an area with a high prevalence of HIV infection, having other STIs, having more than one sexual partner in the past 6 months, exchanging sex for drugs or money, being a male and engaging in sex with other males, or having a sexual partner who is at risk for HIV infection. The frequency of laboratory screening for STIs and HIV depends on the sexual practices and STI history of individual adolescents.

All adolescents should receive medically accurate health guidance regarding responsible sexual behaviors, including abstinence. Adolescents should receive information on how STIs, including HIV and HPV, are transmitted and on possible consequences of infection. Counsel sexually active adolescents about ways to reduce their risk of STIs and unwanted pregnancy, including limiting the number of sexual partners, using condoms and barrier methods consistently, using appropriate methods of birth control, and avoiding substance use in connection with sexual activity. Counseling should include instruction on how to use condoms and other methods of birth control effectively. Despite extensive government funding available to provide "abstinence-only" sexual health education over the past decade, research evidence shows most such programs are not effective in delaying sexual behavior and may actually increase unprotected sex among adolescents once they become sexually active (Breuner, Mattson, American Academy of Pediatrics Committee on Adolescence, et al., 2016). Adolescents should receive positive reinforcement for responsible sexual behaviors, including abstinence, consistent condom use, and appropriate use of birth control. Adolescents should also be counseled on ways to reduce their risk of sexual exploitation. Techniques for counseling adolescents to reduce risky sexual behaviors are discussed in Chapter 18.

Use of Tobacco, Alcohol, and Other Substances

Statistically, experimentation with substances is common among US adolescents. By the twelfth grade, approximately 63% of students have used alcohol, 45% have used electronic vapor products, 32% have tried smoking tobacco, 39% have tried cannabis, and 6% have tried other illicit drugs such as LSD, PCP, acid, or angel dust (Kann, McManus, Harris, et al., 2016). Substance use increases with age, with older teens more likely to use alcohol and cannabis than younger teens. Among twelfth graders, for example, 73% have ever drank alcohol, but only 51% of ninth graders ever tried alcohol (Kann, McManus, Harris, et al., 2016). Furthermore, about 24.6% of twelfth-grade students report binge drinking (having had five or more drinks in a row) at least once in the past month, whereas among ninth graders, 10.4% have done so. The use of electronic vapor products among middle school–age and high school–age persons in the United States is prevalent. Some report that use of electronic vapor product is not harmful, yet there is no evidence that such products enhance smoking cessation or are benign (Drummond & Upson, 2014).

In contemporary US society, adolescents may use tobacco, alcohol, and marijuana because these substances provide an opportunity to challenge authority, demonstrate autonomy, gain entry into a peer group, or simply relieve the stress of growing up. Although use may be accepted among many US teenagers, there are substantive, documented consequences of early experimentation with alcohol, tobacco, and other drugs. Drinking and driving is the leading cause of death among teenagers. Persons who begin smoking at younger ages are more likely to become heavier smokers and are at increased risk for illness and death attributable to smoking. Substance use has also been associated with other health-challenging behaviors, such as delinquency, absenteeism, dropping out of school, lower academic achievement, and early sexual behavior.

In terms of health screening, the nurse can ask adolescents whether they or their friends have ever used tobacco, alcohol, marijuana, or other substances. They should also be asked about their current use and current use patterns among peers. The nurse should assess practices of drinking and driving or riding with someone who has been drinking. If answers to these initial questions indicate some problem use, the nurse should ask about the amount and frequency of use; frequency of getting "high" or "wasted"; use in relation to sexual activity; and difficulties with peers, school, parents, or the law in relation to use.

Adolescents who have begun experimenting or who engage in low-level use need to be made aware of other options that can help them achieve the same goals and of the risks of higher-level use. Furthermore, they need to know the short-term effects of alcohol, tobacco, or other drugs, particularly in relation to driving and school or work performance. Offer cessation plans to adolescents who use tobacco products. Adolescents whose substance use patterns endanger their health should be referred to an appropriate mental health provider. Chapter 18 includes an in-depth discussion of etiology, prevention strategies, and nursing considerations related to adolescent substance use.

Depression and Suicide

A national survey of ninth- through twelfth-grade students found that 34% of boys and 22% of girls reported feeling sad or hopeless almost every day for 2 weeks or longer (Fig. 17.13). Nearly 18% of high school students reported seriously considering suicide during the past year, with female students (23.4%) being more likely than male students

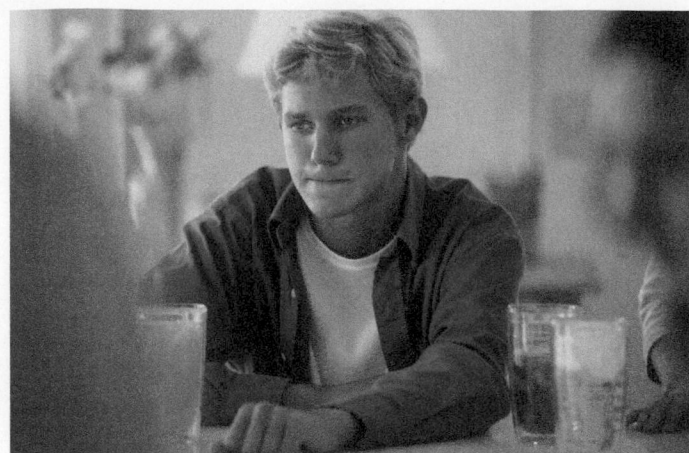

FIG. 17.13 Adolescents use being alone as a method of coping with stress. Health care professionals need to assess whether this also indicates an attempt to cope with depression.

(12.2%) to have considered a suicide attempt (Kann, McManus, Harris, et al., 2016). Around 8.6% of US high school students reported actually having attempted suicide during the previous 12 months, with girls (11.6%) being more likely than boys (5.5%) to have attempted suicide (Kann, McManus, Harris, et al., 2016).

A brief psychologic screening, such as the Psychology Systems Questionnaire (PSQ-2), is necessary during each adolescent health visit. Thorough screening for depression, anxiety, suicidal thoughts, and substance use should be done with adolescents who demonstrate declining school grades, chronic melancholy, or positive score on the brief screen. Most adolescents who are depressed respond affirmatively to the question "Have you been feeling down or blue lately?" although they may not necessarily "look" depressed. Refer nonsuicidal adolescents who report commonly feeling "blue," "down," or "depressed" to a psychologist, psychiatrist, or other mental health professional.

It is crucial to explore thoughts about and possible plans for suicidal acts with all troubled adolescents. Once an assessment of the immediate risk of suicide is completed, the nurse can construct a management scheme that ensures safety. If the adolescent has a specific plan, immediate referral for acute intervention with a psychiatrist or other mental health professional is indicated. (See Chapter 18 for further discussion of suicide.)

Physical, Sexual, and Emotional Abuse

Adolescents who have been physically, sexually, or emotionally abused during childhood or adolescence face challenges to healthy development. Reported cases of physical and sexual abuse declined 56% in physical abuse and 62% in sexual abuse from 1992 to 2010 (Finkelhor & Jones, 2012). Around one in four adolescents reports having been physically abused, primarily by family members and less commonly by someone outside the family. Certain groups of adolescents, such as gay, lesbian, or bisexual youth or those who are developmentally delayed, may be especially vulnerable to abuse.

A common constellation of symptoms among adolescents who have been victims of sexual abuse includes substance abuse, depression, withdrawn mood, violence, and somatic complaints. Adolescents who have been abused are more likely than nonabused adolescents to engage in health-compromising behaviors such as self-mutilation, suicide attempts, injection drug use, and early sexual activity (Ferrara, Guadagno, Sbordone, et al., 2016; Maquire, Williams, Naughton, et al., 2015) and are at higher risk of being sexually exploited.

Early identification of abuse can protect adolescents who have been victims of physical, sexual, and emotional trauma. For this reason, questions about abuse should be part of routine adolescent health visits. Ensure privacy before inquiring about abuse. If an adolescent reports a history of sexual or physical abuse, further questions should be directed toward any ongoing abuse; the circumstances surrounding the abuse incident; and the presence of physical, emotional, or behavioral sequelae, including involvement in risk-taking behaviors. Once a history of maltreatment is suspected or disclosed, health care providers have a legal responsibility to report the case to the appropriate child protection agency. The more acute the problem, the more quickly the report must be made. Adolescents reporting abuse should always be informed about steps in the reporting process before information is disclosed to local authorities.

Adolescents who live in homes where there is constant conflict may run away, sometimes to a friend's home. The conflict may be real (interpersonal) or perceived (intrapersonal), and escalation to abuse or the fear of abuse may prompt the adolescent to leave home. In addition, an adolescent who encounters difficulty with authority figures in the home may leave home believing this will solve the problem. The adolescent may stay in school and maintain close ties with less threatening family members and friends; the term *couch surfing* may be used to refer to the adolescent who spends time at different friends' houses sleeping on the couch or in an available spare room to "crash" temporarily. Such adolescents are often at higher risk for further abuse and neglect.

School and Learning Problems

In 2014, 17% of US youth between 16 and 24 years of age dropped out before completing high school (US Census Bureau, 2016). Dropout rates vary by ethnicity. In 2014, 11% of dropouts were Hispanic, 7% were African American, and 5% were Caucasian (US Census Bureau, 2016). Among in-school adolescents, a low grade point average has been associated with higher levels of emotional distress; cigarette, alcohol, and marijuana use; and earlier onset of sexual activity. School problems and dropping out of school can also be markers for difficulties such as learning disabilities, language barriers, family problems, lack of supportive relationships at school, and employment needs. In contemporary US society, education is critical to economic self-sufficiency. Adolescents who drop out of school can expect to earn approximately $400,000 less over a lifetime than those who graduate (Center for Labor Market Studies, 2011).

Questions about recent grades, school absences, suspensions, and any history of repeating a grade in school can be used to screen for school-related problems. Specific management plans for youth who note school problems should be coordinated with school personnel and with the adolescent's parents or caregivers if possible.

Hypertension

As adolescents experience sexual maturation, along with increases in height and weight, blood pressure increases from the onset of adolescence and continues to rise until the end of pubertal growth. Approximately 1% of adolescents have sustained hypertension, defined as a blood pressure greater than the 95th percentile of standards. The detection of hypertension during adolescence is important because hypertension is one of the major preventable risk factors for adult cardiovascular disease. With increasing levels of obesity, there have been reports of increasing incidence of hypertension among adolescents (Cheung, Bell, Samuel, et al., 2017). Screening for hypertension and associated risk factors should take place annually beginning at age 3 years and emphasized during adolescent health care visits, especially among teens who use tobacco products, a risk for heart disease. Specific guidelines for monitoring and treatment of hypertension in adolescents are found in the 2011 National Heart, Lung, and Blood Institute summary report (see also Chapter 27).

Hyperlipidemia

Along with hypertension, smoking, and obesity, elevated serum cholesterol and triglyceride levels are major risk factors for the development of adult cardiovascular disease. The National Heart, Lung, and Blood Institute (2016) recommends universal lipid (nonfasting or fasting) screening of all children and adolescents between the ages of 9 and 11 years and again between the ages of 17 and 21 years. Low-density lipoprotein (LDL) cholesterol–lowering drug therapy is recommended for children and adolescents 10 years of age and older whose LDL remains elevated after 6 months to 1 year on a restricted-fat diet, lifestyle modification (exercise), and weight management (National Heart, Lung, and Blood Institute, 2016). Additional information and practice guidelines for monitoring cholesterol levels and initiation of cholesterol-lowering medication, as well as specific dietary modifications, are found in the National Heart, Lung, and Blood Institute summary report at http://www.nhlbi.nih.gov/health-pro/guidelines/current/cardiovascular-health-pediatric-guidelines/summary.

Infectious Diseases and Immunizations

An immunization update is an important part of adolescent preventive care. Obtaining a record of the teenager's prior immunizations is important. The tetanus, diphtheria, acellular pertussis (Tdap) vaccine is recommended for adolescents 11 to 18 years old who have not received a tetanus booster (Td) or Tdap dose and have completed the childhood DTaP/DTP series. When the Tdap is used as a booster dose, it may be administered earlier than the previous 5-year interval to provide adequate pertussis immunity (regardless of interval from the last Td dose) (American Academy of Pediatrics, 2015). Meningococcal vaccine (MenACWY-D [Menactra] or MenACWY-CRM [Menveo]) should be given to adolescents 11 to 12 years of age, with a booster dose before age 16 years. If not previously vaccinated, they should receive one dose between 13 and 18 years of age (American Academy of Pediatrics, 2015) (see also Immunizations, Chapter 6).

The quadrivalent HPV vaccine or the bivalent HPV vaccine is recommended for the prevention of cervical precancers and cancers for girls beginning at a minimum age of 9 years. The quadrivalent HPV vaccine is recommended for males ages 9 through 18 years to reduce their likelihood of genital warts (American Academy of Pediatrics, 2015). Each one of the HPV vaccines is administered in a three-dose series; it is important to follow the recommended dose intervals for optimal effectiveness.

All adolescents who have not previously received three doses of hepatitis B vaccine should be vaccinated against hepatitis B virus. The hepatitis A vaccine should be given to adolescents who live in areas where vaccination programs target older children, children who are at increased risk for infection, or children for whom immunity against hepatitis A is desired (American Academy of Pediatrics, 2015). Annual influenza vaccination with the inactivated influenza vaccine is recommended for all children and adolescents (see Chapter 6). All adolescents should also be assessed for previous history of varicella infection or vaccination. Vaccination with the varicella vaccine is recommended for those with no previous history; for those with no previous infection or history, the varicella vaccine may be given in two doses 4 or more weeks apart to adolescents 13 years of age or older (American Academy of Pediatrics, 2015). Adolescents should receive a tuberculin skin test if they have been exposed to active tuberculosis (TB), have lived in or traveled to an area with a high prevalence of TB, have radiographic or clinical findings suggestive of TB, or are infected with HIV (see Chapter 26).

Body Art

Body art (piercing and tattooing) is an aspect of adolescent identity formation. The skin has become the latest source of parent-adolescent conflict. Adolescents often seek body art as an expression of their personal identity and style. Tattoos may mark significant life events such as new relationships, births, and deaths. Piercing the ear, nose, lip, nipple, eyebrow, labia, navel, penis, or tongue may sometimes create a health problem. It is a nursing responsibility to caution girls and boys against having piercing performed by friends, parents, or themselves. Although in most cases piercings have few, if any, serious side effects, there is always a risk for complications such as infection, cyst or keloid formation, bleeding, dermatitis, or metal allergy. Using the same unsterilized needle to pierce body parts of multiple teenagers presents the same risk for HIV, hepatitis C virus, and hepatitis B virus transmission as occurs with other needle-sharing activities. Furthermore, there is a danger of contaminated tattoo ink that occurred in association with skin infections, such as nontuberculous *Mycobacterium chelonae* (Mudedla, Avendano, & Raman, 2015).

Adolescents should be informed about the approximate time for healing after body piercing and the care of the pierced area during and after healing. Some body sites need extra precautions. For example, cartilage (ear, nose) has a poor blood supply and heals slowly and scars easily; nipple piercing puts adolescents at risk for breast abscesses. Finally, migration of the piercing is common with navel and other flat skin surface piercing. Piercing guns should not be used for piercing anything other than the earlobe because guns place the piercing too deeply. The presence of body art in the form of tattoos and branding is common among adolescents and young adults. Professionals as well as amateur artists administer tattoos. The greatest risk is for the tattoo artist, who comes in contact with the client's blood. Adolescents who are amateur tattoo artists benefit from discussions about Standard Precautions and the hepatitis B vaccination. Many states either have no regulations or do not enforce existing regulations of piercing and tattooing facilities. The local health department is a source of information about local regulatory requirements. The Centers for Disease Control and Prevention has a website that outlines safety concerns for persons performing and receiving body art: http://www.cdc.gov/niosh/topics/body_art/.

Sleep Deprivation and Insomnia

The changing social environment of adolescents can often change their sleep patterns at a time when their growth and development require additional sleep for health. Although adolescents should generally get around 9 hours of sleep each night, early-morning school scheduling, extracurricular activities, homework, employment, and desired social time with peers or on the Internet can make it difficult for them to get sufficient sleep. Recent studies into sleep among adolescents have shown that nearly half may not get the recommended amounts of sleep, and as many as one in four are regularly sleep deprived—that is, report 7 hours or less of sleep per night (Kann, McManus, Harris, et al., 2016; Tarokh, Saletin, & Carskadon, 2016). Sleep deprivation can affect physical and mental health and has been associated with higher rates of overweight and obesity, depression, somatic complaints such as headaches and stomachaches, fatigue, and difficulties with concentration. These physical and psychologic effects of inadequate sleep can also affect school performance and thus contribute to school problems. Health teaching and health promotion should include information to promote sufficient sleep.

Homeless and street-involved youth, youth who go to bed hungry because of insufficient access to food, and those with anxiety disorders are all more likely to experience sleep disturbances. However, the high rate of young people who do not get enough sleep and the health consequences of inadequate sleep suggest that nurses should regularly assess all adolescents for the amount and quality of sleep they are getting. Health teaching and health promotion should include information to promote sufficient sleep.

Tanning

The quest for an attractive appearance leads many teenagers to excessive sunbathing and artificial means for tanning. However, this practice has serious long-term risks, and adolescents should be educated regarding the detrimental effects of sunlight on the skin. Long-term effects include premature aging of the skin; increased risk for skin cancer; and, in susceptible individuals, phototoxic reactions.

The popularity of artificial tanning has prompted concern from health care professionals regarding the use of sunlamps and tanning beds. The long-term effects of tanning machines are similar to those of the sun; dermatologists do not recommend tanning by this means. Those who insist on using tanning equipment should be warned that goggles must be worn in tanning booths to prevent serious corneal burning. Education on the use of sunscreens, including hypoallergenic products, with a sun protective factor (SPF) of at least 15 and a non-alcohol base without lanolin, parabens, or fragrance, is important. Broad-spectrum sunscreens that protect against both ultraviolet A and ultraviolet B (UV-A and UV-B) are the most effective. Self-tanning creams safely simulate the appearance of a tan; however, teens using these products should be cautioned that sun protection is still required. Targeting health education messages to adolescents and incorporating educational components relating to sun protection behaviors in school health curricula and in health care visits will increase adolescents' knowledge and awareness. Yet data continue to indicate that adolescents and adults who are in charge of adolescents are disregarding these messages.

HEALTH PROMOTION AMONG SPECIAL GROUPS OF ADOLESCENTS

Certain groups of adolescents experience health problems at disproportionate rates and face barriers to health care because of a lack of financial resources, limited availability of appropriate resources, or other factors.

Minority Adolescents

Minority children (i.e., children of African American, Latino, Asian, Native American, and Alaskan Native descent) are the fastest-growing population within the United States. The population of first- and second-generation immigrant children increased by 66% between 1995 and 2012 and represents one-quarter of all children living in the United States, with the majority being from Mexico (Child Trends, 2013). It is estimated that by 2020 roughly 40% of the US child population will be made up of minorities. In 2012, 38% of African American children, 34% of Latino children, and 14% of Asian children lived in poverty (Child Trends, 2014b).

Most of these children successfully meet growth and development milestones and the challenges of adolescence and young adulthood. Research has begun to identify factors that promote resiliency among minority adolescents from disadvantaged backgrounds, including those who grow up in poverty. Often these young people have come from families and communities that provide nurturing, supportive, and culturally rich environments. To be most effective, future health promotion interventions must include strategies that increase these protective factors in the lives of other adolescents growing up in high-risk environments.

However, too many minority adolescents experience predictable outcomes associated with living in environments where risk factors outweigh protective factors. Compared with nonminority children, higher percentages of minority children and adolescents have learning, emotional, or physical disabilities. They are more likely to drop out of school and have limited opportunities for higher education, become parents at an early age, are incarcerated in youth detention facilities, or die as a result of homicide or unintentional injuries before reaching adulthood. The increase in health risk behaviors during adolescence, in combination with limited access to health care and effective preventive services, places these adolescents at significantly higher risk for adolescent pregnancy, STIs, HIV/AIDS, chronic or other infectious diseases (hypertension, TB, and hepatitis), substance abuse, emotional problems, and violence. All these health problems, which often lead to premature death or chronic disorders, are preventable.

Effective health promotion programs can make important contributions to the prevention of health problems among minority adolescents. A consensus is growing that health promotion programs will be most effective if they are culturally competent. A culturally competent approach is one that recognizes the importance of culture and incorporates—at all levels—the assessment of relations across cultures, with attention to dynamics that result from cultural differences, the expansion of cultural knowledge, and the adaptation of programs to meet culture-specific needs. Nurses, working with other health care professionals and community leaders, can develop or adapt culture-specific health promotion interventions (see Cultural Considerations box).

CULTURAL CONSIDERATIONS

The Adolescent Years

Other societies in which adolescence is seen as part of the life cycle may have ideas very different from those of American culture about how the adolescent years are to be spent. For example, some societies discourage contact between adolescent boys and girls. Sexual experimentation is outlawed, and all grown children, males and females, remain in the homes of their parents until they wed. In America we tend to believe that the way our culture is organized is the way all cultures are or should be organized, but of course, this is not so. Each society is unique. The way we describe adolescence, the way we experience it, and the predisposition of our adolescents toward violence are peculiar to our American culture.

Several basic principles can guide the development of culturally appropriate health promotion efforts (Isaacs, 1993):

- Health promotion messages are most effective when they are conveyed through multiple community institutions. The content of these messages should be consistent across agencies, culturally appropriate, and couched in terms that deal with health-destructive behaviors in a pragmatic rather than a judgmental manner.
- Health promotion efforts should involve peer groups, schools, communities, and families. In particular, families must be recognized as a positive source of cultural strength and a primary source of information, education, and support for young people. Because "family" is defined differently by different cultures, a culture-specific definition of family must be the basis of developing interventions involving families. For example, prevention strategies that involve concerned relatives and friends have proved highly successful in reaching Hispanic youth involved in high-risk behaviors. The willingness of family and friends to be involved is rooted in Hispanic values of familialism and community.
- Those who develop strategies for minority adolescents and communities must draw on community-based values, traditions, and

customs and work with knowledgeable persons from the community in developing focused interventions and communication channels. The challenge for professionals, whose culture may be different from that of the target audience, is to develop collaborative relationships with community members that enable communities to identify health problems and their underlying causes and to design and evaluate programs that address identified needs.

- Health promotion interventions focused on minority adolescents may be most effective if they provide a generic framework and skills for developing relationships and problem solving that can be applied to any health-related decision. There is an emerging belief that this type of generic approach can be more effective than interventions focused on specific problems (e.g., STIs, pregnancy, or substance use) because the behaviors that lead to many adolescent health problems are highly interrelated.
- Health promotion and prevention strategies must be developed and implemented in places where these adolescents are found. Adolescents who have left the school system are often at greater risk for health problems than those who remain in school. Health promotion messages must be incorporated into shelters for homeless and runaway youth, detention centers, residential programs, and community recreation centers to reach young people at highest risk.

To date, there has been little systematic evaluation of the effectiveness of health promotion interventions among minority adolescents. Interventions that work must be documented so that these efforts can be disseminated and adapted for other communities of color.

Lesbian, Gay, Bisexual, and Transgender Adolescents

A recent survey of US high school students revealed that approximately 321,000 are gay or lesbian, 964,000 are bisexual, and 514,000 are unsure of their sexual identity (Zaza, Kann, & Barrios, 2016). These students are as racially, ethnically, and geographically diverse as their heterosexual peers. Although adolescents may participate in same-gender sexual activity or have same-gender attractions, they do not necessarily become lesbian, gay, bisexual, or transgender adults. In 2015 approximately 273,000 high school students had sexual contact only with the same sex and 739,000 students had sexual contact with both sexes (Zaza, Kann, & Barrios, 2016). Assigning sexual orientation labels to adolescents is complex and should be approached cautiously. Nurses confidently and consistently ask teens their gender preference when interviewing them and acknowledge their choice of gender terms. Screening questions regarding sexual attractions and experiences should be phrased in ways that allow adolescents to discuss same- and opposite-gender attractions, such as using the term *partner* rather than *boyfriend* or *girlfriend*.

The population of lesbian, gay, bisexual, and transgender (LGBT) adolescents has unique developmental issues and health challenges. Most of the health challenges of sexual minority teens are responses to negative societal attitudes and messages about homosexual or bisexual orientation. Compared with their heterosexual peers, there is a higher prevalence of being bullied at school or cyberbullied, and experiencing physical or sexual dating violence (Zaza, Kann, & Barrios, 2016). They may use alcohol, marijuana, and other substances to escape their anxieties. They are less likely to participate in sports and belong to exercise facilities, and there is an increased prevalence of eating disorders, especially among lesbians and transgender teens (O'Neill & Wakefield, 2017). Furthermore, they are at much greater risk for suicidal behaviors than their heterosexual peers. Although nurses should screen all youth about suicidal thoughts and history of suicide attempts, it is especially critical for an adolescent who identifies as gay, lesbian, bisexual, or transgender, or one who is questioning his or her sexual orientation. Also, LGBT adolescents need the same sexuality education and information on pregnancy prevention and STI transmission and prevention that is appropriate for all other adolescents.

Publicly disclosing an LGBT orientation during adolescence ("coming out") brings additional challenges. Many adolescents disclose their orientation to a close peer, then a sibling, and finally a parent (Steever, Francis, Gordon, et al., 2014). Adolescents face hostility, violence, and even rejection from their peers and families. Nurses should not encourage teens to disclose their sexual orientation to their families without first forming a safety plan in case the reaction is not supportive. For the majority of young people, referral to an agency providing support services or social opportunities for LGBT adolescents is appropriate. PFLAG is one organization consisting of LGBT people, their family members, and friends, that provides advocacy, education, and support. Parents who seek assistance in adjusting to their son's or daughter's disclosure can be referred to a local chapter of PFLAG (https://www.pflag.org/find-a-chapter).

Adolescents who acknowledge same-gender attractions or relationships are also at risk for violence and harassment from schoolmates, neighbors, and even strangers. Others show rejection in more subtle ways, but even these nonsupportive responses can have an effect on adolescents' healthy development. Sexual minority adolescents fear similar uncaring attitudes among health care providers and avoid disclosing their sexual orientation and emotional health during primary care visits (Snyder, Burack, & Petrova, 2017). To provide sensitive, professional care for gay, lesbian, bisexual, and transgender adolescents, nurses should be sensitive in their choice of language and be nonjudgmental and caring in their communication.

Rural Adolescents

Except for higher rates of accidental injuries (related in part to farm accidents) and lower rates of delinquency among rural adolescents compared with urban ones, few known differences in health problems exist. Research on the health status of rural adolescents is limited, but rural adolescents experience many of the same health problems as adolescents in metropolitan areas. However, rural adolescents face barriers to health promotion because they have more limited access to appropriate health care services.

Rural adolescents' access to health care is limited by shortages of professionally staffed mental and physical health services, inadequately trained providers, transportation problems, and less access to Medicaid in rural states. Rural communities often lack adequately trained nurses, physicians, dentists, psychologists, social workers, and allied health professionals, in addition to modern equipment. Rural health professionals often feel inadequately prepared to address adolescents' physical and psychosocial health issues. In metropolitan areas, providers who are unwilling or unable to address adolescents' concerns can refer to colleagues with expertise in adolescent health issues. The absence of adolescent health specialists, combined with a limited network of agencies focused on adolescent health promotion, exacerbates rural youths' problems in obtaining appropriate services. Finally, rural adolescents who live in poverty are less likely than their low-income urban counterparts to be covered by Medicaid and to have financial coverage for health care services.

In addition to health promotion topics addressed with other populations of adolescents, prevention efforts focused on rural adolescents must include efforts to improve the safety of farm machinery and farming practices. Innovative efforts are needed to increase rural adolescents' access to health care services, including development and funding for school-linked health services, improvements in transportation, use of nonprofessionals and adult community members, better dissemination of information about the availability of local health services, and access to further education in adolescent health for health care providers.

NURSING CARE MANAGEMENT

With continued increases in the numbers of adolescents in the United States and rising rates of health-related problems of youth, there is an unprecedented need for adolescent health promotion. Nursing professionals can make significant contributions to health promotion among adolescents and their families. Because nurses understand the biologic, cognitive, psychosocial, and social transitions of adolescence and their impact on health behavior, they can address adolescents' developmental and health needs. Working with colleagues from other disciplines, community members, parents, and adolescents themselves, nurses must become part of a comprehensive approach that delivers consistent messages across clinical, school, and community-based settings. Nurses should be at the forefront of developing and disseminating culturally appropriate health promotion interventions among special populations, including minority adolescents; gay, lesbian, and bisexual youth; and rural teenagers.

Parents are often confused and perplexed about the changes and behaviors of adolescence. They need support and guidance to help them through this time. They need to understand the changes taking place and to accept the expected behaviors that accompany the process of detachment, to be prepared to "let go," and to promote the changed relationship from one of dependency to one of mutuality. Suggestions for anticipatory guidance of parents of adolescents are listed in the Family-Centered Care box.

FAMILY-CENTERED CARE

Guidance During Adolescence

Encourage parents to:

- Accept adolescent as a unique individual.
- Respect adolescent's ideas, likes and dislikes, and wishes.
- Be involved with school functions and attend adolescent's performances, whether it is a sporting event or a school play.
- Listen and try to be open to adolescent's views, even when they disagree with parental views.
- Avoid criticism about no-win topics.
- Provide opportunity for choosing options and accepting natural consequences of these choices.
- Allow young person to learn by doing, even when choices and methods differ from those of adults.
- Provide adolescent with clear, reasonable limits.
- Clarify house rules and consequences for breaking them.
- Let society's rules and consequences teach responsibility outside the home.
- Allow increasing independence within limitations of safety and well-being.
- Be available for conversation but avoid pressing adolescent too far.
- Respect adolescent's privacy.
- Try to share adolescent's feelings of joy or sorrow.
- Respond to feelings as well as words.
- Be available to answer questions, give information, and provide companionship.
- Try to make communication clear.
- Avoid comparisons with siblings.
- Assist adolescent in selecting appropriate career goals and preparing for adult role.
- Welcome adolescent's friends into the home and treat them with respect.
- Provide unconditional love.
- Be willing to apologize when mistaken.

Be aware that adolescents:

- Are sometimes subject to turbulent, unpredictable behavior.
- Are struggling for independence.
- Are extremely sensitive to feelings and behaviors that affect them.
- May receive a different message from what was sent.
- Consider friends extremely important.
- Have a strong need to belong.

NCLEX REVIEW QUESTIONS

1. Which of the following are the primary causes of mortality among adolescents in the United States? Select all that apply.
   A. Injuries
   B. Suicide
   C. Congenital anomalies
   D. Homicide
   E. Chronic illness
2. Which of the following immunization booster vaccines should be considered for a 13-year-old adolescent who has completed all recommended routine *childhood* vaccinations? Select all that apply.
   A. DTaP vaccine
   B. Tdap vaccine
   C. Meningococcal vaccine
   D. Pneumococcal vaccine
   E. Hepatitis B vaccine
   F. Hib vaccine
3. Which of the following hormones have the most impact on the development of puberty in females and males? Select all that apply.
   A. Follicle-stimulating hormone (FSH)
   B. Insulin
   C. Luteinizing hormone (LH)
   D. Estrogen
   E. Testosterone
4. According to Jean Piaget, adolescent cognitive development is represented by the stage of formal operational thought that includes which of the following? Select all that apply.
   A. Believing that thoughts are all-powerful
   B. Thinking in abstract terms
   C. Thinking about hypotheses
   D. Using a future time perspective
   E. Thinking in the here and now
5. One of the key factors in addressing the health concerns and needs of the adolescent in a clinic or primary care office setting is to:
   A. Provide confidentiality
   B. Include the parent(s) in a discussion about the adolescent's sexual health
   C. Ask the adolescent if she or he is sexually active
   D. Discuss the negative effects of tobacco use

Correct Answers

1. A, B, D; 2. B, C; 3. A, C; 4. B, C, D; 5. A

REFERENCES

Ali, O., & Donohoue, P. A. (2016). Gynecomastia. In R. M. Kliegman, B. F. Stanton, J. W. St. Geme, et al. (Eds.), *Nelson textbook of pediatrics* (20th ed.). Philadelphia: Saunders/Elsevier.

American Academy of Pediatrics. (2017). *Bright futures: Adolescent tools.* https://brightfutures.aap.org/materials-and-tools/tool-and-resource-kit/Pages/adolescence-tools.aspx.

American Academy of Pediatrics, Committee on Infectious Diseases, & Pickering, L., Eds. (2015). *2015 Red book: report of the Committee on Infectious Diseases (30th ed.).* Elk Grove Village, IL, The Academy.

Arain, M., Haque, M., Johal, L., et al. (2013). Maturation of the adolescent brain. *Neuropsychiatric Disease and Treatment, 9*, 449–461.

Breuner, C. C., Mattson, G., American Academy of Pediatrics Committee on Adolescence, et al. (2016). Sexuality education for children and adolescents. *Pediatrics, 138*(2), e1–e11.

Brooks, F. M., Magnusson, J., Spencer, N., et al. (2012). Adolescent multiple risk behaviour: An asset approach to the role of family, school and community. *Journal of Public Health (Oxford, England), 34*(Suppl1), 48–56.

Cabrera, S. M., Bright, G. M., Frane, J. W., et al. (2014). Age of thelarche and menarche in contemporary US females: A cross-sectional analysis. *Journal of Pediatric Endocrinology & Metabolism : JPEM, 27*(0), 47–51.

Center for Labor Market Studies. (2011). *High school dropouts in Chicago and Illinois: the growing labor market, income, civic, social and fiscal costs of dropping out of high school.* http://hdl.handle.net/2047/d20003559.

Centers for Disease Control and Prevention. (2017). *Preventing teen pregnancy.* https://www.cdc.gov/vitalsigns/larc/index.html.

Chase, C. (2014). US state and federal laws targeting distracted driving. *Annals of Advances in Automotive Medicine. Association for the Advancement of Automotive Medicine. Annual Scientific Conference, 58*, 84–98.

Cheung, E. L., Bell, C. S., Samuel, J. P., et al. (2017). Race and obesity in adolescent hypertension. *Pediatrics, 139*(5), e20161433.

Child Trends. (2013). *Immigrant children.* Child Trends Data Bank. Retrieved from http://www.childtrends.org?indicators=immigrant-children.

Child Trends. (2014a). *Overweight children and youth.* Retreived from https://www.childtrends.org/indicators/overweight-children-and-youth/.

Child Trends. (2014b). *Children in poverty.* Retrieved from https://www.childtrends.org/indicators/children-in-poverty/.

Drummond, M. B., & Upson, D. (2014). Electronic cigarettes: Potential harms and benefits. *Annals of the American Thoracic Society, 11*(2), 236–242.

Elkind, D. (1978). Understanding the young adolescent. *Adolescence, 13*(49), 128–134.

Erikson, E. (1968). *Identity: Youth in crisis.* New York: Norton.

Fan, M., Jin, Y., & Khubchandani, J. (2014). Overweight misperception among adolescents in the United States. *Journal of Pediatric Nursing, 29*(6), 536–546.

Ferrara, P., Guadagno, C., Sbordone, A., et al. (2016). Child abuse and neglect: A review of the literature. *Current Pediatric Reviews*, epub ahead of print.

Finkelhor, D., & Jones, L. (2012). *Have sexual abuse and physical abuse declined since the 1990s?* Lebanon: University of New Hampshire, Press.

Fuhrmann, D., Knoll, L., & Blakemore, S. (2015). Adolescence as a sensitive period of brain development. *Trends in Cognitive Sciences, 19*(10), 558–566.

Gao, Z., Chen, S., Pasco, D., et al. (2015). A meta-analysis of active video games on health outcomes among children and adolescents. *Obesity Reviews: An Official Journal of the International Association for the Study of Obesity, 16*(9), 783–794.

Gilligan, C. (1982). *In a different voice.* Cambridge, Mass: Harvard University Press.

Gilligan, C. (1986). Adolescent development reconsidered. Paper presented at Invitational Conference on Health Futures of Adolescents, Daytona Beach, FL.

Haydon, A. A., Herring, A. H., Prinstein, M. J., et al. (2012). Beyond age at first sex: Patterns of emerging sexual behavior in adolescence and young adulthood. *The Journal of Adolescent Health: Official Publication of the Society for Adolescent Medicine, 50*(5), 456–463.

Herman-Giddens, M. E. (2013). The enigmatic pursuit of puberty in girls. *Pediatrics, 132*(6), 1125–1126.

Herman-Giddens, M. E., Steffes, J., Harris, D., et al. (2012). Secondary sexual characteristics in boys: Data from the pediatric research in office settings network. *Pediatrics, 130*(5), e1058–e1068.

Hill, P. L., Duggan, P. M., & Lapsley, D. K. (2012). Subjective invulnerability, risk behavior, and adjustment in early adolescence. *The Journal of Early Adolescence, 32*(4), 489–501.

Horton, S. E. (2015). Religion and health-promoting behaviors among emerging adults. *Journal of Religion and Health, 54*(1), 20–34.

Hoying, J., Melnyk, B. M., & Arcoleo, K. (2016). Effects of the COPE cognitive behavioral skills building TEEN program on the healthy lifestyle behaviors and mental health of Appalachian early adolescents. *Journal of Pediatric Health Care, 30*(1), 65–72.

Isaacs, M. (1993). Developing culturally competent strategies for adolescents of color. In A. Elster, S. Panzarine, & K. Holt (Eds.), *American Medical Association State of the Art Conference on Adolescent Health Promotion: Proceedings, Arlington, VA.* National Center for Education in Maternal and Child Health.

Jacobson, C., Bailin, A., Milanaik, R., et al. (2016). Adolescent health implications of new age technology. *Pediatric Clinics of North America, 63*(1), 183–194.

Kann, L., McManus, T., Harris, W. A., et al. (2016). Youth risk behavior surveillance – United States, 2015. *Morbidity and Mortality Weekly Report. Surveillance Summaries (Washington, D.C.: 2002), 65*, 1–177.

Kohlberg, L., & Gilligan, C. (1972). The adolescent as philosopher: the discovery of the self in a post-conventional world. In J. Kagan & R. Coles (Eds.), *Twelve to sixteen: Early adolescence.* New York: Norton.

Lapsley, D. K. (1993). Toward an integrated theory of adolescent ego development: The "new look" at adolescent egocentrism. *The American Journal of Orthopsychiatry, 63*(4), 562–571.

Lenhart, A. (2015). *Teens, social media & technology overview 2015.* Washington, DC. Pew Research Center. http://www.pewinternet.org/2015/04/09/teens-social-media-technology-2015.

Lofquist, D. A., & Lewis, J. M. (2015). *Improving measurement of same-sex couples.* US Census Bureau, Washington, DC. http://www.census.gov/hhes/samesex/files/Lofquist_Lewis_2015-13.pdf.

Maquire, S. A., Williams, B., Naughton, A. M., et al. (2015). A systematic review of the emotional, behavioural and cognitive features exhibited by school-aged children experiencing neglect or emotional abuse. *Child: Care, Health and Development, 41*(5), 641–653.

McKeever, J. D., Schultheis, M. T., Padmanaban, V., et al. (2013). Driver performance while texting: Even a little is too much. *Traffic Injury Prevention, 14*(2), 132–137.

Meeus, W. (2016). Adolescent psychosocial development: A review of longitudinal models and research. *Developmental Psychology, 52*(12), 1969–1993.

Morelli, M., Bianchi, D., Baiocco, R., et al. (2016). Sexting, psychological distress and dating violence among adolescents and young adults. *Psicothema, 28*(2), 137–142.

Mudedla, S., Avendano, E. E., & Raman, G. (2015). Non-tuberculous mycobacterium skin infections after tattooing in healthy individuals: A systematic review of case reports. *Dermatology Online Journal, 21*(6).

National Center on Addiction and Substance Abuse. *The importance of family dinners VI.* https://www.centeronaddiction.org/addiction-research/reports/importance-of-family-dinners-2010.

National Heart, Lung, and Blood Institute (NHLBI). (2016). *Expert panel on integrated guidelines for cardiovascular health and risk reduction in children and adolescents: summary report.* Bethesda, MD, U.S. Department of Health and Human Services, NHLBI.

Neuman, M. E. (2011). Addressing children's beliefs through Fowler's stages of faith. *Journal of Pediatric Nursing, 26*(1), 44–50.

O'Neill, T., & Wakefield, J. (2017). Fifteen-minute consultation in the normal child: Challenges relating to sexuality and gender identity in children and young people. *Archives of Disease in Childhood. Education and Practice Edition*, epub ahead of print.

Papadimitriou, A. (2016). The evolution of the age of menarche from prehistoric to modern times. *Journal of Pediatric and Adolescent Gynecology, 29*(6), 527–530.

Piaget, J. (1972). Intellectual evolution from adolescence to adulthood. *Human Development, 15*, 1–12.

Reese, B. M., Choukas-Bradley, S., Herring, A. H., et al. (2014). Correlates of adolescent and young adult sexual initiation patterns. *Perspectives on Sexual and Reproductive Health, 46*(4), 211–221.

Snyder, B. K., Burack, G. D., & Petrova, A. (2017). LGBTQ youth's perceptions of primary care. *Clinical Pediatrics, 56*(5), 443–450.

Steever, J., Francis, J., Gordon, L. P., et al. (2014). Sexual minority youth. *Primary Care, 41*(3), 651–669.

Steinberg, L. (1990). Autonomy, conflict and harmony in the family relationship. In S. Feldman & G. Elliot (Eds.), *At the threshold: The developing adolescent*. Cambridge, MA: Harvard University Press.

Sullivan, H. (1953). *The interpersonal theory of psychiatry*. New York: Norton.

Tarokh, L., Saletin, J. M., & Carskadon, M. A. (2016). Sleep in adolescence: Physiology, cognition and mental health. *Neuroscience and Biobehavioral Reviews, 70*, 182–188.

Troop-Gordon, W. (2017). Peer victimization in adolescence: The nature, progression, and consequences of being bullied within a developmental context. *Journal of Adolescence, 55*, 116–128.

US Census Bureau. *School enrollment in the United States: 2016*. https://www.census.gov/newsroom/press-releases/2016/cb16-tps142.html.

US Department of Health and Human Services. (2017). *Healthy people 2020: HIV*. Washington, DC. https://www.healthypeople.gov/2020/topics-objectives/topic/hiv/objectives.

Villanueva, C., & Argente, J. (2014). Pathology or normal variant: What constitutes a delay in puberty? *Hormone Research in Pædiatrics, 82*(4), 213–221.

Walker, L., de Vries, B., & Trevethan, S. (1987). Moral stages and moral orientations in real-life and hypothetical dilemmas. *Child Development, 58*, 842–858.

Zaza, S., Kann, L., & Barrios, L. C. (2016). Lesbian, gay, and bisexual adolescents: Population estimate and prevalence of health behaviors. *JAMA: The Journal of the American Medical Association, 316*(22), 2355–2356.

18

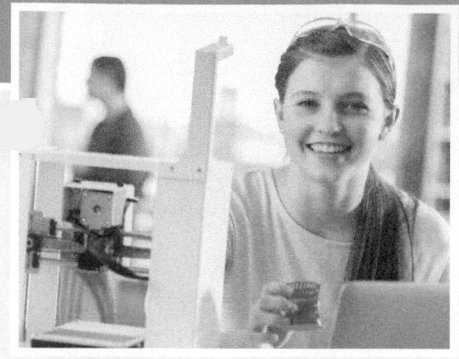

Health Problems of the Adolescent

Cheryl C. Rodgers

http://evolve.elsevier.com/wong/ncic

CONCEPTS

- Reproduction
- Sexuality
- Interpersonal Violence
- Stress
- Addiction
- Safety

HEALTH CONDITIONS OF THE MALE REPRODUCTIVE SYSTEM

PENILE CONDITIONS

Common congenital anomalies of the penis are almost always detected and corrected in infancy or early childhood. In some cases boys who need an operative procedure to repair hypospadias (the most common congenital deformity of the penis) may reach adolescence with a penis that looks different from those of their friends. A few who have received no medical care have uncorrected deformities that can cause serious psychologic problems during this sensitive period of development. These young boys need to be identified for surgical repair of the defect.

Uncircumcised males may encounter some problems during adolescence related to a tight foreskin that cannot be retracted over the enlarging glans (*paraphimosis*). Necrosis and tissue necrosis of the glans may occur if the condition is not treated properly; in most cases the glans edema can be reduced by gentle manual compression, but other noninvasive techniques include the use of ice or compression wraps (Pohlman, Phillips, & Wilcox, 2013). Eventually the foreskin is returned to its original position. Uncircumcised males are at higher risk for infections such as balanitis and prosthitis. Penile carcinoma (penile intraepithelial neoplasia) is associated with numerous human papillomavirus (HPV) types, but only one HPV type, HPV-16, is associated with 76% of penile neoplasias (Diorio & Giuliano, 2016). HPV types 6 and 11 are commonly associated with genital warts, which may be benign or malignant (Diorio & Giuliano, 2016). Although HPV is a common sexually transmitted infection (STI) among American males, penile carcinomas are rare in the United States, and most Western countries account for approximately 1.3% of the malignancies (Diorio & Giuliano, 2016).

Trauma to the penis, including burns and accidental injuries, can occur in various ways. The frenulum (the fold on the lower surface of the glans that connects it with the prepuce) can be torn after retraction of the foreskin, unusually rough masturbation, or coitus. It can be frightening to the young boy but usually heals spontaneously with minimum care. However, any extensive bleeding may require suturing of the tissues. Penile fracture is a rupture of the corpus cavernosum as a result of blunt trauma to the erect penis, usually during vigorous sexual intercourse or masturbation. The condition is considered a urologic emergency, and surgical repair is recommended to prevent further complications (Chahal, Gupta, & Das, 2016).

Drugs such as trazodone (Desyrel), taken alone or in combination with cocaine or Ecstasy (MDMA [3-4 methylenedioxymethamphetamine]), may cause a prolonged erection (priapism), which can be extremely uncomfortable and in some cases may require surgical intervention to release blood trapped in the corpus cavernosum. Drugs available to adults for erectile dysfunction or other drugs not intended for recreational uses may have unintentional and undesirable side effects requiring immediate medical attention. Antidepressant and antipsychotic drugs may also cause an ischemic priapism requiring emergent treatment (Armstrong, Grimsby, & Jacobs, 2015). Other conditions that may be seen include zipper injury or entrapment, entrapment by metal or glass objects, balanitis, prosthitis, and STIs.

VARICOCELE

A varicocele is a congenital condition characterized by elongation, dilation, and tortuosity of the veins of the spermatic cord superior to the testicle. The finding is rare in prepubertal children, but the incidence increases to 5% to 15% in adolescent boys (Elder, 2016). Idiopathic varicocele is the most common treatable cause of male-related impaired fertility, especially if caught and treated early (Elder, 2016). Varicoceles occur most often on the left side because of the greater length of the left spermatic vein and its entry into the left renal artery; the right spermatic vein enters the vena cava directly and at a lesser angle, which may be a source of future difficulty. A varicocele can be palpated as a wormlike mass situated above the testicle that decreases in size when the male is recumbent and becomes distended and tense when he is upright. Some males may experience discomfort during sexual stimulation.

In pubertal boys the left testicle is usually larger than the right. However, when there is an associated varicocele, the left testicle is usually smaller than the right. Testicular size and levels of dihydrotestosterone in seminal plasma decrease with increasing duration of the varicocele. Varicocelectomy is indicated in adolescents when there is growth arrest of the affected testicle or when there is pain associated with the varicocele. Improvement in testicular volume is the main outcome measure after varicocelectomy. There is conflicting evidence if surgical intervention during adolescence allows for catch-up of testicular size (Garcia-Roig & Kirsch, 2015). Varicocele repair has shown improvement in semen parameters among adult patients but there is no established set of semen parameters for adolescents, making semen analysis difficult to interpret (Garcia-Roig & Kirsch, 2015). Varicocelectomy is currently indicated for adolescents based on testicular volume differences and not abnormal semen parameters (Garcia-Roig & Kirsch, 2015).

EPIDIDYMITIS

Epididymitis is an inflammatory reaction of the epididymis of the testicle primarily as a result of an infection (bacterial or viral), a chemical irritant (urine), or a nonspecific cause (local trauma). The clinical presentation is slow and insidious with unilateral scrotal pain, redness, and swelling. Associated symptoms include urethral discharge, dysuria, fever, and pyuria. Epididymitis is not associated with gastrointestinal symptoms as found in testicular torsion. The causative factor in sexually active males 14 to 35 years of age is predominantly *Chlamydia trachomatis* and *Neisseria gonorrhoeae* (McConaghy & Panchal, 2016). Some experts recommend reserving antibiotic therapy only for infants and children under the age of 14 years with piuria or positive urine cultures due to the small amount of those with epididymitis who actually have positive urine cultures (McConaghy & Panchal, 2016). In children 14 years and older, empiric antibiotics are recommended based on the most likely causative organism (McConaghy & Panchal, 2016). Mild presentation of symptoms may mimic testicular torsion, which requires immediate surgical intervention. Therefore immediate evaluation by a practitioner is indicated. Treatment consists of supportive therapy with analgesics, antiinflammatories, and scrotal elevation. If anatomic abnormalities are suspected, refer to a urologist. For adolescent males who test positive for chlamydia or gonorrhea, conduct an assessment for other STIs, and inform the adolescent that his partner will also require treatment.

TESTICULAR TORSION

Torsion of the testicle is a condition in which the tunica vaginalis, which normally encases the testicle, fails to do so and the testis hangs free from its vascular structures. This condition can result in partial or complete venous occlusion with rotation around this vascular axis. In severe torsion the organ can become swollen and painful; the scrotum becomes red, warm, and edematous and appears to be immobile or fixed as a result of spasm of the cremasteric fibers.

Testicular torsion occurs annually in 1 in every 1500 males under the age of 18 years (Afsarlar, Ryan, Donel, et al., 2016). Rapid growth and increasing vascularity of the testicle are thought to be precursors to torsion, accounting for the occurrence at puberty. Typically, the adolescent complains of pain that is severe and acute; nausea, vomiting, and abdominal pain may accompany the pain. On examination, the scrotum is swollen and red, and the cremasteric reflex is often absent. Fever and urinary symptoms are generally not present. If the pain duration is less than 6 hours, manual detorsion may be attempted; however, prompt surgical treatment is necessarily for unsuccessful manual attempts or if pain duration is longer than 6 hours (Elder, 2016).

Nursing Care Management

Nurses should be alert to the possibility of testicular torsion in adolescents who complain of scrotal pain. Because torsion may result from trauma to the scrotum, school nurses are likely to encounter such injuries and should refer the child or adolescent for medical evaluation immediately.

! NURSING ALERT

Refer any male patient with signs of testicular torsion (red, painful, swollen scrotum) for immediate medical evaluation.

GYNECOMASTIA

Some degree of bilateral or unilateral breast enlargement occurs frequently in boys during puberty. Approximately half of adolescent boys have transient gynecomastia, which usually lasts less than 1 year and subsides spontaneously. When gynecomastia has a prepubertal onset, the adolescent should be evaluated for rare adrenal or gonadal tumors, or Klinefelter syndrome. Gynecomastia may also be drug induced; spironolactone, cimetidine, ketoconazole, estrogens, and antiandrogens have all been shown to cause the disorder.

If gynecomastia persists or is extensive enough to cause embarrassment, plastic surgery is indicated for cosmetic and psychologic reasons. Administration of testosterone has no effect on breast development or regression and may even aggravate the condition.

Nursing Care Management

Management usually consists of assuring the adolescent and his parents that this situation is benign and temporary. However, all adolescents with gynecomastia should receive a careful medical evaluation to rule out pathologic causes. The adolescent may benefit from the knowledge that it occurs in up to 70% of his peers.

HEALTH CONDITIONS OF THE FEMALE REPRODUCTIVE SYSTEM

GYNECOLOGIC EXAMINATION

Whether it is her first experience or one of many, adolescent girls are often apprehensive before a pelvic examination. Adolescents are self-conscious about their bodies and the changes taking place. The adolescent needs anticipatory guidance regarding what to expect and what she can do to help herself relax during the procedure. Many fears and apprehensions are a result of information she has obtained from family members and friends. The discussion should begin by addressing these anxieties.

The ideal time to begin preparing a girl for examination of the genitalia is as she is entering puberty. External genitalia examination should always be included as part of a routine physical assessment; excluding the genitalia reinforces the attitude that sexuality is something to be avoided.

The initial reproductive preventive health care visit should occur between 13 and 15 years of age (American College of Obstetricians and Gynecologists, Committee on Adolescent Health Care, 2014). This visit should consist of a general examination, a visual breast examination, an external pelvic examination as indicated, and education regarding healthy behaviors such as normal pubertal development and menstruation. A confidential portion of the visit should include discussion of sexual activity, contraception, and sexually transmitted diseases. Indications for an internal examination are started in asymptomatic women at 21 years of age but should be performed earlier if the adolescent is experiencing any female genital tract, pelvic, urologic, or rectal problems (American College of Obstetricians and Gynecologists, Committee on Adolescent Health Care, 2014). The initial visit provides an excellent opportunity for teaching about hygiene and body functions. Encourage the girl to ask questions about changes in her body and the implications. The pelvic examination should be as nonstressful as possible. Nurses should attempt to make the initial pelvic examination a positive experience for the adolescent because this can increase the likelihood of compliance with annual visits. The teenager should have the option of choosing a supportive person to be present during the examination. Suggested individuals might include a parent, best friend, boyfriend, or other health professional. The use of models and drawings and a display of equipment to be used facilitate understanding. Allowing the adolescent to handle the speculum may help decrease some of the fear. The adolescent is given the choice of wearing a gown or her own clothing during the examination. A description of the examination, including information about the procedure and words that describe anticipated feelings and sensations experienced during the examination, may reduce anxiety. Of major concern to the adolescent is fear of discovery of a pathologic pelvic condition. Reassurance regarding normal physical findings is extremely important.

Most girls favor a semisitting position, which has the additional advantage of allowing eye contact during the procedure. Sometimes a pillow helps the patient feel more comfortable and less vulnerable. The provision of a mirror for the girl to see what is taking place if she so desires helps the examiner explain various aspects of anatomy. When possible, it is important to respect the adolescent's request for a female provider.

Numerous techniques have been described to teach women to relax during a pelvic examination, including breathing exercises, imagery, and other strategies for reducing stress. (See Pain Management, Chapter 5.) When the examination is finished, the provider discusses the findings with the adolescent and makes referrals if indicated. Written materials are useful educational materials.

MENSTRUAL DISORDERS

Amenorrhea

Menarche, or the first menstrual period, occurs relatively late in female pubertal development. Although girls vary in the onset and rate of progression of pubertal development, the sequence and tempo should be the same. When an adolescent is seen with a complaint of absence of menses, a careful history of the timing of her pubertal development will help determine whether there is a need for further evaluation or if reassurance is all that is necessary.

Primary amenorrhea is an absence of any secondary sex characteristics by 13 years old or absence of uterine bleeding with secondary sex characteristics by 15 years old (Sucato & Burstein, 2016). Primary amenorrhea is also characterized when menarche has not occurred 4 years after thelarche (Sucato & Burstein, 2016). The cause of primary amenorrhea may be anatomic, hormonal, genetic, or idiopathic. A thorough patient and family history and physical examination provide clues to the etiology.

Secondary amenorrhea is defined as the absence of menses after menstruation was previously established for more than 3 menstrual cycles or irregular menses for 6 months after the establishment of normal menses (Berz & McCambridge, 2016). Irregular menstrual cycles are common within the first year after menarche because these early cycles may be anovulatory, resulting in regular, irregular, or absent bleeding. Girls with a later onset of menarche take longer to establish regular ovulatory cycles. Pregnancy is the most common cause of secondary amenorrhea and should be ruled out in both types of amenorrhea even if the adolescent denies sexual activity.

Hypogonadotropic Amenorrhea

Functional hypogonadotropic amenorrhea reflects a problem in the central hypothalamic-pituitary axis and often results from hypothalamic suppression as a result of stress (in the home, school, or workplace) or a sudden and severe weight loss, eating disorders, or strenuous exercise (Berz & McCambridge, 2016). Women who are more than 20% underweight for height or who have had rapid weight loss and women with eating disorders such as anorexia nervosa may report amenorrhea.

The **female athlete triad** involves the interrelation of reduced caloric intake, amenorrhea, and low bone mineral density (Berz & McCambridge, 2016) (see http://www.femaleathletetriad.org). Exercise-associated amenorrhea can occur in women undergoing vigorous physical and athletic training and is thought to be associated with many factors, including body composition (height, weight, and percentage of body fat); type, intensity, and frequency of exercise; nutritional status; and presence of emotional or physical stressors. Women who participate in sports emphasizing low body weight are at greatest risk, including the following:

- Sports in which performance is subjectively scored (e.g., dance, gymnastics)
- Endurance sports favoring participants with low body weight (e.g., distance running, cycling)
- Sports in which body contour–revealing clothing is worn (e.g., swimming, diving, volleyball)
- Sports with weight categories for participation (e.g., rowing, martial arts)
- Sports in which prepubertal body shape favors success (e.g., gymnastics, figure skating).

Assessment of amenorrhea begins with a thorough history and physical examination. Specific components of the assessment process depend on a patient's age—adolescent, young adult, or perimenopausal—and whether she has menstruated previously.

An important initial step, often overlooked, is to be sure that the female is not pregnant. Once pregnancy has been ruled out by a β–human chorionic gonadotropin pregnancy test, diagnostic tests may include follicle-stimulating hormone level, thyroid-stimulating hormone and prolactin levels, and screening for an eating disorder (Berz & McCambridge, 2016).

NURSING CARE MANAGEMENT

When amenorrhea is caused by hypothalamic disturbances, the nurse is an ideal health professional to assist women because many of the causes are potentially reversible (e.g., stress, weight loss for nonorganic reasons). Counseling and education are primary interventions and appropriate nursing roles. When a stressor known to predispose a woman to hypothalamic amenorrhea is identified, initial management involves addressing the stressor. Deep-breathing exercises and relaxation techniques are simple yet effective stress reduction measures. Referral for biofeedback or massage therapy also may be useful. In some instances referrals for psychotherapy may be indicated. Together the adolescent and nurse plan how the woman can decrease or discontinue medications known to affect menstruation, correct weight loss, deal more effectively with psychologic stress, address emotional distress, and alter an exercise routine.

If an adolescent's exercise program is thought to contribute to her amenorrhea, several options exist for management. Treatment options include a decrease in the intensity or duration of training or modifications in her diet to include the appropriate nutrition for her age. Accepting the former alternative may be difficult for one who is committed to a strenuous exercise regimen. The adolescent and nurse may have several sessions before the woman elects to try exercise reduction. Many young female athletes may not understand the consequences of low bone density or osteoporosis; nurses can point out the connection between low bone density and stress fractures. The nurse and adolescent should also investigate other factors that may be contributing to the amenorrhea and develop plans for altering lifestyle and decreasing stress.

Although research on effectiveness is inconclusive, a daily calcium intake of 1200 to 1500 mg plus 400 to 800 IU of vitamin D and 60 to 90 mg of potassium are recommended for women experiencing amenorrhea associated with the female athlete triad. Young female athletes can reverse amenorrhea by increasing food intake (a 20% increase in caloric intake). Furthermore, bone mineral dysfunction (the third component of female athlete triad) can be reversed with weight gain and resistance training (Berz & McCambridge, 2016). Oral contraceptives have a positive effect on bone density in amenorrheic women but are usually not used in young women with amenorrhea associated with female athlete triad unless the adolescent is not willing to comply with dietary and exercise recommendations or she continues to be amenorrheic even with compliance (Berz & McCambridge, 2016).

Dysmenorrhea

Dysmenorrhea, pain during or shortly before menstruation, is one of the most common gynecologic problems in women of all ages. Dysmenorrhea begins for most women in adolescence, within the first 3 to 5 years after menarche once ovulation is established (Rani, Sharma, & Singh, 2016). Dysmenorrhea occurs in as many as 90% of adolescents, resulting in missed school or work in 10% to 15% (Yu, 2014). Menstrual problems, including dysmenorrhea, are relatively more common in women who smoke and are obese. Dysmenorrhea is also associated with menarche before 12 years old, nulliparity, and menstrual flow more than 7 days (Yu, 2014). Traditionally dysmenorrhea is differentiated as primary or secondary. Symptoms usually begin with menstruation, although some women have discomfort several hours before onset of flow. The range and severity of symptoms are different from woman to woman and from cycle to cycle in the same woman. Symptoms of dysmenorrhea may last several hours or several days. Pain is usually located in the suprapubic area or lower abdomen. Women describe the pain as sharp, cramping, or a steady, dull ache.

Primary Dysmenorrhea

Primary dysmenorrhea is a condition associated with ovulatory cycles. Primary dysmenorrhea has a biochemical basis and arises from the release of prostaglandins with menses. During the luteal phase and subsequent menstrual flow, prostaglandin F_2-alpha ($PGF_{2\alpha}$) is secreted. Excessive release of $PGF_{2\alpha}$ increases the amplitude and frequency of uterine contractions and causes vasospasm of the uterine arterioles, resulting in ischemia and cyclic lower abdominal cramps. Systemic responses to $PGF_{2\alpha}$ include backache, weakness, sweats, gastrointestinal symptoms, and central nervous system symptoms (dizziness, syncope, headache, and poor concentration). Pain usually begins at the onset of menstruation and lasts 8 to 48 hours.

Nursing Care Management

Management of primary dysmenorrhea depends on the severity of the problem and the individual woman's response to various treatments. Important components of nursing care are information and support. Because menstruation is so closely linked to reproduction and sexuality, menstrual problems such as dysmenorrhea can have a negative influence on sexuality and self-worth. Nurses can correct myths and misinformation about menstruation and dysmenorrhea by providing facts about what is normal. Adolescent and young women need support to foster their feelings of positive sexuality and self-worth.

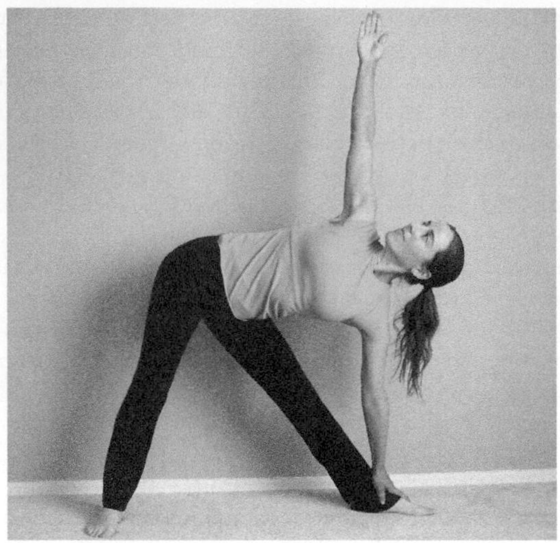

FIG. 18.1 Yoga asana: triangle pose. Helpful for assisting digestion and stretching and strengthening the spine; also used for dysmenorrheal and pelvic congestion. (Courtesy Julie Perry Nelson, Loveland, Colorado.)

Often the nurse can offer more than one alternative for alleviating menstrual discomfort and dysmenorrhea, which gives women options to try to decide which works best for them. Heat (heating pad or hot bath) minimizes cramping by increasing vasodilation and muscle relaxation and minimizing uterine ischemia. Massaging the lower back can reduce pain by relaxing paravertebral muscles and increasing the pelvic blood supply. Soft, rhythmic rubbing of the abdomen (effleurage) is useful because it provides a distraction and an alternative focal point. Transcutaneous electrical nerve stimulation (TENS), progressive relaxation, yoga, acupuncture, herbal preparations, aromatherapy, religious practices, and meditation are also used to decrease menstrual discomfort, although evidence is insufficient to determine their effectiveness (Hofmeister & Bodden, 2016; Midilli, Yasar, & Baysal, 2015) (Fig. 18.1).

Exercise helps relieve menstrual discomfort through increased vasodilation and subsequent decreased ischemia. It also releases endogenous opiates (specifically beta-endorphins), suppresses prostaglandins, and shunts blood flow away from the viscera, resulting in reduced pelvic congestion. Specific dietary changes, such as decreasing salt and refined sugar, and maintaining good nutrition are helpful in decreasing some of the systemic symptoms associated with dysmenorrhea. Medications used to treat primary dysmenorrhea include prostaglandin synthesis inhibitors, primarily nonsteroidal antiinflammatory drugs (NSAIDs) such as ibuprofen or naproxen (Yu, 2014). NSAIDs are most effective if started several days before menses or at least by the onset of bleeding but are associated with many adverse effects, such as drowsiness, dizziness, nausea, and indigestion. NSAIDs should only be used short term.

! NURSING ALERT

If one NSAID is ineffective, often a different one may be effective. If the second drug is unsuccessful after a 6-month trial, combined oral contraceptive pills (OCPs) may be used.

OCPs are a reasonable choice for adolescents who want to use a contraceptive agent. The benefits of their use are attributed to decreased prostaglandin synthesis and endometrial tissue growth (Yu, 2014). Because OCPs have side effects, women may not wish to use them for dysmenorrhea and may be contraindicated for some women.

TABLE 18.1 Herbal Medicinals Taken Orally for Menstrual Disorders

Symptoms or Indications	Herbal Therapy*	Action
Menstrual cramping, dysmenorrhea	Catnip	Uterine antispasmodic
	Dong quai	Uterotonic; antiinflammatory
	Motherwort	Uterotonic
	Passionflower	Uterotonic
	Wild yam	Uterine antispasmodic
	Valerian	Uterine antispasmodic
	Yarrow	Uterine antispasmodic; antiinflammatory
Premenstrual discomfort, tension	Black cohosh root	Estrogen-like luteinizing hormone suppressant; binds to estrogen receptors
Menorrhea, metrorrhagia	Lady's mantle	Uterotonic
	Lemon balm	Uterotonic
	White willow bark	Uterotonic; antiinflammatory

*Many women's herbs do not have rigorous scientific studies backing their use; most uses and properties of herbs have not been validated by the US Food and Drug Administration.

Data from Annie's Remedy. (2016). Dysmenorrhea—Herbs for painful periods. Retrieved from http://www.anniesremedy.com/chart_remedy_dysmenorrhea.php; and National Center for Complementary and Alternative Medicine. (2016). Herbs at a glance. Retrieved from https://nccih.nih.gov/health/herbsataglance.htm.

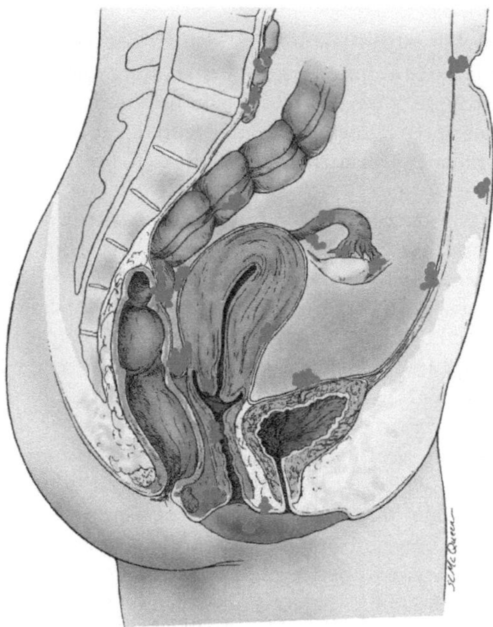

FIG. 18.2 Common sites of endometriosis. (From Lentz, G. M., Lobo, R. A., Gershenson, D. M., et al. [Eds.]. [2012]. *Comprehensive gynecology* [6th ed.]. Philadelphia, PA: Mosby.)

Alternative and complementary therapies are increasingly popular and used in developed countries. Therapies such as acupuncture, acupressure, biofeedback, desensitization, hypnosis, massage, reiki, relaxation exercises, and therapeutic touch have been used to treat pelvic pain. Herbal preparations have long been used for managing menstrual problems, including dysmenorrhea (Table 18.1). Herbal medicines may be valuable in treating dysmenorrhea. However, it is essential that women understand that these therapies are not without potential toxicity and may cause drug interactions.

! NURSING ALERT

Nurses must routinely ask women about the use of herbal and other alternative therapies and document their use.

Secondary Dysmenorrhea

Secondary dysmenorrhea is defined as painful menses associated with a pathologic condition, such as adenomyosis, endometriosis, pelvic inflammatory disease, endometrial polyps, or fibroids. Women with secondary dysmenorrhea often have other symptoms that may suggest the underlying cause. In contrast to primary dysmenorrhea, the pain of secondary dysmenorrhea is often characterized by dull, lower abdominal aching that radiates to the back or thighs and feelings of bloating or pelvic fullness. In addition to a physical examination with a careful pelvic examination, diagnosis may be assisted by ultrasound examination, dilation and curettage, endometrial biopsy, or laparoscopy. Treatment is directed toward removal of the underlying pathology. Many of the measures described for pain relief of primary dysmenorrhea are also helpful for women with secondary dysmenorrhea.

ENDOMETRIOSIS

Endometriosis is characterized by the presence and growth of endometrial tissue outside of the uterus. The tissue may be implanted on the ovaries; anterior and posterior cul-de-sac; broad, uterosacral, and round ligaments; rectovaginal septum; sigmoid colon; appendix; pelvic peritoneum; cervix; and inguinal area (Fig. 18.2). A cystic lesion of endometriosis found in the ovary is sometimes described as a chocolate cyst because of the dark coloring of the contents of the cyst caused by the presence of old blood.

Endometrial tissue contains glands and stoma and responds to cyclic hormone stimulation in the same way that the uterine endometrium does but often out of phase with it. The tissue grows during the proliferative and secretory phases of the cycle. During or immediately after menstruation the tissue bleeds, resulting in an inflammatory response with subsequent fibrosis and adhesions to adjacent organs.

Although the condition usually develops in the third or fourth decade of life, endometriosis has been found in adolescents with disabling pelvic pain or abnormal vaginal bleeding. There appears to be a familial tendency to develop endometriosis and 25% to 30% of adolescents with endometriosis have a first-degree relative with endometriosis (Saridogan, 2017). Impaired fertility may result from adhesions around the uterus that pull the uterus into a fixed, retroverted position. Adhesions around the uterine tubes may block the fimbriated ends or prevent the spontaneous movement that carries the ovum to the uterus.

Symptoms vary among women and range from nonexistent to incapacitating. Severity of symptoms can change over time and may not reflect the extent of the disease. The major symptoms of endometriosis are pelvic pain, dysmenorrhea, and dyspareunia (painful intercourse). Women may also have chronic noncyclic pelvic pain, pelvic heaviness, or pain radiating into the thighs. Many women report bowel symptoms such as diarrhea, pain with defecation, and constipation caused by avoiding defecation because of the pain.

Nursing Care Management

Treatment is based on the severity of symptoms and the goals of the woman or couple. Women without pain who do not want to become pregnant need no treatment. In women with mild pain who may desire a future pregnancy, treatment may be limited to use of NSAIDs during menstruation.

Women who have early symptomatic disease and who can postpone pregnancy may be treated with OCPs that have a low estrogen-to-progestin ratio to shrink endometrial tissue. Any low-dose OCPs can be used if taken for 15 weeks, followed by 1 week of withdrawal. Continuous combined hormone therapy (e.g., OCPs, estrogen/progestin patch, estrogen/progestin vaginal ring) for menstrual suppression and administration of NSAIDs are the usual treatment for adolescents under the age of 16 years who have endometriosis.

Gonadotropin-releasing hormone (GnRH) agonist therapy is reserved for adolescents with severe symptoms due to the adverse effects on bone mineralization (Saridogan, 2017). Treatment is usually limited to 6 months and bone mineral density should be carefully monitored. Although unlikely, it is possible for a woman to become pregnant while taking a GnRH agonist. Because the potential teratogenicity of this drug is unclear, women should use a barrier contraceptive during treatment.

Surgical intervention is often needed for severe, acute, or incapacitating symptoms. Decisions regarding the extent and type of surgery are influenced by a woman's age, desire for children, and location of the disease. For women who do not want to preserve their ability to have children, the only definite cure is total abdominal hysterectomy with bilateral salpingo-oophorectomy (TAH with BSO). In women in their childbearing years who want children and in whom the disease does not prevent bearing children, reproductive capacity should be retained through careful removal by laparoscopic surgery or laser therapy (e.g., coagulation, vaporization, or resection) of all endometrial tissue possible with retention of ovarian function.

Regardless of the type of treatment (except TAH with BSO), endometriosis recurs in approximately 40% of women. Thus for many women endometriosis is a chronic disease with conditions such as chronic pain or infertility. Counseling and education are critical components of nursing care for women with endometriosis. Women need an honest discussion of treatment options, with review of the potential risks and benefits of each option. Because pelvic pain is a subjective, personal experience that can be frightening, support is important. Sexual dysfunction resulting from dyspareunia is common and may necessitate referral for counseling. Support groups for women with endometriosis may be found in some locations. Resolve (http://www.resolve.org), an organization for infertile couples, or the Endometriosis Association (http://www.ivf.com/endohtml.html) may also be helpful. The nursing care discussed in the previous section on dysmenorrhea is appropriate for managing chronic pelvic pain and dysmenorrhea experienced by women with endometriosis.

PREMENSTRUAL SYNDROME

Premenstrual syndrome (PMS) is a complex condition that includes one or more of a large number (more than 150) of physical and psychologic symptoms that can start with ovulation then reoccur during luteal phase of the menstrual cycle and disappear by the end of menstruation (Sucato & Burstein, 2016). All age-groups are affected and up to 30% of adolescents experience PMS (Sucato & Burstein, 2016). Symptoms include fluid retention (e.g., abdominal bloating, pelvic fullness, edema of the lower extremities, breast tenderness, and weight gain), behavioral or emotional changes (e.g., depression, crying spells, irritability, panic attacks, and impaired ability to concentrate), premenstrual cravings (e.g., sweets, salt, increased appetite, and food binges), and headache, fatigue, and backache.

Premenstrual dysphoric disorder (PMDD) is a more severe variant of PMS in which 2% to 6% of women have significant physical and behavioral symptoms that interfere with daily living (Sucato & Burstein, 2016). Based on a large body of evidence, PMDD is included in the *Diagnostic and Statistical Manual of Mental Disorders, Fifth Edition* (DSM-5) as a distinct diagnosis. There are several validated screening tools, such as the Premenstrual Symptoms Screening Tool (PSST), that can help identify PMS and PMDD. To obtain an accurate history, encourage the woman to keep a daily log of her symptoms.

The causes of PMS and PMDD continue to be investigated. A number of biologic and neuroendocrine etiologies have been suggested; however, none has been conclusively substantiated as the causative factor. It is likely that biologic and psychosocial factors contribute to PMS and PMDD (Craner, Sigmon, Martinson, et al., 2014).

Therapeutic and Nursing Care Management

There is little agreement on management. Any changes that help a woman with PMS exert control over her life have a positive effect. For this reason, lifestyle changes are often effective in its treatment.

Nurses can advise women that self-help modalities often result in significant symptom improvement. Regular exercise and regular sleep can provide symptom relief for some women. Nurses can suggest that women not smoke and limit their consumption of refined sugar, salt, red meat, alcohol, and caffeinated beverages. Three small to moderate-size meals and three small snacks a day that are rich in complex carbohydrates and fiber have been reported to relieve symptoms (Akgul & Kanbur, 2015). Calcium, vitamin B_6, and vitamin D have been shown to be moderately effective in relieving symptoms (Akgul & Kanbur, 2015). Supplements of the fruit extract of *Vitex agnus castus* have demonstrated usefulness in relieving some PMS symptoms (Akgul & Kanbur, 2015).

Yoga, acupuncture, hypnosis, light therapy, chiropractic therapy, and massage therapy have all been reported to have a beneficial effect on PMS. Further research is needed for all of these therapies.

Nurses can explain the relation between cyclic estrogen fluctuation and changes in serotonin levels, that serotonin is one of the brain chemicals that assist in coping with normal life stresses, and the ways in which the different management strategies recommended help maintain serotonin levels. Support groups or counseling may be helpful. Stress reduction techniques also may help with symptom management.

If these strategies do not provide significant symptom relief in 1 to 2 months, medication is often added. Many medications have been used in treatment of PMS, but no single medication alleviates all PMS symptoms. Medications often used in the treatment of PMS include diuretics, prostaglandin inhibitors (NSAIDs), and OCPs. However, research with diuretics has only been performed with adults (Akgul & Kanbur, 2015). Studies of progesterone have not shown that it is an effective treatment (Ford, Lethaby, Roberts, et al., 2012). Serotonergic-activating agents, including the selective serotonin reuptake inhibitors (SSRIs), are approved by the Food and Drug Administration (FDA) as first-line pharmacologic therapy for PMS and PMDD (Sucato & Burstein, 2016). The drugs have a rapid onset, so either intermittent or continuous use is effective for symptom relief (Sucato & Burstein, 2016).

ABNORMAL UTERINE BLEEDING

Abnormal uterine bleeding (AUB) is any form of uterine bleeding that is irregular in amount, duration, or timing and is not related to regular menstrual bleeding. Box 18.1 lists possible causes of AUB. Although often used interchangeably, the terms *AUB* and *dysfunctional uterine*

BOX 18.1 Possible Causes of Abnormal Uterine Bleeding

Pregnancy-Related Conditions
- Threatened or spontaneous miscarriage
- Retained products of conception after elective abortion
- Ectopic pregnancy
- Placenta previa/placenta abruptio
- Trophoblastic disease

Lower Reproductive Tract Infections
- Cervicitis
- Endometritis
- Myometritis
- Salpingitis

Benign Anatomic Abnormalities
- Adenomyosis
- Leiomyomata
- Polyps of the cervix or endometrium

Neoplasms
- Endometrial hyperplasia
- Cancer of cervix and endometrium
- Hormonally active tumors (rare)
- Vaginal tumors (rare)

Malignant Lesions
- Cervical squamous cell carcinoma
- Endometrial adenocarcinoma
- Estrogen-producing ovarian tumors
- Testosterone-producing ovarian tumors
- Leiomyosarcoma

Trauma
- Genital injury (accidental, coital trauma, sexual abuse)
- Foreign body
- Lacerations

Systemic Conditions
- Adrenal hyperplasia and Cushings disease
- Blood dyscrasias
- Coagulopathies
- Hypothalamic suppression (from stress, weight loss, excessive exercise)
- Polycystic ovary disease
- Thyroid disease
- Pituitary adenoma or hyperprolactinemia
- Severe organ disease (renal or liver failure)

Iatrogenic Causes
- Medications with estrogenic activity
- Anticoagulants
- Exogenous hormone use (oral contraceptives, menopausal hormone therapy)
- Selective serotonin reuptake inhibitors
- Tamoxifen
- Intrauterine devices
- Herbal preparation (ginseng)

Data from De Silva, N. K. (2016). Abnormal uterine bleeding in adolescents: Evaluation and approach to diagnosis. *UpToDate*. Retrieved from https://www.uptodate.com/contents/abnormal-uterine-bleeding-in-adolescents-evaluation-and-approach-to-diagnosis; American College of Obstetricians and Gynecologists. (2015). Committee Opinion No. 651: Menstruation in girls and adolescents: Using the menstrual cycle as a vital sign. *Obstetrics and Gynecology, 126*(6), e143-e146.

bleeding (DUB) are not synonymous. DUB is any abnormal uterine bleeding that does not have a pathogenic cause (Deligeoroglou, Karountzos, & Creatsas, 2013).

AUB can be anovulatory or ovulatory but is most commonly caused by anovulation. When no surge of LH occurs or if insufficient progesterone is produced by the corpus luteum to support the endometrium, it will begin to involute and shed. This process most often occurs at the extremes of a woman's reproductive years, when the menstrual cycle is just becoming established at menarche or when it draws to a close at menopause. AUB also occurs with any condition that gives rise to chronic anovulation associated with continuous estrogen production. Such conditions include obesity, hyperthyroidism and hypothyroidism, polycystic ovarian syndrome, and any of the endocrine conditions discussed in the sections on amenorrhea. A diagnosis of AUB is made only after ruling out all other causes of abnormal menstrual bleeding.

Therapeutic Management

For mild cases, give iron supplements and ask the adolescent to keep a diary to monitor menstrual patterns (Sucato & Burstein, 2016). The most effective medical treatment of acute bleeding episodes is administration of combined oral contraceptives (estrogen and progestin) (Sucato & Burstein, 2016). For mild bleeding, start with twice-daily dosing of the contraceptives, but adolescents with moderate bleeding should start with 3 to 4 doses per day and taper over 2 weeks (Sucato & Burstein, 2016). Adolescents with severe bleeding may require intravenous estrogen along with a combined oral contraceptive. The oral contraceptive is given for at least 3 to 6 months after the acute phase has passed. Such long-term treatment will help prevent recurrence of the pattern of AUB and hemorrhage. If the woman wants contraception, she should continue to take OCPs. If she has no need for contraception, the treatment may be stopped to assess the woman's bleeding pattern.

Nursing Care Management

Nursing assessments for adolescents or young women who have a menstrual disorder include the following:
- Taking a thorough menstrual, obstetric, sexual, and contraceptive history
- Exploring the adolescent's perceptions of her condition, cultural or ethnic influences, lifestyle, and patterns of coping
- Evaluating the amount of pain or bleeding experienced and its effect on daily activities
- Noting any home remedies and prescriptions to relieve discomfort; a symptom diary, in which the adolescent records emotions, behaviors, physical symptoms, diet, and exercise and rest patterns, is a useful diagnostic tool.

Expected outcomes for the adolescent are that she will do the following:
- Verbalize her understanding of reproductive anatomy, cause of her disorder, medication regimen, and diary use
- Verbalize her understanding and accept her emotional and physical responses to her menstrual cycle
- Develop personal goals that benefit her emotionally and physically
- Choose appropriate therapeutic measures for her menstrual problems
- Adapt successfully to the condition if cure is not possible

In addition to the medical, surgical, and nursing interventions discussed with each problem, additional nursing interventions may include the following:
- Accepting the woman's symptoms as valid
- Correlating data from the daily diary of emotional status, subjective feelings, and physical state with physiologic changes
- Encouraging the woman to express her feelings about her symptoms

- Providing information about therapeutic options (pharmacologic and nonpharmacologic) so the woman or she and her partner can make choices considered best for them
- Providing information about local support groups

Care has been effective when the woman reports improvement in the quality of her life, skill in self-management, and a positive self-concept and body image.

VAGINAL INFECTIONS

Vaginal discharge and itching of the vulva and vagina are among the most common reasons a woman seeks help from a health care provider. More women complain of vaginal discharge than any other gynecologic symptom; however, vaginal discharge resulting from infection must be distinguished from normal secretions. Normal vaginal secretions (or physiologic leukorrhea) are clear to cloudy in appearance, nonirritating, and have a mild, inoffensive odor. The discharge may turn yellow after drying. Normal vaginal secretions are acidic, with a pH range of 4.0 to 5.0. The amount of leukorrhea differs with phases of the menstrual cycle, with greater amounts occurring at ovulation and just before menses. Leukorrhea is also increased during pregnancy. Normal vaginal secretions contain lactobacilli and epithelial cells.

Vaginitis, or abnormal vaginal discharge, is an infection caused by a microorganism. The most common vaginal infections are bacterial vaginosis (BV), candidiasis, and trichomoniasis. Although group B *Streptococcus* is considered normal vaginal flora, it may also cause infection. Vulvovaginitis (i.e., inflammation of the vulva and vagina) may be caused by vaginal infection; copious leukorrhea, which can cause maceration of tissues; and chemical irritants, allergens, and foreign bodies, which may produce inflammatory reactions.

Bacterial Vaginosis

BV is the most common gynecologic infection in the United States (Hilbert, Smith, Chadwick, et al., 2016). It is associated with preterm labor in pregnant women and postoperative infections after a hysterectomy (Hilbert, Smith, Chadwick, et al., 2016). The exact cause of BV is unknown. It is a syndrome in which normal, hydrogen peroxide–producing lactobacilli are replaced with high concentrations of anaerobic and gram-negative bacteria. With the increase of anaerobes, the level of vaginal amines is raised, and the normal acidic pH of the vagina is altered. Epithelial cells slough, and numerous bacteria attach to their surfaces (clue cells). When the amines are volatilized, the characteristic odor of BV occurs. BV discharge is usually profuse, thin, and white, gray, or milky in appearance. Some women also may experience mild irritation or pruritus, although some women with BV remain asymptomatic.

Screening and Diagnosis

A focused history may help distinguish BV from other vaginal infections if the young woman is symptomatic. Reports of fishy odor and increased thin vaginal discharge are most significant, and a report of increased odor after intercourse is also suggestive of BV. You should question women with previous occurrence of similar symptoms, diagnosis, and treatment because women with BV often have been treated incorrectly because of misdiagnosis.

Microscopic examination of vaginal secretions is always performed (Table 18.2). Both normal saline and 10% potassium hydroxide (KOH) smears are made. The presence of clue cells (vaginal epithelial cells coated with bacteria) on wet saline smear is highly diagnostic because the phenomenon is specific to BV. Test vaginal secretions for pH. Nitrazine paper is sensitive enough to detect a pH of 4.5 or greater. In the whiff test, a fishy odor of vaginal discharge will be released when KOH is added to vaginal secretions.

TABLE 18.2 Wet Smear Tests for Vaginal Infections

Infection	Test	Positive Findings
Trichomoniasis	Saline wet smear (vaginal secretions mixed with normal saline on a glass slide)	Presence of many white blood cell protozoa
Candidiasis	Potassium hydroxide (KOH) preparation (vaginal secretions mixed with KOH on a glass slide)	Presence of hyphae and pseudohyphae (buds and branches of yeast cells)
Bacterial vaginosis	Normal saline smear	Presence of clue cells (vaginal epithelial cells coated with bacteria)
	Whiff test (vaginal secretions mixed with KOH)	Release of fishy odor

Therapeutic Management

First-line treatment of BV includes oral metronidazole (Flagyl), although vaginal preparations (e.g., metronidazole gel, clindamycin cream) are also used (Bradshaw & Sobel, 2016). When the woman is taking oral metronidazole, advise her to avoid drinking alcoholic beverages or she will experience severe side effects of abdominal distress, nausea, vomiting, and headache. Treatment of sexual partners is not recommended routinely (Centers for Disease Control and Prevention, 2015).

Candidiasis

Vulvovaginal candidiasis, or yeast infection, is the second most common type of vaginal infection in the United States. The most common organism is *Candida albicans*. It is estimated that 80% to 90% of yeast infections in women are caused by this organism (Mendling, Weissenbacher, Gerber, et al., 2016). The most common non-*albicans Candida* species is *Candida glabrata* (Sobel, 2016).

Numerous factors have been identified as predisposing a woman to yeast infections. These include antibiotic therapy, particularly broad-spectrum antibiotics; diabetes, especially when uncontrolled; pregnancy; obesity; diets high in refined sugars or artificial sweeteners; use of corticosteroids and exogenous hormones; and immunosuppressed states. Clinical observations and research have suggested that tight-fitting clothing and underwear or pantyhose made of nonabsorbent materials create an environment in which a vaginal fungus can grow.

The most common symptom of yeast infection is vulvar and possibly vaginal pruritus. The itching may be mild or intense, interfere with rest and activities, and occur during or after intercourse. Some women report a feeling of dryness. Others may have painful urination as the urine flows over the vulva, especially in women who have excoriations resulting from scratching. Most often the discharge is thick, white, lumpy, and cottage cheese–like. Commonly the vulva is red and swollen, as are the labial folds, vagina, and cervix. Although there is no odor characteristic of yeast infections, sometimes a yeasty or musty smell is noted.

Screening and Diagnosis

In addition to noting the woman's symptoms, their onset, and their course, the history is a valuable screening tool for identifying predisposing risk factors. Physical examination should include a thorough inspection of the vulva and vagina. A speculum examination is always done. Commonly amine (KOH) wet smear and vaginal pH are obtained (see Table 18.2). The amine test is negative and the vaginal pH is normal

(<4.5) with a yeast infection. The characteristic pseudohypha (bud or branching of a fungus) may be seen on a wet smear (Mendling, Weissenbacher, Gerber, et al., 2016).

Therapeutic Management

A number of antifungal preparations are available for the treatment of *C. albicans*. Many topical medications (e.g., miconazole [Monistat] and clotrimazole [Gyne-Lotrimin]) are available as over-the-counter (OTC) agents. Oral medications include a variety of azole medications including fluconazole or itraconazole. Exogenous lactobacillus (in the form of dairy products [yogurt] or powder, tablets, capsules, or suppository supplements) is commonly used among women; however, there is limited evidence providing the effectiveness of this treatment due to poorly designed studies, and most experts provide no recommendations for use (Sobel, 2016). The first time a woman suspects that she may have a yeast infection, she should see a health care provider for confirmation of the diagnosis and treatment recommendation. If she has another infection, she may wish to purchase an OTC preparation and self-treat. Women should always be counseled to seek care for numerous recurrent or chronic yeast infections.

Adolescents who have extensive irritation, swelling, and discomfort of the labia and vulva may find sitz baths helpful in decreasing inflammation and increasing comfort. Adding colloidal oatmeal powder to the bath may also increase the woman's comfort. Not wearing underpants to bed may help decrease symptoms and prevent recurrences. Completing the full course of treatment prescribed, even during menstruation, is essential to removing the pathogen. Adolescent girls should be counseled not to use tampons during menses because the medication will be absorbed by the tampon. If possible, intercourse is avoided during treatment; if this is not feasible, the woman's partner should use a condom to prevent introduction of more organisms. Suggested measures to prevent genital tract infections are in the Nursing Care Guidelines box.

NURSING CARE GUIDELINES

Prevention of Genital Tract Infections in Women

- Choose underwear or hosiery with a cotton crotch.
- Avoid tight-fitting clothing (especially tight jeans).
- Select cloth car seat covers instead of vinyl.
- Limit the time spent in damp exercise clothes (especially swimsuits, leotards, and tights).
- Limit exposure to bath salts or bubble bath.
- Avoid colored or scented toilet tissue.
- If sensitive, discontinue use of feminine hygiene deodorant sprays.
- Use condoms.
- Void before and after intercourse.
- Decrease dietary sugar.
- Do not douche.

SEXUALLY TRANSMITTED INFECTIONS

Sexually transmitted infections (STIs) are infections or infectious disease syndromes transmitted primarily by sexual contact. The term *sexually transmitted infection* includes more than 25 infectious organisms that are transmitted through sexual activity and the dozens of clinical syndromes that they cause (Box 18.2). STIs are among the most common health problems in the United States today, with an estimated 20 million people in the United States being infected with a new STI every year (Centers for Disease Control and Prevention, 2016a). Adolescents and young adults between the ages of 15 and 24 years acquire half of all new STIs each year (Centers for Disease Control and Prevention, 2016a). The following discussion focuses on the most common STIs in adolescents and young women.

BOX 18.2 Sexually Transmitted Infections

Bacteria

- Chlamydia
- Gonorrhea
- Syphilis
- Chancroid
- Lymphogranuloma venereum
- Genital mycoplasmas
- Group B streptococci

Protozoa

- Trichomoniasis

Viruses

- Human immunodeficiency virus
- Herpes simplex virus, types 1 and 2
- Cytomegalovirus
- Viral hepatitis A and B
- Human papillomavirus

Parasites

- Pediculosis (may or may not be sexually transmitted)
- Scabies (may or may not be sexually transmitted)

Prevention

Preventing infection (primary prevention) is the most effective way of reducing the adverse consequences of STIs for adolescents and young women. Risk-free options include complete abstinence from sexual activities that transmit semen, blood, or other body fluids. Involvement in a mutually monogamous relationship with an uninfected partner also eliminates the risk of contracting STIs. Prompt diagnosis and treatment of current infections (secondary prevention) can also prevent personal complications and transmission to others.

Preventing the spread of STIs requires that adolescents at risk for transmitting or acquiring infections change their behavior. A critical first step is to include questions about an adolescent's sexual history, sexual risk behaviors, and drug-related risky behaviors as a part of every assessment (Box 18.3). When the nurse identifies risk factors or risky behaviors, there is an opportunity to provide prevention counseling. Techniques that are effective in providing prevention counseling include using open-ended questions, using understandable language, and reassuring the adolescent that treatment will be provided regardless of consideration such as ability to pay, language spoken, or lifestyle. Prevention messages should include descriptions of specific actions to prevent contracting or transmitting STIs and should be individualized for each adolescent, giving attention to his or her specific risk factors.

To be motivated to take preventive actions, the adolescent must believe that acquiring a disease is serious and that he or she is at risk for infection. Most individuals tend to underestimate their personal risk of infection in a given situation. Thus many adolescents may not perceive themselves as being at risk for contracting an STI, and telling them that they should use protection for STIs may not be well received. Although levels of awareness of STIs are generally high, widespread misconceptions or specific gaps in knowledge also exist. Therefore nurses have a responsibility to ensure that adolescents have accurate, complete

BOX 18.3 Assessing Sexually Transmitted Infection and Human Immunodeficiency Virus Risk Behaviors

Sexual Risk

- Are you sexually active now?
- If no, have you had sex in the past?
- Ever had an oral, vaginal, or anal sexual experience with another person?
- With how many different people? One? Two or three? Four to 10? More than 10?
- Have your partners been men, women, both?
- Ever had sex with a partner who was bisexual?
- Ever shared equipment for tattoo, body piercing?
- Ever had an STI (herpes, gonorrhea, genital warts, chlamydia)?
- Ever had sex against your will?
- What do you do to protect yourself from HIV and STIs?

Drug Use–Related Risk

- Ever injected drugs using shared equipment, including street drugs, steroids?
- Ever had sex with a person who uses drugs or shares equipment?
- Ever had sex while so stoned, high, or drunk that you can't remember the details?
- Ever exchanged sex for drugs, money, shelter?

Other

- Ever had a test for HIV?
- Ever worried about AIDS and would like to talk with someone about it?

AIDS, Acquired immunodeficiency syndrome; *HIV,* human immunodeficiency virus; *STI,* sexually transmitted infection.

knowledge about transmission and symptoms of STIs and the behaviors that place them at risk for contracting an infection.

Sexually Transmitted Infections/Human Immunodeficiency Virus Prevention Strategies

An essential component of primary prevention is counseling the woman regarding sexual practices so she can avoid acquiring or transmitting STIs, including attaining knowledge of her partner, reducing her number of partners, practicing low-risk sex, avoiding the exchange of body fluids, and obtaining vaccinations.

Reducing the number of partners and avoiding partners who have had many previous sexual partners decrease a woman's chances of contracting an STI. Discussing each new partner's previous sexual history and exposure to STIs augments other efforts to reduce risk; however, sexual partners are not always truthful about their sexual history.

Adolescents and young women should be taught low-risk sexual practices and which sexual practices to avoid. Sexual fantasizing is safe, as are caressing, hugging, body rubbing, and massage. Mutual masturbation is low risk as long as there is no contact with a partner's semen or vaginal secretions. All sexual activities are safe when both partners are monogamous, trustworthy, and known (by testing) to be free of disease. Anal-genital intercourse, anal-oral contact, and anal-digital activity are high-risk sexual behaviors and should be avoided.

The physical barrier promoted for the prevention of STIs, including human immunodeficiency virus (HIV), is the latex male condom. The nurse should remind women to use a condom with every sexual encounter; use latex or polyurethane male condoms; use a condom with a current expiration date; use each one only once; and handle it carefully to avoid damaging it with fingernails, teeth, or other sharp objects. Condoms should be stored away from heat, such as in a car; if condoms are stored in a wallet or purse, replace with a new one regularly. Adolescents are taught the differences among condoms and where they can be purchased.

The female condom (i.e., a lubricated polyurethane sheath with a ring on each end that is inserted into the vagina) is an effective mechanical barrier for STIs, including HIV. The consistent use of condoms (male or female) for every act of sexual intimacy when there is the possibility of transmission of disease is stressed by nurses.

Spermicides do not protect against STIs or HIV. Condoms lubricated with nonoxynol-9 are no more effective than nonlubricated condoms; the use of nonoxynol-9 is not recommended (Centers for Disease Control and Prevention, 2011).

Vaccination is an effective method for the prevention of some STIs such as hepatitis B and HPV. Hepatitis B vaccine is recommended for all adolescents. A vaccine is available for HPV types 6, 11, 16, and 18 and is recommended for girls and women 9 to 26 years of age (American Academy of Pediatrics, 2015) (see also Immunizations, Chapter 6).

SEXUALLY TRANSMITTED PROTOZOA INFECTIONS

Trichomoniasis

Trichomonas vaginalis is an STI and is the third most common cause of vaginal infection after BV and candida (Gibson, Bell, & Powerful, 2014). Trichomoniasis is caused by *T. vaginalis,* an anaerobic, one-celled protozoan with characteristic flagella. Although trichomoniasis may be asymptomatic, men present with urethritis whereas women commonly experience characteristically yellowish to greenish, frothy, malodorous discharge. Inflammation of the vulva, vagina, or both may be present, and the woman may complain of irritation. The cervix and vaginal walls may demonstrate characteristic "strawberry spots" or tiny petechiae, and the cervix may bleed on contact. In severe infections the vaginal walls, the cervix, and occasionally the vulva are acutely inflamed.

Screening and Diagnosis

In addition to obtaining a history of current symptoms, obtain a thorough sexual history. Note any history of similar symptoms in the past and the treatment used. Determine whether partners were treated.

Because classic signs may not be present on the woman's physical examination, a speculum examination is always performed, even though it may be uncomfortable. The typical one-celled flagellate trichomonads are easily distinguished on a normal saline wet preparation (see Table 18.2). The pH of the discharge is greater than 5.0. Because trichomoniasis is an STI, once diagnosis is confirmed, the appropriate laboratory studies for other STIs should be carried out.

Therapeutic Management

The recommended treatment is metronidazole or tinidazole orally in a single dose (Gibson, Bell, & Powerful, 2014). Although the male partner is usually asymptomatic, he should receive treatment also because trichomonads often harbor in the urethra or prostate. If partners are not treated, the infection will likely recur.

SEXUALLY TRANSMITTED BACTERIAL INFECTIONS

Chlamydia

Chlamydia trachomatis is the most frequently reported bacterial STI in the United States, yet most cases are still undiagnosed (Centers for Disease Control and Prevention, 2015). Rates are highest among individuals age 15 to 24 years and African Americans (Centers for Disease Control and Prevention, 2015). These infections are often silent and highly destructive; their sequelae and complications are very serious. Chlamydial infections are difficult to diagnose; the symptoms, if present, are nonspecific, and the organism is expensive to culture.

The most serious complication of chlamydial infections is pelvic inflammatory disease leading to infertility, ectopic pregnancy, and chronic pelvic pain (Centers for Disease Control and Prevention, 2015). Chlamydial infection of the cervix causes inflammation, resulting in microscopic cervical ulcerations that may increase the risk of acquiring HIV. Infants born to mothers with chlamydia may develop ophthalmia neonatorum (conjunctivitis) or pneumonia after perinatal exposure (Centers for Disease Control and Prevention, 2015).

Screening and Diagnosis

In addition to obtaining information regarding the presence of risk factors (e.g., younger than 25 years old, no use of barrier contraceptives, new or multiple partners), inquire about the presence of any symptoms (Centers for Disease Control and Prevention, 2015). Although infection is usually asymptomatic, some women may experience vaginal bleeding, mucoid or purulent cervical discharge, abdominal pain, or dysuria; men may report testicular pain, penile discharge, or dysuria.

Laboratory diagnosis of chlamydia is by culture (expensive and labor intensive), DNA probe (relatively less expensive but less sensitive), and nucleic acid amplification tests (NAATs) (expensive but have relatively higher sensitivity) of urine specimens or specimens from the endocervix/vagina (Centers for Disease Control and Prevention, 2015). All pregnant women should have cervical cultures for chlamydia at the first prenatal visit. Screening late in the third trimester (36 weeks) may be carried out if the woman was positive previously or if she is younger than 25 years, has a new sex partner, or has multiple sex partners.

Therapeutic Management

The treatment of chlamydial infections includes doxycycline or azithromycin (Gibson, Bell, & Powerful, 2014). Because chlamydia is often asymptomatic, caution the woman to take all medication prescribed. Azithromycin is often prescribed when compliance is a problem because only one dose is needed. Individuals should abstain from sexual intercourse for 7 days after treatment and all exposed sexual partners should be treated. Adolescents should be screened again in 3 to 6 months after treatment to evaluate for reinfection (Gibson, Bell, & Powerful, 2014).

Gonorrhea

Gonorrhea is probably the oldest communicable disease in the United States. An estimated 820,000 American men and women contract a new gonorrhea infection each year (Centers for Disease Control and Prevention, 2015). The majority of individuals with gonorrhea are young people ages 15 to 24 years old (Centers for Disease Control and Prevention, 2015). The incidence of drug-resistant cases of gonorrhea is increasing dramatically in the United States.

Gonorrhea is caused by the aerobic, gram-negative diplococci *Neisseria gonorrhoeae.* It is almost exclusively transmitted by sexual contact. The bacteria infects mucosal membranes, including the cervix, uterus, fallopian tubes, urethra, rectum, mouth, throat, and eyes (Centers for Disease Control and Prevention, 2015). Although the organism has been recovered from inanimate objects artificially inoculated with the bacteria, there is no evidence that natural transmission occurs this way.

Women are often asymptomatic, but when they are symptomatic, they may have a greenish-yellow purulent endocervical discharge or vaginal bleeding. Women may complain of pain (i.e., chronic or acute severe pelvic or lower abdominal pain). Infected men usually have symptoms and report purulent discharge and dysuria (Gibson, Bell, & Powerful, 2014). Individuals with rectal gonorrhea may be completely asymptomatic or conversely may experience severe symptoms with profuse purulent anal discharge, rectal pain, and blood in the stool. Rectal itching, fullness, pressure, and pain with bowel movements are also common symptoms. Pharyngeal infection is usually asymptomatic but may cause a sore throat. A diffuse vaginitis with vulvitis is the most common form of gonococcal infection in prepubertal girls. There may be few signs of infection, but vaginal discharge, dysuria, or swollen, reddened labia are sometimes present.

Gonococcal infections in pregnancy potentially affect both mother and infant. Perinatal complications of gonococcal infection include premature rupture of the membranes, preterm birth, chorioamnionitis, neonatal sepsis, intrauterine growth restriction, and maternal postpartum sepsis. Amniotic infection syndrome—manifested by placental, fetal, and umbilical cord inflammation after premature rupture of the membranes—may result from gonorrheal infection during pregnancy.

Screening and Diagnosis

Because gonococcal infections are often asymptomatic, the Centers for Disease Control and Prevention recommends screening anyone at risk for gonorrhea (Centers for Disease Control and Prevention, 2015). All pregnant women should be screened at the first prenatal visit, and infected women and those identified with risky behaviors should be rescreened at 36 weeks of gestation.

Gonococcal infection cannot be diagnosed reliably by clinical signs and symptoms alone. Individuals may have "classic" symptoms, vague symptoms that may be attributed to a number of conditions, or no symptoms at all. NAATs are used to diagnose gonorrhea. Vaginal specimens are the preferred testing in women, but urine, oral swabs, or anal swabs can also be used (Gibson, Bell, & Powerful, 2014). Because coinfection is common, any woman suspected of having gonorrhea should have a chlamydial culture and serologic test for syphilis unless one has been done within the past 2 months.

Therapeutic Management

Management of gonorrhea is becoming more challenging as drug-resistant strains are increasing. The treatment of choice for uncomplicated urethral, endocervical, and rectal infections in pregnant and nonpregnant women is ceftriaxone given intramuscularly once. The Centers for Disease Control and Prevention also recommends concomitant treatment for chlamydia because coinfection is common (Centers for Disease Control and Prevention, 2015).

Gonorrhea is highly communicable. Recent (past 60 days) sexual partners should be examined, cultured, and treated with appropriate regimens. Most treatment failures result from reinfection. The adolescent needs to be informed of this and of the consequences of reinfection in terms of chronicity, complications, and potential infertility. Adolescents are counseled to use condoms. All adolescents with gonorrhea should be offered confidential counseling and testing for HIV infection.

Syphilis

Syphilis, one of the earliest described STIs, is caused by *Treponema pallidum,* a motile spirochete. Transmission is thought to be by entry through microscopic abrasions in the subcutaneous tissue, which can occur during sexual intercourse. The disease can also be transmitted through kissing, biting, or oral-genital sex. Transplacental transmission may occur at any time during pregnancy; the degree of risk is related to the quantity of spirochetes in the maternal bloodstream.

Syphilis rates have been decreasing among heterosexual individuals but are increasing among homosexual males (Centers for Disease Control and Prevention, 2015). Rates of congenital syphilis have remained consistent over the years with higher rates among infants born to African American and Hispanic mothers (Centers for Disease Control and Prevention, 2015). Syphilis is a complex disease that can lead to serious systemic disease and even death when untreated. Infection manifests itself in distinct stages with different symptoms and clinical manifestations. Primary syphilis is characterized by a primary lesion, the chancre, which appears 14 to 21 days after infection. This lesion often begins as a painless papule at the site of inoculation and erodes to form a nontender, shallow, ulcer that is accompanied by lymphadenopathy. Secondary syphilis occurs 6 weeks to a few months after the appearance of the chancre. It is characterized by a widespread, symmetric, maculopapular rash on the abdomen and extremities including the palms and soles and generalized lymphadenopathy. The infected individual also may experience fever, headache, and malaise. Condylomata lata (i.e., broad, painless, pink-gray, wartlike infectious lesions) may develop on the vulva, perineum, or anus. If untreated, the individual enters a latent phase that is primarily asymptomatic. Neurologic, cardiovascular, musculoskeletal, or multiorgan system complications can develop in the latent stage.

Screening and Diagnosis

All women who are diagnosed with another STI or with HIV should be screened for syphilis. All pregnant women should be screened for syphilis at the first prenatal visit, again in the late third trimester, and at the time of giving birth if high risk (Centers for Disease Control and Prevention, 2015). A test for antibodies may not be reactive in the presence of active infection because it takes time for the immune system of the body to develop antibodies to any antigens. Up to one-third of people in early primary syphilis may have nonreactive serologic tests. Two types of serologic tests are used: nontreponemal and treponemal. Nontreponemal antibody tests such as Venereal Disease Research Laboratories (VDRL) and rapid plasma reagin (RPR) are used as screening tests. False-positive results are not unusual, particularly with conditions such as acute infection. The treponemal tests, fluorescent treponemal antibody absorbed, and microhemagglutination assays for antibody to *T. pallidum* are more sensitive and used to confirm positive results. Tests (e.g., wet preparations and cultures) for concomitant STIs (e.g., chlamydia and gonorrhea) should be done, and HIV testing offered if indicated.

Therapeutic Management

Penicillin G is the preferred drug for treating patients with all stages of syphilis, including pregnant women (Gibson, Bell, & Powerful, 2014). Individuals with a penicillin allergy should be desensitized rather than offer treatment with an alternative medication (Gibson, Bell, & Powerful, 2014). Specific protocols are recommended by the Centers for Disease Control and Prevention.

> **! NURSING ALERT**
>
> Patients treated for syphilis may experience a Jarisch-Herxheimer reaction. This is an acute febrile reaction often accompanied by headache, myalgias, and arthralgias that develop within the first 24 hours of treatment. The reaction may be treated symptomatically with analgesics and antipyretics. If treatment precipitates this reaction in the second half of pregnancy, women are at risk for preterm labor and birth. They should be advised to contact their health care provider if they notice any change in fetal movement or have any contractions.

Monthly follow-up is mandatory, so repeated treatment may be given if needed. The nurse should emphasize the necessity of long-term serologic testing even in the absence of symptoms. Adolescents are advised to practice sexual abstinence until treatment is completed, all evidence of primary and secondary syphilis is gone, and serologic evidence of a cure is demonstrated. Affected individuals should be told to notify all partners within the previous 90 days before the diagnosis, as they will need treatment.

Pelvic Inflammatory Disease

Pelvic inflammatory disease (PID) is an infectious process that most commonly involves the uterine tubes, causing salpingitis; the uterus, causing endometritis; and, more rarely, the ovaries and peritoneal surfaces. Multiple organisms have been found to cause PID and common agents include *Neisseria gonorrhoeae, C. trachomatis,* and a variety of other aerobic and anaerobic bacteria. It is estimated that each year approximately 1 million women experience an episode of PID, with the highest rates occurring in women ages 15 to 19 years old (Spain & Rheinboldt, 2017). It encompasses a wide variety of pathologic processes; the infection can be acute, subacute, or chronic and can have a wide range of symptoms.

Most PID results from the ascending spread of microorganisms from the vagina and endocervix to the upper genital tract. This spread most commonly happens at the end of or just after menses after reception of an infectious agent. During the menstrual period several factors facilitate the development of an infection: the cervical os is slightly open, the cervical mucus barrier is absent, and menstrual blood is an excellent medium for growth. PID also may develop after a miscarriage or an induced abortion, pelvic surgery, or childbirth.

Risk factors for acquiring PID are those associated with the risk of contracting an STI, including under the age of 25 years, multiple partners, high rate of new partners, and low socioeconomic status (Spain & Rheinboldt, 2017). Women who have a long-term indwelling intrauterine device (IUD) are at increased risk for PID (Spain & Rheinboldt, 2017). PID tends to recur.

Women who have had PID are at increased risk for ectopic pregnancy, infertility, and chronic pelvic pain. Other problems associated with PID include dyspareunia, pyosalpinx (pus in the uterine tubes), tubo-ovarian abscess, and pelvic adhesions.

The symptoms of PID vary, depending on whether the infection is acute, subacute, or chronic; however, pain is common to all types of infection. It may be dull, cramping, intermittent (subacute) or severe, persistent, and incapacitating (acute). Women may also report fever, chills, abdominal pain, nausea and vomiting, increased vaginal discharge, urinary tract infection symptoms, and irregular bleeding.

Screening and Diagnosis

PID is difficult to diagnose because of the accompanying wide variety of symptoms. The Centers for Disease Control and Prevention recommends treatment for PID in all sexually active young women and others at risk for STIs if the following criteria are present and no other cause or causes of the illness are found: lower abdominal tenderness, in combination with adnexal tenderness, uterine tenderness, or cervical motion tenderness. Other criteria to support the diagnosis of PID include an oral temperature of 38.3° C or above, abnormal cervical mucopurulent discharge, microscopic presence of abundant white blood cells in vaginal fluid, elevated erythrocyte sedimentation rate, elevated C-reactive protein, or laboratory documentation of cervical infection with *N. gonorrhoeae* or *C. trachomatis* (Centers for Disease Control and Prevention, 2016b).

Therapeutic and Nursing Care Management

Perhaps the most important nursing intervention is prevention counseling. Primary prevention includes education in avoiding contracting STIs; secondary prevention involves preventing a lower genital tract infection from ascending to the upper genital tract. Instructing women in self-protective behaviors such as practices to avoid contracting STIs and using barrier methods is critical. Women using hormonal contraception or an IUD and those who have chosen tubal ligation must be reminded to use a condom with intercourse when indicated. Also important is the detection of asymptomatic gonorrheal and chlamydial infections through routine screening of women who practice risky behaviors or have specific risk factors such as age.

Although treatment regimens vary with the infecting organism, generally a broad-spectrum antibiotic is used (Spain & Rheinboldt, 2017). Treatment for mild to moderately severe PID may be oral (e.g., ceftriaxone plus doxycycline and metronidazole) or parenteral (e.g., cefotetan or cefoxitin plus doxycycline [oral]), and regimens can be administered in inpatient or outpatient settings. Hospitalization and parenteral antibiotics are recommended for women unresponsive or inability to tolerate an oral regimen, severe illness, pregnancy, tubo-ovarian abscess, or inability to exclude a surgical emergency (Das, Ronda, & Trent, 2016).

The woman with acute PID should be on bed rest in a semi-Fowler's position. Comfort measures include analgesics for pain and all other nursing measures applicable to a patient confined to bed. Few pelvic examinations should be done during the acute phase of the disease. During the recovery phase the woman should restrict her activity and make every effort to get adequate rest and a nutritionally sound diet. Follow-up laboratory work after treatment should include endocervical cultures for a test of cure.

Health education is central to effective management of PID. Nurses should explain the nature of the disease to women and encourage them to comply with all therapy and prevention recommendations, emphasizing the need to take all medication, even if symptoms disappear. Any potential problems (such as a lack of money for prescriptions or a lack of transportation to return for follow-up appointments) that would prevent a woman from completing a course of treatment should be identified, referrals made for assistance as needed, and the importance of follow-up visits stressed. Women should be counseled to refrain from sexual intercourse until their treatment is completed. Contraceptive counseling, including information on barrier methods such as condoms, the contraceptive sponge, and the diaphragm, should be provided.

The potential or actual loss of reproductive capabilities can be devastating and can adversely affect the woman's self-concept. Part of the nurse's role is to help the woman adjust her self-concept to fit reality and accept alterations in a way that promotes health. Because PID is so closely tied to sexuality, body image, and self-concept, the woman diagnosed with it needs supportive care. Her feelings should be discussed, and her partner(s) included when appropriate.

SEXUALLY TRANSMITTED VIRAL INFECTIONS

Human Papillomavirus

HPV infection, also known as *condylomata acuminata,* or *genital warts,* is the most common viral STI in the United States. An estimated 79 million Americans are infected with HPV, and about 14 million new infections occur every year (Centers for Disease Control and Prevention, 2016c). HPV, a double-stranded DNA virus, has more than 40 serotypes that can be sexually transmitted and consists of two categories: low-risk HPVs, which cause skin warts but not cancer, and high-risk HPVs, which cause cancer (Centers for Disease Control and Prevention, 2016c). High-risk HPVs primarily cause cervical, anal, and oropharyngeal cancers (Centers for Disease Control and Prevention, 2016c).

In women HPV lesions are most commonly seen in the posterior part of the introitus. Lesions also are found on the buttocks, vulva, vagina, anus, and cervix. Typically the lesions are small (2 to 3 mm in diameter and 10 to 15 mm in height), soft, papillary swellings occurring singly on the genital and anal-rectal region but may also appear as a cauliflower-like mass. Flat-topped papules, 1 to 4 mm in diameter, are seen most often on the cervix. Often these lesions are visualized only under magnification. The lesions are usually painless, but they may be uncomfortable, particularly when very large, inflamed, or ulcerated. Chronic vaginal discharge, pruritus, or dyspareunia can occur.

Screening and Diagnosis

A woman with HPV lesions may complain of symptoms such as a profuse, irritating vaginal discharge; itching; dyspareunia; or postcoital bleeding. She also may report "bumps" on her vulva or labia. History of a known exposure is important; however, because of the potentially long latency period and the possibility of subclinical infections in men, the lack of a history of known exposure cannot be used to exclude a diagnosis of HPV infection.

Physical inspection of the vulva, the perineum, the anus, the vagina, and the cervix is essential whenever HPV lesions are suspected or seen in one area. Because speculum examination of the vagina may block some lesions, it is important to rotate the speculum blades until all areas are visualized. When lesions are visible, the characteristic appearance previously described is considered diagnostic. However, in many instances cervical lesions are not visible, and some vaginal or vulvar lesions also may be unobservable to the naked eye. Because of the potential spread of vulvar or vaginal lesions to the anus, gloves should be changed between vaginal and rectal examinations.

The only definitive diagnostic test for the presence of HPV is histologic evaluation of a biopsy specimen. The HPV-DNA test can be used to screen for the high-risk types of HPV that are likely to cause cancer.

Therapeutic Management

Many warts may resolve on their own so treatment may not be necessary. Treatment does not eradicate HPV but may reduce the signs and symptoms of warts. Treatment of genital warts should be guided by preference of the patient, number and size of warts, cost of treatment, and provider experience. No one of the treatments is superior to all other treatments, and no one treatment is ideal for all warts (Smith & Angarone, 2015). Imiquimod and podofilox are common treatments but should not be used during pregnancy. Because the lesions can proliferate and become friable during pregnancy, many experts recommend their removal using cryotherapy or various surgical techniques (Centers for Disease Control and Prevention, 2016c).

Women who have discomfort associated with genital warts may find that bathing with an oatmeal solution provides some relief. Keeping the area clean and dry also decreases the growth of the warts. Cotton underwear and loose-fitting clothes that decrease friction and irritation may lessen discomfort. Women should be advised to maintain a healthy lifestyle and be counseled regarding diet, rest, stress reduction, and exercise.

Patient counseling is essential. Women must understand the virus, how it is transmitted, that no immunity is conferred with infection, and that reinfection is likely with repeated contact. Encourage all sexually active women with multiple partners or a history of HPV to use latex condoms for intercourse to decrease acquisition or transmission of the infection. Semiannual or annual health examinations are recommended to assess disease recurrence and screening for cervical cancer. Women who have been treated for HPV infections should have annual Papanicolaou (Pap) tests (Centers for Disease Control and Prevention, 2016c).

Prevention

Preventive strategies that have been suggested include abstinence from all sexual activity, staying in a long-term monogamous relationship, and prophylactic vaccination (Centers for Disease Control and Prevention, 2016c). Three HPV vaccines have been licensed for use in adolescents, but Gardasil 9 is the only available HPV vaccine in the United States

(Centers for Disease Control and Prevention, 2016c). The vaccine is routinely initiated among boys and girls at 11 to 12 years of age but can be given between the ages of 9 and 26 years (Centers for Disease Control and Prevention, 2016c) (see Chapter 6).

Herpes Simplex Virus

Unknown until the middle of the twentieth century, herpes simplex virus (HSV) infection is now widespread in the United States. Although HSV infection is not a reportable disease, it is estimated that 776,000 people in the United States are newly infected with a herpes infection each year (Centers for Disease Control and Prevention, 2016a). Women are more likely than men to become infected, especially if they have multiple partners. Most persons infected with HSV-2 have not been diagnosed, and many infections are transmitted by persons unaware that they are infected.

HSV infection is caused by two different antigen subtypes of HSV: HSV type 1 (HSV-1) and HSV type 2 (HSV-2). HSV-2 is usually transmitted sexually, and HSV-1 nonsexually. Although HSV-1 is more commonly associated with gingivostomatitis and oral labial ulcers (fever blisters) and HSV-2 with genital lesions, neither type is exclusively associated with the respective sites.

Many HSV infections are asymptomatic or have very mild symptoms; however, some may experience one or more painful lesions, fever, chills, malaise, lymphadenopathy, and headaches lasting 2 to 3 weeks. Typically the lesions initially appear as macules and papules that progress to form vesicles, pustules, and ulcers. Women may have a more severe clinical course than do men and may have itching, inguinal tenderness, and vulvar edema. HSV cervicitis is common with initial HSV-2 infections. The cervix may appear normal or be friable, reddened, ulcerated, or necrotic. A heavy, watery-to-purulent vaginal discharge is common. Extragenital lesions may be present because of autoinoculation. Urinary retention and dysuria may occur secondary to autonomic involvement of the sacral nerve root.

Individuals with recurrent episodes of HSV infections commonly have only local symptoms that are usually less severe than those associated with the initial infection. Systemic symptoms are usually absent, although the characteristic prodromal genital tingling is common. Recurrent lesions involve a small number of lesions that are less severe and last 8 to 10 days (Sauerbrei, 2016). Few women with recurrent disease have cervicitis.

The HSV-2 can be passed from the mother to the infant during pregnancy, childbirth, or the newborn period with a higher risk of transmission if the mother is having the first outbreak versus a recurrent outbreak. Exposure to HSV-2 may lead to a potentially fatal neonatal herpes infection (Centers for Disease Control and Prevention, 2016a).

Screening and Diagnosis

Although a diagnosis of herpes infection may be suspected from the history and physical examination, it is confirmed by laboratory studies. A viral culture is obtained by swabbing exudate during the vesicular stage of the disease.

Therapeutic Management

Genital herpes is a chronic and recurring disease for which there is no known cure. Management is directed toward specific treatment during primary and recurrent infections, prevention, self-help measures, and psychologic support.

Oral medications used for treating the first clinical HSV infection include acyclovir, famciclovir, and valacyclovir. These medications are considered for episodic or suppressive therapy for recurrent HSV. Intravenous acyclovir may be used for individuals with a compromised immune system or severe disease (Sauerbrei, 2016). The safety of acyclovir, valacyclovir, and famciclovir therapy during pregnancy has not been established, and benefits of use are considered in relation to the potential harm to the fetus (Sauerbrei, 2016). Continued investigation of these medications during pregnancy is needed.

Cleaning lesions twice a day with saline helps prevent secondary infection. Bacterial infection must be treated with appropriate antibiotics. Measures that may increase comfort for women when lesions are active include warm sitz baths with baking soda; keeping lesions dry by using cool air from a hair dryer or patting dry with a soft towel; wearing cotton underwear and loose clothing; and applying cool, wet black tea bags to lesions. Women can also apply compresses with an infusion of cloves or peppermint oil and clove oil to lesions.

An oral analgesic such as ibuprofen may be used to relieve pain and systemic symptoms associated with initial infections. Because the mucous membranes affected by herpes are extremely sensitive, any topical agents should be used with caution. Nonantiviral ointments, especially those containing cortisone, should be avoided. A thin layer of lidocaine ointment or an antiseptic spray may be applied to decrease discomfort, especially if walking is difficult.

Counseling and education are critical components of the nursing care of women with herpes infections. Information regarding the etiology, signs and symptoms, transmission, and treatment should be provided. The nurse should explain that each woman is unique in her response to herpes and emphasize the variability of symptoms. Women should be helped to understand when viral shedding and thus transmission to a partner are most likely. They should be counseled to refrain from sexual contact from the onset of prodrome until complete healing of lesions.

Some authorities recommend consistent use of condoms for all persons with genital herpes. Condoms may not prevent transmission, particularly male-to-female transmission; however, this does not mean that the partners should avoid all intimacy. Women can be encouraged to maintain close contact with their partners while avoiding contact with lesions. They should be taught how to look for herpetic lesions using a mirror and good light source and a wet cloth or finger covered with a finger cot to rub lightly over the labia. The nurse should ensure that women understand that when lesions are active, sharing intimate articles (e.g., washcloths or wet towels) that come into contact with the lesions should be avoided. Only plain soap and water are needed to clean hands that have come in contact with herpetic lesions; isolation is neither necessary nor appropriate.

Stress, menstruation, trauma, febrile illnesses, chronic illness, and ultraviolet light have all been found to trigger genital herpes. Women may wish to keep a diary to identify stressors that seem to be associated with recurrent herpes attacks so they can avoid these stressors when possible. Referral for stress reduction therapy, yoga, or meditation classes may be indicated. Avoiding excessive heat, sun, and hot baths and using a lubricant during sexual intercourse to reduce friction also may be helpful. Women in their childbearing years should be counseled regarding the risk of herpes infection during pregnancy.

Because neonatal HSV infection is such a devastating disease, prevention is critical. Current recommendations include carefully examining and questioning all women about symptoms at onset of labor (Centers for Disease Control and Prevention, 2016a). If visible lesions are not present at onset of labor, vaginal birth is acceptable. Cesarean birth after labor begins or membranes rupture is recommended if visible lesions are present. Infants who are born through an infected vagina should be observed carefully and cultured. Some experts recommend presumptive treatment of infants who were exposed to HSV during birth (see also Herpes Simplex Virus, Chapter 8). Because HSV infection may be associated with cervical dysplasia, women must be encouraged to have annual Pap tests and gynecologic examinations.

The emotional effect of contracting an incurable STI such as herpes is considerable. At diagnosis many emotions may surface—helplessness, anger, denial, guilt, anxiety, shame, or inadequacy. Women need the opportunity to discuss their feelings and help in learning to live with the disease. Herpes can affect a woman's sexuality, her sexual practices, and her current and future relationships. She may need help in raising the issue with her partner or future partners.

Hepatitis

Five different viruses (hepatitis viruses A, B, C, D, and E) account for almost all cases of viral hepatitis in humans. These are discussed in Chapter 25.

Human Immunodeficiency Virus

Human immunodeficiency virus (HIV) is a bloodborne pathogen and transmission of the virus can occur in the perinatal period, through sexual intercourse with an infected person, or by sharing needles with an infected person. HIV is discussed in Chapter 28.

HEALTH CONDITIONS RELATED TO REPRODUCTION

The biologic maturation that forms the foundation of adolescent development and the transition to adulthood is accompanied by conflicting feelings, attitudes, and social practices related to developing sexuality. During adolescence the sexual drive emerges, and adolescents begin to explore their ability to attract a partner.

The Youth Risk Behavior Surveillance System from the Centers for Disease Control and Prevention conducts a national school-based survey to monitor key health-risk behaviors among youth. The 2015 survey results found that 41.2% of students had had sexual intercourse, with 3.9% having their first sexual encounter before age 13 years. Both of these results have significantly decreased since 1990 when 54.1% of students had sexual intercourse, with 10.2% having their first sexual encounter before age 13 years. Not all young people who have ever had sexual intercourse were currently sexually active; in the survey 30.1% of the students had sexual intercourse with at least one person during the 3 months before the survey. Among those students, 56.2% used a condom during the last sexual intercourse (Kann, McManus, Harris, et al., 2016). The prevalence of being sexually active was higher among white females, black males, and Hispanic males than white males, black females, or Hispanic females (Kann, McManus, Harris, et al., 2016).

The causes of adolescent sexual risk taking are multifactorial. There is great social pressure to experiment with sex, and enticements by the media to enhance physical attractiveness conflict with traditional religious and societal expectations for chastity. Easy access to cars, unsupervised time at home, and changing family composition also contribute to the incidence of sexual experimentation among the adolescent population. Social norms, peer comparison, and situational triggers are environmental circumstances that lead to risk taking and experimentation, and depression, impulsivity, and sensation-seeking attitudes are personality traits that contribute to risk taking and experimentation (Fielder, Walsh, Carey, et al., 2013). In addition, alcohol, marijuana, and cigarette use are strong predictors of initiation of sexual intercourse among adolescents (Fielder, Walsh, Carey, et al., 2013). Family influences can delay the initiation of sexual activity. Adolescents who have at least one warm, supportive parent engage in less risky behavior. Effective parent-child communication about sexual topics can delay the onset of sexual intercourse. In addition, supervision of the adolescent's social activities and peer group, frequently referred to as *parental monitoring,* has consistently been shown to postpone sexual involvement. However, parents may underestimate the level of risk for their child and may not provide the appropriate monitoring and communication to assist in postponing sexual involvement.

Prevention strategies must be comprehensive to decrease high-risk sexual behaviors. Delaying sexual intercourse, using condoms, choosing partners carefully, limiting sexual partners, and using reliable contraception help to reduce the impact of sexual activity on the adolescent. Nurses working with individual adolescents benefit from taking a sexual history so that prevention strategies are appropriate for the level of risk. Questioning adolescents who have not initiated sexual intercourse about their intention to initiate it is helpful because their intentions are positively associated with actual sexual initiation. Instruction in the skills needed to resist sexual intercourse has a stronger influence on reducing sexual activity than simply providing information on STIs or birth control methods.

ADOLESCENT PREGNANCY

Over the last several decades the teenage pregnancy rate in the United States has shown a continual downward trend; however, adolescent pregnancy rates in the United States continue to rank higher than other developed nations. The 2014 teen birth rate was 24.2 per 1000 females ages 15 to 19 years (Centers for Disease Control and Prevention, 2017). The state with the highest teen birth rate is Arkansas (39.5 births per 1000 teens), and the state with the lowest teen birth rate is Massachusetts (10.6 births per 1000 teens) (Centers for Disease Control and Prevention, 2017).

Contraception use among adolescents is variable, with decisions made within the context of the relationship. The less familiar an adolescent is with his or her partner, the less likely it is that they will use contraception during intercourse. One concern is that young adolescent girls are often coerced into having sexual contact by an older partner. Contraception use increases among girls as the duration of the relationship increases. A hormonal method (OCPs, contraceptive patch, injectable progesterone) is more likely to be used in later relationships than in first sexual relationships. Discontinuation of contraception is common; 30% of women age 15 to 19 years old and 47% of women age 20 to 24 years old have discontinued at least one method because of dissatisfaction (Pazol, Whiteman, Folger, et al., 2015).

In most cases, with early prenatal care, teenage pregnancy is no longer considered to be biologically disadvantageous to the child. However, teenage parenting is still regarded as socially, educationally, psychologically, and economically disadvantageous to both mother and child. Predictors of maternal success include participation in a program for pregnant teens, a social support system, and a sense of control over one's life.

Medical Aspects

Adolescents often receive delayed or inadequate prenatal care. Prenatal care may be delayed because the adolescent does not realize she is pregnant or denies the pregnancy until the second or third trimester. Health care providers working with adolescents should have a high index of suspicion for pregnancy. She may or may not have considered the possibility of pregnancy no matter how at risk for pregnancy she is. A pregnant adolescent may give vague reports of irregular periods or missed periods; the bleeding that occurs with implantation may be mistaken for a period, further delaying the diagnosis. Lacking adequate care, adolescent mothers and their unborn infants are at greater risk for low-birth-weight infants and infant deaths. It remains unclear whether this is a result of biologic immaturity or sociodemographic factors. Medical concerns of adolescent pregnancies include gestational diabetes, anemia, preeclampsia, and low platelet syndrome (Kawakita, Wilson, Grantz, et al., 2016).

The obstetric risk and risk to the infant during a second pregnancy for the teenager is much higher. An adolescent with a poor outcome in the first pregnancy has a threefold risk of repeating the poor outcome in the second pregnancy. In teenagers the risk for a preterm delivery recurring is double the rate found in older women.

Diagnosis of Pregnancy

A detailed menstrual and sexual history should be a routine part of health care for adolescents. Review specific symptoms of pregnancy, including amenorrhea, breast tenderness, urinary frequency, fatigue, and nausea. Absence of these symptoms does not exclude pregnancy. It is best not to perform a pregnancy test without the adolescent's knowledge. Before the pregnancy test, discuss with the adolescent what she will do if the test is positive and determine who else is aware she is sexually active and possibly pregnant.

After confirming that a pregnancy test is positive, inform the adolescent privately. Common reactions are ambivalence, shock, fear, or apparent apathy. The nurse should be supportive at this time and assure her the feelings are normal. Review the facts about the pregnancy, including the duration of pregnancy and anticipated due date. The next step is to determine who she plans to inform and, if she is under 18, how she would like to tell her parents. Some girls may want to take some time before notifying their parents. The nurse should schedule a follow-up appointment in 24 to 48 hours to assist with parental notification. Usually, the adolescent informs her parent on her own terms during this period. The nurse can assist with notification by offering to tell the parent for the teen or to be present when she tells her parent. Nonjudgmental support is critical at this time for the safety of the teen and her pregnancy.

Complications of Pregnancy

Bleeding can occur early in pregnancy with an incidence ranging from 7% to 21% (Sapra, Joseph, Galea, et al., 2017). The risk of a spontaneous abortion is higher in women with bleeding than without bleeding (Sapra, Joseph, Galea, et al., 2017). Ultrasound evaluation can assist in determining the prognosis for the pregnancy. Bed rest is usually recommended when bleeding occurs; however, there is little evidence to demonstrate its effectiveness in preventing spontaneous abortions.

When a young woman is seen with bleeding and abdominal pain, an ectopic pregnancy must be ruled out. Ectopic pregnancy occurs when the fertilized egg implants outside of the uterus, usually in the fallopian tube. Impaired tubal transport and alterations in the tubal microenvironment allow for early implantation of the embryo (Horne, Brown, Nio-Kobayashi, et al., 2014). Factors that maintain a normal tubal environment are unknown but ectopic pregnancy is more frequent in women with a history of tubal surgery, PID, and previous ectopic pregnancy. Another risk factor for ectopic pregnancy is smoking, due to changes in the tubal epithelial cell environment caused from the metabolite of nicotine (Horne, Brown, Nio-Kobayashi, et al., 2014). When ectopic pregnancy is suspected, prompt evaluation and treatment are necessary. If the adolescent is seen with hypotension and abdominal pain, the ectopic pregnancy may have ruptured and emergency surgery is indicated.

Structural Factors

Labor may be prolonged in younger teenagers, particularly those 12 to 16 years of age; this is directly related to fetopelvic incompatibility and is a reflection of the teenager's smaller stature and incomplete growth process. The incidence of prolonged labor is highest in girls younger than age 14 years. Girls who are 12 to 13 years old have the highest rate of cesarean births, primarily because of cephalopelvic disproportion. However, older adolescents 15 to 21 years of age, especially those who have previously delivered a baby, often have labors that are shorter than average. The transition between pelvic disproportion and pelvic adequacy appears to occur around 15 years of age in the average adolescent.

Nutritional Needs

Caloric requirements during adolescence closely parallel the growth curve, and the need for protein, calcium, and iron is increased. Young adolescents tolerate caloric restriction poorly, and the anabolic need for calories during pregnancy places an added burden on their bodies. The preconception weight is a major determinant of birth weight for infants born to adolescents. Weight gain recommendations for pregnant girls should be based on their prepregnancy body mass index (BMI), not on their age. A higher weight gain is recommended for thin women and a lower weight gain for women who are overweight or obese (Kominiarek & Rajan, 2016). Primiparous adolescents are more likely than first-time adult pregnant women to gain more than 18 kg (40 lb). Excessive weight gain during pregnancy is associated with labor and delivery complications, preterm labor, maternal anemia, and infant mortality. Excessive weight gain during pregnancy is also linked with postpartum obesity and the associated health risks.

> **! NURSING ALERT**
>
> All pregnant women should take a vitamin and mineral supplement to ensure the recommended dietary allowance for folic acid (0.4 mg [400 mcg] daily) to help prevent neural tube defects. (See Myelomeningocele [Meningomyelocele], Prevention, Chapter 34.) Initiation before pregnancy has shown to have the most benefit. Consider a multivitamin containing folic acid for all sexually active women.

Because of the marked variation in the dietary needs of individual teenagers, there are no hard-and-fast rules to describe an adequate diet for all pregnant girls. The diet must provide sufficient nutrients to meet growth needs of both the prospective mother and the unborn child without the threat of excessive weight gain or fetal malnutrition. To accomplish this the 2009 Institute of Medicine guidelines for weight gain in pregnant females recommend weight gains based on the female's prepregnancy BMI; a female with normal prepregnancy weight and a BMI of 18.5 to 24.9 would be expected to gain 25 to 35 lb, whereas a female with a prepregnancy BMI of 25.0 to 29.9 would be expected gain 15 to 25 lb (Kominiarek & Rajan, 2016). Calcium (Recommended Dietary Allowance 1300 mg/day) and vitamin D (Institute of Medicine recommendation is 600 IU/day; the US Endocrine Task Force recommends 1500 to 2000 IU/day) intake during pregnancy have been shown to have an impact on bone mineral density and growth in the growing fetus; poor intake of these is associated with low birth weight in the newborn. Pregnant adolescents who do not consume dairy products should be taking a calcium supplement to receive adequate intake of this mineral. The best guides for determining nutritional needs for the adolescent and pregnant adolescent are the Recommended Dietary Allowances and the Dietary Guidelines for Americans; the Dietary Reference Intakes (DRIs) from the Institute of Medicine include recommended intakes of vitamins, minerals, and macronutrients for women of all ages and for those who are pregnant.* (See also Nutritional Assessment, Chapter 4.) Pregnant teenagers exhibit food preferences, eating behaviors, and lifestyle habits that are similar to those of their nonpregnant peers. Frequent snacking on foods high in fat and sugar and low in essential nutrients results in less than the recommended intake of calcium; iron;

*See DRIs at the Institute of Medicine home page, http://www.iom.edu.

zinc; folic acid; and vitamins B_{12}, A, D, and K—nutrients of special concern during pregnancy.

Social and Economic Aspects

Poor school performance usually precedes adolescent pregnancy. Unable to achieve academically, the girl views motherhood as a rite of passage into adult status. Adolescents with high educational expectations are less likely than others to become pregnant. Another significant aspect of school dropout and accelerated maturity is the girl's alienation and isolation from her peers during a stage of development when identity formation is closely allied with peer identification. She is deprived of the interrelationship with the adolescent social system that is so essential to the development of a sense of identity. The girl may believe that she no longer "belongs" to the peer group and does not qualify for membership in the older peer group of mothers. On the other hand, the pregnancy may give the adolescent an entrance into a peer group.

FAMILY-CENTERED CARE

Adolescent Pregnancy

The vast majority of adolescent girls who make the decision to continue a pregnancy will choose to parent the infant rather than release the newborn for adoption. Research has demonstrated that many of these young mothers have successful childrearing skills. One key factor is the amount of assistance the mother receives from her family of origin. This assistance may be in the form of financial support or child care assistance. Family support allows the young mother to complete her education and acquire vocational skills while still meeting her child's needs.

Nurses can increase the young mother's sense of competence by providing feedback about positive parenting skills and referring the teenager to community resources, such as parenting classes and infant stimulation programs. Nurses can also initiate and lead support groups for adolescent parents to foster self-confidence and parenting skills.

Mother-Infant Relationship

Adolescents often have unrealistic expectations for the child. The young mother may view the infant as a plaything or a love object for herself. Children of adolescent mothers experience more developmental problems than children of adult mothers. The amount of cognitive stimulation in the child's early home environment is associated with the child's level of cognitive attainment. Children of adolescents may be raised by a grandparent. Although living with a grandparent may have positive effects on child outcomes, coresidence with the grandmother may have negative effects if the mother and grandmother are in conflict. Nurses need to stress the importance of the adolescent caring for the child even when other adults (e.g., mother or grandmother) are involved. The other adults present need education and support to allow optimum development of the infant and adolescent mother.

Several factors influence the mother-infant relationship. Maternal stresses, including changes in circumstances, influence coping ability and sensitivity to the infant's needs. Teenage mothers may consider an argument with a parent, boyfriend, or husband stressful, whereas adult mothers focus on problems directly involving the infant. Vocational and educational disadvantages of both teenage mothers and fathers further affect their coping abilities. It is important to recognize that not all adolescent mothers are alike. Some teenagers adjust well to the stresses and responsibilities of parenting, whereas others may lack the maturity or confidence to nurture optimally. When socioeconomic status is controlled for, it has been found that younger adolescent mothers have lower acceptance of their children compared with older adolescent mothers. A positive correlation exists between the total amount of social support and the frequency of appropriate maternal behavior. An assessment of the individual the adolescent believes is most supportive (e.g., a family member, her partner, a partner's family member, or a close friend) allows the nurse to help the young mother benefit from this support (see Family-Centered Care box).

The cognitive development of the adolescent influences the development of attitudes and realistic expectations regarding childbearing. To cope effectively and solve situational dilemmas, pregnant teenagers must be able to use the problem-solving approach to assess and evaluate consequences. The concrete thought and egocentrism of early adolescence can influence the mother's ability to evaluate the infant's needs. Adolescent mothers may lack knowledge of normal infant growth and development. This deficit may directly affect their perception, interpretation, and responsiveness to infant cues.

Infant characteristics also influence parental behavior. Teenage parents view their children as more temperamentally difficult than do adult parents. Temperamentally difficult infants have an adverse effect on the parents' sensitivity and responsiveness. Parent-infant interaction that is not mutually satisfying can also alter the parents' feelings of effectiveness and self-worth.

Adolescent Fathers

Little information is available about adolescent fathers. Most studies have small sample sizes and rely on reporting from the mother rather than the young man himself. Most teen fathers have a strong emotional commitment to and interest in their child (Lau, 2016). This involvement has positive effects on the mother's self-esteem and decreases her level of distress and depression. The teen mother and her mother largely influence the level of participation a teen father has with his child. Social supports and parenting classes are often lacking for adolescent fathers. The nurse should take advantage of opportunities to involve young fathers in educational programs.

Nursing Care Management

It is evident from the preceding discussion that nurses play a central role in meeting the needs of pregnant teenagers. The nurse may be the one to whom the young girl turns for help and guidance in her dilemma and on whom she relies for support and reassurance.

The first goal in nursing care of the pregnant teenager is to help her obtain health care whether she elects to continue or terminate the pregnancy. Typically, adolescents are reluctant to seek medical help, in part because of anxiety but more often because of a tendency to deny the pregnancy. Early prenatal care is essential for the welfare of both mother and infant. For guidelines, teaching, and general support measures during pregnancy, the reader is directed to the textbooks available on nursing care throughout the maternity cycle.

Basic to the implementation of any care program is communication and the establishment of a trusting relationship. Initially the adolescent may appear apathetic and display little interest in discussing her pregnancy. The nurse must make every effort to put the adolescent at ease and avoid undue pressure. The young girl may have encountered rejection and open criticism from authority figures and peers. Conveying a nonjudgmental and genuine caring acceptance of the adolescent and her goals will assist the nurse in gaining the adolescent's confidence and trust.

Communication takes time and patience. Asking open-ended questions and listening for cues will help identify physical, emotional, social, and cultural influences that might affect the adolescent's progress through the maternity cycle. Factors that might affect her physical status, such as smoking, drug use, and nutritional state, need to be explored and confronted. Each teenager represents a unique situation in terms of background, lifestyle, support structure, and coping mechanisms. Listening to the teenager and understanding the situation from her perspective are essential for a trusting relationship and effective communication.

The adolescent needs help to improve an altered self-image, a crucial factor in adolescence. Giving her as much individual attention as possible; being a sympathetic listener; providing the opportunity for her to know, support, and be supported by other girls in the same situation; and helping her experience success will facilitate progress toward achieving this goal.

The adolescent needs to know what is happening to her, what is expected of her, and how she can help in developing a care plan. Adolescents have their own ideas about the type of help and support they need. Nurses should consult with them and provide them an opportunity to share their ideas. It is important to jointly choose goals that the adolescent believes are beneficial, attainable, and able to be maintained over time. When developing a plan with a teen parent, the nurse should include the family, school, and community; involve the young father early in the relationship; and respect and understand the grandparents' role. The parents of the adolescent mother and the father of the child need to express feelings and attitudes about the situation. The nurse should not make assumptions about whether the girl wishes to have these persons involved in her decisions and care.

Direct postpartum care of adolescents to prevent subsequent pregnancies and enhance life outcomes for the teen parents and child. Health care programs that provide contraceptive services for the young mother at the time of her child's appointment are helpful. Merely dispensing contraception is not enough. Comprehensive programs to promote positive parenting, self-esteem, vocational or academic assessment, career goals, and family cohesiveness are necessary.

ADOLESCENT ABORTION

In 1973 the landmark US Supreme Court case *Roe v. Wade* concluded that individuals had the right to a first-trimester abortion. This right was not absolute but subject to certain state restrictions. Abortion is one of the most controversial moral issues in the United States. For example, many Americans believe that a pregnant woman should be able to obtain an abortion if her own life is endangered, if there is a strong chance that the fetus has a serious defect, or if the pregnancy is a result of a rape. However, some Americans do not believe that a woman should be able to have an abortion for any reason. The right to an abortion is also legally determined by the stage of pregnancy.

Many pregnant adolescents choose to continue their pregnancies and parent the child. From 2004 to 2013, the abortion rate fell more quickly for adolescents ages 15 to 19 years compared with women in any other age-group (Jatlaoui, Ewing, Mandel, et al., 2016). There are many possible explanations for this trend, including the possibility that access to abortion services for teens has decreased, that those who truly do not want to parent are abstaining from intercourse or using more effective methods of contraception, and that there is more social support for parenting among adolescents.

Under current federal constitutional law, minors have the right to obtain first-trimester abortions without parental consent unless otherwise specified by state law. (See the concept of "mature minor" and informed consent in Chapter 22. See also the Alan Guttmacher Institute website [http://www.guttmacher.org] for an update on state policies regarding adolescent abortion and state notification.) Legislation that mandates parental involvement as a requirement for adolescents who seek an abortion has generated considerable controversy. US Supreme Court rulings have held that it is not unconstitutional for states to impose parental notification requirements as long as pregnant adolescents who believe that this involvement would not be in their best interests are allowed to go to court without involving their parents and are legally permitted to make their own decisions. The American Academy of Pediatrics, Committee on Adolescence (2017) and several other health care organizations have reached a consensus that minors should not be compelled or required to involve their parents in this decision but should be encouraged to discuss their pregnancies with their parents and other responsible adults.

Abortion is a controversial and emotional issue and one that frequently confronts health care professionals involved in delivery of services to pregnant adolescents. Because the law in this area is unsettled and varies by state, nurses must stay informed of legal changes as they relate to reproductive rights of minors in the state in which they practice.

Other barriers to receiving an abortion include distance to the clinic, cost, and antiabortion harassment. Abortion services in the United States are offered primarily at freestanding abortion clinics, usually in major population centers. Abortions are not covered by many insurers, and the cost may be prohibitive to many women, especially adolescents.

The medical safety of a legal abortion has been well established. The mortality rate associated with teenage full-term pregnancy is much higher than the rate with abortion. A discussion of surgical procedures available is beyond the scope of this text. First-trimester abortions are performed as outpatient procedures and require local anesthesia or mild sedation only. Complication rates have been reported to be 1% or less. Problems that arise after abortion are endometritis, hemorrhage, Rh sensitization, genital tract injury, retained fetal elements, and (in rare cases) pulmonary embolism or death. Second-trimester abortions are more complicated and are associated with greater risk from hemorrhage. Women who have an induced abortion are no more likely than other women to experience problems in bearing a healthy baby in subsequent pregnancies.

Medical abortions are available for use in the United States for up to 9 weeks after the last menstrual period. Methotrexate, misoprostol, and mifepristone are drugs that have been used to induce early abortion; however, a combination of mifepristone-misoprostol is the preferred form. Misoprostol (Cytotec) is a prostaglandin analog that acts directly on the cervix to soften and dilate and on the uterine muscle to stimulate contractions. Mifepristone, formerly known as RU-486, was approved by the FDA in 2000. It works by binding to progesterone receptors and blocking the action of progesterone, which is necessary for maintaining pregnancy.

With any medical abortion regimen, the woman usually experiences bleeding and cramping. Side effects of the medications include nausea, vomiting, diarrhea, headache, dizziness, fever, and chills. These are attributed to misoprostol and usually subside in a few hours after administration.

Emergency contraception is designed to terminate pregnancy after sexual intercourse has occurred. Emergency contraceptives currently approved by the FDA include oral levonorgestrel, ulipristel acetate, a combination of estrogen and progestin pills (Yuzpe method), and placement of a copper IUD. The American Academy of Pediatrics, Committee on Adolescence (2014) suggests that levonorgestrel is the best emergency contraception method for adolescents because of its low side effect profile and increased effectiveness; however, ulipristel may be more effective in adolescents weighing more than 165 lb. Levonoregestrel is currently available to women age 17 years and older without a prescription and is considered effective when taken within 120 hours of unprotected intercourse (American Academy of Pediatrics, Committee on Adolescence, 2014).

Nursing Care Management

The adolescent considering an abortion will need help to explore the meaning of the various alternatives for elective abortion and consequences to herself and her significant others. It is often difficult for a woman to express her true feelings (e.g., what abortion means to her now and in the future and what support or regret her friends and peers may demonstrate). A calm, matter-of-fact approach on the part of the nurse can be helpful. Clarifying, restating, and reflecting statements; open-ended questions; and feedback are communication techniques that can be used to maintain a realistic focus on the situation and bring the woman's problems into the open. If family or friends cannot be involved, scheduling time for nursing personnel to give the necessary support is an essential component of the care plan.

Information about alternatives to abortion such as referral to adoption agencies or support services if the woman chooses to keep her baby is provided. If a decision is made to have an abortion, the adolescent must be assured of continued support. Information about what is entailed in various procedures, how much discomfort or pain can be expected, and what type of care is needed must be given. A discussion of the various feelings, including depression, guilt, regret, and relief, that the woman might experience after the abortion is needed. Information about community resources for postabortion counseling may be needed.

Most women report relief after an abortion, but some have temporary distress or mixed emotions. Evidence of long-term depression after elective abortion are inconclusive. Guilt and anxiety may occur more with young women, women with poor social support, multiparous women, and women with a history of psychiatric illness. Women having second-trimester abortions may have more emotional distress than women having abortions in the first trimester. Because symptoms can vary among women who have had abortions, nurses must assess women for grief reactions and facilitate the grieving process through active listening and nonjudgmental support and care.

CONTRACEPTION

Family planning services have developed and expanded during recent years, but the need for contraceptive services as part of the health care of adolescents remains great. The birth control pill and condom remain the most popular methods for adolescents; 3-month injectable contraception is more popular among lower-income adolescents. Adolescents commonly delay seeking contraceptive information. The typical interval from onset of sexual intercourse until the first visit for contraception is 1 year. A pregnancy scare is usually the precipitating event for the contraception appointment. Counseling about contraceptive options should be conducted in a manner that is consistent with the cognitive level of the adolescent. The adolescent should be given accurate information about the risks and benefits of each method before making a choice.

Many teenagers feel ambivalent regarding their sexual activity and avoid many contraceptives because their use seems too premeditated and implies that sex is planned rather than a spontaneous activity. Most of these girls believe that sex is all right if it is not planned. This may often play a role in adolescents delaying contraception, waiting for a relationship that is "close enough." A close relationship would allow adolescents to accept and acknowledge their sexual activity.

The choice of a safe and effective contraceptive method must be suited to the individual (Table 18.3). The choice is based on preference after the adolescent is informed of the benefits and disadvantages. Motivation is necessary for most methods. For example, the pill is effective if used correctly, but the adolescent must remember to take the pill at approximately the same time every day. For many young women, a medroxyprogesterone injection (Depo-Provera) is an ideal

TABLE 18.3 Advantages and Disadvantages of Contraceptive Methods in Adolescents

Method	Advantages	Disadvantages
Behavioral Methods		
Abstinence	100% effective in preventing STIs and pregnancy	Peer pressure to conform Relatively high failure rate from noncompliance
Withdrawal (coitus interruptus) Withdrawal of penis before ejaculation	No medical visit necessary	High failure rate Some seminal fluid often released before ejaculation Ejaculate at vaginal orifice may enter vagina No STI protection
Calendar method Refrain from intercourse during fertile period (time of ovulation)	Teaches adolescent girls about their menstrual cycle Encourages couple participation	High failure rate Requires a regular, predictable menstrual cycle (irregular menses are common for first 2 years after menarche) No STI protection
Barrier Methods		
Condom	Minimal side effects Easy to use Available without prescription Portable Provides protection against STIs	Requires consistent use Requires premeditated intent for sexual union May decrease sensation Misuse results in failure Decreased spontaneity
Male—Penile covering to trap sperm	Spermicidal condoms increase effectiveness for pregnancy and STI prevention Inexpensive compared with female condom	Latex sensitivity or allergies in a small percentage of people Improper use may lead to pregnancy or development of STI
Female—Inserted into vagina with base covering part of perineum; may be inserted 8 hours before intercourse	Female participation Made of polyurethane; no latex sensitivities and can be used with oil-based lubricants Provides protection from STIs	May be difficult to insert Noisy

Continued

TABLE 18.3 Advantages and Disadvantages of Contraceptive Methods in Adolescents—cont'd

Method	Advantages	Disadvantages
Diaphragm Cervical covering to prevent sperm from reaching egg Must be used in conjunction with spermicidal jelly May be inserted 4-6 hours before intercourse If inserted early, should be checked for placement before intercourse	Can be fitted in virgins Low failure rate when used correctly Few contraindications May be reused	High failure rate in adolescents because of inconvenience of use Requires consistent use Requires fitting and instruction by medical personnel Requires premeditated intent for sexual union Requires body awareness and comfort with touching oneself for insertion Minimal STI protection May increase incidence of urinary tract infection
Cervical cap Soft rubber dome with a firm but pliable rim; fits over base of the cervix close to the junction of the cervix and vaginal fornices	May be inserted hours before intercourse Insertion and removal similar to diaphragm	Available in only four sizes Must remain in place at least 6 hours after intercourse but no longer than 48 hours Not recommended for women with abnormal Papanicolaou test result, history of toxic shock syndrome, or difficulty with proper fitting No STI protection
Chemicals		
Spermicidal foam, jelly, cream, and suppositories Substance inserted into vagina to kill sperm	Available without prescription Inexpensive Easy to use No major health concerns	High failure rate unless combined with condom Possible for sperm to be ejaculated directly into uterine os, bypassing spermicide in vagina Must be used shortly before coitus; therefore requires interruption of sexual experience Repeated sexual union requires repeated application Requires premeditated intent for sexual union Messy Nonoxynol-9 associated with increased transmission of HIV to women; should not be used with anal sex in male partner sex for same reason No STI protection
Hormonal Methods		
Oral contraceptives Estrogen and progesterone-like compounds Inhibit ovulation by blocking release of gonadotropins from anterior pituitary gland	99% effective if used correctly Safe for adolescents Method of choice for most adolescents Administered by mouth Becomes a ritual not associated with sexual activity Regulates menses, decreases dysmenorrhea and acne, decreases menstrual flow Prevents ovarian and endometrial cancers Prevents functional ovarian cysts	Higher failure rate in adolescents than in older women Need to follow precise instructions; requires continued motivation, consistent use Requires prescription Price substantial for teenager No STI protection Possible side effects include headaches, missed or scanty periods, breakthrough bleeding, blood clot
Medroxyprogesterone acetate (Depo-Provera) Progestin that suppresses hormonal cycle and prevents ovulation Injection given every 3 months	No interruption of intercourse Invisible method	No STI protection Possible side effects include significant weight gain, decreased bone density, decreased HDLs, irregular menses or amenorrhea, decreased libido, depression Fertility perhaps delayed after discontinuation Must return to care provider every 3 months for injection US Food and Drug Administration recommends discontinuation after 2 years because of decreased bone density
Ortho Evra transdermal system 4.5-cm-square patch with norelgestromin and ethinyl estradiol Hormonal patch applied to skin weekly for 3 weeks per month Suppresses ovulation, thickens cervical mucus, and thins endometrium	88.2% effective in perfect users Simple to use Regular menstrual cycles Not associated with sexual activity Avoids first-pass metabolism, resulting in more constant levels	Not recommended for women >90 kg (198 lb) Possible side effects include skin reaction at site, nausea, headache, dysmenorrhea, and breast tenderness Slight increase in risk of blood clot formation over combination oral contraceptive pill Patch may be visible No STI protection

TABLE 18.3 Advantages and Disadvantages of Contraceptive Methods in Adolescents—cont'd

Method	Advantages	Disadvantages
NuvaRing Etonogestrel plus ethinyl estradiol Soft, flexible, transparent ring placed in vagina for 3 weeks Suppresses ovulation	99.3% effective Immediate return to ovulation at discontinuation May leave in place during sexual intercourse Avoids first-pass metabolism, resulting in more constant levels No spermicide needed No vaginal erosion No weight gain	Device may be felt by female or partner during sexual intercourse Device may fall out Possible side effects include headache, vaginitis, leukorrhea, nausea, and breakthrough bleeding May have late withdrawal bleeding requiring placement of ring during menses No STI protection
Levonorgestrel intrauterine system (Mirena) T-shaped intrauterine device that releases 20 mcg/dl of levonorgestrel Inserted within 7 days of menses and remains in place for 5 years Thickens cervical mucus and inhibits sperm mobility and function	>99% effective Effectively prevents fertilization, resulting in low rates of ectopic pregnancy Reduced length and quantity of menstrual bleeding Reduced dysmenorrhea No weight gain	Risk of perforation at time of insertion 2%-12% expulsion rate Not recommended in nulliparous women or women not in monogamous relationships Possible side effects include abdominal pain, headache, vaginal discharge, and breast pain No STI protection
Etonogestrel implant (Implanon) 40 × 2 mm implanted rod Progestin-only method Suppresses ovulation	>99% effective Efficacy not user dependent Provides 3 years of protection Single rod insertion and removal Palpable but not visible after insertion	Irregular menstrual bleeding Other less common side effects include headache, vaginitis, weight gain No STI protection
Emergency or Postcoital Contraception		
Emergency contraception works in one of three ways: by suppressing or delaying ovulation, by preventing the meeting of sperm and egg, or by preventing implantation Progestin-only pill given within 72 hours of intercourse *or* Insertion of a copper-releasing intrauterine device up to 7 days after unprotected intercourse	Useful in unplanned sexual intercourse or contraceptive failure May be given in advance for emergency use Available without prescription for adults	No STI protection May cause nausea if combination method used May change timing of next menstrual cycle

HDL, High-density lipoprotein; *HIV,* human immunodeficiency virus; *STI,* sexually transmitted infection.

choice because it is extremely effective and is administered every 12 weeks, but side effects such as weight gain and decreased bone mineralization may make it undesirable. Sexually active adolescents need to know that contraceptive devices other than condoms do not prevent STIs. Condom use is still important and must be discussed with all sexually and non–sexually active adolescents (see Community and Home Health Considerations box).

Confidentiality is a critical issue when discussing contraception with adolescents. Privacy is important to adolescents as they struggle to forge a personal identity and establish social relationships. Adolescents are particularly concerned about the judgments of others. The predominant belief among many health professionals is that parental notification is important but that the "parents' rights" view is not necessarily sensitive to the health needs and basic rights of youth. No evidence substantiates the belief that providing contraceptive guidance contributes to sexual irresponsibility and promiscuity.

Nursing Care Management

Nurses are often involved in providing education about contraception. Such education is ideally combined with ongoing sex education. Although sexual abstinence is a highly desirable form of contraception for teenagers, nurses working with adolescents must recognize that teens feel multiple pressures to engage in sexual intercourse. Postponing sexual involvement requires effective communication and decision-making skills. Adolescents benefit from role-playing refusal skills and opportunities to practice making decisions in a safe environment. Information about safe sex must be provided, and role-playing how to discuss condom use with a partner is helpful to teenagers.

Education concerning contraception should be provided in both verbal and written form. All available methods, including their benefits, disadvantages, and side effects, should be discussed. Concrete, concise language must be used; demonstrations of how to use the contraceptive

COMMUNITY AND HOME HEALTH CONSIDERATIONS

*Steps for Male Condom Use**

1. Be careful when opening the package; handle the condom gently, and check for breaks or holes in the condom.
2. Squeeze a dab of contraceptive jelly or cream into the tip of the condom.
3. Put on the condom as soon as erection occurs and before any vaginal, anal, or oral contact with the penis.
4. Unroll the condom on the erect penis, leaving about 1.25 cm (0.5 inch) of space at the tip of the condom.
5. Apply some of the contraceptive cream or jelly around the vagina or anus before entry.
6. Hold the rim of the condom in place when withdrawing the penis.
7. Take the condom off away from the partner's genitalia.
8. Throw the used condom away. Never reuse a condom.

*For additional information on acquired immunodeficiency syndrome and human immunodeficiency virus, contact the CDC National Prevention Information Network, PO Box 6003, Rockville, MD 20849; 800-458-5231; email: info@cdcnpin.org; http://www.cdcnpin.org; CDC National AIDS Hotline, 800-342-AIDS, Spanish: 800-344-7432, TTY: 888-480-3739; and National Center for HIV/AIDS, Viral Hepatitis, STD, and TB Prevention, email: cdcinfo@cdc.gov; https://www.cdc.gov/hiv and https://www.cdc.gov/nchhstp.

should be provided; and adolescents should repeat all instructions in their own words. If teenagers are using oral contraceptive pills, they should be encouraged to use a daily activity as a reminder or cue to take the pill. A knowledgeable phone triage person should be available for questions and concerns. Parents or other important adults may be included in all discussions, with the adolescent's permission. An organization that provides education and services for adolescents, including both individual and group counseling, is the Planned Parenthood Federation of America.* It has branches in most cities in the United States.

SEXUAL ASSAULT (RAPE)

Typically, stranger rape is what comes to mind when one thinks of sexual assault; however, more than half of assaults are committed by someone known to the survivor. Although both males and females can be sexually assaulted, females are at greatest risk. Adolescents are at high risk for sexual assault; other high-risk groups include survivors of childhood sexual or physical abuse; persons who are disabled; persons with substance abuse problems; sex workers; persons who are poor or homeless; and persons living in prisons, institutions, or areas of military conflict. Sexual assault remains underreported for multifactorial reasons.

An understanding of the legal definitions of sexual assault, rape, acquaintance rape, and statutory rape is essential for the nurse to identify, treat, and manage adolescent victims (Box 18.4).

Statutory rape laws have been revised in many states across the country. The motivation for tougher laws and greater enforcement is to decrease teen pregnancy, increase male responsibility, and decrease welfare dependency. Traditionally, statutory rape laws have been concerned with the protection of girls. In the past 20 years, many laws have been rewritten to be gender neutral. Statutory rape laws require reporting to child protective services or local law enforcement. One risk of strict

*434 W. 33rd St., New York, NY 10001; 212-541-7800 or 800-230-7526; http://www.plannedparenthood.org.

BOX 18.4 Definitions of Sexual Assaults

Sexual assault—Comprehensive term that includes various types of forced or inappropriate sexual activity. Sexual assault includes both physical and psychologic coercion, as well as touch, penetration, and other sexual contact.

Rape—Forced sexual intercourse that occurs by physical force or psychologic coercion. Rape includes vaginal, anal, or oral penetration by body parts or inanimate objects.

Acquaintance rape (date rape)—Applied to situations in which the assailant and victim know each other.

Statutory rape—Consensual sexual contact by a person 18 years of age or older with a person under the age of consent or unable to consent because of developmental disability. Age of consent varies by state.

statutory rape enforcement is that girls may not seek health care for reproductive care, prenatal care, or domestic violence. Young people may fear not only for themselves but also for their partners. However, sexual coercion of teens by adults remains a problem and results in STIs and adolescent pregnancy.

In the United States the legal age of sexual consent varies among each state but in general, it is illegal for anyone to have sexual intercourse with a child under the age of 16 years. These laws protect the health and safety of children. When consensuality is considered in statutory rape laws and cases, it implies that adolescents are morally and socially responsible for sexual contact that occurs with adults. This does not afford adolescents the same protections provided to children younger than age 12 years (Oudekerk, Guarnera, & Reppucci, 2014).

Nurses can obtain information about their state statutory rape reporting responsibilities from state or local child protective services agencies, legal counsel, rape crisis organizations, state or local law enforcement agencies, or the state nurses' association. The limits of confidentiality should be clearly reviewed with each adolescent patient before beginning the interview about sexual activity.

Diagnostic Evaluation

Rape victims may exhibit a variety of reactions (Box 18.5), and the circumstances of the initial medical evaluation may be frightening and stressful. The initial contact with the rape victim must be supportive because the interrogation and associated activities have the potential to add to the trauma of the sexual assault. First of all, the victim needs to know that she (or he) is (1) all right and (2) not being blamed for the situation.

It is important to obtain a clear account of the circumstances of an alleged rape without forcing the victim to relive a painful experience. Information includes the date, time, location, and an accurate description of any type of sexual contact. The physical examination is carried out as soon as possible because physical evidence deteriorates rapidly. The victim should not bathe or shower before the examination.

NURSING ALERT

It is common for rape victims to delay seeking help, especially in cases of acquaintance or date rape. Nurses can be most supportive by acknowledging the painful and sometimes confusing feelings that surround such experiences and by focusing on the fact that the victim is seeking assistance now.

The young person is always told in advance in understandable terms exactly what to expect in the way of tests and procedures, and the explanation is accompanied by strong emotional support. The victim is examined thoroughly, including nongenital areas, for evidence of injury that might substantiate the use of force.

BOX 18.5 Clinical Manifestations of Rape Victims

May Display a Variety of Emotions and Behaviors:

Hysterical crying
Giggling
Agitation
Feelings of degradation
Anger and rage
Helplessness
Nervousness
Rapid mood swings
Appearing calm and controlled (masking inner turmoil)
Confused
Self-blame
Fear—of the rape and of injury

Evidence of Physical Force From:

Roughness
Nonbrutal beating (slapping)
Brutal beating (slugging, kicking, beating repeatedly with fists)
Choking or gagging

Medical Examination Provides Evidence of:

Penetration
Ejaculation
Use of force

The forensic examination of a sexual assault victim must follow strict legal requirements. The medical record may provide key evidence for the legal case. Practitioners specially trained for rape examination should be used when possible. Nurses are often members of this group and are known as sexual assault nurse examiners (SANEs). Evaluation for STIs is an important part of the evaluation. The following procedures are recommended for the initial examination: NAATs for chlamydia and gonorrhea; wet mount and culture or point-of-care testing of a vaginal swab specimen for trichomoniasis; and a serum sample for HIV infection, hepatitis B, and syphilis. Decisions to perform these tests should be made on an individual basis. Repeat testing for chlamydia and gonorrhea can be done within 1 to 2 weeks and 1 to 2 months, if prophylactic treatment was not administered (Workowski, Bolan, & Centers for Disease Control and Prevention, 2015). Serologic tests for syphilis can be repeated 6 weeks and 3 months, and HIV testing can be repeated at 6 weeks, 3 months, and 6 months after the assault if infection in the assailant could not be ruled out (Workowski, Bolan, & Centers for Disease Control and Prevention, 2015).

Prophylactic treatment for chlamydia, gonorrhea, and trichomoniasis is recommended. Vaccination for hepatitis B should be administered if the patient has not been previously vaccinated. Follow-up doses of vaccine should be administered 1 to 2 and 4 to 6 months after the first dose. Female victims should be provided with emergency contraception. The recommendation for HIV prophylaxis varies depending on the geographic area, the circumstances of the assault, and the known HIV status of the perpetrator. The Centers for Disease Control and Prevention (Workowski, Bolan, & Centers for Disease Control and Prevention, 2015) maintains updates and recommendations for treatment of STIs incurred as a result of sexual assault.*

*https://www.cdc.gov/std/tg2015/.

Therapeutic Management

Adolescents who have been raped arrive at the emergency department or practitioner's office under a variety of circumstances. They are usually brought by parents, friends, or police officers, but some may seek medical help on their own. It is advisable to obtain parental consent for examination, but the examination may be performed without parental consent if the adolescent is mature and the parents are unavailable. A female observer or chaperone should be present during the history and examination of female victims who are examined by a male practitioner. Whether a parent should be present during the examination is determined on an individual basis. The parent's presence is usually encouraged if the parent is supportive and the young person agrees.

Nursing Care Management

Many of the approaches that have been described for sexually abused children (see Chapter 14) also apply to adolescents. Sexual assault is a devastating experience with long-lasting effects. The primary goal of nursing care is to avoid inflicting further stress on the adolescent, who is often angry, confused, frightened, embarrassed, and filled with self-blame. The nurse must do everything possible to reduce the stress of the interrogation and examination. Although most health professionals and law enforcement officers are sensitive to the needs of adolescents and attempt to make the process as nonstressful as possible, the nurse should be alert to cues that indicate the victim is being overstressed.

Follow-up care of the rape victim is essential and extends over a long period. The health-compromising responses to sexual assault include posttraumatic stress disorder (PTSD), anxiety, and depression. PTSD is the most common mental health sequela of sexual violence, with rates of 16% to 60% among women (Ullman & Peter-Hagene, 2016). Aside from the universal need for emotional support, the needs of rape victims vary widely and depend on the nature of the incident, the victim's age when the rape occurred, the physical and emotional injuries sustained by the victim, the legal actions being considered as a result, the resources available for informal support, and the anticipated reactions of persons in the informal support network (see Family-Centered Care box).*

FAMILY-CENTERED CARE

Supporting the Rape Victim's Parents

In addition to the needs of the adolescent rape victim, the nurse should also be sensitive to the needs and reactions of the adolescent's parents. Some parents will be angry and blame the adolescent; others will feel guilty and embarrassed. Many reactions can be expected at the time of the incident, ranging from despair to extreme agitation. Frequently, the parents require as much support and reassurance as the victim. Agitated, angry, or incapacitated parents are unable to provide support for their adolescent. Meeting their needs can foster their ability to support the teenager during the crisis.

HEALTH CONDITIONS WITH A BEHAVIORAL COMPONENT

ANOREXIA NERVOSA AND BULIMIA NERVOSA

Anorexia nervosa (AN) is an eating disorder characterized by a refusal to maintain a minimally normal body weight, intense fear of gaining

*For information about local organizations, contact National Organization for Victim Assistance, Courthouse Square, 510 King St., Suite 424, Alexandria, VA 22314; 800-879-6682 or 703-535-6682; http://www.trynova.org.

weight along with behavior that interferes with weight gain, and a body image disturbance (Herpertz-Dahlmann, 2015). It is a disorder with social, psychologic, behavioral, cultural, and physiologic components resulting in significant morbidity and mortality. AN is characterized by a distorted body image with adolescents' self-confidence relying on their weight and body shape. The disorder is a clinical diagnosis listed in the *Diagnostic and Statistical Manual of Mental Disorders, Fifth Edition* (DSM-5) with two distinct subtypes: restricting type and being-eating/purging type (Herpertz-Dahlmann, 2015). Individuals with AN are described as perfectionists, academically high achievers, conforming, and conscientious.

Bulimia nervosa (from the Greek meaning "ox hunger") refers to an eating disorder similar to AN. Bulimia nervosa (BN) is characterized by repeated episodes of binge eating followed by inappropriate compensatory behaviors, such as self-induced vomiting; misuse of laxatives, diuretics, or other medications; fasting; or excessive exercise (Herpertz-Dahlmann, 2015). The binge behavior consists of secretive, frenzied consumption of large amounts of high-calorie (or "forbidden") foods during a brief time (usually about 2 hours). The binge is counteracted by a variety of weight-control methods (purging), including self-induced vomiting, diuretic and laxative abuse, and rigorous exercise. These binge-purge cycles are followed by self-deprecating thoughts, a depressed mood, and an awareness that the eating pattern is abnormal.

Eating disorder not otherwise specified (EDNOS) is an additional diagnosis for eating disorders. EDNOS includes subthresholds of AN and BN, as well as purging disorder, night eating syndrome, and a residual category for clinically significant problems meeting the definition of a feeding or eating disorder but not satisfying the criteria for any other disorder or condition (American Psychiatric Association, 2013).

One type of EDNOS is **binge eating disorder** (BED), a distinct diagnostic category that is very similar to BN, with the exception that purging is not involved. Binge episodes may be associated with a cluster of symptoms, including eating rapidly; eating until uncomfortably full; eating large amounts in the absence of hunger; eating in secret due to embarrassment; and feeling disgusted, depressed, or guilty after eating.

Epidemiology

Among adolescents in the United States, the incidence of AN is estimated at 0.5% to 2%, and the incidence of bulimia ranges between 0.9% and 3% with up to 10% of cases attributable to males (Campbell & Peebles, 2014). The incidence of BED is not as well documented but estimations range from 1% to 5% with a similar prevalence among males and females (Herpertz-Dahlmann, 2015). The prevalence of disordered eating reaches up to 40% of adolescents (Herpertz-Dahlmann, 2015). The peak age of onset for AN is 13 to 18 years, whereas the onset of BN occurs at an older age of 16 to17 years (Campbell & Peebles, 2014). The frequency of young people under age 12 years who report eating-disordered tendencies is increasing (Herpertz-Dahlmann, 2015).

The epidemiology of these eating disorders is difficult to accurately assess because of changes in diagnostic criteria over time and because the methods of detection, primarily self-report, may not be reliable in an illness characterized by denial and secrecy. Most resources report an increase in the incidence of AN and BN with the use of the diagnosis criteria in DSM-5, with one systematic review reporting a 23% increase in AN and a 28% increase in BN (Herpertz-Dahlmann, 2015).

Pathophysiology

No consensus exists on the pathophysiology of AN and BN. A combination of genetic, neurochemical, psychodevelopmental, sociocultural, and environmental factors appear to cause the disorder (Campbell & Peebles, 2014). Dieting and body dissatisfaction appear to be common to the initiation of both AN and BN. Also characteristic is a childhood preoccupation with being thin reinforced by sociocultural and environmental factors supporting the concepts of ideal body shape. Many sports and artistic endeavors that emphasize leanness (e.g., ballet and running) and sports in which the scoring is partly subjective (e.g., figure skating and gymnastics) or where weight class is prerequisite to participation (e.g., wrestling) have been associated with a higher incidence of eating disorders (Matzkin, Curry, & Whitlock, 2015).

The prominent physiologic changes that occur as a result of weight loss have raised suspicions of a prominent physiologic disturbance as a causative factor. Because most of these physiologic disturbances resolve with the normalization of body weight and healthy eating, this argues against their role as a primary cause. The neurotransmitter serotonin affects appetite control, sexual and social behavior, stress responses, and mood, and possibly accounts for some of the changes seen in patients with AN. BED is also associated with dopamine in the nucleus accumbens portion of the brain that is programmed for reward and motivation. The significance of these changes and their connection to eating disorders are not well understood (Kreipe, 2016).

There are no strong empirical data to indicate that one particular family prototype is responsible for the development of an eating disorder. However, many experts have associated the development of an eating disorder with family characteristics such as an adolescent perception of high parental expectations for achievement and appearance, difficulty managing conflict, poor communication styles, enmeshment and occasionally estrangement from family members, devaluation of the mother or the maternal role, marital tension, and mood and anxiety disorders. Furthermore, a genetic predisposition to anxiety, depression, or obsessive-compulsive disorder may increase the likelihood of developing an eating disorder (Kreipe, 2016). Families struggling with an eating disorder have been characterized as often having difficulties responding positively to the changing physical and emotional needs of the adolescent. Results of twin studies suggest that both genetic and environmental factors contribute to the development of AN. A concordance rate for AN appears higher in monozygotic twins compared with dizygotic twins (Wade, Fairweather-Schmidt, Zhu, et al., 2015). There also appears to be a higher prevalence of affective disorders and alcoholism in first-degree relatives of patients with eating disorders (Trace, Baker, Peñas-Lledó, et al., 2013).

Individuals with eating disorders commonly have psychiatric problems, including affective disorder, anxiety disorder, obsessive-compulsive disorder, and personality disorder. Adult women with eating disorders were found to have higher rates of obsessive-compulsive behavior traits in their childhood. Persons with eating disorders have also been found to have higher reported rates of substance abuse, with alcohol problems being more common in those with BN than AN (Kreipe, 2016). It is important to note that many of the clinical findings are directly related to the state of starvation and improve with weight gain. Research continues in an effort to better understand the etiology and pathogenesis of eating disorders.

Clinical Manifestations

The most obvious manifestation of AN is the severe and profound weight loss induced by self-imposed starvation. The adolescents identify with this skeleton-like appearance and do not regard this body type as abnormal or ugly. Adolescents with AN often eat small amounts of food or play with food on their plates to give the impression that they are eating adequately and not experiencing disturbances in their eating habits. This can lead friends and family to disregard the possibility of AN. The adolescents can display a marked preoccupation with food—preparing meals for others, talking about food, hoarding food.

Many become obsessed with fasting and engage in frequent strenuous exercise. The binge-purge subtype of AN is characterized with chewing then spitting out the food rather than swallowing, or laxative usage to speed up the weight-loss process (Kreipe, 2016) (see Critical Thinking Case Study box).

CRITICAL THINKING CASE STUDY

Anorexia Nervosa

Jane is a 13-year-old girl whose grades have been excellent and whom the teachers describe as a "model student." Recently, Jane's teacher told the nurse practitioner that Jane's parents were in the middle of a "messy divorce." In addition, several of Jane's friends told the nurse practitioner that they are concerned about Jane because she runs every day at lunchtime and seldom eats lunch with them. Jane told her friends that she gained weight over the winter months and that she is running because she wants to qualify for the track team this spring. At the time of her routine health interview and sports physical examination, the nurse practitioner notes that Jane's oral temperature is 36° C (96.8° F) and that she weighs 34 kg (75 lb). Jane has lost 9 kg (20 lb) since her last sports physical.

1. Evidence—Is there sufficient evidence to draw any conclusions about Jane's behavior?
2. Assumptions—Describe some underlying assumptions about the following:
   a. Personality characteristics of individuals with anorexia nervosa (AN)
   b. Factors influencing the development of AN
   c. Clinical manifestations of AN
   d. Treatment of AN
3. What priorities for nursing care should be established for Jane at this time?
4. Does the evidence objectively support your argument (conclusion)?

Answers are available at http://evolve.elsevier.com/wong/ncic.

Young people with AN tend to withdraw from peer relationships and engage in self-imposed social isolation. They continually strive for perfection, which may be demonstrated in other compulsive behaviors. They are usually overachievers, and their schoolwork is very important to them.

In the wake of the severe weight loss, these girls and young women exhibit physical signs of altered metabolic activity. They develop secondary amenorrhea, bradycardia, lowered body temperature, decreased blood pressure, and cold intolerance. They have dry skin and brittle nails and develop lanugo. The changes are usually reversible with adequate weight gain and improved nutritional status.

Bulimia is more common in older adolescent girls and young women; males with bulimia are less common. BN patients may be of average or slightly above-average weight. The diagnosis is confirmed, according to the American Psychiatric Association's DSM-5, by at least one binge-eating episode per week for the preceding 3 months. Although persons with bulimia have many issues in common with those who have other eating disorders, impulse control and satiety regulation are important problems in bulimia. Many individuals with bulimia begin with only occasional binges and purges "just for fun," enjoying the control over their weight while eating amounts of food that would normally produce obesity. As the disease progresses, the frequency of binges increases, the amount of food consumed increases, and they gradually lose control over the binge-purge cycle. The purging provides relief from feelings of guilt resulting from the enormous amounts of food consumed. The family becomes angry, and the individual with bulimia becomes frightened, frustrated, and increasingly guilt ridden, which only increases the symptoms in the self-destructive cycle.

TABLE 18.4 Characteristics of Individuals With Eating Disorders

Factors	Anorexia Nervosa	Bulimia Nervosa
Food	Turns away from food to cope	Turns to food to cope
Personality	Avoids intimacy Introverted Negates feminine role	Seeks intimacy Extroverted Aspires to feminine role
Behaviors	"Model" child Obsessive-compulsive	Often acts out Impulsive
School	High achiever	Variable school performance
Control	Maintains rigid control	Loses control
Body image	Body image distortion	Less frequent body image distortion
Health	Denies illness	Recognizes illness Health fluctuates
Weight	Body weight <85% of expected norm	Within 2.3-7 kg (5-15 lb) of normal body weight or may be overweight
Sexuality	Usually not sexually active	Often sexually active

The frequency of binging can be anywhere from once per week to seven or eight times per day. Because persons with bulimia usually binge on high-calorie foods, especially sweets, ice cream, and pastries, insulin production is stimulated to cope with the added carbohydrates. When the food is vomited, the unused insulin stimulates hunger and the desire to eat.

Diagnostic Evaluation

Diagnosis is made on the basis of clinical manifestations and conformity to the criteria established by the DSM-5 (American Psychiatric Association, 2013). Table 18.4 lists the differences between AN and BN.

History and Physical Examination

A complete history and physical examination are important to rule out other causes for weight loss. The medical assessment of an eating disorder focuses on the complications of altered nutritional status and purging. A careful history assesses weight changes, dietary patterns, and the frequency and severity of purging and excessive exercise. Purging behaviors include vomiting or other methods such as abuse of laxatives, enemas, diuretics, anorexic drugs, caffeine, or other stimulants. Measure the patient's weight and height and evaluate it for appropriateness according to standard weight for height, age, and sex determined according to the percentile of his or her expected body weight or BMI.

Particularly important parts of the physical examination are vital sign measurement (heart rate and blood pressure, both supine and standing, and body temperature). Hypotension, bradycardia, and hypothermia are often seen in association with extremely low weight. Dry skin, lanugo, acrocyanosis, and breast atrophy are findings that have been associated with AN. Distinctive hand lesions (Russell sign) have also been observed; the backs of the hands are often scarred and cut from repeated abrasion of the skin against the maxillary incisors during self-induced vomiting. Other findings include swelling of the parotid and submandibular glands and erosion of the enamel of the anterior teeth because of chronic acid exposure from vomiting.

Prolongation of the QT interval may be detected in some patients. Mitral valve prolapse (MVP) may also develop. An abdominal examination is important to detect intestinal dilation from chronic severe constipation as a result of decreased intestinal motility. Finally, a neurologic examination assesses for other causes of weight loss or vomiting such as evidence of brain tumor.

Screening Tools

All patients in high-risk categories for eating disorders should be screened during routine office visits. The medical history is most important for diagnosing eating disorders because the physical examination may be normal, especially early in the illness. A number of screening questionnaires are available to assist with the interview. For example, with the SCOFF Questionnaire, 1 point is scored for every "yes." A score of 2 or more indicates a likely case of AN or BN. The questions related to the mnemonic SCOFF are as follows (Trent, Moreira, Colwell, et al., 2013):

S—Do you make yourself *sick* because you feel uncomfortably full?
C—Do you worry that you have lost *control* over how much you eat?
O—Have you recently lost more than 6.4 kg (14 lb or *one* stone) in a 3-month period?
F—Do you believe yourself to be *fat* when others say that you are too thin?
F—Would you say that *food* dominates your life?

Laboratory Assessments

The initial laboratory assessment for a patient with an eating disorder should include a complete blood count to evaluate for anemia and other hematologic abnormalities. An erythrocyte sedimentation rate or C-reactive protein may be ordered to detect evidence of inflammation. These levels should be low in an eating disorder. Electrolytes should be measured, along with calcium, magnesium, phosphorus, blood urea nitrogen, and creatinine, as well as urinalysis (including specific gravity) to detect water loading. A human chorionic gonadotropin measurement is assessed to rule out pregnancy in patients with prolonged amenorrhea. In females with amenorrhea, thyroid function tests and measurement of serum prolactin and follicle-stimulating hormone can help rule out prolactinoma (hormone-secreting pituitary tumor), hyperthyroidism, hypothyroidism, or ovarian failure. A bone density study may be ordered to detect bone loss, which is a complication of AN. Other tests are included based on findings of the physical examination.

Complications of Eating Disorders

Many potential complications can occur as a result of starvation and persistent purging. Some of these are osteoporosis, cardiac impairments, cognitive changes, difficulties in psychologic functioning, gastrointestinal dysfunction (e.g., slowed motility, symptoms of nausea and bloating), endocrinologic changes, electrolyte abnormalities (especially hypokalemia and metabolic alkalosis), dental erosions, enlarged salivary glands, and infertility.

AN has been associated with MVP, QT-interval prolongation, and heart failure. MVP is a common finding in patients with AN, affecting 32% to 60% of patients compared with 6% to 22% in the general population. This may be because of an increased ability to detect the disorder in patients with intravascular volume depletion consistent with the state of starvation.

The risk of heart failure is greatest in the first 2 weeks of refeeding in patients with an eating disorder. Patients with moderate to severe AN (e.g., approximately 10% below ideal body weight) are at risk for the refeeding syndrome during the first 2 to 3 weeks of treatment. **Refeeding syndrome** consists of cardiovascular, neurologic, and hematologic complications that occur because of shifts in phosphate from extracellular to intracellular spaces in individuals who have total body phosphorus depletion as a result of malnutrition. Refeeding syndrome can cause cardiac arrest and delirium. The risk is reduced by slower refeeding, replacing phosphorus, and carefully avoiding a high sodium intake. Carefully monitoring serum electrolytes and observing for signs of edema or congestive heart failure are important during refeeding.

Amenorrhea used to be a diagnostic criteria for AN in the DSM-IV; however, many women do not experience amenorrhea and were at risk for being underdiagnosed. In addition, men were excluded from the AN diagnoses with the DSM-IV amenorrhea criteria. Amenorrhea may occur with AN patients as a result of low levels of follicle-stimulating hormone and luteinizing hormone. Menses is usually restored within 6 months of achieving 90% of the ideal body weight.

Therapeutic Management

The treatment and management of AN involve three major thrusts: (1) reinstitution of normal nutrition or reversal of the severe state of malnutrition, (2) resolution of disturbed patterns of family interaction, and (3) individual psychotherapy to correct deficits and distortions in psychologic functioning. Treatment of eating disorders requires interventions of an interdisciplinary team composed of a primary practitioner, nurse, dietitian, and mental health provider with pediatric and adolescent health care experience. Because of the psychogenic nature of the disorder, the treatment may be long.

Many adolescents with AN are treated on an outpatient basis. However, adolescents who have severe malnutrition, electrolyte disturbances, vital sign abnormalities, or psychiatric disturbances (e.g., severe depression or suicidal ideation) may require hospitalization. Persons with BN may benefit from cognitive-behavioral therapy, psychotherapy, family-based therapy, and nutrition counseling (Kreipe, 2016).

Nutrition Interventions

The initial goal is to treat the life-threatening malnutrition and to restore dietary stability and weight gain. This may necessitate intravenous or tube feeding if the malnutrition is severe. The patient should avoid rapid weight gain because it has been associated with severe metabolic abnormalities in some patients, such as refeeding syndrome, which consists of cardiovascular, neurologic, and hematologic complications that occur when nutritional replacement is given too rapidly. This syndrome can be avoided with slow refeeding and the addition of phosphorus when total body phosphorus is depleted. Treatment goal weights are individualized and based on age, height, stage of puberty, premorbid weight, and previous growth charts. In young women who have reached menarche, resumption of menses is an objective measure of return to biologic health.

Dietary interventions are combined with behavioral therapy to improve the underlying psychologic misconception about the weight loss. Another aspect of treatment is to relieve the anxiety related to eating and the depression that accompanies the disorder. Weight gain alone cannot be considered a cure for the disease and is an unreliable sign of progress. Relapses are frequent as the person reverts to previous eating patterns when removed from the therapeutic environment.

The dietitian should be experienced in working with children and adolescents and understand how to implement a dietary plan with sufficient calories needed for weight restoration. The plan needs to be firm but flexible. Letting the patient participate in setting up a food plan through motivational interviewing and teaching food exchanges to patients and parents is important so they can make food choices that will promote weight restoration. The goals of weight restoration are to avoid serious medical complications and restore cognitive functioning to derive the maximum benefit from psychotherapy. The least intrusive method for weight restoration should be used, only resorting to nasogastric or intravenous feeds when other strategies have failed. A reasonable goal for weight gain is approximately 1 kg (2 lb) per week. Pushing for more rapid weight gain can result in increasing anxiety or depression and result in bulimia or more severe relapses.

Psychotherapy

Individual psychotherapy is aimed at helping the young person resolve the adolescent identity crisis, particularly as it relates to a distorted body image. It is essential that adolescents rely on their own thinking, become more realistic in self-appraisal, and become capable of living as self-directed, competent individuals who enjoy life without manipulating the body and its functions. Psychotherapy focuses on helping the young person resolve the adolescent identity crisis, particularly when it results in a distorted body image.

If the disorder is related to a dysfunctional family situation, therapy is most successful when it is started soon after the onset of illness and directed toward disengagement and redirection of malfunctioning processes in the family. The family therapist's goal is to address dysfunctional roles, conflicts, alliances, and patterns that the eating disorder is precipitating or maintaining, while helping family members deal with the eating disorder. Some targets for intervention include control, individuation, communication, expression of feelings, realistic expectations, perfectionism, performance, achievement, marital relationship, and parental attitudes toward dieting and exercise.

Behavioral Therapy

Behavioral modification, usually through cognitive-behavioral therapy or motivational interviewing, has met varying degrees of success. The goal is to increase the patient's feelings of control and responsibility toward achieving recovery. Providing privileges or activities for weight gain or positive eating behaviors may be successful, but treatment should also address the conflict precipitating the disorder. Weight restoration as an outpatient is accomplished with behavioral contracts negotiated between the therapists and patient. The goal is to increase the patient's feelings of control and responsibility toward achieving recovery. The contract can stipulate at what weight tube feedings will be implemented. Realistic goals are set with the patient, including rewards for achievement that include special privileges or outings and consequences such as restrictions on exercise or increased consumption of a feared food. For inpatients, the contract for foods might be negotiated as food exchanges or number of calories. One suggested approach begins with 1200 calories and increases by small calorie increments each day or week. Inpatients need to be closely supervised by the nursing staff during the meal and for 1 to 3 hours after the meal. If the agreed-on number of calories is not consumed, there might be a provision for the intake of a nutritional supplement (Stice, South, & Shaw, 2012). More effectiveness trials and comparative studies are needed to enhance the treatment of eating disorders.

The team responsible for the management of young people with AN arranges a carefully structured environment. First, there must be consistency. The team decides on an approach and adheres to it. The plan is structured with reality testing regarding caloric intake and body image perception as an essential component. The team members provide a unified front to avoid any possibility of manipulation or inconsistency. Second, all team members are involved; responsibility for the program cannot be left to one person. The role and boundaries of each member are clearly spelled out. Third, continuity of team members is important; it is helpful to have the same team members all the time. Fourth, communication among team members is essential. Communication with the patient regarding what is expected is also important. Sometimes the limit setting may seem unreasonable. If the adolescent does not understand the rationale for the limits, he or she may sabotage the entire program. It is also important to communicate with the family. Fifth, the plan must provide for support of the adolescent, the family, and team members. Support the adolescent's efforts, and provide positive feedback for accomplishments made in normalizing eating habits. Meetings are held to discuss the feelings and concerns of the patient, immediate caregivers, and team members.

Pharmacotherapy

Pharmacotherapy in the treatment of eating disorders lacks evidence of efficacy. The few studies that have been done have primarily evaluated medications' efficacy in the treatment of comorbid disorders such as obsessive-compulsive disorders and depression. Anxiolytic medications may be helpful before meals to relieve some AN patients' anxiety.

Tricyclic antidepressants and fluoxetine belong to a group of medications known as selective serotonin reuptake inhibitors (SSRIs), which have been more successful when used with BN. There is also some evidence that tricyclic antidepressants such as desipramine, imipramine, and amitriptyline; monoamine oxidase inhibitors; and buspirone are more effective compared with a placebo in decreasing binging and vomiting in patients with BN (Kreipe, 2016). American Psychiatric Association guidelines have discouraged using medication as the only therapy. Clearly more research is needed to clarify whether medications have a role in the treatment of eating disorders (Frank & Shott, 2016).

Diet

The patient should avoid rapid weight gain because it has been associated with severe metabolic abnormalities in some patients, such as refeeding syndrome as previously described. Lower-calorie refeeding (<1400 kcal/day) should be used for severely malnourished patients, but this practice may be too conservative in mildly and moderately malnourished patients where meals combined with nasogastric tube feeding are used to provide higher caloric intake (Garber, Sawyer, Golden, et al., 2016).

Restoration of body weight to a target weight or BMI should be one of the main goals of nutritional rehabilitation (Makhzoumi, Coughlin, Schreyer, et al., 2017). Establishing a "maintenance weight range" of about 1 kg (2 lb) over or under the target weight helps the adolescent feel in control, encourages maintenance of weight through healthy dietary habits, and teaches the adolescent that uncontrollable weight gain is not inevitable when a normal diet is consumed.

Prognosis

About 50% of people with AN recover completely, 30% recover partially, and 20% remain chronically ill (Harrington, Jimerson, Haxton, et al., 2015). Adolescents with BN have a higher recovery rate with 80% achieving full recovery (Harrington, Jimerson, Haxton, et al., 2015). Predictors of more favorable outcome are having BN rather than AN; having a purging type of AN rather than a restricting type; having a short duration of illness; and having a higher discharge weight after hospitalization. Current research reports that BMI at the start or end of treatment and severity of the eating disorder have no effect on the outcome of individuals with an eating disorder; however, individuals 19 years and older and individuals who participate in an inpatient treatment program have significantly lower rates of relapse (Berends, van Meijel, Nugteren, et al., 2016).

AN has the highest mortality rate of any mental health disorder, with an all-cause mortality rate up to 6% (Harrington, Jimerson, Haxton, et al., 2015). One study found the most common natural causes of mortality to be circulatory collapse, cachexia, and organ failure for patients with AN and pneumonia for patients with BN (Fichter & Quadflieq, 2016). The most common cause of nonnatural mortality was suicide, with higher rates among adolescents with BN compared with AN (Fichter & Quadflieq, 2016). Although the changes associated with AN are often reversible, the physical complications can involve every organ system in the body, and the effects of severe malnutrition are often obvious for many years. For example, adolescents with eating disorders are at risk of developing osteopenia or osteoporosis associated with a twofold to sevenfold higher fracture risk in later life because most of the bone mass is built up during adolescence. Further investigation is necessary to determine the functional significance of these abnormalities and the extent to which they return to normal after nutritional intervention.

Nursing Care Management

Nurses need to adopt and maintain a kind and supportive, yet firm, manner in managing the care of the adolescent with eating disorders without creating a passive-dependent attitude. The individual requires sustained support and reassurance to cope with ambivalent feelings related to body concept and the desire to be seen as cooperative, reliable, and worthy of receiving kindness. Encouraging the adolescent with education and activities that strengthen self-esteem facilitates the resocialization process and promotes social acceptance among peers.

It is important that nurses be aware of the physical side effects of AN. Patients with AN frequently limit their fluid intake. Urinary tract problems are frequent, and ketones and proteins are commonly detected in the urine as a result of fat and protein breakdown. Vital sign instability can be severe and can include orthostatic hypotension; the pulse becomes irregular and may decrease markedly. Bradycardia and hypothermia can result in cardiac arrest.

Eating disorders are complex and multifaceted. Because patients often deny their illness, they may refuse the treatment efforts of health providers. The treatment plan needs to be developed carefully and with patience and empathy. Power struggles with patients may escalate the eating disorder symptomatology in that control issues are often central to the development of eating disorders. Implementing less intrusive interventions first and allowing them time to develop is important before applying more restrictive interventions. If possible, treatment should match patients' readiness to change. The care team needs to agree about the treatment philosophy and protocol to avoid sending mixed messages to the patient. It is important to motivate and treat eating disorder patients with respect and support while being direct with expectations on their eating behaviors (Beukers, Berends, de Man–van Ginkel, et al., 2015).

Nurses, patients, and families can find assistance and information from several organizations. The American Anorexia/Bulimia Association, Inc.,* provides information, referrals, counseling, and activities aimed at combating eating disorders. The National Association of Anorexia Nervosa and Associated Eating Disorders† provides counseling, referral, and self-help programs for young people with AN. The National Eating Disorders Association‡ provides information and support services for both patients and families.

Cost of Care (Insurance)

Treatment programs are characterized by multidisciplinary teams and involve stages and phases over time, which can become expensive. It is up to individual insurance companies or existing state laws if adolescent eating disorders have coverage. More difficult cases require long-term care and can involve multiple hospitalizations and ongoing outpatient care. Families find that insurance companies begin to deny coverage or, in the interest of managing costs, begin to insist on alternative treatment programs that may be inferior. For many families, the costs of care result in serious financial problems. Insufficient treatment may result in chronicity, invalidism, and even death. Nurses must understand the barriers to care and become advocates for their patients. They need to be educated about the unique characteristics of eating disorders in order to advocate for their patients.

*800-522-2230; http://americananorexiabulimiaassociationinc.visualnet.com.

†Hotline 630-577-1330; email: anadhelp@anad.org; http://www.anad.org.

‡603 Stewart St., Suite 803, Seattle, WA 98101; 800-931-2237; http://www.nationaleatingdisorders.org.

BOX 18.6 Early Signs of Anorexia Nervosa

The adolescent:

- Consumes an inappropriate diet (excessively strict) or may refuse to eat altogether
- Develops peculiar eating habits such as toying with food, performing food "rituals," preparing and forcing food on family members without eating any himself or herself
- Denies hunger even after eating very little/almost nothing for days or even weeks
- Engages in excessive exercise, such as compulsive jogging, running up and down stairs, rigorous calisthenics to burn off calories—often to the point of exhaustion
- Takes laxatives, diuretics, or enemas to speed intestinal transit time, to lose added weight, and to empty intestines
- Vomits deliberately; may go to bathroom after a meal and turn on faucets to avoid being heard
- Develops a distorted body image; states she or he "feels fat" as she or he becomes increasingly thin
- Loses weight; fails to achieve the 25th percentile on normal growth curves or jumps across several growth channels on the curve
- Withdraws from social interaction; starts to spend time in room studying, exercising, or otherwise occupied
- Displays personality traits such as perfectionism or obsessive-compulsive disorder tendencies

Prevention

There are no easy ways to prevent an eating disorder. However, public and professional awareness of signs and symptoms can facilitate early identification and treatment to prevent or reduce the long-term adverse consequences. Providing parents with the tools to support positive self-image and tools to create health home environments may help contradict personal or medial influences that lead to eating disorders. Additionally, media literacy on the societal drive for thinness and overall nutrition education may help. Box 18.6 outlines the early signs of AN.

SUBSTANCE ABUSE

Although experimentation with drugs during childhood and adolescence is widespread, most children and teens do not become high-risk users. *Monitoring the Future* has been providing long-term research about the rates of substance use among adolescents, young adults, and adults since 1975 (Johnston, O'Malley, Miech, et al., 2015). The 2014 survey found that marijuana use and acceptance of marijuana use among 12th-graders increased from 2006 to 2011 and then leveled from 2011 to 2013. Binge drinking (five or more alcoholic drinks at least once in the prior 2 weeks) has been on the decline since the early 1980s and reached historically low levels in 2014. Cigarette use has been on a steady decline since the mid-1990s until 2004, which followed a leveling off through 2014. More teens used e-cigarettes in 2014 than any other tobacco product, with a prevalence of 13.6% among 12th-graders (Johnston, O'Malley, Miech, et al,. 2015). The use of illicit drugs other than marijuana has shown minimal change from the late 1990s until 2014 (Johnston, O'Malley, Miech, et al., 2015).

Drug abuse, misuse, and addiction are culturally defined and are voluntary behaviors. Drug tolerance and physical dependence are involuntary physiologic responses to the pharmacologic characteristics of drugs, such as opioids and alcohol. Consequently, an individual can be addicted to a narcotic with or without being physically dependent. A person can also be physically dependent on a narcotic without being addicted (e.g., patients who use opioids to control pain).

MOTIVATION

Most drug use begins with experimentation. The drug may be used only once, may be used occasionally, or may become part of a drug-centered lifestyle. Children and adolescents initiate drug use out of curiosity. Adolescents who use drugs may fall into one of two broad categories—experimenters and compulsive users—or they may fall into a third category somewhere on the continuum between these extremes, referred to as *recreational users,* principally of drugs such as marijuana, cocaine, alcohol, and prescription drugs. For many, the goal is peer acceptance; these users fit more closely with the experimenting, intermittent users. For others, the goal is intoxication or the sustained intense effects from using a particular drug; these users resemble the compulsive users. These users may engage in periodic heavy use, or binges. The groups of greatest concern to health care workers are those whose patterns of use involve high doses or mixed drugs with the danger of overdose and compulsive users with the threat of dependence, withdrawal syndromes, and altered lifestyle.

TYPES OF DRUGS ABUSED

Any drug can be abused, and most are potentially harmful to adolescents still going through formative life experiences. Although rarely considered drugs by society, the chemically active substances frequently abused are the xanthines and theobromines contained in chocolate, tea, coffee, and colas. Ethyl alcohol and nicotine are other drugs that are legal and socially sanctioned. Any of these substances can produce mild to moderate euphoric or stimulant effects and can lead to physical and psychologic dependence.

Drugs with mind-altering abilities that are available on the "street" and are of medical and legal concern are the hallucinogenic, narcotic, hypnotic, and stimulant drugs. In addition, health care professionals are concerned about the use of alcohol and volatile substances that are inhaled to achieve altered sensation (e.g., gasoline, antifreeze, plastic model airplane cement, organic solvents). Cough and cold preparations such as NyQuil, Coricidin, and Robitussin are common substances abused by adolescents and young adults. Many of the medications are often found in the medicine or kitchen cabinet at home and are available at a decreased cost compared with the more exotic drugs of abuse. The abuse of prescription and synthetic drugs such as opioids, benzodiazepines such as Xanax, and stimulants such as Adderall is increasing among adolescents and young people (Stager, 2016). Websites also promote the "safe use" of some psychoactive drugs and supply information on new "designer" drugs that are not detectable on a standard urine drug screening test.

TOBACCO

Cigarette smoking has been on a slow decline since the peak in 1999 despite multiple efforts, including increased costs, changes in community attitudes about smoking, media campaigns with counteradvertising, and tobacco-free environments. However, use of all tobacco products among youth did not change between 2004 and 2014, primarily due to the popularity of electronic cigarettes and hookahs (Johnston, O'Malley, Miech, et al., 2015; Singh, Arrazola, Corey, et al., 2016).

Cigarette smoking is still considered a chief avoidable cause of death. The hazards of smoking at any age are undisputed; however, a preventive approach to teenage smoking is especially important. Because of its addictive nature, smoking begun in childhood and adolescence can result in a lifetime habit, with increased morbidity and early mortality.

The increased popularity of electronic cigarettes has reached into middle- and high-school–age students, and e-cigarettes are the most commonly used tobacco product among middle- and high-school students (Singh, Arrazola, Corey, et al., 2016). There is concern that these products are used to promote smoking cessation, yet there is no evidence to support this claim (Stager, 2016). In fact, a recent study found that 98.7% of flavored e-cigarette products and 99.4% of non-flavored e-cigarette products contained nicotine (Marynak, Gammon, Rogers, et al., 2017). These products can cause nicotine dependency (Stager, 2016).

The effects of secondhand smoke exposure are also well known and include increased incidence of low birth weight and subsequent illness, increased incidence of sudden infant death syndrome (maternal smoking during and after pregnancy), increased incidence of lower respiratory tract infections, exacerbation of asthma symptoms, sleep disturbances, and intellectual impairment (Al-Sayed & Ibrahim, 2014; Homa, Neff, King, et al., 2015).

Etiology

Teenagers begin smoking for a variety of reasons, including imitation of adult behavior; peer pressure; a desire to imitate behaviors and lifestyles portrayed in movies and advertisements; and a desire to control weight, especially among young women. Teenagers who do not smoke usually have family members and friends who do not smoke or who oppose smoking. Most teens who refrain from smoking have a desire to succeed in academics or athletics and plan to go to college (see Community and Home Health Considerations box). Although smoking among college students has increased in recent years, rates of smoking are highest among adolescents who do not complete high school.

Smokeless Tobacco

The term *smokeless tobacco* refers to tobacco products that are placed in the mouth but not ignited (e.g., snuff and chewing tobacco). This substitute for cigarettes continues to pose a hazard to adolescents, although use has steadily declined from 70% in 1999 to 32% in 2015 (Kann, McManus, Harris, et al., 2016). Children and adolescents continue to recognize the risk of smokeless tobacco and have expressed high rates of disapproval (Johnston, O'Malley, Miech, et al., 2015). These products have also been proved to be carcinogenic, and regular use can cause dental problems, foul-smelling breath, and tooth erosion or loss.

Nursing Care Management

Prevention of regular smoking in teenagers is the most effective way to reduce the overall incidence of smoking. A variety of methods have been used. Posters, charts, displays, statistics, and the use of examples of actual damaged lungs to communicate the hazards of smoking all have their supporters and doubters. Some schools also use films and demonstrations in science classes.

For the most part, smoking prevention programs that focus on the negative, long-term effects of smoking on health have been ineffective. Youth-to-youth programs and those emphasizing the immediate effects are more effective but primarily in improving teenagers' attitudes toward not smoking. Because smoking and smoking-related behaviors are social symbols, antismoking campaigns must address the norms of potential

COMMUNITY AND HOME HEALTH CONSIDERATIONS

Early Sexual Maturation, Alcohol, and Cigarettes

Smoking cigarettes and drinking alcohol among adolescents are complex behaviors that are not explained by any one factor. Some theorists and investigators believe there is a relationship between biologic maturation and risk-taking behaviors. For example, young teens who are sexually mature at an earlier age than their peers are often attracted to older girls and boys who may engage in risk-taking behaviors. If older teens smoke, drink, and drive while under the influence of alcohol with no adverse consequences (e.g., no motor vehicle accidents), young teens may believe that they, too, will be safe while smoking, drinking, or riding in an automobile with friends who are drinking.

Although parents and nurses cannot influence the time of biologic maturation, they can identify young teens who are at risk for the initiation of risk-taking behaviors because of early puberty. Parents need to understand that an early-maturing teen might be uncomfortable with his or her body, and they should take advantage of opportunities to build self-esteem. Parental sensitivity to the importance of peer-group acceptance and parental support of a teenager who feels left out or different are crucial. School nurses can provide anticipatory guidance to these teens and help them role-play coping strategies for situations that involve offers to smoke and drink. In addition, school nurses can provide information about physical development during puberty and emphasize that not all teenagers mature at the same time or rate.

Teachers, coaches, and community and church leaders can provide opportunities for these teens to "fit in" with their same-age peers through activities that stress mutual goals. For example, an early-maturing girl is typically taller than her age-mates and can be an asset in sports such as basketball and track-and-field events.

smokers. Anything that ridicules or threatens the social norms of the peer group can be unproductive or counterproductive. Investigators have found that teaching resistance to peer pressure to smoke is effective in early adolescence. Although the effects of these programs may decrease with time, the effects can be enhanced in older adolescents by presenting information in class instead of simply handing out written material to the students.

Two areas of focus for antismoking programs are peer-led programs and use of media in smoking prevention (e.g., CDs, videotapes, and films). Peer-led programs emphasizing the social consequences of smoking have proved most successful. If a significant number of influential peers can "sell" their classmates on the idea that the habit is not popular, the followers will imitate their behavior. Such programs emphasize short-term rather than long-term consequences (e.g., the effects of smoking on personal appearance, such as unattractive stains on teeth and hands and unpleasant odor of breath and clothing).

Pharmacologic agents for smoking cessation include nicotine replacement therapy. Medications such as bupropion and varenicline have been used with success in adults for smoking cessation. Although bupropion has shown some effectiveness in pilot studies among adolescents, this medication is not FDA approved for use in adolescents less than 19 years of age (Stager, 2016). Varenicline now has a black box warning for neuropsychiatric side effects (Stager, 2016).

The impact of school-based antismoking programs can be strengthened by expanding these programs to include parents, mass media, youth groups, and community organizations. For example, mass media efforts that involve antismoking radio campaigns have been identified as the most cost-effective mass media intervention.

Smoking bans in schools also accomplish several goals, including discouraging students from starting to smoke; reinforcing knowledge of the health hazards of cigarette smoking and exposure to environmental tobacco smoke; and promoting a smoke-free environment as the norm (see Community and Home Health Considerations box).

COMMUNITY AND HOME HEALTH CONSIDERATIONS

Nonsmoking Strategies

Nurses who work in schools, hospitals, and community agencies can take advantage of all opportunities to provide education about the dangers of smoking, to discourage smoking initiation by children and adolescents, to encourage smoking cessation, and to promote smoke-free environments. In particular, school nurses must be alert to the vulnerability of young preteens when they enter junior high or middle school. These nurses are in an ideal position to assess stress, personal conflict, weight concerns, peer pressures, and other factors that place preteens at risk for smoking initiation. Nurses should serve as counselors to student, teacher, and parent groups and as advocates for antismoking legislative efforts. The following additional strategies are recommended:*

- Provide brief information about long-term health consequences (e.g., cardiovascular and cancer risks).
- Discuss immediate physiologic consequences (e.g., changes in heart rate, blood pressure, respiratory symptoms, and blood carbon monoxide concentrations).
- Identify alternatives to smoking that also establish a self-image that appears independent, mature, or sophisticated (e.g., weight lifting; jogging; dancing; joining a boys' or girls' club; engaging in volunteer work for a hospital, political, religious, or community group).
- Mention the negative effects in detail (e.g., earlier wrinkling of skin; yellow stains on teeth and fingers; tobacco odor on breath, hair, and clothing).
- State the increasing ostracism of smokers by nonsmokers, both legal and informal, in the workplace and in public places.
- Describe the increasing evidence that secondhand smoke is injurious to the health of nonsmokers who are regularly exposed, especially small children.
- Acknowledge that many adults, who were enticed to start smoking as teenagers because of its social benefits, now wish they could stop smoking.
- Give cooperative adolescents effective arguments to deal with peer pressure (e.g., by not smoking, a teenager demonstrates independence and nonconformity, traits normally prized by youth).
- Request posters or pamphlets from local agencies (e.g., American Cancer Society, American Heart Association, and American Lung Association) to display in prominent places at school.

*The Centers for Disease Control and Prevention has information on the effects of tobacco, smoking cessation, and tobacco control programs; 1600 Clifton Road, Atlanta, GA 30333; 800-232-4636; email: tobaccoinfo@cdc.gov; https://www.cdc.gov/tobacco.

ALCOHOL

Acute or chronic abuse of alcohol (ethanol) is responsible for many acts of violence, suicide, accidental injury, and death. Alcohol drinking is likely to begin in the middle-school years and increases with age. By 18 years of age, 80% to 90% of adolescents have tried alcohol. Ethanol is a depressant that reduces inhibitions against aggressive and sexual acting out. Severe physical and psychologic symptoms accompany abrupt withdrawal, and long-term use leads to slow tissue destruction, especially of the brain and liver cells. The most noticeable effects of alcohol occur within the central nervous system and include changes in cognitive and autonomic functions such as judgment, memory, learning ability, and other intellectual capacities. Young people with alcoholism often drink alone and cannot control their use of alcohol. They often rely on the substance as a defense against depression, anxiety, fear, or anger. Not all of these characteristics are observed in adolescents who are abusing alcohol, but if several signs are evident, the child or adolescent should be considered at risk. Referral to a health care professional and detoxification therapy may be necessary. Information about alcohol and answers to questions are available through the Alcohol Hotline.* Other groups that provide support and counseling for families are Al-Anon, Ala-Teen, Ala-Tot, and Alcoholics Anonymous (an organization that has listings in all local directories).

COCAINE

Although cocaine is not pharmacologically considered a narcotic, it is legally categorized as such. Cocaine is available in two forms: water-soluble cocaine hydrochloride, which is administered by "snorting" or intravenous injection, and nonsoluble alkaloid (freebase) cocaine, which is used primarily for smoking. Crack, or "rock," is a purer, more menacing form of the drug. It can be produced cheaply and smoked in either water pipes or mentholated cigarettes.

Cocaine creates a sense of euphoria, or an indefinable high. Withdrawal does not produce the dramatic symptoms observed in withdrawal from other substances. The effects are those commonly seen in depression, including lack of energy and motivation, irritability, appetite changes, psychomotor delay, and irregular sleep patterns. More serious symptoms include cardiovascular manifestations and seizures. Physical withdrawal should not be confused with the so-called *crash* after a cocaine high, which consists of a long period of sleep. Answers to questions about the risks of using cocaine are available at the National Cocaine Hotline,* which also provides referrals to support groups and treatment centers.

NARCOTICS

Narcotic drugs include opiates, such as heroin and morphine, and opioids (opiate-like drugs), such as hydromorphone (Dilaudid), hydrocodone, fentanyl, meperidine (Demerol), and codeine. These drugs produce a state of euphoria by removing painful feelings and creating a pleasurable experience and a sense of success accompanied by clouding of the consciousness and a dreamlike state. Physical signs of narcotic abuse include constricted pupils, respiratory depression, and, often, cyanosis. Needle marks may be visible on the arms or legs in chronic users. Physical withdrawal from opiates is extremely unpleasant unless controlled with supervised tapering doses of the opioid or substitution of methadone.

As important as the physical effects are the indirect consequences related to the illegal status of narcotic use and the problems associated with securing the drug (e.g., the time-consuming searches to obtain the drug and the often illegal methods used to meet the high cost of purchasing it). Health problems also result from self-neglect of physical needs (e.g., nutrition, cleanliness, dental care); overdose; contamination; and infection, including HIV and hepatitis B and C infection.

CENTRAL NERVOUS SYSTEM DEPRESSANTS

Central nervous system depressants include a variety of hypnotic drugs that produce physical dependence and withdrawal symptoms on abrupt discontinuation. They create a feeling of relaxation and sleepiness but impair general functioning. Drugs in this category include barbiturates, nonbarbiturates, and alcohol. Barbiturates combined with alcohol produce a profound depressant effect. Flunitrazepam (Rohypnol), known as the "date rape drug," is a hypnotic drug abused by adolescents. Many women and men report being raped after unknowingly being given Rohypnol in a drink. Rohypnol is 10 times more powerful than diazepam (Valium). It produces prolonged sedation, a feeling of well-being, and short-term memory loss.

CENTRAL NERVOUS SYSTEM STIMULANTS

Amphetamines and cocaine do not produce strong physical dependence and can be withdrawn without much danger. However, psychologic dependence is strong, and acute intoxication can lead to violent aggressive behavior or psychotic episodes characterized by paranoia, uncontrollable agitation, and restlessness. When combined with barbiturates, the euphoric effects are particularly addictive.

Methamphetamine can be snorted, injected, swallowed, or smoked and produces a burst of energy in its users, along with intense, alternating attacks of boldness and paranoia. It provokes excitement far more intense than that caused by cocaine. The drug, with the street names *crank, meth,* and *crystal,* is inexpensive and has a longer period of action than cocaine. Instead of a short (few minutes) high, as achieved with cocaine, a user can remain "up" for hours on a similar dose of crank.

Health care professionals are concerned about the use of various volatile substances, or inhalants such as gasoline, model cement, and organic solvents; these substances are inhaled by the user to achieve an altered sensation, and the most recent surveillance has indicated a modest increase in use after nearly a decade of decline. Adolescents breathe or place these substances into paper or plastic bags or soda cans from which they rebreathe the fumes to produce a feeling of euphoria and altered consciousness. These substances contain chemical solvents and are extremely hazardous. Dusters contain Freon, a substance that can cause fatal cardiac dysrhythmias. Inhalants are the only substances that have a higher incidence of use among young adolescents. This is probably related to the fact that the products are readily available and may be the only substances available for young teens. Many young children are unaware of the dangers of "sniffing" or "huffing." In addition to rapid loss of consciousness and respiratory arrest, these substances may cause visual scanning problems, language deficiencies, motor instability, memory deficits, and attention and concentration problems.

MIND-ALTERING DRUGS

Hallucinogens (psychedelics, psychotomimetics, psychotropics, or illusionogenics) are drugs that produce vivid hallucinations and euphoria. These drugs do not produce physical dependence, and they can be abruptly withdrawn without ill effect. However, the acute and long-term effects are variable, and in some individuals the dissociative behavior may be prolonged. Cannabis (marijuana, hashish) and lysergic acid diethylamide (LSD) are also included in this category of drugs.

NURSING CARE MANAGEMENT

Nurses who have contact with children and adolescents are in an excellent position to provide information about substance abuse and to serve as patient advocates. Nurses most often encounter young substance abusers when they are (1) experiencing overdose or withdrawal symptoms, (2) manifesting bizarre behavior or confusion secondary to drug ingestion, (3) worried that they are or will become addicted, or (4) worried about a friend or family member who is addicted.

*Toll free 866-925-4030.

*800-COCAINE (800-262-2463).

In particular, nurses who care for hospitalized adolescents need to know if these youths use drugs compulsively. Drug withdrawal can seriously complicate other illnesses. Nurses should be alert for any physical or behavioral clues that indicate the onset of withdrawal or the effects of drugs. School nurses and nurses who work in the community play an essential role in identifying children, adolescents, and families with substance abuse problems. The school nurse may be the first to identify a child or adolescent who has ingested a particular drug by the child's erratic behavior in class or on the school grounds (see Critical Thinking Case Study box). Early identification of those at risk for substance abuse problems is an essential aspect of prevention. Pediatric health care professionals also prevent substance abuse by creating trusting relationships so that children and adolescents feel comfortable asking questions about drugs, and health care professionals can alert them to websites and other aspects of society that encourage experimentation with drugs.

CRITICAL THINKING CASE STUDY

Prescription Medication Abuse in Adolescence

An eighth-grade teacher calls the school nurse, Sally, to her classroom and reports that a girl is behaving "strangely." The girl slept through most of the class before lunch and seldom participates in class discussions. Sally, a registered nurse, takes the girl to her office and performs an initial assessment. On assessment, the girl demonstrates short-term memory lapse, slightly slurred speech, and a delayed pupillary reaction to light. Her blood pressure is 112/68 mm Hg, respirations are 14 breaths/min and regular, and heart rate is 102 beats/min. She denies taking any pills or liquid initially but then states she had a migraine on arrival to school and a friend gave her two blue pills to help with the headache. She refuses to say who gave her the pills and does not know what they were but thought they were Tylenol. She states that she does not know where her mother and father are but thinks they are at work.

1. Evidence—Is there sufficient evidence for Sally to implement a plan of care for this adolescent?
2. What should Sally's next course of action involve? What is her professional responsibility in this case?
3. Assumptions—Describe the underlying assumptions about the following:
   a. The school nurse's physical assessment findings
   b. The misuse of prescription medications by adolescents
4. What nursing priorities and implications for care can be made at this time? What type of care should this eighth-grader receive?

Answers are available at http://evolve.elsevier.com/wong/ncic.

Acute Care

Adolescents experiencing toxic drug effects or withdrawal symptoms are usually seen initially in the emergency department. Experienced emergency department personnel are familiar with the management of acute drug toxicity and the signs, symptoms, and behavioral characteristics associated with a variety of substances. When the drug is questionable or unknown, knowledge of these factors facilitates management and treatment. Often, observation or description of the child's or adolescent's behavior is more valuable than reports by patients or their friends.

The treatment for drug toxicity or withdrawal varies according to the drug and the method used. Every effort is made to determine the type, time of ingestion, amount of drug taken, mode of administration, and factors related to the onset of presenting symptoms. It is helpful to know the individual's pattern of use. For example, if two types of drugs are involved, they may require different treatments. Historically, gastric lavage has been used when the drug has been ingested recently and the cough reflex is intact, but it is of little value when the drug has been administered by the intravenous ("mainlined") or intranasal ("sniffed") route. The administration of a drug antidote such as naloxone and the early (within 1 to 2 hours of ingestion) administration of activated charcoal may be used for opioid overdose. Because the actual content of most street drugs is highly questionable, other pharmaceutic agents are administered with caution, except perhaps the narcotic antagonists in cases of suspected opiate overdoses. It is also necessary to assess for possible trauma sustained while the patient was under the influence of the drug.

Long-Term Management

A major factor in the treatment and rehabilitation of young drug users is careful assessment in the nonacute stage to determine the function that the drug plays in the adolescent's life. The motivation phase is directed toward exploring the factors that influence drug use. It also involves establishing a feeling of self-worth and a commitment to self-help in the teen.

Rehabilitation begins when adolescents decide they can and are willing to change. *Rehabilitation* involves fostering healthy interdependent relationships with caring and supportive adults and exploring alternate mechanisms for problem solving, while simultaneously reducing or eliminating drug use. Persons working with troubled youth must be prepared for *recidivism,* or the tendency to relapse, and maintain a plan for reentry into the treatment process.

Family Support

Most treatment programs for substance abusers are based on adult 12-step models such as Alcoholics Anonymous. Research is needed to determine whether these adult models are effective for adolescents. Tough Love* is one program that is based on the conviction that parents have the right and responsibility to be the policy makers in the family, to set limits on the behavior of their children, and to take control of the household from out-of-control adolescents. The premise is that allowing teenagers to experience the negative consequences of their behavior will bring them closer to accepting help or changing their behavior. Another group that provides support and counseling for families experiencing substance abuse and seeking strategies to cope with their children is Parents Anonymous.† Another source of information is the Substance Abuse and Mental Health Services Administration's National Clearinghouse for Alcohol and Drug Information.‡ The National Institute on Drug Abuse (NIDA) also contains an abundance of information for adolescents on the effects of abused substances, prevention, and treatment (http://www.drugabuse.gov/students-young-adults).

Prevention

Nurses play an important role in education efforts, as well as in individual observation, assessment, and therapy related to substance abuse. In recent years, a variety of educational programs have been applied with promising results. The most effective prevention strategies are those that are part of a broader, more general effort to promote overall health and success. Health-compromising behaviors are often interconnected and have common antecedents. Prevention efforts that focus on changing only one behavior (e.g., alcohol, other drug use) are less likely to be

*http://www.toughlove.com.

†675 W. Foothill Blvd., Suite 220, Claremont, CA 91711; 909-621-6184; http://www.parentsanonymous.org.

‡1 Choke Cherry Road, Rockville, MD 20857; 877-SAMHSA-7; http://ncadi.samhsa.gov.

BOX 18.7 Types of Self-Harm Behaviors

- Cutting
- Poisoning
- Strangulation
- Branding
- Scratching or scraping
- Hitting or banging
- Pulling hair or skin
- Biting
- Burning

successful. Successful programs are those that have promoted parenting skills, social skills among distractible children, academic achievement, and skills to resist peer pressure.

Peer pressure is a powerful tool and can be used effectively in substance abuse prevention. A group that has had some success in reducing injury from drunk driving is Students Against Destructive Decisions (SADD).* Techniques used by this group include peer counseling, parental guidelines for teenage parties, and community awareness. Nurses should encourage the formation of SADD chapters in the high schools in their communities.

SELF-HARM

Self-harm is defined as a direct and intentional damage to one's body without the intent to die (Doyle, Sheridan, & Treacy, 2017). It is also referred to as *self-injury* and *self-mutilation.* This definition excludes indirect self-injury behaviors such as eating disorders or drug abuse and excludes socially accepted behaviors such as tattooing and piercing (Brown & Plener, 2017). The most common methods of self-harm are listed in Box 18.7.

The prevalence of self-harm among adolescents ranges from 1.5% to 65.9%; the wide range of frequencies is due to inconsistencies among researchers on how self-harm is defined, how self-harm is measured, and how age is defined among adolescents (Doyle, Treacy, & Sheridan, 2015). Self-harm peaks at 15 to 16 years of age and starts to decline by 18 years of age. Self-harm is more prominent in females, among individuals with sexual orientation confusion, and among individuals with a history of physical or sexual abuse (Doyle, Treacy, & Sheridan, 2015). Factors associated with self harm include a suicide attempt or self harm among a friend or family member, fighting with parents or friends, and being bullied at school (Doyle, Treacy, & Sheridan, 2015).

ETIOLOGY

Adolescents engage in self-harm to get relief from life stressors or abate emotions such as anger, frustration, or depression. Inflicting physical pain in the form of self-harm provides distraction from stress and feelings. Adolescents also experience euphoria when self-harming. Endorphins are released when the body is injured, resulting in a pleasurable sensation. Self-harming behaviors can become addictive.

Because the hypothalamic-pituitary adrenocortical (HPA) axis is involved in stressful situations, it has been suggested that individuals who self-harm have an altered HPA axis (Brown & Plener, 2017). More research is needed with this association.

*255 Main St., Marlborough, MA 01752; 877-SADD-INC; http://www.sadd.org.

DIAGNOSTIC EVALUATION

Most adolescents who self-harm do not seek treatment because they feel the incident is not serious enough to require help, they do not want any help, or they do not want others to know about their behavior (Doyle, Treacy, & Sheridan, 2015). Adolescents who do seek help primarily go to a friend or family member, thus most self-harm actions are not discussed with health care professionals. Nurses must be aware of the potential for self-harm among adolescents and educate family and friends about warning signs. These signs include the following:

- Multiple cuts/burns on arms, legs, hips, or stomach
- Wearing baggy clothes or long sleeves/pants to conceal wounds
- Finding razors, scissors, lighters, or knives hidden in the adolescent's room
- Spending long periods of time in a locked bedroom or bathroom, especially after conflicts with friends or family

THERAPEUTIC MANAGEMENT

No specific treatment effectively eliminates self-harm behaviors. Adolescents are referred to mental health professionals to confront negative thinking, assist with mood management, and encourage healthy activities to manage stress. The most effective treatment includes family therapy with goals to improve communication, teach conflict-resolution and problem-solving skills, and foster positive relationships.

! NURSING ALERT

The S.A.F.E. Alternatives offers a helpline (1-800-DON'T-CUT [366-8288]) and hosts a website (http://www.selfinjury.com) with information about treatment programs and other resources.

SUICIDE

Suicide is defined as the deliberate act of self-injury with the intent that the injury results in death. Most experts distinguish among suicidal ideation, suicide attempt (or parasuicide), and suicide.

Suicidal ideation involves a preoccupation with thoughts about committing suicide and may be a precursor to suicide. Although it is common for adolescents to experience occasional suicidal thoughts, expressions of preoccupation with suicide should be taken seriously, and an assessment should be conducted for appropriate referral. A **suicide attempt** is intended to cause injury or death. The term *parasuicide* is used to refer to behaviors ranging from gestures to serious attempts to kill oneself. *Parasuicide* is a preferred term because it makes no reference to intent and because a person's motive may be too difficult or complex to determine. However, all parasuicidal activity should be taken seriously.

! NURSING ALERT

A history of a previous suicide attempt is a serious indicator for possible suicide completion in the future. Studies of adolescent suicides have found that as many as half of the adolescents had made previous attempts.

Results from the Youth Risk Behavior Surveillance, 2015, indicated that 8.6% of students nationwide had attempted suicide at least once during the 12 months preceding the survey; the range of suicide attempts by adolescents across the states varied from 5.9% to 12.7% (Kann, McManus, Harris, et al., 2016). The overall incidence of youth suicide has decreased since 1992, yet the Centers for Disease Control and Prevention and other experts note that the incidence is still too high. Approximately 14.6% of the students in this survey reported that they had made a specific plan to attempt suicide in the 12 months preceding the survey. Suicide is currently the third leading cause of death during the teenage years, surpassed only by death from motor vehicle crashes and homicides (see Chapter 17).

ETIOLOGY

Individual, family, and social or environmental factors have all been implicated in suicide. The single most important individual factor is the presence of an active psychiatric disorder (e.g., depression, bipolar disorder, psychosis, substance abuse, or conduct disorder). Alcohol use in particular has been associated with more than 50% of suicides (Thompson & Swartout, 2017). Another strong risk factor for suicide in American high school adolescents is substance abuse; in particular, heroin, methamphetamines, and steroids were found to have the strongest association with four measures of suicidality (suicidal ideation, suicidal plan, suicidal attempt, and severe suicide attempt) (Wong, Zhou, Goebert, et al., 2013). For some teens, suicide becomes the final pathway for release from their psychiatric and social problems. Child and adolescent suicide victims are reported to have higher rates not only of depression but also of conduct disorders, bipolar disorders, substance abuse, and interpersonal problems with parents.

Family factors influencing suicide include parental loss; family disruption; a family history of suicide, depression, substance abuse, or emotional disturbance; child abuse or neglect; unavailable parents; poor communication and isolation within the family; family conflict; and unrealistically high parental expectations or parental indifference with low expectations. Families that respect individuality, are cohesive and caring, balance discipline with a supportive and understanding relationship, have good systems of communication, and have at least one attentive and caring parent available to the child protect adolescents from suicidal outcomes. Social or environmental factors include incarceration, isolation, acute loss of a boyfriend or girlfriend, lack of future options, and availability of firearms in the home.

METHODS

Firearms are by far the most commonly used instruments in completed suicides among adolescent males, whereas cutting or piercing is the most common method among females (Matthews, Woodward, Musso, et al., 2016). For adolescent males, the other common means of suicide are cutting/piercing, jumping, and hanging/suffocating; for females, the other common means are jumping, hanging/suffocating, and firearms.

The most common method of suicide *attempt* is overdose or ingestion of a potentially toxic substance, such as drugs. The second most common method of suicide attempt is self-inflicted laceration.

> **! NURSING ALERT**
>
> Given what is known about youth suicide, nurses should ask parents, especially those with at-risk teenagers, if firearms are available in the house and, if so, recommend their removal. Parents must ensure that their children—especially those who are depressed, have poor problem-solving skills, or use drugs or alcohol—do not have access to firearms. Parents must also be educated on the warning signs of suicide (Box 18.8).

BOX 18.8 Warning Signs of Suicide

- Preoccupation with themes of death—focuses on morbid thoughts
- Wants to give away cherished possessions
- Talks of own death, desire to die
- Loss of energy, loss of interest, listlessness
- Exhaustion without obvious cause
- Changes in sleep patterns—too much or too little
- Increased irritability, argumentativeness, or stubbornness
- Physical complaints—recurrent stomachaches, headaches
- Repeated visits to physician, nurse practitioner, or emergency department for treatment of injuries
- Reckless behavior
- Antisocial behavior—engages in drinking, uses drugs, fights, commits acts of vandalism, runs away from home, becomes sexually promiscuous
- Sudden change in school performance—lowered grades, cutting classes, dropping out of activities
- Resists or refuses to go to school
- Remains distant, sad, remote—flat affect, frozen facial expression
- Describes self as worthless
- Sudden cheerfulness after deep depression
- Social withdrawal from friends, activities, interests that were previously enjoyed
- Impaired concentration
- Dramatic change in appetite

Motivation

Suicidal ideation is common in adolescents. It represents numerous fantasies, such as relief from suffering, a means of gaining comfort and sympathy, or a means of revenge against those who have hurt them. Adolescents have the erroneous perception that the act of suicide will evoke remorse and pity and that they will be able to return and witness the grief. Angry children or adolescents who are unable to directly punish those who have injured or insulted them may take revenge on those who love them through self-destruction ("They'll be sorry when they find me dead"; "They'll be sorry they were mean to me").

For adolescents who are severely depressed, suicide seems to be the only release from their despair. These adolescents rarely provide evidence of their intent and frequently conceal their suicidal thoughts. Many adolescents, however, tell their peers of their suicidal thoughts or plans but avoid telling adults. Social isolation is a significant factor in distinguishing adolescents who will kill themselves from those who will not. It is also more characteristic of those who complete suicide than of those who make attempts or threats.

The frequency of **contagion** or **copycat suicides** (i.e., an increase in youth suicide that occurs after the suicide of one teenager is publicized) is disturbing and may indicate that teenagers perceive suicide as glamorous. In addition, young people may not realize the finality of suicide because they have become desensitized from constantly viewing violence and death on television.

Diagnostic Evaluation

Depression is common among adolescents who attempt suicide. Depression is characterized by both subjective symptoms and objective signs that reflect the adolescent's sadness and despair. Adolescents describe feelings of sadness, despair, helplessness, hopelessness, boredom, loss of interest, and isolation. They may also feel self-reproach, self-deprecation, and guilt. Subjective symptoms of depression or specific changes in behavior place an adolescent at risk for suicide (Box 18.9). Table 18.5

BOX 18.9 Characteristics of Children or Adolescents With Depression

Behavior
- Predominantly sad facial expression with absence or diminished range of affective response
- Solitary play or work; tendency to be alone; lack of interest in play with friends
- Withdrawal from previously enjoyed activities and relationships
- Lowered grades in school; lack of interest in doing homework or achieving in school; refuses to wake up for school
- Diminished motor activity; tiredness
- Tearfulness or crying
- Inability to concentrate
- Dependent and clinging or aggressive and disruptive

Internal States
- Utterance of statements reflecting lowered self-esteem, sense of hopelessness, or guilt
- Suicidal ideations

Physiology
- Constipation
- Loss of energy; fatigue
- Nonspecific complaints of not feeling well
- Change in appetite resulting in weight loss or gain
- Alterations in sleeping pattern, sleeplessness, or hypersomnia

TABLE 18.5 Pediatric Quality Indicator Suicide Risk Assessment for Child and Adolescent Major Depressive Disorder*

Child and Adolescent Major Depressive Disorder: Suicide Risk Assessment	
Measure	Children and adolescents 6-17 years with a diagnosis of major depressive disorder with an assessment for suicide risk
Numerator	Number of children and adolescent visits with an assessment for suicide risk
Denominator	Number of children and adolescent visits with a diagnosis of major depressive disorder

*Endorsed by the National Quality Forum-1365 and 2016 Core Set of Children's Health Care Quality Measures for Medicaid and CHIP.

describes the pediatric quality indicator for suicide risk assessment among children and adolescents with a major depressive disorder.

Therapeutic Management

Threats of suicide should always be taken seriously. There has been a tendency to dismiss suicide attempts as impulsive acts resulting from temporary crises or depression. If a suicide attempt fails to draw attention to their problems or makes them worse, the child or adolescent may conclude that suicide is the only answer. Children and adolescents need to know that someone cares and must be provided with swift and efficient crisis intervention. Although ordinary practitioners can manage an acute depressive reaction without difficulty, the adolescent who has made a serious attempt or has a specific plan for suicide should receive immediate attention and competent psychiatric care.

Youths who are actively suicidal need inpatient care, monitoring, and treatment. Medications for depression and bipolar disorder often take several weeks to reach therapeutic levels. The time until medications and therapy begin to take effect can be trying for the adolescent and the family. It is important to encourage families to support their teen in adherence to the regimen prescribed. The SSRIs are often prescribed for depression, but teens who are taking such medications need careful, frequent monitoring.

! NURSING ALERT

Adolescents who express suicidal feelings and have a specific plan should be monitored at all times. They should not have access to firearms, prescription or over-the-counter drugs, belts, scarves, shoestrings, sharp objects, matches, or lighters. If they are intoxicated, they must be restrained or placed in a protective environment until a psychiatrist or psychologist can assess them.

NURSING CARE MANAGEMENT

Nurses play a pivotal role in reducing adolescent suicide. Nurses have the opportunity to provide anticipatory guidance to parents and adolescents. They can teach parents to be supportive and to develop positive communication patterns that help teens feel connected with and loved by their families. To foster healthy development, parents can be encouraged to provide teens with creative outlets and to assist young people in accepting strong emotions—pain, anger, and frustration—as a normal part of the human experience.

Care of suicidal adolescents includes early recognition, management, and prevention. The most important aspect of management is the recognition of warning signs that indicate that an adolescent is troubled and might attempt suicide. The nurse must take any suicidal remarks seriously and not leave the young person alone until the degree of suicidality is assessed. A mnemonic for the assessment process is ***SLAP***: ***s***pecificity, ***l***ethality, ***a***ccessibility, and ***p***roximity. The first step (specificity) is to ask adolescents whether they feel suicidal or as though they would like to take their own lives. If so, have they chosen a means of suicide and do they have a specific plan? The second stage of assessment (lethality) involves determining the lethality of the methods available to them. Do they plan to use a gun or knife? Have they chosen highly lethal medications, hanging, or carbon monoxide poisoning? The third stage (accessibility) involves determining the availability of the means of suicide, and the fourth stage (proximity) involves assessing whether they have determined a time to commit suicide and when.

Health care professionals must be alert to the signs of depression, and anyone who exhibits such behavior should be referred for thorough psychologic assessment. Depression is manifested differently in children and adolescents than in adults. In teens, it may be masked by impulsive aggressive behaviors. Defiance, disobedience, behavior problems, and psychosomatic disturbances can indicate underlying depression, suicidal ideation, and impending suicide attempts.

! NURSING ALERT

No threat of suicide should be ignored or challenged. Threats are a symptom that must be taken seriously. Too often, suicidal threats or minor attempts are confused with bids for attention. It is also a mistake to be lulled into a false sense of security when an adolescent's depression is apparently relieved. The improvement in attitude may mean that the adolescent has made the decision and found the means to carry out the threat.

Peers and other confidants are valuable observers and excellent sources of information about potential suicide attempts. They may not be able to diagnose depression, but they are able to sense when a friend has undergone a marked personality change. It is important to emphasize that the peer who detects any changes in a friend is a potential rescuer and should not remain silent about the observations. Friendship does not imply collusion. A peer who believes that a friend may be suicidal should alert someone who can help (e.g., a parent, teacher, guidance counselor, school nurse).

Routine health assessments of adolescents should include questions that assess the presence of suicidal ideation or intent. The following questions can be asked (Greydanus & Pratt, 1995):

1. Do you consider yourself a happy person, an unhappy person, or somewhere in the middle?
2. Have you ever been so unhappy or upset that you felt like being dead?
3. Have you ever thought about hurting yourself?
4. Have you ever developed a plan to hurt yourself or kill yourself?
5. Have you ever attempted to kill yourself?

If adolescents answer "yes" to questions 2, 3, or 4, they should be asked if they feel that way now to assess for current suicidality. If teens say they have attempted suicide in the past, assess the number of times and ask them to describe what they were feeling, which method they used, what happened, if they would make a similar attempt, and how they would handle their despair now. Any previous suicide attempt indicates an increased risk for a future attempt. The risk for a suicide attempt in the near future increases as the frequency of suicidal ideation increases. For any expression of suicidal intent, the child or adolescent should receive immediate attention and competent psychiatric care.

! NURSING ALERT

The National Suicide Prevention Lifeline (800-273-TALK [8255]; in Spanish, 888-628-9454) offers someone to talk to 24/7.

Because a suicide attempt is frequently an outgrowth of family distress, it is essential to intervene with the family. It is important to assess family interactions and to recognize disturbed relationships. The most effective approach is recognition of susceptible adolescents during the early stages of family distress so that family counseling can be started. Prevention must be directed toward improving childrearing practices through support and education of parents and changing societal conditions that generate defeat, despair, and maladaptive behavior.

Although confidentiality is an essential part of adolescent counseling, in the case of self-destructive behaviors, confidentiality cannot be honored. Suicidal behavior is reported to the family and other professionals, and adolescents are informed that this will be done. Such action conveys an important message to the youth: that the professionals understand and care.

Many schools have instituted suicide prevention programs. These programs include services such as drop-in counseling and a peer counseling telephone line. Information can also be obtained from the American Association of Suicidology.*

*5221 Wisconsin Ave. NW, Washington, DC 20015; 202-237-2280; http://www.suicidology.org.

NCLEX REVIEW QUESTIONS

1. What is the most common treatable cause of male-related impaired fertility, especially if diagnosed and treated early?
   A. Paraphimosis
   B. Trauma to the penis
   C. Idiopathic varicocele
   D. Epididymitis
2. A 15-year-old female diagnosed previously with anorexia nervosa is admitted to the emergency department. Her mother states that her daughter has not voided in 24 hours and has been lethargic for the last 12 hours. The patient appears cachectic and pale, and her weight is recorded as 78 lb. She is minimally responsive to painful stimulation. A number of diagnostic tests are obtained. Which one of these represents the most immediate threat to her life requiring intervention?
   A. Serum sodium of 149 mEq
   B. Serum potassium of 2.6 mEq
   C. Hemoglobin of 6.8 mg
   D. Arterial pH of 7.30
3. Which of the following scenarios are concerning to health care workers? Select all that apply.
   A. An adolescent using marijuana once to fit in with peers at a party
   B. An adolescent binging on alcohol every weekend
   C. An adolescent using prescription drugs along with alcohol
   D. An adolescent reports feeling jittery until she drinks some alcohol
4. Common causes of pelvic inflammatory disease in the United States include which of the following? Select all that apply.
   A. *Neisseria gonorrhoea*
   B. *Chlamydia trachomatis*
   C. *Treponema pallidum*
   D. Human papillomavirus
5. A warning sign of self-harm includes which one of the following?
   A. Multiple bruises on arms and legs
   B. Poor school performance
   C. Finding tobacco products hidden in the adolescent's room
   D. Spending long periods of time in a locked bedroom or bathroom

Correct Answers

1. C; 2. B; 3. B, C, D; 4. A, B; 5. D

REFERENCES

Afsarlar, C. E., Ryan, S. L., Donel, E., et al. (2016). Standardized process to improve patient flow from the emergency room to the operating room for pediatric patients with testicular torsion. *Journal of Pediatric Urology*, *12*(4), 233.

Akgul, S., & Kanbur, N. (2015). Premenstrual disorder and the adolescent: Clinical case report, literature review, and diagnostic and therapeutic challenges. *International Journal of Adolescent Medicine and Health*, *27*(4), 363–368.

Al-Sayed, E. M., & Ibrahim, K. S. (2014). Second-hand tobacco smoke and children. *Toxicology and Industrial Health*, *30*(7), 635–644.

American Academy of Pediatrics, Committee on Adolescence. (2014). Contraception for adolescents. *Pediatrics*, *134*(4), e1244–e1256.

American Academy of Pediatrics, Committee on Adolescence. (2017). The adolescent's right to confidential care when considering abortion. *Pediatrics*, *139*(2), e20163861.

American Academy of Pediatrics, Committee on Infectious Diseases, & Pickering, L. (Eds.), (2015). *2015 Red book: Report of the Committee on Infectious Diseases* (30th ed.). Elk Grove Village, IL: The Academy.

American College of Obstetricians and Gynecologists, Committee on Adolescent Health Care. (2014). The initial reproductive health visit. *Obstetrics and Gynecology*, *123*, 1143–1147.

American Psychiatric Association (2013). *Diagnostic and statistical manual of mental disorders: DSM-V*. Washington, DC: American Psychiatric Publishing, Inc.

Armstrong, W. R., Grimsby, G. M., & Jacobs, M. A. (2015). Pediatric priapism secondary to psychotherapeutic medications. *Urology*, *86*(2), 376–378.

Berends, T., van Meijel, B., Nugteren, W., et al. (2016). Rate, timing and predictors of relapse in patients with anorexia nervosa following a relapse prevention program: A cohort study. *BMC Psychiatry*, *16*(1), 316.

Berz, K., & McCambridge, T. (2016). Amenorrhea in the female athlete: What to do and when to worry. *Pediatric Annals*, *45*(3), e97–e102.

Beukers, L., Berends, T., de Man–van Ginkel, J. M., et al. (2015). Restoring normal eating behavior in adolescents with anorexia nervosa: A video analysis of nursing interventions. *International Journal of Mental Health Nursing*, *24*(6), 519–526.

Bradshaw, C. S., & Sobel, J. D. (2016). Current treatment of bacterial vaginosis-limitations and need for innovation. *The Journal of Infectious Diseases*, *214*(Suppl. 1), S14–S20.

Brown, R. C., & Plener, P. L. (2017). Non-suicidal self-injury in adolescence. *Current Psychiatry Reports*, *19*(3), 20.

Campbell, K., & Peebles, R. (2014). Eating disorders in children and adolescents: State of the art review. *Pediatrics*, *134*(3), 582–592.

Centers for Disease Control and Prevention: *2015 sexually transmitted diseases treatment guidelines*, 2015. Retrieved from https://www.cdc.gov/std/tg2015/bv.htm.

Centers for Disease Control and Prevention: *2015 sexually transmitted diseases surveillance*, 2016a. Retrieved from https://www.cdc.gov/std/stats15/toc.htm.

Centers for Disease Control and Prevention: *Pelvic inflammatory disease (PID)*, 2016b. Retrieved from https://www.cdc.gov/std/pid/stdfact-pid-detailed.htm.

Centers for Disease Control and Prevention: *Human papillomavirus (HPV)*, 2016c. Retrieved from https://www.cdc.gov/hpv/.

Centers for Disease Control and Prevention: *Reproductive health: teen pregnancy*, 2017. Retrieved from https://www.cdc.gov/teenpregnancy/.

Centers for Disease Control and Prevention: *Sexually transmitted diseases treatment guidelines, 2010*, 2011. Retrieved from https://www.cdc.gov/std/treatment/2010/clinical.htm.

Chahal, A., Gupta, S., & Das, C. (2016). Penile fracture. *BMJ Case Reports*, *2016*.

Craner, J. R., Sigmon, S. T., Martinson, A. A., et al. (2014). Premenstrual disorders and rumination. *Journal of Clinical Psychology*, *70*(1), 32–47.

Das, B. B., Ronda, J., & Trent, M. (2016). Pelvic inflammatory disease: Improving awareness, prevention and treatment. *Infection and Drug Resistance*, *9*, 191–197.

Deligeoroglou, E., Karountzos, V., & Creatsas, G. (2013). Abnormal uterine bleeding and dysfunctional uterine bleeding in pediatric and adolescent gynecology. *Gynecological Endocrinology*, *29*(1), 74–78.

Diorio, G. J., & Giuliano, A. R. (2016). The role of human papilloma virus in penile carcinogenesis and preneoplastic lesions: A potential target for vaccinations and treatment strategies. *The Urologic Clinics of North America*, *43*(4), 419–425.

Doyle, L., Sheridan, A., & Treacy, M. P. (2017). Motivations for adolescent self-harm and the implications for mental health nurses. *Journal of Psychiatric and Mental Health Nursing*, *24*(2–3), 124–142.

Doyle, L., Treacy, M. P., & Sheridan, A. (2015). Self-harm in young people: Prevalence, associated factors, and help-seeking in school-going adolescents. *International Journal of Mental Health Nursing*, *24*(6), 485–494.

Elder, J. S. (2016). Disorders and anomalies of the scrotal contents. In R. M. Kliegman, B. F. Stanton, J. W. St. Geme, et al. (Eds.), *Nelson textbook of pediatrics* (20th ed.). Philadelphia: Saunders/Elsevier.

Fichter, M. M., & Quadflieq, N. (2016). Mortality in eating disorders – results of a large prospective clinical longitudinal study. *The International Journal of Eating Disorders*, *49*(4), 391–401.

Fielder, R. L., Walsh, J. L., Carey, K. B., et al. (2013). Predictors of sexual hookups: A theory-based, prospective study of first-year college women. *Archives of Sexual Behavior*, *42*(8), 1425–1441.

Ford, O., Lethaby, A., Roberts, H., et al. (2012). Progesterone for premenstrual syndrome. *Cochrane Database of Systematic Review*, (3), CD003415.

Frank, G. K., & Shott, M. E. (2016). The role of psychotropic medications in the management of anorexia nervosa: Rationale, evidence and future prospects. *CNS Drugs*, *30*(5), 419–442.

Garber, A. K., Sawyer, S. M., Golden, N. H., et al. (2016). A systematic review of approaches to refeeding in patients with anorexia nervosa. *The International Journal of Eating Disorders*, *49*(3), 293–310.

Garcia-Roig, M. L., & Kirsch, A. J. (2015). The dilemma of adolescent varicocele. *Pediatric Surgery International*, *31*(7), 617–625.

Gibson, E. J., Bell, D. L., & Powerful, S. A. (2014). Common sexually transmitted infections in adolescents. *Primary Care*, *41*(3), 631–650.

Greydanus, D. E., & Pratt, H. D. (1995). Emotional and behavioral disorders of adolescence (Part 2). *Adolesc Health Update*, *8*(1), 1–8.

Harrington, B. C., Jimerson, M., Haxton, C., et al. (2015). Initial evaluation, diagnosis, and treatment of anorexia nervosa and bulimia nervosa. *American Family Physician*, *91*(1), 46–52.

Herpertz-Dahlmann, B. (2015). Adolescent eating disorders: Update on definitions, symptomatology, epidemiology, and comorbidity. *Child & Adolescent Psychiatric Clinics of North America*, *24*(1), 177–196.

Hilbert, D. W., Smith, W. L., Chadwick, S. G., et al. (2016). Development and validation of a highly accurate quantitative real-time assay for diagnosis of bacterial vaginosis. *Journal Clinical Microbiology*, *54*(4), 1017–1024.

Hofmeister, S., & Bodden, S. (2016). Premenstrual syndrome and premenstrual dysphoric disorder. *American Family Physician*, *94*(3), 236–240.

Homa, D. M., Neff, L. J., King, B. A., et al. (2015). Vital signs: Disparities in nonsmokers' exposure to secondhand smoke – United States, 1999–2012. *MMWR. Morbidity and Mortality Weekly Report*, *64*(4), 103–108.

Horne, A. W., Brown, J. K., Nio-Kobayashi, J., et al. (2014). The association between smoking and ectopic pregnancy: why nicotine is BAD for your fallopian tube. *PLoS ONE*, *9*(2), e89400.

Jatlaoui, T. C., Ewing, A., Mandel, M. G., et al. (2016). Abortion surveillance – United States, 2013. *MMWR. Surveillance Summaries: Morbidity and Mortality Weekly Report. Surveillance Summaries / CDC*, *65*(12), 1–44.

Johnston, L. D., O'Malley, P. M., Miech, R. A., et al. (2015). *Monitoring the Future national results on adolescent drug use: 1975-2014: Overview, key findings on adolescent drug use*. Ann Arbor: Institute for Social Research, The University of Michigan.

Kann, L., McManus, T., Harris, W. A., et al. (2016). Youth risk behavior surveillance – United States, 2015. *MMWR. Morbidity and Mortality Weekly Report*, *65*(6), 1–180.

Kawakita, T., Wilson, K., Grantz, K. L., et al. (2016). Adverse maternal and neonatal outcomes in adolescent pregnancy. *Journal of Pediatric and Adolescent Gynecology*, *29*(2), 130–136.

Kominiarek, M. A., & Rajan, P. (2016). Nutrition recommendations in pregnancy and lactation. *The Medical Clinics of North America*, *100*(6), 1199–1215.

Kreipe, R. E. (2016). Eating disorders. In R. M. Kliegman, B. F. Stanton, J. W. St. Geme, et al. (Eds.), *Nelson textbook of pediatrics* (20th ed.). Philadelphia: Saunders/Elsevier.

Lau, C. C. (2016). The lives of young fathers: A review of selected evidence. *Social Policy and Society: A Journal of the Social Policy Association, 15*(1), 129–140.

Makhzoumi, S. H., Coughlin, J. W., Schreyer, C. C., et al. (2017). Weight gain trajectories in hospital-based Treatment of anorexia nervosa. *The International Journal of Eating Disorders, 50*(3), 266–274.

Marynak, K. L., Gammon, D. G., Rogers, T., et al. (2017). Sales of nicotine-containing electronic cigarette products: United States, 2015. *American Journal of Public Health, 107*(5), 702–705.

Matthews, E. M., Woodward, C. J., Musso, M. W., et al. (2016). Suicide attempts presenting to trauma centers: Trends across groups using the national trauma data bank. *The American Journal of Emergency Medicine, 34*(8), 1620–1624.

Matzkin, E., Curry, E. J., & Whitlock, K. (2015). Female athlete triad: Past, present, and future. *The Journal of the American Academy of Orthopaedic Surgeons, 23*(7), 424–432.

McConaghy, J. R., & Panchal, B. (2016). Epididymitis: An overview. *American Family Physician, 94*(9), 723–726.

Mendling, W., Weissenbacher, E. R., Gerber, S., et al. (2016). Use of locally delivered dequalinium chloride in the treatment of vaginal infections: A review. *Archives of Gynecology and Obstetrics, 293*(3), 469–484.

Midilli, T. S., Yasar, E., & Baysal, E. (2015). Dysmenorrhea characteristics of female students of health school and affecting factors and their knowledge and use of complementary and alternative medicine methods. *Holistic Nursing Practice, 29*(4), 194–204.

Oudekerk, B. A., Guarnera, L. A., & Reppucci, N. D. (2014). Older opposite-sex romantic partners, sexual risk, and victimization in adolescence. *Child Abuse and Neglect, 38*(7), 1238–1248.

Pazol, K., Whiteman, M. K., Folger, S. G., et al. (2015). Sporadic contraceptive use and nonuse: Age-specific prevalence and associated factors. *American Journal of Obstetrics and Gynecology, 212*(3), 324.

Pohlman, G. D., Phillips, J. M., & Wilcox, D. T. (2013). Simple method of paraphimosis reduction revisited: Point of technique and review of the literature. *Journal of Pediatric Urology, 9*(1), 104–107.

Rani, A., Sharma, M. K., & Singh, A. (2016). Practices and perceptions of adolescent girls regarding the impact of dysmenorrhea on their routine life. *International Journal of Adolescent Medicine and Health, 28*(1), 3–9.

Sapra, K. J., Joseph, K. S., Galea, S., et al. (2017). Signs and symptoms of early pregnancy loss. *Reproductive Sciences, 24*(4), 502–513.

Saridogan, E. (2017). Adolescent endometriosis. *European Journal of Obstetrics, Gynecology & Reproductive Biology, 209*, 46–49.

Sauerbrei, A. (2016). Optimal management of genital herpes: Current perspectives. *Infection and Drug Resistance, 9*, 129–141.

Smith, L., & Angarone, M. P. (2015). Sexually transmitted infections. *The Urologic Clinics of North America, 42*(4), 507–518.

Sobel, J. D. (2016). Recurrent vulvovaginal candidiasis. *American Journal of Obstetrics and Gynecology, 214*(1), 15–21.

Singh, T., Arrazola, R. A., & Corey, C. G. (2016). Tobacco use among middle and high school students – United States, 2011–2015. *MMWR. Morbidity and Mortality Weekly Report, 65*(14), 361–367.

Spain, J., & Rheinboldt, M. (2017). MDCT of pelvic inflammatory disease: A review of the pathophysiology, gamut of imaging findings, and treatment. *Emergency Radiology, 24*(1), 87–93.

Stager, M. M. (2016). Substance abuse. In R. M. Kliegman, B. F. Stanton, J. W. St. Geme, et al. (Eds.), *Nelson textbook of pediatrics* (20th ed.). Philadelphia: Saunders/Elsevier.

Stice, E., South, K., & Shaw, H. (2012). Future directions in etiologic, prevention, and treatment research for eating disorders. *Journal of Clinical Child and Adolescent Psychology, 41*(6), 845–855.

Sucato, G. S., & Burstein, G. R. (2016). Menstrual problems. In R. M. Kliegman, B. F. Stanton, J. W. St. Geme, et al. (Eds.), *Nelson textbook of pediatrics* (20th ed.). Philadelphia: Saunders/Elsevier.

Thompson, M. P., & Swartout, K. (2017). Epidemiology of suicide attempts among youth transitioning to adulthood. *Journal of Youth and Adolescence*, [epub ahead of print].

Trace, S. E., Baker, J. H., Peñas-Lledó, E., et al. (2013). The genetics of eating disorders. *Annual Review of Clinical Psychology, 9*(1), 589–620.

Trent, S. A., Moreira, M. E., Colwell, C. B., et al. (2013). ED management of patients with eating disorders. *The American Journal of Emergency Medicine, 31*(5), 859–865.

Ullman, S. E., & Peter-Hagene, L. C. (2016). Longitudinal relationships of social reactions, PTSD symptoms, and revictimization in sexual assault survivors. *Journal of Interpersonal Violence, 31*(6), 1074–1094.

Wade, T. D., Fairweather-Schmidt, A. K., Zhu, G., et al. (2015). Does shared genetic risk contribute to the co-occurrence of eating disorders and suicidality? *The International Journal of Eating Disorders, 48*(6), 684–691.

Wong, S. S., Zhou, B., Goebert, D., et al. (2013). The risk of adolescent suicide across patterns of drug use: A nationally representative study of high school students in the United States from 1999 to 2009. *Social Psychiatry and Psychiatric Epidemiology, 48*(12), 1611–1620.

Workowski, K. A., Bolan, G. A., & Centers for Disease Control and Prevention. (2015). Sexually transmitted diseases treatment guidelines, 2015. *MMWR. Recommendations and Reports: Morbidity and Mortality Weekly Report. Recommendations and Reports, 64*(RR–03), 1–137.

Yu, A. (2014). Complementary and alternative treatments for primary dysmenorrhea in adolescents. *The Nurse Practitioner, 39*(11), 1–12.

19

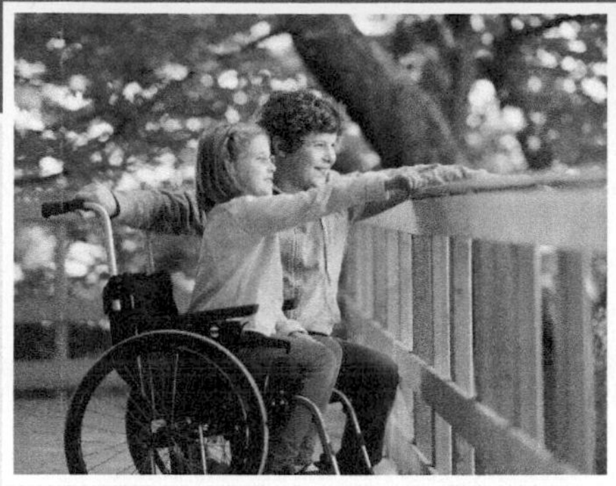

Impact of Chronic Illness, Disability, or End-of-Life Care for the Child and Family

Sharron L. Docherty, Debra Brandon, Alexandra Kathleen Superdock, and Raymond C. Barfield

http://evolve.elsevier.com/wong/ncic

CONCEPTS

Chronic Illness
Palliative Care

PERSPECTIVES ON THE CARE OF CHILDREN AND FAMILIES LIVING WITH OR DYING FROM CHRONIC OR COMPLEX DISEASES

SCOPE OF THE PROBLEM

Advances in medical and nursing care, such as the increasing viability of extremely preterm infants, the portability of life-sustaining technology (e.g., total parental nutrition, ventilatory support), and life-extending treatments for children with conditions that previously would have led to an early death (e.g., malignancies, genetic conditions), have led to an exponential rise in the prevalence of children with complex and chronic diseases (Burke and Alverson, 2010; Simon, Berry, Feudtner, et al, 2010). These children have complex conditions involving several organ systems and require multiple specialists, technologic supports, and community services to assist them to function to their healthiest potential. The complex, high level of skill required to meet their daily health care needs and the continuous nature and potential volatility of the condition sets this group apart from the broader population of children with special health care needs (Cohen, Kuo, Agrawal, et al, 2011; Simon, Berry, Feudtner, et al, 2010; Kuo, Cohen, Agrawal, et al, 2011). A range of terms, such as *complex chronic condition, medically complex, technology dependent,* and *multiply handicapped,* have been used to describe this vulnerable population of children (Cohen, Kuo, Agrawal, et al, 2011; Feudtner, Feinstein, Zhong, et al, 2014). Frequent and prolonged hospitalizations; complex and multisystem health and developmental needs; and reliance on technology and care that cross hospital, clinic, and home settings are the key characteristics that all of these terms seek to signify about the children they are used to represent (Berry, Hall, Hall, et al, 2013; Cohen, Kuo, Agrawal, et al, 2011; Feudtner, Feinstein, Zhong, et al, 2014).

The nature and severity of childhood chronic and complex conditions is widely heterogeneous. Table 19.1 is a non-exhaustive sampling of conditions organized by specialty. However, these children and families are similar in the vulnerability that they experience due to the health and developmental consequences of these diagnoses on the child, such as ongoing functional impairment, neurodevelopmental disability, dependence on medical technology, and the need for ongoing skilled supportive care from health care providers and family members. Although many authors have described the rise in prevalence that has come about because of advances in medical care (Burns, Casey, Lyle, et al, 2010; Simon, Berry, and Feudtner, et al, 2010), accurate estimates of the numbers of affected families are not known. However, the impact of chronic and complex illness in children is wide ranging. The family experiences significant challenges necessitated by the child's care requirements (Goudie, Narcisse, Hall, et al, 2014; Kuo, Cohen, Agrawal, et al, 2011). A child's activity level and developmental opportunities can be affected. Days can be lost from school. Children with complex chronic conditions may be at increased risk for behavior or emotional problems. Parents may lose days from work, experience financial strain, and be challenged both emotionally and physically as they cope with care of the child.

Siblings are also affected by having a "different" brother or sister, and they may simultaneously feel guilt, anger, or jealousy toward their ill sibling. Clinicians need to know that siblings of children with chronic illnesses are at risk for negative psychological effects (Hartling, Milne, Tjosvold, et al, 2014). Parents need encouragement and assistance with

TABLE 19.1 Chronic Conditions of Childhood

Specialty	Examples of Chronic Conditions
Cardiology	Complex congenital heart disease, congestive heart failure, cardiac dysrhythmias, Kawasaki disease, rheumatic fever, hyperlipidemia
Endocrinology	Diabetes, congenital adrenal hyperplasia, Cushing syndrome
Gastroenterology	Short bowel syndrome, biliary atresia, inflammatory bowel disease, hepatitis, cirrhosis, peptic ulcer disease, celiac disease
Hematology	Sickle cell anemia, thalassemia, aplastic anemia, hereditary anemias, hemophilia
Immunology	Immune deficiency, human immunodeficiency virus, Wiskott-Aldrich syndrome, severe combined immunodeficiency disease
Nephrology	Prune belly syndrome, renal disease
Neurology	Cerebral palsy, ataxia telangiectasia, muscular dystrophy, seizure disorder, spina bifida, traumatic brain injury
Oncology	Brain tumor, leukemia, lymphoma, solid tumors, bone tumors, rare tumors
Pulmonology	Asthma, chronic lung disease, cystic fibrosis, tuberculosis
Rheumatology	Systemic lupus erythematosus, juvenile rheumatoid arthritis, dermatomyositis

understanding the reactions of siblings to having a chronically ill family member (e.g., behavioral regression, anxiety, withdrawal, apathy). Additionally, secondary losses (such as, the ability to participate in extracurricular activities or social events) occur because of routines imposed by the affected child's chronic condition.

TRENDS IN CARE

Family-Centered Care

Children's physical and emotional health, as well as their cognitive and social functioning, is strongly influenced by how well their families function (Treyvaud, 2014; Kuhlthau, Bloom, Van Cleave, et al, 2011). The importance of family-centered care—a philosophy that considers the family as the constant in the child's life—is especially evident in the care of children with special needs (see also Family-Centered Care, Chapter 1). As parents learn about the child's health care needs, they often become experts in delivering care. Health care providers, including nurses, are adjuncts to the child's care and need to form partnerships with parents. Effective communication and negotiation between parents and nurses are essential to forming trusting and effective partnerships and finding the best ways to meet the needs of the child and family (Kuo, Houtrow, Arango et al, 2012). Collaborative relationships are characterized by communication, dialogue, active listening, awareness, and acceptance of others' differences (Kuhlthau, Bloom, Van Cleave, et al, 2011).

Family–Health Care Provider Communication

The disclosure of a serious chronic or complex condition of a child is one of the most stressful aspects of communication between families and health care professionals. Often, parents have suspected for some time that something is wrong with their child and believe that their concerns were minimized or ignored by health care professionals (Smaldone and Ritholz, 2011). After a diagnosis is made, factors that influence parent dissatisfaction with the way in which information is communicated include disrespectful attitudes, breaking bad news in an insensitive manner, withholding information, and changing a treatment course without preparing the child and family (Barnes, Gardiner, Gott, et al, 2012). Conversely, parents report satisfaction when they perceived health care providers to be available, demonstrate competence, and engage the child and parent in care decision making (Barnes, Gardiner, Gott, et al, 2012; Kuo, Sisterhen, Sigrest, et al, 2012). Similar factors are important in communication of changes in the child's condition throughout the course of the illness.

Providing information to families with a chronically ill child should be a process of repeated discussions to allow the family to process the information and their reactions to that information and allow them to ask for clarification and further information. Nurses play an important role in ensuring that families' needs are met during discussions related to the child's diagnosis, condition, and treatment. This requires assessment regarding how much information the family is comfortable with, what they understand of the information already given to them, and how they are coping with the information both cognitively and emotionally. Nurses should ensure that the appropriate health care professionals address any concerns or further questions that families may have.

Establishing Therapeutic Relationships

Another important aspect of family-centered care of children with chronic and complex conditions is establishing a therapeutic relationship with the child and family, which has been shown to predict improved health-related outcomes (Kuhlthau, Bloom, Van Cleave, et al, 2011). Families, most often the mother, take on enormous responsibility in providing technical care and symptom management of their child's condition outside of the health care institution (Goudie, Narcisse, Hall, et al, 2014). To build successful therapeutic relationships with families, it is necessary for nurses to recognize parents' expertise with regard to their child's condition and needs. Health care environments for children with serious illnesses are fraught with obstacles that serve as barriers to successful therapeutic relationships with families. Individual discussions, especially with the case manager, primary nurse, clinical nurse specialist, or nurse practitioner, help establish a consistent and flexible care plan that can prevent conflicts or deal with these conflicts before they disrupt care.

The Role of Culture in Family-Centered Care

Issues of culture, ethnicity, and race affect access to services, utilization, and follow-through with referrals and recommendations (Coker, Rodriguez, and Flores, 2010; Toomey, Chien, Elliott, et al, 2013). For some ethnic and minority populations, cultural understandings of illness, the structure of family life, social roles for individuals with disabilities, and other factors related to the perception of children may differ from those of mainstream American culture.

Although culture cannot completely explain how an individual will think and act, understanding cultural perspectives can help the nurse anticipate and understand why families may make certain decisions. Cultural attributes such as values and beliefs regarding illness or chronic condition and its causation, social roles for people who are ill or disabled, family structure, the role of children, childrearing practices, self versus group orientation, spirituality, and time orientation also affect a family's response to illness or chronic condition in a child (Wiener, McConnell, Latella, et al, 2013).

When parents are informed of their child's chronic illness, interpreters familiar with both culture and language should be used. Children, family members, and friends of the family should not be used as translators because their presence may prevent parents from openly discussing the issues. When working with people of cultural backgrounds different from their own, nurses must listen carefully with an initial goal of understanding and articulating the family's perspective. The ability to interpret the mainstream medical culture to the family is also important. Furthermore, every effort is made to incorporate traditional cultural beliefs of a family into treatment plans. It is important to keep in mind that "cultural norms" may not always apply to every family from a shared background. Developing a care plan in conjunction with the family, considering their preferences and priorities, is an important first step in formulating a plan that best meets the family's needs, no matter what their cultural background (Coker, Rodriguez, and Flores, 2010; Wiener, McConnell, Latella, et al, 2013).

Shared Decision Making

Shared decision making among the child, family, and health care team can result from open, honest, culturally sensitive communication and the establishment of a therapeutic relationship among the family and health care providers. In a shared decision-making model, the health care professionals provide honest, clear information regarding diagnosis, prognosis, treatment options, and risk–benefit assessment. The patient and family then share information with the health care team regarding important family values, acceptable levels of discomfort or inconvenience, and the ability to comply with treatments being recommended (Wiener, McConnell, Latella, et al, 2013; Wyatt, List, Brinkman, et al, 2015). This process allows them to discuss all options in terms of the risks and benefits to the child and family, the prognosis or expected course of the illness, and the impact on the family's resources (Box 19.1). Together, the parents and health care team can make decisions that are best for the family and child at the time the decision is made.

Normalization

Normalization refers to the efforts family members make to create a normal family life, their perceptions of the consequences of these efforts, and the meanings they attribute to their management efforts (Knafl, Darney, Gallo, et al, 2010). For chronically ill children, such efforts may include attending school, pursuing hobbies and recreational interests, and achieving employment and a level of independence. For their families, it may entail adapting the family routine to accommodate the ill or disabled child's health and physical needs (Kuo, Cohen, Agrawal, et al, 2011).

Children with chronic and complex conditions and their families face numerous challenges in achieving normalization. Families move between the "normal" of living with the experience of chronic childhood illness and the "normal" of the healthy outside world; they often redefine "normal" based on their particular experiences, needs, and circumstances (Knafl, Darney, Gallo, et al, 2010). Normalization may be an important mediator of illness-related stressors (e.g., treatment demands, uncertainty) on family outcomes.

Nurses can assist families in normalizing their lives by assessing the family's everyday life, social support systems, coping strategies, family cohesiveness, and family and community resources. Interventions include encouraging families to reduce stress through delegation of care and family tasks, identifying ways to incorporate care into current routines, structuring the home environment to encourage the child's engagement in age-appropriate activities, and ensuring families have access to appropriate community support services (Knafl and Santacroce, 2010). Being supportive of the child's illness and treatment and actively including the family in all aspects of care will improve their self-esteem and promote further development (Knafl and Santacroce, 2010).

Home care represents the return to a system and set of priorities in which family values are as important in the care of a child with a chronic health problem as they are in the care of other children. Home care seeks to achieve goals that are consistent with the developmental model (Stein, 1985):

- Normalize the life of the child, including those with technologically complex care, in a family and community context and setting.
- Minimize the disruptive impact of the child's condition on the family.
- Foster the child's maximum growth and development.

With appropriate training and support, families provide complex procedures and treatments in the home. Parents are challenged to retain a homelike setting among monitors, ventilators, and other sophisticated equipment. Throughout the text, home care is discussed as appropriate for specific conditions.

Paralleling normalization and home care is the process of **mainstreaming**, or integrating children with disabilities into regular classrooms. Children who attend school have the advantages of learning and socializing with a wide group of peers. There is an increased focus on individualization as plans are made to meet the academic needs of these children along with those of the rest of the students.

A variety of supplemental programs have been designed in the school system to accommodate special needs, both at school age and younger, through **early intervention**, which consists of any sustained and systematic effort to assist children from birth to 3 years old with disabilities and who are developmentally vulnerable. This change and increasing opportunities for normalization for children with disabilities in large part have resulted from the passage of (1) the Education for All Handicapped Children Act of 1975 (Public Law 94-142) and its 1990 amendments (Public Law 101-476), which changed the name of the Act to the Individuals with Disabilities Education Act (IDEA); (2) the Education of the Handicapped Act Amendments of 1986 (Public Law 99-457), which directs states to develop and implement statewide comprehensive, coordinated, multidisciplinary interagency programs of early intervention services for infants and toddlers with disabilities, as well as support services for their families; and (3) the Americans with Disabilities Act of 1990. Nurses can provide parents with information about these laws and in some cases may participate in the development of individualized educational programs (IEPs) or individualized family service plans (IFSPs) for children with disabilities.

BOX 19.1 Facilitating Shared Decision Making

- Continually assess the impact of the child's illness and treatment on the family.
- Provide honest, accurate information regarding the trajectory of the disease, anticipated complications, and prognostic information.
- Discuss what the family desires for the child's quality of life.
- Avoid personal opinion or judgment of the family's questions and decisions.
- Be aware of nurses' personal and cultural assumptions and the ways these assumptions impact communication, decision making, and judgment.

THE FAMILY OF THE CHILD WITH A CHRONIC OR COMPLEX CONDITION

A major goal in working with the family of a child with chronic or complex illness is to support the family's coping and promote their optimal functioning throughout the child's life. Long-term, comprehensive care involves forming parent–professional partnerships that can support a family's adaptation across the trajectory of the illness to the many changes that may be necessary in day-to-day life, determine

BOX 19.2 Adaptive Tasks of Parents Having Children With Chronic Conditions

1. Accept the child's condition.
2. Manage the child's condition on a day-to-day basis.
3. Meet the child's normal developmental needs.
4. Meet the developmental needs of other family members.
5. Cope with ongoing stress and periodic crises.
6. Assist family members to manage their feelings.
7. Educate others about the child's condition.
8. Establish a support system.

From Canam C: Common adaptive tasks facing parents of children with chronic conditions, *J Adv Nurs* 18:46-53, 1993.

BOX 19.3 Anticipated Parental Stress Points

Diagnosis of the condition: Parents require considerable education while dealing with an emotional response.
Developmental milestones: Times that children normally achieve walking, talking, and self-care are delayed or impossible for the child.
Start of schooling: Particularly stressful are situations in which appropriate schooling will not be in a regular class placement.
Reaching the ultimate attainment: Parents must handle situations such as realizing that ambulation will be impossible or that the child will not learn to read.
Adolescence: Issues such as sexuality and independence become prominent.
Future placement: Decisions about placement must be made when the child becomes an adult or when the parents can no longer care for the child.
Death of the child

expectations of and for the child, and provide a long-term perspective (Box 19.2).

Often the impact of a child's medical or developmental condition is first experienced as a crisis at the time of diagnosis, which may occur at birth, after a long period of diagnostic testing, or immediately after a tragic injury. But the impact may also be felt before the diagnosis is made, when parents are aware that something is wrong with their child but before medical confirmation (Smaldone and Ritholz, 2011).

The diagnosis and initial discharge home are critical times for parents. Several factors can make this particularly difficult, including a long duration of uncertainty in the diagnostic process, negative perceptions of chronic illness, insufficient information, and lack of mutual trust between parents and their child's health care team (Huang, Kenzik, Sanjeev, et al, 2010). Parental feelings of shock, helplessness, isolation, fear, and depression are common.Throughout the first year, parents struggle to accept the child's diagnosis, care, and uncertainty of the future (Coffey, 2006). Optimal support at the time of diagnosis and initial discharge home can be encouraged by providing explicit and uncomplicated information to parents in an empathic way (Nuutila and Salanterä, 2006); assessing the family's daily routine, living conditions, background knowledge, skills and abilities, and coping behaviors; and evaluating the family's understanding of the information. It is also necessary to reassess parents' needs for information and support on a routine basis (Nuutila and Salanterä, 2006).

Other critical times include the exacerbation of the child's physical symptoms, which increases parental care. These crises often involve medical intervention and rehospitalization. Frequently, the child does not return to his or her precrisis level of functioning, and parents and family must adapt to new care needs and schedules. Instability may also follow transition points on the illness trajectory. Supporting parents, respecting their stress and emotions, and acknowledging their role as team members in the care of their child are important aspects of nursing care (Panicker, 2013).

IMPACT OF THE CHILD'S CHRONIC ILLNESS

Each member in the family of a child with a chronic or complex illness is affected by the experience (Goudie, Narcisse, Hall, et al, 2014; Kuo, Cohen, Agrawal, 2011). The effects on the parents and their responses may be so intense that they directly influence the other members' reactions and the child's own coping.

Parents

In addition to the stress of grieving for the loss of hope for a perfect child, parents are affected by whether or not they receive positive feedback from interactions with their child. Many parents feel satisfaction and fulfillment from the parenting role. For others, parenting may be a series of unrewarding experiences that contribute to feelings of inadequacy and failure (Box 19.3). These responses may be most evident in parents who are responsible for the child's care. For example, parents may become preoccupied with their ability to carry out certain procedures, overlooking the child's personal comfort and satisfaction, or failing to offer praise for anything less than perfect cooperation or performance. They may pursue a frustrating activity until they achieve "success"—long after the child has become irritable and uncooperative. As a result, parents can become caught in a pattern of interaction that is mutually unrewarding and minimally productive. This situation may become exacerbated by disagreements or lack of support from other family members and judgment from caregivers and others in the community. For these parents, several strategies may be helpful, including education regarding what can reasonably be expected of their child, assistance in identifying the child's strengths, praise for a parental job well done, and respite care so that parents can renew their energies.

Parental Roles

Parenting a child with a complex chronic condition requires attending to the routine aspects of parenting with the added responsibility of performing complex technical care, symptom management, advocating for their child, and seeking and coordinating health and social services for their ill or disabled child. These added responsibilities must then be balanced with the needs of other family members, extended family and friends, and personal health and obligations to minimize consequences to the overall functioning of the family.

Often one parent or partner remains at home to manage existing family responsibilities while the other remains with the ill child. The partner who is not included in the caregiving activities may feel neglected because all of the attention is directed toward the child and be resentful that he or she is not sufficiently informed to be competent in the care. Without active participation in the child's care, the parent has little appreciation of the time and energy involved in performing these activities. When this partner does attempt to participate, the other parent may criticize the less skillful efforts. As a result, communication and support for each other may be adversely affected.

The nurse can assist parents in avoiding role conflicts by providing anticipatory guidance early on. Teaching should address stressors often identified as having an impact on the marriage, including (1) the burden of care at home assumed by primarily one parent, (2) the financial burden, (3) the fear of the child dying, (4) pressure from relatives, (5) the hereditary nature of the disease (if applicable), and (6) fear of pregnancy. Other causes of tension may center on the inconveniences associated with care, such as long waits for an appointment, lack of parking near care facilities, or lack of overnight accommodations.

Mother–Father Differences

Mothers and fathers of a child with a complex condition often adjust and cope differently. Mothers are often the primary caregiver and are more likely than fathers to give up their jobs to care for their children, often resulting in social isolation (Coffey, 2006). Mothers often have greater needs for social support and positive appraisal of the situation than fathers.

Fathers of children with disabilities struggle with issues that may be distinct from those of the mothers (Swallow, Macfadyen, Santacroce, et al, 2012). Fathers may think that their role as protector is challenged because they do not know how to help and cannot protect their family from the seemingly overwhelming recurring problems. The extensive stresses in the family can leave fathers feeling depressed, weak, guilty, powerless, isolated, embarrassed, and angry. Fearful that they will lose control or be viewed as weak or ineffectual, however, fathers often hide their feelings and display an outward confidence that may lead others to believe that everything is fine. Fathers worry about what the future holds for their children, their ability to manage the increasing financial burden, and the daily disruptions of the entire family (Swallow, Macfadyen, Santacroce, et al, 2012).

Single-Parent Families

Single-parent families are of special concern. As the only parent of a child who may require extensive, sophisticated, and lifelong care, the single parent may feel an enormous burden. Available financial and emotional resources may already be stretched to the limit. A special effort should be made to assist the single parent in finding financial and support services that can ease the burden of care. Nurses can also assist the single parent in identifying helping roles that may be acceptable to relatives and friends.

Siblings

Results of studies are less clear regarding the ways that siblings are affected by having a brother or sister with a complex condition (Anderson and Davis, 2011; Hartling, Milne, Tjosvold, et al, 2014). Most evidence shows a negative effect on siblings of children with chronic illnesses compared with siblings of healthy children (Gold, Treadwell, Weissman, et al, 2011; Hartling, Milne, Tjosvold, et al, 2014). Siblings of children with chronic illnesses report psychosocial problems more often than their peers (Gold, Treadwell, Weissman, et al, 2011). A number of factors increase the risk of negative effects for siblings of ill children. Responsibility for caregiving, differential treatment by parents, and limitations in family resources and recreational time are often the experiences of siblings of ill or disabled children. (Box 19.4).

An important factor in sibling adjustment and coping is information and knowledge regarding their brother's or sister's illness or complex condition. What siblings piece together or overhear is often much worse than the truth. Often they imagine gruesome things regarding the experiences related to the illness, treatment, and hospitalization (Knafl and Santacroce, 2010). Latino siblings have reported less accurate information about their siblings' condition than non-Latino siblings (Lobato, Kao, and Plante, 2005). Parents are usually in the best position to impart information, although they are often overwhelmed with the medical crisis at hand. Nurses can encourage parents to talk with the siblings about how they perceive their sick brother or sister and to be accepting of the siblings' feelings. Nurses can be ideal educators and

BOX 19.4 Supporting Siblings of Children With Special Needs

Promote Healthy Sibling Relationships

- Value each child individually and avoid comparisons. Remind each child of his or her positive qualities and contribution to other family members.
- Help siblings see the differences and similarities between themselves and the child with special needs. Create a climate in which children can achieve successes without feeling guilty.
- Teach siblings ways to interact with the child.
- Seek to be fair in terms of discipline, attention, and resources; require the affected child to do as much for himself or herself as possible.
- Let siblings settle their own differences; intervene only to prevent siblings from hurting one another.
- Legitimize reasonable anger. Even children with special needs behave badly sometimes.
- Respect a sibling's reluctance to be with or to include the child with special needs in activities.

Help Siblings Cope

- Listen to siblings to let them know that their thoughts and suggestions are valued.
- Praise siblings when they have been patient, have sacrificed, or have been particularly helpful. Do not expect siblings to always act in this manner.
- Acknowledge the personal strengths siblings have and their ability to cope with stress successfully.
- Provide age-appropriate information about the child's condition and update it when appropriate.
- Let teachers know what is happening so that they can be understanding and helpful.
- Recognize special stress times for siblings and plan to minimize negative effects.
- Schedule special time with siblings; have a friend or family member substitute when parent is unavailable.
- Encourage siblings to join or help establish a sibling support group.
- Use the services of professionals when needed. If parent feels that such a service is necessary, it should be provided in as vigorous a manner as a service for the child with special needs.

Involve Siblings

- Seek out ways to realistically include siblings in the care and treatment of the child with special needs.
- Limit caregiving responsibilities and give recognition when siblings perform them.
- Develop a library of children's books on special needs.
- Invite siblings to attend meetings to develop plans for the child with special needs (e.g., individualized educational program [IEP], individualized family service plan [IFSP]).
- Discuss future plans with them.
- Solicit their ideas on treatment and service needs.
- Have them visit professionals who work with the child.
- Help them develop competencies to teach the child new skills.
- Provide opportunities for siblings to advocate for the child.
- Allow siblings to set their own pace for learning and involvement.

Data from Powell T, Ogle P: *Brothers and sisters—a special part of exceptional families,* Baltimore, 1985, Paul H Brooks; Spokane Washington Deaconess Medical Center, Pediatric Oncology Unit: Tips for dealing with siblings, *Candlelighters Childhood Cancer Found Q Newslett* 11(3,4):7, 1987; and Carlson J, Leviton A, Mueller M: Services to siblings: an important component of family-centered practice, *ACCH Advocate* 1(1):53-56, 1993.

counselors of siblings during the course of their brother's or sister's illness.

COPING WITH ONGOING STRESS AND PERIODIC CRISES

Professionals can help families cope with stress by providing anticipatory guidance, providing emotional support, assisting the family in assessing and identifying specific stressors, aiding the family in developing coping mechanisms and problem-solving strategies, and working collaboratively with parents so that they become empowered in the process (Anderson and Davis, 2011).

Concurrent Stresses Within the Family

The ability to deal with the overwhelming stress of a chronic illness is challenged further when additional stresses are present. Stressors may be situational or developmental. They may be related to marital difficulties, sibling needs, homelessness, or social isolation. Some families may simultaneously be struggling with a family member's alcohol or other drug problem. Even relatively minor stressors, such as arranging care for siblings, managing the home, and traveling to distant treatment centers, can challenge a family's ability to cope successfully.

Most families, regardless of their income or insurance coverage, have financial concerns. The costs of caring for a child with a complex illness can be overwhelming. Nurses and social workers can help a family review various options for financial assistance, including insurance, managed care, or health maintenance organization policies; Medicaid; Supplemental Security Income; Women, Infants, and Children program; the state Program for Children with Special Health Needs; disease-related associations; and local philanthropic organizations.

Coping Mechanisms

Coping mechanisms are behaviors aimed at reducing the tension caused by a crisis. **Approach behaviors** are coping mechanisms that result in movement toward adjustment and resolution of the crisis. **Avoidance behaviors** result in movement away from adjustment and represent maladaptation to the crisis. Several approach and avoidance behaviors used in coping with a chronic illness are listed in the Nursing Care Guidelines box. Each behavior must be viewed in the context of all of the variables affecting the family. For example, the observation of several avoidance behaviors in an emotionally healthy family may denote significantly less risk to the successful resolution of the crisis than an equal number of avoidance behaviors in an individual who has few available supports.

Parental Empowerment

Empowerment can be seen as a process of recognizing, promoting, and enhancing competence. For parents of children with chronic conditions, empowerment may occur gradually as strength and capabilities are drawn on to master the child's care, manage family life, and plan for the future. Advocating for the child and developing parent–professional partnerships are part of taking charge (Panicker, 2013).

ASSISTING FAMILY MEMBERS IN MANAGING THEIR FEELINGS

Although some previous research has postulated stages of adaptation to a chronic illness, there is a great deal of individual variation in responses to the diagnosis, adjustments made, and time frames for coming to terms with a diagnosis. It is important that professionals recognize and respect a wide range of reactions and coping mechanisms. In fact, members of the family of a child with a complex chronic condition may experience a number of difficult emotions, including fear, guilt, anger, resentment, and anxiety. Learning to manage these emotions promotes adaptive coping. Support from professionals, other family members, and friends can assist family members in managing their feelings. The following discussion examines some common phases of adjustment and emotional reactions.

NURSING CARE GUIDELINES

Assessing Coping Behaviors

Approach Behaviors

Asks for information regarding diagnosis and child's present condition
Seeks help and support from others
Anticipates future problems; actively seeks guidance and answers
Endows the chronic illness or complex condition with meaning
Shares burden of disorder with others
Plans realistically for the future
Acknowledges and accepts child's awareness of diagnosis and prognosis
Expresses feelings (such as, sorrow, depression, and anger) and realizes reason for the emotional reaction
Realistically perceives child's condition; adjusts to changes
Recognizes own growth through passage of time, such as earlier denial and non-acceptance of diagnosis
Verbalizes possible loss of child

Avoidance Behaviors

Fails to recognize seriousness of child's condition despite physical evidence
Refuses to agree to treatment
Intellectualizes about the illness but in areas unrelated to child's condition
Is angry and hostile to members of the staff regardless of their attitude or behavior
Avoids staff, family members, or child
Entertains unrealistic future plans for child with little emphasis on the present
Is unable to adjust to or accept a change in progression of disease
Continually looks for new cures with no perspective toward possible benefit
Refuses to acknowledge child's understanding of disease and prognosis
Uses magical thinking and fantasy; may seek "occult" help
Places complete faith in religion to point of relinquishing own responsibility
Withdraws from outside world; refuses help
Punishes self because of guilt and blame
Makes no change in lifestyle to meet needs of other family members
Resorts to excessive use of alcohol or drugs to avoid problems
Verbalizes suicidal intents
Is unable to discuss possible loss of child or previous experiences with death

Shock and Denial

The initial diagnosis of a chronic illness or complex condition is often met with intense emotion and is characterized by shock, disbelief, and sometimes denial. Denial as a defense mechanism is a necessary cushion to prevent disintegration and is a normal response to grieving for any type of loss. Probably all family members experience various degrees of adaptive denial as they learn of the impact that the diagnosis has on their lives.

Shock and denial can last from days to months, sometimes even longer. Examples of denial that may be exhibited at the time of diagnosis include:

- Physician shopping
- Attributing the symptoms of the actual illness to a minor condition

- Refusing to believe the diagnostic tests
- Delaying consent for treatment
- Acting happy and optimistic despite the revealed diagnosis
- Refusing to tell or talk to anyone about the condition
- Insisting that no one is telling the truth, regardless of others' attempts to do so
- Denying the reason for admission
- Asking no questions about the diagnosis, treatment, or prognosis

Generally, these mechanisms should be respected as short-term responses that allow individuals to distance themselves from the tremendous emotional impact and to collect and mobilize their energies toward goal-directed, problem-solving behaviors.

In children, the importance of denial has repeatedly been demonstrated as a factor in their positive coping with the diagnosis. Denial allows the child to maintain hope in the face of overwhelming odds and to function adaptively and productively. Similar to hope, denial may be an adaptive mechanism for dealing with loss that persists until a family or patient is ready or needs other responses.

Denial is probably the least understood and most poorly dealt-with reaction. If denial is labeled as maladaptive, it can lead to inappropriate attempts to strip away the reaction by repeated and sometimes blunt explanations of the prognosis. However, denial becomes maladaptive only when it prevents recognition of treatment or rehabilitative goals necessary for the child's optimal survival or development.

Adjustment

For most families, adjustment gradually follows shock and is usually characterized by an open admission that the condition exists. This stage may be accompanied by several responses, which are normal parts of the adaptation process. Probably the most universal of these feelings are guilt and self-accusation. Guilt is often greatest when the cause of the disorder is directly traceable to the parent, as in genetic diseases or accidental injury. However, it can occur even without any scientific or realistic basis for parental responsibility. Frequently, the guilt stems from a false assumption that the child's condition is a result of personal failure or wrongdoing, such as not doing something correctly during pregnancy or the birth. Guilt may also be associated with cultural or religious beliefs. Some parents are convinced that they are being punished for some previous misdeed. Others may see the illness as a trial sent by God to test their religious strength and faith. With correct information, support, and time, most parents master guilt and self-accusation.

Children, too, may interpret their serious illness as retribution for past misbehavior. The nurse should be particularly sensitive to the child who passively accepts all painful procedures. This child may believe that such acts are inflicted as deserved punishment. It is vital that parents and health care professionals reassure children that their illnesses are not their fault.

Other common and normal reactions to a diagnosis are bitterness and anger. Anger directed inward may be evident as self-reproaching or punitive behavior, such as neglecting one's health and verbally degrading oneself. Anger directed outward may be manifested in either open arguments or withdrawal from communication and may be evident in the person's relationship with any number of individuals, such as the spouse, the child, and siblings. Passive anger toward the ill child may be evident in decreased visiting, refusal to believe how sick the child is, or an inability to provide comfort. Health care providers are among the most common targets for parental anger. Parents may complain about the nursing care, the insufficient time physicians spend with them, or the lack of skill of those who draw blood or start intravenous infusions.

Children are apt to respond with anger as well, and this includes the affected child and the well siblings. Children are aware of the loss engendered by their illness or complex condition and may react angrily to the restrictions imposed or the feelings of being different. Siblings may also feel anger and resentment toward the ill child and parents for the loss of routine and parental attention. It is difficult for older children and almost impossible for younger children to comprehend the plight of the affected child. Their perception is of a brother or sister who has the undivided attention of their parents, is showered with cards and gifts, and is the focus of everyone's concern.

During the period of adjustment, four types of parental reactions to the child influence the child's eventual response to the disorder:

- **Overprotection:** The parents fear letting the child achieve any new skill, avoid all discipline, and cater to every desire to prevent frustration
- **Rejection:** The parents detach themselves emotionally from the child but usually provide adequate physical care or constantly nag and scold the child
- **Denial:** The parents act as if the disorder does not exist or attempt to have the child overcompensate for it
- **Gradual acceptance:** The parents place necessary and realistic restrictions on the child, encourage self-care activities, and promote reasonable physical and social abilities

Reintegration and Acknowledgment

For many families, the adjustment process culminates in the development of realistic expectations for the child and reintegration of family life with the illness or complex condition in a manageable perspective. Because a large portion of this phase is one of grief for a loss, total resolution is not possible until the child dies or leaves home as an independent adult. Therefore one can regard adjustment as "increased comfort" with everyday living rather than a complete resolution.

This adjustment phase also involves social reintegration in which the family broadens its activities to include relationships outside of the home with the child as an acceptable and participating member of the group. This last criterion often differentiates the reaction of gradual acceptance during the adjustment period from total acceptance or perhaps is more descriptive of the acknowledgment process.

Many parents of children with chronic illnesses experience chronic sorrow, which are feelings of sorrow and loss that recur in waves over time. As the child's condition progresses, parents experience repeated losses that represent further declines and new caregiving demands. Consequently, families must be assessed on an ongoing basis and offered appropriate support and resources as their needs change over time. This represents a critical period of time because the nursing and medical team approach and support provided during this period of time can directly impact the experience of complicated grief after the death of the child. Complicated grief, which is characterized as persistent distress and chronic stress response, may last 6 months or longer after the death of a child and has a significant impact on quality of life of the family left behind (Meert, Shear, Newth, et al, 2011).

ESTABLISHING A SUPPORT SYSTEM

The diagnosis of a child with a complex chronic condition is a major situational crisis that affects the entire family system. However, families can experience positive outcomes as they successfully deal with the many challenges that accompany a child with chronic illness (Hungerbuehler, Vollrath, and Landolt, 2011).

One nursing goal is to assess which families are at risk for succumbing to the effects of the crisis. Several variables—available support system, perception of the event, coping mechanisms, reactions to the child, available resources, and concurrent stresses within the family—influence the resolution of a crisis. Although most families cope well, the needs

BOX 19.5 Concept of Functional Burden

Impact of the Child With Special Needs
The child's need for medical and nursing care
The child's fixed deficits
The child's age-appropriate dependency in activities of daily living
The disruptions in the family routine caused by the care
The psychologic burden of the prognosis on the family

Family Resources and Ability to Cope
The family's physical resources
The family's emotional resources
The family's educational resources
The family's social supports and available help
The competing demands for family members' time and energy

Data from Stein REK: Home care: a challenging opportunity, *Child Health Care* 14(2):90-95, 1985.

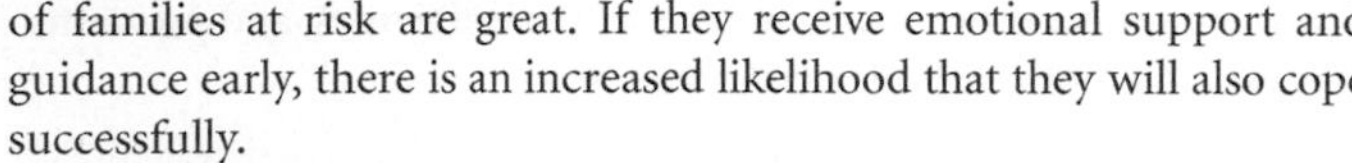

of families at risk are great. If they receive emotional support and guidance early, there is an increased likelihood that they will also cope successfully.

Although it is easy to assume that families of children with the most severe illnesses or disabilities would have the poorest adjustment, the severity of the condition reflects only one part of the overall picture. The level of adjustment is significantly influenced by the **functional burden** on the family (Stein, 1985). This concept considers the issues related to caring for and living with the child in relation to the family's resources and ability to cope (Box 19.5). The family of a child with a high level of technology dependence demanding complex care yet having many resources and coping skills may adjust more successfully to the child's situation than the family of a child with a less serious condition and few resources to counterbalance.

Intrafamilial resources, social support from friends and relatives, parent-to-parent support, parent/professional partnerships, and community resources interweave to provide a flexible web of support for families of children with chronic conditions.

THE CHILD WITH A CHRONIC OR COMPLEX CONDITION

The child's reaction to chronic illness depends to a great extent on his or her developmental level, temperament, and available coping mechanisms; on the reactions of family members or significant others; and, to a lesser extent, on the condition itself. A child's conceptual understanding of his or her own illness is based not only on age and developmental level but also on the duration and type of experience accumulated with the disease. Knowledge of these variables is essential in providing the kind of information and support needed by these children to cope with an often overwhelming situation.

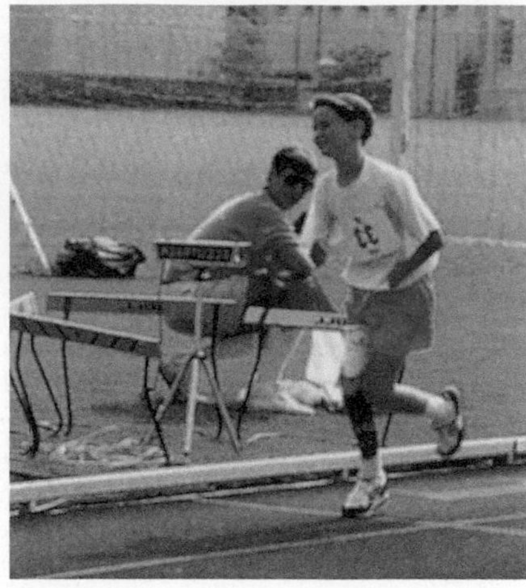

FIG. 19.1 Children with any type of impairment should have the opportunity to develop their skills. (Courtesy of Poyo/Hinton Photography.)

DEVELOPMENTAL ASPECTS

The impact of a complex chronic illness is influenced by the age at onset. Chronic illness affects children of all ages, but the developmental aspects of each age group dictate particular stresses and risks for the child. The nurse must also recognize that children need to redefine their condition and its implications as they develop and grow. For example, appearance, skills, and abilities are highly valued by peers (Fig. 19.1). A teenager who is limited in any of these qualities is subject to rejection. This is especially marked when an illness interferes with sexual attractiveness.

Children's developmental concepts of illness are discussed in Chapter 21. An understanding of these developmental factors facilitates planning care to support the child and minimize the risks. Developmental aspects of chronic illness on children are described in Table 19.2.

TABLE 19.2 Developmental Effects of Chronic Illness or Disability on Children

Developmental Tasks	Potential Effects of Chronic Illness or Disability	Supportive Interventions
Infancy		
Develop a sense of trust	Multiple caregivers and frequent separations, especially if hospitalized	Encourage consistent caregivers in hospital or other care settings.
	Deprived of consistent nurturing	Encourage parental presence, "rooming in" during hospitalization, and participation in care.
Bond, or attach, to parent	Delayed because of separation; parental grief for loss of "dream" child; parental inability to accept the condition, especially a visible defect	Emphasize healthy, perfect qualities of infant. Help parents learn special care needs of infant for them to feel competent.
Learn through sensorimotor experiences	More exposure to painful experiences than pleasurable ones	Expose infant to pleasurable experiences through all senses (touch, hearing, sight, taste, movement).
	Limited contact with environment from restricted movement or confinement	Encourage age-appropriate developmental skills (e.g., holding bottle, finger feeding, crawling).

TABLE 19.2 Developmental Effects of Chronic Illness or Disability on Children—cont'd

Developmental Tasks	Potential Effects of Chronic Illness or Disability	Supportive Interventions
Begin to develop a sense of separateness from parent	Increased dependency on parent for care	Encourage all family members to participate in care to prevent over involvement of one member.
	Over involvement of parent in care	Encourage periodic respite from demands of care responsibilities.
Toddlerhood		
Develop autonomy	Increased dependency on parent	Encourage independence in as many areas as possible (e.g., toileting, dressing, feeding).
Master locomotor and language skills	Limited opportunity to test own abilities and limits	Provide gross motor skill activity and modification of toys or equipment, such as modified swing or rocking horse.
Learn through sensorimotor experience; beginning preoperational thought	Increased exposure to painful experiences	Give choices to allow simple feeling of control (e.g., choice of what book to look at, what kind of sandwich to eat). Institute age-appropriate discipline and limit setting. Recognize that negative and ritualistic behaviors are normal. Provide sensory experiences (e.g., water play, sandbox play, finger painting).
Preschool Age		
Develop initiative and purpose Master self-care skills	Limited opportunities for success in accomplishing simple tasks or mastering self-care skills	Encourage mastery of self-help skills. Provide devices that make tasks easier (e.g., self-dressing).
Begin to develop peer relationships	Limited opportunities for socialization with peers; may appear "like a baby" to age mates Protection within tolerant and secure family, causing child to fear criticism and withdraw	Encourage socialization (e.g., inviting friends to play, daycare experience, trips to park). Provide age-appropriate play, especially associative play opportunities. Emphasize child's abilities; dress appropriately to enhance desirable appearance.
Develop sense of body image and sexual identification	Awareness of body centering on pain, anxiety, and failure Sex-role identification focused primarily on mothering skills	Encourage relationships with same-sex and opposite-sex peers and adults.
Learn through preoperational thought (magical thinking)	Guilt (thinking he or she caused the illness or disability or is being punished for wrongdoing)	Help child deal with criticisms; realize that too much protection prevents child from realities of world. Clarify that cause of child's illness or disability is not his or her fault or a punishment.
School Age		
Develop a sense of accomplishment	Limited opportunities to achieve and compete (e.g., many school absences, inability to join regular athletic activities)	Encourage school attendance; schedule medical visits at times other than school; encourage child to make up missed work.
Form peer relationships	Limited opportunities for socialization	Educate teachers and classmates about child's condition, abilities, and special needs. Encourage sports activities (e.g., Special Olympics). Encourage socialization (e.g., Girl Scouts, Campfire, Boy Scouts, 4-H Club; having a best friend or club membership).
Learn through concrete operations	Incomplete comprehension of the imposed physical limitations or treatment of the disorder	Provide child with information about his or her condition. Encourage creative activities (e.g., VSA Arts).
Adolescence		
Develop personal and sexual identity	Increased sense of feeling different from peers and reduced ability to compete with peers in appearance, abilities, special skills	Help child realize that many of the difficulties the teenager is experiencing are part of normal adolescence (rebelliousness, risk taking, lack of cooperation, hostility toward authority).
Achieve independence from family	Increased dependency on family; limited job or career opportunities	Provide instruction on interpersonal and coping skills. Encourage increased responsibility for care and management of the disease or condition (e.g., assuming responsibility for making and keeping appointment [ideally alone], sharing assessment and planning stages of health care delivery, contacting resources). Discuss planning for future and how condition can affect choices.

Continued

TABLE 19.2 Developmental Effects of Chronic Illness or Disability on Children—cont'd

Developmental Tasks	Potential Effects of Chronic Illness or Disability	Supportive Interventions
Form heterosexual relationships	Limited opportunities for heterosexual friendships; less opportunity to discuss sexual concerns with peers Increased concern with issues such as why did he or she get the disorder and whether he or she will marry and have a family	Encourage socialization with peers, including peers with special needs and those without special needs. Encourage activities appropriate for age (e.g., attending mixed-sex parties, sports activities, driving a car). Be alert to cues that signal readiness for information regarding implications of condition on sexuality and reproduction. Emphasize good appearance and wearing stylish clothes, use of makeup. Understand that adolescent has same sexual needs and concerns as any other teenager.
Learn through abstract thinking	Decreased opportunity for earlier stages of cognition impeding achievement of level of abstract thinking	Provide instruction on decision making, assertiveness, and other skills necessary to manage personal plans.

BOX 19.6 Coping Patterns Used by Children With Special Needs

Develops competence and optimism: Accentuates the positive aspects of the situation and concentrates more on what he or she has or can do than on what is missing or on what he or she cannot do; is as independent as possible

Feels different and withdraws: Sees self as being different from other children because of the chronic health condition; views being different as negative; sees self as less worthy than others; focuses on things he or she cannot do and sometimes over restricts activities needlessly

Is irritable, is moody, and acts out: Uses proactive and self-initiated coping behaviors, although usually counterproductive in that the behaviors are not ego enhancing or socially responsible and do not result in desired outcomes; acts out irritability, which may or may not be associated with condition's symptoms

Complies with treatment: Takes necessary medications, treatments; adheres to activity restrictions; also uses behaviors that indicate developing independence (e.g., assumes responsibility for taking medication)

Seeks support: Talks with adults, children, physicians, and nurses; develops plans to handle problems as they occur; uses downward comparison (i.e., realizes that others have it worse)

Modified from Austin J, Patterson J, Huberty T: Development of the coping health inventory for children, *J Pediatr Nurs* 6(3):166-174, 1991.

COPING MECHANISMS

Children with chronic conditions tend to use five distinct patterns of coping (Box 19.6). Children with more positive and accepting attitudes about their chronic illness use a more adaptive coping style characterized by optimism, competence, and compliance. They show fewer behavior problems at home and at school. The two maladaptive coping patterns—"Feels different and withdraws" and "Is irritable, is moody, and acts out"—are associated with poorer adaptation; children using these strategies have poorer self-concepts, more negative attitudes about their conditions, and more behavior problems at home and at school.

Well-adapted children gradually learn to accept their physical limitations and find achievement in a variety of compensatory motor and intellectual pursuits. They function well at home, at school, and with peers. They have an understanding of their disorder that allows them to accept their limitations, assume responsibility for their care, and assist in treatment and rehabilitation regimens. They express appropriate

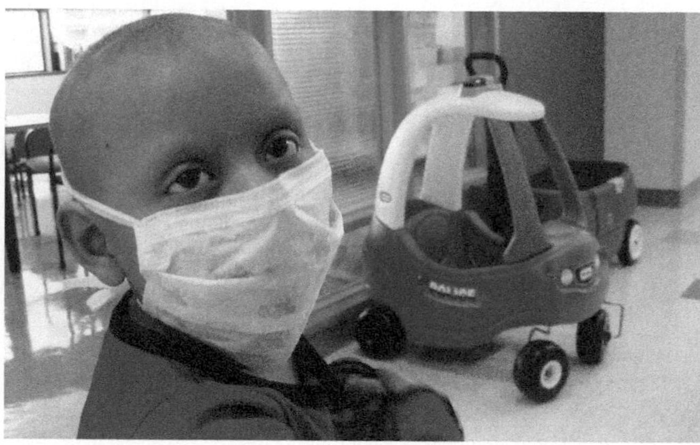

FIG. 19.2 Periods of sadness and anger are appropriate in the child's adjustment to a chronic illness or disability, especially during exacerbations of the disorder.

emotions, such as sadness, anxiety, and anger, at times of exacerbations but confidence and guarded optimism during periods of clinical stability (Fig. 19.2). They are able to identify with other similarly affected individuals, promoting positive self-images and displaying pride and self-confidence in their ability to master a productive, successful life despite their illnesses.

Hopefulness

Children, particularly adolescents, are sensitive to the presence or absence of hope. Hopefulness is an internal quality that mobilizes humans into goal-directed action that may be satisfying and life sustaining. A sense of hopefulness can produce increased participation in health-seeking behaviors and an improved sense of well-being.

Health Education and Self-Care

Health education is an intervention that promotes coping. Children need information about their condition, the therapeutic plan, and how the disease or the therapy might affect their particular situation. Children nearing puberty also need to understand the maturation process and how their chronic illness may alter this event. For example, a youngster with Crohn disease should understand that this disorder is associated with growth failure and delayed puberty, a child with diabetes needs to know that hormonal changes and increased growth needs will alter food and insulin requirements at this time, and a sexually active girl with sickle cell anemia or systemic lupus erythematosus needs to be aware of the risks of pregnancy. The information should not be given all at once but should be timed appropriately to meet their changing needs, and it should be described and repeated as often as the situation demands.

NURSING CARE OF THE FAMILY AND CHILD WITH A CHRONIC OR COMPLEX CONDITION

ASSESSMENT

Because the nurse may meet a family during any phase of the adjustment process, several assessment areas are important. The family's ability to cope with previous stresses influences the current situation, and answers to questions about their usual coping skills are enlightening. Knowledge of concurrent stresses, such as financial, marital or nonmarital, and career or unemployment, helps identify families who may have fewer resources to cope with the child's needs.

Finally, awareness of the family members' reactions to the child and the illness or condition is important. Sample questions that the nurse and family can use to evaluate the support system, perception of the illness, coping mechanisms, resources, and concurrent stresses are listed in Table 19.3. Because factors affecting the family's response may change at any point during the illness, assessment must be a continuous process.

Special challenges exist in assessing the child's feelings about having a chronic condition. Chapter 4 presents several approaches to encourage children to discuss their feelings about their conditions. The nurse should use a variety of communication techniques, such as drawing and play, as assessment tools rather than relying solely on parental reports. Often, children are neglected partners in their care, and their unique needs are not identified.

The needs of working parents and siblings also should be assessed; this is a goal that requires flexibility in scheduling appointments. When working parents know that their input is valuable, they will often change their work schedule to meet with a health professional. Because siblings can be of any age, the use of appropriate communication strategies for assessment must be considered. Nonverbal techniques, such as those discussed in Chapter 4 should be considered for these children.

TABLE 19.3 Assessment of Factors Affecting Family Adjustment

Factors Affecting Adjustment	Assessment Questions
Available Support System	
Status of marital relationship	To whom do you talk when you have something on your mind? (If answer is not the spouse, ask for the reason.)
Alternate support systems	When something is worrying you, what do you do? What helps you most when you are upset?
Ability to communicate	Does talking seem to help when you feel upset?
Perception of the Illness or Disability	
Previous knowledge of disorder	Have you ever heard the word (name of diagnosis) before? Tell me about it (if answer is yes).
Imagined cause of disorder	What are your thoughts about the causes of the disorder?
Effects of illness or disability on family	How has your child's illness or disability affected you and your family? How has your lifestyle changed?
Coping Mechanisms	
Reactions to previous crises	Tell me one time you've had another crisis (problem, bad time) in your family. How did you solve that problem?
Reactions to the child	Do you find yourself being a little more cautious with this child than with your other children?
Childrearing practices	Do you feel as comfortable disciplining this child as your other children?
Influence of religion	Has your religion or faith been of help to you? Tell me how (if answer is yes).
Attitudes	How is this child different from the siblings or other children of similar age? Describe your child's personality. Is it easy, difficult, or in between? When you think of your child's future, what thoughts come to mind?
Available Resources	
	What parts of your child's care are causing the most difficulty for you or your family? What services are available to help? What services do you need that currently are not available?
Concurrent Stresses	
	What other problems are you facing now? (Be specific; ask about financial, marital, sibling, and extended family or friends concerns.)

PROVIDE SUPPORT AT THE TIME OF DIAGNOSIS

The diagnosis is a critical time for parents and can influence how they perceive their health care providers across the trajectory of care. Although they may not hear or remember all that is said to them, they frequently sense a certain attitude of acceptance, rejection, hope, or despair that may influence their ability to absorb the shock and begin adapting to the family's altered future.

Parents may be encouraged to be together when they are informed of their child's condition, thus avoiding the problem of one parent having to interpret complex information and deal with the initial emotional reaction of the other. The informing session should take place in a private, comfortable setting free of distractions and interruptions in an atmosphere in which the parents feel free to express their emotions (Fig. 19.3). Their emotional needs are acknowledged by showing acceptance of expressions, such as crying, sadness, anger, and disappointment. Emotional support is offered by having tissues available if a family member cries and demonstrating through facial and body language that indeed this is a difficult and painful period. Although touching is a powerful expression of empathy, it must be used wisely. For example, it can prematurely terminate free expression of feelings, especially when combined with statements, such as "Everything will be all right." Nurses should also be aware of cultural issues regarding touching (see Chapter 2).

Parents should receive the kind of information they desire. This can be assessed by asking questions, such as "Do you prefer to hear detailed information?" Parents or other family members may have different preferences regarding the amount of information that they wish to hear. Most parents want a clear, simple explanation of the diagnosis; a prediction of possible futures for the child; advice on what to do next;

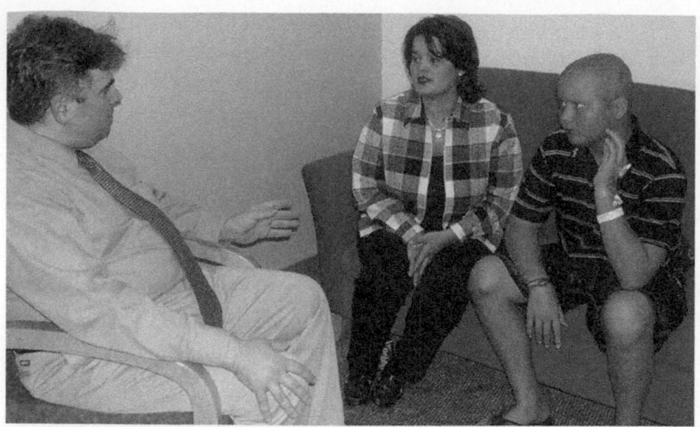

FIG. 19.3 Information sessions should take place in a private, comfortable setting free of distractions and interruptions.

an opportunity to ask questions; a warm, sympathetic listener; and, most important, time. Understanding of explanations is elicited with questions, such as "Do you see what I mean?" or "Is this clear to you?" Technical terms are used with simple definitions. If the parents are unaware of the term, they are given written literature or at least a written summary of the diagnosis.

Finally, the informing conference does not end with the presentation of devastating news. Instead, the child's strengths, appealing behaviors, and potential for development are stressed, as are available rehabilitation efforts or treatments. Parents can be encouraged to view their experiences as a series of challenges that they are capable of handling, particularly with available professional feedback. The parents are assured that the nurse will be available to answer questions and to provide further assistance as needed.

The preceding discussion relates primarily to the initial informing interview. However, because of the need for long-term follow-up, it is only one in a series of continuing discussions. In all interactions, the family's input is solicited and incorporated into the care plan. Some situations require consideration of special problems (see Nursing Care Guidelines box).

SUPPORT THE FAMILY'S COPING METHODS

For the family to meet the stresses of optimally adjusting to the child's condition, each member must be individually supported so that the family system is strong. Although the family can indefinitely support a member who is in need of assistance, its greatest strength lies in every member supporting each other. The nurse should bear in mind that the family member in greatest need is not necessarily the affected child but may be a parent or sibling who is dealing with stresses that require intervention.

Parents

The nurse can provide support by being attentive to families' responses to their children. Mothers and fathers need to experience success, joy, and pride in their children to give the support they need. It is important for nurses to examine their attitudes to determine their ability to engage in parent–professional partnerships. An essential characteristic is the belief that parents are equal to professionals and are experts regarding their child (see Nursing Care Guidelines box).

Parents can be encouraged to discuss their feelings toward the child, the impact of this event on their marriage, and associated stresses such as financial burdens. For most families, regardless of their income or insurance coverage, financial concerns exist. The costs of caring for a child with special needs can be overwhelming. In addition, one or both parents may have to sacrifice job opportunities to remain close to a medical facility or to avoid losing insurance benefits. Numerous volunteer and community resources are available that provide assistance, rehabilitation, equipment, and funding for a variety of health problems. National and local disease-oriented organizations may provide needed assistance and support to families that qualify. Many of these are discussed elsewhere in the text under the specific diagnosis. State and federal departments of health, mental health, social service, and labor may be able to help locate appropriate regional resources. For example, state programs for Children with Special Health Needs provide financial assistance for children with many disabling conditions. Local and national sources of respite care and medical daycare may be useful to families. Nurses should become acquainted with those in their communities and with vocational programs for special groups.

Parent-to-Parent Support

Just being with another parent who has shared similar experiences is helpful. It may not need to be a parent of a child with the same diagnosis because parents in the process of adjusting to a child with special needs—or finding respite services, educational or rehabilitative services, special equipment vendors, and financial counseling—tread a common path. If the agency does not have a parent staff position, the nurse can contact parent groups that will often send a representative. Another strategy is to ask another parent to talk to the parents. The nurse should seek out a parent who is a good listener, has a nonjudgmental approach to differences in families, and possesses good advocacy and problem-solving skills.

The parent self-help group can promote parent-to-parent support.* Group members feel less alone and have the opportunity to observe both coping and mastery role modeling from other members. Parent groups are rich resources for information. Even if parents are unable to attend meetings, they can still benefit from group newsletters and other literature that often accompany membership. Nurses can assist in starting a group by identifying one or two parents as leaders; sharing with them the names, telephone numbers, and addresses of other families who have expressed both an interest and a willingness to release their phone number and address; and guiding them in how to initiate a first meeting.

Advocate for Empowerment

Nurses can advocate for methods that foster opportunities for parent empowerment. For example, nurses can suggest reimbursement for travel and child care plus stipends to enable parents' voices to be heard at meetings and conferences. They can encourage parent membership on committees and advisory boards. They can keep parents informed of pending legislation on child health issues or take action when parents inform them.

The Child

Through ongoing contacts with the child, the nurse (1) observes the child's responses to the disorder, ability to function, and adaptive behaviors within the environment and with significant others; (2) explores the child's own understanding of his or her illness or condition; and (3) provides support while the child learns to cope with his or her feelings. Children are encouraged to express their concerns rather than

*Information about self-help groups and books and pamphlets are available from the National Self-Help Clearinghouse, 365 Fifth Ave., Suite 3300, New York, NY 10016; 217-817-1822; http://www.selfhelpweb.org.

NURSING CARE GUIDELINES

Situations Requiring Special Consideration

Congenital Anomaly

Tension in the delivery room conveys the sense that something is seriously wrong. Communication is often delayed while the physician is involved with the mother's care. The manner in which the infant is presented may well set the tone for the early parent–child relationship.

Clarify role with physician in regard to revealing information to enable immediate parental support.

Explain to parents briefly in simple language what the defect is and something concerning the immediate prognosis before showing them the infant. Later more information can be given when they are more ready to "hear" what is said.

Be aware of nonverbal communication. Parents watch facial expressions of others for signs of revulsion or rejection.

Present infant as something precious.

Emphasize well-formed aspects of infant's body.

Allow time and opportunity for parents to express their initial response.

Encourage parents to ask questions and provide honest, straightforward answers without undue optimism or pessimism.

Cognitive Impairment

Unless cognitive impairment (or mental retardation) is associated with other physical problems, it is often easy for parents to miss clues to its presence or to make defensive excuses regarding the diagnosis.

Plan situations that help parents become aware of the problem.

Encourage parents to discuss their observations of child but withhold diagnostic opinions.

Focus on what the child can do and appropriate interventions to promote progress (e.g., infant stimulation programs) to involve parents in their child's care while helping them gain an awareness of the child's condition.

Physical Disability

If loss of motor or sensory ability occurs during childhood, the diagnosis is readily apparent. The challenge lies in helping the child and parents over the period of shock and grief and toward the phase of acceptance and reintegration.

Institute early rehabilitation (e.g., using a prosthetic limb, learning to read braille, learning to read lips).

Be aware that physical rehabilitation usually precedes psychologic adjustment.

When the cause of the disability is accidental, avoid implying that parents or child was responsible for the injury but allow them the opportunity to discuss feelings of blame.

Encourage expression of feelings (see Communication Techniques, Chapter 4).

Chronic Illness

Realization of the true impact may take months or years. Conflict over parents' versus child's concerns may result in serious problems. When condition is inherited, parents may blame themselves or child may blame the parents.

Help each family member gain an appreciation of the others' concerns.

Discuss hereditary aspect of condition with parents at time of diagnosis to lessen guilt and accusatory feelings.

Encourage child to express feelings by using third-person technique (e.g., "Sometimes when a person has an illness that was passed on by the parents, that person feels angry or bitter toward them").

Multiple Disabilities

The child or parent may require additional time for the shock phase and may be able to attend to only one diagnosis before hearing significant information regarding other disorders.

Acknowledge parents' understanding and acceptance of all diagnoses, especially when an obvious and more hidden disability coexists.

Appreciate the devastating consequences of more than one disability for a child, especially if they interfere with expressive-receptive abilities.

Terminal Illness

Parents require much support to deal with their own feelings and guidance in how to tell the child the diagnosis. They may want to conceal the diagnosis from the child. They may believe that the child is too young to know, will not be able to cope with the information, or will lose hope and the will to live.

Approach the subject of disclosure in a positive way by asking, "How will you tell your child about the diagnosis?"

Help parents understand the disadvantages of not telling the child (e.g., deprives child of the opportunity to discuss feelings openly and ask questions, incurs the risk of child learning the truth from outside and sometimes less tactful sources, may lessen child's trust and confidence in the parents after learning the truth).

Guide parents to see the potential problems involved in fostering a conspiracy.

Offer parents guidelines for how and what to tell the child about the disease or the possibility of death. Explanations should be tailored to child's cognitive ability, be based on knowledge child already has, and be honest. Honesty must be tempered with concern for child's feelings.

Assure parents that telling a child the name of the illness and the reason for treatment instills hope, provides support from others, and serves as a foundation for explaining and understanding subsequent events.

Acknowledge that being honest is not always easy because the truth may prompt the child to ask other distressing questions, such as "Am I going to die?" However, even this difficult question must be answered.

allowing others to express them for them because open discussions may reduce anxiety (see Nursing Care Guidelines box).

One of the most important interventions is alleviating the child's feeling of being different and normalizing his or her life as much as possible (see Nursing Care Guidelines box). Whenever possible, the nurse assists the family in assessing the child's daily routine for indications of a need for normalizing practices. For example, the child who remains in a bedroom all day requires a restructured daily routine to provide activities in different parts of the house, such as eating in the kitchen or dining room with the family. Such children may also be deprived of social, recreational, and academic activities that can be better accommodated by applying normalization practices. For example, home and out-of-home health-related treatments should be planned at times that least interfere with normal daily activities.

Children who are concerned that their condition detracts from their physical attractiveness need attention focused on the normal aspects of appearance and capabilities. Health professionals help strengthen and consolidate the self-image by emphasizing the normal while allowing children to express anger, isolation, fear of rejection, feelings of sadness, and loneliness. The children need positive reinforcement for compliance and any evidence of improvement. Anything that might improve attractiveness and contribute to a positive self-image is used, such as makeup for a teenager with a scar, clothing that disguises a prosthesis, or a hairstyle or wig to cover a deformity or lost hair.

 NURSING CARE GUIDELINES

Developing Successful Parent–Professional Partnerships

Promote primary nursing; in nonhospital settings, designate a case manager.
Acknowledge parents' overall competence and their unique expertise with their child.
Respect parents' time as having value equal to that of other members of child's health care team.
Explain or define any medical, technical, or discipline-specific terms.
Tell families, "I am not sure" or "I don't know" when appropriate.
Facilitate family's effectiveness in team meetings (e.g., provide parents with same information as other participants).

 NURSING CARE GUIDELINES

Encouraging Expression of Emotion

Describe the behavior: "You seem angry at everyone."
Give evidence of understanding: "Being angry is only natural."
Give evidence of caring: "It must be difficult to endure so many painful procedures."
Help focus on feelings: "Maybe you wonder why this happened to you."

 NURSING CARE GUIDELINES

Promoting Normalization

Preparation: Prepare child in advance for changes that may occur from the chronic or complex condition.
Example: Tell the child in advance the possible side effects of drug therapy.
Participation: Include child in as many decisions as possible, especially those relating to his or her care regimen.
Example: The child is responsible for taking medications or scheduling home treatments.
Sharing: Allow both family members and child's peers to be a part of the care regimen whenever possible.
Examples: Give the child his or her medication when the other siblings receive their vitamins.
The parent cooks the same menu for the whole family.
If the child is invited to another's home, the parent advises the family of the child's dietary restrictions.
Control: Identify areas where child can be in control so that feelings of uncertainty, passivity, and helplessness are decreased.
Example: The child identifies activities that are appropriate to his or her energy level and chooses to rest when fatigued.
Expectation: Apply the same family rules to the child with a complex chronic illness as to the well siblings or peers.
Example: The child is disciplined, is expected to fulfill household responsibilities, and attends school in accordance with abilities.

Siblings

The presence of a child with special needs in a family may result in parents paying less attention to the other children. Siblings may respond by developing negative attitudes toward the child or by expressing anger in different forms. The nurse can help by using anticipatory guidance, questioning the parents about what they believe is the best way to have siblings respond to the child, and guiding them through ways to meet their other children's needs for attention. This questioning should take place before serious negative effects occur.

Siblings may also experience embarrassment associated with having a brother or sister with a chronic or complex condition. Parents are then faced with the difficulty of responding to this embarrassment in an understanding and appropriate manner without punishing the siblings for how they feel. Parents are encouraged to talk with the siblings about how they view their affected sibling. For example, siblings of a child with developmental disabilities may express fears about their ability to bear normal children. Adolescents in particular may not be able to discuss these vital issues with their parents and may prefer to consult with the nurse. Many siblings benefit from sharing their concerns with other young people who are experiencing a similar situation. Support groups for siblings can help decrease isolation, promote expression of feelings, and provide examples of effective coping skills.

Many parents express concern about when and how to inform the other children in the family about a sibling's illness or disability. The answer depends on each child's level of sophistication and understanding. However, it is usually best to inform the siblings before a neighbor or other nonfamily member does so. Uninformed siblings may fantasize or develop apprehensions that are out of proportion to the child's actual condition. Furthermore, if parents choose to be silent or deceptive about the issue, they are setting a negative precedent for the siblings to follow rather than encouraging the siblings to cope with the experience in a healthy and nurturing way.

The nurse is sensitive to the reactions of siblings and whenever possible intervenes to promote more positive adjustment. For example, siblings often mention that they are expected to take on additional responsibilities to help the parents care for the child. It is not unusual for them to express a positive reaction to assuming the extra duties but a negative response to feeling unappreciated for doing so. Such feelings can often be minimized by encouraging siblings to discuss this with the parents and by suggesting to parents ways of showing gratitude, such as an increase in allowance; special privileges; and, most significantly, verbal praise.

EDUCATE ABOUT THE DISORDER AND GENERAL HEALTH CARE

Educating the family about the disorder is actually an extension of revealing the diagnosis. Education involves not only supplying technical information but also discussing how the condition will affect the child. Parents may only be able to process limited information at any one time. It may be helpful to provide essential information and then follow by asking, "What else would you like to know about your child's condition?" Responding to parents' questions and concerns ensures that their information needs are met.

Activities of Daily Living

Parents also need guidance in how the condition may interfere with or alter activities of daily living, such as eating, dressing, sleeping, and toileting. One area frequently affected is nutrition. Common problems are undernutrition resulting from food being inappropriately restricted or loss of appetite, vomiting, or motor deficits that interfere with feeding; overnutrition may also occur, usually because of a caloric intake in excess of energy expenditure because of boredom and lack of stimulation in other areas. Although the child requires the same basic nutrients as other children, the daily requirements may differ. Special nutritional considerations are discussed as appropriate throughout the text.

Safe Transportation

Modifications may also be needed regarding car safety. Children with conditions such as low birth weight (see Discharge Planning and Home Care, Chapter 8) or orthopedic, neuromuscular, or respiratory impairments often cannot safely use conventional car restraints. For example, children with hip spica casts cannot sit properly in child safety seats (see Developmental Dysplasia of the Hip, Chapter 33). Modifications can be made to some commercial models, and for older children, a special vest is available that secures the child to the back seat in a lying-down position.*

If a child requires a wheelchair, the family should consult the wheelchair manufacturer for specific instructions regarding safe car transportation. Considerations for wheelchairs used with vehicle transportation must address securing both the wheelchair and the occupant in the wheelchair. Wheelchairs should be secured facing forward with tie downs at four points. The tie-down system should be dynamically crash tested, as should the occupant securement system that secures the child in the wheelchair. For example, use of trays is not recommended for transportation. With children who must travel with additional medical equipment, this equipment (e.g., oxygen, monitors, or ventilators) should be anchored to the floor or underneath the vehicle seat or wheelchair. Soft padding should be added around the equipment to reduce movement. A second adult should be present to monitor the condition of a medically fragile child while traveling.

Primary Health Care

Children with special needs require all the usual health care recommended for any child. Attention to injury prevention, immunizations, dental health, and regular physical examinations is essential. Nurses can play an important role in reminding parents of these aspects of care that are so often neglected when the concern is focused on the child's chronic condition. Specific discussions of nutrition, sleep and activity, dental health, and injury prevention are presented in the chapters on health promotion for specific age groups. Immunizations are discussed in Chapter 10.

Parents also need to be aware of the importance of communicating the child's condition in the event of a medical emergency. Young children are unable to give information about their disorders, and although older children may be reliable sources, after an accident, they may be physically unable to speak. Therefore all children with any type of chronic condition that may affect medical care should wear some type of identification, such as a Medic Alert bracelet,† or carry a card in their wallet that lists the medical condition and a phone number for emergency medical records and other personal information.

PROMOTE NORMAL DEVELOPMENT

Aside from knowledge of the condition and its effect on the child's abilities, the family must be guided toward fostering appropriate development in their child. Although each stage may take longer to achieve, parents are guided toward helping the child fully realize his or her potential in preparation for the next developmental stage. Table 19.2 outlines developmental aspects of complex conditions and supportive interventions. With appropriate planning and knowledge of strategies to improve the child's functional abilities, most children can live fulfilling and productive lives.

One important aspect of promoting normal development is to encourage the child's self-care abilities in both activities of daily living and the medical regimen. An assessment of the child's age and physical, emotional, and mental capacities, as well as the support and structure provided by the family, should be considered in determining the appropriate level of self-care in the medical regimen. Even toddlers can be involved in their own care by holding supplies for the parent during a procedure. Over time, children should be encouraged toward greater autonomy in the self-care arena.

Early Childhood

During infancy, the child is achieving basic trust through a satisfying, intimate, consistent relationship with his or her parents. However, affected children's early existence may be stressful, chaotic, and unsatisfying. Consequently, they may need more parental support and expressions of affection to achieve trust. Likewise, the parents require assistance in finding ways to meet the infant's needs, such as how to hold a rigid or flaccid infant, how to feed a child with tongue thrust or episodes of dyspnea, and how to stimulate a child who seems incapable of achieving any skills. If hospitalizations are frequent or prolonged, every effort is made to preserve the parent–child relationship (see also Chapter 21).

During early childhood, the goal is to adapt to periods of separation from parents, autonomy, and initiative. However, the natural parental response to having a sick child is overprotection (Box 19.7). Parents need help in realizing the importance of brief separations of the child from them and from others involved in the child's care and of providing social experiences outside the home whenever possible. Respite care, which provides temporary relief for family members, can be essential in allowing caregivers time away from the daily burdens.

Young children also need the opportunity to develop independence. Frequently, the child is able to learn self-help skills, such as finger feeding, and removing simple articles of clothing, but the parent continues to perform the act. The nurse can provide parents with anticipatory guidance as to the usual milestones expected from the child. When a child is unable to perform a skill independently, functional aids should be used. With innovation, many adaptations can be implemented in children's environments to increase their mobility and independence

BOX 19.7 Characteristics of Parental Overprotection

- Sacrifices self and rest of family for the child
- Continually helps the child even when the child is capable
- Is inconsistent with regard to discipline or uses no discipline; frequently applies different rules to the siblings
- Is dictatorial and arbitrary, making decisions without considering the child's wishes, such as keeping the child from attending school
- Hovers and offers suggestions; calls attention to every activity; overdoes praise
- Protects the child from every possible discomfort
- Restricts play, often because of fear that the child will be injured
- Denies the child opportunities for growing up and assuming responsibility, such as learning to give own medications or perform treatments
- Does not understand the child's capabilities and sets goals too high or too low
- Monopolizes the child's time, such as sleeping with the child, permitting few friends, or refusing participation in social or educational activities

*Information on car safety restraints for children with special needs is available from the Automotive Safety Program, 1130 West Michigan Street, Fesler Hall Room 207, Indianapolis, IN 46202; 800-543-6227 or 317-274-2997; http://www.preventinjury.org.

†MedicAlert Foundation, 5226 Pirrone Court, Salida, CA 95368; 800-423-5378; http://www.medicalert.org.

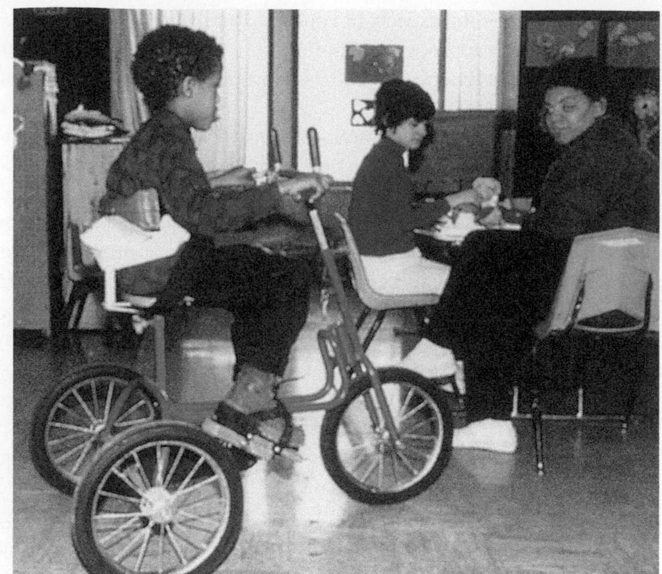

FIG. 19.4 A modified tricycle with block pedals, self-adhesive straps for support, and a modified seat and handle bars can help a child with disabilities gain mobility.

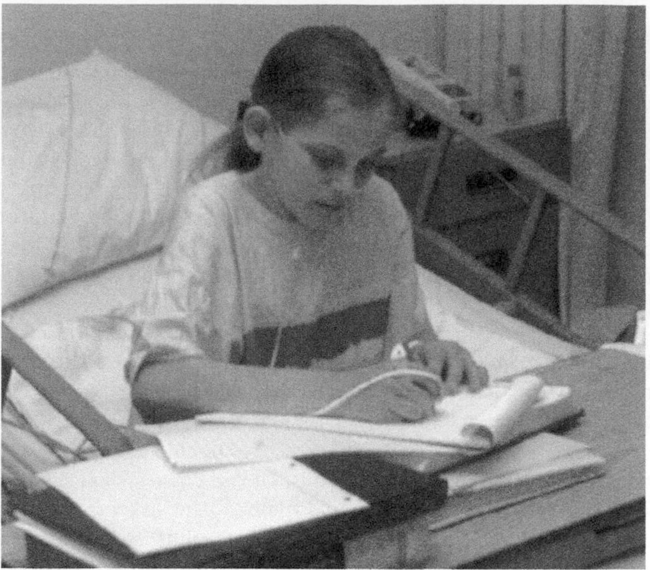

FIG. 19.5 Children with disabilities should continue their schooling as soon as their condition permits.

and allow them to play like other children their age. For example, with slight modifications, a child with physical limitations may be able to ride a tricycle (Fig. 19.4).

Another critical component for normal child development is discipline. Discipline and guidance serve several purposes, such as providing children with boundaries on which to test out their behavior and teaching them socially acceptable behavior. Resentment and hostility can arise among siblings if different standards are applied to each child. The nurse's responsibility is to help parents learn successful methods of managing a child's behaviors before they become problems (see Limit Setting and Discipline, Chapter 2).

School Age

For school-age children, the major tasks are entry into school and achieving a sense of industry. Although the importance of school in the life of all children is well known, school absences are significantly higher among children with chronic illnesses than among their healthy peers. The more school absences the child experiences, the more difficult it is to resume attendance, and school phobia may result. The child should return to school as soon as possible after diagnosis or treatments.

Preparation for entry into or resumption of school is best accomplished through a team approach with the parents, child, teacher, school nurse, and primary nurse in the hospital. Ideally, this planning should begin before hospital discharge, provided that the child is well enough to resume usual activities. A structured plan should be developed, with attention to aspects of care that must be continued during school hours, such as administration of medication or other treatments.

Children also need preparation before entering or resuming school. Having a tutor in the hospital or home as soon as children are physically able helps them realize that school will continue and gives them time to consider this prospect (Fig. 19.5). They need to investigate possible answers to the many questions others will ask. One method of anticipatory preparation is to role-play, with the child as the "returned pupil" and the nurse or parent as "other schoolmates." If the child returns to school with some obvious physical change (such as, hair loss, amputation, or a visible scar), the nurse might also ask questions about these alterations to prompt preparatory responses from the child.

Classroom peers also need preparation, and a joint plan created by the teacher, nurse, and child is best. At a minimum, classmates should be given a description of the child's condition, prepared for any visible changes in the child, and allowed an opportunity to ask questions. The child should have the option of attending this session. As the child's condition changes, particularly if the illness is potentially fatal, school personnel, including the students, need periodic appraisal of the child's status and preparation for what to expect.

Children with special needs are encouraged to maintain or reestablish relationships with peers and to participate according to their capabilities in any age-appropriate activities. Alternative activities may be substituted for those that are impossible or that place a strain on the child's condition. Programs, such as the Special Olympics,* offer children an opportunity to compete with their peers and to achieve athletic skill. Summer camps† allow children to associate with peers and develop a wide variety of skills. Children with special needs can derive enormous benefits from expressive activities, such as art, music, poetry, dance, and drama. With adaptive equipment and imagination, children can participate in a variety of activities. Organizations such as VSA Arts allow children to celebrate and share their accomplishments.‡

*1133 19th St. NW, Washington, DC 20036; 202-628-3630; http://www.specialolympics.org. Several pamphlets on sports and recreation for children with disabilities are available from Easter Seals and American Alliance for Health, Physical Education, Recreation and Dance, 1900 Association Drive, Reston, VA 20191; 703-476-3400 or 800-213-7193; http://www.shapeamerica.org.

†A directory of private and paying camps for children with a variety of chronic illnesses and general physical disabilities is available from the American Camp Association, 5000 State Road 67 North, Martinsville, IN 46151-7902; 765-342-8456; http://www.acacamps.org.

‡VSA Arts has affiliate chapters in all 50 states and in selected sites internationally; yearly festivals are held throughout the world. Information is available from the department of VSA and Accessibility at the Kennedy Center, 2700 F Street, NW, Washington DC 20566; 800-444-1324; http://www.kennedy-center.org/education/vsa.

Children need the opportunity to interact with healthy peers and to engage in activities with groups or clubs composed of similarly affected age-mates. Organizations such as ostomy clubs, diabetes clubs, and cerebral palsy groups share information and provide support related to the special problems the members face.

Adolescence

Adolescence can be a particularly difficult period for the teenager and family. All of the needs discussed previously apply to this age group as well. Developing independence or autonomy, however, is a major task for the adolescent as planning for the future becomes a prominent concern. Although the emphasis in the past has been on achieving independence from physical assistance, recent developments in the fields of special education, adolescent development, and family systems suggest redefining autonomy in terms of individuals' capacities to take responsibility for their own behavior, to make decisions regarding their own lives, and to maintain supportive social relationships. Given this understanding, even individuals with severe impairments can be viewed as autonomous if they perceive their own needs and take responsibility for meeting them, either directly or by engaging the assistance of others. As adolescents become more autonomous, the nurse can help them articulate their needs, participate in developing their own care plans, and discover and express how others can be of greatest assistance.

Physical symptoms are high on teenagers' list of health-related concerns. Because adolescence is a time of enormous physical and emotional changes, it is important for the nurse to distinguish between body changes that are related to the child's complex condition and those that are a result of normal body development. It can be a great comfort for teenagers with disabling conditions to know that many of the changes they experience are normal developmental outcomes.

A sense of feeling different from peers can lead to loneliness, isolation, and depression. Participation in groups of teenagers with chronic conditions or disabilities can alleviate feelings of isolation and smooth the transition to a meaningful relationship with one person in adulthood.

ESTABLISH REALISTIC FUTURE GOALS

One of the most difficult adjustments is setting realistic future goals for the child that are based on the child's own goals and values.

Planning for the future should be a gradual process. All along, the parents should cultivate realistic vocations for the child. For example, if children have physical disabilities, they can be directed toward intellectual, artistic, or musical pursuits. Children with developmental disabilities can be taught manual skills. In this way, the child's development proceeds in the direction of self-support through gainful employment.

With prolonged survival, young people with chronic illnesses must deal with new decisions and problems, such as marriage, employment, and insurance coverage. With appropriate guidance, individuals with disabilities can attain gainful employment, marriage, and a family. For those whose conditions are genetic, counseling is needed regarding future offspring. Prospective spouses often benefit from an opportunity to discuss their feelings regarding marriage to an individual with continued health needs and possibly a limited life span. Health insurance coverage is a critical issue for chronically ill children because of their enormous health care costs over time. The Affordable Care Act allows young adults to remain on their parents insurance until they are 26 years old and prevents private insurance carriers from denying them coverage. Life insurance is another dilemma, especially when children have serious conditions, such as congenital heart anomalies.

PALLIATIVE CARE IN CHILDHOOD TERMINAL ILLNESS

SCOPE OF THE PROBLEM

Although death rates for children have dropped dramatically since the 1980s (64 down to 24/100,00 for ages 1 to 4 years; 31 down to 13/100,000 for ages 5 to 14 years; 98 down to 46/100,000 for ages 15 to 19 years; Child Trends Databank, 2016), the death of a child remains a tragedy to family, friends, and community. Nearly 70% of infant deaths result from congenital malformations, low birth weight, sudden infant death syndrome (SIDS), maternal complications, accidents, cord and placental complications, newborn respiratory distress and bacterial sepsis, neonatal hemorrhage, and circulatory system diseases. Accidents (unintentional injuries), followed by assault (homicide), cancer, and intentional self-harm (suicide), are the leading causes of death for all children 1 to 19 years of age. (See Chapter 1.)

In addition to the children who die each year, approximately another 400,000 children in the United States are living with a life-threatening illness (Burke & Alverson, 2010; Kuo, Cohen, Agrawal, et al., 2011). The number of children living with chronic, life-limiting illnesses has increased exponentially as advances in technology and pharmacology have led to improved treatments (Kuo, Houtrow, & Council on Children with Disability, 2016). These chronic conditions often result in substantial suffering, symptom distress, and health care needs that increase the possibility of death (Box 19.8) (Kuo, Houtrow, & Council on Children with Disability, 2016; Simon, Berry, Feudtner, et al., 2010). The majority of the children who die do so while undergoing intensive treatments in a hospital setting (Keele, Keenan, Sheetz, et al., 2013), having been mechanically ventilated and often experiencing acute and chronic pain

BOX 19.8 Conditions Contributing to Childhood Death

Cancer
Complications of prematurity
Congenital anomalies
- Trisomy 13, 18
- Anencephaly
- Holoprosencephaly
- Lissencephaly
- Inborn errors of metabolism

Cystic fibrosis
Human immunodeficiency virus infection/acquired immunodeficiency syndrome
Major organ dysfunction or failure
- Congenital or acquired heart disease or defects
- Liver defects
- Renal failure

Neurodegenerative diseases
- Muscular dystrophy
- Spinal muscular atrophy
- Adrenoleukodystrophy
- Ataxia-telangiectasia

Severe neurologic and/or physical disability
Severe gastrointestinal disorder or malformation
Epidermolysis bullosa
Severe immunodeficiencies
Severe forms of osteogenesis imperfecta
Trauma
- Accidents

and other distressing symptoms (Pritchard, Burghen, Srivastava, et al., 2008).

There has been growing recognition that the health care system has been failing children and families who are facing a life-threatening illness (Docherty, Brandon, & Miles, 2007; Wolfe, Hammel, Edwards, et al., 2008). Many children suffer from the symptoms of advancing disease and intensive treatments without adequate relief (Keele, Keenan, Sheetz, et al., 2013; Stevenson, Achille, & Lugasi, 2013). For over two decades, the American Academy of Pediatrics, Section on Hospice and Palliative Medicine and Committee on Hospital Care (2013) has provided broad support and guidance regarding principles of palliative care in pediatric practice. In addition, a number of national and international specialty groups have published suggested guidelines for the care of children with life-threatening and terminal illnesses (American Academy of Pediatrics, 2014; National Hospice and Palliative Care Organization, 2016; World Health Organization, 2014). More specifically, the American Academy of Pediatrics and the Institute of Medicine have both called for the integration of palliative care into ongoing medical management of children with life-threatening illnesses from the point of diagnosis to the end of life.

In the decade that followed the American Academy of Pediatrics and Institute of Medicine recommendations, models of integrated pediatric palliative care have been developed in which both curative therapy and palliative care coexist (Kaye, Rubenstein, Levine, et al., 2015). As cure-oriented treatment options decrease, the role of palliative care increases. Hospice services are offered at the end of the continuum of care. In this model, *concurrent care* is defined as the introduction of palliative care principles at the time of a life-threatening diagnosis, with increasing support over time as the disease progresses, including multidimensional assessment to identify, prevent, and alleviate suffering (Bakitas, Lyons, Hegel, et al., 2009; Kaye, Friebert, & Baker, 2016). These models have been supported by studies with adult patients demonstrating that palliative care prolongs life (Temel, Greer, Muzikansky, et al., 2010), improves quality of care (Meyers, Carducci, Loscalzo, et al., 2011), decreases hospital costs, and decreases caregiver burden (Chow & Coyle, 2011). The American Society of Clinical Oncology released a provisional clinical opinion based on available trials advocating for the early integration of palliative care into standard cancer treatment for malignancies with high symptom burden (Smith, Temin, Alesi, et al., 2012).

There remain many challenges to the implementation of integrated models of palliative care, including economic limits within the current health care environment, the lack of necessary tools and skills needed by health care providers, and the misalignment of palliative care exclusively to end-of-life care needs. Palliative care is now widely recognized as a critical part of excellent care for children with complex, chronic, or life-limiting diseases, but patients continue to receive this care very late in their illness trajectory. Many health care professionals lack clinical education in the principles of making the transition with children from curative to palliative care or methods of adequately managing the pain and suffering experienced by children and their families during the dying process (Feudtner, Womer, Augustin, et al., 2013). As our ability to treat disease, disability, and trauma advances, we must also improve our care of those children who live with the specter of chronic, life-threatening illness and premature death.

PRINCIPLES OF PALLIATIVE CARE

Palliative care involves an interdisciplinary approach to the management of a child's life-threatening or life-limiting illness from diagnosis through death and focuses on preventing or relieving the child's symptoms and support of the child and family (American Academy of Pediatrics, 2013). The World Health Organization (2014) defines pediatric palliative care as the "active total care of the child's body, mind, and spirit, and also involv[ing] giving support to the family. It begins when illness is diagnosed, and continues regardless of whether or not a child receives treatment directed at the disease." Palliative care interventions do not serve to hasten death; rather, they provide pain and symptom management, attention to issues faced by the child and family with regard to death and dying, and promotion of optimal functioning and quality of life. The implementation of neonatal and pediatric palliative care consulting services within hospitals has led to enhanced quality of life and end-of-life care for children and their families and support for their care providers (Enguidanos et al., 2014; Younge et al., 2015).

Several principles are hallmarks of palliative care (Levine, Lam, Cunningham, et al., 2013). The child and family are the unit of care in which services are coordinated across all sites of care. An interdisciplinary team of health care professionals consisting of social workers, chaplains, nurses, personal care aides, child life specialists, and physicians skilled in caring for children with life-threatening or life-limiting conditions assists the family by focusing care on the complex interactions between physical, emotional, social, and spiritual needs. In particular, nurses can provide families with the much-needed reassurance that a focus on relief of suffering does not mean that curative or disease-modifying treatments will be abandoned. Rather continued assessment of the appropriateness of disease-focused treatments will direct attention to all of the goals of care including quality of life. If the principles of palliative care are framed in this concurrent care model, unnecessary delays in providing children the treatment they need may be avoided. Multidimensional assessment and open communication among all health care team members including the family will result in early identification of distressing symptoms.

GOALS OF CARE

Palliative care seeks to relieve the physical, emotional, social, and spiritual distress produced by life-limiting conditions, to assist in complex decision making, and to enhance the quality of life (Tamburro, Shaffer, Hahnlen, et al., 2011). To do so most effectively, providers must guide realistic goal setting for the patient. Frequent, periodic, and timely discussions between the health care provider team and parents (and child when developmentally appropriate) regarding the goals of care are critical (Hill, Miller, Walter, et al., 2014). The possibility that a child's illness or condition is not curable and that death may be an inevitable outcome causes everyone involved a great deal of stress (Brandon, Ryan, Sloane, et al., 2014). Physicians, other members of the health care team, and families consider all information regarding the child's situation and make difficult choices regarding treatment options, and these decisions can have a profound impact on the child and family. The goals of care should be frequently revisited to ensure that they are rooted in the personal beliefs of the patient and family and based on realistic assessments of a child's clinical condition. Whenever possible, the goals of the child should be solicited and respected. Establishing goals of care has become an essential component of quality palliative medicine (Hill, Miller, Walter, et al., 2014; Tamburro, Shaffer, Hahnlen, et al., 2011) and should address the physical, emotional, social, and spiritual distress experienced by patients and their families. Nurses are often best situated to evaluate suffering and the impact of the goals of care because of the amount of time they spend with patients and their families compared with other medical team members (Mastro, Johnson, McElvery, et al., 2015). However, for many children goals of care often remain poorly delineated because they are not discussed thoroughly and openly. When asked about obstacles to good palliative care, pediatric nurses have rated "uncertainty about the goals of care" as being second only to "lack of opportunity to debrief after death" (Tubbs-Cooley, Santucci,

Kang, et al., 2011). Successful palliative care requires a candid exchange between the patient, family, and health care team. Unfortunately, such conversation often does not occur early enough to affect outcomes and improve quality of life. In a study investigating the challenges that exist in providing pediatric palliative care to inpatient populations, researchers described providers' hesitation to initiate palliative care discussions and interventions until they were certain that the child was "beginning to die" (Docherty, Brandon, & Miles, 2007). Prognostic uncertainty and the desire to remain hopeful should not prevent the initiation of goals that focus on the relief of symptom distress and suffering even when curative care is still feasible. Common ethical dilemmas facing health care professionals caring for children who are terminally ill are found in Table 19.4.

Physicians often make decisions about care on the basis of the progression of the disease or amount of trauma, the availability of treatment options that would provide cure from disease or restoration of health, the impact of such treatments on the child, and the child's overall prognosis. When the physician discusses this information openly with families, a shared goal-setting process can occur, and potential outcomes can be put on the table. For example, a family and provider discussion may result in the continuation of a particular course of treatment but allow for an important discussion regarding the next step if the child's condition were to continue to decline. Uncertainty about the child's prognosis among health care providers is often a barrier to the provision of optimal palliative care (Friedrichsdorf, 2016; Coad, Patel, & Murray, 2014). As a result, many families have not always received the option of shifting the focus of treatment to the child's comfort and quality of life when cure is unlikely (see Research Focus box). Although current American Academy of Pediatrics (2014) guidelines recommend collaborative integrated care that includes clear and honest discussions with patients and families about the goals of treatment and any concerns they may have, specific discussions about the burden of treatment and the benefits of end-of-life care planning is often absent.

RESEARCH FOCUS

Palliative Care

Results of landmark studies of physician decision making regarding when to change the focus of care to palliation and comfort show high variability across physicians and settings (Randolph, Zollo, Egger, et al., 1999; Thompson, Knapp, Madden, et al., 2009). In one survey of over 300 pediatricians, only 15% of participating physicians would recommend early referral for palliative care for children with cancer. In contrast, 44% would make such a recommendation at end of life (Thompson, Knapp, Madden, et al., 2009). This reluctance to change to a focus on palliative care by physicians occurs for a number of reasons, including the belief that not being able to "save" a child is a "failure." Also, the physician and other members of the health care team may lack knowledge of and experience with the principles of palliative care (Davies, Sehring, Partridge, et al., 2008). Pediatric nurses, empowered with the skills and understanding of quality palliative care, can help the care team focus on palliative care goals and ensure that these principles are integrated into the care model throughout the entire clinical course, even when formal palliative care consultation is not solicited.

TABLE 19.4 Common Ethical Dilemmas in Caring for Terminally Ill Children

Rationale in Providing to Patient	Rationale in Withholding From Patient
Pain Control	
Comfort (the primary goal)	Side effects of opioids
Improved quality of life	Decreased level of cognition
Easier dying process if child is pain free	Fear of addiction (unfounded for terminally ill patients)
Chemotherapy or Experimental Therapy	
Prolonged life span	Decreased blood counts, increased risk of infection, bleeding
Possible increase in quality of life	Side effects of treatment that may be painful, uncomfortable
Provision of sense that family has done everything they can to save the child	
Supplemental Nutrition and Hydration (Intravenous, Nasogastric, Gastrostomy Tube)	
Belief that the child is hungry or thirsty	Supplemental feedings beyond what child can ingest may actually cause nausea or vomiting
Inability or unwillingness of child to eat	Increase in tumor growth (feeding of the tumor)
Fear that child will "starve" to death	Increase in fluid volume may result in congestive heart failure, increased respiratory secretions, and/or pulmonary congestion, which leads to questions of whether to implement diuresis
Primary role of parent to feed and nourish child	Increased risk of skin breakdown if child is incontinent, due to increased urinary output
Parental guilt	Risk of third spacing
	More comfortable and natural death
	Complaint of thirst is associated with dying process, not level of hydration
Resuscitation	
Unwillingness of family to give up	Allows nature to take its course
Conflicts with cultural or religious beliefs	Family believes child has suffered enough, does not want aggressive intervention
Denial that child is actually going to die	Relieves family of responsibility to stop interventions that might prolong life
Autopsy	
Research to help other children	Religious, cultural belief
Ability to check genetic link	Family emotions
	Belief that body will be desecrated for funeral viewing (an unfounded fear)

The current approach by palliative care experts promotes the inclusion of palliative care along the continuum of care from diagnosis through treatment, not merely at the end of life (American Academy of Pediatrics, 2014).

Rarely are families prepared to cope with the numerous decisions that must be made when a child is dying. When the death is unexpected, as in the case of an accident or trauma, the confusion of emergency services and possibly an intensive care setting presents challenges to parents as they are asked to make difficult choices (Von Lützau, Otto, Hechler, et al., 2012). Determination of parental decision-making preferences, which may be active or independent, collaborative or shared between parents and provider, or passive or authoritarian, can help providers support parents. If the child has experienced a life-threatening illness such as cancer or lived with a chronic illness that has now reached its terminal phase, parents are often unprepared for the reality of their child's impending death (see Family-Centered Care box).

FAMILY-CENTERED CARE

Family of the Dying Child

No matter whether you have a PhD or many children, when your child dies, it is a new experience and nothing can prepare you for it. Like so many things in life, experience is the best teacher.

Three of our children have died, and by the time the third was dying, we handled many things differently. We learned a lot about dignity and the rights of the child and family. For example, at first, we didn't know that we had a right to have our child die at home. We also didn't understand pain medications and that if children are taking these medicines and are still in agony, they have not overdosed on the medication.

We learned a lot about case management. With our first two children, lots of different people were making decisions and disagreeing about what was best and what should be done. No one had primary authority. With our third child, one doctor took a primary role. Any questions and problems were handled by one person. I could call him 24 hours a day. It made a lot of difference, and I felt our concerns and needs were better heard and respected.

The nurses caring for our third child at home enabled me to step back and just be his mommy. When I could do this, I realized that we were fighting so hard for his life that we weren't really letting him die. His nurses had worked with him for a long time and really loved him. It was hard for them when we decided to let him die. In his last several days we wanted a lot of family time with our son, and I think the nurses felt left out. Something about their reaction to our increased time with him in the last few days made us feel guilty. If we had all been able to communicate a little more openly, I would have understood that they needed more time with him at the end, too. Everyone's needs could have been met.

Jeni Stepanek
Mother
Upper Marlboro, Maryland

Effective communication is critical for quality palliative care. Barriers to effective communication are among the most important factors perceived to interfere with optimal end-of-life pediatric care (Coad, Patel, & Murray, 2014). Parents almost always want clinicians to discuss advance care options and to assist them in such complex decision making. Although the nurse may not be the one spearheading such discussions, the nurse can be instrumental in advocating for discussions to occur and that patient preferences are verbalized. In a review of the literature on nursing roles and strategies for end-of-life decision making, information broker, supporter, and advocate emerged as key roles that nurses play in the adult acute care setting (Stewart, Pyke-Grimm, & Kelly, 2012). First, as information brokers, pediatric nurses provide information about the child and family to the health care team, provide information to the child and family about treatment plans and goals, and coordinate discussions between the family and health care team. Second, nurses provide an important source of emotional support to the child and family as they attempt to comprehend and assess the impact of the information they are given. Third, nurses actively engage as advocates in palliative care planning by challenging the status quo and by assisting all invested parties to understand the overall patient care mission. This level of advocacy in which the child and family are given assistance with interpreting and understanding goals will lead to valid and shared decision making. The foundation for good decision making depends on establishing clear goals of care based on individual preferences and beliefs that are attainable given a child's clinical condition.

Earlier acknowledgment by both physicians and parents that children have no realistic chance for cure is often associated with implementation of do-not-resuscitate (DNR) orders, and greater provision of palliative care measures, but even when physicians recommend limiting or withdrawing life-sustaining interventions many parents disagree. Current factors influencing physicians' and nurses' resuscitation decisions include (1) patient characteristics (96%), (2) personal experience/biases (85%), (3) family's wishes and desires (81%), (4) disease characteristics (74%), and (5) societal perspectives (36%) (Dupont-Thibodeau, Hindié, Bourque, et al., 2017). Factors found to influence parents' decisions to limit or withdraw life-sustaining measures include parents' prior end-of-life decision making for loved ones; observations of pain and suffering of their child and other hospitalized children; various emotions, including guilt and sorrow; and awareness of their child's desire to forego life-sustaining measures (Sharman, Meert, & Sarnaik, 2005). The use of a pediatric advance directive for older minors may raise awareness of children's wishes as part of the family decision-making process (Knapp, Huang, Madden, et al., 2009; Zinner, 2009), but parents find engagement in advanced care planning to be difficult (Lotz, Daxer, Jox, et al., 2016), especially when they do not agree with their child. Three strategies have been posited for providers to manage differences between parent and child preferences: deference, advocative, and arbitrative. Parental decision-making preferences are deferred to in the deference strategy, whereas child preferences are advocated in the advocative strategy. The arbitrative strategy is used to work to resolve the differences between parents and the child (Sisk, DuBois, Kodish, et al., 2017) (see Research Focus box, Box 19.9, and Table 19.5).

AWARENESS OF DYING IN CHILDREN WITH LIFE-THREATENING ILLNESS

One of the initial reactions of parents (and some health care professionals) to the discovery of a life-threatening illness is to protect the child from

BOX 19.9 Communicating With Families

Listen for an "invitation" to talk about the situation.

"Sometimes I wonder if I am doing the right thing."
"What have other parents done in this situation?"
"Do you know of other children who have survived this?"
"I think the doctor is not telling me everything."

Use open-ended, nonjudgmental questions to explore families' wishes.

"Can you tell me more about how you are feeling?"
"What questions do you (or your child) have that I can answer for you?"
"What are your concerns (or worries, fears) right now?"
"What is important to you (or your child, family) at this time?"

TABLE 19.5 Communicating Bad News to Families

Approach	Effective Techniques
Provide a setting conducive to communication.	Ensure privacy; use appropriate body language; make eye contact. Have parents choose who will attend.
Determine what the parent knows.	Ask questions ("What have you made of all this?" or "What were you told?"). Listen to the vocabulary and comprehension of the parents. Recognize denial but do not acknowledge it at this stage.
Determine what the parent wants to know.	Obtain a clear invitation to share information (if this is what the parent wants). Use questions such as "Are you the sort of person who likes to know every detail or just the basic facts?"
Give information (aligning and educating).	Start at level of parents' comprehension and use the same vocabulary. Give information slowly, concisely, and in simple language. Avoid medical jargon. Check regularly to be certain that content is understood.
Respond to parents' reactions.	Acknowledge all reactions and feelings, particularly using the emphatic response technique (identifying emotion, identifying cause of emotion, and responding appropriately). Expect tears, anger, and other strong emotions.
Close.	Briefly summarize major areas discussed. Ask parents if they have other important issues to discuss at this time. Make an appointment for the next meeting.

RESEARCH FOCUS

Importance of Honest Communication

Numerous studies have found that families facing the impending death of a child depend on information provided to them by the health care team, particularly an honest appraisal of the child's prognosis, to make difficult decisions regarding care options for their child and care measures after life-sustaining measures were eliminated (Sharman, Meert, & Sarnaik, 2005).

As the group of health professionals who are most involved with families, nurses are in an excellent position to ensure that families know the options available to them (see Box 19.2). The nurse's first responsibility is to explore the patient's and family's wishes. This is best done with the physician, but at times nurses need to initiate the process. When discussing difficult issues, nurses are open to the child's or family's indirect comments that communicate uncertainty or concerns about the course of care. Nurses answer questions honestly, and if they do not know the answer, reassure the family that they will arrange for a discussion with the physician. It is important to address any fantasies or misunderstandings by seeking to clarify what the family has heard. Finally, it is important for the nurse to remain neutral and avoid giving personal opinions or experiences. The goal of communication is to facilitate the identification of the family's wishes, based on their unique values and beliefs (see Table 19.2).

the impact of the diagnosis (Bluebond-Langner, 1978; Ferrell, Wittenberg, Battista, et al., 2016a; Larcher, Craig, Bhogal, et al., 2015). However, it is now widely understood that terminally ill children develop an awareness of the seriousness of their diagnosis, even when protected from the truth (Bluebond-Langner, 1978; Jalmsell, Kontio, Stein, et al., 2015; Spinetta, 1974). The avoidance of talking openly and honestly with children with life-threatening illnesses and their siblings can lead to fear, guilt, misconceptions, and the pain of grieving alone. Surviving siblings may experience psychiatric sequelae as children and into adulthood.

Discussing Death With Children

Children need honest and accurate information about their illness, treatments, and prognosis. There is broad consensus across research and practice that it is important to involve children, regardless of age, in discussions about their illness and care plans (Cohen, Mannarino, & Deblinger, 2016; Jacobs, Perez, Cheng, et al., 2015; Taylor, Haase-Casanovas, Weaver, et al., 2010). The appropriate timing and approach for these discussions are less clear (Bluebond-Langner, Belasco, DeMesquita, et al., 2010; Cohen, Mannarino, & Deblinger, 2016). This information needs to be given in clear, simple language. In most situations this best occurs as a gradual process, characterized by increasingly open dialogue among parents, professionals, and the child. Providing an atmosphere of open communication early in the course of an illness facilitates answering difficult questions as the child's condition worsens. Providing appropriate literature about the disease, as well as about the experience of illness and possible death, is also helpful. How and when to involve children in decisions regarding care during their dying process and death are individual matters. In general, the nurse should ask parents how they would like their child to be told of the prognosis and how they want to be included in their child's care. Some parents may request that their child not be told that he or she is dying, even if the child asks. This often places health care providers in a difficult situation. Children, even at a young age, are perceptive. Despite not being told outright that they are dying, they realize that something is seriously wrong and that it involves them. Children deserve to be provided with the truth.

Children and families often have an unspoken anxiety related to the fear of dying and/or the dying process. Children and their families will share some similar fears and worries, but others will be unique (Cohen, Mannarino, & Deblinger, 2016). Identifying the specific fears and fostering candid discussion of them will allow the nurse to minimize the suffering associated with this anxiety as much as possible. The fear of being alone in the face of death is often a contributor to anxiety (Van Breemen, 2009). By reassuring the patient that he or she will not be alone and by creating an environment that avoids isolation, the bedside nurse can combat such worries. The ability of the nurse to facilitate an atmosphere that allows loved ones to be present, encourages candid expression of feelings, and provides a sense of closeness and understanding among family members will do much to minimize the fears associated with dying.

Anxiety and fear may also lead to a range of emotional expressions on the part of the child that may be disturbing to families, particularly if they are not prepared. This may include emotional liability, aggression, and expressions of anger, depression, and withdrawal. Helping families to understand that such expressions are not unexpected or abnormal may ease anxiety for the family and facilitate better coping. The nurse may provide further reassurance by both practicing and introducing families to the concepts of active listening, simple relaxation, and therapeutic touch. The bedside nurse can also structure the hospital or home environment to allow for maximum control and independence within the limitations imposed by the developmental level and physical

TABLE 19.6 Communicating With Dying Children

Approach	Effective Technique
Discuss at the child's level.	Gear information to the child's developmental age, remembering that younger children tend to be concrete thinkers, whereas older children are capable of abstract thought. Begin with the child's experiences ("You've told us how tired you've been lately").
Let the child's questions guide.	Begin the conversation with basic information, and let the child's questions direct the conversation.
Provide opportunities for the child to express feelings.	Look for clues that the child is open to communication. Be accepting of whatever emotion is expressed.
Encourage feedback.	Ask the child to summarize what has been heard. This provides the opportunity to clarify misunderstandings.
Use other resources.	Use books and movies to encourage dialogue. Ask the child to name the people with whom he or she can discuss problems.
Use the child's natural expressive means to stimulate dialogue.	Use books, games, art, play, and music to provide a means of expression.

condition of the child. Nurses can mitigate the suffering of anxiety by explaining all procedures and therapies, detailing the physical effects the child is likely to experience, and answering all questions in a frank, honest manner.

Parents may require professional support and guidance in this process from a nurse, social worker, chaplain, or child life specialist who has a good relationship with the child and family. Certain principles and guidelines can assist nurses and families in determining how to present facts about possible death and hope to a child in a way that fosters trust, enhances meaningful communication, and offers emotional support (Table 19.6 and Box 19.10). Professionals may also provide information to parents about their child's general developmental understanding of and reactions to death and how to explain death in a developmentally appropriate manner, and offer to assist parents when speaking with their terminally ill child and siblings.

- Encourage parents to approach the discussion of death with a child gently. *What* is said is important, but *how* it is said is critical to how a child is able to accept, within his or her ability, the reality of death.
- Advise parents to begin the discussion with a child by using a nonthreatening example such as trees and leaves and how long they live.
- Allow the child's questions to guide the discussion and avoid unnecessary information; speak on the child's developmental level; provide basic information slowly, directly, and honestly, using simple, concrete, age-appropriate words, including "die"; and avoid the use of euphemisms (e.g., "pass away," "lost").
- Clarify misconceptions and let the child know he or she did not cause the illness or impending death; allow the child to express his or her feelings and accept whatever emotions are expressed by the child; provide warmth and support during the discussion; and speak with a calm and reassuring voice.
- Ask the child to repeat what has been discussed to clarify any misunderstandings.

BOX 19.10 The Dying Child's Right to Refuse Treatment

Traditionally, minor children (the age of minority varies with state law) have not had the legal right to give informed consent for treatment or to refuse treatment. One of the major issues is the age at which children have the cognitive ability to understand the medical information, consider and comprehend the consequences of a decision (death), and choose freely among the options. Depending on children's development level, a mature understanding of death does not occur until approximately 9 years of age, but experience with death and an awareness of one's own impending death may affect the ability to understand (Martinson, 1995). These findings are consistent with those of Bluebond-Langner (1978, 1989), who found that fatally ill children progress through a series of stages that shape their understanding of their disease and death.

Other issues raised by opponents include concerns about dispelling hope in the child once death is pronounced as imminent, parents' guilt if they later question the decision, and possible conflict between the child's and parents' wishes. Although there is insufficient research to answer these concerns, it seems unlikely that these situations will occur if the family is allowed to choose therapeutic alternatives in an atmosphere of professional support and with sufficient information. In addition, staff members need to assess each child's capacity to understand the implications of refusing treatment, with documentation of the words and actions of the child that support their conclusions.

- Encourage family members to discuss the child's impending death openly and honestly with the child, siblings, and other family members (Ethier, 2008).

The nurse can facilitate ongoing and open communication about death and dying through the use of various resources, including books (e.g., *The Fall of Freddie the Leaf* by Leo Buscaglia; *I Miss You: A First Look at Death* by Pat Thomas; and *Sad Isn't Bad: A Good-Grief Guidebook for Kids Dealing with Loss* by Michaelene Mundy) and movies (e.g., *The Velveteen Rabbit* by Margery Williams) (Auvrignon, Leverger, & Lasfargues, 2008; Ethier, 2005). Play and art activities (e.g., music, drawing, painting, writing) offer a vehicle for expression of emotions that are often difficult for children to put into words (Rollins & Riccio, 2002).

CHILDREN'S UNDERSTANDING OF AND REACTIONS TO DYING

The use of chronologic age and/or the child's stage of development as a marker for timing and content of discussions about death can be problematic due to the variability in cognitive development within particular ages and stages. Ages and stages may be helpful as a general guide, but communication should be based on the cognitive developmental capabilities of the individual child and his or her readiness for such discussion. This individualized approach not only takes into consideration the cognitive abilities of the child but also includes assessment of potential vulnerabilities, experiences with the illness, readiness for information, and relationships with parents and/or caregivers (Bluebond-Langner, Belasco, DeMesquita, et al., 2010. Influences also include nationality, religion, life-limiting illness, personal experiences with death, and family members' explanations and attitudes surrounding death (Spinetta, 1974; Weaver et al., 2016). By approximately 7 years of age most children understand the key bioscientific components of death (Box 19.11). Studies have found that children ranging in age from 4 to 12 years have an adultlike understanding of death (Wolfelt, 2013). However, anyone working with children must be aware of significant developmental variations related to their understanding and

BOX 19.11 Children's Development of the Subconcepts of Death

Universality
- All living things eventually die.
- Death is all inclusive; everyone dies.
- Death is inevitable, unavoidable.
- Death is unpredictable; exact timing is unknown.

Before Universality
- They themselves, children in general, and/or their family or friends may be viewed as excluded.
- Understanding that *they* will die precedes understanding that *everyone* will die.
- Death is avoidable if you are clever.
- Death occurs in the remote future only.

Irreversibility
- Once the physical body dies, it cannot be made alive again.

Before Irreversibility
- Death is temporary (e.g., falling asleep and waking up, leaving for and returning from a trip) and reversible.

Nonfunctionality
- Once a living thing dies, all life-defining capabilities (e.g., eating, sleeping, seeing, hearing) of the body cease.

Before Nonfunctionality
- The dead continue external functions (e.g., eating, speaking).

Causality
- External and internal events can cause one's death.

Before Causality
- Death results from unrealistic causes (e.g., misbehaving), concrete causes (e.g., poison, guns), or external causes (e.g., accidents, murder).

Noncorporeal Continuation
- Some form of personal continuation exists after death of the physical body (e.g., reincarnation, ascension of the soul to heaven).

Before Noncorporeal Continuation
- Unknown.

fears of death. Cultural, national, and religious differences in beliefs about an afterlife have also been found to influence a child's understanding of death. Sensitive assessment of the child's developmental understanding of death and the family's cultural and spiritual beliefs related to dying and death is an important but often overlooked aspect of care.

Infants and Toddlers

Exactly how preverbal children view death is a mystery because there is no way of reliably assessing their views of death. On the basis of their cognitive abilities, it is likely that they have no concept of death. The egocentricity of toddlers and their vague separation of fact and fantasy make it impossible for them to comprehend absence of life. Although they may repeat what initially sounds like a correct definition of death, such as "Grandpa is dead; he went to heaven," they may expect Grandpa's return for several months before accommodating themselves to the absence. They can perceive events only in terms of their own frame of reference: living.

Reactions to Dying

Separation from parents and alterations in their routine represent threats to the toddler who is seriously ill and to the well-toddler sibling. Behavioral responses may include regression to less independent levels of behavior related to speech, toileting, eating, drinking, crying, clinging, biting, hitting, withdrawal, and physical illness. Toddlers may perceive the seriousness of their condition from the parents' reactions of anxiety, sadness, depression, or anger. Although young children are unaware of the reason for such emotions, they often find their parents' behavior disturbing and upsetting. Helping parents deal with their feelings allows them more emotional reserve to meet the needs of their children. Encouraging parents to stay in the hospital as much as possible and to participate in the child's care promotes the parents' and child's adjustment to a serious, potentially fatal illness or injury. Helpful interventions for infants and toddlers include providing the child with physical comfort (e.g., being held or rocked), consistent providers, consistent routines, and familiar objects (e.g., favorite blanket or toy) (Ethier, 2008).

Preschool Children

Several characteristics of preschoolers' cognitive and psychologic development affect their concept of death. Because they are egocentric at this age, they often have a tremendous sense of self-power and omnipotence. Therefore they believe that their thoughts are sufficient to cause events. The consequence of such magical thinking is feelings of guilt, shame, and punishment.

Concept of Death

Children between 3 and 5 years of age have usually heard the word *death* and have some sense of its meaning. They see death as a departure, possibly as a type of sleep. They may recognize the fact of physical death but do not separate it from living abilities. The dead person in the coffin still breathes, eats, and sleeps. Death is temporary and reversible; life and death can change places with one another. Because of the immature concept of time, they have no real understanding of the universality and inevitability of death. Words such as *forever* and *everyone* have meaning only in the child's egocentric thinking. Waiting until Christmas may be "forever," and anybody the child denotes is "everyone." Children of this age take the literal meaning of words, and euphemisms are avoided. Preschoolers who are told that Grandma has "gone to sleep" may fear going to sleep themselves.

Reactions to Dying

If preschoolers become seriously ill, they may conceive of the illness as punishment for their thoughts or actions. The usual diagnostic and treatment procedures, in combination with enforced hospitalization, can confirm their belief that they are being punished. If their parents do not stay with them during hospitalization or prevent the traumatic procedures, they may believe that the parents are retaliating for previous misdeeds or bad thoughts.

The same principles of magical thinking and omnipotence affect preschoolers when a sibling becomes critically ill or dies. One of the most significant types of death is SIDS. Because it occurs unexpectedly to a healthy infant (who may have been rejected and unwanted by a jealous sibling), preschoolers find no evidence to support a physical cause of death. Indeed, the parents often are unaware of the reason for the fatality and may question any possible cause. If preschoolers are in any way accused or suspected of having harmed the infant, they may feel extremely guilty and responsible for the tragedy. On observing their parents' acute grief, they may interpret the anger or depression as a rejection of them.

When a child becomes ill, the healthy siblings experience the loss of routine and parental attention. It is natural for them to resent such disruptions and blame the changes on the ill child. However, preschoolers have less ability than older children to understand the reasons for the parents' prolonged absence from home. Although parents may explain how ill the sibling is, what the hospital is like, and why they must be there, preschoolers see only the special attention and material rewards that the ill sister or brother is receiving. Because they are also unable to differentiate causes for separation of the parents and ill child, they may fear that the parents will never return. If they should learn that the ill child may not get well or come home, they may interpret this to mean that the parents will also never return. Their greatest fear concerning death is separation from parents. Asking repeated questions; complaining about stomachaches, headaches, and other physical symptoms; displaying intensified fears and emotional outbursts; and showing signs of regression are common behavioral responses to death among preschoolers. They may appear indifferent about the death of a sibling, but this is a normal response related to their limited coping abilities. The well sibling may also engage in "magical thinking," believing that they may have caused their sibling's illness and thus death. Play provides the preschooler with relief from the feelings of grief, but unknowing caregivers may misunderstand this. Helpful interventions for preschoolers include minimizing separation from parents; clarifying misconceptions of illness and death as punishment; using accurate, simple language repeated as often as the child needs; and providing the opportunity to play (Ethier, 2008).

School-Age Children

Although school-age children have a better understanding of causality, less egocentricity, and an advanced perception of time, they may still associate misdeeds or bad thoughts with causing death and feel intense guilt and responsibility for the event. However, because of their higher cognitive abilities, they respond well to logical explanations and comprehend the figurative meaning of words better than children in younger age groups. Although they are less likely to interpret explanations in a purely literal sense, they are still prone to self-referenced definitions. For this reason, it is important for adults to clarify the meanings of statements and to repeatedly ask the children what they think.

Concept of Death

Much of the discussion on the preschool child's understanding of death also relates to the younger school-age child. However, these children have a deeper understanding of death in the concrete sense. Children of this age attempt to ascribe a more comprehensible meaning to the event by personifying death as a devil, God, ghost, or bogeyman. Naturalistic-physiologic explanations of why death occurs and what happens to the dead body may also be a preoccupation in this age group. Factual explanations, such as "When you die, your body decays in the ground" are consistent with their concrete thinking.

By age 7 years, most children have an increasingly adult concept of death. They realize that it is universal, irreversible, and nonfunctional; children with cancer gain a more mature, biologic understanding of death at an earlier age than their well peers. Their attitudes toward death are greatly influenced by the reactions and attitudes of others, particularly their parents.

Reactions to Dying

The increased ability of school-age children to comprehend and reason poses additional risks for them. They may fear the reason for the illness, communicability of the disease to themselves or others, consequences of the disease on their functioning and relationships with others, and the process of dying and death itself. They tend to fear the expectation of the event more than its realization. Their fear of the unknown is greater than that of the known. Like preschoolers, their fantasy explanations for the unexpected or the unknown are usually much more frightening and extreme than the actual situation. For this reason, anticipatory preparation is both necessary and effective. These children respond well to explanations of the disease, names of drugs, and so on. The developmental task of this age is industry; thus helping children who may be facing their own death to maintain control over their body—by understanding what is happening to them and participating in what is done to them—allows them to achieve independence, self-worth, and self-esteem and to avoid a sense of inferiority.

The realization of impending death or failure to recover is a tremendous threat to school-age children's sense of security and ego strength. These children are likely to exhibit their fear more through verbal uncooperativeness. Health care professionals may erroneously interpret this behavior as rude, impolite, insolent, or stubborn. In reality the words are conveying the same meaning as physical attempts to run away or fight off others. This verbal "fight-or-flight" reaction to stress is a plea for some control and power. Additional behavioral responses for the well sibling may include worrying about the health and safety of other family members and having problems in school. Encouraging children to talk about their feelings, allowing control where possible and appropriate, and providing outlets for aggression through play are means of dealing with this expression of anger and fear.

Adolescents

By the time most children reach adolescence, they have a mature understanding of death. As abstract thinking develops, there is more questioning of death and related topics, such as the religious meaning of afterlife. However, other developmental needs, especially formation of the child's own identity, make this an exceptionally difficult time for young people to cope with the loss of a loved one or with their own impending death.

Concept of Death

Although adolescents have a mature understanding of death, they tend to think they will not die as a young person. The search for the spiritual meaning of what follows death is typical at this age.

Reactions to Dying

Adolescents may have a great deal of difficulty in coping with death. Although they have reached the level of adult comprehension of the concept of death, they are least likely of all age groups to accept cessation of life, particularly their own. Developmentally, the rejection of death is understandable because adolescents' tasks are to establish an identity by finding out who they are, what their purpose is, and where they belong.

Adolescents strive for group acceptance and independence from parental constraints. As a result, they rely on peer rules and beliefs for personal direction and reject opposing parental demands. However, when faced with the crisis of serious illness, they may consider themselves alienated from peer associations and unable to communicate with their parents for emotional support. Therefore they may feel virtually alone in their struggle. Support groups or other means of networking with adolescents facing death may be useful.

Healthy adolescents must deal with several maturational crises, such as the acceptance of bodily changes and socialization of intensifying sexual impulses. Any threat to either task increases their vulnerability to the stress of coping with such crises. The devastation of a terminal illness and the effects of chemotherapy may be greater concerns than the prospect of dying. Adolescents' orientation to the present compels them to worry about physical changes even more than the prognosis for future recovery.

Nurses are in a key position in working with terminally ill adolescents. In the hospital setting they spend the greatest amount of time with them. They can structure the hospital admission to allow for maximum self-control and independence while allowing the adolescent the opportunity to get to know the nurse. Answering adolescents' questions honestly; treating them as mature individuals; and respecting their needs for privacy, solitude, and personal expressions of emotions such as anger, sadness, or fear convey to adolescents the adult's true concern for their physical and emotional welfare. Nurses can help parents communicate with adolescents by providing information on typical adolescent responses and coping patterns; acting as role models; avoiding alliances with either parent or child; and allowing parents the opportunity to vent their feelings of frustration, incompetence, or failure in an atmosphere of acceptance and without judgment.

DELIVERY OF PALLIATIVE CARE SERVICES

Once the health care team and family have discussed the likelihood of death as the outcome of a child's medical condition or illness, it is necessary to determine the child's and family's preference for the location of palliative care. The circumstances of the child's illness may influence the location in which palliative care is provided. For instance, traumatic injury or acute illness often leads to death in the emergency department or intensive care unit setting. Children with progressive chronic illnesses or disabilities may initially receive palliative care services through a coordination of services between outpatient visits to their primary physician and care provided by a community agency (home health or hospice) in the home. As the illness progresses, the family may cease to come to the clinic or hospital and depend solely on care provided at home by the community agency as directed by the primary physician. Regardless of the circumstances of the illness or the location of care, it is important to focus on interventions that address all aspects of the child's and family's comfort. This requires attention to the child's physical comfort and the social, emotional, and spiritual needs of the child and family. Based on the decision by the child and family regarding their wishes for care, the family has several options from which to choose.

Hospital

Families may choose to remain in the hospital to receive care if the child's illness or condition is unstable and home care is not an option, or the family is uncomfortable with providing care at home. If a family chooses to remain at the hospital for terminal care, make the setting as homelike as possible. Families can bring familiar items from the child's room at home. In addition, develop a consistent and coordinated care plan for the child's and family's comfort.

Home Care

Some families may prefer to take their child home and receive services from a home care agency. Generally, these services entail periodic nursing visits, medications, equipment, and supplies. The primary physician continues to direct the child's care. Physicians and families often choose home care because of the traditional view that a child must be considered to have a life expectancy of fewer than 6 months to be referred to hospice care. Fortunately, a number of hospice organizations are expanding their services to children, basing admission on the presence of a life-limiting disease process for which a cure is not possible rather than on the sole criterion of a limited 6-month prognosis. Dussell, Kreicbergs, Hilden, and colleagues (2008) found parents whose children received home care had honest, open, end-of-life communication from the physician. Parents were more likely to plan the location of their child's death as the home and to report favorable outcomes. Unfortunately, many families do not have access to palliative care services when their child is dying. Palliative end-of-life care programs for children are becoming more common in hospitals and hospices in the United States, but there is wide variation in the staffing and level of funding of these programs (Feudtner, Womer, Augustin, et al., 2013).

Hospice Care

Hospice care is another option for families who wish to take their child home during the final phases of an illness. Hospice is a community health care program that specializes in the care of dying patients by combining the hospice philosophy with the principles of palliative care. **Hospice philosophy** regards dying as a natural process and views the care of dying patients as including management of the physical, psychologic, social, and spiritual needs of the patient and family. A multidisciplinary group of professionals provide care in the patient's home or an inpatient facility that follows the hospice philosophy. Hospice care for children was introduced in the 1970s (Martinson, 1993), and a number of community hospice organizations now accept children into their care (Ullrich, Sourkes, and Wolfe, 2016).* Collaboration between the child's primary treatment team and the hospice care team is essential to the success of hospice care. Families may continue to see their primary care physicians as they choose.

The goal of hospice care is for children to live life to the fullest without pain, with choices and dignity, in the familiar environment of their homes, and with the support of their families. Hospice care is covered under state Medicaid programs and by most insurance plans. According to the Concurrent Care for Children Requirement in the Patient Protection and Affordable Care Act of 2010, children covered under either Medicaid or the Children's Health Insurance Program are eligible to receive both hospice and curative care (National Consensus Project for Quality Palliative Care, 2013).

The service provides home nursing visits and visits from social workers, chaplains, and, in some cases, physicians. For children, the hospice concept has most commonly been implemented in the home, which benefits the family in a variety of ways. Children who are dying are allowed the opportunity to remain with those they love and with whom they feel secure. Many children who were thought to be in imminent danger of death have gone home and lived longer than expected. Siblings can feel more involved in the care and often have more positive perceptions of the death. In addition to the care and support provided through the dying process to the child and family, hospice is concerned with the family's postdeath adjustment, and bereavement care may continue for a year or more.

Parental adaptation may be more favorable, as is shown by their perceptions of how the experience at home affected their marriage, social reorientation, religious beliefs, and views on the meaning of life and death.

Receiving hospice care in the home does not necessarily mean the child will die in the home. In one study, one-quarter of patients who enrolled with outpatient hospice service were later admitted to the hospital and died in the acute care setting (Thienprayoon, Lee, Leonard, et al., 2015). Reasons for final admission to a hospital vary but may be related to the parents' or siblings' wish to have the child die outside the home; exhaustion on the part of the caregivers; and physical problems such as sudden acute pain or respiratory distress (Knapp, Shenkman, Marcu, et al., 2009).

*National Hospice and Palliative Care Organization, 1731 King St., Suite 100, Alexandria, VA 22314; 703-837-1500; fax: 703-837-1233; http://www.nhpco.org; Children's Hospice International, 500 Montgomery Street, Suite 400, Alexandria, VA 22314; 703-684-0330, 800-2-4-CHILD; http://www.chionline.org.

Location of and Participation in the Child's Care

The location of the child's terminal care and death and the participation of parents in their child's terminal care influence parental bereavement. Parents whose child died in the home rather than the hospital setting and who participated in caring for their child have consistently reported better bereavement outcomes (e.g., adaptive coping; family cohesion; less anxiety, stress, and depression) than parents whose children died in the hospital setting and/or who were not actively involved in their child's care (Goodenough, Drew, Higgins, et al., 2004). The grief work of fathers in particular seems to be facilitated when their children die in the home setting. This finding may be related to the greater opportunity for working fathers to provide care to and spend time with their children at home than in the hospital setting. A recent study suggests that parental opportunity to plan the location of their child's death, whether death occurred in the home or in the hospital, may be a more relevant outcome variable than the child's actual location of death (Dussell, Kreicbergs, Hilden, et al., 2008).

NURSING CARE OF THE CHILD AND FAMILY AT THE END OF LIFE

MANAGEMENT OF PAIN AND SUFFERING

Unfortunately, terminally ill children commonly report the presence of unrelieved pain and other distressing symptoms (Hendricks-Ferguson, 2008; Pritchard, Burghen, Srivastava, et al., 2008). Distressing symptoms can have detrimental effects on the child's quality of life and long-lasting negative effects on the family after the child's death. Parents report that having their child in pain was unendurable and resulted in feelings of helplessness and a sense that they must be present and vigilant to get the necessary pain medications. Persistent pain also has an impact on the family as a whole. Nurses can alleviate the fear of pain and suffering by providing interventions aimed at treating the pain and symptoms associated with the terminal process in children.

Pain and Symptom Management

When the pain and symptoms experienced by dying children are being managed, it is important to clearly communicate the intent of any interventions proposed. For example, many children with progressive cancer may be given "palliative chemotherapy" or "palliative radiotherapy." The health care team and family must understand that the goal of these treatments is either to increase comfort by slowing the progression of an incurable tumor (palliative chemotherapy) or to reduce swelling or pressure from a tumor that is causing pain (palliative radiation). The family should understand that these treatments will not ultimately change the outcome of death for the child. This understanding reduces the chance of confusion among family members and health care providers regarding the focus of care and its aim toward palliation. In addition, providers consider the benefit versus risk of any suggested interventions in relation to the child's current quality of life.

The child's and family's views of quality of life, religious and cultural values, and level of acceptance of the terminal prognosis will shape the types of interventions considered as symptoms occur. One family may choose to continue blood product support if the child is otherwise comfortable and active but has fatigue and shortness of breath related to anemia. Another child and family may forgo transfusions to avoid having to return to the hospital or clinic. The child and family should be aware of potential side effects of any proposed treatments and consequences of choosing not to intervene and are provided with options that are consistent with their values and goals for the child's comfort. Health care practitioners must respect each individual family's choice regarding their child's care.

Nurses should use a holistic approach to symptom management that includes pharmacologic and nonpharmacologic interventions when possible to optimize treatment. For instance, in addition to giving lorazepam for anxiety, instruct the child and family in nonpharmacologic techniques such as distraction or relaxation breathing, and encourage them to explore and communicate fears to further alleviate feelings of anxiety.

Carefully consider the route of medication administration used for pain and symptom management. Generally the nurse should use the least traumatic method of administration. Children may present a special challenge for administration of medication, depending on their age, level of cooperation, and temperament. If taking medicine becomes a struggle, children and parents may underreport the severity of pain and symptoms to avoid the trauma of administering the medication. Most medications can be administered orally, sublingually, intranasally, transdermally, or by intravenous or subcutaneous infusion. Compounding pharmacists can be helpful in making medications in a form that is palatable or can be delivered with less distress.

Give pain control for children in the terminal stages of illness or injury the highest priority. Despite ongoing efforts to educate physicians and nurses on pain management strategies in children, studies have reported that children continue to be undermedicated for their pain (Wolfe, Hammel, Edwards, et al., 2008). Nearly all children experience some amount of pain in the terminal phase of their illness. The current standard for treating children's pain is according to the World Health Organization's analgesic and side-effect stepladder that takes into account the intolerable side effects of opioids (Riley, Ross, Gretton, et al., 2007) (Fig. 19.6). This approach promotes individualizing the pain interventions to children's level of reported pain. Children's pain is assessed frequently, and medications are adjusted as necessary. Pain medications are given on a regular schedule, and extra doses for breakthrough pain are available to maintain comfort. Opioid drugs such as morphine are given for severe pain, and the dosage is increased as necessary to maintain optimum pain relief. Techniques such as distraction, relaxation techniques, and guided imagery are combined with drug therapy to provide the child and family with strategies to control pain (Russell & Smart, 2007). (See Chapter 5 for further discussion of pain assessment and management strategies.)

Occasionally children require very high doses of opioids to control pain. This may occur for several reasons. The child on long-term opioid pain management can become tolerant of the drug, so more drug must be given to maintain the same level of pain relief. This is not to be confused with addiction, which is a psychologic dependence on the side effects of opioids. Addiction is not a factor in managing terminal pain in a child, and the nurse plays an important role in educating parents that their child will not become addicted. Other reasons for increasing dosages of opioids include progression of disease and other physiologic causes of pain. It is important to understand that there is no maximum dosage that can be given to control pain. However, nurses often express concern that administering dosages of opioids that exceed those with which they are familiar will hasten the child's death. The **principle of double effect** addresses such concerns (Box 19.12). It provides an ethical standard that supports the use of interventions that have the intention of relieving pain and suffering even though there is a foreseeable possibility that death may be hastened. In cases in which the child is terminally ill and in severe pain, using large doses of opioids and sedatives to manage pain is justified when no other treatment options are available that would relieve the pain but make the possibility of death less likely. (See Chapter 5 for an extensive discussion of pain assessment and management.)

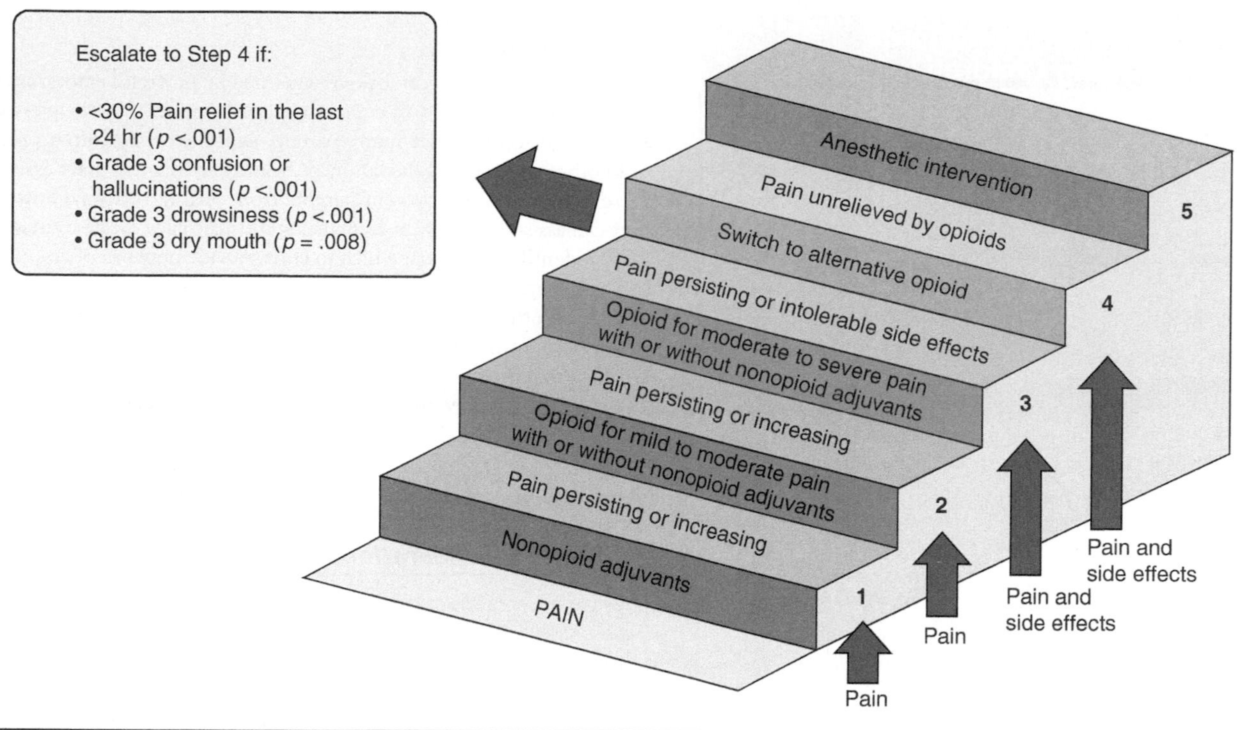

FIG. 19.6 Overview of proposed five-step World Health Organization analgesic and side effect ladder. (From Riley, J., Ross, J. R., Gretton, S. K., et al. [2007]. Proposed five-step World Health Organization analgesic and side effect ladder. *European Journal of Pain* [Suppl S], 23-30.)

BOX 19.12 Ethical Principle of Double Effect

An action that has one good (intended) and one bad (unintended but foreseeable) effect is permissible if the following conditions are met:

- The action itself must be good or indifferent. Only the good consequences of the action must be sincerely intended.
- The good effect must not be produced by the bad effect.
- There must be a compelling or proportionate reason for permitting the foreseeable bad effect to occur.

In addition to medications, nonpharmacologic interventions may also reduce the perception of pain and can sometimes decrease the amount of pain medication that is needed, thereby reducing unwanted side effects. These interventions include providing soothing surroundings, avoiding excessive lighting, ensuring a pleasant room temperature, and having pleasant smells in the room. Other techniques such as music therapy, distraction, and guided imagery should be combined with medications to provide the child and family strategies to control pain. Often families will have insight into the things that comfort their child, and this input should be encouraged because it not only helps the child but may also provide the family comfort (Anderson & Davis, 2011). Better bereavement outcomes (including enhanced family cohesiveness as well as decreased anxiety, stress, and depression) have been reported by parents who were actively involved in the care of their child. Even simple interventions such as placing all commodities within easy reach for the child can contribute to a child's sense of comfort; attentiveness to these details can add much to the quality of nursing care at the end of life. Other simple measures that the bedside nurse may employ to minimize suffering for children with cancer include the use of gentle touch and avoiding pressure on painful areas when required to perform physical procedures. Routine nursing care at the end of life can and should be limited to essential needs. This latter point is easily overlooked in the hospital setting, where, for example, measuring vital signs frequently is a matter of routine and policy.

Children may experience a variety of symptoms besides pain during their terminal course, either as a result of their disease process or as a side effect of medicines used to maintain their comfort (Box 19.13). The underlying disease and previous treatment history will contribute to the types and severity of symptoms the individual child experiences during the dying process. Nurses caring for children who are receiving palliative care for a terminal condition or illness assess frequently for any symptoms that are causing the child physical distress. Assessment includes information regarding the symptom's onset, severity, duration, and effect on the child's quality of life.

These symptoms are consistently managed with appropriate medications or treatments and interventions such as repositioning, relaxation, massage, and other measures to maintain the child's comfort and quality of life. (For further information on pain and symptom management for children, see the Cancer Pain Management in Children [http://www.childcancerpain.org] and End-of-Life Care for Children [http://www.childendoflifecare.org] websites.)

PARENTS' AND SIBLINGS' NEED FOR EDUCATION AND SUPPORT THROUGH THE CAREGIVING PROCESS

Often, as the child's illness worsens, parents and other family members are the primary caregivers while the child is at home. This role can

BOX 19.13 Common Symptoms Experienced by Dying Children

Pain
- Visceral pain
- Bone pain
- Neuropathic pain

Gastrointestinal
- Anorexia
- Nausea and vomiting
- Constipation
- Diarrhea

Genitourinary
- Urinary tract infections
- Urinary retention

Hematologic
- Anemia
- Bleeding

Respiratory
- Cough
- Congestion
- Secretions
- Shortness of breath
- Wheezing

Central Nervous System
- Fatigue
- Fevers, chills
- Sleep disturbance
- Restlessness, agitation
- Seizures

Integumentary
- Dry skin
- Rash, itching
- Pressure sores
- Edema

Emotional
- Fear
- Anxiety
- Depression

create physical, emotional, and financial strain on the larger family system. Therefore parents and other family members caring for dying children have a number of educational and support needs.

Educational Needs

Family caregivers need comprehensive education about various aspects of the care that they are providing to their child. This preparation can ease feelings of helplessness and anxiety and provide a sense of competence as they move from caring for an ill child to caring for a dying child. This education begins early in the transition from curative to palliative care. Table 19.7 provides some common areas of educational needs of family caregivers and suggestions on how nurses can assist families in meeting these needs. Education about physical care is best provided as the need arises. Instructing parents too early in the signs and symptoms of respiratory distress or the method of stopping a nosebleed can increase the parents' anxiety.

Emotional Support

Members of the family can be overwhelmed by powerful emotions that can threaten their ability to cope. Anger, guilt, anxiety, and helplessness are normal feelings that many parents experience and often project onto other members of the family or health care team. Nurses assisting these families cannot prevent parents from feeling this way; however, they can assist the family in recognizing the normalcy of these emotions and in identifying ways in which to cope. A wide network of emotional support is important to parents, such as family members, nurses, physicians, and other health care providers, but parents also find comfort in support from nonfamiliar individuals through social media (Tan, Docherty, Barfield, et al., 2012). Encourage families to seek assistance outside of the family circle and to arrange for periods of respite care when available (see Cultural Considerations box).

CULTURAL CONSIDERATIONS

Cultural Considerations in Dying and Death

Culture influences perceptions, coping styles, and family dynamics in every arena of life. A death in the family is no exception. Language and cultural barriers may impede families from seeking support during the process of dying, death, and bereavement. This can result in unfortunate outcomes, including failure to honor the family's wishes or beliefs regarding end-of-life rituals. To provide optimal support to families, health care providers must have some understanding of cultural influences on family dynamics and the family's perception of an illness, death, and grief, and be willing to invite families to share their wishes and concerns. Serious consideration of language differences and cultural influences is integral to comprehensive care.

Spiritual and Religious Support

Meeting the spiritual or religious needs of the child and family is as important as teaching caregiving techniques. Because many families rely on religion or spirituality for emotional support, the degree to which these needs are met successfully may determine how well the child and family cope with the dying process (Hexem, Mollen, Carroll, et al., 2011). Parents say religion and spirituality both sustain hope for a positive outcome and provide a way to cope with less desirable circumstances and outcomes. Additionally, many families use religion and spirituality as a source of guidance during complex medical decision making. Alongside chaplains, social workers, and community clergy, nurses working with dying children play a key role in addressing spiritual and religious needs. A nurse can participate by assessing the family's spiritual or religious needs, modeling comfort when discussing spiritual matters with the family, facilitating the family's spiritual or religious rituals (e.g., prayer), and informing family members of the hospital's spiritual support resources (e.g. an interfaith chapel, quiet area, or chaplain service). Assessing a family's religious and spiritual needs is complex. Even children and families who do not identify with a particular religion may possess spiritual beliefs and values or experience spiritual distress, especially during times of tribulation. It is therefore reasonable to consider the spiritual needs of all families, regardless of their outward religiosity. Parents' spiritual needs may relate to anger toward God, blame and regret, forgiveness, and needs related to specific ritual or cultural traditions (Ferrell, Wittenberg, Battista, et al., 2016b). Signs of spiritual distress include expressions of doubt, questioning, guilt, and anger (e.g. "Why my child?"; "Why aren't my prayers being answered?"), as well as sudden dramatic increases or decreases in religious practice. Referral to a hospital chaplain is strongly indicated when a family member requests prayers, sacraments, rituals, devotional materials, or a faith

TABLE 19.7 Preparation and Education of Family Caregivers

Needs of Family Caregivers	Professional Interventions
Practical Needs	
Is home care, hospice care, or care in the hospital appropriate for my child?	Explore the family's preferences for home care or hospice as appropriate.
How will we pay for end-of-life care at home, in the hospital, or in hospice?	Evaluate the family's funding source and provide resources and assistance as necessary.
Where do I get equipment and supplies?	Provide the family with appropriate telephone numbers and contact people for questions about equipment and medical care.
How does the equipment work?	
Whom do I call if equipment malfunctions?	
How should we arrange our house to best meet the needs of our child?	Plan for availability of caregivers (i.e., parents, family, friends, professionals) and help coordinate a schedule for provision of care.
Will there be help available to us at home?	
Whom do I call for medical questions?	Provide a contact person for the family to call with concerns or questions.
Personal Care	
How do I give my child a bed bath?	Instruct all caregivers about providing daily care to the child.
How do I wash my child's hair in bed?	Provide written instruction and reference material for caregivers to review.
How do I change linen with my child in bed?	
How do I perform skin care?	
How do I perform mouth care?	
How do I administer medications?	
What do I do if my child does not want to eat?	Assess the child's nutritional status and parents' view on supplemental nutrition.
Is there something I can do to get my child to eat?	Educate the family on decreased nutritional needs and potential complications from overfeeding or overhydration.
Does my child need supplements or a special diet?	
Physical Care	
How do I assess my child's pain?	Assess the child's current comfort status and educate the family on current interventions.
When should I give pain medications?	
What do I do when pain management is ineffective?	Educate the family about assessing the child's comfort level.
	Instruct the family that the child may be uncomfortable for a variety of reasons (e.g., constipation, anxiety, fever, headache, muscle cramp, disease) and educate the family about the appropriate interventions for particular circumstances.
What should I do when our child is constipated or has diarrhea?	Provide an accessible supply of medications that can help alleviate discomfort (i.e., laxatives, sedatives, antipyretics).
How do I control nausea and vomiting?	
What do I do if my child has a fever?	Encourage the caregiver to telephone a contact person about questions or ineffective interventions.
What do I do if my child has seizures?	
What do I do if my child has trouble breathing?	
Activity and Social Interactions	
Can we safely travel and enjoy family gatherings with our child?	Encourage the family to engage in fun and memorable activities with the child.
In which activities can we engage our child?	
Should friends and family be encouraged to visit?	Encourage visitors when appropriate.
What interventions can I do to help my child relax and rest comfortably?	Encourage the family to use relaxation techniques that have previously been beneficial to the child.

perspective about medical decision making, when a family member expresses spiritual or religious objections to a child's treatment, and when a provider notes signs of spiritual distress (by the child or a family member). Religious and spiritual beliefs can be especially relevant to parents' decisions about withholding or withdrawal of life-sustaining therapy (Madrigal, Carroll, Faerber, et al., 2016). In this time, prayer, hope, beliefs about miraculous healing, beliefs about suffering, and specific religious doctrine or tradition may be integral components of parents' decision-making process, and may sometimes directly influence the choices they make.

Sibling Support

It is important to consider the needs of siblings experiencing the death of a brother or sister (Fig. 19.7). As mentioned earlier, the developmental stage and level of maturity of the siblings will have a strong influence on the feelings and behaviors exhibited as their brother's or sister's illness progresses and their care intensifies. Siblings may feel isolated and displaced during the time that a brother or sister is dying. Parents devote the majority of their time to the care and comfort of the dying child, which causes siblings to feel left out. Siblings may become resentful of their sick brother or sister and begin to feel guilty or ashamed about such feelings. Simultaneously, siblings may appreciate having responsibilities in the care of their brother or sister and desire to be included to a greater degree (Russell, Widger, Beaune, et al., 2017). Nurses can assist the family by helping the parents identify ways to involve the siblings in the caring process and provide honest, developmentally appropriate information to siblings (Giovanola, 2005). Encourage parents to spend time with the other children during which the focus is on them. Nurses can assist the parents by helping them identify a trusted friend or family member who can sit with the ill child for a short time. Siblings need

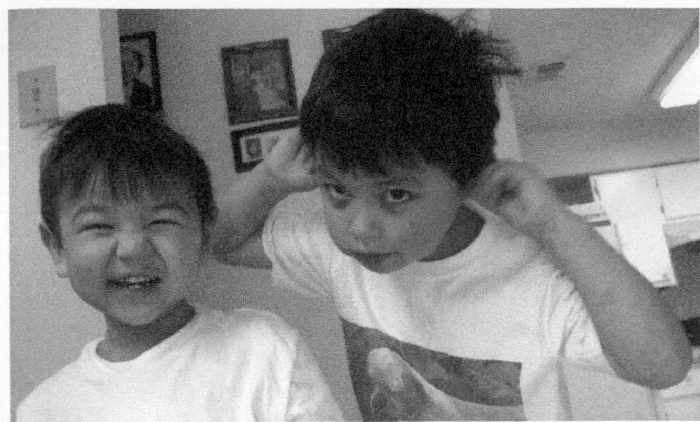

FIG. 19.7 It is important to consider the needs of siblings experiencing the death of a brother or sister.

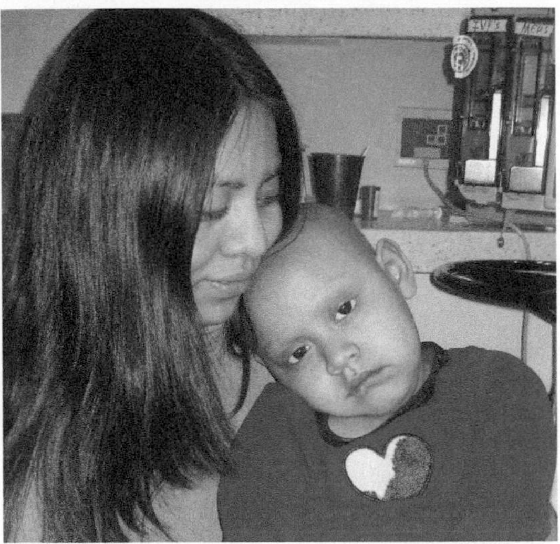

FIG. 19.8 For the dying child there is no greater comfort than the security and closeness of a parent.

for their experiences to be validated and normalized and may sometimes benefit from counseling or support groups, and nurses can help connect parents with these resources (Russell, Widger, Beaune, et al., 2017).

Caregiver Support

As the care of the dying child becomes the primary focus of the parent, personal and household needs often take on secondary significance. These tasks, however, can become burdensome and increase the family's stress if not attended to. Nurses can help the family identify ways for friends, community service organizations, and extended family members to assist with tasks such as household chores, shopping, meal preparation, and laundry.

CARE AT THE TIME OF DEATH

Few parents have cared for a dying child, and thus parents are not prepared to lead their child through the dying process (Fig. 19.8). Awareness that the child's death is near allows the parents and family to determine the location and circumstance of the child's death. This allows the family to create a meaningful death for their child, which improves their ability to cope in the difficult days, weeks, and years after the child has died. Nurses have an important role in helping parents recognize the changes in their child that signal that death may be near (see Applying Evidence to Practice box).

APPLYING EVIDENCE TO PRACTICE

Supporting Grieving Families*

General

Stay with the family; sit quietly if they prefer not to talk; cry with them if desired.

Accept the family's grief reactions; avoid judgmental statements (e.g., "You should be feeling better by now").

Avoid offering rationalizations for the child's death (e.g., "You should be glad your child isn't suffering anymore").

Avoid artificial consolation (e.g., "I know how you feel" or "You are still young enough to have another baby").

Deal openly with feelings such as guilt, anger, and loss of self-esteem.

Focus on feelings by using a feeling word in the statement (e.g., "You're still feeling all the pain of losing a child").

Refer the family to an appropriate self-help group or to professional help if needed.

At the Time of Death

Reassure the family that everything possible is being done for the child, if they wish lifesaving interventions.

Do everything possible to ensure the child's comfort, especially relief of pain.

Provide the child and family the opportunity to review special experiences or memories in their lives.

Express personal feelings of loss or frustration (e.g., "We will miss him so much" or "We tried everything; we feel so sorry that we couldn't save him").

Provide information that the family requests and be honest.

Respect the emotional needs of family members such as siblings, who may need brief respites from being with the dying child.

Make every effort to arrange for family members, especially parents, to be with the child at the moment of death, if they wish to be present.

Allow the family to stay with the dead child for as long as they wish and to rock, hold, or bathe the child.

Provide practical help when possible, such as collecting the child's belongings.

Arrange for spiritual support, such as clergy; pray with the family if they wish it and if no one else can stay with them.

After the Death

Attend the funeral or visitation if there was a special closeness with the family.

Initiate and maintain contact (e.g., send cards, telephone, invite the family back to the unit, or make a home visit).

Refer to the dead child by name; discuss shared memories with the family.

Discourage the use of drugs or alcohol as a method of escaping grief.

Encourage all family members to communicate their feelings rather than remaining silent to avoid upsetting another member.

Emphasize that grieving is a painful process that often takes years to resolve.

*"Family" refers to all significant persons involved in the child's life, such as parents, siblings, grandparents, or other close relatives or friends.

Physical Changes

Physical changes can vary widely among children and are often more pronounced in children dying of prolonged illness or disability. Generally, as the child progresses through the dying process, there is an overall decline in the child's physical condition. This decline may be interspersed with brief spurts of energy or periods of alertness and can cause parents to become exhausted and overwhelmed in "waiting for the inevitable." Often parents ask "how long" their child has to live. Initially this question may represent the parents' attempt to determine what special activities or events the family should try to accomplish. As the dying process progresses, this question may reveal a wish to know how long they and their child will have to endure the dying process.

BOX 19.14 Physical Signs of Approaching Death

Increased sleeping
Loss of sensation and movement in the lower extremities, progressing toward the upper body
Sensation of heat, although body feels cool
Mottling of skin
Loss of senses:
- Tactile sensation decreases
- Sensitivity to light develops
- Hearing is last sense to fail

Confusion, loss of consciousness, slurred speech
Muscle weakness
Decreased urination, more concentrated urine
Loss of bowel and bladder control
Decreased appetite and thirst
Difficulty swallowing
Change in respiratory pattern:
- Cheyne-Stokes respirations (waxing and waning of depth of breathing with regular periods of apnea)
- "Death rattle" (noisy chest sounds from accumulation of pulmonary and pharyngeal secretions)

BOX 19.15 Care During the Terminal Phase

Physical Support

Provide frequent mouth care to prevent drying, cracking, and bleeding of lips and mucous membranes.
Maintain good hygiene by giving bed baths and using skin lotion as tolerated.
Continue necessary medications to manage symptoms and maintain comfort using intravenous infusion (if access is easily established) or subcutaneous infusion.
Discontinue unnecessary medications and procedures (e.g., measuring vital signs).

Emotional Support

Encourage the family to discuss the impending death openly with the child and other family members.
Encourage the family to continue to speak to the child in a calm, reassuring voice.
Provide familiar surroundings or objects.
Encourage caregivers to provide each other with periods of respite.
Allow the performance of spiritual and cultural rituals as desired.
Allow the family time with the child after the death and participation in the preparation of the body if they choose.

As the child moves closer to his or her actual death, some general physical changes are common (Box 19.14). Initially the child may begin to sleep more. Appetite decreases, and the child begins to take only small bites of favorite foods or sips of fluids. As the child begins to eat and drink less, urinary frequency declines and the urine becomes more concentrated. In the final few days before death, the child most likely becomes less responsive. Breathing may become slow and shallow, with periodic deep sighs. Urinary output may decrease or stop. As the child nears the final hours before death, breathing becomes more irregular, deep, and gasping, with long periods of apnea *(Cheyne-Stokes respirations)*, and may be very noisy ("death rattle"), especially if the child is overhydrated. This respiratory pattern can be upsetting for parents to observe, but it is not distressing to the child. The skin may have a pale, grayish-blue color and may be cool to the touch. The child's eyes may be slightly open, with a fixed gaze. It is important to prepare the family for these changes and to provide them with caregiving activities that promote a loving presence in the child's care (Box 19.15). Reassure parents that this is a normal process and that the child is not suffering.

Emotional Changes

As children approach death, they may begin to recall events that were important with their families. They may want to draw pictures or leave messages for important friends and family. Often children begin to reassure their parents and other significant people that they are not afraid and are ready to die.

During the final few days to hours of death, children may experience visions of "angels" or people and talk with them (Ethier, 2005). They may mention that they are not afraid and that someone is waiting for them. Often these visions are of family members or friends who have preceded them in death. In most instances these visions provide a comforting presence and reassurance for the child and family. Not all children will express these types of experiences.

As the child's death approaches, the family may begin the "death vigil," which is a natural phenomenon in which family and friends gather at the bedside. Rarely is the child left alone for any length of time. During this time families may read favorite books, recite prayers, light candles, or play music that is special to the child. Legacy building activities such as hand molds and footprints for infants can also bring special moments of peace for the family. Spiritual, religious, or family rituals surrounding the time of death are important, and nurses involved in the care of the family at this time are sensitive to such needs (Tan, Docherty, Barfield, et al., 2012).

POSTMORTEM CARE

The final moments of a child's life are often extremely stressful as the family waits for the child to die. Families often depend on trusted health care professionals, particularly nurses, to help them recognize the exact moment of the child's death. Once the nurse has observed that the child is no longer showing signs of life, the child is pronounced dead (registered nurse pronouncement is allowed by the State Practice Act). Initially the family may show joy and relief that the child is no longer struggling. They may have many varied emotions in the immediate moments after the child's death, and the nurse must be prepared for a range of reactions. Generally all that is necessary is a supportive presence at this time. In rare instances, particularly in more conflicted families, there may be strong outbursts of anger. It is important for the nurse to be aware of families in which this situation may occur and respond by assuring them that appropriate resources (e.g., social worker, chaplain, security personnel) are readily available to ensure that the situation does not escalate.

Once the initial reaction to the moment of death has occurred, the family may move away from the bedside and enter a phase of relaxation. One or both of the parents may stay with the child, while others in attendance make brief visits to view the child. Nursing care at this time is to facilitate the parents' ability to spend time with their child as they wish. Allow the family the time needed to say good-bye.

When the parents are ready, the nurse offers to bathe and dress the body for removal from the home or hospital room. The parents may wish to undertake this task, may participate with the nurse, or may ask the nurse to do the bathing for them. If the death was at home and the body is prepared for removal and the parents are ready, contact the funeral home. Often hospice organizations have arrangements with the medical examiners in their area that allow the body to be directly removed by a funeral director. In some instances it may be necessary for the police to make a report before the release of the child's body. It is important for the nurse to explain to the parents the requirements of their local area for removal of a body. This allows the parents to be prepared for questions or information that may be required. Hospital deaths require the parents to leave the child, and the body is taken to the morgue. Some parents may ask to go with the body to the morgue, and nurses work within their institutions' regulations to try to honor such requests if possible.

The final separation of the child's body from the parents and family is often the most emotional and traumatic time. The nurse should offer support to the parents and ensure that other family members or friends are available in the coming hours to continue to provide support and assistance to the parents and siblings.

CARE OF THE FAMILY EXPERIENCING UNEXPECTED CHILDHOOD DEATH

In cases of long-term, potentially fatal illnesses, families may experience anticipatory grief. Parents mourn the loss of their child long before the death. They are reminded of their child's uncertain future each time they see the pain the child must endure or experience the sudden loss of hope during a relapse. This prolonged period of anticipatory grief provides families with the opportunity to complete "unfinished business," such as helping the child and siblings understand and cope with a fatal prognosis. Many families reflect on their changed perspective of time after learning of the diagnosis, particularly their heightened awareness of the value of each day.

In contrast, after sudden, unexpected death, the family is deprived of any of the advantages of anticipatory grief. They have no opportunity to prepare themselves or others for the death, and the initial denial may be very strong. Many families feel great guilt and remorse for not having done something additional or different with the child. For example, they may berate themselves for depriving the child of some desired material object or privilege, or, more painfully, for not having prevented the sudden death in some way. "If only I'd been a better parent" is a common feeling at this time. Without proper support, the risk of complicated grief responses may be high. Mothers experiencing the sudden, unexpected death of their child have reported a more prolonged grief response compared with mothers who anticipated their child's death (Meert, Shear, Newth, et al., 2011; Seecharan, Andresen, Norris, et al., 2004).

Death resulting from accident or trauma, or from acute illness in settings such as the emergency department or intensive care unit, often requires the active withdrawal of some form of life-supporting intervention, such as a ventilator or bypass machine. These situations frequently raise difficult ethical issues, and parents are often less prepared for the actual moment of death (Box 19.16). Nurses can assist parents by providing detailed information about what will happen as supportive equipment is withdrawn, ensuring that appropriate pain medications are administered to prevent pain during the dying process, and allowing the parents time to be with and speak to their child before the start of the withdrawal. It is important that the nurse attempt to control the environment around the family at this time. This can be accomplished by providing privacy, playing music that is meaningful to the family, softening lights, monitoring noises, and arranging for any spiritual, religious, or cultural rituals that the family may want performed. After the child's death, allow the family to remain with the body and hold or rock the child if they desire. Once the nurse has removed all tubes and equipment from the body, give parents the option of assisting with the preparation of the body, such as bathing and dressing.

BOX 19.16 Strategies for Intervention With Survivors After Sudden Childhood Death

Arrival of the Family

Meet the family immediately and escort to a private area.

A health care worker with bereavement training should remain with the family.

Provide information about the extent of illness or injury and treatment efforts.

If the health care worker must leave the family or if the family requests privacy, return in 15 minutes so the family does not feel forgotten.

Provide tissues, telephone, coffee, and a Bible.

Pronouncement of Death

When available, the family's own physician should inform them of the child's death.

Alternatively, the physician or nurse should introduce himself or herself and establish calm, reassuring eye contact with the parents.

Honest, clear communication that avoids misinterpretation is essential.

Nonverbal communication such as hugging, touching, or remaining with the family in silence may be most empathetic.

Acknowledge the family's guilt, attempt to alleviate it, and deal openly and nonjudgmentally with anger.

Provide information, answer questions, and offer reassurance that everything possible was done for the child.

Viewing of the Body

Offer the parents the opportunity to see the body; repeat the offer later if they decline.

Before viewing, inform the parents of bodily changes they should expect (tubes, injuries, cold skin).

A single staff member should accompany the family but remain inconspicuous.

Offer the opportunity to hold the child.

Allow the family as much time as they need.

Offer parents the opportunity for siblings to view the body.

Formal Concluding Process

Discuss and answer questions concerning autopsy and funeral arrangements; obtain signatures on the body release and autopsy forms.

Provide anticipatory guidance regarding symptoms of grief response and their normalcy.

Provide written materials about grief symptoms.

Escort the family to the exit or to their car if necessary.

Provide a follow-up phone call in 24 to 48 hours to answer questions and provide support.

Provide referral for community health nursing visit.

Provide referrals to local support and resource groups (e.g., bereavement groups, bereavement counselors, sudden infant death syndrome groups, Parents of Murdered Children, Mothers Against Drunk Driving).

Community-Based Follow-Up

A community health or visiting nurse referral may be helpful after a sudden, unexpected pediatric death. Some families have reported that this was a missing piece in their care. During home visits the nurse can answer the families' questions, provide information about the grief process, assess and support coping mechanisms, and give appropriate referrals to support groups (Box 19.17).

Families who experience a child's sudden death may have recurrent memories of both the child and the death experience and may long grieve over missed opportunities. Support and resource groups that may be useful to families include the First Candle (previously SIDS

BOX 19.17 Aspects of Home Health Nursing Visits for Sudden Infant Death Syndrome

- Express condolences.
- Involve as many family members as possible in the visit.
- Clarify any misconceptions about the circumstances of death.
- Provide and interpret information about sudden infant death syndrome (SIDS).
- Provide information about the grief process.
- Offer suggestions on future coping: holidays, birthdays, anniversaries.
- Evaluate and support coping strategies.
- Assist the family in identifying their support network.
- Reinforce parental ability to care for the other children.
- Offer information about children's grief process.
- Provide information on siblings, risk factors, and monitoring.
- Obtain signatures, if necessary, for autopsy consent form.
- Provide referrals, as desired by family, to crisis intervention, SIDS organizations, and mental health resources.

Alliance),* American SIDS Institute, † Mothers Against Drunk Driving, ‡ and National Organization of Parents of Murdered Children, Inc. §

SPECIAL DECISIONS AT THE TIME OF DYING AND DEATH

People are often unprepared to cope with the numerous decisions that must be made when a loved one is dying or dies. When the death is expected, there is the opportunity to make plans in advance, such as where the child should spend the last days or what types of funeral arrangements are desired. When death is unexpected, the shock is sufficient to render the survivors incapable of making even simple decisions. Those in attendance at the death and those caring for the dying child can be instrumental in initiating decisions that may facilitate the grief process. The following is a brief review of selected instances in which nurses can guide parents in making decisions related to the expected or unexpected death.

RIGHT TO DIE AND DO-NOT-ATTEMPT-RESUSCITATION ORDERS

One of the benefits of hospice has been the recognition of patients' right to die as they wish, with emphasis on the quality of life. Unfortunately, this is not always the focus of care, especially in the traditional hospital setting. Many families are not given the option of terminating treatment when cure is unlikely, and staff may be reluctant to raise the question of "no code" or do-not-attempt-resuscitation (DNAR) orders (i.e., withholding cardiopulmonary resuscitation in response to cardiac arrest).

Guidelines have been established for discontinuing mechanical ventilation and life-support measures for infants whose parents and providers consider care futile (De Lisle-Porter & Podruchny, 2009). Such plans must carefully encompass preplanning, educational, discharge, and postextubation procedures and the needs of the family and health care staff and unit. If parents choose DNAR, they must be aware of exactly what will and will not be done for the child and be assured that this does not mean "no care." For example, the family may wish that oxygen be given to the child for difficult breathing but does not want active resuscitation. Once a decision is made, it must be communicated to all members of the health care team, and a written medical order for the use or withholding of lifesaving measures must be included. An order to "slow" or "delay" code is not legal. Because the child's condition or the family's wishes may change, review DNAR orders regularly. Respect orders even if it is difficult to follow them at the moment of death (Sullivan, Monagle, & Gillam, 2014).

VIEWING OF THE BODY

Although most institutions recognize the need for parents to hold and spend time with the dead child, a dilemma may arise when the body is mutilated. Although the memory of the child's disfigurement can be extremely upsetting and can generate concern regarding how much the child suffered, not seeing the body can leave the parents with imagined ideas of how their child looked. This can be worse than the reality, and it can delay the acceptance of the death. When family members choose to view the body, they need preparation for this upsetting experience. The nurse should inform them about what to expect and why certain parts of the body are covered or bandaged. It is desirable to place the body in a private room, without medical apparatus, and make it as presentable as the situation allows. Some people appreciate the presence of a nurse in the room with them, whereas others desire privacy. Regardless of how badly the body is harmed, parents may want to hold the child. Offer and respect such options. Give family members as much time as they need to say good-bye. For many people, viewing the body is a sign of closure—an opportunity to finish their good-byes and leave the hospital.

ORGAN OR TISSUE DONATION AND AUTOPSY

Many states have legislated a mandatory request for organ or tissue donation when a child dies. For some families this may be a meaningful act—one that benefits another human being despite the loss of their child. Unfortunately, initiating a discussion about tissue donation is often stressful for staff, and there may be confusion regarding whose responsibility this is. In centers in which transplants are performed, a full-time transplant coordinator is usually available to inform the family about organ donation and to take care of details. If such services are not available, the staff determines which members should discuss this topic with the family. Ideally the role is taken by the person who knows the family best, knows when the death is expected, or has the opportunity to spend time with the family when the death is unexpected. Often nurses are in an optimal position to suggest tissue donation after consultation with the attending physician. When possible, the topic is raised before death occurs. Make the request in a private and quiet area of the hospital. Be simple and direct, with questions such as "Are you a donor family?" or "Have you ever considered organ donation?"

Written consent from the family is required before donation can proceed. When requests for organ donation are made, health care practitioners must address common misunderstandings families have about brain death and organ donation (Workman, Myrick, Meyers, et al., 2013). Training of health care professionals regarding sensitive approaches to request organ donation has been shown to increase families' willingness to consent to organ donation (Workman, Myrick, Meyers, et al., 2013). Discussion of the option to donate organs is always separate from communication of impending or actual death.

*49 Locust Avenue, Suite 104, New Canaan, CT 06840; 203-966-1300; http://www.firstcandle.org.

†528 Raven Way, Naples, FL 24110; 239-431-5425; fax: 239-431-5536; http://www.sids.org

‡511 E. John Carpenter Freeway, Suite 700, Irving, TX 75062; 877-ASK-MADD (275-6233); http://www.madd.org.

§635 West 7th Street, Suite 104, Cincinnati, OH 45203; 513-721-5683, 888-818-POMC; fax: 513-345-4489; http://www.pomc.com.

Nurses need to be aware of common questions about organ donation so they can help families make an informed decision. Healthy children who die unexpectedly are excellent candidates for organ donation. Children who have cancer, chronic disease, or infection or who have suffered prolonged cardiac arrest may not be suitable candidates, although this is individually determined. The nurse inquires whether organ donation was discussed with the child or whether the child ever expressed such a wish. Any tissue or combination of tissues and organs can be donated (e.g., skin, corneas, bone, kidney, heart, liver, pancreas). Their removal does not mutilate or desecrate the body, or cause any suffering. The family may have an open casket, and there is no delay in the funeral. There is no cost to the donor family, but organ donation does not eliminate funeral or cremation responsibilities. Most religions permit organ donation as long as the recipient benefits from the transplant, although Orthodox Judaism forbids it.

In cases of unexplained death, violent death, or suspected suicide, autopsy is required by law. In other instances, it may be optional, and the nurse should inform parents of this choice. Explain the procedure, as well as forms that require signing. Inform the family that the child can be in an open casket after an autopsy.

RESEARCH FOCUS

Children's Involvement in the Death Process

Unfortunately, little research has focused on the difference in adjustment between children who do and who do not attend postdeath services. However, one landmark study provided substantial evidence of the benefits of involving children in the experience of their dying sibling. Lauer, Mulhern, Bohne, and colleagues (1985) compared children's perceptions of their sibling's death at home versus death in the hospital. The home care group (ages 5 to 23 years) reported that they were prepared for the impending death, received consistent information and support from their parents, were involved in most activities, found the funeral experience comforting, and viewed their own involvement as the most important aspect of the experience. The non–home care group (ages 2 to 26 years) had opposite perceptions. Another landmark study found that greater participation in the child's care and death, including funeral attendance, was associated with higher self-esteem in the siblings (Michael & Lansdown, 1986). Among adolescents, Kuntz (1991) found that seeing a parent who had died and being involved with the rituals surrounding the death promoted adaptive grieving. Thus it appears that children benefit from increased involvement with the death, rather than isolation and "protection."

SIBLINGS' ATTENDANCE AT FUNERAL SERVICES

One of the most frequent concerns of parents is whether young or school-age children should attend funeral or burial services (see Research Focus box). Sharing moments of deep significance with parents helps children understand the experience and deal with their own feelings, and depriving them of this opportunity may leave children with lifelong regrets (Fig. 19.9). However, a child should never be forced to attend a postdeath service. Children need preparation for postdeath services (Pearson, 2005). They should be told what to expect, particularly how the deceased person will look if the coffin is open. Ideally a parent explains the details to the child. If the parent's grief prevents this communication, a significant family member or friend should substitute.

Children should be prepared for the activities that occur during the services, how long they will last, and what they will see, in particular the casket or child who died. Betty Davies's (1999) book *Shadows in the Sun: The Experiences of Sibling Bereavement in Childhood* is an excellent resource for nurses and families. Bringing children to the service before many visitors arrive may be helpful. They are allowed private time to say good-bye but are spared some of the unpredictable emotional reactions of others, which can be distressing to them. Children are allowed to stay as long as they wish, but respecting their need to leave provides maximum control for them over their ability to grieve comfortably (see Family-Centered Care box).

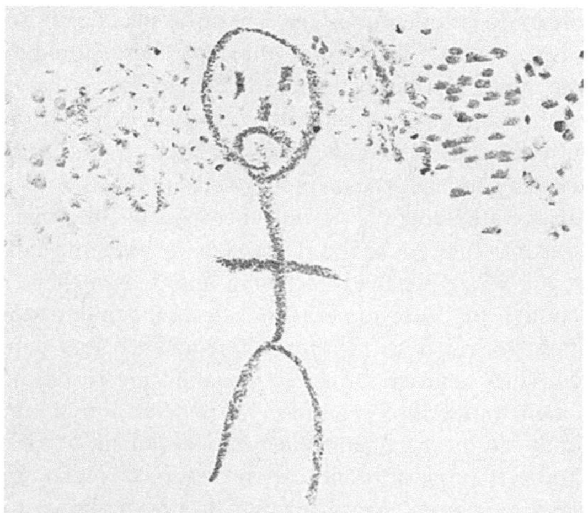

FIG. 19.9 Drawing made by a 7-year-old child whose sister died in a car crash. The drawing shows the boy sad and crying (dots are tears) because he was not allowed to see his dead sibling.

FAMILY-CENTERED CARE

Children Need to Say Good-Bye

Nurse–grief counselors work with children who have experienced the death of someone special, and they use a variety of approaches to allow children to express their feelings. Children often communicate their feelings of being excluded through drawings. They may draw a picture of the dying person in a hospital bed that is raised too high for them to see the person's face clearly. Sometimes children reveal that they did not get to say good-bye because a family member told them, for example, "You don't want to see your grandma this way. She is too sick for you to visit." If the special person died at home, the children had to stay in their room when the funeral home staff took away the body.

Caregivers should not underestimate the importance of allowing children to be involved with the dying person and the significance of a child's loss. When one nurse–grief counselor asked a 6-year-old girl to draw a picture with the theme "This is what I was doing when my _________ died," she drew a picture and completed the sentence with "when my *home* died." Her grandmother had been like her mother. To the child, her home was gone. Children should be given the choice of being included in the family's activities of saying good-bye.

Barbara Bilderback, MS, MA, RN
Bereavement Supervisor
Saint Francis Hospice
Tulsa

CARE OF THE GRIEVING FAMILY

No event is more devastating for families than the threatened or actual loss of a child. Families, especially parents, are deprived of the joy and fulfillment of watching a child grow. All family members are affected by the loss, and their needs must be recognized to facilitate their grief process.

In expected death, the child and family are generally involved in the plan for interventions both before and after the death. In unexpected death, the survivors face the tremendous task of integrating the loss into their lives, with no opportunity for anticipatory grief. In either situation nurses can facilitate the grief process by having a basic understanding of the process. Helpful strategies include being aware of expected reactions, talking with family members, ascertaining their needs, and supporting their efforts to cope, adapt, and grieve (see Applying Evidence to Practice box). Applying the principles of family-centered care is as important at this time as at any other.

GRIEF

Grief is not a single event, but is rather the process of experiencing physiologic, psychologic, behavioral, social, and spiritual reactions to the loss of a child. Grief is highly individualized, encompassing a broad range of manifestations from person to person. It is a natural and expected reaction to loss. It is neither orderly nor predictable. Grieving is often necessary for healing to occur. When death is the expected or a possible outcome of a disorder, the child and family members may experience anticipatory grief. Anticipatory grief may be manifested in varying behaviors and intensities. It may be characterized by denial, anger, depression, and other psychologic and physical symptoms. Anticipatory guidance may assist grieving family members. Health care professionals emphasize that grief reactions such as hearing the dead person's voice, feeling distant from others, or seeking reassurance that they did everything possible for the lost person are normal, necessary, and expected. These reactions in no way signify poor coping, insanity, or an approaching mental breakdown. On the contrary, such behaviors signify that the survivor is working through the acute grief. They are a necessary part of grief work. Anticipatory guidance regarding the mourning process may be helpful to families so that they can recognize the normalcy of their experiences.

It is important to recognize that some family members may experience "complicated" grief. **Complicated grief reactions** (those that continue more than a year after the loss) include such symptoms as intense intrusive thoughts, pangs of severe emotion, distressing yearnings, feelings of being excessively alone and empty, unusual sleep disturbance, and maladaptive levels of loss of interest in personal activities. An unexpected, sudden death is a risk factor for complicated grief (Keesee, Currier, and Neimeyer, 2008). Bereaved persons experiencing such prolonged and complicated grief are referred to an expert in grief and bereavement counseling.

Parental Grief

The grief of parents after the death of a child has been found to be a more intense, complex, long-lasting, and fluctuating grief experience than that of other bereaved individuals. Although parents experience

APPLYING EVIDENCE TO PRACTICE

Communicating With the Bereaved Family

Examples of Nontherapeutic Statements

Advice

You should get out more.
Stop feeling sorry for yourself.
You need to be strong for your family.

Cheerfulness

Now, now, don't cry; cheer up.
Cheer up, you can always have another baby.

Interpretation

It was God's will.
It's better now because she is at peace.

Reassurance

I know how you feel.
God never gives us more than we can handle.
Don't worry, everything will work out.
At least you still have the rest of your family.

Argument

How can you say that?
It's wrong to blame anyone.
You should be glad his suffering is over.

Ignoring the Loss

Remember, you're young and can still have another baby.
It could be worse; he could have lived with severe brain damage.

Examples of Therapeutic Statements

Focus on Feelings

You seem confused and angry.
You are still feeling the pain.
Tell me more about how you are feeling.

Nonjudgmental Questions

Can I be of any help?
Have you decided who the pallbearers will be?

Clarification

Correct me if I'm wrong, but you intend to make all the arrangements.
You believe the accident was your husband's fault?
I'm not sure I understand. Tell me more about __________.

Explanations

You can touch her and hold her if you wish.

Concern, Support, Empathy

Your daughter's birthday is near. That must be painful to deal with.
It's okay to cry.
It sounds like you have been doing some painful thinking.

Support, Silence

I'm here if you want to talk. (Silence)
Hello. (Touch, silence)

Assessment of Coping and Support

Do you have friends and family who can help you now?
You have been through a lot. How are you doing now?
Is there someone who can drive you home?

Validation of Loss

You have been through a very tough time.
He was a special boy to all the staff. I will miss him.

the primary loss of their child, many secondary losses are felt, such as the loss of part of one's self, hopes and dreams for the child's future, the family unit, prior social and emotional community supports, and often spousal support. It is common for parents of the same child to experience different grief reactions.

Studies involving bereaved parents have shown that grieving does not end by the severing of the bond with the deceased child but rather involves a continuing bond between the parent and the dead child (Scholtes & Browne, 2015). Parental resolution of grief is a process of integrating the deceased child into daily life in which the pain of losing a child is never completely gone but lessens. There are occasions of brief relapse but not to the degree experienced when the loss initially occurred. Thus parental grief work is never completed and is a timeless process of accepting the new reality of being without a child, as it changes over time (Davies, 2004). Although parents are expected to grieve the loss of their child, parental grief is often minimized, which leaves parents to work through their grief in isolation and silence.

Parental grief can be stressful on a marriage. As parents become lost in their grief, they are unable to perform many of their roles within the family. For instance, a mother who is generally the nurturing parent might find herself immobilized by grief and unable to nurture and support her husband and surviving children. Her husband, who functions in the family as the provider and protector, was unable to "fix" his dying child. He may now feel the need to "fix" the other members of his family. In addition, he may not have the resources to express his grief, which leads him to postpone his grief by keeping busy at work or around the house. This "tabling" of emotion can lead to outbursts of anger and emotional distancing. Parents often need guidance in understanding each other's needs during their grief process. Not only may the parents be unavailable to each other, but they may also be so lost in their own grief that they cannot easily respond to their children's grief.

Sibling Grief

Each child grieves in his or her own way and on his or her own timeline. Children, even adolescents, grieve differently from adults. Adults and children differ more widely in their reactions to death than in their reactions to any other phenomenon. Children of all ages grieve the loss of a loved one, and their understanding and reactions to death depend on their age and developmental level (Table 19.8). Children

TABLE 19.8 Children's Understanding of and Reactions to Death

Concepts of Death	Reactions to Death	Interventions
Infants and Toddlers		
Death has least significance to children younger than 6 months of age. After parent-child attachment and the development of trust is established, the loss, even if temporary, of the significant person is profound. Prolonged separation during the first several years is thought to be more significant in terms of future physical, social, and emotional growth than at any subsequent age. Toddlers are egocentric and can only think about events in terms of their own frame of reference: living. Their egocentricity and vague separation of fact and fantasy make it impossible for them to comprehend absence of life. Instead of understanding death, this age group is affected more by any change in lifestyle.	With the death of someone else, they may continue to act as though the person is alive. As children grow older, they will be increasingly able and willing to let go of the dead person. Ritualism is important; a change in lifestyle could be anxiety producing. This age group reacts more to the pain and discomfort of a serious illness than to the probable fatal prognosis. This age group also reacts to parental anxiety and sadness.	Help parents deal with their feelings, allowing them more emotional reserve to meet the needs of their children. Encourage parents to remain as near to the child as possible, yet be sensitive to the parents' needs. Maintain as normal an environment as possible to retain ritualism. If a parent has died, encourage the establishment of a consistent caregiver for the child. Promote primary nursing.
Preschool Children		
Children of this age believe their thoughts are sufficient to cause death; the consequence is a feeling of guilt, shame, and punishment. Their egocentricity implies a tremendous sense of self-power and omnipotence. They usually have some sense of the meaning of death. Death is seen as a departure, a kind of sleep. They may recognize the fact of physical death but do not separate it from living abilities. Death is seen as temporary and gradual; life and death can change places with one another. There is no understanding of the universality and inevitability of death.	If they become seriously ill, they conceive of the illness as a punishment for their thoughts or actions. They may feel guilty and responsible for the death of a sibling. Their greatest fear concerning death is separation from their parents. They may engage in activities that seem strange or abnormal to adults. With fewer defense mechanisms to deal with loss, young children may react to a less significant loss with more outward grief than to the loss of a significant person. The loss is so deep, painful, and threatening that the child must deny it for the time being to survive its overwhelming impact. Behavioral reactions such as giggling, joking, attracting attention, or regressing to earlier developmental skills indicate children's need to distance themselves from tremendous loss.	Help parents deal with their feelings, allowing them more emotional reserve to meet the needs of their children. Help parents to understand behavioral reactions of their children. Encourage parents to remain near the child as much as possible, to minimize the child's great fear of separation from parents. If a parent has died, encourage establishment of a consistent caregiver for the child. Promote primary nursing.

TABLE 19.8 Children's Understanding of and Reactions to Death—cont'd

Concepts of Death	Reactions to Death	Interventions
School-Age Children		
These children still associate misdeeds or bad thoughts with causing death and feel intense guilt and responsibility for the event. Because of their higher cognitive abilities, they respond well to logical explanations and comprehend the figurative meaning of words. They have a deeper understanding of death in a concrete sense. They particularly fear the mutilation and punishment they associate with death. They personify death as the devil, a monster, or the bogeyman. They may have naturalistic-physiologic explanations of death. By age 9 or 10, children have an adult concept of death, realizing that it is inevitable, universal, and irreversible.	Because of their increased ability to comprehend, they may have more fears—for example: • The reason for the illness • Communicability of the disease to themselves or others • Consequences of the disease • The process of dying and death itself • Fear of the unknown, which is greater than their fear of the known The realization of impending death is a tremendous threat to their sense of security and ego strength. They are likely to exhibit fear through verbal uncooperativeness rather than actual physical aggression. They are interested in postdeath services. They may be inquisitive about what happens to the body.	Help parents deal with their feelings, allowing them more emotional reserve to meet the needs of their children. Encourage parents to remain near the child as much as possible, yet be sensitive to the parents' needs. Because of children's fear of the unknown, anticipatory preparation is very important. Because the developmental task of this age is industry, interventions of helping children maintain control over their bodies and increasing their understanding allow them to achieve independence, self-worth, and self-esteem and avoid a sense of inferiority. Encourage children to talk about their feelings and provide aggressive outlets. Encourage parents to honestly answer questions about dying rather than avoiding questions or fabricating euphemisms. Encourage parents to share their moments of sorrow with their children. Provide preparation for postdeath services.
Adolescents		
Adolescents have a mature understanding of death. They are still very much influenced by remnants of magical thinking and are subject to feelings of guilt and shame. They are likely to see deviations from accepted behavior as the reason for their illness.	Adolescents straddle transition from childhood to adulthood. They have the most difficulty in coping with death. They are least likely to accept the cessation of life, particularly if it is their own. Concern for the present is much greater than for the past or the future. They may consider themselves alienated from their peers and unable to communicate with their parents for emotional support, feeling alone in their struggle. Adolescents' orientation to the present compels them to worry about physical changes even more than the prognosis. Because of their idealistic view of the world, they may criticize funeral rites as barbaric, money making, and unnecessary.	Help parents deal with their feelings, allowing them more emotional reserve to meet the needs of their children. Avoid alliances with either parent or child. Structure hospital admission to allow for maximum self-control and independence. Answer adolescents' questions honestly, treating them as mature individuals and respecting their needs for privacy, solitude, and personal expressions of emotions. Help the parents understand their child's reactions to death and dying, especially that concern for present crises, such as loss of hair, may be much greater than concern for future ones, including possible death.

often grieve for a longer duration than adults, revisiting their grief as they grow and develop new understandings of death. However, rather than grieving continually, they tend to grieve in spurts, and can be emotional and sad one moment, and then, just as quickly, off and playing.

Children express their grief through play and other behaviors. They can be exquisitely attuned to their parents' grief and try to protect them by not asking questions and avoiding upsetting them. This can set the stage for the sibling to try to become the "perfect child." Children exhibit many of the grief reactions of adults, including physical sensations and illnesses, anger, guilt, sadness, loneliness, withdrawal, acting out, regression, sleep disturbances, isolation, and search for meaning. Again, nurses are attentive for signs that siblings are struggling with their grief and provide guidance to parents when possible.

MOURNING

Shock and Disbelief

Shock, numbness, and disbelief are seen during the immediate phase of grief. As one parent described, "We were as prepared for our son's death as anyone could be, but it was a shock when in a moment his life was finished. I just can't get over the rapidity with which life ends." This temporary numbness protects the survivors from the overwhelming pain associated with grief. Decisions are often made automatically, and only certain details are remembered.

Expression of Grief

When the numbness fades, a period of intense grief begins, characterized by loneliness and yearning for the deceased. During this stage many of the signs of acute grief are evident, and physical complaints such as appetite changes and an inability to sleep are common. There is a tendency to review the events of the deceased's life and to evaluate the relationship with the loved one. Feelings of guilt and anger are common at this time.

Disorganization and Despair

During the stage of disorganization and despair, the pain of the loss is replaced primarily by emptiness, apathy, and deep depression. There is a feeling that life has no meaning and that the pain will never end. This is particularly relevant for parents. For example, mothers often comment that they feel they have suffered a double loss—loss of their child and loss of the mothering role. Feelings of estrangement from other loved ones are common, and social isolation may foster the depression.

Reorganization

Reorganization refers to recovery from the loss. During this gradual process the survivors again find meaning in living, readjust to life without the deceased, develop new or renewed relationships, and learn to live with the memory of the deceased with much less pain. This never means that the loved one is forgotten and the pain is gone. There always remains a deep ache that is never totally replaced with happiness and one that returns more intensely, for example, on holidays or anniversaries.

BEREAVEMENT PROGRAMS

Part of the difficulty in helping the bereaved family is lack of opportunity for follow-up in the traditional health care system. Consequently, many families never receive the support and guidance that could help them in their grief work. At a minimum, one follow-up phone call or meeting with the family is arranged, possibly 1 month after the child's death to give the family time to overcome the phase of shock and disbelief. Families can also be referred to self-help groups, such as the Compassionate Friends,* an international organization for bereaved families, parents, and siblings. When such groups are not available, nurses can be instrumental in helping families network or facilitating parent and sibling groups.

A formal bereavement program or bereavement counseling may help family members work through their grief. Comprehensive bereavement programs begin at the time of the child's death and continue for as long as the family desires. The purpose of a bereavement program is to assist and support families in the process of coping with the devastating impact of the loss of a child and hopefully with grief resolution. The components of such a program include initial contact and support by knowledgeable staff, information and reading materials relevant to the grief process, follow-up contacts by phone or mail, parent and sibling support groups, and referrals for counseling if indicated. Give parents the option of participating in such a program, when available, but do not judge negatively the desire not to participate because grief work is an individual process.

*PO Box 3696, Oak Brook, IL 60522-3696; 630-990-0010, 877-969-0010; fax: 630-990-0246; http://www.compassionatefriends.org. Resolve Through Sharing: 1900 South Ave., AVS-003, La Crosse, WI 54601; 608-775-4747; http://www.bereavementservices.org/RTS.

THE NURSE AND THE CHILD WITH LIFE-THREATENING ILLNESS

NURSES' REACTIONS TO CARING FOR CHILDREN WITH LIFE-THREATENING ILLNESSES

Nurses experience grief and moral distress as they become aware that a child's death is inevitable. Furthermore, nurses experience compassion fatigue as a result of cumulative losses over time as children they care for die and inflict unnecessary pain (Green, Darbyshire, Adams, et al., 2016). Reflection on these experiences and feelings, knowledge of the grief process, and care of oneself are essential for the nurse to provide effective care to dying children and their families (Brandon, Ryan, Sloane, et al., 2014).

Denial

When children are admitted to a pediatric unit with a suspected diagnosis of a serious illness, the initial response from some nurses is shock and denial. However, their behavioral reaction may be withdrawal from the child and family. They choose the "cure" philosophy over the "care" philosophy as a method of distancing themselves from the implications of emotional involvement. Because of their own dependency on denial, some nurses may inappropriately support denial in parents. There are several methods of conveying this message, such as emphasizing only optimistic "survival statistics," negating the seriousness of the illness, focusing on "cheering up" the family, and engaging in casual conversation to avoid meaningful dialogue. Although this increases nurses' comfort in caring for the dying child, it does little to help family members progress beyond denial and begin anticipatory grieving.

Some denial is as important for nurses as it is for the child or parents. It protects nurses from the overwhelming reality of death. It would be extremely difficult to participate in the treatment plan without some expectation of a cure. Denial is also necessary to prevent feelings of failure. In general, nursing and medical goals emphasize curing illness and saving lives, not allowing patients to die. However, denial loses its beneficial functions when nurses refuse to admit the failure of treatment efforts and insist on adhering to the "curing" regimen, regardless of its effectiveness or value. Failure of treatment is not to be equated with personal failure or failure to provide optimum nursing care.

Anger and Depression

Some nurses may be angry for having been assigned to the "leukemia case," for example, because the very exposure to potential failure in a fatal illness is extremely threatening. Others may feel angry for having to subject the child to painful procedures or for being unable to relieve the child's physical and emotional suffering. Instead of anger, some nurses may feel depression for any of these reasons.

Without understanding the reason for the emotion, however, nurses may project the anger onto others, particularly family members. They may be unable to tolerate the child's uncooperative behavior or the parents' continual requests for information. Anger fuels more anger, and parents react with hostility and think the members of the nursing staff are rejecting them. A vicious circle of resentment, mistrust, and frustration may result.

Depression also has adverse effects on the therapeutic relationship because nurses may withdraw from the child and parents as a method of controlling their sadness. Unaware of the reason for the avoidance, family members interpret it as evidence of inadequate care. This reaction also fosters a nonsupportive cycle of avoidance, withdrawal, resentment, and frustration. However, the messages are usually more covert than when the nurses' reaction is anger and may prevent a climax that could result in a solution to the problem.

Guilt

Nurses who feel unable to deal with fatal illness in a child often experience guilt. Nurses who become angry or depressed when caring for a dying child often reveal that they are uncomfortable with this response, but they feel unable to choose a more direct and constructive approach. They express guilt for having been intolerant of the child's or parents' behaviors, and they realize the missed opportunity to provide these individuals with professional support and guidance.

The one important difference between a dying child and an ill child is that there may be no second chance to meet the needs of the dying child. This finality is difficult to comprehend but can lead to a better understanding of one's own responses to dying. For example, when guilt makes an individual uncomfortable enough to seek alternate behavior patterns, there is an opportunity for change, provided the individual is given some assistance and support.

Ambivalence

One of the most universal reactions of nurses is ambivalence in their feelings toward a dying child. There is the fluctuating adherence to hope for a cure and fear of a relapse. Sometimes the motivations for both are more for personal needs. For example, the nurse may hope that the child recovers to avoid readmissions. Or the nurse may wish for a remission so that discharge is ensured. Such thoughts are certainly understandable in light of the emotional toll of nursing a dying child.

Ambivalence may be demonstrated in a particular type of bargaining. Rather than bargaining for extra time, nurses may hope that their colleagues are assigned to the patient or that a death may occur on a shift other than their own. Bargaining for a temporary absence from the dying child is a healthy response because it demonstrates nurses' awareness of their own emotional limits. Nurses who are unable to recognize their personal emotional limits are in danger of seeking to have the professional relationship meet their needs for gratification, achievement, and fulfillment. This results in the loss of an objective evaluation of therapeutic interventions and the increased potential for subjective overinvolvement with the family.

COPING WITH STRESS

Pediatric critical care and oncology nurses surveyed about work stresses ranked patient death as the most stressful, yet one of the most rewarding, experiences. The less experienced the nurse, the more likely that death is rated as a stressor. Furthermore, nurses overestimated the percentage of deaths on their units, which suggests that the experience overwhelms them.

One stress-related outcome of caring for dying children is **burnout**—a state of physical, emotional, and mental exhaustion. It occurs as a result of prolonged involvement with individuals in situations that are emotionally demanding. Nurses working in intensive care units are particularly prone to this occupational hazard, but staff nurses also can experience it when dealing with certain groups of children, such as those who may die. Avoiding burnout and coping constructively, effectively, and therapeutically with children who are dying and their families require a deliberate and concerted effort on the part of the nurse.

Self-Awareness

The initial step in effectively caring for a dying child is making a deliberate choice to become involved. Many nurses react negatively to the word *involvement* because they believe that professionals must remain uninvolved to maintain objectivity. Involvement does not displace objectivity. On the contrary, allowing oneself to feel with the other person expands one's ability to comprehend the meaning and depth of their emotion (see Family-Centered Care box). Ideally the nurse achieves detached concern, which allows sensitive, understanding care because the nurse is sufficiently detached to make objective, rational decisions.

FAMILY-CENTERED CARE

A Dying Child: A Nurse's Perspective

Claire was unresponsive with slow, gasping breathing. Her mother asked me what I thought was happening. I replied honestly, "Your baby is dying because of her brain tumor." The mother put her arms around me and cried. We arranged for Claire to be baptized.

Honesty. Painful as the loss of a child is, my job is to assist the family through this experience. Although I usually wait until a private moment, such as driving home, I found tears streaming down my face as family and friends gathered for Claire's baptism. I went into the kitchen to compose myself, only to find several of my colleagues crying as well. Saying good-bye to a dying child will always be a difficult but shared experience.

Jeanne O'Connor Egan, RN, MSN
Pediatric Clinical Specialist
Children's Hospital
Washington, DC

Knowledge and Practice

Intervening therapeutically with terminally ill children and their families demands more than self-awareness. It also requires that nursing practice be based on sound theoretic formulations and empiric observations that provide a general, concise analysis of the typical reactions of families.

Involvement does carry the potential risk of clouding objectivity, but awareness of one's reactions and investments in the care of a dying child minimize this hazard. Developing awareness requires the willingness to investigate one's motivations for choosing to work in such an area, to understand the stresses inherent in the role, to review one's resolution of past losses, and to contemplate one's own fears of death. Often nurses who have a cold, impersonal reaction to dying patients come to realize that their reaction stems from previous unresolved conflicts or losses. Once they are able to talk about such experiences, they are usually able to gain insight into their behavior and begin to develop alternative methods of reacting.

Nurses also must explore ethical issues surrounding the definition of death, the use of extraordinary and lifesaving measures versus allowing the child to die, and patients' rights to know and choose their own destinies. Once nurses have soundly formulated the principles by which to practice, they need opportunities for decision making. When a team approach is used, nurses can be valuable members of the group if their own values have been clarified and they have critically assessed the family's responses. (See Ethical Decision Making, Chapter 1.)

Support Systems

Support systems are essential to continued functioning in a high-stress environment. They allow nurses to regenerate energies by sharing feelings and concerns with others. Dealing with feelings about death in isolation can lead to repressed feelings such as denial, anger, and depression. These feelings may be manifested in poor interactions among staff, inappropriate or nonsupportive interactions with families, an inability to evaluate care plans or advocate for families, and a need to control. Support is an important catalyst for processing feelings about death.

Social supports may be personal family members such as parents or spouses, extended relatives, and friends. Professional supports include colleagues, consultants, teachers, and supervisors. Peers may be sources of technical and practical advice. Because the death of a patient is more stressful for a less experienced nurse, a mentoring relationship between a senior nurse and the less experienced nurse may provide support and role modeling and assist in the development of effective coping strategies. Forums for staff support and opportunities for debriefing after deaths have been shown to facilitate adaptive coping responses and enhance provider-patient relationships.

Other Strategies

Any number of other strategies may be used to reduce stress. These include maintaining good general health practices, especially regular exercise, and participating in diversionary activities that are of personal interest beyond the workplace. Distancing techniques are also effective, such as leaving work at work, informing other staff not to contact one on one's days off, periodically assuming less demanding assignments, and taking time off when needed (Koy, Yunibhand, Angsuroch, et al., 2017). Mindfulness-based meditation may be another effective strategy to decrease stress and regain a sense of control among nurses experiencing compassion fatigue and burnout.

A final technique is to focus on the positive aspects of the caregiving role. Despite the difficult times in caring for these children and families, many rewarding experiences must be remembered. Dedicated efforts reap numerous rewards, and these must not be forgotten or minimized. Reflection on positive feedback from appreciative families can revitalize self-esteem and job satisfaction.

Some nurses find shared remembrance rituals useful in resolving grief. Similarly, attending the funeral services can be a supportive act for both the family and the nurse and in no way detracts from the professionalism of care. For the family it conveys a sense of worth and caring by the nurse. For the nurse it can provide a sense of closure with the family and facilitate the grief process (Box 19.18).

BOX 19.18 Nurses Experiencing the Stress of Caregiving: Strategies That Help

Recognize the inevitability of the child's death—One's own unrealistic expectations can cause the greatest grief due to the belief that something more should or could have been done to prevent the child's death. Shift the focus of care to providing guidance and comfort for the child and family to increase a sense of accomplishment. Avoid self-blame for situations over which you have no control.

Develop knowledge and apply it—Increase personal knowledge about caring for dying children and their families. Apply this knowledge to provide the best possible care to the patient and family.

Identify ways the work setting can provide support—Ask for relief from highly emotional or conflicted situations, take time off and vacation, seek mentorship, and make use of institutional support services such as multidisciplinary team meetings or employee assistance personnel.

Provide briefings—Inform others involved in the child's care about the child's condition and changes as they occur. After the death, notify caregivers who were closely involved to allow them the opportunity to grieve for the child.

Provide debriefings—Organize staff remembrance services to share experiences and feelings, "bereavement" rounds, and multidisciplinary team review of care.

Find meaning—Accept that even the death of a child is a part of life and find meaning in the caregiving experience with the child and family. Reflect on the experience, what it meant, and how it influenced your view on nursing care.

Separate work and personal life—Develop strategies to leave work behind when at home with family. Avoid trips to the hospital on off days.

Take care of yourself—Recognize the stress of caring for dying children and find healthy activities to help manage that stress. Exercise, good nutrition, and rest are important when work stress is high.

Say good-bye—Identify comfortable ways to say good-bye to the dead child. Attending memorial or funeral services, keeping a memento, journaling, making plantings, and so on are all individual ways to acknowledge the importance of the child to the caregiver.

NCLEX REVIEW QUESTIONS

1. When caring for a 4-year-old with a disability, the nurse notes that while encouraging the child to take part in his care, the mother constantly gives into the child, allowing him to have his own way. What anticipatory guidance can the nurse give to promote normalization in this relationship?
   - **A.** "Giving in" is not a detriment to the child when he or she has a disability and limitations.
   - **B.** Explain that when parents establish reasonable limits, children are likely to develop independence that is appropriate for their age and achievement equal to their limitations.
   - **C.** Advise the parent to wait to explain any procedure to the child until they are at the health care setting or just before the procedure to avoid unduly upsetting the child.
   - **D.** Have the parent realize that it would be unfair to the siblings to expect similar rules to apply to all of the children in the family.
2. Children with disabilities or chronic illness and their families may have different methods of coping than those of healthy children. Often they have a resilience that is to be admired. Which of these statements reflect ways that they foster this resilience? Select all that apply.
   - **A.** Protect the child from having to learn about his or her disability or illness on a repeated basis.
   - **B.** Develop relationships with other children and their families with similar circumstances to build support.
   - **C.** The parents set long-term goals to create a sense of hope.
   - **D.** Focus on the child's strengths and encourage independence.
   - **E.** Accept that chronic illness is part of living.
3. Which of the following factors should a nurse consider when managing the pain of a terminally ill child? Select all that apply.
   - **A.** Pain medications are given on an as-needed schedule, and extra doses for breakthrough pain are available to maintain comfort.
   - **B.** Opioid drugs, such as morphine, are given for severe pain, and the dosage is increased as necessary to maintain optimum pain relief.
   - **C.** Addiction is a factor in managing terminal pain in a child, and the nurse plays an important role in educating parents that their child may become addicted.
   - **D.** Nurses often express concern that administering dosages of opioids that exceed those with which they are familiar will hasten the child's death; in the principle of double effect.

E. In addition to pain medication, techniques such as music therapy, distraction, and guided imagery should be combined with medications to provide the child and family strategies to control pain.

4. It is important to consider the child's developmental understanding of death when working with that child. Which option is the preschool child's developmental stage?
   A. Children of this age believe their thoughts are sufficient to cause death.
   B. They are still very much influenced by remnants of magical thinking and are subject to feelings of guilt and shame.
   C. They have a deeper understanding of death in a concrete sense.
   D. They can perceive events only in terms of their own frame of reference—living.

5. As the nurse caring for a culturally diverse population, it is important to understand cultural health beliefs of families. This can best be accomplished by:
   A. Asking the parents how their extended families feel about their child's illness
   B. Exploring the use of alternative medicines and therapies
   C. Understanding the parents' perception of the seriousness or severity of the illness or disability, as well as concerns and worries they have about the condition
   D. Acknowledging that language constraints may make it necessary for the health care team to make some decisions

Correct Answers

1. B; 2. B, D, E; 3. A, B, D, E; 4. A; 5. C

REFERENCES

Aladangady, N., Shaw, C., Gallagher, K., et al; for Collaborators Group. (2017). Short-term outcome of treatment limitation discussions for newborn infants, a multi-centre prospective observational cohort study. *Archives of Disease in Childhood. Fetal and Neonatal Edition, 102,* 1049.

American Academy of Pediatrics. (2014). Clinical practice guidelines for quality palliative care. *Pediatrics*, Retrieved from http:// www.pediatrics.org/cgi/doi/10.1542/peds.2014-0046.

American Academy of Pediatrics, Section on Hospice and Palliative Medicine and Committee on Hospital Care. (2013). Pediatric palliative care and hospice care commitments, guidelines, and recommendations. *Pediatrics, 132*(5), 966–972.

Anderson, T., & Davis, C. (2011). Evidence-based practice with families of chronically ill children: a critical literature review. *J Evid Based Soc Work, 8,* 416–425.

Auvrignon, A., Leverger, G., & Lasfargues, G. (2008). How to discuss death with a dying child: can a story help? (abstract). *Bulletin de l'Academie Nationale de Medecine, 192*(2), 393–400.

Bakitas, M., Lyons, K. D., Hegel, M. T., et al. (2009). The project ENABLE II randomized controlled trial to improve palliative care for rural patients with advanced cancer: baseline findings, methodological challenges, and solutions. *Palliative and Supportive Care, 7,* 75–86.

Barnes, S., Gardiner, C., Gott, M., et al. (2012). Enhancing patient-professional communication about end-of-life issues in life-limiting conditions: a critical review of the literature. *Journal of Pain and Symptom Management, 44*(6), 866–879.

Berry, J. G., Hall, M., Hall, D. E., et al. (2013). Inpatient growth and resource use in 28 children's hospitals: a longitudinal, multi-institutional study. *JAMA Pediatr, 167*(2), 170–177.

Bluebond-Langner, M. (1978). *The private words of dying children.* Princeton, NJ: Princeton University Press.

Bluebond-Langner, M. (1989). Worlds of dying children and their well siblings. *Death Studies, 13,* 1–16.

Bluebond-Langner, M., Belasco, J. B., & DeMesquita Wander, M. (2010). "I want to live, until I don't want to live anymore": involving children with life-threatening and life-shortening illnesses in decision making about care and treatment. *The Nursing Clinics of North America, 45*(3), 329–343.

Brandon, D. H., Ryan, D., Sloane, R., et al. (2014). Impact of a Pediatric Quality of Life Program on providers' patterns of moral distress. *MCN. The American Journal of Maternal Child Nursing, 39,* 189–197. PMID:24759312.

Burke, R. T., & Alverson, B. (2010). Impact of children with medically complex conditions. *Pediatrics, 126*(4), 789–790.

Burns, K. H., Casey, P. H., Lyle, R. E., et al. (2010). Increasing prevalence of medically complex children in US hospitals. *Pediatrics, 126*(4), 638–646.

Child Trends Databank: *Infant, child, and teen mortality,* 2016. Retrieved from https://www.childtrends.org/?indicators=infant-child-and-teen-mortality.

Chow, K., & Coyle, N. (2011). Providing palliative care to family caregivers throughout the bone marrow transplantation trajectory: research and practice: partners in care. *J Hosp Palliat Nurs, 13,* 7–13.

Coad, J., Patel, R., & Murray, S. (2014). Disclosing terminal diagnosis to children and their families: palliative professionals' communication barriers. *Death Studies, 38*(1–5), 302–307.

Coffey, J. S. (2006). Parenting a child with chronic illness: a metasynthesis. *Pediatric Nursing, 32*(1), 51–59.

Cohen, J. A., Mannarino, A. P., & Deblinger, E. (2016). Treating trauma and traumatic grief in children and adolescents. *Guilford Publications.*

Cohen, E., Kuo, D. Z., Agrawal, R., et al. (2011). Children with medical complexity: an emerging population for clinical and research initiatives. *Pediatrics, 127*(3), 529–538.

Coker, T. R., Rodriguez, M. A., & Flores, G. (2010). Family-centered care for US children with special health care needs: who gets it and why? *Pediatrics, 125*(6), 1159–1167.

Davies, B. (1999). Shadows in the Sun. *New York,* Brunner/Maxel.

Davies, B., Sehring, S. A., Partridge, J. C., et al. (2008). Barriers to palliative care for children: perceptions of pediatric health care providers. *Pediatrics, 121*(2), 282–288.

Davies, R. (2004). New understandings of parental grief: literature review. *Journal of Advanced Nursing, 46*(5), 506–513.

De Lisle-Porter, M., & Podruchny, A. M. (2009). The dying neonate: family-centered end-of-life care. *Neonatal Network, 28*(2), 75–83.

Docherty, S. L., Brandon, D., & Miles, M. S. (2007). Searching for "the dying point": providers' experiences with palliative care in pediatric acute care. *Pediatric Nursing, 33*(4), 335–341.

Dupont-Thibodeau, A., Hindié, J., Bourque, C. J., et al. (2017). Provider perspectives regarding resuscitation decisions for neonates and other vulnerable patients. *The Journal of Pediatrics,* 2017 May 11. pii: S0022-3476(17)30469-9. doi:10.1016/j.jpeds.2017.03.057. [Epub ahead of print].

Dussell, V., Kreicbergs, U., Hilden, J. M., et al. (2008). Looking beyond where children die: determinants and effects of planning a child's location of death. *Journal of Pain and Symptom Management, 37*(1), 33–43.

Enguidanos, S., et al. (2014). Family members' perceptions of inpatient palliative care consult services: a qualitative study. *Palliative Medicine, 28*(1), 42–48.

Ethier, A. M. (2008). Care of the dying child and the family. In D. Tomlinson & N. Kline (Eds.), *Pediatric oncology nursing: advanced clinical handbook* (2nd ed.). New York: Springer-Verlag.

Ethier, A. M. (2005). Death-related sensory experiences. *Journal of Pediatric Oncology Nursing, 22*(2), 104–111.

Ferrell, B. R., Wittenberg, E., Battista, V., et al. (2016a). Exploring the spiritual needs of families with seriously ill children. *International Journal of Palliative Nursing, 22*(8), 388–394.

Ferrell, B., Wittenberg, E., Battista, V., et al. (2016b). Nurses' experiences of spiritual communication with seriously iII children. *Journal of Palliative Medicine, 19*(11), 1166–1170.

Feudtner, C., Feinstein, J. A., Zhong, W., et al. (2014). Pediatric complex chronic conditions classification system version 2: updated for ICD-10 and complex medical technology dependence and transplantation. *BMC Pediatrics, 14*, 199.

Feudtner, C., Womer, J., Augustin, R., et al. (2013). Pediatric palliative care programs in children's hospitals: a cross-sectional national survey. *Pediatrics.*

Friedrichsdorf, S. J. (2016). Contemporary Pediatric Palliative Care: Myths and Barriers to Integration into Clinical Care. *Curr Pediatr Rev.*, [Epub ahead of print]; PMID: 27848889.

Giovanola, J. (2005). Sibling involvement at the end of life. *Journal of Pediatric Oncology Nursing, 22*(4), 222–226.

Gold, J. I., Treadwell, M., Weissman, L., et al. (2011). The mediating effects of family functioning on psychosocial outcomes in healthy siblings of children with sickle cell disease. *Pediatric Blood and Cancer, 57*(6), 1055–1061.

Goodenough, B., Drew, D., Higgins, S., et al. (2004). Bereavement outcomes for parents who lose a child to cancer: are place of death and sex of parent associated with differences in psychological functioning? *Psycho-Oncology, 13*(11), 779–791.

Goudie, A., Narcisse, M. R., Hall, D. E., et al. (2014). Financial and psychological stressors associated with caring for children with disability. *Families, Systems and Health: The Journal of Collaborative Family Healthcare, 32*(3), 280–290.

Green, J., Darbyshire, P., Adams, A., et al. (2016). It's agony for us as well: Neonatal nurses reflect on iatrogenic pain. *Nursing Ethics, 23*(2), 176–190.

Hartling, L., Milne, A., Tjosvold, L., et al. (2014). A systematic review of interventions to support siblings of children with chronic illness or disability. *J Paediatric Child Health, 50*(10), E26–E38.

Hendricks-Ferguson, V. (2008). Physical symptoms of children receiving pediatric hospice care at home during the last week of life. *Oncology Nursing Forum, 35*(6), E108–E115.

Hexem, K. R., Mollen, C. J., Carroll, K., et al. (2011). How parents of children receiving pediatric palliative care use religion, spirituality, or life philosophy in tough times. *Journal of Palliative Medicine, 14*(1), 39–44.

Hill, D. L., Miller, V., Walter, J. K., et al. (2014). Regoaling: a conceptual model of how parents of children with serious illness change medical care goals. *BMC Palliative Care, 13*(1), 9.

Huang, I. C., Kenzik, K. M., Sanjeev, T. Y., et al. (2010). Quality of life information and trust in physicians among families of children with life-limiting conditions. *Patient Relat Outcome Meas, 2010*(1), 141–148.

Hungerbuehler, I., Vollrath, M. E., & Landolt, M. A. (2011). Posttraumatic growth in mothers and fathers of children with severe illnesses. *Journal of Health Psychology, 16*(8), 1259–1267.

Jacobs, S., Perez, J., Cheng, Y. I., et al. (2015). Adolescent end of life preferences and congruence with their parents' preferences: Results of a survey of adolescents with cancer. *Pediatric Blood and Cancer, 62*, 710–714. 2015.

Jalmsell, L., Kontio, T., Stein, M., et al. (2015). On the child's own initiative: Parents communicate with their dying child. *Death Studies, 39*(2), 111–117.

Kaye, E. C., Friebert, S., & Baker, J. N. (2016). Early integration of palliative care for children with high-risk cancer and their families. *Pediatric Blood and Cancer, 63*(4), 593–597.

Kaye, E. C., Rubenstein, J., Levine, D., et al. (2015). Pediatric palliative care in the community. *CA: A Cancer Journal for Clinicians, 65*, 315–333.

Keele, L., Keenan, H. T., Sheetz, J., et al. (2013). Differences in characteristics of dying children who receive and do not receive palliative care. *Pediatrics, 132*(1), 72–78.

Keesee, N. J., Currier, J. M., & Neimeyer, R. A. (2008). Predictors of grief following the death of one's child: the contribution of finding meaning. *Journal of Clinical Psychology, 64*(10), 1145–1163.

Knafl, K. A., & Santacroce, S. J. (2010). Chronic conditions and the family. In P. J. Allen, J. A. Vessey, & N. A. Schapiro (Eds.), *Primary care of the child with a chronic condition* (5th ed.). St Louis: Mosby/Elsevier.

Knapp, C., Huang, I., Madden, V., et al. (2009). An evaluation of two decision-making scales for children with life-limiting illnesses (abstract). *Palliative Medicine, 23*(6), 518–525.

Knapp, C. A., Shenkman, E. A., Marcu, M. I., et al. (2009). Pediatric palliative care: describing hospice users and identifying factors that affect hospice expenditures (abstract). *Journal of Palliative Medicine, 12*(3), 223–229.

Koy, V., Yunibhand, J., Angsuroch, Y., et al. (2017). Relationship between nursing care quality, nurse staffing, nurse job satisfaction, nurse practice environment, and burnout: literature review. *Int J Research in Medical Sciences, 3*(8), 1825–1831.

Kuhlthau, K. A., Bloom, S., Van Cleave, J., et al. (2011). Evidence for family-centered care for children with special health care needs: a systematic review. *Acad Pediatr, 11*(2), 136–143.

Kuntz, B. (1991). Exploring the grief of adolescents after the death of a parent. *Journal of Child and Adolescent Psychiatric and Mental Health Nursing, 4*(3), 105–109.

Kuo, D. Z., Cohen, E., Agrawal, R., et al. (2011). A national profile of caregiver challenges among more medically complex children with special health care needs. *Archives of Pediatrics and Adolescent Medicine, 165*(11), 1020–1026.

Kuo, D. Z., Houtrow, A. J., Arango, P., et al. (2012). Family-centered care: current applications and future directions in pediatric health care. *Maternal and Child Health Journal, 16*(2), 297–305.

Kuo, D. Z. (2016). Houtrow AJ, Council on Children with Disability. Recognition and management of medical complexity. *Pediatrics, 138*(6), pii: e20163021.

Kuo, D. Z., Sisterhen, L. L., Sigrest, T. E., et al. (2012). Family experiences and pediatric health services use associated with family-centered rounds. *Pediatrics, 130*(2), 299–305.

Larcher, V., Craig, F., Bhogal, K., et al. (2015). Making decisions to limit treatment in life-limiting and life-threatening conditions in children: a framework for practice. *Archives of Disease in Childhood, 100*, s1–s23.

Lauer, M. E., Mulhern, R. K., Bohne, J. B., et al. (1985). Children's perceptions of their sibling's death at home or hospital: the precursors of differential adjustment. *Cancer Nursing, 8*(1), 21–27.

Levine, D., Lam, C. G., Cunningham, M. J., et al. (2013). Best practices for pediatric palliative cancer care: a primer for clinical providers. *The Journal of Supportive Oncology, 11*(3), 114–125.

Lobato, D. J., Kao, B. T., & Plante, W. (2005). Latino sibling knowledge and adjustment to chronic illness. *Journal of Family Psychology, 19*(4), 625–632.

Lotz, J. D., Daxer, M., Jox, R. J., et al. (2016). "Hope for the best, prepare for the worst": A qualitative interview study on parents' needs and fears in pediatric advance care planning. *Palliative Medicine*, 2016 Nov 23. pii: 0269216316679913. [Epub ahead of print].

Madrigal, V. N., Carroll, K. W., Faerber, J. A., et al. (2016). Parental sources of support and guidance when making difficult decisions in the pediatric intensive care unit. *The Journal of Pediatrics, 169*, 221–226.

Martinson, I. M. (1995). Improving care of dying children. *The Western Journal of Medicine, 163*, 258–262.

Martinson, I. M. (1993). Hospice care for children: past, present, and future. *Journal of Pediatric Oncology Nursing, 10*(3), 93–98.

Mastro, K. A., Johnson, J. E., McElvery, N., et al. (2015). The benefits of a nurse-driven, patient- and family-centered pediatric palliative care program. *The Journal of Nursing Administration, 45*(9), 423–428.

Meert, K. L., Shear, K., Newth, C. J., et al. (2011). Follow-up study of complicated grief among parents eighteen months after a child's death in the pediatric intensive care unit. *Journal of Palliative Medicine, 14*(2), 207–214.

Meyers, F. J., Carducci, M., Loscalzo, M. J., et al. (2011). Effects of a problem-solving intervention (COPE) on quality of life for patients with advanced cancer on clinical trials and their caregivers: simultaneous care educational intervention (SCEI): linking palliation and clinical trials. *Journal of Palliative Medicine, 14*, 465–473.

Michael, P., & Lansdown, R. G. (1986). Adjustment ot the death of a sibling. *Archives of Disease in Childhood, 61*(3), 278–283.

National Consensus Project for Quality Palliative Care, 2013: *Clinical practice guidelines for quality palliative care, 2013.* Retrieved from http://www.nationalconsensusproject.org/.

National Hospice and Palliative Care Organization (2016). *Children's Project on Palliative/Hospice Services: Compendium of pediatric palliative care.* Alexandria, VA: Author.

Nuutila, L., & Salanterä, S. (2006). Children with a long-term illness: parents' experiences of care. *Journal of Pediatric Nursing, 21*(2), 153–160.

Panicker, L. (2013). Nurses' perceptions of parent empowerment in chronic illness. *Contemporary Nurse: A Journal for the Australian Nursing Profession, 45*(2), 210–219.

Pearson, L. J. (2005). The child who is dying. In J. A. Rollins, R. Bolig, & C. C. Mahan (Eds.), *Meeting children's psychosocial needs across the heath-care continuum*. Austin: Pro-Ed.

Pritchard, M., Burghen, E., Srivastava, D. K., et al. (2008). Cancer-related symptoms most concerning to parents during the last week and day of their child's life. *Pediatrics, 121*(5), e1301–e1309.

Randolph, A. G., Zollo, M. B., Egger, M. J., et al. (1999). Variability in physician opinion on limited pediatric life support. *Pediatr, 103*, e46.

Riley, J., Ross, J. R., Gretton, S. K., et al. (2007). Proposed five-step World Health Organization analgesic and side effect ladder. *European Journal of Pain*, (Suppl.S), 23–30.

Rollins, J. A., & Riccio, L. L. (2002). ART is the heART: a palette of possibilities for hospice care. *Pediatric Nursing, 28*(4), 355–362.

Russell, C., & Smart, S. (2007). Guided imagery and distraction therapy in paediatric hospice care. *Paediatric Nursing, 19*(2), 24–25.

Russell, C. E., Widger, K., Beaune, L., et al. (2017). Siblings' voices: a prospective investigation of experiences with a dying child. *Death Studies*.

Scholtes, D., & Browne, M. (2015). Internalized and externalized continuing bonds in bereaved parents: their relationship with grief intensity and personal growth. *Death Studies, 39*(2), 75–83.

Seecharan, G. A., Andresen, E. M., Norris, K., et al. (2004). Parents' assessment of quality of care and grief following a child's death. *Archives of Pediatrics and Adolescent Medicine, 158*(6), 515–520.

Sharman, M., Meert, K. L., & Sarnaik, A. P. (2005). What influences parents' decisions to limit or withdraw life support? *Pediatric Critical Care Medicine: A Journal of the Society of Critical Care Medicine and the World Federation of Pediatric Intensive and Critical Care Societies, 6*(5), 513–518.

Simon, T. D., Berry, J., Feudtner, C., et al. (2010). Children with complex chronic conditions in inpatient hospital settings in the United States. *Pediatrics, 126*(4), 647–655.

Sisk, B. A., DuBois, J., Kodish, E., et al. (2017). Navigating Decisional Discord: The Pediatrician's Role When Child and Parents Disagree. *Pediatrics*, 2017 May 12. pii: e20170234. doi:10.1542/peds.2017-0234. [Epub ahead of print].

Smaldone, A., & Ritholz, M. D. (2011). Perceptions of parenting children with type 1 diabetes diagnosed in early childhood. *Journal of Pediatric Health Care, 25*(2), 87–95.

Smith, T. J., Temin, S., Alesi, E. R., et al. (2012). American Society of Clinical Oncology provisional clinical opinion: the integration of palliative care into standard oncology care. *Journal of Clinical Oncology : Official Journal of the American Society of Clinical Oncology, 30*, 880–887.

Spinetta, J. J. (1974). The dying child's awareness of death: a review. *Pscyhol Bull, 81*(4), 256–260.

Stein, R. E. K. (1985). Home care: a challenging opportunity. *Children's Health Care: Journal of the Association for the Care of Children's Health, 14*(2), 90–95.

Stevenson, M., Achille, M., & Lugasi, T. (2013). Pediatric palliative care in Canada and the United States: a qualitative metasummary of the needs of patients and families. *Journal of Palliative Medicine, 16*(5), 566–577.

Stewart, J. L., Pyke-Grimm, K. A., & Kelly, K. P. (2012). Making the right decision for my child with cancer: the parental imperative. *Cancer Nursing*, [Epub ahead of print].

Sullivan, J., Monagle, P., & Gillam, L. (2014). What parents want from doctors in end-of-life decision-making for children. *Archives of Disease in Childhood, 99*(3), 216–220.

Swallow, V., Macfadyen, A., Santacroce, S. J., et al. (2012). Fathers' contributions to the management of their child's long-term medical condition: a narrative review of the literature. *Health Expectations: An International Journal of Public Participation in Health Care and Health Policy, 15*(2), 157–175.

Tamburro, R. F., Shaffer, M. L., Hahnlen, N. C., et al. (2011). Care goals and decisions for children referred to a pediatric palliative care program. *Journal of Palliative Medicine, 14*, 607–613.

Tan, J., Docherty, S. L., Barfield, R., et al. (2012). Addressing parental bereavement support needs at the end of life for infants with complex chronic conditions. *Journal of Palliative Medicine, 15*(5), 579–584.

Taylor, S., Haase-Casanovas, S., Weaver, T., et al. (2010). Child involvement in the paediatric consultation: a qualitative study of children and caregivers. *Child: Care, Health and Development, 36*(5), 678–685.

Temel, J. S., Greer, J. A., Muzikansky, A., et al. (2010). Early palliative care for patients with metastatic non-small-cell lung cancer. *The New England Journal of Medicine, 363*, 733–742.

Thienprayoon, R., Lee, S. C., Leonard, D., et al. (2015). Hospice care for children with cancer: where do these children die? *Journal of Pediatric Hematology, 37*(5), 373–377.

Thompson, L. A., Knapp, C., Madden, V., et al. (2009). Pediatricians' perceptions of and preferred timing for pediatric palliative care. *Pediatrics, 123*(5), e777–e782.

Toomey, S. L., Chien, A. T., Elliott, M. N., et al. (2013). Disparities in unmet need for care coordination: the national survey of children's health. *Pediatrics, 131*(2), 217–224.

Treyvaud, K. (2014). Parent and family outcomes following very preterm or very low birth weight birth: a review. *Seminars in Fetal and Neonatal Medicine, 19*(2), 131–135.

Tubbs-Cooley, H. L., Santucci, G., Kang, T. I., et al. (2011). Pediatric nurses' individual and group assessments of palliative, end-of-life, and bereavement care. *Journal of Palliative Medicine, 14*, 631–637.

Ullrich, C. K., Sourkes, B. M., & Wolfe, J. (2016). Palliative care for the child with cancer. In P. A. Pizzo & D. G. Poplack (Eds.), *Principles and practice of pediatric oncology* (7th ed.). Philadelphia/New York: Lippincott-Raven.

Van Breemen, C. (2009). Using play therapy in paediatric palliative care: listening to the story and caring for the body. *International Journal of Palliative Nursing, 15*, 510–514.

Von Lützau, P., Otto, M., Hechler, T., et al. (2012). Children dying from cancer: parents' perspectives on symptoms, quality of life, characteristics of death, and end-of-life decisions. *Journal of Palliative Care, 28*(4), 274–281.

Weaver, M. S., et al. (2016). Establishing psychosocial palliative care standards for children and adolescents with cancer and their families: An integrative review. *Palliative Medicine, 30*(3), 212–223.

Wiener, L., McConnell, D. G., Latella, L., et al. (2013). Cultural and religious considerations in pediatric palliative care. *Palliative and Supportive Care, 11*(1), 47–67.

Wolfe, J., Hammel, J. F., Edwards, K. E., et al. (2008). Easing suffering in children with cancer at the end of life: is care changing? *Journal of Clinical Oncology : Official Journal of the American Society of Clinical Oncology, 26*(10), 1717–1723.

Wolfelt, A. (2013). Helping children cope with grief. *Routledge*.

Workman, J. K., Myrick, C. W., Meyers, R. L., et al. (2013). Pediatric organ donation and transplantation. *Pediatrics, 131*(6), e1723–e1730.

World Health Organization: *WHO definition of palliative care*, 2014. Retrieved from http://www.who.int/cancer/palliative/definition/en/.

Wyatt, K. D., List, B., Brinkman, W. B., et al. (2015). Shared decision making in pediatrics: a systematic review and meta-analysis. *Acad Pediatr, 15*(6), 573–583.

Younge, N., et al. (2015). Impact of a palliative care program on end-of-life care in a neonatal intensive care unit. *Journal of Perinatology, 35*(3), 218–222.

Zinner, S. E. (2009). The use of pediatric advance directives: a tool for palliative care physicians. *Am J Hosp Palliat Med, 25*(6), 427–430.

20

Impact of Cognitive or Sensory Impairment on the Child and Family

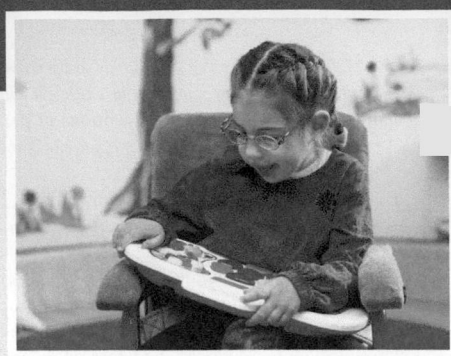

Rosalind Bryant

http://evolve.elsevier.com/wong/ncic

CONCEPTS

- Cognition
- Sensory Perception

COGNITIVE IMPAIRMENT

GENERAL CONCEPTS

Cognitive impairment (CI) is a general term that encompasses any type of intellectual disability and affects from 2.5% to 3% of the population (Ageranioti-Belanger, Brunet, D'Anjou, et al., 2012; Bellman, Byrne, & Sege, 2013; Shapiro & Batshaw, 2016). The term *intellectual disability* (formerly *mental retardation*) has become the most common internationally used term (American Association on Intellectual and Developmental Disabilities, 2013; American Psychiatric Association, 2013; Tasse, Luckasson, & Nygren, 2013). In this chapter, the term *CI* is used synonymously with *intellectual disability.*

Intellectual disability as defined by the American Association on Intellectual and Developmental Disabilities consists of three components: (1) intellectual functioning, (2) adaptive behavior, and (3) age younger than 18 years at time of diagnosis. Intellectual functioning is measured by the intelligence quotient (IQ) test score. CI is considered an umbrella term by the American Association on Intellectual and Developmental Disabilities that is characterized by significant limitations in both intellectual functioning and adaptive behavior (i.e., the inability to reason, plan, solve problems, think abstractly, comprehend complex ideas, learn from experience that is age appropriate, or unable to meet the standards for culturally appropriate demands of daily life) (Tasse, Luckasson, & Nygren, 2013).

The American Psychiatric Association's *Diagnostic and Statistical Manual of Mental Disorders, Fifth Edition* (DSM-5) criteria recommend moving away from exclusively relying on IQ testing toward using additional measures of adaptive functioning (American Psychiatric Association, 2013; Moran, 2013). The DSM-5 is the diagnostic standard and states that the child with CI must demonstrate deficits in adaptive functioning that result in failure to meet developmental and sociocultural standards for personal independence and social responsibility (Moran, 2013).

The American Psychiatric Association's DSM-5 terminology and diagnostic criteria are consistent with those terms established by the American Association on Intellectual and Developmental Disabilities (Tasse, Luckasson, & Nygren, 2013). Careful evaluation to identify the needs of individuals with CI is focused on promoting habilitation for each person. It is anticipated that when appropriate supports are given over a prolonged period, the ability of the person with CI to function each day will generally improve.

Diagnosis and Classification

The diagnosis of CI is usually made after professionals or the family suspects that the child's developmental progress is delayed. In some cases, it is confirmed at birth because of recognition of distinct syndromes. At the other extreme, the diagnosis is made when problems such as speech delays or school problems arouse concern. In all cases a high index of suspicion for developmental delay and behavioral signs is necessary for early diagnosis (Box 20.1), and routine developmental screening can assist in early identification. Delays are typically seen in gross and fine motor and speech development, although the latter is most predictive. Developmental disability can be described as any significant lag or delay in a child's physical, cognitive, behavioral, emotional, or social development when compared against developmental norms. CI is an impairment encompassing intellectual ability and adaptive behavior that are functioning significantly below average (see Box 20.1). In the absence of clear-cut evidence of CI, it is more appropriate to use a diagnosis of developmental disability.

Results of standardized tests are helpful in contributing to the diagnosis of CI. Tests for assessing adaptive behaviors include the Vineland Adaptive Behavior Scale (Vineland-3) and the Adaptive Behavior Assessment System (ABS–third edition). Informal appraisal of adaptive behavior may be made by those fully acquainted with the child (e.g., teachers, parents, other care providers). Frequently, these observations lead parents to seek evaluation of the child's development.

A more useful approach for clinical application is classification based on educational potential or symptom severity. For educational purposes, the mildly impaired group constitutes about 85% of all people with CI, and the group with moderate levels of CI accounts for about 10% of the intellectually disabled population (Shea, 2012) (Table 20.1).

Etiology

The causes of severe CI are primarily genetic, biochemical, and infectious. Although the etiology is unknown in the majority of cases, familial,

BOX 20.1 Early Signs Suggestive of Cognitive Impairment

Dysmorphic syndromes (e.g., Down syndrome, fragile X syndrome)
Irritability or nonresponsiveness to environment
Major organ system dysfunction (e.g., feeding or breathing difficulties)
Gross motor delay
Fine motor delay
Language difficulties or delay
Behavior difficulties

Modified from Shapiro, B., & Batshaw, M. (2016). Intellectual disability. In R. M. Kliegman, B. F. Stantan, J. W. St. Geme III, et al. (Eds.), *Nelson textbook of pediatrics* (20th ed.). Philadelphia, PA: Elsevier; Wilks, T., Gerber, J., & Erdie-Lalena, C. (2010). Developmental milestones: Cognitive development. *Pediatrics in Review, 31*(9), 364-367.

TABLE 20.1 Intensity of Sounds Expressed in Decibels

Decibels	Representative Sound
0	Softest sound normal ear can hear
10	Heartbeat, rustling of leaves
20	Whisper at 1.5 m (5 feet)
30-45	Normal conversation
60	Noise in average restaurant
70-80	Street noises
80	Loud radio in home
90-100	Train
120	Thunder, loud music
140	Jet plane during departure
>140	Pain threshold

social, environmental, and organic causes may predominate. Among individuals with CI, a sizable proportion of the cases are linked to Down syndrome, fragile X syndrome (FXS), or fetal alcohol syndrome. General categories of events that may lead to CI include the following (Gilissen, Hehir-Kwa, Thung, et al., 2014; Hoyme, Kalberg, Elliot, et al., 2016; Katz & Lazcano-Ponce, 2008; Mefford, Batshaw, & Hoffman, 2012):

- Infection and intoxication, such as congenital rubella, syphilis, maternal drug consumption (e.g., fetal alcohol syndrome), chronic lead ingestion, or kernicterus
- Trauma or physical agent (e.g., injury to the brain experienced during the prenatal, perinatal, or postnatal period)
- Inadequate nutrition and metabolic disorders, such as phenylketonuria or congenital hypothyroidism
- Gross postnatal brain disease, such as neurofibromatosis and tuberous sclerosis
- Unknown prenatal influence, including cerebral and cranial malformations, such as microcephaly and hydrocephalus
- Chromosomal abnormalities resulting from radiation; viruses; chemicals; parental age; and genetic mutations that occur in disorders such as Down syndrome and FXS
- Gestational disorders, including prematurity, low birth weight, and postmaturity
- Psychiatric disorders that have their onset during the child's developmental period up to age 18 years, such as autism spectrum disorders (ASDs)
- Environmental influences, including evidence of a deprived environment associated with a history of intellectual disability among parents and siblings

NURSING CARE OF CHILDREN WITH IMPAIRED COGNITIVE FUNCTION

Nurses play a major role in identifying children with CI. In the newborn and early infancy periods, few signs are present, except in such disorders as Down syndrome (discussed later in this chapter). However, delayed developmental milestones are the major clues to CI. In addition, nurses must have a high index of suspicion for early behavior patterns that may suggest CI (see Box 20.1). Parental concerns, such as delayed development compared with siblings, need to be taken seriously. All children should receive regular developmental assessment, and the nurse is often the person responsible for performing such assessments (see Chapter 4). When delays are found, the nurse must use sensitivity and discretion in revealing this finding to parents.

EDUCATE CHILD AND FAMILY

To teach children with CI, one must investigate their learning abilities and deficits. This is important for the nurse who may be involved in a home care program or who may be caring for the child in a school or health care setting. The nurse who understands how these children learn can effectively teach them basic skills or prepare them for various health-related procedures.

Children with CI have a marked deficit in their ability to discriminate between two or more stimuli because of difficulty in recognizing the relevance of specific cues. However, these children can learn to discriminate if the cues are presented in an exaggerated, concrete form and if all extraneous stimuli are eliminated. For example, the use of colors to emphasize visual cues or the use of singing or rhymes to stress auditory cues can help them learn. Their deficit in discrimination also implies that concrete ideas are learned much more effectively than abstract ideas. Therefore demonstration is preferable to verbal explanation, and learning should be directed toward mastering a skill rather than understanding the scientific principles underlying a procedure.

Another cognitive deficit is in short-term memory. Whereas children of average intelligence can remember several words, numbers, or directions at one time, children with CI are less able to do so. Therefore they need simple, one-step directions. Learning through a step-by-step process requires a task analysis in which each task is separated into its necessary components and each step is taught completely before proceeding to the next activity.

One critical area of learning that has had a tremendous impact on education for cognitively impaired individuals is motivation or the use of positive reinforcement to encourage the accomplishment of specific tasks or behaviors. Advances in technology have greatly aided in providing reinforcement, especially in children with severe disabilities and who may have physical disabilities that limit their range of capabilities. For example, with the use of specially designed switches, children are given control of some event in the environment, such as turning on the computer (Fig. 20.1). Activation of the computer becomes the reinforcement for pushing the switch. Repetitive use of these switches provides an early, simplistic association with a technical device that may progress to increasingly complex aids.

Early intervention program is a systematic program of therapy, exercises, and activities designed to address developmental delays in children with disabilities to help achieve their full potentials (Bull & Committee on Genetics, 2011; Crnic, Neece, McIntyre, et al., 2017; Guralnick, 2017; National Down Syndrome Society, 2012a). Considerable evidence indicates that these programs are valuable for cognitively impaired children. Nurses working with these families need to be aware of the types of programs in their community. Under the Individuals with Disabilities Education Act (IDEA) of 1990 (Public Law 101-476),

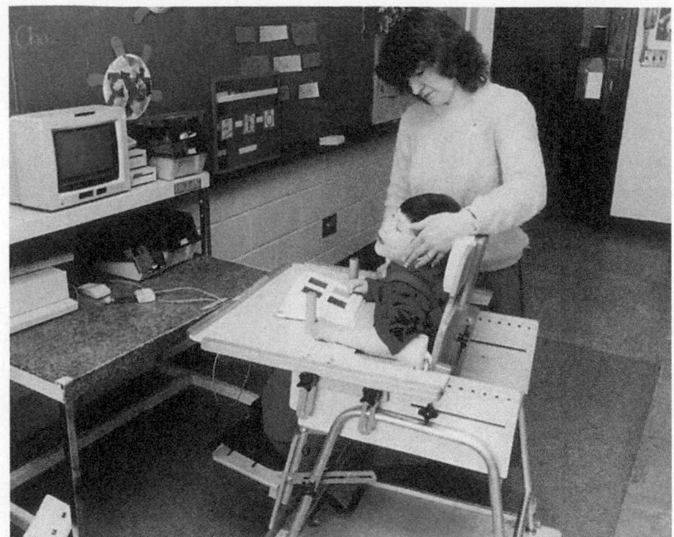

FIG. 20.1 A push panel allows a child with cognitive impairment to turn a computer on and off.

states are encouraged to provide full early intervention services and are required to provide educational opportunities for all children with disabilities from birth to 21 years old. Services may be provided under state programs for Children with Special Health Care Needs (CSHCN) or Head Start, or by private organizations such as National Down Syndrome Society,* Easter Seals,† or The Arc of the United States.‡ Parents should inquire about these programs by contacting the appropriate agencies. Early intervention exposure includes structured educational programs, parent training, and family-intervention training with available family resources that tend to be associated with more positive developmental and behavioral outcomes in children with CI (Crnic, Neece, & McIntyre et al., 2017; Guralnick, 2017; Wallander, Biasini, Thorsten, et al., 2014). As children grow older, their education should be directed toward vocational training that prepares them for as independent a lifestyle as possible within their scope of abilities.

Teach Child Self-Care Skills

When a child with CI is born, parents often need assistance in promoting normal developmental skills that other children learn easily. There is no way to predict when a child should be able to master self-care skills, such as feeding, toileting, dressing, and grooming because a wide age variability exists in the cognitively impaired child who is able to accomplish such functions.

Teaching self-care skills also necessitates a working knowledge of the individual steps needed to master a skill. For example, before beginning a self-feeding program, the nurse performs a task analysis. After a task analysis, the child is observed in a particular situation, such as eating, to determine what skills are possessed and the child's developmental readiness to learn the task. Family members are included in this process because their "readiness" is as important as the child's. Numerous self-help aids are available to facilitate independence and can help eliminate some of the difficulties of learning, such as using a plate with suction cups to prevent accidental spills.*

Promote Child's Optimal Development

Optimal development involves more than achieving independence. It requires appropriate guidance for establishing acceptable social behavior and personal feelings of self-esteem, worth, and security. These attributes are not simply learned through a stimulation program. Rather, they must arise from the genuine love and caring that exist among family members. However, families need guidance in providing an environment that fosters optimal development. Often the nurse can provide assistance in these areas of childrearing.

Another important area for promoting optimal development and self-esteem is ensuring the child's physical well-being. Any congenital defects, such as cardiac, gastrointestinal, or orthopedic anomalies, should be repaired. Plastic surgery may be considered when the child's appearance can be substantially improved. Dental health is significant, and orthodontic and restorative procedures can improve facial appearance immensely.

Encourage Play and Exercise

Children who are cognitively impaired have the same need for play and exercise as any other child. However, because of the children's slower development, parents may be less aware of the need to provide such activities. Therefore the nurse will need to guide parents toward selection of suitable play and exercise activities. Because play has been discussed for children in each age-group in earlier chapters, only the exceptions are presented here (Fig. 20.2).

The type of play is based on the child's developmental age, although the need for sensorimotor play may be prolonged. Parents should use every opportunity to expose the child to as many different sounds, sights, and sensations as possible. Appropriate toys include musical mobiles, stuffed toys, floating toys, a rocking chair or horse, a swing, bells, and rattles. The child should be taken on outings, such as trips to the grocery store or shopping center. Other people should be encouraged to visit in the home, and individuals should relate directly to the child through means such as cuddling, holding, rocking, and talking to the child in the face-to-face fashion.

Toys are selected for their recreational and educational value. For example, a large inflatable beach ball is a good water toy; it encourages interactive play and can be used to learn motor skills, such as balance, rocking, kicking, and throwing. Attractive toys encourage a child to reach, therefore assisting in the development of motor skills (see Fig. 20.2). Musical toys that mimic animal sounds or respond with social phrases are excellent ways of encouraging speech. A doll with removable clothes and different types of closures can help the child learn dressing skills. Toys should be simple in design so that the child can learn to

*Information on early intervention programs in each state is available from the National Down Syndrome Society, 666 Broadway, 8th Floor, New York, NY 10012-2317; 800-221-4602; email: info@ndss.org; http://www.ndss.org; facebook.com/National Down Syndrome Society; twitter.com/NDSS.

†233 South Wacker Drive., Suite 2400, Chicago, IL 60606-4802; 800-221-6827; TTY: 312-726-4258; http://www.easterseals.com; email: info@easterseals.com; facebook.com/easterseals; twitter.com/EasterSealsON.

‡1825 K Street NW, Suite 1200, Washington, DC 20006; 202-534-3700 or 800-433-5255; fax: 202-534-3731; http://www.thearc.org; email: info@thearc.org; facebook.com/thearcus; twitter.com/thearcus; youtube.com/user/thearcoftheus.

*A resource for a variety of self-help equipment is Patterson Medical Corporate Headquarters, 28100 Torch Parkway Suite 700, Warrenville, IL 60555-3938; 800-323-9742; Customer Service: 800-323-5547; http://www.pattersonmedical.com; http://www.facebook.com/PattersonMedical. In Canada: 800-665-9200; 905-858-6000; http://www.pattersonmedical.ca.

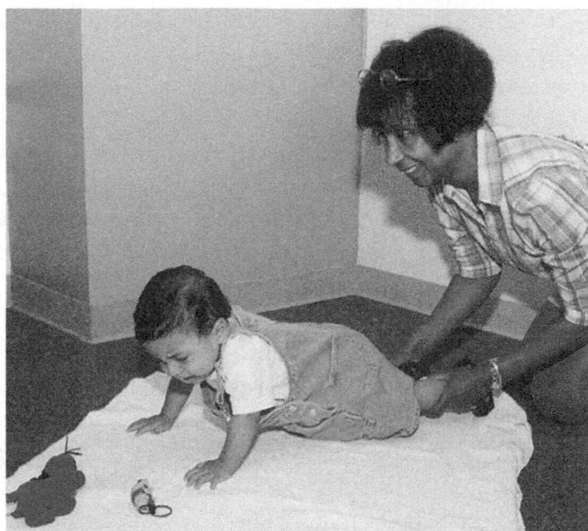

FIG. 20.2 Placing an attractive object outside the child's reach encourages crawling movements. (Courtesy James DeLeon, Texas Children's Hospital, Houston, TX.)

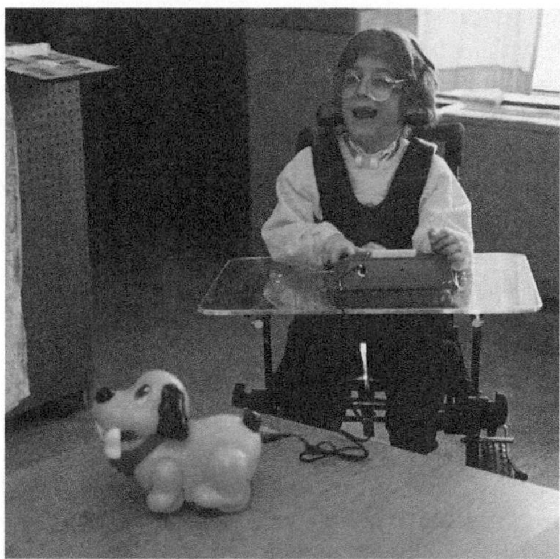

FIG. 20.3 A manual switch allows a child with cognitive impairment to play with a battery-operated toy.

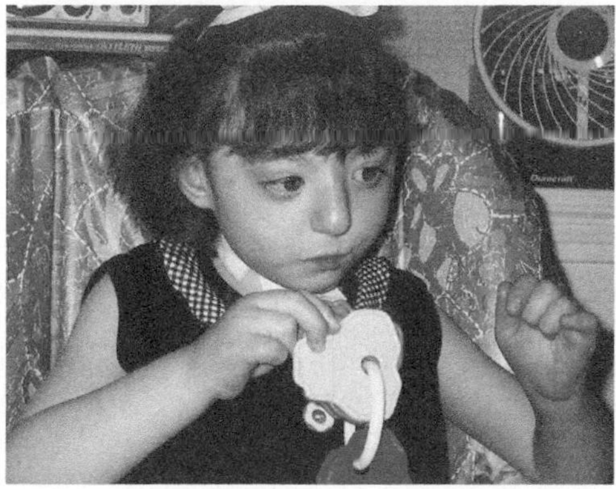

FIG. 20.4 A favorite toy provides stimulation for a young child.

manipulate them without help. For children with severe cognitive and physical impairment, electronic switches can be used to allow them to operate toys (Figs. 20.3 and 20.4).

Suitable activities for physical activity are based on the child's size, coordination, physical fitness and maturity, motivation, and health (see Fig. 20.4). Some children may have physical problems that prevent participation in certain sports, such as atlantoaxial instability in children

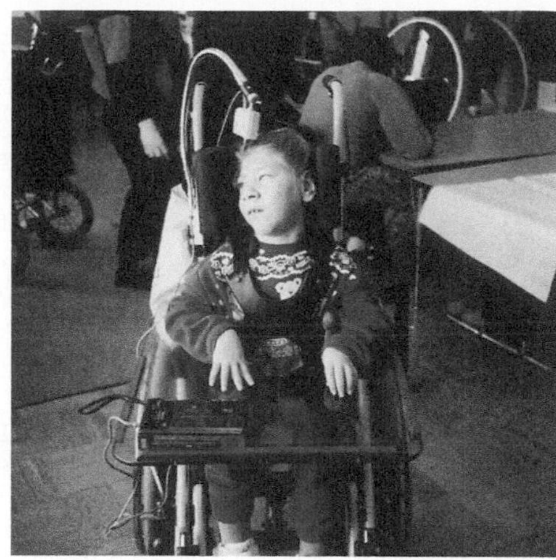

FIG. 20.5 A child with cognitive and physical impairments can activate electronic and communication equipment by moving a device near her head.

with Down syndrome (discussed later in this chapter). These children often have greater success in individual and dual sports than in team sports and enjoy themselves most with children of the same developmental level. The Special Olympics* provides these children with a unique competitive opportunity.

Safety is a major consideration in selecting recreational and exercise activities. For example, toys that may be appropriate developmentally may present dangers to a child who is strong enough to break them or use them incorrectly.

Provide Means of Communication

Verbal skills are typically delayed more than other physical skills. Speech requires adequate hearing and interpretation (receptive skills) and facial muscle coordination (expressive skills). Because both receptive and expressive skills may be impaired, these children need frequent audiometric testing and should be fitted with hearing aids if indicated. In addition, they may need help in learning to control their facial muscles. For example, some children may need tongue exercises to correct the tongue thrust or gentle reminders to keep the lips closed.

Nonverbal communication may be appropriate for some of these children, and various devices are available. For children with physical limitations, several adaptations or types of communication devices are available to facilitate selection of the appropriate picture or word (Fig. 20.5). Some children may be taught sign language or Blissymbols—a highly stylized system of graphic symbols representing words, ideas, and concepts. Although the symbols require education to learn their meaning, no reading skill is required. The symbols are typically arranged on a board, and the person points or uses some type of selector to convey a message.

*1133 19th St. NW, Washington, DC 20036; 800-700-8585 or 202-628-3630; http://www.specialolympics.org; info@specialolympics.org (website includes listing of state offices and 170 countries); http://www.facebook.com>Places>Washington, District of Columbia; twitter.com/SpecialOlympics. In Canada: Special Olympics Canada, 21 St. Clair Ave. E, Suite 600, Toronto, ON M4T 1L9; 416-927-9050 ext. 4388; 888-888-0608; http://www.specialolympics.ca.

Establish Discipline

Discipline must begin early. Limit-setting measures need to be simple, consistently applied, and appropriate for the child's mental age. Control measures are based primarily on teaching a specific behavior rather than on understanding the reasons behind it. Stressing moral lessons is of little value to a child who lacks the cognitive skills to learn from self-criticism or evaluation of previous mistakes. Behavior modification, especially reinforcement of desired actions, and use of time-out procedures are appropriate forms of behavior control.

Encourage Socialization

Acquiring social skills is a complex task, as is learning self-care procedures. Active rehearsals with role-playing and practice sessions and positive reinforcement for desired behavior have been the most successful approaches. Parents should be encouraged early to teach their child socially acceptable behavior: waving goodbye, saying "hello" and "thank you," responding to his or her name, greeting visitors, and sitting modestly. The teaching of socially acceptable sexual behavior is especially important to minimize sexual exploitation. Parents also need to expose the child to strangers so that he or she can practice manners because there is no automatic transfer of learning from one situation to another.

Dressing and grooming are also important aspects of self-esteem and social acceptance. Clothes should be clean, age appropriate, and well fitted with self-adhering fasteners and elastic openings to facilitate self-dressing.

Opportunities for social interaction and infant stimulation programs should began at an early age. As soon as possible, parents should enroll their child in early intervention or other appropriate preschool programs. Not only do these programs provide education and training, but they also offer an opportunity for social interaction with other children and adults. As children grow older, they should have peer experiences similar to those of other children, including group outings, sports, and organized activities, such as scouts and Special Olympics. Nurses should assess the child's abilities and encourage others (e.g., parents, teachers) to promote developmentally appropriate peer interaction, such as classroom and school activities, dance classes, clubs, vacations and family outings (Bull & Committee on Genetics, 2011; National Down Syndrome Society, 2012b; Sanchack & Thomas, 2016; Shapiro & Batshaw, 2016).

Provide Information on Sexuality

Adolescence may be a particularly difficult time for parents, especially in terms of the child's sexual behavior, possibility of pregnancy, future plans to marry, and ability to be independent. Frequently, minimal anticipatory guidance has been offered parents to prepare the child for physical and sexual maturation. The nurse should help in this area by providing parents with information about sexuality education that is geared to the child's developmental level. For example, adolescent girls need a *simple* explanation of menstruation and instructions on personal hygiene during the menstrual cycle.

These adolescents also need practical sexual information regarding anatomy, physical development, and conception.* Because they are easy to persuade and lack judgment, they need a well-defined, concrete code of conduct with specific instructions for handling certain situations. The subtleties of social sexual behavior are less beneficial than specific instructions for handling certain situations. For example, an adolescent should be firmly told never to go alone anywhere with any person that he or she does not know well. To protect the child or adolescent from sexual abuse, parents must closely observe their child's or adolescent's activities and associates. The question of contraceptive protection for these adolescents is often a parental concern (Quint, O'Brien, Committee on Adolescence, et al., 2016).

Parents of these adolescents are often concerned about the advisability of marriage between two individuals with significant CI. There is no conclusive answer; each situation must be judged individually. In some instances, marriage is possible. The nurse should discuss this topic with parents and with the prospective couple, stressing suitable living accommodations and contraceptive methods to prevent pregnancy. If children are conceived, these parents require specialized assistance in learning to meet the needs of their offspring (Bull & Committee on Genetics, 2011; Shea, 2012).

Help Family Adjust to Future Care

Not all families are able to cope with home care of children who are cognitively impaired, especially those who have severe or profound CI or multiple disabilities. Older parents may not be able to continue care responsibilities after they reach retirement or older age. The decision regarding residential placement is a difficult one for families, and the availability of such facilities varies widely. The nurse's role includes assisting parents in investigating and evaluating programs and helping parents adjust to the decision for placement.

Care for the Child During Hospitalization

Caring for the child during hospitalization can be a special challenge. Frequently, nurses are unfamiliar with children who are cognitively impaired, and they may cope with their feelings of insecurity and fear by ignoring or isolating the child. Not only is this approach nonsupportive; it may also be destructive to the child's sense of self-esteem and optimum development, and it may impair the parents' ability to cope with the stress of the experience. To prevent engaging in this nontherapeutic approach, nurses are to use the mutual participation model in planning the child's care. Parents should stay with their child but not be made to feel as if the responsibility is totally theirs.

When the child is admitted, a detailed history is taken (see Chapter 21), with special focus on all self-care abilities. Questions about the child's abilities are approached positively. For example, rather than asking, "Is your child toilet trained yet?" the nurse may state, "Tell me about your child's toileting habits." The assessment should also focus on any special devices that the child uses, effective measures of limit setting, unusual or favorite routines, and any behaviors that may require intervention. If the parent states that the child engages in self-stimulatory or self-injurious activities (e.g., head banging, self-biting), the nurse should inquire about events that precipitate them and techniques (e.g., distraction, medication) that the parents use to manage them (Morano, Ruiz, Hwang, et al., 2017; Oliver & Richards, 2010).

The nurse also assesses the child's functional level of eating and playing; ability to express needs verbally; progress in toilet training; and relationship with objects, toys, and other children. The child is encouraged to be as independent as possible in the hospital.

Realizing that the child may be lonely in the hospital, the nurse makes certain that toys and other activities are provided. The child is placed in a room with other children of approximately the same developmental age, preferably a room with only two beds to avoid overstimulation. The nurse should treat the child with dignity and respect in a manner that promotes acceptance and understanding by

---

*Sources of information on sexuality and conception include Planned Parenthood Federation of America, 123 William St., New York, NY 10038; 212-541-7800 or 800-230-7526; http://www.plannedparenthood.org; http://www.facebook.com/PlannedParenthood/

other children, parents, and those with whom the child comes into contact in the hospital.

Explain procedures to the child using methods of communication that are at the appropriate cognitive level. Generally, explanations should be simple, short, and concrete, emphasizing what the child will physically experience. Demonstration either through actual practice or with visual aids is always preferable to verbal explanation. Include parents in preprocedural teaching to aid in the child's learning and to help the nurse learn effective methods of communicating with the child.

During hospitalization, the nurse should also focus on growth-promoting experiences for the child. For example, hospitalization may be an excellent opportunity to emphasize to parents abilities that the child does have but has not had the opportunity to practice, such as self-dressing. It may also be an opportunity for social experiences with peers, group play, or new educational and recreational activities. For example, one child who had the habit of screaming and kicking demonstrated a definite decrease in those behaviors after he learned to pound pegs and use a punching bag. Through social services, the parents may become aware of specialized programs for the child. Hospitalization may also offer parents a respite from everyday care responsibilities and an opportunity to discuss their feelings with a concerned professional.

Assist in Measures to Prevent Cognitive Impairment

Besides having a responsibility to families with a child with CI, nurses also need to be involved in programs aimed at preventing CI. Many of the familial, social, and environmental factors known to cause mild impairment are preventable. Counseling and education can reduce or eliminate such factors (e.g., poor nutrition, cigarette smoking, chemical abuse), which increase the risk of prematurity and intrauterine growth restriction. Interventions are directed toward improving maternal health by educating women regarding the dangers of chemicals, including prenatal alcohol exposure, which affects organogenesis, craniofacial development, and cognitive ability. Other preventive strategies that play an important role include adequate prenatal care; optimal medical care of high-risk newborns; rubella immunization; genetic counseling; and prenatal screening, especially in terms of Down syndrome or FXS. The use of folic acid supplements prevents neural tube defects during pregnancy and during the childbearing years; the use of newborn screening for treatable inborn errors of metabolism (e.g., congenital hypothyroidism, phenylketonuria, and galactosemia) is appropriate to prevent developmental disabilities in children.

DOWN SYNDROME

Down syndrome is the most common chromosomal abnormality of a generalized syndrome, occurring from 1 in 691 to 733 live births in the United States (Lee, 2016; Weijerman & de Winter, 2010). It occurs in people of all races and economic levels.

Etiology

The cause of Down syndrome is not known, but evidence from cytogenetic and epidemiologic studies supports the concept of multiple causality. Although the cause is unclear, the cytogenetics of the disorder is well established. In most cases, Down syndrome is attributable to an extra chromosome 21 (group G), hence the name nonfamilial trisomy 21. Although children with trisomy 21 are born to parents of all ages, there is a statistically greater risk in older women, particularly those older than 35 years of age. For example, in women 35 years old, the chance of conceiving a child with Down syndrome is about 1 in 350 live births; but in women 40 years old, it is about 1 in 100. However, the majority (approximately 80%) of infants with Down syndrome are born to women younger than 35 years old because younger women have higher fertility rates (Arumugam, Raja, Venugopalan, et al., 2016; Lee, 2016; National Down Syndrome Society, 2012c). About 4% of the cases may be caused by translocation of chromosomes 15 and 21 or 22. This type of genetic aberration is usually hereditary and is not associated with advanced parental age. About 2% to 4% of affected persons demonstrate mosaicism, which refers to a mixture of normal and abnormal chromosomes in the cells. The degree of cognitive and physical impairment has been related to the percentage of cells with the abnormal chromosome makeup. However, numerous other interacting factors are likely to contribute to individual differences and cognitive-level outcomes in Down syndrome, such as early neural development, dietary factors, lifestyle, and the environment (Coppede, 2016; Karmiloff-Smith, Al-Janabi, D'Souza, et al., 2016).

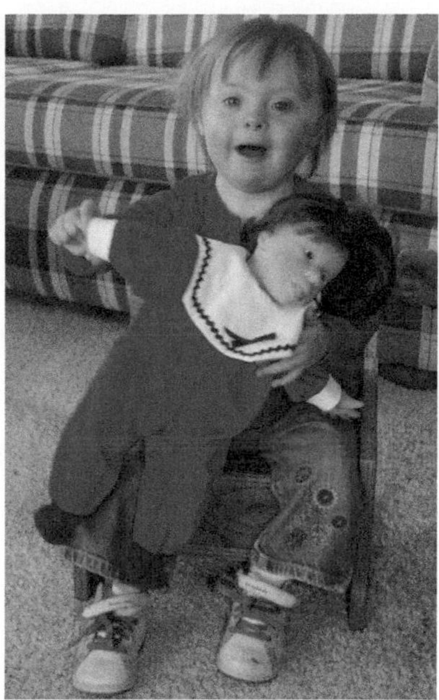

FIG. 20.6 A young child with Down syndrome holding a doll with Down syndrome.

Diagnostic Evaluation

Down syndrome can usually be diagnosed by the clinical manifestations alone (Box 20.2 and Fig. 20.6), but a chromosome analysis should be done to confirm the genetic abnormality.

Several physical problems are associated with Down syndrome. Many of these children have congenital heart malformations, the most common being septal defects. Respiratory tract infections are prevalent and, when combined with cardiac anomalies, are the chief causes of death, particularly during the first year of life. Hypotonicity of chest and abdominal muscles and dysfunction of the immune system probably predispose the child to the development of respiratory tract infection. Other physical problems include thyroid dysfunction, especially congenital hypothyroidism, and an increased incidence of leukemia.

Therapeutic Management

Although no cure exists for Down syndrome, a number of therapies are advocated, such as surgery to correct serious congenital anomalies (e.g., heart defects, strabismus). These children also benefit from evaluative echocardiography soon after birth and regular medical care. Evaluation of sight and hearing is essential, and treatment of otitis media is required to prevent auditory loss, which can influence cognitive function. Periodic testing of thyroid function is recommended, especially if growth is severely delayed.

BOX 20.2 Clinical Manifestations of Down Syndrome

Head and Eyes
Separated sagittal suture
Brachycephaly
Rounded and small skull
Flat occiput
Enlarged anterior fontanel
Oblique palpebral fissures (upward, outward slant)*
Inner epicanthal folds
Speckling of iris (Brushfield spots)

Nose and Ears
Small nose*
Depressed nasal bridge (saddle nose)*
Small ears and narrow canals
Short pinna (vertical ear length)
Overlapping upper helices
Conductive hearing loss

Mouth and Neck
High, arched, narrow palate*
Protruding tongue
Hypoplastic mandible
Delayed teeth eruption and microdontia
Alignment teeth abnormalities (common)
Periodontal disease
Neck skin excess and laxity*
Short and broad neck

Chest and Heart
Shortened rib cage
Twelfth rib anomalies
Pectus excavatum or carinatum
Congenital heart defects (common; e.g., atrial septal defect, ventricular septal defect)

Abdomen and Genitalia
Protruding, lax, and flabby abdominal muscles
Diastasis recti abdominis
Umbilical hernia
Small penis
Cryptorchidism
Bulbous vulva

Hands and Feet
Broad, short hands and stubby fingers
Incurved little finger (clinodactyly)
Transverse palmar crease
Wide space between big and second toes*
Plantar crease between big and second toes*
Broad, short feet and stubby toes

Musculoskeletal and Skin
Short stature
Hyperflexibility and muscle weakness*
Hypotonia
Atlantoaxial instability
Dry, cracked, and frequent fissuring
Cutis marmorata (mottling)

Other
Reduced birth weight
Learning difficulty (average intelligence quotient [IQ] of 50)
Hypothyroidism (common)
Impaired immune function
Increased risk of leukemia
Early-onset dementia (in one-third)

*Most common findings in modified chart (Arumugam, Raja, Venugopalan, et al., 2016; Pueschel, 1999).

About 15% of children with Down syndrome have atlantoaxial instability, but almost all of the children are asymptomatic. The American Academy of Pediatrics no longer recommends screening asymptomatic children with Down syndrome for atlantoaxial instability with cervical spine x-rays due to unproven value of detecting patients at risk of developing spinal cord compression injury (Bull & Committee on Genetics, 2011; National Down Syndrome Society, 2012d). However, the Special Olympics continues to require that all athletes with Down syndrome receive neck x-rays before sports participation because neck x-ray is the only screen available (Lee, 2016; National Down Syndrome Society, 2012d). Surveillance helps define the most appropriate level of physical activity and to identify the small subset of those with either progressive hyperlaxity or instability (O'Toole & Spiegel, 2016). However, recommendations for surveillance of the cervical spine in children with Down syndrome remain varied.

! NURSING ALERT

Immediately report any child with the following signs of spinal cord compression:

- Persistent neck pain
- Loss of established motor skills and bladder or bowel control
- Changes in sensation

Prognosis

Life expectancy for those with Down syndrome has improved in recent years but remains lower than for the general population. The majority of individuals with Down syndrome survive to approximately 60 years old and beyond (Englund, Jonsson, Zander, et al., 2013; National Down Syndrome Society, 2012e; Weijerman & de Winter, 2010). As the prognosis continues to improve for these individuals, it will be important to provide for their long-term health care and social and leisure needs.

Nursing Care Management

Support the Family at the Time of Diagnosis

Because of the unique physical characteristics, infants with Down syndrome are usually diagnosed at birth, and parents should be informed of the diagnosis at this time. Most parents usually prefer that both of them be present during the informing interview so that they can support one another emotionally. Parents appreciate receiving reading material about the syndrome* and being referred to parent groups and/or professional counseling.

*For the ARC and National Down Syndrome Society contact information, see the footnotes earlier in this chapter.

Parental responses to the child may greatly influence decisions regarding future care. Whereas some families willingly take the child home, others consider foster care or adoption. The nurse must answer questions regarding developmental potential carefully because the responses may influence the parents' decision. The nurse should share the available informative sources (e.g., parent groups, professional counseling, and literature) to help the family learn about Down syndrome (see Critical Thinking Case Study box).

CRITICAL THINKING CASE STUDY

Diagnosis of Down Syndrome

The parents of Melissa, a newborn diagnosed as having Down syndrome, ask the nurse, "What are we supposed to do with her?" They further state that they already have three other children at home.

1. What evidence should you consider regarding this condition?
2. What additional information is required at this time?
3. List the nursing intervention(s) that have the highest priority.
4. Identify important patient-centered outcomes with reference to your nursing interventions.

Answers are available at http://evolve.elsevier.com/wong/ncic.

Assist the Family in Preventing Physical Problems

Many of the physical characteristics of infants with Down syndrome present challenges and nursing problems. The hypotonicity of muscles and hyperextensibility of joints complicate positioning. The limp, flaccid extremities resemble the posture of a rag doll; as a result, holding the infant is difficult and cumbersome. Sometimes parents perceive this lack of the infant's molding to their bodies as evidence of inadequate parenting. The extended body position promotes heat loss because more surface area is exposed to the environment. Encourage the parents to swaddle or wrap the infant snugly in a blanket before picking up the child to provide security and warmth. The nurse also discusses with parents their feelings concerning attachment to the child, emphasizing that the child's lack of clinging or molding is a physical characteristic and not a sign of detachment or rejection.

Decreased muscle tone compromises respiratory expansion. In addition, the underdeveloped nasal bone causes a chronic problem of inadequate drainage of mucus. The constant stuffy nose forces the child to breathe by mouth, which dries the oropharyngeal membranes, increasing the susceptibility to upper respiratory tract infections. Measures to lessen these problems include clearing the nose with a bulb-type syringe, rinsing the mouth with water after feedings, increasing fluid intake, and using a cool-mist vaporizer to keep the mucous membranes moist and the secretions liquefied. Other helpful measures include changing the child's position frequently, practicing good hand washing, and properly disposing of soiled articles, such as tissues. If antibiotics are ordered, the nurse stresses the importance of completing the full course of therapy for successful eradication of the infection and prevention of growth of resistant organisms.

Inadequate drainage resulting in pooling of mucus in the nose also interferes with feeding. Because the child breathes by mouth, sucking for any length of time is difficult. When eating solids, the child may gag on the food because of mucus in the oropharynx. Parents are advised to clear the nose before each feeding; give small, frequent feedings; and allow opportunities for rest during mealtime.

The protruding tongue also interferes with feeding, especially of solid foods. Parents need to know that the tongue thrust is not an indication of refusal to feed but a physiologic response. Parents are advised to use a small but long, straight-handled spoon to push the food toward the back and side of the mouth. If food is thrust out, it should be refed.

Dietary intake needs supervision. Decreased muscle tone affects gastric motility, predisposing the child to constipation. Dietary measures, such as increased fiber and fluid, promote evacuation. The child's eating habits may need careful scrutiny to prevent obesity. Height and weight measurements should be obtained on a serial basis. Because the previously used Down syndrome–specific growth charts no longer reflected the current population styles and body proportions, new growth charts were developed to provide indications of how growth of an individual child compares with peers of the same age and sex with Down syndrome (Centers for Disease Control and Prevention, 2016a; Zemel, Pipan, Stallings, et al., 2015).

During infancy, the child's skin is pliable and soft. However, it gradually becomes rough and dry and is prone to cracking and infection. Skin care involves the use of minimum soap and application of lubricants. Lip balm is applied to the lips, especially when the child is outdoors, to prevent excessive chapping.

Assist in Prenatal Diagnosis and Genetic Counseling

Prenatal diagnosis of Down syndrome is possible through chorionic villus sampling and amniocentesis because chromosome analysis of fetal cells can detect the presence of trisomy or translocation. However, advances in development of noninvasive prenatal testing have resulted in a measurement of cell-free deoxyribonucleic acid (DNA) from the plasma of pregnant women, detecting nearly all cases of Down syndrome (Huang, Zheng, Chen, et al., 2014; Lee, 2016; Lewis, Hill, Silcock, et al., 2014; Liao, Chan, Jiang, et al., 2012).

Prenatal testing with genetic counseling should be offered to all women, including those of advanced maternal age (greater than 35 years) and those of younger age (less than 35 years) because most children with Down syndrome are born to younger mothers due to their higher overall birth rate (Lee, 2016). If prenatal testing indicates that the fetus is affected, the nurse must allow the parents to express their feelings concerning elective abortion and support their decision to terminate or proceed with the pregnancy. It is important for nurses to be aware of their own attitudes regarding testing and related decisions.

FRAGILE X SYNDROME

FXS is the most common inherited cause of CI and the second most common genetic cause of CI or intellectual disability after Down syndrome. It has been described in all ethnic groups and races; the incidence of affected boys is 1 in 3600 to 4000, the incidence of affected girls is 1 in 4000 to 6000, the incidence of carrier girls is 1 in 151, and the incidence of carrier boys is 1 in 468 worldwide (Mink, 2016; National Fragile X Foundation, 2017a).

The syndrome is caused by an abnormal gene on the lower end of the long arm of the X chromosome. Chromosome analysis may demonstrate a fragile site (a region that fails to condense during mitosis and is characterized by a nonstaining gap or narrowing) in the cells of affected males and females and in carrier females. This fragile site has been determined to be caused by a gene mutation that results in excessive repeats of nucleotide in a specific DNA segment of the X chromosome. The number of repeats in a normal individual is between 6 and 50. An individual with 50 to 200 base-pair repeats is said to have a permutation and is therefore a carrier. When passed from a parent to a child, these base-pair repeats can expand from 200 or more, which is termed a *full mutation.* This expansion occurs only when a carrier mother passes the mutation to her offspring; it does not occur when a carrier father passes the mutation to his daughters.

The inheritance pattern has been termed X-linked dominant with reduced penetrance. This is in distinct contrast to the classic X-linked recessive pattern in which all carrier females are normal, all affected males have symptoms of the disorder, and no males are carriers. Consequently, genetic counseling of affected families is more complex than that for families with a classic X-linked disorder, such as hemophilia. Both affected sexes are capable of transmitting the fragile X disorder. Prenatal diagnosis of the fragile X gene mutation is possible with direct DNA testing in a family with an established history using amniocentesis or chorionic villus sampling (Finucane, Lincoln, Bailey, et al., 2017; National Fragile X Foundation, 2017b). The FMR1 mutation testing is highly accurate and is being researched regarding the incorporation into the newborn universal screening program (Abrams, Cronister, Brown, et al., 2012; Bagni, Tassone, Neri, et al., 2012; Finucane, Abrams, Cronister, et al., 2012; Sorensen, Gane, Yarborough, et al., 2013). A systematic review of screening technologies found appropriate methods to screen larger populations of males and females at low cost so that early interventions may help prevent or delay the disability of fragile X (Lyons, Kerr, & Mueller, 2015).

Clinical Manifestations

The classic trend of physical findings in adult men with FXS consists of a long face with a prominent jaw (prognathism); large, protruding ears; and large testes (macroorchidism). In prepubertal children, however, these features may be less obvious, and behavioral manifestations may initially suggest the diagnosis (Box 20.3). In carrier females, the clinical manifestations are extremely varied.

Therapeutic Management

FXS has no cure. Medical treatment may include the use of serotonin agents, such as carbamazepine (Tegretol) or fluoxetine (Prozac), to control violent temper outbursts and the use of central nervous system stimulants or clonidine (Catapres) to improve attention span and decrease hyperactivity. Two possible treatments of FXS being investigated are reactivation of the affected gene and protein replacement (Bagni, Tassone, Neri, et al., 2012; Kuehn, 2011).

All affected children require referral to early intervention program that include speech and language therapy, occupational therapy, and special education assistance. A multidisciplinary assessment of common medical problems associated with FXS such as cardiac, neurologic, and orthopedic anomalies and gastrointestinal problems is imperative to improve comprehensive care that may lead to better quality of life for these patients and their families (Kidd, Lachiewicz, Barbouth, et al., 2014).

BOX 20.3 Clinical Manifestations of Fragile X Syndrome

Physical Features

Increased head circumference
Long, wide, or protruding ears
Long, narrow face with prominent jaw
Strabismus
Mitral valve prolapse, aortic root dilation
Hypotonia
In postpubertal males, enlarged testicles

Behavioral Features

Mild to severe cognitive impairment
Speech delay; may be rapid speech with stuttering and word repetition
Short attention span, hyperactivity
Hypersensitivity to taste, sounds, touch
Intolerance to change in routine
Autistic-like behaviors, such as social anxiety and gaze aversion
Possible aggressive behavior

Prognosis

Individuals with FXS are expected to live a normal life span. Their CI may be improved by behavioral and educational interventions that usually begin in preschool-age children.

Nursing Care Management

Because CI is a fairly consistent finding in individuals with FXS, the care given to these families is the same as for any child with intellectual disability. Because the disorder is hereditary, genetic counseling is important to inform parents and siblings of the risks of transmission. In addition, any male or female with unexplained or nonspecific mental impairment should be referred for genetic testing and, if needed, counseling. Families with a member affected by the disorder should be referred to the National Fragile X Foundation.*

SENSORY IMPAIRMENT

HEARING IMPAIRMENT

Hearing impairment is one of the most common disabilities in the United States. An estimated 1 to 6 per 1000 well infants have hearing loss of varying degrees (American Academy of Pediatrics, 2017; Grindle, 2014). For infants admitted to neonatal intensive care units, the incidence rises sharply to approximately 2 to 4 per 100 neonates (American Academy of Pediatrics, Joint Committee on Infant Hearing, 2007; Almadhoob & Ohlsson, 2015; Colella-Santos, Hein, de Souza, et al., 2014). In the United States there are about 1 million children with hearing impairment ranging in age from birth to 21 years old, and almost one-third of these children have other disabilities, such as visual or cognitive deficits.

Definition and Classification

Hearing impairment is a general term indicating disability that may range in severity from slight to profound hearing loss. *Slight to moderately severe hearing loss* describes a person who has residual hearing sufficient to enable successful processing of linguistic information through audition, generally with the use of a hearing aid. *Severe to profound hearing loss* describes a person whose hearing disability precludes successful processing of linguistic information through audition with or without a hearing aid. Hearing-impaired persons who are speech impaired tend not to have a physical speech defect other than that caused by the inability to hear.

Hearing defects may be classified according to etiology, pathology, or symptom severity. Each is important in terms of treatment, possible prevention, and rehabilitation.

Etiology

Hearing loss may be caused by a number of prenatal and postnatal conditions. These may include a family history of childhood hearing impairment, anatomic malformations of the head or neck, low birth weight, severe perinatal asphyxia, perinatal infection (cytomegalovirus,

*2100 M St. NW, Ste. 170, PO Box 302, Washington, DC 20037-1233; 800-688-8765; fax: 202-747-6208; http://www.fragilex.org; email: natlfx@fragilex.org; http://www.facebook.com/natlfragilex; twitter.com/FragileXnews.

rubella, herpes, syphilis, toxoplasmosis, bacterial meningitis), maternal prenatal substance abuse, chronic ear infection, cerebral palsy, Down syndrome, prolonged neonatal oxygen supplementation, or administration of ototoxic drugs (Colella-Santos, Hein, de Souza, et al., 2014; Gan, Rowe, Benton, et al., 2016; Haddad & Keesecker, 2016; Singh, 2015).

In addition, high-risk neonates who survive the once fatal prenatal or perinatal conditions may be susceptible to hearing loss from the disorder or its treatment. For example, sensorineural hearing loss may be a result of continuous humming noises or high noise levels associated with incubators, oxygen hoods, or intensive care units, especially when combined with the use of potentially ototoxic antibiotics.

Environmental noise is a special concern. Sounds loud enough to damage sensitive hair cells of the inner ear can produce irreversible hearing loss. Very loud, brief noise (e.g., gunfire) can cause immediate, severe, and permanent loss of hearing. Longer exposure to less intense but still hazardous sounds (e.g., loud persistent music via headphones, sound systems, concerts, or industrial noises) may also produce hearing loss (Biassoni, Serra, Hinalaf, et al., 2014; Carroll, Eichwald, Scinicariello, et al., 2017; Centers for Disease Control and Prevention, 2016b; Guest, Munro, Prendergast, et al., 2017; Liberman & Kujawa, 2017; Pawlaczyk-Luszczynska, Zamojska-Daniszewska, Dudarewicz, et al., 2017). Hearing loss caused by toxic substances (e.g., smoking or secondhand smoke) or when combined with loud noises, tends to produce a synergistic effect on hearing that causes hearing dysfunction (Fabry, Davila, Arheart, et al., 2011; Talaat, Metwaly, Khafagy, et al., 2014).

TABLE 20.2 Classification of Hearing Impairment Based on Symptom Severity

Hearing Level (dB)	Effect
Slight: 16-25	Has difficulty hearing faint or distant speech Usually is unaware of hearing difficulty Likely to achieve in school but may have problems No speech defects
Mild to moderate: 26-55	May have speech difficulties Understands face-to-face conversational speech at 0.9-1.5 m (3-5 ft)
Moderately severe: 56-70	Unable to understand conversational speech unless loud Considerable difficulty with group or classroom discussion Requires special speech training
Severe: 71-90	May hear a loud voice if nearby May be able to identify loud environmental noises Can distinguish vowels but not most consonants Requires speech training
Profound: 91	May hear only loud sounds Requires extensive speech training

dB, Decibels.

Pathology

Disorders of hearing are divided according to the location of the defect. Conductive or middle-ear hearing loss results from interference of transmission of sound to the middle ear. It is the most common of all types of hearing loss and most frequently a result of recurrent serous otitis media. Conductive hearing impairment involves mainly interference with loudness of sound.

Sensorineural hearing loss involves damage to the inner ear structures or the auditory nerve. The most common causes are congenital defects of inner ear structures or consequences of acquired conditions, such as kernicterus, infection, administration of ototoxic drugs, or exposure to excessive noise. Sensorineural hearing loss results in distortion of sound and problems in discrimination. Although the child hears some of everything going on around him or her, the sounds are distorted, severely affecting discrimination and comprehension.

Mixed conductive-sensorineural hearing loss results from interference with transmission of sound in the middle ear and along neural pathways. It frequently results from recurrent otitis media and its complications.

Central auditory imperception includes all hearing losses that are not linked to defects in the conductive or sensorineural structures. They are usually divided into organic or functional losses. In the organic type of central auditory imperception, the defect involves the reception of auditory stimuli along the central pathways and the expression of the message into meaningful communication. Examples are aphasia, the inability to express ideas in any form, either written or verbal; agnosia, the inability to interpret sound correctly; and dysacusis, difficulty in processing details or discriminating among sounds. In the functional type of hearing loss, no organic lesion exists to explain a central auditory loss. Examples of functional hearing loss are conversion hysteria (an unconscious withdrawal from hearing to block remembrance of a traumatic event), infantile autism, and childhood schizophrenia.

Symptom Severity

Hearing impairment is expressed in terms of a decibel (dB), a unit of loudness (see Table 20.1). Hearing is measured at various frequencies, such as 500, 1000, and 2000 cycles/second, the critical listening speech range. Hearing impairment can be classified according to hearing threshold level (the measurement of an individual's hearing threshold by means of an audiometer) and the degree of symptom severity as it affects speech (Table 20.2). These classifications offer only general guidelines regarding the effect of the impairment on any individual child because children differ greatly in their ability to use residual hearing.

Therapeutic Management

Conductive Hearing Loss

Treatment of hearing loss depends on the cause and type of hearing impairment. Many conductive hearing defects respond to medical or surgical treatment, such as antibiotic therapy for acute otitis media or insertion of tympanostomy tubes for chronic otitis media. When the conductive loss is permanent, hearing can be improved with the use of a hearing aid to amplify sound.

The nurse should be familiar with the types, basic care, and handling of hearing aids, especially when the child is hospitalized.* Types of aids include those worn in or behind the ear, models incorporated into an eyeglass frame, and types worn on the body with a wire connection to the ear (Fig. 20.7). One of the most common problems with a hearing aid is acoustic feedback, an annoying whistling sound usually caused by improper fit of the ear mold. Sometimes the whistling may be at a frequency that the child cannot hear but that is annoying to others. In this case, if children are old enough, they are told of the noise and asked to readjust the aid.

As children grow older, they may be self-conscious about the device. Efforts may be made to make the aid inconspicuous, such as styling the hair to cover behind-the-ear aids or the use of in-the-ear or miniature digital models, or encourage the use of attractive frames for glasses

*Information about hearing aids is available from the International Hearing Society, 16880 Middlebelt Road, Suite 4, Livonia, MI 48154; 800-521-5247 or 734-522-7200; http://www.ihsinfo.org; http://www.facebook.com/ihsinfo; twitter.com/IHSinfo.

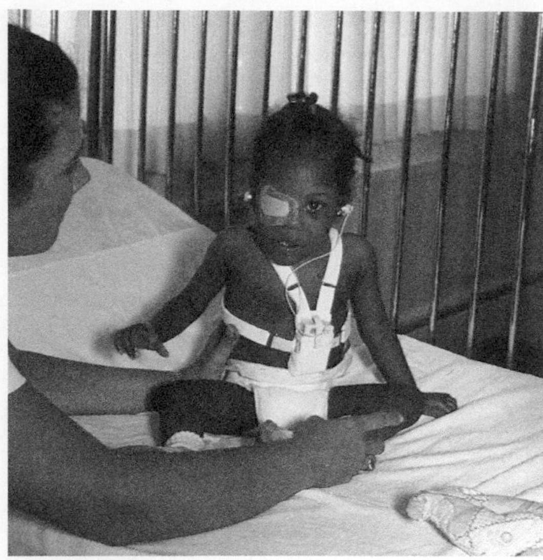

FIG. 20.7 On-the-body hearing aids are convenient for young children, such as this child with severe bilateral hearing loss. Note eye patching for strabismus.

> **! NURSING ALERT**
>
> To reduce or eliminate whistling from a hearing aid, try removing and reinserting the aid, making certain that no hair is caught between the ear mold and the ear canal; cleaning the ear mold or ear; or lowering the volume of the aid.

with connected hearing aids. Give children responsibility for the care of the device as soon as they are able because fostering independence is a primary goal of rehabilitation.

> **! NURSING ALERT**
>
> Stress to parents the importance of storing batteries for hearing aids in a safe location out of reach of children and teaching children not to remove the battery from the hearing aid (or supervising young children when they do so). Battery ingestion requires immediate emergency management.

Sensorineural Hearing Loss

The treatment aim for sensorineural hearing loss is to improve hearing and communication with hearing aids or cochlear implants. Sensorineural hearing loss has been associated with damaged auditory hair cells or nerve fibers or abnormal development of the inner ear structures. Because conventional hearing aids only amplify sound that may not be processed by a damaged inner ear, some children may not benefit from hearing aids and require a referral for a cochlear implant. A cochlear implant bypasses the hair cells to directly stimulate surviving auditory nerve fibers so that they can send signals to the brain. These signals can be interpreted by the brain to produce sound and sensations (Easwar, Yamazaki, Deighton, et al., 2017; Gan, Rowe, Benton, et al., 2016; Grindle, 2014). The cochlear implant* consists of an internal surgically implanted prosthetic device (receiver and electrode array) and external device (microphone, speech processor, and transmitter coil) (Gan, Rowe, Benton, et al., 2016). The cochlear implant provides a sensation of hearing for individuals who have severe or profound hearing loss (Farinetti, Gharbia, Mancini, et al., 2014; Lantos, 2012; Pettinato, De Clerck, Verhoeven, et al., 2017).

Multichanneled implants are sophisticated devices that stimulate the auditory nerve at a number of locations with differently processed signals. This type of stimulation allows a person to use the pitch information present in speech signals, leading to better understanding of speech. The trend is toward early use of cochlear implants, usually by 12 months old, to give the child maximum opportunity to develop listening, language, and speaking skills.

The cochlear implantation is a safe hearing surgical technique associated with a low complication rate. A reported global complication rate comprised minor complications that were mainly infectious in children (acute otitis media) and cochleovestibular in adults (tinnitus and vetigo) and major complications, including mostly reimplantation after revision surgery or device failure (Farinetti, Gharbia, Mancini, et al., 2014). However, cases of meningitis, particularly pneumococcal meningitis, have been reported. Therefore it has been recommended that all children receiving a cochlear implant must be vaccinated with the pneumococcal polyvalent vaccine (Haddad & Keesecker, 2016).

Nursing Care Management

Assess for Hearing Concerns

Assessment of children for hearing impairment is a critical nursing responsibility. Identification of hearing loss before the first 3 months of age with intervention no later than 6 months old is essential to improve the language and educational development for children with hearing impairments (Lammers, Jansen, Grolman, et al., 2015; Rohlfs, Friedhoff, Bohnert, et al., 2017; World Health Organization, 2012). The Joint Committee on Infant Hearing issued guidelines on auditory screening of newborns and infants to detect early hearing loss and implement intervention programs (American Academy of Pediatrics, 2017; American Academy of Pediatrics, Joint Committee on Infant Hearing, 2007; Joint Committee on Infant Hearing of the American Academy of Pediatrics, Muse, Harrison, et al., 2013). Auditory testing is presented in Chapter 4.

At birth, the nurse can observe the neonate's response to auditory stimuli, as evidenced by the startle reflex, head turning, eye blinking, and cessation of body movement. The infant may vary in the intensity of the response, depending on the state of alertness. However, a consistent absence of a reaction should lead to suspicion of hearing loss. Box 20.4 summarizes other clinical manifestations of hearing impairment in infants.

Children who are profoundly hearing impaired are much more likely to be diagnosed during infancy than the child who is less severely affected. If the defect is not detected during early childhood, it likely will become evident during entry into school, when the child has difficulty learning. Unfortunately, some of these children are erroneously placed in special classes for students with learning disabilities or CI. Therefore it is essential that the nurse suspect a hearing impairment in any child who demonstrates the behaviors listed in Box 20.4.

> **! NURSING ALERT**
>
> When parents express concern about their child's hearing and speech development, refer the child for a hearing evaluation. Absence of well-formed syllables *(da, na, yaya)* by 11 months old should result in immediate referral.

*Hearing Enrichment Language Program of the Hough Ear Institute as part INTEGRIS Baptist Medical Center Cochlear Implant Clinic, 3300 N.W. Expressway, Oklahoma City, OK 73112; 405-949-3011 or 888-951-2277; http://integrisok.com/baptist-medical-center-oklahoma-city-ok-services-hearing; facebook.com/integrishealthOK.

BOX 20.4 Clinical Manifestations of Hearing Impairment

Infants

Lack of startle or blink reflex to a loud sound
Failure to be awakened by loud environmental noises
Failure to localize a source of sound by 6 months old
Absence of babble or voice inflections by 7 months old
General indifference to sound
Lack of response to the spoken word; failure to follow verbal directions
Response to loud noises as opposed to the voice

Children

Use of gestures rather than verbalization to express desires, especially after 15 months old
Failure to develop intelligible speech by 24 months old
Monotone and unintelligible speech; lessened laughter
Vocal play, head banging, or foot stamping for vibratory sensation
Yelling or screeching to express pleasure, needs, or annoyance
Asking to have statements repeated or answering them incorrectly
Greater response to facial expression and gestures than to verbal explanation
Avoidance of social interaction; prefer to play alone
Inquiring, sometimes confused facial expression
Suspicious alertness alternating with cooperation
Frequent stubbornness because of lack of comprehension
Irritability at not making themselves understood
Shy, timid, and withdrawn behavior
Frequent appearance of being "in a world of their own" or markedly inattentive

During early childhood, the primary importance of hearing impairment is the effect on speech development. A child with a mild conductive hearing loss may speak fairly clearly but in a loud, monotone voice. A child with a sensorineural defect usually has difficulty in articulation. Communication may be difficult, leading to frustration when words are not understood. For example, an inability to hear higher frequencies may result in the word *spoon* being pronounced "poon." Children with articulation problems need to have their hearing tested.

Lipreading. Although the child may become an expert at lipreading, only about 40% of the spoken word is understood, less if the speaker has an accent, mustache, or beard. Exaggerating pronunciation or speaking in an altered rhythm further lessens comprehension. Parents can help the child understand the spoken word by using the suggestions in the Nursing Care Guidelines box. The child learns to supplement the spoken word with sensitivity to visual cues, primarily body language and facial expression (e.g., tightening the lips, muscle tension, eye contact).

Cued speech. The cued speech method of communication is an adjunct to straight lipreading. It uses hand signals to help the hearing-impaired child distinguish between words that look alike when formed by the lips (e.g., mat, bat). It is most commonly employed by hearing-impaired children who are using speech rather than those who are nonverbal.

Sign language. Sign language, such as American Sign Language (ASL) or British Sign Language (BSL), is a visual-gestural language that uses hand signals that roughly correspond to specific words and concepts in the English language. Encourage family members to learn signing because using or watching hands requires much less concentration than lipreading or talking. Also, a symbol method enables some hearing-impaired children to learn more and to learn faster.

Speech-language therapy. The most formidable task in the education of a child who is profoundly hearing impaired is learning to speak.

NURSING CARE GUIDELINES

Facilitating Lipreading

Attract child's attention before speaking; use light touch to signal speaker's presence.
Stand close to child.
Face child directly or move to a 45-degree angle.
Stand still; do not walk back and forth or turn away to point or look elsewhere.
Establish eye contact and show interest.
Speak at eye level and with good lighting on speaker's face.
Be certain nothing interferes with speech patterns, such as chewing food or gum.
Speak clearly and at a slow and even rate.
Use facial expression to assist in conveying messages.
Keep sentences short.
Rephrase message if child does not understand the words.

Speech is learned through a multisensory approach using visual, tactile, kinesthetic, and auditory stimulation. Encourage parents to participate fully in the learning process.

Additional aids. Everyday activities present problems for older children with hearing impairment. For example, they may not be able to hear the telephone, doorbell, or alarm clock. Several commercial devices are available to help them adjust to these dilemmas. Flashing lights can be attached to a telephone or doorbell to signal its ringing. Trained hearing ear dogs can provide great assistance because they alert the person to sounds, such as someone approaching, a moving car, a signal to wake up, or a child's cry. Special teletypewriters or telecommunications devices for the deaf (TDD or TTY) help hearing-impaired people communicate with each other over the telephone; the typed message is conveyed via the telephone lines and displayed on a small screen.*

Any audiovisual medium presents dilemmas for these children, who can see the picture but cannot hear the message. However, with closed captioning a special decoding device is attached to the television, and the audio portion of a program is translated into subtitles that appear on the screen.†

Socialization. Socialization is extremely important to children's development. If children attend a special school for the hearing impaired, they are able to socialize with peers in that setting. Classmates become a potential source of close friendships because they communicate more easily among themselves. Encourage parents to promote these relationships whenever possible.

---

*Resources and support network information are provided by the Alexander Graham Bell Association for the Deaf and Hard of Hearing, 3417 Volta Place NW, Washington, DC 20007; voice: 202-337-5220; TTY: 202-337-5221; http://www.agbell.org; fax: 202-337-8314; http://www.agbell.org; email: info@agbell.org; facebook.com>...>Washington,District of Columbia>Social Services; https://twitter.com/AGBellAssoc; and Canadian Hearing Society, 271 Spadina Road, Toronto, ON M5R 2V3; voice: 416-928-2500; TTY: 416-964-0023; fax: 416-928-2506; http://www.chs.ca; email: info@chs.ca; https://www.facebook.com>Places>Toronto,Ontario>Medical&Health.

†Additional information is available from the National Captioning Institute, 3725 Concord Pkwy., Suite 100, Chantilly, VA 20151; voice/TTY: 703-917-7600; http://www.ncicap.org.

Children with a hearing impairment may need special help with school or social activities. For children wearing hearing aids, keep background noise to a minimum. Because many of these children are able to attend regular classes, the teacher may need assistance in adapting methods of teaching for the child's benefit. The school nurse is often in an optimal position to emphasize methods of facilitated communication, such as lipreading (see Nursing Care Guidelines box). Because group projects and audiovisual teaching aids may hinder the hearing-impaired child's learning, carefully evaluate the use of these educational methods.

In a group setting, it is helpful for the other members to sit in a semicircle in front of the hearing-impaired child. Because one of the difficulties in following a group discussion is that the hearing-impaired child is unaware of who will speak next, someone should point out each speaker. Speakers can also be given numbers, or their names can be written down as each person talks. If one person writes down the main topic of the discussion, the child is able to follow lipreading more closely. Such practices can increase the child's ability to participate in sports, organizations such as Scouts, and group projects.

Support Child and Family

Once the diagnosis of hearing impairment is made, parents need extensive support to adjust to the shock of learning about their child's disability and an opportunity to realize the extent of the hearing loss. If the hearing loss occurs during childhood, the child also requires sensitive, supportive care during the long and often difficult adjustment to this sensory loss. Early rehabilitation is one of the best strategies for fostering adjustment. Progress in learning communication, however, may not always coincide with emotional adjustment. Depression or anger is common, and such feelings are a normal part of the grieving process.

Care for the Child During Hospitalization

The needs of the hospitalized child with impaired hearing are the same as those of any other child, but the disability presents special challenges to the nurse. For example, verbal explanations must be supplemented by tactile and visual aids, such as books or actual demonstration and practice. Children's understanding of the explanation needs to be constantly reassessed. If their verbal skills are poorly developed, they can answer questions through drawing, writing, or gesturing. For example, if the nurse is attempting to clarify where a spinal tap is done, ask the child to point to where the procedure will be done on the body. Because hearing-impaired children often need more time to grasp the full meaning of an explanation, the nurse needs to be patient, allowing ample time for understanding.

When communicating with the child, the nurse should use the same principles as those outlined for facilitating lipreading. Ideally, nurses without foreign accents should be assigned to the child. The child's hearing aid is checked to ensure that it is working properly. If it is necessary to awaken the child at night, the nurse should gently shake the child or turn on the hearing aid before arousing the child. The nurse should always make certain that the child can see him or her before any procedures, even routine ones such as changing a diaper or regulating an infusion. It is important to remember that the child may not be aware of the nurse's presence until alerted through visual or tactile cues.

Ideally, parents are encouraged to room with the child. However, the nurse must convey to them that this is not to serve as a convenience to the nurse but as a benefit to the child. Although the parents' aid can be enlisted in familiarizing the child with the hospital and explaining procedures, the nurse should also talk directly to the youngster, encouraging expression of feelings about the experience. If the child's speech is difficult to understand, try to become familiar with his or her pronunciation of words. Parents often can be helpful by explaining the child's usual speech habits. Nonverbal communication devices that use pictures or words that the child can point to are also available. The nurse can make boards by using pictures or writing the words on cardboard representing common needs, such as *parent, food, water,* or *toilet.*

The nurse has a special role as child advocate and is in a strategic position to alert other health team members and other patients to the child's special needs regarding communication. For example, the nurse should accompany other practitioners on visits to the child's room to ensure that they speak to the child and that the child understands what is said. Caregivers may forget that the child has the abilities to perceive and learn despite a hearing loss, and consequently they communicate only with the parents. As a result, the child's needs and feelings remain unrecognized and unaddressed.

Because children with impaired hearing may have difficulty forming social relationships with other children, introduced the child to roommates and encourage them to engage in play activities. The hospital setting can provide growth-promoting opportunities for social relationships. With the assistance of a child life specialist, the child can learn new recreational activities, experiment with group games, and engage in therapeutic play. Playing with puppets or dollhouses, role-playing with dress-up clothes, building with blocks or legos, finger painting, and water play can help the child express feelings that previously were suppressed.

Assist in Measures to Prevent Hearing Impairment

A primary nursing role is prevention of hearing loss. Because the most common cause of impaired hearing is chronic otitis media, it is essential that appropriate measures be instituted to treat existing infections and prevent recurrences. Children with a history of ear or respiratory infections or any other condition known to increase the risk of hearing impairment should receive periodic auditory testing.

To prevent the causes of hearing loss that begin prenatally and perinatally, pregnant women need counseling regarding the necessity of early prenatal care, including genetic counseling for known familial disorders; avoidance of all ototoxic drugs, especially during the first trimester; tests to rule out syphilis, rubella, or blood incompatibility; medical management of maternal diabetes; strict control of alcohol intake; adequate dietary intake; and avoidance of smoke exposure. Stress the necessity of routine immunization during childhood to eliminate the possibility of acquired sensorineural hearing loss from rubella, mumps, or measles (encephalitis).

Exposure to excessive noise pollution is a well-established cause of sensorineural hearing loss. The nurse should routinely assess the possibility of environmental noise pollution and advise children and parents of the potential danger. A recent randomized single-blind clinical trial supported the use of earplugs in preventing temporary hearing loss associated with loud music exposure (Ramakers, Kraaijenga, Cattani, et al., 2016). Therefore when individuals engage in activities associated with high-intensity noise (e.g., flying model airplanes, loud music, target shooting, or snowmobiling), they should protect their hearing by wearing ear protection devices, decreasing music volume, and limiting or avoiding exposure to loud sounds (Centers for Disease Control and Prevention, 2016b). Even common household equipment, such as lawn mowers, vacuum cleaners, and telephones, can be harmful.

> **! NURSING ALERT**
>
> Suspect hazardous noise if the listener experiences (1) difficulty in communication while hearing the sound, (2) ringing in the ears (tinnitus) after exposure to the sound, or (3) muffled hearing after leaving the sound.

VISUAL IMPAIRMENT

Visual impairment is a common problem during childhood. In the United States the prevalence of serious visual impairment in the pediatric population is estimated to be between 30 and 64 children per 100,000 population. Vision impairment such as refractive error, strabismus, and amblyopia occur in 5% to 10% of all preschoolers, who are usually identified through vision screening programs (Alley, 2013; American Academy of Pediatrics, 2016; Rahi, Cumberland, Peckham, et al., 2010; US Department of Health and Human Services, Office of Disease Prevention and Health Promotion, 2015; US Preventive Services Task Force, 2011). The nurse's role is one of assessment, detection, prevention, referral, and (in some instances) rehabilitation.

Definition and Classification

Visual impairment is a general term that encompasses both partial sight and legal blindness. *Partial sight* or *partial visual impairment* is defined as a visual acuity between 20/70 and 20/200. The child can generally use normal-sized print because near vision is almost always better than distance vision. *Legal blindness* or *severe permanent visual impairment* is defined as a visual acuity of 20/200 or lower or a visual field of 20 degrees or less in the better eye. It is important to keep in mind that legal blindness is not a medical diagnosis but a legal definition. Educational and governmental agencies in the United States use the legal definition of blindness to determine tax status, eligibility for entrance into special schools, eligibility for financial aid, and other benefits.

Etiology

Visual impairment can be caused by a number of genetic and prenatal or postnatal conditions. These include perinatal infections (herpes, chlamydia, gonococci, rubella, syphilis, toxoplasmosis); retinopathy of prematurity; trauma; postnatal infections (meningitis); and disorders, such as sickle cell disease, juvenile rheumatoid arthritis, Tay-Sachs disease, albinism, and retinoblastoma. In many instances, such as with refractive errors, the cause of the defect is unknown.

Refractive errors are the most common types of visual disorders in children. The term *refraction* means bending and refers to the bending of light rays as they pass through the lens of the eye. Normally, light rays enter the lens and fall directly on the retina. However, in refractive disorders, the light rays either fall in front of the retina (myopia) or beyond it (hyperopia). Other eye problems, such as strabismus, may or may not include refractive errors, but they are important because, if untreated, they result in severe permanent visual impairment from amblyopia. These, along with other less frequent visual disorders, are summarized in Box 20.5. In addition to these disorders, other visual problems can be a result of infection or trauma.

BOX 20.5 Types of Visual Impairment

Refractive Errors

Myopia

Nearsightedness: Ability to see objects clearly at close range but not at a distance

Pathophysiology

Results from eyeball that is too long, causing images to fall in front of the retina

Clinical Manifestations

Headaches
Dizziness
Excessive eye rubbing
Head tilt or forward head thrusts
Difficulty in reading or doing other close work
Clumsiness; walking into objects
Blinking more than usual or irritability when doing close work
Inability to see objects clearly
Poor school performance, especially in subjects that require demonstration, such as arithmetic

Treatment

Corrected with biconcave lenses that focus rays on retina
May be corrected with laser surgery

Hyperopia

Farsightedness: Ability to see objects at a distance but not at close range

Pathophysiology

Results from eyeball that is too short, causing image to focus beyond retina

Clinical Manifestations

Because of accommodative ability, child can usually see objects at all ranges
Most children are normally hyperopic until about 7 years old

Treatment

When required, corrected with convex lenses that focus rays on retina
May be corrected with laser surgery

Astigmatism

Unequal curvatures in refractive apparatus

Pathophysiology

Results from unequal curvatures in cornea or lens that cause light rays to bend in different directions

Clinical Manifestations

Depend on severity of refractive error in each eye
Possible clinical manifestations of myopia

Treatment

Corrected with special lenses that compensate for refractive errors
May be corrected with laser surgery

Anisometropia

Different refractive strength in each eye

Pathophysiology

May develop amblyopia because weaker eye is used less

Clinical Manifestations

Depend on severity of refractive error in each eye
Possible clinical manifestations of myopia

Treatment

Treated with corrective lenses, preferably contact lenses, to improve vision in each eye so that they work as a unit
May be corrected with laser surgery

Continued

BOX 20.5 Types of Visual Impairment—cont'd

Amblyopia

Lazy eye: Reduced visual acuity in one eye

Pathophysiology

Results when one eye does not receive sufficient stimulation
Each retina receives different images, resulting in diplopia (double vision)
Brain accommodates by suppressing less intense image
Visual cortex eventually does not respond to visual stimulation, with resultant loss of vision in that eye

Clinical Manifestations

Poor vision in affected eye

Treatment

Preventable if treatment of primary visual defect, such as anisometropia or strabismus, begins before 6 years old

Strabismus

"Squint" or malalignment of eyes
Esotropia: Inward deviation of eye
Exotropia: Outward deviation of eye

Pathophysiology

May result from muscle imbalance or paralysis, poor vision, or congenital defect
Because visual axes are not parallel, brain receives two images, and amblyopia can result

Clinical Manifestations

Squints eyelids together or frowns
Difficulty in focusing from one distance to another
Inaccurate judgment in picking up objects
Inability to see print or moving objects clearly
Closing one eye to see
Tilting head to one side
If combined with refractive errors, may see any of the manifestations listed for refractive errors
Diplopia
Photophobia
Dizziness
Headaches

Treatment

Depends on cause of strabismus
May involve occlusion therapy (patching stronger eye) or surgery to increase visual stimulation to weaker eye
Early diagnosis essential to prevent vision loss

Cataracts

Opacity of crystalline lens

Pathophysiology

Prevents light rays from entering eye and refracting on retina

Clinical Manifestations

Gradual decrease in ability to see objects clearly
Possible loss of peripheral vision
Nystagmus (with permanent visual impairment)
Gray opacities of lens
Strabismus
Absence of red reflex

Treatment

Requires surgery to remove cloudy lens and replace lens (with intraocular lens implant, removable contact lens, prescription glasses)
Must be treated early to prevent permanent visual impairment from amblyopia

Glaucoma

Increased intraocular pressure

Pathophysiology

Congenital type results from defective development of some component related to flow of aqueous humor
Increased pressure on optic nerve causes eventual atrophy and severe permanent visual impairment

Clinical Manifestations

Loss of peripheral vision—mostly seen in acquired types
Possible bumping into objects
Perception of halos around objects
Possible complaint of pain or discomfort (severe pain, nausea, or vomiting if sudden rise in pressure)
Eye redness
Excessive tearing (epiphora)
Photophobia
Spasmodic winking (blepharospasm)
Corneal haziness
Enlargement of eyeball (buphthalmos)

Treatment

Requires surgical treatment (goniotomy) to open outflow tracts
May require more than one procedure

Trauma

Trauma is a common cause of visual impairment in children. Injuries to the eyeball and adnexa (supporting or accessory structures, such as eyelids, conjunctiva, or lacrimal glands) can be classified as penetrating or nonpenetrating. Penetrating wounds are most often a result of sharp instruments (e.g., sticks, knives, or scissors) or propulsive objects (e.g., firecrackers, guns, arrows, or slingshots). Nonpenetrating injuries may be a result of foreign objects in the eyes, lacerations, a blow from a blunt object such as a ball (baseball, softball, basketball, racquet sports) or fist, or thermal or chemical burns.

Treatment is aimed at preventing further ocular damage and is primarily the responsibility of the ophthalmologist. It involves adequate examination of the injured eye (with the child sedated or anesthetized in severe injuries); appropriate immediate intervention, such as removal of the foreign body or suturing of the laceration; and prevention of complications, such as administration of antibiotics or steroids and complete bed rest to allow the eye to heal and blood to reabsorb (see Emergency Treatment box). The prognosis varies according to the type of injury. It is usually guarded in all cases of penetrating wounds because of the high risk of serious complications.

Infections

Infections of the adnexa and structures of the eyeball or globe may occur in children. The most common eye infection is conjunctivitis. Treatment is usually with ophthalmic antibiotics. Severe infections may

EMERGENCY TREATMENT

Eye Injuries

Foreign Object

Examine eye for presence of a foreign body (evert upper eyelid to examine upper eye).

Remove a freely movable object with pointed corner of gauze pad lightly moistened with water.

Do not irrigate eye or attempt to remove a penetrating object (see Penetrating Injuries).

Caution child against rubbing eye.

Chemical Burns

Irrigate eye copiously with tap water for 20 minutes.

Evert upper eyelid to flush thoroughly.

Hold child's head with eye under a tap of running lukewarm water.

Take child to emergency department.

Have child rest with eyes closed.

Keep room darkened.

Ultraviolet Burns

If skin is burned, patch both eyes (make certain eyelids are completely closed); secure dressing with Kling bandages wrapped around head rather than with tape.

Have child rest with eyes closed.

Refer to an ophthalmologist.

Hematoma ("Black Eye")

Use a flashlight to check for gross hyphema (hemorrhage into anterior chamber; visible fluid meniscus across iris; more easily seen in light-colored than in brown eyes).

Apply ice for first 24 hours to reduce swelling if no hyphema is present.

Refer to an ophthalmologist immediately if hyphema is present.

Have child rest with eyes closed.

Penetrating Injuries

Take child to emergency department.

Never remove an object that has penetrated eye.

Follow strict aseptic technique in examining eye.

Observe for the following:

- Aqueous or vitreous leaks (fluid leaking from point of penetration)
- Hyphema
- Shape and equality of pupils, reaction to light, prolapsed iris (not perfectly circular)

Apply a Fox shield if available (not a regular eye patch) and apply patch over unaffected eye to prevent bilateral movement.

Maintain bed rest with child in a 30-degree Fowler position.

Caution child against rubbing eye.

Refer to an ophthalmologist.

require systemic antibiotic therapy. Steroids are used cautiously because they exacerbate viral infections such as herpes simplex, increasing the risk of damage to the involved structures.

Nursing Care Management

Nursing care of the visually impaired child is a critical nursing responsibility. Discovery of a visual impairment as early as possible is essential to prevent social, physical, and psychologic damage to the child. Assessment involves (1) identifying those children who by virtue of their history are at risk, (2) observing for behaviors that indicate a vision loss, and (3) screening all children for visual acuity and signs of other ocular disorders such as strabismus. This discussion focuses on clinical manifestations of various types of visual problems (see Box 20.5). Vision testing is discussed in Chapter 4.

Infancy. At birth, the nurse should observe the neonate's response to visual stimuli, such as following a light or object and cessation of body movement. The infant may vary in the intensity of the response, depending on the state of alertness.

Of special importance in detecting visual impairment during infancy are the parents' concerns regarding visual responsiveness in their child. Their concerns, such as lack of eye contact from the infant, must be taken seriously. During infancy, the child should be tested for strabismus. Children with lack of binocularity after 2 to 4 months of age or not fixating and following an object by 6 months should be referred to a pediatric ophthalmologist or an eye care specialist (American Academy of Pediatrics, 2016; Rogers & Jordan, 2013).

NURSING ALERT

Suspect visual impairment in an infant who does not react to light and in a child of any age if the parents express concern.

Childhood. Because the most common visual impairment during childhood is refractive error, testing for visual acuity is essential. The school nurse usually assumes major responsibility for vision testing in schoolchildren. In addition to assessing for refractive errors, the nurse should be aware of signs and symptoms that indicate other ocular problems. If the family is given a referral requesting further eye testing, the nurse is responsible for follow-up concerning the recommendation.

Learning that their child is visually impaired precipitates an immense crisis for families. Encourage the family to investigate appropriate early intervention and educational programs for their child as soon as possible. Sources of information include state commissions for the visually impaired, local schools for children with visual impairments, the American Foundation for the Blind,* the National Federation of the Blind,† the National Association for Parents of Children with Visual Impairments,‡ the National Association for Visually Handicapped,§ the American Council of the Blind,¶ and CNIB.¶

Promote Parent-Child Attachment

A crucial time in the life of visually impaired infants is when the infant and the parents are getting acquainted with each other. Pleasurable

*Two Penn Plaza, Suite 1102, New York, NY 10021; 800-232-5463 or 212-502-7600; fax: 888-545-8331; http://www.afb.org; email: afbinfo@afb.net; https://wwwfacebook.com/americanfoundtionfortheblind; https://twitter.com/AFB1921.

†200 E. Wells St., Baltimore, MD 21230; 410-659-9314; fax: 410-685-5653; http://www.nfb.org; office@nfbny.org; http://www.facebook.com/NationalFederationoftheBlind/; https:twitter.com/NFB.

‡PO Box 317, Watertown, MA 02471; 617-972-7441 or 800-562-6265; http://www.spedex.com; napvi@perfins.org.

§111 East 59th St., The Sol and Lillian Goldman Building, New York, NY 10022-1202; 212-821-9200 or 800-284-4422; http://www.lighthouse-guild.org; email: info@lighthouse.org.

¶1703 N. Beauregard St., Suite 420, Alexandria, VA 22311; 800-424-8666; 202-467-5081; fax: 703-465-5085; http://www.acb.org; email: info@acb.org; http://www.facebook.com/AmericanCounciloftheBlindOfficial.

¶1929 Bayview Ave., East York, ON M4G 0A1; Canada: 800-563-2642; fax: 416-480-7700; http://www.cnib.ca.

patterns of interaction between the infant and parents may be lacking if there is not enough reciprocity. For example, if the parent gazes fondly at the infant's face and seeks eye contact but the infant fails to respond because he or she cannot see the parent, a troubled cycle of responses may occur. The nurse can help parents learn to look for other cues that indicate the infant is responding to them, such as whether the eyelids blink; whether the activity level accelerates or slows; whether respiratory patterns change, such as faster or slower breathing, when the parents come near; and whether the infant makes throaty sounds when the parents speak to the infant. In time, parents learn that the infant has unique ways of relating to them. Encourage the parents to show affection using nonvisual methods, such as talking or reading, cuddling, and walking the child.

Promote the Child's Optimal Development

Promoting the child's optimum development requires rehabilitation in a number of important areas. These include learning self-help skills and appropriate communication techniques to become independent. Although nurses may not be directly involved in such programs, they can provide direction and guidance to families regarding the availability of programs and the need to promote these activities in their child.

Development and independence. Motor development depends on sight almost as much as verbal communication depends on hearing. From earliest infancy, parents are encouraged to expose the infant to as many visual-motor experiences as possible, such as sitting supported in an infant seat or swing and being given opportunities for holding up the head, sitting unsupported, reaching for objects, and crawling.

Despite visual impairment, the child can become independent in all aspects of self-care. The same principles used for promoting independence in sighted children apply, with additional emphasis on nonvisual cues. For example, the child may need help in dressing, such as special arrangement of clothing for style coordination and braille tags to distinguish colors and prints.

The child with permanent visual impairment also must learn to become independent in navigational skills. The two main techniques are the tapping method (use of a cane to survey the environment for direction and to avoid obstacles) and guides, such as a sighted human guide or a guide dog. Children who are partially sighted may benefit from ocular aids, such as a monocular telescope.

Play and socialization. Children with severe permanent visual impairments do not learn to play automatically. Because they cannot imitate others or actively explore the environment as sighted children do, they depend much more on others to stimulate and teach them how to play. Parents need help in selecting appropriate play materials, especially those that encourage fine and gross motor development and stimulate the senses of hearing, touch, and smell. Toys with educational value are especially useful, such as dolls with various clothing closures.

Children with severe permanent visual impairments have the same needs for socialization as sighted children. Because they have little difficulty in learning verbal skills, they are able to communicate with age mates and participate in suitable activities. The nurse should discuss with parents the opportunities for socialization outside the home, especially regular preschools. The trend is to include these children with sighted children to help them adjust to the outside world for eventual independence.

To compensate for inadequate stimulation, these children may develop self-stimulatory activities, such as body rocking, finger flicking, or arm twirling. Discourage such habits because they delay the child's social acceptance. Behavior modification is often successful in reducing or eliminating self-stimulatory activities.

Education. The main obstacle to learning is the child's total dependence on nonvisual cues. Although the child can learn via verbal lecturing, he or she is unable to read the written word or to write without special education. Therefore the child must rely on braille, a system that uses raised dots to represent letters and numbers. The child can then read braille with the fingers and can write messages using a braille writer. However, this system is not useful for communicating with others unless others read braille. A more portable system for written communication is the use of a braille slate and stylus or a microcassette tape recorder. A recorder is especially helpful for leaving messages for others and taking notes during classroom lectures. For mathematic calculations, portable calculators with voice synthesizers are available.*

Books on CDs and tapes are significant sources of reading material in addition to braille books, which are large and cumbersome. The Library of Congress† has talking books, and braille books, that are available at many local and state libraries and directly from the Library of Congress. Currently, there are two types of talking books and book players: digital and cassette, though new books are only made in the digital format and recorded cassettes are being phased out (The New York Public Library, 2017). The talking book machine and tape player are provided at no cost to families, and there is no postage fee for returning the materials. Learning Ally (formally known as Recording for the Blind and Dyslexic)‡ also provides texts and CDs and tapes of books, which are helpful for secondary and college students who are visually impaired. A means of writing is learning to use a home computer with a voice synthesizer that can be adapted to speak each letter or word typed.

Children with partial sight benefit from specialized visual aids that produce a magnified retinal image. The basic methods are accommodative techniques, such as bringing the object closer; and devices such as special plus lenses, handheld and stand magnifiers, telescopes, video projection systems, and large-print materials. Special equipment is available to enlarge print. Information about services for the partially sighted is available from the National Association for Visually Handicapped and American Foundation for the Blind. Children with diminished vision often prefer to do close work without their glasses and compensate by bringing the object very near to their eyes. This should be allowed. The exception is children with vision in only one eye, who should always wear glasses for protection.

Care for the Child During Hospitalization

Because nurses are more likely to care for children who are hospitalized for procedures that involve temporary loss of vision than for children who have severe permanent visual impairments, the following discussion concentrates primarily on the needs of such children. The nursing care objectives in either situation are to (1) reassure the child and family throughout every phase of treatment, (2) orient the child to the surroundings, (3) provide a safe environment, and (4) encourage independence. Whenever possible, the same nurse should care for the child to ensure consistency in the approach.

---

*A catalog of numerous products for people with vision problems is available from Lighthouse International: https://www.lighthouseguild.org.

†National Library Service for the Blind and Physically Handicapped, Library of Congress, 1291 Taylor St. NW, Washington, DC 20542-4962; 202-707-5100; 888-657-7323; TTD: 202-707-0744; http://www.loc.gov/nls; nis@loc.gov. (State listings of libraries for visually impaired and physically handicapped readers with severe permanent visual impairments and physical disabilities, as well as other reference circulars, are available from this office.)

‡20 Roszel Road, Princeton, NJ 08540; 800-221-4792 or 866-RFBD-585; http://www.learningally.org; http://www.facebook.com/LearningAlly.org.

When sighted children temporarily lose their vision, almost every aspect of the environment becomes bewildering and frightening. They are forced to rely on nonvisual senses for help in adjusting to the visual impairment without the benefit of any special training. Nurses have a major role in minimizing the effects of temporary loss of vision. They need to talk to the child about everything that is occurring, emphasizing aspects of procedures that are felt or heard. They should always identify themselves as soon as they enter the room and before they approach the child. Because unfamiliar sounds are especially frightening, these are explained. Encourage the parents to room with their child and participate in the care. Familiar objects, such as a teddy bear or doll, should be brought from home to help lessen the strangeness of the hospital. As soon as the child is able to be out of bed, orient the child to the immediate surroundings. If the child is able to see on admission, this opportunity is taken to point out significant aspects of the room. Encourage the child to practice ambulating with the eyes closed to become accustomed to this experience.

The room is arranged with safety in mind. For example, place a stool next to the bed to help the child climb in and out of bed. The furniture is always placed in the same position to prevent collisions. Remind cleaning personnel to keep the room in order. If the child has difficulty navigating by feeling the walls, a rope can be attached from the bed to the point of destination, such as the bathroom. Attention to details (e.g., well-fitting slippers and robes that do not drag on the floor) is important in preventing tripping. Unlike the child who is visually impaired, these children are not familiar with navigating with a cane.

The child is encouraged to be independent in self-care activities, especially if the visual loss may be prolonged or potentially permanent. For example, during bathing, the nurse sets up all of the equipment and encourages the child to participate. At mealtimes, the nurse explains where each food item is on the tray, opens any special containers, prepares cereal or toast, and encourages the child in self-feeding. Favorite finger foods (e.g., sandwiches, hamburgers, hot dogs, or pizza) may be good selections. Praise the child for efforts at being cooperative and independent. Any improvements made in self-care, no matter how small, are stressed.

Appropriate recreational activities are provided, and if a child life specialist is available, such planning is done jointly. Because children with temporary visual impairment have a wide variety of play experiences to draw on, they are encouraged to select activities. For example, if they like to read, they may enjoy listening to books on CD or having someone read to them. If they prefer manual activity, they may appreciate playing with clay or building blocks or feeling different textures and naming them. If they need an outlet for aggression, activities such as pounding or banging on a drum can be helpful. Simple board and card games can be played with a "seeing partner" or an opponent who helps with the game. They should have familiar toys from home to play with because familiar items are more easily manipulated than new ones. If parents want to bring presents, they should be objects that stimulate hearing and touch, such as a radio, music box, or stuffed animal.

Occasionally, children who are visually impaired come to the hospital for procedures to restore their vision. Although this is an extremely happy time, it also requires intervention to help them adjust to sight. They need an opportunity to take in all that they see. They should not be bombarded with visual stimuli. They may need to concentrate on people's faces or their own to become accustomed to this experience. They often need to talk about what they see and to compare the visual images with their mental ones. The children may also go through a period of depression, which must be respected and supported. Encourage the children to discuss how it feels to see, especially in terms of seeing themselves.

Newly sighted children also need time to adjust and engage in activities that were impossible before. For example, they may prefer to use braille to read rather than learning a new "visual approach" because of familiarity with the touch system. Eventually, as they learn to recognize letters and numbers, they will integrate these new skills into reading and writing. However, parents and teachers must be careful not to push them before they are ready. This applies to social relationships and physical activities as well as learning situations.

Assist in Measures to Prevent Visual Impairment

An essential nursing goal is to prevent visual impairment. This involves many of the same interventions discussed for hearing impairments:

- Prenatal screening for pregnant women at risk, such as those with rubella or syphilis infection and family histories of genetic disorders associated with visual loss
- Adequate prenatal and perinatal care to prevent prematurity
- Periodic screening of all children, especially newborns through preschoolers, for congenital and acquired visual impairments caused by refractive errors, strabismus, and other disorders
- Rubella immunization of all children
- Safety counseling regarding the common causes of ocular trauma, including safe practices when working with, playing with, and carrying objects such as scissors, knives, and balls

> **! NURSING ALERT**
>
> A helmet with a face mask should be required for children playing football, hockey, and baseball.

After detection of eye problems, the nurse should encourage the family to prevent further ocular damage by undertaking corrective treatment. For the child with strabismus, this often necessitates occlusion patching of the stronger eye. Compliance with the procedure is greatest during the early preschool years. It is more difficult to encourage school-age children to wear the occlusive patch because the poor visual acuity of the uncovered weaker eye interferes with school work and the patch sets them apart from their peers. In school, they benefit from being positioned favorably (closer to the white board or other visual media) and allowed extra time to read or complete an assignment. If treatment of the eye disorder requires instillation of ophthalmic medication, the family is taught the correct procedure (see Chapter 22).

Children who need glasses to correct refractive errors need time to adjust to wearing glasses. Young children who often pull off glasses benefit from temporal pieces that wrap around the ears or an elastic strap attached to the frames and around the back of the head to hold the glasses on securely. Once children appreciate the value of clear vision, they are more likely to wear the corrective lenses.

Glasses should not interfere with any activity. Special protective guards are available during contact sports to prevent accidental injury, and all corrective lenses should be made from safety glass, which is shatterproof. Often, corrective lenses improve visual acuity so dramatically that children are able to compete more effectively in sports. This in itself is a tremendous inducement to continue wearing glasses.

Contact lenses are a popular alternative to conventional glasses, especially for adolescents. Several types are available, such as hard lenses, including gas-permeable ones, and soft lenses, which may be designed for daily or extended wear. Contact lenses offer several advantages over glasses, such as greater visual acuity, total corrected field of vision, convenience (especially with the extended-wear type), and optimal cosmetic benefit. Unfortunately, they are usually more expensive and require much more care than glasses, including considerable practice to learn techniques for insertion and removal. If they are prescribed, the nurse can be helpful in teaching parents or older children how to care for the lenses.

Because trauma is the leading cause of visual impairment, the nurse has the major responsibility of preventing further eye injury until specific treatment is instituted. The major principles to follow when caring for an eye injury are outlined in the Emergency Treatment box earlier in this chapter. Because patients with a serious eye injury fear visual impairment, the nurse should stay with the child and family to provide support and reassurance.

HEARING–VISUAL IMPAIRMENT

The most traumatic sensory impairment is loss of both vision and hearing, which may have profound effects on the child's development. These losses interfere with the normal sequence of physical, intellectual, and psychosocial growth. Although such children often achieve the usual motor milestones, their rate of development is slower. These children learn communication only with specialized training. Finger spelling is one desirable method often taught to these children. Words are spelled letter by letter into the hearing–visually impaired child's hand, and the child spells into the other person's hand. Some children with residual hearing or visual impairment can learn to speak. Whenever possible, encourage speech because it allows communication with other individuals.

The future prospects for hearing and visually impaired children are, at best, unpredictable. Congenital hearing and visually impairment are accompanied by other physical or neurologic problems, which further diminish the child's learning potential. The most favorable prognosis is for children who have acquired hearing and visual impairments with few, if any, associated disabilities. Their learning capacity is greatly potentiated by their developmental progress before the sensory impairments. Although total independence, including gainful vocational training, is the goal, some children with hearing–visual impairment are unable to develop to this level. They may require lifelong parental or residential care. The nurse working with such families helps them deal with future goals for the child, including possible alternatives to home care during the parents' advancing years.

COMMUNICATION IMPAIRMENT

AUTISM SPECTRUM DISORDERS

ASDs are complex neurodevelopmental disorders of unknown etiology. The American Psychiatric Association's *Diagnostic and Statistical Manual of Mental Disorders, Fifth Edition* (DSM-5) revised the definition for ASD based on two behavior domains that include difficulties in social communication and social interaction, and unusually restricted, repetitive behavior, interest, or activities (American Psychiatric Association, 2013; Brentani, Paula, Bordini, et al., 2013; Lai, Lombardo, & Baron-Cohen, 2014).

ASD is now frequently diagnosed in toddlers because their atypical development is being recognized early (Lai, Lombardo, & Baron-Cohen, 2014; Zwaigenbaum, Bauman, Stone, et al., 2015). It occurs in 1 in 68 children in the United States; is about four times more common in boys than in girls; and is not related to socioeconomic level, race, or parenting style (Christensen, Baio, Braun, et al., 2016; National Autism Association, 2017a).

Etiology

The cause of ASD is unknown. Researchers are investigating a number of theories, including a link between hereditary, genetic, medical, immune dysregulation/neuroinflammation, oxidative stress (damage to cellular tissue), and environmental factors (De Rubeis, He, Goldberg, et al., 2014; Lai, Lombardo, & Baron-Cohen, 2014; Ng, de Montigny, Ofner, et al., 2017; Posar & Visconti, 2016; Wong, Napoli, Krakowiak, et al., 2016). Individuals with ASD may have abnormal electroencephalograms, epileptic seizures, delayed development of hand dominance, persistence of primitive reflexes, metabolic abnormalities (elevated blood serotonin), cerebellar vermis hypoplasia (part of the brain involved in regulating motion and some aspects of memory), and infantile abnormal head enlargement (Raviola, Trieu, DeMaso, et al., 2016; Rutter, 2011).

The strong evidence for a genetic basis in twins is consistent with an autosomal recessive pattern of inheritance. Twin studies demonstrate a high concordance (60% to 96%) for monozygotic (identical) twins and less than 5% concordance for dizygotic (nonidentical) twins. In addition, between 5% and 16% of boys with ASD are positive for the fragile X chromosome (Clifford, Dissanayake, Bui, et al., 2007; Finucane, Lincoln, Bailey, et al., 2017; Grafodatskaya, Chung, Szatmari, et al., 2010).

There is a relatively high risk of recurrence of ASD in families with one affected child (Chawarska, Shic, Macari, et al., 2014; Rutter, 2011; Yoder, Stone, Walden, et al., 2009; Zwaigenbaum, Bauman, Stone, et al., 2015). Several genes have been suggested as possible causative factors in ASD (Talkowski, Minikel, & Gusella, 2014; Willsey & State, 2015; Wong, Napoli, Krakowiak, et al., 2016).

The scientific evidence to date shows no link between measles, mumps, and rubella (MMR) and thimerosal-containing vaccines and ASDs (Barile, Kuperminc, Weintraub, et al., 2012; Goin-Kochel, Mire, Dempsey, et al., 2016; Price, Thompson, Goodson, et al., 2010; Taylor, Swerdfeger, & Eslick, 2014; Uno, Uchiyama, Kurosawa, et al., 2015) (see Translating Evidence into Practice box). ASD has been reported in association with a number of conditions, such as FXS, tuberous sclerosis, Prader-Willie syndrome, metabolic disorders, fetal rubella syndrome, *Haemophilus influenzae* meningitis, and structural brain anomalies (National Autism Association, 2017a; Peterson & Barbel, 2013). Recent reports have retrospectively tied ASD to prenatal and perinatal events, such as maternal and paternal ages over 40 years old (for fathers, 1 in 116 births; for mothers, 1 in 123 births), uterine bleeding during pregnancy, low Apgar score, fetal distress, and neonatal hyperbilirubinemia (Amin, Smith, & Wang, 2011; Kolevzon, Gross, & Reichenberg, 2007; Rutter, 2011). These same researchers, however, urge caution in interpreting these findings.

Clinical Manifestations and Diagnostic Evaluation

Children with ASD demonstrate core deficits primarily in social interactions, communication, and behavior. Failure of social interaction and communication development is the one of the hallmarks of ASD. Parents of autistic children have reported that their child showed less interest in social interaction (e.g., abnormal eye contact, decreased response to own name, decreased imitation, usual repetitive behavior) and had verbal and motor delays (Bolton, Golding, Emond, et al., 2012; National Autism Association, 2017b; Sanchack & Thomas, 2016). Children with ASD may have significant gastrointestinal symptoms. Constipation is a common symptom and can be associated with acquired megarectum in children with ASD (Buie, Campbell, Fuchs, et al., 2010; National Autism Association, 2017a).

Children with ASD do not always have the same manifestations, from mild forms requiring minimal supervision to severe forms in which self-abusive behavior is common. The majority of children with ASD have some degree of CI, with scores typically in the moderate to severe range. Despite their relatively moderate to severe disability, some children with autism (known as savants) excel in particular areas, such as art, music, memory, mathematics, or perceptual skills, such as puzzle building.

TRANSLATING EVIDENCE INTO PRACTICE

Thimerosal-Containing Vaccines and Autism Spectrum Disorders

Ask the Question

Is the incidence of autism spectrum disorders (ASDs) increased in children receiving vaccines containing thimerosal?

Search for the Evidence

Search Strategies

Published studies from 2003 to 2016 focused on the pediatric population and restricted to the English language

Databases Used

PubMed, Cochrane Collaboration, MD Consult, Vaccine Adverse Events Reporting System (VAERS) database, American Academy of Pediatrics, Autism Research Institute

Critically Analyze the Evidence

Grade criteria: Moderate evidence with strong recommendations for practice (Balshem, Helfand, Schünemann, et al., 2011). Evidence does not support an association between the increase incidence of autism and mercury exposure from the pharmaceutical preservative thimerosal.

- A Cochrane systematic review of 64 studies assessing the effectiveness and adverse effects associated with the trivalent measles, mumps, and rubella (MMR) vaccine on healthy patients up to 15 years old found no significant association between MMR with either autism or other conditions (Demicheli, Rivetti, Debalini, et al., 2012). Previously done studies supported the same conclusion because the studies found no association between thimerosal-containing vaccines and ASD (Demicheli, Jefferson, Rivetti, et al., 2005; Hurley, Tadrous, & Miller, 2010; Parker, Schwartz, Todd, et al., 2004; Schultz, 2010; World Health Organization, 2012).
- Two large studies in Europe found no evidence that childhood vaccination with thimerosal-containing vaccines was associated with the development of ASDs. One longitudinal study evaluated more than 14,000 children in the United Kingdom. The mercury exposure from thimerosal-containing vaccines was recorded and calculated at ages 3, 4, and 6 months and compared with cognitive and behavioral developmental assessments performed from 6 to 91 months old (Heron, Golding, & ALSPAC Study Team, 2004). The second study, a cohort of 467,450 children in Denmark, compared the incidence of ASDs in children vaccinated with thimerosal-containing vaccines with the incidence of ASDs in children vaccinated with a thimerosal-free formulation of the same vaccine (Hvid, Stellfeld, & Wohlfahrt, 2003). Another study that evaluated 1047 children from early life to 7 to 10 years old and their biologic mothers found no statistically significant associations between thimerosal exposure from vaccines early in life. It noted a small but statistically significant association between early thimerosal exposure and the presence of tics in boys and recommended there be further research in this area (Barile, Kuperminc, Weintraub, et al., 2012). An evidence-based meta-analysis of case-control and cohort studies reported the components of the vaccines (thimerosal or mercury) or multiple vaccines (MMR) are not associated with the development of autism or ASD (Taylor, Swerdfeger, & Eslick, 2014).
- Case-control studies have also found no relationship between MMR vaccination and the increased risk of ASDs (Price, Thompson, Goodson, et al., 2010; Uno, Uchiyama, Kurosawa, et al., 2015; Yau, Green, Alaimo, et al., 2014). Another small case-control study investigated the mercury level in maternal prenatal serum and early postnatal newborn serum of children with ASD (n = 84) compared with children with intellectual disability or developmental delay (n = 49) and general population (n = 159) and found no significant association with the risk of ASD (Yau, Green, Alaimo, et al., 2014). A similar finding was concluded in a meta-analysis of evidence on the impact of prenatal and early infancy exposures to mercury on autism and attention-deficit/hyperactivity disorder (ADHD) with the recommendation of further study to be conducted on effects of environmental perinatal mercury exposures and increase risk of developmental disorders (Yoshimasu, Kiyohara, Takemura, et al., 2014).

A review study reported 91 studies that examine the potential relationship between mercury and ASD from 1999 to February 2016. Of these studies, the majority (74%) suggest that mercury is a risk factor for ASD, revealing both direct and indirect effects. The evidence indicates that mercury is a risk factor for ASD (Kern, Geier, Sykes, et al., 2016). Conversely, Goin-Kochel, Mire, Dempsey, and colleagues (2016) reported in a cohort study that examined 2755 ASD children based on parental description of ASD onset against vaccine receipt that the findings did not support a connection between regressive-onset ASD and vaccines. Another evidence-based meta-analysis of case-control studies and cohort studies supported the same conclusion; the findings from a large sample of US children (95,727) suggest that vaccinations are not associated with the development of autism or ASD (Taylor, Swerdfeger, & Eslick, 2014).

- In 2004 the Institute of Medicine completed an update to review the evidence and concluded that the epidemiologic evidence supports the rejection of a causal relationship between thimerosal exposure from childhood vaccines and the onset of autism. The Institute of Medicine (2013) review of the evidence reported from January 1990 to May 2013 concluded that the review revealed no evidence that the US childhood immunization schedule is linked to learning or developmental disorders or attention-deficit or disruptive disorders. This was also supported in a report on adverse effects of vaccines by the Institute of Medicine (2011). Based on guidelines established by the US Food and Drug Administration (2014) and other government monitoring agencies, no children will be exposed to excessive mercury from childhood vaccines.

Apply the Evidence: Nursing Implications

There is moderate-quality evidence with a strong recommendation that there is no link between vaccines containing thimerosal and ASDs.

Quality and Safety Competencies: Evidence-Based Practice*

Knowledge

Differentiate clinical opinion from research and evidence-based summaries.

Compare research summaries that provide evidence of the lack of association between vaccines containing thimerosal and autism or other neurodevelopmental disorders.

Skills

Base individualized care plan on patient values, clinical expertise, and evidence.

Integrate evidence into practice by sharing results with parents regarding the benefits of vaccinating their children and the evidence regarding lack of association between immunizations and autism disorders.

Attitudes

Value the concept of evidence-based practice as integral to determining best clinical practice.

Appreciate strengths and weakness of the evidence that confirms the lack of a link between vaccines containing thimerosal and autism or other neurodevelopmental disorders.

Continued

TRANSLATING EVIDENCE INTO PRACTICE—cont'd

Thimerosal-Containing Vaccines and Autism Spectrum Disorders

References

Balshem, H., Helfand, M., Schünemann, H. J., et al. (2011). GRADE guidelines: 3. Rating the quality of evidence. *Journal of Clinical Epidemiology, 64*(4), 401–406.

Barile, J. P., Kuperminc, G. P., Weintraub, E. S., et al. (2012). Thimerosal exposure in early life and neuropsychological outcomes 7-10 years later. *Journal of Pediatric Psychology, 37*(1), 106–118.

Demicheli, V., Jefferson, T., Rivetti, A., et al. (2005). Vaccines for measles, mumps and rubella in children. *Cochrane Database of Systematic Reviews,* (4), CD004407.

Demicheli, V., Rivetti, A., Debalini, M. G., et al. (2012). Vaccines for measles, mumps and rubella in children. *Cochrane Database of Systematic Reviews,* (2), CD004407.

Goin-Kochel, R. P., Mire, S. S., Dempsey, A. G., et al. (2016). Parental report of vaccine receipt in children with autism spectrum disorder: Do rates differ by pattern of ASD onset? *Vaccine, 34,* 1335–1342.

Heron, J., Golding, J., & ALSPAC Study Team. (2004). Thimerosal exposure in infants and developmental disorders: A prospective cohort study in the United Kingdom does not support a causal association. *Pediatrics, 114*(3), 577–583.

Hurley, A. M., Tadrous, M., & Miller, E. S. (2010). Thimerosal-containing vaccines and autism: Review of recent epidemiologic studies. *The Journal of Pediatric Pharmacology and Therapeutics, 15*(3), 173–181.

Hvid, A., Stellfeld, M., & Wohlfahrt, J. (2003). Association between thimersol-containing vaccine and autism. *Journal of the American Medical Association, 290*(13), 1763–1766.

Institute of Medicine. (2004). Immunization safety review:Vaccines and autism. Washington, DC: National Academies Press.

Institute of Medicine. (2011). Adverse effects of vaccines: Evidence and causality, National Academies Press. Retrieved from http://www.iom.edu/Reports/2011/Adverse-Effects-of-Vaccines-Evidence-and-Causality.aspx.

Institute of Medicine. (2013). The childhood immunization schedule and safety: Stakeholders concerns, scientific evidence, and future studies. Washington, DC: National Academies Press.

Kern, J. K., Geier, D. A., Sykes, L. K., et al. (2016). The relationship between mercury and autism: A comprehensive review and discussion. *Journal of Trace Elements in Medicine and Biology, 37,* 8–24.

Parker, S. K., Schwartz, B., Todd, J., et al. (2004). Thimerosal-containing vaccines and autistic spectrum disorder: A critical review of published original data. *Pediatrics, 114*(3), 793–804.

Price, C. S., Thompson, W. W., Goodson, B., et al. (2010). Prenatal and infant exposure to thimerosal from vaccines and immunoglobulins and risk of autism. *Pediatrics, 126*(4), 656–664.

Schultz, S. T. (2010). Does thimerosal or other mercury exposure increase the risk for autism? A review of current literature. *Acta Neurobiologiae Experimentalis, 70*(2), 187–195.

Taylor, L. E., Swerdfeger, A. L., & Eslick, G. D. (2014). Vaccines are not associated with autism: An evidence-based meta-analysis of case-control and cohort studies. *Vaccine, 32*(29), 3623–3629.

Uno, Y., Uchiyama, T., Kurosawa, M., et al. (2015). Early exposure to the combined measles-mumps-rubella vaccine and thimerosal-containing vaccines and risk of autism spectrum disorder. *Vaccine, 33*(21), 2511–2516.

US Food and Drug Administration. (2014). Thimerosal in vaccines. Retrieved from http://www.fda.gov/BiologicsBloodVaccines/SafetyAvailability/vaccineSafety/UCM096228.

World Health Organization. (2012). Global vaccine safety: Global Advisory Committee on Vaccine Safety, report of meeting held 6-June 7, 2012. Retrieved from http://www.who.int/vaccine_safety/committee/reports/Jun_2012/en/.

Yau, V. M., Green, P. G., Alaimo, C. P., et al. (2014). Prenatal and neonatal peripheral blood mercury levels and autism spectrum disorders. *Environmental Research, 133,* 294–303.

Yoshimasu, K., Kiyohara, C., Takemura, S., et al. (2014). A meta-analysis of the evidence on the impact of prenatal and early infancy exposures to mercury on autism and attention deficit/hyperactivity disorder in the childhood. *Neurotoxicology, 44,* 121–131.

Rosalind Bryant

*Based on the Quality and Safety Education for Nurses website at http://www.qsen.org.

! NURSING ALERT

Claims of beneficial results from the use of secretin, a peptide hormone that stimulates pancreatic secretion, have been studied extensively in multiple randomized controlled trials, denoting no clear evidence of any benefit in the treatment of ASD (Krishnaswami, McPheeters, & Veenstra-Vanderweele, 2011; Lee, Oh, & Park, 2014;Williams, Wray, & Wheeler, 2012).*

*Additional information on secretin may be found by contacting the Autism Society, 4340 East-West Hwy., Suite 350, Bethesda, MD 20814-3067; 800-3AUTISM or 301-657-0881; http://www.autism-society.org.

Communication impairments are a common sign in children with ASD that may range from absent to delayed speech. Any child who does not display language skills such as babbling or gesturing by 12 months old, single words by 16 months old, and two-word phrases by 24 months old is recommended for immediate hearing and language evaluation. Autism regression is when the child seems to develop normally but then regresses suddenly; this is a red-flag event that has been frequently displayed in expressive language (Fernell, Eriksson, & Gillberg, 2013; Raviola, Trieu, DeMaso, et al., 2016; Sanchack & Thomas, 2016).

Early recognition, referral, diagnosis, and intensive early intervention tend to improve outcomes for children with ASD (Adelman & Kubiszyn, 2016; National Autism Association, 2017a; Reichow, Barton, Boyd, et al., 2012; Peterson & Barbel, 2013; Zwaigenbaum, Bauman, Stone, et al., 2015). Unfortunately, diagnosis is often not made until 2 to 3 years after symptoms are first recognized. However, in a retrospective study, the majority of parents observed atypical development in their ASD children before 24 months old (Lemcke, Juul, Parner, et al., 2013).

The American Academy of Pediatrics has recommended that pediatric health care providers administer two ASD screenings at ages 18 and 24 months using a valid screening tool. The Modified Checklist for Autism in Toddlers (M-CHAT) as a widely used screening tool for autism accompanied by a follow-up interview (M-CHAT/F) was used in a recent study and demonstrated that minimally trained primary care pediatricians can administer the M-CHAT/F reliably and efficiently during well-child visits (Sturner, Howard, Bergmann, et al., 2016). Children whose screening results are concerning subsequently should receive a comprehensive developmental evaluation from either a developmental pediatrician, child neurologist, child psychiatrist, or child psychologist (Centers for Disease Control and Prevention, 2016c).

Prognosis

Although ASD is usually a lifelong condition with often devastating comorbid conditions, with early and intensive interventions the symptoms associated with autism can be greatly improved, and in some cases reported symptoms were completely overcome (National Autism Association, 2017a; Sanchack & Thomas, 2016; Wodka, Mathy, & Kalb, 2013). Some ultimately achieve independence, but most require lifelong adult supervision. Aggravation of psychiatric symptoms occurs in about half of the children during adolescence, with girls having a tendency for continued deterioration.

Early recognition of behaviors associated with ASD is critical to implement appropriate interventions and family involvement. There is a growing body of evidence that parent-delivered interventions are associated with some improved outcomes, yet further research is needed in this area incorporating consistent measures (Bearss, Burrell, Stewart, et al., 2015; Brentani, Paula, Bordini, et al., 2013; Oono, Honey, & McConachie, 2013). The prognosis is most favorable for children with higher intelligence, functional speech, and less behavioral impairment (Orinstein, Helt, Troyb, et al., 2014; Raviola, Trieu, DeMaso, et al., 2016; Solomon, Buaminger, & Rogers, 2011).

Nursing Care Management

Therapeutic intervention for ASD and associated comorbidities is a specialized area involving professionals with advanced training. Although there is no cure for ASD, numerous therapies have been used. The most promising results have been through highly structured and intensive behavior modification programs. In general, the objective in treatment is to promote positive reinforcement, increase social awareness of others, teach verbal communication skills, and decrease unacceptable behavior. Providing a structured routine for the child to follow is a key in the management of ASD.

ASD is associated with comorbidities (e.g., aggression, explosive outburst, self-injury, asthma, epilepsy, gastrointestinal/digestive disorders, immune disorders, feeding disorders, anxiety disorder, bipolar disorder, sleeping disorders) that have been treated not only with early behavioral modification programs but also with medical management (e.g., aripiprazole [Abilify] and risperidone [Risperdal]) and complementary and alternative medicine (National Autism Association, 2017b; Sanchack & Thomas, 2016). Complementary and alternative medicine has emerged as a treatment of ASD ranging from parent-massage and therapeutic horseback riding to the implementation of elimination diets (e.g., gluten-free diet and casein-free diet); vitamin and omega-3 supplementation; and high-fat, low-carbohydrate ketogenic diet; however, there is a need for further research to validate these therapeutic approaches (Cheng, Rho, & Masino, 2017; Gabriels, Pan, Dechant, et al., 2015; Lee, Oh, & Park, 2014; Lofthouse, Hendren, Hurt, et al., 2012; Ly, Bottelier, Hoekstra, et al., 2017).

When these children are hospitalized, the parents are essential to planning care and ideally should stay with the child as much as possible. Nurses should recognize that not all children with ASD are the same and that they require individual assessment and treatment. Decreasing stimulation by using a private room, avoiding extraneous auditory and visual distractions, and encouraging the parents to bring in possessions the child is attached to may lessen the disruptiveness of hospitalization. Because physical contact often upsets these children, minimal holding and eye contact may be necessary to avoid behavioral outbursts. Take care when performing procedures on, administering medicine to, and feeding these children because they may be either fussy eaters who willfully starve themselves or gag to prevent eating, or indiscriminate hoarders who swallow any available edible or inedible items, such as a thermometer. Eating habits of ASD children may be particularly problematic for families and may involve food refusal accompanied by mineral deficiencies, mouthing objects, eating nonedibles, and smelling and throwing food (Belschner, 2007; Herndon, DiGuiseppi, Johnson, et al., 2009).

Children with ASD need to be introduced slowly to new situations, with visits with staff caregivers kept short whenever possible. Because these children have difficulty organizing their behavior and redirecting their energy, they need to be told directly what to do. Communication should be at the child's developmental level, brief, and concrete.

Family Support

ASD, as with so many other chronic conditions, involves the entire family and often becomes "a family disease." Nurses can help alleviate the guilt and shame often associated with this disorder by stressing what is known from a biologic standpoint and by providing family support. It is imperative to help parents understand that they are not the cause of the child's condition.

Parents need expert counseling early in the course of the disorder and should be referred to the Autism Society website. The society provides information about education, treatment programs and techniques, and facilities such as camps and group homes. Other helpful resources for parents of children with ASD are the local and state departments of mental health and developmental disabilities; these organizations provide important programs and in-school programs throughout the United States for children with ASD.

As much as possible, the family is encouraged to care for the child in the home. With the help of family support programs in many states, families are often able to provide home care and assist with the educational services the child needs. As the child approaches adulthood and the parents become older, the family may require assistance in locating a long-term placement facility.

NCLEX REVIEW QUESTIONS

1. A mother comments to a nurse working on the pediatric unit, "My second child just does not seem to be acting like or responding the same way as my first child." Nursing interventions to respond to this inquiry should include which of the following? Select all that apply.
   A. Assessment for dysmorphic syndromes (e.g., multiple congenital anomalies, microcephaly)
   B. Inquiring about temperament: irritability or lethargy
   C. Explaining that all children are different and that it can be detrimental to compare them
   D. Noting language development appropriate for the child's age
   E. Meeting the siblings to assess similarities that may be familial rather than problematic
2. When interacting with a parent at her child's well visit, which statement by the mother would be an indication for a speech referral? Select all that apply.
   A. Failure to speak any meaningful words spontaneously in a 2-year-old child
   B. Using different words or nicknames for certain people
   C. Failure to use sentences of three or more words in a 3-year-old
   D. Stuttering or any other type of dysfluency
   E. Omission of word endings (e.g., plurals, tenses of verbs) in a 3-year-old
   F. Frequent omission of final consonants in a 3-year-old
3. A mother of a child born with Down syndrome is overwhelmed with the future and asks many questions. Which of the following facts should the nurse be aware of? Select all that apply.
   A. Eighty percent of infants with Down syndrome are born to women younger than 35 years old because younger women have higher fertility rates.
   B. When feeding infants and young children, use a small, straight-handled spoon to push food to the side and back of the mouth. Feeding difficulties occur due to a protruding tongue and hypotonia.
   C. Parents generally believe the experience of having this special child makes them stronger and more accepting of others.
   D. Although some placement in the regular classroom has occurred more recently, this has been found to be detrimental to the child with Down syndrome due to lack of one-on-one teaching.
   E. The child's lack of clinging or molding is a physical characteristic, not a sign of detachment or rejection.

F. Development may be 3 to 4 years beyond the mental age, especially during early childhood.

4. When a child with a visual impairment is hospitalized, the nurse should ensure that which of the following interventions are carried out to decrease stress for the child during the hospitalization? Select all that apply.
   A. Because the child cannot see what may be taking place, the nurse needs to reassure the child and family throughout every phase of treatment.
   B. The nurse will make sure that the parents are comfortable with the placement of objects in the room.
   C. Whenever possible, the same nurse should care for the child to ensure consistency in the approach.
   D. To help the child feel safe, the nurses should take over most of the routine care of the child, unless the parent is present.
   E. Each health care provider should identify himself or herself as soon as entering the child's room.

5. Understanding autism spectrum disorders (ASDs) is very important for those who care for children. Goals of treatment for these children include:
   A. Helping with placement in a long-term care setting because most children cannot remain at home
   B. Putting the child hospitalized with an ASD in a room with another child to help him or her feel more comfortable in the strange environment
   C. Providing a structured routine, whether at home or in the health care setting
   D. Providing comfort for young children by holding or cuddling when able because the disruption of routine can be frightening

Correct Answers

1. A, B, D; 2. A, C, D, F; 3. A, B, C, E; 4. A, C, E; 5. C

REFERENCES

Abrams, L., Cronister, A., Brown, W. T., et al. (2012). Newborn, carrier, and early childhood screening recommendations for fragile X. *Pediatrics, 130*(6), 1126–1135.

Adelman, C. R., & Kubiszyn, T. (2016). Factors that affect age of identification of children with autism spectrum disorder. *Journal of Early Intervention.*

Ageranioti-Belanger, S., Brunet, S., D'Anjou, G., et al. (2012). Behavior disorders in children with an intellectual disability. *Paediatrics & Child Health, 17*(2), 84–88.

Alley, C. L. (2013). Preschool vision screening: Update on guidelines and techniques. *Current Opinion in Ophthalmology, 24*(5), 415–420.

Almadhoob, A., & Ohlsson, A. (2015). Sound reduction management in the neonatal intensive care unit for preterm or very low birth weight infants. *Cochrane Database of Systematic Review,* (1), CD010333.

American Academy of Pediatrics. (2007). Joint Committee on Infant Hearing: Year 2007 position statement: Principles and guidelines for early hearing detection and intervention programs. *Pediatrics, 120*(4), 898–921.

American Academy of Pediatrics. (2017). *Early hearing detection and intervention, a program of the American Academy of Pediatrics.* https://www,aao.org/en-us/advicacy-and-policy/aap-health-initiatives/PEHDIC/pages/early-hearing-detection-and-intervention.aspx.

American Academy of Pediatrics, Committee on Practice and Ambulatory Medicine. (2016). Visual system assessment in infants, children, and young adults by pediatricians. *Pediatrics, 137*(1), 28–30.

American Association on Intellectual and Developmental Disabilities (2013). *Intellectual disability: Definition, classification, and systems of supports* (11th ed.). Washington, DC: Author.

American Psychiatric Association (2013). *Diagnostic and statistical manual of mental disorders* (5th ed.). (DSM-V). Arlington, VA: American Psychiatric Association.

Amin, S. B., Smith, T., & Wang, H. (2011). Is neonatal jaundice associated with autism spectrum disorders: A systematic review. *Journal of Autism and Developmental Disorders, 41*(11), 1455–1463.

Arumugam, A., Raja, K., Venugopalan, M., et al. (2016). Down-syndrome-A narrative review with a focus on anatomical features. *Clinical Anatomy, 29,* 568–577.

Bagni, C., Tassone, F., Neri, G., et al. (2012). Fragile X syndrome: Causes, diagnosis, mechanisms, and therapeutics. *The Journal of Clinical Investigation, 122*(12), 4314–4322.

Barile, J. P., Kuperminc, G. P., Weintraub, E. S., et al. (2012). Thimerosal exposure in early life and neuropsychological outcomes 7-10 years later. *Journal of Pediatric Psychology, 37*(1), 106–118.

Bearss, K., Burrell, T. L., Stewart, L., et al. (2015). Parent training in autism spectrum disorder: What's in a name? *Clinical Child and Family Psychology Review, 18*(2), 170–182.

Bellman, M., Byrne, O., & Sege, R. (2013). Developmental assessment of children. *BMJ (Clinical Research Ed.), 346,* e8687.

Belschner, R. A. (2007). Stop, assess and motivate: The SAM approach to autism spectrum disorder. *The American Journal for Nurse Practitioners, 11*(4), 43–50.

Biassoni, E. C., Serra, M. R., Hinalaf, M., et al. (2014). Hearing and loud music exposure in a group of adolescents at the ages of 14-15 and retested at 17-18. *Noise and Health, 16*(72), 331–341.

Bolton, P. F., Golding, J., Emond, A., et al. (2012). Autism spectrum disorder and autistic traits in the Avon Longitudinal Study of Parents and Children: Precursors and early signs. *Journal of the American Academy of Child and Adolescent Psychiatry, 51*(3), 249–260.

Brentani, H., Paula, C. S., Bordini, D., et al. (2013). Autism spectrum disorders: An overview on diagnosis and treatment. *Revista Brasileira de Psiquiatria (Sao Paulo, Brazil: 1999), 35*(Suppl. 1), S62–S72.

Buie, T., Campbell, D. B., Fuchs, G. J., 3rd, et al. (2010). Evaluation, diagnosis, and treatment of gastrointestinal disorders in individuals with ASDs: A consensus report. *Pediatrics, 125*(Suppl. 1), S1–S18.

Bull, M. J. (2011). Committee on Genetics: Health supervision for children with Down syndrome. *Pediatrics, 128*(2), 393–406.

Carroll, Y., Eichwald, J., Scinicariello, F., et al. (2017). Vital signs: Noise-induced hearing loss among adults-United States 2011-1012. *MMWR. Morbidity and Mortality Weekly Report, 66*(5).

Centers for Disease Control and Prevention. (2016a). *Key findings: Growth charts for children with Down Syndrome in the United States.* Retrieved from https://www.cdc.gov/ncbddd/birthdefects/features/key-findings-new-down-syndrome-growth-charts.html.

Centers for Disease Control and Prevention. (2016b). *Noise-induced hearing loss.* Retrieved from https://www.cdc.gov/ncbddd/hearingloss/niuse.html.

Centers for Disease Control and Prevention. (2016c). Prevalence of autism spectrum disorder among children aged 8 years—autism and developmental disorders monitoring network, 11 sites, United States, 2012. *MMWR. Surveillance Summaries: Morbidity and Mortality Weekly Report. Surveillance Summaries, 65*(3), 1–23.

Cheng, N., Rho, J. M., & Masino, S. A. (2017). Metabolic dysfunction underlying autism spectrum disorder and potential treatment approaches. *Frontiers in Molecular Neuroscience, 10.*

Chawarska, K., Shic, F., Macari, S., et al. (2014). 18-month predictors of later outcomes in younger siblings of children with autism spectrum disorder: A baby siblings research consortium study. *Journal of the American Academy of Child and Adolescent Psychiatry, 53*(12), 1317–1327.

Christensen, D. L., Baio, J., Braun, K. V., et al. (2016). Prevalence and characteristics of autism spectrum disorder among children aged 8 years—Autism and developmental disabilities monitoring network, 11 sites, United States, 2012. *MMWR. Surveillance Summaries: Morbidity and Mortality Weekly Report. Surveillance Summaries, 65*(SS–3), 1–23.

Clifford, S., Dissanayake, C., Bui, Q. M., et al. (2007). Autism spectrum phenotype in males and females with fragile X full mutation and permutation. *Journal of Autism and Developmental Disorders*, *37*(4), 738–747.

Colella-Santos, M. F., Hein, T. A., de Souza, G. L., et al. (2014). Newborn hearing screening and early diagnostic in the NICU. *BioMed Research International*, 845308.

Coppede, F. (2016). Risk factors for Down syndrome. *Archives of Toxicology*, *90*, 2917–2929.

Crnic, K. A., Neece, C. L., McIntyre, L. L., et al. (2017). Intellectual disability and developmental risk: Promoting intervention to improve child and family well-being. *Child Development*, *88*(2), 436–445.

De Rubeis, S., He, X., Goldberg, A. P., et al. (2014). Synaptic, transcriptional and chromatin genes disrupted in autism. *Nature*, *S15*, 209–215.

Easwar, V., Yamazaki, H., Deighton, M., et al. (2017). Cortical representation of interaural time difference is impaired by deafness in development: Evidence from children with early long-term access to sound through bilateral cochlear implants provided simultaneously. *The Journal of Neuroscience*, *37*(9), 2349–2361.

Englund, C. K., Jonsson, B., Zander, C. S., et al. (2013). Changes in mortality and causes of death in the Swedish Down syndrome population. *American Journal of Medical Genetics. Part A*, *161*, 642–649.

Fabry, D. A., Davila, E. P., Arheart, K. L., et al. (2011). Secondhand smoke exposure and the risk of hearing loss. *Tobacco Control*, *20*(1), 82–85.

Farinetti, A., Gharbia, D. B., Mancini, J., et al. (2014). Cochlear implant complications in 403 patients: Compararive study of adults and children and review of the literature. *European Annals of Otorhinolaryngology, Head and Neck Diseases*, *131*, 177–182.

Fernell, E., Eriksson, M. A., & Gillberg, C. (2013). Early diagnosis of autism and impact on prognosis: A narrative review. *Clinical Epidemiology*, *5*, 33–43.

Finucane, B., Abrams, L., Cronister, A., et al. (2012). Genetic counseling and testing for FMRI gene mutations: Practice guidelines of the National Society of Genetic Counselors. *Journal of Genetic Counseling*, *21*(6), 752–760.

Finucane, B., Lincoln, S., Bailey, L., et al. (2017). Prognostic dilemmas and genetic counseling for prenatally detected fragile X gene expansions. *Prenatal Diagnosis*, *37*, 37–42.

Gabriels, R. L., Pan, Z., Dechant, B., et al. (2015). Randomized controlled trial of therapeutic horseback riding in children and adolescents with autism spectrum disorder. *Journal of the American Academy of Child and Adolescent Psychiatry*, *54*(7), 541–549.

Gan, R., Rowe, A., Benton, C., et al. (2016). Management of hearing loss in children. *Paediatrics & Child Health*, *26*(1), 15–20.

Gilissen, C., Hehir-Kwa, J., Thung, D. T., et al. (2014). Genome sequencing identifies major causes of severe intellectual disability. *Nature*, *511*, 344–347.

Goin-Kochel, R. P., Mire, S. S., Dempsey, A. G., et al. (2016). Parental report of vaccine receipt in children with autism spectrum disorder: Do rates differ by pattern of ASD onset? *Vaccine*, *34*, 1335–1342.

Grafodatskaya, D., Chung, B., Szatmari, P., et al. (2010). Autism spectrum disorders and epigenetics. *Journal of the American Academy of Child and Adolescent Psychiatry*, *49*(8), 794–809.

Grindle, C. R. (2014). Pediatric hearing loss. *Pediatrics in Review*, *35*(11), 456–463.

Guest, H., Munro, K. L., Prendergast, G., et al. (2017). Tinnitis with a normal audiogram: Relation to noise exposure but no evidence for cochlear synaptopathy. *Hearing Research*, *344*, 265–274.

Guralnick, M. J. (2017). Early intervention for children with intellectual disabilities: An update. *Journal of Applied Research in Intellectual Disabilities*, *30*, 211–229.

Haddad, J., & Keesecker, (2016). Hearing loss. In R. M. Kliegman, R. F. Stanton, I. I. I. St. Geme, et al. (Eds.), *Nelson textbook of pediatrics* (20th ed.). Philadelphia: Elsevier Inc.

Herndon, A. C., DiGuiseppi, C., Johnson, S. L., et al. (2009). Does nutritional intake differ between children and autism spectrum disorders and children with typical development? *Journal of Autism and Developmental Disorders*, *39*(2), 212–222.

Hoyme, H. E., Kalberg, W. O., Elliot, A. J., et al. (2016). Updated clinical guidelines for diagnosing fetal alcohol spectrum disorders. *Pediatrics*, *138*.

Huang, X., Zheng, J., Chen, M., et al. (2014). Noninvasive prenatal testing of trisomies 21 and 18 by massively parallel sequencing of maternal plasma DNA in twin pregnancies. *Prenatal Diagnosis*, *34*(4), 335–340.

Joint Committee on Infant Hearing of the American Academy of Pediatrics, Muse, C., Harrison, J., et al. (2013). Supplement to the JCIH 2007 position statement: Principles and guidelines for early intervention after confirmation that a child is deaf or hard of hearing. *Pediatrics*, *131*(4), e1324–e1349.

Karmiloff-Smith, A., Al-Janabi, T., D'Souza, H., et al. (2016). The importance of understanding individual differences in Down syndrome[version 1; referees: 2 approved]. *F1000Research*, *5*(F1000 Faculty Rev), 389.

Katz, G., & Lazcano-Ponce, E. (2008). Intellectual disability: Definition, etiological factors, classification, diagnosis, treatment and prognosis. *Salud Publica de Mexico*, *50*(Suppl. 2), S132–S141.

Kidd, S. A., Lachiewicz, A., Barbouth, D., et al. (2014). Fragile X syndrome: A review of associated medical problems. *Pediatrics*, *134*(5), 995–1005.

Kolevzon, A., Gross, R., & Reichenberg, A. (2007). Prenatal and perinatal risk factors for autism: A review and integration of findings. *Archives of Pediatrics and Adolescent Medicine*, *161*(4), 326–333.

Krishnaswami, S., McPheeters, M. L., & Veenstra-Vanderweele, J. (2011). A systematic review of secretin for children with autism spectrum disorders. *Pediatrics*, *127*(5), e1322–e1325.

Kuehn, B. M. (2011). Scientists find promising therapies for fragile X and Down syndromes. *JAMA: The Journal of the American Medical Association*, *305*(4), 344–346.

Lai, M. C., Lombardo, M. V., & Baron-Cohen, S. (2014). Autism. *Lancet*, *383*(9920), 896–910.

Lammers, M. J., Jansen, T. T., Grolman, W., et al. (2015). The influence of newborn hearing screening on the age at cochlear implantation in children. *The Laryngoscope*, *125*(4), 985–990.

Lantos, J. D. (2012). Ethics for the pediatrician: The evolving risk of cochlear implants in children. *Pediatrics in Review*, *33*(7), 323–326.

Lee, B. (2016). Cytogenetics: Down syndrome and other abnormalities of chromosome number. In R. M. Kliegman, R. F. Stanton, I. I. I. St. Geme, et al. (Eds.), *Nelson textbook of pediatrics* (20th ed.). Philadelphia: Elsevier Inc.

Lee, Y. J., Oh, S. H., Park, C., et al. (2014). Advanced pharmacology evidenced by pathogenesis of autism spectrum disorder. *Clinical Psychopharmacology and Neuroscience*, *12*(1), 19–30.

Lemcke, S., Juul, S., Parner, E. T., et al. (2013). Early signs of autism in toddlers: A follow-up study in the Danish National Birth Cohort. *Journal of Autism and Developmental Disorders*, *43*(10), 2366–2375.

Lewis, C., Hill, M., Silcock, C., et al. (2014). Non-invasive prenatal testing for trisomy 21: A cross-sectional survey of service users' views and likely uptake. *BJOG: An International Journal of Obstetrics and Gynaecology*, *121*(5), 582–594.

Liao, G. J., Chan, K. C., Jiang, P., et al. (2012). Noninvasive prenatal diagnosis of fetal trisomy 21 by allelic ratio analysis using targeted massively parallel sequencing of maternal plasma DNA. *PLoS ONE*, *7*(5), e38154.

Liberman, M. C., & Kujawa, S. G. (2017). Cochlear synaptopathy in acquired sensorineural hearing loss: Manifestations and mechanisms. *Hearing Research*.

Lofthouse, N., Hendren, R., Hurt, E., et al. (2012). A review of complementary and alternative treatments for autism spectrum disorders. *Autism Research and Treatment*, article ID 870391.

Ly, V., Bottelier, M., Hoekstra, P. J., et al. (2017). Elimination diet's efficacy and mechanisms in attention deficit hyperactivity disorder and autism spectrum disorder. *European Child and Adolescent Psychiatry*.

Lyons, J. I., Kerr, G. R., & Mueller, P. W. (2015). Fragile X syndrome: Scientific background and screening technologies. *The Journal of Molecular Diagnostics*, *17*(5), 463–471.

Mefford, H. C., Batshaw, M. L., & Hoffman, E. P. (2012). Genomics, intellectual disability, and autism. *The New England Journal of Medicine*, *366*, 733–743.

Mink, J. W. (2016). Congenital, developmental, and neurocutaneous disorders:Fragile X syndrome. In M. K. Crow, J. H. Doroshow, J. M.

Drazen, et al. (Eds.), *Goldman-cecil medicine* (25th ed.). Philadelphia: Elsevier-Saunders.

Moran, M. (2013). DSM-5 provides new take on neurodevelopment disorders. *Psychiatric News, 48*(2), 6–23.

Morano, S., Ruiz, S., Hwang, J., et al. (2017). Meta-analysis of single-case treatment effects on self-injurious behavior for individuals with autism and intellectual disabilities. *Autism & Developmental Language Impairments, 2*, 1–26.

National Autism Association. (2017a). *Autism fact sheet.* Retrieved from http://nationalautismassociation.org/resources/autism-fact-sheet/.

National Autism Association. (2017b). *Medical Intervention.* Retrieved from http://nationalautismassociation.org/resources/signs-of-autism/.

National Down Syndrome Society. (2012a). *Early intervention.* Retrieved from http://www.ndss.org/Resources/Therapies-Development/Early-Intervention/.

National Down Syndrome Society. (2012b). *Recreation and friendship.* Retrieved from http://www.ndss.org/Resources/Wellness/Recreation-Friendship/.

National Down Syndrome Society. (2012c). *Down Syndrome Facts.* Retreived from http://www.ndss.org/Down-Syndrome/Down-Syndrome-Facts/.

National Down Syndrome Society. (2012d). *Atlantoaxial instability and Down syndrome.* Retrieved from http://www.ndss.org/Resources/Health-Care/Associated-Conditions/Atlantoaxial-Instability-Down-Syndrome/.

National Down Syndrome Society. (2012e). *Down syndrome facts.* Retrieved from http://www.ndss.org/Down-Syndrome/Down-Syndrome-Facts/.

National Fragile X Foundation. (2017a). *Prevalence.* Retrieved from https://fragilex.org/fragile-x-associated-disorders/prevalence/.

National Fragile X Foundation. (2017b). *Genetic counselor.* Retrieved from https://fragilex.org/treatment-intervention/genetic-counselor/.

Ng, M., de Montigny, J. G., Ofner, M., et al. (2017). Environmental factors associated with autism spectrum disorder: A scoping review for the years 2003-2013. *Health Promotion and Chronic Disease Prevention in Canada: Research, Policy and Practice, 37*(1), 1–23.

Oliver, C., & Richards, C. (2010). Self-injurious behavior in people with intellectual disability. *Current Opinion in Psychiatry, 23*(5), 412–416.

Oono, I. P., Honey, E. J., & McConachie, H. (2013). Parent-mediated early intervention for young children with autism spectrum disorders (ASD). *Cochrane Database of Systematic Review*, (4), CD009774.

Orinstein, A. J., Helt, M., Troyb, E., et al. (2014). Intervention for optimal outcome in children and adolescents with a history of autism. *Journal of Developmental and Behavioral Pediatrics : JDBP, 35*(4), 247–256.

O'Toole, P., & Spiegel, D. A. (2016). Torticollis. In R. M. Kliegman, B. F. Stanton, I. I. I. St. Geme, et al. (Eds.), *Nelson textbook of pediatrics* (20th ed.). Philadelphia: Elsevier/Saunders.

Pawlaczyk-Luszczynska, M., Zamojska-Daniszewska, M., Dudarewicz, A., et al. (2017). Exposure to excessive sounds and hearing status in academic classical music students. *International Journal of Occupational Medicine and Environmental Health, 30*(1), 55–75.

Pettinato, M., De Clerck, I., Verhoeven, J., et al. (2017). Expansion of prosodic abilities at the transition from babble to words: A comparison between children with cochlear implants and normally hearing children. *Ear and Hearing.*

Peterson, K., & Barbel, P. (2013). On alert for autism spectrum disorders. *Nursing, 43*(4), 28–34.

Posar, A., & Visconti, P. (2016). Autism in 2016: The need for answers. *Jornal de Pediatria.*

Price, C. S., Thompson, W. W., Goodson, B., et al. (2010). Prenatal and infant exposure to thimerosal from vaccines and immunoglobulins and risk of autism. *Pediatrics, 126*(4), 656–664.

Pueschel, S. M. (1999). The child with Down syndrome. In M. D. Levine, W. B. Carey, & A. C. Crocker (Eds.), *Developmental-behavioral pediatrics* (3rd ed.). Philadelphia: Saunders.

Quint, E. H., & O'Brien, R. F. (2016). Committee on Adolescence and The North American Society for Pediatric and Adolescent Gynecology. *Pediatrics, 138*, doi:10.1542/peds.2016-0295.

Rahi, J. S., Cumberland, P. M., Peckham, C. S., et al. (2010). Improving detection of blindness in childhood: The British Childhood Vision Impairment study. *Pediatrics, 126*(4), e895–e903.

Ramakers, G. G. J., Kraaijenga, V. J. C., van Zanten, G. A., et al. (2016). Effectiveness of earplugs in preventing recreational noise-induced hearing loss-A randomized clinical trial. *JAMA Otolaryngology– Head and Neck Surgery, 142*(6), 551–558.

Raviola, G., Trieu, M. L., DeMaso, D. R., et al. (2016). Autism spectrum disorder. In R. M. Kliegman, B. F. Stanton, I. I. I. St. Geme, et al. (Eds.), *Nelson textbook of pediatrics* (p. 20). Philadelphia: Elsevier/Saunders.

Reichow, B., Barton, E. E., Boyd, B. A., et al. (2012). Early intensive behavioral intervention (EIBI) for young children with autism spectrum disorders (ASD). *Cochrane Database of Systematic Review*, (10), CD009260.

Rogers, G. L., & Jordan, C. O. (2013). Pediatric vision screening. *Pediatrics in Review, 34*(3), 126–133.

Rohlfs, A., Friedhoff, J., Bohnert, A., et al. (2017). Unilateral hearing loss in children: A retrospective study and review of the current literature. *European Journal of Pediatrics*, published on line: 28 January.

Rutter, M. L. (2011). Progress in understanding autism: 2007-2010. *Journal of Autism and Developmental Disorders, 41*(4), 395–404.

Sanchack, K. E., & Thomas, C. A. (2016). Autism spectrum disorder: Primary care principles. *American Family Physician, 94*(12), 972–979.

Shapiro, B. K., & Batshaw, M. L. (2016). Intellectual disability. In R. M. Kliegman, B. F. Stanton, I. I. I. St. Geme, et al. (Eds.), *Nelson textbook of pediatrics* (20th ed.). Philadelphia: Elsevier/Saunders.

Shea, S. E. (2012). Intellectual disability (mental retardation). *Pediatrics in Review, 33*(3), 110–121.

Singh, V. (2015). Newborn hearing screening: Present scenario. *Indian Journal of Community Medicine, 40*(1), 62–65.

Solomon, M., Buaminger, N., & Rogers, S. J. (2011). Abstract reasoning and friendship in high functioning preadolescents with autism spectrum disorders. *Journal of Autism and Developmental Disorders, 41*(1), 32–43.

Sorensen, P. L., Gane, L. W., Yarborough, M., et al. (2013). Newborn screening and cascade testing for FMR1 mutations. *American Journal of Medical Genetics. Part A, 161A*(1), 59–69.

Sturner, R., Howard, B., Bergmann, P., et al. (2016). Autism screening with online decision support by primary care pediatricians aided by M-CHAT/F. *Pediatrics, 138*(3), e20153036.

Talaat, H. S., Metwaly, M. A., Khafagy, A. H., et al. (2014). Dose passive smoking induce sensorineural hearing loss in children? *International Journal of Pediatric Otorhinolaryngology, 78*(1), 46–49.

Talkowski, M. E., Minikel, E. V., & Gusella, J. F. (2014). Autism spectrum disorder genetics: Diverse genes with diverse clinical outcomes. *Harvard Review of Psychiatry, 22*(2), 65–75.

Tasse, M. J., Luckasson, R., & Nygren, M. (2013). AAIDD proposed recommendations for ICD-11 and the condition previously known as mental retardation. *Intellectual and Developmental Disabilities, 51*(2), 127–131.

Taylor, L. E., Swerdfeger, A. L., & Eslick, G. D. (2014). Vaccines are not associated with autism: An evidence-based meta-analysis of case-control and cohort studies. *Vaccine, 32*(29), 3623–3629.

The New York Public Library. (2017). *Talking Book Players.* https://www.nypl.org/about/locations/heiskell/digital-player.

Uno, Y., Uchiyama, T., Kurosawa, M., et al. (2015). Early exposure to the combined measles-mumps-rubella vaccine and thimerosal-containing vaccines and risk of autism spectrum disorder. *Vaccine, 33*(21), 2511–2516.

US Department of Health and Human Services, Office of Disease Prevention and Health Promotion. (2015). *Healthy people 2020: vision.* http://www.healthypeople.gov/2020/topics-objectives/topic/vision.

US Preventive Services Task Force. (2011). Vision screening for children 1 to 5 years of age: US Preventive Services Task Force Recommendation statement. *Pediatrics, 127*(2), 340–346.

Wallander, J. L., Biasini, F. J., Thorsten, V., et al. (2014). Dose of early intervention treatment during children's first 36 months of life is associated with developmental outcomes: An observational cohort study in three low/low-middle income countries. *BMC Pediatrics, 14*, 281.

Weijerman, M. E., & de Winter, J. P. (2010). Clinical practice: The care of children with Down syndrome. *European Journal of Pediatrics, 169*(12), 1445–1452.

Williams, K. J., Wray, J. J., & Wheeler, D. M. (2012). Intravenous secretin for autism spectrum disorder (ASD). *Cochrane Database of Systematic Review*, (4), CD003495.

Willsey, A. J., & State, M. W. (2015). Autism spectrum disorders: From genes to neurobiology. *Current Opinion in Neurobiology*, *30*, 92–99.

Wodka, E. L., Mathy, P., & Kalb, L. (2013). Predictors of phrase and fluent speech in children with autism and severe language delay. *Pediatrics*, *131*(4), e1128–e1134.

Wong, S., Napoli, E., Krakowiak, P., et al. (2016). Role of *p*53, mitrochondrial DNA deletions, and paternal age in autism: A case-control study. *Pediatrics*, *137*(4).

World Health Organization. (2012). *Deafness and hearing loss*. http://www.who.int/mediacentre/factsheets/fs300/en/.

Yoder, P., Stone, W. L., Walden, T., et al. (2009). Predicting social impairment and ASD diagnostic in younger siblings of children with autism spectrum disorder. *Journal of Autism and Developmental Disorders*, *39*(10), 1381–1391.

Zemel, B. S., Pipan, M., Stallings, V. A., et al. (2015). Growth charts for children with Down syndrome in the United States. *Pediatrics*, *136*(5).

Zwaigenbaum, L., Bauman, M. L., Stone, W. L., et al. (2015). Early identification of autism spectrum disorder: Recommendations for practice and research. *Pediatrics*, *136*, S10–S40.

21

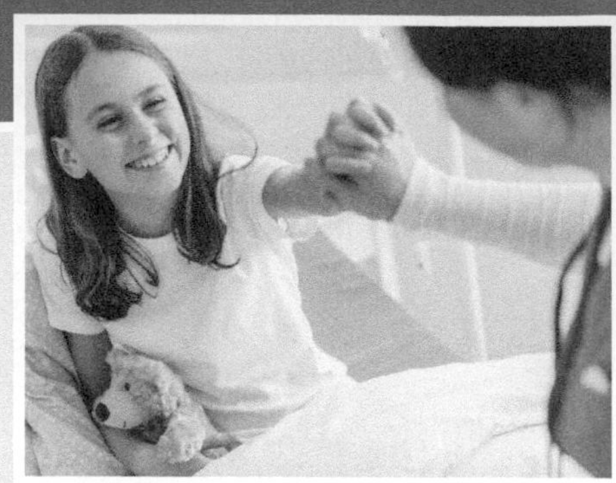

Family-Centered Care of the Child During Illness and Hospitalization

Tara Merck and Patricia Barry McElfresh

http://evolve.elsevier.com/wong/ncic

CONCEPTS

- Stress
- Coping
- Communication
- Family-Centered Care

STRESSORS OF HOSPITALIZATION AND CHILDREN'S REACTIONS

Often, illness and hospitalization are the first crises children must face. Children are particularly vulnerable to these stressors because stress represents a change from the usual state of health and environmental routine and children have a limited number of coping mechanisms to resolve stressors. Major stressors of hospitalization include separation, loss of control, bodily injury, and pain. Children's reactions to these crises are influenced by their developmental age. Previous experience with illness, separation, or hospitalization and innate and acquired coping skills, as well as the seriousness of the diagnosis and current support systems, also affect their reactions. Children express fears caused by the unfamiliar environment or lack of information and control; child-staff relations; and the physical, social, and symbolic environment (Lerwick, 2016).

SEPARATION ANXIETY

The major stress from middle infancy throughout the preschool years, especially for children ages 6 to 30 months, is separation anxiety, also called anaclitic depression. The principal behavioral responses to this stressor during early childhood are summarized in Box 21.1. During the initial stage of protest, children react aggressively to the separation from the parent. They cry and scream for their parents, refuse the attention of anyone else, and are inconsolable in their grief (Fig. 21.1). In contrast, the second stage is the stage of despair. In despair, the crying stops and depression is evident. The child is much less active, is uninterested in play or food, and withdraws from others (Fig. 21.2).

The third stage of detachment is where the child superficially appears to adjust to the loss. The child becomes more interested in the surroundings, plays with others, and seems to form new relationships. However, this behavior is the result of resignation and is not a sign of contentment. The child detaches from the parent in an effort to escape the emotional pain of desiring the parent's presence and copes by forming shallow relationships with others, becoming increasingly self-centered, and attaching primary importance to material objects. This is the most serious stage in that reversal of the potential adverse effects is less likely to occur after detachment is established. The temporary separations imposed by hospitalization do not cause such prolonged parental absences that the child enters into detachment. Although progression to the stage of detachment is uncommon, the initial stages are frequently observed even with brief separations from either parent. Unless health team members understand the meaning of each stage of behavior, they may erroneously label the behaviors as positive or negative. For example, they may see the loud crying of the protest phase as "bad" behavior. Because the protests increase when a stranger approaches the child, they may interpret that reaction as meaning they should stay away. During the quiet, withdrawn phase of despair, health team members may think that the child is finally "settling in" to the new surroundings, and they may see the detachment behaviors as proof of a "good adjustment." The faster this stage is reached, the more likely it is that the child will be regarded as the "ideal patient."

Such reactions are distressing to parents, who are unaware of their meaning (Fig. 21.3). If parents are regarded as intruders, they will see their absence as "beneficial" to the child's adjustment and recovery. They may respond to the child's behavior by staying for only short periods, visiting less frequently, or deceiving the child when it is time

BOX 21.1 Manifestations of Separation Anxiety in Young Children

Stage of Protest

Behaviors observed during later infancy include the following:

- Cries
- Screams
- Searches for parent with eyes
- Clings to parent
- Avoids and rejects contact with strangers

Additional behaviors observed during toddlerhood include the following:

- Verbally attacks strangers (e.g., "Go away")
- Physically attacks strangers (e.g., kicks, bites, hits, pinches)
- Attempts to escape to find parent
- Attempts to physically force parent to stay

Behaviors may last from hours to days.

Protest, such as crying, may be continuous, ceasing only with physical exhaustion.

Approach of stranger may precipitate increased protest.

Stage of Despair

Observed behaviors include the following:

- Is inactive
- Withdraws from others
- Is depressed, sad
- Lacks interest in environment
- Is uncommunicative
- Regresses to earlier behavior (e.g., thumb sucking, bedwetting, use of pacifier, use of bottle)

Behaviors may last for variable length of time.

Child's physical condition may deteriorate from refusal to eat, drink, or move.

Stage of Detachment

Observed behaviors include the following:

- Shows increased interest in surroundings
- Interacts with strangers or familiar caregivers
- Forms new but superficial relationships
- Appears happy

Detachment usually occurs after prolonged separation from parent; it is rarely seen in hospitalized children.

Behaviors represent a superficial adjustment to loss.

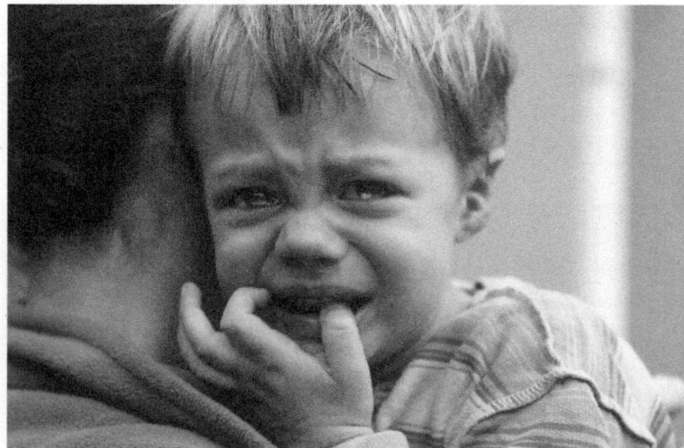

FIG. 21.1 In the protest phase of separation anxiety, children cry loudly and are inconsolable in their grief for the parent.

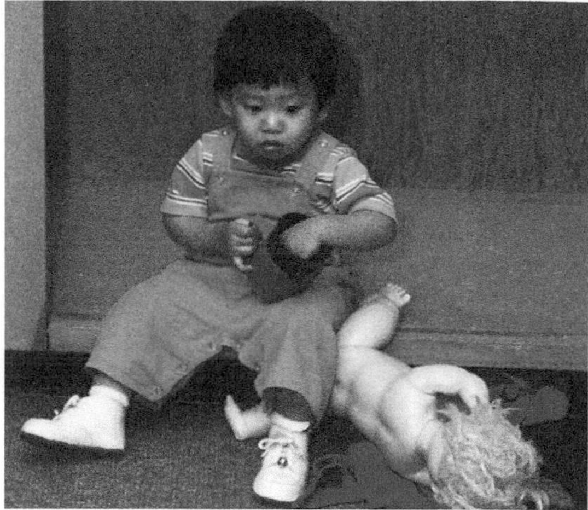

FIG. 21.2 During the despair phase of separation anxiety, children are sad, lonely, and uninterested in food and play.

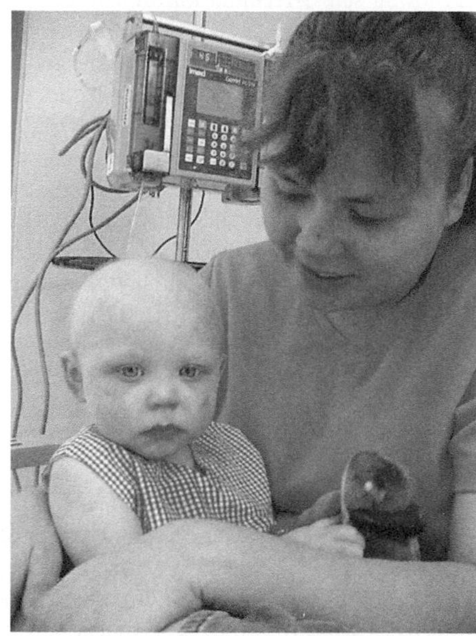

FIG. 21.3 Young children may appear withdrawn and sad even in the presence of a parent. (Courtesy E. Jacob, Texas Children's Hospital, Houston, TX.)

to leave. The result is a destructive cycle of misunderstanding and unmet needs. Considerable evidence suggests that even with stressors, children are remarkably adaptable, and permanent ill effects are rare.

Early Childhood

Separation anxiety is the greatest stress imposed by hospitalization during early childhood. If separation is avoided, young children have a tremendous capacity to withstand any other stress. During this age period, these typical reactions are seen. Children in the toddler stage demonstrate more goal-directed behaviors. For example, they may plead with the parents to stay and physically try to keep the parents with them or try to find parents who have left. They may demonstrate displeasure on the parents' return or departure by having temper tantrums; refusing to comply with the usual routines of mealtime, bedtime, or toileting; or regressing to more primitive levels of development. Temper tantrums, bedwetting, or other behaviors may also be expressions of anger, a physiologic response to stress, or symptoms of illness.

Because preschoolers are more secure interpersonally than toddlers, they can tolerate brief periods of separation from their parents and are more inclined to develop substitute trust in other significant adults. However, the stress of illness usually renders preschoolers less able to cope with separation; as a result, they manifest many of the stage behaviors of separation anxiety, although in general, the protest behaviors are more subtle and passive than those seen in younger children. Preschoolers may demonstrate separation anxiety by refusing to eat, experiencing difficulty in sleeping, crying quietly for their parents, continually asking when the parents will visit, or withdrawing from others. They may express anger indirectly by breaking their toys, hitting other children, or refusing to cooperate during usual self-care activities. Nurses need to be sensitive to these less obvious signs of separation anxiety in order to intervene appropriately.

Later Childhood and Adolescence

In a study that asked children about their fears when hospitalized, children listed their greatest fears regarding hospitalization as being separated from family and friends, being in an unfamiliar environment, receiving treatments, and losing self-determination or choices (Coyne, 2006). In a qualitative study of children 5 to 9 years old, children described hospitalization in stories that focused on being alone and feeling scared, angry, or sad. These children also described the need for protection and companionship while hospitalized (Wilson, Megel, Enenbach, et al., 2010).

Although school-age children are better able to cope with separation in general, the stress and regression imposed by illness or hospitalization may increase their need for parental security and guidance. This is particularly true for younger school-age children who have only recently left the safety of the home and are struggling with the crisis of school adjustment. Older children may react more to the separation from their usual activities and peers than to the absence of their parents. These children may not like school but admit to missing its routine and worry that they will not be able to compete or "fit in" with their classmates when they return. Feelings of loneliness, boredom, isolation, and depression are common. Such reactions may occur more as a result of separation than of concern over the illness, treatment, or hospital setting.

School-age children may need and desire parental guidance or support from adults but may be unable or unwilling to ask for it. Because the goal of attaining independence is so important to them, they are reluctant to seek help directly, fearing that they will appear weak, childish, or dependent. Cultural expectations to "act like a man" or to "be brave and strong" weigh heavily on these children, especially boys, who tend to react to stress with stoicism, withdrawal, or passive acceptance. Often the need to express hostile, angry, or other negative feelings finds outlets in alternate ways, such as irritability and aggression toward parents, withdrawal from hospital personnel, inability to relate to peers, rejection of siblings, or subsequent behavioral problems in school.

For adolescents, separation from home and parents may produce varied emotions. Loss of peer-group contact may pose a severe emotional threat because of loss of group status, inability to exert group control or leadership, and loss of group acceptance. Deviations within peer groups are poorly tolerated, and although group members may express concern for the adolescent's illness or need for hospitalization, they continue their group activities, quickly filling the gap of the absent member. During the temporary separation from their usual group, ill adolescents may benefit from group interactions with other hospitalized teens.

LOSS OF CONTROL

One of the factors influencing the amount of stress imposed by hospitalization is the lack of control. Lack of control increases the perception of threat and can affect children's coping skills. Additional hospital stimuli of sight, sound, and smell may be overwhelming. Without an insight into the type of environment conducive to children's optimal growth, the hospital experience can at best temporarily slow development and at worst permanently restrict it.

EFFECTS OF HOSPITALIZATION ON THE CHILD

Children may react to the stresses of hospitalization before admission, during hospitalization, and after discharge. A recent qualitative study found that children 5 to 6 years of age were able to understand the association between stress and illness; this understanding is related to the child's developmental age and illness experience (Cheetham, Turner-Cobb, & Gamble, 2016). This may or may not be affected by the duration of the condition or prior hospitalizations. Nurses should avoid assuming the child has learned how to cope from prior medical experiences (Box 21.2).

Individual Risk Factors

A number of risk factors make certain children more vulnerable to the stresses of hospitalization, including the environment they live in and their personality traits (Box 21.3). Some children may exhibit significantly greater degrees of psychologic upset than other children. Because

BOX 21.2 Posthospital Behaviors in Children

Young Children

They show initial aloofness toward parents; this may last from a few minutes (most common) to a few days.

This is frequently followed by dependency behaviors:

- Tendency to cling to parents
- Demands for parents' attention
- Vigorous opposition to any separation (e.g., staying at preschool or with a babysitter)

Other negative behaviors include the following:

- New fears (e.g., nightmares)
- Resistance to going to bed, night waking
- Withdrawal and shyness
- Hyperactivity
- Temper tantrums
- Food peculiarities
- Attachment to blanket or toy
- Regression in newly learned skills (e.g., self-toileting)

Older Children

Negative behaviors include the following:

- Emotional coldness followed by intense, demanding dependence on parents
- Anger toward parents
- Jealousy toward others (e.g., siblings)

BOX 21.3 Risk Factors That Increase Children's Vulnerability to the Stresses of Hospitalization

"Difficult" temperament
Lack of fit between child and parent
Age (especially between 6 months old and 5 years old)
Male gender
Below-average intelligence
Multiple and continuing stresses (e.g., frequent hospitalizations)

separation is such an important issue surrounding hospitalization for young children, children who are active and strong willed tend to fare better when hospitalized than those who are passive. Consequently, nurses should be alert to children who passively accept all changes and requests; these children may need more support than "oppositional" children.

The stressors of hospitalization may cause young children to experience short- and long-term negative outcomes. Adverse outcomes may be related to the length and number of admissions, multiple invasive procedures, and the parents' anxiety. Common responses include regression, separation anxiety, apathy, fears, and sleeping disturbances, especially for younger children. Supportive practices, such as family-centered care and frequent family visiting, may lessen the detrimental effects of such admissions.

Changes in the Pediatric Population

The pediatric population in hospitals has changed dramatically over the past two decades. With a growing trend toward shortened hospital stays and outpatient surgery, a greater percentage of the children hospitalized today have more serious and complex problems than those hospitalized in the past. Many of these children are fragile newborns and children with severe injuries or disabilities who have survived because of major technologic advances, yet they have been left with chronic or disabling conditions that require frequent and lengthy hospital stays. The nature of their conditions increases the likelihood that they will experience more invasive and traumatic procedures while they are hospitalized. These factors make them more vulnerable to the emotional consequences of hospitalization and result in their needs being significantly different from those of the short-term patients of the past. The majority of these children are infants and toddlers, which is the age group most vulnerable to the effects of hospitalization. (Refer to Chapter 19 for further discussion on children with special needs.)

Hospitals are looking at ways to decrease length of stay; however, due to complex medical, nursing, and psychosocial needs, this effort has continued to be a challenge. Without special attention devoted to meeting children's psychosocial and developmental needs in the hospital environment, the detrimental consequences of prolonged hospitalization may be severe.

Beneficial Effects of Hospitalization

Although hospitalization is stressful for children, it can also be beneficial. The most obvious benefit is the recovery from illness, but hospitalization also can present an opportunity for children to master stress and feel competent in their coping abilities. The hospital environment can provide children and families with new socialization experiences that can broaden their interpersonal relationships. In addition, hospitalization can provide access to supportive resources that they may never have had access to otherwise. Appropriate nursing strategies to recognize psychologic benefits are presented later in the chapter.

STRESSORS AND REACTIONS OF THE FAMILY OF THE CHILD WHO IS HOSPITALIZED

PARENTAL REACTIONS

The crisis of childhood illness and hospitalization affects every member of the family. Parents' reactions to illness in their child depend on a variety of factors. An association was found between coping abilities and the variables of income range, information provided to the family on admission to the facility, and preparation for hospitalization (Galeano & Carvajal, 2016). A number of factors affecting parent's reactions to variables are identified in Box 21.4.

BOX 21.4 Factors Affecting Parents' Reactions to Their Child's Illness

Seriousness of the threat to the child
Previous experience with illness or hospitalization
Medical procedures involved in diagnosis and treatment
Available support systems
Personal ego strengths
Previous coping abilities
Additional stresses on the family system
Cultural and religious beliefs
Communication patterns among family members
Information and education provided to family throughout hospitalization
Socioeconomic status

Research has identified common themes among parents whose children were hospitalized, including feeling an overall sense of helplessness, questioning the skills of staff, accepting the reality of hospitalization, needing to have information explained in simple language, dealing with fear, coping with uncertainty, and seeking reassurance from caregivers. A qualitative study of parents experiencing care for their child in a pediatric intensive care unit found that they desired continuity of nursing care, needed assurance that the bedside nurse valued their child as an individual, and needed preparation for the complexities of the child's care regimen (Baird, Rehm, Hinds, et al., 2016). Reassurance from the health care team can be in the form of collaboration, information sharing, preparation for procedures, ensuring formal and informal support for the family, and providing information in an unbiased and culturally sensitive manner (Eichner & Johnson, 2012).

SIBLING REACTIONS

Various factors have been identified that influence the effects of the child's hospitalization on siblings. Siblings' reactions to a sister's or brother's illness or hospitalization differ little when a child becomes temporarily ill. Siblings experience loneliness, fear, and worry, as well as anger, resentment, jealousy, and guilt. Illness may also result in children's loss of status within either their family or their social group. It has been found that parents of siblings of children with chronic illness tended to rate sibling health and quality of life better than the siblings' self-reports. The greater disease severity of affected child and older sibling age may be risk factors for impaired well sibling quality of life (Limbers & Skipper, 2014). Although these factors are similar to those seen when a child has a chronic illness, Craft (1993) reported that the following factors regarding siblings are related specifically to the hospital experience and increase the effects on the sibling:

- Being younger and experiencing many changes
- Being cared for outside the home by care providers who are not relatives
- Receiving little information about their ill brother or sister
- Perceiving that their parents treat them differently compared with before their sibling's hospitalization

Parents are often unaware of the number of effects that siblings experience during the sick child's hospitalization and the benefit of simple interventions to minimize such effects, such as explicit explanations about the illness and provisions for the siblings to remain at home. Sibling visitation is usually beneficial to the patient, sibling, and parent but should be evaluated on an individual basis. Siblings should be prepared for the visit with developmentally appropriate information and be given the opportunity to ask questions.

NURSING CARE OF THE CHILD WHO IS HOSPITALIZED

PREPARATION FOR HOSPITALIZATION

Children and families require individualized care to minimize the potential negative effects of hospitalization. One method that can decrease negative feelings and fear in children is preparation for hospitalization. The rationale for preparing children for the hospital experience and related procedures is based on the principle that a fear of the unknown exceeds fear of the known. When children do not have paralyzing fear to cope with, they are able to direct their energies toward dealing with the other, unavoidable stresses of hospitalization.

Although preparation for hospitalization is a common practice, there is no universal standard or program for all settings. The preparation process may be elaborate, with tours, puppet shows, and playtime with miniature hospital equipment; it may involve the use of books, videos, or films; or it may be limited to a brief description of the major aspects of any hospital stay. No consensus exists on the timing of preparation. Some authorities recommend preparing children 4 to 7 years old about 1 week in advance so that they can assimilate the information and ask questions. For older children, the time may be longer. However, for young children, who may begin to wonder about what they observed, 1 or 2 days before admission is sufficient time for anticipatory preparation. The length of the session should be tailored to the children's attention span—the younger the child, the shorter the program. The optimal approach is one that is individualized for each child and family.

Regardless of the specific method of preparation, all children, even those who have been hospitalized before, benefit from an introduction to the environment and routine of the hospital unit. Sometimes it is not possible to prepare children and families for hospitalization, such as in the event of sudden, acute illness. However, care should be taken to orient the child and family to hospital routines, establish expectations, and allow for questions (Abraham & Moretz, 2012).

NURSING TIP

In many hospitals, child life specialists—health care professionals with extensive knowledge of child growth and development and of the special psychosocial needs of children—help prepare children for hospitalization, surgery, and procedures. Although the structure of a program may vary depending on the size of the pediatric facility, the patient population, and the availability of ancillary services, the two primary program objectives for child life interactions are (1) to reduce the stress and anxiety related to the hospitalization or health care–related experiences and (2) to promote normal growth and development in the health care setting and at home (Thompson, 2009).

A collaborative effort between the nurse, child life specialist, and other members of the child's health care team help ensure the best possible hospital experience for the child and family.

Admission Assessment

The nursing admission history refers to a systematic collection of data about the child and family that allows the nurse to plan individualized care. The nursing admission history presented in Box 21.5 is organized according to the Functional Health Patterns outlined by Gordon (2002) (see Nursing Diagnosis, Chapter 1). This assessment framework is a guideline for formulating nursing diagnoses. One of the main purposes of the history is to assess the child's usual health habits at home to promote a more normal environment in the hospital. Therefore questions related to activities of daily living in the nutritional/metabolic, elimination, sleep/rest, and activity/exercise patterns are a major part of the assessment. The questions found under the health perception/health management pattern are directed toward evaluation of the child's preparation for hospitalization and are key factors in determining whether additional preparation is needed. The questions included in the self-perception/self-concept and role/relationship patterns offer insight into the child's potential reaction to hospitalization, especially in terms of separation.

The nurse should also inquire about the use of any medications at home, including complementary medicine practices (Box 21.6). Many families use alternative or complementary therapies simultaneously with or after conventional treatments. It is important that the use of any herbal or complementary therapy be noted in a preoperative assessment because of possible anesthesia or surgical complications related to herbal products (see Critical Thinking Case Study box).

CRITICAL THINKING CASE STUDY

Complementary and Alternative Medicine

Maria, a 13-year-old Hispanic girl, has had severe nosebleeds. She is admitted to the hospital for a complete workup in an attempt to determine the cause. Her parents and grandparents have gathered around her bed. When you enter her room to begin admitting procedures, you notice an unusual scent. Maria's mother is rubbing the contents from an unfamiliar bottle of liquid on Maria. Meanwhile, the grandmother is rubbing Maria's head. She is startled at your entry and drops something on the floor near your feet. You bend over to pick it up and discover that it is a penny.

Questions

1. Evidence: Is there sufficient evidence to draw any conclusions?
2. Assumptions: What are some underlying assumptions that may be drawn from the data about the following:
   a. Complementary or alternative medical remedies
   b. The role of ethnic or folk remedies in modern health care practice
   c. The nurse's role in cases where alternative medicine is practiced (vs. traditional medicine)
3. What implications and priorities for nursing care can be drawn at this time?
4. Does the evidence objectively support your argument (conclusion)?

Answers are available at http://evolve.elsevier.com/wong/ncic.

In addition to completing the nursing admission history, nurses should also perform a physical assessment (see Chapter 4) before planning care. At the very least, the nurse's physical assessment of the child should include observation of the body for any bruises, rashes, signs of neglect, deformities, or physical limitations. The nurse should also listen to the heart and lungs to assess overall physical status. For example, it is impossible to evaluate improvement in respiratory function in a child admitted with pulmonary disease unless there are baseline data with which to compare subsequent findings.

Preparing the Child for Admission

The preparation that children require on the day of admission depends on the kind of prehospital counseling they have received. If they have been prepared in a formalized program, they usually know what to expect in terms of initial medical procedures, inpatient facilities, and nursing staff. However, prehospital counseling does not preclude the need for support during procedures, such as obtaining blood specimens, x-ray tests, or physical examination. For example, undressing young children before they feel comfortable in their new surroundings can be upsetting. Causing needless anxiety and fear during admission may adversely affect the nurse's establishment of trust with these children. Therefore nursing assistance during the admission procedure is vital

BOX 21.5 Nursing Admission History According to Functional Health Patterns*

Health Perception/Health Management Pattern

Why has your child been admitted?

How has your child's general health been?

What does your child know about this hospitalization?

- Ask the child why he or she came to the hospital.
- If the answer is "For an operation or for tests," ask the child to tell you about what will happen before, during, and after the operation or tests.

Has your child ever been in the hospital before?

- How was that hospital experience?
- What things were important to you and your child during that hospitalization? How can we be most helpful now?

What medications does your child take at home?

Why are they given?

When are they given?

How are they given (if a liquid, with a spoon; if a tablet, swallowed with water; or other)?

Does your child have any trouble taking medication? If so, what helps?

Is your child allergic to any medications?

What, if any, forms of complementary medicine practices are being used?

Nutrition/Metabolic Pattern

What is the family's usual mealtime?

Do family members eat together or at separate times?

What are your child's favorite foods, beverages, and snacks?

- Average amounts consumed or usual size of portions
- Special cultural practices, such as family eats only ethnic food

What foods and beverages does your child dislike?

What are your child's feeding habits (bottle, cup, spoon, eats by self, needs assistance, any special devices)?

How does your child like the food served (warmed, cold, one item at a time)?

How would you describe your child's usual appetite (hearty eater, picky eater)?

- Has being sick affected your child's appetite? In what ways?

Are there any known or suspected food allergies?

Is your child on a special diet?

Are there any feeding problems (excessive fussiness, spitting up, colic); any dental or gum problems that affect feeding?

- What do you do for these problems?

Elimination Pattern

What are your child's toileting habits (diaper, toilet trained—day only or day and night, use of word to communicate urination or defecation, potty chair, regular toilet, other routines)?

What is your child's usual pattern of elimination (bowel movements)?

Do you have any concerns about elimination (bedwetting, constipation, diarrhea)?

- What do you do for these problems?

Have you ever noticed that your child sweats a lot?

Sleep/Rest Pattern

What is your child's usual hour of sleep and awakening?

What is your child's schedule for naps; length of naps?

Is there a special routine before sleeping (bottle, drink of water, bedtime story, night light, favorite blanket or toy, prayers)?

Is there a special routine during sleep time, such as waking to go to the bathroom?

What type of bed does your child sleep in?

Does your child have a separate room or share a room; if shares, with whom?

Does your child sleep with someone or alone (e.g., sibling, parent, other person)?

What is your child's favorite sleeping position?

Are there any sleeping problems (falling asleep, waking during night, nightmares, sleep walking)?

Are there any problems in awakening and getting ready in the morning?

- What do you do for these problems?

Activity/Exercise Pattern

What is your child's schedule during the day (preschool, daycare center, regular school, extracurricular activities)?

What are your child's favorite activities or toys (both active and quiet interests)?

What is your child's usual television-viewing schedule at home?

What are your child's favorite programs?

Are there any television restrictions?

Does your child have any illness or disabilities that limit activity? If so, how?

What are your child's usual habits and schedule for bathing (bath in tub or shower, sponge bath, shampoo)?

What are your child's dental habits (brushing, flossing, fluoride supplements or rinses, favorite toothpaste); schedule of daily dental care?

Does your child need help with dressing or grooming, such as hair combing?

Are there any problems with these patterns (dislike of or refusal to bathe, shampoo hair, or brush teeth)?

- What do you do for these problems?

Are there special devices that your child requires help in managing (eyeglasses, contact lenses, hearing aid, orthodontic appliances, artificial elimination appliances, orthopedic devices)?

Note: Use the following code to assess functional self-care level for feeding, bathing and hygiene, dressing and grooming, and toileting:

0: Full self-care

I: Requires use of equipment or device

II: Requires assistance or supervision from another person

III: Requires assistance or supervision from another person and equipment or device

IV: Is totally dependent and does not participate

Cognitive/Perceptual Pattern

Does your child have any hearing difficulty?

- Does the child use a hearing aid?
- Have "tubes" been placed in your child's ears?

Does your child have any vision problems?

- Does the child wear glasses or contact lenses?

Does your child have any learning difficulties?

What is the child's grade in school?

For information on pain, see Chapter 5

Self-Perception/Self-Concept Pattern

How would you describe your child (e.g., takes time to adjust, settles in easily, shy, friendly, quiet, talkative, serious, playful, stubborn, easygoing)?

What makes your child angry, annoyed, anxious, or sad? What helps?

How does your child act when annoyed or upset?

What have your child's experiences been with and reactions to temporary separation from you (parent)?

Does your child have any fears (places, objects, animals, people, situations)?

- How do you handle them?

Do you think your child's illness has changed the way he or she thinks about himself or herself (e.g., more shy, embarrassed about appearance, less competitive with friends, stays at home more)?

Role/Relationship Pattern

Does your child have a favorite nickname?

What are the names of other family members or others who live in the home (relatives, friends, pets)?

Continued

BOX 21.5 Nursing Admission History According to Functional Health Patterns*—cont'd

Who usually takes care of your child during the day and night (especially if other than parent, such as babysitter, relative)?

What are the parents' occupations and work schedules?

Are there any special family considerations (adoption, foster child, stepparent, divorce, single parent)?

Have any major changes in the family occurred lately (death, divorce, separation, birth of a sibling, loss of a job, financial strain, mother beginning a career, other)? Describe child's reaction.

Who are your child's play companions or social groups (peers, younger or older children, adults, or prefers to be alone)?

Do things generally go well for your child in school or with friends?

Does your child have "security" objects at home (pacifier, bottle, blanket, stuffed animal or doll)? Did you bring any of these to the hospital?

How do you handle discipline problems at home? Are these methods always effective?

Does your child have any condition that interferes with communication? If so, what are your suggestions for communicating with your child?

Will your child's hospitalization affect the family's financial support or care of other family members (e.g., other children)?

What concerns do you have about your child's illness and hospitalization?

Who will be staying with your child while hospitalized?

How can we contact you or another close family member outside of the hospital?

Sexuality/Reproductive Pattern

(Answer questions that apply to your child's age group.)

Has your child begun puberty (developing physical sexual characteristics, menstruation)? Have you or your child had any concerns?

Does your daughter know how to do breast self-examination?

Does your son know how to do testicular self-examination?

How have you approached topics of sexuality with your child?

Do you think you might need some help with some topics?

Has your child's illness affected the way he or she feels about being a boy or a girl? If so, how?

Do you have any concerns with behaviors in your child, such as masturbation, asking many questions or talking about sex, not respecting others' privacy, or wanting too much privacy?

Initiate a conversation about an adolescent's sexual concerns with open-ended to more direct questions and using the terms "friends" or "partners" rather than "girlfriend" or "boyfriend":

- Tell me about your social life.
- Who are your closest friends? (If one friend is identified, could ask more about that relationship, such as how much time they spend together, how serious they are about each other, if the relationship is going the way the teenager hoped.)
- Might ask about dating and sexual issues, such as the teenager's views on sexuality education, "going steady," "living together," or premarital sex.
- Which friends would you like to have visit in the hospital?

Coping/Stress Tolerance Pattern

(Answer questions that apply to your child's age group.)

What does your child do when tired or upset?

- If upset, does your child want a special person or object?
- If so, explain.

If your child has temper tantrums, what causes them, and how do you handle them?

Whom does your child talk to when worried about something?

How does your child usually handle problems or disappointments?

Have there been any big changes or problems in your family recently? If so, how have you handled them?

Has your child ever had a problem with drugs or alcohol or tried to commit suicide?

Do you think your child is "accident prone?" If so, explain.

Value/Belief Pattern

What is your religion?

How is religion or faith important in your child's life?

What religious practices would you like continued in the hospital (e.g., prayers before meals or bedtime; visit by minister, priest, or rabbi; prayer group)?

*The focus of the admission history is the child's psychosocial environment. Most of the questions are worded in terms of parental responses. Depending on the child's age, they should be addressed directly to the child when appropriate.

BOX 21.6 Complementary Medicine Practices and Examples

Nutrition, diet, and lifestyle or behavioral health changes: Macrobiotics, megavitamins, diets, lifestyle modification, health risk reduction and health education, wellness

Mind-body control therapies: Biofeedback, relaxation, prayer therapy, guided imagery, hypnotherapy, music or sound therapy, massage, aromatherapy, education therapy

Traditional and ethnomedicine therapies: Acupuncture, ayurvedic medicine, herbal medicine, homeopathic medicine, American Indian medicine, natural products, traditional Asian medicine

Structural manipulation and energetic therapies: Acupressure, chiropractic medicine, massage, reflexology, rolfing, therapeutic touch, Qi Gong

Pharmacologic and biologic therapies: Antioxidants, cell treatment, chelation therapy, metabolic therapy, oxidizing agents

Bioelectromagnetic therapies: Diagnostic and therapeutic application of electromagnetic fields (e.g., transcranial electrostimulation, neuromagnetic stimulation, electroacupuncture)

regardless of how well prepared any child is for the experience of hospitalization. In addition, spending this time with the child gives the nurse an opportunity to evaluate the child's understanding of subsequent procedures (Fig. 21.4). Ideally, a primary nurse is assigned whenever possible to allow for individualized care and to provide an additional support person for the child.

When a child is admitted, nurses follow universal admission procedures (Box 21.7). The minimum considerations for room assignment are age, sex, and nature of the illness. Organizations have developed guidelines regarding patient room placement. Placing children of the same age group and with similar types of illness in the same unit can be both psychologically and medically advantageous. A child who is independent despite physical disabilities may help another child with similar or different limitations, and the parents of the child with disabilities may achieve deeper insight and acceptance of their child's disorder. Age grouping is especially important for adolescents. Many hospitals make an effort to place teenagers on their own unit or in a separate designated section of the pediatric or general unit whenever possible.

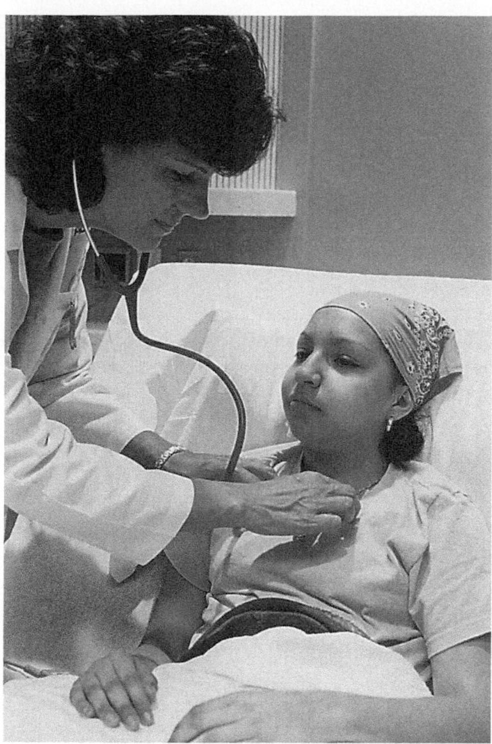

FIG. 21.4 The initial admission procedures give the nurse an opportunity to get to know the child and to assess the child's understanding of the hospital experience.

BOX 21.7 Guidelines for Admission

Preadmission

Assign a room based on developmental age, seriousness of diagnosis, communicability of illness, and projected length of stay.

Prepare roommate(s) for the arrival of a new patient; when children are too young to benefit from this consideration, prepare parents.

Prepare room for child and family, with admission forms and equipment nearby to eliminate need to leave child.

Admission

Introduce primary nurse to child and family.

Orient child and family to inpatient facilities, especially to assigned room and unit; emphasize positive areas of pediatric unit.

Room: Explain call light, bed controls, television, bathroom, telephone, and so on.

Unit: Direct to playroom, desk, dining area, or other areas.

Introduce family to roommate and his or her parents.

Apply identification band to child's wrist, ankle, or both (if not already done).

Explain hospital regulations and schedules (e.g., visiting hours, mealtimes, bedtime, limitations [give written information if available]).

Perform nursing admission history (see Box 21.5).

Take vital signs, blood pressure, height, and weight.

Obtain specimens as needed and order needed laboratory work.

Support child and assist practitioner with physical examination (for purposes of nursing assessment).

NURSING INTERVENTIONS

Preventing or Minimizing Separation

A primary nursing goal is to prevent separation, particularly in children younger than 5 years old. Many hospitals have developed a system of family-centered care. Efforts to collaborate with families and encourage their involvement in the patient's care include optimizing family visitation, family-centered rounding, family presence during procedures or interventions, and opportunities for formal and informal family conferences (Meert, Clark, & Eggly, 2013). Family-centered care started in pediatrics with the increased recognition of child and family separation trauma in the inpatient setting. Policies were adapted first in pediatrics to allow for rooming-in, longer visiting hours, sibling visits, and systems to allow families to accompany patients off the unit for procedures (Institute for Patient- and Family-Centered Care, 2010a, 2010b).

At the very least, most hospitals welcome parents at any time. Many facilities provide sleeping accommodations for at least one person per child. In addition, some units have kitchen privileges and other amenities that create a welcoming atmosphere for parents. However, not all hospitals provide such amenities, and parents' own schedules may prevent rooming-in. In such instances, strategies to minimize the effects of separation must be implemented.

Nurses must have knowledge of the child's separation behaviors. As discussed earlier, the phases of protest and despair are normal. Even if the child rejects strangers, nurses may provide support via their physical presence, using a quiet tone of voice, maintaining eye contact, and using touch in a way that establishes rapport and communicates empathy. If behaviors of detachment are evident, the nurse maintains the child's contact with the parents by frequently talking about them; encouraging the child to remember them; and stressing the significance of their visits, telephone calls, or letters. The use of cellular phones can increase the contact between the hospitalized child and parents or other significant family members and friends.

Parental Absence During Infant Hospitalization

Familiar surroundings also increase the child's adjustment to separation. If the parents cannot stay with the child, they should leave favorite articles from home with the child, such as a blanket or a toy. Children gain comfort and reassurance from holding onto these possessions. They make the association that if the parents left this, the parents will surely return. Placing an identification band on the toy lessens the chances of its being misplaced and provides a symbol that the toy is experiencing the same needs as the child. Other reminders of home include photographs and video recordings of family members reading a story or singing a song. These reminders can be brought out at lonely times, such as on awakening or before sleeping. Some units allow pets to visit, which can have therapeutic benefits for a child. Often the importance of treasured objects to school-age children or adolescents can be overlooked or criticized. However, these older children have a special object to which they formed an attachment in early childhood. Therefore such treasured or transitional objects can help even older children feel more comfortable in a strange environment.

The strange sights, smells, and sounds in the hospital can be frightening and confusing for children. It is important for the nurse to try to evaluate stimuli in the environment from the child's point of view (considering also what the child may see or hear happening to other patients) and to make every effort to protect the child from frightening and unfamiliar sights, sounds, and equipment. The nurse should offer explanations or prepare the child for experiences that are unavoidable. Combining familiar or comforting sights with the unfamiliar can relieve much of the harshness of medical equipment.

Helping children maintain their usual contacts also minimizes the effects of separation imposed by hospitalization. This includes continuing school lessons during the illness and confinement, visiting with friends either directly or through letter writing or telephone calls, and participating in stimulating projects whenever possible (Fig. 21.5). For extended hospitalizations, youngsters enjoy personalizing the hospital room to

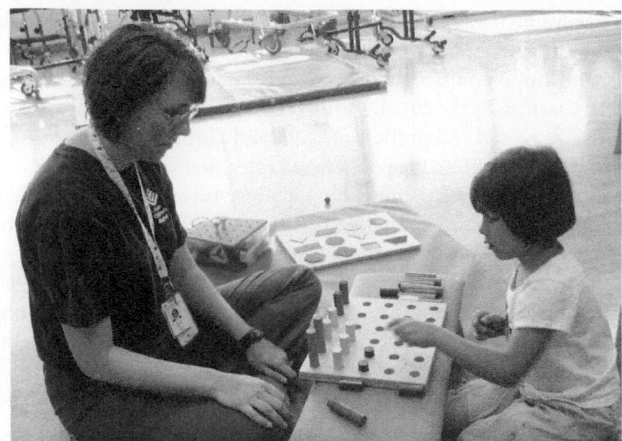

FIG. 21.5 For extended hospitalizations, children enjoy doing projects to occupy time.

Eric's Daily Schedule			
7:30 AM	– Breakfast, morning bath	3:00 PM	– Tutor (M, W, F) – Study time (T, Th)
9:00	– Medications, dressing change	4:00	– Physical therapy
11:00	– Physical therapy	5:30	– Dinner
12:00 PM	– Lunch	9:00	– Medications, dressing change
		9:15	– Bedtime

FIG. 21.6 Time structuring is an effective strategy for normalizing the hospital environment and increasing the child's sense of control.

make it "home" by decorating the walls with posters and cards, rearranging the furniture, and displaying a collection or hobby.

Minimizing Loss of Control

Children feel a loss of control due to physical restrictions, changed routines, and enforced dependency. Some of these stressors cannot be prevented, although most can be minimized through individualized nursing care to can help minimize their impact.

Promoting Freedom of Movement

Younger children react most strenuously to any type of physical restriction or immobilization. Although temporary immobilization may be necessary for some interventions such as maintaining an intravenous line, most physical restrictions can be prevented if the nurse gains the child's cooperation.

For young children, particularly infants and toddlers, preserving parent-child contact is the best means of decreasing the need for restraint. Nearly the entire physical examination can be done in a parent's lap with the parent hugging the child for procedures, such as an otoscopic examination. For painful procedures, the nurse should assess the parents' preferences for assisting, observing, or waiting outside the room.

In some cases, physical restraint or isolation is necessary because of the child's medical diagnosis. Ideas to increase opportunities for movement for those who can be mobile provides a sense of freedom. In these cases, the environment can be altered to increase sensory freedom (e.g., moving the bed toward the window; opening window shades; providing musical, visual, or tactile activities).

Maintaining the Child's Routine

Altered daily schedules and loss of rituals are particularly stressful for toddlers and early preschoolers and may increase the stress of separation. The nursing admission history provides a baseline for planning care around the child's usual home activities. A frequently neglected aspect of altered routines is the change in the child's daily activities. A typical child's day, especially during the school years, is structured with specific times for eating, dressing, going to school, playing, and sleeping. However, this time structure vanishes when the child is hospitalized. Although nurses have a set schedule, the child is frequently unaware of it, and the new schedules that are imposed may be rigid. For example, some units have uniform nap times and bedtimes for all children, but others allow children to stay up late at night. Many children obtain significantly less sleep in the hospital than at home; the primary causes are a delay in sleep onset and early termination of sleep because of hospital routines. Not only are hours of sleep disrupted, but waking hours are spent in passive activities. For example, few institutions impose any limits on the amount of time the child spends watching television. This may lead to children feeling less physically "tired" at bedtime and delay the onset of sleep.

One technique that can minimize the disruption in the child's routine is establishing a daily schedule. This approach is most suitable for non–critically ill school-age and adolescent children who have mastered the concept of time. It involves scheduling the child's day to include all those activities that are important to the child and nurse, such as treatment procedures, schoolwork, exercise, television, playroom, and hobbies. Together, the nurse, parent, and child then plan a written daily schedule with times (Fig. 21.6). The schedule is placed in the child's room, and a clock or watch is available for the child's use. Whenever possible, a calendar is also constructed with special events marked, such as favorite television programs, visits by friends or relatives, events in the playroom, and holidays or birthdays. If specific changes in treatment are expected (e.g., "beginning physical therapy in 2 days"), these are added.

> **! NURSING ALERT**
>
> Ask the young child to select or draw pictures or symbols to represent daily or weekly fun activities (e.g., favorite television programs, family visits, and playroom times). Draw a clock face with the hands of the clock depicting the time each event will occur next to the child's representation. Have the child compare the clock on the schedule with a clock or watch in the room. When the two match, the child knows it is time for a favorite activity.

Encouraging Independence

The dependent role of the hospitalized patient imposes tremendous feelings of loss for older children. Principal interventions should focus on respect for individuality and the opportunity for decision making. Although these sound simple, their efficacy lies with nurses who are flexible and tolerant. It is also important for the nurse to empower the patient while not feeling threatened by a sense of lessened control.

Enabling children's control involves helping them maintain independence and promoting the concept of self-care. Self-care refers to the practice of activities that individuals personally initiate and perform on their own behalf in maintaining life, health, and well-being (Orem, 2001). Although self-care is limited by the child's age and physical condition, most children beyond infancy can perform some activities with little or no help. Whenever possible, these activities are encouraged in the hospital. Other approaches include jointly planning care, time structuring, wearing street clothes, making choices in food selections and bedtime, continuing school activities, and rooming with an appropriate-age child.

BOX 21.8 Bill of Rights for Children and Teens

In this hospital, you and your family have the right to:

- Respect and personal dignity
- Care that supports you and your family
- Information you can understand
- Quality health care
- Emotional support
- Care that respects your need to grow, play, and learn
- Make choices and decisions

From Association for the Care of Children's Health. (1991). *A pediatric bill of rights.* Bethesda, MD: Author.

Promoting Understanding

Loss of control can occur from feelings of having too little influence on one's destiny or from sensing overwhelming control or power over fate. Although preschoolers' cognitive abilities predispose them to magical thinking and delusions of power, all children are vulnerable to misinterpreting causes for stress, such as illness and hospitalization.

Most children feel more in control when they know what to expect because the element of fear of the unknown is reduced. Anticipatory preparation and provision of information help lessen stress and increase understanding (see Chapter 19).

Informing children of their rights while hospitalized fosters greater understanding and may relieve some of the feelings of powerlessness they typically experience. An increasing number of hospitals and organizations have developed a patient "bill of rights" that is prominently displayed throughout the hospital or is presented to children and their families on admission (Box 21.8).

Preventing or Minimizing Fear of Bodily Injury

Beyond early infancy, all children fear bodily injury from mutilation, bodily intrusion, body image change, disability, or death. In general, preparation of children for painful procedures decreases their fears and increases cooperation. Modifying procedural techniques for children in each age group also minimizes fear of bodily injury. For example, because toddlers and young preschoolers are traumatized by insertion of a rectal thermometer, axillary temperatures or temperatures taken with electronic or tympanic membrane devices can effectively be substituted. Whenever procedures are performed on young children, the most supportive intervention is to do the procedure as quickly as possible while maintaining parent-child contact.

Because of toddlers' and preschool children's poorly defined body boundaries, the use of bandages may be particularly helpful. For example, telling children that the bleeding will stop after the needle is removed does little to relieve their fears, but applying a small Band-Aid usually reassures them. The size of bandages is also significant to children in this age group; the larger the bandage, the more importance is attached to the wound. Watching their surgical dressings become successively smaller is one way young children can measure healing and improvement. Prematurely removing a dressing may cause these children considerable concern for their well-being. Specific pain management strategies are discussed in Chapter 5.

For children who fear mutilation of body parts, it is essential that the nurse repeatedly stress the reason for a procedure and evaluate the child's understanding. For example, explaining cast removal to preschoolers may seem simple enough, but children's comprehension of the details may vary considerably from the explanation. Asking the child to draw a picture of what they foresee happening presents substantial evidence of how they perceive events.

Children may fear bodily injury from a great variety of sources. Imaging or diagnostic equipment used for examination, unfamiliar rooms, and awkward positions can be perceived as potentially hazardous. In addition, thoughts and actions can be imagined sources of bodily damage. Therefore it is important to investigate imagined reasons, particularly of a sexual nature, for illness. Because children may fear revealing such thoughts, using techniques such as drawing or doll play may elicit previously undisclosed misconceptions.

Older children fear bodily injury of both internal and external origins. For example, school-age children are aware of the significance of the heart and may fear the actual operation as much as the pain, the stitches, and the possible scar. Adolescents may express concern about the actual procedure but be much more anxious over the resulting scar.

Children can grasp information if it is presented on or close to their level of cognitive development. This necessitates an awareness of the words used to describe events or processes. For example, young children told that they are going to have a "CAT scan" (i.e., CT, computed tomography) may wonder, "Will there be cats or something that scratches?" It is clearer to describe the procedure in simple terms and explain what the letters of the common name stand for. Therefore to prevent or alleviate fears, nurses must be keenly aware of the medical terminology and vocabulary that they use every day.

When children are upset about their illness, their perception can be changed by providing a somewhat different and less negative account of the disease or offering an explanation that is characteristic of the next stage of cognitive development. An example of the first strategy is reassuring a preschooler who fears that after a tonsillectomy, another sore throat means a second operation. Explaining that after tonsils are "fixed" they do not need fixing again can help relieve the fear. An example of the latter strategy is to explain that germs made the tonsils sick and even though germs can cause another sore throat, they cannot cause the tonsils to ever be sick again. This higher-level explanation is based on the school-age child's concept of germs as a cause of disease.

Providing Developmentally Appropriate Activities

A primary goal of nursing care for the child who is hospitalized is to minimize threats to the child's development. Many strategies (e.g., minimizing separation) have been discussed and may be all that the short-term patient requires. However, children who experience prolonged or repeated hospitalization are at greater risk for developmental delays or regression. The nurse who provides opportunities for the child to participate in developmentally appropriate activities further normalizes the child's environment and helps reduce interference with the child's ongoing development.

Interference with normal development may have long-term implications for developing infants and toddlers. The nurse plays a primary role in identifying children at risk and helping plan, implement, and evaluate developmental intervention. (See Chapters 9 and 11.)

School is an integral part of the school-age child's and adolescent's development. Accreditation standards for hospitals serving children consider access to appropriate educational services a key factor in the accreditation decision process when a child's treatment requires a significant absence from school (The Joint Commission, 2011). The nurse can encourage children to resume schoolwork as quickly as their condition permits, help them schedule and protect a selected time for studies, and help the family coordinate hospital educational services with their children's schools. Children should have the opportunity to continue art and music classes, as well as their academic subjects.

To meet the unique developmental needs of adolescents, special units may be developed that provide privacy, increased socialization, and appropriate activities for these young people. Typically, these units can be set apart from the general pediatric facility so that the teenagers do not share space with younger children, who are often perceived as a threat to their maturity.

In caring for adolescent patients, it is essential to provide flexible routines and activities, such as more group activity, wearing of street clothes, and access to the items so critical to adolescents—wireless technology devices, Wi-Fi, smart phones, tablets, DVD players, computers, email, electronic video game systems, and high-definition televisions. Because adolescents' food habits are rarely limited to the three traditional meals a day, a ready supply of snacks should be available. However, the most important benefit of these units is increased socialization with peers. In addition, staff members usually enjoy working with this age group and are able to establish the trust that is so essential for communication.

> **! NURSING ALERT**
>
> When adolescents must share a common activity room with younger patients, referring to the area as the "activity room" rather than the "playroom" may entice them to visit the room and participate in activities.

Although regression is expected and normal for all age groups, nurses have the responsibility for fostering the child's growth and development. Hospitalization can become a significant barrier for learning and advancing. Extended hospitalizations for long-term chronic illness or situations of failure to thrive, abuse, or neglect represent instances in which regression must be seen as an adjustment period to be followed by plans for promoting appropriate developmental skills.

Providing Opportunities for Play and Expressive Activities

Play is one of the most important aspects of a child's life and one of the most effective tools for managing stress. Because illness and hospitalization constitute crises in a child's life and often involve overwhelming stresses, children need to act out their fears and anxieties as a means of coping with these stresses. Play is essential to children's mental, emotional, and social well-being; however, play does not stop when children are ill or in the hospital. On the contrary, play in the hospital serves many functions (Box 21.9). Of all hospital facilities, no room probably alleviates the stressors of hospitalization more than the playroom (or activity room). In the playroom, children temporarily distance themselves from their illness, hospitalization, and the associated stressors. This room should be a safe haven for children, free from medical or nursing procedures (including medication administration), strange faces, and probing questions. The playroom then becomes a sanctuary in an otherwise frightening environment.

Engaging in play activities gives children a sense of control. In the hospital environment, most decisions are made for the child; play and other expressive activities offer the child much-needed opportunities to make choices for themselves. Even if a child chooses not to participate in a particular activity, the nurse has offered the child a choice, perhaps one of only a few real choices the child has had that day.

> **BOX 21.9 Functions of Play in the Hospital**
>
> - Provides diversion and brings about relaxation
> - Helps the child feel more secure in a strange environment
> - Lessens the stress of separation and the feeling of homesickness
> - Provides a means for release of tension and expression of feelings
> - Encourages interaction and development of positive attitudes toward others
> - Provides an expressive outlet for creative ideas and interests
> - Provides a means for accomplishing therapeutic goals (see Use of Play in Procedures, Chapter 19)
> - Places child in active role and provides opportunity to make choices and be in control

Hospitalized children typically have lower energy levels than healthy children of the same age. Therefore children may not appear engaged and enthusiastic about an activity even though they are enjoying the experience. Activities may need to be adjusted or limited based on the child's age, endurance, and any special needs.

Diversional Activities

Almost any form of play can be used for diversion and recreation, but the activity should be selected on the basis of the child's age, interests, and limitations (Fig. 21.7). Children do not necessarily need special direction for using play materials. All they require is the raw materials with which to work and adult approval and supervision to help keep their natural enthusiasm and expression of feelings. Small children enjoy a variety of small, colorful toys that they can play with in bed or in their room or more elaborate play equipment, such as playhouses, sandboxes, rhythm instruments, or large boxes and blocks that may be a part of the hospital playroom.

Games that can be played alone or with another child or an adult are popular with older children, as are puzzles; reading material; quiet, individual activities, such as sewing, stringing beads, and weaving; and Lego blocks and other building materials. Assembling models is an excellent pastime, but one should make certain that all pieces and necessary materials are included in the package so that the child is not disappointed and frustrated.

Well-selected books are of infinite value to children. Children never tire of stories; having someone read aloud gives them endless hours of pleasure and is of special value to children who have limited energy to expend in play. A CD/DVD/radio device, electronic games, and television, included among most hospital room equipment, are useful tools for entertaining children. Computers with access to the Internet can provide diversion, educational opportunities, and online support groups.

When supervising play for ill or convalescent children, it is best to select activities that are simpler than would normally be chosen for the child's specific developmental level. These children usually do not have the energy to cope with more challenging activities. Other limitations also influence the type of activities. Special consideration must be given to children who are confined in terms of movement, have a restricted extremity, or are isolated. Toys for isolated children must be disposable or need to be disinfected after every use.

Toys

Parents of hospitalized children often ask nurses about the types of toys that would be best to bring for their child. Although parents often

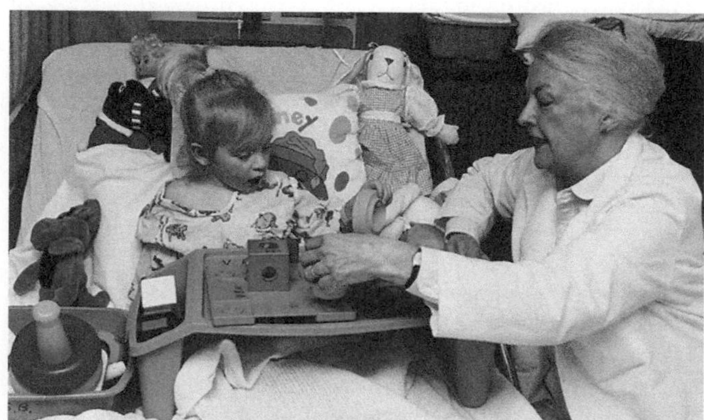

FIG. 21.7 Play materials for children in the hospital need to be appropriate for their age, interests, and limitations.

want to buy new toys for the hospitalized child to offer cheer and comfort, it is often better to wait. Small children need the comfort and reassurance of familiar things, such as the stuffed animal the child hugs for comfort and takes to bed at night. These familiar items are a link with home and the world outside the hospital. All toys brought into the hospital should be assessed for safety.

A highly successful diversion for a child who is hospitalized for a length of time and whose parents are unable to visit frequently is having the parents bring a box with several small, inexpensive, brightly wrapped items with a different day of the week printed on the outside of each package. The child will eagerly anticipate the time for opening each one. If the parents know when their next visit will be, they can provide the number of packages that corresponds to the time between visits. In this way, the child knows that the diminishing packages also represent the anticipated visit from the parent.

Expressive Activities

Play and other expressive activities provide one of the best opportunities for encouraging emotional expression, including the safe release of anger and hostility. Nondirective play that allows children freedom for expression can be tremendously therapeutic. Therapeutic play, however, should not be confused with play therapy, a psychologic technique reserved for use by trained and qualified therapists as an interpretative method with emotionally disturbed children. Therapeutic play, on the other hand, is an effective, nondirective modality for helping children deal with their concerns and fears, and at the same time, it often helps the nurse gain insights into children's needs and feelings.

Tension release can be facilitated through almost any activity; with younger ambulatory children, large-muscle activity such as use of tricycles and wagons is especially beneficial. Much aggression can be safely directed into pounding and throwing games or activities. Beanbags are often thrown at a target or open receptacle with surprising vigor and can help release tension. A pounding board is used with enthusiasm by young children; clay and play dough are beneficial for use at any age.

Creative Expression

Although all children derive physical, social, emotional, and cognitive benefits from engaging in art and other creative activities, children's need for such activities is intensified when they are hospitalized. Drawing and painting are excellent media for expression. Children are more at ease expressing their thoughts and feelings through art because humans think first in images and later learn to translate those images into words. Children need only to be supplied with the raw materials, such as crayons and paper, large brushes and an ample supply of newsprint supported on easels, or materials for finger painting (Fig. 21.8). Children can work individually or work together on a group project, such as a mural painted on a large piece of paper.

Although interpretation of children's drawings requires special training, observing changes in a series of the child's drawings over time can be helpful in assessing psychosocial adjustment and coping. The nurse can use children's drawings, stories, poetry, and other products of creative expression as a springboard for discussion of thoughts, fears, and understanding of concepts or events (see Chapter 4). A child's drawing before surgery, for example, may reveal unvoiced concerns about mutilation, body changes, and loss of self-control.

Nurses can incorporate opportunities for musical expression into routine nursing care. For example, simple musical instruments, such as bracelets with bells, can be placed on infants' legs for them to shake to accompany mealtime music or dressing changes. Dance and movement suggestions may encourage a child to ambulate.

Holidays provide stimulus and direction for unlimited creative projects. Children can participate in decorating the pediatric unit; making pictures and decorations for their rooms gives the children a sense of pride and accomplishment. This is especially beneficial for children who are immobilized and isolated. Making gifts for someone at home helps maintain interpersonal ties.

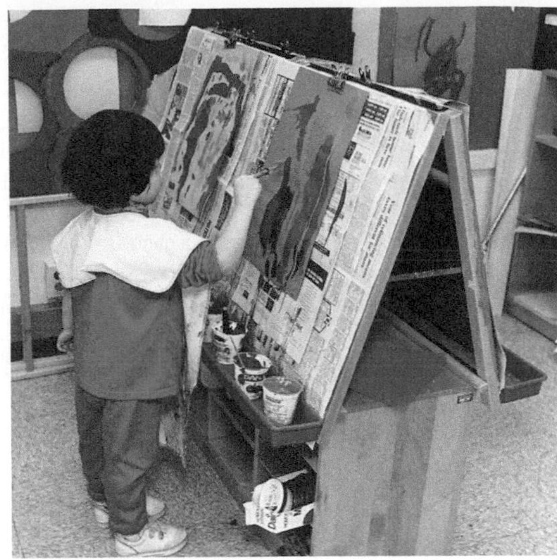

FIG. 21.8 Drawing and painting are excellent media for expression.

Dramatic Play

Dramatic play is a well-recognized technique for emotional release, allowing children to reenact frightening or puzzling hospital experiences. Through use of puppets, replicas of hospital equipment, or some actual hospital equipment, children can act out the situations that are a part of their hospital experience. Dramatic play enables children to learn about procedures and events that concern them and to assume the roles of the adults in the hospital environment.

Puppets are universally effective for communicating with children. Most children see them as peers and readily communicate with them. Children will tell the puppet feelings that they hesitate to express to adults. Puppets can share children's own experiences and help them find solutions to their problems. Puppets dressed to represent figures in the child's environment—for example, a physician, nurse, child patient, therapist, and members of the child's own family—are especially useful. Small, appropriately attired dolls are equally effective in encouraging the child to play out situations, although puppets are usually best for direct conversation.

Play must consider medical needs, but at times, a procedure can be postponed briefly to allow the child to complete a special activity (see Critical Thinking Case Study box). Play must consider any limitations imposed by the child's condition. For example, small children are prone to explore their environment by placing things in their mouth. Therefore a child who is allergic to wheat should not be given modeling dough made with flour. A child on a restricted salt intake should not play with modeling dough because salt is one of its major constituents. At home, the play program can be planned around the therapy regimen. Play can be satisfactorily incorporated into the child's care if the nurse and others involved allow some flexibility and use creativity in planning for play.

Maximizing Potential Benefits of Hospitalization

Although hospitalization generally represents a stressful time for children and families, it also represents an opportunity for facilitating positive change within the child and among family members. For some families, the stress of a child's illness, hospitalization, or both can lead to strengthening of family coping behaviors and the emergence of new coping strategies.

CRITICAL THINKING CASE STUDY

Playroom and Hospital Procedures

Joel, an 8-year-old with cystic fibrosis, has been hospitalized numerous times with complications from the condition. He is playing a board game with his brother, sister, and several other children in the playroom on the pediatric unit. A pediatric phlebotomist enters the playroom and says, "Joel, I need to take some blood. I can see that you are playing a game, so I'll just do it while you play. It will just take a minute." The playroom is usually off limits for invasive procedures. As Joel's nurse, you are aware that Dr. Lung wants the results of the laboratory studies as soon as possible to make a decision about the course of therapy.

Questions

1. Evidence: Is there sufficient evidence to draw any conclusions about this situation at this time?
2. Assumptions: What are some underlying assumptions about the following:
   a. Children and painful procedures, such as venipunctures
   b. The function of play in a hospitalized child
   c. The priority in performing the procedure
   d. Implications of performing the procedure in the playroom
3. What implications and priorities for nursing care can be drawn at this time (i.e., what will you do)?
4. Does the evidence objectively support your argument (conclusion)?

Answers are available at http://evolve.elsevier.com/wong/ncic.

Fostering Parent-Child Relationships

The crisis of illness or hospitalization can mobilize parents into more acute awareness of their child's needs. For example, hospitalization provides opportunities for parents to learn more about their children's growth and development. When parents are helped to understand children's usual reactions to stress, such as regression or aggression, they are not only better able to support the child through the hospital experience but also may extend their insights into childrearing practices once home.

Difficulties in parent-child relationships that existed before hospitalization that are characterized by feeding problems, negative behavior, and sleep disturbances may decrease during hospitalization. The temporary cessation of such problems sometimes alerts parents to the role they may be playing in propagating the negative behavior. With assistance from health professionals, parents can restructure ways of relating to their children to foster more positive behavior.

Hospitalization may also represent a temporary reprieve or refuge from a disturbed home. Typically, abused or neglected children's dramatic physical and social improvement during hospitalization is proof of the benefits and potential growth that can occur during hospitalization. These children temporarily are able to seek support, reassurance, and security from new relationships, particularly with nurses and hospitalized peers.

Providing Educational Opportunities

Illness and hospitalization represent excellent opportunities for children and other family members to learn more about their bodies, each other, and the health professions. For example, during a hospital admission for a diabetic crisis, the child may learn about the disease; the parents may learn about the child's needs for independence, normalcy, and appropriate limits; and each of them may find a new support system in the hospital staff.

Illness or hospitalization can also help older children in choosing a career. Frequently, children have impressions of physicians or nurses that are disproportionately positive or negative. Actual experience with different health professionals can influence their attitude about health professionals and even a decision regarding a career in health care.

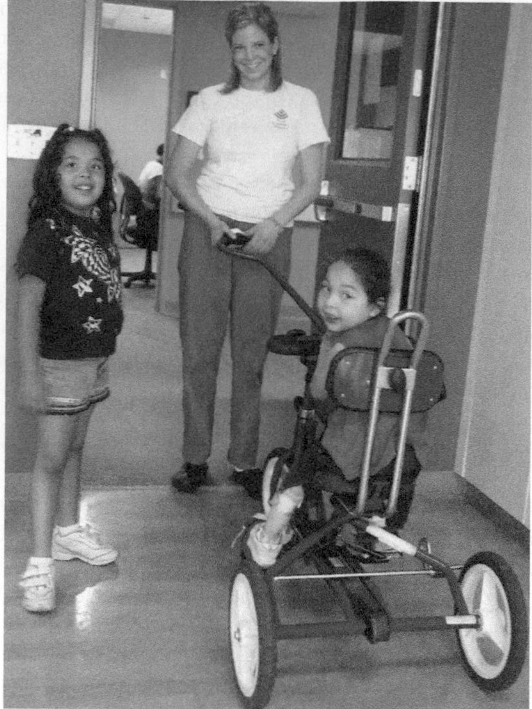

FIG. 21.9 Placing children of the same age group with similar illnesses near each other on the unit is both psychologically and medically supportive. (Courtesy E. Jacob, Texas Children's Hospital, Houston, TX.)

Promoting Self-Mastery

The experience of facing a crisis such as illness or hospitalization can provide an opportunity for self-mastery of coping skills. Younger children have the chance to test fantasy versus reality fears. They realize that they were not abandoned, mutilated, or punished. In fact, they were loved, cared for, and treated with respect for their individual concerns. It is not unusual for children who have undergone hospitalization or surgery to tell others that "it was nothing" or to display proudly their scars or bandages. For older children, hospitalization may represent an opportunity for decision making, independence, and self-reliance. They are proud of having survived the experience and may feel a genuine self-respect for their achievements. Nurses can facilitate such feelings of self-mastery by emphasizing aspects of personal competence in the child and not focusing on uncooperative or negative behavior.

Providing Socialization

Hospitalization may offer children a special opportunity for social acceptance. Lonely, asocial, and even delinquent children find a sympathetic environment in the hospital. Children who have a physical disability or are in some other way "different" from their age mates may find an accepting social peer group (Fig. 21.9). Although this does not always spontaneously occur, nurses can structure the environment to foster a supportive child group. For example, selection of a compatible roommate can help children gain a new friend and learn more about themselves. Forming relationships with significant members of the health care team, such as the physician, nurse, child life specialist, or social worker, can greatly enhance children's adjustment in many areas of life.

Parents may also encounter a new social group in other parents who have similar problems. The waiting room or hallway "self-help" groups are inherent to every institution. Parents meet while in the hospital or clinic and discuss their children's illnesses and treatments. Nurses can capitalize on this informal gathering by encouraging parents to discuss collectively their concerns and feelings. Nurses can also refer parents to organized parent groups or can use the help and support of parents of recovered hospitalized patients. It is important that nurses emphasize to families that each child responds differently to disease, treatments, and care. Any questions should be clarified with the health care team.

NURSING CARE OF THE FAMILY

Although it is not possible to predict exactly which factors are most likely to have an effect on a family's reactions, important variables are the seriousness of the child's illness, the family's previous experience with hospitalization, and the medical procedures involved in the diagnosis and treatment. Nurses can refer to the nursing admission history, which can provide insight into how to care for the child and family. (See Box 19.5.)

SUPPORTING FAMILY MEMBERS

Support involves the willingness to stay and listen to parents' verbal and nonverbal messages. Sometimes the nurse does not give this support directly. For example, the nurse may offer to stay with the child to allow the parents time alone or may discuss with other family members the parents' need for extra relief. Often relatives and friends want to help but do not know how. Suggesting ways, such as babysitting, preparing meals, doing laundry, or transporting the siblings to school, can prompt others to help reduce the responsibilities that burden parents.

Support may also be provided through the clergy. Parents with deep religious beliefs may appreciate the counsel of a clergy member, but because of their stress, they may not have sufficient energy to initiate the contact. Nurses can be supportive by arranging for clergy to visit, upholding parents' religious beliefs, and respecting the individual meaning and significance of those beliefs.

Support involves accepting cultural, socioeconomic, and ethnic values. For example, health and illness are defined differently by various ethnic groups. For some, a disorder that has few outward manifestations of illness, such as diabetes, hypertension, or cardiac problems, is not a sickness. Consequently, a prescribed treatment may be seen as unnecessary. Nurses who appreciate the influences of culture are more likely to intervene therapeutically. (See Chapter 2.)

Parents need help to accept their own feelings toward the ill child. If given the opportunity, parents often disclose their feelings of loss of control, anger, and guilt. They often resist admitting to such feelings because they expect others to disapprove of behavior that is less than perfect. Unfortunately, health personnel, including nurses, sometimes do exercise little tolerance for deviation from the norm. This only increases the psychologic impact of a child's illness on family members. Helping parents identify the specific reason for such feelings and emphasizing that each is a normal, expected, and healthy response to stress may reduce the parents' emotional burden.

Family-centered care also addresses the needs of siblings. Support may involve preparing siblings for hospital visits, assessing their adjustment, and providing appropriate interventions or referrals when needed. The Family-Centered Care box suggests ways that parents can support siblings during hospitalization.

PROVIDING INFORMATION

Important nursing interventions to provide to the family should include information regarding the disease process, its treatment, prognosis, and home care. In addition, anticipatory guidance regarding the child's emotional and physical reactions to illness and hospitalization should be discussed.

For many families, the child's illness is the first contact they have with the hospital experience. Often parents are not prepared for the child's behavioral reactions to hospitalization. Reactions can include separation behaviors, regression, aggression, and hostility. Providing the parents with information about these normal and expected behavioral responses can lessen the parents' anxiety during the hospital admission. The family is equally unfamiliar with hospital rules, which often compounds their confusion and anxiety. Therefore the family needs clear explanations about what to expect and what is expected of them.

Parents also need to be aware of the effects of illness on the family and strategies that prevent negative changes. If appropriate, parents should keep their families well informed and communicate with everyone as much as possible. They should treat all the children equally and as normally as before the illness occurred. Discipline, which initially may not have been a priority for an ill child, should be continued to provide a measure of security and predictability. When ill children know that their parents expect certain standards of conduct from them, they feel certain that they will recover. Conversely, when all limits are removed, they fear that something catastrophic will happen.

Helping parents understand the meaning of posthospitalization behaviors in the sick child is necessary for them to tolerate and support such behaviors. In addition, parents should be forewarned of the common reactions after discharge (see Box 21.2). Parents who do not expect such reactions may misinterpret them as evidence of the child's "being spoiled" and demand perfect behavior at a time when the child is still reacting to the stress of illness and hospitalization. If the behaviors, especially the demand for attention, are dealt with in a supportive manner, most children are able to relinquish them and assume prior levels of functioning.

Nurses should also prepare parents for the reactions of siblings—particularly anger, jealousy, and resentment. Older siblings may deny

FAMILY-CENTERED CARE

Supporting Siblings During Hospitalization

Trade off staying at the hospital with spouse or have a surrogate who knows the siblings well stay in the home.

Offer information about the child's condition to young siblings as well as older siblings; respect the sibling who avoids information as a means of coping with the situation.

Arrange for children to visit their brother or sister in the hospital if possible.

Encourage phone visits and mail between brothers and sisters; provide children with phone numbers, writing supplies, and stamps.

Help each sibling identify an extended family member or friend to be their support person and provide extra attention during parental absence.

Make or buy inexpensive toys or trinkets for siblings, one gift for each day the child will be hospitalized.

- Wrap each gift separately and place them in a basket, box, or other container at the child's bedside.
- Instruct siblings to open one gift at bedtime and to remember that he or she is in their parent's thoughts.

If the child's condition is stable and distance is not prohibitive, plan a special time at home with the siblings or have spouse or another relative or friend bring the children to meet parent(s) at a restaurant or other location near the hospital.

- Have extended family members or friends schedule a visit to the child in the hospital during parental absence.
- Arrange a pass for the child to leave the hospital to join the family if the child's condition permits.

Modified from Craft, M., & Craft, J. (1989). Perceived changes in siblings of hospitalized children: A comparison of sibling and parent reports. *Children's Health Care, 18*(1), 42-48; Rollins, J. (1992). *Brothers and sisters: A discussion guide for families.* Landover, MD: Epilepsy Foundation of America.

such reactions because they provoke feelings of guilt. However, everyone needs outlets for emotions, and the repressed feelings may surface as problems in school or with peers, as psychosomatic illnesses, or in delinquent behavior.

Probably one of the most neglected areas of communication involves giving information to siblings. Frequently, older siblings may begin to ask questions or request explanations. Children in every age group deserve an explanation of the sibling's illness or hospitalization. Nurses can minimize a sibling's fear of also getting sick or that they may have caused the illness.

ENCOURAGING PARENT PARTICIPATION

Preventing or minimizing separation is a key nursing goal with the child who is hospitalized, but maintaining parent-child contact is also beneficial for the family. One of the best approaches is encouraging parents to stay with their child and to participate in the care whenever possible. Although some health facilities provide special accommodations for parents, the concept of rooming-in can be instituted anywhere. The first requirement is the staff's positive attitude toward parents. In a qualitative study of 24 mothers of hospitalized children, mothers expected nurses to provide physical support and emotional support in terms of having a friendly, rather than critical attitude, and being approachable and receptive of mothers' questions and anxieties (Konuk Şener & Karaca, 2017).

When hospital staff members genuinely appreciate the importance of continued parent-child attachment, they foster an environment that encourages parents to stay. When parents are included in the care planning and understand that they are a contributing factor to the child's recovery, they are more inclined to remain with their child and have more emotional reserves to support themselves and the child through the crisis. An empowerment model allows the nurse to focus on parents' strengths and seek ways to promote growth and family functioning so that the parents become empowered in caring for their child. Strategies such as bedside reporting have allowed parents to be involved as active members of the team moving closer to family-centered care. Allowing parents of sick children to participate during rounds can reduce parents' anxiety and improve communication (Blankenship, Harrison, Brandt, et al., 2015).

Because the mother may tend to be the primary family caregiver, she may spend more time in the hospital than the father. Not all parents feel equally comfortable assuming responsibility for their child's care. Some may be under such great emotional stress that they need a temporary reprieve from total participation in caregiving activities. Others may feel insecure in participating in specialized areas of care, such as bathing the child after surgery. On the other hand, some mothers may feel a great need to be in control of their child's care. This seems particularly true of young mothers, mothers of young children, and ethnic or minority mothers. Individual assessment of each parent's preferred involvement is necessary to prevent the effects of separation while supporting parents in their needs as well.

With lifestyles and gender roles changing, fathers may assume all or some of the usual parenting roles in the household. In these cases, it may be the father-child relationship that requires preservation. Fathers need to be included in the care plan and respected for their parental role. For some fathers, the child's hospitalization may represent an opportunity to alter their usual caregiving role and increase their involvement. In single-parent families, the caregiver may not be a parent but an extended family member, such as a grandparent or aunt.

One of the potential problems with continuous parent involvement is neglect of the parent's need for sleep, nutrition, and relaxation. Often the sleeping accommodations are limited to a chair, and sleep is disrupted by nursing procedures. Encouraging the parents to leave for brief periods, arranging for sleeping quarters on the unit but outside the child's room, and planning a schedule of alternating visits with another family member can minimize the stresses for the parent.

Nurses need to structure their roles to complement and augment the caregiving functions of parents. Even in units structured to provide care by parents, parents frequently feel anxiety in their caregiving responsibilities; those more involved in direct care may feel more anxiety than those less involved in direct care. Therefore 24-hour responsibility may be too much for some parents. Assistance and relief by nursing personnel should always be available to these families, and nurses may need to work diligently to establish the strong bond of trust that some parents need to take advantage of these opportunities.

PREPARING FOR DISCHARGE AND HOME CARE

Discharge preparation often involves education of the family for continued care and follow-up in the home. Depending on the diagnosis, this may be relatively simple or highly complex. Preparing the family for home care demands a high degree of competence in planning and implementing discharge instructions.

Nurses are key individuals in the discharge process as they collaborate with others in the planning and implementation phases to ensure appropriate care after hospitalization. Throughout the hospitalization, the nurse should be aware of the need for discharge planning and those factors that affect the family's ability to provide home care. A thorough assessment of the family and home environment should be performed to ensure that the family's emotional and physical resources are sufficient to manage the tasks of home care. (For a discussion of family and home assessment strategies, see Chapter 4.) Consultation with social workers regarding available community services, including respite care, is needed to ensure that appropriate support agencies are available, such as emergency facilities, home health agencies, and equipment vendors. Financial resources are also a consideration. To coordinate the immense task of assessment and to plan implementation, a care coordinator or manager should be included early in the discharge process.

The preparation for hospital discharge and home care begins during the admission assessment. Short- and long-term goals are established to meet the child's physical and psychosocial needs. For children with complex care needs, discharge planning focuses on obtaining appropriate equipment and health care personnel for the home. Discharge planning is also concerned with treatments that parents or children are expected to continue at home. In planning appropriate teaching, nurses need to assess the actual and perceived complexity of the skill, the parents' or child's ability to learn the skill, and the parents' or child's previous or present experience with such procedures.

The discharge teaching plan incorporates levels of learning, such as observing, participating with assistance, and finally acting without help or guidance. The skill is divided into discrete steps, and each step is taught to the family member until it is learned. Return demonstration of the skill is requested before new skills are introduced. A record of teaching and performance provides an efficient checklist for evaluation. All families should receive detailed *written* instructions about home care, with telephone numbers for assistance, before they leave the hospital. Communication between the nurse and home health care, if applicable, is essential for ensuring a smooth transition for the child and family on discharge.

After the family is competent in performing the skill, they are given responsibility for the care. When possible, the family should have a transition or trial period to assume care with minimal health care supervision. This may be arranged on the unit or in a location near the hospital. Such transitions provide a safe practice period for the family, with assistance readily available when needed, and are especially valuable when the family lives far from the hospital.

In many instances, parents need only simple instructions and understanding of follow-up care. However, the overwhelming care assumed by some families, coupled with other stressors that they may be experiencing, necessitates continued professional support after discharge. A follow-up home visit or telephone call gives the nurse an opportunity to individualize care and provide information in perhaps a less stressful learning environment than the hospital. Appropriate referrals and resources may include visiting nurse or home health agencies, private nurse services, school system, physical therapist, mental health counselor, social work, and any number of community agencies. Sharing the important issues surrounding the child's and family's needs is essential. Referral summaries should be concise, specific, and factual. When numerous support services are required, periodic collaboration among the professionals involved and the family is an excellent strategy to ensure efficient usage and comprehensive delivery of services.

CARE OF THE CHILD AND FAMILY IN SPECIAL HOSPITAL SITUATIONS

In addition to a general pediatric unit, children may also receive care in special facilities, such as an intensive care unit, an isolation room, or in the ambulatory setting.

AMBULATORY OR OUTPATIENT SETTING

The ambulatory or outpatient setting provides needed medical services for the child while eliminating the necessity of overnight admission. The benefits of ambulatory care are to minimize stressors of hospitalization, especially separation from the family; reduced chances of infection; and increased cost savings. Admission to the ambulatory or outpatient hospital setting is usually for surgical, therapeutic, or diagnostic procedures, such as insertion of tympanostomy tubes, hernia repair, tonsillectomy, or bronchoscopy.

In the ambulatory or outpatient setting, adequate preparation is particularly challenging. Ideally, the child and parents should receive preadmission preparation, including a tour of the facility and a review of the day's events. Parents need information in advance to help prepare the child and themselves for surgery and enable them to care for the child at home after the procedure. Parents also appreciate suggestions for items to bring to the hospital, such as blankets or stuffed animals. When preadmission preparation is not possible, time should be allowed on the day of the procedure for children to become acquainted with their surroundings and for nurses to assess, plan, and implement appropriate teaching.

Explicit discharge instructions are important after outpatient surgery (refer to Family-Centered Care box and the Preparing for Discharge and Home Care section earlier in this chapter). Parents need guidelines on when to call their health care provider regarding a change in the child's condition. A follow-up telephone call system allows for nurses to check

FAMILY-CENTERED CARE

Discharge From Ambulatory Settings

1. Before beginning, explain that all instructions will also be presented in writing for the family to refer to later.
2. Provide an overview of the typical trajectory (expected pattern) of recovery.
3. Discuss expected progression of the child's activity level during the post-discharge period (e.g., "Mary will probably sleep for the rest of the day and feel kind of tired most of tomorrow but will be back to her usual activities the next day").
4. Explain which activities the child is allowed and what is not permitted (e.g., bed rest, bathing).
5. Discuss dietary restrictions, being very specific and giving examples of "clear fluids" or what is meant by a "full liquid diet."
6. Discuss nausea and vomiting, if applicable, explaining how much is "normal" and what to do if more occurs (e.g., "Juan may be sick to his stomach and vomit. This is normal. However, if he vomits more than three times, please call us at this number right away").
7. Discuss fever and appropriate comfort measures, explaining how much fever is considered "normal," and specifically what to do if the child goes beyond the range.
8. Explain the amount, location, and kind of pain or discomfort the child may experience.
   - Give any prescribed medication before leaving the facility.
   - Send a pain scale home with the family.
   - Explain how much pain and discomfort is "normal" and what to do if the child surpasses that level or if pain management interventions are unsuccessful.
   - Discuss pain management, including dosage for pain medications and details on how to administer them.
   - Describe appropriate nonpharmacologic comfort measures, such as holding, rocking, or swaddling.
9. Provide information about each medication that the child will be taking at home.
   - Review the details, including dose and route.
   - Demonstrate how to administer medications, if necessary (e.g., how to take outer packaging off suppositories, how to insert).
   - Discuss guidelines for requesting other medications.
   - Request that all prescriptions be filled and given to the family before discharge.
10. Make certain the family has all of the equipment and supplies (e.g., gauze and tape for dressing changes) that they will need at home.
11. Discuss complications that may occur and the steps to take if they do.
12. Ensure that appropriate measures are in place for safe transport home.
    - Remind family to use a seat belt or car seat for the child.
    - Determine whether there will be one person whose sole responsibility is helping ensure the child's safety and comfort during transport.
    - Discuss measures the driver may need to take if this is impossible (e.g., be certain a basin is within the child's reach in case vomiting occurs; take a route that permits slower traffic and has places along the roadside to stop if necessary).
    - Determine the availability of a blanket, pillow, and cup with a lid and straw for the child's use in the car.
13. Provide emergency phone numbers for the family to call with any concerns.
14. Explain that the family will be contacted (give an approximate time) to follow up on the child but that they should not hesitate to call if concerns arise before then.
15. Ask the family and child, if appropriate, if they have any questions and problem solve with family members to meet their unique needs.

on the child's progress within 48 to 72 hours after discharge. It also provides an opportunity for the nurse to review discharge information and answer additional questions.

> **! NURSING ALERT**
>
> Help the family prepare for the transportation home by offering these suggestions:
> - Have a blanket and pillow in the car. (Always use the car safety restraint system.)
> - Take a basin or plastic bag in case of vomiting.
> - Use a cup with a cap and straw for the child to drink fluids (except in cases of oral facial surgery in which a straw may be contraindicated).
> - Give any prescribed pain medication before leaving facility.
> - Provide parents verbal and written information regarding potential side effects of pain medication for which they should be vigilant after discharge.
> - Drinks or snacks as appropriate

ISOLATION

Admission to an isolation room increases all of the stressors typically associated with hospitalization. There is further separation from familiar persons; additional loss of control; and added environmental changes, such as sensory deprivation and the strange appearance of visitors. Orientation to time and place is affected. These stressors are compounded by children's limited understanding of isolation. Preschool children have difficulty understanding the rationale for isolation because they cannot comprehend the cause-and-effect relationship between germs and illness. They are likely to view isolation as punishment. Older children understand the causality better but still require information to decrease fantasizing or misinterpretation.

When a child is placed in isolation, preparation is essential for the child to feel in control. With young children, the best approach is a simple explanation, such as "You need to be in this room to help you get better. The germs made you sick, and you could not help that. This is a special place to make all the germs go away."

All children, but especially younger ones, need preparation in terms of what they will see, hear, and feel in isolation. Therefore they are shown the mask, gloves, and gown and are encouraged to "dress up" in them. Playing with the strange apparel lessens the fear of seeing "ghostlike" people walk into the room. Before entering the room, nurses and other health personnel should introduce themselves and let the child see their faces before donning masks. In this way, the child gains a sense of familiarity in an otherwise strange and lonely environment.

When the child's condition improves, appropriate play activities are provided to minimize boredom, stimulate the senses, provide a real or perceived sense of movement, orient the child to time and place, provide social interaction, and reduce depersonalization. For example, the environment can be manipulated to increase sensory freedom by moving the bed toward the door or window. Opening window shades; providing musical, visual, or tactile toys; and increasing interpersonal contact can substitute mental mobility for the limitations of physical movement. Rather than dwelling on the negative aspects of isolation, the child can be encouraged to view this experience as challenging and positive. For example, the nurse can help the child look at isolation as a method of keeping others out and letting only special people in. Children often think of intriguing signs for their doors, such as "Enter at your own risk." These signs also encourage people "on the outside" to talk with the child about the ominous greeting.

> **! NURSING ALERT**
>
> Have the child select a place he or she would like to visit. Help the child decorate the bed and equipment to suit the theme (e.g., truck, circus tent, spaceship, sky). At a set time each day, pretend to go with the child to the special place. Consider including props such as a suitcase or picnic basket.

EMERGENCY ADMISSION

One of the most traumatic hospital experiences for the child and parents is an emergency admission. The sudden onset of an illness or the occurrence of an injury leaves little time for preparation and explanation. Sometimes the emergency admission is compounded by admission to an intensive care unit (ICU) or the need for immediate surgery. However, even in instances requiring only outpatient treatment, the child is exposed to a strange, frightening environment and to experiences that may elicit fear or cause pain.

There is a wide discrepancy between what constitutes a medically defined emergency and a patient-defined emergency. A growing concern is the use of major emergency departments for routine primary care health visits. To offset overcrowding in emergency departments, many facilities have opened urgent care centers for after-hours health care. Telephone triage for minor illnesses for patients is also emerging as a health care delivery mode to differentiate illnesses such as a common cold from true life-threatening conditions that require immediate provider attention and intervention. Other factors contributing to the overuse of emergency departments (as opposed to the primary care provider's office) include the increasing number of uninsured persons and households where both parents work full time and cannot afford to take time off during the day to take the sick child to a health care provider.

In pediatric populations, most visits to an emergency department are for respiratory infections; skin conditions, gastrointestinal disorders, and trauma (e.g., poisoning) account for the remainder of cases. The most common reason parents give for bringing the child to the emergency department is concern about the illness worsening. However, health care providers may not think that the progressive symptoms necessitate immediate or emergency care. One of the nurse's primary goals is to assess the parents' perception of the event and their reasons for considering it serious or life threatening.

Lengthy preparatory admission procedures are often inappropriate for emergency situations. In such instances, nurses must focus their nursing interventions on the essential components of admission counseling (Box 21.10) and complete the process as soon as the child's condition has stabilized.

Unless an emergency is life threatening, children need to participate in their care to maintain a sense of control. Because emergency departments are frequently hectic, there is a tendency to rush through procedures to save time. However, the extra few minutes needed to allow children to participate may save many more minutes of useless resistance and uncooperativeness during subsequent procedures. Other supportive measures include ensuring privacy, accepting various emotional responses to fear or pain, preserving parent-child contact, explaining all events before or as they occur, and personally remaining calm. Pain management strategies are discussed in Chapter 5.

At times, because of the child's physical condition, little or no preparatory counseling for emergency treatment can be done. In such situations, counseling subsequent to the event has therapeutic value. The counseling should focus on evaluating children's thoughts regarding admission and related procedures. It is similar to precounseling

BOX 21.10 Guidelines for Special Hospital Admission

Emergency Admission

Lengthy preparatory admission procedures are often impossible and inappropriate for emergency situations.

Focus assessment on airway, breathing, and circulation; weigh child whenever possible for calculation of drug dosages.

Unless an emergency is life threatening, children need to participate in their care to maintain a sense of control.

Focus on essential components of admission counseling, including the following:

- Appropriate introduction to the family
- Use of child's name, not terms such as "honey" or "dear"
- Determination of child's age and some judgment about developmental age (If the child is of school age, asking about the grade level will offer some evidence of intellectual ability.)
- Information about child's general state of health, any problems that may interfere with medical treatment (e.g., allergies), and previous experience with hospital facilities
- Information about the chief complaint from both the parents and the child

Admission to Intensive Care Unit

Prepare child and parents for elective intensive care unit (ICU) admission, such as for postoperative care after cardiac surgery.

Prepare child and parents for unanticipated ICU admission by focusing primarily on the sensory aspects of the experience and on usual family concerns (e.g., persons in charge of child's care, schedule for visiting, area where family can stay).

Prepare parents regarding child's appearance and behavior when they first visit child in ICU.

Accompany family to bedside to provide emotional support and answer questions.

Prepare siblings for their visit; plan length of time for sibling visitation; monitor siblings' reactions during visit to prevent them from becoming overwhelmed.

Encourage parents to stay with their child:

- If visiting hours are limited, allow flexibility in schedule to accommodate parental needs.
- Give family members a written schedule of visiting times.
- If visiting hours are liberal, be aware of family members' needs and suggest periodic respites.
- Assure family they can call the unit at any time.

Prepare parents for expected role changes and identify ways for parents to participate in child's care without overwhelming them with responsibilities:

- Help with bath or feeding.
- Touch and talk to child.
- Help with procedures.

Provide information about child's condition in understandable language:

- Repeat information often.
- Seek clarification of understanding.
- During bedside conferences, interpret information for family members and child or, if appropriate, conduct report outside room.

Prepare child for procedures even if it involves explanation while procedure is performed.

Assess and manage pain; recognize that a child who cannot talk, such as an infant or child in a coma or on mechanical ventilation, can be in pain.

Establish a routine that maintains some similarity to daily events in child's life whenever possible:

- Organize care during normal waking hours.
- Keep regular bedtime schedules, including quiet times when television or radio is lowered or turned off.
- Provide uninterrupted sleep cycles (60 minutes for infants; 90 minutes for older children).
- Close and open drapes and dim lights to allow for day and night.
- Place curtain around bed for privacy.
- Orient child to day and time; have clocks or calendars in easy view for older children.

Schedule a time when child is left undisturbed (e.g., during naps, visit with family, playtime, or favorite program).

Provide opportunities for play.

Reduce stimulation in environment:

- Refrain from loud talking or laughing.
- Keep equipment noise to a minimum.
- Turn alarms as low as safely possible.
- Perform treatments requiring equipment at one time.
- Turn off bedside equipment that is not in use, such as suction and oxygen.
- Avoid loud, abrupt noises.

techniques; however, instead of supplying information, the nurse listens to the explanations offered by the child. Projective techniques such as drawing, doll play, or storytelling are especially effective. The nurse then bases additional information on what has already been understood.

INTENSIVE CARE UNIT

Admission to an ICU can be traumatic for both the child and parents (Fig. 21.10). The nature and severity of the illness and the circumstances surrounding the admission are major factors. Parents experience significantly more stress when the admission is unexpected rather than expected. Stressors for the child and parent are described in Box 21.11. An effective strategy to help enhance parents' ability to cope is to simply ask them what is stressful and implement interventions specific to their stress. Assessment should be repeated periodically to account for changes in perceptions over time. The use of daily patient goal sheets has been successful in improving communication among health care providers caring for children in the ICU (Agarwal, Frankel, Tourner, et al., 2008). By clearly defining daily patient care goals, health care providers believed that care was improved.

The family's emotional needs are paramount when a child is admitted to an ICU. A major stressor for parents of a child in the ICU is the child's appearance (Latour, van Goudoever, & Hazelzet, 2008). Although the same interventions discussed earlier for the stressors of separation and loss of control apply here, additional interventions may also benefit the family and child (see Box 21.11). Nurse behaviors that exemplified caring and affection were perceived as helpful in decreasing stress (Baird, Rehm, Hinds, et al., 2016). Behaviors perceived as not helpful included separating the child from the parents and communicating poorly with parents. Therefore even critical care must be centered on the family. It is important that visiting hours be liberal and flexible enough to accommodate parental needs and involvement.

Critically ill children become the focus of the parents' lives, and parents' most pressing need is for information. They want to know if their child will live and, if so, whether the child will be the same as before. They need to know why various interventions are being done for the child, that the child is being treated for pain or is comfortable, and that the child may be able to hear them even though not awake. When parents first visit the child in the ICU, they need preparation regarding the child's appearance. Ideally, the nurse should accompany the parents to the bedside to provide emotional support and answer any questions.

Despite the stresses normally associated with ICU admission, a sense of security develops from being carefully monitored and receiving individualized care. Therefore planning for transition to the non-ICU is essential and should include the following:

- Assignment of a primary nurse
- Explanation of the differences between the two units and the rationale for the change to less intense monitoring of the child's physical condition
- Selection of an appropriate room, such as one that is close to the nursing station, and a compatible roommate

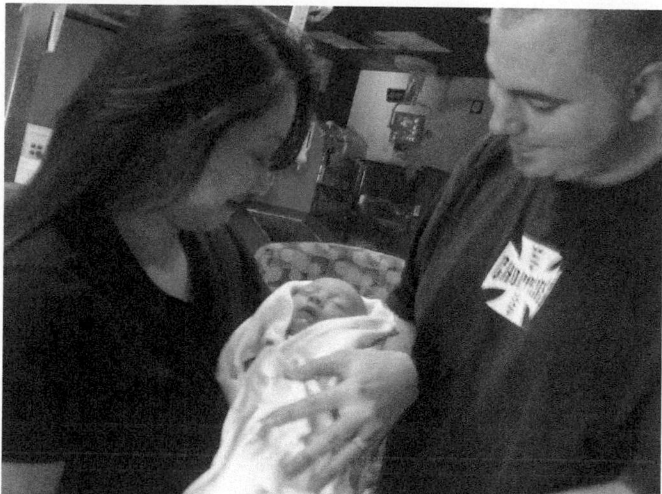

FIG. 21.10 Parental presence during hospitalization provides emotional support for the child and increases the parent's sense of empowerment in the caregiver role. (Courtesy E. Jacob, Texas Children's Hospital, Houston, TX.)

BOX 21.11 Neonatal or Pediatric Intensive Care Unit Stressors for the Child and Family

Physical Stressors

Pain and discomfort (e.g., injections, intubation, suctioning, dressing changes, other invasive procedures)
Immobility (e.g., use of restraints, bed rest)
Sleep deprivation
Inability to eat or drink
Changes in elimination habits

Environmental Stressors

Unfamiliar surroundings (e.g., crowding)
Unfamiliar sounds
- Equipment noise (e.g., monitors, telephone, suctioning, computer printout)
- Human sounds (e.g., talking, laughing, crying, coughing, moaning, retching, walking)

Unfamiliar people (e.g., health care professionals, patients, visitors)
Unfamiliar and unpleasant smells (e.g., alcohol, adhesive remover, body odors)
Constant lights (disturb day/night rhythms)
Activity related to other patients
Sense of urgency among staff
Unkind or thoughtless comments from staff

Psychologic Stressors

Lack of privacy
Inability to communicate (if intubated)
Inadequate knowledge and understanding of situation
Severity of illness
Parental behavior (expression of concern)

Social Stressors

Disrupted relationships (especially with family and friends)
Concern with missing school or work
Play deprivation

Data primarily from Tichy, A. M., Braam, C. M., Meyer, T. A., et al. (1988). Stressors in pediatric intensive care units. *Pediatric Nursing, 14*(1), 40-42.

NCLEX REVIEW QUESTIONS

1. Separation anxiety is something that affects children when they are hospitalized. Each developmental stage has a somewhat different reaction as they deal with this difficulty. Which stage corresponds to the adolescent stage?
   A. May demonstrate separation anxiety by refusing to eat, experiencing difficulty in sleeping, crying quietly for their parents, continually asking when the parents will visit, or withdrawing from others.
   B. Separation anxiety comes in stages: protest, despair, and detachment.
   C. Loss of peer group contact may pose a severe emotional threat because of loss of group status, inability to exert group control or leadership, and loss of group acceptance.
   D. May need and desire parental guidance or support from other adult figures but may be unable or unwilling to ask for it.
2. Play is children's work, even in the hospital. Which of the following are functions of play? Select all that apply.
   A. Provides diversion and brings about relaxation
   B. Keeps the child occupied and directs concerns away from himself or herself
   C. Helps the child feel more secure in a strange environment
   D. Lessens the stress of separation and the feeling of homesickness
   E. Provides a means for release of tension and expression of feelings
   F. Allows the parents to have a break from the unit for a respite period
3. When discharging the pediatric patient from the outpatient setting, the nurse knows that which of the following responses indicate a need for more teaching? Select all that apply.
   A. "The physician said my son can have clear liquids when we return home, which would include Jell-O, pudding, and apple juice."
   B. "The other nurse explained that I can use other things to help with the pain, such as distraction (reading a book, music, or a movie), after the pain medication is given."
   C. "I can get my child's prescription tomorrow, so I can go to my regular pharmacy where they can explain the medication to me."
   D. "I am waiting for my husband to come so he can drive us, and I can watch my son in the car on the way home."

or her acceptance, staff members demonstrate respect for the child. Assent is not a legal requirement but an ethical one to protect the rights of children. Chapter 19 provides further discussion on the dying child's right to refuse treatment.

Eligibility for Giving Informed Consent

Informed Consent of Parents or Legal Guardians

Parents have full responsibility for the care and rearing of their minor children, including legal control over them. As long as children are minors, their parents or legal guardians are required to give informed consent before medical treatment is rendered or any procedure is performed. If the parents are married to each other, consent from only one parent is required for nonurgent pediatric care. If the parents are divorced, consent usually rests with the parent who has legal custody (American Academy of Pediatrics, Committee on Bioethics, 2016). Emergency care of a pediatric patient should never be withheld due to the absence of a parent or legal guardian. Parents also have a right to withdraw consent later. If the legal caregivers disagree on the treatment course, it is within the health care providers' scope to request consultation of a hospital ethics board to determine what care is in the best interest of the patient (Dahl, Sinha, Rosenberg, et al., 2015).

Evidence of Consent

Regulations on obtaining informed consent vary from state to state, and policies differ at each health care facility. It is the physician's legal responsibility to explain the procedure, risks, benefits, and alternatives. The nurse witnesses the patient's, parent's, or legal guardian's signature on the consent form and may reinforce what the patient has been told. A signed consent form is the legal document that signifies that the process of informed consent has occurred. If parents are unavailable to sign consent forms, verbal consent may be obtained via the telephone in the presence of two witnesses. Both witnesses record that informed consent was given and by whom. Their signatures indicate that they witnessed the verbal consent.

Informed Consent of Mature and Emancipated Minors

State laws differ with regard to the age of majority, the age at which a person is considered to have all the legal rights and responsibilities of an adult. In most states, 18 years is the age of majority. Competent adults can give informed consent on their own behalf. An **emancipated minor** is one who is legally under the age of majority but is recognized as having the legal capacity or social status of an adult under circumstances prescribed by state law, such as pregnancy, marriage, high school graduation, independent living, or military service. A **mature minor** exception to consent laws is recognized in a few states for children 14 years and older who possesses the maturity and cognitive abilities to understand all elements of informed consent and make a choice based on the information. Legal action may be required for designation as a mature minor (American Academy of Pediatrics, Committee on Bioethics, 2016).

Treatment Without Parental Consent

Exceptions to requiring parental consent before treating minor children occur in situations in which children need urgent medical or surgical treatment and a parent is not readily available to give consent or refuses to give consent. For example, a child may be brought to an emergency department accompanied by a grandparent, child care provider, teacher, or others. In the absence of parents or legal guardians, persons in charge of the child may be given permission by the parents to give informed consent by proxy. A medical screening examination is required by federal law under the Emergency Medical Treatment and Active Labor Act for all patients presenting to an emergency center. In emergencies, including danger to life or the possibility of permanent injury, appropriate care should not be withheld or delayed because of problems obtaining consent (American Academy of Pediatrics, Committee on Bioethics, 2016). The nurse should document any efforts made to obtain consent.

Parental refusal to give consent for life-saving treatment or to prevent serious harm can occur and requires notification to child protective services to render emergency treatment. For example, Jehovah's Witnesses commonly choose to avoid receiving blood products due to religious beliefs. In cases where a blood product is crucial for the child's survival, it is important to work together with the family, medical team, and child protective services to determine the course of action that is in the best interest of the child. "Parental decision-making should primarily be understood as parents' responsibility to support the interests of their child and to preserve family relationships, rather than being focused on their rights to express their own autonomous choices" (American Academy of Pediatrics, Committee on Bioethics, 2016). Evaluation for child abuse or neglect can occur without parental consent and without notification to the state before evaluation in most states.

Adolescents, Consent, and Confidentiality

The Health Insurance Portability and Accountability Act of 1996 (HIPAA) was passed to help protect and safeguard the security and confidentiality of health information. Because adolescents are not yet adults, parents have the right to make most decisions on their behalf and receive information. Adolescents, however, are more likely to seek care in a setting in which they believe their privacy will be maintained. All 50 states have enacted legislation that entitles adolescents to consent to treatment without the parents' knowledge to one or more "medically emancipated" conditions such as sexually transmitted infections, mental health services, substance abuse and addiction, pregnancy, and contraceptive advice (American Academy of Pediatrics, Committee on Bioethics, 2016). Consent to abortion is controversial, and statutes vary widely by state. The Planned Parenthood Federation of America provides consent and notification law requirements listed by state. State law preempts HIPAA regardless of whether that law prohibits, mandates, or allows discretion about a disclosure.

Informed Consent and Parental Right to the Child's Medical Chart

Some state statutes give parents the unrestricted right to a copy of children's medical records. In states without statutes, the best practice is to allow parents to review or have a copy of minors' charts under reasonable circumstances. Practitioners should avoid restrictive requirements such as review permitted only in the presence of a clinician. Rather, an appropriate practitioner should be available to answer any questions that parents may have during their reviews.

PREPARATION FOR DIAGNOSTIC AND THERAPEUTIC PROCEDURES

Technologic advances and changes in health care have resulted in more pediatric procedures being performed in a variety of settings. Many procedures are both stressful and painful experiences. For many procedures, the focus of care is psychologic preparation of the child and family. However, some procedures require the administration of sedatives and analgesics.

The child life specialist is an especially valued member of the health care team when preparing a child for diagnostic and therapeutic procedures. Child life specialists address the psychosocial concerns that accompany stressful life experiences by promoting optimal child development and minimizing adverse effects. Child life specialists receive advanced education and training in the developmental stages of childhood, as well as strategies to cope with illness and injury. Therapeutic play, procedural preparation and support, developmentally appropriate education, and promoting normalcy are all significant ways the child life specialist can have a positive impact on the health care experience for the child and family. Child life specialists and nursing staff can work together to implement evidence-based interventions to decrease fear, anxiety, and discomfort experienced by children in the health care environment (Association of Child Life Professionals, 2017).

Psychologic Preparation

Preparing children for procedures decreases their anxiety, promotes their cooperation, supports their coping skills and may teach them new ones, and facilitates a feeling of mastery in experiencing a potentially stressful event. Many institutions have developed preadmission teaching programs designed to educate the pediatric patient and family by offering hands-on experience with hospital equipment, the procedure performed, and departments they will visit. Preparatory methods may be formal, such as group preparation for hospitalization. Most preparation strategies are informal, focus on providing information about the experience, and are directed at stressful or painful procedures. The most effective preparation includes the provision of sensory-procedural information and helping the child develop coping skills, such as imagery, distraction, or relaxation.

The Applying Evidence to Practice boxes describe general guidelines for preparing children for procedures along with age-specific guidelines that consider children's developmental needs and cognitive abilities. In addition to these suggestions, nurses should consider the child's temperament, existing coping strategies, and previous experiences in individualizing the preparatory process. Stress point coping can be used to determine the child's most stressful or upsetting part of previous procedural experiences (Thompson, 2009). Once the stress point is identified, coping strategies to address this specific point in the procedure can be discussed with the child. Children who are distractible and highly active or those who are "slow to warm up" may need individualized sessions—shorter for active children and more slowly paced for shy children. Whereas children who tend to cope well may need more emphasis on using their present skills, those who appear to cope less adequately can benefit from more time devoted to simple coping strategies, such as relaxing, breathing, counting, squeezing a hand, or singing. Children with previous health-related experiences still need preparation for repeat or new procedures; however, the nurse must assess what they know, correct their misconceptions, supply new information, and introduce new coping skills as indicated by their previous reactions. Especially for painful procedures, the most effective preparation includes providing sensory-procedural information and helping the child develop coping skills, such as imagery or relaxation (Applying Evidence to Practice boxes).

Children differ in their "information-seeking dimension." Some actively ask for information about the intended procedure, but others characteristically avoid information. Parents can often guide nurses in deciding how much information is enough for the child because parents know whether the child is typically inquisitive or satisfied with short answers. Asking older children their preferences about the amount of explanation is also important.

The exact timing of the preparation for a procedure varies with the child's age, developmental level, and the type of procedure. No exact guidelines govern timing, but in general, the younger the child, the closer the explanation should be to the actual procedure to prevent undue fantasizing and worrying. Concurrent preparation is a strategy that can be used during a procedure to explain what a child can expect to occur and sense immediately before it happens (Thompson, 2009). This can be helpful for emergency procedures, for a highly anxious child, or for younger age-groups where extensive prior preparation is not possible or beneficial. With complex procedures, more time may be needed for assimilation of information, especially with older children. For example, the explanation for an injection can immediately precede the procedure for all ages, but preparation for surgery may begin the day before for young children and a few days before for older children, although the nurse should elicit older children's preferences.

APPLYING EVIDENCE TO PRACTICE

Preparing Children for Procedures

- Determine details of exact procedure to be performed.
- Review parents' and child's present understanding through open-ended questions.
- Base teaching on developmental age and existing knowledge.
- Incorporate parents in the teaching if they desire, especially if they plan to participate in care.
- Inform parents of their supportive role during the procedure, such as standing near child's head or in child's line of vision and talking softly to child, participating in comfort holding positions, and typical responses of children undergoing the procedure.
- Allow for ample discussion to prevent information overload and ensure adequate feedback.
- Use concrete, not abstract, terms and visual aids to describe procedure. For example, use a simple line drawing of a boy or girl and mark the body part that will be involved in the procedure. Use nonthreatening but realistic models.*
- Emphasize that no other body part will be involved.
- If the body part is associated with a specific function, stress the change or noninvolvement of that ability (e.g., after tonsillectomy, child can still speak).
- Use words and sentence length appropriate to child's level of understanding (a rule of thumb for the number of words in a child's sentence is equal to his or her age in years plus 1).
- Avoid words and phrases with dual meanings (see Table 22.1) unless child understands such words.
- Clarify all unfamiliar words (e.g., "Anesthesia is a *different kind of* sleep").
- Emphasize sensory aspects of procedure—what child will feel, see, hear, smell, taste, and touch and what child can do during procedure (e.g., lie still, count out loud, squeeze a hand, hug a doll).
- Allow child to practice procedures that will require cooperation (e.g., turning, deep breathing, using an incentive spirometer).
- Introduce anxiety-inducing information last (e.g., starting an intravenous line).
- Be honest with child about unpleasant aspects of a procedure, but avoid creating undue concern. When discussing that a procedure may be uncomfortable, state that it feels differently to different people.
- Emphasize end of procedure and any pleasurable events afterward (e.g., going home, seeing parents).
- Stress positive benefits of procedure (e.g., "After your tonsils are fixed, you won't have as many sore throats").
- Provide a positive ending, praising efforts at cooperation and coping.

*Soft-sculptured dolls and customized adapters and overlays for preparing children and families about procedures and as teaching models for technical care are available from Legacy Products, Inc., 508 S. Green St., PO Box 267, Cambridge City, IN 47327; 800-238-7951; email: info@legacyproductsinc.com; http://www.legacyproductsinc.com.

Establish Trust and Provide Support

The nurse who has spent time with and established a positive relationship with a child usually finds it easier to gain cooperation. If the relationship

APPLYING EVIDENCE TO PRACTICE

Age-Specific Preparation of Children for Procedures Based on Developmental Characteristics

Infant—Developing Trust and Sensorimotor Thought

Attachment to Parent

Involve parent in procedure if desired.*

Keep parent in infant's line of vision.

If parent is unable to be with infant, place familiar object with infant (e.g., stuffed toy, blanket).

Stranger Anxiety

Have usual caregivers perform or assist with procedure.*

Make advances slowly and in a nonthreatening manner.

Limit number of strangers entering room during procedure.*

Sensorimotor Phase of Learning

During procedure, use sensory soothing measures (e.g., stroking skin, talking softly, giving pacifier, breastfeeding).

Use analgesics (e.g., topical anesthetic, intravenous opioid) to control discomfort.*

Cuddle and hug infant after stressful procedure; encourage parent to comfort infant.

Increased Muscle Control

Expect older infants to resist.

Restrain adequately.

Keep harmful objects out of reach.

Memory for Past Experiences

Realize that older infants may associate objects, places, or persons with prior painful experiences and will cry and resist at the sight of them.

Keep frightening objects out of view.*

Perform painful procedures in a separate room, not in crib (or bed).*

Use nonintrusive procedures whenever possible (e.g., axillary or tympanic temperatures, oral medications).*

Imitation of Gestures

Model desired behavior (e.g., opening mouth).

Toddler—Developing Autonomy and Sensorimotor to Preoperational Thought

Use same approaches as for infant plus the following.

Egocentric Thought

Explain procedure in relation to what child will see, hear, taste, smell, and feel.

Emphasize those aspects of procedure that require cooperation (e.g., lying still).

Tell child it is okay to cry, yell, or use other means to express discomfort verbally.

Designate one health care provider to speak during procedure. Hearing more than one can be confusing and overwhelming to a child.*

Negative Behavior

Expect treatments to be resisted; child may try to run away.

Use firm, direct approach.

Ignore temper tantrums.

Use distraction techniques (e.g., singing a song *with* child).

Restrain adequately using a comfort hold technique.

Animism

Keep frightening objects out of view (young children believe objects have lifelike qualities and can harm them).

Limited Language Skills

Communicate using gestures or demonstrations.

Use a few simple terms familiar to child.

Give child one direction at a time (e.g., "Lie down" and then "Hold my hand").

Use small replicas of equipment; allow child to handle equipment.

Use play; demonstrate on doll but avoid child's favorite doll because child may think doll is really "feeling" procedure.

Prepare parents separately to avoid child's misinterpreting words.

Limited Concept of Time

Prepare child shortly or immediately before procedure.

Keep teaching sessions short (about 5 to 10 minutes).

Have preparations completed before involving child in procedure.

Have extra equipment nearby (e.g., alcohol swabs, new needle, adhesive bandages) to avoid delays.

Tell child when procedure is completed.

Striving for Independence

Allow choices whenever possible but realize that child may still be resistant and negative.

Allow child to participate in care and to help whenever possible (e.g., drink medicine from a cup, hold a dressing).

Preschooler—Developing Initiative and Preoperational Thought

Egocentric

Explain procedure in simple terms and in relation to how it affects child (as with toddler, stress sensory aspects).

Demonstrate use of equipment.

Allow child to play with miniature or actual equipment.

Encourage "playing out" experience on a doll both before and after procedure to clarify misconceptions.

Use neutral words to describe the procedure (see Table 22.1).

Increased Language Skills

Use verbal explanation but avoid overestimating child's comprehension of words.

Encourage child to verbalize ideas and feelings.

Limited Concept of Time and Frustration Tolerance

Implement same approaches as for toddler but may plan longer teaching session (10 to 15 minutes); may divide information into more than one session.

Illness and Hospitalization Viewed as Punishment

Clarify why each procedure is performed; child will find it difficult to understand how medicine can make him or her feel better and can taste bad at the same time.

Ask child thoughts regarding why a procedure is performed.

State directly that procedures are never a form of punishment.

Animism

Keep equipment out of sight except when shown to or used on child.

Fears of Bodily Harm, Intrusion, and Castration

Point out on drawing, doll, or child where procedure is performed.

Emphasize that no other body part will be involved.

Use nonintrusive procedures whenever possible (e.g., axillary temperatures, oral medication).

Apply an adhesive bandage over puncture site.

Encourage parental presence.

Realize that procedures involving genitalia provoke anxiety.

Allow child to wear underpants with gown.

Explain unfamiliar situations, especially noises or lights.

Continued

APPLYING EVIDENCE TO PRACTICE—cont'd

Age-Specific Preparation of Children for Procedures Based on Developmental Characteristics

Striving for Initiative

Involve child in care whenever possible (e.g., hold equipment, remove dressing).

Give choices whenever possible, but avoid excessive delays.

Praise child for helping and attempting to cooperate; never shame child for lack of cooperation.

School-Age Child—Developing Industry and Concrete Thought

Increased Language Skills; Interest in Acquiring Knowledge

Explain procedures using correct scientific and medical terminology.

Explain procedure using simple diagrams and photographs.

Discuss why procedure is necessary; concepts of illness and bodily functions are often vague.

Explain function and operation of equipment in concrete terms.

Allow child to manipulate equipment; use doll or another person as model to practice using equipment whenever possible (doll play may be considered childish by older school-age child).

Allow time before and after procedure for questions and discussion.

Improved Concept of Time

Plan for longer teaching sessions (about 20 minutes).

Prepare up to 1 day in advance of procedure to allow for processing of information.

Increased Self-Control

Gain child's cooperation.

Tell child what is expected.

Suggest several ways of maintaining control the child may select from (e.g., deep breathing, relaxation, counting).

Striving for Industry

Allow responsibility for simple tasks (e.g., collecting specimens).

Include child in decision making (e.g., time of day to perform procedure, preferred site).

Encourage active participation (e.g., removing dressings, handling equipment, opening packages).

Developing Relationships With Peers

Prepare two or more children for same procedure or encourage one to help prepare another.

Provide privacy from peers during procedure to maintain self-esteem.

Adolescent—Developing Identity and Abstract Thought

Increasing Abstract Thought and Reasoning

Discuss why procedure is necessary or beneficial.

Explain long-term consequences of procedures; include information about body systems working together.

Realize adolescent may fear death, disability, or other potential risks.

Encourage questioning regarding fears, options, and alternatives.

Consciousness of Appearance

Provide privacy; describe how the body will be covered and what will be exposed.

Discuss how procedure may affect appearance (e.g., scar) and what can be done to minimize it.

Emphasize any physical benefits of procedure.

Concern More With Present Than With Future

Realize that immediate effects of procedure are more significant than future benefits.

Striving for Independence

Involve adolescent in decision making and planning (e.g., time, place, individuals present during procedure, clothing, whether they will watch procedure).

Impose as few restrictions as possible.

Explore what coping strategies have worked in the past; they may need suggestions of various techniques.

Accept regression to more childish methods of coping.

Realize that adolescent may have difficulty accepting new authority figures and may resist complying with procedures.

Developing Peer Relationships and Group Identity

Same as for school-age child but assumes even greater significance.

Allow adolescents to talk with other adolescents who have had the same procedure.

*Applies to any age.

NURSING TIP

Use photographs or videos of children in different areas of the hospital (e.g., radiology department, operating room) to give children a more realistic idea of equipment they may encounter.

is based on trust, the child will associate the nurse with caregiving activities that give comfort and pleasure most of the time rather than discomfort and stress. If the nurse does not know the child, it is best for the nurse to be introduced by another staff person whom the child trusts. The first visit with the child should not include any painful procedure and ideally should focus on the child first and then on an explanation of the procedure. A simple way to begin the process of creating trust is by engaging in play with the patient through favorite activities or toys. Body language is another key element of promoting trust. Positive body language, such as sitting instead of standing, and avoiding the use of technical medical terminology in conversation can enhance the therapeutic caregiver relationship with the child and family (Lidgett, 2016).

Parental Presence and Support

Children need support during procedures, and for young children, the greatest source of support is the parents. They represent security, protection, safety, and comfort. Parental presence has a positive impact on the level of pain, stress, and negative behavior experienced by the child, as well as parental distress and satisfaction (Matziou, Chrysostomou, Vlahioti, et al., 2013). Additionally, there is no difference in technical complications when parents remain with children. However, controversy exists regarding the role parents should assume during the procedure, especially if discomfort is involved. The nurse should assess the parents' preferences for assisting, observing, or waiting outside the room, as well as the child's preference for parental presence. Respect the child's and parents' choices. Give parents who wish to stay appropriate explanation about the procedure, and coach them about where to sit or stand and what to say or do to help the child through the procedure. Support parents who do not want to be present in their decision, and

TABLE 22.1 Selecting Nonthreatening Words or Phrases

Words and Phrases to Avoid	Suggested Substitutions
Shot, bee sting, stick	Medicine under the skin, poke that will feel like a pinch
Organ	Place in body
Test	To see how (specify body part) is working
Incision, cut	Make an opening
Edema	Puffiness
Stretcher, gurney	Rolling bed, bed on wheels
Stool/urine	Child's usual term
Dye	Medicine to help place in your body show up on a picture
Pain	Hurt, discomfort, "owie," "boo-boo," sore, achy, scratchy, pinch
Deaden, numb	Not feel body part as much
Fix	Make better
Take (as in "take your temperature")	See how warm you are
Take (as in "take your blood pressure")	Check your pressure; hug your arm
Put to sleep, anesthesia	Different kind of sleep so you won't feel anything
Catheter	Soft tube, small straw
Monitor	Television screen
Electrodes	Stickers, ticklers
Specimen	Take some blood

encourage them to remain close by so they can be available to support the child immediately after the procedure. It can be helpful for parents to assist the health care team in identifying an alternative support person for their child, such as a child life specialist or nurse, if they are unable to be present during the procedure. Parents should know that someone will be with their child to provide support. Ideally, this person should inform the parents after the procedure about how the child did.

Provide an Explanation

Age-appropriate explanations are one of the most widely used interventions for reducing anxiety in children undergoing procedures. Before performing a procedure, explain what is to be done, what sensations the child may feel, what is expected of the child, and why the procedure is being done. It is important that the child understand the procedure is not punishment. The explanation should be short, simple, and appropriate to the child's level of comprehension. Long explanations may increase anxiety in a young child. When explaining the procedure to parents with the child present, the nurse uses language appropriate to the child because unfamiliar words can be misunderstood (Table 22.1). If the parents need additional preparation, it is done in an area away from the child. Teaching sessions are planned at times most conducive to the child's learning (e.g., after a rest period) and for the usual span of attention.

Special equipment is not necessary for preparing a child, but for young children who cannot yet think conceptually, using objects to supplement verbal explanation is important. Children often learn through behavior modeling such as seeing a doll experience the procedure, watching a video, or seeing a picture. Additionally, allowing children to handle actual items that will be used in their care, such as a stethoscope, sphygmomanometer, or oxygen mask, helps them develop familiarity with these items and reduces the fear often associated with their use. Miniature versions of hospital items such as gurneys and x-ray and intravenous (IV) equipment can be used to explain what the children can expect and permit them to safely experience situations that are unfamiliar and potentially frightening. Written and illustrated materials are also valuable aids to preparation.*

NURSING TIP

To avoid a delay during a procedure, have extra supplies handy. For example, have tape, bandages, alcohol swabs, and an extra needle when performing an injection or venipuncture.

NURSING TIP

Prepare a basket, toy chest, or cart to keep near the treatment area. Items ideal for the basket include a Slinky; a sparkling "magic" wand (sealed, acrylic tube partially filled with liquid and suspended metallic confetti); a soft foam ball; bubble solution; party blowers; pop-up books with foldout, three-dimensional scenes; real medical equipment, such as a syringe, adhesive bandages, and alcohol packets; toy medical supplies or a toy medical kit; marking pens; a notepad; and stickers. Have the child choose an item to help distract and relax during the procedure. After the procedure, allow the child to choose a small gift, such as a sticker, or to play with items, such as medical equipment. Do not allow a child to keep a syringe to play with because it can cause harm (e.g., air embolism or infection) if connected into a needleless infusion port.

Physical Preparation

One area of special concern is the administration of appropriate sedation and analgesia before stressful procedures.

Performance of the Procedure

Supportive care continues during the procedure and can be a major factor in a child's ability to cooperate. Ideally, the same nurse who explains the procedure should perform or assist with the procedure. The child may also benefit from a parent or trusted caregiver who can offer coaching techniques and support during the procedure. Before beginning, all equipment is assembled, and the room is readied to prevent unnecessary delays and interruptions that increase the child's anxiety. Minimizing the number of people present and allowing one person to speak during the procedure also can decrease the child's anxiety.

To promote long-term coping and adjustment, give special consideration to the patient's age, coping skills, and procedure to be performed in determining where a procedure will occur. Treatment rooms should be used for procedures requiring sedation, such as bone marrow aspirates and lumbar punctures in younger children. Traumatic procedures should never be performed in "safe" areas, such as the playroom. If the procedure is lengthy, avoid conversation that could be misinterpreted by the child. As the procedure is nearing completion, the nurse may inform the child "this is the last piece of tape" or simply inform the child when the procedure is completed.

*Preparatory materials include Hospital Friends, available from Centering Corporation, 7230 Maple St., Omaha, NE 68134; 866-218-0101; https://centering.org/. Other resources include *Berenstain Bears Go to the Doctor* and *Berenstain Bears Visit the Dentist* (New York, Random House).

> **NURSING TIP**
>
> Help the child select and practice a coping technique before the procedure. Consider having the parent or some other supportive person, such as a child life specialist, "coach" the child in learning and using the coping skill.

Expect Success

Nurses who approach children with confidence and who convey the impression that they expect to be successful are less likely to encounter difficulty. It is best to approach a child as though cooperation is expected. Children sense anxiety and uncertainty in an adult and respond by striking out or actively resisting. Although it is not possible to eliminate such behavior in every child, a firm approach with a positive attitude tends to convey a feeling of security to most children.

Involve the Child

Involving children helps gain their cooperation. Permitting choices gives them some measure of control. However, a choice is given only in situations in which one is available. Asking children, "Do you want to take your medicine now?" leads them to believe they have an option and provides them the opportunity to legitimately refuse or delay the medication. This places the nurse in an awkward, if not impossible, position. It is much better to state firmly, "It's time to drink your medicine now." Children usually like to make choices, but the choice must be one that they do indeed have (e.g., "It's time for your medicine. Do you want to drink it plain or with a little water?").

Many children respond to tactics that appeal to their maturity or courage. This also gives them a sense of participation and achievement. For example, preschool children will be proud that they can hold the dressing during the procedure or remove the tape. The same is true for school-age children, who often cooperate with minimal resistance.

Provide Distraction

Distraction is a powerful coping strategy during painful procedures (Matziou, Chrysostomou, Vlahioti, et al., 2013). It is accomplished by focusing the child's attention on something other than the procedure. Singing favorite songs, listening to music with a headset, counting aloud, or blowing bubbles to "blow the hurt away" are effective techniques. (For other nonpharmacologic interventions, see Chapter 20.)

Allow Expression of Feelings

The child should be allowed to express feelings of anger, anxiety, fear, frustration, or any other emotion. It is natural for children to strike out in frustration or to try to avoid stress-provoking situations. The child needs to know that it is all right to cry. Behavior is children's primary means of communication and coping and should be permitted unless it inflicts harm on them or those caring for them. Harmful behavior should be acknowledged and appropriate limitations should be set to promote patient and caregiver safety.

Postprocedural Support

After the procedure, the child continues to need reassurance that he or she performed well and is accepted and loved. If the parents did not participate, the child is united with them as soon as possible so they can provide comfort.

Encourage Expression of Feelings

Planned activity after the procedure is helpful in encouraging constructive expression of feelings. For verbal children, reviewing the details of the procedure can clarify misconceptions and garner feedback for improving the nurse's preparatory strategies. Play is an excellent activity for all children. Infants and young children should have the opportunity for gross motor movement. Older children are able to vent their anger and frustration in acceptable pounding or throwing activities. Play-Doh is a remarkably versatile medium for pounding and shaping. Dramatic play provides an outlet for anger and places the child in a position of control, in contrast to the position of helplessness in the real situation. Puppets also allow the child to communicate feelings in a nonthreatening way. One of the most effective interventions is **therapeutic play**, which includes well-supervised activities such as permitting the child to give an injection to a doll or stuffed toy to reduce the stress of injections (Fig. 22.1).

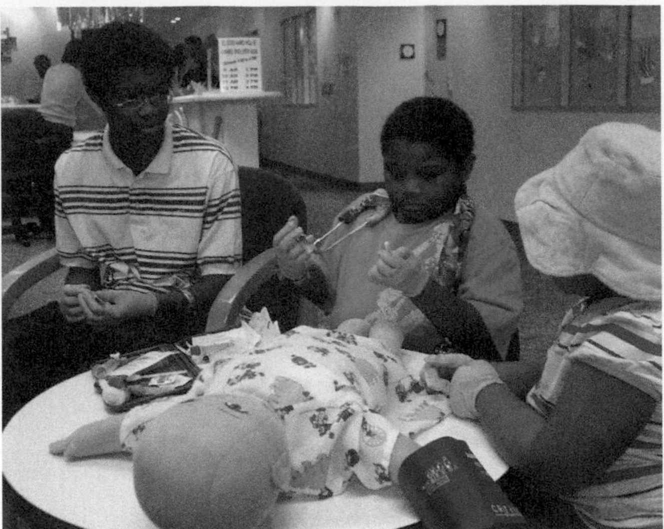

FIG. 22.1 Playing with medical objects provides children with the opportunity to play out fears and concerns with supervision by a nurse or child life specialist.

Positive Reinforcement

Children need to hear from adults that they did the best they could in the situation—no matter how they behaved. There should be specific acknowledgment of what aspect of the procedure the child performed well. It is important for children to know that their worth is not being judged on the basis of their behavior in a stressful situation. Reward systems, such as earning stars, stickers, or a supportive care program such as Beads of Courage that celebrates a child's milestones in medical treatment, are appealing to children.*

Returning to the child a short while after the procedure helps the nurse strengthen a supportive relationship. Relating with the child in a relaxed and nonstressful period allows him or her to see the nurse not only as someone associated with stressful situations but also as someone with whom to share pleasurable experiences.

Use of Play in Procedures

The use of play is an integral part of relationships with children. As such, its value in specific situations is discussed throughout this book, such as in Chapter 21 in relation to hospitalization. Many institutions have elaborate and well-organized play areas and programs under the direction of child life specialists. Other institutions have limited facilities. No matter what the institution provides for children, nurses can include play activities as part of nursing care. Play can be used to teach, express

*Beads of Courage information is available at http://www.beadsofcourage.org/.

BOX 22.1 Play Activities for Specific Procedures

Fluid Intake

Make ice pops using child's favorite juice.
Cut gelatin into fun shapes.
Make a game out of taking a sip when turning page of a book or in games such as Simon Says.
Use small medicine cups; decorate the cups.
Color water with food coloring or powdered drink mix.
Have a tea party; pour at a small table.
Cut straws in half and place in a small container (much easier for child to suck liquid).
Use a "crazy" straw.
Make a "progress poster"; give rewards for drinking a predetermined quantity.

Deep Breathing

Blow bubbles with a bubble blower.
Blow bubbles with a straw (no soap).
Blow on a pinwheel, feather, whistle, harmonica, balloon, or party blower.
Practice band instruments.
Have a blowing contest using balloons,* boats, cotton balls, feathers, marbles, Ping-Pong balls, pieces of paper; blow such objects on a table top over a goal line, over water, through an obstacle course, up in the air, against an opponent, or up and down a string.
Suck paper or cloth from one container to another using a straw.
Dramatize stories such as "I'll huff and I'll puff, and I'll blow your house down" from the "Three Little Pigs."
Do straw-blowing painting.
Take a deep breath and "blow out the candles" on a birthday cake.
Use a little paintbrush to "paint" nails with water and blow nails dry.

Range of Motion and Use of Extremities

Throw beanbags at a fixed or movable target or throw wadded-up paper into a wastebasket.
Touch or kick Mylar balloons held or hung in different positions (if child is in traction, hang balloon from a trapeze).
Play "tickle toes"; have the child wiggle them on request.
Play Twister game or Simon Says.
Play pretend and guessing games (e.g., imitate a bird, butterfly, or horse).
Have tricycle or wheelchair races in safe area.
Play kickball or throw ball with a soft foam ball in a safe area.
Position bed so that child must turn to view television or doorway.
Climb wall with fingers like a "spider."
Pretend to teach aerobic dancing or exercises; encourage parents to participate.
Encourage swimming if feasible.
Play video games or pinball (fine motor movement).
Play hide and seek: hide toy somewhere in bed (or room if ambulatory) and have child find it using specified hand or foot.
Provide clay to mold with fingers.
Paint or draw on large sheets of paper placed on floor or wall.
Encourage combing own hair; play "beauty shop" with "customer" in different positions.

Soaks

Play with small toys or objects (e.g., cups, soap dishes) in water.
Wash dolls or toys.
Pick up marbles or pennies* from bottom of bath container.
Make designs with coins on bottom of container.
Pretend a boat is a submarine by keeping it immersed.
Read to child during soaks; sing with child; or play game, such as cards, checkers, or other board game (if both hands are immersed, move board pieces for child).
Sitz bath: give child something to listen to (e.g., music, stories) or look at (e.g., View-Master, book).
Punch holes in bottom of plastic cup, fill with water, and let it "rain" on child.

Injections

Let child handle syringe, vial, and alcohol swab and give an injection to doll or stuffed animal.
Draw a "magic circle" on area before injection; draw smiling face in circle after injection but avoid drawing on puncture site.
If multiple injections or venipunctures are planned, make a "progress poster"; give rewards for predetermined number of injections.
Have child count to 10 or 15 during injection.

Ambulation

Give child something to push:

- Toddler: push-pull toy
- School-age child: wagon or a doll in a stroller or wheelchair
- Adolescent: decorated intravenous stand

Have a parade; make hats, drums, and so on.

Extending Environment (e.g., for Patients in Traction)

Make bed into a pirate ship or airplane with decorations.
Put up mirrors so patient can see around room.
Move bed frequently to playroom, hallway, or outside.

*Small objects such as marbles and coins, as well as gloves and balloons, are unsafe for young children because of possible aspiration. Latex products also carry the risk of an allergic reaction.

feelings, or achieve a therapeutic goal. Consequently, it should be included in preparing children for and encouraging their cooperation during procedures. Play sessions after procedures can be structured, such as directed toward needle play, or general, with a wide variety of equipment available for children to play with.

Routine procedures such as measuring blood pressure and oral administration of medication may be of concern to children. Box 22.1 describes suggestions for incorporating play into nursing procedures and activities for the hospitalized child that facilitate learning and adjustment to a new situation.

Preparing the Family

The process of patient education involves giving the family information about the child's condition, the regimen that must be followed and why, and other health teaching as indicated. The goal of this education is to enable the family to modify behaviors and adhere to the regimen that has been mutually established (see Applying Evidence to Practice box).

If equipment will be needed at home (e.g., suction machines, syringes), begin making the necessary arrangements in advance so that discharge can proceed smoothly. Whenever possible, make arrangements for the family to use the same equipment in the home that they are using in the hospital. This allows them to become familiar with the items. In addition, the staff can help troubleshoot the equipment in a controlled environment. Plan the teaching sessions well in advance of the time the family will be responsible for performing the care. The more complex the procedure, the more time is needed for training.

Review the instructions with family members (see Applying Evidence to Practice box). Encourage note taking if they desire. Allow ample

APPLYING EVIDENCE TO PRACTICE

General Principles of Family Education

- Establish a rapport with the family.
- Avoid using confusing specialized terms or jargon. Clarify all terms with the family and use the term that is clear to the child.
- When possible, allow family members to decide how they want to be taught (e.g., all at once or over a day or two). This gives the family a chance to incorporate the information at a rate that is comfortable.
- Provide accurate information to the family about the illness.
- Assist family members in identifying obstacles to their ability to comply with the regimen and in identifying the means to overcome those obstacles. Then help family members find ways to incorporate the plan into their daily lives.

practice time under supervision. At least one family member, but preferably two members, should demonstrate the procedure before they are expected to care for the child at home. Provide the family with the telephone numbers of resource individuals who are available to assist them in the event of a problem.

APPLYING EVIDENCE TO PRACTICE

Family Preparation for Procedures

Family education for specific procedures is included throughout this unit. General concepts applicable to most family education sessions include the following:

- Name of the procedure
- Purpose of the procedure
- Length of time anticipated to complete the procedure
- Anticipated effects
- Signs of adverse effects
- Assess the family's level of understanding
- Demonstrate and have family return demonstration (if appropriate)

SURGICAL PROCEDURES

Preoperative Care

Children experiencing surgical procedures require both psychologic and physical preparation. An important concern is restriction of food and fluids before surgery to avoid pulmonary aspiration during anesthesia. Additionally, fasting too long can cause discomfort, headache, dehydration, or hypoglycemia and can delay recovery and hospital discharge (Dolgun, Yavuz, Eroğlu, et al., 2017). Infants require special attention to fluid needs. They should not be without oral fluids for an extended period preoperatively to avoid glycogen depletion and dehydration. If surgical procedures are delayed, it is the nurse's responsibility to communicate with the surgical team to adjust fasting guidelines appropriately (Williams, Johnson, Guzzetta, et al., 2014). Table 22.2 contains current preoperative fasting guidelines.

In general, psychologic preparation is similar to that discussed earlier for any procedure and uses many of the same techniques used in preparing a child for hospitalization, such as films, books, brochures, play, and tours (see Chapter 19). Stress points before and after surgery include the admission process, blood tests, administration of preoperative medication (if prescribed), transport to the operating room, the mask on the face during induction, and the stay in the postanesthesia care unit. Wearing a hospital gown without the security of underpants or pajama bottoms can also be traumatic. Therefore these articles of clothing

TABLE 22.2 Fasting Recommendations to Reduce the Risk of Pulmonary Aspiration*

Ingested Material	Minimum Fasting Period (hr)†
Clear liquids‡	>2
Breast milk	4
Infant formula	6
Nonhuman milk§	6
Light meal¶	6

*These recommendations apply to healthy patients who are undergoing elective procedures. They are not intended for women in labor. Following the guidelines does not guarantee that complete gastric emptying has occurred.
†Fasting periods noted in chart apply to all ages.
‡Examples of clear liquids include water, fruit juices without pulp, carbonated beverages, clear tea, and black coffee.
§Because nonhuman milk is similar to solids in gastric emptying time, the amount ingested must be considered when determining appropriate fasting period.
¶A light meal typically consists of toast and clear liquids. Meals that include fried or fatty foods or meat may prolong gastric emptying time. Both the amount and type of foods ingested must be considered when determining an appropriate fasting period.
From American Society of Anesthesiologists, Committee on Standards and Practice Parameters. (2011). Practice guidelines for preoperative fasting and the use of pharmacological agents to reduce the risk of pulmonary aspiration: Application to healthy patients undergoing elective procedures. *Anesthesiology, 114*(3), 495-511.

should be allowed to be worn into the operating room and removed after induction of anesthesia. Children are at higher risk of ineffective response to anesthesia and complications in the recovery period because of higher anxiety in the preoperative period associated with stranger anxiety (infants), separation anxiety (toddlers and preschoolers), and fear of injury or death (adolescents) (Al-Yateem, Brenner, Shorrab, et al., 2016).

Individualized psychologic intervention consisting of systematic preparation, rehearsal of the forthcoming events, and supportive care at each of these points has shown to be more effective than a single-session preparation or consistent supportive care without systematic preparation and rehearsal (Fortier, Kain, & Morton, 2015). A family-centered preoperative preparation program may consist of a tour of the perioperative areas with short explanations of the events 5 to 7 days before surgery, a video to take home and review a couple of times with additional explanations and demonstrations of perioperative processes, a mask to take home and practice with, pamphlets to guide parents on supporting children during induction, phone calls to coach parents on preparing children 1 or 2 days before surgery, toys and supplies in the holding area, and mobile phone applications with interactive tours and videos. Additionally, the use of interactive electronic games, tablets, or the use of therapy dogs in the preoperative setting can provide effective alternatives or complements to pharmacologic premedication. Therapeutic play is an effective strategy in preparing children, and increased familiarity with medical procedures can decrease anxiety.

Parental Presence

Some institutions support parental presence during induction of anesthesia. Benefits of well-prepared children and parents along with parental presence during induction of anesthesia include reduced anxiety for children and parents, lower doses of postoperative analgesia, lower incidence of severe emergence delirium symptoms, decreased postoperative maladaptive behaviors, and shorter discharge time for short procedures (Fortier, Kain, & Morton, 2015). Other studies have not supported a reduction in children's anxiety (Erhaze, Dowling, & Devane, 2016; Manyande, Cyna, Yip, et al., 2015).

Concern exists regarding the appropriateness of parental presence during induction for all parents. Some parents may become upset by the rapid succession of induction events, by observing their child becoming limp, and by leaving the child in the care of strangers. Although parents who are anxious before surgery tend to become even more anxious after the induction, the reverse is true of parents with little anxiety. There is little evidence to suggest that parental presence during induction provides decreased anxiety for parents and caregivers (Al-Yateem, Brenner, Shorrab, et al., 2016). Appropriate education is essential to help parents understand the stages of anesthesia, what to expect, and how to support their child.

Preoperative Sedation

The goals for using preoperative medications include anxiety reduction, amnesia, sedation, antiemetic effect, and reduction of secretions (Manworren & Fledderman, 2000). (Chapter 5 includes a discussion of pain management strategies for children undergoing surgery.) When drugs are administered, they should be delivered atraumatically via oral, intranasal, or IV routes. Numerous preanesthetic drug regimens are used with children, and no consensus exists on the optimal method. Some institutions promote distraction or parental support instead of medications due to the incidence of postoperative medication delirium (Batawi, 2015).

Intraoperative Care

The role of the pediatric operating room nurse is to advocate for care of the patient in surgery through the verification of procedure and laterality, implants, skin preparation, necessary instrumentation, and supplies. The operating room nurse assesses, recognizes, and intervenes for the pediatric surgical patient at high risk for pressure injury due to patient diagnosis, patient anatomy, general anesthesia, intraoperative positioning, immobility, moisture, and nothing-by-mouth (NPO) status. Clear communication is used through collaboration with the interdisciplinary team (anesthesia, surgeon, scrub technician, nurses, radiology, etc.) to coordinate the intraoperative and postoperative disposition of the surgical patient. Family-centered care is provided through engaging the family in the preoperative procedure verification and updating them throughout the procedure (Herd & Rieben, 2014).

Postoperative Care

Various psychologic and physical interventions and observations help prevent or minimize possible unpleasant effects from anesthesia and the surgical procedure. Although serious postoperative complications in healthy children undergoing surgery are rare, continuous monitoring of the child's cardiopulmonary status is essential during the immediate postoperative period to reduce this risk (Pawar, 2012). Postanesthesia complications such as airway obstruction, postextubation croup, laryngospasm, and bronchospasm make maintaining a patent airway and maximum ventilation critical.

Monitoring the patient's oxygen saturation and providing supplemental oxygen as needed, maintaining body temperature, and promoting fluid and electrolyte balance are important aspects of immediate postoperative care. Vital signs are continuously monitored, and each vital sign is evaluated in terms of side effects from anesthesia, shock, or respiratory compromise (Table 22.3).

A change in vital signs that demands immediate attention in the perioperative period is caused by **malignant hyperthermia (MH)**, a potentially fatal pharmacogenetic disorder of muscle metabolism. In susceptible children, inhaled anesthetics and the muscle relaxant succinylcholine trigger the disorder, producing hypermetabolism. Symptoms of MH include hypercarbia (increasing end-tidal carbon dioxide), elevated temperature, tachycardia, tachypnea, acidosis, muscle rigidity, hyperkalemia, and rhabdomyolysis. A family or previous history of sudden high fever associated with a surgical procedure and myotonia increase the risk for MH. Children who have successfully undergone prior surgery without adverse effects may still be considered susceptible (Salazar, Yang, Shen, et al., 2014).

Treatment of MH includes immediate discontinuation of the triggering agent, hyperventilation with 100% oxygen, and IV dantrolene sodium. If the child is hyperthermic, initiate cooling measures such as ice packs to the groin, axillae, and neck and iced nasogastric (NG) lavage. The surgery may be discontinued, or if it is emergent, it may be continued with a different anesthetic agent. The patient should be transferred to an intensive care unit for at least 36 hours and closely monitored for stabilization of vital signs, metabolic state, and possible recurrence of symptoms.

Managing pain is a major nursing responsibility after surgery. The nurse should assess pain frequently and administer analgesics to provide comfort and facilitate cooperation with postoperative care such as ambulation and deep breathing. Opioids are the most commonly used analgesics. Routinely scheduled IV analgesics, patient-controlled analgesia, regional blocks, and epidural infusions, rather than as-needed orders, provide excellent analgesia in postoperative pediatric patients.

Nonpharmacologic postoperative recovery interventions include the use of distraction, videos, interactive game applications, and therapy dogs. Therapy dogs can facilitate decreased pain perception, increase in activity, and emotional stabilization in the postoperative period (Calcaterra, Veggiotti, Palestrini, et al., 2015).

> **NURSING TIP**
>
> Because deep breathing is usually painful after surgery, be certain that the child has received analgesics. Have the child splint the operative site (depending on its location) by hugging a small pillow or a favorite stuffed animal.

Because respiratory tract infections are a potential complication of anesthesia, make every effort to aerate the lungs and remove secretions. The lungs are auscultated regularly to identify abnormal sounds or any areas of diminished or absent breath sounds. To prevent pneumonia, encourage respiratory movement with incentive spirometers or other motivating activities (see Box 22.1). If these measures are presented as games, the child is more likely to comply. The child's position is changed every 2 hours, and deep breathing is encouraged. Patients with preexisting pulmonary disease may be advised to begin incentive spirometry before the day of surgery (Azhar, 2015). Early respiratory movement can decrease the patient's need for supplemental oxygen and promote discharge home sooner (Shaughnessy, White, Shah, et al., 2015).

During the recovery period, spend some time with the child to assess his or her perceptions of surgery. Play, drawing, and storytelling are excellent methods of discovering the child's thoughts. With such information, the nurse can support or correct the child's perceptions and boost his or her self-esteem for having endured a stressful procedure.

Many pediatric patients are discharged shortly after surgery. Preparation for discharge begins with the preadmission preparation visit. Thorough discharge processes and education can greatly assist in the prevention of unplanned readmissions (Payne & Flood, 2015). The nurse should discuss instructions for postoperative care and review them throughout the perioperative visit. After discharge, the nursing staff often makes phone calls to check the patient's status. Patient

TABLE 22.3 Potential Causes of Postoperative Vital Sign Alterations in Children

Alteration	Potential Cause	Comments
Heart Rate		
Increase	Decreased perfusion (shock) Elevated temperature Pain Respiratory distress (early) Medications (atropine, morphine, epinephrine) Hypoxia	Heart rate may increase to maintain cardiac output.
Decrease	Vagal stimulation Increased intracranial pressure Respiratory distress (late) Medications (neostigmine [Prostigmin])	Bradycardia is of more concern in young child than tachycardia.
Respiratory Rate		
Increase	Respiratory distress Fluid volume excess Hypothermia Elevated temperature Pain	Body responds to respiratory distress primarily by increasing rate.
Decrease	Anesthetics, opioids Pain	Decreased respiratory rate from opioids may be compensated for by increased depth of respiration.
Blood Pressure		
Increase	Excess intravascular volume Increased intracranial pressure Carbon dioxide retention Pain Medication (ketamine, epinephrine)	This is serious in premature infants because it increases risk of intraventricular hemorrhage.
Decrease	Vasodilating anesthetic agents (halothane, isoflurane, enflurane) Opioids (e.g., morphine)	Decreased blood pressure is late sign of shock because of elasticity and constriction of vessels to maintain cardiac output.
Temperature		
Increase	Shock (late sign) Infection Environmental causes (warm room, excess coverings) Malignant hyperthermia	Fever associated with infection usually occurs later than fever of noninfectious origin. Absence of fever does not rule out infection, especially in infants. Malignant hyperthermia requires immediate treatment.
Decrease	Vasodilating anesthetic agents (halothane, isoflurane, enflurane) Muscle relaxants Environmental causes (cool room) Infusion of cool fluids or blood	Neonates are especially susceptible to hypothermia, with serious or fatal consequences.

education and compliance with discharge instructions can also be assessed during these phone calls (Flippo, NeSmith, Stark, et al., 2015) (see Applying Evidence to Practice box).

COMPLIANCE

Compliance, also termed adherence, refers to the extent to which the patient's behavior coincides with the prescribed regimen in terms of taking medication, following diets, or executing other lifestyle changes. In developing strategies to improve compliance, the nurse must first assess level of compliance. Because many children are too young to assume partial or total responsibility for their care, parents are usually primarily responsible for home management.

Factors relating to the care setting are important in ensuring compliance and should be considered in planning strategies to improve compliance. Basically, any aspect of the health care setting that increases the family's satisfaction with the physical setting and the relationship with the provider positively influences adherence to the treatment regimen. However, the more complex, expensive, inconvenient, and disruptive the treatment protocol, the less likely the family is to comply. During long-term conditions that involve multiple treatments and considerable rearrangement of lifestyle, compliance is severely affected.

Although it is helpful to know those factors that influence compliance, assessment must include more direct measurement techniques. When inquiring about a patient's compliance, it can be helpful to ask details about how medication administration or other interventions are carried out instead of asking yes-or-no questions. For example, a health care provider could ask about what time of day patients performs their prescribed interventions, what beverage they prefer to take their medications with, or how many doses were missed this week (Brown & Sinsky, 2013). A number of methods exist, each with advantages and

APPLYING EVIDENCE TO PRACTICE

Postoperative Care

- Ensure that preparations are made to receive child:
  - Bed or crib is ready.
  - Intravenous pumps and poles, suction apparatus, and oxygen flow meter are at bedside.
- Obtain baseline information:
  - Take vital signs, including blood pressure; keep blood pressure cuff in place and deflated to lessen disturbance to child.
  - Take and record vital signs more frequently if any value fluctuates.
- Inspect operative area.
- Check dressing if present.
- Outline any bleeding area on dressing or cast with pen.
- Reinforce, but do not remove, loose dressing.
- Observe areas below surgical site for blood that may have drained toward bed.
- Assess for bleeding and other symptoms in areas not covered with a dressing, such as throat after tonsillectomy.
- Assess skin color and characteristics.
- Assess level of sedation and activity.
- Notify physician of any irregularities in child's condition.
- Assess for evidence of pain. (See Pain Assessment, Chapter 5.)
- Review surgeon's orders after completing initial assessment and check that any preoperative orders, such as seizure or cardiac medications, have been reordered and can be given by available routes (oral preparations may be contraindicated).
- Monitor vital signs as ordered and more often if indicated.
- Check dressings for bleeding or other abnormalities.
- Check bowel sounds.
- Observe for signs of shock, abdominal distention, and bleeding.
- Assess for bladder distention.
- Observe for signs of dehydration.
- Detect presence of infection:
  - Take vital signs every 2 to 4 hours as ordered.
  - Collect or request needed specimens.
  - Inspect wound for signs of infection—redness, swelling, heat, pain, and purulent drainage.

disadvantages. The most successful approach includes a combination of at least two of the following methods:

Clinical judgment—This is subject to bias and inaccuracy unless the nurse carefully evaluates the criteria used in assessment.

Self-reporting—Most people overestimate their compliance even when they admit to lapses.

Direct observation—This is difficult to use outside the health care setting, and awareness of being observed frequently affects performance.

Monitoring appointments—Keeping appointments indirectly indicates compliance with the prescribed care.

Monitoring therapeutic response—Few treatments yield directly measurable results (e.g., decreased blood pressure, weight loss); record on a graph or chart.

Pill counts—The nurse counts the number of pills remaining in the original container and compares the number missing with the number of times the medication should have been taken. Although this is a simple method, families may forget to bring the container or deliberately alter the number of pills to avoid detection. This method is also poorly suited to liquid medication. Another technique is the use of pill container caps that record every opening as a presumptive dose.

Chemical assay—For certain drugs, such as digoxin, measurement of plasma drug levels provides information on the amount of drug recently ingested. However, this method is expensive, indicates only short-term compliance, and requires precise timing of the assay for accurate results.

Compliance Strategies

Strategies to improve compliance involve interventions that encourage families to follow the prescribed treatment regimen. Some evidence suggests that higher levels of self-esteem and increased autonomy favorably affect adolescent compliance (Letitre, DeGroot, Draaisma, et al., 2014). Additionally, anxiety, depression, and self-esteem can be negatively affected when treatment regimens are inadequately followed. However, family factors are important, and characteristics associated with good compliance include family support, family reminders, good communication, and expectations for successful completion of the therapeutic regimen. No one approach is always successful, and the best results occur when at least two strategies are used.

Organizational strategies involve the care setting and the therapeutic plan. This may involve increasing the frequency of appointments, designating a primary provider, reducing the cost of medication by prescribing generic brands, reducing the treatment's disruption of the family's lifestyle, and using "cues" to minimize forgetting. Numerous devices are available commercially or can be improvised for cueing, such as pill dispensers; watches with alarms; charts to record completed therapy; messages on the refrigerator or morning coffee pot; mobile phone applications; and individualistic, self-timed schedules that incorporate the treatment plan into the daily routine, such as physical therapy after the evening bath.

The nurse instructs the family about the treatment plan. Although education is an important factor in enhancing compliance, and patients who are more knowledgeable about their condition are more likely to comply, education alone does not ensure compliant behavior. The nurse should incorporate teaching principles known to enhance understanding and retention of material. Written materials are essential, especially in any regimen requiring multiple or complex treatments, and they need to be understandable to the average individual, who reads at about the fourth-grade level. Learning disabilities can negatively affect medication adherence and should be routinely assessed along with health literacy (Dharmapuri, Best, Kind, et al., 2015). Individualized teaching strategies appropriate for developmental and cognitive levels of the individual, as well as involvement of the immediate and extended family (e.g., grandparents) in education sessions, may enhance compliance.

Treatment strategies relate to the child's refusal or inability to take the prescribed medication. The family may also have difficulty following a prescribed treatment regimen. They may remember and understand the instructions but may not be able to give the medicine as prescribed. Assess the reason for refusal. For example, the child may not be able to swallow pills. In this case perhaps pills could be crushed or a liquid medication substituted (always review medication to ensure that crushing is acceptable before giving this instruction).

Assess the treatment and medication schedule to determine whether it is reasonable for a home situation. Although an every-6-hour or every-8-hour schedule is reasonable for hospitals, a parent would have difficulty getting up once or twice nightly. Instead, the patient could take a medication during the day at times that would be easy to remember.

Behavioral strategies are designed to modify behavior directly. Nurses can use several effective strategies with children to encourage the desired behavior. Positive reinforcement is one strategy that strengthens the behavior. One example of this is the child earning stars or tokens, which can be exchanged for a special privilege or gift. Sticker charts also serve as a visual reminder of positive behavior and motivation to continue compliance. At times, however, disciplinary techniques, such as a time-out for young children or withholding privileges for older children, may be needed to improve compliance. The child life specialist role can be especially helpful in determining behavioral compliance strategies across the developmental spectrum.

SKIN CARE AND GENERAL HYGIENE

MAINTAINING HEALTHY SKIN

Maintaining an IV line, removing a dressing, positioning a child in bed, changing a diaper, using electrodes, and using restraints all have the potential to contribute to skin injury. General guidelines for skin care are listed in the Applying Evidence to Practice box. (Specific guidelines for skin care of neonates are provided in Chapter 7 under Skin Care.)

APPLYING EVIDENCE TO PRACTICE

Skin Care

- Keep skin free of excess moisture (e.g., urine or fecal incontinence, wound drainage, excessive perspiration).
- Cleanse skin with mild nonalkaline soap or soap-free cleaning agents for routine bathing.
- Provide daily cleansing of eyes, oral and diaper or perineal areas, and any areas of skin breakdown.
- Apply non–alcohol-based moisturizing agents after cleansing to retain moisture and rehydrate skin.
- Use minimum amount of tape and adhesives. On very sensitive skin, use a protective, pectin-based or hydrocolloid skin barrier between skin and tape or adhesives.
- Place pectin-based or hydrocolloid skin barriers directly over excoriated skin. Leave barrier undisturbed until it begins to peel off or for 5 to 7 days. With wet, oozing excoriations, place a small amount of stoma powder on site, remove excess powder, and apply skin barrier. Hold barrier in place for several minutes to allow barrier to soften and mold to skin surface.
- Alternate electrode and probe placement sites and thoroughly assess underlying skin typically every 8 to 24 hours.
- Eliminate pressure secondary to medical devices such as tracheostomy tubes, wheelchairs, braces, and gastrostomy tubes.
- Be certain fingers or toes are visible whenever extremity is used for intravenous (IV) or arterial line.
- Use a draw sheet to move child in bed or onto a stretcher; do not drag child from under the arms.
- Position in neutral alignment; pillows, cushions, or wedges may be needed to prevent hip abduction and pressure to bony prominences, such as heels, elbows, and sacral and occipital areas. When child is positioned laterally, pillows or cushions between the knees, under the head, and under the upper arm will help promote neutral body alignment. Avoid donut cushions because they can cause tissue ischemia. Elevate the head of bed 30 degrees or less to reduce pressure unless contraindicated.
- Do not massage reddened bony prominences because this can cause deep tissue damage; provide pressure relief to bony prominences.
- Routinely assess the child's nutritional status. A child who is NPO (nothing by mouth) for several days and is receiving only IV fluid is nutritionally at risk, which can also affect the skin's ability to maintain its integrity. Consider parenteral nutrition.

Assessment of the skin is easiest to accomplish during the bath. Examine for early signs of injury. Risk factors include impaired mobility, protein malnutrition, edema, incontinence, sensory loss, anemia, infection, failure to turn the patient, and intubation. Identification of risk factors helps determine children who need a more thorough skin assessment. Several risk assessment scales are available for use in pediatrics, such as the Braden Q Scale, the Neonatal Skin Risk Assessment Scale, the Waterlow Scale, and the Glamorgan Scale (Razmus & Bergquist-Beringer, 2017). Initial assessment should occur on admission to identify pressure ulcers and wounds that occurred before admission.

Pressure ulcers, a form of pressure injuries, are localized damage to the skin and/or underlying soft tissue due to decreased perfusion as a result of increased pressure. Pressure ulcers most often occur over bony prominences or related to medical or other devices. Pressure injuries are staged to classify the amount of tissue damage that has occurred.* Necrotic tissue must be removed so the tissue depth can accurately be assessed. Accurate documentation of redness or obvious skin breakdown is essential. Color, size (diameter and depth), location, presence of sinus tracts, odor, exudate, and response to treatment are observed and recorded at least daily.

Pressure ulcers in children typically occur on the occiput, ear lobes, sacrum, heels, and scapula (Schober-Flores, 2012); the heels and sacrum are common sites in adults. Critically ill children, children with sensory deficits, mobility deficits, cardiopulmonary abnormalities, and bariatric patients are at a higher risk of pressure ulcers and skin breakdown because they often have several risk factors combined. Although pressure ulcers in hospitalized children are generally uncommon, the incidence in critically ill children can be significantly higher. In a multisite study, risk factors associated with pressure ulcers in pediatric intensive care unit patients included age 2 years or less, length of stay 4 or more days, and ventilatory support (Schindler, Mikhailov, Kuhn, et al., 2011). Interventions found to prevent pressure ulcers in critically ill children include the following:

- Assessing the patient's skin from head to toe on admission and each shift
- Turning children every 2 hours
- Using pillows, blanket rolls, and positioning devices
- Using draw sheets to minimize shear
- Using pressure reduction surfaces (e.g., foam overlays, gel pads, specialty beds)
- Allowing moisture reduction through the use of dry-weave diapers and disposable underpads
- Using skin moisturizers
- Conducting nutrition consults

Medical devices such as pulse oximeter probes, bilevel and continuous positive airway pressure masks, oxygen cannulas, orthotics, and casts can also cause pressure ulcers. Additionally, both medical devices and special garments such as shoes, slippers, jewelry, hair ties, and restraints should be removed and to inspect skin at least every shift.

Friction and shear contribute to pressure ulcers. **Friction** occurs when the surface of the skin rubs against another surface, such as bed sheets. The skin may have the appearance of an abrasion. The skin damage is usually limited to the epidermal and upper layers. It most often occurs over the elbows, heels, or occiput. Prevention of friction injury includes the use of customized splinting or foam-padded boots over the heels; gel pillows under the heads of infants and toddlers; moisturizing agents; protective, transparent barrier dressings over susceptible areas; and soft, smooth bed linens and clothing (Schober-Flores, 2012). By

*Staging of pressure ulcers and guidelines for prevention and management of pressure ulcers are available online from the National Pressure Ulcer Advisory Panel.

itself, friction does not cause tissue necrosis, but when it acts with gravity, it results in shear injury.

Shear is the result of the force of gravity pushing down on the body and friction of the body against a surface, such as the bed or chair. For example, when a patient is in the semi-Fowler position and begins to slide to the foot of the bed, the skin over the sacral area remains in the same place because of the resistance of the bed surface. The blood vessels, bone, and muscle in the area are stretched and slide parallel to the stationary skin, which may cause small-vessel thrombosis and tissue death (Schober-Flores, 2012). Prevention of shear injury includes using lift sheets when repositioning a patient, elevating the bed no more than 30 degrees for short periods, and elevating the knees to interrupt the pull of gravity on the body toward the foot of the bed.

Epidermal stripping results when the epidermis is unintentionally removed when tape is pulled off the skin. These lesions are usually shallow and irregularly shaped. Babies are at increased risk for epidermal injury. Prevention includes using no tape when possible or securing dressings with laced binders (Montgomery straps) or stretchy netting (Spandage or stockinette). Using porous or low-tack tapes (e.g., Medipore, paper, hydrogel), using alcohol-free skin sealants (No Sting Barrier Film), or picture framing wounds with hydrocolloid or wafer barriers (e.g., DuoDERM, Coloplast, Stomahesive) and then taping on top of the barrier also will reduce epidermal stripping.

Tape should be placed so there is no tension, traction, or wrinkles on the skin. To remove tape, slowly peel the tape away, while stabilizing the underlying skin. Adhesive remover may be used to break the adhesive bond but may be drying to the skin. Avoid adhesive removers in preterm neonates because absorption rates vary and toxicity may occur. Remove the adhesive with water to prevent absorption and irritation. Wetting the tape with water or alcohol-based foam hand cleansers may facilitate removal.

Chemical factors can also lead to skin damage. Fecal incontinence, especially when mixed with urine; wound drainage; or gastric drainage around gastrostomy tubes can erode the epidermis. The skin can quickly progress from redness to denudement if exposure continues. Moisture barriers, gentle cleansing with alcohol-free cleansers or wipes as soon after exposure as possible, and skin barriers can be used to prevent damage caused by chemical factors. For nonintact skin, a barrier cream with zinc oxide should be applied (Schober-Flores, 2012). It is important to only cleanse the stool and urine during diaper changes, not the paste. In addition, foam dressings that wick moisture away from the skin are helpful around gastrostomy tubes and tracheostomy sites.

BATHING

Most infants and children can be bathed at the bedside or in a standard bathtub or shower. Assess the child and family's preferences for bath time frequency and family involvement. For infants and young children confined to bed, use commercially available bath cloths or the towel method. Immerse two towels in a dilute soap solution and wring them damp. With the child lying supine on a dry towel, place one damp towel on top of the child and use it to gently clean the body. Discard the towel and dry the child and turn him or her prone. Repeat the procedure using the second damp towel. If bar soap is used, discard the basin and bar soap after a single bath (Marchaim, Taylor, Hayakawa, et al., 2012) because they can serve as a reservoir for pathogens in the hospital setting. Chlorhexidine is much less likely to harbor microbes (Powers, Peed, Burns, et al., 2012; Rupp, Huerta, Yu, et al., 2013), but it is generally not approved for use in infants less than 2 months of corrected gestational age. Daily chlorhexidine gluconate bathing in the pediatric population can reduce bacteremia and prevent hospital-acquired infections (Karcz, Kelley, Conrad, et al., 2015; Milstone, Elward, Song, et al., 2013).

Infants and small children are never left unattended in a bathtub, and infants who are unable to sit alone are securely held with one hand during the bath. The nurse securely supports the infant's head with one hand or grasps the infant's farther arm while the head rests comfortably on the nurse's arm. Children who are able to sit without assistance need only close supervision and a pad placed in the bottom of the tub to prevent slipping and loss of balance.

School-age children and adolescents may shower or bathe. Nurses need to use judgment regarding the amount of supervision the child requires. Some can assume this responsibility unaided, but others need someone in constant attendance. Children with cognitive impairments, physical limitations such as severe anemia or leg deformities, or suicidal or psychotic problems (who may commit bodily harm) require close supervision.

Areas that require special attention are the ears, between skinfolds, the neck, the back, and the genital area. The genital area should be carefully cleansed and dried, with particular care given to skinfolds. In uncircumcised boys under 3 years of age the foreskin is not fully retractile. For older males, the foreskin should be gently retracted, the exposed surfaces cleansed, and the foreskin then replaced. If the condition of the glans indicates inadequate cleaning, such as accumulated smegma, inflammation, phimosis (condition in which the foreskin cannot be retracted), or foreskin adhesions, teaching proper hygiene is indicated. Do not forcibly retract the foreskin to avoid trauma and further complications (Hunter, 2012). Notify the provider of abnormal clinical findings during genitourinary assessment. In the Vietnamese and Cambodian cultures, the foreskin is traditionally not retracted until adulthood. Older children have a tendency to avoid cleaning the genitalia; therefore they may need a gentle reminder.

ORAL HYGIENE

Mouth care is an integral part of daily hygiene and should be continued in the hospital. Oral hygiene can prevent infection and promote comfort, adequate nutrition, and verbal communication. For some young children, this is their first introduction to the use of a toothbrush. Infants and debilitated children require the nurse or a family member to perform mouth care. For infants who do not yet have teeth, a soft moistened cloth or swab can be used to gently clean the gums. Children should begin brushing their teeth after the first teeth emerge around 6 months of age. For children less than 3 years of age, a grain-sized amount of fluoride toothpaste should be used. For children 3 to 6 years of age, a pea-sized amount of fluoride toothpaste should be used (American Dental Association, 2017). Although young children can manage a toothbrush and are encouraged to use it, most need assistance to perform satisfactorily. Older children, although capable of brushing and flossing without assistance, sometimes need to be reminded.

HAIR CARE

Children should have their hair brushed and combed at least once daily. The hair is styled for comfort and in a manner pleasing to the child and parents. The hair should not be cut without parental permission, although clipping hair to provide access to a scalp vein for IV insertion may be necessary.

If children are hospitalized for more than a few days, the hair may need shampooing. With infants, the hair may be washed during the daily bath or less frequently. For most children, washing the hair and scalp once or twice weekly is sufficient unless there is an indication for more frequent washing, such as after a high fever and profuse sweating. Adolescents normally have increased oily sebaceous secretions that require frequent hair care and more frequent shampoos.

Almost any child can be transported to an accessible sink for shampooing. Inspect the hair and scalp before shampooing using a fine toothcomb to assess for the presence of lice or other scalp abnormalities. Nits will be a gray-white color, the size of a knot of thread, and difficult to remove from the scalp in comparison to dandruff. Adult lice are a red-black color and the size of a sesame seed (Eisenhower & Farrington, 2012). If lice is suspected, an order for a pediculicide treatment and nit combing must be obtained. It is important for the nurse to don personal protective equipment including a gown and cap during the lice removal process. Additionally, other members of the household should be evaluated for the presence of lice and the family educated on the importance of individual hair care products.

Patients who are unable to be transported can receive a shampoo in their beds with adequate protection, specially adapted equipment or positioning, or dry shampoo caps. Comb or brush the hair before washing. When necessary, a shampoo basin may be used or the child may be positioned near the edge of the bed, towels placed under the shoulders and neck, a large plastic garbage bag draped at the edge of the bed with one open end under the shoulders, and the hair placed inside the opening. The other end is opened and placed in a collection container. Water can be transported in a basin.

For African American children with curly hair, most standard combs are inadequate and may cause hair breakage and discomfort. Use a special comb with widely spaced teeth. It is also much easier to comb the hair after shampooing when it is wet. Use a special hair dressing or pomade, which usually has a coconut oil base. Rub the preparation on the hands and then transfer it to the hair to make it more pliable and manageable. Consult the child's parents regarding the preparation to use on the child's hair and ask if they can provide some for use during the child's hospitalization. Petroleum jelly should not be used. If braiding or plaiting the hair, weave it loosely while the hair is damp. The hair tightens as it dries, which could result in tension folliculitis. Tight braids should be avoided as braiding can increase pressure on the scalp or hide pressure injuries.

FEEDING THE SICK CHILD

Loss of appetite is a symptom common to most childhood illnesses. Decreased appetite can be a result of pain or discomfort, nausea and vomiting, emotional concerns, or loss of control. Because an acute illness is usually short, the nutritional state is seldom compromised. Urging food on the sick child may precipitate nausea and vomiting. In most cases, children can usually determine their own need for food.

Refusing to eat may also be one way children can exert power and control in an otherwise helpless situation. For young children, loss of appetite may be related to depression caused by separation from their parents. Parents' concern with eating can intensify the problem. Forcing a child to eat meets with rebellion and reinforces the behavior as a control mechanism. Encourage parents to relax any pressure during an acute illness. Although it is best to provide high-quality, nutritious foods, the child may desire foods and liquids that contain mostly empty or nonnutritional calories. Some well-tolerated foods include gelatin, diluted clear soups, carbonated drinks, flavored ice pops, dry toast, and crackers. Even though these substances are not nutritious, they can provide necessary fluid and calories.

Dehydration is always a hazard when children have a fever or anorexia, especially when accompanied by vomiting or diarrhea. Fluids should not be forced, and the child should not be awakened to take fluids. Forcing fluids may create the same difficulties as urging the child to eat unwanted food. Gentle persuasion with preferred beverages will usually meet with success. Using play techniques can also be effective (see Applying Evidence to Practice box).

APPLYING EVIDENCE TO PRACTICE

Feeding a Sick Child

Take a dietary history (see Chapter 4) and use information to make eating time as similar to eating at home as possible.

Encourage parents or other family members to feed child or to be present at mealtimes.

Make mealtimes pleasant; avoid any procedures immediately before or after eating; make certain child is rested and pain free.

Serve small, frequent meals rather than three large meals or serve three meals and nutritious between-meal snacks.

Provide finger foods for young children.

Involve children in food selection and preparation whenever possible.

Serve small portions and serve each course separately, such as soup first, followed by meat, potatoes, and vegetables and ending with dessert. With young children, camouflage size of food by cutting meat thicker so less appears on plate or by folding a cheese slice in half. Offer second helpings.

Ensure a variety of foods, textures, and colors.

Provide food selections that are favorites of most children, such as peanut butter and jelly sandwiches, hot dogs, hamburgers, macaroni and cheese, pizza, spaghetti, tacos, fried chicken, corn, and fruit yogurt.

Avoid foods that are highly seasoned, have strong odors, or are all mixed together unless typical of cultural practices.

Provide fluid selections that are favorites of most children, such as fruit punch, cola, ginger ale, sweetened tea, flavored ice pops, sherbet, ice cream, milk, milkshakes, pudding, gelatin, clear broth, or creamed soups.

Offer nutritious snacks, such as frozen yogurt or pudding, ice cream, oatmeal or peanut butter cookies, hot cocoa, cheese slices, pieces of raw vegetable or fruit, and dried fruit or cereal.

Make food attractive and different—for example:

- Serve a "picnic lunch" in a paper bag.
- Pack food in a Chinese takeout container; decorate container.
- Put a "face" or a "flower" on a hamburger or sandwich with pieces of vegetable.
- Use a cookie cutter to shape a sandwich.
- Serve pudding, yogurt, or juice frozen as an ice pop.
- Make Slurpies or snow cones by pouring flavored syrup on crushed ice.
- Serve fluids through brightly colored or unusually shaped straws.
- Make "bowtie" sandwiches by cutting them in triangles and placing two points together.
- Slice sandwiches into "fingers."
- Grate mounds of cheese.
- Cut apples horizontally to make circles.
- Put a banana on a hot dog bun and spread with peanut butter.
- Break uncooked spaghetti into toothpick lengths and skewer cheese, cold meat, vegetables, or fruit chunks.

Praise children for what they do eat.

Do not punish children for not eating by removing their dessert or putting them to bed.

An understanding of children's feeding habits can also increase food consumption. For example, if children are given all their food at one time, they generally eat the dessert first. Likewise, if they are presented with large portions, they often push the food away because the amount overwhelms them. If young children are not supervised during mealtime, they tend to play with the food rather than eat it. Therefore nurses should present food in the usual order, such as soup first followed by small portions of meat, potatoes, and vegetables, and ending with dessert.

When the child is feeling better, appetite usually begins to improve. It is best to take advantage of any hungry period by serving high-quality foods and snacks. If the child still refuses to eat, offer nutritious fluids, such as prepared breakfast drinks. Parents can help by bringing in food items from home, especially if the family's cultural eating habits differ from the hospital food. A clinical dietitian may be consulted for alternative food choices.

When children are placed on special diets, such as clear liquids after surgery or during episodes of diarrhea, assessment of their intake and readiness to advance to more complex foods is essential.

Regardless of the type of diet, charting the amount consumed is an important nursing responsibility. Descriptions need to be detailed and accurate, such as "4 ounces of orange juice, one pancake, and 8 ounces of milk." Comments such as "ate well" or "ate poorly" are inadequate. Charting the percentage of the meal eaten is also inadequate unless food is measured before serving. For infants, assess the duration, amount, and frequency of breastfeeding or bottle-feeding and the possible addition of solid foods to determine whether nutrition is adequate.

If the parents are involved in the child's care, encourage them to keep a list of everything the child eats. Using a premeasured cup for fluids ensures a more accurate estimate of intake. A comparison of the intake at each meal can isolate food deficiencies, such as insufficient intake of meat or vegetables. Behaviors associated with mealtime also identify possible factors influencing appetite. For example, the observation "Child eats well when with other children but plays with food if left alone in room" helps the nurse plan mealtime activities that stimulate the child's appetite.

Although sick children's appetites may be poor and not characteristic of their home eating habits, the hospital stay provides numerous opportunities for nurses to assess the family's knowledge of good nutrition and to implement teaching as needed to improve nutritional intake.

CONTROLLING ELEVATED TEMPERATURES

An elevated temperature, most frequently from fever but occasionally caused by hyperthermia, is one of the most common symptoms of illness in children. This manifestation is a great concern to parents. To facilitate an understanding of fever versus hyperthermia, the following terms are defined:

Set point—The temperature around which body temperature is regulated by a thermostat-like mechanism in the hypothalamus

Fever (hyperpyrexia)—An elevation in set point such that body temperature is regulated at a higher level; may be arbitrarily defined as rectal temperature above 38°C (100.4°F)

Hyperthermia—Body temperature exceeding the set point, which usually results from the body or external conditions creating more heat than the body can eliminate, such as in heat exhaustion, heatstroke, aspirin toxicity, seizures, or hyperthyroidism

Body temperature is regulated by a thermostat-like mechanism in the hypothalamus. This mechanism receives input from centrally and peripherally located receptors. When temperature changes occur, these receptors relay the information to the thermostat, which either increases or decreases heat production to maintain a constant set point temperature. However, during an infection, pyrogenic substances cause an increase in the body's normal set point, a process that is mediated by prostaglandins. Consequently, the hypothalamus increases heat production until the core temperature reaches the new set point.

During the fever (febrile) state, shivering and vasoconstriction generate and conserve heat during the chill phase of fever, raising central temperatures to the level of the new set point. The temperature reaches a plateau when it stabilizes in the higher range. When the temperature is greater than the set point or when the pyrogen is no longer present, a crisis, or defervescence, of the temperature occurs.

Most fevers in children are of brief duration with limited consequences and are viral in origin. Children may experience warm, flushed skin, chills, aches, malaise, or irritability during a fever. However, children who appear very ill, immunocompromised children, and neonates are at high risk for serious bacterial illness, such as urinary tract infections or bacteremia, and will likely receive a sepsis workup, antibiotics, and hospitalization (Sahib El-Radhi, Carroll, & Klein, 2009).

Fever has physiologic benefits, including increased white blood cell activity, interferon production and effectiveness, and antibody production and enhancement of some antibiotic effects such as penicillin (Patricia, 2014). Contrary to popular belief, neither the rise in temperature nor its response to antipyretics indicates the severity or etiology of the infection, which casts doubt on the value of using fever as a diagnostic or prognostic indicator.

Therapeutic Management

Treatment of elevated temperature depends on whether it is attributable to a fever or hyperthermia. Because the set point is normal in hyperthermia but increased in fever, different approaches must be used to lower body temperature successfully.

Fever

The principal reason for treating fever is the relief of discomfort. However, children with cardiopulmonary disease or immunocompromised children may not tolerate the increase in metabolic demand from a fever and should receive antipyretic therapy. Relief measures include pharmacologic and environmental intervention. The most effective intervention is the use of antipyretics to lower the set point.

Antipyretics include acetaminophen, aspirin, and nonsteroidal antiinflammatory drugs (NSAIDs). Acetaminophen is the preferred drug. Aspirin should not be given to children because of its association in children with influenza virus or chickenpox and Reye syndrome. One nonprescription NSAID, ibuprofen, is approved for fever reduction in children as young as 6 months of age.

Another antipyretic, acetaminophen can be given every 4 hours but no more than five times in 24 hours due to the risk of hepatotoxicity. Because body temperature normally decreases at night, three or four doses in 24 hours will control most fevers. The temperature is usually retaken 30 to 60 minutes after the antipyretic is given to assess its effect but should not be repeatedly measured. The child's level of discomfort is the best indication for continued treatment.

The nurse can use environmental measures to reduce fever if they are tolerated by the child and if they do not induce shivering. Shivering is the body's way of maintaining the elevated set point by producing heat. Compensatory shivering greatly increases metabolic requirements above those already caused by the fever.

Traditional cooling measures, such as wearing minimum clothing; exposing the skin to air; reducing room temperature; increasing air circulation; and applying cool, moist compresses to the skin (e.g., the forehead), are effective if used approximately 1 hour after an antipyretic is given so the set point is lowered. Cooling procedures such as sponging or tepid baths are ineffective in treating febrile children (these measures are effective for hyperthermia) either when used alone or in combination with antipyretics, and they cause considerable discomfort (Monsma, Richerson, & Sloand, 2015).

Seizures associated with a fever occur in 2% to 5% of all children, usually in those between 6 months and 5 years of age. About 30% to 50% of children have subsequent febrile seizures; a younger age at onset and a family history of febrile seizures are associated with increased incidence of recurring episodes. Evidence does not support the use of antipyretic drugs or anticonvulsants to prevent a second febrile seizure. Nursing interventions should focus on ways to provide care and comfort during a febrile illness (Rosenbloom, Finkelstein, Adams-Webber, et al., 2013). Simple febrile seizures lasting less than 10 minutes do not cause brain damage or other debilitating effects (Patricia, 2014). (See Febrile Seizures, Chapter 30.)

Hyperthermia

Unlike in fever, antipyretics are of no value in hyperthermia because the set point is already normal. Consequently, cooling measures are used. If a child is severely hyperthermic with a core temperature above 40°C, it may be necessary to perform continuous monitoring of vital signs including core temperature and urinary output and administer intravenous fluids in a critical care environment (Chan & Mamat, 2015). Cool applications to the skin help reduce the core temperature. Cooled blood from the skin surface is conducted to inner organs and tissues, and warm blood is circulated to the surface, where it is cooled and recirculated. The surface blood vessels dilate as the body attempts to dissipate heat to the environment and facilitate this cooling process.

Commercial cooling devices, such as cooling blankets or mattresses, are available to reduce body temperature. Place the patient on the bed and cover with a sheet or lightweight blanket. Frequent temperature monitoring is essential to prevent excessive cooling of the body.

Traditionally, cool compresses decrease high temperature. For tepid tub baths, it is usually best to start with warm water and gradually add cool water until the desired water temperature of 37°C (98.6°F) is reached to acclimate the child to the lower water temperature. Generally, the temperature of the water only has to be 1°C (or 2°F) less than the child's temperature to be effective. The child is placed directly in the tub of tepid water for 15 to 20 minutes, while water is gently squeezed from a washcloth over the back and chest or gently sprayed over the body from a sprayer. In the bed or crib, cool washcloths or towels are used, exposing only one area of the body at a time. Continue sponging for approximately 20 minutes.

After the tub or sponge bath, the child is dried and dressed in lightweight pajamas, a nightgown, or a diaper and placed in a dry bed. The child is dried by gently rubbing the skin surface with a towel to stimulate circulation. The temperature is retaken 30 minutes after the tub or sponge bath. The tub or sponge bath should not be continued or restarted until the skin surface is warm or if the child feels chilled. Chilling causes vasoconstriction, which defeats the purpose of the cool applications. In this condition, little blood is carried to the skin surface; the blood remains primarily in the viscera to become heated.

Whether a temperature elevation in the critically ill child is caused by fever or hyperthermia, it should be treated aggressively. The metabolic rate increases 10% for every 1°C increase in temperature and three to five times during shivering, thus increasing oxygen, fluid, and caloric requirements. If the child's cardiovascular or neurologic system is already compromised, these increased needs are especially hazardous. In all children with an elevated temperature, attention to adequate hydration is essential. Most children's needs can be met through additional oral fluids.

FAMILY TEACHING AND HOME CARE

Fever is one of the most common problems for which parents seek health care. High levels of parental anxiety (fever phobia) surrounding potential complications of fever such as seizures and dehydration are prevalent and can result in overusing antipyretics. Parents need to know that sponging is indicated for elevated temperatures from hyperthermia rather than fever and that ice water and alcohol are inappropriate, potentially dangerous solutions (Monsma, Richerson, & Sloand, 2015). Parents should know how to take the child's temperature, how to read the thermometer accurately, and when to seek professional care (see Family-Centered Care box). A dedicated thermometer should be used for rectal route. Oral temperatures should not be taken within 15 minutes of the child eating or drinking hot or cold food. Some of the newer temperature-measuring devices, such as plastic strip or digital thermometers, may be better suited for home use. (See Temperature, Chapter 4.) If the use of acetaminophen or ibuprofen is indicated, the parents need instructions in administering the drug. Emphasize accuracy in both the amount of drug given and the time intervals at which the drug is administered. Along with reduced activity, encourage small, frequent sips of clear liquids. Dress the child in light clothing; use a light blanket for children who are cold or shivering (Monsma, Richerson, & Sloand, 2015).

FAMILY-CENTERED CARE

The Child With Fever

Call the Doctor Immediately If

Your child is younger than 3 months old and has a temperature of 100.4°F or higher.

The fever is over 40°C (104°F).

Your child looks or acts very sick or sleepy, or has a stiff neck, severe headache, severe ear pain, severe sore throat, repeated vomiting or diarrhea, unexplained rash on the skin, confusion, trouble breathing, or inability to be comforted.

Your child has had a recent seizure.

Your child has a history of immune system problems such as cancer or sickle cell disease.

Your child has been in a very hot place such as a car.

Your child has taken steroid medication

The fever continues for more than 24 hours in a child younger than 2 years or more than 3 days in a child older than 2 years.

Modified from American Academy of Pediatrics. (2015). When to call the pediatrician: Fever. Retrieved from https://www.healthychildren.org/English/health-issues/conditions/fever/Pages/When-to-Call-the-Pediatrician.aspx.

SAFETY

Safety is an essential component of any patient's care, but children have special characteristics that require an even greater concern for safety. Because small children in the hospital are separated from their usual environment and do not possess the capacity for abstract thinking and reasoning, it is the responsibility of everyone who comes in contact with them to maintain protective measures throughout their hospital stay. Nurses need to understand the age level at which each child is operating and plan for safety accordingly.

Identification bands and the use of two patient identifiers are particularly important for children. Infants and unconscious patients are unable to tell or respond to their names. Toddlers may answer to any name or to a nickname only. Older children may exchange places, give an erroneous name, or choose not to respond to their own names as a joke, unaware of the hazards of such practices. Additionally, allergy bands for medications and food should be worn by all patients.

ENVIRONMENTAL FACTORS

All of the environmental safety measures for the protection of adults apply to children, including good illumination, floors that are clear of fluid and objects that might contribute to falls, and nonskid surfaces in showers and tubs. All staff members should be familiar with the area-specific fire plan. Elevators and stairways should be made safe.

All windows should be secured. Window blind and curtain cords should be out of reach, with split cords to prevent strangulation. Pacifiers should not be tied around the neck or attached to an infant by a string.

Electrical equipment should be in good working order and used only by personnel familiar with its use. It should not be in contact with moisture or situated near tubs. Electrical outlets should have covers to prevent burns in small children, whose exploratory activities may extend to inserting objects into the small openings.

Staff members should practice proper care and disposal of small objects such as syringe caps, needle covers, and temperature probes. Staff also must carefully check bathwater before placing the child in it and never leave children alone in a bathtub. Infants are helpless in water, and small children (and some older ones) may turn on the hot water faucet and be severely burned.

Furniture is safest when it is scaled to the child's proportions, is sturdy, and is well balanced to prevent its being easily tipped over. A special hazard for children is the danger of entrapment under an electronically controlled bed when it is activated to descend. Infants and small children must be securely strapped into infant seats, feeding chairs, and strollers. Baby walkers should not be used because they provide access to hazards, resulting in burns, falls, and poisonings. Infants; young children; and children who are weak, paralyzed, agitated, confused, sedated, or cognitively impaired should never be left unattended on treatment tables, on scales, or in treatment areas. Even premature infants are capable of surprising mobility; therefore portholes in incubators must be securely fastened when not in use.

Crib sides up should always be raised and fastened securely. Use cribs that meet federal safety standards (https://www.cpsc.gov/safety-education/safety-education-centers/cribs). Anyone attending an infant or small child on a stretcher or table should never turn away without maintaining hand contact with the child—that is, keeping one hand on the child's back or abdomen to prevent rolling, crawling, or jumping from the open crib (Fig. 22.2). A child who is likely to climb over the sides of the crib is safest when placed in a specially constructed crib with a cover over the top. Never tie nets to the movable crib sides or use knots that do not permit quick release.

The safest sleeping position to prevent sudden infant death syndrome is wholly supine until at least 1 year of age (American Academy of Pediatrics, Task Force on Sudden Infant Death Syndrome, 2016). No pillows should be placed in a young infant's crib while the infant is sleeping. A firm sleep surface with no other bedding or any soft items in the crib in a shared room (not a shared bed) and the avoidance of overheating, exposure to tobacco smoke, alcohol, and illicit drugs further increase the safety of an infant's sleeping environment. The use of car seats, strollers, swings, or other sitting devices should not be used for routine sleep. Additionally, swaddling is not recommended for infants over 2 months of age due to the risk of death if the infant rolls into the prone position. In accordance with the American Academy of Pediatric guidelines to avoid extra bedding in the crib, many institutions recommend an infant sleep sack for adequate warmth and safety.

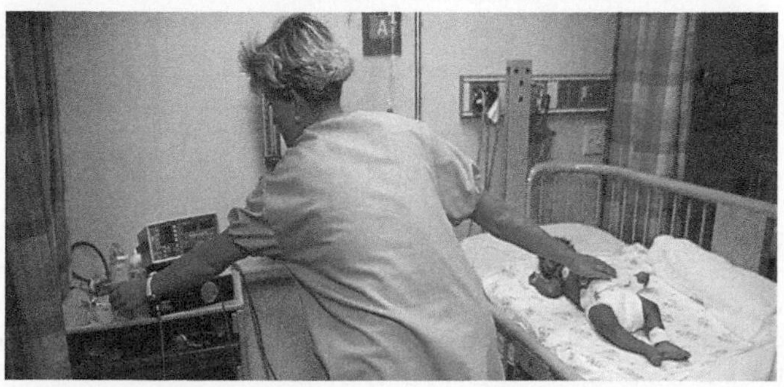

FIG. 22.2 The nurse maintains hand contact when her back is turned.

Toys

Toys play a vital role in the everyday lives of children, and they are no less important in the hospital setting. Nurses are responsible for assessing the safety of toys brought to the hospital by well-meaning parents and friends. Toys should be appropriate to the child's age, condition, and treatment. For example, if the child is receiving oxygen, electrical or friction toys or equipment are not safe because sparks can cause oxygen to ignite. Inspect toys to ensure they are nonallergenic, washable, and unbreakable and that they have no small, removable parts that can be aspirated or swallowed or can otherwise inflict injury on a child. All objects within reach of children younger than 3 years of age should pass the choke tube test. A toilet paper roll is a handy guide. If a toy or object fits into the cylinder (items less than $1\frac{1}{4}$ inches across or balls less than $1\frac{3}{4}$ inches in diameter), it is a potential choking danger to the child. Latex balloons pose a serious threat to children of all ages. If the balloon breaks, a child may put a piece of the latex in his or her mouth. If it is aspirated or swallowed, the latex piece is difficult to remove, resulting in choking. Latex balloons should never be permitted in the hospital setting.

Preventing Falls

Although children have a known predisposition to falls based on normal growth and development, falls risk identification and prevention for children with medical conditions is especially important due to greater risk for injury from a fall (Murray, Edlund, & Vess, 2016). Falls prevention begins with identification of children most at risk for falls. Pediatric hospitals use various methods to identify a child's risk of falls. After a risk assessment is performed, multiple interventions are needed to minimize pediatric patients' risk of falling, including education of patient, family, and staff.

To identify children at risk of falling, perform a fall risk assessment on patients on admission and throughout hospitalization. Risk factors for hospitalized children include the following:

- **Medication effects**—Postanesthesia or sedation; analgesics or narcotics, especially in those who have never had narcotics in the past and in whom effects are unknown
- **Altered mental status**—Secondary to seizures, brain tumors, or medications
- **Altered or limited mobility**—Reduced skill at ambulation secondary to developmental age, disease process, tubes, drains, casts, splints, or other appliances; new to ambulation with assistive devices such as walkers or crutches
- **Postoperative children**—Risk of hypotension or syncope secondary to large blood loss, a heart condition, or extended bed rest
- History of falls
- Infants or toddlers in cribs with side rails down or on the daybed with family members
- Changes to the patient's environment

Once children at risk of falls have been identified, alert other staff members by posting signs on the door and at the bedside, applying a special-colored armband labeled "Fall Precautions," labeling the chart with a sticker, or documenting information on the chart.

Prevention of falls requires alterations in the environment, including the following:

- Keep the bed in the lowest position with the breaks locked and the side rails up.

- Place the call bell within reach and orient the patient and caregivers to the bed and room.
- Ensure that all necessary and desired items are within reach (e.g., water, glasses, tissues, snacks).
- Offer toileting on a regular basis, especially if the patient is taking diuretics or laxatives.
- Keep lights on at all times, including dim lights while sleeping.
- Lock wheelchairs before transferring patients.
- Ensure that the patient has an appropriate-size gown and nonskid footwear. Do not allow gowns or ties to drag on the floor during ambulation.
- Keep the floor clean and free of clutter. Post a "wet floor" sign if the floor is wet.
- Ensure that the patient has glasses on if he or she normally wears them.
- Use a gait belt during ambulation.
- Keep the patient's door open unless isolation status prohibits.

Preventing falls also relies on age-appropriate education of patients. Assist the child with ambulation even though he or she may have ambulated well before hospitalization. Patients who have been lying in bed need to get up slowly, sitting on the side of the bed before standing.

The nurse also needs to educate family members:

- Call the nursing staff for assistance, and do not allow patients to get up independently.
- Keep the side rails of the crib or bed up whenever patient is in the crib or bed.
- Do not leave infants on the daybed; put them in the crib with the side rails up.
- When all family members need to leave the bedside, notify the staff, and ensure that the patient is in the bed or crib with the side rails up and call bell within reach (if appropriate).

In the event of a fall, it is important to immediately respond to the needs of the patient; notify appropriate personnel, including caregivers; and document the event.

INFECTION CONTROL

According to the Centers for Disease Control and Prevention, nosocomial (health care–associated) infections pose a significant threat to patient safety. These infections occur when there is interaction among patients, health care personnel, equipment, and bacteria. Health care–associated infections include infections such as *Clostridium difficile* or hospital-onset methicillin-resistant *Staphylococcus aureus,* as well as central line–associated bloodstream infections (CLABSIs), catheter-associated urinary tract infections (CAUTIs), and some surgical site infections. Health care–associated infections can be preventable if caregivers practice meticulous cleaning and disposal techniques.

Standard Precautions synthesize the major features of Universal (blood and body fluid) Precautions (designed to reduce the risk of transmission of blood-borne pathogens) and body substance isolation (designed to reduce the risk of transmission of pathogens from moist body substances). Standard Precautions involve vigilant hand hygiene and the use of barrier protection, such as gloves, goggles, gown, or mask, to prevent contamination from (1) blood; (2) all body fluids, secretions, and excretions except sweat, regardless of whether they contain visible blood; (3) nonintact skin; and (4) mucous membranes. Standard Precautions are designed for the care of all patients to reduce the risk of transmission of microorganisms from both recognized and unrecognized sources of infection.

Transmission-Based Precautions are designed for patients with documented or suspected infection or colonization (i.e., presence of microorganisms in or on patient but without clinical signs and symptoms of infection) with highly transmissible or epidemiologically important pathogens for which additional precautions beyond Standard Precautions are needed to interrupt transmission in hospitals. There are three types of Transmission-Based Precautions: Airborne Precautions, Droplet Precautions, and Contact Precautions. They may be combined for diseases that have multiple routes of transmission (Box 22.2). They are to be used in addition to Standard Precautions.

Airborne Precautions reduce the risk of airborne transmission of infectious agents. Airborne transmission occurs by dissemination of either airborne droplet nuclei (small-particle residue [<5 mm] of evaporated droplets that may remain suspended in the air for long periods) or dust particles containing the infectious agent. Microorganisms carried in this manner can be dispersed widely by air currents and may become inhaled by or deposited on a susceptible host within the same room or over a longer distance from the source patient, depending on environmental factors. Individuals may become infected who have not had direct face-to-face contact with the source individual. Special air handling and ventilation are required to prevent airborne transmission. Airborne Precautions apply to patients with known or suspected infection with pathogens transmitted by the airborne route such as measles, varicella, and tuberculosis.

Droplet Precautions reduce the risk of droplet transmission of infectious agents. Droplet transmission involves contact of the conjunctivae or the mucous membranes of the nose or mouth of a susceptible person with large-particle droplets (>5 mm) containing microorganisms generated from a person who has a clinical disease or who is a carrier of the microorganism. Droplets are generated from the source person primarily during coughing, sneezing, or talking and during procedures such as suctioning and bronchoscopy. Transmission requires close contact between source and recipient persons because droplets do not remain suspended in the air and generally travel only short distances, usually 3 feet or less but up to 10 feet, through the air. Because droplets do not remain suspended in the air, special air handling and ventilation are not required to prevent droplet transmission. Droplet Precautions apply to any patient with known or suspected infection with pathogens that can be transmitted by infectious droplets (see Box 22.2).

Contact Precautions reduce the risk of transmission of microorganisms by direct or indirect contact. Direct-contact transmission involves skin-to-skin contact and physical transfer of microorganisms to a susceptible host from an infected or colonized person, such as occurs when turning or bathing patients. Direct-contact transmission also can occur between two patients (e.g., by hand contact). Indirect contact transmission involves contact of a susceptible host with a contaminated intermediate object, usually inanimate, in the patient's environment. Contact Precautions apply to specified patients known or suspected to be infected or colonized with microorganisms that can be transmitted by direct or indirect contact.

> **! NURSING ALERT**
>
> The most common piece of medical equipment, the stethoscope, can be a potent source of harmful microorganisms and nosocomial infections.

Nurses caring for young children are frequently in contact with body substances, especially urine, feces, and vomitus. Nurses need to exercise judgment concerning those situations when gloves, gowns, or masks are necessary. For example, wear gloves and possibly gowns for changing diapers when there are loose or explosive stools. Otherwise, the plastic lining of disposable diapers provides a sufficient barrier between the hands and body substances. During feedings or oral

BOX 22.2 Types of Precautions and Patients Requiring Them

Standard Precautions for Prevention of Transmission of Pathogens

Use Standard Precautions for the care of all patients.

Airborne Precautions

In addition to Standard Precautions, use Airborne Precautions for patients known or suspected to have serious illnesses transmitted by airborne droplet nuclei. Examples of such illnesses include measles, varicella (including disseminated zoster), and tuberculosis.

Droplet Precautions

In addition to Standard Precautions, use Droplet Precautions for patients known or suspected to have serious illnesses transmitted by large-particle droplets. Examples of such illnesses include the following:

- Invasive *Haemophilus influenzae* type b disease, including meningitis, pneumonia, epiglottitis, and sepsis
- Invasive *Neisseria meningitidis* disease, including meningitis, pneumonia, and sepsis
- Other serious bacterial respiratory tract infections spread by droplet transmission, including diphtheria (pharyngeal), mycoplasma pneumonia, pertussis, pneumonic plague, streptococcal pharyngitis, pneumonia, and scarlet fever in infants and young children
- Serious viral infections spread by droplet transmission, including adenovirus, influenza, mumps, parvovirus B19, and rubella

Contact Precautions

In addition to Standard Precautions, use Contact Precautions for patients known or suspected to have serious illnesses easily transmitted by direct patient contact or by contact with items in the patient's environment. Examples of such illnesses include the following:

- Gastrointestinal, respiratory, skin, or wound infections or colonization with multidrug-resistant bacteria judged by the infection control program, based on current state, regional, or national recommendations, to be of special clinical and epidemiologic significance
- Enteric infections with a low infectious dose or prolonged environmental survival, including *Clostridium difficile;* for diapered or incontinent patients: enterohemorrhagic *Escherichia coli* O157:H7, *Shigella* organisms, hepatitis A, or rotavirus
- Respiratory syncytial virus, parainfluenza virus, or enteroviral infections in infants and young children
- Skin infections that are highly contagious or that may occur on dry skin, including diphtheria (cutaneous), herpes simplex virus (neonatal or mucocutaneous), impetigo, major (noncontained) abscesses, cellulitis or decubitus, pediculosis, scabies, staphylococcal furunculosis in infants and young children, zoster (disseminated or in the immunocompromised host)
- Multidrug-resistant organisms, infection, or colonization (methicillin-resistant *Staphylococcus aureus,* vancomycin-resistant enterococci)
- Viral or hemorrhagic conjunctivitis
- Viral hemorrhagic infections (Ebola, Lassa, or Marburg)

A complete list of the guidelines for isolation precautions for the prevention of transmission of infections agents in health care can be found at https://www.cdc.gov/infectioncontrol/guidelines/isolation/index.html.

medication administration, wear gowns if the child is likely to vomit or spit up, which often occurs during burping. When wearing gloves, wash the hands thoroughly after removing the gloves because gloves fail to provide complete protection. The absence of visible leaks does not indicate that gloves are intact.

Another essential practice of infection control is that all needles (uncapped and unbroken) are disposed of in a rigid, puncture-resistant container located near the site of use. Consequently, these containers are installed in patients' rooms. Because children are naturally curious, extra attention is needed in selecting a suitable type of container and a location that prevents access to the discarded needles. The use of needleless systems allows secure syringe or IV tubing attachment to vascular access devices without the risk of needlestick injury to the child or nurse.

TRANSPORTING INFANTS AND CHILDREN

Infants and children need to be transported within the unit and to areas outside the pediatric unit. Infants and small children can be carried for short distances within the unit, but for more extended trips, the child should be securely transported in a suitable conveyance.

Small infants can be held or carried in the horizontal position with the back supported and the thigh grasped firmly by the carrying arm (Fig. 22.3, *A*). In the football hold, the infant is carried on the nurse's arm with the head supported by the hand and the body held securely between the nurse's body and elbow (Fig. 22.3, *B*). Both of these holds leave the nurse's other arm free for activity. The infant also can be held in the upright position with the buttocks on the nurse's forearm and the front of the body resting against the nurse's chest. The infant's head and shoulders are supported by the nurse's other arm in case the infant moves suddenly (Fig. 22.3, *C*). Older infants are able to hold their heads erect but are still subject to sudden movements. Medically stable infants can be carried in a variety of ways for transport as long as the infants head is supported at all times.

The method of transporting children depends on their age, condition, and destination. Older children are safe in wheelchairs or on stretchers. Younger children can be transported in a crib, on a stretcher, in a wagon with raised sides, or in a wheelchair with a safety belt. Stretchers should be equipped with high sides and a safety belt, both of which are secured during transport.

Special care is needed in transporting critically ill patients in the hospital. Critically ill children should always be transported on a stretcher or bed (rather than carried) by at least two appropriately trained staff members with monitoring continued during transport. A blood pressure monitor (or standard blood pressure cuff), pulse oximeter, and cardiac monitor/defibrillator should accompany every patient (Alamanou & Brokalaki, 2014). Airway equipment, oxygen, and emergency medications should accompany the patient. The monitoring and staff members required for transport will vary depending on the acuity and clinical status of the patient. Additionally, it is important for the nurse to be familiar with emergency transport of patients in the event of severe weather, fire, or security threats when power or elevators may be unavailable.

RESTRAINING METHODS

The Centers for Medicare and Medicaid Services (2015) has established regulations to minimize the use and ensure safety of patients in restraints. It defines *restraint* as "any manual method, physical or mechanical device, material, or equipment that immobilizes or reduces the ability of a patient to move his or her arms, legs, body, or head freely ... or a drug or medication when it is used as a restriction to manage the patient's

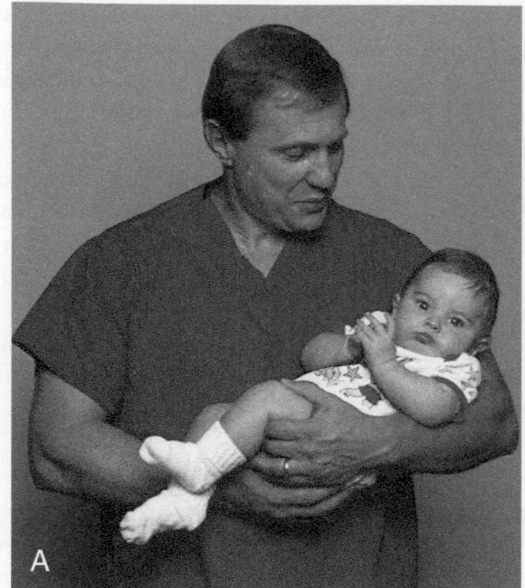

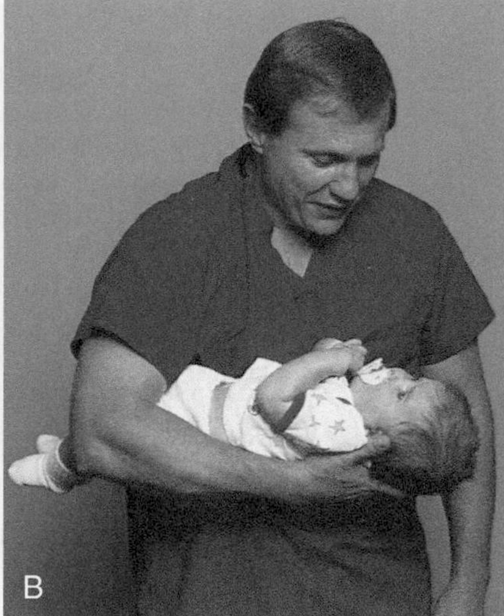

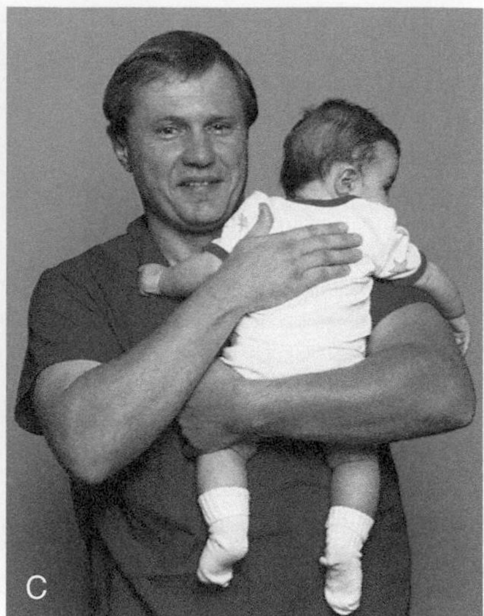

FIG. 22.3 Transporting infants. **A,** The infant's thigh firmly grasped in the nurse's hand. **B,** Football hold. **C,** Back supported.

behavior or restrict the patient's freedom of movement and is not a standard treatment or dosage for the patient's condition." A restraint should only be applied by a health care team member with demonstrated competency in restraint management. The physical force may be human, mechanical devices, or a combination of the two. Examples of restraints include limb restraints, elbow restraints, vest restraints, and tight tucking of sheets to prevent movement in bed.

Mechanical supports such as immobilizers for fractures, orthopedic devices to maintain proper body alignment, leg braces, protective helmets, and surgical dressings are not considered restraints. An armboard to secure a peripheral IV line is not considered a restraint unless it is tied down to the bed or immobilizes the entire limb such that the patient cannot access his or her body. Hand mitts are not considered a restraint unless tied down to the bed or used in conjunction with a wrist restraint. Developmentally age-appropriate safety interventions for infants, toddlers, and preschoolers, such as net enclosures on beds, crib domes, crib side rails, and high chair lap safety belts, are generally not considered restraints. Picking up, redirecting, or holding an infant, toddler, or preschooler is not considered restraint. Interventions that would typically be employed by a child care provider outside of a health care environment to ensure safety in young children are not considered restraints.

Before initiating restraints, the nurse completes a comprehensive assessment of the patient to determine whether the need for a restraint outweighs the risk of not using one. Restraints can result in loss of dignity, violation of patient rights, psychologic harm, physical harm, and even death. Consider alternative methods first and document them in the patient's record. Some examples of alternative measures include bringing a child to the nurses' station for continuous observation, providing diversional activities such as music, and encouraging the participation of the parents. The use of restraints can often be avoided with adequate preparation of the child; parental or staff supervision of the child; or adequate protection of a vulnerable site, such as an infusion device.

The nurse needs to assess the child's development, mental status, potential to hurt others or self, and safety. The nurse is responsible for selecting the least restrictive type of restraint. Using less restrictive restraints is often possible by gaining the cooperation of the child and parents. An order must be obtained as soon as possible (during application or within a few minutes) after the initiation of restraints and specify the timeframe they can be used, the reason they are being used, and reasons for discontinuation. Discontinuation of restraints should occur as soon as it is safe, even if the order timeframe has not expired.

Restraints for violent, self-destructive behavior are limited to situations with a significant risk of patients physically harming themselves or others because of behavioral reasons and when nonphysical interventions are not effective. Before initiating a behavioral restraint, the nurse should assess the patient's mental, behavioral, and physical status to determine the cause for the child's potentially harmful behavior. If behavioral restraints are indicated, a collaborative approach involving the patient (if appropriate), the family, and the health care team should be used. Behavioral restraints can include personal restraints, such as a physical hold, or mechanical restraints such as secured anklets and wristlets or bilateral arm immobilizers.

Unless state law is more restrictive, behavioral restraints for children must be reordered every 15 minutes for a personal restraint, every 1 hour for children under 9 years of age, and every 2 hours for children 9 to 17 years old; orders for adults 18 and older are required every 4 hours. A licensed independent practitioner or specially trained nurse must conduct an in-person evaluation within 1 hour and at least every 24 hours to continue restraints.

Children in behavioral restraints must be observed and assessed according to facility policy—typically continuously, every 15 minutes, or every 2 hours. Assessment components include signs of injury associated with applying restraint, nutrition and hydration, circulation and range-of-motion of extremities, vital signs, hygiene and elimination, physical and psychologic status and comfort, and readiness for discontinuation of restraint. The nurse must use clinical judgment in setting a schedule within the facility's policy for when each of these parameters needs to be evaluated.

Nonviolent/non–self-destructive patients may also require restraints to support medical healing. Examples of situations where a nonbehavioral restraint may be necessary for the patient's safety include removal of an artificial airway or airway adjunct for delivery of oxygen, indwelling catheters, tubes, drains, lines, pacemaker wires, or disruption of suture sites. The medical-surgical restraint is used to ensure that safe care is given to the patient. Patient confusion, agitation, unconsciousness, and developmental inability to understand direct requests or instructions may warrant the use of nonbehavioral restraints to maintain patient safety. The potential risks of the restraint are offset by the potential benefit of providing safer care.

Nonbehavioral restraints can be initiated by an individual order or by protocol; the use of the protocol must be authorized by an individual order. The order for continued use of restraints must be renewed each day. Patients are monitored per facility policy, typically at least every 2 hours.

Restraints with ties must be secured to the stationary bed or crib frame, not the side rails. Suggestions for increasing safety and comfort while the child is in a restraint include leaving one finger breadth between skin and the device and tying knots that allow for quick release. The nurse can also increase safety by ensuring the restraint does not tighten as the child moves and decreasing wrinkles or bulges in the restraint. Placing jacket restraints over an article of clothing; placing limb restraints below waist level, below knee level, or distal to the IV; and tucking in dangling straps also increase safety and comfort. Do not place objects over a patient's face to protect staff from being spit on or bitten. Masks and face shields should be readily available for staff to wear; some facilities also provide bite gloves and arm/hand wraps made of strong barrier materials such as Kevlar for staff to wear to prevent injury from bites and scratches.

Mummy Restraint or Swaddle

When an infant or small child requires short-term restraint for examination or treatment that involves the head and neck (e.g., venipuncture, throat examination, gavage feeding), a papoose board with straps or a mummy wrap effectively controls the child's movements. When used only for the duration of the test or procedure, this is not considered a restraint. The mummy restraint or swaddle should not be used for behavior or long-term restraint. A blanket or sheet is opened on the bed or crib with one corner folded to the center. The infant is placed on the blanket with the shoulders at the fold and feet toward the opposite corner. With the infant's right arm straight down against the body, the right side of the blanket is pulled firmly across the infant's right shoulder and chest and secured beneath the left side of the body. The left arm is placed straight against the infant's side, and the left side of the blanket is brought across the shoulder and chest and locked beneath the body on the right side. The lower corner is folded and brought over the body and tucked or fastened securely with safety pins. Safety pins can be used to fasten the blanket in place at any step in the process. To modify the mummy restraint for chest examination, bring the folded edge of the blanket over each arm and under the back and then fold the loose edge over and secure it at a point below the chest to allow visualization and access to the chest (Fig. 22.4, *A*).

Arm and Leg Restraints

Occasionally, the nurse needs to restrain one or more extremities or limit their motion. Several commercial restraining devices are available,

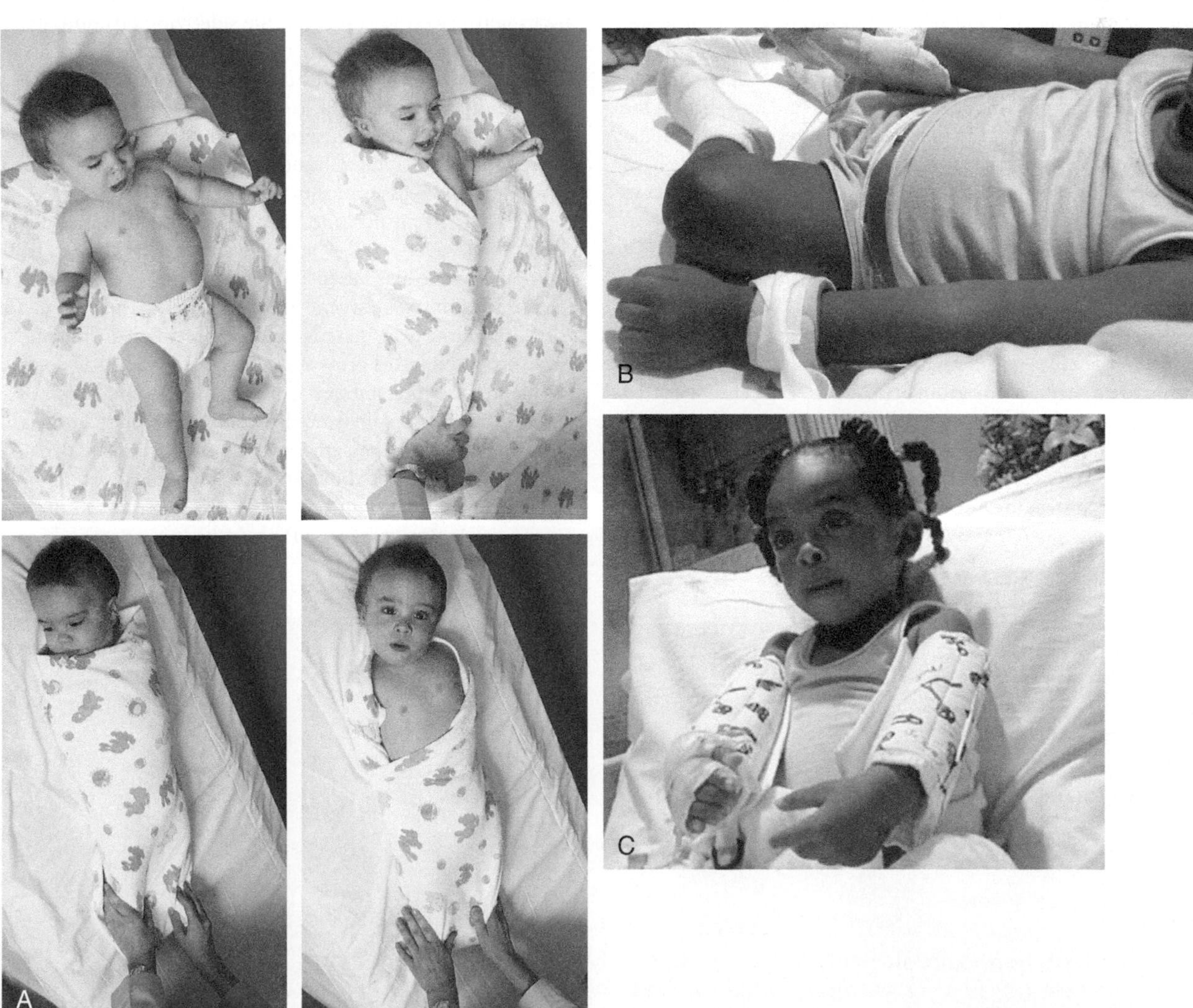

FIG. 22.4 Restraint examples from most restrictive to least restrictive. **A,** Mummy restraint. **B,** Wrist restraints. **C,** Elbow restraints.

including disposable wrist and ankle restraints (Fig. 22.4, *B*). Restraints must be appropriate to the child's size and padded to prevent undue pressure, constriction, or tissue injury, and the extremity must be observed frequently for signs of irritation or impaired circulation. The ends of the restraints are never tied to the side rails because lowering the rail will disturb the extremity, frequently with a jerk that may hurt or injure the child.

Elbow Restraint

Sometimes it is important to prevent the child from reaching the head or face (e.g., after cleft lip or palate surgery, when a scalp vein infusion is in place, or to prevent scratching in skin disorders). Bilateral elbow restraints fashioned from a variety of materials function well (Fig. 22.4, *C*). Commercial elbow restraints or immobilizers are available. They extend from just below the axilla to the wrist and are sometimes referred to as "no-no's." A shoulder strap to prevent slipping may be used in an awake, active older infant or toddler to prevent slippage but should not be used when sleeping.

POSITIONING FOR PROCEDURES

Infants and small children are unable to cooperate for many procedures. Therefore the nurse is responsible for minimizing their movement and discomfort with proper positioning. It can also be helpful to involve the caregivers or child life specialists during procedures to minimize distress in the child. Older children usually need only minimal, if any, positioning hold or movement restrictions. Careful explanation and preparation beforehand and support and simple guidance during the procedure are usually sufficient. For painful procedures, the child should receive adequate analgesia and sedation to minimize pain and the need for excessive restraint. For local anesthesia, use buffered lidocaine to reduce the stinging sensation or a topical anesthetic. (See Pain Management, Chapter 5.)

FEMORAL VENIPUNCTURE

The nurse places the child supine with the legs in a frog position to provide extensive exposure of the groin area. A towel can also be placed under the hips. The infant's legs can be effectively controlled by the nurse's forearms and hands (Fig. 22.5). Only the side used for the venipuncture is uncovered, so the practitioner is protected if the child urinates during the procedure. Apply pressure to the site to prevent oozing from the site.

EXTREMITY VENIPUNCTURE OR INJECTION

The most common sites of venipuncture are the veins of the extremities, especially the arm and hand. A convenient position is to place the child in the parent's (or assistant's) lap with the child facing the parent and in the straddle position. Next, place the child's arm for venipuncture on a firm surface, such as a treatment table. The nurse can partially stabilize the child's outstretched arm and have the parent hug the child's upper body, preventing movement; the nurse can then use the parent's arm to immobilize the venipuncture site. This type of comfort hold also comforts the child because of the close body contact, allows for distraction techniques for the child, and allows each person to maintain eye contact (Fig. 22.6).

LUMBAR PUNCTURE

Pediatric lumbar puncture (LP) sets contain smaller spinal needles, but sometimes the provider will specify a different size or type of needle depending on the child's size or obesity. The technique for the LP procedure in infants and children is similar to that in adults, although modifications are suggested in neonates, who have less distress in a side-lying position with modified neck extension than in flexion or a sitting position.

Children can be positioned in a side-lying or sitting position. Children are usually easiest to control in the side-lying position, with the head flexed and the knees drawn up toward the chest. Even cooperative children need to be held gently under the knees and around the shoulders to prevent possible trauma from unexpected, involuntary movement. They can be reassured that, although they are trusted, holding will serve as a reminder to maintain the desired position. It also provides a measure of support and reassurance to them (Fig. 22.7).

A flexed sitting position may be used, depending on the child's ability to cooperate and whether sedation will be used. In the sitting position with the hips flexed and spine curved forward, the interspinous space is maximized between L3 and L5 (Ford, 2016). The child is placed with the buttocks at the edge of the table. For an infant, the nurse's hands immobilize the arms and legs. Neck flexion has not been shown to enhance the interspinous space opening in children.

Specimens and spinal fluid pressure are obtained, measured, and sent for analysis in the same manner as for adult patients. Take vital signs as ordered throughout and after the procedure, and observe the child for any changes in level of consciousness, motor activity, and other neurologic signs. Post-LP headache may occur and can be related

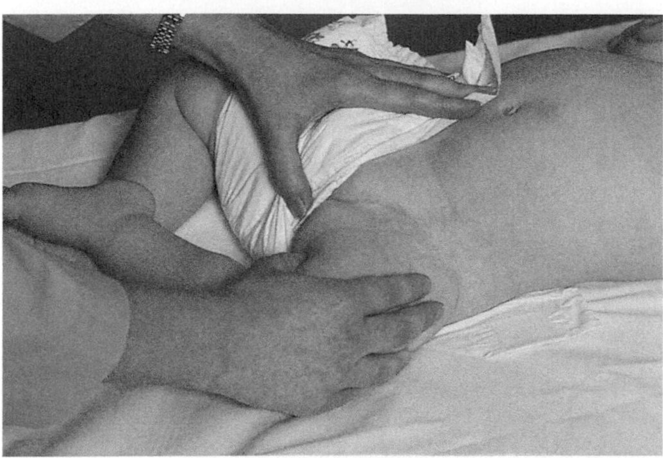

FIG. 22.5 Positioning infant for femoral venipuncture.

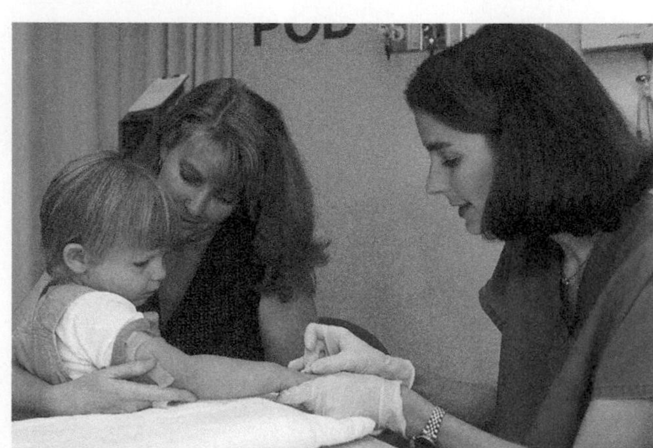

FIG. 22.6 Therapeutic comfort hold of child for extremity venipuncture with parental assistance.

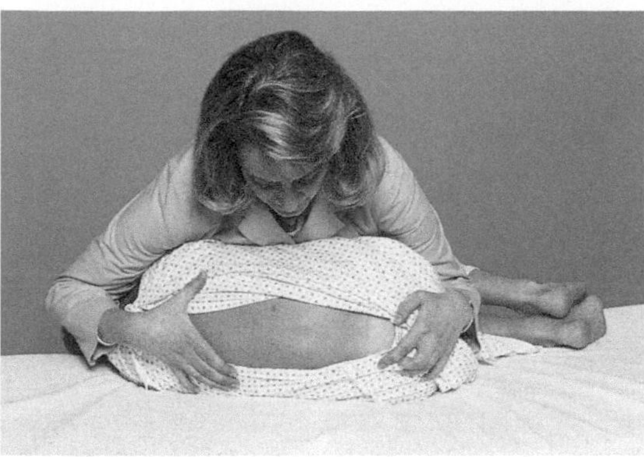

FIG. 22.7 Side-lying position for lumbar puncture.

to larger needle size, prior history of headaches, and postural changes. There is insufficient evidence to support the use of bed rest after LP to reduce post-LP headaches (Rusch, Schulta, Hughes, et al., 2014). Treatment generally includes rest and oral analgesics that do not inhibit platelet function.

BONE MARROW ASPIRATION OR BIOPSY

The position for a bone marrow aspiration or biopsy depends on the chosen site. In children, the posterior or anterior iliac crest is most frequently used, but in infants less than 18 months old, the tibia may be selected because the iliac crest has not yet ossified.

If the posterior iliac crest is used, the child is positioned prone, and if the anterior iliac crest is used, the child is typically positioned side-lying or supine. Sometimes a small pillow or folded blanket is placed under the hips to facilitate obtaining the bone marrow specimen. Children should receive adequate analgesia or anesthesia to relieve pain and should be monitored appropriately throughout the procedure. If the child might awaken, he or she may need to be held, preferably by two people—one person to immobilize the upper body and a second person to immobilize the lower extremities. A pressure dressing is applied to the puncture site on completion of the procedure and maintained for 24 hours.

COLLECTION OF SPECIMENS

Many of the specimens needed for diagnostic examination of children are collected in much the same way as they are for adults. Older children are able to cooperate if given proper instruction regarding what is expected of them. Infants and small children, however, are typically unable to follow directions or control body functions sufficiently to help in collecting some specimens.

FUNDAMENTAL STEPS COMMON TO ALL PROCEDURES

The following steps are very important for every procedure and should be considered fundamental aspects of care. These steps, although important, are not listed in each of the specimen collection procedures.

1. Assemble the necessary equipment.
2. The staff member should introduce himself or herself to the family and verify the specimen that is to be collected.
3. Identify the child using two patient identifiers (e.g., patient name and medical record or birth date; neither can be a room number). Compare the same two identifiers with the specimen container and order.
3. Perform hand hygiene, maintain aseptic technique, and follow Standard Precautions.
4. Explain the procedure to parents and child according to the developmental level of the child; reassure the child that the procedure is not a punishment.
5. Provide atraumatic care and position the child securely.
6. Prepare area with antiseptic agent.
7. Place specimens in appropriate containers with appropriate collection information such as date and time and apply a patient identification label to the specimen container in the presence of the child and family.
8. Discard puncture device in puncture-resistant container near the site of use.
9. Wash the procedural preparation agent off if povidone-iodine is used, if skin is sensitive, and for infants. Check that all collection supplies have been removed from the patient's bed space area to ensure patient safety.
10. Remove gloves and perform hand hygiene after the procedure. Have children wash their hands if they have helped.
11. Praise the child for helping.
12. Document pertinent aspects of the procedure, such as number of attempts, site, and amount of blood or urine withdrawn, as well as type of test performed.

URINE SPECIMENS

There are many diagnostic situations that warrant urine specimens. The age of the child will affect the collection technique, as well as developmental considerations. Children will better understand what is expected if the nurse uses familiar terms, such as "pee-pee," "wee-wee," or "tinkle." Preschoolers and toddlers are usually unable to void on request. It is often best to offer them water or other liquids that they enjoy and wait about 30 minutes until they are ready to void voluntarily. Some have difficulty voiding in an unfamiliar receptacle. Potty chairs or a potty hat placed on the toilet is usually satisfactory. Toddlers who have recently acquired bladder control may be especially reluctant because they undoubtedly have been admonished for "going" in places other than those approved by parents. Enlisting the parents' help usually leads to success. School-age children are generally cooperative with collection methods but curious. They are concerned about the reasons behind things and are likely to ask questions regarding the disposition of their specimen and what one expects to discover from it. Self-conscious adolescents may be reluctant to carry a specimen through a hallway or waiting room and appreciate a paper bag for disguising the container. The presence of menses may be an embarrassment or a concern to teenage girls; therefore it is a good idea to ask them about this and make adjustments as necessary. The specimen can be delayed or a notation made on the laboratory slip to explain the presence of red blood cells.

At times, parents may be asked to bring a urine sample to a health care facility for examination, especially when infants are unable to void during an outpatient visit. In these instances, parents need instructions on applying the collection device and storing the specimen. Ideally, the specimen should be brought to the designated place as soon as possible. If there is a delay, the sample should be refrigerated and the lapsed time reported to the examiner.

Although it is a convenient and noninvasive collection method, direct urine aspiration from a diaper can alter the specimen results. Superabsorbent gel disposable diapers may absorb all urine and may also produce a false crystalluria. Direct aspiration from the diaper may not be suitable for all urine specimen tests. Nurses should verify collection procedures with the laboratory before collection.

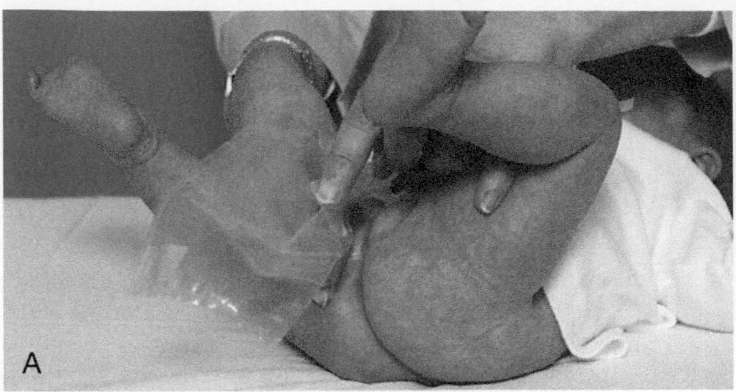

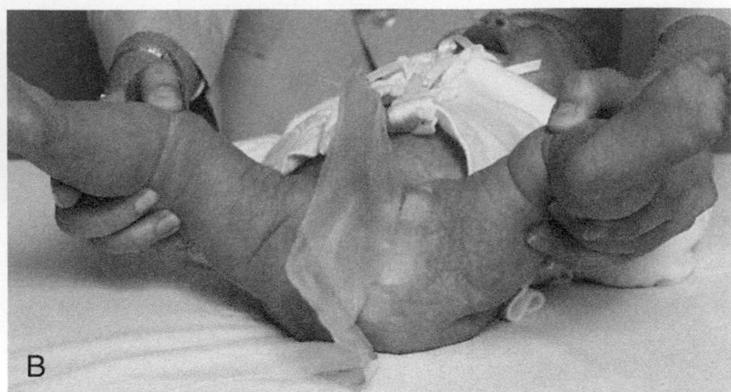

FIG. 22.8 Application of urine collection bag. **A,** On female infants, the adhesive portion is applied to the exposed and dried perineum first. **B,** The bag adheres firmly around the perineal area to prevent urine leakage.

Urine Collection Bags

For infants and toddlers who are not toilet trained, special urine collection bags with self-adhering material around the opening at the point of attachment may be used. To prepare the infant, the genitalia, perineum, and surrounding skin are washed and dried thoroughly because the adhesive will not stick to a moist, powdered, or oily skin surface. The collection bag is easiest to apply if attached first to the perineum, progressing to the symphysis pubis (Fig. 22.8). With girls, the perineum is stretched taut during application to ensure a leakproof fit. With boys, the penis and sometimes the scrotum are placed inside the bag. The adhesive portion of the bag must be firmly applied to the skin all around the genital area to avoid leakage. The bag is checked frequently and removed as soon as the specimen is available because the moist bag may become loosened on an active child.

The American Academy of Pediatrics guidelines (American Academy of Pediatrics, Subcommittee on Urinary Tract infections, Steering Committee on Quality Improvement and Management, 2011) for diagnosis and management of urinary tract infections in infants 2 to 24 months old recommend that any positive screen obtained from a bag specimen be confirmed by culture via bladder catheterization or suprapubic aspiration due to an unacceptably high rate of false-positive results. Although the bag specimen collection method is less invasive and traumatic to an infant, some families and clinicians may prefer to collect only one definitive specimen and avoid additional delay in obtaining a second specimen. Urine bag specimens may be most appropriate for a urine dipstick or urinalysis, not urine cultures (Stein, Dogan, Hoebeke, et al., 2015).

NURSING TIP

In infants, wipe the abdomen with an alcohol pad, and fan it dry; the cooling effect often causes voiding within 2 minutes. Apply pressure over the suprapubic area or stroke the paraspinal muscles (along the spine) to elicit the Perez reflex. In infants 4 to 6 months of age, this reflex causes crying, extension of the back, flexion of the extremities, and urination.

Clean-Catch Specimens

Clean-catch specimen traditionally refers to a urine sample obtained for culture after the urethral meatus is cleaned and the first few milliliters of urine are voided (midstream specimen). In girls, the perineum is wiped with an antiseptic pad from front to back. In boys, the tip of the penis is cleansed. If the boy is uncircumcised, the foreskin is retracted and the glans is cleansed. It is important that the inside of the specimen cup or lid is not touched or contaminated during collection to ensure accurate results.

NURSING TIP

When using a urine collection bag, cut a small slit in the diaper and pull the bag through to allow room for urine to collect and to facilitate checking on the contents. To obtain small amounts of urine, use a syringe without a needle to aspirate urine directly from the diaper. If diapers with absorbent gelling material that trap urine are used, place a small gauze dressing, some cotton balls, or a urine collection device inside the diaper to collect urine, and aspirate the urine with a syringe.

Twenty-Four-Hour Collection

For a 24-hour collection, collection bags are required in infants and small children. Older children require special instruction about notifying someone when they need to void or have a bowel movement so that urine can be collected separately and is not discarded. Some older school-age children and adolescents can take responsibility for collection of their own 24-hour specimens and can keep output records and transfer each voiding to the 24-hour collection container.

The collection period always starts and ends with an empty bladder. At the time the collection begins, instruct the child to void and discard the specimen. All urine voided in the subsequent 24 hours is saved in a container with a preservative or is placed on ice. Twenty-four hours from the time the precollection specimen was discarded, the child is again instructed to void, the specimen is added to the container, and the entire collection is taken to the laboratory.

Infants and small children who are bagged for 24-hour urine collection require a special collection bag. Frequent removal and replacement of adhesive collection devices can produce skin irritation. A thin coating of sealant, such as Skin-Prep, applied to the skin helps protect it and aids adhesion (unless its use is contraindicated, such as in premature infants or children with irritated skin). Plastic collection bags with collection tubes attached are ideal when the container must be left in place for a time. These can be connected to a collecting device or emptied periodically by aspiration with a syringe. When such devices are not available, a regular bag with a feeding tube inserted through a puncture hole at the top of the bag serves as a satisfactory substitute. However, take care to empty the bag as soon as the infant urinates to prevent leakage and loss of contents. An indwelling catheter may also be placed for the collection period.

Bladder Catheterization and Other Techniques

Bladder catheterization or suprapubic aspiration is used when a specimen is urgently needed or a child is unable to void or otherwise provide an adequate specimen. The American Academy of Pediatrics recommends

TABLE 22.4 Straight Catheter or Foley Catheter*

	Size (Length of Insertion [cm]) for Girls	Size (Length of Insertion [cm]) for Boys
Term neonate	5-6 (5)	5-6 (6)
Infant to 3 yr	5-8 (5)	5-8 (6)
4-8 yr	8 (5-6)	8 (6-9)
8 yr to prepubertal	10-12 (6-8)	8-10 (10-15)
Pubertal	12-14 (6-8)	12-14 (13-18)

*Foley catheters are approximately 1 Fr size larger because of the circumference of the balloon. Example: 10-Fr Foley catheter = approximately 12-Fr calibration.

that a urine specimen be obtained by bladder catheterization or suprapubic aspiration in ill-appearing febrile infants with no apparent source of infection before antimicrobial administration and to confirm a positive screen for infection (American Academy of Pediatrics, Subcommittee on Urinary Tract Infections, Steering Committee on Quality Improvement and Management, 2011).

Catheterization is a sterile procedure, and Standard Precautions for body substance protection should be followed. If the catheter is to remain in place, a Foley catheter is used. Table 22.4 gives guidelines for choosing the appropriate-size catheter and length of insertion. The supplies needed for this procedure include sterile gloves, sterile lubricant anesthetic, the appropriate-size catheter, povidone-iodine (Betadine) swabs or an alternative cleansing agent and 4 × 4–inch gauze squares, a sterile drape, and a syringe with sterile water if a Foley catheter is used. It may also be helpful to ensure an extra catheter is readily available if needed. Many manufacturers no longer recommend testing the balloon of the Foley catheter by injecting sterile water before catheter insertion due to risk of weakening the balloon.

Adolescent boys and children with a history of urethral surgery may be catheterized with a curved, coudé-tipped catheter to assist with guiding the catheter past tight or partially blocked urethral openings. Children with myelodysplasia and those who have been identified as being sensitive or allergic to latex are catheterized with catheters manufactured from an alternative material. When an indwelling catheter is indicated for urinary drainage, a lubricious-coated or silicone catheter is selected because these materials produce less irritation of the urethral mucosa compared with Silastic or latex catheters when left in place for more than 72 hours.

A 2% lidocaine lubricant with applicator is assembled according to the manufacturer's instructions, and several drops of the lubricant are placed at the meatus. The child is advised that the lubricant is used to reduce any discomfort associated with inserting the catheter and that introduction of the catheter into the urethra will produce a sensation of pressure and a desire to urinate (Gray, 1996) (see Translating Evidence into Practice box).

NURSING TIP

Although lidocaine lubricant may reduce discomfort during urinary catheterization, it is important for the nurse to weigh the benefit of analgesia against a prolonged procedure time. Lidocaine gel lubricant takes approximately 5 to 10 minutes for the anesthetic benefit to take effect. This increase in procedure length may significantly increase the anxiety of a young child. Thus the lidocaine lubricant may be more appropriate in the older child or adolescent age-groups.

In male patients, grasp the penis with the nondominant hand and retract the foreskin. In uncircumcised newborns and infants, the foreskin may be adhered to the shaft; use care when retracting. If the penis is pendulous, place a sterile drape under the penis. Using the sterile hand, swab the glans and meatus three times with povidone-iodine beginning at the meatus and moving outward toward the edge of the glans. If appropriate to use lidocaine lubricant based on the child's age, developmental level, and preference, apply a small amount of lidocaine jelly to the tip of the penis over the urethra. Gently introduce the tip of the lidocaine jelly applicator into the urethra 1 to 2 cm (0.4 to 0.8 inch) so that the lubricant flows only into the urethra; insert 5 to 10 ml 2% lidocaine lubricant into the urethra and hold it in place for 2 to 5 minutes by gently squeezing the distal penis. Lubricate the catheter and insert it into the urethra while gently stretching the penis and lifting it to a 90-degree angle to the body. Resistance may occur when the catheter meets the urethral sphincter. Ask the patient to inhale deeply and advance the catheter. Do not force a catheter that does not easily enter the meatus, particularly if the child has had corrective surgery. For indwelling catheters, after urine is obtained, advance the catheter to the hub, inflate the balloon with sterile water, pull it back gently to test inflation, and connect it to the closed drainage system. Cleanse the glans and meatus, and replace the retracted foreskin. If blood is seen at any time during the procedure, discontinue the procedure and notify the provider.

In female patients, place a sterile drape under the buttocks. Use the nondominant hand to gently separate and pull up the labia minora to visualize the meatus. Swab the meatus from front to back three times using a different povidone-iodine swab each time. If appropriate to use lidocaine lubricant based on the child's age, developmental level, and preference, place 1 to 2 ml 2% lidocaine lubricant on the periurethral mucosa and insert the lubricant 1 to 2 ml into the urethral meatus. Delay catheterization for 2 to 5 minutes to maximize absorption of the anesthetic into the periurethral and intraurethral mucosa. Add lubricant to the catheter and gently insert it into the urethra until urine returns; then advance the catheter an additional 2.5 to 5 cm (1 to 2 inches). When using an indwelling Foley catheter, inflate the balloon with sterile water and gently pull back; then connect to a closed drainage system. Cleanse the meatus and labia (see Cultural Considerations box). Because the use of lidocaine jelly can increase the volume of intraurethral lubricant, urine return may not be as rapid as when minimal lubrication is used. For both male and female patients, apply a securement device from the catheter tubing to the patient's thigh to avoid kinks and painful pulling on the catheter. Ensure that the patient can move his or her thigh without pulling on the catheter tubing.

! NURSING ALERT

Do not advance the catheter too far into the bladder to prevent knotting of catheters and tubes within the bladder. Feeding tubes should not be used for urinary catheterization because they are more flexible, longer, and prone to knotting compared with commercially designed urinary catheters.

CULTURAL CONSIDERATIONS

Bladder Catheterization

Parents may be upset when their child is catheterized. Aside from the trauma the child experiences, some parents may fear that the procedure affects the daughter's virginity. To correct this misconception, the family may benefit from a detailed explanation of the genitourinary anatomy, preferably with a model that shows the separate vaginal and urethral openings. The nurse can also indicate that catheterization has no effect on virginity.

TRANSLATING EVIDENCE INTO PRACTICE

The Use of Lidocaine Lubricant for Urethral Catheterization

Ask the Question

PICOT Question

In children, does a lidocaine lubricant decrease the pain associated with urethral catheterization?

Search for the Evidence

Search Strategies

Search selection criteria included English-language publications, research-based studies, and review articles on the use of the lidocaine lubricant before urethral catheterization.

Databases Used

Cochrane Collaboration, PubMed, MD Consult, BestBETs, American Academy of Pediatrics

Critically Analyze the Evidence

- Gray (1996) published a review of strategies to minimize distress associated with urethral catheterization in children and supported intraurethral instillation of a local anesthetic that contains 2% lidocaine before catheter insertion.
- One prospective, double-blind, placebo-controlled trial evaluated the use of lidocaine lubricant for discomfort in 20 children before urethral catheterization. Two doses of lidocaine lubricant instilled into the urethra 5 minutes apart significantly reduced pain and distress during urethral catheterization (Gerard, Cooper, Duethman, et al., 2003).
- Boots and Edmundson (2010) conducted a randomized controlled trial in 200 children in a follow-up to the study by Gerard and colleagues. Conclusions were that a topical application of 2% lidocaine gel followed by urethral instillation of lidocaine gel is effective in reducing discomfort before urinary catheterization, and two urethral instillations offered no significant difference over a single instillation.
- Mularoni, Cohen, DeGuzman, and colleagues (2009) found in a three-armed placebo-controlled, double-blind, randomized controlled trial of 43 children younger than 2 years of age that topical and intraurethral lidocaine lubricant was superior to the placebos of topical aqueous lubricant alone and topical and intraurethral aqueous lubricant in lowering distress, but it did not fully alleviate pain.
- A placebo-controlled, double-blind, randomized controlled trial of 115 children younger than 2 years of age found no significant difference when 2% lidocaine gel was compared with a nonanesthetic lubricant. The lubricant was applied to the genital mucosa for 2 to 3 minutes and liberally applied to the catheter but not instilled into the urethra (Vaughn, Paton, Bush, et al., 2005).
- A randomized controlled trial of 126 children ages 4 days to 23 months found a significant decrease in pain response in children who received topical and intraurethral 2% lidocaine gel compared with children who received a non-anesthetic lubricant (Castelo, Li, Taddio, et al., 2014).
- A randomized controlled trial of 133 children ages 0 to 24 months found no difference in pain response in children who received intraurethral 2% lidocaine gel lubricant compared with children who received a nonanesthetic lubricant during urethral catheterization. However, there was significantly increased pain response in children during instillation of the lidocaine lubricant compared with the nonanesthetic lubricant. Additionally, there was no difference in parent satisfaction scores between the nonanesthetic lubricant and lidocaine lubricant (Poonai, Li, Langford, et al., 2015).

Apply the Evidence: Nursing Implications

There is moderate-quality evidence with strong recommendations (Guyatt, Oxman, Vist, et al., 2008) for using a lidocaine lubricant to decrease pain associated with urethral catheterization.

Four published research studies were found to support the use of anesthetic before urethral catheterization, one found topical application alone insufficient to reduce pain, and one found no difference in pain response between anesthetic and nonanesthetic application. Several publications support the effectiveness of lidocaine gel lubricant in clinical practice. Topical application followed by one or two transurethral instillations of 2% lidocaine gel before urethral catheterization minimizes distress and reduces pain before urinary catheterization.

Quality and Safety Competencies: Evidence-Based Practice*

Knowledge

Differentiate clinical opinion from research and evidence-based summaries.

Describe use of lidocaine gel for pain reduction during urethral catheterization.

Skills

Base individualized care plan on patient values, clinical expertise, and evidence.

Integrate evidence into practice by using lidocaine gel for pain reduction during urethral catheterization in children.

Attitudes

Value the concept of evidence-based practice (EBP) as integral to determining best clinical practice.

Appreciate the strengths and weakness of evidence for using lidocaine gel for pain reduction during urethral catheterization in children.

References

Boots, B. K., & Edmundson, E. E. (2010). A controlled, randomised trial comparing single to multiple application lidocaine analgesia in paediatric patients undergoing urethral catheterisation procedures. *Journal of Clinical Nursing, 19*(5–6), 744–748.

Castelo, M., Li, J., Taddio, A., et al. (2014). A randomized controlled trial of 2% lidocaine gel compared to current standard of care in infants undergoing urinary catheterization. *Annals of Emergency Medicine, 64*(Suppl. 4), S105.

Gerard, L. L., Cooper, C. S., Duethman, K. S., et al. (2003). Effectiveness of lidocaine lubricant for discomfort during pediatric urethral catheterization. *Journal of Urology, 170*, 564–567.

Gray, M. (1996). Atraumatic urethral catheterization of children. *Pediatric Nursing, 22*(4), 306–310.

Guyatt, G. H., Oxman, A. D., Vist, G. E., et al. (2008). GRADE: An emerging consensus on rating quality of evidence and strength of recommendations. *British Medical Journal, 336*, 924–926.

Mularoni, P. P., Cohen, L. L., DeGuzman, M., et al. (2009). A randomized clinical trial of lidocaine gel for reducing infant distress during urethral catheterization. *Pediatric Emergency Care, 25*(7), 439–443.

Poonai, N., Li, J., Langford, C., et al. (2015). Intraurethral lidocaine for urethral catheterization in children: A randomized controlled trial. *Pediatrics, 136*(4), 880–886.

Vaughn, H., Paton, E. A., Bush, A., et al. (2005). Does lidocaine gel alleviate the pain of bladder catheterization in young children? A randomized, controlled trial. *Pediatrics, 116*(4), 917–920.

*Adapted from the QSEN at http://www.qsen.org.

Suprapubic aspiration is mainly used when the bladder cannot be accessed through the urethra (e.g., with some congenital urologic birth defects, severe phimosis, or labial adhesions) or to reduce the risk of contamination that may be present when passing a catheter. With the advent of small catheters (5- and 6-French straight catheters), the need for suprapubic aspiration has decreased. Access to the bladder via the urethra has a much higher success rate than suprapubic aspiration, in which success depends on the practitioner's skill at assessing the location of the bladder and the amount of urine in the bladder. However, suprapubic aspiration remains a more accurate specimen collection method for urine cultures and should be considered for infants who have unsatisfactory urine collection or inconclusive results (Eliacik, Kanik, Yavascan, et al., 2016).

Suprapubic aspiration involves aspirating bladder contents by inserting a 20- or 21-gauge needle in the midline approximately 1 cm (0.4 inch) above the symphysis pubis and directed vertically downward. The nurse prepares the skin as for any needle insertion, and the bladder should contain an adequate volume of urine. This can be assumed if the infant has not voided for at least 1 hour or the bladder can be palpated above the symphysis pubis or verified via ultrasound. This technique is useful for obtaining sterile specimens from young infants because the bladder is an abdominal organ and is easily accessed. Suprapubic aspiration is painful; therefore pain management during the procedure is important (see Atraumatic Care box).

ATRAUMATIC CARE

Bladder Catheterization or Suprapubic Aspiration

- Use distraction to help the child relax (e.g., blowing bubbles, deep breathing, singing a song).
- Use lidocaine jelly to anesthetize the area before insertion of the catheter. EMLA cream (a eutectic mix of lidocaine and prilocaine) or LMX cream (lidocaine) may lessen an infant's discomfort as the needle passes through the skin for suprapubic aspiration, but care should be taken that the site is thoroughly cleaned and prepped before the procedure.
- Children often become agitated at being restrained for either procedure. Use comfort measures through touch and voice, both during and after the procedure, to help reduce the child's distress.

STOOL SPECIMENS

Stool specimens are frequently collected from children to identify parasites and other organisms that cause diarrhea, assess gastrointestinal function, and check for occult (hidden) blood. Ideally, stool should be collected without contamination with urine, but in children wearing diapers, this is difficult unless a urine bag is applied. Children who are toilet trained should urinate first, flush the toilet, and then defecate into a bedpan (preferably one that is placed on the toilet to avoid embarrassment) or a commercial potty hat over the toilet. Stool specimens should never be contaminated with toilet water to avoid inaccurate results.

Stool specimens should be large enough to obtain an ample sampling, not merely a fecal fragment. Specimens are placed in an appropriate container, which is covered and labeled. If several specimens are needed, mark the containers with the date and time and keep them in a specimen refrigerator. Exercise care in handling the specimen because of the risk of contamination. If a stool specimen cannot be obtained, some laboratory tests may allow for internal rectal swab.

NURSING TIP

To obtain a stool specimen, use a tongue depressor or disposable spoon or knife to collect the stool.

BLOOD SPECIMENS

Whether the blood specimen is collected by the nurse or by others, the nurse is responsible for making certain that specimens such as serial examinations and fasting specimens are collected on time and that the proper equipment is available. Collecting, transporting, and storing specimens can have a major impact on laboratory results. For accurate results, blood must be collected in the proper tube for the test. When preparing for blood specimen collection, the nurse should consult the institution's laboratory reference guide to determine appropriate tubes for specimen collection, as well as the volume of blood required for the test. Inadequate sample size will result in rejected specimens and may require repeat venipuncture in order to obtain accurate samples, causing additional discomfort for the patient. When multiple blood tests are ordered for a patient, and there is concern about the total volume of blood that may be needed, the nurse should be aware that the World Health Organization advises that the maximum volume of blood collected over any 24-hour period should not exceed 3 ml/kg (Clinical Laboratory Standards Institute, 2017; Howie, 2011). When collecting multiple samples via vacutainer system, the order of sample collection also has an impact on test results because the additive from one tube may inadvertently be transferred to subsequent tubes, affecting sample integrity (Clinical Laboratory Standards Institute, 2017). See Fig. 22.9 for proper order of collection. The order of collection is different if collecting blood in capillary tubes or microtainers.

Venous blood samples can be obtained by direct venipuncture or by aspiration from a peripheral venous catheter or central venous access device. Evidence for best practice supports use of direct venipuncture as the preferred method for venous blood collection because it minimizes risk for hemolysis of specimen (Heyer, Derzon, Winges, et al., 2012). However, when venous access is difficult or repeated specimens are necessary, sampling blood from an indwelling catheter may be warranted. Benefits of using an existing catheter include decreased anxiety, decreased discomfort, and improved patient/caregiver satisfaction (Infusion Nurses Society, 2016). Withdrawing blood specimens through peripheral lock devices in small peripheral veins has varying degrees of success. Although it avoids an additional venipuncture for the child, attempting to aspirate blood from the peripheral lock may shorten the life of the device and may cause hemolysis of the blood specimen, leading to ambiguous

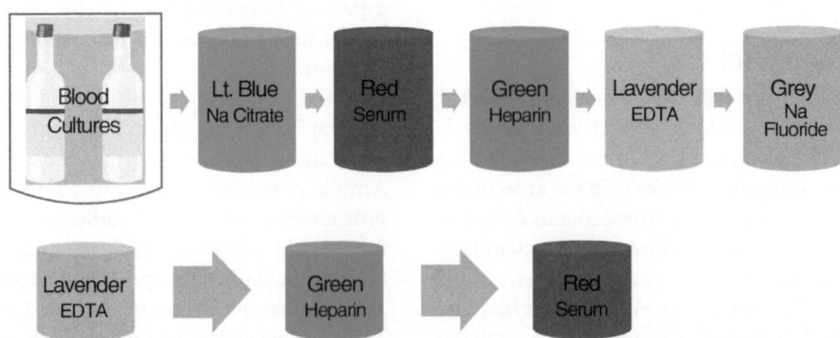

FIG. 22.9 Order of draw for blood collection by vacutainer and microtainer. (Courtesy Cook Children's Medical Center Laboratory.)

results. Factors to consider when deciding to use an IV catheter for blood collection include difficulty of venous access, vein size, location of existing IV catheter, catheter size, type of IV fluid infusing, ease of aspiration, and frequency of blood sampling. Any of these factors may increase the risk of hemolysis of the specimen (Halm & Gleaves, 2009). Before obtaining laboratory specimens, 1 to 2 ml of blood must be withdrawn from the catheter to clear any saline, heparin, or IV fluids from the tubing. When using an IV infusion site for specimen collection, pause the infusion before collecting the blood sample because the type of fluid being infused may affect test results. For example, a specimen collected for glucose determination would be inaccurate if removed from a catheter through which glucose-containing solution was infusing.

Blood Collection From Central Venous Catheters

Central lines can be used to withdraw blood specimens; however, risks include catheter occlusion and catheter-associated bloodstream infection. When collecting blood specimens from a central line, a small volume of blood must first be withdrawn and discarded to clear the line of any IV fluids, heparin, or other fluids that might erroneously affect test results. The Infusion Nurses Society (2011) recommends withdrawing and discarding 1.5 to 2 times the fill volume of the central venous access device (CVAD) before obtaining laboratory specimens. Limited research supports using the initial discard volume as a blood culture specimen (see Research Focus box). Some facilities allow reinfusion of the blood initially withdrawn from the CVAD, especially when blood conservation is essential. Another technique that conserves blood is the push-pull method in which blood is withdrawn into a syringe and reinfused into the CVAD three times. A new sterile syringe is then attached and the laboratory specimen is withdrawn; no blood is discarded. If drawing blood from a multilumen central line, ensure that all lumens are clamped, except for the lumen being used to draw blood.

RESEARCH FOCUS

Central Venous Access Device

In 62 pediatric oncology emergency patients, the initial 5 ml of blood drawn from a central venous access device (CVAD) was used to inoculate blood culture bottles instead of the usual practice of discarding this first 5 ml of blood. A second specimen was obtained (as per standard of care) and used to inoculate separate blood culture bottles. In the 186 paired blood cultures, 4.8% were positive. In all positive cultures, both specimens contained the same organism. In 4 pairs, the first specimen (the one that is usually discarded) grew organisms earlier than the standard of care specimen, allowing for earlier administration of definitive antibiotics. The results of this study could lead to a change in practice, allowing the first 5 to 10 ml of blood obtained from CVADs to be used for blood cultures, rather than discarding this initial sample (Winokur, Pai, Rutledge, et al., 2014).

Blood Collection From Peripheral Veins

When venipuncture is performed, the needed specimens are collected as quickly as possible, and after the needle is withdrawn, pressure is applied to the puncture site with dry gauze until bleeding stops (see Atraumatic Care box). When the venipuncture site is in the antecubital fossa, pressure should be applied with the arm extended, not flexed, to reduce bruising. The nurse then covers the site with an adhesive bandage. In young children, adhesive bandages pose an aspiration hazard, so avoid using them, or remove the adhesive bandage as soon as the bleeding stops. If bruising or hematoma develops after venipuncture, applying warm compresses to the ecchymotic area increases circulation, helps remove extravasated blood, and decreases pain.

Blood Collection From Arterial Vessels

Arterial blood samples are sometimes needed for blood gas measurement, although noninvasive techniques, such as transcutaneous oxygen monitoring and pulse oximetry, are used frequently. Arterial samples may be obtained by arterial puncture using the radial, brachial, or femoral arteries or from indwelling arterial catheters. Assess adequate circulation before arterial puncture by observing capillary refill or performing the Allen test, a procedure that assesses the circulation of the radial, ulnar, or brachial arteries. When collecting a blood sample from an established arterial line, use the in-line sampling port, and follow institutional policy. Because unclotted blood is required, use only heparinized collection tubes or syringes for arterial blood samples. In addition, no air bubbles should enter the collection tube or syringe because they can alter blood gas concentration. Crying, fear, and agitation can also affect blood gas values; therefore make every effort to comfort the child. Pack arterial blood samples in ice to reduce blood cell metabolism and transport to the laboratory immediately.

Blood Collection by Capillary Methods

Take capillary blood samples from children by fingerstick or heelstick. When using a finger for capillary blood collection, use the second or third finger. Cleanse the area with alcohol or chlorhexidine and allow to dry. After performing the fingerstick, wipe once with dry gauze before beginning collection. Gently massage the entire finger to maintain blood flow. Avoid squeezing just the tip of the finger. Hold the fingerstick site facing downward to facilitate blood collection. A common method for taking peripheral blood samples from infants younger than 6 months of age is by heelstick. Before the blood sample is taken, cleanse the area with alcohol or chlorhexidine. Holding the infant's foot firmly with the free hand, the nurse then punctures the heel with an automatic lancet device. An automatic device delivers a more precise puncture depth and is less painful than using a manual lancet (Sorrentino, Fumagalli, Milani, et al., 2017). Several studies demonstrate that the automatic lancet is safer and has been shown to require fewer heel punctures, less collection time, and lower recollection rates (Sorrentino, Fumagalli, Milani, et al., 2017). A surgical blade of any kind is contraindicated. Although obtaining capillary blood gases is a common practice, this method may not accurately reflect arterial values.

The most serious complications of infant heel puncture are necrotizing osteochondritis from lancet penetration of the underlying calcaneus bone, resulting in infection, and abscess of the heel. To avoid osteochondritis, the puncture should be no deeper than 2 mm and should be made at the outer aspect of the heel. The boundaries of the calcaneus can be marked by an imaginary line extending posteriorly from a point between the fourth and fifth toes and running parallel with the lateral aspect of the heel and another line extending posteriorly from the middle of the great toe and running parallel with the medial aspect of the heel (Fig. 22.10). Repeated trauma to the walking surface of the heel can cause fibrosis and scarring that may interfere with locomotion.

Children do not like the discomfort associated with venous, arterial, and capillary punctures. These procedures have been identified by children as the most frequent causes of pain during hospitalization. Arterial puncture was identified as being one of the most painful of all procedures experienced. Toddlers are most distressed by venipuncture, followed by school-age children and then adolescents. Consequently, nurses should use developmentally appropriate language when preparing a child for venipuncture (see Table 22.1 and Applying Evidence to Practice box on p. 681) and use developmentally appropriate pain reduction techniques to lessen the discomfort of these procedures. (See Pain Management, Chapter 5.)

ATRAUMATIC CARE

Guidelines for Skin and Vessel Punctures

To Reduce Pain From Heel, Finger, Venous, or Arterial Punctures

- Apply EMLA cream (a eutectic mix of lidocaine and prilocaine) topically over the site if time permits (>60 minutes). LMX cream (lidocaine) also may be used and requires a shorter application time (30 minutes). The cream should be covered with a small transparent dressing or a piece of plastic wrap (e.g., Press'n Seal) for the specified time interval. To remove the transparent dressing atraumatically, grasp opposite sides of the film and pull the sides away from each other to stretch and loosen the film. After the film begins to loosen, grasp the other two sides of the film and pull. If unable to wait 30 to 60 minutes for topical creams to be effective, use a vapocoolant spray or buffered lidocaine (injected intradermally near the vein with a 30-gauge needle) to numb the skin more quickly.
- Use nonpharmacologic methods of pain and anxiety control (e.g., ask the child to take a deep breath when the needle is inserted and again when the needle is withdrawn, to exhale a large breath or blow bubbles to "blow hurt away," or to count slowly and then faster and louder if pain is felt).
- Keep all equipment out of sight until used.
- Encourage parental presence or assistance, if they wish.
- Restrain the child *only as needed* to perform the procedure safely; use comfort positioning (see p. 700).
- Allow the skin preparation agent to dry completely before penetrating the skin.
- Use the smallest-gauge needle (e.g., 25 gauge) that permits free flow of blood; for neonates and infants, a 27-gauge needle may be sufficient for obtaining 1 to 1.5 ml of blood and for prominent veins (needle length is only 1.25 cm [0.5 inch]).
- If possible, avoid putting an IV line in the dominant hand or the hand the child uses to suck the thumb.
- Use an automatic lancet device for precise puncture depth of the finger or heel; press the device lightly against the skin; avoid steadying the finger against a hard surface.
- Have a "two-try-only" policy to reduce excessive insertion attempts—two operators each have two insertion attempts. If insertion is not successful after four punctures, consider alternative venous access, such as a PICC.
- Have a policy for proactively identifying children with difficult access and appropriate interventions (e.g., most experienced operator for the first attempt, use transilluminator or ultrasonography for insertion guidance).

For Multiple Blood Samples

- Use an intermittent infusion device (e.g., saline lock) to collect additional samples from an existing IV line.
- Consider PICC lines early, not as a last resort.
- Coordinate care to allow several tests to be performed on one blood sample; use micromethods of collection whenever possible.
- Cluster orders for bloodwork to minimize painful venipunctures and/or line entries.
- Anticipate tests (e.g., drug levels, chemistry, immunoglobulin levels) and ask the laboratory to save blood for additional testing.
- Maximum blood collection volumes for any 24-hour period should not exceed 3 ml/kg; limits should be lower for children who are acutely or chronically ill (Clinical Laboratory Standards Institute, 2017; Howie, 2011).

For Heelsticks in Newborns

- Heelsticks have been shown to be more painful than venipuncture (Shah & Ohlsson, 2011).
- Kangaroo care (placing the diapered newborn against the parent's bare chest in skin-to-skin contact) 10 to 15 minutes before and during heelstick reduces pain (Johnston, Campbell-Yeo, Disher, et al., 2017).
- Breastfeeding during a neonatal heelstick is effective in reducing pain and has been found to be more effective than sucrose in some studies (Benoit, Martin-Misener, Latimer, et al., 2017).
- If breast milk is unavailable, administer sucrose and encourage the newborn to suck a pacifier (Stevens, Yamada, Ohlsson, et al., 2016). When commercially manufactured 24% sucrose solution is unavailable, add 1 teaspoon of sugar to 4 teaspoons of sterile water. Use this solution to coat the pacifier, or administer 2 ml to the tongue 2 minutes before the procedure.
- Although safe for use in preterm infants when applied correctly, EMLA has been found to be no more effective than placebo in preventing pain during heelsticks (Anand & Hall, 2006).

IV, Intravenous; *PICC*, peripherally inserted central catheter.

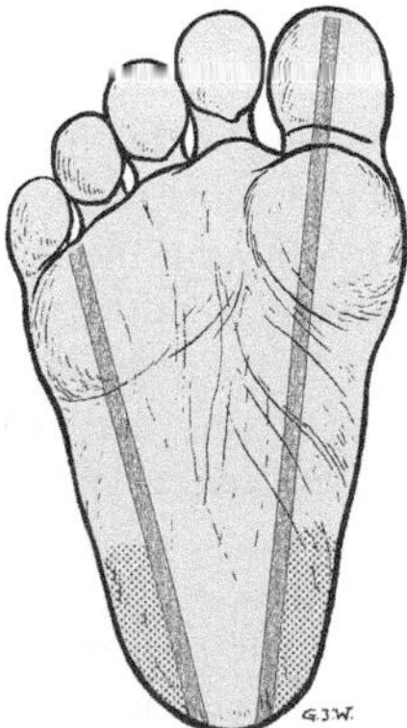

FIG. 22.10 Puncture site *(colored stippled area)* on the sole of an infant's foot.

RESPIRATORY SECRETION SPECIMENS

Collection of sputum is sometimes required for the diagnosis of respiratory infections, especially tuberculosis. Because the infectious organisms are in the lungs and lower airways, the sputum specimen must be produced by deep cough, not just spitting oral secretions into a container. Older children and adolescents are able to cough forcefully and supply sputum specimens when given proper directions. The nurse must make it clear to the child that a coughed specimen is needed, not merely mucus cleared from the throat. It is helpful to demonstrate a deep cough. Infants and small children are unable to follow directions to cough on demand. However, younger children usually swallow any sputum produced; therefore gastric washings (lavage) may be used to collect a sputum specimen. Gastric washing specimens should be collected in early morning for best results. Sometimes a satisfactory sputum specimen can be obtained using a suction device such as a mucus trap, if the catheter is inserted into the trachea and the cough reflex elicited. This procedure can be uncomfortable for the child, so the nurse should be sure to provide developmentally appropriate comfort measures. A catheter inserted into the back of the throat is not sufficient. For children with a tracheostomy, a specimen is easily aspirated from the trachea or major bronchi by attaching a collecting device to the suction apparatus.

Viral pathogens, such as influenza or respiratory syncytial virus, may be detected by nasal washings or by nasopharyngeal swab. However, these two collection methods are not always interchangeable and the nurse must clarify the proper collection method for the test ordered. A specimen collected by an improper method will be rejected by the laboratory and the patient will have to endure the discomfort of repeat collection.

To collect a specimen by nasal wash, the child is placed supine, and 1 to 3 ml of sterile normal saline is instilled by syringe (without needle) into one nostril. The contents of the nasal passage are aspirated using a small, sterile bulb syringe and placed in a sterile container. As an alternative method, the syringe with normal saline can be attached to a short length (5 cm or 2 inches) of 18- to 20-gauge tubing. The tubing is placed into the nostril, then the saline is quickly instilled and then the tubing is slowly withdrawn while gently aspirating to recover the nasal specimen. To prevent any additional discomfort, all of the equipment should be ready before beginning the procedure.

Other respiratory secretion collection methods include nasopharyngeal and oropharyngeal swabs used to test for strep pharyngitis, bordetella, and other pathogens. Swab sticks should have plastic, not wooden, shafts. The nurse swabs both tonsils and the posterior pharynx when obtaining an oropharyngeal specimen. Touching the teeth, gums, and tongue with the swab stick should be avoided. The swab stick is immediately inserted into the culture tube, taking care that the swab does not come in contact with the outside of the container or the hands of the nurse collecting the sample. Some culture kits require squeezing an ampule within the culture tube to release the culture medium. Viral testing usually requires that the specimen be placed in a special container and be transported on ice, so the nurse should ensure that the correct container is on hand before obtaining the specimen.

ADMINISTRATION OF MEDICATION

DETERMINATION OF DRUG DOSAGE

Nurses must have an understanding of the safe dosages of the medications they administer to children, as well as the expected actions, possible side effects, and signs of toxicity. Unlike the standardized doses for adult medications, dosing for pediatric medications is usually presented as a recommended dose range, based on age, weight, or body surface area. Differences between adult and pediatric dosing of medications are related to physiologic differences. Factors related to growth and maturation affect an individual's capacity to metabolize and excrete drugs. Immaturity or defects in any of the important processes of absorption, distribution, biotransformation, or excretion can significantly alter the pharmacodynamics of a drug, resulting in increased toxicity or inadequate effect. Newborn and premature infants are particularly vulnerable to the harmful effects of drugs due to immature enzyme systems in the liver (where most drugs are broken down and detoxified), lower concentrations of plasma proteins (necessary for binding and transporting drugs), and immature functioning of kidneys (where most drugs are excreted). Children metabolize many drugs more rapidly than adults. Consequently, children may require larger doses (per weight) than adults and/or more frequent administration to achieve a therapeutic effect. This is particularly important in pain control, when the dosage of analgesics may need to be increased or the interval between doses decreased in order to meet the needs of the child.

Nurses are accountable for the medications that they administer. An important part of that responsibility is having a working knowledge of drug actions and potential side effects. In addition, nurses should know the safe dose ranges for the drugs with which they work. Before giving any medication, the pediatric nurse must be vigilant to verify that the drug has been dispensed in a dose that is within the recommended range for the child. Pediatric dosages are most often expressed in units of measure per body weight (mg/kg). Some medications, such as chemotherapy, are more precisely dosed using body surface area (BSA), which historically is believed to be a more accurate reflection of metabolic rate and less affected by adipose tissue than weight-based calculations. The ratio of BSA to weight varies inversely with length; therefore an infant who is shorter and weighs less than an older child or adult has relatively more BSA than would be expected from the weight. BSA can be determined by using the West nomogram or the commonly used Mosteller formula: square root of [ht (cm) × wt (kg)] ÷ 3600. Conversion programs are also widely available on the Internet.

Checking Dosage

Administering the correct dosage of a drug is a shared responsibility between the provider who orders the drug and the nurse who carries out that order. Children react with unexpected severity to some drugs, and ill children may be especially sensitive to drugs. When a dose is ordered that is outside the usual range, or when there is some question regarding the preparation or the route of administration, the nurse should check with the prescribing provider before proceeding with the administration because the nurse is legally liable for any drug administered.

Even when given at the correct dosage, many drugs are potentially hazardous or lethal. For this reason, the Institute for Safe Medical Practice has identified a list of "high-alert" medications (see http://www.ismp.org/Tools/highalertmedicationLists.asp). Most facilities have regulations requiring that these high-alert medications be double checked by another nurse before giving them to the child. Among drugs that require such safeguards are antiarrhythmics, anticoagulants, chemotherapeutic agents, and insulin. Other high-alert medications include epinephrine, opioids, and sedatives. A misplaced decimal point placement could result in a 10-fold or greater dosing error. So even if this precaution is not mandatory, nurses are wise to incorporate this safe practice and take the additional time to independently check and recheck drug dose calculations.

Another category of high-alert medications are the "look-alike, sound-alike" drugs that have similar names but significantly different doses and side effects. To emphasize these differences, Tall Man lettering is recommended by the Institute for Safe Medication Practices and the Food and Drug Administration (Institute for Safe Medication Practices, 2016). Examples of Tall Man lettering include DOBUTamine and DOPamine, and predniSONE and prednisoLONE.

Identification

Before the administration of any medication, the child must be correctly identified using two identifiers (e.g., name and medical record number or birth date). With an infant, young child, or nonverbal child, the parent or guardian (if present) can verify the child's identity. After verbal verification of the child's identity (by the parent, guardian, or child), the identification band should be verified using two identifiers. Bedside computers and handheld barcode scanners can be used to verify the ID bracelet directly with the patient's electronic record.

Preparing the Parents

Nearly all parents have given some type of medication to their child and can describe the approaches they have found successful. In some cases, it is less traumatic for the hospitalized child if a parent gives the medication, provided that the nurse prepares the medication and supervises its administration. Children that take daily medications at home are accustomed to the parent functioning in this capacity and may be less likely to fuss than if a stranger administers the medication. Individual decisions need to be made regarding parental presence and participation for other procedures, such as holding the child during injections.

Preparing the Child

Every child requires developmentally appropriate preparation for parenteral administration of medication and supportive care during the procedure (see p. 680). Even if the child has received several injections, rarely does a child become accustomed to the discomfort. With every dose of medication, the nurse should be cognizant of the developmental needs of the child, whether it is the first dose or the 200th dose for that child.

ORAL ADMINISTRATION

The oral route is preferred for giving medications to children because of the ease of administration. Oral medications are available in a variety of dosing formulations, including tablets, capsules, chewable tablets, orally dissolving tablets, sprinkles, and oral liquids. Although some children are able to swallow or chew solid medications at an early age, solid preparations are not recommended for younger children because of the danger of aspiration. Determining when a child is old enough to swallow pills depends on the developmental age of the child, the size of the pill, and the child's past experiences with medications. The nurse should ensure that the formulation of any prescribed medication will be appropriate for the child, based on developmental level, swallowing ability, and available formulations of the medication.

Many pediatric medications come in liquid preparations for added ease of administration. Some liquids may have an unpleasant aftertaste. The taste can be camouflaged whenever necessary, by mixing the medication with a small amount of juice or applesauce. In the hospital, pharmacies can provide flavored syrup, known as syrpalta, for this purpose (see Atraumatic Care box).

Preparation

The most accurate means for measuring small amounts of medication is the plastic disposable calibrated oral syringe. Not only does the syringe provide a reliable measure, but it also serves as a convenient means for transporting and administering the medication. The medication can be placed directly into the child's mouth from the syringe.

A device called the Rx Medibottle (The Medicine Bottle Co., Hinsdale, Illinois; http://www.medibottle.com) has shown to be more effective in delivering unpleasant-tasting oral medication to infants than an oral syringe (Purswani, Radhakrishnan, Irfan, et al., 2009). This device allows an infant to suck juice or other liquids from a nipple attached to a specially designed bottle, while receiving undiluted medication dispensed in spurts from a syringe inserted into a central sleeve of the bottle.

Paper cups are totally unsuitable for liquid medications because they collapse easily, are likely to have irregularly shaped or crumpled bottoms, and retain considerable amounts of thick medication. Molded plastic cups with measuring lines are often supplied with over-the-counter medications for cough and fever, but the vast majority of families in one study could not measure a 5-ml dose within 0.5 ml (Ryu & Lee, 2012; Yin, Parker, Sanders, et al., 2016). Measures less than 1 teaspoon are impossible to determine accurately with a medicine cup. The teaspoon is also an inaccurate measuring device and is subject to error. Teaspoons vary greatly in capacity, and different persons using the same spoon will pour different amounts, resulting in potentially dangerous dosing errors (Beckett, Tyson, Carroll, et al., 2012; Torres, Parker, Sanders, et al., 2017).

Because of the risk of inaccurate dosing when using medicine cups and teaspoons, a policy statement issued by the American Academy of Pediatrics recommends that all liquid oral medications, over-the-counter and prescription, should be dosed only in milliliters and never in teaspoons or other nonmetric units (American Academy of Pediatrics, 2015). Syringes are the preferred device for dosing accuracy. Measuring cups with metric markings may be used as an alternative. A convenient hollow-handled medicine spoon, calibrated in milliliters, is available to accurately measure and administer the drug. Household spoons, including measuring spoons, should be avoided.

Another unreliable device for measuring liquids is the dropper, which varies to a greater extent than the teaspoon or measuring cup. The volume of a drop varies according to the viscosity (thickness) of the liquid measured (Peacock, Parnapy, Raynor, et al., 2010). Viscous fluids produce much larger drops than thin liquids. Many medications are supplied with caps or droppers designed for measuring each specific preparation. These are accurate when used to measure that specific medication but are not reliable for measuring other liquids. Emptying dropper contents into a medicine cup invites additional error. Because some of the liquid clings to the sides of the cup, a significant amount of the drug can be lost.

Young children and some older children have difficulty swallowing tablets or pills. For these children, tablets may need to be crushed. Commercial devices* are available, or simple methods can be used for crushing tablets. Some pills can be crushed and mixed with applesauce or a small amount of juice. Some drugs, such as medication with an enteric or protective coating or formulated for slow release should not be crushed because crushing will alter the amount of drug that is absorbed. In some cases this might result in overdose of medication. The Institute for Safe Medication Practices (ISMP) maintains a list of oral medications that should not be crushed (http://www.ismp.org/tools/DoNotCrush.pdf). In addition, some drugs may be hazardous if the powder becomes aerosolized with crushing. These drugs should be prepared in a pharmacy, or consult the pharmacist or drug label for recommendations.

*Several styles of pill crushers are available in local drug stores and from Trademark Medical, 449 Sovereign Court, St. Louis, MO 63011; 800-325-9044; http://www.trademarkmedical.com.

ATRAUMATIC CARE

Encouraging a Child's Acceptance of Oral Medication

- Mix the drug with a small amount (about 5 ml) of a sweet-tasting substance, such as flavored syrups, jam, fruit purees, sherbet, or applesauce; avoid essential food items because the child may later refuse to eat them.
- Give a "chaser" of water, juice, or child's drink of choice, or ice pop or frozen juice bar after the drug.
- Avoid dairy products with medication administration due to risk of interfering with absorption
- If nausea is a problem, give a carbonated beverage poured over finely crushed ice before or immediately after the medication.
- When medication has an unpleasant taste, have the child pinch the nose and drink the medicine through a straw. Much of what we taste is associated with smell.
- Commercially available flavorings such as apple, banana, and bubble gum (e.g., FLAVORx) can be added to liquid medications at many pharmacies for a nominal additional cost. As an alternative, some pharmacies may be able to prepare the drug in a flavored, chewable troche or lozenge.*
- Infants will suck medicine from a needleless syringe or dropper in small increments (0.25 to 0.5 ml) at a time. Use a nipple or special pacifier with a reservoir for the drug.

*For information about compounding drugs, contact Technical Staff, Professional Compounding Centers of America, 9901 S. Wilcrest Drive, Houston, TX 77099; 800-331-2498; http://www.pccarx.com.

When children need to take solid oral medication for an extended period, the nurse can help teach the child how to swallow tablets or capsules. Training sessions include using verbal instruction, demonstration, reinforcement for swallowing progressively larger candy or capsules, no attention for inappropriate behavior, and gradual withdrawal of guidance after children can swallow their medication. Helpful tips for patients of all ages can be found at http://www.pillswallowing.com.

In some situations, pediatric doses may require splitting pills or tablets. The nurse should be vigilant to ensure that the divided dose is accurate. With tablets, only those that are scored can be halved or quartered accurately. If the medication is soluble, the tablet or contents of a capsule can be mixed in a small premeasured amount of liquid and the appropriate portion given (Valizadeh, Rasekhi, Hamishehkar, et al., 2015). For example, if half a dose is required, the tablet is dissolved in 5 ml of water, and 2.5 ml is given.

Administration

Although administering liquids to infants is relatively easy, the nurse must take care to prevent aspiration. While holding the infant in a semireclining position, place the medication in the mouth using an oral syringe (without a needle). It is best to place the syringe along the side of the infant's tongue and administer the liquid slowly in small amounts, waiting for the child to swallow between increments.

NURSING TIP

In infants up to 11 months of age and children with neurologic impairments, blowing a small puff of air in the face frequently elicits a swallow reflex.

Medicine cups can be used effectively for children, toddlers, and older infants who are able to drink from a cup. Because of the natural outward tongue thrust in infancy, medications may need to be retrieved from the lips or chin and refed. Allowing the infant to suck the medication that has been placed in an empty nipple or inserting the syringe or dropper into the side of the mouth, parallel to the nipple, while the infant nurses is another convenient method for giving liquid medications to infants. Medication is not added to the infant's formula feeding because the child may subsequently refuse the formula. Dispose of any plastic covers that may be on the ends of syringes because these covers are choking hazards.

Children are more likely to take their oral medication willingly if they can be feel involved in the process (as opposed to being forced). Giving choices to a child helps them feel involved. Although taking the medicine is not a choice, the child can be offered other options such as whether they want to take the medicine before or after a specific activity, or what they would like to drink with their medicine, or if they want to help give the medicine. Allowing a child to push the plunger of the syringe of oral medication while the caregiver holds the syringe in the mouth may improve adherence.

When giving oral liquids from a syringe, it is often helpful to give the dose in several small increments and allow the child to swallow between squirts. Place the tip of the syringe into the pocket formed between the lower teeth and cheek. Aiming at the back of the throat increases the risk of aspiration. Children who refuse to cooperate or who resist consistently despite explanation and encouragement may require physical holding. If holding is necessary, it should be done in a position of comfort, sitting up or semireclining. Make every effort to reassure the child that holding is for his or her well-being and is not a form of punishment.

There is always a risk in using even mild forceful techniques. A crying child can aspirate a medication, particularly when lying on the back. If the nurse or caregiver holds the child in the lap with the child's right arm behind the nurse/caregiver, the left hand firmly grasped by the nurse's left hand, and the head securely cradled between the nurse's arm and body, the medication can be slowly administered into the mouth (Fig. 22.11). Never give oral medication with a child lying flat, due to increased risk of aspiration.

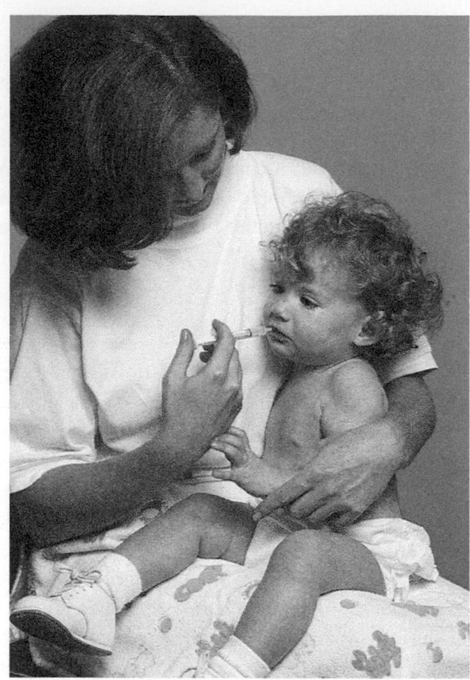

FIG. 22.11 A nurse partially restrains a child for easy and comfortable administration of oral medication.

If part of a dose of oral medication is lost due to spitting, drooling, or vomiting, the nurse should discuss with a provider before readministering the dose. There are no evidence-based recommendations regarding a specific time frame for repeating a dose of medication after a patient has vomited (Kendrick, Ma, Dezorzi, et al., 2012). Because it is difficult to accurately estimate the amount of dose that was actually received, giving additional amounts may result in overdose.

INTRAMUSCULAR ADMINISTRATION

Selecting the Syringe and Needle

The volume of medication prescribed for intramuscular injections in small children necessitates selection of a syringe that can measure small amounts of solution. For volumes less than 1 ml, the tuberculin syringe, calibrated in 0.01-ml increments, is appropriate. Doses smaller than 0.5 ml may be facilitated by the use of a 0.5-ml, low-dose syringe. These syringes, along with specially constructed needles, minimize the possibility of inadvertently administering incorrect amounts of a drug because of dead space, which allows fluid to remain in the syringe and needle after the plunger is pushed completely forward. A minimum of 0.2 ml of solution remains as dead space in a standard needle hub; therefore when very small amounts of two drugs are combined in the syringe, such as mixtures of insulin, the ratio of the two drugs can be altered significantly, due to dead space. Measures that minimize the effect of dead space are (1) when two drugs are combined in the syringe, always draw them up in the same order to maintain a consistent ratio between the drugs; (2) use the same brand of syringe (dead space may vary between brands); and (3) use one-piece syringe units (needle permanently attached to the syringe).

Dead space is also an important factor to consider when injecting medication because flushing the syringe with an air bubble adds an additional amount of medication to the prescribed dose. This can be hazardous when very small amounts of a drug are given. Consequently, flushing is not recommended, especially when less than 1 ml of medication is given. Syringes are calibrated to deliver a prescribed drug dose, and the amount of medication left in the hub and needle is not part of the syringe barrel calibrations.

Certain drugs such as iron dextran and diphtheria and tetanus toxoid may cause irritation when tracked into the subcutaneous tissue. The Z-track method is recommended for use in infants and children rather than an air bubble. In the Z-track method, slight traction is applied to the skin over the injection site, so that it shifts slightly; while maintaining the skin taut, the injection is administered, skin traction is released, and the needle is removed. The skin shifts back to its original location, sealing off the needle track over the muscle and preventing leakage into subcutaneous layer of skin. Changing the needle after withdrawing the fluid from the vial is another technique to minimize tracking.

The needle length must be sufficient to penetrate the subcutaneous tissue and deposit the medication into the body of the muscle. The needle gauge should be as small as possible to deliver the fluid safely. Smaller-diameter (25- to 30-gauge) needles cause the least discomfort, but larger gauges are needed for viscous medication and prevention of accidental bending of longer needles.

Determining the Site

Factors to consider when selecting a site for an intramuscular (IM) injection on an infant or child include the following:

- The amount and viscosity of the medication to be injected
- The amount and general condition of the muscle mass
- The frequency or number of injections to be given during the course of treatment
- The type of medication being given
- Factors that may impede access to or cause contamination of the site
- The child's ability to assume the required position safely

Older children and adolescents usually pose few problems in selecting a suitable site for IM injections, but infants, with their small and underdeveloped muscles, have fewer available options. It is sometimes difficult to assess the amount of fluid that can be safely injected into a single site. Usually 1 ml is the maximum volume that should be administered in a single IM site to small children and older infants. The muscles of small infants may not tolerate more than 0.5 ml. As the child approaches adult size, the nurse can use volumes approaching those given to adults. However, the larger the amount of solution, the larger the muscle at the injection site must be.

Injections must be administered in muscles large enough to accommodate the quantity of medication, while avoiding major nerves and blood vessels. The IM immunization site recommended by the Centers for Disease Control and Prevention, World Health Organization, and American Academy of Pediatrics for infants is the anterolateral thigh or vastus lateralis (Table 22.5 and Fig. 22.12). However, immunizations at the ventrogluteal site have been found to have fewer local reactions

TABLE 22.5 Intramuscular Injection Sites in Children

	Vastus Lateralis (Fig. 22.12, *A*)	Ventrogluteal (Fig. 22.12, *B*)	Deltoid (Fig. 22.12, *C*)
Location*	Palpate to find greater trochanter and knee joints; divide vertical distance between these two landmarks into thirds; inject into middle third	Palpate to locate greater trochanter, anterior superior iliac tubercle (found by flexing thigh at hip and measuring up to 1-2 cm [0.4-0.8 inch] above crease formed in groin), and posterior iliac crest; place palm of hand over greater trochanter, index finger over anterior superior iliac tubercle, and middle finger along crest of ileum posteriorly as far as possible; inject into center of V formed by fingers	Locate acromion process; inject only into upper third of muscle that begins about two finger breadths below acromion
Needle Insertion and Size	Insert needle perpendicular to knee in infants and young children or perpendicular to thigh or slightly angled toward anterior thigh. 22-25 gauge (⅝-1 inch)	Insert needle perpendicular to site but angled slightly toward iliac crest. 22-25 gauge (½-1 inch)	Insert needle perpendicular to site but angled slightly toward shoulder. 22-25 gauge (½-1 inch)
Advantages	Large, well-developed muscle that can tolerate larger quantities of fluid (0.5 ml [infant] to 2.0 ml [child]) Easily accessible if child is supine, side lying, or sitting	Free of important nerves and vascular structures Easily identified by prominent bony landmarks Thinner layer of subcutaneous tissue than in dorsogluteal site, thus less chance of depositing drug subcutaneously rather than intramuscularly Can accommodate larger quantities of fluid (0.5 ml [infant] to 2.0 ml [child]) Easily accessible if child is supine, prone, or side lying Less painful than vastus lateralis	Faster absorption rates than gluteal sites Easily accessible with minimal removal of clothing Less pain and fewer local side effects from vaccines compared with vastus lateralis
Disadvantages	Thrombosis of femoral artery from injection in midthigh area Sciatic nerve damage from long needle injected posteriorly and medially into small extremity More painful than deltoid or gluteal sites	Health professionals' unfamiliarity with site	Small muscle mass; only limited amounts of drug can be injected (0.5-1.0 ml) Small margins of safety with possible damage to radial nerve and axillary nerve (not shown; lies under deltoid at head of humerus)

*Locations are indicated by asterisks in Fig. 22.12.

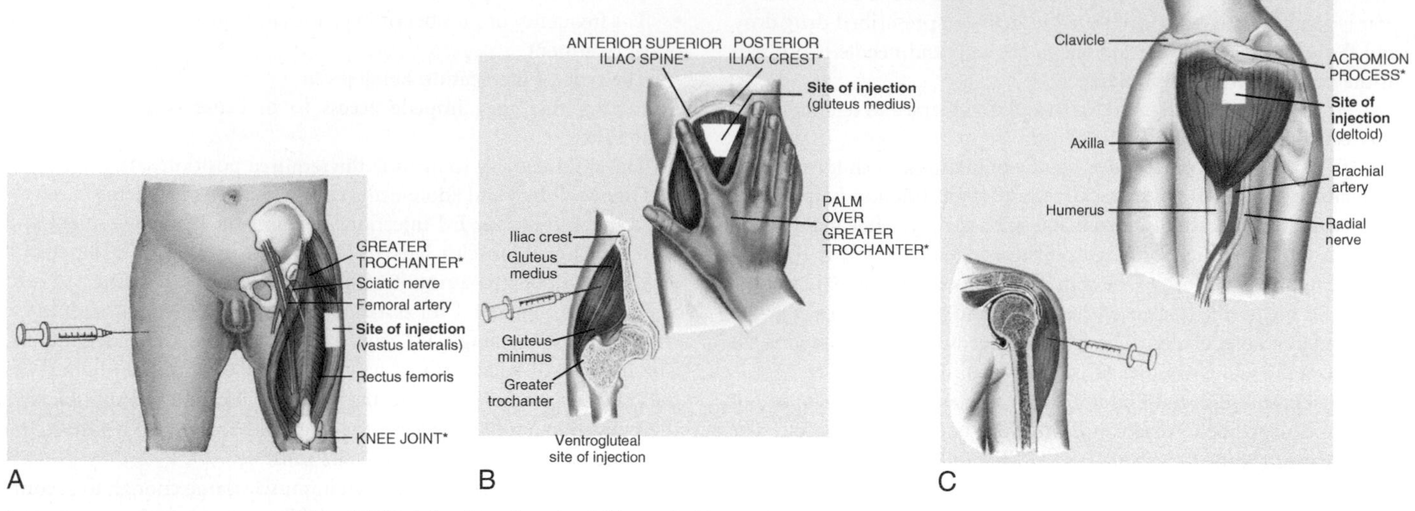

FIG. 22.12 Injection sites in children. **A,** Vastus lateralis. **B,** Ventrogluteal. **C,** Deltoid.

and fever (Junqueira, Tavares, Martins, et al., 2010). Studies have also found fewer systemic reactions (e.g., irritability and persistent crying or screaming) and greater parental acceptance for the ventrogluteal site. The ventrogluteal site is relatively free of major nerves and blood vessels, is a relatively large muscle with less subcutaneous tissue than the dorsal site, has well-defined landmarks for safe site location, and is easily accessible in several positions. Distraction and prevention of unexpected movement may be more easily achieved by placing the child supine on a parent's lap for ventrogluteal site use (Cook & Murtagh, 2006).

The deltoid muscle, a small muscle near the axillary and radial nerves, can be used for small volumes of fluid in children as young as 18 months of age. Its advantages are less pain and fewer side effects from the injectate (as observed with immunizations), compared with the vastus lateralis. Table 22.5 summarizes the three major injection sites, and Fig. 22.12 illustrates the location of the preferred IM injection sites for children.

Administration

Although injections that are executed with care seldom cause trauma to children, there have been reports of serious disability related to IM injections in children. Repeated use of a single site has been associated with fibrosis of the muscle with subsequent muscle contracture. Injections close to large nerves, such as the sciatic nerve, have been responsible for permanent disability, especially when potentially neurotoxic drugs are administered. For this reason, the dorsogluteal site (buttocks) is no longer recommended as a site for IM injections for children under the age of 10 years (Brown, Gillespie, & Chard, 2015). When such drugs are injected, use great care in locating the correct site.

Aspiration during intramuscular vaccine administration is no longer recommended by the Centers for Disease Control and Prevention, World Health Organization, American Academy of Pediatrics, or Immunization Action Coalition (Kroger, Duchin, & Vazquez, n.d.; Sisson, 2015). Aspiration for routine injections into deltoid or vastus lateralis is not indicated because there are no large blood vessels in these locations. Aspiration may still be indicated before injection of medications such as penicillin into larger muscle groups such as the ventrogluteal site (Crawford & Johnson, 2012). One study of IM injection techniques revealed that the straighter the path of needle insertion (e.g., 90-degree angle), the less displacement and shear to tissue, causing less discomfort.

When preparing medication from a glass ampule, a reported potential hazard is the inadvertent creation of glass particles that fall into the medication solution when the ampule is broken open. When the medication is withdrawn into the syringe, the glass particles are also withdrawn and subsequently injected into the patient. As a precaution, medication from glass ampules must be withdrawn through a needle with a filter.

Most children are unpredictable, and few are totally cooperative when receiving an injection. Even children who appear to be relaxed and constrained can become nervous under the stress of the procedure and find it difficult to sit still for an injection. It is advisable to have someone available to help hold the child during an injection, if needed. Because children often jerk or pull away unexpectedly, the nurse should carry an extra needle to exchange for the contaminated one so that delay is minimal. The child, even a small one, is told that he or she is receiving an injection (preferably using a phrase such as "putting the medicine under the skin"), and then the procedure is carried out as quickly and skillfully as possible to avoid prolonging the stressful experience. Invasive procedures such as injections are especially anxiety provoking in young children, who may associate any painful procedure with punishment. Because injections are painful, the nurse should use excellent injection techniques and developmentally appropriate pain reduction measures to reduce discomfort (see Applying Evidence to Practice box).

Small infants can usually be restrained without assistance. A larger infant's body can be securely restrained between the nurse's arm and body. To inject into the body of a muscle, the nurse firmly grasps the muscle mass between the thumb and fingers to isolate and stabilize the site (Fig. 22.13). However, in obese children it is preferable to first spread the skin with the thumb and index finger to localize the muscle by then grasping the muscle deeply on each side.

If medication is given around the clock, the nurse must wake the child. Although it may seem easier to surprise the sleeping child and do it quickly, this can cause the child to fear going back to sleep. When awakened first, children will know that nothing will be done to them unless they are forewarned. The Applying Evidence to Practice box summarizes administration techniques that maximize safety and minimize the discomfort often associated with injections.

APPLYING EVIDENCE TO PRACTICE

Intramuscular Administration of Medication

Apply EMLA (a eutectic mix of lidocaine and prilocaine) or LMX cream (lidocaine) topically over site if time permits. (See Pain Management, Chapter 5.)

- Prepare medication.
- Select appropriately sized needle and syringe.
- If withdrawing medication from an ampule, use a needle equipped with a filter that removes glass particles; then use a new, nonfilter needle for injection.
- Maximum volume to be administered in a single site is 1 ml for older infants and small children.
- Have medication at room temperature before injection.
- Determine site of injection (see Table 22.5); make certain that muscle is large enough to accommodate volume and type of medication.
- For infants and small or debilitated children, use the vastus lateralis or ventrogluteal muscles; the dorsogluteal muscle is insufficiently developed to be a safe site for infants and small children.
- Obtain sufficient help in restraining child.
- Explain briefly what is to be done and, if appropriate, what child can do to help.
- Expose injection area for unobstructed view of landmarks.
- Select a site where skin is free of irritation and danger of infection; palpate for and avoid sensitive or hardened areas.
- With multiple injections, rotate sites. When giving multiple injections at the same time (immunizations, for example), the Centers for Disease Control and Prevention recommends that injection sites in the same muscle group must be at least 1 inch apart.
- Place child in a lying or sitting position; child is not allowed to stand because landmarks are more difficult to assess, restraint is more difficult, and the child may faint and fall.
- **Ventrogluteal**—on side with upper leg flexed and placed in front of lower leg
- **Vastus lateralis**—supine, lying on side, or sitting

Use a new, sharp needle (not one that has pierced rubber stopper on vial) with smallest diameter that permits free flow of the medication.

Grasp muscle firmly between thumb and fingers to isolate and stabilize muscle for deposition of drug in its deepest part; in obese children, spread skin with thumb and index finger to displace subcutaneous tissue and grasp muscle deeply on each side.

Allow skin preparation to dry completely before penetrating skin.

Decrease perception of pain.

- Distract child with conversation.
- Give child something on which to concentrate (e.g., squeezing a hand or side rail, pinching own nose, humming, counting, yelling "Ouch!").
- Spray vapocoolant on site before injection, place a cold compress or wrapped ice cube on site about 1 minute before injection, or apply cold to contralateral site.
- Studies have shown that applying manual pressure to the injection site for 10 seconds before injection can reduce postinjection pain (Derya, Ukke, Taner, et al., 2015; Öztürk, Baykara, Karadag, et al., 2017).
- Have child hold a small adhesive bandage and place it on puncture site after intramuscular injection is given.
- Insert needle quickly using a dartlike motion at a 90-degree angle unless contraindicated.

Avoid tracking any medication through superficial tissues:

- Replace needle after withdrawing medication.
- Use the Z-track or air-bubble technique as indicated.
- Avoid any depression of the plunger during insertion of the needle.
- The Centers for Disease Control and Prevention no longer recommends aspiration before intramuscular injections (Thomas, Mraz, & Rajcan, 2016).
- Remove needle quickly; hold gauze firmly against skin near needle when removing it to avoid pulling on tissue.
- Apply firm pressure to site after injection; massage site to hasten absorption unless contraindicated, as with irritating drugs.
- Place a small adhesive bandage on puncture site; with young children, decorate it by drawing a smiling face or other symbol of acceptance.
- Hold and cuddle young child and encourage parents to comfort child; praise older child.
- Allow expression of feelings.
- Discard syringe and uncapped, uncut needle in puncture-resistant container located near site of use.
- Record time of injection, drug, dose, and injection site.

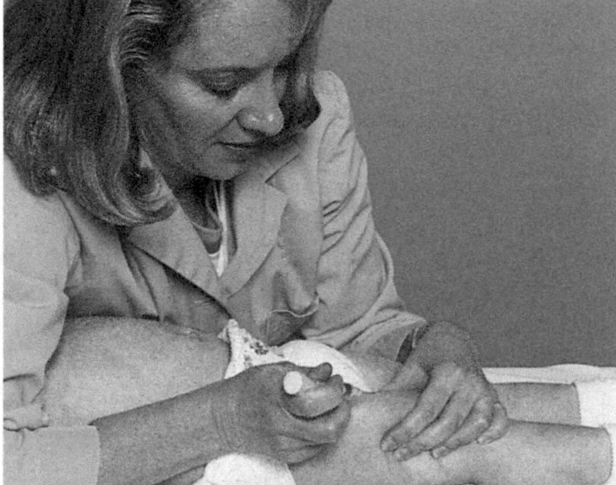

FIG. 22.13 Holding a small child for intramuscular injection. Note how the nurse isolates and stabilizes the muscle.

SUBCUTANEOUS AND INTRADERMAL ADMINISTRATION

Subcutaneous and intradermal injections are frequently administered to children, but the technique differs little from the method used with adults. Examples of **subcutaneous injections** include insulin, hormone replacement, allergy desensitization, and some vaccines. Tuberculin testing, local anesthesia, and allergy testing are examples of frequently administered **intradermal injections**.

Techniques to minimize the pain associated with these injections include changing the needle if it pierced a rubber stopper on a vial, using 26- to 30-gauge needles (only to inject the solution), and injecting small volumes (≤0.5 ml). The angle of the needle for the subcutaneous injection is typically 90 degrees. In children with little subcutaneous tissue, some practitioners insert the needle at a 45-degree angle. However, the benefit of using the 45-degree angle rather than the 90-degree angle remains controversial.

Although subcutaneous injections can be given anywhere there is subcutaneous tissue, common sites include the center third of the lateral aspect of the upper arm, the abdomen, and the center third of the anterior thigh. Some providers believe it is not necessary to aspirate before injecting subcutaneously; for example, this is an accepted practice in the administration of insulin. Automatic injector devices do not aspirate before injecting.

When giving an intradermal injection into the volar surface of the forearm, the nurse should avoid the medial side of the arm, where the skin is more sensitive.

NURSING TIP

Families often need to learn injection techniques to administer medications, such as insulin, at home. Begin teaching as early as possible to allow the family the maximum amount of practice time.

INTRAVENOUS ADMINISTRATION

The IV route for administering medications is frequently used in pediatric therapy. For some drugs, it is the only effective route. This method is used for giving drugs to children who

- Have poor absorption as a result of diarrhea, vomiting, or dehydration
- Need a high serum concentration of a drug
- Have resistant infections that require parenteral medication over an extended time
- Need continuous pain relief
- Require emergency treatment

The nurse needs to consider several factors in relation to IV medication. When a drug is administered intravenously, the effect is almost instantaneous, and further control of side effects is limited. Most drugs for IV administration require a specified minimum dilution, rate of flow, or both, and many drugs are highly irritating or toxic to tissues outside the vascular system. In addition to the precautions and nursing observations commonly related to IV therapy, factors to consider when preparing and administering drugs to infants and children by the IV route include the following:

- Amount of drug to be administered
- Minimum dilution of drug and whether child is fluid restricted
- Type of solution in which drug can be diluted
- Length of time over which drug can be safely administered
- Rate limitations of child, vascular system, and infusion equipment
- Time that this or another drug is to be administered
- Compatibility of all drugs that child is receiving intravenously
- Compatibility with infusion fluids

Before any IV infusion, check the site of insertion for patency, which includes flushing easily without resistance and brisk blood return. Never flush against resistance and if encountered, the integrity of the access should be further evaluated (Gorski, Hadaway, Hagle, et al., 2016). Never administer medications in the same IV tubing with blood products. Only one antibiotic should be administered at a time. Extra fluids needed to administer IV medications can be problematic for infants and fluid-restricted children. Syringe pumps are often used to deliver IV medication because they minimize fluid requirements and more precisely deliver small volumes of medication compared with large-volume infusion pumps. Regardless of the technique, the nurse must know the minimum dilutions for safe administration of IV medications to infants and children.

Peripheral Intermittent Infusion Device

When extended access to a vein is required without the need for continuous fluid, a **peripheral lock**, also known as an **intermittent infusion device** or **saline** or **heparin lock**, is an alternative. The peripheral lock allows a child more freedom than being connected to a continuous IV infusion. It is most frequently used for intermittent infusion of medication, such as antibiotics, via peripheral venous route. A short, flexible catheter is used as the lock device, and a site is selected where there will be minimal movement, such as the forearm. The catheter is inserted and secured in the same manner as for any peripheral IV infusion device, but the hub is capped with a stopper or injection cap. When it is time for medication administration, the injection cap is disinfected, the lock is flushed to ensure patency, and then IV tubing, primed with either normal saline or medication, is connected.

TABLE 22.6 Intravenous Catheter Flushes for Lines Without Continuous Fluid Infusions

Peripheral lines (Hep-Lock or saline locks)	NS* after medications or every 8 hours for dormant lines; instill 2½ times tubing volume 24-g catheters: NS* or heparin 2 units/ml
Midline	Heparin 10 units/ml; 3 ml in a 10-ml syringe† after medications or every 8 hours if dormant Newborns: heparin 1-2 units/ml to run continuously at ordered rate
External central line (nonimplanted, nontunneled, tunneled, or PICC)	Heparin 10 units/ml; 3 ml in a 10-ml syringe† after medications or once daily if dormant Newborns: heparin 2 units/ml; 2-3 ml after medications or to check line patency, OR heparin 1-2 units/ml to run continuously at ordered rate
Totally implanted central line (TIVAS, implanted port)	Heparin 10 units/ml; 5 ml after medications or once daily if dormant and accessed; if not accessed, heparin 100 units/ml; 5 ml every month
Arterial and central venous pressure continuous monitored lines	Heparin 2 units/ml in 55-ml syringe to run continuously at 1 ml/hr

*Use 5% dextrose in water when medication is incompatible with saline.
†Smaller syringes may be used when flush is delivered by a pump.
NS, Normal saline; *PICC*, peripherally inserted central catheter; *TIVAS*, totally implantable venous access device.

The type of device used may vary, and the care and use of the peripheral lock are carried out according to the protocol of the institution or unit. However, the general concept is the same. The catheter remains in place and is flushed with saline before and after infusion of the medication, to maintain patency. See the Translating Evidence into Practice box and Table 22.6 on flushing with normal saline or heparin.

Children who require medications on a short-term basis may be discharged from the hospital with a peripheral lock in place to continue receiving IV medications at home under the care of a home health infusion company. When IV therapy is needed for more than 6 days, use of a midline catheter or peripherally inserted central catheter is recommended (O'Grady, Alexander, Burns, et al., 2011). Midline catheters are peripheral catheters that are placed in one of the larger veins of the upper arm, with the catheter tip terminating below the axilla. Midline catheters are appropriate for short-term use, usually lasting 2 to 6 weeks (Adams, Little, Vinsant, et al., 2016). A midline catheter is not considered a central venous catheter, so total parenteral nutrition (TPN) or any other drug known to irritate a peripheral vein (e.g., chemotherapy

TRANSLATING EVIDENCE INTO PRACTICE

Normal Saline or Heparinized Saline Flush Solution in Pediatric Intravenous Lines

Ask the Question

PICOT Question

Is there a significant difference in the longevity of IV intermittent infusion locks in children when NS is used as a flush instead of an HS solution?

Search for the Evidence

Search Strategies

Selection criteria included evidence during the years 2006 to 2017 with the following terms: *saline versus heparin intermittent flush, children's heparin lock flush, heparin lock patency, peripheral venous catheter in children.*

Databases Used

CINAHL, PubMed

Critical Appraisal of the Evidence

- No differences in patency were established in a double-blind prospective randomized study in neonates. Saline flush was deemed preferable to heparin in peripheral intravenous locks in neonates, in consideration of complications associated with heparin (Arnts, Heijnen, Wilbers, et al., 2011).
- Increased patency or longer dwell times were found with HS solutions versus NS (Kumar, Vandermeer, Bassler, et al., 2013; Tripathi, Kaushik, & Singh, 2008).
- Younger children and preterm neonates with lower gestational ages were associated with shorter patency of IV catheters (Tripathi, Kaushik, & Singh, 2008).
- Infusion devices flushed with NS lasted longer than those flushed with HS (Cook, Bellini, & Cusson, 2011).
- Injection of 0.9% sodium chloride is safe for maintaining patency of peripheral locks in adults and children older than age 12 years (American Society of Hospital Pharmacists Commission on Therapeutics, 2006).
- Either preservative-free heparin or preservative-free 0.9% sodium chloride may be used to flush a peripheral IV line (Arnts, Heijnen, Wilbers, et al., 2011; Bellini, 2012; Cook, Bellini, & Cusson, 2011; White, Crawley, Rennie, et al., 2011); however, catheter patency may be maintained by flushing with saline when converting from continuous to intermittent use (Infusion Nurses Society, 2011).
- Low-dose heparin may prolong duration of catheter patency and decrease the incidence of phlebitis, without increase in heparin-related side effects; however, the results are not statistically significant (Kumar, Vandermeer, Bassler, et al., 2013).
- After each catheter use, peripheral catheters should be locked with preservative-free 0.9% sodium chloride (Infusion Nurses Society, 2011).
- Intermittent flushing with normal saline results in fewer complications, lower cost, and less time compared with continuous infusion (Stok & Wieringa, 2016).
- The Centers for Disease Control and Prevention recommends use of NS for intermittent flushing to avoid complications (O'Grady, Alexander, Burns, et al., 2011).
- Switching from heparin to saline involves educational and administrative interventions (Thamlikitkul & Indranoi, 2006).
- NS is more cost effective (Thamlikitkul & Indranoi, 2006).
- NS flush has fewer side effects. Heparin flush can be associated with anti-coagulation, thrombocytopenia, drug interactions, and hypersensitivity (Arnts, Heijnen, Wilbers, et al., 2011).
- NS flushes once a day maintained patency of pediatric peripheral IV locks, resulting in reduced costs and increased patient satisfaction (Schreiber, Zanchi, Ronfani, et al., 2015).
- Nurses in Italy tend to use heparin with smaller-gauge (24-gauge) catheters when access is less frequent (12 hours or more between doses) and when patients are on specific units (hematology/oncology, pediatric surgery, and short-stay units) (Bisogni, Guisti, Ciofi, et al., 2014).

Apply the Evidence: Nursing Implications

There is low-quality evidence with a weak recommendation (Guyatt, Oxman, Vist, et al., 2008) for using NS versus HS flush solution in pediatric IV lines. Further research is still needed with larger samples of children, especially preterm neonates, using small-gauge catheters (24 gauge) and other catheters flushed with NS and HS as intermittent infusion devices only (no continuous infusions). Variables to be considered include catheter dwell time; medications administered; period between regular flushing and flushing associated with medication administration; pain, erythema, and other localized complications; concentration and amount of HS used; flush method (positive-pressure technique vs. no specific technique); reason for IV device removal; and complications associated with either solution. NS is a safe alternative to HS flush in infants and children with intermittent IV locks larger than 24 gauge; smaller neonates may benefit from HS flush (longer dwell time), but the evidence is inconclusive for all weight ranges and gestational ages.

Quality and Safety Competencies: Evidence-Based Practice*

Knowledge

Differentiate clinical opinion from research and evidence-based summaries.

Describe methods for using NS or HS flush solution in pediatric IV lines.

Skills

Base individualized care plan on patient values, clinical expertise, and evidence.

Integrate evidence into practice on NS or HS flush solution in pediatric IV lines.

Attitudes

Value the concept of evidence-based practice as integral to determining best clinical practice.

Appreciate the strengths and weakness of evidence for NS or HS flush solution in pediatric IV lines.

References

American Society of Hospital Pharmacists Commission on Therapeutics. (2006). ASHP therapeutic position statement on the institutional use of 0.9% sodium chloride injection to maintain patency of peripheral indwelling intermittent infusion devices. *American Journal of Health-System Pharmacy, 63*(13), 1273–1275.

Arnts, I. J., Heijnen, J. A., Wilbers, H. T., et al. (2011). Effectiveness of heparin solution versus normal saline in maintaining patency of intravenous locks in neonates: A double blind randomized controlled study. *Journal of Advanced Nursing, 67*(12), 2677–2685.

Bellini, S. (2012). Flushing of intravenous locks in neonates: No evidence that heparin improves patency compared with saline. *Evidence-Based Nursing, 15,* 86–87.

Bisogni, S., Guisti, F., Ciofi, D., et al. (2014). Heparin solution for maintaining peripheral venous catheter patency in children: A survey of current practice in Italian pediatric units. *Issues in Comprehensive Pediatric Nursing, 37*(2), 122–135.

Cook, L., Bellini, S., & Cusson, R. M. (2011). Heparinized saline vs normal saline for maintenance of intravenous access in neonates: An evidence-based practice change. *Advances in Neonatal Care, 11,* 208–215.

Guyatt, G. H., Oxman, A. D., Vist, G. E., et al. (2008). GRADE: An emerging consensus on rating quality of evidence and strength of recommendations. *British Medical Journal, 336*(7650), 924–926.

Infusion Nurses Society. (2011). Infusion nursing standards of practice. *Journal of Infusion Nursing, 34*(Suppl. 1), S63–S64.

Kumar, M., Vandermeer, B., Bassler, D., et al. (2013). Low dose heparin use and the patency of peripheral intravenous catheters in children: A systematic review. *Pediatrics, 131*(3), e864–e872.

Continued

TRANSLATING EVIDENCE INTO PRACTICE—cont'd

Normal Saline or Heparinized Saline Flush Solution in Pediatric Intravenous Lines

O'Grady, N. P., Alexander, M., Burns, L. A., et al. (2011). Guidelines for the prevention of intravascular catheter-related infections. Atlanta, GA: Healthcare Infection Control Practices Advisory Committee of the Centers for Disease Control and Prevention.

Schreiber, S., Zanchi, C., Ronfani, L., et al. (2015). Normal saline flushes performed once daily maintain peripheral intravenous catheter patency: A randomized controlled trial. *Archives of Disease in Children, 100*(7), 700–703.

Stok, D., & Wieringa, J. W. (2016). Continuous infusion versus intermittent flushing: Maintaining peripheral intravenous access in newborn infants. *Journal of Perinatology, 36*(10), 870–873.

Thamlikitkul, V., & Indranoi, A. (2006). Switching from heparinized saline flush to normal saline flush for maintaining peripheral venous catheter patency. *International Journal for Quality in Health Care, 18*(3), 183–185.

Tripathi, S., Kaushik, V., & Singh, V. (2008). Peripheral IVs: Factors affecting complications and patency—A randomized controlled trial. *Journal of Infusion Nursing, 31*(3), 182–188.

White, M. L., Crawley, J., Rennie, E. A., et al. (2011). Examining the effectiveness of 2 solutions used to flush capped pediatric peripheral intravenous catheters. *Journal of Infusion Nursing, 34*, 260–270.

*Adapted from the QSEN at http://www.qsen.org.
HS, Heparinized saline; *IV*, intravenous; *NS*, normal saline.

drugs) should not be administered through it. The high concentration of glucose in TPN is irritating to the vessel; therefore TPN should always be infused through a central catheter.

Central Venous Catheters

Children with acute or chronic illnesses who require repeated blood sampling or medications, long-term chemotherapy, intensive care, or frequent hyperalimentation or antibiotic therapy are best managed with a central venous catheter. Because the large central veins (such as the subclavian, femoral, or superior vena cava) allow more rapid diffusion of fluids and medications, they offer a more durable venous access than peripheral IV catheters. However, central venous catheters also have a greater risk of bloodstream infection.

Short-term or nontunneled central venous catheters are used in acute care, emergency, and intensive care units. These catheters are made of polyurethane and are placed in large veins such as the subclavian, femoral, or jugular. Insertion is by surgical incision or percutaneous threading. A chest radiograph should be taken to verify that the catheter tip is properly located in a large central vein before administration of fluids or medications.

Peripherally inserted central catheters (PICCs) can be used for short-term and moderate-length therapy. These catheters consist of silicone or polymer material and are placed by specially trained nurses, physicians, or interventional radiologists. The most common insertion site is above the antecubital area using the median, cephalic, or basilic vein. The catheter is threaded either with or without a guidewire into the superior vena cava.

The decision to insert a PICC needs to be made before several attempts at peripheral IV insertion are made. When the antecubital veins have been punctured repeatedly, they are not considered candidates for this type of catheter. Because this catheter is the least costly and has less chance of complications than other CVADs, it is an excellent choice for many pediatric patients who require IV therapies for weeks or months.

Children with chronic illnesses who require long-term venous access, for months or years, are best managed with a central venous access device (CVAD). CVADs have several different characteristics. They can be tunneled or nontunneled, external or internal, inserted peripherally or centrally. Factors that influence selection of the type of CVAD for a child include the reason for placement of the catheter (diagnosis), length of therapy, risk to the patient in placement of the catheter, and availability of resources to assist the family in maintaining the catheter.

! NURSING ALERT

Most PICC lines are not sutured into place, so care is needed when changing the dressing.

Long-term CVADs include tunneled catheters and implanted infusion ports (Table 22.7 and Fig. 22.14). They may have single, double, or triple lumens. Several lumen (multilumen) catheters allow more than one therapy to be administered at the same time. Reasons to use multilumen catheters include repeated blood sampling, TPN, administration of blood products or infusion of large quantities or concentrations of fluids, administration of incompatible drugs or fluids at the same time (through different lumens), and central venous pressure monitoring.

With any of the central venous catheters, medication is easily instilled through the injection cap. Maintenance of the catheter includes dressing changes, flushing to maintain patency, and prevention of occlusion or dislodgment.

! NURSING ALERT

When working with tunneled catheters, PICCs, and peripheral IV catheters, avoid the use of any scissors around the tubing or dressing. Removal is best accomplished using fingers and much patience. In the event that a tunneled catheter is cut, use a padded clamp to occlude the catheter between the exit site and the site of damage to avoid blood loss. Repair kits are available, which may save the catheter and avoid surgery to replace a damaged catheter.

NURSING TIP

To minimize risk of pulling and infection, tubing of external central lines should not be allowed to dangle. Tucking tubing into a swim suit top, sports bra, or a pocket sewn on the inside of a T-shirt provides a place in which to coil the catheter tubing of tunneled external CVAD while the child is at play. Central line wraps are also commercially available.

To access the implanted CVAD, the port must be palpated and stabilized. The overlying skin should be cleansed. The port should only be accessed with a special noncoring Huber needle. The needle is inserted through the diaphragm of the port, which is usually located on the top or side, depending on the style. If the port needs to be accessed for several days, a special infusion set with a Huber needle and extension tubing with a Luer connection can be inserted and an occlusive dressing applied to keep the needle in place (see Fig. 22.14). When the infusion set is used, the procedure for administration of fluids and medications is the same as for an intermittent infusion device or a central venous catheter. To prevent infection, meticulous aseptic technique must be used any time the CVAD is entered, including instillation of heparin or saline to prevent clotting. Huber needles need to be changed at established intervals, usually 5 to 7 days (see Research Focus box).

TABLE 22.7 Comparison of Long-Term Central Venous Access Devices

Description	Benefits	Care Considerations
Tunneled Catheter (e.g., Hickman or Broviac Catheter)		
Silicone, radiopaque, flexible catheter with open ends or VitaCuffs (biosynthetic material impregnated with silver ions) on catheter(s) enhances tissue ingrowth May have more than one lumen	Reduced risk of bacterial migration after tissue adheres to cuff One or two Dacron cuffs Easy to use for self-administered infusions Removal requires pulling catheter from site (nonsurgical procedure)	Requires daily heparin flushes Requires semipermeable dressing over exit site at all times; dressing must be changed regularly and whenever it becomes wet or loose Must be clamped or have clamp nearby at all times Must keep exit site dry Heavy activity restricted until tissue adheres to cuff Water sports may be restricted (risk of infection) Risk of infection still present Protrudes outside body; susceptible to damage from sharp instruments and may be pulled out; may affect body image More difficult to repair Patient or family must learn catheter care
Groshong Catheter		
Clear, flexible, silicone, radiopaque catheter with closed tip and two-way valve at proximal end Dacron cuff or VitaCuff on catheter enhances tissue ingrowth May have more than one lumen	Reduced time and cost for maintenance care; no heparin flushes needed Reduced catheter damage; no clamping needed because of two-way valve Increased patient safety because of minimal potential for blood backflow or air embolism Reduced risk of bacterial migration after tissue adheres to cuff Easily repaired Easy to use for self-administered intravenous infusions	Requires weekly irrigation with normal saline Must keep exit site dry Heavy activity restricted until tissue adheres to cuff Water sports may be restricted (risk of infection) Risk of infection still present Protrudes outside body; susceptible to damage from sharp instruments and may be pulled out; can affect body image Patient or family must learn catheter care
Implanted Ports (e.g., Port-a-Cath, Infus-a-Port, Mediport, Norport, Groshong Port)		
Totally implantable metal or plastic device that consists of self-sealing injection port with top or side access with preconnected or attachable silicone catheter that is placed in large blood vessel	Reduced risk of infection Placed completely under the skin and therefore much less likely to be pulled out or damaged No maintenance care and reduced cost for family Heparinized monthly and after each infusion to maintain patency (only Groshong port requires saline) No limitations on regular physical activity, including swimming Dressing needed only when port accessed with Huber needle that is not removed No or only slight change in body appearance (slight bulge on chest)	Must pierce skin for access; pain with insertion of needle; can use local anesthetic (EMLA, LMX) or intradermal buffered lidocaine before accessing port Special noncoring needle (Huber) with straight or angled design must be used to inject into port Skin preparation needed before injection Difficult to manipulate for self-administered infusions Catheter may dislodge from port, especially if child "plays" with port site (twiddler syndrome) Vigorous contact sports generally not allowed Removal requires surgical procedure

EMLA, Eutectic mix of lidocaine and prilocaine; *LMX,* lidocaine.

RESEARCH FOCUS

Dressing Changes

Semipermeable transparent dressings should be changed at least every 5 to 7 days; the interval depends on the dressing material, age, and condition of the patient; infection rate reported by the organization; environmental conditions; and manufacturer-labeled uses and directions (Infusion Nurses Society, 2011). In children older than 2 months of age, use of chlorhexidine-impregnated dressing (i.e., BioPatch) should be considered as an extra prevention measure for catheter-related bloodstream infection (Infusion Nurses Society, 2011).

The children and parents are taught the procedure for care of the CVAD before discharge from the hospital, including preparation and injection of the prescribed medication, the flush, and dressing changes. A protective device may be recommended for some active children to prevent their accidentally dislodging the needle. Many children take responsibility for preparing and administering medications. Both verbal and written step-by-step instructions are provided for the learners.

Infection and catheter occlusion are two of the most common complications of central venous catheters. They require treatment with antibiotics for infection and a fibrinolytic agent, such as alteplase, for thrombus formation (Blaney, Shen, Kerner, et al., 2006). When the line is not in use, the catheter should be clamped. The parents are cautioned to keep scissors away from the child to prevent accidental cutting of the catheter. If the catheter leaks, the parents are instructed to tape it above the leak and then clamp the catheter at the taped site. The child should be taken to the provider as soon as possible to prevent infection or clotting after a catheter leak.

! NURSING ALERT

If a central venous catheter is accidentally removed, apply pressure to the entry site to the vein, not the exit site on the skin.

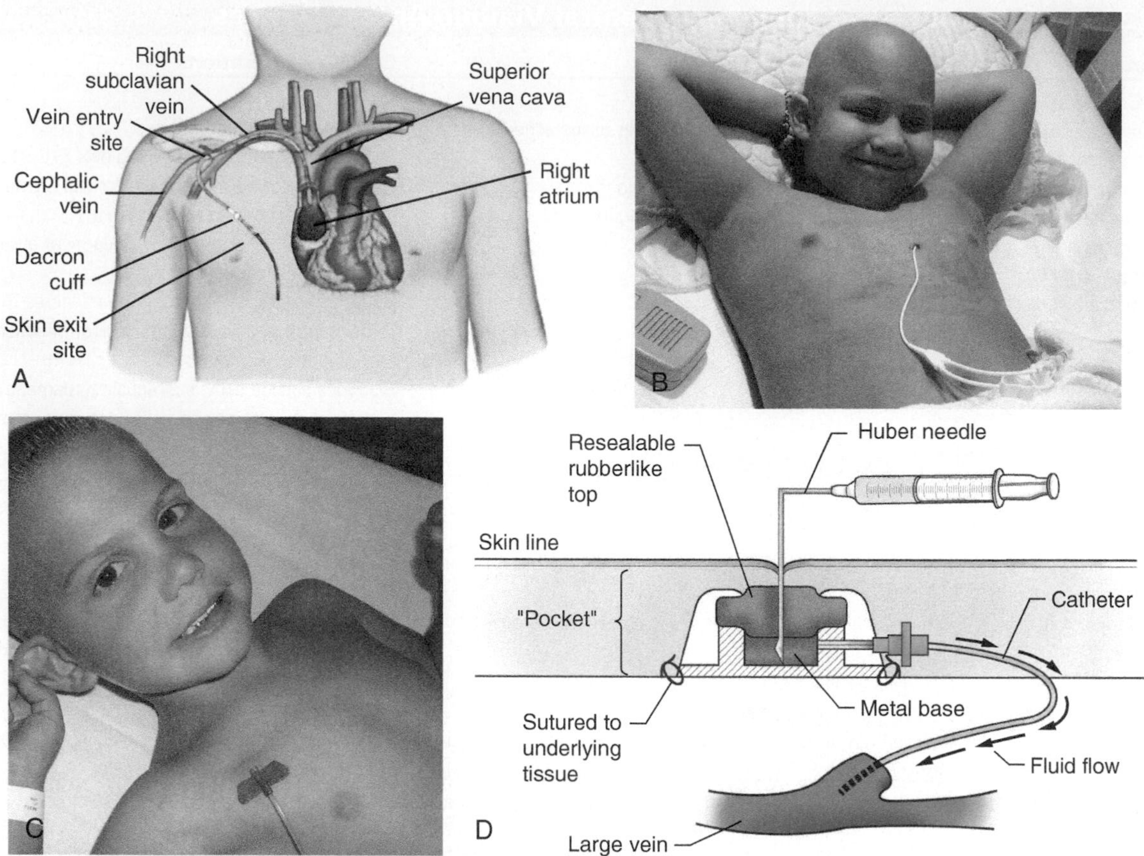

FIG. 22.14 Venous access devices. **A,** External central venous catheter insertion and exit site. **B,** Child with an external central venous catheter (dressing removed for photo). **C,** Child with an implanted port with a Huber needle in place (dressing removed for photo). **D,** Side view of an implanted port.

Intraosseous Infusion

Situations may occur in which rapid establishment of systemic access is vital and venous access is complicated by peripheral circulatory collapse, hypovolemic shock (secondary to vomiting or diarrhea, burns, or trauma), cardiopulmonary arrest, or other conditions. It is recommended that intraosseous access be obtained if venous access cannot be readily achieved after three unsuccessful attempts or 90 seconds in a pediatric resuscitation (Chameides, Samson, Schexnayder, et al., 2012; Tobias & Ross, 2010). Intraosseous infusion provides a rapid, safe, and lifesaving alternate route for administration of fluids and medications until intravascular access is possible. Health care providers, including physicians, nurses, and paramedics, can secure intraosseous cannulation within 30 to 60 seconds. Some hospitals recommend pediatric advanced life support training before performing this procedure. This procedure is usually reserved for children who are unconscious or for those receiving analgesia because the procedure is painful. Local anesthesia should be used for a semiconscious patient. Contraindications for placement of an intraosseous catheter include concurrent problems involving that extremity, such as skin rash, bone fracture, osteogenesis imperfecta, or osteosarcoma.

A large-bore rigid needle such as an intraosseous needle (e.g., Cook) or a bone marrow aspiration needle (e.g., Jamshidi) is inserted into the medullary cavity of a long bone. The anteromedial aspect of the tibia—1 to 3 cm (0.4 to 1.2 inch) below the tibial tuberosity—is the preferred site for children of all ages because it is flat and has a large marrow cavity. In newborns, the distal third of the femur may be used. The distal tibia is an alternative site. A battery-powered intraosseous needle driver (EZ-IO) is also available for use in prehospital and hospital settings and has a high rate of success in pediatric resuscitation and stabilization (Greene, Bhananker, & Ramaiah, 2012).

Once established, the intraosseous route can be used during resuscitation to administer the same medications that could be given through the IV route. During infusion through an intraosseous needle, monitor the extremity closely for swelling or oozing of fluid at the insertion site. Give particular attention to the dependent tissue of the leg. Extravasation of fluid from the bone marrow may be hidden under the leg. Check for swelling of the entire lower leg when the intraosseous bone marrow needle is in the tibia or ankle, and check the entire upper leg when the intraosseous needle is in the femur. Compartment syndrome has resulted from an infiltrated intraosseous line. Other complications, although rare, include fractures, skin necrosis, osteomyelitis, and cellulitis (Tobias & Ross, 2010).

Once the intraosseous needle is in place, it should stand alone and feel secure. The needle should be secured using tape and gauze. If a bone marrow aspirate needle is used, gauze should be built up around the needle to provide support and prevent trauma or dislodgment. Drugs may be pushed and fluids delivered via an infusion pump. The intraosseous line may be discontinued after IV access has been achieved.

MAINTAINING FLUID BALANCE

MEASUREMENT OF INTAKE AND OUTPUT

Accurate measurements of fluid intake and output (I&O) are essential to the assessment of fluid balance. Measurements from all sources—including gastrointestinal, parenteral, urine, stools, vomitus, fistulas, NG suction, sweat, and drainage from wounds—must be included in assessment of fluid balance. Although the provider usually indicates when I&O measurements are to be recorded, it is a nursing responsibility to keep an accurate I&O record on children in certain situations, including the following:

- Receiving IV therapy
- Recently underwent major surgery
- Receiving diuretic or corticosteroid therapy
- With severe thermal burns or injuries
- With renal disease or damage
- With congestive heart failure
- With dehydration
- With diabetes mellitus
- With oliguria
- In respiratory distress
- With chronic lung disease

Infants and small children who are unable to use a bedpan and those who have bowel movements with every voiding require the application of a collecting device. If collecting bags are not used, wet diapers or pads are carefully weighed to ascertain the amount of fluid lost. This includes liquid stool, vomitus, and other losses. The volume of fluid in milliliters is equivalent to the weight of the fluid measured in grams. The specific gravity as a measure of osmolality assists in assessing the degree of hydration.

NURSING TIP

Remember: 1 g of wet diaper weight = 1 ml of urine.

In infants with diapers, weigh all dry diapers to be used and note in an indelible marker the dry weight of the diaper; when there is fluid (urine or liquid stool) in the diaper, the amount of output can be approximated by subtracting the weight of the dry diaper from the weighed amount of the wet diaper.

Disadvantages of the weighed-diaper method of fluid measurement include (1) an inability to differentiate one type of loss from another because of admixture, (2) loss of urine or liquid stool from leakage or evaporation (especially if the infant is under a radiant warmer), and (3) additional fluid in the diaper (superabsorbent disposable type) from absorption of atmospheric moisture (in high-humidity incubators).

Special Needs When the Child Is Not Permitted to Take Fluids by Mouth

Infants or children who are unable or not permitted to take fluids by mouth (NPO) have special needs. To ensure that they are not inadvertently given oral fluids, a sign can be placed in some obvious place, such as over their beds or on their shirts, to alert caregivers and other hospital personnel to the NPO status. To prevent the temptation to drink, fluids should not be left at the bedside. Older children may try to sneak a drink when out of sight of caregivers, so nurses would be wise to keep an eye on NPO children if they go into bathrooms or other locations where they are not easily observed.

Oral hygiene, a part of routine hygienic care, is especially important when fluids are restricted or withheld. For young children who cannot brush their teeth or rinse their mouth without swallowing fluid, the mouth and teeth can be cleaned and kept moist by swabbing with saline-moistened gauze.

NURSING TIP

To keep the mouth feeling moist when the child is NPO, give ice chips (if this is permitted by the provider) or spray the mouth from an atomizer. To meet the need to suck, infants are provided with a safe commercial pacifier.

The child who is fluid restricted presents an equal challenge. Limiting fluids is often more difficult for the child than being NPO, especially when IV fluids are also eliminated. To make certain the child does not drink the entire allotted amount early in the day, the total daily amount is calculated, then divided to provide fluids at periodic intervals throughout the child's waking hours. Serving the fluids in small containers gives the illusion of larger servings. No extra liquid is left at the bedside.

PARENTERAL FLUID THERAPY

Site and Equipment

The site selected for peripheral IV infusion depends on accessibility and convenience. Although it is possible to use any accessible site in older children, the child's developmental, cognitive, and mobility needs must be considered when selecting a site. Ideally, in older children, the superficial veins of the forearm should be used, leaving the hands free. An older child can help select the site and thereby maintain some measure of control. For veins in the extremities, it is best to start with the most distal site and avoid the child's favored hand to reduce the disability related to the procedure. Restrict the child's movements as little as possible, and avoid a site over a joint in an extremity, such as the antecubital space. In small infants, a superficial vein of the hand, wrist, forearm, foot, or ankle is usually most convenient and most easily stabilized (Fig. 22.15). Foot veins should be avoided in children learning to walk and in children already walking. Superficial veins of the scalp have no valves, insertion is easy, and they can be used in infants up to about 9 months of age, but they should be used only when other site attempts have failed.

A transilluminator (Fig. 22.16), also known as near-infrared imaging, aids in finding and evaluating veins for access. Although not as powerful as ultrasound, a transilluminator requires minimal training and experience to use (Bahl, Pandurangadu, Tucker, et al., 2016). Small veins that may not be visible or palpable (especially in infants and toddlers) are often more readily visualized using a transilluminator. The cephalic vein in the proximal forearm may be the optimal vein for ultrasound-guided placement (Takeshita, Nakayama, Nakajima, et al., 2015). Because veins stand out so clearly with transillumination, they appear more superficial than they are. Although visualization of veins is improved with transillumination, an increase in successful venipuncture is not guaranteed (Rothbart, Yu, Müller-Lobeck, et al., 2015). Some devices require assistance to hold in place. Commercial devices have not caused burns in infants or children. Practice in this technique is necessary for optimal outcomes (Stolz, Cappa, Minckler, et al., 2016).

Selection of a scalp vein may require clipping the hair in the area around the site to better visualize the vein and provide a smoother surface on which to tape the catheter hub and tubing. Clipping a portion of the infant's hair may be upsetting to parents; therefore they should be told what to expect and be reassured that the hair will grow back. Remove as little hair as possible directly over the insertion site and taping surface. Save the clipped hair because parents often wish to keep it. A rubber band slipped onto the head from brow to occiput will

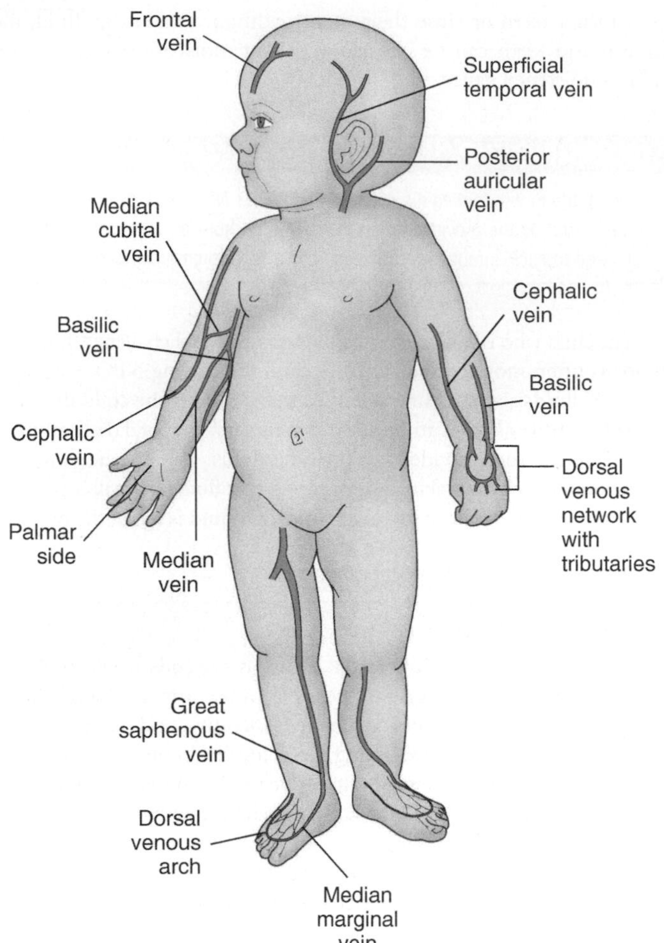

FIG. 22.15 Preferred sites for venous access in infants.

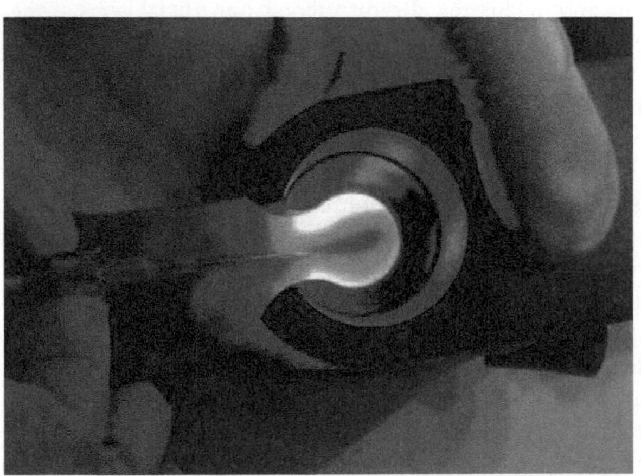

FIG. 22.16 Transilluminator: low-heat light-emitting diode (LED) light placed on the skin to illuminate veins; an opening allows cannulation of vein. (Professor Mark Waltzman, Children's Hospital, Boston.)

usually suffice as a tourniquet, although if the vessel is visible, a tourniquet may not be necessary.

For most IV infusions in children, a 22- to 24-gauge catheter may be used if therapy is expected to last 6 days or less. The smallest-gauge and shortest-length catheter that will accommodate the prescribed therapy should be chosen. The length of the catheter may be directly related to infection or embolus formation; the shorter the catheter, the fewer the complications. The gauge of the catheter should be sufficient to maintain adequate flow of the IV fluids into the cannulated vein, while allowing adequate blood flow around the catheter walls to promote proper hemodilution of the infusate.

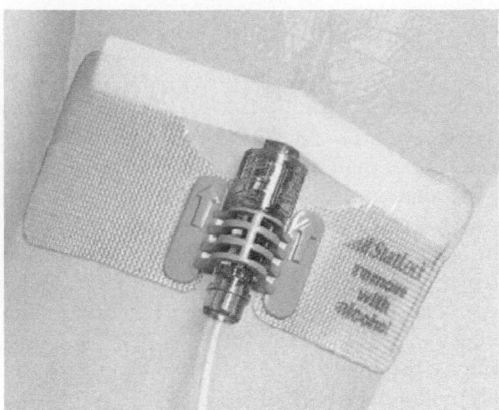

FIG. 22.17 StatLock securement devices enhance peripheral intravenous line dwell time and decrease phlebitis.

NURSING TIP

A tab of tape should be placed on the rubber band to help grasp it when removing it from the infant's head. The rubber band should be cut to avoid accidentally dislodging the catheter when moving the rubber band over the IV insertion site. The tape tab will lift the rubber band and allow it to be cut. Hold the rubber band in two places and cut between these areas to prevent the rubber band from snapping on the head.

Determining the best catheter for the patient early in the therapy provides the best chance of avoiding catheter-related complications. As the duration of therapy increases, decisions regarding the type of infusion device (short peripheral, midline, PICC, or central venous catheter) should be explored. Guidelines such as flowcharts and algorithms are available to help in these decisions.

SECUREMENT OF A PERIPHERAL INTRAVENOUS LINE

Catheters must be stabilized for easy monitoring and evaluation of the access site, to promote delivery of therapy, and to prevent damage, dislodgement, or migration of the catheter (Infusion Nurses Society, 2011; Registered Nurses' Association of Ontario, 2008).

To maintain the integrity of the IV line, adequate protection of the site is required. The catheter hub is firmly secured at the puncture site with a transparent dressing and commercial securement device (e.g., StatLock) (Fig. 22.17) or clear nonallergenic tape. Transparent dressings are ideal because the insertion site is easily observed. Minimal tape should be used at the puncture site and on 1 to 2 inches of skin beyond the site to avoid obscuring the insertion site for early detection of infiltration. The catheter insertion site and 1 to 2 inches along the vein proximal to the site should be readily visible so the area can be monitored for signs of infiltration, irritation, or leakage.

A protective cover is applied directly over the catheter hub at the insertion site to protect the catheter from accidental dislodgement. Easy access to the IV site for frequent (hourly) assessments must be considered (Infusion Nurses Society, 2011). Improvised plastic cups that are cut in half with tape-covered edges should not be used because they have injured patients. A commercial site protector (e.g., I.V. House) is available in different sizes (Fig. 22.18). Its ventilation holes prevent moisture

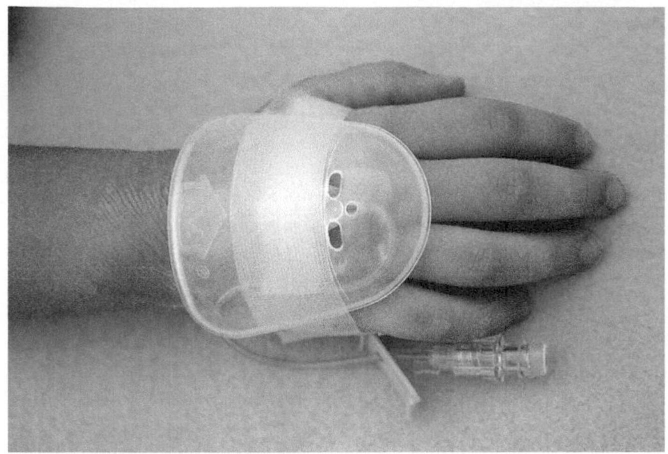

FIG. 22.18 I.V. House used to protect the intravenous site.

from accumulating under the dome. This device is designed to protect the IV site and allow for visibility of the site. The device also minimizes use of padded boards, splints, or other restraints and tape and maintains skin integrity. The connector tubing or extension tubing can be looped to make it small enough to fit under the protective cover to prevent accidental snagging of the catheter. It is important to safely secure the IV tubing to prevent infants and children from becoming entangled in the tubing and accidentally pulling out the catheter or needle. Securing the tubing in this manner also eliminates movement of the catheter hub at the insertion site (mechanical manipulation). A colorful and interesting sticker can be applied to the protecting device to add a positive note to the procedure.

Finger and toe areas are left uncovered by dressings or tape to allow for assessment of circulation. The thumb is never immobilized because of the risk of developing contractures with prolonged limitation of movement. An extremity should never be encircled with tape. The use of roll gauze, self-adhering stretch bandages (Coban), and Ace bandages should also be avoided because these products can cause constriction and hide signs of infiltration.

! NURSING ALERT

Opaque covering should be avoided; however, if any type of opaque covering is used to secure the IV line, the insertion site and extremity distal to the site should be visible to detect an infiltration. If these sites are not visible, they must be checked frequently to detect problems early.

Traditionally, padded boards and splints have been used to partially immobilize the IV site. Padded boards and splints and restraints were appropriate when metal needles were inserted into the vein to prevent the sharp end from puncturing the vessel, especially at a joint. With the more recent use of soft, pliable catheters, arm or leg boards may not be necessary and have several disadvantages. They can obscure the IV site, can constrict the extremity, may excoriate the underlying tissue and promote infection, can cause a contracture of a joint, can restrict useful movement of the extremity, and are uncomfortable. Unfortunately, no research has been conducted to demonstrate the proposed benefit of increasing dwell time (patency of the IV line). Adequate securement should eliminate the need for padded boards in most circumstances. Older children who are alert and cooperative can usually be trusted to protect the IV site.

SAFETY CATHETERS AND NEEDLELESS SYSTEMS

Needlestick injuries are a serious risk for nurses and other health care professionals who provide IV therapy to their patients. Current technologies, including safety catheters and needleless systems, have minimized the risk of exposure to blood-borne pathogens by needlestick injury. Safety catheters employ retractable needle mechanisms to prevent accidental needlesticks when using over-the-needle peripheral IV catheters.

Needleless IV systems are designed to prevent needlestick injuries during administration of IV push medications and IV piggyback medications. There are three general types of needleless systems, based on how the connector displaces fluid:

- Negative displacement systems, including blunt-tip cannulas for use with preslit injection caps; these cause a backflow of blood into the catheter when a syringe is disconnected.
- Positive displacement systems—a valve system that pushes a small amount of IV fluid back into the cap when disconnecting. This action prevents inadvertent catheter occlusion.
- Neutral displacement systems.

Flushing and disconnection procedures are different for each type of system. There is no way to know which type of mechanism is used by simply looking at the connectors. Therefore the nurse must have an understanding of the mechanics of the system in use at the institution. Some needleless devices can be used with any tubing, but other devices can only be used with compatible IV delivery systems. There is some evidence that positive-pressure systems (blunt cannula systems) are associated with lower CLABSI rates and decrease the risk of catheter-related clots.

! NURSING ALERT

Misconnections of tubing have occurred, resulting in patient deaths. Many needleless IV systems allow other types of tubing such as blood pressure and oxygen tubing to connect and instill air directly into the IV line. Before tubing is connected or reconnected to a patient, trace it completely from the patient to the point of origin for verification.

INFUSION PUMPS

A variety of infusion pumps are available and used in nearly all pediatric infusions to accurately administer medication and minimize the possibility of overloading the circulation. It is important to calculate the amount to be infused in a given length of time, set the infusion rate, and monitor the apparatus frequently (at least every 1 to 2 hours) to make certain that the desired rate is maintained, the integrity of the system remains intact, the site remains intact (free of redness, edema, infiltration, or irritation), and the infusion does not stop. Smart infusion pump technology provides built-in safety features that can alert nurses when pump settings are outside of programmed parameters, thereby reducing infusion errors and improving patient safety. Smart pump software within the infusion pump is programmed with dose and infusion rate information for commonly used drugs. The smart pump can recognize drug information in its database, check dosing, calculate infusions, monitor line pressure, and report errors back to nursing.

Continuous infusion pumps, although convenient and efficient, are not without risks. Overreliance on the accuracy of the machine can cause either too much or too little fluid to be infused; therefore its use does not eliminate careful periodic assessment by the nurse. Excess pressure can build up if the machine is set at a rate faster than the vein is able to accommodate (or if the machine continues to pump when the catheter is no longer in the vein).

> **! NURSING ALERT**
>
> Consider the child's age, development, and neurologic status, as well as the predictability of the child (how the child responds to painful treatments), when determining the need for assistance to maintain safety. Manual removal of tape is the preferred method. Only if absolutely necessary should a small cut be made in the tape, using bandage scissors, to facilitate its removal. Before cutting the tape:
>
> - Ensure that all fingers and toes are visible.
> - Remove any barrier that hinders visibility, such as a protective covering.
> - Protect the child's skin and digits by sliding your own finger(s) between the tape and the child's skin so the scissors do not touch the patient.
> - Cut on the tape on the medial aspect (thumb side) of the extremity.

MAINTENANCE

In a consensus guideline of 16 organizations and professional associations, the following maintenance recommendations were made for central venous catheters (O'Grady, Alexander, Burns, et al., 2011):

- Use transparent dressings to allow site visualization. If diaphoresis, bleeding, or oozing prevents adequate adhesion, gauze dressings can be used.
- Replace any dressing when damp, visibly soiled, or loose. Routinely replace transparent dressings every 7 days and gauze dressings every 2 days unless the risk of central catheter dislodgement outweighs the benefits of the dressing change.
- During dressing changes, use chlorhexidine to cleanse skin surrounding central lines and use chlorhexidine, tincture of iodine, an iodophor, or alcohol surrounding peripheral lines. No recommendations can be made for the use of chlorhexidine in infants younger than 2 months of age.
- Chlorhexidine-impregnated sponge dressings should be used for short-term central catheters in patients older than 2 months when central line–associated bloodstream rates are not decreasing with other efforts, such as chlorhexidine skin cleansing, maximum sterile barrier precautions during insertion, and staff education.
- Do not apply ointments to the insertion site; they promote fungal growth and antimicrobial resistance.
- Replace IV administration sets at the following frequencies:
  - Continuous infusions of crystalloids at no less than 96-hour intervals, but at least every 7 days
  - Blood product or lipid emulsion sets within 24 hours of starting the infusion
  - Propofol sets every 6 to 12 hours and when the vial is changed
- No recommendation was made on the frequency of intermittent set changes.
- Include all needleless components (including injection caps at the catheter hub) in administration set changes.
- In pediatric patients, peripheral IV catheters may remain in place until a complication occurs or the therapy is complete.
- Promptly remove temporary central catheters or peripheral IV catheters as soon as they are no longer needed.

COMPLICATIONS

The same precautions regarding maintenance of asepsis, prevention of infection, and observation for infiltration are carried out with patients of any age. However, infiltration is more difficult to detect in infants and small children than in adults. The increased amount of subcutaneous fat and the amount of tape used to secure the catheter often obscure the early signs of infiltration. When the fluid appears to be infusing too slowly or ceases, the usual assessment for obstruction within the apparatus—kinks, screw clamps, shutoff valve, and positioning interference (e.g., a bent elbow)—often locates the difficulty. When these actions fail to detect the problem, it may be necessary to carefully remove some of the dressing to obtain a clear view of the venipuncture site. Dependent areas, such as the palm and undersides of the extremity or the occiput and behind the ears, should be examined because infiltrations in these areas may not be readily visible.

Whenever possible, the hospital identification (ID) band (or bracelet) should not be placed on the same extremity where a peripheral IV site is located. The ID band can act like a tourniquet, preventing adequate venous return, resulting in serious circulatory impairment. To check for return blood flow through the catheter, the tubing is removed from the infusion pump, and the bag is lowered below the level of the infusion site. Resistance during flushing or aspiration for blood return also indicates that the IV infusion may have infiltrated surrounding tissue. A good blood return, or lack thereof, is not always an indicator of infiltration in small infants. Flushing the catheter and observing for edema, redness, or streaking along the vein are appropriate methods for assessment of the IV patency.

IV therapy in pediatrics can be difficult to maintain because of mechanical factors such as vascular trauma resulting from the catheter, the insertion site, vessel size, vessel fragility, pump pressure, the patient's activity level, operator skill and insertion technique, forceful administration of boluses of fluid, and infusion of irritants or vesicants through a small vessel. These factors cause infiltration and extravasation injuries. **Infiltration** is defined as inadvertent administration of a nonvesicant solution or medication into surrounding tissue. **Extravasation** is defined as inadvertent administration of vesicant solution or medication into surrounding tissue (Infusion Nurses Society, 2011). A **vesicant** or **sclerosing agent** causes varying degrees of cellular damage when even minute amounts escape into surrounding tissue. Guidelines are available for determining the severity of tissue injury by staging characteristics, such as the amount of redness, blanching, the amount of swelling, pain, the quality of pulses below infiltration, capillary refill, and warmth or coolness of the area (Infusion Nurses Society, 2011).*

Treatment of infiltration or extravasation varies according to the type of drug involved. Guidelines are available outlining the sequence of interventions and specific treatment of infiltration or extravasation with antidotes.

> **! NURSING ALERT**
>
> When infiltration or extravasation is observed (signs include erythema, pain, edema, blanching, streaking on the skin along the vein, and darkened area at the insertion site), immediately stop the infusion, elevate the extremity, notify the provider, and initiate the ordered treatment as soon as possible. Remove the IV line when it is no longer needed (e.g., after infusing an antidote).

Phlebitis, or inflammation of the vessel wall, may also develop in children who require IV therapy. There are three types of phlebitis: mechanical (caused by rapid infusion rate, manipulation of the IV), chemical (caused by medications), and bacterial (caused by staphylococcal organisms). The initial sign of phlebitis is erythema (redness) at the insertion site. Pain may or may not be present.

---

*Guidelines for determining tissue injury severity are available from the Infusion Nurses Society, 315 Norwood Park South, Norwood, MA 02062; 781-440-9408; http://www.ins1.org.

Peripheral IV catheters are the most commonly used intravascular device. Heavy cutaneous colonization of the insertion site is the single most important predictor of catheter-related infection with all types of short-term, percutaneously inserted catheters. Phlebitis, largely a mechanical rather than infectious process, remains the most important complication associated with the use of peripheral venous catheters.*

! NURSING ALERT

The most effective ways to prevent infection of an IV site are to cleanse hands between each patient, wear gloves when inserting a catheter, and closely inspect the insertion site and physical condition of the dressing. Proper education of the patient and family regarding signs and symptoms of an infected site can help with early detection of infection.

REMOVAL OF A PERIPHERAL INTRAVENOUS LINE

When the time comes to discontinue an IV infusion, many children are distressed by the thought of catheter removal. Therefore they need a careful explanation of the process and suggestions for helping. Encouraging children to remove or help remove the tape from the site provides them with a measure of control and often fosters their cooperation. The procedure consists of turning off any pump apparatus, occluding the IV tubing, removing the tape, pulling the catheter out of the vessel in the opposite direction of insertion, and exerting firm pressure at the site. A dry dressing (adhesive bandage strip) is placed over the puncture site. The use of adhesive-removal pads can decrease the pain of tape removal, but the skin should be washed after use to avoid irritation. To remove transparent dressings (e.g., OpSite, Tegaderm), pull the opposing edges parallel to the skin to loosen the bond. Hand sanitizer can be applied over the top of the dressing to help loosen the adhesive and allow the dressing to come off more easily. Inspect the catheter tip after removal, to ensure that the catheter is intact and that no portion remains in the vein.

When removing the needle from an implanted port, the line should be flushed with 5 ml of heparin, 100 units/ml, before removal of the needle, to ensure patency during the interim between accesses.

Nontunneled central lines can be removed by specially trained nurses with orders by provider. Tunneled lines and implanted ports should be removed by the surgical team.

RECTAL ADMINISTRATION

The rectal route for administration of medications is useful when a child is unable to take oral medications due to vomiting, altered gastrointestinal motility, or altered mental status. Advantages to medication administration via the rectal route include no need to coax a child to swallow unpleasant tasting medications, and relative ease of accessibility for giving medications during an emergency if the patient is unconscious or vomiting and there is no venous access. Some of the drugs available in suppository form are acetaminophen, aspirin, sedatives, analgesics (morphine), antiemetics, and laxatives. Absorption by rectal mucosa is dependent on several factors, including gut motility, amount of time that the drug remains in the rectum, and amount of stool present at time of drug administration. The difficulty in using the rectal route is that unless the rectum is empty at the time of insertion, the absorption of the drug may be delayed, diminished, or prevented by the presence of feces. Sometimes the drug is later evacuated, securely surrounded by stool. If the patient is neutropenic, immunosuppressed, or thrombocytopenic, the rectal route may be contraindicated due to risk of introducing bacteria into the bloodstream.

When preparing to administer medication by the rectal route, first remove the wrapping on the suppository and lubricate the suppository with warm water (water-soluble jelly may hinder medication absorption). Have the child lie on the side with top leg flexed; alternatively, the child can lie prone. Provide developmentally appropriate distraction for the child during the procedure. Rectal suppositories are traditionally inserted with the apex (pointed end) foremost. Reverse contractions or the pressure gradient of the anal canal may help the suppository slip higher into the canal. Using a gloved hand or finger cot, quickly but gently insert the suppository into the rectum beyond both of the rectal sphincters. Then hold the buttocks together firmly to relieve pressure on the anal sphincter until the urge to expel the suppository has passed, which occurs within 5 to 10 minutes. Sometimes the amount of drug ordered is less than the dose available. The irregular shape of most suppositories makes the process of dividing them into a desired dose difficult if not dangerous. If the suppository must be halved, it should be cut lengthwise. However, there is no guarantee that the drug is evenly dispersed throughout the glycerin base.

If medication is administered via a retention enema, the same procedure is used. Drugs given by enema are diluted in the smallest amount of solution possible to minimize the likelihood of being evacuated.

OPTIC, OTIC, AND NASAL ADMINISTRATION

There are few differences in administering eye, ear, and nose medication to children and to adults. The major difficulty is in gaining children's cooperation. Older children need only an explanation and direction. Although the administration of optic, otic, and nasal medication is not painful, these drugs can cause unpleasant sensations, which can be eliminated with various techniques.

To instill eye medication, place the child supine or sitting with the head extended and ask the child to look up. Use one hand to pull the lower eyelid downward; the hand that holds the dropper rests on the head so that it may move synchronously with the child's head, thus reducing the possibility of trauma to a struggling child or dropping medication on the face (Fig. 22.19). When the lower eyelid is pulled down, a small conjunctival sac is formed; apply the solution or ointment to this area rather than directly on the eyeball. If applying an ointment, start at the inner canthus and move outward. Another effective technique is to pull the lower eyelid down and out to form a cup effect, into which the medication is dropped. Take care not to touch the tip of the dropper to the eyeball. Gently close the eyelids to prevent expression of the medication. Wipe excess medication from the inner canthus outward to prevent contamination to the contralateral eye.

NURSING TIP

To reduce unpleasant sensations when administering medications:

- **Eye**—Apply finger pressure to the lacrimal punctum at the inner aspect of the eyelid for 1 minute to prevent drainage of medication to the nasopharynx and the unpleasant "tasting" of the drug.
- **Ear**—Allow medications stored in the refrigerator to warm to room temperature before instillation.
- **Nose**—Position the child with the head hyperextended to prevent strangling sensations caused by medication trickling into the throat rather than up into the nasal passages.

*Guidelines for prevention of intravascular device–related infections are available from the Centers for Disease Control and Prevention, 1600 Clifton Road, Atlanta, GA 30333; 404-639-1515; http://www.cdc.gov/ncidod/dhqp/gl_intravascular.html.

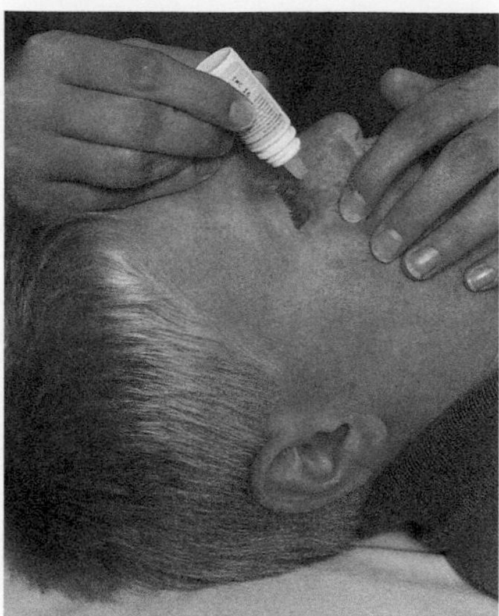

FIG. 22.19 Administering eye drops.

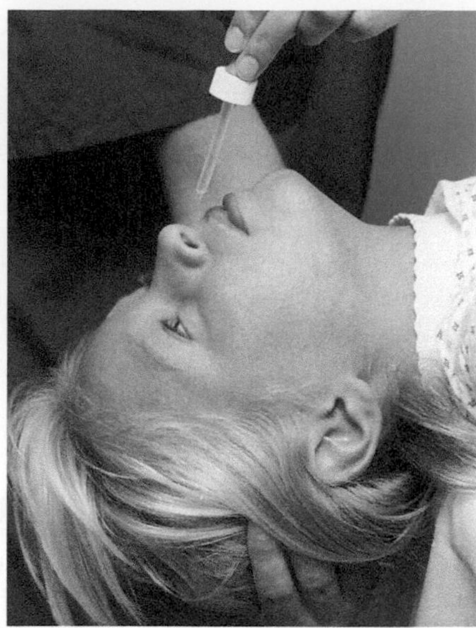

FIG. 22.20 Proper position for instilling nose drops.

Instilling eye drops in infants can be difficult because they often clench the eyelids tightly closed. One approach is to place the drops in the nasal corner where the eyelids meet. The medication pools in this area, and when the child opens the eyelids, the medication flows onto the conjunctiva. For young children, playing a game can be helpful, such as instructing the child to keep the eyes closed to the count of three and then open them, at which time the drops are quickly instilled. Ointment can be applied by gently pulling down the lower eyelid and placing the ointment in the lower conjunctival sac.

DRUG ALERT

If both eye ointment and drops are ordered, give drops first, wait 3 minutes, and then apply the ointment to allow each drug to work. When possible, administer eye ointments before bedtime or naptime because the child's vision will be blurred temporarily.

Ear drops are instilled with the child in the prone or supine position and the head turned to the appropriate side. To avoid uncomfortable stimulation of vertigo, ensure that ear medications are at room temperature before instilling. For children younger than 3 years of age, the external auditory canal is straightened by gently pulling the pinna downward and straight back. The pinna is pulled upward and back in children older than 3 years of age. To place the drops deep into the ear canal without contaminating the tip of the dropper, place a disposable ear speculum in the canal and administer the drops through the speculum. Position the bottle so that the drops fall against the side of the ear canal. After instillation, the child should remain lying on the unaffected side for a few minutes. Gentle massage of the area immediately anterior to the ear facilitates the entry of drops into the ear canal. The use of cotton pledgets prevents medication from flowing out of the external canal. However, they should be loose enough to allow any discharge to exit from the ear. Premoistening the cotton with a few drops of medication prevents the wicking action from absorbing the medication instilled in the ear.

Nose drops are instilled in the same manner as in the adult patient. Remove mucus from the nose with a clean tissue or a washcloth. Unpleasant sensations associated with medicated nose drops are minimized when care is taken to position the child with the head extended well over the edge of the bed or pillow (Fig. 22.20). Depending on size, infants can be positioned in the football hold (see Fig. 22.4, *B*), in the nurse's arm with the head extended and stabilized between the nurse's body and elbow and the arms and hands immobilized with the nurse's hands, or with the head extended over the edge of the bed or a pillow. Insert nasal spray dispensers into the naris vertically and then angle them to avoid trauma to the septum and to direct medication toward the inferior turbinate. After instillation of the drops, the child should remain in position for 1 minute to allow the drops to come in contact with the nasal surfaces.

AEROSOL THERAPY

Aerosol therapy can be an effective method for administering medication directly into the airway. Bronchodilators, steroids, mucolytics, and antibiotics, suspended in particulate form, can be inhaled so that the medication reaches the small airways. This route of administration can be useful in avoiding the systemic side effects of certain drugs and in reducing the amount of drug necessary to achieve the desired effect. Aerosol therapy is particularly challenging in children who are too young to cooperate with controlling the rate and depth of breathing. Administration of aerosolized medications to children requires skill, patience, and creativity. Because many children with airway diseases, such as asthma, use aerosol therapies on a regular basis, it is important for families to have an understanding of the home plan of care, including drugs to use for maintenance and drugs to use for rescue.

Breath sounds and work of breathing should be assessed before and after treatments. Young children who become upset by having a mask held close to the face may become fatigued with fighting the procedure and may actually appear worse during and immediately after the therapy. It may be necessary to spend a few minutes calming the child after the procedure and allowing the vital signs to return to baseline to accurately assess changes in breath sounds and work of breathing.

FAMILY TEACHING AND HOME CARE

The nurse usually assumes responsibility for preparing families to administer medications at home. The family should understand why the child is receiving the medication and the effects that might be

DRUG ALERT

Medications can be aerosolized or nebulized with air or with oxygen-enriched gas. The **metered-dose inhaler (MDI)** is a self-contained, handheld device that allows for intermittent delivery of a specified amount of medication. Many bronchodilators are available in this form and are successfully used by children with asthma. A **spacer device** attached to the MDI can help with coordination of breathing and aerosol delivery. It also allows the aerosolized particles to remain in suspension longer. For nebulized administration, a handheld nebulizer discharges a medicated mist through a mouthpiece or a small plastic mask, which the child holds over the nose and mouth. To avoid particle deposition in the nose and pharynx, the child is instructed to take slow, deep breaths through an open mouth during the treatment. For home use, an air compressor is necessary to force air through the liquid medication to form the aerosol. Compact, portable units can be obtained from health equipment companies.

expected, as well as the amount, frequency, and length of time the drug is to be administered. Instruction should be carried out in an unhurried, relaxed manner, preferably in an area away from a busy ward or office.

Instruct the caregiver carefully regarding the correct dosage. Some persons have difficulty understanding medical terminology, and just because they nod or otherwise indicate they understand, the nurse should not assume that the message is clear. It is important to be certain they have acceptable devices for measuring the drug. If the drug is packaged with a dropper, syringe, or plastic cup, the nurse should show or mark the point on the device that indicates the prescribed dose and demonstrate how the dose is drawn up into a dropper or syringe, measured, and the bubbles eliminated. To allow an opportunity to demonstrate their understanding of the skills required, caregivers should always perform return demonstration before returning home. This is essential when the drug has potentially serious consequences from incorrect dosage, such as insulin or digoxin, or when more complex administration is required, such as parenteral injections. When teaching a parent to give an injection, the nurse must ensure that the caregivers have adequate time for instruction and practice.

Home modifications are often necessary because the availability of equipment or assistance can differ from the hospital setting. For example, the parent may need guidance in devising methods that allow one person to hold the child and safely give the drug.

NURSING TIP

To administer oral, nasal, or optic medication when only one person is available to hold the child, and the child is unable to cooperate, use the following procedure:

- Place child supine on a flat surface (e.g., bed, couch, floor).
- Sit facing child so child's head is between operator's thighs and child's arms are under operator's legs.
- Place lower legs over child's legs to restrain lower body, if necessary.
- To administer oral medication, place a small pillow under child's head to reduce risk of aspiration.
- To administer nasal medication, place a small pillow under child's shoulders to aid flow of liquid through nasal passages.

The nurse should clarify with parents the time that the drug is to be administered. For instance, when a drug is prescribed in association with meals, the number of meals that the family is accustomed to eating influences the amount of drug the child receives. Does the family have meals twice a day or five times a day? When a drug is to be given several times during the day, together the nurse and parents can work out a schedule that accommodates the family's routine. This is particularly significant if a drug must be given at equal intervals throughout a 24-hour period. For example, telling parents that the child needs 1 tsp of medicine four times a day is subject to misinterpretation because the parents may routinely schedule the doses at incorrect times. Instead, a preplanned schedule based on 6-hour intervals should be set up with the number of days required for the therapeutic dosage listed. Modification should also be made to accommodate sleep schedules. Written instructions should accompany all drug prescriptions.

NURSING TIP

If parents have difficulty reading or if there is a language barrier, use colors and/or pictures to convey instructions. For example, mark each drug with a color and place the appropriate color on a calendar chart or on a drawing of a clock to identify when the drug needs to be given. If a liquid medication and syringe are used, also mark the syringe at the place the plunger needs to be with color-coded tape. Several websites and phone applications are available to help create patient-specific medication calendars.

NASOGASTRIC, OROGASTRIC, AND GASTROSTOMY ADMINISTRATION

When a child has an indwelling feeding tube or a gastrostomy, oral medications are usually given via that route. An advantage of this method is the ability to administer oral medications around the clock without disturbing the child. A disadvantage is the risk of occluding, or clogging, the tube, especially when giving viscous solutions through small-bore feeding tubes. The most important preventive measure is adequate flushing after the medication is instilled (see Applying Evidence to Practice box).

ALTERNATIVE FEEDING TECHNIQUES

Some children are unable to take nourishment by mouth because of anomalies of the throat, esophagus, or bowel; impaired swallowing capacity; severe debilitation; respiratory distress; or unconsciousness. These children are frequently fed by way of a tube inserted orally or nasally into the stomach (**orogastric** [OG] or **NG gavage**) or duodenum-jejunum (**enteral gavage**) or by a tube inserted directly into the stomach (**gastrostomy**) or jejunum (**jejunostomy**). Such feedings may be intermittent or by continuous drip. Feeding resistance, a problem that may result from any long-term feeding method that bypasses the mouth, is discussed in Chapter 8. During gavage or gastrostomy feedings, infants are given a pacifier. Nonnutritive sucking has several advantages, such as increased weight gain and decreased crying. However, only pacifiers with a safe design can be used to prevent the possibility of aspiration. Using improvised pacifiers made from bottle nipples is not a safe practice.

When a child is concurrently receiving continuous-drip gastric or enteral feedings and parenteral (IV) therapy, the potential exists for inadvertent administration of the enteral formula through the circulatory system. The possibility for error increases when the parenteral solution is a fat emulsion, a milky-appearing substance. Safeguards to prevent this potentially serious error include the following:

- Be sure that the feeding bag and all tubings are cleaned on a regular basis, according to the manufacturer's recommendations.
- Use enteral-specific connectors (ENFit) that are not compatible with Luer or needleless connections used for IV tubing (Guenter & Lyman, 2016).

APPLYING EVIDENCE TO PRACTICE

Nasogastric, Orogastric, or Gastrostomy Medication Administration in Children

Use elixir or suspension (rather than tablet) preparations of medication whenever possible.
Dilute viscous medication or syrup with a small amount of water if possible.
If administering tablets, crush tablet to a fine powder and dissolve drug in a small amount of warm water.
Never crush enteric-coated or sustained-release tablets or capsules.
Avoid oily medications because they tend to cling to side of tube.
Do not mix medication with enteral formula unless fluid is restricted. If adding a drug:
- Check with pharmacist for compatibility and appropriateness of route (some medications, such as tacrolimus and ursodiol, cannot be given via enteral feeding route).
- Shake formula well and observe for any physical reaction (e.g., separation, precipitation).
- Label formula container with name of medication, dosage, date, and time infusion started.

Check for correct placement of nasogastric or orogastric tube (see Translating Evidence into Practice box).
Attach syringe (with adaptable tip but without plunger) to tube.
Pour medication into syringe.
Unclamp tube and allow medication to flow by gravity.
Adjust height of container to achieve desired flow rate (e.g., increase height for faster flow).
As soon as syringe is empty, pour in water to flush tubing.
- Amount of water depends on length and gauge of tubing.
- Determine amount before administering any medication by using a syringe to fill completely an unused nasogastric or orogastric tube with water. Amount of flush solution is usually 1.5 times this volume.
- With certain drug preparations (e.g., suspensions), more fluid may be needed.

If administering more than one drug at the same time, flush tube between each medication with clear water.
Clamp tube after flushing unless tube is left open.

- Use a separate, specifically designed enteral feeding pump mounted on a separate pole for continuous-feeding solutions.
- Label all tubing of continuous enteral feeding with brightly colored tape or labels.
- Use specifically designed continuous-feeding bags to contain the solutions instead of parenteral equipment, such as a burette.
- Whenever access or connections are made, trace the tubing all the way from the patient to the bag to ensure that the correct tubing source is selected.

GAVAGE FEEDING

Infants and children can be fed simply and safely by a tube passed into the stomach through either the nares or the mouth. The tube can be left in place or inserted and removed with each feeding. In older children, it is usually less traumatic to tape the tube securely in place between feedings. For long-term enteral tube feedings, the tube should be removed and replaced with a new tube according to hospital policy, manufacturer recommendations, specific orders, and the type of tube used. Meticulous hand washing is practiced during the procedure to prevent bacterial contamination of the feeding, especially during continuous-drip feedings.

Preparations

The equipment needed for gavage feeding includes the following:

- A suitable tube selected according to the child's size, the viscosity of the solution being fed, and anticipated duration of treatment
- A receptacle for the fluid; for small amounts, a 10- to 30-ml syringe barrel or Asepto syringe is satisfactory; for larger amounts, a 60-ml syringe with a catheter tip is more convenient
- A 10-ml barrel syringe to aspirate stomach contents after the tube has been placed
- Water or water-soluble lubricant to lubricate the tube; sterile water is used for infants
- Paper or other nonallergenic tape to mark the tube and to attach the tube to the infant's or child's cheek (and nose, if placed through the nares)
- pH paper to determine the correct placement in the stomach
- The solution for feeding

Not all feeding tubes are the same. Polyethylene and polyvinylchloride types lose their flexibility and need to be replaced frequently, usually every 3 or 4 days. Polyurethane and silicone tubes remain flexible, so they can remain in place up to 30 days. Advantages of small-bore tubes include a reduced incidence of pharyngitis, otitis media, aspiration, and discomfort. Disadvantages include difficulty during insertion (may require a stylet or metal guide wire), collapse of the tube during aspiration of gastric contents to test for correct placement, dislodgment during forceful coughing, migration out of position, knotting, occlusion, and unsuitability for thick feedings.

Procedure

Infants are easier to control if they are first wrapped in a mummy restraint (see Fig. 22.5, *A*). Even tiny infants with random movements can grasp and dislodge the tube. Preterm infants do not ordinarily require restraint, but if they do, a small blanket folded across the chest and secured beneath the shoulders is usually sufficient. Be careful so that breathing is not compromised.

Whenever possible, the infant should be held and provided with a means for nonnutritive sucking during the procedure to associate the comfort of physical contact with the feeding. When this is not possible, gavage feeding is carried out with the infant or child lying supine or on the right side; the head and chest should be elevated. Feeding the child in a sitting position helps maintain placement of the tube in the lowest position, thus increasing the likelihood of correct placement in the stomach.

Although the most accurate method for testing tube placement is radiography, this practice is not always possible before each feeding. Research indicates that bedside assessment of gastrointestinal aspirate color and pH is useful in predicting feeding tube placement (see Translating Evidence into Practice box). If doubt exists regarding correct placement, consult the provider. The Applying Evidence to Practice box describes the procedure for gavage feeding.

Studies evaluating NG and OG tube length in infants and children found that age-specific methods for predicting the distance based on height are more accurate estimates of internal distance to the stomach (Beckstrand, Ellett, & McDaniel, 2007). A convenient morphologic measurement, the nose-ear-midxiphoid-umbilicus (NEMU) span, approached the accuracy of the age-specific prediction equations and is easy to use in a clinical setting. The best option for older children and when an accurate height is unavailable is to adapt the nose-ear-midxiphoid-umbilicus measurement for NG or OG tube length (Fig. 22.22, *A*) (see Translating Evidence into Practice box).

Ellet and Beckstrand (1999) found significant tube placement errors (43.5%) in a study of 39 hospitalized children. Children who were

TRANSLATING EVIDENCE INTO PRACTICE

Confirming Nasogastric Tube Placement in Pediatric Patients

Ask the Question

PICOT Question

In children, how should correct placement of NG tubes be assessed during hospitalization?

Search for Evidence

Search Strategies

Search selection criteria included English, research-based articles, and children and adolescents requiring NG tube placement. Search areas included aspirate, auscultation and radiology methods, NG tube length prediction methods, age-related height-based methods, and accurate NG tube placement. Searches excluded newborns and preterm infants.

Databases Used

PubMed, Cochrane Collaboration, MDConsult, Joanna Briggs Institute, AHRQ–National Guideline Clearinghouse, TRIP database Plus, PedsCCM, BestBETS

Critical Appraisal of the Evidence

Studies compared various methods used to evaluate correct placement of the NG tube.

Accurate NG tube length measurement:

- Children 8 years, 4 months of age or younger: use age-related height-based (AHRB) equation for NG length predictions.
- Children older than 8 years, 4 months of age; short stature; or when you cannot obtain accurate height: use nose-ear-midxiphoid-umbilicus (NEMU) (Beckstrand, Cirgin Ellett, & McDaniel, 2007).
- No significant difference between AHRB and NEMU methods of tube placement; using nose-ear-xiphoid only resulted in increased risk of misplaced tube (Cirgin Ellet, Cohen, Perkins, et al., 2012).

Radiographs

- Although abdominal x-ray provides confirmation of enteral tube location, the results can sometimes be equivocal. In addition, this method cannot be used for ongoing, frequent placement verification basis due to the risk of radiation exposure to the child (Irving, Lyman, & Northington, 2014). Alternate methods of verification have evidence-based support in the literature (Cincinnati Children's Hospital Medical Center, 2011).

Nonradiologic Verification Methods

- A pH of 5 or less supports that the tip of the tube is in the gastric location (Ellett, Croffie, Cohen, et al., 2005; Huffman, Pieper, Jarczyk, et al., 2004; Nyqvist, Sorell, & Ewald, 2005; Phang, Marsh, Barlows, et al., 2004; Society of Pediatric Nurses Clinical Practice Committee, SPN Research Committee, & Longo, 2011; Westhus, 2004).
- A pH greater than 5 does not reliably predict correct distal tip location. This may indicate respiratory or esophageal placement or the presence of medications to suppress acid secretion. Gastric aspirate pH means are statistically significantly lower compared with means from intestinal and respiratory pH aspirates (Ellett, Croffie, Cohen, et al., 2005; Gilbertson, Rogers, & Ukoumunne, 2011; Phang, Marsh, Barlows, et al., 2004; Society of Pediatric Nurses Clinical Practice Committee, SPN Research Committee, & Longo, 2011; Westhus, 2004).

Visual Inspection of Aspirate

- Visual inspection is less accurate than pH to confirm placement. Aspirate colors are specific to the intended placement location. Gastric contents are clear, off-white, or tan or may be brown-tinged if blood is present. Respiratory secretions may look the same. Intestinal contents are often bile stained, light to dark yellow, or greenish-brown (Phang, Marsh, Barlows, et al., 2004; Society of Pediatric Nurses Clinical Practice Committee, SPN Research Committee, & Longo, 2011; Westhus, 2004).

Enzyme Testing

- Aspirate testing of enzyme levels for bilirubin, pepsin, and trypsin is highly accurate but limited to laboratory assessment (Ellett, Croffie, Cohen, et al., 2005; Westhus, 2004).

CO_2 Monitoring

- CO_2 monitoring is a reliable method to determine incorrect tube placement in the respiratory tract; it requires a capnograph monitor (Ellett, Croffie, Cohen, et al., 2005).
- CO_2 monitoring is useful to determine whether or not the enteral tube is in the respiratory tract; however, CO_2 monitoring does not provide information for determining whether the tube is in the intestines, stomach, or esophagus (Cirgin Ellet, Cohen, Perkins, et al., 2012).

Gastric Auscultation

- Auscultation as a verification tool is reliable only 60% to 80% of the time and should not be used without additional methods (Neumann, Meyer, Dutton, et al., 1995).
- Although evidence shows auscultation alone is not a reliable confirmatory test, it is still widely used by nurses for evaluation of enteral tube placement (Lyman, Kemper, Northington, et al., 2016; Northington, Lyman, Guenter, et al., 2017).
- Using aspirate and nonaspirate NG tube placement verification methods in combination increases the likelihood for accurate NG tube placement to 97% to 99%, similar to the radiologic chest radiography gold standard of 99% (Ellett, Croffie, Cohen, et al., 2005; Phang, Marsh, Barlows, et al., 2004; Society of Pediatric Nurses Clinical Practice Committee, SPN Research Committee, & Longo, 2011; Westhus, 2004).

Electromagnetic Device

- An electromagnetic tracing device demonstrated 100% accuracy in enteral feeding tubes in a study of both adults and children; however, the device requires special training for use and cannot detect enteral tubes smaller than 8 French (Bourgault, Heath, Hooper, et al., 2015; Powers, Luebbehusen, Spitzer, et al., 2011).

Apply the Evidence: Nursing Implications

There is good evidence with strong recommendations (Guyatt, Oxman, Vist, et al., 2008) that a combination of verification methods to confirm NG tube placement will reduce the required number of x-rays in children (Society of Pediatric Nurses Clinical Practice Committee, SPN Research Committee, & Longo, 2011). These methods include pH testing and visual inspection of the pH aspirate. There is also good evidence that improving the accuracy of predicting NG tube length before insertion will enhance the precision of successful NG tube placement. Auscultation is used in combination with other NG tube verification methods. Further investigation of additional noninvasive, user-friendly, portable verification methods is warranted, including ultrasound and electromagnetic tracer (Powers, Luebbehusen, Spitzer, et al., 2011).

Quality and Safety Competencies: Evidence-Based Practice*

Knowledge

Differentiate clinical opinion from research and evidence-based summaries.

Describe the various verification methods to confirm NG tube placement.

Skills

Base individualized care plan on patient values, clinical expertise, and evidence.

Integrate evidence into practice by using the techniques for NG and OG tube placement verification in clinical care.

Continued

TRANSLATING EVIDENCE INTO PRACTICE—cont'd

Confirming Nasogastric Tube Placement in Pediatric Patients

Attitudes

Value the concept of evidence-based practice as integral to determining best clinical practice.

Appreciate the strengths and weakness of evidence for confirming NG tube placement.

NG, Nasogastric; *OG*, orogastric.

References

Beckstrand, J., Cirgin-Ellett, M., & McDaniel, A. (2007). Predicting internal distance to the stomach for positioning nasogastric and orogastric feeding tubes in children. *Journal of Advanced Nursing, 59*, 274–289.

Bourgault, A. M., Heath, J., Hooper, V., et al. (2015). Methods used by critical care nurses to verify feeding tube placement in clinical practice. *Critical Care Nurse, 35*(1), e1–e7.

Cincinnati Children's Hospital Medical Center. (2011). Confirmation of nasogastric/orogastric tube (NGT/OGT) placement—BeST Evidence Statement. Retrieved from https://www.childrensmn.org/departments/webrn/pdf/ng-og-verification-clinical-standard-preview-2015.pdf.

Cirgin Ellett, M. L., Cohen, M. D., Perkins, S. M., et al. (2012). Comparing methods of determining insertion length for placing gastric tubes in children 1 month to 17 years of age. *Journal for Specialists in Pediatric Nursing, 17*(1), 19–32.

Ellett, M. L., Croffie, J. M., Cohen, M. D., et al. (2005). Gastric tube placement in young children. *Clinical Nursing Research, 14*, 238–252.

Gilbertson, H. R., Rogers, E. J., & Ukoumunne, O. C. (2011). Determination of a practical pH cutoff level for reliable confirmation of nasogastric tube placement. *Journal of Parenteral and Enteral Nutrition, 35*(4), 540–544.

Guyatt, G. H., Oxman, A. D., Vist, G. E., et al. (2008). GRADE: An emerging consensus on rating quality of evidence and strength of recommendations. *British Medical Journal, 336*, 924–926.

Huffman, S., Pieper, P., Jarczyk, K. S., et al. (2004). Methods to confirm feeding tube placement: Application of research in practice. *Pediatric Nursing, 30*, 10–13.

Irving, S. Y., Lyman, B., Northington, L., et al. (2014). Nasogastric tube placement and verification in children: Review of the current literature. *Critical Care Nurse, 34*(3), 67–78.

Society of Pediatric Nurses Clinical Practice Committee, SPN Research Committee, & Longo, M. A. (2011). Best evidence: Nasogastric tube placement verification. *Journal of Pediatric Nursing, 26*(4), 373–376.

Lyman, B., Kemper, C., Northington, L., et al. (2016). Use of temporary enteral access devices in hospitalized neonatal and pediatric patients in the United States. *Journal of Parenteral and Enteral Nutrition, 40*(4), 574–580.

Neumann, M. J., Meyer, C. T., Dutton, J. L., et al. (1995). Hold that x-ray: Aspirate pH and auscultation prove tube placement. *Journal of Clinical Gastroenterology, 20*, 293–295.

Northington, L., Lyman, B., Guenter, P., et al. (2017). Current practices in home management of nasogastric tube placement in pediatric patients: A survey of parents and homecare providers. *Journal of Pediatric Nursing, 33*, 46–53.

Nyqvist, K. H., Sorell, A., & Ewald, U. (2005). Litmus tests for verification of feeding tube location in infants: Evaluation of their clinical use. *Journal of Clinical Nursing, 14*, 486–495.

Phang, J. S., Marsh, W. A., Barlows, T. G., et al. (2004). Determining feeding tube location by gastric and intestinal pH values. *Nutrition in Clinical Practice, 19*, 640–644.

Powers, J., Luebbehusen, M., Spitzer, T., et al. (2011). Verification of an electromagnetic device compared with abdominal radiograph to predict accuracy of feeding tube placement. *Journal of Parenteral and Enteral Nutrition, 35*(4), 535–539.

Westhus, N. (2004). Methods to test feeding tube placement in children. *MCN The American Journal of Maternal Child Nursing, 29*, 282–291.

*Adapted from the QSEN at http://www.qsen.org.

APPLYING EVIDENCE TO PRACTICE

Nasogastric Tube Feedings in Children

Place child supine with head slightly hyperflexed or in a sniffing position (nose pointed toward ceiling).

Measure the tube for approximate length of insertion and mark the point with a small piece of tape.

Consider using lidocaine nasal spray to numb the nostril before tube insertion.

Insert a tube that has been lubricated with sterile water or water-soluble lubricant through either the mouth or one of the nares to the predetermined mark. Because most young infants are obligatory nose breathers, insertion through the mouth causes less distress and helps stimulate sucking. In older infants and children, the tube is passed through the nose and alternated between nostrils. An indwelling tube is almost always placed through the nose.

- When using the nose, slip the tube along the base of the nose and direct it straight back toward the occiput.
- When entering through the mouth, direct the tube toward the back of the throat (see Fig. 22.21, *B*).
- If the child is able to swallow on command, synchronize passing the tube with swallowing.

Confirm placement (see Translating Evidence into Practice: Confirming Nasogastric Tube Placement in Pediatric Patients box).

Stabilize the tube by holding or taping it to the cheek, not to the nose or forehead because of possible damage to the nostril. To maintain correct placement, measure and record the amount of tubing extending from the nose or mouth to the distal port when the tube is first positioned. Recheck this measurement before each feeding.

Warm the formula to room temperature. Do *not* microwave! Pour formula into the barrel of the syringe attached to the feeding tube. To start the flow, give a gentle push with the plunger but then remove the plunger and allow the fluid to flow into the stomach by gravity. The rate of flow should not exceed 5 ml every 5 to 10 minutes in premature and very small infants and 10 ml/min in older infants and children to prevent nausea and regurgitation. The rate is determined by the diameter of the tubing and the height of the reservoir containing the feeding and is regulated by adjusting the height of the syringe. A usual feeding may take 15 to 30 minutes to complete.

Flush the tube with sterile water (1 or 2 ml for small tubes to 5 to 15 ml or more for large ones), or see discussion of flushing for administering medication through nasogastric tubes in the Translating Evidence into Practice box to clear it of formula.

Cap or clamp indwelling tubes to prevent loss of feeding.

- If the tube is to be removed, first pinch it firmly to prevent escape of fluid as the tube is withdrawn. Withdraw the tube quickly.

Position the child with the head elevated 30 to 45 degrees or on the right side for 30 to 60 minutes in the same manner as after any infant feeding to minimize the possibility of regurgitation and aspiration. If the child's condition permits, bundle the youngster after the feeding.

Record the feeding, including the type and amount of residual, the type and amount of formula, and how it was tolerated.

- For most infant feedings, any amount of residual fluid aspirated from the stomach is refed to prevent electrolyte imbalance, and the amount is subtracted from the prescribed amount of feeding. For example, if the infant is to receive 30 ml and 10 ml is aspirated from the stomach before the feeding, the 10 ml of aspirated stomach contents is refed along with 20 ml of feeding. Another method can be used in children. If residual fluid is more than one-fourth of the last feeding, return the aspirate and recheck in 30 to 60 minutes. When residual fluid is less than one-fourth of the last feeding, give the scheduled feeding. If large amounts of aspirated fluid persist and the child is due for another feeding, notify the provider.

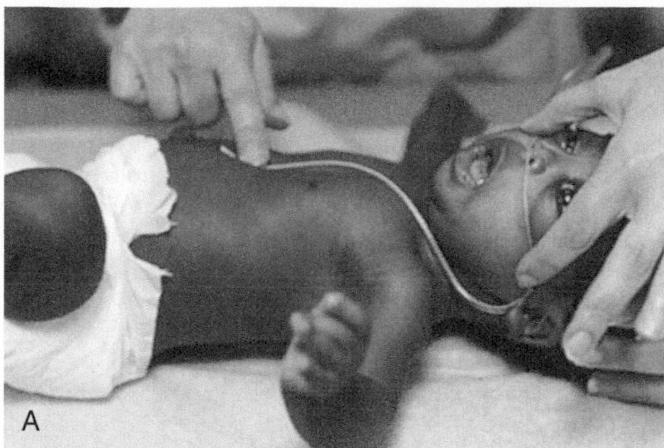

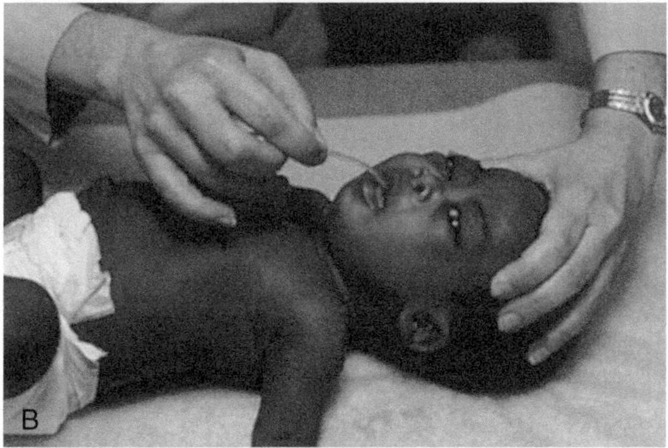

FIG. 22.21 Gavage feeding. **A,** Measuring the tube for orogastric feeding from the tip of the nose to the earlobe and to the midpoint between the end of the xiphoid process and the umbilicus. **B,** Inserting the tube.

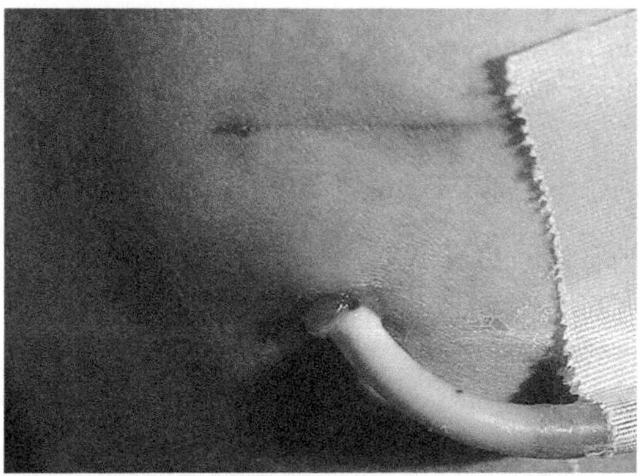

FIG. 22.22 Appearance of healthy granulation tissue around a stoma.

comatose or semicomatose, were inactive, had swallowing difficulty, or had Argyle tubes experienced increased tube placement errors. Findings supported the effectiveness of radiographs in documenting tube placement.

GASTROSTOMY FEEDING

Feeding by way of gastrostomy, or G tube, is often used for children in whom passage of a tube through the mouth, pharynx, esophagus, and cardiac sphincter of the stomach is contraindicated or impossible. It is also used to avoid the constant irritation of an NG tube in children who require tube feeding over an extended period. A gastrostomy tube may be placed with the child under general anesthesia or percutaneously using an endoscope with the patient sedated and under local anesthesia (percutaneous endoscopic gastrostomy). The tube is inserted through the abdominal wall into the stomach about midway along the greater curvature and secured by a purse-string suture. The stomach is anchored to the peritoneum at the operative site. The tube used can be a Foley, wing-tip, or mushroom catheter. Immediately after surgery, the catheter may be left open and attached to gravity drainage for 24 hours or more.

Direct postoperative care of the wound site toward prevention of infection and irritation. Cleanse the area with soap and water at least daily or as often as needed to keep the area free of drainage. After healing, meticulous care is needed to keep the area surrounding the tube clean and dry to prevent excoriation and infection. Exercise care to prevent excessive pull on the catheter that might cause widening of the opening and subsequent leakage of highly irritating gastric juices. Use barrier ointments such as zinc oxide, petrolatum-based ointment, and nonalcohol skin barrier film to control leakage; add absorptive powders and pectin-based skin barrier wafers if skin irritation is present (Wound Ostomy and Continence Nurses Society, 2011). Secure the tube to the abdomen using a commercial stabilizer, polyurethane foam, or the H tape method, and leave a small loop of tubing at the exit site to prevent tension on the site.

Granulation tissue may grow around a gastrostomy site (Fig. 22.22). This moist, beefy-red tissue is not a sign of infection. However, if it continues to grow, the excess moisture can irritate the surrounding skin. The use of hydrogen peroxide for routine site cleansing has been identified as one of the possible causes of hypergranulation tissue (Wound Ostomy and Continence Nurses Society, 2011), corrosion and excessive drying of the tissue, and disruption of wound healing. Clinical guidelines issued by the Wound Ostomy and Continence Nurses Society (2011) recommend managing hypergranulation by stabilizing the tube, keeping the peristomal area dry by applying polyurethane foam, and using triamcinolone (0.5%) three times a day. Silver nitrate may also be used for hypergranulation.

For children receiving long-term gastrostomy feeding, a **skin-level device** (e.g., MIC-KEY, Bard Button) offers several advantages. The small, flexible silicone device protrudes slightly from the abdomen, is cosmetically pleasing, affords increased comfort and mobility to the child, is easy to care for, and is fully immersible in water. The one-way valve at the proximal end minimizes reflux and eliminates the need for clamping. However, the skin-level device requires a well-established gastrostomy site and is more expensive than the conventional tube. In addition, the valve may become clogged. When functioning, the valve prevents air from escaping; therefore the child may require frequent bubbling. With some devices, during feedings, the child must remain fairly still because the tubing easily disconnects from the opening if the child moves. With other devices, extension tubing can be securely attached to the opening (Fig. 22.23). The feeding is instilled at the other end of the tubing in a manner similar to that for a regular gastrostomy. The extension tubing may also have a separate medication port. Both the feeding and the medication ports have plugs attached. Some skin-level devices require a special tube to be able to decompress the stomach (to check residual or decompress air).

Feeding of water, formula, or pureed foods is carried out in the same manner and rate as for gavage feeding. A mechanical pump may be used to regulate the volume and rate of feeding. After feedings, the infant or child is positioned on the right side or in the Fowler position, and the tube may be clamped or left open and suspended between feedings, depending on the child's condition. A clamped tube allows more mobility but is only appropriate if the child can tolerate intermittent feedings without vomiting or prolonged backup of feeding into the tube. Sometimes a Y tube is used to allow for simultaneous decompression during feeding. If a Foley catheter is used as the gastrostomy tube, apply

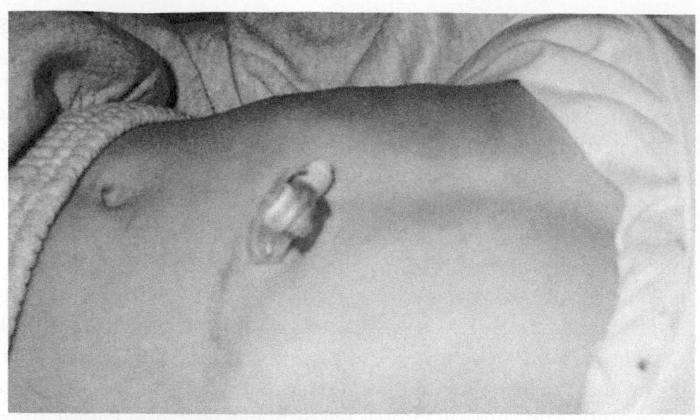

FIG. 22.23 Child with a skin-level gastrostomy device (MIC-KEY), which provides for secure attachment of extension tubing to the gastrostomy opening.

very slight tension. The tube is securely taped to maintain the balloon at the gastrostomy opening and prevent leakage of gastric contents and the tube's progression toward the pyloric sphincter, where it may occlude the stomach outlet. As a precaution, the length of the tube is measured postoperatively and then remeasured each shift to be certain it has not slipped. The nurse can make a mark above the skin level to further ensure its placement. When the gastrostomy tube is no longer needed, it is removed; the skin opening usually closes spontaneously by contracture.

> **NURSING TIP**
>
> In the event that a gastrostomy button or tube is accidentally pulled out, a Foley catheter can be gently inserted in the tract to maintain patency until a new tube can be inserted.

NASODUODENAL AND NASOJEJUNAL TUBES

Children at high risk for regurgitation or aspiration, such as those with gastroparesis, mechanical ventilation, or brain injuries, may require placement of a postpyloric feeding tube. A trained provider inserts the nasoduodenal or nasojejunal tube because of the risk of misplacement and potential for perforation in tubes requiring a stylet. Accurate placement is verified by radiography. Small-bore tubes may easily clog. Flush the tube when feeding is interrupted, before and after medication administration, and routinely every 4 hours or as directed by institutional policy. Tube replacement should be considered monthly to ensure optimal tube patency. Continuous feedings are delivered by a mechanical pump to regulate their volume and rate. Bolus feeds are contraindicated. Tube displacement is suspected in children showing signs of feeding intolerance such as vomiting. In these cases, stop the feedings and notify the provider.

TOTAL PARENTERAL NUTRITION

Total parenteral nutrition (TPN) provides for the total nutritional needs of infants and children whose lives are threatened because feeding by way of the gastrointestinal tract is impossible, inadequate, or hazardous.

Total parenteral nutrition therapy involves IV infusion of highly concentrated solutions of protein, glucose, and other nutrients. The solution is infused through conventional tubing with a special filter attached to remove particulate matter or microorganisms that may have contaminated the solution. The highly concentrated solutions require infusion into a vessel with sufficient volume and turbulence to allow for rapid dilution. The wide-diameter vessels selected are the superior vena cava and innominate or intrathoracic subclavian veins approached by way of the external or internal jugular veins. The highly irritating nature of concentrated glucose precludes the use of the small peripheral veins in most instances. However, dilute glucose-protein hydrolysates that are appropriate for infusing into peripheral veins are being used with increasing frequency. When peripheral veins are used, intralipid becomes the major calorie source. For long-term alimentation, central venous catheters are usually used.

The major nursing responsibilities are the same as for any IV therapy and include control of sepsis, monitoring of the infusion rate, and assessment of the patient. The TPN solution must be prepared under rigid aseptic conditions, which is best accomplished by specially trained technicians. Nurses should change the TPN, lipids, and tubing on a frequent basis. More frequent tubing changes are required for TPN and lipids because these solutions can increase risk of microbial growth. Meticulous aseptic precautions should be used whenever the line is entered or changed. In some institutions, this may be a nursing responsibility. If so, the procedure is carried out according to hospital protocol.

The infusion is maintained at a constant rate by means of an infusion pump to ensure the proper concentrations of glucose and amino acids. Accurate calculation of the rate is required to deliver a measured amount in a given length of time. Because alterations in flow rate are relatively common, the drip should be checked frequently to ensure an even, continuous infusion. The TPN infusion rate should not be increased or decreased without the provider being informed because alterations can cause hyperglycemia or hypoglycemia.

General assessments, such as vital signs, I&O measurements, and checking results of laboratory tests, facilitate early detection of infection or fluid and electrolyte imbalance. Additional amounts of potassium and sodium chloride are often required in hyperalimentation; therefore observation for signs of potassium or sodium deficit or excess is part of nursing care. This is rarely a problem except in children with reduced renal function or metabolic defects. Hyperglycemia may occur during the first day or two as the child adapts to the high-glucose load of the hyperalimentation solution. Although hyperglycemia occurs infrequently, insulin may be required to help the body adjust. When this occurs, nursing responsibilities include blood glucose testing. To prevent hypoglycemia when the hyperalimentation is disconnected, the rate of the infusion and the amount of insulin are decreased gradually.

FAMILY TEACHING AND HOME CARE

When alternative feedings are needed for an extended period, the family needs to learn how to feed the child with an NG, gastrostomy, or TPN feeding regimen. The same principles apply as discussed earlier in this chapter for compliance, especially in terms of education, and in Chapter 21 for discharge planning and home care. Plan ample time for the family to learn and perform the procedures under supervision before they assume full responsibility for the child's care. Refer the family to community agencies that provide support and practical assistance. The Oley Foundation (http://www.oley.org) is a nonprofit research and education organization that assists persons receiving enteral nutrition and home TPN.

PROCEDURES RELATED TO ELIMINATION

ENEMA

The procedure for giving an enema to an infant or child does not differ essentially from that for an adult except for the type and amount of

TABLE 22.8 Administration of Enemas to Children

Age	Amount (ml)	Insertion Distance
Infant	120-240	2.5 cm (1 inch)
2-4 years	240-360	5 cm (2 inch)
4-10 years	360-480	7.5 cm (3 inch)
11 years	480-720	10 cm (4 inch)

fluid administered and the distance for inserting the tube into the rectum (Table 22.8). Depending on the volume, use a syringe with rubber tubing, an enema bottle, or an enema bag.

An isotonic solution is used in children. Plain water is not used because, being hypotonic, it can cause rapid fluid shift and fluid overload. The Fleet enema (pediatric or adult sized) is not advised for children because of the harsh action of its ingredients (sodium biphosphate and sodium phosphate). Commercial enemas can be dangerous to patients with megacolon and to dehydrated or azotemic children. The osmotic effect of the Fleet enema may produce diarrhea, which can lead to metabolic acidosis. Several case studies have reported additional complications such as extreme hyperphosphatemia, hypernatremia, and hypocalcemia, which may lead to neuromuscular irritability and coma.

NURSING TIP

If prepared saline is not available, the nurse can make some by adding 1 tsp of table salt to 500 ml (1 pint) of tap water.

The enema may be administered with the child positioned on the left side, while lying on absorbent chux pads. Because it is difficult for infants and young children to retain the solution after it is administered, the buttocks may be held together for a short time to retain the fluid. Older children are ordinarily able to hold the solution if they understand what to do and if they are not expected to hold it for too long. The nurse should have the bedpan handy or, for ambulatory children, ensure that the bathroom is available before beginning the procedure. An enema is an intrusive procedure and thus can be threatening to children of all ages; therefore developmentally appropriate preparation and distraction is especially important for the comfort of the child.

A preoperative bowel preparation solution given orally or through an NG tube is increasingly being used instead of an enema. The polyethylene glycol–electrolyte lavage solution (GoLYTELY) mechanically flushes the bowel without significant absorption, thereby avoiding potential fluid and electrolyte imbalances. NuLYTELY, a modification of GoLYTELY, has the same therapeutic advantages as GoLYTELY and was developed to improve on the taste. Another effective oral cathartic is magnesium citrate solution.

OSTOMIES

Children may require stomas for various health problems. The most frequent causes in infants are necrotizing enterocolitis and imperforate anus and, less often, Hirschsprung disease. In older children, the most frequent causes are inflammatory bowel disease, especially Crohn disease (regional enteritis), and ureterostomies for distal ureter or bladder defects.

Care and management of ostomies in older children differ little from the care of ostomies in adult patients. The major emphasis in pediatric care is preparing the child for the procedure and teaching care of the ostomy to the child and family. The basic principles of preparation are the same as for any procedure (see p. 680). Simple, straightforward language is most effective together with the use of illustrations and a replica model (e.g., drawing a picture of a child with a stoma on the abdomen and explaining it as "another opening where bowel movements [or any other term the child uses] will come out"). At another time, the nurse can draw a pouch over the opening to demonstrate how the contents are collected. Using a doll to demonstrate the process is an excellent teaching strategy, and special books are available.

Children with ileostomies are fitted immediately after surgery with an appliance to protect the skin from the proteolytic enzymes in the liquid stool. Infants may not be fitted with a pouch in the immediate postoperative period. When stomal drainage is minimal, as is often the case in small or preterm infants, a gauze dressing will suffice. Give the parents a choice of caring for the colostomy with or without an appliance. Pediatric appliances are available in a variety of sizes to ensure an adequate fit.

Ostomy equipment consists of a one- or two-piece system with a hypoallergenic skin barrier to maintain peristomal skin integrity. The pouch should be large enough to contain a moderate amount of stool and flatus but not so large as to overwhelm the infant or child. A backing helps minimize the risk of skin breakdown from moisture trapped between the skin and pouch. Avoid small clips and rubber bands to prevent choking in young children.

Protection of the peristomal skin is a major aspect of stoma care. Well-fitting appliances are important to prevent leakage of contents. Before applying the appliance, prepare the skin with a skin sealant that is allowed to dry. Then apply stoma paste around the base of the stoma or to the back of the wafer. The sealant and paste work together to prevent peristomal skin breakdown.

In infants with a colostomy left unpouched, skin care is similar to that of any diapered child. However, protect the peristomal skin with a barrier substance (e.g., zinc oxide ointment [Sensi-Care] or a mixture of zinc oxide ointment and stoma powder [Stomahesive]). A diaper larger than the one usually worn may be needed to extend upward over the stoma and absorb drainage. If the skin becomes inflamed, denuded, or infected, the care is similar to the interventions used for diaper dermatitis. A zinc-based product helps protect healthy skin, heal excoriated skin, and minimize pain associated with skin breakdown. The skin protectant adheres to denuded, weeping skin. The nurse can apply zinc-based products over topical antifungal and antibacterial agents if infection is present. No-sting barrier film is a skin sealant that has no alcohol base and can be used on open skin without stinging.

With young children, preventing them from pulling off the pouch is also an important consideration. One-piece outfits keep exploring hands from reaching the pouch, and the loose waist avoids any pressure on the appliance. Keeping the child occupied with toys during the pouch change is also helpful. As children mature, encourage their participation in ostomy care. Even preschoolers can assist by holding supplies, pulling paper backings from the appliance, and helping clean the stoma area. Toilet training for bladder control needs to begin at the appropriate time as for any other child.

Older children and adolescents should eventually have total responsibility for ostomy care just as they would for usual bowel function. During adolescence, concerns for body image and the ostomy's impact on intimacy and sexuality emerge. The nurse should stress to teenagers that the presence of a stoma need not interfere with their activities. Children and adolescents can choose which ostomy equipment is best suited to their needs. Attractively designed and decorated pouch covers are well liked by teenagers.

Children with familial adenomatous polyposis may require a colectomy with ileoanal reservoir to prevent or treat carcinoma of the colon. Peristomal skin care for these children is particularly challenging because of increased liquid stools, increased digestive enzymes that may cause skin breakdown, and the stoma being at skin level rather than raised. Additional care with this condition includes close monitoring of fluid and electrolyte status and increased incidence of bowel obstruction.

An enterostomal therapy nurse specialist is an important member of the health care team and will have additional suggestions and assistance with skin care information and ostomy pouching options. The nurse can obtain further information by contacting the Wound, Ostomy and Continence Nurses Society (http://www.wocn.org).

FAMILY TEACHING AND HOME CARE

Because these children are almost always discharged with a functioning colostomy, preparation of the family should begin as early as possible in the hospital. The nurse instructs the family in the application of the device (if used), care of the skin, and appropriate action in case skin problems develop. Early evidence of skin breakdown or stomal complications, such as ribbonlike stools, excessive diarrhea, bleeding, prolapse, or failure to pass flatus or stool, is brought to the attention of the physician, nurse, or stoma specialist. The same principles are applied as discussed earlier in this chapter for compliance, especially in terms of education, and in Chapter 21 for discharge planning and home care.

NCLEX REVIEW QUESTIONS

1. When administering a medication to a child, the nurse knows that:
   A. The most accurate means for measuring small amounts of medication is the plastic disposable calibrated oral syringe.
   B. A teaspoon is often the unit of measurement for pediatric medication and is especially helpful when working with families.
   C. Using a dropper is also acceptable, remembering that thick fluids are easier to measure than viscous fluids.
   D. For more exact measuring, emptying dropper contents into a medicine cup can be helpful.
2. During hospitalization, there may be a reason to use restraints. Protocol for using restraints may include which of the following? Select all that apply.
   A. One finger breadth should be left between the skin and the device, and knots should be tied to allow for quick release.
   B. Elbow restraints fashioned from a variety of materials function well when a child's hands must be kept from his or her face—for example, after cleft lip or palate surgery.
   C. A papoose board with straps or a mummy wrap effectively controls the child's movements when an infant or small child requires short-term restraint for examination or treatment that involves the head and neck.
   D. Before initiating a behavioral restraint, the nurse should assess the patient's mental, behavioral, and physical status to determine the cause for the child's potentially harmful behavior.
   E. Unless state law is more restrictive, behavioral restraints for children must be reordered every 2 hours for children under 9 years of age and every 3 hours for children 9 to 17 years old.
3. You are working with a new nurse to give an intramuscular injection. Which principles do you want to include when doing this teaching? Select all that apply.
   A. Usually 2 ml is the maximum volume that should be administered in a single site to small children and older infants.
   B. New evidence suggests that immunizations at the ventrogluteal site have been found to have fewer local reactions and fever.
   C. Distraction and prevention of unexpected movement may be more easily achieved by placing the child supine on a parent's lap for ventrogluteal site use.
   D. The deltoid muscle advantages are less pain and fewer side effects from the injectate compared with the vastus lateralis.
   E. Aspiration during intramuscular vaccine administration is always recommended.
4. When obtaining a heelstick for laboratory results:
   A. The heelstick is performed because it is less invasive and less painful than a venipuncture.
   B. Breastfeeding during a neonatal heelstick is effective in reducing pain and has been found to be more effective than sucrose in some studies.
   C. Although safe for use in preterm infants when applied correctly, EMLA has been found to be much more effective than placebo in preventing pain during heel lancing.
   D. To avoid osteochondritis (underlying calcaneus bone, infection, and abscess of the heel), the puncture should be no deeper than 1 mm and should be made at the inner aspect of the heel.
5. Children and adolescents should be prepared for procedures according to their level of development and understanding. Which interventions by the nurse would be helpful? Select all that apply.
   A. Explain procedure in relation to what the child will see, hear, taste, smell, and feel.
   B. Although older children may associate objects, places, or persons with prior painful experiences, infants will not have a memory of past experiences.
   C. For school-age children, preparation can take several days in advance of the procedure to allow for processing of information.
   D. Provide privacy; describe how the body will be covered and what will be exposed.
   E. Allowing adolescents to talk with other adolescents who have had the same procedure may increase their level of anxiety and is not recommended.

Correct Answers

1. A; 2. A, B, C, D; 3. B, C, D; 4. B; 5. A, D

REFERENCES

Adams, D. Z., Little, A., Vinsant, C., et al. (2016). The midline catheter: A clinical review. *Journal of Emergency Medicine, 51*(3), 252–258.

Alamanou, D. G., & Brokalaki, H. (2014). Intrahospital transport policies: The contribution of the nurse. *Health Science Journal, 8*(2), 166–178.

Al-Yateem, N., Brenner, M., Shorrab, A. A., et al. (2016). Play distraction versus pharmacological treatment to reduce anxiety levels in children undergoing day surgery: A randomized controlled non-inferiority trial. *Child: Care, Health and Development, 42*(4), 572–581.

American Academy of Pediatrics. (2011). Subcommittee on Urinary Tract Infections: Urinary Tract Infection: Clinical practice guideline for the diagnosis and management of the initial UTI in febrile infants and children 2 to 24 months. *Pediatrics, 128*(3), 595–610.

American Academy of Pediatrics. (2015). *When to call the pediatrician: fever.* American Academy of Pediatrics, https://www.healthychildren.org/

English/health-issues/conditions/fever/Pages/When-to-Call-the-Pediatrician.aspx.

American Academy of Pediatrics. (2016). Task Force on Sudden Infant Death Syndrome: SIDS and other sleep-related infant deaths: Evidence base for 2016 updated recommendations for a safe infant sleeping environment. *Pediatrics, 138*(5), e1–e34.

American Academy of Pediatrics, Committee on Bioethics. (2016). Informed consent in decision-making in pediatric practice. *Pediatrics, 138*(2), e1–e9.

American Dental Association. (2017). *Mouth healthy: Babies and kids.* Mouth Healthy, http://www.mouthhealthy.org/en/babies-and-kids.

Anand, K. J., & Hall, R. W. (2006). Pharmacological therapy for analgesia and sedation in the newborn. *Archives of Diseases in Childhood Fetal and Neonatal Edition, 91*(6), 448–453.

Association of Child Life Professionals. (2017). *Mission, values, vision.* Association of Child Life Professionals, http://www.childlife.org/child-life-profession/mission-values-vision.

Azhar, N. (2015). Pre-operative optimisation of lung function. *Indian Journal of Anaesthesia, 59*(9), 550–556.

Bahl, A., Pandurangadu, A. V., Tucker, J., et al. (2016). a randomized controlled trial assessing the use of ultrasound for nurse-performed IV placement in difficult access ED patients. *The American Journal of Emergency Medicine, 34*(10), 1950–1954.

Batawi, H. E. (2015). Effect of preoperative oral midazolam sedation on separation anxiety and emergence delirium among children undergoing dental treatment under general anesthesia. *Journal of International Society of Preventive & Community Dentistry, 5*(2), 88–94.

Beckett, V. L., Tyson, L. D., Carroll, D., et al. (2012). Accurately administering oral medication to children isn't child's play. *Archives of Disease in Childhood, 97*(9), 838–841.

Beckstrand, J., Ellett, M. L. C., & McDaniel, A. (2007). Predicting internal distance to the stomach for positioning NG and OG feeding tubes in children. *Journal of Advanced Nursing, 59*(3), 274–289.

Benoit, B., Martin-Misener, R., Latimer, M., et al. (2017). Breast-feeding analgesia in infants: An update on the current state of evidence. *The Journal of Perinatal & Neonatal Nursing, 31*(2), 145–159.

Blaney, M., Shen, V., Kerner, J. A., et al. (2006). Alteplase for the treatment of central venous catheter occlusion in children: Results of a prospective, open-label, single-arm study (the Cathflo Activase Pediatric Study). *Journal of Vascular and Interventional Radiology, 17*(11 Pt. 1), 1745–1751.

Brown, J., Gillespie, M., & Chard, S. (2015). The dorso-ventro debate: In search of empirical evidence. *The British Journal of Nursing, 24*(22), 1132–1139.

Brown, M., & Sinsky, C. A. (2013). Medication adherence: We didn't ask and they didn't tell. *Family Practice Management, 20*(2), 23–30.

Calcaterra, V., Veggiotti, P., Palestrini, C., et al. (2015). Post-operative benefits of animal-assisted therapy in pediatric surgery: A randomised study. *PLoS ONE, 10*(6), 1–13.

Centers for Medicare and Medicaid Services. (2015). *State Operations Manual Appendix A Survey Protocol, Regulations and Interpretive Guidelines for Hospitals.* Revision 151, 11-20-15. http://www.cms.gov/Regulations-and-Guidance/Guidance/Manuals/downloads/som107ap_a_hospitals.pdf.

Chameides, L., Samson, R. A., Schexnayder, S. M., et al. (Eds.), (2012). *Pediatric advanced life support provider manual.* American Heart Association.

Chan, Y. K., & Mamat, M. (2015). Management of heat stroke. *Trends in Anaesthesia and Critical Care, 5*(2–3), 65–69.

Clinical Laboratory Standards Institute (2017). Collection of diagnostic venous blood specimens. In *CLSI standard GP41* (7th ed.). Wayne, PA: Clinical and Laboratory Standards Institute.

Cook, I. F., & Murtagh, J. (2006). Ventrogluteal area—a suitable site for intramuscular vaccination of infants and toddlers. *Vaccine, 24*(13), 2403–2408.

Crawford, C. L., & Johnson, J. A. (2012). To aspirate or not: An integrative review of the evidence. *Nursing, 42*(3), 20–25.

Dahl, A., Sinha, M., Rosenberg, D. I., et al. (2015). Assessing physician-parent communication during emergency medical procedures in children: An observational study in a low-literacy Latino patient population. *Pediatric Emergency Care, 31*(5), 339–342.

Derya, E. Y., Ukke, K., Taner, Y., et al. (2015). Applying manual pressure before benzathine penicillin injection for rheumatic fever prophylaxis reduces pain in children. *Pain Management Nursing, 16*(3), 328–335.

Dharmapuri, S., Best, D., Kind, T., et al. (2015). Health literacy and medication adherence in adolescents. *The Journal of Pediatrics, 166*(2), 378–382.

Dolgun, E., Yavuz, M., Eroğlu, B., et al. (2017). Investigation of preoperative fasting times in children. *Journal of Perianesthesia Nursing, 32*(2), 121–124.

Eisenhower, C., & Farrington, E. A. (2012). Advancements in the treatment of head lice in pediatrics. *Journal of Pediatric Health Care, 26*(6), 451–461.

Eliacik, K., Kanik, A., Yavascan, O., et al. (2016). A comparison of bladder catheterization and suprapubic aspiration methods for urine sample collection from infants with a suspected urinary tract infection. *Clinical Pediatrics, 55*(9), 819–824.

Erhaze, E. K., Dowling, M., & Devane, D. (2016). Parental presence at anaesthesia induction: A systematic review. *International Journal of Nursing Practice, 22*(4), 397–407.

Firdouse, M., Wajchendler, A., Koyle, M., et al. (2017). Checklist to improve informed consent process in pediatric surgery: A pilot study. *Journal of Pediatric Surgery, 52*(5), 859–863.

Flippo, R., NeSmith, E., Stark, N., et al. (2015). Reduction of 30-day preventable pediatric readmission rates with postdischarge phone calls utilizing a patient- and family-centered care approach. *Journal of Pediatric Health Care, 29*(6), 492–500.

Ford, J. M. (2016). *Lumbar puncture (Pediatric).* Elsevier. https://lms.elsevierperformancemanager.com/ContentArea/NursingSkills/GetNursingSkillsDetails?skillid=CCP_081&skillkeyid=809&searchTerm=lumbar%20puncture&searchContext=nursingskills.

Fortier, M. A., Kain, Z. N., & Morton, N. (2015). Treating perioperative anxiety and pain in children: A tailored and innovative approach. *Pediatric Anesthesia, 25*(1), 27–35.

Gorski, L. A., Hadaway, L., Hagle, M., et al. (2016). 2016 infusion therapy standards of practice. *Journal of Infusion Nursing, 39*(Suppl. 1), S1–S159.

Greene, N., Bhananker, S., & Ramaiah, R. (2012). Vascular access, fluid resuscitation, and blood transfusion in pediatric trauma. *International Journal of Critical Illness and Injury Science, 2*(3), 135–142.

Guenter, P., & Lyman, B. (2016). ENFit enteral nutrition connectors. *Nutrition in Clinical Practice, 31*(6), 769–772.

Halm, M. A., & Gleaves, M. (2009). Obtaining blood samples from peripheral intravenous catheters: Best practice. *American Journal of Critical Care, 18*(5), 474–478.

Herd, H. A., & Rieben, M. A. (2014). Establishing the surgical nurse liaison role to improve patient and family member communication. *AORN Journal, 99*(5), 594–599.

Heyer, N. J., Derzon, J. H., Winges, L., et al. (2012). Effectiveness of practices to reduce blood sample hemolysis in EDs: A laboratory medicine best practices systematic review and meta-analysis. *Clinical Biochemistry, 45*(13–14), 1012–1032.

Howie, S. R. C. (2011). Blood sample volumes in child health research: Review of safe limits. *Bulletin of the World Health Organization, 89*, 46–53.

Hunter, D. (2012). Conditions affecting the foreskin. *Nursing Standard, 26*(37), 35–39.

Infusion Nurses Society. (2011). Infusion nursing standards of practice. *Journal of Infusion Nursing, 34*(Suppl. 1), S63–S64.

Infusion Nurses Society. (2016). *Policies and procedures for infusion therapy* (5th ed.). Infusion Nurses Society. author.

Institute for Safe Medication Practices. (2016). *FDA and ISMP lists of look-alike drug names with recommended Tall Man letters.* From https://www.ismp.org/Tools/tallmanletters.pdf.

Johnston, C., Campbell-Yeo, M., Disher, T., et al. (2017). Skin-to-skin care for procedural pain in neonates. *Cochrane Database of Systematic Reviews,* (2), CD008435.

Junqueira, A. L., Tavares, V. R., Martins, R. M., et al. (2010). Safety and immunogenicity of hepatitis B vaccine administered into ventrogluteal vs. anterolateral thigh sites in infants: A randomized controlled trial. *International Journal of Nursing Studies, 47*(9), 1074–1079.

Karcz, A., Kelley, K., Conrad, J., et al. (2015). Daily bathing of pediatric inpatients with chlorhexidine gluconate to prevent hospital acquired infections. *American Journal of Infection Control, 43*(6), S8.

Kendrick, J. G., Ma, K., DeZorzi, P., et al. (2012). Vomiting of oral medications by pediatric patients: Survey of medication redosing practices. *The Canadian Journal of Hospital Pharmacy, 65*(3), 196–201.

Kroger, A. T., Duchin, J., & Vazquez, M. *General best practice guidelines for immunization: best practice guidance of the Advisory Committee on Immunization Practices (ACIP)*. https://www.cdc.gov/vaccines/hcp/acip-recs/general-recs/downloads/general-recs.pdf.

Letitre, S. L., DeGroot, E. P., Draaisma, E., et al. (2014). Anxiety, depression and self-esteem in children with well-controlled asthma: Case-control study. *Archives of Disease in Childhood, 99*(8), 744–748.

Lidgett, C. D. (2016). Improving the patient experience through a commit to sit service excellence initiative. *Journal of Patient Experience, 3*(2), 67–72.

Manworren, R., & Fledderman, M. (2000). Preparation of the child and family for surgery. In B. V. Wise, C. McKenna, G. Garvin, et al. (Eds.), *Nursing care of the general pediatric surgical patient*. Gaithersburg, MD: Aspen.

Manyande, A., Cyna, A. M., Yip, P., et al. (2015). Non-pharmacological interventions for assisting the induction of anaesthesia in children. *The Cochrane Database of Systematic Reviews, 7*, 1–73.

Marchaim, D., Taylor, A. R., Hayakawa, K., et al. (2012). Hospital bath basins are frequently contaminated with multidrug-resistant human pathogens. *American Journal of Infection Control, 40*(6), 562–564.

Matziou, V., Chrysostomou, A., Vlahioti, E., et al. (2013). Parental presence and distraction during painful childhood procedures. *The British Journal of Nursing, 22*(8), 470–475.

Milstone, A. M., Elward, A., Song, X., et al. (2013). Daily chlorhexidine bathing to reduce bacteraemia in critically ill children: A multicentre, cluster-randomised, crossover trial. *Lancet, 381*(9872), 1099–1106.

Monsma, J., Richerson, J., & Sloand, E. (2015). Empowering parents for evidence-based fever management: An integrative review. *Journal of the American Association of Nurse Practitioners, 27*(4), 222–229.

Murray, E., Edlund, B. J., & Vess, J. (2016). Implementing a pediatric fall prevention policy and program. *Pediatric Nursing, 42*(5), 256–259.

O'Grady, N. P., Alexander, M., Burns, L. A., et al. (2011). Guidelines for the prevention of intravascular catheter-related infections. *Clinical Infectious Diseases, 52*(9), e162–e193.

Ozturk, D., Baykara, Z. G., Karadag, A., et al. (2017). The effect of the application of manual pressure before the administration of intramuscular injections on students' perceptions of postinjection pain: A semi-experimental study. *Journal of Clinical Nursing, 26*(11–12), 1632–1638.

Patricia, C. (2014). Evidence-based management of childhood fever: What pediatric nurses need to know. *Journal of Pediatric Nursing, 29*(4), 372–375.

Pawar, D. (2012). Common post-operative complications in children. *Indian Journal of Anaesthesia, 56*(5), 496–501.

Payne, N. R., & Flood, A. (2015). Preventing pediatric readmissions: Which ones and how? *The Journal of Pediatrics, 166*(3), 519–520.

Peacock, G., Parnapy, S., Raynor, S., et al. (2010). Accuracy and precision of manufacturer-supplied liquid medication administration devices before and after patient education. *Journal of the American Pharmacists Association, 50*(1), 84–86.

Poston, R. D. (2016). Assent described: Exploring perspectives from the inside. *Journal of Pediatric Nursing, 31*(6), 353–365.

Powers, J., Peed, J., Burns, L., et al. (2012). Chlorhexidine bathing and microbial contamination in patients' bath basins. *American Journal of Critical Care, 21*(5), 338–342.

Purswani, M. U., Radhakrishnan, J., Irfan, K. R., et al. (2009). Infant acceptance of a bitter-tasting liquid medication: A randomized controlled trial comparing the Rx Medibottle with an oral syringe. *Archives of Pediatrics & Adolescent Medicine, 163*(2), 186–188.

Razmus, I., & Bergquist-Beringer, S. (2017). Pressure ulcer risk and prevention practices in pediatric patients: A secondary analysis of data from the national database of nursing quality indicators. *Ostomy/Wound Management, 63*(2), 26–36.

Registered Nurses' Association of Ontario. (2008). *Care and maintenance to reduce vascular access complications, guideline supplement*. Toronto: Author.

Rosenbloom, E., Finkelstein, Y., Adams-Webber, T., et al. (2013). Do antipyretics prevent the recurrence of febrile seizures in children? A systematic review of randomized controlled trials and meta-analysis. *European Journal of Paediatric Neurology*, [Epub ahead of print]; May 21.

Rothbart, A., Yu, P., Müller-Lobeck, L., et al. (2015). Peripheral intravenous cannulation with support of infrared laser vein viewing system in a pre-operation setting in pediatric patients. *BMC Research Notes, 8*, 463.

Rupp, M. E., Huerta, T., Yu, S., et al. (2013). Hospital basins used to administer chlorhexidine baths are unlikely microbial reservoirs. *Infection Control & Hospital Epidemiology, 34*(6), 643–645.

Rusch, R., Schulta, C., Hughes, L., et al. (2014). Evidence-based practice recommendations to Prevent/Manage post-lumbar puncture headaches in pediatric patients receiving intrathecal chemotherapy. *Journal of Pediatric Oncology Nursing, 31*(4), 230–238.

Ryu, G. S., & Lee, Y. J. (2012). Analysis of liquid medication dose errors made by patients and caregivers using alternative measuring devices. *Journal of Managed Care Pharmacy, 18*(6), 439–445.

Sahib El-Radhi, A., Carroll, J., & Klein, N. (2009). *Clinical manual of fever in children*. Springer.

Salazar, J. H., Yang, J., Shen, L., et al. (2014). Pediatric malignant hyperthermia: Risk factors, morbidity, and mortality identified from the nationwide inpatient sample and kids' inpatient database. *Pediatric Anesthesia, 24*(12), 1212–1216.

Schindler, C., Mikhailov, T., Kuhn, E., et al. (2011). Protecting fragile skin: Nursing interventions to decrease development of pressure ulcers in pediatric intensive care. *American Journal of Critical Care, 20*(1), 26–34.

Schober-Flores, C. (2012). Pressure ulcers in the pediatric population. *Journal of the Dermatology Nurses' Association, 4*(5), 295–306.

Shah, V., & Ohlsson, A. (2011). Venepuncture versus heel lance for blood sampling in term neonates. *Cochrane Database of Systematic Reviews*, (5), CD001452.

Shaughnessy, E. E., White, C., Shah, S. S., et al. (2015). Implementation of postoperative respiratory care for pediatric orthopedic patients. *Pediatrics, 136*(2), 505–512.

Sisson, H. (2015). Aspirating during the intramuscular injection procedure: A systematic literature review. *Journal of Clinical Nursing, 24*(17–18), 2368–2375.

Sorrentino, G., Fumagalli, M., Milani, S., et al. (2017). The impact of automatic devices for capillary blood collection on efficiency and pain response in newborns: A randomized controlled trial. *International Journal of Nursing Studies, 72*, 24–29.

Stein, R., Dogan, H. S., Hoebeke, P., et al. (2015). Urinary tract infections in children: EAU/ESPU guidelines. *European Urology, 67*(3), 546–558.

Stevens, B., Yamada, J., Ohlsson, A., et al. (2016). Sucrose for analgesia in newborn infants undergoing painful procedures. *Cochrane Database of Systematic Reviews*, (7), CD001069.

Stolz, L. A., Cappa, A. R., Minckler, M. R., et al. (2016). Prospective evaluation of the learning curve for ultrasound-guided peripheral intravenous placement. *The Journal of Vascular Access, 17*(4), 366–370.

Takeshita, J., Nakayama, Y., Nakajima, Y., et al. (2015). Optimal site for ultrasound-guided venous catheterisation in paediatric patients. *Critical Care, 19*(1), 15.

Thomas, C. M., Mraz, M., & Rajcan, L. (2016). Blood aspiration during IM injection. *Clinical Nursing Research, 25*(5), 549–559.

Thompson, R. H. (2009). *The handbook of child life: A guide for pediatric psychosocial care*. Springfield IL: Charles C Thomas Publisher.

Tobias, J. D., & Ross, A. K. (2010). Intraosseous infusions: A review for the anesthesiologist with a focus on pediatric use. *Anesthesia and Analgesia, 110*(2), 391–401.

Torres, A., Parker, R. M., Sanders, L. M., et al. (2017). Parent preferences and perceptions of milliliters and teaspoons: Role of health literacy and experience. *Academic Pediatrics*, pii: S1876-2879(17)30147 [Epub ahead of print].

Valizadeh, S., Rasekhi, M., Hamishehkar, H., et al. (2015). Medication errors in oral dosage form preparation for neonates: The importance of preparation technique. *Journal of Research in Pharmacy Practice*, *4*(3), 147–152.

Williams, C., Johnson, P. A., Guzzetta, C. E., et al. (2014). Pediatric fasting times before surgical and radiologic procedures: Benchmarking institutional practices against national standards. *Journal of Pediatric Nursing*, *29*(3), 258–267.

Winokur, E. J., Pai, D., Rutledge, D. N., et al. (2014). Blood culture accuracy: Discards from central venous catheters in pediatric oncology patients in the emergency department. *Journal of Emergency Nursing*, *40*(4), 323–329.

Wound Ostomy and Continence Nurses Society. (2011). *Pediatric Ostomy Care: Best Practice for Clinicians*. From http://www.wocn.org/WOCN_Library.

Yin, H. S., Parker, R. M., Sanders, L. M., et al. (2016). Liquid medication errors and dosing tools: A randomized controlled experiment. *Pediatrics*, *138*(4), e20160357.

23

The Child With Fluid and Electrolyte Imbalance

Mary A. Mondozzi, Rose Ann Urdiales Baker, and Marilyn J. Hockenberry

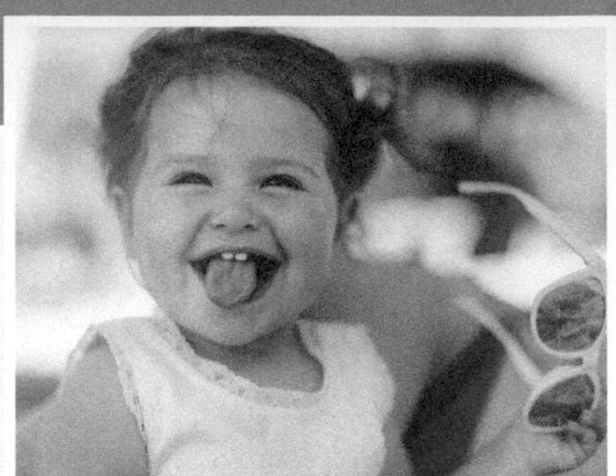

http://evolve.elsevier.com/wong/ncic

CONCEPTS

- Fluid and Electrolyte Balance
- Acud-Base Balance
- Cellular Regulation

DISTRIBUTION OF BODY FLUIDS

The distribution of body fluids, or total body water (TBW), involves the presence of intracellular fluid (ICF) and extracellular fluid (ECF). Water is the major constituent of body tissues, and the TBW in an individual ranges from 45% (in late adolescence) to 75% (in term newborn) of total body weight.

The ICF refers to the fluid contained within the cells, whereas the ECF is the fluid outside the cells. The ECF is further broken down into several components: intravascular (contained within the blood vessels), interstitial (surrounding the cell; the location of most ECF), and transcellular (contained within specialized body cavities such as cerebrospinal, synovial, and pleural fluid). In the newborn about 50% of the body fluid is contained within the ECF, whereas 30% of the toddler's body fluid is contained within the ECF.

Body water is important in body function not only because of its abundance but also because it is the medium in which body solutes are dissolved and all metabolic reactions take place. Because even small alterations in fluid composition affect these metabolic processes, precise regulation of the volume and composition of the fluid is essential. In healthy individuals, body water remains singularly constant, but marked alterations in either its volume or distribution, which occur in many disease states, can produce severely damaging physiologic consequences.

WATER BALANCE

Under normal conditions the amount of water ingested closely approximates the amount of urine excreted in a 24-hour period, and the water in food and from oxidation approximates the amount lost in feces and through evaporation. In this way, the body maintains equilibrium.

Mechanisms of Fluid Movement

Water is retained in the body in a relatively constant amount and, with few exceptions, is freely exchangeable among all body fluid compartments. The proximity of the extravascular compartment to the cells allows for continuous change in volume and distribution of fluids, largely determined by solutes (especially sodium) and physical forces (Fig. 23.1). Transport mechanisms are the basis for all activity within the cells, and because the cells have limited ability to store materials, movement in and out of cells must be rapid. Internal control mechanisms are responsible for distribution and maintenance of fluid balance (Box 23.1).

Maintaining Water Balance

Maintenance water requirement is the volume of water needed to replace obligatory fluid loss such as that from insensible water loss (through the skin and respiratory tract), evaporative water loss, and losses through urine and stool formation. The amount and type of these losses may be altered by disease states such as fever (with increased sweating), diarrhea, gastric suction, and pooling of body fluids in a body space (often referred to as third spacing).

Nurses should be alert for altered fluid requirements in various conditions:

Increased requirements:

- Fever (add 12% per rise of 1°C)
- Vomiting, diarrhea
- High-output kidney failure
- Diabetes insipidus
- Diabetic ketoacidosis
- Burns
- Shock
- Tachypnea
- Radiant warmer (preterm infant)
- Phototherapy (infants)
- Postoperative bowel surgery (e.g., gastroschisis)

Decreased requirements:

- Heart failure
- Syndrome of inappropriate antidiuretic hormone
- Mechanical ventilation

PATHOPHYSIOLOGY REVIEW

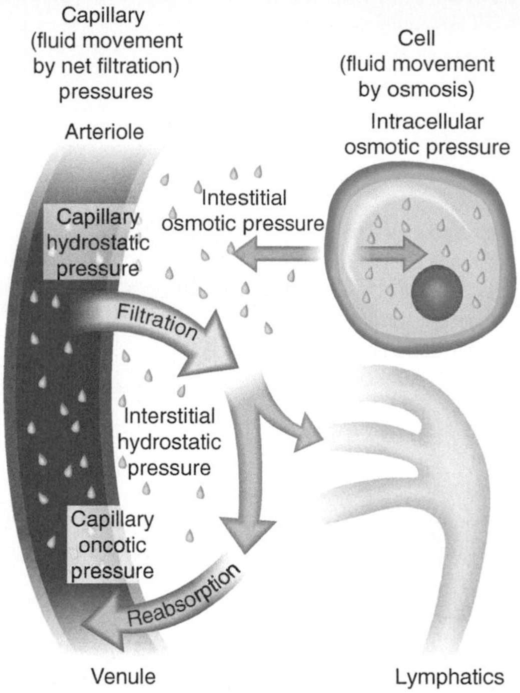

Arterial Capillary Pressures	
Capillary hydrostatic pressure	35 mm Hg
Interstitial fluid hydrostatic pressure	2 mm Hg
Net hydrostatic pressure	**33 mm Hg**
Capillary oncotic pressure	24 mm Hg
Interstitial fluid oncotic pressure	0 mm Hg
Net oncotic pressure	**24 mm Hg**
Net filtration pressure	**+9 mm Hg**

Venous Capillary Pressures	
Capillary hydrostatic pressure	18 mm Hg
Interstitial fluid hydrostatic pressure	1 mm Hg
Net hydrostatic pressure	**17 mm Hg**
Capillary oncotic pressure	25 mm Hg
Interstitial fluid oncotic pressure	0 mm Hg
Net oncotic pressure	**25 mm Hg**
Net filtration pressure	**–8 mm Hg**

FIG. 23.1 Pathophysiology Review. Capillary filtration forces. Water, electrolytes, and small molecules exchange freely between the vascular compartment and the interstitial space at the site of capillaries and small venules. The rate and amount of exchange are driven by the physical forces of hydrostatic and oncotic pressures and the permeability and surface area of the capillary membranes. The two opposing hydrostatic pressures are capillary hydrostatic pressure and interstitial hydrostatic pressure. The two opposing oncotic pressures are capillary oncotic pressure and interstitial oncotic pressure. The *forces that favor filtration* from the capillary are capillary hydrostatic pressure and interstitial oncotic pressure, and the *forces that oppose filtration* are capillary oncotic pressure and interstitial hydrostatic pressure. The sum of their effects is known as *net filtration pressure.* In the example of normal exchange above, a small amount of fluid moves to the lymph vessels, which accounts for the net filtration difference between the arterial and venous ends of the capillary. (From McCance, K., & Huether, S. [2014]. *Pathophysiology: The biological basis for disease in adults and children* [7th ed.]. St. Louis, MO: Mosby.)

- After surgery
- Oliguric renal failure
- Increased intracranial pressure

Basal maintenance calculations for required body water are based on the body's requirements for water in a normometabolic state, at rest; estimated fluid requirements are then increased or decreased from these parameters based on increased or decreased water losses, such as with elevated body temperature or congestive heart failure. Daily maintenance fluid requirements are listed in Table 23.1.

Maintenance fluids contain both water and electrolytes and can be estimated from the child's age, body weight, degree of activity, and body temperature. Basal metabolic rate (BMR) is derived from standard tables and adjusted for the child's activity, temperature, and disease state. For example, for afebrile patients at rest, the maintenance water requirement is approximately 100 ml for each 100 kcal expended. Children with fluid losses or other alterations require adjustment of these basic needs to accommodate abnormal losses of both water and electrolytes as a result of a disease state. For example, insensible losses increase

BOX 23.1 Internal Control Mechanisms Influencing Fluid Balance

Thirst—The impetus to ingest water is stimulated by increased solute concentration (osmolality) of extracellular fluid and/or diminished intravascular volume.

Antidiuretic hormone (ADH)—ADH is released from the posterior pituitary gland in response to increased osmolality and decreased volume of intravascular fluid; it promotes water retention in the renal system by increasing the permeability of renal tubules to water.

Aldosterone—Aldosterone is secreted by the adrenal cortex; it enhances sodium reabsorption in renal tubules, thus promoting osmotic reabsorption of water.

Renin-angiotensin system—Diminished blood flow to the kidneys stimulates renin secretion, which reacts with plasma globulin to generate angiotensin, a powerful vasoconstrictor. Angiotensin also stimulates the release of aldosterone.

TABLE 23.1 Daily Maintenance Fluid Requirements*

Body Weight	Amount of Fluid Per Day
1-10 kg	100 ml/kg
11-20 kg	1000 ml plus 50 ml/kg for each kg >10 kg
>20 kg	1500 ml plus 20 ml/kg for each kg >20 kg

*Not appropriate for neonatal use.

when basal expenditure increases by fever or hypermetabolic states. Hypometabolic states, such as hypothyroidism and hypothermia, decrease the BMR.

Changes in Fluid Volume Related to Growth

The percentage of TBW varies among individuals, and in adults and older children, it is related primarily to the amount of body fat. Consequently, females, who have more body fat than males, and obese persons tend to have less water content in relation to weight.

The fetus is composed primarily of water, with little tissue substance. As the organism grows and develops, a progressive decrease occurs in TBW, with the fastest rate of decline taking place during fetal life. The changes in water content and distribution that occur with age reflect the changes that take place in the relative amounts of bone, muscle, and fat making up the body. At maturity the percentage of TBW is somewhat higher in the male than in the female and is probably a result of the differences in body composition, particularly fat and muscle content (Fig. 23.2).

Another important aspect of growth change as it corresponds to water distribution is related to the ICF and ECF compartments. In the fetus and prematurely born infant, the largest proportion of body water is contained in the ECF compartment. As growth and development proceed, the proportion within the ECF compartment decreases as the ICF and cell solids increase. The ECF diminishes rapidly from approximately 40% of body weight at birth to less than 30% at 1 year of age. The different effects on males and females become apparent at puberty.

Water Balance in Infants

Because of several characteristics, infants and young children have a greater need for water and are more vulnerable to alterations in fluid and electrolyte balance. Compared with older children and adults, they have a greater fluid intake and output relative to size. Water and electrolyte disturbances occur more frequently and more rapidly, and children adjust less promptly to these alterations.

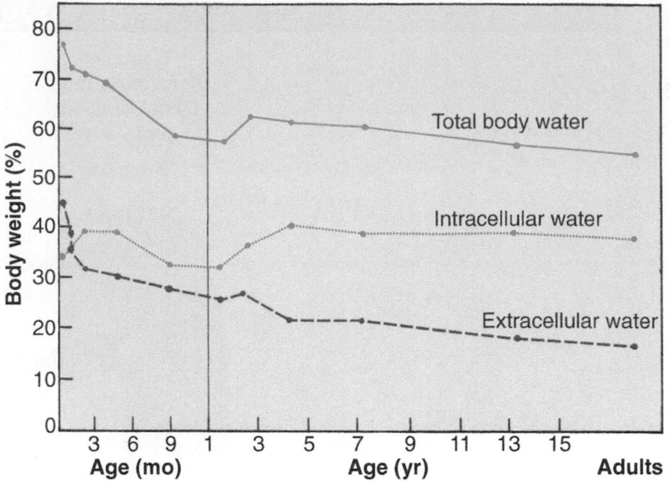

FIG. 23.2 Changes in total body water, intracellular water, and extracellular water in percentages of body weight. (Based on data from Friis-Hansen, B. [1961]. Body water compartments in children: Changes during growth and related changes in body composition. *Pediatrics, 28,* 169-181.)

The fluid compartments in the infant vary significantly from those in the adult, primarily because of an expanded extracellular compartment. The ECF compartment constitutes more than half of the TBW at birth and has a greater relative content of extracellular sodium and chloride. The infant loses a considerable amount of fluid in the first few days after birth and still maintains a larger amount of ECF than the adult until about 2 to 3 years of age. This contributes to greater and more rapid water loss during this age period.

Fluid losses create compartment deficits that reflect the duration of dehydration. In general, approximately 60% of fluid is lost from the ECF, and the remaining 40% comes from the ICF. The amount of fluid lost from the ECF increases with acute illness and decreases with chronic loss.

Fluid losses may be divided into insensible, urinary, and fecal losses and vary with the patient's age. Approximately two-thirds of insensible water losses occurs through the skin, and the remaining one-third is lost through the respiratory tract. Environmental heat and humidity, skin integrity, body temperature, and respiratory rate all influence insensible fluid loss. Infants and children have a much greater tendency to become highly febrile than do adults. Fever increases insensible water loss by approximately 7 ml/kg/24 hr for each 1°F rise in temperature above 37.2°C (99°F). Fever and increased surface area relative to volume both contribute to greater insensible fluid losses in young patients.

Body Surface Area

The infant's relatively greater body surface area (BSA) allows larger quantities of fluid to be lost through the skin. It is estimated that the BSA of the premature neonate is five times more, and that of the newborn is two or three times more, than that of the older child or adult. The proportionately longer gastrointestinal tract in infancy is also a source of relatively greater fluid loss, especially from diarrhea.

Metabolic Rate

The rate of metabolism in infancy is significantly higher than in adulthood because of the larger BSA in relation to the mass of active tissue. Consequently, infants have a greater production of metabolic wastes that the kidneys must excrete. Any condition that increases metabolism causes greater heat production, with its concomitant insensible fluid loss and an increased need for water for excretion. The BMR in infants and children is higher to support cellular and tissue growth.

Kidney Function

The infant's kidneys are functionally immature at birth and are therefore inefficient in excreting waste products of metabolism. Of particular importance for fluid balance is the inability of the infant's kidneys to concentrate or dilute urine, to conserve or excrete sodium, or to acidify urine. Therefore the infant is less able to handle large quantities of solute-free water than is the older child and is more likely to become dehydrated when given concentrated formulas or overhydrated when given excessive free water or dilute formula.

Fluid Requirements

As a result of these characteristics, infants ingest and excrete a greater amount of fluid per kilogram of body weight than do older children. Because electrolytes are excreted with water and the infant has limited ability for conservation, maintenance requirements include both water and electrolytes. The daily exchange of ECF in the infant is much greater than that of older children, which leaves the infant little fluid volume reserve in dehydrated states. Fluid requirements depend on hydration status, size, environmental factors, and underlying disease.

DISTURBANCES OF FLUID AND ELECTROLYTE BALANCE

Disturbances of fluids and their solute concentration are closely interrelated. Alterations in fluid volume affect the electrolyte component, and changes in electrolyte concentration influence fluid movement. Because intracellular water and electrolytes move to and from the ECF compartment, any imbalance in the ICF is reflected by an imbalance in the ECF. Disturbances in the ECF involve either an excess or a deficit of fluid or electrolytes. Of these, fluid loss occurs more frequently.

Sodium is the chief solute in ECF and the primary determinant of ECF volume. It is considered a unique electrolyte in that water balance determines sodium concentration; when water is lost and sodium concentration becomes elevated, compensatory mechanisms in the kidney stop ADH secretion so water is retained. The thirst mechanism (not fully functional in infants) is also stimulated so water is replaced, thus increasing the total body water content and returning sodium to a normal level (Greenbaum, 2015). Sodium depletion in diarrhea occurs in two ways: out of the body in stool and into the ICF compartment to replace potassium to maintain electrical equilibrium. Potassium is found primarily inside the cell (intracellular), but small amounts are also found in ECF.

Depletion of ECF, usually caused by gastroenteritis, is one of the most common problems encountered in infants and children. (See Chapter 25.) Until modern techniques for fluid replacement were perfected, gastroenteritis was one of the chief causes of infant mortality. Fluid and electrolyte problems related to specific diseases and their management are discussed throughout the book where appropriate. The major fluid disturbances, their usual causes, and clinical manifestations are listed in Table 23.2; the most common fluid disturbances, dehydration and edema, are elaborated further in the following sections. Problems of fluid and electrolyte disturbance always involve both water and electrolytes; therefore replacement includes administration of both, calculated on the basis of ongoing processes and laboratory serum electrolyte values.

In conditions that involve alterations in the amount and composition of body fluid compartments, nurses consider many factors when planning management (Box 23.2). The following discussion is concerned with the general concepts of two common fluid volume disturbances, dehydration and edema, which are features of a variety of conditions.

TABLE 23.2 Disturbances of Fluid and Electrolyte Balance

Mechanisms and Situations	Manifestations	Management and Nursing Care
Water Depletion		
Failure to absorb or reabsorb water Complete or sudden cessation of intake or prolonged diminished intake: • Neglect of intake by self or caregiver—confused, psychotic, unconscious, or helpless • Loss from gastrointestinal tract—vomiting, diarrhea, nasogastric suction, fistula Disturbed body fluid chemistry: inappropriate ADH secretion Excessive renal excretion: glycosuria (diabetes) Loss through skin or lungs: • Excessive perspiration or evaporation—febrile states, hyperventilation, increased ambient temperature, increased activity (basal metabolic rate) • Impaired skin integrity—transudate from injuries • Hemorrhage Iatrogenic: • Overzealous use of diuretics • Improper perioperative fluid replacement • Use of radiant warmer or phototherapy	General symptoms dependent to some extent on proportion of electrolytes lost with water Thirst Variable temperature—increased (infection) Dry skin and mucous membranes Poor skin turgor Poor perfusion (decreased pulse, slowed capillary refill time) Weight loss Fatigue Diminished urinary output Irritability and lethargy Tachycardia Tachypnea Altered level of consciousness, disorientation Laboratory findings: • High urine specific gravity • Increased hematocrit • Variable serum electrolytes • Variable urine volume • Increased blood urea nitrogen • Increased serum osmolality	Provide replacement of fluid losses commensurate with volume depletion. Provide maintenance fluids and electrolytes. Determine and correct cause of water depletion. Measure fluid intake and output. Monitor vital signs. Monitor urine specific gravity. Monitor body weight. Monitor serum electrolytes.

Continued

TABLE 23.2 Disturbances of Fluid and Electrolyte Balance—cont'd

Mechanisms and Situations	Manifestations	Management and Nursing Care
Water Excess		
Water intake in excess of output: • Excessive oral intake • Hypotonic fluid overload • Plain water enemas Failure to excrete water in presence of normal intake: • Kidney disease • Congestive heart failure • Malnutrition	Edema: • Generalized • Pulmonary (moist rales or crackles) • Intracutaneous (noted especially in loose areolar tissue) Elevated central venous pressure Hepatomegaly Slow, bounding pulse Weight gain Lethargy Increased spinal fluid pressure Central nervous system manifestations (seizures, coma) Laboratory findings: • Low urine specific gravity • Decreased serum electrolytes • Decreased hematocrit • Variable urine volume	Limit fluid intake. Administer diuretics. Monitor vital signs. Monitor neurologic signs as necessary. Determine and treat cause of water excess. Analyze serum electrolytes frequently. Implement seizure precautions.
Sodium Depletion (Hyponatremia)		
Prolonged low-sodium diet Decreased sodium intake Fever Excess sweating Increased water intake without electrolytes Tachypnea (infants) Cystic fibrosis Burns and wounds Vomiting, diarrhea, nasogastric suction, fistulas Adrenal insufficiency Renal disease Diabetic ketoacidosis (DKA) Malnutrition	Associated with water loss: • Same as with water loss—dehydration, weakness, dizziness, nausea, abdominal cramps, apprehension • Mild—apathy, weakness, nausea, weak pulse • Moderate—decreased blood pressure, lethargy Laboratory findings: • Sodium concentration <130 mEq/L (may be normal if volume loss) • Urine specific gravity depends on water deficit or excess	Determine and treat cause of sodium deficit. Administer IV fluids with appropriate saline concentration. Monitor fluid intake and output.
Sodium Excess (Hypernatremia)		
High salt intake—enteral or IV Renal disease Fever Insufficient breast milk intake in neonate (dehydration hypernatremia) High insensible water loss: • Increased temperature • Increased humidity • Hyperventilation • Diabetes insipidus • Hyperglycemia	Intense thirst Dry, sticky mucous membranes Flushed skin Temperature possibly increased Hoarseness Oliguria Nausea and vomiting Possible progression to disorientation, convulsions, muscle twitching, nuchal rigidity, lethargy at rest, hyperirritability when aroused Laboratory findings: • Serum sodium concentration ≤150 mEq/L • High plasma volume • Alkalosis	Determine and treat cause of sodium excess. Administer IV fluids as prescribed. Measure fluid intake and output. Monitor laboratory data. Monitor neurologic status. Ensure adequate intake of breast milk and provide lactation assistance with new mother-baby pair before hospital discharge.

TABLE 23.2 Disturbances of Fluid and Electrolyte Balance—cont'd

Mechanisms and Situations	Manifestations	Management and Nursing Care
Potassium Depletion (Hypokalemia)		
Starvation Clinical conditions associated with poor food intake Malabsorption IV fluid without added potassium Gastrointestinal losses—diarrhea, vomiting, fistulas, nasogastric suction Diuresis Administration of diuretics Administration of corticosteroids Diuretic phase of nephrotic syndrome Healing stage of burns Potassium-losing nephritis Hyperglycemic diuresis (e.g., diabetes mellitus) Familial periodic paralysis IV administration of insulin in DKA Alkalosis	Muscle weakness, cramping, stiffness, paralysis, hyporeflexia Hypotension Cardiac arrhythmias, gallop rhythm Tachycardia or bradycardia Ileus Apathy, drowsiness Irritability Fatigue Laboratory findings: • Decreased serum potassium concentration ≥3.5 mEq/L • Abnormal ECG—notched or flattened T waves, decreased ST segment, premature ventricular contractions	Determine and treat cause of potassium deficit. Monitor vital signs, including ECG. Administer supplemental potassium. Assess for adequate renal output before administration. For IV replacement, administer potassium slowly. Always monitor ECG for IV bolus potassium replacement. For oral intake, offer high-potassium fluids and foods. Evaluate acid-base status.
Potassium Excess (Hyperkalemia)		
Renal disease Renal failure Adrenal insufficiency (Addison disease) Associated with metabolic acidosis Too-rapid administration of IV potassium chloride Transfusion with old donor blood Severe dehydration Crushing injuries Burns Hemolysis Dehydration Potassium-sparing diuretics Increased intake of potassium (e.g., salt substitutes)	Muscle weakness, flaccid paralysis Twitching Hyperreflexia Bradycardia Ventricular fibrillation and cardiac arrest Oliguria Apnea—respiratory arrest Laboratory findings: • High serum potassium concentration ≤5.5 mEq/L • Variable urine volume • Flat P wave on ECG, peaked T waves, widened QRS complex, increased PR interval	Determine and treat cause of potassium excess. Monitor vital signs, including ECG. Administer exchange resin, if prescribed. Administer IV fluids as prescribed. Administer IV insulin (if ordered) to facilitate movement of potassium into cells. Monitor potassium levels. Evaluate acid-base status.
Calcium Depletion (Hypocalcemia)		
Inadequate dietary calcium Vitamin D deficiency Rapid transit through gastrointestinal tract Advanced renal insufficiency Administration of diuretics Hypoparathyroidism Alkalosis Calcium trapped in diseased tissues Increased serum protein (albumin) Cow's milk—tetany of the newborn (inappropriate calcium/phosphorus ratio in whole milk for newborn) Exchange transfusion with citrated blood Inadequate parenteral administration in diseased status	Neuromuscular irritability Tingling of nose, ears, fingertips, toes Tetany Laryngospasm Generalized convulsions May be changes in clotting Positive Chvostek and Trousseau signs Hypotension Cardiac arrest Laboratory findings: • Decreased serum calcium concentration (8.8-10.8 mEq/L) or increased serum protein levels • Prolonged QT interval	Determine and treat cause of calcium deficit. Administer oral calcium supplements as prescribed; administer IV slowly and diluted. Monitor IV site; calcium may cause vascular irritation. Monitor serum calcium, vitamin D, and parathyroid levels. Monitor serum protein levels. Avoid cow's milk in infants younger than 12 months.

Continued

TABLE 23.2 Disturbances of Fluid and Electrolyte Balance—cont'd

Mechanisms and Situations	Manifestations	Management and Nursing Care
Calcium Excess (Hypercalcemia)		
Acidosis Prolonged immobilization Conditions associated with increased bone catabolism Hypoproteinemia Kidney disease Hypervitaminosis D Hyperparathyroidism Hyperthyroidism Excessive IV or oral administration	Constipation Weakness, fatigue Nausea, vomiting Anorexia Dry mouth (thirst) Muscle hypotonicity Bradycardia or cardiac arrest Increased calcium concentration in urine, causing formation of kidney stones Laboratory findings: • Increased serum calcium levels or decreased serum protein levels • Prolonged QRS complex or PR interval, shortened QT interval	Determine and treat cause of calcium excess. Monitor serum calcium levels. Monitor ECG.

ADH, Antidiuretic hormone; *ECG,* electrocardiogram; *IV,* intravenous.

BOX 23.2 Areas of Concern in Planning Management of Fluid Problems

- Volume of body fluids (e.g., water content of the patient)
- Osmolality of the body fluids, which affects the distribution of body water among the various compartments
- Hydrogen ion status (i.e., whether there has been a disturbance in the pH of body fluids or a disturbance in the homeostatic mechanisms that maintain the pH)
- Electrolyte deficits from cells and extracellular water
- Disturbances in the equilibrium between the mineral skeleton and body fluids
- Length of time alteration in fluid status has existed

Specific disorders are discussed in Chapter 25 and elsewhere in the book where appropriate.

DEHYDRATION

Dehydration is a common body fluid disturbance encountered in the nursing care of infants and young children; it occurs whenever the total output of fluid exceeds the total intake, regardless of the underlying cause. Dehydration is also commonly referred to as volume depletion. Although dehydration can result from lack of oral intake (especially in elevated environmental temperatures), more often it is a result of abnormal losses, such as those that occur in vomiting or diarrhea, when oral intake only partially compensates for the abnormal losses. Other significant causes of dehydration are diabetic ketoacidosis and extensive burns.

! NURSING ALERT

In a child with a history of fluid loss and potential or actual dehydration, gear nursing assessment toward the possibility of impending shock.

In early dehydration (during the first 2 days), fluid loss is derived from both the ECF and the ICF because the increased osmolality of the diminished ECF volume causes fluid from the ICF compartment to move into the ECF compartment. As dehydration becomes chronic, the cellular losses become greater.

Types of Dehydration

Because sodium is the primary osmotic force that controls fluid movement between the major fluid compartments, dehydration is often described according to plasma sodium concentrations (e.g., isonatremic, hyponatremic, or hypernatremic). Other osmotic forces, however, such as glucose in diabetic ketoacidosis and protein in nephrotic syndrome, may also play a dominant role. Consequently, dehydration is conventionally classified as isotonic, hypotonic, or hypertonic.

Isotonic (isosmotic or isonatremic) dehydration occurs in conditions in which electrolyte and water deficits are present in approximately balanced proportions. This is the primary form of dehydration occurring in children. The observable fluid losses are not necessarily isotonic, but losses from other avenues make adjustments so that the sum of all losses, or the net loss, is isotonic. Because no osmotic force is present to cause a redistribution of water between the ICF and ECF, the major loss is sustained from the ECF compartment. This significantly reduces the plasma volume and thus the circulating blood volume, with its effect on the skin, muscles, and kidneys. Shock is the greatest threat to life in isotonic dehydration, and the child with isotonic dehydration displays symptoms characteristic of hypovolemic shock. Plasma sodium remains within normal limits, between 130 and 150 mEq/L (Friedman, Beck DeGroot, et al., 2015; Huether, 2014).

Hypotonic (hyposmotic or hyponatremic) dehydration occurs when the electrolyte deficit exceeds the water deficit. Because ICF is more concentrated than ECF in hypotonic dehydration, water transfers from the ECF to the ICF to establish osmotic equilibrium. This movement further increases the ECF volume loss, and shock is a frequent result. Because there is a greater proportional loss of ECF in hypotonic dehydration, the physical signs tend to be more severe with smaller fluid losses than in isotonic or hypertonic dehydration. Plasma sodium concentrations are typically less than 130 mEq/L (Huether, 2014).

Hypertonic (hyperosmotic or hypernatremic) dehydration results from water loss in excess of electrolyte loss and is usually caused by a proportionately larger loss of water or a larger intake of electrolytes. This type of dehydration is the most dangerous and requires much more specific fluid therapy. This sometimes occurs in infants with diarrhea who are given fluids by mouth that contain large amounts of solute or in children receiving high-protein nasogastric tube feedings that place an excessive solute load on the kidneys. In hypertonic dehydration, fluid shifts from the lesser concentration of the ICF to the ECF. Plasma sodium concentration is greater than 150 mEq/L (Huether, 2014).

Because the ECF volume is proportionately larger, hypertonic dehydration consists of a greater degree of water loss for the same intensity of physical signs. Shock is less apparent in hypotonic dehydration. However, neurologic disturbances, such as seizures, are more likely to occur. Cerebral changes are serious and may result in permanent damage. These include disturbance of consciousness, poor ability to focus attention, lethargy, increased muscle tone with hyperreflexia, and hyperirritability to stimuli (e.g., tactile, auditory, bright lights).

Degree of Dehydration

A determination of the type and degree of dehydration is necessary to develop an effective plan of therapy. The degree of dehydration has been described as a percentage of body weight dehydrated: mild—less than 3% in older children or less than 5% in infants; moderate—5% to 10% in infants and 3% to 6% in older children; and severe—more than 10% in infants and more than 6% in older children (Carson, Mudd, & Madati, 2016; Greenbaum, 2015). Water constitutes only 60% to 70% of the infant's weight. However, adipose tissue contains little water and is highly variable in individual infants and children. A more accurate means of describing dehydration is to reflect acute fluid loss (time frame of ≥48 hours) in milliliters per kilogram of body weight. For example, a loss of 50 ml/kg is considered to be a mild fluid loss, whereas a loss of 100 ml/kg produces severe dehydration.

Weight is the most important determinant of the percent of total body fluid loss in infants and younger children. However, often the preillness weight is unknown. Other predictors of fluid loss include a changing level of consciousness (irritability to lethargy), altered response to stimuli, decreased skin elasticity and turgor, prolonged capillary refill (>2 seconds), increased heart rate, and sunken eyes and fontanels.

Clinical signs provide clues to the extent of dehydration (Table 23.3). The earliest detectable sign is usually tachycardia, followed by dry skin and mucous membranes, sunken fontanels, signs of circulatory failure (coolness and mottling of extremities), loss of skin elasticity, and prolonged capillary filling time (see Table 23.4 for clinical manifestations of dehydration and Fig. 23.3 for signs of dehydration). There is evidence that the clinical signs of abnormal capillary refill, abnormal skin turgor, and abnormal respiratory pattern are the most useful in predicting dehydration of 5% or more in children (Carson, Mudd, & Madati, 2017).

Compensatory mechanisms attempt to maintain fluid volume by adjusting to these losses. Interstitial fluid moves into the vascular compartment to maintain the blood volume in response to hemoconcentration and hypovolemia, and vasoconstriction of peripheral arterioles helps maintain pumping pressure. When fluid losses exceed the body's ability to sustain blood volume and blood pressure, circulation is seriously compromised and the blood pressure falls. This results in tissue hypoxia with accumulation of lactic acid, pyruvate, and other acid metabolites, which contribute to the development of metabolic acidosis.

Renal compensation is impaired by reduced blood flow through the kidneys, and little urine is formed. Increased serum osmolality stimulates the secretion of antidiuretic hormone (ADH) to conserve fluid and initiates the renin-angiotensin mechanisms in the kidney, causing further vasoconstriction. Aldosterone is released to promote sodium retention and conserve water in the kidneys. If dehydration increases in severity, urine formation is greatly diminished and metabolites and hydrogen ions that are normally excreted by this route are retained.

Shock, a common manifestation of severe depletion of ECF volume, is preceded by tachycardia and signs of poor perfusion and tissue oxygenation (by pulse oximeter readings). Peripheral circulation is poor as a result of reduced blood volume; therefore the skin is cool and mottled with decreased capillary filling. Impaired kidney circulation often leads to oliguria and azotemia. Although low blood pressure may accompany other symptoms of shock, in infants and young children it is usually a late sign and may herald the onset of cardiovascular collapse (see p. 967, Congestive Heart Failure).

Diagnostic Evaluation

To initiate a therapeutic plan, several factors must be determined:

- The degree of dehydration based on physical assessment
- The type of dehydration based on the pathophysiology of the specific illness responsible for the dehydrated state
- Specific physical signs other than general signs
- Initial plasma sodium concentrations
- Serum bicarbonate concentration
- Any associated electrolyte (especially serum potassium) and acid-base imbalances (as indicated)

TABLE 23.3 Evaluating Extent of Dehydration

	LEVEL OF DEHYDRATION		
Clinical Signs	**Mild**	**Moderate**	**Severe**
Weight loss—infants	3%-5%	6%-9%	≤10%
Weight loss—children	3%-4%	6%-8%	10%
Pulse	Normal	Slightly increased	Very increased
Respiratory rate	Normal	Slight tachypnea (rapid)	Hyperpnea (deep and rapid)
Blood pressure	Normal	Normal to orthostatic (>10 mm Hg change)	Orthostatic to shock
Behavior	Normal	Irritable, more thirsty	Hyperirritable to lethargic
Thirst	Slight	Moderate	Intense
Mucous membranes*	Normal (moist)	Dry	Parched
Tears	Present	Decreased	Absent, sunken eyes
Anterior fontanel	Normal	Normal to sunken	Sunken
External jugular vein	Visible when supine	Not visible except with supraclavicular pressure	Not visible even with supraclavicular pressure
Skin*	Capillary refill >2 sec	Slowed capillary refill (2-4 sec [decreased turgor])	Very delayed capillary refill (>4 sec) and tenting; skin cool, acrocyanotic or mottled
Urine	Decreased	Oliguria	Oliguria or anuria

*These signs are less prominent in patients who have hypernatremia.

Data from Jospe, N., & Forbes, G. (1996). Fluids and electrolytes—clinical aspects. *Pediatrics in Review, 17*(11), 395-403; and Steiner, M. J., DeWalt, D. A., & Byerly, J. S. (2004). Is this child dehydrated? *Journal of the American Medical Association, 291*(22), 2746-2754.

TABLE 23.4 **Clinical Manifestations of Dehydration**

Manifestation	Isotonic (Loss of Water and Salt)	Hypotonic (Loss of Salt in Excess of Water)	Hypertonic (Loss of Water in Excess of Salt)
Skin			
• Color	Gray	Gray	Gray
• Temperature	Cold	Cold	Cold or hot
• Turgor	Poor	Very poor	Fair
• Feel	Dry	Clammy	Thickened, doughy
Mucous membranes	Dry	Slightly moist	Parched
Tearing and salivation	Absent	Absent	Absent
Eyeball	Sunken	Sunken	Sunken
Fontanel	Sunken	Sunken	Sunken
Body temperature	Subnormal or elevated	Subnormal or elevated	Subnormal or elevated
Pulse	Rapid	Very rapid	Moderately rapid
Respirations	Rapid	Rapid	Rapid
Behavior	Irritable to lethargic	Lethargic or comatose; convulsions	Marked lethargy with extreme hyperirritability on stimulation

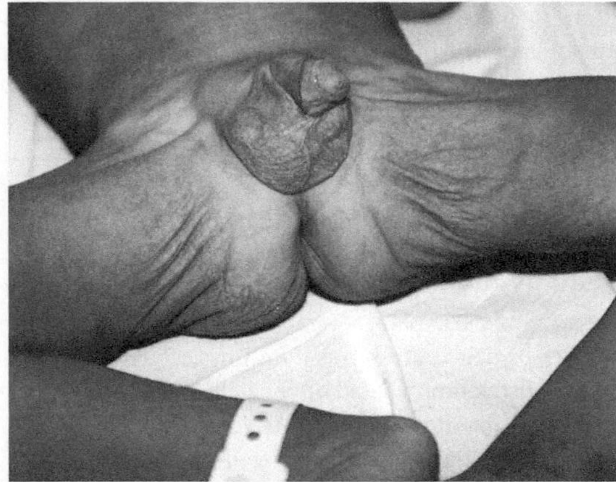

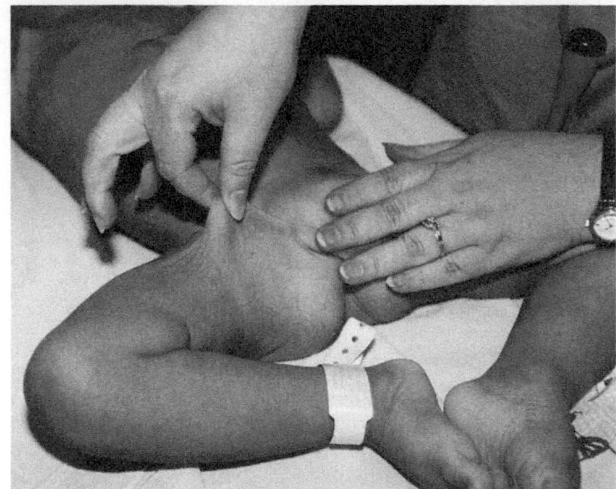

FIG. 23.3 Loss of skin elasticity because of dehydration.

Initial and regular, ongoing evaluations assess the patient's progress toward equilibrium and the effectiveness of therapy.

In the examination of an infant or younger child, one of the most important determinants of the extent of dehydration is body weight because this can assist in determining the percentage of total body fluid lost; however, because the preillness weight is often unknown, clinical manifestations must be evaluated (see Research Focus box). Important clinical manifestations include changing sensorium (irritability to lethargy); decreased response to stimuli; integumentary changes (decreased elasticity and turgor); prolonged capillary refill; increased heart rate; sunken eyes; and, in infants, sunken fontanels. Using multiple predictors increases the sensitivity of assessing the fluid deficit, and studies have shown a reasonably high degree of agreement between experienced observers in assessment of the level of dehydration. Objective signs of dehydration are present at a fluid deficit of less than 5%.

RESEARCH FOCUS

Pediatric Dehydration

In past reviews of pediatric dehydration assessment, the best three individual examination signs for assessing dehydration were prolonged capillary refill time (>2 seconds), abnormal skin turgor, and abnormal respiratory pattern (Emond, 2009). A recent meta-analysis of 9 studies of over 1000 children revealed that clinical dehydration assessment scales provide some improved diagnostic accuracy, but it is still suboptimal. Current evidence form this review did not support the routine use of ultrasound or urinalysis to determine dehydration severity (Freedman, Vandermeer, Milne, et al., 2015). There is some evidence to support serum urea and creatinine as markers for dehydration along with bicarbonate that is consistently decreased in moderate to severe dehydration (Hoxha, Azemi, Avdiu et al., 2014; Whitney, Santucci, Hsiao, et al., 2016).

Therapeutic Management

Medical management is directed at correcting the fluid imbalance and treating the underlying cause. When the child is alert, awake, and not in danger, correction of dehydration may be attempted with oral fluid administration. Most cases of dehydration are mild and can be managed at home by this method. Several commercial rehydration fluids are available for use (see Table 25.3). Oral rehydration management consists of replacement of fluid loss over 4 to 6 hours, replacement of continuing losses, and provision for maintenance fluid requirements. In general, the mildly dehydrated child may be given 50 ml/kg of **oral rehydration solution (ORS)**, whereas the child with moderate dehydration may be given 100 ml/kg of ORS. The child with fluid losses from diarrhea may be given an additional 10 ml/kg for each stool (Greenbaum, 2015). Amounts and rates are determined from body weight and severity of dehydration and are increased if rehydration is incomplete or if excess losses continue, until the child is well hydrated and the basic problem is under control.

The child may not be thirsty even though dehydrated and may refuse oral fluids initially for fear of continued emesis (if occurring) or because of decreased strength, oral stomatitis, or thrush. In such children rehydration may proceed by administering 2 to 5 ml of ORS by a syringe or small medication cup every 2 to 3 minutes until the child is able to tolerate larger amounts; if the child has emesis, administering small amounts (5 ml) of ORS every 5 minutes or so may help overcome fluid deficit, and the emesis will often lessen over time (Hendrickson, Zaremba, Wey, et al., 2017). Evidence indicates that oral administration of ondansetron (Zofran) to children with acute gastroenteritis and vomiting reduces emesis and increases time to oral rehydration, thus preventing intravenous (IV) therapy (Carter & Fedorowicz, 2012; Hendrickson, Zaremba, Wey, et al., 2017). Oral rehydration therapy (ORT) is effective for treating mild or moderate dehydration in children, is less expensive, and involves fewer complications than therapy (Carson, Mudd, Madati, 2016; Kleinman & Greer, 2014). ORSs enhance and promote the reabsorption of sodium and water. These solutions greatly reduce vomiting and the need for IV infusions (Hendrickson, Zaremba, Wey, et al., 2017). ORSs, including lower-osmolarity ORS (224 mmol/L), are available in the United States as commercially prepared solutions and are successful in treating the majority of infants with dehydration. See the Quality Patient Outcomes box. (See Diarrhea, Chapter 25, for a complete discussion of fluid replacement therapy for dehydration.)

QUALITY PATIENT OUTCOMES

Fluid Volume Deficit

- Moist mucous membranes
- Sodium and potassium within normal limits
- Voiding (>1 ml/kg/hr)
- Capillary refill of 2 seconds or less
- Skin turgor brisk
- Fluid intake and output balanced

NURSING TIP

Enhance the flavor of an ORS such as Pedialyte (unflavored) by adding a teaspoon of unsweetened powder Kool-Aid to each 60 to 90 ml of ORS. Older children may take a small Popsicle orally instead of fluids that require drinking. Many commercially available Popsicles are relatively inexpensive, contain small amounts of sucrose, and contain approximately 40 to 50 ml of fluid. Frozen oral hydration may be accepted by some children when conventional ORS is rejected (see Box 25.7 and Table 25.3 for models of rehydration and composition of ORS).

Parenteral Fluid Therapy

Parenteral fluid therapy is initiated whenever the child is unable to ingest sufficient amounts of fluid and electrolytes to meet ongoing daily physiologic losses, replace previous deficits, and replace ongoing abnormal losses. Patients who usually require IV fluids are those with severe dehydration, those with uncontrollable vomiting, those who are unable to drink for any reason (e.g., extreme fatigue, coma), or those with severe gastric distention.

Because dehydration (volume depletion) constitutes a great threat to life, the first priority is the restoration of circulation by rapid expansion of the ECF volume to treat or prevent shock. IV administration of fluid begins immediately, although the exact nature of the dehydration and the serum electrolyte values are not known. The solution selected is based on what is known regarding the probable type and cause of the dehydration. This usually involves an isotonic solution such as 0.9% sodium chloride or lactated Ringer, both of which are close to the body's serum osmolality of 285 to 300 mOsm/kg and do not contain dextrose (which is contraindicated in the early treatment stages of rehydration, but especially in diabetic ketoacidosis).

Parenteral rehydration therapy has three phases. The initial therapy is used to expand ECF volume quickly and to improve circulatory and renal function. During initial therapy, an isotonic electrolyte solution is used at a rate of 20 ml/kg, given as an IV bolus over 5 to 20 minutes and repeated as necessary after assessment of the child's response to therapy. In a meta-analysis of 10 randomized clinical trials, isotonic fluids were found safer than hypotonic fluids in preventing severe hyponatremia following administration (Wang, Xu, & Xiao, 2014). Subsequent therapy is used to replace deficits, meet maintenance water and electrolyte requirements, and catch up with ongoing losses. Water and sodium requirements for the deficit, maintenance, and ongoing losses are calculated at 8-hour intervals, taking into consideration the amount of fluids given with the initial boluses and the amount administered during the first 24-hour period. With improved circulation during this phase, water and electrolyte deficits can be evaluated, and acid-base status can be corrected either directly through the administration of fluids or indirectly through improved renal function. Potassium is withheld until kidney function is restored and assessed and circulation has improved.

The final phase of therapy allows the patient to return to normal and begin oral feedings, with a gradual correction of total body deficits. The potassium loss in ICF is replaced slowly by way of the ECF. The body fat and protein stores are replaced through diet. If the child is unable to eat or if feeding aggravates a chronic condition, IV maintenance fluids are provided.

Although the initial phase of fluid replacement is rapid in both isotonic and hypotonic dehydration, it is contraindicated in hypertonic dehydration because of the risk of water intoxication, especially in the brain cells, specifically the central pontine cells. Central pontine myelinolysis may occur with an overcorrection of fluid deficit and an overly rapid correction of serum sodium concentration (Greenbaum, 2015). There is an apparent lag time for sodium to reach a steady state when diffusing in and out of brain cells, whereas water diffuses almost instantaneously. Consequently, rapid administration of fluid will cause equally rapid diffusion of water into the dehydrated brain cells, causing marked cerebral edema. Because ECF volume is maintained relatively well in hypertonic as opposed to the other types of dehydration, shock is not a usual manifestation.

WATER INTOXICATION

Water intoxication, or water overload, is observed less often than dehydration. However, it is important that nurses and others who care for children be alert to this possibility in certain situations. Children who ingest excessive amounts of electrolyte-free water develop a concurrent decrease in serum sodium accompanied by central nervous system (CNS) symptoms. There is a large urinary output, and because water moves into the brain more rapidly than sodium moves out, the child may also exhibit irritability, somnolence, headache, vomiting, diarrhea, or generalized seizures. The affected child usually appears well hydrated but may be edematous or even dehydrated.

Fluid intoxication can occur during acute IV water overloading, too-rapid dialysis, tap water enemas, feeding of incorrectly mixed infant formula, or excess water ingestion, or with too rapid reduction of glucose levels in diabetic ketoacidosis (Greenbaum, 2015). Patients with CNS infections occasionally retain excessive amounts of water. Administration of inappropriate hypotonic solutions (e.g., 0.45% sodium chloride) may cause a rapid reduction in sodium and result in symptoms of water overload.

Infants are especially vulnerable to fluid overload. Their thirst mechanism is not well developed; therefore they are unable to "turn off" fluid intake appropriately. A decreased glomerular filtration rate does not allow for repeated excretion of a water load, and ADH levels may not be maximally reduced. Consequently, infants are unable to excrete a water overload effectively.

Administration of inappropriately prepared formula is one of the more common causes of water intoxication in infants (Greenbaum, 2015). Families who cannot afford to buy enough formula may dilute the formula to increase the volume or even substitute water for the formula. A family may run out of formula and dilute the remaining amount to make it last until they are able to purchase more. In addition, water is sometimes used for pacification. Water intoxication can also occur in infants who receive overly vigorous hydration during a febrile illness.

A number of clinicians have reported water intoxication in infants after swimming lessons, in water births (Byard & Zuccollo, 2010), with excessive enema administration, and with gastric lavage (Manz, 2007). Although they hold their breath, some infants apparently swallow a large amount of water during repeated submersion. Anticipatory guidance to parents should include a discussion of swimming instruction and advice to stop a lesson if the child swallows unusual amounts of water or exhibit any symptoms of hyponatremia.

EDEMA

Edema represents an abnormal accumulation of fluid within the interstitial tissue and subsequent tissue expansion and develops when a defect in the normal cardiovascular circulation or a failure in the lymphatic drainage to remove the increased amounts occurs. The processes responsible for fluid removal include venous hydrostatic pressure, oncotic pressure of intravascular and interstitial spaces, an intact semipermeable capillary wall, tissue tension, and lymphatic flow.

Mechanisms of Edema Formation

A defect of any of the homeostatic mechanisms maintaining fluid balance can cause accumulation of interstitial fluid. Disequilibrium results from anything that (1) alters the retention of sodium, such as renal disease or hormonal influences; (2) affects the formation or destruction of plasma proteins, such as starvation or liver disease; or (3) alters membrane permeability, such as minimal change nephrotic syndrome or trauma.

Edema may be localized to a small or large area, such as that occurring in urticaria, infection, and pulmonary congestion, or it can be generalized, as in the hypoproteinemia of the nephrotic syndrome and starvation. A severe, generalized accumulation of great amounts of fluid in all body tissues is termed anasarca.

Increased Venous Pressure

The colloidal osmotic pressure of the plasma proteins draws fluid back into the vascular system as long as this force is greater than the venous hydrostatic pressure. However, when the venous pressure increases, fluid tends to be retained in the interstitial spaces. This can occur when an individual remains in the same position for a long time, such as swollen ankles and feet after standing or sitting for long periods. Constrictive dressings or restraints applied too tightly to extremities will obstruct venous return, increase venous and capillary pressure, and cause edema. The most graphic pathologic illustrations are pulmonary edema caused by pulmonary circulation overload in cardiac defects with a left-to-right shunt and ascites caused by portal hypertension. Edema from any cause is increased in dependent areas because of this added factor of increased venous hydrostatic pressure and the gravitational effects in these areas.

Capillary Permeability

Damage to capillary walls or alteration in their permeability permits exudation of plasma protein into the interstitial space. Most often this occurs as local edema, such as that manifested in inflammatory and hypersensitivity reactions. Capillary damage from burns allows extensive exudation of protein-rich fluid into the interstitial spaces to compound edema formation.

Diminished Plasma Proteins

A fall in plasma protein levels hampers the osmotic pull back into the vessels. Consequently, fluid remains in the interstitial spaces. Although other factors play a role, such as hydrostatic pressure of both the arterial vascular system and the tissues and sodium concentration, significantly low protein levels (<4.5 mg/dl) are associated with edema. Examples of this are the massive albumin losses of the minimal change nephrotic syndrome, diminished serum protein from insufficient dietary protein, and (sometimes) hemodilution of plasma proteins from IV fluid administration in chronic dehydration.

Lymphatic Obstruction

Obstruction of lymph flow creates edema high in protein content. This occurs infrequently in childhood but can result from trauma to the lymphatic glands or from removal of lymph nodes.

Tissue Tension

Tissue hydrostatic pressure is ordinarily of little consequence. However, it plays a significant role in determining distribution of edema fluid in certain pathologic conditions. Loose tissues allow a greater amount of fluid accumulation than tissues that are tightly bound by dense fibrous bands in which tissue pressure rapidly increases to limit further extravasation of fluid. Edema appears earlier and more readily in loose structures such as those in the periorbital and genital tissues. The alveolar structure of lung tissue is probably a contributing factor in pulmonary edema, as well as in increased hydrostatic pressure in the pulmonary vessels.

Other Factors in Edema Formation

Any factor that causes sodium retention by the kidneys will produce or augment edema formation. This includes stimulation of the renin-angiotensin-aldosterone mechanisms for sodium reabsorption created by the diminished plasma volume in edema, which resulted from primary causes. The salt-retaining property of steroids is responsible for the edema associated with their administration.

Several types of edema exist, all of which can provide a palpable swelling of the interstitial space that is either localized or generalized. These include the following:

- Peripheral edema, or localized or generalized palpable swelling of the interstitial space
- Ascites, or the accumulation of fluid in the abdominal cavity (usually associated with renal or liver abnormalities)
- Pulmonary edema, which occurs when interstitial volume increases
- Cerebral edema, which is a particularly threatening form of edema caused by trauma, infection, or other etiologic factors, including vascular overload or injudicious IV administration of hypotonic solutions
- Overall fluid gain, especially seen in patients with kidney disease

Assessment

Generalized edema resulting from any of the previously listed types is manifested by swelling in the extremities, face, perineum, and torso. Loss of normal skin creases may be assessed. Daily weights are more sensitive indicators of water gain or loss and should be obtained.

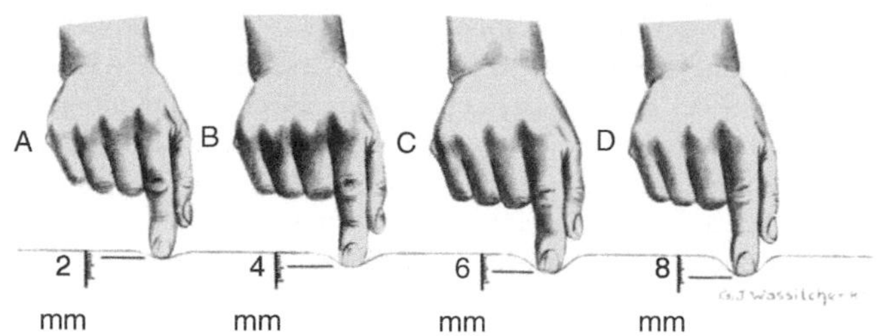

FIG. 23.4 Assessment of pitting edema. **A,** +1. **B,** +2. **C,** +3. **D,** +4. (From Lowdermilk, D. L., & Perry, S. E. [2007]. *Maternity and women's health care* [9th ed.]. St. Louis, MO: Mosby.)

Abdominal girth measurement changes may also be an indicator of edema in children. Pitting edema may occur and can be assessed by pressing the fingertip against a bony prominence for 5 seconds. If the tissue rebounds immediately on removing the finger, the patient does not have pitting edema. A quick way to determine the severity is to measure the degree of pitting edema (Fig. 23.4).

Therapeutic Management

The primary goal in the management of edema is treatment of the underlying disease process, which is discussed elsewhere in relation to the specific disorder. However, an essential aspect in the management of any fluid overload is early recognition, in which nurses play a vital role. The management of edema is discussed throughout the text with specific conditions. See the Quality Patient Outcomes box.

QUALITY PATIENT OUTCOMES

Fluid Volume Excess

- Fluid intake and output balanced
- No edema
- No weight gain
- No respiratory distress related to fluid volume excess

NURSING RESPONSIBILITIES IN FLUID AND ELECTROLYTE DISTURBANCES

Nursing observation and intervention are essential to the detection and therapeutic management of disturbances in fluid and electrolyte balance. Imbalances may be precipitated by a variety of circumstances, and the balance may be so precarious, especially in newborns and infants, that changes can take place in a very short time. Therefore an important nursing responsibility is anticipation and perceptive observation for any signs of imbalance, particularly in those situations and conditions in which imbalance is likely to occur. Conditions in which changes can develop with surprising rapidity in young children include diarrhea; vomiting; sweating; fever; disorders such as type 1 diabetes, bowel surgery, renal disease, and cardiac anomalies; administration of certain drugs such as diuretics and steroids; and trauma, such as major surgery, burns, and other extensive injury.

Nurses must be comfortable with equipment used to deliver fluids to infants and children and be familiar with the information and techniques for physical assessment of each age-group. An understanding of normal serum chemistry levels provides additional data on which to base assessments and interventions and to validate observations. Data that are helpful in assessment related to fluid and electrolyte balance include the proposed treatment plan, including medications and fluid therapies, laboratory reports, history of illness, and records of fluid intake and output (I&O). An important nursing role is teaching parents to recognize early signs of dehydration and how to know when to start oral rehydration when the child is mildly dehydrated. Anticipatory guidance is also given to parents regarding acceptable oral fluid intake in infants (preferably no water), caution against dilution of formula with extra water, and avoiding the administration of water enemas.

ASSESSMENT

Whether the child is at home, in the practitioner's office or clinic, or in the hospital, nursing assessment is an essential part of the nursing care plan. The assessment of suspected or potential fluid and electrolyte disturbance begins with the observation of general appearance. Ill children usually have drawn expressions, have dry mucous membranes and lips, and "look sick." Loss of appetite is one of the first behaviors observed in most childhood illnesses, and the infant's or child's activity level is diminished from baseline or usual activities. The child is irritable, seeks the parent's comfort and attention, and displays purposeless movements and inappropriate responses to people and familiar objects. In some cases the child may not protest advances by the health care worker and procedures such as taking vital signs or starting an IV infusion. These are signs that the child truly feels bad and that the condition is serious and immediate intervention is necessary. As the child's illness and level of dehydration become more severe, irritability progresses to lethargy and even unconsciousness.

History

The nurse can obtain much of the information regarding the child's behavior from the parent or primary caregiver. In addition to initial observations, a good history is extremely valuable to the assessment. The amount and type of fluid I&O (especially abnormal output) are important. An accurate estimate of fluid losses is beyond the capacity of history givers, but rough estimates of excessive fluid losses or diminished output can usually be obtained from information such as the number and consistency of stools the child has passed in the past 24 hours, the number of times the child voided, and the type and amount of food and fluid ingested or vomited. For an infant, ask about the number of wet diapers in the past 24 hours. Parents frequently omit this information from their discussion with the health professional. Having the parents estimate the amount of urine in the diaper at each void is of little value because of the absorbent diaper material, which pulls fluids away from the child's skin. Encourage new parents of a newborn to record on a piece of paper the number of wet diapers and the times the infant has breastfed or bottle-fed. In general the number of days in life (up to 6 to 10 days of age) should equal the number of wet diapers per day. For example, a 4-day-old infant who is breastfeeding can be expected to have a minimum of 4 wet diapers in the 24-hour period. It may be more difficult to tell if a female infant has voided if stooling also occurs; one easy way to tell with absorbent diapers is to pull apart the crotch of the diaper from the outside and inspect the absorbent granules for signs of urine.

Both the type and the amount of fluid intake provide valuable information. The quality and quantity can be determined—is intake sustained, excessive, or curtailed? Loss early in diarrheal illness progresses rapidly, and the water losses can exceed sodium losses, leading to hypernatremia. Hypernatremic dehydration indicates a significant interference with water intake. Also important is a history of normal or increased intake of fluids containing caffeine (e.g., tea) which may cause diuresis, or fluids containing high amounts of sucrose (e.g., cola, sports drinks, fruit-flavored drinks), an alternative home remedy fluid, or other solute-containing fluids, which can contribute to hyponatremic dehydration in the face of abnormal losses.

A history of gradual weight gain and observations of any puffiness, especially in areas with less dense tissues (periorbital, scrotal), or "clothes fitting tighter" offer early clues to edema. A history of excessive water intake, especially when associated with diminished output, is important in assessing edema and water intoxication.

Clinical Observations

Fever and infection can also produce tachycardia, the earliest manifestation of dehydration. Therefore these are considered in the assessment of hydration status. Dry skin and mucous membranes (oral) usually appear early. A sunken fontanel is a useful observation if the status of the fontanel is known when the infant is healthy. Signs of circulatory failure usually indicate severe dehydration because compensatory mechanisms are able to sustain blood pressure in the low-normal range for some time. Loss of skin elasticity, generally manifested in children less than 2 years of age, is measured by the time it takes for pinched abdominal skin to recoil. This sign is also observed in undernourished children. Also, in hypertonic dehydration the skin has a smooth, velvety feel before it develops disturbed elasticity.

Assess capillary filling time by pinching a toe or a thumb or lightly pressing the abdominal skin and estimating the time it takes for the blood to return. Capillary filling time in mild dehydration is less than 2 seconds, increasing to more than 4 seconds in severe dehydration. The technique is effective in children of all ages. However, it can be altered in the presence of heart failure, which affects circulation time, and hypertonic dehydration, in which fluid loss is primarily intracellular. Additional clinical signs observed in children with dehydration include cool mottled extremities, sunken eyes, tachypnea, and changes in sensorium.

When caring for the acutely ill child, assess vital signs frequently, and record weight frequently during the initial phase of therapy. It is important to use the same scale each time the child is weighed and to predetermine the weight of any equipment or devices that must remain attached during the weighing process, including arm boards, and any clothing the child might be wearing. Take routine weights at the same time each day. One of the nurse's most important roles in fluid and electrolyte disturbance is related to I&O. Accurate measurements are essential to the assessment of fluid balance. Measurements from all sources—including gastrointestinal and parenteral I&O from urine, stools, vomitus, fistulas, nasogastric suction, sweat, and drainage from wounds—must be taken into consideration (see also Chapter 22).

SHOCK

Shock, or **circulatory failure**, is a complex clinical syndrome characterized by inadequate tissue perfusion to meet the metabolic demands of the body, resulting in cellular dysfunction and eventual organ failure. Although the causes are different, the physiologic consequences are the same and include hypotension, tissue hypoxia, and metabolic acidosis. Circulatory failure in children is a result of hypovolemia, altered peripheral vascular resistance, or pump failure.

Etiology

The most common type of circulatory failure in infants and children is **hypovolemic shock**, which follows a reduction in circulating blood volume related to blood loss (e.g., trauma, major bleeding), plasma losses (e.g., burns, peritonitis), or extracellular fluid losses (e.g., diarrhea, dehydration) beyond the child's physiologic ability to compensate. **Cardiogenic shock** results from impaired cardiac muscle function that leads to decreased cardiac output. This type of shock may be seen after cardiac surgery and in children with acute dysrhythmias, congestive heart failure, trauma, or cardiomyopathy. **Distributive shock**, or vasogenic shock, results from a vascular abnormality that produces maldistribution of blood supply throughout the body. This classification includes (1) neurogenic shock, characterized by massive vasodilation resulting from the loss of sympathetic nervous system tone, which can occur with spinal cord injuries; (2) anaphylactic shock, characterized by a hypersensitivity reaction that causes massive vasodilation and capillary leak and may occur with drug or latex allergy, insect stings, or blood transfusion; and (3) septic shock, characterized by a decreased cardiac output and derangements in the peripheral circulation in response to a severe, overwhelming infection. **Obstructive shock** may resemble hypovolemic shock but is caused by cardiac tamponade, tension pneumothorax, ductal-dependent congenital heart lesions, or massive pulmonary embolism (Perkin, de Caen, Berg, et al., 2013). The types of shock are described in Box 23.3. *Neurogenic shock* occurs in association with spinal cord injury and is discussed in Chapter 30

Pathophysiology

The circulatory system of the healthy child is able to transport oxygen and nutrients to meet the essential needs of body tissues and can respond to increased demands resulting from an elevated metabolic rate. The cardiac output and distribution to the various body tissues can change rapidly in response to intrinsic (myocardial and intravascular) or extrinsic (neuronal) control mechanisms. In shock states these mechanisms are altered or challenged.

Reduced blood flow, as in hypovolemic shock, causes diminished venous return to the heart, low central venous pressure (CVP), low cardiac output, and hypotension. The reduced intravascular volume triggers a chain of compensatory mechanisms. Fluid is mobilized from the extracellular fluid compartment. Vasomotor centers in the medulla are signaled, causing depressed vagal activity and increased sympathetic activity, which increase the force and rate of cardiac contraction and constrict the arterioles and veins, thereby increasing peripheral vascular resistance.

Simultaneously the lowered blood volume also leads to the release of large amounts of catecholamines, antidiuretic hormone, adrenocorticosteroids, and aldosterone in an effort to conserve body fluids. The catecholamines augment the vasomotor activity to produce vasoconstriction and reduce blood flow to the skin, kidneys, muscles, and splanchnic viscera in order to shunt the available blood to the brain and heart. Consequently, the skin feels cold and clammy, there is poor capillary filling, and glomerular filtration and urinary output are significantly reduced.

Impaired perfusion to the peripheral tissues also produces metabolic alterations. Oxygen depletion causes the cells to revert to anaerobic glycolytic metabolism, forming pyruvic acid; pyruvic acid is then converted to lactic acid, producing lactic acidosis. The acidosis places an extra burden on the lungs as they attempt to compensate for the metabolic acidosis by increasing the respiratory rate. Impaired cellular uptake and metabolism of glucose create an early, transient hyperglycemia. When plasma fluid is lost, hemoconcentration and diminished blood flow increase the viscosity of the blood and further impair perfusion.

Prolonged vasoconstriction results in fatigue, and the release of vasodilator substances such as histamine leads to vasodilation. Venules, which are less sensitive to vasodilator substances, remain constricted for a time. This causes massive pooling in the capillary and venular beds and transudation of plasma fluid into the tissues, which further depletes blood volume.

Complications of shock create further hazards. Central nervous system hypoperfusion may eventually lead to cerebral edema, cortical infarction, or intraventricular hemorrhage. Renal hypoperfusion causes renal ischemia with possible tubular or glomerular necrosis and renal vein thrombosis. Reduced blood flow to the lungs can interfere with

BOX 23.3 Types of Shock

Hypovolemic

Characteristics

Reduction in size of vascular compartment
Falling blood pressure
Poor capillary filling
Low CVP

Most Frequent Causes

Blood loss (hemorrhagic shock)—Trauma, gastrointestinal bleeding, intracranial hemorrhage
Plasma loss—Increased capillary permeability associated with sepsis and acidosis, hypoproteinemia, burns, peritonitis
Extracellular fluid loss—Vomiting, diarrhea, glycosuric diuresis, heatstroke

Distributive

Characteristics

Reduction in peripheral vascular resistance
Profound inadequacies in tissue perfusion
Increased venous capacity and pooling
Acute reduction in return blood flow to the heart
Diminished cardiac output

Most Frequent Causes

Anaphylaxis (anaphylactic shock)—Extreme allergy or hypersensitivity to a foreign substance
Sepsis (septic shock, bacteremic shock, endotoxic shock)—Overwhelming sepsis and circulating bacterial toxins
Loss of neuronal control (neurogenic shock)—Interruption of neuronal transmission (spinal cord injury)
Myocardial depression and peripheral dilation—Exposure to anesthesia or ingestion of barbiturates, tranquilizers, opioids, antihypertensive agents, or ganglionic blocking agents

Cardiogenic

Characteristic

Decreased cardiac output

Most Frequent Causes

After surgery for congenital heart disease
Primary pump failure—Myocarditis, myocardial trauma, biochemical derangements, heart failure
Dysrhythmias—Supraventricular tachycardia, atrioventricular block, and ventricular dysrhythmias; secondary to myocarditis or biochemical abnormalities (occasionally)

Obstructive

Characteristic

Mechanical obstruction of blood flow to or from the heart

Most Frequent Causes

Tension pneumothorax
Cardiac tamponade
Pulmonary embolism
Congenital cardiac defects with left ventricular outflow tract obstruction (e.g., coarctation of the aorta, interrupted aortic arch, critical aortic stenosis)

CVP, Central venous pressure.
Modified from Ralston, M., Hazinski, M. F., & Zaritsky, A. L. (Eds.). (2006). *Pediatric advanced life support: Provider manual.* Dallas, TX: American Heart Association; Perkin, R. M., de Caen, A. R., Berg, M. D., et al. (2013). Shock, cardiac arrest, and resuscitation. In M. F. Hazinski (Ed.), *Nursing care of the critically ill child.* St. Louis, MO: Elsevier Mosby.

surfactant secretion and result in shock lung or acute respiratory distress syndrome (ARDS). ARDS is characterized by sudden pulmonary congestion and atelectasis with formation of a hyaline membrane and subsequent lung tissue injury. (See Chapter 26.) Gastrointestinal (GI) tract bleeding and perforation are always a possibility following splanchnic ischemia and necrosis of intestinal mucosa. Metabolic complications of shock may include hypoglycemia, hypocalcemia, and other electrolyte disturbances.

Shock states characterized by vascular abnormalities (distributive shock) have a somewhat different pathophysiologic pattern of hemodynamic collapse. In neurogenic shock, the sympathetic nervous system mechanisms that maintain vascular tone are interrupted, causing reduced vascular resistance and peripheral pooling of blood; with this increased vascular capacity there is loss of effective circulating blood volume. Septic shock produces a hyperdynamic state in which there is often an elevated plasma volume and reduced peripheral resistance that lead to widespread vasodilation. In many cases there is a high cardiac output caused by the vasodilation in infected tissues and elsewhere, plus a high metabolic rate resulting from the elevated body temperature. Degenerating tissues cause aggregation of red blood cells and sludging of the blood. Development of disseminated intravascular coagulation, triggered by either the degenerating tissue or bacterial toxins, consumes the clotting factors and produces widespread hemorrhages. (See Chapter 28.)

Clinical Manifestations

Shock can be regarded as a form of compensation for circulatory failure and because of its progressive nature, can be divided into two stages or phases: **compensated** and **hypotensive** (previously referred to as decompensated). Cardiac arrest represents irreversible shock. At all stages the principal differentiating signs are the degree of tachycardia and perfusion to extremities, the level of consciousness, and blood pressure (BP). Additional signs or modifications of these more universal signs may be present, depending on the type and cause of the shock. Initially, the child's ability to compensate is effective; therefore early signs are subtle. As the shock state advances, signs are more obvious and indicate early decompensation (Table 23.5).

In early septic shock, there are chills, fever, and vasodilation, with increased cardiac output that results in warm, flushed skin (hyperdynamic, or "warm" shock). A later and ominous development is disseminated intravascular coagulation (see Chapter 28), the major hematologic complication of septic shock. Anaphylactic shock is frequently accompanied by urticaria and angioneurotic edema, which is life threatening when it involves the respiratory passages (see Anaphylaxis, later in this chapter).

Compensated Shock

When vital organ function is maintained by intrinsic mechanisms and the child's ability to compensate is effective, cardiac output and systemic arterial BP are usually normal or increased. However, blood flow is generally uneven or maldistributed in the microcirculation. Early clinical signs are subtle and include apprehension, irritability, normal BP, narrowing pulse pressure, thirst, pallor, and diminished urinary output.

! NURSING ALERT

Unexplained mild tachycardia and a decrease in perfusion of the hands and feet are differentiating features of compensated shock.

Hypotensive (Decompensated) Shock

As shock progresses, perfusion in the microcirculation becomes marginal despite compensatory adjustments, and the signs are more obvious and

TABLE 23.5 Clinical Signs of Shock

Clinical Signs	Hypovolemic Shock	Distributive Shock	Cardiogenic Shock	Obstructive Shock
Respiratory rate	Normal to increased	Normal to increased	Labored	Labored
Breath sounds	Normal	Normal (crackles may/ may not be present)	Crackles, grunting	Crackles, grunting
Systolic blood pressure	Compensated-normal	Compensated-normal	Hypotensive-low	Hypotensive-low
Pulse pressure	Narrow	Variable	Narrow	Narrow
Heart rate	Tachycardia	Tachycardia	Tachycardia	
Peripheral pulses	Weak	Bounding or weak	Weak	
Skin	Pale, cool	Warm or cool	Pale, cool	
Capillary refill	Delayed (>2 sec)	Variable	Delayed (>2 sec)	
Urine output	Decreased (<1 ml/kg/hr [<30 kg; 66 lb]; <30-50 ml/kg/hr [>30 kg, 66 lb])			
Level of consciousness	Irritable early	Late, lethargic		

Data from Chameides, L., Samson, R., Schexnayder, S. M., et al. (Eds.). (2011). *Pediatric advanced life support: Provider manual.* Dallas, TX: American Heart Association. Part 6: Recognition of Shock (Figure 2, p. 83, Recognition of Shock Flowchart).

indicate early decompensation. These signs are tachypnea; moderate metabolic acidosis; oliguria; and cool, pale extremities with decreased skin turgor and poor capillary filling. Hypotensive shock may be differentiated from compensated shock by evaluating blood pressure; the child in hypotensive shock will have a low blood pressure, but hypotension is a late finding. Another clinical sign of hypotensive shock is a change in level of consciousness as brain perfusion declines. The outcomes of circulatory failure that progress beyond the limits of compensation are tissue hypoxia, metabolic acidosis, and eventual dysfunction of all organ systems.

! NURSING ALERT

In hypotensive shock, tachycardia is pronounced and pulse pressure (difference between systolic and diastolic BP) becomes narrowed. There is poor capillary filling, and the child exhibits confusion, sleepiness, and decreased responsiveness.

As hypotensive shock progresses along a physiologic continuum, clinical signs indicate a progression of circulatory damage. With the progression of shock there is damage to vital organs (e.g., the heart or brain) of such magnitude that the entire system is disrupted regardless of therapeutic intervention. There is pronounced systemic vasoconstriction and hypoxia of visceral and cutaneous circulations with hypotension, acidosis, lethargy or coma, and oliguria or anuria. The child is totally obtunded. A thready and weak pulse, hypotension, periodic breathing or apnea, anuria, and stupor or coma are signs of impending cardiac arrest. Death occurs even if cardiovascular measurements return to normal levels with therapy.

! NURSING ALERT

Hypotension is a late and poor prognostic sign of shock, so signs of shock must be recognized and appropriate interventions implemented before hypotension is evident.

Irreversible or **terminal shock** is the end point of the physiologic continuum if interventions are not effective in reversing the effects of shock. Damage to vital organs, such as the heart or brain, is of such magnitude that the entire organism will be disrupted regardless of therapeutic intervention. Death occurs even if cardiovascular measurements return to normal levels with therapy.

Diagnostic Evaluation

The nurse can discern the cause of shock from the history and physical examination. The severity of shock is determined by measurement of vital signs, including CVP and capillary filling. Laboratory tests that assist in assessment are blood gas measurements, pH, and sometimes liver function tests. Coagulation tests are evaluated when there is evidence of bleeding, such as oozing from a venipuncture site, bleeding from any orifice, or petechiae. Cultures of blood and other sites are indicated when there is a high suspicion of sepsis. Renal function tests are performed when impaired renal function is evident.

Therapeutic Management

Treatment of shock consists of three major components: oxygenation and ventilation, fluid administration, and improvement of the pumping action of the heart (vasopressor support). The first priority is to establish an airway and administer oxygen. Once the airway is ensured, circulatory stabilization is the major concern. Placement of one or more multilumen central lines, preferably above the diaphragm (to deliver drugs closer to the heart and limit tissue injury from caustic medications), is a priority in shock (Perkin, de Caen, Berg, et al., 2013). These lines are needed for rapid volume replacement, administration of vasoactive drugs, and hemodynamic monitoring. However, if immediate intravenous access cannot be accomplished an intraosseous device should be inserted to administer medications and fluids (see Chapter 22).

Oxygenation and Ventilatory Support

Oxygen is the first drug to be administered to an infant or child in shock (Perkin, de Caen, Berg, et al., 2013). The lung is very sensitive to shock. The decrease in or redistribution of blood flow to respiratory muscles plus the increased work of breathing can rapidly lead to respiratory failure. Critically ill patients are unable to maintain an adequate airway. To place the lung at rest and improve ventilation, endotracheal intubation is initiated early with positive-pressure ventilation and supplemental oxygen. Blood gases, oxygen saturation (using pulse oximetry), and pH are monitored frequently.

Increased extravascular lung fluid caused by edema—both hydrostatic and permeable—contributes to the development of respiratory complications. Hydrostatic edema occurs from the elevation of pulmonary microvascular pressure as a result of left ventricular dysfunction; permeable edema occurs when damage to alveolar cell and pulmonary capillary epithelium causes fluid to leak into the interstitial space, resulting in

ARDS. (See Chapter 26.) Direct therapy toward maintaining normal arterial blood gas measurements, normal acid-base balance, and circulation, and make efforts to remove fluid and prevent its accumulation by increasing oncotic pressure and decreasing microvascular hydrostatic pressure. Promote elevated oncotic pressure by diuresis with furosemide or mannitol, colloid administration, or both.

Cardiovascular Support

In many cases rapid restoration of blood volume is the main therapy needed in the resuscitation of the child in shock. An isotonic crystalloid solution (0.9% normal saline or lactated Ringer solution) is usually the first choice for fluid replacement. Crystalloid is given in IV boluses of 20 ml/kg over 5 to 20 minutes and repeated as necessary. Blood products may also be given if acute blood loss is the cause of hypovolemia. The child's response is assessed after each bolus. An increase in BP and a decrease in heart rate indicate successful resuscitation. An increased cardiac output results in improved capillary circulation and skin color. Colloids (protein-containing fluids) are often administered to children in shock; albumin is the most common. Because albumin is a protein solution, it remains in the vascular space much longer than crystalloid fluids. A smaller volume of albumin can be given to increase intravascular volume and support cardiac output; with crystalloid fluids, a larger volume is needed to achieve the same effect. Fresh-frozen plasma is used to correct coagulopathies, not as volume replacement. Additional volume expanders include dextrans and hydroxyethyl starch (hetastarch).

For the critically ill child with shock and multisystem organ dysfunction, more aggressive monitoring is necessary. CVP measurements of right atrial pressure or pulmonary wedge pressure help guide fluid therapy. In children with persistent shock, place a pulmonary artery catheter for more accurate monitoring. Determination of arterial blood gases, hematocrit, serum electrolytes, glucose, and calcium concentrations provides additional information concerning composition of circulating blood. Correction of acidosis, hypoxemia, and any metabolic derangements is mandatory.

Inotropic Support

Temporary pharmacologic support may be required to enhance myocardial contractility, reverse metabolic or respiratory acidosis, and maintain arterial pressure. The principal agents used to improve cardiac output and circulation are the exogenous catecholamines, administered by constant infusion pump. Dopamine is the preferred drug in most situations because it also improves renal perfusion. Other agents (e.g., dobutamine, milrinone, epinephrine, norepinephrine) may be used to improve cardiac output, depending on the situation. Vasopressin has been used in adults to increase systemic vascular resistance and blood pressure, but its use in pediatric shock may be limited to vasodilatory (warm) shock (Perkin, de Caen, Berg, et al., 2013).

Metabolic acidosis is usually corrected with adequate tissue perfusion and improved renal function. This is accomplished with adequate ventilatory support, including oxygen, and restoration of blood volume and peripheral circulation. Calcium chloride may be administered to improve cardiac function and to offset the reduced ionized calcium associated with large amounts of albumin, whole blood, or fresh-frozen plasma. Routine administration of calcium in a pediatric cardiac arrest is not recommended unless there is documented evidence of hypocalcemia, hyperkalemia, hypermagnesemia, or calcium channel blocker overdose (de Caen, Berg, Chameides, et al., 2015). Diuretics, such as furosemide (Lasix), cause a reduction in ventricular filling pressures without changing cardiac output or heart rate and promote sodium and water excretion by the kidney in cases in which pulmonary congestion is a problem.

Nursing Care Management

The child in shock requires observation and care, preferably in an intensive care environment. The initial action in caring for the child in shock is ensuring adequate tissue oxygenation (see Emergency Treatment and Quality Patient Outcome boxes). The nurse should be prepared to administer oxygen by the appropriate route and to assist with any indicated intubation and ventilation procedures. Other procedures and activities that require immediate attention are establishing an IV line, estimating body weight (for calculating weight-based drug dosages), obtaining baseline vital signs, placing an indwelling urinary catheter, obtaining blood gas and other measurements, and administering medications as indicated.

EMERGENCY TREATMENT

Shock

Ventilation

Establish airway; be prepared for intubation.

Administer 100% oxygen.

Fluid Administration

Restore vascular volume.

Cardiovascular Support

Administer inotropes and vasopressors.

General Support

Keep child flat with legs raised above level of heart.

Keep child warm and calm.

Monitor and treat pain.

QUALITY PATIENT OUTCOMES

Shock

- Oxygen content of blood optimized
- Cardiac output improved
- Oxygen demand reduced
- Metabolic abnormalities corrected
- Type of shock identified and treated

NURSING ALERT

Early clinical signs of shock include apprehension, irritability, normal BP, narrowing pulse pressure (difference between diastolic and systolic BP), thirst, pallor, diminished urinary output, unexplained mild tachycardia, and decreased perfusion of the hands and feet.

The nurse's primary responsibilities are to monitor vital signs (systolic BP in particular), central venous pressure, intake and output, oxygenation status, and cardiac output and mean arterial pressure and to perform a general assessment of the level of consciousness, circulatory perfusion, and parenteral infusion sites. The nurse titrates IV medications according to patient responses and obtains vital signs every 15 minutes during the critical periods and thereafter as needed. Urinary output should be measured hourly; blood gases, lactate, hematocrit, pH, and electrolytes should be monitored frequently to assess the child's status and the efficacy of therapy. Cardiorespiratory monitors are attached and monitored continuously. Oxygen saturation monitors provide continuous measurement of oxygenation, and a central venous (Cvo_2) or mixed venous (Svo_2) oxygen saturation monitor may also be used. In the initial stages of acute shock, care of the child often requires a team of nurses due to the number of activities that must be carried out simultaneously.

Children may be sedated in the acute phase of shock, depending on the precipitating cause, the child's age, and the ability to implement therapeutic interventions such as endotracheal intubation and placement of central venous and arterial lines for continuous monitoring of cardiopulmonary status. Parents will require additional reassurance that their child's comfort and pain needs are being adequately addressed. The acutely ill child requires close observation for complications related to immobilization, including deep vein thrombosis prophylaxis, skin care, tissue edema, muscle atrophy, constipation, and bone demineralization. (See Chapter 33, Immobilization.) Special efforts are made to prevent skin breakdown and ventilator-associated pneumonia and to maintain adequate nutritional status in the child who must be on mechanical ventilation for a prolonged period.

Family Support

Throughout the intense activity, do not overlook the parents. A member of the staff, such as a nurse, social worker, or clergy, may be called to provide comfort and support. If the family is not at the hospital, someone should contact them at frequent intervals to inform them about what is being done and whether there is any improvement. Ideally, someone should remain with the parents to serve as a liaison between them and the intensive care team. However, this is not always feasible in such a critical situation. As soon as possible, the parents should be allowed to see the child.

SEPTIC SHOCK

Sepsis and septic shock are caused by an infectious organism and the patient's immune, inflammatory, and coagulation responses to the infecting organism (Perkin, de Caen, Berg, et al., 2013). Normally an infection triggers an inflammatory response in a local area, which results in vasodilation, increased capillary permeability, and eventually elimination of the infectious agent. The widespread activation and systemic release of inflammatory mediators is called the systemic inflammatory response syndrome (SIRS) (Boehne, Sasse, Karch, et al., 2017). Box 23.4 provides the exact definitions for SIRS, infection, sepsis, and severe sepsis. SIRS can occur in response to both infectious and noninfectious (e.g., trauma, burns) causes. When caused by infection, it is called *sepsis.* Septic shock is sepsis with organ dysfunction and hypotension and SIRS in children with pneumonia should be identified early because they will need more intense monitoring and treatment (Frazier, Sepanski, Mangum, et al., 2015). Most of the physiologic effects of shock occur because the exaggerated immune response triggers more than 30 different mediators, which results in diffuse vasodilation, increased capillary permeability, and maldistribution of blood flow. This impairs oxygen and nutrient delivery to the cells, resulting in cellular dysfunction. If the process continues, multiple organ dysfunction occurs and may result in death. Table 23.6 includes the age-specific vital signs and laboratory values reflective of septic shock in children.

The incidence of septic shock is increasing in adults and children (Martin, 2012), possibly as a result of greater numbers of immunosuppressed patients, more widespread use of invasive devices in the seriously ill, increased awareness of the diagnosis, and a growing number of resistant microorganisms.

Three stages have been identified in septic shock. In early septic shock the patient has chills, fever, and vasodilation with increased cardiac output, which results in warm, flushed skin that reflects vascular tone

BOX 23.4 Definitions of Systemic Inflammatory Response Syndrome, Infection, Sepsis, and Severe Sepsis

SIRS—The presence of at least two of the following four criteria, one of which must be abnormal temperature or leukocyte count:

Core temperature of more than 38.5°C (101.3°F) or less than 36°C (96.8°F).

Tachycardia, defined as a mean heart rate more than 2 SD above normal for age in the absence of external stimulus, chronic drugs, or painful stimuli; or otherwise unexplained persistent elevation over a 0.5- to 4-hour period; or, for children younger than 1 year old: bradycardia, defined as a mean heart rate less than the 10th percentile for age in the absence of external vagal stimulus, β-blocker drugs, or congenital heart disease; or otherwise unexplained persistent depression over a 0.5-hour period.

Mean respiratory rate more than 2 SD above normal for age or mechanical ventilation for an acute process not related to underlying neuromuscular disease or the receipt of general anesthesia.

Leukocyte count elevated or depressed for age (not secondary to chemotherapy-induced leukopenia) or more than 10% immature neutrophils.

Infection—A suspected or proven (by positive culture, tissue stain, or PCR test) infection caused by any pathogen; or a clinical syndrome associated with a high probability of infection. Evidence of infection includes positive findings on clinical examination, imaging, or laboratory tests (e.g., white blood cells in a normally sterile body fluid, perforated viscus, chest radiograph consistent with pneumonia, petechial or purpuric rash, or purpura fulminans).

Sepsis—SIRS in the presence of or as a result of suspected or proven infection.

Severe sepsis—Sepsis plus cardiovascular organ dysfunction or ARDS or two or more other organ dysfunctions.

ARDS, Acute respiratory distress syndrome; *PCR,* polymerase chain reaction; *SD,* standard deviations; *SIRS,* systemic inflammatory response syndrome.

From Goldstein, B., Giroir, B., Randolph, A., et al. (2005). International Pediatric Sepsis Consensus Conference: Definitions for sepsis and organ dysfunction in pediatrics. *Pediatric Critical Care Medicine, 6*(1), 2-8; used with permission.

abnormalities and hyperdynamic, warm, or hyperdynamic-compensated responses. Blood pressure and urinary output are normal. The patient has the best chance for survival in this stage. The second stage—the normodynamic, cool, or hyperdynamic-decompensated stage—lasts only a few hours. The skin is cool, but pulses and BP are still normal. Urinary output diminishes, and the mental state becomes depressed. With advancing disease, certain signs of circulatory decompensation that deteriorate to signs of circulatory collapse are indistinguishable from late shock of any cause. In the hypodynamic, or cold, stage of shock, cardiovascular function progressively deteriorates, even with aggressive therapy. The patient has hypothermia, cold extremities, weak pulses, hypotension, and oliguria or anuria. Patients are severely lethargic or comatose. Multiorgan failure is common. This is the most dangerous stage of shock.

Management of septic shock involves measures to provide hemodynamic stability and adequate oxygenation to the tissues and the use of antimicrobials to treat the infectious organism (Perkin, de Caen, Berg, et al., 2013). As with other forms of shock, hemodynamic stability is achieved with fluid volume resuscitation and inotropic agents as needed (Table 23.7). Providing adequate oxygenation often requires supplemental oxygen, intubation and mechanical ventilation, sedation, and paralysis to decrease the work of breathing. Septic shock involves activation of

TABLE 23.6 Age-Specific Vital Signs and Laboratory Variables in Septic Shock*

	HEART RATE (BEATS/MIN)		Respiratory Rate	Leukocyte Count	Systolic Blood
Age-Group	Tachycardia	Bradycardia	(Breaths/Min)	(Leukocytes × 10^3/mm^3)	Pressure (mm Hg)
0 days-1 wk	>180	<100	>50	>34	<65
1 wk to 1 mo	>180	<100	>40	>19.5 or <5	<75
1 mo to 1 yr	>180	<90	>34	>17.5 or <5	<100
2-5 yr	>140	N/A	>22	>15.5 or <6	<94
6-12 yr	>130	N/A	>8	>13.50 or <4.5	<105
13-<18 yr	>110	N/A	>4	>11 or <4.5	<117

*Lower values for heart rate, leukocyte count, and systolic blood pressure are for 5th percentile, and upper values for heart rate, respiratory rate, or leukocyte count are for 95th percentile.

N/A, Not applicable.

From Goldstein, B., Giroir, B., & Randolph, A. (2005). International pediatric sepsis consensus conference: Definitions for sepsis and organ dysfunction in pediatrics. *Pediatric Critical Care Medicine, 6*(1), 2-8; used with permission.

TABLE 23.7 Pediatric Septic Shock Goal-Directed Therapy

Physiologic Parameter	Therapeutic Goal	Monitoring Method	Manipulation
Tissue perfusion	Capillary refill: <2 seconds Mean arterial pressure: 65-70 mm Hg Urinary output: >0.5 ml/kg/hr CVP: 8-12 mm Hg	Capillary refill Mean arterial pressure Urinary output CVP	Fluids (crystalloids, colloids): 20 ml/kg bolus; 40-60 ml/kg in 1st hour Sympathomimetics: dopamine (first line), norepinephrine or epinephrine (second line) Vasodilators: nitroprusside
Oxygenation	O_2 saturation: >93% Central venous O_2 saturation: >70% Hemoglobin within normal range for age Hematocrit: 30% O_2 extraction: 0.3-0.6 Serum lactate: <2 mmol/L	O_2 saturation Central venous O_2 saturation Hemoglobin concentration Hematocrit Arterial blood gases O_2 extraction: $(CaO_2\text{-}CvO_2)/CaO_2$ Serum lactate	FiO_2 PEEP Mean arterial pressure Transfusion (blood, PRBCs) if hemoglobin <10 mg/dl
Urinary output and renal perfusion	Urinary output: >0.5 ml/kg/hr	Urinary output Creatinine clearance BUN	Continuous renal replacement therapy: CVVHD at 10% fluid overload or acute renal failure Dialysis
Metabolic and nutritional support	Glucose: 80-110 mg/dl iCa^{++}: 1.14-1.29 Positive nitrogen balance	Serum glucose Serum iCa^{++} Healing of wounds and overall status Weight Albumin-prealbumin, total protein, albumin/globulin ratio Indirect calorimetry	Dextrose Insulin iCa^{++} Enteral feeding Total parenteral nutrition Micronutrients: vitamins (vitamin K), minerals
Adrenal support	Prevention of adrenal insufficiency and refractory hypotension	Cortisol level Blood pressure Therapeutic trial	Hydrocortisone

BUN, Blood urea nitrogen; *CVP,* central venous pressure; *CVVHD,* continuous venovenous hemofiltration/dialysis; *iCa^{++}*, serum ionized calcium; *PEEP,* positive end-expiratory pressure; *PRBCs,* packed red blood cells.

From Arnal, L. E., & Stein, F. (2003). Pediatric septic shock. *Seminars in Pediatric Infectious Diseases, 14*(2), 165-172; used with permission.

complement proteins that promote clumping of the granulocytes in the lung. The granulocytes can release chemicals that can cause direct lung injury to the pulmonary capillary endothelium. This causes a fluid leak into the alveoli, which causes stiff, noncompliant lungs. Disseminated intravascular coagulation and multiorgan dysfunction may also occur and require prompt assessment and management.

Newer therapies are being developed to modify the host immune response by attempting to block various mediators, thereby interrupting the inflammatory cascade. Evidence-based management protocols for the management of adult and pediatric septic shock have recently been published (deCaen, Berg, Chameides, et al., 2015; Dellinger, Levy, Rhodes, et al., 2013).

Nursing Care Management

Early identification of the symptoms of septic shock is critical to patient survival. A high index of suspicion is required in all critically ill patients who are at greater risk for sepsis because of multiple invasive lines and devices, poor nutrition, and impaired immune function. Subtle alterations in tissue perfusion and unexplained tachypnea and tachycardia often are early warning signs. Identification of the infectious agent and prompt treatment are also critical to patient survival. Patients should receive broad-spectrum antibiotics, and the nurse should remove the site of infection if possible (e.g., indwelling central lines). Patients should be managed in an intensive care unit (ICU) in which continuous monitoring and sophisticated cardiac and respiratory support are available. Multidisciplinary collaboration is essential in managing these critically ill patients.

> **! NURSING ALERT**
>
> To aid in early identification and management, nurses caring for children at risk for septic shock should be alert to early signs: fever, tachycardia, and tachypnea.

ANAPHYLAXIS

Anaphylaxis is the acute clinical syndrome resulting from the interaction of an allergen and a patient who is hypersensitive. This antigen-antibody (immunoglobulin E [IgE]) reaction stimulates the release of chemical substances, primarily histamine, from mast cells (Perkin, de Caen, Berg, et al., 2013). Histamine release causes vasodilation and increases capillary permeability, allowing fluid to leak into the interstitial space. Severe reactions are immediate, often life threatening, and often involve multiple systems, primarily the cardiovascular, respiratory, GI, and integumentary systems. Exposure to the antigen can be through ingestion, inhalation, skin contact, or injection. Food allergy is the most common cause of anaphylaxis outside the hospital, whereas medication and latex allergies are more common in the hospital (Sampson, Wang, & Sicherer, 2016). The most common allergens are listed in Box 23.5.

Prevention of a reaction is the primary goal. Preventing exposure is more easily accomplished in children known to be at risk, including those with a history of a previous allergic reaction to a specific antigen, a history of allergy (atopy), a history of severe reactions in immediate family members, and a reaction to a skin test (although skin tests are not available for all allergens).

BOX 23.5 Common Allergens Associated With Anaphylaxis

Drugs and Medical Products

Antibiotics (penicillin, cephalosporins, tetracycline, aminoglycosides, streptomycin, amphotericin B)
Analgesics (aspirin, indomethacin, phenylbutazone)
Local anesthetics (lidocaine, procaine, bupivacaine, tetracaine)
Chemotherapeutic agents (bleomycin, cisplatin, carboplatin, l-asparaginase, etoposide)
Antiepileptic drugs
Diagnostic contrast media (sulfobromophthalein sodium dye, dehydrocholic acid [Decholin], iodinated contrast media, iopanoic acid [Telepaque])
Latex (gloves, urinary catheters) (see Latex Allergy, Chapter 32)
Blood products

Foods (see Chapter 11)

Milk and milk products
Nuts and seeds
Legumes (peanuts, soybeans, beans, lentils)
Eggs
Seafood (fish, shellfish)
Wheat
Citrus fruits, strawberries
Chocolate

Venoms

Hymenopteran (bee, yellow jacket, hornet, wasp, fire ant)
Snake
Jellyfish
Spider

Biologic Agents

Allergen extracts
Antisera (snake, tetanus, diphtheria)
Enzymes
Hormones
Immunoglobulin
Blood and blood products

Pathophysiology

An anaphylactic reaction occurs as a result of an interaction between an allergen and a preexisting specific IgE. When the antigen enters the circulatory system, a generalized reaction rapidly occurs. Vasoactive amines (principally histamine or histamine-like substances) are released from mast cells and cause vasodilation, bronchoconstriction, and increased capillary permeability. Consequently, there is increased venous capacity and pooling, reduced arterial pressure, and rapid loss of fluid into interstitial spaces, causing a marked decrease in venous return to the heart.

Clinical Manifestations

The onset of clinical symptoms usually occurs within seconds or minutes of exposure to the antigen. The rapidity of the reaction is directly related to its intensity—the sooner the onset, the more severe the reaction. However, the onset may be delayed for as long as 2 hours. Typically the reaction is preceded by one or more prodromal signs and symptoms, including vague complaints of uneasiness or impending doom, restlessness, irritability, severe anxiety, headache, dizziness, paresthesia, and disorientation. The patient may lose consciousness.

Cutaneous signs of flushing and urticaria are common early signs followed by angioedema, most notable in the eyelids, lips, tongue, hands, feet, and genitalia. Bronchiolar constriction may follow, causing narrowing of the airway; pulmonary edema and hemorrhage also may occur. Laryngeal edema with severe acute upper airway obstruction may be life threatening and requires rapid intervention. Shock occurs as a result of mediator-induced vasodilation, which causes capillary permeability and loss of intravascular fluid into the interstitial space. Sudden hypotension and impaired cardiac output with poor perfusion are seen. As outlined in Box 23.6, any or all of several reactions may affect one or more organ systems.

> **! NURSING ALERT**
>
> Penicillin allergy is associated with immediate onset (within 1 hour of administration) or accelerated onset (1 to 72 hours after administration) of skin eruption, especially a urticarial rash, or more serious symptoms such as laryngeal edema or anaphylactic shock.

Therapeutic Management

Successful outcome of anaphylactic reactions depends on rapid recognition of their severity and prompt treatment. The goals of treatment are providing ventilation, restoring adequate circulation, and preventing further exposure by identifying and removing the cause when possible.

BOX 23.6 Possible Manifestations of Anaphylactic Reaction

Cardiovascular
Tachycardia
Dysrhythmia
Hypotension
Relative hypovolemia

Respiratory
Rhinitis (sneezing, nasal itching, rhinorrhea)
Laryngeal edema (stridor)
Bronchospasm (cough, wheezing)

Gastrointestinal
Nausea and vomiting
Abdominal pain
Diarrhea

Cutaneous (Skin)*
Diffuse flushing, feeling of warmth
Urticaria (itching of skin and raised rash [hives])
Angioedema (periorbital, perioral)

Central Nervous System, Other
Sense of impending doom*
Sometimes loss of consciousness*
Headache*
Seizures

*Early signs.

A biphasic reaction may occur within 4 hours after symptoms have originally subsided, so it is important to monitor the child closely for this reaction (Sampson, Wang, & Sicherer, 2016). Additional interventions such as fluid resuscitation, oxygen administration, beta-agonists, antihistamines, and corticosteroids should be considered in the child who experiences a moderate to severe anaphylactic reaction.

If this is the initial anaphylactic reaction, it is especially important to identify the allergen and implement measures to prevent any future reaction. The patient should carry medical identification at all times. Desensitization by a pediatric allergist may be recommended in certain cases.

The nurse can manage a mild cutaneous reaction with no evidence of respiratory distress or cardiovascular compromise with antihistamines, such as diphenhydramine (Benadryl) or cetirizine. Moderate or severe distress presents a life-threatening emergency and requires immediate intervention (see also Food Sensitivity, Chapter 11).

Nursing Care Management

Major nursing responsibilities in anaphylaxis include anticipating which children are likely to develop a reaction, recognizing the early signs, and intervening appropriately. When an anaphylactic reaction is suspected, nursing responsibilities include immediate intervention and preparation for medical therapy. If emergency supplies such as epinephrine are not immediately available, emergency medical services should be accessed. Ventilation is ensured by placing the child in a head-elevated position, unless contraindicated by hypotension, to facilitate breathing and administer oxygen. If the child is not breathing, cardiopulmonary resuscitation (CPR) is initiated and emergency medical services are summoned. (See Quality Patient Outcomes box.)

QUALITY PATIENT OUTCOMES

Anaphylaxis

- Early recognition of symptoms
- Airway patency maintained
- Adequate circulation restored and maintained
- Further exposure to allergic agent prevented

If the cause can be determined, implement measures to slow the spread of the offending substance. For example, discontinue an IV medication or contrast dye infusion. If the cause can be determined, measures are implemented to slow the spread of the offending substance. An IV infusion is established immediately. Emergency medications are given intravenously whenever possible; however, epinephrine may be given intramuscularly (see Drug Alert box). Vital signs and urinary output are monitored frequently. Medications are administered as prescribed, with regular assessment to monitor effectiveness and to detect signs of side effects of medication and fluid overload.

DRUG ALERT

Epinephrine

Intramuscular administration of epinephrine (0.01 mg/kg up to 0.3 mg) is the first line of therapy, and administration should never be delayed. Two premixed preparations are available: EpiPen Jr (0.15 mg) for children 8 to 25 kg (3.5 to 11.25 lb) and EpiPen (0.3 mg) for children over 25 kg (11.25 lb). As in any shock state, the airway is the first concern, followed by assessment of breathing and then circulation (ABCs).

To prevent an anaphylactic reaction, parents are always asked about possible allergic responses to foods, medications, products such as latex, and environmental conditions. (See Latex Allergy, Chapter 32.) These are displayed prominently on the patient's chart and an allergy alert wristband. Note the specific allergen and the type and severity of the reaction. Parents are excellent historians, especially when the child has displayed a dramatic reaction to a substance. Drugs, including related drugs (e.g., penicillin and nafcillin), that have produced a previous reaction are never given.

! NURSING ALERT

Families should always inform other caregivers (e.g., day care staff) and school personnel, especially the school nurse, of their children's allergies. These individuals should be prepared to respond immediately to a severe reaction.

The child and the parents need as much reassurance as can be provided without giving false hope. Keep them informed of the child's progress, the reasons for the therapies, and what they can reasonably expect. This is a frightening experience and one that the family will remember and make every effort to prevent from recurring. The use of a convenient and visible method of conveying medical information, such as a bracelet or necklace, is encouraged. For the child who is allergic to insect venom, prescribe the family an emergency kit to be kept with the child at all times (e.g., EpiPen or EpiPen Jr). Teach both the family and the child, if the child is old enough and is likely to be away from the family (e.g., at school), how to use the equipment. (See Chapter 22)

TOXIC SHOCK SYNDROME

Toxic shock syndrome (TSS) is a relatively rare condition caused by the toxins produced by the *Staphylococcus* bacteria. *S. aureus* is the most commonly found cause of TSS. First described in the late 1970s, TSS can cause acute multisystem organ failure and a clinical picture that resembles septic shock. TSS became well known in 1980 because of the striking relationship between the disease and tampon use. An aggressive health education campaign about the dangers of prolonged tampon use and a change in the chemical composition of tampons have markedly reduced the incidence of TSS in menstruating women. Cases of TSS have also been reported in men, older women, and children.

Pathophysiology

Evidence from several sources suggests that TSS occurs secondary to infection with *S. aureus*—namely, toxic shock syndrome toxin–1 (TSST-1) (Gaensbauer & Todd, 2016). Enterotoxin A and enterotoxin B may be associated with nonmenstrual TSS (Gaensbauer & Todd, 2016). The organism is believed to produce an epidermal toxin, but the precise mode of transmission is not known.

In approximately half the cases, TSS is seen in menstruating women and is usually associated with tampon use. The tampon may carry the organism from the fingers or vulva into the vagina during insertion, may traumatize the vaginal wall, or may provide a favorable environment for growth of the organism. TSS has also been associated with other bacterial infections, such as sinusitis or pneumonia, catheter site infections, skin infections, postoperative wound infections, and infection related to foreign bodies such as nasal packing or contraceptive diaphragms (Gaensbauer & Todd, 2016).

Clinical Manifestations

The sudden development of high fever, vomiting and diarrhea, profound hypotension, shock, oliguria, and an erythematous macular rash with subsequent desquamation are characteristic manifestations of TSS. Other manifestations include headache, blurred vision, purulent conjunctivitis, abdominal guarding, and purulent vaginal discharge.

Complications of TSS include respiratory distress, cardiac dysfunction, abnormal coagulation (particularly disseminated intravascular coagulation), and abnormal liver function. Impaired perfusion to the extremities may become severe, with eventual necrosis and loss of extremities.

Diagnostic Evaluation

The diagnosis is established on the basis of criteria in the TSS case definition of the Centers for Disease Control and Prevention (Box 23.7). A history of tampon use contributes to the diagnosis. Laboratory tests may include cultures from blood, vagina, cervix, and discharge from any suspected source of infection. Other laboratory tests are those that facilitate the management of shock.

Therapeutic Management

The management of TSS is the same as management of shock of any cause. Because the disease is highly varied in intensity, therapy toward supportive care for mild cases should be directed to hospitalization and for severe cases to intensive care. Appropriate parenteral antibiotics are usually administered after cultures are obtained. Preventing complications of impaired circulation demands constant observation and immediate therapeutic intervention for hypotension, pulmonary dysfunction, acidosis, hematologic changes, and renal impairment.

Nursing Care Management

Nursing care and observation of the acutely ill patient are the same as those described for shock of any cause. Because the disease is relatively rare, major nursing efforts should be directed toward prevention. The association between TSS and tampon use provides some direction for education. Avoiding the use of tampons offers the most certain preventive measure, although this approach is probably unacceptable to most adolescent girls, who prefer the freedom, comfort, and inconspicuousness that tampons afford.

Adolescent girls who use tampons can be taught general hygiene measures, such as good hand washing and careful insertion to avoid vaginal abrasion. It is wise to modify their use, alternating with sanitary napkins—perhaps using the napkins during the night, when at home during the day, and when flow is slight. Young girls are advised not to use superabsorbent tampons and not to leave any tampon in the body for more than 4 to 6 hours.

BOX 23.7 Criteria for Definition of *S. Aureus* Toxic Shock Syndrome

Fever of 38.9°C (102°F) or higher

Presence of diffuse macular erythroderma

Desquamation, particularly of palms and soles, 1 to 2 weeks after onset of illness

Hypotension, defined as a systolic blood pressure of 90 mm Hg or less for adults and below the 5th percentile for children younger than 16 years of age; or an orthostatic drop in diastolic blood pressure of 15 mm Hg or more with a change from lying to sitting; or orthostatic syncope; or orthostatic dizziness

Involvement of three or more of the following organ systems: GI, muscular, mucous membrane, renal, hepatic, hematologic, or CNS

Toxic shock syndrome is probable when four of the five major criteria are fulfilled. In addition, if blood and cerebrospinal fluid cultures are obtained, they must be negative for any organisms other than *Staphylococcus aureus*. Serologic tests for Rocky Mountain spotted fever, leptospirosis, and measles also must be negative.

CNS, Central nervous system; *GI*, gastrointestinal.
Adapted from Wharton, M., et al. (1990). Case definitions for public health surveillance. *MMWR Recommendations and Reports, 39*(RR-13), 1-43.

! NURSING ALERT

Patients who use tampons need to understand that they should remove the tampon and consult their health care professional if they develop a sudden high fever, vomiting, diarrhea, muscle pain, dizziness, fainting or near-fainting when standing up, or a rash that resembles a sunburn.

BURNS

OVERVIEW

Burn injuries are usually attributed to extreme heat sources but may also result from exposure to cold, chemicals, electricity, or radiation. Most burns are relatively minor and do not require definitive medical treatment. However, burns involving a large body surface area, critical body parts, or the pediatric or geriatric population often benefit from treatment in specialized burn centers. The American Burn Association (2016) has established criteria to guide decisions regarding the severity of injury and the need for transfer for specialized care.

Epidemiology and Etiology

Burn injuries represent one of the most severe traumas a body can sustain. Ongoing efforts toward education, burn prevention, safer home and work environments, and new methods of firefighting have significantly decreased burn injuries. Scald burns (e.g., hot water, grease, hot foods, etc.) are most common among young children, whereas flame burns are more prevalent among older children. The bathroom is the area where scald burns from tap water most often occur, and these injuries tend to be more severe covering a larger portion of the body. The death rate from fire and burn injury has declined by 53% from 1999 to 2013 (Safe Kids Worldwide, 2015). Fire and burns are the fifth leading cause of unintentional injury and child injury death in the United States. Approximately 250 children 14 years of age and under died from fire or burn injuries in 2014 (Centers for Disease Control and Prevention, 2016).

Children playing with matches or other ignition devices accounted for 64% of home fires between 2007 and 2011 (National Fire Protection Agency, 2014). Boys 2 to 5 years of age have the highest rate of nonfatal burns, and children younger than 9 years old cause most fire-related deaths and injuries due to playing with fire. Careless smoking is associated with the majority of fatal house fires and is the most common cause of residential fire deaths. The use of heating sources is another common cause of house fires. The source of ignition is often a combustible material stored near the furnace or device, buildup of creosote in the chimney, spillage of fuel, or use of the wrong fuel. Many of these fires result in multiple deaths and injuries, especially in rural areas. The majority of fatal house fires occur during the cold winter months, most commonly in the eastern part of the United States, from December through February. The single most important element in the decrease in fire-related deaths seen since 1978 is the use of smoke alarms (Pruitt, Wolf, & Mason, 2012).

The use of alternative heating devices such as kerosene heaters, wood-burning stoves, and glass-front fireplaces has increased the risk of contact burns in all age-groups. Most contact burns result from the lack of shielding to prevent contact with hot surfaces. Flame burns involving flammable liquids such as gasoline account for approximately 30% of injuries seen in the pediatric population, especially in children over 8 years of age. The ignition of clothing is the second leading cause of burn admissions. In the past, girls were more susceptible, but the incidence has decreased significantly, and clothing ignition deaths have decreased as clothing styles have changed; such injuries are now rare among children, with little overall gender difference. Between 1975, when it was mandated that sleepwear in sizes 0 to 6x had to successfully pass a standard flame test, and 1999, when the law was repealed, the percentage of clothing burns caused by sleepwear in children ages 0 to 12 decreased from 55% to 27%. Sleepwear-related burns are still being closely monitored to assess the effect of deregulation of sleepwear garments on related burns (Pruitt, Wolf, & Mason, 2012).

Electrical injuries caused by household current are seen often when young children insert conductive objects into electrical outlets or bite or suck on connected electrical cords in sockets. They occur most commonly during the spring and summer months and are also associated with risk-taking behaviors in young boys. Direct contact with high- or low-voltage current and lightning strikes are the most frequent mechanism of injury. The resistance of the tissue and the path of the electric current are responsible for the damage incurred. Electric current travels through the body on the path of least resistance (e.g., tissue, fluid, blood vessels, and nerves). A more localized burn is produced if skin resistance is high at the area of contact, whereas a more systemic pattern of injury is produced if the skin resistance is low. Often compared with a crush injury, serious electrical trauma results from current passing through vital organs, muscle compartments, and nerve or vascular pathways. Loss of limbs, cardiac fibrillation, respiratory collapse, and burns are common after exposure to electrical energy.

Chemical burns can cause extensive injury. The severity of injury is related to the chemical agent (e.g., acid, alkali, or organic compound) and the duration of contact. The mechanism of injury differs from that in other burns in that there is a chemical disruption and alteration of the physical properties of the exposed body area. Noxious agents exist in many common household cleaning products used in the home. In addition to concern for localized damage, the potential for systemic toxicity must also be addressed. Of particular concern are the exposure of the eyes to chemical agents and the ingestion of caustic substances. Although radiation injuries are rare, the most common sources in pediatrics are related to radiation exposure from medical therapies and ultraviolet light.

Nonaccidental trauma, which is a leading cause of traumatic injury in children, is another source of burn injury. These sources that result in burn injuries most commonly occur to children 3 years of age and younger. Nonaccidental trauma is most likely to occur when parents perceive there is little community support or to those who live in poverty-level households headed by a young, single parent. Approximately 8% to 12% of all forms of nonaccidental trauma cases in the United States are caused by burning (Wibbenmeyer, Liao, Heard, et al., 2014). With nonaccidental burn injury, scald burns are the most common, followed by contact burns from hot objects. Nonaccidental burn trauma should be suspected if the burn distribution on the body is inconsistent with the reported incident, the injury is not consistent with the child's developmental level, and there was a delay in seeking treatment. It is also important to explore any history of family instability and an inability to deal with stress in crisis situations. Laws now exist in all states requiring health care workers to report suspected child abuse.

The causative agent in all burns has important implications for the treatment and prognosis of the pediatric patient. The nurse uses knowledge of the pathophysiologic processes of each type of injury in assessing the trauma and in planning, implementing, and evaluating care. Psychosocial issues are also important considerations in planning for the optimum long-term outcome.

BURN WOUND CHARACTERISTICS

The child's physiologic responses, therapy, prognosis, and physical disposition are directly related to the amount of tissue destroyed; therefore the severity of the burn injury is assessed on the basis of the percentage of body surface area burned and the depth of the burn. Also important in determining the seriousness of injury are the location of the wounds, the child's age and general health, the causative agent, respiratory involvement, and concomitant injuries.

Extent of Injury

The extent of the burn is expressed as a percentage of total body surface area (TBSA) injured. The child has different body proportions than the adult, resulting in an inaccurate estimation of injury if the standard adult rule of nines is used. The proportions of the child's trunk and arms are roughly the same as those of the adult. However, the infant's head and neck make up 18% of the TBSA and each lower extremity accounts for 14% of the TBSA. A modified rule of nines for the pediatric population proposes that for each year of life after age 2 years, 1% is deducted from the head and 0.5% is added to each leg (American Burn Association, 2016). It is generally more efficient to use any of a variety of charts designed to assign body proportions to children of different ages (Fig. 23.5).

Depth of Injury

A thermal injury is a three-dimensional wound and is also assessed in relation to the depth of injury. Traditionally the terms *first, second, third,* and *fourth degree* have been used to describe the depth of tissue injury. However, with the current emphasis on wound healing, this traditional terminology is being replaced by more descriptive terms related to the extent of destruction to the epithelializing elements of the skin. In general, first-degree burns are classified as superficial, and second-degree burns as partial-thickness. Third- and fourth-degree wounds are classified as

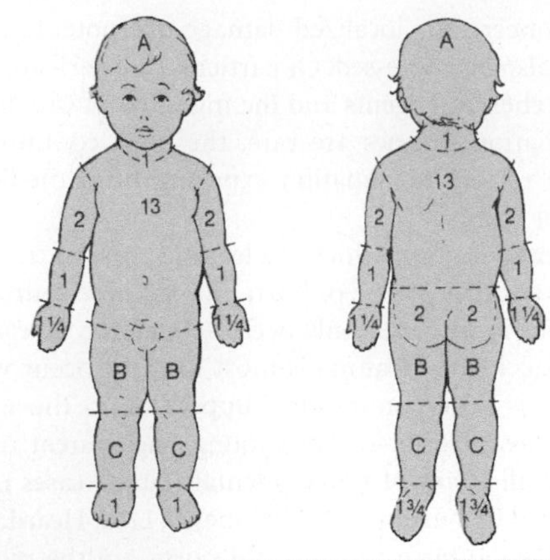

RELATIVE PERCENTAGES OF AREAS AFFECTED BY GROWTH

AREA	BIRTH	AGE 1 YR	AGE 5 YR
A = ½ of head	9½	8½	6½
B = ½ of one thigh	2¾	3¼	4
C = ½ of one leg	2½	2½	2¾

A

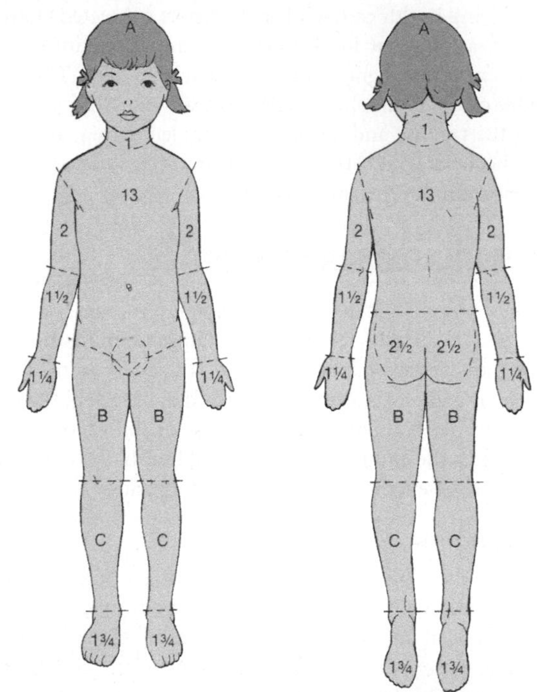

RELATIVE PERCENTAGES OF AREAS AFFECTED BY GROWTH

AREA	AGE 10 YR	AGE 15 YR	ADULT
A = ½ of head	5½	4½	3½
B = ½ of one thigh	4½	4½	4¾
C = ½ of one leg	3	3¼	3½

B

FIG. 23.5 Charts for estimation of distribution of burns in children. **A,** Children from birth to age 5 years. **B,** Older children.

full-thickness wounds. Partial-thickness wounds are further classified as superficial or deep in relation to the time required for healing to occur and the functional and cosmetic results anticipated. Because both terminologies are often used interchangeably, they are both presented in Fig. 23.6, which describes the characteristics of burn wounds.

Superficial (first-degree) burns are usually of minor significance. This type of injury involves the epidermal layer only. There is often a latent period followed by erythema due to vasodilation, tissue damage is minimum, the protective functions of the skin remain intact, and systemic effects are rare. Pain is the predominant symptom, and blisters do not form. The dead epidermis sloughs and is replaced by regenerating keratinocytes within 3 or 4 days without scarring (Pastar, Stojadinovic, Yin, et al., 2014). The burning sensation and pain usually resolve in 48 to 72 hours, and in 3 to 6 days the damaged epithelium peels off in small scales or sheets (Carrougher, 1998). An example of a superficial first-degree burn is a mild sunburn, without any blistering.

Partial-thickness (second-degree) injuries involve the epidermis and varying degrees of the dermal layer where the skin barrier is disrupted. These wounds are painful, moist, red, and blistered. Keratinocytes at the wound edge loose adhesion to each other, develop flexibility, migrate over the wound bed, and proliferate (Pastar, Stojadinovic, Yin, et al., 2014).With superficial partial-thickness burns, dermal elements are intact, and the wound should heal in approximately 14 days with variable amounts of scarring. The wound is extremely sensitive to temperature changes, exposure to air, and light touch. Although classified as second-degree or partial-thickness, deep dermal burns resemble full-thickness injuries in many respects, except the sweat glands and hair follicles remain intact. The burn may appear mottled, with pink, red, or white areas exhibiting blisters and edema formation (Fig. 23.7). Systemic effects are similar to those encountered with full-thickness burns. Although these wounds heal spontaneously in approximately 21 days, they do so with extensive scarring.

Full-thickness (third-degree) burns are serious injuries that involve the entire epidermis and dermis and extend into the subcutaneous tissue. Thrombosed vessels can be seen beneath the surface of the wound, and nerve endings, sweat glands, and hair follicles are destroyed. The burn varies in color from red to tan, waxy white, brown, or black and is distinguished by a dry, leathery appearance (Fig. 23.8). Normally, full-thickness burns lack sensation in the area of injury because of the destruction of nerve endings. However, most full-thickness burns have superficial and partial-thickness burned areas at the periphery of the wound, where nerve endings are intact and exposed. Also, excised eschar and donor sites contain exposed nerve fibers, causing pain. Finally, as peripheral fibers regenerate, painful sensation returns. Consequently, children often experience severe pain related to the size and depth of the burn. Full-thickness wounds are not capable of reepithelialization and require surgical excision and grafting to close the wound.

Fourth-degree burns are also full-thickness injuries and involve underlying structures such as muscle, fascia, and bone. The wound appears dull and dry, and ligaments, tendons, and bone may be exposed. Most often in the case of an extremity, it must be amputated due to the extensive damage and inability to repair the area. In some instances a plastic reconstruction procedure called a flap can be performed. A flap is where varying composites of different types of tissue components (e.g., skin, muscle, fat, etc.) with its blood supply intact are taken from one area of the person's body to cover the damaged area.

Severity of Injury

Burns are classified as major, moderate, or minor, which is useful in determining the patient's disposition for treatment. Burn patients can usually be distinguished as (1) those with a major burn injury that require the services and facilities of a specialized burn center; (2) those with a moderate burn who may be treated in a hospital with expertise in burn care; and (3) those with minor injuries, who can be treated on an outpatient basis (Table 23.8). The severity of the injury depends on the extent and depth of the burn, the causative agent, body area involved, patient's age, and concomitant injuries and illnesses.

The nurse makes an initial assessment of the extent of skin damage by observation and simple diagnostic techniques. The extent of body surface area involvement is readily calculated, and the appearance of the wound provides clues as to whether the injury involves the full

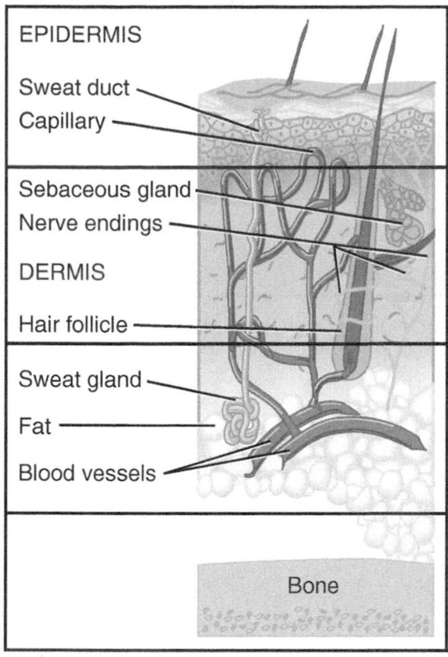

Skin layers	Burn thickness	Degree	WOUND APPEARANCE	WOUND SENSATION	COURSE OF HEALING
EPIDERMIS Sweat duct Capillary	PARTIAL-THICKNESS BURN	1st-degree	Epidermis remains intact and without blisters Erythema; skin blanches with pressure	Painful	Discomfort lasts 48-72 hours. Desquamation occurs in 3-7 days.
Sebaceous gland Nerve endings DERMIS Hair follicle	PARTIAL-THICKNESS BURN	2nd-degree	Wet, shiny, weeping surface Blisters Wound blanches with pressure	Painful Very sensitive to touch, air currents	Superficial partial-thickness burn heals in <21 days. Deep partial-thickness burn requires >21 days for healing. Healing rates vary with burn depth and presence/absence of infection.
Sweat gland Fat Blood vessels	FULL-THICKNESS BURN	3rd-degree	Color variable (i.e., deep red, white, black, brown) Surface dry Thrombosed vessels visible No blanching	Insensate (↓ pinprick sensation)	Autografting is required for healing.
Bone	FULL-THICKNESS BURN	4th-degree	Color variable Charring visible in deepest areas Extremity movement limited	Insensate	Amputation of extremities is likely. Autografting is required for healing.

FIG. 23.6 Classification of burn depth according to depth of injury. (From Black, J. M. [2008]. *Medical-surgical nursing: Clinical management for positive outcomes* [8th ed.]. Philadelphia, PA: Saunders.)

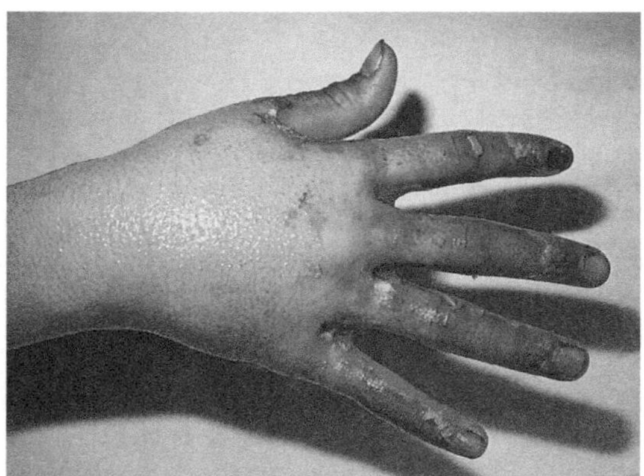

FIG. 23.7 Deep partial-thickness burn.

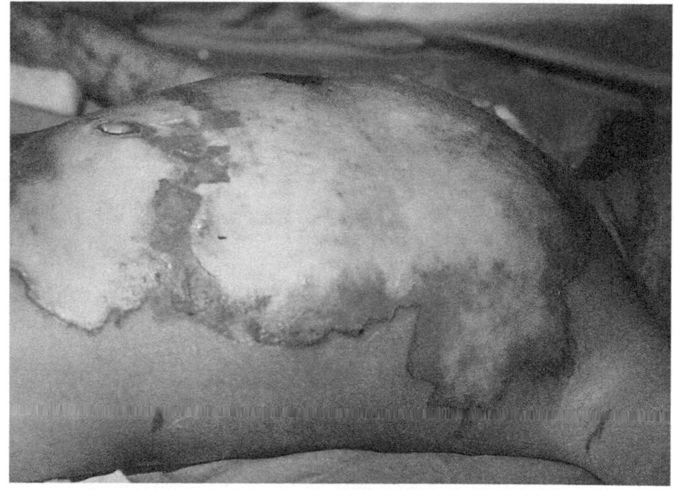

FIG. 23.8 Full-thickness thermal injury.

thickness of the skin or only a portion of the skin layers. Touching injured surfaces to test for blanching and capillary refill indicates whether circulation to the area is intact.

It is important to consider the cause of injury and the duration of contact with the burning agent. In general with burn injuries, the more intense the heat source and the longer the contact, the deeper the resulting injury. Hot liquids may result in partial-thickness burns, whereas full-thickness injuries are associated with flame burns. This may vary with the child's age. Very young children are likely to sustain deeper injuries because of the thin nature of infant skin. This makes estimation of burn depth difficult in young children, especially after scald injuries. Also in all burns, there can be cellular death at the wound site for up to 48 hours postinjury resulting in an expanded area and depth than what was originally calculated (Nielson, Duethman, Howard, et al., 2017). Nonaccidental burn injuries tend to be more severe than accidental burns because contact with the burning agent is prolonged. Electrical injuries may also be difficult to assess initially. Visible tissue destruction may appear to be minimal and the extent of damage to underlying structures may not be evident. The circumstances of the burn may also suggest the presence of associated injuries.

Certain areas of the body carry a higher risk of complications and therefore require specialized care. Burns of the hands and feet and across joints may not necessarily involve a large body surface area, but injury and scar formation may interfere with normal growth and development. Specialized care is required to preserve maximum function. Burns to the face and neck, along with a history of the injury occurring in an enclosed space, raise a high index of suspicion of inhalation injury. In addition, airway compromise and hypoxia may result from edema formation and pulmonary injury. Damage to the delicate cartilage of the nose and ears can result in facial deformities. Perineal burns are prone to infection and maceration in all patients, especially in young children who are not toilet trained. Scar bands and contractures in the perineal area may interfere with hygiene and mobility.

TABLE 23.8 Severity Grading System Adopted by American Burn Association

	Minor*	Moderate	Major
Partial-thickness burns	<10% of total body surface area (TBSA)	10%-20% of TBSA	>20% of TBSA
Full-thickness burns			All
Treatment	Usually outpatient; may require 1- to 2-day admission	Admission to hospital, preferably one with expertise in burn care	Admission to burn center

*Minor burns exclude any burn involving the face, hands, feet, perineum, or crossing joints; circumferential burns; electrical injuries; any injury complicated by inhalation injury or concomitant trauma; and children with psychosocial factors affecting the injury.
From Vaccaro, P., & Trofino, R. B. (1991). Care of the patient with minor to moderate burns. In R. B. Trofino (Ed.), *Nursing care of the burn-injured patient.* Philadelphia, PA: FA Davis.

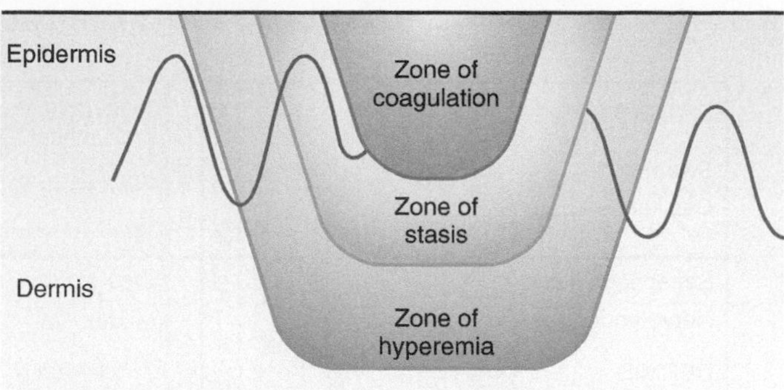

FIG. 23.9 Zones of injury in burn. (From Townsend, C. M. [2007]. *Sabiston textbook of surgery* [18th ed.]. Philadelphia, PA: Saunders.)

BOX 23.8 Zones of Burn Injury

Zone of coagulation (necrosis)—Area beneath obviously destroyed tissue. Capillary flow has ceased and tissue destruction is irreversible; tissue is dead.

Zone of stasis—Area beneath and surrounding zone of coagulation; markedly reduced capillary flow; tissue severely damaged from heat but not coagulated. Tissue in this zone can be saved with prevention of further injury and with adequate perfusion.

Zone of hyperemia—Area metabolically active; displays usual response to tissue injury.

Children younger than 2 years of age have a significantly higher mortality rate than older children with burns of a similar magnitude. The infant has minimum protein stores, which are rapidly depleted during burn shock; an immature immune response, which increases the risk of infection and sepsis; and a greater amount of body water in proportion to size that is intolerant of rapid fluid shifts. In addition, the child has not achieved mature renal function. This negatively affects the ability to retain sodium and water. These considerations combined with the previously discussed fragility of the skin in the very young, increase the severity of injury.

Many patients sustaining thermal injuries may also suffer associated trauma. The circumstances of the accident may offer clues to related trauma. Children involved in house fires may have jumped from a window, sustaining fractures. Motor vehicle accidents and electrical injuries often result in concomitant injuries. Any suspicion of nonaccidental burn trauma should alert the health care team to rule out other injuries.

PATHOPHYSIOLOGY

A burn injury represents a catastrophic insult that involves all organ systems. Understanding the pathophysiology underlying thermal trauma is essential to provide appropriate nursing care to the pediatric burn victim.

Local Response

Damage to human skin by heat results in two types of injury: an immediate direct cellular response and a delayed response caused by dermal ischemia. Irreversible cellular damage from protein denaturation occurs at temperatures exceeding 45°C (113°F). Three zones of injury demonstrate the evolution of local tissue damage (Fig. 23.9). The unstable area of injured cells, which may survive under ideal conditions, is designated the zone of stasis. Progressive injury caused by dermal ischemia may occur in this zone (Box 23.8).

Edema Formation

Thermal injury to the vessels in the two outer zones results in increased capillary permeability. At the same time, vasodilation causes an increase in hydrostatic pressure within the capillaries. The increased hydrostatic pressure, combined with the increased capillary permeability, causes loss of water, protein, and electrolytes from the circulating volume into the interstitial spaces.

To understand the physiologic mechanism of the formation of burn edema, an understanding of the microvascular fluid balance is necessary. Burn injury not only causes edema at the site, but extravasated and sequestered fluid and protein also enter nonburned tissue. The directly injured cells have a damaged cell membrane that leads to an increase in sodium and potassium shift, resulting in cell swelling. Intracellular water and sodium increase. This process occurs not only in injured cells but also with those that are not directly heat injured. Edema develops when the rate of fluid being filtered from the microvessels exceeds that of the lymph flow. The edema in the interstitial space develops rapidly over the first 8 to 12 hours following the injury and is dependent on the depth and extent of the burn injury (Rowan, Cancio, Elster, et al., 2015).

Fluid Loss

Fluid transport across the microcirculatory wall in normal and pathologic states is quantitatively described by the Landis-Starling equation. This equation describes the physical forces and physiologic mechanisms that govern fluid transfer between vascular and extravascular compartments. Normal capillary barriers that separate the intravascular and interstitial compartments are disrupted, which results in severe depletion of plasma volume and an increase in extracellular fluid. This rapid and extensive fluid shift is manifested as hypovolemia (Rae, Fidler, & Gibran, 2016).

Circulatory Status

Significant circulatory alterations take place in the zone of stasis located around the dead coagulated tissue. Heated red blood cells become spherical. These heat-damaged cells, together with hemoconcentration from fluid shifts, depressed cardiac output, and tissue edema, reduce the blood flow in the burned area, resulting in capillary stasis. Thrombi develop which further impedes circulation and produces tissue ischemia and necrosis. Hyperviscosity and impaired blood flow are attributed to the release of substances such as thromboplastin and clot-activating factors from damaged cells. These substances cause the production of microemboli, platelet adhesion and aggregation, and increased pain and edema. Circulation in the area around partial-thickness wounds ceases immediately after injury but is usually restored within 24 to 48 hours. In full-thickness burns, however, the vascular supply is completely occluded, and no appreciable circulation is reestablished until granulation takes place at the interface between burned and unburned skin.

Tissue Repair

With reasonable care, superficial partial-thickness injuries heal spontaneously and uneventfully through the generative capacity of the stratum germinativum and epithelial cells of the lining of skin appendages. Deep partial-thickness burns heal more slowly by regeneration from the epithelial lining of skin appendages, sweat glands, and hair follicles. Infection, trauma, or severe hypothermia easily converts a partial-thickness wound to a full-thickness injury, especially in the normally thinner skin of young children. Fluid loss and metabolic consequences may be considerable.

Cell destruction by coagulation necrosis occurs in full-thickness burns. Dead tissue and exudate convert to a thick, leathery eschar in 48 to 72 hours; the eschar liquefies and begins to separate in 12 to 21 days if not surgically excised. This process is a result of autolysis, leukocyte digestion, and disintegration of collagen fibers. The dead avascular tissue provides an ideal environment for bacterial growth. If tissue is not grafted, new granulation tissue forms on the wound bed. The wound heals slowly by granulation from the edges, with a high risk of infection and severe scarring. Full-thickness burns result in severe edema with fluid and electrolyte shifts and extensive metabolic changes.

Systemic Responses

Cardiovascular System

The immediate postburn period is marked by dramatic alterations in circulation, known as burn shock. A precipitous drop in cardiac output precedes any change in circulating blood or plasma volumes. This initial decrease in cardiac output (approximately 50% of normal resting values) is attributed to a circulating myocardial depressant factor that is associated with severe burn injury and directly affects the contractility of the heart muscle. As a result of fluid losses through denuded skin, increased capillary permeability, and vasodilation, the circulating volume decreases rapidly; cardiac output is reduced even further, usually leveling off at approximately 20% of normal resting values. After adequate fluid resuscitation, cardiac output spontaneously returns to normal in 24 to 36 hours. If fluid is not replaced, cardiac output continues to decrease, resulting in inadequate perfusion, organ dysfunction, and ultimately death.

Capillary permeability with leakage of fluid takes place both in uninjured areas and in the burn wound. Together with the shrinkage of drying eschar, severe edema caused by the rapid fluid shift to the interstitial spaces may produce a tourniquet effect, resulting in compartment syndrome. Compartments are composed of groups of muscles in the extremities and are surrounded by fibrous tissue. The inability of the fascia to expand in the presence of massive edema increases the pressure in the compartment, compromising circulation and entrapping nerves. Treatment is required during the acute phase and consists of a surgical incision of the burned tissue (escharotomy) to restore distal circulation. If the escharotomy is not sufficient, an incision of the muscle sheath (fasciotomy) is performed (Fig. 23.10).

Edema fluid accumulates rapidly in the first 18 hours after injury and reaches a maximum in approximately 48 hours. Capillary permeability returns to normal, and fluid is reabsorbed, chiefly by way of the lymphatics. Reabsorption usually proceeds at the rate of fluid accumulation, although it may persist longer. Redistribution of fluid is often complex and unpredictable and is marked by diuresis.

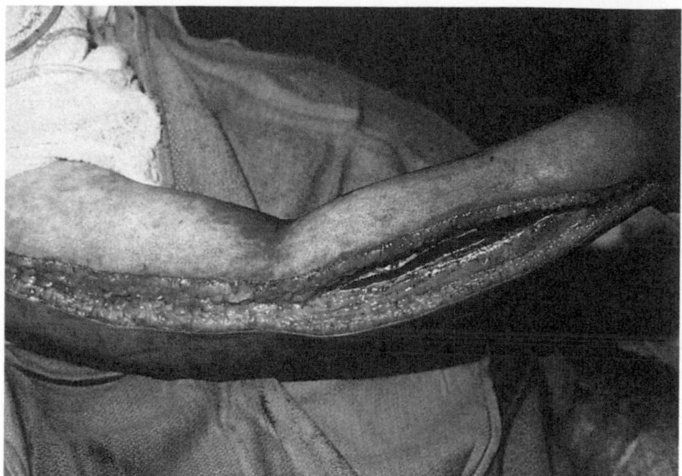

FIG. 23.10 Escharotomy and fasciotomy in severely burned arm.

In most children the cardiovascular system is able to withstand the demands placed on it, although shock is a prominent feature of large thermal injuries. Some children are prone to congestive heart failure and pulmonary edema. In addition, peripheral circulation in infants is less efficient and more labile, which complicates the burn response and therapy in this age-group.

Renal System

Children younger than 2 years of age lack the ability to concentrate urine because of the immaturity of their renal system and are therefore at an increased risk for dehydration. In addition, the child has a relatively larger TBSA in relation to weight than an adult. These issues, combined with limited physiologic reserves, increase the fluid requirements for children during burn shock resuscitation and in compensating for evaporative water losses (American Burn Association, 2016). Loss of fluid from the intravascular compartment causes renal vasoconstriction that in turn leads to reduced renal plasma flow and depressed glomerular filtration. When adequate fluids are provided, the glomerular filtration rate returns to normal, and by the third or fourth postburn day, urinary output increases as edema fluid is mobilized and eliminated. In the first few days, oliguria is more commonly the result of inadequate fluid replacement than of acute renal failure. If the child does not respond to treatment or if there is inadequate fluid resuscitation, acute renal failure may develop, with significant kidney damage.

Blood urea nitrogen (BUN) and creatinine levels are elevated as a result of tissue breakdown, decreased circulating volume, and oliguria. Hematuria may also be evident from the hemolysis of red blood cells, and oliguria may develop as a consequence of the increased pigment load. Myoglobinuria is especially common after extensive electrical injury or burn injuries with deep muscle destruction. Cell destruction releases large amounts of myoglobin, which occludes the kidney tubules and places these victims, especially those of electrical trauma at high risk for renal failure.

Gastrointestinal System

The GI system has been recognized as a target of systemic shock. After a burn injury, blood flow decreases to the GI system by one-third even though cardiac output is maintained by resuscitation fluids. Ischemia results and can produce ulcer formation, enterocolitis (severe enough to cause full-thickness necrosis), and even intestinal perforation. Poor perfusion to the kidney and the liver can ensue, resulting in organ dysfunction. The GI tract functions as a barrier to contain GI bacteria within it. Disruption of the GI mucosal integrity is possibly a focus for sepsis in the burn patient.

Depending on the proportion of burn size, atrophy of the GI tract mucosa can occur immediately after injury. The atrophy results in gut barrier dysfunction, leading to increased bacterial translocation and ultimately sepsis. Within hours after injury, enteral nutrition can be started safely. Implementing this practice assists in maintaining caloric goals and may also reduce infection for the burn patient. Intestinal motility returns as fluid losses are replaced unless irreversible necrosis of the bowel has occurred as a result of insufficient perfusion (Colon, Schlegel, & Chung, 2012).

The greatly accelerated metabolic rate in burn patients is supported by protein and lipid catabolism. The child has limited glycogen stores to provide energy, which therefore accelerates the protein and lipid breakdown. No other disease state produces as great a hypermetabolism as the burn injury. Therefore protein breakdown in the muscle and also in other organs can lead to multiple organ dysfunction (Jeschke, 2016). When the burn injury is extensive (>50% of TBSA), energy needs may approach twice the predicted basal requirements.

The stress of injury places high demands on the body. Stress-invoked glycogen breakdown depletes the energy stores in 12 to 24 hours, after which the body resorts to glyconeogenesis for high-energy needs. Blood glucose levels may be elevated as a result of insulin resistance. Rapid protein breakdown and muscle wasting occur if sufficient protein replacement is not provided.

Body temperature reflects the net balance between heat production and heat loss. As a result of the accelerated metabolism, children with burn injuries typically exhibit an elevated body temperature, even in the absence of infection. The thermoregulatory response is activated and results in an elevation of core body temperature. Burn-injured patients strive for a core body temperature of about 38°C (100.4°F). Low or "normal" temperature may indicate overwhelming sepsis or a fatigued physiologic capability to maintain temperature and should be viewed with concern. Routine methods of heat conservation after a major burn injury are inadequate because of excessive heat loss through evaporation and convection (Saffle, Graves, & Cochran, 2012). Heat is lost as a result of the energy-consuming process of water evaporation from the damaged skin surface. The body tries to raise the core and skin temperature to offset heat losses secondary to evaporation through the burn eschar (Gauglitz, Finnerty, Herndon, et al., 2012). Infants and young children are especially vulnerable because of the large surface area relative to metabolically active tissue. Burning destroys a lipid layer and converts skin that is normally impermeable to water to a state that transmits water vapor at least four times as rapidly as unburned skin. In partial-thickness burns this loss is greatest on the day of injury; in full-thickness burns it rises slowly at first and rapidly increases to reach a peak approximately the fourth day after the burn. Evaporative losses continue until partial-thickness wounds are healed and full-thickness burns are grafted. Therefore body stores of energy are rapidly depleted unless sufficient replacement is provided or losses are reduced.

Medications that affect metabolic rate may be used to prevent loss of body protein stores, thus protecting immunity, wound healing, muscle integrity, and organ function. Oxandrolone is an anabolic steroid that works to maintain and restore muscle mass, increase weight gain, and promote wound healing. Supplements of essential amino acids such as glutamine and arginine provide an anticatabolic effect, support wound healing, indirectly preserve lean body mass, improve immune function, and provide an antioxidant quality (Demling, 2005).

Neuroendocrine System

As a systemic response to stress from the burn injury, adrenal activity is markedly increased and catecholamines, such as epinephrine and norepinephrine, are released, which initiates vasoconstriction. Soon after, other local mediators are released, such as histamine, bradykinin, serotonin, prostaglandins, and many others. This induces vasodilation and increased cell permeability, resulting in local edema and the development of capillary leakage, requiring fluid resuscitation (Rae, Fidler, & Gibran, 2016).

Anemia and Metabolic Acidosis

The hematocrit is initially elevated because of hemoconcentration resulting from fluid shifts to the interstitial spaces, red blood cell destruction, and increased blood viscosity. A combination of heat-damaged red blood cells, blood loss at the wound sites, and dilution from resuscitation fluids results in anemia for the burn patient (Fidkowski & Fuzaylov, 2012). In addition, a reduced red blood cell half-life results from increased cell fragility. A significant loss of circulating red blood cell mass is predominantly associated with major burns.

Most burn patients exhibit some degree of metabolic acidosis as a result of the disruption of the body's buffering action because of the fluid shift to the extravascular spaces and the altered concentrations of potassium, sodium, chloride, and bicarbonate ions. Reduced blood volume and cardiac output, result in diminished perfusion and tissue hypoxia, with a shift to anaerobic metabolism. The resultant formation of metabolic acids is usually sufficiently compensated by respiratory mechanisms. Renal compensatory activities are impaired by the decreased blood flow.

Growth and Development

Children may demonstrate postburn growth restriction. Regular height and extremity assessments are necessary to detect subtle deformities until development is normalized.

Complications

Thermally injured children are subject to a number of serious complications, both from the wound and from systemic alterations resulting from the injury. The immediate threat to life is related to airway compromise and profound shock. During healing, infection—both local and systemic sepsis—is the primary complication. Mortality associated with thermal trauma in children increases with the severity of injury and decreases as age advances. In children older than 3 years, the mortality rate is similar to that of adults. Below this age, the rate of survival from the burn and its associated complications lessens considerably.

Pulmonary System

The impact of thermal injury on pulmonary function includes a full range of respiratory dysfunctions including inhalation injury, disruption of the oxygen supply to the body, aspiration of gastric contents, bacterial pneumonia, pulmonary edema and insufficiency, and emboli. In every age and burn size category, pneumonia is associated with a high risk of mortality and can cause a secondary insult leading to further toxic damage even days after the injury. Inhalation of carbonaceous debris impairs function of the cilia and results in a release of inflammatory mediators that are chemotactic to neutrophils and destroys alveolar-based macrophages, leading to a proliferation of bacteria (Nielson, Duethman, Howard, et al., 2017).

The mortality rate of children with isolated burns is 1% to 2%, but it increases to 40% when smoke inhalation is a factor (Lee, Norbury, & Herndon, 2012). Inhalation injuries result from trauma to the tracheobronchial tree after inhalation of the heated gases and toxic chemicals produced during combustion. Although direct thermal injury to the upper airway may occur, heat damage below the vocal cords is rare. Inspired heated air is cooled in the upper airway before reaching the trachea. Reflex closure of the cords and laryngeal spasm prevent full inhalation. Evidence of direct thermal injury to the upper airway includes burns of the face and lips, singed nasal hairs, and laryngeal edema. Clinical manifestation may be delayed as long as 24 to 48 hours (Woodson, Talon, Traber, et al., 2012). Wheezing, increasing secretions, hoarseness, wet rales, and carbonaceous secretions are signs of respiratory tract involvement. Upper airway obstruction is often associated with burn shock and fluid resuscitation. In such situations endotracheal intubation may be necessary to preserve a patent airway.

Suspect inhalation of carbon monoxide when the injury has occurred in an enclosed space. (See Smoke Inhalation Injury, Chapter 26, for a discussion of carbon monoxide inhalation.) Inhalation of other products of combustion, such as smoke and toxic chemicals, can produce varying degrees of pulmonary damage. Smoke from burning wood is extremely irritating; burning plastic materials, especially polyvinyl chloride, release smoke with gases containing chlorine, sulfuric acid, and cyanide. Respiratory injury is manifested by mucosal erythema and edema, followed by sloughing of the mucosa. A mucopurulent membrane replaces the mucosal lining and seriously compromises respiration and ventilation.

A common etiologic factor in respiratory failure in the pediatric population is bacterial pneumonia, which may be secondary to airway injury or contamination from intubation or may be acquired through hematogenous spread of bacteria. Early in the postburn period the largest percent of pulmonary infections result from nosocomial exposure, immobility, and abdominal distention. The hematogenous variety occurs later and is related to the septic burn wound or other foci, such as phlebitis at the site of an invasive IV line. A less common complication is pulmonary edema resulting from fluid overload or ARDS in association with gram-negative sepsis. (See Chapter 26.) This syndrome results from pulmonary capillary damage and leakage of fluid into the interstitial spaces of the lung. A loss of compliance and interference with oxygenation are the consequences of pulmonary insufficiency in conjunction with systemic sepsis.

Deep burns, especially those encircling the thorax, may cause restriction of chest excursion as a result of edema and inelastic eschar formation. Young children are particularly at risk because of the pliability of the skeletal structure. Hypoxia is relieved by an escharotomy of longitudinal incisions along the anterior axillary lines, combined with a transverse incision at the costal level. This procedure allows expansion of the chest wall to facilitate ventilation.

Wound Sepsis

Sepsis is a critical problem in the treatment of burns and is an ever-present threat after the shock phase. Initially, burn wounds are relatively pathogen free unless contaminated with potentially infectious material such as dirt or polluted water. However, dead tissue and exudate provide a fertile field for bacterial growth. On approximately the third postburn day, early colonization of the wound surface by a preponderance of gram-positive organisms (primarily staphylococci) changes to predominantly gram-negative opportunistic organisms, particularly *Pseudomonas aeruginosa*. By the fifth postburn day, bacterial invasion is well underway beneath the surface of the burn wound.

Characteristics of the burn wound contribute to the proliferation of pathogenic organisms. Vascular supply to full-thickness burns is occluded immediately, and no appreciable blood is supplied to the area for approximately 3 weeks after the injury. In partial-thickness wounds the circulation to the injured area is suspended for 24 to 48 hours; circulation is then restored unless infection supervenes. Thrombosis from bacterial invasion will impair circulation sufficiently to convert partial-thickness wounds to full-thickness injuries. These large amounts of nonviable tissue also provide an excellent medium for the growth of microorganisms. Hence the burn wound serves as the site of primary invasion for instances of localized or generalized infection. Because the burned child is immunosuppressed for many weeks after the burn injury, maintaining the wound at low contamination levels by meticulous wound care and vigilance for signs of infection can decrease the frequency of septic episodes caused by wound flora (Rowan, Cancio, Elster, et al., 2015).

Occlusion of the local blood supply impairs the delivery of both humoral and cellular defense mechanisms to the burned area. Initially there is a decrease in inflammatory and phagocytic cells to the wound, but the number of phagocytes gradually increases until they are present in abundance by the third postburn week, when granulation tissue is forming. Granulation tissue, with its rich blood supply, affords increasing resistance to infection. Organisms are normally a part of skin flora, so cultures with an organism concentration of $<10^5$ bacteria/g tissue has been arbitrarily chosen as the level of burn wound invasion.

Microflora present is influenced by the treatment modalities and choice of antibiotics. During the past 30 years there has been a reduction in the percentage of specific bacteria and fungi recovered from burn wounds. This reduction reflects improvements in patient management, nutritional support, aggressive excision and grafting of wounds, topical antimicrobial therapy, and wound dressings. Sepsis, in burn injury, is a major complication and a significant factor in morbidity and mortality among pediatric patients (Vyles, Sinha, Rosenberg, et al., 2014).

! NURSING ALERT

Disorientation in the burned patient is one of the first signs of overwhelming sepsis. A spiking fever and diminished bowel sounds accompanied by paralytic ileus occur and progressively increase over 48 to 72 hours, after which the temperature falls to subnormal limits. Other factors suggesting sepsis include hyperglycemia, insulin resistance, thrombocytopenia, abdominal distention, enteral feeding intolerance, and diarrhea. At this time the wound deteriorates, the white blood cell count is depressed, and septic shock becomes manifest.

Gastrointestinal System

GI dysfunction is common after burn injury as evidenced by feeding intolerance, mucosa ulceration, and bleeding, particularly in the stomach and duodenum. Within 72 hours of a major burn injury a significant number of patients may develop mucosal changes. This may progress to ulceration with septic episodes and hypoxemia. Potential causes of stress ulcers in burn patients include mucosal ischemia, increased acid production, increased acid back-diffusion, energy depletion, bile reflux, and direct mucosal injury with placement of intraluminal tubes.

Excessive fluid volume and burns to the chest or abdomen decrease compliance and can contribute to a serious complication (increased intraabdominal pressure) that may have an underestimated incidence in burned individuals. Although children with increased intraabdominal pressure readings tended to be younger, larger TBSA injuries and full-thickness components were significantly associated with elevated pressures and can result in tissue ischemia (Strang, Van Lieshout, Breederveld, et al., 2014). Increased intraabdominal pressure has the potential to impair hemodynamics, renal function, hepatic malperfusion, and pulmonary dysfunction. Despite maintaining cardiac output with fluid replacement, renal function remains impaired in the presence of increased intraabdominal pressure. To restore perfusion in children who have developed increased abdominal pressure a decompressive laparotomy is necessary.

Enteral feeding is one of the most important means of providing nutrition and has led to a decrease in mortality. Early enteral feeding often prevents some of these potential complications. Aggressive fluid resuscitation aids in maintaining adequate mucosal blood flow. Antacid and H_2 receptor antagonist therapy can effectively prevent ulceration of the stomach and duodenum.

Ileus is also a common complication after a burn injury. Sepsis, electrolyte imbalance, narcotics, and renal failure are common causes. Patients experience abdominal distention and pain. Early enteral feeding again can assist in avoiding intestinal complications (Tran & Chin, 2014).

THERAPEUTIC MANAGEMENT

Emergency Care

The initial management of the burn patient begins at the scene of injury. The first priority is to stop the burning process. The child should then be transported immediately to the nearest medical facility for definitive treatment and evaluation for transfer to a burn center. The child and the family will be extremely frightened and anxious; sensitivity to their emotional state provides reassurance during the transport process.

Stop the Burning Process

The chief aim of rescue in flame burns is to smother the fire, not fan it. Children tend to panic and run, which serves only to spread the flames and make assistance more difficult. Place the injured child in a horizontal position and rolled in a blanket, rug, or similar article, taking care to not cover the head and face because of the danger of inhaling toxic fumes. If nothing is available, the victim should lie down, cover the mouth with the hands, and roll over slowly to extinguish the flames. Remaining in the vertical position may cause the hair to ignite or may lead to the inhalation of flames, heat, or smoke.

Major burn injuries with large amounts of denuded skin should briefly be cooled with a single application of tepid water. Heat is rapidly lost from burned areas, and additional cooling leads to a drop in core body temperature and potential circulatory collapse. Continuous wet dressings or the application of ice promotes vasoconstriction because of cooling, resulting in impaired circulation to the burned area and increased tissue damage. Chemical burns present special circumstances and require flushing with copious amounts of water during transport to a medical facility. The use of neutralizing agents on the skin is contraindicated because a chemical reaction is initiated and further injury may result. If the chemical is in powder form, the addition of water may spread the caustic agent. The powder should be brushed off if possible. If the chemical burn produces a blister, it is advisable to open the blister with a sterile object to remove any chemical present.

Remove burned clothing to prevent further damage from smoldering fabric and hot beads of melted synthetic materials. If the clothing adheres, do not pull to remove. Trim around the clothing. This prevents removal of good skin cells with the damaged skin cells. Also remove jewelry to eliminate the transfer of heat from the metal and constriction from edema formation. These steps also provide better access to the burn and preclude more painful removal later on.

Assess the Victim's Condition

As soon as the flames are extinguished, assess the victim's condition. Airway, breathing, and circulation are the priority concerns. Cardiopulmonary and cerebral emergencies are always a consideration after trauma. Cardiopulmonary complications may result from inhalation of toxic fumes and smoke, exposure to electric current, hypovolemia, and shock. Institute emergency measures as appropriate (e.g., CPR, etc.).

Cover the Burn

Cover the burn with a clean, dry cloth to prevent contamination and alleviate pain by eliminating air contact. Cover the child who has extensive burns to prevent hypothermia. No attempt should be made to treat the burn. Debridement of the burn at this time is unnecessary. The application of topical ointments, oils, or other home remedies immediately postburn is contraindicated because these applications may intensify the burn.

Transport the Child to Medical Aid

Do not give the child with an extensive burn anything by mouth to avoid aspiration in the presence of paralytic ileus and upper airway edema and to prevent water intoxication. The child is transported to the nearest medical facility. If this cannot be accomplished within a relatively short time, establish IV access if possible with a large-bore catheter. Oxygen, if available, is administered at 100%. Give a report of the initial assessment and any interventions implemented to the medical facility assuming responsibility for the child's care.

Provide Reassurance

Providing reassurance and psychologic support to both the family and the child helps immeasurably during postinjury crisis. Reducing anxiety helps conserve the energy needed to cope with the physiologic and emotional stress of a traumatic injury.

Management of Minor Burns

Treatment of burns classified as minor can usually be managed adequately on an outpatient basis when the caregiver is reliable and able to carry out instructions for care and observation. Patients with less than optimum circumstances may require close follow-up to ensure compliance with the treatment program.

Cleanse the burn with mild soap and tepid water. Debridement of the burn includes removal of any embedded debris, devitalized tissue, and chemicals. Removal of intact blisters remains controversial. Some authorities argue that blisters provide a barrier against infection; others maintain that blister fluid is an effective medium for the growth of microorganisms (Smith, 2000). Most practitioners favor covering the burn with an antimicrobial ointment to reduce the risk of infection and provide some pain relief. The dressing consists of a fine-mesh gauze placed over the ointment and a light wrap of gauze dressing that avoids interference with movement. This helps keep the burn clean and protect it from trauma. Instruct the caregiver to wash the burn, reapply the dressing, and return the child to the office or clinic as directed for observation of signs of infection, progression of healing, or any other related complications (e.g., ineffectiveness of pain medication, decreased appetite, etc.). The frequency of dressing changes can vary.

Some practitioners prefer an occlusive dressing, such as a hydrocolloid or a silver wound dressing, which is placed over the burn after cleansing. This method eliminates the discomfort associated with frequent dressing changes but impairs visualization of the burn surface.

If there is a high probability of infection or other complications or if there is doubt about the ability to carry out instructions, direct the parents to return daily or every other day for dressing changes and inspection, or a nurse may be assigned to make a home visit for that purpose. Frequent removal of the dressing is an effective mode of debridement. Soaking the dressing in tepid water before removal helps loosen the dressing and debris as well as reduces discomfort. Burns of the face and ears are usually treated by an open method (Carrougher, 1998). The burn is washed and debrided in the same manner, and a thin film of antimicrobial ointment is applied to the skin without a dressing twice a day.

Obtain a tetanus history on admission. Administer tetanus prophylaxis if there is no history of immunization or if more than 5 years have passed since the last immunization. Administration of antibiotics for minor burns is controversial. A mild analgesic such as acetaminophen is usually sufficient to relieve discomfort; the antipyretic effect of the drug also alleviates the sensation of heat.

Most minor burns heal without difficulty, but hospitalization is indicated if the burn margin becomes erythematous, gross purulence is noted, or the child develops evidence of systemic reaction (e.g., fever or tachycardia). Evaluate the child for functional impairment, and instruct the caregiver in the exercise and ambulation program. After healing, an evaluation of scar maturation and range of motion will indicate any need for further therapy.

Management of Major Burns

When a child with extensive burns is admitted to the hospital for treatment, a variety of assessments are conducted and therapies initiated. Of these, the priority concerns include the establishment and maintenance of an adequate airway, initiation of fluid administration, and evaluation and treatment of the burn. Although the order of implementation may vary from institution to institution and the condition of the child, a number of procedures and activities are generally initiated on admission. Some are carried out simultaneously (Box 23.9).

Other therapies, including nutritional support, positioning and splinting to prevent contractures, treatment of anemia and hypoproteinemia, psychosocial support, and rehabilitative aspects of burn management, are initiated as appropriate throughout the course of treatment.

Establishment of an Adequate Airway

The first priority of care is airway maintenance. Thermal injuries to the face, nares, and upper torso; a history of injury in an enclosed space; carbonaceous sputum; an examination of the oral and nasal membranes that reveals edema, hyperemia, and blisters; and evidence of trauma to the upper respiratory passages all suggest inhalation of noxious agents or respiratory burns. If there is evidence of respiratory involvement, administer 100% oxygen and determine blood gas values, including carbon monoxide levels.

If the child exhibits changes in sensorium, air hunger, nasal flaring, grunting, or other signs of respiratory distress insert an endotracheal tube to maintain the airway. When severe edema of the face and neck is anticipated, perform intubation before swelling makes it difficult or impossible. A controlled intubation is preferred to an emergency procedure. Intubation allows for the delivery of humidified oxygen, the removal of secretions from respiratory passages, and the provision of ventilatory support.

Treatment may include bronchodilators (e.g., albuterol) to reduce bronchospasm. Bronchopulmonary hygiene to prevent atelectasis and pooling of secretions reduces the risk of pneumonia. Therapies include percussion and postural drainage, frequent position changes, and suctioning to remove secretions. Placing the child in a semi-Fowler position with high-flow oxygen and maximum humidity is often sufficient to relieve bronchospasm produced by trauma to the bronchial mucosa.

When full-thickness burns encircle the chest, constricting eschar may limit chest wall excursion. The child becomes increasingly difficult to ventilate. Escharotomy of the chest, where the eschar is incised through the fatty tissue, relieves this pressure and improves ventilation.

BOX 23.9 Major Burn Management

- Ascertain the adequacy of the airway, and provide oxygen, intubation, and ventilatory support as indicated.
- Assess breathing rate and depth. Note any use of accessary muscles, nasal flaring, or grunting which may indicate respiratory compromise.
- Insert a large-bore intravenous (IV) line, preferably through unburned skin, to deliver fluids at a sufficiently rapid rate to effect resuscitation.
- Remove clothing and jewelry, and examine for secondary trauma.
- Evaluate the burn wound, and determine the extent and depth of injury.
- Obtain an admission weight.
- Calculate fluid requirements, and establish the appropriate regimen.
- Obtain baseline laboratory studies.
- Provide IV medication for control of pain and anxiety only after adequate oxygenation is ensured and fluid resuscitation is initiated.
- Insert a nasogastric tube to empty stomach contents and maintain gastric decompression.
- Insert an indwelling Foley catheter to obtain specimens and monitor hourly output.
- Perform escharotomy or fasciotomy to the chest and extremities for constricting circumferential eschar, elevated compartment pressures, or impaired circulation.
- Apply topical antimicrobials and dressings to the burn wounds.
- Obtain a history regarding the injury and other pertinent data.
- Administer appropriate tetanus prophylaxis.
- Prophylactic antibiotic administration is not recommended.

Fluid Replacement Therapy

The objectives of fluid therapy are compensation for water and sodium losses to the traumatized area and the interstitial spaces, replenishment of sodium deficits, restoration of circulating volume, provision of adequate perfusion, correction of acidosis, and improvement of renal function. The volume of fluids should be just enough to provide adequate vital organ perfusion without producing unintentional (iatrogenic) pathologic changes. Initiate treatment for burn shock in children with burns in excess of 15% of TBSA.

Types of fluid and electrolyte therapy in the first 24 hours after injury remain controversial. Lactated Ringer solution appears to be the most common resuscitation fluid currently used. Proponents of crystalloids alone for resuscitation report that other solutions, specifically colloids, are no better and certainly more expensive than crystalloids for maintaining intravascular volume after burn injury. No consensus has been made to the use of colloids within the first 24 hours and further research is necessary.

The composition of the fluid administered varies with the philosophy of the individual practitioner and may consist of an isotonic saline solution, a near-isotonic solution, or even a hypertonic saline solution. Children's decreased tolerance to hypertonic solutions may result in hypernatremia, hyperosmolality, and intracellular dehydration. Many formulas have been proposed as guidelines for fluid administration after burn injury. The most commonly employed regimen is the Parkland formula. It is important to remember that any formula used during resuscitation serves only as a guideline; individual adjustments must be made based on the patient's response to therapy to avoid under or over resuscitation. Over resuscitation can cause a condition called "fluid creep" that can produce significant complications such as pulmonary edema, acute respiratory distress syndrome, abdominal and extremity compartment syndrome, and multiple organ dysfunction. Fluid replacement is maintained at a rate that provides an hourly urinary output of 30 ml in older children and 0.5 to 1 ml/kg in children weighing less than 30 kg (66 lb) (American Burn Association, 2016). Other parameters monitored during fluid resuscitation include vital signs, capillary refill, and sensorium.

Some common reasons for patients to require fluids well in excess of the calculated volume include underestimation of burn size (particularly in pediatric patients), pulmonary injury that sequesters resuscitation fluid in the lung, electrical injury with greater tissue destruction than is visible, and delay in the initiation of fluid resuscitation (Smith, 2000). Irreversible burn shock that persists despite aggressive fluid resuscitation remains a significant cause of death in the immediate postburn period.

> **! NURSING ALERT**
>
> Capillary refill, alterations in sensorium, and urinary output are the most reliable indicators for assessing the adequacy of fluid resuscitation in burned children. Blood pressure can remain normotensive even in a state of hypovolemia.

After the initial 24 to 48 hours, the capillary seal is restored. Fluid requirements decrease to a constant that persists until wound coverage is achieved. Colloid solutions such as albumin or plasma are useful to maintain plasma volume. Fluid balance may continue to be a problem throughout the course of treatment, especially during periods of increased evaporative loss from the burn wound. Approximately 48 to 72 hours after injury, interstitial fluid returns to the vascular compartment and diuresis occurs to eliminate excess fluids. During this phase, increasing intake to match urinary output can result in circulatory overload.

Nutrition

For 2 or 3 days immediately after injury, burn patients experience a hypometabolic phase when their metabolic rate and cardiac output decrease. Following this phase patients experience a hypermetabolic phase. This hypermetabolism is characterized by a hyperdynamic circulatory response with increased body temperature, oxygen and glucose consumption, carbon dioxide production, glycogenolysis, proteolysis, and lipolysis. This response begins on the fifth postburn day and continues up to 9 months after the burn, causing erosion of lean body mass, muscle weakness, immunodepression, and poor wound healing (Jeschke, 2016) This hypermetabolism is thought to be directly and indirectly associated with poor outcomes after a burn and can lead to slow wound healing, loss of lean body mass, and increased morbidity (Jeschke, 2016). Nutritional support, particularly through enteral feedings and initiated early in the burn patient's course, has become more aggressive. The continuity of these feedings is important.

Some burn patients are able to eat. Encourage a high-protein, high-calorie diet as soon as possible after resolution of paralytic ileus. However, many have poor appetites and are unable to meet energy requirements solely by oral feeding. Most children with burns in excess of 25% TBSA require supplementation with tube feeding. An absence of bowel sounds does not preclude enteral nutrition. Because the small bowel maintains motility and absorptive capabilities, the placement of a small-bore feeding tube into the duodenum allows for the safe delivery of enteral nutrition during periods of paralytic ileus associated with trauma, sepsis, and anesthesia. A nasogastric tube that decompresses the stomach protects the patient from aspiration.

Use of total parenteral nutrition has essentially been replaced by enteral nutrition for both theoretic and practical reasons and only used for those children who are unable to tolerate enteral support due to risks. Enteral nutrition directly nourishes the bowel mucosa with nutrients (e.g., glutamine). Small amounts of these nutrients within the bowel lumen stimulate the function of intestinal cells and normal mucosa function. This may help preserve normal blood supply to the intestines. Maintaining intestinal integrity may reduce bacterial translocation and sepsis, as well as preserve immune function. Along with the hazards of central venous access, total parenteral nutrition appears to be associated with increased secretion of tumor necrosis factor and other proinflammatory mediators (Saffle, Graves, & Cochran, 2012).

Specific guidelines for vitamin and micronutrient supplementation for the burn patient have not been established. Although supplementation with a variety of micronutrients is common practice, limited research has been done in burn patients on the homeostasis of vitamins and trace elements after burn injury (Nordlund, Pham, & Gibran, 2014).

Medication

Antibiotics are usually not administered prophylactically. The administration of systemic antibiotics to control wound colonization is not indicated because decreased circulation to the injured area prevents delivery of the medication to areas of deepest injury. Surveillance cultures and monitoring of the clinical course provide the most reliable indicators of developing infection. Appropriate antibiotics can then be instituted to treat the identified organism. Group B streptococci cultured from the throat or wounds are particularly destructive to grafted tissue. Do not overlook otitis media as a source of fever in the pediatric population.

Pain management presents a significant challenge and provisions of some form of sedation and analgesia is necessary. Effective pain management can lead to better outcomes due to the reduction in physiologic demands caused by stress on the body and a decrease in psychologic disorders such as depression and posttraumatic stress (Meyer, Wiechman, Woodson, et al., 2012). During the initial resuscitation period, IV administration of narcotics, along with anxiolytics, is required for baseline and procedural pain management. Morphine, fentanyl (Sublimaze), and midazolam (Versed) are the most commonly used agents (Singleton, Preston, & Cochran, 2015). (See Pain Management, Chapter 5.)

Anesthetic agents such as nitrous oxide, propofol, and ketamine also are used to control procedural pain. A major drawback with nitrous oxide is that staff is exposed to the gas because it is self-administered by the patient. Propofol, a nonbarbiturate hypnotic agent without analgesic activity, has advantages of rapid onset and little cumulative effect after extended infusion periods. It can cause depressed respiratory drive, loss of airway reflexes, and hypertension. Propofol must be given in doses large enough to cause loss of consciousness to prevent response to painful procedures. Even though this drug has a 'black box' warning of increased morbidity when used for the pediatric population, it is perceived as effective and safe and ranks high in use (Singleton, Preston, & Cochran, 2015). Ketamine has been widely used in burn patients and may preserve airway reflex; however, side effects may be noted, such as production of copious upper airway secretions, tachycardia, and hypertension. Ketamine can produce post administration hallucinations, particularly in adolescent boys. Repeated use may produce tolerance, so increased doses are required over time. To avoid volatile anesthetics, a combination of midazolam and fentanyl can be given intravenously (Meyer, Wiechman, Woodson, et al., 2012).

Management of the Burn Wound

After the initial period of shock and restoration of fluid balance, the primary concern is the burn wound. The primary goal for burn wound management is to close the burn as soon as possible (Rowan, Cancio, Elster, et al., 2015). The objectives of burn wound management include prevention of infection, removal of devitalized tissue, and closure of the wound. The application of dressings and topical antimicrobial therapy reduces pain by minimizing air exposure.

Primary Excision

In children with large, full-thickness burn wounds, excision is performed as soon as the patient is hemodynamically stable after initial resuscitation. Because the burn wound is precipitating the exaggerated physiologic response, many associated complications do not resolve until the eschar is excised and the wound is closed. One of the most effective therapies for decreasing mortality from major burn injuries is the early excision of the burn wound and its coverage by various techniques (Rowan, Cancio, Elster, et al., 2015).

Wound Hygiene

Hydrotherapy is used to cleanse the burn and assist with separating eschar. This involves either showering (spraying off the burn) or immersion (soaking in a tub) at least once a day. There are variances from institution to institution on the particular method, however, immersion therapy is becoming less common and being replaced by shower hydrotherapy. Hydrotherapy helps cleanse not only the wound but the entire body and also aids in maintenance of range of motion. Partial-thickness burns require debridement of devitalized tissue to promote healing. Debridement is very painful and requires some type of analgesia and anxiolytic before the procedure. The water acts to loosen and remove sloughing tissue, exudate, and topical medications. Mesh gauze entraps the exudative slough and is readily removed during hydrotherapy (Fig. 23.11). Any loose tissue is carefully trimmed away before the burn is redressed (Fig. 23.12).

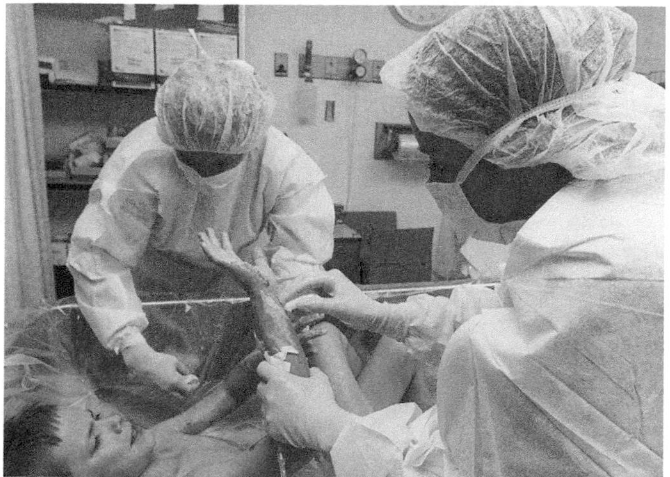

FIG. 23.11 Removal of dressing during hydrotherapy. (Courtesy CR Boeckman Regional Burn Center, Akron, Ohio.)

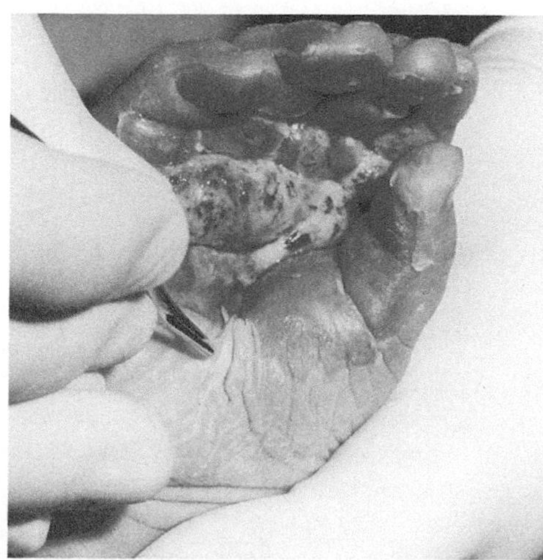

FIG. 23.12 Dead skin and debris are carefully trimmed away before dressing is applied. (Courtesy CR Boeckman Regional Burn Center, Akron, Ohio.)

Burn Wound Dressings

Daily dressing changes of the burn wound are recommended to allow for inspection and cleansing of the burn. Dressing changes offer an opportunity to meticulously observe the burn for infection. The volume of draining and the physical condition of the dressing also dictate frequency of dressing change. Often burn dressings become saturated, soiled, or disheveled, indicating that additional dressing changes may be required (Hartford, 2012).

Topical Antimicrobial Agents

Several methods are used for covering the burn wound (Box 23.10 and Fig. 23.13). All meet the objective of preparation for permanent wound coverage, and all use some type of topical agent. Before the development of effective topical agents for reducing the incidence of invasive organisms, wound sepsis was the major cause of mortality from burn injury. The goal is to minimize wound colonization. A variety of specific agents are available; examples include silver sulfadiazine (Thermazene), Santyl (Collagenese), andmafenide acetate (Sulfamylon). Topical agents do not eliminate organisms from the wound but can effectively inhibit bacterial growth. To be effective, a topical application must be nontoxic, capable of diffusing through eschar, harmless to viable tissue, inexpensive, and easy to apply. It should not encourage

BOX 23.10 Methods of Burn Wound Management

Exposure—Wounds are left open to air; crust forms on partial-thickness wounds, and eschar forms on full-thickness burns.

Open—A thin layer of topical antimicrobial agent is applied directly to the wound surface, and the wound is left uncovered.

Modified—Antimicrobial is applied directly or impregnated into thin gauze and applied to the wound; gauze or net secures the area (see Fig. 23.14).

Occlusive—Antimicrobial is impregnated in gauze or applied directly to the wound; multiple layers of bulky gauze are placed over the primary layer and secured with gauze or net. Occlusive methods may impede joint movement due to bulky gauze wraps. Advantages include reduction of evaporative heat loss from the wound, comfort, and protection.

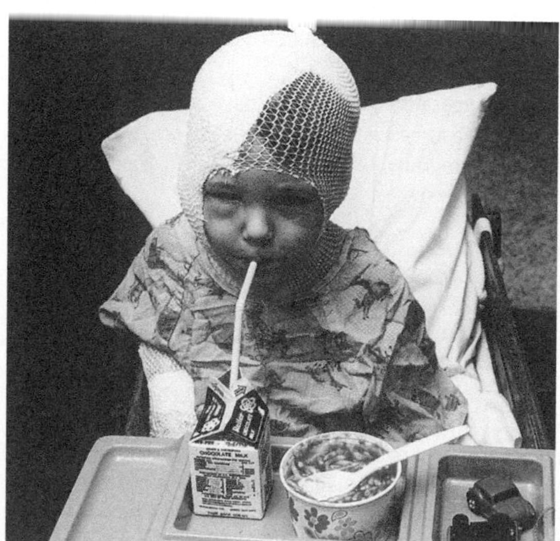

FIG. 23.13 Burn wound covered with gauze dressings and secured with tubular elastic netting. (Courtesy CR Boeckman Regional Burn Center, Akron, Ohio.)

the development of resistant strains of bacteria and should produce minimum electrolyte derangement.

Some topical agents are packaged and prepared on a fine-mesh gauze, which allows ease of application (Fig. 23.14). The gauze provides necessary protection for the wound, maximizes patient comfort, increases the rate of healing, reduces the necessity for frequent dressing changes, and is cost-effective. Examples include a nanocrystalline film of pure silver (Acticoat and Silverlon), a hydrofiber with ionic silver (Aquacel Ag), a silver silicone foam dressing (Mepilex Ag), and a wound contact layer with glycosaminoglycan hydrogel (Mepitel). Most often these gauzes are used on superficial second-degree burns, on donor sites, and for graft care, except for Acticoat, which can also be used for full-thickness wounds.

Temporary Skin Substitutes

Permanent coverage of extensive burns is a prolonged process that requires repeated operations for debridement and grafting. Transient physiologic wound closure is achieved by temporary skin substitutes, thereby helping control pain, absorb wound exudates, and prevent wound desiccation (Rowan, Cancio, Elster, et al., 2015). Temporary skin substitutes markedly reduce pain and facilitate movement of joints to retain range of motion.

Allograft (homograft) skin comes from human cadavers and is processed by commercial skin banks (Box 23.11). These skin banks screen donors for communicable diseases and track the skin much like blood transfusions. Allograft skin is particularly useful in the coverage of surgically excised, deep partial-thickness and full-thickness wounds in extensive burns when available donor sites are limited. Severe immunosuppression occurs in massively burned children, and the allograft becomes adherent (Fig. 23.15). The allograft can remain in place until suitable donor sites become available. Typically rejection occurs approximately 14 days after application. The use of an allograft is limited by the availability of tissue banks and the supply of suitable donors.

Although various animal skins have been used to provide temporary coverage of wounds, only porcine xenograft is widely used today. Porcine xenograft does not vascularize, but it will adhere to a clean superficial burn and provide excellent pain control while the burn heals (Vloemans, Hermans, van der Wal, et al., 2014). Pigskin dressings are replaced daily or every 2 or 3 days. They are particularly effective in children with partial-thickness scald burns of the hands and face because they allow relatively pain-free movement, which reduces contracture formation and has the added benefit of improving appetite and morale (Fig. 23.16).

When applied early to a superficial partial-thickness injury, biologic dressings appear to accelerate burn wound healing. They create an environment at the burn surface that is conducive to epithelial growth; this is in contrast to topical antimicrobial agents, which may slow epithelialization. Biologic dressings must be applied to clean burns. If the dressing covers areas of heavy microbial contamination, infection occurs beneath the dressing. In the case of partial-thickness burns, such an infection may convert the burn to a full-thickness injury. It is important to observe the burn wound daily for any signs of an infectious process.

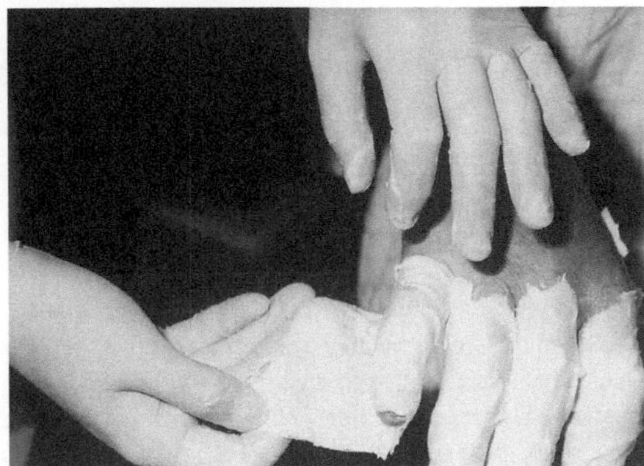

FIG. 23.14 Gauze impregnated with ointment applied to burn wound. Note how each finger is wrapped separately. (Courtesy CR Boeckman Regional Burn Center, Akron, Ohio.)

BOX 23.11 Types of Skin Grafts

Temporary Grafts

Allografts (homografts)—Skin that is obtained from genetically different members of the same species who are free of disease

Xenografts (heterografts)—Skin that is obtained from members of a different species, primarily pigskin

Permanent Grafts

Autografts—Tissue obtained from undamaged areas of the patient's own body

Isografts—Histocompatible tissue obtained from genetically identical individuals

Methods of Applying Split-Thickness Grafts

Sheet graft—A sheet of skin, removed from the donor site, is placed intact over the recipient site and sutured in place (see Fig. 23.18).

Mesh graft—A sheet of skin is removed from the donor site and passed through a mesher, which produces tiny slits in the skin. The meshing allows the expansion of the skin to cover 1½ to 9 times the area of the sheet graft (see Fig. 23.19).

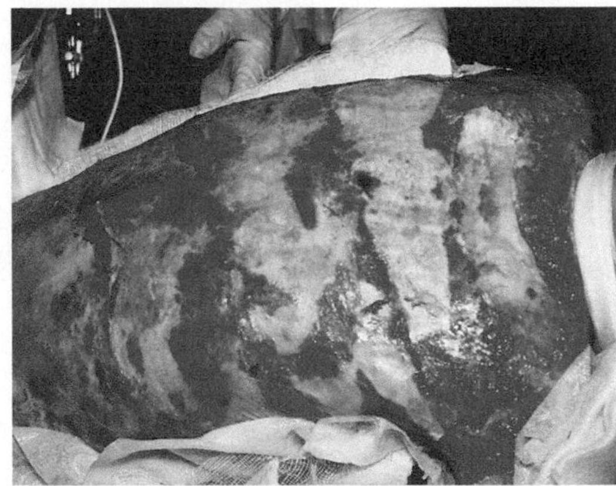

FIG. 23.15 Adherent allograft applied to excised full-thickness wound.

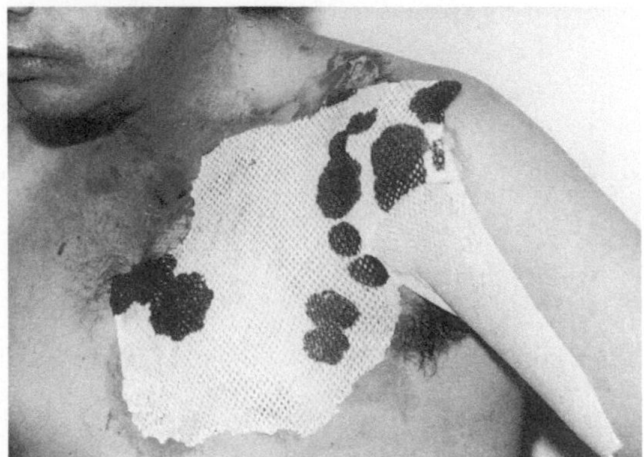

FIG. 23.16 Porcine xenograft applied to partial-thickness burn. (Courtesy CR Boeckman Regional Burn Center, Akron, Ohio.)

Synthetic Skin Coverings

A number of satisfactory skin substitutes are available for the management of partial-thickness burns. Ideally, the dressing should provide many of the properties of human skin: adherence, elasticity, durability, and hemostasis. Synthetic skin substitutes are readily available, have varied shelf lives, and are relatively expensive.

Synthetic dressings are composed of a variety of materials and can be used successfully in the management of superficial partial-thickness burns and donor sites. These dressings do not contain antimicrobial properties. Examples include a pertrolatum dressing (Xeroform), a hydrocolloid dressing (DuoDERM), and transparent adhesive films (OpSite and Tegaderm). As with biologic dressings, it is important that the burn is free of debris before applying the dressing. Body temperature elevation or evidence of purulence, erythema, or cellulitis around the burn edges may indicate that the burn has become infected beneath the dressing. Prompt discontinuance of the synthetic dressing is indicated. All synthetic dressings are reputed to hasten burn wound healing and reduce discomfort.

Dermal Replacements

The development of products that replace or allows the dermis to regenerate has significantly improved burn wound healing and decreased scar formation. Integra Dermal Regeneration Template (Integra) is a two-layer product that can be applied to partial- and full-thickness burns. The inner layer is a porous matrix made of cross-linked fibers (designed to induce better regeneration of the patient's normal tissue by acting as a scaffold. The outer layer is a soft silicone membrane that protects the wound from infection and holds moisture for 2 to 3 weeks acting like the skin's epidermis. The silicone layer is peeled off after the dermis is formed. The application of artificial skin does not replace the grafting procedure, but it prepares the burn wound to accept an ultrathin autograft. Advantages include faster healing of the burn wound when integrity of the dermis is restored, faster healing of donor sites with the use of ultrathin grafts, and restoration of sweat glands and hair follicles. Integra must be observed for submembrane infection. A disadvantage is its high cost.

AlloDerm is another, newer covering to promote dermal replacement. It is created from donated human skin that has been processed to remove all cells but maintains the important biochemical and structural components. This process makes AlloDerm an acellular tissue that will not result in rejection. The donated skin is screened and tested for any type of transmittable disease. When used on the burn, it provides a foundation for new tissue regeneration.

Permanent Skin Coverings

Permanent coverage of deep partial- and full-thickness burns is usually accomplished with a split-thickness skin graft. This graft consists of the epidermis and a portion of the dermis removed from an intact area of skin by a special instrument: the dermatome (Fig. 23.17). If all the wounds cannot be grafted at once, there are priority areas for coverage: the face, hands, joint surfaces, and neck. These preferential sites are chosen to hasten healing, establish function, and improve the patient's sense of well-being.

With extensive burns it is often difficult to find enough viable skin to cover the wounds; therefore available donor sites are used to the best advantage by special techniques. Box 23.11 describes the various types of split-thickness skin grafts. Sheet grafts (Fig. 23.18) are used in areas where cosmetic results are most visible; mesh grafts (Fig. 23.19) result in a less desirable cosmetic and functional outcome. Requirements for the successful vascularization of any graft are listed in Box 23.12.

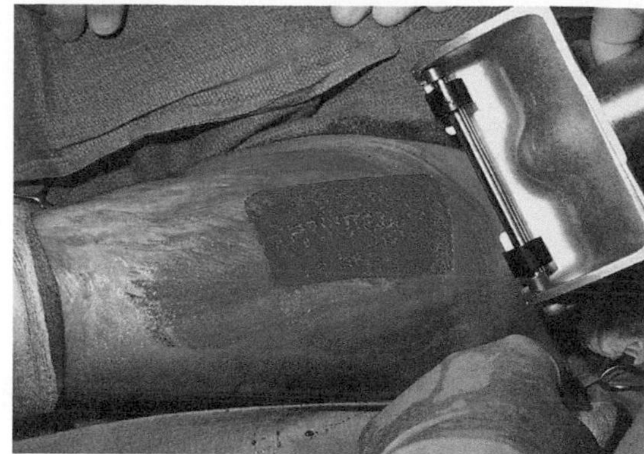

FIG. 23.17 Removal of split-thickness skin graft with a dermatome.

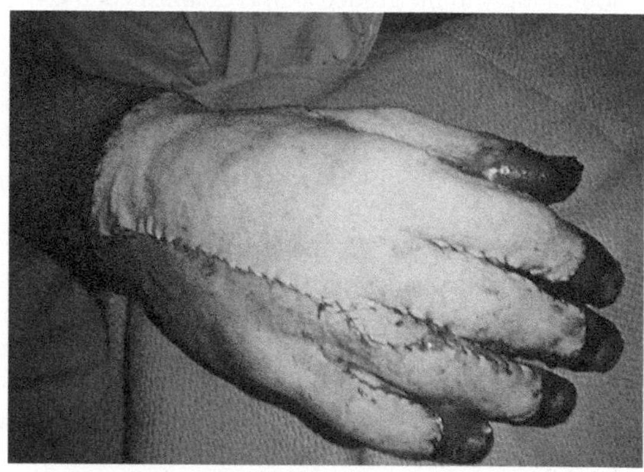

FIG. 23.18 Sheet graft.

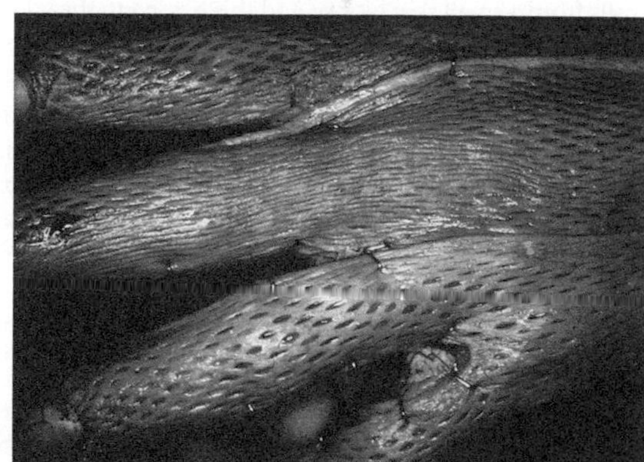

FIG. 23.19 Mesh graft.

BOX 23.12 Requirements for a Successful Graft

- Sufficient nourishment until the new blood supply is established from the base of the recipient bed
- Primary tissue contact (e.g., actual contact between the surface of the graft and a recipient bed that is free of bacteria and necrotic skin)
- Avoidance of bleeding, hematoma formation, and fluid accumulation beneath the graft
- Prevention of infection
- Prevention of mechanical trauma

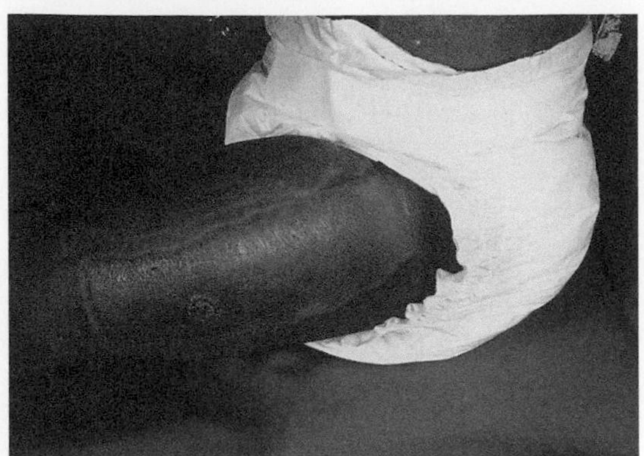

FIG. 23.20 Healed donor site.

Until blood supply to the grafted skin is established, it is nourished by osmotic interchange with the recipient bed. Wound healing occurs as the area releases fibrin, which attaches the graft to the bed. The fibrin is infiltrated by leukocytes, fibroblasts, and the capillary buds of the granulation tissue. This process begins within hours of grafting, and vascularization is established after 3 days. Within 2 weeks the graft is attached to the recipient bed by connective tissue.

The donor site is dressed with synthetic wound coverings or fine-mesh gauze until the dressing separates at 10 to 14 days, when the wound is healed. Dressings are not changed on donor sites to avoid damage to newly healed, delicate epithelium. Healed donor sites are available for reharvesting in patients with extensive burns and limited undamaged skin (Fig. 23.20). The quality of skin from donor sites is decreased when multiple grafts are taken.

Cultured Epithelium

For more than 30 years it has been possible to culture vast numbers of epithelial cells from a small skin biopsy, and this has led to the widespread use of cultured epithelial grafts to cover burns. Colonies of epithelial cells expand into broad sheets of undifferentiated epithelial cells. The resulting sheets are attached to a petrolatum gauze carrier to ease handling. Many of the imperfections associated with epithelial cell wound closure may be attributed to the lack of dermis. Despite scattered cases, application of cultured epithelial grafts onto dermal replacement products that have been vascularized, can improve short- and long-term results (Kagan, Peck, Ahrenholz, et al., 2013). High cost is a disadvantage of using both applications. (See Quality Patient Outcomes box.)

QUALITY PATIENT OUTCOMES

Acute Management of Burns

- Stable body temperature
- Adequate fluid replacement and urinary output
- Adequate nutrition and reduction of metabolic losses
- No evidence of acute complications
- Pain controlled
- Evidence of wound healing
- No evidence of contractures
- Adequate emotional support

NURSING CARE MANAGEMENT

Nursing care of the pediatric burn patient represents a challenge to the nurse's knowledge of anatomy and physiology, the behavioral sciences, and pathophysiology. Patient outcome after thermal injury is the result of the collaboration of an interprofessional burn team using a family-centered care approach. In addition to providing nursing care, the nurse functions as the patient care advocate to coordinate the efforts of the interprofessional burn team.

Because the care of burned children encompasses such a broad range of skills and foci, it has been divided into segments that correspond to the major phases of burn treatment. The acute phase, also referred to as the emergent or resuscitative phase, involves the first 24 to 48 hours. The management phase extends from the completion of adequate resuscitation through wound coverage. The rehabilitative phase begins once the majority of the wounds have healed and rehabilitation becomes the predominant focus of the care plan. This phase continues until all reconstructive procedures and corrective measures have been accomplished, which often extends over a period of months or years.

Acute Phase

The primary emphasis during the emergent phase is the treatment of burn shock and management of pulmonary status. Monitoring vital signs, output, fluid infusion, and respiratory parameters are ongoing activities in the hours immediately after injury. IV infusion begins immediately and is regulated to maintain a urinary output of at least 0.5 to 1 ml/kg in children weighing less than 30 kg (66 lb). Expect an output of 30 to 50 ml/hr in children weighing more than 30 kg. Urinary output, vital signs, laboratory data, and objective signs of adequate hydration guide the rate of fluid administration.

! NURSING ALERT

Early indicators for the adequacy of hydration are level of consciousness and capillary refill.

The nurse observes patients for changes in all parameters. They require constant observation and assessment, with special attention given to signs of respiratory, cardiac, and renal complications. Alterations in electrolyte balance can produce clinical symptoms of confusion, weakness, cardiac irregularities, and seizures. Changes in respiratory function and gas exchange are reflected clinically by restlessness, irritability, increased work of breathing, and alterations in blood gas values. The loss of the skin's protective function exposes burned children to an increased risk of hypothermia.

Care of the burn wound is secondary to the more critical problems of respiratory and cardiac failure. When transfer to a special burn care facility is anticipated, it is important to cover the wounds with clean dry sheets and wrap the child in blankets to maintain body temperature during transfer. The burn can be evaluated and dressed after arrival at the burn center. If no burn unit is available, the burn is cleansed and dressed in the emergency department. Many burn centers maintain a pictorial record of the burn to record progress and for legal purposes, especially in cases of suspected nonaccidental burn trauma. The burn is treated according to the protocol of the specific burn facility. The burn team implements infection control procedures and ensures that staff and visitors comply with established protocols to prevent cross-contamination in the burn unit.

Throughout the acute phase of care, do not overlook the psychosocial needs of the children and their families. The child is frightened, uncomfortable, and often confused. Children may be isolated from familiar persons and surroundings, and the often overwhelming physical needs at this time are the primary focus of the staff and parents. In addition to feeling concern for their child, the parents experience guilt, which is related to the fact they did not or could not protect their child. Consistency in the information presented and the attitude of the staff creates a sense of familiarity and stability during the emergent phase.

Management and Rehabilitative Phases

After the patient's condition is stabilized, the management phase begins. The multidisciplinary team concentrates on preventing infections, closing the burn wound as quickly as possible, and managing the numerous complications that may occur. Although the rehabilitative phase begins when permanent burn closure has been achieved, rehabilitation issues are identified on admission and are included in the care plan throughout the hospital course.

The management phase of burn care involves intensive nursing care, which is often difficult for the patient, family, and nursing staff. Except for minor burn injuries, care should take place in a burn center and involve a variety of disciplines, such as respiratory care, nutrition, physical therapy, occupational therapy, child life specialist, and social services.

Comfort Management

The severe pain of the burn and resultant therapies, the anxiety generated by these experiences, sleep deprivation, itching related to healing, and the conscious and unconscious interpretations of traumatic events contribute to the psychologic reactions and behaviors commonly observed in children with burns. It is important to assess the individual experiences and needs of the burn-injured child. A common myth in pediatrics is that children do not feel pain as intensely as adults do. What may be more accurate is that children do not always express their pain in the same way as adults. Children may display pain through behaviors of fear, anxiety, agitation, anger, aggression, tantrums, depression, withdrawal, and regression.

How the child's experience of pain from the burn injury and anxiety from the hospitalization are managed have lasting psychologic effects. Pain appears to increase the risk for children for the development of anxiety symptoms and anxiety disorders. A careful nursing history that includes the child's past experiences with pain and ways that caregivers successfully handled those events may provide clues to the control of current pain. Caregiver involvement is especially important for a child (Lee, Norbury, & Herndon, 2012). Interventions may include medications (including IV morphine, Fentanyl and short-term anesthetics such as propofol or ketamine), relaxation techniques, distraction therapy, cutaneous stimulation by touching, and family participation. Nonpharmacologic therapies may be used as adjuncts in the treatment of pain. In the pediatric population, distraction and imagery work well and augment pharmacologic interventions (Jeffs, Dorman, Brown, et al., 2014).

To reduce the anxiety associated with an unfamiliar environment and frightening treatments, it is important to offer thorough, age-appropriate explanations to the child before procedures. Compounding the pain is the child's interpretation of it and of the procedure; this is closely related to the child's developmental level. Children often feel anger, guilt, and depression; as in all illnesses, they may also exhibit regressive behavior. When children appear to accept pain with little or no response, psychologic consultation is in order.

Care of the Burn Wound

Closing the burn is the primary goal of burn wound care. The nurse has a major responsibility for cleansing, debriding, and applying topical medications and dressings to the burn. Because dressing removal is a painful procedure and causes anxiety, children should receive adequate analgesia along with anxiolytics, before the scheduled dressing change. The nurse should administer medication so that the drug's peak effect coincides with the procedure. Children who have an understanding of the procedure to be performed and some perceived control demonstrate less maladaptive behavior. Children respond well to participating in decisions and the actual procedure as their condition allows.

With some children, nonpharmacologic interventions are effective means of coping with pain. Distraction therapy, deep breathing, relaxation techniques, and involvement of child life may facilitate the procedure. Most children also benefit from parental participation. Medical play is often effective in helping the younger child gain some mastery over the procedure. Incorporate those techniques that work best for the individual patient into the care plan and consistently implement them during the dressing change procedure.

Outer dressings are removed; any dressings that have adhered to the burn are easier to remove by applying tepid water. Loose or easily detached tissue is also debrided during the cleansing process. Encourage children to participate in dressing removal. Giving them something constructive to do helps them focus on something other than the procedure. In providing coverage for the burn, it is important that all areas be clean, the medication be amply applied or dressing covers the entire burn, and that no two burned surfaces touch each other (e.g., fingers or toes, or ears touching the side of the head). If touching, the burned surfaces will heal together, causing deformity or dysfunction.

Topical medications are applied directly to the burn with a clean gloved hand or impregnated into fine-mesh gauze before application. Prepackaged dressings already come prepared. Apply the dressings to assist in exudate absorption, wound debridement, and increased patient comfort. All dressings applied circumferentially should be wrapped in a distal-to-proximal manner. Apply the dressing with sufficient tension to remain in place without impairing circulation or limiting motion. A stable dressing is especially important when the child is ambulatory.

Another challenge for nurses is preventing graft loss. After a graft is applied in surgery, there is usually a period of immobility for the child. Positioning must be maintained in order to prevent graft loss from shearing forces of movement. Grafted joint areas may be splinted to maintain range of motion or prevent contracture formation, and this may cause discomfort. Dressings protect the grafts and must be monitored for increased drainage or odors that are signs of infection. The child must also be instructed not to pick under the dressings, which could result in graft loss or infection.

Burns that involve the eyelids require special care to prevent corneal ulceration. No solution other than saline should come in contact with the eyes during the cleansing process. Avoid vigorous debridement in this area of thin, delicate tissue. Assess the patient throughout the healing process for the ability to close the eyes. Inability to close the eyes because of contracture formation, administration of paralytic agents, or corneal burns requires instilling ophthalmic ointment. A patch is not used over the affected eye because it is not found to improve healing or reduce pain (Flynn, D'Amico, & Smith, 1998).

Universal Precautions, including the use of personal protective equipment (PPE) and barrier techniques should be followed when caring for all patients with thermal injuries. Frequent hand and forearm washing is the single most important element of the infection control program. Implement strict policies for cleaning the environment and patient care equipment to minimize the risk of cross-contamination. All visitors and members of other departments should be oriented to the infection control policies, including the importance of hand and forearm washing and use of PPE when needed. Screen all visitors for infection and contagious diseases before patient contact.

Nutrition

Oral feedings are common unless the child is intubated or paralytic ileus persists. Because children often lack an appetite, the nursing staff must patiently provide a great deal of encouragement and help. Consultation between the parents and dietitian helps determine food preferences. Children who are old enough should participate in meal planning.

Nourishing snacks are provided between scheduled meals. Painful procedures should not be scheduled around meals; most children are too physically exhausted and emotionally upset to eat at this time. Many children eat better in an atmosphere more nearly like what they are accustomed to at home. When their condition allows, children enjoy sitting at a table for meals and interacting with other children.

Children who require enteral supplementation by tube feeding must be monitored on an ongoing basis for feeding intolerance and tube malposition. The nurse should monitor and record any indications of abdominal distention, diarrhea, or electrolyte and metabolic derangement. Accurate documentation of oral, parenteral, and enteral nutritional intake is essential to evaluate the adequacy of nutritional support.

Prevention of Complications: Acute Care

The maintenance of body temperature is important to the child with burns. Reduction of heat loss is imperative to decrease energy demands and evaporative water loss. Ambient temperatures and humidity should be maintained at 28° to 33°C (82.4° to 91.4°F) and 80%, respectively, to control heat loss (Lee, Norbury, & Herndon, 2012). Large areas of the body should not be exposed simultaneously during dressing changes. Warmed solutions, linens, occlusive dressings, heat shields, a radiant warmer, and warming blankets assist in preventing hypothermia. The optimum environment for the child with burns can be uncomfortable for persons attending the child.

The chief danger during acute care is infection—burn wound infection, generalized sepsis, or bacterial pneumonia. The burn should be assessed for changes indicative of infection, which include conversion of a partial-thickness to a full-thickness burn injury, early eschar separation, subeschar hemorrhage, degeneration of granulation tissue, discoloration of unburned skin at the wound margins, or green discoloration of subcutaneous fat (indicative of *Pseudomonas* and other gram-negative organisms). In addition to the signs of developing burn wound infection, the child with systemic sepsis may have a core temperature of more than 38.5° C (101.3°F) or less than 36° C (96.8°F), tachycardia, tachypnea, and leukocytosis or leukopenia. Tachycardia and tachypnea are common presenting symptoms in many pediatric diseases. Children with septic shock often maintain a normal BP until they are severely ill. Shock may occur long before hypotension in children and is a late sign leading to decompensated shock. Meticulous assessment should include signs of decreased perfusion (including decreased peripheral pulses), altered alertness, prolonged capillary refill (>2 seconds), mottled or cool extremities, or decreased urinary output.

Children are reluctant to move when doing so causes pain, and they are likely to assume a position of comfort. Unfortunately, the most comfortable position is flexion, which encourages the formation of contractures and loss of function. Ongoing efforts to prevent contractures include the positioning and splinting of involved extremities in extension, active and passive physical therapy, and the encouragement of spontaneous movement when feasible. In addition to maintenance of proper body alignment, frequent position changes are important to improve bronchopulmonary hygiene and capillary perfusion to common pressure areas. Low–air loss beds are beneficial for the morbidly obese or for children with posterior grafts. Areas of particular concern for pressure area development in the pediatric population are the posterior scalp, heels, and areas exposed to mechanical irritation from splints and dressings.

Prevention of Complications: Long-Term Care

The rehabilitative phase of care begins once burn wound coverage has been achieved. Scar formation becomes a major problem as healing occurs (Fig. 23.21). The scar tissue is metabolically active and highly vascular; collagen is deposited in an undefined pattern. Contractile properties of the scar tissue can result in disabling contractures, deformity, and disfigurement. As long as the scar is raised, red, and firm, it is considered active (Fig. 23.22). Hypertrophic scarring typically reaches a peak approximately 4 to 6 months after burn wound healing, and most scars mature or become inactive in 1 to 2 years. The mature scar is characterized by pigmented color, flattening, and increased suppleness of the tissue (Fig. 23.23).

Uniform pressure applied to the scar decreases the blood supply and forces the collagen into a more normal alignment. When pressure is removed, blood supply to the scar is immediately increased; therefore periods without pressure should be brief to avoid nourishment of the hypertrophic tissue. Continuous pressure to areas of scarring can be achieved by elastic bandages or commercially available pressure garments.

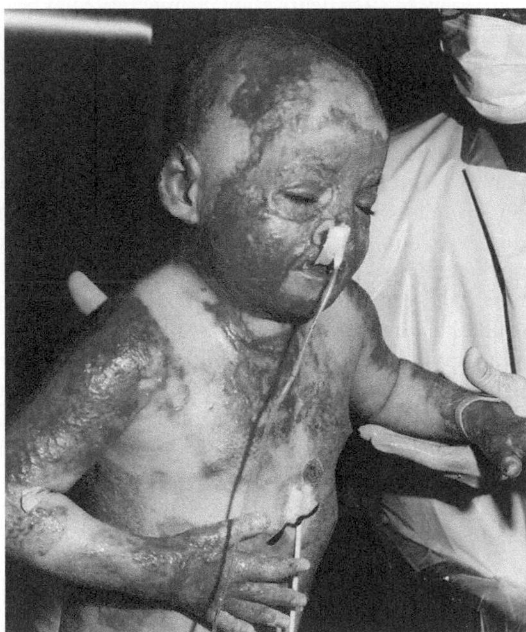

FIG. 23.21 Extensive scars from flame burn. (Courtesy CR Boeckman Regional Burn Center, Akron, Ohio.)

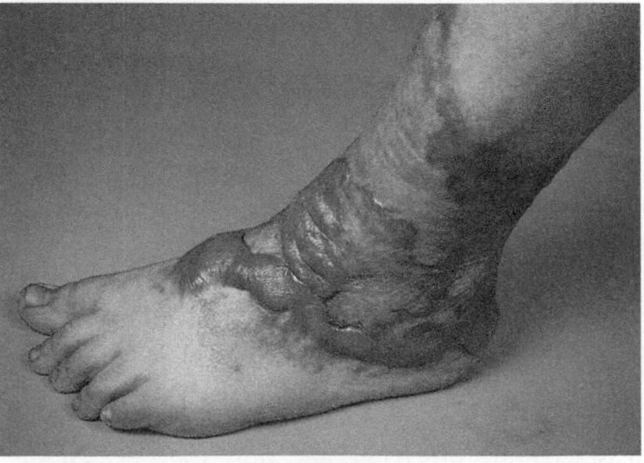

FIG. 23.22 Hypertrophic immature scar.

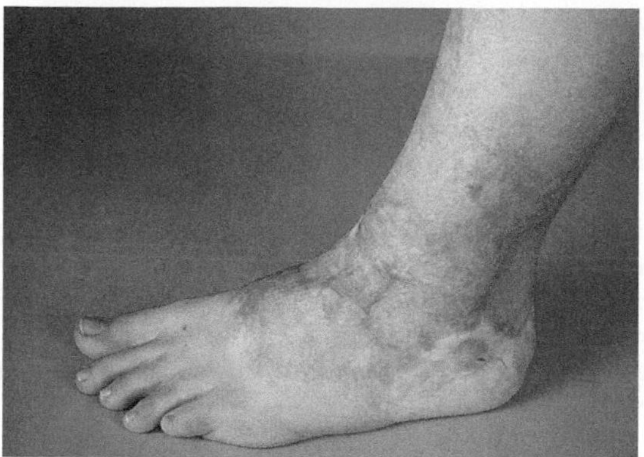

FIG. 23.23 Flat, mature scar after pressure.

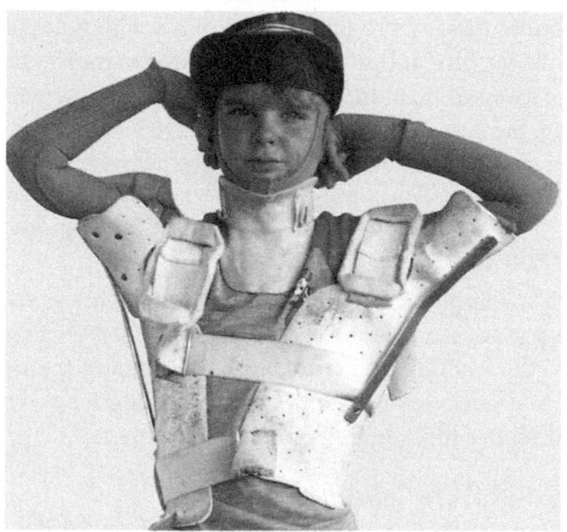

FIG. 23.24 Child in elasticized (Jobst) garment and "airplane" splints.

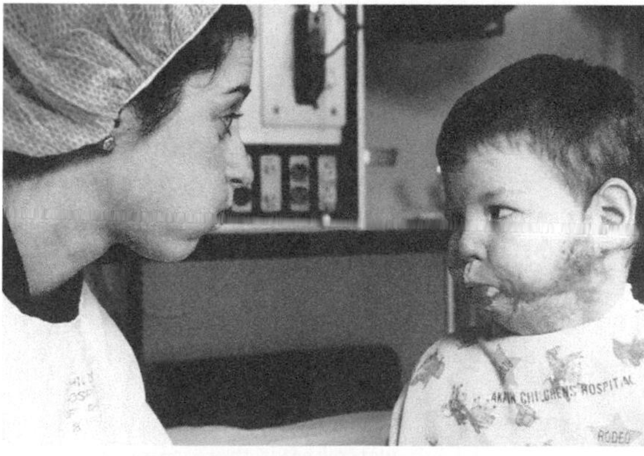

FIG. 23.25 Daily physical therapy to prevent contracture deformity is continued at home or in an outpatient setting. Note how nurse encourages child to imitate her facial action. (Courtesy CR Boeckman Regional Burn Center, Akron, Ohio.)

Because these custom-made garments are often worn for months, revision may be required as the child grows. It is much easier to prevent scarring and contracture of the burn than to resolve an existing problem. Splints and appliances may also be necessary until burn maturation occurs (Fig. 23.24). Part of outpatient and home care often includes the continuation of regular physical therapy (Fig. 23.25).

Scar tissue has certain significant properties, particularly for growing children. Intense itching occurs in healing burn wounds and scar tissue until the scar is no longer active. Itching is usually treated with

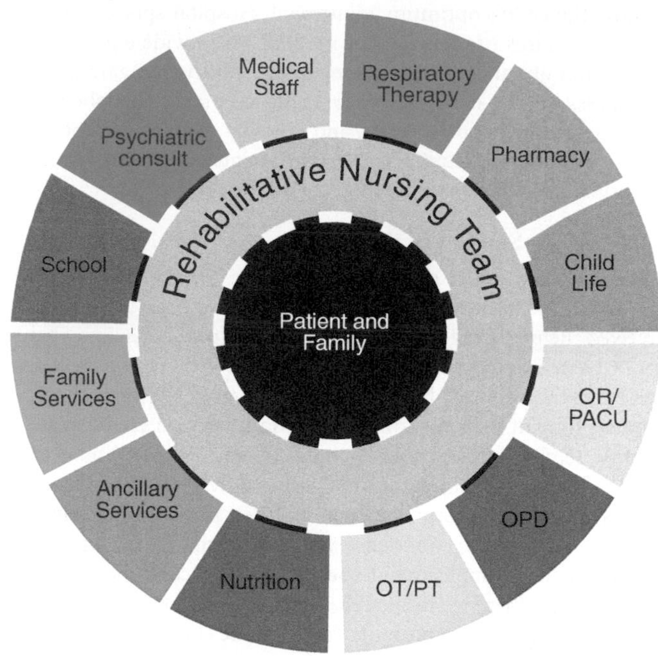

FIG. 23.26 Multidisciplinary approach to rehabilitation of pediatric burn patient.

hydroxyzine (Atarax) or diphenhydramine and frequent applications of a moisturizer, such as Eucerin, cocoa butter, Vasoline Intensive Care, or Nivea. Massage therapy during the application of moisturizers is also beneficial to stretch scar tissue and help prevent contracture. Scar tissue has no sweat glands, and children with extensive scarring may experience difficulty during hot weather. Alert caregivers to this possibility and make sure they are prepared to institute alternate methods of cooling when necessary.

Scar tissue does not grow and expand like normal tissue, which may create difficulties, especially in functional areas such as the hands and over joints. Additional surgery is sometimes required to allow independent functioning in daily activities, to improve cosmetic appearance, or to restore anatomic integrity. Reconstructive surgery employs various techniques, including local or distant flaps, full- or partial-thickness grafts, tissue expanders, or pedicle flaps.

The nursing activities in the rehabilitative phase of treatment focus on the child's and family's adaptation to the burn injury and their ability to reintegrate into the community. The multidisciplinary team approach remains the model for support of the child and family (Fig. 23.26).

The psychologic pain and impact of severe burn injury are as intense as the physical trauma. The impact of severe burns taxes the capabilities at all ages. Very young children, who suffer acutely from separation anxiety, and adolescents, who are developing an identity, are probably the most affected psychologically. Toddlers cannot understand why the parents they love and who have protected them can leave them in such a frightening and unfamiliar place. Adolescents, in the process of achieving independence from the family, find themselves in a dependent role with a damaged body. Being different from others at a time when conformity with peers is so important is difficult to accept.

Anticipation of the return to school can be overwhelming and frightening. It is essential that health care professionals recognize the importance of preparing teachers and classmates for the child's return. Provide teachers with information to assist the child and family and to promote the child's optimum adjustment. Hospital-sponsored school reentry programs use a variety of methods to provide education and information about the implications of the injury, the garments and appliances, and the need for support and acceptance. Telephone calls, videotapes, information packets, and visits by members of the health care team offer opportunities to help with reintegration into the school environment—a focal point of the child's life.

Psychosocial Support of the Child

Children should begin early to do as much for themselves as possible and to be active participants in their care. Loss of control and perceived helplessness may result in acting-out behaviors. Nurses should be sensitive to these feelings and allow the child the opportunity for choices and decision making as the condition allows. At the same time, it is important to set boundaries and establish a daily schedule to provide a sense of predictability, security, and control. During illness, children regress to a previous developmental level that allows them to deal with stress. As children begin to participate in their care, they gain in confidence and self-esteem. Fears and anxieties diminish with accomplishment and self-confidence. If the child demonstrates nonadherence in the rehabilitative phase, initiate a behavior modification program to promote or reward the child's accomplishment in care.

Select and encourage activities on the basis of each child's developmental level and interest. Quiet activities such as reading, coloring, and games are always appropriate. Critically ill children enjoy tapes and stories, even though they may not be able to actively participate in play. Television is a satisfactory diversion but should not replace contact with others. Play that encourages the expression of anger, frustration, and guilt is especially therapeutic. Medical play is a valuable tool to teach children what to expect and their role in the treatment process. School-age children benefit by continuing study activities as they are able.

Children need to feel that they look nice. The burns, dressings, and medical equipment do little to foster a positive self-image. Small things, such as careful hair combing, a bright ribbon or pajamas, a pretty blanket, or colorful stickers will help them feel better about themselves and feel worthwhile to others.

Children need to know that their injury and the treatments are not punishment for real or imagined transgressions and that the nurse understands their fear, anger, and discomfort. They also need body contact. This is often difficult to arrange for the child with massive burns; stroking areas of unburned skin is comforting. Even older children enjoy sitting on the nurse's, parent's, or caregiver's lap and being cuddled and hugged. This can be a reward or a comfort in times of stress, but most of all it is a natural part of childhood.

Psychosocial Support of the Family

There is a growing recognition that trauma affects not only the victim but also those closest to the child. Severe trauma challenges the belief that the world is safe and predictable. Parents, caregivers, and other family members are concerned about the child's survival, recovery, and future potential. Recognizing and respecting each family's strengths, differences, and methods of coping allow the nurse to respond to their unique needs by implementing a family-centered approach to care. It is the family, particularly the parents or caregiver, who are the most significant persons in the child's life.

As in any emergency situation, all attention is focused on the child, and the parents or caregiver feel powerless and ineffectual. Most parents or caregivers feel overwhelming guilt, whether or not the guilt is justified. They feel responsible for the injury. These feelings may have a negative effect on the child's rehabilitation. For example, parents or caregivers may indulge the child and allow poor behavior that affects physical and emotional recovery.

Nurses have the opportunity to assist parents or caregivers in coping with the stresses of the child's illness and with their own feelings of guilt and helplessness. The parents or caregiver need to be informed of the child's progress and assisted in coping with their feelings while providing support to their child. The nurse can help them understand that it is not selfish to look after themselves and their own needs to better meet the needs of their child. Definitive professional help may be needed for parents or caregivers whose response to the injury is severe or whose response to stress is manifested in destructive behavior.

The parents or caregivers are members of the interprofessional burn team and participate in the development of the care plan. It is important to address their input to consider all aspects of the physical, emotional, social, and cultural factors affecting the child and family and to establish a realistic home therapy program. The family's willingness to assume responsibility for care and their ability to implement the therapeutic regimen are assessed. Explore home, school, and other environmental factors with the family, as well as financial concerns and available community resources. The nurse can then develop a specific care plan, with an anticipated follow-up program.

Caring for the Caregiver

Burn care is a complex and demanding specialty. Nurses who choose this field reap many rewards and endure many stresses. Ongoing support from peers, the multidisciplinary team, and nursing management is important to assist burn nurses in caring for themselves so they can continue to render high-quality care to their patients.

Prevention of Burn Injury

Burn prevention is the responsibility of all members of the community. Nurses have an obligation to participate in educational efforts directed at parents, caregivers, children, and others regarding the prevention of burn injuries and fire-related deaths. The best cure is prevention.

Infants and toddlers are most commonly injured by hot liquids in the kitchen and bathroom. These injuries often occur as a result of inadequate supervision of this curious and energetic age-group. Target prevention efforts at parents and other caregivers; education includes the importance of adequate supervision and the establishment of safe play areas in the home. Hot liquids should be kept out of reach; tablecloths and dangling appliance cords are often pulled by toddlers, spilling hot grease and liquids on them. Electrical cords and outlets represent a potential risk to small children, who may chew on accessible cords and insert objects into outlets.

Since 1974 the Consumer Product Safety Commission has recommended a reduction of hot water heater thermostats to a maximum of 49°C (120°F). This recommendation has been supported by utility companies, burn treatment centers, medical personnel, and others interested in public safety. Established plumbing standards for newly constructed homes and residential units require antiscald technology and a maximum water heater temperature of 120°F. However, many hot water heaters remain set at levels well above the safe level. Small children are especially at risk for scald injuries from hot tap water because of their decreased reaction time and agility, their curiosity, and the thermal sensitivity of their skin (Fig. 23.27). Educate caregivers about never leaving a child in a bath without adult supervision. Caregivers should also test the water before placing a child in the tub or shower.

Microwave ovens, although perceived by many as safer than conventional ovens and stoves, heat foods and liquids to high temperatures that can result in burns from spills, splashes, and the release of steam (Box 23.13). Young children operating the microwave or getting food out of them account for a majority of these injuries.

As children mature, risk-taking behaviors increase. Matches and lighters are dangerous in the hands of the young. Between 2007 and 2011, an estimated 7100 home structural fires occurred per year and 43% occurred as a result of children under the age of 6 years playing with fire (National Fire Protection Association, 2014). Adults must remember to keep potentially hazardous items out of the reach of children; a lighter, like a match, is a tool for adult use. Children with conduct disorders, such as attention-deficit/hyperactivity disorder, are at a greater risk of fire interest and fire-setting activities. Counseling or intervention programs aimed to prevent fire-setting activity can deter this type of behavior. Education related to fire safety and survival should begin with the very young. They can practice "stop, drop, and roll" to extinguish a fire and the fire escape route, including a safe meeting place away from the home in case of fire. Materials such as coloring books are available from many fire departments and burn foundations. Community burn prevention programs also provide opportunities to educate children and parents about fire, burn hazards, and prevention behaviors.

Community activities are helpful in the effort to support burn survivors and prevent burns. The Aluminum Cans for Burned Children is an exemplary effort based in the Paul and Carol David Foundation Burn Institute, Akron, Ohio. Activities funded by Aluminum Cans for Burned Children include the Burn Survivors Support Group, Burn Camp, and meetings of Juvenile Firestoppers (for children with fire-setting behavior). Adult weekend retreats and school and family education sessions are a part of this program. Burn center staff and fire department staff present the programs. Additional information on burn care and prevention can be obtained from the American Burn Association.*

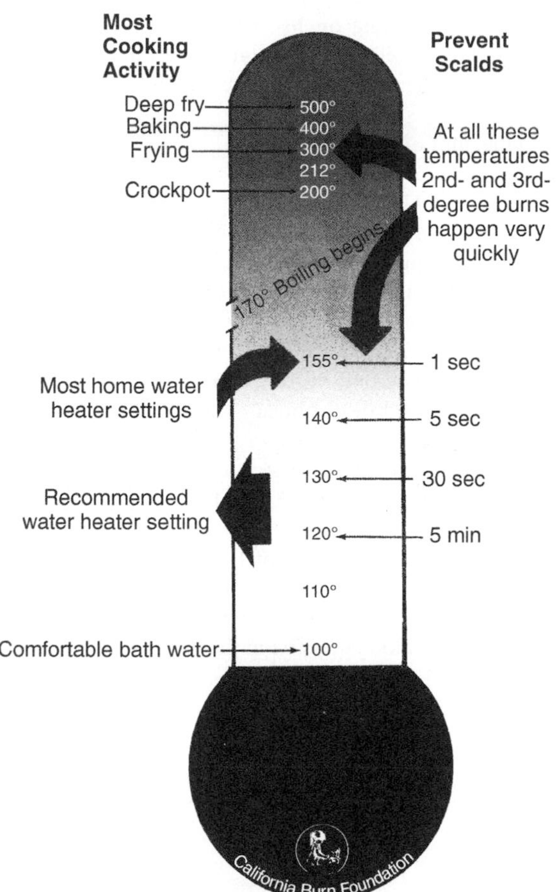

FIG. 23.27 Temperatures associated with common burn injuries in the home. All temperatures given in Fahrenheit. Note: Most authorities recommend that water heaters be kept at 120°F (49°C). (Courtesy California Burn Foundation, Canoga Park, California.)

BOX 23.13 Microwave Safety

- Do not let small children operate the microwave.
- Place microwave ovens at a safe height (but higher than children's faces) and within easy reach to avoid spills.
- Never leave a young child alone while food is heating in the microwave.
- For food heated in containers, puncture plastic wrap, use vented lids, or wait 1 minute before removing a sealed covering; then lift the covering from the corner farthest away from face or arm.
- Never heat baby formula or milk in a plastic bottle liner because it may burst.
- Before adding a cold liquid to a liquid that has been heated in the microwave, insert a spoon to prevent bubbling over of the hot liquid.
- Stir food well or let it stand for 1 minute before tasting it so the heat can distribute evenly.

FUTURE RESEARCH NEEDS

Many advances in burn prevention have reduced the occurrence of burn injury. Early excision and grafting of the burn wound, with control of infection, have improved survival rates for burn injury. Research in 2014 included areas in epidemiology, burn resuscitation, infection, critical care, nutrition and metabolism, pain management, rehabilitation, psychology, reconstruction, prevention, and fire fighter safety. A few examples of progress in research and the pediatric population resulted. It was found in the pediatric population that changes in fat metabolism, elevated fasting glucose, and possible insulin resistance continue for months after the injury. Risk factors include age, percentage of burn injury, and total body fat. In regard to increased body fat, it was found that this factor has a significant impact on a child's recovery from severe burn injury. Compared with nonobese pediatric burn patients, obese pediatric burn patients with comparable burn sizes suffered more pulmonary infections, required longer mechanical ventilation, and sustained a lengthier ICU admission (Sen, Palmieri, & Greenhalgh, 2015). Areas for future research include multidisciplinary and holistic care needed to improve not only the physical recovery, but also the psychologic recovery to treat this type of challenging trauma. Evidence for improvement of burn nursing care is best organized with research findings (Carrougher, 1998). Evidence-based practice integrates the nurse's clinical expertise with the best methods. It helps structure how to make accurate and timely decisions for care of the patient.

*625 North Michigan Ave., Suite 2550, Chicago, IL 60611; 312-642-9260; fax: 312-642-9130; email: info@ameriburn.org; http://www.ameriburn.org.

NCLEX REVIEW QUESTIONS

1. The most common type of dehydration in children occurs when electrolyte and water deficits are present in approximately balanced proportions. This is called ____________ dehydration.
   A. Hypotonic
   B. Hypertonic
   C. Isotonic
   D. Hyponatremic
2. The greatest threat to life as a result of dehydration in children is:
   A. Oliguria
   B. Shock
   C. Arrhythmia
   D. Hypotension
3. A 3-year-old boy is seen in the clinic at 8:30 pm with a history of vomiting for 2 days and poor oral intake; he has voided once since the previous day. Examination reveals a lethargic child sitting on the mother's lap. He has a capillary refill of 4 seconds, apical heart rate of 128, respiratory rate of 32, and poor skin turgor. Stated body weight is 25 kg. Based on this information, the nurse anticipates performing which of the following?
   A. Demonstrating to the mother how to give 5 to 10 ml of Pedialyte by mouth every 5 to 10 minutes
   B. Administering an intravenous fluid bolus of 450 ml of 5% dextrose in water over 60 minutes
   C. Administering an intravenous fluid bolus of 500 ml of 0.9% normal saline over 20 minutes
   D. Administering an intravenous fluid bolus of 1000 ml of 5% dextrose and 0.45% normal saline over 30 minutes
4. A 4-day-old infant is seen in the emergency department for a possible seizure earlier in the day. The infant was being breastfed but without much success, so an aunt gave him a bottle of water. The infant continued to cry, and the mother was too exhausted to breastfeed, so another bottle of water was given while someone went to the store to purchase infant formula. The pregnancy, delivery, and postpartum history reveal no particular problems for this term infant that might contribute to seizures. The physical examination is unremarkable, with the exception of hypertonic reflexes. The infant is awake, alert, and sucking on his fists. Diagnostic studies are obtained, including an electrocardiogram. The nurse anticipates which of the following as the possible explanation for the infant's condition?
   A. Serum potassium of 3.9 mEq
   B. Serum glucose of 69 mg
   C. Serum sodium of 118 mEq
   D. Arterial pH of 7.34
5. A burn injury involving the epidermis and varying degrees of the dermal layer that is painful, moist, red, and blistered describes which of the following?
   A. Superficial or first-degree burn
   B. Partial-thickness or second-degree burn
   C. Full-thickness or third-degree burn
   D. Fourth-degree burn
6. A 10-year-old child suffered extensive second- and third-degree burns in an apartment fire. His weight is 75 lb (34 kg). Fluid replacement therapy will optimally:
   A. Result in an hourly urine output of 1 ml/kg
   B. Result in an hourly urine output of 20 ml/kg
   C. Result in an hourly urine output of 30 ml/kg
   D. Maintain a systolic blood pressure in the 95th percentile for the child's weight

Correct Answers

1. C; 2. B; 3. C; 4. C; 5. B; 6. C

REFERENCES

American Burn Association (ABA). (2016). *Advanced burn life support provider manual 2016 update*. Chicago: ABA.

Boehne, M., Sasse, M., Karch, A., et al. (2017). Systemic inflammatory response syndrome after pediatric congenital hearth surgery: In cadence risk factors, and clinical outcome. *Journal of Cardiac Surgery, 32*, 116–125.

Byard, R. W., & Zuccollo, J. M. (2010). Forensic issues in cases of water birth fatalities. *The American Journal of Forensic Medicine and Pathology, 31*(3), 258–260.

Carrougher, G. (1998). *Burn care and therapy*. St. Louis, MO: Mosby.

Carson, R. A., Mudd, S. S., & Madati, J. (2016). Clinical practice guideline for the treatment of pediatric acute gastroenteritis in the outpatient setting. *Journal of Pediatric Health Care: Official Publication of National Association of Pediatric Nurse Associates & Practitioners, 30*(6), 610–616.

Carson, R. A., Mudd, S. S., & Madati, J. (2017). Clinical practice guideline for the treatment of pediatric acute gastroenteritis in the outpatient setting. *Journal of Emergency Nursing*, http://www.jenonline.org.

Carter, B., & Fedorowicz, Z. (2012). Antiemetic treatment for acute gastroenteritis in children: An updated Cochrane systematic review with meta-analysis and mixed treatment comparison in a Bayesian framework. *BMJ Open, 2*(4), e000622.

Center for Disease Control (CDC). (2016). *Ten leading causes of death by age groups highlighting unintentional injury deaths, United States-2014*, Atlanta, GA. Retrieved from https://www.cdc.gov/injury/wisqars/leadingcauses.html.

Colon, N. C., Schlegel, C., & Chung, D. H. (2012). Surgical management of complications of burn injury. In D. N. Herndon (Ed.), *Total burn care*. Philadelphia: Saunders.

de Caen, A. R., Berg, M. D., Chameides, L., et al. (2015). Pediatric advanced life support: 2015 American Heart Association guidelines for cardiopulmonary resuscitation and emergency cardiovascular care. *Circulation, 132*(Suppl. 2), S526–S542.

Dellinger, R. P., Levy, M. M., Rhodes, A., et al. (2012). Surviving sepsis campaign: International guidelines for management of severe sepsis and septic shock. *Critical Care Medicine, 41*(2), 58–637, 2013.

Demling, R. H. (2005). The role of anabolic hormones for wound healing in catabolic states. *Journal of Burns and Wounds, 4*, e2.

Emond, S. (2009). Dehydration in infants and young children. *Annals of Emergency Medicine, 53*(3), 395–397.

Fidkowski, C., & Fuzaylov, G. (2012). Anesthesia for pediatric burn patients. In B. J. Phillips (Ed.), *Pediatric burns*. Amherst, MA: Cambria.

Flynn, C. A., D'Amico, F., & Smith, G. (1998). Should we patch corneal abrasions? A meta-analysis. *The Journal of Family Practice, 47*(4), 246–270.

Frazier, S. B. N., Sepanski, R., Mangum, C., et al. (2015). Association of systemic inflammatory response syndrome with clinical outcomes of pediatric patients with pneumonia. *Southern Medical Journal, 108*(11), 665–669.

Freedman, S. B., Vandermeer, B., Milne, A., et al. (2015). Diagnosing clinically significant dehydration in children with acute gastroenteritis using noninvasive methods: A meta-analysis. *Journal of Pediatrics, 166*(4), 908–916.

Friedman, J. N., Beck, C. E., DeGroot, J., et al. (2015). Comparison of isotonic and hypotonic intravenous maintenance fluids: A randomized clinical trial. *JAMA Pediatr*, *169*(5), 445–451.

Gaensbauer, J. T., & Todd, J. K. (2016). Toxic shock syndrome. In R. M. Kliegman, B. F. Stanton, J. W. St. Geme, et al. (Eds.), *Nelson textbook of pediatrics* (20th ed.). Philadelphia: Saunders.

Gauglitz, G. G., Finnerty, C. C., Herndon, D. N., et al. (2012). Modulation of the hypermetabolic response after burn. In D. N. Herndon (Ed.), *Total burn care*. Philadelphia: Saunders.

Greenbaum, L. A. (2015). Electrolyte and acid-base disorders. In R. M. Kliegman, B. F. Stanton, J. W. St. Geme, et al. (Eds.), *Nelson textbook of pediatrics* (20th ed.). Philadelphia: Saunders.

Hartford, C. E. (2012). Care of outpatient burns. In D. N. Herndon (Ed.), *Total burn care*. Philadelphia: Saunders.

Hendrickson, M. A., Zaremba, J., Wey, A. R., et al. (2017). The use of a triage-based protocol for oral rehydration in a pediatric emergency department. *Pediatric Emergency Care*, pec-online.com.

Hoxha, T. F., Azemi, M., Avdiu, M., et al. (2014). The usefulness of clinical and laboratory parameters for predicting severity of dehydration in children with acute gastroenteritis. *Medicinski Arhiv*, *68*(5), 304–307.

Huether, S. E. (2014). The cellular environment: Fluids and electrolytes, acids and bases. In K. L. McCance, S. E. Huether, V. L. Brashers, et al. (Eds.), *Pathophysiology: The biologic basis for disease in adults and children* (7th ed.). St. Louis: Mosby.

Jeffs, D., Dorman, D., Brown, S., et al. (2014). Effect of virtual reality on adolescent pain during burn wound care. *Journal of Burn Care and Research*, *35*(5), 395–408.

Jeschke, M. G. (2016). Postburn hypermetabolism: Past, present, and future. *Journal of Burn Care and Research*, *37*(2), 86–96.

Kagan, R. J., Peck, M. D., Ahrenholz, D. H., et al. (2013). Surgical management of the burn wound and use of skin substitute: An expert panel white paper. *Journal of Burn Care and Research*, *34*(2), e60–e79. doi:10.1097/BCR.0b013e31827039a6.

Kleinman, R. E., & Greer, F. R. (2014). *Pediatric nutrition* (7th ed.). Elk Grove Village, IL: American Academy of Pediatrics.

Lee, J. O., Norbury, W. B., & Herndon, D. N. (2012). Special considerations of age: The pediatric burned patient. In D. N. Herndon (Ed.), *Total burn care*. Philadelphia: Saunders.

Manz, F. (2007). Hydration in children. *Journal of the American College of Nutrition*, *26*(Suppl. 5), S562–S569.

Martin, G. S. (2012). Sepsis, severe sepsis and septic shock: Changes in incidence, pathogens and outcomes. *Expert Review of Anti-infective Therapy*, *10*(6), 701–706.

Meyer, W. J., Wiechman, S., Woodson, L., et al. (2012). Management of pain and other discomforts in burned patients. In D. N. Herndon (Ed.), *Total burn care*. Philadelphia: Saunders.

National Fire Protection Association (NFPA). (2014). *Playing with fire*. Retrieved from http://www.nfpa.org/news-and-research/fire-statistics-and-reports/fire-statistics/fire-causes/arson-and-juvenile-firesetting/children-playing-with-fire.pdf.

Nielson, C. B., Duethman, N. C., Howard, J. M., et al. (2017). Burns: Pathophysiology of systemic complications and current management. *Journal of Burn Care and Research*, *38*(1), e469–e481. doi:10.1097/BCR.0000000000000355.

Nordlund, M. J., Pham, T. N., & Gibran, N. S. (2014). Micronutrients after burn injury: A review. *Journal of Burn Care and Research*, *35*(2), 121–133.

Perkin, R. M., de Caen, A. R., Berg, M. D., et al. (2013). Shock, cardiac arrest, and resuscitation. In M. F. Hazinski (Ed.), *Nursing care of the critically ill child*. St. Louis, MO: Elsevier Mosby.

Pastar, I., Stojadinovic, O., Yin, N. C., et al. (2014). Epithelialization in wound healing: A comprehensive review. *Advances in Wound Care*, *3*(7), 445–464.

Pruitt, B. A., Wolf, S. E., & Mason, A. D. (2012). Epidemiological, demographic, and outcome characteristics of burn injury. In D. N. Herndon (Ed.), *Total burn care*. Philadelphia: Saunders.

Rae, L., Fidler, P., & Gibran, N. (2016). The physiologic basis of burn shock and need for aggressive fluid resuscitation. *Critical Care Clinics*, *32*(4), 491–505.

Rowan, M. P., Cancio, L. C., Elster, E. A., et al. (2015). Burn wound healing and treatment: Review and advancements. *Critical Care*, *19*, 243.

Safe Kids Worldwide (SKW). (2015). *Burn and scalds safety*. Washington, DC. Retrieved from http://www.safekids.org/fact-sheet/burns-and-fire-safety-fact-sheet-2015-pdf.

Saffle, J. R., Graves, C., & Cochran, A. (2012). Nutritional support of the burned patient. In D. N. Herndon (Ed.), *Total burn care*. Philadelphia: Saunders.

Sampson, H. A., Wang, J., & Sicherer, S. H. (2016). Anaphylaxis. In R. M. Kliegman, B. F. Stanton, J. W. St. Geme, et al. (Eds.), *Nelson textbook of pediatrics* (20th ed.). Philadelphia: Saunders.

Sen, S., Palmieri, T., & Greenhalgh, D. (2015). Review of burn research for year 2014. *Journal of Burn Care and Research*, *36*(6), 587–594.

Singleton, A., Preston, R. J., & Cochran, A. (2015). Sedation and analgesia for critically ill pediatric burn patients: The current state of practice. *Journal of Burn Care and Research*, *36*(3), 440–445.

Smith, M. L. (2000). Pediatric burns: Management of thermal, electrical, and chemical burns and burn-like dermatologic conditions. *Pediatric Annals*, *29*(6), 367–378.

Strang, S. G., Van Lieshout, E. M. M., Breederveld, R. S., et al. (2014). A systematic review on intra-abdominal pressure in severely burned patients. *Burns: Journal of the International Society for Burn Injuries*, *40*, 9–16.

Tran, S., & Chin, A. C. (2014). Burn sepsis in children. *Clinical Pediatric Emergency Medicine*, *15*(2), 149–157.

Whitney, R. E., Santucci, K., Hsiao, A., et al. (2016). Cost effectiveness of point-of-care testing for dehydration in the pediatric ED. *The American Journal of Emergency Medicine*, *34*, 1573–1575.

Wibbenmeyer, L., Liao, J., Heard, J., et al. (2014). Factors related to child maltreatment in children presenting with burn injuries. *Journal of Burn Care and Research*, *35*(5), 374–381.

Woodson, L. C., Talon, M., Traber, D. L., et al. (2012). Diagnosis and treatment of inhalation injury. In D. N. Herndon (Ed.), *Total burn care*. Philadelphia: Saunders.

Vloemans, A. F., Hermans, M. H., van der Wal, M. B., et al. (2014). Optimal treatment of partial thickness burns in children: A systematic review. *Burns: Journal of the International Society for Burn Injuries*, *40*, 177–190.

Vyles, D., Sinha, M., Rosenberg, D. I., et al. (2014). Predictors of serious bacterial infections in pediatric burn patients with fever. *Journal of Burn Care and Research*, *35*(4), 291–295.

Wang, J., Xu, E., & Xiao, Y. (2014). Isotonic versus hypotonic maintenance IV fluids in hospitalized children: A meta-analysis. *Pediatrics*, *133*(1), 105–113.

24

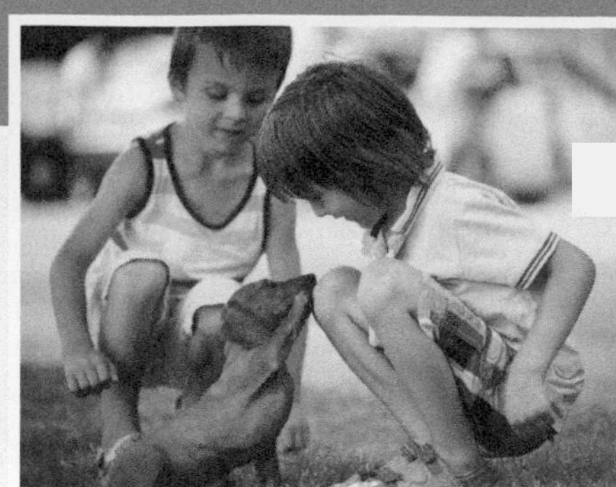

The Child With Renal Dysfunction

Patricia A. Ring and Cynthia J. Camille

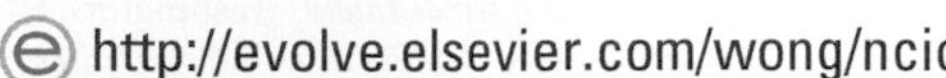

CONCEPTS

- Infection
- Acid-Base Balance
- Fluid Regulation

RENAL STRUCTURE AND FUNCTION

The kidney's primary responsibility is to maintain the composition and volume of the body fluids in equilibrium. To maintain this constant internal environment, the kidney must respond appropriately to alterations in the internal environment caused by variations in dietary intake and extrarenal losses of water and solutes. This is accomplished by the formation of urine (the product of glomerular filtration), tubular reabsorption, and tubular secretion. **Reabsorption** is the transport of a substance from the tubular lumen to the blood in surrounding vessels. **Secretion** is transport in the opposite direction (i.e., from the blood to the lumen). These processes are either active or passive. **Excretion** is the elimination of a substance from the body, in this case urine.

A secondary function of the kidney is the production of certain humoral substances. One such substance is an enzyme, erythropoietin-stimulating factor (or erythrogenin), which acts on a plasma globulin to form erythropoietin, which in turn stimulates erythropoiesis in the bone marrow. Its production increases in the presence of hypoxia and androgens. Few red blood cells form in the absence of erythropoietin, which accounts somewhat for the anemia associated with advanced kidney disease. The kidney also secretes another enzyme, renin, in response to reduced blood volume, decreased blood pressure, or increased secretion of catecholamines. Renin stimulates the production of the angiotensins, which produce arteriolar constriction and an elevation in blood pressure and stimulate the production of aldosterone by the adrenal cortex.

RENAL PHYSIOLOGY

The structural and functional unit of the kidney is the **nephron**, which contains a complex system of tubules, arterioles, venules, and capillaries (Fig. 24.1, *A*). The nephron consists of the Bowman capsule, which encloses a tuft of capillaries and is joined successively to the proximal convoluted tubule, the loop of Henle, the distal convoluted tubule, and the straight or collecting duct (Fig. 24.1, *B*). Collecting tubules join larger ducts, and all the larger collecting ducts of one renal pyramid join to form a single duct that opens into a minor calyx. A number of calyces empty into one of several major calyces that converge into the renal pelvis. The renal pelvis narrows after it leaves the kidney and forms what then becomes a ureter, through which urine drains into the urinary bladder.

The blood supply to the kidneys constitutes approximately one fifth of the total cardiac output; therefore profuse bleeding can accompany renal trauma. Because interstitial tissue is sparse, individual nephrons with their blood vessel component are closely packed together. A sizable afferent arteriole, which separates into capillary loops that constitute the glomerular tuft, supplies each nephron. Blood leaves by a smaller efferent arteriole. From there the efferent arterioles branch into a peritubular capillary network and hairpin loops called the vasa recta, which parallel the loops of Henle and collecting ducts. The total surface area of the renal capillaries is approximately equal to the total surface area of the tubules.

The Bowman capsule is composed of two cellular layers that separate the blood from the glomerular filtrate: the capillary endothelium and a layer of tubular epithelial lining cells. Situated between these layers is the basal lamina, or basement membrane. This glomerular membrane is permeable because the capillary endothelium is fenestrated with pores, or fenestrae. Also, the outer surface of the glomerular epithelium consists of fingerlike projections (pseudopodia, or podocytes) that cover the entire surface to form slits called slit pores. The basement membrane has no visible openings but behaves as though it contains pores or channels. Consequently, the glomerular filtrate (which has essentially the same composition as plasma except for the large protein molecules and cellular elements) passes through these three layers at a rapid rate. The structure of these layers becomes altered in kidney disease.

Glomerular Filtration

Filtration through the glomerular capillaries is governed by the same mechanism as filtration across other capillaries in the body (i.e., the size of the capillary bed, the permeability of the capillaries, and the hydrostatic and osmotic pressure gradients across the capillaries). The filtration capacity of the glomerulus is the product of permeability of the glomerular capillaries and three pressure forces: glomerular hydrostatic pressure, colloidal osmotic (oncotic) pressure (COP), and intracapsular pressure.

PATHOPHYSIOLOGY REVIEW

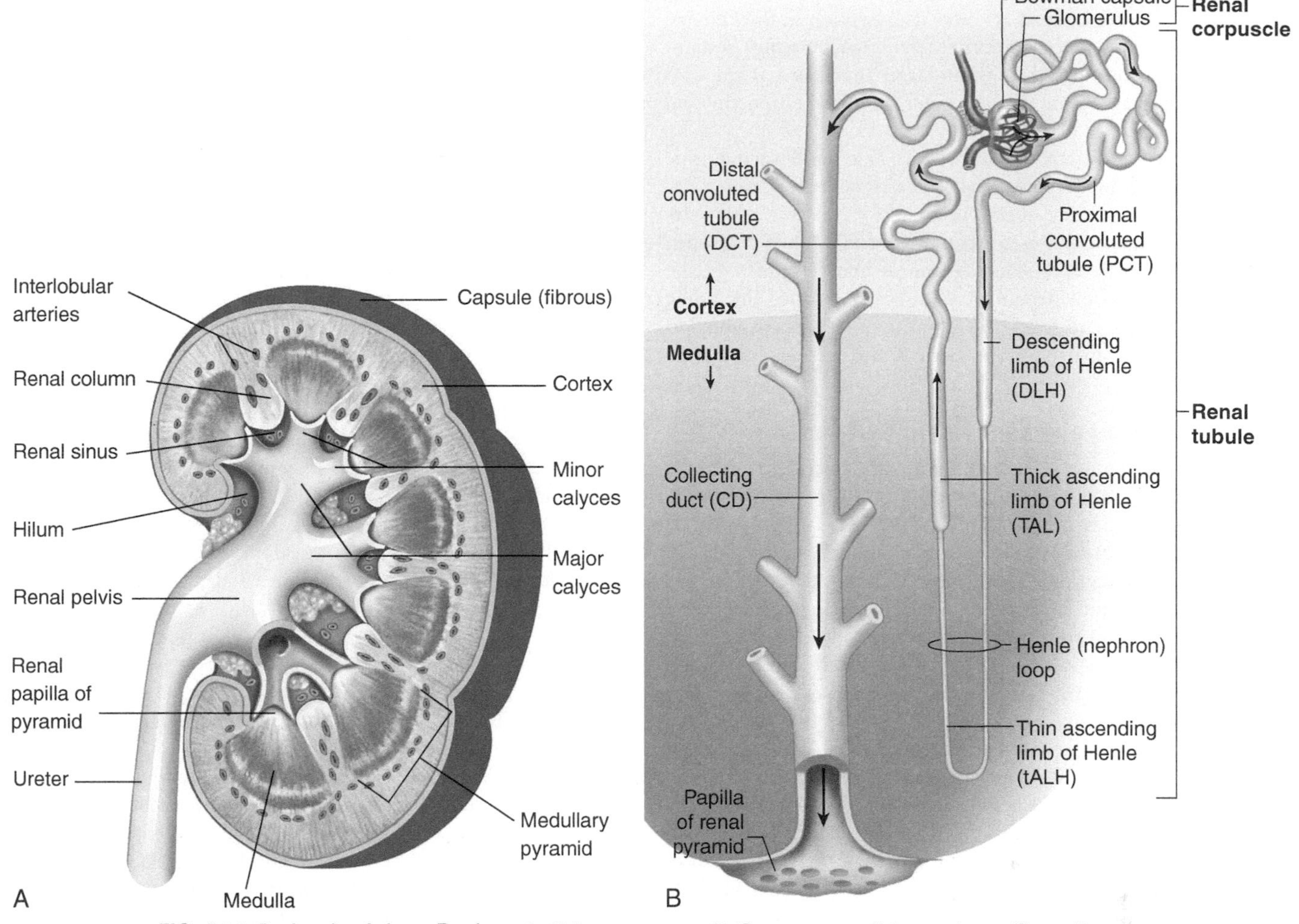

FIG. 24.1 Pathophysiology Review. A, Kidney structure. **B,** Components of the nephron. (From Patton, K. T., & Thibodeau, G. A. [2010]. *Anatomy and physiology* [7th ed.]. St. Louis, MO: Mosby.)

Blood enters the nephron at a substantial pressure. This hydrostatic pressure forces plasma fluid and solutes through the capillary membrane and into the unit's collecting apparatus. As this filtrate travels through the renal tubules, water and solutes are selectively reabsorbed back into the vascular compartment. That which is not reabsorbed is excreted as urine. Filtration takes place as long as hydrostatic pressure within the glomerular capillaries exceeds the opposing COP of the plasma proteins. If the pressure becomes equal through decreased hydrostatic pressure or decreased COP, no further filtration takes place. In a state of dehydration, more water is reabsorbed; when water intake is increased, more is excreted as urine. In conditions that produce osmotic diuresis (i.e., when large solutes, such as glucose, are filtered through the capillaries in such excessive amounts that they cannot be reabsorbed), the osmotic attraction of the solute causes less water to be reabsorbed, resulting in water being excreted in the urine with the solute.

Tubular Function

The function of the renal tubules is to modify the glomerular filtrate. Tubular cells may add more of a substance to the filtrate (tubular secretion), remove some or all of a substance from the filtrate (tubular reabsorption), or both. The reabsorption is selective and discriminating for substances essential to body processes and equilibrium, whereas nonessential substances are eliminated as waste. The substances are secreted or reabsorbed in the tubules by osmosis, passive movement down a chemical or electric gradient, or are actively transported against these gradients. These processes operate throughout the length of the tubules, but there are variations in the types, amounts, and mechanisms by which substances are secreted or reabsorbed in the different tubular segments. The cellular characteristics of each segment are largely responsible for these variations (see Fig. 24.1).

Active transport mechanisms move vital substances both inward and outward from the tubular filtrate. For example, the proximal tubule reabsorbs essential substances such as glucose, amino acids, and sodium ions and returns them directly to the blood. Active transport mechanisms here, as elsewhere, have a limited capacity, or threshold, for moving the solute. When the maximum of the transport mechanism is reached, no more substance is reabsorbed, and the remainder is excreted in the urine. For example, when blood glucose concentrations exceed their transport capacity, the surplus remains in the filtrate to be excreted in the urine (glycosuria). When two substances share a common transport mechanism, the first substance may be blocked by the addition of a second substance (selective inhibition). The effect of many therapeutic agents (e.g., diuretics) depends on this process.

Electrolytes are moved by both active transport and diffusion; the transport of certain electrolytes, particularly sodium, has important effects on other substances. For example, sodium is actively transported from all parts of the nephron. The movement of sodium ions produces both an electric and an osmotic gradient, which causes chloride ions and water to diffuse from the tubules in an effort to establish equilibrium. This is the obligatory water reabsorption in the kidneys. There is a limit to the concentration gradient against which sodium can be transported out; therefore when larger than normal amounts of sodium ions remain in the tubules, water is obliged to remain with the sodium.

Under normal conditions the kidneys are able to adjust the urine and solute excretion in response to the requirements for body water and electrolyte balance. They are able to excrete or conserve both water and most electrolytes in addition to excreting the end products of protein metabolism, principally urea. The volume of urine excreted by the kidneys in a given period depends on the water balance (including intravascular filtration pressure), the quantity of solutes presented to the kidneys, and the capacity of the kidneys to dilute or concentrate the filtrate.

Renal Development and Function in Early Infancy

Development of the kidney begins within the first weeks of embryonic life but is not completed until about the end of the first year after birth. The nephrons increase in number and reach their full complement by 34 to 46 weeks of gestation. However, at this point they are immature and less efficient than at later ages. Many of the tubular sections are not fully formed, and the glomeruli enlarge considerably after birth.

Glomerular filtration and absorption are relatively low in the infant and do not reach adult values until between 1 and 2 years of age. Consequently, the newborn is unable to dispose of excess water and solutes rapidly or efficiently.

The tubular length of nephrons is highly variable. Glomerular size is less variable. The juxtaglomerular nephrons show more advanced development than the cortical nephrons. The loop of Henle (the site of the urine-concentrating mechanism) is short in the newborn, which reduces the ability to reabsorb sodium and water and therefore produces very dilute urine; however, the newborn pituitary gland secretes adequate amounts of antidiuretic hormone. The length of tubules gradually increases until concentrating ability reaches adult levels by approximately the third month of life. Urea synthesis and excretion are slower during this time, and the newborn retains large quantities of nitrogen and essential electrolytes to meet the needs for growth in the first weeks of life. Consequently, the excretory burden is minimized. The lower concentration of urea, the principal end product of nitrogen metabolism, also reduces concentrating capacity because it contributes to the concentration mechanism.

Other characteristics of the newborn's kidneys result in renal function that differs from that of older children and adults. Newborn infants are unable to excrete a water load at rates similar to those of older persons. Hydrogen ion excretion is reduced, acid secretion is lower for the first year of life, and plasma bicarbonate levels are low. Because of these inadequacies of the kidney and because of less efficient blood buffers, the newborn is more liable to develop severe metabolic acidosis. Sodium excretion is reduced in the immediate newborn period, and the kidneys are less able to adapt to sodium deficiencies and excesses. For example, an isotonic saline infusion may produce edema because of impaired ability to eliminate excess sodium. Conversely, inadequate reabsorption of sodium from the tubules may increase sodium losses in disorders such as vomiting or diarrhea. Moreover, infants have a diminished capacity to reabsorb glucose and, during the first few days, to produce ammonium ions.

The kidney functions during fetal life and produces urine that contributes to the amniotic fluid volume. The 24-hour urine volume is low at birth, rapidly increases in the neonatal period, and steadily increases with normal growth. The kidneys continue to grow in size until body growth is complete in adolescence.

RENAL PELVIS AND URETERS: STRUCTURE AND FUNCTION

The renal pelvis is a funnel-shaped structure that originates at the major calyces and terminates in the funnel-shaped ureteropelvic junction. The ureter is a thin mucomuscular tube that extends from the ureteropelvic to the ureterovesical junction in the base of the bladder.

The principal function of the renal pelvis and ureter is the transport of urine from the kidney to the bladder. Urine is moved via a process called **peristalsis**, whereby muscular movements originating in the renal pelvis propel a bolus of urine toward the urinary bladder for storage and eventual evacuation when the child urinates. The renal pelvis stores only a relatively small volume of urine (approximately 15 ml in adults) before a contraction is triggered that pushes the urine toward the bladder. The forward movement of urine from the kidney to the bladder is called **efflux**, whereas abnormal (or backward) urine movement is termed **reflux**. Aside from mechanical stretching, neurogenic and hormonal factors modulate ureteral peristalsis.

The ureterovesical junction joins the ureters and bladder. It is made up of three principal components: the lowest segment of the ureter, the trigone muscle, and the adjacent bladder wall. The ureters allow the passage of urine from the upper urinary tracts while preventing backflow of urine from the bladder to the ureters. During bladder filling, intravesical pressure remains relatively low and the detrusor muscle remains in a relaxed state. A peristaltic contraction of the ureter propels urine into the bladder. During micturition, there is an increase in intravesical pressure as the detrusor muscle contracts; this raises the potential for harmful reflux into the upper urinary tracts. The normal ureterovesical junction has several mechanisms to prevent reflux. The terminal (intravesical) ureteral segment tunnels through the bladder wall at an oblique angle. During bladder contraction, tension in the detrusor muscle squeezes the intravesical ureter closed. The trigone muscle that surrounds the ureteral orifice of the terminal ureter enhances this process. In addition, the longitudinally arranged muscle of the intravesical ureter contracts, providing further resistance to reflux. Anatomic defects of the ureterovesical junction, such as lateral displacement of the ureter or reduced length of the intravesical ureter, predispose the child to primary reflux. Secondary reflux can result from high pressure in the bladder causing failure of the ureteral vesical junction to close during bladder contraction. There is a recognized correlation between lower urinary tract dysfunction and persistent reflux and evidence suggesting that reflux in older children with lower urinary tract dysfunction is secondary rather than primary (Fast, Nees, Van Batavia, et al., 2013).

URETHROVESICAL UNIT: STRUCTURE AND FUNCTION

The urethrovesical unit consists of the bladder, urethra, and pelvic muscles; it is also called the lower urinary tract. The urinary bladder is a muscle-lined sac that stores and empties itself of urine. In the infant the bladder lies entirely in the abdomen. The bladder assumes its place in the true pelvis shortly before puberty. This change in position is due to the maturation of the pelvic bone rather than migration of the bladder and urethra.

The bladder has two inlets (the ureteral orifices) and a single outlet (the urethral orifice). The base of the bladder is a relatively fixed, triangular area consisting of the bladder neck and trigone. In contrast, the body of the bladder is distensible, changing from a tetrahedron (four-sided shape) when relatively empty to a nearly spherical shape as the bladder fills.

One of the four layers of the bladder wall consists of smooth muscle bundles that promote bladder evacuation via micturition. Collectively this muscular tunic is called the **detrusor**. The muscular tunic of the bladder wall also contains **collagen**, a tough, nonelastic substance that maintains the integrity of the bladder wall while also preventing overdistention. Certain pathologic factors, including denervation of the bladder and obstruction of the outlet, may cause an overabundance of collagen in the detrusor muscle. This causes a loss of bladder compliance (distensibility), abnormally high filling pressures, and trabeculation (irregularity) of the bladder wall.

The urethra is a mucomuscular tube that connects the external meatus and the bladder. The male urethra originates at the bladder neck, piercing the prostate and pelvic floor before tunneling through the posterior portion of the penis and terminating at the glans penis. The proximal portion of the urethra comprises the sphincter mechanism, whereas the distal portion serves as a conduit for the passage of urine or semen. The urethral meatus is a vertical slit located at the summit of the glans penis.

The female urethra follows a relatively short, straight course compared with the male. It originates at the bladder base and terminates at an external meatus located immediately superior to the vaginal orifice. The distal two-thirds of the female urethra are fused with the vaginal wall.

The primary responsibilities of the bladder are to store urine manufactured by the kidneys and to evacuate this urine at regular intervals via the process of micturition. During infancy the bladder is expected to empty spontaneously; by the fourth year of life (or earlier) the child is expected to gain control of detrusor and urethral sphincter function. Control of the urethrovesical unit is referred to as **urinary continence**. Continent individuals are expected to hold their urine for at least 2 hours while awake. During sleeping hours they may arise once to urinate, although many children and young adults sleep for 8 hours or more without interruption. Three factors—anatomic integrity of the lower urinary tract, detrusor control, and competence of the urethral sphincter mechanism—must function normally for an individual to achieve and maintain continence.

Detrusor control requires successful integration of neurologic structures in the brain, spinal cord, and peripheral nervous systems. The brain influences bladder function via its inhibitory role on detrusor contractions. The stable detrusor contracts only when its owner gives permission and several areas of the brain work together to control detrusor stability. A pathologic condition of one of these areas may produce detrusor overactivity, or the loss of control over detrusor contractions.

The spinal cord influences lower urinary tract function because it transmits messages between the brain and the target organ. Two areas in the spinal cord are particularly significant. The thoracolumbar cord (spinal levels T10–L2) influences bladder and urethral sphincter function. Sympathetic impulses from the brain travel to the bladder body and smooth muscle of the urethra, causing relaxation of the detrusor muscle and contraction of urethral smooth muscle. This combination of actions promotes bladder filling and storage of urine. The sacral spinal cord (spinal segments S2–S4) influences the bladder muscle, promoting micturition. Parasympathetic impulses travel from these nuclei, causing contraction of the detrusor muscle and indirectly promoting relaxation of smooth muscle in the urethra.

Two peripheral nerve plexuses directly influence control of the detrusor muscle. The pelvic plexus provides parasympathetic innervation to the bladder and urethra, and the inferior hypogastric plexus provides sympathetic innervation (Gray & Moore, 2009).

The final mechanism responsible for the attainment and maintenance of continence is the urethral sphincter mechanism. Traditionally two sphincters are described. The internal sphincter consists of the smooth muscle of the bladder and proximal urethra, and the external sphincter consists of the periurethral striated muscle. However, it is better to describe a single mechanism consisting of elements of compression and elements of tension.

Elements of compression are necessary for the urethra to form a watertight seal between episodes of urination. The softness (collapsibility) of the urethral wall is important for continence, particularly when a catheter alters urethral integrity. The mucus produced by the epithelium further enhances the watertight seal of the urethra. The mucus reduces surface tension, promoting collapse of the walls and sealing the microscopic fissures against urinary leakage.

The vascular cushion also acts as an element of compression (in addition to producing tension), contributing to urethral closure during physical stress. The vascular cushion, or network of the arterioles, venules, and arteriovenous communications in the urethra, promotes urethral compression by transmitting pressure from the muscles surrounding the urethra and those intrinsic to its walls. The vascular cushion contributes to urethral closure pressure because it is filled with an incompressible fluid that has its own intrinsic pressure.

The elements of tension in the urethral sphincter mechanism consist of the vascular cushion, intrinsic smooth and skeletal muscles, and periurethral striated muscle. These muscles are specially innervated to maintain the tension needed for urethral closure between episodes of micturition and to provide an extra measure of urethral tension, which is needed when significant physical exertion stresses sphincter closure. The pelvic muscles receive somatic innervation, which allows voluntary interruption of the urinary stream and provides added protection against precipitous rises in abdominal pressure.

Clinical Manifestations

As in most disorders of childhood, the incidence and type of kidney or urinary tract dysfunction change with the age and maturation of the child. In addition, the presenting complaints and the significance of these complaints vary with age. For example, a complaint of enuresis has greater significance at 8 years old than at 4 years old. In newborns, renal abnormalities may be associated with a number of other malformations, for example, obvious neural tube defects to the subtle abnormal shape or position of the outer ear. Failure to thrive in children may be a sign of impaired renal function.

Many of the clinical manifestations of renal disease are common to a variety of childhood disorders, but their presence is an indication to obtain further information from the child's history, family history, and laboratory studies as part of a complete physical examination. Important signs and symptoms that suggest possible renal or genitourinary tract disease in children at different ages are outlined in Box 24.1. Suspected renal disease can be further evaluated by means of laboratory tests, radiographic studies, and renal biopsy.

Laboratory Tests

Both urine and blood studies contribute vital information for the detection of renal problems. The single most important test is probably routine urinalysis. Specific urine and blood tests provide additional information.

Glomerular filtration rate (GFR) is generally accepted as the best overall index of kidney function. Though the gold standard for measurement of GFR has been the filtration of the small carbohydrate inulin, this is not a practical test clinically. The kidney handles creatinine, an end product of protein metabolism in muscle, in a similar way so that its plasma concentration can be used to estimate GFR. Creatinine clearance tends to slightly overestimate GFR. Serum creatinine is a function

BOX 24.1 Signs and Symptoms of Urinary Tract Disorders or Disease

Neonatal Period (Birth to 1 Month)
Poor feeding
Vomiting
Failure to gain weight
Rapid respiration (acidosis)
Respiratory distress
Spontaneous pneumothorax or pneumomediastinum
Frequent urination
Screaming on urination
Poor urinary stream
Jaundice
Seizures
Dehydration
Other anomalies or stigmata
Enlarged kidneys or bladder

Infancy (1 to 24 Months)
Poor feeding
Vomiting
Failure to gain weight
Excessive thirst
Frequent urination
Straining or screaming on urination
Foul-smelling urine
Pallor
Fever
Persistent diaper rash
Seizures (with or without fever)
Dehydration
Enlarged kidneys or bladder

Childhood (2 to 14 Years)
Poor appetite
Vomiting
Growth failure
Excessive thirst
Enuresis, incontinence, frequent urination
Painful urination
Swelling of face
Seizures
Pallor
Fatigue
Blood in urine
Abdominal or back pain
Edema
Hypertension
Tetany

of both creatinine excretion and production, so it varies, depending on muscle mass. Equations have been developed to estimate kidney function using serum creatinine and variables such as age, sex, race, and body size. In the past, 12- or 24-hour urine collections have been used routinely to measure creatinine clearance, and therefore GFR, but studies have shown these difficult to obtain urine collections do not provide a better estimate of GFR than the equations (Webster, Nagler, Morton, et al., 2017). In the case where a 24-hour urine collection is indicated, the nurse is responsible for assisting in obtaining a complete and accurate collection.

Table 24.1 outlines the major urine and blood tests. Radiologic and other tests of urinary system function are described in Table 24.2. Blood tests of renal function are outlined in Table 24.3.

Nursing Care Management

Nursing responsibilities in the assessment of renal disorders and diseases begin with observation of the child for any manifestations that might indicate dysfunction. The most significant ongoing assessments in children with renal conditions are accurate measurement and recording of weight and height, intake and output, and blood pressure. (See Chapter 4.) These assessments are necessary not only for children with known renal dysfunction but also for those children at risk for developing renal complications (e.g., children in shock, postoperative patients).

In addition to the general manifestations of renal conditions, many conditions have specific characteristics that distinguish them from other disorders. These are discussed as appropriate throughout the chapter.

The nurse is generally responsible for preparing infants, children, and parents for tests and collection of urine and (sometimes) blood specimens. (See Preparation for Diagnostic and Therapeutic Procedures, and Collection of Specimens, Chapter 22.) Nurses observe the characteristics of the urine collected, often perform any of a number of tests on urine specimens (e.g., urine specific gravity, protein, blood, glucose, ketones), and assist with more complex diagnostic tests. Nurses must be familiar with significant laboratory tests, their implications, and preprocedural care.

DRUG ALERT

Fleet Enemas

Use of Fleet enemas in children with acute or chronic renal failure is potentially lethal because of the risk of hyperphosphatemia. Requests for Fleet enemas in this situation should not be implemented without careful investigation.

GENITOURINARY TRACT DISORDERS

URINARY TRACT INFECTION

Urinary tract infection (UTI) is a common and potentially serious problem in children. The overall prevalence is approximately 400,000 are diagnosed annually in young children (Bunting-Early, Shaikh, Woo, et al., 2017). Caucasians, females, and uncircumcised boys have the highest rates. Specifically, girls have a twofold to fourfold higher prevalence than do circumcised boys. Uncircumcised males younger than 3 months old and females younger than 12 months old have the highest baseline prevalence of UTI (Schlager, 2016). UTI may involve the urethra and bladder (lower urinary tract) or the ureters, renal pelvis, calyces, and renal parenchyma (upper urinary tract). Because of the difficulty in distinguishing upper from lower tract infection, particularly in young children, UTI is often broadly defined. Upper UTIs or kidney infection (pyelonephritis) tend to present with fever and may lead to renal scarring that may be associated with decreased kidney function, hypertension and renal disease over time. It is important to note that UTI's in neonates (infants ≤30 days of age) are often associated with congenital anomalies of the kidney and urinary tract (CAKUT) and resulting bacteremia. The typical time of presentation of UTI in term infants is in the second or third week of life (Bonadio & Maida, 2014). Diagnosis of UTI is made based on the presence of both pyuria and at least 50,000 colonies per ml of a single uropathic organism in an appropriately collected specimen (American Academy of Pediatrics Subcommittee on Urinary Tract Infection, 2016). Various terms related to urinary tract infections are defined in Box 24.2.

TABLE 24.1 Urine Tests of Renal Function

Test	Normal Range	Deviations	Significance of Deviations
Physical Tests			
Volume	Age related	Polyuria	Osmotic factors (urinary glucose level in diabetes mellitus)
	Newborn: 30-60 ml	Oliguria	Retention caused by obstructive disease
	Children: Bladder capacity (oz) = Age (yr) + 1		Inadequate bladder emptying caused by neurogenic bladder or obstructive disorder
		Anuria	Obstruction of urinary tract; acute renal failure
Specific gravity	With normal fluid intake: 1.016-1.022	High	Dehydration
			Presence of protein or glucose
	Newborn: 1.001-1.020		Presence of radiopaque contrast medium after radiologic examinations
	Others: 1.001-1.030	Low	Excessive fluid intake
			Distal tubular dysfunction
			Insufficient antidiuretic hormone
			Diuresis
		Fixed at 1.010	Chronic glomerular disease
Osmolality	Newborn: 50-600 mOsm/L	High or low	Same as for specific gravity
	Thereafter: 50-1400 mOsm/L		More sensitive index than specific gravity
Appearance	Clear pale yellow to deep gold	Cloudy	Contains sediment
		Cloudy reddish-pink to reddish-brown	Blood from trauma or disease
			Myoglobin after severe muscle destruction
		Light	Dilute
		Dark	Concentrated
		Red	Trauma
Chemical Tests			
pH	Newborn: 5-7	Weak acid or neutral	If associated with metabolic acidosis, suggests tubular acidosis
	Thereafter: 4.8-7.8		If associated with metabolic alkalosis, suggests potassium deficiency
	Average: 6		Urinary tract infection
		Alkaline	Metabolic alkalosis
Protein level	Absent	Present	Abnormal glomerular permeability (e.g., glomerular disease, changes in blood pressure)
			Most kidney disease
			Orthostatic in some individuals
Glucose level	Absent	Present	Diabetes mellitus
			Infusion of concentrated glucose-containing fluids
			Impaired tubular reabsorption
Ketone levels	Absent	Present	Conditions of acute metabolic demand (stress)
			Diabetic ketoacidosis
Leukocyte esterase	Absent	Present	Can identify both lysed and intact white blood cells via enzyme detection
Nitrites	Absent	Present	Most species of bacteria convert nitrates to nitrites in the urine
Microscopic Tests			
White blood cell count	<1-2	>5 polymorphonuclear leukocytes/field	Urinary tract inflammatory process
		Lymphocytes	Allograft rejection
			Malignancy
Red blood cell count	<1-2	4-6/field in centrifuged specimen	Trauma
			Stones
			Glomerular injury
			Infection
			Neoplasms
Presence of bacteria	Absent to a few	>100,000 organisms/ml in centrifuged specimen	Urinary tract infection
Presence of casts	Occasional	Granular casts	Tubular or glomerular disorders
			Degenerative process in advanced renal disease
		Cellular casts	Pyelonephritis
		White blood cell	Glomerulonephritis
		Red blood cell	Proteinuria; usually transient
		Hyaline casts	

TABLE 24.2 **Radiologic and Other Tests of Urinary System Function**

Test	Procedure	Purpose	Comments and Nursing Responsibilities
Urine culture and sensitivity	Collection of sterile specimen	Determines presence of pathogens and drugs to which they are sensitive	Send specimen to laboratory immediately after collection. Catheterization, clean-catch, or suprapubic specimen.
Renal bladder ultrasound	Transmission of ultrasonic waves through renal parenchyma, along ureteral course, and over bladder	Allows visualization of renal parenchyma, renal pelvis without exposure to external beam radiation or radioactive isotopes. Visualization of dilated ureters and bladder wall also possible. Can show renal cysts and stones, though less sensitive than CT. Doppler ultrasonography can be used to evaluate renal vascular flow.	Noninvasive procedure.
Testicular (scrotal) ultrasound	Transmission of ultrasonic waves through scrotal contents and testis	Allows visualization of scrotal contents, including testis. Testicular ultrasound used to identify masses, and Doppler-enhanced ultrasound used to differentiate hyperemia of epididymoorchitis from ischemia or torsion	Noninvasive procedure.
Plain film of the abdomen (KUB)	Flat plate x-ray film of abdomen and pelvis	Can identify certain types of stones that are calcium containing as well as calculi or opaque foreign bodies in bladder (diagnostic choice for nephrolithiasis is noncontrast helical CT) Assess stool burden	Prepare for routine x-ray film.
VCUG	Contrast medium injected into bladder through urethral catheter until bladder is full; films taken before, during, and after voiding	Visualizes bladder outline and urethra, reveals reflux of urine into ureters. Provides information on bladder emptying. Used to diagnose PUV	Prepare child for catheterization.
Radionuclide (nuclear) cystogram	Radionuclide-containing fluid injected through urethral catheter until bladder is full; images generated before, during, and after voiding	Alternative to voiding cystourethrography to evaluate reflux, although visualization of anatomic details is relatively poor. Used in some institutions for follow up of initial VCUG due to less radiation.	Prepare child for catheterization.
Radioisotope imaging studies (renal scans)	Contrast medium injected intravenously; computer analysis to measure uptake or washout (excretion) for analysis of organ function	DMSA radioisotope to visualize renal scars and differential renal function; does not visualize ureters and bladder. MAG-3 radioisotope assesses obstruction and shows differential function between the two kidneys. DTPA is an alternative to MAG-3 but imaging is limited because it is only filtered at the glomerulus.	Insert or assist with insertion of IV. Monitor IV infusion. Urethral catheterization may accompany MAG-3 or DTPA scan; prepare child for catheterization when indicated.
MRI	Uses strong magnetic fields and radio waves to form images	MRI of kidneys used to evaluate renal mass. Magnetic resonance angiography used to evaluate renovascular hypertension and has reduced need for renal angiography. Magnetic resonance urogram used to detect specific urologic abnormalities, such as ectopic ureter.	MRI often requires sedation in infants and children due to need to stay still, typically in an enclosed space. Follow NPO guidelines depending on timing of study. Assist with IV access if indicated. Magnetic devices or implants may be unsafe for MRI, including cochlear implants and permanent pacemakers.
CT	Narrow-beam x-rays and computer analysis provide precise reconstruction of area	Visualizes vertical or horizontal cross section of kidney Especially valuable to distinguish tumors, cysts, and stones. Noncontrast helical CT is gold standard for radiologic diagnosis of renal stone disease. Renal CT angiogram used to evaluate blood flow in hypertensive patients and is now used more commonly than renal arteriography.	Noncontrast scan is noninvasive. Contrast-enhanced CT scan preparation may require child be NPO for a few hours. With speed of newer scans, the need for sedation is decreased, but if required will also require NPO. Assist with IV access if needed. *Used selectively due to higher radiation exposure.*

TABLE 24.2 Radiologic and Other Tests of Urinary System Function—cont'd

Test	Procedure	Purpose	Comments and Nursing Responsibilities
Cystoscopy	Direct visualization of bladder and lower urinary tract through small scope inserted via urethra	Investigation of bladder and lower tract lesions; visualizes urethral openings, bladder wall, trigone, and urethra	NPO orders per protocol, typically no solid food after midnight, liquids until 4-6 hours before procedure. Carry out preoperative preparations; cystoscopy is done under anesthesia in children.
Renal biopsy	Removal of kidney tissue by open or percutaneous technique for study by light, electron, or immunofluorescent microscopy	Yields histologic and microscopic information about glomeruli and tubules; helps distinguish between types of nephritic syndromes Distinguishes other renal disorders	Nothing orally 4-6 hours before test. Premedicate as ordered. Prepare setup for procedure. Assist with procedure. Take vital signs. Apply pressure to area with pressure dressing and, if feasible, a sandbag. Bed rest for 24 hours. Observe for abdominal pain, tenderness. Monitor intake and output. Surgical incision may be required in infants.
Urodynamics	Set of tests to measure bladder filling, storage, and evacuation functions: Uroflowmetry—Test to determine efficiency of urination Cystometrography: Graphic comparison of bladder pressure as a function of volume Voiding pressure study: Comparison of detrusor contraction pressure, sphincter EMG, and urinary flow	Determine characteristic of voiding dysfunction Used to identify type (cause) of incontinence or urinary retention Especially valuable for voiding dysfunction complicated by urinary tract infection, urinary retention, or neurogenic bladder dysfunction	Prepare child for urinary catheterization. The bladder will be filled with contrast, sterile water, or saline solution. The child may experience fullness, coolness from the fluid, and urine leakage during the study Insertion of rectal tube will produce feelings of rectal fullness or pressure. Insertion of needles may be required for sphincter EMG. (Institution specific, often use electrode patches.)

CT, Computed tomography; *DMSA,* dimercaptosuccinic acid; *DTPA,* diethylenetriamine pentaacetic acid; *EMG,* electromyography; *IV,* intravenous; *KUB,* kidney, ureters, and bladder; *MAG-3,* mercaptoacetyltriglycine or mertiatide; *MRI,* magnetic resonance imaging; *NPO,* nothing by mouth; *PUV,* posterior urethral valve; *VCUG,* voiding cystourethrogram.

TABLE 24.3 Blood Tests of Renal Function

Test	Normal Range (mg/dl)	Deviations	Significance of Deviations
Blood urea nitrogen (BUN)	Newborn: 4-18 Infant, child: 5-18	Elevated	Renal disease—acute or chronic (the higher the BUN, the more severe the disease) Increased protein catabolism Dehydration Hemorrhage High protein intake Corticosteroid therapy
Uric acid	Child: 2.0-5.5	Increased	Severe renal disease
Creatinine	Infant: 0.2-0.4 Child: 0.3-0.7 Adolescent: 0.5-1.0	Increased	Severe renal impairment

BUN, Blood urea nitrogen.

BOX 24.2 Classifications of Urinary Tract Infections or Inflammations

Bacteriuria—Presence of bacteria in the urine

Asymptomatic bacteriuria—Significant bacteriuria with no evidence of clinical infection (usually defined as >100,000 colony-forming units/mm^3)

Symptomatic bacteriuria—Bacteriuria accompanied by physical signs of urinary infection (dysuria, suprapubic discomfort, hematuria, fever)

Recurrent urinary tract infection (UTI)—Repeated episode of bacteriuria or symptomatic UTI

Persistent UTI—Persistence of bacteriuria despite antibiotic treatment

Febrile UTI—Bacteriuria accompanied by fever and other physical signs of UTI; presence of a fever typically implies pyelonephritis

Cystitis—Inflammation of the bladder

Urethritis—Inflammation of the urethra

Pyelonephritis—Inflammation of the upper urinary tract and kidneys

Urosepsis—Febrile UTI coexisting with systemic signs of bacterial illness; blood culture reveals presence of urinary pathogen

Single and recurrent UTI can develop in children with normal urinary tracts as well as those with congenital anomalies. An initial UTI is often in the first year of life and has been associated with an increased risk of renal scarring. Recent studies have identified risk factors for renal scarring in children and adolescents. These include an abnormal renal ultrasound or a combination of high fever (≥39°C) and causative organism other than *Escherichia coli.* (Shaikh, Craig, Rovers, et al., 2014). Though vesicoureteral reflux is a known risk factor for recurrent UTI and renal scarring, it is not always a factor, as febrile UTI can occur in the absence of reflux.

Etiology

A variety of organisms can be responsible for UTI. *Escherichia coli* remains the most common uropathogen overall, but the prevalence is higher in females (83%) than males (50%) (Edlin, Shapiro, Hersh, et al., 2013). Other gram-negative organisms associated with UTI include *Proteus mirabilis, Pseudomonas aeruginosa, Klebsiella,* and *Enterobacter.* Gram-positive bacterial pathogens include *Enterococcus, Staphylococcus saprophyticus,* and, rarely, *Staphylococcus aureus* (Schlager, 2016). Viruses and fungi are uncommon causes of UTI in children. Most uropathogens originate in the gastrointestinal tract, migrate to the periurethral area, and ascend to the bladder. A number of factors contribute to the development of UTI, including anatomic, physical, and chemical conditions or properties of the host's urinary tract.

Pathogenesis and Host Factors. Evidence suggests that most UTIs after the newborn period result from ascending infection from uropathogens on the periurethral mucosa. A variety of virulence factors allow the bacteria to attach and ascend to the bladder and kidney. Host factors influence the risk of development of UTI and include urologic abnormalities, genetic factors, and functional abnormalities such as bowel bladder dysfunction.

After invasion by bacteria, the first line of defense in the lower urinary tract is complete evacuation by voiding. Inflammation in the bladder and urethral walls is apparent within 30 minutes of invasion by a bacterial pathogen. Polymorphonuclear leukocytes rapidly migrate to the bladder wall, which becomes completely injected within 2 hours. Complete evacuation of the bladder is particularly important for the eradication of bacteria from the urine. Urination not only helps remove bacteria and associated toxins contained in the urine but also allows more efficient destruction of the bacteria remaining on the thin film of urine that is adherent to the vesical wall.

The structure of the lower urinary tract has traditionally been thought to account for the increased incidence of bacteriuria in females. The short urethra, which measures approximately 2 cm (0.75 inch) in young girls and 4 cm (1.5 inches) in mature women, provides a ready pathway for invasion of organisms. In addition, the closure of the urethra at the end of micturition may return contaminated bacteria to the bladder. The longer male urethra (20 cm or 8 inches) and the antibacterial properties of prostatic secretions inhibit the entry and growth of pathogens. The importance of the length of the urethra in the pathogenesis of UTI has been questioned because of the high incidence of UTI in male neonates. The presence or absence of the foreskin has been shown to be a significant factor, with prevalence of UTI in infant males with 11% of uncircumcised male infants developing a UTI in the first year of life compared with 0.1% of circumcised male infants (Schlager, 2016). The presence of a foreskin is associated with increased periurethral colonization with uropathogens, providing a plausible explanation for the increased association between UTI in infancy in the uncircumcised male (American Academy of Pediatrics Task Force on Circumcision, 2012). Virulence factors are important in the pathogenesis of UTIs and, coupled with the propensity of bacteria to adhere to the female periurethral mucosa, may explain the increased incidence of UTI in females. The single most important host factor influencing the occurrence of UTI is urinary stasis. New research has shown that urine is not sterile, but bacterial communities or microbiota have been found in the female bladder, leading to ongoing research in this area (Wolfe & Brubaker, 2015). Under normal conditions the act of completely and repeatedly emptying the bladder flushes away organisms before they have an opportunity to multiply and invade surrounding tissue. However, urine that remains in the bladder provides an excellent culture medium for most uropathogens.

Incomplete bladder emptying (stasis) may result from reflux (see p. 790 for a discussion of reflux), anatomic abnormalities (especially those involving the ureters), or extrinsic ureteral or bladder compression. The pressure of overdistention within the bladder may increase the risk of infection by decreasing host resistance, probably as a result of lessened blood flow to the mucosa. This often occurs in a neurogenic bladder or as a consequence of voluntarily holding back urine (Vasudeva & Madersbacher, 2014).

Incomplete bladder emptying may also result from dysfunctional voiding, where a child habitually contracts the urethral sphincter during voiding. Because of the close association of bowel and bladder function, *bowel and bladder dysfunction* has become the term referring to a constellation of associated symptoms caused by difficulty relaxing the pelvic floor muscles. Common symptoms include urinary frequency, urgency, incontinence, enuresis, incomplete bladder emptying, constipation, and encopresis. UTI is frequently seen in these children, who are typically otherwise healthy children who develop abnormal voiding habits during or after toilet training.

Extrinsic factors that may be responsible for functional bladder neck obstruction are pregnancy and chronic and intermittent constipation. In both conditions the full uterus or rectum displaces the bladder and posterior urethra in the fixed and limited space of the bony pelvis, causing obstruction, incomplete micturition, and urinary stasis. Treating constipation and administering antibiotic therapy for UTI reduces the recurrence of infection. Failure to relieve the fecal retention in spite of adequate treatment of the UTI may result in recurrence.

Other extrinsic factors that can contribute to UTI include catheters, especially short-term indwelling catheters, and administration of antimicrobial agents. Antimicrobials alter the host's normal perineal flora, allowing easier colonization of uropathogens. Poor hygiene, local inflammation from vaginitis, masturbation, or pinworm infestation may also increase the risk of ascending infection. The essential oils in bubble baths and shampoos can irritate the urethra of both boys and girls, causing painful and frequent urination. There is no evidence that plain tub baths increase the risk of UTI, but infections have been related to the use of hot tub or whirlpool baths. Sexual intercourse may produce transient bacteriuria in females and is associated with an increased risk of UTI.

Clinical Manifestations

The clinical manifestations of UTIs depend on the child's age. Infants and toddlers under 2 years of age have nonspecific symptoms, such as fever, irritability, lethargy, poor feeding, vomiting, and diarrhea. Newborns may have fever, hypothermia, jaundice, tachypnea, or cyanosis, and they appear quite ill. The classic symptoms of UTI are often observed in children over 2 years of age. These include enuresis or daytime incontinence in the child who has been toilet trained, fever, foul-smelling urine, increased frequency of urination, dysuria, or urgency. Symptoms of dysfunctional voiding are found in Box 24.3. Children may also complain of abdominal pain or costovertebral angle tenderness

BOX 24.3 Symptoms of Dysfunctional Voiding

- Urinary tract infection without fever
- Changes in urinary frequency
- Constipation
- Squatting or holding to stay dry
- Daytime or nighttime wetting
- Straining to void
- Urgency to void

(flank pain). Some patients have hematuria or vomiting. Infants and young boys may develop obstructive-like symptoms, with dribbling of urine, straining with urination, or a decrease in the force and size of the urinary stream. High fever and chills accompanied by flank pain, severe abdominal pain, and leukocytosis suggest pyelonephritis. However, flank pain and tenderness may be the only indication of pyelonephritis on physical examination.

Manifestations in older children and adolescents are more specific. Symptoms of lower tract infections include frequency and painful urination of a small amount of turbulent urine that may be grossly bloody. Fever is usually absent or low grade. Upper tract infection is characterized by fever (>38°C), chills, and flank pain, often in addition to lower tract symptoms.

Many UTIs in children are asymptomatic or atypical in clinical presentation, and complaints may be unrelated to the urinary tract. Many are treated as respiratory or gastrointestinal tract infections. It is important to identify these children so treatment can be initiated. Significant renal scarring can occur, especially in infants and young children.

Diagnostic Evaluation

The diagnosis of UTI depends on a high degree of suspicion, evaluation of the history and physical examination, and urinalysis and culture. Urine with a possible infection may appear cloudy, hazy, or thick, with noticeable strands of mucus and pus; it also may have an unpleasant odor, even when fresh. A presumptive UTI diagnosis can be made on the basis of microscopic examination of the urine, which often reveals pyuria (at least 10 white blood cells/ml of uncentrifuged urine) and the presence of at least one bacterium on Gram stain. However, a normal urinalysis may also be present in conditions of asymptomatic bacteriuria. The key to distinguishing true UTI from asymptomatic bacteriuria is the presence of pyuria (American Academy of Pediatrics, Subcommittee on Urinary Tract Infection, 2016).

Detection of bacteria in a urine culture confirms the diagnosis of UTI, but urine collection is often difficult, especially in infants and small children. (See Collection of Specimens, Chapter 22.) Several factors may alter a urine specimen. Contamination of a specimen by organisms from sources other than the urine is the most common cause of false-positive results. Bag urine specimens are commonly contaminated by perineal and perianal flora and are usually considered inadequate for a definitive diagnosis. The American Academy of Pediatrics guidelines for evaluating febrile infants and children from 2 to 24 months recommends obtaining a urine specimen for culture and urinalysis before an antimicrobial agent is administered and obtaining it by catheterization or suprapubic aspiration (American Academy of Pediatrics, Subcommittee on Urinary Tract Infection, 2016). If a urinalysis obtained by a bag specimen is negative, that may be sufficient, but if it is positive, a specimen still needs to be obtained by catheterization or suprapubic aspiration.

NURSING TIP

Clean-catch urine specimen collection from a young girl is easier when the child sits on the toilet facing the tank. In this position the child (especially the toddler) is more stable and relaxed. The labia are naturally separated, decreasing the likelihood of contamination. This position is also useful for older girls who perform clean, intermittent self-catheterization.

Unless the specimen is a first morning sample, a recent high fluid intake may indicate a falsely low organism count. Therefore do not encourage children to drink large volumes of water in an attempt to obtain a specimen quickly.

The most accurate tests of bacterial content are suprapubic aspiration (for children <2 years of age) and properly performed bladder catheterization (as long as the first few milliliters are excluded from collection). Care of a urine specimen obtained for culture is an important nursing responsibility related to diagnosis. The specimen must be fresh (<1 hour after voiding with storage at room temperature or <4 hours after voiding with refrigeration) to ensure sensitivity and specificity of the urinalysis and to prevent growth of organisms (American Academy of Pediatrics, Subcommittee on Urinary Tract Infection, 2016) (see Translating Evidence into Practice box).

Because urine culture results are not available for at least 24 hours, predictive tests are utilized to direct therapy. Urine dipsticks indicate the presence of leukocyte esterase and nitrites, and urine microscopic examination allows for detection of bacteria and white blood cells. Leukocyte esterase is a surrogate marker for pyuria, and nitrite is converted from dietary nitrates in the presence of most gram-negative enteric bacteria in the urine. Because the conversion of dietary nitrates to nitrites takes 4 hours in the bladder, it is not a sensitive marker for infants or children who empty their bladder frequently. The test is helpful if positive but not if negative. Also, not all urinary pathogens reduce nitrate to nitrite (American Academy of Pediatrics, Subcommittee on Urinary Tract Infection, 2016).

Therapeutic Management

The goals of treatment of children with UTI are to eliminate the acute infection, prevent complications, and reduce the likelihood of renal damage (American Academy of Pediatrics, Subcommittee on Urinary Tract Infection, 2016). Antibiotic therapy depends on laboratory culture and sensitivity tests. Nonetheless, empiric therapy on the basis of the child's history and presenting symptoms may be necessary when fever or systemic illness complicates UTI. Common antiinfective agents used for UTI include the penicillins, sulfonamide (including trimethoprim-sulfamethoxazole), the cephalosporins, and nitrofurantoin. All antibiotics may cause side effects or prove ineffective because of bacterial resistance (Table 24.4).

Infants and young children with suspected pyelonephritis and fever may require admission to the hospital for intravenous antibiotics and hydration. Blood and urine cultures may be obtained on admission and after therapy. Nitrofurantoin is not used for treatment of febrile infants or patients where pyelonephritis is suspected because it is excreted in the urine and does not achieve therapeutic concentrations in the blood or kidney (American Academy of Pediatrics, Subcommittee on Urinary Tract Infection, 2016).

Historically, all children with a febrile UTI were evaluated for vesicoureteral reflux (VUR) because of concern of renal scarring with recurrent kidney infections (Schaeffer, Greenfield, Ivanova, et al., 2016). Controversy continues regarding appropriate evaluation with newer guidelines recommending a renal ultrasound after an initial febrile UTI in a child age 2 to 24 months of age. An abnormal renal ultrasound or

TRANSLATING EVIDENCE INTO PRACTICE

Urinary Specimen Collection in Infants and Children 2 to 24 Months With Suspected Urinary Tract Infection

Ask the Question

PICOT Question

In infants or children with a possible urinary tract infection (UTI), what is the preferred method for collecting a urine specimen?

Search for the Evidence

Search Strategies

Search criteria included English-language publications within the past 15 years and research-based articles on infants or children with signs or symptoms of UTI.

Databases Used

Cochrane Collaboration, Joanna Briggs Institute, National Guideline Clearinghouse (AHRQ), PubMed

Critically Analyze the Evidence

GRADE criteria: Evidence quality moderate; recommendation strong (Guyatt, Oxman, Vist, et al., 2008)

A review of the literature revealed several studies evaluating specimen collection techniques in infants and children. In 2016 the American Academy of Pediatrics reaffirmed the clinical practice guideline for diagnosis and management of the initial UTI in febrile infants and children ages 2 to 24 months. There is a strong recommendation that a urine specimen should be obtained for culture and urinalysis before prescribing an antibiotic. The new guideline recommends that when the degree of illness warrants immediate antibiotic therapy, then urine specimens should be obtained through catheterization or suprapubic aspiration (SPA) of urine (American Academy of Pediatrics, Subcommittee on Urinary Tract Infection, 2016). When the degree of illness does not require immediate antibiotic therapy, a urine specimen evaluation within 1 hour of voiding can be evaluated for leukocyte esterase and nitrite using urine dipstick testing (American Academy of Pediatrics, Subcommittee on Urinary Tract Infection, 2016; Mori, Yonemoto, Fitzgerald, et al., 2010). A systematic review comparing dipstick testing and microscopy showed that dipstick testing performed well for determining UTI in children over 2 years of age (Mori, Yonemoto, Fitzgerald, et al., 2010). Dipstick testing for leukocyte esterase or nitrite was not helpful when negative. For children younger than 2 years, microscopy showed the best diagnostic accuracy.

- Urine culture specimen in 599 children less than 2 years revealed contamination rates of 26% using clean-catch urine, 12% in catheter specimen urine, and 1% in suprapubic aspirated urine. Authors recommend that when clean-catch specimens are necessary, the collection procedure needs to be optimized for all collections in this manner (Tosif, Baker, Oakley, et al., 2012).
- An observational study of 3066 infants less than 93 days old evaluated specimen collection via urinary catheterization compared with a urine bag. Results showed that bag specimens sent for urine culture were more likely to have two organisms, nonpathogenic bacteria, and ambiguous results. Although parents prefer the urine bag method of specimen collection, culture results are more accurate when specimens are collected via urinary catheterization (Schroeder, Newman, Wasserman, et al., 2005).
- McGillivray, Mok, Mulrooney, and colleagues (2008) compared sensitivity and specificity of specimens collected via "clean-void" bag technique versus specimens collected via urinary catheterization to diagnose UTIs. The authors concluded that urine samples should be collected via catheterization in infants less than 90 days old due to low sensitivity of bag specimens. Bag specimens are an acceptable method of collecting urine to screen for UTI but can miss up to 12% of UTIs.

Apply the Evidence: Nursing Implications

- Urine specimens should be collected by catheterization or suprapubic aspiration in infants and children less than 2 years of age whose illness warrants immediate antibiotic therapy.
- When an infant or child less than 2 years of age is not assessed to appear ill and there is a low likelihood of UTI, a urine specimen can be obtained using the most convenient method for urinalysis. If the results are positive for leukocyte esterase or nitrite or there is microscopic evidence for leukocytes or bacteremia, a urine specimen should be obtained through catheterization or suprapubic aspirate.
- When a noninvasive method is used to obtain urine for UTI screening, meticulous methods for collection should be followed. The specimen should be evaluated within 1 hour of voiding.

References

American Academy of Pediatrics, Subcommittee on Urinary Tract Infection. (2016). Reaffirmation of AAP clinical practice guideline: The diagnosis and management of the initial urinary tract infection in febrile infants and young children 2–24 months of age. *Pediatrics,* e20163026.

Guyatt, G. H., Oxman, A. D., Vist, G. E., et al. (2008). GRADE: An emerging consensus on rating quality of evidence and strength of recommendations. *British Medical Journal, 336,* 924–926.

McGillivray, D., Mok, E., Mulrooney, E., et al. (2008). A head-to-head comparison: "Clean-void" bag versus catheter urinalysis in the diagnosis of urinary tract infection in young children. *Journal of Pediatrics, 147*(4), 451–456.

Mori, R., Yonemoto, N., Fitzgerald, A., et al. (2010). Diagnostic performance of urine dipstick testing in children with suspected UTI: A systematic review of relationship with age and comparison with microscopy. *Acta Paediatrica, 99,* 581–583.

Schroeder, A. R., Newman, T. B., Wasserman, R. C., et al. (2005). Choice of urine collection methods for the diagnosis of urinary tract infection in young, febrile infants. *Archives of Pediatrics and Adolescent Medicine, 159*(10), 915–922.

Tosif, S., Baker, A., Oakley, E., et al. (2012). Contamination rates of different urine collection methods for the diagnosis of urinary tract infections in young children: An observational cohort study. *Journal of Paediatrics and Child Health, 48,* 659–664.

Originally Developed by Ashley R. Breland

NURSING TIP

For best results, cleanse, rinse, and dry the perineal area thoroughly before applying the urine collection bag, and remove the bag promptly after voiding occurs. Even if contamination from the perineal skin is minimized, there may be significant contamination, but leaving the urine at room temperature for more than 1 hour is more likely to yield a contaminated urine specimen (American Academy of Pediatrics, Subcommittee on Urinary Tract Infection, 2016).

a second febrile UTI warrants a VCUG according to these guidelines (American Academy of Pediatrics, Subcommittee on Urinary Tract Infection, 2016). The Randomized Intervention for Vesicoureteral Reflux (RIVUR) trial was a multicenter, randomized, placebo-controlled trial comparing placebo and antibiotic prophylaxis in children with grade I to IV VUR. Results of this study showed substantially reduced risk of recurrence of UTI with urinary prophylaxis, but no significant effect on renal scarring (Hoberman, Chesney, et al., 2014; Schaeffer, Greenfield, Ivanova, et al., 2016). The finding that urinary prophylaxis is effective has challenged the recommendation to limit VCUG use, which was based in part by the argument that prophylaxis was not effective and doing the study would not affect the treatment (Lee, Lorenzo, & Koyle,

TABLE 24.4 Common Side Effects of Urinary Antiinfective Agents

Drug	Side Effects	Nursing Interventions
Trimethoprim-sulfamethoxazole (Bactrim, Septra)	Rash, urticaria, photosensitivity, nausea, bone marrow depression (long-term use)	Maintain adequate fluid intake. Advise parents and child to use sunscreen. May perform periodic blood counts in long-term use.
Amoxicillin (Amoxil, Polymox, Trimox)	Nausea, vomiting, diarrhea	Refrigerate suspension; discard suspension after 14 days.
Nitrofurantoin (Macrodantin, Furadantin)	Nausea, pneumonitis or pulmonary fibrosis (long-term use)	Administer with food or milk.
Cephalexin (Keflex)	Nausea, diarrhea	Administer with food or milk.
Ceftazidime (Fortaz)	Renal toxicity	
Gentamicin (Garamycin)	Renal toxicity, ototoxicity	Keep child well hydrated. Monitor urinary output, blood urea nitrogen, creatinine. Monitor serum levels, especially in infants.

2016). There is not yet consensus, and research is ongoing, with assessment and management individualized for the specific patient. VUR is neither necessary nor sufficient to cause acute pyelonephritis and renal scarring in children, but compelling evidence shows that VUR is strongly associated with renal damage (Routh, Bogaert, Kaefer, et al., 2012).

Anatomic defects such as primary reflux or bladder neck obstruction may require surgical correction to prevent recurrent infection or may indicate the need for prophylactic antibiotics and careful follow-up monitoring. Follow-up is an important component of medical management because the relapse rate is high and recurrent infection tends to occur 1 to 2 months after termination of treatment. The aim of therapy and careful follow-up in such cases is to prevent morbidity and reduce the chance of renal scarring.

Prognosis. With prompt and adequate treatment at the time of diagnosis, the long-term prognosis for UTIs is usually excellent. Evidence shows that delay in treatment initiation of 72 hours or more increases risk of permanent renal scars after the first episode of febrile UTI (Karavanaki, Soldatou, Koufadaki, et al., 2017; Shakih, Mattoo, Keren, et al., 2016). The hazard of progressive renal injury is greatest when infection occurs in young children (especially <2 years of age) and is associated with congenital renal malformations and reflux. Therefore early diagnosis of children at risk is particularly important during infancy and toddlerhood. (See Quality Patient Outcomes box.)

QUALITY PATIENT OUTCOMES

Urinary Tract Infections

- Treatment based on culture and sensitivity
- Renal function maintained
- Appropriate diagnosis of renal abnormalities

Nursing Care Management

Objectives of nursing care include identification of children with UTI and education of parents and children regarding prevention and treatment of infection. Aside from the influence of renal abnormalities, girls between the ages of 2 and 6 years are in general a high-risk group. This is a common age for development of constipation and stool and urine withholding behaviors as children learn bowel and bladder control. Encouragement of good toilet habits and dietary intake of fluid and fiber can help avoid these problems. Parents should be aware of signs and symptoms of UTI, and a routine urinalysis should be performed if there are concerns. Nurses should instruct parents to observe for signs of UTI, which are not always as obvious as those of upper respiratory tract infection.

! NURSING ALERT

A child who exhibits the following should be evaluated for UTI:
- Incontinence in a toilet-trained child
- Strong-smelling urine
- Frequency or urgency
- Pain with urination

Because infants and young children are unable to accurately express their symptoms verbally, it may be difficult to detect discomfort they may be experiencing from dysuria. A careful history regarding voiding habits, stooling patterns, and episodes of unexplained irritability may assist in detecting less obvious cases of UTI. Encourage parents to observe for specific clues of UTI in suspected cases (see Critical Thinking Case Study box).

CRITICAL THINKING CASE STUDY

Urinary Tract Infection and Constipation

During your assessment of Ginger, a 4-year-old admitted to the hospital for a severe urinary tract infection, her mother tells you that Ginger has bowel movements every third or fourth day. They are usually large, hard-formed stools, and Ginger sometimes has trouble evacuating the stool.

Questions

1. What evidence should you consider regarding Ginger's UTI and constipation?
2. What additional information is required at this time?
3. Describe the nursing interventions that have the highest priority.
4. Identify important patient-centered outcomes with reference to your nursing interventions.

Answers are available at http://evolve.elsevier.com/wong/ncic.

Collecting an appropriate specimen is essential when an infection is suspected. It is the nurse's responsibility to take every precaution to obtain acceptable specimens depending on the patient's age, toilet training status, and symptoms.

Other tests are often performed to detect anatomic defects. Prepare children for these tests as appropriate for their age. Children who are old enough to understand need an explanation of the procedure, its purpose, and what they will experience. (See Preparation for Diagnostic and Therapeutic Procedures, Chapter 22.) Sometimes a simple description of the urinary system is helpful. For children under 3 to 4 years of age, the nurse can explain the procedure using a doll. For those who are older, a simple drawing of the bladder, urethra, ureters, and kidneys makes the explanation more understandable. Especially with preschool children, the nurse must clarify that the urinary tract is separate from any sexual function and that the test is for a problem that they did not cause. It is not uncommon for children to associate blame for perceived wrongdoing (e.g., masturbation) or unacceptable thoughts with the reason for the illness or tests.

Testing is usually done on an outpatient basis, so it is easier to overlook the need for adequate preparation. If surgery is subsequently indicated, the child will need continued explanations at the child's level to decrease fear and anxiety.

Because antiinfective drugs are indicated in the treatment of UTI, the nurse teaches the patient and parents the appropriate dosage and scheduling and provides suggestions for administration. Certain drugs are available in liquid form; others are available only in capsule or pill form. In general, capsules are separated and pills are crushed, with their contents mixed into a small volume of food, such as yogurt or applesauce, or chilled liquid to mask a disagreeable taste. Encourage brushing the teeth after administering medication at bedtime because there is often sugar in liquid formulations. Reinforce compliance with medication regimens and completion of therapy. Nurses may be instrumental in assisting parents with suggestions to help them incorporate medication administration into their routine, particularly when the child is on long-term urinary prophylaxis requiring daily medication.

Encourage adequate fluid intake for the prevention and treatment of UTI because this helps prevent risk factors such as constipation and urinary stasis. Fluid requirements are dependent on body size and fluid losses, but maintenance can be calculated based on the Holliday-Segar method, shown in Box 24.4. Using this formula, a 25-kg child should have 1600 ml or 53 ounces per day (Hines, 2012). This formula is used for parenteral fluid replacement in children who are hospitalized. Fluid is also obtained from food, so this may be an overestimate of actual fluid intake. Have children avoid bladder irritants such as caffeinated or carbonated beverages. The child who is febrile and unable to drink liquids is given intravenous (IV) hydration until the fever resolves and oral liquids are tolerated.

Prevention. Prevention is the most important goal in both primary and recurrent infection. Most preventive measures are simple, ordinary hygienic habits that should be a routine part of daily care. Investigate any signs of intestinal parasites (e.g., scratching between the legs and around the anal area) and treat them appropriately. Advise sexually active adolescent girls to urinate as soon as possible after intercourse to flush out bacteria introduced during sex. Also teach parents and older children health practices that prevent UTI (Box 24.5).

BOX 24.4 Fluid Requirements in Children

Example: Determine fluid requirements for a 7-year-old child weighing 25 kg:
- First 10 kg: 100 ml/kg/day × 10 kg = 1000 ml/day
- Second 10 kg: 50 ml/kg/day × 10 kg = 500 ml/day
- Each additional 1 kg: 20 ml/kg/day × 5 kg = 100 ml/day

Answer: 1600 ml/day

Children who experience recurrent febrile UTIs or recurrent infections complicated by VUR may be given a suppressive or prophylactic antibiotic for a period of months or several years. The medication is commonly administered once a day; the patient and parents are typically advised to give the antibiotic before sleep because this represents the longest period without voiding. Commonly used antibiotics for urinary prophylaxis include sulfamethoxazole and trimethoprim, trimethoprim, nitrofurantoin, or first-generation cephalosporins.

VESICOURETERAL REFLUX

VUR refers to the retrograde flow of urine from the bladder into the upper urinary tract. Reflux increases the chance for febrile UTI but does not cause it. When bladder pressure is high enough, refluxing urine can fill the ureter and renal pelvis. This is identified most often at peak bladder pressure during voiding, but it can occur as the bladder fills and remain after voiding, even draining down into the bladder, leaving residual urine until the next void. The International Classification System describes the degree of reflux from the bladder into upper genitourinary tract structures (Fig. 24.2).

Primary reflux results from a congenital anomaly that affects the ureterovesical junction. Normally the ureter has a segment within the bladder wall that is compressed during a bladder contraction. This

BOX 24.5 Preventing Measures for UTI

Factors Predisposing to Development	Measures of Prevention
Short female urethra close to vagina and anus	Perineal hygiene—wipe from front to back. Wear cotton panties rather than nylon.
Incomplete emptying and overdistention of bladder	Encourage toilet posture to relax the pelvic floor: knees separated and feet supported for girls. Avoid "holding" urine; encourage child to void frequently, especially before a long trip or other circumstances in which toilet facilities are not available. Take time to relax and empty bladder completely with each void.

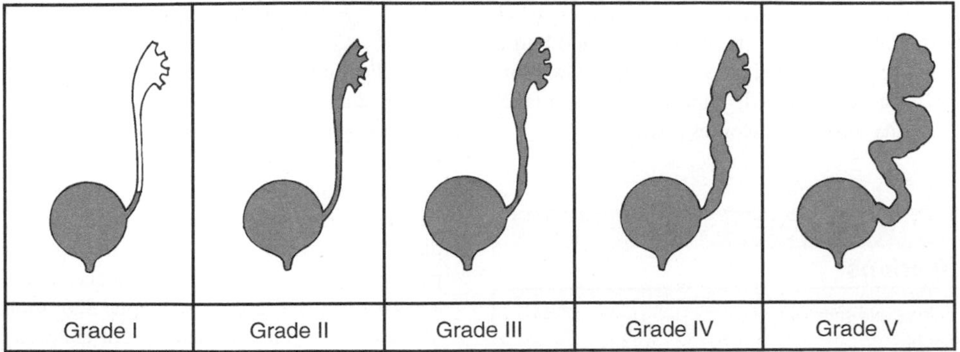

FIG. 24.2 Grades of reflux. (From Retik, A. B., & Cukier, J. [Eds.]. [1987]. *Pediatric urology.* Baltimore, MD: Williams & Wilkins.)

"antireflux" mechanism does not work if that segment is shortened and not able to be compressed by the bladder muscle, allowing for backflow of urine. It is well recognized that children with UTI and VUR are at increased risk for pyelonephritis, as well as renal scarring (Schlager, 2016).

Secondary reflux occurs as a result of abnormally high pressure in the bladder, typically from anatomic (e.g., posterior urethral valves) or functional bladder obstruction (e.g., dysfunctional voiding or neurogenic bladder). It is a common finding in children with neurogenic bladder secondary to spina bifida. The severity of the bladder abnormality affects the degree of VUR, and treatment is typically focused on the underlying problem and not correction of the VUR in these cases.

Reflux with infection is the most common cause of pyelonephritis in children. There has been long-standing consensus that reflux of infected urine into the renal parenchyma results in renal scarring and predisposes to kidney disease. This belief has been increasingly questioned with the view that VUR is a sign of abnormal renal development that results in decreased formation of renal parenchyma, referred to as primary renal scarring. Current management is based on the premise that VUR is a risk factor for renal scarring because it allows bacteria to ascend from the bladder to the kidney and cause pyelonephritis. Because of the lack of conclusive evidence and the known association between VUR and renal scarring that can lead to chronic kidney disease, VUR is still regarded as a risk factor, and recommendations include performing an initial evaluation of renal status, growth, and blood pressure on any child with VUR (Schlager, 2016).

Therapeutic Management

In most cases of VUR, conservative, nonoperative therapy is effective in controlling infection. There is a high rate of spontaneous resolution over time. Factors associated with spontaneous resolution included diagnosis at less than 1 year of age, lower grades of VUR, prenatal hydronephrosis, and unilateral reflux. The correlation of grade to rate of spontaneous resolution is 82%, 80%, 46%, 30%, and 13% for grades I, II, III, IV, and V, respectively (Schlager, 2016). Other factors that may affect resolution rates are coexisting anomalies, voiding dysfunction, timing of reflux, and gender (Kirsch, Arlen, Leong, et al., 2014). Medical therapy consists of continuous antibiotic prophylaxis (CAP), based on the assumption that this will keep bacteria from multiplying and causing infection and that reflux of noninfected urine does not cause renal damage. The most common antibiotics used for this purpose are trimethoprim and sulfamethoxazole, trimethoprim, or nitrofurantoin given once daily at bedtime. Amoxicillin is used in infants less than 2 months of age but is not otherwise used because of the increased likelihood of resistant organisms. Traditionally CAP has been used until documentation of resolution of VUR. This approach is being reconsidered, and the use of CAP is being individualized, with children often coming off after toilet training if they have no evidence of voiding dysfunction. Risks and benefits are discussed with parents with consideration of grade of reflux, rates of spontaneous resolution, elimination habits, and family preferences. This long-term therapy requires medical supervision and reliable, cooperative parents who can be compliant with CAP recommendations and seek medical attention if there are symptoms suggestive of UTI or unexplained fever. Urine cultures are not recommended routinely but should be obtained if there are symptoms or unexplained fever because breakthrough infections can occur despite CAP.

Surgical management of VUR corrects the anatomy at the insertion of the refluxing ureter into the bladder and consists of open surgical correction with reimplantation of the ureter(s) or endoscopic correction. Surgical intervention is indicated in patients who are unlikely to resolve their reflux and are at risk for renal damage; including those with grade V reflux with scarring, grade V reflux over 6 years of age, and children who fail medical therapy. Again, families play a role in the decision, both in their preferences and their ability to follow through with recommendations. For example, a child with recurrent UTIs whose parents are not compliant with CAP may be a candidate for surgical correction regardless of the grade of reflux.

Renal ultrasonography is performed 1 month postoperatively to check for ureteral obstruction. The option of endoscopic correction is a minimally invasive alternative where injection of a bulking agent beneath the mucosa of the ureterovesical junction to change the angle of the ureter is performed during cystoscopy. The substance currently used is dextranomer/hyaluronic acid or Deflux, which has a success rate of upward of 80%, depending on grade of reflux. There is no incision, and it is an outpatient procedure, whereas reimplantation requires a brief hospital stay. There is some evidence that the results may not be durable, with recurrence of reflux over time, so studies are ongoing (Routh, Bogaert, Kaefer, et al., 2012).

Nursing Care Management

The primary nursing goal in children receiving medical therapy is encouraging compliance. Emphasize the importance of maintaining the medical regimen to parents and older children. The medications prescribed are usually well tolerated by children, but parents may need advice regarding encouraging children to take the medication. The methods described in Chapter 22 provide some guidelines for administration and encouraging compliance. The importance of hygiene and a frequent voiding schedule are also discussed. Parents need to know that breakthrough infections can occur despite CAP, so being aware of symptoms of UTI and seeking medical attention are critical.

Because siblings are at risk for VUR, nurses should encourage parents to be aware of this and discuss whether their other children should be screened using renal ultrasonography with cystography if the ultrasound is abnormal. Screening with VCUG was previously recommended for all siblings, but currently it is offered and encouraged if there is a history of UTI in a sibling. Awareness of the increased risk also leads to appropriate assessment of the urine in a child with fever or urinary tract symptoms. All children require age-appropriate preparation for the tests and consideration of use of lidocaine jelly before catheterization. (See Collection of Specimens, Chapter 22.)

GLOMERULAR DISEASE

ACUTE GLOMERULONEPHRITIS

Acute glomerulonephritis (AGN) as a classification includes a number of distinct entities. It may be a primary event or a manifestation of a systemic disorder (Table 24.5), and the disease can range from mild to severe. The common features include oliguria, edema, hypertension and circulatory congestion, hematuria, and proteinuria. Many cases are postinfectious and have been associated with pneumococcal, streptococcal, and viral infections. Postinfectious diseases are presumed to result from immune complex formation and glomerular deposition, and the clinical presentations may be indistinguishable. Postinfectious glomerulonephritis exhibits a better clinical course than other acute proliferative glomerulonephritis.

Acute poststreptococcal glomerulonephritis (APSGN), also known as postinfectious glomerulonephritis, is the most common of the noninfectious renal diseases in childhood although the incidence in developed countries has declined over the past few decades (Stratta, Musetti, Barreca, et al., 2014). APSGN can occur at any age but primarily affects early school-age children, with a median age of onset between 3 and 12 years (Dagan, Cleper, Davidovits, et al., 2016). It is uncommon in children younger than 3 years of age.

TABLE 24.5 Renal Involvement Associated With Systemic Disease Process

Disease	Mechanism	Renal Manifestation	Comments
Systemic lupus erythematosus (SLE)	Deposition of autoantibody-antigen complexes in kidney	Variable degrees of hematuria and proteinuria More severe—Nephrotic syndrome, hypertension, renal insufficiency	Responsive to corticosteroid and antimetabolite therapy Renal failure most common cause of death from SLE Rare before adolescence but may occur in school-age children
Anaphylactoid (Schönlein-Henoch) purpura	Deposition of immunoglobulin (primarily IgA) in the glomerular mesangium	Hematuria (gross or microscopic) Less common—Edema, hypertension, Nephrotic syndrome with oliguria and hypertension, indicate severe involvement Rarely—Acute renal failure	Renal involvement in 20%-70% of cases Renal involvement most serious manifestation of the disease More common in children >6 years old Immunosuppression medication may be beneficial in severe cases
Sickle cell disease	Infarction of renal vessels by sickle cells (especially medullary) Results in decreased circulation in vasa recta and impaired sodium and chloride ion reabsorption in collecting ducts	Hematuria Nephrotic syndrome Defective urine concentration Progressive glomerulonephritis	Irreversible with increasing age Severe urinary tract infections with bacteremia not uncommon
Polyarteritis nodosa	Fibroid necrosis of arterial walls Large vessels—Patchy renal infarction Microscopic vessels—Necrotizing glomerulitis	Proteinuria Hematuria Severe hypertension	Kidney function usually normal, but multiple renal infarcts may decrease renal function
Bacterial endocarditis	Focal or diffuse, immune-complex deposition related to chronic bacteremia Some embolization of glomeruli by bacteria and fibrin from endocardial vegetations	Proteinuria Hematuria	Renal involvement seen in approximately 50% of cases Renal involvement seldom of major significance
Prolonged bacteremia (infected atrioventricular shunts)	Immune-complex deposition with exudation and cellular proliferation	Variable degrees of persistent nephrotic syndrome	Vigorous antibiotic therapy or removal of infected shunt required

IgA, Immunoglobulin A.

Etiology

It is generally accepted that APSGN is an immune-complex disease—that is, a reaction that occurs as a by-product of an antecedent streptococcal infection with certain strains of the group A β-hemolytic streptococci, although other bacteria and viruses have also been implicated (VanDe-Voorde, 2015). Most streptococcal infections do not cause APSGN. A latent period of 1 to 2 weeks occurs between a streptococcal infection of the throat, or 3 to 6 weeks between a skin infection and the onset of clinical manifestations. The peak incidence of disease corresponds to the incidence of streptococcal infections. Disease secondary to streptococcal pharyngitis is more common in the winter or spring. However, when associated with pyoderma (principally impetigo), it may be more prevalent in late summer or early fall, especially in warmer climates. Multiple cases tend to occur in families. Second attacks are rare.

Pathophysiology

The mechanism by which the reaction takes place is still speculative. One proposal to explain the pathologic process is that the streptococcal infection is followed by the release of a membrane-like material from the specific organism into the circulation. Because it is antigenic, antibodies are formed and an immune-complex reaction occurs after the appropriate period. These immune complexes become trapped in the glomerular capillary loop.

The kidney itself appears normal or moderately enlarged, but microscopic examination reveals a diffuse proliferative and exudative process. Glomerular capillary loops are almost obliterated by swelling, and infiltration with polymorphonuclear leukocytes adds to the appearance of increased cellularity. Consequently, the glomeruli appear dense and lobulated. Examination with the electron microscope reveals discrete nodules or "humps" in the basement membrane, which is identified as deposits of immune complexes. These deposits are not evident after approximately 6 weeks.

Endothelial cell proliferation and edema occlude the capillary lumen of affected glomeruli, and the afferent arteriole is probably constricted by vasospasm, both of which significantly reduce the glomerular filtration rate. This occurs without a proportional decrease in renal blood flow and results in a reduced capacity to form filtrate from the glomerular plasma flow. Vascular and tubular changes are mild and nonspecific; therefore tubular function is less severely impaired.

The decreased filtration of plasma results in an excessive accumulation of water and retention of sodium. These cause expanded plasma and interstitial fluid volumes that lead to circulatory congestion, edema and hypertension. It is unclear whether a decreased glomerular filtration rate, increased capillary permeability, or vascular spasm is responsible for these various manifestations.

Clinical Manifestations

Typically, affected children are in good health until they experience the antecedent infection. In some instances there is no history of an infection, or it is described as only a mild cold. The onset of nephritis appears after a latent period. Because the child appears well during this time, parents may not recognize the association.

Initial signs of nephritic reaction include puffiness of the face, especially around the eyes (periorbital edema); anorexia; and the passage

TABLE 24.6 Comparison of Poststreptococcal Glomerulonephritis and Nephrotic Syndrome

Manifestations	Acute Poststreptococcal Glomerulonephritis	Minimal Change Nephrotic Syndrome
Streptococcal antibody titers	Elevated	Normal
Blood pressure	Elevated	Normal or decreased
Edema	Primarily periorbital and peripheral	Generalized, severe
Circulatory congestion	Common	Absent
Proteinuria	Mild to moderate	Massive
Hematuria	Gross or microscopic	Microscopic or none
Red blood cell casts	Present	Absent
Azotemia	Present	Absent
Serum potassium levels	Normal or increased	Normal
Serum protein levels	Minimum reduction	Markedly decreased
Serum lipid levels	Normal	Elevated
Peak age at onset (yr)	5-7	2-3

of cola-colored urine. The edema is more prominent in the face in the morning but spreads during the day to involve the extremities, genitalia, and abdomen. The edema is usually only moderate and may not be appreciated by someone unfamiliar with the child's normal appearance. The urine is cloudy, smoky brown, or what parents describe as resembling tea or cola, and it is severely reduced in volume.

! NURSING ALERT

Evaluate a child who exhibits the following for possible AGN:

- Periorbital, gonadal, abdominal, or lower extremity edema
- Loss of appetite
- Decreased urinary output
- Cola- or tea-colored urine
- Antecedent streptococcal infection (other bacteria and viruses may also be responsible)

The child is pale, irritable, and lethargic and appears unwell but seldom expresses specific complaints. Older children may complain of headaches, abdominal discomfort, or dysuria. On examination there is usually a mild to moderate elevation in blood pressure compared with normal values for age, although severe hypertension may be present. Occasionally a child will have an onset with severe symptoms such as seizures from hypertensive encephalopathy, pulmonary and circulatory congestion, or hematuria in the absence of hypertension and edema. Table 24.6 compares APSGN and minimal change nephrotic syndrome (MCNS).

Clinical Course. The acute edematous phase of glomerulonephritis usually persists from 4 to 10 days but may persist for 2 or 3 weeks, during which time the child remains listless, anorexic, and apathetic. The weight fluctuates, the urine remains smoky brown, and the blood pressure may suddenly reach dangerously high levels at any time during this phase.

The first sign of improvement is an increase in urinary output with a corresponding decrease in body weight as edema resolves. With diuresis the child begins to feel better, the appetite improves, and the blood pressure decreases to normal. Gross hematuria diminishes, however microscopic hematuria and proteinuria may persist for months to years (Dagan, Cleper, Davidovits, et al., 2016). Renal function and hypocomplementemia usually normalize by 8 weeks.

Prognosis. Almost all children correctly diagnosed as having APSGN recover completely, and specific immunity is conferred so that subsequent recurrences are uncommon (Kim, 2016). Deaths from complications can occur but fortunately are rare. A few children may develop chronic kidney disease.

Complications. The major complications that may develop during the acute phase of glomerulonephritis are hypertensive encephalopathy, acute cardiac decompensation, and acute kidney injury (AKI). Normally, cerebral blood flow responds to acute arterial hypertension by vasoconstriction. However, acute and severe hypertension may cause this protective autoregulation of cerebral blood flow to fail, leading to hyperperfusion of the brain and cerebral edema. The premonitory signs of encephalopathy are headache, dizziness, abdominal discomfort, and vomiting. If the condition progresses, there may be transient loss of vision or hemiparesis, disorientation, and generalized tonic-clonic seizures.

Hypervolemia, not cardiac failure, causes cardiac decompensation during the acute edematous phase of nephritis. However, signs of circulatory congestion are evident. The heart is enlarged, and increased pulmonary vascular markings are evident on x-ray examination. Increased pulmonary capillary permeability is also believed to be an important factor in the development of pulmonary edema. AKI with persistent oliguria or anuria is an uncommon complication but one that requires an appropriate treatment regimen.

Diagnostic Evaluation

Urinalysis during the acute phase characteristically shows hematuria, proteinuria, and increased specific gravity. Proteinuria generally parallels the hematuria but is not usually the massive proteinuria seen in nephrotic syndrome. Gross discoloration of urine reflects its red blood cell and hemoglobin content. Microscopic examination of the sediment shows many red blood cells, leukocytes, epithelial cells, and granular and red blood cell casts. Bacteria are not seen, and urine cultures are negative.

Cultures of the pharynx are positive for streptococci in only a few cases, and the numbers are not significantly greater than the normal carrier incidence in many communities. Positive cultures help establish a diagnosis. Cultures should be obtained from other household members, and persons positive for group A streptococci should receive a course of antistreptococcal therapy.

Unless the disease has progressed to renal failure, the blood examination reveals normal electrolyte (sodium, potassium, and chloride ions) and carbon dioxide levels. Azotemia resulting from impaired glomerular filtration is reflected in elevated blood urea nitrogen (BUN) and creatinine levels in at least 50% of cases. When proteinuria is heavy, there may be changes associated with nephrotic syndrome (i.e., transient hypoproteinemia and hyperlipidemia).

Serologic tests are needed for diagnosis. Antibody responses to the extracellular products of the streptococci provide indirect evidence of previous streptococcal infection. These include antistreptolysin O (ASO), antistreptokinase (ASKase), antihyaluronidase (AHase), antideoxyribonuclease B (ADNase-B), and antinicotyladenine dinucleotidase (ANADase). The ASO titer is the most familiar and readily available test for streptococcal antibodies. ASO appears in the serum approximately 10 days after the initial infection; however, there is no correlation between the degree of elevation and the severity or prognosis of the glomerulonephritis. It is a useful diagnostic tool when nephritis follows a pharyngeal infection but is of less value after pyoderma. An ASO titer of 250 Todd units or higher is of diagnostic significance, as is a rising titer in two samples taken 1 week apart. More consistent and reliable antibody tests after streptococcal skin infections are elevated AHase and ADNase-B titers.

Of more importance for clinical serologic diagnosis is measurement of the C3 serum complement level. The serum C3 level is decreased initially but returns to normal within 8 to 10 weeks after onset of the glomerulonephritis. Other studies include a chest x-ray examination, which shows characteristic generalized cardiac enlargement, pulmonary congestion, and pleural effusion during the edematous phase of acute disease. Renal biopsy for diagnostic purposes is seldom required but may be useful in the diagnosis of atypical cases.

Therapeutic Management

No specific treatment is available for APSGN. Recovery is spontaneous and uneventful in most cases. Management consists of general supportive measures and early recognition and treatment of complications. Children who have normal blood pressure and a satisfactory urinary output can generally be treated at home but must be closely monitored. Those with substantial edema, hypertension, gross hematuria, or significant oliguria are often hospitalized because of the unpredictability of complications. Short hospitalization may be necessary in uncomplicated cases; prolonged hospitalization is required only for children with severely impaired renal function.

General Measures. Bed rest is not necessary during the acute phase because ambulation does not seem to have an adverse effect on the course of the disease. Because they are generally listless and experience fatigue and malaise, most children voluntarily restrict their activities during the most active phase of the disease.

Fluid Balance. Regular measurement of vital signs, body weight, and intake and output is essential to monitor the disease's progress and detect complications that may appear at any time during the course of the disease. A record of daily weight is the most useful means to assess fluid balance and should be kept for children treated at home and for those who are hospitalized. Sodium and water restriction is useful when the output is significantly reduced (<2 to 3 dl/24 hr). In these children the water allowed is equivalent to the calculated insensible loss plus the volume of urine excreted.

Diuretics are of limited value when severe renal failure is present because little sodium reaches the distal tubules as a result of the reduced filtration rate. However, when renal failure is not severe, diuretic therapy (usually furosemide [Lasix]) is helpful if significant edema and fluid overload are present. Rarely, children with ASPGN develop AKI with oliguria that significantly alters the fluid and electrolyte balance. These children require careful management that may include peritoneal dialysis (PD) or hemodialysis (HD).

Loss of glomerular filtration in children with severe forms of APSGN may produce electrolyte imbalances, especially hyperkalemia, acidosis, hypocalcemia, and hyperphosphatemia. Management of these electrolyte disturbances is described under Acute Kidney Injury.

Hypertension. Acute hypertension must be anticipated and identified early. Blood pressure measurements are taken at least every 4 to 6 hours. Significant but not severe hypertension is controlled with thiazide or loop diuretics. Other antihypertensive drugs, such as calcium channel blockers, beta blockers, or angiotensin-converting enzyme inhibitors, may be needed in severe cases. Seizure activity associated with hypertensive encephalopathy requires anticonvulsant therapy and antihypertensive agents (see Renal Failure, p. 802, for management of severe hypertension).

Nutrition. Dietary restrictions depend on the stage and severity of the disease, especially the extent of edema. A regular diet is permitted in uncomplicated cases, but sodium intake is usually limited (no salt is added to foods) for children with hypertension or edema. Foods with substantial amounts of potassium are generally restricted during the period of oliguria. Protein restriction is reserved only for children with severe azotemia resulting from prolonged oliguria. The loss of appetite associated with the disease usually limits the protein intake sufficiently.

Antibiotics. Antibiotic therapy is indicated only for those children with evidence of persistent streptococcal infections. Antibiotics do not alter the course of the disease but are often recommended to prevent transmission of nephritogenic streptococci to other family members. Authorities are divided on the use of prophylactic antimicrobials for other family members.

Nursing Care Management. Nursing care of the child with glomerulonephritis involves careful assessment of the disease status, with regular monitoring of vital signs (including frequent measurement of blood pressure), fluid balance, and behavior. Vital signs provide clues to the severity of the disease and early signs of complications. The nurse carefully measures them and records and reports any abnormalities. The nurse notes the volume and character of urine and weighs the child daily. Assessment of the child's appearance for signs of cerebral complications is an important nursing function because the severity of the acute phase is variable and unpredictable. The child with edema, hypertension, and gross hematuria may be subject to complications, and anticipatory preparations are important nursing care responsibilities.

For most children a regular diet is allowed but should contain no added salt. Foods high in sodium and salted treats are eliminated, and the nurse should advise parents and friends against bringing items such as potato chips or pretzels. However, the total amount of salt ingested is usually less than prescribed because of poor appetite. Fluid restriction, if prescribed, is more difficult; the amount permitted should be evenly divided throughout the waking hours and served in small cups to give the illusion of larger servings. Meal preparation and service require special attention because the child has a poor appetite and is indifferent to meals during the acute phase. Collaboration with parents and the dietitian and special consideration for food preferences will facilitate meal planning.

During the acute phase children are generally content to lie in bed. As they begin to feel better and their symptoms subside, they will want to be up and about. Activities should be planned to allow for frequent rest periods and avoidance of fatigue.

Children with mild edema and no hypertension, as well as convalescent children being treated at home, need follow-up care. Parents are instructed regarding general measures, including activity, diet, and prevention of infection. Strenuous activity is usually restricted until there is no evidence of proteinuria or macroscopic hematuria. Health supervision is continued with weekly, followed by monthly, visits for evaluation and urinalysis. Parent education and support in preparation for discharge and home care include education in home management and the need for follow-up care and health supervision.

CHRONIC OR PROGRESSIVE GLOMERULONEPHRITIS

The majority of cases of renal glomerular disease are AGN, MCNS, and glomerulonephritis associated with systemic diseases. These pose relatively few problems of diagnosis, and their natural course is fairly predictable. Some result in a prolonged course and a poor ultimate prognosis. They are defined by correlating the clinical manifestations, pathologic conditions, and natural course of the individual diseases.

Chronic glomerulonephritis (CGN) describes a variety of different disease processes that may be distinguished from one another by renal biopsy. These include membranoproliferative glomerulonephritis (MPGN), membranous glomerulonephritis, focal segmental glomerulosclerosis (FSGS), and immunoglobulin A nephropathy (IgA nephropathy). In CGN tissue damage and progression to fibrosis are related to the immune response that brings about inflammation, failure to activate glomerular repair, and excessive fibrogenic activity *Rapidly progressive glomerulonephritis* is the term used to describe an acute illness with severe, acute onset that causes rapidly progressive deterioration of renal function in weeks to months. Renal biopsy of these patients shows a variety of diseases, with the common feature of greater than 50% glomerular crescents found in the biopsy section.

Pathophysiology

In most cases of CGN, immunologic mechanisms can be implicated either through direct attack on the kidney or secondary to the accumulation of immune complexes in the glomerular filter or fibrin deposition from previously damaged glomeruli. Either can contribute to further glomerular damage and can initiate chronic changes in the glomerular structure (Niaudet, 2016a). In many cases there is no history of an acute glomerular disease. In other cases CGN may represent one of a succession of exacerbations of a preexisting disease. CGN that is not associated with other diseases may go undetected for years and be relatively asymptomatic until kidney destruction produces marked reduction in renal function. Consequently, the disease is more common in adolescents than in younger children. Renal insufficiency with all its manifestations occurs as the ultimate event.

Clinical Manifestations

Early in the disease, clinical symptoms may be limited to proteinuria or microscopic hematuria detected on a routine examination. Laboratory findings may indicate decreased renal function. Nephrotic range proteinuria may be present. Symptoms vary based on the cause for the CGN but may include hypertension, edema, intermittent gross hematuria, and other manifestations of chronic kidney disease.

Diagnostic Evaluation

Laboratory findings may include proteinuria, with casts and red and white blood cells. Elevated BUN, creatinine, and uric acid levels are evidence of decreased renal function. Electrolyte alterations include metabolic acidosis, elevated potassium, elevated phosphorus, and decreased calcium levels. The renal insufficiency may extend from 5 to 15 years and even longer, or rapid deterioration may progress to end-stage renal disease (ESRD).

Therapeutic Management

Early in the course of the disease, treatment is appropriate to the underlying disease and is largely symptomatic in most cases. Nursing efforts should be directed toward providing optimum conditions for the child's physical, psychologic, and social development. As few restrictions as feasible should be imposed, and the child should be allowed to live as normal a life as possible for as long as possible. Some forms of CGN are treated with corticosteroids or cytotoxic agents. Marked hypertension is controlled with antihypertensive agents, and anemia may require recombinant erythropoietin and iron supplements. Ultimately, dialysis or transplantation may be needed to restore relatively good health; however, these alternatives are reserved until renal failure is far advanced. (See Chronic Kidney Disease, p. 806 for more detailed management of specific problems.) Children with rapidly progressive glomerulonephritis should be referred to a center specializing in renal disease.

Nursing Care Management

The problems of CGN and those encountered in chronic renal insufficiency from any cause are discussed under Chronic Renal Failure.

NEPHROTIC SYNDROME

Nephrotic syndrome is the most common presentation of glomerular injury in children. It is defined as massive proteinuria, hypoalbuminemia, hyperlipidemia, and edema and is a clinical manifestation of a large number of distinct glomerular disorders in which increased glomerular permeability to plasma protein results in massive urinary protein loss. After a description of the three major forms of nephrotic syndrome, the remainder of the discussion is devoted to minimal change disease (also known as idiopathic nephrosis, minimal lesion nephrosis, nil disease, childhood nephrosis, lipoid nephrosis, or uncomplicated nephrosis).

Types of Nephrotic Syndrome

Nephrotic syndrome can be classified as primary, when the syndrome is restricted to glomerular injury, or secondary, when it develops as part of a systemic illness. Although it may have several different histologic variations, the most common form of the primary disease is MCNS. A congenital form is also recognized.

Minimal Change Nephrotic Syndrome. Approximately 80% of cases of nephrotic syndrome in children result from MCNS. MCNS can be seen at any age but is predominantly a disease of the preschool child. Diagnosis of MCNS is rare in children younger than 6 months of age, uncommon in infants younger than 1 year of age, and unusual after the age of 8 years. The incidence of the disease in the United States is approximately 2 to 7 per 100,000 children per year. In younger children males outnumber females 2:1. In adolescence the ratio is 1:1 (Lane, 2016).

A nonspecific illness, usually a viral upper respiratory tract infection, often precedes the manifestations by 4 to 8 days but is considered to be a precipitating factor rather than a cause.

Secondary Nephrotic Syndrome. Nephrotic syndrome may occur after or in association with glomerular damage of known or presumed cause. Prominent among causes of glomerular damage is AGN or CGN. Less commonly, secondary nephrotic syndrome occurs during the course of collagen vascular diseases (such as disseminated lupus erythematosus or anaphylactoid purpura) or as a result of toxicity to drugs (such as trimethadione and heavy metals), stings, or venom. Nephrotic syndrome

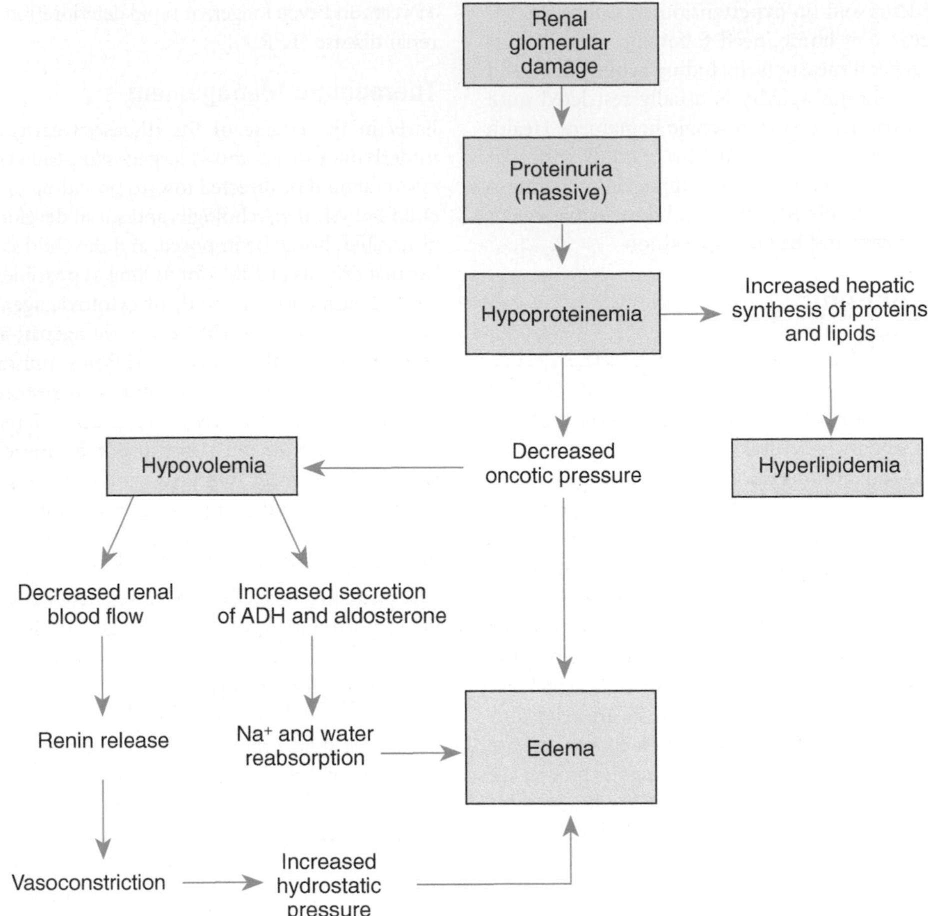

FIG. 24.3 Sequence of events in nephrotic syndrome. *ADH,* Antidiuretic hormone.

is the major presenting symptom of renal disease in pediatric patients with acquired immunodeficiency syndrome. Rare causes are sickle cell disease, hepatitis, malaria, cyanotic heart disease, tuberculosis, infected ventriculojugular shunts, renal vein thrombosis, or malignancies.

Congenital Nephrotic Syndrome–Finnish Type. A recessive gene on an autosome causes the hereditary form of nephrotic syndrome. Infants who have congenital nephrotic syndrome–Finnish type are small for gestational age, and proteinuria and edema manifest within the first few days to months of age. The disease does not respond to the usual therapy. Death in the first year or two of life is possible if the infant does not receive treatment, including IV administration of albumin, nutritional support, dialysis, or a kidney transplant (Spahiu, Merovci, Jashari, et al., 2016).

Pathophysiology

The pathogenesis of MCNS is not completely understood. A metabolic, biochemical, or physiochemical disturbance in the basement membrane of the glomeruli may lead to increased permeability to protein, but the causes and mechanisms are only speculative

The glomerular membrane, which is normally impermeable to albumin and other large proteins, becomes permeable to proteins, especially albumin, that leak through the membrane and are lost in urine (hyperalbuminuria). This reduces the serum albumin level (hypoalbuminemia), which decreases the COP in the capillaries As a result, the hydrostatic pressure exceeds the pull of the COP, and fluid accumulates in the interstitial spaces and body cavities, particularly the abdominal cavity (ascites). The shift of fluid from the plasma to the interstitial spaces reduces the vascular fluid volume (hypovolemia), which in turn stimulates the renin-angiotensin system and the secretion of antidiuretic hormone and aldosterone. Tubular reabsorption of sodium and water increases in an attempt to increase intravascular volume. The elevation of serum cholesterol, phospholipids, and triglycerides is not fully understood. The sequence of events in nephrotic syndrome is shown in Fig. 24.3.

Clinical Manifestations

A previously well child begins to gain weight, which progresses over a period of days or weeks. Puffiness of the face, especially around the eyes, is apparent on arising in the morning but subsides during the day, when swelling of the abdomen, genitalia, and lower extremities is more prominent. Generalized edema (anasarca) may develop gradually or rapidly. Edema of the intestinal mucosa may cause diarrhea, loss of appetite, and poor intestinal absorption. The volume of urine is decreased, and it appears darkly opalescent and frothy.

The child often has extreme skin pallor and may experience skin breakdown during periods of severe edema. The child may be irritable and more easily fatigued or lethargic but does not appear seriously ill. Weight loss from poor appetite and loss of protein is not uncommon, although it is often obscured by edema. Changes in the nails appear as white (Muehrcke) lines parallel to the lunula, which are caused by prolonged hypoalbuminemia. The blood pressure is usually normal or slightly decreased. The child is more susceptible to infection, especially cellulitis, pneumonia, peritonitis, or sepsis.

> **! NURSING ALERT**
>
> Evaluate a child who exhibits the following for the possibility of nephrotic syndrome:
> - Periorbital, abdominal, gonadal, or lower extremity edema
> - Weight gain greater than that expected based on previous pattern
> - Decreased urinary output
> - Pallor, fatigue

In rare cases children with MCNS have significant or persistent hypertension, gross or persistent hematuria, or significant or persistent azotemia (i.e., increased nitrogenous products in the blood).

Diagnostic Evaluation

The diagnosis of MCNS in children is based on the history and clinical manifestations (e.g., edema, proteinuria, hypoalbuminemia, and hypercholesterolemia in the absence of significant hematuria and hypertension). Massive proteinuria is reflected in urinary excretion of protein that often reaches levels in excess of 2 g/m^2 of body surface/day, with relatively greater clearance of low-molecular-weight proteins. Hyaline casts from high protein levels and sluggish flow and oval fat bodies, as well as a few red blood cells, can be found in the urine of most affected children, although there is seldom gross hematuria. Specific gravity is high and proportionate to the amount of protein concentration. If hypovolemia is not significant and the child is well hydrated, the glomerular filtration rate is usually normal.

Total serum protein concentrations are reduced, with the albumin fractions significantly reduced (<2 g/dl) and plasma lipids elevated. Serum cholesterol may be as high as 450 to 1500 mg/dl. Hemoglobin and hematocrit are usually normal or elevated, and the platelet count is high (500,000 to 1,000,000/mm^3) as a result of hemoconcentration. Serum sodium concentration is usually low, approximately 130 to 135 mEq/L. Total calcium levels are low due to albumin binding, so ionized calcium is a more reliable measure of calcium levels.

If renal biopsy is performed, it provides information regarding the glomerular status and type of nephrotic syndrome, the likely response to drugs, and the probable course of the disease. Under the microscope the foot processes of the basement membrane appear fused in a child with MCNS. The major focuses in differential diagnosis are to establish the edema as renal in origin and to distinguish MCNS from other glomerulopathies with nephrotic syndrome as a manifestation.

Therapeutic Management

Medical management consists of both immunosuppressive and nonimmunosuppresive measures. The primary objective is to reduce the excretion of urinary protein and maintain protein-free urine. Additional objectives include prevention or treatment of acute infection, control of edema, establishment of good nutrition, and readjustment of any disturbed metabolic processes. Children with severe symptoms may be hospitalized for assessment and observation for evidence of infection, response to therapy, and parental education.

General Measures. General treatment is principally supportive. During the edema phase the child is often limited to quiet activities. Acute and intercurrent infections are treated with appropriate antibiotics, and providers make efforts to minimize the risk of infection. In addition to the usual vaccinations, children with nephrotic syndrome should receive the pneumococcal conjugate vaccine (PCV13) and pneumococcal polysaccharide vaccine (PPSV23). Live vaccines should not be given while the child is on steroid therapy (Banerjee, Dissanayake, & Abeyagunawardena, 2016).

Diet. The child in remission maintains a regular diet. However, salt is restricted during periods of massive edema and while on corticosteroid therapy; no salt is added at the table, and foods with very high salt content are excluded. Although a low-sodium diet will not remove edema, its rate of increase may be reduced. Water is seldom restricted. A diet generous in protein is logical, but there is no evidence that it is beneficial or alters the outcome of the disease. The presence of azotemia and renal failure is a contraindication for high-protein intake.

Corticosteroid Therapy. The response of most affected children to corticosteroids has established these drugs as the primary therapeutic agents in the management of nephrotic syndrome. Corticosteroid therapy begins as soon as the diagnosis has been determined and is administered orally in a dosage of 60 mg/m^2/day (with a maximum dose of 60 mg/day). Prednisone is the steroid of choice. The drug is continued daily for 4 to 6 weeks and then reduced to 40 mg/m^2 (with a maximum dose of 40 mg) on alternate days for 2 to 5 months with taper (Lombel, Gipson, & Hodson, 2013). Studies suggest that the duration of steroid treatment for the initial episode should be at least 3 months.

The course of the disease is fairly predictable. There is little change during the first few days of therapy. In most patients, diuresis occurs as the urinary protein excretion diminishes within 7 to 21 days after the initiation of steroid therapy. Other clinical manifestations stabilize or return to normal shortly thereafter. Approximately 90% of patients will achieve remission during the initial course of prednisone treatment. If the child has not responded to therapy within 28 days of daily steroid administration, the likelihood of subsequent response diminishes.

Children with MCNS are often described according to their response to corticosteroid therapy (Box 24.6). Children with MCNS typically relapse one to three times per year. Steroid-dependent children tend to have frequent relapses over many years and receive large amounts of steroids, which results in cushingoid features and may cause growth retardation. They may also require supportive treatment (e.g., diuretics, diet). Steroid-resistant children are thought to have a high risk of developing chronic kidney disease (Lombel, Hodson, & Gipson, 2013).

> **DRUG ALERT**
>
> ***Steroids***
>
> Children who require frequent courses of steroid therapy are highly susceptible to complications of steroids, such as growth retardation, behavior changes, cataracts, increased appetite, obesity, hypertension, gastrointestinal bleeding, bone demineralization, infections, and hyperglycemia. Children who do not respond to steroid therapy, those who have frequent relapses, and those in whom the side effects threaten their growth and general health may be considered for a course of therapy using other immunosuppressant medications.

BOX 24.6 Classification of Nephrotic Syndrome According to Steroid Response

Steroid sensitive—Responds to steroids; relapses may occur after illness

Frequent relapse—Two or more relapses within 6 months of initial response; four or more relapses within a 12-month period

Steroid dependent—Two consecutive relapses while on steroid therapy or within 2 weeks of steroid cessation

Steroid resistant—Does not enter remission after 4 weeks of prednisone therapy

Modified from Bagga, A., & Mantan, M. (2005). Nephrotic syndrome in children. *Indian Journal of Medical Research, 122,* 13-28.

Immunosuppressant Therapy. It is possible to reduce the relapse rate and induce long-term remission in children with frequent relapsing or steroid-resistant nephrotic syndrome with the administration of an oral alkylating agent, usually cyclophosphamide (Cytoxan) given orally for 12 weeks (Niaudet, 2016b). Prolonged courses of cyclosporine or mycophenolate mofetil reduce the risk of relapse in children compared with corticosteroids alone (Lombel, Hodson, & Gipson, 2013).

Rituximab, a monoclonal antibody, has been shown to be an effective treatment for some children with steroid resistant/dependent or frequently relapsing nephrotic syndrome (Iijima, Sako, & Nozu, 2016).

The nurse and family must be aware of the potential side effects associated with the use of the immunosuppressant drugs. Complications associated with the use of cyclophosphamide include neutropenia, infection, gonadal toxicity, malignancy, and hemorrhagic cystitis. Cyclosproine and mycophenolate mofetil can cause nephrotoxicity and an increased risk of infections. Close monitoring of children on these medications is critical.

Diuretics. Oral diuretics may have a blunted effectiveness in treating the edema of nephrotic syndrome (Ellis, 2016). Loop diuretics, usually furosemide, alone or in combination with metolazone, are sometimes useful in cases in which edema interferes with respiration or ambulation or there is hypertension or significant edema in the scrotum or labia. In addition, plasma expanders such as salt-poor human albumin may be administered to severely edematous children requiring prompt control; however, they must be administered frequently because the glomeruli are readily permeable to albumin in the acute stage.

Prognosis. The prognosis for ultimate recovery in most cases is good. For children who respond to steroid therapy the tendency to relapse decreases with time. With early detection and prompt implementation of therapy to eradicate proteinuria, progressive basement membrane damage is minimized so that renal function is usually normal or near normal when the tendency for relapses is past. It is estimated that approximately 80% of affected children have this favorable prognosis, although more than 20% will continue to have relapses in adulthood (Hjorten, Anwar, & Reidy, 2016). (See Quality Patient Outcomes box.)

QUALITY PATIENT OUTCOMES

Nephrotic Syndrome

- Protein-free urine
- Acute infections prevented
- Edema absent or minimal
- Nutrition maintained
- Metabolic abnormalities controlled

Nursing Care Management

Daily monitoring of intake and output is an important nursing function. Strict and accurate measurement is essential but may be difficult in very young children. In these cases the nurse can measure for output by methods such as weighing diapers. Other methods of monitoring progress include examination of the urine for albumin, daily weight, and measurement of abdominal girth. Assessment of edema, such as increased or decreased swelling around the eyes and dependent areas, the degree of pitting (if noted), and color and texture of the skin, is part of nursing care. The nurse monitors vital signs to detect any early signs of complications such as shock or an infectious process.

In children hospitalized with MCNS, elevating edematous parts may be helpful to shift fluid to more comfortable distributions, but diuresis with medications and salt and water restriction to remove edema fluid are the best therapies. Areas that are particularly edematous, such as the scrotum, abdomen, and legs, may require support. Clean skin surfaces and separate them with clothing, cotton, or antiseptic powder to prevent intertrigo.

Because these children are particularly vulnerable to upper respiratory tract infection, protect them from contact with infected roommates, family, or visitors. Spontaneous peritonitis can occur secondary to migration of intestinal bacteria across the bowel wall and into the peritoneum. Monitor vital signs to detect any early signs of an infectious process.

Loss of appetite that accompanies active nephrosis creates a perplexing problem for nurses. During this time the combined efforts of the nurse, dietitian, parents, and child are necessary to formulate a nutritionally adequate and attractive diet. Small, frequent meals may be best tolerated. Salt and fluids are restricted during the edema phase. (See Feeding the Sick Child, Chapter 22.)

As the edema subsides, children are allowed increased fluids. Suitable recreational and diversional activities are also an important part of their care. Once the edema fluid has been lost, children can usually resume their normal activities without problems. Irritability and mood swings accompanying the disease process and steroid therapy are not unusual manifestations in these children and create an additional challenge to the nurse and the family.

Family Support and Home Care. Most children are treated at home during relapses unless the edema and proteinuria are severe. Teach parents to detect signs of relapse and to notify the health care provider if they occur. Nurses should instruct parents in urine testing for albumin, administration of medications, and general care. Urine is usually tested

CRITICAL THINKING CASE STUDY

Nephrotic Syndrome

Reese is an 8-year-old boy with relapsing nephrotic syndrome who has become steroid dependent. During your initial assessment in the outpatient clinic, you identify the following: (1) weight has increased 2 kg (4.4 lb) in the past 2 weeks; (2) blood pressure is 100/70 mm Hg; (3) mother reports that Reese is not urinating very much, and she does not know how much he has been drinking; (4) while you are measuring Reese's abdominal girth, he guards his abdomen and complains of a stomachache; and (5) his temperature is 38°C (100.4°F) orally.

Questions

1. What evidence should you consider regarding Reese's condition?
2. What additional information is required at this time? Which of the following actions should you do first?
   a. Examine Reese's abdomen, while eliciting from his mother a thorough history of illness symptoms for the past 24 hours.
   b. Elicit a 24-hour recall of food and fluid intake from both Reese and his mother.
   c. Obtain a clean-catch urine specimen. Divide the specimen so you can perform a dipstick analysis immediately, and retain the rest of the specimen for possible urinalysis and culture after consultation with the primary health practitioner.
   d. Explore the mother's understanding of Reese's illness and its relationship to his current condition to begin outlining your teaching plan for this family.
3. List the nursing interventions that have the highest priority.
4. Identify important patient-centered outcomes with reference to your nursing interventions.

Answers are available at http://evolve.elsevier.com/wong/ncic.

daily for albumin while the child is receiving medicine for nephrotic syndrome or if the child has an illness, and twice a week during remission. Salt is restricted to no additional salt during relapse and steroid therapy, but a regular diet is suitable for the child in remission. Nurses should instruct parents regarding avoiding contact with infected playmates, but the child may attend school. It is important for parents of children on corticosteroid therapy to be aware of the common side effects of steroid therapy (e.g., rounding of the face, increased appetite, behavior changes, abdominal distention, and hirsutism) and to distinguish some of these from the edema formation of the disease. Reassure parents that the symptoms will disappear gradually after discontinuation of the drug. The child should receive close medical or nursing observation to detect unusual but more serious side effects (see Critical Thinking Case Study box).

The prolonged course of the relapsing form of nephrotic syndrome is taxing to both the child and the family. In the worst cases of frequent remissions and relapses with periodic disruption of family life by hospitalization, a severe strain is placed on the child and the family, both psychologically and financially. Parents of children with frequent relapses who respond poorly to medications need reassurance regarding this characteristic of the disease so they do not become discouraged. At the same time, impress on them the importance of long-term care to gain their cooperation. A satisfactory response is more likely when relapses are detected and therapy is instituted early, and remissions are prolonged when instructions are carried out faithfully. For example, stopping the prednisone before completion of treatment because the edema has resolved increases the risk of relapse.

Social isolation may be a problem for these children. Isolation is related to frequent hospitalization or confinement during relapse, the risk of infection that may precipitate an exacerbation, lack of energy, and the child's reluctance to face friends at home or school because of the changes in appearance resulting from the disease or the medication. Both the parents and the child need someone to listen to their complaints, to assist them in coping with both short- and long-term problems associated with the disease, and to find solutions to their problems. Continuous support of the child and family is one of the major nursing considerations.

RENAL TUBULAR DISORDERS

Disorders of renal tubular function include a variety of conditions involving one or more abnormalities in specific mechanisms of tubular transport or reabsorption. Glomerular function is normal or mildly impaired. Eventually more widespread kidney destruction with renal failure may occur. In some cases the dysfunction has little, if any, effect on renal function. These disorders may be permanent or transient and may originate as primary defects or arise as a secondary effect of metabolic disease or exogenous toxins. Renal tubular disorders may be congenital (usually displaying characteristic patterns of genetic transmission), appear without evidence of hereditary transmission, or be acquired as a result of known or unknown causes.

Unlike the classic manifestations of glomerular diseases, edema and hypertension are absent, and the BUN level and routine urinalysis are usually normal. Tubular proteinuria may be demonstrated. Manifestations of tubular disorders are primarily metabolic disturbances or deficiencies, such as failure to thrive, metabolic bone disease, or persistent acidosis. The variety of these disorders is extensive, and the incidence is rare.

TUBULAR FUNCTION

The function of the proximal tubules is the reabsorption of substances from the glomerular filtrate, including sodium, potassium, chloride, bicarbonate, glucose, phosphate, and amino acids. A number of disorders feature impairment of reabsorption of one or more filtrate constituents, and most involve defects in the transport mechanisms for these substances. Impaired tubular reabsorption of any specific substance causes that substance to appear in the urine, sometimes with reduced levels in the blood. Examples include bicarbonate and phosphate.

The primary functions of the distal renal tubules are acidification of urine; potassium secretion; and selective and differential reabsorption of sodium, chloride, and water, which determines the final urinary concentration. Because the contribution of the distal tubule to urine composition depends in part on the volume and composition of the filtrate from the proximal tubule, the net contribution of the distal tubule is related to proximal tubular function and glomerular filtration.

RENAL TUBULAR ACIDOSIS

Renal tubular acidosis (RTA) is a syndrome of sustained metabolic acidosis in which there is impaired reabsorption of bicarbonate or excretion of net hydrogen ion but in which glomerular function is normal. On the basis of underlying pathophysiology, renal tubular acidosis is divided into proximal renal tubular acidosis and distal renal tubular acidosis. Proximal renal tubular acidosis results from a defect in bicarbonate reabsorption, whereas distal renal tubular acidosis results from an inability to establish an adequate gradient of pH between blood and tubular fluid. A number of genetic abnormalities have been identified for all types of primary RTA (Santos, Ordóñez, Claramunt-Taberner, et al., 2015).

Proximal Tubular Acidosis (Type II)

Impaired bicarbonate reabsorption in the proximal tubule causes proximal tubular acidosis. It may occur as an isolated defect (primary), but more often it appears in association with other proximal tubular disorders (secondary). As a result of a depressed renal threshold, bicarbonate reabsorption in the proximal tubule is incomplete, causing the plasma concentration of bicarbonate to stabilize at a lower level than normal. This results in a hyperchloremic metabolic acidosis. There is no impairment of distal tubular integrity or, in most cases, of the distal acidifying mechanism.

A more complex abnormality in the proximal tubules is Fanconi syndrome, in which transport mechanisms are damaged by the accumulation of toxic metabolites or the tubular epithelium is damaged by heavy metals such as lead, cadmium, or platinum. Fanconi syndrome can be part of a number of hereditary diseases, be acquired, or be idiopathic (with a cause that is not identifiable). The major clinical manifestation and presenting symptom of Fanconi syndrome is growth failure. Tachypnea from hyperchloremic metabolic acidosis is also evident. Dehydration, vomiting, episodic fever, nephrolithiasis secondary to hypercalciuria, muscle weakness or paralysis as a result of hypokalemia, and episodes of severe life-threatening acidemia (sometimes triggered by a concurrent infection) may also be seen. The disorder may be transient or permanent.

Distal Tubular Acidosis (Type I)

Distal tubular acidosis is caused by the kidney's inability to establish a normal pH gradient between tubular cells and tubular contents. The most characteristic feature is the inability to produce a urinary pH below 6.0 despite the presence of severe metabolic acidosis.

Distal renal tubular acidosis usually occurs as a primary, isolated defect but may also occur in association with other diseases or disorders (Gomez, Gil-Peña, & Santos, 2016). Most secondary causes are rare. The primary disorder is usually considered to be a hereditary defect with a variable degree of expression and a greater penetrance in females. After the age of 2 years, the child usually has growth failure, often with a history of vomiting, polyuria, dehydration, anorexia, and failure to thrive. Evidence of bone demineralization may be present, along with the occasional formation of renal calculi in older children.

The inability to secrete hydrogen ions causes an accumulation of the ions in the body, which soon depletes the available hydrogen buffer and produces a sustained acidosis. Acidosis slows normal somatic growth, and demineralization of bone occurs as bone salts are mobilized to buffer the excessive hydrogen ions. Increased serum levels of both calcium and phosphorus contribute to the development of stones within the renal system. Both sodium and potassium are secreted in larger amounts. Serum potassium levels are depleted as the distal tubules excrete large amounts of potassium ions in an attempt to conserve sodium because hydrogen ions are unable to participate in the exchange. Hyponatremia stimulates increased aldosterone secretion, which further aggravates the hypokalemia. With the depletion of bicarbonate ions, more chloride is reabsorbed in the proximal tubule to create a hyperchloremia.

Prognosis. The primary disorder is usually permanent. However, secondary effects on growth and stone formation can be avoided with early diagnosis and therapy. When the disorder occurs as a secondary complication and renal damage is prevented, the prognosis is good (Gil-Peña, Mejía, & Santos, 2014).

Therapeutic Management

Treatment of both proximal and distal disorders consists of the administration of sufficient bicarbonate or citrate to balance metabolically produced hydrogen ions; to maintain the plasma bicarbonate level within normal range; and to correct associated electrolyte disorders, especially hypokalemia. Proximal disorders require large volumes of bicarbonate to compensate for urinary losses; in distal disorders the alkali required to maintain a normal plasma concentration is low. Most authorities favor a mixture of sodium and potassium bicarbonate (or citrate) to prevent deficiencies of either cation. The citrate solutions (Bicitra, Polycitra, or Shohl solution) are usually more easily tolerated than bicarbonate solutions.

Nursing Care Management

Nursing goals include recognizing the possibility of renal tubular acidosis in children who fail to thrive or who display other symptoms suggestive of the disorders and referring these children for medical evaluation. Helping parents understand the importance of adhering to the medication plan as a long-term goal is essential. (See Compliance and Administration of Medication, Chapter 22.) Children who must continue the medication indefinitely need to learn the importance of taking the medications as soon as they are old enough to assume responsibility for their own care.

NEPHROGENIC DIABETES INSIPIDUS

Nephrogenic diabetes insipidus (NDI) is the major disorder associated with a defect in the ability to concentrate urine. In this disorder the distal tubules and collecting ducts are insensitive to the action of antidiuretic hormone or its exogenous counterpart, vasopressin. Although several inheritance patterns have been identified, more than 90% of patients have an X-linked defect of the vasopressin receptor (Bichet & Bockenhauer, 2016). The disease is more variable in female carriers of the defective gene, who may exhibit only a mild defect in urine-concentrating ability. The differential diagnosis for NDI should include chronic obstructive renal disorders, sickle cell disease, renal tuberculosis, and other renal disorders that may cause high urinary output with failure of the kidney to respond to vasopressin.

Clinical Manifestations and Diagnostic Evaluation

NDI is manifested in the newborn period by vomiting, unexplained fever, failure to thrive, and severe recurrent dehydration with hypernatremia. The passage of copious amounts of dilute urine, which produces severe dehydration and hypoelectrolytemia, is a serious threat to life during this period and may be responsible for the high incidence of cognitive impairment and motor retardation found in affected persons. Growth retardation is probably related to diminished food intake and poor general health because of uncontrolled polydipsia. Diagnosis is suspected on the basis of the patient and family history and confirmed by a urine osmolality value consistently below that of plasma. Lack of response to vasopressin administration rules out other causes.

Therapeutic Management

Therapy involves provision of adequate volumes of water to compensate for urinary losses and minimization of urine output through diet and medication. As a result of an insatiable thirst, most of the child's time is spent drinking and voiding, with decreased time for activity and stimulation. These children may go to great lengths to satisfy their thirst. A low-sodium, low-solute diet and the use of hydrochlorothiazide with or without amiloride to increase the reabsorption of sodium and water in the proximal tubule help reduce the amount of tubular fluid delivered to the distal tubules and to diminish the volume of water excreted (Dabrowski, Kadakia, & Zimmerman, 2016). Urinary output may be reduced when nonsteroidal antiinflammatory drugs (NSAIDs) are administered in conjunction with hydrochlorothiazide. Supplemental potassium may be required to prevent hypokalemia as a result of thiazide therapy. Normal growth and a normal life span are possible if the disease is recognized early and treatment is instituted and maintained.

Nursing Care Management

Nursing goals for children with NDI and their families are to recognize signs of the disorder early and assist them in coping with the long-term inconvenience of the continual thirst and elimination problems. Families need to learn to administer medications and help with diet planning for those on sodium restriction and needing supplemental potassium. The problem of ensuring adequate hydration is lifelong, and families need to adapt to away-from-home fluid needs and avoid activities that contribute to dehydration when fluids may not be available. Genetic counseling is recommended.

MISCELLANEOUS RENAL DISORDERS

HEMOLYTIC UREMIC SYNDROME

Hemolytic uremic syndrome (HUS) is an acute renal disease characterized by a triad of manifestations: AKI, hemolytic anemia, and thrombocytopenia. HUS occurs primarily in infants and small children between the ages of 6 months and 3 years. It has been recognized predominantly in Caucasians and, although it occurs worldwide, is more prevalent in South Africa, Argentina, and the west coasts of North and South America. HUS represents one of the main causes of AKI in early childhood.

Etiology

Diarrhea-positive (D+) HUS accounts for more than 90% of cases and is caused by ingestion of Shiga toxin producing *Escherichia coli. E. coli* O157:H7 is the most common pathogen, although other serotypes have also been reported (Karpman, Loos, Tati, et al., 2016). Occurrences tend to occur in scattered outbreaks and have been traced to undercooked meat, especially ground beef; unpasteurized apple juice; alfalfa sprouts; and public pools. Diarrhea negative (D–) or atypical HUS may be due to a number of causes, including nonenteric infections, disturbances in the complement system, malignancies, or genetic disorders (Loirat, Fakhouri, Ariceta, et al., 2016).

Pathophysiology

The primary site of injury appears to be the endothelial lining of the small glomerular arterioles, but other organs and tissues may be involved (e.g., the liver, brain, heart, pancreatic islet cells, and muscles). The endothelium becomes swollen and occluded with the deposition of platelets and fibrin clots (intravascular coagulation). Red blood cells are damaged as they move through the partially occluded blood vessels. The spleen removes these fragmented red blood cells, causing acute hemolytic anemia. Fibrinolytic action on the precipitated fibrin causes these fibrin-split products to appear in the serum and urine. The characteristic thrombocytopenia is produced by the platelet aggregation within damaged blood vessels or the damage and removal of platelets.

Clinical Manifestations

The disease occurs after a prodromal period, during which there is an episode of diarrhea and vomiting. Less often the preceding illness is an upper respiratory tract infection or, occasionally, varicella, measles, or a UTI.

The hemolytic process persists for several days to 2 weeks. During this time the child is anorexic, irritable, and lethargic. There is marked and rapid onset of pallor accompanied by hemorrhagic manifestations such as bruising, purpura, or rectal bleeding. Severely affected patients are anuric and often hypertensive. Seizures and stupor suggest central nervous system involvement, and there may be signs of acute heart failure. Mild cases demonstrate anemia, thrombocytopenia, and azotemia; urinary output may be reduced or increased.

Diagnostic Evaluation

The triad of anemia, thrombocytopenia, and renal failure is sufficient for diagnosis. Proteinuria, hematuria, and urinary casts are evidence of renal involvement; BUN and serum creatinine levels are elevated. Low hemoglobin and hematocrit and a high reticulocyte count confirm the hemolytic nature of the anemia.

Therapeutic Management

Treatment is symptomatic and directed toward control of the complications and hematologic manifestations of renal failure. The initial supportive measures for most children are those used in managing renal failure: fluid replacement (calculated with great care), treatment of hypertension, and correction of acidosis and electrolyte disorders (Karpman, Loos, Tati, et al., 2016). The most consistently effective treatment is early hemodialysis, PD, or continuous hemofiltration, which is instituted in any child who has been anuric for 24 hours or who demonstrates oliguria with uremia or hypertension and seizures. Blood transfusions with fresh, washed packed cells are administered for severe anemia but are used with caution to prevent circulatory overload from added volume.

Once vomiting and diarrhea have resolved, the child is restarted on enteral nutrition. Sometimes parenteral nutrition is required for children with severe, persistent colitis and for those in whom tissue catabolism is marked. There is no substantial evidence that heparin, corticosteroids, or fibrinolytic agents are beneficial, and in some instances they may aggravate the condition. Ecluzimab, a monoclonal antibody, has shown promise in treating and minimizing recurrences of D-HUS (Loirat, Fakhouri, Ariceta, et al., 2016).

Prognosis. With prompt treatment the survival rate of D+ HUS is approximately 95% (Mody, Gu, Griffin, et al., 2015), but residual renal impairment ranges from 10% to 50%. Death is usually caused by residual renal impairment or central nervous system injury. D– HUS has a less favorable outcome, varying according to cause (Durkan, Kim, Craig, et al., 2016).

Nursing Care Management

Nursing care is the same as that provided in AKI and, for children with continued impairment, includes management of chronic disease. Because of the sudden and life-threatening nature of the disorder in a previously well child, parents are often ill prepared for the impact of hospitalization and treatment. Therefore support and understanding are especially important aspects of care.

> **! NURSING ALERT**
>
> To prevent infection from contaminated meat, the internal temperature of the food, such as hamburger, should be at least 74°C (165°F). Cooking the ground beef until no pink color is seen may not be sufficient to kill the bacteria. Therefore a meat thermometer is needed to ensure a safe product. Discourage parents from giving children unpasteurized apple juice and unwashed raw vegetables. Also discourage the use of antimotility drugs for diarrhea.

FAMILIAL NEPHRITIS (ALPORT SYNDROME)

Alport syndrome (AS) is a hereditary disease characterized by high-tone sensorineural deafness, ocular disorders, and chronic kidney disease caused by mutations in type IV collagen. Most people with AS have the X-linked form of the condition. Less common are autosomal recessive and dominant forms.

Hematuria presents during infancy in affected boys. Gross hematuria may be associated with acute respiratory tract infections. Proteinuria and progressive renal failure begin in childhood. The progression rate to end-stage kidney disease depends on the form of AS. Females may have only microhematuria or progress to ESRD, again depending on the form of the condition they have (Savige, Colville, Rheault, et al., 2016).

Treatment is symptomatic and supportive. Dialysis and kidney transplantation are ultimate therapeutic measures for ESRD. Hearing loss and ocular disorders should receive appropriate attention, and families should be counseled regarding the genetic implications of the disease.

UNEXPLAINED PROTEINURIA

Often apparently healthy children with no suggestion of renal disease demonstrate proteinuria on routine urinalysis. The percentage of children with unexplained proteinuria ranges from 1% at 6 years of age to 11% at puberty, reaching a maximum prevalence at age 13 in girls and age 16 in boys.

Unexplained proteinuria can be categorized as transient (inconstant), persistent, or orthostatic or postural. Transient proteinuria is a common finding with no known cause but sometimes increases with febrile illness, exercise, or dehydration. Persistent proteinuria usually signifies renal disease. Orthostatic proteinuria is seen in 3% to 5% of adolescents and young adults; although proteinuria is evident in both the recumbent and the erect position, it is quantitatively greater in the erect position. The cause is unknown, but minor glomerular changes occur in many instances. The condition is benign and generally resolves over time.

In cases of unexplained proteinuria, it is important to confirm or exclude renal disease with appropriate diagnostic tests. Repeated

BOX 24.7 Classification of Renal Injury

Grade I—Renal contusion or subcapsular hematoma; gross or microscopic hematuria
Grade II—Parenchymal laceration <1.0 cm deep; nonexpanding perirenal hematoma
Grade III—Parenchymal laceration >1.0 cm deep; no urinary extravasation
Grade IV—Laceration extending from parenchyma into collecting system and/or injury to main renal artery or vein
Grade V—Shattered kidney; devascularization of kidney due to avulsion of renal hilum

Data from American Association for the Surgery of Trauma (http://www.aast.org/Library/TraumaTools.aspx).

examination for proteinuria, an orthostatic test, urine culture, and (if proteinuria is persistent) more definitive tests—including 24-hour protein excretion, renal ultrasound, and renal scan—are indicated.

RENAL TRAUMA

Serious injuries of the genitourinary tract are not uncommon in the pediatric age-group, with a peak incidence between ages 10 and 20 years. Despite their relatively protected location, the kidneys in children are more mobile than they are in adults, and the outer borders are less well protected. They are separated from the skin surface by only 2 to 3 cm (0.75 to 1.2 inches) in young children. This results in an increased risk of renal trauma in children as opposed to adults.

Most injuries are of the nonpenetrating or blunt type and usually involve falls, recreational motor vehicles such as dirt bikes, bicycle accidents, and motor vehicle accidents (Dangle, Fuller, Gaines, et al., 2016). Penetrating trauma (e.g., gunshot or stab wound) is much less common in children. Some children have preexisting renal abnormalities, particularly congenital anomalies associated with mild to moderate hydronephrosis that were unrecognized before the injury.

The nurse should suspect renal injury in children who complain of flank pain and have abrasions or contusions on the overlying skin. Hematuria is present, but the amount of blood in the urine is not a reliable indicator of the seriousness of the injury. Many relatively insignificant injuries are associated with grossly bloody urine, whereas some of the most severe injuries are found in children with only microscopic hematuria (Box 24.7).

Renal rupture involves the actual splitting open of the kidney capsule, causing extravasation of blood or a mixture of blood and urine into the surrounding retroperitoneal space. Renal vascular injury, although unusual, requires immediate recognition and surgical intervention. Because the volume-per-minute blood flow through the kidney is greater (25% of cardiac output) than to any other abdominal organ, injury to the kidney may result in a rapid loss of blood.

Active children may or may not have a history of unusual trauma. Abdominal or flank pain and tenderness are caused by bleeding around the kidney and may or may not be associated with fever. Clots passing down the ureter may cause pain similar to that of renal colic, and dysuria is common. Patients with more severe injuries may complain of nausea or abdominal pain. There may be a palpable abdominal mass caused by loss of blood or urine into the retroperitoneum. The fibrous capsule enclosing the kidney prevents expansion of a hematoma; therefore exsanguination and shock are seldom observed, even in severe renal trauma.

Diagnosis is made on the basis of intravenous pyelography, angiography, or retrograde pyelography. Unsuspected hydronephrosis often is first detected as a result of traumatic injury.

Therapeutic Management

Severe injury requires close observation in the hospital intensive care unit and blood replacement if there is severe internal or external bleeding. In most cases bleeding subsides spontaneously. Surgical exploration is indicated if there are multiple injuries, extravasation of blood around the kidneys, or disruption of the major vessels or the collecting system. Children with less severe injuries, such as contusions only, are placed on bed rest. They should remain on bed rest for 3 days after cessation of gross bleeding because the substance released from injured renal tissue (urinary urokinase) has strongly fibrinolytic properties that may precipitate serious bleeding. The prognosis depends on the nature and extent of the injury.

Nursing Care Management

Nursing management is directed toward recognizing and assisting in the diagnosis of renal injury. Care of both the child and the family is primarily supportive. The nurse implements all the concepts related to emergency hospitalization and care. (See Chapter 22.) Postsurgical care, if indicated, is the same as for any other surgical patient. Recommendations for children with a solitary kidney participating in sports are varied. Each child should be individually assessed and advised on the need for protective equipment before engaging in contact, collision, or limited contact activities (Psooy, 2014).

RENAL FAILURE

Renal failure is the inability of the kidneys to excrete waste material, concentrate urine, and conserve electrolytes. The disorder can be acute or chronic and affects most of the systems in the body. Two terms that are often used in relation to renal failure need some clarification: azotemia is the accumulation of nitrogenous waste within the blood, whereas uremia is a more advanced condition in which retention of nitrogenous products produces toxic symptoms. Azotemia is not life threatening, whereas uremia is a serious condition that often involves other body systems.

ACUTE KIDNEY INJURY

AKI is said to exist when the kidneys suddenly are unable to appropriately regulate the volume and composition of urine in response to food and fluid intake and the needs of the organism. The principal feature is oligoanuria* associated with azotemia, acidosis, and diverse electrolyte disturbances. AKI is not common in childhood. The outcome depends on the cause, associated findings, and prompt recognition and treatment.

Etiology

AKI can develop as a result of a large number of related or unrelated clinical conditions: poor renal perfusion, acute renal injury, or the final expression of chronic renal disease. The most common cause in children is transient renal failure resulting from dehydration or other causes of poor perfusion that respond to restoration of fluid volume. Causes of AKI are usually classified as prerenal, intrinsic renal, and postrenal. Severe or long-standing prerenal or postrenal causes can produce severe secondary renal damage.

Prerenal Causes. Prerenal causes of AKI are most common in children and are related to the reduction of renal perfusion in an anatomically

*The definition of oligoanuria varies extensively in the literature—from 1.8 to 4 dl/m^2/24 hr.

and physiologically normal kidney and collecting system. Dehydration secondary to diarrheal disease or persistent vomiting is the most common cause of prerenal failure in infants and children. Surgical shock and trauma (including burns) are also common causes. Hypovolemia and decreased renal perfusion cause a decreased glomerular filtration rate and stimulate the secretion of renin, aldosterone, and antidiuretic hormone, which further diminish urine flow. Extended and severe hypoperfusion (secondary to procedures such as cardiac surgery) can produce cortical or tubular necrosis. Increasing awareness of the potential for the development of AKI allows for earlier detection and treatment should it occur (Jefferies & Devarajan, 2016). In general, the azotemia that accompanies this type of renal failure is rapidly reversible with prompt attention to expansion of the extracellular fluid volume. Prerenal failure is often difficult to distinguish from tubular or cortical necrosis. Renal artery stenosis, altered peripheral vascular resistance related to sepsis, and hepatorenal syndrome are less common causes.

Intrinsic Renal Causes. Intrinsic renal causes of AKI constitute the largest group that requires extended management. These include diseases and nephrotoxic agents that damage the glomeruli, tubules, or renal vasculature. Glomerular disease is the most common cause of glomerular damage, whereas tubular destruction is more often caused by ischemia or nephrotoxins. Vascular damage is an uncommon cause of renal failure in childhood. The type and extent of damage determine the degree and duration of renal insufficiency, and it is difficult to predict in any given case whether acute necrosis will develop.

Postrenal Causes. AKI resulting from obstructive uropathy is uncommon in children except during the first year of life. Relief of the obstruction can restore renal function. The degree of recovery depends on the duration of the renal failure.

Pathophysiology

AKI is usually reversible, but the deviations of physiologic function can be extreme, and mortality in the pediatric age-group is still high. There is severe reduction in the glomerular filtration rate, an elevated BUN level, and decreased tubular reabsorption of sodium from the proximal tubule. Consequently, there is increased concentration of sodium in the distal tubule, which causes stimulation of the renin mechanism. The local action of angiotensin causes vasoconstriction of the afferent arteriole, which further reduces glomerular filtration and prevents urinary losses of sodium. There is a significant reduction in renal blood flow.

The pathologic conditions that produce AKI caused by glomerulonephritis, HUS, and other renal disorders are discussed in relation to those disease processes. The necrotic processes within the nephron can be cortical, tubular, or both.

Cortical Necrosis. Complete cortical necrosis usually results from severe ischemia, infection, or intravascular coagulation and represents a severe cause of AKI. In the pediatric age-group this occurs most commonly during the neonatal period as a result of hypoxia and shock. When cortical destruction is incomplete, some recovery of renal function may occur.

Tubular Necrosis. Damage to the renal tubules can be broadly classified as secondary to renal ischemia and associated with the ingestion or inhalation of substances toxic to the kidneys. Renal tubules are particularly vulnerable to a wide variety of toxic agents that produce vasoconstriction and to focal patches of ischemia that cause a necrosis of the tubular epithelium down to, but not including, the basement membrane. A lesion produced by sustained reduction in renal blood flow also involves the basement membrane, which may become fragmented and ruptured to the extent that the continuity of tubular structure is disrupted. The lesions may affect any segment of the tubules, appearing at irregular intervals along with normal segments throughout the kidney.

Reepithelialization in the areas with intact basement membrane heals tubular lesions. Such healing is unable to take place in areas in which the basement membrane has been disrupted; connective tissue grows through the ruptured membrane, thus preventing reestablishment of tubular integrity. Individual cells within the nephron, but not the entire nephron, are capable of regeneration.

Clinical Course. The clinical course of the child with AKI is variable and depends on the cause. In reversible AKI there is a period of severe oliguria, or a low-output phase, followed by an abrupt onset of diuresis, or a high-output phase; this phase is followed by a gradual return to, or toward, normal urine volumes. The length of the oliguric phase in older children and adolescents is 10 to 14 days but is highly variable at all ages depending on the cause of the AKI. The onset of the diuretic phase appears unexpectedly, and over several days it proceeds in stepwise fashion from very low to above-normal urine volumes. During the oliguric phase, manifestations of uremia are present but may also be accompanied by other clinical disorders that make assessment difficult, such as infection, anoxia, and shock.

Clinical Manifestations

In many instances of AKI the infant or child is already critically ill with the precipitating disorder, and the explanation for development of oliguria may or may not be readily apparent. The underlying illness often overshadows the renal failure and often assumes the priority of care (e.g., the patient who is in shock from endotoxemia, the infant who is severely dehydrated from gastroenteritis, or a child who is subject to seizures as a result of hypertensive encephalopathy associated with AGN).

The prime manifestation of AKI is oliguria, generally a urinary output of less than 1 ml/kg/hr. Anuria (no urinary output in 24 hours) is uncommon, except in obstructive disorders. Other symptoms related to AKI include edema, drowsiness, circulatory congestion, and cardiac arrhythmia from hyperkalemia. Seizures may be caused by hyponatremia or hypocalcemia and tachypnea from metabolic acidosis. With continued oliguria, biochemical abnormalities can develop rapidly, and circulatory and central nervous system manifestations appear.

Diagnostic Evaluation

When a previously well child develops AKI without obvious cause, a careful history is obtained to reveal symptoms that may be related to glomerulonephritis; obstructive uropathy; or exposure to nephrotoxic chemicals, such as ingestion of heavy metals or inhalation of carbon tetrachloride or other organic solvents or drugs (e.g., methicillin, sulfonamides, NSAIDs, neomycin, polymyxin, and kanamycin). Laboratory data reflect the kidney dysfunction: hyperkalemia, hyponatremia, metabolic acidosis, hypocalcemia, anemia, or azotemia (Table 24.7).

Therapeutic Management

The most effective management of AKI is prevention. The development of AKI is a known risk in certain situations. This should be anticipated and recognized, and adequate therapy should be implemented (e.g., fluid therapy for children with hypovolemia in conditions such as dehydration, burns, and hemorrhage). Nephrotoxic drugs should be used with caution or avoided in children with renal disease, and all personnel should be knowledgeable about precautions related to their administration. For example, a generous fluid intake is needed for children receiving antimetabolite drugs and after radiotherapy.

TABLE 24.7 Laboratory Findings Associated With Acute Renal Failure

Clinical Problem	Mechanism	Clinical Considerations
Azotemia	Ongoing protein catabolism	Lower rate of production in neonates and persons with depleted protein stores
Elevated blood urea nitrogen levels	Significantly decreased excretion	Increased in situations involving large amounts of necrotic tissue or extravasated blood
Elevated plasma creatinine levels	Continued production Significantly decreased excretion	Production less affected by other factors More sensitive measure of intensity of azotemia Low in neonate because of small muscle mass relative to size
Metabolic acidosis	Continued endogenous acid production Significantly decreased excretion Depletion of extracellular and intracellular fluid buffers	Compensatory hyperventilation Opisthonos Major threat to life
Hyponatremia	Dilution of extracellular fluid Decreased excretion of water	May develop cerebral signs
Hyperkalemia	Ongoing protein catabolism Decreased excretion compounded by metabolic acidosis	Most important electrolyte to be considered in acute renal failure May contribute to cardiac arrhythmia With electrocardiogram changes, major threat to life Loss may be from gastrointestinal tract
Hypocalcemia	Associated with metabolic acidosis and hyperphosphatemia	During alkali therapy, may cause tetany

The treatment of AKI is directed toward treatment of the underlying cause, management of the complications of renal failure, and provision of supportive therapy within the constraints imposed by the renal failure. Treatment of poor perfusion resulting from dehydration consists of volume restoration as described in the treatment of dehydration. (See Chapter 23.) If oliguria persists after restoration of fluid volume or if the renal failure is caused by intrinsic renal damage, the physiologic and biochemical abnormalities that have resulted from kidney dysfunction must be corrected or controlled. Central venous pressure monitoring is usually implemented.

Initially a catheter is inserted to rule out urine retention, to collect available urine for electrolytes and analysis, and to monitor the results of diuretic administration. The catheter may or may not be removed. Some clinicians believe that it serves little purpose during the oliguric phase and predisposes the patient to bladder infections. Others maintain a catheter for hourly urine measurements.

The use of mannitol, loop diuretics such as furosemide and other medications in the prevention and treatment of AKI have been studied. The 2012 KDIGO Guidelines on Acute Kidney Injury state that the use of mannitol in the prevention of AKI is not scientifically justified due to inadequate studies. They do not recommend the use of diuretics to prevent or treat AKI except as an aid in the management of volume overload.

Fluid and Calories. The amount of exogenous water provided should not exceed the amount needed to maintain zero water balance. It is calculated on the basis of estimated endogenous water formation and losses from sensible (primarily gastrointestinal) and insensible sources. No allotment is calculated for urine as long as oliguria persists.

The child with AKI has a tendency to develop water intoxication and hyponatremia, both of which make it difficult to provide calories in sufficient amounts to meet the child's needs and reduce tissue catabolism, metabolic acidosis, hyperkalemia, and uremia. If the child is able to tolerate oral foods, concentrated food sources that are high in carbohydrates and fat but low in protein, potassium, and sodium may be provided. However, many children have functional disturbances of the gastrointestinal tract, such as nausea and vomiting. Therefore the IV route is generally preferred, and nourishment usually consists of essential amino acids or a combination of essential and nonessential amino acids administered by the central venous route.

Control of water balance in these patients requires careful monitoring of feedback information, such as accurate intake and output, body weight, and electrolyte measurements. In general, during the oliguric phase, no sodium, chloride, or potassium is given unless there are other large, ongoing losses. Regular measurement of plasma electrolytes, pH, BUN, and creatinine levels is required to assess the adequacy of fluid therapy and to anticipate complications that require specific treatment.

Hyperkalemia. An elevated serum potassium level is the most immediate threat to the life of the child with AKI. Potassium ions are not being excreted, while at the same time the release of potassium from cells is accelerated by acidosis, stress, and tissue breakdown in cases associated with internal bleeding or trauma. Because cardiac arrhythmia and cardiac arrest may result, electrocardiograms (ECGs) and serum potassium ion levels are monitored regularly. Hyperkalemia can be minimized and sometimes avoided by eliminating potassium from all food and fluids, by reducing tissue catabolism, and by correcting acidosis.

! NURSING ALERT

Any of the following signs of hyperkalemia constitute an emergency and should be reported immediately:

- Serum potassium concentrations in excess of 7 mEq/L
- Presence of ECG abnormalities, such as loss of P wave, prolonged RS complex, depressed ST segment, tall and tented T waves, bradycardia, or heart block

Several measures are available to reduce the serum potassium concentration, and the priority of implementation is usually based on the rapidity with which the measures are effective. Temporary measures that produce a rapid but transient effect are as follows:

- Calcium gluconate administered intravenously over 2 to 4 minutes with continuous ECG monitoring, exerts a protective effect on cardiac conduction.
- Sodium bicarbonate administered intravenously over 30 to 60 minutes, elevates the serum pH to cause a transient shift of extracellular fluid potassium into the intracellular fluid. However, there is a risk of hypocalcemia, tetany, and fluid overload.

- Glucose and insulin administered intravenously, accelerate glycogen synthesis, causing glucose and potassium to move into the cells. Insulin facilitates the entry of glucose into cells.

These effects produce only transient protection by redistributing existing potassium stores; they do not remove potassium from the body. However, they provide relief while more definitive but slower-acting measures are being implemented. Potassium can be removed by either of two methods:

1. Administration of a cation exchange resin such as sodium polystyrene sulfonate (Kayexalate), 1 g/kg, administered orally or rectally, to bind potassium and remove it from the body. This requires time to be effective, and a sodium ion is exchanged for each potassium ion. This increased sodium concentration adds to the body fluids, which may contribute to fluid overload, hypertension, and cardiac failure.
2. Dialysis or continuous hemofiltration (see p. 810). Hemodialysis is efficient but requires specialized facilities. PD is simpler and can be carried out in almost any hospital setting. Indications for dialysis in AKI are continued oliguria associated with any of the following:
   - Severe, persistent acidosis
   - Inability to reduce serum potassium levels to a safe range with other methods
   - Clinical uremic syndrome consisting of nausea and vomiting, drowsiness, and progression to coma
   - Circulatory overload, hypertension, and evidence of cardiac failure

The optimal timing for initiation of renal replacement therapy is controversial. One strategy is to institute renal replacement therapy within hours of the diagnosis of severe AKI being made, regardless of other symptoms. Another strategy is to delay renal replacement therapy until any of the previously listed symptoms presents. Differences in mortality have not been demonstrated between the two approaches (Gaudry, Hajage, Schortgen, et al., 2016).

Hypertension. Hypertension is a common and serious complication of AKI, and blood pressure determinations are taken at least every 4 to 6 hours to detect it early. The most common cause of hypertension in AKI is overexpansion of the extracellular fluid and plasma volume, together with activation of the renin-angiotensin system. The goal of therapy is to prevent hypertensive encephalopathy and avoid overtaxing the cardiovascular system.

When there is a threat of encephalopathy, labetalol (a beta and alpha blocker) may be administered intravenously as bolus infusions or a continuous drip. Sodium nitroprusside may be given but requires close monitoring. For less urgent situations, hydralazine, clonidine, or verapamil may be given intravenously. Oral drugs used for acute hypertension include nifedipine, captopril, minoxidil, hydralazine, propranolol, or furosemide.

Other Complications. Other complications that may occur with AKI are anemia, seizures and coma, cardiac failure, and pulmonary edema. Anemia is commonly associated with AKI, but transfusion is not recommended unless the hemoglobin level drops below 6 g/dl. Transfusions consist of fresh, packed red blood cells given slowly to reduce the likelihood of increasing blood volume, hypertension, and hyperkalemia.

Seizures occur often when renal failure progresses to uremia and are also related to hypertension, hyponatremia, and hypocalcemia. Treatment is directed toward the specific cause when known. More obscure causes are managed with antiepileptic drugs.

Cardiac failure with pulmonary edema is almost always associated with hypervolemia. Treatment is directed toward reduction of fluid volume, with water and sodium restriction and administration of diuretics. Digitalis is ineffective and can be hazardous.

Diuretic, or High-Output, Phase. When the output begins to increase, either spontaneously or in response to diuretic therapy, the nurse should monitor the intake of fluid, potassium, and sodium, and provide adequate replacement to prevent depletion and its consequences. In some cases the high-output phase is mild and lasts only a few days; in others enormous amounts of electrolyte-rich urine are passed.

Prognosis. The prognosis of AKI depends largely on the nature and severity of the causative factor or precipitating event and the promptness and competence of management. The mortality rate is less than 20%. The outcome is least favorable in children with rapidly progressive nephritis and cortical necrosis. Children in whom AKI is a result of HUS or AGN may recover completely, but residual renal impairment or hypertension is more often the rule. Complete recovery is usually expected in children whose renal failure is a result of dehydration, nephrotoxins, or ischemia. AKI after cardiac surgery has a less favorable prognosis. It is often impossible to assess the extent of recovery for several months. (See Quality Patient Outcomes box.)

QUALITY PATIENT OUTCOMES

Acute Kidney Injury

- Underlying cause of acute kidney injury identified and treated
- Water balance maintained
- Hypertension controlled
- Electrolyte balance maintained
- Diet maintains calories while minimizing tissue catabolism, metabolic acidosis, hyperkalemia, and uremia

Nursing Care Management

Nursing care of the infant or child with AKI involves addressing the underlying cause plus carefully observing and managing the renal status. The major goal is reestablishment of renal function (with emphasis on providing an adequate caloric intake to minimize reduction of protein stores); prevention of complications; and monitoring of fluid balance, laboratory data, and physical manifestations. The probability of dialysis or continuous hemofiltration is high, and the nurse must anticipate the availability of the necessary equipment. Because the child requires intensive observation and often specialized equipment, the usual disposition is admission to an intensive care unit where equipment and trained personnel are available.

The major nursing tasks in the care of the infant or child with AKI are monitoring and assessing fluid and electrolyte balance. Limiting fluid intake requires ingenuity on the part of caregivers to cope with the child who is thirsty. One strategy involves rationing the daily intake with small amounts of fluid served in containers that give the impression of larger volumes. Older children who understand the rationale of fluid limits can help determine how their daily ration should be distributed.

Meeting nutritional needs is sometimes a problem because the child may be nauseated and because getting the child to eat concentrated foods without fluids may be difficult. When nourishment is provided by the IV route, careful monitoring is essential to prevent fluid overload. This can become a major challenge in the face of nutritional requirements and administration of IV medications. The IV drugs being used may be nephrotoxic, which can require a specified volume of solution for delivery. In some instances blood products must also be delivered. Preventing fluid overload while delivering medications and calories requires concerted collaboration. In addition, nursing measures such as maintaining an optimum thermal environment, reducing any elevation of body temperature, and reducing restlessness and anxiety are used to decrease the rate of tissue catabolism.

The nurse must be continually alert for behavior changes that indicate the onset of complications. Infection from reduced resistance, anemia, and general morbidity is a constant threat. Fluid overload and electrolyte disturbances can precipitate cardiovascular complications such as hypertension and cardiac failure. Fluid and electrolyte imbalances, acidosis, and accumulation of nitrogenous waste products can produce neurologic involvement manifested by coma, seizures, or alterations in sensorium.

Although children with AKI are usually quite ill and voluntarily diminish their activity, infants may become restless and irritable, and children are often anxious and frightened. Frequent, painful, and stress-producing treatments and tests must be performed. A supportive, empathetic nurse can provide comfort and stability in a threatening and unnatural environment.

Family Support. Providing support and reassurance to parents is among the major nursing responsibilities. The seriousness and emergency nature of AKI are stressful to parents, and most feel some degree of guilt regarding the child's condition, especially when the illness is the result of ingestion of a toxic substance, dehydration, or a genetic disease. They need reassurance and an empathetic listener. They also need to be kept informed of the child's progress and provided explanations regarding the therapeutic regimen. The equipment and the child's behavior are sometimes frightening and anxiety provoking. Nurses can do much to help parents comprehend and deal with the stresses of the situation.

CHRONIC KIDNEY DISEASE

The kidneys are able to maintain the chemical composition of fluids within normal limits until more than 50% of functional renal capacity is destroyed by disease or injury. Chronic kidney disease (CKD) occurs when the diseased kidneys can no longer maintain the normal chemical structure of body fluids under normal conditions. Progressive deterioration over months or years produces a variety of clinical and biochemical disturbances that conclude in the clinical syndrome known as uremia. The final stage of CKD, ESRD, is irreversible. Treatment with dialysis or transplantation is required when the glomerular filtration rate decreases below 10% to 15% of normal. The pattern of renal dysfunction is remarkably uniform no matter what disease process initiates the advanced disease.

Etiology

A variety of diseases and disorders can result in CKD. The most common causes of CKD before age 5 years are congenital renal and urinary tract malformations (particularly renal hypoplasia and dysplasia and obstructive uropathy) and VUR. Glomerular and hereditary renal diseases predominate in children 5 to 15 years of age. The glomerular diseases that most commonly lead to CKD are chronic pyelonephritis, CGN, and glomerulonephropathy associated with systemic diseases such as anaphylactoid purpura and lupus erythematosus. Hereditary nephritis, congenital nephrotic syndrome, Alport syndrome, polycystic kidney, and several other hereditary disorders result in renal failure in childhood. Renal vascular disorders such as HUS, vascular thrombosis, or cortical necrosis are less common causes.

Pathophysiology

Early in the course of progressive nephron destruction, the child remains asymptomatic with only minimum biochemical abnormalities. Unless its presence is detected in the process of routine assessment, signs and symptoms that indicate advanced renal damage often emerge only late in the course of the disease. Midway in the disease process, as increasing numbers of nephrons are totally destroyed, and most others are damaged to varying degrees; the few that remain intact are hypertrophied but functional. These few normal nephrons are able to make sufficient adjustments to stresses to maintain reasonable degrees of fluid and electrolyte balance. Definitive biochemical examination at this time reveals restricted tolerance to excesses or restrictions. As the disease progresses to the end stage because of severe reduction in the number of functioning nephrons, the kidneys are no longer able to maintain fluid and electrolyte balance, and the features of uremia appear.

The following sections briefly summarize the pathophysiology of specific biochemical abnormalities.

Retention of Waste Products. Serum creatinine and BUN levels are utilized to evaluate renal function. Creatinine is a waste product of muscle catabolism. Because muscle mass is relatively stable, creatinine production is also stable. Most creatinine is filtered out by the kidneys and expelled in the urine. BUN (a by-product of protein breakdown) levels also increase as kidney function declines. BUN is a less precise marker than creatinine as is not produced at a stable rate and can be influenced by protein intake, hydration status and other factors (Lopez-Giacoman & Madero, 2015).

Water and Sodium Retention. The damaged kidneys are able to maintain sodium and water balance under normal circumstances, although the few remaining functional nephrons are required to increase their rate of filtration and reabsorption in proportion to their numbers. The limitations of this capacity become apparent under stress. The nature of abnormalities in adjustment depends on the underlying renal disease. Infants and small children with kidney dysplasia or urinary obstructive disease tend to excrete large volumes of dilute urine low in sodium content. Children with glomerular disease tend to retain both sodium and water as a result of a greater reduction of glomerular filtration than of tubular reabsorption. Children with defective sodium reabsorption from tubular disease tend to lose sodium, with a corresponding osmotic water loss. Consequently, sodium excesses may cause edema and hypertension, whereas sodium deprivation can result in hypovolemia and circulatory failure. Only in ESRD is markedly reduced glomerular filtration inadequate to handle normal amounts of sodium and water. Retention of these substances leads to edema and vascular congestion.

Hyperkalemia. Dangerous hyperkalemia is uncommon in CKD until the end stage. However, the kidneys are unable to adjust readily to increased ingestion of potassium, and they require a longer period to rid the body of this excess.

Acidosis. A sustained metabolic acidosis is characteristic of CKD; it results from the damaged kidney's inability to excrete a normal load of metabolic acids generated by normal metabolic processes. There is reduced capacity of the distal tubules to produce ammonia and impaired reabsorption of bicarbonate. Despite continuous hydrogen ion retention and bicarbonate loss, the plasma pH is maintained at a level compatible with life by other buffering mechanisms, particularly the bone salt (see the following sections).

Calcium and Phosphorus Disturbances. Calcium and phosphorus homeostasis are affected by CKD. Profound and complex disturbances in the metabolism of these substances result in significant bone demineralization and impaired growth. This appears to be related to several factors (Box 24.8). These complex disturbances in calcium, phosphorus, and bone metabolism produce growth arrest or delay; bone pain; and

BOX 24.8 Factors Related to Bone Demineralization in Chronic Renal Failure

- In a state of acidosis there is dissolution of the alkaline salts of bone, which serve as buffers, and the release of phosphorus and calcium into the bloodstream.
- Reduced glomerular filtration and excretion of inorganic phosphate lead to an elevation of plasma phosphate with a concomitant decrease in serum calcium.
- Decreased serum calcium concentration stimulates the secretion of parathyroid hormone, which results in reabsorption of calcium from bones. Under normal circumstances parathyroid hormone inhibits the tubular reabsorption of phosphates.
- Diseased kidneys are unable to complete the synthesis of vitamin D to its most active form, 1,25-dihydroxycholecalciferol, which is necessary for the absorption of calcium from the gastrointestinal tract and deposition of calcium in bone. This acquired resistance to vitamin D decreases calcium absorption, permits retention of phosphorus, and contributes to secondary hyperparathyroidism.

BOX 24.9 Causes of Anemia in Chronic Renal Failure

- Shortened life span of red blood cells caused by some extracorpuscular factor associated with the uremic state
- Impaired red blood cell production resulting from decreased production of erythropoietin
- Blood loss related to increased tendency to bleed, associated with a prolonged bleeding time, probably related to impaired platelet function and laboratory blood samples
- Hyperparathyroidism
- Hypersplenism, which may be related to silicone deposition (from dialysis blood lines) and granuloma formation in the spleen
- Diseases related to hemolytic anemia, such as systemic lupus erythematosus and sickle cell disease

deformities known as renal osteodystrophy, sometimes called renal rickets, because the disorganization of bone growth and demineralization are similar to that caused by vitamin D–resistant rickets.

Anemia. A consistent feature of CKD is anemia, which appears to result from several factors (Box 24.9).

Growth Disturbance. One of the most striking effects of CKD in childhood, and one that can have profound psychologic and social consequences for the developing child, is delayed growth. The cause is poorly understood but may be related to nutritional and biochemical factors (Box 24.10).

Sexual maturation may be delayed or may not occur in children with CKD, and secondary amenorrhea commonly develops in girls past puberty. CKD can also cause sexual dysfunction by creating imbalances in gonadal hormone levels. Decreased testosterone levels impair spermatogenesis in males; decreased estrogen, luteinizing hormone, and progesterone cause anovulation and menstrual irregularities (usually amenorrhea) in females. Autonomic neuropathy and anemia are also factors that can alter sexual function.

Other Disturbances. Children with CKD are more susceptible to infection, especially pneumonia, UTI, and septicemia, although the reason for this is not entirely clear. Hyperventilation, a manifestation of the respiratory compensatory mechanism for metabolic acidosis, and pulmonary edema may contribute to upper respiratory tract infection. These children become extraordinarily sensitive to changes in vascular volume that may cause, in addition to pulmonary overload, cerebral symptoms and circulatory manifestations such as hypertension and cardiac failure.

BOX 24.10 Probable Causes of Growth Failure in Chronic Renal Failure

- Renal osteodystrophy
- Poor nutrition associated with dietary restrictions (especially protein) and loss of appetite
- Biochemical abnormalities associated with renal failure, such as sustained acidosis or renal sodium wasting
- Hypertension
- Corticosteroid treatment
- Tissue resistance to growth hormone
- Trace mineral and vitamin deficiencies

Numerous neurologic manifestations appear with advanced renal failure, although no specific toxin or biochemical defect has been identified. However, disturbances in enzyme function, disturbances in water and electrolyte balance, altered calcium ion concentration, hypertension, and accumulation of various "uremic toxins" have been implicated.

Clinical Manifestations

The first symptom of CKD may be loss of normal energy and increased fatigue on exertion. For example, the child may prefer quiet, passive activities rather than participation in more active games and outdoor play. The child is usually somewhat pale, but the change is often so subtle that it may not be evident to parents or others. Blood pressure is sometimes elevated. Growth is affected early in the development of CKD, and falling behind on the growth chart is often the first measurable sign.

Other manifestations may appear as the disease progresses. The child does not eat as well (especially breakfast), shows less interest in normal activities such as schoolwork or play, and has a decreased or increased urinary output and a compensatory intake of fluid. For example, a child who has achieved bladder control may wet the bed at night. Pallor becomes more evident as the skin develops a characteristic sallow, muddy appearance as a result of anemia and deposition of urochrome pigment in the skin. The child may complain of headache, muscle cramps, and nausea. Other signs and symptoms include weight loss, facial puffiness, malaise, bone or joint pain, growth retardation, dryness or itching of the skin, bruised skin, and sometimes sensory or motor loss. Amenorrhea is common in adolescent girls.

Therapy is generally initiated before the appearance of the uremic symptoms, although on some occasions the symptoms may be observed. Manifestations of untreated uremia reflect the progressive nature of the homeostatic disturbances and general toxicity. Gastrointestinal symptoms include loss of appetite, nausea, and vomiting. Bleeding tendencies are apparent in bruises, bloody diarrheal stools, stomatitis, and bleeding from the lips and mouth. Intractable itching occurs, probably related to a number of factors, including dry skin and hyperparathyroidism (Wojtowicz-Prus, Kiliś-Pstrusińska, Reich, et al., 2016). Deposits of urea crystals may appear on the skin as uremic frost but are seldom seen because of the availability of dialysis and transplantation. There may be an unpleasant uremic odor to the breath. Respirations become deeper as a result of metabolic acidosis, and circulatory overload is manifested by hypertension, congestive heart failure, and pulmonary edema. Progressive confusion, dulling of the sensorium, and ultimately coma are signs of neurologic involvement. Other signs may include tremors, muscular twitching, and seizures.

Diagnostic Evaluation

The diagnosis of CKD is usually suspected on the basis of any of a number of clinical manifestations, a history of prior renal disease, or biochemical findings. The onset is usually gradual, and the initial signs and symptoms are vague and nonspecific. Laboratory and other diagnostic tools and tests are of value in assessing the extent of renal damage, biochemical disturbances, and related physical dysfunction. Often, they can help establish the nature of the underlying disease and differentiate between other disease processes and the pathologic consequences of renal dysfunction.

Therapeutic Management

Classification of CKD as stage 1 (GFR ≥90) through stage 5 (GFR <15 or dialysis) helps with evaluation and management decisions through the use of medical protocols such as the National Kidney Foundation Kidney Disease Outcomes Quality Initiative evidence-based clinical practice guidelines (http://www.kidney.org/professionals/KDOQI). The goals of management are to maximize effective renal function, maintain body fluid and electrolyte balance within acceptable limits, treat systemic complications, and promote as active and normal a life as possible for the child for as long as possible. This becomes increasingly difficult as the disease progresses toward end stage. Therapeutic measures designed to relieve one manifestation may negatively affect another. For example, antihypertensive agents may further impair renal function.

Activity. Allow children unrestricted activity and to set their own limits regarding rest and extent of exertion. Encourage them to attend school. If the effort is too great, home tutoring can be arranged.

Diet. Regulation of diet has been seen as the most effective means, short of dialysis, for reducing the quantity of materials that require renal excretion. The goal of the diet in renal failure is to provide sufficient calories and protein for growth while minimizing the excretory demands made on the kidney, to limit metabolic bone disease (osteodystrophy), and to minimize fluid and electrolyte disturbances. Dietary protein intake is limited to the recommended dietary allowance (RDA) for the child's age. Restriction of protein intake below the RDA is believed to negatively affect growth and neurodevelopment. Dietary phosphorus may need to be restricted. Remember that any attempt to restrict dietary intake in children potentially restricts caloric intake and can limit growth.

Protein in the diet should include foods of high biologic value. When given with meals, substances that bind phosphorus in the intestines prevent its absorption and allow a more liberal intake of phosphorus-containing protein. Sodium and water are not usually limited unless there is evidence of edema or hypertension.

Potassium is not restricted as long as creatinine clearance remains at acceptable limits (30 to 35 ml/min). However, restrictions are instituted for patients with oliguria or anuria. Restrictions of any or all of these minerals may be imposed in later stages or at any time in which factors cause abnormal serum concentrations.

Because of modified dietary intake, altered metabolism, and poor appetite, some dietary supplementation is usually needed. Because fat-soluble vitamins can accumulate in patients with CKD, vitamins A, E, and K are not supplemented beyond normal dietary intake. Active and/or inactive forms of vitamin D are prescribed, and water-soluble vitamin supplementation may be required if the diet is inadequate. Other dietary needs are discussed in relation to osteodystrophy and anemia. Dietary management of the child with renal failure is a difficult and complex problem that necessitates collaboration with a registered dietitian who is knowledgeable about pediatric nutrition and the impact of renal failure.

Osteodystrophy. Measures directed at prevention or correction of the calcium/phosphorus imbalance are reduction of dietary phosphorus, administration of a phosphorus-binding agent, provision of supplemental calcium, control of acidosis, and administration of an active and/or inactive form of vitamin D.

The reduction of protein and milk intake can control dietary phosphorus. Oral administration of phosphorus-binding agents, which combine with the phosphorus to decrease gastrointestinal absorption and thus the serum levels of phosphate, can further reduce phosphorus levels. Calcium carbonate preparations can be used as phosphorus binders. These medications act as phosphate binders, calcium supplements, and alkalizing agents. Calcium carbonate preparations can be given with meals to bind phosphorus if the child is hyperphosphatemic or mildly hypocalcemic. If given 1 to 2 hours after meals, they act as calcium supplements for children with stable phosphorus but low calcium levels. Calcium acetate can also be used. Newer, iron-based binders can be used when there is concern for hypercalcemia (Stormont, McCoy, Bashir, et al., 2016). Aluminum hydroxide gels are effective phosphorus binders but have been shown to cause aluminum loading when used in children with renal failure. Aluminum intoxication leads to altered sensorium, an inability to talk, ataxia, seizures, and severe bone disease.

Secondary hyperparathyroidism (evidenced by an elevated intact PTH level), in a child with normal phosphate, calcium and 25OH vitamin D levels requires treatment with an active form of vitamin D. Oral medications such as calcitriol (Rocaltrol) increase absorption of calcium through the gastrointestinal tract. The serum calcium level is monitored frequently during periods when the drugs are being initiated or changed to detect hypercalcemia. Intact parathyroid hormone levels are measured every 2 to 3 months with target levels based on the stage of CKD.

Osseous deformities that result from renal osteodystrophy, especially those related to ambulation, are troublesome and require correction if they occur. Careful attention to the management of osteodystrophy and bone growth can prevent deformities in some children.

Acidosis. Pharmacologic treatment of acidosis is initiated early in children who have chronic renal insufficiency. In addition to reducing the formation of metabolic acids by avoiding excessive dietary protein intake, alkalizing agents such as sodium bicarbonate or a combination of sodium and potassium citrate (Bicitra, Polycitra, or Shohl solution) alleviate acidosis. Correction of acidosis is best attempted after calcium levels are elevated because rapid correction may precipitate tetany in a hypocalcemic child.

Anemia. Because the anemia associated with renal failure is related to decreased production of erythropoietin, it usually cannot be successfully managed with hematinic agents. Provide sufficient sources of folic acid and iron in the diet, although this is difficult when protein sources are restricted. Inadequate intake and iron losses that may occur are managed by supplemental iron, usually ferrous sulfate. Providing adequate sources of ascorbic acid at the same time that iron-rich foods or supplements are given enhances the absorption.

The medication recombinant human erythropoietin (r-HuEPO) corrects anemia (improving energy level and general well-being) and eliminates the need for frequent blood transfusions in patients with CKD. To support the formation of new red blood cells before r-HuEPO therapy, iron stores must be adequate. Iron supplements are required in conjunction with r-HuEPO.

Hypertension. Hypertension of advanced renal disease may be managed initially by cautious use of a low-sodium diet, fluid restriction, and perhaps diuretics such as thiazides or furosemide. Strict restriction of sodium intake may be necessary in patients with oliguria. Severe hypertension may require the combination of a beta blocker and a vasodilator (propranolol and hydralazine). Other drugs that may be used include nifedipine, atenolol, minoxidil, prazosin, captopril, or labetalol, either singly or in combinations.

Growth Retardation. One major consequence of CKD is growth retardation. Children with onset of renal failure earlier in life have more severe growth impairment than those diagnosed later (Rodig, McDermott, Schneider, et al., 2014). These children grow poorly both before and after initiation of dialysis. Assurance of adequate nutritional intake, correction of fluid and electrolyte imbalances, anemia, and metabolic acidosis should be undertaken. The use of recombinant human growth hormone has shown marked acceleration in growth velocity in children with growth retardation secondary to CKD (Rees, 2016).

Miscellaneous Complications. Intercurrent infections are treated with appropriate antimicrobials. Most of these drugs are excreted through the kidneys; therefore the dosage is usually reduced in proportion to the decrease in renal function, and the interval between doses is extended in these children to avoid possible toxic effects from accumulation. Any drug eliminated through the kidneys is administered with caution. Serum levels of ototoxic or nephrotoxic drugs (e.g., aminoglycosides or vancomycin) are assessed regularly to ensure a safe, nontoxic level.

Dental defects are common in children with chronic kidney disease; the earlier the onset of the disease, the more severe the dental manifestations. These defects include hypoplasia, hypomineralization, tooth discoloration, alteration in the size and shape of teeth, malocclusion (secondary to deficient skeletal growth), ulcerative stomatitis, occasional oral hematomas, and an increase in calcific deposits around the teeth. Regular dental care is especially important in these children. Other nondental complications are treated symptomatically—for example, chlorpromazine (Thorazine) or prochlorperazine (Compazine) is given for nausea, antiepileptics are given for seizures, and diphenhydramine (Benadryl) is given for pruritus. Once a child reaches CKD stage 5, death can occur unless waste products and toxins are removed from body fluids by dialysis or kidney transplantation. Since the adaptation of these techniques for infants and small children, the outlook for these patients has improved remarkably. In cases in which the patient has other serious illnesses or organ system failures and aggressive care is considered futile, the appropriate end-of-life recommendation may be for palliative care and comfort measures only. (See Quality Patient Outcomes box.)

QUALITY PATIENT OUTCOMES

Chronic Renal Failure

- Sufficient calories and protein for growth maintained
- Excretory demands made on the kidney are limited
- Metabolic bone disease (osteodystrophy) minimal
- Fluid and electrolyte disturbances managed
- Hypertension managed
- Growth retardation treated

Nursing Care Management

The child with CKD has a life maintained by drugs and artificial means, and the multiple stresses placed on these children and their families are often overwhelming. Progressive deterioration of renal function occurs at varying rates. As the affected child progresses from renal insufficiency to uremia and then to dialysis or transplantation, the need for supportive nursing care is intensified. Team effort is more important than ever and involves coordination of personnel from medicine, nursing, social services, child life, physical and occupational therapy, dietetics, and psychologic or psychiatric specialties.

Progressive disease places a number of stresses on the child and family. There is a continuing need for repeated examinations that often entail painful procedures, side effects, and occasional hospitalizations. Diet therapy can become progressively more restrictive and intense, and parents may need help in learning to select appropriate foods, read labels carefully for sodium and potassium content, and modify meals to accommodate the child's special needs. The child is required to take a variety of medications. Compliance is difficult when long-term therapies are involved. Ever present in all aspects of the treatment regimen is the agonizing realization that, without treatment, death is inevitable.

CKD presents the same nonspecific stresses on child and family as any other chronic or life-threatening illness. (See Chapters 22 and 24) The reactions and adaptation of the child and family depend on the child's age and developmental stage, the family's cultural and socioeconomic background, the quality of the interpersonal relationships of family members, and the communication patterns within the family. In general, the problems observed and the emotional responses to the stress of the illness are influenced less by the nature of the illness than by the family relationships and personalities (see Family-Centered Care box).

FAMILY-CENTERED CARE

Family Priorities

Families who have children with long-term chronic illnesses, such as end-stage renal disease, spend a lot of time in hospitals, outpatient clinics, and primary health care facilities. When they miss appointments or respond less quickly than anticipated, sometimes they are quickly labeled *noncompliant.* It is important to remember that families have to develop priorities for the unit as a whole. Sometimes the family may decide that it is more important for the parent to go to work or to attend a sibling's school performance than to attend an appointment scheduled for them by health care personnel. The chronically ill child cannot and should not always be the number-one priority for the family. The professional staff who work with the family can help the parents prioritize the needs of the ill child within the needs of the family constellation.

Teresa Hall, MS, RN
Hathaway Children's Services
Sylmar, California

One of the first and most noticeable changes is the alteration in physical appearance—fluctuations in weight, anemia, and failure to grow. Children must adjust to the fact that they will always be different from their peers in some ways. They may be shorter, often more tired, and unable to participate in all the activities that are attractive to young people. Children who have had diversion procedures, dialysis, and other surgeries or who urinate into a bag need to learn positive coping strategies for the alterations in their body image and for the questions and potential teasing of peers. It is not unusual for children with chronic conditions to exhibit behavioral regression. This is particularly so for children with renal failure because their appearance is often of a child much younger than their chronologic age.

School is often difficult for these children. Frequent absences for illnesses, evaluations, or treatments disrupt the educational process and socialization. Teachers and school systems are not always sympathetic to the rights and needs of a child with a chronic illness (e.g., the right

BOX 24.11 Processes of Fluid and Electrolyte Movement

Osmosis—Passive movement of water from a solution of lower concentration to a solution of higher concentration of particles
Diffusion—Random movement of particles from an area of greater concentration to an area of lower concentration
Ultrafiltration—Process by which plasma water is removed because of a pressure gradient between the blood and dialysate compartments

to equal education and the need for flexibility and special help at times), which places an additional burden on the parents.

In some families illness and stressful experiences act as a unifying force; in other families stress aggravates preexisting problems and contributes to family disharmony. The relentless nature of the disease and its therapies not only places physical and emotional stresses on the family but is also a chronic drain on the family finances. Insurance rarely covers the full cost of the multiple hospitalizations and outpatient expenses. The federal Medicare program, for which most children qualify, funds ESRD care. However, there are many hidden costs, such as transportation to special treatment centers, meals, and sometimes lodging away from home. Some private foundations, churches, and community groups provide temporary assistance, and nurses should become familiar with those in the area of their practice that can offer financial and educational services to these families. For example, the National Kidney Foundation* and numerous other agencies provide services and information for families, including pamphlets and descriptive literature. Particularly useful are booklets written for children with renal disease.

Certain specific stresses related to CKD and its treatment are predictable. When it first becomes apparent that kidney failure is inevitable, both the child and the parents often experience depression and anxiety. Acceptance is particularly difficult if renal failure progresses rapidly after the diagnosis. Children, and especially parents, usually express denial and disbelief. Denial can also develop when progression toward dialysis or transplant has been prolonged and both the child and the parents come to believe it will never occur.

Once the renal failure is established and the symptoms become progressively more distressing, parents usually perceive the initiation of dialysis or kidney transplantation as a positive experience. After the initial concerns of implementing the treatment, the child begins to feel better, and parental anxiety is relieved for a time.

RENAL REPLACEMENT THERAPY

Technologic advances in the care of children with AKI and CKD provide several renal replacement therapies for maintaining excretory function in acute disease and for prolonging life in those with CKD stage 5. The primary modalities are hemodialysis, peritoneal dialysis (PD), hemofiltration, and transplantation.

Dialysis is the process of separating colloids and crystalline substances in solution by the difference in their rate of diffusion through a semipermeable membrane. Three processes accomplish this movement across the membrane: osmosis, diffusion, and ultrafiltration (Box 24.11). Methods of dialysis currently available for clinical management of renal failure are as follows:

- Hemodialysis, in which blood is circulated outside the body through artificial cellophane membranes that permit a similar passage of water and solutes
- PD, wherein the abdominal cavity acts as a semipermeable membrane through which water and solutes of small molecular size move by osmosis and diffusion according to their respective concentrations on either side of the membrane
- Hemofiltration, in which blood filtrate is circulated outside the body by hydrostatic pressure exerted across a semipermeable membrane and replaced (simultaneously) by electrolyte solution

The choice of whether to use hemodialysis, PD, or hemofiltration depends on the nature of the renal failure (acute versus chronic) and the cause of the renal failure. For chronic dialysis, family lifestyles and preferences are considered in choice of treatment. Hemodialysis is more efficient than PD but is technically more difficult in infants and very young children. In these children hemofiltration may be a viable substitute for dialysis. As a rule, dialysis is reserved for children who are in end-stage renal failure because it requires creation of an access and special equipment. It may be used acutely for conditions such as severe metabolic acidosis, accidental poisoning, chronic heart failure with fluid overload, hyperkalemia, severe hypernatremia, severe hyperphosphatemia, and tumor lysis syndrome.

The absolute indications for dialysis are life-threatening electrolyte abnormalities; severe volume overload; and bilateral neoplastic disease or bilateral nephrectomies performed for various reasons, including intractable hypertension. Although each child is assessed on an individual basis, indications for instituting dialysis in CKD are biochemical abnormalities, including elevated BUN, acidosis, severe hyperphosphatemia, and elevated potassium. Other indications include deteriorating central nervous system function or congestive heart failure that is unresponsive to other therapy. Growth failure, severe osteodystrophy, insufficient caloric intake, and an inability to carry out normal activities are sometimes criteria for dialysis.

Most children show rapid clinical improvement with the implementation of dialysis, although it is directly related to the duration of uremia before dialysis and the extent to which dietary regulations are followed. Growth rate and skeletal maturation improve, but recovery of normal growth is uncommon. In many cases sexual development, although delayed, has progressed to completion.

HEMODIALYSIS

Hemodialysis is the preferred dialytic method for children with acute conditions such as life-threatening hyperkalemia or poisoning with dialyzable compounds. Protein loss is less extensive than with PD. However, hemodialysis is technically difficult in small children less than 20 kg (44 lb) because their delicately balanced cardiovascular dynamics may be upset by the rapid changes in blood volume and systemic blood pressure that may occur with this method. In addition, it may be difficult to place vascular access for hemodialysis in small children.

Hemodialysis is the preferred form of dialysis for certain family situations in which any one person is unable to take the time and responsibility to perform the procedures at home. It is best suited to children who live close to the dialysis center because they must come to the center as often as three or more times a week for treatments. Children who are not good candidates for PD because of family noncompliance, recurrent peritoneal infections, or unstable living conditions are treated with hemodialysis.

Procedure

Hemodialysis requires special dialysis equipment: the hemodialyzer, or so-called artificial kidney (Figs. 24.4 and 24.5). Hemodialyzers are

*30 E. 33rd St., New York, NY 10016; 212-889-2210 or 800-622-9010; http://www.kidney.org.

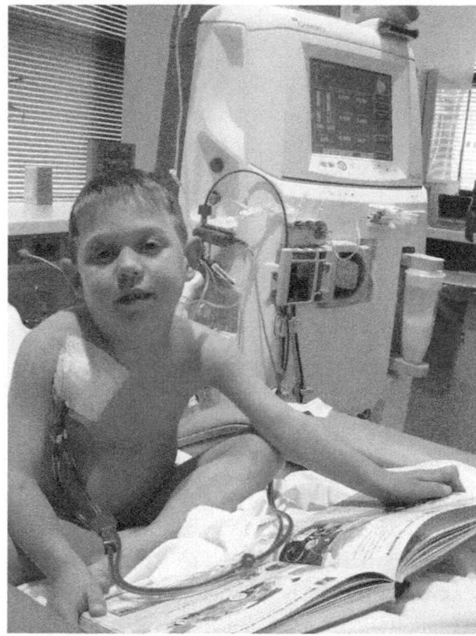

FIG. 24.4 Diversional activities help lessen the boredom children can experience during hemodialysis.

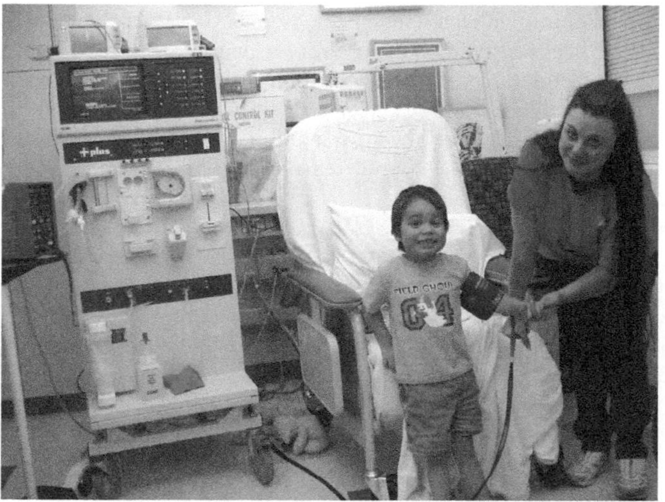

FIG. 24.5 Young child receiving hemodialysis.

available in two forms: parallel flow (plate) and hollow fiber. Hollow fiber dialyzers are preferable for children because their blood compartment is rigid and available in relatively small volumes. Pediatric dialysis can be safely carried out when the total dialysis circuit volume does not exceed 10% of the child's estimated blood volume.

Hemodialysis also requires one of three means of blood access: grafts, fistulas, or external access devices. An arteriovenous fistula is an access in which a vein and artery are connected surgically. The preferred site is the radial artery and a forearm vein. The creation of a subcutaneous (internal) arteriovenous fistula by anastomosing a segment of the radial artery and brachiocephalic vein produces dilation and thickening of the superficial vessels of the forearm to provide easy access for repeated venipuncture. Fewer complications and less restriction of activity are observed with the use of a fistula. If vessels are inadequate for an autogenous fistula, a synthetic graft may be placed in the arm or thigh with either a loop or straight configuration. Both the graft and the fistula require needle insertion at each dialysis session. For short-term external vascular access, percutaneous catheters are inserted in the femoral or internal jugular veins, even in very small children. Avoid subclavian access because of the potential complication of stenosis. For long-term external vascular access, cuffed, dual-lumen (single-lumen for infants) catheters can be surgically placed similarly to other central venous access devices. They are ready to be used immediately and do not require needles.

Various hemodialysis schedules are used, but most centers recommend dialysis three times a week for 3 to 5 hours, depending on the child's size. Some centers have initiated intensified dialysis (4 to 7 days per week) programs (Thumfart, Pommer, Querfeld, et al., 2014).

The length of a hemodialysis treatment, the blood flow rate, and dialyzer characteristics contribute to adequacy of treatment. The current target level for adequacy is a Kt/V (clearance × time/volume) of 1.4 or higher. For a complete description of the highly specialized process of hemodialysis, see the numerous references available on this topic. Dietary limitations are necessary in chronic dialysis to avoid biochemical complications. Fluid and sodium are restricted to prevent fluid overload and its associated symptoms of hypertension, cerebral manifestations, and congestive heart failure. Potassium is restricted to prevent complications related to hyperkalemia; phosphorus restriction helps prevent parathyroid hyperactivity and its attendant risk of abnormal calcification in soft tissues. Adequate protein intake is necessary to maximize growth potential. Fluid limitations are determined by residual urinary output and the need to limit intradialytic weight gain.

Seizures during or after hemodialysis are now uncommon. With the current practice of hemodialysis, cerebral edema caused by alterations in osmolality in the brain when the BUN level is lowered rapidly (associated with dialysis disequilibrium syndrome) is rare.

Home Hemodialysis

With appropriate cannulization and proper training and education of both the child and the parents, hemodialysis can be performed at home. Benefits include less absence from school, more flexibility with dialysis timing, and improved quality of life (Hothi, Stronach, & Sinnott, 2016). Home hemodialysis is especially advantageous for children that live a great distance from the dialysis center.

Home hemodialysis units are available to some children, and the preparation and management are similar to those required for hemodialysis in the hospital. The patient is equipped with a dialysis unit that is used with the vascular access established for outpatient dialysis. Parents of children on home hemodialysis must know how to operate the equipment, connect the unit to the vascular access, and assess the child's status. Home hemodialysis is more prevalent in sparsely populated regions of the country.

Nursing Care Management

Initiating a hemodialysis regimen is a traumatic and anxiety-provoking experience for most children. After surgery for implantation of the graft, fistula, or long-term external access device, the initial experience with the hemodialysis machine and its implication can be frightening. They need reassurance about the preparations for dialysis and the conduct of the treatment. They are anxious about repeated venipunctures (with implanted shunts and for blood chemistries) and about the sight of their blood leaving their body and entering the machine (see Atraumatic Care box). The child's physiologic response to the treatment (e.g., nausea and vomiting, cramps, or seizures) can also cause anxiety. These are usually individual responses related to the child's overall well-being and degree of compliance with the total medical regimen. Once the initial fear of the machine has been resolved, the nurse can help children develop strategies for dealing with restricted activity and movement for the duration of each treatment (see Fig. 24.5).

ATRAUMATIC CARE

Minimizing Pain of Access for Hemodialysis

Buffered lidocaine or a more rapid onset local anesthetic (e.g., procaine) with a small-gauge needle (30 gauge) should be used to anesthetize the area before venipuncture of the graft or fistula. An anesthetizing topical preparation such as EMLA (a eutectic mixture of local anesthetics [lidocaine and prilocaine]) also can be applied 1 hour before venipuncture. (See Pain Management, Chapter 5.)

With their increased need for independence and their urge for rebellion, adolescents may not adapt well to dialysis. They resent dependency on a machine, parents, professional staff, and an unrelenting therapy program. Depression, hostility, or both are common in adolescents undergoing hemodialysis. The adverse consequences of the disease include the need for diet restrictions, limitations in physical activity (resulting from lack of energy, frequent illnesses, and specific restrictions related to access), and the sense of being different from other children. Withdrawal from peers and social isolation may occur, and noncompliance with the therapeutic regimen is not uncommon.

Body changes related to the disease process, such as growth retardation, skin color changes, and lack of sexual maturation, are stress provoking. Dietary restrictions are particularly burdensome for both children and parents. Children feel deprived when unable to eat foods previously enjoyed and unrestricted for other family members. Consequently, failure to cooperate is common. Diet restrictions can be interpreted as punishment if children are unable to fully understand the purpose of the restrictions. Some children will sneak forbidden food items at every opportunity. Allowing children, especially adolescents, maximum participation in and responsibility for their own treatment program is helpful. The extent of adherence and adjustment depends on the personalities of the involved persons, the quality of their relationships, and their coping mechanisms.

After weeks, months, or years of hemodialysis, the parents and the child feel anxiety associated with the prognosis and continued pressures of the treatment. The relentless need for treatment interferes with family plans and activities, including school. Graft and fistula problems are a common source of aggravation. Most families and children on hemodialysis look to kidney transplantation as a desirable alternative to long-term treatment.

PERITONEAL DIALYSIS

For acute conditions, PD is quick, relatively easy to learn, safe to perform and requires minimum equipment with specially trained nurses. PD is a slow, gentle process that decreases the stress on body organs that can occur with the rapid chemical and volume changes of hemodialysis. The procedure is indicated for neonates, children with severe cardiovascular disease, or those who are poor risks for vascular access.

Chronic PD is the preferred form of dialysis for children and parents who are independent; families who live a long distance from the medical center; infants; school-age children; and adolescents, who prefer fewer dietary restrictions and a gentler form of dialysis. Chronic PD is most often performed at home.

Contraindications for the use of PD include recent abdominal surgery or peritoneal adhesions and scarring. A higher rate of infection (peritonitis) is observed with this modality.

Procedure

In acute situations PD catheter insertion may be accomplished at the bedside; catheters for long-term use are placed surgically in the operating room with the patient under anesthesia. A catheter is inserted through the anterior abdominal wall, and the catheter cuff is sutured into place. Chronic PD catheters are tunneled through a subcutaneous tract before exiting the skin in a manner similar to implantation of central venous access devices. At the time of dialysis a commercially prepared dialysis solution is allowed to flow by gravity through the catheter and into the peritoneal cavity, where it remains while equilibrium between plasma and dialysis fluid takes place. Approximately 30 to 50 ml/kg, or 1100 ml/m^2, of dialysis solution are instilled at each cycle. The fluid is then allowed to flow by gravity drainage into a receptacle, and fresh dialysis solution is again instilled.

In PD each pass or cycle is characterized by inflow time, dwell time, and drain time. The length of each portion of the cycle is part of the dialysis prescription. The dwell time and type of solution used varies according to the goals of the treatment (i.e., removal of water, solute, electrolyte, or all of these). The procedure is usually continued until renal function is restored, waste products are reduced, or (in prolonged need) the patient is switched to a form of chronic PD, such as continuous ambulatory peritoneal dialysis (CAPD) or continuous cycling peritoneal dialysis (CCPD). An acute PD catheter may remain in place for several weeks, provided that all who enter the system adhere to aseptic technique.

Home Dialysis

The development of satisfactory methods for CAPD and its alternative, CCPD, has provided additional means for managing ESRD at home. In both methods, commercially available sterile dialysis solution is instilled into the peritoneal cavity through the surgically implanted indwelling catheter. The warmed solution is allowed to enter the peritoneal cavity by gravity and remains a variable length of time according to the procedure used. Dialysis solution is infused and dialysate drained through a single catheter.

In CAPD the dialysis solution is instilled and the line is clamped off and worn attached to the abdomen or thigh, or even placed in a pocket. Manufacturers offer a variety of disconnect devices (e.g., Y set), all of which minimize the connectivity and amount of tubing the patient carries between exchanges. The solution remains in the peritoneum for 4 to 6 hours. The dialysate is then drained via gravity into a bag. Another warmed bag is infused, and the process is repeated so that there is fluid in the abdomen continuously. The procedure is performed a minimum of three times during the day and once at night. For an active child CAPD has proved to be a satisfactory alternative to hemodialysis.

CCPD is a modification of CAPD and intermittent PD. The dialysis exchange is usually performed at night using a PD machine that warms the dialysis fluid and automates the cycles of inflow of dialysis fluid and outflow of dialysate. As with CAPD, the CCPD system is opened during the day but is opened only twice as opposed to multiple times. Nighttime dialysis allows the child more freedom during the day and relieves parents of the need to perform multiple exchanges.

The care and management of the procedure are the responsibility of the parents of young children. Older children and adolescents are able to carry out the procedure themselves, thus providing them with some control and less dependency. This is especially important for adolescents.

Complications. CAPD and CCPD are currently considered the methods of choice for most children who require dialysis because they are easier to initiate and maintain than hemodialysis. Peritonitis is the major complication of home PD. The patients are treated intraperitoneally with antibiotics, and some may require catheter replacement. Although the risk of infection is continuously present, most practitioners believe it is not great enough to discourage the use of these methods.

However, other complications have been noted in patients on home PD. Tunnel infections are evidenced by swelling, warmth, and tenderness along the subcutaneous catheter tract; such infections are managed with administration of antibiotics or catheter replacement. Peritoneal leaks and ventral hernias caused by the sustained intraabdominal pressure that develops within the peritoneum have also been found in a significant number of children. Few of these patients respond to a reduction in dialysis solution volume, and many require surgical intervention.

! NURSING ALERT

Observe for changes in the color of the dialysis solution draining from the child. The solution should be straw colored and clear. If the color is pink, bright yellow, or brown, or if the solution is cloudy, notify the practitioner immediately.

Nursing Care Management

The availability of home dialysis has offered a greater degree of freedom for persons undergoing long-term dialysis. It eliminates the need for a residence convenient to a dialysis unit and for frequent trips to the unit, except for monthly evaluations. The nurse is responsible for teaching the family. Education focuses on the disease, its implications, and the therapeutic plan; the possible psychologic effects of the disease and the treatment; and the technical aspects of the procedure.

The family must learn how to take vital signs before and after the dialysis and how to interpret the significance of blood pressure and temperature variations. They need to know how to vary the composition of the dialysis solution to compensate for variations in the vital signs and to maintain an accurate record of all aspects of the treatment.

Parents of the young child using CAPD need to learn how to exchange bags and manage the procedure at home. Even newborn infants are able to benefit from PD. Older children can learn to take responsibility for their own treatments as much as possible. Encourage the family to ask questions throughout the preparation time, including those that clarify anatomy and physiology, mechanical functioning, and side effects of the disease and the treatment. The PD schedule is outlined to meet the individual needs of the patient and family. Most schedules are arranged for uninterrupted sleep at night and coordination of the dialysis with school and other activities. The nurse discusses diet, medication, and activity and explores feelings about the entire therapeutic program with the child and family.

Infection is the greatest hazard of PD; therefore instruct the family to contact the appropriate persons at the earliest evidence of peritonitis. In most instances peritonitis can be controlled with antibiotics. Unfortunately, there is a high incidence of peritonitis, and repeated infections may necessitate replacement of the catheter or its removal and abandonment of the peritoneum as an access route.

The importance of emotional and material support cannot be overemphasized. The National Kidney Foundation, mentioned previously, provides a number of services and information for families of children with renal disease. A relatively new organization, the American Association of Kidney Patients,* has been organized to promote the interest and welfare of kidney patients. It provides education and support for patients and public education regarding all areas of kidney disease.

CONTINUOUS VENOVENOUS HEMOFILTRATION

A third type of "dialysis" or renal replacement therapy used primarily in acute care settings is continuous venovenous hemofiltration (CVVH). This type of therapy uses specialized equipment (e.g., hemofilter, blood pump, tubing connected to a vascular access) to ultrafiltrate blood continuously at a very slow rate. With this procedure, fluid balance may be achieved within 24 to 48 hours after initiation. Continuous venovenous hemodialysis (CVVHD) is used to remove excess fluid from patients with severe oliguric fluid overload.

CVVHD is an ideal form of renal replacement therapy for children with fluid overload from surgical procedures (e.g., cardiovascular surgery) who do not have severe biochemical abnormalities. It is commonly used for critically ill children who require volume-expanding fluids such as hyperalimentation solution, albumin, or packed red cells. It creates space for the infusion of these replacement solutions in fluid-sensitive patients. CVVHD has proved to be a highly successful alternative form of dialysis for critically ill children who might not survive the rapid volume changes that occur with hemodialysis and PD.

TRANSPLANTATION

Kidney transplantation is the preferred means of renal replacement therapy in the pediatric age-group. Although PD and hemodialysis are life preserving and are able to be carried out in the home in a large number of cases, neither method is compatible with a normal lifestyle. Transplantation, on the other hand, offers the opportunity for a relatively normal life.

Kidneys for transplant are available from two sources: a living donor, usually a parent, grandparent, or sibling, or a deceased donor, wherein the family of a dead or brain-dead patient consents to donation of a healthy kidney. The criteria for selection of kidney recipients are liberal, but uniform criteria have not been established among the various centers that specialize in the procedure. In general, there is no limit to age. In some cases a person's mental status (e.g., emotional instability or nonadherence to drug therapy) may be a reason to defer transplantation until the recipient's psychoemotional status improves and it is reasonable to assume that the recipient will carry out the posttransplant regimen (see Family-Centered Care box).

FAMILY-CENTERED CARE

Medical Care Rationing

The criteria for selection of renal transplant recipients sometimes create dilemmas for professionals. In most cases the decision is simply a matter for the transplant team and the family to resolve for the benefit of the child involved. However, in some situations the solution is less clear, especially in view of the scarcity of donor kidneys and the expense of the procedure. The matter creates more questions than answers.

For example, should a child without a severe mental or physical disability take priority over one with these disabilities? Should financial responsibility be a consideration? Some youngsters with kidney transplants have discontinued their medications, thereby either causing damage to their kidney or losing the graft. Should these youngsters receive a second transplant? Should very young children whose families have proved unreliable in adhering to a therapeutic regimen be given a transplant when the success of the graft depends on following a prescribed therapeutic plan? Are young, single, adolescent mothers likely to be less adherent in following the prescribed medical regimen? Can persons on limited incomes manage to acquire the costly medications? If not, should the government subsidize payment?

What solutions to these dilemmas are available, and how do providers justify decisions? Should hospital ethics committees make the decisions?

*3505 E. Frontage Road, Suite 315, Tampa, FL 33607; 800-749-2257; http://www.aakp.org.

Children who have ESRD secondary to malignancy must be cancer free for a specified time before transplantation (depending on the type of malignancy). Generalized infection must be eradicated before attempted transplantation, and the recipient should have adequate bladder capacity. Some children may have bladder augmentation or other genitourinary surgery as preparation for transplantation. Children with abnormal urinary tracts may be subject to more posttransplant urologic complications and infection than they would be otherwise.

Procedure

The kidney graft is placed in the extraperitoneal space, usually the anterior iliac fossa; the renal artery is anastomosed to the internal iliac or hypogastric artery; the renal vein is anastomosed to the hypogastric vein; and the ureter is implanted into the bladder or anastomosed to the recipient's ureter. Small children receiving a large donor kidney may require placement within the abdomen with vessel anastomoses to the aorta and inferior vena cava. Unless there is medical contraindication, the recipient's failed kidneys are left in place. Severe hypertension, neoplasm, large and continuous protein losses, and persistent severe VUR are the usual reasons for nephrectomy.

The primary goal in transplantation is the long-term survival of the grafted tissue. The means by which this is attempted include securing tissues that are antigenically similar to that of the recipient and suppressing the recipient's immune mechanism.

Selection of Donor Tissue

The source of a donor kidney is either a live person or a deceased donor. The closer the genetic relationship between the donor and the recipient, the better the possibility of long-term survival. The only truly compatible tissue match is that between identical twin siblings. The next best possible match is a sibling, followed by a parent or grandparent. In some states the use of siblings is impossible until the possible donor is of age to give consent for removal of a kidney. Unrelated donors are least likely to be compatible. Careful immunologic studies are carried out to determine the donor whose kidney is least likely to be rejected by the recipient.

Suppression of the Immune Response

After the best possible tissue match is obtained for a transplant, suppressing the recipient's immune response can significantly lengthen the survival time. The immunosuppressant therapy of choice varies by institution. A combination of prednisone, tacrolimus, and mycophenolate is commonly used. Other therapies include antilymphocyte globulin or monoclonal antibodies, administered intravenously either for induction or rescue from rejection.

The administration of these drugs is not without hazard. The major problem encountered with nonspecific immunosuppression is that it not only suppresses the immune response to the grafted tissue but also suppresses the body's capacity to respond to other antigenic stimuli. Consequently, the child is vulnerable to overwhelming infections.

Prednisone is an immunosuppressant and antiinflammatory agent that acts to stabilize cell walls, reduce migration of white blood cells into the inflamed area, and inhibit deposition of fibrin and collagen. It also depresses T cells, B cells, and phagocytes. A number of complications from corticosteroid therapy are cause for concern. Interference with linear growth has led many centers to use alternate-day administration in an effort to improve growth rates and to decrease other long-term side effects such as cataracts, fluid and sodium retention, hypertension, gastric ulcer, and obesity. Researchers are studying steroid-free and early steroid withdrawal treatment protocols with the goal of minimizing side effects without compromising graft survival (Haller, Royuela, Nagler, et al., 2016).

Rejection

Rejection of a transplanted kidney is the most common cause of transplant failure. Rejection can be one of three types: hyperacute, acute, or chronic. Hyperacute rejection is irreversible, develops immediately or within a few hours after revascularization, and is related to circulating antibodies preformed in the recipient against the donor tissue antigens.

Acute rejection usually occurs between the first few days and months after transplantation but may occur years later, especially if the patient becomes poorly compliant with immunosuppressant medications. Both biochemical and clinical abnormalities are evidence of rejection. The most common finding is an elevated serum creatinine and BUN. Fever, which is usually accompanied by swelling and tenderness over the graft; hypertension; and diminished urinary output may occur. Most acute rejection episodes respond to IV administration of methylprednisolone sodium succinate (Solu-Medrol), antilymphocyte globulin, or monoclonal antibodies.

! NURSING ALERT

The child with a kidney transplant who exhibits any of the following should be evaluated immediately for possible rejection:

- Fever
- Swelling and tenderness over graft area
- Diminished urinary output
- Elevated blood pressure
- Elevated serum creatinine

Slow, gradual deterioration of renal function that typically begins 6 months or more after transplantation characterizes chronic rejection. Elevations of serum creatinine, proteinuria, or hematuria are signs of rejection. In addition, the rejection may have symptomatology indistinguishable from that of the original kidney disease. No present therapy can halt the process, which inevitably leads to loss of the implanted kidney.

Prognosis

According to the 2014 annual report of the North American Pediatric Renal Trials and Collaborative Studies the overall graft survival rate for kidneys at 1 and 3 years is 96% and 93% respectively from living donors and 96% and 90% respectively from deceased donors. Predictors of graft survival for children include age at transplantation, pretransplantation dialysis, early rejection, and race. Infections, cancer/malignancy, and cardiovascular causes are the most life-threatening problems after transplantation (Holmberg & Jalanko, 2016). Long-term graft survival is not guaranteed, and many children require a second or third transplant. Successful kidney transplantation does improve rehabilitation of children with kidney failure, both educationally and psychologically.

Nursing Care Management

The possibility of kidney transplantation often comes as a hope for relief from the rigors of dialysis or the restriction of a conservative management regimen. Most children and families respond well to a kidney transplant. Children with successful kidney transplants are usually able to resume life activities similar to those of their unaffected peers. The rehabilitation of children with kidney transplants is influenced primarily by their pattern of functioning before becoming ill. It is important to remember that transplantation is a treatment that has a far less negative impact on the child's normal life activities than dialysis, although multiple medications and clinic visits remain a part of their life. Stresses remain for the child and family in relation to the uncertainty of the future, the child's health and well-being, social isolation, and financial burdens.

A variety of serious emotional and psychologic conflicts may arise as a consequence of donor selection, including ambivalence of donors faced with surgery and relinquishing a kidney, feelings of guilt if one should prove to be unacceptable as a donor, and the emotional impact of having a live relative–donated kidney rejected by the recipient. This especially can result in guilt feelings when a parent is the donor.

The child recipient responds in various ways to a kidney transplant. The concept of having a foreign body, especially a deceased donor kidney, inside their own body is sometimes disturbing to children. They often speculate about the age, sex, personality, and physical characteristics of the donor. They may fear that the kidney will wear out if it came from an older person. Some children are distressed to find that their donor kidney came from a person of the opposite sex. Corticosteroid therapy, necessary in kidney transplants, creates undesirable side effects (e.g., growth failure, obesity, characteristics of Cushing syndrome, acne, and hirsutism) that are often a source of emotional and social problems for older children. Gum hyperplasia, brittle fingernails, and hair breakage can also occur.

DRUG ALERT

Patient Education

Providing patient education is a critical role for nursing staff. The nurse must be aware of the potential side effects of every medication the child is taking and provide appropriate surveillance and education. Children who are concerned about changes in their body due to the immunosuppressant medications may stop taking them. Surveillance for the development of a number of conditions, including the BK polyoma virus, lymphoproliferative disease, diabetes mellitus, hypertension, dyslipidemias, and skin changes, is required (Holmberg & Jalanko, 2016). Education for minimizing the risk of developing these and other conditions is necessary.

DRUG ALERT

Medication Noncompliance After Kidney Transplant

The most common reason for poor medication adherence in childhood kidney transplant recipients is dislike of undesirable side effects. The cosmetic implications of the side effects can be overwhelming, especially to adolescent girls. Deliberate discontinuation of the drugs is most common in teenage girls. Poor medication knowledge, number of medications, and length of time since transplant can negatively affect medication adherence (Loghman-Adham, 2003). (See Compliance, Chapter 22.)

Working with children and their families during the various stages of renal failure, dialysis, and transplantation is a difficult, challenging and rewarding experience. Nurses must become familiar with the family; assess family strengths, weaknesses, and coping mechanisms; and be prepared to provide intensive support and guidance during the prolonged experience. The child and family need help accepting what is happening to them. They also need help in following the nurse's anticipatory guidance regarding predictable stresses and in dealing constructively with the physical, emotional, and financial burdens that are an ongoing part of this prolonged disability.

DEFECTS OF THE GENITOURINARY TRACT

PHIMOSIS

Phimosis is a narrowing or stenosis of the preputial opening of the foreskin that prevents retraction of the foreskin over the glans penis. It is a normal finding in infants and young boys and usually disappears as the child grows and the distal prepuce dilates. Occasionally the narrowing obstructs the flow of urine, resulting in a dribbling stream or even ballooning of the foreskin with accumulated urine during voiding.

Balanitis is an inflammation or infection of the phimotic foreskin, which occurs occasionally and is managed as any other inflammation or infection. Phimosis is often treated effectively by application of steroid cream twice a day for 1 month, with the option for surgical treatment with circumcision in severe cases.

Nursing Care Management

Proper hygiene of the phimotic foreskin in infants and young boys consists of external cleansing during routine bathing. The foreskin should not be forcibly retracted because it may create scarring that can prevent future retraction. Furthermore, retraction of the tight foreskin can result in paraphimosis, a condition in which the retracted foreskin cannot be replaced in its normal position over the glans. This causes edema and venous congestion created by constriction by the tight band of foreskin—a urologic emergency that requires immediate evaluation.

HYDROCELE

Hydrocele is the presence of peritoneal fluid in the scrotum between the parietal and visceral layers of the tunica vaginalis and is the most common cause of painless scrotal swelling in children and adolescents, along with nonincarcerated inguinal hernia. Hydroceles may be communicating or noncommunicating. A communicating hydrocele usually develops when the process vaginalis does not close during development, allowing for communication with the peritoneum. Noncommunicating hydroceles have no connection to the peritoneum with fluid coming from the mesothelial lining of the tunica vaginalis. Hydroceles are common in newborns and often resolve spontaneously, usually by 12 months of age. In older children, noncommunicating hydroceles may be idiopathic or a result of trauma, epididymitis, orchitis, testicular torsion, torsion of the appendix testis or appendix epididymis, or tumor.

Communicating hydroceles may change in size during the day or with straining, whereas noncommunicating hydroceles are not reducible and so do not change in size with crying or straining. Surgical repair is indicated for communicating hydroceles persisting past 1 year of age because of the increased risk of development of an incarcerated inguinal hernia. Idiopathic hydroceles are repaired if symptomatic and reactive hydroceles usually resolve with treatment of the underlying cause, such as epididymitis.

Nursing Care Management

Surgical treatment is an outpatient procedure. Advise parents that there is often temporary swelling and discoloration of the scrotum that resolves spontaneously. Straddle toys are avoided for 2 to 4 weeks and strenuous activities in older boys may be avoided for 1 month. If a dressing is used, it is removed in 2 to 3 days and typically the child may bathe in 3 days.

CRYPTORCHIDISM

Cryptorchidism is failure of one or both testes to descend normally through the inguinal canal into the scrotum. Absence of testes within the scrotum can be a result of undescended (cryptorchid) testes, retractile testes, or absent testes. There is also the potential for ascending testes, where testes were in the scrotum in early childhood and then "ascended," also known as acquired undescended testes. Undescended testes can be located in the abdomen, the inguinal canal, the upper scrotum or, rarely, in an ectopic location outside of the normal pathway of descent.

The prevalence of cryptorchidism is reported to be 30% in preterm boys and 3% in full-term boys; with spontaneous descent probable during the first 6 months of life with correction for prematurity. If persistent after 6 months, probability of spontaneous descent decreases. The prevalence of acquired cryptorchidism is 1% to 7% and peaks around 8 years of age (Kolon, Herndon, Baker, et al., 2014).

Pathophysiology

Testicular development is influenced by a number of genes, but the dominant one is located on the Y chromosome. This gene stimulates the medullary sex cords of the embryonic gonad to differentiate into secretory Sertoli cells. Beginning around week 7, these cells secrete a glycoprotein, müllerian inhibiting substance that leads to development of a male genital system. Testicular descent is a critical element of the development of the male genital system. This descent occurs in two phases; the first is dominated by müllerian inhibiting substance and the second phase by testosterone. Between weeks 8 and 15 a cordlike structure, the gubernaculum, extends from the developing testis (located in the lower abdomen) to the labioscrotal swelling. The fetus grows, but the length of this gubernaculum remains relatively fixed, anchoring the testis to the developing inguinal canal (transabdominal migration) in preparation for the second phase of descent. This second phase begins around weeks 25 to 30 and is characterized by shrinkage of the gubernaculum under the influence of testosterone, causing the testis to migrate down the inguinal canal and into a scrotal position (transinguinal migration). Descent is also characterized by protrusion of peritoneum, the processus vaginalis that closes before birth.

Cryptorchidism occurs when one or both testes fail to descend through the inguinal canal and into the scrotum. Several processes may slow or arrest testicular descent, including endocrine abnormalities affecting the hypothalamic-pituitary-testicular axis, denervation of the genitofemoral nerve, traction of the gubernaculum, abnormal development of the epididymis, or preterm birth. Congenital hernias and abnormal testes often accompany cryptorchid testes, and they are at risk for subsequent torsion.

An ectopic testis emerges outside the inguinal ring into the perineum or femoral area, or lies in a transverse scrotal or prepenile location. The most common site is the superficial inguinal pouch. Ectopia is postulated to occur because of obstruction of the scrotal inlet, scarring (fibrosis) of the gubernaculum, or other mechanical anomalies.

Absent testis may be due to agenesis or atrophy from loss of blood supply secondary to prenatal testicular torsion. This has been termed the *vanishing testis syndrome or testicular regression syndrome.* **Anorchism** is absence of both testes and may be associated with genotypic and phenotypic abnormalities such as congenital adrenal hyperplasia (CAH). A newborn with a male phallus and bilateral nonpalpable testes may be a genetic female with CAH. Failure to diagnose CAH can result in life-threatening electrolyte imbalances. Disorders of sexual development or other abnormalities should also be considered, especially if there are also noted abnormalities of the phallus such as severe hypospadias or micropenis (Kolon, Herndon, Baker, et al., 2014).

Associated conditions and complications resulting from undescended testes include inguinal hernia, testicular torsion, testicular trauma, subfertility, and testicular cancer. Surgical repositioning the testes may reduce but not prevent the potential long-term issues of infertility and testis cancer (Kolon, Herndon, Baker, et al., 2014).

Retractile testes can be found at any level within the path of testicular descent, but they are most commonly identified in the groin. Fortunately, they are not truly cryptorchid. Instead, they are introverted to an inguinal or abdominal position because of an overactive cremasteric reflex. The cremasteric reflex, observed as withdrawal of the testis above the scrotum and into the inguinal canal in response to various stimuli, including exposure to cool temperatures, is active during infancy and peaks around age 4 to 5 years. Unlike the cryptorchid testis, the retractile testis can be gently moved into the scrotum without residual tension and does not require treatment. Retractile testes can become ascending testes and require annual monitoring.

Clinical Manifestations

A nonpalpable testis is typically observed by the parent or detected during routine physical examination. If one testis is not palpable, the affected hemiscrotum will appear smaller than the other. With bilateral nonpalpable testes, both hemiscrota appear small. In the case of retractile testes, the parents may report intermittently observing the testes in the scrotum, interspersed with periods when they cannot be visualized or palpated. Frequently, the retractile testis will be observed in the scrotum when the child is in a warm bath.

Diagnostic Evaluation

It is important to differentiate the true undescended testis from the more common retractile testis. Retractile testes can be "milked" or pushed back into the scrotum, but truly undescended ones cannot. For examination, the examiner can obviate the cremasteric reflex by placing the child in a cross legged position or by applying firm finger pressure on the external ring before palpating the abdomen or genitalia. (See Fig. 4.39.)

Undescended testes are palpable along the inguinal canal, but those in the abdominal cavity usually are not. Imaging is not routinely used to locate nonpalpable testes. Exploratory surgery is used for both diagnosis and treatment, beginning with examination under anesthesia and progressing to laparoscopy or open inguinal approach.

Therapeutic Management. Current evidence based recommendations state that if spontaneous testicular descent does not occur by 6 months of age in congenital undescended testes, that surgical correction should be performed within the next year. (Kolon, Herndon, Baker, et al., 2014). Previously utilized hormonal therapy to induce testicular descent is no longer recommended due to low response rates. **Orchiopexy** is the procedure for repositioning undescended testes that are palpable and is performed through an inguinal or scrotal incision. The goal is to place and fix the testes in a normal scrotal position to decrease the risk of testicular torsion and traumatic injury to a testis in the inguinal canal. Placement allows for easier examination to monitor for testicular cancer and early correction may reduce the risk of infertility.

The timing of the surgery is important, as it is in any genital surgery. Orchiopexy is usually performed between 6 and 24 months of age in the case of congenital cryptorchidism. Fewer psychologic effects and a higher rate of fertility may be achieved when repair takes place at an early age. Having both testes in the scrotum by school age prevents psychologic problems related to body image and peer group embarrassment because the empty scrotum is smaller in size and altered in shape.

In the routine surgical procedure for undescended testes, the testes are brought down into the scrotum and secured in that position without tension or torsion. A simple orchiopexy for a palpable testis can usually be performed in an outpatient surgical unit. Diagnostic laparoscopic surgery is utilized by the surgeon with laparoscopic experience for exploration of boys with nonpalpable testes. If an intraabdominal testis is identified, this permits planning for a more definitive procedure, which may be open or laparoscopic.

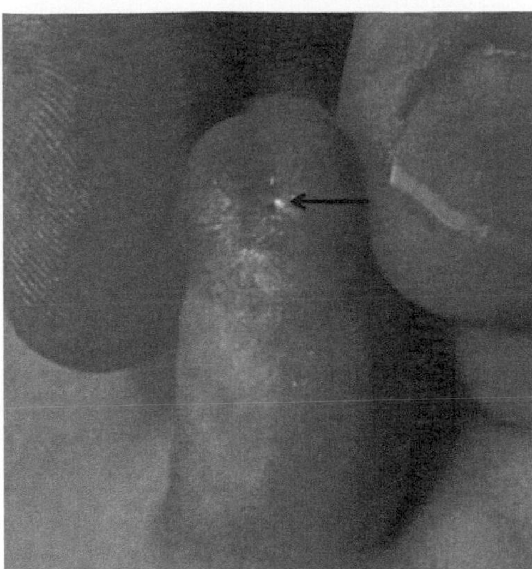

FIG. 24.6 Distal hypospadias with a stenotic meatus *(arrow)* located on the glans with no chordee. (From Holcomb, G. W., Murphy, J. P., & Ostlie, D. J. [2014]. *Ashcraft's pediatric surgery* [6th ed.]. Philadelphia, PA: Elsevier.)

Nursing Care Management

Postoperative nursing care is directed toward preventing infection and instructing parents in home care of the child, including pain control. Infection is prevented by carefully cleansing the operative site of stool and urine. Observation of the wound for complications and activity restrictions are discussed. The child should avoid vigorous sports activities and use of toys that are straddled for 2 weeks postoperatively. All boys with cryptorchidism should learn to perform testicular self-examination starting at puberty.

HYPOSPADIAS

Hypospadias is a congenital anomaly of the male urethra that results in abnormal ventral placement of the urethral opening on the underside of the penis, ranging from the glans to the perineum (Fig. 24.6). It is one of the most common congenital anomalies with an incidence reported to be 1 in 300 males (0.3%). Recurrence rate is approximately 13 times greater in first-degree relatives, including brother, father, or son (Snodgrass & Bush, 2016). Both genetic and environmental factors have been associated with hypospadias. Severity of hypospadias is based on the position of the urethral opening and the degree of chordee, or ventral curvature of the penis. The more distant the opening from the normal position at the tip of the glans and the more marked curvature increases the severity and the need for more extensive surgical correction. In mild cases the meatus is just below the tip of the penis. In the most severe malformations the meatus is located on the perineum between the halves of the scrotum (bifid scrotum). In addition, the foreskin is usually absent ventrally and, when combined with chordee, gives the organ a hooded and crooked appearance. In severe cases the altered appearance may leave the infant's gender in doubt at birth because of the perineal position of the meatus and small penis. In any case of ambiguous genitalia, additional evaluation is essential. Cryptorchidism is present in about 10% of infants with hypospadias and increases with more proximal hypospadias with the meatus at the scrotum or perineum. There is an increased risk of disorders of sex development in patients with severe hypospadias, both with and without cryptorchidism.

Surgical Correction

The principal objectives of surgical correction are (1) to enhance the child's ability to void in the standing position with a straight stream, (2) to improve the physical appearance of the genitalia for psychologic reasons, and (3) to preserve a sexually adequate organ. The choice of surgical procedure is affected primarily by the severity of the defect and the presence of associated anomalies. Numerous techniques are utilized in repair of hypospadias and are performed under general anesthesia typically as an outpatient procedure.

Hypospadias repair may be done by primary tubularization for milder forms in which a new urethra is made by rolling a ventral strip of penile shaft skin that normally would have formed the urethra. For more severe hypospadias, an onlay island flap is used to create the urethra, transferring a strip of inner foreskin onto the ventral urethral plate. In severe forms, including those with significant chordee, a two-stage repair is used to straighten the penis and create a new urethra. These are typically performed at least 6 months apart. There is no consensus on the best surgical approach for correcting severe hypospadias and complication rates are high; specifically development of urethrocutaneous fistula, urethral stricture or meatal stenosis, and urethral diverticulum (Prat, Natasha, Polak, et al., 2012).

The chordee that often coexists with a hypospadias defect is repaired by release of the ventral skin. When the chordee persists, additional procedures may be indicated. In many cases, a single operation will be all that is needed to correct hypospadias and chordee.

The preferred time for surgical repair is 6 to 12 months of age, before the child has developed body image. Occasionally a short course of testosterone is administered preoperatively to achieve additional penile size to facilitate the surgery.

Nursing Care Management

Neonatal circumcision should be avoided in hypospadias where there is incomplete foreskin because this is not conducive to a safe clamp or Plastibell circumcision. In severe cases, the foreskin may be used in reconstruction. In mild hypospadias, the foreskin is not incomplete and the abnormality may not be noted until after circumcision. This does not affect future successful reconstruction if it is needed. In most cases, the appearance after reconstruction will be of a circumcised normal penis.

Frequently parents are informed of what is to be surgically corrected but are not advised of what to expect as a reasonable consequence. More refined surgical techniques performed by surgeons specializing in pediatric urologic conditions have improved cosmetic and functional outcomes in these boys. If children are old enough to understand what is occurring, the nurse also prepares them for the operation and the expected outcome.

Hypospadias repair may require some type of urinary diversion with a silicone stent or feeding tube to promote optimum healing and to maintain the position and patency of the newly formed urethra. This is left in the bladder to drain urine for 5 to 10 days. In most infants and children who are not toilet trained, the catheter drains directly into the diaper. In older children, the catheter is connected to a leg bag or a larger bedside bag at night. Drainage bags should always be positioned below the bladder level for proper drainage. Tub baths are avoided until the catheter is removed. Most children will have a caudal or penile nerve block in addition to general anesthesia, which lasts 6 to 8 hours. Appropriate administration of prescribed pain medications for 48 to 72 hours after surgery will help control discomfort. When a catheter is left in place, bladder spasms are common and are very uncomfortable. Anticholinergic medications, such as oxybutynin, are typically used to prevent spasms. Parents should be advised of the possibility of bladder spasms, which are usually brief and intense. The child may arch his back and bring his knees to his chest and may leak urine around the catheter with a spasm. Oxybutynin is given every 8 hours typically and may require dosing adjustment, such as increasing the frequency to every 6 hours to control bladder spasms. Once the catheter is removed, the medication is no longer needed. Often a prophylactic antibiotic is given until shortly after catheter removal. Anticholinergic medication is constipating, and this is a common problem in the postoperative period and may be avoided with preventative measures, such as giving adequate fluid and a stool softener or laxative if needed. Preparing patients for these potential problems is an important nursing responsibility. Patients usually go home with a dressing that often comes off in 1 to 2 days and typically is removed in the bath in 3 days if there is no stent in place. If the dressing is soiled, it can be cleaned gently. The parent should be prepared that the appearance of the penis postoperatively is often swollen, discolored, and /or bruised. This is expected and will resolve with time. While healing, applying petroleum jelly to the diaper to prevent the penis from sticking can help prevent bleeding and increase comfort.

The child should avoid straddle toys, sandboxes, swimming, and rough activities until allowed by the surgeon.

EPISPADIAS AND EXSTROPHY COMPLEX

Bladder exstrophy is a severe defect involving the musculoskeletal system and the urinary, reproductive, and in some cases, the intestinal tract. It is one of three anomalies that define the exstrophy-epispadias complex (EEC). Epispadias is the least severe of the complex and is due to failure of the urethra to close normally, resulting in an exposed or open dorsal urethra. Bladder exstrophy is a more severe defect characterized by an open, "inside-out bladder" with the inner surface exposed and the dorsal urethra (epispadias) on the lower abdominal wall (Figs. 24.7 and 24.8). Classic bladder exstrophy typically includes findings of diastasis (separation) of the symphysis pubis (pelvic bone), low set umbilicus, anteriorly displaced anus, defects of the genitalia, and inguinal hernia. The third and most severe defect is cloacal exstrophy, which includes both bladder exstrophy and exstrophy of the large intestine (hindgut) through an abdominal wall defect. In addition, there is anal atresia, omphalocele, hypoplasia of the colon, anomalous genitalia, and often spinal dysraphism. There may be abnormalities of one or both kidneys. The International Clearinghouse for Birth Defects Surveillance and Research reports a prevalence of cloacal exstrophy at 1 in 131, 579 live births with higher rates in females (Feldkamp, Botto, Amar, et al., 2011) and bladder exstrophy at 2.07 per 100,000 live births and nearly twice as common in males than females (Siffel, Correa, Amar, et al., 2011).

Pathophysiology

The pathogenesis of bladder exstrophy appears to be due to a complex embryologic defect in abdominal wall development. The extent of the defect and the stage of development when the rupture occurs affect the extent of the anomaly will be seen within the EEC.

In males with bladder exstrophy, the defect of the genitalia includes epispadias and upward curvature of a shortened penis and may include other abnormalities, such as undescended testes and inguinal hernias. In females, there is epispadias, a bifid clitoris, and small labia minora. The vagina is shortened compared with normal. In cloacal exstrophy patients, there are often more severe anomalies, such as bifid or duplicated uterus, split clitoris, completely separated labia, and a duplicate or absent vagina in females. Males may have a split penis and scrotum or a short, flat penis with hypospadias. In either sex, separation of the pubic bones is generally corrected by pelvic osteotomy, particularly if there is extreme diastasis, as this increases the likelihood of successful bladder closure.

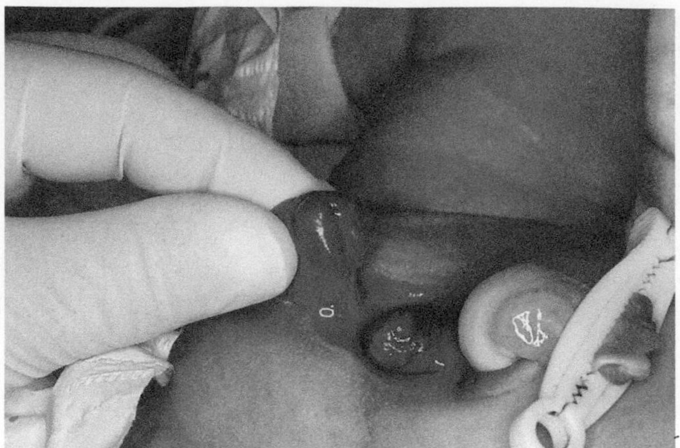

FIG. 24.7 Newborn with bladder exstrophy and epispadias. (Courtesy Tim Yankee, St. Francis Hospital, Tulsa, Oklahoma.)

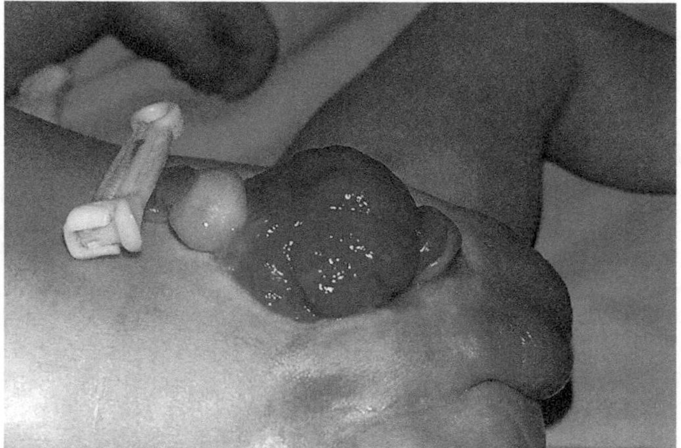

FIG. 24.8 Exstrophy of bladder. (Courtesy H. Gil Rushton, MD, Children's National Medical Center, Washington, DC.)

In bladder exstrophy patients, the upper urinary tract is usually normal. Fertility is possible in females but decreased in males, possibly because of semen abnormalities, abnormal ejaculation, or a combination of both. Assisted reproductive techniques remain a viable option for patients with infertility. Recent studies indicate good long-term outcomes on erectile and general sexual function in both men and women with epispadias and bladder exstrophy (Suominen, Santtila, & Taskinen, 2015).

Therapeutic Management

The objectives of treatment are (1) preservation of renal function, (2) attainment of urinary control, (3) adequate reconstructive repair for acceptable appearance, (4) prevention of UTIs, and (5) preservation of optimum external genitalia with continence and sexual function. There are two surgical approaches currently utilized to correct bladder exstrophy. One is termed *modern staged repair of bladder exstrophy* (MSRBE), typically involving three surgeries beginning with closure of the bladder and abdominal wall. Complete primary repair of bladder exstrophy (CPRBE) is a single stage surgical closure combining closure of the bladder, abdominal wall, partial tightening of the bladder neck, and in some cases, bilateral ureteral reimplantation to correct reflux. Often, pelvic osteotomies are performed at the time of primary closure to deepen the flattened pelvis, close the pubic diastasis, and release tension on the abdominal wall to improve success of primary closure (Inouye, Tourchi, & Di Carlo, 2014).

For the child with bladder exstrophy, CPRBE may be performed within the first 72 hours of life or as a delayed procedure at about 2 months of age. For the child with cloacal exstrophy, pelvic osteotomies are needed because of the wide pelvic diastasis and surgery is done within 48 to 72 hours of life to close the bladder and omphalocele and perform intestinal diversion (Inouye, Tourchi, & Di Carlo, 2014).

In some children, reconstruction (tightening) of the bladder neck may not provide sufficient resistance to achieve urinary continence. In these cases, further intervention may be needed.

Abnormalities of the genitalia are addressed to ensure optimal sexual function. In boys the testes are typically cryptorchid, and bilateral orchiopexy is combined with reconstruction of the bifid scrotum to preserve testicular function. In girls, surgical enlargement of the vaginal introitus may be needed to permit intercourse. In both genders, plastic surgery to reduce scarring of the genital area or to create an umbilicus may significantly improve the child's body image and emerging sexual identity.

Nursing Care Management

In bladder exstrophy the everted bladder appears bright red through the abdominal opening. It is important to prevent trauma to the exposed mucosa. After delivery of an infant with bladder exstrophy, the umbilical cord is clamped with the usual plastic clamp, but the clamp is exchanged for a soft umbilical tape or silk suture material to limit trauma to the exposed bladder. The bladder is covered with plastic wrap or a transparent adhesive dressing for protection. Specifics of care reflect surgeon preference. Some prefer the transparent adhesive dressing that adheres to the intact skin but not the bladder. The bladder may be irrigated intermittently with sterile saline during diaper changes, although this is not absolutely necessary.

Nursing care after the complete primary repair is focused on pain management and maintenance of immobilization. Around the clock IV pain medications are important for several days after surgery as keeping the infant quiet is important to success of the bladder closure. This is extremely important in these cases, as achieving a successful initial closure is one of the best indicators for a good prognosis long term. Nasogastric tube decompression may be used to prevent abdominal distention. Dehiscence may occur postoperatively, and signs of suture separation or wound problems are promptly reported to the practitioner. Immobilization of the pelvis with traction for 2 to 4 weeks is typical even if osteotomies are not performed. A common form of traction for newborns is modified Bryant's traction, though spica casting and other alternatives are used. Chapter 34 discusses nursing care of the child in a spica cast. The child is kept supine and lifted to assess skin with sufficient help to manage lines and keep the patient in good alignment. If orthopedic pins are in place, the care of pins and adjacent skin should be performed according to orthopedic surgeon instructions. Prevention of skin breakdown is important and adhesive foam dressings over pressure areas such as the sacrum or heels or where skin comes in contact with equipment may be helpful. Fluidized positioners are also used and replaced with a reshaped positioner daily.

Postoperative nursing care after bladder neck reconstruction and antireflux surgery (ureteral reimplantation) includes routine wound care and careful monitoring of urinary output from the bladder and ureteral drainage tubes. The nurse should ensure the catheters are intact and are not twisted or kinked. Care after a penile lengthening, chordee release, and urethral reconstruction is similar to care after hypospadias repair.

Children who fail to attain continence after bladder neck reconstruction may require further surgical intervention including bladder augmentation or bladder removal with a continent diversion.

Family Support and Home Care. Bladder exstrophy and other disorders of the EEC are significant congenital abnormalities that require lifelong care by a team of specialists. Improvement in surgical techniques has helped achieve better outcomes, specifically that of the goal of continence. Parental stress is significant, and support services may be helpful. Patients may also benefit from psychologic support as adjustment problems are common, particularly in adolescents. Parents should receive teaching and practice on care of the infant or child at home and have access to resources to call if there are questions. Allowing time for the parent to voice concerns can facilitate evaluation of their understanding and help direct discharge needs.

When the infant is discharged with an unrepaired defect, plastic wrap is placed over the defect to prevent irritation of the exposed bladder from abrasive diapers. Current practice typically allows for the bladder to be immersed in water for a tub bath, cleansed with mild soap, and rinsed with clean water. With these complex patients, post op care is individualized and may vary with physician preference. Urinary tract infections are common in these patients and parents learn to recognize the signs of urinary tract infection and to report a suspected infection to the practitioner.

DISORDERS OF SEX DEVELOPMENT

Infants born with a discrepancy between external genitalia, gonadal and chromosomal sex, are currently referred to as having a **disorder of sex development (DSD)**. The presentation at birth may be a genital appearance that does not permit gender declaration and this is termed **ambiguous genitalia**. These may include bilateral cryptorchidism, perineal hypospadias with bifid scrotum, clitoromegaly, posterior labial fusion, phenotypic female appearance with a palpable gonad, and hypospadias and unilateral nonpalpable gonad. Also included in the DSD category are infants with discordant genitalia and sex chromosomes. Turner syndrome (45, XO) and Klinefelter syndrome (47, XXY) are also DSDs that do not present with ambiguous genitalia.

PATHOPHYSIOLOGY

Normal sexual differentiation starts at 7 weeks of gestation when fetuses with a Y chromosome begin developing testes. Early on both female (XX) and male (XY) fetuses have a similar reproductive structure. Multiple genes contribute to this process and mutations in these genes can lead to various DSDs. Congenital malformation of the genitalia are most frequently because of androgen deficiency in XY individuals and androgen excess in XX patient, though in many cases no endocrine etiology can be found (Grinspon & Rey, 2014).

Initial evaluation includes karyotype and assessment of adrenal and gonadal function, and this information can be used to categorize the infant into one of three categories:

- Virilized XX (XX DSD)
- Undervirilized XY (XY DSD)
- Mixed sex chromosome pattern

THERAPEUTIC MANAGEMENT

The most common cause of ambiguous genitalia is **congenital adrenal hyperplasia (CAH)**, which can lead to life-threatening salt-wasting adrenal insufficiency in the first weeks of life. Though now a part of neonatal screening in the United States, any infant with genital ambiguity should be evaluated urgently. Laboratory testing includes a measurement of 17-hydroxyprogesterone in addition to karyotype with immediate probe for SRY (sex-determining region on the Y chromosome). Serum electrolytes are monitored as signs and symptoms of adrenal insufficiency may include hypoglycemia, hypovolemia, hyponatremia, hyperkalemia, vomiting, and diarrhea. Fluids and electrolytes need to be replaced urgently, and the nurse plays a key role in assessing the infant and providing prescribed therapy. Additional laboratory testing may be indicated, as well as pelvic and abdominal ultrasonography to evaluate for gonads, uterus, and vagina.

FAMILY SUPPORT

The birth of a child with ambiguous genitalia has been termed a psychosocial emergency for the family. They require support because the answers to a seemingly simple question as to what sex is their child requires evaluation and time. Involvement in a multidisciplinary team that may include endocrinology, urology, genetics, surgeons, in addition to nurses and social workers can make clear communication challenging and the nurse may be instrumental in coordinating family meetings with the team.

The infant and child with DSD pose very complex and controversial management questions, including sex assignment and potential genital surgery. Traditional approaches are being questioned and continue to evolve. Referral to a specialized center for children with DSD is recommended.

OBSTRUCTIVE UROPATHY

Congenital urinary obstruction may be best defined as urinary flow impairment that has limited or may potentially limit normal renal development (Peters, 2016). Urinary obstruction in children includes a wide spectrum and is one of the most common conditions affecting the urinary tract. Obstruction can be congenital or acquired, unilateral or bilateral, and complete or incomplete (Fig. 24.9). Prenatal ultrasound has allowed for diagnosis of potential obstructive conditions before birth. **Hydronephrosis**, which is a dilation of the renal pelvis, with or without dilation of the calyces, is a common finding on fetal ultrasound and may be due to a transient dilation of the collecting system, upper or lower urinary tract obstruction, or nonobstructive processes such as vesicoureteral reflux, megaureter, and prune belly syndrome. It is important to realize that not all hydronephrosis represents obstruction. The most common causes of hydronephrosis are transient hydronephrosis, ureteropelvic junction obstruction (UPJO), and vesicoureteral reflux. Hydronephrosis is graded based on severity, and the likelihood of having obstruction or a significant renal anomaly correlates with the severity. Though there are different grading systems, a commonly used one is the Society of Fetal Urology that grades hydronephrosis based on the degree of pelvic dilation, number of calyces seen, and the appearance of the renal parenchyma on ultrasound. The grading is from 0 to IV, with 0 being normal, without dilation of the renal pelvis. Grade I has mild dilation of the renal pelvis only, grade II, moderate dilation of the renal pelvis including a few calyces, grade III has dilation of the renal pelvis with visualization of all the dilated calyces and normal renal parenchyma. Grade IV has a similar appearance as grade III, but with thinning of the renal parenchyma.

Bilateral involvement increases the risk of significant renal abnormality and impaired renal function. Obstruction may occur at any level of the urinary tract, causing dilation above the obstruction. For example, when the bladder outlet is obstructed, the bladder, kidneys, and both

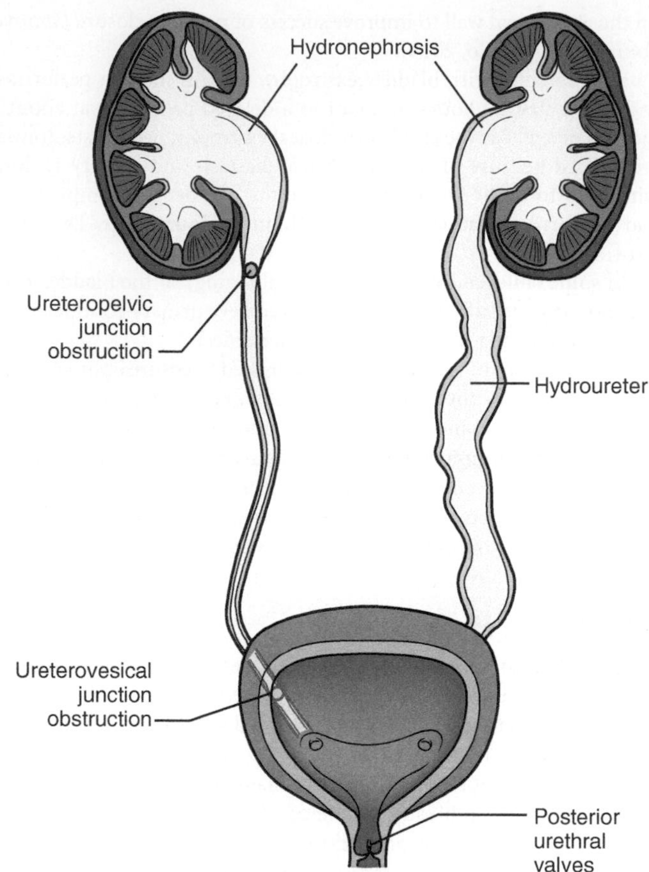

FIG. 24.9 Major sites of urinary tract obstruction.

ureters may become distended. When both ureter and renal pelvis are distended, it is termed **hydroureteronephrosis**. If there is obstruction at the ureterovesical junction (UVJ), the ureter and renal pelvis of that side will be dilated and the contralateral (opposite) side may remain normal in appearance and function. Similarly, if the ureteropelvic junction (UPJ) becomes obstructed, the renal pelvis and calyces will become dilated. The ureteropelvic junction is the most common site of obstruction. Less common causes of obstruction include congenital megaureter, which is an enlarged ureter that may or may not be obstructed and also may or may not reflux. A **ureterocele** is an abnormality of ureteral development where the distal end of the ureter is dilated, forming a bulge that is usually in the bladder (intravesical) or partially extending beyond the bladder neck (ectopic). Though rare, urethral obstruction can result from a prolapsed ureterocele. Ureteroceles are commonly associated with the upper pole of a duplex system and if not detected by prenatal ultrasound, commonly present with urinary tract infection in the first few months of life.

Obstruction is the single largest entity leading to renal insufficiency in boys younger than 1 year and is the largest single cause of renal failure requiring transplantation (Peters, 2016). Posterior urethral valves are obstructing membranes in the urethra that occur only in boys and are the most common cause of bladder outlet obstruction. Because the blockage is low, it affects everything "upstream" and causes the bladder to become thick-walled, as well as causing bilateral hydroureteronephrosis. **Oligohydramnios** (low amniotic fluid volume) occurs because most of the amniotic fluid volume depends on fetal urine production and thus is an indicator of poor renal function or bilaterally obstructed kidneys. Severe oligohydramnios also affects lung development in the fetus and resulting pulmonary hypoplasia with poor postnatal outcomes. Although valves can be treated with ablation, there is commonly some degree of renal damage that decreases the renal reserve, affecting long-term function and resulting in renal insufficiency and renal failure when the child "outgrows" his kidney function. The obstruction also may result in significant bladder dysfunction, referred to as "valve bladder syndrome."

Pathophysiology

The effects of obstruction on the developing kidney depend on when it occurs and the severity of obstruction. Because it occurs when the kidney is forming, it is very different from an acquired obstruction of a mature kidney. Obstruction during development alters the growth regulation, tissue differentiation, and function. These changes can result in poorly functioning renal tissue called dysplasia. There may also be progression of renal dysfunction. Two forms of progressive renal dysfunction include an uncorrected partial obstruction, such as a UPJ obstruction; and a previously obstructed but corrected obstruction with some degree of renal damage, such as posterior urethral valves (PUVs). Structural alterations caused by obstruction are evident in significant hydronephrosis as a distortion in normal architecture and relative alterations in the amount of renal tissue elements. Subtle changes are functionally important and include fibrosis and increased interstitial tissue, as well as abnormal tubules and glomeruli (Peters, 2016).

The pathophysiologic changes produced by obstruction are influenced by the location and severity of the blockage and by the presence of complicating factors, such as infection. With obstruction, or in the event of a solitary kidney, compensatory renal growth occurs in the contralateral kidney. This is from cellular hypertrophy (enlargement) rather than hyperplasia or increase in nephrons (Meldrum, 2016). The detrusor muscle of the bladder is also affected by obstruction of the bladder outlet and becomes thickened and trabeculated, with compromise in effectiveness and function.

Clinical Manifestations

The clinical manifestations of obstructive uropathy depend on the location of the obstructing lesion, its severity, and the underlying cause. The most common presentation is the finding of abnormalities, typically hydronephrosis, on fetal ultrasound. If not diagnosed in utero, an infant may be noted to have an abdominal mass or develop urinary tract infection. Congenital obstruction is often asymptomatic, as in the case of the most common obstruction of the upper urinary tract, UPJO. In older children with UPJO, abdominal or flank pain, often with chronic nausea, is more common. Urinary tract infections or hematuria are more common presentations of ureterocele or megaureter. Maternal oligohydramnios may signal a significant obstruction or renal problem in the developing fetus. This can lead to respiratory distress due to pulmonary hypoplasia and is life threatening. Although posterior urethral valves are diagnosed prenatally in most cases; respiratory distress, sepsis, abdominal distention, not voiding in the first 48 hours of life, and renal failure can be manifestations. Depending on the spectrum of this disease, it may not be diagnosed until voiding problems are persistent later in childhood.

Urolithiasis, formation of calculi (stones) in the urinary tract, has increased in children in recent years and can cause obstruction of the renal pelvis or ureter. It is associated with underlying metabolic conditions and urinary tract malformation. Stones can produce a characteristic pain called renal colic, which is more common in adolescents than young children. This pain is characterized by discomfort in the flank, lower back, or lower abdomen. The discomfort is typically intense and it is not relieved by changes in position.

Obstruction of the bladder produces lower urinary tract symptoms. These symptoms are closely related to those produced by other dysfunctional voiding conditions, including detrusor overactivity and urinary retention. Symptoms include poor force of urinary stream, intermittency of voided stream, feelings of incomplete bladder emptying, and post void dribbling. In addition, children with obstruction of the bladder or urethra may experience frequency of urination, nocturia, nocturnal enuresis, urgency, and urge incontinence.

Although primary hypertension is increasingly present in the pediatric population, the most common cause of secondary hypertension seen in urology is obstructive uropathy, specifically UPJO and PUV (Norwood & Peters, 2016).

Diagnostic Evaluation

Imaging studies are used to assess for obstruction. Ultrasonography is the initial test to assess kidneys, including size, hydronephrosis, dilated ureters, bladder wall, and bladder emptying. Stones may be visualized on ultrasound, although a plain film of the abdomen can show certain types of stones. Noncontrast helical computed tomography is the gold standard for diagnosis of stones, but is used selectively due to the greater radiation exposure. A VCUG is performed to rule out vesicoureteral reflux and assess for posterior urethral valves. Assessment of renal function is most commonly determined by a radionuclide scan, specifically a MAG-3 renal scan, which assesses the differential function between the kidneys and the uptake and excretion of radioisotope for analysis of function. A DMSA scan can assess differential function and renal scars, but does not visualize the ureters and bladder (see Table 24.2).

Prenatal detection of significant lower urinary tract obstruction has resulted in prenatal intervention in severe cases to drain the obstructed bladder into the amniotic fluid via a vesico-amniotic shunt. This is a specialized procedure with high risk of complications, and studies are ongoing as to the overall effectiveness. A recent review of the effect on perinatal and postnatal survival showed improvement in perinatal survival, but 1 to 2 year survival and renal function outcome were still uncertain, with no difference in renal function in those fetuses that underwent fetal intervention and those that did not (Nassr, Shazly, Abdelmagied, et al., 2016).

Therapeutic Management. The management of obstructive uropathy depends on the degree of the obstruction and the likelihood that renal function will be compromised unless aggressive intervention is undertaken. For example, UPJ obstruction causing hydronephrosis in the neonate may or may not require surgical intervention. In contrast, PUV obstruction requires aggressive intervention to optimize renal function.

With the wide spectrum of obstructive changes, criteria for intervention remain somewhat controversial. Careful monitoring with intervention when indicated is more common in some of the conditions that in previous years would have always warranted surgery. In the case of severe obstructive uropathy with renal insufficiency, intervention is needed. The most common example of this is PUV, where primary valve ablation is done endoscopically to relieve the obstruction. In some cases, often in a premature infant with a very small urethra, a cutaneous vesicostomy is performed to allow urine to drain from the bladder via an incontinent stoma from the dome of the bladder to the abdominal wall and into the diaper. In some cases, transient diversion of the upper urinary tract is indicated, with ureterostomies brought out to the skin or nephrostomy tubes for temporary drainage. When surgical correction is indicated for a UPJO, the preferred procedure is a dismembered pyeloplasty, which allows for excision of the pathologic segment. Laparoscopic pyeloplasties are more commonly used with the technical challenges facilitated by robotic assistance. There is a trend toward nonoperative management of megaureter, depending on the type and symptoms. If there are recurrent UTIs, pyelonephritis, persistent flank pain, or hematuria, surgical correction is warranted. The procedure involves excision of the distal stenotic ureter with tapering and reimplantation into the bladder.

Permanent urinary diversion may involve a continent urinary diversion that incorporates a segment of bowel or ureter to increase bladder capacity (bladder augmentation), if needed, and creation of a stoma that allows the bladder to be emptied by placing a catheter through the stoma into the bladder. In contrast to transient diversions, this procedure is reserved for older children and requires ongoing intermittent catheterization.

Prognosis. The prognosis depends on the type of obstruction, the degree of irreversible renal damage, whether renal dysplasia is present, the age at diagnosis, and the severity of complications. Despite improvements in corrective surgery, some patients develop renal failure, which may evolve over a highly variable period that can extend into adulthood. Careful follow-up care should extend throughout childhood and adolescence, especially when any degree of renal insufficiency is present.

Nursing Care Management

Nursing goals in urinary tract obstruction include helping identify cases, assisting with diagnostic procedures, and caring for children with complications. Preparing parents and children for procedures, especially urinary diversion procedures, is a major nursing responsibility. (See Preparation for Diagnostic and Therapeutic Procedures, Chapter 22.)

Parents and children need emotional support and counseling during the potentially lengthy management of these disorders. Parents are the primary caregivers during infancy and early childhood, when most reparative surgery is performed. They need assistance in learning to manage the care of the child and in detecting subtle signs of urinary tract infection or complications of procedures. Parents may perform intermittent catheterization until the child is mature enough to perform their own. Anticholinergics may also be used to decrease pressure in the bladder and parents should be aware of the side effects of these medications. (See also Management of Genitourinary Function, p. 821.)

Children and adolescents who require intermittent catheterization need psychologic support and guidance. Noncompliance with care can be risky and is not uncommon when adolescents assert their independence and try to be "like everyone else" and skip catheterizations and medications. Those with progressive renal deterioration may face the prospect of dialysis or transplantation and the emotional turmoil that accompanies these procedures.

NCLEX REVIEW QUESTIONS

1. The nurse is caring for a 4-year-old girl with a history of frequent urinary tract infections. What should the nurse be aware of before obtaining a urine sample? Select all that apply.
   A. To obtain a clean-catch urine specimen, have the child sit on the toilet facing backward toward the tank.
   B. Because children who have a UTI will have painful urination, have the child drink a large amount of fluid before obtaining the sample.
   C. The specimen must be fresh—less than 1 hour after voiding with storage at room temperature or less than 4 hours after voiding with refrigeration.
   D. If a urinalysis obtained by a bag specimen is negative, a specimen still needs to be obtained by catheterization or suprapubic aspiration.
   E. The key to distinguishing a true UTI from asymptomatic bacteriuria is the presence of pyuria.
   F. Because the child is febrile, the nurse should immediately start an antimicrobial and then obtain a urine culture.
2. A child with periorbital edema, decreased urine output, pallor, and fatigue is admitted to the pediatric unit. The child is being examined for acute glomerulonephritis. Which of the following nursing measures should be considered? Select all that apply.
   A. On examination there is usually a mild to moderate elevation in blood pressure compared with normal values for age, although severe hypertension may be present.
   B. Urinalysis during the acute phase characteristically shows hematuria, proteinuria, and increased specific gravity.
   C. The primary objective is to reduce the excretion of urinary protein and maintain protein-free urine.
   D. Assessment of the child's appearance for signs of cerebral complications is an important nursing function because the severity of the acute phase is variable and unpredictable.
   E. Because these children are particularly vulnerable to upper respiratory tract infection, protect them from contact with infected roommates, family, or visitors.
3. When caring for a child with acute renal failure, which nursing measure requires immediate attention?
   A. Serum potassium concentrations in excess of 7 mEq/L
   B. Sodium level of 135
   C. Transfusion for hemoglobin of 8
   D. Mannitol and furosemide for a urine output of 2 ml/kg/hr
4. When giving discharge instructions to a parent post hypospadias repair, the nurse recognizes a need for more teaching when the mother says which of the following? Select all that apply.
   A. "I know I should never clamp off the catheter."
   B. "My child can take a tub bath when we arrive home because it will soothe the area."
   C. "An antibacterial ointment may be applied to the penis daily for infection control."
   D. "Fluids should be monitored and rationed to prevent fluid overload."
   E. "My child should avoid straddle toys, sandboxes, swimming, and rough activities until allowed by the surgeon."
5. What is the 24-hour fluid requirement for a child weighing 32 kg?
   A. 1920 ml/day
   B. 1740 ml/day
   C. 1840 ml/day
   D. 1620 ml/day

Correct Answers

1. A, C, E; 2. A, B, D; 3. A; 4. A, C, E; 5. B

REFERENCES

American Academy of Pediatrics, Subcommittee on Urinary Tract Infection. (2016). Reaffirmation of AAP clinical practice guideline: The Diagnosis and Management of the Initial Urinary Tract Infection in Febrile Infants and Young Children 2–24 Months of Age. *Pediatrics*, e20163026.

American Academy of Pediatrics Task Force on Circumcision. (2012). Circumcision policy statement. *Pediatrics, 130*(3), 585–586.

Banerjee, S., Dissanayake, P. V., & Abeyagunawardena, A. S. (2016). Vaccinations in children on immunosuppressive medications for renal disease. *Pediatric Nephrology (Berlin, Germany), 31*(9), 1437–1448.

Bichet, D. G., & Bockenhauer, D. (2016). Genetic forms of nephrogenic diabetes insipidus (NDI): Vasopressin receptor defect (X-linked) and aquaporin defect (autosomal recessive and dominant). *Best Practice and Research. Clinical Endocrinology and Metabolism, 30*(2), 263–276.

Bonadio, W., & Maida, G. (2014). Urinary tract infection in outpatient febrile infants younger than 30 days of age: A 10-year evaluation. *The Pediatric Infectious Disease Journal, 33*(4), 342–344.

Bunting-Early, T. E., Shaikh, N., Woo, L., et al. (2017). The need for improved detection of urinary tract infections in young children. *Frontiers in Pediatrics, 5*, 24. [Published online Feb 21, 2017].

Dabrowski, E., Kadakia, R., & Zimmerman, D. (2016). Diabetes insipidus in infants and children. *Best Practice and Research. Clinical Endocrinology and Metabolism, 30*(2), 317–328.

Dagan, R., Cleper, R., Davidovits, M., et al. (2016). Post-infectious glomerulonephritis in pediatric patients over two decades: Severity-associated features. *The Israel Medical Association journal: IMAJ, 18*(6), 336–340.

Dangle, P. P., Fuller, T. W., Gaines, B., et al. (2016). Evolving mechanisms of injury and management of pediatric blunt renal trauma-20 years of experience. *Urology, 90*, 159–163.

Durkan, A. M., Kim, S., Craig, J., et al. (2016). The long-term outcomes of atypical haemolytic uraemic syndrome: A national surveillance study. *BMJ (Clinical Research Ed.), 101*(4), 387–391.

Edlin, R. S., Shapiro, D. J., Hersh, A. L., et al. (2013). Antibiotic resistance patterns of outpatient pediatric urinary tract infections. *Journal of Urology, 190*(1), 222–227.

Ellis, D. (2016). Pathophysiology, evaluation and management of edema in childhood nephrotic syndrome. *Frontiers in Pediatrics, 3*, 111.

Fast, A. M., Nees, S. N., Van Batavia, J. P., et al. (2013). Outcomes of targeted treatment for vesicoureteral reflux in children with nonneurogenic lower urinary tract dysfunction. *Journal of Urology, 190*(3), 1028–1033.

Feldkamp, M. L., Botto, L. D., Amar, E., et al. (2011). Cloacal exstrophy: An epidemiologic study from the International Clearinghouse for Birth Defects Surveillance and Research. *American Journal of Medical Genetics. Part C, Seminars in Medical Genetics, 157C*(4), 333–343.

Gaudry, S., Hajage, D., Schortgen, F., et al. (2016). Initiation strategies for renal-replacement therapy in the intensive care unit. *New England Journal of Medicine, 375*(2), 122–133.

Gil-Peña, H., Mejía, N., & Santos, F. (2014). Renal tubular acidosis. *The The Journal of Pediatrics, 164*(4), 691–697.

Gomez, J., Gil-Peña, H., Santos, F., et al. (2016). Primary distal renal tubular acidosis: Novel findings in patients study by next-generation sequencing. *Pediatric Research, 79*, 496–501.

Gray, M., & Moore, K. N. (2009). Atlas of genitourinary anatomy and physiology. In *Urologic disorders: Adult and pediatric care*. St. Louis: Mosby.

Grinspon, R. P., & Rey, R. A. (2014). When hormone defects cannot explain it: Malformative disorders of sex development. *Birth Defects Research. Part C, Embryo Today: Reviews, 102*(4), 359–373.

Haller, M. C., Royuela, A., Nagler, E. V., et al. (2016). Steroid avoidance or withdrawal for kidney transplant recipients (Review). *Cochrane Database of Systematic Reviews*, (8), CD005632, http://onlinelibrary.wiley.com/doi/10.1002/14651858.CD005632.pub3/full.

Hines, E. Q. (2012). Fluids and electrolytes. In M. M. Tschudy & K. M. Arcara (Eds.), *The Harriet Lane handbook* (ed. 19). Philadelphia: Elsevier Mosby.

Hjorten, R., Anwar, Z., & Reidy, K. J. (2016). Long-term outcomes of childhood onset nephrotic syndrome. *Frontiers in Pediatrics, 4*(53).

Hoberman, A., Chesney, R. W., & RIVUR Trial Investigators. (2014). Antimicrobial prophylaxis for children with vesicoureteral reflux. *The New England Journal of Medicine, 371*(11), 1072–1073.

Holmberg, C., & Jalanko, H. (2016). Long-term effects of paediatric kidney transplantation. *Nature Reviews. Nephrology, 12*(5), 301–311.

Hothi, D. K., Stronach, L., & Sinnott, K. (2016). Home hemodialysis in children. *Hemodialysis International, 20*(3), 349–357.

Iijima, K., Sako, M., & Nozu, K. (2016). Rituximab for nephrotic syndrome in children. *Clinical and Experimental Nephrology*, http://link.springer.com/article/10.1007/s10157-016-1313-5.

Inouye, B. M., Tourchi, A., Di Carlo, H. N., et al. (2014). Modern management of the exstrophy-epispadias complex. *Surgery Research and Practice, 2014*, 58764.

Jefferies, J. L., & Devarajan, P. (2016). Early detection of acute kidney injury after pediatric cardiac surgery. *Progress in Pediatric Cardiology, 41*, 9–16.

Karavanaki, K. A., Soldatou, A., Koufadaki, A. M., et al. (2017). Delayed treatment of the first febrile urinary tract infection in early childhood increased the risk of renal scarring. *Acta paediatrica, 106*, 149–154.

Karpman, D., Loos, S., Tati, R., et al. (2016). Haemolytic uraemic syndrome. *Journal of Internal Medicine, 281*(2), 123–148.

(2012). KDIGO Clinical Practice Guideline for Acute Kidney Injury. *Kidney International. Supplement, 2*(1), http://www.sciencedirect.com/science/journal/21571716/2/1.

Kim, K. H. (2016). Clinical manifestation patterns and trends in poststreptococcal glomerulonephritis. *Child Kidney Disease, 20*(1), 6–10.

Kirsch, A. J., Arlen, A. M., Leong, T., et al. (2014). Vesicoureteral reflux index (VURx): A novel tool to predict primary reflux improvement and resolution in children less than 2 years of age. *Journal of Pediatric Urology, 10*(6), 1249–1254.

Kolon, T. F., Herndon, C. D. A., Baker, L. A., et al. (2014). Evaluation and treatment of cryptorchidism: AUA guideline. *Journal of Urology, 192*, 337–345.

Lane, J. C. (2016). Pediatric nephrotic syndrome. In C. B. Langman (Ed.), *Medscape*. http://emedicine.medscape.com/article/982920-overview.

Lee, L. C., Lorenzo, A. J., & Koyle, M. A. (2016). The role of voiding cystourethrography in the investigation of children with urinary tract infections. *Canadian Urological Association Journal, 10*(5–6), 210–214.

Loghman-Adham, M. (2003). Medication noncompliance in patients with chronic disease: Issues in dialysis and renal transplantation. *The American Journal of Managed Care, 9*(2), 15–171.

Loirat, C., Fakhouri, F., Ariceta, G., et al. (2016). An international consensus approach to the management of atypical hemolytic uremic syndrome in children. *Pediatric Nephrology (Berlin, Germany), 31*(1), 15–39.

Lombel, R. M., Gipson, D. S., & Hodson, E. M. (2013). Treatment of steroid-sensitive nephrotic syndrome: New guidelines from KDIGO. *Pediatric Nephrology (Berlin, Germany), 28*(3), 415–426.

Lombel, R. M., Hodson, E. M., & Gipson, D. S. (2013). Treatment of steroid-resistant nephrotic syndrome in children: New guidelines from KDIGO. *Pediatric Nephrology (Berlin, Germany), 28*(3), 409–414.

Lopez-Giacoman, S., & Madero, M. (2015). Biomarkers in chronic kidney disease, from kidney function to kidney damage. *World Journal of Nephrology, 4*(1), 57–73.

Meldrum, K. K. (2016). Pathophysiology of urinary tract obstruction. In A. J. Wein, L. R. Kavoussi, A. W. Partin, et al. (Eds.), *Campbell-Walsh Urology*. Philadelphia: Elsevier.

Mody, R. K., Gu, W., Griffin, P. M., et al. (2015). Postdiarrheal hemolytic uremic syndrome in United States children: Clinical spectrum and predictors of in-hospital death. *The Journal of Pediatrics, 166*(4), 1022–1029.

Nassr, A. A., Shazly, S. A., Abdelmagied, A. M., et al. (2016). Effectiveness of vesico-amniotic shunt in fetuses with congenital lower urinary tract obstruction: An updated systematic review and meta-analysis. *Ultrasound in Obstetrics and Gynecology*, doi:10.1002/uog.15988.

Niaudet, P. (2016a). Overview of the pathogenesis and causes of glomerulonephritis in children. In F. B. Stapleton & M. S. Kim (Eds.), *UpToDate*. https://www.uptodate.com/contents/overview-of-the-pathogenesis-and-causes-of-glomerulonephritis-in-children.

Niaudet, P. (2016b). Treatment of idiopathic nephrotic syndrome in children. In T. K. Mattoo & M. S. Kim (Eds.), *UpToDate*. https://www.uptodate.com/contents/treatment-of-idiopathic-nephrotic-syndrome children/print?source=search_result&search=treatment%20of%20idiopathic%20nephrotic%20sydnrome%20in%20children&selectedTitle=1~51.

North American Pediatric Renal Trials and Collaborative Studies (NAPRTCS). *NAPRTCS 2014 Annual Transplant Report*. North American Pediatric Renal Trials and Collaborative Studies. https://web.emmes.com/study/ped/annlrept/annualrept2014.pdf.

Norwood, V. F., & Peters, C. A. (2016). Disorders of renal functional development in children. In A. J. Wein, L. R. Kavoussi, A. W. Partin, et al. (Eds.), *Campbell-Walsh Urology*. Philadelphia: Elsevier.

Peters, C. A. (2016). Congenital urinary obstruction: Pathophysiology. In A. J. Wein, L. R. Kavoussi, A. W. Partin, et al. (Eds.), *Campbell-Walsh Urology*. Philadelphia: Elsevier.

Prat, D., Natasha, A., Polak, A., et al. (2012). Surgical outcome of different types of primary hypospadias repair during three decades in a single center. *Urology*, *79*(6), 1350–1353.

Psooy, K. (2014). Sports and the solitary kidney: What parents of a young child with a solitary kidney should know. *Canadian Urological Association Journal*, *8*(7–8), 233–235.

Rees, L. (2016). Growth hormone therapy in children with CKD after more than two decades of practice. *Pediatric Nephrology (Berlin, Germany)*, *31*(9), 1421–1435.

Rodig, N. M., McDermott, K. C., Schneider, M. F., et al. (2014). Growth in children with chronic kidney disease: A report from the Chronic Kidney Disease in Children Study. *Pediatric Nephrology (Berlin, Germany)*, *29*(10), 1987–1995.

Routh, J. C., Bogaert, G. A., Kaefer, M., et al. (2012). Vesicoureteral reflux: Current trends in diagnosis, screening, and treatment. *European Urology*, *61*, 773–782.

Santos, F., Ordóñez, F. A., Claramunt-Taberner, D., et al. (2015). Clinical and laboratory approaches in the diagnosis of renal tubular acidosis. *Pediatric Nephrology (Berlin, Germany)*, *30*(12), 2099–2107.

Savige, J., Colville, D., Rheault, M., et al. (2016). Alport syndrome in women and girls. *Clinical Journal of the American Society of Nephrology : CJASN*, *11*(9), 1713–1720.

Schaeffer, A. J., Greenfield, S. P., Ivanova, A., et al. (2016). Reliability of grading of vesicoureteral reflux and other findings on voiding cystourethrography. *Journal of Pediatric Urology*, http://dx.doi.org/10.1016/j.jpurol.2016.06.020.

Schlager, T. A. (2016). Urinary tract infections in infants and children. *Microbiology Spectrum*, *4*(5), UTI-0022.

Shakih, N., Mattoo, T. K., Keren, R., et al. (2016). Early antibiotic treatment for pediatric febrile urinary tract infection and renal scarring. *Journal of the American Medical Association Pediatrics*, *170*(9), 848–854.

Shaikh, N., Craig, J. C., Rovers, M. M., et al. (2014). Identification of children and adolescents at risk for renal scarring after a first urinary tract infection: A meta-analysis with individual patient data. *Journal of the American Medical Association Pediatrics*, *168*(10), 893–900.

Siffel, C., Correa, A., Amar, E., et al. (2011). Bladder exstrophy: An epidemiologic study from the International Clearinghouse for Birth Defects Surveillance and Research, and an overview of the literature. *American Journal of Medical Genetics. Part C, Seminars in Medical Genetics*, *157C*(4), 321–332.

Snodgrass, W. T., & Bush, N. C. (2016). Hypospadias. In A. J. Wein, L. R. Kavoussi, A. W. Partin, et al. (Eds.), *Campbell-Walsh Urology*. Philadelphia: Elsevier.

Spahiu, L., Merovci, B., Jashari, H., et al. (2016). Congenital nephrotic syndrome-Finish type. *Medical Archives (Sarajevo, Bosnia and Herzegovina)*, *70*(3), 232–234.

Stratta, P., Musetti, C., Barreca, A., et al. (2014). New trends of an old disease: The acute post infectious glomerulonephritis at the beginning of the new millennium. *Journal of Nephrology*, *27*(3), 229–239.

Stormont, R., McCoy, R., Bashir, K., et al. (2016). New pharmacotherapy options for hyperphosphatemia. *U. S. Pharmacist*, *41*(3), HS18–HS22.

Suominen, J. S., Santtila, P., & Taskinen, S. (2015). Sexual function in patients operated for bladder exstrophy and epispadias. *Journal of Urology*, *194*(1), 195–199.

Thumfart, J., Pommer, W., Querfeld, U., et al. (2014). Intensified hemodialysis in adults, and in children and adolescents. *Deutsches Ärzteblatt International*, *111*(14), 237–243.

VanDeVoorde, R. G. (2015). Acute poststreptococcal glomerulonephritis: The most common acute glomerulonephritis. *Pediatrics in Review*, *36*(1), 3–13.

Vasudeva, P., & Madersbacher, H. (2014). Factors implicated in pathogenesis of urinary tract infections in neurogenic bladders: Some revered, few forgotten, others ignored. *Neurourology and Urodynamics*, *33*(1), 95–100.

Webster, A. C., Nagler, E. V., Morton, R. L., et al. (2017). Chronic kidney disease. *Lancet*, *389*(10075), 1238–1252.

Wojtowicz-Prus, E., Kiliś-Pstrusińska, K., Reich, A., et al. (2016). Chronic kidney disease-associated pruritus in children. *Acta Dermato-Venereologica*, *96*(7), 938–942.

Wolfe, A. J., & Brubaker, L. (2015). "Sterile urine" and the presence of bacteria. *European Urology*, *68*(2), 173–174.

25

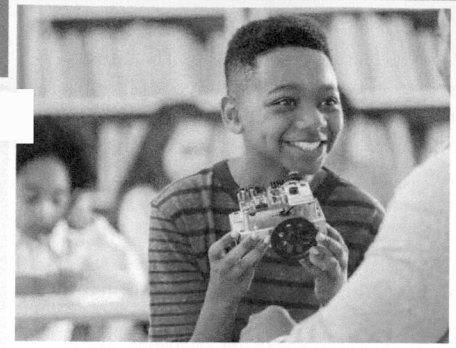

The Child With Gastrointestinal Dysfunction

Cheryl C. Rodgers

http://evolve.elsevier.com/wong/ncic

CONCEPTS

- Elimination
- Nutrition
- Fluid and Electrolyte Balance
- Inflammation
- Infection
- Tissue Integrity
- Patient Education

GASTROINTESTINAL STRUCTURE AND FUNCTION

The primary function of the gastrointestinal (GI) tract is the digestion and absorption of nutrients. The GI tract also has secretory, barrier, endocrine, and immunologic functions (Box 25.1). The extensive surface area of the GI tract and its digestive function represent the major means of exchange between the human organism and the environment. Thus any dysfunction of the GI tract can cause significant problems with the exchange of fluids, electrolytes, and nutrients.

DEVELOPMENT OF THE GASTROINTESTINAL TRACT

The development of the GI tract (from mouth to anus) occurs in several stages from conception through birth. The GI tract may be divided into three parts in intrauterine life: foregut (esophagus, stomach, and proximal duodenum), midgut (distal duodenum, jejunum, ileum, cecum, and proximal colon), and hindgut (distal colon and rectum). The salivary glands, liver, gallbladder, and pancreas are outgrowths of the foregut and midgut.

The esophagus develops from the foregut and can be identified by 4 weeks of gestation. It elongates rapidly after the fourth week to a length of approximately 10 cm (4 inches) at term. The stomach also develops from the primitive foregut and can be identified by the fourth week of gestation. It continues to develop in the second trimester. From the fifth week of gestation until term, the intestine lengthens a thousandfold.

The third trimester is the period of most extensive and rapid growth of the gut. At full term, the small intestine is approximately 250 to 300 cm (98 to 118 inches) and will grow to approximately 2 to 4 m (6.5 to 13 feet) in the adult. The large intestine develops from the midgut and the hindgut and is approximately 30 to 50 cm (12 to 20 inches) at term.

During pregnancy the fetus receives nutrients via the placenta. At birth the full-term infant is capable of adaptation to extrauterine nutrition. This adaptation process includes coordinated sucking and swallowing, efficient gastric emptying and intestinal motility, regulation of digestive secretions and enzymes, efficient digestion and absorption, and excretion of waste products. The infant's capacity to adapt to enteral nutrition depends on the gestational age at birth and the type of nutrients to which the GI tract is exposed.

Movement of nutrients through the GI tract occurs as a result of contraction of the intestinal smooth muscles. A combination of myogenic, neural, and neuroendocrine input during fasting and digestion regulates GI movement. By 26 weeks of gestation, uncoordinated contractions occur, but gastric emptying is slow. By 36 weeks of gestation, motility is similar to that of the full-term infant, and coordinated sucking and swallowing allow preterm infants to feed orally. Intestinal motility improves with gestational age, but it is not known whether the introduction of enteral feeding initiates coordinated motor activity. **Meconium**, a thick, greenish-black material consisting of epithelial cells, digestive tract secretions, and residue of swallowed amniotic fluid, is normally expelled from the intestine shortly after birth and provides evidence of patency of the GI tract.

At term the mechanical functions of digestion are relatively immature. Swallowing is an automatic reflex action for the first 3 months, and the infant has no voluntary control of swallowing until the striated muscles in the throat establish their cerebral connections. This begins at approximately 6 weeks of age. By 6 months the infant is capable of swallowing, holding food in the mouth, or spitting it out at will. The mechanism of sucking is also a reflexive activity in the newborn, and the muscular action of the tongue has a typical forward thrust. With neural and muscular development, the infant gradually acquires the ability to perform the coordinated muscular action typical of the adult type of swallowing. (See Chapter 10.) The eruption of the primary teeth facilitates chewing. The timing of dietary changes closely parallels these progressive developmental capabilities. First foods are those that require merely swallowing; these are followed by foods that need no mastication and finally those that require biting and chewing.

BOX 25.1 Functions of the Gastrointestinal Tract

- Process and absorb nutrients necessary to maintain metabolic processes and to support growth and development.
- Perform an excretory function for both digestive residue and other waste products that pour into the intestine from the blood or are excreted in the bile.
- Provide detoxification while other routes of elimination (e.g., kidneys, liver, skin) are still immature.
- Participate in maintaining fluid and electrolyte balance in infancy.
- Serve a lymphoid function by providing a barrier to bacteria, viruses, and parasites. The liver also processes antigens and produces immunoglobulins.

The stomach, which lies horizontally, is round until the child is approximately 2 years of age. It then gradually elongates until approximately 7 years of age, when it assumes the shape and anatomic position of the adult stomach. This anatomic placement of the stomach in infancy influences positioning practices during and after feeding. (See Chapter 7.) At birth the stomach capacity is small, but it increases rapidly with age.

The frequency and character of stools are affected by the rate of peristalsis and the nature of ingested food. The frequent, yellow stools of the neonate gradually assume a more adult regularity and character in the infant. When compared with the older child, the capacity of the infant's stomach is smaller, but the emptying time is faster. Both the stomach capacity and the emptying time have implications for the amount and frequency of feedings during infancy.

The secretory cells of the GI tract are believed to be functional at birth. However, because most of the digestive enzymes depend on a specific pH, their efficiency may be impaired. The newborn produces only small amounts of saliva, which contains the starch-splitting enzyme amylase. Therefore its primary purpose at this time is to moisten the mouth and throat. By the end of the second year, the salivary glands have increased in size about five times to reach their full size and function.

DIGESTION

Three processes—digestion, absorption, and metabolism—are necessary for the body to convert nutrients into forms it can use. Nutrients are composed of six major substances: carbohydrates, proteins, fats, vitamins, minerals, and water. Digestion is the initial preparation of food for use by the body. Two basic activities are involved: mechanical or muscular activity producing GI motility (movement) and chemical or enzymatic activity resulting from GI secretions.

Mechanical digestion occurs through a series of neuromuscular actions that move and mix food along the GI tract at a rate suitable for digestion and absorption. Three types of muscles in the stomach and intestines contribute to this motility: (1) circular muscles churn and mix food particles; (2) longitudinal muscles propel the food mass; and (3) sphincter muscles (the lower esophageal, pyloric, ileocecal, and anal sphincters) control passage of the food mass to the next segment. The nervous system regulates these muscular actions. The intramural plexus forms the complex network of nerves within the GI wall that control smooth muscle contractions.

Chemical digestion involves five types of GI secretions: (1) enzymes (specific actions on degradation of nutrients), (2) hormones (stimulate or inhibit GI secretions), (3) hydrochloric acid (produces the pH necessary for the activity of specific enzymes), (4) mucus (lubricates and protects the GI tract), and (5) water and electrolytes (transport nutrients for digestion and absorption). Numerous cells and glands produce these secretions. The cells that secrete mucus and GI hormones are found primarily in the mucosa of the stomach and small intestine. The salivary glands and pancreas secrete enzymes, the gastric glands secrete enzymes and hydrochloric acid, and the liver secretes bile.

Mechanical and chemical digestion begins in the mouth. Biting and chewing mix food with saliva and reduce the food into a bolus. The saliva moistens the food to aid in swallowing. Salivary amylase begins the process of digestion of complex carbohydrates, or starches.

The next phase of digestion is swallowing, or deglutition. Safe swallowing requires coordination of the oral and pharyngeal phases of swallowing to prevent food material from entering the airway. The coordination of swallowing is controlled by the interaction of the cranial nerves and the muscles of the mouth, pharynx, and esophagus. The oral phase of swallowing is voluntary. The pharyngeal phase is involuntary and consists of elevation of the palate, uvula, and larynx, followed by a peristaltic wave. The upper esophageal sphincter then relaxes to allow passage of the bolus into the esophagus. Peristalsis (wavelike movements that squeeze food along the entire length of the alimentary tract) moves the food through the esophagus, and the lower esophageal sphincter (LES) relaxes to allow the food to enter the stomach.

Once a bolus of food has entered the stomach, the LES contracts to prevent food from refluxing (returning) into the esophagus. The stomach stores, mixes, and empties the food during digestion. The gastric glands secrete enzymes, hydrochloric acid, and mucus, which mix with the food to continue the process of digestion. The enzyme pepsin, formed from pepsinogen, begins the breakdown of whole proteins into polypeptides. Hydrochloric acid, secreted by the parietal cells, aids in the digestion of proteins. The hormone gastrin is released in the stomach in response to food. Gastrin stimulates the parietal cells to produce more hydrochloric acid. When the pH is very low, a feedback mechanism stops secretion of gastrin to prevent excessive acid formation. The mucus serves primarily to form a protective barrier between the acid and the gastric mucosa.

Partially digested food and watery secretions (chyme) are delivered to the small intestine. Up to this time, most of the digestion has been mechanical. The major part of chemical digestion, as well as several types of movement that aid in mechanical digestion, occurs in the small intestine. The small intestine secretes a large number of enzymes, each of which is specific for one of the fundamental types of nutrients. The mucosa of the small intestine secretes disaccharidases (maltase, lactase, and sucrase) that convert maltose, lactose, and sucrose to monosaccharides (glucose, fructose, and galactose). Aminopeptidase and dipeptidase convert polypeptides to smaller peptides and amino acids.

Secretions from the liver and pancreas complete the process of chemical digestion. The pancreas produces insulin (a hormone necessary for the metabolism of carbohydrates, fats, and proteins) and several enzymes that digest nutrients. Amylase converts starch to disaccharides. Trypsin and chymotrypsin convert proteins and polypeptides to smaller polypeptides. Lipase converts fats to glycerides and fatty acids. These pancreatic enzymes become active only after the inactive forms are secreted into the small intestine. For example, the enzyme enterokinase, secreted by the intestinal mucosal glands, is necessary for trypsinogen to be converted into trypsin. Otherwise, activated enzymes would digest the pancreas and pancreatic duct.

Another important aid in digestion and absorption in the small intestine is bile. Bile is produced in the liver and stored by the gallbladder. When fat enters the small intestine, the hormone cholecystokinin, which stimulates the gallbladder to release bile, is secreted by the intestinal mucosal glands. Bile, an emulsifying agent for fats that facilitates the digestion of fats by lipase, is necessary for the absorption of the fat-soluble vitamins A, D, E, and K. Absence of bile causes increased amounts of ingested fat to appear in the feces (steatorrhea), as well as a deficiency of these vitamins.

PATHOPHYSIOLOGY REVIEW

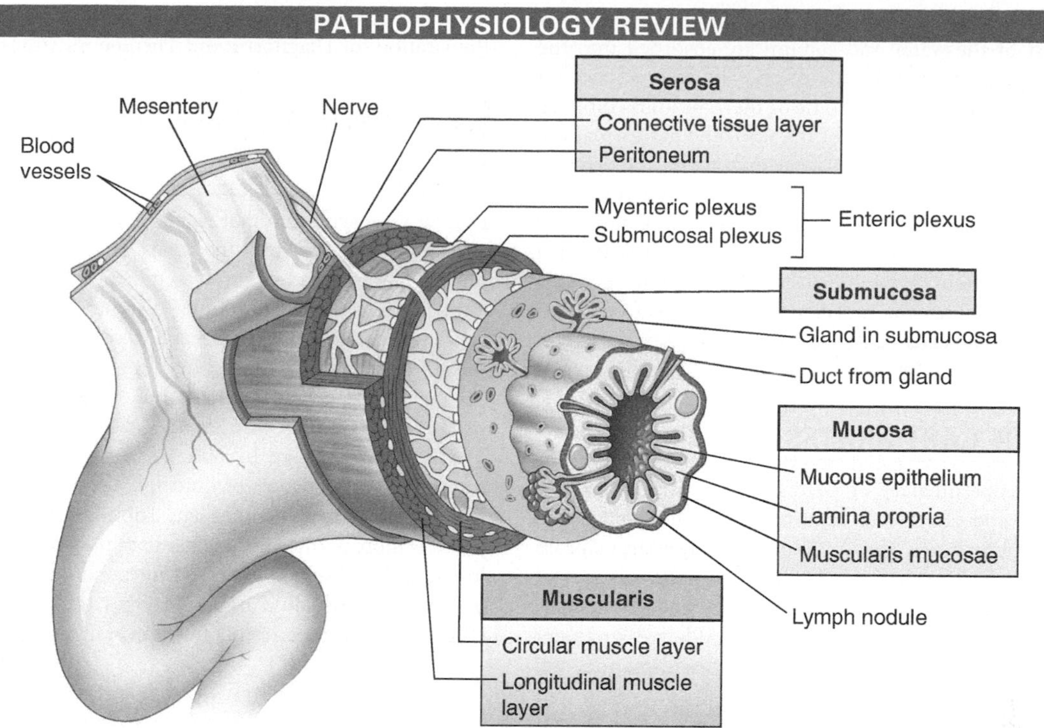

FIG. 25.1 Wall of the gastrointestinal (GI) tract. The wall of the GI tract is made up of four layers with a network of nerves between the layers. Shown here is a generalized diagram of a segment of the GI tract. Note that the serosa is continuous with a fold of serous membrane called a *mesentery*. Note also that digestive glands may empty their products into the lumen of the GI tract by way of ducts. (From Patton, K. T., & Thibodeau, G. A. [2010]. *Anatomy and physiology* [7th ed.]. St. Louis, MO: Mosby.)

ABSORPTION

After digestion of the food is complete, the simplified nutrient end products—monosaccharides (glucose, fructose, and galactose) from carbohydrates, fatty acids and glycerides from fats, and small peptides and amino acids from proteins—are ready for absorption. Vitamins and minerals are also released as a result of digestion. Water and electrolytes contribute to the fluid food mass that is finally absorbed.

The principal site for absorption of nutrients in the GI tract is the small intestine. The wall of the GI tract consists of folds and projections that are progressively smaller (Fig. 25.1). These mucosal folds, villi, and microvilli increase the inner surface area approximately 600 times over the outer serosa, yielding an extremely large surface for absorption.

The mucosal folds are elevated folds along the mucosa. The villi can be seen by light microscope and are small, fingerlike projections covering the mucosal folds. The villi increase the surface area further. Each villus has a vascular supply, including venous and arterial capillaries and lacteals (lymphatic vessels in the small intestine that contain the substance chyle). The microvilli, numerous minute projections on the surface of each villus (visible by electron microscope), form the brush border.

The small intestine has several mechanisms of absorption, including passive diffusion, carrier-mediated diffusion, active energy-driven transport, and engulfment. Passive diffusion (osmosis) occurs across the epithelial membrane in the direction from higher concentration to lower concentration. Carrier-mediated diffusion occurs as molecules are carried across the epithelial cells of microvilli by a molecule that serves as a vehicle. Large molecules must be combined with a smaller molecule to pass from a greater pressure gradient to a lesser one. For example, vitamin B_{12} requires intrinsic factor to be carried into the intestinal circulation.

In active energy-driven transport, nutrients require energy to be absorbed and to cross the intestinal epithelial membrane. This mechanism is referred to as a *pump*. The pump transports molecules across the membrane by means of energy supplied by the cell's metabolism. The sodium pump, which transports glucose, is an example of this mechanism.

Engulfment, or pinocytosis, is the process that allows large macromolecules to be absorbed by the epithelial cells of the villi. The epithelial cell engulfs the macromolecule and opens to allow the particle to enter the interior of the cell. The particle then enters the capillary blood. This mechanism transports some whole proteins and fat droplets.

After absorption by these mechanisms, the end products of carbohydrates and proteins are absorbed into the intestinal capillaries and enter the portal blood circulation of the liver, where further metabolic conversion occurs. The transfer of the end products of fat digestion is unique in that the fat molecules pass between the cells of the intestinal mucosa and into the lacteals of the villi. From there, they enter the larger lymph vessels and then the portal blood flow at the thoracic duct. Exceptions include the medium- and short-chain fatty acids, which can be absorbed directly into the blood circulation of the villi. Most of the fats commonly consumed are long-chain fatty acids, which are transported by way of the lacteals.

Fat-soluble vitamins are absorbed with digested fats in the presence of bile. Water-soluble vitamins, vitamin B complex, and vitamin C are absorbed in the small intestine. Absorption of vitamin B_{12} takes place only in the ileum. The majority of water and electrolyte absorption also takes place in the small intestine.

The large intestine completes the process of absorption and functions primarily to absorb sodium and additional water. The remainder of the products of digestion passes into the large intestine through the ileocecal valve. The muscular activity of the large intestine propels the mass forward. Most of the water and sodium are absorbed into the bloodstream in the proximal half of the colon. The colonic bacteria synthesize vitamin K, vitamin B_{12}, and some of the vitamin B complex. Bacteria also affect the color and odor of the stool and gas formation. The odor is primarily caused by products of bacterial action and depends on the type of colonic flora and ingested food. Defects in digestion or absorption notably alter the odor and appearance of feces. Color is the result of bilirubin end products converted by bacteria to urobilinogen and then oxidized to urobilin (stercobilin). The feces that are excreted consist of undigested residue, water, bacteria, and mucus. Defecation occurs when the internal and external anal sphincters relax after distention of the rectum by feces.

ASSESSMENT OF GASTROINTESTINAL FUNCTION

The most common consequences of GI disease in children include malabsorption, fluid and electrolyte disturbances, malnutrition, and poor growth. (See Dehydration, Chapter 23, and Acute Diarrhea Disease later). A thorough GI assessment includes history questions, general observations, clinical examination, and specific tests and procedures. The most important basic nursing assessments include measurement of intake and output, height and weight, abdominal examination, and simple stool and urine tests.

Numerous clinical manifestations provide clues to specific GI problems (Box 25.2). Some cases involve only one manifestation, whereas others may involve several signs and symptoms as part of the disease complex or syndrome.

A number of tests assess GI function (Table 25.1). Nurses are often responsible for collecting specimens. (See Collection of Specimens, Chapter 22.) Because children may refuse to drink contrast media, generally dislike enemas, and are frightened by unfamiliar equipment, they need preparation for procedures and collection of specimens. (See Preparation for Diagnostic and Therapeutic Procedures, Chapter 22.)

GASTROINTESTINAL DISORDERS

DIARRHEA

Diarrhea is a symptom that results from disorders involving digestive, absorptive, and secretory functions. Diarrhea is caused by abnormal intestinal water and electrolyte transport. Worldwide, there are an estimated 1.7 billion episodes of diarrhea each year (Leung, Chisti, & Pavia, 2016). The incidence and morbidity of diarrhea are more prominent in low-income countries such as areas of Asia and Africa (Leung, Chisti, & Pavia, 2016), and among children younger than 5 years of age (Leung, Chisti, & Pavia, 2016).

Diarrhea is caused by abnormal intestinal water and electrolyte transport. The transport of fluid and electrolytes in the developing GI tract is related to the child's age. The intestinal mucosa of the young infant is more permeable to water than that of an older child. Therefore in young infants with increased intestinal luminal osmolality caused by diarrhea, more fluid and electrolytes are lost than in older children (Box 25.3). Diarrhea results from several pathophysiologic processes.

Types of Diarrhea

Diarrheal disturbances involve the stomach and intestines (gastroenteritis), the small intestine (enteritis), the colon (colitis), or the colon and intestines (enterocolitis). Diarrhea is classified as acute or chronic.

Acute diarrhea is defined as a sudden increase in frequency and a change in consistency of stools, often caused by an infectious agent in the GI tract (Box 25.4). It may be associated with upper respiratory or urinary tract infections, antibiotic therapy, or laxative use. Acute diarrhea is usually self-limited (14 days' duration) and subsides without specific

BOX 25.2 Clinical Manifestations of Gastrointestinal Dysfunction in Children

Failure to thrive—Deceleration from established growth pattern or consistently remaining below the 5th percentile for height and weight on standard growth charts; sometimes accompanied by developmental delays

Spitting up or regurgitation—Passive transfer of gastric contents into the esophagus or mouth

Vomiting—Forceful ejection of gastric contents; involves a complex process under central nervous system control that causes salivation, pallor, sweating, and tachycardia; usually accompanied by nausea

Projectile vomiting—Vomiting accompanied by vigorous peristaltic waves; typically associated with pyloric stenosis or pylorospasm

Nausea—Unpleasant sensation vaguely referred to the throat or abdomen with an inclination to vomit

Constipation—Passage of firm or hard stools or infrequent passage of stool with associated symptoms such as difficulty expelling the stools, blood-streaked stools, and abdominal discomfort

Encopresis—Overflow of incontinent stool causing soiling; often caused by fecal retention or impaction

Diarrhea—Increase in the number of stools with increased water content as a result of alterations of water and electrolyte transport by the gastrointestinal (GI) tract; may be acute or chronic

Hypoactive, hyperactive, or absent bowel sounds—Evidence of intestinal motility problems that may be caused by inflammation or obstruction

Abdominal distention—Protuberant contour of the abdomen that may be caused by delayed gastric emptying, accumulation of gas or stool, inflammation, or obstruction

Abdominal pain—Pain associated with the abdomen that may be localized or diffuse, acute or chronic; often caused by inflammation, obstruction, or hemorrhage

Gastrointestinal bleeding—Bleeding from an upper or lower GI source; may be acute or chronic

Hematemesis—Vomiting of bright red blood or denatured blood that results from bleeding in the upper GI tract or from swallowed blood from the nose or oropharynx

Hematochezia—Passage of bright red blood per rectum, usually indicating lower GI tract bleeding

Melena—Passage of dark-colored, tarry stools caused by denatured blood, suggesting upper GI tract bleeding or bleeding from the right colon

Jaundice—Yellow coloration of the skin and sclerae associated with liver dysfunction

Dysphagia—Difficulty swallowing caused by abnormalities in the neuromuscular function of the pharynx or upper esophageal sphincter or by disorders of the esophagus

Dysfunctional swallowing—Impaired swallowing resulting from central nervous system defects or structural defects of the oral cavity, pharynx, or esophagus; can cause feeding problems or aspiration

Fever—Common manifestation of illness in children with GI disorders; usually associated with dehydration, infection, or inflammation

TABLE 25.1 Gastrointestinal Diagnostic Procedures

Test	Description	Purpose	Comments
Stool examination	Gross, microscopic, and chemical examination of stool specimen	To detect normal and abnormal constituents	Explain process for collecting samples. Fresh specimen is optimum.
Ova and parasites (O&P)	Microscopic examination of stool contents for parasites or their eggs	To aid in diagnosis of parasitic infections	Requires several fresh specimens placed in special preservative. Obtaining three samples improves probability of detection of organism.
Bacterial culture	Sample contents grown on culture medium	To detect bacterial pathogens in stool	Fresh specimen is important to improve probability of detection of organism. Serologic tests determine presence of bacterial toxins.
Stool assay for vital pathogens	Enzyme-linked immunosorbent assay (ELISA)	To detect viral pathogens in stool	Standard ELISA test is available for detection of rotavirus and adenovirus.
Giardia antigen	ELISA	To detect presence of *Giardia* organisms	This is more sensitive than single stool for O&P.
Quantitative fat	Detection of abnormal quantities of fat in stool	To aid in diagnosis of pancreatic insufficiency or malabsorption by measuring stool-reducing substances	This requires 72-hour collection of stool and simultaneous food intake record. Instruct patient to consume >50 g of fat.
Reducing substances	Unabsorbed sugars measured in stool (glucose, fructose, lactose, galactose, and pentose)	To detect elevated levels of reducing substances in stool, which are abnormal and suggest carbohydrate malabsorption	This requires random fresh stool specimen delivered immediately to laboratory. Fermentation by bacteria can give false low if stool is not tested immediately.
pH	Stool pH <5 suggestive of carbohydrate malabsorption; colonic bacterial fermentation produces short-chain fatty acids, which lower stool pH	To detect carbohydrate malabsorption	Obtain random fresh stool and refrigerate. Avoid barium procedures and laxatives before study. These can alter test results.
Occult blood guaiac test	Stool smeared on guaiac-impregnated paper, and 2 drops of developing solution added to reverse side; blue color indicates hemoglobin	To detect presence of blood in stool	This is an easily and quickly measured screening test. Small amounts of blood (e.g., from bleeding mouth, gums, nose) may give positive results.
***Helicobacter pylori* Testing**			
Serology test	Blood test for antibody to *H. pylori* (anti-Hg IgG)	To assess for exposure to *H. pylori*	This test does not determine whether infection is acute or chronic.
C urea breath test	Collection of breath after ingestion of isotopic urea with either carbon 14 or carbon 13; measures labeled carbon dioxide in expired air	To determine if there is active infection with *H. pylori* in the stomach	This is one of most accurate methods to determine *H. pylori* infection in children ages 2 years or older. Carbon 13 is nonradioactive (preferred), and carbon 14 has low level of radioactivity.
Urease test	Biopsy of stomach, which is stained and placed in Christensen urea medium which turns color in presence of *H. pylori*	To determine presence of *H. pylori* in stomach	Sample must be obtained during endoscopy.
Radiography			
Plain films	Anteroposterior and lateral radiographs of abdomen and pelvis	To detect foreign body or mass, reveal bowel gas patterns, and detect obstruction or perforation in GI tract	Prepare family and child for study. No special physical preparation is required.
Contrast studies—upper GI and lower GI series	Radiopaque media (barium or water-soluble contrast) or air swallowed or administered as enema	To assess structure and function of GI tract and to detect luminal defects, or masses	Barium enema sometimes requires cleansing enemas and oral cathartics before procedure. Contrast material may be given by nasogastric (NG) or gastrostomy tube. Contrast enemas may reduce intussusception. Prepare family and child for swallowing contrast media, NG tube insertion, or enema. Encourage fluids after procedure.

Continued

TABLE 25.1 Gastrointestinal Diagnostic Procedures—cont'd

Test	Description	Purpose	Comments
Ultrasonography (sonography)	Measures and records reflection of pulsed or continuous high-frequency sound waves	To locate, measure, and delineate abdominal organs	Prepare family and child for study. This is noninvasive, with no radiation involved. Doppler studies demonstrate presence and direction of blood flow; often require intravenous (IV) contrast material.
Computed tomography (CT)	Pinpoint x-ray directed on horizontal or vertical plane to provide series of "cuts" or "slices" that are fed into computer and assembled in image displays on video screen and transferred to permanent record	To visualize horizontal and vertical cross section of abdomen at any axis To distinguish density of various tissue structure of organs To detect blunt trauma to internal organs and masses	Prepare family and child for study. CT is usually noninvasive, but may require oral or IV contrast material and may require sedation.
Magnetic resonance imaging (MRI)	Images formed by reemission of radio signals by atomic nuclei stimulated in magnetic field	To visualize internal body structures in any plane; permits soft tissue discrimination unavailable with many techniques	Prepare family and child for procedure. MRI is usually noninvasive, but may require oral or IV contrast material. MRI may require sedation for lengthy procedure. Patient remains NPO 3 to 4 hours before study; patient is immobilized, and test takes long time. MRI does not expose patient to ionizing radiation. No magnetic material can be present in scanner.
Manometry			
Esophagus	Multilumen catheter inserted into esophagus, and water perfusion or solid state sensed by transducer and recorded	To evaluate dysphagia, esophageal spasm, achalasia, dysmotility	Teach and prepare child and family before procedure. Patient remains NPO 6 to 8 hours before procedure. Patient cooperation is required.
Rectal	Records reflex responses of anal sphincter to transient distention of rectal balloon	To measure sphincter function, especially to screen for constipation and Hirschsprung disease	Teach and prepare child and family before procedure. Administer enema to clear rectum before procedure.
Biopsy			
Liver	Removal of small piece of living tissue for microscopic examination by needle or surgically General sedation or local anesthesia used	To evaluate for biliary obstruction, hepatitis, metabolic disease To assess response to treatment interventions	Teach and prepare patient and family before procedure. Preliminary laboratory studies are needed. Liver biopsy is contraindicated with prolonged bleeding or clotting times, anemia, infection, or obstructive jaundice.
Esophagus, stomach, intestine	Small sample of mucosal tissue taken for microscopic evaluation	To evaluate for infection, inflammation, mucosal abnormalities	Teach and prepare patient and family before procedure. This biopsy requires conscious or general sedation. It is usually obtained with endoscopy.
Endoscopy			
Upper GI, colonoscopy, flexible sigmoidoscopy, anoscopy	Endoscope introduced into area to be examined Endoscope has flexible-tip light source and aspiration and instrument channel	To directly visualize GI tract to evaluate abnormalities, detect lesions, obtain biopsies To perform therapeutic procedures—polypectomies, removal of foreign bodies, sclerotherapy of esophageal varices, placement of feeding tubes or percutaneous catheters	Teach and prepare patient and family before procedure. Patient remains NPO 4 to 8 hours before procedure. Lower GI requires bowel cleansing. Patient requires conscious or general sedation.
Esophageal pH monitoring	Probe that measures pH placed through nose into distal esophagus and records pH over time	To determine frequency and duration of gastric acid refluxed into the esophagus (GER) To establish association between patient symptoms (e.g., pain, apnea, failure to thrive, asthma, wheezing, hoarseness) and acid reflux	Teach and prepare patient and family before procedure. This is usually done over 24-hour period, along with events diary to determine association or relation between symptoms and acid/GER. Patient remains NPO 4 hours before tube is passed; discontinue antacids and other medications 24 hours to 7 days (omeprazole) before study.

TABLE 25.1 **Gastrointestinal Diagnostic Procedures—cont'd**

Test	Description	Purpose	Comments
Breath hydrogen test	Noninvasive study to assess for carbohydrate intolerance Hydrogen generated in colon by bacterial fermentation of undigested carbohydrates and then absorbed into blood, where it diffuses into expired air via lungs	To evaluate for bacterial overgrowth, lactase or sucrase-isomaltase deficiency To evaluate for malabsorption or bacterial overgrowth by detecting rise in expired hydrogen after oral loading with specific carbohydrate	Teach and prepare patient and family before procedure. Patient remains NPO 12 hours before test. Previous night's dinner should consist of meat, rice, and water; avoid other starches. Antibiotics may reduce hydrogen levels.
d-xylose absorption test	d-Xylose solution administered orally; serum levels of d-xylose measured at 30, 60, 90, and 120 minutes Urine collected for total of 5 hours to measure d-xylose excretion	To evaluate absorptive capacity of small intestinal mucosa To diagnose small-bowel malabsorption caused by celiac disease	Teach and prepare patient and family before procedure. Patient remains NPO 4 to 8 hours before test. Test is used less often, largely replaced by endoscopic biopsies to evaluate for villous atrophy.
Hepatobiliary scintigraphy	Nuclear medicine study Radiopharmaceutical administered intravenously, then sequential images of liver, biliary system, and bowel obtained	To evaluate conditions of liver and biliary tract abnormalities and gallbladder disease To aid in diagnosis and monitoring of these conditions, such as biliary atresia	Prepare family and child for study. Images may be obtained for up to 24 hours if excretion is delayed.

GER, Gastroesophageal reflux; *GI,* gastrointestinal; *NPO,* nothing by mouth.

BOX 25.3 **Consequences of Fluid and Electrolyte Loss**

Dehydration
- Voluminous losses of fluid in frequent, watery stools
- Losses when there is also vomiting
- Reduced fluid intake resulting from nausea or anorexia
- Increased insensible losses from fever, hyperpnea, and, sometimes, high environmental temperature
- Continued (although diminished) obligatory renal losses

Electrolyte Imbalance
- Losses of sodium, chloride, potassium, and, in some cases, bicarbonate
- Inadequate replacement of electrolytes when hypotonic or hypertonic solutions are used

Metabolic Acidosis
- Increased absorption of short-chain fatty acids produced in the colon from bacterial fermentation of unabsorbed dietary carbohydrates
- Accumulation of lactic acid from tissue hypoxia secondary to hypovolemia
- Loss of bicarbonate in stools
- Ketosis from fat metabolism when glycogen stores are depleted in untreated diarrheal dehydration or inadequate carbohydrate intake; may result in malnutrition

BOX 25.4 **Causes of Acute Diarrhea**

Infection and Parasitic Infestation
Bacteria—*Salmonella, Shigella, Campylobacter, Escherichia coli, Yersinia, Aeromonas, Clostridium difficile, Staphylococcus aureus*
Viruses—Rotavirus, Norovirus, small and round viruses, adenovirus, pestivirus, astrovirus, parvovirus
Parasites—*Giardia lamblia, Cryptosporidium, Isospora belli, Microsporidia, Strongyloides, Entamoeba histolytica*

Associated Conditions
Upper respiratory tract infections
Urinary tract infections
Otitis media

Dietary Causes
Overfeeding
Introduction of new foods
Reinstituting milk too soon after diarrheal episode
Osmotic diarrhea from excess sugar in formula or juice
Excessive ingestion of sorbitol or fructose

Medications
Antibiotics
Laxatives

Toxic Causes
Ingestion of
- Heavy metals (arsenic, lead, mercury)
- Organic phosphates

Functional Causes
Irritable bowel syndrome

Other Causes
Pseudomembranous enterocolitis
Hirschsprung enterocolitis

treatment. Acute infectious diarrhea (infectious gastroenteritis) is caused by a variety of viral, bacterial, and parasitic pathogens (Table 25.2).

Chronic diarrhea is an increase in stool frequency and increased water content with duration of more than 14 days. It is often caused by chronic conditions such as malabsorption syndromes, inflammatory bowel disease (IBD), immunodeficiency, food allergy, lactose intolerance, or chronic nonspecific diarrhea, or as a result of inadequate management of acute diarrhea.

Intractable diarrhea of infancy is a syndrome that occurs in the first few months of life, persists for longer than 2 weeks with no recognized

TABLE 25.2 Infectious Causes of Acute Diarrhea

Agents	Pathology	Characteristics	Comments
Viral			
Rotavirus Incubation—48 hours Diagnosis—EIA	Fecal-oral transmission 8 groups (A-H)—Most group A virus replicates in mature villus epithelial cells of small intestine; leads to (1) imbalance in ratio of intestinal fluid absorption to secretion and (2) malabsorption of complex carbohydrates	Mild to moderate fever Vomiting followed by onset of watery stools Fever and vomiting generally abate in approximately 2 days, but diarrhea persists 5 to 7 days	Most common cause of diarrhea in children <5 years old; infants 6 to 12 months old most vulnerable; affects all ages; usually milder in children >3 years old Immunocompromised children at greater risk for complications Peak occurrences in winter months Important cause of nosocomial infections
Norovirus Incubation—12 to 48 hours Diagnosis—PCR assays	Fecal-oral; contaminated water Pathology similar to that of rotavirus; affects villus epithelial cells of small intestine, leading to (1) imbalance in ratio of intestinal fluid absorption to secretion and (2) malabsorption of complex carbohydrates	Abdominal cramps, nausea, vomiting, malaise, low-grade fever, watery diarrhea without blood; duration 2 to 3 days; tends to resemble so-called food poisoning symptoms with nausea predominating	Affects all ages Multiple strains often named for the location of outbreak (e.g., Norwalk, Sapporo, Snow Mountain, Montgomery)
Bacterial			
Escherichia coli Incubation—3 to 4 days; variable depending on strain Diagnosis—Sorbitol MacConkey (SMAC) agar positive for blood, but fecal leukocytes absent or rare	*E. coli* strains produce diarrhea as result of enterotoxin production, adherence, or invasion (enterotoxigenic-producing *E. coli*, enterohemorrhagic *E. coli*, enteroaggregative *E. coli*)	Watery diarrhea 1 to 2 days, then severe abdominal cramping and bloody diarrhea Can progress to hemolytic uremic syndrome	Food-borne pathogen Traveler's diarrhea Cause of nursery epidemics Symptomatic treatment Antibiotics may worsen course Avoid antimotility agents and opioids
***Salmonella* groups** (nontyphoidal) Gram-negative rods, nonencapsulated nonsporulating Incubation—6 to 72 hours Diagnosis—Gram stain, stool culture	Invasion of mucosa in the small and large intestine, edema of the lamina propria, focal acute inflammation with disruption of the mucosa and microabscesses	Nausea, vomiting, colicky abdominal pain, bloody diarrhea, fever; symptoms variable (mild to severe) May have headache and cerebral manifestations (e.g., drowsiness confusion, meningismus, seizures) Infants may be afebrile and nontoxic May result in life-threatening septicemia and meningitis Nausea and vomiting typically of short duration; diarrhea may persist as long as 2 to 3 weeks Typically shed virus for average of 5 weeks; cases reported up to 1 year	Incidence highest in summer months; food-borne outbreaks common Usually transmitted person to person but may transmit via undercooked meats or poultry; about half the cases caused by poultry and poultry products In children, related to pets (e.g., dogs, cats, hamsters, turtles) Communicable as long as organisms are excreted Antibiotics not recommended in uncomplicated cases Antimotility agents also not recommended—prolong transit time and carrier state
Salmonella typhi Produces enteric fever—systemic syndrome Incubation—usually 7 to 14 days, but could be 3 to 30 days, depending on size of inoculum Diagnosis—positive blood cultures; also sometimes positive stool and urine cultures Late stage—positive bone marrow culture	Bloodstream invasion; after ingestion, organism attaches to microvilli of ileal brush borders and bacteria invade the intestinal epithelium via Peyer patches Next, organism is transported to intestinal lymph nodes and enters bloodstream via thoracic ducts, and circulating organism reaches reticuloendothelial cells, causing bacteremia	Manifestations dependent on age Abdominal pain, diarrhea, nausea, vomiting, high fever, lethargy Must be treated with antibiotics	Incidence much lower in developed countries; about 400 cases/year in United States; 65% of US cases acquired via international cases Ingestion of foods and water contaminated with human feces is most common mode of transmission Congenital and intrapartum transmission possible Two vaccines available

TABLE 25.2 **Infectious Causes of Acute Diarrhea—cont'd**

Agents	Pathology	Characteristics	Comments
***Shigella* groups** Gram-negative nonmotile anaerobic bacilli Incubation—1 to 7 days Diagnosis—stool culture loaded with polymorphonuclear leukocytes	Enterotoxins—invade the epithelium with superficial mucosal ulcerations	Children appear sick Symptoms begin with fever, fatigue, anorexia Crampy abdominal pain preceding watery or bloody diarrhea Symptoms usually subside in 5 to 10 days	Most cases in children younger than 9 years old, with about one-third of cases in children ages 1 to 4 weeks old Antibiotics shorten illness and lower mortality All patients at risk for dehydration Acute symptoms may persist for ≤1 week Antidiarrheal medications not recommended because they may predispose patient to toxic megacolon
***Yersinia* enterocolitis** Incubation—dose dependent, 1 to 3 weeks Diagnosis—stool culture, ELISA Patients have leukocytosis, elevated sedimentation rate	Pathology poorly understood; possibly caused by production of enterotoxin	Mucoid diarrhea, sometimes bloody; abdominal pain suggestive of appendicitis; fever, vomiting	Seen more frequently in the winter months Transmitted by pets and food Antibiotics usually do not alter the clinical course in uncomplicated cases; antibiotics used in complicated infections and compromised hosts
Campylobacter jejuni Microaerophilic, motile, gram-negative bacilli Incubation—1 to 7 days Ability to cause illness appears dose related Diagnosis—stool culture, sometimes blood culture Commonly found in GI tract of wild or domestic animals	Not fully understood, possibly (1) adherence to intestinal mucosa by toxin, (2) invasion of the mucosa in the terminal ileum and colon, (3) translocation in which the organisms penetrate the mucosa and replicate in the lamina propria	Fever, abdominal pain, diarrhea that can be bloody, vomiting Watery, profuse, foul-smelling diarrhea Clinically similar to infection by *Salmonella* or *Shigella* organisms Fecal-oral transmission	Most infections in humans relate to consumption of contaminated foods or water, such as undercooked meats, particularly chicken Also acquired from contaminated household pets (e.g., dogs, cats, hamsters) Bimodal peaks in infants <1 year old and again at ages 15 to 29 years old Antibiotics do not prolong the carriage of bacteria and may eliminate organism more quickly Erythromycin is the drug of choice Antimotility agents not recommended because they tend to prolong symptoms
Vibrio cholerae Gram-negative, motile, curved bacillus living in bodies of salt water Incubation—1 to 3 days Diagnosis—stool culture	Enters via oral route in contaminated food or water; if survives acid stomach environment, travels to the small intestine, adheres to the mucosa, and produces toxin	Onset abrupt; vomiting, watery diarrhea without cramping or tenesmus Dehydration can occur quickly	More prevalent in developing countries Rehydration most important treatment Antibiotics can shorten diarrhea Despite continued efforts, still no vaccine
Clostridium difficile Gram-positive anaerobic bacillus with the ability to produce spores Diagnosis—by detecting *C. difficile* toxin in stool culture	Produces two important toxins (A and B) Toxin binds to the enterocyte surface receptor, resulting in alteration permeability, protein synthesis, and direct cytotoxicity	Mostly mild watery diarrhea lasting a few days Some prolonged diarrhea and illness May cause pseudomembranous colitis Some individuals extremely ill with high fever, leukocytosis, hypoalbuminemia	Associated with alteration of normal intestinal flora by antibiotics Adults tend to have more severe symptoms than children Treatment with antibiotics (metronidazole) in mildly to moderately symptomatic patients; for nonresponders, give vancomycin Resistant strains have developed Relapse common
Clostridium perfringens Anaerobic, gram-positive, spore-producing bacilli Incubation—8 to 24 hours	Toxins produced in the intestine after ingestion of organism	Acute onset—watery diarrhea, crampy abdominal pain Fever, nausea, and vomiting are rare Duration of illness usually 24 hours	Transmitted by contaminated food products, most often meats and poultry Usually self-limiting and medical intervention not needed Oral rehydration usually sufficient Antibiotics serve no purpose and should not be used

Continued

TABLE 25.2 Infectious Causes of Acute Diarrhea—cont'd

Agents	Pathology	Characteristics	Comments
Clostridium botulinum Gram-positive anaerobic spore-producing bacilli Incubation—12 to 26 hours (range, 6 hours to 8 days) Diagnosis—To detect toxin, submit blood and stool culture to special laboratory (usually state health department)	Botulism caused by binding of toxin to the neuromuscular junction	Clinical presentation related to age and the strain of the botulism GI—abdominal pain, cramping, and diarrhea Other strains—respiratory compromise, CNS symptoms	Transmitted in contaminated food products Can be acquired via wound infection Treatment is supportive care and neutralization of the toxin
***Staphylococcus* organisms** Gram-positive nonmotile, aerobic or facultative anaerobic bacteria Incubation—generally short, 1 to 8 hours Diagnosis—identify organism in food, blood, pus, aspirate	Direct tissue invasion and production of toxin	Clinical presentation dependent on site of entry In food poisoning, profuse diarrhea, nausea, and vomiting	Transmitted in inadequately cooked or refrigerated foods Self-limiting Symptomatic treatment

CNS, Central nervous system; *EIA,* enzyme immunoassay; *ELISA,* enzyme-linked immunosorbent assay; *GI,* gastrointestinal; *PCR,* polymerase chain reaction.

BOX 25.5 Factors That Predispose to Diarrhea

Age—As a rule, the younger the child, the greater the susceptibility and the more severe the diarrhea. Diarrhea occurs more commonly in infancy, is a lesser threat in early childhood, and usually constitutes only a minor problem in older children.

Impaired health—Malnourished or immunocompromised children are more susceptible and tend to have more severe diarrhea.

Environment—Diarrhea occurs with greater frequency where there is crowding, substandard sanitation, poor facilities for preparation and refrigeration of food, and generally inadequate health care education. The frequency of diarrhea in infancy is closely related to the ingestion of contaminated milk; breastfed infants have a lower incidence of diarrhea.

pathogens, and is refractory to treatment. The most common cause is acute infectious diarrhea that was not managed adequately.

Chronic nonspecific diarrhea (CNSD), also known as *irritable colon of childhood* and *toddlers' diarrhea,* is a common cause of chronic diarrhea in children 6 to 54 months of age. These children have loose stools, often with undigested food particles, and diarrhea lasting longer than 2 weeks' duration. Children with CNSD grow normally and have no evidence of malnutrition, no blood in their stool, and no enteric infection. Poor dietary habits and food sensitivities have been linked to chronic diarrhea. The excessive intake of juices and artificial sweeteners such as sorbitol, a substance found in many commercially prepared beverages and foods, may be a factor. Box 25.5 lists other factors that predispose patients to chronic diarrhea.

Etiology

Most pathogens that cause diarrhea are spread by the fecal-oral route through contaminated food or water or are spread from person to person where there is close contact (e.g., day care centers). Lack of clean water, crowding, poor hygiene, nutritional deficiency, and poor sanitation are major risk factors, especially for bacterial or parasitic pathogens. Infants are often more susceptible to frequent and severe bouts of diarrhea because their immune system has not been exposed to many pathogens and has not acquired protective antibodies (Box 25.6). Worldwide, the most common causes of acute gastroenteritis are infectious agents, viruses, bacteria, and parasites.

Rotavirus is the most important cause of serious gastroenteritis among children, with 28% of all cases causing fatality (Lamberti, Ashraf, Walker, et al., 2016). The virus is spread through the fecal-oral route or by person-to-person contact, and almost all children are infected with rotavirus at least once by the age of 5 years (Bass, 2016). Rotavirus is the most common cause of diarrhea-associated hospitalization, with an estimated 80,000 hospitalizations occurring annually in the United States in children less than 5 years of age (Bass, 2016).

Salmonella, Campylobacter, Yersinia, and *Shigella* organisms are the most frequently isolated bacterial pathogens in the United States (Kotloff, 2017). These organisms are gram-negative bacteria and can be contracted through raw or undercooked food, contaminated food or water, or through the fecal-oral route. Among children and adults in the United States annually, *Salmonella* occurs in approximately 8172 people; *Campylobacter* occurs in 8547 people; *Shigella* occurs in 2913 people; and *Yersinia* occurs in 302 people (Marder, Cieslak, Cronquist, et al., 2017). (See also Intestinal Parasitic Diseases, Chapter 6.)

Antibiotic administration is frequently associated with diarrhea because antibiotics alter the normal intestinal flora, resulting in an overgrowth of other bacteria. *Clostridium difficile* is the most common bacterial overgrowth with a 12-fold increases in pediatric incidence from 1991 to 2009 (McFarland, Ozen, Dinleyici, et al., 2016). Children acquire most *C. difficile* infections in health care facilities, but 41% are acquired from the community, such as day care centers (McFarland, Ozen, Dinleyici, et al., 2016).

Pathophysiology

Invasion of the GI tract by pathogens results in increased intestinal secretion as a result of enterotoxins, cytotoxic mediators, or decreased intestinal absorption secondary to intestinal damage or inflammation.

BOX 25.6 Causes of Chronic Diarrhea

Malabsorptive Causes
Celiac disease
Pancreatic insufficiency (cystic fibrosis, chronic pancreatitis, Shwachman syndrome)
Short-bowel syndrome
Lactose intolerance
Congenital enzyme deficiency (sucrase-isomaltase deficiency)

Allergic Causes
Allergic gastroenteropathy
Eosinophilic gastroenteritis

Immunodeficiency
Acquired hypoglobulinemia
Wiskott-Aldrich syndrome
Agammaglobulinemia
Severe combined immunodeficiency disease
Thymic hypoplasia
Selective immunoglobulin A deficiency
Human immunodeficiency virus or acquired immunodeficiency syndrome

Inflammatory Bowel Disease
Ulcerative colitis
Crohn disease

Endocrine Causes
Hyperthyroidism
Congenital adrenal hyperplasia
Addison disease

Motility Disorders
Hirschsprung disease
Intestinal pseudoobstruction

Parasitic Infestations
Ascaris organisms
Giardia organisms

Other Causes
Radiation enteritis
Protein-losing enteropathy (Ménétrier disease, intestinal lymphangiectasia)
Abdominal tumors

Enteric pathogens attach to the mucosal cells and form a cuplike pedestal on which the bacteria rest. The pathogenesis of the diarrhea depends on whether the organism remains attached to the cell surface, resulting in a secretory toxin (noninvasive, toxin-producing, noninflammatory-type diarrhea), or penetrates the mucosa (systemic diarrhea). Noninflammatory diarrhea is the most common diarrheal illness, resulting from the action of enterotoxin that is released after attachment to the mucosa. The most serious and immediate physiologic disturbances associated with severe diarrheal disease are dehydration, acid-base imbalance with acidosis, and shock that occurs when dehydration progresses to the point that circulatory status is seriously impaired.

Diagnostic Evaluation

Evaluation of the child with acute gastroenteritis begins with a careful history that seeks to discover the possible cause of diarrhea, to assess the severity of symptoms and the risk of complications, and to elicit information about current symptoms indicating other treatable illnesses that could be causing the diarrhea. The history should include questions about recent travel, exposure to untreated drinking or washing water sources, contact with animals or birds, day care center attendance, recent treatment with antibiotics, or recent diet changes. History questions should also explore the presence of other symptoms such as fever and vomiting, frequency and character of stools (e.g., watery, bloody), urinary output, dietary habits, and recent food intake.

Extensive laboratory evaluation is not indicated in children who have uncomplicated diarrhea and no evidence of dehydration because most diarrheal illnesses are self-limiting. Laboratory tests are indicated for children who are severely dehydrated and receiving intravenous (IV) therapy. Watery, explosive stools suggest glucose intolerance; foul-smelling, greasy, bulky stools suggest fat malabsorption. Diarrhea that develops after the introduction of cow's milk, fruits, or cereal may be related to enzyme deficiency or protein intolerance. Neutrophils or red blood cells in the stool indicate bacterial gastroenteritis or IBD. The presence of eosinophils suggests protein intolerance or parasitic infection. Stool cultures should be performed only when blood, mucus, or polymorphonuclear leukocytes are present in the stool; when symptoms are severe; when there is a history of travel to a developing country; and when a specific pathogen is suspected. Gross blood or occult blood may indicate pathogens such as *Shigella, Campylobacter,* or hemorrhagic *Escherichia coli* strains. Providers may use an enzyme-linked immunosorbent assay (ELISA) to confirm the presence of rotavirus or *Giardia* organisms. If there is a history of recent antibiotic use, test the stool for *C. difficile* toxin. When bacterial and viral cultures are negative and when diarrhea persists for more than a few days, examine stools for ova and parasites. A stool specimen with a pH of less than 6 and the presence of reducing substances may indicate carbohydrate malabsorption or secondary lactase deficiency. Stool electrolyte measurements may help identify children with secretory diarrhea.

Determine urine specific gravity if dehydration is suspected. Obtain a complete blood count, serum electrolytes, creatinine, and blood urea nitrogen (BUN) in the child who has moderate to severe dehydration or who requires hospitalization. The hemoglobin, hematocrit, creatinine, and BUN levels are usually elevated in acute diarrhea and should normalize with rehydration.

Therapeutic Management

The major goals in the management of acute diarrhea include assessment of fluid and electrolyte imbalance, rehydration, maintenance fluid therapy, and reintroduction of an adequate diet. Treat infants and children with acute diarrhea and dehydration first with **oral rehydration therapy (ORT)**. ORT is one of the major worldwide health care advances. It is more effective, safer, less painful, and less costly than IV rehydration. The American Academy of Pediatrics, World Health Organization, and Centers for Disease Control and Prevention all recommend ORT as the treatment of choice for most cases of dehydration caused by diarrhea (Box 25.7). **Oral rehydration solutions (ORSs)** enhance and promote the reabsorption of sodium and water. These solutions greatly reduce vomiting, duration of illness, and the need for intravenous infusions (Dekate, Jayashree, & Singhi, 2013). ORSs, including reduced osmolarity ORS, are available in the United States as commercially prepared solutions (Table 25.3) and are successful in treating the majority of infants with dehydration. Guidelines for rehydration recommended by the American Academy of Pediatrics are given in Table 25.4. (See Quality Patient Outcomes box.)

After rehydration, ORS may be used during maintenance fluid therapy by alternating the solution with a low-sodium fluid such as breast milk, lactose-free formula, or half-strength lactose-containing formula. In older children, ORS can be given and a regular diet continued. Ongoing stool losses should be replaced on a 1:1 basis with ORS. If the stool volume is not known, approximately 10 ml/kg (4 to 8 oz) of ORS should be given for each diarrheal stool.

BOX 25.7 Model for Rehydration

- For mild to moderate dehydration, rehydration solution should consist of 50 mEq of sodium per liter. In infants who are breastfed, breastfeeding should continue.
- For mild to moderate dehydration, give 50 ml/kg of oral rehydration solution to children.
- For severe dehydration, give 30 ml/hr of oral rehydration for infants, 60 ml/hr for toddlers, and 90 ml/hr for older children. There is a high likelihood for intravenous fluid when children cannot tolerate these oral intake requirements.
- Add 10 ml/kg of fluid for every loose stool or episode of vomiting.
- Reevaluate the need for further rehydration; initiate maintenance therapy using maintenance formulations.
- In children with diarrhea without significant dehydration, the maintenance phase may be initiated without the need for rehydration solution.
- As soon as adequate rehydration has been achieved, start a regular diet along with fluid therapy and wean intravenous fluids.

Modified from Churgay, C. A., & Aftab, A. (2012). Gastroenteritis in children: part II, prevention and management. *American Family Physician, 85*(11), 1066-1070.

QUALITY PATIENT OUTCOMES

Diarrhea

- Adequate hydration maintained during illness
- Appropriate diagnostic tests performed
- Antibiotics given only if appropriate
- No repeat visits to the emergency department or pediatrician during the course of the illness
- No tissue breakdown
- Normal elimination returns

Solutions for oral hydration are useful in most cases of dehydration, and vomiting is not a contraindication. Give a child who is vomiting an ORS at frequent intervals and in small amounts. For young children, the caregiver may give the fluid with a spoon or small syringe in 5- to 10-ml increments every 1 to 5 minutes. An ORS may also be given via nasogastric or gastrostomy tube infusion. Infants without clinical signs of dehydration do not need ORT. They should, however, receive the same fluid recommended for infants with signs of dehydration in the maintenance phase and for ongoing stool losses. Probiotics when used in conjunction with ORS reduces the duration of antibiotic-associated diarrhea in children (Barnes & Yeh, 2015).

Early reintroduction of nutrients is desirable and has gained more widespread acceptance. Continued feeding or early reintroduction of a normal diet after rehydration has no adverse effects and actually lessens the severity and duration of the illness and improves weight gain when compared with the gradual reintroduction of foods (Bhutta,

TABLE 25.3 Composition of Some Oral Rehydration Solutions

Formula	NA (mEq/L)	K (mEq/L)	Cl (mEq/L)	Base (mEq/L)	Glucose (g/L)
Pedialyte (Abbott)*	45	20	35	30 (citrate)	25
Rehydralyte (Abbott)	75	20	65	30 (citrate)	25
Enfalyte (Mead Johnson)	50	25	45	34 (citrate)	30
World Health Organization†	90	20	80	30 (bicarbonate)	20

*Note that many generic products are available with compositions identical to Pedialyte.
†Must be reconstituted with 1 L water.
Cl, Chloride; *K,* potassium; *Na,* sodium.

TABLE 25.4 Treatment of Acute Diarrhea

Degree of Dehydration	Signs and Symptoms	Rehydration Therapy*	Replacement of Stool Losses	Maintenance Therapy
Mild (5% to 6%)	Increased thirst Slightly dry buccal mucous membranes	ORS, 50 ml/kg within 4 hours	ORS, 10 ml/kg (for infants) or 150 to 250 ml at a time (for older children) for each diarrheal stool	Breastfeeding, if established, should continue; give regular infant formula if tolerated. If lactose intolerance suspected, give undiluted lactose-free formula (or half-strength lactose-containing formula for brief period only); infants and children who receive solid food should continue their usual diet.
Moderate (7% to 9%)	Loss of skin turgor, dry buccal mucous membranes, sunken eyes, sunken fontanel	ORS, 100 ml/kg within 4 hours	Same as above	
Severe (>9%)	Signs of moderate dehydration plus 1 of following: rapid thready pulse, cyanosis, rapid breathing, lethargy, coma	Intravenous fluids (Ringer lactate), 40 ml/kg until pulse and state of consciousness return to normal; then 50 to100 ml/kg or ORS	Same as above	

*If no signs of dehydration are present, rehydration therapy is not necessary. Proceed with maintenance therapy and replacement of stool losses.
ORS, Oral rehydration solution.

! NURSING ALERT

Encouraging intake of clear fluids by mouth, such as fruit juices, carbonated soft drinks, and gelatin, does not help diarrhea. These fluids usually have a high carbohydrate content, a very low electrolyte content, and a high osmolality. Have patients avoid caffeinated beverages because caffeine is a mild diuretic and may lead to increased loss of water and sodium. Chicken or beef broth is not given because it contains excessive sodium and inadequate carbohydrate. A BRAT diet (bananas, rice, applesauce, and toast or tea) is contraindicated for the child and especially for the infant with acute diarrhea because this diet has little nutritional value (low in energy and protein), is high in carbohydrates, and is low in electrolytes.

2016). Infants who are breastfeeding should continue to do so, and ORS should be used to replace ongoing losses in these infants. Formula-fed infants should resume their formula; if it is not tolerated, a lactose-free formula may be used for a few days. In toddlers there is no contraindication to continuing soft or pureed foods. In older children a regular diet, including milk, can generally be offered after rehydration has been achieved. In cases of severe dehydration and shock, IV fluids are initiated whenever the child is unable to ingest sufficient amounts of fluid and electrolytes to (1) meet ongoing daily physiologic losses, (2) replace previous deficits, and (3) replace ongoing abnormal losses. Patients who usually require IV fluids are those with severe dehydration, uncontrollable vomiting, inability to drink for any reason (e.g., extreme fatigue, coma), and severe gastric distention.

Select the IV solution on the basis of what is known regarding the probable type and cause of the dehydration. The type of fluid normally used is a saline solution containing 5% dextrose in water. Sodium bicarbonate may be added because acidosis is usually associated with severe dehydration. Although the initial phase of fluid replacement is rapid in both isotonic and hypotonic dehydration, rapid replacement is contraindicated in hypertonic dehydration because of the risk of water intoxication.

After the severe effects of dehydration are under control, begin specific diagnostic and therapeutic measures to detect and treat the cause of the diarrhea. Because of the self-limiting nature of vomiting and its tendency to improve when dehydration is corrected, the use of antiemetic agents is usually not needed; however, ondansetron has few side effects and may be administered if vomiting persists and interferes with ORT (Bhutta, 2016).

The use of antibiotic therapy in children with acute gastroenteritis is controversial. Antibiotics may shorten the course of some diarrheal illnesses (e.g., those caused by *Shigella* organisms). However, most bacterial diarrheas are self-limiting, and the diarrhea often resolves before the causative organism can be determined. Antibiotics may prolong the carrier period for bacteria such as *Salmonella*. Antibiotics may be considered, however, in patients who are less than 3 months of age or on immunosuppressive medication, or who have clinical signs of shock, severe malnutrition, dysentery, suspected cholera, or suspected giardiasis (Wen, Best, & Nourse, 2017). (See Intestinal Parasitic Diseases, Chapter 6.)

Nursing Care Management

The management of most cases of acute diarrhea takes place in the home with education of the caregiver. Teach caregivers to monitor for signs of dehydration (especially the number of wet diapers or voidings) and the amount of fluids taken by mouth, and to assess the frequency and amount of stool losses. Education relating to ORT, including the administration of maintenance fluids and replacement of ongoing losses, is important (see Critical Thinking Case Study box). ORS should be administered in small quantities at frequent intervals. Vomiting is not a contraindication to ORT unless it is severe. Information concerning the introduction of a normal diet is essential. Parents need to know that a slightly higher stool output initially occurs with continuation of a normal diet and with ongoing replacement of stool losses. The benefits of a better nutritional outcome with fewer complications and a shorter duration of illness outweigh the potential increase in stool frequency. Address parents' concerns to ensure adherence to the treatment plan.

? CRITICAL THINKING CASE STUDY

Diarrhea

A mother brings her 8-month-old infant, Mary, to the primary care clinic. The mother reports that Mary has had a "cold" for about 2 days, and this morning she began to vomit and has had diarrhea for the past 8 hours. Mary's mother states that she is still breastfeeding, but Mary is not taking as much fluid as usual and she is having three times as many stools as usual (the stools are watery). When the nurse practitioner examines Mary, she notes that her temperature is 38°C (100.4°F), her pulse and blood pressure are in the normal range, her mucous membranes are slightly dry, but she has tears when she cries. The nurse practitioner also notes that Mary's weight has not changed from what it was when she was seen in the clinic 2 weeks ago for her well-child visit. What interventions should the nurse practitioner include in her initial management of Mary?

1. Evidence—Is there sufficient evidence for the nurse practitioner to draw any conclusions for her initial plan of management?
2. Assumptions—Describe some underlying assumptions about the following:
   a. Clinical manifestations of various levels of dehydration
   b. Management of acute diarrhea
   c. Breastfeeding and the management of acute diarrhea
   d. Use of antidiarrheal medications for acute diarrhea
3. What nursing interventions should the nurse practitioner implement at this time?
4. Does the evidence support your conclusion?

Answers are available at http://evolve.elsevier.com/wong/ncic.

If the child with acute diarrhea and dehydration is hospitalized, the nurse must obtain an accurate weight and carefully monitor intake and output. The child may be placed on parenteral fluid therapy with nothing by mouth (NPO) for 12 to 48 hours. Monitoring the IV infusion is an important nursing function. The nurse must ensure that the correct fluid and electrolyte concentration is infused, that the flow rate is adjusted to deliver the desired volume in a given time, and that the IV site is maintained.

Accurate measurement of output is essential to determine whether renal blood flow is sufficient to permit the addition of potassium to the IV fluids. The nurse is responsible for examination of stools and collection of specimens for laboratory examination. (See Collection of Specimens, Chapter 22.) Take care when obtaining and transporting stools to prevent possible spread of infection. Use a clean tongue depressor to obtain specimens for laboratory examination or as an applicator for transfer to a culture medium. Transport stool specimens to the laboratory in appropriate containers and media according to hospital policy.

Diarrheal stools are highly irritating to the skin, and extra care is necessary to protect the skin of the diaper region from excoriation. (See Diaper Dermatitis, Chapter 32.) Avoid taking temperatures rectally because they stimulate the bowel, increasing passage of stool.

Support for the child and family involves the same care and consideration given to all hospitalized children. (See Chapter 21.) Keep parents informed of the child's progress and instruct them in the use of frequent and proper hand washing and the disposal of soiled diapers, clothes, and bed linen. Everyone caring for the child must be aware of "clean" areas and "dirty" areas, especially in the hospital, where the sink in the child's room is used for many purposes. Discard soiled diapers and linen in receptacles close to the bedside.

Prevention. The best intervention for diarrhea is prevention. The fecal-oral route spreads most infections, and parents need information about preventive measures such as personal hygiene, protection of the water supply from contamination, and careful food preparation.

> **! NURSING ALERT**
>
> To reduce the risk of bacteria transmitted via food, encourage parents to do the following:
> - Quickly freeze or refrigerate all ground meat and other perishable foods.
> - Never thaw food on the counter or let it sit out of the refrigerator for more than 2 hours.
> - Wash hands, utensils, and work areas with hot, soapy water after contact with raw meat to keep bacteria from spreading.
> - Check ground meat with a fork to make certain no pink is showing before taking a bite.
> - Cook all dishes made with ground meat until brown or gray inside or to an internal temperature of 71°C (160°F).

Meticulous attention to perianal hygiene, disposal of soiled diapers, proper hand washing, and isolation of infected persons also minimize the transmission of infection. (See Infection Control, Chapter 22.)

Parents need information about preventing diarrhea while traveling. Caution them against giving their children adult medications that are used to prevent traveler's diarrhea. The best measure during travel to areas where water may be contaminated is to allow children to drink only bottled water and carbonated beverages (from the container through a straw supplied from home). Children should also avoid tap water, ice, unpasteurized dairy products, raw vegetables, unpeeled fruits, meats, and seafood.

Vaccines can protect children from some diarrhea-related diseases. The rotavirus vaccine was integrated into the national immunization program in the United States in 2006, and subsequently the rotavirus season was noted to be shorter, along with a 76% decline in diarrhea hospitalization rates among children less than 5 years of age (Lamberti, Ashraf, Walker, et al., 2016).

CONSTIPATION

Constipation is an alteration in the frequency, consistency, or ease of passing stool. It is defined as unsatisfactory defecation due to infrequent stools, difficult stool passage, or perceived incomplete defecation (Bruce, Bruce, Short, et al., 2016). Constipation is an alteration in the frequency, consistency, or ease of passing stool. The frequency of bowel movements varies by age, but children 4 years and older can be diagnosed with constipation if they have less than three stools per week (Poddar, 2016). Constipation is often associated with painful bowel movements, blood-streaked or retained stool, abdominal pain, lack of appetite, and stool incontinence (i.e., soiling) (Bruce, Bruce, Short, et al., 2016). Having extremely long intervals between defecation is **obstipation**. Constipation with fecal soiling is **encopresis**.

Constipation may arise secondary to a variety of organic disorders or in association with a wide range of systemic disorders. Structural disorders of the intestine, such as strictures, ectopic anus, and Hirschsprung disease (HD), may be associated with constipation. Systemic disorders associated with constipation include hypothyroidism, hypercalcemia resulting from hyperparathyroidism or vitamin D excess, and chronic lead poisoning. Constipation is also associated with drugs such as antacids, diuretics, antiepileptics, antihistamines, opioids, and iron supplementation. Spinal cord lesions may be associated with loss of rectal tone and sensation. Affected children are prone to chronic fecal retention and overflow incontinence.

The majority of children have **idiopathic** or **functional constipation** because no underlying cause can be identified. Chronic constipation may occur as a result of environmental or psychosocial factors, or a combination of both. Transient illness, withholding and avoidance secondary to painful or negative experiences with stooling, and dietary intake with decreased fluid and fiber all play a role in the etiology of constipation.

Newborn Period

Normally, newborn infants pass a first meconium stool within 24 to 36 hours of birth. Any newborn that does not do so should be assessed for evidence of intestinal atresia or stenosis, HD, hypothyroidism, meconium plug, or meconium ileus. **Meconium plug** is caused by meconium that has reduced water content and is usually evacuated after digital examination but may require irrigations with a hypertonic solution or contrast medium. **Meconium ileus**, the initial manifestation of cystic fibrosis, is the luminal obstruction of the distal small intestine by abnormal meconium. Treatment is the same as for a meconium plug; early surgical intervention may be needed to evacuate the small intestine.

Infancy

The onset of constipation frequently occurs during infancy and may result from organic causes such as HD, hypothyroidism, and strictures. It is important to differentiate these conditions from functional constipation. Constipation in infancy is often related to dietary practices. It is less common in breastfed infants, who have softer stools than bottle-fed infants. Breastfed infants may also have decreased stools because of more complete use of breast milk with little residue. When constipation occurs with a change from human milk or modified cow's milk to whole cow's milk, simple measures such as adding or increasing the amount of vegetables and fruit in the infant's diet and increasing fluids such as sorbitol-rich juices usually correct the problem. When a bottle-fed infant passes a hard stool that results in an anal fissure, stool-withholding behaviors may develop in response to pain on defecation (see Critical Thinking Case Study box).

> **? CRITICAL THINKING CASE STUDY**
>
> ***Constipation***
>
> Harry, an 8-month-old infant, is seen by the pediatric nurse practitioner for his well-child visit. Harry's mother states that he usually has one hard stool every 4 or 5 days, which causes discomfort when the stool is passed. He has also had one episode of diarrhea and two episodes of ribbon-like stools. Abdominal distention and vomiting have not accompanied the constipation, and Harry's growth has been appropriate for his age. Currently, his diet consists of cow's milk–based formula only. Harry's mother reports that the infrequent passage of hard stools began approximately 6 weeks ago when she stopped breastfeeding. Which interventions should the nurse practitioner include in the initial management of Harry's problem?
>
> 1. Evidence—Is there sufficient evidence for the nurse practitioner to draw any conclusions about the management of Harry's problem?
> 2. Assumptions—Describe some underlying assumptions about the following:
>   a. Causes of constipation in infants
>   b. Factors associated with functional constipation in infants
>   c. Management of functional constipation in infants
> 3. What interventions should the nurse practitioner implement at this time?
> 4. Does the evidence support these interventions?

Answers are available at http://evolve.elsevier.com/wong/ncic.

Childhood

Most constipation in early childhood is due to environmental changes or normal development when a child begins to attain control over bodily functions. A child who has experienced discomfort during bowel movements may deliberately try to withhold stool. Over time, the rectum accommodates to the accumulation of stool, and the urge to defecate passes. When the bowel contents are ultimately evacuated, the accumulated feces are passed with pain, thus reinforcing the desire to withhold stool.

Constipation in school-age children may represent an ongoing problem or a first-time event. The onset of constipation at this age is often the result of environmental changes, stresses, and changes in toileting patterns. A common cause of new-onset constipation at school entry is fear of using the school bathrooms, which are noted for their lack of privacy. Early and hurried departure for school immediately after breakfast may also impede bathroom use.

Therapeutic Management

Treatment of constipation depends on the cause and duration of symptoms. A complete history and physical examination are essential to determine appropriate management. It may be necessary to facilitate passage of the obstruction by irrigation with a hypertonic solution or water-soluble enema. If the constipation is due to HD, surgical treatment may include resection of the intestine and saline irrigations.

Management of the infant should include education of the parents concerning normal bowel habits. Short, transient periods of constipation usually require no intervention. Mild constipation usually resolves as solid food is introduced in the diet. Stool softeners such as malt extract or lactulose may be used for hard stools or anal fissures. The persistent use of rectal stimulation with thermometers or cotton-tipped applicators is discouraged because these methods often result in anal fissures and increased pain that may trigger stool withholding.

The management of simple constipation consists of a plan to promote regular bowel movements. Often this is as simple as changing the diet to provide more fiber and fluids, eliminating foods known to be constipating, and establishing a bowel routine that allows for regular passage of stool. Stool-softening agents such as docusate or lactulose may also be helpful. Polyethylene glycol (PEG) 3350 without electrolytes (MiraLax) is a chemically inert polymer that has been introduced as a new laxative in recent years. Children tolerate it well because it can be mixed in any beverage of choice. If other symptoms such as vomiting, abdominal distention, or pain and evidence of growth failure are associated with the constipation, investigate the condition further.

Management of chronic constipation requires an organized and ongoing approach. It is important for families to realize that it usually requires months or years to resolve, and relapse is common. The goals for management include restoring regular evacuation of stool, shrinking the distended rectum to its normal size, and promoting a regular toileting routine. This requires a combination of therapies and should include bowel cleansing, maintenance therapy to prevent stool retention, modification of diet, bowel habit training, and behavioral modification (Box 25.8).

BOX 25.8 Treatment for Organic Causes of Constipation

Phase I: Clean-Out and Disimpaction (3 to 5 Days)

Oral clean-out method preferred for children older than 4 years
- High-dose mineral oil
- Polyethylene glycol
- Magnesium hydroxide

Enema clean-out
- Milk and molasses
- Normal saline solution
- Microlax, mineral oil, or hypertonic phosphate

Nasogastric lavage (hospitalization)
- Polyethylene glycol electrolyte solution

Phase 2: Maintenance (6 to 12 Months)

Oral laxatives
- Polyethylene glycol
- Mineral oil
- Lactulose
- Magnesium hydroxide

High-fiber diet
Increased fluid intake
Behavioral training

Phase 3: Weaning

Gradual tapering of laxatives
Continue high-fiber diet, fluid intake, behavior modification

Adapted from Tobias, N., Mason, D., Lutkenhoff, M., et al. (2008). Management principles of organic causes of childhood constipation. *Journal of Pediatric Health Care, 22*(1), 12-23.

DRUG ALERT

Mineral Oil

Mineral oil must be given carefully to avoid the risk of aspiration. It should not be used in children younger than 1 year (Podder, 2016).

After the impaction is removed, maintenance therapy often lasting for 6 to 12 months is necessary to promote easy passage of stool and to prevent stool retention. Maintenance therapy includes stool softeners and laxatives. Stool softeners are often ineffective for severe constipation; laxative therapy may be necessary to return the rectum to its normal size. Because of the minimal side effects, taste, and efficacy, PEG is a more favorable constipation intervention than lactulose (Podder, 2016). PEG increases fluid in the colon. The additional volume of fluid stimulates the urge to defecate.

Changes in the diet may be helpful but are usually not effective alone. Encouraging the intake of fiber ultimately helps maintain regular elimination once the rectum returns to normal size and the laxatives are tapered. Recommended daily fiber intake is age in years + 5 grams of fiber per day (Podder, 2016). Effective counseling is an essential element of the treatment plan for children with chronic constipation. Explain normal bowel function, the purpose of interventions, and the need for persistence to the child and family.

Retraining therapy involves habit training, reinforcement for sitting on the toilet and defecating, and emotional support. Parents should establish a regular toilet time once or twice a day, preferably after a meal. A reasonable amount of time (5 to 10 minutes) should be spent attempting to defecate completely. Biofeedback may be indicated as a form of behavior modification and as a means to teach children to relax the anal sphincter during defecation.

Nursing Care Management

Unfortunately, constipation tends to be self-perpetuating. A child who has difficulty or discomfort when attempting to evacuate the bowels has a tendency to retain the bowel contents, and thus constipation becomes a chronic problem. Nursing assessment begins with a history of bowel habits; diet; events that may be associated with the onset of constipation; drugs or other substances that the child may be taking;

TABLE 25.5 Fiber Content of Select Foods

Food	Serving Size	Grams of Fiber
Apple, raw, with skin	1 apple	3.3
Bananas, ripe, raw	1 small-sized banana	3.1
Beans, baked, canned	1 cup	10.4
Beans, pinto, mature seeds*	1 cup	15.4
Beets*	1 cup	3.4
Blackberries, raw	1 cup	7.6
Blueberries, raw	1 cup	3.5
Bread, mixed grain (includes whole grain)	1 slice	1.6
Broccoli*	1 cup	5.1
Brussels sprouts*	1 cup	4.1
Carrots*	1 cup	4.7
Cereals, ready-to-eat, General Mills, Cheerios	1 cup	3.6
Cereals, ready-to-eat, General Mills, Raisin Nut Bran	1 cup	5.1
Cereals, ready-to-eat, Kellogg's All Bran, original	½ cup	8.8
Cereals, ready-to-eat, Kellogg's Raisin Bran	1 cup	7.3
Collards*	1 cup	5.3
Dates, daglet noor	1 cup	14.2
Lentils, mature seeds*	1 cup	15.6
Lima beans, large, mature*	1 cup	13.2
Oat bran, cooked	1 cup	5.7
Oranges, raw	1 orange	3.1
Pears, raw	1 pear	5.1
Peas, green, frozen*	1 cup	8.8
Raisins, seedless	1 cup	5.4
Spinach*	1 cup	4.3
Vegetables, mixed, frozen*	1 cup	8.0
Wheat flour, whole grain	1 cup	14.6
Wheat flour, white, all-purpose, enriched	1 cup	3.5

*Cooked, boiled, drained, no salt.
From Perry, S. E., Hockenberry, M. J., Lowdermilk, D. L., et al. (2014). *Maternal child nursing care* (5th ed.). St. Louis, MO: Mosby.

and the consistency, color, frequency, and other characteristics of the stool. If there is no evidence of a pathologic condition that requires further investigation, the nurse's major task is to educate the parents regarding normal stool patterns and to participate in the education and treatment of the child.

Dietary modifications are helpful in preventing constipation. Fiber is an important part of the diet. Parents benefit from guidance about foods high in fiber (Table 25.5) and ways to promote healthy food choices in children. If bran is added to the diet, creative ways to disguise the consistency, such as adding it to cereal, peanut butter, mashed potatoes, fruit shakes, and baked goods, are helpful. Beans are often found in Mexican dishes children enjoy and can be added to soups, salads, and stews. Beyond the age when foreign body aspiration is a hazard, a good source of fiber is corn and popcorn.

Parents need reassurance concerning the prognosis for establishing normal bowel habits. Many parents are concerned about constipation and view the condition as dangerous. Families need thorough instructions about the treatment plan. If the child needs enemas or medication, give the family the appropriate instructions. It is important to discuss attitudes and expectations regarding toilet habits and the treatment plan.

VOMITING

Vomiting is the forceful ejection of gastric contents through the mouth. It is a well-defined, complex, coordinated process that is under central nervous system control and is often accompanied by nausea and retching. In contrast, regurgitation is a simpler, more passive, and effortless phenomenon. Vomiting has many causes, including acute infectious diseases, increased intracranial pressure, toxic ingestions, food intolerances and allergies, mechanical obstruction of the GI tract, adrenal insufficiency, nephrologic disease, pregnancy, and psychogenic problems (Sreedharan & Liacouras, 2016). Vomiting is common in childhood, is usually self-limiting, and requires no specific treatment. However, complications can occur in children, including acute fluid volume loss (dehydration) and electrolyte disturbances, malnutrition, aspiration, and Mallory-Weiss syndrome (small tears in the distal esophageal mucosa).

Etiology

The child's age, pattern of vomiting, and duration of symptoms help determine the cause. For example, chronic and intermittent episodes of vomiting may indicate malrotation, whereas vomiting on a specific day at the same time before school is not likely to be a result of organic disease. The color and consistency of the emesis vary according to the cause. Green, bilious vomiting suggests bowel obstruction. Curdled stomach contents, mucus, or fatty foods that are vomited several hours after ingestion suggest poor gastric emptying or high intestinal obstruction. Gastric irritation by certain medicines, foods, or toxic substances may cause vomiting. Forceful vomiting is associated with pyloric stenosis.

Associated symptoms also help identify the cause. Fever and diarrhea accompanying vomiting suggest an infection. Constipation associated with vomiting suggests an anatomic or functional obstruction. Localized abdominal pain and vomiting often occur with appendicitis, pancreatitis, or peptic ulcer disease. A change in the level of consciousness or a headache associated with vomiting indicates a central nervous system or metabolic disorder.

Pathophysiology

The act of vomiting, including nausea and retching, is under the control of the central nervous system. Two areas of the medulla are involved as the vomiting center. The medullary center is also activated by impulses from a second center, the chemoreceptor trigger zone, which is located in the floor of the fourth ventricle (Box 25.9). **Nausea** is a sensation that may be induced by visceral, labyrinthine (inner ear), or emotional stimuli. It is characterized by the desire to vomit, with discomfort felt in the throat or abdomen. Nausea is often associated with autonomic symptoms such as salivation, pallor, sweating, and tachycardia. Retching may occur with or without vomiting. **Retching** involves a series of spasmodic movements during inspiration, creating a negative intrathoracic pressure, and contraction of the abdominal muscles. Projectile vomiting is preceded and accompanied by vigorous peristaltic waves.

Vomiting is a well-recognized response to psychologic stress. During stress, adrenaline levels rise and may stimulate the chemoreceptor trigger zone. Nausea and vomiting are likely a protective mechanism to remove toxins from the system. Vomiting may follow GI infection or toxic ingestion, or it can be a learned behavioral response.

BOX 25.9 Sources of Vomiting Stimuli

Higher cortical centers—Either deep-seated or superficial psychologic disturbances. Stimuli include those associated with unpleasant sights, repugnant odors, and fright.

Chemoreceptor trigger zone—Transmits impulses to cortical center; located on the floor of the fourth ventricle. Stimuli include chemical stimulation by drugs (e.g., apomorphine, morphine, ipecac, and some digitalis derivatives), toxins (e.g., from uremia, infections, or radiation), cerebral hypoxia, increased intracranial pressure, and disturbances of the semicircular canals of the inner ear.

Reflex excitement (vagal and sympathetic afferent nerves)—Results from disturbed gastrointestinal and other viscera. Stimuli include irritation, inflammation, or mechanical disturbance in gastrointestinal tract (e.g., distention or obstruction); irritation of other viscera (e.g., heart, renal pelvis, bladder); and pain.

Cyclic vomiting syndrome is a rare disorder, affecting approximately 2% of children in the United States, and is characterized by bouts of vomiting that can last from hours to several days (Sreedharan & Liacouras, 2016). The cause of this syndrome is unknown, although a family history of migraines is usually present in at least 80% of the patients (Sreedharan & Liacouras, 2016).

Diagnostic Evaluation

The diagnostic evaluation includes a thorough history and physical examination. The description of the vomitus; relationship to meals or specific foods; behavior; and presence of pain, constipation, diarrhea, or jaundice are important components of the history. Physical examination should include an assessment of the hydration status and an abdominal examination.

Further evaluation may include analysis of urine for protein or blood, serum electrolytes, and radiographic studies. A plain radiograph of the chest or abdomen or ultrasonography may reveal anatomic abnormalities. Brain scans are used to when tumors are considered. Endoscopy of the upper GI tract may be a valuable diagnostic procedure if the provider suspects esophagitis. A psychiatric evaluation may be indicated if cyclic vomiting, anorexia nervosa, bulimia, or self-poisoning is present. Self-induced vomiting and rumination may be a self-stimulation or gratification activity.

Therapeutic Management

Management is directed toward detection and treatment of the cause of the vomiting and prevention of complications, such as dehydration and malnutrition. Vomiting is often a symptom of a common infectious illness that is self-limiting and resolves with no specific treatment. Further investigation is indicated if there is dehydration, progressively severe vomiting, or persistent vomiting for more than 24 hours, or if the history and physical examination fail to suggest a diagnosis. If vomiting leads to dehydration, oral rehydration or parenteral fluids may be required.

Antiemetic drugs may be indicated when the child is not able to tolerate anything orally or in the cases of postoperative vomiting, chemotherapy-induced vomiting, cyclic vomiting syndrome, or acute motion sickness (Sreedharan & Liacouras, 2016). Adverse effects with earlier-generation antiemetics (such as promethazine and metoclopramide) include somnolence, nervousness, irritability, and dystonic reactions, and they should not be routinely administered to children. Ondansetron (Zofran) is an antiemetic with limited adverse effects and is beneficial when the child is not able to tolerate anything orally or in the case of postoperative vomiting, chemotherapy-induced vomiting, cyclic vomiting syndrome, or acute motion sickness (Sreedharan & Liacouras, 2016). For children who are prone to motion sickness, it is often helpful to administer an appropriate dose of dimenhydrinate (Dramamine) before a trip (see Translating Evidence into Practice box).

Nursing Care Management

The major emphasis of nursing care of the vomiting infant or child is on observation and reporting of vomiting behavior and associated symptoms and on the implementation of measures to reduce the vomiting. Accurate assessment of the type of vomiting, appearance of the emesis, and the child's behavior in association with the vomiting greatly aids in establishing a diagnosis.

The cause of the vomiting determines the nursing intervention. When the vomiting is a manifestation of improper feeding methods, establishing proper techniques through teaching and example ordinarily corrects the situation. If the vomiting is a probable sign of GI obstruction, the nurse usually withholds food or implements special feeding techniques. The nurse should direct efforts toward maintaining hydration and preventing dehydration in a vomiting child.

The thirst mechanism is the most sensitive guide to fluid needs, and ad libitum administration of a glucose-electrolyte solution to an alert child restores water and electrolytes satisfactorily. It is important to include carbohydrates to spare body protein and to avoid ketosis resulting from exhaustion of glycogen stores. Small, frequent feedings of fluids or foods are preferable and more effective. Once vomiting has abated, offer more liberal amounts of fluids, followed by gradual resumption of the regular diet.

Position the infant or child upright who is vomiting to prevent aspiration and observe him or her for evidence of dehydration. Carefully monitor fluid and electrolyte status to avoid the possibility of electrolyte imbalance. It is important to emphasize the need for the child to brush the teeth or rinse the mouth after vomiting to dilute the hydrochloric acid that comes in contact with the teeth.

INGESTION OF FOREIGN SUBSTANCES

Children are prone to ingesting foreign substances because they frequently put their hands or other objects or substances in their mouth. Infants and small children in particular instinctively explore items with the mouth. Older children often place items in their mouth and accidentally swallow them. Rarely, a child deliberately swallows unusual objects or substances. Hands come into contact with dirt and contaminated objects that may contain lead, bacteria, or parasites.

PICA

Pica is an eating disorder characterized by the compulsive and excessive ingestion of both food and nonfood substances for at least 1 month (Katz, Kitts, & DeMaso, 2016). Food picas include the excessive eating of ordinary foods or unprepared food substances, such as coffee grounds or uncooked cereals. Nonfood picas include the ingestion of substances such as clay, soil, stones, paint, ice, hair, paper, rubber, and feces. Pica is more common in children, women (especially during pregnancy), individuals who have autism or cognitive impairment, and those with anemia or chronic renal failure. In some cultures pica is an accepted practice based on the presumed nutritional or therapeutic properties or on religious or superstitious beliefs.

There are several theories on the cause of pica, including psychologic theories (compulsive neurosis) and nutritional theories (craving caused by a nutrient deficiency). Pica is clearly associated with both iron and zinc deficiencies, although controversy exists regarding whether pica is

TRANSLATING EVIDENCE INTO PRACTICE

Use of Antiemetics in Children With Acute Gastroenteritis

Ask the Question

In children with acute gastroenteritis (AGE), should antiemetics be used?

Search for the Evidence

Search Strategies

Search criteria included English-language publications within the past 6 years (2011 to 2017), research-based articles (level 3 or higher) regarding antiemetic use among children with AGE.

Databases Used

PubMed/Medline, CINAHL, Cochrane, National Guideline Clearinghouse (AHRQ), American Academy of Pediatrics, National Institute of Health and Clinical Excellence, European Society for Paediatric Gastroenterology, Hepatology, and Nutrition, Joanna Briggs Institute

Critically Analyze the Evidence

GRADE criteria: Evidence quality moderate; recommendation strong (Balshem, Hefland, Schunemann, et al., 2011)

A review of the literature revealed two systematic reviews and three randomized control trials from 2011 to 2017 that evaluated the use of antiemetics in the treatment of children with AGE.

- A Cochrane review in 2011 revealed 7 randomized controlled trials (1020 patients) evaluating the safety and efficacy of antiemetics to treat gastroenteritis-induced vomiting in children (Fedorowicz, Jagannath, & Carter, 2011). Ondansetron was found more effective than placebo in studies evaluating hospital admission rates, need for intravenous (IV) rehydration therapy, and resolution of vomiting. When comparing placebo, dimenhydrinate was found more effective in one study, and metoclopramide was more effective in another single study.
- A systematic review from 1980 to 2012 revealed 10 studies (1479 participants) evaluating the evidence of safety and effectiveness of antiemetics (dexamethasone, dimenhydrinate, granisetron, metoclopramide, and ondansetron) for gastroenteritis-induced vomiting in children and adolescents (Carter & Fedorowicz, 2012). There is clear evidence from 9 studies that ondansetron is more effective than placebo in resolving vomiting, reducing the need for IV rehydration therapy, and reducing the hospital admission rate. A single study showed a reduction in mean vomiting days among children receiving dimenhydrinate versus placebo and among granisteron versus placebo. Studies of metoclopramide were underpowered, and a single study of dexamethasone versus placebo showed no statistically significant difference in vomiting.
- A group of 144 children diagnosed with acute gastroenteritis were randomized to receive dimenhydrinate or placebo in a pediatric emergency department (Gouin, Vo, Roy, et al., 2012). No statistically significant difference regarding the frequency of vomiting was noted between the two groups.
- A group of 76 children diagnosed with acute gastroenteritis were randomized to receive an orally disintegrating ondansetron tablet or domperidone suspension (dosing based on body weight), then evaluated for vomiting for the next 24 hours (Rerksuppaphol & Rerksuppaphol, 2013). Sixty-two percent of patients in the ondansetron group and 44% of patients in the domperidone group had no vomiting after treatment, although no statistically significant difference was noted ($p = 0.16$).
- Another study randomized 356 children to receive ondansetron ($n = 119$) versus domperiodone ($n = 119$) versus placebo ($n = 118$) for treatment of acute gastroenteritis who failed oral rehydration in an emergency department (Marchetti, Bonati, Maestro, et al., 2016). Fourteen children (12%) needed IV rehydration in the ondansetron group compared with 30 children (25%) in the domperidone and 34 (29%) children in the placebo group.

Apply the Evidence: Nursing Implications

Ondansetron reduces the duration of vomiting in children with AGE and ondansetron and domperidone relieves the incidence of vomiting in children with AGE. There is limited evidence for dimenhydrinate and metoclopramide, and no evidence for other antiemetics in children with AGE who are vomiting. The number of children requiring IV rehydration and hospital admission for AGE is reduced with administration of ondansetron.

References

Balshem, H., Hefland, M., Schunemann, H. J., et al. (2011). GRADE guidelines: Rating the quality of evidence. *Journal of Clinical Epidemiology, 64*(4), 401–406.

Carter, B., & Fedorowicz, Z. (2012). Antiemetic treatment for acute gastroenteritis in children: An updated Cochrane systematic review with meta-analysis and mixed treatment comparison in a Bayesian framework. *BMJ Open, 2*, 1–11.

Fedorowicz, Z., Jagannath, V. A., & Carter, B. (2011). Antiemetics for reducing vomiting related to acute gastroenteritis in children and adolescents. *Cochrane Database of Systematic Reviews*, (9), CD005506.

Gouin, S., Vo, T., Roy, M., et al. (2012). Oral dimenhydrinate versus placebo in children with gastroenteritis: A randomized controlled trial. *Pediatrics, 129*, 1050–1055.

Marchetti, F., Bonati, M., Maestro, A., et al. (2016). Oral ondansetron versus domperidone for acute gastroenteritis in pediatric emergency departments: Multicenter double blind randomized controlled trial. *PLoS ONE, 11*(11), e0165441.

Rerksuppaphol, S., & Rerksuppaphol, L. (2013). Randomized study of ondansetron versus domperidone in the treatment of children with acute gastroenteritis. *Journal of Clinical Medicine Research, 5*(6), 460–466.

the cause or the result of the deficiency. Pica has also been reported as the presenting symptom in children with celiac disease thought to be caused by iron deficiency. Pica for dirt (geophagia) is the principal risk factor for visceral larva migrans (a common parasite in children and adults) (Katz, Kitts, & DeMaso, 2016).

In some instances pica is relatively harmless. However, when the ingested substance contains a toxic ingredient (e.g., lead in paint), the consequences can be serious. Other significant consequences of pica include intestinal obstruction or perforation, dental injury, and malnutrition (Katz, Kitts, & DeMaso, 2016).

The nurse can detect pica by the history, physical examination, and radiologic studies. However, it is often unrecognized, and children may deny any unusual eating behaviors. The nurse should consider pica when children known to be at risk for this condition develop abdominal pain, other GI symptoms, or anemia. Children exhibiting signs of this disorder should be evaluated, and if a potentially harmful substance is involved, it should be removed from the child's environment. Nursing education regarding the dangers of pica, especially lead, and assistance in helping families remove the substance are important. (See Chapter 14.)

FOREIGN BODIES

Foreign body ingestion is a preventable cause of mortality and morbidity in children. Annually 1500 children die in the United States from foreign body aspiration (Laya, Restrepo, & Lee, 2017). Most foreign body ingestions occur in children younger than 3 years old, with the peak incidence between 10 and 24 months of age (Laya, Restrepo, & Lee, 2017). The predisposition is due to the tendency to explore by placing objects in their mouth, immature swallowing coordination, and inability to adequately chew certain foods due to lack of molars (Laya, Restrepo, & Lee, 2017). Nuts and seeds are the most commonly aspirated foods, but other items include coins, hot dogs, whole grapes, marshmallows, round candy, and metal or plastic objects.

Where the foreign bodies are retained depends on the GI tract's size, shape, diameter, and motility. Foreign bodies tend to become impacted at normally narrow sites of the GI tract. Pathologic narrowing of the intestine or intestinal stomas can also be a cause of foreign body obstruction. Foreign bodies in the stomach or intestine usually pass on their own. However, if they do become impacted, this generally occurs in the esophagus; other common sites include the ileocecal valve, pylorus, duodenum, or appendix.

Signs and Symptoms

A history of choking followed by an acute episode of vigorous coughing is the most common presentation of foreign body ingestion. Initial signs and symptoms also may include dyspnea and wheezing. Aspirated foreign bodies that lodge in the larynx or trachea cause stridor. When these are in the large bronchi, crepitation and wheezes can be found. Wheezes and crepitation can be heard in both lungs, but unilateral findings have a higher specificity for foreign body aspiration (Khan & Orenstein, 2016a).

Other symptoms may be those that are common with GI complaints in general (e.g., dysphagia, excessive drooling, poor feeding, vomiting, gagging, anorexia, neck or throat pain, sensation of a foreign object, and refusal to eat or drink).

Complications

Foreign bodies are generally classified as sharp or dull, pointed or blunt, and toxic or nontoxic. Some foreign bodies are ingested and may be excreted without complications, but other foreign bodies, especially those that are pointed, toxic, or aspirated, require immediate treatment. Complications from foreign bodies include pneumonia, perforation, obstruction, pneumothorax, and pneumomediastinum (Berdan & Sato, 2017). Foreign bodies should be immediately removed if the child is in severe distress and unable to swallow secretions. Disc batteries are a medical emergency because the composition of the batteries can cause damage to the mucosa within 1 hour of aspiration/ingestion (Khan & Orstein, 2016a). Single battery ingestion can be monitored closely with conservative management, but ingestion of multiple magnets has a high risk of complications, and they must be removed promptly. Sharp objects (e.g., straight pins, needles, straightened paper clips) need to be removed without delay if lodged in the esophagus.

Diagnostic Evaluation

As mentioned, there may be no signs or symptoms, but some children come to the physician for evaluation because of problems. The nurse should perform a complete history and physical examination. Assess the airway and breathing first. Findings on the chest evaluation might include inspiratory stridor or expiratory wheezing. Findings on an abdominal examination could be hypoactive or absent bowel sounds. The physical examination might demonstrate swelling, erythema, or crepitus suggestive of esophageal perforation.

Assessment often involves radiologic evaluation. A plain x-ray film of the neck, chest, and abdomen may be ordered. Biplane radiographic studies identify radiopaque esophageal foreign bodies. Flat objects such as coins may be visible in the coronal plane. Objects in the trachea generally orient into the sagittal plane and are easiest to see in the lateral projection. Handheld metal detectors have been used to detect coins. Endoscopy should be done in patients with symptoms suggestive of obstruction, even if the radiographic evidence is negative.

Therapeutic Management

Intervention is urgent when a child has sharp objects, magnets, or disc batteries lodged in the esophagus because of the risk of perforation or acid burns (Berdan & Sato, 2017). Urgent intervention is also important anytime the airway is compromised. If the child is asymptomatic and the foreign body does not carry an emergent risk, it is reasonable to wait 24 hours to see if it will pass. Foreign objects should not be allowed to remain in the esophagus for more than 24 hours because of the potential for complications such as erosion, perforation, or formation of fistulas.

Flexible endoscopy allows direct visualization of the esophagus, stomach, and duodenum. It is the best approach for removing a foreign object. It involves passing a narrow tube with a camera on the end through the mouth into the esophagus, stomach, and duodenum with the patient under sedation. The foreign object can be detected and removed. Rigid endoscopy is used to remove sharp objects at the level of the hypopharynx and cricopharyngeal muscle.

Another technique that has been used to remove foreign bodies is bougienage (Khan & Orstein, 2016a). This involves passing a dilator to push objects into the stomach. The drawback is that this method does not allow inspection of the esophagus to assess for injury or damage, and it increases the risk of perforation of the esophagus.

Another method involves passing a Foley catheter into the esophagus, inflating it distal to the obstruction, and then withdrawing it (Khan & Orstein, 2016a). However, there is a risk of airway obstruction and an inability to directly visualize the esophagus.

Coins have been removed using the penny pincher technique, which involves passing grasping forceps through a nasogastric (NG) tube using fluoroscopic guidance. This method allows for direct control of the object, but again it does not permit inspection of the esophagus.

Important variables in the application of treatment guidelines include the type of foreign object, its location in the GI tract, and whether the patient is symptomatic. Of all foreign bodies that reach the stomach, 80% to 90% pass spontaneously (Laya, Restrepo, & Lee, 2017). The progress of a foreign body may be followed radiographically. Examine all stools to detect the passage of the object. The child should be fed the usual diet. Sharp objects such as long pins or chicken or fish bones should be removed endoscopically rather than risk perforation by allowing them to pass spontaneously (Berdan & Sato, 2017). Endoscopic or surgical intervention should be implemented if the object fails to progress through the GI tract.

Nursing Care Management

The primary nursing intervention is prevention of foreign body ingestion through family teaching. All children who are old enough to understand are taught not to put anything in their mouth except food. Infants and young children who cannot follow such advice must have their environment protected.

Prevention includes supervision and ongoing education as the child matures. Any small items, diaper pins, or sharp objects are placed out of the area where an infant is usually cared for, plays, or sleeps. As the infant becomes more mobile, the environment is inspected carefully for hazardous objects. Any potentially dangerous items are placed out of reach of a young child or discarded where they cannot be retrieved easily. Toys are carefully examined for small or removable parts that could be accidentally ingested. If infants and small children wear earrings, the earrings should have screw backs to prevent them from falling off. Infants and small children who wear other jewelry should be carefully supervised. Infants or young children should not be allowed to play with marbles, coins, or objects with small batteries.

Once an object is swallowed, parents need guidelines on seeking treatment (see Emergency Treatment box). When no treatment is advised and the object is left to pass spontaneously, parents should examine all stools for verification that the object has passed safely through the GI tract, usually within 3 or 4 days. For children in diapers this is easily accomplished by squeezing the stool between the diaper to locate the object. For toilet-trained children a piece of plastic wrap placed across the toilet bowl to collect the stool makes it easier to examine the feces. A tongue blade or similar disposable object may be needed to break up the stool for inspection.

EMERGENCY TREATMENT

Foreign Body Ingestion

Seek medical treatment immediately if
- Any sharp or large object or a battery was ingested.
- There are signs that the object may have been aspirated (i.e., coughing, choking, inability to speak, or difficulty breathing). (See Chapter 26.)
- There are signs of gastrointestinal perforation (i.e., chest or abdominal pain; evidence of bleeding in vomitus, stool, hematocrit, or vital signs).
- There are signs that the object may be lodged in the esophagus (i.e., increased salivation, drooling, gagging, or difficulty swallowing).
- There are signs that the object may be lodged in the pharynx (i.e., discomfort in the throat or chest—more likely with a fish or chicken bone or large piece of meat).

Seek medical advice even if the object is smooth and small (usually less than the size of a nickel).

If no treatment is advised, check the stool for passage of the object; do not give laxatives.

DISORDERS OF MOTILITY

HIRSCHSPRUNG DISEASE (CONGENITAL AGANGLIONIC MEGACOLON)

Hirschsprung disease (HD) is a congenital anomaly that results in mechanical obstruction from inadequate motility of part of the intestine. It accounts for about one-fourth of all cases of neonatal intestinal obstruction. The incidence is 1 in 5000 live births (Fiorino & Liacouras, 2016). It is four times more common in males than in females and follows a familial pattern in a small number of cases. Mutations in the *RET* protooncogene have been found in children with HD (Fiorino & Liacouras, 2016).

Pathophysiology

The pathology of HD relates to the absence of ganglion cells in the affected areas of the intestine, resulting in a loss of the rectosphincteric reflex and an abnormal microenvironment of the cells of the affected intestine. The term *congenital aganglionic megacolon* describes the primary defect, which is the absence of ganglion cells in the myenteric plexus of Auerbach and the submucosal plexus of Meissner (Fig. 25.2).

The absence of ganglion cells in the affected bowel results in a lack of enteric nervous system stimulation, which decreases the internal sphincter's ability to relax. Unopposed sympathetic stimulation of the intestine results in increased intestinal tone. In addition to the contraction of the abnormal bowel and the resulting lack of peristalsis, there is a loss of the rectosphincteric reflex. Normally, when a stool bolus enters the rectum, the internal sphincter relaxes and the stool is evacuated. In HD, the internal sphincter does not relax. In about 80% of the cases, the aganglionic segment includes only the rectum and some portion of the distal colon, termed *short-segment disease* (Fiorino & Liacouras, 2016). However, the entire colon or part of the small intestine may be involved; this is considered *long-segment HD*. Occasionally, skip segments or total intestinal aganglionosis may occur. Approximately 15% have long-segment disease, and 5% have total intestinal aganglionosis (Fiorino & Liacouras, 2016).

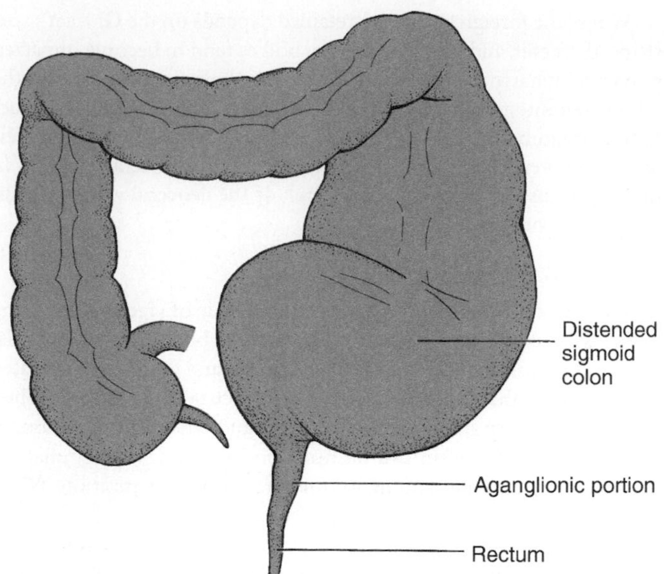

FIG. 25.2 Hirschsprung disease.

BOX 25.10 Clinical Manifestations of Hirschsprung Disease

Newborn Period

Failure to pass meconium within 24 to 48 hours after birth
Refusal to feed
Bilious vomiting
Abdominal distention

Infancy

Failure to thrive
Constipation
Abdominal distention
Episodes of diarrhea and vomiting
Signs of enterocolitis
- Explosive, watery diarrhea
- Fever
- Appears significantly ill

Childhood

Constipation
Ribbonlike, foul-smelling stools
Abdominal distention
Visible peristalsis
Easily palpable fecal mass
Undernourished, anemic appearance

Clinical Manifestations

Most children with HD are diagnosed in the first few months of life. Clinical manifestations vary according to the age when symptoms are recognized and the presence of complications, such as enterocolitis (Box 25.10). A neonate usually is seen with a distended abdomen, feeding intolerance with bilious vomiting, and a delay in the passage of meconium. Typically, 99% of term infants pass meconium in the first 48 hours of life, whereas few infants with HD do so (Fiorino & Liacouras, 2016).

Diagnostic Evaluation

In the neonate the diagnosis is suspected on the basis of clinical signs of intestinal obstruction or failure to pass meconium. In infants and children the history is an important part of diagnosis and typically includes a chronic pattern of constipation. On examination the rectum is empty of feces, the internal sphincter is tight, and leakage of liquid stool and accumulated gas may occur if the aganglionic segment is short. A contrast enema often demonstrates the transition zone between the dilated proximal colon (megacolon) and the aganglionic distal segment. However, this typical megacolon and narrow distal segment may not develop until age 2 months or later.

To confirm the diagnosis, rectal biopsy is performed either surgically to obtain a full-thickness biopsy specimen or by suction biopsy for histologic evidence of the absence of ganglion cells. A noninvasive procedure that may be used is anorectal manometry, in which a catheter with a balloon attached is inserted into the rectum. The test records the reflex pressure response of the internal anal sphincter to distention of the balloon. A normal response is relaxation of the internal sphincter, followed by a contraction of the external sphincter. In HD the external sphincter contracts normally but the internal sphincter fails to relax.

Therapeutic Management

The majority of children with HD require surgery rather than medical therapy. One of three operative procedures is performed: a Soave pull-through, the Swenson procedure, and the Duhamel procedure (Fiorino & Liacouras, 2016). Once the child is stabilized with fluid and electrolyte replacement and colonic cleansing with enemas, if needed, surgery is performed, usually with a high rate of success. Surgical management consists primarily of the removal of the aganglionic portion of the bowel to relieve obstruction, restore normal motility, and preserve the function of the external anal sphincter. The transanal Soave endorectal pull-through procedure consists of pulling the end of the normal bowel through the muscular sleeve of the rectum, from which the aganglionic mucosa has been removed. With earlier diagnosis the proximal bowel may not be extremely distended, thus allowing for a primary pull-through or one-stage procedure and eliminating the need for a temporary colostomy. Simpler operations, such as an anorectal myomectomy, may be indicated in very short-segment disease.

After the pull-through procedure, the majority of children achieve fecal continence. However, some children may experience anal stricture, recurrent enterocolitis, prolapse, or perianal abscess, and incontinence may occur and require further therapy, including dilations or bowel retraining therapy (Fiorino & Liacouras, 2016).

Nursing Care Management

The nursing concerns depend on the child's age and the type of treatment. If the disorder is diagnosed during the neonatal period, the main objectives are to help the parents adjust to a congenital defect in their child, foster infant-parent bonding, prepare the parents for the medical-surgical intervention, and prepare the parents to assume the care of the child after surgery.

The child's preoperative care depends on the age and clinical condition. A child who is malnourished may not be able to withstand surgery until his or her physical status improves. Often this involves symptomatic treatment with enemas and a low-fiber, high-calorie, high-protein diet. Physical preoperative preparation includes the same measures that are common to any surgery. (See Surgical Procedures, Chapter 22.) In the newborn, whose bowel is presumed sterile, no additional preparation is necessary. However, in other children, preparation for the pull-through procedure involves emptying the bowel with repeated saline enemas and decreasing bacterial flora with oral or systemic antibiotics and colonic irrigations using antibiotic solution. Enterocolitis is the most serious complication of HD. Emergent preoperative care includes frequent monitoring of vital signs and blood pressure for signs of shock; monitoring fluid and electrolyte replacements, as well as plasma or other blood derivatives; and observing for symptoms of bowel perforation, such as fever, increasing abdominal distention, vomiting, increased tenderness, irritability, dyspnea, and cyanosis.

Because progressive distention of the abdomen is a serious sign, the nurse measures abdominal circumference with a paper tape measure, usually at the level of the umbilicus or at the widest part of the abdomen. The point of measurement is marked with a pen to ensure reliability of subsequent measurements. Abdominal measurement can be obtained with the vital sign measurements and is recorded in serial order so that any change is obvious. To reduce stress to the acutely ill child when frequent measurements of abdominal circumference are needed, the tape measure can be left in place beneath the child rather than removed each time.

Postoperative care is the same as that for any child or infant with abdominal surgery. (See Surgical Procedures, Chapter 22.) The nurse involves the parents in the care of the child, allowing them to help with feedings and observe for signs of wound infection or irregular passage of stool. After surgery, parents need instruction concerning the development of complications such as enterocolitis, fecal incontinence, and obstruction. Some children will require daily anal dilations in the postoperative period to avoid anastomotic strictures; parents are often taught to perform the procedure in the home and will need encouragement and detailed instructions to perform these dilations. Although less common, a diverting colostomy may be performed in some children with HD. Parents are taught how to care for the colostomy and how to provide meticulous skin care to prevent skin breakdown; the assistance of a wound and skin care specialist is essential for optimal follow-up and consistent skin care.

Parents may need to bring the child with an ostomy to an outpatient clinic for support, encouragement, and additional instructions on skin and ostoma care after the child is discharged. In general the prognosis for the infant or child with HD is positive and most live a normal life. In a few cases problems with fecal incontinence may persist. A long-term study of children with HD for 1 to 19 years reported satisfying bowel control among 53% of the sample, soiling with 13%, constipation among 6%, and abdominal distention with 26% (Muller, Rossignol, Montalva, et al., 2016).

GASTROESOPHAGEAL REFLUX

Gastroesophageal reflux (GER) is defined as the transfer of gastric contents into the esophagus. This phenomenon is physiologic, occurring throughout the day, most frequently after meals and at night; therefore it is important to differentiate GER from gastroesophageal reflux disease (GERD). GERD represents symptoms or tissue damage that results from GER. The peak incidence of GER occurs at 4 months of age and generally resolves spontaneously in most infants by 1 year of age (Mousa & Hassan, 2017). GER becomes a disease when complications such as failure to thrive, respiratory problems, or dysphagia develop.

Certain conditions predispose children to a high prevalence of GERD, including neurologic impairment, chronic respiratory disorders, esophageal atresia, and obesity (Mousa & Hassan, 2017). Family clustering has also been identified; therefore a genetic predisposition to GERD is also likely (Khan & Orenstein, 2016b). Sandifer syndrome is an uncommon condition, usually occurring in young children, that is characterized by repetitive stretching and arching of the head and neck that can be mistaken for a seizure. This maneuver likely represents a physiologic neuromuscular response attempting to prevent acid refluxate from reaching the upper portion of the esophagus (Khan & Orenstein, 2016b).

Infants who are prone to develop GER include premature infants and infants with bronchopulmonary dysplasia. Children who have had tracheoesophageal or esophageal atresia repairs, neurologic disorders, scoliosis, asthma, cystic fibrosis, or cerebral palsy are also prone to develop GER.

Pathophysiology

Although the pathogenesis of GER is multifactorial, its primary causative mechanism likely involves inappropriate transient relaxation of the LES. Factors that increase abdominal pressure (e.g., coughing and sneezing, scoliosis, and overeating) may contribute to GER. Esophageal symptoms are caused by inflammation from the acid in the gastric refluxate, whereas reactive airway disease may result from stimulation of airway reflexes by the acid refluxate.

Clinical Manifestations

During infancy the most common clinical manifestation of GER is passive regurgitation. Regurgitation generally resolves spontaneously in most infants by 12 months and almost all infants by 24 months (Khan & Orenstein, 2016b). Clinical manifestations of GER are listed in Box 25.11. GER is one of the causes of apparent life-threatening events and has also been associated with chronic respiratory disorders, including reactive airway disease, recurrent stridor, chronic cough, and recurrent pneumonia in infants. Esophagitis can also cause discomfort in the chest area, which may be manifested as unusual irritability or poor intake of nutrients. Poor weight gain and poor growth may occur in a child with an insufficient intake of nutrients or with a large amount of regurgitation.

For preschool children GER may occur with intermittent vomiting. Older children tend to initially come to the physician with a more adult-like pattern of heartburn, regurgitation, and reswallowing. GERD may cause severe inflammation, chronic blood loss with anemia and hematemesis, hypoproteinemia, or melena. If the inflammation goes untreated, scarring and strictures may form. Barrett mucosa, another potential finding in the presence of chronic inflammation, is characterized by changes in the distal esophageal mucosa with metaplastic potentially malignant epithelium.

GER is common in children with asthma, but recurrent pneumonia caused by GER is uncommon except in children with neurologic impairments. Hoarseness has also been associated with GER in children.

BOX 25.11 Clinical Manifestations and Complications of Gastroesophageal Reflux

Symptoms in Infants

- Spitting up, regurgitation, recurrent vomiting (may be forceful)
- Excessive crying, irritability, arching of the back, stiffening
- Poor weight gain
- Respiratory problems (e.g., cough, wheeze, stridor, gagging, choking with feedings)
- Feeding refusal

Symptoms in Children

- Heartburn
- Abdominal pain
- Chronic cough, hoarse voice
- Dysphagia
- Asthma
- Recurrent vomiting

Complications

- Esophagitis
- Esophageal stricture
- Laryngitis
- Recurrent pneumonia
- Anemia
- Barrett esophagus

Adapted from Lightdale, J. R., Gremse, D. A., & Section on Gastroenterology, Hepatology, and Nutrition. (2013). Gastroesophageal reflux: Management guidance for the pediatrician. *Pediatrics, 131*(5), e1684–e1695.

Diagnostic Evaluation

The history and physical examination are usually sufficiently reliable to establish the diagnosis of GER. Standardized questionnaires, such as the Infant Gastroesophageal Reflux Questionnaire, are commonly used to assist with the diagnosis (Khan & Orenstein, 2016b). An upper GI series is helpful in evaluating the presence of anatomic abnormalities (e.g., pyloric stenosis, malrotation, annular pancreas, hiatal hernia, esophageal stricture). The 24-hour intraesophageal pH monitoring study was the gold standard in the diagnosis of GER; however, this test is a poor detector of weakly acidic (pH 4 to 7) reflux, which is prevalent in infants and children (Mousa & Hassan, 2017). Endoscopy with biopsy may be helpful to assess the presence and severity of esophagitis, strictures, and Barrett esophagus and to exclude other disorders such as Crohn disease. Scintigraphy detects radioactive substances in the esophagus after a feeding of the compound and assesses gastric emptying. It can differentiate between aspiration of gastric contents from reflux and aspiration from poor oropharyngeal muscle coordination.

Therapeutic Management

Therapeutic management of GER depends on its severity. No therapy is needed for the infant who is thriving and has no respiratory complications. Avoidance of certain foods that exacerbate acid reflux (e.g., caffeine, citrus, tomatoes, alcohol, peppermint, spicy or fried foods) can improve mild GER symptoms. Lifestyle modifications in children (e.g., weight control if indicated; small, more frequent meals) and feeding maneuvers in infants (e.g., thickened feedings; upright positioning) can help as well.

Feedings thickened with 1 teaspoon to 1 tablespoon of rice cereal per ounce of formula may be recommended. This may benefit infants who are underweight as a result of GERD; however, the additional calories are not beneficial among infants who are overweight. These infants may benefit from prethickened formulas that are now commercially available. Constant NG feedings may be necessary for the infant with severe reflux and failure to thrive until surgery can be performed. Elevating the head of the bed and weight loss, if applicable, can reduce GER symptoms. Prone positioning of infants also decreases episodes of GER; however, due to the risk of sudden infant death syndrome, all infants should sleep in the supine position (Khan & Orenstein, 2016b). The American Academy of Pediatrics continues to recommend supine positioning for sleep. (See Chapter 11.)

Pharmacologic therapy may be used to treat infants and children with GERD. Both H_2-receptor antagonists (cimetidine [Tagamet], ranitidine [Zantac], or famotidine [Pepcid]) and proton pump inhibitors (PPIs; esomeprazole [Nexium], lansoprazole [Prevacid], omeprazole [Prilosec], pantoprazole [Protonix], and rabeprazole [Aciphex]) reduce gastric hydrochloric acid secretion and may stimulate some increase in the lower esophageal sphincter tone. Use of metoclopramide for GERD in infants and children is no longer recommended due to the common incidence of side effects without significant benefit (Cohen, Bueno de Mesquita, & Mimouni, 2015).

Surgical management of GER is reserved for children with severe complications such as recurrent aspiration pneumonia, apnea, severe

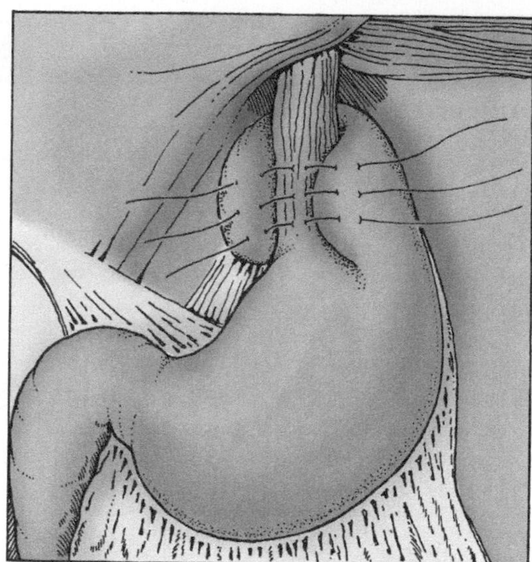

FIG. 25.3 Nissen fundoplication sutures passing through esophageal musculature. (Redrawn from Campbell, A., & Ferrara, B. [1993]. Toupet partial fundoplication. *AORN Journal, 57,* 671-679.)

esophagitis, or failure to thrive, and for children who have failed to respond to medical therapy. The **fundoplication** (Fig. 25.3) is a common surgical procedure for the treatment of GERD in children who have failed medical therapy or have life-threatening complications of GERD (Mousa & Hassan, 2017). This surgery involves passage of the gastric fundus behind the esophagus to encircle (i.e., wrap) the distal esophagus. Complications after fundoplication include a wrap that is too tight, causing dysphagia, small bowel obstruction, or gas-bloat; or a wrap that is too loose, causing continuation of symptoms (Khan & Orenstein, 2016b).

Prognosis. The majority of infants with GER have a mild problem that generally improves by 12 to 18 months of age and requires only conservative lifestyle changes or medical therapy. If GER is severe and remains unsuccessfully treated, multiple complications can occur. Esophageal strictures caused by persistent esophagitis with scarring are one of the most significant complications. Recurrent respiratory distress with aspiration pneumonia, another serious complication, is an indication for surgery. Failure to thrive caused by GER can often be managed with medical therapy and nutritional support. (See Quality Patient Outcomes box.)

QUALITY PATIENT OUTCOMES

Gastroesophageal Reflux

- Adequate weight gain
- Limited spitting up or vomiting
- Good sleep habits
- No recurrent pneumonias

Nursing Care Management

Nursing care is directed at identifying children with symptoms suggestive of GER; educating parents regarding home care, including feeding, positioning, and medications when indicated; and caring for the child undergoing surgical intervention. For the majority of infants, parental reassurance of the benign nature of the condition and its relationship to physiologic maturity is the most important intervention. To help parents cope with the inconvenience of dealing with a child who spits up or regurgitates frequently, simple tips such as using bibs and protective clothes during feeding and prone positioning when holding the infant after feeding are beneficial.

It is important to educate and reassure parents about positioning. In the past, recommendations encouraged upright positioning during sleeping for both infants and older children. The supine position for sleeping continues to be the recommended infant sleeping position. Parents should not place infants on their sides as an alternative to fully supine sleeping, and avoidance of soft bedding and soft objects in the bed is important. Rescheduling of the family's routine may be required to accommodate more frequent feeding times. If parents use thickened formula, they should also enlarge the nipple opening for easier sucking. Usually breastfeeding may continue, and the mother may provide more frequent feeding times or express the milk for thickening with rice cereal. Parents should avoid feeding the child spicy foods or any foods that they find aggravate symptoms in general and should avoid caffeine, chocolate, tobacco smoke, and alcohol when breastfeeding. Other practical advice includes advising the parents to avoid vigorous play after feedings and to avoid feeding just before bedtime.

When regurgitation is severe and growth is a problem, continuous NG tube feedings may decrease the amount of emesis and provide constant buffering of gastric acid. Special preparation of caregivers is required when this type of nutritional therapy is indicated.

The nurse can support the family by providing information about all aspects of treatment. Parents often require specific information about the medications given for GER. PPIs are most effective when administered 30 minutes before breakfast so that the peak plasma concentrations occur with mealtimes. If they are given twice a day, the second best time for administration is 30 minutes before the evening meal. Parents need to be reassured because it takes several days of administration to achieve a steady state of acid suppression. They may not see the results that they expect right away. A number of formulations available in PPIs allow for more efficient administration. Some preparations are available in dissolvable pills. There are powder and granule preparations as well. Many pharmacies will compound the medication in a liquid form for administration.

Postoperative nursing care after the Nissen fundoplication is similar to that for other types of abdominal surgery. (See Chapter 22.) Gastric decompression by an NG tube or gastrostomy must be maintained to avoid distention in the immediate postoperative period. Usually the NG tube should not be replaced by the nurse if it is accidentally removed because of the risk of injury to the operative site. When postoperative ileus resolves, the NG tube is removed or the gastrostomy tube is elevated in preparation for feeding. If bolus feedings are initiated through the gastrostomy, the tube may need to remain vented for several days or longer to avoid gastric distention from swallowed air. Edema surrounding the surgical site and a tight gastric wrap may prohibit the infant from expelling air through the esophagus. Some infants benefit from clamping of the tube for increasingly longer intervals until they are able to tolerate continuous clamping between feedings. During this time, if the infant displays increasing irritability and evidence of cramping, some relief may be provided by venting the tube.

Preparation for Home Care. If medical management is prescribed or surgery is performed, nursing responsibilities include educating caregivers about administering drugs at home, special feeding regimens or formula preparation, gastrostomy care, and postoperative care. (See Chapter 22.) After surgery, reflux is completely controlled in most cases, with these children attaining normal health and growth. If a gastrostomy tube is inserted during surgery, it may be removed after several months unless nutritional supplementation is needed. In severe cases of bloating or dumping syndrome, continuous tube feedings may be better tolerated. Caregivers should be aware of potential postoperative problems, such as difficulty vomiting, bloating symptoms, or discomfort with large solid-food meals, and seek guidance from their health care provider as needed.

IRRITABLE BOWEL SYNDROME

Irritable bowel syndrome (IBS) is classified as a functional GI disorder. IBS occurs more frequently in adolescents than children, 22% to 35% versus 6% to 14%, respectively (Giannetti, Maglione, Sciorio, et al., 2017). Children with IBS often have alternating diarrhea and constipation, flatulence, bloating or a feeling of abdominal distention, lower abdominal pain, a feeling of urgency when needing to defecate, and a feeling of incomplete evacuation of the bowel. Abdominal pain should be present for at least 4 days per month over the last 2 months plus either a change in frequency or appearance of stool (Chopra, Patel, Basude, et al., 2017). IBS has been identified as a cause of recurrent abdominal pain in 68% of children (Giannetti, Maglione, Sciorio, et al., 2017).

The cause of IBS is not clear, but it is believed to involve a combination of genetic and environmental factors. Strong predictors for the development of IBS in a child include having a mother, father, or twin with IBS (Kridler & Kamat, 2016). In addition, children with IBS have been noted to be less confident in their ability to deal with daily stress and have higher prevalence of anxiety, depression, introverted personalities, and difficulty sleeping (Kridler & Kamat, 2016). The intestinal microbiome is the focus of IBS research to evaluate whether inflammation may trigger nerves in the gut to cause IBS symptoms (Chopra, Patel, Basude, et al., 2017; Kridler & Kamat, 2016).

Children with IBS are evaluated to rule out organic causes for their symptoms, such as inflammatory bowel disease (IBD), lactose intolerance, and parasitic infections. A comprehensive history is obtained, including features and triggers of the symptoms, as well as associated symptoms such as headaches, recent infections, diet history, family history, and social history. Typically there are no abnormal physical findings on examination. Many children with symptoms appear active and healthy and have normal growth.

Therapeutic Management

There is no cure for IBS, so management involves controlling the child's symptoms. The long-range goal of treatment is development of regular bowel habits and relief of symptoms. Management depends on whether IBS is constipation or diarrhea predominant. Constipation-predominant IBS is managed by increasing fiber with diet changes and supplements, whereas diarrhea-predominant IBS is managed with diet changes, PPIs, and loperamide (Chopra, Patel, Basude, et al., 2017; Kridler & Kamat, 2016). A recent Cochrane systematic review found evidence suggesting that probiotics are effective in relieving recurrent abdominal pain (Newlove-Delgado, Martin, Abbott, et al., 2017).

Psychosocial interventions including cognitive-behavioral therapy and hypnotherapy can decrease abdominal pain in children (Abbott, Martin, Newlove-Delgado, et al., 2017; Chopra, Patel, Basude, et al., 2017). Cognitive-behavioral therapy provides stress management and coping skills that may lessen IBS symptoms.

Nursing Care Management

The primary nursing goal is family support and education. The disorder is stressful to children and parents. The nurse can help by providing support and reassurance that, although the symptoms are difficult to deal with, the disorder is not generally a threat to the child's health (see Community and Home Health Considerations box).

COMMUNITY AND HOME HEALTH CONSIDERATIONS

Irritable Bowel Syndrome

Parents, school nurses, and teachers frequently interact with children and adolescents who complain of abdominal pain. Complaints of abdominal pain can lead to interruption of activities and absence from school. Those caring for children should be aware of this symptom complex and become skilled in the identification of its manifestations. If the student has other worrisome features, such as weight loss, rectal bleeding, or significant fatigue, further diagnostic evaluation may be necessary. However, many students with uncomplicated abdominal pain and irritable bowel syndrome benefit from reassurance, diet counseling, and stress management. Parents, school nurses, and teachers should also remember that helping adolescents learn to cope with life events may influence their anxiety and depression and ultimately reduce the symptoms of abdominal pain and irritable bowel syndrome.

INFLAMMATORY CONDITIONS

ACUTE APPENDICITIS

Appendicitis, inflammation of the **vermiform appendix** (blind sac at the end of the cecum), is the most common cause of emergency abdominal surgery in childhood. In the United States 100,000 cases are diagnosed each year (Aiken & Oldham, 2016a). The peak incidence of appendicitis is between 12 and 18 years, with boys affected slightly more often than girls (Aiken & Oldham, 2016a). Classically, the first symptom of appendicitis is periumbilical pain, followed by nausea, right lower quadrant pain, and, later, vomiting with fever (Rentea, Peter, & Snyder, 2017). Perforation occurs in up to 82% of children under 5 years of age, likely due to an inability to verbalize their symptoms (Aiken & Oldham, 2016a). Perforation of the appendix can occur within approximately 48 hours of the initial complaint of pain (Aiken & Oldham, 2016a). Complications from appendiceal perforation include major abscess, phlegmon, enterocutaneous fistula, peritonitis, and partial bowel obstruction. A **phlegmon** is an acute suppurative inflammation of subcutaneous connective tissue that spreads.

Etiology

The cause of appendicitis is obstruction of the lumen of the appendix, usually by hardened fecal material (fecalith). Swollen lymphoid tissue, frequently occurring after a viral infection, can also obstruct the appendix. Another rare cause of obstruction is a parasite such as *Enterobius vermicularis,* or pinworms, which can obstruct the appendiceal lumen.

Pathophysiology

With acute obstruction, the outflow of mucus secretions is blocked and pressure builds within the lumen, resulting in compression of blood vessels. The resulting ischemia is followed by ulceration of the epithelial lining and bacterial invasion. Subsequent necrosis causes perforation or rupture with fecal and bacterial contamination of the peritoneal cavity. The resulting inflammation spreads rapidly throughout the abdomen (**peritonitis**), especially in young children, who are unable to localize infection. Progressive peritoneal inflammation results in functional intestinal obstruction of the small bowel (**ileus**) because intense GI reflexes severely inhibit bowel motility. Because the peritoneum represents a major portion of total body surface, the loss of extracellular fluid to the peritoneal cavity leads to electrolyte imbalance and hypovolemic shock.

BOX 25.12 Clinical Manifestations of Appendicitis

- Right lower quadrant abdominal pain
- Fever
- Rigid abdomen
- Decreased or absent bowel sounds
- Vomiting (typically follows onset of pain)
- Constipation or diarrhea
- Anorexia
- Tachycardia
- Rapid, shallow breathing
- Pallor
- Lethargy
- Irritability
- Stooped posture

Clinical Manifestations. The first symptom of appendicitis is usually colicky, cramping, abdominal pain located around the umbilicus (Box 25.12). **Referred pain** is the term used for this vague periumbilical localization. The midgut shares the same T10 dermatome, so pain is often perceived to be coming from this area. Generally, this pain progresses and becomes constant. The most important physical finding is focal abdominal tenderness. As the inflammation progresses to involve the serosa of the appendix and the peritoneum of the abdominal wall, the pain may shift to the right lower quadrant. The **McBurney point**, located two-thirds the distance along a line between the umbilicus and the anterosuperior iliac spine, is the most common point of tenderness. Localized peritoneal signs may occur with gentle percussion or maneuvers such as heel strike or shaking the bed. Other helpful findings are Rovsing sign, tenderness in the right lower quadrant that occurs during palpation or percussion of other abdominal quadrants; obturator sign, pain with flexion and internal rotation of the right hip; psoas sign, pain with left side with right hip extension; and Dunphy sign, pain with coughing (Rentea, Peter, & Snyder, 2017). Rebound tenderness—pain on deep palpation with sudden release—may be present, but it is not a finding specific to appendicitis (Aiken & Oldham, 2016a). Nausea, vomiting, and anorexia typically occur after the pain starts. Diarrhea, as well as other common signs of childhood illness such as upper respiratory tract congestion, poor feeding, lethargy, or irritability, may accompany appendicitis.

The child may not be able to walk well and may complain of pain in the right hip caused by inflammation in the psoas or iliopsoas muscles. Low-grade fever (38°C [100.4°F]) may occur with the initial presentation; however, the absence of fever does not exclude appendicitis. Because of the great variability in the presentation and location of appendicitis, any child with focal tenderness, regardless of the location, should be considered to potentially have acute appendicitis (see Community and Home Health Considerations box).

Diagnostic Evaluation

Diagnosis is not always straightforward. Fever, vomiting, abdominal pain, and an elevated white blood cell count are associated with appendicitis but are also seen in IBD, pelvic inflammatory disease, gastroenteritis, urinary tract infection, right lower lobe pneumonia, mesenteric adenitis, Meckel diverticulum, and intussusception. Prolonged symptoms and delayed diagnosis often occur in younger children, in whom the risk of perforation is greatest because of their inability to verbalize their complaints.

COMMUNITY AND HOME HEALTH CONSIDERATIONS

Acute Appendicitis

Abdominal pain is a common complaint among school-age children, but in some cases it may indicate acute appendicitis. School nurses and nurse practitioners in school-based clinics should become familiar with the "typical" pattern of symptoms in acute appendicitis and how to assess and evaluate an acute abdomen. School nurses also need to impress on teachers and coaches the importance of early referral to the health suite for further assessment. Early referral to the health suite and an alert school nurse or nurse practitioner may make the difference between an uncomplicated appendectomy and a delayed diagnosis of a perforated appendix with peritonitis.

NURSING ALERT

Signs of peritonitis in addition to fever usually include sudden relief from pain after perforation; subsequent increase in pain, which is usually diffuse and accompanied by rigid guarding of the abdomen; progressive abdominal distention; tachycardia; rapid, shallow breathing as the child refrains from using abdominal muscles; pallor; chills; irritability; and restlessness.

The diagnosis is based primarily on the history and physical examination (see Box 25.12). Pain, the cardinal feature, is initially generalized (usually periumbilical). However, it usually descends to the lower right quadrant. The most intense site of pain may be at the McBurney point. Rebound tenderness is not a reliable sign and is extremely painful to the child. Referred pain, elicited by light percussion around the perimeter of the abdomen, indicates peritoneal irritation. Movement, such as riding over bumps in an automobile or gurney, aggravates the pain. In addition to pain, significant clinical manifestations include fever, a change in behavior, anorexia, and vomiting.

Laboratory studies usually include a complete blood count (CBC); urinalysis (to rule out a urinary tract infection); and, in adolescent females, serum human chorionic gonadotropin (to rule out an ectopic pregnancy). A white blood cell count greater than 10,000/mm^3 and an elevated C-reactive protein (CRP) are common but are not necessarily specific for appendicitis. An elevated percentage of bands (often referred to as "a left shift") may indicate an inflammatory process. CRP is an acute-phase reactant that rises within 12 hours of the onset of infection.

Ultrasound is the imaging technique of choice in diagnosing appendicitis, although a computed tomography (CT) scan may be used. Ultrasound is considered positive in the presence of enlarged appendiceal diameter; appendiceal wall thickening; and periappendiceal inflammatory changes, including fat streaks, phlegmon, fluid collection, and extraluminal gas (Aiken & Oldham, 2016a). The accuracy of imaging for diagnosing appendicitis is 95% (Rentea, Peter, & Snyder, 2017).

Therapeutic Management

The treatment for appendicitis before perforation is surgical removal of the appendix (appendectomy). Usually antibiotics are administered preoperatively. IV fluids and electrolytes are often required before surgery, especially if the child is dehydrated as a result of the marked anorexia characteristic of appendicitis.

The operation is usually performed through a right lower quadrant incision (open appendectomy). Laparoscopic surgery is commonly used to treat nonperforated acute appendicitis in pediatric patients. Three cannulas are inserted in the abdomen: one in the umbilicus, one in the left lower abdominal quadrant, and one in the suprapubic area. A small telescope is inserted through the left lower quadrant cannula, and an endoscopic stapler is inserted through the umbilical cannula. The appendix is ligated with the stapler and removed through the umbilical cannula. Advantages of laparoscopic appendectomy include reduced time in surgery and under anesthesia and reduced risk of postoperative wound infection (Aiken & Oldham, 2016b).

Ruptured Appendix. Management of the child diagnosed with peritonitis caused by a ruptured appendix often begins preoperatively with IV administration of fluid and electrolytes, systemic antibiotics, and NG suction. Postoperative management includes IV fluids, continued administration of antibiotics, and NG suction for abdominal decompression until intestinal activity returns. Sometimes surgeons close the wound after irrigation of the peritoneal cavity. Other times, they leave the wound open (delayed closure) to prevent wound infection.

The treatment of a localized perforation with an appendiceal abscess is controversial. Some surgeons prefer to treat these children with antibiotics and IV fluids and allow the abscess to drain spontaneously. An elective appendectomy is then performed 2 to 3 months later.

Prognosis. Complications are uncommon after a simple appendectomy, and recovery is usually rapid and complete. The mortality rate from perforating appendicitis has improved from nearly certain death a century ago to less than 1% at the present time (Rentea, Peter, & Snyder, 2017). Complications, however, including wound infection and intraabdominal abscess, are not uncommon. Early recognition of the illness is important to prevent complications.

! NURSING ALERT

In any instance in which severe abdominal pain is observed, the nurse must be aware of the danger of administering laxatives or enemas. Such measures stimulate bowel motility and increase the risk of perforation.

Nursing Care Management

Because successful treatment of appendicitis is based on prompt recognition of the disorder, an important nursing objective is to assist in establishing a diagnosis. Because abdominal pain is a common childhood complaint, the nurse needs to make some preliminary assessment of the severity of the pain. (See Chapter 5.) One of the most reliable estimates is the degree of change in behavior. A child who stays home from school and voluntarily lies down or refuses to play is much more likely to have considerable pain than a child who is absent from school but plays contentedly at home. Younger, nonverbal children will assume a rigid, side-lying position with the knees flexed and have decreased range of motion of the right hip.

For nurses involved in primary ambulatory care, the responsibility of recognizing a possible case of appendicitis and prompt medical or surgical referral is particularly important. The importance of a detailed history and thorough abdominal examination cannot be overemphasized. Palpating the abdomen should be delayed until all other assessments have been made. Instruct the child to point with one finger to the site of the abdominal pain. Rebound tenderness may be present but is not always a sufficiently reliable test in children. Light palpation will satisfactorily elicit pain without causing excessive trauma (see Atraumatic Care box). Ask the child with mild pain to lift the heels and drop them to the floor two or three times, to hop on one foot, or to "puff out" or "pull in" the abdomen to check for tenderness without more painful probing. Chapter 4 discusses other techniques for assessment of the abdomen.

ATRAUMATIC CARE

Palpating the Abdomen for Abdominal Pain

Because children associate the stethoscope with listening, use the bell piece for initial palpation of the abdomen for tenderness. Children usually endure pressure from the stethoscope that they would not tolerate from a probing hand. Follow with manual palpation, using a gentle touch without lifting the hand from the abdomen while observing the child's face for signs of discomfort, such as a grimace and watchful eyes on the examination of the abdomen.

Physical preparation of the child with appendicitis is similar to that for any child undergoing surgery. (See Chapter 22.) In situations in which medical treatment is required to correct problems associated with peritonitis, the nurse must anticipate procedures and set up equipment as quickly as possible to avoid any delay in preparing the child for surgery. Psychologic preparation of the child and parents is similar to that used in other emergency situations. (See Chapter 22.)

Postoperative care for the nonperforated appendix is the same as for most abdominal operations. Care of the child with a ruptured appendix and peritonitis is more complex. The child may need to remain in the hospital for several days or may be discharged with home care services to provide IV antibiotics and dressing changes.

Postoperatively the child is maintained on IV fluids and antibiotics and is allowed nothing by mouth (NPO). The child also remains on low, intermittent gastric decompression until there is evidence of return of intestinal motility. Listening for bowel sounds and observing for other signs of bowel activity (such as passage of stool) are part of the routine assessment.

A drain may be placed in the wound during surgery, and frequent dressing changes with meticulous skin care are essential to prevent excoriation of the surgery area. If the wound is left open, moist dressings (usually saline-soaked gauze) and wound irrigations with antibacterial solution are used to provide an optimum healing environment.

Pain management is an essential part of the child's care. Not only is the incision painful, but the repeated dressing changes and irrigations also cause considerable distress. Because pain is continuous during the first few postoperative days, analgesics are given regularly to control pain. Procedures are performed when the analgesics are at peak effect. (See Chapter 5.)

Psychosocial care after surgery is also important. Sudden, acute illnesses cause unique stress because there is little time for preparation or planning. Parents and older children need an opportunity to express their feelings and concerns regarding the events surrounding the illness and hospitalization. The nurse can provide important education and psychosocial support to promote adequate coping, with alleviation of anxiety for both the child and the family (see Nursing Care Plan box).

MECKEL DIVERTICULUM

Meckel diverticulum is a remnant of the fetal omphalomesenteric duct, which connects the yolk sac with the primitive midgut during fetal life (Kennedy & Liacouras, 2016a). Normally the structure is obliterated between the fifth and seventh week of gestation, when the placenta replaces the yolk sac as the source of nutrition for the fetus. Failure of obliteration may result in an omphalomesenteric fistula (a fibrous band connecting the small intestine to the umbilicus), umbilical cyst, vitelline duct remnant, mesodiverticular bands, and Meckel diverticula (Bagade & Khanna, 2015).

Meckel diverticulum is a true diverticulum because it arises from the antimesenteric border of the small intestine and includes all layers

NURSING CARE PLAN

The Child With Appendicitis

Case Study

Lisa is a 10-year-old girl who has a 2-day history of generalized periumbilical pain and anorexia. Today she developed a fever and vomiting, so her parents took her to her pediatrician. On examination, Lisa was febrile with abdominal pain midway between the anterior superior iliac crest and umbilicus. The pain intensifies with any activity or deep breathing. Blood work was performed and a complete blood count (CBC) with differential shows a white blood cell (WBC) count of 21,000/mm^3, 79% bands, 14% lymphocytes, 6% eosinophils, and a normal hemoglobin and platelet count. With Lisa's history and physical findings, she was referred to a local emergency department.

Assessment

Based on Lisa's history, what are the most important signs and symptoms that you need to be aware of?

Appendicitis Defining Characteristics

History of abdominal pain for 2 days that started around the umbilicus and has now progressed to the lower right abdomen (McBurney point)

Fever

Anorexia

Nausea and vomiting

Elevated WBC count (>10,000/mm^3) along with a high percentage of bands (left shift)

Elevated C-reactive protein (CRP)

Nursing Interventions

What are the most appropriate nursing interventions for a child with appendicitis?

Nursing Interventions	Rationale
Close monitoring of the patient's status. Follow clinical and laboratory findings. Blood studies included CBC, CRP, and electrolytes.	To identify infection, signs of inflammation, changes in fluid and electrolyte status which require additional treatment
Close monitoring of diagnostic evaluation studies (i.e., computed tomography [CT] scan and/or ultrasound).	To confirm diagnosis of appendicitis
Administer intravenous (IV) fluids.	To correct fluid deficit and electrolyte imbalances
Administer analgesics as ordered.	To reduce pain
Administer antiemetics as ordered.	To reduce nausea and alleviate vomiting
Monitor temperature and vital signs.	To observe for signs of infection
Administer antipyretic medication as indicated.	To reduce fever
Administer antibiotics as ordered.	To treat infection
Maintain nothing-by-mouth (NPO) status.	To keep stomach empty in anticipation of possible surgery
Identify patient and family stressors that may accompany a diagnosis of appendicitis.	Providing financial and emotion support for family can help decrease some of the stressors associated with this condition
Review disease, medication, dietary restrictions.	Understanding the medical condition and therapies allows family to make informed decisions about care

Expected Outcomes

Lisa will exhibit decreased pain.

Lisa will exhibit no evidence of nausea or vomiting.

The temperature will remain within normal limits.

Sufficient fluid and electrolytes are maintained.

Patient/family indicate understanding of appendicitis and treatment.

Case Study (Continued)

Results of the CT scan demonstrate a ruptured appendix. Lisa is now being prepared for surgery. The nurse performing the assessment finds Lisa's temperature to be elevated. Lisa reports the pain had initially resolved but she now reports increasing pain (rated 9 out of 10) and nausea.

Assessment

What concerns you most based on the scenario?

Lisa's appendix has ruptured and the recurrence of pain and fever is likely related to an infection or possible abscess.

What immediate steps should be taken to further evaluate Lisa's status?

Check CBC and differential.

Document temperature and vital signs (pulse, respirations, blood pressure).

Assess and document location and rating of pain.

Administer antipyretic agent, analgesic, antiemetic, and IV fluids.

The following laboratory results have returned from Lisa's blood work:

CBC: WBC 24,000/mm^3, bands 81%, lymphocytes 12%, eosinophils 5%, normal hemoglobin, and normal platelets

Electrolytes and kidney function: potassium 3.4, sodium 135, blood urea nitrogen (BUN) 25, serum creatinine 1.2

Nursing Interventions

What are the most appropriate nursing interventions for Lisa before and after surgery?

Nursing Interventions	Rationale
Administer antibiotics as ordered. IV antibiotics are given for a minimum of 3 days postoperatively in children with complicated appendicitis then transitioned to oral antibiotics at discharge.	To treat infection
Administer analgesics as ordered.	To reduce pain
Administer antiemetics as ordered.	To reduce nausea and alleviate vomiting
Monitor temperature and vital signs.	To observe for signs of infection and shock
Administer IV fluids and monitor electrolytes.	To correct fluid deficit and electrolyte imbalances
Follow laboratory findings. Blood studies including CBC, CRP, and intraoperative cultures if obtained.	To identify infection, and signs of inflammation
Advance diet as tolerated postoperatively.	To maintain nutritional status

Expected Outcome

Lisa will exhibit no signs of infection.

Pain is controlled initially with IV analgesics then transitioned to oral analgesics.

Continued

NURSING CARE PLAN—CONT'D

The Child With Appendicitis

Lisa will exhibit no evidence of nausea or vomiting and tolerate a regular diet.
The temperature is within normal limits.
Sufficient fluid and electrolytes are maintained.

Case Study (Continued)

Lisa's parents are anxious and upset with the urgent need for surgery and hospitalization. You are concerned that they do not understand what is happening to their daughter.

Assessment

What are the most important aspects of Lisa's care to discuss with her parents at this time?

Family's Knowledge of Illness-Defining Characteristics

Understands definition of appendicitis and ruptured appendix
Describes rationale for urgent surgery
Describes rationale for subsequent hospitalization and need for IV antibiotics
Expresses fears and concerns
Shows appropriate reactions to child's illness

Nursing Interventions

What are the most appropriate nursing interventions for this diagnosis?

Nursing Interventions	Rationale
Review disease and treatment before surgery.	Understanding the medical condition and therapies allow families to make informed decisions about care
Review disease and treatment after surgery.	To increase knowledge and compliance with treatment plan to control pain, treat infection, maintain adequate fluid and electrolyte balance, and maximize nutrition
Arrange for social worker to meet with family to assess emotional and financial needs.	To identify and modify stressors associated with urgent and prolonged hospitalization
As child nears discharge, arrange for discussions with parents to discuss home care.	Family must be aware of necessary treatment and monitoring to be compliant with care

Expected Outcome

Parents indicate understanding of appendicitis and treatment.
Parents verbalize understanding the signs and symptoms of infection and understand the actions to treat infection.
Parents verbalize understanding of the plan for managing postsurgical treatment at home.

of the intestinal wall. Meckel diverticulum is often referred to by the "rule of 2s" because it occurs in 2% of the population, has a 2:1 male-to-female ratio, is located within 2 feet of the ileocecal valve, is commonly 2 cm in diameter and 2 inches in length, contains 2 types of ectopic tissue (pancreatic and gastric), and is more common before age 2 (Kennedy & Liacouras, 2016a).

Pathophysiology

Bleeding, obstruction, or inflammation causes the symptomatic complications of Meckel diverticulum (Lin, Huang, Bao, et al., 2017). Bleeding, which is the most common problem in children, is caused by peptic ulceration or perforation because of the unbuffered acidic secretion. Several mechanisms may cause obstruction such as intussusception or entanglement of the small intestine.

Clinical Manifestations

Signs and symptoms are based on the specific pathologic process, such as inflammation, bleeding, or intestinal obstruction (Box 25.13). The most common clinical presentation is rectal bleeding caused by ulceration at the junction of the ectopic gastric mucosa and normal ileal mucosa. The bleeding is usually painless and may be dramatic and occur as bright red or currant jelly–like stools, or it may occur intermittently and appear as tarry stools. The bleeding may be significant enough to cause hypotension. Volvulus and intussusception are common obstructive mechanisms in children with Meckel diverticulum, and these children present with symptoms of abdominal pain, distention, nausea, and vomiting (Kennedy & Liacouras, 2016a).

BOX 25.13 Clinical Manifestations of Meckel Diverticulum

Abdominal Pain

Similar to appendicitis
May be vague and recurrent

Bloody Stools*

Painless
Bright or dark red with mucus (currant jelly–like stool)
In infants, bleeding sometimes accompanied by pain

Occasional

Severe anemia
Shock

*Often a presenting sign.

Diagnostic Evaluation

Diagnosis is usually based on the history, physical examination, and radiographic studies. Meckel diverticulum is often a diagnostic challenge. A technetium-99 pertechnetate scan (Meckel scan) is the most effective diagnostic testing, especially for a bleeding diverticulum, with sensitivity ranging from 80% to 90% and a specificity of 95% (Lin, Huang, Bao, et al., 2017). Laboratory studies such as a CBC and a basic metabolic panel are usually part of the general workup to rule out any bleeding disorder and to evaluate for dehydration.

Therapeutic Management

The standard treatment for symptomatic Meckel diverticulum is surgical removal. In instances in which severe hemorrhage increases the surgical risk, medical intervention to correct hypovolemic shock (e.g., blood replacement, IV fluids, and oxygen) may be necessary. Antibiotics may be used preoperatively to control infection. If intestinal obstruction has occurred, appropriate preoperative measures are used to correct fluid and electrolyte imbalances and prevent abdominal distention.

Prognosis. If symptomatic Meckel diverticulum is diagnosed and treated early, full recovery is likely. Because of the potential for surgical complications, resection of asymptomatic Meckel diverticulum remains controversial.

Nursing Care Management

Nursing objectives are the same as for any child undergoing surgery. (See Chapter 22.) When intestinal bleeding is present, specific preoperative considerations include frequent monitoring of vital signs and blood pressure, keeping the child on bed rest, and recording the approximate amount of blood lost in stools.

Postoperatively the child requires IV fluids and an NG tube for decompression and evacuation of gastric secretions. Because the onset of illness is usually rapid, psychologic support is important, as in other acute conditions, such as appendicitis. It is important to remember that massive rectal bleeding is usually traumatic to both the child and the parents and may significantly affect their emotional reaction to hospitalization and surgery.

INFLAMMATORY BOWEL DISEASE

Inflammatory bowel disease (IBD) should not be confused with IBS. *IBD* is a term used to refer to three major forms of chronic intestinal inflammation: Crohn disease (CD), ulcerative colitis (UC), and inflammatory bowel disease unspecified (IBDU). CD and UC have similar epidemiologic, immunologic, and clinical features, but they are distinct disorders. The diagnosis of IBDU is used for patients with colonic disease, but their features are not specific to UC or CD; it is very rare (Conrad & Rosh, 2017).

Approximately 70,000 children in the United States have IBD (Rosen, Dhawan, & Saeed, 2017). Over the past 30 years the incidence of CD has risen, whereas the incidence of UC in children has remained stable (Grossman & Baldassano, 2016). Both CD and UC tend to be more aggressive if the onset occurs in childhood (Conrad & Rosh, 2017). Exacerbations and remissions without complete resolution of symptoms are also characteristics of IBD.

Etiology

Despite decades of research, the etiology of IBD is not completely understood, and there is no known cure. There is evidence to indicate a multifactorial etiology. Genetic, environmental, and microbial factors are associated with IBD, and research focuses on genetic associations and theories of defective immunoregulation of the inflammatory response to bacteria or viruses in the GI tract (Rosen, Dhawan, & Saeed, 2017). Genome-wide studies have confirmed at least 150 genes that increase the risk for IBD in individuals (Rosen, Dhawan, & Saeed, 2017). Furthermore, children who immigrate from developing countries to Western countries show an incidence of IBD similar to that of Western populations, confirming an environmental factor with the disease (Rosen, Dhawan, & Saeed, 2017). Finally, most individuals have 10 trillion bacteria and fungi in their intestinal microbiome, but children and adults with IBD have small diversity of intestinal bacterial species with an overrepresentation and underrepresentation of some species (Rosen, Dhawan, & Saeed, 2017).

Pathophysiology. The inflammation found with UC is limited to the colon and rectum, with the distal colon and rectum the most severely affected. Inflammation affects the mucosa and submucosa and involves continuous segments along the length of the bowel with varying degrees of ulceration, bleeding, and edema. Thickening of the bowel wall and fibrosis are unusual, but long-standing disease can result in shortening of the colon and strictures. Toxic megacolon is the most dangerous form of severe colitis.

The chronic inflammatory process of CD involves any part of the GI tract from the mouth to the anus but most often affects the terminal ileum. The disease involves all layers of the bowel wall (transmural) in a discontinuous fashion, meaning that between areas of intact mucosa, there are areas of affected mucosa (skip lesions). The inflammation may result in ulcerations; fibrosis; adhesions; stiffening of the bowel wall; stricture formation; and fistulas to other loops of bowel, bladder, vagina, or skin.

Clinical Signs and Symptoms

Children with UC may experience mild, moderate, or severe symptoms, depending on the extent of mucosal inflammation and systemic symptoms. UC often manifests with the insidious onset of diarrhea, possibly with hematochezia, and usually without fever or weight loss. The course of the disease may remain mild with intermittent exacerbations. Some children and adolescents are seen with grossly bloody diarrhea, cramps, urgency with defecation, mild anemia, fever, anorexia, weight loss, and moderate signs of systemic illness. Severe UC is characterized by frequent bloody stools, abdominal pain, significant anemia, fever, and weight loss. Extraintestinal manifestations are not common in UC. Enlarged lymph nodes (lymphadenopathy), arthritis, and the skin lesions of erythema nodosum may be present.

Common presenting manifestations of CD include diarrhea, abdominal pain with cramps, fever, and weight loss. Extraintestinal manifestations, including aphthous ulcers, peripheral arthritis, erythema nodosum, digital clubbing, renal stones, and gallstones, are more common with CD than UC (Grossman & Baldassano, 2016). Growth failure and delayed sexual maturation are often present for several years before overt GI symptoms are present (Conrad & Rosh, 2017). Both malabsorption and anorexia are factors that contribute to the growth problems that are prevalent in CD. Children with CD may have perianal disease, including tags, fissures, fistulas, or abscesses (Rosen, Dhawan, & Saeed, 2017). The effects of UC and CD are listed in Fig. 25.4. Table 25.6 provides a comparison of UC and CD.

Diagnostic Evaluation

The diagnosis of UC and CD comes from the history, physical examination, laboratory evaluation, and other diagnostic procedures. Laboratory tests include a CBC to evaluate anemia and an erythrocyte sedimentation rate (ESR) or CRP to assess the systemic reaction to the inflammatory process. The ESR or CRP may be elevated, indicating a systemic response to an inflammatory process. Levels of total protein, albumin, iron, zinc, magnesium, vitamin B_{12}, and fat-soluble vitamins may be low in children with CD. Stools are examined for blood, leukocytes, and infectious organisms. A serologic panel is often used in combination with clinical findings to diagnose IBD and to differentiate between CD and UC.

In patients with CD, an upper GI series with small bowel follow-through assists in assessing the existence, location, and extent of disease. Upper endoscopy and colonoscopy with biopsies are an integral part of diagnosing IBD (Rosen, Dhawan, & Saeed, 2017). Endoscopy allows direct visualization of the surface of the GI tract so that the extent of inflammation and narrowing can be evaluated. CT and ultrasound also may be used to identify bowel wall inflammation, intraabdominal abscesses, and fistulas. Colonoscopy can confirm the diagnosis and evaluate the extent of the disease. Discrete ulcers are commonly seen in patients with CD, whereas microulcers and diffuse abnormalities and inflammation are seen in patients with UC (Grossman & Baldassano, 2016). CD lesions may pierce the walls of the small intestine and colon, creating tracts called *fistulas* between the intestine and adjacent structures such as the bladder, anus, vagina, or skin.

Therapeutic Management

The natural history of the disease continues to be unpredictable and characterized by recurrent flare-ups that can severely impair patients' physical and social functioning (Grossman & Baldassano, 2016). The goals of therapy are to control the inflammatory process to reduce or

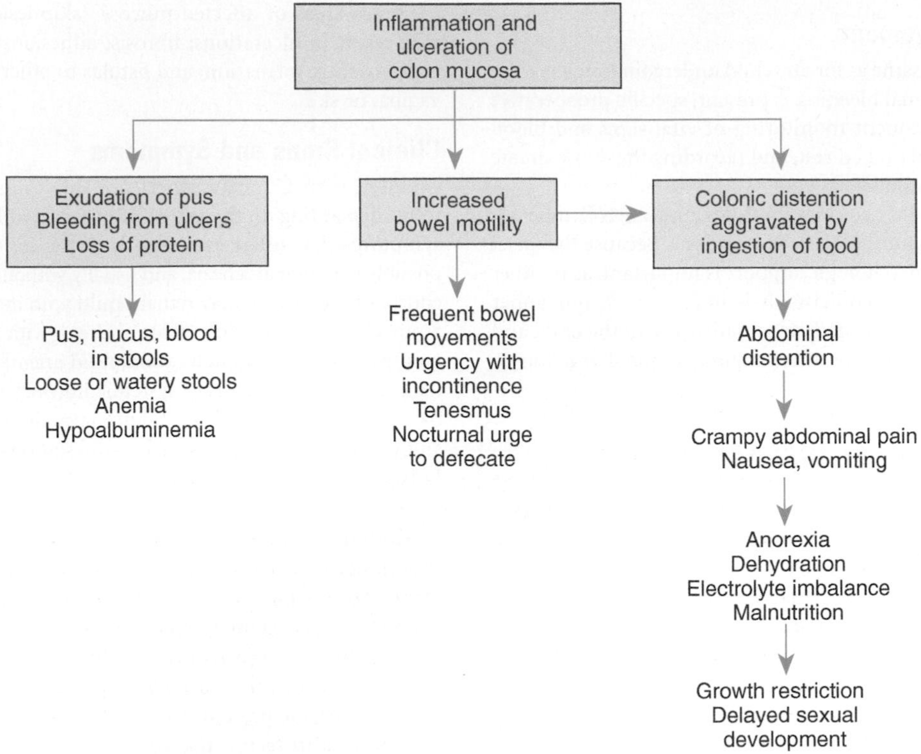

FIG. 25.4 Effects of ulcerative colitis or Crohn disease.

TABLE 25.6 Clinical Manifestations of Inflammatory Bowel Diseases

Characteristics	Ulcerative Colitis	Crohn Disease
Rectal bleeding	Common	Uncommon
Diarrhea	Often severe	Moderate to severe
Pain	Less frequent	Common
Anorexia	Mild or moderate	May be severe
Weight loss	Moderate	May be severe
Growth retardation	Usually mild	May be severe
Anal and perianal lesions	Rare	Common
Fistulas and strictures	Rare	Common
Rashes	Mild	Mild
Joint pain	Mild to moderate	Mild to moderate

eliminate the symptoms, obtain long-term remission, promote normal growth and development, and allow as normal a lifestyle as possible. Treatment is individualized and managed according to the type and the severity of the disease, its location, and the response to therapy. CD is more disabling, has more serious complications, and is often less amenable to medical and surgical treatment than is UC. Because UC is confined to the colon, a colectomy may cure UC.

Medical Treatment. The goal of any treatment regimen is first to induce remission of acute symptoms and then to maintain remission over time. 5-Aminosalicylates (5-ASAs) are effective in the induction and maintenance of remission in mild to moderate UC. Mesalamine, olsalazine, and balsalazide are preferred over sulfasalazine because of reduced side effects (e.g., headache, nausea, vomiting, neutropenia, and oligospermia). Suppository and enema preparations of mesalamine are used to treat left-sided colitis. These drugs decrease inflammation by inhibiting prostaglandin synthesis. 5-ASAs can be used to induce remission in mild CD.

Corticosteroids, such as prednisone and prednisolone, are indicated in induction therapy in children with moderate to severe UC and CD. These drugs inhibit the production of adhesion molecules, cytokines, and leukotrienes. Although these drugs reduce the acute symptoms of IBD, they are not commonly used for maintenance therapy because of their long-term side effects including growth suppression (adrenal suppression), weight gain, and decreased bone density (Rosen, Dhawan, & Saeed, 2017). High doses of IV corticosteroids may be administered in acute episodes and tapered according to clinical response. Budesonide, a synthetic corticosteroid, is designed for controlled release in the ileum and is indicated for ileal and right-sided colitis; budesonide has fewer side effects than prednisone and prednisolone but is also less effective (Rosen, Dhawan, & Saeed, 2017).

Immunomodulators, such as azathioprine and its metabolite 6-mercaptopurine (6-MP), are used to induce and maintain remission in children with IBD who are steroid resistant or steroid dependent and in treating chronic draining fistulas. They block the synthesis of purine, thus inhibiting the ability of deoxyribonucleic acid (DNA) and ribonucleic acid (RNA) to hinder lymphocyte function, especially that of T cells. Side effects include infection, pancreatitis, hepatitis, bone marrow toxicity, arthralgia, and malignancy. Methotrexate is also useful in inducing and maintaining remission in CD patients who are unresponsive to standard therapies. Cyclosporine and tacrolimus have both been effective in inducing remission in severe steroid-dependent UC. 6-MP or azathioprine is then used to maintain remission. Patients on immunomodulating medications require regular monitoring of their CBC and differential to assess for changes that reflect suppression of the immune system because many of the side effects can be prevented or managed by dose reduction or discontinuation of medication.

Antibiotics, such as metronidazole and ciprofloxacin, may be used as an adjunctive therapy to treat complications such as perianal disease or small bowel bacterial overgrowth in CD. Side effects of these drugs are peripheral neuropathy, nausea, and a metallic taste.

Biologic therapies act to regulate inflammatory and anti-inflammatory cytokines. The use of anti–tumor necrosis factor-α (TNF-α) agents such as infliximab and adalimumab decrease active inflammation and are effective in healing the intestinal mucosal lining and perianal fistulas, and have even improved linear growth in children (Grossman & Baldassano, 2016; Rosen, Dhawan, & Saeed, 2017). These agents are now being used as front-line therapy in children with CD with severe deep mucosal ulcerations, perianal fistulas, or growth failure (Rosen, Dhawan, & Saeed, 2017).

Nutritional Support. Nutritional support is important in the treatment of IBD. Growth failure is a common serious complication, especially in CD. Growth failure is characterized by weight loss, alteration in body composition, retarded height, and delayed sexual maturation. Malnutrition causes the growth failure, and its etiology is multifactorial. Malnutrition occurs as a result of inadequate dietary intake, excessive GI losses, malabsorption, drug-nutrient interaction, and increased nutritional requirements. Inadequate dietary intake occurs with anorexia and episodes of increased disease activity. Excessive loss of nutrients (e.g., protein, blood, electrolytes, and minerals) occur secondary to intestinal inflammation and diarrhea. Carbohydrate, lactose, fat, vitamin, and mineral malabsorption, as well as vitamin B_{12} and folic acid deficiencies, occur with disease episodes and with drug administration and when the terminal ileum is resected. Finally, nutritional requirements are increased with inflammation, fever, fistulas, and periods of rapid growth (e.g., adolescence).

The goals of nutritional support include correction of nutrient deficits and replacement of ongoing losses, provision of adequate energy and protein for healing, and provision of adequate nutrients to promote normal growth. Nutritional support includes both enteral and parenteral nutrition. A well-balanced, high-protein, high-calorie diet is recommended for children whose symptoms do not prohibit an adequate oral intake. There is little evidence that avoiding specific foods influences the severity of the disease. Supplementation with multivitamins, iron, and folic acid is recommended.

Special enteral formulas, given either by mouth or continuous NG infusion (often at night), may be required. Elemental formulas are completely absorbed in the small intestine with almost no residue. A diet consisting only of elemental formula not only improves nutritional status but also induces disease remission, either without steroids or with a diminished dosage of steroids required. An elemental diet is a safe and potentially effective primary therapy for patients with CD. Unfortunately, remission is not sustained when NG feedings are discontinued unless maintenance medications are added to the treatment regimen.

Total parenteral nutrition (TPN) has also improved nutritional status in patients with IBD. Short-term remissions have been achieved after TPN, although complete bowel rest has not reduced inflammation or added to the benefits of improved nutrition by TPN. Nutritional support is less likely to induce a remission in UC than in CD. Improvement of nutritional status is important, however, in preventing deterioration of the patient's health status and in preparing the patient for surgery.

Surgical Treatment. Surgery is indicated for UC when medical and nutritional therapies fail to prevent complications. Surgical options include a subtotal colectomy and ileostomy that leaves a rectal stump as a blind pouch. A reservoir pouch is created in the configuration of a J or an S to help improve continence postoperatively. An ileoanal pull-through preserves the normal pathway for defecation. Pouchitis, an inflammation of the surgically created pouch, is the most common late complication of this procedure. In many cases UC can be cured with a total colectomy.

Surgery may be required in children with CD when complications cannot be controlled by medical and nutritional therapy. Segmental intestinal resections are performed for small bowel obstructions, strictures, or fistulas. Diversion of the fecal stream, such as a colostomy, allows the colon to be less active and causes the disease to become dormant but on reconnection of the colon, disease often reoccurs (Grossman & Baldassano, 2016).

Prognosis. IBD is a chronic disease. Relatively long periods of quiescent disease may follow exacerbations. The outcome is influenced by the regions and severity of involvement, as well as by appropriate therapeutic management. Malnutrition, growth failure, and bleeding are serious complications. The overall prognosis for UC is good.

The development of colorectal cancer (CRC) is a long-term complication of IBD. Because the risk for CRC occurs 8 to 10 years after diagnosis, surveillance colonoscopy with multiple biopsies should begin approximately 7 to 10 years after diagnosis of UC or CD (Rosen, Dhawan, & Saeed, 2017). In CD, surgical removal of the affected colon does not prevent cancer from developing elsewhere in the GI tract.

Nursing Care Management

The nursing considerations in the management of IBD extend beyond the immediate period of hospitalization. These interventions involve continued guidance of families in terms of (1) managing diet; (2) coping with factors that increase stress and emotional lability; (3) adjusting to a disease of remissions and exacerbations; and (4) when indicated, preparing the child and parents for the possibility of diversionary bowel surgery. (See Quality Patient Outcomes box.)

QUALITY PATIENT OUTCOMES

Inflammatory Bowel Disease

- Remission without symptoms of abdominal pain, bloating, diarrhea, and rectal bleeding
- Optimum quality of life maintained by minimizing impairment of daily activities

Because nutritional support is an essential part of therapy, encouraging the anorexic child to consume sufficient quantities of food is often a challenge. Successful interventions include involving the child in meal planning; encouraging small, frequent meals or snacks rather than three large meals a day; serving meals around medication schedules when diarrhea, mouth pain, and intestinal spasm are controlled; and preparing high-protein, high-calorie foods such as eggnog, milkshakes, cream soups, puddings, or custard (if lactose is tolerated). (See Feeding the Sick Child, Chapter 22.) Using bran or a high-fiber diet for active IBD is questionable. Bran, even in small amounts, has been shown to worsen the patient's condition. Occasionally the occurrence of aphthous stomatitis further complicates adherence to dietary management. Mouth care before eating and the selection of bland foods help relieve the discomfort of mouth sores.

When NG feedings or TPN is indicated, nurses play an important role in explaining the purpose and the expected outcomes of this therapy. The nurse should acknowledge the anxieties of the child and family members and give them adequate time to demonstrate the skills necessary to continue the therapy at home, if needed (see Critical Thinking Case Study box).

The importance of continued drug therapy despite remission of symptoms must be stressed to the child and family members. Failure to adhere to the pharmacologic regimen can result in exacerbation of the disease. (See Compliance, Chapter 22.) Unfortunately, exacerbation of IBD can occur even if the child and family are compliant with the treatment regimen; this is difficult for the child and family to cope with.

CRITICAL THINKING CASE STUDY

Inflammatory Bowel Disease

Susan, a 13-year-old girl, was admitted to the hospital because of bloody diarrhea, abdominal pain, and weight loss. After a thorough evaluation, including laboratory tests, radiographic studies, and gastrointestinal endoscopy procedures, the diagnosis of Crohn disease (CD) was made. Medical treatment, including corticosteroid drugs and nutritional support, was implemented during this hospitalization.

Susan has improved considerably and is to be discharged home this week. Enteral formula administered by continuous nighttime nasogastric (NG) tube infusion will be continued at home, and both Susan and her family are eager to learn how to perform these feedings. You are the nurse responsible for Susan's discharge planning. Which interventions relating to these feedings should you include in Susan's preparations for discharge?

1. Evidence—Are there sufficient data to formulate any specific interventions for discharge?
2. Assumptions—Describe some underlying assumptions about the following:
   a. The goals of nutritional support for children with CD
   b. Teaching required by an adolescent or family member who is administering NG tube feedings at home
   c. Psychosocial issues related to CD
3. What are the priorities for discharge planning at this time?
4. Does the evidence support your conclusion?

Answers are available at http://evolve.elsevier.com/wong/ncic.

Emotional Support. The nurse should attend to the emotional components of the disease and assess any sources of stress. Frequently, the nurse can help children adjust to problems of growth retardation, delayed sexual maturation, dietary restrictions, feelings of being "different" or "sickly," inability to compete with peers, and necessary absence from school during exacerbations of the illness.

If a permanent colectomy-ileostomy is required, the nurse can teach the child and family how to care for the ileostomy. The nurse can also emphasize the positive aspects of the surgery, particularly accelerated growth and sexual development, permanent recovery, and the normality of life despite bowel diversion. Introducing the child and parents to other ostomy patients, especially those who are the same age, is effective in fostering eventual acceptance. Whenever possible, offer continent ostomies as options to the child, although they are not performed in all centers in the United States.

Because of the chronic and often lifelong nature of the disease, families benefit from the educational services provided by organizations such as the Crohn's and Colitis Foundation of America (CCFA).* If diversionary bowel surgery is indicated, United Ostomy Associations of America† and the Wound, Ostomy and Continence Nurses Society‡ are available to assist with ileostomy care and provide important psychologic support through their self-help groups. Adolescents often benefit by participating in peer-support groups, which are sponsored by the CCFA.

*386 Park Ave. S., 17th Floor, New York, NY 10016; 800-932-2423; http://www.ccfa.org. In Canada: Crohn's and Colitis Foundation of Canada, http://www.ccfc.ca.

†PO Box 512, Northfield, MN 55057-0512; 800-826-0826; http://www.ostomy.org. In Canada: United Ostomy Association of Canada, 344 Bloor St. W., Suite 501, Toronto, Ontario M5S 3A7; 1-888-969-9698; http://www.ostomycanada.ca.

‡15000 Commerce Pkwy., Suite C, Mt. Laurel, NJ 08054; 888-224-9626; http://www.wocn.org.

PEPTIC ULCER DISEASE

Peptic ulcer disease (PUD) is a chronic condition that affects the stomach or duodenum. Ulcers are described as gastric or duodenal and as primary or secondary. A **gastric ulcer** involves the mucosa of the stomach; a **duodenal ulcer** involves the pylorus or duodenum. Most **primary ulcers** are idiopathic or associated with *Helicobacter pylori* infection and tend to be chronic, occurring more frequently in the duodenum (Blanchard & Czinn, 2016). **Secondary ulcers** result from the stress of a severe underlying disease or injury (e.g., severe burns, sepsis, increased intracranial pressure, severe trauma, multisystem organ failure) and are more frequently gastric with an acute onset (Blanchard & Czinn, 2016).

Etiology

The exact cause of PUD is unknown, although infectious, genetic, and environmental factors are important. There is an increased familial incidence, likely due to *H. pylori*, which is known to cluster in families (Blanchard & Czinn, 2016). *H. pylori* is a microaerophilic, gram-negative, slow-growing, spiral-shaped, and flagellated bacterium known to colonize the gastric mucosa in about half of the population of the world (Blanchard & Czinn, 2016). *H. pylori* synthesizes the enzyme urease, which hydrolyses urea to form ammonia and carbon dioxide. Ammonia then absorbs acid to form ammonium, thus raising the gastric pH. *H. pylori* may cause ulcers by weakening the gastric mucosal barrier and allowing acid to damage the mucosa. It is believed that it is acquired via the fecal-oral route, and this hypothesis is supported by finding viable *H. pylori* in feces.

In addition to ulcerogenic drugs, both alcohol and smoking contribute to ulcer formation. There is no conclusive evidence to implicate particular foods, such as caffeine-containing beverages or spicy foods, but polyunsaturated fats and fiber may play a role in ulcer formation. Psychologic factors may play a role in the development of PUD, and stressful life events, dependency, passiveness, and hostility have all been implicated as contributing factors.

Pathophysiology

Most likely, the pathology is due to an imbalance between the destructive (cytotoxic) factors and defensive (cytoprotective) factors in the GI tract. The toxic mechanisms include acid, pepsin, medications such as aspirin and nonsteroidal antiinflammatory drugs (NSAIDs), bile acids, and infection with *H. pylori.* The defensive factors include the mucus layer, local bicarbonate secretion, epithelial cell renewal, and mucosal blood flow. Prostaglandins play a role in mucosal defense because they stimulate both mucus and alkali secretion. The primary mechanism that prevents the development of peptic ulcer is the secretion of mucus by the epithelial and mucus glands throughout the stomach. The thick mucus layer acts to diffuse acid from the lumen to the gastric mucosal surface, thus protecting the gastric epithelium. The stomach and the duodenum produce bicarbonate, decreasing acidity on the epithelial cells and thereby minimizing the effects of the low pH. When abnormalities in the protective barrier exist, the mucosa is vulnerable to damage by acid and pepsin. Exogenous factors, such as aspirin and NSAIDs, cause gastric ulcers by inhibition of prostaglandin synthesis.

Zollinger-Ellison syndrome is rare but may occur in children who have multiple, large, or recurrent ulcers. This syndrome is characterized by hypersecretion of gastric acid, intractable ulcer disease, and intestinal malabsorption caused by a gastrin-secreting tumor of the pancreas. The pathogenesis, manifestations, and complications of PUD are outlined in Fig. 25.5.

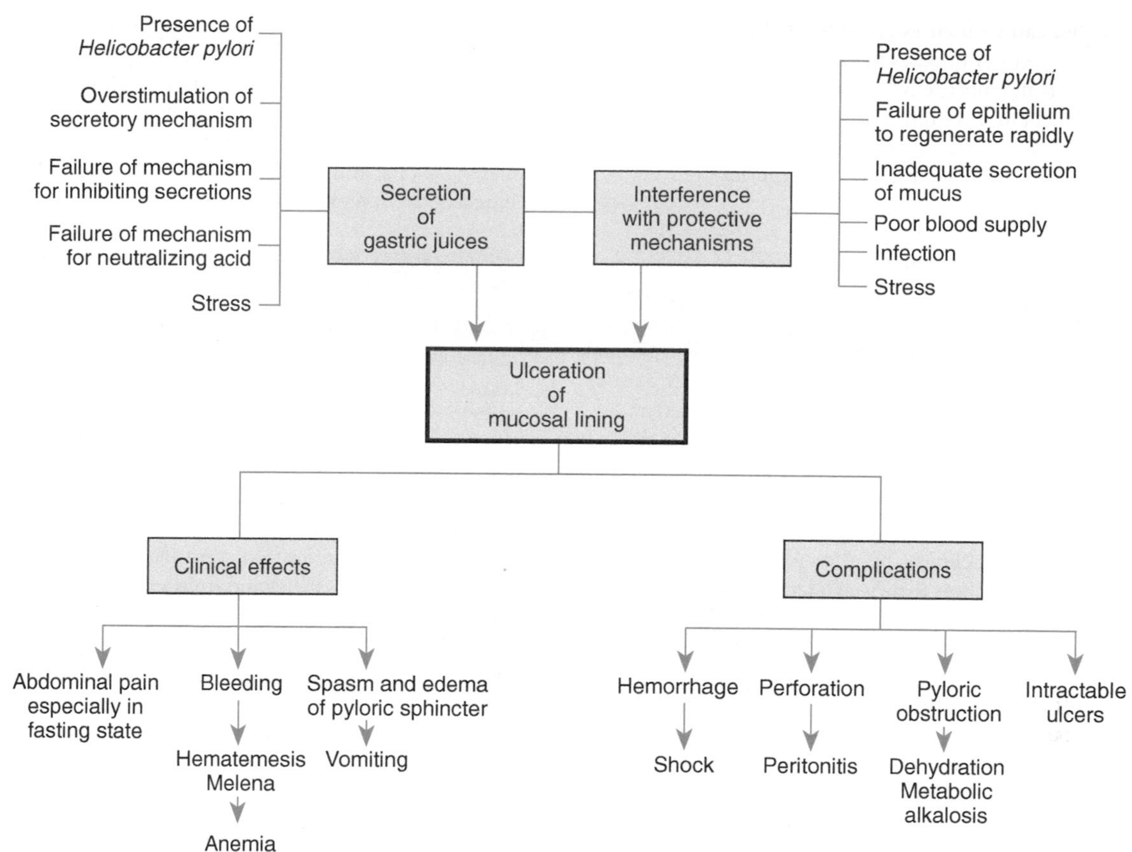

FIG. 25.5 Possible causes and effects of peptic ulcer.

Clinical Manifestations

The clinical manifestations of PUD vary according to the child's age and the ulcer's location. Common clinical manifestations include chronic abdominal pain, especially when the stomach is empty, such as during the night or early morning; recurrent vomiting; hematemesis; melena; chronic anemia; and abdominal tenderness (Box 25.14).

Diagnostic Evaluation

Diagnosis is based on the history of symptoms, physical examination, and diagnostic testing. The focus is on symptoms such as epigastric abdominal pain, nocturnal pain, oral regurgitation, heartburn, weight loss, hematemesis, and melena. History should include questions relating to the use of potentially causative substances such as NSAIDs, corticosteroids, alcohol, and tobacco. Frequently a history of epigastric and periumbilical pain accompanies PUD. However, children often find it difficult to describe the location of their pain and frequently indicate the location by moving their hand in a circular movement all around the stomach area. Asking the child to take one finger and point to the area where it hurts the most often helps identify the location of the pain. Pain may also be elicited during the examination with palpation.

Laboratory studies may include a CBC to detect anemia, stool analysis for occult blood, liver function tests (LFTs), ESR, or CRP to evaluate IBD; amylase and lipase to evaluate pancreatitis; and gastric acid measurements to identify hypersecretion. Stool analysis is performed to rule out infection. Polyclonal and monoclonal stool antigen tests are an accurate, noninvasive method both for the initial diagnosis of *H. pylori* and for the confirmation of its eradication after treatment (Yang, 2016). A C^{13} urea breath test measures bacterial colonization in

BOX 25.14 Characteristics of Peptic Ulcers

Neonates

Usually gastric and secondary ulcers

Commonly a history of prematurity, respiratory distress, sepsis, hypoglycemia, or an intraventricular hemorrhage

Perforation possibly leading to massive bleeding

Infants to 2-Year-Old Children

Most likely to have a secondary ulcer located equally in the stomach or duodenum

Primary ulcers less common and usually located in stomach

Likely to be noticed in relation to illness, surgery, or trauma

Hematemesis, melena, or perforation

2- to 6-Year-Old Children

Primary or secondary ulcers

Located equally in stomach and duodenum

Perforation more likely in secondary ulcers

Periumbilical pain, poor eating, vomiting, irritability, nighttime wakening, hematemesis, melena

Children Over 6 Years

Usually primary and most often duodenal ulcers

More typical of adult type

Chance of recurrence greater

Often associated with *Helicobacter pylori*

Epigastric pain or vague abdominal pain

Nighttime wakening, hematemesis, melena, and anemia possible the gastric mucosa and can be used as an additional noninvasive test to determine the presence of antibodies to *H. pylori.*

An upper GI series is the most reliable way to detect and diagnose PUD in children (Blanchard & Czinn, 2016). Direct visualization of the gastric and duodenal mucosa helps identify specific lesions, and biopsy specimens can determine the presence of *H. pylori.*

Therapeutic Management

The major goals of therapy for children with PUD are to relieve discomfort, promote healing, prevent complications, and prevent recurrence. Management is primarily medical and consists of administration of medications to treat the infection and to reduce or neutralize gastric acid secretion. Antacids are beneficial medications to neutralize gastric acid. Histamine (H_2) receptor antagonists (antisecretory drugs) act to suppress gastric acid production. These medications have few side effects. PPIs, such as omeprazole, lansoprazole, pantoprazole, and esomeprazole, act to inhibit the hydrogen ion pump in the parietal cells, thus blocking the production of acid. Although these drugs have not been well studied in children, they are used in clinical practice to treat ulcers, GER, esophagitis, and gastritis and appear to be well tolerated with infrequent side effects (e.g., headache, diarrhea, nausea) (Blanchard & Czinn, 2016).

Mucosal protective agents, such as sucralfate and bismuth-containing preparations, may be prescribed for PUD. Sucralfate is an aluminum-containing agent that forms a barrier over ulcerated mucosa to protect against acid and pepsin. Bismuth compounds are sometimes prescribed for the relief of ulcers, but they are used less frequently than PPIs. Although these compounds inhibit the growth of microorganisms, the mechanism of their activity is poorly understood. In combination with antibiotics, bismuth is effective against *H. pylori.* Although concern has been expressed about the use of bismuth salts in children because of potential side effects, none of these side effects has been reported when these compounds have been used in the treatment of *H. pylori* infection. These agents are available in both pill and liquid forms. Because they block the absorption of other medications, they should be given separately from other medications.

Triple-drug therapy is the standard first-line treatment regimen for *H. pylori* and has demonstrated 90% efficacy in the eradication of *H. pylori* (Kalach, Bontems, & Cadranel, 2015). Examples of drug combinations used in triple therapy are (1) bismuth, clarithromycin, and metronidazole; (2) lansoprazole, amoxicillin, and clarithromycin; and (3) metronidazole, clarithromycin, and omeprazole. Common side effects of medications include diarrhea, nausea, and vomiting.

In addition to medications, the child with PUD should have a nutritious diet and avoid caffeine. Warn adolescents about gastric irritation associated with alcohol use and smoking.

Children with an acute ulcer who have developed complications, such as massive hemorrhage, require emergency care. The administration of IV fluids, blood, or plasma depends on the amount of blood loss. Replacement with whole blood or packed cells may be necessary for significant loss.

Surgical intervention may be required for complications such as hemorrhage, perforation, or gastric outlet obstruction. Ligation of the source of bleeding or closure of a perforation is performed. A vagotomy and pyloroplasty may be indicated in children with bleeding ulcers despite aggressive medical treatment (Patel, Bommayya, Choudhry, et al., 2015).

Prognosis. The long-term prognosis for PUD is variable. Many ulcers are successfully treated with medical therapy; however, primary duodenal peptic ulcers often recur. Complications such as GI bleeding can occur and extend into adult life. The effect of maintenance drug therapy on long-term morbidity remains to be established with further studies.

Nursing Care Management

The primary nursing goal is to promote healing of the ulcer through compliance with the medication regimen. If an analgesic-antipyretic is needed, acetaminophen, not aspirin or NSAIDs, is used. Critically ill neonates, infants, and children in intensive care units should receive H_2 blockers to prevent stress ulcers.

DRUG ALERT

H_2 Blockers

Critically ill children receiving IV H_2 blockers should have their gastric pH values checked at frequent intervals.

For nonhospitalized children with chronic illnesses, consider the role stress plays. In children, many ulcers occur secondary to other conditions, and the nurse should be aware of family and environmental conditions that may aggravate or precipitate ulcers. Children may benefit from psychologic counseling and from learning how to cope constructively with stress.

OBSTRUCTIVE DISORDERS

Obstruction in the GI tract occurs when the passage of nutrients and secretions is impeded by a constricted or occluded lumen or when there is impaired motility (paralytic ileus). Obstructions may be congenital or acquired. Congenital obstructions, such as esophageal or intestinal atresias, imperforate anus, and meconium ileus, usually appear in the neonatal period. Other obstructions of congenital etiology (e.g., malrotation, HD, pyloric stenosis, volvulus, incarcerated hernia, and Meckel diverticulum) appear after the first few weeks of life. Intestinal obstruction from acquired causes such as intussusception and tumors may occur in infancy or childhood.

Acute intestinal obstruction is commonly characterized by abdominal pain, nausea, vomiting, abdominal distention, and a change in stooling patterns (Box 25.15). Pain is caused by intermittent muscular contractions proximal to the obstruction as the bowel attempts to move luminal contents along the normal path. It may also be due to

BOX 25.15 Clinical Manifestations of Mechanical (Paralytic) Intestinal Obstruction

Colicky abdominal pain—From peristalsis attempting to overcome the obstruction
Abdominal distention—As a result of accumulation of gas and fluid above the level of the obstruction
Vomiting—Often the earliest sign of a high obstruction; a later sign of lower obstruction (may be bilious or feculent)
Constipation and obstipation—Early signs of low obstructions; later signs of higher obstructions
Dehydration—From losses of large quantities of fluid and electrolytes into the intestine
Rigid and boardlike abdomen—From increased distention
Bowel sounds—Gradually diminish and cease
Respiratory distress—Occurs as the diaphragm is pushed up into the pleural cavity
Shock—Caused by plasma volume diminishing as fluids and electrolytes are lost from the bloodstream into the intestinal lumen
Sepsis—Caused by bacterial proliferation with invasion into the circulation

both water and electrolytes from extensive and prolonged vomiting. There are decreased serum levels of both sodium and potassium, although these may be masked by the hemoconcentration from extracellular fluid depletion. Of greater diagnostic value are a decrease in serum chloride levels and increases in pH and bicarbonate (carbon dioxide content), indicative of metabolic alkalosis. The blood urea nitrogen will be elevated as evidence of dehydration. However, in those cases diagnosed early, laboratory findings may not be significant.

Therapeutic Management

Surgical relief of the pyloric obstruction by pyloromyotomy is the standard therapy for this disorder. Preoperatively the infant must be rehydrated and metabolic alkalosis corrected with parenteral fluid and electrolyte administration. Replacement fluid therapy usually delays surgery for 24 to 48 hours. The stomach is decompressed with an NG tube if the infant continues with vomiting. In infants with no evidence of fluid and electrolyte imbalance, surgery is performed without delay.

The surgical procedure is often performed by laparoscope and consists of a longitudinal incision through the circular muscle fibers of the pylorus down to, but not including, the submucosa (**pyloromyotomy**, or the Fredet-Ramstedt operative procedure) (see Fig. 25.6, *B*). The procedure has a high success rate. Laparoscopic surgery may result in a shorter surgical time, more rapid postoperative feeding, and shorter hospital stay (Hunter & Liacouras, 2016).

Feedings are usually begun 4 to 6 hours postoperatively, beginning with small, frequent feedings of water or electrolyte solution. If clear fluids are retained, about 24 hours after surgery formula is started in the same small increments. The amount and the interval between feedings are gradually increased until a full feeding schedule is reinstated, which usually takes about 48 hours.

Prognosis. The prognosis for infants and small children with HPS is excellent when the diagnosis is confirmed early, and the mortality rate is low (0% to 0.5%). A small percentage of children with HPS will have GER.

Nursing Care Management

Nursing care involves primarily observation for clinical features that help establish the diagnosis, careful regulation of fluid therapy, and reestablishment of normal feeding patterns. Nurses must be alert to signs of HPS in infants and refer them for medical evaluation. HPS should be considered a possibility in the very young infant who appears alert but fails to gain weight and has a history of vomiting after feedings. Assessment is based on observation of eating behaviors and evidence of other characteristic clinical manifestations, hydration, and nutritional status.

Preoperatively, the emphasis is on restoring hydration and electrolyte balance. The infant is kept NPO and given IV fluids with glucose and electrolytes based on serum electrolyte values and clinical appearance. Careful monitoring of the IV fluids and strict monitoring of intake and output are important. Record accurate description of any vomiting and the number and character of stools.

Observations include assessment of vital signs, particularly those that indicate fluid or electrolyte imbalances. These infants are especially prone to metabolic alkalosis from loss of hydrogen ions and depletion of potassium, sodium, and chloride, all of which are contained in gastric secretions. Assess the skin and mucous membranes for alterations in hydration status. (See Chapter 23 for manifestations of fluid and electrolyte disturbances.)

If stomach decompression and gastric lavage are part of preoperative management, the nurse is responsible for ensuring that the NG tube is patent and functioning properly and for measuring and recording the type and amount of drainage. Encourage parents to visit and become involved in the child's care. Most parents need support and reassurance that the condition is caused by a structural problem and is not a reflection of their parenting skills and capacities.

Postoperative vomiting is common, and most infants, even with successful surgery, exhibit some vomiting during the first 24 to 48 hours. IV fluids are administered until the infant is taking and retaining adequate amounts by mouth. Much of the same care that was instituted before surgery is continued postoperatively, including observation of vital signs, monitoring of IV fluids, and careful monitoring of intake and output. In addition, the infant is observed for responses to the stress of surgery and for evidence of pain. Appropriate analgesics should be given around the clock because pain is continuous. The surgical incision(s) is inspected for drainage or erythema, and any signs of infection are reported to the surgeon. A surgical adhesive may be used for incision closure, and parents are instructed regarding the care of the incision and any dressings before discharge.

Feedings are usually instituted within 12 to 24 hours postoperatively, beginning with clear liquids. They are offered in small quantities at frequent intervals. If the infant has been breastfed, breast milk expressed by the mother may be given by bottle when the infant is able to tolerate feedings, or the mother is instructed to limit nursing time and gradually increase the time to previous patterns. Observation and recording of feedings and the infant's responses to feedings are a vital part of postoperative care. Care of the operative site consists of observation for any drainage or signs of inflammation and care of the incision.

INTUSSUSCEPTION

Intussusception is the most common cause of intestinal obstruction in children between 3 months and 6 years old (Carroll, Kavanagh, Ni Leidhin, et al., 2017). Intussusception is more common in males than in females and is more common in children younger than 2 years old. Although specific intestinal lesions occur in a small percentage of the children, generally the cause is not known. Only 12.5% to 25% of intussusception cases have a pathologic lead point, such as a polyp, lymphoma, or Meckel diverticulum (Carroll, Kavanagh, Ni Leidhin, et al., 2017). The idiopathic cases may be caused by hypertrophy of intestinal lymphoid tissue secondary to viral infection.

Pathophysiology

Intussusception occurs when a proximal segment of the bowel telescopes into a more distal segment, pulling the mesentery with it. The mesentery is compressed and angled, resulting in lymphatic and venous obstruction. As the edema from the obstruction increases, pressure within the area of intussusception increases. When the pressure equals the arterial pressure, arterial blood flow stops, resulting in ischemia and the pouring of mucus into the intestine. Venous engorgement also leads to leaking of blood and mucus into the intestinal lumen, forming the classic currant jelly–like stools. The most common site is the ileocecal valve (ileocolic), where the ileum invaginates into the cecum and then further into the colon (Fig. 25.7). Other forms include ileoileal (i.e., one part of the ileum invaginates into another section of the ileum) and colocolic (i.e., one part of the colon invaginates into another area of the colon) intussusceptions, usually in the area of the hepatic or splenic flexure or at some point along the transverse colon.

Clinical Manifestations

Intussusception usually manifests with the sudden onset of crampy abdominal pain, inconsolable crying, and a drawing up of the knees to the chest in an otherwise healthy child (Box 25.17). Between episodes the child appears normal. As the obstruction progresses, bilious vomiting severe abdominal distention, which results from accumulation of gas and fluid above the level of the obstruction. As abdominal distention progresses, the abdomen may become extremely tender, rigid, and firm.

When abdominal contents continue to accumulate, nausea and vomiting occur. Vomiting of gastric contents is often the first sign of a high obstruction, such as obstruction of the pylorus, and vomiting of bile-stained material is a sign of obstruction of the small intestine. Persistent vomiting can lead to dehydration and electrolyte disturbances. Constipation and obstipation (prolonged absence of defecation) are early signs of low obstructions and later signs of higher obstructions. In acute conditions such as intussusception, the clinical manifestations are apparent within a few hours of the onset of the disorder. In other conditions such as hypertrophic pyloric stenosis the signs and symptoms may have a more gradual onset. Bowel sounds may initially be hyperactive, then diminish or cease. Respiratory distress may occur when the diaphragm is pushed up into the pleural cavity as a result of severe abdominal distention.

HYPERTROPHIC PYLORIC STENOSIS

Hypertrophic pyloric stenosis (HPS) occurs when the circumferential muscle of the pyloric sphincter becomes thickened, resulting in elongation and narrowing of the pyloric canal. This produces an outlet obstruction and compensatory dilation, hypertrophy, and hyperperistalsis of the stomach. This condition usually develops in the first few weeks of life, causing nonbilious vomiting, which occurs after a feeding; projectile vomiting may develop and the infant is fussy and hungry after vomiting. If the condition is not diagnosed early, dehydration, metabolic alkalosis, and failure to thrive may occur. The precise etiology of HPS is not known. Boys are affected four to six times more frequently than girls (Hunter & Liacouras, 2016). It is more common in white infants and is seen less frequently in African American and Asian infants (Hunter & Liacouras, 2016).

Pathophysiology

The circular muscle of the pylorus thickens as a result of hypertrophy. This produces severe narrowing of the pyloric canal between the stomach and the duodenum. Consequently, the lumen at this point is partially obstructed. Over time, inflammation and edema further reduce the size of the opening, resulting in complete obstruction. The hypertrophied pylorus may be palpable as an olive-like mass in the upper abdomen (Fig. 25.6).

Pyloric stenosis is not a congenital disorder. It is believed that local innervation may be involved in the pathogenesis. In most cases, HPS is an isolated lesion; however, it may be associated with intestinal malrotation, esophageal and duodenal atresia, and anorectal anomalies.

Clinical Manifestations

Infants with HPS have nonbilious vomiting in the early stages (Box 25.16). Vomiting usually begins at 3 weeks of age but can start as early as 1 week and as late as 5 months. Vomiting usually occurs 30 to 60 minutes after feeding and becomes projectile as the obstruction progresses. Initially the infant is hungry and irritable, but prolonged vomiting may lead to dehydration, weight loss, and failure to thrive. Gastric peristalsis may be visible on examination, and the olive-shaped mass in the epigastrium just to the right of the umbilicus may be palpated (see Fig. 25.6, *A*). Indirect (unconjugated) hyperbilirubinemia may be present in a small percentage of affected infants; this usually resolves with surgical correction and is reported to occur as a result of a decreased level of glucuronyl transferase (see also Chapter 8).

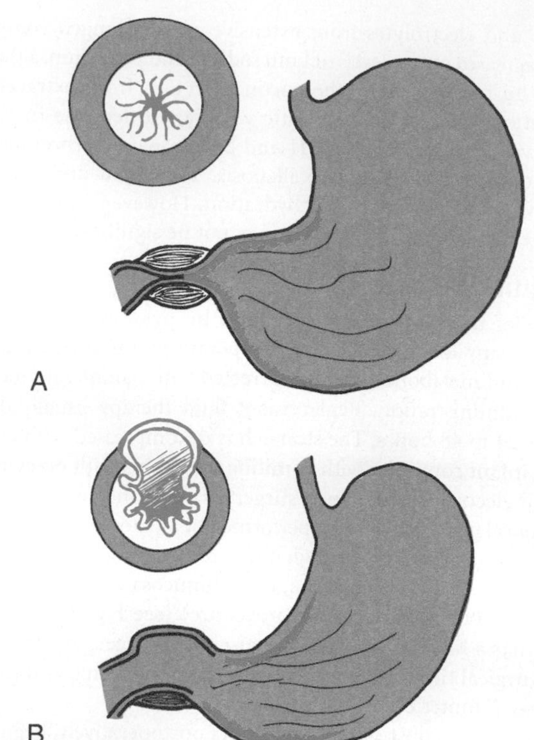

FIG. 25.6 Hypertrophic pyloric stenosis. **A,** Enlarged muscular tumor nearly obliterates pyloric canal. **B,** Longitudinal surgical division of muscle down to submucosa establishes adequate passageway.

BOX 25.16 Clinical Manifestations of Hypertrophic Pyloric Stenosis

Projectile vomiting
- May be ejected 3 to 4 feet from the child when in a side-lying position, 1 foot or more when in a back-lying position
- Usually occurs shortly after a feeding, but may not occur for several hours
- May follow each feeding or appear intermittently
- Nonbilious vomitus that may be blood tinged

Infant hungry, avid nurser; eagerly accepts a second feeding after vomiting episode
No evidence of pain or discomfort except that of chronic hunger
Poor weight gain
Signs of dehydration
Distended upper abdomen
Readily palpable olive-shaped tumor in the epigastrium just to the right of the umbilicus
Visible gastric peristaltic waves that move from left to right across the epigastrium

Diagnostic Evaluation

The diagnosis of HPS is often made after the history and physical examination. The olive-like mass is most easily palpated when the stomach is empty, the infant is quiet, and the abdominal muscles are relaxed. If the diagnosis is inconclusive from the history and physical examination, ultrasonography will demonstrate an elongated mass surrounding a long pyloric canal. If ultrasonography does not demonstrate a hypertrophied pylorus, upper GI radiography should be done to rule out other causes of vomiting.

If the condition is not diagnosed early, laboratory findings reflect the metabolic alterations created by moderate to severe depletion of

PATHOPHYSIOLOGY REVIEW

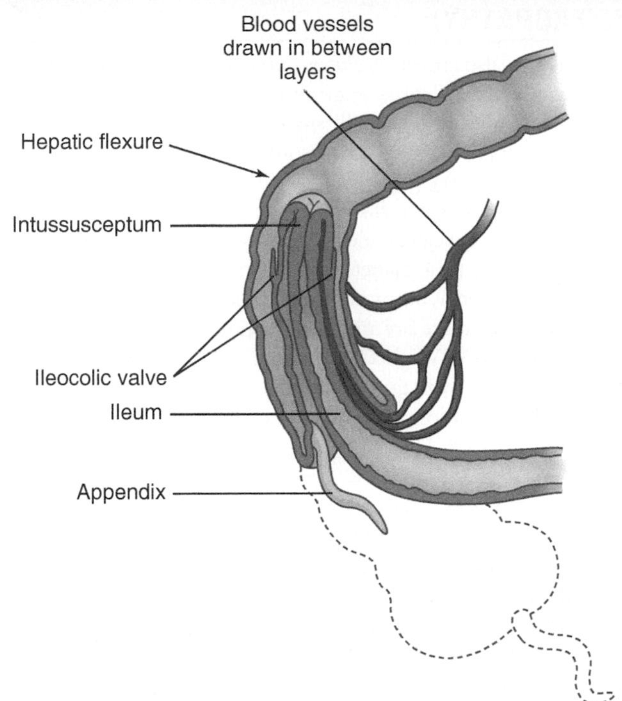

FIG. 25.7 Ileocecal valve (ileocolic) intussusception.

BOX 25.17 Clinical Manifestations of Intussusception

- Sudden acute abdominal pain
- Child screaming and drawing the knees onto the chest
- Child appearing normal and comfortable between episodes of pain
- Vomiting
- Lethargy
- Passage of red, currant jelly–like stools (stool mixed with blood and mucus)
- Tender, distended abdomen
- Palpable sausage-shaped mass in upper right quadrant
- Empty lower right quadrant (Dance sign)
- Eventual fever, prostration, and other signs of peritonitis

may occur and lethargy increases. The classic triad of intussusception symptoms (abdominal pain, abdominal mass, bloody stools) is present in less than 30% of children (Kennedy & Liacouras, 2016b). A more chronic case may be presented, characterized by diarrhea, anorexia, weight loss, occasional vomiting, and periodic pain. Because intussusception is potentially life threatening, be aware of such signs, and closely observe and refer these children for further medical evaluation. With atypical cases, lethargy may be the primary symptom. If the distal bowel remains distended, necrosis and perforation are possible.

Diagnostic Evaluation

Frequently, subjective findings lead to the diagnosis. However, definitive diagnosis is based on ultrasonography that reveals a characteristic heterogenous mass and a "bull's-eye." A rectal examination reveals mucus, blood, and occasionally a low intussusception itself.

Therapeutic Management

Conservative treatment consists of radiologist-guided pneumoenema (gas enema) or ultrasound-guided hydrostatic enema, the advantage of the latter being that no ionizing radiation is needed (Kennedy & Liacouras, 2016b). Recurrence of intussusception after conservative treatment is rare; however, this procedure should not be attempted with prolonged intussusception, signs of shock, peritoneal irritation, or intestinal perforation (Kennedy & Liacouras, 2016b).

IV fluids, NG decompression, and antibiotic therapy may be used before hydrostatic reduction is attempted. If these procedures are not successful, the child may require surgical intervention. Surgery involves manually reducing the invagination and, when indicated, resecting any nonviable intestine.

Prognosis. Nonoperative reduction is successful in the majority of stable cases. Gas enema is slightly more successful with reduction compared to a hydrostatic enema (83% versus 70%, respectively) (Carroll, Kavanagh, Ni Leidhin, et al., 2017). Surgery is required for patients in whom the reduction is unsuccessful or for patients who are unstable. With early diagnosis and treatment, serious complications and death are uncommon.

Nursing Care Management

The nurse can help establish a diagnosis by listening to the parent's description of the child's physical and behavioral symptoms. It is not unusual for parents to state that they thought something was seriously wrong before others shared their concerns. The description of the child's severe colicky abdominal pain combined with vomiting is a significant sign of intussusception.

As soon as a possible diagnosis of intussusception is made, the nurse prepares the parents for the immediate need for hospitalization, the nonsurgical technique of hydrostatic reduction, and the possibility of surgery. It is important to explain the basic defect of intussusception. The nurse can easily demonstrate this by creating a model of the defect. Use the example of a telescoping rod, or push the end of a finger on a rubber glove back into itself. Then demonstrate the principle of reduction by hydrostatic pressure by filling the glove with water, which pushes the "finger" into a fully extended position.

Physical care of the child does not differ from that for any child undergoing abdominal surgery. Even though nonsurgical intervention may be successful, the usual preoperative procedures, such as maintenance of NPO status, routine laboratory testing (CBC and urinalysis), signed parental consent, and preanesthetic sedation, are performed. Children with perforation will require IV fluids, systemic antibiotics, and bowel decompression before undergoing surgery. Fluid volume replacement and restoration of electrolytes may be required in such children before surgery. Before surgery the nurse monitors all stools.

! NURSING ALERT

Passage of a normal brown stool usually indicates that the intussusception has reduced itself. This is immediately reported to the practitioner, who may choose to alter the diagnostic and therapeutic care plan.

Postprocedural care includes observations of vital signs, blood pressure, intact sutures and dressing, and the return of bowel sounds. After spontaneous or hydrostatic reduction, the nurse observes for passage of water-soluble contrast material (if used) and the stool patterns because the intussusception may recur. Children may be admitted to the hospital or monitored on an outpatient basis. A recurrence of intussusception is treated with the conservative reduction techniques described previously, but a laparotomy is considered for multiple recurrences.

MALROTATION AND VOLVULUS

Malrotation of the intestine is caused by the abnormal rotation of the intestine around the superior mesenteric artery during embryologic development. Malrotation may manifest in utero or at any age, but the majority of patients (80%) present in the first month of life (Carroll, Kavanagh, Ni Leidhin, et al., 2017). Infants may have intermittent bilious vomiting, recurrent abdominal pain, distention, or lower GI bleeding. Malrotation is the most serious type of intestinal obstruction because if the intestine undergoes complete volvulus (i.e., the intestine twisting around itself), compromise of the blood supply will result in intestinal necrosis, peritonitis, perforation, and death.

Diagnostic Evaluation

It is imperative that malrotation and volvulus be diagnosed promptly and surgical treatment instituted quickly. In addition to a history and physical, a plain abdominal radiograph and lateral decubitus view are obtained; bowel distention will be present proximal to the distention on plain radiograph, and a lateral view will demonstrate air-fluid levels in the distended bowel (Bales & Liacouras, 2016). An upper GI series is the most accurate imaging study (Carroll, Kavanagh, Ni Leidhin, et al., 2017).

Therapeutic Management

Surgery is indicated to remove the affected area. Because of the extensive nature of some lesions, short-bowel syndrome (SBS) is a postoperative complication.

Nursing Care Management

Preoperatively the nursing care is the same as that provided to an infant or child with intestinal obstruction. IV fluids, NG decompression, and systemic antibiotics are implemented. In the rapidly deteriorating infant, fluid volume resuscitation and vasopressors may be required for preoperative stabilization. Postoperatively, the nursing care is similar to that provided to the infant or child who has undergone abdominal surgery.

MALABSORPTION SYNDROMES

Chronic diarrhea and malabsorption of nutrients characterize malabsorption syndromes. An important complication of malabsorption syndromes in children is failure to thrive. Most cases are classified according to the location of the supposed anatomic or biochemical defect. The term **celiac disease** is often used to describe a symptom complex with four characteristics: (1) steatorrhea (fatty, foul, frothy, bulky stools), (2) general malnutrition, (3) abdominal distention, and (4) secondary vitamin deficiencies.

Digestive defects are conditions in which the enzymes necessary for digestion are diminished or absent, such as (1) cystic fibrosis, in which pancreatic enzymes are absent; (2) biliary or liver disease, in which bile flow is affected; or (3) lactase deficiency, in which there is congenital or secondary lactose intolerance.

Absorptive defects are conditions in which the intestinal mucosal transport system is impaired. This may occur because of a primary defect (e.g., celiac disease) or secondary to inflammatory disease of the bowel that results in impaired absorption because bowel motility is accelerated (e.g., ulcerative colitis). Obstructive disorders (e.g., Hirschsprung disease) also cause secondary malabsorption from enterocolitis.

Anatomic defects, such as extensive resection of the bowel or SBS, affect digestion by decreasing the transit time of substances and affect absorption by severely compromising the absorptive surface.

CELIAC DISEASE (GLUTEN-SENSITIVE ENTEROPATHY)

Celiac disease, also known as *gluten-induced enteropathy, gluten-sensitive enteropathy,* and *celiac sprue,* is an autoimmune disorder triggered by the ingestion of gluten in genetically susceptible individuals (Fok, Holland, Gil-Zaragozano, et al., 2016). The disorder results in permanent intestinal intolerance to dietary gluten, a protein present in wheat, barley, and rye that causes damage to the villi in the small intestine. Children with unexplained iron deficiency anemia, recurrent aphthous stomatitis, dental enamel defects, type 1 diabetes, Down syndrome, selective immunoglobulin A deficiency, autoimmune thyroid disease, Turner syndrome, or Williams syndrome are more susceptible to being diagnosed with the disease (Paul, McVeigh, Gil-Zaragozano, et al., 2016). The disease is seen more frequently in Europe and the United States in approximately 1% of these populations, and it is rarely reported in Asians or African Americans (Branski, Troncone, & Fasano, 2016).

Pathophysiology

Celiac disease is characterized by villous atrophy in the small intestine in response to the protein gluten. When individuals are unable to digest the gliadin component of gluten, an accumulation of a toxic substance occurs that is damaging to the mucosal cells. Damage to the mucosa of the small intestine leads to villous atrophy, hyperplasia of the crypts, and infiltration of the epithelial cells with lymphocytes. Villous atrophy leads to malabsorption due to the reduced absorptive surface area (see Fig. 25.1).

Genetic predisposition is an essential factor in the development of celiac disease. Membrane receptors involved in preferential antigen presentation to $CD4^+$ T cells play a crucial role in the immune response characteristic of celiac disease. Children with genetic susceptibilities, namely *HLA-DQ2* or *HLA-DQ8,* are more susceptible to being diagnosed with celiac disease (Lebwohl, Sanders, & Green, 2017).

Clinical Manifestations

Symptoms of celiac disease appear when solid foods such as beans and pasta are introduced into the child's diet between the ages of 1 and 5 years (Box 25.18). There is usually an interval of several months between the introduction of gluten into the diet and the onset of symptoms. Intestinal symptoms are common in children diagnosed within the first 2 years of life. Other symptoms include failure to thrive, chronic diarrhea, abdominal distention and pain, muscle wasting, aphthous ulcers, and fatigue.

Diagnostic Evaluation

Gluten should not be excluded from the diet until the diagnostic evaluation is complete so proper identification can occur. The first step is a serologic blood test for tissue transglutaminase and antiendomyseal antibodies in children 18 months of age or older (Branski, Troncone, & Fasano, 2016). Positive serologic markers should be followed by an upper GI endoscopy with biopsy. The diagnosis of celiac disease is based on a biopsy of the small intestine demonstrating the characteristic changes of mucosal inflammation, crypt hyperplasia, and villous atrophy (Branski, Troncone, & Fasano, 2016).

Therapeutic Management

Treatment of celiac disease consists primarily of dietary management. Although a gluten-free diet is prescribed, it is actually low in gluten because it is impossible to remove every source of this protein. Because gluten is found primarily in wheat and rye, but also in smaller quantities in barley and oats, these four foods are eliminated. Corn, rice, and millet are substitute grain foods.

BOX 25.18 Clinical Manifestations of Celiac Disease

Impaired Fat Absorption
Steatorrhea (excessively large, pale, oily, frothy stools)
Exceedingly foul-smelling stools

Impaired Nutrient Absorption
Malnutrition
Muscle wasting (especially prominent in legs and buttocks)
Anemia
Anorexia
Abdominal distention

Behavioral Changes
Irritability
Uncooperativeness
Apathy

Celiac Crisis*
- Acute, severe episodes of profuse watery diarrhea and vomiting
- May be precipitated by
  - Infections (especially gastrointestinal)
  - Prolonged fluid and electrolyte depletion
  - Emotional disturbance

*In very young children.

Children with untreated celiac disease may have lactose intolerance, especially if their mucosal lesions are extensive. Lactose intolerance usually improves as the mucosa heals with gluten withdrawal. Specific nutritional deficiencies, such as iron, folic acid, and fat-soluble vitamin deficiencies, are treated with appropriate supplements.

Prognosis. Celiac disease is regarded as a chronic disease; its severity varies greatly among children. The most severe symptoms usually occur in early childhood and again in adult life. Most children who comply with dietary management are healthy and remain free of symptoms and complications; however, children should be evaluated annually for nutritional deficiencies, impaired growth, delayed puberty, and reduced bone mineral density (Fok, Holland, Gil-Zaragozano, et al., 2016).

Nursing Care Management

The main nursing consideration is helping the child adhere to the dietary regimen. Considerable time is involved in explaining the disease process to the child and parents, the specific role of gluten in aggravating the disorder, and those foods that must be restricted. It is difficult to maintain a diet indefinitely when the child has no symptoms and temporary transgressions result in no difficulties. However, the majority of individuals who relax their diet will experience a relapse of their disease.

Although the chief source of gluten is cereal and baked goods, grains are frequently added to processed foods as thickeners or fillers. To compound the difficulty, gluten is added to many foods as hydrolyzed vegetable protein, which is derived from cereal grains. The nurse must advise parents of the necessity of reading all label ingredients carefully to avoid hidden sources of gluten.

Many of children's favorite foods contain gluten, including bread, cake, cookies, crackers, donuts, pies, spaghetti, pizza, prepared soups, hot dogs, luncheon meats, and some prepared hamburgers. Many of these products can be eliminated from the infant's or young child's diet fairly easily, but monitoring the diet of the school-age child or adolescent is more difficult. Luncheon preparation away from home is particularly difficult because bread, luncheon meats, and instant soups are not allowed. For families on restricted food budgets, the diet adds an additional financial burden because many inexpensive or convenient foods cannot be used.

In addition to restricting gluten, other dietary alterations may be necessary. For example, in some children who have more severe mucosal damage, the digestion of disaccharides is impaired, especially in relation to lactose. Therefore these children often need a temporarily lactose-free diet, which necessitates eliminating all milk products. In general, dietary management includes a diet high in calories and proteins with simple carbohydrates such as fruits and vegetables, but low in fats. Because the bowel is inflamed as a result of the pathologic processes in absorption, the child must avoid high-fiber foods such as nuts, raisins, raw vegetables, and raw fruits with skin until inflammation has subsided.

It is important to stress long-range complications and to remind parents of the child's physical status before dietary treatment and the dramatic improvement after treatment. The nurse can be instrumental in allowing the child to express concerns and frustration while focusing on ways in which the child can still feel normal. Encourage the child and parents to find new recipes using suitable ingredients, such as Mexican or Chinese dishes that use corn or rice. Consult a registered dietitian to provide children and their families with detailed dietary instructions and education.

Several resources are available to assist children and parents in all aspects of coping with celiac disease. The National Celiac Association* provides support and guidance to families and supplies educational materials concerning a gluten-free diet, food sources, recipes, and travel information.

SHORT-BOWEL SYNDROME

Short-bowel syndrome (SBS) is a malabsorptive disorder that occurs as a result of decreased mucosal surface area, usually because of extensive resection of the small intestine. Malabsorption may be exacerbated by other factors, such as bacterial overgrowth and dysmotility. The most common congenital causes of SBS in children are short-bowel syndrome, multiple atresias, and gastroschisis; other causes resulting in bowel resection include necrotizing volvulus, meconium peritonitis, Crohn disease, and trauma (Vanderhoof & Branski, 2016).

The definition of SBS includes two important findings: (1) decreased intestinal surface area for absorption of fluid, electrolytes, and nutrients; and (2) a need for parenteral nutrition (PN) (Martin, Ladd, Werts, et al., 2017). The prognosis for infants with SBS has improved dramatically, but the mortality rate within 5 years after diagnosis remains at 27% to 37% (Martin, Ladd, Werts, et al., 2017).

Therapeutic Management

The goals of therapy for infants and children with SBS include (1) preserving as much length of bowel as possible during surgery; (2) maintaining optimum nutritional status, growth, and development while intestinal adaptation occurs; (3) stimulating intestinal adaptation with enteral feeding; and (4) minimizing complications related to the disease process and therapy (Vanderhoof & Branski, 2016).

Nutritional Support. Nutritional support is the long-term focus of care for children with SBS. The initial phase of therapy includes PN as

*PO Box 600066, Newton, MA 02460; 1-888-4CELIAC or 617-262-5422; http://www.nationalceliac.org. In Canada: Canadian Celiac Association, 5025 Orbitor Drive, Suite 400, Mississauga, Ontario, Canada, L4W 4Y5; 1-800-363-7296; http://www.celiac.ca.

the primary source of nutrition. The second phase is the introduction of enteral feeding, which usually begins as soon as possible after surgery. Elemental formulas containing glucose, sucrose and glucose polymers, hydrolyzed proteins, and medium-chain triglycerides facilitate absorption. Usually these formulas are given by continuous infusion through an NG or gastrostomy tube. As the enteral feedings are advanced, the PN solution is decreased in terms of calories, amount of fluid, and total hours of infusion per day. If enteral feedings are tolerated, oral feedings should be attempted to minimize oral aversion and preserve oral skills (Vanderhoof & Branski, 2016).

The final phase of nutritional support occurs when growth and development are sustained. When PN is discontinued, there is a risk of nutritional deficiency secondary to malabsorption of fat-soluble vitamins (A, D, E, and K) and trace minerals (iron, selenium, zinc). Serum vitamin and mineral levels should be monitored closely and supplemented enterally, if needed. Pharmacologic agents have been used to reduce secretory losses. H_2 blockers, PPIs, and octreotide inhibit gastric or pancreatic secretion. Cholestyramine is often prescribed to improve diarrhea that is associated with bile salt malabsorption.

Numerous complications are associated with SBS and long-term PN. Infectious, metabolic, and technical complications can occur. Sepsis can occur after improper care of the catheter. The GI tract can also be a source of microbial seeding of the catheter. Bowel atrophy may foster increased intestinal permeability of bacteria. A lack of adequate sites for central lines may become a significant problem for the child in need of long-term PN. Hepatic dysfunction and cholestasis may also occur (Cohran, Prozialeck, & Cole, 2017).

Bacterial overgrowth is likely to occur when the ileocecal valve is absent or when stasis exists as a result of a partial obstruction or a dilated segment of bowel with poor motility. Alternating cycles of broad-spectrum antibiotics are used to reduce bacterial overgrowth. This treatment may also decrease the risk of bacterial translocation and subsequent central venous catheter infections. A high-fat and low-carbohydrate diet may be helpful in reducing bacterial overgrowth (Vanderhoof & Branski, 2016). Other complications of bacterial overgrowth and malabsorption include metabolic acidosis and gastric hypersecretion.

Many surgical interventions, including intestinal valves, tapering enteroplasty or stricturoplasty, intestinal lengthening, and interposed segments, have been used to slow intestinal transit, reduce bacterial overgrowth, or increase mucosal surface area. Intestinal transplantation has been performed successfully in children. Children with a permanent dependence on PN or severe complications of long-term PN are candidates for transplantation.

Prognosis. The prognosis for infants with SBS has improved with advances in PN and with the understanding of the importance of intraluminal nutrition. Improved supportive care for the management of therapy-related problems and the development of more specific immunosuppressive medications for transplantation have all contributed to improved management. The prognosis depends in part on the length of the residual small intestine. An intact ileocecal valve also improves the prognosis. Infants and children with SBS die from PN-related problems, such as fulminant sepsis or severe PN cholestasis.

Nursing Care Management

The most important components of nursing care are administration and monitoring of nutritional therapy. During PN therapy, care must be taken to minimize the risk of complications related to the central venous access device (i.e., catheter infections, occlusions, dislodgment, or accidental removal). Care of the enteral feeding tubes and monitoring of enteral feeding tolerance are also important nursing responsibilities.

When hospitalization is prolonged, the child's developmental and emotional needs must be met. This often requires special planning to promote normal family adjustment and adaptation of the hospital routines. Family members require psychosocial support and education to cope successfully with SBS.

Many infants with SBS have an intestinal ostomy performed at the time of the initial bowel resection. Routine ostomy care is another important nursing responsibility. Because infants and children with SBS have chronic diarrhea, perineal skin irritation is often a problem after ostomy closure. Frequent diaper changes, gentle perineal cleansing, and protective skin ointments help prevent skin breakdown. (See Diaper Dermatitis, Chapter 32.)

Home Care. When long-term PN is required, preparation of the family for home care of the child is a major nursing responsibility. Preparation for home nutritional support begins as early as possible to prevent lengthy hospitalizations with subsequent problems such as developmental delays and family stresses. Many infants and children can be successfully cared for at home with enteral and parenteral nutrition if the family is thoroughly prepared and provided with adequate support services. Most families benefit from home nursing care to assist with and supervise therapy. Careful follow-up care by a multidisciplinary nutritional support service is essential. Most home health agencies now provide portable enteral and parenteral equipment, which enables the child and family to maintain a more normal and active lifestyle. The nurse plays an active and important role in the success of a home nutrition program. Home infusion companies provide portable equipment, which enables the child and family to maintain a more normal lifestyle.

GASTROINTESTINAL BLEEDING

GI bleeding in infants and children is an uncommon but potentially serious problem (Casciani, Nardo, Chin, et al., 2017). Most actual or apparent instances of GI bleeding cause great anxiety for the parents or caregivers. Blood may be vomited or passed per rectum, but the origin of the blood may not be the GI tract. In the newborn, swallowed maternal blood at the time of delivery may account for some episodes of apparent GI bleeding. A bleeding site on the nipple of a nursing mother may lead to heme-positive stools in the breastfed infant. Finally, blood can be swallowed during epistaxis and then passed as hematemesis or melena.

Once it has been established that the cause of bleeding is from a source in the GI tract, further investigation for the source and cause is undertaken. Upper GI bleeding is defined as bleeding from a site above the ligament of Treitz, which is attached to the duodenum at its junction with the jejunum. Lower GI bleeding comes from a source distal to the ligament of Treitz. Diagnostic studies such as endoscopy, scintigraphy, and angiography have improved the ability to localize the site of bleeding.

Etiology

The esophagus is a common site of upper GI bleeding. Esophagitis caused by GER may lead to chronic and often occult blood loss. Esophageal varices secondary to portal hypertension may cause massive bleeding. Peptic inflammation (gastritis and duodenitis) or ulceration is the most common cause of upper GI bleeding in children. Hemorrhagic gastritis may occur in the newborn infant after a difficult delivery or asphyxia. In this circumstance gastric perforation is a serious complication that requires emergent treatment. Less common causes of upper GI bleeding include bleeding disorders, vascular malformations, GI duplications, Mallory-Weiss syndrome (an esophageal tear caused by protracted vomiting), and hematobilia (bleeding into biliary passages).

In lower GI bleeding, small amounts of bright red blood in the stool of a healthy child may be due to an anal fissure. Colonic polyps are another cause of passage of bright red blood per rectum in toddlers and older children. Bleeding associated with diarrhea may indicate a serious problem. Enteric infections remain the leading cause, but the nurse should consider necrotizing enterocolitis, hemolytic uremic syndrome, IBD, and food allergy. Other causes are intussusception with the passage of blood per rectum (see earlier in this chapter) or Meckel diverticulum with the painless passage of currant jelly–like stools (see earlier in this chapter).

Pathophysiology

The GI tract has an extensive surface area and a rich vascular supply. Bleeding can occur anywhere along the GI tract from a vein, artery, or vascular malformation. In an otherwise healthy newborn infant, hemophilia or inherited coagulation-factor deficits are rarely accompanied by bleeding unless other conditions are superimposed. Children with liver disease may also have deficient coagulation factors because of poor synthesis and malabsorption of vitamin K, which is a risk factor for GI bleeding.

Portal hypertension may lead to GI bleeding because the formation of portosystemic shunts can result in dilated venous channels in vulnerable locations such as the esophagus and stomach. These dilated venous channels (varices) may bleed, causing severe GI hemorrhage.

Diagnostic Evaluation

The diagnosis of GI bleeding is often made on the basis of the history and physical examination. Hematemesis is the vomiting of bright red blood or denatured blood that looks like coffee grounds, usually representing an upper GI source of bleeding. Hematochezia is the passage of bright red blood per rectum, indicating lower GI bleeding. This blood may precede or follow a bowel movement or be mixed with or coat the stool. Bright red blood that coats the stool may be due to a hard bowel movement, hemorrhoids, or anal fissures. Blood mixed with stool indicates a bleeding source proximal to the rectum. Blood passed alone after a bowel movement is most likely due to bleeding in the perianal or rectal area, possibly caused by a polyp. Blood with mucus in the stool indicates an inflammatory or infectious condition, and currant jelly–like stools indicate vascular compromise, such as intussusception. Melena is the passage of black, tarry stools that contain denatured (digested) blood and suggests an upper GI source of bleeding. Occasionally, bright red blood may be passed per rectum from an upper GI source of bleeding when the bleeding is massive. It is important to test emesis or stool for occult blood to differentiate true bleeding from the ingestion of food containing food coloring. In older children, false-positive stool tests for occult blood can also occur with the ingestion of red meats and iron preparations.

Laboratory studies are determined on the basis of the history and physical examination. In many instances, a CBC with platelet quantification, prothrombin, partial thromboplastin, and coagulation studies will be done. Children who have acute illness, fever, and joint pain in addition to GI bleeding need an ESR and stool studies with culture to evaluate for enteric pathogens, ova and parasites, and *C. difficile*. When IBD is suspected, a metabolic panel to determine total protein and albumin may be added to a CBC, ESR, and LFTs. The child with massive painless rectal bleeding may require a nuclear medicine scan to rule out Meckel diverticulum. If there is evidence of portal hypertension or chronic liver disease, LFTs, liver imaging studies, and a liver biopsy may be necessary. A barium enema is performed if intussusception is suspected.

Imaging studies help differentiate among several suspected diagnoses. CT of the sinuses helps localize bleeding that is coming from the nasopharynx or sinuses. A chest radiograph may distinguish hemoptysis related to cystic fibrosis, bronchiectasis, or other chronic lung conditions from hematemesis. Angiography can be used to identify the source of bleeding and to allow embolization or vasopressin infusion for treatment. Endoscopy is the diagnostic method chosen when the source of bleeding is thought to be secondary to gastritis, esophagitis, PUD, colitis, or polyps. Endoscopic examinations also permit visualization of the intestinal mucosa and collection of biopsy specimens and cultures.

Therapeutic Management

Treatment of GI bleeding in children depends on its severity and cause. The first step in management of acute GI bleeding is to assess the magnitude of blood loss and restore the child's hemodynamic stability. Severe bleeding necessitates hospitalization. IV fluids (normal saline or lactated Ringer solution) are administered rapidly. Oxygen therapy is indicated if the bleeding is severe. Transfusion of blood products may be required if the blood loss is significant, and any existing coagulopathy should be corrected.

Upper GI mucosal lesions are usually treated with H_2-receptor antagonists (e.g., cimetidine, ranitidine, or famotidine) or PPIs (e.g., omeprazole, lansoprazole, pantoprazole, or esomeprazole) and antacids to reduce acidity and promote mucosal healing. Variceal hemorrhage can be treated with peripheral vasopressin infusion and endoscopic sclerotherapy to hasten tissue fibrosis. Balloon tamponade to place pressure on the bleeding area may be performed as a temporary measure until endoscopic sclerotherapy can be done.

Therapy for lower GI bleeding is directed toward the primary underlying condition. The treatment may include medical or surgical management. Surgery may be required if the bleeding is severe despite aggressive medical intervention.

Nursing Care Management

The infant or child with acute and severe GI bleeding requires emergency care. Initial management includes assessment of the magnitude of bleeding and hemodynamic status and assistance with resuscitation efforts (see Critical Thinking Case Study box).

CRITICAL THINKING CASE STUDY

Hematemesis

A 6-month-old infant is seen in the emergency department. The parents brought the infant to the hospital because he spit up formula with blood streaks. In the emergency department the infant has tachypnea, tachycardia, and a fever of 39°C (102.2°F). A chest x-ray film shows pneumonia. The infant is admitted to the hospital to receive antibiotics and for observation. Several hours after admission to the inpatient unit, the mother calls the nurse when the infant vomits a large amount of bright red blood. The infant is pale and lethargic. Which of the following should *not* be included in the initial nursing actions?

1. Call for assistance and estimate the amount of blood loss.
2. Obtain vital signs and monitor capillary refill, skin color, and behavior.
3. Prepare to pass a nasogastric tube, obtain blood for laboratory analyses, and start an intravenous line.
4. Test stool for blood (Hematest or Hemoccult).

Questions

1. Evidence—Are there sufficient data to support your decision?
2. Assumptions—Describe some underlying assumptions about the following:
   a. Hematemesis in an infant
   b. The diagnosis of hematemesis
3. What are the priorities for this child at this time?
4. What are the nursing actions that need to be implemented?

Answers are available at http://evolve.elsevier.com/wong/ncic.

> **! NURSING ALERT**
>
> Monitor closely for signs of shock: restlessness; increased respiratory and heart rate; poor capillary refill; pallor; cool, clammy extremities; and decreased blood pressure (a late sign). Call for assistance immediately if these signs are observed.

Make certain oxygen and suction equipment is available. An IV line should be inserted and preparation made for the administration of IV fluids, usually normal saline or lactated Ringer solution. Draw blood for laboratory analysis, including hemoglobin, hematocrit, blood urea nitrogen, creatinine, coagulation studies, and type and crossmatch. The nurse should be prepared to insert an NG tube to help locate the site of bleeding and to lavage the stomach with normal saline at room temperature if upper GI bleeding is suspected. Avoid taking rectal temperatures to prevent further irritation or damage to the rectal mucosa of a child suspected of having rectal bleeding or fissures. After the child is stabilized, ongoing monitoring in an intensive care setting may be indicated.

In cases of mild or chronic bleeding, there is more time for a thorough history and diagnostic evaluation, often in an outpatient setting. Important nursing responsibilities include assisting with the history and physical examination, diagnostic procedures, and education regarding the therapeutic plan.

The parents or caregivers of a child with GI bleeding may be extremely anxious and panic stricken. They need reassurance that most instances of bleeding are self-limiting and can be treated successfully. In life-threatening situations, special emotional support is required. Keep the family informed about the source, cause, and treatment of the bleeding.

HEPATIC DISORDERS

The liver is a vital organ whose functions can be divided into several groups: (1) vascular functions of storing and filtering blood; (2) secretory function of producing bile; (3) metabolism of carbohydrate, protein, and fat; (4) synthesis of blood-clotting components and storage of iron and vitamins (A, D, B_{12}, and K); and (5) detoxification and excretion of certain drugs and metabolic substances. Many disorders, including biliary atresia, hepatitis, and cirrhosis, can cause liver dysfunction in children.

ACUTE HEPATITIS

Hepatitis is an acute or chronic inflammation of the liver that can result from infectious or noninfectious reasons. Viruses such as hepatitis viruses, Epstein-Barr virus (EBV), and cytomegalovirus (CMV) are common causes of many types of hepatitis. Other causes of hepatitis are nonviral (e.g., abscess, amebiasis), autoimmune, metabolic, drug induced, anatomic (e.g., choledochal duct cyst and biliary atresia), hemodynamic (e.g., shock, congestive heart failure), and idiopathic (e.g., sclerosing cholangitis and Reye syndrome). Determining the cause of acute or chronic hepatitis is important in determining the treatment and prognosis for the child. Epidemiologic features and serologic testing are used to differentiate the causes. Table 25.7 compares the features of hepatitis A, B, and C viruses.

Hepatitis A Virus

Hepatitis A virus (HAV) incidence in the United States has declined since the introduction of a vaccine in 1995. There were approximately 1390 new cases in the United States in 2015 (Centers for Disease Control and Prevention, 2017). The virus is spread directly or indirectly by the fecal-oral route by ingestion of contaminated foods, direct exposure to infected fecal material, or close contact with an infected person. The virus is particularly prevalent in developing countries with poor living conditions, inadequate sanitation, crowding, and poor personal hygiene practices. The spread of HAV has been associated with improper food handling and high-risk areas such as households with infected persons, residential centers for the disabled, and day care centers. The average incubation period is about 21 days (Jensen & Balistreri, 2016). Fecal shedding of the virus can occur for 2 weeks before and for 1 week after the onset of jaundice. During this time, although the individual is asymptomatic, the virus is most likely to be transmitted. Infants with HAV infection are likely to be asymptomatic (anicteric hepatitis). Children often have diarrhea, and their symptoms are frequently attributed to gastroenteritis. Younger children rarely develop jaundice; however, 70% of older children and adults infected with HAV develop clinical signs with icteric hepatitis that typically lasts 7 to 14 days (Jensen & Balistreri, 2016). The prognosis of HAV infection is usually good, and complications are rare.

Hepatitis B Virus

Although the incidence of hepatitis B virus (HBV) is declining after the introduction of a universal immunization program, approximately 1.25 million people in the United States are infected with HBV, with 400 million HBV cases worldwide (Jensen & Balistreri, 2016). HBV can be an acute or chronic infection, ranging from an asymptomatic, limited infection to fatal, fulminant (rapid and severe) hepatitis (Jensen & Balistreri, 2016). There are no environmental or animal reservoirs for HBV. Humans are the main source of infections. HBV may be transmitted parenterally, percutaneously, or transmucosally. Hepatitis B surface antigen (HBsAg) has been found in all body fluids, including feces, bile, breast milk, sweat, tears, vaginal secretions, and urine, but only blood, semen, and saliva have been found to contain infectious HBV particles. HBV infection from human bites has been documented, but transmission from feces has not. HBV has been acquired after blood transfusion, but the likelihood of this has been reduced through blood product–screening procedures. Adults whose occupations are associated with considerable exposure to blood or blood products, such as health care workers, are at an increased risk of contracting HBV.

Most HBV infections in children are acquired perinatally. Transmission from mother to infant during the perinatal period (i.e., blood exposure during delivery) results in chronic infection in up to 90% of infants if the mother is positive for HBsAg and HBeAg (Jensen & Balistreri, 2016). HBsAg has been inconsistently detected in breast milk, but no increased risk of transmission has been found, and breastfeeding is currently recommended after infant immunization (Jensen & Balistreri, 2016). Infants and children who are not infected during the perinatal period remain at high risk for acquiring person-to-person transmission from their mother.

HBV infection occurs in children and adolescents in the following specific high-risk groups: (1) individuals with hemophilia or other disorders who have received multiple transfusions, (2) children and adolescents involved in IV drug abuse, (3) institutionalized children, (4) preschool children in endemic areas, and (5) individuals engaged in sexual activity with an infected partner. The incubation period for HBV infection ranges from 45 to 160 days, with an average of 120 days (Jensen & Balistreri, 2016). HBV infection can cause a carrier state and lead to chronic hepatitis with eventual cirrhosis or hepatocellular carcinoma in adulthood.

Hepatitis C Virus

Hepatitis C virus (HCV) is the most common cause of chronic liver disease, with an estimated 4 million people in the United States and

TABLE 25.7 Comparison of Hepatitis Types A, B, and C

Characteristics	Type A	Type B	Type C
Incubation period	15 to 50 days, average 28 days	45 to 160 days, average 120 days	2 to 24 weeks, average 7 to 9 weeks
Period of communicability	Believed to be latter half of incubation period to first week after onset of clinical illness	Variable Virus in blood or other body fluids during late incubation period and acute stage of disease; may persist in carrier state for years to lifetime	Begins before onset of symptoms May persist in carrier state for years
Mode of transmission	Principal route—fecal-oral Rarely—parenteral	Principal route—parenteral Less frequent route—oral, sexual, any body fluid Perinatal transfer—transplacental blood (last trimester), at delivery, or during breastfeeding, especially if mother has cracked nipples	Principal route—parenteral Nonparenteral spread possible
Clinical features			
• Onset	Usually rapid, acute	More insidious	Usually insidious
• Fever	Common and early	Less frequent	Less frequent
• Anorexia	Common	Mild to moderate	Mild to moderate
• Nausea and vomiting	Common	Sometimes present	Mild to moderate
• Rash	Rare	Common	Sometimes present
• Arthralgia	Rare	Common	Rare
• Pruritus	Rare	Sometimes present	Sometimes present
• Jaundice	Present (many cases anicteric)	Present	Present
Immunity	Present after one attack; no crossover to type B or C	Present after one attack; no crossover to type A or C	Present after one attack; no crossover to type A or B
Carrier state	No	Yes	Yes
Chronic infection	No	Yes	Yes
Prophylaxis			
• Immune globulin (IG)	Passive immunity Successful, especially in early incubation period and preexposure prophylaxis	Passive immunity Inconsistent benefits; probably of no use	Not currently recommended by Centers for Disease Control and Prevention
• HAV vaccine	Two inactivated vaccines administered to all children ages 12 to 23 months old: Havrix and Vaqta; given in a 2-dose schedule (6 months between doses)		
• HBV immune globulin (HBIG)	No benefit	Postexposure protection possible if given immediately after definite exposure	No benefit
• HBV vaccine		Provides active immunity Universal vaccination recommended for all newborns	
Mortality rate	0.1% to 0.2%	0.5% to 2.0% in uncomplicated cases; may be higher in complicated cases	1% to 2% in uncomplicated cases; may be higher in complicated cases

HAV, Hepatitis A virus; *HBV*, hepatitis B virus.

170 million people worldwide infected (Jensen & Balistreri, 2016). HCV is transmitted parenterally through exposure to blood and blood products from HCV-infected persons, whereas perinatal transmission is the most common mode of transmission among children (Jensen & Balistreri, 2016). Recent improvements in donor screening and inactivation procedures for blood products, such as the factor concentrates used for hemophilia patients, have significantly reduced the risk of transmission through blood products. Currently the most common cause of HCV infection is illegal drug use with exposure to blood or blood products from an HCV-infected individual, and sexual transmission is the second most common cause of HCV infection (Jensen & Balistreri, 2016).

The clinical course is variable. The incubation period for HCV ranges from 2 to 24 weeks, with an average of 7 to 9 weeks (Jensen & Balistreri, 2016). The natural history of the disease in children is not well defined. Some children may be asymptomatic, but HCV can become a chronic condition and can cause cirrhosis and hepatocellular carcinoma. About 85% of individuals infected with HCV develop chronic disease (Jensen & Balistreri, 2016).

Hepatitis D Virus

Hepatitis D virus (HDV) rarely occurs in children and must occur in individuals already infected with HBV (Jensen & Balistreri, 2016). HDV is a defective RNA virus that requires the helper function of HBV. The incubation period is 2 to 8 weeks, but with coinfection of HBV the incubation period is similar to an HBV infection (Jensen & Balistreri, 2016). HDV infection occurs through blood and sexual contact and commonly occurs among drug abusers, individuals with hemophilia, and persons immigrating from endemic areas.

Hepatitis E Virus

Hepatitis E virus (HEV) was formerly known as non-A, non-B hepatitis. Transmission may occur through the fecal-oral route or from contaminated water. The incubation period ranges from 15 to 60 days, with an average of 40 days (Jensen & Balistreri, 2016). This illness is uncommon in children, does not cause chronic liver disease, is not a chronic condition, and has no carrier state. However, it can be a devastating disease among pregnant women, with an unusually high fatality rate.

Pathophysiology

Pathologic changes occur primarily in the parenchymal cells of the liver and result in variable degrees of swelling; infiltration of liver cells by mononuclear cells; and subsequent degeneration, necrosis, and fibrosis. Structural changes within the hepatocyte account for altered liver functions, such as impaired bile excretion, elevated transaminase levels, and decreased albumin synthesis. The disorder may be self-limiting, with regeneration of liver cells without scarring, leading to a complete recovery. However, some forms of hepatitis do not result in complete return of liver function. These include fulminant hepatitis, which is characterized by a severe, acute course with massive destruction of the liver tissue causing liver failure and high mortality risk within 1 to 2 weeks; and subacute or chronic active hepatitis, which is characterized by progressive liver destruction, uncertain regeneration, scarring, and potential cirrhosis.

The progression of liver disease is characterized pathologically by four stages: (1) stage one is characterized by mononuclear inflammatory cells surrounding small bile ducts, (2) in stage two there is proliferation of small bile ductules, (3) stage three is characterized by fibrosis or scarring, and (4) stage four is cirrhosis.

Clinical Manifestations

The clinical manifestations and course of uncomplicated acute viral hepatitis are similar for most of the hepatitis viruses. Usually the prodromal, or anicteric, phase (absence of jaundice) lasts 5 to 7 days. Anorexia, malaise, lethargy, and easy fatigability are the most common symptoms. Fever may be present, especially in adolescents. Nausea, vomiting, and epigastric or right upper quadrant abdominal pain or tenderness may occur. Arthralgia and skin rashes may occur and are more likely in children with hepatitis B than those with hepatitis A. The transaminases, rather than the bilirubin, are often be elevated in acute hepatitis, and hepatomegaly may be present. Some mild cases of acute viral hepatitis do not cause symptoms or can be mistaken for influenza.

In young children most of the prodromal symptoms disappear with the onset of jaundice, or the icteric phase. Many children with acute viral hepatitis, however, never develop jaundice. If jaundice occurs, it is often accompanied by dark urine and pale stools. Pruritus may accompany jaundice and can be bothersome for children.

Children with chronic active hepatitis may be asymptomatic but more commonly have nonspecific symptoms of malaise, fatigue, lethargy, weight loss, or vague abdominal pain. Hepatomegaly may be present, and the transaminases are often very high, with mild to severe hyperbilirubinemia.

Fulminant hepatitis is due primarily to HBV or HCV. Many children with fulminant hepatitis develop characteristic clinical symptoms and rapidly develop manifestations of liver failure, including encephalopathy, coagulation defects, ascites, deepening jaundice, and an increasing white blood cell count. Changes in mental status or personality indicate impending liver failure. Although children with acute hepatitis may have hepatomegaly, a rapid decrease in the size of the liver (indicating loss of tissue due to necrosis) is a serious sign of fulminant hepatitis. Complications of fulminant hepatitis include GI bleeding, sepsis, renal failure, and disseminated coagulopathy.

Diagnostic Evaluation

Diagnosis is based on the history, physical examination, and serologic markers for hepatitis A, B, and C. No LFT is specific for hepatitis, but serum aspartate aminotransferase (AST) and serum alanine aminotransferase (ALT) levels are markedly elevated. Serum bilirubin levels peak 5 to 10 days after clinical jaundice appears. Histologic evidence from liver biopsy may be required to establish the diagnosis and to assess the severity of the liver disease. Serologic markers indicate the antibodies or antigens formed in response to the specific virus and confirm the diagnosis. Serum immunologic tests are not available to detect HAV antigen, but there are two HAV antibody tests: anti-HAV immunoglobulin G (IgG) and immunoglobulin M (IgM). Anti-HAV antibodies are present at the onset of the disease and persist for life. A positive anti-HAV antibody test can indicate acute infection, immunity from past infection, passive antibody acquisition (e.g., from transfusion, serum immunoglobulin infusion), or immunization. To diagnose an acute or recent HAV infection, a positive anti-HAV IgM test that is present with the onset of the disease and that persists for only 2 or 3 days is required.

Diagnosis of hepatitis B is confirmed by the detection of various hepatitis virus antigens and the antibodies that are produced in response to the infection. These antibodies and antigens and their significance include the following:

HBsAg—Hepatitis B surface antigen (found on the surface of the virus), indicating ongoing infection or carrier state

Anti-HBs—Antibody to surface antigen HbsAg, indicating resolving or past infection

HBcAg—Hepatitis B core antigen (found on the inner core of the virus), detected only in the liver

Anti-HBc—Antibody to core antigen HbcAg, indicating ongoing or past infection

HBeAg—Hepatitis B antigen (another component of the HBV core), indicating active infection

Anti-HBe—Antibody to HbeAg, indicating resolving or past infection

IgM anti-HBc—IgM antibody to core antigen

Tests are available for detection of all the HBV antigens and antibodies except HBcAg. HBsAg is detectable during acute infection. Presence of HBsAg indicates that the individual has been infected with the hepatitis virus. If the infection is self-limiting, HBsAg disappears in most patients before serum anti-HBs can be detected (termed the *window phase of infection*). IgM anti-HBc is highly specific in establishing the diagnosis of acute infection, as well as during the window phase in older children and adults. However, IgM anti-HBc usually is not present in perinatal HBV infection. Clinical improvement is usually associated with a decrease in or disappearance of these antigens, followed by the appearance of their antibodies. For example, anti-HBc of the IgM class often occurs early in the disease, followed by a rise in anti-HBc of the IgG class. Because the antibodies persist indefinitely, they are used to identify the carrier state (i.e., individuals with HBV who have no clinical disease but are able to transmit the organism). Persons with chronic HBV infection have circulating HBsAg and anti-HBc, and on rare occasions anti-HBsAg is present. Both anti-HBs and anti-HBc are detected in persons with resolved infection, but anti-HBs alone are present in individuals who have been immunized with the HBV vaccine.

HCV-RNA is the earliest serologic marker for HCV. HCV-RNA can be detected during the incubation period before symptoms of HCV disease are expressed. A positive HCV-RNA result indicates active infection, and persistence of HCV-RNA indicates chronic infection. A negative test correlates with resolution of the disease. HCV-RNA is also used to determine patient response to antiviral therapy for HCV.

The history of all patients should include questions to seek evidence of (1) contact with a person known to have hepatitis, especially a family member; (2) unsafe sanitation practices, such as contaminated drinking water; (3) ingestion of certain foods, such as clams or oysters (especially from polluted water); (4) multiple blood transfusions; (5) ingestion of hepatotoxic drugs, such as salicylates, sulfonamides, antineoplastic agents, acetaminophen, and anticonvulsants; and (6) parenteral administration of illicit drugs or sexual contact with a person who uses these drugs.

Therapeutic Management

The goals of management include early detection, support and monitoring of the disease, recognition of chronic liver disease, and prevention of spread of the disease. Special high-protein, high-carbohydrate, low-fat diets are generally not of value. The use of corticosteroids alone or with immunosuppressive drugs is not advocated in the treatment of chronic viral hepatitis. However, steroids have been used to treat chronic autoimmune hepatitis. Hospitalization is required in the event of coagulopathy or fulminant hepatitis.

Therapy for hepatitis depends on the severity of inflammation and the cause of the disorder. HAV is treated primarily with supportive care. The US Food and Drug Administration approved several medications for treatment of children with HBV and HCV. Human interferon-alpha is being used successfully in the treatment of chronic hepatitis B and C in children. Lamivudine is used for the treatment of HBV. It is well tolerated with no significant side effects and is approved for children older than 2 years of age (Jensen & Balistreri, 2016). Combined therapy with lamivudine and interferon-alpha does not improve response rates (Jensen & Balistreri, 2016). Adefovir is used to treat HBV in children older than 12 years of age. Entecavir and tenofovirhave recently been approved for HBV treatment in adolescents ages 16 years or older (Jensen & Balistreri, 2016). Peginterferon-α2b has not been approved for use in children in the United States but has been used to treat HBV in people in other countries (Jensen & Balistreri, 2016).

Prevention. Proper hand washing and Standard Precautions prevent the spread of viral hepatitis. Prophylactic use of standard immune globulin is effective in preventing hepatitis A in situations of preexposure (such as anticipated travel to areas where HAV is prevalent) or within 2 weeks of exposure.

Hepatitis B immune globulin (HBIG) is effective in preventing HBV infection after one-time exposures such as accidental needle punctures or other contact of contaminated material with mucous membranes and should be given to newborns whose mothers are HbsAg positive. HBIG is prepared from plasma that contains high titers of antibodies against HBV. HBIG should be given within 72 hours of exposure.

Vaccines have been developed to prevent HAV and HBV infection (see Table 25.7). HBV vaccination is recommended for all newborns and children who did not receive the vaccination as a newborn. (See Immunizations, Chapter 6.) Because HDV cannot be transmitted in the absence of HBV infection, it is possible to prevent HDV infection by preventing HBV infection. Routine serologic testing for anti-HCV of children older than 12 months of age who were born to women previously identified as being infected with HCV is also recommended (Jensen & Balistreri, 2016).

Prognosis. The prognosis for children with hepatitis is variable and depends on the type of virus and the child's age and immunocompetency. Hepatitis A and E are usually mild, brief illnesses with no carrier state. Hepatitis B can cause a wide spectrum of acute and chronic illness. Infants are more likely than older children to develop chronic hepatitis. Hepatocellular carcinoma during adulthood is a potentially fatal complication of chronic HBV infection. Hepatitis C frequently becomes chronic, and cirrhosis may develop in these children.

Nursing Care Management

Nursing objectives depend largely on the severity of the hepatitis, the medical treatment, and factors influencing the control and transmission of the disease. Because children with mild viral hepatitis are frequently cared for at home, it is often the nurse's responsibility to explain any medical therapies and infection control measures. When further assistance is needed for parents to comply with instructions, a public health nursing referral is necessary.

Encourage a well-balanced diet and a schedule of rest and activity adjusted to the child's condition. Because the child with HAV is not infectious within 1 week after the onset of jaundice, the child may feel well enough to resume school shortly thereafter. Caution parents about administering any medication to the child because normal doses of many drugs may become dangerous because of the liver's inability to detoxify and excrete them.

Standard Precautions are followed when children are hospitalized. However, these children are not usually isolated in a separate room unless they are fecally incontinent or their toys and other personal items are likely to become contaminated with feces. Discourage children from sharing their toys.

Hand washing is the single most effective measure in prevention and control of hepatitis in any setting. Parents and children need an explanation of the usual ways in which hepatitis is spread (fecal-oral route and parenteral route). Parents should also be aware of the recommendation for universal vaccination against HBV for newborns and adolescents. (See Chapter 6.)

In young people with HBV infection who have a known or suspected history of illicit drug use, the nurse has the responsibility of helping them realize the associated dangers of drug abuse, stressing the parenteral mode of transmission of hepatitis, and encouraging them to seek counseling through a drug program.

BILIARY ATRESIA

Biliary atresia (BA), or extrahepatic biliary atresia (EHBA), is a progressive inflammatory process that causes both intrahepatic and extrahepatic bile duct fibrosis, resulting in eventual ductal obstruction. The incidence of BA is approximately 1 in 10,000 to 15,000 live births (Hassan & Balistreri, 2016). Associated malformations include polysplenia and malrotation of the intestine. BA, if untreated, usually leads to cirrhosis, liver failure, and death.

Pathophysiology

The exact cause of BA is unknown, although immune- or infection-mediated mechanisms may be responsible for the progressive process that results in complete obliteration of the bile ducts. BA is not seen in the fetus or stillborn or newborn infant. This suggests that BA is acquired late in gestation or in the perinatal period and is manifested a few weeks after birth.

Congenital infections have been implicated as a cause of hepatocellular damage leading to BA, yet no specific agent is identified in every case. Immune-mediated bile duct injury from viral exposure and immaturity of the neonatal immune system may play a role in the destruction of bile ducts and development of EHBA. Other potential causes include an early first trimester insult to the developing bile ducts or a postnatal viral insult (Hassan & Balistreri, 2016). Early in the course of the disease, the intrahepatic ducts are patent from the interlobular ductules to the porta hepatis. The size of these structures is variable and is correlated with the infant's age and with bile excretion after surgical treatment. These structures are present in most affected infants under 2 months of age but gradually disappear over the next few months and by 4 months are completely replaced by fibrous tissue.

The degree of involvement of the extrahepatic biliary ducts is also variable. The majority of cases of BA (85%) have a complete obliteration of the extrahepatic biliary tree at or above the porta hepatis (Hassan & Balistreri, 2016). But some infants have a patent proximal portion of the extrahepatic duct or patency of the gallbladder, cystic duct, and common bile duct. Microscopic examination of the liver tissue reveals cholestasis with absent or diminished bile duct proliferation and fibrosis.

Clinical Manifestations

Many infants with BA are full term and appear healthy at birth. If jaundice persists beyond 2 weeks of age, especially if the direct (conjugated) serum bilirubin is elevated, the nurse should suspect BA. The urine may be dark, and the stools often become progressively acholic or gray, indicating absence of bile pigment. Hepatomegaly is present early in the course of the disease, and the liver is firm on palpation.

Diagnostic Evaluation

Early diagnosis is critical to the child with EHBA; the outcome in children surgically treated before 2 months of age is much better than in patients with delayed treatment. The diagnosis of BA is suspected on the basis of the history, physical findings, and laboratory studies. Laboratory tests include a CBC, bilirubin levels, and liver function studies. Additional laboratory analyses, including α_1-antitrypsin level, TORCH titers and other intrauterine infections (see Maternal Infections, Chapter 9), hepatitis serology, and urine cytomegalovirus, may be indicated to rule out other conditions that cause cholestasis and jaundice. An abdominal ultrasound is usually performed to identify potential causes of extrahepatic obstruction, such as a choledochal cyst. The patency of the extrahepatic biliary system is demonstrated by a nuclear scintiscan using technetium 99m iminodiacetic acid (^{99m}Tc-IDA, or HIDA; HIDA scan). If there is no evidence of radioactive material excreted into the duodenum, BA is the most probable diagnosis. Because the nuclear scan may take up to 5 days for the results, a percutaneous liver biopsy is probably the most useful method of diagnosing BA (Govindarajan, 2016). The definitive diagnosis of BA is further established during an exploratory laparotomy and an intraoperative cholangiogram that demonstrates complete obstruction at some level of the biliary tree.

Therapeutic Management

Medical management of BA is primarily supportive. It includes nutritional support with infant formulas that contain medium-chain triglycerides and essential fatty acids. Supplementation with fat-soluble vitamins (A, D, E, and K); a multivitamin; and minerals, including iron, zinc, and selenium, is usually required. Aggressive nutritional support in the form of continuous gastrostomy feedings or TPN may be indicated for moderate to severe growth failure; the enteral solution should be low in sodium. Phenobarbital may be prescribed after hepatic portoenterostomy to stimulate bile flow, and ursodeoxycholic acid may be used to decrease cholestasis and the intense pruritus from jaundice. In cases of advanced liver dysfunction, management is the same as in infants with cirrhosis.

The primary surgical treatment of BA is hepatic portoenterostomy (Kasai procedure), which a segment of intestine is anastomosed to the resected porta hepatis to attempt bile drainage (Fig. 25.8). A Roux-en-Y jejunal limb is then anastomosed to the porta hepatis (a Y-shaped anastomosis performed to provide bile drainage without reflux). Complications after portoenterostomy include ascending cholangitis, cirrhosis, portal hypertension, and GI bleeding. Prophylactic antibiotics are given after the Kasai procedure to minimize the risk of ascending cholangitis. After the Kasai procedure approximately one-third of infants become jaundice free and regain normal liver function. Another one-third of infants demonstrate liver damage; however, they may be supported by medical and nutritional interventions. A final third require liver transplantation. Liver transplantation is required for children who cannot regain bile flow and for those with end-stage liver disease or severe portal hypertension. Complications after liver transplantation include obstruction and bile leaks at the biliary anastomosis, portal hypertension, hemorrhage, infection, and rejection. Immunosuppressive drugs are required after transplantation.

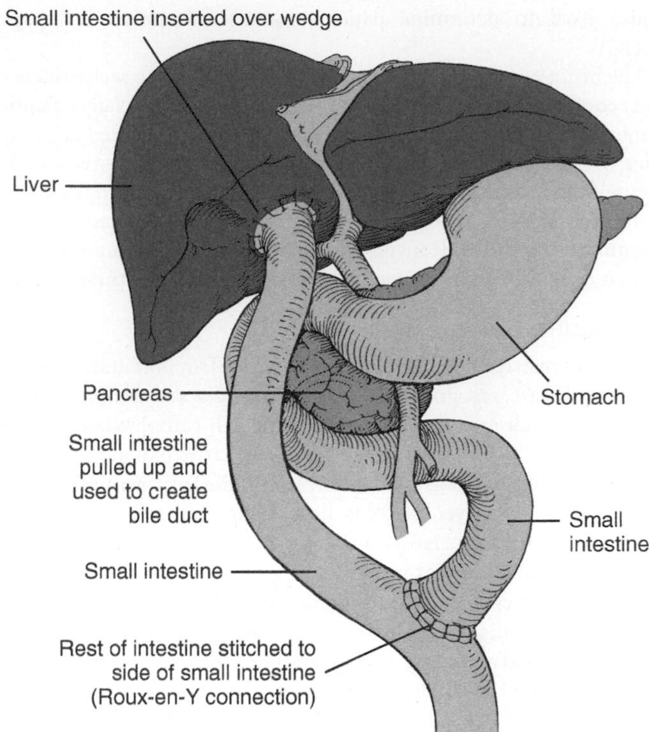

FIG. 25.8 Biliary atresia—Kasai procedure.

Prognosis. Untreated BA results in progressive cirrhosis and death in most children by 3 years of age (Govindarajan, 2016). The Kasai procedure improves the prognosis but is not a cure. There is only 20% survival in patients 20 years after the Kasai procedure and only 10% survival in patients 30 years after the procedure (Govindarajan, 2016).

Biliary drainage can often be achieved if the surgery is performed before the intrahepatic bile ducts are destroyed; the success rate is much higher, up to 90%, if surgery is performed in an infant younger than 2 months of age (Hassan & Balistreri, 2016). Long-term survival rates of 64% to 92% have been noted in children after portoenterostomy (Govindarajan, 2016). However, even with successful bile drainage, many children ultimately develop liver failure and require liver transplantation.

The advances in surgical techniques for liver transplantation and the development of immunosuppressive and antifungal drugs have significantly improved the success of transplantation. Surgical techniques and immunosuppression have contributed to survival rates of 83% to 91% in children who underwent transplant (Yanagi, Matsuura, Hayashida, et al., 2017). The major obstacle remains the shortage of suitable infant donors.

Liver disease progresses in infants with delayed diagnosis or in children in whom surgery has failed to provide adequate bile drainage. Cirrhosis and splenomegaly occur with hypoalbuminemia, ascites, and coagulopathy. Malabsorption of fat and fat-soluble vitamins and malnutrition result in severe growth failure. Retained bile salts and cholesterol further contribute to pruritus (itching) and xanthomas, often requiring the administration of ursodeoxycholic acid. The severity of pruritus intensifies as the jaundice progresses as the result of disease advancement.

Nursing Care Management

There are many important nursing interventions for the child with BA. The nurse should educate family members regarding all aspects of the treatment plan and the rationale for therapy. Immediately after a hepatic portoenterostomy, nursing care is similar to that after any major abdominal surgery. If an interrupted jejunal conduit has been performed, the family needs to learn how to care for the two stomas and how to refeed the bile after feedings. Teaching includes the proper administration of medications. Administration of nutritional therapy, including special formulas, vitamin and mineral supplements, gastrostomy feedings, or parenteral nutrition, is an essential nursing responsibility. Growth failure in such infants is common, and increased metabolic needs combined with ascites, pruritus, and nutritional anorexia constitute a challenge for care. The nurse teaches caregivers how to monitor and administer nutritional therapy in the home. Pruritus may be a significant problem that is addressed by drug therapy or comfort measures such as baths in colloidal oatmeal compounds and trimming of fingernails. The risk of complications of BA, such as cholangitis, portal hypertension, GI bleeding, and ascites, should be explained to the caregivers.

These children and their families require special psychosocial support. The uncertain prognosis, discomfort, and waiting for transplantation can produce considerable stress. (See Cirrhosis, next.) In addition, extended hospitalizations, as well as pharmacologic and nutritional therapy, can impose significant financial burdens on the family, as with any chronic condition. The expertise of a multidisciplinary health care team, including surgeons, gastroenterologists, pediatricians, nurses, nutritionists, pharmacists, child life specialists, and social workers, is often necessary. Parent support groups can be beneficial as well. The Children's Liver Association for Support Services (C.L.A.S.S.)* and the American Liver Foundation† provide educational materials, programs, and support systems for parents of children with liver disease.

CIRRHOSIS

Cirrhosis occurs as an end stage of many chronic liver diseases, including BA and chronic hepatitis. Infectious, autoimmune, toxic injury, and chronic diseases such as hemophilia and cystic fibrosis can cause severe liver damage. A cirrhotic liver is irreversibly damaged.

Pathophysiology

Cirrhosis occurs as a result of hepatocyte injury with necrosis, fibrosis, regeneration, and eventual degeneration. The diminished parenchymal cell mass causes regeneration of tissue with nodular areas of proliferating hepatocytes that stretch the surrounding connective tissue. Hepatocytes respond to injury with deposition of collagen that forms fibrous connective tissue. This scar tissue and nodular areas of regeneration impair the intrahepatic blood flow. Ongoing necrosis and self-perpetuation of this pathologic process are the result of cirrhosis.

Failure of hepatocellular function and portal hypertension occur and often lead to complications, including ascites, severe cholestasis, encephalopathy (hepatic coma), and GI bleeding.

Clinical Manifestations

Clinical manifestations of cirrhosis include jaundice, poor growth, anorexia, muscle weakness, and lethargy. Ascites, edema, GI bleeding, anemia, and abdominal pain may be present in children with impaired intrahepatic blood flow. Pulmonary function may be impaired because of pressure against the diaphragm due to hepatosplenomegaly and ascites. Dyspnea and cyanosis may occur, especially on exertion. Intrapulmonary arteriovenous shunts may develop, which can also cause hypoxemia. Spider angiomas and prominent blood vessels on the upper torso are often present.

Diagnostic Evaluation

The diagnosis of cirrhosis is based on (1) the history, especially in regard to prior liver disease, such as hepatitis; (2) physical examination, particularly hepatosplenomegaly; (3) laboratory evaluation, especially LFTs, such as bilirubin and transaminases, ammonia, albumin, cholesterol, and prothrombin time; and (4) liver biopsy for characteristic changes. Doppler ultrasonography of the liver and spleen is useful to confirm ascites, to evaluate the blood flow through the liver and spleen, and to determine the patency and size of the portal vein if liver transplantation is considered.

! NURSING ALERT

The most common complication from percutaneous liver biopsy is internal bleeding. Vital signs and laboratory values, especially hematocrit, should be monitored for evidence of hemorrhage and shock.

Therapeutic Management

Unfortunately, there is no successful treatment to arrest the progression of cirrhosis. The goals of management include monitoring liver function and managing specific complications such as esophageal varices and malnutrition. Assessment of the child's degree of liver dysfunction is important so that the child can be evaluated for transplantation at the appropriate time.

Liver transplantation has improved the prognosis substantially for many children with cirrhosis. Pediatric liver transplantation is one of the most successful solid organ transplants with a 1-year survival rate of 83% to 91%, depending on the age at transplant (Yanagi, Matsuura, Hayashida, et al., 2017). The policy governing the allocation of livers for transplantation by the United Network for Organ Sharing allows pediatric patients less than 12 years of age, those with acute fulminant liver failure, or those with chronic liver disease to be placed at the top of the network's transplantation lists (United Network for Organ Sharing, 2017). Although this change has benefited many pediatric patients, the shortage of available donors for children continues to dictate transplantation decisions, and many children continue to die while waiting for a suitable donor.

Nutritional support is an important therapy for children with cirrhosis and malnutrition. Supplements of fat-soluble vitamins are often required, and mineral supplements may be indicated. In some instances aggressive nutritional support in the form of enteral feeding or PN may be necessary.

*25379 Wayne Mills Place, Suite 143, Valencia, CA 91355; 877-679-8256; http://www.classkids.org.

†39 Broadway, Suite 2700, New York, NY 10006; 212-668-1000; http://www.liverfoundation.org.

Esophageal and gastric varices can be a life-threatening complication of portal hypertension. Acute hemorrhage is managed with IV fluids; blood products; vitamin K, if needed to correct coagulopathy; vasopressin or somatostatin; and gastric lavage. If acute hemorrhage persists, the most common secondary approach is endoscopic sclerotherapy or endoscopic banding ligation (Choudhary, Puri, Saigal, et al., 2016). Balloon tamponade with a Sengstaken-Blakemore tube may be indicated for the unstable patient with acute hemorrhage (Choudhary, Puri, Saigal, et al., 2016). Ascites is managed by sodium and fluid restrictions and diuretics. Severe ascites with respiratory compromise is managed with albumin infusions or by paracentesis.

Although the full mechanism of hepatic encephalopathy is unknown, failure of the damaged liver to remove endogenous toxins, such as ammonia, plays a role. Treatment is directed at limiting the ammonia formation and absorption that occur in the bowel, especially with the drugs neomycin and lactulose. Because ammonia is formed in the bowel by the action of bacteria on ingested protein, neomycin reduces the number of intestinal bacteria so less ammonia is produced. The fermentation of lactulose by colonic bacteria produces short-chain fatty acids, which lower the colonic pH, thereby inhibiting bacterial metabolism. This decreases the formation of ammonia from bacterial metabolism of protein.

Prognosis. The success of liver transplantation has revolutionized the approach to liver cirrhosis. Liver failure and cirrhosis are indications for transplantation. Careful monitoring of the child's condition and quality of life is necessary to evaluate the need for and timing of transplantation.

Nursing Care Management

Several factors influence nursing care of the child with cirrhosis, including the cause of the cirrhosis, the severity of complications, and the prognosis. The prognosis is often poor unless successful liver transplantation occurs. Therefore nursing care of this child is similar to that for any child with a life-threatening illness. (See Chapter 19.) Hospitalization is required when complications such as hemorrhage, severe malnutrition, or hepatic failure occur. Nursing assessments are directed at monitoring the child's condition, and interventions are aimed at treatment of specific complications. If liver transplantation is an option, the family needs support and assistance to cope (see Family-Centered Care box).

FAMILY-CENTERED CARE

End-Stage Liver Disease

In many cases the child with liver disease and the family must cope with an uncertain progression of the disease. The only hope for long-term survival may be liver transplantation. Transplantation can be successful, but the waiting period may be long because there are many more children in need of organs than there are donors. The procedure is expensive and is only performed at designated medical centers, which are often far from the family's home. The nurse should recognize the unique stresses of coping with end-stage liver disease and waiting for transplantation, and should offer support and assistance to the family in coping with these stressors. The assistance of social workers and support from other parents can also be beneficial.

STRUCTURAL DEFECTS

Congenital defects of the GI tract can involve any portion from the mouth to the anus. Most are apparent at birth or shortly thereafter and are anomalies in which normal growth ceased at a crucial stage of embryonic development, leaving the structure in an embryonic form or only partially completed. The result may be atresia, malposition, nonclosure, or any number of variations.

Atresia is absence of a normal opening or normally patent lumen. Atresia at any point along the length of the GI tract creates an obstruction to the normal progress of nutrients and secretions. The most common anomalies requiring surgical intervention are atresias of the esophagus, intestine, and anus. The congenital defects considered in this chapter include abnormalities of the lip, palate, trachea, esophagus, and anus.

ESOPHAGEAL ATRESIA AND TRACHEOESOPHAGEAL FISTULA

Congenital esophageal atresia (EA) and tracheoesophageal fistula (TEF) are rare malformations that represent a failure of the esophagus to develop as a continuous passage and a failure of the trachea and esophagus to separate into distinct structures. These defects may occur as separate entities or in combination, and without early diagnosis and treatment they pose a serious threat to the infant's well-being.

The incidence of EA is estimated to be approximately 1 in 3000 neonates (Wu, Kuang, Lv, et al., 2017). There appears to be a slightly higher incidence in males, and the birth weight of most affected infants is significantly lower than average, with an unusually high incidence of preterm birth in infants with EA and a subsequent increase in mortality. A history of maternal polyhydramnios is common.

Approximately 50% of the cases of EA/TEF are a component of VATER or VACTERL association, acronyms used to describe associated anomalies (VATER for *V*ertebral defects, imperforate *A*nus, *T*racheo*e*sophageal fistula, and *R*adial and *R*enal dysplasia; and VACTERL for *V*ertebral, *A*nal, *C*ardiac, *T*racheal, *E*sophageal, *R*enal, and *L*imb) (Khan & Orenstein, 2016c). Cardiac anomalies may also occur with EA/TEF; therefore all patients should undergo a workup for associated anomalies.

Pathophysiology

The esophagus develops from the first segment of the embryonic gut. During the fourth and fifth weeks of gestation, the foregut normally lengthens and separates longitudinally. Each longitudinal portion fuses to form two parallel channels (the esophagus and the trachea) that are joined only at the larynx. Anomalies involving the trachea and esophagus are caused by defective separation, incomplete fusion of the tracheal folds after this separation, or altered cellular growth during embryonic development.

The most commonly encountered form of EA and TEF (80% to 90% of cases) is one in which the proximal esophageal segment terminates in a blind pouch and the distal segment is connected to the trachea or primary bronchus by a short fistula at or near the tracheal bifurcation (Fig. 25.9, *C*). The second most common type (7% to 8%) consists of a blind pouch at each end, widely separated and with no communication to the trachea (Fig. 25.9, *A*). An H-type EA refers to an otherwise normal trachea and esophagus connected by a fistula (4% to 5%) (Fig. 25.9, *E*). Extremely rare anomalies involve a fistula from the trachea to the upper esophageal segment (0.8%) (Fig. 25.9, *B*) or to both the upper and lower segments (0.7% to 6%) (Fig. 25.9, *D*).

Clinical Manifestations

The presence of EA is suspected in a newborn with frothy saliva in the mouth and nose, drooling, choking, and coughing. Respiratory distress may be mild or significant, depending on the type of defect and the infant's gestational age. If fed, the infant may swallow normally but suddenly cough and gag, with return of fluid through the nose and mouth. The infant may become cyanotic and apneic because of aspiration of breastmilk or saliva.

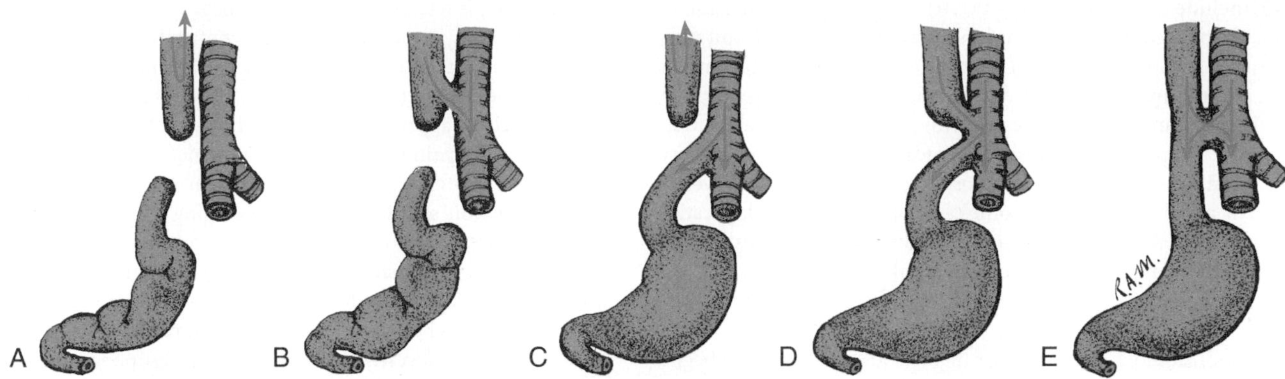

FIG. 25.9 **A–E,** Five most common types of esophageal atresia and tracheoesophageal fistula. (See text for discussion.)

In the infant who has EA with a distal TEF (type C), the stomach becomes distended with air, and thoracic and abdominal compressions (especially during crying) cause the gastric contents to be regurgitated through the fistula and into the trachea, producing a chemical pneumonitis. When the upper segment of the esophagus opens directly into the trachea (types B and D), the infant is in danger of aspirating any swallowed material. Cyanosis or choking during feeding may be the only symptom of type H fistula (see Fig. 25.9, *E*). The child with this type of EA may not manifest symptoms until later in life when he or she shows signs of chronic respiratory problems, recurrent pneumonia, and signs of GER (Khan & Orenstein, 2016c).

Diagnostic Evaluation

Although the diagnosis is established on the basis of clinical signs and symptoms, the exact type of anomaly is determined by radiographic studies. A radiopaque catheter is inserted into the hypopharynx and advanced until it encounters an obstruction. Chest radiographs are taken to ascertain esophageal patency or the presence and level of a blind pouch. Films that show air in the stomach indicate a connection between the trachea and the distal esophagus in types C, D, and E. Complete absence of air in the stomach is seen in types A and B. Occasionally, fistulas are not patent, which makes their presence more difficult to diagnose. A careful bronchoscopic examination may be performed in an attempt to visualize the fistula.

The presence of polyhydramnios (accumulation of 2000 ml of amniotic fluid) prenatally is a clue to the possibility of EA in the unborn infant, especially with defect type A, B, or C. With these types of EA/TEF, amniotic fluid normally swallowed by the fetus is unable to reach the GI tract to be absorbed and excreted by the kidneys. The result is an abnormal accumulation of amniotic fluid, or polyhydramnios.

Therapeutic Management

The treatment of EA and TEF includes maintenance of a patent airway, prevention of pneumonia, gastric or blind pouch decompression, supportive therapy, and surgical repair of the anomaly.

When EA with a TEF is suspected, the infant is immediately deprived of oral intake, IV fluids are initiated, and the infant is positioned to facilitate drainage of secretions and decrease the likelihood of aspiration. Accumulated secretions are suctioned frequently from the mouth and pharynx. A double-lumen catheter should be placed into the upper esophageal pouch and attached to intermittent or continuous low suction. The infant's head is kept upright to facilitate removal of fluid collected in the pouch and to prevent aspiration of gastric contents. Broad-spectrum antibiotic therapy is often instituted if there is a concern about aspiration of gastric contents.

Most malformations can be corrected surgically in one operation or in two or more staged procedures. The success depends on early diagnosis before complications occur and on the presence and severity of associated anomalies and illness factors, including preterm birth. With measures instituted to prevent aspiration pneumonia and to ensure adequate hydration and nutrition, surgery may be postponed to allow for more effective treatment of pneumonia and physiologic stabilization so that the infant can better withstand the complex surgery. The delay also offers an opportunity for further evaluation and assessment to rule out any associated anomalies and to optimize respiratory support.

Thoracoscopic repair of EA/TEF is being used successfully, thus negating the need for a thoracotomy and minimizing associated postoperative complications and morbidities (Khan & Orenstein, 2016c). The surgery consists of a thoracotomy with division and ligation of the TEF and an end-to-end or end-to-side anastomosis of the esophagus. A chest tube may be inserted to drain intrapleural air and fluid. For infants who are not stable enough to undergo definitive repair or those with a lengthy gap (>3 to 4 cm) between the proximal and distal esophagus, a staged operation is preferred that involves gastrostomy, ligation of the TEF, and constant drainage of the esophageal pouch (Khan & Orenstein, 2016c). A delayed esophageal anastomosis is usually attempted after several weeks to months.

A primary anastomosis may be impossible because of insufficient length of the two segments of esophagus. This occurs if the distance between the two segments is 3 to 4 cm (1.2 to 1.6 inches) (approximately 3 vertebral bodies) or greater; this is often referred to as *long-gap EA* (Khan & Orenstein, 2016c). In these cases an esophageal replacement procedure using a part of the colon or gastric tube interposition may be necessary to bridge the missing esophageal segment. Further surgical techniques may be performed later to facilitate esophageal lengthening.

Tracheomalacia may occur as a result of weakness in the tracheal wall that exists when a dilated proximal pouch compresses the trachea early in fetal life. It may also occur as a result of inadequate intratracheal pressure causing abnormal tracheal development. Clinical signs of tracheomalacia include barking cough, stridor, wheezing, recurrent respiratory tract infections, cyanosis, and sometimes apnea.

Prognosis. The survival rate is nearly 100% in otherwise healthy children. Most deaths are the result of extreme prematurity or other lethal associated anomalies.

Potential complications after the surgical repair of EA and TEF depend on the type of defect and surgical correction. Complications of repair include an anastomotic leak, strictures caused by tension or ischemia, esophageal motility disorders causing dysphagia, respiratory compromise, scoliosis, chest wall deformity, and GER. Anastomotic esophageal strictures may cause dysphagia, choking, and respiratory distress. The strictures are often treated with routine esophageal dilation. Feeding difficulties are often present for months or years after surgery, and the infant must be monitored closely to ensure adequate weight gain, growth, and development. In some cases laparoscopic fundoplication may be required. At times the infant must be fed via gastrostomy or jejunostomy to provide adequate caloric intake.

Nursing Care Management

Nursing responsibility for detection of this serious malformation begins immediately after birth. For the infant with the classic signs and symptoms of EA (see Nursing Alert) the major concern is the establishment of a patent airway and prevention of further respiratory compromise. Cyanosis is usually a result of laryngeal spasm caused by overflow of saliva into the larynx from the proximal esophageal pouch or aspiration; it normally resolves after removal of the secretions from the oropharynx by suctioning. The passage of a small-gauge orogastric (OG) feeding tube via the mouth into the stomach during the initial nursing physical assessment is helpful to determine the presence of EA or other obstructive defects.

> **! NURSING ALERT**
>
> Any infant who has an excessive amount of frothy saliva in the mouth or difficulty with secretions and unexplained episodes of apnea, cyanosis, or oxygen desaturation should be suspected of having an EA/TEF and referred immediately for medical evaluation.

Preoperative Care. The nurse carefully suctions the mouth and nasopharynx and places the infant in an optimum position to facilitate drainage and avoid aspiration. The most desirable position for a newborn who is suspected of having the typical EA with a TEF (e.g., type C) is supine (or sometimes prone) with the head elevated on an inclined plane of at least 30 degrees. This positioning minimizes the reflux of gastric secretions at the distal esophagus into the trachea and bronchi, especially when intraabdominal pressure is elevated.

It is imperative to immediately remove any secretions that can be aspirated. Until surgery the blind pouch is kept empty by intermittent or continuous suction through an indwelling double-lumen catheter passed orally or nasally to the end of the pouch. In some cases a percutaneous gastrostomy tube is inserted and left open so that any air entering the stomach through the fistula can escape, thus minimizing the danger of gastric contents being regurgitated into the trachea. The gastrostomy tube is emptied by gravity drainage. Feedings through the gastrostomy tube and irrigations with fluid are contraindicated before surgery in the infant with a distal TEF.

Nursing interventions include respiratory assessment, airway management, thermoregulation, fluid and electrolyte management, and parenteral nutritional support.

Often the infant must be transferred to a hospital with a specialized care unit and pediatric surgical team. The nurse advises the parents of the infant's condition and provides them with necessary support and information.

Postoperative Care. Postoperative care for these infants is the same as for any high-risk newborn. Adequate thermoregulation is provided, the double-lumen NG catheter is attached to low-suction or gravity drainage, parenteral nutrition is provided, and the gastrostomy tube (if applicable) is returned to gravity drainage until feedings are tolerated. If a thoracotomy is performed and a chest tube is inserted, attention to the appropriate function of the closed drainage system is imperative. Pain management in the postoperative period is important even if only a thoracoscopic approach is used. In the first 24 to 36 hours the nurse should provide pain management for the neonate just as for an adult undergoing a similar procedure. (See Pain in Neonates, Chapter 5.) Tracheal suction should only be done using a premeasured catheter and with extreme caution to avoid injury to the suture line.

If tolerated, gastrostomy feedings may be initiated and continued until the esophageal anastomosis is healed. Before oral feedings are initiated and the chest tube (if applicable) is removed, a contrast study or esophagram will verify the integrity of the esophageal anastomosis.

The nurse must carefully observe the initial attempt at oral feeding to make certain the infant is able to swallow without choking. Oral feedings are begun with sterile water, followed by frequent small feedings of breast milk or formula. Until the infant is able to take a sufficient amount by mouth, oral intake may need to be supplemented by bolus or continuous gastrostomy feedings. Ordinarily infants are not discharged until they can take oral fluids well. The gastrostomy tube may be removed before discharge or maintained for supplemental feedings at home.

Special Problems. Upper respiratory tract complications are a threat to life in both the preoperative and postoperative periods. In addition to pneumonia, the infants are in constant danger of respiratory distress resulting from atelectasis, pneumothorax, and laryngeal edema. Any persistent respiratory difficulty after removal of secretions must be reported to the surgeon immediately. The infant should be monitored for anastomotic leaks and signs of infection such as purulent chest tube drainage, an increased white blood cell count, and temperature instability.

For the infant who requires esophageal replacement, nonnutritive sucking should be provided with a pacifier. Infants who are on NPO status for an extended period and have not received oral stimulation frequently have difficulty eating by mouth after corrective surgery and may develop oral hypersensitivity and feeding aversion. They require patient, firm guidance in learning the techniques of taking food into the mouth and swallowing after repair. A referral to a multidisciplinary feeding behavior team may be necessary.

One of the difficulties in TEF is the immediate transfer of the sick infant to the intensive care unit and sometimes lengthy hospitalization. Parent-infant bonding is facilitated by encouraging parents to visit the infant, participate in his or her care when appropriate, and express their feelings regarding the infant's condition. The nurse in the intensive care unit should assume responsibility for ensuring that the parents are fully informed of the infant's progress.

Family Support, Discharge Planning, and Home Care. Some infants with EA/TEF may require periodic esophageal dilations on an outpatient basis. Discharge education should include instructions about feeding techniques in the child with a repaired esophagus, including a semiupright feeding position, small feedings, and observation for adequacy of swallowing (e.g., regurgitation, cyanosis, choking). Tracheomalacia is often a complication; parents are educated about the signs and symptoms of this condition, which include a barking cough, stridor, wheezing, recurrent respiratory tract infections, cyanosis, and sometimes apnea. GER may also occur when feedings resume and may contribute to reactive airway disease with wheezing and labored respirations as the prominent clinical manifestations. Problems with thriving and gaining weight may occur in the first 5 years of life in the child with EA/TEF, especially if the infant is born preterm. The nurse should be alert to the achievement of developmental milestones that indicate a need for early intervention and multidisciplinary referral.

Preparing parents for discharge of their infant involves teaching the techniques that will be continued at home. The parents learn signs of respiratory difficulty and of esophageal stricture (e.g., poor feeding, choking, dysphagia, drooling, regurgitating undigested food) and GER.

Parents must be aware of feeding restrictions. Remind parents that it is particularly important to guard against the infant swallowing foreign objects. They should cut solid food into small pieces, teach the child to chew thoroughly, give frequent sips of liquid to help swallow food, and avoid foods such as whole hot dogs or large pieces of meat that may become lodged in the esophagus. (See Safety Promotion and Injury Prevention, Chapter 10.)

Discharge planning should include attainment of needed equipment and home nursing services to assist with ongoing assessment of the child and continuity of care.

ABDOMINAL WALL DEFECTS

Gastroschisis and omphalocele are two of the more common forms of congenital abdominal wall defects. Gastroschisis occurs in varying incidences worldwide from about 3 to 4 in 10,000 births, and omphalocele occurs in approximately 1 to 2 in 10,000 live births (St. Louis, Kim, Browne, et al., 2017). Numerous reports cite an increase in the incidence of gastroschisis, although the cause of this increased incidence is unknown (St. Louis, Kim, Browne, et al., 2017). An omphalocele occurs when the abdominal contents herniate through the umbilical ring (hernia of the umbilical cord), usually with an intact peritoneal sac, whereas gastroschisis occurs when the herniation of intestine is lateral to the umbilical ring. This herniation is usually to the right of the umbilicus, and a peritoneal sac is not present.

Omphalocele

Omphalocele is related to a true failure of embryonic development. It occurs when there is failure of the caudal or lateral in folding of the abdominal wall at approximately the third week of gestation. With the deficiency in the abdominal wall, the bowel is unable to complete its return to the abdomen between the tenth and twelfth weeks of gestation.

The omphalocele is usually covered only by a translucent peritoneal sac (Fig. 25.10). The sac may contain only a small portion of the bowel or most of the bowel and other abdominal viscera, such as the liver. If the sac ruptures, the abdominal contents become exposed. Omphalocele often is associated with other anomalies (50% to 70% incidence of anomalies), including cardiac, neurologic, skeletal, and genitourinary (GU) anomalies; imperforate anus; ileal atresia; and bladder exstrophy.

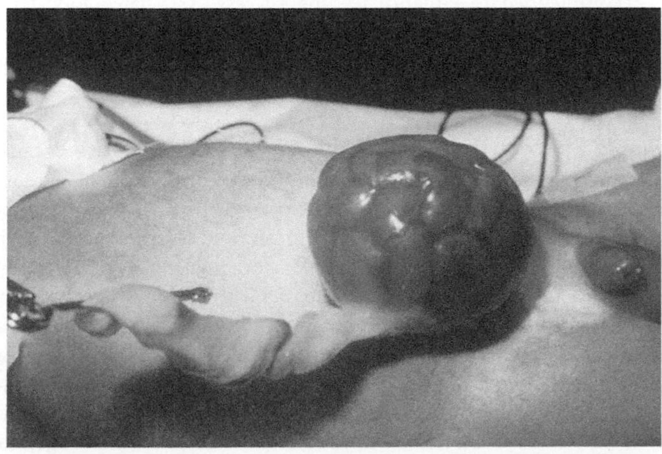

FIG. 25.10 Omphalocele in membranous sac.

Omphalocele is also associated with trisomies 18, Beckwith-Wiedemann syndrome, congenital heart disease, Meckel diverticulum, inguinal hernias, renal or limb deformities, and closed gastroschisis (Watanabe, Suzuki, Hara, et al., 2017).

A small omphalocele may go undetected at first glance and appear as a bulge in the umbilical cord. It is therefore imperative to inspect an unusually large umbilical cord for omphalocele before clamping to prevent possible damage to bowel tissue. (See Care of the Umbilicus, Chapter 7.)

With the increasing frequency of and improvements in prenatal ultrasonography, many abdominal wall defects are being diagnosed prenatally. The benefits of prenatal ultrasonographic diagnosis include the ability to transfer the mother to a tertiary care center, where pediatric surgeons and a neonatal intensive care unit are available to assist with care after delivery.

Initial management after delivery includes inspection of the defect and any associated anomalies. If the bowel covering is intact, a nonadherent dressing is placed over the defect to prevent injury; if the bowel is exposed, the exposed abdominal contents and membranes are covered with a bowel bag or moist dressings and a plastic drape to prevent excessive fluid loss, drying, and temperature instability. IV fluids and antibiotics are administered, and a further evaluation for other associated anomalies is completed. Placement of a Silastic double-lumen catheter (NG-OG) is performed to accomplish gastric bowel decompression.

After initial medical management and stabilization, several surgical options may be carried out, depending on the size of the defect, associated medical problems, and surgeon preference. Primary closure of the omphalocele is one option if the defect is small. The sac is resected, contents are reduced into the abdominal cavity, and an attempt is made to close the abdominal fascia with sutures. The abdominal wall may need to be stretched. If an intestinal atresia exists, a bowel resection may be performed, possibly involving a diverting stoma.

When primary closure of the defect is not possible because of the small size of the abdominal cavity or an extremely large omphalocele, staged reduction is accomplished. One nonoperative approach with a large omphalocele is to treat the omphalocele sac with a topical substance such as silver sulfadiazine to enhance epithelialization of the membrane (Ledbetter, 2012). Additional reduction of the defect may be used by applying a compression dressing or elastic bandage. This process may take up to 12 months and the infant can be started on regular feedings; parents can be taught to apply the topical ointment or dressings at home (Ledbetter, 2012). Another approach involves closure with skin flaps from the lateral abdominal wall. In the event that the sac has been disrupted, a silo mesh may be used to house the omphalocele as described in the care of the gastroschesis.

Postoperatively these infants may require mechanical ventilation and parenteral nutrition. Intraabdominal compression may prevent effective respiration and restrict blood flow to the lower extremities and abdominal organs. Feedings may resume once adequate bowel function is established. Postoperatively the infant is monitored for complications seen with abdominal surgery, including infection, evisceration, intestinal volvulus, obstruction, and a ventral hernia.

Long-term complications include GER, failure to thrive (growth failure), ventral hernia, and feeding issues if the infant has been on NPO status for a lengthy period. Additional complications may occur related to the presence of associated conditions such as Beckwith-Wiedemann syndrome.

Gastroschisis

Gastroschisis occurs when the bowel herniates through a defect in the abdominal wall to the right of the umbilical cord and through the rectus muscle (Fig. 25.11). There is no membrane covering the exposed

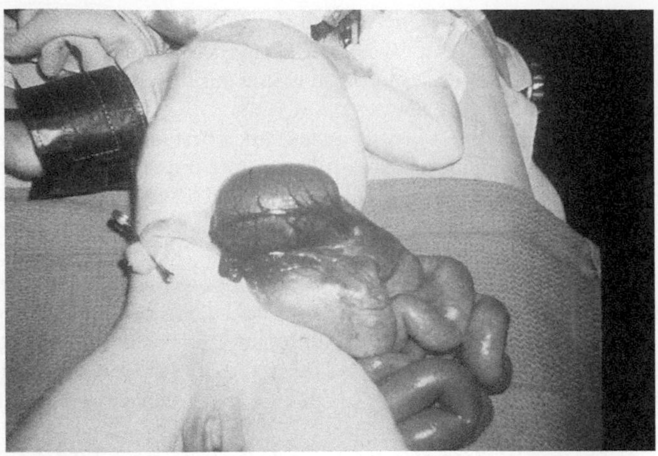

FIG. 25.11 Gastroschisis with exposed bowel (uncovered for photo purposes only).

bowel. Controversy exists regarding the etiology of gastroschisis. It has been suggested that at some point between the bowel's stay in the umbilical cord and the completion of fixation, a tear occurs at the base of the umbilical cord, allowing the intestine to herniate. The gap between the cord and the tear is filled in by skin, giving the appearance of a defect in the abdominal wall to the right of the umbilical cord. The base of the defect is narrow, and the lack of membranes results in thickening and foreshortening of the bowel. Gastroschisis is usually not associated with other major congenital anomalies (10% to 20% incidence of associated anomalies); however, jejunoileal atresia, ischemic enteritis, and malrotation may occur as a result of the defect itself. Gastroschisis has been classified as simple and complicated; those within the latter category may involve bowel atresia, perforation, ischemia, or necrosis (Lakshminarayanan & Lakhoo, 2014). Prenatal management of gastroschesis is evolving with emphasis on protection of the bowel from the effects of amniotic fluid, but there is no evidence-based consensus on prenatal management at this time.

Initial management involves covering the exposed bowel with a transparent plastic bowel bag or loose, moist dressings. If the opening in the abdominal cavity through which the bowel is protruding is small and strangulation of the bowel is possible, the abdominal opening is enlarged at the bedside. IV fluids and antibiotics are administered, and a double-lumen NG tube is inserted for bowel decompression. Fluid replacement for gastroschisis is increased twofold to threefold because of large losses from the exposed viscera.

Adequate thermoregulation and fluid management are extremely important for both omphalocele and gastroschisis. During surgery the abdominal wall is stretched and the mass of bowel is replaced in the abdomen. If primary closure is not possible, a prefabricated, spring-loaded Silastic silo is placed over the unprotected bowel in labor and delivery or in the neonatal intensive care unit shortly after birth to protect the bowel and decrease fluid loss; primary surgical closure is attempted at a later date once the bowel is reduced. The silo is reduced over several days or weeks, at which time it is removed surgically and the defect is closed. Infection is a concern during this period.

Infants with gastroschisis have traditionally been operated on within 24 hours of birth because of temperature instability, risk of infection in the unprotected bowel, and fluid loss. Studies have shown that outcomes vary in regards to early surgical closure versus silo management and later surgical closure; some outcomes are heavily dependent on the amount of bowel to be replaced into the abdominal cavity and subsequent intraabdominal pressure with primary closure. However, simple gastroschisis when the bowel is in good condition is usually treated with immediate closure (Lakshminarayanan & Lakhoo, 2014).

Postoperatively most infants require mechanical ventilation because of respiratory distress secondary to increased abdominal pressure. Pain management is imperative, especially in the first 72 hours. Morphine and fentanyl are effective opioid analgesics. Many infants also require prolonged nutritional support (parenteral and enteral) because of poor bowel function. Prolonged parenteral nutrition may cause liver failure. Exposure of the bowel to amniotic fluid in utero predisposes the infant to prolonged paralytic ileus and hypomotility. Other complications include infection, transient renal impairment, intestinal obstruction, vena cava compression, and a subsequent decrease in blood flow to the lower extremities.

Prognosis

Advanced surgical techniques, improved parenteral nutrition delivery systems, and better medical management have improved the prognosis for the newborn with an abdominal wall defect. Survival estimates for infants with gastroschisis range from 96% for simple gastroschisis to 89% for complex gastroschisis (Lakshminarayanan & Lakhoo, 2014). Because many newborns with omphalocele often have serious associated congenital anomalies, the prognosis for survival of such infants is often not as predictable or as positive as it is for those with gastroschisis (Watanabe, Suzuki, Hara, et al., 2017).

Nursing Care Management

Nursing care is similar to that for any high-risk infant. Infection is a constant threat before surgery, and careful positioning and handling are necessary to prevent rupture of the omphalocele sac or herniated bowel, or disturbance of the Silastic material used for gradual silo reduction. Viscera should be protected with moist dressings or a silo as described previously. Heat and fluid loss from the exposed viscera are major concerns in the preoperative period. Therefore thermoregulation and attention to adequate fluid volume are critical. Fluid replacement is vital and must compensate for losses. The GI tract is decompressed via an NG tube before surgery to aid in bowel reduction.

Postoperative care includes monitoring for signs of complications and assessment of bowel function; pain management with an opioid is also important in the recovery of the infant. Parenteral nutritional support may be necessary when ileus persists. It may require several days or weeks for normal bowel function to return and before full feedings can be achieved. Infants with a prolonged bowel recovery phase are prime candidates for the development of feeding resistance; therefore consultation with a feeding specialist in the early postoperative period is recommended to enhance feeding success. Associated long-term problems with gastroschisis include bowel adhesions, bowel obstruction, necrotizing enterocolitis, parenteral nutrition–related cholestasis, and poor weight gain (Lakshminarayanan & Lakhoo, 2014).

Family Support, Discharge Planning, and Home Care. Because these abdominal defects are visible and may be shocking to parents, immediate emotional support at the time of birth is essential. The family needs a brief explanation of the defect and reassurance that their child is in no immediate danger (unless circumstances are different). After the parents have had time to interact with their newborn, inform them about the surgical treatment and postoperative care. At the time of discharge from the hospital, many of these infants are receiving oral feedings, but extended parenteral nutrition may be required if malabsorption and poor bowel function occur. The nurse can ensure continuity of care by referral to a home health care agency, especially if long-term nutritional support is required.

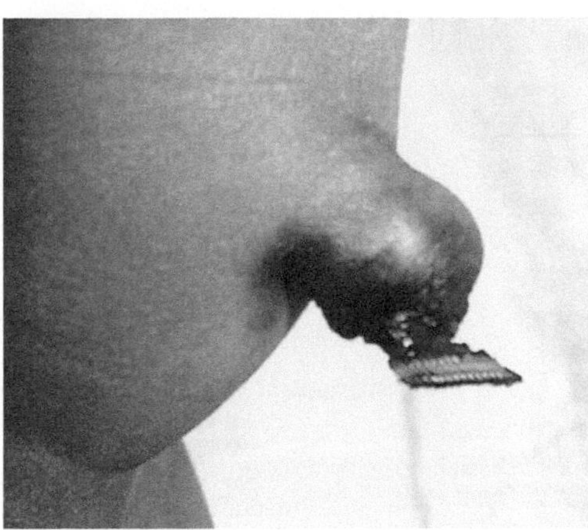

FIG. 25.12 Newborn with umbilical hernia. (From Zitelli, B. J., & Davis, H. W. [2007]. *Atlas of pediatric physical diagnosis* [5th ed.]. St. Louis, MO: Mosby).

HERNIAS

A **hernia** is a protrusion of a portion of an organ or organs through an abnormal opening. The danger of herniation arises when the protrusion is constricted, impairing circulation, or when the protrusion interferes with the function or development of other structures. The herniations discussed in this section are those that protrude through the diaphragm, the abdominal wall, or the inguinal canal.

UMBILICAL HERNIA

The **umbilical hernia** is a common hernia observed in infants. It occurs when fusion of the umbilical ring is incomplete at the point where the umbilical vessels exit the abdominal wall. It affects low-birth-weight and preterm infants more often than full-term infants. An umbilical hernia usually is an isolated defect, but it may be associated with other congenital anomalies, such as Down syndrome (trisomy 21) and trisomies 13 and 18. The size of the defect is variable, and the protrusion is more prominent when the infant is crying (Fig. 25.12). **Incarceration**, in which the hernia is constricted and cannot be reduced manually, is rare. Hernias usually resolve spontaneously by 3 to 5 years of age. If the hernia persists beyond this age, it is usually surgically corrected on an elective basis.

Nursing Care Management

The appearance of an umbilical hernia may be disconcerting to parents. Therefore they need reassurance that the defect usually is not harmful. Taping or strapping the abdomen to flatten the protrusion does not aid in resolution and can produce skin irritation.

Nursing care of the child with an umbilical hernia repair is essentially the same as that for other minor GI surgery. The procedure may be performed on an outpatient basis. Observe the child for complications related to a hematoma or infection. The child may resume a normal diet and activity postoperatively; however, strenuous activity or play is restricted for 2 to 3 weeks.

INGUINAL HERNIA

Inguinal hernias account for approximately 80% of all childhood hernias and occur more frequently in boys than in girls (approximately 6:1). An incidence of 0.8% to 5% is reported in term newborns and up to 30% in low-birth-weight and preterm infants (Abdulhai, Glenn, & Ponsky, 2017).

Pathophysiology

Inguinal hernia comes from persistence of all or part of the processus vaginalis, the tube of peritoneum that precedes the testicle through the inguinal canal into the scrotum (in boys), or the round ligament into the labia (in girls), during the eighth month of gestation. After descent of the testicle, the proximal portion of the processus vaginalis normally atrophies and closes, whereas the distal portion forms the tunica vaginalis, which envelops the testicle in the scrotum. When the upper portion fails to atrophy, the abdominal fluid or an abdominal structure (e.g., bowel, ovary, fallopian tubes) can be forced into it, creating a palpable bulge or mass. The persistent sac may end at any point along the inguinal canal; it may stop at the inguinal ring or extend all the way into the scrotum or labia (Fig. 25.13).

Clinical Manifestations

This common defect is usually asymptomatic unless the abdominal contents are forced into the patent sac. Most often it appears as a painless inguinal swelling that varies in size. It disappears during periods of rest or is reducible by gentle compression. It appears when the infant cries or strains or when the older child strains, coughs, or stands for a long time. The defect can be palpated as a thickening of the cord in the groin, and the silk glove sign can be elicited by rubbing together the sides of the empty hernial sac.

Sometimes the herniated loop of intestine becomes partially obstructed, producing variable symptoms that may include irritability, tenderness, anorexia, abdominal distention, and difficulty defecating. Occasionally the loop of bowel becomes **incarcerated** (irreducible) or strangulated (loss of blood supply), with symptoms of complete intestinal obstruction that, left untreated, will progress to strangulation and necrotic bowel. Incarceration occurs more often in infants under 12 months of age. The incidence of incarceration is reported to be 3% to 16% but as high as 30% in premature infants (Abdulhai, Glenn, & Ponsky, 2017).

Therapeutic Management

The treatment for hernias is prompt, elective surgical repair in the healthy child as soon as the defect is diagnosed. However, an incarcerated hernia requires emergent surgical care. Because there was believed to be a significant incidence of bilateral involvement, many surgeons advocated exploration of both sides; however, this practice has gained disfavor due to complications occurring with open exploration (Aiken & Oldham, 2016b). Laparoscopic exploration of the contralateral side may be performed without risk of injury to the vas deferens (Aiken & Oldham, 2016b).

Nursing Care Management

Prompt recognition of an inguinal hernia is imperative. The hernia may first be noticed when the infant is crying or straining to stool (Valsalva maneuver). Nursing care of the infant or child with an inguinal hernia involves preoperative preparation of the infant and appropriate explanation to the parents of the child's expected postoperative status. Most hernia repairs can be managed on an outpatient basis. The preterm infant usually has hernia repair several days before discharge. The former preterm infant diagnosed after discharge is admitted the day of surgery and, after repair, is observed for 12 to 24 hours for apnea and bradycardia.

Postoperatively the incision is kept clean and dry, and the infant's pain is managed appropriately. In infants and small children who are not yet toilet trained, the wound may be covered with an occlusive dressing or left without a dressing. Changing diapers as soon as they become damp helps reduce the chance of irritation or infection of the incision.

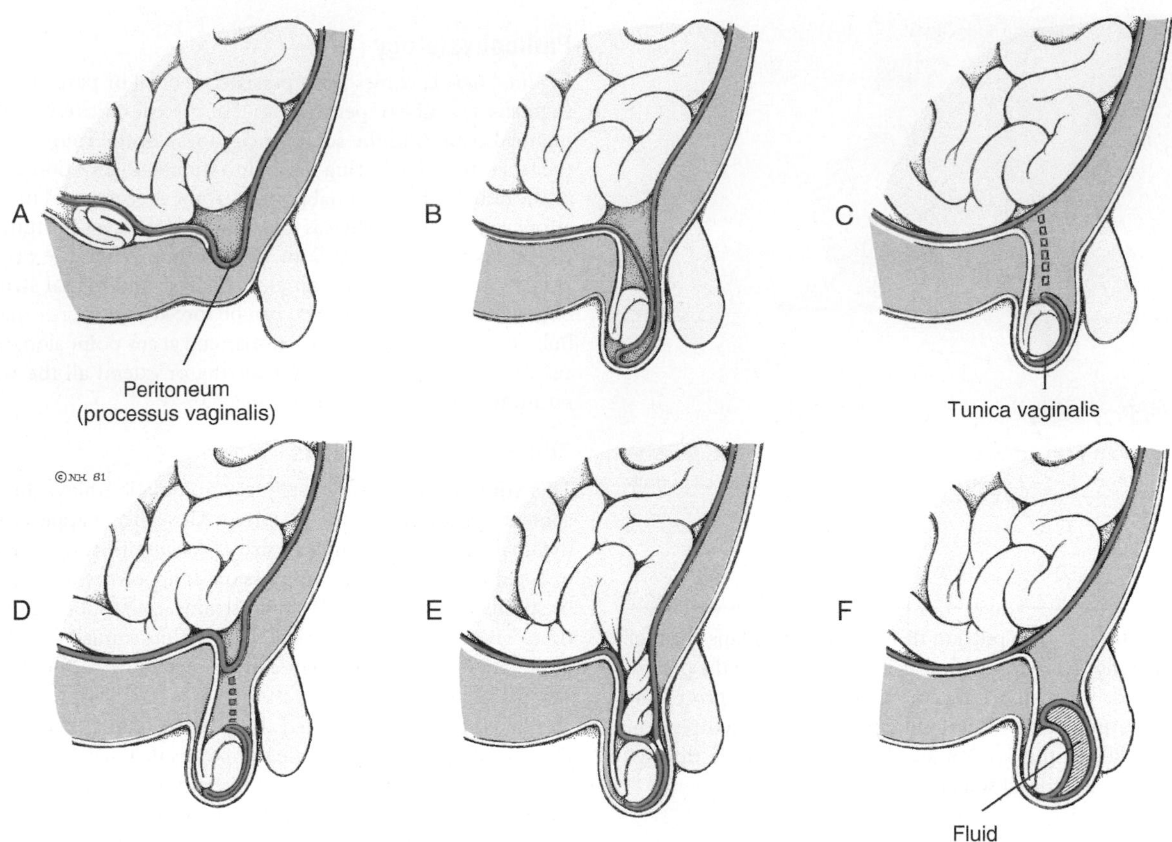

FIG. 25.13 Development of inguinal hernias. **A** and **B,** Prenatal migration of processus vaginalis. **C,** Normal. **D,** Partially obliterated processus vaginalis. **E,** Hernia. **F,** Hydrocele.

No restrictions are placed on activity for the infant or toddler, but older children are cautioned against lifting, pushing, wrestling or fighting, bicycle riding, and participation in sporting events for about 3 weeks.

If surgery is postponed, parents need to learn the signs of incarcerated hernia, simple measures to reduce it (e.g., a warm bath, avoidance of upright positioning, and comfort measures to reduce crying), and where to call for assistance if relief is not obtained in a reasonably short time.

FEMORAL HERNIA

Femoral hernias are rare in children, with a reported incidence of less than 1% (Abdulhai, Glenn, & Ponsky, 2017). The incidence is higher in girls than in boys. The hernia may manifest as a recurrent hernia after inguinal hernia repair. Initial symptoms are swelling in the groin area associated with severe abdominal pain and cramping. Treatment and management are the same as for inguinal hernia. Incarceration and strangulation are frequent complications.

ANORECTAL MALFORMATIONS

Anorectal malformations (ARMs) are among the more common congenital malformations caused by abnormal development, with an incidence of approximately 1 in 3000 births (Akay & Klein, 2016). These malformations may range from simple imperforate anus to other associated complex anomalies of GU and pelvic organs, which may require extensive treatment for fecal, urinary, and sexual function. Anorectal malformations may occur in isolation or as a part of the VACTERL association (see earlier in this chapter). These anomalies are classified according to the newborn's gender and abnormal anatomic features, including GU defects (Box 25.19). More than half of all ARMs are associated with other anomalies.

BOX 25.19 Classification of Anorectal Malformations

Male Defects

Perineal fistula
Rectourethral bulbar fistula
Rectourethral prostatic fistula
Rectovesicular (bladder neck) fistula
Imperforate anus without fistula
Rectal atresia

Female Defects

Perineal fistula
Rectovestibular fistula
Imperforate anus without fistula
Rectal atresia
Rectovaginal fistula
Cloaca

From Gangopadhyay, A. N., & Pandey, V. (2015). Anorectal malformations. *Journal of Indian Association of Pediatric Surgeons, 20*(1), 10-15.

Rectal atresia and stenosis occur when the anal opening appears normal, there is a midline intergluteal groove, and usually no fistula exists between the rectum and urinary tract. **Rectal atresia** is a complete obstruction (inability to pass stool) and requires immediate

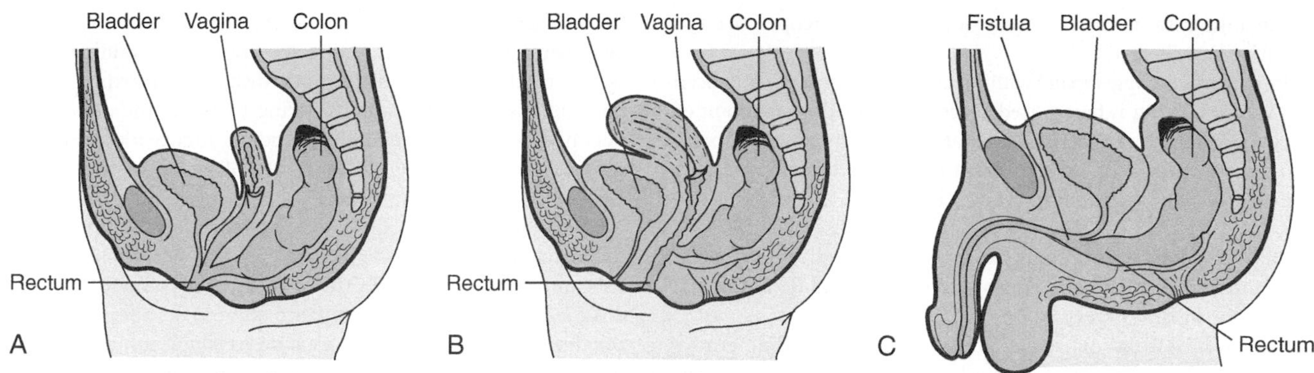

FIG. 25.14 Anorectal malformations. **A,** Typical cloaca (female). **B,** Low rectovaginal fistula (female). **C,** Rectourethral bulbar fistula (male).

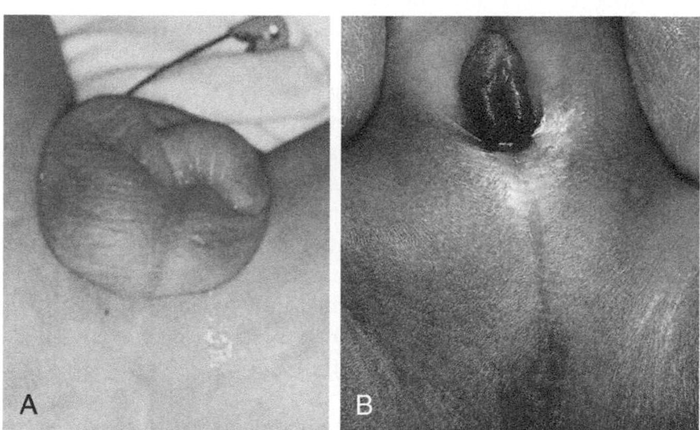

FIG. 25.15 A, No visible external opening is consistent with high imperforate anus defect; absence of intergluteal cleft is also common. **B,** Imperforate anus in female, commonly associated with cloacal anomaly, which manifests as a single perineal opening on perineum. (From Zitelli, B. J., & Davis, H. W. [2007]. *Atlas of pediatric physical diagnosis* [5th ed.]. St. Louis, MO: Mosby.)

surgical intervention. Rectal stenosis may not become apparent until later in infancy when the infant has a history of difficult stooling, abdominal distention, and ribbonlike stools. A persistent cloaca is a complex anorectal malformation in which the rectum, vagina, and urethra drain into a common channel opening into the perineum (Fig. 25.14, *A*).

Imperforate anus includes several forms of malformation without an obvious opening (Fig. 25.15). Frequently a fistula (an abnormal communication) leads from the distal rectum to the perineum or GU system (see Fig. 25.14, *B* and *C*). The fistula may be evidenced when meconium is evacuated through the vaginal opening, the perineum below the vagina, the male urethra, or the perineum under the scrotum. The presence of meconium on the perineum does not indicate anal patency. A fistula may not be apparent at birth, but as peristalsis increases, meconium is forced through the fistula into the urethra or onto the newborn's perineum.

Pathophysiology

During embryonic development the cloaca becomes the common channel for the developing urinary, genital, and rectal systems. The cloaca is divided at the sixth week of gestation into an anterior urogenital sinus and a posterior intestinal channel by the urorectal septum. After the lateral folds join the urorectal septum, separation of the urinary and rectal segments takes place. Further differentiation results in the anterior GU system and the posterior anorectal channel. An interruption of this development leads to incomplete migration of the rectum to its normal perineal position.

Diagnostic Evaluation

The diagnosis of an anorectal malformation is based on the physical finding of an absent anal opening. Other symptoms may include abdominal distention, vomiting, absence of meconium passage, or presence of meconium in the urine. Additional physical findings with an anorectal malformation are a flat perineum and the absence of a midline intergluteal groove. The appearance of the perineum alone does not accurately predict the extent of the defect and associated anomalies. GU and spinal-vertebral anomalies associated with anorectal malformations should be considered when an anomaly is noted. EA with or without TEF, cardiac defects, and spinal or vertebral anomalies may occur in association with anorectal malformations, and the infant should be carefully evaluated for the presence of these and other anomalies. Although rare, some ARMs may not be diagnosed until later in infancy or early childhood.

A perineal fistula (see Box 25.19) may be diagnosed by clinical observation. The presence of a prominent anal dimple and a band of skin tissue commonly known as a bucket handle is indicative of a perineal fistula. Abdominal and pelvic ultrasonography is performed to further evaluate the infant's anatomic malformation. An IV pyelogram and a voiding cystourethrogram are performed to evaluate associated anomalies involving the urinary tract. Other diagnostic examinations that may be performed include pelvic magnetic resonance imaging, radiography, ultrasound, and fluoroscopic examination of pelvic anatomic contents and lower spinal anatomy.

Therapeutic Management

The primary management of anorectal malformations is surgical. Once the defect is identified, take steps to rule out associated life-threatening defects, which need immediate surgical intervention. Provided no immediate life-threatening problems exist, the newborn is stabilized and kept NPO for further evaluation. IV fluids are provided to maintain glucose and fluid and electrolyte balance. Current recommendation is that surgery be delayed at least 24 hours to properly evaluate for the presence of a fistula and possibly other anomalies (Akay & Klein, 2016).

The surgical treatment of anorectal malformations varies according to the defect but usually involves one, or possibly a combination of several, of the following procedures: anoplasty, colostomy, posterior sagittal anorectoplasty (PSARP) or other pull-through with colostomy, and colostomy (take-down) closure. The Nursing Care

Management discussion below outlines some aspects of preoperative and postoperative care.

A primary laparoscopic repair (without colostomy) of some anorectal malformations is being is being used successfully for the treatment of ARMs. This minimizes surgical risks, associated morbidity, and postoperative pain management with no significant risk for rectal prolapse, anal stenosis, or anorectal manometry (Han, Xia, Guo, et al., 2017).

Prognosis. The long-term prognosis depends on such factors as the type of defect, anatomy of the sacrum and vertebrae, quality of muscles, and the success of the surgery.

The presence of a flat or "rocker" bottom and no midline groove usually carries a poor prognosis for bowel continence because of associated neurologic, muscular, and anatomic problems. When the internal anal sphincter is absent, incontinence is a common long-term problem. These children may achieve socially acceptable continence over time with the aid of a bowel management program. Other potential complications after surgical treatment of anorectal anomalies include strictures, recurrent rectourinary fistula, mucosal prolapse, and constipation. Long-term outcomes in adults with surgically treated ARM are reported to be positive, depending on the type and severity of the defect, as well as associated anomalies (Gangopadhyay & Pandey, 2015). Constipation, fecal soiling, and fecal incontinence are problems that such children and adults must deal with on a regular basis, but the functional outcome is reported to be excellent (Gangopadhyay & Pandey, 2015).

Nursing Care Management

The first nursing responsibility is assisting in identification of anorectal malformations. A newborn who does not pass stool within 24 hours after birth or has meconium that appears at a location other than the anal opening requires further assessment. Preoperative care includes diagnostic evaluation, GI decompression, bowel preparation, and IV fluids.

For the newborn with a perineal fistula, an **anoplasty** is performed, which involves moving the fistula opening to the center of the sphincter and enlarging the rectal opening. Postoperative nursing care after anoplasty is primarily directed toward healing the surgical site without other complications. A program of anal dilations is usually initiated when the child returns for the 2-week checkup. Feedings are started soon after surgical repair, and breastfeeding is encouraged because it causes less constipation.

In neonates with anomalies such as **cloaca** (female), rectourethral prostatic fistula (male), and vestibular fistula (female), a descending colostomy is performed to allow fecal elimination and avoid fecal contamination of the distal imperforate section and subsequent urinary tract infection in infants with urorectal fistulas. With a colostomy, postoperative nursing care is directed toward maintaining appropriate skin care at the stoma sites (both distal and proximal), managing postoperative pain, and administering IV fluids and antibiotics. Postoperative NG decompression may be required with laparotomy, and nursing care focuses on maintenance of appropriate drainage. (See Chapter 22 for colostomy care.)

The PSARP is a common surgical procedure for the repair of anorectal malformations in infants approximately 1 to 2 months after the initial colostomy. Preoperative PSARP care often involves irrigation of the distal stoma to prevent fecal contamination of the operative site. During this time parents must be given accurate yet simple information regarding the infant's appearance postoperatively and expectations as to their level of involvement in the child's care.

In the PSARP procedure the repair is made via a posterior midline sacral approach to dissect the different muscle groups involved without damaging strategic innervation of pelvic structures so optimum postoperative bowel continence is achieved. A laparotomy may be required if the rectum is unidentifiable by the posterior approach. Additional management after successful repair involves a program of anal dilations, colostomy closure, and a bowel management program.

Parents are instructed in perineal and wound care or care of the colostomy as needed. Anal dilations may be necessary for some infants. Parents should observe stooling patterns and observe for signs of anal stricture or complications. Information on dietary modifications and administration of medications is included in counseling. Nurses have a vital role in helping families of a child with anorectal malformations provide optimum care so bowel management is successful and quality of life enhanced for the child and family.

Family Support, Discharge Planning, and Home Care. Long-term follow-up care is essential for children with complex malformations. Parents need reassurance when a colostomy is performed regarding the child's appearance and their ability to care for the child at home. With much patience and reassurance, parents learn how to provide optimum care of the skin and the appliance, while maintaining an appropriate bond with the child.

After the definitive pull-through procedure, toilet training may be delayed. Complete continence is seldom achieved at the usual age of 2 to 3 years. Bowel habit training, bowel management irrigation programs, diet modification, and administration of stool softeners or fiber help children improve bowel function and social continence. Some children never achieve bowel continence and must rely on daily bowel irrigations. Support and reassurance during the slow progression to normal, socially acceptable function are essential.

NCLEX REVIEW QUESTIONS

1. A 16-month-old has a history of diarrhea for 3 days with poor oral intake. He received intravenous fluids, has tolerated some oral fluids in the emergency department, and is being discharged home. Instructions for diet for this child should include:
   A. BRAT diet (bananas, rice, applesauce, and toast) for 24 hours, then a soft diet as tolerated
   B. Chicken or beef broth for 24 hours, then resume a soft diet
   C. Offer a regular diet as child's appetite warrants
   D. Keep on clear liquids and toast for 24 hours
2. A 5-month-old infant is seen in the well-child clinic for a complaint of vomiting and failure to grow. His birth weight was 7 lb, and he now weighs 8 lb, 10 oz. The infant's mother reports that he is taking 4 to 7 oz of formula every 4 to 5 hours, but he "spits up a lot after eating and then is hungry again." The child is noted to be alert but appears malnourished. The mother reports that his stools are brown in color, and he has 1 to 2 bowel movements every day. Based on these findings, the nurse anticipates the infant has:
   A. Meckel diverticulum
   B. Hypertrophic pyloric stenosis
   C. Intussusception
   D. Hirschprung disease

3. Because children with celiac disease must limit their intake of products containing gluten in wheat, rye, oats, and barley, they are at risk for which of the following nutritional deficiencies? Select all that apply.
   A. Iron deficiency anemia
   B. Folic acid deficiency
   C. Zinc deficiency
   D. Vitamin A, D, E, and K deficiency
   E. Vitamin B_{12} deficiency
4. A formerly preterm infant who had surgery for necrotizing enterocolitis is now 6 months old and has short-bowel syndrome. He is unable to absorb most nutrients taken by mouth and is totally dependent on parenteral nutrition, which he receives via a central venous catheter. The clinic nurse following this infant is aware that this infant should be closely observed for the development of:
   A. Gastroesophageal reflux
   B. Chronic diarrhea
   C. Cholestasis
   D. Failure to thrive
5. The nurse caring for a 4-month-old infant with biliary atresia and significant urticaria can anticipate administering:
   A. Diphenhydramine
   B. Ursodiol (ursodeoxycholic acid)
   C. Loratidine
   D. Zantac
6. Hepatitis A virus is transmitted by which of the following? Select all that apply.
   A. Breast milk from mother with HAV
   B. Ingestion of contaminated food
   C. Fecal-oral route
   D. Casual contact with infected person
   E. Blood transfusion

Correct Answers

1. C; 2. B; 3. A, B, D; 4. C; 5. B; 6. B, C

REFERENCES

Abbott, R. A., Martin, A. E., Newlove-Delgado, T. V., et al. (2017). Psychosocial interventions for recurrent abdominal pain in childhood. *Cochrane Database of Systematic Review*, (3), CD010973.

Abdulhai, S. A., Glenn, I. C., & Ponsky, T. A. (2017). Incarcerated pediatric hernias. *The Surgical Clinics of North America, 97*(1), 129–145.

Akay, B., & Klein, M. D. (2016). Surgical conditions of the anus and rectum. In R. M. Kliegman, B. F. Stanton, J. W. St. Geme, et al. (Eds.), *Nelson textbook of pediatrics* (20th ed.). Philadelphia: Elsevier/Saunders.

Aiken, J. J., & Oldham, K. T. (2016a). Acute appendicitis. In R. M. Kliegman, B. F. Stanton, J. W. St. Geme, et al. (Eds.), *Nelson textbook of pediatrics* (20th ed.). Philadelphia: Elsevier/Saunders.

Aiken, J. J., & Oldham, K. T. (2016b). Inguinal hernias. In R. M. Kliegman, B. F. Stanton, J. W. St. Geme, et al. (Eds.), *Nelson textbook of pediatrics* (20th ed.). Philadelphia: Elsevier/Saunders.

Bagade, S., & Khanna, G. (2015). Imaging of omphalomesenteric duct remnants and related pathologies in children. *Current Problems in Diagnostic Radiology, 44*(3), 246–255.

Bales, C., & Liacouras, C. A. (2016). Intestinal atresia, stenosis, and malrotation. In R. M. Kliegman, B. F. Stanton, J. W. St. Geme, et al. (Eds.), *Nelson textbook of pediatrics* (20th ed.). Philadelphia: Elsevier/Saunders.

Barnes, D., & Yeh, A. M. (2015). Bugs and guts: Practical applications of probiotics for gastrointestinal disorders in children. *Nutrition in Clinical Practice, 30*(6), 747–759.

Bass, D. M. (2016). Rotaviruses, caliciviruses, and astroviruses. In R. M. Kliegman, B. F. Stanton, J. W. St. Geme, et al. (Eds.), *Nelson textbook of pediatrics* (20th ed.). Philadelphia: Elsevier/Saunders.

Berdan, E. A., & Sato, T. T. (2017). Pediatric airway and esophageal foreign bodies. *The Surgical Clinics of North America, 97*(1), 85–91.

Bhutta, Z. A. (2016). Acute gastroenteritis in children. In R. M. Kliegman, B. F. Stanton, J. W. St Geme, et al. (Eds.), *Nelson textbook of pediatrics* (20th ed.). Philadelphia: Saunders/Elsevier.

Blanchard, S. S., & Czinn, S. J. (2016). Peptic ulcer disease in children. In R. M. Kliegman, B. F. Stanton, J. W. St. Geme, et al. (Eds.), *Nelson textbook of pediatrics* (20th ed.). Philadelphia: Elsevier/Saunders.

Branski, D., Troncone, R., & Fasano, A. (2016). Celiac disease. In R. M. Kliegman, B. F. Stanton, J. W. St. Geme, et al. (Eds.), *Nelson textbook of pediatrics* (20th ed.). Philadelphia: Elsevier/Saunders.

Bruce, J. S., Bruce, C. S., Short, H., et al. (2016). Childhood constipation: Recognition, management and the role of the nurse. *British Journal of Nursing (Mark Allen Publishing), 25*(22), 1231–1242.

Carroll, A. G., Kavanagh, R. G., Ni Leidhin, C., et al. (2017). Comparative effectiveness of imaging modalities for the diagnosis and treatment of intussusception: A critically appraised topic. *Academic Radiology, 24*(5), 521–529.

Casciani, E., Nardo, G. D., Chin, S., et al. (2017). MR enterography in paediatric patients with obscure gastrointestinal bleeding. *European Journal of Radiology, 93*, 209–216.

Centers for Disease Control and Prevention. (2017). *Surveillance for viral hepatitis – United States, 2015*. https://www.cdc.gov/hepatitis/statistics/2015surveillance/index.htm.

Chopra, J., Patel, N., Basude, D., et al. (2017). Abdominal pain-related functional gastrointestinal disorders in children. *British Journal of Nursing (Mark Allen Publishing), 26*(11), 624–631.

Choudhary, N. S., Puri, R., Saigal, S., et al. (2016). Innovative approach of using esophageal stent for refractory post-band ligation esophageal ulcer bleed following liver donor liver transplantation. *Journal of Clinical and Experimental Hepatology, 6*(2), 149–150.

Cohen, S., Bueno de Mesquita, M., & Mimouni, F. B. (2015). Adverse effects reported in the use of gastroesophageal reflux disease treatments in children: A 10 years literature review. *British Journal of Clinical Pharmacology, 80*(2), 200–208.

Cohran, V. C., Prozialeck, J. D., & Cole, C. R. (2017). Redefining short bowel syndrome in the 21st century. *Pediatric Research, 81*(4), 540–549.

Conrad, M. A., & Rosh, J. R. (2017). Pediatric inflammatory bowel disease. *Pediatric Clinics of North America, 64*(3), 577–591.

Dekate, P., Jayashree, M., & Singhi, S. (2013). Management of acute diarrhea in emergency room. *Indian Journal of Pediatrics, 80*(3), 235–246.

Fiorino, K., & Liacouras, C. A. (2016). Congenital aganglionic megacolon (Hirschsprung disease). In R. M. Kliegman, B. F. Stanton, J. W. St. Geme, et al. (Eds.), *Nelson textbook of pediatrics* (20th ed.). Philadelphia: Elsevier/Saunders.

Fok, C. Y., Holland, K. S., Gil-Zaragozano, E., et al. (2016). The role of nurses and dieticians in managing paediatric coeliac disease. *British Journal of Nursing (Mark Allen Publishing), 25*(8), 449–455.

Gangopadhyay, A. N., & Pandey, V. (2015). Anorectal malformations. *Journal of Indian Association of Pediatric Surgeons, 20*(1), 10–15.

Giannetti, E., Maglione, M., Sciorio, E., et al. (2017). Do children just grow out of irritable bowel syndrome? *The Journal of Pediatrics, 183*, 122–126.

Govindarajan, K. K. (2016). Biliary atresia: Where do we stand now? *World Journal of Hepatology, 8*(36), 1593–1601.

Grossman, A. B., & Baldassano, R. N. (2016). Chronic ulcerative colitis. In R. M. Kliegman, B. F. Stanton, J. W. St. Geme, et al. (Eds.), *Nelson textbook of pediatrics* (20th ed.). Philadelphia: Elsevier/Saunders.

Han, Y., Xia, Z., Guo, S., et al. (2017). Laparoscopically assisted anorectal pull-through versus posterior sagittal anorectoplasy for high and intermediate anorectal malformations: A systematic review and meta-analysis. *PLoS ONE, 12*(1), e0170421.

Hassan, H. H., & Balistreri, W. F. (2016). Cholestasis. In R. M. Kliegman, B. F. Stanton, J. W. St Geme, et al. (Eds.), *Nelson textbook of pediatrics* (20th ed.). Philadelphia: Saunders/Elsevier.

Hunter, A. K., & Liacouras, C. A. (2016). Pyloric stenosis and other congenital anomalies of the stomach. In R. M. Kliegman, B. F. Stanton, J. W. St. Geme, et al. (Eds.), *Nelson textbook of pediatrics* (20th ed.). Philadelphia: Elsevier/Saunders.

Jensen, M. K., & Balistreri, W. F. (2016). Viral hepatitis. In R. M. Kliegman, B. F. Stanton, J. W. St Geme, et al. (Eds.), *Nelson textbook of pediatrics* (20th ed.). Philadelphia: Elsevier/Saunders.

Kalach, N., Bontems, P., & Cadranel, S. (2015). Advances in the treatment of Helicobacter pylori infection in children. *Annals of Gastroenterology, 28*(1), 10–18.

Katz, E. R., Kitts, R. L., & DeMaso, D. R. (2016). Pica. In R. M. Kliegman, B. F. Stanton, J. W. St. Geme, et al. (Eds.), *Nelson textbook of pediatrics* (20th ed.). Philadelphia: Elsevier/Saunders.

Kennedy, M., & Liacouras, C. A. (2016a). Intestinal duplications, Meckel diverticulum, and other remnants of the omphalomesenteric duct. In R. M. Kliegman, B. F. Stanton, J. W. St. Geme, et al. (Eds.), *Nelson textbook of pediatrics* (20th ed.). Philadelphia: Elsevier/Saunders.

Kennedy, M., & Liacouras, C. A. (2016b). Intussusception. In R. M. Kliegman, B. F. Stanton, J. W. St. Geme, et al. (Eds.), *Nelson textbook of pediatrics* (20th ed.). Philadelphia: Elsevier/Saunders.

Khan, S., & Orenstein, S. R. (2016a). Ingestions. In R. M. Kliegman, B. F. Stanton, J. W. St. Geme, et al. (Eds.), *Nelson textbook of pediatrics* (20th ed.). Philadelphia: Elsevier/Saunders.

Khan, S., & Orenstein, S. R. (2016b). Gastroesophageal reflux disease. In R. M. Kliegman, B. F. Stanton, J. W. St. Geme, et al. (Eds.), *Nelson textbook of pediatrics* (20th ed.). Philadelphia: Elsevier/Saunders.

Khan, S., & Orenstein, S. R. (2016c). Esophageal atresia and tracheoesophageal fistula. In R. M. Kliegman, B. F. Stanton, J. W. St. Geme, et al. (Eds.), *Nelson textbook of pediatrics* (20th ed.). Philadelphia: Elsevier/Saunders.

Kotloff, K. L. (2017). The burden and etiology of diarrheal illness in developing countries. *Pediatric Clinics of North America, 64*(4), 799–814.

Kridler, J., & Kamat, D. (2016). Irritable bowel syndrome: A review for general pediatricians. *Pediatric Annals, 45*(1), e30–e33.

Lakshminarayanan, B., & Lakhoo, K. (2014). Abdominal wall defects. *Early Human Development, 90*(12), 917–920.

Lamberti, L. M., Ashraf, S., Walker, C. L., et al. (2016). A systematic review of the effect of rotavirus vaccination on diarrhea outcomes among children younger than 5 years. *The Pediatric Infectious Disease Journal, 35*(9), 992–998.

Laya, B. F., Restrepo, R., & Lee, E. Y. (2017). Practical imaging evaluation of foreign bodies in children: An update. *Radiologic Clinics of North America, 55*(4), 845–867.

Lebwohl, B., Sanders, D. S., & Green, P. H. R. (2017). *Coeliac disease, Lancet epub ahead of print.*

Ledbetter, D. J. (2012). Congenital abdominal wall defects and reconstruction in pediatric surgery: Gastroschesis and omphalocele. *The Surgical clinics of North America, 92*(3), 713–727.

Leung, D. T., Chisti, M. J., & Pavia, A. T. (2016). Prevention and control of childhood pneumonia and diarrhea. *Pediatric Clinics of North America, 63*(1), 67–79.

Lin, X. K., Huang, X. Z., Bao, X. Z., et al. (2017). Clinical characteristics of Meckel diverticulum in children: A retrospective review of a 15-year single-center experience. *Medicine, 96*(32), e7760.

Marder, E. P., Cieslak, P. R., Cronquist, A. B., et al. (2017). Incidence and trends of infections with pathogens transmitted commonly through food and the effect of increasing use of culture-independent diagnostic tests on surveillance – foodborne disease active surveillance network, 10 U.S. sites, 2013-2016. *MMWR. Morbidity and Mortality Weekly Report, 66*(15), 397–403.

Martin, L. Y., Ladd, M. R., Werts, A., et al. (2017). Tissue engineering for the treatment of short bowel syndrome in children. *Pediatric Research*, epub ahead of print.

McFarland, L. V., Ozen, M., Dinleyici, E. C., et al. (2016). Comparison of pediatric and adult antibiotic-associated diarrhea and Clostridium dificile infections. *World Journal of Gastroenterology : WJG, 22*(11), 3078–3104.

Mousa, H., & Hassan, M. (2017). Gastroesophageal reflux disease. *Pediatric Clinics of North America, 64*(3), 487–505.

Muller, C. O., Rossignol, G., Montalva, L., et al. (2016). Long-term outcome of laparoscopic Duhamel procedure for extended Hirschsprung's disease. *Journal of Laparoendoscopic and Advanced Surgical Techniques. Part A, 26*(12), 1032–1035.

Newlove-Delgado, T. V., Martin, A. E., Abbott, R. A., et al. (2017). Dietary interventions for recurrent abdominal pain in childhood. *Cochrane Database of Systematic Review*, (3), CD010972.

Patel, R., Bommayya, N., Choudhry, M., et al. (2015). Bleeding duodenal ulcer in a healthy infant presenting with rectal bleeding and requiring surgical treatment. *Journal of Pediatric Surgical Special, 9*, 38–40.

Paul, S. P., McVeigh, L., Gil-Zaragozano, E., et al. (2016). Diagnosis and nursing management of coeliac disease in children. *Nursing Children and Young People, 28*(1), 18–24.

Poddar, U. (2016). Approach to constipation in children. *Indian Pediatrics, 53*(4), 319–327.

Rentea, R. M., Peter, D., & Snyder, C. L. (2017). Pediatric appendicitis: State of the art review. *Pediatric Surgery International, 33*(3), 269–283.

Rosen, M. J., Dhawan, A., & Saeed, S. A. (2017). Inflammatory bowel disease in children and adolescents. *JAMA Pediatrics, 169*(11), 1053–1060.

Sreedharan, R., & Liacouras, C. A. (2016). Major symptoms and signs of digestive tract disorders. In R. M. Kliegman, B. F. Stanton, J. W. St. Geme, et al. (Eds.), *Nelson textbook of pediatrics* (20th ed.). Philadelphia: Elsevier/Saunders.

St Louis, A. M., Kim, K., Browne, M. L., et al. (2017). Prevalence trends of selected major birth defects: A multi-state population-based retrospective study, United States, 1999 to 2007. *Birth Defects Research*, epub ahead of print.

United Network for Organ Sharing. (2017). *Questions and answers for transplant candidates about liver allocation.* https://www.unos.org/wp-content/uploads/unos/Liver_patient.pdf.

Vanderhoof, J. A., & Branski, D. (2016). Short bowel syndrome. In R. M. Kliegman, B. F. Stanton, J. W. St. Geme, et al. (Eds.), *Nelson textbook of pediatrics* (20th ed.). Philadelphia: Elsevier/Saunders.

Watanabe, S., Suzuki, T., Hara, F., et al. (2017). Omphalocele and gastroschisis in newborns: Over 16 years of experience from a single clinic. *Journal of Neonatal Surgery, 6*(2), 27.

Wen, S. C., Best, E., & Nourse, C. (2017). Non-typhoidal Salmonella infections in children: Review of literature and recommendations for management. *Journal of Paediatrics and Child Health*, epub ahead of print.

Wu, Y., Kuang, H., Lv, T., et al. (2017). Comparison of clinical outcomes between open and thoracoscopic repairfor esophageal atresia with tracheoesophageal fistula: A systematic review and meta-analysis. *Pediatric Surgery International*, epub ahead of print.

Yanagi, Y., Matsuura, T., Hayashida, M., et al. (2017). Bowel perforation after liver transplantation for biliary atresia: A retrospective study of care in the transition from childhood to adulthood. *Pediatric Surgery International, 33*(2), 155–163.

Yang, H. R. (2016). Updates on the diagnosis of Helicobacter pylori infection in children: What are the differences between adults and children? *Pediatric Gastroenterology, Hepatology & Nutrition, 19*(2), 96–103.

26

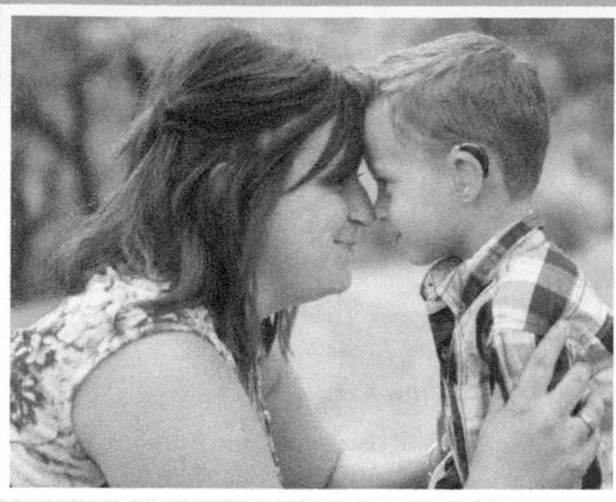

The Child With Respiratory Dysfunction

Patricia Conlon

http://evolve.elsevier.com/wong/ncic

CONCEPTS

- Gas Exchange
- Inflammation
- Infection
- Fluid and Electrolyte Balance
- Patient Education

RESPIRATORY TRACT STRUCTURE

The thoracic cavity, located in the bony framework provided by the ribs, vertebrae, and sternum, consists of three major sections: the three-lobed lung on the right; the two-lobed lung on the left; and the mediastinum, or the space between the lungs. The mediastinum contains the esophagus, trachea, large blood vessels, and heart. Smooth parietal pleura line the entire thoracic cavity and adhere to the ribs and superior surface of the diaphragm. Each lung is encased in a separate visceral pleural sac that, when inflated, lies against the parietal pleura. Normally the two pleural membranes are separated by only enough fluid to lubricate the surface for painless movement during filling and emptying of the lungs.

The two cone-shaped lungs consist of the bronchi, bronchioles, and innumerable small air sacs, or alveoli. Through these thin-walled sacs, gas exchange occurs by simple diffusion between the inspired air and the bloodstream. The amount of gas exchanged depends on many factors, including the amount and composition of air inhaled, thickness of the alveolar wall, adequacy of circulation to the alveoli, and substances within the alveoli that either prevent their inflation (e.g., surface-active surfactant) or prevent gas exchange (e.g., fluids).

With age, changes take place in the air passages that increase the respiratory surface area. The major changes are in the number and size of alveoli and in the increased branching of terminal bronchioles. Although the number of conducting airways is complete early in fetal life, the air sacs are shallow with wide necks and have few shared walls, or septa, at birth. This promotes patency but limits surface area for gas exchange. The alveoli are large with thick septa that have little elastic recoil (not unlike the emphysemic lung). During the first year, bronchioles continue to branch, and the globular alveoli formed earlier in the terminal units rapidly increase in number with each generation. These alveoli partition and divide existing alveoli to form smaller lobular units separated by thinner septa, thus enlarging the area available for gas exchange.

Alveoli increase steadily in number, but it is unclear when septal division ceases and an increase in size begins. It appears to occur sometime during middle childhood, although evidence indicates that an increase in the number of alveoli for each terminal airway takes place at puberty. Approximately nine times more alveoli are present at age 12 years than at birth. In later stages of growth, the structures lengthen and enlarge. In addition, collateral pathways of ventilation develop, including pores through alveolar walls and possibly pathways between bronchioles.

RESPIRATORY FUNCTION

Respiratory movements are first evident at approximately 20 weeks of gestation, and throughout fetal life amniotic fluid is exchanged in the alveoli. In the neonate the respiratory rate is rapid to meet the needs of a high metabolism. During growth the respiratory rate steadily decreases until it levels off at maturity. The volume of air inhaled increases with the growth of the lungs and is closely related to body size. In addition, a qualitative difference exists in expired air at different ages. During growth the amount of oxygen in the expired air gradually decreases and the amount of carbon dioxide increases.

Ventilation, the exchange of gases in the lung, results from changes in pressure gradients created by changes in the size of the thoracic cavity. Contraction of the diaphragm and external intercostal muscles increases the size of the thorax and decreases the intrathoracic pressure. As a result, air moves from the atmosphere, which has a higher pressure, into the lungs, which have a lower pressure. The principles of artificial or mechanical ventilation are based on this concept. Mechanical (artificial) respiratory devices increase the pressure entering the air passages (positive pressure breathing devices) or lowers the pressure around the body (negative pressure ventilator).

The two primary forces that affect the mechanics of breathing are compliance and resistance. Compliance is a measure of chest wall and lung distensibility. It represents the relative ease with which the chest and lungs expand with increasing volume and then collapse away from the pleural wall with decreasing volume (elastic recoil). The two major factors determining compliance are alveolar surface tension, which is lowered by surfactant, a lipoprotein at the air-fluid interface that allows alveolar expansion and prevents alveolar collapse, and elastic recoil, the tendency of the lungs to return to the resting state after inspiration (a passive process that requires no muscular effort). Other factors influencing compliance include the degree of tissue hydration, lung blood volume, surface forces at the air-fluid interface, and chest or lung tissue pathologic state (e.g., fibers of elastin or collagen). Factors that interfere with compliance and recoil increase the work of breathing.

Compliance is normally high in the newborn and infant because of a more pliant (flexible) rib cage. This greater compliance causes the rib cage to be easily distorted with increased negative pressure in the pleural cavity or when factors inhibit the stabilizing action of the intercostal muscles. As the child grows, chest wall compliance decreases and elastic recoil increases; therefore ventilation becomes progressively more efficient. In pathologic states an increase in compliance indicates that the lungs or chest wall is abnormally easy to inflate and has lost some elastic recoil, such as in asthma. A decrease in compliance indicates that the lungs or chest wall is abnormally stiff or difficult to inflate.

Any condition that decreases or increases compliance or increases airway resistance results in increased work of breathing (e.g., increased respiratory rate, retractions, nasal flaring, and use of accessory muscles). When respiratory muscle fatigue develops, respiratory failure can occur. Resistance is determined primarily by airway size. The body must overcome three sources of resistance during breathing: tissue resistance in the chest wall (about 20% resistance); tissue resistance in the lungs (about 15% resistance); and, most important, flow resistance in the airways (which often increases with respiratory disease). The four factors determining resistance are flow rate velocity, gas viscosity, length of airway, and airway diameter. If any of the first three variables increases, resistance to airflow also increases. If airway diameter decreases, resistance increases exponentially.

The diameter of the airways and thus the airflow are determined by the balance of forces that tend to widen or narrow the airways. One of these is neural regulation of bronchial smooth muscles mediated through autonomic nerves. Sympathetic impulses relax the airways, and parasympathetic impulses constrict them. Reflex constriction occurs in response to irritating inhalants such as dust, smoke, or sulfur dioxide; arterial hypoxemia and hypercapnia; cold air; and some drugs, such as acetylcholine and histamine. Other factors that alter airway size are peribronchial pressure, which tends to narrow the airways, and intraluminal pressure, which tends to keep the airways open. For example, forced expiration causes increased peribronchial pressure and thus narrowing of the airways; a positive pressure breathing apparatus increases intraluminal pressure, keeping the airways open.

ASSESSMENT OF RESPIRATORY FUNCTION

PHYSICAL ASSESSMENT

Information about the child's respiratory status is obtained from observations of physical signs and behavior. However, to make a useful assessment, the nurse must know what to look for and how to interpret findings. (See Physical Examination, Chapter 4.) Auscultation of the lung fields is helpful in identifying specific pathologic conditions and in assessing the child's responses to treatment. Auscultation is essential when determining airway patency. Palpation and percussion provide information regarding areas of pain and tissue density. Chapter 4 describes breath sounds and their terminology.

Respiration

The nurse should assess the configuration of the chest and the pattern of respiratory movement, including rate, regularity, symmetry of movements, depth, effort expended in respiration, and use of accessory muscles of respiration. To determine deviations, the nurse must know the normal type and rate of respiration in relation to the child's size and age. (See inside cover.) Respirations (ventilations) are best determined when the child is sleeping or quietly awake. They should be counted while the child is unaware because an alteration in breathing rate may occur.

Tachypnea (rapid respirations) often occurs with anxiety, excitement, elevated temperature, severe anemia, and metabolic acidosis. It may also be associated with respiratory alkalosis. By observing changes in respiratory rate, the nurse can follow and evaluate the progress of disorders.

Alterations in the depth of respirations—too deep (hyperpnea) or too shallow (hypopnea)—are often recognized as abnormal only in the extremes. Hyperpnea is noted with fever, severe anemia, respiratory alkalosis associated with psychosis, central nervous system (CNS) disturbances, and respiratory acidosis that accompanies disorders such as diabetic ketoacidosis or diarrhea. Hypoventilation may occur with metabolic alkalosis. Hypoventilation in preterm infants may occur as a result of pulmonary immaturity, absence of adequate substrate to support respiratory muscle activity, neurologic insult, and neurologic immaturity.

Associated Observations

Retractions, or a sinking in of soft tissues relative to the cartilaginous and bony thorax, may occur in some pulmonary disorders. In disease states (particularly in severe airway obstruction), retractions become extreme. Subcostal retraction, observed anteriorly at the lower costal margins, indicates a flattened diaphragm because it not only lowers the floor of the thorax but also pulls on the rib cage in response to a greater than normal decrease in intrathoracic pressure. In severe airway obstruction, retractions extend to the supraclavicular areas and the suprasternal notch.

Nasal flaring is a sign of respiratory distress and a significant finding in an infant. The enlargement of the nostrils helps reduce nasal resistance and maintains airway patency. Nasal flaring may be intermittent or continuous and should be described as minimum or marked.

Head bobbing in a sleeping or exhausted infant is a sign of dyspnea. The head, supported on the caregiver's arm only at the suboccipital area, bobs forward with each inspiration. This is caused by neck flexion resulting from contraction of the scalene and sternocleidomastoid muscles.

Noisy breathing such as "snoring" is frequently associated with hypertrophied adenoidal tissue, choanal obstruction, polyps, or a foreign body in the nasal passages.

Stridor, which is a high-pitched, noisy respiration, is usually an indication of narrowing of the upper airway, either as a result of edema and inflammation or in association with an upper airway obstruction, often from mucus secretions or possibly from a foreign object. Stridor may be inspiratory or expiratory. Common causes in children include croup, epiglottitis, foreign body, or tracheitis.

Grunting is frequently a sign of pain in older children, suggesting acute pneumonia or pleural involvement. It is also observed in pulmonary edema and is a characteristic of respiratory distress in newborns and infants. It is the body's attempt at more efficient respirations. Grunting serves to increase end-respiratory pressure and thus prolong the period of oxygen and carbon dioxide exchange across the alveolocapillary membrane.

Wheezing is a continuous musical sound originating from vibrations in narrowed airways. Wheezing is primarily heard on expiration. Infants may have wheezing as a result of increased airway resistance and a compliant chest wall. Older children often have wheezing with a lower respiratory tract infection as a result of inflammation, bronchospasm, and accumulated secretions.

Color changes of the skin, especially mottling, pallor, and cyanosis, are important. Except for the peripheral bluish discoloration (acrocyanosis) resulting from circulatory stasis in the newborn or the mottling resulting from a cool environment, mottling and cyanosis are significant and usually indicate cardiopulmonary disease.

Chest pain may be a complaint of older children and may have a variety of causes, both pulmonary and nonpulmonary. It may be caused by disease of any of the chest structures. Most pleural pain is related to respiration; therefore respiratory movements are shallow and rapid and may be accompanied by grunting, especially in the younger patient.

Clubbing, or proliferation of tissue about the terminal phalanges, accompanies a variety of conditions, frequently those associated with chronic hypoxia, primarily cardiac defects, and chronic pulmonary disease (e.g., cystic fibrosis). Although clubbing often worsens with lung disease, it does not accurately reflect disease progression. The degree of clubbing depends on the extent to which the nail base is lifted on the dorsal surface of the phalanx by the tissue proliferation. The greater the angle formed above the finger or toe at the skin-nail junction, the more pronounced the clubbing, especially when there is a decided curvature to the nail.

Cough is often associated with respiratory disease, although it may suggest other disorders. It serves as a protective mechanism and an indicator of irritation. Some types of cough are characteristic of specific diseases. For example, a severe cough is associated with measles and cystic fibrosis, and the paroxysmal cough accompanied by an inspiratory "whoop" is typical of pertussis in infants and small children. A brassy, nonproductive cough is part of the symptomatology of croup and foreign body aspiration. Because there are no cough receptors in the alveoli, a cough may be absent in a child with pneumonia in the early stages of the disease but is a common feature during active pneumonia and recovery.

DIAGNOSTIC PROCEDURES

Several procedures are available for assessing respiratory function and diagnosing respiratory disease. All these procedures require preparation and support of the child and the family to ensure cooperation and accurate results.

Pulmonary Function Tests

Noninvasive pulmonary mechanics are often measured at the bedside of infants and children with the use of pneumotachography or spirometry. However, information obtained limits diagnosis because the same functional abnormality may occur in different diseases. These tests are useful to evaluate the severity and course of a disease and to study the effects of treatment.

Radiology and Other Diagnostic Procedures

Radiography is used frequently in diagnostic evaluation of children. When possible, technicians and others try to prevent unnecessary exposure of the child (and nursing personnel), and they protect the more radiosensitive areas (such as the patient's immature gonads and thyroid gland) with a lead shield. Lead shields, correctly placed and consistently applied to areas not needed for diagnostic purposes, are essential. Play and modification of methodology effectively reduce the trauma sometimes associated with the procedure and gain the child's cooperation. Nurses, regardless of age and pregnancy status, should use protective equipment to guard against unnecessary radiation exposure during diagnostic examinations.

Blood Gas Determination

Blood gas measurements are sensitive indicators of change in respiratory status in acutely ill patients. They provide valuable information regarding lung function, lung adequacy, and tissue perfusion and are essential for monitoring conditions involving hypoxemia, carbon dioxide retention, and pH. For the acutely ill patient, this information also guides decisions regarding therapeutic interventions, such as adjusting mechanical ventilator settings, modifying chest physiotherapy (CPT), administering oxygen/continuous positive airway pressure (CPAP)/bilevel positive airway pressure (BiPAP), or positioning the child for maximum ventilation.

Arterial blood gas (ABG) sampling helps evaluate gas exchange and oxygenation and may be performed on blood from an artery or a capillary. Historically, some controversy surrounds the collection of "arterialized" capillary blood for blood gas measurements. However, many believe it to be a safe and relatively accurate method and that capillary blood gas (CBG) can accurately reflect the arterial pH and Pco_2 in most pediatric disease states. The blood samples are obtained by a heel stick after dilation of the vascular bed by warming. ABG samples may also be obtained through an indwelling arterial catheter, arterial puncture, or the neonate's umbilical artery. An accurate ABG or CBG requires unclotted whole or capillary blood; therefore use a heparinized syringe or capillary tube to draw blood samples. Do not allow air bubbles to enter the sample because air alters the blood gas concentration. Depending on the laboratory facilities, as little as 0.1 ml may be sufficient in small infants.

Although ABG values are similar for children and adults, newborns can have slightly lower values and still be considered normal. For example, normal pH values for a newborn range from 7.26 to 7.29, the average PaO_2 is 70 mm Hg, the average $Paco_2$ is 33 mm Hg, and the average bicarbonate is 20 mEq/L. ABG values also depend on the concentration of oxygen the child is breathing. The arterial PaO_2 should rise in proportion to the oxygen concentration being inhaled. Therefore when evaluating ABG values, consider the percentage of oxygen administered (if any), the child's body temperature (as little as 1°F can alter the blood gas values 5% to 8%), and the presence of anxiety (if children hyperventilate, $Paco_2$ may be reduced) or crying (can cause breath holding, resulting in decreased PaO_2).

One approach to determine a simple acid-base disturbance:

- Evaluate the pH to determine whether acidemia or alkalemia is present.
- Evaluate the Pco_2 to determine whether the imbalance is respiratory.
- Evaluate the bicarbonate levels to determine whether the imbalance is metabolic.

Noninvasive Monitoring

Pulse oximetry provides a continuous or intermittent noninvasive method of determining oxyhemoglobin saturation (Sao_2). Applying the sensor correctly is essential for accurate Sao_2 measurements. Because the sensor must identify every pulse beat to calculate the Sao_2, movement can interfere with sensing. Some devices synchronize the oxygen saturation reading with the heartbeat, thereby reducing the interference caused by motion. Sensors are not placed on extremities used for blood pressure monitoring or with indwelling arterial catheters because pulsatile blood flow can be affected. It is recommended that the probe site be changed according to manufacturer guidelines.

Ambient light from ceiling lights and phototherapy or high-intensity heat and light from radiant warmers can interfere with readings. Therefore cover the sensor to block these light sources. Intravenous dyes; green, purple, or black nail polish; nonopaque synthetic nails; and possibly ink used for footprinting can also cause inaccurate Sao_2 measurements. The nurse should remove the dyes or, in the case of porcelain nails, use a different area used for the sensor. Skin color, thickness, and edema do not affect the readings.

Elevated levels of carboxyhemoglobin, methemoglobin, and fetal hemoglobin affect the accuracy of the device because it can only distinguish between oxyhemoglobin and deoxyhemoglobin; therefore the child with carbon monoxide poisoning may have a normal Sao_2 reading but an abnormal (low) Pao_2. Oximetry is insensitive to hyperoxia because hemoglobin approaches 100% saturation for all Pao_2 readings above approximately 100 mm Hg, which is a potentially dangerous situation for the preterm infant at risk for developing oxidative stress. Oxidative stress may lead to complications such as bronchopulmonary dysplasia and retinopathy of prematurity. Therefore the preterm infant being monitored with oximetry should have a range of upper and lower limits identified, such as 90% to 93%, and a protocol should be established for decreasing oxygen when saturations are high.

NURSING TIP

For the infant—Secure the sensor to the great toe and tape the wire to the sole of the foot (or use a commercial holder that fastens with a self-adhering closure). Placing a snugly fitting sock over the foot may help anchor the device, but the site should be checked frequently for color, temperature, and pulses.

For the child—Secure the sensor to the index finger and tape the wire to the back of the hand. Use a self-adhering, Ace type of wrap (e.g., Coban) around the finger or hand to further secure the sensor and wire. For the child with compromised skin, the site should be checked periodically for color, temperature, and pulses.

Another noninvasive method is **transcutaneous monitoring** (TCM), which provides continuous monitoring of transcutaneous partial pressure of oxygen in arterial blood ($tcPao_2$) and, with some devices, of carbon dioxide in arterial blood ($tcPaco_2$). An electrode is attached to the warmed skin to facilitate arterialization of cutaneous capillaries. The site of the electrode must be changed every 3 to 4 hours (or more frequently according to skin status) to avoid burning the skin, and the machine must be calibrated with every site change. This monitoring is used in neonatal intensive care units, but it may not reflect an accurate Pao_2 in infants with impaired local circulation.

End-tidal carbon dioxide monitoring ($ETCO_2$) measures exhaled carbon dioxide noninvasively. Capnometry provides a numeric display, and capnography provides a graph over time. Continuous capnometry is available in many bedside physiologic monitors, as well as standalone monitors. $ETCO_2$ differs from pulse oximetry in that it is more sensitive to the mechanics of ventilation rather than oxygenation. Hypoxic episodes can be prevented through the early detection of hypoventilation, apnea, or airway obstruction.

$ETCO_2$ monitoring is obtained by measuring exhaled CO_2 and provides real-time evidence of ventilation. The use of capnography provides a noninvasive method for measuring the partial pressure of CO_2 during inspiration and expiration; the $ETCO_2$ waveform (capnograph) provides information about expired CO_2, as well as any underlying physiologic conditions or disease processes. Measurement of Pco_2 at end expiration ($P_{ET}CO_2$) approximates alveolar Pco_2 in patients with normal lungs and pulmonary blood flow. $ETCO_2$ can be monitored with or without an artificial airway in place. A sudden decrease in $ETCO_2$ in an intubated patient may indicate endotracheal tube obstruction, extubation, esophageal malposition, or a leak or disruption in the system. In a nonintubated patient, a decrease in $ETCO_2$ may be indicative of hypoventilation, sepsis, or malignant hypothermia.

Children who are experiencing an asthma exacerbation, receiving procedural sedation, or are mechanically ventilated may have $ETCO_2$ monitoring. Although $ETCO_2$ monitoring is not a substitute for ABGs, it does have the advantage of providing ventilation information continuously and noninvasively. Normal $ETCO_2$ values are 30 to 43 mm Hg, which is slightly lower than normal arterial Pco_2 of 35 to 45 mm Hg. During cardiopulmonary resuscitation (CPR), $ETCO_2$ values consistently below 15 mm Hg indicate ineffective compressions or excessive ventilation. Changes in waveform and numeric display follow changes in ventilation by a very few seconds and precede changes in respiratory rate, skin color, and pulse oximetry values.

When there is a change in the $ETCO_2$ value or waveform, assess the patient quickly for adequate airway, breathing, and circulation. Sedated patients may be hypoventilating and need stimulation. Intubated patients may need suctioning, may have self-extubated or dislodged the tube, or may have equipment failure or disconnection. Patients with asthma may have a worsening condition. Problems with the $ETCO_2$ monitoring system can include a kink in the sample line or disconnection. In general, check the patient first and then the equipment.

DEFENSES OF THE RESPIRATORY TRACT

The respiratory tract has several anatomic and biochemical characteristics that provide natural defenses against the many biologic and inanimate agents that can damage respiratory tissues. Intact defenses help repel and resist the impact of injurious agents; factors that reduce the integrity of these mechanisms increase the vulnerability of these tissues to invasion and disease. Respiratory tract defenses include the following:

- **Lymphoid tissues**—Faucial, lingual, and pharyngeal tonsils (adenoids) and other pharyngeal lymphoid tissues form a protective circle around the entrance to the respiratory tract. These help localize and contain invading organisms so they can be destroyed by the body's humoral defense mechanisms.
- **Mucous blanket**—The epithelium of the respiratory tract secretes sticky mucus to which airborne organisms adhere.
- **Ciliary action**—The mucus secreted by the columnar epithelium of the respiratory tract is kept flowing, carrying microorganisms and other foreign agents away from the lungs to be coughed or swallowed.
- **Epiglottis**—The epiglottis and the epiglottis reflex protect the respiratory tract from invading material, including infectious exudate from the upper tract, and prevent such material from being aspirated into the lower tract.
- **Cough**—The expulsive force of the cough reflex propels foreign material out of the lower tract.
- **Position changes**—Changes in body position encourage drainage of tracheobronchial passages.
- **Lymphatics**—Lymphatics draining the terminal bronchi and bronchioles remove invading organisms, which are filtered and destroyed in the regional lymph nodes.
- **Humoral defenses**—Organisms and other foreign material are removed or destroyed by phagocytes, enzymes, and immunoglobulins, especially immunoglobulin A, secreted by the bronchial epithelium.

Some children have conditions (e.g., chronic asthma, cystic fibrosis, and the various immunodeficiency disorders) that predispose them to infection as a result of interference with the efficiency of these mechanisms. Frequent, intense exposure to organisms that accompany conditions of crowding or continual exposure to irritating substances in the air results in breakdown of healthy defenses. Concurrent illness, malnutrition, or fatigue reduces the efficiency of natural defenses. Drying of the mucous membranes also inhibits the activity of humoral defenses, such as immunoglobulins.

GENERAL ASPECTS OF RESPIRATORY TRACT INFECTIONS

Infections of the respiratory tract are described according to the areas of involvement. The upper respiratory tract, or upper airway, consists of the oronasopharynx, pharynx, larynx, and upper part of the trachea. The lower respiratory tract consists of the lower trachea, bronchi, bronchioles, and alveoli. The bronchi and bronchioles are the reactive portion of the lower respiratory tract because they have smooth muscle content and the ability to constrict. Respiratory tract infections spread from one structure to another because of the contiguous nature of the mucous membrane lining the entire tract. Consequently, infections of the respiratory tract involve several areas rather than a single structure, although the effect on one may predominate in any given illness.

ETIOLOGY AND CHARACTERISTICS

Respiratory tract infections account for the majority of acute illnesses in children. The age of the child, season, living conditions, and preexisting medical problems influence the cause and course of these infections.

Infectious Agents

The respiratory tract is subject to a wide variety of infective organisms. Most infections are caused by viruses, particularly respiratory syncytial virus (RSV), rhinovirus, nonpolio enteroviruses (coxsackievirus A and B), parainfluenza virus, influenza virus, adenoviruses, and human metapneumovirus. Other agents involved in primary or secondary invasion include group A β-hemolytic streptococci (GABHS), *Bordetella pertussis,* staphylococci, *Haemophilus influenzae, Chlamydia trachomatis, Mycoplasma* organisms, and pneumococci.

Age

Healthy full term infants younger than 3 months are presumed to have a lower infection rate because of the protective function of maternal antibodies. However, infants are susceptible to respiratory infections, such as pertussis, during this time. The infection rate increases from 3 to 6 months old, which is the period between the disappearance of maternal antibodies and the infant's own antibody production. The viral infection rate continues to remain high during the toddler and preschool years. By 5 years old, viral respiratory tract infections are less frequent, but the incidence of *Mycoplasma pneumoniae* and GABHS infections increases. The amount of lymphoid tissue increases throughout middle childhood, and repeated exposure to organisms confers increasing immunity as children grow older.

Some viral and bacterial agents produce a mild illness in older children but cause severe lower respiratory tract illness or croup in infants. For example, RSV causes a relatively harmless tracheobronchitis in childhood but is a serious disease in infancy.

Size

Anatomic differences influence the response to respiratory tract infections. The diameter of the airways is smaller in young children and subject to considerable narrowing from edematous mucous membranes and increased production of secretions. In addition, the distance between structures within the tract is shorter in the young child. Therefore organisms move more rapidly down the respiratory tract for more extensive involvement. The relatively short and open eustachian tube in infants and young children allows pathogens easy access to the middle ear.

Resistance

The ability to resist pathogens depends on several factors. Deficiencies of the immune system place the child at risk for infection. Other conditions that decrease resistance are malnutrition, anemia, and fatigue. Conditions that weaken defenses of the respiratory tract and predispose a child to infection include allergies (e.g., allergic rhinitis), bronchopulmonary dysplasia (BPD), asthma, history of RSV infection, cardiac anomalies that cause pulmonary congestion, and cystic fibrosis (CF). Day care attendance and exposure to secondhand smoke also increases the likelihood of infection.

Seasonal Variations

The most common respiratory tract pathogens appear in epidemics during the winter and spring months, but mycoplasmal infections occur more often in autumn and early winter. Infection-related asthma (e.g., asthmatic bronchitis) occurs more frequently during cold weather. Winter and spring are typically RSV season, when children are indoors in close contact and more likely to spread the disease to one another.

CLINICAL MANIFESTATIONS

Infants and young children, especially those between 6 months and 3 years of age, react more severely to acute respiratory tract infection than do older children. Young children display a number of generalized signs and symptoms and local manifestations that differ from those seen in older children and adults. Signs and symptoms associated with respiratory tract illnesses are outlined in Box 26.1. Box 26.2 lists components for assessing respiratory function.

NURSING CARE OF THE CHILD WITH A RESPIRATORY TRACT INFECTION

Assessment

Assessment of the respiratory system follows the guidelines described in Chapter 4 (for nose, mouth and throat, chest, and lungs). The assessment should include heart rate, respiratory rate, depth and rhythm, oxygenation, hydration status, body temperature, level of consciousness, activity level, and level of comfort. Special attention is given to the observations outlined in Box 26.1, the components in Box 26.2, and assessment of the following:

- Respiratory effort (respiratory rate, rhythm and depth; accessory muscle use; retractions; nasal flaring)
- Oxygenation (pulse oximetry, skin color)
- Body temperature
- Child's activity level
- Child's level of comfort

> **! NURSING ALERT**
>
> A noninvasive pulse oximeter (oxygen saturation) measurement should be performed on *all* children with a respiratory illness as part of the routine physical assessment.

BOX 26.1 Signs and Symptoms Associated With Respiratory Tract Infections in Infants and Small Children

Fever
May be absent in neonates (<28 days)
Greatest at ages 6 months to 3 years
Temperature may reach 103° to 105°F (39.5° to 40.5°C) even with mild infections
Often appears as first sign of infection
May leave child listless and irritable or somewhat euphoric and more active than normal, temporarily; leads some children to talk with unaccustomed rapidity
Tendency to develop high temperatures with infection in certain families
May precipitate febrile seizures (see Chapter 30)

Meningismus
Meningeal signs without infection of the meninges
Occurs with abrupt onset of fever
Accompanied by
- Headache
- Pain and stiffness in the back and neck
- Presence of Kernig and Brudzinski signs

Subsides as the temperature drops

Anorexia
Common with most childhood illnesses
Frequently the initial evidence of illness
Persists to a greater or lesser degree throughout febrile stage of illness; often extends into convalescence

Vomiting
Occurs readily in small children with illness
A clue to the onset of infection
May precede other signs by several hours
Usually short lived but may persist during the illness
Is frequent cause of dehydration

Diarrhea
Usually mild, transient diarrhea, but may become severe
Often accompanies viral respiratory tract infections

Abdominal Pain
Common complaint
Sometimes indistinguishable from pain of appendicitis in older child
May be caused by mesenteric lymphadenitis
May represent referred pain (e.g., chest pain associated with pneumonia)
May be related to muscle spasms from vomiting, especially in nervous, tense children

Nasal Blockage
Small nasal passages of infants easily blocked by mucosal swelling and exudation
Can interfere with respiration and feeding in infants
May contribute to the development of otitis media and sinusitis

Nasal Discharge
Common feature
May be thin and watery (rhinorrhea) or thick and purulent
Depends on the type and stage of infection
Associated with itching
May irritate upper lip and skin surrounding the nose

Cough
Common feature
May be evident only during the acute phase
May persist several months after a disease

Respiratory Sounds
Sounds associated with respiratory disease:
- Cough
- Hoarseness
- Grunting
- Stridor
- Wheezing

Findings on auscultation:
- Wheezing
- Crackles
- Absence of air movement

Sore Throat
Frequent complaint of older children
Young children (unable to describe symptoms) may not complain even when highly inflamed
Increased drooling noted by parents
Refusal by child to take oral fluids or solids

The nursing care of the child with a respiratory tract infection follows established guidelines based on the child's and family's individualized needs (see Nursing Care Plan box).

Ease Respiratory Efforts

Many acute respiratory tract infections are mild and cause few symptoms. Although children may feel uncomfortable and have a stuffy nose and some mucosal swelling, acute respiratory distress occurs infrequently. Interventions delivered at home are usually sufficient to relieve minor discomfort and ease respiratory efforts. However, in some cases, the infant or child may require hospitalization for observation and therapy.

Warm or cool mist is a common therapeutic measure for symptomatic relief of respiratory discomfort. The moisture soothes inflamed membranes and is beneficial when there is hoarseness or laryngeal involvement. Mist tents have been used in the hospital for humidifying the air and relieving discomfort but are seldom used in developed countries. The use of steam vaporizers in the home is often discouraged because of the hazards related to their use and limited evidence to support their efficacy (Lonie, Baker, & Teixeira, 2016; Verma, Lodha, & Kabra, 2013).

A time-honored method (but not evidence based) of producing steam is the shower. Running a shower of hot water into the empty bathtub or open shower stall with the bathroom door closed produces a quick source of steam. Keeping a child in this environment for 10 to 15 minutes may help ease respiratory efforts. A small child can sit on the lap of a parent or other adult. The use of kettles or bowls of boiling water are strongly discouraged due to the risk of accidental scalding.

Promote Rest

Children who have an acute febrile illness should be encouraged to rest and engage in quiet activities. Most children limit activities when febrile and increase activity as the fever subsides.

BOX 26.2 Components for Assessing Respiratory Function

Pattern of Respirations

Rate—Rapid (tachypnea), normal, or slow for the particular child

Depth—Normal depth, too shallow (hypopnea), too deep (hyperpnea); usually estimated from the amplitude of thoracic and abdominal excursion (age dependent)

Ease—Effortless, labored (dyspnea), orthopnea, associated with intercostal or substernal retractions (inspiratory "sinking in" of soft tissues in relation to the cartilaginous and bony thorax), pulsus paradoxus (blood pressure falling with inspiration and rising with expiration), nasal flaring, head bobbing (head of sleeping child with suboccipital area supported on caregiver's forearm bobbing forward in synchrony with each inspiration), grunting, or wheezing

Labored breathing—Continuous, intermittent, becoming steadily worse, sudden onset, at rest or on exertion, associated with wheezing, grunting, associated with chest pain

Rhythm—Variation in rate and depth of respirations

Other Observations

Evidence of infection—Check for elevated temperature; enlarged cervical lymph nodes; inflamed mucous membranes; and purulent discharges from the nose, ears, or lungs (sputum).

Cough—Observe the characteristics of the cough (if present): when the cough is heard (e.g., night only, on arising), the nature of the cough (paroxysmal with or without wheeze, "croupy" or "brassy"), frequency of the cough, association with swallowing or other activity, character of the cough (moist or dry), productivity.

Wheeze—Note whether it is expiratory or inspiratory, high pitched or musical, prolonged, slowly progressive or sudden, associated with labored breathing.

Cyanosis—Note distribution (peripheral, perioral, facial, trunk as well as face), degree, duration, association with activity.

Chest pain—Older children may complain of this. Note location and circumstances: localized or generalized; referred to base of neck or abdomen; dull or sharp; deep or superficial; associated with rapid, shallow respirations or grunting.

Sputum—Older children may provide sputum sample by coughing, whereas young children may need use of bulb suction or gastric lavage in early morning to provide a sample. Note volume, color, viscosity, and odor.

Bad breath—May be associated with some throat and lung infections.

NURSING CARE PLAN

The Child With Acute Respiratory Tract Infection

Case Study

Sarah is a 7-month-old who is being evaluated in the emergency department for fever and cough. Mom reports over the past 2 days that Sarah has not been as active as usual and has been eating less. She started coughing during the night and upon awakening was noted to have a temperature of 103°F (39.4°C). She has been diagnosed with bronchiolitis.

Assessment

Based on these events, what are the most important subjective and objective data that should be assessed?

Acute Respiratory Tract Infection Defining Characteristics

Usually high fever, tachypnea, tachycardia
Retractions
Nasal flaring
Dyspnea (reported by older children)
Breath sounds—usually rhonchi or fine crackles
Cough—productive or nonproductive
Skin color—pallor or cyanosis depending on severity
Irritable, restless, or lethargic
Poor appetite

Nursing Interventions

What are the most appropriate nursing interventions for this infant with acute respiratory tract infection?

Nursing Interventions	Rationale
Position infant for maximum ventilation and airway patency	To allow for increased chest expansion
Monitor vital signs, including temperature, respiratory, cardiac, and oxygen status	To quickly identify alterations in temperature, respiratory status, or circulation and determine the need for additional interventions
Provide humidified oxygen as prescribed	To improve oxygenation and minimize drying of nasal mucous membranes
Suction airway (external nose, mouth, nasopharynx) as indicated	To remove secretions and maintain airway patency
Administer antipyretics as indicated	To reduce fever and promote comfort
Administer antibiotics as indicated	To treat infection source
Obtain specimens (i.e., secretions, blood) as indicated	To identify infective organisms
Maintain appropriate precautions such as standard precautions, droplet isolation, and frequent hand washing	To prevent spread of infection
Monitor hydration status through strict intake and output and daily weights	To prevent dehydration or fluid overload
Implement comfort measures such as allowing parent presence, parent holding infant, and comfort item such as favorite blanket or stuffed animal	To reduce anxiety and promote comfort

Expected Outcomes

Respiration rate will be in an acceptable range and nonlabored
Airway will remain patent
Body temperature will remain in acceptable range
Infection will resolve
Adequate hydration status will be maintained

Case Study (Continued)

Sarah's parents are anxious and upset about their daughter's condition and hospitalization. You want to educate them on what is happening to their daughter.

Continued

NURSING CARE PLAN—CONT'D

The Child With Acute Respiratory Tract Infection

Assessment

What are the most important aspects of care to discuss with her parents at this time?

Family's Knowledge of Illness Defining Characteristics

Defining acute respiratory tract infection
Description of treatment regimen including rationale for medications
Expression of fears and concerns
Display of appropriate reactions to child's condition

Nursing Interventions

What are the most appropriate nursing interventions for this diagnosis?

Nursing Interventions	Rationale
Educate family about characteristics of acute respiratory tract infection.	To promote understanding of etiology and symptoms of respiratory infections
Educate family about strategies to facilitate ventilation (i.e., sitting up) and encourage secretion clearance (i.e., instilling saline drops and nasal suctioning).	To promote understanding of measures to enhance ventilation and airway clearance
Educate family about Sarah's hospital and discharge medications including antipyretics and antibiotics as prescribed.	To promote understanding of treatment regimen
Allow family to remain with infant and encourage family's involvement in the infant's care.	To decrease effects of separation and promote family sense of control and involvement in care
Arrange for social worker to meet with family to assess emotional and financial needs as indicated.	To identify and modify stressors associated hospitalization

Expected Outcomes

Parents verbalize characteristics of acute respiratory tract infection.
Parents verbalize treatment including medication and strategies to promote ventilation and airway clearance.
Parents verbalize discharge medications including antipyretics and antibiotics.
Parents remain involved in patient's care.
Parents verbalize resources available for emotional and financial support as indicated.

Promote Comfort

Older children are usually able to manage nasal secretions with little difficulty. Instruct parents in the correct administration of nose drops or throat gargles, if ordered. For very young infants, who normally breathe through their noses, an infant nasal aspirator or a rubber ear syringe is helpful in removing nasal secretions before feeding. This practice, in addition to instillation of saline nose drops, may clear nasal passages and promote feeding. Saline nose drops can be prepared at home by dissolving ½ to 1 tsp of salt in 1 cup of warm water. Two to three drops of saline can be put into the nostril and a bulb syringe used to suction it out.

> **! NURSING ALERT**
>
> To avoid rebound nasal congestion, vasoconstrictive nose drops or sprays should not be administered for more than 3 days.

Topical vapor rubs could be considered for children older than age 2 years, to ease nasal congestion. A recent study found that people with the common cold had significantly improved sleep quality when using a vapor rub containing camphor, menthol, and eucalyptus oils compared with placebo (Santhi, Ramsey, Phillipson, et al., 2017). These vapor rubs never should be given orally or placed beneath the nose.

Prevent Spread of Infection

Perform careful hand washing when caring for children with respiratory tract infections. Children and families should use a tissue or their elbow when they cough or sneeze. Used tissues should be immediately thrown into the wastebasket and not allowed to accumulate in a pile. Children with respiratory tract infections should not share drinking cups, eating utensils, washcloths, or towels. To decrease contamination with respiratory viruses, wash hands frequently and do not touch eyes or nose with hands.

Parents should try to remove affected children from contact with other children when possible. An effort should be made to teach well children to stay away from ill children, to wash their hands frequently, and to avoid eating or drinking from the same utensils or cups.

Reduce Body Temperature

If the child has a significantly elevated temperature, controlling the fever is important to ensure comfort. Nurses should verify that family members have a thermometer and know how to take a child's temperature and read the thermometer accurately.

If the practitioner has prescribed an antipyretic such as ibuprofen (for infants and children 6 months and older) or acetaminophen, parents may need help administering the drug. Most parents can read the label and calculate the desired dose, but some may require careful instruction. It is important to emphasize accuracy in both the amount of drug given and the time intervals for drug administration to avoid cumulative effects. Encourage cool liquids to reduce the temperature and minimize the chances of dehydration (see Controlling Elevated Temperatures, Chapter 22.)

> **! NURSING ALERT**
>
> Parents are cautioned regarding over-the-counter combination "cold" remedies because these often include acetaminophen. Careful calculation of both the acetaminophen given separately and the acetaminophen in combination medications is necessary to avoid an overdose.

Promote Hydration

Dehydration is a potential complication when children have respiratory tract infections and are febrile or anorexic, especially when vomiting or diarrhea is present. Infants are especially prone to fluid and electrolyte deficits when they have a respiratory illness because a rapid respiratory rate that accompanies such illnesses precludes adequate fluid intake. In addition, the presence of fever increases the total body fluid turnover in infants. If the infant has nasal secretions, this further prevents adequate respiratory effort by blocking the narrow nasal passages when the infant reclines to bottle-feed or breastfeed and ceases the compensatory mouth breathing effort, thus causing the child to limit intake of fluids. Parents encourage adequate fluid intake by offering small amounts of favorite fluids (clear liquids if vomiting) at frequent intervals. High-calorie or thick fruit juices may not be tolerated if the child is having vomiting and diarrhea. Oral rehydration solutions, such as Infalyte or Pedialyte, are beneficial for infants and young children, and water or a low-carbohydrate flavored drink are appropriate for older children. Popsicles and flavored ice are other options to consider. Fluids with caffeine (tea, coffee) are avoided because these may act as diuretics and promote fluid loss. Carbonated drinks, fruit drinks, and energy drinks are not recommended for oral rehydration (Davies, 2015). Infants who are breastfeeding should continue to be breastfed because human milk confers some degree of protection from infection (see Chapter 7). Fluids should not be forced, and children should not be awakened to take fluids unless the practitioner advises it. Forcing fluids may create the same difficulties as urging unwanted food (discussed later). Gentle persuasion with preferred beverages is usually successful. (See Chapter 23 for instructions on oral hydration.)

Intravenous (IV) fluids may be required short term to reestablish hydration if the child is dehydrated and not drinking. A nasogastric tube may be placed to provide enteral hydration using Infalyte or Pedialyte.

To assess their child's level of hydration (see Chapter 23), advise parents to observe the frequency of voiding and to notify the nurse or practitioner if there is insufficient voiding.

> **! NURSING ALERT**
>
> Counting the number of wet diapers in a 24-hour period is a satisfactory method of assessing output in nonhospitalized infants and toddlers who are not acutely ill. Otherwise urinary output should be approximately 0.5 to 1 ml/kg/hr in a child who weighs less than 30 kg (66 lb) and 30 ml/hr for children 30 kg and larger. The practitioner should be notified if the urine output is low.

Observe for Deterioration

Signs of clinical deterioration include increasing respiratory distress, increasing respiratory rate, increasing heart rate, worsening hypoxia, poor perfusion, reduced level of consciousness, and lethargy. Any deterioration is notified to the primary service.

Provide Nutrition

Loss of appetite is characteristic of children with acute infections. In most cases children can be permitted to determine their own need for food. Urging foods on anorexic children may precipitate nausea and vomiting and cause an aversion to feeding that can extend into the convalescent period and beyond. Many children show no decrease in appetite, and others respond well to foods such as gelatin, popsicles, soup, and puddings (See Feeding the Sick Child, Chapter 22.) In the acute period of the illness, maintaining hydration with encouragement of fluids is of greater importance.

Provide Family Support and Home Care

Young children with respiratory tract infections may be irritable and difficult to comfort. Therefore the family needs support, encouragement, and practical suggestions concerning comfort measures and administration of medication.

In addition to antipyretics and nose drops, the child may require antibiotic therapy. Parents of children receiving oral antibiotics need to understand the importance of administering the drug regularly and continuing it for the prescribed length of time, regardless of whether the child appears ill. Parents are cautioned against giving the child any medications that are not approved by the practitioner or prescribed for another child. (See Chapter 22 for administration of medications and teaching parents.) Adverse effects have occurred in children who have received preparations intended for adults (e.g., some long-acting nose drops and dextromethorphan cough squares [mistaken for candy]).

UPPER RESPIRATORY TRACT INFECTIONS

ACUTE VIRAL NASOPHARYNGITIS

A number of viruses, usually rhinoviruses, RSV, adenovirus, influenza virus, and parainfluenza virus, cause acute nasopharyngitis (the equivalent of the "common cold").

Clinical Manifestations

Symptoms of nasopharyngitis are more severe in infants and children than in adults. Fever is common, especially in young children. Older children may have low-grade fevers, which appear early in the illness. In children 3 months to 3 years, fevers occur suddenly and are associated with irritability, restlessness, decreased appetite and fluid intake, and decreased activity. Nasal inflammation may lead to obstruction of passages, producing open-mouth breathing. Vomiting and diarrhea may also be present.

The initial symptoms in older children are dryness and irritation of nasal passages and the pharynx, followed by chilling sensations, muscular aches, an irritating nasal discharge, and, occasionally, coughing or sneezing. Nasal inflammation may lead to obstruction. Continual wiping away of secretions causes skin irritation to nares.

The disease is self-limiting and symptoms last 10 to 14 days with a peak on day 2 to 3 of illness. Occasionally fever recurs and a child (particularly an infant) might experience otitis media (OM), usually early or after the initial phase of nasopharyngitis is past. Pneumonia is less frequent but may be observed in some infants.

Therapeutic Management

Children with nasopharyngitis are managed at home. There is no specific treatment, and effective vaccines are not available. Antipyretics may be prescribed for fever and discomfort. (See Chapter 22 for management of fever.) Fluids and rest are recommended.

Decongestants result in vasoconstriction of the nasal mucosa and are available orally and topically as nose drops, but there is little evidence to show efficacy in children. They may be more effective and "safe" with children over 12 but can be used in children over 6 years. They may be administered 15 to 20 minutes before feeding and at bedtime. Spray bottles and bottles of nose drops should be used only for one child and only for one illness because they become easily contaminated with bacteria or viruses. Side effects can include nosebleeds, drying of the nasal membranes, and rebound nasal congestion. To avoid rebound congestion, nose drops or sprays should not be administered for more than 3 days. Because these drugs affect all vascular beds, they should be given with caution to children with diabetes.

> **! NURSING ALERT**
>
> To prevent cross-contamination with nose drops, draw about 0.25 ml of nose spray solution into a clean needleless tuberculin syringe. Instill a small amount of the nose spray solution into the child's nostrils using the blunt syringe.

Over-the-counter cough suppressants are not routinely recommended and should be prescribed with caution (cough is a protective way of clearing secretions) (Lowry & Leeder, 2015). A cough is normal when the airway is irritated and suppressing it may result in adverse outcomes. Products containing dextromethorphan or codeine may be prescribed for a dry, hacking cough, especially at night. Some preparations contain up to 22% alcohol and can cause confusion, hyperexcitability, dizziness, nausea, and sedation. They should not be administered to young children continuously and must be stored securely away.

Recent concerns regarding serious side effects of cough and cold preparations in young children, particularly infants, and lack of convincing evidence that such medications are effective in reducing symptoms have prompted recommendations by health experts to carefully evaluate the benefits and risks of recommending such preparations for children (Lowry & Leeder, 2015). The American Academy of Pediatrics states that over-the-counter cough and cold medications do not work for children under 6 years and in some cases may pose a health risk (Clarke, 2017).

Antihistamines are largely ineffective in treatment of nasopharyngitis. These drugs have a weak atropine-like effect that dries secretions, but they can cause drowsiness or, paradoxically, have a stimulatory effect on children. There is no support for the usefulness of expectorants, and antibiotics are usually not indicated. The pediatric quality indicator for the appropriate treatment of children with upper respiratory infection is listed in Table 26.1.

DRUG ALERT

Over-the-Counter Cold Preparations

Over-the-counter cold preparation such as pseudoephedrine and some antihistamines are not appropriate for the treatment of the common cold in infants and toddlers; these may cause serious side effects in such children and have been associated with death in infants (Lowry & Leeder, 2015). Advise parents to consult the primary care provider before using these drugs in infants and toddlers.

Prevention

Nasopharyngitis is so widespread in the general population that it is impossible to prevent. The best methods for preventing transmission of these viruses are frequent hand washing and avoiding touching one's eyes, nose, and mouth. Children are more susceptible to colds because they have not yet developed resistance to many types of viruses. Very young infants are subject to relatively serious complications; therefore they should be protected from exposure.

Nursing Care Management

A cold is often the parents' first introduction to an illness in their infants. Most discomfort of nasopharyngitis is related to the nasal obstruction, especially in small infants. Elevating the head of the bed or crib mattress assists with drainage of secretions; suctioning and vaporization may also provide relief. Saline nose drops and gentle suction with a bulb syringe, particularly before feeding, are useful.

Maintaining adequate fluid intake is essential during any infectious process. Although a child's appetite for solid foods is usually diminished for several days, it is important to offer favorite fluids to prevent dehydration. Fluids can be cool (e.g., gelatin, popsicles) or warm (e.g., soups, broths), depending on individual preference.

Because nasopharyngitis is spread from secretions, the best means for prevention is avoiding contact with affected persons. This goal is difficult when large numbers of people are confined in a small area for a long time, such as day care centers and classrooms. Family members with a cold should try to "keep it to themselves" by carefully disposing of tissues and not sharing towels, glasses, or eating utensils. They should also cover the mouth and nose with tissues when coughing or sneezing and wash hands thoroughly after nose blowing or sneezing. The most frequent carriers of infection are the human hands, which deposit viruses on doorknobs, faucets, and other everyday objects. Children should wash their hands thoroughly or use hand sanitizer before touching their nose, mouth, or eyes.

Family Support

Support and reassurance are important elements of care for families of young children with recurrent upper respiratory tract infections (URIs). Because URIs are so frequent in children less than 3 years of age, families may feel they are on an endless roller coaster of illness. Reassure them that frequent colds are a normal part of childhood, there are hundreds of viruses that cause them, and that by 5 years of age most children will have developed immunity to many viruses. Parents who work outside the home should expect to take time off to care for ill children during the fall and winter months. Parents should know the signs of respiratory complications and should notify a health professional if any signs of complications appear, if signs of dehydration are present, or if the child does not improve within 2 or 3 days (Box 26.3).

TABLE 26.1 Pediatric Quality Indicator: Treatment for Children With Upper Respiratory Infection*

Appropriate Treatment for Children With Upper Respiratory Infection	
Measure	Children 3 months to 18 years of age who were diagnosed with upper respiratory infection (URI) and were not dispensed an antibiotic prescription on or 3 days after the episode.
Numerator	Number of children who were not prescribed or dispensed a prescription for antibiotic medication on or within 3 days after the URI Episode date during the measurement time.
Denominator	Number of children who had an outpatient or emergency department visit with only a diagnosis of URI.

*Endorsed by the National Quality Forum-0069 and Center for Medicare and Medicaid Services-154v1.

BOX 26.3 Early Evidence of Respiratory Complications

Parents are instructed to notify the health professional if they note any of the following:

- Evidence of earache
- Respirations faster than 50 to 60 beats/min
- Fever over 101°F (38.3°C)
- Listlessness
- Increasing irritability with or without fever
- Persistent cough for 2 days or more
- Wheezing
- Crying
- Refusal to eat
- Restlessness and poor sleep patterns

Modified from National Association of Pediatric Nurse Associates and Practitioners. (1989). *Baby's first cold.* New York: Winthrop Consumer Products.

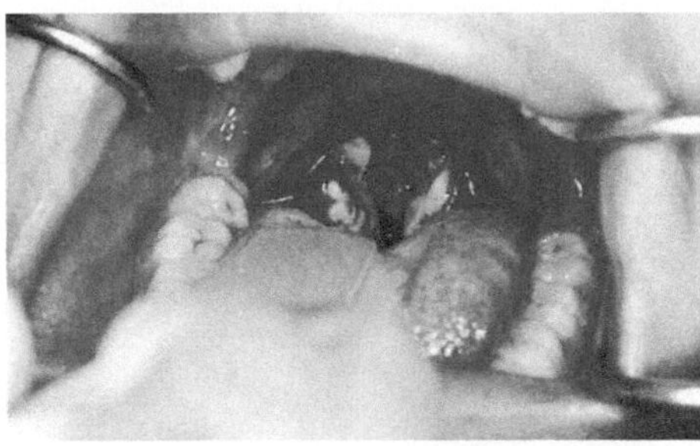

FIG. 26.1 Tonsillitis and pharyngitis. (Courtesy Dr. Edward L. Applebaum, Head, Department of Otolaryngology, University of Illinois Medical Center, Chicago.)

TABLE 26.2 Evaluation of Child With Suspected GABHS

When to Consider Checking for GABHS	When Suspicion of GABHS Is Considered Low
Acute onset of sore throat	Children under 3 years
Exudate on pharynx	Children with symptoms more suggestive of viral cause (e.g., nasal discharge, conjunctivitis, hoarse, cough, diarrhea, mouth ulcers, stomatitis)
Fever	
Enlarged anterior cervical lymph nodes	
History of exposure to GABHS	

GABHS, Group A β-hemolytic streptococcus.

ACUTE STREPTOCOCCAL PHARYNGITIS

Group A β-hemolytic streptococci (GABHS) infection of the upper airway (strep throat) is not in itself a serious disease, but affected children are at risk for serious sequelae: acute rheumatic fever, which is an inflammatory disease of the heart, joints, and CNS (see Chapter 27), and acute glomerulonephritis, which is an acute kidney infection (see Chapter 24). Permanent damage can result from these sequelae, especially acute rheumatic fever. GABHS may also cause skin manifestations, including impetigo and pyoderma.

Scarlet fever may also occur as a result of a strain of group A streptococcus. The clinical manifestations of scarlet fever include pharyngitis and a characteristic erythematous sandpaper-like rash; otherwise scarlet fever shares the same clinical manifestations as those mentioned for GABHS, and treatment and sequelae are the same. Severe scarlet fever is rarely seen in the United States.

Clinical Manifestations

GABHS infection is generally a relatively brief illness that varies in severity from subclinical (no symptoms) to severe toxicity. The onset is often abrupt and characterized by pharyngitis, headache, fever, and abdominal pain. The tonsils and pharynx may be inflamed and covered with exudate (50% to 80% of cases) (Fig. 26.1), which usually appears by the second day of illness. However, streptococcal infections should be suspected in children over the age of 2 years who have pharyngitis even if no exudate is present.

Anterior cervical lymphadenopathy (30% to 50% of cases) usually occurs early, and the nodes are often tender. Pain can be relatively mild to severe enough to make swallowing difficult. Clinical manifestations usually subside in 3 to 5 days unless complicated by sinusitis or parapharyngeal, peritonsillar, or retropharyngeal abscess. Nonsuppurative complications may appear after the onset of GABHS—acute nephritis in about 10 days and rheumatic fever in an average of 18 days.

Children who are GABHS carriers may have a positive throat culture but often experience a coincidental viral illness. Although antibiotic administration is not indicated for most GABHS carriers, some conditions require antibiotic therapy; these are published in the American Academy of Pediatrics, Report of the Committee on Infectious Diseases (2015) *Red Book.* Transmission to others from a carrier is reportedly minimal.

Diagnostic Evaluation

Although 80% to 90% of all cases of acute pharyngitis are viral, a throat culture and/or rapid antigen testing (obtained by vigorous swabbing of both tonsils and the posterior pharynx) may be performed to rule out GABHS (Academy of Pediatrics, Report of the Committee on Infectious Diseases, 2015). Rapid identification of GABHS with diagnostic test kits is possible in the office or clinic setting. However, because these kits have questionable sensitivity and depend on a high-quality swab being obtained, a confirmatory throat culture is recommended in patients who have a negative test result with a rapid diagnostic test kit and classic signs of the infection are present (Academy of Pediatrics, Report of the Committee on Infectious Diseases, 2015) (Table 26.2).

Because some children normally harbor streptococci in their throats, a positive culture or antigen test is not always conclusive evidence of active disease. Most streptococcal infections are short-term illnesses, and antibody (antistreptolysin O) responses appear later than symptoms and are useful only for retrospective diagnosis.

Therapeutic Management

If streptococcal sore throat infection is present, oral penicillin or other related medications such as ampicillin and amoxicillin is prescribed for 10 days to control the acute local manifestations and to maintain an adequate level to eliminate organisms that might remain to initiate rheumatic fever symptoms. Penicillin does not prevent the development of acute glomerulonephritis in susceptible children. However, it may prevent the spread of a nephrogenic strain of GABHS to others in the family. Penicillin usually produces a prompt response within 24 hours. Some patients require retreatment if the organism is not eradicated. Amoxicillin given once a day for 10 days is as effective as penicillin given multiple times per day (Academy of Pediatrics, Report of the Committee on Infectious Diseases, 2015).

Intramuscular (IM) penicillin G benzathine is also an appropriate therapy. This drug ensures adequate blood concentrations and avoids the problem of compliance, yet it is painful. Some preparations contain penicillin G procaine as well to decrease the pain. An oral macrolide (erythromycin, azithromycin, clarithromycin) or a cephalosporin (cephalexin) is indicated for children who are allergic to penicillin (Academy of Pediatrics, Report of the Committee on Infectious Diseases, 2015). The pediatric quality indicator for the testing and treatment of the child with pharyngitis is listed in Table 26.3.

Nursing Care Management

The nurse often obtains a throat swab for culture and instructs the parents about administering the antibiotic and analgesics as prescribed. Some children may prefer quiet activities during the acute phase of the illness, whereas others may limit activity only if the temperature is elevated. Cold or warm compresses to the neck may provide relief. In children old enough to cooperate, warm saline gargles offer some relief of throat discomfort. Pain may interfere with oral intake, and the child should not be forced to eat. Instead, encourage cool liquids or ice chips, which are usually more acceptable than solids.

Special emphasis is placed on correctly administering oral medication and completing the course of antibiotic therapy. (See Administration of Medication, and Compliance, Chapter 22.) If an antibiotic injection

TABLE 26.3 Pediatric Quality Indicator: Pharyngitis Testing/Treatment*

Testing/Treatment for Children With Pharyngitis	
Measure	Children 2-18 years of age who were diagnosed with pharyngitis, ordered an antibiotic, and received a group A streptococcus (strep) test for the episode.
Numerator	Number of children who had a group A streptococcus test in the 7-day period from 3 days prior through 3 days after the diagnosis of pharyngitis during the measurement time.
Denominator	Number of children who had an outpatient or emergency department visit with a diagnosis of pharyngitis during the measurement period and an antibiotic ordered on or 3 days after the visit.

*Endorsed by the National Quality Forum-0002 and Center for Medicare and Medicaid Services-146v1.

is required, it must be administered deep into a large muscle mass (e.g., the vastus lateralis or ventrogluteal muscle). Parents need to be aware of the residual tenderness. Local applications of heat are helpful in relieving discomfort. (For other atraumatic strategies to reduce injection pain, such as application over the site of EMLA [a eutectic mix of lidocaine and prilocaine] 1 hour before the injection or LMX-4 [lidocaine 4%] 30 minutes beforehand; see Administration of Medication: Intramuscular Administration, Chapter 22.) If the child continues to be febrile, has not improved within 24 to 48 hours, or appears toxic, further evaluation by the health care provider is important.

DRUG ALERT

Administration of Procaine or Benzathine Penicillin

Never administer penicillin G procaine or penicillin G benzathine suspensions intravenously; they may cause embolism or toxic reaction with ensuing death in minutes. Instead, administer these medications deep into the muscle tissue to decrease localized reactions and pain.

Prevention

No immunization is available for prevention of streptococcal disease. The organism is spread by close contact with affected persons—direct projection of large droplets or physical transfer of respiratory secretions containing the organism. Children with streptococcal infection are noninfectious to others 24 hours after initiation of antibiotic therapy. It is generally recommended that children not return to school or day care until they have been taking antibiotics for a full 24-hour period.

Nurses should remind children with a streptococcal throat infection to discard their toothbrush and replace it with a new one after they have been taking antibiotics for 24 hours. Orthodontic appliances must be washed thoroughly because they may harbor organisms. Parents are cautioned to prevent other household members, especially if immunocompromised, from having close contact with the sick child and avoid sharing towels, drinking or eating items.

TONSILLITIS

The tonsils are masses of lymphoid tissue located in the pharyngeal cavity. The tonsils filter and protect the respiratory and alimentary tracts from invasion by pathogenic organisms. They also play a role in antibody formation. Although the size of tonsils varies, children generally have larger tonsils than adolescents or adults. This difference is thought to be a protective mechanism because young children are especially susceptible to URIs.

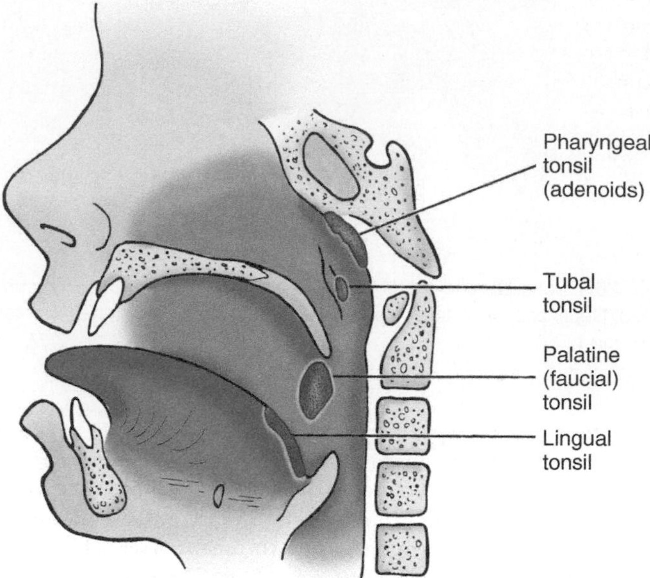

FIG. 26.2 Location of various tonsillar masses.

Pathophysiology

Several pairs of tonsils are part of a mass of lymphoid tissue encircling the nasopharynx and oropharynx, known as the Waldeyer tonsillar ring (Fig. 26.2). The palatine, or faucial, tonsils are located on either side of the oropharynx, behind and below the pillars of the fauces (opening from the mouth). A surface of the palatine tonsils is usually visible during oral examination. The **palatine tonsils** are those removed during tonsillectomy. The pharyngeal tonsils, also known as the **adenoids**, are located above the palatine tonsils on the posterior wall of the nasopharynx. Their proximity to the nares and eustachian tubes causes difficulties in instances of inflammation. The lingual tonsils are located at the base of the tongue. The tubal tonsils, found near the posterior nasopharyngeal opening of the eustachian tubes, are not part of the Waldeyer tonsillar ring.

Etiology

Tonsillitis often occurs with pharyngitis. Because of the abundant lymphoid tissue and the frequency of URIs, tonsillitis is a common cause of illness in young children. The causative agent may be viral or bacterial.

Clinical Manifestations

The manifestations of tonsillitis are caused by inflammation. As the palatine tonsils enlarge from edema, they may meet in the midline (kissing tonsils), obstructing the passage of air or food. The child has difficulty swallowing and breathing. When enlargement of the adenoids occurs, the space behind the posterior nares may become blocked, making it difficult or impossible for air to pass from the nose to the throat. As a result, the child breathes through the mouth. Chronic enlargement of the tonsils and adenoids may result in obstruction of breathing during sleep.

If mouth breathing is continuous, the mucous membranes of the oropharynx become dry and irritated. There may be an offensive mouth odor and impaired senses of taste and smell. Because air cannot be trapped for proper speech sounds, the voice has a nasal and muffled quality. A persistent cough is also common. Because of the proximity of the adenoids to the eustachian tubes, this passageway is frequently blocked by swollen adenoids, interfering with normal drainage and frequently resulting in OM or difficulty hearing.

Therapeutic Management

Medical Treatment

Because the illness is self-limiting, treatment of viral pharyngitis is symptomatic. Throat cultures positive for GABHS infection require antibiotic treatment. It is important to differentiate between viral and streptococcal infection in febrile, exudative tonsillitis. Because the majority of infections are of viral origin, early rapid tests can eliminate unnecessary antibiotic administration.

Surgical Treatment

Surgical treatment of chronic tonsillitis is controversial. Except in documented cases of recurrent, frequent streptococcal infection or a history of development of a peritonsillar abscess, tonsillectomy is not indicated in the child who has recurrent pharyngitis.

Tonsillectomy (surgical removal of the palatine tonsils) may be indicated for massive hypertrophy that results in difficulty breathing or eating. Absolute indications are peritonsillar abcess; PFAPA: periodic fever, aphthous stomatitis, pharyngitis, and cervical adenitis; airway obstruction, chronic tonsillitis unresponsive to antimicrobials, multiple antibiotic allergies, and tonsils requiring tissue pathology (Ingram & Friedman, 2015). Consideration of tonsillectomy include: at least seven episodes of tonsillitis in the previous year, or at least five tonsillitis episodes in each of the previous 2 years, or at least three episodes of tonsillitis in each of the previous 3 years (Ingram & Friedman, 2015). One episode of tonsillitis consists of a sore throat plus at least one of the following: temperature greater than 100.9°F (38.3°C), cervical adenopathy (>2 cm or tender nodes), exudate on the tonsils, or positive culture for GABHS.

Adenoidectomy (the surgical removal of the adenoids) is recommended for children who have hypertrophied adenoids that obstruct nasal breathing or a history of four or greater episodes of recurrent purulent rhinorrhea in the previous 12 months in a child under 12 years of age (one episode should be documented by intranasal examination or imaging, American Academy of Otolaryngology—Head and Neck Surgery, 2011). Other indications include persisting symptoms of adenoiditis after 2 courses of antibiotics, sleep disturbance with nasal obstruction lasting over 3 months, hyponasal speech, otitis media with effusion (OME) greater than 3 months, dental malocclusion or orofacial growth disturbance as validated by an orthodontist/dentist, OME with effusion in a child at least 4 years old, or cardiopulmonary complications associated with adenoid hypertrophy (American Academy of Otolaryngology—Head and Neck Surgery, 2011).

For some children the effectiveness of tonsillectomy or adenoidectomy is modest and may not justify the risk of surgery. In practice, most providers rely on individualized decision making and do not subscribe to an absolute set of eligibility criteria for these surgical procedures.

A Cochrane review (Burton, Glasziou, Chong, et al., 2014) concluded there was a modest benefit to adenotonsillectomy in children with recurrent sore throats; others have reached similar conclusions (Morad, Sathe, Francis, et al., 2017).

Contraindications to either tonsillectomy or adenoidectomy are (1) cleft palate because both tonsils help minimize escape of air during speech; (2) acute infections at the time of surgery because the locally inflamed tissues increase the risk of bleeding; and (3) uncontrolled systemic diseases or blood dyscrasias.

Generally, removal of the tonsils should not occur until after 3 or 4 years of age because of the problem of excessive blood loss in young children and the possibility of regrowth or hypertrophy of lymphoid tissue. The tubal and lingual tonsils often enlarge to compensate for the lost lymphoid tissue, resulting in continued pharyngeal and eustachian tube obstruction.

Nursing Care Management

Nursing care of the child with tonsillitis involves providing comfort and minimizing activities or interventions that precipitate bleeding. A soft to liquid diet is generally preferred. Warm saltwater gargles, warm fluids, throat lozenges, and analgesic-antipyretic drugs such as acetaminophen are useful to promote comfort. Often opioids are needed to reduce pain for the child to drink. Combination nonopioid and opioid elixirs such as hydrocodone (Lortab) relieve pain. Analgesics should be given routinely every 4 hours while symptoms persist.

If surgery is needed, the child requires the same psychologic preparation and physical care as for any procedure. (See Chapter 22.) The following discussion focuses on specific nursing care for tonsillectomy and adenoidectomy (T&A), although both procedures may not be performed.

The nurse takes a complete history, with special notation of any bleeding tendencies because the operative site is highly vascular. Baseline vital signs are important for postoperative monitoring and observation. Signs of any URI are noted and reported, and bleeding and clotting times may be obtained with the usual laboratory work requests. During physical assessment the presence of any loose teeth is noted. (See Surgical Procedures, Chapter 22.)

After the surgery, until they are fully awake, children are positioned to facilitate drainage of secretions. Suctioning is performed carefully to avoid trauma to the oropharynx. When alert, children may prefer sitting up, although they should remain in bed for the remainder of the day. They are discouraged from coughing frequently, clearing their throat, blowing their nose, or any activities that could aggravate the operative site.

Some secretions, particularly dried blood from surgery, are common. Inspect all secretions and vomitus for evidence of fresh bleeding (some blood-tinged mucus is expected). Dark brown (old) blood is usually present in the emesis, as well as in the nose and between the teeth. If parents are not prepared for this, they may be frightened at a time when they need to be calm and reassuring.

The throat is very sore after surgery. An ice collar may provide relief, but many children find it bothersome and refuse to use it. Most children experience moderate pain after a T&A and need pain medication at regular intervals for at least the first 24 to 48 hours. Analgesics may need to be given intravenously to avoid the oral route, however liquid analgesics may be given as tolerated. Local anesthetics, such as tetracaine lollipops or ice pops, and antiemetics, such as ondansetron (Zofran), or Scopolamine transdermal patch (ages 12 and older) may be administered postoperatively. (See Pain Management, Chapter 5.)

A recent integrative review of pain management for pediatric tonsillectomy revealed that preoperative education (child and parent) regarding anxiety and pain were important in the management of the child's postoperative pain (Howard, Finn Davis, Phillips, et al., 2014). In addition, family education regarding both pharmacologic and nonpharmacologic pain management in the home setting was viewed as being crucial to successful outcomes. An optimal pharmacologic postoperative pain medication regimen was not described, however reviews suggest that acetaminophen and hydrocodone may be safe and effective for postoperative pain (Howard, Finn Davis, Phillips, et al., 2014).

DRUG ALERT

Codeine

Codeine is contraindicated in pediatric patients post tonsillectomy and adenoidectomy. In 2012 the US Food and Drug Administration issued a Drug Safety Communication that codeine use in certain children after tonsillectomy and/or adenoidectomy may lead to rare but life-threatening adverse events or death. In 2013 a boxed warning (the Food and Drug Administration's strongest) was added to codeine drug labels to warn about the risks associated with it and to contraindicate its use in this population. Some institutions have removed codeine from its formulary for pediatric patients, and others have issued restrictions on its use.

Codeine is converted to morphine in the liver by the enzyme cytochrome P450 2D6 (CYP2D6). Some patients are very slow metabolizers and do not convert adequate amounts of codeine to morphine and do not experience any analgesia; others are ultrarapid metabolizers and will produce approximately three to four times as much morphine from a given dose of codeine as expected. As reported by the Food and Drug Administration, this has led to hypopnea, apnea, and death in a number of pediatric patients. At least four cases of death or severe respiratory depression have occurred after tonsillectomy among toddlers and children given codeine who were either ultrarapid or extensive metabolizers. The deaths may be the result of genetically based differences in clinical response to codeine that are not detected without specific testing or the occurrence of an adverse event. Parents should seek immediate help if sleepiness, confusion, or difficult or noisy breathing occurs (US Food and Drug Administration, 2013).

Food and fluid are restricted until children are able to swallow them and are alert with no signs of hemorrhage. Cool water, crushed ice, flavored ice pops, or diluted fruit juice is given; fluids with a red or brown color are generally avoided to distinguish fresh or old blood in emesis from the ingested liquid. Straws should be avoided because they may damage the surgical site and cause subsequent bleeding. Citrus juice may cause discomfort and is usually poorly tolerated. Milk, ice cream, or pudding is not usually offered until clear fluids are retained because milk products coat the mouth and throat, causing the child to clear the throat, which may initiate bleeding.

Children often begin soft foods, particularly gelatin, cooked fruits, sherbet, soup, and mashed potatoes, on the first or second postoperative day or as the child tolerates feeding. The pain from surgery often inhibits oral intake, reinforcing the need for adequate pain control.

NURSING ALERT

The most obvious early sign of bleeding is the child's continuous swallowing of the trickling blood. While the child is sleeping, note the frequency of swallowing. If continuous bleeding is suspected, notify the surgeon immediately.

Postoperative hemorrhage is unusual but can occur. The nurse observes the throat directly for evidence of bleeding, using a good source of light and, if necessary, carefully inserting a tongue depressor. Other signs of hemorrhage are tachycardia, pallor, frequent clearing of the throat or swallowing by a younger child, and vomiting of bright red blood. Restlessness, an indication of hemorrhage, may be difficult to differentiate from general discomfort after surgery. Decreasing blood pressure is a much later sign of shock. A cream-colored membrane is often visible on the tonsillar bed postoperatively for 5 to 10 days postsurgery; reassure parents this is an expected finding.

Surgery may be required to cauterize or ligate a bleeding vessel. Airway obstruction may also occur as a result of edema or accumulated secretions and is indicated by signs of respiratory distress, such as stridor, drooling, restlessness, agitation, increasing respiratory rate, and progressive cyanosis. Suction equipment and oxygen should be available after tonsillectomy.

Family Support and Home Care

Discharge instructions include (1) avoiding foods that are irritating or highly seasoned, (2) avoiding the use of gargles or vigorous toothbrushing, (3) discouraging the child from coughing or clearing the throat or putting objects in the mouth, (4) using analgesics and opioids for pain, and (5) limiting activity to decrease the potential for bleeding. Hemorrhage may occur up to 10 days after surgery as a result of tissue sloughing from the healing process. Any sign of bleeding warrants immediate medical attention. Objectionable mouth odor and slight ear pain with a low-grade fever are common for a few days postoperatively. However, persistent severe earache, fever, or cough requires medical evaluation. Most children are ready to resume normal activity within 1 to 2 weeks after the operation.

Most children are admitted to a same-day surgery or ambulatory surgery unit and discharged home after a recovery period. T&A often represents the first hospitalization experience for the child and family. Because the surgery is usually an elective procedure, there is ample opportunity to prepare both children and parents for this event. Both need reassurance about what to expect at the time of admission, before and after surgery, and at discharge. Children are informed about postoperative discomfort and reassured that they will be able to talk. Some children believe the procedure will immediately "make the throat all better" and are dismayed to find that it still hurts after the surgery.

INFECTIOUS MONONUCLEOSIS

Infectious mononucleosis is an acute, self-limiting infectious disease that is common among young people under 25 years old. Symptoms include fever, exudative pharyngitis with petechiae, lymphadenopathy, hepatosplenomegaly, and an increase in atypical lymphocytes. The course is usually mild but occasionally can be severe or, rarely, accompanied by serious complications.

Etiology and Pathophysiology

The Epstein-Barr virus is the principal cause of infectious mononucleosis. It appears in both sporadic and epidemic forms, but the sporadic cases are more common. The virus is believed to be transmitted by direct contact with oral secretions (close personal contact is needed to transmit the virus), blood transfusion, or transplantation. It is mildly contagious, and the period of communicability is unknown. The incubation period after exposure in adolescents is estimated to be 30 to 50 days (American Academy of Pediatrics, Report of the Committee on Infectious Diseases, 2015).

Clinical Manifestations

Symptoms of infectious mononucleosis can appear 10 days to 6 weeks after exposure and may be acute or insidious. The common presenting symptoms vary greatly in type, severity, and duration. The characteristics of the disease are malaise, sore throat, and fever with generalized lymphadenopathy and splenomegaly that may persist for several months. Often the symptoms appear insidiously with fatigue, lack of energy, and sore throat. The child's chief complaint is difficulty in maintaining the usual level of activity. This is often attributed to lack of sleep or a URI. In many instances the manifestations never arouse enough concern to bring the affected individual to medical attention. The clinical manifestations of infectious mononucleosis are usually less severe (often subclinical or unapparent), and the recovery phase is shorter in younger children than in older children and young adults. Many young children do not develop all the expected clinical and laboratory findings. Often an insidious symptom is the only or the presenting symptom.

A skin rash that involves a discrete macular eruption is present in some cases and is often associated with the administration of ampicillin or amoxicillin (Jenson, 2016). Other symptoms include headache, epistaxis, and a severe sore throat. The tonsils may be enlarged, reddened, and sometimes covered with a diphtheria-like membrane. In some cases airway compromise may occur with tonsillar swelling. In about half the cases the spleen is enlarged to 2 to 3 cm below the costal margin (Jenson, 2016). The extensive mononuclear infiltration produces symptoms related to any body tissue, and the clinical picture can resemble that of many conditions, including neurologic manifestations and cardiac involvement.

Diagnostic Evaluation

The diagnosis is established on the basis of clinical manifestations, increase in atypical leukocytes in a peripheral blood smear, and a positive heterophil agglutination test. Differential diagnosis depends on the clinical symptoms present. For example, the pharyngitis may simulate symptoms of diphtheria and streptococcal pharyngitis. Lymphadenopathy, fever, malaise, CNS manifestations, and skin eruptions may be similar to symptoms seen in a variety of conditions. The leukocyte count may be normal or low, but usually lymphocytic leukocytosis develops.

The nonspecific heterophil antibody tests (Monospot or Paul-Brunell) determine the extent to which the patient's serum will agglutinate sheep red blood cells. The response is mainly to immunoglobulin M that is present in the first 2 weeks and may last 6 months (American Academy of Pediatrics, Report of the Committee on Infectious Diseases, 2015). In infectious mononucleosis a titer of 1:160 is considered diagnostic, although a rising titer during the earlier stages is the best indicator. Because children less than age 4 years have a lower rate of heterophil antibody responses, the diagnosis may be overlooked in this group.

The spot test (Monospot) is a slide test of high specificity for the diagnosis of infectious mononucleosis. It is rapid, sensitive, inexpensive, and easy to perform, and it has the advantage that it can detect significant agglutinins at lower levels, thus permitting earlier diagnosis. Blood is usually obtained for the test by finger puncture and is placed on special paper. If the blood agglutinates, forming fragments or clumps, the test is positive for the infection.

Therapeutic Management

No specific treatment exists for infectious mononucleosis. A mild analgesic is usually sufficient to relieve the bothersome symptoms of headache, fever, and malaise. Rest is encouraged for fatigue but is not imposed for any specified time. Affected children and adolescents should regulate activities according to their own tolerance unless complicating factors are present. If the spleen is enlarged, contact and collision sports are discouraged until it resolves (American Academy of Pediatrics, Report of the Committee on Infectious Diseases, 2015).

A short course of corticosteroids may assist in decreasing some of the complications (e.g., airway obstruction) of the illness. Administration of ampicillin or amoxicillin frequently precipitates a maculopapular rash in affected persons (80% of cases); therefore their use may be contraindicated. Gargles, warm drinks, analgesic or anesthetic troches, or analgesics, including opioids, can relieve a sore throat. Although corticosteroids have been used to treat respiratory distress from tonsillar hypertrophy, hemolytic anemia, thrombocytopenia, and neurologic complications, the routine use of steroids is not recommended (American Academy of Pediatrics, Report of the Committee on Infectious Diseases, 2015).

Prognosis

The course of infectious mononucleosis is self-limiting and usually uncomplicated. Contrary to popular belief, mononucleosis is not necessarily a difficult, prolonged, or disabling disease, and the prognosis is generally good. Acute symptoms usually disappear within 7 to 10 days, and the persistent fatigue subsides within 2 to 4 weeks. A number of affected children or adolescents may need to restrict activities for 2 to 3 months; the disease rarely extends for longer periods. The child is encouraged to maintain limited activities to prevent deconditioning.

Complications are uncommon but can be serious and require appropriate management. Neurologic complications occur in some outbreaks and vary in severity and outcome. These include seizures, ataxia, aseptic meningitis, encephalitis, optic neuritis, cranial nerve palsies, and perceptual distortions of shapes, spatial relationships, and sizes. Other complications include pneumonitis, orchitis, myocarditis, transverse myelitis, hemolytic anemia, agranulocytosis, thrombocytopenia, hemophagocytic lymphohistiocytosis, and ruptured spleen. Some evidence indicates a depressed cellular immune reactivity during the course of the disease and for some time afterward. Thus it is best to avoid live vaccines until several months after recovery. The Epstein-Barr virus can replicate in B lymphocytes, resulting in T-lymphocyte growth, and lymphomas can occur.

Nursing Care Management

Direct nursing responsibilities toward providing comfort measures to relieve the symptoms and helping affected children and adolescents and their families determine appropriate activities for the stage of the disease and their interests. Airway assessment for impending obstruction during the acute phase of the illness is imperative. The adolescent with infectious mononucleosis may not be able to swallow secretions and may be in considerable pain. The child or adolescent is encouraged to increase clear fluid intake and decrease solid foods that may exacerbate the pain. In addition, the nurse should encourage the affected individual to curtail activities that are strenuous until splenomegaly is resolved. Pain medications in elixir form such as acetaminophen, ibuprofen, or hydrocodone may be required during the acute phase so the adolescent can swallow liquids. Make every effort to prevent a secondary infection by counseling the adolescent to limit exposure to persons outside the family, especially during the acute phase of illness.

! NURSING ALERT

Advise the family to seek medical evaluation of the child or adolescent if

- Breathing becomes difficult
- Severe abdominal pain develops
- Sore throat pain is so severe that the child is unable to eat or drink
- Respiratory stridor is observed

INFLUENZA

Influenza (the "flu") is caused by the orthomyxoviruses and classified into three distinct groups: types A and B, which cause epidemic disease (and are included in the vaccine), and type C, which causes milder illness and is not included in the vaccine. The viruses undergo significant changes from time to time. Major changes that occur at intervals of usually 5 to 10 years are called **antigenic shift**; minor variations within the same subtypes, **antigenic drift**, occur almost annually. Consequently, antigenic drift can alter the virus sufficiently to result in susceptibility of individuals to a type for which they were previously immunized or infected.

The disease is spread from one individual to another by direct contact (large-droplet infection) usually occurring during talking, sneezing or coughing, or by articles recently contaminated by nasopharyngeal secretions. There is no predilection for a specific age-group, but attack rates are highest in young children who have not had previous contact with a strain, as well as patients with chronic medical conditions (e.g., diabetes, asthma) and pregnant women. It is frequently most severe in infants and older adults. During epidemics, infection among school-age children is believed to be a major source of transmission in a community. Influenza is more common during the winter months.

The disease has a 1- to 4-day incubation period (average of 2 days), and affected persons are most infectious for 24 hours before and 5 to 7 days after the onset of symptoms (Centers for Disease Control and Prevention, 2017). The virus has a peculiar affinity for epithelial cells of the respiratory tract mucosa, where it destroys ciliated epithelium with metaplastic hyperplasia of the tracheal and bronchial epithelium with associated edema. The alveoli may also become distended with a hyaline-like material. The viruses can be isolated from nasopharyngeal secretions early after the onset of infection, and serologic tests identify the type by complement fixation or the subgroups by hemagglutination inhibition. Outbreaks in the community can last many weeks.

H1N1 (swine flu) is a subtype of influenza type A. In 2009 a pandemic of H1N1 caused significant morbidity and mortality, particularly in Mexico and the United States, lasting until the end of August 2010. A pandemic is defined by the World Health Organization (WHO) as the spread of a new disease to which the population has little or no immunity and that spreads rapidly from human to human. The H1N1 vaccine has been included in the seasonal influenza vaccination since the 2011–2012 season.

Occasionally influenza type A disease can be caused by a virus that had a swine or avian origin. Any influenza virus that is novel in nature is reportable to the Centers for Disease Control and Prevention (American Academy of Pediatrics, Report of the Committee on Infectious Diseases, 2015).

Clinical Manifestations

The manifestations of influenza may be subclinical, mild, moderate, or severe. In most cases, there is a dry cough and a tendency toward hoarseness. A sudden onset of fever and chills is accompanied by flushed face, photophobia, myalgia, sore throat, headaches, hyperesthesia, and sometimes prostration. Children may have vomiting or diarrhea. Subglottal croup is common, especially in infants. The symptoms last 4 or 5 days. Complications include severe viral pneumonia (often hemorrhagic), febrile seizures, encephalitis, encephalopathy, dehydration, and secondary bacterial infections, such as myocarditis, OM, sinusitis, or pneumonia. Diagnosis is confirmed by analyzing nasopharyngeal secretions for viral culture or rapid detection testing. Influenza A and B can be rapidly detected by direct fluorescent antibody and indirect immunofluorescent antibody staining.

Therapeutic Management

Uncomplicated influenza in children usually requires only symptomatic treatment: acetaminophen or ibuprofen for fever and sufficient fluids to maintain hydration. Oseltamivir, zanamivir, and peramivir are recommended to treat influenza for patients at high risk of complications from the flu (American Academy of Pediatrics, Report of the Committee on Infectious Diseases, 2015). Amantadine hydrochloride (Symmetrel) had been effective in reducing symptoms associated with type A disease but there has been an increase in influenza strains resistant to amantadine, and thus the neuraminidase inhibitors, oseltamivir and zanamivir, have been recommended for influenza treatment (American Academy of Pediatrics, Report of the Committee on Infectious Diseases, 2015). A small number of influenza strains are resistant to oseltamivir.

Zanamivir can be used to treat patients ages 7 years and older or as prophylaxis for patients ages 5 years and older (American Academy of Pediatrics, Report of the Committee on Infectious Diseases, 2015). It is an inhaled medication effective for types A and B influenza. The drug is taken twice daily for 5 days and is administered by a specially designed oral inhaler (Diskhaler); bronchospasm may occur in children with an underlying airway disease. Bronchospasm and a decline in lung function can occur when zanamivir is used in patients with underlying airway disease such as asthma or chronic obstructive pulmonary disease.

Oseltamivir is a neuroaminidase inhibitor that may be administered orally for 5 days to decrease the flu symptoms. The medication can be used for infants and children of any age and is effective for types A and B influenza (American Academy of Pediatrics, Report of the Committee on Infectious Diseases, 2015). As with other antiviral drugs, for best results the medication should be started within 2 days of the onset of symptoms. Children should not receive aspirin because of its possible link with Reye syndrome.

Prevention

The influenza vaccine is recommended annually for children 6 months to 18 years. Influenza vaccine (inactivated influenza vaccine) may be given to any healthy children ages 6 months and older. An intradermal preparation of influenza vaccination is available for people 18 to 64 years old. During the 2016–2017 influenza season, the live attenuated influenza vaccine, administered intranasally, was discontinued due to concerns about its effectiveness (Belongia, Karron, Reingold, et al., 2018).

The influenza vaccine is administered yearly because different strains of influenza are used each year in the manufacture of the vaccine. It is safe and effective provided the antigens in the vaccine correlate with the circulating influenza viruses. The influenza vaccine may be given simultaneously with other vaccines but at a separate site. Two doses are needed at least 28 days apart to all children 6 months to 9 years in their first or second vaccination seasons to adequately protect them against influenza. A topical analgesic cream such as LMX4 or EMLA should be applied to the site beforehand to reduce pain. See Chapter 6 for guidelines for influenza vaccine to patients with a hypersensitivity to eggs.

Nursing Care Management

Nursing care is the same as for any child with a URI, including helping the family implement measures to relieve symptoms. Prolonged fever or appearance of fever during early convalescence is a sign of secondary bacterial infection and should be reported to the practitioner for antibiotic therapy. In addition to the measures mentioned previously, nursing care of the child with influenza includes educating the parents regarding the prevention of the spread of the disease to other individuals, especially those who are at higher risk for complications, and educating the parents about the use of antiviral medications. Many institutions have developed protocols to allow nurses to screen patients for eligibility to receive the influenza vaccine. The protocol then functions as an order to administer it to those who are eligible.

OTITIS MEDIA

Otitis media (OM) is the presence of fluid in the middle ear along with acute signs of illness and symptoms of middle ear inflammation (Venekamp, Damoiseaux, & Schilder, 2017). It is one of the most prevalent illnesses of early childhood. Its incidence is highest in the winter months. Many cases of bacterial OM are preceded by a viral respiratory tract infection. The two viruses most likely to precipitate OM are RSV and

BOX 26.4 Standard Terminology for Otitis Media

Otitis media (OM)—An inflammation of the middle ear without reference to etiology or pathogenesis

Acute otitis media (AOM)—An inflammation of the middle ear space with a rapid onset of the signs and symptoms of acute infection—namely, fever and otalgia (ear pain)

Otitis media with effusion (OME)—Fluid in the middle ear space without symptoms of acute infection

BOX 26.5 Factors Predisposing Children to Development of Otitis Media

- The eustachian tubes are short, wide, and straight and lie in a relatively horizontal plane (see Fig. 26.3).
- The cartilage lining is undeveloped, making the tubes more distensible and therefore more likely to open inappropriately.
- The normally abundant pharyngeal lymphoid tissue readily obstructs the eustachian tube openings in the nasopharynx.
- Immature humoral defense mechanisms increase the risk of infection.
- The usual lying-down position of infants favors the pooling of fluid, such as formula or exudate, in the pharyngeal cavity.

influenza. Most episodes of *acute otitis media* (AOM) occur in the first 24 months of life, but the incidence decreases with age, except for a small increase at age 5 or 6 years when children enter school. OM occurs infrequently in children older than 7 years of age. Children who have siblings or parents with a history of chronic OM have a higher incidence of OM. Out-of-home day care is a significant risk factor for OM.

Children living in households with many members are more likely to have OM than those living with fewer persons. Passive smoking increases the risk of persistent middle ear effusion by enhancing attachment of the pathogens that cause otitis to the respiratory epithelium in the middle ear space, prolonging the inflammatory response and impeding drainage through the eustachian tube (Kerschner & Preciado, 2016). Family socioeconomic status is another important risk factors for the occurrence of OM (Kerschner & Preciado, 2016).

A relationship has been observed between the incidence of OM and infant feeding methods. Infants fed breast milk have a lower incidence of OM compared with formula-fed infants. Breastfeeding may protect infants against respiratory viruses and allergy because it contains secretory immunoglobulin A, which limits the exposure of the eustachian tube and middle ear mucosa to microbial pathogens and foreign proteins. Reflux of milk up the eustachian tubes is less likely in breastfed infants because of the semivertical positioning during breastfeeding compared with bottle-feeding. Breastfeeding should be encouraged for at least 6 months (Korvel-Hanquist, Djurhuus, & Homoe, 2017).

OM has been defined in a variety of ways. The standard terminology is given in Box 26.4, and AOM and OM with effusion (OME) guidelines have been published (Siddiq & Grainger, 2015; Rosenfeld, Shin, Schwartz, et al., 2016).

Etiology

AOM is frequently caused by *Streptococcus pneumoniae, H. influenzae,* and *Moraxella catarrhalis.* The two viruses most likely to precipitate OM are RSV and influenza, although the adenoviruses, human metapneumoviruses, and picornaviruses (rhinovirus and enterovirus) also cause a significant number of URIs and OM. The etiology of the noninfectious type is unknown, although it is frequently the result of blocked eustachian tubes from the edema of URIs, allergic rhinitis, or hypertrophic adenoids. *Chronic OM* is frequently an extension of an acute episode.

Pathophysiology

OM is primarily a result of a dysfunctioning eustachian tube. The eustachian tube is part of a contiguous system composed of the nares, nasopharynx, eustachian tube, middle ear, and mastoid antrum and air cells. Mechanical or functional obstruction of the eustachian tube causes accumulation of secretions in the middle ear. Infection or allergy can cause intrinsic obstruction. Extrinsic obstruction is usually a result of enlarged adenoids or nasopharyngeal tumors. Eustachian tube obstruction results in negative middle ear pressure and, if persistent, produces a transudative middle ear effusion. Sustained negative pressure and impaired ciliary transport within the tube inhibit drainage. When the passage is not totally obstructed, contamination of the middle ear can take place by reflux, aspiration, or insufflation during crying, sneezing, nose blowing, and swallowing when the nose is obstructed. Several factors predispose infants and young children to development of OM (Box 26.5 and Fig. 26.3).

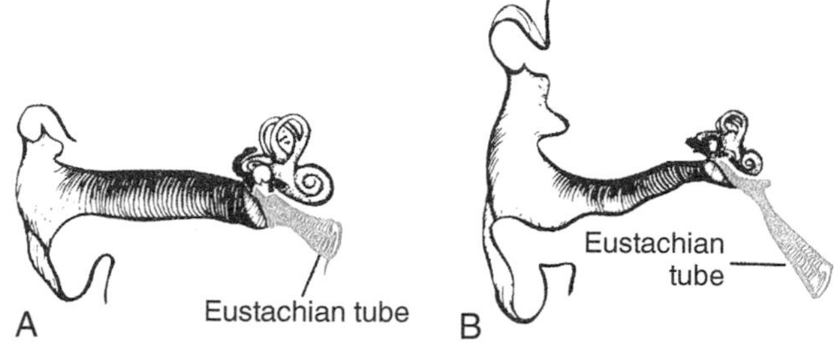

FIG. 26.3 Comparison of anatomic position of eustachian tube in a child **(A)** and an adult **(B)**. Eustachian tube is shorter, wider, straighter, and more horizontal in a child than in an adult.

Complications

The consequences of prolonged middle ear disorders can be either functional or structural. The principal functional consequence is hearing loss, although loss in most children is conductive in nature and mild in severity. The causes of hearing loss are negative middle ear pressure, effusion in the middle ear, involvement of the eighth cranial nerve, and structural damage to the tympanic membrane. However, the most feared consequence of hearing loss is its adverse effect on development of speech, language, and cognition. Children who have prolonged periods of middle ear effusion perform less well on speech and language tests than those who have few or no middle ear diseases.

Structural complications or sequelae involve primarily the tympanic membrane. Tympanic membrane retraction or retraction pockets occur in areas of low tensile strength or atrophic segments of the drum head when continued negative middle ear pressure draws the tympanic membrane inward. This retraction may result in impaired sound transmission, perforation of the thinned-out areas, or infection in the pockets and, later, cholesteatoma.

Tympanosclerosis (eardrum scarring) is the deposition of hyaline material into the fibrous layer of the tympanic membrane. It often occurs in children with inflammatory middle ear disease or those with repeated tympanoplasty tube placement. Eardrum perforation is a common complication in AOM and often accompanies chronic disease. Persistent perforation is a complication of tympanostomy tube placement. Surgery is required to close some perforations.

Adhesive OM (glue ear) is a thickening of the mucous membrane by proliferation of fibrous tissue that can cause fixation of the ossicles with a resultant hearing loss. Chronic suppurative OM, an inflammation of the middle ear and mastoid, is evidenced by perforation and discharge (otorrhea) for up to 6 weeks' duration. Labyrinthitis, infection of the inner ear, and mastoiditis, infection of the mastoid sinus, are rare since the advent of antibiotic therapy. Meningitis and other suppurative intracranial conditions are possible complications of extension of infection from the middle ear or mastoid. However, these complications occur infrequently when adequate antibiotic therapy is implemented. Vestibular dysfunction or labyrinthitis may result in impaired balance and motor problems.

Cholesteatoma is the least common but most potentially dangerous sequela of OME. A cholesteatoma forms when the keratinizing, stratified, squamous epithelial cell lining desquamates to form scales that accumulate within the middle ear space. As it enlarges, the cholesteatoma erodes all structures it encounters, especially bone, destroying the ossicles and gaining entry to the inner ear and meninges. Clinical signs are a foul-smelling, grayish-yellow discharge; sometimes pain; and permanent, progressive hearing loss. Treatment is surgical excision of the entire cholesteatoma.

Clinical Manifestations

As purulent fluid accumulates in the small space of the middle ear chamber, pain results from the pressure on surrounding structures. Infants become irritable and can indicate their discomfort by holding or pulling at their ears and rolling their head from side to side. Young children usually verbally complain of the pain. A temperature as high as 104°F (40°C) is common, and postauricular and cervical lymph glands may be enlarged. Rhinorrhea, vomiting, diarrhea, and signs of concurrent respiratory tract or pharyngeal infection may also be present. Loss of appetite typically occurs, and sucking or chewing tends to aggravate the pain. In children with OME, exudate accumulates and pressure increases, with the potential for tympanic membrane rupture. As a result of rupture, there is immediate relief of pain, a gradual decrease in temperature, and the presence of purulent discharge in the external auditory canal.

Severe pain or fever is usually absent in OME, and the child may not appear ill. Instead there is a feeling of "fullness" in the ear, a popping sensation during swallowing, and a feeling of "motion" in the ear if air is present above the level of fluid. Because chronic serous OM is the most frequent cause of conductive hearing loss in young children, audiometry may reveal deficient hearing.

Diagnostic Evaluation

Careful assessment of tympanic membrane mobility with a pneumatic otoscope is essential to differentiate AOM from OME (Kerschner & Preciado, 2016). If an accumulation of cerumen prevents adequate visualization of the tympanic membrane, the cerumen should be removed before inspection of the membrane. A diagnosis of AOM is made with moderate to severe bulging of the tympanic membrane, acute onset of ear drainage not due to acute otitis externa, mild bulging of the tympanic membrane with onset of pain occurring less than 48 hours, and intense erythema of the tympanic membrane (Kerschner & Preciado, 2016). An immobile tympanic membrane or an orange-colored membrane indicates OME. In OME these symptoms may be absent, and other nonspecific symptoms such as rhinitis, cough, or diarrhea are often present.

Several tests provide an assessment of mobility of the tympanic membrane. Chapter 4 discusses pneumatic otoscopy and tympanometry. Acoustic reflectometry measures the level of sound transmitted and reflected from the middle ear to a microphone located in a probe tip placed against the ear canal opening and directed toward the tympanic membrane. The information provides a measure of canal length and presence of effusion. The greater the cancellation of transmitted sound by reflected sound, the greater the probability of middle ear effusion.

Therapeutic Management: Acute Otitis Media

Treatment for AOM is one of the most common reasons for antibiotic use in the ambulatory setting. However, recent concerns about drug-resistant strains have led infectious disease authorities to recommend careful and judicious use of antibiotics for treatment of this illness. The American Academy of Pediatrics and the Centers for Disease Control and Prevention have initiated a Get Smart campaign to educate families about judicious use of antibiotics (American Academy of Pediatrics, Report of the Committee on Infectious Diseases, 2015). Current recommendations regarding antibiotic administration to children with AOM are as follows (American Academy of Pediatrics, Report of the Committee on Infectious Diseases, 2015):

- Definitive diagnosis of AOM (middle ear effusion, bulging tympanic membrane, or new otorrhea not due to otitis externa)
- Mild bulging of the tympanic membrane with recent erythema or ear pain

The latest American Academy of Pediatrics recommendations also place emphasis on assessment and management of pain in children with AOM. For fever or discomfort associated with OM, analgesic-antipyretic drugs such as acetaminophen or ibuprofen may be given. The health care practitioner may prescribe topical pain relief drops such as benzocaine or lidocaine. A narcotic analgesic may be required for children with severe pain, but side effects are common and the child should be closely monitored for gastrointestinal (GI) upset, constipation, respiratory depression, and altered mental status.

When antibiotics are necessary, oral amoxicillin in high doses (80 to 90 mg/kg/day, divided twice daily) is recommended for 5 to 7 days with children 2 years and older, and 10 days with younger children, children with underlying medical conditions, craniofacial anomalies, tympanic membrane perforation or children with chronic otitis media.

Second-line antibiotics used to treat OM include amoxicillin-clavulanate (Augmentin) (which is recommended if conjunctivitis is also present); azithromycin; and cephalosporins such as cefdinir, cefuroxime, and cefpodoxime. IM ceftriaxone is used if the causative organism is a highly resistant pneumococcus or if there is noncompliance with the therapy. An important consideration with the use of single-dose IM injections is the pain involved in this therapy. One strategy to minimize pain at the injection site is to reconstitute the cephalosporin with 1% lidocaine (without epinephrine). A topical anesthetic cream such as EMLA or LMX4 can be applied to the site beforehand to reduce pain. The use of steroids, decongestants, and antihistamines to treat AOM is not recommended.

Supportive care or symptomatic treatment of AOM includes treating the fever and pain. For fever or discomfort associated with OM, analgesic-antipyretic drugs such as acetaminophen or ibuprofen (ibuprofen only if over 6 months of age) may be given. Topical pain relief is recommended by external application of heat or cold, or the practitioner may prescribe topical pain relief drops such as benzocaine drops. Antibiotic ear drops have no value in treating AOM. Decongestants and antihistamines are not recommended for children with ear infections.

Children with AOM may be seen after antibiotic therapy is complete to evaluate the effectiveness of the treatment and to identify potential complications, such as effusion or hearing impairment.

Myringotomy, a surgical incision of the eardrum, may be necessary to alleviate the severe pain of AOM. A myringotomy is also performed to drain infected middle ear fluid in the presence of complications (e.g., mastoiditis, labyrinthitis, or facial paralysis) or to allow purulent middle ear fluid to drain into the ear canal for culture. A minimally invasive laser-assisted myringotomy procedure may be performed in outpatient settings. These procedures should only be performed by ear, nose, and throat specialists.

Therapeutic Management: Recurrent Otitis Media

Therapy for recurrent AOM includes surgery. Chemoprophylaxis is no longer recommended because of the cost of therapy, potential adverse effects of therapy (e.g., allergic reaction, GI upset), and most importantly contribution to bacterial resistance (Kerschner & Preciado, 2016). Tympanostomy tube placement may be indicated with chronic OM (three episodes in 6 months or four episodes in 1 year, with one episode during the preceding 6 months) (Kerschner & Preciado, 2016). Tympanostomy tubes are pressure equalization devices (grommets) that facilitate drainage and ventilation of the middle ear.

Therapeutic Management: Otitis Media With Effusion

In some children, residual middle ear effusions remain after episodes of AOM. Management options for OM with residual effusion include observation, antibiotics alone, or a combination of antibiotic and corticosteroid therapy. Antibiotics are not required for initial treatment of OME (Kerschner & Preciado, 2016). Hearing testing is performed in children who have OME for 3 months or more.

Some children have fluid that persists in the middle ear for weeks or months. OME is frequently associated with mild to moderate hearing impairment. The major goal of therapy is to establish and maintain an aerated middle ear that is free of fluid with a normal mucosa and ultimately to achieve normal hearing.

Placement of tympanostomy tubes is recommended after a total of 3 to 6 months of bilateral effusion with a bilateral hearing deficit (Kerschner & Preciado, 2016). This therapy allows for mechanical drainage of the fluid, which promotes healing of the membrane and prevents scar formation and loss of elasticity. The primary objective is to allow the eustachian tube a period of recovery while the surgically placed tube performs its functions. The surgery is relatively benign; however, sometimes the tubes become plugged, and they often require reinsertion. Complications of repeated or long-term tube placement are tympanosclerosis, localized or diffuse atrophy of the membrane, persistent perforation, or, rarely, cholesteatoma. Myringotomy with or without insertion of PE tubes should *not* be performed for initial management of OME but may be recommended for children who have recurrent episodes of OME with a long cumulative duration. A recent meta-analysis concluded that tympanostomy tubes had a significant improvement in hearing and a decrease in the incidence of AOM compared with watchful waiting (Steele, Adam, Di, et al., 2017).

Tonsillectomy, either alone or with adenoidectomy, is not considered an effective treatment of OME. Steroids are not recommended for treatment of OME in children of any age.

Prevention

Routine immunization with the pneumococcal vaccine has reduced the incidence of AOM in some infants and children, especially those with frequent episodes of AOM (Kerschner & Preciado, 2016). A new conjugate vaccine, Prevnar 13, replaces Prevnar (PCV 7) and is approved for use in patients 6 weeks to 17 years old (American Academy of Pediatrics, Report of the Committee on Infectious Diseases, 2015). The vaccine is administered as a four-dose series beginning at 2 months of age. Influenza vaccination to children over 6 months is also important.

Parents are encouraged to reduce risk factors for AOM by breastfeeding infants for at least the first 6 months of life, avoiding propping the formula bottle, decreasing or discontinuing pacifier use after 6 months, and preventing exposure to tobacco smoke (Kerschner & Preciado, 2016).

Prognosis

Most cases of OM resolve without any residual effects. However, varying degrees of hearing loss can occur. Although conductive hearing loss is most often associated with OM, sensorineural hearing loss may also be present, especially in severe forms of chronic or recurrent OM because of the passage of toxic products from fluids into the cochlea through the tympanic membrane. The longer the fluid is present, the greater the sensorineural hearing loss. Children who are prone to OM should be referred to a pediatric otolaryngologist and possibly a pediatric allergist for identification and treatment of the cause of their eustachian tube dysfunction. They should also be referred to a speech and language pathologist for primary prevention counseling. In addition, the child should ideally be monitored by an audiologist to evaluate the adequacy of hearing.

Nursing Care Management

Nursing objectives for the child with AOM include relieving pain, facilitating drainage when possible, preventing complications or recurrence, educating the family in care of the child, and providing support to the child and family.

Analgesics are helpful to reduce severe earache, as well as control fever (ibuprofen and acetaminophen). Ibuprofen has a longer duration of action (about 6 hours) and is especially beneficial for nighttime comfort but should not be used in children under 6 months of age unless directed by a provider. The application of heat over the ear while the child lies on the affected side may reduce pain in some children but may aggravate discomfort in others. This position also facilitates drainage of the exudate if the eardrum has ruptured or if myringotomy was performed.

If the ear is draining, the external canal may be cleaned with sterile cotton swabs coupled with topical antibiotic treatment, as directed by the provider. If ear wicks or lightly rolled sterile gauze packs are placed in the ear after surgical treatment, they should be loose enough to allow accumulated drainage to flow out of the ear; otherwise the infection may be transferred to the mastoid process. Parents should keep these wicks dry during shampoos or baths. Occasionally drainage is so profuse that the pinna and surrounding skin become excoriated from exudate. Frequent cleansing and application of various moisture barriers (e.g., Proshield Plus Skin Protectant), zinc oxide–based products, or petrolatum jelly (e.g., Vaseline) can prevent or treat this.

Preventing recurrence requires adequate parent education regarding antibiotic therapy. Because the symptoms of pain and fever usually subside within 24 to 48 hours, nurses must emphasize that although the child may appear well, the infection is not completely eradicated until all the prescribed medication is taken. It is important to stress the potential complications of OM, especially hearing loss, which can be prevented with adequate treatment and follow-up care. (See Administration of Medication, and Compliance, Chapter 22.)

Tympanostomy tubes may be indicated to allow ventilation into the middle ear to equalize middle ear pressure. Most children's hearing improves right after surgery and ear drainage is common up to 1 week after insertion. The tympanostomy tube is eventually pushed out of the eardrum usually 8 to 18 months after tube placement. Parents should be aware of the appearance of a tympanostomy tube (usually a tiny plastic spool-shaped tube) so they can recognize it if it falls out. They are reassured that this is normal and requires no immediate intervention, although they should notify the practitioner.

Tympanostomy tubes may allow water to enter the middle ear, but recommendations for earplugs are inconsistent. Most patients, including very young children, often need no special water precautions. Recent research has indicated that there is no need for water precautions unless the child develops recurrent drainage after swimming (Moualed, Masterson, Kumar, et al., 2016). Healthcare providers offer recommendations for water precautions.

Reducing the chances of OM is possible with simple measures, such as sitting or holding an infant upright for feedings. Propping bottles is discouraged to avoid pooling of milk while the child is in the supine position and to encourage human contact during feeding. Eliminating tobacco smoke and known allergens is also recommended. Forceful nose blowing during a URI is discouraged to avoid forcing organisms to ascend through the eustachian tube. Early detection of middle ear effusion is essential in prevention of complications. Infants and preschool children should be screened for effusion, and all schoolchildren, especially those with learning disabilities, should be tested for middle ear effusion. Frequent audiologic evaluations, medical consultation, and education of parents and children are advised when middle ear effusion is detected.

ACUTE OTITIS EXTERNA

AOE is commonly caused by *Pseudomonas aeruginosa* or *Staphylococcus aureus* but may include other pathogens such as aspergillus and candidal species. Ordinarily the external ear canal is protected by a waxy, water-repellent coating composed of highly viscid secretions of the sebaceous glands and the watery, pigmented secretions of apocrine glands, in combination with exfoliated surface cells. Inflammation occurs when this environment is altered by swimming, bathing, or increased environmental humidity; by infection, dermatoses, or insufficient cerumen; or by trauma from a foreign body (FB) or a finger. The ear canal becomes irritated, and maceration takes place. It is most common in 5 to 14 year olds and peaks in summer (American Academy of Pediatrics, Report of the Committee on Infectious Diseases, 2015). It is commonly referred to as swimmer's ear.

The predominant symptom of external ear infection is ear pain accentuated by manipulation of the pinna, especially pressure on the tragus. The pain often appears to be out of proportion to the degree of inflammation. Conductive hearing loss may be present as a result of the edema, secretions, and accumulation of debris within the canal. Edema, erythema, a cheesy green-blue-gray discharge, and tenderness appear as the infection progresses. The external canal may be so tender and swollen that visualization is difficult. There may be a fever. In advanced cases the pain is intense, constant, and aggravated by jaw motion or ear manipulation.

Therapeutic objectives include relief of pain, edema, and itching, as well as restoration of normal flora, cerumen, and canal epithelium. Analgesics are prescribed for pain. Debris is removed with gentle suction and wisps of cotton on metal cotton carriers. Otic preparations such as polymyxin-B sulfate/neomycin sulfate, ciprofloxacin and gentamycin sulfate, with or without corticosteroids, are instilled in the canal for a 7 to 10 days. If the child has tympanostomy tubes, polymyxin-B sulfate, neomycin sulfate, or gentamycin should not be used because of the risk of ototoxicity. A gauze wick may be inserted if edema is present to facilitate the medication reaching the site of inflammation. The wick is removed after swelling and pain have subsided, but the drops are continued for at least 3 days after relief of pain. The best management for external ear inflammation is prevention.

Nursing Care Management

Nurses can teach parents or patients simple steps to prevent recurrent infections. Children should limit their stay in the water to less than an hour, if possible, and ears should dry completely (1 to 2 hours) before entering the water again. Placing a combination of acetic acid (white vinegar) and rubbing alcohol (50:50) in both ear canals on arising, at bedtime, and at the end of each swim is effective in restoring pH and preventing recurrence. This mixture must not be used if tympanostomy tubes are present. The solution should remain in the canal for 5 minutes. The child should be cautioned not to submerge his or her head in water for 7 to 10 days, but well-fitting earplugs can be used if this is not possible.

Caution children not to pick at the ears with a pencil, cotton swab, bobby pin, or other object, which can injure or infect the ear canal.

NURSING TIP

In an older child (usually older than 3 years of age), to keep the ear dry, pull the auricle up and out to straighten the canal, and then use a conventional hair dryer, set on low or no heat, held at a distance of 18 to 24 inches for 30 seconds, three times a day if tolerated.

CROUP SYNDROMES

Croup is a general term applied to a group of symptoms characterized by hoarseness, a resonant cough described as "barking" or "brassy" (croupy), varying degrees of inspiratory stridor, and varying degrees of respiratory distress resulting from swelling or obstruction in the region of the larynx and subglottic airway. Acute infections of the larynx are of greater importance in infants and small children than they are in older children because of the increased incidence in children in this age-group and the smaller diameter of the airway, which renders it subject to significantly greater narrowing with the same degree of inflammation (Fig. 26.4). With widespread immunization programs aimed at preventing *H. influenzae* type B, most cases of croup in the United States are attributed to viruses—namely, influenza types A and B, adenovirus, RSV, and measles (Roosevelt, 2016). Bacteria such as *Mycoplasma pneumonia* can also cause croup.

Croup is a common respiratory disease of childhood and occurs more often in boys than in girls. The number of croup cases increases in the late autumn through early winter months. It occurs primarily in children 6 months to 3 years of age and is rare after 6 years of age. Hospitalization may be necessary for some children with croup, and a small percentage of hospitalized children require positive airway pressure or intubation.

Croup syndromes affect to varying degrees the larynx, trachea, and bronchi. However, laryngeal involvement often dominates the clinical picture because of the severe effects on the voice and breathing. Croup syndromes are usually described according to the primary anatomic area affected (i.e., epiglottitis [or supraglottitis], laryngitis, laryngotracheobronchitis [LTB], and tracheitis). In general, LTB tends to occur

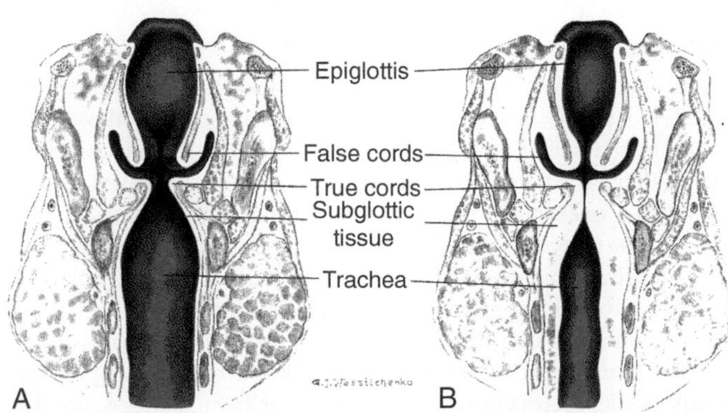

FIG. 26.4 A, Normal larynx. **B,** Obstruction and narrowing resulting from edema of croup.

TABLE 26.4 Comparison of Croup Syndromes

	Acute Epiglottitis	Acute LTB	Acute Spasmodic Laryngitis	Acute Tracheitis
Age-group affected	2-5 years but varies	Infant or child <5 years	1-3 years	1 months to 6 years
Etiologic agent	Bacterial	Viral	Viral with allergic component	Viral or bacterial with allergic component
Onset	Rapidly progressive	Slowly progressive	Sudden; at night	Moderately progressive
Major symptoms	Dysphagia Stridor aggravated when supine Drooling High fever Toxic appearance Rapid pulse and respirations	URI Stridor Brassy cough Hoarseness Dyspnea Restlessness Irritability Low-grade fever Nontoxic appearance	URI Croupy cough Stridor Hoarseness Dyspnea Restlessness Symptoms awakening child Symptoms disappearing during day Tendency to recur	URI Croupy cough Purulent secretions High fever No response to LTB therapy
Treatment	Airway protection, possible intubation, tracheotomy Humidified oxygen Fluids Antibiotics Reassurance	Corticosteroids Fluids Reassurance Nebulized epinephrine (possible short-term improvement) Heliox—moderate-to-severe croup	Cool mist Reassurance	Antibiotics Fluids

LTB, Laryngotracheobronchitis; *URI*, upper respiratory tract infection.

in very young children, whereas epiglottitis is more characteristic of older children. Table 26.4 provides a comparison of croup syndromes.

Because croup is one of the most benign conditions causing upper airway obstruction, it is vitally important to correctly identify it and distinguish the type of croup syndrome or condition (i.e., spasmodic croup or LTB as opposed to a potentially life-threatening condition such as epiglottitis, bacterial tracheitis, FB aspiration, or a peritonsillar abscess). The key differences between LTB and epiglottitis are the absence of cough, the presence of dysphagia, and the high degree of toxicity in children with epiglottitis. Children with epiglottitis usually look worse than they sound, in contrast to children with LTB, who sound worse than they look (see Critical Thinking Case Study box).

CRITICAL THINKING CASE STUDY

Croup

Kim, a 4-year-old, is admitted to the emergency department with a sore throat, pain on swallowing, drooling, and a fever of 102.2°F (39°C). She looks ill, is agitated, and prefers to sit up and lean over. What nursing interventions should the nurse implement in this situation?

1. Evidence—Is there sufficient evidence to draw any conclusions about Kim's condition at this time?
2. Assumptions—Describe some underlying assumptions about each of the following:
   a. Epiglottitis in children
   b. Symptoms of epiglottitis
   c. Precautions to be taken when a child has suspected epiglottitis
   d. Immediate nursing interventions when caring for a child with epiglottitis
3. Identify priorities for nursing care of this child in the emergency department.
4. Does the evidence objectively support your argument (conclusion)?

Answers are available at http://evolve.elsevier.com/wong/ncic.

ACUTE EPIGLOTTITIS

Acute epiglottitis, or acute supraglottitis, is a medical emergency. It is a serious obstructive inflammatory process that occurs principally in children between 2 and 5 years of age but can occur from infancy to adulthood. The disorder is a medical emergency and requires immediate medical attention. The obstruction is supraglottic, as opposed to the subglottic obstruction of laryngitis. The causative agent is usually *H. influenzae.* LTB and epiglottitis do not occur together. Epiglottitis (noninfectious) may also be caused by ingestion of caustic agents, smoke inhalation, or foreign bodies (Abdallah, 2012).

Clinical Manifestations

The onset of epiglottitis is abrupt, less often preceded by cold symptoms and more often by a sore throat. It can rapidly progress to severe respiratory distress. The child usually goes to bed asymptomatic to awaken later complaining of sore throat and pain on swallowing. The child has a fever and appears sicker than clinical findings suggest. The child insists on sitting upright and leaning forward (tripod position), with the chin thrust out, mouth open, and tongue protruding. Drooling of saliva is common because of the difficulty or pain on swallowing and excessive secretions.

NURSING ALERT

Three clinical observations that are predictive of epiglottitis are absence of spontaneous cough, presence of drooling, and agitation.

The child is irritable and extremely restless and has an apprehensive and frightened expression. The voice is thick and muffled, with a froglike croaking sound on inspiration. The child is not hoarse. Suprasternal and substernal retractions may be visible. Slow, quiet breathing provides better air exchange. The sallow color of mild hypoxia may progress to frank cyanosis if treatment is delayed. The throat is red and inflamed, and a distinctive, large, cherry red, edematous epiglottis is visible on careful throat inspection.

> **! NURSING ALERT**
>
> Throat inspection should only be performed when immediate endotracheal intubation or an emergency tracheotomy can be performed if needed.

Therapeutic Management

Epiglottitis may develop suddenly, with respiratory obstruction appearing rapidly. Progressive obstruction leads to hypoxia, hypercapnia, and acidosis, followed by decreased muscular tone, reduced level of consciousness, and, when obstruction becomes more or less complete, sudden death.

A lateral neck radiograph of the soft tissues is indicated for diagnosis. Experienced personnel with advanced airway management skills should accompany the child to the radiology department. For a young child who is likely to become more agitated by the procedure, it is preferable that the child remain on the parent's lap if content there during transportation and in the examination area during portable radiology.

Endotracheal intubation is usually considered for the child with epiglottitis with severe respiratory distress. Nasotracheal intubation is sometimes preferred. It is recommended that the intubation or any invasive procedure, such as starting an IV infusion, be performed in an area where emergency airway maintenance can be easily and quickly accomplished. For patients who are not intubated, humidified oxygen is administered as necessary either via mask in older children or as blow-by in younger children to avoid further agitation. Whether or not there is an artificial airway, the child requires intensive observation by experienced personnel. The epiglottal swelling usually decreases after 24 hours of antibiotic therapy, and the epiglottis is near normal by the third day. It is recommended that diagnostic tests and invasive procedures be postponed on the child with suspected epiglottitis until an airway has been established.

Children with suspected bacterial epiglottitis are given antibiotics intravenously, followed by oral administration to complete a 7- to 10-day course. Ceftriaxone/cefotaxime and vancomycin are generally the first antibiotics started. A blood culture and epiglottic culture for intubated patients should be considered before antibiotic administration. The use of corticosteroids for reducing edema may be beneficial during the early hours of treatment.

Prevention

It is recommended that all children receive the *H. influenzae* type B conjugate vaccine beginning at 2 months old (American Academy of Pediatrics, Report of the Committee on Infectious Diseases, 2015). Since administration of the vaccine has become a routine part of the immunization schedule, the incidence of epiglottitis has declined. The disease now tends to be caused by viral agents. (See Immunizations, Chapter 6.)

Nursing Care Management

Epiglottitis is a serious and frightening disease for the child, family, and health professionals. It is important to act quickly but calmly and provide support without unduly increasing anxiety. The child is allowed to remain in the position that provides the most comfort and security, and parents are reassured that everything possible is being done to obtain relief for their child. Droplet isolation precautions are indicated for 24 hours after initiation of effective antibiotic therapy to control spread of respiratory organisms. Prophylactic antibiotic treatment of household and other contacts may be indicated. Continuous monitoring of respiratory status, including pulse oximetry (or blood gases if the patient is intubated), is part of nursing observations, and the IV infusion is maintained. (See Chapter 22.)

> **! NURSING ALERT**
>
> Nurses who suspect epiglottitis should not attempt to visualize the epiglottis directly with a tongue depressor or take a throat culture but should have the child seen by the provider immediately. Resuscitation equipment and suction should be immediately available and ready at the child's bedside.

ACUTE LARYNGITIS

Acute infectious laryngitis is a common illness in older children and adolescents. Infants and smaller children experience more generalized involvement. (See next section on LTB.) Viruses are the usual causative agents, and the principal complaint is hoarseness, which may be accompanied by other upper respiratory symptoms (e.g., coryza, sore throat, cough, nasal congestion) and systemic manifestations (e.g., fever, headache, myalgia, malaise). Other complaints vary with the infecting virus. For example, adenoviruses and influenza viruses are responsible for more systemic involvement; parainfluenza virus, rhinoviruses, and RSV cause more mild illness.

Therapeutic and Nursing Care Management

The disease is almost always self-limiting without long-term sequelae. Treatment is supportive with fluids and humidified air.

ACUTE LARYNGOTRACHEOBRONCHITIS

Acute *laryngotracheobronchitis* (LTB) is the most common type of croup experienced by children admitted for hospitalization and primarily affects children 6 to 36 months old. Organisms responsible for LTB are the parainfluenza virus types 1, followed by parainfluenza virus types 2 and 3, adenoviruses, RSV, and *M. pneumoniae.* Less common causative organisms include influenza A and B, rhinoviruses, enteroviruses, herpes simplex virus. *Staphylococcus aureus, Streptococcus pyogenes,* and *Streptococcus pneumoniae.* The illness is usually preceded by a URI, which gradually descends to adjacent structures. It is characterized by the gradual onset of low-grade fever, and the parents often report that the child went to bed and later awoke with a barky, brassy cough and at times inspiratory stridor. Symptoms are typically worse at night, and agitation and crying tend to exacerbate the symptoms.

Inflammation of the mucosa lining the larynx and trachea causes a narrowing of the airway. When the airway is significantly narrowed, the child struggles to inhale air past the obstruction and into the lungs, producing the characteristic inspiratory stridor and suprasternal retractions. Other classic manifestations include cough and hoarseness. Respiratory distress in infants and toddlers may be manifested by nasal flaring, intercostal retractions, tachypnea, and continuous stridor. The typical child with LTB is a toddler who develops the classic barking or seal-like cough and acute stridor after several days of rhinitis. The degree of respiratory distress varies; hypoxia and decreased oxygen saturations are observed primarily when the obstruction is severe enough to prevent adequate ventilation and CO_2 removal. This can lead to respiratory acidosis and respiratory failure.

Therapeutic Management

The major objective in medical management of infectious LTB is maintaining an airway and providing for adequate respiratory exchange. Children with mild croup (no stridor at rest) are managed at home. Parents need to learn the signs of respiratory distress so that they can call professional help if needed. Children whose symptoms progressively get worse should receive medical attention.

Cool mist may provide relief for children with mild croup, although there is no substantial evidence to its efficacy (Petrocheilou, Tanou, Kalampouka, et al., 2014). In the hospital, mist may be provided with a face mask or as blow-by. The cool-temperature therapy modalities assist by constricting edematous blood vessels. In the home environment, suggestions to provide cool air include taking the child outside to breathe in cool night air, using a cold-water vaporizer or humidifier, standing in front of the open freezer, or taking the child to a cool basement or garage. Although these are often recommended, there is no evidence to unconditionally support their use. However, a ride in the car with the window down may help relieve symptoms, and the child often improves on the way to the emergency department (ED) due to exposure to cool air.

Nebulized racemic epinephrine is administered as quickly as possible for moderate to severe cases. The beta-adrenergic effects cause mucosal vasoconstriction and subsequent decreased subglottic edema. The onset of action is rapid. Peak effect is observed in less than 2 hours. Additional doses may be administered every 20 to 30 minutes as needed. A Cochrane review found that children receiving nebulized epinephrine showed improvement in croup severity scores within 30 minutes of treatment; however, the effects were transient (Bjornson, Russell, Vandermeer, et al., 2013). The authors concluded that neither racemic epinephrine, inhaled L-epinephrine, or intermittent positive pressure breathing had a significant advantage over simple nebulization (Bjornson et al., 2013). Close observation of patients receiving nebulized racemic epinephrine is critical to detect the reappearance of symptoms, monitor the response to therapy, and note any deterioration in respiratory status. The patient who has received nebulized epinephrine for croup should be observed for 3 to 4 hours for any visible signs of respiratory distress.

The use of corticosteroids is beneficial because the antiinflammatory effects decrease subglottic edema. Oral steroids (dexamethasone) have proven effective in the treatment of croup (as a single dose) and are considered standard treatment for this condition; IV or IM dexamethasone may be given to children who are unable to tolerate oral dosing. The onset of action is clinically detectable as early as 6 hours after administration, with continued improvement over a period of 12 to 24 hours.

Supplemental oxygen with mist may be needed if hypoxemic. On occasion, intubation and ventilation may be required when airway obstruction becomes more severe.

It is essential to allow children with mild croup to continue to drink beverages they like and to encourage parents to use comforting measures with their child (e.g., holding, rocking, walking, singing, reading books). If the child is unable to take oral fluids, IV fluid therapy may be indicated.

> **! NURSING ALERT**
>
> Children with severe respiratory distress (traditionally, a respiratory rate >60 breaths/min for infants) should not be given anything by mouth to prevent aspiration and increased work of breathing.

Nursing Care Management

The most important nursing function in the care of children with LTB is continuous, vigilant observation and accurate assessment of respiratory status. Cardiac, respiratory, and pulse oximetry monitoring supplement visual observations. Changes in therapy are frequently based on nurses' observations and assessment of a child's status, response to therapy, and tolerance of procedures. The trend away from early intubation of children with LTB emphasizes the importance of nursing observation and the ability to recognize impending respiratory failure so that intubation can be implemented without delay. Intubation equipment and bag and valve mask equipment should be readily accessible and taken with the child during transport to other areas (e.g., pediatric intensive care if intubation and further observation are required). A croup scoring system may be used to determine severity of symptoms.

> **! NURSING ALERT**
>
> Early signs of impending airway obstruction include increased pulse and respiratory rate; substernal, suprasternal, and intercostal retractions; nasal flaring; and increased restlessness.

To conserve energy, children are given every opportunity to rest. Infants or small children find that being placed on a face mask, coughing, having laryngeal spasms, and needing IV therapy are additional sources of distress. Infants and small children prefer sitting upright, and most want to be held. Blow-by mist can be administered by a parent while the child is being held. Children need the security of the parent's presence. Because crying increases respiratory distress and hypoxia, the nurse needs to assess a child's individual tolerance for these therapies. An extremely fussy child may do better when held in the parent's lap with cool mist directed toward the child's face.

The rapid progression of croup, the alarming sound of the cough and stridor, and the child's apprehensive behavior and ill appearance combine to create a frightening experience for the parents. They need reassurance regarding the child's progress and an explanation of treatments. The family should be encouraged to remain with the child as much as possible, especially when this decreases the child's distress.

Fortunately, as the crisis subsides and the child responds to therapy, breathing becomes easier and recovery is generally prompt. Home care after discharge includes monitoring for worsening symptoms, continued humidity, adequate hydration, and nourishment. Encourage parents to ask questions about home care and preparation for discharge.

ACUTE SPASMODIC LARYNGITIS

Acute spasmodic laryngitis (spasmodic croup, "midnight croup," or "twilight croup") is distinct from laryngitis and LTB and characterized by paroxysmal attacks of laryngeal obstruction that occur chiefly at night. Signs of inflammation are absent or mild, and there is often a history of previous attacks lasting for 2 to 5 days, followed by an uneventful recovery. It usually affects children ages 1 to 3 years old. Some children appear to be predisposed to the condition; allergy and psychogenic factors contribute to some cases.

The child goes to bed well or with some mild respiratory symptoms but awakes suddenly with the characteristic barking, metallic cough; hoarseness; noisy inspirations; and restlessness. The child appears anxious and frightened. However, there is no fever, the episode subsides in a few hours, and the child appears well the next day with the exception of slight hoarseness.

Therapeutic and Nursing Care Management

Children with spasmodic croup are managed at home. Cool mist is recommended for the child's room. Warm mist provided by steam from hot running water in a closed bathroom may be helpful. Sometimes sudden exposure to cold air relieves the spasm (as when the child is taken out into the night air to seek medical care). Parents are usually advised to have the child sleep in humidified air until the cough has subsided to prevent subsequent episodes. Children with moderately severe symptoms may be hospitalized for observation and therapy with

TABLE 26.5 Comparison of Conditions Affecting the Bronchi

	Asthma	Bronchitis	Bronchiolitis
Description	Exaggerated response of bronchi to a trigger such as URI, dander, cold air, exercise bronchospasm, exudation, and edema of bronchi	Usually occurs in association with URI Seldom an isolated entity	Most common infectious disease of lower airways Maximum obstructive impact at bronchiolar level
Age-group affected	Infancy to adolescence or adulthood	First 4 years of life	Usually children 2-12 months of age; rare after age 2 years Peak incidence approximately age 6 months
Etiologic agents	Most often viruses such as RSV in infants but may be any of a variety of URI pathogens	Usually viral Other agents (e.g., bacteria, fungi, allergic disorders, airborne irritants) can trigger symptoms	Viruses, predominantly RSV; also adenoviruses, parainfluenza viruses, human metapneumovirus, and *Mycoplasma pneumoniae*
Predominant characteristics	Wheezing, cough, labored respirations	Persistent dry, hacking cough (worse at night), becoming productive in 2-3 days	Labored respirations, poor feeding, cough, tachypnea, retractions, flaring nares, emphysema, increased nasal mucus, wheezing, may have fever
Treatment	Inhaled corticosteroids, bronchodilators, leukotriene modifiers, allergen, and control of triggers	Cough suppressants if needed	Provide supplemental oxygen if saturations ≤ 90%; bronchodilators (optional) Suction nasopharynx Ensure adequate fluid intake Maintain adequate oxygenation

RSV, Respiratory syncytial virus; *URI*, upper respiratory tract infection.

cool mist and racemic epinephrine, as for LTB. Patients may respond to corticosteroid therapy. The disease is usually self-limiting.

BACTERIAL TRACHEITIS

Bacterial tracheitis, an infection of the mucosa and soft tissues of the upper trachea, is a distinct entity with features of both croup and epiglottitis. The disease occurs typically at a mean age between 5 and 7 years and may cause severe airway obstruction (Roosevelt, 2016). It is believed to be a complication of LTB or other viral upper respiratory infections, and although *Staphylococcus aureus* is the most frequent bacterial organism responsible, *M. catarrhalis, S. pneumoniae, S. pyogenes,* alpha-hemolytic streptococci, and *H. influenzae* have also been implicated. Causes of bacterial tracheitis are often polymicrobial. Viruses such as influenza A and B, RSV, parainfluenza, measles, and enteroviruses have been associated with bacterial tracheitis.

Anteroposterior or lateral neck x-rays show narrowing (Steeple sign), and infiltrates may be seen. An endoscopy of the airway performed in the operating room (OR) or intensive care unit (ICU) is usually indicated to remove secretions and obtain cultures.

Many of the manifestations of bacterial tracheitis are similar to those of LTB but are unresponsive to LTB therapy. There is a history of previous URI with croupy cough, stridor unaffected by position, toxicity, absence of drooling, respiratory distress, and high fever. A prominent manifestation is the production of thick, purulent tracheal secretions. Respiratory difficulties are secondary to these copious secretions. If not treated, children with this condition quickly develop a life-threatening respiratory failure and/or acute respiratory distress syndrome (ARDS) (Griffin & Young, 2015).

Therapeutic and Nursing Care Management

Bacterial tracheitis requires vigorous management with antipyretics, fluid status, and antibiotics (10-day course). A trial of inhaled bronchodilators may be performed but is generally not beneficial. Many children require endotracheal intubation and mechanical ventilation; patients are closely monitored for impending respiratory failure if not intubated. Early recognition to prevent life-threatening airway obstruction is essential.

INFECTIONS OF THE LOWER AIRWAYS

The reactive portion of the lower respiratory tract includes the bronchi and bronchioles in children. Cartilaginous support of the large airways is not fully developed until adolescence. Consequently, the smooth muscle in these structures represents a major factor in constriction of the airway, particularly in the bronchioles—the portion that extends from the bronchi to the alveoli. Table 26.5 compares some of the major features of bronchial and bronchiolar infections.

BRONCHITIS

Bronchitis (sometimes referred to as tracheobronchitis) is an inflammation of the large airways (trachea and bronchi) that is frequently associated with a URI. Viral agents are the primary cause of the disease, including influenza A and B, parainfluenza, coronavirus (types 1 to 3), rhinovirus, respiratory syncytial virus, and human metapneumovirus. The condition is characterized by a dry, hacking, and nonproductive cough that is worse at night, lasting more than 5 days but can persist for 1 to 3 weeks.

Bronchitis is a mild, self-limiting disease that requires only symptomatic treatment, including analgesics, antipyretics, and humidity. Cough suppressants may be useful to allow rest, especially at night, but can interfere with clearance of secretions. Most patients recover uneventfully in 5 to 10 days. Adolescents with chronic bronchitis (>3 months) should be screened for tobacco or marijuana use. Chronic bronchitis can be associated with underlying conditions such as CF and bronchiectasis.

RESPIRATORY SYNCYTIAL VIRUS AND BRONCHIOLITIS

Bronchiolitis is an acute viral infection with maximum effect at the bronchiolar level. The infection occurs primarily in winter and spring. Most cases of bronchiolitis are caused by RSV, adenoviruses, parainfluenza viruses, and human metapneumovirus, but RSV is the most common cause, resulting in more than 57,000 hospitalizations and 2.1 million outpatient visits each year (Smith, Seales, & Budzik, 2017).Occasionally,

M. pneumoniae has been associated with bronchiolitis in children. RSV occurs less frequently in breastfed infants, and more frequently in children who live in crowded conditions. RSV infection is the most frequent cause of hospitalization in children less than 2 years old. In addition, severe RSV infections in the first year of life represent a significant risk factor for the development of asthma that can persist into adulthood (Smith, Seales, & Budzik, 2017). The precise link between RSV and asthma is unknown. RSV can also be associated with ongoing wheezing and impaired respiratory function (American Academy of Pediatrics, Report of the Committee on Infectious Diseases, 2015). It is important to note that not all infants and children with RSV will develop a bronchiolitis (Coates, Camarda, & Goodman, 2016). Occasionally, infants with RSV may have a concurrent viral or bacterial infection (e.g., otitis media, pertussis). Subsequent reinfections are common but they are usually less severe (American Academy of Pediatrics, Report of the Committee on Infectious Diseases, 2015).

Etiology

RSV is a paramyxovirus containing a single strand of RNA and is part of the Paramyxoviridae family. RSV strains have two major subgroups: A and B. More children develop bronchiolitis and pneumonia from RSV subgroup A infections than from subgroup B infections during major outbreaks. The disease usually begins in the fall, reaches a peak during the winter, and then decreases during the spring. Children who are preterm, have cyanotic or complicated congenital heart disease (CHD), or are immunosuppressed often have more severe illness.

BOX 26.6 Signs and Symptoms of Respiratory Syncytial Virus

Initial

Rhinorrhea
Pharyngitis
Coughing, sneezing
Wheezing
Possible ear or eye infection
Intermittent fever

With Progression of Illness

Increased coughing and wheezing
Fever
Tachypnea and retractions
Refusal to nurse or bottle feed
Copious secretions

Severe Illness

Tachypnea >70 breaths/min
Listlessness
Apneic spells
Poor air exchange; poor breath sounds
Cyanosis

Pathophysiology

RSV infection affects the epithelial cells of the respiratory tract. The ciliated cells swell, protrude into the lumen, and lose their cilia. The infection produces a fusion of the infected cell membrane with cell membranes of adjacent epithelial cells, thus forming a giant cell with multiple nuclei. At the cellular level this fusion results in multinucleated masses of protoplasm, or syncytia.

The bronchiolar mucosa swells, and lumina are subsequently filled with mucus and exudate. The walls of the bronchi and bronchioles are infiltrated with inflammatory cells, and peribronchiolar interstitial pneumonitis is usually present. Because luminal epithelial cells are shed into the bronchioles when they die, the lumina are frequently obstructed, particularly on expiration. The varying degrees of obstruction produced in small air passages lead to hyperinflation, obstructive emphysema resulting from partial obstruction, and patchy areas of atelectasis. Dilation of bronchial passages on inspiration allows sufficient space for intake of air, but narrowing of the passages on expiration prevents air from leaving the lungs. Thus air is trapped distal to the obstruction and causes progressive overinflation (emphysema).

Transmission

The transmission of RSV is predominantly through direct contact with respiratory secretions (less than 3 to 6 feet), mainly as a result of inoculation from hand to eye, nose, or other mucous membranes. It can also occur by direct inoculation by large-particle aerosols or by self-inoculation from contaminated fomites. RSV in secretions can survive for several hours on countertops, gloves, paper tissues, and cloth, and for 30 minutes on skin; it remains infectious when transferred from hands or objects. There is no documentation of distant spread of RSV by small-particle aerosols (airborne transmission). The incubation period is 2 to 8 days, but viral shedding can last 3 to 4 weeks.

Clinical Manifestations

The younger the infant, the greater the likelihood that severe lower respiratory tract disease requiring hospitalization will occur. The peak incidence for RSV is less than 3 months of age, but can occur at all ages. Higher rates occur in children who attend a day care home or day care center. The severity of RSV tends to diminish with age and repeated infections.

Symptoms such as rhinorrhea and low-grade fever often appear first. In time, a cough may develop. If the disease progresses, it becomes a lower respiratory tract infection and manifests typical symptoms (Box 26.6). Infants and preterm infants may have several days of URI symptoms or no symptoms except slight lethargy, poor feeding, or irritability (American Academy of Pediatrics, Report of the Committee on Infectious Diseases, 2015).

Once the lower airway is involved, classic manifestations include signs of altered air exchange, such as wheezing, retractions, crackles, dyspnea, tachypnea, and diminished breath sounds. Bronchiolitis peaks on day 3 to 5 (Pedra & Stark, 2017). Pneumonia may occur in conjunction with bronchiolitis.

Diagnostic Evaluation

Because RSV infection may be manifested as a URI, it is often difficult to identify the specific etiologic agent by clinical criteria alone. The most difficult distinction is between RSV and asthma because both conditions involve the lower airway and have similar symptoms.

Routine testing for specific viruses is no longer recommended because bronchiolitis may be caused by many viruses (Smith, Seales, & Budzik, 2017). Routine x-rays are also not indicated (Smith, Seales, & Budzik, 2017). If identification is necessary, rapid immunofluorescent antibody–direct fluorescent antibody staining or enzyme-linked immunosorbent assay techniques for RSV antigen detection are performed on nasopharyngeal secretions. The more traditional viral culture is becoming obsolete because it takes several days to get a result.

Other simultaneous viral or bacterial infections may occur with RSV. The infant should be carefully evaluated for the presence of urinary tract infection, meningitis, and bacteremia; antibiotics are prescribed only for a coexisting bacterial infection.

Therapeutic Management

Most children with bronchiolitis can be managed at home. Uncomplicated cases of bronchiolitis are treated symptomatically with adequate fluid intake, airway maintenance, and medications. Hospitalization is usually recommended for children with respiratory distress or those with poor feeding, lethargy, dehydration, moderate to severe respiratory distress, apnea, or hypoxemia. Other reasons for hospitalization include complicating conditions, such as underlying lung or heart disease (e.g., prematurity), or caregiver inability to provide adequate care during illness.

The American Academy of Pediatrics recommends continuous pulse oximetry and supplemental oxygen are not necessary if oxygen saturations are 90% or higher (Smith, Seales, & Budzik, 2017). Heated, high-flow nasal cannula (HHFNC) has been increasingly used for hospitalized infants and young children with bronchiolitis who are at risk of respiratory failure. HHFNC allows extra humidity blended with oxygen administration and continuous positive airway pressure to be administered. The provider indicates the flow rate and percentage of the oxygen therapy. The HHFNC improves functional residual capacity, reducing the work of breathing. If respiratory acidosis is present CPAP, BiPAP, or intubation may be required.

Routine chest percussion and drainage is not recommended (Smith, Seales, & Budzik, 2017). Infants with abundant nasal secretions benefit from regular suctioning, especially before feeding. Nasal aspiration of the external nares using an aspirator may be sufficient to remove most secretions. Nasopharyngeal suctioning is traumatic to the airways but can be considered if there are signs of respiratory distress or deoxygenation. Researchers found that the use of deep suctioning in the first day of admission and not suctioning the nose at least every 4 hours resulted in a longer length of stay for infants (Mussman, Parker, Statile, et al., 2013).

Fluids by mouth may be contraindicated because of tachypnea, weakness, and fatigue. Therefore IV fluids are preferred until the acute stage of the disease has passed. Nasogastric fluids may be required if the infant is unable to tolerate oral fluids and a peripheral IV is difficult to establish.

Clinical assessments, noninvasive oxygen monitoring, and, in severe cases, blood gas values guide therapy. Medical therapy for bronchiolitis is primarily supportive and aimed at decreasing airway hyperresonance and inflammation, and promoting adequate fluid intake. Bronchodilators are not recommended and are rarely beneficial. The use of 3% nebulized (hypertonic) saline is associated with an increase in mucociliary clearance in children with RSV when used greater than 24 hours, but it is recommended for use only in patients hospitalized for more than 3 days (Smith, Seales, & Budzik, 2017).

The use of systemic corticosteroids is controversial but may be used in some centers. Some studies have reported prolonged viral shedding with corticosteroid use. Antibiotics are not part of the treatment of RSV unless there is a coexisting bacterial infection such as OM or pneumonia. Additional treatment recommendations are to encourage breastfeeding, avoid passive tobacco smoke exposure, and promote preventive measures, including hand washing and the administration of palivizumab (Synagis) to high-risk infants.

Ribavirin, an inhaled antiviral agent (synthetic nucleoside analog), is the only specific therapy approved for hospitalized children. However, use of this drug in infants with RSV is controversial because of concerns about the high cost, aerosol route of administration, potential toxic effects among exposed health care personnel, and conflicting results of efficacy trials (Chu & Englund, 2013; Mejias & Ramilo, 2015).

The only product available in the United States for prevention of RSV is palivizumab, a humanized mouse monoclonal antibody that is given once every 30 days (15 mg/kg/dose) between November and March. It is usually given as an IM injection but may also be given IV. Candidates for this drug include the following (Smith, Seales, & Budzik, 2017):

- Infants born before 29 weeks of gestation
- Infants in the first year of life with hemodynamically significant heart disease
- Infants in the first year of life for preterm infants (<32 weeks gestation) with chronic lung disease or children in the second year of life with chronic lung disease who require continued medical intervention

Some children acquire the illness despite palivizumab prophylaxis.

DRUG ALERT

Palivizumab Administration

The lyophilized powder form of palivizumab should be administered within 6 hours of being reconstituted with sterile water because it is preservative free.

QUALITY PATIENT OUTCOMES

Bronchiolitis

- Oxygen saturation 90% or higher
- Respiratory rate less than 60 breaths/min
- Adequate oral fluid intake

Nursing Care Management

Children admitted to the hospital with suspected RSV infection may need separate rooms or may cohort with other RSV-infected children. Contact and Standard Precautions are used with hospitalized patients and some institutions use Droplet precautions in addition. Hand washing is essential to reduce spread of the illness. Other isolation procedures of potential benefit are those aimed at diminishing the number of hospital personnel, visitors, and uninfected children in contact with the child. In some cases, visitors, especially children, may be screened for illness before being allowed to visit high-risk infants. Another measure is to make patient assignments so that nurses assigned to children with RSV are not caring for other patients who are considered high risk. Staff must be careful to avoid touching the nasal mucosa or conjunctiva.

Infants with RSV infection often have copious nasal secretions, making breathing and nursing or bottle-feeding difficult. This engenders concerns that the child will lose weight or stop breastfeeding altogether. Encourage breastfeeding mothers to pump their milk and store appropriately for later use. (See Chapter 7.) Parents should learn how to instill normal saline drops into the nares and suction the mucus with a bulb syringe before feedings and before bedtime so the child may eat and rest better; unfortunately no medications appropriate for infants can help with these symptoms. To address the issue of decreased fluid intake, parents may offer small amounts of fluids, 5 to 10 ml at a time, with a medication syringe every 10 minutes or so. Infants may cough or vomit as the secretions settle in the stomach and make them prone to emesis of such secretions.

The nurse aims additional interventions at monitoring oxygenation with pulse oximetry when clinically indicated, monitoring IV fluids or NG fluids, monitoring for fever and administering antipyretics, and providing information for the parent regarding the infant's status. Inform the parents that the infant's cough may persist for a few weeks.

The critically ill infant with RSV may be placed in the pediatric ICU for continuous monitoring of respiratory status, cardiac output, and maintenance of adequate systemic pressure. IV fluids, antibiotics, positive airway pressure or mechanical ventilation, and inotropes may be required if the child is unstable. Parents and family members need emotional support and information regarding the child's status during this crisis.

The unpredictability of the infant's individual response to the disease compounds parental anxiety. However, in most cases the infant recovers quickly from the disease and resumes normal daily activities, including fluid intake.

PNEUMONIA

Pneumonia, an inflammation of the pulmonary parenchyma, is common in childhood, occurring more frequently in infancy and early childhood. Clinically, pneumonia may occur either as a primary disease or as a complication of another illness.

Pneumonia can be classified according to morphology, etiologic agent, or clinical form. Although morphologic classification is typically used (Box 26.7), the most useful classification is based on the etiologic agent (i.e., viral, bacterial, mycoplasmal, or aspiration of foreign substances) (Table 26.6). The causative agent is usually introduced into the lungs through inhalation or from the bloodstream. Pneumonia may be caused by histomycosis, coccidioidomycosis, and other fungi. Other terms that describe pneumonias are *hemorrhagic, fibrinous,* and *necrotizing.* Pneumonitis is a localized acute inflammation of the lung without the toxemia associated with lobar pneumonia.

The clinical manifestations of pneumonia vary depending on the etiologic agent, the child's age, the child's systemic reaction to the infection, the extent of the lesions, any underlying conditions, and the degree of bronchial and bronchiolar obstruction. The clinical history, the child's age, the general health history, the physical examination, radiography, and the laboratory examination can help identify the etiologic agent. Many organisms can cause pneumonia, and they vary according to the age of the child (see Table 26.6).

BOX 26.7 Types of Pneumonia

Lobar pneumonia—All or a large segment of one or more pulmonary lobes is involved. When both lungs are affected, it is known as *bilateral* or *double pneumonia.*

Bronchopneumonia—Begins in the terminal bronchioles, which become clogged with mucopurulent exudate to form consolidated patches in nearby lobules; also called *lobular pneumonia.*

Interstitial pneumonia—Inflammatory process more or less confined within the alveolar walls (interstitium) and the peribronchial and interlobular tissues.

TABLE 26.6 Organisms Causing Pneumonia in Children*

Microbial Agent	Susceptible Hosts
Bacteria	
Chlamydia trachomatis	Primarily infants ≤ 3 months
Mycoplasma hominis	Primarily infants ≤ 3 months
Treponema pallidum	Primarily infants ≤ 3 months
Ureaplasma urealyticum	Primarily infants ≤ 3 months
Staphylococcus aureus	Primarily children <5 years
Streptococcus pyogenes	Primarily children <5 years
Chlamydophila pneumoniae	Primarily children ≥5 years
Mycoplasma pneumoniae	Primarily children ≥5 years
Streptococcus pneumoniae	All
Viruses	
Adenovirus	Primarily children <5 years
Human metapneumovirus	Primarily children <5 years
Influenza A and B	Primarily children <5 years
Parainfluenza 1, 2, and 3	Primarily children <5 years
Respiratory syncytial virus	Primarily children <5 years
Rhinovirus	Primarily children <5 years

*Excluding neonatal pneumonia (in infants <28 days of age).
Adapted from Barson, W. J. (2017). Pneumonia in children: Epidemiology, pathogenesis, and etiology. *UpToDate.* https://www.uptodate.com/contents/pneumonia-in-children-epidemiology-pathogenesis-and-etiology.

VIRAL PNEUMONIA

Viral pneumonias occur more frequently than bacterial pneumonias and are seen in children of all age-groups. They are often associated with viral URIs, and the pathologic changes involve interstitial pneumonitis with inflammation of the mucosa and the walls of bronchi and bronchioles. There could also be parenchymal involvement. There are few clinical symptoms to distinguish among the responsible organisms, and only laboratory examination can differentiate among specific viruses.

Clinical Manifestations

The onset may be acute or insidious, and symptoms vary from mild fever, slight cough, and malaise to high fever, severe cough, and fatigue. Early in the illness, the cough is likely to be unproductive or productive of small amounts of whitish sputum. Radiography reveals diffuse or patchy infiltration with a peribronchial distribution.

Therapeutic and Nursing Care Management

The prognosis is generally good, although viral infections of the respiratory tract render the affected child more susceptible to secondary bacterial invasion. Treatment is usually symptomatic and includes measures to promote oxygenation and comfort, such as oxygen administration, chest percussion and postural drainage, antipyretics for fever management, monitoring fluid intake, and family support. Antibiotics are reserved for children in whom the presence of a bacterial infection is demonstrated.

PRIMARY ATYPICAL PNEUMONIA

Atypical pneumonia refers to pneumonia that is caused by pathogens other than the traditionally most common and readily cultured bacteria (e.g., *S. pneumoniae*). In the category of atypical pneumonias, *M. pneumoniae* is the most common bacterial pathogen of community-acquired pneumonia in children 5 years of age or older (Jain, Williams, Arnold, et al., 2015). Community-associated methicillin-resistant *Staphylococcus aureus* (CA-MRSA) has become prevalent in certain areas. Community acquired pneumonia occurs principally in the fall and winter months and is more prevalent in crowded living conditions. Most affected persons recover from acute illness at home in 7 to 10 days with symptomatic treatment, followed by 1 week of convalescence. The incubation period is 2 to 3 weeks, but the cough may last several weeks.

Clinical Manifestations

The onset may be sudden or insidious and is usually accompanied by general systemic symptoms, including fever, chills (in older children), headache, malaise, anorexia, and muscle pain (myalgia). These symptoms are followed by rhinitis, sore throat, and a dry, hacking cough. The cough, initially nonproductive, produces seromucoid sputum that later becomes mucopurulent or blood streaked. The degree of fever varies widely, from several days to 2 weeks. Dyspnea occurs infrequently.

Radiographic examination reveals evidence of pneumonia before physical signs are apparent. There may be fine crepitant crackles over various areas of the lung fields, but consolidation is usually not demonstrated. The pathologic process consists of interstitial round cell infiltration and edema of alveolar septa and varying distribution of areas of inflammation, necrosis, and ulceration of the mucosal lining of bronchi and bronchioles. Areas of consolidation and emphysema are present.

Therapeutic and Nursing Care Management

Most affected persons recover from acute illness in 7 to 10 days with symptomatic treatment, followed by a week of convalescence. Hospitalization is rarely necessary. Erythromycin, azithromycin, and clarithromycin are the primary agents used for treating atypical pneumonia.

BACTERIAL PNEUMONIA

Bacterial pneumonia is often a serious infection. The pathogenetic mechanisms involved are often aspiration or hematogenous dissemination. The cause varies, depending on the child's age, underlying illness, and degree of immunosuppression or immunocompetence.

Etiology and Epidemiology

S. pneumoniae is the most common bacterial pathogen responsible for community-acquired pneumonia in both children and adults. Other bacteria that cause pneumonia in children are group A streptococci, *S. aureus, M. catarrhalis, M. pneumoniae,* and *C. pneumoniae.*

Beyond the neonatal period, bacterial pneumonias display distinct clinical patterns that facilitate their differentiation from other forms of pneumonia. The onset of illness is abrupt and generally follows a viral infection that disturbs the natural defense mechanisms of the upper respiratory tract. In the 3-month to 5-year age-group, *S. pneumoniae, M. catarrhalis,* and group A streptococci are common causes. *H. influenzae* type B is causing fewer infections because of the Hib vaccine. *S. aureus* pneumonia is also now rarely seen in infants and toddlers.

Clinical Manifestations

The child with bacterial pneumonia usually appears ill. Symptoms include fever, malaise, rapid and shallow respirations, cough, and chest pain. The older child may complain of headache, chills, abdominal pain, chest pain, or meningeal symptoms (meningism) (Box 26.8). Respiratory distress may or may not be present. In some cases the only finding is an increased respiratory rate. The pain of pneumonia may be referred to the abdomen and confused with appendicitis.

Infants and young children develop more severe symptoms than older children. Cyanosis and apnea are common, and the parent may report the infant's activity and eating pattern was decreased for a few days. Additional clinical manifestations in infants include abrupt fever, vomiting, diarrhea, and abdominal distention. Because pneumonia in newborns carries a high morbidity and mortality rate, bacterial infection should be suspected in all neonates with respiratory symptoms.

Initially, the cough is usually hacking and nonproductive, and breath sounds are diminished or heard as scattered crackles. When consolidation is present, breath sounds may be tubular in quality with no adventitious noises. As the infection resolves, coarse crackles and wheezing are heard, and the cough becomes productive with purulent sputum.

Staphylococcal pneumonia is rare but particularly progressive and must be treated aggressively. The onset is rapid, with rapid deterioration. Conjunctivitis and furuncles are signs of a probable staphylococcal infection.

BOX 26.8 General Signs of Pneumonia

Fever—Usually quite high

Respiratory signs

- Cough: unproductive to productive with whitish sputum
- Tachypnea
- Breath sounds: rhonchi or fine crackles
- Dullness with percussion
- Chest pain
- Retractions
- Nasal flaring
- Pallor to cyanosis (depends on severity)

Chest x-ray—Diffuse or patchy infiltration, with peribronchial distribution

Behavior—Irritable, restless, lethargic

Gastrointestinal signs—Anorexia, vomiting, diarrhea, abdominal pain

Diagnostic Evaluation

The key to a preliminary diagnosis is finding pulmonary infiltrates on radiographic examination, usually revealing lobar consolidation and, in some severe cases, pleural effusion. Laboratory studies include Gram stain and culture of sputum in older children, nasopharyngeal specimens, blood cultures, and, on occasion, lung aspiration and biopsy. The white blood cell count may be elevated, but it may be normal for infants with staphylococcal disease. Children with streptococcal disease usually have an elevated antistreptolysin O titer. The infant or child with recurrent pneumonia should be further evaluated for CF or an immunodeficiency disease. Diagnostic evaluation should include ruling out aspiration pneumonia as a potential cause.

Therapeutic Management

Antimicrobial therapy has significantly reduced the morbidity and mortality from bacterial pneumonia. Oral high-dose amoxicillin (90 mg/kg/day) in 2 to 3 doses is widely used for outpatient management of infants and children younger than 5 years of age. Amoxicillin-clavulanate (Augmentin) or a second-generation cephalosporin (e.g., cefuroxime, cefadroxil) may otherwise be used. If the child is not tolerating oral medication, a dose of Ceftriaxone intramuscularly may be considered to begin treatment. Erythromycin is the drug of choice for older children and adolescents because of its activity against *M. pneumoniae.* In the hospital, medications are given parenterally for rapid action and maximum effect. IV cefuroxime, cefotaxime, and ceftriaxone are considered the primary antibacterial agents for bacterial pneumonia in the hospitalized child. Parenteral or oral erythromycin should be added for children older than 5 years of age until *M. pneumoniae* is ruled out. Chest percussion with postural drainage may be helpful in clearing secretions in some cases.

Most older children with pneumonia can be treated at home, especially if the condition is recognized and treatment initiated early. Antibiotic therapy, rest, liberal oral intake of fluids, and administration of antipyretics for fever are the principal therapeutic measures. Hospitalization is indicated when pleural effusion or empyema accompanies the disease, when compliance with therapy is estimated to be poor, when there are chronic illnesses such as congenital heart disease or bronchopulmonary dysplasia, and it may be indicated in infants less than 3 months old. Other indicators for hospitalization include dehydration, respiratory distress (moderate to severe), hypoxemia, or failure of outpatient therapy, or the presence of secondary comorbidities that generally result in a more severe infection (immunocompromised, cardiac disease, pulmonary disease).

Prognosis

The prognosis for pneumonia is generally good, with rapid recovery when it is recognized and treated early. The course of staphylococcal pneumonia is generally prolonged. The prognosis varies with the length of the illness before treatment, although early recognition and treatment are usually beneficial.

Prevention

The use of the pneumococcal conjugate vaccine (PCV13; Prevnar 13) is recommended for infants and children at 2, 4, 6, and between 12 and 15 months. Prevnar 13 is also recommended for children ages 24 to 71 months with underlying medical conditions who are at high risk for the development of pneumococcal disease or complications. High-risk groups include children who have anatomic or functional asplenia, sickle cell disease, and other hemoglobinopathies; immunocompromising conditions, including human immunodeficiency virus (HIV) infection; diabetes mellitus, chronic renal failure, nephrotic syndrome, chronic heart disease, chronic lung disease, or a cochlear implant; or a cerebrospinal fluid leak. (See Immunizations, Chapter 6.)

Complications

At present the classic features and clinical course of pneumonia are rarely seen because of early and vigorous antibiotic and supportive therapy. However, some children, especially infants, with staphylococcal pneumonia develop empyema, pyopneumothorax, or tension pneumothorax (Fig. 26.5). AOM and pleural effusion are common in children with pneumococcal pneumonia (Box 26.9).

When fluid is either suspected or identified by radiograph in the pleural cavity, a needle aspiration or thoracentesis may be performed. Nonpurulent effusions do not require surgical drainage.

Continuous closed chest drainage may be instituted with a complicated pleural effusion. Closed drainage is continued until drainage fluid is free of pathogens, which rarely requires more than 5 to 7 days. If a large amount of purulent drainage is obtained, an appropriate antibiotic can be instilled into the pleural space and chest drainage is stopped for about an hour after instillation. Rarely, a thoracotomy with debridement of infected lung tissue is needed.

Additional therapies for empyema may involve instillation of intrapleural fibrinolytics such as urokinase or streptokinase or video-assisted thoracoscopy (Livingston, Colozza, Vogt, et al., 2016; van Loo, van Loo, Selvadurai et al., 2014). These may preclude the need for open debridement and thoracotomy.

BOX 26.9 Pneumothorax

Pneumothorax occurs when air accumulates in the pleural space; this air increases intrapleural pressure, making it more difficult to expand the affected lung. This leads to the clinical manifestations of chest pain, dyspnea, and often back pain, labored respirations, tachycardia, and decreased oxygen saturation. In neonates and infants on mechanical ventilation the first clinical signs of a pneumothorax are oxygen desaturation and hypotension. The three major types of pneumothorax are tension, spontaneous, and traumatic. The definitive diagnosis of pneumothorax is a chest radiograph. The emergent treatment involves needle aspiration of the air within the pleural space; subsequently a chest tube to closed drainage is usually inserted to prevent the reaccumulation of air.

Pleural effusion occurs when there is an excessive accumulation of fluid in the pleural space. The diagnosis is made by chest radiograph, and the treatment involves evacuation of the fluid by needle aspiration followed by insertion of a chest tube to closed drainage.

PATHOPHYSIOLOGY REVIEW

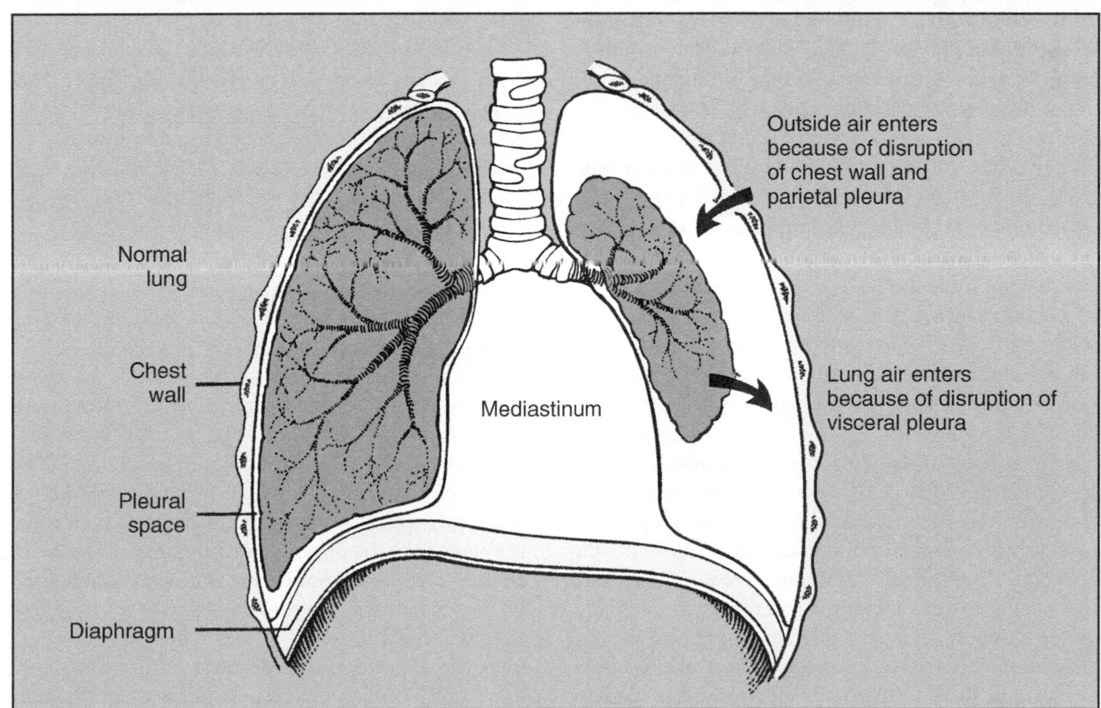

FIG. 26.5 Pneumothorax. Air in the pleural space causes the lung to collapse around the hilus and may push mediastinal contents (heart and great vessels) toward the other lung. (From McCance, K. L., & Huether, S. E. [2010]. *Pathophysiology: The biological basis for disease in adults and children* [6th ed.]. St. Louis, MO: Mosby.)

Thoracentesis

Dyspnea resulting from pressure from fluid accumulation in the pleural cavity requires removal by thoracentesis. Thoracentesis involves insertion of a needle percutaneously into the pleural space to remove pleural fluid and can be performed to obtain fluid for culture or to instill antibiotics directly into the pleural cavity. Nursing responsibilities include obtaining and setting up equipment, preparing the child physically and psychologically, monitoring the sedated child's vital signs after the procedure and recovery, and assisting with the procedure. Many institutions utilize sedation teams to sedate patients for procedures. If this is not available, the nurse monitors the child throughout the procedure also. If continuous closed chest drainage is anticipated, this equipment should also be available. Adequate pain management is imperative. Nurses who perform procedural sedation should receive additional education and demonstrate competency before administering sedation medications. Additional nursing responsibilities may include documenting the patient's tolerance of procedure, as well as managing pain after the procedure.

In addition, the nurse makes the child comfortable and records observations and physical and emotional responses. Specimens are sent to the laboratory for culture. Continuous closed chest drainage is managed according to the same protocol as for the child with a thoracotomy.

Nursing Care Management

Nursing care of the child with pneumonia is primarily supportive and symptomatic but necessitates thorough respiratory assessment and administration of supplemental oxygen (as required) and antibiotics. The child's respiratory rate and status, oxygenation, general disposition, and level of activity are frequently assessed. To prevent dehydration, fluids are frequently administered intravenously during the acute phase. A nasogastric tube may be placed to provide hydration and antibiotics if oral intake is poor.

Nursing care of the child with a chest tube requires close attention to respiratory status, as noted previously. The chest tube and drainage device used are monitored for proper function (i.e., drainage is not impeded, vacuum setting is correct, tubing is free of kinks, dressing covering chest tube insertion site is intact, water seal is maintained [if used], drainage tube is below the chest tube entry site, and chest tube remains in place). Movement in bed and ambulation with a chest tube are encouraged according to the child's respiratory status, but children require frequent doses of analgesics such as acetaminophen and ibuprofen or ketoralac because having a chest tube in place can be painful.

If needed, supplemental oxygen may be administered by nasal cannula, face-mask, blow-by, or face tent. Children are usually more comfortable in a semierect position but should be allowed to determine the position of comfort. Lying on the affected side ("good lung up") splints the chest on that side and reduces pleural rubbing that often causes discomfort. Fever is controlled by cooling the environment and administering antipyretic drugs as prescribed. Temperature is monitored regularly.

Vital signs and oxygenation are monitored to assess the progress of the disease and to detect early signs of complications. Children with ineffectual cough or those with difficulty handling secretions, especially infants, may require suctioning to maintain a patent airway. A simple bulb suction syringe is usually sufficient for clearing the nares and nasopharynx of infants, but mechanical suction should be readily available if needed. A nasal aspirator device can be attached to wall suction to remove secretions from nares without causing trauma to the nasal mucosa. Older children can usually handle secretions without assistance. Postural drainage, chest percussion, and nebulized bronchodilator therapy may be prescribed, depending on the child's condition. However, there is a lack of empirical support about the benefit of chest percussion in children with community-acquired pneumonia.

The nurse educates the family about observing for worsening symptoms, completing antibiotic therapy if prescribed, using antipyretics, encouraging oral fluids, and not being concerned if the child has a poor appetite for a few days.

The hospitalized child may be apprehensive, and the treatments and tests are frightening and stress producing. It is important to involve the entire family in the care as appropriate and to encourage questions and facilitate effective communication. Reducing the child's anxiety, apprehension, and psychologic distress leads to relaxation and decreased respiratory efforts. Easing respiratory efforts further reduces the child's apprehension. Encouraging the presence of the caregiver provides the child with a source of comfort and support.

NEONATAL PNEUMONIA

Pneumonia in the immediate neonatal period is different from other types of pneumonia described. If infection occurs within 3 to 5 days of birth, the pathogen is usually obtained from the mother transplacentally, or through aspiration of infected amniotic fluid intrauterine, or during or after birth. Group B hemolytic streptococcus may be present in the mother's vagina and asymptomatic but can cause a serious pneumonia to a newborn.

C. trachomatis, an intracellular microorganism similar to gram-negative bacteria, is responsible for one of the most common sexually transmitted infections. Chlamydial pneumonia is usually an afebrile illness that occurs in the newborn between 2 and 19 weeks after delivery (American Academy of Pediatrics, Report of the Committee on Infectious Diseases, 2015). It is characterized by a persistent cough, tachypnea, and sometimes rales. Radiographs show nonspecific abnormalities. Oral azithromycin given for 3 days is the treatment of choice; alternatively, erythromycin base or ethylsuccinate is administered for 14 days (American Academy of Pediatrics, Report of the Committee on Infectious Diseases, 2015).

Herpes simplex virus (HSV) may also be transmitted at the time of birth and can result in fatal pneumonia (Speer, 2017). Other viral or fungal infections can be transmitted intrauterine. Early symptoms of neonatal pneumonia can be nonspecific but may include respiratory distress. IV acyclovir is started if HSV infection is suspected. A 10- to 14-day treatment course is usually indicated (Speer, 2017).

OTHER INFECTIONS OF THE RESPIRATORY TRACT

PERTUSSIS (WHOOPING COUGH)

Pertussis, or whooping cough, is an acute respiratory tract infection caused by *Bordetella pertussis* that occurs primarily in children younger than 4 years of age who have not been immunized. It is highly contagious and is particularly threatening in young infants, who have a higher morbidity and mortality rate. Infants less than 6 months of age may not come in to the practitioner with the typical cough; in this age-group, apnea is a common presenting manifestation. Likewise, older children often manifest the disease with a persistent cough and the absence of the characteristic whoop. (See Table 6.2 for signs, symptoms, and management of pertussis.) It presents as a URI, and cough symptoms develop. The cough can be mild but is generally more severe in unimmunized children. It persists 6 to 10 weeks and can result in encephalopathy, seizures, pneumonia, rib fractures (adolescents), bleeding into the conjunctiva, or even death (infants). The incubation period is 7 to 10 days but can be as long as 21 days (American Academy of Pediatrics,

Report of the Committee on Infectious Diseases, 2015). The incidence is highest in the summer and fall months, and a single attack confers lifetime immunity.

Pertussis is diagnosed via culture or polymerase chain reaction assay using nasopharyngeal secretions. Most children can be cared for at home on oral antibiotics (e.g., erythromycin, azithromycin, clarithromycin). Antibiotics in the early stage may result in a milder form of the infection, but they also limit its spread to others. Household members, high-risk individuals (immunodeficiency, pregnancy, chronic lung conditions, infants, or those who care for infants), and close contacts (within 3 feet of a person who has symptoms) may be treated to prevent them from developing the infection (American Academy of Pediatrics, Report of the Committee on Infectious Diseases, 2015).

The resurgence of pertussis in the United States, particularly among children 10 years old and older, has prompted concerns over the long-term effects of the pertussis vaccine. Consequently a new booster vaccine for pertussis has been approved for children. Boostrix contains acellular pertussis, diphtheria toxoid, and tetanus toxoid and is indicated as a booster for children 11 years and older (American Academy of Pediatrics, Report of the Committee on Infectious Diseases, 2015). (See also Immunizations, Chapter 6.)

TUBERCULOSIS

Tuberculosis (TB) infections and mortality from TB have been declining since 1990 (World Health Organization, 2017). However, it is one of the leading causes of death worldwide. In 2015 approximately 1 million children developed TB infection and 170,000 children died from the disease (World Health Organization, 2017). In the United States, approximately 4.6% of TB cases were reported among children younger than 15 years of age with more cases occurring in children under 5 years of age (Centers for Disease Control and Prevention, 2016).

Etiology

TB is caused by *Mycobacterium tuberculosis,* an acid-fast bacillus not readily decolorized by acids after staining. Children are susceptible to the human *(M. tuberculosis)* and the bovine *(Mycobacterium bovis)* organisms. In parts of the world where TB in cattle is not controlled or milk is not pasteurized, the bovine type is a common source of infection.

Although the causative agent for TB is the tubercle bacillus, other factors influence the degree to which the organism produces an altered state in the host. These include heredity (resistance to the infection may be genetically transmitted), gender (higher rates in adolescent girls), age (lower resistance in infants, higher incidence during adolescence), stress (emotional or physical), nutritional state, immunodeficiency (HIV, immunosuppressive medications), intravenous drug abuse, medical conditions (diabetes mellitus, chronic renal failure, malnutrition), and intercurrent infection (measles and pertussis) (American Academy of Pediatrics, Report of the Committee on Infectious Diseases, 2015). The risk is increased for individuals who are born in another country, have a parent who was born in another country, lived outside the United States for 2 months or more, or who use tobacco (World Health Organization, 2017). Adolescents and adults being treated with tumor necrosis factor–α (TNF-α) antagonists for conditions such as inflammatory bowel disease or arthritis have been identified as having contracted TB; therefore it is recommended that screening for TB occur in such persons before the use of TNF-α antagonists (American Academy of Pediatrics, Report of the Committee on Infectious Diseases, 2015).

Children with HIV infection have an increased incidence of TB disease, and all children with TB should be tested for HIV (Box 26.10).

BOX 26.10 Factors Affecting Resistance to Tuberculosis

Heredity

No evidence of hereditary tendency

Evidence that resistance to infection may be genetically transmitted

Sex

Early years: no sex differences in incidence

Later childhood and adolescence: morbidity and mortality higher in girls than in boys

Age

Diminished resistance to infection in infancy

- Delay in development of acquired immunity
- Diminished capacity to resist extension of infective process

Increased tendency to develop disease during puberty and adolescence

- New infection superimposed on a previous one
- Increased contacts
- Indigenous reinfection stimulated by metabolic changes or suboptimum diets during a period of rapid growth

Stress States

Temporary stressful circumstances (e.g., injury or illness, undernutrition, emotional distress, chronic fatigue) increasing susceptibility to infection

Increased secretion of adrenal steroids suppressing protective inflammatory response and permitting infection to spread

Therapeutic administration of corticosteroids (similar effect)

Nutrition

Active disease inversely proportional to state of nutrition

Excellent nutrition essential to young children's recovery from disease

Intercurrent Infection

Infectious diseases (especially human immunodeficiency virus, measles, pertussis) activating latent tuberculosis

Noncompliance with therapy

TB is the leading cause of the mortality of persons infected with HIV. All contacts of an affected child are examined for the disease.

Pathophysiology

The source of infection in children is usually an infected member of the household or any frequent visitor to the household. Transmission of *M. tuberculosis* occurs when the child inhales microdroplets (usually 1 to 5 mm in size) into the respiratory tract after someone has coughed or sneezed. Although the lung is the most frequent portal of entry in humans, the organism *M. bovis* can be ingested via infected milk (unpasteurized milk or fresh cheese). When the *M. tuberculosis* droplet is inhaled, it passes down the bronchial tree, implants in either a bronchiole or alveolus, and starts to multiply. *M. bovis* typically causes cervical lymphadenitis, meningitis, and intestinal TB disease and is more common in adults and children from countries where *M. bovis* is prevalent (American Academy of Pediatrics, Report of the Committee on Infectious Diseases, 2015).

Epithelial cells surround and encapsulate the multiplying bacilli in an attempt to wall off the invading organisms, thus forming the typical tubercle. During the inflammatory process, some bacilli leave the focal area and are carried to the regional lymph nodes that drain the area; as a result, the child develops a fever. The tuberculin skin test is positive, and radiography findings may or may not be evident.

Extension of the primary lesion at the original site causes progressive tissue destruction as it spreads within the lung, discharges material from foci to other areas of the lungs (e.g., bronchi or pleura), or produces pneumonia. Erosion of blood vessels by the primary lesion can cause widespread dissemination of the tubercle bacillus to near and distant sites (miliary TB). Organisms deposited in the upper lung zones, bones, kidneys, and brain may find favorable environments for growth, but organs and tissue such as bone marrow, liver, and spleen appear to inhibit multiplication of the bacilli.

Extrapulmonary TB may be manifested as meningitis or inflammation of the lymph nodes, middle ear, mastoid, bones, joints, and on the skin (American Academy of Pediatrics, Report of the Committee on Infectious Diseases, 2015). With the exception of meningitis, treatment for extrapulmonary TB may be the same drug regimen as for pulmonary TB. Renal TB is rare in children but may occur in adolescents.

Clinical Manifestations

Clinical manifestations of pulmonary TB in children are extremely variable and are present in approximately one-third of cases. The disease may be asymptomatic or produce a broad range of symptoms, including general responses such as fever, cough, night sweats, chills, delayed growth, and weight loss or more specific symptoms related to the site of infection (e.g., lungs, bone, brain, kidneys) within 1 to 6 months after infection (American Academy of Pediatrics, Report of the Committee on Infectious Diseases, 2015). Lung disease may or may not include cough (which progresses slowly over weeks to months), aching pain and tightness in the chest, and (rarely) hemoptysis.

As increasing amounts of lung tissue become involved, the respiratory rate increases, the lung on the affected side does not expand as well as the other, auscultation reveals diminished breath sounds and crackles, and there is dullness to percussion. In children (usually infants) who are unable to contain the spread of infection, the fever persists; the generalized symptoms are present; and the patient develops pallor, anemia, weakness, and weight loss.

Diagnostic Evaluation

Diagnosis is based on information derived from physical examination, history, reaction to a tuberculin test, organism cultures, and radiographic examinations. In addition, it must be determined whether the lesion is in the active, quiescent, or healed stage.

The American Academy of Pediatrics (American Academy of Pediatrics, Report of the Committee on Infectious Diseases, 2015) does not recommend universal testing of all children for TB. Instead, a targeted testing method is used, wherein only children and adolescents at high risk for contracting the disease and those patients at risk for progression to TB disease are screened. A risk factor questionnaire facilitates screening of children at first contact with the care provider, every 6 months for the first year of life, and then annually. Recommendations for tuberculin skin testing of children are listed in Box 26.11.

The Xpert MTB/RIF rapid molecular test performed on sputum is used to diagnose TB and determine Rifampin resistantance. Results are available in less than 2 hours, and are endorsed by the World Health Organization. The test is a nucleic acid amplification that can diagnose multidrug resistant TB (Centers for Disease Control and Prevention, 2016). Reporting of confirmed cases of TB is a requirement in all states.

Tuberculin Test

The tuberculin skin test (TST) is the most common test used to determine whether a child has been infected with the tubercle bacillus. A primary infection initiates a hypersensitivity reaction to the protein fraction of the tubercle bacillus, which can be detected 2 to 10 weeks after the infection. Bacille Calmette-Guerin immunization can result in a positive TST. The TST should not take place within 6 weeks of administration of a live vaccine (American Academy of Pediatrics, Report of the Committee on Infectious Diseases, 2015).

The standard dose of purified protein derivative (PPD) is 5 tuberculin units in 0.1 ml of solution, which is administered using a 27-gauge needle and a 1-ml syringe intradermally into the volar aspect of the forearm. The tuberculin is injected intradermally with the bevel of the needle pointing upward in the volar or dorsal aspect of the forearm. A wheal 6 to 10 mm in diameter should form between the layers of the skin when the solution is injected properly. If the wheal does not form, the procedure is repeated. The reaction to the skin test is determined in 48 to 72 hours; reactions occurring after 72 hours should be measured and considered to be the result. The size of the transverse diameter of induration, not the erythema, is measured.

A positive TST reaction indicates that the person has been infected and has developed sensitivity to the protein of the tubercle bacillus; it does not, however, confirm the presence of active disease. Once individuals react positively, they will always react positively. Any negative reaction

BOX 26.11 Tuberculin Skin Test Recommendations for Infants, Children, and Adolescents

Children for Whom Immediate Tuberculin Skin Test Is Indicated

Contacts of persons with confirmed or suspected contagious tuberculosis (TB; contact investigation)

Children with radiographic or clinical findings suggesting TB disease

Children immigrating from endemic countries (e.g., Asia, Middle East, Africa, Latin America, countries of the former Soviet Union), including international adoptees

Children with travel histories to endemic countries or significant contact with indigenous persons from such countries*

Children Who Should Have Annual Tuberculin Skin Test†

Children infected with human immunodeficiency virus (HIV)

Children at Increased Risk for Progression of Infection to Disease

Children with other medical risk factors, including diabetes mellitus, chronic renal failure, malnutrition, and congenital or acquired immunodeficiencies, deserve special consideration. Without recent exposure, these people are not at increased risk of acquiring TB infection. Underlying immune deficiencies associated with these conditions theoretically would enhance the possibility for progression to severe disease. Initial histories of potential exposure to TB should be included for all of these patients. If these histories or local epidemiologic factors suggest a possibility of exposure, immediate and periodic TST should be considered. An initial TST should be performed before initiation of immunosuppressive therapy, including prolonged systematic corticosteroid administration, organ transplantation, use of TNF-α antagonists or blockers, or other immunosuppressive therapy.

*If child is well, TST should be delayed for up to 10 weeks after return.

†Initial tuberculin skin testing is done at the time of diagnosis or circumstance, beginning as early as 3 months old.

TB, Tuberculosis; *TNF-α,* tumor necrosis factor–α; *TST,* tuberculin skin test.

From American Academy of Pediatrics, Committee on Infectious Diseases, Pickering, L. (Ed.). (2015). *Red book: 2015 report of the Committee on Infectious Diseases* (29th ed.). Elk Grove Village, IL: Author.

BOX 26.12 Definition of Positive Tuberculin Skin Test Results in Infants, Children, and Adolescents

Induration ≥5 mm

Children in close contact with known or suspected contagious cases of tuberculosis (TB) disease

Children suspected to have TB disease:

- Findings on chest radiography consistent with active or previously active TB
- Clinical evidence of TB disease[†]

Children receiving immunosuppressive therapy, including immunosuppressive doses of corticosteroids or who have immunosuppressive conditions, including human immunodeficiency virus (HIV) infection

Induration ≥10 mm

Children at increased risk of disseminated disease:

- Children younger than 4 years old
- Children with other medical risk conditions, including Hodgkin disease, lymphoma, diabetes mellitus, chronic renal failure, or malnutrition

Children at increased risk of exposure to TB:

- Children born in high-prevalence (TB) regions of the world
- Children frequently exposed to adults who are HIV infected, homeless, users of illicit drugs, residents of nursing homes, incarcerated or institutionalized
- Children who travel to high-prevalence (TB) regions of the world

Induration ≥15 mm

Children 4 years old or older without any risk factors

From American Academy of Pediatrics, Committee on Infectious Diseases, Pickering, L. (Ed.). (2015). *Red book: 2015 report of the Committee on Infectious Diseases* (29th ed.). Elk Grove Village, IL: Author.

does not exclude active disease because false negatives can occur due to immunosuppression or certain medications. Guidelines for interpreting the TST are listed in Box 26.12. A clinical examination and a chest x-ray are recommended if the child has a positive TST reaction.

A negative reaction does not exclude the presence of latent tuberculosis infection or active disease. Children with immunosuppression, concurrent viral infection (e.g., measles, varicella, influenza), HIV, disseminated TB disease, and recent TB infection may have decreased TST reactivity. Several factors can produce false-negative results (Box 26.13). Prompt radiographic evaluation of all children with a positive TST is recommended.

A finding of latent tuberculosis infection (LTBI) indicates infection in a person who has a positive TST, no physical findings of disease, and normal chest radiograph findings. A diagnosis of LTBI or TB disease in a young child represents a public health sentinel event indicating recent transmission of the *M. tuberculosis* organism (American Academy of Pediatrics, Report of the Committee on Infectious Diseases, 2015). The term *tuberculosis disease* is used when a child has clinical symptoms or radiographic manifestations caused by the *M. tuberculosis* organism.

Bacteriologic Examination

A definitive diagnosis is made by demonstrating the presence of mycobacteria in culture. The organism is identified from microscopic examination of properly prepared and stained smears from early-morning gastric washings or from sputum, pleural fluid, urine, spinal fluid, draining lymph nodes, and other body fluids. Induced sputum and

BOX 26.13 Circumstances Producing False-Negative Reactions to Tuberculin Tests

Tuberculin reaction suppressed by

- Intercurrent diseases (e.g., viral diseases such as measles, rubella, influenza, mumps, varicella, and probably others [about 4 weeks])
- Live-virus vaccines (e.g., measles, mumps, and rubella vaccines [about 4 weeks])
- Corticosteroids and other immunosuppressive agents
- Immunodeficiency disease
- Severe malnutrition
- Malignancies (leukemia, lymphoma, Hodgkin disease)

Testing before the body develops a sensitivity to the protein fraction of the tubercle bacillus (e.g., newborn or child younger than 2 years)

Use of outdated testing material; mixture that has been prepared for too long or has been exposed to sunlight

Faulty technique (e.g., deep injection, no wheal formed, improper measurement of solution, or leaking of solution from a defective or loosely fitting syringe)

Overwhelming tuberculosis infections; end-stage and terminal miliary disease

Improper reading (interpretation of results)

Early tuberculosis infection (<12 weeks)

gastric lavage sputum specimens are often obtained for culture from children who are unable to expectorate a sputum specimen.

Immunologic Testing

The QuantiFERON-TB Gold and T-SPOT TB are tests of interferon quantification (interferon gamma release assay [IGRA]). They are the preferred tests to perform on asymptomatic children over 5 years of age who have received the bacille Calmette-Guérin (BCG) vaccine and have a borderline positive or negative TST (American Academy of Pediatrics, Report of the Committee on Infectious Diseases, 2015). These tests cannot determine latent infection but children with a positive IGRA test are considered to be infected with the *M tuberculosis* bacterium.

Radiographic Studies

Radiographic examinations may be normal or may show lymphadenopathy, pleural effusion, or cavitary TB. However, the lesions of numerous chronic intrathoracic diseases resemble tuberculous lesions, therefore chest radiography is not diagnostic by itself.

Therapeutic Management

Medical management of tuberculous lesions in children consists of adequate nutrition, antimicrobial therapy, general supportive measures, prevention of unnecessary exposure to other infections that further compromise the body's defenses, prevention of reinfection, and sometimes surgical procedures.

A child with LTBI is treated with antimicrobial drugs to decrease the risk of acquiring active TB disease in the years after the initial acquisition and to reduce the lifelong chance of developing TB disease. The recommended drug regimen for LTBI in children and adolescents includes a daily dose of isoniazid (INH) for 9 months or alternatively twice a week with directly observed therapy (DOT) for 9 months. If the child has isoniazid-resistant disease, rifampin once daily for 4 months can be used, or alternatively, DOT twice a week can be done for 4 months (American Academy of Pediatrics, Report of the Committee on Infectious Diseases, 2015).

DOT means that a health care worker or other responsible, mutually agreed-on individual is present when medications are administered to the patient. If the reliability of self-administration of medications is in doubt, directly observed, twice-weekly therapy must be administered by a health care professional. DOT decreases the rates of relapse, treatment failures, and drug resistance and is recommended for treatment of children and adolescents with TB in the United States.

Pulmonary and Extrapulmonary Tuberculosis

For the child with clinically active pulmonary and extrapulmonary TB, the goal is to achieve sterilization of the tuberculous lesion. A combination of isoniazid, pyrazinamide, and ethambutol daily or twice weekly for 2 months is recommended, followed by isoniazid and rifampicin for 4 months (American Academy of Pediatrics, Report of the Committee on Infectious Diseases, 2015). Alternatively, DOT with isoniazid, rifampin, and pyrazinamide two to three times per week for 6 months is recommended (American Academy of Pediatrics, Report of the Committee on Infectious Diseases, 2015). Alternative treatment regimens may be used when managed by a TB specialist. Infection with *M. bovis* is treated with isoniazid and rifampin for 9 to 12 months.

Tuberculosis Meningitis

The same antimicrobial medications are used in the treatment of TB meningitis, but the duration is different. For *M. tuberculosis,* a 2-month treatment with isoniazid, pyrazinamide, and aminoglycoside or ethionamide daily, followed by a 7- to 10-month course of daily or twice-a-week isoniazid and rifampin, for 9 to 12 months in total, is recommended. Treatment for *M. bovis* lasts 12 months and pyrazamide is not used. The duration of therapy is also longer for patients who have HIV infection or who have cavitary lesions or positive sputum analysis after 2 months of antimicrobial therapy (American Academy of Pediatrics, Report of the Committee on Infectious Diseases, 2015).

When drug resistance is suspected, other antimicrobials are added to the therapeutic regimen until drug susceptibility results are available. It is not within the scope of this text to outline the treatment regimen for multiple drug–resistant and extensively drug–resistant TB.

Surgical procedures may be required to remove the source of infection in tissues that are inaccessible to antimicrobial therapy or that are destroyed by the disease. Orthopedic procedures for correction of bone deformities, bronchoscopy for removal of a tuberculous granulomatous polyp, or resection of a portion of a diseased lung may also be performed.

Prognosis

Most children recover from primary TB infection and may be unaware of its presence. However, very young children have a higher incidence of disseminated disease. It is a serious disease during the first 2 years of life and in children infected with HIV. Except in cases of tuberculous meningitis, death seldom occurs in treated children. Antibiotic therapy has decreased mortality and hematogenous spread from primary lesions.

Prevention

The only certain means to prevent TB is to avoid contact with the tubercle bacillus. Maintaining an optimum state of health with adequate nutrition and avoiding debilitating infections promote natural resistance but do not prevent infection.

Pasteurization of milk and routine testing and elimination of diseased cattle have helped reduce the incidence of bovine TB. Infants and children should be given only pasteurized milk from TB-free cattle.

A source of concern is that the infected child or family members may spread the disease when visiting in the hospital. Most children with TB, especially under 10 years of age, are not contagious and can be hospitalized on an open unit if they are receiving therapy. Children with no cough and a negative sputum smear can also be cared for without isolation. Children and adolescents with infectious pulmonary TB (i.e., those whose sputum smears show acid-fast bacilli) should be on Isolation Precautions until effective therapy has been initiated, their sputum smears show a diminishing number of organisms, and their cough is improving. Ideally, they should be cared for in an Airborne Isolation room (American Academy of Pediatrics, Report of the Committee on Infectious Diseases, 2015). Staff should be fitted for appropriately sized N-95 or higher-level particulate-filtering respirator.

Masks are indicated when children are coughing and not reliably covering their mouths. Family members should be managed with Airborne Precautions when visiting until they are demonstrated not to have infectious TB.

Limited immunity can be produced by administration of BCG. The freshly prepared vaccine, injected intradermally, produces definite, although incomplete, protection against TB (ranging from 50% to 80%). In most instances, positive tuberculin reactions develop after inoculation. BCG vaccination is not generally recommended for use in the United States but is used in many other countries. In the United States it may be recommended for long-term protection of infants and children with negative TST who are not infected with HIV and who (1) are at high risk for continuing exposure to persons with infectious pulmonary TB, or (2) are continuously exposed to persons with TB who have bacilli resistant to both INH and rifampin (American Academy of Pediatrics, Report of the Committee on Infectious Diseases, 2015). The BCG is a very painful vaccination.

Nursing Care Management

Hospitalization for TB is seldom necessary in the United States. Only children with the more serious forms of the disease are placed in the hospital. The major nursing care of children with TB involves nurses in ambulatory settings: outpatient departments, schools, and public health agencies.

Asymptomatic children can lead an essentially unrestricted life. They can and should attend school (or day care) once they have started therapy and clinical symptoms have been reduced. Older children are restricted from vigorous activities such as competitive games and contact sports during the active stage of primary TB. They should also continue the regular immunization schedule and maintain optimum health with proper diet, adequate rest, and avoidance of infection. Nurses assume several roles in management of the disease, including helping the family understand the rationale for diagnostic procedures, assisting with radiographic examinations, performing and interpreting skin tests correctly, obtaining specimens for laboratory examination, and educating about the antimicrobial regimen.

Sputum specimens are difficult or impossible to obtain from an infant or young child because they swallow any mucus coughed from the lower respiratory tract. The best means for obtaining material for smears or culture is by gastric washing (i.e., aspiration of lavaged contents from the fasting stomach with a nasogastric tube). The procedure is carried out and the specimen obtained early in the morning before the customary breakfast time. In some cases, an induced sputum specimen may be obtained by administering aerosolized normal saline for 10 to 15 minutes, followed by CPT and suctioning of the nasopharynx for sputum collection.

Ambulatory Care

Nursing supervision of the child at home involves teaching the parents and child about the disease and its ramifications. Historically the disease has been regarded with fear, and numerous misconceptions need to be addressed. Reducing parental anxieties helps them deal with the illness more constructively and collaborate more effectively in planning the child's continued care. Because the success of therapy depends on compliance with drug therapy, instruct the parents regarding the importance of giving the medication as often and as long as it is ordered. (See Compliance, Chapter 22.) Promoting optimum general health and preventing intercurrent infections and reinfections with the tubercle bacillus are important. The American Lung Association has excellent patient education materials.*

Case Finding

Case finding and follow-up of known contacts are important nursing responsibilities. Every case of TB identified in the community involves nurses in follow-up of known contacts—individuals from whom the affected person may have acquired the disease and persons who may have been exposed to the diseased individual. Early diagnosis affords a means for early protection or treatment and prevents further spread of the disease. Cases are notified to the health department.

RESPIRATORY DISTURBANCE CAUSED BY NONINFECTIOUS IRRITANTS

FOREIGN BODY INGESTION AND ASPIRATION

Foreign body (FB) aspiration is a life-threatening event due to potential airway obstruction and inability to adequately oxygenate the body. Small children characteristically explore objects with their hands and mouth and are prone to place FBs into the air passages (nose and mouth). They also place objects such as beads, paper clips, plastic toys, small magnets, or food items in the nose or mouth, which can easily be aspirated into the trachea. Small items may also be placed into the external ear canal; small rocks and pebbles appear to be a favorite item for boys, whereas girls prefer colorful beads.

When such objects are placed into the nose or mouth, they can be aspirated into the airway, causing subsequent obstruction. Ingestion or aspiration of an FB can occur at any age but is most common in older infants and children ages 1 to 3 years. Severity depends on the location, type of object aspirated, and extent of obstruction. For example, dry vegetable matter, such as a seed, nut, piece of carrot, or popcorn, that does not dissolve and that may swell when moistened creates a particularly difficult problem. The high fat content of potato chips and peanuts may cause the added risk of lipoid pneumonia. "Fun foods" such as hard candy and hot dogs are among the worst offenders. Offending foods include nuts, hot dogs, round candy, peanuts and other types of nuts, grapes, cookies or biscuits, pieces of meat, caramels, carrots, apples, peas, celery, popcorn, fruit and vegetable seeds, cherry pits, gum, and peanut butter. Round foods are the most frequent offenders. The first four items together make up more than 40% of all aspirated food items. Other items include plastic or glass beads, button or disk batteries, burst latex balloons, pen or marker caps, and coins. Objects such as small lithium or cadmium batteries may cause esophageal or tracheal corrosion. Magnets can trap tissue/mucosa in between them, which can result in necrosis of that area. Aspiration of certain medications can cause inflammation and stenosis.

A sharp or irritating object produces irritation and edema. A round, pliable object that does not readily break apart is more likely to occlude an airway than an object with a different shape. A small object may cause little if any pathologic change, whereas an object of sufficient size to obstruct a passage can produce various changes, including atelectasis, emphysema, inflammation, and abscess.

*American Lung Association, 55 W. Wacker Drive, Suite 1150, Chicago, IL 60601; 800-548-8252; http://www.lungusa.org.

Pathophysiology

Most inhaled FBs lodge in a mainstem or lobar bronchus, a few find their way into more distal portions of the lung field, and the remaining FBs lodge in the trachea. They also may shift over time so symptoms can change. The site is determined by the object's size, weight, and configuration. For example, heavy objects such as bullets, coins, and nails are more likely to drop into the dependent portions of the tracheobronchial tree. The object may remain in the same location or move in the airway. It can be coughed from a smaller to a larger airway and reaspirated in a different passage—or it might be ejected forcefully into the mouth and subsequently swallowed.

Signs of obstruction caused by an FB in a bronchus are explained by the same mechanisms that control the flow of fluids in pipes (Fig. 26.6). During normal respiration the caliber of bronchi and bronchioles becomes larger during inspiration and smaller during expiration. When a small object partially obstructs a passage, air passes around the obstruction during both inspiration and expiration (bypass valve). In this type of obstruction a wheeze is heard. A somewhat larger obstruction will allow air to enter the distal portion when bronchioles enlarge during inspiration, but when they diminish in caliber during expiration, the lumen becomes occluded and air becomes trapped distal to the obstruction (check valve). This type of obstruction produces obstructive hyperinflation. When there is complete blockage of the bronchus by an FB or by the FB and swollen mucosa, air is unable to move in either direction (stop valve), and the air distal to the obstruction is absorbed, leaving an area of obstruction atelectasis. The right bronchus, with its shorter length and straighter angle, is the usual site of bronchial obstruction.

Clinical Manifestations

Initially, an FB in the air passages produces choking, gagging, or coughing, but symptoms depend on the site of obstruction and on the interval between aspiration and presentation. Up to half of all children with FB ingestion may be asymptomatic. Laryngotracheal obstruction most commonly causes dyspnea, cough, stridor, and hoarseness because of a decreased air entry. Cyanosis may also occur if the obstruction becomes worse. Bronchial obstruction usually produces cough (frequently paroxysmal), wheezing, asymmetric breath sounds, decreased airway entry, and dyspnea. In some cases, a FB obstruction may be mistaken for croup or asthma.

If the obstruction progresses, the child's face may become livid, and sometimes the child becomes unconscious and dies of asphyxiation if the object is not removed. If obstruction is partial, hours, days, or even weeks may pass without symptoms after the initial period. Secondary symptoms are related to the anatomic area in which the FB is lodged and are usually caused by a persistent respiratory tract infection located distal to the obstruction. A history of recurrent intractable pneumonia is reason to consider an FB in an airway. Often, by the time secondary symptoms appear, the parents have forgotten the initial episode of coughing and gagging. The most common symptoms observed in children brought to medical attention are stridor, wheezing, sternal retraction, and cough. When an object is lodged in the larynx, the child is unable to speak or breathe.

Diagnostic Evaluation

The diagnosis of FB obstruction is usually suspected on the basis of the history and physical signs. Radiographic examination reveals opaque FBs but is of limited value in localizing vegetable matter and some plastic items. Up to half of children with tracheal foreign bodies have a normal chest radiography study. Bronchoscopy is required for a definitive diagnosis and removal of objects in the larynx and trachea.

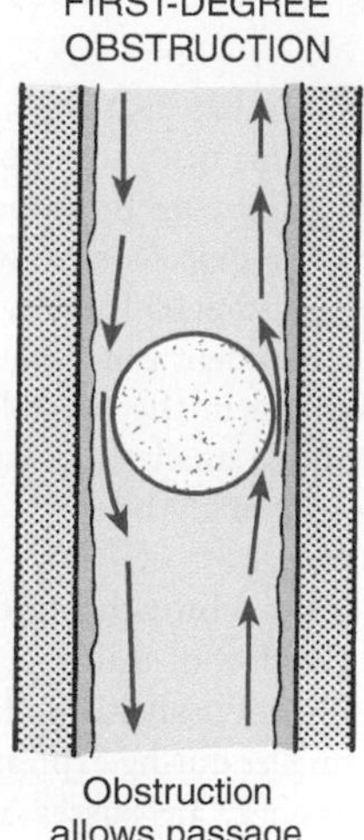
FIRST-DEGREE
OBSTRUCTION
Obstruction allows passage of air in both directions

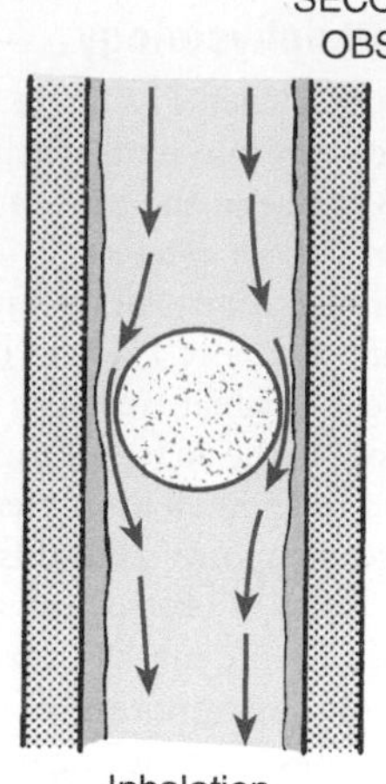
SECOND-DEGREE
OBSTRUCTION
Inhalation

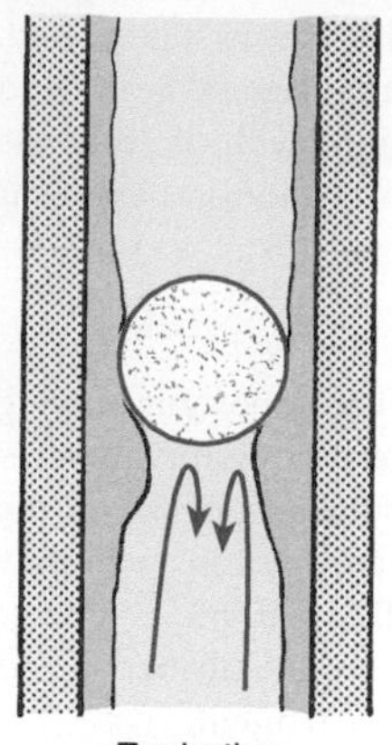
Expiration
Air able to move past the obstruction in one direction only. Air passages enlarge during inspiration and diminish during expiration.
COMPLETE
OBSTRUCTION
Air unable to move in either direction. FB and edematous mucosa obliterate passage.

FIG. 26.6 Mechanisms of airway obstruction by foreign body.

Fluoroscopic examination is valuable in detecting FBs in the bronchi. On fluoroscopy, a check-valve–obstructed lung remains expanded, the diaphragm remains low and fixed on the obstructed side, and the heart and mediastinum shift to the unobstructed side during expiration. In a stop-valve obstruction, the heart and mediastinum are drawn to the obstructed side and remain there during both inspiration and expiration. The diaphragm on the obstructed side remains high, whereas that on the unobstructed side moves normally.

The mainstay of diagnosis and management of foreign bodies is endoscopy and bronchoscopy. If there is doubt about the presence of an FB, these procedures can be diagnostic and therapeutic.

Therapeutic Management

FB aspiration may result in life-threatening airway obstruction, especially in infants because of the small diameters of their airways. Current recommendations for the emergency treatment of the choking child include the use of abdominal thrusts for children over 1 year old and back blows and chest thrusts for children less than 1 year old. An FB is rarely coughed up spontaneously; therefore it must be removed by endoscopy or bronchoscopy. Removal of the FB must be done as soon as possible because the progressive local inflammatory process triggered by the foreign material hampers removal. In addition, a chemical pneumonia soon develops, and vegetable matter begins to macerate within a few days, further complicating its removal.

Nursing Care Management

A major role of nurses is to recognize the signs of FB aspiration and implement immediate measures to relieve the obstruction. All persons working with children should be prepared to deal effectively with aspiration of an FB. Choking on food or other material should not be fatal. Two simple procedures—back blows and the abdominal thrust, which can be used by both health professionals and lay persons—can save lives. It is the nurse's obligation to learn these techniques and teach them to parents and other groups. To aid a child who is choking, nurses need to recognize the signs of distress. Not every child who gags or coughs while eating is truly choking.

! NURSING ALERT

The child in distress (1) cannot speak, (2) becomes cyanotic, and (3) collapses. These three signs indicate that the child is truly choking and requires immediate and quick action. The child can die within 4 minutes. Follow-up care after the FB is removed includes monitoring for respiratory distress and educating the parents.

Prevention

Small children should not be allowed access to small objects that they might place in their nose or mouth. Anticipatory guidance for parents of small children is essential. Nurses are in a position to teach prevention in a variety of settings (see Community and Home Health Considerations box). They can educate parents singly or in groups about hazards of aspiration in relation to the developmental level of their children and encourage them to teach their children safety. Caution parents about behaviors that their children might imitate (e.g., holding foreign objects, such as pins, nails, and toothpicks, in their lips or mouth). (Chapters 10 and 12 discuss prevention based on the child's age.)

COMMUNITY AND HOME HEALTH CONSIDERATIONS

Foreign Body Aspiration

Everyone who has contact with young children between the ages of 9 months and 3 years should be on guard for potential situations in which these children could aspirate small pieces of food, toys, or other objects. In general, pediatric nurses should teach parents about the dangers of aspiration and how to keep their children safe. In addition, pediatric nurses are in an excellent position to educate ancillary health personnel, day care providers, and babysitters. In the school setting, nurses should also be alert to situations in which younger siblings might be at risk for aspiration of small objects found in the school. Nurses can become active in their communities by alerting toy manufacturers of potentially unsafe toys and games.

FOREIGN BODY IN THE NOSE

Children sometimes place foreign objects, such as food (peanuts are a favorite), crayons, small plastic toys, pieces of plastic, beans, beads, erasers, wads of paper, peas, and small stones, into their nose. An FB is suspected when there is unilateral nasal discharge that is foul smelling, local obstruction with sneezing, mild discomfort, and (rarely) pain. The irritation produces local mucosal swelling if the items increase in size as they absorb moisture (hygroscopic). Signs of obstruction and discomfort may increase with time. Infection usually follows, as evidenced by foul breath and a purulent or bloody discharge from one nostril.

Although the object is usually situated anteriorly, unskilled attempts at removal may move it further posteriorly. Removal should occur as soon as possible to prevent the risk of aspiration and local tissue necrosis. Removal usually occurs easily with either forceps, suction or inflation of a balloon catheter behind the obstruction. In some cases mild sedation may be necessary.

! NURSING ALERT

Parental report of a small child swallowing an item or placing it into the nose requires careful evaluation of the child's airway, even if the child is asymptomatic. The child may insert an object in the nose that may not be visible, but during play or other activities the object may be aspirated into the trachea, causing obstruction and distress.

ASPIRATION PNEUMONIA

Aspiration pneumonia occurs when food, secretions, vomitus, medications, inert materials, volatile compounds, hydrocarbons (e.g., kerosene, gasoline, solvents, lighter fluid, furniture polish, and mineral oil), or liquids enter the lung and cause inflammation and a chemical pneumonitis. Many conditions increase the risk of aspiration (Box 26.14). Aspiration of fluid or food substances is particularly hazardous in the child who has difficulty swallowing or is unable to swallow because of paralysis, weakness, debility, congenital anomalies such as cleft palate or tracheoesophageal fistula, or absent cough reflex (unconsciousness), or if the child is force-fed, especially while crying or breathing rapidly.

BOX 26.14 Conditions That Increase Risk of Aspiration

Altered Level of Consciousness

Central nervous system injury or disease (e.g., meningitis, seizures, paralysis, trauma, poisoning, toxic ingestion)
Sedation
General anesthesia

Dysphagia

Esophageal dysmotility
Neurologic deficit
Gastroesophageal reflux

Mechanical Disruption of Defensive Barriers

Endotracheal tube
Tracheostomy
Feeding tube (orogastric or nasogastric)

Persistent Vomiting

Modified from Hazinski, M. F. (Ed.). (2013). *Nursing care of the critically ill child* (3rd ed.). St. Louis, MO: Elsevier/Mosby.

Clinical signs of the aspiration of oral secretions may not be distinguishable from other forms of acute bacterial pneumonia. For example, if vegetable matter has been aspirated, manifestations may not appear for several weeks after the event. Classic symptoms include an increasing cough or fever, foul-smelling sputum, deteriorating chest radiographs, and other signs of lower airway involvement. These deviations may persist for weeks, while the child starts to feel better. The irritated mucosa can be a site for bacterial infection. Aspiration can result in death from asphyxia.

Pathogenesis

The severity of the lung injury depends on the pH of the aspirated material, the presence of bacteria, and the volatility and viscosity of the substance. Irritation from aspiration during swallowing, vomiting, or gastric lavage may also cause pulmonary involvement. Pathologic changes include signs of inflammation (e.g., edema, hyperemia, infiltration of polymorphonuclear cells); vascular thrombosis and hemorrhage; and necrosis of bronchial, bronchiolar, and alveolar tissues. Other reactions are bronchospasm, atelectasis, emphysema, pulmonary hemorrhage, necrosis, surfactant impairment, and pulmonary edema. Aspiration of inert fluids may not produce a chemical or bacterial pneumonia, but these fluids can decrease lung compliance and cause hypoxemia.

Clinical Manifestations

Acid aspiration may produce immediate pulmonary symptoms that worsen over the first 24 hours. Coughing and vomiting, which occur almost immediately after ingestion, contribute to the aspiration. CNS symptoms include agitation, restlessness, confusion, drowsiness, and coma. The temperature is elevated (100° to 104°F [37.8° to 40°C]). (See Ingestion of Injurious Agents, Chapter 14.)

After swallowing, coughing, and choking, the child becomes short of breath, and older children complain of dyspnea. There are varying degrees of cyanosis, tachycardia, tachypnea, nasal flaring, and retractions. Intercostal retractions, grunting, cough, and fever may appear within 30 minutes or be delayed for a few hours. Localized areas of dullness are felt on percussion, and moderately intense wheezes and crackles are heard. Severe injury causes hemoptysis, pulmonary edema, severe cyanosis, and death within 24 hours of aspiration.

Therapeutic Management

Inducing the child to vomit is contraindicated because of the renewed danger of aspiration. Bronchitis or pneumonia usually develops early (within the first 24 hours) but may be delayed. Recovery from pulmonary involvement occurs in most instances despite a severe clinical course. Treatment is the same as for any lower respiratory tract inflammation and consists of high humidity, supplemental oxygen, hydration, and treatment of any secondary infection. Endotracheal intubation may be required if the child develops respiratory failure.

Hydrocarbon Aspiration Pneumonia

Children frequently develop pneumonia secondary to the ingestion of various forms of hydrocarbons (e.g. gasoline, motor oil, lamp oil, lighter fluid, mineral spirits), which are commonly found in the home or garages. Petroleum distillates are generally impure substances contaminated with heavy metals or other toxic chemicals that cause systemic, as well as local, effects.

Hydrocarbons are usually packaged in attractive containers, and some have a pleasant aroma; consequently, they are frequently ingested accidentally by young children. On average, children swallow less than 30 ml (often about 3 to 4 ml). They begin coughing severely and do not ingest any more of the contents. Although CNS abnormalities, GI irritation, cardiomyopathy, and renal toxicity can occur, the most serious complication is pneumonitis. Distillates that have high volatility (evaporate quickly), decreased viscosity (thinner solution), and low surface tension are more likely to be aspirated and produce respiratory complications. Decreased viscosity enhances penetration into distal airways. Lower surface tension facilitates spread over a larger area of lung surface. Consequently, ingestion of lighter fluid, kerosene, or gasoline is more likely to cause a pathologic condition than substances that have high viscosity (e.g., petroleum jelly, tar, or lubricating oil).

Even in small amounts, hydrocarbons spread over the surface of tissues and the lungs and interfere with gas exchange. They are readily absorbed by the GI tract and excreted by the lungs.

Lipoid Pneumonia

Oily substances aspirated into the respiratory passages initially cause an interstitial proliferative inflammation that may include an exudative pneumonia. The next stage involves a diffuse, chronic, proliferative fibrosis that is often complicated by acute bronchopneumonia. The final stage features multiple localized nodules or tumor-like paraffinomas. There are no characteristic manifestations. Cough is usually present, and dyspnea occurs in severe cases. Secondary bronchopneumonia is common. The outcome depends on the extent of pulmonary damage, the general condition of the infant or child, and discontinuation of the oily inhalation. No specific treatment exists.

Powder Inhalation

A significant number of infants suffer talcum powder aspiration. Commercial talcum powder is predominantly a mixture of talc (hydrous magnesium silicate) and other silicates. Severe respiratory distress occurs immediately as a result of an inflammatory reaction in small bronchioles initiated by deep inhalation of the extremely light powder.

Nursing Care Management

Care of the child with aspiration pneumonia is the same as that described for the child with pneumonia from other causes. However, the major focus of nursing care is on *prevention* of aspiration. Proper feeding techniques should be carried out for weak, debilitated, and uncooperative children, and measures should be taken to prevent aspiration of any material that might enter the nasopharynx. Nasogastric tubes used for feedings are checked before the initiation of bolus feedings; continuous nasogastric tube feedings are also evaluated periodically for proper tube placement. The child should be maintained with the head elevated during feeding and for 30 minutes after it if possible.

Children who are at risk for swallowing difficulties as a result of illness, physical debilitation, anesthesia, or sedation are kept on nothing-by-mouth status until they can properly swallow fluids effectively. An evaluation by an occupational therapist or speech therapist may be indicated to assess ability to swallow effectively. The child who is at risk for vomiting and is incapable of protecting the airway should be positioned in a side-lying position.

Oily nose drops and oil-based medications are not ideal for infants and small children. Solvents, lighter fluid, and other hydrocarbon substances should be kept away from older infants and small children, who are likely to put anything in their mouth and who may be attracted by the slightly sweet smell. Talcum powder is not necessary for newborn hygiene and should be avoided.

PULMONARY EDEMA

Pulmonary edema (PE) is the movement of excess fluid into the alveoli and interstitium of the lungs caused by extravasation from the pulmonary vasculature (Mazor & Green, 2016). It can cause respiratory compromise, which can be life threatening. The two main types of PE are cardiogenic and noncardiogenic.

Cardiogenic (hydrostatic, hemodynamic) PE is caused by an increase in pulmonary capillary pressure because of an increase in pulmonary venous pressure. It can be caused by excessive IV fluid administration, renal failure, left ventricular failure, heart valve disorder (e.g., aortic regurgitation, aortic stenosis, mitral regurgitation), myocardial ischemia, myocarditis, acute tachydysrhythmia, or coronary artery disease (Powell, Graham, O'Reilly, et al., 2016). Noncardiogenic PE is caused by various conditions that result in increased pulmonary capillary permeability. Some subtypes of noncardiogenic PE include permeability PE (caused by ARDS or acute lung injury [ALI]), high-altitude PE (caused by rapid ascension to heights above 12,000 feet), or neurogenic PE (after CNS insult, such as seizures, head injury, or cerebral hemorrhage). Some less common forms of PE are reperfusion PE (after removal of thromboemboli from the lung or a lung transplant); reexpansion PE (caused by rapid reexpansion of a collapsed lung); or PE that results from opiate overdose (methadone or heroin), salicylate toxicity (chronic), aspiration (FB inhalation), inhalation injuries, submersion injury, pulmonary embolism, viral infections, or pulmonary veno-occlusive disease. Other causes include traumatic injury, organ dysfunction caused by sepsis, multiorgan failure, alcoholism or substance abuse, pregnancy (eclampsia), chronic renal impairment, malnutrition, hypertension, or a blood transfusion (transfusion-related ALI).

Pathophysiology

Fluid flows from the pulmonary vasculature into the alveolar interstitial space and then returns to the systemic circulation in a normal lung. Movement of this fluid is controlled by the net difference between hydrostatic and osmotic pressures and the permeability of the capillary membrane (Mazor & Green, 2016). Increased pulmonary hydrostatic pressure or increased permeability of the vascular membrane results in movement of fluid into the alveoli and interstitium of the lung. The pulmonary lymph system normally drains away any fluid from the alveoli, but when the amount of fluid present in the alveoli exceeds lymph drainage, PE occurs.

Symptoms include extreme shortness of breath, cyanosis, tachypnea, diminished breath sounds, anxiety, agitation, confusion, diaphoresis, orthopnea, respiratory crackles, expiratory wheezing (in young infants), heart murmur, third heart sound (S_3) gallop, cool peripheries, jugular venous distention, nocturnal dyspnea, cough, pink frothy sputum (if severe), tachycardia, hypertension, or hypotension (if caused by left ventricle dysfunction).

Therapeutic Management

Management of PE depends on the cause but can include oxygen therapy, peak end-expiratory pressure (PEEP) via CPAP, and intubation with ventilatory support if respiratory failure occurs. If ventricular failure is the cause, medications such as diuretics, digoxin, positive inotropes, and vasodilators (nitroglycerin) may be started, and the child may be placed on a fluid and sodium restriction. Morphine may be prescribed to relieve dyspnea. The primary goal of management is to determine why PE occurred and treat the underlying condition.

Nursing Care Management

Nursing care of the child with PE is similar to that for any other acute respiratory condition. Pulse oximetry is monitored, and vital signs are observed closely for any deterioration. The nurse should note changes in Sao_2, $ETCO_2$, and ABG values. An ongoing assessment of the child's cardiopulmonary status is needed by checking lung sounds and observing respiratory rate, rhythm, depth, and effort. Oxygen, medications, and other respiratory treatments are administered as prescribed. Close monitoring of intake and output, electrolytes, and comfort is important. The child should be monitored for restlessness, anxiety, and air hunger.

Placing the child in a high-Fowler position may help with lung expansion. Because this position places pressure on bony prominences in the sacrum and hips, pressure areas must be relieved at intervals. Most of the care of PE occurs in the ICU, which is anxiety provoking for the child and family. They should be given the opportunity to express their fears and anxieties and to ask questions. (For other nursing care activities, see the following section on ARDS and ALI.)

ACUTE RESPIRATORY DISTRESS SYNDROME AND ACUTE LUNG INJURY

Acute respiratory distress syndrome (ARDS) and *acute lung injury* (ALI) are potentially life-threatening inflammatory lung conditions that may occur in children and adults. They are caused by direct injury to the lungs or by systemic insults that lead indirectly to lung injury with subsequent hypoxemia and respiratory failure due to noncardiogenic pulmonary edema. Sepsis, trauma, viral pneumonia, aspiration, fat emboli, drug overdose, reperfusion injury after lung transplantation, smoke inhalation, and submersion injury, among others, have been associated with ARDS and ALI. Both are characterized by respiratory distress and hypoxemia that occur within 72 hours of a serious injury or surgery in a person with previously normal lungs. ALI involves a spectrum of inflammatory disease responses to a precipitating event, with ARDS being the more severe form of ALI.

Animation—Bag Ventilation

The diagnostic criteria established by the American European Consensus Conference (Bernard, Artigas, Brigham, et al., 1994) have been superseded by the Berlin definition of ARDS (ARDS Definition Task Force, Ranieri, Rubenfeld, et al., 2012). According to the Berlin definition, ARDS occurs within 1 week of a known clinical insult or new or worsening respiratory symptoms; is characterized by bilateral opacities on chest imaging not fully explained by effusions, lobar/lung collapse, or nodules; and manifests as respiratory failure not fully explained by cardiac failure or fluid overload. Hypoxemia is expressed in terms of the ratio of partial pressure of oxygen (Pa_{O_2}) to the fraction of inspired oxygen (Fi_{O_2}) (P/F ratio). In the setting of a PEEP or CPAP $\geq$5 cm H_2O, mild, moderate, and severe ARDS are defined by P/F ratios between 200 and 300, between 100 and 200, and $\leq$100 mm Hg, respectively. In 2015 the Pediatric Acute Lung Injury Consensus Conference Group published pediatric-specific definitions, recommendations regarding treatment, and future research priorities.

Pathologically, the hallmark of ARDS is increased permeability of the alveolar-capillary membrane that results in pulmonary edema (Fig. 26.7). During the acute phase of ARDS, inflammatory mediators cause damage to the membrane, with consequent increase in pulmonary capillary permeability and the development of interstitial edema. Later stages are characterized by pneumocyte and fibrin infiltration of the alveoli, with the start of either the healing process or fibrosis. When fibrosis occurs, the child may demonstrate respiratory distress and the need for mechanical ventilation. In ARDS, the lungs become stiff as a result of surfactant inactivation; gas diffusion is impaired; and eventually, bronchiolar mucosal swelling and congestive atelectasis occur. The net effect is decreased functional residual capacity, pulmonary hypertension, and increased intrapulmonary right-to-left shunting of blood. Surfactant secretion is reduced, and the atelectasis and fluid-filled alveoli provide an excellent medium for bacterial growth. Hypoxemia or increased work of breathing may require ventilatory support.

The child with ARDS may first demonstrate only symptoms caused by an injury or infection, but as the condition deteriorates, tachypnea, increasing respiratory effort, cyanosis, and decreasing oxygen saturation occur. The hypoxemia may be refractory to oxygen administration.

Therapeutic Management

Treatment involves supportive measures to ensure adequate oxygenation and pulmonary perfusion, treatment of infection (or the precipitating cause), maintenance of adequate cardiac output and vascular volume, hydration, adequate nutritional support, comfort measures, prevention of complications such as GI ulceration and aspiration, and psychologic support. Specific treatment should be directed against the underlying cause (e.g., antibiotics and source control for infection).

Definitive therapy is directed toward improvement of oxygenation. The use of endotracheal intubation, PEEP, and low tidal volume may be required to ensure maximum oxygen delivery by increasing functional residual capacity, reducing intrapulmonary shunting, and reducing pulmonary fluid. Inappropriate use of mechanical ventilation may worsen the lung injury, resulting in volutrauma, barotrauma, atelectrauma, and biotrauma to the injured lungs. Ventilation with low tidal volume (6 ml/kg of ideal body weight) has been associated with lower mortality rates in children with ALI (Wong, Jit, Sultana, et al., 2017). Other supportive strategies include use of the prone position, pharmacologic neuromuscular blockade to facilitate ventilation, administration of inhaled nitric oxide or prostaglandins, and high-frequency oscillatory ventilation. The evidence to support these therapies is variable and evolving. Extracorporeal membrane oxygenation (ECMO) should be considered in cases of severe ARDS when the cause of respiratory failure is believed to be reversible or if the child is likely to be suitable for consideration for lung transplantation (Pediatric Acute Lung Injury Consensus Conference Group, 2015).

Fluid administration to maintain adequate intravascular volume and end-organ perfusion must be balanced against the desire to decrease lung fluid to improve oxygenation. The provision of adequate nutrition, maintenance of patient comfort, and prevention of complications such as GI ulceration are essential. Psychologic support of the patient and family is also important.

Prognosis

The prognosis for patients with ARDS is improving. Nonetheless, the mortality rate remains high and ranges from 14% to 45% in children (Lopez-Fernandez, Azagra, de la Oliva, et al., 2012). The precipitating disorder influences the outcome; the worst prognosis is associated with uncontrolled sepsis, bone marrow transplantation, cancer, and multisystem involvement with hepatic failure. Children who recover may have persistent pulmonary function test abnormalities, cough, and exertional dyspnea.

Nursing Care Management

The child with ARDS is cared for in the ICU during the acute stages of illness. Nursing care involves close monitoring of oxygenation and respiratory status, as well as assessment of cardiac output, perfusion, fluid and electrolyte balance, and renal function (urinary output). Blood gas analysis, acid-base status, and pulse oximetry are important evaluation tools. Most children with ARDS require invasive monitoring via arterial and central venous catheters. Diuretics may be administered to reduce pulmonary fluid, and vasodilators may be administered to decrease pulmonary vascular pressure. Nutritional support is often required because of the prolonged acute phase of the illness. Nursing management also includes monitoring the effects of the numerous parenteral fluids and drugs used to stabilize the child and monitoring for changes in the child's hemodynamic status. To prevent superimposed ventilator-associated pneumonia (VAP), nursing care includes elevation of the head of the bed to between 30 and 35 degrees (crib at 20 degrees) unless contraindicated and frequent oral care at least every 4 hours. Additional strategies to prevent VAP include use of a closed suctioning

PATHOPHYSIOLOGY REVIEW

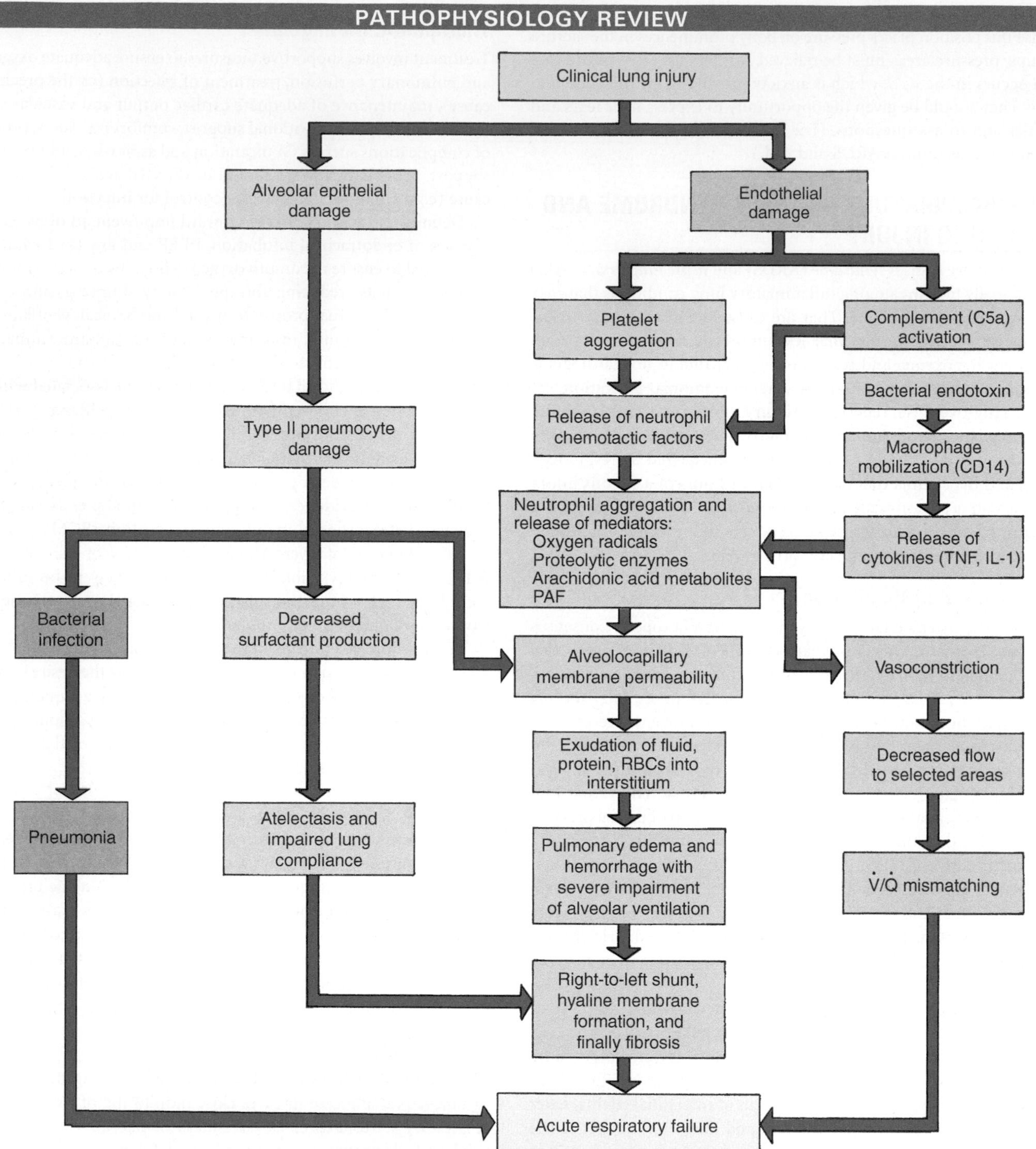

FIG. 26.7 Pathogenesis of acute respiratory distress syndrome. *IL-1,* Interleukin-1; *PAF,* platelet-activating factor; *RBCs,* red blood cells; *TNF,* tumor necrosis factor; *V/Q,* ventilation-perfusion. (From McCance, K. L., & Huether, S. E. [2010]. *Pathophysiology: The biological basis for disease in adults and children* [6th ed.]. St. Louis, MO: Mosby.)

system, removal of oropharyngeal secretions, draining breathing circuit condensate periodically, and avoiding reintubation (Garland, 2010). The risk of pressure ulcers is greater with the head of the bed in an elevated position, and this must be balanced with the risk of VAP. Careful and ongoing skin assessment and pressure area observation are essential. The multidisciplinary care team performs a daily assessment of readiness to wean or liberate from mechanical ventilation. The child must also be assessed for risk of deep-vein thrombosis, and appropriate prophylactic strategies must be initiated (e.g., passive range of motion exercises as able, sequential compression devices, anticoagulant therapy, and early ambulation). Respiratory distress is a frightening situation for both the child and the parents, and attention to their psychologic needs is a major element in the care of these children. The child is often sedated during the acute phase of the illness, and weaning from sedation requires close monitoring and interventions to promote comfort.

SMOKE INHALATION INJURY

A number of noxious substances that may be inhaled are toxic to humans. They are primarily products of incomplete combustion and cause more deaths from fires than flame injuries. The severity of the injury depends on the nature of the substances generated by the material being burned, whether the victim is confined in a closed space, and the duration of contact with the smoke.

General Aspects

Possible inhalation injury is suspected when there is a history of flames or smoke in a closed space, whether or not burns are present. Sooty material around the nose or in the sputum; singed nasal hairs; or mucosal burns of the nose, lips, mouth, or throat are all signs that the affected person requires observation for possible pulmonary injury from inhalants. A hoarse voice and cough are further evidence of airway involvement, and increased inspiratory and expiratory stridor indicates severe damage to the upper passages. Signs of respiratory distress also include tachypnea, tachycardia, and diminished or abnormal breath sounds, including crackles and wheezes.

Three distinct syndromes of pulmonary complications may occur in the child suffering from inhalation injury: early carbon monoxide poisoning, airway obstruction, and pulmonary edema; ARDS occurring at 24 to 48 hours, or later in some cases; and late complications of pneumonia and pulmonary emboli (Antoon & Donovan, 2016). Strangulation may also occur from the cervical eschar secondary to a severe burn. Smoke inhalation causes three different types of injury: heat, local chemical, and systemic.

Heat Injury

Heat causes thermal injury to the upper airway, but because air has low specific heat, the injury goes no farther than the upper airway. Reflex closure of the glottis prevents injury to the lower airway. Heat may reach the middle airway occasionally, but it rarely penetrates to the lungs.

Chemical Injury

The combustion of materials such as clothing, furniture, and floor coverings can generate a wide variety of gases. Acids, alkalis, and their precursors in smoke can produce chemical burns. These substances can be carried deep into the respiratory tract, including the lower respiratory tract, in the form of insoluble gases. Soluble gases tend to dissolve in the upper respiratory tract.

Synthetic materials are especially toxic, producing gases such as oxides of sulfur and nitrogen, acetaldehyde, formaldehyde, hydrocyanic acid, and chlorine. Heated plastics are the source of extremely toxic vapors, including chlorine and hydrochloric acid from polyvinylchloride, and hydrocarbons, aldehydes, ketones, and acids from polyethylene. Irritant gases such as nitrous oxide or carbon dioxide combine with water in the lungs to form corrosive acids. Aldehydes cause denaturation of proteins, cellular damage, and edema of pulmonary tissues. Chemical burns to the airways are similar to burns on the skin, except they are painless because the tracheobronchial tree is relatively insensitive to pain.

Inhalation of small amounts of noxious irritants produces alveolar and bronchiolar damage that can lead to obstructive bronchiolitis. Severe exposure causes further injury, including alveolocapillary damage with hemorrhage, necrotizing bronchiolitis, inhibited secretion of surfactant, and formation of hyaline membranes, all manifestations of ARDS.

Systemic Injury

Systemic injury occurs from gases that are nontoxic to the airways (e.g., carbon monoxide, hydrogen cyanide). They can result in injury and death by interfering with or inhibiting cellular respiration. Carbon monoxide (CO) is a colorless, odorless, tasteless gas with an affinity for hemoglobin 230 times greater than that of oxygen. When CO enters the bloodstream, it readily binds with hemoglobin to form carboxyhemoglobin (COHb). Because CO combines more readily and is released less readily than oxygen, very low levels of tissue oxygen must be reached before appreciable amounts of oxygen are released from the hemoglobin. Therefore tissue hypoxia reaches dangerous levels before oxygen is available to meet tissue needs.

> **! NURSING ALERT**
>
> With carbon monoxide poisoning, the oxygen saturation (Sa_{O_2}) obtained by pulse oximetry will be normal because the device measures only oxygenated and deoxygenated hemoglobin; it does not measure dysfunctional hemoglobin, such as COHb.

Accidental CO poisoning is most often a result of exposure to fumes from heaters or smoke from structural fires, although poorly ventilated recreational vehicles with improperly operated or maintained gas lamps or stoves and cooking in underventilated areas with charcoal grills or hibachis are also frequent causes. Intentional CO poisoning may occur in an attempted suicide in a vehicle parked in a closed garage for a long period. Accidental CO poisoning may also occur in a vehicle with inadequate vented exhaust that leaks into the vehicle's passenger (or closed truck bed) compartment. CO is produced by incomplete combustion of carbon or carbonaceous material, such as wood or charcoal.

The signs and symptoms of CO poisoning are secondary to tissue hypoxia and vary with the level of COHb. Younger children may display symptoms before older children and adults after exposure due to their increased oxygen use and respiratory rate. Mild manifestations include headache, visual disturbances, irritability, and nausea, whereas more severe intoxication causes confusion, hallucinations, ataxia, and coma. CO may increase cerebral blood flow, increase cerebral capillary permeability, and increase cerebrospinal fluid pressure, all of which contribute to the CNS signs observed. The bright, cherry-red lips and skin often described are less common than pallor and cyanosis. Patients who have significant exposure to CO can develop a delayed neurologic deficit, which can occur 3 to 240 days after initial exposure. The deficits can last up to a year.

Therapeutic Management

The treatment of children with smoke toxicity is largely symptomatic. The most widely accepted treatment is placing the child on humidified 100% oxygen as quickly as possible and monitoring for signs of respiratory distress and impending failure. Baseline blood gases and COHb levels are drawn. Arterial oxygen partial pressure may be within normal limits unless there is marked respiratory depression. If CO poisoning is confirmed, 100% oxygen is continued until COHb levels fall to the nontoxic range of about 10%. CO is removed by the lung circulation due to oxygen combining competitively with hemoglobin and displacing the CO.

Respiratory distress may occur early in the course of smoke inhalation as a result of hypoxia, or patients who are breathing well on admission may suddenly develop respiratory distress. Therefore endotracheal intubation equipment should be readily available. Transient edema of the airways can occur at any level in the tracheobronchial tree. Assessment and localization of the obstruction should be accomplished before severe swelling of the head, neck, or oropharynx occurs. Intubation is often necessary when (1) severe burns in the area of the nose, mouth, and face increase the likelihood of developing oropharyngeal edema and obstruction; (2) vocal cord edema causes obstruction; (3) the patient has difficulty handling secretions; and (4) progressive respiratory distress requires artificial ventilation. Controversy surrounds tracheotomy, but many prefer this procedure when the obstruction is proximal to the larynx and reserve nasotracheal intubation for lower tract involvement. An electrocardiogram should be considered with significant exposure to rule out myocardial ischemia.

Pulmonary care may be facilitated by bronchodilators, inhaled corticosteroids, humidification, and CPT to enhance the removal of necrotic material, minimize bronchoconstriction, and avoid atelectasis. Bronchoscopy may be needed to clear heavy secretions.

CO is excreted primarily through the lungs. Treatment of CO intoxication with 100% oxygen via nonrebreathing face mask reduces the COHb level by one-half in 40 to 60 minutes. Hyperbaric oxygen therapy (HBOT) may be required for severe carbon monoxide poisoning (COHb level >25% in children, end-organ ischemia, loss of consciousness) to dissolve additional oxygen from COHb in the blood (Kostic, 2016). HBOT significantly decreases the half-life of COHb compared with 100% oxygen treatment alone.

Nursing Care Management

Nursing care of the child with inhalation injury is the same as that for any child with respiratory distress. The initial goal is to maintain a patent airway and effective ventilation status; endotracheal intubation may be required early, depending on the patient's respiratory status and the progression of airway and pulmonary edema. (See also Respiratory Failure, later in this chapter.) In the acute phase, the nurse should monitor vital signs, oxygenation, work of breathing, and other respiratory assessments frequently. The administration of nebulized bronchodilators, humidified oxygen, and inhaled corticosteroids is often part of the nursing care. Chest percussion and postural drainage are often required. Fluid requirements for children experiencing inhalation injury are greater than for those with surface burns alone, and IV fluids are generally prescribed. However, one concern is the development of pulmonary edema; therefore accurate monitoring of intake and output is essential. (See also Nursing Care Management earlier in this chapter for mechanical ventilation care.)

In addition to the observation and management of the physical aspects of inhalation injury, the nurse also deals with the psychologic needs of a frightened child and distraught parents. Parents need support, reassurance, and information about their child's condition, treatment, and progress. The nurse also can provide anticipatory guidance and educate families on prevention of inhalation injuries and the importance of CO detectors in the home.

ENVIRONMENTAL TOBACCO EXPOSURE

Numerous investigations indicate that parental or family smoking is an important cause of morbidity in children. Children exposed to passive or environmental tobacco smoke have an increased number of respiratory illnesses, increased respiratory symptoms (e.g., cough, sputum, and wheezing), and reduced performance on pulmonary function tests. AOM and OME are also increased in children who have smoking family members. Indoor exposure to tobacco smoke has been linked to asthma in children (Makadia, Roper, Andrews, et al., 2017). Among children with asthma, there is an association between parental/family member cigarette smoking and asthma exacerbations, trips to the ED, medication use, and impaired recovery after hospitalization for acute asthma. Children and infants exposed to secondhand smoke experience more wheezing episodes. Maternal cigarette smoking is associated with increased respiratory symptoms and illnesses in children; decreased fetal growth; increased deliveries of low-birth-weight, preterm, and stillborn infants; and a greater incidence of sudden infant death syndrome (SIDS). Antenatal maternal smoking is a significant risk factor for SIDS (Friedmann, Dahdouh, Kugler, et al., 2017). The risk for diagnosis of early-onset asthma in the first 3 years of life is associated with in utero exposure to maternal smoking.

State, federal, and local governments have enacted legislation prohibiting smoking in public and workplaces. Children experience more secondhand smoke exposure in the home setting than anywhere else. The impact of tobacco smoke also contributes to an increase in childhood deaths attributed to residential fires in households where adults smoke. The financial impact of secondhand smoke exposure is significant. In 2010 the average annual smoking-attributable health care expenditures were $170 billion (Xu, Bishop, Kennedy, et al., 2015).

Electronic cigarettes have increased in popularity among adults as well as middle school–age and teenage children. Regular use of electronic cigarettes has increased tenfold among high-school students, from 1.5% in 2011 to 16% in 2015 (Chun, Moazed, Calfee, et al., 2017), and 5% of middle school students reported regular use of electronic cigarettes in 2015 (Chun et al., 2017). This increase may be due to adolescents' belief that electronic cigarettes are less harmful and less addictive than cigarettes (Amrock, Lee, & Weitzman, 2016). Although these products are advertised as being safe because they are smokeless, the battery-powered cigarettes still contain nicotine and other chemicals. Recent studies have shown toxic effects on the pulmonary system, including altered airways, increased oxidative stress, interference in lung development, and impaired immune defense against bacterial and viral pathogens (Chun, Moazed, Calfee, et al., 2017). Electronic cigarettes can also increase the risk for cancer (Canistro, Vivarelli, Cirillo, et al., 2017).

Secondhand smoke consists of passive smoke exposure emitted from a tobacco product. The amount of passive smoke exposure in infants and children is directly related to the number of smokers in a household. Cotinine, a by-product of nicotine, is considered a valid biochemical marker for smoke exposure. Cotinine levels are increased in children who live in homes with smokers, and these levels increase proportionately with the number of smokers in the home. Cotinine levels have also been used to document exposure to passive smoke in the fetus and newborn (Evlampidou, Bagkeris, Vardavas, et al., 2015).

In recent years, concern has grown regarding "thirdhand" tobacco exposure—the tobacco toxins that remain in the environment long after the smoker has stopped smoking (Samet, Chanson, & Wipfli, 2015). Such toxins may be found in cars, homes, clothing, and hands.

Nursing Care Management

Passive smoke exposure during childhood may also contribute to the development of bronchopulmonary dysplasia in adulthood, and some have attributed infertility in adults to exposure to secondhand smoke as children. Nurses and other health care professionals need to include assessments of passive smoke exposure in all children, especially those with respiratory illnesses. In families where smokers refuse to quit, house rules should be established for reducing smoke in the child's environment, such as smoking outside of the home, wearing removable clothing while smoking, and not smoking in vehicles. Nurses should also inform caregivers of the health hazards of children's exposure to tobacco smoke*; set an example for children and families; and become

*For a copy of the Environmental Protection Agency report Respiratory Health Effects of Passive Smoking, visit http://cfpub.epa.gov/ncea/CFM/recordisplay.cfm?deid=2835.

advocates for "no smoking" ordinances in public places, prohibition of advertising tobacco products in the media, and inclusion of health warnings of sidestream smoke on tobacco products. Nurses have an important role in offering tobacco smoking cessation counseling and in teaching such classes in the community at large. The role of the nurse in promoting smoking cessation among adolescents is discussed in Chapter 18. Adolescents should be screened for inhalation of tobacco products or marijuana and counseling on cessation should be offered.

STRUCTURAL DEFECTS

CONGENITAL DIAPHRAGMATIC HERNIA

Congenital diaphragmatic hernia (CDH) results when the diaphragm does not form completely, resulting in an opening between the thorax and the abdominal cavity. The diaphragm forms at 4 to 8 weeks of gestation when two membranes close together to separate the abdominal and thoracic cavities. The most common type of CDH (90%) is a left posterolateral defect, also known as a Bochdalek hernia because the herniation occurs through the foramen of Bochdalek (Fig. 26.8). The less common type is the hernia of Morgagni, which is more anterior and often not detected until adulthood. With the Bochdalek hernia, the intestines and other abdominal structures, such as the stomach, liver, or bowel, can enter the thoracic cavity, compressing the lung. Lung hypoplasia may occur on the affected side and to a lesser degree on the contralateral side. Ventilation is further compromised by hypoplasia and compression of the lung, including the airways and blood vessels. In addition to the anatomic defect, pulmonary hypoplasia and pulmonary hypertension have also been recently recognized as components in the pathology of CDH.

This serious defect requires prompt recognition (usually in utero) and aggressive treatment to reduce its high mortality risk. The incidence of CDH is approximately 1 in 2000 to 5000 live births and females are affected twice as often as males (Maheshwari & Carlo, 2016). CDH occurs more commonly on the left side (Maheshwari & Carlo, 2016). Associated anomalies have occurred in 10% to 20% of cases, and CDH is observed in several chromosomal syndromes.

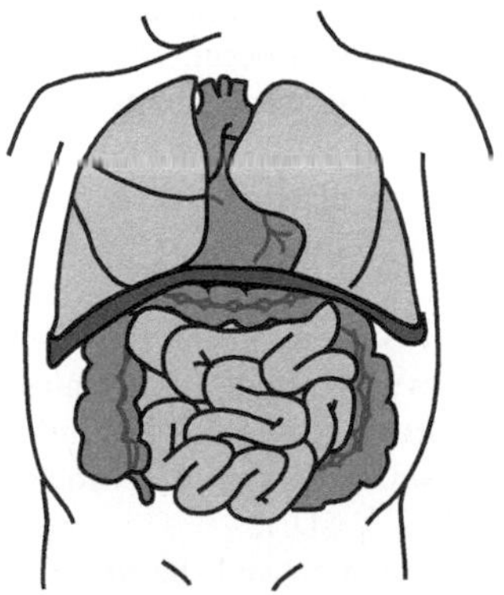

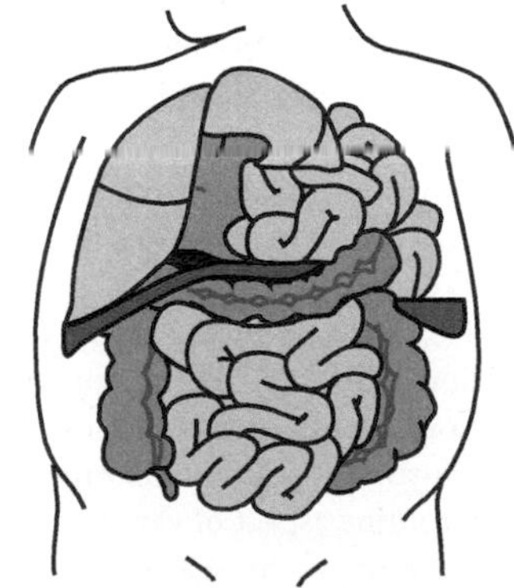

FIG. 26.8 A, Normal diaphragm separating the abdominal and thoracic cavities. **B,** Diaphragmatic hernia with a small lung and abdominal contents in the thoracic cavity. (From Ehrlich, P. F., & Coran, A. G. [2011]. Diaphragmatic hernia. In R. M. Kliegman, B. F. Stanton, J. W. St. Geme, et al. [Eds.], *Nelson textbook of pediatrics* [19th ed.]. Philadelphia, PA: Saunders.)

Clinical Manifestations

The most common manifestation of CDH is acute respiratory distress in the newborn. Infants with a CDH may be dyspneic and cyanotic and have a scaphoid abdomen (because of abdominal contents in the chest). Cardiac output is impaired, and the infant exhibits signs and symptoms of shock. Some infants with small defects may not exhibit respiratory symptoms until later in infancy.

Diagnostic Evaluation

Prenatal diagnosis of CDH as early as the twenty-fourth week of gestation is possible. The three main features detected by ultrasonography that confirm the diagnosis are polyhydramnios, mediastinal shift, and loops of bowel in the chest cavity. In severe cases fetal hydrops is evident. Low maternal serum alpha-fetoprotein levels are seen in cases of CDH; however, the finding is not specific for this anomaly.

Antenatal diagnosis of CDH has the advantages of counseling the family regarding pregnancy alternatives and potential problems of the neonatal period (especially if other syndromes or chromosomal abnormalities are present); continuing the pregnancy and further management, including possible antenatal treatment; and transporting the fetus with a CDH in utero to a tertiary center for management. A multidisciplinary team of neonatologists, neonatal nurses, respiratory therapists, and pediatric surgeons can intervene early in the acute phase to improve the infant's chances for survival and a positive outcome. After birth, the diagnosis of CDH may depend on the type of hernia present. In the majority of cases the diagnosis is suspected on the basis of the clinical manifestations and is confirmed by a chest radiograph. The chest radiograph shows fluid- and air-filled loops of intestine in the affected side of the chest. The mediastinum may be shifted to the unaffected side, and auscultation may reveal decreased breath sounds on the affected side. The presence or absence of liver herniation is a predictive indicator of postnatal survivability, as well as lung-to-head ratio and fetal lung volume (Oluyomi-Obi, Kuret, Puligandla, et al., 2017).

Therapeutic Management

Fetal Surgery

Fetoscopic endoluminal tracheal occlusion has been performed in cases of severe CDH to expand the lungs and push the abdominal contents back into the abdomen, thus producing larger, functional lungs.

After Birth

The severity of symptoms depends on the size of the defect in the diaphragm, how much of the abdominal contents are present in the chest, the size of the lungs, and at what stage of gestation the herniation occurred. Many infants with a CDH have respiratory distress and require immediate respiratory assistance, which includes endotracheal intubation and GI decompression with a double-lumen catheter to decompress the stomach and reduce compression of the lung. At birth, bag and mask ventilation is contraindicated to prevent air from entering the stomach and especially the intestines, further compromising pulmonary function. When the newborn cries at birth, air is swallowed and the bowel becomes inflated, so its presence in the chest cavity can further compromise lung function. Close attention to the infant's acid-base status is imperative in the management and prevention of pulmonary hypertension. Low ventilatory positive pressure and the lowest mean airway pressure possible, combined with rapid ventilatory rates (80 to 120 breaths/min), may reduce the incidence of pulmonary leaks from overinflation of the unaffected lung. ECMO may also be indicated after birth if severe.

An umbilical arterial catheter will help monitor postductal arterial oxygen tension (Pao_2) and allow infusion of IV fluids, glucose, and electrolytes. Bicarbonate-containing IV fluids may be administered to maintain a pH between 7.5 and 7.6 to prevent acidosis. A transcutaneous oxygen pressure monitor or pulse oximeter may be placed preductally (right hand) and postductally (left hand, arm, or either foot) to monitor the amount of ductal shunting through the patent ductus arteriosus. Ductal shunting of deoxygenated blood occurs when pressure in the pulmonary artery is equal to or less than peripheral blood pressure. If pulmonary hypertension is severe with decreased pulmonary venous return, right atrial pressure will be greater than left atrial pressure, resulting in right-to-left shunting of blood through the foramen ovale. The net results of these events cause further hypoxia, hypercarbia, and acidosis. (See Persistent Pulmonary Hypertension of the Newborn, Chapter 9.) Echocardiography is performed to determine any cardiac anomalies, as well as to detect any pulmonary hypertension and ductal shunting. Survival rates are lower with underlying cardiac disease, such as hypoplastic left heart syndrome.

Because acidosis increases pulmonary hypertension and consequently shunting of unoxygenated blood away from the lungs, it is imperative to monitor acid-base status closely. Close attention to the infant's thermoregulatory status (maintaining a neutral thermal environment) and glucose requirements during the acute phase is another priority of care. Ventilatory management should be individualized on the basis of the infant's response and requirements.

Surfactant replacement therapy may also be used to stabilize neonates with CDH, but outcomes have not demonstrated an overall advantage in relation to ECMO requirements and mortality rate (Garcia & Stolar, 2012). The use of inhaled nitric oxide to relieve pulmonary hypertension of CDH has also been used in some cases, with mixed results (Maheshwari & Carlo, 2016). (See Nitric Oxide, Surfactant, and Persistent Pulmonary Hypertension of the Newborn, Chapter 9.)

Another strategy that has demonstrated considerable success in the management of CDH is the use of permissive hypercapnia wherein hyperventilation is not employed in order to reduce iatrogenic lung injury and barotrauma. Preductal Spo_2 is maintained at 85 to 90, Pco_2 is ignored, and metabolic acidosis is corrected with buffers instead of hyperventilation. Using lung-protective ventilation (gentle ventilation) strategies aimed at decreasing mean inflation pressures (<25 cm H_2O) and avoiding hyperventilation have demonstrated better overall outcomes and have significantly decreased pulmonary complications such as pneumothorax. Allowing slight hypercapnia has been associated with decreased mortality rate, a longer period of ventilation before repair, a shorter period of ventilation after repair, and a lower rate of ECMO use (Guidry, Hranjec, Rodgers, et al., 2012).

Operative treatment involves returning the abdominal organs to the abdomen and repairing the diaphragmatic defect. The timing of surgical repair may vary. With milder symptoms, such as no pulmonary hypertension or pulmonary hypoplasia, surgical correction occurs 2 to 3 days after birth. Most repairs occur 5 to 10 days after birth in the absence of severe pulmonary hypoplasia and pulmonary hypertension.

Postoperative management involves continuation of ventilatory therapy, monitoring of acid-base balance, and allowing slight hypercapnia. In addition, gastric decompression, thermoregulation, sedation, and maintenance of adequate cardiac output and peripheral perfusion are continued. If the infant is too unstable for surgical repair, ECMO is considered.

Prognosis

CDH is a complex problem of pulmonary hypoplasia, immature lungs, and other associated problems. The overall mortality rates for CDH are decreasing, as the pathophysiology is better understood in relation to current treatment modalities. Current data suggest overall survival rates of 70% to 92%; however, survival rates vary according to CDH severity and associated conditions such as esophageal atresia and cardiac anomalies (Burgos, Modee, Osy et al., 2017). Surgical repair of the defect alone does not resolve the infant's problems related to organ immaturity. Long-term complications of CDH include chronic lung disease, gastroesophageal reflux, feeding problems, recurrent diaphragmatic herniation, pneumonia, failure to grow, sensorineural hearing loss, scoliosis, and impaired motor and cognitive function.

Nursing Care Management

Assessment of the infant at birth is an integral component of nursing care. Prompt recognition of neonatal respiratory distress, cyanosis, a scaphoid abdomen, and a possible mediastinal shift would alert the nurse to investigate possible causes of these symptoms. Any one or a combination of these signs may signal the presence of CDH. A newborn in respiratory distress at birth who does not initially respond to resuscitation is further evaluated for CDH; endotracheal intubation is an option for providing adequate oxygenation until CDH is ruled out. If CDH is diagnosed prenatally and the infant is in distress, endotracheal intubation is required to prevent further accumulation of air in the stomach and intestines and subsequent respiratory compromise.

! NURSING ALERT

Any newborn infant with a scaphoid abdomen, moderate to severe respiratory distress, decreased breath sounds unilaterally, and a history of polyhydramnios should be suspected of having a CDH. Ventilation should not be given with bag and mask to prevent further intestinal air and subsequent respiratory compromise.

Preoperative care involves prompt recognition, resuscitation, and stabilization of the infant, including ventilatory support, blood gas monitoring, fluid volume maintenance, and administration of IV fluids and electrolytes. Gastric decompression is achieved with a double-lumen tube, and the infant is observed for signs of impaired cardiac output, acidosis, and hypoxemia.

Postoperative care includes the routine observations discussed in the care of the high-risk infant. Close observation to detect signs of respiratory distress or fluid and electrolyte imbalances is an important nursing function. The infant should be closely monitored for signs of mediastinal shift, pulmonary air leak, and infection. Hypovolemia as a result of third spacing of intravascular fluids may occur. The nurse should also pay attention to skin care because these infants often experience prolonged sedation, an increase in skin moisture, tubes and drains coming in contact with the skin, altered nutrition, and altered hemodynamics, all of which place the infant at risk for skin breakdown.

Nursing care of the infant with a CDH is also aimed at reducing noxious stimulation either from care activities such as routine suctioning or from environmental factors such as environmental noise. Measures that further reduce infant stress, such as management of pain, should be a routine aspect of care for the infant with a CDH.

Because of the serious nature of the condition and the urgency of treatment, the parents are in great need of ongoing support and education regarding postoperative care. The infant with a CDH may require long-term hospitalization and care. As soon as medically possible, the parents should be involved in the daily care of their child, and every effort must be made to promote bonding.

PIERRE ROBIN SEQUENCE

Pierre Robin sequence (PRS), which is also known as Pierre Robin syndrome, is a defect characterized by mandibular hypoplasia, retroposition of the tongue and mandible, and cleft palate, which often results in airway obstruction, respiratory distress, and feeding problems. The condition has an incidence of 1 in 8500 live births and is often associated with other congenital anomalies (Ren, Gao, Li, et al., 2017). The tongue may be large (glossoptosis) and frequently falls over the neonate's airway, causing occlusion and respiratory distress. In severe upper airway obstruction, a tracheostomy and a feeding tube may be required. From a lateral view the infant's lower jaw can be seen to be positioned posterior (micrognathia) to the upper jaw. PRS may be diagnosed in the nursery when the infant has apnea and cyanosis, due primarily to the upper airway obstruction. The neonate is positioned to facilitate an open airway (ideally not supine), and the practitioner is notified immediately.

A tongue-lip adhesion is a common surgical procedure that repositions the tongue anteriorly (Ren, Gao, Li, et al., 2017). A nasal trumpet may be indicated to maintain an open airway, but ultimately, surgical distraction of the mandible is required. There are usually no associated neurocognitive defects in isolated PRS.

Nursing care is aimed at early recognition of the infant with PRS, positioning to maintain an open airway, and providing parents with information and reassurance.

CHOANAL ATRESIA

Choanal atresia, the most common congenital anomaly of the nose, is a bony and/or membranous septum located between the nose and the pharynx. The atresia may be unilateral or bilateral. Because most infants are preferential nasal breathers, bilateral choanal atresia may be associated with apnea and cyanosis when the infant is at rest. When the infant cries, he or she breathes in through the mouth and pinks up. Unilateral choanal atresia may not be associated with apnea. Inability to pass a suction catheter through the nose into the pharynx or cyanosis without obvious respiratory distress usually leads to its detection. Nearly half of the infants with choanal atresia have other anomalies (CHARGE syndrome, Treacher Collins syndrome, and Tessier syndrome). Surgical correction is required.

LONG-TERM RESPIRATORY DYSFUNCTION

ALLERGIC RHINITIS

Allergic rhinitis affects as many as 20% to 40% of the pediatric population and is associated with numerous airway disorders, including asthma, OME, and chronic sinusitis (Milgrom & Sicherer, 2016). Seasonal allergic rhinitis (also known as hay fever) usually follows a spring-fall pattern and is caused by tree, grass, and weed pollens. Seasonal allergic rhinitis usually does not develop until the individual has been sensitized by two or more pollen seasons. Year-round or perennial allergic rhinitis is more common and is triggered by household inhaled allergens such as feathers, household dust, animal dander, air pollutants, and molds. The risk for allergic rhinitis is increased in infants exposed to tobacco smoke, heavy exposure to indoor allergens, and delivery by cesarean section if there is a family history of allergies or asthma (Milgrom & Sicherer, 2016). However, early exposure to dogs and cats appears to be a protective factor (Milgrom & Sicherer, 2016).

Allergic rhinitis is classified as seasonal allergic rhinitis (SAR) or perennial allergic rhinitis (PAR). SAR has a cyclic, well-defined course, and PAR causes year-round symptoms (Milgrom & Sicherer, 2016). Allergic rhinitis may also be classified as mild intermittent, moderate-severe intermittent, mild persistent, or moderate-severe persistent. Symptoms of intermittent allergic rhinitis occur less than 4 days per week or less than 4 consecutive weeks, whereas persistent occurs more than 4 days per week or more than 4 consecutive weeks (Milgrom & Sicherer, 2016).

Pathophysiology

Allergic rhinitis requires two conditions: a familial predisposition to develop allergy and exposure of a sensitized person to the allergen. Inhalants in the form of microscopic airborne particles (e.g., pollens, mold, animal danders, and environmental dusts) enter the upper respiratory tract with inhalation and bind to submucosal mast cells in the respiratory tract epithelium.

In the allergic child, symptoms are mediated by immunoglobulin E (IgE), which is produced by the child's B lymphocytes. The IgE molecules on the cell surfaces trigger the rapid release of mast cell mediators (e.g., histamine, prostaglandins, and leukotrienes), as well as the slower synthesis of cell interactive compounds called cytokines; this action is often called the **early-phase response**. Histamine, a potent vasodilator, acts directly on local receptors to produce vasodilation, mucosal edema, and increased production of mucus. The cytokines summon cells to the area and are responsible for the slower **late-phase allergic** reaction of inflammation and destruction of the mucosal surface, which progresses to chronic nasal obstruction. The late-phase response typically occurs 4 to 8 hours after antigen exposure as a result of the migration of neutrophils, basophils, eosinophils, macrophages, and T lymphocytes into the nasal mucosa (Milgrom & Sicherer, 2016). Repeated exposure of these sensitized membranes to specific aeroallergens results in clinical allergic disease. Allergic rhinitis is rare in children under 2 years of age because repeated exposure to the allergen is needed to develop the allergy.

Clinical Manifestations

Children who have allergic rhinitis have a history of watery rhinorrhea, nasal obstruction, sneezing, itchy throat, or nasal pruritus. Symptoms may be chronic, recurrent, or acute and include itching of the nose, eyes, palate, pharynx, and conjunctiva. The nasal stuffiness sometimes progresses to partial or total obstruction of airflow, and mucus secretion with postnasal drainage can occur. Nasal itching is troublesome, and the affected child attempts to alleviate the symptoms by rubbing the nose—the "allergic salute" (Fig. 26.9). The presence of nasal itching helps identify allergic rhinitis from other types of rhinitis. Other symptoms include throat clearing, irritability, snoring during sleep, fatigue, malaise, headache, and poor school performance.

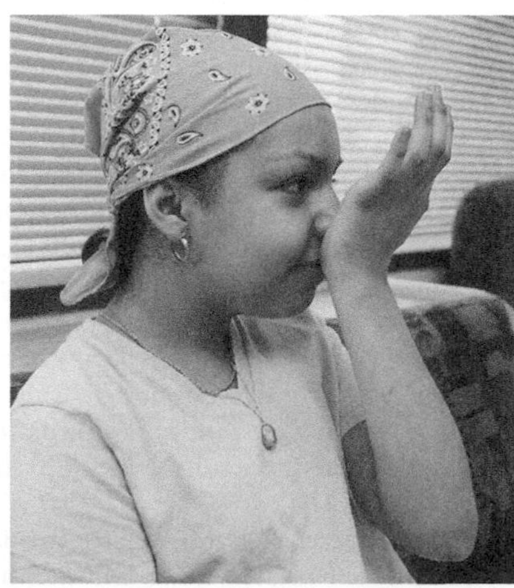

FIG. 26.9 "Allergic salute." (Courtesy Paul Vincent Kuntz, Texas Children's Hospital, Houston.)

On physical examination, children may display dark circles beneath their eyes, or "allergic shiners," secondary to obstruction of normal outflow from regional lymphatics and veins. If the nasal obstruction is severe, the child becomes an obligate mouth breather and is seen with an open mouth, or "allergic gape." Facial findings include a horizontal nasal crease across the lower third of the nose caused by frequent rubbing induced by the nasal pruritus, and Dennie-Morgan lines, or extra wrinkles below the lower eyelids. The child may develop facial tics and mannerisms in an attempt to avoid scratching the nose. Examination of the child's nose often reveals a pale, boggy nasal mucosa with enlarged nasal turbinates.

Symptoms that appear during peak symptom periods include tearing and soreness of the eyes and gelatinous conjunctival discharge in the morning, irritability, fatigue, depression, and loss of appetite.

When the nurse suspects allergic rhinitis, it is important to obtain information regarding clinical signs of related disorders, including middle ear disease, ear pain, delayed speech or language development, chronic cough, wheezing, exercise intolerance, eczema, or urticaria. It is also important to ask about any family history of allergies and to obtain information about specific triggers or environmental changes that may have precipitated an episode of rhinitis, such as seasonal pollens (e.g., tree, grass, weed), feathers, mold, pets, fungi, dust mites, cockroaches, rodents, cigarette smoking, or the use of a woodburning stove. Chronic rhinitis with significant nasal obstruction can lead to various abnormalities in growth and in physical, psychosocial, and intellectual development. It can also lead to social stigmatization related to ongoing symptoms.

Diagnostic Evaluation

Diagnosis of allergic rhinitis is based on a thorough history and physical examination. Because allergic rhinitis is often associated with atopic dermatitis or asthma, examination of the skin and chest is indicated. Diagnostic tests include a nasal smear to determine the number of eosinophils in the nasal secretions, blood examination for total IgE and elevated eosinophils, skin tests, and various challenge tests.

Skin testing is a useful adjunct in establishing a definitive diagnosis for allergic rhinitis. Skin testing involves the injection of specific allergens and should be performed by a practitioner educated in allergy treatment who has access to reliable reagents, experience in interpreting results, and adequate facilities to treat adverse reactions to the procedure. The allergenic extract is introduced into the epidermis (on arm or back usually) by scratch, prick, or puncture; a single intradermal injection of a dilute concentration of specific allergen; or serial dilution (threefold or tenfold) injections to determine the end point of reactivity. After a suitable time (10 to 30 seconds), the size of the resultant wheal and flare reaction is measured to assess the patient's sensitivity. The magnitude of the wheal and flare response correlates roughly with the severity of symptoms produced by natural exposure to the same allergen. However, a positive skin test does not always indicate the presence of clinical reactivity. Before skin testing occurs, the patient should withhold medications such as montelukast (Singulair) (1 day), antihistamines (7 days), antihistamine nasal sprays (3 days), decongestants (4 days), and antacids (3 days) to prevent false-negative results. Tricyclic antidepressants can interfere with skin reactions for 2 weeks but stopping the medication can have detrimental effects, so testing occurs while the patient continues the medication; however, it is important to realize that the results can be affected (Isik et al., 2011).

Skin testing and immunotherapy (see discussion later in this chapter) are generally safe procedures, but they are not without risk. Severe and even fatal reactions can occur within a short time, depending on the type of extract used and individual sensitivity.

> **! NURSING ALERT**
>
> The onset of a reaction is often insidious. Mild initial symptoms may include local pruritus, pallor, flushing, cyanosis, shortness of breath, dyspnea, cough, malaise, or abdominal pain. Later developments include hypotension, airway obstruction, chest pain, ventricular fibrillation, and loss of consciousness. Nurses need to recognize these symptoms, solicit urgent provider assistance, and be able to initiate emergency treatment.

Therapeutic Management

Therapy is directed toward avoidance of offending allergens and the use of medication and immunotherapy (hyposensitization or desensitization). Avoidance measures involve removing allergens from the environment and are usually effective for allergies to foods, drugs, and animals. If a patient is unable to avoid allergens, symptoms can be controlled with medication, but treatment should be individualized. For mild symptoms or intermittent symptoms with exposure to a known allergen, a second-generation oral antihistamine such as cetrizine, fexofenadine, or loratadine is recommended. An antihistamine (azelastine), glucocorticoid (fluticasone), or cromolyn nasal spray could also be considered. If the allergic rhinitis symptoms are more persistent, the glucocorticoid nasal sprays are first-line treatment and may even be used in combination sprays with an antihistamine twice daily.

Topical nasal corticosteroids are safe and effective therapies and are more effective than oral antihistamines for symptom relief. First-generation agents include beclomethasone (Vancenase and Beconase), flunisolide (Nasalide), and budesonide (Rhinocort or Pulmicort). Second-generation agents are fluticasone (Flovent) and mometasone (Nasonex). Dry powder preparations are also available (beclomethasone furoate or ciclesonide). Inhaled corticosteroids are administered with the nasal tip pointing away from the nasal septum (cartilage) to prevent nasal perforation (a rare but reported complication). Experts have expressed concerns in relation to possible decreased linear growth in children who take intranasal corticosteroids. To date, studies have not conclusively demonstrated growth failure. It may take several days or weeks to see relief of symptoms, especially if the child had been symptomatic for a long time. Side effects are minimal, with occasional nasal irritation, epistaxis, and changes in smell or taste.

Antihistamines reduce sneezing, rhinorrhea, and nasal itching but have less effect on nasal stuffiness than nasal corticosteroids. Antihistamines act by inhibiting the effects of histamine by binding to H_1 receptors. Classic first-generation antihistamines such as diphenhydramine (Benadryl) and chlorpheniramine (Chlor-Trimeton) are effective but may produce undesirable side effects such as dry mouth, urinary retention, constipation, and sedation or restlessness that results in impaired school performance. The second-generation antihistamines such as desloratadine (Clarinex), cetirizine (Zyrtec), and fexofenadine hydrochloride (Allegra) are approved for use in children 6 months and older (Milgrom & Sicherer, 2016). Azelastine is a topically active antihistamine available in nasal spray for children over 5 years old. These drugs are nonsedating and have few cardiovascular adverse effects.

If nasal obstruction is a prominent feature, children may use oral α-adrenergic decongestants, such as pseudoephedrine, in combination with an antihistamine (fexofenadine-pseudoephedrine, loratadine-pseudoephedrine) to relieve nasal stuffiness. Take caution, however, with long-term use because of rebound effects (return of symptoms) and habituation (lessened effectiveness). Other side effects of these drugs include nervousness, irritability, headache, insomnia, hypertension, and tachycardia.

Cromolyn sodium is a mast cell stabilizer used prophylactically on a regular basis and is effective in preventing both the early and the late responses to antigen by preventing release of histamine and other inflammatory mediators. Its usefulness is limited by the fact that it must be taken four times a day, a schedule that is difficult to maintain in children. It can also be used before expected exposure to an allergen, such as a pet. Ipratropium bromide (Atrovent), available as a nasal spray, may be used for serious rhinorrhea but should be limited to less than 5 days per month to avoid rebound nasal congestion (Milgrom & Sicherer, 2016).

The leukotriene modifier, montelukast, is approved for patients 6 months or older with perennial allergic rhinitis. This class of drugs inhibits mucosal edema and mucus production and decreases bronchoconstriction. The Food and Drug Administration issued a warning regarding cases of neuropsychiatric side effects in children taking the leukotriene modifier montelukast. Adverse effects include agitation, aggression, anxiety, hallucinations, depression, insomnia, and suicidal thoughts (US Food and Drug Administration, 2013).

Allergen immunotherapy may be necessary if drug therapy and avoidance of allergens are ineffective in controlling symptoms or if drugs evoke undesirable side effects. Before allergen immunotherapy is begun, a positive skin test reaction to the allergen should be confirmed. Allergen immunotherapy is used to desensitize the child to the allergen over time and can be accomplished by sublingual administration or by subcutaneous injection of the allergen. With the sublingual form, a portion of the allergen is placed under the tongue, and symptom relief is achieved in 2 years (Lin, Erekosima, Kim, et al., 2013). In 2016 three products for sublingual therapy were approved to treat allergic rhinitis due to short ragweed pollen and some grass pollens (Food and Drug Administration, 2016). In 2017 Odactra was approved to treat house-mite allergies, with or without conjunctivitis in patients ages 18 through 65 years old (Food and Drug Administration, 2017). Allergen immunotherapy is also performed using increasing doses of allergen extracts given subcutaneously. This process takes about 4 to 8 months to complete, and then maintenance treatment is continued every 3 to 4 weeks for 3 to 5 years. Infants under 1 year rarely mount an appropriate response to allergens. Allergen immunotherapy is most effective in reducing symptoms caused by seasonal pollen-related allergy (see also Food Sensitivity, Chapter 11).

Nursing Care Management

An important aspect in nursing care of the child with allergic rhinitis is to counsel the parents and patient about the causes of the condition, or triggers, and assist in the implementation of steps to avoid the triggers. Environmental modification in the home is important (see Allergen Control, later in this chapter). Nurses can also help by recognizing rhinitis and referring children for diagnosis and therapy.

Another important aspect of caring for the child with allergic rhinitis is preparation for skin tests and allergen immunotherapy injections. These procedures are a source of stress and discomfort for many children. Young children, in particular, cannot understand how uncomfortable injections that must be given regularly over a long period will make them feel better. The use of a vapocoolant spray and distraction can be considered in with these procedures. All children who receive skin tests need an explanation of the procedure.

Children with allergic rhinitis and their family members need specific and detailed information relating to their medications. Having poorly controlled allergies can result in poor sleep, fatigue, decreased cognitive functioning, and a decreased quality of life. In the case of seasonal rhinitis, antihistamines or topical antiinflammatory medications are often started approximately 2 weeks before the allergy season begins. Phone or mailed reminders to families to start their medications are helpful in preventing lower respiratory tract complications of allergic rhinitis. In addition, some nasal sprays may not reach their maximum effect or improve symptoms until a week after they are started. First-generation antihistamines that have sedation as a side effect should not be given to teenagers who are driving, and children should be cautioned to avoid hazardous activities such as bicycling or skating if drowsiness occurs; these are often best taken at night to minimize daytime drowsiness. School nurses, teachers, and parents should monitor children receiving sedating antihistamines for any changes in learning or cognitive functioning in school. Follow-up monitoring is essential to be sure children do not exceed the correct dosage and that correct administration procedures are followed, especially with inhaled medications.

NURSING TIP

To distinguish allergies from colds, be aware that

- Allergies occur repeatedly and are often seasonal.
- Allergies are seldom accompanied by fever.
- Allergies often involve itching in the eyes and nose.
- Allergies usually trigger constant and consistent bouts of sneezing.
- Allergies are often accompanied by ear and eye problems.

ASTHMA

Asthma is a chronic inflammatory disorder of the airways characterized by recurring symptoms, airway obstruction, and bronchial hyperresponsiveness (Pinfield, Gaskin, Bentley, et al., 2015). In susceptible children, inflammation causes recurrent episodes of wheezing, breathlessness, chest tightness, and cough, especially at night or in the early morning. These asthma episodes are associated with airflow limitation or obstruction that is reversible either spontaneously or with treatment. The inflammation also causes an increase in bronchial hyperresponsiveness to a variety of stimuli. Asthma is the most common chronic disease of childhood, the primary cause of school absences, and the third leading cause of hospitalizations in children under the age of 15 years. More than 25 million people are known to have asthma, and about 7 million of them are children (National Heart, Lung, and Blood Institute, 2014). Although the onset of asthma may occur at any age, 80% to 90% of children have their first symptoms before 4 or 5 years of age.

Based on the symptom indicators of disease severity, asthma is classified into four categories: intermittent, mild persistent, moderate persistent, and severe persistent. Symptoms increase in frequency or intensity until the last category of severe persistent asthma (Box 26.15). These categories provide a stepwise approach to the pharmacologic management, environmental control, and educational interventions needed for each category. For example, if control of asthma is not maintained at one level or step, pharmacologic therapy for the next step up should be considered. If control is adequate at one step, a gradual stepwise reduction in therapy may be possible. The stepwise approach is a guide to assist clinical decision making, but it is not a specific prescription. Therapy and management should be reviewed every 1 to 6 months and should be individualized to the patient. In addition to pharmacologic management, environmental control and educational interventions are essential at each step (Pinfield, Gaskin, Bentley, et al., 2015).

Etiology

Studies of children with asthma indicate that allergy influences both the persistence and the severity of the disease. In fact, **atopy**, or the genetic predisposition for the development of an IgE-mediated response

BOX 26.15 Asthma Severity Classification in Children: Ages 0 to 11*

Step 5 or 6: Severe Persistent Asthma

Continual symptoms throughout the day
Frequent nighttime symptoms
Peak expiratory flow (PEF): <60%
Forced expiratory volume in 1 second (FEV_1): <75% of predicted value
Interference with normal activity: Extremely limited
Use of short-acting β-agonist for symptom control: Several times a day

Step 3 or 4: Moderate Persistent Asthma

Daily symptoms
Nighttime symptoms three or four times a month (ages 0 to 4); more than once per week but not nightly (ages 5 to 11)
PEF: 60% to 80% of predicted value
FEV_1: 75% to 80%
PEF variability: >30%
Interference with normal activity: Some limitation
Use of short-acting β-agonist for symptom control: Daily

Step 2: Mild Persistent Asthma

Symptoms more than two times a week, but less than one time a day
Nighttime symptoms: One or two times a month (ages 0 to 4); three or four times a month (ages 5 to 11)
PEF or FEV_1: ≥ 80% of predicted value
PEF variability: 20% to 30%
Interference with normal activity: Minor limitation
Use of short-acting β-agonist for symptom control: More than 2 days a week but not daily

Step 1: Intermittent Asthma

Symptoms less than 2 days a week
Nighttime symptoms (awakenings): None (ages 0 to 4); less than two times a month (ages 5 to 11)
PEF or FEV_1: ≥ 80% of predicted value
PEF variability: <20%
Interference with normal activity: None
Use of short-acting β-agonist for symptom control: Less than 2 days a week

*The presence of one clinical feature of severity is sufficient to place a patient in that category. An individual should be assigned to the most severe grade in which any feature occurs. The characteristics in this table are general and may overlap because asthma is highly variable. An individual's classification may change over time. Risk factors for each category are not presented in this table. See the original table referenced above for additional classification data. Asthma treatment should not be based on this table.

From National Asthma Education and Prevention Program. Guidelines for the diagnosis and management of asthma: Summary report 2007. Retrieved from https://www.nhlbi.nih.gov/guidelines/asthma/index.htm.

to common aeroallergens, is the strongest identifiable predisposing factor for developing asthma (Pinfield, Gaskin, Bentley, et al., 2015). Although allergens play an important role in asthma, 20% to 40% of children with asthma have no evidence of allergic disease. The allergic reaction in the airways is significant because it can cause an immediate reaction, with obstruction, and it can precipitate a late bronchial obstructive reaction several hours after the initial exposure. This delayed bronchial response is associated with an increase in the airway hyperresponsiveness to nonimmunologic stimuli and can persist for several weeks or more after a single allergen exposure.

BOX 26.16 Triggers Tending to Precipitate or Aggravate Asthmatic Exacerbations

Allergens:
- Outdoor—Trees, shrubs, weeds, grasses, molds, pollens, air pollution, spores
- Indoor—Dust or dust mites, mold, cockroach antigen
- Irritants—Tobacco smoke, wood smoke, odors, sprays

Exposure to occupational chemicals
Exercise
Cold air
Changes in weather or temperature
Environmental change—Moving to new home, starting new school
Colds and infections
Animals—Cats, dogs, rodents, horses
Medications—Aspirin, nonsteroidal antiinflammatory drugs, antibiotics, beta blockers
Strong emotions—Fear, anger, laughing, crying
Conditions—Gastroesophageal reflux, tracheoesophageal fistula
Food additives—Sulfite preservatives
Foods—Nuts, milk and dairy products
Endocrine factors—Menses, pregnancy, thyroid disease

In addition to allergens, other substances and conditions can serve as triggers that may exacerbate asthma (Box 26.16). Asthma is a complex disorder involving biochemical, genetic, immunologic, environmental, infectious, endocrine, and psychologic factors. Evidence shows that viral respiratory tract infections may have a significant role in the development and expression of asthma (National Heart, Lung, and Blood Institute, 2014).

Risk factors for asthma include the following:

- Atopy (includes a history of allergies or atopic dermatitis)
- Heredity (e.g., parent/sibling with asthma)
- Gender (boys are affected more frequently than girls until adolescence, when the trend reverses)
- Smoking or exposure to secondhand smoke
- Maternal smoking during pregnancy
- Ethnicity (African Americans at greatest risk)
- Low birth weight
- Being overweight

Pathophysiology

There is general agreement that inflammation contributes to heightened airway reactivity in asthma. Multiple mechanisms contribute to airway inflammation, involving a number of different pathways. It is unlikely that asthma is caused by either a single cell or a single inflammatory mediator. Rather, it appears that asthma results from complex interactions among inflammatory cells, mediators, and the cells and tissues present in the airways (Fig. 26.10) (Liu, Covar, Spahn, et al., 2016). However, recognition of the importance of inflammation has made the use of antiinflammatory agents, such as steroids, a key component of asthma therapy.

Another important component of asthma is bronchospasm and obstruction. The mechanisms responsible for the obstructive symptoms in asthma (Fig. 26.11) include inflammatory response to stimuli; airway edema and accumulation and secretion of mucus; spasm of the smooth muscle of the bronchi and bronchioles, which decreases the caliber of the bronchioles; and airway remodeling, which causes cellular changes (Pinfield, Gaskin, Bentley, et al., 2015).

Airflow is determined by the size of the airway lumen, degree of bronchial wall edema, mucus production, smooth muscle contraction,

PATHOPHYSIOLOGY REVIEW

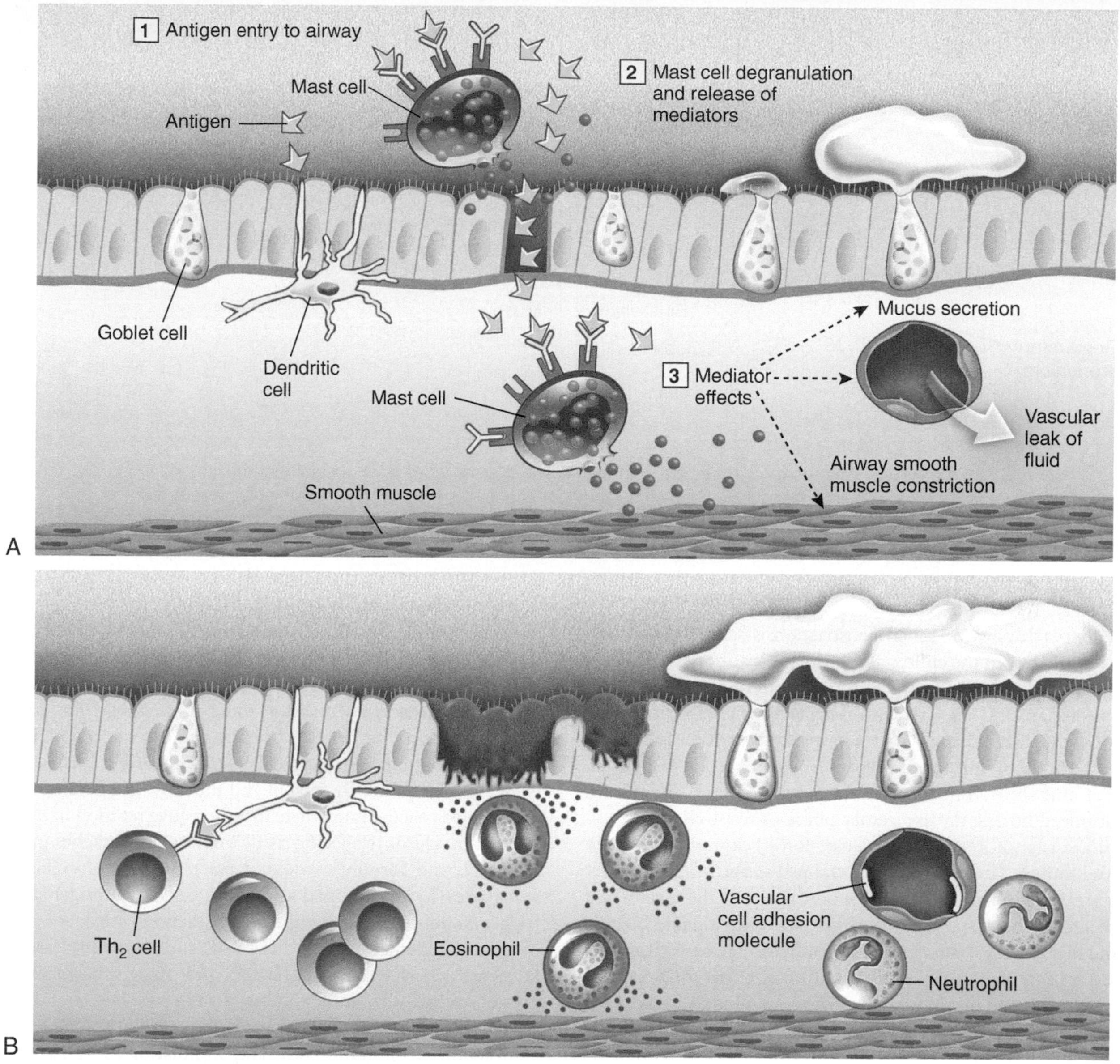

FIG. 26.10 Asthmatic responses. **A,** In the early asthmatic response, inhaled antigen (1) binds to preformed immunoglobulin E (IgE) on mast cells. Mast cells degranulate (2) and release mediators such as histamine, leukotrienes, prostaglandin D_2, platelet-activating factor, and others. Acute inflammation opens intercellular tight junctions, allowing antigen to penetrate and activate submucosal mast cells. Secreted mediators (3) induce active bronchospasm, edema, and mucus secretion. Inflammatory responses are set in motion by chemotactic factors and upregulation of adhesion molecules (not shown). At the same time, as shown on the left, antigen may be received by dendritic cells that process and later present it, either in regional lymph nodes to naive (Tho) T lymphocytes or locally to memory Th_2 cells in the airway mucosa (see **B**). **B,** In the late asthmatic response, areas of epithelial damage are caused at least in part by toxicity of eosinophil products (major basic protein, eosinophilic cationic protein, eosinophil-derived neurotoxin, and eosinophil peroxidase). Many inflammatory cells have been recruited by chemokines and upregulation of vascular cell adhesion molecules. Local T lymphocytes display a predominant Th_2 cytokine profile. They produce interleukin-4 (IL-4) and IL-13, which promote switching of B cells to favor IgE production, and IL-3, IL-5, and granulocyte-macrophage colony–stimulating factor, which encourage eosinophil differentiation and survival. (From McCance, K. L., & Huether, S. E. [2010]. *Pathophysiology: The biological basis for disease in adults and children* [6th ed.]. St. Louis, MO: Mosby.)

PATHOPHYSIOLOGY REVIEW

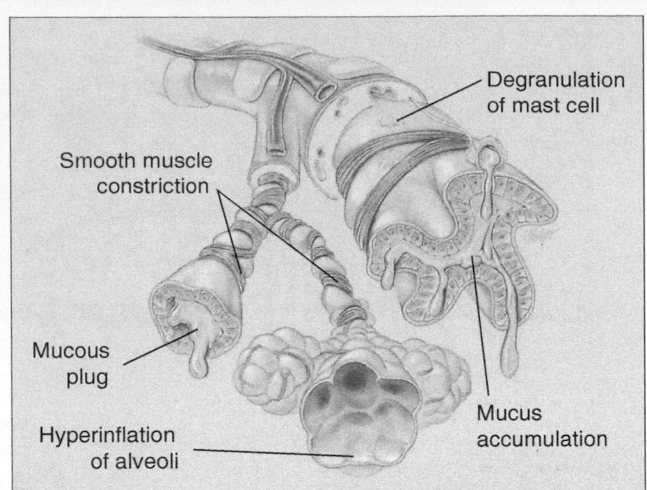

FIG. 26.11 Airway obstruction caused by asthma. **A,** The normal lung. **B,** Bronchial asthma: thick mucus, mucosal edema, and smooth muscle spasm causing obstruction of small airways; breathing becomes labored and expiration is difficult. (Modified from Des Jardins, T., & Burton, G. G. [1995]. *Clinical manifestations and assessment of respiratory disease* [3rd ed.]. St. Louis, MO: Mosby.)

and muscle hypertrophy. Bronchial constriction is a normal reaction to foreign stimuli, but in the child with asthma it is abnormally severe, producing impaired respiratory function. The smooth muscle arranged in spiral bundles around the airway causes narrowing and shortening of the airway, which significantly increases airway resistance to airflow.

Because the bronchi normally dilate and elongate during inspiration and contract and shorten on expiration, the respiratory difficulty is more pronounced during the expiratory phase of respiration.

Increased resistance in the airway causes forced expiration through the narrowed lumen. The volume of air trapped in the lungs increases as airways are functionally closed at a point between the alveoli and the lobar bronchi. This trapping of gas forces the individual to breathe at higher and higher lung volumes. Consequently, the person with asthma fights to inspire sufficient air. This expenditure of effort for breathing causes fatigue, decreased respiratory effectiveness, and increased oxygen consumption. The inspiration occurring at higher lung volumes hyperinflates the alveoli and reduces the effectiveness of the cough. As the severity of obstruction increases, there is reduced alveolar ventilation with carbon dioxide retention, hypoxemia, respiratory acidosis, and eventually respiratory failure. Chronic inflammation may also cause permanent damage (airway remodeling) to airway structures and is difficult to successfully treat with current therapies.

Exacerbations are episodes of progressively worsening shortness of breath, cough, wheezing, or chest tightness, or some combination of these changes. A decrease in expiratory airflow is also characteristic. Airways narrow because of bronchospasm, mucosal edema, and mucus plugging, with air being trapped behind occluded or narrowed airways. Functional residual capacity rises because the child is breathing close to total lung capacity; hyperinflation enables the child to keep the airways open and permits gas exchange to occur. Hypoxemia can occur during such episodes because of the mismatching of ventilation and perfusion. This is seen with increasing carbon dioxide tension and decreasing oxygen tension levels.

Allergies and Asthma

Having an allergy is the strongest epidemiologic risk factor for chronic asthma morbidity and mortality. Many substances in the environment can induce an asthmatic response, but the most significant are those that are antigenic (i.e., that evoke the immune response). The antigen (or foreign substance) is deposited on the respiratory mucosa, where lysozymes immediately digest its outer coating, releasing fragments of foreign protein that initiate the immune sequence. The antibody (immunoglobulin) most active in allergic disorders, including asthma, is IgE, located primarily in skin and mucous membranes.

IgE mediates the immediate hypersensitive reaction in the bronchial mucosa that leads to specific tissue binding. IgE attaches to surfaces of mast cells and basophils, where it reacts with the specific antigen to which they have developed a bonding capacity. Antigenic substances trigger an immediate hypersensitivity reaction with subsequent release of chemical mediators from mast cells and basophils: histamine; leukotrienes; platelet-activating factor; and other substances, including prostaglandins, serotonin, and various kinins. The major effects of the mediators in the airways are increased permeability of the blood vessels, contraction of smooth muscle, and stimulation of mucus secretion.

Clinical Manifestations

The classic manifestations of asthma are dyspnea, wheezing, and coughing. However, children may experience symptoms that range from acute episodes of shortness of breath, wheezing, and cough followed by a quiet period to a relatively continuous pattern of chronic symptoms that fluctuate in severity. Older children may complain of chest tightness and an intermittent generalized chest pain. An attack may develop gradually or appear abruptly and may be preceded by a URI. Symptoms are often worse at night or during exercise. The child's age is often a significant factor because the first attack frequently occurs between ages 3 and 8 years. In infancy, an attack usually follows a respiratory tract infection. Bronchoconstriction in response to an allergen can have an immediate, histamine type of pattern or a late response with airway hypersensitivity lasting for days, weeks, or months. A second wave of symptoms can occur 6 to 8 hours after the initial antigen exposure.

Children may experience a prodromal itching localized at the front of the neck or over the upper part of the back. An asthmatic episode usually begins with children feeling uncomfortable or irritable and increasingly restless. They may also complain of having a headache, feeling tired, or feeling tightness in the chest. Respiratory symptoms include a hacking, paroxysmal, irritative, and nonproductive cough caused by bronchial edema. Accumulated secretions, acting as a foreign body, stimulate the cough. As the secretions become more profuse, the cough becomes rattling and productive of frothy, clear, gelatinous sputum. Bronchial spasm and mucosal edema reduce the size of the bronchial lumen, and the bronchi may be occluded by mucous plugs.

A common symptom of asthma is coughing in the absence of respiratory tract infection, especially at night. This may disrupt sleep, leading to excessive fatigue during the day and poor school performance. Wheezing may be mild or discernible only on auscultation at the end of expiration, or severe enough to be audible.

Younger children have a tendency to assume the tripod sitting position, whereas older children have a tendency to sit upright with shoulders hunched over, hands on the bed or chair, and arms braced to facilitate the use of accessory muscles of respiration. The child may speak with short, panting, broken phrases. Infants and small children are restless, irritable, and unable to be comforted. If hypoxemia develops, the child may become agitated, confused, and more irritable.

Infants may display supraclavicular, intercostal, suprasternal, subcostal, and sternal retractions. However, clinical symptoms of asthma may be less obvious in infancy. Because infants have a more pliant (flexible) chest, a prolonged expiratory phase may not be easy to observe. Wheezing, a characteristic symptom often associated with asthma, may occur in infants with respiratory tract infections, cardiac defects, and aspiration pneumonia.

Examination of the chest reveals hyperresonance on percussion. Breath sounds are coarse and loud, with sonorous crackles throughout the lung fields. Expiration is prolonged. Coarse rhonchi can be heard, as well as generalized inspiratory and expiratory wheezing that becomes more high pitched as obstruction progresses. With minimum obstruction, wheezing may be mild (discernible only on auscultation at the end of expiration) or even absent.

With severe spasm or obstruction, breath sounds and crackles may be inaudible. Cough is ineffective despite repeated hacking maneuvers. This represents a lack of air movement and may be misinterpreted as improvement by unknowing examiners.

> **! NURSING ALERT**
>
> Shortness of breath with air movement in the chest restricted to the point of absent breath sounds accompanied by a sudden rise in respiratory rate is an ominous sign indicating respiratory failure and imminent asphyxia.

Children with chronic asthma develop generalized vascularization, mucosal thickening, and hypertrophy of the mucous glands and fibers of the bronchial musculature. With repeated episodes the thoracic cavity becomes fixed in a hyperaerated state (barrel chest), with a depressed diaphragm, elevated shoulders, and increased use of accessory muscles of respiration.

Diagnostic Evaluation

The diagnosis is determined primarily on the basis of clinical manifestations, history, physical examination, and to a lesser extent laboratory tests. Generally, chronic cough in the absence of infection or diffuse wheezing during the expiratory phase of respiration is sufficient to establish a diagnosis.

Pulmonary function tests (PFTs) provide an objective method of evaluating the presence and degree of lung disease and the response to therapy. Spirometry can generally be performed reliably on children by the age of 5 or 6 years and includes either the traditional and simple mechanical spirometer often used in clinics, offices, and the home or new computerized versions. The National Asthma Education and Prevention Program (2007) recommends that spirometry testing be done at the time of initial assessment of asthma, after treatment is initiated and symptoms have stabilized, and at least every 1 to 2 years to assess the maintenance of airway function.

Bronchoprovocation testing (i.e., direct exposure of the mucous membranes to a suspected antigen in increasing concentrations) helps identify inhaled allergens. Exposure to methacholine (methacholine challenge), histamine, or cold or dry air may be performed to assess airway responsiveness or reactivity. Exercise challenges may be used to identify children with exercise-induced bronchospasm (EIB) (Liu, Covar, Spahn, et al., 2016). Although these tests are highly specific and sensitive, they place the child at risk for an asthmatic episode and should be done under close observation in a qualified laboratory or clinic.

The **peak expiratory flow rate** (PEFR) can be measured using a peak expiratory flow meter (PEFM). The PEFR is the maximum flow of air that can be forcefully exhaled in 1 second and is measured in liters per minute. Three zones of measurement, patterned after a traffic light, are typically used to interpret the PEFR (see Applying Evidence to Practice box). Each child needs to establish his or her own personal best value during a 2- to 3-week period when the child's asthma is stable. During this time, the PEFR is recorded at least twice a day. The personal best value can be used to determine the severity of asthma symptoms present. PEFR monitoring can be used for short-term monitoring, managing exacerbations, and daily long-term monitoring. However, PEFM should not be used to diagnose asthma severity. The Expert Panel (National Asthma Education and Prevention Program, 2007) recommends either PEFM or symptom monitoring or a combination of both.

> **APPLYING EVIDENCE TO PRACTICE**
>
> ***Interpreting Peak Expiratory Flow Rates****
>
> - Green (80% to 100% of personal best) signals all clear. Asthma is under reasonably good control. No symptoms are present, and the routine treatment plan for maintaining control can be followed.
> - Yellow (50% to 79% of personal best) signals caution. Asthma is not well controlled. An acute exacerbation may be present. Maintenance therapy may need to be increased. Call the practitioner if the child stays in this zone.
> - Red (below 50% of personal best) signals a medical alert. Severe airway narrowing may be occurring. A short-acting bronchodilator should be administered. Notify the practitioner if the peak expiratory flow rate does not return immediately and stay in yellow or green zone.
>
> *These zones are guidelines only. Specific zones and management should be individualized for each child.
>
> Modified from American Lung Association. (2017). Measuring your peak flow rate. Washington, DC: American Lung Association. Retrieved from http://www.lung.org/lung-health-and-diseases/lung-disease-lookup/asthma/living-with-asthma/managing-asthma/measuring-your-peak-flow-rate.html.

Because measurement of PEFR depends on effort and technique, children need instructions, demonstrations, and frequent reviews of technique (see Family-Centered Care box). In some cases, a low PEFR may not truly mean that the child's asthma is poorly controlled. Each individual child's PEFR varies according to age, height, sex, and race.

A variety of easy-to-use, inexpensive PEFMs are available for use in the home and at school to assess changes in pulmonary function. In general, children 5 years of age and older are able to use a PEFM successfully. However, young children need to be supervised while they

FAMILY-CENTERED CARE

Use of a Peak Expiratory Flow Meter

1. Before each use, make certain the sliding marker or arrow on the peak expiratory flow meter is at the bottom of the numbered scale.
2. Stand up straight.
3. Remove gum or food from your mouth.
4. Close your lips tightly around the mouthpiece. Be certain to keep your tongue away from the mouthpiece.
5. Blow out as hard and as quickly as you can, a "fast, hard puff."
6. Note the number by the marker on the numbered scale.
7. Repeat entire routine three times, but wait at least 30 seconds between each routine.
8. Record the highest of the three readings, not the average.
9. Measure your peak expiratory flow rate (PEFR) close to the same time and same way each day (e.g., morning and evening; before and 15 minutes after taking medication).
10. Keep a record of your PEFRs.

are learning to use their PEFM. Children should use the same PEFM over time, and they should bring it for use at every follow-up visit. Using the same brand of meter is recommended because different brands can give significantly different values. The use of a PEFM provides objective monitoring regarding the severity of asthma and can decrease asthma episodes, health care visits, and missed school days. Similarly, studies show that PEFM use can improve quality of life and asthma health outcomes in children with asthma (Walter, Sadeque-Igbal, Ulysse, et al., 2015).

Skin testing is useful in identifying specific allergens, and those obtained by the puncture technique correlate better than intracutaneous tests with symptoms and measurements of specific IgE antibody. It is recommended that all patients with year-round asthma symptoms be tested with skin tests or laboratory blood analysis to determine sensitization to perennial allergens (e.g., house dust mites, cats, dogs, cockroaches, molds, and fungus) (National Heart, Lung, and Blood Institute, 2014).

In addition to these tests, other important tests include laboratory tests (complete blood count with differential) and chest radiographs. The complete blood count may show a slight elevation in the white blood cell count during acute asthma, but elevations to more than 12,000/mm^3 or an increased percentage of band cells (immature neutrophils) may indicate respiratory tract infection. Eosinophilia results greater than 500/mm^3 tend to suggest an allergic or inflammatory disorder.

Frontal and lateral radiographs show infiltrates and hyperexpansion of the airways, with the anteroposterior diameter on physical examination indicating an increased diameter (suggestive of barrel chest). Additional diagnostic tests for conditions such as gastroesophageal reflux may be carried out to determine whether they may contribute to asthma symptoms. Radiography may assist in ruling out a respiratory tract infection.

Therapeutic Management: General

The overall goals of asthma management are to maintain normal activity levels, maintain normal pulmonary function, prevent chronic symptoms and recurrent exacerbations, provide optimal drug therapy with minimal or no adverse effects, and assist the child in living as normal and happy a life as possible. This includes facilitating the child's social adjustments in the family, school, and community and normal participation in recreational activities and sports. To accomplish these goals, several treatment principles need to be followed (Pinfield, Gaskin, Bentley, et al., 2015):

- Regular contact with the health care provider is necessary to control symptoms and prevent exacerbations. Registered nurse (RN) care coordinators or case managers can often assist with this and troubleshoot symptoms via phone.
- Prevention of exacerbations includes avoiding triggers, avoiding allergens, and using medications as needed.
- Therapy includes efforts to reduce underlying inflammation and relieve or prevent symptomatic airway narrowing.
- Therapy includes patient education, environmental control, pharmacologic management, and the use of objective measures to monitor the severity of disease and guide the course of therapy.

Allergen Control

Nonpharmacologic therapy is aimed at the prevention and reduction of exposure to airborne allergens and irritants. House dust mites and other components of house dust are frequent agents identified in children who are allergic to inhalants. The cockroach, another common household inhabitant, is an important allergen in many locations. Exterminating live cockroaches, carefully cleaning kitchen floors and cabinets, putting food away after eating, and taking trash out in the evening are essential measures to control cockroaches. Other animal-related allergens include mice (especially in the homes of inner-city children), cat dander, and dog dander. Sensitized persons should carefully evaluate having such pets in the household, but there are inconclusive data on the effects of cat or dog dander on asthma development (Kanchongkittiphon, Mendell, Gaffin, et al., 2015). Additional sources of pollutants include particulate matter produced by tobacco smoke, wood-burning stoves, pesticides, lead, mold spores, and nitrogen dioxide (from burning fuels or vehicle emissions); these are believed to contribute to asthma morbidity in children and should be avoided or minimized (Kanchongkittiphon, Mendell, Gaffin, et al., 2015). Exposure to tobacco smoke is a significant contributing factor in the development and triggering of asthma in infants and children (Makadia, Roper, Andrews, et al., 2017). Living in damp homes also can be factors in the development of asthma in infants and small children (Kanchongkittiphon, Mendell, Gaffin, et al., 2015).

Skin testing can identify specific allergens. Steps are then taken to eliminate or avoid them. Often, simply removing the offending environmental allergens or irritants (e.g., removing carpeting from the home of a child who is sensitive to mold and dust mites) decreases the frequency of asthma episodes. Dehumidifiers or air conditioners control nonspecific factors, such as extremes of temperature, that trigger an episode. Avoiding known outdoor allergens such as tree, grass, and weed pollen when these are high may reduce asthma exacerbations as well. Additional suggestions include the following:

- Cover pillows and mattresses with dustproof covers.
- Wash bedding in hot water once a week. Dry completely.
- Avoid using feather- or down-filled pillows and mattresses.
- Keep child indoors while lawn is being mowed, bushes and trees are being trimmed, or pollen count is high.
- Keep windows and doors closed during pollen season; use air conditioner if possible, or go to places that are air conditioned, such as libraries and shopping malls, when the weather is hot.
- The child should not be present during cleaning activities.
- Wet-mop bare floors weekly; wet-dust and clean child's room weekly.
- Vacuum carpet and fabric-covered furniture every week to reduce dust buildup, using a high-efficiency particulate air filter.
- Limit or prevent child's exposure to tobacco and wood smoke; do not allow cigarette smoking in the house or car; select day care centers, play areas, and shopping malls that are smoke free.
- Use air conditioners with high-efficiency particulate air filters.

- Use indoor air purifiers with high-efficiency particulate air filters.
- Choose stuffed toys that can be washed in hot water. Dry completely before the child plays with the toy.

Despite the proven association between the incidence of asthma and exposure to these residential hazards, little evidence-based research exists that demonstrates an overall reduction in symptoms, even with significant interventions aimed at environmental (housing) modifications such as removal of carpeting, cleaning, and extermination (Kanchongkittiphon, Mendell, Gaffin, et al., 2015) (see Community and Home Health Considerations box).

COMMUNITY AND HOME HEALTH CONSIDERATIONS

Herbal Treatment of Asthma

Herbs and plants are often used by adults and children to treat asthma; however, the safety and effectiveness of such therapies have been controversial. The US Food and Drug Administration has cautioned against relying on the use of homeopathic remedies to treat asthma because they have not been assessed by the Food and Drug Administration.

Drug Therapy

Pharmacologic therapy is used to prevent and control asthma symptoms, reduce the frequency and severity of asthma exacerbations, and reverse airflow obstruction. A stepwise approach is recommended based on the severity of the child's asthma. Appropriate medications for asthma is a pediatric quality indicator listed in Table 26.7. Because inflammation is considered an early and persistent feature of asthma, therapy is directed toward long-term suppression of inflammation.

Asthma medications are categorized into two general classes: long-term control medications (preventive medications) to achieve and maintain control of inflammation, and quick-relief medications (rescue medications) to treat symptoms and exacerbations.

Quick-relief and long-term medications are often used in combination. Inhaled corticosteroids, cromolyn sodium and nedocromil, long-acting β_2-agonists, methylxanthines, and leukotriene modifiers are used as long-term control medications. Short-acting β_2-agonists, anticholinergics, and systemic corticosteroids are used as quick-relief (or rescue) medications. Bronchodilators that relax bronchial smooth muscle and dilate the airways include β_2-agonists, methylxanthines, and anticholinergics that can be used as both quick-relief and long-term medications.

Many asthma medications are given by inhalation with a nebulizer or a **metered-dose inhaler (MDI)**. The MDI should always be attached to a spacer when an inhaled corticosteroid is administered to prevent yeast infections in the mouth. Spacers are also important for children who have difficulty coordinating or learning proper inhalation technique. The spacer and holder can be equipped with a mask or a mouthpiece (Fig. 26.12) (see Family-Centered Care box later in this chapter). Metered-dose inhalers that contain propellant chlorofluorocarbons (CFCs) have been banned in the United States due to their linkage with depletion of the earth's ozone level. An alternative propellant, hydrofluoroalkane, does not cause ozone depletion, delivers more fine particles of the medication, and has less oral deposition. The Diskus inhaler and the Turbuhaler are a dry powder inhaler. These devices are breath activated, and the child needs to inhale as quickly and as deeply as possible to use them effectively. The Diskhaler and Aerosolizer are similar, but with the Aerosolizer the medication must be loaded into the inhaler before use. Infants and young children who have difficulty using MDIs or other inhalers can receive their asthma medications via a **handheld nebulizer** (Fig. 26.13). When this device is used, the medication is mixed with saline (also available in premixed form) and nebulized with compressed air. Children should breathe normally with the mouth open to provide a direct route to the trachea.

Corticosteroids are antiinflammatory drugs used to treat reversible airflow obstruction and control symptoms and reduce bronchial hyperresponsiveness in chronic asthma. Inhaled corticosteroids should be used as first-line therapy in children over 5 years of age. Clinical studies of corticosteroids have indicated significant improvement of all asthma parameters, including decreases in symptoms, emergency visits, hospitalizations, and medication requirements (Falk, Hughes, & Rodgers, 2016).

Corticosteroids may be administered parenterally, orally, or by inhalation. Oral medications are metabolized slowly, with an onset of action up to 3 hours after administration and peak effectiveness occurring within 6 to 12 hours. Oral systemic steroids may be given for short periods (e.g., 3- or 10-day "bursts") to gain prompt control of inadequately controlled persistent asthma or to manage severe persistent asthma. These drugs should be given in the lowest effective dose. They have few side effects (cough, dysphonia, and oral thrush), and there is evidence that they improve the long-term outcomes for children of all ages with mild or moderate persistent asthma. Evidence from clinical trials that monitored children for 6 years indicates that the use of inhaled

TABLE 26.7 Pediatric Quality Indicator: Appropriate Medications for Asthma*

Appropriate Medications for Asthma	
Measure	Children who were identified as having moderate to severe persistent asthma and were appropriately prescribed medication during the measurement period.
Numerator	Number of children who were dispensed at least one prescription for a preferred asthma therapy during the measurement time.
Denominator	Number of children who were identified as having asthma.

*Endorsed by the National Quality Forum-0036 and Center for Medicare and Medicaid Services-126v1.

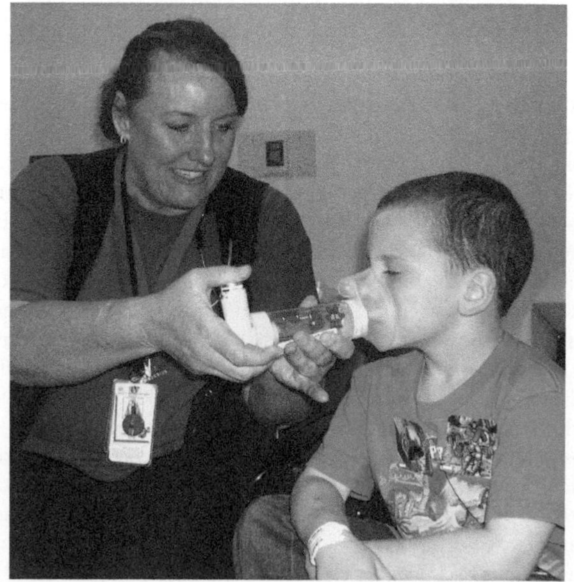

FIG. 26.12 Child using metered-dose inhaler with aerochamber and face mask.

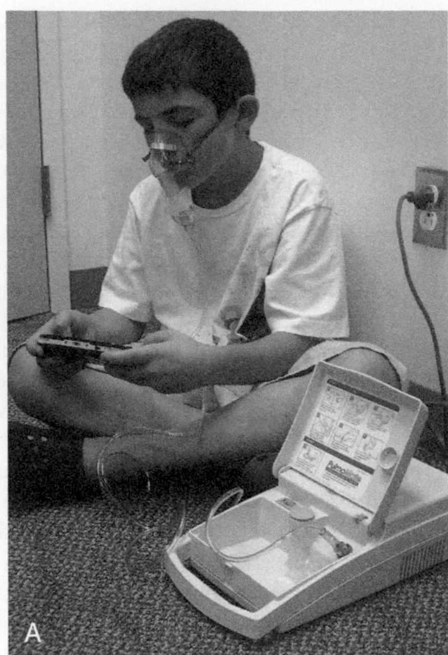
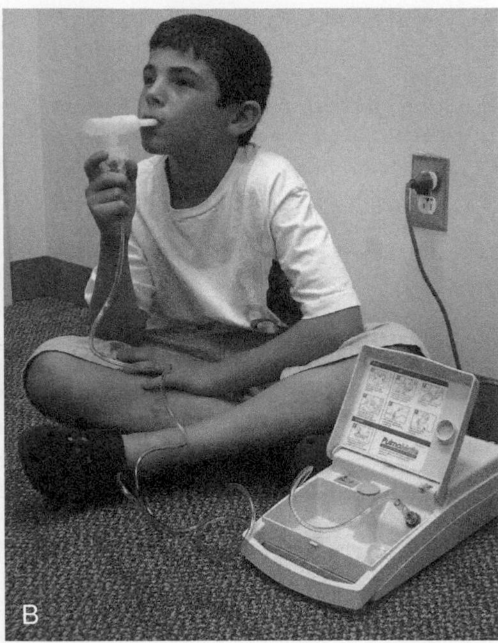

FIG. 26.13 Child with asthma may take a nebulized aerosol treatment with **(A)** a mask or **(B)** a mouthpiece. (Courtesy Texas Children's Hospital, Houston.)

corticosteroids at recommended dosages does not have long-term significant effects on growth, bone mineral density, or suppression of the adrenal-pituitary axis (Falk, Hughes, and Rodgers, 2016). However, primary care providers should frequently monitor (at least every 3 to 6 months) the growth of children and adolescents taking corticosteroids to assess the systemic effects of these drugs and make appropriate reductions in dosages or changes to other types of asthma therapy when necessary. The inhaled corticosteroids include budesonide and fluticasone.

β-Adrenergic agonists (short acting) (primarily albuterol, levalbuterol [Xopenex], and terbutaline) are used for treatment of acute exacerbations and for the prevention of EIB. These drugs bind with the β-receptors on the smooth muscle of airways, where they activate adenylate cyclase and convert adenosine monophosphate (AMP) to cyclic AMP (cAMP). The increased cAMP enhances binding of intracellular calcium to the cell membrane, reducing the availability of calcium and thus allowing smooth muscle to relax. Other effects of the drug help stabilize mast cells to prevent release of mediators. Most β-adrenergics used in asthma therapy affect predominantly the β_2-receptors, which help eliminate bronchospasm. β_1-adrenergic effects such as increased heart rate and GI disturbances have been minimized. Albuterol is given orally, via inhaler or via nebulizer, whereas levalbuterol is given via inhaler or nebulizer only. Levalbuterol is more expensive than albuterol but reportedly causes fewer side effects than albuterol. There continues to be some discussion about the administration of β_2-agonists via an MDI versus a nebulizer. However, administration via an MDI is as effective to delivery of medication by a small-volume nebulizer in reversing bronchospasm (Mitselou, Hedlin, & Hederos, 2016).

Long-acting β_2-agonists (LABAs) are approved as single-ingredient products (Serevent and Foradil) and in combination products containing inhaled corticosteroids (Advair and Symbicort). The National Asthma Education and Prevention Program (2007) recommends use of a long-acting β_2-agonist (LABA) with low- or medium-dosage inhaled corticosteroid to improve lung function and asthma symptoms, as well as reduce use of short-acting β_2-agonists. They are used for patients whose symptoms cannot be adequately controlled on asthma controller medications.

LABAs must be added to antiinflammatory therapy and never as monotherapy (Liu, Covar, Spahn, et al., 2016). Inhaled β-adrenergic agents should not be taken more than three or four times daily for acute symptoms without medical supervision. LABAs can increase the risk of severely worsening asthma symptoms, potentially leading to hospitalizations and death. The Food and Drug Administration has required LABA manufacturers to conduct studies to evaluate the safety of using them with inhaled corticosteroids versus inhaled corticosteroids alone. Salmeterol and Foradil are not used for patients younger than 4 years of age.

DRUG ALERT

Salmeterol and Foradil Precautions

Salmeterol and Foradil are *never* used to treat acute symptoms or exacerbations.

Theophylline was used for decades to relieve symptoms and prevent asthma attacks; however, it is now used primarily when the child is not responding to maximal therapy (Liu, Covar, Spahn, et al., 2016). Therapeutic levels should be monitored closely with this drug because it has a narrow therapeutic window. Theophylline is not recommended for acute asthma exacerbations.

Cromolyn sodium is medication used as maintenance therapy for asthma in children over 2 years of age. It stabilizes mast cell membranes; inhibits activation and release of mediators from eosinophil and epithelial cells; and inhibits the acute airway narrowing after exposure to exercise; cold, dry air; and sulfur dioxide. It does not result in immediate relief of symptoms and has minimal side effects (occasional cough from inhalation of the powder formulation). It is only available as an oral preparation or via nebulizer. Cromolyn sodium and nedocromil sodium inhaler preparations were discontinued in 2010.

Leukotrienes are mediators of inflammation that cause increases in airway hyperresponsiveness. Leukotriene modifiers (such as zafirlukast [Accolate] and montelukast sodium) block inflammatory and bronchospasm effects. These drugs are not used to treat acute episodes but are given orally in combination with β-agonists and steroids to provide long-term control and prevent symptoms in mild persistent asthma. Montelukast is approved to treat asthma in children 12 months old and older, whereas zafirlukast is approved for children 5 years and older.

Anticholinergics (atropine and ipratropium) help relieve acute bronchospasm. However, these drugs have adverse side effects that include drying of respiratory secretions, blurred vision, and cardiac and CNS stimulation. The primary anticholinergic drug used is ipratropium, which does not cross the blood-brain barrier and therefore elicits no CNS effects (as does atropine). Ipratropium, when used in combination with albuterol, has been effective during acute severe asthma in significantly improving lung function and reducing hospitalizations in children coming to the ED (Liu, Covar, Spahn, et al., 2016).

Omalizumab (Xolair) is a monoclonal antibody that is used for patients with moderate to severe persistent allergic asthma whose asthma symptoms are not controlled by inhaled corticosteroids. It blocks the binding of IgE to mast cells to inhibit the inflammation associated with asthma. Many patients with asthma are atopic and possess specific IgE antibodies to allergens responsible for airway inflammation. It has been approved for use in children 12 years and older. IgE levels are measured before beginning treatment. Dosage and frequency of administration of Xolair are dependent on the serum total IgE level and body weight. The drug is administered once or twice a month by subcutaneous injection. Efficacy of omalizumab is not immediate and takes 12 to 16 weeks. It is expensive, and there have been reported cases of severe immediate or delayed anaphylactic reactions. In early 2007 the Food and Drug Administration added a black box warning to the drug that highlights the risk of anaphylaxis. Anaphylaxis was observed in 0.14% of patients receiving omalizumab in clinical trials, and 60% occurred within 2 hours of administration; therefore recommendations include observing the recipient for 2 hours after the first three doses are administered and 30 minutes thereafter for subsequent doses (Thomson & Chaudhuri, 2012).

Some children with severe asthma and a history of severe life-threatening episodes may need a prescription for an EpiPen (subcutaneous injectable epinephrine).

Magnesium sulfate, a potent muscle relaxant that acts to decrease inflammation and improves pulmonary function and peak flow rate, may be used in pediatric patients treated in the ED or ICU with moderate to severe asthma. Studies on the use of intravenous and inhaled magnesium sulfate offer significant benefits for children with acute asthma exacerbations (Griffiths, Kew, & Normansell, 2016; Schuh, Sweeney, Freedman, et al., 2016).

Antibiotics should not be used to treat acute asthma attacks except when a bacterial infection resulting from another condition such as pneumonia or sinusitis is present.

Breathing Exercises and Physical Training

These therapies help produce physical and mental relaxation, improve posture, strengthen respiratory musculature, and develop more efficient patterns of breathing. For the motivated child, breathing exercises and controlled breathing help prevent overinflation and improve efficiency of the cough. However, these exercises are not recommended during acute exacerbations of asthma.

Hyposensitization

The role of hyposensitization in childhood asthma is somewhat controversial. In the past, *allergen immunotherapy* was used for seasonal allergies and when single substances were identified as the offending allergen. It is not recommended for allergens that can be eliminated, such as foods, drugs, and animal dander.

The National Asthma Education and Prevention Program guidelines (2007) recommend allergen immunotherapy for asthma patients in the following situations:

- When there is evidence of a relationship between asthma symptoms and unavoidable exposure to an allergen to which the patient is sensitive
- When symptoms occur all year or at least during a major portion of the year
- When symptom control is difficult with drug therapy because multiple medications are required, the patient is not responsive to available drugs, or the patient refuses to take the medications

Injection therapy is usually limited to clinically significant allergens. The initial dose of the offending allergen(s), based on the size of the skin reaction, is injected subcutaneously. The amount is increased at weekly intervals until a maximum tolerance is reached, after which a maintenance dose is given at 4-week intervals. This may be extended to 5- or 6-week intervals during the off-season for seasonal allergens. Successful treatment is continued for a minimum of 3 years and then stopped. If no symptoms appear, acquired immunity is assumed; if symptoms recur, treatment begins again. Hyposensitization injections should be administered by specifically educated personnel and only with emergency equipment and medications readily available in the event of an anaphylactic reaction.

Exercise and Exercise-Induced Bronchospasm

Exercise and exercise-induced bronchospasm (EIB) is an acute, reversible, usually self-terminating airway obstruction that develops during or after vigorous activity, reaches its peak 5 to 10 minutes after stopping the activity, and usually stops in another 20 to 30 minutes. Patients with EIB have cough, shortness of breath, chest pain or tightness, wheezing, and endurance problems during exercise, but an exercise challenge test in a laboratory is necessary to make the diagnosis.

The problem occurs rarely in activities that require short bursts of energy (e.g., baseball, sprints, gymnastics) and more commonly in those that involve endurance exercise (e.g., soccer, basketball, distance running). Swimming is well tolerated by children with EIB because they are breathing air fully saturated with moisture and because of the type of breathing required in swimming.

Parents, teachers, and practitioners often exclude children with asthma from exercise, and the children themselves are reluctant to participate because it may provoke an attack. However, doing so can seriously hamper peer interaction and physical health. Exercise is advantageous for children with asthma, and most children can participate in activities at school and in sports with minimal difficulty, provided their asthma is under control. Evaluate participation on an individual basis. Appropriate prophylactic treatment with short-acting β-adrenergic agents or cromolyn sodium before exercise usually permits full participation in strenuous exertion.

Therapeutic Management: Specific

Children with asthma have exacerbations at varying intervals, with severity ranging from wheezing to life-threatening status asthmaticus (Table 26.8). Protocols have been developed for treating the child experiencing an asthmatic episode at home or in the ED (National Asthma Education and Prevention Program, 2007).

Successful home management of acute asthma begins before symptoms develop. All patients and family members should learn how to monitor symptoms to recognize early signs of deterioration. Children with moderate to severe persistent asthma and those with a history of

TABLE 26.8 Estimating Severity of Asthma Exacerbations

Sign and Symptom Assessment	Mild	Moderate	Severe	Respiratory Arrest Imminent
Breathless	While walking Can lie down	While at rest (infant: softer, shorter cry; difficulty feeding) Prefers sitting	While at rest (infant: stops feeding) Sits upright	
Talks in:	Sentences	Phrases	Words	Not talking
Alertness	May be agitated	Usually agitated	Usually agitated	Drowsy or confused
Respiratory rate	Increased	Increased	Often >30 breaths/min	
Accessory muscle used; suprasternal retractions	Usually not present	Commonly present	Usually present	Paradoxic thoracoabdominal movement
Wheeze	Moderate, often only end expiratory	Loud, throughout exhalation	Usually loud throughout inhalation and exhalation	Absence of wheeze
Pulse (beats/min)	<100	100-120	>120	Bradycardia
Pulsus paradoxus	Absent or <10 mm Hg	May be present 10-25 mm Hg	Often present 20-40 mm Hg (child)	Absence suggests respiratory muscle fatigue
PEF (percent predicted or percentile personal best)	≥ 70%	About 50%-69% or response lasts <2 hr	About 50%	<25% PEF testing may not be appropriate in severe attacks
Oxygen saturation (Sa_{O_2}), (on room air) at sea level	>95%	90%-95%	<90%	
Pa_{O_2} (on room air)	Normal	≥ 60 mm Hg	<60 mm Hg; possible cyanosis	
Pco_2	<42 mm Hg	<42 mm Hg	≤42 mm Hg; possible respiratory failure	

NOTE: Hypoventilation develops more rapidly in children than adults or adolescents.
PEF, Peak expiratory flow.
From The National Asthma Education and Prevention Program. (2007). *Expert Panel Report 3: Guidelines for diagnosis and management of asthma.* Bethesda, MD: National Heart, Lung, and Blood Institute, National Institutes of Health.

severe exacerbations should learn how to monitor their peak flow rate to assess the severity of the exacerbation and the response to therapy. All children should be given a written action plan to follow in the event of symptoms or an exacerbation. This plan should include information on how to adjust medications in response to signs, symptoms, and peak flow measurements and when to seek medical help. School-age children should have a written action plan that is appropriate for the school setting.

Status Asthmaticus

Status asthmaticus is a medical emergency that can result in respiratory failure and death if unrecognized and untreated. Children who continue to display respiratory distress despite vigorous therapeutic measures, especially the use of sympathomimetics (e.g., albuterol, epinephrine), are in status asthmaticus. The condition may develop gradually or rapidly, often coincident with complicating conditions, such as pneumonia or a respiratory virus, which can influence the duration and treatment of the exacerbation.

! NURSING ALERT

The child with asthma who sweats profusely, remains sitting upright, and refuses to lie down is in severe respiratory distress. Also, the child who suddenly becomes agitated, or the agitated child who suddenly becomes quiet, may be seriously hypoxic and requires immediate intervention.

Therapy for status asthmaticus is aimed at improving ventilation, decreasing airway resistance and relieving bronchospasm, correcting dehydration and acidosis, allaying child and parent anxiety related to the severity of the event, and treating any concurrent infection. Humidified oxygen is recommended and should be given to maintain an oxygen saturation greater than 90%. Inhaled aerosolized short-acting β_2-agonists are recommended for all patients. Three treatments of β_2-agonists spaced 20 to 30 minutes apart are usually given as initial therapy, and continuous administration of β_2-agonists may be initiated. A systemic corticosteroid (oral, IV, or IM) may also be given to decrease the effects of inflammation. An anticholinergic such as ipratropium bromide may be added to the aerosolized solution of the β_2-agonist. Anticholinergics have resulted in additional bronchodilation in patients with severe airflow obstruction. An IV infusion is often initiated to provide a means for hydration and to administer medications. Correction of dehydration, acidosis, hypoxia, and electrolyte disturbance is guided by frequent determination of arterial pH, blood gases, and serum electrolytes.

Additional therapies in acute asthma attacks may include the use of IV magnesium sulfate, a potent muscle relaxant that decreases inflammation and improves pulmonary function and peak flow rate among pediatric patients with moderate to severe asthma when treated in the ED or ICU. Heliox (a mixture of 70% to 80% helium and 20% to 30% oxygen) may be administered to decrease airway resistance and thereby decrease the work of breathing; it can be delivered via a nonrebreathing face mask from premixed tanks, which may be blended in a standalone unit or within a ventilator. It may be used in acute exacerbations as an adjunct to β_2-agonist and IV corticosteroid therapy to improve pulmonary function until the two latter medications have time to take full effect in decreasing bronchospasm; the effects of heliox are usually seen within 20 minutes of administration, whereas other drugs may take longer to exert the desired effect. Ketamine, a dissociative anesthetic, is believed to cause smooth muscle relaxation and decrease airway resistance caused by severe bronchospasm in acute asthma; it may be administered as an adjunct to other therapies mentioned previously.

A child suspected of having status asthmaticus is usually seen in the ED and is often admitted to a pediatric ICU for close observation and continuous cardiorespiratory monitoring. A key component in the prevention of morbidity is helping the child, parents, teachers, coaches, and other adults to recognize features of deteriorating respiratory status, use the correct rescue drugs effectively, and immediately place the child with deteriorating respiratory status into the care of trained health care professionals instead of waiting to see if the asthma gets better on its own. For the child going into early status asthmaticus, immediate medical care is required to prevent irreversible respiratory failure and possible death.

Prognosis

Although deaths from asthma have been relatively uncommon since the 1980s, the rate of death from asthma increased steadily in the United States until it peaked in the mid-1990s and then slowly decreased over the next 10 years. In 2015, 3615 children younger than 18 years old died from asthma (Centers for Disease Control and Prevention, 2017). In 2011, 14% of all children in the United States were diagnosed with asthma and 70% of these children had recurrent asthma (Liu, Covar, Spahn, et al., 2016). There has been a significant increase in asthma-related ED visits and hospitalizations. Mortality and morbidity rates for asthma are especially high among black children, whose hospitalization and death rates are two to seven times higher than nonblack children (Liu, Covar, Spahn, et al., 2016). Most asthma deaths in children occur in the home, school, or community before lifesaving medical care can be administered.

Some children's asthma symptoms may improve at puberty, but up to two-thirds of children with asthma continue to have symptoms through puberty and into adulthood. The prognosis for control or disappearance of symptoms varies in children from those who have rare and infrequent attacks to those who are constantly wheezing or are subject to status asthmaticus. In general, when symptoms are severe and numerous, when symptoms have been present for a long time, and when there is a family history of allergy, there is a greater likelihood of a poor prognosis. Risk factors that may predict persistence of symptoms into childhood (from infancy) include atopy, male gender, exposure to environmental tobacco, and maternal history of asthma. Many children who outgrow their exacerbations continue to have airway hyperresponsiveness and cough as adults. Furthermore, airway hyperresponsiveness in adults appears to be associated with decreased lung function.

The adolescent age-group appears to be the most vulnerable, with the greatest increase in mortality from the condition occurring in children 10 to 14 years of age. No reliable data exist to explain this increase. Factors that have been postulated include exposure of atopic persons to more allergens (particularly in large urban centers), change in severity of the disease, abuse of drug therapy (toxicity), failure of families and practitioners to recognize the severity of asthma, failure to take asthma controller medications daily, and psychologic factors such as denial and refusal to accept the disease. Risk factors for asthma deaths include early onset, frequent attacks, difficult-to-manage disease, adolescence, history of respiratory failure, psychologic problems (refusal to take medications), dependency on or misuse of asthma drugs (high use), presence of physical stigmata (e.g., barrel chest, intercostal retractions), and abnormal PFTs.

Nursing Care Management

Acute Asthma Care

Children who are admitted to the hospital with acute asthma are ill, anxious, and uncomfortable. The progression or resolution of status asthmaticus is variable. Continual observation and assessment are essential (see Nursing Care Plan box).

NURSING CARE PLAN

The Child With Acute Asthma Exacerbation

Case Study

Jeremy is a 17-year-old male with a history of asthma. His asthma symptoms have been controlled with use of a long-acting inhaler twice daily but an increase in seasonal allergies and a recent upper respiratory infection has caused an exacerbation of his symptoms. Jeremy rarely uses his peak expiratory flow meter (PEFM); instead, he waits until his symptoms become severe before starting to use his rescue medications. He now presents to his primary care provider with his mother to seek further treatment as his symptoms are not resolving with his current treatment.

Assessment

Based on these events, what are the most important subjective and objective data that should be assessed?

Acute Asthma Exacerbation Defining Characteristics

Dyspnea
Shortness of breath
Diminished breath sounds and/or adventitious breath sounds (wheezing)
Increased respiratory rate
Use of accessory muscles (retractions)
Dry cough
Chest tightness or chest pain

Nursing Interventions

What are the most appropriate nursing interventions for a child with acute respiratory tract infection?

Nursing Interventions	Rationale
Monitor circulation, airway, and breathing (CABs) closely.	To provide supportive measures as needed to maintain circulation, airway, and breathing
Allow patient to assume position of comfort.	To promote maximum ventilator function
Administer humidified oxygen to maintain oxygen saturation (Sa_{O_2}) above 90%.	To enhance oxygenation of tissues and minimize drying of the nasal mucous membranes
Administer rescue medications (as prescribed) that can include inhalers, nebulization, and/or oral or intravenous (IV) steroids.	To open constricted airways and allow air exchange and to enhance tissue oxygenation
Assess patient's response to rescue medications.	To determine need for more aggressive interventions
Assist patient in recognizing factors that trigger asthma symptoms.	To enhance patient's awareness of factors that exacerbates asthma
Assist patient to understand the purpose and use of the PEFM.	To allow early recognition of asthma symptoms before acute exacerbation
Observe technique for use of PEFM, inhaler, and/or nebulizer.	To ensure appropriate technique to maximize accuracy and effectiveness

Expected Outcomes

Respirations will be easy and nonlabored at a rate within normal limits for age.
Airway will remain patent.

Continued

NURSING CARE PLAN—CONT'D

The Child With Acute Asthma Exacerbation

Jeremy will verbalize health maintenance measures (i.e., avoiding triggers, use of peak flow meter, use of inhalers).

Case Study (Continued)

Jeremy had no improvement with the nebulized treatment provided in the primary care office and his symptoms worsened. He was transferred to a nearby hospital for further evaluation. On arrival to the emergency department (ED), Jeremy is unable to answer questions, refuses to lie down, and displays short rapid breaths with significant retractions. His mother is concerned about what is happening to him.

Assessment

What are the most important signs and symptoms based on this scenario?

Status Asthmaticus Defining Characteristics

Inability to speak in full sentences
Agitation, confusion
Rapidly progressive shortness of breath
Tachypnea and tachycardia
Chest tightness
Retractions
Cyanosis

Nursing Interventions

What are the most appropriate nursing interventions for this child?

Nursing Interventions	Rationale
Monitor CABs closely.	To provide supportive measures as needed to maintain circulation, airway, and breathing
Allow patient to assume position of comfort.	To promote maximum ventilator function
Administer humidified oxygen to maintain oxygen saturation (Sao_2) above 90%.	To enhance oxygenation of tissues and minimize drying of nasal mucous membranes
Administer short-acting β-agonist medications continuously via nebulizer as prescribed.	To open constricted airways and allow air exchange and to enhance tissue oxygenation
Obtain blood specimen for electrolytes, complete blood count, renal function tests, and arterial blood gases.	To determine current status of patient and institute therapy based on results
Obtain IV access and administer corticosteroid, hydration, and electrolytes as prescribed.	To decrease inflammation and correct dehydration, acidosis, and electrolyte disturbances
Educate family about status asthmaticus and treatment underway to resolve condition.	To promote awareness of characteristics and treatment for status asthmaticus
Arrange for social worker to meet with family to assess emotional and financial needs.	To identify and modify stressors associated with acute exacerbation of illness and sudden hospitalization
Transfer patient from the ED to the pediatric intensive care unit.	To allow for continuous cardiorespiratory monitoring and further treatment

Expected Outcome

Respirations will be easy and nonlabored at a rate within normal limits for age.
Airway will remain patent.
Gas exchange will remain adequate.
Family will verbalize an accurate interpretation of Jeremy's condition and treatment.

When β_2-agonists and corticosteroids are given, the child is monitored closely and continuously for relief of respiratory distress and signs of side effects or toxicity (e.g., tachycardia, restlessness, irritability, hyperactivity). Although food may not be well tolerated in the acute phase, the child may avoid upset stomach associated with corticosteroids by taking small amounts of a food, such as a few crackers, once the respiratory status has stabilized somewhat. Pulse oximetry is monitored along with rate and depth of breathing, auscultation of air movement, adventitious sounds, and any signs of respiratory distress (e.g., nasal flaring, tachypnea, retractions). The child on supplemental oxygen requires intermittent or continuous oxygenation monitoring, depending on the severity of respiratory compromise and initial oxygenation status. The child in status asthmaticus should be placed on continuous cardiorespiratory (including blood pressure) and pulse oximetry monitoring.

If required, IV access is usually initiated once the child has been placed on oxygen. The child may respond well to topical anesthesia for the procedure (e.g., EMLA or LMX4). Oral fluid intake may be limited during the acute phase; IV fluid replacement may be required to provide adequate hydration. Endotracheal intubation equipment should be readily available. Medications administered intravenously are monitored for their desired effect and for any untoward effects.

Children with acute asthma are apprehensive and anxious, and they often hyperventilate as a result of the anxiety. Calm coaching to increase depth and slow rate of respirations while administering oxygen with a simple mask may alleviate the child's fears. The calm, efficient presence of a nurse helps reassure the child that he or she is safe and will be cared for during this stressful period. Assure children that they will not be left alone and that their parents are allowed to remain with them.

Parents need reassurance and want to be informed of their child's condition and therapies. They may believe that they have in some way contributed to the child's condition or could have prevented the episode. Reassurance regarding their efforts expended on the child's behalf and their parenting capabilities can help alleviate their stress. Efforts to reduce parental apprehension also reduce the child's distress. Anxiety is easily communicated to the child from parents and members of the staff.

General Care

The nursing care of the child with asthma begins with a review of the child's health history; the home, school, and play environment; the parents' and child's attitudes about the child's condition; and a comprehensive physical assessment with focus on the respiratory system. Nursing care of children with asthma involves both acute and long-term care. Nurses who are involved with children in the home, hospital, school, outpatient clinic, or practitioner's office play an important role in helping children and their families learn to live with the condition. The disease can be managed so that it does not require ED visits or hospitalization and does not interfere with family life, physical activity, or school attendance. The nursing process in the care of the child with asthma is outlined in the Nursing Care Plan box.

Physical assessment of asthma involves the same observations and techniques described in Chapter 4. In addition, the nurse notes and evaluates physical characteristics of chronic respiratory involvement, including chest configuration (e.g., barrel chest), posturing (tripod), and type of breathing. A history of the current and previous episodes and precipitating factors or events provides important information. An asthma scoring system may be used to determine severity of symptoms. The nursing assessment should include questions about nighttime waking related to symptoms, frequency of use of the quick-acting bronchodilator, ability to participate in school or other activities, PEFR scores, any medication side effects and other visits to a provider related to asthma symptoms.

Nurses perform a variety of vital functions in asthma care, including asthma education in the primary care setting and in schools and other community settings, care of the child with asthma in the acute care setting, ambulatory care, and intensive care. Nurses also obtain information on how asthma affects the child's everyday activities and self-concept, the child's and family's adherence to the prescribed therapy, and their personal treatment goals. Assess the child's and family's satisfaction with asthma control, the quality of care, their perception of the severity of the disease, and their level of social support.

One of the major emphases of nursing care is outpatient management by the family. Parents are taught how to recognize and respond to symptoms of bronchospasm, maintain health and prevent complications, and promote normal activities. The child's asthma action plan should be reviewed periodically at least every 6 months in children with moderate to severe disease; precipitating factors, illness management, and medication use should be discussed. The nurse determines any cultural or ethnic beliefs or practices that influence self-management and that may necessitate modifications in educational approaches to meet the family's needs.

Avoid Allergens

One goal of asthma management is avoidance of an acute exacerbation. Parents and children need to know how to avoid allergens that precipitate asthma episodes. The nurse educates the parent and child on how to modify the environment to reduce contact with the offending allergen(s). Caution the parents to avoid exposing a sensitive child to excessive cold, wind, or other extremes of weather; smoke; sprays; and other irritants. Parents should also eliminate from the diet any foods known to provoke symptoms.

Approximately 2% to 6% of children with asthma are sensitive to aspirin; therefore nurses should caution parents to use analgesic-antipyretic drugs for discomfort or fever and to read package labeling. Parents are taught to avoid administering aspirin to *any* child because of its association with Reye syndrome unless specifically recommended by and under the supervision of a health practitioner. Salicylate compounds are in other common medicines such as Pepto-Bismol, which should be avoided. Children with aspirin-induced asthma may also be sensitive to nonsteroidal antiinflammatory drugs (NSAIDs) and tartrazine (yellow dye number 5, a common food coloring). Acetaminophen is safe for children and is the analgesic of choice.

Relieve Bronchospasm

Teach parents and older children to recognize early signs and symptoms of an impending attack so that it can be controlled before symptoms become distressing. Most children can recognize prodromal symptoms well before an attack (about 6 hours) and implement preventive therapy. Objective signs that parents may observe include rhinorrhea, cough, low-grade fever, irritability, itching (especially in front of the neck and chest), apathy, anxiety, sleep disturbance, abdominal discomfort, and loss of appetite.

Children who use a nebulizer, MDI, Diskus, or Turbuhaler to deliver drugs need to learn how to use the device correctly. The MDI device delivers medication directly to the airways; therefore the child needs to learn to breathe slowly and deeply for better distribution to narrowed airways (see Family-Centered Care box). Use of a spacer or AeroChamber slows down the delivery of those particles to assist with their inhalation. It is recommended for all patients who use MDIs because less medication is lost in the air and more enters the lungs.

Young children and those who are unable to manipulate the MDI or hold their breath for 10 seconds should use a spacer. A spacer is a 4- to 8-inch tube that fits on the end of the MDI mouthpiece. These devices allow the parent or child to deliver the medication from the MDI into the spacer, from which the child then inhales the medication, while taking slow, steady breaths at his or her own pace. Spacers also help prevent yeast infections in the mouth when corticosteroids are inhaled via an MDI.

The nurse also needs to caution the child and parents about the adverse effects of prescribed drugs and the dangers of overuse of β_2-agonists. They should know that it is important to use these drugs when needed but not indiscriminately or as a substitute for avoiding the symptom-provoking allergen. Caution parents against purchasing over-the-counter preparations because these medications can place the children at risk for increased dosage of a drug and toxicity. Educate parents on how to read labels on prepared foods and snacks to determine the presence of allergens.

The family should obtain a PEFM and learn to use this device to monitor the child's asthma. A written asthma action plan that includes the three peak flow meter zones and the child's asthma medications may be obtained from the child's primary care provider (Fig. 26.14).

A written asthma action plan can significantly reduce the risk of asthma death (Liu, Covar, Spahn, et al., 2016). Medications used for asthma exacerbations are also included in the asthma plan. This action plan should be used to make decisions about asthma management at home and at school. The nurse may assist the child and family in preparing this plan, emphasizing that they determine the success of the plan and not the health professionals.

Maintain Health and Prevent Complications

The child should be protected from a respiratory tract infection that can trigger an attack or aggravate the asthmatic state, especially in young children whose airways are mechanically smaller and more reactive. Annual influenza vaccinations are recommended for all children over 6 months. Vaccination against pneumococcal infection is part of the routine childhood vaccination schedule, and children with asthma should be immunized, especially those on prolonged high-dose corticosteroids (American Academy of Pediatrics, Report of the Committee on Infectious Diseases, 2015). The pneumococcal vaccine is also recommended for patients ages 19 through 64 years who are smokers or have asthma (American Academy of Pediatrics, Report of the Committee on Infectious Diseases, 2015). Equipment used for the child, such as nebulizers, must be kept absolutely clean to decrease the chances of contamination with bacteria and fungi.

Teach and encourage breathing exercises and controlled breathing for motivated children, and provide information concerning activities that promote diaphragmatic breathing, side expansion, and improved mobility of the chest wall. Play techniques that can be used for younger children to extend their expiratory time and increase expiratory pressure include blowing cotton balls or a Ping-Pong ball on a table, blowing a pinwheel, blowing bubbles, or preventing a tissue from falling by blowing it against the wall.

Promote Self-Care and Normalization

Self-care and asthma self-management programs are important in helping the child and family cope with asthma. Most asthma self-management programs for children convey several principles. First, asthma is a common disease that can be controlled with appropriate drug therapy, environmental control, education, and management skills. Second, it is much easier to prevent than to treat an asthma episode; adherence

FAMILY-CENTERED CARE

Use of a Metered-Dose Inhaler

Steps for Checking How Much Medicine Is in the Canister

1. If the canister is new, it is full.
2. Check product label to see how many inhalations should be in each canister.
3. The most accurate way to determine how many doses remain in a metered-dose inhaler (MDI) is to count and record each dose as it is used.
4. Many dry powder inhalers have a dose-counting device or dose indicator on the canister to let you know when the canister is empty.
5. Placing dry powder inhalers or MDIs with hydrofluoroalkanes in water will destroy these inhalers.

Steps for Using the Inhaler With Mouthpiece

1. Remove the cap and hold inhaler upright.
2. Shake the inhaler.
3. Attach spacer, as appropriate.
4. Tilt the head back slightly and breathe out slowly.
5. With the inhaler in an upright position, insert the mouthpiece:
   a. About 3 to 4 cm (1 to 1½ inches) from the mouth, or
   b. Into the mouth, forming an airtight seal between the lips and the mouthpiece
6. At the end of a normal expiration, depress the top of the inhaler canister firmly to release the medication (into the mouth), and breathe in slowly (about 3 to 5 seconds). Relax the pressure on the top of the canister.
7. Hold the breath for at least 5 to 10 seconds to allow the aerosol medication to reach deeply into the lungs.
8. Remove the inhaler and breathe out slowly through the nose.
9. Wait 1 minute between puffs (if an additional puff is needed) when using a bronchodilator.

NOTE: Inhaled dry powder such as budesonide (Pulmicort) requires a different inhalation technique. To use a dry powder inhaler, the base of the device is turned until a click is heard. It is important to close the mouth tightly around the mouthpiece of the inhaler and inhale rapidly.

Steps for Using the Inhaler With an AeroChamber (see Fig. 26.12)

The AeroChamber comes with a mask (small, medium, and large sizes) or a mouthpiece attached.

1. Remove the cap and hold inhaler upright.
2. Shake the inhaler.
3. Attach AeroChamber.
4. For AeroChambers with a mouthpiece, with the inhaler in an upright position, insert the mouthpiece into the mouth, forming an airtight seal between the lips and the mouthpiece.
5. For AeroChambers with a mask, apply AeroChamber mask to child's face and make sure there is a good seal.
6. Have child breathe slow, regular breaths. Depress the top of the inhaler canister firmly to release the medication (into the AeroChamber) as the child breathes slowly in and out. Relax the pressure on the top of the canister.
7. Hold the AeroChamber in place over the child's face until six breaths have been taken. Give one puff at a time.
8. Wait 1 minute between puffs when using a bronchodilator.
9. Remove the inhaler and the AeroChamber.

The AeroChamber is washed weekly using soap and water.

Common Problems for Children Using Inhalers

- Child refuses or resists treatment.
- Inhalation is too rapid.
- Child is unable to coordinate the spray with inhalation.
- Breath is not held long enough after inhalation.

Modified from Nurses' Asthma Education Working Group. (1998). *Nurses: Partners in asthma care.* NIH Pub No 98-3308. Bethesda, MD: National Heart, Lung, and Blood Institute, National Institutes of Health.

to a therapeutic program is necessary to prevent exacerbations. Third, children with asthma can live full and active lives. Although a visit to the ED or hospital due to an asthma exacerbation is undesirable, it also presents an opportunity to assess the child's/family's current knowledge about asthma, its triggers, prevention, and treatment to prevent future visits. The technique used for MDI or nebulizer administration should be observed and education provided when needed.

Asthma camps provide an opportunity for children with asthma to engage in physical activity while learning about their disease in a controlled environment with their peers and health professionals. Children who attend asthma camps often demonstrate improved asthma self-management skills.

Self-contained programs and brochures for patient education are available from the Asthma and Allergy Foundation of America* and the American Lung Association.† The National Heart, Lung, and Blood Institute‡ provides educational materials for asthma education in the school setting and also copies of the *Guidelines for the Diagnosis and Management of Asthma* (National Asthma Education and Prevention Program, 2007).

*8201 Corporate Drive, Suite 1000, Landover, MD 20785; 800-727-8462; http://www.aafa.org.

†1301 Pennsylvania Ave., NW, Washington, DC 20004; 202-785-3355, 800-548-8252; http://www.lungusa.org.

‡NHLBI Health Information Center, PO Box 30105, Bethesda, MD 20824-0105; 301-592-8573; fax: 240-629-3246; http://www.nhlbi.nih.gov.

Child and Family Support

The nurse working with children with asthma can provide support in a number of ways. Many children voice frustration because their exacerbations interfere with their daily activities and social lives. These children also need reassurance from the health team that they can learn to control and cope with their asthma and live a normal life. Be aware of children, especially adolescents, who demonstrate signs of depression and may not comply with therapy.

Children in disruptive family situations (e.g., divorce, separation, violence, custodial battles) may disregard their daily asthma medication regimen or may be at higher risk as a result of neglect by adults who are in charge of their care. Adolescents struggling with a sense of identity and body image often regard asthma as a condition that will "go away," especially if there is a time lapse between symptoms, and may abandon the therapeutic regimen. They also have a sense of invincibility and may not recognize the future impact of poor adherence to their treatment regimen. In some cases adolescents find themselves in charge of other siblings in blended family situations and may ignore their own health needs. Referral for counseling and guidance is appropriate when the child's or adolescent's life is potentially in danger and the therapeutic

Asthma Action Plan

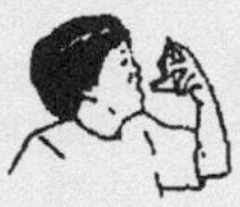

Name: ______________________________

Doctor: ______________________ **Date:** __________

Phone for doctor or clinic: ______________________

Emergency contact phone and name: ______________________

You can use the colors of a traffic light to help learn about your asthma medicines.

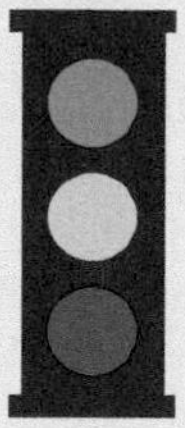

1. **Green** means **Go.** Use preventive medicine.
2. **Yellow** means **Caution.** Use quick-relief medicine.
3. **Red** means **Stop.** Get help from a doctor.

1. Green — Go

- Breathing is good
- No cough or wheeze
- Can work and play

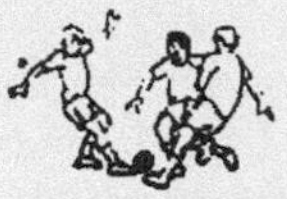

Peak flow number

______ to ______

Personal best peak flow __________

Use preventive medicine.

Medicine	How much to take	When to take it

5 to 60 minutes before exercise, use this medicine:

____

2. Yellow — Caution

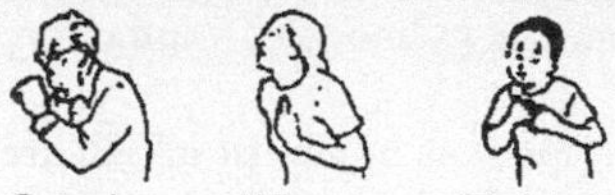

Cough Wheeze Tight chest

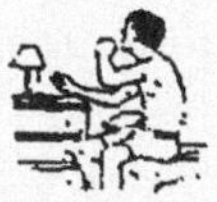

Wake up at night

Peak flow number

______ to ______

(50% to 80% of my best peak flow)

Take quick-relief medicine to keep an asthma attack from getting bad

Medicine	How much to take	When to take it
(short-acting beta$_2$ agonist)		

If symptoms return to Green Zone after 1 hour of taking above quick-relief medication, take __________ (medicine) and __________ (medicine).

If symptoms **do not** return to Green Zone after 1 hour of taking the quick-relief medication, take __________ (short-acting beta$_2$ agonist) (medicine) and add __________ (oral steroid) (medicine).

Call your doctor if symptoms do not improve within _____ hours after taking the oral steroid or if your symptoms are in the Red Zone.

3. Red — Stop — Danger

- Medicine is not helping
- Breathing is hard and fast
- Nose opens wide
- Can't walk
- Ribs show
- Can't talk well

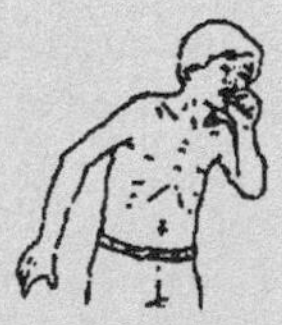

Peak flow number

______ to ______

(50% or less of personal best)

Get help from a doctor now!
Take these medicines until you talk with the doctor.

Medicine	How much to take	When to take it
(short-acting beta$_2$ agonist)		
(oral steroid)		

Go to the emergency department immediately or call the ambulance if you cannot reach your doctor and you are still in the Red Zone after 15 minutes.

These signs signal **DANGER**:

- Difficulty walking or breathing
- Mental confusion
- Fingernails or lips are blue

Call the ambulance.

FIG. 26.14 Asthma action plan. (Redrawn from the National Asthma Education and Prevention Program, National Heart, Lung, and Blood Institute. [1995]. *Asthma management and prevention: Global initiative for asthma.* NIH Publication No. 96-3659A. Washington, DC: National Institutes of Health.)

regimen for asthma is abandoned due to other crises. Nurses and other caregivers are mandated reporters of medical neglect in these situations.

The short- and long-term adaptation of children with asthma often depends on the family's acceptance of the disorder. The task of living day to day with affected children involves the entire family. There are periodic crises and the ever-present threat of a crisis, requiring parental vigilance; sleepless nights; frequent trips to the physician, ED, or hospital; and often overwhelming medical expenses. Throughout, these stresses encourage parents to promote as normal a life as possible for their children.

CYSTIC FIBROSIS

Cystic fibrosis (CF) is a condition characterized by exocrine (or mucus-producing) gland dysfunction that produces multisystem involvement. CF is the most common lethal genetic illness among Caucasian children, adolescents, and young adults. It is estimated that 1 in 29 Caucasians in the United States is a symptom-free carrier. More than 95% of the documented cases of CF occur in Caucasians (1 in 3500 live births); the incidence in other ethnic groups varies, affecting African Americans in 1 in 15,000 live births and Hispanics in 1 in 9200 live births (Egan, Green, & Voynow, 2016).

Etiology

CF is inherited as an autosomal recessive trait. The affected child inherits the defective gene from both parents, with an overall incidence of 1 in 4 births if both parents carry the gene. The mutated gene responsible for CF is located on the long arm of chromosome 7. This gene codes a protein of 1480 amino acids called the cystic fibrosis transmembrane regulator (CFTR). The CFTR protein is related to a family of membrane-bound glycoproteins. The glycoproteins constitute a cAMP-activated chloride channel and also regulate other chloride and sodium channels at the surfaces of the epithelial cells.

Functional expression of the CF defect reduces the ability of the epithelial cells in the airways and pancreas to transport chloride. Abnormal transport of sodium and chloride across the epithelium leads to increased viscosity of airway mucus, abnormal mucociliary clearance, and lung disease. The severity of lung disease and presence of hepatic disease cannot be predicted by genotype, which suggests a major environmentally acquired component of organ system dysfunction or another gene that modifies the CF phenotype (Egan, Green, & Voynow, 2016).

The *ΔF508* gene mutation is the most common alteration found in CF. It occurs in 70% of all known CF chromosomes and is closely related to pancreatic insufficiency. Most of the remaining cases of CF are explained by more than 1500 other mutations. CFTR may be divided into five classes based on the type of defect. Individuals in the first three classes have more severe pulmonary disease and pancreatic insufficiency, whereas those in classes 4 and 5 have milder pulmonary symptoms and better weight gain. However, experts emphasize that even within each class there is substantial phenotype variability (Egan, Green, & Voynow, 2016).

Pathophysiology

With the discovery of the CFTR gene, research is continuing to determine its multisystem effects on the body. Several clinical features characterize CF: increased viscosity of mucous gland secretions, a striking elevation of sweat electrolytes, an increase in several organic and enzymatic constituents of saliva, and abnormalities in autonomic nervous system function. Although both sodium and chloride are affected, the defect appears to be primarily a result of abnormal chloride movement; the CFTR appears to function as a chloride channel.

Children with CF demonstrate decreased pancreatic secretion of bicarbonate and chloride and an increase in sodium and chloride in both saliva and sweat. This last characteristic is the basis for the sweat chloride diagnostic test. The sweat electrolyte abnormality is present from birth, continues throughout life, and is unrelated to the severity of the disease or the extent to which other organs are involved. The sodium and chloride content of sweat in 98% to 99% of children with CF is two to five times greater than that of children without CF.

The primary factor, and the one responsible for many of the clinical manifestations of the disease, is mechanical obstruction caused by the increased viscosity of mucous gland secretions (Fig. 26.15). Instead of forming a thin, freely flowing secretion, the mucous glands produce a thick, heavy mucoprotein that accumulates and dilates them. Small passages in organs such as the pancreas and bronchioles become obstructed as secretions precipitate or coagulate to form concretions in glands and ducts.

Because of the increased viscosity of bronchial mucus, there is greater resistance to ciliary action (probably secondary to infection and ciliary destruction); a slower flow rate of mucus; and incomplete expectoration, which also contributes to the mucus obstruction. This retained mucus serves as an excellent medium for bacterial growth. Reduced oxygen–carbon dioxide exchange causes variable degrees of hypoxia, hypercapnia, and acidosis. In severe, progressive lung involvement, compression of pulmonary blood vessels and progressive lung dysfunction frequently lead to pulmonary hypertension, cor pulmonale, respiratory failure, and death.

Pulmonary complications are present in almost all children with CF, but the onset and extent of involvement are variable. Symptoms are produced by stagnation of mucus in the airways, with eventual bacterial colonization leading to destruction of lung tissue. The abnormally viscous and tenacious secretions are difficult to expectorate and gradually obstruct the bronchi and bronchioles, causing scattered areas of bronchiectasis, atelectasis, and hyperinflation. The stagnant mucus also provides an optimal environment for bacterial growth.

The most common pathogens are *P. aeruginosa, B. cepacia,* methicillin-resistant *S. aureus* (MRSA), *B. dolosa, S. aureus, H. influenzae, Escherichia coli,* and *K. pneumoniae.* Children with CF who are chronically colonized with these organisms have poorer survival rates than children who are not colonized. Fungal colonization with *Candida* or *Aspergillus* organisms in the respiratory tract is also common.

The pseudomonal strains are particularly pathogenic for children with CF because in most patients the alveolar macrophages cannot destroy *Pseudomonas* organisms. The pseudomonal strains also quickly develop resistance to most medications by developing mucoid strains, and once a person with CF is colonized with these organisms, they are difficult to eradicate. *P. aeruginosa* infection is not specific for CF but occurs much more frequently in CF than in other diseases characterized by chronic airway obstruction.

B. cepacia is especially worrisome because this organism is extremely virulent, produces bacteremia, and has been associated with rapid pulmonary function deterioration and death in a significant number of CF patients. Methicillin-sensitive *S. aureus* is the most common organism to colonize the respiratory tract and likely to occur with coinfection of *P. aeruginosa, A. fumigatus,* or *H. influenzae* (Sobin, Kawai, & Irace, 2017).

Gradual progression of pulmonary disease follows chronic infection. Bronchial epithelium is destroyed, and infection spreads to peribronchial tissues, resulting in weakening of bronchial walls and peribronchial fibrosis. The pattern is chronic, progressive fibrosis with decreased oxygen–carbon dioxide exchange and a concurrent alteration in pulmonary vasculature. Chronic hypoxemia causes contraction and hypertrophy of medial muscle fibers in pulmonary arteries and arterioles,

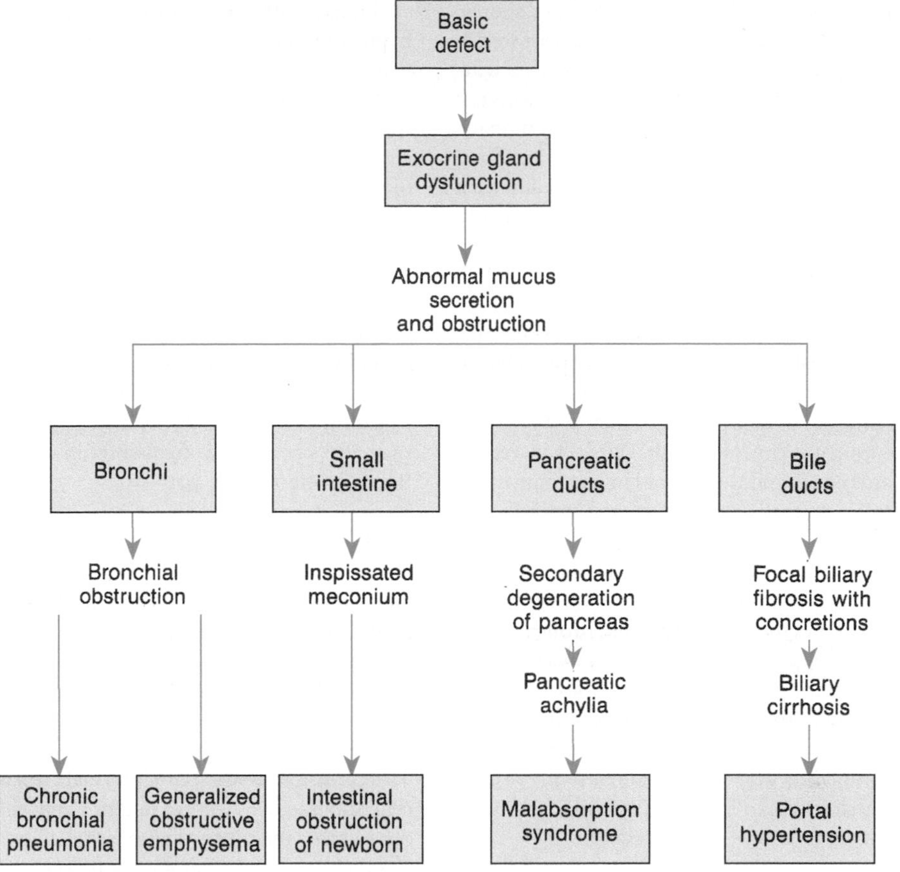

FIG. 26.15 Various effects of exocrine gland dysfunction in cystic fibrosis.

leading to pulmonary hypertension and eventual cor pulmonale. Pneumothorax may occur when peripheral bullae rupture; hemoptysis can occur with the erosion of bronchial arteries into a bronchus.

The paranasal sinuses are often filled with secretions and inflammatory products. Nasal and sinus polyps are common, sometimes resulting in bone erosion. Treatment for chronic sinusitis may involve oral antibiotics, decongestants, nasal saline lavage, nasal sinus washout under anesthesia, and nasal corticosteroids.

The extent of GI involvement varies. In the pancreas of many patients, thick secretions block the ducts, leading to cystic dilations of the acini (small lobes of the gland), which then undergo degeneration and progressive diffuse fibrosis. This event prevents essential pancreatic enzymes from reaching the duodenum, which causes marked impairment in the digestion and absorption of nutrients, particularly fats, proteins, and, to a lesser degree, carbohydrates. Disturbed absorption is reflected in excessive stool fat (steatorrhea) and foul smells from putrefied protein (azotorrhea).

The endocrine function of the pancreas often remains unchanged because the islets of Langerhans are normal but may decrease in number as pancreatic fibrosis develops and progresses. The incidence of diabetes mellitus (cystic fibrosis–related diabetes [CFRD]) is greater in children with CF than in the general population, which may be caused by changes in pancreatic architecture and diminished blood supply over time. Consequently, with increased survival, and primarily in adolescents and adults, CFRD has been reported to be the most common complication associated with CF. Around 50% of people with CF develop diabetes by 30 years of age. It is associated with increased morbidity, and mortality. Severe insulin deficiency occurs as a result of β islet cell dysfunction, and severe insulin resistance may occur, especially during an acute illness. Consequently, CFRD has characteristics of both types 1 and 2 diabetes mellitus. Adequate insulin is needed to maintain a high nutritional status, and this correlates with optimal lung function.

In the liver, focal biliary obstruction and fibrosis are common and become more extensive with time, eventually giving rise to a distinctive type of multilobular biliary cirrhosis. Some children develop extensive liver involvement with fatty infiltration despite adequate nutrition. The gallbladder is small and contains a firm, gelatinous material that also fills the cystic duct. Findings similar to those in the pancreas are found in the salivary glands and contribute to a dry mouth and susceptibility to infection as a result of interference with salivation.

The reproductive systems of both males and females are adversely affected with CF. The glands of the uterine cervix are often filled with mucus, and copious amounts of mucus may block the cervical canal and prevent sperm entry. More than 95% of males with CF are sterile due to obliteration or atresia of the epididymis, vas deferens, and seminal vesicles, resulting in decreased or absent sperm production (Egan, Green, & Voynow, 2016).

Clinical Manifestations

The clinical manifestations vary widely and change as the disease progresses. The most common symptoms are (1) progressive chronic obstructive lung disease associated with infection; (2) maldigestion from exocrine pancreatic insufficiency; (3) growth failure from malabsorption and anorexia; and (4) diabetes symptoms of hyperglycemia, polyuria, glycosuria, and weight loss from pancreatic insufficiency. The usual pattern is one of growth failure (failure to thrive), with an increased weight loss despite an increased appetite and gradual deterioration of the respiratory system. The diagnosis may not be readily apparent, especially when there is no familial evidence of CF. Some children display symptoms at birth. Others may not develop symptoms for weeks, months, or years. Some show only mild forms of the disease, with limited impairment of digestion and respiratory problems, whereas others have severe malabsorption and life-threatening pulmonary complications. Although most affected children display both pulmonary and GI symptoms, a few have only enzyme deficiency without pulmonary disease, and a few have only pulmonary disease without pancreatic insufficiency.

Respiratory Tract

Initial pulmonary manifestations are often wheezing respirations and a dry, nonproductive cough. Eventually diffuse bronchial and bronchiolar obstruction leads to irregular aeration with progressive pulmonary disturbance and secondary infection. The most prominent and constant feature of pulmonary involvement is chronic cough. Dyspnea increases, the cough often becomes paroxysmal, and the mucoid impactions within the small air passages cause a generalized obstructive hyperinflation and patchy areas of atelectasis.

Progressive pulmonary involvement with hyperaeration of functioning alveoli produces the overinflated, barrel-shaped chest in which the anteroposterior diameter approaches the lateral diameter. Bronchiectatic cysts and subpleural blebs in the upper lobes occur in advanced disease and may rupture, causing pneumothorax. When ventilation and subsequent diffusion and gas exchange are significantly impaired, cyanosis and clubbing of the fingers and toes may occur. The child or adolescent has repeated episodes of bronchitis and bronchopneumonia and is subject to chronic nasal congestion, rhinitis, chronic sinusitis, and nasal polyps. Ear, nose, and throat surgeries are often needed.

Gastrointestinal Tract

The earliest postnatal manifestation of CF is meconium ileus, which occurs in 10% to 15% of newborns with the disease (Egan, Green, & Voynow, 2016). Thick, putty-like, tenacious, mucilaginous meconium blocks the lumen of the small intestine, usually at or near the ileocecal valve, which gives rise to signs of intestinal obstruction, including abdominal distention, vomiting, failure to pass stools, and rapid development of dehydration with associated electrolyte imbalance. Thick intestinal secretions continue to be problematic throughout life. Children of all ages are subject to intestinal obstruction (distal ileum) from heavy or impacted feces. Gumlike masses in the cecum can obstruct the bowel, causing pain, nausea, and vomiting. This is referred to as *meconium ileus equivalent. Distal intestinal obstruction syndrome* is partial or complete intestinal obstruction that occurs in some children with CF.

As the disease progresses, obstruction of pancreatic ducts prevents digestive enzymes (e.g., trypsin, chymotrypsin, amylase, lipase) from being released into the duodenum, which prevents conversion of ingested food into compounds that can be absorbed by the intestinal mucosa. Consequently, the undigested food (chiefly unabsorbed fats and proteins) is excreted, increasing the bulk of feces to two or three times the normal amount. The bulky nature of the stools may go unnoticed at first, but usually by 6 months of age the child passes large, loose stools with normal frequency or has chronic diarrhea with unformed stools. As solid foods are added to the diet, the excessively large stools become frothy and extremely foul smelling (steatorrhea).

Because so little is absorbed from the intestine, affected children have difficulty maintaining weight despite a healthy appetite and diet. Unable to compensate for the fecal losses, many children lose weight and exhibit marked wasting of tissues and growth failure. Growth failure (failure to thrive) is common due to decreased absorption of nutrients, vitamins, and fat; increased oxygen demands for pulmonary function; and delayed bone growth.

Infants with CF who have growth failure frequently demonstrate hypoalbuminemia resulting from diminished absorption of protein, which in severe cases causes generalized edema. The abdomen is distended, the extremities are thin, and the sallow skin droops from wasted buttocks. The impaired ability to absorb fats results in a deficiency of the fat-soluble vitamins A, D, E, and K, which may cause bleeding problems if vitamin K deficiency is significant. Anemia is a common complication. Growth failure may be an initial diagnosis in young children with previously undiagnosed CF. Many older children with CF have an increased prevalence of gastroesophageal reflux.

Another common GI complication is prolapse of the rectum, which occurs in infancy and early childhood and is related to large, bulky stools; malnutrition; and increased intraabdominal pressure secondary to paroxysmal cough. Appendicitis, intussusception, and constipation may also occur more frequently in children with CF (Demeyer, De Boeck, Witters, et al., 2016).

Reproductive System

Delayed puberty in girls with CF is common even when their nutritional and clinical status is good. Women with CF who become pregnant have an increased incidence of premature labor and delivery and low birth weight in the infant. Favorable nutritional status and pulmonary function are positively correlated with favorable pregnancy outcomes.

Integumentary System

The consistent finding of abnormally high sodium and chloride concentrations in the sweat is a unique characteristic of CF. Parents frequently observe that their infants taste "salty" when they kiss them. The chloride channel defect in sweat glands prevents reabsorption of sodium and chloride, which leaves the affected person at risk for abnormal salt loss, dehydration, and hypochloremic and hyponatremic alkalosis during hyperthermic conditions. This is especially important to the infant because of limited fluid stores and the potential for inadequate sodium intake with most commercially prepared infant formulas. The disease is sometimes expressed in other ways (e.g., hyponatremia caused by massive losses through sweat, especially in high environmental temperatures or febrile episodes).

Diagnostic Evaluation

Traditionally, the diagnosis of CF was based on a positive sweat chloride test, absence of pancreatic enzymes, radiography, chronic obstructive pulmonary disease, and family history. Newer diagnostic methods make it possible to diagnose CF early in infancy so therapies can be implemented to increase the child's overall survival and quality of life. In addition to the sweat chloride test and factors listed previously, diagnosis may be confirmed by newborn screening, deoxyribonucleic acid (DNA) identification of mutant genes, or abnormal nasal potential difference measurement.

The quantitative sweat chloride test (pilocarpine iontophoresis) involves stimulating the production of sweat with a special device (involving stimulation with 3-mA electric current), collecting the sweat on filter paper, and measuring the sweat electrolytes. The quantitative analysis requires a sufficient volume of sweat (>75 mg). Two separate samples are collected to ensure the reliability of the test. Normally sweat chloride content is less than 40 mEq/L, with a mean of 18 mEq/L. A chloride concentration greater than 60 mEq/L is diagnostic of CF; in infants younger than 3 months, a sweat chloride concentration greater than 40 mEq/L is highly suggestive of CF. In some situations DNA testing may be substituted for the sweat test.

The presence of a mutation known to cause CF on the CFTR gene predicts with a high degree of certainty that the individual has CF;

however, multiple CFTR mutations may also be present and detected with DNA assay. Chest radiography reveals characteristic patchy atelectasis and obstructive emphysema. PFTs are sensitive indices of lung function, providing evidence of abnormal small airway function in CF. Radiographs, including contrast enema, are used for diagnosis of meconium ileus.

Other diagnostic tools that may aid in diagnosis include stool fat or enzyme analysis. Stool analysis requires a 72-hour sample with accurate recording of food intake during that time. In some cases, CF may go undiagnosed until the child is older and is seen with clinical manifestations that previously were not acute.

Screening

Early detection of CF is associated with better clinical outcomes and fewer hospitalizations. All 50 states screen newborns for CF (Egan, Green, & Voynow, 2016). The newborn screening test consists of an immunoreactive trypsinogen analysis performed on a dried spot of blood, which may be followed by direct analysis of DNA for the presence of the *ΔF508* mutation or other mutations on the same dried blood spot. Benefits of early screening and detection include earlier nutritional intervention and preservation of lung function for identified infants. Perceived disadvantages of early screening include the parental anxiety that false-positive results may generate. Children who were identified and treated early in infancy with aggressive nutritional support had improved growth and cognitive function well into adolescence (Egan, Green, & Voynow, 2016). Although the technology is available to conduct carrier screening for the general population, this issue remains controversial, and widespread implementation of carrier screening programs is not recommended. An in utero diagnosis of CF is also possible based on detection of two CF mutations in the fetus.

Therapeutic Management

Improved survival among patients with CF during the past 2 decades is attributable largely to antibiotic therapy and improved nutritional and respiratory management. The goals of CF therapy are to prevent or minimize pulmonary complications, ensure adequate nutrition for growth, encourage appropriate physical activity, and promote a reasonable quality of life for the child and the family. A multidisciplinary system approach is needed to accomplish these goals. Current research and modern technologies are exploring methods to attack the genetic defect. For example, a number of clinical trials are underway to examine the feasibility of correcting the underlying genetic defect using gene therapy where patients inhale the CF gene monthly via a nebulizer.

CFTR modulator therapies are available to patients who have specific mutations in the CFTR gene. The Food and Drug Administration has two approved medications for this: ivacaftor (Kalydeco), which is available for children ages 2 years and older, and lumacaftor/ivacaftor (Orkambi), which is available to children ages 6 years and older. The medications last 12 hours, so twice-daily dosing is required. These medications regulate the flow of sodium and fluids in cell linings in the affected organs, reducing the likelihood of the development of sticky mucus in organs.

Management of Pulmonary Problems

Management of pulmonary problems is directed toward prevention and treatment of pulmonary infection by improving ventilation, removing mucopurulent secretions, and administering antimicrobial agents. Many children develop respiratory symptoms by 3 years of age. The large amounts and viscosity of respiratory secretions in children with CF contribute to the likelihood of respiratory tract infections. Recurrent pulmonary infections in the child with CF result in greater damage to the airways; small airways are destroyed, causing bronchiectasis.

Airway Clearance Therapy

CPT has been the cornerstone of airway clearance therapy (ACT) in the prevention of pulmonary infection for many years. Several other ACT strategies are now available to assist with removal of secretions, including percussion and postural drainage, positive expiratory therapy (PEP), active-cycle-of-breathing technique, autogenic drainage, oscillatory PEP, high-frequency chest compressions, and exercise. The decision on which technique to use is based on the child and the family. Several techniques may be used, and they are usually adapted over time. It is importance to foster adherence to ACTs from a young age. They are usually performed on average twice daily (on rising and in the evening) and more frequently if needed, especially during pulmonary infection. Percussion and postural drainage is especially useful for infants and young children but is often not adequate for older children.

PEP is performed by breathing out with a moderate force through a device. This creates resistance and a positive pressure in the airways, helping keep them open. It allows airflow to get around the mucus and moves it toward the larger airways, where it can be expectorated. Three devices that help accomplish this are PEP valves, Flutters, and acapellas. The PEP valve allows air to be inhaled through a one-way valve and blown out through a hole or resistance. The Flutter mucus clearance device is a small, handheld plastic pipe with a stainless-steel ball on the inside (Fig. 26.16). An acapella provides high-frequency oscillation as well as PEP.

The active-cycle-of-breathing technique is a series of breathing techniques that help clear secretions. Examples include forced expiration, or "huffing," with the glottis partially closed; thoracic expansion exercises; and relaxation and breathing control. Young children can be taught games with breathing that can develop into these techniques as they get older.

Autogenic drainage involves a variety of breathing techniques that the older child can use to force mucus in lower lobes up into the airways so it can be successfully expelled. Handheld percussors or electronic chest vibrators may be used to loosen secretions but may not be as effective as some of the other techniques described.

High-frequency chest compression (HFCC) is accomplished by use of a mechanical chest device that is worn for periodic treatments during the day (Fig. 26.17). HFCC provides rapid entry and exit of air in the lungs and assists with mucus breakdown and clearance. It is a common ACT used in patients with CF. Nebulization therapies are generally administered during the vest therapy. Some studies have reported more

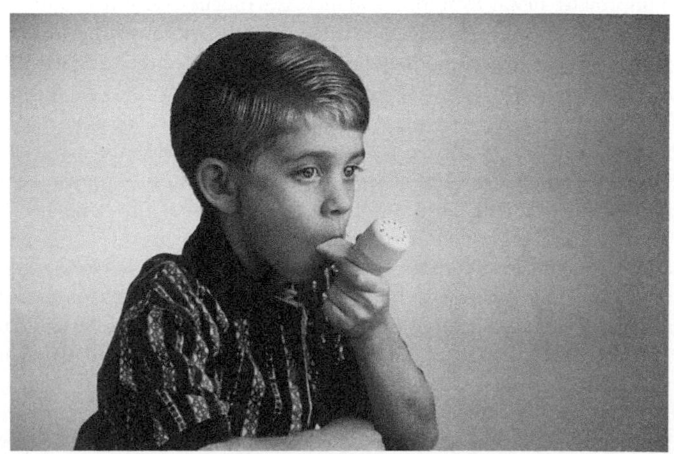

FIG. 26.16 Child using Flutter mucus clearance device. (Courtesy Scandipharm, Inc.)

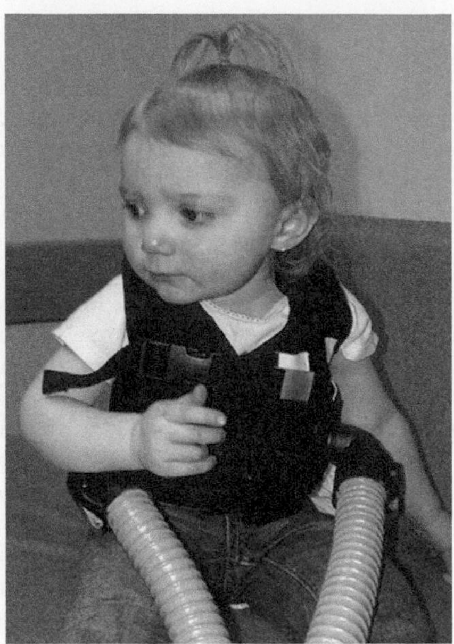

FIG. 26.17 An 18-month-old female cystic fibrosis patient wearing a high-frequency chest compression (HFCC) vest (the *inCourage System*). (From Des Jardins, T, & Burton G. [2011]. *Clinical manifestations and assessment of respiratory disease* [6th ed.]. St. Louis, MO: Mosby.)

effective mucus clearance with this treatment than with other conventional treatments. Some children and adolescents with an implantable vascular access port may experience localized pain with the vest.

Patients with CF have been found to regress when conventional ACT is discontinued. Therefore although it is time consuming for the child and family, it is an essential part of care.

Bronchodilator medication delivered in an aerosol opens bronchi for easier expectoration and is administered before ACTs when the patient exhibits evidence of reactive airway disease or wheezing. Another aerosolized medication is recombinant human deoxyribonuclease (DNase, known generically as dornase alfa [Pulmozyme]), which decreases the viscosity of mucus. It is well tolerated and has no major adverse effects; minor reactions are voice alterations and laryngitis. This medication, given once or twice daily via nebulization, has resulted in improvements in spirometry, PFTs, dyspnea scores, and perceptions of well-being and has reduced the viscosity of sputum (Yang, Chilvers, Montgomery, et al., 2016).

Nebulized hypertonic saline (6% to 7%) has shown some effectiveness in improving airway hydration and increases mucus clearance in patients with CF who are 6 years of age and older; this treatment, however, causes bronchospasm and may not be recommended for patients with severe disease (Goralski & Donaldson, 2014).

Clinical trials are in progress to examine the effects of inhaled dry powdered mannitol for improving mucociliary clearance in CF by rehydrating the airway. Initial reports showed significant improvement in lung function and sputum (De Boeck, Haarman, Hull, et al., 2017).

Physical exercise is an important adjunct to daily ACT. Exercise stimulates mucus excretion and provides a sense of well-being and increased self-esteem. Any aerobic exercise that the patient enjoys should be encouraged. The ultimate aim of exercise is to increase lung vital capacity, remove secretions, increase pulmonary blood flow, and maintain healthy lung tissue for effective ventilation.

Colonization with *P. aeruginosa* and *B. cepacia* signals progressive involvement. Although the bacteria are impossible to eradicate, they can be successfully controlled. Patients with CF metabolize antibiotics more rapidly than normal; therefore drug dosage is often higher than would be expected. Depending on its sensitivity, *P. aeruginosa* is usually treated with either piperacillin-tazobactam, ceftazidime, cefepime, imipenem-cilastin, meropenem or ticaracillin-clavulanate, ciprofloxacin, levofloxacin, tobramycin, or amikacin. Antibiotic treatment of *B. cepacia* and *S. aureus* should be based on susceptibility and synergy testing. The duration of therapy depends on the patient's response, which is measured by clinical indicators, including cough, fatigue, and exercise intolerance, in addition to tests such as PFTs, chest radiography, and oxygen measurements.

The Cystic Fibrosis Foundation's core principles of Infection Prevention and Control advise that staff, people with CF, and their families need regular and ongoing education that all patients with CF have some colonization of the secretions in the respiratory tract. As a result, individuals with CF should separate from others with CF by at least 6 feet to reduce the chance of cross-infection and contact precautions are needed for all patients, regardless of what pathogens are present in their sputum (Cystic Fibrosis Foundation, 2013). Patients with CF are advised to wear a mask in common areas of health care facilities, but health care workers are not required to wear a mask routinely in the care of these patients (Saiman, Siegel, LiPuma, et al., 2014).

Pulmonary infections are treated as soon as they are recognized. In patients with CF, characteristic signs of pulmonary infection—fever, tachypnea, and chest pain—may be absent. Therefore a careful history and physical examination are essential. The presence of anorexia, weight loss, and decreased activity alerts the practitioner to pulmonary infection and the need for an antibiotic regimen. Aerosolized tobramycin is beneficial for patients with frequent pulmonary exacerbations (Egan, Green, & Voynow, 2016). This medication is usually administered by jet or ultrasonic nebulizers after ACT is performed. This type of delivery system allows for direct antimicrobial application with little systemic absorption. It is not uncommon for the child with CF to be placed on as many as two or three antibiotics and one antifungal medication to treat coexisting pulmonary infections.

IV antibiotics may be administered at home as an alternative to hospitalization. The use of peripherally inserted central catheters (PICCs) for the administration of antibiotics in children with CF is a viable option with limited complications and fewer needle punctures to obtain blood specimens and to maintain often lengthy treatment with parenteral antibiotics. Alternatively, an implanted vascular access device offers the advantage of access for blood draws and antibiotic infusion. Patients may receive antibiotic therapy at home and continue daily activities with minimum disruptions. However, when pulmonary function does not improve with outpatient management, hospitalization may be recommended for continued antibiotic therapy and vigorous ACT. Some children with CF are hospitalized for IV antibiotic therapy and ACT periodically (a "tune-up") to keep them well. Oxygen administration may be used for children with acute episodes but must be used cautiously because many children with CF have chronic carbon dioxide retention, and the unsupervised use of oxygen can be harmful. With repeated infection and inflammation, bronchial cysts and emphysema may develop. These cysts may rupture, resulting in a pneumothorax (see Box 26.9).

! NURSING ALERT

Signs of a pneumothorax are usually nonspecific and include tachypnea, tachycardia, dyspnea, pallor, and cyanosis. A subtle drop in oxygen saturation (measured by pulse oximetry) may be an early sign of pneumothorax.

Blood streaking of the sputum is usually associated with increased pulmonary infection, or advanced lung disease. Hemoptysis greater than 250 ml/24 hr for the older child (less for a younger child) indicates a potentially life-threatening event and needs to be treated immediately.

Sometimes bleeding can be controlled with bed rest, IV antibiotics, replacement of acute blood loss, IV conjugated estrogens (Premarin) or vasopressin (Pitressin), and correction of any coagulation defects with vitamin K or fresh frozen plasma. If hemoptysis persists, the site of bleeding should be localized via bronchoscopy and cauterized or embolized. Children and adolescents with CF should be given the age-appropriate immunizations, including the annual trivalent inactivated influenza virus vaccine. Treatment of nasal polyps includes intranasal corticosteroids, oral antihistamines, and decongestants. If these measures are ineffective, surgical interventions may be necessary. Patients with hemoptysis should not receive nonsteroidal antiinflammatory medications.

Long-term daily ibuprofen (NSAID) given in a dose sufficient to achieve a peak plasma concentration between 50 and 100 mcg/ml has been shown to slow the rate of decline in pulmonary function and to decrease the need for IV antibiotics in young patients with mild pulmonary involvement. Although this therapy is generally well tolerated, careful monitoring for adverse effects (GI bleeding) is essential. Lung transplantation is a final therapeutic option for many CF patients with severe disease. Heart-lung and double-lung procedures have been successfully performed in children with advanced pulmonary vascular disease and hypoxia; however, whether such procedures significantly improve quality of life and survival rates in children with CF is debated in the current literature. The obstacles surrounding this technique are availability of donated organs; complications from surgery; and recurrence of pulmonary infections and obstructive bronchiolitis, which decreases transplanted lung function. Some experts state that infections such as *B. cepacia,* diabetes, and older age represent a negative factor for long-term survival after transplant (Egan, Green, & Voynow, 2016).

Management of Gastrointestinal Problems

The principal treatment for pancreatic insufficiency is replacement of pancreatic enzymes, which are administered with meals and snacks to ensure that digestive enzymes are mixed with food in the duodenum. Enteric-coated products prevent the neutralization of enzymes by gastric acids, thus allowing activation to occur in the alkaline environment of the small bowel. The amount of enzymes depends on the severity of the insufficiency, the child's response to enzyme replacement, and published guidelines. A dosing schedule is based on grams of consumed fat or body weight. Usually one to five capsules are administered with a meal, and fewer are taken with snacks. To avoid overdosing, enzyme replacement should not exceed 2500 units lipase/kg/meal for children over 12 months of age (Egan, Green, & Voynow, 2016). Capsules can be swallowed whole or taken apart and the contents sprinkled on a small amount of food to be taken at the beginning of the meal. The amount of enzyme is adjusted to achieve normal growth and a decrease in the number of stools to one or two per day. Pancreatic enzymes should be taken within 30 minutes of eating. The enteric-coated beads should not be chewed or crushed because destroying the enteric coating can lead to inactivation of the enzymes and excoriation of oral mucosa. The powder form is used with infants and young children; caregivers must prevent inhalation of the powder, which may precipitate acute bronchospasm. The powder may also start to predigest the food, making it unpalatable. Enzymes are mixed into cereal or fruit such as applesauce for small children or into a small amount of breast milk or formula for infants. Enzyme dosing may need to be adjusted by the provider if abdominal side effect occurs such as flatus, pain, loose stools, bloating, or steatorrhea.

One issue of concern with pancreatic enzymes is that generic enzymes are not considered adequate and only proprietary enzymes should be given to children with CF. Because the uptake of fat-soluble vitamins is decreased, water-miscible forms of these vitamins (A, D, E, and K) are given, along with multivitamins and the pancreatic enzymes. When high-fat foods are eaten, the child is encouraged to add extra enzymes.

Children with CF require a well-balanced, high-protein, high-caloric diet, with unrestricted fat (because of the impaired intestinal absorption). Improved nutrition in children with CF has been associated positively with improved lung function. To meet his or her energy requirements, the patient with mild pulmonary disease must consume 5% to 10% more than the recommended dietary allowance (RDA); for those with moderate-to-severe lung disease, energy requirements may be as high as 20% to 50% or more of the RDA (Kleinman & Greer, 2014). Persons with CF also require an intake of fat (35% to 40% of calories) in comparison to the recommendation for the general population (20% to 30%) (Turck, Braegger, Colombo, et al., 2016). A group of experts recommends that children and adolescents with CF 2 to 20 years of age should have an energy intake of 110% to 200% of standards for healthy persons (Turck, Braegger, Colombo, et al., 2016).

Regular nutritional monitoring should be a standard part of the medical care of the child with CF and should occur every month from birth to 6 months, then every 2 months until 12 months of age; during the second year of life growth assessments should take place every 2 to 3 months and between 2 years of age and 18 years every 3 months (Turck, Braegger, Colombo, et al., 2016). The weight-for-length goal for growth in the first 2 years of life should be above the 50th percentile on World Health Organization standard growth charts, and in children 2 to 18 years a body mass index (BMI) above the 50th percentile should be the goal for growth (Turck, Braegger, Colombo, et al., 2016). Breastfeeding with enzyme supplementation should be continued as long as possible and, when necessary, supplemented with a higher-calorie-per-ounce (e.g., 24 kcal/oz) formula to achieve adequate growth. For formula-fed infants, commercial cow's milk–based formulas may be adequate to achieve desired growth. There is no evidence to support the use of high-energy or hydrolyzed formula (Turck, Braegger, Colombo, et al., 2016). Growth failure despite adequate nutritional support may indicate deterioration of pulmonary status. Data indicate that better forced expiratory volume in 1 second (FEV_1) status (≤80%) strongly correlates with BMI percentiles above the 50th percentile; therefore as noted earlier, the target weight for children with CF ages 2 to 20 years should be ideally maintained above the 50th percentile (Turck, Braegger, Colombo, et al., 2016). Patients with CF may experience frequent anorexia as a result of the copious amounts of mucus produced and expectorated, persistent cough, effects of medications, fatigue, and sleep disruption. They may be placed on oral nutritional supplements, nighttime (or continuous) supplemental nasogastric/gastrostomy feedings, or, rarely, parenteral alimentation in an effort to build up nutritional reserves if there has been a history of inability to maintain weight. An enzyme supplement is encouraged with enteric feedings; these may be given at the initiation of the infusion, at bedtime, and at the conclusion of the feeding infusion.

Meconium ileus and meconium ileus equivalent, or total or partial intestinal obstruction, can occur at any age. Constipation is often the result of a combination of malabsorption (either from inadequate pancreatic enzyme dosage or a failure to take the enzymes), decreased intestinal motility, and abnormally viscous intestinal secretions. These problems usually do not require surgical interventions and may be treated with Miralax, GoLYTELY or Colyte (osmotic solutions given orally or by nasogastric tube), other laxatives, stool softeners, or rectal administration of diatrizoate meglumine (Gastrografin).

Rectal prolapse occurs in a small number of children with CF. The first episode of rectal prolapse is frightening to both parents and child. Its reduction usually requires immediate guidance and intervention, which is managed by simply guiding the rectum back into place with a gloved, lubricated finger with the child lying on her or his side. Further management usually involves attempting to decrease the bulk of daily stools through pancreatic enzyme replacement.

Children with CF often experience transient or chronic gastroesophageal reflux, which should be treated with the appropriate histamine-receptor antagonist and GI motility drug, dietary modifications, and an upright position after feedings or meals.

Management of Endocrine Problems

The management of CFRD is critical in the therapeutic treatment of the child with CF. CFRD presents a combination of insulin resistance and insulin deficiency, with unstable glucose homeostasis in the presence of acute lung infection and treatment. Children with CF may be at increased risk for glucose management problems as a result of decreased nutrient absorption, anorexia, and severity of pulmonary illness. Diagnosis of CFRD is made using an oral glucose tolerance test. Children with CFRD require close monitoring of blood glucose, administration of insulin injections, diet and exercise management, and quarterly glycosylated hemoglobin (A1c) monitoring. The prevalence of CFRD increases with age, and there is increased morbidity and mortality among children with CFRD compared with those without (Castellani & Assael, 2017). Microvascular complications such as retinopathy and nephropathy may occur in children and adolescents with CFRD (Egan, Green, & Voynow, 2016). However, ketoacidosis is reported to be rare in individuals with CFRD (Egan, Green, & Voynow, 2016).

Children with CFRD should perform blood glucose checks three times daily, preferably before meals, and should be on an insulin regimen. With mild CFRD, a single daily dose of long acting insulin may be sufficient for glycemic control. During illness exacerbations, hyperglycemia may be prevalent.

Bone health is of concern in children and adults with CF. The pancreatic insufficiency of CF and chronic steroid use present potential risks for less than optimum bone growth in such children. Assessment of bone health by history and bone mass density evaluation should be considered in assessing the child's (≤8 years old) health status to detect and prevent osteoporosis or osteopenia.

The administration of recombinant human growth hormone is being used for children with CF who have growth delay to achieve optimum growth. A Cochrane review reported human growth hormone benefits for children with CF are increased height, weight, and lean tissue mass, and improved lung functioning (Thaker, Haagensen, Carter, et al., 2015). However, there is no evidence that it improves clinical status or health-related quality of life.

Prognosis

The median survival age for CF patients is 37 years (Egan, Green, & Voynow, 2016). Despite considerable progress and a recent surge in new treatment modalities, CF remains a progressive and incurable disease. The pulmonary involvement ultimately determines the patient's outcome because pancreatic enzyme deficiency is less of a problem if adequate nutrition is ensured. With advances in technology, parents and adolescents are challenged to set future goals that may include college, careers, social relationships, and marriage. Concurrently they are faced with increasing morbidity and higher rates of CF complications as they grow older.

Nursing Care Management

Assessment of the child with CF involves comprehensive assessment of all affected systems, with special focus on pulmonary and GI systems. Pulmonary assessment is the same as that described for asthma, with special attention to lung sounds, observation of cough, and evidence of decreased activity or fatigue. GI assessment primarily involves observing the frequency and nature of the stools and abdominal distention. The observer is also alert to evidence of growth failure or failure to thrive (e.g., weight loss, muscle wasting, pallor, anorexia, decreased activity [from baseline norm]). Family members are interviewed to determine the child's eating and eliminating habits and confirm a history of frequent respiratory tract infections or bowel obstruction in infancy.

The nurse assesses the newborn for feeding and stooling patterns, which may indicate a potential problem such as meconium ileus. The nurse also participates in diagnostic testing such as the initial newborn screening, immunoreactive trypsinogen, DNA analysis, or sweat chloride test.

Parents are often anxious and puzzled about the diagnostic tests and the possible implications of the test results. They need careful explanations of the disease, how it might affect their family, and what they can do to provide the best possible care for their child. It is crucial to involve the parents in the follow-up for early diagnostic testing; the neonate may require several follow-up visits in the first few weeks of life if initial test results are not conclusive.

The uncertainty, fear, and initial shock associated with the diagnosis are overwhelming to parents. They must face the impact of the chronic, life-threatening nature of the disease and the prospect of intensive treatment, for which they must assume a major part of the responsibility and for which they are ill prepared. They often fear that they will be unable to provide the care the child needs. One of the most difficult aspects of the diagnosis is the implications inherent in its etiology (i.e., the recognition that each parent contributed the gene responsible for the defect).

Hospital Care

Most patients with CF require hospitalization only for treatment of pulmonary infection (exacerbation of their pulmonary symptoms), uncontrolled diabetes, or a coexisting medical problem that cannot be treated on an outpatient basis. All patients with CF require contact isolation for their own protection and wear a mask in communal areas of the hospital.

When the child with CF is hospitalized for diagnosis or treatment of pulmonary complications, aerosol therapy, chest percussion therapy, and postural drainage are instituted or continued. Respiratory therapists often initiate, supervise, and provide these treatments; however, it is the nurse's responsibility to monitor the patient's tolerance to the procedure and evaluate its effectiveness in relation to treatment goals. The nurse may, at times, administer aerosol therapy, perform CPT, assist with ACTs such as the mechanical vest, and teach breathing exercises. ACT should not be performed before or immediately after meals. Planning ACT so that it does not coincide with meals is difficult in the hospital situation but is essential to the effectiveness of this treatment.

Nursing assessments, including observation of respiratory pattern, work of breathing, and lung auscultation, are vital. Noninvasive pulse oximetry provides valuable data about the patient's oxygenation status. Supplemental oxygen therapy may be administered to the child with mild or moderate respiratory distress. One of the nursing challenges in the care of the child with CF is encouraging compliance with the therapeutic regimen, which often involves taking a significant number of medications; pancreatic enzymes; vitamins A, D, E, and K; oral antifungals for *Candida* infection; antihistamines; antiinflammatory agents; and oral antibiotics. This may be overwhelming to the child. Factor in multiple inhaled bronchodilators, ACT and aerosol treatments, potential blood glucose monitoring and insulin administration, various other medications, and increased mucus production during the acute phase, and it is not uncommon for the child with CF to rebel with this regimen and refuse some interventions. Gentle coaxing, positive reinforcement, and frank negotiation may be required to enlist cooperation for effective medication compliance.

The child's sleep is disrupted frequently by hospital routines; therefore nursing care should be flexible enough to allow him or her some quiet time without affecting vital care. In some cases a daily schedule of events, including medication administration, CPT, aerosolized therapy, and dressing changes, may need to be mutually developed with the child, nurses, and physician so that the child feels he or she has some control of the care.

The diet for the child with CF represents another challenge; careful planning with a pediatric dietitian and the child's input may help decrease the loss of appetite and weight loss that are often part of the condition. Patients with CF, especially adolescents, enjoy foods brought from home. Children in the early stages of CF often have a good appetite. With infection and increased lung involvement, their appetite diminishes, and eventually it becomes a challenge to tempt failing appetites. Age-appropriate nutrition education with specific nutritional goals for CF patients may increase compliance with prescribed enzyme therapy and nutritional supplements.

When dietary intake fails to meet the child's needs for growth, enteral feedings or supplements may be considered. These feedings may be administered via an enteric tube during the night to minimize the disruption of daily activities, including school. A low-profile gastrostomy tube affords the child few activity restrictions and minimum disruption of body image in comparison to a nasogastric tube or conventional gastrostomy tube. The child and parents are encouraged to perceive this therapy not as a last-ditch effort but as an adjunct therapy to maintain optimum growth and prevent excessive weight loss. In some cases the nurse shows adolescents how to insert a nasogastric tube for nighttime supplemental feedings; the tube may then be removed in the morning.

The child needs support during the many treatments and tests that are a part of the hospitalization. Blood tests, IV fluids and medications, PICC line and vascular access placement and site care, and vascular access device accessing or deaccessing are almost always a part of the acute care treatment, and the child soon associates hospitalization with these stress-provoking procedures.

Depression, anxiety, and disturbed self-image may occur in children and adolescents with CF. Older adolescents and young adults are especially prone to depression due to the realization of the poor prognosis and unmet life expectations and goals.

Providing support to both the child and the family is essential. The progressive nature of the disease makes each illness requiring hospitalization a potentially life-threatening event. Skilled nursing care and sympathetic attention to the emotional needs of the child and family help them cope with the stresses associated with repeated respiratory tract infections and hospitalizations.

Home Care

Most children and adolescents with CF can be managed at home. The goals of care include normalization and daily activities, including school and peer involvement. The care plan should be flexible so that family activities are disrupted as little as possible. Parents may initially require assistance finding and contacting durable medical equipment companies that provide home care equipment. They also need opportunities to learn how to use the equipment and to solve problems they may encounter while delivering therapy at home.

Patients and family members need education about the preferred diet of nutritious meals with tolerated fat, increased protein and carbohydrate, and the administration of pancreatic enzymes and nutritional supplements. It is important to stress to parents that the enzymes, in the amount regulated to the child's needs, should be administered at the beginning of all meals and snacks.

One of the most important aspects of educating parents for home care is teaching ACTs. The success of a therapy program depends on conscientious performance of these treatments regularly as prescribed. The number of times these therapies are performed each day is determined on an individual basis, and often parents readily learn to adjust the number and intensity of the treatments to the child's needs.

For pulmonary infection, home IV antibiotics may be prescribed. Home IV care may be preferred for willing and competent families because it reduces tension and usually brings a sense of belonging to the family members; however, this option depends on a number of factors, including availability of an agency with adequate staff to perform multiple daily home antibiotic infusions, willingness of the family to assist with infusions, and adherence to therapy at home. With the use of venous access devices such as PICC lines or vascular access devices, the parents and child learn the technique of direct administration into the IV line. Around-the-clock administration may be difficult for families and requires certain adjustments such as waking at least once during the night to give the drug. Occasionally infusion through an ambulatory infusion pump may be beneficial.

For the child or adolescent with chronic sinusitis, daily or twice-daily nasal lavage may be helpful. Caution parents to avoid commercial saline preparations with benzyl alcohol because these may burn the nasal mucosa. At home, Neilmed Salt or a mixture of noniodized salt and baking soda is frequently used in boiled/distilled water. Adolescents need instruction on performing this procedure themselves.

Families also need information about medications and possible side effects. If a child is receiving ibuprofen, observations for side effects such as GI irritation are essential. Children receiving antibiotics may require serum drug levels and other routine blood tests to ensure therapeutic dosing.

Children and adolescents with CF should receive routine primary care with special attention to diet, growth and development, and immunizations. Primary care providers should be alert to any weight loss or flattening in the growth curve associated with loss of appetite, which could indicate a pulmonary exacerbation in children with CF. Anticipatory guidance concerning issues of discipline, how to incorporate aspects of the treatment regimen into the school environment, and delayed pubertal development are also important considerations for the primary care provider. Home palliative care for the child or adolescent with CF who is in the terminal stages may be carried out with the assistance of hospice. (See Chapter 19.)

Family Support

The most challenging aspect of providing care for the family of a child or adolescent with CF is meeting the emotional needs of the child and family. The diagnosis, treatment, and prognosis for CF are often associated with many problems and frustrations. The diagnosis can evoke feelings of guilt and self-recrimination in parents.

The long-range problems for an infant, child, or adolescent with CF are those encountered in any chronic illness. (See Chapter 19.) Both the child and the family must make many adjustments, the success of which depends on their ability to cope and also on the quality and quantity of support they receive from outside sources. Combined efforts of a variety of health professionals are needed to provide the most comprehensive services to families. It is often the nurse who assesses the home situation, organizes and coordinates these services, and collects the data needed to evaluate the effectiveness of the services.

The persistent need for treatment several times a day places tremendous strain on the family. Children often balk at these treatments, and the parents are in the position of insisting on adherence. The stress and anxiety related to this routine may produce feelings of resentment in both the child and the family members. When possible, occasional trusted respite care should be available to allow parents to leave the situation for short periods without undue anxiety about the child's welfare.

The affected child or adolescent may become resentful about the disease, its relentless routine of therapy, and the necessary restrictions it places on activities and relationships. The child's activities are interrupted or built around treatments, medications, and diet. This imposes hardships and influences his or her quality of life. The nurse should encourage the child to attend school and join age-appropriate peer groups to live as normally and productively as possible. Sports are often an important part of the child's and adolescent's life; interaction with peers is a valuable life experience, especially to adolescents. The child or adolescent with CF should be encouraged to participate in sports activities as much as physical and pulmonary health allows. Exercise is encouraged to increase pulmonary vital capacity, promote muscle development, and enhance cardiovascular function.

Nurses should monitor adolescents with CF for signs of eating disturbances. The topic of eating disorders is understudied in patients with CF; however, several factors create a predisposition for the disorder. The need for high calorie consumption along with early satiety and a potential body image disorder leaves adolescents vulnerable to eating disorders (Quick, Byrd-Bredbenner, & Neumark-Sztainer, 2013). In addition, depression in CF patients has been associated with worse health outcomes, adherence, and quality of life (Smith, Georgiopoulos, & Quittner, 2016). As the disease progresses, however, family stress should be expected, and the patient may become angry and noncompliant. It is important for the nurse to recognize the family's changing needs and the grief they may experience as the CF worsens. Families should be made aware of resources for counseling. Patients need to be guided into activities that enable them to express anger, sorrow, and fear without guilt.

The nurse can assist the family in contacting resources that provide help to families with affected children. Various special child health services, many local clinics, private agencies, service clubs, and other community groups offer equipment and medications either free or at reduced rates. The Cystic Fibrosis Foundation* has chapters throughout the United States to provide education and services to families and professionals.

Transition to Adulthood

As life expectancy continues to rise for children and adolescents with CF, issues related to marriage, sexuality, childbearing, and career choice become more pressing. Males must be informed at some point that they will often be unable to produce offspring. It is important that the distinction be made between sterility and impotence. Normal sexual relationships can be expected. Female patients may be able to bear children but should be informed of the possible harmful effects on the respiratory system created by the burden of pregnancy. They also need to know that their children will be carriers of the CF gene; therefore genetic counseling for those planning on having children is essential. Adolescent females should be offered counseling concerning the use of oral contraceptives and other contraceptive options.

Adolescents with CF should take personal ownership and management of the illness to maximize their life's potential. Many adolescents and young persons with the illness enroll in college or vocational and technical training school and complete degrees by either distance learning or attending a local school. Young people should set life goals and live normal lives to the extent their illness allows. Adolescents who have had lung transplantation are encouraged to continue taking antirejection medications even though they may feel as though their respiratory status has improved to the point that these medications are no longer necessary.

Life as an independent adult should be encouraged for children with CF. From the time that children can take partial responsibility for their own care (e.g., ACT and taking pancreatic enzymes), independence and accountability should be fostered. Although the prognosis for these children has improved, many will need continued support as they cope with the demands of surviving with CF.

Anticipatory grieving and other aspects related to care of a child with a terminal illness are also part of nursing care. For example, it is important to prepare the child and family members for end-of-life decisions and care. Families may need information about specific interventions such as hospice and treatments for pain and dyspnea. (See Chapter 19.)

OBSTRUCTIVE SLEEP APNEA

Pediatric obstructive sleep-disordered breathing reportedly affects between 1% and 6% of all children and up to 59% of obese children (Schwengel, Dalesio, & Stierer, 2014). Sleep-disordered breathing problems in this spectrum range from partial obstruction of the upper airway to continuous episodes of complete upper airway obstruction, with the most severe form being obstructive sleep apnea (OSA) (Owens, 2016).

Obstructive sleep apnea is defined by the American Thoracic Society (1996) as a disorder of breathing during sleep with prolonged partial upper airway obstruction and/or complete obstruction that disrupts normal respiration during sleep and normal sleep patterns. Adenotonsillar hypertrophy is a common cause of OSA, but tonsil size does not correlate with the degree of OSA (Owens, 2016). Other causes of OSA include allergies associated with chronic rhinitis/nasal obstruction, craniofacial abnormalities, gastroesophageal reflux, nasal septal deviation, and cleft palate repair (Owens, 2016). OSA in children is a distinctly separate condition from OSA in adults with regard to etiology, clinical manifestations, and treatment. Common symptoms of OSA include nightly snoring, breathing pauses, choking or gasping on arousal, disturbed sleep patterns, secondary enuresis, daytime sleepiness, and daytime neurobehavioral problems (Owens, 2016). OSA is to be distinguished from primary snoring, which is snoring without obstructive apnea or abnormalities in gas exchange. If left untreated, OSA may result in complications such as growth failure, cor pulmonale, hypertension, poor attention span, behavioral problems (impulsiveness, hyperactivity, rebelliousness and aggression), attention-deficit/hyperactivity disorder, hypertension, cardiac ventricle dysfunction, and death.

The diagnosis of OSA is made by an overnight sleep study (polysomnography), which provides evidence of sleep disturbance, respiratory pauses, and changes in oxygenation. The six-channel polysomnography can be performed in children of all ages with videotaping and audiotaping. Polysomnography can distinguish between OSA and primary snoring (Owens, 2016).

Therapeutic Management

Adenotonsillectomy is now recommended as the first-line treatment of children with adenotonsillar hypertrophy (Owens, 2016). Cure rates after adenotonsillectomy are reported to range between 70% and 90%

*6931 Arlington Road, 2nd floor, Bethesda, MD 20814-3205; 301-951-4422 or 800-344-4422; http://www.cff.org. In Canada: Canadian Cystic Fibrosis Foundation, 2221 Yonge St., Suite 601, Toronto, Ontario M4S 2B4; http://www.cysticfibrosis.ca.

in uncomplicated cases (Owens, 2016). However, more recent evidence indicates that it may not be as effective in children with obesity (Boudewyns, Abel, Alexopoulos, et al., 2017).

CPAP and BiPAP (cycles between high and low pressure) may be helpful in older children with OSA whose condition persists after surgical intervention or in children who are not good candidates for surgical intervention. CPAP is a long-term therapy with frequent assessments to evaluate the required amount of pressure and the overall effectiveness of the intervention. Many children resist wearing the CPAP or BiPAP devices. Gentle coaxing, patience, reassurance, and gradually building up the duration of time on the therapies may help when possible.

Surgical interventions such as tracheotomy or mandibular distraction may be required for children with craniofacial syndromes such as Goldenhar, Pierre Robin, Apert, and Crouzon, in which there is partial or complete upper airway obstruction (Schwengel, Dalesio, & Stierer, 2014).

Nursing Care Management

Nursing care of the child with OSA involves early detection by observation of the infant's or child's sleep patterns, active participation in the diagnostic polysomnography, observation of oxygenation and vital signs, application of CPAP when indicated, and monitoring the patient's response to diagnostic therapy. Counseling families of children with OSA may involve dietary counseling for exercise programs and weight management, use of the CPAP or BiPAP equipment, and direct postoperative care after the surgical intervention of tonsillectomy or adenoidectomy. The nurse can be instrumental in helping the child and family cope with the chronic illness diagnosis should intervention such as CPAP or BiPAP be required.

RESPIRATORY EMERGENCY

RESPIRATORY FAILURE

Effective pulmonary gas exchange requires clear airways, normal lungs and chest wall, and adequate pulmonary circulation. Anything that affects these functions or their relationships can compromise respiration. In general, the term **respiratory insufficiency** is applied to two conditions: when there is increased work of breathing but gas exchange function remains near normal and when normal blood gas tensions cannot be maintained and hypoxemia and acidosis develop secondary to carbon dioxide retention. **Respiratory failure** is the inability of the respiratory apparatus to maintain adequate gas exchange. This process involves pulmonary dysfunction that generally results in impaired alveolar-capillary gas exchange, which can lead to hypoxemia or hypercapnia. **Respiratory arrest** is the cessation of respiration. Respiratory failure is the most common cause of cardiopulmonary arrest in children.

Apnea is generally defined as cessation of breathing for more than 20 seconds, or for a shorter period when associated with hypoxemia or bradycardia (Kline-Tilford, Sorce, Levin, et al., 2013). Apnea can be (1) central, in which both airflow and chest wall movement are absent; (2) obstructive, in which airflow is absent but chest wall motion is present; and (3) mixed, in which both central and obstructive components are present.

Respiratory dysfunction may have an abrupt or an insidious onset. Respiratory failure can occur as an emergency situation or may be preceded by gradual and progressive deterioration of respiratory function. Most clinical manifestations are nonspecific and are affected by variations among individual patients and differences in the severity and duration of inadequate gas exchange.

Conditions That Predispose to Respiratory Failure

Respiratory disorders are classified according to three dominant functional abnormalities, although all three types may be present in the disease. In **obstructive lung disease** there is increased resistance to airflow in either the upper or the lower respiratory tract. Obstruction can result from anomalies (e.g., tracheomalacia, choanal atresia, vocal paralysis), aspiration (e.g., meconium, mucus, vomitus, FB), infection (e.g., epiglottitis, pneumonia, pertussis, severe tonsillitis), tumors (e.g., hemangioma, cystic hygroma), anaphylaxis, and laryngospasm from local irritation (e.g., intubation, drowning, aspiration).

In **restrictive lung disease**, impaired lung expansion results from loss of lung volume, decreased distensibility, or chest wall disturbance. Causes of pulmonary restriction include respiratory distress syndrome, pneumonia, cystic fibrosis, pneumothorax, pulmonary edema, pleural effusion, submersion injury, congenital diaphragmatic hernia, abdominal distention, muscular dystrophy, paralytic conditions (e.g., poliomyelitis, botulism), and severe structural obstructions such as severe scoliosis.

In **primary inefficient gas transfer** there is insufficient alveolar ventilation for carbon dioxide removal or impaired oxygenation of pulmonary capillary blood as a result of dysfunction of the respiratory control mechanism or a diffusion defect. Causes of respiratory center depression include cerebral trauma (e.g., birth injuries, shaken baby syndrome); intracranial tumors; CNS infection (e.g., meningitis, encephalitis); overdose with barbiturates, opioids, or benzodiazepines; severe asphyxia (e.g., hypercapnia, hypoxemia); and tetanus. Pulmonary diffusion defects include pulmonary edema, fibrosis, embolism, or hypertension; collagen disorders; *Pneumocystis carinii* pneumonia; anemia; and hemorrhage.

Recognition of Respiratory Failure

Respiratory failure that occurs as a result of acute obstruction of a major airway or cardiac arrest is sudden and readily apparent. Gradual and more covert development of signs and symptoms is less easily recognized. Evaluation of respiratory adequacy is based on both clinical assessment and laboratory studies.

Unless respiratory arrest occurs suddenly, signs of hypoxemia and hypercapnia are usually subtle in their development, becoming more obvious as respiratory failure progresses. The unknowing observer may attribute early signs such as mood changes and restlessness to other causes, and some signs can be altered by other factors. Clinical manifestations of respiratory failure are listed in Box 26.17.

In clinical situations in which impaired ventilation can be anticipated or clinical manifestations indicate impending hypoxemia, serial measurements of blood gases should be obtained and monitored to detect impending respiratory failure, and therapy should be implemented before respiratory acidosis becomes extreme.

NURSING CARE MANAGEMENT

Nursing observation and judgment are vital to successful management of respiratory failure. The interventions used in the management of respiratory failure are often dramatic, requiring special skills, and are frequently emergency procedures. If respiratory arrest occurs, the primary objectives are to recognize the situation and immediately initiate resuscitative measures, such as opening the airway and positioning, administering supplemental oxygen and positive pressure ventilation, suctioning, performing CPR, or intubating if the child's status continues to deteriorate.

When the situation is not an arrest, the suspicion of respiratory failure is confirmed by assessment, and the severity is defined by capillary

BOX 26.17 Clinical Manifestations of Respiratory Failure

Cardinal Signs
Restlessness
Tachypnea
Tachycardia
Diaphoresis

Early but Less Obvious Signs
Mood changes, such as euphoria or depression
Headache
Altered depth and pattern of respirations (increased work of breathing)
Hypertension
Exertional dyspnea
Anorexia
Increased cardiac output and urinary output
Central nervous system symptoms (e.g., decreased efficiency, impaired judgment, anxiety, confusion, restlessness, irritability, depressed level of consciousness)
Nasal flaring
Retractions
Expiratory grunting
Wheezing or prolonged expiration

Signs of More Severe Hypoxia
Hypotension
Depressed respirations
Dimness of vision
Bradycardia
Arrhythmias
Somnolence
Cyanosis, peripheral or central
Stupor
Coma
Dyspnea

or arterial blood gas analysis. Interventions such as administering supplemental oxygen, opening the airway, positioning, stimulation, suctioning, and early intubation may avert an arrest. When severity is established, an attempt is made to determine the underlying cause by thorough evaluation.

The principles of management are to (1) maintain ventilation and maximize oxygen delivery, (2) correct hypoxemia and hypercapnia, (3) treat the underlying cause, (4) minimize extrapulmonary organ failure, (5) apply specific and nonspecific therapy to control oxygen demands, and (6) anticipate complications. Monitoring the patient's condition is critical.

Observation and Monitoring

The nurse monitors the child to anticipate respiratory failure, determine a course of action, and assess the patient's response to treatment. Often the child is transferred to a pediatric ICU. The child is kept as comfortable as possible, and observation is geared toward general appearance, responsiveness, pulse oximetry, and vital signs. The child is positioned to allow maximum lung expansion and comfort, such as sitting upright or leaning forward (depending on respiratory status).

The nurse closely monitors the child's cardiac and respiratory status by observation and by electronic means. Because one goal of therapy is to control the body's oxygen demands, assessments of fever and pain should be frequent. Both conditions (as well as cold stress) can dramatically increase oxygen requirements, especially in younger children, and therefore increase respiratory effort. Measure oxygenation by the use of pulse oximetry or blood gas monitoring.

Family Support

Children who are in respiratory distress often relax after an airway is established and their respiratory effort is assisted. However, they are anxious and frightened when they are unable to communicate; therefore it is important to effectively manage the child's anxiety. This may be accomplished initially with mild sedation until the child's ventilatory status has improved. It is also stressful to parents to watch their child's inability to vocalize and helplessness. It is important to talk to the child and parents to reassure them that the child's voice will return when the breathing tube (endotracheal tube or tracheostomy) is removed. Assistive communication devices should be offered as appropriate to age and development (e.g., electronic pads, paper and pen, picture boards).

Parents are often concerned about the (often) life-threatening implications generated by the need for the procedure and the possible long-term residual effects on the brain and on the child's psychologic status. For families whose child had a respiratory arrest, support focuses on keeping the family informed of the child's status and helping them cope with a near-death experience or an actual death. (See Chapter 19.) Knowing that their child requires CPR is a frightening and often overwhelming experience for parents. Uncertainty regarding outcome—both mortality and morbidity—is a primary concern.

NCLEX REVIEW QUESTIONS

1. A 12-year-old child is in the urgent care clinic with a complaint of fever, headache, and sore throat. A diagnosis of group A β-hemolytic streptococcus (GABHS) pharyngitis is established with a rapid-strep test, and oral penicillin is prescribed. The nurse knows that which of the following statements about GABHS is correct?
   A. Children with a GABHS infection are less likely to contract the illness again after the antibiotic regimen is completed.
   B. A follow-up throat culture is recommended after the completion of antibiotic therapy.
   C. Children with a GABHS infection are at increased risk for the development of rheumatic fever and glomerulonephritis.
   D. Children with a GABHS infection are at increased risk for the development of rheumatoid arthritis in adulthood.
2. A 5-year-old is recovering from a tonsillectomy and adenoidectomy and is being discharged home with his mother. Home care instructions should include which of the following? Select all that apply.
   A. Observe the child for continuous swallowing.
   B. Encourage the child to take sips of cool, clear liquids.
   C. Administer codeine elixir as necessary for throat pain.
   D. Observe the child for restlessness or difficulty breathing.
   E. Encourage the child to cough every 4 to 5 hours to prevent pneumonia.
   F. Administer an analgesic such as acetaminophen for pain.
3. A 3-month-old infant is seen in the clinic with the following symptoms: irritability, crying, refusal to nurse for more than 2 to 3 minutes, rhinitis, and a rectal temperature of 101.8°F (38.8°C). The

labor, delivery, and postpartum history for this term infant is unremarkable. The nurse anticipates a diagnosis of:

A. Acute otitis media (AOM)
B. Otitis media with effusion (OME)
C. Otitis externa
D. Respiratory syncitial virus (RSV)

4. A 5-year-old is seen in the urgent care clinic with the following history and symptoms: sudden onset of severe sore throat after going to bed, drooling and difficulty swallowing, axillary temperature of 102.2°F (39.0°C), clear breath sounds, and absence of cough. The child appears anxious and is flushed. Based on these symptoms and history, the nurse anticipates a diagnosis of:

A. Group A β-hemolytic streptococcus (GABHS) pharyngitis
B. Acute tracheitis
C. Acute epiglottitis
D. Acute laryngotracheobronchitis

5. A 2-month-old formerly healthy infant born at term is seen in the urgent care clinic with intercostal retractions, respiratory rate of 62, heart rate of 128, refusal to breastfeed, abundant nasal secretions, and a pulse oximeter reading of 88% in room air. The diagnosis of respiratory syncytial virus is made. The infant's oxygen saturation remains 95% in room air, and the respiratory rate is 54, with intercostal retractions; heart rate is 120 beats per minute. After 2 hours of observation and an intravenous bolus of fluids, the infant is being discharged home. The nurse provides which of the following home care instructions for this infant? Select all that apply.

A. Continue breastfeeding infant.
B. Discontinue breastfeeding and administer Pedialyte for 24 hours.
C. Observe infant for labored breathing or apnea (cessation of breathing).
D. Instill normal saline drops in both nares and suction thoroughly before feeding and before placing to sleep.
E. Place infant to sleep on his side with the head of bed slightly elevated to facilitate breathing.
F. Keep the infant out of day care or nursery.

Correct Answers

1. C; 2. A, B, D, F; 3. A; 4. C; 5. A, C, D, F

REFERENCES

Abdallah, C. (2012). Acute epiglottitis: trends, diagnosis and management. *Saudi J Anaesth, 6*(3), 279–281.

American Academy of Otolaryngology—Head and Neck Surgery. (2011). Clinical practice guideline: tonsillectomy in children. *Bulletin, 19*, 6.

American Academy of Pediatrics, *Report of the Committee on Infectious Diseases, Pickering L, editor: 2015 Red book: Report of the Committee on Infectious Diseases, ed 30, Elk Grove Village, Ill*, 2015.

American Thoracic Society. (1996). Standards and indications for cardiopulmonary sleep studies in children. *American Journal of Respiratory and Critical Care Medicine, 153*(2), 866–878.

Amrock, S. M., Lee, L., & Weitzman, M. (2016). Perceptions of e-cigarettes and noncigarette tobacco products among US youth. *Pediatrics, 138*(5), e20154306.

Antoon, A. Y., & Donovan, M. K. (2016). Burn injuries. In R. M. Kliegman, B. F. Stanton, J. W. St. Geme, et al. (Eds.), *Nelson textbook of pediatrics* (20th ed.). Philadelphia: Saunders.

ARDS Definition Task Force, Ranieri, V. M., Rubenfeld, G. D., et al. (2012). Acute respiratory distress syndrome: the Berlin definition. *JAMA: The Journal of the American Medical Association, 307*(23), 2526–2533.

Belongia, E. A., Karron, R. A., Reingold, A., et al. (2018). The Advisory Committee on Immunization Practices recommendation regarding the use of live influenza vaccine: A rejoinder. *Vaccine, 36*(3), 343–344.

Bernard, G. R., Artigas, A., Brigham, K. L., et al. (1994). The American-European Consensus Conference on ARDS. Definitions, mechanisms, relevant outcomes, and clinical trial coordination. *American Journal of Respiratory and Critical Care Medicine, 149*(3 Pt. 1), 818–824.

Bjornson, C., Russell, K., Vandermeer, B., et al. (2013). Nebulized epinephrine for croup in children. *Cochrane Database of Systematic Review*, (10), CD006619.

Boudewyns, A., Abel, F., Alexopoulos, E., et al. (2017). Adenotonsillectomy to treat obstructive sleep apnea: is it enough? *Pediatric Pulmonology, 52*(5), 699–709.

Burgos, C. M., Modee, A., Ost, E., et al. (2017). Addressing the causes of later mortality in infants with congenital diaphragmatic hernia. *J Pediatric Surgery, 52*(4), 526.

Burton, M. J., Glasziou, P. P., Chong, L. Y., et al. (2014). Tonsillectomy or adenotonsillectomy versus non-surgical treatment for chronic/recurrent acute tonsillitis. *Cochrane Database of Systematic Review*, (11), CD001802.

Canistro, D., Vivarelli, F., Cirillo, S., et al. (2017). E-cigarettes induce toxicological effects that can raise the cancer risk. *Scientific Reports, 7*(1), 2028.

Castellani, C., & Assael, B. M. (2017). Cystic fibrosis: a clinical view. *Cellular and Molecular Life Sciences, 74*(1), 129–140.

Centers for Disease Control and Prevention: *Most recent asthma data*, 2017. Retrieved from https://www.cdc.gov/asthma/most_recent_data.htm.

Centers for Disease Control and Prevention: *Epidemiology of pediatric tuberculosis in the United States, 1993-2015*, https://www.cdc.gov/tb/publications/slidesets/pediatrictb/, 2016.

Chu, H. Y., & Englund, J. A. (2013). Respiratory syncytial virus disease: prevention and treatment. *Current Topics in Microbiology and Immunology, 372*, 235–258.

Chun, L. F., Moazed, F., Calfee, C. S., et al. (2017). Pulmonary toxicity of e-cigarettes. *American Journal of Physiology. Lung Cellular and Molecular Physiology, 313*(2), L193–L206.

Clarke, K. E. N. (2017). Can I give my 5-year-old over-the-counter cough medicine? *American Academy of Pediatrics*, Retrieved from https://healthychildren.org/English/tips-tools/ask-the-pediatrician/Pages/Can-I-give-my-5-year-old-cough-medicine.aspx.

Coates, B. M., Camarda, L. E., & Goodman, D. M. (2016). Wheezing, bronchiolitis, and bronchitis. In R. M. Kliegman, B. F. Stanton, J. W. St. Geme, et al. (Eds.), *Nelson textbook of pediatrics* (20th ed.). Philadelphia: Elsevier/Saunders.

Cystic Fibrosis Foundation: *Infection prevention and control clinical care guidelines*, 2013. Retrieved from https://www.cff.org/Care/Clinical-Care-Guidelines/Infection-Prevention-and-Control-Clinical-Care-Guidelines/Infection-Prevention-and-Control-Clinical-Care-Guidelines/.

Davies, A. (2015). Management of gastroenteritis in children under five years. *Nursing Standard, 29*(27), 51–57.

De Boeck, K., Haarman, E., Hull, J., et al. (2017). Inhaled dry powder mannitol in children with cystic fibrosis: a randomised efficacy and safety trial. *Journal of Cystic Fibrosis, 16*(3), 380–387.

Demeyer, S., De Boeck, K., Witters, P., et al. (2016). Beyond pancreatic insufficiency and liver disease in cystic fibrosis. *European Journal of Pediatrics, 175*(7), 881–894.

Egan, M., Green, D. M., & Voynow, J. A. (2016). Cystic fibrosis. In R. M. Kliegman, B. F. Stanton, J. W. St. Geme, et al. (Eds.), *Nelson textbook of pediatrics* (20th ed.). Philadelphia: Elsevier/Saunders.

Evlampidou, I., Bagkeris, M., Vardavas, C., et al. (2015). Prenatal second-hand smoke exposure measured with urine cotinine may reduce gross motor development at 18 months of age. *The Journal of Pediatrics, 167*(2), 246–252.

Falk, N. P., Hughes, S. W., & Rodgers, B. C. (2016). Medications for chronic asthma. *American Family Physician, 94*(6), 454–462.

Food and Drug Administration: *Safety: Singulair (montelukast sodium) tablets, chewable tablets, and oral granules: safety labeling changes*, 2013. Retrieved from http://www.fda.gov/Safety/MedWatch/SafetyInformation/ucm285264.htm.

Food and Drug Administration News Release: *FDA approves Odactra for house dust mite allergies*, 2017. Retrieved from https://www.fda.gov/NewsEvents/Newsroom/PressAnnouncements/ucm544330.htm.

Food and Drug Administration Briefing Document: *Allergenic Products Advisory Committee: Clinical Development of Allergen Immunotherapies for the treatment of Food Allergy*, 2016. Retrieved from https://www.fda.gov/downloads/AllergenicProductsAdvisoryCommittee/UCM482114.pdf.

Friedmann, I., Dahdouh, E. M., Kugler, P., et al. (2017). Maternal and obstetrical predictors of sudden infant death syndrome (SIDS). *The Journal of Maternal-fetal and Neonatal Medicine*, *30*(19), 2315–2323.

Garcia, A., & Stolar, C. J. H. (2012). Congenital diaphragmatic hernia and protective ventilation strategies in pediatric surgery. *Surg Clin N Am*, *92*(3), 659–668.

Garland, J. S. (2010). Strategies to prevent ventilator-associated pneumonia in neonates. *Clinics in Perinatology*, *37*(3), 629–643.

Goralski, J. L., & Donaldson, S. H. (2014). Hypertonic saline for cystic fibrosis: worth its salt? *Expert Rev Respir Med*, *8*(3), 267–269.

Griffin, E. S., & Young, T. M. (2015). Bacterial tracheitis in a 9-month-old child. *Journal of Emergency Nursing*, *41*(2), 109–112.

Griffiths, B., Kew, K. M., & Normansell, R. (2016). Intravenous magnesium sulfate for treating children with acute asthma in the emergency department. *Paediatric Respiratory Reviews*, *20*, 45–47.

Guidry, C. A., Hranjec, T., Rodgers, B. M., et al. (2012). Permissive hypercapnia in the management of congenital diaphragmatic hernia: our institutional experience. *Journal of the American College of Surgeons*, *214*(4), 640–645, 647.

Howard, D., Finn Davis, K., Phillips, E., et al. (2014). Pain management for pediatric tonsillectomy: an integrative review through the perioperative and home experience. *J Specialist Pediatr Nurs*, *19*(1), 5–16.

Ingram, D. G., & Friedman, N. R. (2015). Toward adenotonsillectomy in children: as review for the general pediatrician. *JAMA Pediatr*, *169*(12), 1155–1161.

Isik, S. R., Ceilkel, S., Karakaya, G., et al. (2011). The effects of antidepressants on the results of skin prick tests used in the diagnosis of allergic diseases. *International Archives of Allergy and Immunology*, *154*(1), 63–68.

Jain, S., Williams, D. J., Arnold, S. R., et al. (2015). Community-acquired pneumonia requiring hospitalization among U.S. children. *The New England Journal of Medicine*, *372*(9), 835–845.

Jenson, H. (2016). Epstein-Barr virus. In R. M. Kliegman, B. F. Stanton, J. W. St. Geme, et al. (Eds.), *Nelson textbook of pediatrics* (20th ed.). Philadelphia: Elsevier/Saunders.

Kanchongkittiphon, W., Mendell, M. J., Gaffin, J. M., et al. (2015). Indoor environmental exposures and exacerbation of asthma: an update to the 2000 review by the Institute of Medicine. *Environmental Health Perspectives*, *123*(1), 6–20.

Kerschner, J. E., & Preciado, D. (2016). Otitis media. In R. M. Kliegman, B. F. Stanton, J. W. St. Geme, et al. (Eds.), *Nelson textbook of pediatrics* (20th ed.). Philadelphia: Elsevier/Saunders.

Kleinman, R. E., & Greer, F. R. (Eds.), (2014). *Pediatric nutrition* (7th ed). Elk Grove Village, IL: American Academy of Pediatrics.

Kline-Tilford, A. M., Sorce, L. R., Levin, D. L., et al. (2013). Pulmonary disorders. In M. F. Hazinski (Ed.), *Nursing care of the critically ill child* (3rd ed.). St. Louis: Elsevier.

Korvel-Hanquist, A., Djurhuus, B. D., & Homoe, P. (2017). The effect of breastfeeding on childhood otitis media. *Current Allergy and Asthma Reports*, *17*(7), 45.

Kostic, M. A. (2016). Poisonings. In R. M. Kliegman, B. F. Stanton, J. W. St. Geme, et al. (Eds.), *Nelson textbook of pediatrics* (20th ed.). Philadelphia: Elsevier/Saunders.

Lin, S. Y., Erekosima, N., Kim, J. M., et al. (2013). Sublingual immunotherapy for the treatment of allergic rhinoconjunctivitis and asthma: a systematic review. *JAMA: The Journal of the American Medical Association*, *309*(12), 1278–1288.

Liu, A. H., Covar, R. A., Spahn, J. D., et al. (2016). Childhood asthma. In R. M. Kliegman, B. F. Stanton, J. W. St. Geme, et al. (Eds.), *Nelson textbook of pediatrics* (20th ed.). Philadelphia: Saunders.

Livingston, M. H., Colozza, S., Vogt, K. N., et al. (2016). Making the transition from video-assisted thoracoscopic surgery to chest tube with fibrinolytics for empyema in children: any change in outcomes? *Canadian Journal of Surgery. Journal Canadien de Chirurgie*, *59*(3), 167–171.

Lonie, S., Baker, P., & Teixeira, R. (2016). Steam vaporizers: a danger for paediatric burns. *Burns: Journal of the International Society for Burn Injuries*, *42*(8), 1850–1853.

Lopez-Fernandez, Y., Azagra, A. M., de la Oliva, P., et al. (2012). Pediatric acute lung injury epidemiology and natural history study: Incidence and outcome of the acute respiratory distress syndrome in children. *Critical Care Medicine*, *40*(12), 3238–3245.

Lowry, J. A., & Leeder, J. S. (2015). Over-the-counter medications: update on cough and cold preparations. *Pediatrics in Review*, *36*(7), 286–297.

Maheshwari, A., & Carlo, W. A. (2016). Diaphragmatic hernia. In R. M. Kliegman, B. F. Stanton, J. W. St. Geme, et al. (Eds.), *Nelson textbook of pediatrics* (20th ed.). Philadelphia: Elsevier/Saunders.

Makadia, L. D., Roper, P. F., Andrews, J. O., et al. (2017). Tobacco use and smoke exposure in children: new trends, harm, and strategies to improve health outcomes. *Current Allergy and Asthma Reports*, *17*(8), 55.

Mazor, R., & Green, T. P. (2016). Pulmonary edema. In R. M. Kliegman, B. F. Stanton, J. W. St. Geme, et al. (Eds.), *Nelson textbook of pediatrics* (20th ed.). Philadelphia: Elsevier/Saunders.

Mejias, A., & Ramilo, O. (2015). New options in the treatment of respiratory syncytial virus disease. *The Journal of Infection*, *71*(Suppl1), S80–S87.

Milgrom, H., & Sicherer, S. H. (2016). Allergic rhinitis. In R. M. Kliegman, B. F. Stanton, J. W. St. Geme, et al. (Eds.), *Nelson textbook of pediatrics* (20th ed.). Philadelphia: Elsevier/Saunders.

Mitselou, N., Hedlin, G., & Hederos, C. A. (2016). Spacers versus nebulizers in treatment of acute asthma – a prospective randomized study in preschool children. *The Journal of Asthma*, *53*(10), 1059–1062.

Morad, A., Sathe, N. A., Francis, D. O., et al. (2017). Tonsillectomy versus watchful waiting for recurrent throat infection: a systematic review. *Pediatrics*, *139*(2), e20163490.

Moualed, D., Masterson, L., Kumar, S., et al. (2016). Water precautions for preventon of infection in children with ventilation tubes (grommets). *Cochrane Database of Systematic Review*, CD010375.

Mussman, G. M., Parker, M. W., Statile, A., et al. (2013). Suctioning and lengths of stay in infants hospitalized with bronchiolitis. *JAMA Pediatr*, *167*(5), 414–421.

National Asthma Education and Prevention Program (2007). *Expert Panel Report 3: guidelines for the diagnosis and management of asthma*. Bethesda, MD: National Heart Lung and Blood Institute, National Institutes of Health. Retrieved from https://www.nhlbi.nih.gov/guidelines/asthma/01_front.pdf.

National Heart, Lung, and Blood Institute: *What is asthma?* 2014. Retrieved from https://www.nhlbi.nih.gov/health/health-topics/topics/asthma/.

Oluyomi-Obi, T., Kuret, V., Puligandla, P., et al. (2017). Antenatal predictors of outcome in prenatally diagnosed congenital diaphragmatic hernia (CDH). *Journal of Pediatric Surgery*, *52*(5), 881–888.

Owens, J. A. (2016). Sleep medicine. In R. M. Kliegman, B. F. Stanton, J. W. St. Geme, et al. (Eds.), *Nelson textbook of pediatrics* (20th ed.). Philadelphia: Elsevier/Saunders.

Pedra, P. A., & Stark, A. R.: *Bronchiolitis in infants and children: Treatment outcome and prevention, In UpToDate, Mallory GB and Edwards MS (Ed), UpToDate, Waltham MA*, 2017.

Petrocheilou, A., Tanou, K., Kalampouka, E., et al. (2014). Viral croup: diagnosis and a treatment algorithm. *Pediatric Pulmonology*, *49*, 421–429.

Pinfield, J., Gaskin, K., Bentley, J., et al. (2015). Recognition and management of asthma in children and young people. *Nursing Standard*, *39*(3), 50–58.

Powell, J., Graham, D., O'Reilly, S., et al. (2016). Acute pulmonary oedema. *Nursing Standard*, *39*(23), 51–59.

Quick, V. M., Byrd-Bredbenner, C., & Neumark-Sztainer, D. (2013). Chronic illness and disordered eating: a discussion of the literature. *Advances in Nutrition*, *4*(3), 277–286.

Ren, X. C., Gao, Z. W., Li, Y. F., et al. (2017). The effects of clinical factors on airway outcomes of mandibular distraction osteogenesis in children with Pierre Robin sequence. *International Journal of Oral and Maxillofacial Surgery*, *46*(7), 805–810.

Roosevelt, G. E. (2016). Acute inflammatory upper airway obstruction. In R. M. Kliegman, B. F. Stanton, J. W. St. Geme, et al. (Eds.), *Nelson textbook of pediatrics* (20th ed.). Philadelphia: Elsevier/Saunders.

Rosenfeld, R. M., Shin, J. J., Schwartz, S. R., et al. (2016). Clinical practice guideline: otitis media with effusion (update). *Otolaryngology–Head and Neck Surgery: Official Journal of American Academy of Otolaryngology-Head and Neck Surgery, 154*(2), 201–214.

Saiman, L., Siegel, J. D., LiPuma, J. T., et al. (2014). Infection prevention and control guideline for cystic fibrosis: 2013 update. *Infection Control & Hospital Epidemiology, 35*(S1), S1–S67.

Samet, J. M., Chanson, D., & Wipfli, H. (2015). The challenges of limiting exposure to THS in vulnerable populations. *Curr Environ Health Rep, 2*(3), 215–225.

Santhi, N., Ramsey, D., Phillipson, G., et al. (2017). Efficacy of a topical aromatic rub (Vicks VapoRub) on effects on self-reported and actigraphically assessed aspects of sleep in common cold patients. *Open Journal of Respiratory Diseases, 7*, 83–101.

Schuh, S., Sweeney, J., Freedman, S. B., et al. (2016). Magnesium nebulization utilization in management of pediatric asthma (MagNUM PA) trial: study protocol for a randomized controlled trial. *Trials, 17*(1), 261.

Schwengel, D. A., Dalesio, N. M., & Stierer, T. L. (2014). Pediatric obstructive sleep apnea. *Anesthesiology Clinics, 32*(1), 237–261.

Siddiq, S., & Grainger, J. (2015). The diagnosis and management of acute otitis media: American Academy of Pediatrics guidelines 2013. *Arch Dis Child Educ Pract Ed, 100*(4), 193–197.

Smith, B. A., Georgiopoulos, A. M., & Quittner, A. L. (2016). Maintaining mental health and function for the long run in cystic fibrosis. *Pediatric Pulmonology, 51*(S44), S71–S78.

Smith, D. K., Seales, S., & Budzik, C. (2017). Respiratory syncytial virus bronchiolitis in children. *American Family Physician, 95*(2), 94–99.

Sobin, L., Kawai, K., Irace, A. L., et al. (2017). Microbiology of the upper and lower airways in pediatric cystic fibrosis patients. *Otolaryngology–Head and Neck Surgery: Official Journal of American Academy of Otolaryngology-Head and Neck Surgery, 157*(2), 302–308.

Speer, M. E.: *Neonatal pneumonia*, In J.A. Barcia-Prats and M.S. Edwards (Eds.), Up to Date, 2017.

Steele, D. W., Adam, G. P., Di, M., et al. (2017). Effectiveness of tympanostomy tubes for otitis media: a meta-analysis, *Pediatrics* epub ahead of print.

Thaker, V., Haagensen, A. L., Carter, B., et al. (2015). Recombinant growth hormone therapy for cystic fibrosis in children and young adults. *Cochrane Database of Systematic Review*, (5), CD008901.

The Pediatric Acute Lung Injury Consensus Conference Group. (2015). Pediatric acute respiratory distress syndrome: consensus recommendations from the pediatric acute lung injury consensus conference. *Pediatric Critical Care Medicine Journal, 16*(5), 428–439.

Thomson, N. C., & Chaudhuri, R. (2012). Omalizumab: clinical use for the management of asthma. *Clin Med Insights Circ Respir Pulm Med, 6*(1), 27–40.

Turck, D., Braegger, C. P., Colombo, C., et al. (2016). ESPEN-ESPGHAN-ECFS guidelines on nutrition care for infant, children, and adults with cystic fibrosis. *Clinical Nutrition: Official Journal of the European Society of Parenteral and Enteral Nutrition, 35*(3), 557–577.

van Loo, A., van Loo, E., Selvadurai, H., et al. (2014). Intrapleural urokinase versus surgical management of childhood empyema. *Journal of Paediatrics and Child Health, 50*(10), 823–826.

Venekamp, R. P., Damoiseaux, R. A., & Schilder, A. G. (2017). Acute otitis media in children. *American Family Physician, 95*(2), 109–110.

Verma, N., Lodha, R., & Kabra, S. K. (2013). Recent advances in management of bronchoiolitis. *Indian Pediatrics, 50*(10), 939–949.

Walter, H., Sadeque-Igbal, F., Ulysse, R., et al. (2015). The effectiveness of school-based family asthma educational programs on the quality of life and number of asthma exacerbations of children aged five to 18 years diagnosed with asthma: a systematic review protocol. *JBI Databased System Rev Implement Rep, 13*(10), 69–81.

Wong, J. J., Jit, M., Sultana, R., et al. (2017). Mortality in pediatric acute respiratory distress syndrome: a systematic review and meta-analysis. *Journal of Intensive Care Medicine*, epub ahead of print.

World Health Organization: *TB: global tuberculosis report* 2017. Retrieved from http://www.who.int/mediacentre/factsheets/fs104/en/.

Xu, X., Bishop, E. E., Kennedy, S. M., et al. (2015). Annual healthcare spending attributable to cigarette smoking: an update. *American Journal of Preventive Medicine, 48*(3), 326–333.

Yang, C., Chilvers, M., Montgomery, M., et al. (2016). Dornase alfa for cystic fibrosis. *Cochrane Database of Systematic Review*, (4), CD001127.

27

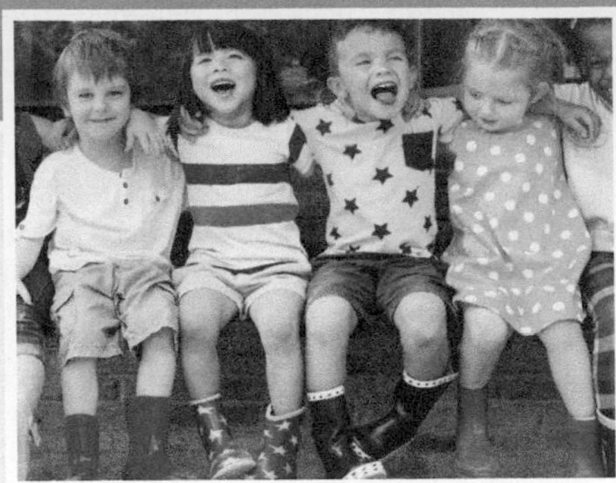

The Child With Cardiovascular Dysfunction

Margaret L. Schroeder, Annette L. Baker, Heather Bastardi, and Patricia O'Brien

http://evolve.elsevier.com/wong/ncic

CONCEPTS

- Perfusion
- Hemodynamics

CARDIAC STRUCTURE AND FUNCTION

Cardiovascular disorders in children are divided into two major groups: congenital cardiac defects and acquired heart disorders. Congenital heart defects are anatomic abnormalities present at birth that result in abnormal cardiac function. The clinical consequences of congenital heart defects fall into two broad categories: heart failure (HF) and hypoxemia. *Acquired cardiac disorders* refer to disease processes or abnormalities that occur after birth and can be seen in the normal heart or in the presence of congenital heart defects. They result from various factors, including infection, autoimmune responses, environmental factors, and familial tendencies.

Understanding the effects of congenital and acquired heart defects requires knowledge of the normal heart's structure and function, including embryologic development, fetal circulation, and postnatal changes. Basic cardiac physiology is presented in this section; altered hemodynamics are discussed on p. 967.

CARDIAC DEVELOPMENT AND FUNCTION

The heart is a muscular four-chambered organ whose primary purpose is to pump blood throughout the body. It is located slightly to the left of the sternum in the space between the two pleural cavities, called the **mediastinum**. The main mass of the heart is formed by the muscular tissue, the myocardium. Lining the inner surface of the myocardium is the endocardium, a thin layer of endothelial tissue. The heart also has its own special covering, a double-walled membrane called the **pericardium**. Between the two layers is a slight space (pericardial space), which is filled with a few drops of serous fluid (pericardial fluid). These layers provide for frictionless movement of the heart muscle.

The interior of the heart is divided into four chambers. The two upper chambers are called **atria**, and the two bottom chambers are called **ventricles**. The atria are divided into the right atrium (RA) and the left atrium (LA) by the atrial septum. The ventricles are divided into the right ventricle (RV) and the left ventricle (LV) by the ventricular septum. Located within the heart are four valves, whose main function is to prevent the backflow of blood. The tricuspid valve, so named because it has three leaflets, or cusps, of endocardial tissue projecting into the ventricles, is located between the RA and the RV. The mitral valve has two leaflets and is located between the LA and the LV. Together these two valves are often termed **atrioventricular (AV) valves**. The valve leaflets are attached to the heart muscle by several cordlike structures called **chordae tendineae**. The semilunar valves are located in the pulmonary artery (pulmonic valve) and the aorta (aortic valve). Heart sounds (S_1 and S_2) are related to the vibrations that result during closing of these valves. (See Chapter 4.)

Embryologic Development

The heart and other components of the circulatory system (blood, blood vessels, lymph) begin to develop from the mesoderm during the fourth week of gestation and are completely formed by the eighth week.

During the third week, two endocardial tubes fuse to become the heart tube. As the tube elongates, it begins to coil to the right (dextro- or d-looping). This looping occurs by approximately the twenty-eighth day, when the heart begins to beat. Concentrations of mesenchymal cells enlarge and cause their lining (endocardium) to bulge into the heart lumen. These internal bulges are called *endocardial cushions* and eventually merge to divide the heart chambers. During the fifth week, the midcardiac tube grows rapidly and assumes a characteristic convoluted shape with identifiable structures. These structures ultimately give rise to the heart chambers and great vessels and include (1) a common atrium; (2) a common ventricle; (3) the bulbus cordis, which eventually helps form the outflow tracts of the ventricles; (4) the sinus venosus, which develops into the inferior and superior vena cava and coronary sinus; and (5) the truncus arteriosus, which divides into the pulmonary artery and aorta and also gives rise to the aortic arch.

The atrial septum is formed by the growth of both the septum primum and the septum secundum at about the fourth week of fetal development. Overlapping of the septum primum and septum secundum before fusion occurs results in a temporary flap opening known as the foramen ovale. The ventricular septum develops from the joining of the muscular and membranous ventricular septa during the fourth to eighth weeks of growth (Fig. 27.1). Congenital defects may result if disturbances occur in the formation of various structures during this partitioning process.

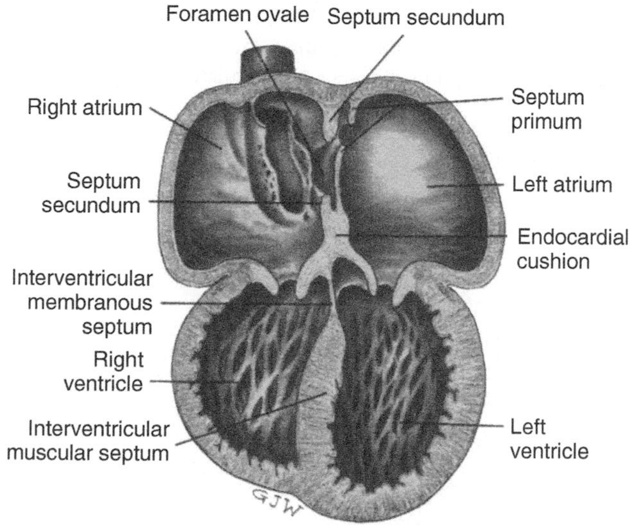

FIG. 27.1 Septal development of the heart.

Fetal Circulation

The fetal circulation directs the maximum concentration of oxygenated blood to the most vital organ, the brain. During fetal life, the lungs are essentially nonfunctional, and the liver is only partially functional so the fetus needs less blood directed to these organs.

Blood carrying oxygen and nutritive materials from the placenta enters the fetal system through the umbilicus via the large umbilical vein (Fig. 27.2, *A*). The blood then travels to the liver, where it divides. Part of the blood enters the portal and hepatic circulation of the liver, and the remainder travels directly to the inferior vena cava (IVC) by way of the ductus venosus. Because of the higher pressure of blood entering the RA from the IVC, it is directed in a straight pathway across the RA and through the foramen ovale to the LA. In this way, the better-oxygenated blood enters the LA and LV to be pumped through the aorta to the head and upper extremities. Blood from the head and upper extremities entering the RA from the superior vena cava (SVC) is directed downward through the tricuspid valve into the RV. From there it is pumped through the pulmonary artery, where the major portion is shunted to the descending aorta via the ductus arteriosus. A small amount flows to and from the nonfunctioning fetal lungs. Blood is returned to the placenta from the descending aorta through the two umbilical arteries.

Before birth, the high pulmonary vascular resistance created by the collapsed fetal lung causes greater pressures in the right side of the heart and the pulmonary artery. At the same time, the free-flowing placental circulation and the ductus arteriosus produce a low systemic vascular resistance in the remainder of the fetal vascular system.

Postnatal Circulation

With the clamping of the umbilical cord and the expansion of the lungs at birth, the hemodynamics of the fetal vascular system undergoes pronounced and abrupt changes. The low-pressure placenta is removed from the circulation, the heart takes over pumping blood around the

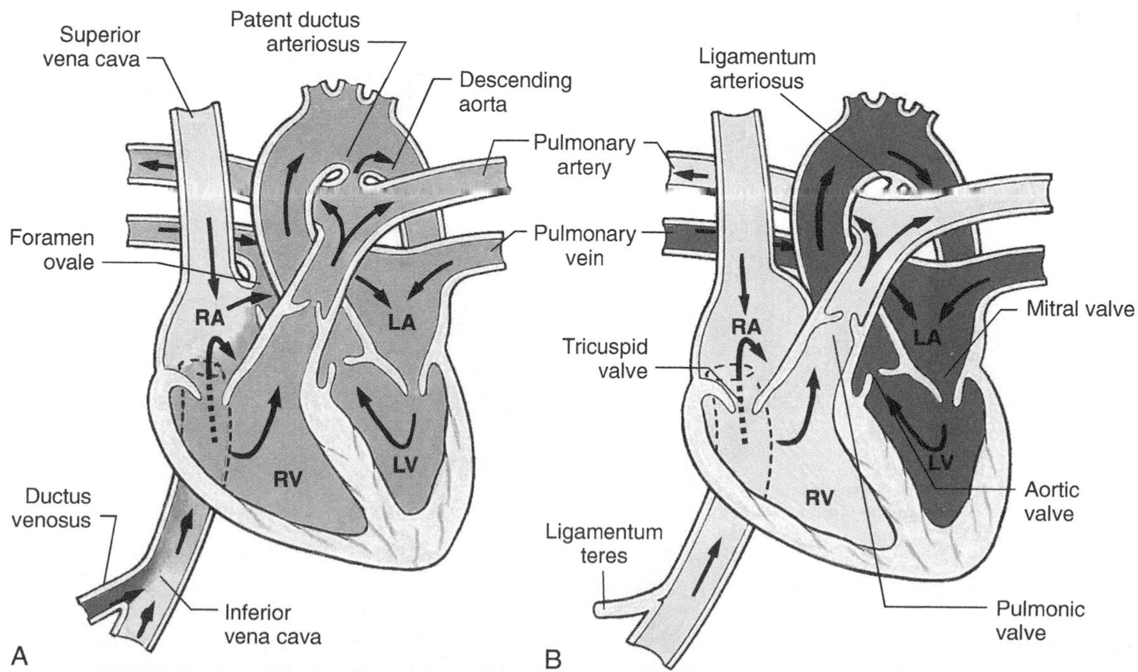

FIG. 27.2 Changes in circulation at birth. **A,** Prenatal circulation. **B,** Postnatal circulation. *Arrows* indicate direction of blood flow. Although four pulmonary veins enter the LA, for simplicity this diagram shows only two. *RA,* Right atrium; *LA,* left atrium; *RV,* right ventricle; *LV,* left ventricle.

body, and systemic vascular resistance starts to rise. With the postnatal rise in systemic vascular resistance, the LV walls become thicker than the walls of the RV, and the pressures on the left side of the heart rise. The lungs expand and take over oxygenation; the increased oxygen has a vasodilating effect on the pulmonary bed, causing a fall in pulmonary vascular resistance. Pressures on the right side of the heart decrease because the RV is pumping blood to the low-pressure pulmonary bed. The transition to a high-pressure systemic circulation and low-pressure pulmonary circulation (seen throughout life) usually takes 6 to 8 weeks.

The patent ductus arteriosus (PDA) starts to close within the first day after birth by constriction of smooth muscle in the vessel. Closure is influenced by oxygen levels, prostaglandin levels, and maturity. The PDA in a preterm infant responds differently, with less responsiveness to oxygen and higher levels of prostaglandins, both of which can cause delayed ductal closure. The PDA usually closes completely by 2 to 3 weeks of age (Park, 2014).

After birth, the normal adult blood flow patterns within the heart begin. Blood returning from the body via the SVC and IVC is received in the RA. It flows to the RV through the tricuspid valve. The RV pumps the blood through the pulmonic valve into the pulmonary artery and then to the lungs, where the blood becomes saturated with oxygen. The blood is then returned from the lungs via the pulmonary veins into the LA, where it flows through the mitral valve to the LV, and finally through the aortic valve to the aorta and into the systemic circulation (see Fig. 27.2, *B*).

Arteries are thicker-walled blood vessels with thin muscular layers that carry highly oxygenated blood away from the heart to the capillary bed, which supplies oxygen and nutrients to the tissues. Veins are thin-walled blood vessels that return desaturated blood to the heart. The arterial system provides resistance to blood flow to maintain blood pressure (BP) and circulation. The venous system acts as a collecting system and a reservoir to accommodate changes in circulating blood volume. Both work together to provide equilibrium and maintain BP.

The heart muscle receives its blood supply through the coronary circulation during diastole. The right and left coronary arteries, which arise above the aortic valve, supply all of the myocardium. The heart is the first organ to receive blood with each heartbeat; the brain is next. These two organs depend most on adequate oxygen levels for normal function. Coronary veins collect the blood and return it to the RA directly or through the coronary sinus, which drains into the RA. The flow of blood throughout the systemic circulatory system is shown in Fig. 27.3.

Conduction System

To maintain an orderly and effective pumping action, the heart has a specialized electrical conduction system. Electrical impulses generated

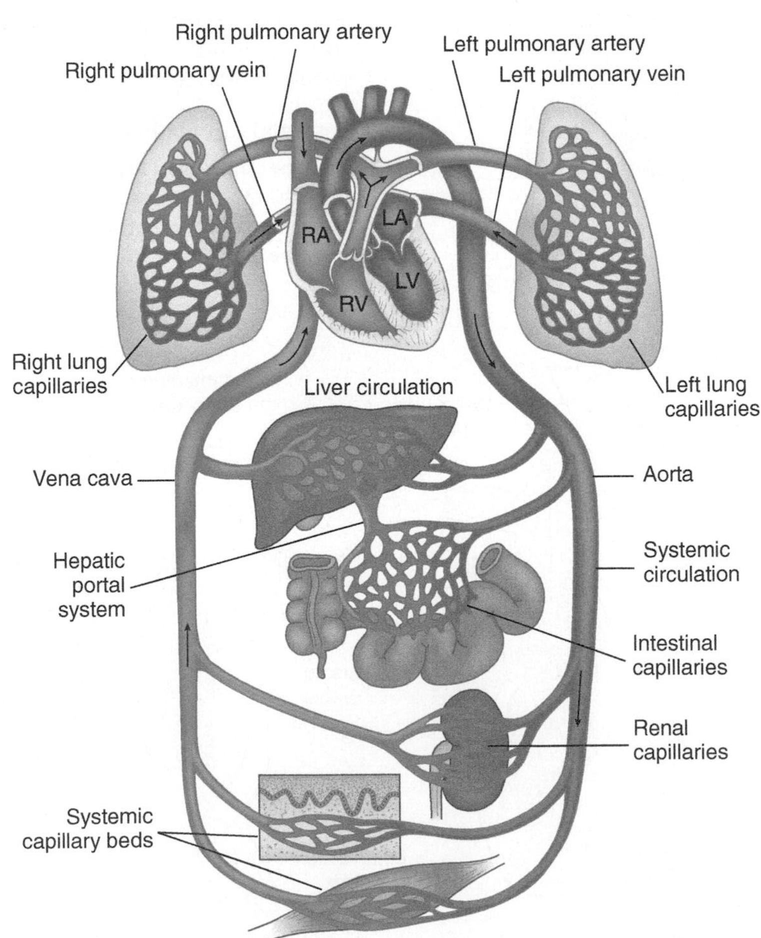

FIG. 27.3 Diagram showing serially connected pulmonary and systemic circulatory systems and how to trace the flow of blood. Right heart chambers propel unoxygenated blood through the pulmonary circulation, and the left side of the heart propels oxygenated blood through the systemic circulation. See Fig. 27.2 for abbreviations. (From McCance, K. L., & Huether, S. E. [2010]. *Pathophysiology: The biological basis for disease in adults and children* [6th ed.]. St. Louis, MO: Mosby.)

within the heart initiate the mechanical contraction that leads to the circulation of blood. Although all myocardial cells are capable of developing an action potential and depolarizing without external stimulation, certain specialized cells make up the heart's normal conduction system. These structures include the following:

- **Sinoatrial (SA) node,** located within the RA wall near the opening of the SVC
- **AV node,** also located within the RA but near the lower end of the septum
- **AV bundle (bundle of His),** which extends from the AV node along each side of the interventricular septum and then divides into right and left bundle branches
- **Purkinje fibers,** which extend from the AV bundle into the walls of the ventricles

The SA node is normally the heart's pacemaker and initiates an impulse. The impulse spreads from the SA node throughout the atria to cause depolarization. As the atria depolarize, impulses spread to the AV node to conduct to the ventricles. The AV node is the major pathway by which the impulses from the atria can be transmitted to the ventricles. The impulses then spread to the AV bundle and Purkinje fibers to cause simultaneous depolarization of the ventricles.

A cardiac cycle is composed of sequential contraction (systole) and relaxation (diastole) of both the atria and the ventricles. First, the atria contract, ejecting blood into the relaxed ventricles. Then, as the atria relax, the ventricles contract to eject blood into the pulmonary artery and aorta. During diastole, blood enters the atria from the systemic and pulmonary veins, which completes one cardiac cycle. The coronary arteries fill in diastole.

Basic Cardiac Physiology

The heart is basically a complex pump, ejecting blood throughout the body. The heart and lungs function together to deliver oxygen to the tissues and remove waste products such as carbon dioxide. The primary function of the cardiopulmonary system is to provide effective oxygen transport to meet the body's metabolic needs. To perform this function, the heart must maintain an adequate cardiac output. By definition, cardiac output is the volume of blood ejected by the heart in 1 minute. This is calculated by multiplying the heart rate (number of beats per minute) by the stroke volume. Stroke volume is the amount of blood ejected by the heart in any one contraction. Three factors influence stroke volume: preload, afterload, and contractility.

Cardiac output = Heart rate × Stroke volume

↑

Preload

Afterload

Contractility

The autonomic nervous system influences heart rate. The sympathetic fibers increase heart rate, and the parasympathetic fibers, acting through the vagus nerve, decrease heart rate. Levels of circulating catecholamines and other hormones also influence heart rate. Generally, an increase in heart rate increases cardiac output, and a decrease or irregularity in heart rate (bradycardia, dysrhythmia) impairs cardiac output. However, a very fast heart rate shortens diastole and impairs coronary artery perfusion, which causes eventual impairment of cardiac muscle function.

In simple terms, preload is the volume of blood returning to the heart, or the circulating blood volume. In physiologic terms, preload refers to myocardial fiber length. If the amount of blood delivered to the heart increases, the myocardial fibers lengthen, and a greater amount of blood is pumped out of the heart. The circulating blood volume is easiest to assess clinically using the central venous pressure (CVP).

Afterload refers to the resistance against which the ventricles must pump when ejecting blood (ventricular ejection). Conditions that make it more difficult for the heart to pump blood forward into the circulation (e.g., severe hypertension) increase the afterload. Afterload is determined by several complex factors, primarily the relative resistances of the systemic circulation (systemic vascular resistance) and the pulmonary circulation (pulmonary vascular resistance). Clinically, in the absence of hemodynamic monitoring, measurement of arterial BP gives some indication of afterload. Higher BP indicates greater afterload.

Contractility refers to the efficiency of myocardial fiber shortening, or the ability of the cardiac muscle to act as an efficient pump. There is no simple bedside technique to assess contractility, although an echocardiogram may be useful. Contractility is often inferred in clinical practice. Assessments of peripheral tissue perfusion (pulses, warmth of extremities, and capillary refill) and urinary output can be helpful. Decreased contractility is suspected if the extremities are cool with thready pulses and urinary output is diminished. Certain states are known to depress contractility (e.g., hypoxia, acidosis).

Adequate systemic perfusion depends on an appropriate heart rate, adequate circulating blood volume, efficient pump function, appropriate systemic and pulmonary vascular resistances, capillary permeability, and tissue utilization of oxygen. The body makes frequent adjustments in the various determinants of cardiac output to maintain a steady state. Cardiac output is often low in the early postoperative period after cardiac surgery.

Several clinical examples are useful to illustrate these principles. The Starling law (Frank-Starling curve) demonstrates that an increase in ventricular end-diastolic volume (caused by an increased preload) somewhat increases stroke volume. Because the myocardial fibers can stretch only to a certain point and still function effectively, any increase in volume beyond this point impairs cardiac output. When decreased cardiac output results from decreased preload (e.g., in hypovolemia due to blood loss), treatment involves providing volume, either with intravenous (IV) fluids or blood products. If decreased cardiac output results from a dramatic increase in afterload (e.g., severe hypertension) that increases the myocardial workload, treatment involves reducing afterload with vasodilating drugs. Medications such as digoxin (Lanoxin) or IV inotropic agents such as dopamine (Intropin) or dobutamine (Dobutrex) enhance contractility. Adjustments in heart rate are the most common response to changes in cardiac output. The heart rate is slowest during sleep and can more than double with strenuous physical exercise.

ASSESSMENT OF CARDIAC FUNCTION

History

Taking an accurate health history is an important first step in assessing an infant or child for possible heart disease. Parents may have specific concerns, such as poor feeding or fast breathing in their infant or the inability of their 7-year-old to keep up with his friends on the soccer field. Other parents may not realize that their child has a medical problem; the child may always have been pale and a fussy baby.

Asking details about the mother's health history, pregnancy, and birth history is important in assessing infants. Mothers with chronic health conditions, such as diabetes or lupus erythematosus, are more likely to have infants with heart disease. Some medications, such as phenytoin (Dilantin), are teratogenic to the fetus. Maternal alcohol use or illicit drug use increases the risk of congenital heart defects. Exposure to infection, such as rubella, early in pregnancy may result in congenital anomalies. Infants with low birth weight because of intrauterine growth restriction are more likely to have congenital anomalies. High-birth-weight infants, often offspring of diabetic mothers, also have an increased incidence of heart disease.

A detailed family history is also important. There is an increased incidence of congenital cardiac defects if either parent or a sibling has a heart defect. Some diseases, such as Marfan syndrome and hypertrophic cardiomyopathy, are hereditary. A family history of frequent fetal loss, sudden infant death, and sudden death in adults may indicate heart disease. Congenital heart defects occur in many disorders such as Down syndrome and Turner syndrome.

The health history of an infant should include details about feeding patterns, weight gain, and development. Feeding difficulties accompanied by fatigue, rapid breathing, and sweating with feeds and poor weight gain are common in infants with heart disease. The incidence of frequent respiratory infections and breathing problems should be noted. Parents should be asked about color changes, particularly cyanosis or pallor.

With older children and adolescents, history taking should include questions about exercise tolerance and activities, edema and respiratory problems, chest pain, palpitations, and neurologic problems such as fainting or headaches. Recent infections or toxic exposures may precede the development of heart diseases such as cardiomyopathy or rheumatic fever.

In all patients, a review of all other health problems and the presence of other congenital anomalies are important. All medications taken, including over-the-counter medications and herbal supplements, should be reviewed because prolonged or incorrect use of many medications can cause cardiac symptoms.

Physical Examination

Assessment of vital signs is helpful in screening patients for diseases of the cardiovascular system. A normal pulse rate varies with age. The younger the patient, the faster the rate. A heart rate that is abnormally fast (tachycardia) or abnormally slow (bradycardia) may indicate cardiac disease. It is important to note that an acceleration of the heart rate with inspiration is normal. A fast respiratory rate (tachypnea) may indicate HF. Hypertension is diagnosed by serial BP measurements.

> **! NURSING ALERT**
>
> A systolic BP difference between the upper and lower extremities with upper extremity hypertension and bounding pulses in the arms and reduced pulses in the legs is suggestive of coarctation of the aorta.

Several aspects of physical examination may yield evidence of heart disease. (See Chapter 4 for a general discussion of physical assessment of the heart.) During inspection, perform a general assessment of skin color (particularly the presence of cyanosis), position of comfort, and overall nutritional status. During palpation, establish the point of maximum intensity and the apical impulse because they may offer clues to the position of the heart. Note the presence of a thrill, a soft vibration over the heart that reflects the transmitted sound of a heart murmur. Assess the quality of chest activity ("active precordium"), quality and symmetry of all pulses, warmth of extremities, and presence or absence of edema. Locating the hepatic and splenic borders for evidence of organ enlargement is also important.

Auscultation of heart sounds begins with assessment of heart rate and rhythm. The normal heart sounds S_1 and S_2 are auscultated, and the normal physiologic splitting of S_2 is noted. This splitting is caused by the normal closure of the aortic valve before the pulmonic valve. The presence of additional heart sounds, such as a gallop or a murmur, is noted. Auscultation of lung sounds, in particular crackles, wheezing, grunting, or decreased or absent breath sounds in some areas, is also important in the assessment of cardiovascular disease.

Murmurs are heart sounds that reflect the flow of blood within the heart. They may occur in either systole or diastole or in both (a continuous murmur). They may reflect blood flow through a normal heart (particularly during periods of increased cardiac output such as fever, anemia, or rapid growth) or indicate abnormalities within the heart or the great arteries. (See Chapter 4 for a more detailed discussion of heart murmurs.) About 80% of children have an innocent murmur of one type at some point during childhood (Park, 2014). Innocent murmurs are present in infants and children with normal cardiac anatomy and heart function.

TESTS OF CARDIAC FUNCTION

A variety of invasive and noninvasive tests may be employed in the diagnosis of heart disease. Table 27.1 briefly outlines cardiac diagnostic procedures. The more frequently conducted tests are described here.

Electrocardiography

Electrocardiography (ECG or EKG) measures the electrical activity of the heart displayed in graphic form and provides information on heart rate and rhythm, abnormal rhythms or conduction, ischemic changes, and other information (Fig. 27.4). The normal ECG consists of the following:

P wave—Represents the spread of the impulse over the atria (atrial depolarization). The sinus node's electrical activity is not represented in the ECG.

P-R interval—Represents the time that elapses from the beginning of atrial depolarization to the beginning of ventricular depolarization. It is termed P-R instead of P-Q because the Q wave is frequently absent.

QRS complex—Represents ventricular depolarization. It is actually composed of three separate waves—the Q, the R, and the S—that result from the currents generated when the ventricles depolarize before their contraction.

T wave—Represents ventricular repolarization.

Q-T interval—Represents ventricular depolarization and repolarization. This interval varies with heart rate; the faster the rate, the shorter the Q-T interval. Therefore in children this interval is normally shorter than in adults.

ST segment—Represents the time that the ventricles are in the absolute refractory period, the period between ventricular depolarization and repolarization.

An ECG is taken by placing leads or electrodes on the skin to transmit electrical impulses back to a recording machine. Usually the electrodes are attached to the extremities and chest with an adhesive, such as hydrogel, or with a suction bulb. An electrolyte lubricant is placed between the skin and the lead to increase conductivity. Chest leads must be positioned correctly because even minor misplacement can cause considerable inaccuracy in the recording. The standard adult ECG is measured using 12 leads (6 limb leads and 6 chest leads). The standard pediatric ECG is measured using 15 leads, with leads added on the right side of the chest and on the left lateral chest area.

An ECG takes about 15 minutes to perform and the child must remain still while the tracing is done. Infants and young children may be fussy with lead placement. The leads can be frightening and may pull at the skin when being placed and removed. Infants and young children may be more cooperative if they can rest in the parent's lap during the procedure.

ECG has been adapted for ambulatory use to diagnose and monitor patients with arrhythmias. Continuous ambulatory monitoring is done

TABLE 27.1 Procedures for Cardiac Diagnosis

Procedure	Description
Chest radiography (x-ray)	Provides information on heart size and pulmonary blood flow patterns
Electrocardiography (ECG)	Graphic measure of electrical activity of heart
Holter monitoring	24-hour continuous ECG recording used to assess dysrhythmias
Echocardiography	Uses high-frequency sound waves obtained by a transducer to produce an image of cardiac structures
Transthoracic	Done with transducer on chest
M-mode	Provides one-dimensional graphic view to estimate ventricular size and function
Two-dimensional	Provides real-time, cross-sectional views of heart to identify cardiac structures and cardiac anatomy
Doppler	Shows blood flow patterns and pressure gradients across structures
Fetal	Images fetal heart in utero
Transesophageal	Uses transducer placed in esophagus behind heart to obtain images of posterior heart structures or improve views in patients with poor images from chest approach
Cardiac catheterization	Uses radiopaque catheters placed in a peripheral blood vessel and advanced into heart to measure pressures and oxygen levels in heart chambers and visualize heart structures and blood flow patterns
Hemodynamics	Measures pressures and oxygen saturations in heart chambers
Angiography	Involves injection of contrast material to illuminate heart structures and blood flow patterns
Biopsy	Employs special catheter to remove tiny samples of heart muscle for microscopic evaluation; used in assessing infection, inflammation, or muscle dysfunction disorders and to evaluate for rejection after heart transplantation
Electrophysiologic study	Employs special catheters with electrodes to record electrical activity from within heart; used to diagnose rhythm disturbances
Exercise stress test	Monitors heart rate, blood pressure, ECG, and oxygen consumption at rest and during progressive exercise on a treadmill or bicycle
Cardiac magnetic resonance imaging	Noninvasive imaging technique; allows evaluation of vascular anatomy outside of heart (e.g., coarctation of the aorta, vascular rings) and estimation of ventricular mass and volume

with a Holter monitor, a transistorized tape recorder attached to chest leads. Holter recording, often used when a child is having daily symptoms of a potential arrhythmia, records the heart rhythm continuously for 24 to 72 hours. The recording is then sent to a pediatric cardiologist to interpret. The child and the parents are instructed to keep a diary of activities so that any correlation between activity and any rhythm event may be interpreted. For intermittent rhythm events, an event monitor, which can be used when a child feels an abnormal rhythm, is often used. Implantable loop recorders can be placed under the skin for months to capture infrequent symptoms. There are now smart phone applications that can detect some arrhythmias (Haberman, Jahn, Bose, et al., 2015).

Bedside ECG cardiac monitoring is commonly used in pediatrics, especially in the care of children with heart disease. The bedside monitor provides valuable information about heart rate and rhythm through a graphic display of the ECG tracing and a digital display. An alarm can be set with parameters matched to individual patient requirements and will sound if the heart rate is above or below the set parameters. Gelfoam electrodes are commonly used and are placed on the right side of the chest (above the level of the heart) and on the left side of the chest; a ground electrode is placed on the abdomen (Fig. 27.5). Electrodes should be changed every 1 or 2 days because they irritate the skin. Bedside monitors are an adjunct to patient care and should never be substituted for direct assessment and auscultation of heart sounds. The nurse should assess the patient, not the monitor.

Echocardiography

Echocardiography is one of the most frequently used procedures for detecting cardiac dysfunction in children. Echocardiography involves the use of ultra-high-frequency sound waves to produce an image of the heart's structure. A transducer placed directly on the chest wall delivers repetitive pulses of ultrasound and processes the returned signals (echoes).

Recent improvements in echocardiographic technology allow the diagnosis of most congenital heart defects by noninvasive echo imaging. Many defects are now diagnosed prenatally with fetal echocardiography, and the number of infants diagnosed with heart defects in utero is rising.

There are three types of transthoracic echocardiography. Motion-mode (M-mode) echocardiography provides a one-dimensional view of the heart and is useful in determining its size, the presence or absence of structures, and their relationship to one another. Two-dimensional (2D), or cross-sectional, echocardiography provides information about spatial relationships between structures. Pulse, or continuous Doppler, echocardiography is generally used with 2D "echo" to provide information about volume flow rate. Three-dimensional (3D) imaging is used primarily to assess valve anatomy and function.

Although the test is noninvasive, painless, and associated with no known side effects, it can be stressful for children. The child must lie quietly for up to an hour for a full anatomic study. Lack of cooperation can limit the ability to obtain all the needed images. Infants and young children may need a mild sedative (see Preoperative Sedation, p. 687) or anesthesia. Older children benefit from preparation for the test. The distraction of a videotape or music is often helpful.

Transesophageal echocardiography (TEE) is performed with the transducer passed into the esophagus to an area behind the atria. It can provide information in cases in which it is difficult to obtain images using the transthoracic approach. In pediatrics, the most common use is in the operating room to assess the cardiac repair before the patient comes off cardiopulmonary bypass. Patients require IV sedation or general anesthesia, and often intubation, for a TEE.

Cardiac Magnetic Resonance Imaging

Cardiac magnetic resonance imaging (MRI) uses magnetic field and pulses of radio wave energy to produce real-time 3D images of the intracardiac and extracardiac vascular structures and assessments of ventricular function. It is often used in older children and adolescents when more quantitative information (e.g., volume of ventricular

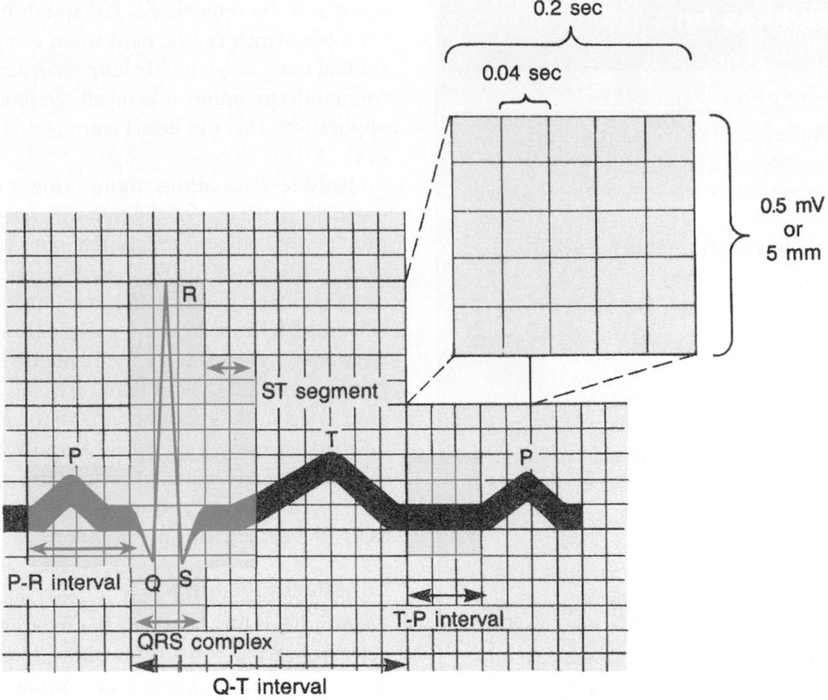

FIG. 27.4 Normal electrocardiogram pattern. Inset *(upper right)* shows conventional time and voltage or amplitude (height) calibrations.

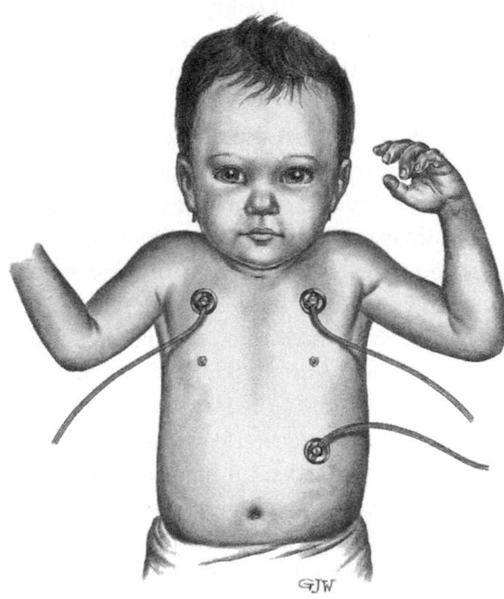

FIG. 27.5 Electrode placement for standard chest lead II in cardiac monitoring.

chambers, measurement of valve regurgitation) is needed that cannot be obtained by echo or if echo imaging windows have become limited. The use of MRI has rapidly expanded in the last decade. Although MRI is noninvasive, it can take an hour or more and patients have to lie still inside the scanner. Children under age 7 years, patients with claustrophobia, and those with developmental delays or other issues that limit cooperation will require anesthesia, deep sedation, or conscious sedation (depending on institutional preferences). Because the MRI is a magnet, patients with metal implants such as pacemakers, implantable cardioverter-defibrillators, or cochlear implants cannot be scanned and all patients are carefully screened for safety compatibility.

Cardiac Catheterization

Cardiac catheterization is an invasive diagnostic procedure, in which a radiopaque catheter is inserted through a peripheral blood vessel into the heart. It is usually combined with angiography (angiocardiography), in which a radiopaque contrast material is injected through the catheter and into the circulation. Cardiac catheterization provides information regarding the following:

- Oxygen saturation of blood within the chambers and great vessels
- Pressure changes within these structures
- Cardiac output or stroke volume (the amount of blood pumped out of the LV into the aorta with each contraction)
- Anatomic abnormalities, such as septal defects or obstruction to flow

The catheter is usually introduced through a percutaneous puncture into the femoral vein (the catheter is threaded over a guide wire inserted through a large-bore needle). Other blood vessels are sometimes used if femoral access is not possible. Once the vessel is entered, the catheter is guided through the heart with the aid of fluoroscopy. As the tubing is advanced, the child may feel pressure at the insertion site and vasospasm (fluttering) of the small vessels. Once the catheter is within the heart, blood samples and pressure readings are taken for analysis. Then contrast material may be injected and films taken of the dilution and circulation of the material.

Cardiac catheterization may be performed for diagnostic, interventional, or electrophysiologic purposes (Table 27.2). The two types of diagnostic cardiac catheterization are right-sided, or venous, catheterization, in which the catheter is introduced from a vein into the RA, and left-sided, or arterial, catheterization, in which the catheter is threaded by way of a systemic artery retrograde into the aorta and LV, from a right-sided approach across the LA by means of a septal puncture, or through an existing abnormal septal opening. In children, the most common method is right-sided catheterization because septal defects permit entry into the left side of the heart. The number of

TABLE 27.2 Common Intervnetional Cardiac Catheterization Procedures in Children and Adolescents

Intervention	Diagnosis
Balloon atrial septostomy	Transposition of the great vessels Other complex defects
Balloon dilation	Valvar pulmonary stenosis Branch pulmonary artery stenosis Congenital valvar aortic stenosis Rheumatic mitral stenosis Recurrent coarctation of the aorta
Stent placement	Pulmonary artery stenosis Coarctation of the aorta in adolescents
Coil occlusion	Small patent ductus arteriosus Collateral vessels in single ventricle patients
Transcatheter device closure	Some atrial septal defects (secundum type) Larger patent ductus arteriosus Fenestrations after Fontan procedures
Transcatheter Pulmonary Valve replacement	Incompetent pulmonary valves after surgery to repair right ventricular outflow tract
Radiofrequency ablation	Some tachydysrhythmias

All patients are evaluated for suitability for a catheter-based intervention (age, size, and location of defect, risk and benefits of procedure, etc.). Surgery may be indicated for some patients (Feltes, Bacha, Beekman, et al., 2011; Holzer & Hijazi, 2016).

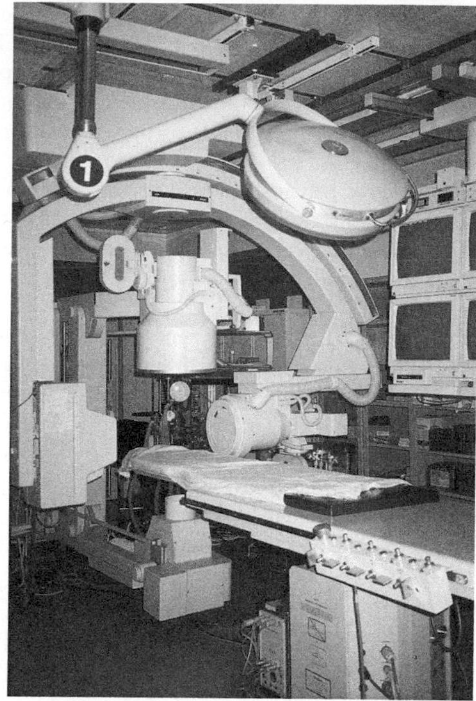

FIG. 27.6 Cardiac catheterization laboratory.

diagnostic catheterizations is decreasing as improvements in echocardiography and other noninvasive imaging methods allow more accurate noninvasive diagnosis.

Interventional cardiac catheterization is the use of a catheter-delivered device to treat heart disease, such as use of a balloon catheter to dilate narrowed valves and vessels and catheter delivery of devices to close some simple defects. It has rapidly expanded in the last 30 years as new techniques, devices, and applications have been developed. It has replaced surgical treatment for some congenital heart defects, such as isolated valvular pulmonary artery stenosis, and has become an alternate therapy for others, such as closing patent ductus arteriosus or atrial septal defects in some patients with favorable anatomy. In a large multicenter experience evaluating more than 3800 cases, adverse events are more common during interventional catheterizations, about 20%, compared with 10% for diagnostic cases (Bergersen, Marshall, Gavreau, et al., 2010). Deaths (most in newborns) and serious adverse events were less than 1% (Bergersen, Marshall, Gavreau, et al., 2010). Complications include balloon or device damage to vessels or valves and damage to structures due to thrombus or embolization (Lock, 2006).

Electrophysiologic studies are used to evaluate and treat dysrhythmias. Diagnostic electrophysiologic catheterization employs catheters with tiny electrodes that record the heart's electrical impulses directly from the conduction system. Interventional electrophysiologic catheterization uses radiofrequency ablation to destroy abnormal accessory pathways. Some pacemakers can be placed in the catheterization laboratory.

Nursing Care Management

Cardiac catheterization has become a routine procedure and may be done on an outpatient basis. Catheterization is not without risks, however, especially in neonates and seriously ill infants and children. Patients are exposed to radiation, general anesthesia for many cases, and contrast materials and medications that can cause allergic reactions or renal insufficiency. Possible complications include acute hemorrhage from the entry site requiring transfusion (more likely with interventional procedures because larger catheters are used), loss of a pulse due to vascular injury in the catheterized extremity (usually transient, resulting from a clot, hematoma, or intimal tear), and transient dysrhythmias (generally catheter induced). Serious complications such as valve damage, perforation of the heart, central nervous system (CNS) injury, stroke, or death are rare (Feltes, Bacha, Beekman, et al., 2011).

Preprocedural care. A complete nursing assessment is necessary to ensure a safe procedure with minimum complications. This assessment should include accurate height (essential for correct catheter selection) and weight. Obtaining a history of allergic reactions is important because some of the contrast agents are iodine based. Specific attention to signs and symptoms of infection is crucial. Severe diaper rash may be a reason to cancel the procedure if femoral access is required. Because assessment of pedal pulses is important after catheterization, the nurse should assess and mark the pulses (dorsalis pedis, posterior tibial) before the child goes to the catheterization room. Baseline oxygen saturation using pulse oximetry in children with cyanosis is also recorded.

Preparing the child and family for the procedure is the joint responsibility of the health care team. School-age children and adolescents benefit from a description of the catheterization laboratory (Fig. 27.6) and a chronologic explanation of the procedure, emphasizing what they will see, feel, and hear. They may bring earphones so that they can listen to music during the catheterization procedure. Preparation materials such as picture books, videotapes, or tours of the catheterization laboratory may be helpful. Preparation should be geared to the child's developmental level.

The child's caregivers often benefit from the same explanations. Additional information, such as the expected length of the catheterization, description of the child's appearance after catheterization, and usual postprocedure care, should be outlined (also see the Prepare the Child and Family for Invasive Procedures section later in this chapter).

Methods of sedation vary among institutions and may include oral or IV medications (see Chapter 22). The child's age, heart defect, clinical status, and type of catheterization procedure planned are considered when sedation is determined. General anesthesia is needed for most interventional procedures. Children are allowed nothing by mouth (NPO) for 6 to 8 hours or more before the procedure except for clear liquids, which stop 2 hours before the procedure. Infants and patients with polycythemia may need IV fluids to prevent dehydration and hypoglycemia.

Postprocedural care. Patients may recover from the catheterization procedure in a recovery unit or in their hospital rooms. Some may require care in the intensive care unit (ICU). Patients are placed on a cardiac monitor and a pulse oximeter for the first few hours after catheterization.

The most important nursing assessments include the following:

- Pulses, especially below the catheterization site, for equality and symmetry (Pulse distal to the site may be weaker for the first few hours after catheterization but should gradually increase in strength.)
- Temperature and color of the affected extremity because coolness or blanching may indicate arterial obstruction
- Vital signs, which may be taken as frequently as every 15 minutes, with special emphasis on the heart rate, which is counted for 1 full minute for evidence of dysrhythmias or bradycardia
- BP, especially for hypotension, which may indicate hemorrhage from cardiac perforation or bleeding at the site of initial catheterization
- Dressing, for evidence of bleeding or hematoma formation in the femoral or antecubital area
- Fluid intake, both IV and oral, to ensure adequate hydration (Blood loss in the catheterization laboratory, the child's preprocedure NPO status, and diuretic actions of contrast material used during the procedure put the child at risk for hypovolemia and dehydration.)

Infants are particularly at risk for hypoglycemia. They should receive dextrose-containing IV fluids, and blood glucose levels should be checked.

! NURSING ALERT

If bleeding occurs, direct, continuous pressure is applied 2.5 cm (1 inch) above the percutaneous skin site to localize pressure over the vessel puncture (Bergersen, Foerster, Marshall, et al., 2009).

Depending on hospital policy, the child may remain in bed with the affected extremity maintained straight for 4 to 6 hours after venous catheterization and 6 to 8 hours after arterial catheterization to facilitate healing of the cannulated vessel. If younger children have difficulty complying, they can be held in the parent's lap with the leg maintained in the correct position. The child's usual diet can be resumed as soon as tolerated, beginning with sips of clear liquids and advancing as the condition allows it. Generally there is only slight discomfort at the percutaneous site. Acetaminophen (Tylenol) or ibuprofen is usually adequate to treat pain. The catheterization site is covered with an occlusive dressing to prevent bleeding and contamination that could cause infection. Home care instructions are listed in the Family-Centered Care box.

CONGENITAL HEART DISEASE

The incidence of congenital heart disease (CHD) in children is approximately 1 in 110 live births in the United States (Reller, Strickland, Riehle-Colarusso, et al., 2008). Of these, approximately 25% infants have a critical congenital heart defect (Box 27.1) and will require treatment within the first year of life (Botto, Correa, & Erickson, 2001; Hoffman & Kaplan, 2002). In the neonatal period, 4.2% of all neonatal deaths were due to CHD (Petrini, Broussard, Gilboa, et al., 2010). Nearly half (48%) of deaths due to CHD occur during infancy (younger than 1 year of life) (Gilboa, Salemi, Nembhard, et al., 2010). Despite these statistics, mortality due to congenital heart disease has improved over the last few decades due to surgical and catheter interventions, early detection (see Research Focus box), and ongoing pharmaceutical advancements. In 2010 it was estimated that there were approximately 2.4 million people living with CHD in the United States, 1 million of whom were children (Gilboa, Devine, Kucik, et al., 2016).

BOX 27.1 Critical Congenital Cardiovascular Defects

Coarctation of the aorta
Double-outlet right ventricle
d-Transposition of the great arteries
Ebstein anomaly
Hypoplastic left heart syndrome
Interrupted aortic arch
Pulmonary atresia (with intact septum)
Single ventricle
Total anomalous pulmonary venous return
Tetralogy of Fallot
Tricuspid atresia
Truncus arteriosus

From Centers for Disease Control and Prevention (CDC). (2018). Facts about critical congenital heart defects. Retrieved from https://www.cdc.gov/ncbddd/heartdefects/cchd-facts.html.

FAMILY-CENTERED CARE

After Cardiac Catheterization

- Remove pressure dressing the day after catheterization. Cover site with an adhesive bandage strip for several days. Put a new bandage on every day for the next 2 days.
- Keep site clean and dry. Avoid tub baths for the first 3 days; older children may shower the first day after catheterization.
- Observe site for redness, swelling, drainage, and bleeding. Monitor the child for fever. Observe the catheter leg for coolness. Notify practitioner if these occur.
- The child should avoid strenuous exercise for several days but may attend school.
- The child can resume regular diet without restrictions.
- Use acetaminophen or ibuprofen for pain.
- Keep follow-up appointments per practitioner's instructions.

RESEARCH FOCUS

Pulse Oximetry Screening for Critical Congenital Heart Defects

Using pulse oximetry screening in a newborn infant can assist in early detection of critical congenital heart defects (CCHDs), thereby prompting timely intervention and potentially improving outcomes for the infant. In a systematic review and meta-analysis of screening for CCHDs in asymptomatic newborn babies, researchers looked at 13 eligible studies to assess the performance of pulse oximetry. The overall sensitivity of pulse oximetry was 76.5%. The specificity was 99.9% with a false-positive rate of 0.14% that was even lower when pulse oximetry screening was performed 24 hours after birth versus before (0.05% vs. 0.5%, $p = 0.0017$). Pulse oximetry then is highly specific for detecting CCHDs with moderate sensitivity (Thangaratinam, Brown, Zamora, et al., 2012). In 2015 the Centers for Disease Control and Prevention noted that 43 states have legislation, regulations, or hospital guidelines supporting the use of pulse oximetry in the screening for CCHDs in the newborn (Glidewell, Olney, Hinton, et al., 2015).

A congenital heart defect can be a single defect in the septum, a heart valve, or the arteries and veins, but it is often a combination of defects in one or more of these areas. The exact cause of most congenital cardiac diseases is unknown. Most are thought to be a result of multiple factors—a complex interaction of genetic and environmental influences. Some risk factors are known to be associated with increased incidence of congenital heart defects. Maternal risk factors include chronic illnesses such as diabetes or poorly controlled phenylketonuria, alcohol consumption, and exposure to environmental toxins and infections. Family history of a cardiac defect in a parent or sibling increases the likelihood of a cardiac anomaly. The risk of CHD increases if a first-degree relative (parent or sibling) is affected. The familial risk is higher with left-sided obstructive lesions.

Congenital heart anomalies are often associated with chromosomal abnormalities, specific syndromes, or congenital defects in other body systems. Down syndrome (trisomy 21) and trisomy 13 and 18 are highly correlated with congenital heart defects. Syndromes associated with heart defects include DiGeorge syndrome, also known as 22q11 deletion syndrome (heart defects, poor immune system function, a cleft palate, complications related to low levels of calcium in the blood, and delayed development with behavioral and emotional problems), Noonan syndrome (pulmonic valve anomalies and cardiomyopathy), Williams syndrome (aortic and pulmonic stenosis), and Holt-Oram syndrome (upper limb anomalies and atrial septal defect). Extracardiac defects such as tracheoesophageal fistula, renal abnormalities, and diaphragmatic hernia are seen in association with heart anomalies.

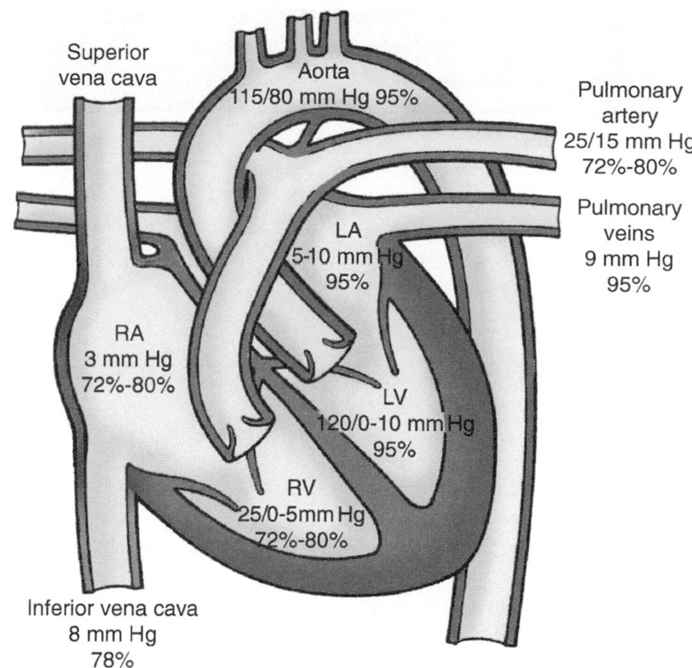

FIG. 27.7 Normal chamber pressures (mm Hg) and oxygen saturations (SaO_2) in cardiac chambers and great arteries. For simplicity, only two of the four pulmonary veins are shown. See Fig. 27.2 for abbreviations.

ALTERED HEMODYNAMICS

The physiology of heart defects is to defined by pressure gradients, blood flow, and resistance within the circulation. Blood flows because of pressure gradients in different parts of the body and because of the heart's pumping action. Like any fluid, blood flows from an area of high pressure to one of low pressure and takes the path of least resistance. The rate of flow is directly proportional to the pressure gradient (i.e., the higher the pressure gradient, the greater the rate of flow) and inversely proportional to the resistance (i.e., the higher the resistance, the lower the rate of flow). However, increased resistance does not always decrease flow. If the proximal cardiac chamber can increase the driving pressure proportionally, flow can remain unchanged.

Normally the pressure on the right side of the heart is lower than that on the left side, and the resistance in the pulmonary circulation is less than that in the systemic circulation. Likewise, vessels entering or exiting these chambers have corresponding pressures (e.g., lower pressure in the pulmonary artery and higher pressure in the aorta). Therefore if an abnormal connection exists between the heart chambers, such as a septal defect, blood flows from an area of higher pressure (left side) to one of lower pressure (right side). This directional flow of blood is termed a *left-to-right shunt.* If the opening is small, the amount of blood shunted to the atrium or ventricle may be minimal.

An understanding of saturations within the heart is also helpful in understanding CHD. The blood returning to the heart via the great veins (the SVC and the IVC) should have the lowest oxygen saturation because the tissues should have extracted oxygen, leaving the venous blood desaturated. Saturations in the RA, RV, and pulmonary artery should be equal. Blood returning from the lungs to the heart through the pulmonary veins should be fully saturated, the most oxygen-rich blood in the body. Saturations on the left side of the heart should all be equal, with fully saturated blood entering the aorta and first supplying the heart muscle through the coronary arteries and then supplying the brain (Fig. 27.7). Normally, saturated blood circulates separately from desaturated blood. Depending on the type of defect, saturated and desaturated blood may be mixed. The amount of mixed blood that reaches the systemic circulation is a significant feature of several cardiac anomalies, and varying degrees of hypoxemia and cyanosis result.

CLINICAL CONSEQUENCES OF CONGENITAL HEART DISEASE

Depending on the severity of the cardiac defect and the altered hemodynamics, two principal clinical consequences can occur: congestive heart failure (CHF) and hypoxemia. Defects that result in left-to-right shunting of blood cause symptoms of CHF. Defects that result in decreased pulmonary blood flow cause cyanosis. The conditions can occur alone or together. They can also occur both before surgical repair and after surgical intervention in some cases. Advanced heart failure, a situation in which heart failure persists despite surgical and medical interventions, is addressed later in this chapter. Pulmonary hypertension, an uncommon condition, may occur as a result of congenital heart defects and is included in this section. Pulmonary hypertension as a congenital condition is discussed later in this chapter. Nursing care plays a critical role in the early identification and supportive management of these conditions.

CONGESTIVE HEART FAILURE

Congestive heart failure is the inability of the heart to pump an adequate amount of blood to the systemic circulation at normal filling pressures to meet the body's metabolic demands. It can be referred to as either *congestive heart failure* (CHF) or *heart failure* (HF). Causes of CHF can be classified in terms of the following changes:

- Volume overload, especially with left-to-right shunts that may cause the RV to hypertrophy to compensate for the additional blood volume
- Pressure overload, primarily resulting from obstructive lesions, such as valvular stenosis or coarctation of the aorta
- Decreased contractility, primarily decreased contractility of the myocardium, caused by factors such as cardiomyopathy or myocardial

BOX 27.2 Etiologies of Heart Failure in Newborns, Infants, Children, and Adolescents

Newborn or Infant

Normal Cardiac Structure

Anemia
Dysrhythmias
Cardiomyopathy
Electrolyte imbalances
Endocrinopathies
Extracardiac shunts
Hypertension
Hypoxic-ischemic events
Kawasaki disease
Sepsis

Congenital Heart Disease

Obstruction to flow out of the left ventricle (e.g., aortic stenosis, coarctation of the aorta)
Obstruction to flow into the left ventricle (e.g., mitral stenosis)
Pulmonary vein stenosis
Total anomalous pulmonary venous connection
Systemic ventricular volume overload (e.g., aortic or mitral valve regurgitation, patent ductus arteriosus, atrioventricular canal defect, ventricular septal defect)
Single ventricle
Truncus arteriosus

Child or Adolescent

Normal Cardiac Structure

Anemia
Dysrhythmias
Cardiomyopathy
Hypertension
Inherited
Kawasaki disease
Medications
Myocarditis
Renal failure
Other noncardiac diseases (e.g., muscular dystrophy, cystic fibrosis)

Congenital Heart Disease

Aortic regurgitation
Mitral regurgitation
Mitral stenosis
Pulmonary vein stenosis
Failed palliation procedures

ischemia from severe anemia or asphyxia; heart block; acidemia; and low levels of potassium, glucose, calcium, or magnesium

- High cardiac output demands, in which the body's need for oxygenated blood exceeds the heart's cardiac output (even though the volume may be normal), such as in sepsis, hyperthyroidism, and severe anemia

The etiology of HF varies according to the age of onset; CHF occurs in children with both CHD and normal cardiac structure (Box 27.2). CHF occurs most frequently secondary to congenital heart defects in which structural abnormalities result in an increased volume load or increased pressure load on the ventricles. For example, septal defects can cause large left-to-right shunts, which result in a volume load on the RV. Obstruction to flow out of the LV, such as narrowing of the aorta (coarctation of the aorta), can cause increased pressure inside the ventricle. HF can also be a result of an excessive workload on a normal myocardium. Myocardial failure, in which the contractility of the heart muscle is impaired, can result from cardiomyopathy, drugs, electrolyte imbalances, dysrhythmias, and other causes. Diseases in other organ systems, particularly the lungs, also can cause CHF. Obstructive changes in the lungs result in increased pulmonary vascular resistance, which increases the RV workload. In time, the right side of the heart has difficulty pumping blood forward to the lungs, becomes dilated, and hypertrophies; then signs and symptoms of right-sided heart failure are seen. *Cor pulmonale* is the term for CHF resulting from obstructive lung diseases such as cystic fibrosis or bronchopulmonary dysplasia.

Altered Hemodynamics

Theoretically, HF may be divided into two types: right-sided failure and left-sided failure. In right-sided failure, RV function is reduced. RV end-diastolic pressure rises, causing increased CVP and systemic venous engorgement. Systemic venous hypertension causes hepatomegaly and may cause edema in the extremities. In left-sided failure, LV dysfunction occurs and LV end-diastolic pressure rises; the result is increased pressure in the LA and also in the pulmonary veins. The lungs become congested with blood, which leads to elevated pulmonary pressures and pulmonary edema.

Although each type of HF produces different signs and symptoms, clinically it is unusual to observe solely right- or left-sided failure in children. Because each side of the heart depends on adequate functioning of the other side, failure of one chamber causes a reciprocal change in the opposite chamber.

Compensatory Mechanisms

The heart initially tries to meet the body's demand for increased cardiac output through several compensatory mechanisms called the cardiac reserve. These include hypertrophy and dilation of the cardiac muscle and stimulation of the sympathetic nervous system (Fig. 27.8).

Hypertrophy and dilation of the cardiac muscle. In response to the need to increase cardiac output, the cardiac muscle hypertrophies, developing greater tension. It is able to generate increased pressure within the ventricle, pumping blood out of the heart at a higher pressure. Also, the cardiac muscle can dilate and increase the stretch of its fibers, which increases the force of contraction. However, both hypertrophy and dilation have potentially negative effects. Hypertrophy may result in decreased ventricular compliance over time. When compliance decreases, a higher filling pressure is required to produce the same stroke volume. The increased muscle mass impairs oxygenation to the heart muscle. Beyond a certain amount of dilation, the force of contraction decreases and the heart fails. (See discussion of the Starling law, p. 961.)

Stimulation of the sympathetic nervous system. When cardiac output begins to fall, stretch receptors and baroreceptors in the blood vessels stimulate the sympathetic nervous system, releasing catecholamines. Catecholamines increase the force and rate of myocardial contraction, as manifested by tachycardia. They cause peripheral vasoconstriction, which results in increased systemic vascular resistance; increased venous return; and reduced blood flow to the limbs, viscera, and kidneys. Sympathetic cholinergic fibers cause sweating.

Although initially successful in increasing cardiac output, prolonged sympathetic stimulation also has negative effects. By shortening the diastolic period, tachycardia increases oxygen consumption by the heart muscle, eliminates the heart's resting phase, and impairs coronary artery

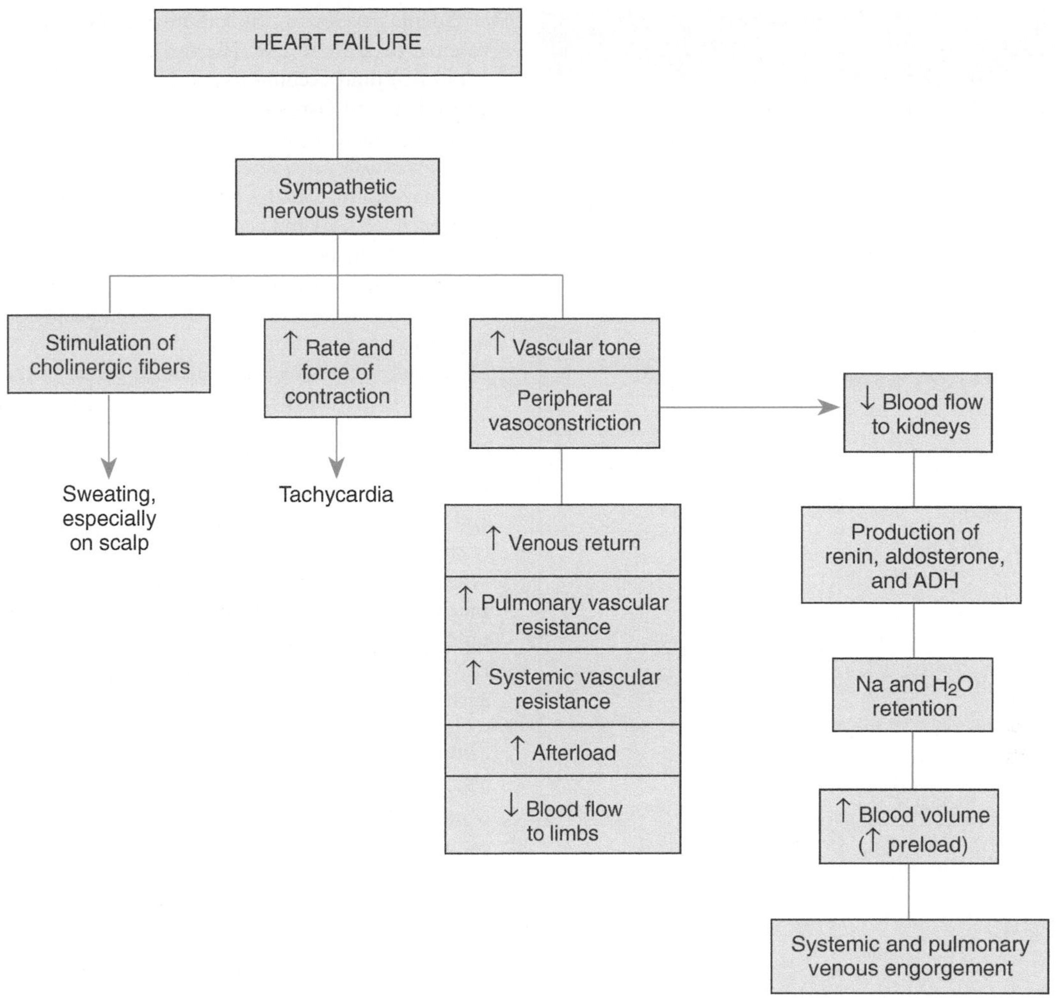

FIG. 27.8 Pathophysiology of heart failure. *ADH,* Antidiuretic hormone.

perfusion. A continued increase in systemic vascular resistance increases the afterload on the heart muscle, which requires extra work by the heart muscle and reduces systemic blood flow.

The renal system is particularly sensitive to reductions in blood flow and renal perfusion, which activate the renin-angiotensin-aldosterone mechanism. Renin angiotensin secretion causes vasoconstriction and leads to an increase in aldosterone secretion, which causes retention of salt and water. Retention of salt and water causes an increase in preload. Although at first helpful to the failing heart, the sodium and water retention becomes excessive, resulting in signs of systemic venous congestion and fluid overload.

Clinical Manifestations

As the capacity of the compensatory mechanisms is exceeded, the child exhibits signs of HF because of decreased myocardial contraction, increased preload, and increased afterload. The signs and symptoms of CHF can be divided into three groups: (1) impaired myocardial function, (2) pulmonary congestion, and (3) systemic venous congestion (Box 27.3). Because these hemodynamic changes occur from different causes and at different times, the clinical presentation may vary among children.

Impaired Myocardial Function

One of the earliest signs of CHF is tachycardia (sleeping heart rate >160 beats/min in infants) as a direct result of sympathetic stimulation. Heart rate is elevated even during rest but becomes extremely rapid with the slightest exertion. Ventricular dilation and excess preload result in extra heart sounds S_3 and S_4, referred to as gallop rhythm. Diaphoresis often occurs, especially on the head during exertion. Children are easily fatigued, have poor exercise tolerance, and are often irritable. Decreased cardiac output results in poor perfusion, manifested by cold extremities, weak pulses, slow capillary refill, low BP, and mottled skin. Extreme pallor or duskiness is an ominous sign.

Pulmonary Congestion

Tachypnea (respiratory rate >60 breaths/min in infants) occurs in response to decreased lung compliance (ability to expand). Tachypnea can lead to hypoxemia because oxygen does not reach the alveoli for gas exchange in adequate amounts with fast breathing rates. Mild cyanosis results from impaired gas exchange and is relieved by oxygen administration. Dyspnea is caused by a decrease in the distensibility of the lungs. Inability to feed with resultant poor weight gain is primarily a result of tachypnea and dyspnea on exertion. Costal retractions occur as the pliable chest wall in the infant is drawn inward during attempts to ventilate the noncompliant lungs. Initially dyspnea may be evident only on exertion, but it may progress to the point that even slight activity results in labored breathing. In infants dyspnea at rest is a prominent sign and may be accompanied by flaring nares.

As the LV fails, blood volume and pressure increase in the LA, pulmonary veins, and lungs. Eventually the pulmonary capillary

BOX 27.3 Clinical Manifestations of Heart Failure

Impaired Myocardial Function
Tachycardia
Sweating (inappropriate)
Decreased urinary output
Fatigue
Weakness
Restlessness
Anorexia
Pale, cool extremities
Weak peripheral pulses
Decreased blood pressure
Gallop rhythm
Cardiomegaly

Pulmonary Congestion
Tachypnea
Dyspnea
Retractions (infants)
Flaring nares
Exercise intolerance
Orthopnea
Cough, hoarseness
Cyanosis
Wheezing
Grunting

Systemic Venous Congestion
Weight gain
Hepatomegaly
Peripheral edema, especially periorbital
Ascites
Neck vein distention (children)

pressure exceeds the plasma osmotic pressure, which forces fluid into the interstitial space and finally causes pulmonary edema. Increased interstitial lung water also decreases the compliance of the lungs and increases the work of breathing.

Orthopnea (dyspnea in the recumbent position) is caused by increased blood flow to the heart and lungs from the extremities. It is relieved by sitting up because then blood pools in the lower extremities, which decreases venous return. In addition, this position decreases pressure from the abdominal organs on the diaphragm. In infants orthopnea may be evident in the inability to lie supine and the desire to be held upright.

Edema of the bronchial mucosa may produce wheezing from obstruction to airflow. Mucosal swelling and irritation result in a persistent, dry, hacking cough. As pulmonary edema increases, the cough may be productive due to increased secretions. Pressure on the laryngeal nerve results in hoarseness. A late sign of HF is gasping and grunting respirations.

Systemic Venous Congestion

Systemic venous congestion from right-sided failure results in increased pressure and pooling of blood in the venous circulation. Hepatomegaly occurs from pooling of blood in the portal circulation and transudation of fluid into the hepatic tissues. The liver may be tender on palpation, and its size is an indication of the course of HF.

Edema develops as the sodium and water retention causes systemic vascular pressure to rise. The earliest sign is weight gain. However, as additional fluid accumulates, it leads to swelling of soft tissue that is dependent and favors the flow of gravity, such as the sacral area and scrotum (when recumbent) and loose periorbital tissues. In infants edema is usually generalized and difficult to detect. Gross fluid accumulation may produce ascites and pleural effusions.

Distended neck and peripheral veins result from consistently elevated CVP. Normally neck and hand veins collapse when the head or hands are raised above the level of the heart because the blood drains by gravity back to the heart. When the venous pressure is high, however, it slows venous return, which causes the veins to remain distended. Distended neck veins are difficult to detect in the short, fat necks of infants and are usually observed only in older children.

Diagnostic Evaluation

Diagnosis is made on the basis of clinical symptoms such as tachypnea and tachycardia at rest, dyspnea, retractions, activity intolerance (especially during feeding in infants), weight gain caused by fluid retention, and hepatomegaly. A chest x-ray film demonstrates cardiomegaly and increased pulmonary vascular markings due to increased pulmonary blood flow. Signs of ventricular hypertrophy appear on the ECG. Echocardiography is performed to determine the cause of HF, such as a congenital heart defect or poor ventricular function.

Therapeutic Management

The goals of treatment are to (1) improve cardiac function (increase contractility and decrease afterload), (2) remove accumulated fluid and sodium (decrease preload and minimize fluid overload), (3) decrease cardiac demands, and (4) improve tissue oxygenation and decrease oxygen consumption. For most infants diagnosed with CHF the cause is a congenital heart defect. Infants are stabilized on medical therapy and then referred for surgical repair. Today many children are being surgically repaired in the neonatal and early infancy stages before the onset of CHF symptoms (Margossian, 2008). In infants who do manifest these symptoms, medical and nutrition management are optimized preoperatively. For children newly diagnosed with CHF, the cause may be worsening ventricular function after a previous cardiac repair, cardiomyopathy, arrhythmia, or other condition. In addition to management of the CHF, the underlying cause is treated if possible.

Remove Accumulated Fluid and Sodium

Treatment to remove accumulated fluid and sodium consists of administration of diuretics, possible fluid restriction, and possible sodium restriction. Diuretics are the mainstay of therapy to eliminate excess water and salt and to prevent reaccumulation. The most commonly used agents are listed in Table 27.3. Because furosemide (Lasix) and the thiazides cause potassium depletion, oral potassium supplements and rich dietary sources are often necessary.

Fluid restriction may be required in the acute stages of CHF and must be carefully calculated to avoid dehydrating the child, especially if cyanosis and significant polycythemia are present. Infants rarely need fluid restriction because CHF makes feeding so difficult that they struggle to take maintenance fluids.

Sodium-restricted diets are used less often in children than in adults to control CHF because of their potential negative effects on the child's appetite and ultimate growth. If salt intake is restricted, the diet usually focuses on avoiding additional table salt and highly salted foods. Low-salt formulas are available but are used infrequently because infants need a normal sodium source to offset the sodium depletion of chronic diuretic therapy. Most infant formulas have slightly more sodium than does breast milk.

TABLE 27.3 Diuretics Used in Heart Failure

Actions	Comments	Nursing Care Management
Furosemide (Lasix)		
Blocks reabsorption of sodium and water in proximal renal tubule and interferes with reabsorption of sodium in the loop of Henle and in the most proximal portion of distal tubule	Drug of choice in severe heart failure Causes excretion of chloride and potassium (hypokalemia may precipitate digitalis toxicity)	Begin to record output as soon as drug is given. • Observe for dehydration caused by profound diuresis. • Observe for side effects (e.g., nausea and vomiting, diarrhea, ototoxicity, hypokalemia, dermatitis, postural hypotension). • Encourage consumption of foods high in potassium and/or give potassium supplements. • Monitor chloride and acid-base balance with long-term therapy. • Observe for signs of digoxin toxicity.
Chlorothiazide (Diuril)		
Acts directly on distal tubules to decrease sodium, water, potassium, chloride, and bicarbonate absorption	Less frequently used drug Causes hypokalemia, acidosis in large doses	Observe for side effects (e.g., nausea, weakness, dizziness, paresthesia, muscle cramps, skin eruptions, hypokalemia, acidosis). Encourage consumption of foods high in potassium and/or give potassium supplements.
Spironolactone (Aldactone)		
Blocks action of aldosterone, which promotes retention of sodium and excretion of potassium	Weak diuretic Has potassium-sparing effect; frequently used with thiazides, furosemide Poorly absorbed from gastrointestinal tract Takes several days to achieve maximum actions	Observe for side effects (e.g., skin rash, drowsiness, ataxia, hyperkalemia). Do not administer potassium supplements.

Improve Cardiac Function

Two groups of drugs are used to enhance myocardial function in CHF: digitalis glycosides (digoxin), which improve contractility, and angiotensin-converting enzyme (ACE) inhibitors, which reduce the afterload on the heart and thus make it easier for the heart to pump. Myocardial efficiency is improved through administration of digitalis glycosides. The beneficial effects are increased cardiac output, decreased heart size, decreased venous pressure, and relief of edema. In children, digoxin (Lanoxin) is used almost exclusively because of its more rapid onset of action and decreased risk of toxicity as a result of its relatively short half-life (1½ days) compared with other digitalis preparations. It is available as an elixir (50 mcg/ml) for oral administration. For infants the dose is often calculated in micrograms (1000 mcg = 1 mg). Because digoxin has a very narrow margin of safety, the dosage must be calculated exactly. Premature infants are more sensitive to digoxin and require smaller dosages because their impaired renal excretion causes the drug to accumulate in the blood faster than in full-term infants and children.

Treatment consists of a digitalizing dose, given intravenously or orally in divided doses over 24 hours to produce optimal cardiac effects, and a maintenance dose, given orally twice a day to maintain blood levels. During digitalization, the child is monitored by means of an ECG to observe for the desired effects (prolonged PR interval and reduced ventricular rate) and detect side effects, especially dysrhythmias.

> **! NURSING ALERT**
>
> A fall in the serum potassium level enhances the effects of digoxin, increasing the risk of digoxin toxicity. Increased serum potassium levels diminish digoxin's effect. Therefore serum potassium levels (normal range, 3.5 to 5.5 mmol/L) must be carefully monitored.

Digoxin is the only oral inotropic agent generally available for infants and children, although other oral inotropic agents are being used in clinical trials in adults. For patients with severe HF, IV inotropic agents such as dopamine or milrinone are used to improve contractility. They are generally given in ICU settings.

Reduce Afterload

Another group of drugs used in the treatment of HF is the ACE inhibitors. Common medications in this class are captopril (Capoten), given three times a day; enalapril (Vasotec), given twice a day; and lisinopril, given once daily. ACE inhibitors inhibit the normal function of the renin-angiotensin system in the kidney. The production of renin triggers the production of angiotensin I and angiotensin II, which causes vasoconstriction and aldosterone secretion. The ACE inhibitors block the conversion of angiotensin I to angiotensin II so that, instead of vasoconstriction, vasodilation occurs. Vasodilation results in decreased pulmonary and systemic vascular resistance, decreased BP, a reduction in afterload, and decreased RA and LA pressures. It also reduces the secretion of aldosterone, which reduces preload by preventing volume expansion from fluid retention and decreases the risk of hypokalemia. Renal blood flow is improved, which enhances diuresis. The principal side effects of ACE inhibitors are hypotension, renal dysfunction, hyperkalemia, and cough.

> **DRUG ALERT**
>
> ***ACE Inhibitors***
>
> Because ACE inhibitors also block the action of aldosterone, the addition of potassium supplements or spironolactone (Aldactone) to the drug regimen of patients taking diuretics and an ACE inhibitor may cause hyperkalemia.

Decrease Cardiac Demands

To lessen the workload on the heart, metabolic needs are minimized by (1) providing a neutral thermal environment to prevent cold stress in infants, (2) treating any existing infections, (3) reducing the effort of breathing (by placement in semi-Fowler position), (4) using medication to sedate an irritable child, and (5) providing for rest and decreasing environmental stimuli.

Improve Tissue Oxygenation

All the preceding measures serve to increase tissue oxygenation, either by improving myocardial function or by lessening tissue oxygen demands. In addition, supplemental cool humidified oxygen may be administered to increase the amount of available oxygen during inspiration. Oxygen administration is especially helpful in patients with pulmonary edema, intercurrent respiratory tract infections, and increased pulmonary vascular resistance (oxygen is a vasodilator that decreases pulmonary vascular resistance).

> **! NURSING ALERT**
>
> Oxygen is a drug and is administered only with an appropriate order.

An oxygen hood, face tent, or nasal cannula is used to deliver supplemental oxygen. Nasal cannulas are ideal for long-term oxygen administration because the child can be ambulatory and can easily eat and drink. Cool humidification is necessary to counteract the drying effect of oxygen. The amount of cool humidity is carefully regulated to prevent chilling.

Nursing Care Management

Infants or children with CHF may be acutely ill, and some may require intensive care until their symptoms improve. Expert nursing care is essential to reduce the cardiac demands that strain the failing heart muscle (see Nursing Care Plan box). During this time the child and family require emotional support; for some children, severe HF represents end-stage cardiac disease (see Advanced Heart Failure, later in this chapter). Although the objectives of nursing care are the same, interventions for infants often differ from interventions for older children. (See Quality Patient Outcomes box.)

Minimize Fluid Overload

Diuresis assists in decreasing preload and minimizing volume overload. When diuretics are given, the nurse records fluid intake and output and monitors body weight at the same time each day to evaluate the benefit of the drug. Because profound diuresis may cause dehydration and electrolyte imbalance (e.g., loss of sodium, potassium, chloride, bicarbonate), the nurse observes for signs indicating one of these complications, as well as signs and symptoms suggesting reactions to the drugs. Give diuretics early in the day to children who are toilet trained to avoid the need to urinate at night. If potassium-losing diuretics are given, the nurse encourages consumption of foods high in potassium, such as bananas, oranges, whole grains, legumes, and leafy vegetables, and administers prescribed supplements.

NURSING CARE PLAN

The Child With Heart Failure

Case Study

George is a 2-week-old boy with congenital heart disease. At birth he initially showed no signs or symptoms but within the first week he developed symptoms of heart failure. He was found to have coarctation of the aorta and is now under the care of the cardiology team and scheduled for surgery. George is experiencing more signs of heart failure and the care is now focused on preventing further symptoms before he goes to surgery.

Assessment

What are the most important signs of heart failure that you need to look for in a young infant?

Heart Failure Defining Characteristics (Subjective and Objective Data)

Tachycardia
Tachypnea
Ineffective peripheral circulation, cool extremities
Hypotension
Rapid, weak peripheral pulses
Prolonged capillary refill, longer than 2 or 3 seconds
Narrow pulse pressure
Distended neck veins in older children
Cardiomegaly revealed on chest radiograph
Gallop rhythm
Edema
Rapid weight gain
Feeding difficulty
Irritability

Nursing Interventions and Rationales

What are the most appropriate nursing interventions for an infant in heart failure?

Nursing Interventions	Rationales
Assess and record heart rate, respiratory rate, blood pressure, and any signs or symptoms of decreased cardiac output every 2 to 4 hours and as necessary.	To detect change in vital signs and infant's physical status that reflect altered cardiac output and cardiogenic shock
Administer cardiac drugs on schedule. Assess and record any side effects or any signs and symptoms of toxicity. Follow hospital protocol for administration.	To avoid dangers inherent in failure to administer cardiac drugs as prescribed and to perform careful assessment before administration
Keep accurate record of intake and output.	To detect heart failure, which causes decreased urinary output
Weigh infant on same scale at same time of day as previously. Document results and compare to previous weight.	To monitor for weight increases, which may indicate excess fluid accumulation
Administer diuretics on schedule. Assess and record effectiveness and any side effects noted.	To eliminate excess water and salt because fluid retention commonly occurs with heart failure
Offer small, frequent feedings to infant's tolerance.	To increase caloric intake and compensate for fatigue during feeding and increased metabolic rate because of poor cardiac function
Organize nursing care to allow infant uninterrupted rest.	To allow adequate rest because poor cardiac output decreases energy level and lowers tolerance to activity

NURSING CARE PLAN—CONT'D

The Child With Heart Failure

Expected Outcome

George's cardiac function will be protected by decreasing cardiac demands, improving respiratory function, and preventing fluid excess.

Infant will have adequate cardiac output as evidenced by the following:

Heart rate within acceptable range (state specific range)
Respiratory rate within acceptable range (state specific range)
Skin warm to touch
Strong and equal peripheral pulses
Blood pressure normal for age
Brisk capillary refill within 2 or 3 seconds
Lack of distended neck veins
Normal sinus rhythm
Lack of edema
Adequate urinary output (state specific; 1 to 2 ml/kg/hr)
Age-appropriate weight gain on standardized growth curve
Successful feeding

Case Study (Continued)

George's blood pressure is increased and the pulses in his arms are bounding. You find weak femoral pulses and his extremities are cool to touch. George's breathing appears labored and you note nasal flaring but no intercostal retractions at this time. His color is pale and slightly mottled.

Assessment

What are the most important signs and symptoms of impaired breathing in this infant?

Impaired Breathing Defining Characteristics (Subjective and Objective Data)

Tachypnea
Dyspnea
Retractions
Crackles
Shortness of breath
Cyanosis
Pallor
Mottling
Nasal flaring
Grunting
Head bobbing
Cough
Use of accessory muscles
Activity intolerance

Do the findings described in the case study concern you?

The effect of the coarctation of the aorta causes a narrowing within the aorta that increases pressure proximal to the defect (upper extremities) and a decreased pressure distal to it (lower extremities). It is not surprising to find high blood pressure, bounding upper extremity pulses, and weak or even absent femoral pulses and cool extremities in these infants. You should follow his breathing patterns closely and observe for breathing changes.

How would you assess the effectiveness of these interventions?

Evaluate for changes in breathing patterns, respiratory rate, labored breath sounds; observe for nasal flaring or change in color to dusky or blue.

Why are breathing pattern changes a concern?

Coarctation of the aorta can cause pulmonary congestion as a result of decreased cardiac output. Breathing difficulties can be a sign of progression of heart failure.

Nursing Interventions and Rationales

What are the most appropriate nursing interventions for this diagnosis?

Nursing Interventions	Rationales
Assess and record oxygen saturation every 2 to 4 hours or more often as needed.	To evaluate pulmonary effectiveness
Elevate head of bed at a 30- to 45-degree angle.	To promote maximum chest expansion
Assess and record respiratory rate, breath sounds, and any signs or symptoms of ineffective pattern every 2 to 4 hours and as needed.	To detect indicators of worsening heart failure
Administer humidified oxygen in correct amount and route of delivery. Record percent of oxygen and route of delivery. Assess and record child's response to therapy.	To reduce respiratory distress by easing respiratory effort
Suction if infant has ineffective cough or is unable to manage secretions. Assess and record amount and characteristics of secretions.	To maintain patent airway to promote respiratory expansion

Expected Outcome

George will have an effective breathing pattern and maintain stable respiratory pattern until surgery as evidenced by respiratory rate within acceptable limits for age.

Infant will have effective breathing pattern as evidenced by the following:

Respiratory rate within acceptable range (state specific range)
Clear and equal breath sounds bilaterally anteriorly and posteriorly
Pink or tan color
Absence of nasal flaring, retractions, cough, and head bobbing
Unlabored breath sounds

Case Study (Continued)

George's parents ask you what you have found in your initial assessment. They ask about why he seems to be having problems breathing. What should you say to the parents?

Assessment

What are the most important aspects of George's care to discuss with his parents at this time?

Family's Knowledge of Illness—Defining Characteristics (Subjective and Objective Data)

Understands definition of heart failure
States four characteristics of signs of heart failure
Describes medications the infant is taking
Expresses fears and concerns
Shows appropriate reactions to infant's illness

Nursing Interventions and Rationales

What are the most appropriate nursing interventions for this diagnosis?

Continued

NURSING CARE PLAN—CONT'D

The Child With Heart Failure

Nursing Interventions	Rationales
Educate family about characteristics of heart failure. Assess and record effectiveness of teaching session.	To promote understanding of measures to improve cardiac function and decrease demands
Educate family about George's daily care such as medication administration. Assess and record results and family's participation in care.	To promote understanding of disease and medication side effects
Educate family regarding illness factors that should prompt them to take George to the primary care practitioner (fever, blue skin color, poor eating).	To prevent further compromise of cardiac and respiratory status

Expected Outcome

George's parents will understand the signs and symptoms of heart failure and will understand the actions being taken by the health care team.

QUALITY PATIENT OUTCOMES

Heart Failure

- Adequate cardiac output
- Decreased cardiac demands
- Improved respiratory function
- No evidence of fluid excess
- Adequate support and education

NURSING ALERT

Observe for signs of hypokalemia (muscle weakness, hypotension, dysrhythmias, tachycardia or bradycardia, irritability, drowsiness) or hyperkalemia (muscle weakness, twitching, bradycardia, ventricular fibrillation, oliguria, apnea) from supplement overdose.

Fluid restriction is rarely necessary in infants because of their difficulty in feeding. However, if fluids are restricted, the nurse plans fluid intake schedules for a 24-hour period, allowing for administration of most fluids during waking hours. With toddlers and preschoolers it is psychologically advantageous to give small amounts of liquid in small cups so that the containers appear full. Suitable containers are decorated medicine cups, small paper cups, doll-sized teacups, and measuring cups. It is also important to avoid leaving extra fluids at the bedside because older children may help themselves to additional servings. Placing them in charge of recording fluid intake will help gain their cooperation.

If salt intake is to be limited, the nurse discusses food sources of sodium with the family and discourages their bringing salt-containing treats to the child. At mealtime check the child's tray to make sure the appropriate diet is provided.

Improve Cardiac Function

Digoxin is used to improve cardiac function. Digoxin is a potentially dangerous drug because the margin of safety between therapeutic, toxic, and lethal doses is very narrow. Many toxic responses are extensions of its therapeutic effects. The nurse's responsibility in administering digoxin includes calculating and giving the correct dosage and observing for signs of toxicity. The child's apical pulse is always checked before administering digoxin. As a rule, the drug is not given if the pulse is below 90 to 110 beats/min in infants and young children or below 70 beats/min in older children (the cutoff point for adults is 60 beats/min). The nurse should also use judgment in evaluating the pulse rate. If it is significantly lower than the previous recording, the dose should be withheld until the practitioner is notified.

The apical rate is measured because a pulse deficit (radial pulse rate lower than apical) may be present with decreased cardiac output. The pulse is auscultated for 1 full minute to evaluate alterations in rhythm. If the child is monitored by ECG, a rhythm strip is obtained and attached to the chart for rate and rhythm analysis, such as abnormal lengthening of the P-R interval (>50% increase over the predigitalization interval) and dysrhythmias.

The most common signs of digoxin toxicity in infants and children are bradycardia (although other dysrhythmias may occur), anorexia, nausea, and vomiting. Although vomiting should alert the nurse to observe for other evidence of cardiac toxicity, one episode of vomiting does not warrant cessation of the drug because vomiting from other causes frequently occurs, especially in infants. Vomiting associated with digoxin toxicity is often unrelated to feedings, and infants are usually less interested in feeding and show a recent decrease in oral intake. When in doubt regarding what caused the vomiting and whether another dose of digoxin should be given, the nurse should seek the practitioner's advice before administering the next dose. When concerned about possible digoxin toxicity, the nurse should check the digoxin drug level.

DRUG ALERT

Digoxin Toxicity

Therapeutic serum digoxin levels range from 0.8 to 2 mcg/L. Observe for signs of toxicity, especially bradycardia and vomiting.

Other extracardiac signs of toxicity are neurologic and visual disturbances, which are extremely difficult to identify in children and consequently are of little value in assessing toxicity in infants.

Because digoxin toxicity can occur from accidental overdose, great care must be taken in properly calculating and measuring the dosage. When converting milligrams to micrograms to milliliters, the nurse carefully checks the placement of the decimal point because an error causes a significant change in dosage. For example, 0.1 mg is 10 times the dosage of 0.01 mg.

DRUG ALERT

Digoxin Dosing

Infants rarely receive more than 1 ml (50 mcg, or 0.05 mg) in one dose; a higher dose is an immediate warning of a dosage error. To ensure safety, compare the calculation with that of another staff member before giving digoxin.

If digoxin toxicity occurs, especially as a result of a drug overdose, withhold all subsequent doses. The nurse monitors the child closely for dysrhythmias, which are treated appropriately if they occur. Digoxin immune Fab fragment (Digiband) is used as an antidote to digoxin in cases of severe digitalis toxicity. Because of the long half-life of digoxin

(18 to 35 hours in infants and children with normal renal function; longer in those with renal impairment and in premature infants and adults), it may be several days before the blood level returns to normal (Taketomo, Hodding, & Kraus, 2009).

These same principles are taught to parents in preparation for the child's discharge, although the correct dose in milliliters is usually specified on the container, which reduces potential errors in calculation. The nurse observes the parent measuring the elixir in the dropper and stresses that the level mark is the meniscus of the fluid observed at eye level. Other instructions for administering digoxin are listed in the Family-Centered Care box. Nurses should also advise parents of the signs of digoxin toxicity.

FAMILY-CENTERED CARE

Administering Digoxin

- Give digoxin at regular intervals, usually every 12 hours, such as at 8 AM and 8 PM.
- Administer the drug carefully by slowly directing it to the side and back of the mouth.
- Do not mix the drug with foods or other fluids because refusal to consume these would result in inaccurate intake of the drug.
- If the child has teeth, give water after administering the drug; whenever possible, brush the teeth to prevent tooth decay from the sweetened liquid.
- If a dose is missed, do not give an extra dose or increase the dose. Stay on the same medication schedule.
- If the child vomits, do not give a second dose.
- If more than two consecutive doses have been missed, notify the physician or other designated practitioner.
- Frequent vomiting, poor feeding, or slow heart rate can be signs of digoxin toxicity; if they occur, contact the physician.
- If the child becomes ill, notify the physician or other designated practitioner immediately.
- Keep digoxin in a safe place, preferably in a locked cabinet.
- In case of accidental overdose of digoxin, call the nearest poison control center immediately.

Reduce Afterload

For patients receiving ACE inhibitors for afterload reduction, the nurse should carefully monitor BP before and after dose administration, observe for symptoms of hypotension, and notify the practitioner if BP is low. Monitor serum electrolyte levels. Because ACE inhibitors also block the action of aldosterone, they act as potassium-sparing agents. Most patients do not need potassium supplements or spironolactone while receiving these medications. Numerous medications affecting the kidney can potentiate renal dysfunction, so children taking multiple diuretics along with an ACE inhibitor require accurate measurement of urine output.

Decrease Cardiac Demands

The infant requires rest and conservation of energy for feeding. Make every effort to organize nursing activities to allow for uninterrupted periods of sleep. Whenever possible, encourage parents to stay with their infant to provide the holding, rocking, and cuddling that help children sleep more soundly. To minimize disturbing the infant, changing bed linen and complete bathing are done only when necessary. Plan feeding to accommodate the infant's sleep and wake patterns. The child is fed when hungry, such as when sucking on fists, rather than when crying for a bottle because the stress of crying exhausts the limited energy supply. Because infants with HF tire easily and may sleep through feedings, smaller feedings every 3 hours may be helpful. Gavage feedings may be instituted to provide adequate nutrition and allow the infant to rest.

Make every effort to minimize unnecessary stress. With infants this primarily involves preserving the parent-child relationship and meeting the infant's needs to reduce frustration. Older children need an explanation of what is happening to them to decrease anxiety about their illness and necessary treatments, such as cardiac monitoring, oxygen administration, and medications. Outlining a plan for the day, preparing the child for tests and procedures, providing quiet activities, and providing adequate rest periods are all helpful interventions with older children. Some infants and children require sedation during the acute phase of illness to allow them to rest.

Carefully monitor temperature for hyperthermia (a sign of infection) or hypothermia (loss of heat to ambient air). Report fevers because infection must be treated promptly. Fever increases oxygen demands and is poorly tolerated. If body temperature is low, keep the child warm with additional blankets or a radiant heater. Maintaining body temperature is important for children who are receiving cool, humidified oxygen and for children who tend to be diaphoretic, losing heat via evaporation.

Prevent skin breakdown from edema with frequent change of position and the use of pressure-relieving or pressure-reducing mattresses or beds. The skin, especially over the sacrum, is checked for evidence of redness from pressure.

Reduce Respiratory Distress

Careful assessment, positioning, and oxygen administration can reduce respiratory distress. Respirations are counted for 1 full minute during a resting state. Any evidence of increased respiratory distress is reported because this may indicate worsening HF. The infant or child is often given humidified supplemental oxygen via an oxygen hood or tent, nasal cannula, or mask. The child's response to oxygen therapy is carefully evaluated by noting the respiratory rate; ease of respiration; color; and especially oxygen saturations, as measured by oximetry.

Respiratory tract infections can exacerbate CHF and should be appropriately treated and prevented if possible. The child should be protected from persons with respiratory tract infections and should have a noninfectious roommate. Practice good hand-washing technique before and after caring for any hospitalized child. Antibiotics may be given to combat respiratory tract infection. The nurse ensures that the drug is given at equal intervals over a 24-hour period to maintain high blood levels of the antibiotic.

Maintain Nutritional Status

Meeting the nutritional needs of infants with CHF or serious cardiac defects is a nursing challenge. The metabolic rate of these infants is greater because of poor cardiac function and increased heart and respiratory rates. Their caloric needs are greater than those of the average infant because of their increased metabolic rate, yet fatigue limits their ability to take in adequate calories. For a fragile infant with serious CHD, feeding is similar to exercise in an adult, and the infant often does not have the energy or cardiac reserve to do extra work. The nurse seeks measures to enable the infant to feed easily without excess fatigue and to increase the caloric density of the formula.

The infant should be well rested before feeding and fed soon after awakening so as not to expend energy on crying. A 3-hour feeding schedule works well for many infants. (Feeding every 2 hours does not provide enough rest between feedings, and a 4-hour schedule requires an increased volume of feeding, which many infants are unable to take.) The feeding schedule should be individualized to the infant's needs. Infants should be well supported and fed in a semiupright position. The infant may need to rest frequently and may need to have the jaw and cheeks stroked to encourage sucking. Generally, giving an infant about a half-hour to complete a feeding is reasonable. Prolonging the feeding time can exhaust the infant and decrease the rest period between feedings.

Infants with feeding difficulties are often gavage fed using a nasogastric tube to supplement oral feedings and ensure adequate caloric intake. If they are stressed and fatigued, in respiratory distress, or tachypneic at 80 to 100 breaths/min, oral feedings may be withheld and all nutrition given by gavage feedings. Gavage feedings are usually a temporary measure until the infant's medical status improves and nutritional needs can be met through oral feedings. Some infants with severe CHF, neurologic deficits, or significant gastroesophageal reflux may need placement of a gastrostomy tube to allow adequate nutrition.

The caloric density of formulas is frequently increased by concentration and then the addition of Polycose (or, less commonly, corn oil or medium-chain triglycerides oil). Infant formulas provide 20 kcal/oz, and the use of additives can increase the calories to 30 kcal/oz or more. This allows the infant to obtain more calories despite intake of a smaller volume of formula. The caloric density of the formula must be increased slowly (by 2 kcal/oz/day) to prevent diarrhea or formula intolerance. Encourage breastfeeding mothers to provide the infant with alternating feedings of breast milk and high-calorie formula. Some lactating mothers prefer to feed the child expressed breast milk that has been fortified with Similac or Enfamil powder, Polycose, or corn oil to increase caloric intake. A diet plan specific to the individual infant's needs is calculated and prescribed by the nutritionist in collaboration with the other health care personnel.

Support the Child and Family

HF is a serious complication of heart disease. Parents and older children are usually acutely aware of the critical nature of the condition. Because stress places additional demands on cardiac function, the nurse should focus on reducing anxiety through anticipatory preparation, frequent communication with the parents regarding the child's progress, and constant reassurance that everything possible is being done.

Home care involves many of the same interventions discussed later in this chapter under Plan for Discharge and Home Care. The nurse teaches the family about the medications that need to be administered and alerts them to the signs of worsening HF that require medical attention, such as increased sweating, decreased urinary output, or poor feeding. Compliance can be a major issue because patients are often prescribed multiple medications, and the medication regimen can change frequently. Facilitate the family's adherence to the medication schedule by adapting the schedule to their usual home routines, avoiding medication administration at night, and providing charts or visual aids to help them remember when to give medications. (See Chapter 23.)

Hypoxemia

Hypoxemia refers to an arterial oxygen tension (or pressure, Pao_2) that is lower than normal and can be identified by measuring arterial oxygen saturation (Sao_2) or Pao_2 to detect decreased levels. Hypoxia is a reduction in tissue oxygenation that is caused by low Sao_2 and Pao_2 and results in impaired cellular processes. Cyanosis is a blue discoloration of the mucous membranes, skin, and nail beds of the child with reduced oxygen saturation. It results from the presence of deoxygenated hemoglobin (hemoglobin not bound to oxygen) at a concentration of 5 g/dl of blood or more. Cyanosis is usually apparent when Sao_2 is 85% or lower. Determination of cyanosis is subjective. Its appearance can vary depending on skin pigment, quality of light, color of the room, and clothing worn by the child. The presence of cyanosis may not accurately reflect arterial hypoxemia because both Sao_2 and the amount of circulating hemoglobin are involved. Children with severe anemia may not be cyanotic despite severe hypoxemia because the hemoglobin level may be too low to produce the characteristic blue color. Conversely, patients with polycythemia may appear cyanotic despite a near-normal Pao_2. Finally, infants and children with some complex cardiac anomalies, such as single ventricle defects and transposition of the great arteries with a ventricular septal defect, can be both hypoxemic and cyanotic and have symptoms of HF.

Altered Hemodynamics

Heart defects that cause hypoxemia and cyanosis are those that allow desaturated venous blood (blue blood) to enter the systemic circulation without passing through the lungs. Three types of defect cause cyanosis in infants. The first involves severe obstruction to pulmonary blood flow and blood shunting from the right side to the left side of the heart, or right-to-left shunting. Tetralogy of Fallot is the most common example. The second is mixing of arterial and venous blood within the chambers of the heart itself; a single ventricle is an example. The third defect, transposition of the great arteries, presents a unique situation in which the pulmonary and systemic circulations are parallel rather than in sequence. Fully oxygenated blood returns to the lungs, and desaturated blood returns to the body. Newborns with transposition of the great arteries depend on intracardiac mixing from a patent foramen ovale, septal defect, or ductus arteriosus to allow oxygenation.

Clinical Manifestations

Over time, two physiologic changes occur in the body in response to chronic hypoxemia: polycythemia and clubbing. Persistent hypoxemia stimulates erythropoiesis, which results in polycythemia, an increased number of red blood cells. Theoretically a greater number of red blood cells increase the oxygen-carrying capacity of the blood. However, this increased red blood cell formation may result in anemia if iron is not readily available for the formation of hemoglobin. In addition, polycythemia increases the viscosity of the blood, and platelets and other coagulation factors tend to be crowded out. These hematologic changes increase the likelihood of postoperative bleeding. Clubbing, a thickening and flattening of the tips of the fingers and toes, is thought to occur because of chronic tissue hypoxemia and polycythemia (Fig. 27.9).

Infants with mild hypoxemia may be asymptomatic except for cyanosis and exhibit near-normal growth and development. Those with more severe hypoxemia may exhibit fatigue with feeding, poor weight gain, tachypnea, and dyspnea. Children who are cyanotic from birth are generally smaller than their peers, exhibit poor weight gain, have dyspnea on exertion, fatigue easily, and have poor exercise tolerance.

Severe hypoxemia resulting in tissue hypoxia is manifested by clinical deterioration and signs of poor perfusion. The infant is pale and dusky with increased cyanosis; cool to the touch with diminished pulses; and lethargic with signs of respiratory distress, including hyperpnea and gasping respirations. Tissue hypoxia causes metabolic acidosis, which

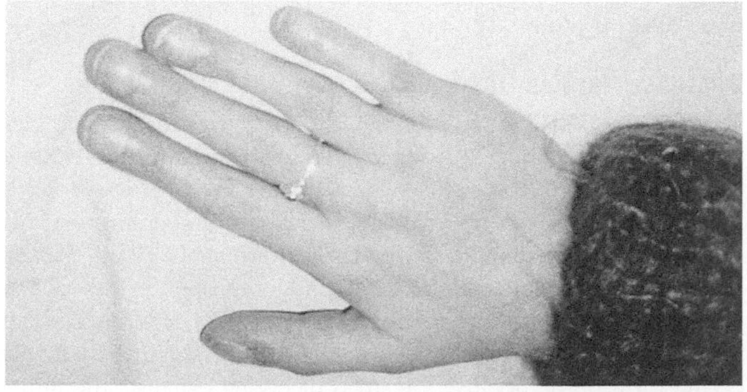

FIG. 27.9 Clubbing of the fingers.

leads to hyperventilation and a rapidly worsening clinical course unless prompt treatment is instituted.

Hypercyanotic spells, also referred to as *blue spells* or *tet spells* because they are often seen in infants with tetralogy of Fallot, may occur in any child whose heart defect includes obstruction to pulmonary blood flow and communication between the ventricles (see Fig. 27.11). When sudden infundibular spasms decrease pulmonary blood flow there is an increase in right-to-left shunting (the proposed mechanism in tetralogy of Fallot), and the infant becomes acutely cyanotic and hyperpneic. This then leads to hypoxia. Hypoxia causes acidosis, which further increases pulmonary vascular resistance; this, in turn, further decreases pulmonary blood flow. Thus a vicious cycle ensues. Spells, rarely seen before 2 months of age, occur most frequently in the first year of life and more often in the morning, and they may be preceded by feeding, crying, or defecation. Because profound hypoxemia causes cerebral hypoxia, hypercyanotic spells require prompt assessment and treatment to prevent brain damage or possibly death.

Patients with persistent right-to-left shunts as a result of CHD are at risk for significant neurologic complications. Polycythemia and the resultant increased viscosity of the blood increase the risk of thromboembolic events. Small blood clots in the venous system reach the right side of the heart and can enter the systemic circulation and travel to the brain through the right-to-left shunt. The presence of poor ventricular function and atrial arrhythmias further increases the risk of cerebrovascular accidents (CVAs), or strokes. More common in patients with severe cyanosis, thromboembolic events may occur spontaneously but often follow an acute febrile illness, a hypoxic spell, cardiac catheterization, or cardiac surgery, including the Fontan procedure with fenestration (Fig. 27.10). Patients who are cyanotic, especially those with systemic-to-pulmonary shunts, are at increased risk of bacterial endocarditis (BE; infective) (see p. 994).

Negative developmental consequences, particularly in the area of motor and cognitive development, may occur from chronic hypoxemia. Fifty percent of postnatal brain growth takes place in the first year of life, so chronic hypoxemia, poor growth, and poor nutrition during this period can have significant adverse effects. In addition, the risks of CVA; periods of profound cyanosis and hypoxia during hypercyanotic spells; and multiple surgeries, hospitalizations, and cardiac catheterizations significantly increase the possibility of neurologic insult, resulting in developmental delays. The desire to minimize these risks is an important factor in the trend toward early corrective surgical repair of cyanotic defects in infancy.

Diagnostic Evaluation

Cyanosis in the newborn can be a result of cardiac, pulmonary, metabolic, or hematologic disease, although cardiac and pulmonary causes occur most often. To distinguish between the two, a hyperoxia test may be helpful. The infant is placed in a 100% oxygen environment, and blood parameters are monitored. A $Pa{O_2}$ of 100 mm Hg or higher suggests lung disease, and a $Pa{O_2}$ lower than 100 mm Hg suggests cardiac disease (the problem is related to inadequate perfusion of the pulmonary bed) (Park, 2014). An accurate history, a chest radiograph (demonstrating reduced pulmonary blood flow), and especially an echocardiogram contribute to the diagnosis of cyanotic heart disease.

Therapeutic Management

Newborns generally exhibit cyanosis within the first few days of life as the ductus arteriosus, which provided pulmonary blood flow, begins to close. Prostaglandin E_1, which causes vasodilation and smooth muscle relaxation and thus increases dilation and patency of the ductus arteriosus, is administered intravenously to reestablish pulmonary blood flow. The use of prostaglandins has been lifesaving for infants with ductus-dependent cardiac defects. The increase in oxygenation allows the infant's condition to be stabilized and a complete diagnostic evaluation to be performed before further treatment is needed.

Hypercyanotic spells occur suddenly, and prompt recognition and treatment are essential. In the hospital setting, spells are often seen during blood drawing or IV line insertion, when the child is highly agitated, or after cardiac catheterization. Treatment of a hypercyanotic spell is outlined in the Applying Evidence to Practice box. Placing an infant in the knee-chest position reduces the venous return from the legs (which is desaturated) and increases systemic vascular resistance, which diverts more blood into the pulmonary artery (Fig. 27.11). Morphine, administered subcutaneously or through an existing IV line, is helpful in reducing infundibular spasm. A spell may indicate the need for prompt surgical treatment. In rare cases, propranolol (Inderal) may be given in the interim to prevent infundibular spasm.

The cyanotic infant or child is well hydrated to keep the hematocrit and blood viscosity within acceptable limits to reduce the risk of CVA. Monitor the infant closely for anemia because of the risk of CVAs and the reduced arterial oxygen-carrying capacity that occurs. Iron supplementation and possibly blood transfusion are used as needed.

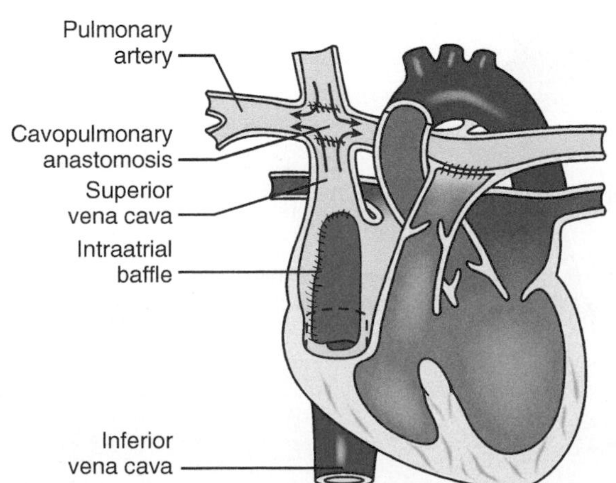

FIG. 27.10 Fontan procedure: third stage of single ventricle palliation.

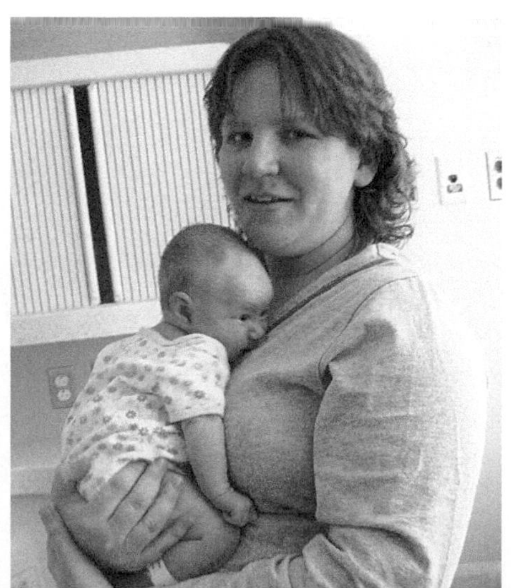

FIG. 27.11 Infant held in the knee-chest position.

APPLYING EVIDENCE TO PRACTICE

Guidelines for Treating Hypercyanotic Spells

- Place infant in knee-chest position (see Fig. 27.11).
- Employ a calm, comforting approach.
- Administer 100% oxygen by face mask.
- Give morphine subcutaneously or through existing intravenous line.
- Begin intravenous fluid replacement and volume expansion, if needed.
- Repeat morphine administration.

Respiratory tract infections or reduced pulmonary function from any cause can worsen hypoxemia in the cyanotic child. Aggressive pulmonary hygiene, chest physiotherapy, administration of antibiotics, and use of oxygen to improve arterial saturations are important interventions.

Surgical Intervention

Many cardiac causes of hypoxemia can be repaired surgically and are described in the discussion of the particular cardiac defect (see Boxes 27.4 to 27.7 later in this chapter). However, some severely hypoxemic

Text continued on p. 985

BOX 27.4 Defects With Increased Pulmonary Blood Flow

Atrial Septal Defect (see Fig. 27.13, *A*)

Description—Abnormal opening between the atria, allowing blood from the higher-pressure left atrium to flow into the lower-pressure right atrium. There are three types of atrial septal defect (ASD):

Ostium primum (ASD 1)—Opening at lower end of septum; may be associated with mitral valve abnormalities

Ostium secundum (ASD 2)—Opening near center of septum

Sinus venosus defect—Opening near junction of superior vena cava and right atrium; may be associated with partial anomalous pulmonary venous connection

Pathophysiology—Because left atrial pressure slightly exceeds right atrial pressure, blood flows from the left to the right atrium, causing an increased flow of oxygenated blood into the right side of the heart. Despite the low pressure difference, a high rate of flow can still occur because of low pulmonary vascular resistance and the greater distensibility of the right atrium, which further reduces flow resistance. This volume is well tolerated by the right ventricle because it is delivered under much lower pressure than with a ventricular septal defect. Although there is right atrial and ventricular enlargement, cardiac failure is unusual in an uncomplicated ASD. Pulmonary vascular changes usually occur only after several decades if the defect is left unrepaired.

Clinical manifestations—Patients may be asymptomatic. Spontaneous closure of ASDs are most likely to occur in younger patients and those with small defects (Vick & Bezold, 2017). They may develop heart failure (HF), particularly in the third or fourth decade of life if the ASD goes undiagnosed, as the pulmonary artery pressure then begins to rise. There is a characteristic murmur. Patients are at risk for atrial dysrhythmias (probably caused by atrial enlargement and stretching of conduction fibers) and pulmonary vascular obstructive disease and emboli formation later in life from chronically increased pulmonary blood flow.

Surgical closure—Surgical patch closure (pericardial patch or Dacron patch) is done for moderate to large defects. Open repair with cardiopulmonary bypass

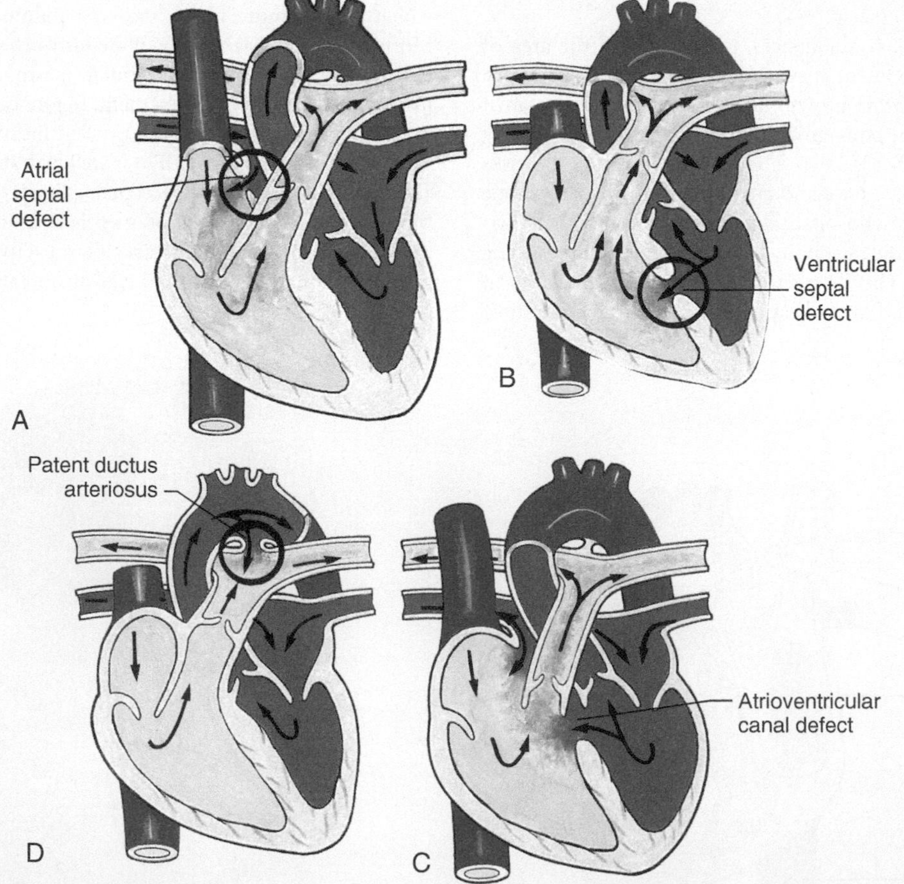

FIG. 27.13 **A,** Atrial septal defect. **B,** Ventricular septal defect. **C,** Atrioventricular canal defect. **D,** Patent ductus arteriosus.

BOX 27.4 Defects With Increased Pulmonary Blood Flow—cont'd

is usually performed before school age. In addition, the sinus venosus defect requires patch placement, so the anomalous right pulmonary venous return is directed to the left atrium with a baffle. The ASD 1 type may require mitral valve repair or, rarely, replacement of the mitral valve.

Transcatheter closure—ASD 2 closure with a device during cardiac catheterization is becoming commonplace and can be done as an outpatient procedure. The Amplatzer septal occluder is most commonly used. Smaller defects that have a rim around them for attachment of the device can be closed with a device; large, irregular defects without a rim require surgical closure. Successful closure in appropriately selected patients yields results similar to surgery but involves shorter hospital stays and fewer complications. Patients receive low-dose aspirin for 6 months (Moore, Hegde, El-Said, et al., 2013).

Prognosis—Outcomes for both treatment options is very good. Limited data also suggest that the rates of procedural success may be comparable to or possibly better with surgery vs. transcatheter closure, but that there may be an increased rate of reintervention associated with percutaneous closure (Du, Hijazi, Kleinman, et al., 2002).

Ventricular Septal Defect (see Fig. 27.13, *B*)

Description—Abnormal opening between the ventricles. May be classified according to location: membranous (accounting for 80%) or muscular. May vary in size from a small pinhole to absence of the septum, which results in a common ventricle. Ventricular septal defects (VSDs) are frequently associated with other defects, such as pulmonic stenosis, transposition of the great vessels, patent ductus arteriosus, atrial defects, and coarctation of the aorta. Many VSDs (20% to 60%) close spontaneously. Spontaneous closure is most likely to occur during the first year of life in children having small or moderate defects.

Pathophysiology—Because of the higher pressure within the left ventricle and because the systemic arterial circulation offers more resistance than the pulmonary circulation, blood flows through the defect into the pulmonary artery. The increased blood volume is pumped into the lungs, which may eventually result in increased pulmonary vascular resistance. Increased pressure in the right ventricle as a result of left-to-right shunting and pulmonary resistance causes the muscle to hypertrophy. If the right ventricle is unable to accommodate the increased workload, the right atrium may also enlarge as it attempts to overcome the resistance offered by incomplete right ventricular emptying.

Clinical manifestations—HF is common. There is a characteristic murmur.

Surgical treatment

Palliative—Pulmonary artery banding (placement of a band around the main pulmonary artery to decrease pulmonary blood flow) may be done in infants with multiple muscular VSDs or complex anatomy. Improvements in surgical techniques and postoperative care make complete repair in infancy the preferred approach.

Complete repair (procedure of choice)—Small defects are repaired with sutures. Large defects usually require sewing a knitted Dacron patch over the opening. Cardiopulmonary bypass is used for both procedures. The approach for the repair is generally through the right atrium and the tricuspid valve. Postoperative complications include residual VSD and conduction disturbances.

Transcatheter closure—Catheter closure of muscular, postoperative, or fenestrated defects is also widely used in centers nationwide. Device closures of VSDs carry more risk than with ASDs. The most common complication noted in one study was complete atrioventricular (AV) block requiring pacemaker placement in 5.7% of the subjects (Butera, Carminati, Chessa, et al., 2007).

Prognosis—Risks depend on the location of the defect, the number of defects, surgical vs. transcatheter closure, and the presence of other associated cardiac defects. Single membranous defects are associated with low mortality risk (<2%); multiple muscular defects can carry a higher risk (Jacobs, Mavroudis, Jacobs, et al., 2004).

Atrioventricular Canal Defect (see Fig. 27.13, *C*)

Description—Also referred to as *AV septal defects* or *endocardial cushion defects.* Incomplete fusion of the endocardial cushions. Consists of a low ASD that is continuous with a high VSD and clefts of the mitral and tricuspid valves, which creates a large central AV valve that allows blood to flow between all four chambers of the heart. The directions and pathways of flow are determined by pulmonary and systemic resistance, left and right ventricular pressures, and the compliance of each chamber, although flow is generally from left to right. It is the most common cardiac defect in children with Down syndrome.

Pathophysiology—The alterations in hemodynamics depend on the severity of the defect and the child's pulmonary vascular resistance. Immediately after birth, while the newborn's pulmonary vascular resistance is high, there is minimum shunting of blood through the defect. Once this resistance falls, left-to-right shunting occurs and pulmonary blood flow increases. The resultant pulmonary vascular engorgement predisposes the child to development of HF.

Clinical manifestations—Patients usually have moderate to severe HF. There is a characteristic murmur. There may be mild cyanosis that increases with crying. Patients are at high risk for developing pulmonary vascular obstructive disease.

Surgical treatment

Palliative—Pulmonary artery banding is occasionally done in small infants with severe symptoms. Single ventricle palliation is necessary for some infants who have a right or left ventricle dominant canal defect (see p. 987).

Complete repair—Surgical repair consists of patch closure of the septal defects and reconstruction of the AV valve tissue (either repair of the mitral valve cleft or fashioning of two AV valves). Postoperative complications include heart block, HF, mitral regurgitation, dysrhythmias, and pulmonary hypertension.

Prognosis—Operative mortality rate is generally low with patients who are younger (>2.5 months) and smaller (<3.5 kg) having worse outcomes (Jacobs, Mavroudis, Jacobs, et al., 2004; St. Louis, Jodhka, Jacobs, et al., 2014). A potential later problem is mitral regurgitation, which may require valve replacement.

Patent Ductus Arteriosus (see Fig. 27.13, *D*)

Description—Failure of the fetal ductus arteriosus (artery connecting the aorta and pulmonary artery) to close within the first weeks of life. The continued patency of this vessel allows blood to flow from the higher-pressure aorta to the lower-pressure pulmonary artery, which causes a left-to-right shunt.

Pathophysiology—The hemodynamic consequences of patent ductus arteriosus (PDA) depend on the size of the ductus and the pulmonary vascular resistance. At birth the resistance in the pulmonary and systemic circulations is almost identical, so the resistance in the aorta and pulmonary artery is equalized. As the systemic pressure comes to exceed the pulmonary pressure, blood begins to shunt from the aorta across the duct to the pulmonary artery (left-to-right shunt). The additional blood is recirculated through the lungs and returned to the left atrium and left ventricle. The effect of this altered circulation is increased workload on the left side of the heart, increased pulmonary vascular congestion and possibly resistance, and potentially increased right ventricular pressure and hypertrophy.

Clinical manifestations—The amount of shunting will determine the degree of clinical manifestations. There is a characteristic machinery-like murmur. Patients may be asymptomatic or show signs of HF. Moderate to large PDAs may present as left-sided volume overload or reversible pulmonary arterial hypertension.

Medical management—Administration of indomethacin (prostaglandin inhibitor) has proved successful in closing a patent ductus in premature infants and some newborns.

Surgical treatment—Surgical division or ligation of the patent vessel is performed via a left thoracotomy. In video-assisted thoracoscopic surgery, a thoracoscope and instruments are inserted through three small incisions on the left side of the chest to place a clip on the ductus. The surgical approach are dependent on the size and age of the patient.

Transcatheter treatment—Coils to occlude the PDA are placed in the catheterization laboratory in many centers. Premature or small infants (with small-diameter femoral arteries) and patients with large or unusual PDAs may require surgery.

Prognosis—Both surgical and nonsurgical procedures can be done at low risk with less than 1% mortality rate. PDA closure in very premature infants has a higher mortality rate because of the additional significant medical problems.

BOX 27.5 Obstructive Defects

Coarctation of the Aorta (see Fig. 27.14, *A*)

Description—Localized narrowing near the insertion of the ductus arteriosus, which results in increased pressure proximal to the defect (head and upper extremities) and decreased pressure distal to the obstruction (body and lower extremities).

Pathophysiology—The effect of a narrowing within the aorta is increased pressure proximal to the defect (upper extremities) and decreased pressure distal to it (lower extremities).

Clinical manifestations—There may be high blood pressure and bounding pulses in the arms, weak or absent femoral pulses, and cool lower extremities with lower blood pressure. There are signs of heart failure in infants. In infants with critical coarctation, the hemodynamic condition may deteriorate rapidly with severe acidosis and hypotension. Mechanical ventilation and inotropic support are often necessary before surgery. Older children may experience dizziness, headaches, fainting, and epistaxis resulting from hypertension. Patients are at risk for hypertension, ruptured aorta, aortic aneurysm, and stroke.

Surgical treatment—Surgical repair is the treatment of choice for infants younger than 6 months of age and for patients with long-segment stenosis or complex anatomy. Repair is by either (1) resection of the narrowed portion with an end-to-end anastomosis of the aorta or (2) enlargement of the section using a graft of prosthetic material or portion of the left subclavian artery. Because this defect is outside the heart and pericardium, cardiopulmonary bypass is not required, and a thoracotomy incision is used. Postoperative hypertension is treated with intravenous sodium nitroprusside, esmolol, or milrinone, followed by oral medications, such as angiotensin-converting enzyme inhibitors or beta blockers. Residual permanent hypertension after repair of coarctation of the aorta (COA) seems to be related to age and time of repair. To prevent both hypertension at rest and exercise-provoked systemic hypertension after repair, elective surgery for COA is advised within the first 2 years of life. Percutaneous balloon angioplasty techniques have proved to be very effective in relieving residual postoperative coarctation gradients.

Transcatheter treatment—Balloon angioplasty is a primary intervention for COA in older infants and children. In adolescents, stents may be placed in the aorta to maintain patency. The goal of the procedure is to achieve a reduction in gradient to less than 10%, or more than 90% relief of obstruction angiographically. Dilation and/or stent implantation for native or recurrent coarctation seems to immediately relieve obstruction in more than 90% of cases (Holzer, Chisolm, Hill, et al., 2008).

Prognosis—There are low rates of morbidity, mortality, and reintervention for infants and children who underwent COA repair via a left thoracotomy (Mery, Guzmán-Pruneda, Trost, et al., 2015). Major long-term complications include recoarctation, aortic aneurysm, and systemic hypertension (Brown, Burkhart, Connolly, et al., 2013).

Aortic Stenosis (see Fig. 27.14, *B*)

Description—Narrowing or stricture of the aortic valve, causing resistance to blood flow in the left ventricle, decreased cardiac output, left ventricular hypertrophy, and pulmonary vascular congestion. Valvular aortic stenosis (AS), the most common type, is usually caused by malformed cusps that result in a bicuspid rather than tricuspid valve or fusion of the cusps. Subvalvular stenosis is a stricture caused by a fibrous ring below a normal valve; supravalvular stenosis occurs infrequently. Valvular AS is a serious defect because (1) the obstruction tends to be progressive; (2) sudden episodes of myocardial ischemia, or low cardiac output, can result in sudden death; and (3) surgical repair rarely results in a normal valve. This is one of the rare instances in

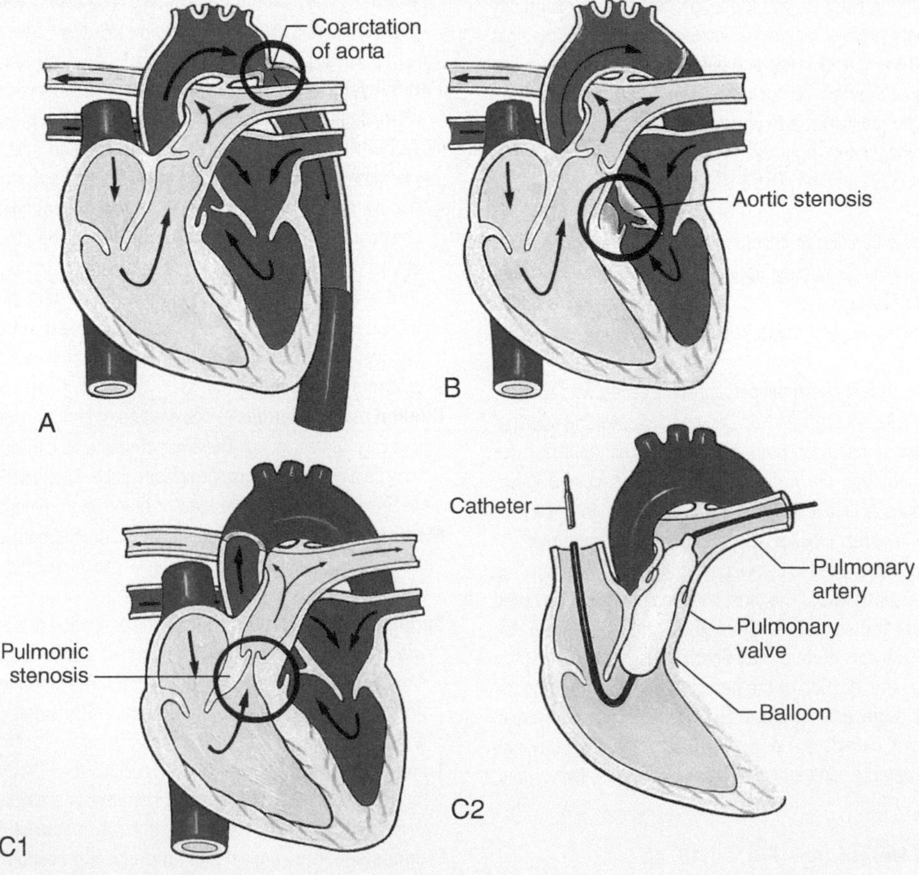

FIG. 27.14 A, Coarctation of the aorta. **B,** Aortic stenosis. **C,** Pulmonary stenosis.

BOX 27.5 Obstructive Defects—cont'd

which strenuous physical activity may be curtailed because of the cardiac condition.

Pathophysiology—A stricture in the aortic outflow tract causes resistance to ejection of blood from the left ventricle. The extra workload on the left ventricle causes hypertrophy. If left ventricular failure develops, left atrial pressure will increase; this causes increased pressure in the pulmonary veins, which results in pulmonary vascular congestion (pulmonary edema).

Clinical manifestations—Newborns with critical AS demonstrate signs of decreased cardiac output with faint pulses, hypotension, tachycardia, and poor feeding. Children show signs of exercise intolerance, chest pain, and dizziness when standing for a long period. There is a characteristic murmur. Patients are at risk for infective endocarditis, coronary insufficiency, and ventricular dysfunction.

Valvular Aortic Stenosis

Surgical treatment—Aortic valvotomy is performed under inflow occlusion. Used rarely because balloon dilation in the catheterization laboratory is the first-line procedure. Newborns with critical AS and small left-sided structures may undergo a stage 1 Norwood procedure (see Hypoplastic Left Heart Syndrome, page 984).

Prognosis—Aortic valvotomy remains a palliative procedure and the patient may require further surgery to repair or even replace the aortic valve. An aortic homograft with a valve may also be used (extended aortic root replacement), or the pulmonic valve may be moved to the aortic position and replaced with a homograft valve (Ross procedure). If the obstruction is at the subvalvular region and results from narrowing of the left ventricular outflow tract with a small aortic valve annulus, a patch may be required to enlarge the entire left ventricular outflow tract and annulus and replace the aortic valve, an approach known as the Konno procedure. Patients that have obstruction at both the valvular and subvalvular regions may undergo a combination of these two procedures, also called a Ross-Konno procedure.

Nonsurgical treatment—The narrowed valve is dilated using balloon angioplasty in the catheterization laboratory. This procedure is usually the first intervention.

Prognosis—Complications include aortic insufficiency or valvular regurgitation, tearing of the valve leaflets, and loss of pulse in the catheterized limb.

Pulmonary Stenosis (see Fig. 27.14, *C*)

Description—Narrowing at the entrance to the pulmonary artery. Resistance to blood flow causes right ventricular hypertrophy and decreased pulmonary blood flow. Pulmonary atresia is the extreme form of pulmonic stenosis (PS) in that there is total fusion of the commissures and no blood flows to the lungs. The right ventricle may be hypoplastic.

Pathophysiology—When PS is present, resistance to blood flow causes right ventricular hypertrophy. If right ventricular failure develops, right atrial pressure increases, and this may result in reopening of the foramen ovale, shunting of deoxygenated blood into the left atrium, and systemic cyanosis. If PS is severe, HF occurs, and systemic venous engorgement is noted. An associated defect such as a patent ductus arteriosus partially compensates for the obstruction by shunting blood from the aorta to the pulmonary artery and into the lungs.

Clinical manifestations—Patients may be asymptomatic; some have mild cyanosis or HF. Progressive narrowing causes increased symptoms. Newborns with severe narrowing are cyanotic. There is a characteristic murmur. Cardiomegaly is evident on chest radiographic films. Patients are at risk for infective endocarditis.

Surgical treatment—Need for surgical treatment is rare with widespread use of balloon angioplasty techniques, but in some cases pulmonary valvotomy with cardiopulmonary bypass is necessary.

Transcatheter treatment—Balloon angioplasty in the cardiac catheterization laboratory to dilate the valve. A catheter is inserted across the stenotic pulmonic valve into the pulmonary artery, and a balloon at the end of the catheter is inflated and rapidly passed through the narrowed opening. The procedure is associated with few complications and has proved to be highly effective. It is the treatment of choice for discrete PS in most centers and can be done safely in neonates.

Prognosis—Risk is low for both surgical and transcatheter procedures; mortality rate is low, slightly higher in neonates. Both balloon dilation and surgical valvotomy leave the pulmonary valve incompetent because they involve opening the fused valve leaflets; however, these patients are clinically asymptomatic. Long-term problems with restenosis or valve incompetence may occur.

BOX 27.6 Defects With Decreased Pulmonary Blood Flow

Tetralogy of Fallot (see Fig. 27.15, *A*)

Description—The classic form includes four defects: (1) ventricular septal defect (VSD), (2) pulmonic stenosis, (3) overriding aorta, and (4) right ventricular hypertrophy.

Pathophysiology—The alteration in hemodynamics varies widely, depending primarily on the degree of pulmonary stenosis, but also on the size of the VSD and the pulmonary and systemic resistance to flow. Because the VSD is usually large, pressures may be equal in the right and left ventricles. Therefore the shunt direction depends on the difference between pulmonary and systemic vascular resistance. If pulmonary vascular resistance is higher than systemic resistance, the shunt is from right to left. If systemic resistance is higher than pulmonary resistance, the shunt is from left to right. Pulmonary stenosis decreases blood flow to the lungs and consequently the amount of oxygenated blood that returns to the left side of the heart. Depending on the position of the aorta, blood from both ventricles may be distributed systemically.

Clinical manifestations—Some infants may be acutely cyanotic at birth; others have mild cyanosis that progresses over the first year of life as the pulmonary stenosis worsens. There is a characteristic murmur. There may be acute episodes of cyanosis and hypoxia, called *blue spells* or *tet spells*. Anoxic spells occur when the infant's oxygen requirements exceed the blood supply, usually during crying or after feeding. Patients are at risk for emboli, seizures, and loss of consciousness or sudden death after an anoxic spell.

Surgical treatment—Elective repair is usually performed in the first year of life. Indications for repair include increasing cyanosis and the development of hypercyanotic spells. Complete repair involves closure of the VSD and resection of the infundibular stenosis, with placement of a pericardial patch to enlarge the right ventricular outflow tract. In some repairs, the patch may extend across the pulmonic valve annulus (transannular patch), making the pulmonic valve incompetent. The procedure requires a median sternotomy and the use of cardiopulmonary bypass.

Prognosis—The operative mortality rate for total correction of tetralogy of Fallot is less than 3% (Jacobs, Mavroudis, Jacobs, et al., 2004). Long-term complications include chronic pulmonary regurgitation with right ventricular enlargement and decreased function requiring pulmonary valve replacement, residual right ventricular outflow tract obstruction, aortic root dilation and aortic valve insufficiency, arrhythmias, and sudden cardiac death. Pulmonary valve replacement is performed either surgically or in the catheterization laboratory using a transcatheter approach (Doyle, Kavanaugh-McHugh, & Fish, 2016).

Continued

BOX 27.6 Defects With Decreased Pulmonary Blood Flow—cont'd

Tricuspid Atresia (see Fig. 27.15, *B*)

Description—The tricuspid valve fails to develop; consequently, there is no communication from the right atrium to the right ventricle. Blood flows through an atrial septal defect (ASD) or a patent foramen ovale to the left side of the heart and through a VSD to the right ventricle and out to the lungs. The condition is often associated with pulmonary stenosis and transposition of the great arteries. There is complete mixing of deoxygenated and oxygenated blood in the left side of the heart, which results in systemic desaturation, and varying amounts of pulmonary obstruction, which causes decreased pulmonary blood flow.

Pathophysiology—At birth the presence of a patent foramen ovale (or other atrial septal opening) is required to permit blood flow across the septum into the left atrium; the patent ductus arteriosus allows blood flow to the pulmonary artery into the lungs for oxygenation. A VSD allows a modest amount of blood to enter the right ventricle and pulmonary artery for oxygenation. Pulmonary blood flow is often diminished.

Clinical manifestations—Cyanosis is usually seen in the newborn period. There may be tachycardia and dyspnea. Older children have signs of chronic hypoxemia with clubbing.

Therapeutic management—For the neonate whose pulmonary blood flow depends on the patency of the ductus arteriosus, a continuous infusion of prostaglandin E_1 is started at 0.1 mcg/kg/min until surgical intervention can be arranged.

Surgical treatment—Patients with tricuspid atresia follow the staged surgical approach for single ventricle anatomy (see p. 987) with the left ventricle becoming the ventricular pump.

Prognosis—Surgical mortality rate is less than 5% (Jacobs, Mavroudis, Jacobs, et al., 2004); the rate increases when the anatomy is more complex and other risk factors are present. Postoperative complications include dysrhythmias, systemic venous hypertension, pleural and pericardial effusions, and ventricular dysfunction.

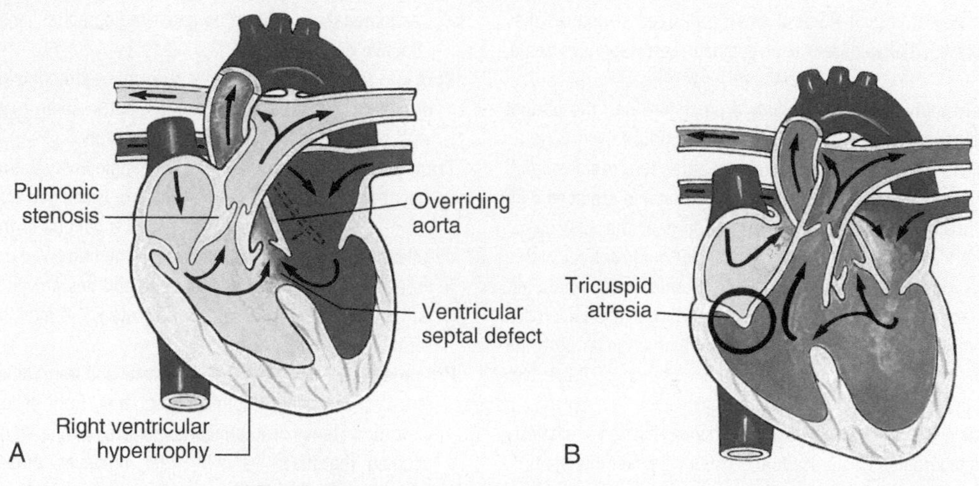

FIG. 27.15 A, Tetralogy of Fallot. **B,** Tricuspid atresia.

BOX 27.7 Mixed Defects

Transposition of the Great Arteries or Transposition of the Great Vessels (see Fig. 27.16, *A*)

Description—The pulmonary artery leaves the left ventricle, and the aorta exits from the right ventricle, with no communication between the systemic and pulmonary circulations.

Pathophysiology—Associated defects such as septal defects or patent ductus arteriosus must be present to permit blood to enter the systemic circulation or the pulmonary circulation for mixing of saturated and desaturated blood. The most common defect associated with transposition of the great arteries (TGA) is a patent foramen ovale. At birth there is also a patent ductus arteriosus, although in most instances this closes after the neonatal period. Another associated defect may be a ventricular septal defect (VSD). The presence of a VSD increases the risk of heart failure (HF) because it permits blood to flow from the right to the left ventricle, into the pulmonary artery, and finally to the lungs. However, it also produces increased pulmonary blood flow under high pressure, which can result in high pulmonary vascular resistance.

Clinical manifestations—Vary according to the type and size of the associated defects. Newborns with minimum communication are severely cyanotic and have depressed function at birth. Those with large septal defects or a patent ductus arteriosus may be less cyanotic but have symptoms of HF. Heart sounds vary according to the type of defect present. Cardiomegaly is usually evident a few weeks after birth.

Therapeutic management (to provide intracardiac mixing)—Intravenous prostaglandin E_1 may be administered preoperatively to maintain ductal patency and ensure adequate systemic blood flow. During cardiac catheterization or under echocardiographic guidance, a balloon atrial septostomy (Rashkind procedure) may also be performed to increase mixing by opening the atrial septum.

Surgical treatment—An arterial switch operation (ASO; also called a Jatene procedure) is the procedure of choice performed in the first weeks of life. It involves transecting the great arteries and anastomosing the main pulmonary artery to the proximal aorta (just above the aortic valve) and anastomosing the ascending aorta to the proximal pulmonary artery. The coronary arteries are switched from the proximal aorta to the proximal pulmonary artery to create a new aorta. Reimplantation of the coronary arteries is critical to the infant's survival, and they must be reattached without torsion or kinking to provide the heart with its supply of oxygen. The advantage of the arterial switch procedure is the reestablishment of normal circulation, with the left ventricle acting as the systemic pump. Potential complications of the arterial switch include narrowing at the great artery anastomoses and coronary artery insufficiency.

BOX 27.7 Mixed Defects—cont'd

Intraatrial baffle repairs—Intraatrial baffle repairs are rarely performed, although many adolescents and adults survive today with repairs that were done more than 15 years ago. An intraatrial baffle is created to divert venous blood to the mitral valve and pulmonary venous blood to the tricuspid valve using the patient's atrial septum (Senning procedure) or a prosthetic material (Mustard procedure). A disadvantage is the continuing role of the right ventricle as the systemic pump and the late development of right ventricular failure and rhythm disturbances. Other potential postoperative complications include loss of normal sinus rhythm, baffle leaks, and ventricular dysfunction.

Rastelli procedure—This procedure is the operative choice in infants with TGA, VSD, and severe pulmonary stenosis. It involves closure of the VSD with a baffle so left ventricular blood is directed through the VSD into the aorta. The pulmonary valve is then closed, and a conduit is placed from the right ventricle to the pulmonary artery to create a physiologically normal circulation. Unfortunately, this procedure requires multiple conduit replacements as the child grows.

Prognosis—Outcomes after the ASO are quite good. There are some long-term complications, including neoaortic, pulmonary, and coronary artery complications, but most patients maintain normal cardiovascular function and exercise capacity (Khairy, Clair, Fernandes, et al., 2013). Patients who undergo a Senning or Mustard procedure demonstrate diminished long-term survival rates and substantial morbidity (Cuypers, Eindhoven, Slager, et al., 2014).

Total Anomalous Pulmonary Venous Connection (see Fig. 27.16, *B*)

Description—Rare defect characterized by failure of the pulmonary veins to join the left atrium. Instead, the pulmonary veins are abnormally connected to the systemic venous circuit via the right atrium or various veins draining toward the right atrium, such as the superior vena cava. The abnormal attachment results in mixed blood being returned to the right atrium and shunted from the right to the left through an atrial septal defect (ASD). Total anomalous pulmonary venous connection (TAPVC; also called *total anomalous pulmonary venous return* or *total anomalous pulmonary venous drainage*) is classified according to the pulmonary venous point of attachment as follows:

Supracardiac—Attachment above the diaphragm, such as to the superior vena cava (most common form) but not directly to the heart (see Fig. 27.16, *B*)

Cardiac—Direct attachment to the heart, such as to the right atrium or coronary sinus

Infradiaphragmatic—Attachment below the diaphragm, such as to the inferior vena cava (most severe form)

Pathophysiology—The right atrium receives all the blood that normally would flow into the left atrium. As a result, the right side of the heart hypertrophies, whereas the left side, especially the left atrium, may remain small. An associated ASD or patent foramen ovale allows systemic venous blood to shunt from the higher-pressure right atrium to the left atrium and into the left side of the heart. As a result, the oxygen saturation of the blood in both sides of

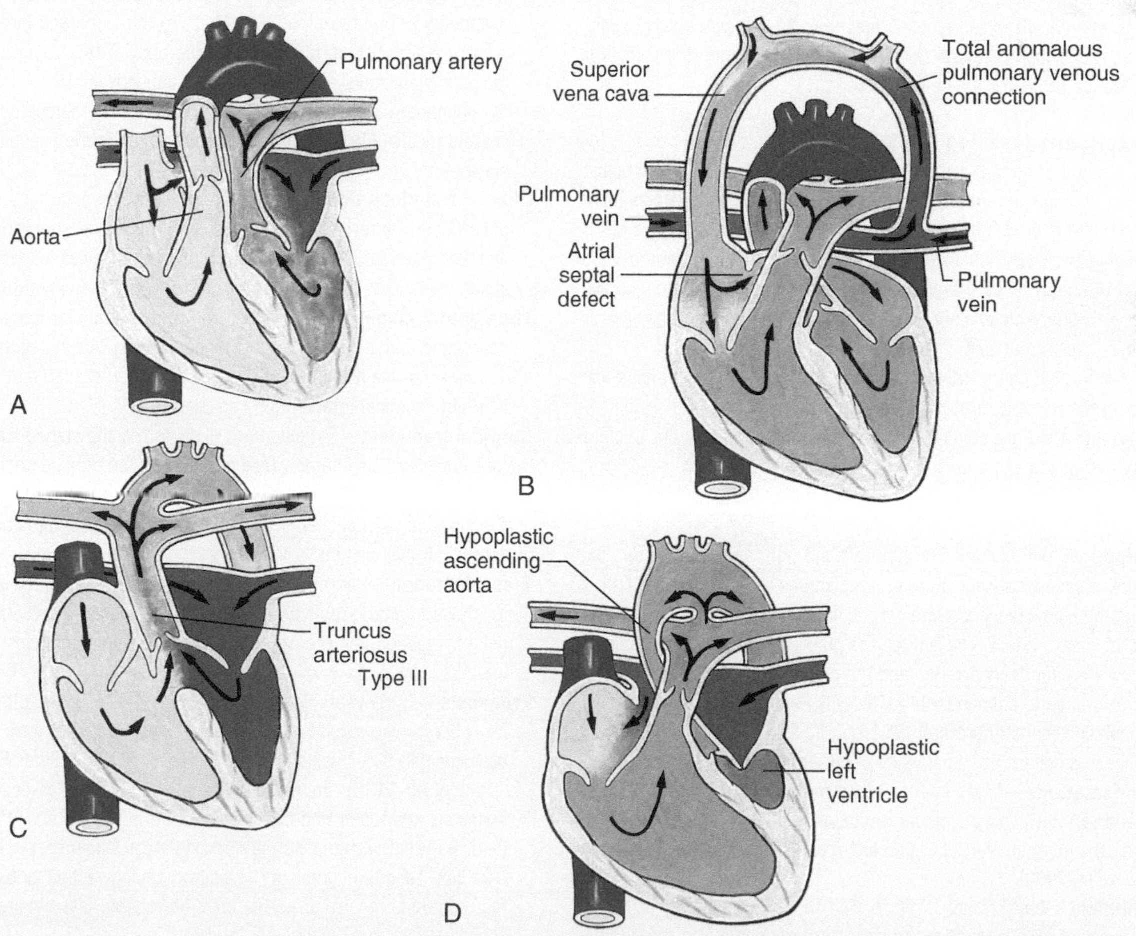

FIG. 27.16 A, Transposition of the great arteries or transposition of the great vessels. **B,** Total anomalous pulmonary venous connection. **C,** Truncus arteriosus. **D,** Hypoplastic left heart syndrome.

Continued

BOX 27.7 Mixed Defects—cont'd

the heart (and ultimately in the systemic arterial circulation) is the same. If the pulmonary blood flow is large, pulmonary venous return is also large, and the amount of saturated blood is relatively high. However, if there is obstruction to pulmonary venous drainage, pulmonary venous return is impeded, pulmonary venous pressure rises, and pulmonary interstitial edema develops and eventually contributes to HF. Infradiaphragmatic TAPVC is often associated with obstruction to pulmonary venous drainage and is a surgical emergency.

Clinical manifestations—Most infants develop cyanosis early in life. The degree of cyanosis is inversely related to the amount of pulmonary blood flow—the more pulmonary blood, the less cyanosis. Children with unobstructed TAPVC may be asymptomatic until pulmonary vascular resistance decreases during infancy, increasing pulmonary blood flow, with resulting signs of HF. Cyanosis becomes worse with pulmonary vein obstruction; once obstruction occurs, the infant's condition usually deteriorates rapidly. Without intervention, cardiac failure progresses to death.

Surgical treatment—Corrective repair is performed in early infancy. The surgical approach varies with the anatomic defect. In general, however, the common pulmonary vein is anastomosed to the back of the left atrium, the ASD is closed, and the anomalous pulmonary venous connection is ligated. The cardiac type is most easily repaired; the infradiaphragmatic type carries the highest morbidity and mortality rates because of the higher incidence of pulmonary vein obstruction. Potential postoperative complications include reobstruction; bleeding; dysrhythmias, particularly heart block; pulmonary artery hypertension; and persistent heart failure.

Prognosis—Mortality rate for all types is less than 10% (Jacobs, Mavroudis, Jacobs, et al., 2004) and is lowest for the cardiac type; morbidity increases with the presence of pulmonary vein obstruction.

Truncus Arteriosus (see Fig. 27.16, *C*)

Description—Failure of normal septation and division of the embryonic bulbar trunk into the pulmonary artery and the aorta, which results in development of a single vessel that overrides both ventricles. Blood from both ventricles mixes in the common great artery, which leads to desaturation and hypoxemia. Blood ejected from the heart flows preferentially to the lower-pressure pulmonary arteries, so pulmonary blood flow is increased and systemic blood flow is reduced. There are three types:

Type I—A single pulmonary trunk arises near the base of the truncus and divides into the left and right pulmonary arteries.

Type II—The left and right pulmonary arteries arise separately but in close proximity and at the same level from the back of the truncus.

Type III—The pulmonary arteries arise independently from the sides of the truncus.

Pathophysiology—Blood ejected from the left and right ventricles enters the common trunk, so pulmonary and systemic circulations are mixed. Blood flow is distributed to the pulmonary and systemic circulations according to the relative resistances of each system. The amount of pulmonary blood flow depends on the size of the pulmonary arteries and the pulmonary vascular resistance. Generally, resistance to pulmonary blood flow is less than systemic vascular resistance, which results in preferential blood flow to the lungs. Pulmonary vascular disease develops at an early age in patients with truncus arteriosus.

Clinical manifestations—Most infants are symptomatic with moderate to severe HF and variable cyanosis, poor growth, and activity intolerance. There is a characteristic murmur. Thirty-five percent of patients have 22q11 deletions (Goldmuntz & Lin, 2008).

Surgical treatment—Early repair is performed in the first month of life. It involves closing the VSD so that the truncus arteriosus receives the outflow from the left ventricle, excising the pulmonary arteries from the aorta and attaching them to the right ventricle using a right ventricle to pulmonary artery conduit and possible repair of the truncal valve. Postoperative complications include truncal valve insufficiency, persistent heart failure, bleeding, pulmonary artery hypertension, dysrhythmias, and residual VSD. Because conduits are not living tissue, they will not grow along with the child and may also become narrowed with calcifications. One or more conduit replacements will be needed in childhood.

Prognosis—Per-operative mortality rate is about 10%, with highest mortality rate in patients who required repair for both truncal valve and aortic arch interruption (Russell, Pasquali, Jacobs, et al., 2012). Long-term complications include truncal valve regurgitation and conduit stenosis.

Hypoplastic Left Heart Syndrome (HLHS) (see Fig. 27.16, *D*)

Description—Underdevelopment of the left side of the heart with significant hypoplasisa of the left ventricle including atresia, stenosis, or hypoplasia of the aortic and/or mitral valves and hypoplasia of the ascending arota and arch. Most blood from the left atrium flows across the patent foramen ovale to the right atrium, to the right ventricle, and out the pulmonary artery. The descending aorta receives blood from the patent ductus arteriosus supplying systemic blood flow.

Pathophysiology—An ASD or patent foramen ovale allows saturated blood from the left atrium to mix with desaturated blood from the right atrium and to flow through the right ventricle and out into the pulmonary artery. From the pulmonary artery, the blood flows both to the lungs and through the ductus arteriosus into the aorta and out to the body. The amount of blood flow to the pulmonary and systemic circulations depends on the relationship between the pulmonary and systemic vascular resistances. The coronary and cerebral vessels receive blood by retrograde flow through the hypoplastic ascending aorta.

Clinical manifestations—There is mild cyanosis and signs of HF until the patent ductus arteriosus closes, then progressive deterioration with cyanosis and decreased cardiac output, leading to cardiovascular collapse. The condition is usually fatal in the first months of life without intervention.

Therapeutic management—Neonates require stabilization with mechanical ventilation and inotropic support preoperatively. A prostaglandin E_1 infusion is needed to maintain ductal patency and ensure adequate systemic blood flow until surgical intervention can occur.

Surgical treatment—Patients with HLHS follow the staged surgical approach for single ventricle anatomy (see p. 987) with the right ventricle becoming the ventricular pump. Postoperative complications include dysrhythmias, systemic venous hypertension, pleural and pericardial effusions, thrombotic events, and ventricular dysfunction.

Transplantation—Heart transplantation in the newborn period is another option for these infants. Problems include the shortage of newborn organ donors, risk of rejection, long-term problems with chronic immunosuppression, and infection.

Prognosis—Thirty years ago a diagnosis of HLHS was uniformly fatal. Today, for children who survive to the age of 12 months, long-term survival is now approximately 90% (Alsoufi, Mori, Gillespie, et al., 2015; Siffel, Riehle-Colarusso, Oster, et al., 2015). Improved outcomes have been associated with early diagnosis and repair and increased monitoring in the hospital and at home, particularly between the first- and second-stage surgeries (see Family-Centered Care box). Long-term problems include worsening ventricular function, tricuspid regurgitation, recurrent aortic arch narrowing, dysrhythmias, thrombotic complications, and developmental delays.

newborns have cardiac defects, particular those with single ventricle anatomy, which are not amenable to corrective repair and may undergo a palliative surgical procedure to establish a shunt. The shunt serves the same purpose as the ductus arteriosus: to increase blood flow to the lungs through a systemic artery–to–pulmonary artery connection. Currently, a modified Blalock-Taussig operation, in which a Gore-Tex or Impra tube graft is placed to create a communication between the right or left subclavian artery and the pulmonary artery on the same side, is the preferred procedure. The original Blalock-Taussig shunt procedure directly anastomosed the subclavian artery to the pulmonary artery to provide pulmonary blood flow and was the first operation devised for patients with cyanotic heart disease. Because of the higher resistance in the systemic circulation, blood flows from the subclavian artery to the pulmonary artery and to the lungs for oxygenation. The small diameter of the subclavian artery and the shunt (often 3.5 or 4 mm) automatically restricts the volume of blood flow to the pulmonary artery, which prevents severe pulmonary overcirculation and HF. Table 27.4 outlines the most commonly performed shunt procedures today. More detailed discussion of surgical palliation for the infant with single ventricle anatomy is on p. 987.

After a shunt procedure, assess the infant for signs of increased or decreased pulmonary blood flow. If the shunt is too small or has narrowed, the newborn may remain severely hypoxemic, with oxygen saturations below 70%. Surgical revision of the shunt or placement of an additional shunt may be needed. In some patients, the shunt is too large, causing increased pulmonary blood flow resulting in signs and symptoms of HF and oxygen saturations above 85%. The infant may require diuretic therapy, afterload reduction, and increased calories (see discussion of HF). Most surgeons place infants on low-dose aspirin therapy for several months to prevent platelet aggregation and subsequent narrowing of the shunt. Acute cyanosis and signs of tissue hypoxia may occur if the shunt is occluded and pulmonary blood flow is severely limited; shunt occlusion is a medical emergency. The presence of prosthetic material puts patients at risk for infective (bacterial) endocarditis.

TABLE 27.4 Selected Shunt Procedures for Children With Cardiac Defects

Shunt Type	Comments
Modified Blalock-Taussig shunt—Subclavian artery to pulmonary artery using Gore-Tex or Impra tube graft	Shunt flow sometimes excessive, requiring use of diuretics Possibility of thrombosis; aspirin usually prescribed postoperatively Easy to ligate at time of definitive correction Shunt size fixed and may become too small as child grows
Sano modification—Right ventricular to pulmonary artery conduit using Gore-Tex	Prevents diastolic runoff of systemic blood into the pulmonary arteries Provides a higher diastolic blood pressure and seemingly better coronary perfusion Used in place of the modified Blalock-Taussig shunt in the Norwood procedure
Bidirectional Glenn shunt (cavopulmonary anastomosis)—Superior vena cava to side of right pulmonary artery; blood flow to both lungs	Done as a second shunt, often used as a staging step to a Fontan procedure Can be incorporated into eventual modified Fontan procedure Relieves severe cyanosis and decreases volume overload on ventricle Carries risk of embolic events (mixing defect); aspirin often prescribed Pulmonary arteriovenous fistulas may occur months or years later, causing desaturation (uncommon finding)
Central shunt—Ascending aorta to main pulmonary artery using Gore-Tex graft	Length of shunt acts to restrict blood flow; symptoms of heart failure may occur; diuretic therapy may be required Uncommon; used when modified Blalock-Taussig shunt cannot be used Easy to insert and remove at time of repair Possibility of thrombosis; aspirin usually prescribed postoperatively

Nursing Care Management

The general appearance of infants and children with significant cyanosis poses unique concerns. Blue lips and fingernails are obvious signs of the hidden cardiac defect. Clubbing and small, thin stature in older children further indicate severe heart disease. Body image concerns are important. These children are often teased about their appearance and singled out as different. Adolescents are especially concerned about their body image, and cyanosis can become a particular issue for them. Many children, when asked what surgery will do, reply, "make me pink." Accentuating the normal and positive and being careful not to call attention to their cyanosis are helpful interventions. Meeting other children who are cyanotic in the clinic or hospital reassures them that they are not the only ones who are blue.

Parents are often fearful of their child's bluish color because cyanosis is usually associated with lack of oxygen and severe illness. They also must deal with comments from relatives, friends, and strangers in the community about their child's abnormal color. They need a simple explanation of hypoxemia and cyanosis and reassurance that cyanosis does not imply a lack of oxygen to the brain. Their questions and fears need to be addressed in a calm, supportive manner, and positive aspects of their child's growth and development must be emphasized. Teach parents the treatment for hypercyanotic spells. (See Applying Evidence to Practice box, p. 978.)

Dehydration must be prevented in hypoxemic children because it increases the risk of CVAs. Fluid status is carefully monitored through accurate intake and output and daily weight measurements. Maintenance fluid therapy is the minimum requirement; supplemental fluids should be readily available, and gavage feeding or IV hydration is given to children unable to take in adequate fluids orally. Fever, vomiting, and diarrhea can cause dehydration and require prompt treatment. Instruct parents in the importance of adequate fluid intake and measures to prevent dehydration. An oral electrolyte solution such as Pedialyte should be available at home in the event that the infant is unable to tolerate the usual formula. The practitioner should be notified of fever, vomiting, diarrhea, or other problems.

Preventive measures and accurate assessment of respiratory infection are important nursing considerations. Any compromise in pulmonary function increases the infant's hypoxemia. Good hand washing and protection from individuals with an obvious respiratory tract infection are important. Aggressive pulmonary hygiene, treatment with antibiotics or antiviral agents as indicated, and delivery of supplemental oxygen to decrease hypoxemia are necessary measures. Infants may need to be gavage fed or given parenteral nutrition if respiratory distress prevents oral feeding.

CLASSIFICATION OF CONGENITAL HEART DEFECTS

Congenital heart defects have been classified into several categories. Traditionally a physical characteristic, cyanosis, has been used as the

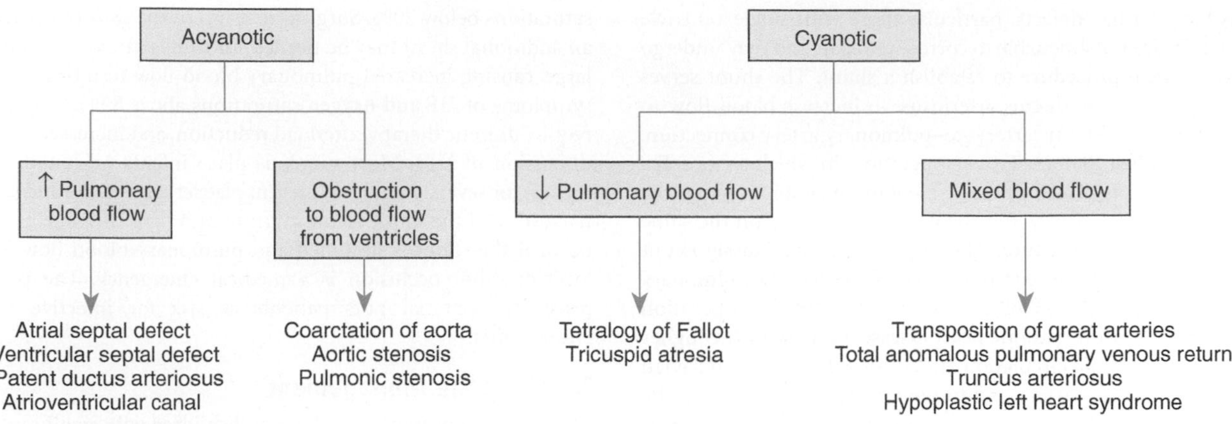

FIG. 27.12 Comparison of acyanotic-cyanotic and hemodynamic classification systems for congenital heart disease.

! NURSING ALERT

Intracardiac shunting of blood from the right side (desaturated) to the left side of the heart allows air in the venous system to go directly to the brain, which results in an air embolism. Therefore all IV lines should have filters in place to prevent air from entering the system, and the entire tubing and any syringes used for flushing or medication administration are checked for air. Any air is removed, and all connections are secured.

distinguishing feature, so the anomalies have been divided into acyanotic and cyanotic defects. In clinical practice this system is problematic because children with acyanotic defects may develop cyanosis. Also, more often, those with cyanotic defects may be pink and have more clinical signs of HF. Because of the complexity of many defects and the variability of their clinical manifestations, the cyanotic-acyanotic classification system has proven to be inadequate and misleading.

A more useful classification system is based on hemodynamic characteristics, or movements involved in the circulation of blood. The defining characteristic is blood flow patterns: (1) increased pulmonary blood flow; (2) decreased pulmonary blood flow; (3) obstruction to blood flow out of the heart; and (4) mixed blood flow, in which saturated and desaturated blood mix within the heart or great arteries. Fig. 27.12 outlines both classification systems.

With the hemodynamic classification system, the clinical manifestations of each group are more uniform and predictable. Defects that allow blood flow from the high-pressure left side of the heart to the lower-pressure right side (left-to-right shunt) result in increased pulmonary blood flow and cause HF. Obstructive defects impede blood flow out of the ventricles; obstruction on the left side of the heart results in HF, whereas severe obstruction on the right side causes cyanosis. Defects that cause decreased pulmonary blood flow result in cyanosis. Mixed lesions present a variable clinical picture based on the degree of mixing and amount of pulmonary blood flow; hypoxemia (with or without cyanosis) and HF usually occur together. (For more detailed explanations, see discussions of specific defects later in this chapter.)

More than 35 types of congenital heart defect have been identified, and some patients have multiple defects. Although some defects are common and fairly uniform, such as atrial septal defects or pulmonic stenosis, others are uncommon and highly variable, such as single ventricle anomalies. The more common defects require no intervention or are treated with a single surgical intervention. Severe critical congenital heart defects (see Box 27.1) often require multiple surgical and catheterization interventions and lifelong management by a cardiologist. Severe

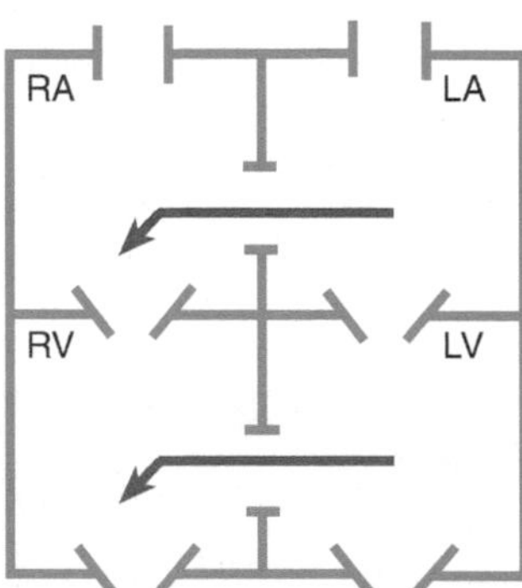

FIG. 27.17 Hemodynamics in defects with increased pulmonary blood flow. See Fig. 27.2 for abbreviations.

defects include all cyanotic heart disease and other complex defects such as AV canal, critical aortic stenosis, critical coarctation of the aorta, and complex ventricular septal defects. Most patients with these defects are identified during the newborn period or early infancy, are severely ill, and require surgical treatment. The clinical presentation and management of the most common defects are outlined in the following sections, Boxes 27.4 to 27.7, and Figs. 27.13 to 27.16.

The outcomes of surgical treatment for patients with moderate to severe disease are variable. Patient risk factors for increased morbidity and mortality include prematurity or low birth weight, a genetic syndrome, multiple cardiac defects, a noncardiac congenital anomaly, and age at the time of surgery (neonates are a higher-risk group). For example, aortic stenosis and coarctation presenting in the first week of life are more severe and carry a higher mortality risk than if they manifest at 1 year of age. In general, the outcomes of surgical procedures have steadily improved, with mortality rates for many severe defects below 10%, and the incidence of complications and length of hospital stay have declined.

DEFECTS WITH INCREASED PULMONARY BLOOD FLOW

In cardiac defects with increased pulmonary blood flow, intracardiac communications along the septum or an abnormal connection between the great arteries allows blood to flow from the high-pressure left side of the heart to the lower-pressure right side of the heart (Fig. 27.17). Increased blood volume on the right side of the heart increases pulmonary blood flow at the expense of systemic blood flow. Clinically patients demonstrate signs and symptoms of HF. Atrial and ventricular septal

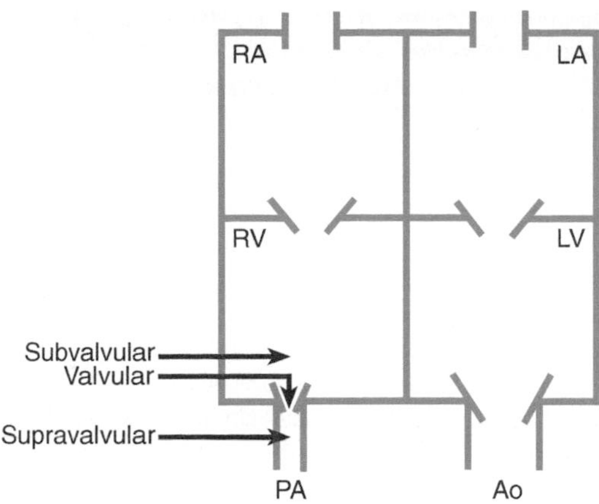

FIG. 27.18 Obstruction to ventricular ejection can occur at the valvular level (shown), below the valve (subvalvular), or above the valve (supravalvular). Pulmonic stenosis is shown here. *Ao,* Aorta; *PA,* pulmonary artery. See Fig. 27.2 for other abbreviations.

defects and patent ductus arteriosus are typical anomalies in this group (see Box 27.4).

OBSTRUCTIVE DEFECTS

Obstructive defects are those in which blood exiting the heart meets an area of anatomic narrowing (stenosis), which causes obstruction to blood flow. The pressure in the ventricle and in the great artery before the obstruction is increased, and the pressure in the area beyond the obstruction is decreased. The location of the narrowing is usually near the valve (Fig. 27.18):

Valvar—Narrowing at the site of the valve itself

Subvalvar—Narrowing in the ventricle below the valve (also referred to as the *ventricular outflow tract*)

Supravalvar—Narrowing in the great artery above the valve

Coarctation of the aorta (narrowing of the aortic arch), aortic stenosis, and pulmonic stenosis are typical defects in this group (see Box 27.5). Hemodynamically there is a pressure load on the ventricle and decreased cardiac output. Clinically infants and children exhibit signs of HF. Children with mild obstruction may be asymptomatic. Rarely, as in severe pulmonic stenosis, hypoxemia may occur.

DEFECTS WITH DECREASED PULMONARY BLOOD FLOW

In defects with decreased pulmonary blood flow, there is obstruction of pulmonary blood flow and an anatomic defect (atrial septal defect or ventricular septal defect) between the right and left sides of the heart (Fig. 27.19). Because blood has difficulty exiting the right side of the heart via the pulmonary artery, pressure on the right side increases, exceeding left-side pressure. This allows desaturated blood to shunt right to left, which causes desaturation in the left side of the heart and in the systemic circulation. Clinically these patients are hypoxemic and usually appear cyanotic. Tetralogy of Fallot and tricuspid atresia are the more common defects in this group (see Box 27.6).

MIXED DEFECTS

Many complex cardiac anomalies are classified together in the mixed category (see Box 27.7) because survival in the postnatal period depends on mixing of blood from the pulmonary and systemic circulations within the heart chambers. Hemodynamically, fully saturated systemic blood mixes with the desaturated pulmonary blood, which causes a relative desaturation of the systemic blood. Pulmonary congestion occurs because the differences in pulmonary artery pressure and aortic pressure favor pulmonary blood flow. Cardiac output decreases because of a volume load on the ventricle. Clinically these patients have a variable picture that combines some degree of desaturation (although cyanosis is not always visible) and signs of CHF, often requiring multiple surgical interventions, the first being in the first week of life.

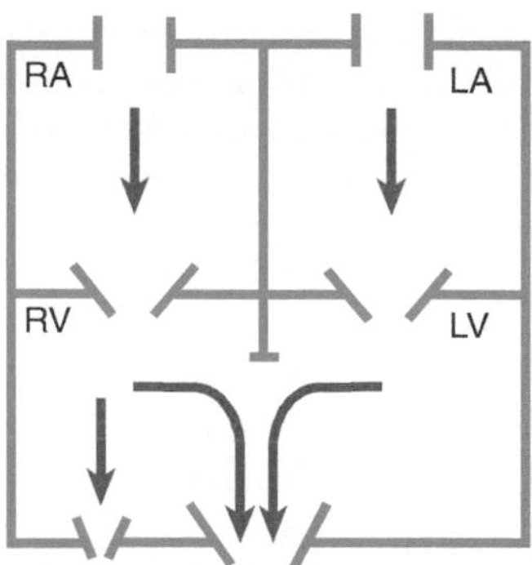

FIG. 27.19 Hemodynamic defects with decreased pulmonary blood flow. See Fig. 27.2 for abbreviations.

BOX 27.8 Single Ventricle Congenital Heart Defects

Hypoplastic left heart syndrome
Unbalanced complete atrioventricular canal
Double-inlet left ventricle
Tricuspid atresia
Pulmonary atresia with intact ventricular septum

SINGLE VENTRICLE ANATOMY

Many of the mixed defects are cardiac anomalies that have a single functioning ventricle. These defects (Box 27.8) require a staged approach to single ventricle palliation, allowing the single functioning ventricle to do the work normally done by two ventricles and separating oxygenated blood from deoxygenated blood.

Stage I or Norwood (first week of life)—(1) Establishes systemic blood flow by connecting the RV to the aorta, (2) rebuilds a small aorta and connects it to the ventricle, and (3) creates pulmonary blood flow either through a modified Blalock-Taussig shunt (3- to 4-mm Gore-Tex tube from the subclavian artery to the pulmonary artery) or a Sano modification (conduit from the RV to the pulmonary artery [PA]). (See Table 27.4.)

Stage II or bidirectional Glenn (3 to 8 months of age)—Creates a direct connection between the superior vena cava and the pulmonary artery, allowing half of the systemic deoxygenated blood to return passively, but directly, to the lungs. (See Table 27.4.)

Stage III or Fontan (2 to 4 years of age)—Directs systemic venous return to the lungs without a ventricular pump through surgical connections between the right atrium and the pulmonary artery (see Fig. 27.15). A fenestration (opening) is sometimes made in the right atrial baffle to relieve pressure. The patient must have normal ventricular function and a low pulmonary vascular resistance for the procedure to be successful. The modified Fontan procedure separates oxygenated and deoxygenated blood inside the heart and eliminates the excess volume load on the ventricle but does not restore normal anatomy or hemodynamics.

Between the first- and second-stage surgeries, the cardiac circulation is particularly fragile and the infant requires extra care and careful monitoring (see Family-Centered Care box, following). Long-term concerns for individuals who have completed single ventricle palliation and are living with Fontan physiology include the development of protein-losing enteropathy, atrial dysrhythmias, late ventricular dysfunction, and developmental delays. They will need lifelong care, including frequent follow-ups, procedures, and medications for most of their life.

FAMILY-CENTERED CARE HOME MONITORING PROGRAM

The heart of a baby with single ventricle anatomy has an abnormal circulation compared with a typical heart, which has two ventricles. For a baby with single ventricle anatomy, the ventricle has to pump blood to both the lungs and the body. Following the first surgery, there remains an imbalance between blood flow to the lungs and blood flow to the body. The heart is doing more work than in a normal circulation and is always near the maximum amount of work it can do. Because of this, an infant with a single ventricle requires extra care and careful monitoring during the interstage period, the time between the first and second surgeries. When they are discharged home after the first surgery they are followed by a home monitoring program, which is now a standard of care for cardiac centers across the United States and plays a key role in decreasing interstage mortality and improving outcomes after the stage II surgery (Ghanayem, Hoffman, Mussatto, et al., 2003; Petit, Fraser, Mattamal, et al., 2011).

In the home monitoring program, parents track oxygen saturations, weight gain, and feeding trends on a daily basis. Before discharge, nurses teach families how to check oxygen saturations and use an infant scale. Families receive comprehensive education on breaches or "red flag" events (decreased saturations, weight loss, intercurrent illness) that they should report to the cardiology team. Nurse practitioners and dietitians contact families weekly to assess progress, evaluate possible breaches, and discuss parental concerns.

NURSING CARE OF THE CHILD WITH CONGENITAL HEART DISEASE AND HIS OR HER FAMILY

When a child is born with a severe cardiac anomaly, parents face the immense psychologic and physical tasks of adjusting to the birth of a child with special needs. Family issues and nursing interventions to support the family are similar to those described in Chapters 9 and 19. This section focuses primarily on (1) educating the family about the disorder, (2) management of the illness at home, and (3) care and support of the child and his or her family during an invasive procedure such as cathereterization or surgery. For nursing care related specifically to the child with hypoxemia and CHF, the reader should refer to earlier discussions of these topics.

Nursing care of the child with a congenital heart defect begins as soon as the diagnosis is suspected. The rate of prenatal diagnosis of congenital heart disease is variable, ranging from 28% to 33% in some centers to as high as 74% in other centers (Friedberg, Silverman, Moon-Grady, et al., 2009; Levy, Pretorius, Rothman, et al., 2013; Sklansky, Berman, Pruetz, et al., 2009). As the rate of prenatal diagnosis increases, new demands are being placed on nurses to counsel and support families as they prepare for the birth of these infants. Once the infant is born, the unremitting stresses of care—physical exhaustion, financial costs, emotional upset, fear of death, and concern for the child's future—are frequently not fully appreciated by those caring for the family. Even when the child's condition is stabilized or corrected, the family may need to make new adjustments in their lifestyle (see Family-Centered Care box).

FAMILY-CENTERED CARE

The Diagnosis of Heart Disease

Remember, we don't have your experience. We don't see children every day who have heart disease. We would have been upset finding out our child had to have his tonsils out. How could we ever be prepared for this? Please remember, we only know people who have trivial heart murmurs. How could we ever expect this to happen? And to us, this is the worst problem we've ever heard of.

We still fear most what we don't know and understand. Be honest with us. If you don't know either, tell us. But at least don't leave us wondering about what you know and we don't. Not knowing anything really can be worse than knowing something bad. Be honest, but don't strip us of hope.

Please, remember we are trying to absorb complex information in a short period of time. And we are trying to understand it in a context of great pain and emotional investment. This is our lives you're talking about. Please be thorough, but keep it simple. Tell us again—maybe even again and again—when we can concentrate a little better.

Educate the Family About the Disorder

When parents learn of the heart defect, they are often initially in a period of shock, followed by high anxiety, especially fear of the child's death. Once parents are ready to hear about their child's heart condition, it is essential that they receive a clear explanation based on their level of understanding. A review of normal cardiac anatomy is helpful before explaining the anatomic defect. A simple diagram, pictures, or a model of the heart can be most helpful in visualizing the heart and the congenital defect. Parents appreciate receiving written information about the specific condition.* Health care professionals should take advantage of subsequent encounters with the family to assess parental understanding of the condition and clarify information as needed.

Different health personnel may convey the same information using different diagrams and medical terms. To prevent this from becoming a problem, the same type of diagram should be used by all, and the parents should write down any unclear terms or ask for clarification. Sometimes it is helpful to provide the family with a glossary of frequently used words for reference.

Parents often use multiple resources, particularly the Internet, to obtain information about their child's heart defect. Locating information can be easy with helpful information located at national organizations and large parent support groups.† Parents also find support through contacts with other parents and parent groups. Social media plays an important role for many families affected by congenital anomalies and offers a place for them to provide support, seek education, and make friends with other families sharing similar experiences (Jacobs, Boyd, Brennan, et al., 2016). It is important for parents to realize that not all

*American Heart Association, http://www.heart.org; National Association for Children's Heart Disorders, http://kidswithheart.org; Little Hearts, http://www.littlehearts.org. Many major medical centers that perform pediatric heart surgery also have information on their websites.

†Congenital Heart Information Network, http://tchin.org; Heart Rhythm Society (information on arrhythmias), http://www.hrsonline.org; Adult Congenital Heart Association, http://www.achaheart.org; National Pediatric Cardiology Quality Improvement Collaborative, https://npcqic.org; Children's Heart Foundation, http://www.childrensheartfoundation.com; Sisters By Heart, http://www.sistersbyheart.org.

websites offer medically accurate information and that information from other parents may not be applicable to their own situation. Some children with rare, complex heart defects require individualized treatment plans, and general information on the Internet or in books may not apply to them. Parents should talk to their health care team, in particular their cardiologist, about information they have received from other sources.

The nurse must give information to the child in a manner that is appropriate to the child's developmental age. As the child matures, the level of information is revised to match the child's new cognitive level. Preschoolers need basic information about what they will experience more than what is actually occurring physiologically. School-age children benefit from a concrete explanation of the defect. Preadolescents and adolescents often appreciate a more detailed description of how the defect affects their heart. Children of all ages need to be able to express their feelings concerning the diagnosis.

Help the Family Manage the Illness at Home

Parents are the child's principal caregivers and need to develop a positive, supportive working relationship with the health care team. Because most children spend the majority of their time at home with episodic trips to the hospital, parents manage their child's illness on a daily basis. They monitor for signs of illness, give medications and treatments, bring their child to appointments, work with a variety of caregivers, and alert the team to problems. Successful relationships are a partnership between parents and caregivers that is built on mutual trust and respect. Good communication between the family, the cardiology specialists, and the primary care provider is essential. As children reach adolescence, they begin to take a larger role in managing their illness and making decisions about their care.

Parents should be aware of the symptoms of their child's cardiac condition and signs of worsening clinical status. They should know how to contact their child's cardiologist at all times and know what to do in an emergency. Parents of children who may develop CHF should be familiar with the symptoms (see Box 27.3) and know when to contact the practitioner. Parents of children with cyanosis should be informed about fluid management and hypercyanotic spells (see p. 977). Parents should have an information sheet with their child's diagnosis, significant treatments such as surgical procedures, allergies, other health care problems, current medications, and health care providers' contact numbers available in case of emergencies and to share with other caregivers such as teachers, babysitters, or day care providers.

The family also needs to be knowledgeable regarding the therapeutic management of the disorder and the role that surgery, other procedures, medications, and a healthy lifestyle play in maintaining good health. Medications play a critical role in the management of some cardiac conditions such as arrhythmias and severe HF, in anticoagulation after implantation of artificial valves, and in antirejection treatment after heart transplantation. Some patients must take multiple medications daily for life. Many medications can be dangerous if taken incorrectly and require close monitoring. Teach parents the correct procedure for giving medications and caution them to keep them in a safe area to prevent accidental ingestion (see Family-Centered Care box, p. 994).

Another area of parental concern is the child's level of physical activity. Most children do not need to restrict activity, and the best approach is to treat the child normally and allow self-limited activity. Exceptions primarily involve strenuous recreational and competitive sports in children with specific cardiac problems. Discuss activities and exercise restrictions with the child's cardiologist. Avoid deliberately attempting to prevent crying because it can establish a maladaptive parental pattern of relating to the infant.

Infants and children with congenital heart disease (CHD) require good nutrition. Breastfeeding is possible for many infants with CHD. Countering a common misconception that breastfeeding would not be possible for these infants because they would get tired or exhibit poor growth, Barbas and Kelleher (2004) found that breastfeeding could be successful with adequate support and education of the mother. Providing adequate nutrition to infants with HF or complex congenital defects is especially difficult due to their high caloric requirements and inability to suck effectively because of fatigue and tachypnea. Instructing parents in feeding methods that decrease the work of the infant and giving high-calorie formula are important interventions.

Infants with heart disease should be immunized according to the current guidelines. Immunization schedules may need to be modified around times of acute illness or surgical procedures (Smith, 2001). Infants and children younger than 2 years of age with unrepaired heart defects, cyanotic lesions, pulmonary hypertension, or a history of prematurity should receive the vaccine for respiratory syncytial virus (RSV) according to the American Academy of Pediatrics recommendations, which are updated annually. Use of the RSV vaccine palivizumab has been shown to reduce hospitalization due to RSV infection in infants and young children with hemodynamically significant CHD (Feltes, Cabalka, Meissner, et al., 2003). (See Chapter 26.)

Infants and children who have serious heart disease are at risk for developmental delays (Majnemer, Limperopoulos, Shevell, et al., 2009). There is growing interest in characterizing and mitigating these outcomes through early identification and initiation of integrated developmental services. Multiple factors can influence neurodevelopmental outcomes, including genetics (e.g., chromosomal abnormalities and microdeletions), family background (e.g., parental intelligence quotient [IQ] and socioeconomic status), preoperative factors (including prematurity, cyanosis, shock), intraoperative factors (e.g., use of cardiopulmonary bypass, deep hypothermic circulatory arrest), and postoperative factors (e.g., hemodynamic instability, hypoxia, acidosis, cardiac arrest, stroke, ischemic events). In 2012 the American Heart Association published guidelines for the evaluation and management of neurodevelopment outcomes in children with congenital heart disease (Marino, Lipkin, Newburger, et al., 2012). These guidelines outline an algorithm for surveillance, screening, evaluation, reevaluation, and management of developmental disorder or disability to supplement the 2006 American Academy of Pediatrics statement on developmental surveillance and screening.

Prepare the Child and Family for Invasive Procedures

Chapter 22 provides an extensive discussion of the principles for preparing children for invasive procedures. In 2003 the American Heart Association published a scientific statement, "Recommendations for Preparing Children and Adolescents for Invasive Cardiac Procedures" (LeRoy, Elixson, O'Brien, et al., 2003), that addresses issues specific to the child with heart disease. The reader is referred to these resources for a complete review of the topic. The following discussion highlights some important aspects of preparation for cardiac catheterization and cardiac surgery.

The expected outcomes for preprocedure preparation include reducing anxiety, improving patient cooperation with procedures, enhancing recovery, developing trust with caregivers, and improving long-term emotional and behavioral adjustment after procedures (LeRoy, Elixson, O'Brien, et al., 2003). Important factors to consider in planning preparation strategies are the child's cognitive developmental level, previous hospital experiences, temperament and coping style, the timing of the preparation, and the involvement of the parents. The most beneficial preparation strategies usually combine information giving and training in coping skills such as conscious breathing exercises, distraction techniques, guided imagery, and other behavioral interventions.

Handling preoperative and precatheterization workups on an outpatient basis is common for most elective procedures. Children are then admitted on the morning of the procedure. Preprocedure teaching is often done in the clinic setting or at home, and a tour of the ICU and the inpatient facilities may be added. Children of different ages and developmental levels require different amounts of information and different approaches. Young children should be prepared close in time to the event; older children and adolescents may benefit from teaching several weeks in advance. Include parents in the preparation session to support their child and learn about upcoming events.

The preoperative or precatheterization preparation should include information on the environment, equipment, and procedures that the child will encounter during and after the procedure. The nurse can use many educational techniques, such as verbal and written information, hospital tours, preoperative classes, and picture books or videos. Information about what the child will see, hear, and feel should be included, especially for older children and adolescents. Some of the sensory experiences of being in an ICU or catheterization laboratory include sights (e.g., monitors, many people, lots of equipment), sounds (e.g., beeping noises, alarms, voices), and sensations (e.g., lines and dressings, tape, feelings of discomfort, thirst). Familiar aspects of the environment, such as BP cuffs, stethoscopes, or oximeter probes, are reviewed, and new equipment such as monitors, IV lines, and oxygen masks are described. Comforting aspects of the environment are emphasized, such as play areas, chairs for parents, and televisions. Many patients who will be sedated during catheterization or receive narcotic pain relievers after surgery will have minimal recall of that period and will not need detailed information about the equipment or procedures used. Information should be specific to the planned procedure for each patient.

Discuss ways the child can cope with the experience and be helped to recover. For young children, bringing a familiar stuffed animal or comfort object with them will help relieve anxiety, whereas for older children bringing music with headphones to the catheterization laboratory will help distract them during the procedure. Topics to discuss regarding recovery after catheterization include the need to lie still to prevent bleeding at the catheter site, progression of the diet, pain control measures, and monitoring methods. Review the importance of ambulation, coughing and deep breathing, and drinking and eating after surgery, and describe pain management and monitoring routines. Review simple coping strategies for use during painful procedures, including distraction techniques such as counting, blowing, singing, or telling stories.

Children and their families should have a choice about an ICU tour. Exposure to the ICU environment can actually increase anxiety in some children, particularly young children, those with previous hospital experiences, and those who are highly anxious (LeRoy, Elixson, O'Brien, et al., 2003). If a visit to the recovery room and ICU is planned, it should take place when there is minimal activity in the area, when the parents can accompany the child, and when the child is well rested. Usually the day before the procedure is ample time to allow the child to ask questions and to prevent undue fantasizing about the experience. Protect the child from frightening sights in the unit. The child and parents are encouraged to ask questions and to explore further any equipment in the room, but they should not be pushed to assimilate more information than they are able.

Preoperative physical care differs little, if any, from that provided for any other surgery and is discussed in Chapter 22. Assure the child that the parents will be there when the child wakes up. Also allow the parents to accompany the child as far as possible to the operating suite. After all of the equipment and procedures have been explained, it is important to talk about "getting well" and going home.

Provide Postoperative Care

Immediate postoperative care is usually provided by specially trained nurses in the ICU. Performing many of the procedures, specialized monitoring and observations related to vital functions, requires advanced educational training (the reader should refer to critical care texts for further information). However, nurses caring for the child before surgery and during the convalescent period need to be familiar with the major principles of care.

Observe Vital Signs and Arterial and Venous Pressures

During the immediate postoperative period, record vital signs frequently, including BP, until the child's condition is stable. The heart rate and respirations are counted for 1 full minute, compared with the values on the ECG monitor. The heart rate is normally increased after surgery. The nurse observes cardiac rhythm and notifies the practitioner of any changes in regularity. Dysrhythmias may occur postoperatively secondary to administration of anesthetics, acid-base and electrolyte imbalance, hypoxia, surgical intervention, or trauma to conduction pathways.

At least hourly, auscultate the lungs for breath sounds. Diminished or absent breath sounds may indicate an area of atelectasis, pleural effusion, or pneumothorax. All such cases require further assessment. Auscultation guides the nurse's selective use of postural drainage and percussion to those pulmonary lobes most in need. It also allows a more objective evaluation of effective ventilation.

Temperature changes are typical during the early postoperative period. Hypothermia is expected immediately after surgery due to hypothermia procedures, effects of anesthesia, and loss of body heat to the cool environment. During this period the child is kept warm to prevent additional heat loss. Infants may be placed under radiant heat warmers. During the next 24 to 48 hours the body temperature may rise to 100°F (37.8°C) or slightly higher as part of the inflammatory response to tissue trauma. After this period an elevated temperature is most likely a sign of infection and warrants immediate investigation for probable cause.

Intraarterial monitoring of BP is almost always done after open-heart surgery. Residual vasoconstriction after cardiopulmonary bypass makes indirect BP readings less reliable, and intraarterial monitoring permits continuous rather than intermittent observation. A catheter is passed into the radial artery or the dorsalis pedis or posterior tibial artery. The other end is attached to an electronic monitoring system, which provides a continuous recording of the BP. The intraarterial line is maintained with a low-rate, constant infusion of heparinized saline to prevent clotting, and the amount of irrigant is recorded as intake fluid. Continuous BP readings are compared with those taken indirectly using a sphygmomanometer or oscillometric device (Dinamap). A discrepancy between the two may indicate a change in peripheral vascular resistance, a malfunction in the electronic device, or human error in using the wrong-size BP cuff. The nurse also observes for potential complications of intraarterial monitoring, such as arterial thrombosis, infection, air emboli, or blood loss through the catheter. Prevention of each of these hazards is similar to care for any other type of infusion line.

Several IV lines are inserted preoperatively, including a peripheral IV to give fluids and medications and a CVP line that is usually inserted in a large vessel in the neck. Intracardiac monitoring lines are placed intraoperatively in the RA, LA, or pulmonary artery. Intracardiac lines allow assessment of pressures inside the cardiac chambers, which give vital information on blood volume, cardiac output, ventricular function, pulmonary artery pressures, and responses to drug therapy in the immediate postoperative period. The RA and CVP lines may also be used to infuse fluids and medications. LA lines and pulmonary artery lines are used with more complex repairs. Intracardiac lines are used only in the ICU, although CVP lines may remain for use as a central IV line outside the ICU. All lines must be cared for using strict aseptic technique to prevent infection. Patients must be carefully assessed for bleeding at the time of line removal. See critical care texts for a more complete discussion of intracardiac lines.

Maintain Respiratory Status

Infants usually require mechanical ventilation in the immediate postoperative period. Children may be extubated in the operating room or in the first few postoperative hours, especially if cardiopulmonary bypass was not required. Once extubated, humidified O_2 via nasal cannula or mask prevents drying of mucosa and helps bridge to room air. Encourage the child to turn and deep breathe at least hourly. When developmentally appropriate, encourage the use of incentive spirometry. Every means is employed to enhance ventilation and decrease pain, such as splinting of the operative site and use of analgesics.

For the intubated patient, suctioning is performed only as needed and is done carefully to avoid vagal stimulation (which can trigger cardiac dysrhythmias) and laryngospasm, especially in infants. Suctioning is intermittent and is maintained for no more than 5 seconds to prevent depleting the oxygen supply. Supplemental oxygen is administered with a manual resuscitation bag before and after the procedure to prevent hypoxia. The heart rate is monitored after suctioning to detect changes in rhythm or rate, especially bradycardia. The child should always be positioned facing the nurse to permit assessment of the child's color and tolerance of the procedure.

! NURSING ALERT

During suctioning, observe for signs and symptoms of respiratory distress, such as tachypnea, use of accessory muscles for breathing, restlessness, and acute onset of hypoxia.

Chest tubes are inserted into the pleural or mediastinal space during surgery or in the immediate postoperative period to remove pleural drainage and air. The chest tube is attached to a disposable water-seal drainage system. The underwater drainage prevents air from traveling up the tube into the pleural space and causing a pneumothorax. Nursing considerations include never interrupting water-seal drainage unless the chest tube is clamped, checking for tube patency (fluctuation in the water-seal chamber), and maintaining sterility.

Check drainage hourly for color and quantity. Immediately postoperatively the drainage may be bright red, but afterward it should be serous. The largest volume of drainage occurs in the first 12 to 24 hours, and drainage is greater after extensive heart surgery.

! NURSING ALERT

Chest tube drainage of more than 3 ml/kg/hr for more than 3 consecutive hours or 5 to 10 ml/kg in any 1 hour is excessive and may indicate postoperative hemorrhage. Notify the surgeon immediately because cardiac tamponade can develop rapidly and is life threatening.

Chest radiographs are taken when the tubes are inserted to check their location and after they are removed to evaluate the inflation of the lungs. Chest tubes are usually removed on the first to third postoperative day when drainage has diminished.

Removal of chest tubes can be an uncomfortable, frightening experience (see Atraumatic Care box). Warn children that they will feel a sharp, momentary pain. After the suture is cut, the tubes are quickly pulled out at the end of full inspiration in the extubated patient to prevent intake of air into the pleural cavity. (In the intubated patient, the tubes are pulled out on inspiration because the lungs are stented open with the positive pressure ventilation.) A purse-string suture (placed when the tubes were inserted) is pulled tight to close the opening. A petrolatum-covered gauze dressing is immediately applied over the wound and securely taped to the skin on all four sides so that an airtight seal is formed. The dressing is checked for signs of drainage and is removed the next day. Breath sounds are auscultated because pneumothorax is a possible complication of chest tube removal. A chest x-ray film is usually obtained after removal to assess for pneumothorax or pleural effusion.

ATRAUMATIC CARE

Chest Tube Removal

Intravenous (IV) analgesics such as morphine sulfate (0.1 mg/kg), often in combination with midazolam (Versed), may be given before the procedure. Oral analgesics and sedatives are an alternative to IV medications.

Provide Maximum Rest

After heart surgery maximum rest should be provided to decrease the workload of the heart and to promote healing. Nursing care is planned according to the child's usual activity and sleep patterns. The simplest way to ensure individualized, efficient, high-quality care is to plan at the beginning of the shift the nursing procedures to be done. Identify periods of rest and discuss the schedule with the parents.

Provide Comfort

Heart surgery is both painful and frightening for children, and providing comfort is a primary nursing concern. Several incisions are used for heart surgery. A median sternotomy following the sternum down the center of the chest is most common. A ministernotomy opens the lower sternum. A thoracotomy incision is most uncomfortable because it goes through muscle tissue. It allows access to the side of the chest through an incision that runs from under the arm around the back to the scapula.

Adequate pain control decreases postoperative complications such as atelectasis, pneumonia, and deep vein thrombosis by improving coughing and ambulation. Pain level is now considered the fifth vital sign. Many pain assessment tools are available for infants and children of different ages. (See Pain Assessment, Chapter 5.)

Continuous IV infusion of opioids, particularly morphine and fentanyl, is a safe and effective method of pain control. Patient-controlled analgesia may be used with children old enough to understand the concept. Children receiving opioid infusions for a prolonged period are weaned slowly from the medication to prevent withdrawal symptoms. Nonsteroidal antiinflammatory drugs (NSAIDs) such as IV ketorolac (Toradol) or oral ibuprofen may provide relief of moderate postoperative pain.

Most patients need IV analgesics for pain control during the 24- to 48-hour postoperative period. After lines and tubes have been removed and when patients are tolerating oral fluids, pain may be controlled with oral narcotics such as oxycodone, often combined with acetaminophen or an oral NSAID such as ibuprofen, or with acetaminophen alone. As noted earlier, thoracotomy incisions are usually more painful than sternotomies because the incision is through muscle. Acetaminophen or ibuprofen alone is usually adequate for pain control after discharge. (See Pain Management, Chapter 5.)

In addition to providing pharmacologic pain control, make every effort to minimize the discomfort of procedures by other means, such as by placing a firm pillow or favorite stuffed animal against the chest incision during coughing and performing treatments after pain medication is given, preferably at a time that coincides with the drug's peak effect. Employ nonpharmacologic measures to lessen the perception of pain, and encourage parents to comfort their child as much as possible. (See Pain Management, Chapter 5.)

Monitor Fluids

Intake and output of all fluids must be accurately calculated. Intake is primarily IV fluids; however, the nurse also needs to keep a record of fluid used to flush the arterial, CVP, and intracardiac lines or to dilute medications. Monitoring of output includes hourly recordings of urine (usually a Foley catheter is inserted and attached to a closed collecting device), drainage from chest and nasogastric tubes, and blood drawn for analysis. Low cardiac output is common after open heart surgery and is characterized by low urine output. This places the patient at a higher risk for renal failure.

> **! NURSING ALERT**
>
> The signs of renal failure are decreased urinary output (<1 ml/kg/hr) and elevated levels of blood urea nitrogen and serum creatinine.

During open-heart surgery, the cardiopulmonary pump is primed with a large volume of fluid (usually electrolyte solution), which may greatly dilute the patient's blood. The large amount of fluid also diffuses into the interstitial spaces, causing total-body edema and pulmonary edema. Patients return from the operating room with fluid overload. Fluids are restricted to less than maintenance level during the first postoperative day, and drugs are used to promote diuresis. A return to maintenance fluid levels then occurs over the next few days. Electrolyte levels are closely monitored because electrolyte imbalances, especially hypokalemia, are a common result of diuresis and fluid shifts, and electrolytes may need replacement.

Fluid requirements are based on the child's weight and body surface area. Weights are obtained daily at the same time of day. Oral fluids are usually withheld until the child is extubated. Patients begin taking clear liquids when bowel sounds are heard and advance slowly to a regular diet. Nausea and vomiting are common in the first few days after surgery, likely a side effect of anesthesia and analgesics. Providing adequate nutrition, ideally by oral intake, becomes important by the fourth or fifth postoperative day. Consider nasogastric tube feedings or parenteral nutrition for patients who are unable to tolerate oral feedings.

Plan for Progressive Activity

Fatigue and weakness are common after heart surgery. However, moderate activity is essential to prevent pulmonary and vascular complications. Initially, turning, coughing, and deep breathing are sufficient to promote respiratory expansion. Passive range-of-motion exercises, especially to the lower extremities, are instituted to prevent venous stasis.

A progressive schedule of ambulation and activity is planned, based on the child's preoperative activity patterns and postoperative cardiovascular and pulmonary function. Provide the child with toys to encourage movement. It is important to plan the activity at times when the child is well rested, is comfortable (usually has had analgesic medication), and is not scheduled for any strenuous procedure or treatment immediately afterward.

Once extubated, ambulation is initiated early. Patients progress from sitting on the edge of the bed and dangling the legs to standing up and to sitting in a chair while being assisted and assessed by the nursing staff. Carefully monitor the heart rate, oxygen saturation, and respirations to assess the degree of cardiac demand imposed by each activity. Tachycardia, dyspnea, cyanosis, desaturation, progressive fatigue, or dysrhythmias indicate the need to limit further energy expenditure.

Observe for Complications of Heart Surgery

Several complications can occur after heart surgery, most of which are related to open-heart surgery and the use of cardiopulmonary bypass. Many of the procedures discussed in the preceding paragraphs are aimed at preventing these problems. Only those that have not already been discussed are included here. A serious complication, infective endocarditis (bacterial), is discussed on p. 994.

Cardiac changes. Preoperatively the workload of the heart is increased because of the abnormal hemodynamics caused by the congenital defect. In the initial postoperative period the heart is under increased stress because of the effects of surgery and the use of the heart-lung machine. In some cases cardiac function can actually be worse in the early postoperative period despite repair of the congenital defect. HF, hypoxia, low cardiac output, dysrhythmias, and tamponade are all potential postoperative problems.

HF may occur postoperatively because of excessive pulmonary blood flow or fluid overload (see p. 970 for assessment and management of HF). Hypoxia may occur because of inadequate pulmonary blood flow or because of respiratory problems. Rapid assessment of the causes of hypoxia and appropriate interventions to improve ventilation and perfusion are vital because hypoxia can rapidly lead to acidosis, which can impair ventricular function.

Low cardiac output syndrome and decreased peripheral perfusion can occur from hypothermia or inability of the LV to maintain systemic circulation. It affects up to 25% of infants and young children after cardiac surgery (Hoffman, Wernovsky, Atz, et al., 2003). The most important signs of adequate peripheral perfusion are rapid capillary refill, good skin color, warm extremities, and strong pulses. Indications of low cardiac output are similar to signs of shock (i.e., decreased BP, decreased pulse pressure, cool extremities, metabolic acidosis, and oliguria). Low cardiac output states are aggressively treated with IV inotropic medications such as dopamine, dobutamine, epinephrine, and milrinone. Milrinone, widely used in pediatrics, has also been shown to prevent low cardiac output syndrome (Hoffman, Wernovsky, Atz, et al., 2003). If maximum medical therapy is failing, cardiac assist methods such as extracorporeal membrane oxygenation or a ventricular assist device may be used.

Dysrhythmias are common in the early postoperative period and can result from electrolyte imbalance, especially hypokalemia, and surgical intervention to the septum or myocardium. The heart rate and rhythm are carefully monitored by observing the ECG pattern and by counting the apical pulse for 1 full minute. In some children, a faster than normal rate may be required to maintain an adequate cardiac output in the postoperative period, and a slower than normal rhythm can impair cardiac output. Epicardial pacing wires may be inserted during surgery for managing cardiac dysrhythmias postoperatively.

Cardiac tamponade is compression of the heart by blood and other effusion (clots) in the pericardial sac, which severely restricts the normal heart movement. Signs include rising and equalizing RA and LA filling pressures, narrowing pulse pressure, tachycardia, dyspnea, apprehension, and an abrupt stop to chest tube drainage from mediastinal tubes. The nurse immediately reports any evidence of this potentially fatal complication. An echocardiogram confirms the diagnosis. Treatment consists of prompt pericardiocentesis to remove the blood or fluid. If active hemorrhage and coagulopathy are present, steps are taken to enhance blood clotting.

Pulmonary changes. Areas of atelectasis are common immediately after surgery as a result of deflation of the lung during cardiopulmonary bypass. Other pulmonary complications include pneumothorax, especially caused by faulty chest tubes; pulmonary edema from increased pulmonary blood flow or HF; and pleural effusion caused by persistent venous congestion. Signs of pneumothorax are persistent decreased breath sounds, sudden dyspnea, tachycardia, rapid shallow respirations, cyanosis, and sometimes sharp chest pain. Signs of pulmonary edema are tachypnea, rales, wheezing, moist dyspneic respirations, tachycardia, cyanosis, and restlessness. Signs and symptoms of pleural effusions include increased respiratory rate, vomiting, decreased breath sounds, fatigue, irritability, and decreased oxygen saturation. Chest radiography is important in the accurate diagnosis of pulmonary complications and is done frequently postoperatively.

Neurologic changes. Neurologic complications such as seizures, strokes, cerebral edema, and hypoxic or ischemic brain injury are uncommon after open-heart surgery but can be devastating when they occur. Nurses are alert to the possibility of neurologic symptoms and perform ongoing neurologic assessments, including evaluation of the equality of strength and reflexes in both extremities for evidence of paralysis; pupil size, equality, reaction to light, and accommodation; and the child's orientation to the environment. The nurse also observes for focal or generalized seizure activity. Any evidence of cerebral damage is reported immediately. Further neurologic evaluation and management are needed for all abnormalities.

Seizures are the most common neurologic condition, seen most often in infants. Longer periods of deep hypothermic cardiopulmonary bypass (>40 minutes), sometimes needed in complex repairs on neonates, have been associated with an increased risk of seizure activity and later developmental delays (Wypij, Newberger, Rappaport, et al., 2003). Significant improvements in cardiopulmonary bypass techniques, arterial filters, and equipment and a better understanding of neuroprotection during heart surgery have resulted in a reduced incidence of seizures, movement disorders, and coma (Menasche, DuPlessis, Wessel, et al., 2002).

Infection. All patients are at risk for infections postoperatively; especially vulnerable are infants, those with poor cardiac function, and those who require multiple invasive lines and procedures for a prolonged period. Prophylactic antibiotics are given for the first 1 or 2 days. All dressings are applied and changed using aseptic technique. Good hand washing, careful use of aseptic technique when placing and accessing lines, and close attention to surgical wounds are all important to prevent infection. Monitor patients closely for fever and signs of infection. Monitor all IV sites for signs of infection or phlebitis. Appropriate treatment is instituted if an infection is identified.

Hematologic changes. While passing through the heart-lung machine, blood is exposed to substantial trauma because of mechanical action and direct contact with oxygen, foreign substances, and massive doses of anticoagulants. The result of mechanical trauma is red blood cell hemolysis and potential renal tubular necrosis. Heparinization of the blood during extracorporeal circulation can result in clotting abnormalities from decreased thrombin and prothrombin levels, decreased levels of platelets, and altered platelet aggregation. Because blood-clotting mechanisms are affected, signs of hemorrhage, especially bleeding from the chest tubes and a fall in arterial and venous pressures, are important observations.

Hemolysis of red blood cells leads to blood loss and anemia, which may require packed red blood cell transfusion. The nurse monitors results of complete blood counts to identify the severity of the hemolysis. Urine is tested for blood. If transfusions are required, the child is closely observed for signs of reaction and fluid overload. The need to measure urinary output hourly has already been discussed.

Normally the filter and bubble trap on the heart-lung machine remove air emboli, tiny clots, fat debris, and organisms from the arterialized (oxygenated) blood before its return to the body. However, the entry of impure blood into the systemic circulation can cause fat embolism, thromboembolism, and infection anywhere in the body and, most important, in the brain.

Postpericardiotomy syndrome. The postpericardiotomy syndrome of fever, leukocytosis, pericardial friction rub, or pericardial and pleural effusion can occur anytime the pericardium is opened, either in the immediate postoperative period or after surgery, typically around day 7 to 21. The cause is unknown, although etiologic theories include viral infection, autoimmune response to myocardial tissue, and a reaction to blood in the pericardium. The syndrome is self-limiting and is treated with rest, salicylates, NSAIDs, and sometimes steroids. Pericardiocentesis or pleurocentesis may be needed to treat large effusions.

Provide Emotional Support

Children may become depressed after surgery. This is thought to be caused by preoperative anxiety, postoperative psychologic and physiologic stress, and sensory overstimulation. Typically the child's disposition improves on leaving the ICU. (See Chapter 21.)

Children may also be angry and uncooperative after surgery as a response to the physical pain and to the loss of control imposed by the surgery and treatments. They need an opportunity to express feelings, either verbally or through activity. Nurses can praise children for their efforts to cooperate and should refrain from expecting too much courage or bravery. Children often regress in their behavior during the stress of surgery and hospitalization. Children also may express feelings of anger or rejection toward parents. The nurse must reassure parents that this is normal and that with continued support the anger will subside.

The nurse can support the parents by being available to provide information and explaining all the procedures to them. The first few postoperative days are particularly difficult because parents see their child in pain and realize the potential risks from surgery. They often are overwhelmed by the physical environment of the ICU and feel useless because they can do so little for their child. The nurse can minimize such feelings by including parents in caregiving activities and comfort and play activities; by providing information about the child's condition; and by being sensitive to their emotional and physical needs. The importance of their presence in making the child feel more secure is stressed, even if they do not provide physical care.

Plan for Discharge and Home Care

Assessment of discharge needs should begin at admission so parents and health care providers have ample time to plan for a safe discharge and arrange for necessary equipment and supports. The family needs verbal and written instructions on medication, nutrition, activity restrictions, wound care, pain management, and signs and symptoms of infection or complications. Other discussion topics may include return to school and work, special medication teaching for warfarin (Coumadin) or other drugs that require detailed home management, and infective endocarditis (subacute bacterial endocarditis [SBE]) prophylaxis. Referrals to community agencies may be necessary to assist parents in the transition from hospital to home and to reinforce the teaching (see Family-Centered Care box).

The parents also need clear instructions on when to seek medical care for complications and how to contact the health care provider. Follow-up with the cardiologist and primary care provider is also arranged before discharge. Encourage parents to keep an updated summary of their child's diagnosis, surgical procedures, allergies, medications, health care providers with contact information, and other health problems readily available for emergencies and to share this

FAMILY-CENTERED CARE

Discharge Teaching After Cardiac Surgery

- Medication teaching
- Activity restrictions
- Diet and nutrition
- Wound care (include dressings, if any, suture removal, bathing)
- Infective endocarditis (bacterial) prophylaxis
- Follow-up appointments: cardiologist, primary care provider
- Contact information for community agencies as needed: visiting nurse service, early developmental intervention, home supply companies
- When to call the cardiologist or primary care provider
- Signs and symptoms of postoperative problems
- Review of cardiac defect and surgical repair

summary with school personnel, babysitters, and others. Appropriate medical identification, such as a MedicAlert bracelet, is indicated for children with a pacemaker or a heart transplant and for those receiving anticoagulation therapy or antidysrhythmic medication.

The nurse also discusses common behavior disturbances that may occur after discharge, such as nightmares, sleep disturbances, separation anxiety, and overdependence. A supportive, consistent response is essential to allow the child to overcome the surgical experience. The child may work out feelings and fears through therapeutic play, and this should be encouraged.

Although surgical correction of heart defects has improved dramatically, it is still not possible to totally repair many complex anomalies. Some repairs require several operations over a period of years. For many children, repeat procedures are required to replace conduits or valves or to manage complications such as restenosis. Consequently, the long-term prognosis is uncertain, and full recovery is not always possible. For these families, close medical follow-up and continued emotional support are essential.

ACQUIRED CARDIOVASCULAR DISORDERS

Acquired cardiac disorders include disease processes or abnormalities that occur after birth and can be seen in the otherwise normal heart or in the presence of congenital heart defects. They occur for a variety of reasons, including infection, autoimmune response, environmental factors, and familial tendencies. Nursing care often plays a critical role in the identification and supportive management of these cardiovascular disorders.

BACTERIAL (INFECTIVE) ENDOCARDITIS

Infective endocarditis (IE) (also called *bacterial endocarditis* or *subacute bacterial endocarditis [SBE]* in the past) is an infection of the inner lining of the heart (endocardium), generally involving the valves. The incidence of IE is much less in children than adults but increasing in both groups (Gupta, Sakhuja, McGrath, et al., 2016). In the past, it was most often a result of bacteremia in children with acquired or congenital anomalies of the heart or great vessels, particularly those with valvular abnormalities, prosthetic valves, shunts, recent cardiac surgery with invasive lines, and rheumatic heart disease (RHD) with valve involvement. More recently, only half the cases were in children with underlying heart disease (Gupta, Sakhuja, McGrath, et al., 2016). The increased incidence of IE in children without cardiac abnormalities is likely related to the increased use of indwelling central lines to treat other serious diseases (Bragg & Alvarez, 2014). The incidence of neonatal IE has also increased because of the increased use of indwelling lines and fewer than a third of the IE cases seen in neonates occur in those with congenital heart disease (Day, Gauvreau, Shulman, et al., 2009). Endocarditis can also occur without any known risk factors, commonly affecting the mitral or aortic valve.

The most common causative agents are *Streptococcus viridans* and *Staphylococcus aureus*. Gram-negative bacterias known as HACEK, and fungi such as *Candida* and *Aspergillus* are also causes of IE (Baltimore, Gewitz, Baddour, et al., 2015). Positive blood cultures are present in most patients; however, endocarditis can also be present despite negative blood cultures, especially if antibiotics have already been given. Culture-negative endocarditis has been reported in 5% to 10% of IE cases (Bragg & Alvarez, 2014) and up to 30% in other studies (Gupta, Sakhuja, McGrath, et al., 2016).

Pathophysiology

Organisms may enter the bloodstream from any site of localized infection. Endocarditis may occur from routine exposure to bacteremia associated with usual daily activities such as brushing teeth although it can also occur after procedures such as dental work, invasive procedures involving the gastrointestinal and genitourinary tracts, cardiac surgery, especially if synthetic material is used (valves, patches, conduits); or from long-term indwelling catheters. The microorganisms grow on the endocardium, forming vegetations (verrucae), deposits of fibrin, and platelet thrombi. The lesion may invade adjacent tissues, such as the aortic and mitral valves, and may break off and embolize elsewhere, especially to the spleen, kidney, and CNS.

Clinical Manifestations

The onset of symptoms is usually insidious, with unexplained low-grade, intermittent fever. Other common nonspecific symptoms are malaise, anorexia, HF symptoms, arthralgias, and weight loss (Baltimore, Gewitz, Baddour, et al., 2015). IE should be considered in at-risk patients who have any of these symptoms. Patients can also present acutely with high fevers and rapidly declining health, requiring immediate hospitalization and treatment.

The presentation in newborns and infants can be nonspecific with signs of sepsis or HF. Feeding intolerance, respiratory distress, tachycardia, and hypotension may be seen. Septic emboli are more common in infants resulting in infection outside the heart (osteomyelitis, meningitis, pneumonia) (Baltimore, Gewitz, Baddour, et al., 2015).

The clinical findings of IE in children are seen in four areas: bacteremia (or fungemia), valvulitis, immunologic responses, and emboli (Baltimore, Gewitz, Baddour, et al., 2015). A new murmur or a change in a previously existing one is frequently found as a result of damage to valves or perforation of the myocardium. Symptoms of HF may be present. Signs that result from embolus formation elsewhere in the body include splinter hemorrhages (thin black lines) under the nails, Osler nodes (red, painful intradermal nodes with white centers found on the pads of the phalanges), Janeway spots (painless hemorrhagic areas on the palms and soles), petechiae on the oral mucous membranes, and splenomegaly, although all these signs are less common in children than in adults (Baltimore, Gewitz, Baddour, et al., 2015).

Diagnostic Evaluation

Definitive diagnosis can be made after growth of the organism and identification of the causative agent in the blood. Several blood specimens (three are recommended) are drawn for culture to rule out contamination during venipuncture and dilution. Because the most common organisms causing IE, staphylococci and streptococci, are found on the skin, strict sterile technique is practiced in obtaining cultures to avoid contamination. Obtaining an adequate blood volume for culture is also important.

When an organism is identified, sensitivity studies are done to determine appropriate antibiotic therapy. Echocardiographic findings include new or increasing valvular insufficiency, vegetations, abscesses, and decreased ventricular function. Vegetations cannot always be visualized with echo imaging. Other findings may support the diagnosis of IE, such as ECG changes (AV block), anemia, an elevated erythrocyte sedimentation rate, leukocytosis, microscopic hematuria, and radiographic evidence of cardiomegaly. A diagnosis of culture-negative endocarditis is made when the patient has echocardiographic or clinical evidence of IE but no organism can be cultured (Baltimore, Gewitz, Baddour, et al., 2015).

The Duke criteria provide guidelines for the diagnosis of IE in adults and are useful in the diagnosis of childhood endocarditis as well. These criteria divide signs and symptoms into major and minor criteria. IE can be diagnosed if the child has two major criteria, or one major and three minor, or five minor criteria. The two major criteria include positive blood culture results and echocardiographic evidence of endocardial involvement (vegetations or new valvular regurgitation). Minor criteria include fever, predisposing risk factors of congenital heart disease, presence of a central venous line, or IV drug use; vascular phenomena that include major arterial emboli, septic pulmonary infarcts, mycotic aneurysm, intracranial hemorrhage, conjunctival hemorrhage, or Janeway lesions; and immunologic phenomena such as glomerulonephritis, Osler's nodes, Roth spots, and rheumatoid factor (Li, Sexton, Mick, et al., 2000).

Therapeutic Management

Treatment for IE includes the administration of high-dose antibiotics given intravenously for 2 to 8 weeks to completely eradicate the infecting microorganism (Bragg & Alvarez, 2014). Infectious disease specialists should be consulted to assist in determining the appropriate regimen for each patient. Blood cultures are performed periodically to evaluate the response to antibiotic therapy. Serial echocardiograms are done to evaluate for ventricular function, vegetations, and valve damage. Cardiac surgery may be indicated to repair or replace damaged valves.

Early medical treatment for IE is successful in many patients. However, patients diagnosed late, patients with underlying heart disease or a clinical course complicated by HF, embolic events, or significant valvular dysfunction, or IE caused by antibiotic-resistant organisms or fungi carry a mortality rate of 5% to 10% (Baltimore, Gewitz, Baddour, et al., 2015). Infections with *Staphylococcus aureus* have a higher mortality rate in the modern era than those caused by streptococci (Gupta, Sakhuja, McGrath, et al., 2016). Nonfatal complications result from embolism to other structures, especially to the CNS (causing hemiplegia, aphasia, meningitis, convulsions), kidney (resulting in hematuria, proteinuria), spleen, and bowel.

Prevention of Endocarditis

Prevention involves administration of prophylactic antibiotic therapy to high-risk patients before dental procedures that are associated with the risk of entry of organisms (Box 27.9). Drugs of choice for prophylaxis, given 1 hour before the procedure, include amoxicillin, ampicillin, and clindamycin in penicillin-allergic patients (Wilson, Taubert, Gewitz, et al., 2007).

Additional procedures that require prophylaxis (only in the high-risk group) include invasive procedures of the respiratory tract and procedures on infected skin or musculoskeletal tissue. Maintenance of excellent oral hygiene and prevention of oral disease is still of utmost importance, especially in children with CHD. The 2015 American Heart Association Scientific Statement shifted the focus from antibiotic prophylaxis for dental work to an emphasis on excellent oral hygiene and prevention of oral diseases as being more effective in preventing IE (Baltimore, Gewitz, Baddour, et al., 2015).

BOX 27.9 Patients at High Risk for Endocarditis

Artificial heart valves
Previous diagnosis of infective endocarditis
Congenital heart disease (CHD), including only the following:*

- Unrepaired cyanotic CHD, including palliative shunts and conduits
- Repaired CHD using prosthetic material or device during the first 6 months after the procedure (including surgical or catheterization placement of these materials)
- Residual defects after CHD repair at the site or adjacent to the site of a prosthetic patch or prosthetic device (inhibiting endothelialization)

Cardiac transplantation recipients with cardiac valvulopathy

*Other than these high-risk patients, antibiotic prophylaxis is no longer routinely recommended.
Adapted from Wilson, W., Taubert, K. A., Gewitz, M., et al. (2007). Prevention of infective endocarditis: Guidelines from the American Heart Association. *Circulation, 116*(15), 1736–1754; Kimberlin, D. W., Long, S. S., Brady, M. T., et al. (2015). Prevention of bacterial endocarditis. In *2015 red book: Report of the committee on infectious diseases* (30th ed.). Elk Grove Village, IL: American Academy of Pediatrics.

Nursing Care Management

Nurses counsel parents of high-risk children concerning the signs and symptoms of endocarditis and the need for prophylactic antibiotic therapy before dental work. The family's dentist should be advised of the child's cardiac diagnosis as an added precaution to ensure preventive treatment. It is important that all children with congenital or acquired heart disease maintain the highest level of oral health to reduce the chance of bacteremia from oral infections. (See Chapter 12.)

Parents should also have a high index of suspicion regarding potential infections. Without unduly alarming them, the nurse stresses that any unexplained fever, weight loss, or change in behavior (lethargy, malaise, anorexia) must be brought to the practitioner's attention. Children at risk (e.g., those with CHD) should have blood drawn for culture if they have a fever without an obvious source. Early diagnosis and treatment are important in preventing further cardiac damage, embolic complications, and growth of resistant organisms. (See Quality Patient Outcomes box.)

QUALITY PATIENT OUTCOMES

Infective Endocarditis

- Prevention in high-risk patients with antibiotic prophylaxis
- Early recognition and treatment

Treatment of endocarditis requires long-term parenteral drug therapy. In many cases, IV antibiotics may be administered at home via a peripherally inserted central catheter (PICC line) with nursing supervision. Nursing goals during this period are (1) preparation of the child for IV infusion, usually with an intermittent-infusion device and several venipunctures for blood cultures; (2) observation for side effects of antibiotics, especially inflammation along venipuncture sites; (3) observation for complications, including embolism and HF; and (4) education regarding the importance of follow-up visits for cardiac evaluation, echocardiographic monitoring, and blood cultures. Some children may need preparation for surgery and, later, postoperative care.

ACUTE RHEUMATIC FEVER AND RHEUMATIC HEART DISEASE

Acute rheumatic fever (ARF) is a result of an abnormal immune response to a group A streptococci (GAS) infection, usually pharyngitis, in a genetically susceptible host (Marijon, Mirabel, Celermajer, et al., 2012). It occurs most often in late school-age children and adolescents and is rare in adults. ARF is a self-limited illness that occurs after untreated pharyngitis and involves inflammation of connective tissues: the joints, skin, brain, and heart. Cardiac valve damage, which is referred to as rheumatic heart disease (RHD), the most significant complication of ARF, occurs in more than half the cases. The mitral valve is most often affected.

In developed countries, ARF and RHD have become uncommon, probably as a result of improved hygiene, improved access to medical care and antibiotic drugs, and a change in the organism itself (Gewitz, Baltimore, Tani, et al., 2015). However, ARF remains a devastating problem in developing (third world) countries because of overcrowded living conditions and poor access to medical care, and among some ethnic and socioeconomic groups in developed countries (Marijon, Mirabel, Celermajer, et al., 2012). In the developing world, ARF and resulting RHD is the leading cause of HF in young people (Remenyi, Carapetis, Wyber, et al., 2013).

Etiology

Strong evidence supports a relationship between upper respiratory tract infection with GAS and subsequent development of ARF (usually within 2 to 6 weeks). Prevention or treatment of GAS infection prevents ARF. If the GAS infection is untreated, antibodies are produced to fight the infection, which can also act against the heart valves causing damage. If children have one strep infection, they are at greater risk for repeated infections and recurrent infections cause the cumulative valve damage of RHD.

Pathophysiology and Clinical Manifestations

ARF is the result of an immune response after infection with GAS, which can be asymptomatic and often go untreated. The diagnosis is based on a set of diagnostic criteria first described by Dr. T. Duckett Jones in 1944 and known as the Jones criteria. Endorsed by the American Heart Association and the World Heart Federation, the most recent revision was completed in 2015 and added evidence supporting the use of Doppler echocardiogram in the diagnosis of carditis (Gewitz, Baltimore, Tani, et al., 2015). The Jones criteria are outlined in Box 27.10.

The most significant manifestation of ARF is carditis. Carditis is the only manifestation of ARF that leads to permanent damage (Narula, Chandrasekhar, Rahimtoola, et al., 1999). In the acute illness, clinical signs and symptoms reflect valvulitis, myocarditis, and pericarditis. Clinically, rheumatic carditis is most commonly associated with the left-sided valves, especially the mitral valve. The classic presentation of carditis was the auscultation of a new regurgitant murmur. Increasingly, as echocardiography is more available in the developing world, ARF and RHD is diagnosed by echo Doppler before the murmur is present. It is now recommended that echocardiograms be performed in all suspected and confirmed cases of ARF (Gewitz, Baltimore, Tani, et al., 2015). Patients with valve involvement may experience progressive valvular damage as time passes.

The second major manifestation is polyarthritis caused by edema, inflammation, and effusions in joint tissue. Joint manifestations usually accompany the acute febrile period, most often in the first 1 to 2 weeks; however, they can persist for 4 weeks in untreated patients.

Chorea reflects CNS involvement. It is usually exaggerated by anxiety and attempts at deliberate fine motor activity and is relieved by rest, especially sleep. The time course of symptoms of chorea is variable and may occur later in the illness—up to 6 months after exposure.

The other manifestations, erythema marginatum and subcutaneous nodules, are uncommon but are highly specific for ARF.

In addition to these major manifestations, minor manifestations that may support the diagnosis include arthralgia and fever, which may be low grade and which often spikes in the late afternoon. Laboratory findings reflect an inflammatory process. Other vague signs and symptoms include unexplained epistaxis, abdominal pain that may be severe enough to simulate appendicitis, weakness, fatigue, pallor, anorexia, and weight loss.

BOX 27.10 Clinical Manifestations of Acute Rheumatic Fever (Jones Criteria, 2015 Revision)

Major Manifestations

Carditis (seen in 50% to 70% of cases)
- New murmur of valve regurgitation (mitral valve most common)
- Echo Doppler evidence of cardiac involvement
- Tachycardia out of proportion to fever
- Pericardial friction rub
- Chest pain
- Muffled heart sounds
- Cardiomegaly on chest x-ray
- Prolonged PR interval on electrocardiogram

Polyarthritis (seen in 35% to 66%)
- Swollen, hot, red, very painful joint pain
- Migratory: affects one joint for 1 to 2 days, then another is affected
- Large joints: knees, elbows, hips, shoulders, wrists

Chorea (seen in 10% to 30%) (also called Sydenham's chorea or St. Vitus dance)
- Sudden aimless irregular movements of extremities, exacerbated by stress
- Profound muscle weakness
- Emotional lability
- Facial grimaces and speech disturbances
- More common in females

Subcutaneous nodules (0% to 10%)
- Nontender swelling over bony prominences
- May persist for many weeks and then resolve

Erythema marginatum (less than 6%)
- Pink rash with pale center and wavy, well-demarcated borders
- Seen on trunk and extremities
- More prominent with heat, blanches with pressure
- Nonpruritic

Minor Manifestations

Arthralgias
Fever (greater than 38.5°C)
ESR above 60 mm and/or CRP greater than 3 mg/dl
Prolonged PR interval

CRP, C-reactive protein; *ESR,* erythrocyte sedimentation rate.
Adapted from Gewitz, M. H., Baltimore, R. S., Tani, L. Y., et al. (2015). Revision of the Jones criteria for the diagnosis of acute rheumatic fever in the era of Doppler echocardiography: A scientific statement from the American Heart Association. *Circulation, 131,* 1806–1818.

Diagnostic Evaluation

No single symptom or laboratory test can provide a definitive diagnosis of ARF. Rather, the diagnosis is based on a set of diagnostic criteria known as the Jones criteria, which were recently updated in 2015 (Gewitz, Baltimore, Tani, et al., 2015). Clinical and laboratory findings are divided into major and minor manifestations (see Box 27.10). Patients must have two major manifestations or one major and two minor manifestations for diagnosis. Some recurrent episodes of ARF in high-risk populations may only have three minor manifestations (Gewitz, Baltimore, Tani, et al., 2015). Age of the patient (5 to 15 years) and preceding sore throat are also important diagnostic clues.

Laboratory tests are done to confirm the clinical diagnosis. Rapid antigen detection test and a throat culture are done to assess for GAS colonization. Streptolysin O is a streptococcal extracellular product that produces lysis of the red blood cells. Antistreptolysin O (ASLO) titers measure the concentration of antibodies formed in the blood against this product. Normally, the titers begin to rise about 7 days after onset of the infection and reach maximum levels in 4 to 6 weeks. Therefore a rising titer demonstrated by at least two ASLO tests is the most reliable evidence of recent streptococcal infection. Elevated titers are seen in at least 80% of patients with ARF (Steer & Gibofsky, 2017). Tests to assess for inflammation include a complete blood count, erythrocyte sedimentation rate (ESR), and C-reactive protein levels (CRP). An electrocardiogram is done to assess for a prolonged PR interval. A chest radiograph is done to assess cardiomegaly and signs of cardiac involvement. An echocardiogram with Doppler to confirm the presence of carditis is done in all patients, even those without clinical signs of carditis. Echo Doppler has been found to be more sensitive than auscultatory findings of a new murmur in identifying cardiac valve dysfunction (Gewitz, Baltimore, Tani, et al., 2015). In high-risk populations, a lower threshold for fever (38°C) and lower inflammatory markers (ESR above 30, CRP above 3) are considered diagnostic (Gewitz, Baltimore, Tani, et al., 2015).

Therapeutic Management

Primary prevention involves prompt diagnosis and treatment of strep throat infections so that ARF does not occur. Oral penicillin is the drug of choice or an alternative in penicillin-sensitive children (Gerber, Baltimore, Eaton, et al., 2009).

For children with ARF, treatment includes antibiotics, antiinflammatory therapy and supportive care and management of HF in some. Antibiotics are given to treat the GAS infection and begin long-term prophylactic treatment to prevent future infections. Penicillin is the drug of choice. Salicylates are used to control the inflammatory process, especially in the joints, and reduce the fever and discomfort. The diagnosis must be confirmed before aspirin therapy is started so clinical signs are not masked by the therapy. The World Health Organization (2004) recommends 100 mg/kg/day of aspirin divided equally into 4 or 5 doses as initial therapy. After 2 weeks with symptomatic improvement, the dose is reduced to 50 to 60 mg/kg/day and discontinued when the patient has been symptom free for 2 weeks. Administration of prednisone may be indicated in patients with pericarditis or HF and in patients who do not respond to aspirin therapy. Neither salicylates nor prednisone has been shown to affect cardiac sequelae.

Supportive care involves initial bed rest during the acute illness and then quiet activities as symptoms subside. Good nutrition is important. Care for children with significant carditis includes HF therapies such as supplemental oxygen, diuretics, fluid and salt restriction, digoxin, or ACE inhibitors. Children with chorea with motor impairment must be protected from injury and eliminate physical and emotional stress, which can exacerbate their symptoms.

Children who have had ARF are susceptible to recurrent infections that are likely to result in RHD and further damage to the heart valves. Prophylactic treatment against recurrence of ARF (secondary prevention) is started after the acute therapy. The treatment of choice is intramuscular injections of benzathine penicillin G every 28 days because it is most effective. Alternative therapy includes oral doses of penicillin or erythromycin twice a day, or one daily dose of sulfadiazine. The duration of secondary prophylaxis is based on the presence of residual heart disease. If ARF occurs without carditis, prophylaxis is recommended for 5 years or until age 21 years, whichever is longer. In patients with carditis, 10 years is recommended or until 21 years old. In patients with RHD, prophylaxis can continue until the age of 40 years and may be indicated indefinitely depending on the individual's risk (Gerber, Baltimore, Eaton, et al., 2009).

Patients with significant cardiac valve damage will need ongoing medical management for HF. They are also at risk for atrial fibrillation and embolic events. Management of RHD may require surgical valve repair or replacement. Valve replacement with a mechanical valve requires lifelong anticoagulation with warfarin.

Nursing Care Management

The objective of nursing care is, first, prevention. Clinicians need to be aware that untreated or undertreated strep throat infections can cause ARF. Rapid strep tests or throat cultures should be done and prompt treatment with antibiotics and follow-up is important. Parents need to be clear that all the antibiotic medicine must be finished. Repeat strep pharyngitis infections may have fewer symptoms or be asymptomatic and trigger ARF or cause further valve damage so a high index of suspicion is important. All patients with ARF receive antibiotic prophylaxis to prevent future infections.

For the child with ARF, nursing care goals include (1) encouraging compliance with drug regimens, (2) facilitating recovery from the illness, and (3) providing emotional support. Nurses play an important role in secondary prevention by educating parents about ARF and RHD and working with patients and families to ensure follow-up with antibiotic prophylaxis. Because compliance is a major concern in long-term drug therapy, every effort is made to encourage adherence to the therapeutic plan (see Compliance, Chapter 22). A community-based approach including health care facilities, schools, and families with excellent communication among them and a personalized approach has been most successful in gaining compliance with years of antibiotic medications (Bono-Neri, 2016). Dedicated health teams to deliver secondary prophylaxis have been most successful (Remond, Coyle, Mills, et al., 2016).

Interventions for ARF are primarily concerned with providing rest, adequate nutrition, and management of cardiac symptoms or chorea. HF management may entail multiple medications, oxygen, fluid restrictions, and careful education about home care management. One of the most disturbing manifestations of ARF is chorea. The onset is gradual and may occur weeks to months after the illness. Sometimes mistaken for nervousness, clumsiness, or inattentiveness, it is usually a source of great frustration to the child because the movements, incoordination, and weakness severely limit physical ability. It is important that parents and teachers are aware of the involuntary, sudden nature of the movements and that the movements are transitory and will eventually disappear. Safety precautions to protect the child from harm or falls are instituted.

Children with RHD will need lifelong follow-up, education, and management of HF and monitoring for progressive valve disease. If surgery is required, preparation for the procedure is provided. An important aspect of postoperative care is education about anticoagulation medications and follow-up. (See Quality Patient Outcomes box.)

QUALITY PATIENT OUTCOMES

Acute Rheumatic Fever

- Group A β-hemolytic streptococcus tonsillopharyngitis identified and treated
- Early recognition and treatment to prevent cardiac valve damage
- Recurrence prevented with prophylaxis compliance

KAWASAKI DISEASE

Kawasaki disease (KD) is an acute systemic vasculitis of unknown cause. The illness is self-limiting and resolves in 6 to 8 weeks. Without treatment, however, approximately 20% to 25% of children develop cardiac sequelae. Damage to the coronary arteries (the blood vessels that supply the heart muscle) is the most common sequelae and involves dilation of the coronary arteries and/or coronary artery aneurysm formation. Infants younger than 1 year of age are at the greatest risk for heart involvement. Children older than 5 years of age are also at increased risk of developing coronary sequelae, perhaps because KD is often not suspected in older children, which may lead to delayed diagnosis and treatment. KD has become a leading cause of acquired heart disease in children in the United States.

KD is seen in children of most racial and ethnic backgrounds. The incidence rate is estimated at 112 cases per 100,000 children less than 5 years of age. KD occurs 1.5 to 1.7 times more frequently in males than in females, and approximately 76% of affected children are younger than 5 years of age, with peak incidence in the toddler age-group (Holman, Curns, Belay, et al., 2003).

The etiology of KD remains unconfirmed. Although KD is not spread by person-to-person contact, several factors support an infectious cause or trigger. KD is often seen in geographic and seasonal outbreaks, with more cases reported in the late winter and early spring. KD is also a pediatric illness, which suggests the development of passive immunity. Some experts believe that the illness may represent a final common pathway triggered by an infectious agent or more than one potential agent. Genetic studies are ongoing in order to ascertain why some children are more likely to get KD than others (i.e., the possibility that the illness represents a final common pathway in a genetically susceptible host).

Pathophysiology

KD involves widespread inflammation of the small and medium-sized blood vessels with the coronary arteries being the most susceptible to damage. During the acute stage of the illness there is progressive inflammation of the small vessels (capillaries, venules, arterioles) along with pancarditis. This inflammation is reflected in the clinical signs and symptoms and in laboratory test results. Inflammatory markers (C-reactive protein level and erythrocyte sedimentation rate) are elevated in the acute illness. The vasculitis can progress to the medium-sized muscular arteries, potentially damaging the walls of the vessels and leading to the formation of coronary artery aneurysms in some children. Initial evidence of enlargement of the coronary arteries by echocardiogram can be detected as early as day 7 of illness. Affected vessels can continue to enlarge for several weeks and generally reach their largest diameter approximately 4 to 6 weeks from the onset of fever. Longer duration of fever is associated with the development of aneurysms (Wilder, Palinkas, Kao, et al., 2007). Aneurysms of the peripheral vessels (axillary, brachial, iliac, cervical, and renal arteries) can occur, although this is rare and usually is seen only in children who have the large/giant coronary aneurysms. In the acute phase, myocarditis (inflammation of the myocardium) is common. Decreased LV function may be evident on echocardiogram; however, the majority of children do not have clinical signs of HF. Ventricular function usually improves after the administration of IV immune globulin (IVIG). Occasionally, however, a child will present with severe ventricular dysfunction and/or cardiogenic shock. The systemic inflammation gradually subsides and eventually ceases with normalization of inflammatory markers 6 to 8 weeks from the onset of fever.

Over time, aneurysmal vessels try to heal through multiplication of cells in the vessels in an attempt to restore a "normal" lumen diameter. This process is called myointimal proliferation. The smaller the initial dilation, the more likely the vessel lumen diameter will regress to a normal size. However, even if the lumen size is restored, the affected vessel may not be completely normal. The walls of these vessels are thicker and may be subject to scarring and calcification (potentially causing stenosis), especially at the distal ends of the aneurysm in patients with large/giant aneurysms.

Almost all of the morbidity and mortality resulting from KD are due to cardiac complications and mainly occur in patients who have giant aneurysms. Coronary thrombosis may result from sluggish blood flow in a dilated or aneurysmal vessel. Over the years, in patients with large aneurysms, stenosis and scarring may lead to impeded blood flow, which can result in myocardial ischemia or infarction.

Clinical Manifestations

The course of KD can be divided into three phases: acute, subacute, and convalescent. The acute phase begins with an abrupt onset of high fever that is unresponsive to antibiotics and antipyretics. Over the first week or so, the diagnostic symptoms become evident. The bulbar conjunctivae of the eyes become reddened, with clearing around the iris (limbal sparing). The eyes are generally dry, without significant drainage. Inflammation of the pharynx and the oral mucosa develops, with red, cracked lips and the characteristic "strawberry tongue" (i.e., the normal coating of the tongue sloughs off, leaving the large papillae exposed, so the tongue resembles a strawberry). The rash of KD differs from child to child but is never vesicular and is most often accentuated in the perineum. Often the groin area may desquamate early in the illness. The child's hands and feet become edematous, and the palms and soles become erythematous. The child may have cervical lymphadenopathy (usually unilateral ≤1.5 cm). The node is not usually very tender or red. To meet "classic" criteria, children have prolonged fever (≤4 days) along with four out of five of the diagnostic criteria. During the acute stage, the child is typically very irritable and inconsolable. This behavior may continue for several weeks and is often one of the last features to improve. Approximately one-third of patients develop a temporary arthritis beginning in the small joints. Cardiac manifestations during this period may include myocarditis, decreased LV function, pericardial effusion, and mitral regurgitation. Generally, these findings are subclinical, but occasionally children with poor ventricular function present with symptoms of cardiogenic shock. On physical examination, the child may be tachycardic with a gallop rhythm. The coronary arteries may begin to show enlargement during this phase.

The subacute phase begins with resolution of the fever and lasts until all outward clinical signs of KD have disappeared. If changes in the coronary arteries occur, enlargement or dilation is generally evident by echocardiography during the second week of illness. Damaged vessels can continue to enlarge and reach their maximum diameter approximately 4 to 6 weeks from the onset of illness. Thrombocytosis and hypercoagulability in a child with expanding aneurysms and disrupted blood flow place him or her at risk for coronary thrombosis. During the subacute period, the child may develop periungual desquamation (peeling that begins under the fingertips and toes) of the hands and feet. A temporary arthritis may be evident during this phase and can affect the larger weight-bearing joints. Irritability persists during this period.

In the convalescent phase, the clinical signs of KD have mostly resolved, but the laboratory values may still be abnormal. Arthritis may continue into this stage. Coronary dimensions peak approximately 4 to 6 weeks from the onset of illness. The convalescent phase is complete when all laboratory values return to normal (6 to 8 weeks after onset). At the end of this stage, most parents report that the child appears to have returned to baseline in terms of temperament, energy, and appetite.

Cardiac Involvement

The most serious complication of KD is the development of coronary artery aneurysms and the potential for myocardial infarction in children who have developed aneurysm formation. Any vessel that has a z-score ≥2.5 (standard deviations above the mean) is considered to be outside the normal range. A small aneurysm is defined as having a z-score of 2.5 to 5.0 and a medium aneurysm is defined as having a z-score of ≥5 to <10, and an absolute dimension <8 mm. Although giant aneurysms have traditionally been defined as those measuring greater than 8 mm in diameter, recent data suggest that coronary dimensions should be standardized for body mass index (BMI) using z-scores (standard deviations above/below mean). The rationale for this relates to the theory that an 8-mm vessel in a 4-month-old is relatively larger than an 8-mm vessel in a 12-year-old. Therefore the new American Heart Association guidelines define a large or giant aneurysm as having a coronary measurement that has a z-score >10 (standard deviations above the mean), or having an absolute dimension of >8 mm (McCrindle, Rowley, Newburger, et al., 2017). As would be expected, blood flow is extremely abnormal in large/giant aneurysms, placing these patients at highest risk for thrombus formation. Myocardial ischemia can result from thrombotic occlusion or stenotic occlusion of a coronary aneurysm. Symptoms of acute myocardial infarction in young children can be subtle and may include abdominal pain, vomiting, restlessness, inconsolable crying, pallor, and shock. Complaints of actual chest pain or pressure are more typical in older children (Kato, Ichinose, & Kawasaki, 1986).

Diagnostic Evaluation

Currently no specific diagnostic test exists for KD. Therefore the diagnosis is established on the basis of clinical findings and associated laboratory results that support the diagnosis. The clinical criteria in Box 27.11 should be used as guidelines. Many children with KD do not meet standard diagnostic criteria, and infants often have an incomplete presentation. It is therefore important to consider KD as a possible diagnosis in any infant or child with prolonged elevated temperature that is unresponsive to antibiotics and is not attributable to another cause. The American Heart Association has provided a diagnostic algorithm to guide the evaluation and treatment of patients with incomplete symptoms who have prolonged fever or other features of KD (Fig. 27.20).

Associated laboratory findings, when combined with clinical data, can be helpful in making the diagnosis of KD. The typical child with KD is somewhat anemic and has a leukocytosis with a "shift to the left" (increased immature white blood cells) during the acute phase.

BOX 27.11 Clinical Criteria for Diagnosis of Kawasaki Disease

Fever for at least 5 days

Presence of at least four of the five following symptoms:

1. Changes in extremities
   Acute—Erythema of palms and soles, edema of hands and feet
   Subacute—Periungual peeling of fingers and toes in second and third week
2. Polymorphous exanthem
3. Bilateral bulbar conjunctival injection without exudate
4. Erythema and cracking of lips, strawberry tongue, and/or erythema of oral and pharyngeal mucosae
5. Cervical lymphadenopathy (node >1.5 cm in diameter), usually unilateral

Patients with fever for at least 5 days and fewer than four symptoms described above can be diagnosed as having Kawasaki disease when coronary artery abnormalities are detected by two-dimensional echocardiography or angiography. When four or more principal features are present, the diagnosis of Kawasaki disease can be made on day 4 of illness. In very rare occurrences, with an experienced clinician, diagnoses can be made on day 3.

NOTE: These criteria should be used as a guideline; however, not all of the symptoms need to be present at once. In addition, atypical or incomplete Kawasaki disease should be considered in patients with some features, prolonged fever, and no alternative diagnosis (see algorithm for incomplete Kawasaki disease, Fig. 27.16).

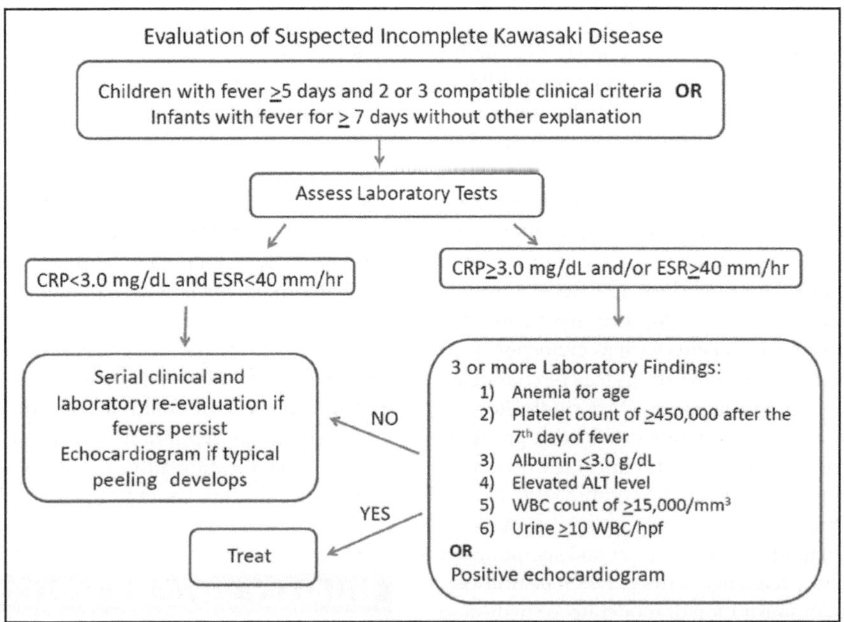

FIG. 27.20 Evaluation of suspected incomplete Kawasaki disease *(KD). CRP,* C-reactive protein; *echo,* echocardiography; *ESR,* erythrocyte sedimentation rate. (From McCrindle, B. W., Rowley, A. H., Newburger, J. W., et al. [2017]. Diagnosis, treatment, and long-term management of Kawasaki disease: A scientific statement of health professionals from the American Heart Association. *Circulation, 135,* 1379–1381.)

Thrombocytosis with hypercoagulability becomes evident in the subacute phase with peak platelet counts occurring approximately 3 weeks after the onset of fever. An elevated erythrocyte sedimentation rate and C-reactive protein level reflect ongoing inflammation and can persist for 6 to 8 weeks. The erythrocyte sedimentation rate can be further elevated by the administration of IVIG; therefore it is better to measure the C-reactive protein level as an indicator of inflammation after IVIG administration. Microscopic urinalysis reveals a sterile pyuria with mononuclear cells that will not be evident with a regular dipstick test because the white blood cells are not polymorphonuclear neutrophils. Transient elevation of liver enzymes may occur during the acute phase, reflecting inflammation of the liver. Examination of cerebrospinal fluid may show aseptic meningitis (presence of inflammatory cells). Albumin levels may be lower than normal, particularly in the sickest children (Newburger, de Ferranti, & Fulton, 2016). Some children experience a temporary arthritis during the illness that resolves over time. Both small and large joints may be affected in the short term. A rare sequela can be sensorineural hearing loss. If decreased hearing is suspected, the child should undergo audiologic testing.

Echocardiograms are used to monitor myocardial function and coronary artery dimensions. A baseline echocardiogram is obtained at the time of diagnosis to evaluate coronary size and ventricular and valvar function. Common findings on echocardiogram during the acute phase may include pericardial effusions, mitral regurgitation, and decreased ventricular function. Follow-up echocardiograms should be performed within 1 to 2 weeks after diagnosis and again 4 to 6 weeks after treatment. More frequent echocardiograms to assess coronary dimensions are indicated in patients who have continued fever, those who require retreatment with IVIG, and those with coronary dilation on baseline or other studies. In these patients, echocardiograms may be performed twice a week until coronary dimensions stabilize.

Therapeutic Management

The standard treatment of KD includes high-dose IVIG along with salicylate therapy. High-dose IVIG has been shown to reduce the duration of fever and the incidence of coronary artery abnormalities when given within the first 10 days of illness and optimally within the first 7 days (Newburger, Takahashi, Burns, et al., 1986). A single large infusion of 2 g/kg over 8 to 12 hours is recommended (McCrindle, Rowley, Newburger, et al., 2017). Approximately 10% to 20% of children continue to have fever after the initial treatment with IVIG and may be candidates for retreatment or adjunctive therapies (Tremoulet, Best, Song, et al., 2008). In addition, patients with coronary dilation or aneurysm formation are candidates for additional treatment focused on decreasing inflammation. Retreatment with a second dose of IVIG is often given for patients with persistent or recrudescent fever without other cause 36 hours after the completion of the initial dose of IVIG. Additional therapies such as steroids and infliximab (Remicade) have also been used after IVIG failure. The use of other agents such as cyclosporine or cyclophosphamide and other antiinflammatory drugs may be considered in the sickest patients with developing aneurysms (McCrindle, Rowley, Newburger, et al., 2017). However, the best therapy for this group of high-risk patients is still unknown and warrants continued research.

Aspirin is given initially in an antiinflammatory/antipyretic dosages (ranging from moderate to high dose, 30 to 50 mg/kg/day or 80 to 100 mg/kg/day) divided every 6 hours to control fever and symptoms of inflammation. Practice as to dose preference varies between institutions. It is important to note that the administration of moderate- or high-dose aspirin has not been shown to make a difference in the incidence of coronary artery sequelae. Once fever has subsided, the aspirin dosage is decreased to an antiplatelet dosage (3 to 5 mg/kg/day). Low-dose aspirin therapy is continued in patients without echocardiographic evidence of coronary abnormalities until the platelet count has returned to normal (4 to 6 weeks). If the child develops coronary abnormalities, low-dose (antiplatelet) salicylate therapy is continued. Additional anticoagulation therapy, such as clopidogrel or warfarin administration, is indicated in children with medium or large/giant coronary enlargement, respectively. In infants, lovenox may be used instead of warfarin because it is easier to maintain a steady state.

Prognosis

The vast majority of children with KD recover fully after treatment without cardiovascular sequelae. When cardiovascular complications occur, however, serious morbidity may result. Death occurs very rarely (<0.1% to 0.2%) and is almost always a result of ischemia caused by coronary thrombosis or stenosis. The long-term prognosis for a particular child depends on whether or not a child develops coronary enlargement, and, if so, the extent of the coronary damage (i.e., how large the enlargement is). Children with coronary abnormalities are followed closely. Long-term testing may include periodic ECGs, echocardiography, stress testing (stress echoes and/or myocardial perfusion scans) at rest and during exercise, and cardiac computed tomography angiogram (CTA) and/or MRI. The frequency and type of testing depends on individual risk, as well the availability of various testing modalities at the individual centers (Baker & Newburger, 2008; Newburger, Takahashi, Gerber, et al., 2004). Although echocardiography is sensitive in visualizing coronary dilation in the proximal coronaries, it does not detect stenoses of the coronary arteries. Cardiac catheterization or cardiac CTA may be performed to obtain a more complete picture of the full coronary system in children who still have significant abnormalities 6 months to 1 year after illness onset. In addition, these tests may be indicated in situations in which stenosis or thrombosis and/or myocardial ischemia is suspected from the results of noninvasive testing. Both of these modalities can visualize the proximal and distal vessels, and decisions as to the best imaging technique are made on an individual basis.

Children without coronary artery aneurysms have now been followed for more than 40 years in Japan and the United States and do not show an increased incidence of accelerated atherosclerosis or premature heart disease. Recent studies have suggested that peripheral vessels are not stiffer in patients who have had KD without aneurysms and those children have an excellent long-term prognosis (McCrindle, Rowley, Newburger, et al., 2017). Nonetheless, it is recommended that children who have had KD have as few other risk factors for coronary disease as possible. Cholesterol levels and BP should be monitored as per the general population guidelines, and children should be encouraged to lead a heart-healthy lifestyle in terms of diet, exercise, and avoidance of smoking. Children without coronary enlargement may be discharged from cardiology follow-up between 1 month and 1 year after initial onset, depending on practice variations (McCrindle, Rowley, Newburger, et al., 2017).

Nursing Care Management

The nursing care of children with KD can be challenging. Inpatient care focuses on symptomatic relief, emotional support, diagnostic assistance, medication administration, and education of the child and family. (See Quality Patient Outcomes box.)

QUALITY PATIENT OUTCOMES

Kawasaki Disease

- Early diagnosis and treatment
- Prevention of cardiovascular complications

In the initial phase of illness, the nurse must monitor the child's cardiac status carefully. Intake and output and daily weight measurements are recorded. The child may be reluctant to eat and may be partially dehydrated. IV fluids need to be administered with care because of the usual finding of myocarditis. The child should be assessed frequently for signs of HF, including decreased urinary output, gallop rhythm, tachycardia, and respiratory distress. Close cardiac monitoring is indicated during the infusion of IVIG (because of the large fluid load), particularly in children younger than 1 year of age, and in any child with cardiac symptoms. Sedation is generally required before echocardiography in children younger than 2½ to 3 years of age because the child must remain still in order to obtain adequate visualization of the coronary arteries, cardiac structures, and function.

Nursing care for patients with KD is focused primarily on symptomatic relief. To minimize skin discomfort, application of cool cloths and unscented lotions and use of soft, loose clothing are helpful. During the acute phase, mouth care, including application of lubricating ointment to the lips, is important for the mucosal inflammation. The nurse should offer clear liquids and soft foods and monitor temperature carefully. It is important to document temperature just before aspirin administration because fever reflects ongoing inflammation and may indicate the need for further treatment. If the temperature is very high, acetaminophen may be given in addition to high-dose aspirin. (See Controlling Elevated Temperatures, Chapter 23.) If arthritis develops, passive range-of-motion exercises may help maintain mobility and can be done most easily during the child's bath.

The administration of IVIG should follow the same guidelines as for administration of any blood product, with frequent monitoring of vital signs. Patients must be watched for allergic reactions and are often premedicated with Benadryl and Tylenol. The nurse must monitor cardiac status because of the large fluid volume being administered to patients who may have subclinical myocarditis or diminished LV function. Check patency of the IV line because extravasation can result in tissue damage. Hypercoagulability and venous fragility often make it difficult to maintain IV access in children with KD.

Patient irritability is perhaps the most challenging problem for parents of children with KD. These children need to be placed in a quiet environment that promotes adequate rest. Their parents need to be supported in their efforts to comfort an often inconsolable child. They may need time away from their child, and nurses can often provide respite care for the family. Parents need to understand that irritability is a hallmark of KD and that they need not feel guilty or embarrassed about their child's behavior.

Discharge Teaching

Parents need accurate information about the usual course of KD, including the importance of follow-up monitoring and the circumstances under which they should contact their practitioner. Irritability is likely to persist for up to 2 months after the onset of symptoms. Peeling of the hands and feet is painless and occurs primarily in the second and third weeks. Arthritis, especially of the larger weight-bearing joints, may persist for several weeks. Affected children are typically most stiff in the mornings, during cold weather, and after naps. Passive range-of-motion exercises in the bathtub are often helpful in increasing flexibility. Although the arthritis in KD is always temporary, it can be severe and may interfere with walking. (Note: Other high-dose NSAIDs should not be given with high-dose salicylates, and the use of NSAIDs may interfere with the antiplatelet effects of low-dose aspirin.)

Most important, parents should be educated about the potential for recrudescent illness after discharge. Persistent or recrudescent fever 36 hours after IVIG completion should prompt reevaluation and possible additional treatments. Instruct the parents to take the child's temperature daily after discharge and to contact their clinician if the child has a fever.

Parents should be instructed about the administration of salicylates. It is rare to give high-dose aspirin for a prolonged length of time in this era. However, if the child is receiving high dosages, parents should be aware of the signs of aspirin toxicity: ringing in the ears (tinnitus), headache, dizziness, and confusion. The main side effect of low-dose aspirin is easy bruising. In addition, aspirin should be temporarily discontinued and the practitioner notified if the child is exposed to chickenpox or influenza because of the drug's possible association with Reye syndrome.

All parents should understand the unlikely but real possibility of myocardial infarction and the signs and symptoms of cardiac ischemia in a child. At the time of hospital discharge, the final cardiac sequelae are often evolving, as changes in the coronary arteries occur over the first 4 to 6 weeks after the onset of KD. Because coronary artery changes take place over the initial 4 to 6 weeks after illness onset, it is important that follow-up planning includes an echocardiogram and cardiology appointment approximately 1 to 2 weeks after hospital discharge and again in 4 to 6 weeks. More frequent echocardiograms are indicated for patients with coronary dilation or aneurysm formation and may include twice-weekly echocardiograms until vessel dimensions stabilize (McCrindle, Rowley, Newburger, et al., 2017). If the child has developed coronary artery aneurysms, parents should be taught cardiopulmonary resuscitation.

Finally, children with coronary abnormalities may require indefinite antiplatelet therapy with low-dose aspirin or other anticoagulants. In such cases children should avoid contact sports and have yearly influenza vaccines. The administration of measles-mumps-rubella vaccine should be delayed for 11 months after the administration of IVIG because the body might not produce the appropriate number of antibodies. In addition, the varicella vaccine should not be given for at least 11 months after IVIG therapy (Kimberlin, Long, Brady, et al., 2015).

SYSTEMIC HYPERTENSION

Hypertension is the most common cause of CVA and is a major contributor to atherosclerotic disease in adults. Traditionally, primary hypertension has been considered a disease of older adults. However, in recent years there has been increasing evidence that primary hypertension does occur in children and adolescents, posing long-term health risks. End-organ effects can be seen in young children as a result of chronic hypertension. These findings emphasize the importance of BP evaluation for all individuals beginning at age 3 years (younger if additional risk factors). A working group of the American Academy of Pediatrics has published new clinical practice guidelines for clinicians for the screening and management of high BP in children and adolescents (Flynn, Kaelber, Baker-Smith, et al., 2017). This publication updated the normative tables for BP and modified the cutpoints for what is considered to be elevated BP and hypertension. The 2017 normative tables are now based solely on normal-weight children (excluding those with elevated BMI). In addition, categorical cut points (rather than percentiles) are now used for teenagers ≥13 years old to define normal, elevated, and hypertensive values (see inside back cover).

The definition for the diagnosis of hypertension has been modified in the new guidelines. The category of prehypertension is now renamed "elevated blood pressure." As in prior guidelines, the extent of the diagnostic workup for hypertension depends on the degree of BP elevation.

For children ages 1 to 13 years old, the following definitions are now used:

- *Elevated blood pressure* is defined as a systolic or diastolic BP that falls at or above the 90th percentile for age and height but is under the 95th percentile or 120/80 mm Hg to less than the 95th percentile (whichever is lower).
- Stage 1 hypertension is classified as BPs that fall persistently at or above the 95th percentile to less than the 95th percentile + 12 mm Hg or 130/80 to 139/89 (whichever is lower).
- Stage 2 hypertension is defined as BPs that are persistently at or above the 95th percentile plus 12 mm Hg or ≥140/90.

For children ≥13 years old, the following definitions are currently used:

- Elevated BP is defined simply as 120 to 129/<80 mm Hg.
- Stage 1 hypertension is defined as 130 to 139/80 to 89 mm Hg.
- Stage 2 hypertension is defined as ≥140/90 mm Hg.

White-coat hypertension is diagnosed when the patient's BP is higher than the 95th percentile in the clinician's office but falls under the 95th percentile outside of this setting.

Etiology

Hypertension in young children, compared with older adolescents and adults, was thought to occur more commonly secondary to a structural abnormality or an underlying pathologic process. However, the results of screening programs of relatively healthy children have challenged this view. When secondary hypertension is diagnosed, the most common causes in young children is renal disease, followed by cardiovascular, endocrine, or some neurologic disorders. In older children/adolescents, stress/anxiety and/or effects from pharmacologic agents may play a role (Mattoo, 2017). As a rule, the younger the child and the more severe the hypertension, the more likely it is to be due to a secondary cause. The conditions associated with secondary hypertension in children and adolescents are listed in Box 27.12.

The causes of primary or idiopathic hypertension are undetermined. There is evidence that both genetic and environmental factors play a role. The incidence of hypertension is greater in children with a family history of hypertension. African Americans have a higher incidence of hypertension than Caucasians. In the African American population, hypertension seems to develop earlier and is frequently more severe. Environmental factors that contribute to the risk of developing hypertension may include obesity; salt ingestion; smoking; lead exposure; medications, including certain stimulant drugs and toxins; and stress.

Clinical Manifestations

Clinical manifestations associated with hypertension depend largely on the underlying cause and the degree of hypertension. Adolescents and older children with significant hypertension may complain of frequent headaches, dizziness, or changes in vision. In infants or young children who cannot communicate symptoms, observation of behavior may provide clues, although gross behavioral changes may not be apparent until complications are present. Parents of infants and small children who have been treated for hypertension report that their child had previously been irritable and often indulged in an abnormal degree of head banging or rubbing.

Diagnostic Evaluation

It is clear from the increasing numbers of cases of hypertension and prehypertension being identified in children and adolescents that a BP determination should be a routine part of annual assessment. Current guidelines recommend BP ascertainment in all children older than 3 years of age and earlier in children with individual risk factors or health conditions. Measure BP in children of any age if they are diagnosed as having or are suspected of having coarctation of the aorta, unexplained HF, unexplained heart murmurs, prematurity, unexplained seizures or other neurologic signs, an abdominal mass or masses, edema, ascites, evidence of renal failure, hypernatremia, failure to thrive, possible obstructive sleep apnea, respiratory distress, hyperlipidemia, or unexplained headaches. Because hypertension is strongly associated with obesity, a BMI should be calculated for each child at the routine physical examination.

BOX 27.12 Conditions Associated With Secondary Hypertension in Children

Renal Disorders

Congenital defects
- Polycystic kidney, ectopic kidney, horseshoe kidney
- Obstructive anomalies
- Hydronephrosis

Renal tumor
- Wilms tumor
- Renovascular tumor

Abnormalities of renal arteries

Renal vein thrombosis

Acquired disorders
- Glomerulonephritis—acute or chronic
- Pyelonephritis
- Nephritis associated with collagen disease

Cardiovascular Disease

Coarctation of aorta

Arteriovenous fistula

Aortic or mitral insufficiency

Metabolic and Endocrine Diseases

Adrenal tumors
- Adenoma
- Pheochromocytoma
- Neuroblastoma

Cushing syndrome

Adrenogenital syndrome

Hyperthyroidism

Aldosteronism

Hypercalcemia

Diabetes mellitus

Neurologic Disorders

Space-occupying lesions of the cranium (increased intracranial pressure)
- Tumors, cysts, hematoma
- Cerebral edema
- Encephalitis (including Guillain-Barré and Reye syndromes)

Miscellaneous Causes

Drugs (corticosteroids, oral contraceptives, pressor agents, stimulant drugs, amphetamines)

Burns

Genitourinary surgery

Trauma (e.g., stretching of femoral nerve with leg traction)

Insect bites (e.g., scorpion)

Intravascular overload (blood, fluid)

Hypernatremia

Toxemia of pregnancy

Heavy metal poisoning

Licorice

Mattoo, T. K. (2017). Evaluation of hypertension in children and adolescents. *UpToDate*. Retrieved from https://www.uptodate.com/contents/evaluation-of-hypertension-in-children-and-adolescents.

Before initiating a workup for hypertension, BP should be measured several times in the sitting position. If BP readings are in the elevated range, they should be repeated at three separate times. Automated BPs should be taken several times, the first one discarded and the next three averaged. Ideally, elevated automated BP readings should be repeated by auscultation. *Note:* BP norms are based on auscultated pressures. To obtain an accurate reading, take care to quiet the child or relax the adolescent while the measurement is recorded to avoid false readings. The chief cause of falsely elevated BP readings is the use of improperly fitting, narrow cuffs. Therefore attention to correct measurement technique is essential. (See Blood Pressure, Chapter 4.) Note that a child who is large for his or her age may normally have a higher BP than a child who is of average size. Upper and lower extremity BP in the supine position should always be assessed when hypertension is suspected, along with the presence of femoral pulses because of the possibility of secondary hypertensions from undiagnosed coarctation of the aorta. Twenty-four-hour BP (ambulatory BP [AMBP]) monitoring devices detect changes in pressure throughout the day and night, and thus may give a more realistic picture. These devices are especially helpful in diagnosing white-coat hypertension and can be used with older children or adolescents, who are able to tolerate being attached to an ambulatory monitor (Flynn, Daniels, Hayman, et al., 2014). To be the least intrusive, it is recommended that the 24-hour BP monitor be worn on the nondominant arm. The child or parent should keep a log during AMBP monitoring to document level of activity or, at a minimum, sleeping and waking times. AMBP monitors should document readings at least hourly and ideally more often (every 20 minutes).

Evaluation of the child with high BP includes a thorough assessment of lifestyle and additional risk factors, detection of potential secondary causes, and documentation of the presence or absence of end-organ effects. For children whose BP falls in the elevated range, weight management and lifestyle modifications (e.g., regular moderate to vigorous exercise, DASH diet [see later discussion], stress reduction, adequate sleep, and avoidance of smoking) should be reviewed, and BPs should be repeated in 6 months. Upper and lower BPs (right arm, left arm, and one leg) should be measured if a patient continues to have elevated BPs at the 6-month check with reinforcement of lifestyle counseling. If auscultated BP is still elevated at three separate visits in 12 months, an AMBP should be obtained (if child old enough to cooperate) and further testing should be done. The workup occurs more quickly in patients with stage 1 or 2 hypertension. Lifestyle modification is recommended for all. In addition, in patients with stage 1 hypertension, BP is rechecked by auscultation in 1 to 2 weeks (with upper and lower BPs) and again at 3 months. If still elevated, AMBP is obtained and further diagnostic workup is indicated with possible specialty referral and initiation of treatment. For stage 2 hypertension, upper and lower BP should be checked immediately, with repeat BP measurements within 1 week or referral to specialist promptly (within 1 week). If still high, AMBP and diagnostic evaluation should begin and treatment initiated. In severe cases of very high BP the patient should be referred to an emergency department for immediate evaluation. Table 27.5 outlines the recommended workup for patients with persistent elevated BP or stage 1 or 2 hypertension (Flynn, Kaelber, baker-Smith, et. al., 2017).

The nurse should take a careful medical history of the child or adolescent, including perinatal and all past medical history and current medications, drug use (particularly stimulant drugs), or smoking. In addition, the nurse should obtain a thorough family history to screen for other relatives with hypertension or other cardiovascular risk factors, including age of onset in first- or second-degree relatives. Psychosocial history including stressors should be documented, as well as lifestyle habits (diet, physical activity, sleep habits, smoking, alcohol, drugs).

As mentioned, the timing and extent of additional testing is driven by the degree of BP elevation. Initial testing includes urinalysis, renal function studies such as creatinine and blood urea nitrogen levels, a lipid profile, and electrolyte levels. Additional laboratory data may include additional laboratory work and/or imaging depending on age and history. In young children or children who have significant hypertension, secondary causes should be investigated thoroughly. A renal ultrasonographic scan provides a first-line screen for renovascular hypertension or other renal disease and should be obtained in children with hypertension under age 6 years. A renal ultrasound may be indicated in older children if their history, laboratory work, or urinalysis shows concern for renal origin. Additional renovascular imaging may be indicated in some cases. Testing may include a renal magnetic resonance angiogram or renal CTA. Echocardiography is used to rule out structural heart problems, such as coarctation of the aorta, and to assess for end-organ damage such as the presence of LV hypertrophy. A finding that the child's LV mass is higher than normal would support the presence of chronically elevated BP because the heart muscle thickens in response to chronic hypertension.

Therapeutic Management

Therapy for secondary hypertension involves diagnosis and treatment of the underlying cause. In those cases amenable to surgical repair, the nature of the condition, the type of surgery, and the child's age are all important considerations. Children or adolescents with consistently elevated BP readings from no known cause (primary or idiopathic hypertension) or those with secondary hypertension not amenable to surgical correction may be treated with a combination of nonpharmacologic and pharmacologic interventions.

Dietary practices and lifestyle changes are important in the control of hypertension for both children and adults and should be instituted first, except in severe cases. In salt-sensitive children, high salt intake increases the risk of hypertension for those genetically predisposed and aggravates existing hypertension unless salt intake is limited. The DASH diet provides a lower-salt diet that has been associated with improvement in BP and is thought to be beneficial for all patients with hypertension. *DASH* stands for *D*ietary *A*pproaches to *S*top *H*ypertension. The DASH diet consists of vegetables, fruits, whole grains, and low-fat dairy products, and it is low in sugar and salt.

Because obesity and hypertension are closely related, a weight-reduction program is recommended for overweight youngsters. Regular aerobic exercise augments weight reduction and improves BP measurements. Ideally, children should be counseled to obtain 3 to 5 days of moderate or vigorous exercise (30 to 60 minutes each time). The exercise regimen is most effective if it can be individualized to the child's interest. It is helpful to quantify how much time is spent in sedentary activities (e.g., overall screen time) compared with how much time daily is spent in aerobic activities. Regular sleep habits are important. In addition, stress reduction strategies may be beneficial and may include biofeedback, yoga, and relaxation. Smoking should be avoided.

Drug therapy is initiated with caution in children. Because the long-term effects of antihypertensive agents on children are not known, drug treatment of asymptomatic children with mild or borderline hypertension is not recommended. However, antihypertensive drug therapy is indicated for treating those patients who have significant elevations of BP despite nonpharmacologic intervention. This includes children and adolescents with persistent hypertension (stage 1 or higher), symptomatic hypertension, secondary hypertension, end-organ evidence of hypertension (e.g., increased LV mass), and/or significant additional risk factors, such as diabetes.

The American Academy of Pediatrics recommends initiating pharmacologic therapy with one drug (recommendations for drugs for initial

TABLE 27.5 Childhood Hypertension Evaluation

Diagnostic Procedures or Tests	Rationale	Indications
Thorough history, including the following: • Detailed past medical history • Family history • Lifestyle factors: diet, exercise, smoking, alcohol, drugs • Assess sleep habits	Help focus further evaluation	All patients with elevated BP or higher
Laboratory evaluation: • Electrolytes, blood urea nitrogen, creatinine, urinalysis, fasting lipid panel	Identify concerns for secondary causes	Children with the following: • Persistent elevated BP after 1 year • Stage 1 hypertension over 3 visits in 3 months • Stage 2 hypertension for 2 visits in 1 week or sooner depending on severity
HgbA1C AST, ALT	Screening for diabetes, fatty liver	Obese children/adolescents with persistently elevated or stage 1 or 2 BP (in addition to above laboratory evaluation)
Renal ultrasonography	Assess renal size, Doppler gradient, congenital anomaly	Children ≤6 years old Children >8 years old if suspected of having renovascular hypertension
Complete blood count	Identify anemia, chronic renal disease	Patients with abnormal renal function
Polysomnography	Identify sleep disorder associated with hypertension	Children with history of loud, frequent snoring
Drug screen	Identify substances that cause hypertension	Children with history suggestive of possible contribution by substances or drugs
Echocardiography	Identify left ventricular hypertrophy, LV geometry, rule out coarctation	Assess before considering medication; if normal, reassess yearly in patients with stage 2 hypertension or incompletely treated stage 1; in abnormal, reassess every 6-12 months; obtain in all patients with BP gradient (upper to lower)
Additional Evaluation as Indicated		
Magnetic resonance angiography or computed tomography Arteriography	Identify renovascular disease	Patients suspected of having renal artery stenosis
Ambulatory BP monitoring	Identify white-coat hypertension, abnormal diurnal BP pattern, BP load	Children >5 years old in whom white-coat hypertension is suspected and those for whom other information on BP pattern is needed after elevated BP for ≥1 year or stage 1 after 3 clinic visits; in addition, obtain for surveillance on patients with high-risk conditions such as repaired coarctation
Plasma and urine catecholamine levels	Identify catecholamine-mediated hypertension	If concern for catecholamine excess based on family history, patient history or physical examination (flushing, palpitations, headache, sweating), abdominal mass
Plasma and urine steroid levels	Identify steroid-mediated hypertension	If concern for congenital adrenal hyperplasia
Plasma renin level Plasma aldosterone	Identify low renin level or elevated aldosterone	If concern for mineralocorticoid-related disease

ALT, Alanine aminotransferase; *AST,* aspartate aminotransferase; *BP,* blood pressure; *HgbA1C,* hemoglobin A1C; *LV,* left ventricle.
Modified from Flynn, J. T., Kaelber, D. C., Baker-Smith, C. M., Blowey, D., Carroll, A. E., Daniels, S. R. ... Subcommittee on Screening and Management of High Blood Pressure in Children: Clinical practice guideline for screening and management of high blood pressure in children and adolescents. *Pediatrics, 140*(3), e20171904, 2017.

therapy include an ACE inhibitor, angiotensin receptor blocker, long-acting calcium channel blocker, or thiazide diuretic). Additional agents may be added if adequate BP control is not obtained. The goal of therapy is to reduce BP levels below the 90th percentile and less than 130/80 mm Hg (in adolescents ≥13 years old).

The oral antihypertensive drugs used most often in children include ACE inhibitors (lisinopril, captopril, enalapril, fosinopril), long-acting calcium channel blockers (amlodipine [Norvasc]), angiotensin receptor blockers (losartan [Cozaar]), and thiazide diuretics (hydrochlorothiazide [HydroDIURIL]), to mention a few.

Pharmacologic intervention needs to be tailored to meet the needs of the individual child and is determined by the hypotensive effect produced and the appearance of any side effects. For example, ACE inhibitors and angiotensin receptor blockers have been effective in children with diabetes or certain renal diagnoses, whereas beta blockers and calcium channel blockers are often used by children with a history of migraine headaches. The goal of treatment is to use the lowest dose

DRUG ALERT

ACE Inhibitors and Angiotensin Receptor Blockers

ACE inhibitors and angiotensin receptor blockers are teratogenic and therefore should not be used during pregnancy. Adolescent girls should be counseled regarding this precaution.

of medication to achieve a normotensive state throughout the day without accompanying side effects. For many antihypertensive drugs, minimal data are available regarding side effects in children. Therefore the nurse should consider any behavioral or physical changes that occur after institution of therapy as possible side effects and should revise therapy as needed.

Nursing Care Management

The nurse is a valuable link in the delivery of health care for hypertension in the pediatric age-group. Active in detection, diagnosis, and therapy in any setting—hospital, school, clinic, private office, public health service, and private practice—nurses are frequently the primary contact in well-child care and follow-up clinics. They are often the liaison between the family and the health care services. (See Quality Patient Outcomes box.)

QUALITY PATIENT OUTCOMES

Hypertension

- Underlying cause of hypertension identified
- Blood pressure control maintained
- Dietary practices (DASH diet) and lifestyle changes (regular exercise, no smoking, optimize body mass index) effectively used to control hypertension
- Compliance with medication regimen, if prescribed

DASH, Dietary approaches to stop hypertension.

A BP measurement should be part of the routine physical examination in children over age 3 years and in younger children who have individual risk factors for hypertension. In carrying out the procedure, it is important for the nurse to use the correct cuff size. Any questionable reading is repeated by auscultation and average BPs determined. Ideally, the BP should be assessed with the child in the sitting position with both feet on the floor. The arm should be at the level of the heart. The right arm is used for consistency in measurements. In addition, initial comparisons should be made between the upper and lower extremities. This is best performed in the supine position.

Nursing counseling and guidance of affected children can be challenging. Education aimed at understanding hypertension and its implications over the life span is essential in promoting patient and family compliance with both nonpharmacologic and pharmacologic therapies. (See Compliance, Chapter 22.)

Home BP and 24-hour ambulatory BP measurement can facilitate surveillance in children with chronic hypertension and can also provide documentation of the effectiveness of therapy. A family member can be instructed in how to take and record accurate BP measurements, which can decrease the number of trips to a health care facility. Parameters should be reviewed and should include instructions on when to contact the practitioner regarding elevated values. When this option is not feasible, the school nurse can often be a valuable resource in monitoring BP.

The nurse plays an important role in assessing individual families and providing targeted information regarding nonpharmacologic modes of intervention, such as reviewing the DASH diet, weight loss, smoking cessation, and exercise programs. If extensive dietary counseling is required, the child should be referred to a registered dietitian with expertise in working with children and adolescents. Exercise regimens should be individualized. Children and young adolescents generally prefer team sports rather than individual training, which they may view as a burden rather than an enjoyable activity. If peers and family members can participate in any of the management strategies, the child is more likely to comply with the plan. In recent years, many health-related exercise applications (apps) have become available for computers, phones, and handheld devices. These apps may be of interest for children/adolescents who prefer to exercise at home and/or use technology. It also gives the child/adolescent some autonomy in deciding what type of activity to do.

If drug therapy is prescribed, the nurse needs to provide information to the family regarding the reasons for drug therapy, how the drug works, frequency of BP monitoring, and possible side effects of the medication (Box 27.13). Explain that the drug needs to be taken consistently to achieve any prolonged control of BP. Stress the need for close follow-up, especially because antihypertensive therapy can sometimes be safely decreased or discontinued if BP remains under control over time.

Learning needs vary greatly depending on developmental levels and individual differences. Some children and families require a great deal of support, education, and guidance, whereas others need only education and periodic follow-up. A positive approach is essential; negative feedback will only alienate the family. Exploring the reasons for difficulty in compliance can often provide realistic alternatives. Continued education, support, and reinforcement for positive behavior are major nursing responsibilities.

DYSLIPIDEMIA (ABNORMAL LIPID METABOLISM)

Hyperlipidemia is a general term for excessive lipids (fat and fatlike substances). *Dyslipidema* refers to all disorders of lipid metabolism resulting in abnormalities in the lipid profile that can include elevated total cholesterol, low-density lipoprotein (LDL) cholesterol or triglycerides, and/or low levels of high-density lipoprotein (HDL) cholesterol. Dyslipidemia plays an important role in producing atherosclerosis (buildup of fatty plaques in the arteries), which eventually can lead to coronary artery disease (CAD), the leading cause of morbidity and mortality in the adult population in the United States. The risk of premature CAD has been shown to increase with elevated plasma concentrations of total cholesterol and LDL cholesterol and with low levels of HDL cholesterol. Elevated non-HDL cholesterol (LDL + very-low-density lipoprotein [VLDL]) is also associated with an increased incidence of atherosclerosis. In adults, interventions that decrease LDL levels and increase HDL levels have been shown to lower the risk for CAD. See Table 27.6 for normal cholesterol values. In addition to abnormal cholesterol levels, known risk factors correlating with the development CAD include the following:

- Positive family history of elevated cholesterol and/or early heart disease
- Cigarette smoking
- Obesity
- Sedentary lifestyle
- Nutritional factors
- Older age
- Male gender
- Hypertension
- Type 1 or type 2 diabetes

In addition to these risk factors, the American Heart Association has categorized patients with certain comorbid conditions as higher risk. These include the following (Kavey, Allada, Daniels, et al., 2006):

- Chronic inflammatory diseases
- Cancer survivors
- Transplant patients
- Congenital heart disease
- Coronary artery aneurysms from KD

Research to date indicates that a presymptomatic phase of atherosclerosis begins in childhood with the development of fatty streaks evident in autopsies of children who died of noncardiac causes (McGill,

BOX 27.13 Antihypertensive Drugs Commonly Used in the Treatment of Pediatric Hypertension, With Blood Pressure Goal and Nursing Interventions

BP Goal for Pharmacologic Prescription

Attain BP below 90th percentile or 130/80 mm Hg, whichever is lower.
Increase every 2 to 4 weeks (can use home BP measurements).
Add second agent if needed (thiazide diuretic often used as second agent).

Choice of Agents

Initial therapy: ACE inhibitor, ARB, long-acting calcium channel block, or thiazide diabetic. Beta-blocker is not recommended for initial therapy (due to side-effect profile).
Note: For children with CKD, proteinuria, or diabetes, first-line therapy should be an ACE inhibitor or ARB unless contraindicated.

Angiotensin-Converting Enzyme Inhibitors

Action: Act primarily by interfering with the production of angiotensin II, a potent vasoconstrictor.

Common ACE Inhibitors Used in Children

Lisinopril, fosinopril, enalapril, captopril
- Monitor blood pressure and pulse.
- Take 1 hour before meals to increase absorption.
- Monitor laboratory values before and after initiation: serum potassium, creatinine, CBC.
- Contraindicated in pregnancy.
- Side effects may include a cough, headache, dizziness (advise to avoid rapid position changes).
- African Americans may require higher doses for efficacy.
- Stay well hydrated.

Angiotensin Receptor Blockers

Actions: Block angiotensin-causing vasodilation.

Common ARBs

Losartan [Cozaar]), valsartan
- Contraindicated in pregnancy.
- Can cause elevated potassium; check serum potassium and creatinine levels.
- Not used in children with decreased creatinine clearance.
- Potential side effects: headache, dizziness.

Calcium Channel Blockers

Actions: Block the movement of calcium, thereby dilating arteries and lowering BP.

Amlodipine (Norvasc)/Nifedipine (Extended Release)

- May increase heart rate.
- Do not crush nifedipine.
- Side effects may include peripheral edema, constipation, flushing, dizziness.

Thiazide Diuretics

Actions: Lower BP by increasing removal of salt and water from the body.

Hydrochlorothiazide, Chlorthalidone

- Monitor electrolytes on a regular basis.
- Use chlorthalidone with caution in patients with chronic renal disease.
- Often used in combination therapy.
- Side effects may include dizziness, hypokalemia.

ACE, Angiotensin-converting enzyme; *ARB,* angiotensin receptor blocker; *BP,* blood pressure; *CBC,* complete blood count; *CKD,* chronic kidney disease.

TABLE 27.6 Lipid Values in Children/Adolescents

Category	Normal mg/dl	Borderline High mg/dl	Elevated g/dl
TC	<170	170-199	≤200
LDL	<110	110-120	≤130
Non-HDL	<120	120-144	≤145
HDL*	>45	N/A	N/A

*Borderline-low HDL 40-45; low HDL <40.
HDL, High-density lipoprotein; *LDL,* low-density lipoprotein; *TC,* total cholesterol.
Data adapted from National Heart, Lung, and Blood Institute. (2011). Expert panel on integrated guidelines for cardiovascular health and risk reduction in children and adolescents: Summary report. *Pediatrics, 128*(Suppl 5), S213-S256.

McMahan, & Gidding, 2008). The extent of atherosclerosis is positively associated with the number of adult risk factors. Higher levels of total cholesterol, LDL cholesterol, and non-HDL cholesterol and low levels of HDL cholesterol are associated with more severe atherosclerosis. Lipid values show trends from childhood to adulthood, particularly in children with the most severely abnormal lipid values (Zachariah & de Ferranti, 2013). These children with elevated lipids are more likely to become adults with elevated lipids. In addition, recent studies support a relationship between the presence of risk factors in young people and subclinical markers of atherosclerosis (Kusters, Wiegman, Kastelein, et al., 2014), supporting the rationale for universal screening and management of lipid levels and cardiovascular risk factors (National Heart, Lung, and Blood Institute, 2011). The benefits of statin therapy are well documented in the adult population in the reduction of CAD. The goal of lipid screening is to identify children and adolescents with familial hyperlipidemia (FH) and/or other types of dyslipidemias early in life so that treatment can begin in those patients at increased risk.

FH is a genetic defect that causes significant elevation of LDL cholesterol and is associated in an increased risk of premature CAD. Homozygous FH is very rare (1 in 1 million) and is known to cause CAD during childhood. This condition is usually diagnosed in the first year or two of life by the appearance of xanthomas on the skin. Treatment options are limited as these patients do not have the LDL receptors necessary to respond to statin therapy. Patients with this rare condition may require more invasive treatments, such as plasmapheresis, to control LDL levels. New medications are being trialed in this population. In contrast to homozygous FH, the incidence of heterozygous FH is much more common (with a reported incidence of 1 in 200 to 500 people). Untreated heterozygous FH results in elevated LDL cholesterol (>160 to 190 mg/dl) and is associated with a significant increase in early coronary disease in young to middle adult years, supporting the recommendation for early screening and interventions aimed at lowering LDL cholesterol (Watts, Gidding, Wierzbicki, et al., 2014).

Lifestyle modification comprises the first line of treatment for the vast majority of patients with dyslipidemia. In addition to lifestyle, patients with heterozygous FH generally require lipid-lowering medications (statin therapy) to attain adequate LDL reduction.

Box 27.14 provides the definitions of cholesterol.

BOX 27.14 What Is Cholesterol?

Cholesterol, a fatlike steroid alcohol, is part of the lipoprotein complex in plasma that is essential for cellular metabolism. Triglycerides, natural fats synthesized from carbohydrates, are used for energy. Both are major lipids transported on lipoproteins, a combination of lipids and proteins, which include the following:

Chylomicrons—Produced in the intestine in response to the intake of dietary fat. These are the principal transporters of dietary fat (triglycerides) from the intestine to the blood and ultimately to the fatty tissue. Chylomicrons are usually not present in the blood after a 12- to 14-hour fast.

Very-low-density lipoproteins (VLDLs)—Contain high concentrations of triglycerides, moderate concentrations of cholesterol, and little protein.

Low-density lipoproteins (LDLs)—Contain low concentrations of triglycerides, high levels of cholesterol, and moderate levels of protein. The end product of VLDL synthesis, LDLs are the major carriers of cholesterol to the cells. Cells use cholesterol for synthesis of membranes and steroid production. Elevated levels of circulating LDL are a strong risk factor for cardiovascular disease.

High-density lipoproteins (HDLs)—Contain very low concentrations of triglycerides, relatively little cholesterol, and high levels of protein. HDLs transport free cholesterol to the liver for secretion in the bile. High levels of HDL are thought to protect against cardiovascular disease, whereas low levels of HDLs are considered an independent risk factor.

The cholesterol profile includes the following:

$$\text{Total cholesterol} = \text{LDL} + \text{HDL} + \text{VLDL}$$

Levels of total cholesterol, triglycerides, and HDL cholesterol are measured directly via a blood test. In the fasting state, LDL concentration is calculated using the following formula:

$$\text{LDL} = \text{Total cholesterol} - [\text{HDL} + (\text{Triglycerides}/5)]$$

A calculated LDL is considered accurate as long as the fasting triglyceride level is below 350 to 400 mg/dl. If triglycerides are higher than this, LDL cholesterol can be measured directly using a more specialized test.

Diagnostic Evaluation/Screening

The diagnosis of dyslipidemia is based on analysis of blood. A blood specimen for determination of a full lipid profile should ideally be drawn after a 12-hour fast. However, a non-HDL cholesterol value (total cholesterol minus HDL cholesterol) can be obtained in the nonfasting state. It is important to note that lipid values can be affected by significant febrile illnesses, and therefore lipids should not be measured within 3 weeks of a febrile illness. Average lipid values vary by age and gender, with HDL values decreasing in males as they go through puberty. Total cholesterol and LDL cholesterol may also decrease during puberty. Children/adolescents are considered to have elevated cholesterol if their total cholesterol value is over 200 mg/dl and/or their LDL cholesterol value is over 130 mg/dl or if their non-HDL cholesterol is over 145 mg/dl. Higher HDL values are desirable. HDL values below 40 mg/dl are considered to be low with an average HDL being approximately 55 mg/dl. Triglycerides should be less than 100 mg/dl in young children (under 10) and less than 130 mg/dl in older children and adolescents. It is common to see elevated triglycerides in the setting of elevated BMI. Triglyceride values respond well to dietary modifications, particularly a low-glycemic diet.

Current national guidelines recommend universal screening of lipid values in childhood, regardless of family history. The recommendations call for lipid screening to be performed at healthy physical examinations twice: between 9 and 11 years of age and again between 17 and 21 years of age (National Heart, Lung, and Blood Institute, 2011). This recommendation is in addition to the previously recommended selective screening, which targets children at an earlier age who are considered to be at high risk based on family history and/or individual risk factors. Historically, ascertaining only family history misses many "at-risk" children, as many families do not know their full genetic history and many parents do not know their own lipid values. Selective screening is recommended earlier for those children over 2 years old who have a first- or second-degree relative with a total cholesterol greater than 240 or known dyslipidemia, or if there is a history of early cardiovascular disease (less than 55 years in a male and less than 65 years in a female). In addition, early screening should be done in children with individual health risk factors such as diabetes. In children with abnormal lipid values, a screening thyroid-stimulating hormone should be obtained to rule out hypothyroidism as a secondary cause of dyslipidemia.

Current guidelines recommend obtaining a total cholesterol and HDL cholesterol as an initial screen so that a non-HDL level (total cholesterol minus HDL cholesterol) can be calculated (National Heart, Lung, and Blood Institute, 2011; Zachariah & de Ferranti, 2013). This method of screening provides the clinician more information than total cholesterol alone and is still practical in that it is accurate in the nonfasting state. If the non-HDL level is elevated, the child is referred for a full fasting lipid profile.

Therapeutic Management

Regardless of the cause of high cholesterol (genetic or lifestyle factors, or a combination), the treatment of high cholesterol levels in pediatrics begins with lifestyle modification. Lifestyle habits, including diet, exercise patterns, and smoking—all known to be risk factors for cardiovascular disease—are normally established at a young age. The American Heart Association, American Academy of Pediatrics, and National Heart, Lung, and Blood Institute recommend a heart-healthy diet for all American children, with dietary counseling recommended for those children with known elevated cholesterol values (National Heart, Lung, and Blood Institute, 2011; Zachariah & de Ferranti, 2013). Dietary management is tailored to the individual patient, depending on his or her specific dyslipidemia. A heart-healthy diet focuses on a balanced intake of nutrients for children over 2 years of age, favoring low-fat dairy products, avoiding trans fats, decreasing saturated fats, and reducing sweetened beverages and simple sugars. The recommended diet for all children and adolescents is one that is rich in fruits and vegetables and whole grains.

For families to understand the recommendations for lifestyle modification, it is important to schedule enough time in the visit to provide accurate dietary information to families, as food labeling can be confusing. Without counseling, patients tend to replace foods high in fat with foods low in fat but high in simple sugars, which can raise triglyceride values, decrease the effectiveness of nutritional interventions, and provide wasted calories (Box 27.15).

Current research favors a "Mediterranean"-type diet. Whole grains, fruits, and vegetables form the foundation of this diet. In addition, this diet favors the use of monounsaturated fats, such as nuts, fish, avocadoes, olive oil, and canola oil, which have beneficial effects on HDL cholesterol values.

For patients with elevated LDL cholesterol, total fat should be limited to 30% of calories. In addition, children with abnormal LDL cholesterol levels are advised to reduce saturated fat intake to 7% to 10% of calories and dietary cholesterol intake to less than 300 mg/day. Dietary recommendations can be confusing, and individualized guidelines should ideally be provided by a certified dietitian with expertise in lipid management for children and adolescents.

BOX 27.15 Recommendations for Dietary/Lifestyle Management of Dyslipidemia for Children/Adolescents Over the Age of 2 Years

For All Children/Adolescents

- Obtain 1 hour of moderate or vigorous physical activity at least 5 days a week.
- Ideally less than 2 hours per day of sedentary screen time.
- Avoid firsthand and secondhand smoke exposure.
- Eat a diverse diet rich in fruits, vegetables, whole grains, lean meats, and fish.
- Refer to a registered dietitian for individual nutritional counseling.

Elevated LDL Cholesterol

- Obtain 25% to 30% of calories from fat.
- Less than 7% of calories from saturated fats (approximately 12 to 15 g/day).
- Avoid trans fats.
- Favor monounsaturated fats.
- Less than 200 mg/day of dietary cholesterol.

Elevated Triglycerides or Non-HDL Cholesterol

- Decrease intake of simple sugars.
- Avoid white bread, white pasta, white potatoes, white rice, sugary cereals, cookies, cakes, and candy.
- Do not drink sugar-sweetened beverages.
- Replace simple sugars with complex carbohydrates.
- Should get only 25% to 30% of calories from fat.
- Should get less than 7% of calories from saturated fats.
- Favor monounsaturated fats (beneficial effects on HDL cholesterol).
- Use olive oil and canola oil, and consume avocados, nuts, and fish.
- Avoid trans fats.
- Increase dietary fish intake for omega-3 fatty acids.

HDL, High-density lipoprotein; *LDL*, low-density lipoprotein.
Adapted from National Heart, Lung, and Blood Institute. (2011). Expert panel on integrated guidelines for cardiovascular health and risk reduction in children and adolescents: Summary report. *Pediatrics, 128*(Suppl 5), S213-S256.

HDL cholesterol responds to an increase in monounsaturated fats such as those mentioned previously. Avoidance of smoking and increased physical exercise also raise HDL values and should be encouraged.

If triglyceride levels are elevated, specific dietary recommendations include a low-glycemic diet, decreasing the intake of foods high in simple carbohydrates such as white flour, white rice, white bread, white pasta, sugary cereals, juice, and soda. Weight management should be addressed if the child has an elevated BMI. In addition to food choice, portion size may also be an issue for these children, and the "plate method" is often recommended (½ fruits and vegetables, ¼ protein, and ¼ complex carbohydrates).

Dietary supplements such as plant stanols reduce LDL and may be beneficial in lowering LDL cholesterol. Data are mixed as to the benefit of fiber supplementation. Many clinicians favor obtaining fiber from natural dietary sources—whole grains, fruits, and vegetables—rather than from supplements.

Population recommendations intended to decrease cardiovascular risk have been in place for several decades, yet the incidence of childhood obesity in the United States has increased significantly during this time period. Education and programs aimed at decreasing this trend and increasing heart-healthy living (e.g., diet and exercise, avoidance of smoking) are extremely important to decrease cardiovascular risk for the next generation. Assessment of BMI, targeted nutritional and lifestyle education, referral to programs geared to achieving weight loss if indicated, and follow-up of abnormal parameters should be an integral part of every well-child visit. Moderate or vigorous exercise of at least 300 minutes per week is recommended for children and adolescents. The use of screen time for computers, video games, TV, and phones has increased sedentary time periods in this population. Ideally, recreational screen time should be limited to less than 2 hours daily, and physical exercise should be encouraged instead. However, technology can also be used in a positive way: there are many applications for devices that provide exercise classes online and are readily available for use at home. In addition, patients can use devices to track lifestyle (diet, exercise, sleep). These options may be appealing to young people and should be incorporated into counseling.

Dietary changes alone can decrease LDL values 10% to 15%; however, it is quite likely that despite lifestyle changes, children with severe genetic hypercholesterolemia such as FH and those with individual risk factors will ultimately meet the recommendations for the use of lipid-lowering medication (McCrindle, Urbina, Dennison, et al., 2007).

The most common medications include the class of drugs know as "statins" or hydroxymethylglutaryl–coenzyme A (HMG-CoA) reductase inhibitors. Some of the more common statins include atorvastatin, simvastatin, rosuvastatin, and pravastatin. In young children, some clinicians may use bile acid–resin binders such as cholestyramine (Questran) and colestipol (Colestid) before beginning statin therapy. Nicotinic acid can help raise HDL cholesterol but is rarely used in pediatrics because of symptoms of flushing and documentation of elevated liver transaminases. Fish oil supplementation may be helpful in situations with very high triglyceride levels.

Pharmacologic Intervention

The recent National Heart, Lung, and Blood Institute guidelines recommend waiting until age 10 years to consider lipid-lowering medication unless the child has severe individual risk factors or homozygous hyperlipidemia, in which case medication may be indicated earlier (National Heart, Lung, and Blood Institute, 2011; Zachariah & de Ferranti, 2013). The current guidelines recommend the initiation of lipid-lowering medications if, after 6 months of lifestyle modification, cholesterol values are still elevated.

- LDL-C over 190 mg/dl in patients without a positive history of early heart disease
- LDL-C over 160 mg/dl with a positive family history of early heart disease or with one high-level risk condition or two moderate-level risk factors
- LDL-C over 130 mg/dl in very high-risk patients

The target level for LDL-C in childhood is aimed at the 95th percentile or less than 130 mg/dl and ideally less than 110 mg/dl, which is the 75th percentile. Clinicians start at the lowest dose of medication initially, increasing as required to obtain goal LDL values. Certain individual risk factors, such as diabetes, hypertension, history of childhood cancer, inflammatory disorders, transplant, or coronary artery aneurysms from KD, lower the threshold for pharmacologic intervention and lower the LDL goal as well.

HMG-CoA reductase inhibitors (statins) continue to be the most effective medication for lipid lowering. The use of statins is approved by the Food and Drug Administration for boys and girls over the age of 10 years, and their use is endorsed in the most severely affected patients. Before initiation of statin therapy, baseline liver function tests (alanine aminotransferase [ALT]) and creatine kinase (CK) levels are generally obtained. Clinical practice varies but ALT, along with a fasting lipid profile, is generally repeated approximately 1 to 2 months after the initiation of therapy and with any dosage changes. Once the patient is taking a stable dosage, laboratory tests are repeated at 6- to 12-month intervals, depending on the individual practice. Some clinicians measure CK in routine follow-up, whereas others only measure this parameter in the setting of clinical complaints of muscle aches. Side effects may include elevation of liver transaminase levels but are generally well tolerated in an otherwise healthy child/adolescent. Potential side effects should be reviewed with patients/families, including rhabdomyolysis. This is a very rare occurrence, particularly in young people, but when it happens, it is serious and can cause renal failure. Patients should be instructed to discontinue the medication and contact their clinician if they experience the new onset of muscle aches or dark brown urine. In addition, female patients need to be educated that statins are considered teratogenic and cannot be taken during pregnancy. Oral contraceptives may be given in conjunction with lipid-lowering medication; however, they may increase lipid values, potentially necessitating modification of the statin dose.

Ezetimibe works by inhibiting cholesterol absorption. It lowers LDL levels by preventing intestinal uptake of dietary and biliary cholesterol. It is generally used in combination therapy with a statin, with the goal of further lowering LDL values. This medication is approved for children older than 10 years of age.

Bile acid–resin binders act by binding bile acids in the intestinal lumen. Because they are not absorbed by the intestine, they do not produce systemic toxicity and are safe for children. Cholestyramine and colestipol are both powders that are mixed with water or juice just before ingestion. Many patients cannot tolerate resin binders because the powder has a gritty texture and does not dissolve completely in liquid. Colestid also comes in a tablet form but the tablet is quite large. Side effects may include constipation, abdominal pain, gastrointestinal bloating, flatulence, and nausea.

Patients who take resin binders should be instructed to take one multivitamin supplement daily because bile acid–binding agents may interfere with the absorption of fat-soluble vitamins. Because they can interfere with absorption of other medications, any other medications should be given at least 1 hour before or 6 hours after the bile acid–binding agent is ingested. The results of a complete blood count, chloride and folate levels, and serum concentrations of vitamins A, D, and E should be evaluated yearly.

Nursing Care Management

Nurses play an important role in the screening, education, and support of children with hyperlipidemia and their families. When a child is referred to a preventive cardiology or lipid clinic, it is essential that the family be adequately prepared for the visit. Generally the parents/child will be asked to keep some type of dietary history before this visit. Families are instructed to keep their child fasting for at least 12 hours before blood tests. Therefore it is important to schedule the blood test early in the morning. At the visit, a complete individual and family health history is taken. The family history should include both biologic parents and all first- and second-degree relatives. Questions are asked about the presence of early heart disease, hypertension, CVAs, sudden death, hyperlipidemia, diabetes, metabolic syndrome, and endocrine abnormalities. Nurses may also uncover risk factors when obtaining a health history for other purposes in their general practice. It is therefore important that nurses be familiar with current screening practices and with the availability of resources for children with concerning family histories.

At the visit, parents and extended families are informed about cholesterol and hyperlipidemia. This education should include a brief introduction to the different lipoprotein categories, including cholesterol, HDL, LDL, and triglycerides. In addition, behavioral risk factors for heart disease, such as smoking and lack of exercise, are reviewed. For management to be effective, parents, as well as the child (particularly older children), should understand the rationale for dietary and pharmacologic intervention in the prevention of future cardiovascular disease.

Nutritional education is an important part of the treatment of any child or teenager with high cholesterol. Ideally, dietary counseling should be provided by a dietitian with expertise in pediatric lipid disorders/management. Dietary compliance may become an issue of control and a source of great stress for many families. Children with high cholesterol levels should not be viewed as having a disease. Rather, the positive aspects of healthy eating, regular exercise, and avoiding smoking are emphasized. Basic dietary changes are encouraged for the whole family so the affected child is not singled out. The focus is positive, with emphasis on making healthy dietary choices, such as substituting chicken and fish for hot dogs and hamburgers. Children can learn to participate in food preparation and decision making. (See Cultural Considerations box.)

CULTURAL CONSIDERATIONS

Cultural Food Differences

Cultural differences must be considered and recommendations individualized. For example, it is more realistic to suggest frying food in a monounsaturated oil such as canola oil than to forbid frying food altogether in families where this is common practice. Substitution rather than elimination needs to be emphasized. Visual aids are often helpful, especially for children (e.g., test tubes depicting the amount of fat in a hot dog, or the number of packets of sugar in a fruit-flavored yogurt or in a soda). Diets should be flexible and individually tailored by a dietitian experienced in combining recommendations that meet both the nutritional demands of the growing child and lipid modifications. Parents are encouraged to participate in dietary and educational sessions, ask questions, and share ideas and experiences.

Parents often feel guilty about the hereditary component of hyperlipidemia. Many of these same parents are frustrated if diet alone is not making a significant enough difference in their child's lipid profile. However, it is important to discuss the fact that a dietary approach alone is often not sufficient, especially for children with FH who have LDL values greater than the 95th percentile.

If pharmacologic therapy is recommended, parents and patients should receive counseling as to the rationale, current knowledge of benefit, dosage, and possible side effects of the drug. Medication schedules should remain flexible and should not interfere with the child's daily activities. Follow-up phone calls by the nurse between visits allow parents to discuss their concerns and ask any questions that may have arisen.

! NURSING ALERT

The recommendations for fat intake for the general population are intended for children over 2 years of age. It is generally thought that children under the age of 2 years require a higher percentage of calories from fat. However, recent studies have supported the safety of low-fat dairy products in younger children. Therefore low-fat dairy products are appropriate for children less than 1 year old who are obese or who have additional cardiovascular risk factors (American Academy of Pediatrics, 2008).

CARDIAC DYSRHYTHMIAS

Dysrhythmias, or abnormal heart rhythms, can occur in children with structurally normal hearts, as features of some congenital heart defects, and in patients after surgical repair of congenital heart defects. They occur in patients with cardiomyopathy and cardiac tumors. They can occur secondary to metabolic and electrolyte imbalances. Childhood dysrhythmias can have a genetic or familial etiology. Dysrhythmias can be classified in several ways, such as by heart rate characteristics (bradycardia and tachycardia) or by the origin of the dysrhythmia in the atria or ventricles. Most are due to abnormalities in impulse generation in the RA or to abnormalities in the conduction pathways.

Some dysrhythmias are well tolerated and self-limiting. Others may cause decreased cardiac output with associated symptoms. Some dysrhythmias can cause sudden death. Treatment depends on the cause of the dysrhythmia and its severity. Underlying causes are treated if possible (as with electrolyte imbalances). Some dysrhythmias (such as bradycardia caused by congenital heart block) are well tolerated and may not require treatment for many years. Others may require medications, radiofrequency ablation, or pacemaker placement. Some can be difficult to treat and require multiple therapies.

Many advances have been made in the diagnosis and treatment of pediatric dysrhythmias. Improvements in technology have allowed better diagnosis, the development of ablation techniques, and the expansion of pacemaker capabilities. New antidysrhythmic medications have proven safe and effective in children. Radiofrequency ablation has offered a cure for some dysrhythmias. Pediatric electrophysiology has become a highly specialized field, and the student is referred to more detailed sources for an in-depth discussion. The following sections describe diagnostic studies and provide a general discussion of the most common tachycardia (supraventricular tachycardia) and the most common bradycardia (complete heart block) that require treatment in the pediatric population.

Diagnostic Evaluation

Before diagnosing an infant or child with an abnormal heart rate, nurses must be familiar with the standards for normal heart rate in the particular age-group. (See inside back cover.) Heart rate patterns considered normal for a particular child can vary tremendously. An initial nursing responsibility is recognition of an abnormal heartbeat, in either rate or rhythm. When a dysrhythmia is suspected, the apical rate is counted for 1 full minute and compared with the radial rate, which may be lower because not all of the apical beats are felt. Consistently high or low heart rates should be regarded as suspicious. Accurate nursing assessment is essential. The patient should be placed on a cardiac monitor with recording capabilities. A 12-lead ECG yields more information than the monitor recording and should be taken as soon as possible. Recent advances in bedside telemetry allow storage of ECG tracings for later analysis.

Several advances in the diagnosis of cardiac dysrhythmias have greatly improved the understanding and treatment of these conditions in children. The basic diagnostic procedure is the ECG, including 24-hour Holter monitoring. However, more definitive procedures include both noninvasive and invasive techniques.

Electrophysiologic cardiac catheterization allows identification of conduction disturbances and immediate investigation of drugs that may control the dysrhythmia. Electrode catheters are introduced intravenously and directed toward the right side of the heart. The heart is then selectively stimulated to induce dysrhythmias. Once a dysrhythmia occurs, different antidysrhythmic drugs are administered intravenously to monitor which pharmacologic agent is most successful in terminating the dysrhythmia.

Another procedure that may be employed is transesophageal recording. An electrode catheter is passed to the lower esophagus and, when in position at a point proximal to the heart, is used to stimulate and record dysrhythmias.

The onset and diagnosis of a cardiac dysrhythmia are frightening experiences for parents and older children. Sometimes the dysrhythmia rapidly leads to HF and a medical crisis. In this situation parents need much support to express their feelings and to understand the diagnosis and its treatment. Often parents and children have an unspoken fear of potential death even if the dysrhythmia is benign, and repeated explanations are needed to relieve anxiety.

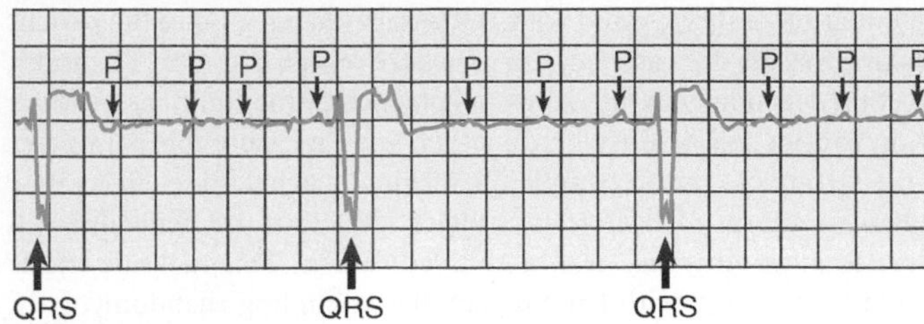

FIG. 27.21 Complete heart block. Note slow rhythm and several P waves not followed by a QRS complex.

Bradydysrhythmias

Sinus bradycardia in children can be due to the influence of the autonomic nervous system, as with hypervagal tone, or can be in response to hypoxia and hypotension. Once the infant receives adequate oxygenation and any acidosis is eliminated, the heart rate often returns to baseline. Sinus bradycardias are also known to develop after atrial repairs involving atrial suture lines such as in the Fontan procedure.

Complete AV block is also referred to as *complete heart block* (Fig. 27.21). This can be either congenital (occurring in children with structurally normal hearts) or acquired after surgery to repair cardiac defects. AV blocks are most often related to edema around the conduction system and resolve without treatment. Temporary epicardial wires are placed in most patients at surgery; if a rhythm disturbance occurs, temporary pacing can be employed. Just before discharge the health practitioner removes the wires by pulling slowly and deliberately down on them from the site of insertion.

A permanent pacemaker may be needed in some children, such as those with postsurgical AV block or, less frequently, congenital AV block. The pacemaker takes over or assists in the heart's conduction function. The surgical implantation of a pacemaker is usually a low-risk procedure. Once the wire has been introduced, a small incision is made and a pocket is formed under the muscle to house and protect the generator. The generator is placed under the abdominal muscle in infants and young children and in the upper chest below the clavicle in older children and adolescents. Depending on patient size and cardiac anatomy, some pacemakers can be placed transvenously in the catheterization laboratory, rather than in the operating room. Continuous ECG monitoring is necessary during the recovery phase to assess pacemaker function. The nurse should be aware of the programmed rate and expected individual generator variations. A baseline ECG and chest x-ray film are obtained for future comparison. The pacemaker pocket site is monitored for signs of infection. Analgesics are given for pain.

Pacemaker functions have become dramatically more sophisticated; pacemakers can control heart rate according to activity, cardiac output, and respirations. In addition, some models can be programmed for overdrive pacing or cardioversion when the generator detects accelerated rates beyond established normal values.

When a pacemaker is implanted, the education of the parents and child includes an explanation of the device, a description of the component parts, an explanation of the surgical procedure, and discharge teaching. The pacemaker is made up of two basic parts: the pulse generator and the lead. The pulse generator is composed of the battery and the electronic circuitry. The function is to produce the electrical impulse sent to the heart and to receive and respond to signals produced by the heart. The lead is an insulated, flexible wire that conducts the electrical impulse from the pulse generator to the heart. Two types of leads are available: transvenous and epicardial. The child's size and the heart's structure determine which lead is more appropriate. Transvenous leads are inserted into a large vein, often the subclavian, and advanced into the right side of the heart. Placement is secured by engaging a small corkscrew or fishhook attachment at the end of the lead into the endocardium. Epicardial leads are attached directly to the epicardial layer of the heart. Parents should be aware of which type of lead is in place in their child.

Discharge teaching includes information about the signs and symptoms of infection, general wound care, and activity restrictions. Parents, and patients if they are old enough, should learn to take the pulse and should know the settings of the pacemaker. If the patient's low rate is set at 80 beats/min and the heart rate is only 68 beats/min, there is a possible problem with the pacemaker that needs to be investigated. Instructions for telephone transmission of ECG readings are also given. Telephone connections can be used to transmit ECG data and also to monitor battery life and pacemaker function. The pacemaker generator has to be replaced periodically because of battery depletion. Children with pacemakers should wear a medical alert device, and their parents should have a paper identification card with specific pacemaker data in case of an emergency. Cardiopulmonary resuscitation instruction is suggested for parents.

Tachydysrhythmias

Sinus tachycardia (abnormally fast heart rate) secondary to fever, anxiety, pain, anemia, dehydration, or any other etiologic factor requiring increased cardiac output should be ruled out first before diagnosing it as pathologic. Supraventricular tachycardia (SVT), the most common tachydysrhythmia found in children, refers to a rapid regular heart rate of 200 to 300 beats/min (Fig. 27.22). The two most common forms of SVT are atrioventricular reentrant tachycardia (AVRT), including the Wolff-Parkinson-White (WPW) syndrome, and atrioventricular nodal reentrant tachycardia (AVNRT). The more common form, AVRT, occurs in about 73% of the population (Ko, Deal, Strasburger, et al., 1992). The rapid rhythm originates above the ventricle and is most commonly caused by a reentry mechanism that involves an accessory pathway or the AV conduction system. The onset and termination of SVT are abrupt. The QRS complex is usually narrow (in contrast with ventricular tachycardia, in which the QRS complexes are typically wide), and the P waves are often absent. Infants and young children with SVT may be unable to compensate for the rapid heart rate, and the clinical course can progress to HF. Important signs in the infant and young child are poor feeding, extreme irritability, and pallor. Older children may experience palpitations, dizziness, chest pain, diaphoresis, and syncope.

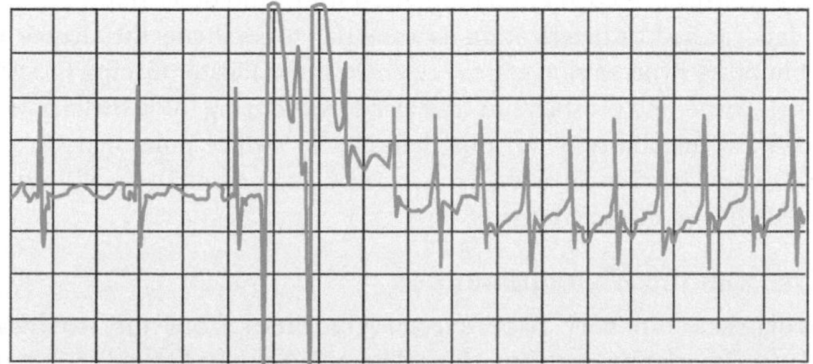

FIG. 27.22 Supraventricular tachycardia (SVT). Note normal sinus rhythm (three PQRST complexes) on the left and abrupt onset of a very fast rhythm (SVT) on the right.

The treatment of SVT depends on the degree of compromise imposed by the dysrhythmia. In some instances, vagal maneuvers, such as applying ice to the face, massaging the carotid artery (on one side of the neck only), or having an older child perform a Valsalva maneuver (e.g., exhaling against a closed glottis, blowing on the thumb as if it were a trumpet for 30 to 60 seconds), can reverse the SVT. When vagal maneuvers fail, adenosine may be used to end the episode of SVT by impairing AV node conduction. IV adenosine is the first-line pharmacologic measure for termination of SVT in infants and children in the emergency setting. Adenosine must be given by rapid IV push with a saline bolus immediately after the drug. Incrementally increasing doses given about 2 minutes apart may be needed. The desired effect usually occurs in 10 to 20 seconds. Synchronized shock with a defibrillator is also used for cardioversion for patients that are hemodynamically unstable with a tachyarrythmia such as SVT with a palpable pulse, or electively in patients with hemodynamically stable SVT, under the direction of a pediatric cardiologist (American Heart Association, 2016).

Traditional first-line medical management of chronic SVT is a beta blocker or digoxin. Digoxin should not be used in patients with WPW syndrome because it can accelerate conduction across the accessory pathway in this particular group of patients. Choice of beta blockers is based on age, using propranolol, a shorter-acting agent for infants, and atenolol, a longer-acting beta blocker for older children. More aggressive pharmacologic treatment with amiodarone or flecainide may be needed for those with more severe symptoms or recurrence of SVT.

If cardiac output is significantly compromised or signs of HF exist, esophageal overdrive pacing or synchronized cardioversion can be employed in the intensive care setting. Transesophageal atrial overdrive pacing is accomplished through placement of a protected lead into the esophagus, behind the LA of the heart. The lead is then attached to a stimulator capable of pacing at very rapid rates to interrupt the tachydysrhythmia. Synchronized cardioversion is the timed delivery of a preset amount of energy through the chest wall in an attempt to reestablish an organized rhythm. Sedation is needed for both procedures. Cardioversion should never be performed on a conscious patient.

Radiofrequency ablation has become first-line therapy for some types of SVT. The procedure is done in the cardiac electrophysiology catheterization laboratory and begins with mapping of the conduction system to identify the dysrhythmia focus. A catheter delivering radiofrequency current is directed at the site, and the identified area is heated to destroy the tissue in the area. Success rates vary but can be as high as 90% (Dubin, 2016). A successful ablation is curative, and antidysrhythmic medications can be discontinued.

Another procedure, cryoablation, is also used in treatment of SVT, particularly the AVNRT form. Liquid nitrous oxide is used to cool a catheter to subfreezing temperatures, which then destroys the tissue of target by freezing. This procedure also takes place in the cardiac electrophysiology catheterization laboratory.

Preparation is similar to that for cardiac catheterization and other electrophysiologic studies. The risks and benefits of ablation need to be reviewed. These are lengthy procedures, often 6 to 8 hours, and sedation or general anesthesia is required. Postprocedure care is similar to that for cardiac catheterization, with the addition of careful dysrhythmia monitoring. Patients and their families often have great hope for a cure and are disappointed if the ablation is unsuccessful.

A primary focus of nursing care is education of the family regarding the symptoms of SVT and the treatment. SVT may occur again despite therapy. After the first episode of SVT, parents should learn to take a radial pulse for 1 full minute. If medication is prescribed, instructions regarding accurate dosage and the importance of administering the correct dose at specified intervals are stressed (see Critical Thinking Case Study box).

CRITICAL THINKING CASE STUDY

Infant With a Tachydysrhythmia

You are working in the emergency department when a father comes through the doors, carrying his 1-month-old crying infant. The infant is awake and very irritable. Father reports that the infant has not been feeding well for the past 6 hours, and he has noticed sweating (diaphoresis) with attempted feedings. No history of fever is noted. Further assessment reveals a diaphoretic infant, crying, with a respiratory rate of 60, blood pressure 60/40 mm Hg, and a heart rate that is too fast to count by auscultation. When the infant is attached to the cardiorespiratory monitor, the heart rate is 220 beats/min, nonvariable, with an oxygen saturation of 97%. Capillary refill time is slightly prolonged at 3 seconds, and femoral pulses are palpable but weak.

1. What evidence should you consider regarding this condition?
2. What additional information is required at this time?
3. List the nursing intervention(s) that have the highest priority.
4. Identify important patient-centered outcomes with reference to your nursing interventions.

Answers are available at http://evolve.elsevier.com/wong/ncic.

PULMONARY HYPERTENSION

Pulmonary hypertension (PH) is a pulmonary vascular disease associated with diverse cardiac, lung, and systemic diseases, as well as familial and idiopathic etiologies. The pulmonary arteries are described as having vascular narrowing due to decreased vascular growth and surface area and intraluminal obstruction, and they undergo structural remodeling of the vessel wall (Abman & Ivy, 2011). It is defined by a mean pulmonary arterial pressure (mPAP) ≥25 mm Hg in children over 3 months of age and is categorized based on the World Health Organization classification system (Table 27.7). In the pediatric population, there are three causes of PH: (1) increased pulmonary venous pressures (e.g., mitral stenosis, LV noncompliance); (2) posttricuspid cardiac shunts (e.g., large ventricular septal defect, large PDA); and (3) small PAs, that is, too few or too narrow (e.g., idiopathic pulmonary arterial hypertension, persistent pulmonary hypertension of the newborn, connective tissue disorders, hypoxia, drugs, toxins). There is no cure for PH and there is significant morbidity and mortality. Advancements in therapeutic management in the last 10 to 15 years, however, are helping to slow the progression of the disease and improve quality of life.

TABLE 27.7 World Health Organization Classification of Pulmonary Hypertension (Nice)

1. Pulmonary arterial hypertension (PAH)
   1. Idiopathic pulmonary arterial hypertension (IPAH)
   2. Heritable
   3. Drug and toxin induced
   4. Associated pulmonary arterial hypertension (APAH; pulmonary arterial hypertension associated with other disease, e.g., connective tissue disorder, human immunodeficiency virus, portal hypertension, congenital heart disease, schistosomiasis)

1′. Pulmonary veno-occlusive disease (PVOD)

1″. Persistent pulmonary hypertension of the newborn (PPHN)

2. Pulmonary hypertension (PH) due to left-sided heart disease (e.g., left ventricular dysfunction, mitral valve disease)
3. PH due to lung disease or hypoxemia (e.g., chronic obstructive pulmonary disease)
4. Chronic thromboembolic disease
5. Unclear multifactorial mechanisms

Adapated from Simonneau, G., Gatzoulis, M. A., Adatia, I., et al. (2013). Updated clinical classification of pulmonary hypertension. *Journal of the American College of Cardiology, 62*(25 Suppl), D34–D41.

Pathophysiology

No one knows what causes the pathologic changes for PH, but the pathophysiology is likely multifactorial. Proliferative vasculopathy of the small pulmonary arterioles characterized by hypertrophy and hyperplasia of the intima, as well as smooth muscle contraction, contribute to increasing pulmonary vascular resistance. High pulmonary vascular resistance causes progressive right-sided heart failure, low cardiac output, and high mortality rates.

Although seen less often today due to early surgical intervention, congenital heart defects with a large left-to-right shunt (such as a ventricular septal defect, PDA, or complete AV canal), which cause increased pulmonary blood flow, may result in pulmonary hypertension. If these defects are not repaired early, the high pulmonary flow will cause changes in the pulmonary artery vessels and the vessels will lose their elasticity. This causes increased resistance in the pulmonary bed and results in eventual right-sided heart failure because the heart cannot pump against the greater resistance. The flow of blood becomes right to left, and cyanosis is seen. This is known as Eisenmenger syndrome. Because of surgical repair of these defects early in life, this occurs infrequently now.

Clinical Manifestations

The clinical manifestations include dyspnea with exercise, chest pain, and syncope. Dyspnea is the most common symptom and is caused by impaired oxygen delivery. Chest pain is the result of coronary ischemia in the RV from severe hypertrophy. Syncope reflects a limited cardiac output, leading to decreased cerebral blood flow. Right-sided heart dysfunction is steadily progressive as the pulmonary vessels become obstructed and the pulmonary artery pressure increases. The RV hypertrophies to attempt to maintain a normal cardiac output. With time and continued increases in pulmonary vascular resistance, the cardiac output decreases. When signs of right-sided heart failure with systemic venous congestion and edema are evident, the prognosis is poor.

Diagnostic Evaluation

Initial evaluation consists of physical examination, chest radiography, ECG, echocardiography, and cardiac catheterization (Abman, Hansmann, Archer, et al., 2015). An extensive workup is needed to better characterize the causes, associated factors, hemodynamics, and disease severity. It includes evaluation of cardiac and pulmonary function, coagulation tests, collagen vascular evaluation, sleep study, and other studies. Right-sided cardiac catheterization is essential to evaluate the degree of pulmonary hypertension and the response to vasodilator therapy. Oxygen, nitric oxide, and prostacyclin may all be used during the catheterization to assess the ability of various therapies to reduce pulmonary artery pressure. Exercise capacity, as assessed by the 6-minute walk test, is predictive of disease severity.

Therapeutic Management

Pediatric pulmonary hypertension guidelines from the American Heart Association and American Thoracic Society outline treatment recommendations for conditions specific to the pediatric population, including persistent pulmonary hypertension of the newborn, congenital diaphragmatic hernia, bronchopulmonary dysplasia, and CHD (Abman,

TABLE 27.8 Pharmacological Therapy for Pediatric Pulmonary Hypertension

Drug Class	Agent	Dose Form	Adverse Effects	Comments
Calcium channel blocker	Nifedipine, diltiazem	Oral	Bradycardia, decreased cardiac output, peripheral edema, rash, gum hyperplasia, constipation	Only effective for PH if patient is responsive to vasodilator testing in the catheterization laboratory. Requires high (maximal) dosing to achieve desired vasodilation.
PDE5 inhibitor	Sildenafil, tadalafil	Oral	Flushing, hypotension, headache, priapism	
Endothelin receptor antagonists	Bosentan, ambrisentan	Oral	Hepatotoxic, peripheral edema, teratogenic	Requires monthly LFTs; birth control is important for adolescents and young women.
Prostacylin	Epoprostenol (Flolan), treprostinil (Remodulin)	IV/SC	Headache, flushing, hypotension, site pain (subcutaneous form), cellulitis, central line complications, jaw pain, nausea/diarrhea	Flolan has an extremely short half-life (2-5 minutes) and PH crisis occurs rapidly if infusion is stopped. Dosing is complex and there is a high risk of error.
Prostacylin	Treprostinil (Remodulin)	Oral	Headache, flushing, pain in extremeties, jaw pain, nausea/diarrhea (gastrointestinal side effects can be greater than other dose forms)	Transition from IV/SC form occurs over days in the hospital. Timing of dosing is critical; if 2 doses are missed, need IV/SC form. Cannot be crushed, chewed, or compounded.
Prostacylin	Treprostinil (Remodulin)	Inhaled	Headache, flushing, pain in extremeties, jaw pain, nausea/diarrhea	Must be inhaled one to nine times every 6 hours. Can worsen reactive airway symptoms.

IV/SC, Intravenous/subcutaneous; *LFTs,* liver function tests; *PH,* pulmonary hypertension.
Adapted from Abman, S. H., Hansmann, G., Archer, S. L., et al. (2015). Pediatric pulmonary hypertension: Guidelines from the American Heart Association and American Thoracic Society. *Circulation, 132*(21), 2037–2099.

Hansmann, Archer, et al., 2015). The discussion here focuses on pharmacotherapy, supportive therapy, and, briefly, invasive interventions.

There are three classes of drugs that are used extensively in the treatment of pediatric PH: PDE5 inhibitors (sildenafil, tadalafil), endothelin receptor antagonists (bosentan, ambrisentan), and prostanoids or PGI_2 analogs (epoprostenol, treprostinil). Vasoconstriction is a primary component of PH and these drugs work on different aspects to promote vasodilation and smooth muscle relaxation. For patients who are responsive to inhaled nitric oxide (iNO) or vasodilator drug testing during cardiac catheterization, oral calcium channel blockers (nifedipine and diltiazem) have been successful and are the treatment of choice. Table 27.8 reviews the common pulmonary hypertension drugs, dose form availability, and adverse side effects, and comments on important aspects in the administration of these medications. Choice of treatment is determined by the severity of the disease, and all of these medications carry adverse effects.

In general, situations that may exacerbate the disease and cause hypoxia are avoided. Exercise prescriptions are specific to each patient. Patients should avoid high altitudes because of the relative hypoxia, and some patients have moved to sea level to slow the progress of the disease. Supplemental oxygen is commonly used to relieve hypoxia, especially at night while sleeping. Patients with pulmonary artherial hypertension (PAH) are at risk for thromboembolic events. Anticoagulation therapy has been shown to increase survival in adults. Many patients are treated with warfarin to prevent pulmonary embolism, which can be fatal. Digoxin and diuretics are often used to treat right-sided heart failure.

Some patients fail to respond to medical management and disease progression leads to severe RV dysfunction. In these cases, there are two potential options available. Creation of an atrial septostomy or communication between the two atria can be done in the catheterization laboratory. This often increases cardiac output and thus results in some improvement in function and quality of life. Lung transplantation may be another treatment option for children, primarily those with severe disease. Patients with PAH and Eisenmenger syndrome have had a higher early mortality rate after lung transplantation than other lung transplant patients.

Nursing Care Management

The diagnosis of PH is devastating for the child and family. There is no known cure, and the treatments require significant lifestyle changes and commitment on the part of patient and family to make them successful. Anxiety, depression, and fear of the future are common. Patients and families require extensive education about the disease and its management. They need emotional support to cope with a poor prognosis and make decisions about treatment options.

The medical treatment is complex and involves different medications and therapies. Families are often referred to a specialized center that has experience in the management of PH. This may involve travel far from home with associated emotional and financial hardships. The patient and family must cope with the symptoms of the disease and the side effects of the treatment. Dealing with a continuous IV infusion or continuous oxygen administration requires a major adjustment in lifestyle to accommodate the therapy. The prostacyclin infusion cannot be interrupted at any time because symptoms can worsen and cause acute pulmonary hypertensive crisis, which can be fatal. Backup systems must be in place at all times. The patient and family must make a commitment to adhere to a complex regimen of preparing the infusion, maintaining the equipment, and maintaining sterility of the central line. Treatments are expensive, so insurance coverage and financial issues are critical. Nurses have an important role in educating and preparing families to perform these complex therapies. Discharge planning involves many team members and outside agencies. The nurse has a pivotal role in coordinating the child's care in the hospital and the transition to home.

CARDIOMYOPATHY

Cardiomyopathy refers to abnormalities of the myocardium in which the cardiac muscles' ability to contract or relax is impaired. Cardiomyopathies are relatively rare in children. Possible causes include familial or genetic factors, infection, deficiency states, metabolic abnormalities, and collagen vascular diseases. Most cardiomyopathies in children are considered primary or idiopathic disorders, in which the cause is unknown and the cardiac dysfunction is not associated with systemic disease. Abnormalities of the cardiac myocyte and essential cellular functions underlie the clinical manifestations of organ dysfunction. Some of the known causes of secondary cardiomyopathy are toxicity from anthracyclines (e.g., the antineoplastic agents doxorubicin [Adriamycin]), hemochromatosis (from excessive iron storage), Duchenne muscular dystrophy, KD, collagen diseases, and thyroid dysfunction.

Cardiomyopathies can be divided into three broad clinical categories according to the type of abnormal structure and dysfunction present: dilated cardiomyopathy, hypertrophic cardiomyopathy, and restrictive cardiomyopathy. Dilated cardiomyopathy is characterized by ventricular dilation and greatly decreased contractility, which result in symptoms of HF. This is the most common type of cardiomyopathy in children. Its cause is often unknown, although carnitine deficiency, metabolic diseases, drug toxicities, dysrhythmias, and infection causing myocarditis should be considered. The clinical findings are of HF with tachycardia, dyspnea, hepatosplenomegaly, fatigue, and poor growth. Dysrhythmias may be present and may be more difficult to control with worsening HF. Chest radiography demonstrates cardiomegaly and congested lung fields. The echocardiogram demonstrates poor ventricular contractility, dilated LV, and reduced shortening and ejection fraction. Cardiac catheterization with endomyocardial biopsy is usually performed for diagnosis and identification of a possible infectious cause.

Hypertrophic cardiomyopathy is characterized by an increase in heart muscle mass without an increase in cavity size. It usually occurs in the LV and is associated with abnormal diastolic filling. Mutations of several genes that encode proteins of the cardiac sarcomere have been identified. The expression of clinical disease varies greatly among patients. Infants of diabetic mothers may have a hypertrophic cardiomyopathy that resolves with time. Clinical symptoms usually appear in the school-age period or adolescence and may include anginal chest pain, dysrhythmias, and syncope. Sudden death is possible. One study confirmed that unexplained syncope in the childhood age-group (<18 years of age) with known hypertrophic cardiomyopathy had a 60% cumulative risk of sudden death within 5 years of the syncopal event (Spirito, Autore, Rapezzi, et al., 2009). Presentation in infancy includes signs of HF and carries a poor prognosis. Chest radiography shows a mildly enlarged heart. The ECG demonstrates LV hypertrophy, often with ST-T changes. The echocardiogram is most helpful and demonstrates asymmetric septal hypertrophy and an increase in LV wall thickness, with a small LV cavity.

Restrictive cardiomyopathy, rare in children, involves a restriction to ventricular filling caused by endocardial or myocardial disease or both. RA or LA enlargement or both, apparent on the ECG, are often seen. The chest radiograph shows an enlarged heart. The echocardiogram reveals atrial dilation. Systolic function, the ability of the heart to squeeze, is often normal or mildly impaired, whereas diastolic function, the ability of the heart to relax, is very abnormal. Patients are at risk for embolic events and the development of pulmonary hypertension. Symptoms are dizziness, exercise intolerance, and dry cough and can progress to those of HF (see p. 1012).

Therapeutic Management

Treatment is directed at correcting the underlying cause whenever feasible. In most affected children, however, this is not possible, and treatment is aimed at managing HF (see p. 970) and dysrhythmias. Administration of digoxin and diuretics and aggressive use of afterload-reduction agents have been found to be helpful in managing symptoms in those with dilated cardiomyopathy. Carvedilol (Coreg), a beta blocker, is the newest medication to be added to the treatment of some children with chronic HF. The α- and β-adrenergic receptors are blocked, causing decreased heart rate, decreased BP, and vasodilation. In addition, beta blockers have antiarrhythmic effects, coronary artery vasodilatory effects, and negative chronotropic effects (Moffett & Chang, 2006). Carvedilol is used in compensated HF, not in the acute diagnostic or decompensated HF phase (Rossano & Shaddy, 2014). Practice guidelines for the management of HF in children have been outlined and provide an in-depth review of available therapies (Rosenthal, Chrisant, Edens, et al., 2004). Digoxin and inotropic agents are usually not helpful in the other forms of cardiomyopathy because increasing the force of contraction may exacerbate the muscular obstruction and actually impair ventricular ejection. Beta blockers such as propranolol or calcium channel blockers such as verapamil have been used to reduce LV outflow obstruction and improve diastolic filling in those with hypertrophic cardiomyopathy.

Careful monitoring and effective treatment of dysrhythmias are essential. The placement of an implantable defibrillator should be considered for patients at high risk of sudden death due to ventricular arrhythmias. Anticoagulants may be given to reduce the risk of thromboembolism, a complication of the sluggish circulation through the heart.

ADVANCED HEART FAILURE

HF is a syndrome that results from ventricular dysfunction, volume overload, or pressure overload and is a complex disorder that can result from structural or functional abnormalities. In children, it leads to characteristic signs and symptoms such as poor growth, feeding difficulties, respiratory distress, exercise intolerance, and fatigue. For the pediatric population, a four-tiered standard classification system, the Ross Heart Failure Classification System, stratifies the levels of HF based on these signs and symptoms from Level I (no limitations or symptoms) to the most advanced HF, Level IV (symptomatic at rest with tachypnea, retractions, grunting, or diaphoresis) (Francis, Greenberg, Hsu, et al., 2010; Ross, 2012). Interventions and therapies are advanced if patients progress to higher levels of HF.

Cardiac resynchronization therapy (CRT) using biventricular pacing is an effective treatment in adult patients with HF and is beginning to be applied in the pediatric population. With pharmacologic therapies discussed earlier, CRT has the potential to improve cardiac function in this group of patients. The causes for HF in the young are more varied and often include patients with a single ventricle, making CRT more challenging. Initial studies of CRT in this population demonstrate improved outcomes in those with adequate follow-up (Cecchin, Frangini, Brown, et al., 2009; Dubin, Janousek, Rhee, et al., 2005).

For worsening HF and signs of poor perfusion, severely ill children may benefit from mechanical ventilation, oxygen administration, IV inotropic support, and IV administration of afterload-reduction agents such as milrinone. Mechanical support devices such as extracorporeal membrane oxygenation or ventricular assist devices may be used in patients with progressive decline in cardiac status. Extracorporeal membrane oxygenation is employed primarily for infants and younger patients. Its use is limited to several weeks or less because of complications such as bleeding and infection. Ventricular assist devices, currently standard for older children and adolescents and becoming more readily available for infants and younger children, can be used for longer periods (Cassidy, Dominguez, Haynes, et al., 2013). Risks include infection and embolic complications. Both devices can be used as a bridge to heart transplantation to allow more time to wait for a donor organ. Heart transplantation may be a treatment option for patients who have worsening symptoms despite maximum medical therapy (see below).

Nursing Care Management

Because of the poor prognosis for many children with cardiomyopathy, nursing care is consistent with that for any child with a life-threatening disorder (see Chapter 19). One of the most difficult adjustments for the child may be the realization of failing health and the need for restricted activity, especially if the child is a normally active youngster. Include the child in decisions regarding activity and allow him or her to discuss feelings, particularly if the disease follows a progressive and fatal course. Once symptoms of HF or dysrhythmias develop, implement the same nursing care as discussed on p. 970. If cardiac transplantation is being considered, the child and family have great needs in terms of psychologic preparation and postoperative care. The nurse plays an important role in assessing the family's understanding of the procedure and long-term consequences. Children of school age and older should be fully informed to give their consent to the procedure (see Informed Consent, Chapter 22).

HEART TRANSPLANTATION

Heart transplantation has become a treatment option for infants and children with worsening HF and a limited life expectancy despite maximum medical and surgical management. Indications for cardiac transplantation in children are cardiomyopathy and end-stage CHD. It is also an option for patients with some forms of complex congenital cardiac defects, such as hypoplastic left heart syndrome, for which conventional surgical approaches have a high mortality risk or they have experienced severe complications such as valve regurgitation, ventricular dysfunction, or dysrhythmias.

The heart transplant procedure may be orthotopic or heterotopic. **Orthotopic** heart transplantation refers to removal of the recipient's own heart and implantation of a new heart from a donor who has experienced brain death but whose heart is healthy. The donor and recipient are matched by weight. In **heterotopic** heart transplantation, the recipient's own heart is left in place and a new heart is implanted to act as an additional pump or "piggyback" heart; this type of transplantation is rarely done in children.

Before transplantation, potential recipients undergo a careful cardiac evaluation to determine whether any other medical or surgical options could improve the patient's cardiac status. Other organ systems are assessed to identify problems that might preclude or increase the risk of transplantation. A psychosocial evaluation of the patient and family is done to assess family function, support systems, and ability to comply with the complex medical regimen after the transplant. Support services to help the family successfully care for their child are provided when possible. Parents and older adolescents need extensive education about the risks and benefits of transplantation so they can make an informed decision.

Patients are listed on a national computer network organized by the United Network for Organ Sharing (2001) to match donors and recipients. (See Organ or Tissue Donation and Autopsy, Chapter 19.) The Pediatric Heart Transplant Study (PHTS) was founded in 1991 as a not-for-profit organization dedicated to the advancement of the science and treatment of children during listing for and after heart transplantation. A report from the PHTS reviewed the last decade of pediatric patients listed for heart transplant and summarized the changes, trends, and outcomes of the decade from January 2000 to December 2009. As of December 31, 2009, there were 35 institutions with 4319 pediatric patients listed and 3100 transplanted patients in the database (Dipchand, Kirk, Mahle, et al., 2013). Current survival rates for pediatric heart transplant patients are 86%, 77.9%, 70.3%, and 63% at 1, 3, 5, and 10 years, respectively (United States Department of Health and Human Services, 2016).

Wait list mortality rate remains high, particularly in the smallest children. Progress in suitable ventricular assist devices for use in children as a bridge to transplantation has made outcomes to survival for cardiac transplantation more successful (Blume, Naftel, Bastardi, et al., 2006). A multicenter study using the US Scientific Registry of Transplant Recipients was conducted (Almond, Thiagarajian, Piercy, et al., 2009). Among 3098 children listed for a heart transplant between 1999 and 2006, the median age was 2 years. Sixty percent of patients were listed as top status (30% ventilated and 18% on supportive measures), and of those children, 17% died, 63% received transplants, 8% recovered, and 12% remained listed. These numbers indicate that waiting time in the United States remains high, and high-risk groups in these categories could benefit from emerging cardiac assist devices, such as extracorporeal membrane oxygenation and ventricular assist devices. One retrospective study reported that biventricular support offered an additional means to reverse extremely elevated pulmonary vascular resistance and explored options for a total implantable system for patients not eligible for heart transplantation (Brancaccio, Filippelli, Michielon, et al., 2012). In addition, ABO-incompatible heart transplants are being performed successfully in the younger population (Henderson, Canter, Mahle, et al., 2012).

The posttransplantation course is complex. Overall causes of death within the PHTS data set include rejection (8%), infection (12%), early graft failure (10%), sudden cardiac death (9%), and myocardial infarction (8%), as well as smaller numbers of multisystem causes. Although heart function is greatly improved or normal after transplantation, the risk of rejection is serious. The leading cause of death in the first 3 years after heart transplantation is rejection, with the greatest risk in the first 6 months. Rejection of the heart is diagnosed primarily by endomyocardial biopsy in children. Serial echocardiograms are often used in infants to reduce the need for invasive biopsies. Immunosuppressants must be taken for life and have many systemic side effects. Induction followed by double-drug therapy for immunosuppression with a calcineurin inhibitor (tacrolimus) and mycophenolate mofetil is most commonly used in pediatric patients. Steroids are used with induction at the time of transplant and are commonly discontinued with induction or weaned off over several months unless the patient is highly sensitized at the time of transplant.

Potential long-term problems that may limit survival include coronary artery disease, often termed *chronic rejection;* renal dysfunction; lymphoma; and infection. In the short term, after successful transplantation, children are able to return to full participation in age-appropriate activities and appear to adapt well to their new lifestyle. Transplantation is not a cure because patients must live with the lifetime consequences of chronic immunosuppression. It is to be expected that pediatric patients will require a second heart transplant in their lifetime.

Nursing Care Management

Nursing care after transplantation is complex, demanding careful attention to both the physical needs of the child and the emotional needs of the child and family. Successfully caring for a child after heart transplantation requires the expertise and dedication of many members of the health care team. Nurses play vital roles in assessment, coordination of care, psychosocial support, and patient and family education. The nurse must monitor the heart transplant recipient carefully for signs of rejection, infection, and the side effects of the immunosuppressant medications. Optimizing long-term health includes managing cholesterol levels, participating in routine exercise, refraining from smoking, aggressively controlling BP, and optimizing bone health. The nurse also needs to assess the patient's and family's psychosocial well-being to identify issues such as increased family stress, depression, substance abuse, and school problems. Noncompliance with an intense medication regimen, especially during adolescence, can lead to serious medical problems and can be fatal. Some patients and families need psychiatric support, and many patients need supportive services for learning problems. Chapter 24 discusses immunosuppressants and their nursing implications in relation to renal transplantation. Chapter 29 reviews care of the immunosuppressed child. Chapter 19 presents psychosocial concerns and appropriate interventions for the child with a life-threatening disorder.

The first 6 months to 1 year after transplantation are most intense because the risk of complications is greatest and the patient and family are adjusting to a new lifestyle. Parents of heart transplant recipients also have a high incidence of posttraumatic stress symptoms, and the transplant team should routinely assess the parent's or caretaker's psychologic functioning (Farley, DeMaso, D'Angelo, et al., 2007). The health care team monitors patients closely, with frequent visits and laboratory tests. Care is usually shared between local health care providers and the transplant center. Many patients are able to return to school and other age-appropriate activities within 2 to 3 months after the transplant.

NCLEX REVIEW QUESTIONS

1. You are working with a new graduate on the pediatric unit and your patient is returning from the cardiac catheterization laboratory. You feel the graduate understands the important nursing interventions when she says which of the following? Select all that apply.
   A. "Check pulses, especially below the catheterization site, for equality and symmetry."
   B. "Check vital signs, which may be taken as frequently as every 30 to 45 minutes, with special emphasis on the heart rate, which is counted for 1 full minute for evidence of dysrhythmias or bradycardia."
   C. "Special attention needs to be given to the BP, especially for hypertension, which may indicate hemorrhage or bleeding from the catheterization site."
   D. "Check the dressing for evidence of bleeding or hematoma formation in the femoral or antecubital area."
   E. "Allow the child to ambulate because this will prevent skin breakdown from lying so long in one place."
2. You are working with a family with a child who has a congenital heart defect. Future surgery is planned, and you are teaching the parent how to reduce cardiac demands. The parent needs more teaching when she says which of the following?
   A. "I will wake my child for feeding every 2 hours so he can get enough calories to gain weight."
   B. "When I give the digoxin, I will listen to the pulse for 1 full minute."
   C. "I should protect my child from people who have respiratory infections."
   D. "I will count the number of wet diapers to be sure my child is not getting too much or too little fluid."
3. Which heart defect and hemodynamic change pairing is correct?
   A. Aortic stenosis and obstruction to blood flow out of the heart
   B. Ventricular septal defect and decreased pulmonary blood flow
   C. Tricuspid atresia and increased pulmonary blood flow
   D. Atrioventricular canal and mixed blood flow, in which saturated and desaturated blood mix within the heart or great arteries
4. You are discharging a 5-week-old infant with a congenital heart defect who will be going home on digoxin. Which of the following answers by the father indicate the need for more teaching? Select all that apply.
   A. "I know I give the drug carefully by slowly directing it to the side and back of the mouth."
   B. "I give the medication every 12 hours, and I can place it in a bit of formula so I know the baby will take it."
   C. "If I miss a dose, I don't give an extra dose, but I give the next dose as ordered."
   D. "If the baby vomits, I should give a second dose."
   E. "If more than two doses have been missed, I should call the doctor."
5. You are working in the pediatric clinic, and a child presents with symptoms that are suspicious of the acute phase of Kawasaki disease. Which of the following symptoms are included? Select all that apply.
   A. Periungual desquamation (peeling that begins under the fingertips and toes) of the hands and feet is present.
   B. The bulbar conjunctivae of the eyes become reddened, with clearing around the iris.
   C. A temporary arthritis is evident, which may affect the larger weight-bearing joints.
   D. Inflammation of the pharynx and the oral mucosa develops, with red, cracked lips and the characteristic "strawberry tongue."
   E. Loud pansystolic murmur along with ECG changes are present.

Correct Answers

1. A, D; 2. A; 3. A; 4. A, C, E; 5. B, D

REFERENCES

Abman, S. H., Hansmann, G., Archer, S. L., et al. (2015). Pediatric pulmonary hypertension: Guidelines from the American Heart Association and American Thoracic Society. *Circulation, 132*(21), 2037–2099.

Abman, S. H., & Ivy, D. D. (2011). Recent progress in understanding pediatric pulmonary hypertension. *Current Opin in Pediatrics, 23*(3), 298–304.

Almond, C., Thiagarajian, R. R., Piercy, G. E., et al. (2009). Waiting list mortality among children listed for heart transplantation in the United States. *Circulation, 119,* 717–727.

Alsoufi, B., Mori, M., Gillespie, S., et al. (2015). Impact of patient characteristics and anatomy on results of Norwood operation for Hypoplastic Left Heart Syndrome. *The Annals of Thoracic Surgery, 100*(2), 591–598.

American Academy of Pediatrics. (2008). Lipid screening and cardiovascular health in childhood. *Pediatrics, 122,* 198–208.

American Heart Association. (2016). *Pediatric advanced life support: Provider manual.* Dallas, TX: American Heart Association.

Baker, A. L., & Newburger, J. W. (2008). Kawasaki disease. *Circulation, 118,* e110–e112.

Baltimore, R. S., Gewitz, M., Baddour, L. M., et al. (2015). Infective endocarditis in childhood: 2015 update. Scientific statement from the American Heart Association. *Circulation, 132,* 1487–1515.

Barbas, K. H., & Kelleher, D. K. (2004). Breastfeeding success among infants with congenital heart disease. *Pediatric Nursing, 30,* 285–289.

Bergersen, L., Foerster, S., Marshall, A. C., et al. (2009). *Congenital heart disease: The catheterization manual.* New York: Springer.

Bergersen, L., Marshall, A. C., Gavreau, K., et al. (2010). Adverse event rates in congenital cardiac catheterization – a multicenter experience. *Catheterization and Cardiovascular Interventions, 75*(3), 389–400.

Blume, E. D., Naftel, D. C., Bastardi, H. J., et al. (2006). Outcomes of children bridged to heart transplantation with ventricular assist devices: A multi-institutional study. *Circulation, 113,* 2313–2319.

Bono-Neri, F. (2016). Acute rheumatic fever: Global persistence of a preventable disease. *Journal of Pediatric Health Care, 31*(3), 275–284.

Botto, L. D., Correa, A., & Erickson, J. D. (2001). Racial and temporal variations in the prevalence of heart defects. *Pediatrics, 107*(3), E32.

Bragg, L., & Alvarez, A. (2014). Endocarditis. *Pediatrics in Review, 35*(4), 162–167.

Brancaccio, G., Filippelli, S., Michielon, R., et al. (2012). Ventricular assist devices as a bridge to heart transplantation or as destination therapy in pediatric patients. *Transplantation Proceedings, 44*(7), 2007–2012.

Brown, M. L., Burkhart, H. M., Connolly, H. M., et al. (2013). Coarctation of the aorta: Lifelong surveillance is mandatory following surgical repair. *Journal of the American College of Cardiology, 62*(11), 1020–1025.

Butera, G., Carminati, M., Chessa, M., et al. (2007). Transcatheter closure of perimembranous ventricular septal defects: Early and long-term results. *Journal of the American College of Cardiology, 50*(12), 1189–1195.

Cassidy, J., Dominguez, T., Haynes, S., et al. (2013). A longer waiting game: Bridging children to heart transplant with the Berlin Heart EXCOR device – the United Kingdom experience. *The Journal of Heart and Lung Transplantation, 32*(11), 1101–1106.

Cecchin, F., Frangini, P. A., Brown, D. W., et al. (2009). Cardiac resynchronization therapy (and multisite pacing) in pediatrics and congenital heart disease: Five years experience in a single institution. *Journal of Cardiovascular Electrophysiology, 20*(1), 58–65.

Cuypers, J. A., Eindhoven, J. A., Slager, M. A., et al. (2014). The natural and unnatural history of the Mustard procedure: Long-term outcome up to 40 years. *European Heart Journal, 35*(25), 1666–1674.

Day, M. D., Gauvreau, K., Shulman, S., et al. (2009). Characteristics of children hospitalized with infective endocarditis. *Circulation, 119*(6), 865–870.

Dipchand, A. I., Kirk, R., Mahle, W. T., et al. (2013). Ten year report of pediatric heart transplantation: A report from the Pediatric Heart Transplant Study. *Pediatric Transplantation, 17*, 99–111.

Doyle, T., Kavanaugh-McHmugh, A., & Fish, F. A. (2016). *Management and outcome of tetralogy of Fallot*. UpToDate. https://www.uptodate.com/contents/management-and-outcome-of-tetralogy-of-fallot.

Du, Z. D., Hijazi, Z. M., Kleinman, C. S., et al. (2002). Comparison between transcatheter and surgical closure of secundum atrial septal defect in children and adults: Results of a multicenter nonrandomized trial. *Journal of the American College of Cardiology, 39*(11), 1836–1844.

Dubin, A. M. (2016). *Management of supraventricular tachycardia in children*. UpToDate. https://www.uptodate.com/contents/management-of-supraventricular-tachycardia-in-children.

Dubin, A. M., Janousek, J., Rhee, E., et al. (2005). Resynchronization therapy in pediatric and congenital heart disease patients. *Journal of the American College of Cardiology, 46*(12), 2277–2283.

Farley, L. M., DeMaso, D. R., D'Angelo, E., et al. (2007). Parenting stress and parental post-traumatic stress disorder in families after pediatric heart transplantation. *The Journal of Heart and Lung Transplantation, 2*, 120–126.

Feltes, T. F., Bacha, E., Beekman, R. H., et al. (2011). Indications for cardiac catheterization and intervention in pediatric cardiac disease: A scientific statement from the American Heart Association. *Circulation, 123*, 2607–2652.

Feltes, T. F., Cabalka, A. K., Meissner, H. C., et al. (2003). Palivizumab prophylaxis reduces hospitalization due to respiratory syncytial virus in young children with hemodynamically significant congenital heart disease. *The Journal of Pediatrics, 143*, 532–540.

Flynn, J. T., Daniels, S. R., Hayman, L. L., et al. (2014). Update: Ambulatory blood pressure monitoring in children and adolescents: A scientific statement from the American Heart Association. *Hypertension, 63*(5), 1116–1135.

Flynn, J. T., Kaelber, D. C., Baker-Smith, C. M., et al. (2017). Subcommittee on Screening and Management of High Blood Pressure in Children: Clinical practice guideline for screening and management of high blood pressure in children and adolescents. *Pediatrics, 140*(3), e20171904.

Francis, G. S., Greenberg, B. H., Hsu, D. T., et al. (2010). ACCF/AHA/ACP/HFSA/ISHLT 2010 Clinical competence statement on management of patients with advanced heart failure and cardiac transplant: A report of the ACCF/AHA/ACP Task Force on Clinical Competence and Training. *Journal of the American College of Cardiology, 56*(5), 424–453.

Friedberg, M. K., Silverman, N. H., Moon-Grady, A. J., et al. (2009). Prenatal detection of congenital heart disease. *The Journal of Pediatrics, 155*(1), 26–31.

Gerber, M. A., Baltimore, R. S., Eaton, C. B., et al. (2009). Prevention of rheumatic fever and diagnosis and treatment of acute streptococcal pharyngitis: A scientific statement from the American Heart Association. *Circulation, 119*, 1541–1551.

Gewitz, M. H., Baltimore, R. S., Tani, L. Y., et al. (2015). Revision of the Jones Criteria for the diagnosis of acute rheumatic fever in the era of Doppler echocardiography: A scientific statement from the American Heart Association. *Circulation, 131*, 1806–1818.

Ghanayem, N. S., Hoffman, G. M., Mussatto, K. A., et al. (2003). Home surveillance program prevents interstage mortality after the Norwood procedure. *The Journal of Thoracic and Cardiovascular Surgery, 126*, 1367–1377.

Gilboa, S. M., Devine, O. J., Kucik, J. E., et al. (2016). Congenital heart defects in the United States: Estimating the magnitude of the affected population in 2010. *Circulation, 134*, 101–109.

Gilboa, S. M., Salemi, J. L., Nembhard, W. N., et al. (2010). Mortality resulting from congenital heart disease among children and adults in the United States, 1999 to 2006. *Circulation, 122*, 2254–2263.

Glidewell, J., Olney, R. S., Hinton, C., et al. (2015). State legislation, regulations, and hospital guidelines for newborn screening for critical congenital heart defects – United States, 2011 to 2014. *MMWR. Morbidity and Mortality Weekly Report, 64*(23), 625–630.

Goldmuntz, E., & Lin, A. (2008). Genetics of congenital heart defects. In H. D. Allen, D. J. Driscoll, R. E. Shaddy, et al. (Eds.), *Moss and Adams' Heart Disease in infants, children, and adolescents* (7th ed.). Philadelphia, PA: Lippincott Williams & Wilkins.

Gupta, S., Sakhuja, A., McGrath, E., et al. (2016). Trends, microbiology, and outcomes of infective endocarditis in children during 2000 to 2010 in the United States. *Congenital Heart Disease, 12*(2), 196–201.

Haberman, Z. C., Jahn, R. J., Bose, R., et al. (2015). Wireless Smartphone ECG enables large scale screening in diverse populations. *Journal of Cardiovascular Electrophysiology, 26*(5), 520–526.

Henderson, H. T., Canter, C. E., Mahle, W. T., et al. (2012). ABO-incompatible heart transplantation: Analysis of the Pediatric Heart Transplant Study (PHTS) database. *The Journal of Heart and Lung Transplantation, 31*(2), 173–179.

Hoffman, J. I. E., & Kaplan, S. (2002). The incidence of congenital heart disease. *Journal of the American College of Cardiology, 39*, 1890–1900.

Hoffman, T. M., Wernovsky, G., Atz, A. M., et al. (2003). Efficacy and safety of milrinone in preventing low cardiac output syndrome in infants and children after corrective surgery for congenital heart disease. *Circulation, 107*, 996–1002.

Holman, R. C., Curns, A. T., Belay, E. D., et al. (2003). Kawasaki syndrome hospitalizations in the United States, 1997 and 2000. *Pediatrics, 112*(3 Pt. 1), 495–501.

Holzer, R. J., Chisolm, J. L., Hill, S. L., et al. (2008). Stenting complex aortic arch obstructions. *Catheterization and Cardiovascular Interventions, 71*(3), 375–382.

Holzer, R. J., & Hijazi, Z. M. (2016). Transcatheter pulmonary valve replacement: State of the art. *Catheterization and Cardiovascular Interventions, 87*(1), 117–128.

Jacobs, R., Boyd, L., Brennan, K., et al. (2016). The importance of social media for patients and families affected by congenital anomalies: A Facebook cross-sectional analysis and user survey. *Journal of Pediatric Surgery, 51*, 1766–1771.

Jacobs, J. P., Mavroudis, C., Jacobs, M. L., et al. (2004). Lessons learned from the data analysis of the second harvest (1998-2001) of the Society of Thoracic Surgeons (STS) Congenital Heart Surgery Database. *European Journal of Cardio-throacic Surgery, 26*(1), 18–37.

Kato, H., Ichinose, E., & Kawasaki, T. (1986). Myocardial infarction in Kawasaki disease: Clinical analysis in 195 cases. *The Journal of Pediatrics, 108*(6), 923–927.

Kavey, R. W., Allada, V., Daniels, S. R., et al. (2006). Cardiovascular risk reduction in high-risk pediatric patients: A scientific statement for the

American Heart Association expert panel on population and prevention science. *Circulation, 114*, 2710–2738.

Khairy, P., Clair, M., Fernandes, S. M., et al. (2013). Cardiovascular outcomes after the arterial switch operation for D-transposition of the great arteries. *Circulation, 127*(3), 331–339.

Kimberlin, D. W., Long, S. S., Brady, M. T., et al. (2015). Kawasaki disease. In *2015 Red Book: Report of the committee on infectious diesases* (30th ed.). Elk Grove Village, IL: American Academy of Pediatrics.

Ko, J. K., Deal, B. J., Strasburger, J. F., et al. (1992). Supraventricular tachycardia mechanisms and their age. *American Journal of Cardiology, 69*(12), 1028.

Kusters, D. M., Wiegman, A., Kastelein, J. J., et al. (2014). Carotid-intima thickness in children with familial hypercholesterolemia. *Circulation Research, 114*, 307–310.

LeRoy, S. S., Elixson, E. M., O'Brien, P., et al. (2003). Recommendations for preparing children and adolescents for invasive cardiac procedures: A statement from the American Heart Association Pediatric Nursing Subcommittee of the Council on Cardiovascular Nursing in collaboration with the Council on Cardiovascular Diseases of the Young. *Circulation, 108*, 2550–2564.

Levy, D. J., Pretorius, D. H., Rothman, A., et al. (2013). Improved prenatal detection of congenital heart disease in an integrated health care system. *Pediatric Cardiology, 34*(3), 670–679.

Li, J. S., Sexton, D. J., Mick, N., et al. (2000). Proposed modifications to the Duke criteria for the diagnosis of infective endocarditis. *Clinical Infectious Diseases, 30*(4), 633–638.

Lock, J. E. (2006). Cardiac catheterization. In J. F. Keane, J. Lock, & D. F. Fyler (Eds.), *Nadas' pediatric cardiology* (2nd ed.). Philadelphia, PA: Saunders.

Majnemer, A., Limperopoulos, C., Shevell, M. I., et al. (2009). A new look at outcomes of infants with congenital heart disease. *Pediatric Neurology, 40*, 197–204.

March of Dimes. (2013). *Congenital heart disease and CCHD*. http://www.marchofdimes.org/complications/congenital-heart-defects.aspx.

Margossian, R. (2008). Contemporary management of pediatric heart failure. *Expert Review of Cardiovascular Therapy, 6*(2), 187–197.

Marijon, E., Mirabel, M., Celermajer, D. S., et al. (2012). Rheumatic heart disease. *Lancet, 379*, 953–964.

Marino, B. S., Lipkin, P. H., Newburger, J. W., et al. (2012). Neurodevelopmental outcomes in children with congenital heart disease: Evaluation and management: A scientific statement from the American Heart Association. *Circulation, 126*, 1143–1172.

Mattoo, T. K. (2017). *Evaluation of hypertension in children and adolescents*, UpToDate. https://www.uptodate.com/contents/evaluation-of-hypertension-in-children-and-adolescents.

McCance, K. L., & Huether, S. E. (2010). *Pathophysiology: The biological basis for disease in adults and children* (6th ed.). St. Louis, MO: Mosby.

McCrindle, B. W., Rowley, A. H., Newburger, J. W., et al. (2017). Diagnosis, treatment, and long-term management of Kawasaki Disease: A scientific statement of health professionals from the American Heart Association. *Circulation, 135*, 1379–1381.

McCrindle, B. W., Urbina, E. M., Dennison, B. A., et al. (2007). Drug therapy of high-risk lipid abnormalities in children and adolescents: A scientific statement from the American Heart Association Atherosclerosis, Hypertension, and Obesity in Youth Committee, Council of Cardiovascular Disease in the Young, with the Council on Cardiovascular Nursing. *Circulation, 115*(14), 1948–1967.

McGill, H. C., McMahan, A., & Gidding, S. S. (2008). Preventing heart disease in the 21st century: Implication of the pathobiological determinants of atherosclerosis in youth (PDAY) study. *Circulation, 117*, 1216–1227.

Menasche, C. C., DuPlessis, A. J., Wessel, D. L., et al. (2002). Current incidence of acute neurological complications after open heart operations in children. *The Annals of Thoracic Surgery, 73*, 1752–1758.

Mery, C. M., Guzmán-Pruneda, F. A., Trost, J. G., et al. (2015). Contemporary results of aortic coarctation repair through left thoracotomy. *The Annals of Thoracic Surgery, 100*(3), 1039–1046.

Moffett, B. S., & Chang, A. C. (2006). Future pharmacologic agents for treatment of heart failure in children. *Pediatric Cardiology, 27*, 533–551.

Moore, J., Hegde, S., El-Said, H., et al. (2013). Transcatheter device closure of atrial septal defects: A safety review. *JACC. Cardiovascular Interventions, 6*(5), 433-42.

Narula, J., Chandrasekhar, Y., Rahimtoola, S., et al. (1999). Diagnosis of acute rheumatic carditis. *Circulation, 100*, 1576–1581.

National Heart, Lung, and Blood Institute. (2011). Expert panel on integrated guidelines for cardiovascular health and risk reduction in children and adolescents: Summary report. *Pediatrics, 128*(Suppl. 5), S213–S256.

Newburger, J. W., de Ferranti, S. D., & Fulton, D. R. (2016). *Cardiovascular sequelae of Kawasaki disease*. UpToDate. http://www.uptodate.com/contents/cardiovascular-sequelae-of-kawasaki-disease.

Newburger, J. W., Takahashi, M., Burns, J. C., et al. (1986). The treatment of Kawsaki syndrome with intravenous gamma gobulin. *The New England Journal of Medicine, 315*(6), 341–347.

Newburger, J. W., Takahashi, M., Gerber, M. A., et al. (2004). Diagnosis, treatment, and long-term management of Kawasaki disease: A statement for health professionals from the Committee on Rheumatic Fever, Endocarditis, and Kawasaki Disease, Council on Cardiovascular Disease in the Young, American Heart Association. *Circulation, 110*(17), 2747–2771.

Park, M. K. (2014). *Pediatric cardiology for practitioners* (6th ed.). Philadelphia, PA: Elsevier/Saunders.

Petit, C. J., Fraser, C. D., Mattamal, R., et al. (2011). The impact of a dedicated single-ventricle home-monitoring program on interstage somatic growth, interstage attrition, and 1-year survival. *The Journal of Thoracic and Cardiovascular Surgery, 142*, 1358–1366.

Petrini, J. R., Broussard, C. S., Gilboa, S. M., et al. (2010). Racial differences by gestational age in neonatal deaths attributable to congenital heart defects – United States, 2003 to 2006. *MMWR. Morbidity and Mortality Weekly Report, 59*(37), 1208–1211.

Reller, M. D., Strickland, M. J., Riehle-Colarusso, T., et al. (2008). Prevalence of congenital heart defects in metropolitan Atlanta, 1998 to 2005. *The Journal of Pediatrics, 153*(6), 807–813.

Remenyi, B., Carapetis, J., Wyber, R., et al. (2013). Position statement of the World Heart Federation on the prevention and control of rheumatic heart disease. *Nature Reviews Cardiology, 10*(5), 284–292.

Remond, M. G., Coyle, M. E., Mills, J. E., et al. (2016). Approaches to improving adherence to secondary prophylaxis for rheumatic fever and rheumatic heart disease: A literature review with global perspective. *Cardiology in Review, 24*(2), 94–98.

Rosenthal, D., Chrisant, M. R., Edens, E., et al. (2004). International Society for Heart and Lung Transplantation: Practice guidelines for management of heart failure in children. *The Journal of Heart and Lung Transplantation, 23*, 1313–1333.

Ross, R. D. (2012). The Ross classification for heart failure in children after 25 years: A review and age stratified revision. *Pediatric Cardiology, 33*, 1295.

Rossano, J. W., & Shaddy, R. E. (2014). Heart failure in children: Etiology and treatment. *The Journal of Pediatrics, 165*(2), 228–233.

Russell, H. M., Pasquali, S. K., Jacobs, J. P., et al. (2012). Outcomes of repair of common arterial trunk with truncal valve surgery: A review of the Society of Thoracic Surgeons congenital heart surgery database. *The Annals of Thoracic Surgery, 93*(1), 164–169.

Siffel, C., Riehle-Colarusso, T., Oster, M. E., et al. (2015). Survival of children with hypoplastic left heart syndrome. *Pediatrics, 136*(4), e864–e870.

Simonneau, G., Gatzoulis, M. A., Adatia, I., et al. (2013). Updated clinical classification of pulmonary hypertension. *Journal of the American College of Cardiology, 62*(Suppl.25), D34–D41.

Sklansky, M. S., Berman, D. P., Pruetz, J. D., et al. (2009). Prenatal screening for major congenital heart disease: Superiority of outflow tracts over the 4-chamber view. *Journal of Ultrasound in Medicine, 28*(7), 889–899.

Smith, P. A. (2001). Primary care in children with congenital heart disease. *Journal of Pediatric Nursing, 16*, 308–319.

Spirito, P., Autore, C., Rapezzi, C., et al. (2009). Syncope and risk of sudden death in hypertrophic cardiomyopathy. *Circulation, 1109*, 1703–1710.

St Louis, J. D., Jodhka, U., Jacobs, J. P., et al. (2014). Contemporary outcomes of complete atrioventricular septal defect repair: Analysis of the Society of Thoracic Surgeons congenital heart surgery database. *The Journal of Thoracic and Cardiovascular Surgery, 148*(6), 2526–2531.

Steer, A., & Gibofsky, A. (2017). *Acute rheumatic fever: clinical manifestations and diagnosis.* UpToDate. https://www.uptodate.com/contents/acute-rheumatic-fever-clinical-manifestations-and-diagnosis.

Taketomo, C., Hodding, J., & Kraus, D. (2009). *Pediatric dosage handbook* (16th ed.). Hudson, OH: Lexi-Comp.

Thangaratinam, S., Brown, K., Zamora, J., et al. (2012). Pulse oximetry screening for critical congenital heart defects in asymptomatic newborn babies: A systematic review and meta-analysis. *Lancet, 379,* 2459–2464.

Tremoulet, A. H., Best, B. M., Song, S., et al. (2008). Resistance to intravenous immunoglobulin in children with Kawasaki disease. *The Journal of Pediatrics, 153*(1), 117–121.

United Network for Organ Sharing. (2001). *UNOS Scientific Registry Annual Report*, Richmond, VA, The Network.

United States Department of Health and Human Services. (2016). *Organ Procurement and Transplantation Network (OPTN).* http://www.unos.org/data/.

Vick, G. W., & Bezold, L. I. (2017). *Classification of atrial septal defects (ASDs), and clinical features and diagnosis of isolated ASDs in children*, UpToDate. http://www.uptodate.com/contents/classification-of-atrial-septal-defects-asds-and-clinical-features-and-diagnosis-of-isolated-asds-in-children.

Watts, G. F., Gidding, S., Wierzbicki, A. S., et al. (2014). Integrated guidance on the care of familial hypercholesterolemia from the International FH Foundation. *Journal of Clinical Lipidology*, *8*(2), 148–172.

Wilder, M. S., Palinkas, L. A., Kao, A. S., et al. (2007). Delayed diagnosis by physicians contributes to the development of coronary artery aneurysms in children with Kawasaki syndrome. *Pediatric Infectious Disease*, *26*(3), 256–260.

Wilson, W., Taubert, K. A., Gewitz, M., et al. (2007). Prevention of infective endocarditis: Guidelines from the American Heart Association. *Circulation, 116*(15), 1736–1754.

World Health Organization. (2004). *Rheumatic Fever and Rheumatic Heart Disease: a report of a WHO expert consultation.* http://www.who.int/cardiovascular_diseases/publications/trs923/en/.

Wypij, D., Newberger, J. W., Rappaport, L. A., et al. (2003). The effect of duration of deep hypothermic circulatory arrest in infant heart surgery on late neurodevelopment: The Boston Circulatory Arrest Trial. *The Journal of Thoracic and Cardiovascular Surgery, 126,* 1397–1403.

Zachariah, J. P., & de Ferranti, S. D. (2013). NHLBI integrated pediatric guidelines: Battle for a future free of cardiovascular disease. *Future Cardiology, 9*(1), 13–22.

28

The Child With Hematologic or Immunologic Dysfunction

Rosalind Bryant

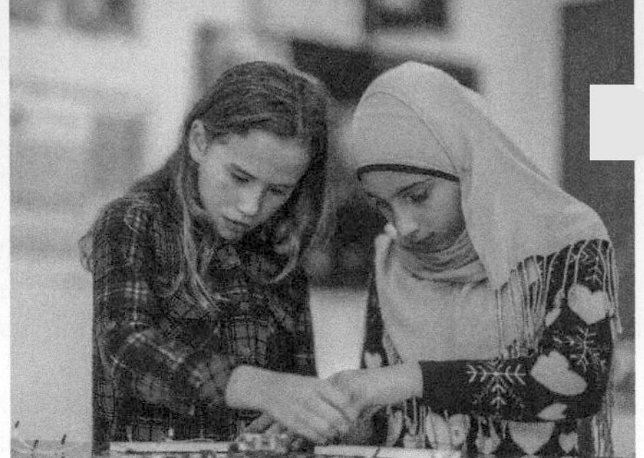

http://evolve.elsevier.com/wong/ncic

CONCEPTS

- Perfusion
- Clotting

THE HEMATOLOGIC SYSTEM AND ITS FUNCTION

ORIGIN OF FORMED ELEMENTS

Blood is composed of a fluid portion called plasma and a cellular portion known as the formed elements of the blood. The two components are approximately equal in volume. Plasma is about 90% water and 10% solutes. The principal solutes are albumin, electrolytes, and proteins. Among the proteins are clotting factors, globulins, circulating antibodies, and fibrinogen. The cellular elements sequentially develop into mature red blood cells (RBCs, erythrocytes), white blood cells (WBCs, leukocytes), and platelets (thrombocytes).

The major hematopoietic (blood-forming) organs of the body are the red bone marrow (myeloid tissue) and the lymphatic system, which consists of lymph (fluid), lymphatic vessels, and lymphoid structures (the lymph nodes, spleen, thymus, and tonsils). Although the lymphatic system plays an important role in regulating blood cells, the lymph vessels and fluids do not produce cells. The lymph nodes regulate the manufacture of WBCs. The spleen and liver are the primary organs for hematopoiesis in the young fetus and for cell removal in postnatal life. Macrophages (formerly called *reticular cells*) are cells of mesodermal origin that are widely dispersed in the lining of the vascular and lymph channels. Macrophages form a network and are capable of phagocytosis (ingestion and digestion of foreign substances); formation of immune bodies; and differentiation into other cells, such as hemocytoblasts, myeloblasts, and lymphoblasts.

All of the formed elements of the blood, except to some extent the agranulocytes, are produced in myeloid tissue during postnatal life. During embryonic development the mesenchyme, spleen, liver, thymus, and yolk sac serve as additional sites of blood cell formation. In individuals with certain blood disorders, these sites, particularly the spleen, can be stimulated to produce blood cells and constitute extramedullary hematopoiesis. In infants and young children all of the bone contains red marrow (so-called because of its color from the formation of erythrocytes), but as bone growth ceases near the end of adolescence, only the ribs, sternum, vertebrae, and pelvis continue to produce blood cells. The remainder of the bone marrow becomes yellow from deposition of fat. However, in conditions of increased demand for blood cells, the yellow marrow can revert to red marrow and become another hematopoietic source.

Although the progressive development of each blood cell is fairly well delineated, there is considerable controversy regarding the origin of the blood cell. One of the most widely held theories (monophyletic theory) is that each blood cell originates from a primordial (primitive) cell called a blast, or totipotential stem cell, which has the ability to self-replicate and transform into all the blood components.

The second-generation stem cell, called the pluripotent stem cell, is committed to produce erythroblast, myeloblast, monoblast, lymphoblast, or megakaryoblast. The blast cells sequentially develop into mature RBCs (erythrocytes), WBCs (leukocytes), platelets (thrombocytes), and other cells (such as mast cells and macrophages).

Red Blood Cells (Erythrocytes)

The erythrocyte is formed from the hemocytoblast in the red bone marrow. The pluripotential stem cell forms the proerythroblast. The initial cell of this series has a deep blue–staining (basophilic) cytoplasm and therefore is called a basophilic erythroblast. The chief change in the erythroblast is accumulation of hemoglobin in the cytoplasm. As the basophilic material decreases and the amount of hemoglobin increases, the cell comes to be called a polychromatic erythroblast, which describes its mixture of staining properties. At the same time that the nucleus decreases in size, the basophilic material disappears, so the cell is uniformly stained by eosin dye—hence the name *orthochromatic erythroblast,* or *normoblast.* Finally, the normoblast completely loses its nucleus by a process of extrusion as it squeezes through the pores of the membrane into the capillary. Because of the loss of its nucleus, the cell caves in on both sides, which gives the mature erythrocyte its characteristic appearance as a biconcave disk. During each of these stages the different cells continue to undergo mitosis so that increasingly greater numbers of cells are produced. Because the mature RBC does not have a nucleus, it is unable to multiply.

The reticulocyte is the last stage of development before the mature erythrocyte. Reticulocytes are slightly larger than erythrocytes, and their presence indicates active RBC production (erythropoiesis). Ordinarily the total proportion of circulating reticulocytes is between 0.5% and

1.5%. The reticulocyte, or "retic," count is a simple laboratory test frequently used to indirectly analyze hematopoiesis.

Regulation of Erythrocyte Production

The usual life span of the mature erythrocyte is 120 days. Apparently, as RBCs grow old, their membranes become fragile and eventually rupture. The contents of the cell fragment as they circulate through the blood vessels and are phagocytized by the macrophages in the spleen, liver, and bone marrow. The hemoglobin is broken down into the iron-containing pigment hemosiderin and the bile pigments biliverdin and bilirubin. Most of the iron is reused by the bone marrow for production of new RBCs or stored in the liver and other tissues for future use. The bile pigments are excreted by the liver in bile.

Normally there is a homeostatic balance between RBC production and destruction. This balance ensures adequate tissue oxygenation and a blood viscosity that allows the blood to flow freely through the vessels. The basic regulator of erythrocyte production is tissue oxygenation and renal production of erythropoietin (also called erythropoietic stimulating factor). In states of tissue hypoxia, the kidney releases erythropoietin into the bloodstream. As a result the bone marrow is stimulated to produce new RBCs. The major activity seems to be an increase in both maturation rate and mitosis at all stages of erythrocyte production but primarily at the stem cell level.

During this rapid increase in RBC production, the circulating erythrocytes may not be totally mature. Consequently, the number of reticulocytes may increase dramatically (as high as 30% or more of the total RBC count). Even normoblasts or nucleated RBCs may appear in the blood. A failure of this rise in erythrocyte and reticulocyte count to occur may indicate bone marrow failure.

Once tissue oxygenation is adequate, the production of erythropoietin ceases. Thus tissue oxygen requirements control both the stimulation and termination of erythrocyte production. Note that the basic regulatory mechanism is the ability of RBCs to transport oxygen to the tissues in response to their needs, not the circulating numbers of erythrocytes. Oxygen transport depends on both the number of circulating RBCs and the amount of normal hemoglobin in the cell. This explains why **polycythemia** (increase in the number of erythrocytes) occurs in conditions characterized by prolonged tissue hypoxia, such as cyanotic heart defects. (See Chapter 27.) If the circulating numbers of erythrocytes controlled erythropoietin release, this feedback mechanism would maintain erythrocyte production at a constant level (4.5 to 5.5 million/mm^3 of blood) regardless of existing tissue hypoxia.

Functions of Erythrocytes

The major function of RBCs is to transport hemoglobin, which in turn carries oxygen to all cells of the body. However, erythrocytes have other significant functions: they contain carbonic anhydrase, an enzyme that catalyzes the reaction between carbon dioxide and water, which allows large quantities of carbon dioxide to react with blood for transportation to the lungs, and the hemoglobin, a protein, serves as an acid-base buffer, which, in combination with carbon dioxide, maintains the blood pH at a constant level.

Hemoglobin

Hemoglobin is a complex molecule composed of four globin chains. The type of hemoglobin in the cells depends on both the stage of life and the presence of any abnormalities in the genes that regulate the production of hemoglobin. Fetal hemoglobin, composed of two α and two γ chains, has a greater affinity for oxygen and is best suited to the fetal environment. During the latter part of pregnancy, the fetus begins developing adult hemoglobin (two α and two β chains). When a defect in hemoglobin synthesis is present (e.g., sickle cell disease [SCD] or thalassemia), fetal hemoglobin may be produced into adulthood. Research is currently underway to develop cell-free hemoglobin that can be used for oxygen and carbon dioxide transport. Hemoglobin values vary according to the child's age.

Several tests offer important information about hemoglobin. The hematocrit, which is approximately three times the concentration of hemoglobin (in grams per deciliter), indicates the percentage volume of circulating packed RBCs in the total blood. Under normal conditions, hemoglobin and the hematocrit are in a fixed relationship with each other and vary according to the child's age and sex (Lerner, 2016).

RBC indices are based on ratios of packed RBC volume, hemoglobin concentration, and RBC count, and they are a useful way of designating different types of anemias. Values for mean corpuscular volume (MCV) and mean corpuscular hemoglobin (MCH) do not stay constant during infancy and childhood. MCH concentration (MCHC) values, however, are more constant.

MCV is the average (mean) volume or size of a single RBC. The normal range for RBCs is given in Table 28.1.

MCH is the average weight of hemoglobin in each RBC (see Table 28.1). Normochromic cells are those with a normal hemoglobin content or normal MCH. Cells with below-normal MCH are termed *hypochromic,* and those with above-normal MCH are termed *hyperchromic.*

MCHC is the average concentration of hemoglobin in the RBC. MCHC is calculated from the amount of hemoglobin in 100 ml of RBCs rather than the amount of hemoglobin in whole blood. The mean MCV value of 77 g/dl and MCHC value of 33 g/dl is reached at approximately 6 months of age (Lerner, 2016). Fig. 28.1 shows how RBC indices are used as indicators of different types of anemia.

White Blood Cells (Leukocytes)

The term *leukocyte* encompasses a number of cells with similar yet distinct functions. They are divided into two major classes—granulocytes and agranulocytes—based on the presence or absence, respectively, of granules within the cytoplasm of the cells.

Granulocytes

There are three types of granulocytes: neutrophils, basophils, and eosinophils. The name of each of these refers to the characteristic staining property of the granule during laboratory analysis. Neutrophils stain neutral to the dyes, whereas basophils stain purple to the basic methylene blue dye, and eosinophils take on a red color from acidic eosin dye. Because the nuclei of neutrophils have two or more lobules that are connected by fine chromatin strands, the term **polymorphonuclear leukocytes** (cells with many-formed nuclei), or simply *polys,* or *segs* (segmented or mature neutrophils) and *bands* (immature neutrophils with the nuclei connected) may be used collectively to refer to the neutrophils.

The granulocytes, like erythrocytes, are produced in the bone marrow. For this reason, these cells are sometimes referred to as *myelogenous leukocytes.* These cells, in theory, originate from primitive stem cells, which develop into myeloblasts. The genesis of neutrophils, basophils, and eosinophils is similar to the stages observed during erythrocyte production. The differentiation of myeloblasts into various mature WBCs is primarily a result of specialization within the cytoplasm and degeneration of the nucleus. Unlike erythrocytes, however, all WBCs are nucleated.

Accelerated production of immature granulocytes leads to increased numbers of bands in the peripheral circulation (referred to as a shift to the left in the complete blood count [CBC]), which is indicative of a bacterial infection. The absolute neutrophil count (ANC) reflects the body's ability to handle bacterial infections. If the ANC is less than 500/mm^3, a severe risk of infection is present.

TABLE 28.1 Tests Performed as Part of a Complete Blood Count

Test (Average Value)	Description, Comments
Red blood cell (RBC) count (4.5-5.5 million/mm^3)	Number of RBCs/mm^3 of blood Indirectly estimates Hgb content of blood Reflects function of bone marrow
Hemoglobin (Hgb) determination (11.5-15.5 g/dl)	Amount of Hgb (g)/dl of whole blood Total blood Hgb primarily depends on number of circulating RBCs but also on amount of Hgb in each cell
Hematocrit (Hct) (35%-45%)	Percent volume of packed RBCs in whole blood Indirectly measures Hgb content Is approximately three times Hgb content
RBC indices	
Mean corpuscular volume (MCV) (77-95 fl)	Average or mean volume (size) of a single RBC MCV values are expressed as femtoliters (fl) or cubic microns (mm^3)
Mean corpuscular hemoglobin (MCH) (25-33 pg/cell)	Average or mean quantity (weight) of Hgb in a single RBC MCH values are expressed as picograms (pg) or micromicrograms (mmcg)
Mean corpuscular hemoglobin concentration (MCHC) (31%-37% Hgb [g]/dl RBC)	Average concentration of Hgb in a single RBC MCHC values are expressed as percent Hgb (g)/cell or Hgb (g)/dl RBC MCV and MCH depend on accurate counts of RBCs, whereas MCHC does not; therefore MCHC is often more reliable All indices depend on average cell measurements and do not show individual RBC variations (anisocytosis)
RBC volume distribution width (RDW) (13.4% ± 1.2%)	Average size of RBCs Differentiates some types of anemia
Reticulocyte count (0.5%-1.5% erythrocytes)	Percent reticulocytes in RBCs Index of production of mature RBCs by bone marrow Decreased count indicates depressed bone marrow function Increased count indicates erythrogenesis in response to some stimulus When reticulocyte count is extremely high, other forms of immature RBCs (normoblasts, even erythroblasts) may be present Indirectly estimates hypochromic anemia Usually elevated in patients with chronic hemolytic anemia
WBC count (4.5-13.5 × 10^3 cells/mm^3)	Number of WBCs/mm^3 of blood Total number of WBCs less important than differential count
Differential WBC count	Inspection and quantification of WBC types present in peripheral blood Values are expressed as percentages; to obtain absolute number of any type of WBC, multiply its respective percentage by total number of WBCs
Neutrophils (polys) (54%-62%) (3-5.8 × 10^3 cells/mm^3)	Primary defense in bacterial infection; capable of phagocytizing and killing bacteria
Bands (3%-5%) (0.15-0.4 × 10^3 cells/mm^3)	Immature neutrophil Increased numbers in bacterial infection Also capable of phagocytosis and killing
Eosinophils (1%-3%) (0.05-0.25 × 10^3 cells/mm^3)	Named for their staining characteristics with eosin dye Increased in allergic disorders, parasitic diseases, certain neoplasms, and other diseases
Basophils (0.075%) (0.015-0.030 × 10^3 cells/mm^3)	Named for their characteristic basophilic stippling Contain histamine, heparin, and serotonin; believed to cause increased blood flow to injured tissues while preventing excessive clotting
Lymphocytes (25%-33%) (1.5-3.0 × 10^3 cells/mm^3)	Involved in development of antibody and delayed hypersensitivity
Monocytes (3%-7%)	Large phagocytic cells that are involved in early stage of inflammatory reaction
ANC >1000/mm^3)	Percent neutrophils/bands times WBC count Indicates body's capability to handle bacterial infections
Platelet count (150-400 × 10^3/mm^3)	Number of platelets/mm^3 of blood Cellular fragments that are necessary for clotting to occur
Stained peripheral blood smear	Visual estimation of amount of Hgb in RBCs and overall size, shape, and structure of RBCs Various staining properties of RBC structures may be evidence of immature forms of erythrocytes Shows variation in size and shape of RBCs: microcytic, macrocytic, poikilocytic (variable shapes)

ANC, Absolute neutrophil count; *Hct,* hematocrit; *Hgb,* hemoglobin; *MCH,* mean corpuscular hemoglobin; *MCHC,* mean corpuscular hemoglobin concentration; *MCV,* mean corpuscular volume; *RBC,* red blood cell; *WBC,* white blood cell.

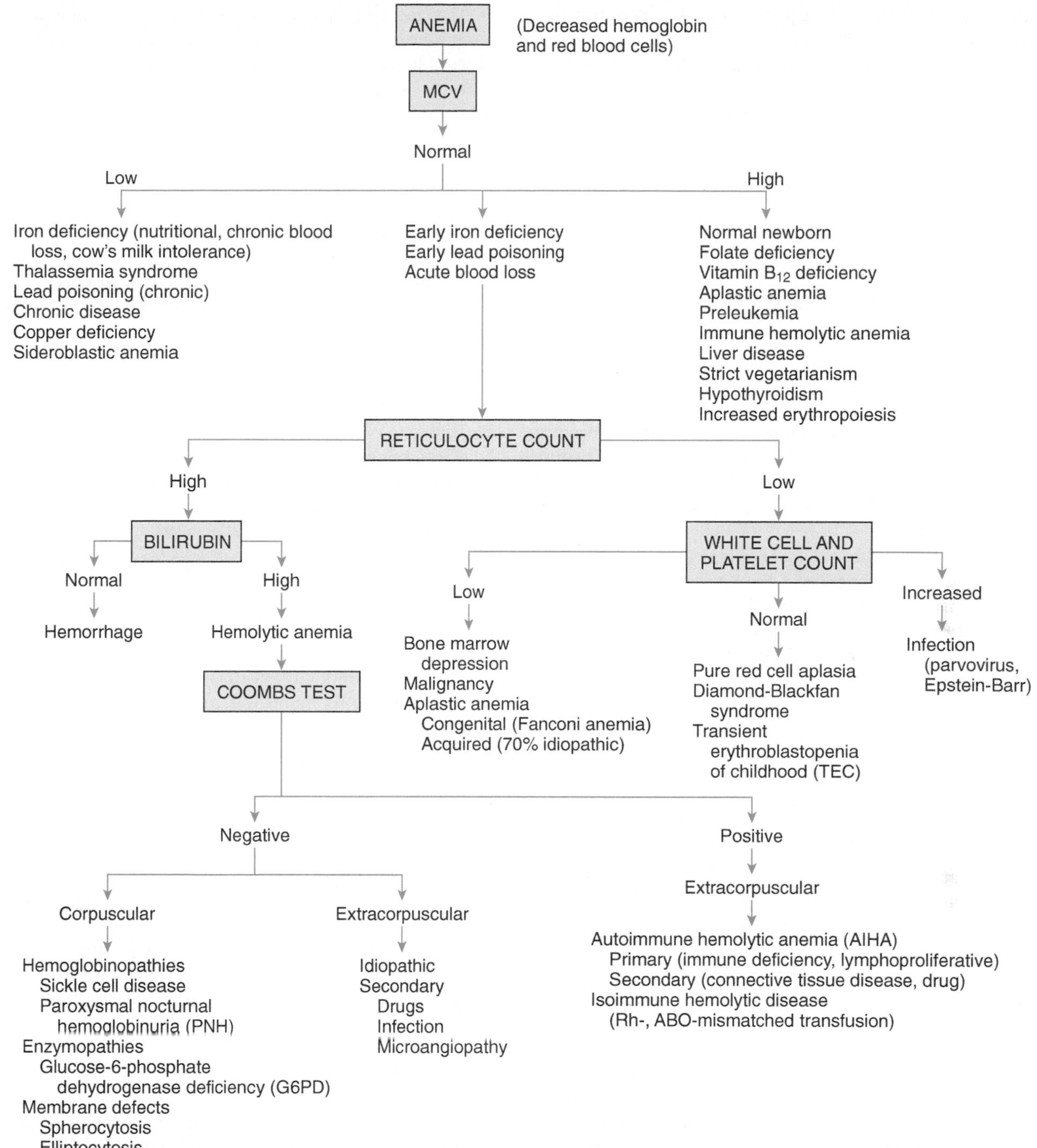

FIG. 28.1 Approach to the diagnosis of anemia by mean corpuscular volume (MCV) and reticulocyte count. (Modified data from Brugnara, C., Oski, F. A., & Nathan, D. G. [2015]. Diagnostic approach to the anemic patient. In S. H. Orkin, D. E. Fisher, D. Ginsburg, et al. [Eds.], *Nathan and Oski's hematology of infancy and childhood* [8th ed.]. Philadelphia, PA: Saunders; Lanzkowsky, P. [2016]. Classification and diagnosis of anemia in children. In P. Lanzkowsky, J. M. Lipton, & J. D. Fish: *Lanzkowsky's manual of pediatric hematology and oncology* [6th ed.]. San Diego, CA: Elsevier; Lerner, N. [2016]. The anemias. In R. M. Kliegman, B. F. Stanton, J. W. St. Geme III, et al. [Eds.], *Nelson textbook of pediatrics* [20th ed.]. Philadelphia, PA: Elsevier.)

Agranulocytes

The agranulocytes include two cell types: monocytes and lymphocytes. Characteristically these cells do not develop granules, and the nuclei are not lobulated. They originate in various lymphogenous organs, and for this reason they are sometimes referred to as **lymphogenous leukocytes**. However, because stem cells and reticular cells are capable of differentiating into monocytes or lymphocytes, the origin of these cells is frequently designated as the *lymphomyeloid complex,* which includes bone marrow, lymph nodes, spleen, liver, thymus, subepithelial lymphoid tissue (tonsils, vermiform appendix, and intestinal lymphoid tissues), and connective tissues (mesenchymal cells of the reticuloendothelial system).

The monocytes follow the same sequence of development from the stem cell as the granulocytes. The monocytes in turn have the ability to exit the vessels and develop into macrophages, large cells that are highly effective phagocytes. Kupffer cells are macrophages located in the liver. Histiocytes are macrophages in the connective tissue. These names are remnants of the old reticular endothelial system designations.

Lymphocytopoiesis (lymphocyte formation) takes place anywhere in the lymphomyeloid complex. Lymphocytes develop from blast (stem) cells. The lymphocyte has the potential to develop into other cells, such as T cells or B cells (see p. 1059).

Regulation of Leukocyte Production

The exact life span of the leukocytes is not as clearly defined as that of the erythrocytes because they exist in the circulation primarily for transport to extravascular areas, where they reside in reservoirs or where they are needed to resist infection. Therefore their survival rate is described in terms of three phases: (1) the hematopoietic phase, extending from the development of the blast cell to the delivery of the mature leukocyte into the circulation; (2) the intravascular phase, the period within the circulation; and (3) the extravascular phase, the time spent in the viscera or tissues.

Granulocytes have a half-life of 6 to 8 hours in the blood and, after entering the tissues, die over a period of 4 to 5 days. Agranulocytes live for an extended period because they remain in inflamed tissue areas longer than the granulocytes. Monocytes wander back and forth between the blood and tissues and are capable of becoming macrophages; their half-life in the blood is 8 to 10 hours, but their half-life in the tissue is 60 to 90 days.

The regulation of leukocytes is based on the body's need for them. Tissue damage from bacterial or viral agents promotes leukocyte circulation and production. However, **leukocytosis** (increase in leukocytes) results from tissue destruction from almost any source, such as hemorrhage, neoplastic disease, toxicity, operative procedures, chemical and thermal injury, and tissue ischemia.

The leukocytes probably die as a result of their activity at the site of injury and are phagocytized by other newly formed WBCs. Effective control of the inflammatory process with subsequent tissue recovery most likely results in feedback to the bone marrow and causes lymphogenous organs to cease increased production of WBCs.

Functions of Leukocytes

Although all of the leukocytes play some role in the immune process, each of the WBCs has a specific role. Neutrophils and monocytes are effective phagocytes and as a result are primarily involved in inflammatory reactions. **Neutrophilia** (increased numbers of neutrophils) is most evident in an acute inflammation, whereas **monocytosis** (increased numbers of monocytes) is more evident in chronic conditions. The reason is that as the affected area becomes acidic from tissue necrosis, neutrophils, which prefer a neutral environment, become less efficient, and monocytes, which become macrophages, become more powerful. These cells also increase in number during chronic inflammation. The other functions of lymphocytes in terms of the immune process are discussed on p. 1059.

The function of eosinophils is still not completely known. They seem to have parasiticidal properties because they can selectively destroy parasites. They may also function in the immediate type of allergic or anaphylactic hypersensitivity reaction because **eosinophilia** (increased numbers of eosinophils) is well documented in such conditions. Eosinophils also are thought to release a substance called profibrinolysin, which, when activated to form fibrinolysin, digests fibrin and thereby helps dissolve a clot.

The function of basophils is also not completely understood, although **basophilia** (increased numbers of basophils) occurs during the healing phase of inflammation and during prolonged inflammation. Basophils in the blood exit the vessels and become mast cells in the tissue. They are responsible for histamine release, which results in increased permeability of the vessels to allow WBCs to exit the vessels at the site of injury.

Platelets

Platelets are actually small fragments of megakaryocytes. They are smaller than blood cells, do not possess a cellular structure, and consist of a clear substance containing granules. Platelets originate from part of the myelogenous group of WBCs. Platelets are formed when the megakaryocytic membrane invaginates, fuses within the cell to separate the cytoplasm, and then fragments.

Regulation of Platelet Production

The life span of platelets is estimated as 8 to 10 days. Apparently the body regulates platelet levels to maintain a fairly constant level (between 150,000 and 400,000/mm^3). Platelet production is probably regulated by a hormone, thrombopoietin, but the source and mode of action of this substance are unknown. Old platelets are most likely removed by the liver and spleen.

Function of Platelets

The term **thrombocyte** means "clot" *(thrombo)* and "cell" *(cyte)* and accurately describes the main function of platelets. When there is a break in the continuity of a blood vessel, the platelets, which are normally flat and round or oval, come in contact with the wet vessel surface and dramatically change their shape to become swollen spheres with long, irregular projections called pseudopodia (false feet). As a result, the platelets begin to adhere to the wet endothelium and to one another. The first platelets at the site of injury release substances that attract other thrombocytes to the area. This causes a layering of platelets, which eventually forms a plug. This plug is large enough to partially or totally occlude the opening in the vessel wall but small enough to allow blood flow to continue unimpaired through the vessel.

In small vessel tears the platelet plug is sufficient to produce hemostasis, and additional blood coagulation is not necessary. When platelet counts are low, however, these numerous small ruptures, which occur continually in the body as a result of general functioning, are not repaired. Consequently, small hemorrhagic areas called **petechiae** form under the skin. They are similar in appearance to reddish freckles or tiny spiderwebs.

Platelets also influence hemostasis by releasing a substance called serotonin at the site of injury. Serotonin is a vasoconstrictor that produces vascular spasm to decrease the blood flow to the injured area.

ASSESSMENT OF HEMATOLOGIC FUNCTION

Several tests assess hematologic function, and additional procedures can identify the cause of the dysfunction. The following discussion is limited to a description of the most common and one of the most valuable tests, the CBC. Other procedures, such as those related to iron, coagulation, and immune status, are discussed throughout the chapter as appropriate.

The CBC with differential (CBCD) consists of the following determinations: RBC count, WBC count, hematocrit, hemoglobin level, differential WBC count, RBC indices (MCV, MCH, and MCHC), and peripheral smear. Additional tests may be included, such as the reticulocyte count, RBC volume distribution width, and platelet count. Table

28.1 describes each of these. Most of the determinations can be performed on a small quantity of blood (micromethod), and values are computed automatically. The nurse should be familiar with the significance of the findings from the CBCD (see Table 28.1) and should be aware of the normal values for age.

The history and physical examination are essential to the identification of hematologic dysfunction, and the nurse is often the first person to suspect a problem based on information from these sources. Comments by the parent regarding the child's lack of energy, food diary showing decreased sources of iron, frequent infections, and bleeding that is difficult to control offer clues to the more common disorders affecting the blood. A careful physical appraisal can reveal findings such as persistent fatigue, pallor, petechiae, or bruising that may indicate minor or serious hematologic conditions. Nurses need to be aware of the clinical manifestations of blood diseases to assist in recognizing symptoms and establishing a diagnosis.

RED BLOOD CELL DISORDERS

ANEMIA

Anemia is a reduction in RBCs mass and/or hemoglobin concentration compared with normal values for age (Brugnara, Oski, & Nathan, 2015; Lerner, 2016). The anemias are the most common hematologic disorders of infancy and childhood and are not diseases but manifestations of underlying pathologic processes (see Fig. 28.1).

Classification

The anemias can be classified using two basic approaches: etiology as manifested by erythrocyte or hemoglobin depletion and morphology, the characteristic changes in RBC size, shape, and color (Box 28.1).

Although the morphologic classification is useful in the laboratory evaluation of anemia, the etiology provides direction for planning nursing care. For example, anemia with reduced hemoglobin concentration may be caused by a dietary depletion of iron, and the principal intervention is replenishing iron stores.

The main causes of anemia are inadequate production of RBCs or RBC components, increased destruction of RBCs, and excessive loss of RBCs through hemorrhage. Each of these factors affects the amount of hemoglobin that is available to carry oxygen to the cells (see Box 28.1). Therefore the classification is based on the various conditions that can result from any of these physiologic changes.

Pathophysiology and Clinical Manifestations

The basic physiologic defect caused by anemia is a decrease in the oxygen-carrying capacity of blood and consequently a reduction in the amount of oxygen available to the cells. When the anemia has developed slowly, the child usually adapts to the declining hemoglobin level. Most children seem to have a remarkable ability to function well despite low levels of hemoglobin. Also, compensatory mechanisms such as a shift in the oxyhemoglobin dissociation curve may delay the development of any obvious signs.

When the hemoglobin level falls sufficiently to produce clinical manifestations, the signs and symptoms (e.g., weakness, fatigue, and a waxy pallor in severe anemia) are due to tissue hypoxia (Box 28.2). Cyanosis, which results from an increased quantity of deoxygenated hemoglobin in arterial blood, is typically not evident. Anemia is caused by decreased levels of hemoglobin or RBCs, not inadequate oxygen saturation of existing hemoglobin.

Central nervous system manifestations include headache, dizziness, lightheadedness, irritability, slowed thought processes, decreased attention span, apathy, and depression. Growth retardation resulting from decreased cellular metabolism, and coexisting anorexia is a common finding in chronic severe anemia. It is frequently accompanied by delayed sexual maturation in the older child.

The effects of anemia on the circulatory system can be profound. A reduction in hemoglobin concentration that results in decreased oxygen-carrying capacity of the blood is associated with a compensatory increase in heart rate and cardiac output (see Box 28.2). Initially this greater cardiac output compensates for the lower oxygen-carrying capacity of the blood because blood replenished with oxygen returns to the

BOX 28.1 Red Blood Cell Morphology

Size (Cell Size)
Variation in red blood cell (RBC) sizes (anisocytosis)
- Normocytes (normal cell size)
- Microcytes (smaller than normal cell size)
- Macrocytes (larger than normal cell size)

Shape (Cell Shape)
Variation in RBC shapes (poikilocytosis)
- Spherocytes (globular cells)
- Drepanocytes (sickle-shaped cells)
- Numerous other irregularly shaped cells

Color (Cell Staining Characteristics)
Variation in hemoglobin concentration in the RBC
- Normochromic (sufficient or normal amount of hemoglobin per RBC)
- Hypochromic (reduced amount of hemoglobin per RBC)
- Hyperchromic (increased amount of hemoglobin per RBC)

RBC, Red blood cell.

BOX 28.2 Signs and Symptoms of Anemia

Decreased Red Blood Cell Production
Pallor
Tachycardia
Fatigue, headache
Muscle weakness
Systolic heart murmur
Frontal bossing

Increased Red Blood Cell Destruction
Icteric sclera, jaundice
Fatigue, headache
Tachycardia
Dark urine
Splenomegaly
Hepatomegaly
Low blood pressure (late sign of shock)

Increased Red Blood Cell Loss
Pallor
Fatigue, headache
Muscle weakness
Cool skin
Tachycardia
Decreased peripheral pulses
Low blood pressure (late sign of shock)

tissues at a faster than normal rate. The increased circulation and turbulence within the heart may produce a heart murmur. Because the cardiac workload increases during exercise, infection, or emotional stress, cardiac failure may occur.

Acute or chronic hemorrhage results in loss of plasma and all formed elements of the blood. After acute hemorrhage the body replaces plasma within 1 to 3 days, maintaining blood volume. However, this results in a low concentration of RBCs, which are gradually replaced within 3 to 4 weeks. During this period there is usually a normocytic normochromic anemia, provided that iron stores are sufficient for hemoglobin synthesis.

In chronic blood loss the actual number of RBCs may be normal because of continuous replacement. However, insufficient iron is available to form hemoglobin as quickly as it is lost. As a result, erythrocytes are usually microcytic and hypochromic.

Routine Screening

The major authorities cite the following recommendations:

American Academy of Family Physicians and US Preventive Services Task Force—All children should be screened for anemia once during infancy (US Department of Health and Human Services, 2009). Current evidence is insufficient to assess the balance of benefits (e.g., growth, cognition, psychomotor, or neurodevelopmental outcomes) and harms (e.g., false-positive results, anxiety, and cost) of screening for iron deficiency anemia in asymptomatic children ages 6 to 24 months with the measurement of serum hemoglobin or hematocrit as the usual first step (US Preventive Services Task Force, 2015; Siu, 2015).

American Academy of Pediatrics—Hemoglobin concentration or hematocrit should be measured once during infancy (between 9 and 12 months), early childhood (between 1 and 5 years), late childhood (between 5 and 12 years), and adolescence (between 14 and 20 years).

Canadian Task Force on the Periodic Health Examination—Hemoglobin concentration screening should be performed on children at high risk for iron deficiency anemia: preterm infants, infants born of a multiple pregnancy or to an iron deficient woman, infants with cow milk consumption greater than 500 ml/day, bottle use beyond 12 months, and children in low socioeconomic groups (Hartfield, 2010; Hepburn & Thibodeau, 2016).

Diagnostic Evaluation

In general, anemia may be suspected from findings on the history and physical examination, such as lack of energy, easy fatigability, and pallor. Unless the anemia is severe, however, another clue to the disorder may be alterations in the CBC, such as decreased numbers of RBCs and decreased hemoglobin and hematocrit levels. Although anemia is sometimes defined as a hemoglobin level below 10 or 11 g/dl, this arbitrary cutoff is inappropriate for all children because hemoglobin levels normally vary with age.

Various findings of the CBC are also significant, such as increased reticulocyte levels, which indicate the body's response to an increased demand for RBCs. A peripheral smear may demonstrate significant changes in the shape of RBCs, such as sickled cells. Tests to measure the amount of hemoglobin in a single cell are helpful in determining the cause of the anemia (see Table 28.1 and p. 1024). Sometimes a bone marrow aspiration may be necessary to evaluate the body's ability to produce normal cells. For example, in leukemia the bone marrow is hyperplastic (producing increased numbers of cells), whereas in aplastic anemia (see Aplastic Anemia, later in this chapter) the bone marrow is hypoplastic (producing decreased numbers of cells) or aplastic (producing no cells).

Tests for hematologic function do not always reflect the immediate changes occurring in the blood. For example, in acute massive hemorrhage the hemoglobin and hematocrit values may not be reliable because the plasma volume may not increase for several hours. Without the hemodilution caused by the reexpansion of the vascular space, the hemoglobin and hematocrit may be close to normal, and the RBC loss may not be apparent. Consequently, assessing the quantity of blood loss in a seriously ill child may be difficult. The estimated volume of blood loss must be analyzed in conjunction with the child's total blood volume to determine the percentage of blood loss. Blood specimens obtained from central lines may more accurately reflect the patient's status than specimens obtained from an extremity because of the vasoconstriction of the peripheral vasculature. Decreased blood pressure changes are a late sign because of the compensatory mechanisms.

Therapeutic Management

The objective of medical management is to reverse the anemia by treating the underlying cause. In nutritional anemias the specific deficiency is corrected. In blood loss from acute hemorrhage, RBC transfusion may be given. In patients with severe anemia, supportive medical care may include oxygen therapy, bed rest, and replacement of intravascular volume with intravenous (IV) fluids. In addition to these general measures, the nurse may implement more specific interventions, depending on the cause. The next sections discuss these interventions.

Nursing Care Management

The physical examination yields valuable evidence regarding the severity of the anemia and some indication of its possible cause (see Fig. 28.1 and Box 28.2). In interviewing the family, the nurse stresses the following areas: (1) nutrition, especially if the child is lactose intolerant or has inadequate intake of iron; (2) past history of chronic, recurrent infection; (3) eating habits, particularly pica (consumption of nonnutritive substances such as dirt, starch, lead-based paint chips, paper); (4) bowel habits and presence of frank blood in stools or black, tarry stools as a result of chronic blood loss; and (5) familial history of hereditary diseases, such as SCD or thalassemia.

The nurse should also be aware of the importance of taking a thorough history to obtain pertinent information that may aid in identifying the cause of the anemia. For example, statements such as "My child drinks a lot of milk" or "My teenager is on a liquid or vegetarian diet" are clues to possible iron deficiency.

Prepare the Child and Family for Laboratory Tests

Several blood tests may be ordered sequentially. Therefore the child may undergo multiple finger or heel sticks or venipunctures enduring repeated puncture trauma. These invasive procedures may be better tolerated with the application of a topical anesthetic known as EMLA (a eutectic mixture of lidocaine and prilocaine) or ELA-LMX (lidocaine) cream before needle punctures.

The nurse is responsible for preparing the child for the tests by (1) explaining the significance of each test, particularly why the tests are not all done at one time; (2) encouraging parent(s) or another supportive person to be with the child during the procedure; and (3) allowing the child to play with the equipment on a doll or to participate in the actual procedure (e.g., by holding the Band-Aid).

Older children may appreciate the opportunity to observe the blood cells under a microscope or in photographs. This experience is especially important if a serious blood disorder, such as aplastic anemia, is suspected because it serves as a foundation for explaining the pathophysiology of the disorder.

Bone marrow aspiration is not a routine hematologic test but is essential for definitive diagnosis of the certain anemias such as severe aplastic anemia. (Chapter 22 presents information on preparing the child.)

NURSING TIP

Suggested explanations to use in teaching children about blood components are as follows:

Red blood cells—Carry the oxygen you breathe from your lungs to all parts of your body

White blood cells—Help keep germs from causing infection

Platelets—Small parts of cells that help make bleeding stop by forming a clot (scab) over the hurt area

Plasma—The liquid portion of blood; has clotting factors that help make bleeding stop

Decrease Tissue Oxygen Needs

Because the basic pathology in anemia is a decrease in the oxygen-carrying capacity of the RBCs, an important nursing responsibility is to minimize tissue oxygen needs by continual assessment of the child's energy level. In most instances of anemia this is not necessary, but when it is, the nurse must implement several important interventions. These same interventions apply to any child with a nursing diagnosis of fatigue or activity intolerance.

! NURSING ALERT

Signs of exertion include tachycardia, palpitations, tachypnea, dyspnea, hyperpnea, dizziness, lightheadedness, diaphoresis, and change in skin color. The child looks fatigued (e.g., sagging, limp posture; slow, strained movements; inability to tolerate additional activity; difficulty sucking in infants).

Assess the child's level of tolerance for activities of daily living and play, and make adjustments to allow as much self-care as possible without undue exertion. During periods of rest the nurse measures vital signs and observes behavior to establish a baseline of nonexertion energy expenditure. During periods of activity the nurse repeats these measurements and observations to compare them with resting values.

Once a baseline of physical tolerance has been established, the nurse anticipates which activities will be physically taxing, such as dressing, feeding, or getting out of bed, and allows for conservation of energy by assisting the child as needed. Because dependency can be threatening, however, allow the child as much control in the environment as possible. For example, a child with severe anemia may be unable to walk to the bathroom but may be able to use a bedside commode or be transported in a wheelchair to the lavatory rather than having to use a bedpan. Scheduling activities throughout the day with planned rest periods in between maximizes the child's energy potential without causing undue exertion. Anticipate and implement necessary safety measures (e.g., staying with the child when the child is out of bed and raising side rails when the child is in the bed to prevent falls).

Plan diversional activities that promote rest but prevent boredom and withdrawal. Because short attention span, irritability, and restlessness are common in anemia and increase stress demands on the body, plan appropriate activities such as the following:

- Listening to music, using earphones, wireless earbuds, or headsets
- Watching television or playing video games
- Reading or listening to stories
- Continuing a favorite hobby, such as stamp or rock collecting
- Coloring or drawing
- Playing board and card games
- Being transported in wheelchair or stroller

Choosing the appropriate roommate, such as a child of similar age with a diagnosis that also requires restricted activity, is another helpful intervention.

If infants or young children are hospitalized, consider the importance of preventing separation from parents. Crying and fretfulness place greater stress demands on the body, which increase oxygen needs. Parents may need help in understanding the importance of their presence and the basis for their child's mood changes.

Prevent Complications

Children with anemia are prone to infection because tissue hypoxia causes cellular dysfunction, and the disturbed metabolic processes weaken the host's defenses against foreign agents. Infection also worsens the anemia by increasing metabolic needs and, in instances of chronic infection, also interferes with erythropoiesis and shortens the survival time of RBCs. Take all of the usual precautions to prevent infection, such as practicing thorough hand washing, selecting an appropriate room in a noninfectious area, restricting visitors or hospital personnel with active infection, and maintaining adequate nutrition. The nurse also observes for signs of infection, particularly temperature elevation and leukocytosis. However, an elevated WBC count sometimes occurs in anemia without the presence of systemic or local infection.

Drawing multiple blood samples may present a problem with cumulative blood loss and necessitate blood replacement. This situation occurs most often in infants with severe anemia. To prevent this situation, blood may be withdrawn through a continuous IV line and replaced after the exact amount needed has been tested and discarded. As a precaution, keep a record of the volume of blood withdrawn. Using micromethods of testing whenever possible minimizes the amount of blood required for the test. The nurse needs to observe for cumulative effects of blood loss, particularly signs of shock and increased hypoxia, and to explain to parents the necessity for taking multiple blood samples and the reason for blood replacement.

The main complication of anemia is cardiac decompensation, which can result from excessive demands on the heart due to increased metabolic needs or cardiac overload. The nurse should observe for signs and symptoms of heart failure such as tachycardia, dyspnea, rales, moist respirations, cough, and sweating. Obviously, preventing heart failure by minimizing hypoxia and closely monitoring IV infusions is of first priority. Packed RBCs are usually administered to prevent circulatory hypervolemia. When blood transfusions are required in severe anemia to increase the hemoglobin level, follow all of the usual precautions for administering blood and observe for signs of transfusion reactions (Table 28.2).

BLOOD TRANSFUSION THERAPY

Technologic advances in blood banking and transfusion medicine allow the administration of only the blood component needed by the child, such as packed RBCs in anemia or platelets for bleeding disorders (Table 28.3). Regardless of the blood component administered, the nurse must be aware of the possibility of transfusion reactions.

Although hemolytic reactions are rare, ABO incompatibility remains the most common cause of death from blood transfusion, and human error is usually responsible (e.g., administration of blood of the wrong type to the patient or mislabeling of a blood product) (Pahuja, Puri, Mahajan, et al., 2017; Strauss, 2016). Blood is usually matched between the donor and recipient for blood group (A, B, AB, or O) and Rh factor (positive or negative). However, AB-type RBCs can be transfused into individuals with blood types A, B, and AB, and Rh-negative RBCs can be given to Rh-positive individuals.

TABLE 28.2 Nursing Care of the Child Receiving Blood Transfusions

Complication	Signs and Symptoms	Precautions and Nursing Responsibilities
Immediate Reactions		
Hemolytic reactions		
Most severe type, but rare Incompatible blood Incompatibility in multiple transfusions	Sudden severe headache Chills Shaking Fever Pain at needle site and along venous tract Nausea and vomiting Sensation of tightness in chest Red or black urine Flank pain Progressive signs of shock or renal failure	Identify donor and recipient blood types and groups before transfusion is begun; verify with another nurse or practitioner. Transfuse blood slowly for first 15-20 min and/or initial 20% of blood volume; remain with patient. Stop transfusion immediately in event signs or symptoms occur, maintain patent intravenous line, and notify practitioner. Save donor blood to recrossmatch with patient's blood. Monitor for evidence of shock. Insert urinary catheter and monitor hourly outputs. Send sample of patient's blood and urine to laboratory for presence of hemoglobin (indicates intravascular hemolysis). Observe for signs of hemorrhage resulting from disseminated intravascular coagulation. Support medical therapies to reverse shock.
Febrile reactions		
Leukocyte or platelet antibodies Plasma protein antibodies	Fever Chills	May give acetaminophen for prophylaxis. Leukocyte-poor red blood cells (RBCs) are less likely to cause reaction. Stop transfusion immediately; report to practitioner for evaluation.
Allergic reactions		
Recipient reaction to allergens in donor's blood	Urticaria Pruritus Flushing Asthmatic wheezing Laryngeal edema	Give antihistamines for prophylaxis to children with tendency to allergic reactions. Stop transfusion immediately. Administer epinephrine for wheezing or anaphylactic reaction.
Circulatory overload		
Too rapid transfusion (even a small quantity) Transfusion of excessive quantity of blood (even slowly)	Precordial pain Dyspnea Rales Cyanosis Dry cough Distended neck veins Hypertension	Transfuse blood slowly. Prevent overload by using packed RBCs or administering divided amounts of blood. Use infusion pump to regulate and maintain flow rate. Stop transfusion immediately if signs of overload. Place child upright with feet in dependent position to increase venous resistance.
Air emboli		
May occur when blood is transfused under pressure	Sudden difficulty in breathing Sharp pain in chest Apprehension	Normalize pressure before container is empty when infusing blood under pressure. Clear tubing of air by aspirating air with syringe at nearest Y connector if air is observed in tubing; disconnect tubing and allow blood to flow until air has escaped only if a Y connector is not available.
Hypothermia		
	Chills Low temperature Irregular heart rate Possible cardiac arrest	Allow blood to warm at room temperature (<1 hour). Use approved mechanical blood warmer or electric warming coil to warm blood rapidly; never use microwave oven. Take temperature if patient complains of chills; if subnormal, stop transfusion.
Electrolyte disturbances		
Hyperkalemia (in massive transfusions or in patients with renal problems)	Nausea, diarrhea Muscular weakness Flaccid paralysis Paresthesia of extremities Bradycardia Apprehension Cardiac arrest	Use washed RBCs or fresh blood if patient is at risk.
Delayed Reactions		
Transmission of infection		
Hepatitis Human immunodeficiency virus (HIV) infection Malaria Syphilis Other bacterial or viral infection	Signs of infection (e.g., jaundice) Toxic reaction—High fever, severe headache or substernal pain, hypotension, intense flushing, vomiting or diarrhea	Blood is tested for antibodies to HIV, hepatitis C virus, and hepatitis B core antigen; in addition, blood is tested for hepatitis B surface antigen and alanine aminotransferase, and a serologic test is performed for syphilis. Units that test positive are destroyed. Individuals at risk for carrying certain viruses are deterred from donation. Report any sign of infection and, if it occurs during transfusion, stop transfusion immediately, send sample for culture and sensitivity testing, and notify practitioner.

TABLE 28.2 Nursing Care of the Child Receiving Blood Transfusions—cont'd

Complication	Signs and Symptoms	Precautions and Nursing Responsibilities
Alloimmunization		
Antibody formation Occurs in patients receiving multiple transfusions	Increased risk of hemolytic, febrile, and allergic reactions	Use limited number of donors. Observe carefully for signs of reactions.
Delayed hemolytic reaction		
	Destruction of RBCs and fever 5-10 days after transfusion	Observe for posttransfusion anemia and decreasing benefit from successive transfusion.

TABLE 28.3 Nursing Administration of Blood Components

Component and Indications	Dosage	Nursing Administration
Packed red blood cells (PRBCs) Symptomatic anemia Renal or liver disease Hemolysis Decreased erythropoiesis Splenic or liver sequestration **Whole blood** (rarely used) Acute massive blood loss	Volume packed RBCs = Weight (kg) × Change in hematocrit (Hct) desired Volume of whole blood = Weight (kg) × Change in Hct desired × 2	1. Assess for PRBC reaction (e.g., pruritus, rash, cough, fever). 2. Regulate infusion rate using microaggregate filter via infusion pump to 5 ml/kg/hr over 2-4 hours (usual rate). Do not use the tubing to infuse more than 1 unit of blood. 3. Monitor vital signs before transfusion, 15 minutes after initiation, hourly during transfusion, and on completion of transfusion. 4. Do not refrigerate blood in the nursing unit. Use only the blood bank refrigerator. 5. Ensure that each unit is infused ≤4 hours. If a longer infusion time is needed, the unit must be divided in the blood bank. 6. Do not infuse solutions other than normal saline in the line with RBCs.
Fresh frozen plasma (FFP) Deficiencies of plasma clotting factors in bleeding patients (e.g., disseminated intravascular coagulation [DIC]); liver failure; vitamin K deficiency with bleeding; or replacement of antithrombin III (ATIII), protein C, or protein S	10-15 ml/kg (use within 6-24 hours of thawing)	1. Assess for FFP reaction (e.g., pain, bleeding, swelling). 2. Regulate infusion rate using microaggregate filter to 20 ml/min over 1-2 hours q 12-24 hours until hemorrhage stops. 3. Monitor prothrombin time (PT) and partial thromboplastin time (PPT) before and after FFP infusion. 4. Monitor levels of other coagulation factors (e.g., fibrinogen, fibrin split products, D-dimer, ATIII, protein C, and protein S).
Platelets (plt) Active hemorrhage, DIC Thrombocytopenia with bleeding or if indicated by clinical status	1 unit/10 kg or 6 unit/m^2 intravenously (IV)	1. Assess for plt reaction (e.g., pruritus, rash, fever, bleeding). 2. Regulate infusion rate using 170-mm microaggregate filter to 10 ml/kg/hr, IV push or over 1 hour or as fast as patient can tolerate. 3. Monitor vital signs before transfusion, 15 minutes after initiation, and at the end of infusion. 4. Obtain postplatelet count 60 minutes to 24 hours after infusion.
Granulocytes (rarely used) As adjunct with other measures in treatment of severe infections in the septic neonate or high-risk patient (e.g., proven bacterial infection in severely neutropenic patient unresponsive to antibiotic therapy)	10-15 ml/kg IV usually daily × 4 days	1. Assess for granulocyte reaction (e.g., chills, rash, dyspnea). 2. Monitor vital signs before transfusion, 15 minutes after initiation, and at the end of transfusion. 3. Premedicate 1 hours before transfusion, usually with antihistamines, acetaminophen, or steroids. 4. Infuse at slow rate (2-4 hours) using 170-mm blood filter within a 24-hour period. 5. Minimum of 4-6 hours between amphotericin B and granulocyte infusion recommended.
Factor VIII (plasma derived or recombinant) Hemophilia A Acquired factor VIII deficiency **Factor IX (plasma derived or recombinant)** Hemophilia B **FEIBA (factor eight inhibitor bypass activity), plasma derived** Hemophilia A or B with inhibitors (antibodies) **Factor VIIa (recombinant)** Hemophilia A or B with inhibitors	1 unit/kg IV of factor VIII = 2% of factor activity 35-50 units/kg IV of factor VIII q 12-24 hours 1 unit/kg of factor IX = 1% of factor activity 30-50 units/kg IV q 24 hours 75-100 units/kg IV q 8-24 hours (maximum dose 200 units/kg/day) 90 mcg/kg IV q 2 hours (35-120 mcg/kg dosage range)	1. Assess adverse reaction (e.g., hives, itchy wheals with redness, tightness in chest, wheezing, low blood pressure, or dyspnea). Notify health care provider immediately if symptoms are present. 2. Use reconstituted factor within 3 hours of mixing. 3. Inject reconstituted factor intravenously over 2-5 minutes.
Cryoprecipitate (CRYO) (rarely used) Control bleeding in patients with DIC Hypofibrinogenemia	4 bags CRYO/10 kg IV	1. Assess CRYO reaction (e.g., rash, bleeding). 2. Monitor closely PT/PPT and levels of fibrinogen, fibrinogen split products, D-dimer. 3. Use a filter needle to draw up and administer within 15-30 minutes.

DIC, Disseminated intravascular coagulation; *HIV,* human immunodefiency virus; *RBC,* red blood cell.

When blood is mismatched, the A or B antiagglutinin is mixed with RBCs containing A or B agglutinogens, respectively, and agglutination (clumping) of the RBCs occurs. The agglutinins, which are bivalent, attach themselves to two different erythrocytes at the same time, causing the cells to clump together and clog small blood vessels. Over a few hours to days, the entrapped cells degenerate and hemolyze, liberating excessive quantities of hemoglobin into the circulation. The eventual hemolysis of large numbers of RBCs decreases the blood volume, which causes circulatory failure and shock. Treatment is aimed at replacing lost blood and using plasma volume expanders.

Acute kidney shutdown and eventual renal failure are the result of renal vasoconstriction caused by antigen-antibody complexes derived from the RBC surface. The greatly reduced blood flow leads to complete renal failure and death within 7 to 12 days. Treatment involves promoting diuresis with rapid administration of dilute IV fluids and diuretics such as furosemide and mannitol, and alkalinizing body fluids, which renders hemoglobin more soluble.

Another consequence of hemolysis is the release of large quantities of phospholipids, which are capable of stimulating disseminated intravascular coagulation (DIC) (see p. 1056). As a result, the plasma is depleted of the coagulation factors needed to prevent hemorrhage. Without treatment with heparin to prevent the coagulation and with blood components to initiate clotting, death from generalized hemorrhage can occur.

In addition to the nursing precautions and responsibilities outlined in Table 28.2, other general guidelines that apply to all transfusions include the following:

- Take vital signs, including blood pressure, before administering blood to establish baseline data for intratransfusion and posttransfusion comparison: 15 minutes after initiation, hourly while blood is infusing, and on completion of the transfusion.
- Check the blood type and group of the recipient against the donor's, regardless of the blood product used.
- Administer the first 50 ml of blood or initial 20% of volume (whichever is smaller) slowly and stay with the child.
- Administer with normal saline in a piggyback setup or have normal saline available.
- Administer blood through an appropriate filter to eliminate particles in the blood and prevent the precipitation of formed elements; gently shake the container frequently.
- Use blood within 30 minutes of its arrival from the blood bank. If it is not used, return it to the blood bank; do not store it in a regular unit refrigerator.
- Infuse a unit of blood (or the specified amount) within 4 hours. If the infusion will exceed this time, divide the blood into appropriate-size quantities by the blood bank, with the unused portion refrigerated under controlled conditions.
- If a reaction of any type is suspected, stop the transfusion, take vital signs, maintain a patent IV line with normal saline and new tubing, notify the practitioner, and do not restart the transfusion until the child's condition has been medically evaluated.

Blood is usually administered to children by infusion pump; therefore the usual precautions and management related to pumps apply. When the blood infusion begins with a standard transfusion set, the filter chamber is filled to allow the total filter to be used. The drip chamber is partially filled with blood to permit counting of the drops. When the flow rate is adjusted, remember that blood administration sets do not use microdrops (60 drops/ml) but regular drops (usually 10 or 15 drops/ml). The nurse must consider this when calculating the flow rate.

Oxygen may be administered to provide optimum environmental conditions for hemoglobin saturation. Oxygen administration is of limited value, however, because each gram of hemoglobin is able to carry a limited amount of the gas. In addition, prolonged use of supplemental oxygen can decrease erythropoiesis. Therefore monitor the child closely for evidence of decreasing benefit from oxygen. One of the first signs of hypoxia is restlessness.

ANEMIA CAUSED BY NUTRITIONAL DEFICIENCIES

IRON DEFICIENCY ANEMIA

Anemia caused by an inadequate supply or loss of iron is the most prevalent nutritional disorder worldwide and the most preventable mineral disturbance. Over the past decade, the prevalence of iron deficiency anemia has declined during infancy in the United States (Mahoney, 2017). The reduced prevalence of iron deficiency anemia in infants has been partly attributed to American Academy of Pediatrics' promotion of iron-fortified formula instead of cow's milk during the first year of life in conjunction with the US Special Supplemental Nutrition Program for Women, Infants, and Children (WIC) that provides iron-fortified formula and routine screening of Hgb levels during early childhood (Baker, Greer, & Committee on Nutrition, 2010; Fleming, 2015; Powers & Buchanan, 2014). The promotion of iron supplement in the exclusively breastfed infant, introduction of iron-fortified infant formula and cereal, weaning from the bottle by 1 year of age, limiting intake of cow's milk to 16 to 24 oz/day, and delayed introduction of cow's milk into the diet have also contributed to the decreased incidence of iron deficiency anemia in infants and young children (Fleming, 2015; Sills, 2016). Adolescent are also at risk for iron deficiency because of their rapid growth rate, menses, poor eating habits, obesity, and strenuous activities (Fleming, 2015; Sills, 2016). However, iron deficiency both with and without anemia still remains to be a relatively common health problem, especially among at-risk children (Fleming, 2015; Mahoney, 2017; Miller, 2013).

Etiology

Iron deficiency anemia can be caused by any number of factors that decrease the supply of iron, impair its absorption, increase the body's need for iron, or affect the synthesis of hemoglobin (Box 28.3). Although the clinical manifestations and diagnostic evaluation are similar regardless of the cause, the therapeutic and nursing care management depends on the specific reason for the iron deficiency. The following discussion is limited to iron deficiency anemia resulting from inadequate iron in the diet.

At birth the full-term infant has approximately a 0.5 g supply of iron, and an average of 0.8 mg of iron must be absorbed each day during the first 15 years of life (Sills, 2016). During the last trimester of pregnancy, iron is transferred from the mother to the fetus at the rate of 4 mg/day. Most of the iron is stored in the circulating hemoglobin of the erythrocytes, and the remainder is deposited in the liver, spleen, and bone marrow. Along with maternal iron supplements, delayed umbilical clamping for 1 to 3 minutes can improve iron status and reduce the risk of iron deficiency in the newborn (Anderson, Domeliof, Anderson, et al., 2014; Mercer, Erickson-Owens, Collins, et al., 2017; Miller, 2013; Sills, 2016). Maternally derived iron stores are adequate for the first 5 to 6 months in the full-term infant but for only about 2 to 3 months in premature infants or infants of multiple births. If dietary sources of iron are not supplied to meet the infant's growth demands after depletion of fetal iron stores, iron deficiency anemia results. Physiologic anemia should not be confused with iron deficiency anemia resulting from nutritional causes.

Vegetarian diets, popular among teenage girls, have been associated with nutritional deficiencies. Some infants and toddlers who have been

BOX 28.3 Causes of Iron Deficiency Anemia

Inadequate Supply of Iron

Deficient dietary intake

- Rapid growth rate
- Excessive milk intake, delayed addition of solid foods
- Poor general eating habits
- Exclusive breastfeeding of infant after 6 months of age

Inadequate iron stores at birth

- Low birth weight, prematurity, multiple births
- Severe iron deficiency in mother (hemoglobin level <9 g/dl)
- Fetal blood loss at or before delivery

Impaired Iron Absorption

Presence of iron inhibitors

- Phytates, phosphates, or oxalates
- Gastric alkalinity

Malabsorption disorders

- Lactose intolerance
- Inflammatory bowel disease

Chronic diarrhea

Blood Loss

Acute or chronic hemorrhage

Parasitic infestation

Excessive Demands for Iron Required for Growth

Prematurity

Adolescence

Pregnancy

fed inappropriate vegetarian diets have had severe protein-energy malnutrition, as well as deficiencies of iron, vitamin B_{12}, and vitamin D. Unrefined cereals contain substances that modify the absorption of minerals such as zinc, calcium, and iron. Individuals consuming strict vegetarian diets that include a large amount of unrefined cereals could be at a greater risk of rickets, vitamin B_{12} and folate deficiency, and iron deficiency anemia (Camaschella, 2015; Renda & Fischer, 2009).

Pathophysiology

Iron is required for the production of hemoglobin. One molecule of hemoglobin consists of protein (globin) combined with four molecules of a pigmented compound (heme). Each molecule of heme contains one atom of iron. When iron stores are deficient, the production of hemoglobin is reduced. Consequently, the main effect of iron deficiency is decreased hemoglobin level and reduced oxygen-carrying capacity of the blood.

Clinical Manifestations

The clinical manifestations are directly attributable to the reduction in the amount of oxygen available to the tissues and resemble those seen in any type of anemia. Usually the signs are insidious and obscure, and the severity is directly related to the duration of the dietary deficiency.

Although infants with iron deficiency anemia tend to be underweight, many are overweight because of excessive milk ingestion (known as *milk baby*). These children become anemic for two reasons: milk, a poor source of iron, is given almost to the exclusion of solid foods, and increased fecal loss of blood occurs in 50% of iron deficient infants fed cow's milk. This asymptomatic loss of hemoglobin causes iron deficiency (Griebler, Bruckmuller, Kien, et al., 2015; Richardson, 2007; Sills, 2016). Although chubby, these infants are pale (sometimes porcelain-like), usually demonstrate poor muscle development, and are prone to infection.

Although the mechanism is unknown, iron deficiency anemia enhances the leakage of plasma proteins, which causes edema; retarded growth; and decreased serum concentration of the proteins albumin, gamma globulin, and transferrin (a protein that binds iron and transports it through the plasma). Other manifestations of iron deficiency include irritability, tachycardia, fatigue, glossitis, angular stomatitis, and koilonychia (concave or "spoon" fingernails). The association between iron deficiency anemia and impaired neurocognitive function (e.g., attention span, memory, alertness, learning and behavioral problems) in both infants and adolescents has been established, but the mechanism by which iron deficiency anemia impairs neurologic function is unknown (Fleming, 2015; Sills, 2016).

Diagnostic Evaluation

Laboratory tests that measure or describe hemoglobin, the morphologic changes in the RBC, and iron concentration are usually performed (see Table 28.1). The RBC count may be normal, borderline, or moderately reduced in the child with iron deficiency anemia. Typically, the nearly normal number of erythrocytes is strikingly out of proportion to the low hemoglobin concentration. RBCs are typically small (microcytic), so that MCV is decreased (see Box 28.1). For infants 1 year of age, an MCV below 70 femtoliters (fl) is considered diagnostic. In children from 1 to 10 years of age, an MCV value of 70 fl plus the child's age in years is a quick calculation of the lower limit of normal.

The reticulocyte count is usually normal or slightly reduced because of decreased stores of iron (see Table 28.1). However, in severe anemia, when tissue hypoxia elicits an erythropoietic response, the reticulocyte count may be elevated to 3% or 4%. The level of erythrocyte protoporphyrin, the immediate precursor of heme, becomes elevated in RBCs whenever heme synthesis is disturbed.

In terms of differential diagnosis, a stool analysis for occult blood (guaiac test) is commonly performed to confirm or rule out the possibility of chronic fecal blood loss, especially from milk intolerance or structural anomalies such as diverticulitis.

Iron Studies

In addition to tests that indirectly indicate the level of iron by revealing the effects of iron deficiency on the RBCs, several other tests are usually performed that more directly measure the amount of circulating iron. The serum iron concentration (SIC) is the amount of circulating iron and is normally about 70 mcg/dl in infants and slightly higher in older children. Lower limits of SIC vary not only with age but also with the time of day; they are highest in the morning, when the test should be performed.

The total iron-binding capacity (TIBC) is the amount of transferrin (iron-binding globulin), which is necessary for the transport of iron in the bloodstream. When combined with transferrin, the iron is loosely bound to the globulin molecule so that it can be released easily to tissue cells anywhere in the body. In iron deficiency anemia TIBC is elevated above the normal range of 350 mcg/dl (6 months to 2 years) or 450 mcg/dl (children >2 years and adults). The elevated TIBC represents the body's compensatory mechanism to absorb more iron from exogenous sources than normally during states of deficiency. Transferrin saturation is calculated by dividing the SIC by the TIBC and multiplying the result by 100 to express the value as a percentage. A transferrin saturation of 10% suggests anemia.

These biochemical tests (ferritin, TIBC, SIC) are acute phase reactants, which means in an inflammatory setting a positive acute phase reactant may overestimate iron stores (Fleming, 2015; Sills, 2016). It has been recommended that the ferritin level be used simultaneously with measurement of C-reactive protein (CRP) to identify false-negative results associated with inflammation (Baker, Greer, & Committee on Nutrition, 2010; Sills, 2016). Other tests not affected by inflammation that are available in some clinical laboratories are the serum transferrin receptor (validated only in adults as elevated in iron deficiency) and reticulocyte hemoglobin content used in all ages, which has been used to accurately assess iron status (Baker, Greer, & Committee on Nutrition, 2010; DeLoughery, 2014; Fleming, 2015; Sills, 2016).

Therapeutic Management

Prevention is the primary goal and is achieved through optimum nutrition and appropriate iron supplementation. In infants, the following guidelines are recommended to prevent iron deficiency (American Academy of Pediatrics, Committee on Nutrition, 1999; Baker, Greer, & Committee on Nutrition, 2010; Sills, 2016):

- Use only breast milk or iron-fortified formula (containing 10 to 12 mg/L for full-term infants and 15 mg/L for preterm infants of iron) for the first 12 months.
- Iron supplementation of 1 mg/kg/day should be provided by 4 to 6 months of age in full-term infants and 2 mg/kg/day by 2 months of age in preterm infants.
- Administer iron drops at a dosage of 2 to 3 mg/kg/day to a maximum of 15 mg/day of elemental iron to breastfed preterm infants after 2 months of age, and give iron-fortified infant cereal when solid foods are introduced.
- Limit the amount of formula to no more than 1 L/day to encourage intake of iron-rich solid foods.
- Universal screening for anemia should be performed at approximately 12 months of age with determination of Hgb concentration and assessment of risk factors associated with iron deficiency anemia.

After the diagnosis of iron deficiency anemia is made, therapeutic management focuses on increasing the amount of supplemental iron the child receives. This is usually done through dietary counseling and the administration of oral iron supplements. In formula-fed infants the most convenient and best sources of supplemental iron are iron-fortified commercial formula and iron-fortified infant cereal (Baker, Greer, & Committee on Nutrition, 2010; National Institutes of Health, 2016). Iron-fortified formula provides a relatively constant and predictable amount of iron and is not associated with an increased incidence of gastrointestinal (GI) symptoms, such as colic, diarrhea, or constipation. Infants younger than 12 months old should *not* be given fresh cow's milk because it may increase the risk of GI blood loss occurring from exposure to a heat-labile protein in cow's milk or cow's milk–induced GI mucosal damage resulting from a lack of cytochrome iron (heme protein) (Kett, 2012; Subramaniam & Girish, 2015). If GI bleeding is suspected, several stool analyses for occult blood known as *guaiac tests* are performed to identify any intermittent blood loss.

If the addition of iron-rich foods to the diet does not provide sufficient supplemental quantities of the mineral, oral iron supplements are prescribed. Ferrous iron is more readily absorbed than ferric iron and results in higher hemoglobin levels. Ingested iron is absorbed largely from the duodenum, and absorption is facilitated by an acid environment. Children normally absorb an average of 10% to 20% of the iron in oral supplements, but during periods of iron deficiency they absorb an additional 5% to 10%. Oral iron supplementation is prescribed as 3 to 6 mg of elemental iron per kilogram per day. Lower dosages of iron are associated with fewer side effects. Ideally the daily dose of iron should be given in two or three divided doses between meals. Ascorbic acid (vitamin C) appears to facilitate absorption of iron and may be given as vitamin C–enriched foods and juices with the iron preparation. Side effects of oral iron therapy include nausea, gastric irritation, diarrhea or constipation, and anorexia, but these occur infrequently, especially in infants. If the iron produces vomiting and diarrhea, it should be administered with meals and in gradually increasing doses.

The response to oral iron therapy is reflected in a peak increase in the reticulocyte count by the fifth to tenth day of administration. After the reticulocyte rise, the hemoglobin and hematocrit levels and RBC count increase. The hemoglobin level rises from 0.1 to 0.4 g/dl/24 hr depending on anemia severity; therefore a substantial increase should occur by the end of 1 month (Richardson, 2007; Sills, 2016).

If the hemoglobin level fails to rise after 1 month of oral therapy, it is important to assess noncompliance, persistent bleeding, iron malabsorption, improper iron administration, or other causes of anemia. Parenteral (IV or intramuscular) iron administration is safe and effective but is painful, expensive, and occasionally associated with regional lymphadenopathy, transient arthralgias, or serious allergic reaction (Bregman & Goodnough, 2014; Fleming, 2015). Therefore parenteral iron administration is reserved for children who have iron malabsorption, chronic hemoglobinuria, or intolerance to oral preparations. The deep intramuscular injection route for iron administration is discouraged because it is painful and may leak into the subcutaneous tissue causing skin discoloration at the injection site. Careful observation with IV iron administration is required because of the risk of anaphylaxis, so a test dose is recommended before use. Several IV iron preparations (e.g., ferumoxytol, ferric carboxymaltose, iron sucrose complex, iron isomaltoside) show promise in complete replacement of iron with little toxicity (Auerbach, 2011; DeLoughery, 2014; Smith, 2012). Transfusions are indicated for the most severe anemia and in cases of serious infection, cardiac dysfunction, or surgical emergency when anesthesia is required. Packed RBCs (2 to 3 ml/kg), not whole blood, are used to minimize the chance of circulatory overload. Supplemental oxygen is administered when tissue hypoxia is severe.

As macrocytic anemias, both folate and vitamin B_{12} deficiencies result in defective ribonucleic acid (RNA) and deoxyribonucleic acid (DNA) synthesis (Carmel, Watkins, & Rosenblatt, 2015; Lerner, 2016). Folate deficiency is a common micronutrient disorder that is caused by inadequate diet, overcooking of vegetables with loss of folates, and/or malabsorption. The deficiency is treated with correctly prepared and intake of folate-enriched foods and/or 1 mg of folate daily (Carmel, Watkins, & Rosenblatt, 2015; Smith, 2012).

Vitamin B_{12} deficiency commonly develops when the gastric mucosa fails to secrete sufficient intrinsic factor, which is essential for absorption of vitamin B_{12}. Deprived of vitamin B_{12}, the bone marrow produces fewer but macrocytic RBCs. The erythrocytes are usually immature and, because of their extremely fragile cell membranes, are rapidly destroyed during circulation. Treatment initially involves the administration of a 100-mcg or higher dose of vitamin B_{12} parenteral therapy for several days, followed by injections of 500 or 1000 mcg of vitamin B_{12} every 1 to 2 months. Researchers compared oral and parenteral vitamin B_{12} therapy and found that they yielded comparable benefits (Chan, Low, & Lee, 2016; Smith, 2012; Vidal-Alaball, Butler, Cannings-John, et al., 2016).

Prognosis

Prognosis for a child with iron deficiency anemia, folate deficiency, or vitamin B_{12} deficiency is very good. There is evidence that if the anemia is severe and long-standing, diminished cognitive function, behavioral changes, delayed infant growth and development, decreased exercise tolerance, and impaired immune function may develop (Angulo-Barroso, Li, Santos, et al., 2016; Fleming, 2015; Jauregui-Lobera, 2014). However, there is lack of convincing evidence that iron treatment of young children with iron deficiency anemia or nonanemic iron deficiency has an effect on psychomotor development or cognitive function (Abdullah, Thorpe, Mamak, et al., 2015; McDonagh, Blazina, Dana, et al., 2015; Thompson, Biggs, & Pasricha, 2013; Wang, Zhan, Gong, et al., 2013). However, there is need for further large long-term follow-up randomized interventional studies to be conducted.

Nursing Care Management

A primary nursing objective is to prevent nutritional anemia through family education. Nurses need to be aware of recommendations regarding iron supplementation during infancy and appropriate sources of dietary iron. The nurse should encourage parents to limit the quantity of milk, to use iron-fortified infant formulas, and to introduce solid foods. This may be difficult when parents believe milk is best for the infant and equate the resultant weight gain with "healthiness." Although milk is an excellent food, it is deficient in iron, vitamin C, zinc, and fluoride. Sources of each of these nutrients and the role they play in preventing deficiencies need to be discussed with the family, especially the person responsible for feeding the infant. For example, the mother may have less decision-making power regarding feeding than the grandmother who cares for the child.

Also stress that overweight is not synonymous with good health. If the infant has obvious signs of anemia, such as pallor, listlessness, frequent infections, and muscular weakness, point these out as evidence of suboptimum health. In some instances, it is helpful to chart the hemoglobin or hematocrit values to visually impress on parents the change in iron levels. Often, increased blood values correspond to improved physical status and reinforce the benefit of dietary or oral iron supplementation. It should be stressed with the family that the iron medication must continue for 2 to 3 months after blood values normalize to replenish the body's iron stores.

Instructing parents regarding proper administration of oral iron supplements is an essential nursing responsibility. Several factors, such as stomach acidity, affect the absorption of iron (see Quality Patient Outcomes box).

QUALITY PATIENT OUTCOMES

Iron Deficiency Anemia

- Early recognition of signs and symptoms of iron deficiency anemia
- Appropriate quantity of milk, use of iron-fortified infant formula, and introduction of solid foods
- Adherence to oral iron supplement and appropriate administration
- Hemoglobin increase within 1 month and anemia resolved within 6 months

DRUG ALERT

Iron Supplements

Ideally iron supplements are administered in two divided doses between meals, when the presence of free hydrochloric acid is greatest, and are accompanied by a citrus fruit or juice, which helps reduce iron to its most soluble state.

An adequate dosage of oral iron turns the stools a tarry green or black color. The nurse advises parents of this normally expected change and inquires about its occurrence on follow-up visits. Absence of the greenish-black stool may be a clue to poor compliance. If compliance is an issue, make every effort to institute strategies to improve adherence to the medication regimen, such as administering the drug once a day at the most convenient time. (See Compliance, Chapter 22)

Oral iron supplements are available in liquid or tablet form. Liquid preparations may temporarily stain the teeth. If possible, take the medication through a straw or give it through a syringe or medicine dropper placed toward the back of the mouth. Brushing the teeth after administration of the drug lessens the discoloration.

NURSING ALERT

Because iron ingested in excessive quantities is toxic, even fatal, parents should keep no more than a 1-month supply in the home and store it safely away from the reach of children.

Counseling families whose children are anemic is often a difficult and challenging task. Meal planning must be based on the family's budget, cultural pattern, and food preferences (see Cultural Considerations box). Often this requires more than a brief discussion with the mother or usual caregiver about foods high in iron. For teaching to be effective, the nurse may need to offer recipes, assist in planning a shopping list, and investigate food prices for economy. Because the physical effects of anemia are insidious, parents may not consider their child ill and consequently may view the medication and diet changes as unnecessary. Stressing the physical and behavioral improvements and what effect the improved diet will have on all family members may encourage parents to adhere to the treatment plan.

CULTURAL CONSIDERATIONS

Tea Drinking and Nonheme Iron Absorption

In cultures in which tea is drunk as a common beverage, administer iron with some other liquid because the tannins in tea form an insoluble complex with nonheme iron that is from foods other than meat. In addition, the phytates in legumes and maize and the phenolic compounds in herbal teas may adversely affect the uptake of iron (Baird-Gunning & Bromley, 2016; Camaschella, 2015). There is clear evidence to show that tea drinking limits the absorption of nonheme iron, whereas ascorbic acid enhances iron absorption (Fan, 2016; Nelson & Poulter, 2004; Thankachan, Walczyk, Muthayya, et al., 2008).

Diet education of teenagers is difficult, especially because teenage girls are particularly prone to following weight-reduction diets. Emphasizing the effect of anemia on appearance (pallor) and energy level (difficulty maintaining popular activities) may be useful.

ANEMIAS CAUSED BY INCREASED DESTRUCTION OF RED BLOOD CELLS

Excessive destruction or hemolysis of erythrocytes can occur from a defect in the RBC (intracorpuscular defect) that shortens the life span of the cell so that production cannot keep pace with destruction. In sickle cell anemia and thalassemia, erythrocyte life spans are decreased because of a hemoglobin defect, whereas in spherocytosis erythrocyte life span is decreased due to a defective red cell membrane. Extracorpuscular factors are those conditions that cause hemolysis in otherwise normal RBCs. A classic example is blood group incompatibility, such as hemolytic disease of the newborn or incompatibility secondary to mismatched blood transfusion. Damage to a normal red cell may be caused by toxic drugs, burns, poisonings (such as from lead), infections (such as malaria), and splenic sequestration (hypersplenism).

HEREDITARY SPHEROCYTOSIS

Hereditary spherocytosis (HS), a common hemolytic disorder, is caused by a defect in the proteins that form the RBC membrane (Lux, 2015; Segel & Casey, 2016). It occurs in most ethnic groups, but it is primarily prevalent in persons of northern European heritage, with a reported incidence of 1 in 2000 to 3000 (DaCosta, Galimand, Fenneteau, et al., 2013; Lux, 2015; Segel & Casey, 2016).

The condition is transmitted in an autosomal dominant pattern. However, 25% of cases are thought to represent new mutations or inheritance through an autosomal recessive mode or autosomal dominant mode with reduced penetrance (Bolton-Maggs, Langer, Iolascon, et al., 2011; Segel & Casey, 2016). The affected cells have a smaller surface area relative to their volume than normal RBCs so they become inflexible spheres known as spherocytes. The inflexibility of these cells makes it difficult for them to circulate through the spleen and leads to their early destruction.

Clinical manifestations vary widely from very mild to severe that includes anemia, splenomegaly (usually modest and does not correlate with the severity of disease), and jaundice (most often scleral icterus). HS frequently manifests in the first 24 hours of the newborn's life as severe hyperbilirubinemia. Folic acid supplementation should be given to these children to prevent deficiency due to the rapid cell turnover. Laboratory findings include a hemoglobin level between 7 and 10 g/dl, a reticulocyte count of 6% to 20% (inversely correlated with hemoglobin level), high MCHC, and an increase in osmotic fragility.

Aplastic crisis, which results in a sudden cessation of RBC production by the bone marrow, is a serious complication. Hemoglobin and hematocrit values drop rapidly, which results in severe anemia. Transfusion support may be needed, and close monitoring of the child's cardiovascular status is necessary.

Splenectomy, a treatment for HS, is generally reserved for children older than 5 years of age with symptomatic anemia. The splenectomy corrects the hemolysis but not the RBC defect. Occasionally splenectomy is performed in children younger than 5 years of age who are severely anemic and are showing signs of failure to thrive. Children who are scheduled to undergo a splenectomy should be evaluated for the presence of gallstones before surgery. If gallstones are present, a cholecystectomy is performed at the time of splenectomy.

Because of the risk of life-threatening bacterial infection after splenectomy, these children are immunized with the pneumococcal, meningococcal, and *Haemophilus influenzae* type b vaccines before surgery and receive prophylactic penicillin for several years after splenectomy. The parents should be instructed on the importance of seeking immediate medical attention if their child develops a fever of 101.3°F (38.5°C) or higher as a common sign of infection or postsplenectomy sepsis (DaCosta, Galimand, Fenneteau, et al., 2013; Lux, 2015). Given the lifelong increased risk of severe infection and thromboembolic complications in splenectomized children, partial splenectomy may be useful for selected patients with HS, with the goal of decreasing hemolysis while maintaining splenic phagocytic function (Lux, 2015; Rosman, Broens, Trzpis, et al., 2017).

SICKLE CELL ANEMIA

Sickle cell anemia (SCA) is one of a group of diseases collectively termed hemoglobinopathies, in which normal adult hemoglobin (hemoglobin A [HgbA]) is partly or completely replaced by abnormal sickle hemoglobin (HgbS). SCD refers to a group of hereditary disorders, all of which are related to the presence of HgbS. Although the name *SCD* is sometimes used to refer to SCA, this usage is incorrect. The correct terms for SCA are *HgbSS disease* and *homozygous sickle cell disease.* In the United States the most common forms of SCD are as follows:

SCA—The homozygous form of the disease (HgbSS), in which valine, an amino acid, is substituted for glutamic acid at the sixth position of the β chain.

Sickle cell C disease—A heterozygous variant of SCD (HgbSC), characterized by the presence of both HgbS and hemoglobin C (HgbC), in which lysine is substituted for glutamic acid at the sixth position of the β chain.

Sickle thalassemia disease—A combination of sickle cell trait and β-thalassemia trait. In the β^+ (beta plus) form, some normal adult hemoglobin can still be produced. In the β^0 (beta zero) form, there is no ability to produce normal adult hemoglobin.

Of the SCDs, SCA is the most common form in African Americans in the United States, followed by sickle cell C disease and sickle β-thalassemia. Numerous other sickle syndromes exist in which HgbS is paired with rare mutant globins.

SCD is one of the most common genetic diseases worldwide, affecting approximately 100,000 Americans; other nationalities, such as Africans, Hispanics, Italians, Greeks, Iranians, and Turks; and individuals of Arab, Caribbean, and Asian Indian descent. The incidence of the disease varies in different geographic locations. Among African Americans, the incidence of sickle cell trait is about 8%, whereas among inhabitants of West Africa the frequency of sickle cell trait is reportedly as high as 40%. The high incidence of sickle cell trait in these individuals is believed to be a selective protection against malaria caused by endemic *Plasmodium falciparum* infection (Driscoll, 2007; McCavit, 2012; Nussbaum, McInnes, & Willard, 2016). The physiologic basis for the influence of malaria on the sickle gene (so-called balanced polymorphism) is known but not well understood (Azar & Wong, 2016; Nussbaum, McInnes, & Willard, 2016).

Mode of Transmission

The gene that determines the production of HgbS is situated on an autosome. When both parents have sickle cell trait, there is a 25% chance with each pregnancy of producing an offspring with SCA. In the United States it is estimated that 1 in 12 African Americans carry the trait; therefore the risk of two African American parents having a child with the disease is 0.7%. Other forms of SCD occur through the union of two individuals who carry the heterozygous form of hemoglobin variants.

Basic Defect

The basic defect responsible for the sickling of erythrocytes is contained in the globin fraction of hemoglobin, which is composed of 574 amino acids. Under conditions of dehydration, acidosis, hypoxia, and temperature elevation, the relatively insoluble HgbS changes its molecular structure to form long, slender crystals. These filamentous crystals cause distortion of the cell membrane, so the cell changes from a pliable disk to a crescent- or sickle-shaped RBC. The filamentous forms are associated with much greater viscosity than those with the normal holly leaf structure of HgbA.

In most instances the sickling response is reversible under conditions of adequate oxygenation and hydration. During this time the RBCs are indistinguishable from normal erythrocytes on peripheral examination. RBCs with HgbS can sickle and unsickle under appropriate conditions. After repeated cycles of sickling and unsickling, the RBCs become irreversibly sickled.

Although the defect is inherited, the sickling phenomenon is usually not apparent until later in infancy because of the presence of fetal hemoglobin (HgbF). HgbF is composed of two α and two γ polypeptide chains. At 32 weeks of gestation, the production of β and δ chains begins. These combine with α chains to form the major adult hemoglobins: HgbA (two α and two β chains) and $HgbA_2$ (two α and two δ chains). The newborn with SCD is generally asymptomatic because of the protective effect of HgbF (60% to 80%), but this rapidly decreases during the first year, so the child is at risk for sickle cell–related complications (Driscoll, 2007; Ellison, 2012; Heeney & Ware, 2015).

Sickle Cell Trait

Persons with sickle cell trait have the same basic defect, but only about 35% to 45% of the total hemoglobin is HgbS. The remainder is HgbA. Normally these individuals are asymptomatic. Although complications are rare, they have been described in individuals with sickle cell trait. Nonpainful gross hematuria is the major complication, seen primarily in the teenage and adult years. Under conditions of extreme or prolonged deoxygenation, such as riding in a nonpressurized aircraft or undergoing military training, splenic sequestration with profound anemia can occur, resulting in death.

Pathophysiology and Clinical Manifestations

The clinical manifestations of SCA are primarily the result of (1) obstruction caused by the sickled RBCs, (2) vascular inflammation, and (3) increased RBC destruction. The abnormal adhesion, entanglement, and enmeshing of rigid sickle-shaped cells accompanied by the inflammatory process intermittently blocks the microcirculation, causing vasoocclusion (Fig. 28.2). The resultant absence of blood flow to adjacent tissues causes local hypoxia, which leads to tissue ischemia and infarction (cellular death) (Box 28.4). Most of the complications seen in SCA can be traced to this process and its impact on various organs of the body (Fig. 28.3).

Initially the spleen may become enlarged from congestion and engorgement with sickled cells. This repeated insult to the splenic sinuses results in infarction. The functioning cells are gradually replaced by fibrotic tissue until, by the age of 5 years, the spleen has decreased in size and has been totally replaced by a fibrous mass (functional asplenia). Without the spleen to filter bacteria and to promote the release of large numbers of phagocytic cells, these individuals are highly susceptible to infection.

The liver is also altered in form and function. Liver failure and necrosis are the result of severe impairment of hepatic blood flow from anemia and capillary obstruction. Moderate hepatomegaly is common by the age of 1 year and usually persists throughout childhood and early adulthood. The rapid destruction of RBCs often results in the development of pigmented gallstones. Obstruction of the common bile duct by gallstones is uncommon; therefore cholecystectomy is

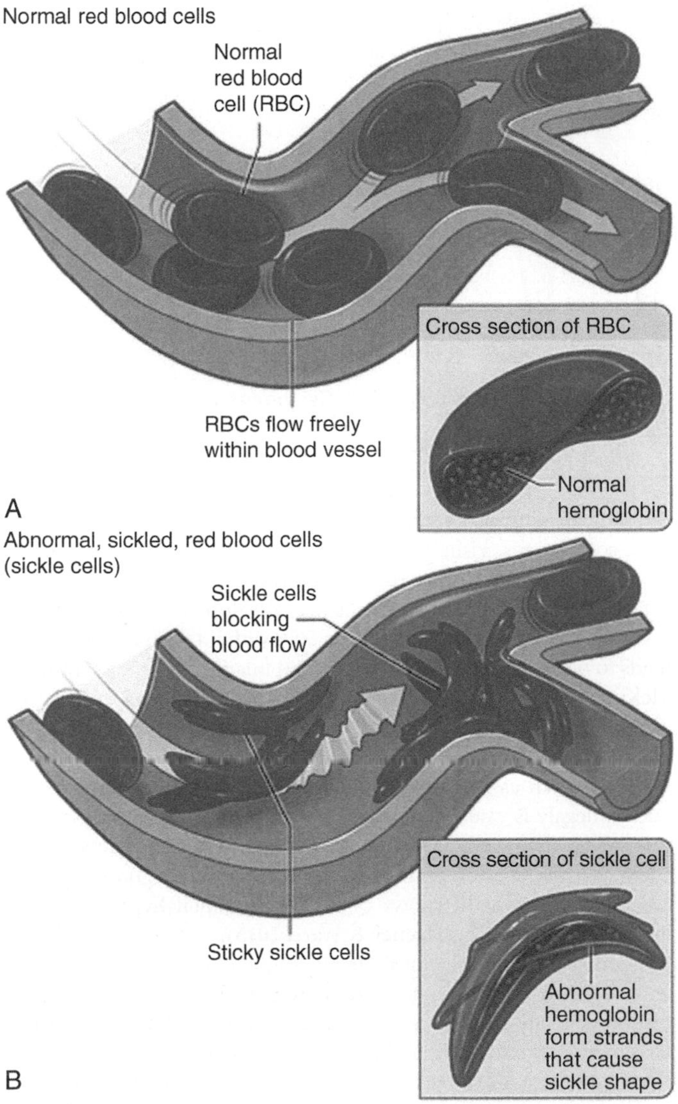

FIG. 28.2 A, Normal red blood cells (RBCs) flowing freely in a blood vessel. The inset image shows a cross section of a normal red blood cell with normal hemoglobin. **B,** Abnormal, sickled red blood cells clumping and blocking blood flow in a blood vessel. (Other cells also may play a role in this clumping process.) The inset image shows a cross section of a sickle cell with abnormal hemoglobin. (From National Heart, Lung, and Blood Institute. [2016, Aug]. *What is sickle cell anemia?* Bethesda, MD: National Institutes of Health.)

BOX 28.4 Clinical Manifestations of Sickle Cell Anemia

General

Possible growth retardation
Chronic anemia (hemoglobin level of 6 to 9 g/dl)
Possible delayed sexual maturation
Marked susceptibility to sepsis

Vasoocclusive Crisis

Pain in area(s) of involvement
Manifestations related to ischemia of involved areas:

- **Extremities**—Painful swelling of hands and feet (sickle cell dactylitis, or hand-foot syndrome), painful joints
- **Abdomen**—Severe pain resembling acute surgical condition
- **Cerebrum**—Stroke, visual disturbances
- **Chest**—Symptoms resembling pneumonia, protracted episodes of pulmonary disease
- **Liver**—Obstructive jaundice, hepatic coma
- **Kidney**—Hematuria
- **Genitals**—Priapism (painful penile erection)

Sequestration Crisis

Pooling of large amounts of blood

- Hepatomegaly
- Splenomegaly
- Circulatory collapse

Effects of Chronic Vasoocclusive Phenomena

Heart—Cardiomegaly, systolic murmurs
Lungs—Altered pulmonary function, susceptibility to infections, pulmonary insufficiency
Kidneys—Inability to concentrate urine, enuresis, progressive renal failure
Liver—Hepatomegaly, cirrhosis, intrahepatic cholestasis
Spleen—Splenomegaly, susceptibility to infection, functional reduction in splenic activity progressing to autosplenectomy
Eyes—Intraocular abnormalities with visual disturbances, sometimes progressive retinal detachment and blindness
Extremities—Avascular necrosis of hip or shoulder; skeletal deformities, especially lordosis and kyphosis; chronic leg ulcers; susceptibility to osteomyelitis
Central nervous system—Hemiparesis, seizures

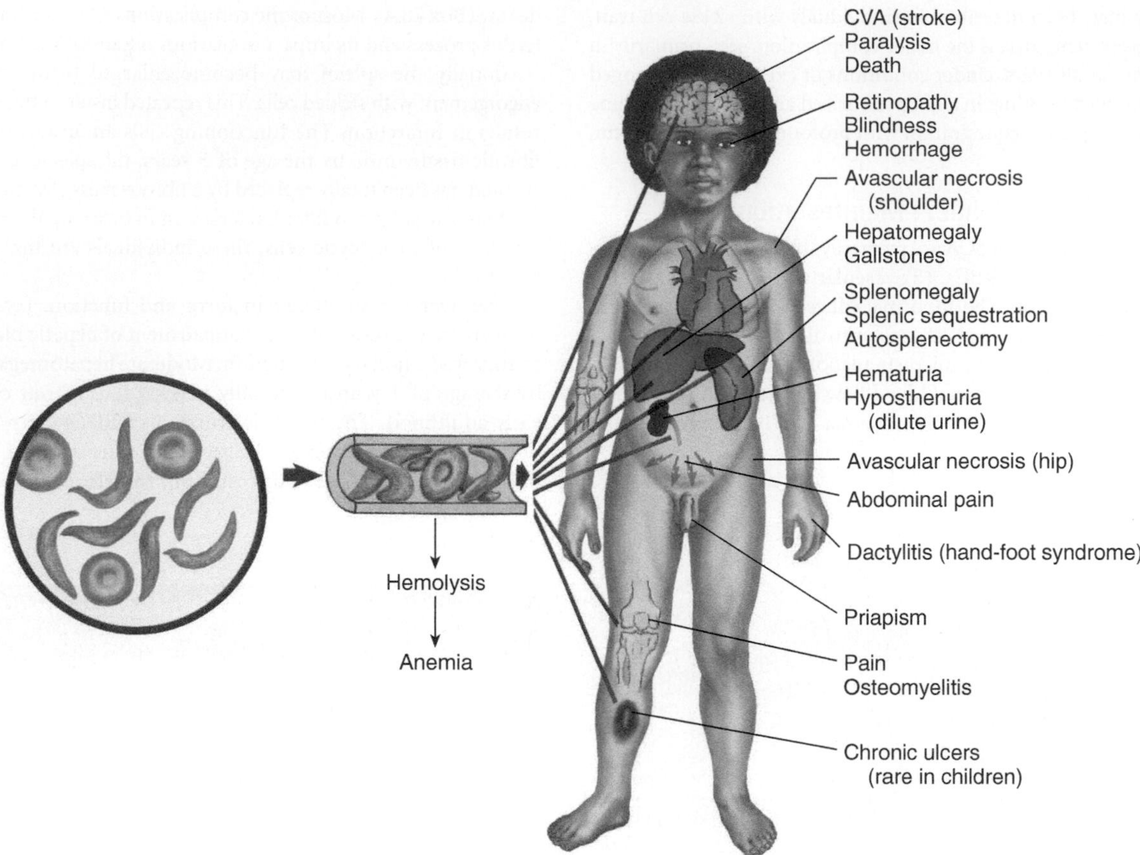

FIG. 28.3 Effects of sickled red blood cells on circulation with related complications. *CVA,* Cerebrovascular accident.

generally not recommended for asymptomatic patients. If recurrent episodes of right upper abdominal pain occur, cholecystectomy may be indicated.

Kidney abnormalities are probably the result of the same cycle of congestion of glomerular capillaries and tubular arterioles with sickle cells and hemosiderin, tissue necrosis, and eventual scarring. The principal results of kidney ischemia are hematuria, inability to concentrate urine, enuresis, and occasionally nephrotic syndrome.

Bone changes include hyperplasia and congestion of the bone marrow, which result in osteoporosis, widening of the medullary spaces, and thinning of the cortices. As a result of the weakening of bone, especially in the lumbar and thoracic regions, skeletal deformities, particularly lordosis and kyphosis, may occur. Because of chronic hypoxia, the bone becomes susceptible to osteomyelitis, frequently from *Salmonella* organisms. Aseptic necrosis of the femoral head from chronic ischemia is an occasional problem.

Changes in the central nervous system are primarily vascular and result from the same cyclic reaction of occlusion, ischemia, and infarction. Stroke, or cerebrovascular accident, is a major complication occuring in approximately 11% of children with SCD before the ages of 18 to 20 years who present with focal neurologic findings lasting greater than 24 hours and abnormal brain neuroimaging that can result in permanent paralysis or death (DeBaun, Frei-Jones, & Vichinsky, 2016; Driscoll, 2007; Estcourt, Fortin, Hopewell, et al., 2017). Silent cerebral infarct occurs in 20% of SCA children who lack focal neurologic findings lasting greater than 24 hours and are diagnosed as an abnormality on magnetic resonance imaging (DeBaun, Frei-Jones, & Vichinsky, 2016; Driscoll, 2007; McCavit, 2012). Any number of neurologic symptoms can indicate a minor cerebral insult, such as headache, aphasia, weakness, convulsions, visual disturbances, or unilateral hemiplegia. Loss of vision is usually the result of progressive retinopathy and retinal detachment. Cognitive impairment (e.g., developmental delays, poor or declining school performances) from SCA without any other overt signs tends to be associated with silent cerebral infarct (DeBaun, Armstrong, McKinstry, et al., 2012; Driscoll, 2007; Yawn, Buchanan, Afenyl-Annan, et al., 2014).

Heart problems are mainly attributable to the stress of chronic anemia, which can eventually result in decompensation and failure. Cardiomegaly is visualized on chest radiographic examination, and a systolic flow murmur is frequently present as a consequence of the anemia. An echocardiogram may be necessary to diagnose abnormal cardiac structure as it shows cardiomegaly, septal hypertrophy, and impaired contractility (Heeney & Ware, 2015).

Cardiac dysfunction with sickle-related pulmonary arterial restriction tend to cause pulmonary hypertension that is routinely screened and diagnosed in adult sickle cell patients using echocardiogram. However, screening asymptomatic children for pulmonary hypertension with echocardiogram for elevated pulmonary arterial pressure is controversial.

With the formation of sickled erythrocytes, mechanical fragility increases, which decreases the life span of the RBC. Hemolysis occurs both during intravascular circulation and as a result of stagnation of sickled cells in the congested spleen (see Fig. 28.2). Although the body attempts to compensate through stimulated erythropoietic activity, as evidenced by a hyperplastic bone marrow, the rate of destruction exceeds the rate of production. A normocytic normochromic anemia results. With increased hemolysis, hemosiderosis (increased storage of iron) is present in the liver, spleen, bone marrow, kidneys, and lymph nodes (see Box 28.4).

Other Signs and Symptoms

In addition to the effects of sickling on various organ structures, the child with SCA may have a variety of complaints such as exercise intolerance, anorexia, jaundiced sclera, and gallstones. Chronic leg ulcers are common in adolescents and adults and are thought to be a result of decreased circulation due to vasoocclusion and tissue ischemia. Other generalized effects include retardation of growth in both height and weight, delayed sexual maturation, and decreased fertility. When the child reaches adulthood, full sexual development and adult height are usually achieved.

Sickle Cell Crises

The clinical manifestations of SCA vary markedly in severity and frequency. The most acute symptoms of the disease occur during periods of exacerbation called *crises.* There are several types of episodic crises: vasoocclusive, acute splenic sequestration, aplastic, hyperhemolytic, stroke, chest syndrome, and infection related. The crises may occur individually or concomitantly with one or more other crises.

Vasoocclusive crisis (VOC), preferably called a *painful episode* or *event,* is the most common type of non–life-threatening crisis. It is characterized by ischemia that causes mild to severe pain that may last from minutes to days. A child experiencing a VOC alone may have localized or generalized pain, acute abdominal pain from visceral hypoxia or gallstones, priapism (an unwanted painful penile erection), and arthralgia. The pain is often migratory, with the presence of a low-grade fever.

VOCs can result in a variety of skeletal problems. One of the more frequent is hand-and-foot syndrome (dactylitis), which occurs primarily in young children ages 6 months to 2 years. It is caused by infarction of short tubular bones and is characterized by pain and swelling of the soft tissue over the hands and feet. It usually resolves spontaneously within a couple of days to weeks. Localized swelling over joints with arthralgia can occur from erythrostasis with sickle cells.

Sequestration crisis is caused by the pooling of large quantities of blood, usually in the spleen and infrequently in the liver, which causes a decrease in blood volume and ultimately shock. The splenic crisis may be acute or chronic. The chronic manifestation is termed hypersplenism. The acute form occurs most commonly in children between 2 months and 5 years of age and may result in death from profound anemia and cardiovascular collapse. Splenic sequestration has occurred in older children and adolescents with sickle cell C disease or sickle β-thalassemia.

Aplastic crisis is diminished RBC production, usually triggered by infection with a virus (especially the human parvovirus) or other organism. When it is superimposed on the rapid destruction of RBCs, a profound anemia results. Packed RBC transfusion is occasionally required in children exhibiting signs and symptoms of congestive heart failure.

Megaloblastic anemia is attributed to an excessive nutritional need for folic acid and/or vitamin B_{12} during periods of pronounced erythropoiesis. Because infection is not always antecedent to aplastic or hypoplastic crises, it is possible that folic acid deficiency is a causative agent.

Hyperhemolytic crisis is an accelerated rate of RBC destruction characterized by anemia, jaundice, and reticulocytosis. This complication frequently suggests other coexisting conditions, such as viral illness; transfusion reactions to alloantibodies; or glucose-6-phosphate dehydrogenase (G6PD) deficiency, which is also common in African Americans.

A cerebrovascular accident (CVA, stroke) is a sudden and severe complication, often with no related illnesses. Sickled cells block the major blood vessels in the brain, which results in cerebral infarction causing variable degrees of neurologic impairment. Repeat CVA causes progressive brain damage in the majority of children who have already experienced one stroke and did not receive monthly transfusions because long-term red cell transfusions reduce the risk of CVA as supported by a moderate quality of evidence (DeBaun & Kirkham, 2016; Estcourt, Fortin, Hopewell, et al., 2017; Heeney & Ware, 2015; Wang & Dwan, 2013).

Another serious complication is acute chest syndrome (ACS), which is clinically similar to pneumonia. ACS is defined as a new pulmonary infiltrate on chest x-ray of a SCD patient that may be accompanied by chest pain, fever, cough, tachypnea, wheezing, and hypoxia (Dastgiri & Dolatkhah, 2016; Driscoll, 2007; Heeney & Ware, 2015; Meier & Miller, 2012). Researchers believe that a VOC or infection results in sickling in the small blood vessels of the lungs, with ensuing occlusion, stasis, and anemia. Repeated episodes of chest syndrome may cause restrictive lung disease and pulmonary hypertension.

Overwhelming infection, especially with *Streptococcus pneumoniae* and *H. influenzae* type b as a result of defective splenic function, is the major cause of death in children with SCD under the age of 5 years. Repeated insults on the splenic sinuses by sickled cells result in impaired filtration and function, which allows the development of septicemia and possibly subsequent death.

Diagnostic Evaluation

Although SCA is usually reported during the neonatal period and early part of infancy, it may not be recognized until the toddler or preschool period during a crisis precipitated by an acute upper respiratory tract or GI infection. However, early diagnosis (before 2 months of age) facilitates initiation of appropriate interventions to minimize complications. Several specific tests detect abnormal hemoglobin in the homozygous or heterozygous form of the disease.

Examination of a stained blood smear may reveal a few sickled RBCs. Because the erythrocyte assumes its normal discoid shape under adequate oxygenation, however, no sickled cells may be present even in the homozygous form of the disease. Whenever sickle cells are found, diagnostic test results are usually positive for SCA, not sickle cell trait.

For screening purposes the sickle turbidity test (Sickledex) is used because it can be performed on blood from a finger or heel stick and yields accurate results in 3 minutes. If the test result is positive, however, hemoglobin electrophoresis is necessary to distinguish between those children with the trait and those with the disease. In hemoglobin electrophoresis, the blood is specially prepared and separated into various hemoglobins by high-voltage electrophoresis. The resulting pattern of the separated peptides as it appears on paper is referred to as *fingerprinting* of the protein. This test is accurate, rapid, and specific for detecting the homozygous and heterozygous forms of the disease, as well as the percentages of the various hemoglobins and used as the initial screening test increasingly in centers within the United States. Certain states also provide confirmation of an SCD electrophoresis by DNA sequencing as the initial screening test (Therrell, Padilla, Loeber, et al., 2015; McCavit, 2012).

Screening of Newborns

Universal screening of newborns for SCD has become standard in all 50 US states and territories and has expanded globally (Kuznik, Habib, Manube, et al., 2016; Therrell, Padilla, Loeber, et al., 2015; McCavit, 2012; McGann, 2016; Meier & Miller, 2012). The screening provides early identification of these children before complications develop. At birth, infants have up to 80% of HbF, which does not carry the defect. Because levels of HgbS are low at birth, Hgb electrophoresis or other tests that measure Hgb concentrations are indicated. Early diagnosis (before 2 months of age) facilitates parental education regarding the importance of maintaining current immunizations, taking prophylaxtic antibiotics, detecting splenomegaly, and recognizing of early signs of infection and other SCD complications.

The death rate from splenic sequestration and septicemia has decreased. Nurses should teach parents to palpate the child's spleen and seek medical attention at the first sign of complications (DeBaun, Frei-Jones, & Vichinsky, 2016; Heeney & Ware, 2015). Penicillin prophylaxis is started by 2 months of age, and parents are instructed to seek medical attention if their child develops a fever of 101.3°F (38.5°C) or higher (see Translating Evidence into Practice box).

TRANSLATING EVIDENCE INTO PRACTICE

Sickle Cell Anemia and Penicillin Prophylaxis

Ask the Question

In children with sickle cell anemia (SCA), does prophylaxis with penicillin reduce the risk of pneumococcal infection?

Search for the Evidence

Search Strategies

Search selection criteria included English-language publications within the past 25 years, research-based articles (level 3 or lower), and child populations.

Databases Used

PubMed, Cochrane Collaboration, MD Consult

Critically Analyze the Evidence

- Hirst and Owusu-Ofori (2014) published an updated systematic Cochrane review of three trials that met the inclusion criteria and showed a reduced incidence of infection in children with SCD receiving prophylactic penicillin. Two trials looked at whether treatment was effective. The third trial continued one of the early trials and looked at when it was safe to stop treatment. Adverse drug effects were rare and minor. Researchers found that penicillin given preventively reduces the rate of pneumococcal infections in children with SCD under 5 years old. Further research may help determine the ideal age to safely withdraw penicillin. A systematic review (Gwaram & Gwaram, 2014) supported the conclusion that there is strong evidence that daily oral penicillin prophylaxis greatly reduces the risk of pneumococcal infection in children with SCA younger than 3 years old.

Researchers combined the clinical experiences of three sickle cell programs in the eastern United States in an attempt to determine the age and disease-specific risk of *Streptococcus pneumoniae* bacteremia and meningitis in children with SCD at a time when penicillin prophylaxis was routine (Hord, Byrd, Stowe, et al., 2002). Forty-seven pneumococcal infections (44 bacteremia, 3 meningitis) among 40 patients with SCD were observed. Most children who developed infections were reportedly taking prophylactic penicillin and received pneumococcal vaccine (Pneumovax) at age 24 months. The observed severe pneumococcal infection rate in HgbSS children younger than 5 years was less than that reported before penicillin prophylaxis in this specific population.

Administration of oral prophylactic penicillin was compared with the 14-valent pneumococcal vaccine in preventing pneumococcal infection in 242 children between the ages of 6 months and 3 years with HgbSS (John, Ramlal, Jackson, et al., 1984). In the first 5 years of the trial, there were 11 pneumococcal infections in the pneumococcal vaccine group and higher infection rates in those given the vaccine before 1 year of age. No pneumococcal isolates were found in the group receiving penicillin, although four pneumococcal isolates were found in this group within 1 year of stopping the penicillin prophylaxis at age 3 years. This study supported the use of penicillin prophylaxis to prevent pneumococcal infection in children younger than 3 years of age.

In a multicenter, randomized, double-blind, placebo-controlled clinical trial, 105 children received penicillin twice daily; a control group of 110 children received a placebo twice daily (Gaston, Verter, Woods, et al., 1986). The trial was terminated 8 months early when an 84% reduction in the incidence of pneumococcal infections was observed in the group treated with penicillin compared with the placebo group. There were no deaths in the penicillin group, but three deaths from infection occurred in the placebo group. Researchers stressed the importance of screening children during the neonatal period and prescribing prophylactic penicillin to decrease the morbidity and mortality associated with pneumococcal infection.

Zarkowsky, Gallagher, Gill, and colleagues (1986) conducted a retrospective analysis of 178 episodes of bacteremia in children with sickle hemoglobinopathies that occurred during 13,771 patient-years of follow-up ($N = 3451$). The predominant pathogen in patients younger than 6 years of age was *S. pneumoniae* (66%), and gram-negative organisms were responsible for 50% of the bacteremias in patients 6 years and older. The incidence of pneumococcal bacteremia in children with sickle cell anemia younger than 3 years of age was 6.1 events per 100 patient-years. The results of this study supported prophylactic administration of penicillin for prevention of pneumococcal bacteremia in children younger than 3 years of age.

A cohort study of 315 patients with HgbSS who lived in Jamaica was conducted between June 1973 and December 1981 (Lee, Thomas, Cupidore, et al., 1995). The patients were divided into three groups to determine whether interventions such as penicillin prophylaxis, parental education in early diagnosis of acute splenic sequestration, and close monitoring in a sickle cell clinic improved survival. A significant decline in deaths from acute splenic sequestration and pneumococcal septicemia and meningitis was found. The research indicated that early detection of sickle cell disease and prophylactic measures could significantly reduce deaths associated with HgbSS.

Riddington and Owusu-Ofori (2002) conducted a systematic review of randomized controlled trials evaluating the effectiveness of prophylactic antibiotic administration in preventing pneumococcal infection in children with SCD. The review of published research found that penicillin prophylaxis significantly reduced the risk of pneumococcal infection in children with HgbSS with minimal adverse reactions.

McCavit, Gilbert, and Buchanan (2013) conducted a cross-sectional electronic survey of 106 pediatric hematologists with expertise in SCD regarding their practices related to penicillin prophylaxis in children with SCD after 5 years of age. Eighty-four percent of pediatric hematologists from 76 centers competed the survey, and 76% routinely recommended cessation of penicillin prophylaxis after 5 years of age.

Apply the Evidence: Nursing Implications

There is good evidence with strong recommendation (Guyatt, Oxman, Vist, et al., 2008) that penicillin prophylaxis significantly reduces the risk of pneumococcal infection in children with sickle cell anemia. The epidemiologic studies strongly suggest that all children with sickle cell anemia should be started on prophylactic penicillin at 2 months of age. Parents and children with sickle cell anemia should be instructed in the importance of taking the prophylactic penicillin twice daily and seeking medical attention immediately for acute illness, especially if the temperature exceeds 101.3°F (38.5°C), regardless of the use of prophylaxis. Most pediatric hematologists with SCD expertise recommend cessation of prophylactic penicillin after 5 years of age.

TRANSLATING EVIDENCE INTO PRACTICE—CONT'D

Sickle Cell Anemia and Penicillin Prophylaxis

QSEN Quality and Safety Competencies: Evidence-Based Practice*

Knowledge

Differentiate clinical opinion from research and evidence-based summaries.

Summarize the epidemiologic studies that strongly suggest that children with SCA should be started on prophylactic penicillin. A survey of pediatric experts recommends stopping prophylactic penicillin after 5 years of age.

Skills

Base individualized care plan on patient values, clinical expertise, and evidence.

Integrate evidence into practice by making sure infants with SCD are started on penicillin at 2 months of age. Most pediatric SCD experts recommend stopping prophylactic penicillin in children with SCD after 5 years of age.

Attitudes

Value the concept of evidence-based practice as integral to determining best clinical practice.

Appreciate strengths and weaknesses of evidence for preventing pneumococcal infection in children with SCD.

HgSS, Homozygous sickle cell disease; *SCA,* sickle cell anemia; *SCD,* sickle cell disease.

References

Gaston, M. H., Verter, J. I., Woods, G., et al. (1986). Prophylaxis with oral penicillin in children with sickle cell anemia: A randomized trial. *New England Journal of Medicine, 314*(25), 1593–1599.

Guyatt, G. H., Oxman, A. D., Vist, G. E., et al. (2008). GRADE: An emerging consensus on rating quality of evidence and strength of recommendations. *British Medical Journal, 336,* 924–926.

Gwaram, H. A., & Gwaram, B. A. (2014). A systematic review of effectiveness of daily oral penicillin v prophylaxis in the prevention of pneumococcal infection in children with sickle cell anaemia. *Nigerian Journal of Medicine, 23*(2), 118–129.

Hirst, C., & Owusu-Ofori, S. (2014). Prophylactic antibiotics for preventing pneumococcal infection in children with sickle cell disease. *Cochrane Database of Systematic Reviews,* (11), CD003427, doi:10.1002/14651858.CD003427.pub3.

Hord, J., Byrd, R., Stowe, L., et al. (2002). *Streptococcus pneumoniae* sepsis and meningitis during the penicillin prophylaxis era in children with sickle cell disease. *Journal of Pediatric Hematology/Oncology, 24*(6), 470–472.

John, A. B., Ramlal, A., Jackson, H., et al. (1984). Prevention of pneumococcal infection in children with homozygous sickle cell disease. *British Medical Journal, 288*(6430), 1567–1570.

Lee, A., Thomas, P., Cupidore, L., et al. (1995). Improved survival in homozygous sickle cell disease: Lessons from cohort study. *British Medical Journal, 311*(7020), 1600–1602.

McCavit, T. L., Gilbert, M., & Buchanan, G. R. (2013). Prophylactic penicillin after 5 years of age in patients with sickle cell disease: A survey of sickle cell disease experts. *Pediatric Blood & Cancer, 60,* 935–939.

Riddington, C., & Owusu-Ofori, S. (2002). Prophylactic antibiotics for preventing pneumococcal infection in children with sickle cell disease. Retrieved from http://www.cochrane.org/reviews/en/ab003427.html.

Zarkowsky, H. S., Gallagher, D., Gill, F. M., et al. (1986). Bacteremia in sickle hemoglobinopathies. *The Journal of Pediatrics, 109*(4), 579–585.

*Adapted from the QSEN at http://www.qsen.org.

Therapeutic Management

The aims of therapy are to prevent the sickling phenomenon, which is responsible for the pathologic sequelae, and to treat the medical emergency of sickle cell crisis. The successful achievement of these aims depends on prompt nursing interventions and medical therapies, child and family preventive measures, and innovative treatment interventions.

Medical management of a crisis is directed at supportive, symptomatic, and specific treatments. The main objectives are to provide (1) bed rest to minimize energy expenditure and to improve oxygen utilization; (2) hydration through oral and IV therapy; (3) electrolyte replacement because hypoxia results in metabolic acidosis, which also promotes sickling; (4) analgesia for severe pain from vasoocclusion; (5) blood replacement to treat anemia and to reduce the viscosity of the sickled blood; and (6) antibiotic therapy to treat any existing infection.

Administration of pneumococcal, *H. influenzae* type b, and meningococcal vaccines is recommended for these children because of their susceptibility to infection from functional asplenia. (See Immunizations, Chapter 10.) Oral penicillin prophylaxis is recommended by 2 months of age to reduce the chance of pneumococcal sepsis (see Translating Evidence into Practice box). The nurse assumes an important role in helping the family comply with a medication regimen and seek medical attention immediately when the child has a fever of 101.3°F (38.5°C) or higher, an increase in spleen size, or severe pallor (Driscoll, 2007; Heeney & Ware, 2015; Yawn & John-Sowah, 2015; Yawn, Buchanan, Afenyl-Annan, et al., 2014).

Oxygen therapy is of little therapeutic value unless the patient is hypoxic (Heeney & Ware, 2015). Oxygen administration is usually not effective in reversing sickling or reducing pain because the oxygen is not able to reach the enmeshed sickled RBCs through the clogged vessels.

Another important component of care is the use of blood transfusions. An RBC transfusion is used in aplastic, hyperhemolytic, and splenic sequestration crises; in stroke prevention; and before general surgery. Exchange transfusion (erythrocytapheresis) is a successful, rapid method of reducing the number of circulating sickle cells and therefore slowing down the vicious circle of hypoxia, tissue ischemia, and injury. It is used in ACS and after a stroke to prevent recurrence and further tissue damage. Routine transfusions to maintain the hemoglobin value between 9 and 10 g/dl in children with central nervous system disease can minimize the chances of further neurologic problems. In the event of major surgery, exchange or partial exchange transfusions may be given preoperatively to prevent anoxia and suppress the formation of new sickle cells. A simple packed RBC transfusion to raise the hemoglobin value to 10 g/dl, as well as maintenance hydration preoperatively and postoperatively, should be sufficient to prevent sickling complications secondary to anesthesia (DeBaun, Frei-Jones, & Vichinsky, 2016; Heeney & Ware, 2015; McCavit, 2012). However, sickle cell patients with a higher surgical risk, which may include a history of pulmonary disease, previous ACS, stroke, or multiple hospitalizations, should undergo exchange transfusion or multiple simple transfusions to reduce the chance of SCD complications by decreasing the level of HgbS to less than 30%. Simple and exchange transfusions are also used in life-threatening ACS and after acute overt stroke to prevent recurrence and further tissue damage (Azar & Wong, 2016; Meier & Miller, 2012; Wang & Dwan, 2013).

Multiple transfusions carry the risk of transmission of viral infection, hyperviscosity, transfusion reactions, alloimmunization, hemosiderosis, and transfusion-related acute lung injury (Heeney & Ware, 2015; Pahuja, Puri, Mahajan, et al., 2017; Secher, Stensballe, & Afshari, 2013). To reduce iron overload from chronic transfusion therapy, chelation therapy may be started. Currently, there are three chelators available in the United States. Deferoxamine (Desferal), an effective parenteral chelator, has been the standard treatment for over 40 years and is usually administered at 30 to 40 mg/kg over 8 to 10 hours for 5 or 7 nights per week. Deferiprone and deferasirrox are oral chelators approved by the US Food and Drug Administration that are becoming more commonly used (Fortin, Madgwick, Trivella, et al., 2016; Vichinsky, El-Beshlawy, Al Zoebie, et al., 2017) . The oral iron chelators are used alone or in combination with deferoxamine. The chelator selection tend to be based on availability and cost of chelator, age of patient, drug side effects, patient comorbidities, local experience, and preference (Azar & Wong, 2016; Fortin, Madgwick, Trivella, et al., 2016).

The appropriate time for beginning treatment is controversial, but chelation is often initiated when the ferritin level is higher than 1000 ng/ml or after a year or more of monthly transfusions. Ferritin level is also an acute phase reactant that is recognized as an ineffective or inaccurate test to determine iron overload; however, it is widely used to monitor effectiveness of chelation (Azar & Wong, 2016; DeBaun, Frei-Jones, & Vichinsky, 2016; Kahnooji, Rashidinejad, Yazdanpanah, et al., 2016; Yawn & John-Sowah, 2015). In contrast, liver biopsy testing allows a direct measurement of hepatic iron concentration but does not accurately estimate total body iron deposition in other affected organs (e.g., heart, spleen) and also has a risk of hemorrhage, infection, and discomfort (DeBaun, Frei-Jones, & Vichinsky, 2016). Noninvasive alternatives for liver biopsy are based on the magnetic properties of iron. Initially, *magnetic susceptometry* and *superconducting quantum interference devices* were used and provided an accurate measurement of hepatic iron; however, recently more practical and precise *tissue magnetic resonance relaxation rates* (T1/T2*) are now available that provide an accurate and reliable measurement of cardiac, hepatic, and splenic iron deposition (DeBaun, Frei-Jones, & Vichinsky, 2016). However, these specialized devices are not readily available in all centers.

Children with HgbSS disease and HgbS-β^0-thalassemia have the highest risk of stroke and should be monitored with annual transcranial Doppler ultrasonography (TCD) (Driscoll, 2007; Heeney & Ware, 2015; McCavit, 2012). TCD is a cost-effective, noninvasive ultrasound technique that screens for stroke risk in children who have SCD. TCD is performed on children with SCD from 2 to 16 years of age and measures the average velocity of intracranial vascular flow within the large cerebral arteries (DeBaun, Frei-Jones, & Vichinsky, 2016; Yawn, Buchanan, Afenyl-Annan, et al., 2014; Yawn & John-Sowahm, 2015). The recommended treatment for children with confirmed abnormal TCD findings is chronic transfusion therapy (Armstrong-Wells, Grimes, Sidney, et al., 2009; DeBaun, Frei-Jones, & Vichinsky, 2016). The duration of transfusion is indefinite, although current studies are addressing whether patients may be transitioned safely from red cell transfusions and chelation to hydroxyurea and phlebotomy to prevent stroke and decrease iron concentration (Estcourt, Fortin, Hopewell, et al., 2017; McCavit, 2012). Multiple transfusions carry the risk of transmission of viral infection, hyperviscosity, transfusion reactions, alloimmunization, and hemosiderosis, which must be discussed with the parents or legal guardian before the initiation of a transfusion program.

In children with recurrent life-threatening splenic sequestration, splenectomy may be a lifesaving measure. However, the spleen usually atrophies on its own through progressive fibrotic changes (functional asplenia) by 6 years of age in children with SCA. Surgical splenectomy or autosplenectomy has several benefits because the spleen is the major site of sickling, sequestration, and destruction of RBCs.

Prognosis

The prognosis varies, but most patients live into their fifth decade. The greatest risk is usually in children younger than 5 years of age, and the majority of deaths in these children are caused by overwhelming infection. As the child grows older, however, the crises may become less severe and less frequent, although death in early adulthood is not uncommon. Consequently, SCA is a chronic illness with a potentially terminal outcome. Physical and sexual maturation are delayed in adolescents with SCA. Although adults achieve normal height, typically below normal weight, and normal sexual function, the delay may present problems to the adolescent (Heeney & Ware, 2015; Redding-Lallinger & Knoll, 2006).

Individuals with SCD who have higher levels of HbF tend to have a milder disease with fewer complications than those with lower levels (Adewoyin, 2015; Driscoll, 2007; Meier & Miller, 2012). Hydroxyurea is a US Food and Drug Administration–approved medication that increases the production of HbF, reduces endothelial adhesion of sickle cells, improves the sickle cell hydration and cell size, increases nitric oxide production (a vasodilator), and lowers leukocyte and reticulocyte counts (National Institutes of Health, National Heart, Lung, and Blood Institute, 2014; Nevitt, Jones, & Howard, 2017; Yawn, Buchanan, Afenyi-Annan, et al., 2014). Long-term follow-up of patients taking hydroxyurea alone revealed a 40% reduction in mortality rate and decreased frequency of VOC, ACS, hospital admissions, and abnormal transcranial Doppler; stroke prevention; and decreased need for transfusions, thus making SCD crises milder (DeBaun, Frie-Jones, & Vichinsky, 2016; DeBaun & Kirkham, 2016; Gjamila, Chaturvedi, Rodeghier, et al., 2016; Nevitt, Jones, & Howard, 2017). Pediatric studies have shown that hydroxyurea can be used safely and effectively in children (Wang, Ware, Miller, et al., 2011).

Hematopoietic stem cell transplantation (HSCT) from a human leukocyte antigen (HLA)–matched sibling or unrelated donor is the only potential cure of SCD, with a high risk of neurologic complications (Azar & Wong, 2016; Driscoll, 2007; Heeney & Ware, 2015; Locatelli & Pagliara, 2012). In some young people chronic pain becomes a significant problem. Allogeneic HSCT offers a curative approach for some children with SCD, with overall survival 92% to 95% and event-free survival of 82% to 86% (Driscoll, 2007; Hsieh, Fitzhugh, Weitzel, et al., 2014; Lacatelli & Pagliara, 2012).

Children and adolescents younger than 16 years of age who have severe complications (e.g., stroke, recurrent ACS, or refractory pain) and have an HLA-matched donor available were offered HSCT as a treatment modality, but this has been relatively slow to gain widespread acceptance (DeBaun, Frei-Jones, & Vichinsky, 2016; Haining, Duncan, El-haddad, et al., 2015; Lucarelli, Isgro, Sodani, et al., 2012). Eventually, improved survival with other HSCT modalities, such as umbilical cord blood transplantation, haploidentical transplants, and nonmyeloablative conditioning regimens, may augment sibling donor protocols and widen the availability of HSCT as a potential cure to SCD patients (Driscoll, 2007; Lucarelli, Isgro, Sodani, et al., 2012).

For those patients who lack a suitable HLA-matched donor, ex vivo gene therapy autologous hematopoietic stem cell transplantation brings hope of a potential curative treatment option (Negre, Eggimann, Beuzard et al., 2016). Gene therapy for hemoglobin disorders has made major progress from the early discovery of β-globin regulatory elements to the development of lentiviral vectors, including HPV569 and BB305 vectors, with early clinical benefit observed in SCD (Negre, Eggimann, Beuzard et al., 2016). Recently a patient with SCD was treated with lentiviral vector-mediated addition of an antisickling β-globin gene into autologous hematopoietic stem cells that engrafted and produced normal blood cell counts in all lineages (Ribeil, Hacein-Bey-Abina, Payen, et al., 2017).

Nursing Care Management

Many nurses are involved in SCA screening programs to identify persons with the abnormal hemoglobin so that therapy can be implemented for homozygotes and genetic counseling provided for heterozygotes. The nurse should seek medical attention immediately for young children who exhibit any of the signs previously described and whose families belong to a racial or geographic group known to be at risk for SCD. (See Quality Patient Outcomes box.)

Assessment of the child in sickle cell crisis includes all areas and systems that can be affected by circulatory obstruction, including vital signs; neurologic signs; vision; hearing; and the respiratory, GI, renal, and musculoskeletal systems. It is also important to identify the location and intensity of pain.

QUALITY PATIENT OUTCOMES

Sickle Cell Disease

- Early recognition of signs and symptoms of sickle cell anemia
- Tissue deoxygenation minimized
- Sickle cell crisis prevented or quickly managed
- Pain appropriately managed
- Stroke prevented
- Prophylactic penicillin regimen followed
- Hypoxia prevented when surgery is necessary
- Pneumococcal, *H. influenzae* type b, and meningococcal vaccines administered

Minimize Tissue Deoxygenation

Anything that increases cellular metabolism also results in tissue hypoxia. For the child, minimization of tissue deoxygenation includes (1) taking frequent rest breaks during physical activities; (2) avoiding contact sports if the spleen is enlarged because rupture will cause massive internal hemorrhage; (3) avoiding environments with low oxygen concentration, such as high altitudes or nonpressurized airplane flights; and (4) avoiding known sources of infection. If the child has even a mild infection, the parents must seek medical attention at once.

Promote Hydration

The nurse emphasizes the importance of adequate hydration to prevent sickling and delay the vasoocclusion and hypoxia-ischemia cycle. The nurse calculates the child's fluid requirements (approximately 1600 ml/m^2/day), which is the minimum daily fluid intake. The nurse also assesses the child's usual fluid consumption to evaluate its adequacy and makes adjustments based on this knowledge. It is not sufficient to advise parents to "force fluids" or "encourage drinking." They need specific instructions on how many glasses or bottles of fluid are required. Many foods are also a source of fluid, particularly soups, popsicles, yogurt, ice cream, sherbet, gelatin, and puddings.

Encourage children to drink by giving them a special cup, thermos, or water bottle with a straw from which to drink throughout the day. The nurse advises parents to take advantage of times of thirst, such as on awakening or after playing; to serve frequent small portions; and to leave the cup within easy reach for self-service. Flavored ice pops and crushed ice "slurpies" are sources of fluid commonly accepted by children.

Because the kidneys' ability to concentrate urine is impaired, the child is especially prone to dehydration. Dilute urine or urine of low specific gravity is no longer a valid sign of adequate hydration. Parents should observe for other indications of fluid loss, such as dry mucous membranes, dry diapers, weight loss, and a sunken fontanel in infants. In addition, without the ability to conserve water by concentrating urine, the child is prone to dehydration from environmental factors, particularly overheating. The nurse alerts parents to the need for the child to wear proper indoor and outdoor clothing and avoid excessive exposure to the sun.

Increased fluid intake combined with impaired kidney function results in the problem of enuresis. Parents who are unaware of this fact frequently employ the usual measures to discourage bed-wetting, such as limiting fluids at night, and may resort to punishment and shaming to force bladder control. The nurse discusses this problem with the parents, stressing that the child's ability to concentrate urine is impaired. Reminding the child to urinate frequently during the day is helpful, and waking the child during the night may prove beneficial if the child's sleep patterns are not disturbed. Parents who are toilet training their toddlers should be aware of the more frequent pattern of urination and increased difficulty in learning control. Enuresis is treated as a complication of the disease to alleviate parental pressure on the child and to prevent any fluid restriction.

Minimize Crises

Because infection is the major cause of death due to the body's inability to resist infection, the nurse stresses to parents the importance of adequate nutrition, frequent medical supervision, proper hand washing, and isolation from known sources of infection. Keep in mind that children also need to live a normal life. Overprotection can be as devastating emotionally as an infection is physically. Parents need to be aware of the need to seek prompt medical care at the first sign of any infection.

Teach the family the signs and symptoms of crises and advise them to seek medical attention immediately when any are present. Teaching parents spleen palpation for earlier detection of splenic sequestration can reduce mortality risk from this serious complication.

Promote Supportive Therapies

The success of many of the medical therapies relies heavily on nursing implementation. Management of pain is an especially difficult problem and often involves experimenting with various analgesics, including opioids, and various schedules before relief is achieved. Unfortunately, these children tend to be undermedicated, which results in "clock watching" and demands for additional doses sooner than might be expected. Often this incorrectly raises suspicion of drug addiction, when in fact the problem is one of inadequate pain control (see Family-Centered Care box). In choosing and scheduling analgesics, the goal is prevention of pain.

Medication given by mouth can be as effective as IV medication when equianalgesic dosages are prescribed. The nurse should combine any pain management program with psychologic support to help the child deal with the depression, anxiety, and fear that accompany the disease. This includes regular visits with the child to discuss his or her concerns during the hospitalization and positive reinforcement of adaptive coping skills, such as successful methods of dealing with the pain and compliance with treatment prescriptions. To reduce the negative connotation associated with the term *crisis,* it is best to say "pain episode."

Frequently, heat to the affected area is soothing. Cold compresses are not applied to the area because doing so enhances vasoconstriction and occlusion. Bed rest is usually well tolerated during a crisis, although the actual rest obtained depends a great deal on pain alleviation and the use of organized schedules of nursing care. Although the objective of bed rest is to minimize oxygen consumption, some activity, particularly passive range-of-motion exercises, is beneficial to promote circulation. Usually the best course is to let children determine their activity tolerance.

If blood transfusions or exchange transfusions are given, the nurse has the responsibility of observing for signs of transfusion reaction (see Table 28.2). Because hypervolemia from too-rapid transfusion can

FAMILY-CENTERED CARE

Fear of Addiction

Although the pain during a sickle cell crisis is usually severe and opioids are needed, many families fear that their child will become addicted to the narcotic. Unfortunately, misinformed health professionals may foster this unfounded fear, which results in needless suffering. Extremely few children with SCD who receive opioids for severe pain become behaviorally addicted to the drug (DeBaun, Frei-Jones, & Vichinsky, 2016). Families and older children, especially adolescents, need to be reassured that opioids are medically indicated, high doses may be needed, and children rarely become addicted.

VOC, as the clinical hallmark, is the most common, severe, and debilitating painful episode experienced by patients with SCD (Driscoll, 2007; McCavit, 2012; Yawn & John-Sowah, 2015) (see Fig. 28.3). The chronic nature of the pain can greatly affect the child's development. A multidisciplinary team (e.g., physician, psychologist, child life specialist, family, nurse, social worker) approach is best for vasoocclusive pain management that includes pharmacologic treatments, hydration, physical therapy, and nonpharmacologic and complementary treatment (e.g., prayer, spiritual healing, massage, heating pads, herbs, relaxation, breathing exercises, distraction, music, guided imagery, self-motivation, acupuncture, and biofeedback) (Adewoyin, 2015; Ballas, 2011; Brandow, Weisman, & Panepinto, 2011; Meier & Miller, 2012).

When mild to moderate VOC is reported, nonsteroidal antiinflammatory medication (e.g., ibuprofen, ketorolac) or nonopioids (e.g., acetaminophen) are used initially. If these drugs are not effective alone, an opioid may be added. The dosages of both drugs are titrated (adjusted) to a therapeutic level. Opioids such as immediate- and sustained-release morphine, oxycodone, hydrocodone, hydromorphone (Dilaudid), and methadone are administered intravenously or orally for severe pain and are given around the clock. In conjunction with the opioid, intravenous ketorolac for a maximum of a 5-day course is commonly used to enhance the pain management effect. Patient-controlled analgesia (PCA) has been used successfully for sickle cell–related pain. PCA reinforces the patient's role and responsibility in managing the pain and provides flexibility in dealing with pain, which may vary in severity over time (see Pain Management, Chapter 5).

SCD, Sickle cell disease; *VOC,* vasoocclusive crisis.

DRUG ALERT

Meperidine

Meperidine (pethidine [Demerol]) is not recommended. Normeperidine, a metabolite of meperidine, is a central nervous system stimulant that produces anxiety, tremors, myoclonus, and generalized seizures when it accumulates with repetitive dosing. Patients with SCD are particularly at risk for normeperidine-induced seizures (Ellison, 2012; National Institutes of Health and National Heart, Lung, and Blood Institute, Division of Blood Diseases and Resources, 2014).

increase the workload of the heart, the nurse also must be alert to signs of cardiac failure.

In splenic sequestration, gently measure the size of the spleen because increasing splenomegaly is an ominous sign. A decrease in the size of the spleen denotes response to therapy. The nurse also closely monitors vital signs and blood pressure to detect impending shock. Anemia is typically not a presenting complication in VOCs but is a critical problem in other types of crisis. The nurse monitors for evidence of increasing anemia and institutes appropriate nursing intervention.

Oxygen administration is not beneficial in vasoocclusive episodes unless hypoxemia is present (Heeney & Ware, 2015). It does not reverse sickled RBCs, and if used in a nonhypoxic patient, it decreases erythropoiesis. Because prolonged oxygen therapy can aggravate the anemia, report any signs of lack of therapeutic benefit, such as restlessness, increased pallor, and continued pain.

Record intake, especially of IV fluids, and output. The child's weight should be taken on admission because it serves as a baseline for evaluating hydration. Because diuresis can result in electrolyte loss, the nurse observes for signs of hypokalemia and should be familiar with normal serum electrolyte values to report changes. Nurses also need to be aware of the signs of chest syndrome and stroke, both potentially fatal complications (see Nursing Alert, p. 1043).

Decrease Surgical Risks

The main surgical risk is hypoxia from anesthesia. However, emotional stress, the demands of wound healing, and infection potentially increase the sickling phenomenon, both in children with the disease and in those with the trait. The primary nursing objectives are to minimize each of these threats preoperatively and postoperatively by keeping the child well hydrated, preparing the child psychologically, and preventing infection.

Encourage Screening and Genetic Counseling

Screening is recommended during the neonatal period because early diagnosis allows earlier, more prevention-oriented treatment, such as prophylactic antibiotic therapy and parent education about potential complications. The advantages of trait identification lie in selective reproduction of offspring not afflicted with HgbS. Alternate methods of childbearing include artificial insemination, adoption, and abortion of affected fetuses. However, for some, these alternatives are unacceptable.

To be effective, the nurse should combine screening with genetic counseling and long-term follow-up. The nurse can be instrumental in such programs by conducting parent education sessions, providing follow-up for the family in the home, disseminating correct information about the disease and trait to the community, and rendering support to parents of children newly diagnosed with the trait or the disease. A primary consideration in genetic counseling is informing parents of the 25% chance with each pregnancy of having a child with the disease when both parents carry the trait. (See Chapter 3)

NURSING TIP

One simple yet graphic way of illustrating the difference between normal discoid RBCs and sickle cells is to roll round or oval objects, such as marbles, through a tube to demonstrate normal blood cell circulation and then roll pointed objects such as screws or jacks through the tube. The effect of sickling and clumping of the pointed objects is especially noticeable at a bend or slight narrowing of the tube. This same idea can be expanded to discuss the importance of increased fluid in keeping the pointed objects suspended away from one another to prevent concentration.

Prenatal diagnosis is possible through amniocentesis or fetoscopy and fetal blood sampling during the sixteenth week of gestation. Analysis of amniotic cells for a DNA fragment associated with the gene responsible for sickled β-globulin chain synthesis can be performed as early as the twelfth week with chorionic sampling. In the event the fetus is affected, the decision regarding termination of the pregnancy should be left to the couple.

Explain the Disease

Because SCA may be recognized in the young child, most of the nurse's counseling is directed at the parents. The nurse explains to parents the basic effect of tissue hypoxia on RBCs and the effect of sickling on the circulation (see Fig. 28.2). Taking time to establish a sound basis of understanding regarding why certain measures are beneficial to the child encourages parents to practice them.*

The nurse advises the parents to inform all treating practitioners of the child's condition. The use of a medical identification bracelet is another way of ensuring awareness of the disease. The nurse can stress the benefits of displaying this information, especially in emergencies when anesthesia may be required.

! NURSING ALERT

Report signs of the following immediately:

Acute chest syndrome

- Severe chest pain, back pain, or abdominal pain
- Fever of 101.3°F (38.5°C) or higher
- Cough
- Dyspnea, tachypnea
- Retractions
- Declining oxygen saturation (oximetry)

Stroke

- Severe, unrelieved headaches
- Severe vomiting
- Jerking or twitching of the face, legs, or arms
- Seizures
- Strange, abnormal behavior
- Inability to move an arm or a leg
- Stagger or an unsteady walk
- Stutter or slurred speech
- Weakness in the hands, feet, or legs
- Changes in vision

Support the Family

Families need the opportunity to discuss their feelings regarding transmitting a potentially fatal, chronic illness to their child. Some parents are able to cope with this fact; some feel great guilt and remorse for giving their child the disease, whereas others regret not knowing that they carried the trait. For many parents, decision making regarding subsequent pregnancies is fraught with doubt and ambivalence.

Because of the widely publicized prognosis for children with SCA, many parents express their fear of death. The prognosis varies; with early diagnosis and treatment these children are living longer. Previously identified predictors of a severe course of SCA included low hemoglobin level (approximately 7 g/dl), dactylitis or painful episode, and elevated WBC count exhibited before the age of 24 months (Miller, Sleeper, Pegelow, et al., 2000). However, a recent systematic review determined that the only predictive tests consistently associated with severe SCA outcome are elevated TCD velocities and increased reticulocyte count (Meier, Fasano, & Levett, 2017). All of the other predictors had mixed results, which was attributed to improved supportive care with reduction in infectious deaths and stroke rate. The nurse should care for the family as for any family with a child who has a chronic and life-threatening illness, and give some consideration to the siblings' reactions, the stress on the marital relationship, and the childrearing attitudes displayed toward the child (see Nursing Care Plan box).

BETA-THALASSEMIA (β-THALASSEMIA OR COOLEY ANEMIA)

Worldwide, thalassemia is a common monogenic disorder affecting as many as 15 million people (Yaish, 2015). In the United States an estimated 2000 persons have β-thalassemia major (DeBaun, Frei-Jones, & Vichinsky, 2016). The term *thalassemia* comes from the Greek word *thalassa*, meaning "sea," and is applied to a variety of inherited blood disorders characterized by deficiencies in the rate of production of specific globin chains in hemoglobin. The name appropriately refers to people living near the Mediterranean Sea—namely, Italians, Greeks, and Syrians, or to their descendants. Evidence suggests that the high incidence of the disorder among these groups is a result of selective advantage of the trait in protecting against malaria, as is postulated for SCD. The disorder has a wide geographic distribution, however, probably as a result of genetic migration through intermarriages or possibly as a result of spontaneous mutation.

The thalassemias are classified according to the hemoglobin chain affected and the amount of the globin chain that is synthesized. The two major categories are α-thalassemia and β-thalassemia. Thalassemia is seen in various population groups in India, Asia, Africa, and inhabitants of the Mediterranean and Middle Eastern regions, and the majority of births of affected individuals occur in these groups (Choudhry, 2017; Higgs, Engel, & Stamatoyannopoulos, 2012). However, in the past few decades, there has been an influx of migrants from these high-prevalence countries, mainly into North America and Central and North Europe, with rapid increases in thalassemia populations.

β-Thalassemia is the most common of the thalassemias and occurs in four forms: two heterozygous forms, *thalassemia minor* (generally an asymptomatic silent carrier state) and *thalassemia trait* (which produces a mild microcytic anemia); *thalassemia intermedia*, which may involve either homozygous or heterozygous abnormalities and is manifested as splenomegaly and moderate to severe anemia; and a homozygous form, *thalassemia major* (also known as Cooley anemia), which results in a severe anemia that is not compatible with life without transfusion support.

Mode of Transmission

Thalassemia is an autosomal recessive disorder with varying expressivity. Both parents must be carriers to produce a child with β-thalassemia major. The typical mode of transmission is between parents who are heterozygous for thalassemia.

Pathophysiology and Clinical Manifestations

Normal postnatal HgbA is composed of two α and two β polypeptide chains. In β-thalassemia there is a partial or complete deficiency in the synthesis of the β chain of the hemoglobin molecule. Consequently, there is a compensatory increase in the synthesis of α chains, and γ-chain production remains activated, which results in formation of defective hemoglobin. This unbalanced polypeptide unit is unstable; when it

*Sickle Cell Disease Association of America, Inc., 231 E. Baltimore St., Suite 800, Baltimore, MD 21202; 410-528-1555, 800-421-8453; fax: 410-528-1495; e-mail: scdaa@sicklecelldisease.org; http://www.sicklecell-disease.org; https://www.facebook.com/sicklecellcampaign; Sickle Cell Information Center, PO Box 109, Grady Memorial Hospital, 80 Jesse Hill Jr. Drive SE, Atlanta, GA 30303; 404-616-3572; fax: 404-616-5998; e-mail: aplatt@emory.edu; http://www.scinfo.org; National Heart, Lung, and Blood Institute Health Information Center, PO Box 30105, Bethesda, MD 20824-0105; 301-592-8573; fax: 301-592-8563; https://www.nhlbi.nih.gov. Guideline for the Management of Acute and Chronic Pain in Sickle-Cell Disease is available from the American Pain Society, 4700 W. Lake Ave., Glenview, IL 60025-1485; 847-375-4715; fax: 866-572-2654; e-mail: info@ampainsoc.org, http://www.ampainsoc.org; https://www.facebook.com/americanpainsociety.

NURSING CARE PLAN

The Child With Sickle Cell Anemia

Case Study

Donny is a 2-year-old boy with sickle cell anemia (HgbSS). He returns to the hematology clinic this morning after being seen last night in the emergency department (ED) for pain. His mother states that he is having more pain in his feet over the past several hours and he no longer wants to walk. The mother has been giving Donny the pain medications as prescribed by the ED doctor, but she feels his pain is getting worse. On examination, you find that his feet and hands are swollen and he cries out when you touch them.

Assessment

What are the most important signs of acute pain that you need to look for in a young child with sickle cell disease (SCD)?

Sickle Cell Vasoocclusive Pain Defining Characteristics

Pain can be in any location in the body; can be rapid in onset and severe; and may be localized or generalized

Low-grade fever may be present

Localized swelling over joints with arthralgia can occur

Nursing Interventions and Rationales

What are the most appropriate nursing interventions for a child with SCD experiencing pain?

Nursing Interventions	Rationales
Discuss schedule of medication around the clock with parents.	To control pain
Encourage high level of fluid intake.	To ensure hydration
Recognize that various analgesics, including opioids and medication schedules, may need to be tried.	To ensure satisfactory pain relief
Reassure child and family that analgesics, including opioids, are medically indicated, that high doses may be needed, and that children rarely become addicted.	To avoid needless suffering because of unfounded fears
Apply heat application or massage to affected area. Avoid applying cold compresses.	To prevent vasoconstriction that may enhance sickling

Case Study (Continued)

Donny's pain is not being controlled by oral pain medications, and the plan is to begin intravenous (IV) pain medications to control his pain. What is the most appropriate IV medication for Donny at this time?

A dose of morphine (0.1 to 0.2 mg/kg/dose) is given every 10 minutes for three doses.

What important nursing interventions should be implemented at this time?

Give both the morphine and ketorolac. If pain is still not relieved after three doses of morphine, switch to patient-controlled analgesia (PCA) and admit. Give ketorolac 1 mg/kg for first dose, then 0.5 mg/kg /dose IV every 6 hours; not to exceed 5 days (maximum of 30 mg/dose).

Nursing Interventions	Rationales
Administer morphine and ketorolac safely.	To prevent adverse effects and overdose
Monitor for side effects of morphine; assess respiratory status closely and prevent constipation.	To prevent discomfort and adverse effects after administration
Monitor for side effects of ketorolac; assess for bleeding (gastrointestinal [GI] or renal) closely.	
Educate parents on the safety and effectiveness of morphine and ketorolac as pain-relieving medications.	To reduce unfounded fears
Reassess the child's pain level after administering morphine and ketorolac continue to assess frequently.	To ensure satisfactory pain relief
Recognize that various analgesics and doses may need to be tried.	To ensure optimal pain relief

Case Study (Continued)

Because Donny is only 2 years old, what kind of pain assessment tool is most appropriate for a child this age?

Because Donny is in a great deal of pain, the FLACC Pain Assessment Tool is an appropriate observational tool to use at this time. The FLACC is an interval scale that includes the five categories of behavior: facial expression (F), leg movement (L), activity (A), cry (C), and consolability (C). See Chapter 5 for more discussion of this tool.

How frequently should Donny's pain be assessed?

Donny's pain should be assessed frequently to determine whether the IV morphine is providing enough pain relief. Morphine (0.1 to 0.2 mg/kg/dose) is given every 10 minutes for three doses. After this initial intervention, pain assessment will help determine what to do next. Donny may require additional medications to control his pain. If the IV morphine provided relief, discharge on oral morphine (0.2 to 0.5 mg/kg) or convert to home opioid equivalent with ibuprofen every 6 hours. Instruct to continue around-the-clock medications at home, emphasize increased fluid intake, and start bowel regimen to prevent constipation. If is pain is still not under control after three doses of IV morphine, initiate morphine PCA and admit to hospital.

PCA: Loading dose of 0.1 mg/kg (maximum 8 mg); basal rate of 0.01 mg/kg and intermittent dose 0.035 mg/kg (maximum 8 mg) with the interval lockout approximately 10 minutes. A 4-hour limit 0.5 to 0.75 mg/kg with IV fluids at 1½ maintenance rate is administered unless history of acute chest syndrome, then IV is at maintenance rate.

Once the pain is controlled (e.g., decrease swelling, using extremities, no crying when touch extremities), gradually decrease IV analgesic. If drinking orally, at least maintenance and half fluids daily, and then may convert to home oral opioid equivalent with ibuprofen every 6 hours and discharge home. If pain remains under control and Donny is drinking fluids adequately at home, instruct the parents to continue home oral opioid every 24 hours, then stop opioid and continue to observe for any signs of pain. Continue ibuprofen for 24 hours after stopping the opioid and then stop ibuprofen with no signs of pain observed.

Expected Outcome

Donny's pain will be controlled in a timely manner.

Case Study (Continued)

Donny is not eating or drinking this morning and appears lethargic in the examination room. When you question his mother regarding the last time he drank something, she remembers it was over 12 hours ago.

Assessment

What are the most important signs and symptoms of dehydration in a child with SCD?

Deficient Fluid Volume Defining Characteristics

Dry mucous membranes

Loss of skin turgor

NURSING CARE PLAN—CONT'D

The Child With Sickle Cell Anemia

Sunken eyes
No or diminished tears
Sunken fontanel
Dark urine
Rapid, thready pulse
Rapid breathing

Nursing Interventions and Rationales

What are the most appropriate nursing interventions for dehydration in a young child with sickle cell anemia who is experiencing a vasoocclusive crisis?

Nursing Interventions	Rationales
Calculate recommended daily fluid intake (1600 ml/m^2/day) and base child's fluid requirements on this amount.	To ensure adequate hydration
Increase fluid intake above minimum requirements during physical exercise or emotional stress and during a crisis.	To compensate for additional fluid needs
Give parents written instructions regarding specific quantity of fluid required daily.	To encourage compliance
Encourage child to drink.	To ensure adequate hydration
Increase fluid intake above minimum requirements during physical exercise or emotional stress and during a crisis.	To compensate for additional fluid needs

Expected Outcome

Donny will receive appropriate hydration and will demonstrate electrolyte and fluid stability.

Case Study (Continued)

Donny's parents ask you what you have found in your initial assessment. They ask about why he has swollen hands and feet and how that causes pain from SCD. They are very worried and think it is their fault that this happened.

Assessment

What are the most important aspects of Donny's care to discuss with his parents at this time? What should be included regarding SCD in a young child?

Family's Knowledge of Illness: Defining Characteristics

Lack of understanding
Inability to identify signs and symptoms of painful crises
Inability to follow disease management guidelines
Difficulty describing treatment plan

Nursing Interventions and Rationales

What are the most appropriate nursing interventions to help a family manage a young child with SCD?

Nursing Interventions	Rationales
Explain signs of developing complications, such as fever, pallor, respiratory distress, persistent headaches, and pain. Discuss dactylitis in the young child.	To ensure prompt and appropriate treatment
Reinforce basic information regarding trait transmission and refer to genetic counseling services if appropriate.	To allow for informed decision making
Provide information on what to do when complications occur, such as fever, pallor, respiratory distress, persistent headaches, and pain.	To ensure prompt and appropriate treatment
Stress importance of adequate nutrition; routine immunizations, including pneumococcal and meningococcal vaccinations; protection from known sources of infection; and frequent health evaluation and regularly scheduled comprehensive evaluation.	To encourage preventive measures and decrease risk for infection exposure

Expected Outcome

Donny's parents will state the signs and symptoms of SCD and will understand the actions being taken by the health care team. His parents will be prepared to manage his disease at home.

disintegrates, it damages the RBCs, which causes severe anemia. To compensate for the hemolytic process, an overabundance of erythrocytes is formed unless transfusion therapy suppresses the bone marrow. Excess iron from packed RBC transfusions and from the rapid destruction of defective cells is stored in various organs (hemosiderosis).

The onset of clinical manifestations in thalassemia major may be insidious and not recognized until late infancy or early toddlerhood (Box 28.5). The clinical effects of thalassemia major are primarily attributable to defective synthesis of HgbA, structurally impaired RBCs, and the shortened life span of the erythrocyte. The major consequences of thalassemia are caused by the pathologic condition, resultant chronic hypoxia, and iron overload from the supportive treatment of multiple blood supplements (Fig. 28.4 and see Box 28.5).

Anemia results from the body's inability to maintain a level of erythropoiesis commensurate with hemolysis. The bone marrow compensates by producing large numbers of immature cells, such as normoblasts and erythroblasts; large cells that are extremely thin and form bizarre shapes; and target cells, which have abnormal staining properties. As a result of the excessive production of abnormal RBCs, their life span is severely shortened.

Aplastic crises after infection, folic acid deficiencies from the demands of bone marrow hyperplasia, and progressive hemolysis from repeated blood transfusions all worsen anemia. The spleen becomes greatly enlarged as a result of extramedullary hematopoiesis, rapid destruction of the defective erythrocytes, and, rarely, progressive fibrosis from hemochromatosis. Splenomegaly may progress until the organ's very size interferes with the function of other abdominal organs and respiratory expansion.

With progressive anemia, signs of chronic hypoxia—namely, headache, irritability, precordial and bone pain, decreased exercise tolerance, listlessness, and anorexia—may develop. Another common symptom in these children is frequent epistaxis, although the exact reason is unknown. Hyperuricemia and gout from rapid cellular catabolism also occur.

Hemosiderosis refers to excess iron storage in various tissues of the body, especially the spleen, liver, lymph glands, heart, and pancreas,

BOX 28.5 Clinical Manifestations of β-Thalassemia

Anemia (Before Diagnosis)
Pallor
Unexplained fever
Poor feeding
Enlarged spleen or liver

Progressive Anemia
Signs of chronic hypoxia
Headache
Precordial and bone pain
Decreased exercise tolerance
Listlessness
Anorexia

Other Features
Small stature
Delayed sexual maturation
Bronzed, freckled complexion (if not receiving chelation therapy)

Bone Changes (Older Children If Untreated)
Enlarged head
Prominent frontal and parietal bosses
Prominent malar eminences
Flat or depressed bridge of the nose
Enlarged maxilla
Protrusion of the lip and upper central incisors and eventual malocclusion
Generalized osteoporosis

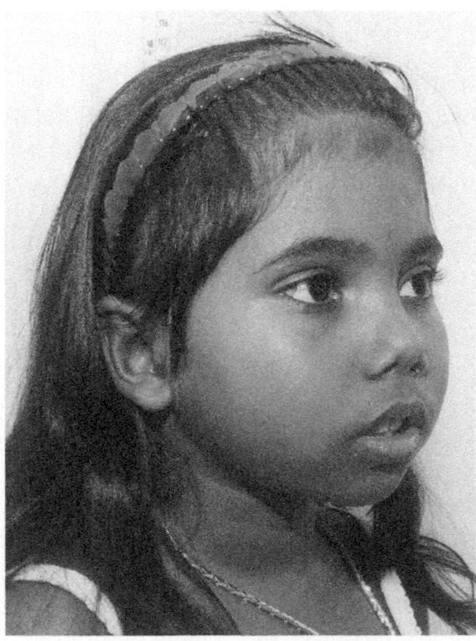

FIG. 28.4 A young girl with β-thalassemia demonstrating mild frontal bossing of the right forehead and mild maxillary prominence. (Courtesy James DeLeon, Texas Children's Hospital, Houston.)

but without associated tissue injury. Hemochromatosis refers to excess iron storage that results in cellular damage. It is not known how iron storage causes tissue destruction. Chronic hypoxia is believed to be an important contributing factor.

In thalassemia, excess of hemosiderin, the iron-containing pigment from the breakdown of hemoglobin, results from decreased hemoglobin synthesis and increased hemolysis of transfused erythrocytes. Decreased production of hemoglobin results in an excess supply of available iron. In addition, the body probably responds to the anemia by increasing the rate of GI absorption of dietary iron because ineffective erythropoiesis is a potent controlling factor in exogenous iron use. However, the primary source of additional iron is from the hemolysis of supplemental erythrocytes and the rapid destruction of defective RBCs. With the prophylactic use of deferoxamine and/or oral chelators (deferiprone and deferasirox) to minimize excess iron storage, the characteristic changes in body structures from hemochromatosis have been greatly reduced.

Retarded growth and, especially, delayed sexual maturation are common findings. There is evidence that both may also be caused by pituitary failure, although the exact reasons for this are unclear, but the impaired growth is probably also related to hemochromatosis. It is possible that the endocrine glands are extremely sensitive to iron toxicity and that even small amounts of deposited iron can produce organ dysfunction. Children with severe disease usually exhibit significant growth retardation. The development of secondary sexual characteristics is delayed or absent in many adolescents (Chatterjee & Bajoria, 2010; Sankaran, Nathan, & Orkin, 2015; Nienhuis & Nathan, 2012).

Diagnostic Evaluation

Hematologic studies reveal characteristic changes in the RBCs (e.g., microcytosis, hypochromia, anisocytosis, poikilocytosis, target cells, and basophilic stippling of various stages). Low hemoglobin and hematocrit levels often occur in severe anemia, although they are typically less pronounced than the reduction in the RBC count because of the proliferation of immature erythrocytes.

Hemoglobin electrophoresis confirms the diagnosis and is helpful in distinguishing the type and severity of the thalassemia because it analyzes the quantity and kind of hemoglobin variants found in the blood. In β-thalassemia, levels of HgbF and $HgbA_2$ (a type of normal adult hemoglobin) are elevated because neither depends on β-chain polypeptides for synthesis.

Therapeutic Management

The objective of supportive therapy is to maintain sufficient hemoglobin levels to prevent bone marrow expansion and bony deformities and to provide sufficient RBCs to support growth and normal physical activity. Transfusions are the foundation of medical management, with a goal of maintaining the hemoglobin level above 9.5 g/dl, an aim that may require transfusions as often as every 3 weeks. The advantages of this therapy include (1) improved physical and psychologic well-being because of the ability to participate in normal activities, (2) decreased cardiomegaly and hepatosplenomegaly, (3) fewer bone changes, (4) normal or near-normal growth and development until puberty, and (5) fewer infections.

One of the potential complications of frequent blood transfusions is iron overload (hemosiderosis). Each milliter of packed red blood cells contains 1 milligram of iron. Because the body has no effective means of eliminating the excess iron, the mineral is deposited in body tissues. To minimize the development of hemosiderosis and hemochromatosis in thalassemia major patient, there are three approved iron-chelating agents (deferoxamine, deferasirox, and deferiprone); each varies in its route of administration, pharmacokinetics, adverse events, and efficacy (DeBaun, Frei-Jones, & Vichinsky, 2016). Deferoxamine is given intravenously or subcutaneously at home via a portable infusion pump over a period of 12 to 14 hours daily. Deferoxamine side effects may include bradycardia, headache, rigors, hypotension, local pain, visual problems, and hearing problems. Vitamin C should be given orally only to patients who are ascorbate depleted and only while deferoxamine is being administered. Administration of vitamin C significantly augments iron excretion in response to deferoxamine, particularly in patients with vitamin C deficiency (Choudhry, 2017; Sankaran, Nathan, & Orkin, 2015). As postulated, vitamin C may delay the conversion of ferritin to hemosiderin, which allows more iron to remain in chelatable form.

Significant liver fibrosis, cardiac dysfunction, and growth impairment may be prevented if chelation therapy is adequate (Sankaran, Nathan, & Orkin, 2015). Therefore adherence to an intensive schedule is required for substantial chelation therapy. The availability of oral chelators (deferiprone and deferasirox) is a major advance in the care of patients undergoing long-term transfusion therapy that is used individually or in combination with another chelator. Deferasirox was approved by the Food and Drug Administration in 2005 for the treatment of patients 2 years and older with chronic iron overload secondary to recurrent blood transfusions (Cappellini, Bejaoui, Agaoglu, et al., 2011; Sankaran, Nathan, & Orkin, 2015). A daily dose of 30 to 40 mg/kg of deferasirox is generally well tolerated, with mild GI events and rash as common toxicities. Because Deferasirox has once-daily dosing with mild side effects and is twice as effective as desferrioxamine, it is considered the gold-standard chelating agent (Aydinok, 2012; Choudhry, 2017). Deferiprone was licensed in 2011 and is administered two to three times daily, with side effects of nausea, vomiting, abdominal pain, diarrhea, and arthropathy. The most serious toxicity of deferiprone is the occurrence of agranulocytosis in 1.1% and neutropenia in 4.9% of the patients that necessitates monitoring blood counts (Choudhry, 2017; DeBaun, Frei-Jones, & Vichinsky, 2016; Higgs, Engel, & Stamatoyannopoulos, 2012). Deferoxamine, in combination with deferiprone, is routinely used in patients with increased cardiac iron (DeBaun, Frei-Jones, & Vichinsky, 2016). Combination therapy of deferoxamine and deferasirox may also be efficacious in similar patients.

DRUG ALERT

Chelation

Chelation strategies, such as oral chelator, combination parenteral and oral chelation therapy, and organ-targeted chelation, may have a considerable impact on the quality of life of patients with thalassemia (Choudhry, 2017; Sankaran, Nathan, & Orkin, 2015).

Magnetic resonance imaging is used to evaluate the iron content of the liver, heart, and other organs and has become the method of choice for guiding iron chelating therapy in combination with laboratory measurement of serum ferritin levels and, in certain circumstances, liver biopsy (Kahnooji, Rashidlinejad, Yazdanpanah, et al., 2016).

To reduce the requirement of blood transfusions in patients with thalassemia, a few investigations and protocols reported that hydroxyurea may reduce the need for transfusions and recommended the need for well-designed randomized controlled trials to establish high-quality evidence (Ansari, Lassi, Ali, et al., 2016; Foong, Ho, Loh, et al., 2016). A recent meta-analysis reported that hydroxyurea is potentially effective in management of non–transfusion-dependent β-thalassemia patients; however, more randomized evidence is needed to further validate this meta-analysis (Algiraigri, Wright, Paolucci, et al., 2017).

In some children with severe splenomegaly who require repeated transfusions, a splenectomy may be necessary to decrease the disabling effects of abdominal pressure and to increase the life span of supplemental RBCs. Over time the spleen may accelerate the rate of RBC destruction and therefore increase transfusion requirements. After a splenectomy, children generally require fewer transfusions, although the basic defect in hemoglobin synthesis remains unaffected. A major postsplenectomy complication is severe and overwhelming infection. Therefore these children are often on prophylactic antibiotics with close medical supervision for many years and should receive the pneumococcal and meningococcal vaccines in addition to regularly scheduled immunizations. (See Immunizations, Chapter 10.)

Prognosis

Most children treated with blood transfusions and early chelation therapy have a remarkably improved life span as they survive well into adulthood (Higgs, Engel, & Stamatoyannopoulos, 2012; Sankaran, Nathan, & Orkin, 2015). The most common causes of death are heart disease, liver damage with cirrhosis, postsplenectomy sepsis, and multiorgan failure secondary to hemochromatosis (Choudhry, 2017; Sankaran, Nathan, & Orkin, 2015; Yaish, 2015). The three adverse prognostic factors for event-free survival are presence of heptomegaly (2 cm below costal margin), iron overload (serum ferritin greater than 1000 ng/ml), and portal fibrosis (Choudhry, 2017). Children with the absence of these adverse prognostic factors have greater than 97% event-free survival (Choudhry, 2017). A curative treatment for some children is HSCT. Children younger than 16 years of age who undergo allogeneic HSCT have a high rate of complication-free survival; approximately 80% to 97% of these children are cured (DeBaun, Frei-Jones, & Vichinsky, 2016; Issaragrisil & Kunacheewa, 2016; Lucarelli, Isgro, Sodani, et al., 2012). Also, related cord-blood transplantation has a disease-free survival of about 90% (Higgs, Engel, & Stamatoyannopoulos, 2012; Issaragrisil & Kunacheewa, 2016). Children without a matched donor may benefit from haploidentical family member transplant, which has shown encouraging results (Lucarelli, Isgro, Sodani, et al., 2012; Locatelli, Merli, & Strocchio, 2016). New approaches for correction of thalassemia through the introduction of gene therapy strategies, including the use of lentiviral vectors, generation of pluripotent stem cells, and gene targeting, are ongoing but continue to have concerns (Arlet, Dussiot, Moura, et al., 2016; Raja, Rachchh, & Gokani, 2012; Sankaran, Nathan, & Orkin, 2015).

Nursing Care Management

The objectives of nursing care are to (1) promote compliance with transfusion and chelation therapy, (2) assist the child in coping with the anxiety-provoking treatments and the effects of the illness, (3) foster the child's and family's adjustment to a chronic illness, and (4) observe for complications of multiple blood transfusions. Basic to each of these goals is explaining to parents and older children the defect responsible for the disorder, its effect on RBCs, and the potential effects of untreated hemosiderosis (such as delayed growth and maturation and heart disease). Because this condition is prevalent among families of Mediterranean descent, the nurse also inquires about the family's previous knowledge about thalassemia. All families with a child with thalassemia should be tested for the trait and referred for genetic counseling.

Support the Family

As with any chronic illness, the family's needs must be met for optimum adjustment to the stresses imposed by the disorder. (See Chapter 21.) Sources of information for the family are the Cooley's Anemia Foundation* and the Thalassemia Action Group. Genetic counseling for the parents and fertile offspring is mandatory, and both prenatal diagnosis using amniocentesis or fetal blood sampling and screening for thalassemia

*330 Seventh Ave., No. 200, New York, NY 10001; 800-522-7222; fax: 212-279-5999; e-mail: info@cooleysanemia.org; http://www.thalassemia.org; https://www.facebook.com/pages/Thalassemia-org/162500870481012.

trait are available. There has been a marked decline in the number of new cases of thalassemia worldwide. This may be a result of education and testing of parents.

Assist in Coping With the Effects of the Disorder

Body image alterations, decreased growth, and sexual immaturity are frequently difficult adjustment problems for older children. These children feel different from their peers, and the delayed sexual development is a major issue for the maturing adolescent with an improved life expectancy. Adolescents need an opportunity to express their thoughts and feelings about these complex issues. They can learn grooming measures that make them appear more sexually mature, such as wearing up-to-date clothing, adopting new hairstyles, and wearing well-applied makeup. Children with the characteristic bone changes may benefit from surgery or use of orthodontic appliances to improve facial structure.

With frequent transfusion therapy there is less restriction on physical activity because of severe anemia, and the nurse should encourage these children to pursue activities that they are able to tolerate. The frequency of treatment, however, can interfere with a normal lifestyle. To minimize disruptions and improve cooperation, the nurse can help arrange for blood transfusions and medical supervision at times that interfere least with the child's regular activities, especially school.

ANEMIAS CAUSED BY IMPAIRED OR DECREASED PRODUCTION OF RED BLOOD CELLS

Impaired or decreased production of RBCs can occur as a result of either bone marrow failure or deficiency of essential nutrients. Bone marrow failure may be caused by (1) replacement of bone marrow by fibrous tissue or by neoplastic cells, as in leukemia; (2) depression of marrow activity by irradiation, chemicals, or drugs; and (3) interference with bone marrow activity caused by systemic disorders such as severe infection, chronic renal disease, widespread malignancy (without marrow infiltration), collagen diseases, or hypothyroidism. When depression of the hematologic system is extensive, aplastic anemia develops.

The reason systemic disorders affect erythrocyte production varies according to the condition. For example, in severe chronic infection there is evidence that depression of erythropoiesis is caused by a defect in the conversion of protoporphyrin into hemoglobin. In addition, there is some degree of hemolysis, although the exact mechanism is not known.

APLASTIC ANEMIA

Aplastic anemia (AA) is a rare and life-threatening disorder that affects approximately 2 to 6 in 1 million children and adults each year (Hord, 2016; Korthof, Bekassy, & Hussein, 2013). AA refers to a condition in which production of the formed elements of the blood is simultaneously depressed. The peripheral blood smear demonstrates cytopenia, including at least two of the triad that consists of leukopenia, thrombocytopenia, and profound anemia. Hypoplastic anemia is characterized by a profound depression of RBC formation but normal or slightly decreased production of WBCs and platelets. One type of hypoplastic anemia is pure RBC aplasia, which can be congenital or acquired. The acquired defect in erythropoiesis is an autoimmune condition that occurs mostly in adults. The congenital condition (Diamond-Blackfan syndrome) is marked by complete or almost complete absence of all cells of the erythroid series with normal production of the other myeloid cells. Its treatment, which consists of transfusions, splenectomy, and administration of corticosteroids, is similar to that for other diseases that result in profound anemia. The prognosis varies, although long-term survival is possible. The principal causes of death are cardiac failure, hepatitis from transfusion therapy, and sepsis. Hemosiderosis and hemochromatosis (see p. 1046) also affect vital tissues necessary for survival.

BOX 28.6 Common Causes of Acquired Aplastic Anemia

- Human parvovirus infection, hepatitis, or overwhelming infection
- Irradiation
- Immune disorders such as eosinophilic fasciitis and hypoimmunoglobulinemia
- Drugs such as certain chemotherapeutic agents, anticonvulsants, and antibiotics
- Industrial and household chemicals, including benzene and its derivatives, which are found in petroleum products, dyes, paint remover, shellac, and lacquers
- Infiltration and replacement of myeloid elements, such as in leukemia or the lymphomas
- Idiopathic (in most cases no identifiable precipitating cause found)

AA can be primary (congenital, or present at birth) or secondary (acquired). The best-known congenital disorder of which AA is an outstanding feature is Fanconi anemia syndrome, a rare hereditary disorder that is characterized by pancytopenia, hypoplasia of the bone marrow, and patchy brown discoloration of the skin due to the deposition of melanin. It is associated with multiple congenital anomalies of the musculoskeletal and genitourinary systems. The syndrome appears to be inherited as an autosomal recessive trait with varying penetrance; therefore affected siblings may demonstrate different combinations of defects.

Several factors contribute to the development of acquired hypoplastic anemia; however, most of the cases are considered idiopathic (Box 28.6). The following discussion focuses on acquired severe AA, which carries a poorer prognosis and follows a more rapidly fatal course than the primary types.

Diagnostic Evaluation

The onset of clinical manifestations, which include anemia, leukopenia, and decreased platelet count, is usually insidious, not unlike that seen in leukemia. Definitive diagnosis is determined from bone marrow examination, which demonstrates the conversion of red bone marrow to yellow, fatty bone marrow. Severe AA is based on the Camitta's criteria, which is less than 25% bone marrow cellularity with at least two of the following findings: absolute neutrophil count (ANC) less than 500/mm^3, platelet count less than 20,000/mm^3, and absolute reticulocyte count less than 40,000/mm^3 (Miano & Dufour, 2015; Passweg & Marsh, 2010). However, a study evaluated the Camitta's criteria and suggested the criteria be modified to include the ANC as an essential criterion rather than optional (Yoon, Huh, Lee, et al., 2012). Yoon, Huh, Lee, and colleagues (2012) recommended the need for further large studies to possibly modify the Camitta's criteria. Moderate AA is defined as less than 50% bone marrow cellularity with presence of mild to moderate cytopenia (Shimamura & Williams, 2015).

Therapeutic Management

The objectives of treatment are based on the recognition that the underlying disease process is failure of the bone marrow to carry out its hematopoietic functions. Therefore therapy is directed at restoring function to the marrow and involves two main approaches: immunosuppressive therapy to counter the presumed immunologic responses that prolong aplasia and replacement of the bone marrow through transplantation. Bone marrow transplantation is the treatment of choice for severe AA when an HLA-matched sibling donor exists.

Immunosuppressive therapy (IST) is an alternative preferred line of treatment for children with acquired AA who do not have a matched sibling bone marrow donor (Shimamura & Williams, 2015; Young, Bacigalupo, & Marsh, 2010). Antithymocyte globulin (ATG) or anti-lymphocyte globulin (ALG) is the principal drug treatment used for AA. The rationale for using ATG is based on the theory that AA may be a result of autoimmunity.

IST is a combination of ATG and cyclosporine that suppress T cell–dependent autoimmune responses by recognizing human lymphocyte cell surface antigen and decreasing the lymphocytes without causing bone marrow suppression (Peinemann & Labeit, 2014). Cyclosporine is administered orally for several weeks to months. ATG usually is administrated intravenously over 12 to 16 hours for 4 days after a test dose to check for hypersensitivity. Response to IST is typically delayed and responses generally do not start before 3 to 4 months after treatment (Samarasinghe & Webb, 2012; Shimamura & Williams, 2015). An IST course may be repeated, depending on the reduction in circulating lymphocytes and the patient's response (see Nursing Care Management). Because of the hypersensitivity response associated with ATG (i.e., fever, chills, myalgias), methylprednisolone is given intravenously to prevent these side effects. Growth factors, given parenterally, may be used to prevent neutropenic infection and enhance bone marrow production (Passweg & Marsh, 2010).

DRUG ALERT

Antithymocyte Globulin, Cyclosporin A, and Granulocyte-Macrophage Colony-Stimulating Factor

In children who fail to respond to IST, success has been achieved by repeating a second course of ATG/cyclosporine, or using high-dose cyclophosphamide as an effective immunosuppressive agent or using androgens or considering an unrelated HLA-matched hematopoietic stem-cell transplant. Androgens no longer have a primary role in the management of aplastic anemia, unless the other therapies discussed are unavailable or unsuccessful (Shimamura & Williams, 2015). However, androgens have been used effectively to stimulate erythropoiesis in treating some patients with aplastic anemia as an adjunct to ATG (Shimamura & Williams, 2015).

Although IST is effective in ameliorating the pancytopenia of aplastic anemia, IST has a significant risk in development of somatic mutations that may evolve into myelodysplastic syndrome (MDS) or acute myeloid leukemia (AML) (Georges & Srorb, 2016). Although unrelated HLA-matched bone marrow transplant can be successfully performed after the IST failure or after evolution to MDS/AML, recent studies suggest that first-line treatment with an HLA-matched unrelated bone marrow should be strongly considered for children with acquired severe AA who lack an HLA-identical sibling donor (Dufour, Veys, Carraro, et al., 2015).

HSCT should be considered early in the course of the disease if a compatible donor can be found. Transplantation is more successful if performed before multiple transfusions have sensitized the child to leukocytes and HLAs. Children who are eligible for transplantation should be transferred to one of the medical centers that specialize in this procedure. Many different preparative regimens are available, and all aim to decrease the rate of graft-versus-host disease. All regimens include immunosuppressive therapy, and some also include irradiation (either total body or thoracoabdominal). Patients who have received a large number of transfusions before bone marrow transplantation have a higher rejection rate and lower survival rate (Scheinberg, 2012). With the use of immunosuppressive therapy and HLA-identical sibling donor, the allogeneic bone marrow transplantation offers 90% chance of long-term survival (Hord, 2016; Scheinberg, 2012). Recently survival outcomes from unrelated HLA-matched bone marrow transplantation are approaching the success seen with HLA-identical sibling bone marrow transplant (Georges & Storb, 2016).

Nursing Care Management

The care of the child with AA is similar to the care of the child with leukemia and includes preparing the child and family for the diagnostic and therapeutic procedures, preventing complications from the severe pancytopenia, and emotionally supporting the family in the face of potentially fatal outcome. Information and support are available from the Aplastic Anemia and MDS International Foundation, Inc.*

DRUG ALERT

Antithymocyte Globulin

During administration of ATG, whether into a central venous catheter or peripheral vein, the nurse must pay special attention to the infusion to prevent extravasation. Meticulous care of the venous access catheter is essential because of the child's susceptibility to infection. Although anaphylactic reactions to ATG are rare, make emergency preparations in advance, and have epinephrine and oxygen readily available. The nurse should observe for immediate reactions to ATG, which include fever and skin rash. Delayed reactions (serum sickness) may also occur within 7 to 14 days of a course of ATG, and the manifestations are similar to those in immediate reactions. The symptoms are reversed, and in the case of serum sickness may be prevented, with corticosteroids.

The aspects of nursing care are discussed in the section on leukemia, so the only interventions specific to AA are presented here. Because growth factors are usually given subcutaneously over several days, an anesthetic cream, EMLA or LMX, may be used to minimize pain at the injection site. Chemotherapeutic agents have been used in relapsed AA patients who have been treated with ATG and colony-stimulating factor (CSF) therapy. Many of the side effects associated with chemotherapy, such as nausea and vomiting, alopecia, and mucosal ulceration, are experienced by children receiving treatment for AA. Specialized care required for AA children who have HSCT is discussed in the section on HSCT.

DEFECTS IN HEMOSTASIS

Hemostasis is the process that stops bleeding when a blood vessel is injured. Vascular and plasma clotting factors, as well as platelets, are required. A complex system of clotting, anticlotting, and clot breakdown (**fibrinolysis**) mechanisms exists in equilibrium to ensure clot formation only in the presence of blood vessel injury and to limit the clotting process to the site of vessel wall injury. Dysfunction in these systems leads to bleeding or abnormal clotting.

MECHANISMS INVOLVED IN NORMAL HEMOSTASIS

Understanding the role that factor deficiencies play in promoting bleeding tendencies requires a review of the normal coagulation process of the

*100 Park Avenue, Suite 108, Rockville, MD 20850; 800-747-2820; 301-279-7202; fax 301-279-7205; e-mail: help@aamds.org; http://www.aamds.org; https://www.facebook.com/aamds.

blood. Although the coagulation process is complex, clotting depends on three main elements: vascular events, platelets, and clotting factors.

Vascular Events

At the time and site of injury, several events occur to initiate hemostasis: local vasoconstriction, compression of the blood vessels by extravasated blood, and release of von Willebrand factor by endothelial walls. Collagen present in exposed subendothelial cells acts as a site for platelet adhesion.

Platelets

Normally the platelets do not adhere to one another or to normal endothelium. However, when a blood vessel is injured, certain events take place. First, platelet adhesion occurs at the site of the injury, providing a plug. The platelets change shape, develop pseudopods, and release a variety of chemicals to stimulate vasoconstriction and vessel repair and to activate and recruit more platelets to the injury site. Receptor sites are located on the platelets for fibrinogen and other adhesive proteins, which cause the platelets to stick together (aggregation). As the membranes of the platelets change, the phospholipids necessary for blood coagulation are exposed so that fibrin, which secures the platelet plugs to the site, can be produced. Finally, the clot compresses and is secured to the injury.

Defects in platelets and clotting factors are the most common causes of bleeding during childhood. The following discussion focuses on the major conditions that require nursing intervention.

Clotting Factors

The clotting factors (Table 28.4 and Fig. 28.5) are activated in sequence to develop a fibrin clot. Two mechanisms exist that can generate prothrombin to produce thrombin:

1. **Intrinsic pathway**—Factor XII, high-molecular-weight kininogen (HMK, Fitzgerald factor), and prekallikrein (KAL, Fletcher factor) react on a negatively charged surface (contact activation reaction) to activate factor XI (PTA, plasma thromboplastin antecedent). The partial thromboplastin time measures abnormalities in the intrinsic pathway (abnormalities in factors I, II, V, VIII, IX, X, XII, HMK, and KAL).
2. **Extrinsic pathway**—A lipoprotein tissue factor stimulates activation of factor VII. The prothrombin time measures abnormalities of the extrinsic pathway (abnormalities in factors I, II, V, VII, and X). Table 28.5 presents laboratory tests to assess hemostasis.

HEMOPHILIA

The term *hemophilia* refers to a group of bleeding disorders resulting from congenital deficiency, dysfunction, or absence of specific coagulation proteins or factors (Di Paola, Montgomery, Gill, et al., 2015; Sharathkumar & Pipe, 2008). Although the symptomatology is similar regardless of which clotting factor is deficient, the identification of specific factor deficiencies has allowed definitive treatment with replacement agents.

In about 80% of all cases of hemophilia, the inheritance pattern is demonstrated as X-linked recessive. (See Chapter 3.) The two most

TABLE 28.4 Blood-Clotting Factors

Factor Number	Synonyms
I	Fibrinogen
II	Prothrombin
III	Platelet factor 3, thromboplastin
IV	Calcium
V	Labile factor, proaccelerin, Ac globulin
VII	Serum prothrombin conversion accelerator (SPCA), proconvertin, stable factor
VIII	Antihemophilic factor (AHF)
IX	Plasma thromboplastin component (PTC), Christmas factor
X	Stuart-Prower factor
XI	Plasma thromboplastin antecedent (PTA)
XII	Hageman factor
XIII	Fibrin-stabilizing factor (FSF)
KAL	Prekallikrein, Fletcher factor
HMK	High-molecular-weight kininogen, Fitzgerald factor

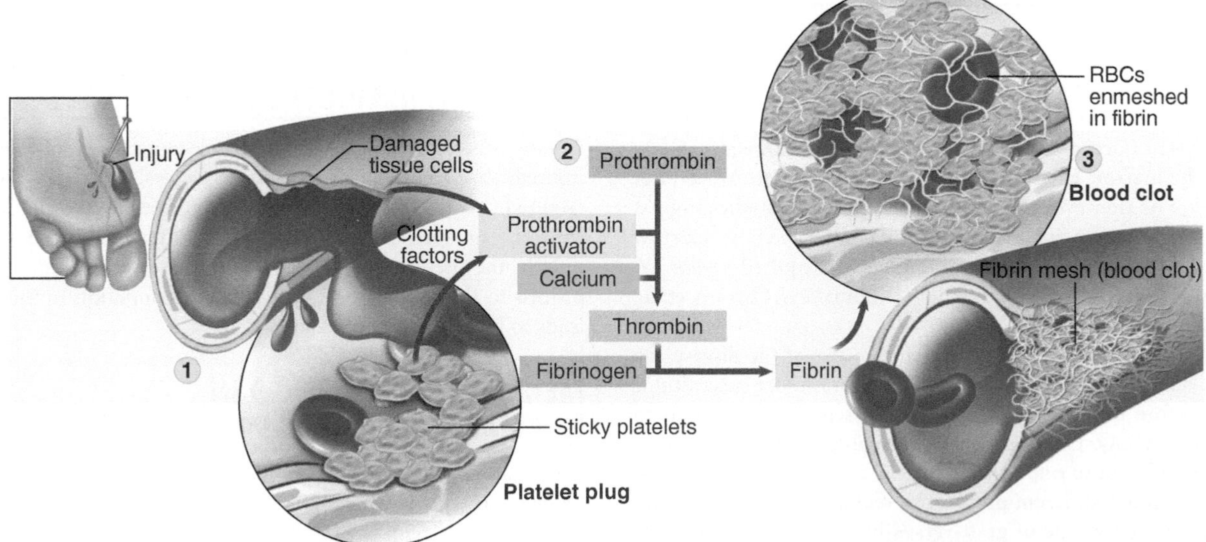

FIG. 28.5 Blood clotting. The extremely complex clotting mechanism can be distilled into three basic steps: release of clotting factors from both injured tissue cells and sticky platelets at the injury site (which form a temporary platelet plug); series of chemical reactions that eventually result in the formation of thrombin; and formation of fibrin and trapping of red blood cells (RBCs) to form a clot. (From Thibodeau, G. A., & Patton, K. T. [2010]. *The human body in health and disease* [5th ed.]. St. Louis, MO: Mosby.)

TABLE 28.5 Laboratory Tests to Assess Hemostasis

Test	Description	Comments
Platelet Function		
Platelet function analyzer (PFA 100)	Measures platelet function and interaction with von Willebrand factor Has replaced bleeding time in some centers	Results are altered with intake of NSAIDs, anticoagulants, ASA, or ASA-containing products
Bleeding time	Measures time it takes for bleeding from small superficial wound to cease	Function depends on platelet aggregation and vasoconstriction; two common methods used are Ivy (incision made on the forearm) and Duke (incision made on the earlobe)
Tourniquet test	Measures platelet function and capillary fragility; pressure applied to forearm with tourniquet for 5-10 minutes	Normal response is absence of petechiae or <10 petechiae Abnormal in platelet and connective tissue disorders
Clot retraction test	Measures degree to which clot shrinks and expresses serum	Depends on platelet function
Blood-Clotting Mechanisms		
Whole blood clotting time	Measures time it takes for clot to form *within* blood	Prolonged clotting time indicates problem in thrombin-to-fibrin phase or in any factor in intrinsic clotting mechanism; difficult test to standardize; therefore often unreliable results
Prothrombin time (PT)	Measures activity of prothrombin and factors necessary for its conversion to thrombin and fibrinogen	Actually measures not prothrombin levels but activity; because it bypasses intrinsic-extrinsic mechanism, detects deficiencies of factors V, VII, X, and fibrinogen as well as prothrombin
Partial thromboplastin time (PPT)	Similar to PT but measures activity of thromboplastin, which depends on intrinsic clotting factors	Specific for factor deficiencies, except factor VII, which results in a normal PTT but prolonged PT
Thromboplastin generation test	Measures blood's ability to generate thromboplastin	Allows for determination of specific factor deficiencies, especially distinguishing between factors VII and IX
Prothrombin consumption test	Indirectly measures thromboplastin generation and prothrombin response	Normally, as blood clots, prothrombin is converted to thrombin so that serum is depleted of prothrombin; if thromboplastin is decreased (as a result of extrinsic factor deficiencies), not all prothrombin will be converted and removed from serum
Fibrinogen level	Directly measures fibrinogen levels in blood	Not dependent on phase I or II deficiencies

ASA, Acetylsalicylic acid; *NSAIDs*, nonsteroidal antiinflammatory drugs.

common forms of the disorder are factor VIII deficiency (hemophilia A, or classic hemophilia) and factor IX deficiency (hemophilia B, or Christmas disease), with prevalence of approximately 1 in 5000 and 1 in 20,000 to 30,000 live male births, respectively (Centers for Disease Control and Prevention, 2017a; National Hemophilia Foundation, 2017a; Marcdante & Kliegman, 2015; Sharathkumar & Carcao, 2011). Von Willebrand disease (vWD) is another hereditary bleeding disorder characterized by a deficiency, abnormality, or absence of the protein called *von Willebrand factor (vWF)*. The following discussion is primarily concerned with factor VIII deficiency, which accounts for 80% to 85% of all cases.

Modes of Transmission

Hemophilia is transmitted as an X-linked recessive disorder, but only about 60% of affected children have a positive family history for the disease. Up to one-third of all hemophilia cases may be caused by a gene mutation. The most frequent pattern of transmission is through the union of an unaffected male with a trait-carrier female. Because the treatment of persons with hemophilia has improved, the results of a union between an affected male and a normal female or a carrier female must also be considered. For example, the chances are equal (e.g., 1 in 4) that an offspring of an affected male and a carrier female will be an affected son, an affected daughter, a carrier daughter, or a normal son. Such parentage is one of the few ways in which a female inherits the disorder. Female carriers may have low levels of factor VIII and be symptomatic.

Pathophysiology and Clinical Manifestations

The basic defect of hemophilia A is a deficiency of factor VIII (antihemophilic factor). Factor VIII is produced by the liver and is necessary for the formation of thromboplastin in phase I of blood coagulation. The less factor VIII that is found in the blood, the more severe the disease.

A major feature of hemophilia is that its expression varies markedly with regard to the degree of bleeding severity. Hemophilia is generally classified into three groups according to the severity of the factor deficiency; 60% to 70% of children with hemophilia demonstrate the severe form of the disorder (Table 28.6).

The effect of hemophilia is prolonged bleeding anywhere from or in the body. With severe factor deficiencies, hemorrhage can occur as a result of minor trauma, such as after circumcision, during loss of deciduous teeth, or as a result of a slight fall or bruise. In children with less severe deficiencies, however, the bleeding tendency may not be noted until the onset of walking.

Subcutaneous and intramuscular hemorrhages are common. Hemarthrosis, which refers to bleeding into the joint cavities, especially the knees, elbows, and ankles, is the most frequent form of internal bleeding. Bony changes and crippling deformities occur after repeated bleeding episodes over several years. Early signs of hemarthrosis are a feeling of stiffness, tingling, or ache in the affected joint, followed by a decrease in the ability to move the joint. Obvious signs and symptoms are warmth, redness, swelling, and severe pain, with considerable loss of movement.

TABLE 28.6 Clinical Severity of Hemophilia

Clinical Severity	Factor VIII Activity	Bleeding Tendency
Severe	<1%	Spontaneous bleeding without trauma
Moderate	1%-5%	Bleeding with trauma
Mild	>5%-40%	Bleeding with severe trauma or surgery

Spontaneous hematuria is not uncommon. Epistaxis may occur but is not as frequent as other kinds of hemorrhage. Petechiae are uncommon in persons with hemophilia because repair of small hemorrhages depends on platelet function, not on blood-clotting mechanisms.

Bleeding into the tissue can occur anywhere but is serious if it occurs in the neck, mouth, or thorax because the airway can become obstructed. Intracranial hemorrhage can have fatal consequences and is one of the major causes of death. Hemorrhage anywhere along the GI tract can lead to anemia, and bleeding into the retroperitoneal cavity is especially hazardous because of the large space for blood to accumulate. Hematomas in the spinal cord can cause paralysis.

Diagnostic Evaluation

The diagnosis is usually made from a history of bleeding episodes, evidence of X-linked inheritance (only one-third of cases are new mutations), and laboratory findings. To understand the significance of various tests of hemostasis, it is helpful to recall the usual mechanisms to control bleeding (e.g., the function of platelets and clotting factors). The results of tests that measure platelet function, such as the bleeding time, are all normal in persons with hemophilia, whereas the results of tests that assess clotting factor function may be abnormal (see Table 28.5). The tests specific for hemophilia include factor VIII and IX assays, procedures normally done by specialized laboratories. Other tests are those that depend on specific factors for a reaction to occur, especially the partial thromboplastin time. Carrier detection is possible in classic hemophilia using DNA testing and is an important consideration in families in which female offspring may have inherited the trait.

Therapeutic Management

The primary therapy for hemophilia is replacement of the missing clotting factor. The products currently available are factor VIII concentrates, either produced through genetic engineering (recombinant form) or derived from pooled plasma, which are reconstituted with sterile water immediately before use. A synthetic form of vasopressin, 1-deamino-8-D-arginine vasopressin (DDAVP), is the treatment of choice in mild hemophilia and vWD (types I and IIA only) if the child shows an appropriate response. After DDAVP administration a threefold to fourfold rise in factor VIII activity should occur. Because the goal is to raise the factor VIII level at least 30%, patients with moderate factor VIII deficiency do not benefit. In addition, various therapies are employed when bleeding occurs or is anticipated (Table 28.7).

DRUG ALERT

Cryoprecipitate

Cryoprecipitate is no longer recommended for use in treating factor VIII deficiency. Since the availability of highly purified factor VIII concentrate (monoclonal) in 1988 and the licensing of recombinant factor VIII concentrate in 1992 (marketed not as a blood product but as a drug), the National Hemophilia Foundation has advised practitioners to use only these products. Cryoprecipitate cannot be treated to safely eliminate hepatitis or human immunodeficiency virus (HIV).

TABLE 28.7 Adjunct Therapies for Hemophilia A

Site of Bleed	Treatment
Joint	Rest, ice, elevation Splint, elastic wrap, crutches Physical therapy
Soft tissue	Ice, elevation Splint or elastic wrap
Muscle	Rest, ice, elevation Splint, elastic wrap, crutches Physical therapy Complete bed rest for iliopsoas muscle bleed
Mucous membrane (e.g., nose, mouth)	Pressure to nares (for nosebleed) Topical antifibrinolytic agent (ε-aminocaproic acid) Nasal pack (sometimes necessary)

Aggressive factor concentrate replacement therapy is initiated to prevent chronic crippling effects from joint bleeding. If replacement therapy begins immediately, local measures such as ice applications and splinting are seldom needed. Other drugs may be included in the therapy plan, depending on the source of the hemorrhage. Corticosteroids are given for hematuria, acute hemarthrosis, and chronic synovitis. It is recommended that patients with hemophilia avoid aspirin and nonsteroidal antiinflammatory drugs (NSAIDs) because they inhibit platelet function (National Hemophilia Foundation, 2016; Scott, 2016a). However, NSAIDs such as ibuprofen are effective in relieving pain caused by synovitis and are occasionally used with caution (Hermans, De Moerloose, Fischer et al., 2011; National Hemophilia Foundation, 2016). Oral use of ε-aminocaproic acid (EACA, Amicar) prevents clot destruction. Its use is limited to mouth trauma or surgery, with a dose of factor concentrate given first. The child may rinse the mouth with this medication and then swallow it.

In some children with hemophilia, the factor replacement is seen by the body as a foreign protein when it is administered and the body produces an antibody (inhibitor) that destroys the factor. When individuals are resistant to first-line therapy, they are treated with one of two equally effective agents, recombinant activated factor VIIa or human activated prothrombin complex concentrate (Guelcher, 2016; Matino, Makris, Dwan, et al., 2015).

A regular program of exercise and physical therapy is an important aspect of management. If started early and continued throughout adulthood, planned, individualized physical activity strengthens muscles around joints and may decrease the number of spontaneous bleeding episodes.

! NURSING ALERT

Passive range-of-motion exercises should never be part of an exercise regimen after an acute episode because the joint capsule could easily be stretched and bleeding could recur. Active range-of-motion exercises are best so that the patient can gauge his or her own pain tolerance.

Treatment without delay results in more rapid recovery and a decreased likelihood of complications; therefore most children are treated at home. The family is taught how to perform venipuncture and how to administer factor VIII to children over 2 to 3 years of age. The child learns the procedure for self-administration at 8 to 12 years of age. Home treatment is highly successful, and the rewards, in addition to the immediacy, are less disruption of family life, fewer school or work days missed, and enhancement of the child's self-esteem and independence. Although home treatment for hemophilia promotes freedom, flexibility, and autonomy for the boys and the family, mothers or caregivers who usually provide the daily childcare may view the treatment experience as a burden (von der Lippe, Frich, Harris, et al., 2017). It is important for the health professionals to provide practical and emotional support for the caregivers of these boys.

Prophylactic therapy is periodic factor replacement for children with severe hemophilia to prevent bleeding complications, including arthropathy and spontaneous and life-threatening bleeding events (Di Paola,Montgomery, Gill, et al., 2015; Scott, 2016a; von der Lippe, Frich, Harris, et al., 2017). Primary prophylaxis in patients with severe hemophilia has been practiced for many years in developed countries and has proved to be effective in preventing naturopathy. In primary prophylaxis, factor VIII concentrate is infused on a regular basis before the onset of joint damage. Secondary prophylaxis involves the infusion of factor VIII concentrate on a regular basis after the child experiences his or her first joint bleed. The infusions are given every other day or three times a week for several weeks to promote healing. Episodic factor replacement may be a cost-effective alternative to primary prophylaxis, but prophylaxis decreases the development of joint disease compared with on-demand treatment (Manco-Johnson, Abshire, Shapiro, et al., 2007). However, prompt appropriate treatment of hemorrhage and prophylactic therapy are key to excellent care and prevention of long-term morbidity in patients with hemophilia (Di Paola, Montgomery, Gill, et al., 2015; Lillicrap, 2013).

Prognosis

The progress made in hemophilia care over the years has been striking. The institution of home infusion therapy and the use of safer, more effective factor concentrates, coupled with the establishment of comprehensive treatment centers and the adoption of prophylactic treatment regimens, have revolutionized the treatment and management of hemophilia (Di Paola, Montgomery, Gill, et al., 2015; Sharathkumar & Carcao, 2011). Early recognition of joint and muscle bleeds is emphasized because immediate adequate treatment with clotting factor is possible using home infusion therapy. Early treatment has significantly reduced the morbidity formerly associated with hemophilia. The availability of comprehensive hemophilia treatment centers offers the child with hemophilia and the family a coordinated multidisciplinary approach to meeting their needs and improving the child's health and well-being.

Although there is no cure for hemophilia, its symptoms can be controlled and its potentially crippling deformities markedly reduced or even avoided. Today many children with hemophilia function with minimal or no joint damage. They have an average life expectancy and are normal in every aspect but one: they have a tendency to bleed, which is a significant inconvenience but not necessarily a life-threatening event.

Unfortunately, those individuals with hemophilia who were treated before the development of current purification techniques for factor VIII concentrate (between 1979 and 1985) may have been exposed to HIV. It is estimated that 90% of severe hemophiliacs seroconverted to HIV-positive status, and 30% developed acquired immunodeficiency syndrome (AIDS) (National Hemophilia Foundation, 2017b). Individuals with hemophilia diagnosed since the 1990s and treated with recombinant factor products are at virtually no risk for developing HIV infection from treatment. Recombinant factor VIII and factor IX products that are devoid of human protein materials have become the treatment of choice for children and previously untreated hemophilia patients (Di Paola, Montgomery, Gill, et al., 2015).

Gene therapy may prove to be a treatment option in the future. Techniques are under development to introduce the factor VIII or IX genes into hepatocytes, fibroblasts, endothelial cells using adeno-associated viral vectors, and other novel ideas for genetic correction (Branchford, Monahan, & Di Paola, 2013; Nienhuis, Nathwani, & Davidoff, 2017; Walsh & Batt, 2013). The scientific community remains undaunted in its attempt to make gene-addition therapy a 21st-century reality for patients with hemophilia A and B. Efforts are underway to improve viral vector strategies, including selection of both appropriate vectors and the appropriate cell in which to express the gene, and to obtain a better understanding of the immune consequences of gene transfer (Di Paola, Montgomery, Gill, et al., 2015; Lytle, Brown, Paik, et al., 2016; Nienhuis, Nathwani, & Davidoff, 2017).

Nursing Care Management

The earlier a bleeding episode is recognized, the more effectively it can be treated. Signs that indicate internal bleeding are especially important to recognize. Children are aware of internal bleeding and are reliable in telling the examiner the location of an internal bleed. In addition, the nurse maintains a high level of suspicion when a child with hemophilia shows signs such as headache; slurred speech; loss of consciousness (from cerebral bleeding); and black, tarry stools (from GI bleeding). (See Quality Patient Outcomes box.)

QUALITY PATIENT OUTCOMES

Hemophilia

- Early recognition of signs and symptoms of hemophilia
- Bleeding episodes prevented
- Bleeding episodes treated early with factor replacement
- Adherence to prophylactic factor replacement program when indicated
- Hemarthrosis prevented when possible with limited joint damage
- Exercise program and physical therapy ongoing

Prevent Bleeding

The goal of prevention of bleeding episodes is directed toward decreasing the risk of injury. Prevention of bleeding episodes is geared mostly toward appropriate exercises to strengthen muscles and joints and to allow age-appropriate activity. During infancy and toddlerhood, the normal acquisition of motor skills creates innumerable opportunities for falls, bruises, and minor wounds. Restraining the child from mastering motor development can bring more serious long-term problems than allowing the behavior. However, the environment should be made as safe as possible, with close supervision maintained during playtime to minimize incidental injuries.

For older children the family usually needs assistance in preparing the child for school. A nurse who knows the family can be instrumental in discussing the situation with the school nurse and in joint planning of an appropriate activity schedule. Because almost all individuals with hemophilia are boys, the physical limitations in regard to active sports may be a difficult adjustment, and activity restrictions must be tempered with sensitivity to the child's emotional and physical needs. Use of protective equipment, such as helmets, face masks, shin/wrist/forearm guards, kneepads, and other equipment appropriate for the type of athletic activity, is encouraged to prevent injury. Children and adolescents with severe hemophilia can participate in noncontact sports such as swimming, golf, walking, jogging, fishing, and bowling. Contact sports such as football, boxing, hockey, wrestling, and rugby are strongly discouraged because the risk of injury outweighs the physical and psychosocial benefits of participating in these sports (Anderson & Forsyth, 2017; Polus, 2016; Scott, 2016a). However, studies have reported that the absolute increase in risk of bleeds associated with regular participation in high-impact athletic activities (e.g., basketball, football, hockey, gymnastics, karate, soccer, skateboarding) that is supported by adult coaching and supervision of school-age hemophiliac children who received routine prophylactic factor replacement is small and is accompanied with improved quality of life and joint health (Broderick, Herbert, Latimer, et al., 2012; Cuesta-Barriuso, Torres-Ortuno, Perez-Alenda, et al., 2016).

To prevent oral bleeding, some readjustment in terms of dental hygiene may be needed to minimize trauma to the gums, such as using a water irrigating device, softening the toothbrush in warm water before brushing, or using a sponge-tipped disposable toothbrush. A regular toothbrush should be soft-bristled and small. Adolescents also need to be advised of the dangers of using safety razors with blades and should use an electric shaver.

Because any trauma can lead to a bleeding episode, all persons caring for these children must be aware of their disorder. These children should wear medical identification, and older children should be encouraged to recognize situations in which disclosing their condition is important, such as during dental extractions or injections. Health personnel need to take special precautions to prevent the use of procedures that cause bleeding such as intramuscular injection. The subcutaneous route is substituted for intramuscular injection whenever possible. Venipunctures for blood samples are usually preferred by children. There is usually less bleeding after venipuncture than after finger or heel puncture. Neither aspirin nor any aspirin-containing compound should be used. Acetaminophen is a suitable aspirin substitute, especially for use during control of pain at home.

Recognize and Control Bleeding

As noted, the earlier a bleeding episode is recognized, the more effectively it can be treated. Factor replacement therapy should be instituted according to established medical protocol, and supportive measures may be implemented, such as RICE, which is the mnemonic for rest, ice, compression, and elevation. When parents and older children are taught such measures beforehand, they can be prepared to initiate immediate treatment. Plastic bags of ice or cold packs should be kept in the freezer for such emergencies. However, such measures do not take the place of factor replacement.

Prevent Crippling Effects of Bleeding

As a result of repeated episodes of hemarthrosis, incompletely absorbed blood in the joints, and limitation of motion, bone and muscle changes occur that may result in flexion contractures and joint fixation. Obviously prevention of bleeding is the ideal goal. However, because spontaneous bleeding is not uncommon in persons with severe hemophilia, definitive measures, including replacement therapy and physical therapy, are necessary to limit joint damage.

During bleeding episodes, the joint is elevated and immobilized. Active range-of-motion exercises are usually instituted after the acute phase. This allows the child to control the degree of exercise according to the level of discomfort. Physical therapy is beneficial to promote maximum function of the joint and unaffected body parts. Success of a physical therapy plan involves control of pain by administering analgesics before therapy and adjusting the dose to provide maximum benefit.

If an exercise program is initiated in the home, a physical therapist or public health nurse may need to supervise compliance with the regimen. Rarely, orthopedic intervention, such as casting, application of traction, or aspiration of blood, may be necessary to preserve joint function. Diet is also an important consideration because excessive body weight can increase the strain on affected joints, especially the knees, and predispose the child to hemarthrosis. Consequently, children need calories that meet their energy requirements.

Support the Family and Prepare for Home Care

Factor concentrates have greatly changed the outlook for these children by minimizing the bleeding and allowing the child to live a normal, unrestricted life. Children are taught to take responsibility for their disease at an early age. They learn their limitations, preventive measures, and self-administration of the factor replacement.

The needs of families who have children with hemophilia are best met through a comprehensive team approach of physicians (e.g., pediatrician, hematologist, orthopedist), nurse practitioner, nurse, social worker, and physical therapist.

Parent-group discussions are beneficial in meeting the needs of similarly affected families. For example, with the improved prognosis for these children, adolescents with hemophilia and their parents face vocational and financial problems in addition to concern over future childbearing. After children reach 21 years of age, many insurance companies will no longer insure them. This can be disastrous because of the cost of treatment, which can exceed $100,000 per year. The National Hemophilia Foundation* and the Canadian Hemophilia Society† provide numerous services and publications for both health care providers and families.

Individuals who have become infected with HIV through transfusions and factor replacement products face the consequences of this dreaded disease. Consequently, they need the support of health professionals, especially in areas of safe sexual practices to avoid disease transmission and public education regarding AIDS and ways to deal with public reactions to those who have AIDS.

Identify Persons at Risk

Genetic counseling is essential as soon as possible after diagnosis. Unlike in many other disorders in which both parents carry the trait, the feeling of responsibility for this condition usually rests with the mother. Unless she has an opportunity to discuss her feelings, the couple's relationship may suffer. Prenatal DNA testing can identify affected fetuses and identify carriers in most cases.

VON WILLEBRAND DISEASE

Von Willebrand disease (vWD) is a hereditary bleeding disorder characterized by a deficiency of or defect in a protein called *von Willebrand factor* (vWF). The vWF protein contributes to the adherence of platelets to damaged endothelium and serves as a carrier protein for factor VIII (Flood & Scott, 2016; Marcdante & Kliegman, 2015; Neutze & Roque, 2016). This results in prolonged bleeding time because platelets fail to adhere to the walls of the ruptured vessel to form a platelet plug. Even though bleeding time is insensitive to platelet function defects, it is still used by some centers. The platelet function analyzer (PFA-100) is a rapid, accurate detection of platelet dysfunction and vWD used by many centers, but its results may be affected by some conditions (e.g., sepsis, pregnancy, certain medications) and therefore requires the need for further platelet aggregation testing (Flood & Scott, 2016; Kehrel &

*116 W. 32nd St., 11th floor, New York, NY 10001; 212-328-3700, 800-42-HANDI; fax: 212-328-3777; e-mail: handi@hemophilia.org; http://www.hemophilia.org; https://www.facebook.com/NationalHemophiliaFoundation.

†400-1255 University St., Montreal, Quebec, Canada H3B 3B6; 514-848-0503, 800-668-2686; fax: 514-848-9661; e-mail: chs@hemophilia.ca; http://www.hemophilia.ca; https://www.facebook.com/CanadianHemophiliaSociety.

Brodde, 2013; Sarangi & Acharya, 2017) (see Table 28.5). The disease can cause mild, moderate, or severe bleeding. Most cases of vWD are mild and require intervention only for dental and surgical procedures.

The most characteristic clinical feature of vWD is an increased tendency toward bleeding from mucous membranes. The most common symptom is frequent nosebleeds, followed by gingival bleeding, easy bruising, and excessive menstrual bleeding (menorrhagia) in females. Unlike hemophilia, vWD affects both males and females because its inheritance shows an autosomal dominant pattern. However, the treatment and final outcome are similar in both disorders. Treatment of bleeding is with DDAVP and/or a specially concentrated clotting factor such as Humate-P. Currently, a recombinate vWD preparation is undergoing clinical trials (Flood & Scott, 2016).

Nursing Care Management

The nursing goals are similar to those for hemophilia, with special considerations related to epistaxis. Nosebleeds are often a frightening experience for the child and parents. A calm, reassuring manner can alleviate anxiety and promote the child's cooperation. Because most of the nosebleeding originates in the anterior part of the nasal septum, bleeding can be controlled by applying pressure to the tip of the nose with the thumb and forefinger (see Emergency Treatment box). During this time the child breathes through the mouth. If local measures are not successful at stopping the bleeding, DDAVP is used to treat mild and moderate vWD (Ben-Ami & Revel-Vilk, 2013; Marcdante & Kliegman, 2015). DDAVP increases vWF and factor VIII secretion from storage in the endothelial cells (Castaman & Linari, 2017; Flood & Scott, 2016; Marcdante & Kliegman, 2015).

EMERGENCY TREATMENT

Epistaxis

- Have child sit up with neck forward or erect (not lie down).
- Apply continuous pressure to tip of nose with thumb and forefinger for at least 10 minutes.
- Do not insert cotton or wadded tissue into nostril or blow nose because this may dislodge clot.
- Apply ice or cold cloth to bridge of nose if bleeding persists.
- Keep child calm and quiet.

For menorrhagia, factor replacement therapy or the administration of DDAVP may be beneficial on the first day of the menstrual cycle to lessen the flow. Teaching the adolescent methods to prevent embarrassing accidents during menstruation, such as using double sanitary pads, helps her adjust to the inconvenience. Interestingly, some women do not experience excessive bleeding during vaginal childbirth; however, the risk of hemorrhage tends to increase during the postpartum period (Buga-Corbu, Arion, Davila, et al., 2014; Castaman, 2013). This is thought to be due to the increased levels of factor VIII and von Willebrand factor during pregnancy with levels decreasing after giving birth (Buga-Corbu, Arion, Davila, et al., 2014). Decisions regarding childbearing are difficult because of the dominant pattern of inheritance.

IMMUNE THROMBOCYTOPENIA (IDIOPATHIC THROMBOCYTOPENIC PURPURA)

Idiopathic or immune thrombocytopenic purpura (ITP), the formerly used term because purpura is an infrequent sign at presentation, is being referred to as immune thrombocytopenia by some expert sources (Rodeghiero, Stasi, Gernsheimer, et al., 2009). ITP is an acquired hemorrhagic disorder that is characterized by thrombocytopenia, (e.g., easy bruising, mucosal bleeding, petechiae, menorrhagia), and normal bone marrow with a normal or increased number of immature megakaryocytes and eosinophils. Although the causes are not known, it is understood that ITP involves the evolution of antibodies against multiple platelet antigens, leading to reduced platelet survival and impaired platelet production (Consolini, 2011; McCrae, 2011; Scott, 2016b; Wilson, 2015). ITP is the most common thrombocytopenia of childhood and usually presents 1 to 4 weeks after a viral illness, with the majority of cases in children younger than 10 years of age with peak incidence between ages 1 and 6 years (Consolini, 2011; McCrae, 2011; Scott, 2016b; Wilson, 2015).

The disease occurs in one of two forms: an acute, self-limiting course or a chronic course (>12 months' duration). The acute form occurs most commonly after upper respiratory tract infections; after the childhood diseases of measles, rubella, mumps, or chickenpox; or after infection with human parvovirus.

Clinical symptoms include petechiae, bruising, bleeding from mucous membranes, and prolonged bleeding from abrasions. Symptomatic bleeding does not usually occur until the platelet count is lower than 20,000/mm^3. Fatal hemorrhages have been reported in less than 1% of all patients.

Diagnostic Evaluation

In ITP the platelet count is reduced to less than 20,000/mm^3; therefore results of tests that depend on platelet function, such as the tourniquet test, bleeding time, and clot retraction time, are abnormal. There is no definitive test that establishes a diagnosis of ITP; several tests are usually performed to rule out other disorders of which thrombocytopenia is a manifestation, such as systemic lupus erythematosus, lymphoma, and leukemia.

Therapeutic Management

Management of ITP is primarily supportive because the disease is self-limiting in the majority of cases. Activity is restricted at the onset while the platelet count is low and while active bleeding or progression of lesions is occurring. Treatment for acute presentation is symptomatic and has included prednisone, IV immune globulin (IVIG), and anti-D antibody. These are not curative therapies. Some experts suggest that no therapy is necessary for asymptomatic patients because there is no difference in the recovery time of platelet counts with and without treatment (Kuhne & Imbach, 2013; Scott, 2016b; Wilson, 2015). Anti-D antibody is a plasma-derived immunoglobulin that causes a transient hemolytic anemia in Rh(D)-positive patients with ITP. With the clearance of antibody-coated RBCs, there is prolonged survival of platelets due to the anti-D antibody blockade of the Fc receptors on the reticuloendothelial cells. The platelet count usually increases approximately 48 hours after an infusion of anti-D antibody; therefore it is not appropriate therapy for patients who are actively bleeding. The benefits of choosing anti-D antibody IV therapy over prednisone or IVIG are that anti-D antibody can be given in one dose over a period of 5 to 10 minutes, and it is significantly less expensive than IVIG. Historically patients who were treated with prednisone first underwent a bone marrow examination to rule out leukemia, but this is now controversial because leukemia rarely manifests with a low platelet count alone (Marcdante & Kliegman, 2015; Wilson, 2015). Therefore the use of anti-D antibody and IVIG alleviates the need for a bone marrow examination. Before receiving the initial dose of anti-D antibody, patients must meet certain criteria. Premedication with acetaminophen 5 to 10 minutes before infusion is recommended.

Splenectomy is for patients who have chronic severe ITP that is not responsive to pharmacologic management and have increased risk of severe hemorrhage. It is the only treatment associated with long-term

DRUG ALERT

Anti-D Antibody

After administration of anti-D antibody, observe the child for a minimum of 1 hour and maintain a patent IV line. Obtain baseline vital sign measurements before the infusion and again 5, 20, and 60 minutes after beginning the infusion. If fever, chills, or headache occurs during or shortly after the infusion, the nurse should administer acetaminophen, diphenhydramine (Benadryl), and/or hydrocortisone (Solu-Cortef). Observe the patient for an additional hour after the anti-D antibody infusion is complete.

remission for the majority of children with chronic ITP and therefore removes the risk of hemorrhage (Marcdante & Kliegman, 2015; McCrae, 2011; Wilson, 2015). Before splenectomy is considered, it is generally recommended to wait until the child is older than 5 years of age because of the increased risk of bacterial infection. Administration of pneumococcal, meningococcal, and *H. influenzae* vaccines before splenectomy is recommended (if they were not previously administered). The child also receives penicillin prophylaxis after splenectomy. The appropriate length of prophylactic therapy is controversial, but in general, a minimum of 3 years of therapy is recommended.

Prognosis

The majority of children with ITP have a self-limiting course without major complications. Some children develop chronic ITP and require ongoing therapy. A splenectomy may modify the disease process, and the child may be asymptomatic. Splenectomy is associated with a lifelong risk of overwhelming infection caused by encapsulated organisms, increased risk of thrombosis, and the potential development of pulmonary hypertension in adulthood. As an alternative to splenectomy, rituximab has been used off-label (currently unapproved for treating ITP) in children to treat chronic ITP, with 30% to 40% of children obtaining a partial or complete remission (Scott, 2016b). Two effective agents that act to stimulate thrombopoiesis, romiplastin and eltrombopag, are approved by the Food and Drug Administration to treat adults with chronic ITP, with preliminary encouraging data using these thrombopoietic agents in children (Scott, 2016b).

Nursing Care Management

Nursing care is largely supportive and should include teaching regarding the possible side effects of therapy and restriction of contact sports while the child's platelet count is less than 50,000/mm^3 as some experts recommend (Consolini, 2011; Kumar, Lambert, Breakey, et al., 2015). Children with ITP should not participate in any contact sports, bike riding, skateboarding, in-line skating, gymnastics, climbing, or running. Parents are encouraged to engage their children in quiet activities and to prevent any injuries to the child's head (e.g., by having the child wear protective headgear). Instruct the parents to obtain prompt medical evaluation if the child sustains head or abdominal trauma. As with any condition with an uncertain outcome, the family needs emotional support. (See Quality Patient Outcomes box.)

QUALITY PATIENT OUTCOMES

Immune Thrombocytopenic Purpura

- Serious bleeding episode prevented
- Activities that increase risk for serious bleeding avoided
- Treatment administered without serious side effects

DRUG ALERT

NSAIDs

Using aspirin or other NSAIDs to control pain has critical harmful effects for these children; therefore it is recommended to use substitutes (such as acetaminophen).

DISSEMINATED INTRAVASCULAR COAGULATION

Disseminated intravascular coagulation (DIC), also known as consumption coagulopathy, is characterized by diffuse fibrin deposition in the microvasculature, consumption of coagulation factors, and endogenous generation of thrombin and plamin. DIC is a secondary disorder of coagulation that occurs as a complication of a number of pathologic processes such as hypoxia, acidosis, shock, endothelial damage (burns), and many severe systemic disease states (e.g., congenital heart disease, necrotizing enterocolitis, gram-negative bacterial sepsis, rickettsial infections, and some severe viral infections). The hallmarks of this disorder are bleeding and clotting, which occur simultaneously.

Pathophysiology

DIC occurs when the first stage of the coagulation process is abnormally stimulated (Fig. 28.6). Although there is no well-defined sequence of events, two distinct phases can be identified. First, when the clotting mechanism is triggered in the circulation, thrombin is generated in greater amounts than the body neutralizes. Consequently, there is rapid conversion of fibrinogen to fibrin, with aggregation and destruction of platelets. Local and widespread fibrin deposition occurs in blood vessels. The thrombi impede the blood flow, with eventual necrosis of tissues. Concurrently, the fibrinolytic mechanism is activated, which causes extensive destruction of clotting factors. With a deficiency of clotting factors, the child is vulnerable to uncontrollable hemorrhage into vital organs. An additional complication is damage to and hemolysis of RBCs.

Clinical Manifestations

The signs and symptoms of DIC are the same as those of many other diseases, which often confuses the diagnosis. There is evidence of bleeding—petechiae, purpura, bleeding from openings in the skin (e.g., a venipuncture site or surgical incision), hypotension, and dysfunction of organs from infarction and ischemia.

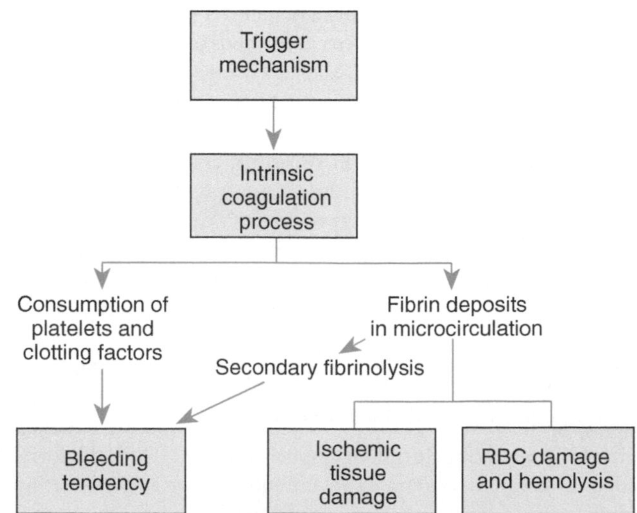

FIG. 28.6 Effects of disseminated intravascular coagulation. *RBC,* Red blood cell.

BOX 28.7 Clinical Manifestations of Disseminated Intravascular Coagulation

Petechiae
Purpura
Bleeding from openings in the skin
- Venipuncture site
- Surgical incision

Bleeding from umbilicus, trachea (newborn)
Evidence of gastrointestinal bleeding
Hypotension
Organ dysfunction from infarction and ischemia

Diagnostic Evaluation

DIC is suspected when there is an increased tendency to bleed (Box 28.7). Hematologic findings include prolonged prothrombin, partial thromboplastin, and thrombin times. There is a profoundly depressed platelet count, fragmented RBCs, and depleted fibrinogen levels.

Therapeutic Management

Treatment of DIC is directed toward control of the underlying or initiating cause, which in most instances stops the coagulation problem spontaneously. Platelets and fresh frozen plasma may be needed to replace lost plasma components, especially in the child whose underlying disease remains uncontrolled. Extremely ill newborn infants may require exchange transfusion with fresh blood. The administration of IV heparin to inhibit thrombin formation is most often restricted to cases in which there has been no response to treatment of the underlying disease or replacement of coagulation factors and platelets.

Nursing Care Management

The goals of nursing care are to be aware of the possibility of DIC in the severely ill child and to recognize signs that might indicate its presence. The skills needed to monitor IV infusion and blood transfusions and to administer heparin are the same as for any child receiving these therapies. Because the child is usually cared for in an intensive care unit, the special needs of the family must be considered. (See Chapter 21.)

OTHER HEMATOLOGIC DISORDERS

NEUTROPENIA

Neutropenia is a reduction in the absolute number of circulating neutrophils and band forms in the blood that is below the normal level by age and race (Dale, 2017; Dinauer, Newburger, & Borregaard, 2015; Walkovich & Newburger, 2016). Neutropenia is usually defined as an ANC of less than 1000/mm^3 in infants 2 weeks to 1 year of age or less than 1500/mm^3 in children older than 1 year of age. African Americans have ANCs that are 200 to 600/mm^3 lower than those of Caucasians (Dinauer, Newburger, & Borregaard, 2015; Walkovich & Newburger, 2016). The ANC is calculated by multiplying the total WBC count by the percentage of neutrophils and bands in the differential count (see Table 28.1). When the ANC is less than 500/mm^3, it is defined as severe neutropenia with an increased risk of life-threatening infection (Celkan & Koc, 2015; Walkovich & Newburger, 2016). Several different types of neutropenia occur in children (Table 28.8). This discussion focuses on the most common type: chronic benign neutropenia.

Diagnostic Evaluation

Chronic benign neutropenia generally represents disorders characterized by mild to moderate neutropenia that are not associated with an increase in infections and often have spontaneous remissions (Celkan & Koc, 2015; Walkovich & Newburger, 2016). Neutropenia is often detected as an incidental finding during the evaluation of a child with fever. The ANC is usually below 500/mm^3, and the only physical findings (if any) are those related to infection. Oral ulcerations and skin infections are the most common manifestation of chronic benign neutropenia. However, most children have no infections despite the markedly reduced ANC. Examination of bone marrow aspirates shows normal cellularity with absence of mature neutrophils. Antineutrophil antibodies are usually present, but their absence does not exclude the diagnosis.

To determine a child's neutrophil response during times of infection, a steroid stimulation test may be performed. The child is given a dose of IV steroid, and the neutrophil count is measured at hourly intervals for 4 to 5 hours. If the ANC increases to more than 1000/mm^3 after the dose of steroid, the child will have the same response during times of infection. Failure of the ANC to rise is an indication for increased vigilance and medical attention if the child develops a fever of 101.3°F (38.5°C) or higher. These children may require hospitalization and aggressive treatment with broad-spectrum IV antibiotics, depending on the severity of the illness.

Therapeutic Management

Therapy to increase the ANC is rarely required. Children who have recurrent or severe infections, however, may benefit from the administration of granulocyte colony-stimulating factor (G-CSF). CSFs are a naturally occurring group of glycoproteins. They were first discovered and characterized because of their effect on growth and differentiation of marrow cells. Recombinant DNA technology has enabled the production of large quantities of highly purified CSFs that are nearly identical to the naturally occurring substances and have successfully increased the neutrophil count in a wide variety of neutropenic conditions (Celkan & Koc, 2015; Dale, 2017; Walkovich & Newburger, 2016).

Children with chronic benign neutropenia have normal cellular immunity; therefore they should receive their routine childhood immunizations.

Nursing Care Management

The care of the child with neutropenia primarily focuses on educating the parents. Instruct parents to keep their child away from large indoor crowds (e.g., grocery store on Saturday morning, movie theaters, day care centers, church nursery) and individuals who are ill. Parents also need to seek medical attention if their child has a fever of 101.3°F (38.5°C) or higher, or if skin lesions develop. Because G-CSF is administered parenterally only, parents need to know how to administer subcutaneous injections.

Support the Family

Neutropenia can have many effects on family life. Some parents must quit their jobs to avoid sending their child to day care. Provide financial counseling as indicated. Parents of children with neutropenia need a listening ear for their frustrations and continued reassurance that these children usually recover by the age of 4½ years.

HENOCH-SCHÖNLEIN PURPURA

Henoch-Schönlein purpura (HSP), also referred to as allergic vasculitis, allergic purpura, and anaphylactoid purpura, is a relatively common acquired disorder in children characterized by a nonthrombocytopenic purpura, arthritis, nephritis, and abdominal pain.

The etiology is unknown, but the disease often follows an upper respiratory tract infection, and allergy or drug sensitivity plays a role in some instances. The disease occurs in children ages 6 months to 16

TABLE 28.8 Clinical and Hematologic Features of Some Congenital Neutropenias

Feature	Severe Congenital Neutropenia (Kostmann Disease)	Familial Benign Neutropenia	Chronic Benign Neutropenia; Idiopathic Autoimmune Neutropenia	Reticular Dysgenesis
Etiology	Autosomal recessive (occasionally autosomal dominant) inheritance pattern	Dominant inheritance pattern	Antineutrophil antibodies detected in almost all cases	Failure of stem cells to produce myeloid and lymphoid cells
Severity	Severe illness Life-threatening pyogenic infections in first months of life	Variable; benign to severe infections	Benign	Severe, fatal thymic dysplasia; lymphoid hypoplasia
Clinical findings	Skin infection Aphthous ulcers Septicemia Meningitis Peritonitis Lung abscess Lymphadenopathy Splenomegaly (20%)	Less troublesome infection to severe infection	Paronychia Gingivitis Impetigo—mild infections, localized	Severe bacterial and viral infection Neonatal death
Hematologic findings	Anemia Neutropenia, <200/mm^3 Monocytosis Eosinophilia Risk of leukemia	Neutropenia, usually <300/mm^3 Monocytosis	No anemia Absent mature PMN Some band forms Monocytosis	Neutropenia Lymphopenia
Marrow findings	↑ Promyelocytes Absent MM, B, PMN ↑ Monocytes ↑ Eosinophils ↑ Plasma cells	↓ MM, B, PMN "Maturation arrest"	Absent PMN Normal myeloid cells to band stage; lymphocytes increased	Absent myeloid and absent lymphoid cells Normal thrombopoiesis and erythropoiesis
Treatment	Antibiotics Supportive measures G-CSF Bone marrow transplantation	No therapy G-CSF, if indicated	Antibiotics, as indicated G-CSF, if indicated	Bone marrow transplantation

B, Bands; *G-CSF,* granulocyte colony-stimulating factor; *MM,* metamyelocytes; *PMN,* polymorphonuclear leukocytes.
Modified data from Fioredda, F., Calvillo, M., Bonanomi, S., et al. (2012). Congenital and acquired neutropenias consensus guidelines on therapy and follow-up in childhood from the neutropenia committee of the marrow failure syndrome group of the AIEOP (Associiazione Italiana Emato-Oncologia Pediatrica). *American Journal of Hematology, 87*(2), 238-243; and modified data from Lanzkowsky, P. (2016). *Lanzkowsky's manual of pediatric hematology and oncology.* San Diego, CA: Academic Press.

years but more frequently in children ages 2 to 11 years. It is observed more often in Caucasian children than in those of other races and almost twice as often in boys than in girls.

Pathophysiology

The disease is characterized by inflammation of small blood vessels, and the manifestations observed are influenced by the size and distribution of the affected vessels. A generalized vasculitis of dermal capillaries (and to a lesser extent small arterioles and veins), causing extravasation of RBCs, produces the petechial skin lesions. Inflammation and hemorrhage may also occur in the GI tract, synovium, glomeruli, and central nervous system.

Clinical Manifestations

The onset of the disease may be abrupt, with the simultaneous appearance of several manifestations, or gradual, with the sequential appearance of different manifestations. The primary feature, however, is a symmetric purpura that involves the buttocks and lower extremities but may extend to include the extensor surfaces of the upper extremities and, less commonly, the upper trunk and face. The rash may be associated with maculopapular lesions, urticaria, and erythema. There is often marked edema of the scalp, eyelids, lips, ears, and dorsal surfaces of the hands and feet, especially in infants and younger children. In severe cases the skin may slough, leaving denuded areas that are similar in appearance and treatment to partial-thickness burns.

Arthritic effects are evident in two-thirds of affected children and range from asymptomatic swelling around a single joint to painful, tender swelling of several joints, most often the knees and ankles. The involvement is periarticular and resolves in a few days without permanent damage or deformity.

Two-thirds of affected children have GI involvement manifested by recurrent colicky midabdominal pain, often associated with nausea and vomiting. The stools contain gross or occult blood and mucus.

Renal involvement occurs in up to 50% of affected children and is potentially the most serious long-term complication. Initially the nephritis is manifested as blood, casts, and protein in the urine. Although the majority of children with renal involvement recover completely, some develop chronic renal disease with eventual renal failure.

Diagnostic Evaluation

Diagnosis is usually established on the basis of the history and clinical manifestations. Laboratory tests are used to assess GI and renal involvement and to determine adequacy of hemostatic function. Tests for occult blood in the stool are performed. Increased levels of immunoglobulin A are a frequent finding.

Therapeutic Management

Management is primarily supportive, with close observation for signs of renal or GI involvement. Edema, rash, malaise, and arthralgia are usually managed with appropriate analgesics such as NSAIDs and mild sedation if necessary. Corticosteroids may be prescribed for relief of more severe edema, arthralgia, and colicky abdominal pain. The nephropathy requires careful monitoring of fluid and electrolyte balance, salt intake, and blood pressure. Antihypertensive agents may be needed.

The majority of children recover without the need for hospitalization, and in most instances a single acute episode clears spontaneously within a month. Others may have periodic recurrences for as long as 2 to 3 years before attaining permanent remission from symptoms. Rarely, death occurs from severe GI complications, acute renal failure, or central nervous system involvement. Children with HSP nephritis should receive long-term follow-up because renal involvement is evident in 40% of the patients, many of whom exhibit severe proteinuria (Wilson, 2015).

Nursing Care Management

Nursing care of the child hospitalized with HSP is primarily supportive, with vigilant observation for signs of complications. The nurse should measure vital signs and record them at regular intervals, obtain specimens for laboratory examination, and administer medication as prescribed. Carefully observe urine and stools for fresh and occult blood.

If the child suffers from joint pain, proper positioning, careful movement, and administration of analgesics, including opioids, helps reduce discomfort. More severe involvement, such as GI symptoms and nephritis, is managed as for any such disorder.

Concern about the unsightly appearance of the rash is common. Inform the child and parents that it is only a temporary phenomenon and that the child can wear clothing that helps hide the rash, such as a long-sleeved shirt, long pants, or a robe. Emphasizing good grooming and attractive apparel helps promote a more positive self-image. If the skin surface is denuded, treatment may involve débridement and dressing changes similar to that in the care of burns. (See Chapter 23.)

IMMUNOLOGIC DEFICIENCY DISORDERS

A number of disorders can cause profound, often life-threatening, alterations in the body's immune system. The most serious are those conditions that completely depress immunity, such as severe combined immunodeficiency disease (SCID). However, the one disorder that generates the most anxiety in both the family and the community is HIV infection and the subsequent development of AIDS.

Several classifications of immune dysfunction exist. AIDS, SCID, and Wiskott-Aldrich syndrome are disorders in which the body is unable to mount an immune response. The immune response can also be misdirected. In autoimmune disorders, antibodies, macrophages, and lymphocytes attack healthy cells. Some such disorders and their target organs are myasthenia gravis (muscle cells), Graves disease (thyroid cells), and type 1 diabetes (B cells in the pancreas). AIDS, SCID, and Wiskott-Aldrich syndrome are discussed here; the other disorders are covered elsewhere in this book.

MECHANISMS INVOLVED IN IMMUNITY

The function of the immune system is to differentiate "self" from "nonself" and to initiate a response to eliminate the "nonself" or foreign substance, known as an antigen. All cells in the body have specific cell surface markers unique to the individual. These cell surface markers are known as the **major histocompatibility complex (MHC)**. Because the markers were first identified on human leukocytes, they are commonly referred to as **human leukocyte antigens (HLAs)**.

The body's protective mechanisms consist of complex, overlapping defense systems. Intact skin serves as the first line of protection for the body. Body secretions such as saliva, sweat, and tears contain chemicals that can kill many organisms. The stomach contains acids that can destroy swallowed pathogens. Organisms trapped in the mucus of the nose and mouth are expelled by sneezing or coughing. If the foreign substance has penetrated these barriers, cellular elements are mobilized.

The immune system is composed of the primary lymphoid organs (thymus, bone marrow, and probably liver) and the secondary lymphoid organs (lymph nodes, spleen, and gut-associated lymphoid tissue). The immune system has two types of function: nonspecific and specific. Nonspecific immune defenses are activated on exposure to any foreign substance but react similarly regardless of the type of antigen; they are unable to identify the antigen, except to know that it is "nonself." The principal activity of this system is phagocytosis, the process of ingesting and digesting foreign substances. Phagocytic cells include neutrophils and monocytes (see p. 1024). Specific defenses are discussed in the following section.

Specific Immune Mechanisms

Specific (adaptive) defenses are those that have the ability to recognize the antigen and respond selectively. The components of adaptive immunity are humoral immunity and cell-mediated immunity. The cells responsible for these two forms of immunity are the lymphocytes, specifically B lymphocytes and T lymphocytes.

Humoral immunity involves antibody production and complement and is concerned with immune processes occurring outside the cells, such as on cell surfaces or in body fluids. The principal cell involved in antibody production is the B lymphocyte, which is probably produced in the bone marrow. When challenged with an antigen, B cells divide and differentiate into plasma cells. The plasma cells produce and secrete large quantities of antibodies specific to the antigen. Five classes of immunoglobulin (Ig) antibodies have been identified: IgG, IgM, IgA, IgD, and IgE, each serving a specific function.

On initial exposure to an antigen, the B-lymphocyte system begins to produce antibody, predominantly IgM, which appears in 2 to 3 days. This process is referred to as the primary antibody response. With subsequent exposure to the antigen, a secondary antibody response occurs. Specific IgG antibodies are formed within 4 to 10 days. An example of the secondary response is the response that occurs with repeat administration of an immunization agent, often called a booster. Memory B cells allow the immune system to recognize the same antigen for months or years.

When antibody reacts with antigen, they bind to form an antigen-antibody complex. This binding serves several functions. Antibody aids in the phagocytosis of antigen by sensitizing it in such a manner that it is more readily destroyed by phagocytes, a process known as opsonization.

Antibody also activates or fixes complement, the second component of humoral immunity. The complement system is a series of proteins (C1 to C9) present in serum that results in a cascade of enzymatic actions and death of a viable antigen. After being activated by antibody, complement produces a chemotactic factor that summons T lymphocytes and macrophages to the antigen site.

Cell-mediated immunity involves a variety of specific functions mediated by the T lymphocyte and occurs within the cell. T lymphocytes do not carry typical immunoglobulins on their surfaces as do the B cells. Microscopically, T cells appear identical, but they are functionally heterogeneous, and there are several subsets, including cytotoxic T cells, helper T cells, and suppressor T cells. T cells may also be classified structurally by the distinctive molecules on their surfaces, known as cluster designations (CDs). Once mature, T cells carry markers known as T2 (CD2), T3 (CD3), T5 (CD5), and T7 (CD7). Helper T cells carry a T4 (CD4) marker and a suppressor, and cytotoxic T cells carry a T8 (CD8) marker.

Specific functions of cell-mediated immunity include protection against most viral, fungal, and protozoan infections and slow-growing bacterial infections, such as tuberculosis; rejection of histoincompatible grafts; mediation of cutaneous delayed hypersensitivity reactions, such as in tuberculin testing; and probably immune surveillance for malignant cells. In addition, T lymphocytes also have regulatory functions within the immune system. For example, helper T lymphocytes help B lymphocytes and other types of T cells to mount an optimum immune response. The cellular immune response is initiated when a T lymphocyte is sensitized by antigen. In response to this contact, the T cell releases numerous humoral factors called **lymphokines**, which eventually bring about the death of the antigen. Interferons are a group of proteins secreted by leukocytes and infected host cells that nonspecifically inhibit viral replication, promote phagocytosis, and stimulate the killer activity of sensitized lymphocytes.

HUMAN IMMUNODEFICIENCY VIRUS INFECTION AND ACQUIRED IMMUNODEFICIENCY SYNDROME

HIV infection and AIDS have generated intense investigation and constitute one of the world's most serious medical, public health, and social challenges of our time (Grace, 2015; United Nations AIDS, 2016). In the early 1980s the first cases of AIDS were identified in adult men in urban coastal communities; eventually AIDS affected women and children and broader social and geographic groups. Advances in research and major improvements in the treatment and management of HIV infection have stabilized the incidence of new HIV infections and AIDS globally, with disproportionate distribution of HIV infections and AIDS deaths occurring among people of sub-Saharan Africa (United Nations AIDS, 2016).

Worldwide, from 1999 to 2002 it was estimated that 60% of the 42 million HIV-infected individuals were women, and 2.7 million children younger than 15 years of age were living with HIV/AIDS (Centers for Disease Control and Prevention, 2013). The estimated rate of persons living with HIV/AIDS globally in 2015 declined to approximately 36.7 million (34 to 39.8 million) HIV-infected individuals; approximately 77% of pregnant women living with HIV had access to antiretroviral medicines to prevent transmission to their babies, and approximately 150,000 children became newly infected with HIV, decreased from 290,000 in 2010 (United Nations AIDS, 2016).

The Centers for Disease Control and Prevention (2013) estimate that approximately 200 infants with HIV infection are born in the United States annually. The majority of these children acquired the disease perinatally from their mothers. The rate of mother-to-child transmission of HIV continues to decrease due to prenatal screening, elective cesarean, and use of antiretroviral treatment of HIV-infected mothers and infants (Centers for Disease Control and Prevention, 2017b; Paintsil & Andiman, 2009; Yogev & Chadwick, 2016). Transmission from mother to child can be significantly reduced by the use of preventive interventions, especially antiretroviral therapy during pregnancy, labor, and the neonatal period (Centers for Disease Control and Prevention, 2017b; Grace, 2015; Yogev & Chadwick, 2016).

Children of minority populations in the United States are disproportionately affected by the HIV epidemic. Of the children diagnosed with AIDS, the majority were African American, followed by Hispanic and Caucasian. In the United States from the beginning of the epidemic through 2014, it was reported that of the more than 5000 individuals who acquired HIV/AIDS through perinatal transmission, 82% of the deaths were among HIV-infected children less than 13 years old (Centers for Disease Control and Prevention, 2017b).

Although adolescents ages 13 to 24 years with AIDS account for only approximately 4% of the cumulative total of AIDS cases in the United States, they are one of the growing groups of newly infected persons in the country (Yogev & Chadwick, 2016). The rising AIDS rate among adolescents may be attributed to increased participation in high-risk behaviors such as unprotected sexual contact and IV drug use. More than 50% of HIV-positive youth report being unaware of their diagnosis (Centers for Disease Control and Prevention, 2016). Considering the long latency period of 8 to 12 years between the time of infection and the development of clinical symptoms, it is estimated that 15% to 20% of all AIDS cases were acquired between 13 and 19 years of age (Yogev & Chadwick, 2016).

Etiology

HIV is a retrovirus that is the primary cause of AIDS. There are different strains of HIV. HIV-2 is prevalent in Africa, whereas HIV-1 is the more common form in the United States and elsewhere. Horizontal transmission of HIV occurs through intimate sexual contact or parenteral exposure to blood or body fluids containing visible blood. Perinatal (vertical) transmission occurs when an HIV-infected pregnant woman passes the infection to her infant. There is no evidence that casual contact between infected and uninfected individuals can spread the virus.

The majority of children with HIV infection are younger than 7 years of age. Children with HIV fall into two subpopulations: infants born to HIV-infected women and adolescents infected as a result of high-risk behaviors.

Perinatal transmission accounts for almost all HIV infections in young children in the United States (Centers for Disease Control and Prevention, 2016; Yogev & Chadwick, 2016). Rates of transmission of HIV from mother to child have varied among countries; the United States and Europe have documented transmission rates in untreated women between 12% and 30%, whereas transmission rates in Africa and Haiti have been higher (25% to 52%), likely because of more advanced maternal disease and the presence of coinfections (Yogev & Chadwick, 2016). There has been a significant decrease in perinatal transmission to less than 1% to 2% with the use of active antiretroviral combination therapy, elective cesarean delivery, and avoidance of breastfeeding for HIV-infected mothers and their newborns (Centers for Disease Control and Prevention, 2017b; Yogev & Chadwick, 2016).

It has been recommended that all pregnant women be tested for HIV and if positive, treated with antiretroviral regimen, irrespective of viral load or CD4 count (Centers for Disease Control and Prevention, 2017a; Ishikawa, Dalai, Johnson, et al., 2016; Yogev & Chadwick, 2016). Antiretroviral regimen administered to the pregnant mother and to the infant within 48 to 72 hours of life is the most popular regimen in the developing world because of its ease of administration, low cost, and decreased risk of transmitting HIV (Centers for Disease Control and Prevention, 2017b; Paintsil & Andiman, 2009). The World Health Organization has recommended that pregnant women be treated with an antiretroviral regimen appropriate for their own health that should be continued at least throughout breastfeeding (in resource-limited areas) and for the remainder of their lives (Yogev & Chadwick, 2016). Because breastfeeding is essential for infant survival in developing countries, HIV mothers on antiretroviral treatment who exclusively breastfed for a duration of their own choosing had lower HIV-1 breast milk concentrations than mothers who abruptly weaned the infant at approximately 4 months of age (Kuhn, Kim, Walter, et al., 2013). Culturally appropriate opportunities for HIV testing, diagnosis, and access to early treatment and prevention services to reduce further HIV transmission are key to reducing new infections and ultimately decreasing HIV prevalence in the United States and globally (Centers for Disease Control and Prevention, 2017b; United Nations AIDS, 2016).

Transfusion of infected blood or blood products has accounted for 3% to 6% of all pediatric AIDS cases to date (Yogev & Chadwick, 2016). Before donor blood started to be routinely tested for HIV in 1985, children with hemophilia were especially at risk because factor concentrates were prepared from pooled plasma. Since the initiation of donor blood screening and development of purification techniques for factor concentrates, transfusion-associated HIV infection has become virtually nonexistent. Major advances in screening and testing of the blood supply in the United States have reduced the risk of receiving a contaminated single transfusion to 1 in approximately 1.5 to 2 million (Strauss, 2016).

Sexual contact is the leading source of exposure to HIV in the United States. In the young pediatric population this is an infrequent route of transmission; a small number of children have been infected through sexual abuse. In contrast, sexual activity is a major cause of HIV infection in adolescents. Adolescents commonly take risks and experiment; participation in high-risk behaviors, including IV drug use and unsafe sexual practices, increases their risk of becoming infected with HIV. Studies have reported that male circumcision reduces heterosexually acquired HIV infections in adolescent boys and men; however, it was emphasized that this offers only partial protection, and it remains critical to promote the practice of safe sex (Lawal & Olapade-Olaopa, 2017; Tobian, Serwadda, Quinn, et al., 2009).

Pathophysiology

HIV primarily infects a specific subset of T lymphocytes, the $CD4^+$ T cells, but it can also invade cells of the monocyte-macrophage lineage. The virus takes over the machinery of the $CD4^+$ lymphocyte, using it to replicate itself and rendering the $CD4^+$ cell dysfunctional. With suppression of cell-mediated immunity, the person is at risk for opportunistic infections. HIV also causes dysfunction of B cells and antigen-presenting cells, which results in suppression of humoral immunity.

Although the course of HIV infection varies among individuals, a common progression of events has been recognized. Immediately after primary infection, there is dissemination of virus and seeding of lymphoid organs, along with a transient decrease in the number of $CD4^+$ lymphocytes in peripheral blood. An immune response follows, and the resulting level of plasma virus is generally maintained for years. A period of clinical latency ensues that may be longer than 10 years in adults. The $CD4^+$ lymphocyte count gradually decreases over time; at some point, physical symptoms appear. The count eventually reaches a critical level below which there is substantial risk of opportunistic illnesses, followed by death.

A more rapid progression of disease tend to occur in perinatally infected children. This is primarily due to the naiveté and immaturity of the developing immune system. Rapid progression of HIV infection in infants and children is also correlated with higher viral burden and faster depletion of infected CD4 lymphocytes than in adults (Yogev & Chadwick, 2016). Perinatally acquired HIV has declined with the use of preventive measures such as HIV counseling, voluntary testing practices, and highly active antiretroviral therapy (HAART). HAART, typically a combination of two nucleoside analog reverse transcriptase inhibitors and a protease inhibitor, is the current standard for treatment of HIV-infected pregnant women and has significantly reduced the transmission of HIV to their babies 99% of the time (Hayden, 2013; Siberry, 2014). Routine HIV counseling and voluntary testing using the opt-in (must agree) or opt-out (right of refusal) approach is the recommended standard of care for pregnant women in the United States (American Academy of Pediatrics Committee on Pediatric AIDS, 2008; Centers for Disease Control and Prevention, 2017b; Siberry, 2014; Simpkins, Siberry, & Hutton, 2009).

BOX 28.8 Common Clinical Manifestations of Human Immunodeficiency Virus Infection in Children

- Lymphadenopathy
- Hepatosplenomegaly
- Oral candidiasis
- Chronic or recurrent diarrhea
- Failure to thrive
- Developmental delay
- Parotitis

BOX 28.9 Common Defining Conditions for Acquired Immunodeficiency Syndrome in Children

- *Pneumocystis carinii* pneumonia
- Lymphoid interstitial pneumonitis
- Recurrent bacterial infections
- Wasting syndrome
- Candidal esophagitis
- Human immunodeficiency virus encephalopathy
- Cytomegalovirus disease
- *Mycobacterium avium-intracellulare* complex infection
- Pulmonary candidiasis
- Herpes simplex disease
- Cryptosporidiosis

Clinical Manifestations

The majority of infants with perinatally acquired HIV infection are clinically normal at birth. Common clinical manifestations of HIV infection in children (Box 28.8) vary and include such signs as lymphadenopathy, hepatosplenomegaly, and unexplained diarrhea. Diarrhea may be a result of pathogens or HIV itself due to malabsorption of carbohydrate, protein, and fat (Yogev & Chadwick, 2016). HIV-infected children often do not grow normally; they may be proportionally smaller in both length and weight for age.

The diagnosis of AIDS in children may be associated with the occurrence of certain AIDS-related illnesses or conditions (Centers for Disease Control and Prevention, 2017b). Common AIDS-defining conditions observed among American children are listed in Box 28.9.

Recurrent bacterial infections, parotitis, lymphoid interstitial pneumonitis (LIP), and early onset of progressive neurologic deterioration are characteristic of children with HIV infection but are rarely seen in affected adults. Kaposi sarcoma, one of the hallmarks of adult disease, is found in fewer than 1% of affected children.

Central nervous system abnormalities considered to be the direct effects of HIV infection occur in most children with AIDS. Secondary infections with opportunistic and common pathogens are infrequent in this population. Either global or specific neuropsychologic deficits may occur at random intervals. Many affected children display evidence of developmental disability. Deficits in motor skills, communication, and behavioral functioning are common. Expressive language (use of language) is more frequently impaired than receptive language (understanding of language).

Diagnostic Evaluation

For children 18 months of age and older, the HIV enzyme-linked immunosorbent assay (ELISA) and Western blot immunoassay are performed to determine HIV infection. In infants born to HIV-infected mothers, results of these assays are positive because of the presence of maternal antibodies derived transplacentally. Maternal antibodies may persist in the infant for up to 18 months. Therefore other diagnostic tests are used, most commonly the HIV polymerase chain reaction (PCR) for detection of proviral DNA.

Currently, there are several inexpensive rapid HIV tests available with sensitivity and specificity better than those of the standard enzyme immunoassay with only a single step that allows test results to be reported within less than 30 minutes (Yogev & Chadwick, 2016). A positive rapid test is either confirmed by Western blot testing or two different positive rapid tests (testing different HIV-associated antibodies). Viral diagnostic assays, such as HIV DNA or RNA PCR or HIV culture, are considerably more useful in young infants, allowing a definitive diagnosis in most infected infants by 1 to 6 months of age (Yogev & Chadwick, 2016). In the United States HIV tests approved by the Food and Drug Administration include (1) combination tests that detect both HIV antigen and antibody, and (2) tests that accurately differentiate HIV-1 from HIV-2 antibodies (Centers for Disease Control and Prevention, 2017b). With the identification of HIV antigen, individuals may be diagnosed with HIV infection before development of symptoms.

As mentioned, the diagnosis of HIV infection can be obtained from positive results on two separate virologic tests performed on separate blood specimens. Infants born to HIV-infected women are also considered HIV infected if they meet the Centers for Disease Control and Prevention surveillance case definition for AIDS. Before testing, provide counseling to the parent or guardian, including an explanation of HIV infection, the reason for the test, implications of positive test results, confidentiality issues, risk reduction behaviors, and beneficial effects of early intervention.

The Centers for Disease Control and Prevention (1994, 2008) has developed a classification system to describe the spectrum of HIV disease in children (Table 28.9). The system indicates the severity of clinical signs and symptoms and the degree of immunosuppression. Mild signs and symptoms include lymphadenopathy, parotitis, hepatosplenomegaly, and recurrent or persistent sinusitis or otitis media. Moderate signs and symptoms include LIP and a variety of organ-specific dysfunctions or infections. Severe signs and symptoms include AIDS-defining illnesses with the exception of LIP. Children with LIP have a better prognosis than those with other AIDS-defining illnesses.

The clinical and immunologic classification categories are mutually exclusive. Once classified, an infant or child may not be reclassified into a less severe category, even if clinical or immunologic status improves in response to antiretroviral therapy or other factors. For children whose HIV infection is not yet confirmed, the letter *E* (vertically exposed) is placed in front of the classification. The immune categories are based on $CD4^+$ lymphocyte counts and percentages. Age adjustment of these numbers is necessary because normal counts, which are relatively high in infants, decline steadily until 6 years of age, when they reach adult norms.

Therapeutic Management

The goals of therapy for HIV infection include slowing the growth of the virus, preventing and treating opportunistic infections, and providing nutritional support and symptomatic treatment. Antiretroviral drugs work at various stages of the HIV life cycle to prevent reproduction of functional new virus particles. Antiretroviral therapy regimens are continually evolving. Although antiretroviral drugs are not a cure, they can delay progression of the disease (Centers for Disease Control and Prevention, 2016; Yogev & Chadwick, 2016). Classes of antiretroviral agents include nucleoside reverse transcriptase inhibitors (e.g., zidovudine, didanosine, stavudine, lamivudine, abacavir); nonnucleoside reverse transcriptase inhibitors (e.g., nevirapine, delavirdine, efavirenz); and protease inhibitors (e.g., indinavir, saquinavir, ritonavir, nelfinavir, amprenavir, lopinavir, ritonavir). Combinations of antiretroviral drugs are used to stall the emergence of drug resistance, including the addition of other Food and Drug Administration–approved drug classes (e.g., fusion inhibitors, entry inhibitors, integrase inhibitors, pharmacokinetic enhancers) (Appadurai & Senapati, 2017; Huang, Chen, Dolan, et al., 2017; US Department of Health and Human Services, 2017). Antiretroviral therapy regimens and guidelines are continually evolving. Therapy is lifelong, making adherence difficult. Laboratory markers (e.g., $CD4^+$ lymphocyte count, viral load) assist in monitoring both disease progression and response to therapy.

Strict scheduling requirements, side effects, and need for multiple medications, which at times are not very palatable, make it difficult for children and adolescents to take their medications at the right time and in proper coordination with their meals. Yet adhering to the medication schedule is critical to preventing the development of resistant forms of HIV (Yogev & Chadwick, 2016). Clinical improvements include weight

TABLE 28.9 Pediatric Human Immunodeficiency Virus Infection Classification*

Immunologic Category	N: No Signs/ Symptoms	A: Mild Signs/ Symptoms	B: Moderate Signs/ Symptoms†	C: Severe Signs/ Symptoms†
No evidence of suppression	N1	A1	B1	C1
Evidence of moderate suppression	N2	A2	B2	C2
Severe suppression	N3	A3	B3	C3

*Children whose human immunodeficiency virus infection status is not confirmed are classified by using the above table with the letter *E* (for perinatally exposed) placed before the appropriate classification code (e.g., EN2).

†Both category C and lymphoid interstitial pneumonitis in category B are reportable to state and local health departments as acquired immunodeficiency syndrome.

From Centers for Disease Control and Prevention. (1994). 1994 revised classification system for human immunodeficiency virus infection in children less than 13 years of age. *MMWR Recommendations and Reports, 43*(RR-12), 1-10; Centers for Disease Control and Prevention. (1994). Revised surveillance case definitions for HIV infection among adults, adolescents, and children aged <18 months and for HIV infection and AIDS among children aged 18 months to <13 years—United States, 2008. *MMWR Recommendations and Reports, 57*(10), 1-12. (No changes have been made to the HIV infection classification system with revised case definitions for public health surveillance only and not as a guide for clinical diagnosis.)

gain in children with previous growth retardation, decreased hepatosplenomegaly, improvement in symptoms of HIV-associated encephalopathy, and improvement in immune system function.

Pneumocystis carinii pneumonia (PCP) is the most common opportunistic infection in children infected with HIV. It occurs most frequently between 3 and 6 months of age, when HIV status may be unclear. All infants born to HIV-infected women should receive prophylaxis until HIV infection is reasonably excluded (Siberry, 2014; Simpkins, Siberry, & Hutton, 2009). For children older than 1 year of age, the need for prophylaxis depends on the presence of severe immunosuppression or a history of PCP. Trimethoprim-sulfamethoxazole is the agent of choice. If adverse effects are experienced with this medication, dapsone, atovaquone, or pentamidine may be used.

Prophylaxis is often given for other opportunistic infections, such as disseminated *Mycobacterium avium-intracellulare* complex infection, candidiasis, and herpes simplex. However, prophylaxis may be discontinued if the patients have experienced sustained (>6 months' duration) immune reconstitution with HAART, regardless of a history of opportunistic infection (Yogev & Chadwick, 2016). Administration of IVIG has been helpful in preventing recurrent or serious bacterial infections in some HIV-infected children.

Immunization against common childhood illnesses, including the pneumococcal and influenza vaccines, is recommended for all children exposed to and infected with HIV. The varicella and measles-mumps-rubella (MMR) vaccine can be administered if there is no evidence of severe immunocompromise (Yogev & Chadwick, 2016). Because antibody production to vaccines may be poor or decrease over time, immediate prophylaxis after exposure to several vaccine-preventable diseases (e.g., measles, varicella) is warranted. It should be recognize that children receiving IV gamma globulin prophylaxis may not respond to the MMR vaccine if given in close proximity to the IVGG dose (McLean, Fiebelkorn, Temte, et al., 2013).

HIV infection often leads to marked failure to thrive and multiple nutritional deficiencies. Nutritional management may be difficult because of recurrent illness, diarrhea, and other physical problems. The nurse should implement intensive nutritional interventions if the child's growth begins to slow or weight begins to decrease. Children with opportunistic infections (e.g., *Pneumocystis* pneumonia), encephalopathy and regressing developmental milestones, or wasting syndrome have the worst prognosis, with 75% dying before 3 years of age (Yogev & Chadwick, 2016).

Prognosis

Early recognition and improved medical care have changed HIV infection from a rapidly fatal disease to a chronic one. After the introduction of combination antiretroviral therapy, the numbers of new AIDS cases and deaths declined substantially. In United States, from 2009 to 2013 the annual estimated number and rate of deaths of HIV-infected children younger than 13 years old remained stable (Centers for Disease Control and Prevention, 2015; Simpkins, Siberry, & Hutton, 2009). In contrast, adolescents and young adults (13 to 24 years old) with AIDS that represent a minority of cases in the United States (about 4%) constitute one of the growing groups of newly infected persons in the country (Simpkins, Siberry, & Hutton, 2009; Yogev & Chadwick, 2016).

The most accurate prognostic indicators of a poor outcome are a CD4 lymphocyte percentage of less than 15% and a high viral load of more than 100,000 copies/ml (Yogev & Chadwick, 2016). A growing number of countries worldwide have committed to ending the AIDS epidemic by 2030 by achieving the 90-90-90 treatment target by 2020, whereby 90% of people living with HIV know their HIV status, 90% of people who know their HIV-positive status are accessing treatment, and 90% of people on treatment have suppressed viral loads (Paintsil & Andiman, 2009; United Nations AIDS, 2016). This would change a fatal disease to a chronic disease for HIV-positive adults and children worldwide. Also recent discoveries of new antiretroviral drugs, new vaccines, and advances in gene therapy are encouraging as the focus is on the elimination of HIV/AIDS (Huang,Tomitaka, Raymond, et al., 2017; Yogev & Chadwick, 2016).

Nursing Care Management

Education concerning the transmission and control of infectious diseases, including HIV infection, is essential for children with HIV infection and anyone involved in their care. The basic tenets of standard precautions should be presented in an age-appropriate manner, with careful consideration of the educational level of the individual. (See Infection Control, Chapter 6.) To reduce the incidence of opportunistic infections, parents and children should be counseled about (1) the importance of good hand washing, (2) avoiding raw or undercooked food *(Salmonella)*, (3) avoiding drinking or swimming in lake or river water or being in contact with young farm animals *(Cryptosporidium)*, and (4) the risk of playing with pets (*Toxoplasma* and *Bartonella* from cats, *Salmonella* from reptiles) (Yogev & Chadwick, 2016). Safety issues, including appropriate storage of special medications and equipment (e.g., needles and syringes), are emphasized. Unfortunately, relatives, friends, and others in the general public may be fearful of contracting HIV infection, and criticism and ostracism of the child and family may occur. In an effort to protect the child and deal with the community's fear, the family may limit the child's activities outside the home. Although certain precautions are justified in limiting exposure to sources of infections, they must be tempered with concern for the child's normal developmental needs. Both the family and the community need ongoing education about HIV to dispel many of the myths that have been perpetuated by uninformed persons.

Prevention is a key component of HIV education. Educating adolescents about HIV is essential in preventing HIV infection in this age-group. Education should include information on the routes of transmission, the hazards of IV and other recreational drug use, and the value of sexual abstinence and safe sex practices (United Nations AIDS, 2016; Yogev & Chadwick, 2016). Such education should be a part of anticipatory guidance provided to all adolescent patients. Nurses should also encourage adolescents at risk to undergo HIV counseling and testing. In addition to identifying infected teenagers and getting them into care, such counseling affords adolescents an opportunity to learn about, and possibly change, their risk behaviors. (See Quality Patient Outcomes box.)

QUALITY PATIENT OUTCOMES

Human Immunodeficiency Virus

- Early recognition of signs and symptoms of human immunodeficiency virus (HIV)
- HIV infection slowed or maintained
- Growth and development promoted
- No infectious complications or cancer development
- Adherence to antiretroviral therapy
- Prolonged survival
- Quality of life supported

The nurse's role in the care of the child with HIV is multifaceted. The nurse serves as educator, direct care provider, case manager, and advocate. As with all children with chronic illnesses, these children have much involvement with the health care system. Clinic visits and hospitalizations may become frequent as the disease progresses. The physiologic care of the child is directed at minimizing exposure to infections; delaying the development of viral resistance; supplying nutritional support; providing comfort measures, including pain management; and assessing and recognizing changes in status that may indicate new complications. The scope of nursing care changes with new symptoms, changes in treatment, and disease progression. Psychologic interventions vary with the unique circumstances of each child and family.

Common psychosocial concerns include disclosing the diagnosis to the child, making custody plans when the parent is infected, and anticipating the loss of a family member. Other stressors may include financial difficulties, HIV-associated stigma, attempts to keep the diagnosis a secret, infection of other family members, and any losses associated with HIV. Most mothers of these children are single mothers who are also HIV infected. As primary caretakers, they often attend to the needs of their child first, neglecting their own health in the process. The nurse can encourage the mother to receive regular health care. Family members are often involved in the care of the child, particularly if the mother has symptomatic illness. The nurse is an integral part of the multidisciplinary team necessary for the successful management of the complex medical and social problems of these families.

The multiple complications associated with HIV disease may be potentially painful. Aggressive pain management is essential for these children to have an acceptable quality of life. Their pain may be caused by infections (e.g., otitis media, dental abscess), encephalopathy (e.g., spasticity), adverse effects of medications (e.g., peripheral neuropathy), or an unknown source (e.g., deep musculoskeletal pain). Pain is related not only to disease processes but also to the various treatments these children often undergo, including venipunctures, lumbar punctures, biopsies, and endoscopies. Ongoing assessment of pain is crucial and is most easily accomplished in older children who are able to communicate. Nonverbal and developmentally delayed children are more difficult to assess. The nurse should be alert for other signs of pain: emotional detachment, lack of interactive play, irritability, and depression. Effective pain management depends on the appropriate use of pharmacologic agents, including EMLA or LMX cream, acetaminophen, NSAIDs, muscle relaxants, and opioids. Tolerance to opioids may indicate the need for increased dosing; monitoring of use ensures safety. Nonpharmacologic interventions (e.g., guided imagery, hypnosis, relaxation, and distraction techniques) are useful adjuncts.

Children with HIV infection attend day care centers and school. It is well established that the risk of HIV transmission in school settings is minimal. These institutions are required to follow Centers for Disease Control and Prevention and Occupational Safety and Health Administration (OSHA) guidelines for infection control measures. Standard Precautions describing proper management of blood and body fluids are followed. It is recommended that school personnel receive current HIV information and include it in the health education curriculum from kindergarten through twelfth grade (American Academy of Pediatrics, Committee on Nutrition, 1999; American Academy of Pediatrics, Committee on Pediatric AIDS, 2000; National Association of School Psychologists, 2012). School nurses play a vital role in educating the school staff, students, and parents. They also are invaluable in monitoring the needs of known affected children.

Confidentiality is another major issue in day care and school attendance. Parents and legal guardians have the right to decide whether they inform a school or day care agency of a child's HIV diagnosis.* Unfortunately, myths about HIV infection continue to exist, and the family often wishes to avoid any potential criticism or ostracism of the child.

*Additional information is available from the National AIDS hotline, 800-342-AIDS (2437); TTY/TDD 800-243-7889.

WISKOTT-ALDRICH SYNDROME

Wiskott-Aldrich syndrome (WAS) is a congenital X-linked recessive disorder characterized by a triad of abnormalities: thrombocytopenia with small platelets, eczema, and immunodeficiency involving selective functions of B and T lymphocytes.

Pathophysiology

An abnormal gene that was identified on the proximal arm of the X chromosome was designated the WAS protein (Bonilla & Notarangelo, 2015; Buckley, 2016). The exact defect is unknown. A variety of pathologic findings are evident. The platelets are abnormally small and have a shortened life span, possibly because of a metabolic defect in their synthesis. The primary immunologic defect consists of the inability of phagocytes (macrophages) to process foreign antigens, particularly polysaccharides such as pneumococci. As a result, immunologically competent cells fail to produce normal immunoglobulin patterns. The level of IgM is diminished early in the course of the disease, whereas levels of IgA and IgE may be elevated with a normal or slightly low IgG concentration (Bonilla & Notarangelo, 2015; Buckley, 2016). Typically, isohemagglutinins (anti-A and anti-B agglutinins in the blood) are decreased or absent. There is a defect in antibody production that progresses to an antibody deficiency with a decrease in T suppressor lymphocytes that explains the increased susceptibility to opportunistic infections (Bonilla & Notarangelo, 2015; Fleisher, 2006).

The thymus and lymph nodes are normal at birth but become progressively dysfunctional with age until a profound cellular immunodeficiency results. Consequently, these children are highly susceptible to infection and malignancy, especially lymphoma and leukemia.

Clinical Manifestations

At birth, the presenting feature may be increased bleeding at the circumcision site or bloody diarrhea because of the thrombocytopenia (Bonilla & Notarangelo, 2015; Buckley, 2016). As the child grows older, recurrent infection and eczema become more severe, and the bleeding becomes less frequent.

Eczema is typical of the allergic type and readily becomes superinfected. Chronic infection with herpes simplex is a frequent problem and may lead to chronic keratitis of the eye with loss of vision. Chronic pulmonary disease, sinusitis, and otitis media result from repeated infections. In children who survive the bleeding episodes and overwhelming infections, malignancy presents an additional risk to survival.

Diagnostic Evaluation

The diagnosis can usually be made during the neonatal period because of the thrombocytopenia. Specific tests for immunologic function confirm the diagnosis. Carrier detection is also possible.

Therapeutic Management

Medical treatment primarily involves counteracting the bleeding tendencies with platelet transfusions, giving IVIG to provide passive immunity, using G-CSF to correct neutropenia and prevent infections, administering prophylactic antibiotics to prevent and control infection, and providing aggressive local therapy for the eczema (Bonilla & Notarangelo, 2015; Buckley, 2016; Dale, 2017). Splenectomy may improve the platelet count, although the risk of asplenic sepsis in these infants is extremely high. These children require the same prophylactic antibiotics and appropriate immunizations as does any child with asplenia. Despite their immunodeficiency, they are able to mount an adequate immunologic response to the inactivated vaccines. When an HLA-matched donor exists, WAS is usually cured with HSCT and should be performed as early as possible (Albert, Notarangelo, & Ochs, 2010; Buckley, 2016; Mahlaoui, Pellier, Mignot, et al., 2012). The 5-year survival rate after HSCT for WAS approximates 90% for transplants performed after year 2000 (Bonilla & Notarangelo, 2015). Shin, Kim, Li, and colleagues (2012) reported excellent results after unmanipulated unrelated donor HSCT in 47 patients with WAS that were transplanted over 20 years ago. Several clinical trials worldwide have focused on replacing the WAS gene using lentiviral vector effectively in more than 20 patients (Albert, Notarangelo, & Ochs, 2010; Thrasher & Williams, 2017).

Nursing Care Management

Without HSCT, survival beyond adolescence is uncommon. Because of the guarded prognosis for these children, the main nursing consideration is supporting the family in the care of a potentially fatally ill child. (See Chapter 19.) Physical care should be directed at controlling the problems that are imposed by the disorder. The measures used to control bleeding are similar to those used in hemophilia and vWD. Another major goal is to prevent or control infection. Because eczema is a troublesome problem, nursing measures specific to this condition are especially important.

The genetic implications of this X-linked recessive disorder differ little from those for any other X-linked disease. However, the multiplicity of defects tends to affect emotional adjustment and physical care to a greater degree than in other X-linked disorders. The nurse must be especially supportive by providing short-term goals during periods of hospitalization and by focusing on long-range needs through coordinated efforts with a public health nurse.

SEVERE COMBINED IMMUNODEFICIENCY DISEASE

SCID is a defect characterized by the absence of both humoral and cell-mediated immunity (Bonilla & Notarangelo, 2015; Buckley, 2016). The terms *Swiss-type lymphopenic agammaglobulinemia,* which refers to the autosomal recessive form of the disease, and *X-linked lymphopenic agammaglobulinemia* have been used to describe this disorder, which, as the names imply, can follow either mode of inheritance.

Pathophysiology

The exact cause of SCID is unknown. Theories include a defective stem cell that is incapable of differentiating into B or T cells; defects in the organs responsible for the differentiating process, primarily the thymus and lymphoid complex; or an enzymatic defect that suppresses lymphocytic cell function.

The consequence of the immunodeficiency is an overwhelming susceptibility to infection and to the graft-versus-host reaction, which can occur when any histoincompatible (unmatched) tissue from an immunocompetent donor is infused into the immunodeficient recipient. Because of its immunodeficiency, the body is unable to reject the foreign, incompatible tissue. Therefore the antigenic donor cells attack the host's tissues. The graft-versus-host reaction is a serious complication in the treatment of SCID with HSCT.

Clinical Manifestations

The most common manifestation is susceptibility to infection early in life, most often in the first month. Specifically, the disorder in children is characterized by chronic infection, failure to completely recover from an infection, frequent reinfection, and infection with unusual agents. In addition, the history reveals no logical source of infection. Failure to thrive is a consequence of the persistent illness.

If the child should receive blood products containing viable lymphocytes, signs of graft-versus-host reaction, such as fever, skin rash, alopecia, hepatosplenomegaly, and diarrhea, are expected (Bonilla & Notarangelo, 2015). Because tissue damage does not become evident in the reaction for 7 to 20 days, the symptoms may be mistaken for an infection. However, the presence of a graft-versus-host reaction increases the child's susceptibility to overwhelming infection and therefore is a grave complication.

Diagnostic Evaluation

Diagnosis is usually based on a history of recurrent, severe infections from early infancy; a familial history of the disorder; and specific laboratory findings, which include lymphopenia, lack of lymphocyte response to antigens, and absence of plasma cells in the bone marrow. Documentation of immunoglobulin deficiency is difficult during infancy because of the normally delayed response of infants in producing their own immunoglobulins and maternal transfer of IgG. Currently newborn screening for SCID can be performed by quantifying levels of T-cell receptor (TCR) excision circles (TRECs) in dried blood spots collected at birth (Cross, 2013; Centers for Disease Control and Prevention, 2015; Dorsey, Dvorak, Cowan, et al., 2017; Puck, 2012). TRECs are a by-product of rearrangement of TCR genes during intrathymic T-cell development and the TREC levels are extremely low or absent in patients with SCID. Since newborn screening for SCID has been started in various parts of the United States, including 32 states and the District of Columbia, several cases of SCID have been identified at birth in otherwise healthy-looking newborns (Centers for Disease Control and Prevention, 2015; Dorsey, Dvorak, Cowan, et al., 2017). Quantification of TRECs represents an important, yet nonspecific, indicator of a possible severe T-cell immunodeficiency, the diagnosis of which must be confirmed by appropriate immunophenotypic, functional, and molecular tests (Bonilla & Notarangelo, 2015).

Therapeutic Management

The definitive treatment is a histocompatible HSCT. If the condition is diagnosed at birth or within the first 3 months of life, more than 95% of cases can be treated successfully with HLA-identical or T-cell–depleted haploidentical (usually a parent) related bone marrow stem cells (Buckley, 2016; Dorsey, Dvorak, Cowan, et al., 2017). The most suitable donor is a sibling with HLA-matched bone marrow followed by the use of other stem cell sources such as haploidentical related donor, HLA-matched unrelated donor, and cord blood donor. Because SCID is inherited, an identical twin, who usually is a perfect donor, is not a candidate because he or she would also display the disorder.

Before newborn screening for SCID became a reality, most patients were infected when initially diagnosed and required immediate aggressive interventions (Bonilla & Notarangelo, 2015). Approaches to manage SCID patients included providing passive immunity with IVIG and maintaining the child in a sterile environment. The latter is effective only if the measure is instituted before any infectious process takes hold in the infant, and it represents an extreme effort to prevent life-threatening infections. Other transplant procedures include nonidentical-HLA bone marrow grafting and fetal liver or thymus transplantation. The results of these procedures are still uncertain, although they provide potential hope for future children born with the disorder. Several investigators used hematopoietic stem and progenitor cell gene therapy successfully, with many challenges (e.g., safer retroviral and lentiviral vectors, optimization of methods to preserve viability and function during product manufacture), but there is a need to overcome these challenges before gene therapy can be offered as a standard of care (Bonilla & Notarangelo, 2015; Dorsey, Dvorak, Cowan, et al., 2017).

Nursing Care Management

Nursing care focuses on preventing infection and supporting the child and family. If bone marrow transplantation is attempted, the care is consistent with that needed by patients undergoing bone marrow transplantation for any condition. (See Chapter 29.) To prevent infection, implement all interventions aimed at protecting the immunocompromised child. However, even with exacting environmental control, these children are prone to opportunistic infection. Chronic fungal infections of the mouth and nails with *Candida albicans* are frequent problems despite vigorous efforts at prevention or treatment. A hoarse voice may result from repeated esophageal and vocal cord erosions from the fungus. It is important to stress to parents that such conditions are not a result of laxity on their part in preventing them but are a result of the severe immunologic disorder. Encourage parents to immediately notify a physician regarding any evidence of a worsening infection.

Although newborn screening optimizes the chances of successful treatment, newborns present new issues in their management, including parental emotional difficulties (e.g., shock, guilt, apprehension regarding losing the child), as well as defining the best treatment regimen (Dorsey, Dvorak, Cowan, et al., 2017). Nursing care should be directed at supporting the family in caring for a child with a potential fatal illness. (See Chapter 19.) Genetic counseling is essential because of the modes of transmission in either form of the disorder.

NCLEX REVIEW QUESTIONS

1. A child is admitted to the pediatric unit. The mother reports that the doctor says her son is anemic. What laboratory findings/manifestations would the nurse expect to see to confirm iron deficiency anemia?
   A. Cyanosis, due to inadequate oxygen saturation of existing hemoglobin
   B. A decreased reticulocyte count
   C. A total iron-binding capacity (TIBC) that is elevated above the normal range
   D. Decreased blood pressure changes, which are an early sign because of the compensatory mechanisms
2. A child with sickle cell anemia is admitted in a vasoocclusive crisis. Which of the following interventions should the nurse expect to see ordered? Select all that apply.
   A. Cold compresses to painful joints
   B. IV fluids started, and oral fluids encouraged
   C. Meperidine ordered every 4 hours for pain
   D. High-calorie, high-protein diet
   E. Antibiotics ordered for any existing infection
3. You are working with a recent graduate on the pediatric unit. You are assigned to take care of an adolescent with β-thalassemia. The nurse needs more information about this disease if she states which of the following? Select all that apply.
   A. "We need to check the patient's iron level to make sure he is not anemic."
   B. "I believe this is most common in those of Hispanic descent, although this patient is Mediterranean."
   C. "The doctor will be prescribing deferasirox (Exjade) or defoxamine (Desferal) for chelation therapy."
   D. "This patient looks much younger than I would expect. I guess he's just a late bloomer."
   E. "I think a transfusion will be ordered, since his hemoglobin level is 9.0."
4. Which is the most accurate genetic explanation for a family with hemophilia?
   A. It is a Y-linked dominant disorder.
   B. It is equally distributed among males and females.
   C. It is an X-linked recessive disorder.
   D. It is an autosomal recessive disorder.
5. You are discharging a patient with hemophilia. Which of the following responses by the parents indicate an understanding of this disorder? Select all that apply.
   A. "My child should remain active to decrease joint problems, and most children with hemophilia can participate in the same activities as peers."
   B. "Care should be taken to avoid bleeding of gums, and softening the toothbrush in warm water before brushing or using a sponge-tipped disposable toothbrush may be helpful."
   C. "Signs of internal bleeding should be recognized, such as headache, slurred speech, loss of consciousness (from cerebral bleeding), and black, tarry stools (from gastrointestinal bleeding)."
   D. "If there is bleeding in a joint, elevation, ice, and rest should help and may prevent the need for factor VIII replacement."
   E. "All of my son's teachers need to be aware of what to do if he gets a bloody nose."

Correct Answers

1. C; 2. B, D, E; 3. A, B, D; 4. C; 5. B, C, E

REFERENCES

Abdullah, K., Thorpe, K. E., Mamak, E., et al. (2015). Optimizing early child development for young children with non-anemic iron deficiency in primary care practice setting (OptEC): Study protocol for a randomized controlled trial. *Trials, 16*, 132.

Adewoyin, A. S. (2015). Management of sickle cell disease: A review for physician education in Nigeria (Sub-Saharan Africa). *Anemia, 2015*, Article ID 791498, 21 pages.

Albert, M. H., Notarangelo, L. D., & Ochs, H. D. (2010). Clinical spectrum, pathophysiology and treatment of Wiskott-Aldrich syndrome. *Current Opinion in Hematology, 18*, 42–48.

Algiraigri, A. H., Wright, N. A. M., Paolucci, E. O., et al. (2017). Hydroxyurea for nontransfusion-dependent β-thalassemia: A systematic review and meta-analysis. *Hematology/Oncology and Stem Cell Therapy, 10*(3), 116–125.

American Academy of Pediatrics, Committee on Nutrition. (1999). Iron fortification of infant formulas. *Pediatrics, 104*(1), 119–123.

American Academy of Pediatrics, & Committee on Pediatric AIDS. (2000). Identification and care of HIV-exposed and HIV-infected infants, children and adolescents in foster care. *Pediatrics, 106*(1), 149–153.

American Academy of Pediatrics Committee on Pediatric AIDS. (2008). HIV testing and prophylaxis to prevent mother-to-child transmission in the United States. *Pediatrics, 122*(5), 1127–1134.

Anderson, O., Domeliof, M., Anderson, D., et al. (2014). Effect of delayed vs early umbilical cord clamping on iron status and neurodevelopment at age 12 months: A randonmized clinical trial. *JAMA Pediatrics, 168*(6), 547–554.

Anderson, A., & Forsyth, A. (2017). *Playing it safe: bleeding disorders, sports and exercise*, The National Hemophilia Foundation.

Angulo-Barroso, R. M., Li, M., Santos, D. C. C., et al. (2016). Iron supplementation in pregnancy or infancy and motor development: A randomized controlled trial. *Pediatrics, 137*.

Ansari, S. H., Lassi, Z. S., Ali, S. M., et al. (2016). Hydroxyurea for β-thalassemia major. *Cochrane Database of Systematic Reviews*, (1), Art. No.: CD012064.

Appadurai, R., & Senapati, S. (2017). *How mutations can resist drug binding yet keep HIV-1 protease functional*, Biochemistry ACS Publications,pubs.acs.org/biochemistry.

Arlet, J., Dussiot, M., Moura, I. C., et al. (2016). Novel players [beta]-thalassemia dyserythropoiesis and new therapeutic strategies. *Current Opinion in Hematology*, *23*(3), 181–188.

Armstrong-Wells, J., Grimes, S., Sidney, D., et al. (2009). Utilization of TCD screening for primary stroke prevention in children with sickle cell disease. *Neurology*, *72*, 1316–1321.

Auerbach, M. (2011). Should intravenous iron be upfront therapy for iron deficiency anemia? *Pediatric Blood and Cancer*, *56*, 511–512.

Aydinok, Y. (2012). Thalassemia. *Hematology (Amsterdam, Netherlands)*, *17*, S28–S31.

Azar, S., & Wong, T. E. (2016). Sickle cell disease: A brief update. *The Medical Clinics of North America*.

Ballas, S. K. (2011). Update on pain management in sickle cell disease. *Hemoglobin*, *35*(5–6), 520–529.

Baird-Gunning, J., & Bromley, J. (2016). Correcting iron deficiency. *Australian Prescriber*, *39*, 193–199.

Baker, R. D., Greer, F. R., & Committee on Nutrition. (2010). Diagnosis and prevention of iron deficiency and iron-deficiency anemia in infants and young children (0-3 years of age). *Pediatrics*, *126*, 1040–1050.

Ben-Ami, T., & Revel-Vilk, S. (2013). The use of DDAVP in children with bleeding disorders. *Pediatric Blood and Cancer*, *60*, S41–S43.

Bolton-Maggs, P. H. B., Langer, J. C., Iolascon, A., et al. (2011). Guidelines for the diagnosis and management of hereditary spherocytosis—2011 update. *British Journal of Haematology*, *156*, 37–49.

Bonilla, F. A., & Notarangelo, L. D. (2015). Primary immunodeficiency diseases. In S. H. Orkin, D. E. Fisher, D. Ginsburg, et al. (Eds.), *Nathan and Oski's hematology of infancy and childhood* (8th ed.). Philadelphia: Saunders.

Branchford, B. R., Monahan, P. E., & Di Paola, J. (2013). New developments in the treatment of pediatric hemophilia and bleeding disorders. *Current Opinion in Pediatrics*, *25*, 23–30.

Brandow, A. M., Weisman, S. J., & Panepinto, J. A. (2011). The impact of a multidisciplinary pain management model on sickle cell disease pain hospitalizations. *Pediatric Blood and Cancer*, *56*(5), 789–793.

Bregman, D. B., & Goodnough, L. T. (2014). Experience with intravenous ferric carboxymaltose in patients with iron deficiency anemia. *Therapeutic Advances in Hermatology*, *5*(2), 48–60.

Broderick, C. R., Herbert, R. D., Latimer, J., et al. (2012). Association between physical activity and risk of bleeding in children with hemophilia. *JAMA: The Journal of the American Medical Association*, *308*(14), 1452–1459.

Brugnara, C., Oski, F. A., & Nathan, D. G. (2015). Diagnostic approach to the anemic patient. In S. H. Orkin, D. E. Fisher, D. Ginsburg, et al. (Eds.), *Nathan and Oski's hematology of infancy and childhood* (8th ed.), Philadelphia: Saunders.

Buckley, R. H. (2016). Primary combined antibody and cellular immunodeficiencies. In R. M. Kliegman, B. F. Stanton, J. W. St.Geme III, et al. (Eds.), *Nelson textbook of pediatrics* (20th ed.). Philadelphia: Elsevier Inc.

Buga-Corbu, I., Arion, C., Davila, C., et al. (2014). Current therapy in children and adolescents with von Willebrand disease. *Journal of Medicine and Life*, *7*(2), 264–269.

Camaschella, C. (2015). Iron-deficiency anemia. *The New England Journal of Medicine*, *372*, 1832–1843.

Cappellini, M. D., Bejaoui, M., Agaoglu, L., et al. (2011). Iron chelation with deferasirox in adult and pediatric patients with thalassemia major: Efficacy and safety during 5 years' follow-up. *Blood*, *118*, 884–893.

Carmel, R., Watkins, D., & Rosenblatt, D. S. (2015). Megaloblastic anemia. In S. H. Orkin, D. E. Fisher, D. Ginsburg, et al. (Eds.), *Nathan and Oski's hematology of infancy and childhood* (8th ed.). Philadelphia: Saunders.

Castaman, G. (2013). Changes of von Willebrand factor during pregnancy in women with and without von Willebrand disease. *Meditterranean Journal of Hematology and Infectious Diseases*, *5*(1), e2013052.

Castaman, G., & Linari, S. (2017). Diagnosis and treatment of von Willebrand Disease and rare bleeding disorders. *Journal of Clinical Medicine*, *6*, 45.

Celkan, T., & Koc, B. S. (2015). Approach to the patient with neutropenia in childhood. *Türk pediatri arşivi*, *50*, 136–144.

Centers for Disease Control and Prevention. (1994). 1994 Revised classification system for human immunodeficiency virus infection in children less than 13 years of age. *MMWR. Recommendations and Reports: Morbidity and Mortality Weekly Report. Recommendations and Reports*, *43*(RR–12), 1–10.

Centers for Disease Control and Prevention. (2008). Revised Surveillance Case Definitions for HIV Infection Among Adults, Adolescents, and Children Aged <18 Months and for HIV Infection and AIDS Among Children Aged 18 Months to <13 Years—United States. *MMWR. Recommendations and Reports: Morbidity and Mortality Weekly Report. Recommendations and Reports*, *57*(10), 1–12.

Centers for Disease Control and Prevention. (2013). *HIV prevention: Progress to date*, https://www.cdc.gov/nchhstp/newsroom/docs/HIVFactSheets/Progress-508.pdf.

Centers for Disease Control and Prevention. (2015). *Severe combined immunodeficiency (SCID)*, https://www.cdc.gov/newbornscreening/scid.html.

Centers for Disease Control and Prevention. (2016). *HIV in the United States: At a glance*, https://www.cdc.gov/statistics/overview/ataglance.html.

Centers for Disease Control and Prevention. (2017a). *Hemophilia Facts—United States*, https://www.cdc.gov/ncbddd/hemophilia/facts.html.

Centers for Disease Control and Prevention. (2017b). *HIV among pregnant women, infants and children*, https://www.cdc.gov/hiv/group/gender/pregnant women/index.html.

Chan, C. Q. H., Low, L. L., & Lee, K. H. (2016). Oral vitamin B12 replacement for the treatment of pernicious anemia. *Frontiers in Medicine*, *3*, 38.

Chatterjee, R., & Bajora, R. (2010). Critical appraisal of growth retardation and pubertal disturbances in thalassemia. *Annals of the New York Academy of Sciences*, *1202*, 100–114.

Choudhry, V. P. (2017). Thalassemia minor and major: Current management. *Indian Journal of Pediatrics*, *84*(8), 607–611.

Consolini, D. M. (2011). Thrombocytopenia in infants and children. *Pediatrics in Review*, *32*, 135–151.

Cross, C. (2013). Ontario newborns now screened for SCID. *CMAJ*, *185*(13), E616.

Cuesta-Barriuso, R., Torres-Ortuno, A., Perez-Alenda, S., et al. (2016). Sporting activities and quality of life in children with hemophilia: An observational study. *Pediatric Physical Therapy*, *28*, 453–459.

DaCosta, L., Galimand, J., Fenneteau, O., et al. (2013). Hereditary spherocytosis, elliptocytosis, and other red cell membrane disorders. *Blood Reviews*, *27*, 167–178.

Dale, D. C. (2017). How I manage children with neutropenia. *British Journal of Haematology*, *178*(3), 351–363.

Dastgiri, S., & Dolatkhah, R. (2016). Blood transfusions for treating acute chest syndrome in people with sickle cell disease. *Cochrane Database of Systematic Reviews*, (8), Art.No.: CD007843.

DeBaun, M. R., Armstrong, F. D., McKinstry, R. C., et al. (2012). Silent cerebral infarcts: A review on a prevalent and progressive cause of neurologic injury in sickle cell anemia. *Blood*, *17*, 4587–4596.

DeBaun, M. R., Frei-Jones, M., & Vichinsky, E. (2016). Hemoglobinopathies. In R. M. Kliegman, B. F. Stanton, I. I. I. St. Geme, et al. (Eds.), *Nelson textbook of pediatrics* (20th ed.). Philadelphia: Elsevier.

DeBaun, M. R., & Kirkham, F. J. (2016). Central nervous system complications and management in sickle cell disease. *Blood*, *127*(7), 829–838.

DeLoughery, T. G. (2014). Microcytic Anemia. *The New England Journal of Medicine*, *371*, 1324–1331.

Dinauer, M. C., Newburger, P. E., & Borregaard, N. (2015). Phagocyte system and disorders of granulopoiesis and granulocyte function. In S. H. Orkin, D. E. Fisher, D. Ginsburg, et al. (Eds.), *Nathan and Oski's hematology of infancy and childhood* (8th ed.). Philadelphia: Saunders.

Di Paola, J., Montgomery, R. R., Gill, J. C., et al. (2015). Hemophilia and von Willebrand disease. In S. H. Orkin, D. E. Fisher, D. Ginsburg, et al. (Eds.), *Nathan and Oski's hematology of infancy and childhood* (8th ed.). Philadelphia: Elsevier Saunders.

Dorsey, M. J., Dvorak, C. C., Cowan, M. J., et al. (2017). Treatment of infants identified as having severe combined immunodeficiency by means of newborn screening. *Journal of Allergy and Clinical Immunology*, *139*, 733–742.

Driscoll, M. C. (2007). Sickle cell disease. *Pediatrics in Review*, *28*, 259–268.

Dufour, C., Veys, P., Carraro, E., et al. (2015). Similar outcome of upfront-unrelated and matched sibling stem cell transplantation in idiopathic paediatric aplastic anaemia. A study on behalf of the UK Paediatric BMT Working Party, Paediatric Diseases Working Party and Severe Aplastic Anaemia Working Party of EBMT. *British Journal of Haematology*, *171*, 585–594.

Ellison, A. M. (2012). Sickle cell disease: Advice on handling emergencies. *Contemporary Pediatrics*, 18–27.

Estcourt, L. J., Fortin, P. M., Hopewell, S., et al. (2017). Blood transfusion for preventing primary and secondary stroke in people with sickle cell disease. *Cochrane Database of Systematic Reviews*, (1), Art.No.:CD003146.

Fan, F. S. (2016). Iron deficiency anemia due to excessive green tea drinking. *Clinical Case Reports*, *4*(11), 1053–1056.

Fleisher, T. A. (2006). Primary immune deficiencies: Windows into the immune system. *Pediatrics in Review*, *27*(10), 363–372.

Fleming, M. D. (2015). Disorders of iron and copper metabolism, the sideroblastic anemias and lead toxicity. In S. H. Orkin, D. E. Fisher, D. Ginsburg, et al. (Eds.), *Nathan and Oski's hematology of infancy and childhood* (8th ed.). Philadelphia: Saunders.

Flood, V. H., & Scott, J. P. (2016). Von willebrand disease. In R. M. Kliegman, B. F. Stanton, J. W. St.Geme III, et al. (Eds.), *Nelson textbook of pediatrics* (20th ed.). Philadelphia: Elsevier, Inc.

Foong, W. C., Ho, J. J., Loh, C. K., et al. (2016). Hydroxyurea for reducing blood transfusion in non-transfusion dependent beta thalassaemias. *Cochrane Database of Systematic Reviews*, (10), Art.No.:CD011579.

Fortin, P. M., Madgwick, K. V., Trivella, M., et al. (2016). Invention for improving adherence to iron chelation therapy in people with sickle cell disease or thalassaemia. *Cochrane Database of Systematic Reviews*, (9), Art. No.:CD012349.

Georges, G. E., & Storb, R. (2016). Hematopoietic stem cell transplantation for acquired aplastic anemia. *Current Opinion in Hematology*, *23*(6), 495–500.

Ghafuri, D. L., Chaturvedi, S., Rodeghier, M., et al. (2016). Secondary benefit of maintaining normal transcranial Doppler velocities when using hydroxyurea for prevention of severe sickle cell anemia. *Pediatric Blood and Cancer*, *00*, 1–4.

Grace, R. F. (2015). Hematologic manifestations of systemic diseases. In S. H. Orkin, D. E. Fisher, D. Ginsburg, et al. (Eds.), *Nathan and Oski's hematology of infancy and childhood* (8th ed.). Philadelphia: Saunders.

Griebler, U., Bruckmuller, M. U., Kien, C., et al. (2015). Health effects of cow's milk consumption in infants up to 3 years of age: A systematic review and meta-analysis. *Public Heath Nutrition*, *19*(2), 293–307.

Guelcher, C. J. (2016). Evolution of the treatments for hemophilia. *Journal of Infusion Nursing*, *39*(4), 218–224.

Haining, W. N., Duncan, C., El-haddad, A, et al. (2015). Principles of bone marrow and stem cell transplantation. In S. H. Orkin, D. E. Fisher, D. Ginsburg, et al. (Eds.), *Nathan and Oski's hematology of infancy and childhood* (8th ed.). Philadelphia: Saunders.

Hartfield, D. (2010). Iron deficiency is a public health problem in Canadian infants and children. *Paediatr & Child Health*, *15*(6), 347–350.

Hayden, E. C. (2013). Bid to cure HIV ramps up. *Nature*, *498*, 417–418.

Heeney, M., & Ware, R. (2015). Sickle cell disease. In S. H. Orkin, D. E. Fisher, D. Ginsburg, et al. (Eds.), *Nathan and Oski's hematology of infancy and childhood* (8th ed.). Philadelphia: Saunders.

Hepburn, C. M., & Thibodeau, M. L. (2016). The CPSP: An active surveillance program protecting and promoting the health of Canadian children and youth. *Paediatr & Child Health*, *21*(5), 263–264.

Hermans, C., De Moerloose, P., Fischer, K., et al. (2011). Management of acute haemarthrosis in haemophilia A without inhibitors: Literature review, Europen survey and recommendations. *Haemophilia*, *17*, 383–392.

Higgs, D. R., Engel, J. D., & Stamatoyannopoulos, G. (2012). Thalassaemia. *Lancet*, *379*, 373–383.

Hord, J. D. (2016). The acquired pancytopenias. In R. M. Kliegman, B. F. Stanton, J. W. St.Geme III, et al. (Eds.), *Nelson textbook of pediatrics* (20th ed.). Philadelphia: Elsevier Inc.

Hsieh, M. M., Fitzhugh, C. D., Weitzel, R. P., et al. (2014). Nonmyeloablative HLA-matched sibling allogeneic hematopoietic stem cell transplantation for severe sickle cell phenotype. *JAMA: The Journal of the American Medical Association*, *312*(1), 48–56.

Huang, R., Chen, Z., Dolan, S., et al. (2017). The dual modulatory effects of efavirenz on GABAa receptors are mediated via two distinct sites*. *Neuropharmacology*, *121*, 167–178.

Huang, Z., Tomitaka, A., Raymond, A., et al. (2017). Current application of CRISPR/Cas9 gene-editing technique to eradicate HIV/AIDS. *Gene Therapy*, *24*(7), 377–384.

Issaragrisil, S., & Kunacheewa, C. (2016). Matched sibling donor hematopoietic stem cell transplantation for thalassemia. *Current Opinion in Hematology*, *23*(6), 508–514.

Ishikawa, N., Dalal, S., Johnson, C., et al. (2016). *Should HIV testing for all pregnant women continue? Cost-effectiveness of universal testing compared to focused approaches across high to very low HIV prevalence settings, JIAS 19*, http://www.jiasociety.org/index.php/jas/article/view/21212.

Jauregui-Lobera, I. (2014). Iron deficiency and cognitive functions. *Neuropsychiatric Disease and Treatment*, *10*, 2087–2095.

Kahnooji, M., Rashidinejad, H. R., Yazdanpanah, M. S., et al. (2016). Myocardial iron load measured by cardiac magnetic resonance imaging to evaluate cardiac systolic function in thalassemia. *ARYA Atherosclerosis*, *12*(5), 226–230.

Kehrel, B. E., & Brodde, M. F. (2013). State of the art in platelet function testing. *Transfusion Medicine and Hemotherapy: Offizielles Organ der Deutschen Gesellschaft fur Transfusionsmedizin und Immunhamatologie*, *40*, 73–86.

Kett, J. C. (2012). Anemia in infancy. *Pediatrics in Review*, *33*(4), 186–187.

Korthof, E. T., Bekassy, A. N., & Hussein, A. A. (2013). Management of acquired aplastic anemia in children. *Bone Marrow Transplantation*, *48*(2), 191–195.

Kuhn, L., Kim, H.-Y., Walter, J., et al. (2013). HIV-1 concentrations in human breast milk before and after weaning. *Science Translational Medicine*, *5*, 213.

Kuhne, T., & Imbach, P. (2013). Management of children and adolescents with primary immune thrombocytopenia: Controversies and solutions. *Vox Sanguinis*, *104*, 55–66.

Kumar, M., Lambert, M. P., Breakey, V., et al. (2015). Sports participation in children and adolescents with immune thrombocytopenia (ITP). *Pediatric Blood and Cancer*, *62*, 2223–2225.

Kuznik, A., Habib, A. G., Munube, D., et al. (2016). Newborn screening and prophylactic intervention for sickle cell disease in 47 countries in sub-saharan Africa: A cost-effectiveness analysis. *BMC Health Service Research*, *16*(304), 1572–1576.

Lawal, T. A., & Olapade-Olaopa, E. O. (2017). Circumcision and its effects in Africa. *Translational Andrology and Urology*, *6*(2), 149–151.

Lerner, N. (2016). The anemias. In R. M. Kliegman, B. F. Stanton, J. W. St. Geme III, et al. (Eds.), *Nelson textbook of pediatrics* (20th ed.). Philadelphia: Elsevier Inc.

Lillicrap, D. (2013). The future of hemostasis management. *Pediatric Blood and Cancer*, *60*(Suppl. 1), S44–S447.

Locatelli, F., Merli, P., & Strocchio, L. (2016). Transplantation for thalassemia major: Alternative donors. *Current Opinion in Hematology*, *23*(6), 515–523.

Locatelli, F., & Pagliara, D. (2012). Allogenic hematopoietic stem cell transplantation in children with sickle cell disease. *Pediatric Blood and Cancer*, *59*(2), 372–376.

Lucarelli, G., Isgro, A., Sodani, P., et al. (2012). Hematopoietic stem cell transplantation in thalassemia and sickle cell anemia. *Cold Spring Harbor Perspectives in Medicine*, *2*(5), a011825. Published online April 4, 2012.

Lux, S. E. (2015). Disorders of the red cell membrane. In S. H. Orkin, D. E. Fisher, D. Ginsburg, et al. (Eds.), *Nathan and Oski's hematology of infancy and childhood* (8th ed.). Philadelphia: Saunders.

Lytle, A. M., Brown, H. C., Paik, N. Y., et al. (2016). Effects of FVIII immunity on hepatocyte and hematopoietic stem cell-directed gene therapy of murine hemophilia A, Molecular Therapy- Methods and Clinical

Development. *Molecular Therapy. Methods & Clinical Development, 10*(3), 15056.

Mahlaoui, N., Pellier, I., Mignot, C., et al. (2012). Characteristics and outcome of early-onset, severe forms of Wiskott-Aldrich syndrome. *Blood, 121*(9), 1510–1516.

Mahoney, D. H. (2017). Iron deficiency in infants and young children: Screening, prevention, clinical manifestations, and diagnosis, *UpToDate*, http://www.uptodate.com.

Manco-Johnson, M. J., Abshire, T. C., Shapiro, A. D., et al. (2007). Prophylaxis versus episodic treatment to prevent joint disease in boys with severe hemophilia. *The New England Journal of Medicine, 357*, 535–544.

Marcdante, K. J., & Kliegman, R. M. (2015). Hemostatic Disorders. In K. J. Mardante & R. M. Kliegman (Eds.), *Nelson essentials of pediatrics* (20th ed.). Philadelphia: Elsevier Saunders.

Matino, D., Makris, M., Dwan, K., et al. (2015). Recombinant (non-human) factor VIIa clotting factor concentrates versus plasma concentrates for acute bleeds in people with haemophilia and inhibitors. *Cochrane Database of Systematic Reviews*, (12), Art. No.:CD004449.

McCavit, T. L. (2012). Sickle cell disease. *Pediatrics in Review, 33*, 195–206.

McCrae, K. (2011). Immune thrombocytopenia: No longer "idiopathic. *Cleveland Clinic Journal of Medicine, 78*(6), 358–373.

McDonagh, M. S., Blazina, I., Dana, T., et al. (2015). Screening and routine supplementation for iron deficiency anemia: A systematic review. *Pediatrics, 135*(4), 723–733.

McGann, P. T. (2016). Time to invest in sickle cell anemia as a global health priority. *Pediatrics, 137*(6), 210160348.

McLean, H. Q., Fiebelkorn, A. P., Temte, J. L., et al. (2013). Prevention of measles, rubella, congenital rubella syndrome, and mumps, 2013: Summary recommendations of the Advisory Committee on Immunization Practices (ACIP). *MMWR. Recommendations and Reports: Morbidity and Mortality Weekly Report. Recommendations and Reports, 62*(RR–04), 1–34.

Meier, E. M., Fasano, R. M., & Levett, P. R. (2017). A systematic review of the literature for severity predictors in children with sickle cell anemia. *Blood Cells, Molecules & Diseases*, Feb 2. pii: S1079-9 796(16)30138—3.

Meier, E. R., & Miller, J. L. (2012). Sickle cell disease in children. *Drugs, 72*, 895–906.

Mercer, J. S., Erickson-Owens, D. A., Collins, J., et al. (2017). Effects of delayed cord clamping on residual placental blood volume, hemoglobin and bilirubin levels in term infants: A randomized controlled trial. *Journal of Perinatology, 37*(3), 260–264.

Miano, M., & Dufour, C. (2015). The diagnosis and treatment of aplastic anemia: A review. *International Journal of Hematology, 101*(6), 527–535.

Miller, J. L. (2013). Iron deficiency anemia: A common and curable disease. *Cold Spring Harbor Perspectives in Medicine, 3*(3), Published online April 23, 2013.

Miller, S. T., Sleeper, L. A., Pegelow, C. H., et al. (2000). Prediction of adverse outcomes in children with sickle cell disease. *The New England Journal of Medicine, 342*, 83–89.

National Association of School Psychologists (2012). *Supporting students with HIV/AIDS (position statement)*. Bethesda MD: Author.

National Hemophilia Foundation. (2016). *Steps for living: Pain management*, https://stepsforliving.hemophilia.org/step-out/non-factor-treatment/pain-management.

National Hemophilia Foundation. (2017a). *Fast Facts*, https://www.hemophilia.org/About-Us/Fast-Facts.

National Hemophilia Foundation. (2017b). *HIV/AIDS*, https://www.hemophilia.org/Bleeding-Disorders/Blood-Safety/HIV/AIDS.

National Institutes of Health; National Heart, Lung, and Blood Institute. (2014). *Division of Blood Disease and Resources: Evidence-based management of sickle cell disease, Expert Panel Report*, https://www.nhlbi.nih.gov/guildelines.

National Institutes of Health, Office of Dietary Supplements. (2016). *Iron dietary supplement fact sheet*, https//ods.od.nih.gov/factsheets/Iron-HealthProfessional/.

Negre, O., Eggimann, A. V., Beuzard, Y., et al. (2016). Gene therapy of the β-hemoglobinopathies by lentiviral transfer of the βA(T87Q)-globin gene. *Human Gene Therapy, 15*, 64–81.

Nelson, M., & Poulter, J. (2004). Impact of tea drinking on iron status in the UK: A review. *Journal of Human Nutrition and Dietetics, 17*, 43–54.

Neutze, D., & Roque, J. (2016). Clinical evaluation of bleeding and bruising in primary care. *American Family Physician, 93*(4), 279–286.

Nevitt, S. J., Jones, A. P., & Howard, J. (2017). Hydroxyurea (hydroxycarbamide) for sickle cell disease. *The Cochrane Database of Systematic Reviews*, (4), Art.No.:CD002202.

Nienhuis, A. W., & Nathan, D. (2012). Pathophysiology and clinical manifestations of the β-thalassemias. *Cold Spring Harbor Perspectives in Medicine, 2*(12), a011726. Published online December 1, 2012.

Nienhuis, A. W., Nathwani, A. C., & Davidoff, A. M. (2017). Gene therapy for hemophilia. *Molecular Therapy, 25*(5), 1163–1167.

Nussbaum, R. L., McInnes, R. R., & Willard, H. F. (2016). Genetic variation in populations. In R. L. Nussbaum, R. R. McInnes, & H. F. Willard (Eds.), *Thompson and Thompson Genetics in Medicine* (8th ed.). Philadelphia: Elsevier.

Pahuja, S., Puri, V., Mahajan, G., et al. (2017). Reporting adverse transfusion reactions: A retrospective study from tertiary care hospital from New Delhi, India. *Asian Journal of Transfusion Science, 11*(1), 6–12.

Paintsil, E., & Andiman, W. A. (2009). Update on successes and challenges regarding mother-to-child transmission of HIV. *Current Opinion in Pediatrics, 21*, 94–101.

Passweg, J. R., & Marsh, J. C. W. (2010). Aplastic anemia: First-line treatment by immunosuppressive and sibling marrow transplantation. *Hematology, 2010*, 36–42.

Peinemann, F., & Labeit, A. M. (2014). Stem cell transplantation of matched sibling donors compared with immunosuppressive therapy for acquired severe aplastic anaemia: A Cochrane systematic review. *BMJ Open, 4*(7), e005039.

Polus, A. (2016). *Information on sports selection for people with haemophilia, Haemophiia Heath-Sports and Exercise*, https://www.haemophiliahealth.com.au/sports-and-exercise/information-on-sports-selection.

Powers, J. M., & Buchanan, G. R. (2014). Diagnosis and management of iron deficiency anemia. *Hematology/Oncology Clinics of North America, 28*(4), 729–745.

Puck, J. M. (2012). Laboratory technology for population-based screening for severe combined immunodeficiency in neonates: The winner is T-cell receptor excision circles. *Journal of Allergy and Clinical Immunology, 129*(3), 607–617.

Raja, J. V., Rachchh, M. A., & Gokani, R. H. (2012). Recent advances in gene therapy for thalassemia. *Journal of Pharmacy & Bioallied Sciences, 4*, 194–201.

Redding-Lallinger, R., & Knoll, C. (2006). Sickle cell disease—pathophysiology and treatment. *Current Problems in Pediatric and Adolescent Health Care, 36*(10), 346–376.

Renda, M., & Fischer, P. (2009). Vegetarian diets in children and adolescents. *Pediatrics in Review, 30*, e1–e8.

Ribeil, J. A., Hacein-Bey-Abina, S., Payen, E., et al. (2017). Gene therapy in a patient with sickle cell disease. *The New England Journal of Medicine, 376*(9), 848–855.

Richardson, M. (2007). Microcytic anemia. *Pediatrics in Review, 28*, 5–14.

Rodeghiero, F., Stasi, R., Gernsheimer, T., et al. (2009). Standardization of terminology, definitions and outcome criteria in immune thrombocytopenic purpura of adults and children: Report from an international working group. *Blood, 113*(11), 2386–2393.

Rosman, C. W. K., Broens, P. M. A., Trzpis, M., et al. (2017). A long term follow-up study of subtotal splenectomy in children with hereditary spherocytosis. *Pediatric Blood and Cancer, 64*(10).

Samarasinghe, S., & Webb, D. K. (2012). How I manage aplastic anaemia in children. *British Journal of Haematology, 157*(1), 26–40.

Sankaran, V. G., Nathan, D. G., & Orkin, S. H. (2015). The thalassemias. In S. H. Orkin, D. E. Fisher, D. Ginsburg, et al. (Eds.), *Nathan and Oski's hematology of infancy and childhood* (8th ed.). Philadelphia: Saunders.

Sarangi, S. N., & Acharya, S. S. (2017). Bleeding disorders in congenital syndromes. *Pediatrics, 139*(2).

Scheinberg, P. (2012). Aplastic anemia: Therapeutic updates in immunosuppressive and transplantation. *Hematology / the Education*

Program of the American Society of Hematology. American Society of Hematology. Education Program, 1, 292–300.

Scott, J. P. (2016a). Platelet and blood vessel disorders. In R. M. Kliegman, B. F. Stanton, J. W. St.Geme, et al. (Eds.), *Nelson textbook of pediatrics* (20th ed.). Philadelphia: Elsevier.

Scott, J. P. (2016b). Hereditary clotting factor deficiencies: Factor VIII or factor IX deficiency (hemophilia A or B). In R. M. Kliegman, B. F. Stanton, J. W. St.Geme, et al. (Eds.), *Nelson textbook of pediatrics* (20th ed.). Philadelphia: Elsevier.

Secher, E. L., Stensballe, J., & Afshari, A. (2013). Transfusion in critically ill children: An ongoing dilemma. *Acta Anaesthesiologica Scandinavica, 57*, 684–691.

Segel, G. B., & Casey, D. (2016b). Hereditary spherocytosis. In R. M. Kliegman, B. F. Stanton, J. W. St.Geme III, et al. (Eds.), *Nelson textbook of pediatrics* (20th ed.). Philadelphia: Elsevier.

Sharathkumar, A. A., & Carcao, M. (2011). Clinical advances in hemophilia management. *Pediatric Blood and Cancer, 57*, 910–920.

Sharathkumar, A. A., & Pipe, S. W. (2008). Post-thrombotic syndrome in children: A single center experience. *Journal of Pediatric Hematology, 30*(4), 261–266.

Shimamura, A., & Williams, D. A. (2015). Aquired aplastic anemia and pure red cell aplasia. In S. H. Orkin, D. E. Fisher, D. Ginsburg, et al. (Eds.), *Nathan and Oski's hematology of infancy and childhood* (8th ed.). Philadelphia: Saunders.

Shin, C. R., Kim, M.-O., Li, D., et al. (2012). Outcomes following hematopoietic cell transplantation of Wiskott-Aldrich syndrome. *Bone Marrow Transplantation, 47*, 1428–1435.

Simpkins, E. P., Siberry, G. K., & Hutton, N. (2009). Thinking about HIV infection. *Pediatrics in Review, 30*, 337–349.

Siberry, G. K. (2014). Preventing and managing HIV infection in infants, children, and adolescents in the United States. *Pediatrics in Review, 35*(7), 268–286.

Sills, R. (2016). Iron-deficiency anemia. In R. M. Kliegman, B. F. Stanton, J. W. St.Geme III, et al. (Eds.), *Nelson textbook of pediatrics* (20th ed.). Philadelphia: Elsevier.

Siu, A. L. (2015). Screening for iron deficiency anemia in young children: USPSTF recommendation statement. *Pediatrics, 136*(4), 746–752.

Smith, A. (2012). Guide to evaluation and treatment of anaemia in general practice. *Drug Review, 5*, 25–42.

Strauss, R. G. (2016). Risk of blood transfusions. In R. M. Kliegman, B. F. Stanton, J. W. St.Geme III, et al. (Eds.), *Nelson textbook of pediatrics* (20th ed.). Philadelphia: Elsevier.

Subramaniam, G., & Girish, M. (2015). Iron deficiency anemia in children. *Indian Journal of Pediatrics, 82*(6), 558–564.

Thankachan, P., Walczyk, T., Muthayya, S., et al. (2008). Iron absorption in young Indian women: The interaction of iron status with the influence of tea and ascorbic acid. *The American Journal of Clinical Nutrition, 87*, 881–886.

Therrell, B. L., Padilla, C. D., Loeber, J. G., et al. (2015). Current status of newborn screening worldwide: 2015. *Seminars in Perinatology, 39*, 171–187.

Thompson, J., Biggs, B. A., & Pasricha, S. R. (2013). Effects of daily iron supplementation in 2- to 5-year-old children: Systematic review and meta-analysis. *Pediatrics, 131*, 739–753.

Thrasher, A. J., & Williams, D. A. (2017). Evolving gene therapy in primary immunodeficiency. *Molecular Therapy, 25*(5), 1132–1141.

Tobian, A. A. R., Serwadda, D., Quinn, T. C., et al. (2009). Male circumcision for the prevention of HSV-2 and HPV infections and syphilis. *The New England Journal of Medicine, 360*, 1298–1309.

United Nations AIDS. (2016). *Global AIDS update*. Retrieved from http://www.unaids.org/en/resources/documents/2016/Global-AIDS-update-2016.

US Department of Health and Human Services, Agency for Healthcare Research and Quality. (2009). *Guide to clinical preventive services: recommendations of the US Preventive Services Task Force*, (AHRQ Publication No. 09-IP006), Rockville, Md, 2009, The Agency. Retrieved from http://www.ahrq.gov/clinic/pocketgd09.

US Department of Health and Human Services. (2017). *AIDS info: Understanding HIV/AIDS*, https://aidsinfo-nih-gov./understanding-hiv-aids/fact-sheets/21/58/fda-approved-hiv-medicines.

US Preventive Services Task Force. (2015). Screening for iron deficiency anemia in young children: Recommendation statement. *American Family Physician, 92*(12), 1097A–1097B.

Vichinsky, E., El-Beshlawy, A., Al Zoebie, A., et al. (2017). Long-term safety and efficacy of desferasirox in young pediatric patients with transfusional hemosiderosis:Results from a 5-year observational study (ENTRUST). *Pediatric Blood & Cancer, 00*, e26507.

Vidal-Alaball, J., Butler, C. C., Cannings-John, R., et al. (2016). Oral vitamin B12 versus intramuscular vitamin B12 for vitamin B12 deficiency. *Cochrane Database of Systematic Review*, (3), CD004655.

von der Lippe, C., Frich, J. C., Harris, A., et al. (2017). Treatment of hemophilia: A qualitative study of mothers' perspectives. *Pediatric Blood and Cancer, 64*, 121–127.

Walkovich, K., & Newburger, P. E. (2016). Leukopenia. In R. M. Kliegman, B. F. Stanton, J. W. St.Geme III, et al. (Eds.), *Nelson textbook of pediatrics* (20th ed.). Philadelphia: Elsevier.

Walsh, C. E., & Batt, K. M. (2013). Hemophilia clinical gene therapy: Brief review. *Translational Research: The Journal of Laboratory and Clinical Medicine, 161*, 307–312.

Wang, W. C., & Dwan, K. (2013). Blood transfusion for preventing primary and secondary stroke in people with sickle cell disease. *Cochrane Database of Systematic Review*, (11), CD003146.

Wang, W. C., Ware, R. E., Miller, S. T., et al. (2011). Hydroxycarbamide in very young children with sickle-cell anaemia: A multicenter, randomised, controlled trial (BABY HUG). *Lancet, 377*(9778), 1663–1672.

Wang, B., Zhan, S., Gong, T., et al. (2013). Iron therapy for improving psychomotor development and cognitive function in children under the age of three with iron deficiency anaemia. *Cochrane Database of Systematic Review*, (6), CD001444, 1–50.

Wilson, D. B. (2015). Acquired platelet defects. In S. H. Orkin, D. E. Fisher, D. Ginsburg, et al. (Eds.), *Nathan and Oski's hematology of infancy and childhood* (8th ed.). Philadelphia: Saunders.

Yaish, H. M. (2015). *Pediatric thalassemia*, http://emedicine.medscape.com/article/958850-overview.

Yawn, B. P., Buchanan, G. R., Afenyl-Annan, AN, et al. (2014). Management of sickle cell disease: Summary of the 2014 evidence-based report by expert panel members. *JAMA: The Journal of the American Medical Association, 312*(10), 1033–1048.

Yawn, B. P., & John-Sowah, J. (2015). Management of sickle cell disease: Recommendations from the 2014 expert panel report. *American Family Physician, 92*(12), 1069–1076.

Yogev, R., & Chadwick, E. G. (2016). Acquired immunodeficiency syndrome (human immunodeficiency virus). In R. M. Kliegman, B. F. Stanton, J. W. St.Geme III, et al. (Eds.), *Nelson textbook of pediatrics* (20th ed.). Philadelphia: Elsevier.

Yoon, H. H., Huh, S. J., Lee, J. H., et al. (2012). Should we still use Camitta's criteria for severe aplastic anemia? *The Korean Journal of Hematology, 47*(2), 126–130.

Young, N. S., Bacigalupo, A., & Marsh, J. C. W. (2010). Aplastic anemia: Pathophysiology and treatment. *Biology of Blood and Marrow Transplantation: Journal of the American Society for Blood and Marrow Transplantation, 16*, S119–S125.

29

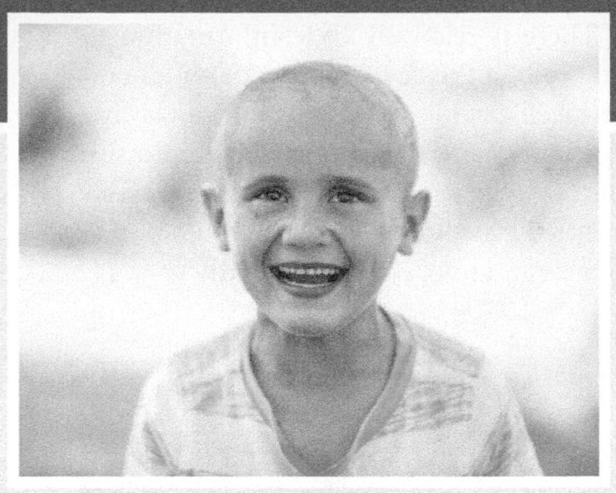

The Child With Cancer

Kathleen S. Ruccione

http://evolve.elsevier.com/wong/ncic

CONCEPTS

- Cellular Regulation
- Family Dynamics
- Patient/Family Education
- Nutrition
- Infection

CANCER IN CHILDREN

Few situations in nursing exceed the challenges of caring for a child with cancer. Despite dramatic improvements in survival rates, the family's informational and support needs are great as they cope with a serious physical illness and the fear that the child will not be cured. Nurses should base support of patients and their families on the premise that effective communication promotes understanding and clarity. With informed communication and compassionate care, fear diminishes, hope emerges, and the cancer journey feels less overwhelming.

This chapter summarizes clinical overviews and nursing care issues for the most common types of pediatric cancer. Chapter 19 discusses situations when the disease is life threatening and the general psychologic needs of these children and their families in terms of chronic illness.

EPIDEMIOLOGY

Childhood cancer is rare; approximately 16,400 cases of cancer are diagnosed in children younger than 20 years of age in the United States each year (Scheurer, Lupo, & Bondy, 2016). Despite the relatively low incidence, approximately 1300 children younger than 15 years of age die of their disease each year, making cancer the leading cause of death from disease in this age-group (Scheurer, Lupo, & Bondy, 2016).

The incidence of specific subtypes of childhood cancer varies according to age, sex, and race/ethnicity. For example, males have a higher overall incidence of cancer compared with females, with a ratio of 1.1 : 1 (Scheurer, Lupo, & Bondy, 2016). This reflects the higher incidence of acute lymphoblastic leukemia (ALL), non-Hodgkin lymphoma (NHL), and central nervous system (CNS) tumors—the most common types of childhood cancer—in young boys. Caucasian children have an overall higher incidence of cancer compared with African American children. This is accounted for by the higher incidence in ALL, Ewing sarcoma, and melanoma in Caucasian children. The incidence of cancer is more pronounced in children from infancy to 4 years of age and in adolescents ages 15 to 19 years; however, the types of cancers occurring among these two groups are very distinct, with neuroblastoma and retinoblastoma more common in young children, and lymphoma and sarcoma more common in adolescents (Scheurer, Lupo, & Bondy, 2016). (See Research Focus box.)

RESEARCH FOCUS

Childhood Cancer Survival Rates

Childhood cancer survival has dramatically increased over the past 5 decades since chemotherapy was first given to children. In the 1960s, the overall survival rate of childhood cancer was 28% compared with 3-year survival rates that now exceed 80% (Scheurer, Lupo, & Bondy, 2016). Improvement in survival among the adolescent group has lagged behind younger age groups, although that is changing. The cancers demonstrating the greatest improvement in survival rates are acute lymphoblastic leukemia, non-Hodgkin lymphoma, and Wilms tumor. A general definition of "cure" in childhood cancer includes completion of all therapy, no clinical and radiologic evidence of disease, and a period of 5 years since diagnosis.

ETIOLOGY

Often the first question asked by parents of children newly diagnosed with cancer is, "How did my child get this, and did I do something to cause it?" Parents are also understandably concerned about whether their other children also will get cancer. Although there are numerous hypotheses concerning what causes childhood cancer, the most enduring theory is that genetic alteration results in the unregulated proliferation of cells. Significant advances have been made in our understanding of cell proliferation, programmed cell death (**apoptosis**), genes that activate tumor growth (**oncogenes**), genes that keep tumor growth in check (**tumor suppressor genes**), and changes in gene expression without gene alteration (**epigenetics**). Cancer is the result of multiple genetic events, but it is not necessarily hereditary. Overall, the incidence of cancers caused by direct inheritance is low, but much has been learned about cancer by studying its inherited forms.

In the early 1970s Alfred Knudson proposed the "two-hit hypothesis." This explanation of cancer inheritance is best illustrated in the inherited form of retinoblastoma. Like most genes, the retinoblastoma gene *(Rb1)* is normally present in two copies on each cell. *Rb1* is a tumor suppressor gene responsible for controlling cell growth. When just one of the gene copies is lost—the "first hit"—the cell remains normal. However, if the second copy is lost—the "second hit"—abnormal cell proliferation occurs and retinoblastoma develops (Knudson, Hethcote, & Brown, 1975). A child can inherit one altered copy of the retinoblastoma gene from either mother or father. When this happens, it takes only one more hit (e.g., an environmental exposure) for retinoblastoma to develop.

Chromosome abnormalities have been identified in many childhood malignancies and are important in the development of various types of cancer. Chromosome abnormalities can be confined to the tumor or can be present in all cells; the latter are called **germ-line mutations**. Chromosome abnormalities can be due to **translocations** (a rearrangement of information between two chromosomes) or **abnormal numbers** of chromosomes. (See Research Focus box.)

RESEARCH FOCUS

Chromosome Abnormalities and Cancer

The Philadelphia chromosome was the first chromosomal abnormality to be identified in a malignancy. It occurs as a result of a translocation between chromosomes 9 and 22 and is observed in almost all patients with a type of leukemia (chronic myeloid leukemia) (Rau & Loh, 2016). In recent years, many well-established chromosome translocations have been identified in childhood leukemia and some solid tumors. In addition, children with certain types of congenital chromosome abnormalities, especially those with syndromes caused by abnormal numbers of chromosomes, have an increased incidence of cancer. For example, children with Down syndrome (trisomy 21) have a much higher risk of developing leukemia compared with the general population (Plon & Malkin, 2016).

Perhaps the most well-known inherited cancer predisposition syndrome is Li-Fraumeni syndrome, which is mainly due to constitutional (in all cells) mutation in the tumor suppressor gene, *p53.* This syndrome is characterized by early incidence of brain tumors, premenopausal breast cancer, soft tissue and bone sarcomas, leukemias, and lymphomas (Plon & Malkin, 2016). Other genetic syndromes that can affect genes or chromosomes and are associated with a predisposition to cancer include Fanconi anemia, Bloom syndrome, Beckwith-Weidemann syndrome, neurofibromatosis type 1, ataxia-telangiectasia, and Klinefelter syndrome.

Children with immunodeficiencies, such as Wiskott-Aldrich syndrome or acquired immunodeficiency syndrome, or children whose immune system has been suppressed, such as after transplant procedures, are at a greater risk for developing various cancers. Of major concern is the increased risk of developing second malignant neoplasms (SMNs) after curative treatment for childhood cancer.

Risk Factors

Lifestyle-related behaviors are the main factors that increase the risk of cancer in adults, but as far as is now known, they have little to no effect on cancer in children. There is relatively little information to support a major environmental role in the development of childhood cancer. However, there are a few well-established risk factors, including exposure to ionizing radiation, carcinogenic drugs, immunosuppressive therapy, certain viral infections (e.g., Epstein-Barr virus, human papillomavirus [HPV]), race/ethnicity, and genetic conditions or chromosomal abnormalities (Table 29.1) (Scheurer, Lupo, & Bondy, 2016).

TABLE 29.1 Known Risk Factors for Childhood Cancers

Cancer Type	Risk Factors
Acute lymphoblastic leukemia	• Ionizing radiation (primarily of historical importance) • Race (i.e., White) • Genetic conditions (i.e., Down syndrome, Bloom syndrome, and others) • Birth weight more than 400 g
Acute myeloid leukemia	• Chemotherapeutic agents (i.e., alkylating agents and epipodophyllotoxins) • Genetic conditions (i.e., Down syndrome and neurofibromatosis 1)
Brain tumors	• Therapeutic radiation to the head • Genetic conditions (i.e., neurofibromatosis 1, tuberous sclerosis, and others)
Hodgkin disease	• Family history (i.e., monozygotic twins) • Infections (i.e., Epstein-Barr virus)
Non-Hodgkin lymphoma	• Immunodeficiency (i.e., acquired and congenital immunodeficiency, immunosuppressive therapy) • Infections (i.e., Epstein-Barr virus associated with Burkitt lymphoma in African countries)
Osteosarcoma	• Ionizing radiation (i.e., cancer radiation therapy and high radium exposure) • Chemotherapy (i.e., alkylating agents) • Genetic conditions (i.e., Li-Fraumeni syndrome, hereditary retinoblastoma)
Ewing sarcoma	• Race (White)
Neuroblastoma	• None known
Retinoblastoma	• No known nonhereditary risk factors
Wilms tumor	• Congenital anomalies (i.e., aniridia, Beckwith-Wiedemann syndrome, other congenital and genetic conditions) • Race (White and Black)
Rhabdomyosarcoma	• Congenital anomalies and genetic conditions (i.e., Li-Fraumeni syndrome and neurofibromatosis 1)
Hepatoblastoma	• Genetic conditions (i.e., Beckwith-Wiedemann syndrome, hemihypertrophy, Gardner syndrome, family history of adenomatous polyposis)
Malignant germ cell tumors	• Cryptorchidism associated with testicular germ cell tumors

From Scheurer, M. E., Lupo, P. J., & Bondy, M. L. (2016). Epidemiology of childhood cancer. In P. A. Pizzo & D. G. Poplack (Eds.), *Principles and practice of pediatric oncology* (7th ed.). Philadelphia, PA: Lippincott.

Prevention

Knowledge of the risk factors that increase the likelihood of cancer holds the promise of prevention. Unfortunately, because few carcinogens are associated with cancer in children, there are no generally recognized preventive measures for childhood cancer.

Nevertheless, pediatric health professionals have another role in cancer prevention, namely educating parents and children about the hazards of known carcinogens associated with adult-type cancers. This is particularly true for the effects of cigarette smoking (and exposure to secondhand smoke) and excessive exposure to ultraviolet radiation (e.g., exposure to sunlight and tanning) because lung cancer is the leading cause of death from cancer in adults, and malignant melanoma is the leading cause of death from diseases of the skin. Children at higher risk for skin cancer are those with sun or tanning bed exposure; light-colored eyes, complexion, and hair; a history of sunburn; skin that burns, freckles, and reddens easily; and certain types of moles (Centers for Disease Control and Prevention, 2017). Not only these children but all children should be protected from overexposure to the sun and to tanning beds. To provide early detection of other types of cancer, clinicians have historically recommended that males learn testicular self-examination, and that females learn breast self-examination. However, teaching breast and testicular self-examination is no longer supported by the US Preventive Services Task Force (2016a, 2016b). Children and teens should have periodic health examinations by a health care professional, including a Papanicolaou smear for females and testicular examination for males when developmentally appropriate. In addition, to prevent HPV-associated malignancies, HPV vaccine is recommended for routine vaccination at age 11 or 12 years (Centers for Disease Control and Prevention, 2016).

DIAGNOSTIC EVALUATION

The evaluation of a child suspected of having cancer may take several days to complete. The essential components of a comprehensive evaluation include complete history and review of symptoms, physical examination, laboratory tests, diagnostic imaging, diagnostic procedures (e.g., lumbar puncture [LP], bone marrow aspirate, and biopsy), and surgical pathology depending on whether biopsy/surgical resection is performed.

Complete History

History of present illness—Onset of symptoms, severity and duration, alleviating or potentiating factors

History of previous illnesses and comorbidities—Communicable diseases, infections, medication history, previous hospitalizations or surgeries, exposure to blood products, immunization status, comorbid conditions, disabilities

Family history—Family members with prior cases of cancer: type, age at diagnosis, treatment, and outcome

Present health status of family members—History of illness or disease in other family members

Developmental factors—Milestones obtained, recent regression in any milestones

Psychosocial factors—Include family concerns or problems, culture/language

Review of Symptoms

Skin—History of bruising or bleeding, lesions, lumps, open sores

Head, eyes, ears, nose, and throat (HEENT)—History of trauma, vision disturbances, proptosis, pupil discoloration, unequal pupils, eye muscle weakness, infection, difficulty swallowing

Heart—History of murmur or congenital heart defect

Lungs—History of infection, asthma or reactive airway disease, cough, wheezing, shortness of breath, dyspnea

Abdomen—History of abdominal swelling, pain, mass, change in bowel or bladder patterns

Musculoskeletal—History of weakness in extremities, limited range of motion, tenderness or swelling, joint pain

Neurologic—Loss of developmental milestones, altered consciousness, decreased sensations, abnormal reflexes, abnormal cerebellar functions, headaches, seizures

Lymphatic—History of enlarged lymph nodes, frequent infections

Hematologic—History of bruising, nosebleeds or gum bleeding, paleness, fatigue, bloody or tarry-colored stools

Physical Examination

See Physical Examination, Chapter 4.

General—Orientation, general state of health

Skin—Petechiae or ecchymosis, lesions or sores, presence of blood from gum or nose, color of skin

HEENT—Macrocephaly, bulging fontanel, evidence of infection, proptosis, pupil discoloration, anisocoria, extraocular movements not intact, limited peripheral vision, nystagmus, leukocoria

Heart—Murmur or thrill, peripheral pulses

Lungs—Evidence of infection, rales or rhonchi, decreased breath sounds, dyspnea, tachypnea

Abdomen—Hepatosplenomegaly, mass, decreased bowel sounds, striae

Neurologic—Altered consciousness, altered sensation, abnormal reflexes, abnormal cerebellar functions, unstable gait, dysarthria, cranial nerve deficits

Lymphatic—Enlarged lymph nodes

Laboratory Tests

Several laboratory tests must be performed to accurately diagnose and treat children with cancer. The majority of patients have a complete blood count (CBC), serum chemistries, liver function tests, coagulation studies, and urinalysis done on initial presentation. For example, the CBC for patients with leukemia often reveals low hemoglobin; low platelet count; and low, normal, or high white blood cell counts. In addition, these patients may have elevated lactate dehydrogenase, creatinine, and uric acid, which require close monitoring when therapy is initiated. Frequent CBCs are necessary to monitor effects of therapy and, in some hematologic malignancies, response to therapy.

Blood chemistry yields important information with regard to kidney, liver, and bone function and electrolyte balance. These tests are important to help detect the extent of disease and also to monitor for side effects during therapy. For example, a patient with bone metastasis may have elevated alkaline phosphatase. Elevations in blood urea nitrogen and creatinine may reflect kidney damage from chemotherapy agents. Consequently, regular blood chemistries and urinalysis are standard procedures throughout the course of the disease and its treatment.

Diagnostic Procedures

An LP is a routine test employed in leukemia, brain tumors, and other cancers that may metastasize to the CNS. An LP is also used to administer intrathecal drugs in patients with various malignancies, such as leukemia.

A bone marrow test is performed by aspirating marrow with a large- or fine-bore needle. A bone marrow biopsy is performed by obtaining a piece of bone through a special type of needle. These tests are performed to determine the presence or absence of cancer cells or response to therapy in the bone marrow. For example, the type of leukemia can be identified by examination of the patient's bone marrow and core biopsy. Also, patients with other solid tumors, such as neuroblastoma, may have spread of disease to the bone marrow, which can be determined by these procedures.

Diagnostic Imaging

Modern diagnostic imaging has greatly improved the ability to accurately diagnose childhood cancers. The most commonly employed modes of imaging include x-rays, computed tomography (CT), magnetic resonance imaging (MRI), and positron emission tomography (PET); in addition, metaiodobenzylguanidine (MIBG) scan is used in certain pediatric malignancies such as neuroblastoma and soft tissue tumors. Interventional radiology uses imaging to guide diagnostic and treatment procedures in the diagnosis and management of pediatric malignancies. The nurse should be aware of the Image Gently campaign to improve safe and effective imaging care of children. Parents who have heard of this effort may have questions about radiation exposure in the imaging of their children (Image Gently, 2014).

Pathologic and Molecular Evaluation

For most types of childhood cancer, a biopsy is necessary to establish the diagnosis. Besides determining what type of cancer the patient has, this tissue sample can also be sent for various biologic studies that help define the patient's risk of relapse or recurrence and allow the health care team to plan risk-adapted therapy. For example, a bone marrow biopsy determines whether the patient has acute lymphoblastic leukemia or acute myeloid leukemia, and indicates the specific leukemia subtype that is the basis for how aggressively it should be treated. Similarly, patients with neuroblastoma undergo a biopsy of the tumor to establish the diagnosis and to evaluate the tumor for amplification of an oncogene, *MYCN*, which is a prognostic factor considered for treatment planning. Increasingly, the diagnostic evaluation includes molecular genetic testing (e.g., deoxyribonucleic acid [DNA] sequencing, reverse transcription-polymerase chain reaction [RT-PCR], fluorescence in situ hybridization [FISH]) to find the biologic abnormalities of the tumor. As more is learned about these cell changes in cancer, it is becoming possible to design therapies that target these abnormalities or block their effects; this is called **targeted therapy**, which is the basis of precision medicine.

TREATMENT MODALITIES

Survival of children with cancer has greatly improved through the use of (1) multimodal therapy consisting of surgery, chemotherapy/biotherapy, blood or marrow transplant (now referred to as hematopoietic stem cell transplant [SCT]), and radiation therapy; (2) enrollment of large numbers of children in cooperative group clinical trials or protocols; and (3) improvements in supportive care.

Current efforts are aimed at increasing the survival of patients with high-risk malignancies, decreasing the acute and long-term side effects of treatment, and studying the biology and genomics of the diseases to better identify patients who are at different risk levels for disease recurrence and can therefore benefit from risk-adapted and targeted therapies.

Surgery

The main goal of surgery, besides obtaining biopsies, is to remove the tumor and restore normal body functioning to the greatest extent possible. Surgery is most successful when the tumor is encapsulated and localized (confined to the site of origin). Surgery may be used for palliation when the cancer is regional (metastasized to an area adjacent to the original site) or advanced (widespread throughout the body). Generally, the best prognosis is directly related to early detection of the tumor because that facilitates surgical removal.

Because the majority of pediatric cancers respond well to chemotherapy, more conservative surgical excision is increasingly used in a variety of tumors in an attempt to preserve function and cosmesis. For example, in some types of bone cancer, such as osteosarcoma, patients are successfully treated with resection of the diseased portion of the bone rather than amputation.

Radiation Therapy

Radiation therapy is frequently used in the treatment of childhood cancer, usually in conjunction with chemotherapy or surgery. It can be used for curative purposes and for palliation to relieve symptoms by shrinking the size of the tumor. Recent advances in radiation therapy that allow the beam to be aimed precisely have optimized its beneficial effects and minimized many of the undesirable side effects by sparing normal tissue.

Ionizing radiation is cytotoxic in at least three different ways: (1) damaging the pyrimidine bases cytosine, thymine, and uracil needed for the synthesis of nucleic acids; (2) causing single-strand breaks in the DNA or ribonucleic acid (RNA) molecule; or (3) causing double helical-strand breaks in these molecules. Disturbing cellular metabolic and reproductive functions causes lethal or sublethal damage. *Lethal damage* refers to the death of the cell. *Sublethal damage* refers to injured cells that may subsequently be repaired. Many of the acute side effects are the result of lethal damage to radiosensitive tissue, particularly proliferating cells such as those of the bone marrow, gastrointestinal tract, and hair follicles. Late effects (late-occurring or long-term effects) are usually the result of cell death.

The acute untoward reactions from radiation therapy depend primarily on the area being irradiated. Total-body irradiation is associated with the most severe reactions and is employed to prepare the immune system for SCT. Table 29.2 summarizes the acute effects of radiation therapy and nursing interventions that may be helpful in mitigating or preventing them.

In some areas of the United States, proton beam radiation is available. Protons are positively charged subatomic particles. Protons deposit energy differently than x-ray beams. There is no "exit dose" beyond the tumor involved in proton radiation therapy; therefore local control of the tumor is a major benefit with no long-term effects to organs surrounding the target area (Hill-Kayser, Tochner, Both, et al., 2013). For example, some brain tumor patients receive radiation to the spine. With traditional forms of radiation therapy, lasting damage to nearby vital organs such as the heart and lungs is possible; however, with proton therapy the heart and lungs would not be affected, avoiding long-term cardiac and pulmonary damage.

Chemotherapy

Chemotherapy may be the primary form of treatment, or it may be an adjunct to surgery, radiation therapy, or SCT. The majority of chemotherapy agents work by interfering with the function or production of nucleic acids, DNA, or RNA. Although several drugs have been effective in treating different forms of cancer as single agents, the remarkable increase in survival rates has been the result of improved combination drug regimens. Combining drugs allows for optimum cell cycle destruction with minimum toxic effects and decreased resistance by the cancer cells to the agent. For example, a treatment regimen called VAC (vincristine [Oncovin], doxorubicin [Adriamycin], and cyclophosphamide [Cytoxan]) combines complementary cytotoxic effects with distinct side effects. Doxorubicin and cyclophosphamide are myelosuppressive, whereas vincristine is neurotoxic.

In addition to more effective combinations of drugs, several advances in the administration of chemotherapy have permitted continuous or intermittent intravenous (IV) administration without multiple

TABLE 29.2 **Early Side Effects of Radiotherapy**

Site	Effects	Nursing Interventions
Gastrointestinal tract	Nausea and vomiting	Give antiemetic on schedule around the clock. Measure amount of emesis to assess for dehydration.
	Anorexia	Encourage fluids and foods best tolerated, usually light, soft, small, and frequent meals. Monitor weight.
	Mucosal ulceration	Use frequent mouth rinses and oral hygiene to prevent mucositis.
	Diarrhea	Control with antispasmodics and kaolin pectin preparations. Observe for signs of dehydration.
Skin	Alopecia (occurs within 2 weeks; hair may regrow by 3-6 months)	Introduce idea of wig. Stress necessity of scalp hygiene and need for head covering in sun and cold weather.
	Dry or moist desquamation	Do not refer to skin change as a "burn" (implies use of too much radiation). Avoid lotions and other creams to skin. Wash daily, using soap (e.g., Dove) sparingly. Do not remove skin marking for radiation fields. Avoid exposure to sun. For desquamation, consult practitioner for skin hygiene and care.
Head	Nausea and vomiting (from stimulation of vomiting center in brain)	Same as for gastrointestinal tract.
	Alopecia	Same as for skin.
	Mucositis	Encourage regular dental care, fluoride treatments.
	Potential effects: • Parotitis • Sore throat • Loss of taste	Provide analgesics as needed to relieve discomfort
	• Xerostomia (dry mouth)	Combat severe dryness of mouth with oral hygiene and liquid diet..
Urinary bladder	Rarely cystitis	Encourage liberal fluid intake and frequent voiding. Monitor for hematuria.
Bone marrow	Myelosuppression	Observe for fever (temperature >101°F [38.3°C]). Initiate workup for sepsis as ordered. Administer antibiotics as prescribed. Avoid use of suppositories, rectal temperatures. Institute bleeding precautions. Observe for signs of anemia.

venipunctures. The use of venous access devices (e.g., catheters and implantable infusion ports) has greatly facilitated safe and effective drug administration with minimum discomfort for the child. (See Chapter 22.) Continuous infusions over an extended period using syringe pumps have made possible the administration of certain drugs, such as cytosine arabinoside, in higher doses with less toxicity than when the drug is administered intermittently.

Chemotherapeutic agents can be classified according to their primary mechanism of action. Alkylating agents replace a hydrogen atom of a molecule by an alkyl group. The irreversible combination of alkyl groups with nucleotide chains, particularly DNA, causes unbalanced growth of unaffected cell constituents so that the cell eventually dies. These agents have a steep dose-response curve and, for this reason, can be used in high-dose therapy regimens. Examples of alkylating agents include cyclophosphamide, ifosfamide, cisplatin, and dacarbazine. Antimetabolites resemble essential metabolic elements needed for cell growth but are sufficiently altered in molecular structure to inhibit further synthesis of DNA or RNA; their maximum effect occurs in cells that are actively producing DNA. Examples of antimetabolites include methotrexate and mercaptopurine. Plant alkaloids arrest cells in metaphase (a phase of mitosis) by binding to microtubular protein needed for spindle formation. Examples include vincristine and vinblastine. Antitumor antibiotics are natural products that interfere with cell division by reacting with DNA in such a way as to prevent further replication of DNA and transcription of RNA. Examples include doxorubicin and daunomycin.

Both adrenal and gonadal hormones have antineoplastic properties, although the precise mechanism of action is still unclear. In theory, adrenocorticosteroids bind with DNA and alter the transcription process. Although there are a number of cortisone preparations, dexamethasone and prednisone are most often used in cancer therapy.

A number of agents are not categorized according to the preceding classifications. For example, L-asparaginase is an enzyme isolated from extracts of bacterial cultures of *Escherichia coli* or *Erwinia carotovora*. It hydrolyzes L-asparagine, an amino acid, to L-aspartic acid, which prevents the cell from synthesizing protein needed for DNA and RNA synthesis. Because L-asparagine is synthesized by normal cells but must be exogenously supplied to certain leukemic and lymphoma cells, administration of the enzyme destroys the essential exogenous supply while sparing normal cells of untoward effects.

An understanding of the actions and side effects of these drugs is essential to nursing care of children with cancer. Unfortunately, almost all standard chemotherapy drugs are not selectively cytotoxic for malignant cells, and other cells with a high rate of proliferation, such as the bone marrow elements, hair, skin, and epithelial cells of the gastrointestinal tract, are also affected. Frequently the problems related to the destruction of these normal cells require more nursing care than those related to the disease itself.

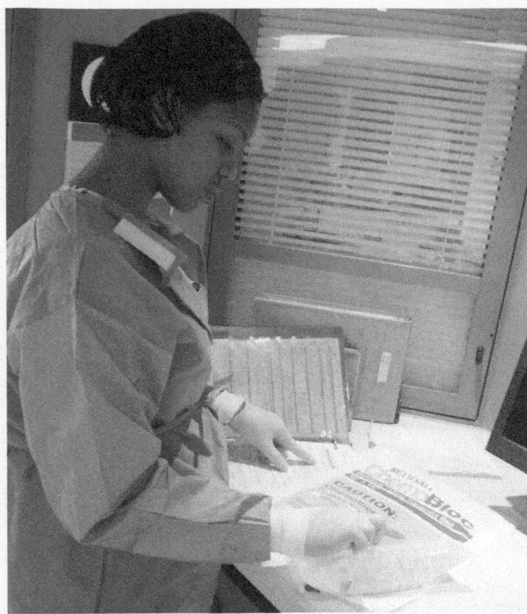

FIG. 29.1 Nurses caring for children with cancer require expertise in the safe administration of chemotherapy.

Precautions in Administering and Handling Chemotherapeutic Agents

Many chemotherapeutic agents are vesicants (sclerosing agents) that can cause severe cellular damage if even minute amounts of the drug infiltrate surrounding tissue. Only nurses experienced with chemotherapeutic agents should administer vesicants (Fig. 29.1). Standards are available* and must be followed meticulously to prevent tissue damage to patients. Interventions for extravasation vary, but each nurse should be aware of the institution's policies before giving any vesicant, and implement them at once if indicated.

! NURSING ALERT

Chemotherapeutic drugs must be given through a free-flowing IV line. The infusion is stopped immediately if any sign of infiltration (e.g., pain, stinging, swelling, or redness at needle site) occurs.

In addition to extravasation, a potentially fatal complication is anaphylaxis, especially from L-asparaginase, bleomycin, cisplatin, or etoposide. (See Anaphylaxis, Chapter 23.) Hypersensitivity reactions to these chemotherapeutic agents are characterized by urticaria, angioedema, flushing, rashes, difficulty breathing, hypotension, and nausea or vomiting. Nursing responsibilities include prevention, recognition, and preparation for serious reactions. Prevention begins with a careful history of known allergies, and recognition includes education of the patient and family regarding signs and symptoms to report. (See Chapter 4.) If a reaction is suspected, the nurse discontinues the drug, flushes and maintains the IV line with saline, and monitors the child's vital signs and subsequent responses.

*_2016 Updated American Society of Clinical Oncology/Oncology Nursing Society Chemotherapy Administration Safety Standards, Including Standards for Pediatric Oncology_ is available from the Oncology Nursing Society, 125 Enterprise Drive, Pittsburgh, PA 15275; 412-859-6100, 866-257-4667; http://www.ons.org/practice-resources/standards-reports/chemotherapy.

! NURSING ALERT

When chemotherapy or immunotherapy agents with known anaphylactic potential are given, it is standard practice to observe the child for 1 hour after the infusion for signs of anaphylaxis (e.g., rash, urticaria, hypotension, wheezing, nausea, vomiting). Emergency equipment (especially blood pressure monitor, bag and valve mask, and suction) and emergency drugs (especially oxygen, epinephrine, antihistamine, aminophylline, corticosteroids, and vasopressors) must be readily available.

In addition to the many patient-focused responsibilities during chemotherapy administration, nurses must also use safeguards to protect themselves. Handling chemotherapeutic agents may present risks to handlers and to their offspring, although the exact degree of risk is not known. The Oncology Nursing Society has published comprehensive guidelines for safe practice issues related to administration of chemotherapy.* The Oncology Nursing Society also has established safe management procedures for chemotherapy administered in the home.* Basic nursing guidelines are in the Nursing Care Guidelines box.

NURSING CARE GUIDELINES

Handling Chemotherapeutic Agents

- Use great care and strict aseptic technique in handling chemotherapeutic agents to prevent any physical contact with the substance.
- Drugs are prepared in a properly ventilated room (which incorporates a protective front panel and vertical laminar airflow to reduce potential for inhalation during preparation).
- Wear disposable gloves and protective clothing and discard in special container after each use.
- Wear face and eye protection when splashing is possible, and wear a respirator when the risk of inhalation is possible.
- Use a sterile gauze pad when priming intravenous (IV) tubing, connecting and disconnecting tubing, inserting syringes into vials, breaking glass ampules, or performing any other procedure in which antineoplastic drugs may be inadvertently discharged.
- Dispose of all contaminated needles, syringes, IV tubing, and other contaminated equipment in a leak-proof and puncture-resistant container; do not recap or break needles.

Biologic Therapy

Biologic therapy, also called biotherapy, uses substances made from living organisms, derived from living organisms, or laboratory-produced versions of these substances to treat cancer (Ceppi, Beck-Popovic, Bourquin, et al., 2017). Biotherapies can be grouped into three main types: (1) those that do not target cancer cells directly, but stimulate the body's immune system to act against cancer cells, and are collectively referred to as immunotherapy or biologic response modifier therapy; (2) those that use antibodies or segments of genetic material to target cancer cells directly; and (3) therapies that interfere with specific molecules involved in tumor growth and progression and are referred to as targeted therapies (Ceppi, Beck-Popovic, Bourquin, et al., 2017).

*_Chemotherapy and Biotherapy Guidelines and Recommendations for Practice (4th Edition)_ can be obtained from the Oncology Nursing Society, 125 Enterprise Drive, Pittsburgh, PA 15275; 866-257-4667, 412-859-6100; http://www.ons.org.

Immunotherapy works by stimulating the activity of the immune system against cancer cells or by counteracting signals produced by cancer cells that suppress immune responses (US Food and Drug Administration, 2016). Immunotherapy includes the use of monoclonal antibodies that attach to proteins on cancer cells so the immune system can find and destroy the cells. Other antibodies block pathways that allow cancer cells to escape the immune system; these are called checkpoint inhibitors. Nonspecific immunotherapies include two types of cytokines: interferons and interleukins. Other immunotherapies include oncolytic virus therapy and chimeric antigen receptor (CAR) T-cell therapy. CAR T-cell therapy is being studied in childhood acute leukemia that does not respond to traditional chemotherapy. Surveillance for and management of side effects of immunotherapy are critical nursing responsibilities. Side effects may range from mild to severe. For example, with CAR T-cell therapy, adverse events may include cytokine release syndrome, neurologic symptoms, tumor lysis syndrome, and graft-versus-host disease (Becze, 2017).

Targeted therapies are substances that interfere with specific molecules involved in cancer. They are different from standard chemotherapy in two ways (National Institutes of Health, 2017a): (1) they act on molecular targets, rather than affecting all rapidly dividing normal and malignant cells; and (2) they are selected or designed to affect their target, compared with chemotherapy drugs that were identified because they kill cells. Previously, targeted therapies have had limited use in pediatric patients but are now being evaluated in clinical trials. Careful monitoring of side effects is essential because the profile of adverse events may be different than that seen in adults, and because these agents may affect the process of growth and development in pediatric patients in unexpected ways (Gore, DiGregori, & Porter, 2013).

Hematopoietic Stem Cell Transplant

Another approach to the treatment of childhood cancer is transplantation of hematopoietic (blood-forming) stem cells. Stem cell transplant (SCT) restores stem cells in children who have diseases that require high doses of chemotherapy or radiation therapy and/or replacement of dysfunctional bone marrow. Blood-forming stem cells from bone marrow, peripheral blood, or cord blood can be sources for SCT. The main types of SCT are allogeneic, where cells are obtained from a family member or volunteer donor, and autologous, where cells previously stored from the patient are given back to the patient by IV infusion. In either type of SCT, if it is successful, the newly transfused cells begin to produce functioning nonmalignant blood cells. In essence, the recipient accepts a new blood-forming organ.

Children receiving an allogeneic SCT undergo a pretransplant conditioning regimen consisting of radiation therapy and/or high-dose chemotherapy to rid the body of malignant cells and suppress the immune system to prevent rejection of the transplanted marrow. (See Family-Centered Care box.)

FAMILY-CENTERED CARE

Decision for Transplant

A family's decision for a child to undergo a stem cell transplant (SCT) is fraught with uncertainties. Often the child faces certain death from the malignancy without the SCT. The preparation of the child for the transplant also places the patient at great medical risk.

Once the preparatory regimen begins and the child's immune system is destroyed, there is no turning back. Unlike kidney transplantation, SCT does not have a "rescue" procedure, such as dialysis, for supportive therapy. If the donor is a sibling, the expectation that his or her marrow will "save" the brother or sister can be a concern, especially if the transplant fails. Parents often must leave home to stay at the transplant center and encounter additional stressors such as arranging child care, taking leave from work, and managing finances. If old enough to understand the risks, the patient faces the greatest stress, such as fear of SCT failure or life-threatening complications.

The selection process for a suitable donor and the potential complications in allogeneic transplantation are related to the human leukocyte antigen (HLA) system complex. Some of the major HLA antigens are A, B, C, D, DR, and DQ. There is wide diversity for each of these HLA loci. For example, more than 20 different HLA-A antigens and more than 40 different HLA-B antigens can be inherited. The genes are inherited as a single unit, or haplotype. A child inherits one unit from each parent; thus a child and each parent have one identical and one nonidentical haplotype. Because the possible haplotype combinations among siblings follow the laws of Mendelian genetics, there is a 1 in 4 chance that two siblings have identical haplotypes and are perfectly matched at the HLA loci.

The importance of HLA matching is to prevent the serious complication of graft-versus-host disease (GVHD) after allogeneic transplant. Because the child's immune system is essentially rendered nonfunctional, the recipient is unlikely to reject the bone marrow. However, the donor's marrow may contain antigens not matched to the recipient's antigens, which begin attacking body cells. The more closely the HLA systems match, the less likely GVHD is to develop. However, GVHD can occur even with a perfect HLA match because of unidentified and thus unmatched histocompatibility antigens (Gottschalk, Naik, Hegde, et al., 2016).

Umbilical cord blood or haploidentical family donors (i.e., parents) are additional sources of hematopoietic stem cells for use in children with cancer (Gottschalk, Naik, Hegde, et al., 2016). The benefit of using umbilical cord blood is the blood's relative immunodeficiency at birth, allowing for partially matched, unrelated cord blood transplants to be successful, with a lower risk of GVHD-related problems (Sarvaria, Jawdat, Madrigal, et al., 2017). A benefit of using a haploidentical family member is the immediate availability of the donor, which is especially important when children urgently need SCT.

Autologous Transplantation

Autologous transplants use the patient's own marrow that was collected from disease-free tissue, frozen, and may have been treated to remove malignant cells. Peripheral blood stem cell transplant (PBSCT) is also used in children with cancer. This type of transplant differs in the way stem cells are collected. Most commonly, colony-stimulating factor (CSF) is first given to stimulate the production of many stem cells (Karakukcu & Unal, 2015). Once the white blood cell count is high enough, the stem cells are collected by an apheresis machine. This machine filters out peripheral stem cells from whole blood and returns the remainder of the blood cells and plasma to the child. Stem cells have been collected without problems in even very small children weighing 20 kg (44 lb) or less (Gottschalk, Naik, Hegde, et al., 2016). The peripheral stem cells are then frozen until the patient is ready for the PBSCT. Children with solid tumors such as neuroblastoma, Hodgkin lymphoma, NHL, rhabdomyosarcoma, Ewing sarcoma, and Wilms tumor have been treated with autologous transplants.

COMPLICATIONS OF THERAPY

Although great advances have been achieved through current modes of cancer therapy, the successes are not without consequences. Numerous acute side effects are commonly expected with chemotherapy/biotherapy and radiation therapy. Several other complications that are less frequent, but generally more serious, are described here.

Pediatric Oncologic Emergencies

Tumor Lysis Syndrome

Life-threatening conditions may develop in children with cancer as a result of the malignancy and/or aggressive treatment modalities. Acute tumor lysis syndrome has hallmark metabolic abnormalities that are the direct result of rapid release of intracellular contents during the lysis of malignant cells. This typically occurs in patients with acute lymphoblastic leukemia or Burkitt lymphoma during the initial treatment period, but may occur spontaneously before onset of therapy. Tumor lysis syndrome also may occur in other malignancies that have a large tumor burden, are very sensitive to chemotherapy, or have a rapid proliferative rate. The metabolic abnormalities of tumor lysis syndrome include hyperuricemia, hypocalcemia, hyperphosphatemia, and hyperkalemia. The crystallization of uric acid that can occur with hyperuricemia can lead to acute renal failure (Freedman, Rheingold, & Fisher, 2016).

Risk factors for development of tumor lysis syndrome include high white blood cell count at diagnosis, large tumor burden, cancer cell sensitivity to chemotherapy, and high proliferative rate. In addition to the described metabolic abnormalities, children may develop a spectrum of clinical symptoms, including flank pain, lethargy, nausea and vomiting, muscle cramps, pruritus, tetany, and seizures.

Management of tumor lysis syndrome consists of early identification of patients at risk, prophylactic measures, and early interventions. Patients at risk for tumor lysis syndrome should have serum chemistries and urine pH monitored frequently, strict recording of intake and output, and aggressive administration of IV fluids. Medications, such as allopurinol, that reduce uric acid formation and promote excretion of by-products of purine metabolism are often used. If tumor lysis syndrome occurs, IV hydration continues and the specific metabolic abnormalities are treated. Hyperuricemia is now effectively treated with recombinant urate oxidase, or rasburicase. This medication converts uric acid to allantoin, which is more soluble in urine. Exchange transfusions are sometimes necessary to reduce the metabolic consequences of massive tumor lysis, especially in children with a high tumor burden.

Hyperleukocytosis

Hyperleukocytosis, defined as a peripheral white blood cell count greater than 100,000/mm^3, can lead to capillary obstruction, microinfarction, and organ dysfunction. Children often experience respiratory distress and cyanosis. They also experience neurologic changes, including altered level of consciousness, visual disturbances, agitation, confusion, ataxia, and delirium. Management consists of rapid cytoreduction by chemotherapy, hydration, urinary alkalinization, and allopurinol. Leukapheresis or exchange transfusion may be necessary.

Superior Vena Cava Syndrome

Space-occupying lesions located in the chest, especially from Hodgkin disease and NHL, may cause superior vena cava syndrome (SVCS), leading to airway compromise and potentially to respiratory failure. The second leading cause of SVCS is thrombotic complications of implantable IV devices, such as central venous catheters and port catheters (Freedman, Rheingold, & Fisher, 2016).

Children are initially seen with cyanosis of the face, neck, and upper chest; facial and upper extremity edema; and distended neck and chest veins. They may be anxious and have dyspnea, wheezing, or a frequent cough from airway obstruction. Management consists of airway protection and alleviation of respiratory distress. Rapid treatment is initiated, and symptoms typically improve as the disease is effectively treated.

Spinal Cord Compression

Malignancies can invade or impinge on the spinal cord, causing acute symptoms of cord compression. Primary CNS tumors can originate or spread to the spinal cord. Other solid tumors, such as neuroblastoma or rhabdomyosarcoma, can metastasize to the spinal cord and cause compression. Back pain is a common initial manifestation, but other symptoms can include sensation change, extremity weakness, loss of bowel and bladder function, and respiratory insufficiency. Careful physical examination is essential in early detection of symptoms, and MRI is the gold standard for diagnosis (Freedman, Rheingold, & Fisher, 2016). Treatment may include high-dose steroids to reduce associated edema and alleviate symptoms and rapid initiation of treatment such as emergent radiation or laminectomy if indicated.

Disseminated Intravascular Coagulation

Overwhelming infections in the immunocompromised child constitute an emergency situation. Sepsis from bacteria or fungus can result in numerous complications, including disseminated intravascular coagulation (DIC). Children with DIC form excessive microthrombi throughout the vascular system due to hyperactivation of the clotting cascade, downregulation of anticoagulants, and impaired fibrinolysis, which leaves the child susceptible to hemorrhage. Life-threatening hemorrhage can occur from DIC with thrombocytopenia (platelet count of less than 20,000/mm^3) (Andrews, Galel, Wong, et al., 2016). Treatment is focused on identifying and treating the underlying cause, along with infusing heparin to minimize microthrombi and cryoprecipitate to replace fibrinogen.

NURSING CARE MANAGEMENT

This section presents an overview of general nursing concepts that apply to most childhood cancers. Specific nursing care for children with a particular type of cancer is discussed under each disease section later in this chapter. This discussion focuses on the physical aspects of care. In addition, refer to Chapter 21 for family-centered care and Chapter 19 for end of life care. (See Quality Patient Outcomes box.)

QUALITY PATIENT OUTCOMES

The Child With Cancer

- Child and family educated about disease and treatment
- Child and family safely perform self-care as appropriate
- Treatment administered on schedule with appropriate drug doses
- Side effects of treatment managed
- Treatment complications prevented
- Child and family strengths and coping skills supported
- Quality of life during treatment maintained
- Child and family adjusted to chronic illness
- Growth and development maintained during treatment

SIGNS AND SYMPTOMS OF CANCER IN CHILDREN

Early detection is critical to starting treatment with the best prospect for eventual cure. Cancers in children are often difficult to recognize. Therefore being alert to the persistence of possible signs and symptoms is essential (Box 29.1). This section discusses some of the more significant clues leading to a diagnosis of pediatric cancer.

Pain may be an early or late initial sign of cancer and requires a careful history of its onset, characteristics, location, intensity, and alleviating factors. Pain may be generalized or present at a specific

BOX 29.1 Possible Signs and Symptoms of Childhood Cancer

- Unusual mass or swelling
- Unexplained paleness and loss of energy
- Easy bruising
- Persistent, localized pain or limping
- Prolonged, unexplained fever or illness
- Frequent headaches, often with vomiting
- Sudden eye or vision changes
- Unexplained, rapid weight loss

Data from American Cancer Society. (2016). Finding cancer in children. Retrieved from https://www.cancer.org/cancer/cancer-in-children/finding-childhood-cancers-early.html.

location. For example, bone pain occurs in approximately 20% of children with leukemia. Pain, swelling, and tenderness at the tumor site may be initial signs in solid tumors. In addition, a mass is a typical finding in children with solid tumors. An abdominal mass in a child must be evaluated for a malignancy, such as Wilms tumor or neuroblastoma.

Fever is a frequent occurrence during childhood and is caused by numerous illnesses, including cancer. The cause of fever in cancer patients is infection or the malignant process itself. This is often referred to as tumor-associated fever. The exact mechanism by which the malignancy causes a fever is not completely understood. Cytokines (e.g., interleukin, tumor necrosis factor) are known to be involved, and are thought to be released either directly from tumor cells or from macrophages responding to tumor (Foggo & Cavenagh, 2015).

A careful skin assessment will reveal signs of a low platelet count. Ecchymosis and petechiae are most commonly found on the child's extremities and under constricting parts of clothing like waistbands. Spontaneous gum or nose bleeding may occur when the platelet count falls below 20,000/mm^3.

The child with malignant invasion of the bone marrow often appears pale, with symptoms of lethargy, weight loss, and malaise. These symptoms may be attributed to anemia caused by the replacement of normal cells with malignant cells in the bone marrow. The nurse should assess for signs and symptoms of anemia. (See Chapter 28.)

Swollen lymph nodes are another common finding in children. However, enlarged, firm lymph nodes in a child with fever for more than 1 week, a recent history of weight loss, or an abnormal chest x-ray film may indicate a serious disease and should be evaluated further.

Recognizing one sign is facilitated by the widespread use of cell phone photography. Leukocoria or white eye reflex can be seen as a yellow "glow" in the pupil, as opposed to the normal red pupillary reflex, in photographs. It can be a sign of retinoblastoma that needs prompt medical attention. Squinting, strabismus, or swelling can indicate other solid tumors of the eye.

The child with a brain tumor develops signs and symptoms related to the area of the brain involved. The nurse's thorough physical assessment can indicate the likely area of tumor involvement.

MANAGING SIDE EFFECTS OF TREATMENT

Cancer care encompasses more than treatments aimed at eliminating the malignant cells. Because of the delicate balance between killing malignant cells and preserving functional cells, supportive therapy usually is needed during those times that serious damage occurs to normal body tissues. A major concern for the child receiving treatment for cancer is the risk for the development of complications secondary to the treatment.

Infection

The nurse caring for the child with fever must be aware of the signs and symptoms of septic shock, as discussed in Chapter 23. The child with fever who has an absolute neutrophil count (ANC) lower than 500/mm^3 is at risk for the following (See Nursing Care Guidelines box):

- Overwhelming infection
- Malaise
- Dehydration
- Seizures (young infants and children)
- Invasion of organisms producing secondary infections

NURSING CARE GUIDELINES

Calculating the Absolute Neutrophil Count (ANC)

1. Determine the total percentage of neutrophils ("polys, or segs," and "bands").
2. Multiply white blood cell (WBC) count by percentage of neutrophils.

Example: WBC = 1000/mm^3, neutrophils = 7%, nonsegmented neutrophils (bands) = 7%

Step 1: 7% + 7% = 14%

Step 2: 0.14 × 1000 = 140/mm^3 ANC

The child with fever is evaluated for potential sites of infection, such as from a needle puncture, mucosal ulceration, minor abrasion, or skin tears (e.g., a hangnail). Although the body may not be able to produce an adequate inflammatory response to the infection and the usual clinical signs of infection may be partially expressed or absent, fever will occur. Therefore the child's temperature is monitored closely. To identify the source of infection, the health care team takes blood, stool, urine, and nasopharyngeal cultures and chest x-rays.

Once infection is suspected, broad-spectrum IV antibiotic therapy is begun before the organism is identified and may be continued for 7 to 10 days. If the child does not have a venous access device, a heparin lock peripheral IV should be inserted to prevent the inconvenience and discomfort of multiple venipunctures in administering antibiotic therapy.

The organisms most lethal to these children are (1) viruses, particularly varicella (chickenpox), herpes zoster, herpes simplex, respiratory syncytial virus, influenza, cytomegalovirus; (2) protozoan, *Toxoplasma gondii;* (3) fungi, especially *Pneumocystis jiroveci* (formally known as *carinii*) and *Candida albicans;* (4) gram-negative bacteria, such as *Pseudomonas aeruginosa, E. coli,* and *Klebsiella* organisms; and (5) gram positive bacteria, especially *Staphylococcus* and *Enterococcus* species (Ardura & Koh, 2016).

Prophylaxis against *Pneumocystis* pneumonia, such as trimethoprim-sulfamethoxazole, is routinely given to most children during treatment for cancer (Ardura & Koh, 2016). Colony-stimulating factors (CSFs), a family of glycoprotein hormones that regulate the reproduction, maturation, and function of blood cells, are now routinely used as supportive measures to prevent the side effects caused by low blood counts. CSFs promote stem cell proliferation and stimulate a more rapid maturation of the cells, allowing them to enter the bloodstream earlier. Granulocyte colony-stimulating factor (G-CSF; filgrastim [Neupogen], pegfilgrastim [Neulasta]) directs granulocyte development and can decrease the duration of neutropenia. This reduces the incidence and duration of infection in children receiving treatment for cancer. G-CSF is also being used to decrease the bone marrow recovery time after SCT (Ardura & Koh, 2016). G-CSF is usually administered intravenously or subcutaneously 24 hours after chemotherapy is discontinued and is given for 10 to 14 days. G-CSF is discontinued when the ANC surpasses 10,000/mm^3. The pegylated or long-acting form of G-CSF, pegfilgrastim, is given only once after completion of therapy and typically has its peak efficacy (highest white blood cell count) about 8 to 10 days after administration. During G-CSF therapy, children may experience bone pain, fever, rash, malaise, and headaches.

Prevention of infection continues as a priority after discharge from the hospital. Some institutions allow the child to return to school when the ANC is above 500/mm^3. Other institutions place no restrictions on the child, regardless of the blood count. If the ANC falls below 500/mm^3, cautious isolation from crowded areas, such as shopping centers or subways, is advisable. At all times, family members should be encouraged to practice good hand washing to avoid introducing pathogens into the home, and they should know how to take a temperature and who to call in the event of fever (see Critical Thinking Case Study box).

CRITICAL THINKING CASE STUDY

Fever and Neutropenia

Billy, 9 years old, is undergoing chemotherapy for high-risk acute lymphoblastic leukemia (ALL) and recently hospitalized with a fever of 103°F (39.5°C). He last received chemotherapy 10 days ago with vincristine, doxorubicin, and peg-L-asparaginase and is currently taking oral dexamethasone for 21 days. His white blood cell count is 0.1/mm^3, with an absolute neutrophil count (ANC) of 0. His platelet count is 31,000/mm^3, and his hemoglobin is 8.1 g/dl. He has noticeable petechiae on his arms and legs with multiple bruises in various stages of healing.

After your morning report, you visit Billy, start your assessment, and note the following: Billy is an alert and oriented 9-year-old boy. His tongue and oral mucosa are covered with a white plaque. Vital signs are as follows: temperature, 102.6°F (39.2°C), axial; respiratory rate, 24 breaths/min; heart rate, 140 beats/min; blood pressure, 100/56 mm Hg. Further observation of the patient and his surroundings reveals (1) a sign over his bed that reads "no needle punctures"; (2) he is currently getting 5 L of oxygen via nasal cannula; (3) the port-a-cath is accessed with intravenous fluids infusing; and (4) the dressing is clean and dry.

1. What evidence should you consider regarding this condition?
2. What additional information is required at this time?
3. List the nursing intervention(s) that have the highest priority.
4. Identify important patient-centered outcomes with reference to your nursing interventions.

Answers are available at http://evolve.elsevier.com/wong/ncic.

Hemorrhage

Before the use of transfused platelets, hemorrhage was a leading cause of death in children with some types of cancer. Now most bleeding episodes can be prevented or controlled with judicious administration of platelet concentrates or platelet-rich plasma. The incidence of severe spontaneous internal hemorrhage varies, but usually does not occur until the platelet count is 20,000/mm^3 or less (Hockenberry, Kline, & Rodgers, 2016).

Because infection increases the tendency toward hemorrhage, and because bleeding sites become more easily infected, take special care to avoid performing skin punctures whenever possible. When performing finger sticks, venipunctures, intramuscular injections, and bone marrow tests, employ aseptic technique with continued observation for bleeding. Meticulous mouth care is essential because gingival bleeding with resultant mucositis is a frequent problem. Because the rectal area is prone to ulceration from various drugs, hygiene is essential. To prevent additional trauma, avoid rectal temperatures and suppositories. Frequent turning and the use of a pressure-reducing mattress under bony prominences prevent development of pressure sores and decubital ulcers.

Platelet transfusions are generally reserved for active bleeding episodes that do not respond to local treatment and that may occur during induction or relapse therapy. Epistaxis and gingival bleeding are the most common. The nurse teaches parents and children measures to control nose bleeding. Applying pressure at the site without disturbing clot formation is the general rule. Platelet concentrates normally do not have to be cross-matched for blood group or type. However, because platelets contain specific antigen components similar to blood group factors, children who receive multiple transfusions may become sensitized to a platelet group other than their own. Therefore platelets are cross-matched with the donor's blood components whenever possible.

Transfused platelets generally survive in the body for 1 to 3 days. The peak effect is reached in about 1 hour and decreased by half in 24 hours. After a transfusion, the nurse observes and records the approximate time when hemostasis of bleeding sites occurs. Delayed hemostasis is evidence of platelet destruction. For long-term patients, multiple transfusion therapy becomes progressively less effective.

During bleeding episodes the parents and child need much emotional support (see Critical Thinking Case Study box). The sight of oozing blood is upsetting. Often parents request a platelet transfusion, unaware of the necessity of trying local measures first. The nurse can help calm their anxiety by explaining the reason for delaying a platelet transfusion until absolutely necessary. Because compatible donors decrease the risk of antigen formation in the recipient, the nurse should encourage parents to locate suitable donors for eventual blood use.

CRITICAL THINKING CASE STUDY

Bleeding

Paul, 14 years old, is undergoing chemotherapy for non-Hodgkin lymphoma but has recently been hospitalized with an infection. He last received chemotherapy 12 days ago. His current platelet count is 28,000/mm^3. He has noticeable petechiae on his arms and legs with multiple bruises in various stages of healing. After your morning report, you visit Paul, start your assessment, and note the following: Paul is alert and oriented. The right sclera has a hemorrhage, and multiple petechiae and bruises are on the arms and legs. Petechiae are noted on the buccal mucosa and palate. Further observation of the patient and his surroundings reveals (1) a sign over his bed that reads "no needle punctures"; (2) he is currently getting 5 L of oxygen via nasal cannula; (3) the port-a-cath is accessed with intravenous fluids infusing; and (4) the dressing is clean and dry.

1. What evidence should you consider regarding this condition?
2. What additional information is required at this time?
3. List the nursing intervention(s) that have the highest priority.
4. Identify important patient-centered outcomes with reference to your nursing interventions.

Answers are available at http://evolve.elsevier.com/wong/ncic.

Children at home who have low platelet counts (usually <100,000/mm^3) should avoid activities that might cause injury or bleeding, such as riding bicycles or skateboards, skating, climbing trees or playground equipment, and contact sports such as football or soccer. Once the platelet count rises, these restrictions are not necessary. In addition, aspirin and aspirin-containing products are not used; for mild pain or significantly elevated temperature, acetaminophen is substituted.

Anemia

Initially anemia may be profound if there is complete replacement of the bone marrow by cancer cells. During induction therapy, blood transfusions with packed red blood cells may be necessary to raise the hemoglobin to levels approaching 10 g/dl. The usual precautions in caring for the child are instituted. (See Chapter 28.)

Anemia is also a consequence of drug-induced myelosuppression. Although not as severely affected as the white blood cells, erythrocyte production may be delayed. Because children have an amazing capacity to withstand low hemoglobin levels, the best approach is to allow the child to regulate activity with reasonable adult supervision. It may be necessary for the parents to alert the schoolteacher to the child's physical limitations, particularly in terms of strenuous activity.

Nausea and Vomiting

The nausea and vomiting that occur shortly after administration of several of the drugs and as a result of cranial or abdominal irradiation can be profound and debilitating. The advent of serotonin receptor blockers (5-hydroxytryptamine-3 or 5-HT3 receptor antagonists) has greatly improved management of nausea and vomiting caused by chemotherapy and radiation therapy. The advantage of these agents over conventional drugs is that they produce no extrapyramidal side effects, such as difficulty speaking or swallowing, shuffle walk, slow movements, trembling, stiffness of the arms and legs, or loss of balance. Published guidelines recommend 5-HT3 antagonists and corticosteroids for children receiving highly or moderately emetogenic chemotherapy (Patel, Robinson, Thackray et al., 2017).

For mild to moderate vomiting, phenothiazine-type drugs remain the mainstay of therapy. Promethazine (Phenergan), prochlorperazine (Compazine), or trimethobenzamide (Tigan) may be effective agents. Metoclopramide is a more effective antiemetic for acute nausea or vomiting. Unfortunately, the drug causes a number of side effects in children, particularly extrapyramidal reactions, such as muscle tremors or twitching, agitation, grimacing, dysarthria, and oculogyric crisis (fixation of eyes in one position for minutes or hours). Prophylaxis with diphenhydramine (Benadryl) is recommended to reduce the incidence of extrapyramidal symptoms when metoclopramide is given (Krane, Casillas, & Zeltzer, 2016).

Synthetic cannabinoids are now being used in adolescents undergoing chemotherapy. A drug that has yielded promising results is tetrahydrocannabinol, or dronabinol. Dronabinol helps control nausea and vomiting and also is an effective appetite stimulant (Feyer & Jordan, 2011).

The most beneficial regimen for antiemetic control has been the administration of the antiemetic before chemotherapy begins (30 minutes to 1 hour before) and regular (not as-needed) administration for at least 24 hours after chemotherapy. The goal is to prevent the child from ever experiencing nausea or vomiting because this can prevent the development of anticipatory symptoms (the conditioned response of developing nausea and vomiting before receiving the drug). Other nonpharmacologic interventions (similar to those discussed for pain management in Chapter 5) can be useful in controlling posttherapy and anticipatory nausea and vomiting. Giving the antineoplastic drug with a mild sedative at bedtime is also helpful for some children, and there is evidence that nighttime administration of drugs such as methotrexate and 6-mercaptopurine may be more effective than morning administration.

Altered Nutrition

Altered nutrition is a common side effect of treatment. Continued assessment of the child's nutritional status, child's intake, and energy expenditure must occur throughout treatment. The child's height, weight, and head circumference (for children younger than 3 years old) must be measured routinely during visits to the hospital or clinic. Energy reserves should be evaluated with routine skinfold measurements. Biochemical assays such as serum prealbumin, transferrin, and albumin may be helpful to evaluate nutritional status in some children, but a single assay should not be used alone for a nutritional evaluation (Lawson, Daley, Sams, et al., 2013). There are no specific criteria that mandate nutritional interventions in children undergoing cancer treatment. Instead each child should have an individualized nutritional care plan based on routine assessments. Most pediatric cancer treatment centers have a nutritionist who can be consulted to develop the nutritional care plan and revise it as needed. Nutritional status is important to maintain because a compromised nutritional status can contribute to reduced tolerance to treatment, altered metabolism of chemotherapy drugs, prolonged episodes of neutropenia, and increased risk for infection.

> **! NURSING ALERT**
>
> Some children develop aversions to certain foods if they are eaten during chemotherapy. It is best to refrain from offering the child's favorite foods while the child is receiving chemotherapy.

Supportive nutrition measures include oral supplements with high-protein and high-calorie foods. Ways to increase calories include using whole milk, adding tofu (high in protein) to most meals, and serving full-fat yogurt, ice cream, and milk instead on nonfat or low-fat items. Cooking with butter; putting sugar on cereal; and making high-calorie snacks such as trail mix, peanut butter, or dried fruit readily available for the child are other ways to increase calories. Enteral feeding may be necessary when children are unable to maintain the necessary calories to prevent weight loss. Parenteral hyperalimentation is used most frequently for children who have digestive problems, after surgery, or with SCT. Chapter 22 discusses these interventions in more detail.

Despite such approaches, some children still do not eat. Theories to explain persistent anorexia include the following: (1) a physical effect related to the cancer that is nonspecific; (2) a conditioned aversion to food from nausea and vomiting during treatment; (3) a response to stress in the environment, related to eating or to the child's condition; (4) a result of depression; and (5) a control mechanism when so much else has been imposed on the child. When loss of appetite and weight decline persists, the nurse should investigate the family situation to determine whether any of these variables are contributing to the problem, and discuss with the treatment team.

Mucosal Ulceration

One of the most distressing side effects of several drugs is gastrointestinal mucosal cell damage, which results in ulcers anywhere along the alimentary tract. Oral ulcers (stomatitis) are red, eroded, painful areas in the mouth or pharynx. (See Stomatitis, Chapter 6.) Similar lesions may extend along the esophagus and occur in the rectal area. They greatly compound anorexia because eating is extremely uncomfortable.

> **! NURSING ALERT**
>
> Viscous lidocaine is not recommended for young children. If applied to the pharynx, it may depress the gag reflex, increasing the risk of aspiration. Seizures have also been associated with the use of oral viscous lidocaine, most likely as a result of the rapid absorption into the bloodstream via the oral lesions (Lutwak, Howland, Gambetta, et al., 2013).

Some helpful interventions when oral ulcers develop are feeding a bland, moist, soft diet; using a soft sponge toothbrush (Toothette) instead of a toothbrush; frequently rinsing the mouth with chlorhexidine mouthwash or sodium bicarbonate and salt mouth rinses (using a solution of 1 tsp of baking soda and ½ tsp of table salt in 1 quart of water); using sucralfate; and administering local anesthetics without alcohol, such as a solution of diphenhydramine and Maalox (aluminum and magnesium hydroxide) or UlcerEase (Chaveli-Lopez & Bagan-Sebastian, 2016). Although local anesthetics are effective in temporarily relieving the pain, many children dislike the taste and numb feeling they produce.

! NURSING ALERT

Avoid agents such as lemon glycerin swabs and hydrogen peroxide because of their drying effects on the mucosa. In addition, the acidity of lemon may be very irritating, especially on eroded tissue.

Administering mouth care is particularly difficult in infants and toddlers. A satisfactory method of cleaning the gums is to wrap a piece of gauze around a finger; soak it in saline or plain water; and swab the gums, palate, and inner cheek surfaces with the finger. Children should perform mouth care routinely before and after any feeding and as often as every 2 to 4 hours to rid mucosal surfaces of debris, which becomes an excellent medium for bacterial and fungal growth if left undisturbed.

Dental hygiene can become a serious problem if the child wears an orthodontic appliance. The accumulated debris on braces is difficult to remove without vigorous brushing, and the appliance itself traumatizes the gums. For this reason, sometimes braces are removed before starting chemotherapy treatment.

Difficulty eating is a major problem with stomatitis and may warrant hospitalization if the child refuses fluids. The child usually chooses the foods that are best tolerated. Surprisingly, some children prefer salty foods to bland ones. Drinking can usually be encouraged if a straw is used to bypass the ulcerated oral mucosa. The nurse should encourage parents to relax any eating pressures because the anorexia accompanying stomatitis is well justified. In addition, because it is a temporary condition, once the ulcers heal, the child can resume good food habits. Ordinarily, severe mucosal ulceration indicates a need for decreased chemotherapy until complete healing takes place, usually within a week. Analgesics, including opioids, may be needed when treatment cannot be altered, such as during SCT.

If rectal ulcers develop, meticulous toilet hygiene, warm sitz baths after each bowel movement, and an occlusive ointment applied to the ulcerated area promote healing; the use of stool softeners is necessary to prevent further discomfort. The child may avoid defecation to prevent discomfort; for this reason, parents should record bowel movements to keep track. Rectal temperatures and suppositories are always avoided because they may traumatize the area.

Neurologic Problems

Vincristine, and to a lesser extent vinblastine, can cause various neurotoxic effects. One of the more common neurotoxic effects is severe constipation caused from decreased bowel innervation. Administration of opioids can further aggravate constipation. The nurse advises parents to record bowel movements and to notify the practitioner of a change in stool habits. Physical activity and stool softeners are helpful in preventing the problem, but laxatives, such as polyethylene glycol, are often necessary to stimulate evacuation. Dietary changes such as increased fiber may not be effective because the increased bulk tends to increase fecal distention and discomfort without producing the necessary mechanical stimulation.

Footdrop and weakness and numbness of the extremities may cause difficulty in walking or fine hand movement. The nurse should observe for these problems and warn parents of these side effects, which are reversible once the drug is stopped. Wearing high-top tennis shoes or using a footboard in bed may help preserve proper alignment. If weakness occurs while the child is attending school, temporary alteration of activity may be necessary. Parents should inform the teacher of the situation to avoid unrealistic expectations of the child's abilities.

Another neurotoxic effect is severe jaw pain. Analgesics may help relieve the discomfort. Children may avoid movement by not talking or chewing, although continuous chewing, such as with gum, may actually reduce the pain.

A neurologic syndrome, postirradiation somnolence, may develop 5 to 8 weeks after CNS irradiation and last for 4 to 15 days. It is characterized by somnolence with or without fever, anorexia, and nausea and vomiting. Parents should be warned of the possibility of such symptoms and be encouraged to seek medical evaluation because somnolence may be an early indicator of long-term neurologic sequelae after cranial irradiation.

Hemorrhagic Cystitis

Sterile hemorrhagic cystitis is a side effect of chemical irritation to the bladder from chemotherapy or radiation therapy. It can be prevented by (1) a liberal oral or parenteral fluid intake (at least 1.5 times the recommended daily fluid requirement [2 L/m^2/day]); (2) frequent voiding immediately after feeling the urge, including immediately before bed, one nighttime void, and on arising; (3) administration of the drug early in the day to allow for sufficient fluids and frequent voiding; and (4) administration of mesna, a drug that inhibits the urotoxicity of cyclophosphamide and ifosfamide (Freedman, Rheingold, & Fisher, 2016).

! NURSING ALERT

If signs of cystitis such as burning on urination occur, prompt medical evaluation is needed. Hemorrhagic cystitis warrants a full workup and timely intervention.

In most cases IV fluids are given before, during, and after the drug to ensure adequate hydration, thereby eliminating the need for the child to drink large amounts of fluid. If oral home administration is prescribed, the family needs specific instructions on exactly how much fluid the child must have.

Alopecia

Hair loss is a side effect of several chemotherapeutic drugs and cranial irradiation. Not all children lose their hair during chemotherapy, and some children may experience thinning of the hair rather than baldness. However, retaining hair is the exception rather than the rule. It is better to warn children and parents of this side effect to allow them some time to adapt to hair loss.

The family should know that the hair falls out in clumps, causing patchy baldness. To lessen the trauma of seeing large amounts of hair on bed linen or clothing, the child can wear a disposable surgical cap to collect the shed hair during the period of greatest hair loss, or the hair can be cut short or the head shaved. Families should also be aware that wigs are a tax deductible expense. Hair typically regrows in 3 to 6 months, and it is often a different color and texture than before cancer treatment.

NURSING TIP

Encouraging children to choose a wig similar to their own hairstyle and color before the hair falls out is helpful in fostering later adjustment to hair loss.

If the child chooses not to wear a wig, attention to some type of head covering is important, especially in cold or sunny climates. Scalp hygiene is also important. The scalp should be washed regularly as with any other body part.

Steroid Effects

Short-term steroid therapy produces physical changes and alterations in body image, which, although not clinically significant, can be extremely distressing to older children. One of these is cushingoid appearance. The child's face becomes rounded and puffy (see Fig. 31.5). Unlike hair loss, little can be done to camouflage this obvious change, although careful avoidance of salt and salt-containing foods can help reduce fluid accumulation. It is not unusual for other children to tease the child. It is helpful to reassure the child that, after cessation of the drug, the facial contours will return to normal. The use of loose-fitting clothes, such as warm-up outfits, can help camouflage the change in weight.

Children receiving steroid therapy look healthy. The moon face, red cheeks, supraclavicular fat pads, protuberant abdomen, and fluid retention indicate weight gain. However, the actual weight gain resulting from increased muscle mass and subcutaneous tissue may be small. Therefore the nurse should evaluate weight gain by observing the extremities and measuring skinfold thickness and arm circumference during steroid therapy to determine whether the weight gain is a result of increased dietary intake.

Shortly after beginning steroid therapy, children may experience mood changes, which range from feelings of well-being and euphoria to depression and irritability. If parents are unaware of these drug-induced changes, they may become unduly concerned. Therefore the nurse should warn them of the reactions and encourage them to discuss the behavioral changes with each other and the child.

NURSING CARE DURING HEMATOPOIETIC STEM CELL TRANSPLANTATION

Because of the aggressive preconditioning therapy used to remove the marrow and the potential for complications while waiting for engraftment of transplanted stem cells, children undergoing SCT are usually hospitalized for several weeks. SCT patients must have numerous procedures performed, such as the insertion of a venous access device, administration of intensive chemotherapy and irradiation, and strict infection precautions. During the period after transplantation and before the new marrow begins adequately replacing granulocytes, the child is extremely susceptible to infection, and any infection can be life threatening. In addition, many of the side effects previously discussed occur in the child undergoing SCT.

The most common complication in allogeneic transplants is acute GVHD, which can affect the skin, gastrointestinal tract, and liver. The characteristics and severity of the manifestations vary according to the severity and area affected. Emphasis is now placed on the prevention of GVHD, using various agents such as a calcineurin inhibitor in conjunction with mycophenolate mofetil, methotrexate, or sirolimus (Gottschalk, Naik, Hegde, et al., 2016).Treatment involves the use of steroids or other immunosuppressive medications. However, this treatment further increases the risk of infection in the already susceptible patient. All blood products are irradiated to minimize the introduction of additional antigens.

Skin breakdown and delayed wound healing frequently occur in the patient undergoing SCT. Preventive interventions to minimize pressure on dependent areas of the skin include the use of pressure-relieving or pressure-reducing beds or mattresses and frequent movement. Measures to promote healing when breakdown occurs include frequent sitz baths to the perianal area and protective skin barriers, such as hydrocolloid dressings or occlusive ointments.

Throughout this long ordeal the family is worried about successful engraftment and possible fatal complications. An unfortunate post-transplant possibility is recurrence of the disease after engraftment. Consequently, nurses need to provide sensitive care and maintain a supportive attitude during the many crises that may arise. If the procedure is not successful, the care needed by these families is consistent with that required by the family of any child with a life-threatening disorder (see Chapter 19).

PREPARATION FOR PROCEDURES

Children in particular need psychologic preparation for the various treatment interventions, which often involve surgery, IV injections, bone marrow aspirations, and LPs. The diagnostic procedures initially employed to confirm the diagnosis and those that are repeated to monitor treatment can be a source of discomfort and stress to the child and family. Even noninvasive procedures such as imaging and radiologic tests are frightening to a young child. Some of these tests require the child to lie motionless for a prolonged time in a confined space with little or no communication. Consequently, infants and young children are usually sedated, and older children need an explanation of what to expect and reminders during the test of how much longer they must remain still. The same principles for preparing children for procedures that are discussed in Chapter 22 apply here, including the option of having parents stay with the child whenever possible. Children who undergo repeated tests need additional preparation and emotional support to manage their stress.

Two procedures, bone marrow studies and LPs, are so commonly performed in many types of childhood cancer that they deserve special consideration in preparing children (Fig. 29.2). Both tests can be frightening to children because they are done behind the child's field of vision. Professionals caring for children with cancer recommend the use of developmentally appropriate support using both pharmacologic and nonpharmacologic approaches and sedation if required (see Chapter 22).

Topical anesthetics such as eutectic mixture of local anesthetics (EMLA) and LMX4 creams are used as a local anesthetic before intrusive procedures, including venipunctures, implanted port access, LPs, and subcutaneous or intramuscular injections (Hockenberry, Kline, & Rodgers, 2016). Local intradermal anesthesia with lidocaine is frequently used for LP and bone marrow examination. To reduce the stinging

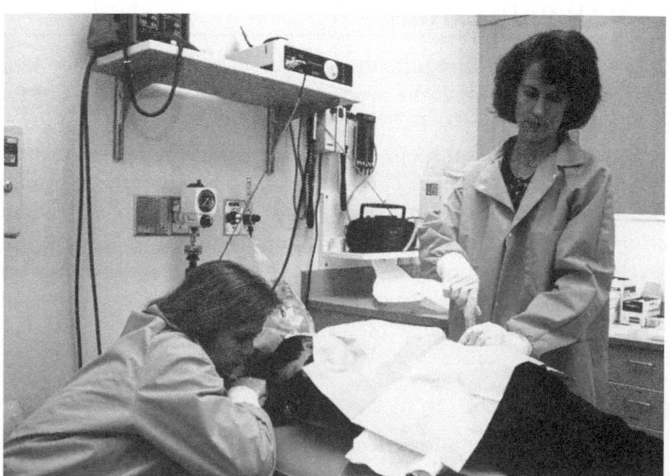

FIG. 29.2 Child with leukemia undergoing bone marrow aspiration.

sensation from lidocaine, sodium bicarbonate should be added (see Pain Management, Chapter 5.) Deeper infiltration of the muscle and periosteum of the bone with buffered lidocaine further reduces the pain from the large-bore aspiration or biopsy needle entering the bone.

For bone marrow studies, LPs, and other procedures, children of preschool age and older should be prepared beforehand. Physical care after the procedures is minimal. A small pressure bandage is applied to the bone marrow puncture site, and an adhesive bandage is applied to the LP site. No activity restriction is necessary after the bone marrow test, although the site is usually sore and the child may prefer to remain quiet. Recommendations after LP vary. If medication was instilled, the child may be placed in a slight Trendelenburg position to facilitate circulation of the medicated spinal fluid.

PAIN MANAGEMENT

Nurses must be knowledgeable about the basic pathophysiology of cancer pain and treatment-related side effects. The World Health Organization's three-step analgesic pain ladder should be incorporated into the approach to pain management for every child with cancer (Ullrich, Sourkes, & Wolfe, 2016). Nurses must acquire extensive knowledge of nonopioid and opioid analgesics, as well as nonpharmacologic approaches used in pediatric pain management (see Chapter 5.) Interdisciplinary pain management teams are used in many pediatric cancer centers. These teams serve as consultants and provide expertise in the assessment and management of pain. The nurse often serves as the coordinator of care, playing a key role in cancer pain management and implementing the pain team's plan of care.

Pharmacologic management of disease-related pain involves a variety of methods. It may take more than one trial of one type of medication to find the appropriate agent to manage a patient's pain. The route of administration must be considered as well. Providing "pain relief" by administering painful intramuscular injections as an alternative to the IV route is not appropriate therapy because many oral preparations are now available with comparable efficacy. Furthermore, children may refuse needed pain medication if it involves an injection. Nonsteroidal antiinflammatory drugs (NSAIDs), acetaminophen with codeine, oxycodone, and morphine are commonly used agents in the management of disease-related pain (Fielding, Sanford, & Davis, 2013). All are available in the oral form, and morphine and the NSAID ketorolac (Toradol) are available as IV preparations. Appropriate dosing is imperative. Doses are titrated to increase the amount of analgesia and minimize side effects.

HEALTH PROMOTION

Children with cancer require the same basic health supervision as do any children. Sometimes the overwhelming needs and demands placed on the family, coupled with the singular concern focused on the cancer by both family and health care professionals, result in a lack of attention to typical health care needs. Nurses should monitor the type of primary care the child receives, using guidelines for recommended medical supervision. Areas of particular concern are growth, physical and cognitive development, and neurologic status. Two other areas are also important: (1) dental care because of potential side effects from treatment, and (2) immunizations because of concern with live virus vaccines and immunosuppression.

Dental Care

Irradiation to the head and neck can cause a number of late complications (Landier, Armenian, Meadows, et al., 2016). Some are irreversible, such as facial asymmetry, but those affecting the teeth and gums (e.g., caries, periodontal disease) benefit from excellent oral hygiene, including regular use of systemic and topical fluoride and regular dental examinations and cleaning. (See Dental Health, Chapter 12.) Delayed or absent development of the permanent teeth can occur (Effinger, Migliorati, Hudson, et al., 2014). Depending on the child's age, this can be a source of acute psychologic distress, especially during early school-age years, when "losing a tooth" is a status symbol. Children need to be aware of this possibility and need help to explain the delay to peers.

Daily toothbrushing and flossing are encouraged in children with granulocyte counts in excess of $500/mm^3$ and platelet counts above $40,000/mm^3$. Fluoride rinses are used as discussed in Chapter 12. Oral hygiene for children whose counts are below these parameters is limited to wiping the teeth with moistened gauze sponges or Toothettes.

Immunizations

Viral replication after the administration of live vaccine for polio, measles, rubella, and mumps can cause serious disease in immunocompromised children. The child receiving chemotherapy for cancer should not receive live, attenuated vaccines. Inactivated vaccines can be given to immunosuppressed children. Siblings and other family members can receive the live measles, mumps, and rubella vaccine and the varicella vaccine without risk to the child who is immunosuppressed. Guidelines for immunization of children receiving chemotherapy and SCT patients have been published (Ardura & Koh, 2016).

An important indication for isolation is an outbreak of childhood communicable disease, especially chickenpox. Ideally the school nurse should work with the treating practitioner to decide the optimum time for school attendance. Parents should be taught to work with the school or day care staff to be sure they understand the risk to the child being treated for cancer and that they notify the parents immediately of any exposure. If the child has been exposed to the varicella virus, varicella-zoster immune globulin given within 96 hours may favorably alter the course of the disease. Antiviral agents, such as acyclovir, should be given if the child develops varicella. Without treatment, death from disseminated varicella can occur due to disease in the liver, lung, and CNS (Ardura & Koh, 2016). (See also Immunizations, Chapter 6.)

> **! NURSING ALERT**
>
> Children vaccinated 2 weeks before or during chemotherapy should be considered unimmunized and should be revaccinated or receive live virus vaccines 6 months after chemotherapy has stopped (American Academy of Pediatrics, 2015). Most institutions have individual guidelines regarding vaccinations in a child undergoing immunosuppressive therapy. The nurse should be aware of these guidelines and educate patients and families about the need for and timing of immunizations.

FAMILY EDUCATION

Nurses working with children who have cancer have a significant supportive role in helping the family understand the various therapies, preventing or managing expected side effects or toxicities, and observing for late effects of treatment. Helping families learn what they need to know is a constant feature of the nursing role, especially in terms of new treatments, clinical trials, home care, and transition to off-therapy and adult-focused health care. Nurses must stay well informed themselves to be able to help families learn as they establish a "new normal" in their lives. Several excellent resources are available to use in family education. The National Cancer Institute (https://www.cancer.gov/) and the Children's Oncology Group (https://www.childrensoncologygroup.org/) websites are reliable sources of regularly updated information concerning childhood cancer research and care. The Association of Pediatric Hematology/Oncology Nurses* has developed a portfolio of educational materials for family education. The American Childhood Cancer Organization† is an international organization providing support, education, and advocacy programs for children with cancer and their families. Similarly, the Coalition Against Childhood Cancer (CAC2)‡ is composed of numerous foundations that provide advocacy and resources focused on childhood cancer.

Instruction regarding home care frequently involves teaching about medication schedules, observing for side effects or toxicities that require further evaluation, taking measures to prevent or manage these problems, and caring for special devices such as central venous catheters.§ Medication adherence is an important issue because poor adherence to treatment regimens can result in disease relapse or serious medical complications (Gupta & Bhatia, 2017). Every effort must be made to ensure that the family understands the importance of adhering to the prescribed treatment schedule and follow-up care. Finding methods to identify and minimize nonadherence is an active area of current research. (See Chapter 22.)

Many families use complementary and alternative medicine (CAM), primarily for symptom relief. CAM includes therapies that are not thought of as standard medical care. Complementary therapies are used along with standard medical treatment; alternative therapies are used instead of standard medical treatment. There are many different types of CAM therapy available. A few examples include dietary supplements, homeopathy, and acupuncture. Most families using CAM therapies do not abandon standard care, but often they do not tell their physician about CAM use (McLean & Kemper, 2016). Undisclosed use of alternative therapies may interfere with the effectiveness of the prescribed treatment. Reasons given by families for not communicating about their use of CAM therapies include anticipation of negative response from their physician, believing that physicians do not need to know, and that they are not asked (McLean & Kemper, 2016).

Nurses are instrumental in building trusting relationships with families to facilitate discussion of concerns and questions openly with their physician who can guide them. To provide family education, nurses should familiarize themselves with reliable resources about CAM, such as the American Academy of Pediatrics guidelines (Kemper, Vohra, & Walls, 2008) for counseling families about CAM therapies and the factsheets on CAM posted on the cancer.gov website. Many treatment centers have developed integrative medicine programs, which combine state-of-the art medical therapy with evidence-based CAM practices. Nurses should be aware of how to access these programs in their institutions on behalf of patients and families.

COMPLETION OF THERAPY

Care does not end when the child completes therapy. With the increasing awareness of late effects, nurses have an important role in the assessment of the child for problems such as delayed growth, secondary malignancies, and disturbances in body systems. The family needs to be aware of the importance of continued medical supervision, for both primary care and survivorship care. Other health care professionals caring for the child, such as school nurses, family physicians, and dentists, should be informed of the child's cancer diagnosis. As children reach adulthood, transition services may be available in the treatment center to help ease the transfer of primary care to adult health care professionals in the community. Adolescents/young adults may benefit from genetic counseling regarding cancers that are likely to be inherited. If the possibility of infertility exists, fertility options should be discussed for pubertal males and females before the start of treatment, and readdressed during survivorship care. The Children's Oncology Group has developed guidelines for long-term follow-up care for pediatric cancer survivors.* Nurses involved with these children should be familiar with these guidelines and use all opportunities to help patients and families access needed survivorship and transition care.

*8735 W. Higgins Road, Suite 300, Chicago, IL 60631; 847-375-4724; fax: 847-375-6478; http://www.aphon.org.

†PO Box 498, Kensington, MD 20895; 855-858-2226 or 301-962-3520; fax: 301-962-3521; http://www.acco.org.

‡Coalition Against Childhood Cancer (CAC2), https://cac2.org/.

§Home care instructions for giving medications to children and caring for a central venous catheter are available in Wilson, D., & Hockenberry, M. J. (2008). *Wong's clinical manual of pediatric nursing* (7th ed.). St. Louis, MO: Mosby.

CANCERS OF BLOOD AND LYMPH SYSTEMS

ACUTE LEUKEMIAS

Leukemia is a broad term given to a group of malignant diseases of the bone marrow, blood, and lymphatic system. In healthy children, the bone marrow makes blood stem cells that mature to become lymphoid or myeloid stem cells. Myeloid cells differentiate into red blood cells, platelets, and white blood cells. Lymphoid stem cells become lymphoblasts that differentiate into B lymphocytes, T lymphocytes, and natural killer cells (National Institutes of Health, 2017b). In acute leukemias, immature cells predominate that cannot function effectively. Two types of leukemia are seen most often in children: acute lymphoblastic leukemia (ALL) and acute myeloid leukemia (AML).

Acute Lymphoblastic Leukemia

Older synonyms for ALL include acute lymphatic, lymphocytic, and lymphoid leukemia. ALL is the most common form of childhood cancer, with an annual incidence of approximately 4900 new cases annually in the United States (Rabin, Gramatges, Margolin, et al., 2016). It occurs more often in boys than in girls and in Caucasians more than in African Americans (Rabin, Gramatges, Margolin, et al., 2016). The peak age of onset is between 2 and 5 years old. Risk factors for ALL include prenatal exposure to x-rays, previous treatment with chemotherapy, and certain genetic conditions (e.g., Down syndrome, Bloom syndrome, Fanconi anemia) (National Institutes of Health, 2017b). Various chromosomal abnormalities also have been identified in leukemic cells of children with ALL (Rabin, Gramatges, Margolin, et al., 2016).

Clinical Staging and Prognosis

In the past, the standard ways to classify ALL were with the French-American-British (FAB) morphologic system and cytochemical stains. Now the standard accepted method is immunophenotyping in which panels of monoclonal antibodies are used to determine T-lineage, B-lineage, and myeloid antigens (Rabin, Gramatges, Margolin, et al., 2016). In addition, chromosomal number (ploidy) and structural rearrangements are evaluated using molecular genetic analyses. The most important prognostic factors in determining long-term survival for children with ALL (Table 29.3) include the child's age, initial white

*Long-Term Follow-up Guidelines for Survivors of Childhood, Adolescent, and Young Adult Cancers (Version 4). Retrieved from http://www.survivorshipguidelines.org/.

TABLE 29.3 Selected Prognostic Factors for Acute Lymphoblastic Leukemia

Factor	Criteria
Age	Favorable: >1 year or ≤10 years at diagnosis.
Initial white blood cell count	Favorable: <50,000/mm^3 (B-cell ALL; association not seen in T-cell ALL).
Sex	Favorable: Female.
Race and ethnicity	Poorer outcomes associated with African American and Hispanic children than with Caucasian and Asian children. These differences likely reflect effects of multifactorial influences, such as socioeconomic status, access to care, treatment adherence, and host pharmacokinetic factors.
Immunophenotype	Survival is better in B-cell ALL than in T-cell ALL. (Specific immunophenotypic markers are no longer used to determine prognosis, but are important as targets for therapeutic agents.)
Cytogenetics/genomic alterations	Favorable: high hyperdiploidy (50-65 chromosomes); *ETV6-RUNX1* gene fusion. Unfavorable: Philadelphia chromosome; *MLL* gene rearrangements; hypodiploidy; intrachromosomal amplification of *AML1* gene.
Treatment response	Favorable: rapid response to treatment (best prognosis associated with undetectable levels of minimal residual disease or at least <10^{-4} at the end of standard induction).
Nutritional status	Unfavorable: malnutrition or obesity at diagnosis, and ongoing poor nutritional status throughout intensive postinduction treatment.

ALL, Acute lymphoblastic leukemia.
Adapted from Rabin, K. R., Gramatges, M. M., Margolin, J. F., & Poplack, D. G. (2016). Acute lymphoblastic leukemia. In P. A. Pizzo & D. G. Poplack (Eds.), *Principles and practice of pediatric oncology* (7th ed.). Philadelphia, PA: Lippincott; National Institutes of Health, National Cancer Institute. (2017). Childhood acute lymphoblastic leukemia treatment. Retrieved from https://www.cancer.gov/types/leukemia/hp/child-all-treatment-pdq.

blood cell count, CNS involvement, testicular involvement, Down syndrome, sex, race and ethnicity, and nutritional status; leukemic cell characteristics that affect prognosis include morphology, immunophenotype, and cytogenetics/genomic alterations such as ploidy and structural rearrangements (National Institutes of Health, 2017b). ALL has demonstrated dramatic improvements in survival rates such that current long-term disease-free survival rates for children with ALL approach 90% in major pediatric cancer treatment centers.

Clinical Manifestations

The onset of leukemia varies from acute to insidious. In most instances the child displays remarkably few symptoms. For example, leukemia may be diagnosed when a minor infection, such as a cold, fails to completely disappear. The child continues to be pale, listless, irritable, febrile, and anorexic. Parents often suspect some underlying problem when they observe the child's weight loss, petechiae, bruising without cause, and continued complaints of bone and joint pain. At other times there may be an extended history of signs and symptoms mimicking such conditions as rheumatoid arthritis or mononucleosis. Sometimes leukemia is an incidental finding on a routine physical examination or during treatment for an injury.

Signs and symptoms of ALL reflect infiltration of the bone marrow by nonfunctional leukemic cells ("blasts"). The three main consequences of bone marrow infiltration are (1) anemia from decreased erythrocytes, (2) infection from neutropenia, and (3) bleeding from decreased platelet production. Approximately half of patients have an elevated white blood cell count at presentation (>10,000/mm^3). Other signs and symptoms indicate leukemic cell infiltration of other organs; highly vascular organs, such as the spleen and liver, are most severely affected. Commonly seen are hepatosplenomegaly (68% of patients), splenomegaly (63%), fever (61%), lymphadenopathy (50%), bleeding (e.g., petechiae or purpura, 48%), and bone pain (23%) (Rabin, Gramatges, Margolin, et al., 2016). Two important sites of extramedullary disease are the CNS and testes because they can serve as "sanctuaries" for leukemic cells that require specific therapy.

Diagnostic Evaluation

Leukemia is usually suspected from the history, physical manifestations, and a peripheral blood smear that contains leukemic blasts, frequently in combination with low blood counts. The diagnostic evaluation includes a thorough history and physical examination, laboratory tests (CBC with differential, blood chemistries), and bone marrow aspiration/biopsy (cytogenetic analysis, immunophenotyping). Definitive diagnosis is based on analysis of the bone marrow sample. Typically the bone marrow of a child with ALL shows a monotonous infiltrate of blast cells. Once the diagnosis is confirmed, an LP is performed to determine whether there is any CNS involvement. Although only a small number of children have CNS involvement at diagnosis, they are usually asymptomatic.

Therapeutic Management

Treatment of ALL is based on risk groups defined by clinical and laboratory findings. Children with a higher risk of relapse/recurrence are treated with the most intensive therapy. Although specifics for various risk groups vary, treatment is generally divided into phases: induction, CNS preventive therapy/consolidation, interim maintenance, delayed intensification, maintenance or continuation therapy, and remission.

Almost immediately after confirmation of the diagnosis, induction therapy begins and lasts for 4 to 5 weeks (Rabin, Gramatges, Margolin, et al., 2016). The principal drugs are the corticosteroids (dexamethasone or prednisone), vincristine, and L-asparaginase, with or without an anthracycline. A complete remission is determined by the presence of less than 5% blast cells in the bone marrow and no detectable leukemia in extramedullary sites.

Because many of the drugs also cause myelosuppression of normal blood elements, the period immediately after a remission can be critical. The body is defenseless against invading organisms (especially normal bacterial flora) and susceptible to spontaneous hemorrhage. Consequently, supportive therapy during this time is essential. Supportive care consists of transfusion support and use of antibacterial and antifungal agents.

CNS preventive therapy is based on the understanding that leukemic cells could be present in the CNS where they are protected from many systemic chemotherapy drugs by the blood-brain barrier. For this reason, all children receive CNS prophylactic therapy. The combination of intrathecal chemotherapy (either methotrexate alone or in combination with cytarabine and hydrocortisone) plus CNS-directed systemic chemotherapy (dexamethasone, L-asparaginase, and high-dose methotrexate with leukovorin rescue) is standard; cranial radiation may be used for children at highest risk for CNS relapse (National Institutes of Health, 2017b).

Past clinical trials have shown that postinduction therapy is needed to maintain remission. Treatment regimens vary, but all patients receive consolidation/intensification after achieving a complete remission. Most commonly used is the Berlin, Frankfurt, Münster (BFM) "backbone" (a very intensive chemotherapy regimen from the International BFM Study Group that greatly increased ALL survival). This backbone includes consolidation with cyclophosphamide, cytarabine, and mercaptopurine given initially, followed by interim maintenance with high-dose methotrexate with or without leukovorin rescue. Next, delayed intensification is given using drugs and schedules similar to those used in the induction and consolidation phases. This is followed by maintenance therapy with daily mercaptopurine and weekly low-dose methotrexate; vincristine and a corticosteroid may be given, as well as continued intrathecal therapy (National Institutes of Health, 2017b; Rabin, Gramatges, Margolin, et al., 2016). A critical challenge during maintenance therapy is medication adherence because it has been shown that anything less than 95% adherence increases the risk of relapse (Bhatia, Landier, Shangguan, et al., 2012).

Although the optimum duration of therapy is not known, current practice is to continue treatment for 2 to 3 years. After cessation of therapy all children require regular medical follow-up to observe for relapse and late effects of treatment.

Acute Myeloid Leukemia

AML accounts for 20% of all cases of childhood leukemia and has an annual incidence of approximately 730 new cases in the United States (Arceci & Meshinchi, 2016). The incidence is similar for males and females, and higher rates are seen during the first year of life. AML is associated with a variety of predisposition syndromes, including constitutional chromosome abnormalities, inherited single gene mutations, and inherited cytopenias (Arceci & Meshinchi, 2016; National Institutes of Health, 2017c). In addition, therapy-related AML can be caused by treatment with certain chemotherapeutic drugs and/or radiation therapy (National Institutes of Health, 2017c).

Clinical Staging and Prognosis

There is no established clinical staging system for AML; it is considered disseminated at diagnosis. The World Health Organization (WHO) classification system is used to categorize subtypes of AML. These subtypes have distinguishing chromosomal changes, as well as changes in morphology, histochemistry, immunophenotype, and molecular characteristics; some specific subtypes are associated with prognosis (Arceci & Meshinchi, 2016).

Favorable prognosis is associated with Down syndrome in children who are less than 4 years of age at diagnosis, no minimal residual disease (MRD) findings after initial therapy, and certain cytogenetic and genetic abnormalities. Unfavorable prognosis is associated with an initial white blood cell count greater than 100,000/mm^3, presence of MRD after initial therapy, and specific cytogenetic and genetic abnormalities (Arceci & Meshinchi, 2016).

Progress in the management of AML has improved the 5-year survival rate to 68% for children younger than 15 years and to 57% for adolescents in the 15- to 19-year-old age-group (National Institutes of Health, 2017c). However, there is a wide range in outcome for different biologic subtypes of AML, which needs to be taken into account when considering prognosis for an individual patient. Research is focused on improving the survival rates and defining risk groups to enable risk-adapted therapy.

Clinical Manifestations

Many signs and symptoms of AML are similar to those of ALL and reflect infiltration of the bone marrow or extramedullary sites by myeloblasts. Typical signs and symptoms include fever with or without an infection, night sweats, shortness of breath, weakness or fatigue, easy bruising/bleeding, petechiae, bone or joint pain, and an eczema-like skin rash. In AML, painless lumps (leukemia cutis) that may be blue or purple in color may appear in the neck, underarm, abdomen, groin, or elsewhere. Other painless lumps, blue-green in color and called chloromas, may be found around the eyes.

Diagnostic Evaluation

With a few differences, the workup for AML is similar to that for ALL. Procedures and tests include physical examination and history, CBC with differential, blood chemistries, chest x-ray, bone marrow aspiration/biopsy, cytogenetic analysis, RT-PCR test, immunophenotyping, molecular testing, and an LP. A chloroma may be biopsied if present.

Therapeutic Management

Treatment for AML is generally more intense and of shorter duration than treatment for ALL. Chemotherapy is the main treatment modality for AML and is generally given in two phases: induction followed by postremission consolidation/intensification (National Institutes of Health, 2017c). For most subtypes of AML, maintenance therapy has not been shown to improve outcome and is therefore not used in most treatment regimens. Typically children are given two courses of induction chemotherapy and two courses of intensification. Standard remission induction consists of a three-drug regimen of cytarabine, daunorubin, and etoposide. CNS treatment with intrathecal medication is usually included in treatment regimens; CNS irradiation is not usually used in AML treatment. Once remission is achieved (no signs of leukemia detected), SCT may be performed. Alternatively, intensive chemotherapy may be given and SCT reserved in case the AML relapses. Intensification chemotherapy usually consists of high-dose cytarabine with or without daunorubicin; intrathecal chemotherapy is given every 1 to 2 months during intensification. The following discussion elaborates on the pathologic process and related clinical manifestations in the most susceptible organs of the body (Fig. 29.3).

Nursing Care Management

Nursing care of the child with acute leukemia, ALL or AML, is directly related to the regimen of therapy. Myelosuppression, drug toxicity, and leukemic infiltration cause secondary complications that necessitate supportive physical care. This discussion focuses on supportive interventions for the child with leukemia and the family. General aspects of care appropriate for the child with leukemia are discussed earlier under Nursing Care of the Child with Cancer.

Prepare the Family for Diagnostic and Therapeutic Procedures

From the time before diagnosis to cessation of therapy, children must undergo several tests, the most traumatic of which are bone marrow aspiration or biopsy and LP. Multiple finger sticks and venipunctures for blood analysis and drug infusion are common occurrences for several years after the diagnosis. Therefore children need an explanation of the rationale for each procedure, what can be expected, and what they can do to help. (See Preparation for Diagnostic and Therapeutic Procedures, Chapter 22.)

Depending on the child's age, one way of beginning diagnostic preparation is to explain the tests, procedures, and treatment plan. Using a drawing or letting the child look at a drop of blood under a microscope not only teaches but also fosters trust between the nurse and the child. It also allows the nurse to assess the child's level of understanding. An error many health professionals make is to overestimate children's knowledge about their bodies. For example, a bone marrow aspiration makes sense only when it is clarified that the center of a bone contains the cells that later become "working" blood cells or leukemic cells.

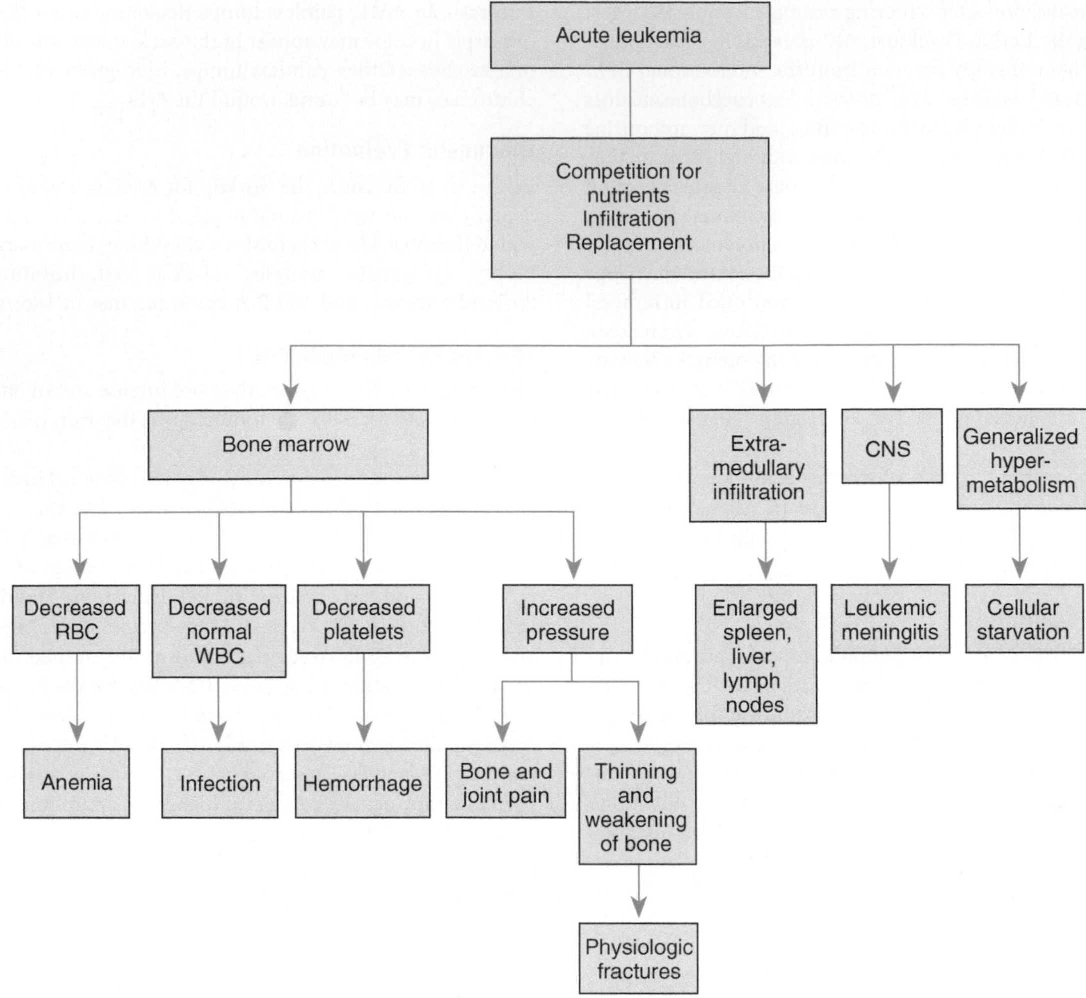

FIG. 29.3 Principal sites of tissue involvement in leukemia. *CNS,* Central nervous system; *RBC,* red blood cell; *WBC,* white blood cell.

Provide Continued Emotional Support

Nursing care of the child with leukemia is based on typical problems the family confronts during the treatment phases and afterward. Therefore the nurse's role is one of continual support, guidance, clarification, and clinical judgment. Parents need to know how to recognize symptoms that demand medical attention. Although some of the reactions discussed are expected, parents should still report them to their practitioner. Warning parents of their possible occurrence beforehand also allows parents to prepare. At the same time, it reassures them that these reactions are not caused by a return of leukemic cells.

The nurse must also use judgment in recognizing which side effects are normal reactions and which indicate toxicity. Frequently it is the office or clinic nurse who screens such telephone calls and gives advice, when appropriate. Usually nausea and vomiting are not indications for drug cessation. However, severe vomiting may require immediate intervention to prevent dehydration. Signs of infection, mucosal ulceration, hemorrhagic cystitis, peripheral neuropathy, and constipation require medical evaluation.

Another aspect of continued emotional support involves prognosis. Leukemia is not invariably fatal, but present statistics must be correctly interpreted. Although almost 80% of children with ALL live 5 years or longer, these are average estimates that apply to those children treated with the most successful protocols since diagnosis. For the high-risk child with ALL or the child with AML, the prognosis may be significantly poorer. Of those who do survive after completing therapy, some will relapse.

The nurse must be familiar with survival statistics to interpret them correctly to parents. At the same time, the nurse must realize that a realistic understanding of the chances for survival requires an adjustment period. During the initial diagnosis or when a relapse occurs, parents may find it difficult to hear the facts.

Statistics are numbers. Sometimes they bring hope, and at other times they bring despair. Although they are important in terms of research, better treatment, and identification of high- or low-risk populations, they present a general picture of what to expect. The nurse who is working with family members must individualize the numbers to relate to the people. An understanding of each member's emotional needs, as well as competent care of physical ones, is essential to the positive, growth-promoting support of the family. Comprehensive emotional support for the family of a child with a chronic illness and of a child at end of life in Chapter 19.

LYMPHOMAS

The lymphomas, a group of neoplastic diseases that arise from the lymphoid and hematopoietic systems, are divided into Hodgkin disease and NHL. These diseases are further subdivided according to tissue

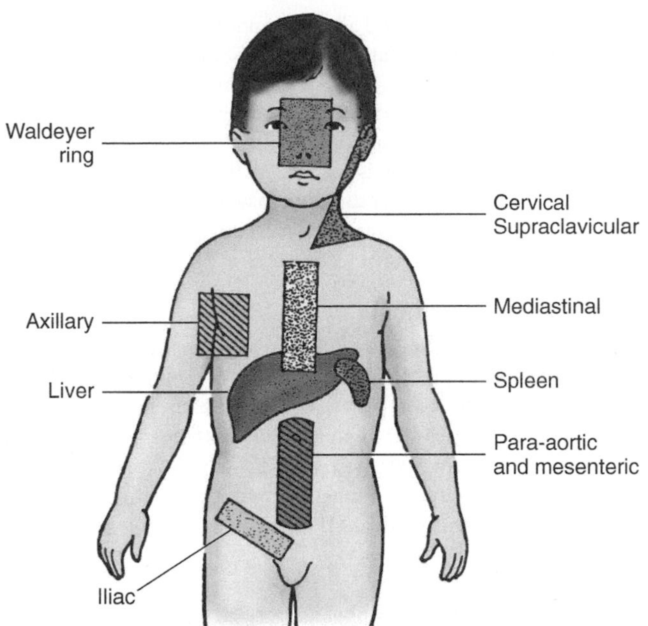

FIG. 29.4 Main areas of lymphadenopathy and organ involvement in Hodgkin disease.

type and extent of disease. In children NHL is more common than Hodgkin disease. Although Hodgkin disease is extremely rare before 5 years of age, there is a striking increase in children ages 15 to 19 years, when it occurs with almost the same frequency as leukemia. Epstein-Barr virus is thought to have a role in the causation of Hodgkin lymphoma (National Institutes of Health, 2017d).

Hodgkin Lymphoma

Hodgkin lymphoma affects about 29 in 1 million children (National Institutes of Health, 2017d). Hodgkin lymphoma has a childhood form, a young adult form, and an older adult form. In the United States the highest incidence is among adolescents. The malignancy originates in the lymphoid system and primarily involves the lymph nodes. It predictably metastasizes to nonnodal or extra lymphatic sites, especially the spleen, liver, bone marrow, lungs, and mediastinum (i.e., mass of tissues and organs separating the lungs, including the heart and its vessels, trachea, esophagus, thymus, and lymph nodes), although no tissue is exempt from involvement (Fig. 29.4). It is classified according to four histologic types: (1) lymphocytic predominance, (2) nodular sclerosis, (3) mixed cellularity, and (4) lymphocytic depletion.

Clinical Staging and Prognosis

Accurate staging of the extent of disease is the basis for treatment protocols and expected prognosis. More than one staging system exists; Box 29.2 shows the Ann Arbor Staging Classification.

Each stage is further subdivided into A, B, E, S, or X. Stage A denotes absence of associated general symptoms. Stage B indicates presence of symptoms, such as night sweats, fever (100.4°F [38°C]), or weight loss of 10% or more during the preceding 6 months. Stage E represents extra lymphatic disease beyond the contiguous nodal disease. Stage S indicates splenic involvement, and stage X indicates mediastinal bulky disease.

The prognosis for patients with Hodgkin lymphoma has improved dramatically, largely as a result of systematic staging, risk group stratification, and improved treatment protocols. The prognosis is excellent in children with localized disease. Overall survival rates for patients with Hodgkin lymphoma are as high as 95%; however, the survival rate is dependent on histology and staging (Frew, Lewis, & Lucraft, 2013).

BOX 29.2 Ann Arbor Staging of Hodgkin Disease

Stage I: Lesions are limited to one lymph node area or only one additional extralymphatic site (I_E), such as the liver, lungs, kidney, or intestines.
Stage II: Two or more lymph node regions on the same side of the diaphragm or one additional extralymphatic site or organ (II_E) on the same side of the diaphragm is involved.
Stage III: Lymph node regions on both sides of the diaphragm are involved with spread to one extralymphatic site (III_E), spleen (III_S), or both (III_{SE}).
Stage IV: Diffuse spread throughout the body to one or more extralymphatic sites with or without involvement of associated lymph nodes.

Even in those with disseminated disease, long-term remissions are possible in more than half the patients. For relapses, complete remission may occur in 30% to 60% of patients undergoing autologous SCT (Metzger, Krasin, Choi, et al., 2016).

Clinical Manifestations

Hodgkin lymphoma is characterized by painless enlargement of lymph nodes. The most common finding is enlarged, firm, nontender, movable nodes in the supraclavicular or cervical area. In children the lymph node located near the left clavicle may be the first enlarged node, which is referred to as the sentinel node. Enlargement of axillary and inguinal lymph nodes is less frequent.

Other signs and symptoms depend on the extent and location of involvement. Mediastinal lymphadenopathy may cause a persistent, nonproductive cough. Enlarged retroperitoneal nodes may produce unexplained abdominal pain. Systemic symptoms include low-grade or intermittent fever (Pel-Ebstein disease), anorexia, nausea, weight loss, night sweats, and pruritus. Generally, such symptoms indicate advanced lymph node and extralymphatic involvement.

Diagnostic Evaluation

The history and physical examination often yield important clues to the disease, such as a history of systemic symptoms, presence of a mediastinal mass, and enlargement of lymph nodes, spleen, or liver. Because multiple organs can become involved, the diagnostic evaluation requires several tests to confirm the diagnosis and assess the extent of involvement for accurate staging. Tests include CBC, biochemistry profile (lactate dehydrogenase, albumin, renal and hepatic function studies, alkaline phosphatase), erythrocyte sedimentation rate, C-reactive protein, and serum ferritin. Imaging tests include chest radiography, CT of neck and chest, and CT or MRI of abdomen and pelvis (Metzger, Krasin, Choi, et al., 2016).

A lymph node biopsy is essential to establish histologic diagnosis and staging. The presence of Hodgkin and Reed-Sternberg cells is considered diagnostic of Hodgkin disease because it is absent in the other lymphomas; however, it may occur in infectious mononucleosis. A bone marrow aspiration or biopsy also is usually performed.

Therapeutic Management

The primary treatment modalities for Hodgkin lymphoma are chemotherapy and irradiation. The length and intensity of therapy are based on disease-related factors (e.g., stage, number of involved nodal regions, tumor bulk, B symptoms, and early response); other factors that may be considered are age, sex, and histology (National Institutes of Health, 2017d). The goal of treatment is cure; however, aggressive therapy increases the chances of complications that can seriously compromise quality of life. One of the major concerns with combined radiation and cytotoxic drug therapy is the risk of serious late effects in children with an excellent prognosis. Consequently, treatment that is risk adapted and response based aims to minimize long-term complications. Because of the diversity of approaches to treatment, the following is an overview of general principles that may not apply to all children.

Most newly diagnosed children are treated with risk-adapted chemotherapy alone or in combination with radiation therapy. Radiation may entail involved field radiation, extended field radiation (involved areas plus adjacent nodes), or total nodal irradiation (the entire axial lymph node system), depending on the extent of involvement. Various combinations of chemotherapy drugs may be used, based on the most effective combinations used in the past: MOPP (methotrexate, vincristine [Oncovin], procarbazine, and prednisone) and ABVD (doxorubicin [Adriamycin], bleomycin, vinblastine, and dacarbazine). Today, COPP (substituting cyclophosphamide for methotrexate) has generally replaced MOPP. In addition, etoposide has been included in chemotherapy regimens in place of alkylating agents to reduce gonadal toxicity (National Institutes of Health, 2017d).

Follow-up care of children who have completed therapy is essential to identify relapse and long-term complications, especially SMNs. Children without a functioning spleen are at increased risk of infection; therefore prophylactic antibiotics are administered for an indefinite period, and survivors are advised to seek immediate medical care if they develop symptoms of infection even if they are taking antibiotics. Also, pneumococcal, meningococcal, and HIB immunizations are recommended. (See Chapter 6.)

Nursing Care Management

Nursing care involves preparation for diagnostic and operative procedures, explanation of treatment side effects, and child and family support. Once the child is hospitalized for suspected Hodgkin lymphoma, a battery of diagnostic tests is ordered. The family and child need an explanation of why each test is performed because many of them, such as bone marrow aspiration and lymph node biopsy, are invasive procedures. (See Chapter 22.)

Explanations of chemotherapeutic reactions are based on the specific drug regimen. The most common side effects, such as nausea and vomiting, body image changes, neuropathy, and mucosal ulceration, are discussed the Nursing Care Management section. Involved field radiation results in few side effects, sometimes consisting only of a mild skin reaction. With extended field radiation to the chest and abdomen, nausea and vomiting, weight loss, and mucosal ulceration (esophagitis, gastric ulcers) are common. The usual measures for providing relief are discussed previously in this chapter and outlined in Table 29.2.

The most common side effect of extensive irradiation is malaise, which may result from damage to the thyroid gland, causing hypothyroidism. Lack of energy is particularly difficult for adolescents because it prevents them from keeping up with their peers. Sometimes adolescents push themselves to the point of physical exhaustion rather than admit fatigue and give in to their decreased activity tolerance. Parents should observe for such behavior, such as extreme fatigue at the end of the day, falling asleep at the dinner table, inability to concentrate on homework, or an increased susceptibility to infection. Regular bedtimes and periodic rest times are important for these children, especially during chemotherapy, when myelosuppression increases the risk of infection and debilitation. Before discharge (if the child has been hospitalized), the nurse should discuss a feasible school schedule with the parents and child. If alterations are necessary, such as elimination of strenuous physical education, they are discussed with the teacher, school nurse, and principal. Follow-up care is essential to diagnose hypothyroidism early and institute thyroid replacement.

An area of concern for adolescents is the high risk of sterility from irradiation and chemotherapy. Both irradiation to the gonads and drugs, particularly procarbazine and alkylating agents, may lead to infertility. Younger patients with a greater complement of oocytes are more likely to retain ovarian function. Adolescents should be informed of these side effects, and any options for fertility preservation, early in the course of the diagnosis and treatment.

Although sexual function is not altered, the appearance of secondary sexual characteristics and menstruation may be delayed in the pubescent child. Delayed sexual maturation may be an extremely sensitive and painful area for children. (See Chapter 17.)

Non-Hodgkin Lymphoma

Approximately 750 to 800 new cases of NHL are diagnosed each year in the United States, with an incidence of 10 children per 1 million under the age of 20 years (Allen, Kamdar, Bollard, et al., 2016). The etiology of NHL is basically unknown, but possible risk factors include past cancer treatment, infection with Epstein-Barr virus or human immunodeficiency virus, and inherited or acquired immunodeficiency (National Institutes of Health, 2017e).

Staging and Prognosis

NHL exhibits a variety of morphologic, cytochemical, and immunologic features. Classification is based on immunophenotype, molecular biology, and clinical response to treatment, with the majority of cases categorized as lymphoblastic, mature B-cell (including Burkitt lymphoma), and anaplastic large cell lymphoma (National Institutes of Health, 2017e). Immunologically these cells are also classified as T cells; B cells (an example of which is Burkitt lymphoma); or non-T, non-B cells, which lack specific immunologic properties.

A favorable prognosis is defined by young age, low stage without mediastinal involvement, low tumor burden, and good response to initial therapy (Allen, Kamdar, Bollard, et al., 2016). The staging system used for Hodgkin lymphoma is not used for NHL. Box 29.3 presents the most commonly used NHL staging system.

The use of aggressive combination chemotherapy has had a major impact on NHL survival rates in children. The most effective treatment regimens result in cure in 85% to 95% of children with limited disease involvement, and 70% to 90% of children with extensive disease are cured (Allen, Kamdar, Bollard, et al., 2016).

Clinical Manifestations

Clinical manifestations depend on the anatomic site and extent of involvement. Many of the signs and symptoms seen in Hodgkin lymphoma may be present in NHL, although it is rare for a single symptom to lead to the diagnosis. Rather, metastasis to the bone marrow or CNS

BOX 29.3 St. Jude Staging of Non-Hodgkin Lymphoma

Stage I: Disease limited to one lymph node area or only one additional extralymphatic site (excluding thoracic or abdomen).

Stage II: Single tumor with regional lymph node involvement; two or more lymph node regions on the same side of the diaphragm; two single tumors with/without regional involvement on the same side of the diaphragm; or primary resectable gastrointestinal tumor with/without involvement of adjacent mesenteric nodes.

Stage III: Two single tumors on opposite sides of diaphragm; two nodal areas above/below the diaphragm; primary intrathoracic tumor or extensive intraabdominal disease; or paraspinal or epidural tumors.

Stage IV: Tumor has spread into central nervous system and/or bone marrow may produce signs and symptoms typical of leukemia. Lymphoid tumors compressing various organs may cause intestinal or airway obstruction, cranial nerve palsies, or spinal paralysis.

The exception to the usual presentation of NHL is Burkitt lymphoma, a type of cancer that is rare in the United States but endemic in parts of Africa. It is a rapidly growing neoplasm that is most commonly seen as a mass in the jaw, abdomen, or orbit. However, no anatomic site appears exempt from involvement. Peripheral lymphadenopathy, hepatosplenomegaly, or signs of conversion to leukemia are rarely seen.

Diagnostic Evaluation

Current recommendations for diagnostic evaluation and staging include history and physical examination; blood chemistries; total body imaging (CT, PET, MRI); LP; bone marrow aspiration; and biopsy. Cancer cells are examined by immunophenotyping (immunohistochemistry, flow cytometry), cytogenetics, and/or FISH (National Institutes of Health, 2017e).

Therapeutic Management

Because NHL is generally considered to be widespread at diagnosis, most children are treated with combination chemotherapy. The role of radiation is limited, although it may be used in children who do not have a complete response to chemotherapy (National Institutes of Health, 2017e). Treatment for NHL is based on histologic subtype. Lymphoblastic lymphoma therapy is similar to leukemia therapy; the protocols include induction, consolidation, and maintenance phases, some with intrathecal chemotherapy with or without cranial-spinal radiation therapy. The most commonly used chemotherapy regimens for newly diagnosed lymphoblastic lymphoma include prednisone, dexamethasone, vincristine, daunorubicin, doxorubicin, L-asparaginase, cyclophosphamide, cytarabine, methotrexate, 6-mercaptopurine, 6-thioguanine, and intrathecal treatments during maintenance. Newly diagnosed children with diffuse mature B-cell lymphoma are treated with surgery (stage I and II only) and chemotherapy; those with anaplastic large cell lymphoma are treated with surgery (stage I) and chemotherapy. These multiagent regimens are administered for 6 to 24 months.

Nursing Care Management

Nursing care of the child with NHL is similar to the care discussed under Nursing Care of the Child with Cancer. With intensive chemotherapy, nursing care is primarily directed toward managing the side effects of these agents.

NERVOUS SYSTEM TUMORS

BRAIN TUMORS

Tumors of the CNS are the most common solid tumor in children and account for about 25% of all childhood cancers, with an annual incidence of 5 per 100,000 children less than 20 years of age in the United States (Crawford, 2013). About 60% of the tumors are infratentorial (below the tentorium cerebelli), which means they occur in the posterior part of the brain, primarily in the cerebellum or brainstem. This anatomic distribution accounts for the frequency of symptoms resulting from increased intracranial pressure (ICP). The other tumors are supratentorial or lie within the midbrain structures. Fig. 29.5 shows the major brain tumors of childhood.

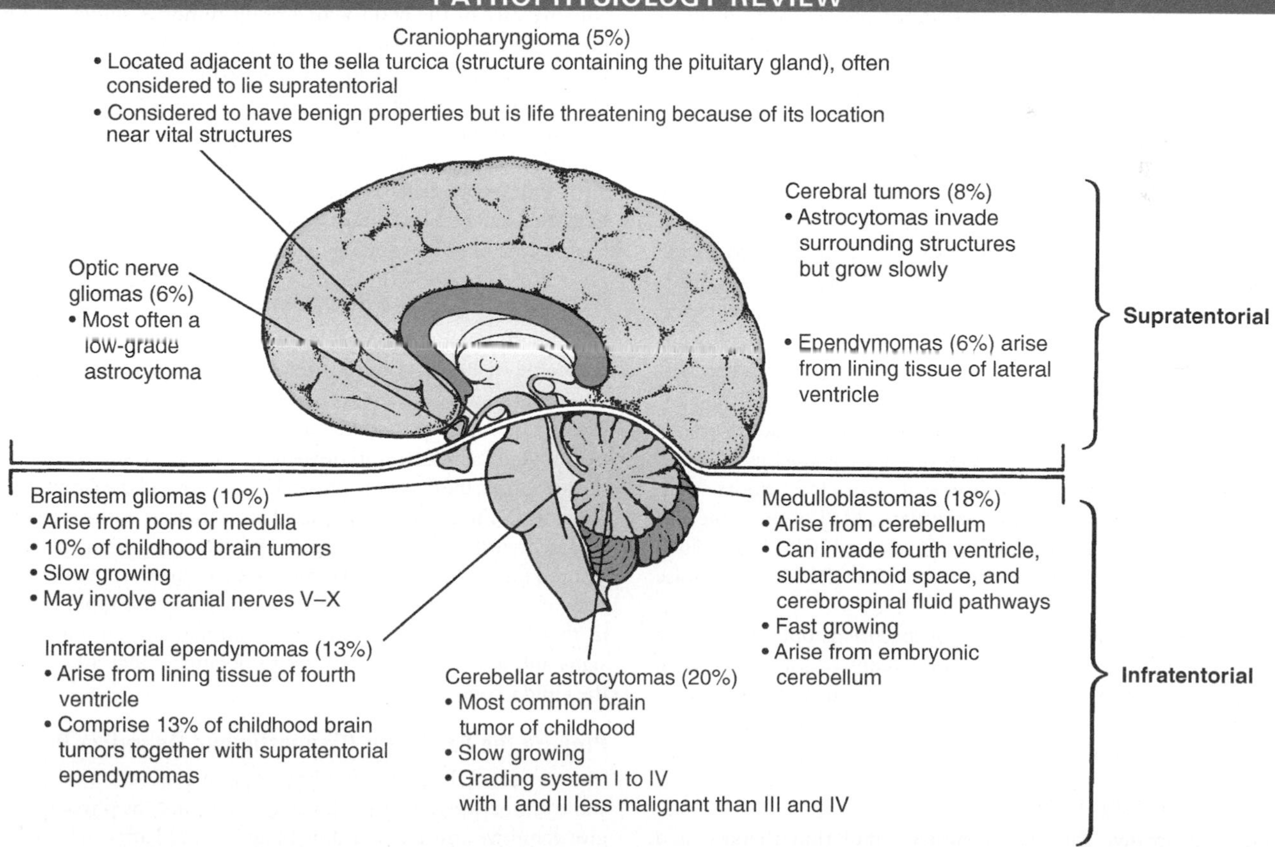
PATHOPHYSIOLOGY REVIEW
Craniopharyngioma (5%)
• Located adjacent to the sella turcica (structure containing the pituitary gland), often considered to lie supratentorial
• Considered to have benign properties but is life threatening because of its location near vital structures
Optic nerve gliomas (6%)
• Most often a low-grade astrocytoma
Cerebral tumors (8%)
• Astrocytomas invade surrounding structures but grow slowly
• Ependymomas (6%) arise from lining tissue of lateral ventricle
Supratentorial
Brainstem gliomas (10%)
• Arise from pons or medulla
• 10% of childhood brain tumors
• Slow growing
• May involve cranial nerves V–X
Infratentorial ependymomas (13%)
• Arise from lining tissue of fourth ventricle
• Comprise 13% of childhood brain tumors together with supratentorial ependymomas
Cerebellar astrocytomas (20%)
• Most common brain tumor of childhood
• Slow growing
• Grading system I to IV with I and II less malignant than III and IV
Medulloblastomas (18%)
• Arise from cerebellum
• Can invade fourth ventricle, subarachnoid space, and cerebrospinal fluid pathways
• Fast growing
• Arise from embryonic cerebellum
Infratentorial

FIG. 29.5 Location of brain tumors in children. (From McCance, K. L., & Huether, S. E. [2014]. *Pathophysiology: The biological basis for disease in adults and children* [7th ed.]. St. Louis, MO: Elsevier.)

Because brain tumors can arise from any cell within the cranium, it is possible to have tumors originating from the glial cells, nerve cells, neuroepithelium, cranial nerves, blood vessels, pineal gland, and hypophysis. Within each of these structures, specific cells may be involved that provide a histologic classification. For example, astrocytes, cells that form most of the supportive tissue for the neurons, may form astrocytomas, the most common glial tumor. Brain tumors may be benign or malignant, although what matters the most is location, given the vital functions the brain controls. A small percentage of childhood brain tumors is associated with genetic predisposition; examples include Li-Fraumeni syndrome and neurofibromatosis. Other known risk factors include cranial irradiation and immunosuppression (Parsons, Pollack, Hass-Kogan, et al., 2016). Genomic studies of brain tumors are an active area of research.

Clinical Manifestations

The signs and symptoms of brain tumors are directly related to their anatomic location, tumor size, and to some extent the child's age. For instance, in infants whose sutures are still open, a bulging fontanel indicates hydrocephalus. Head circumference measurements allow for detection of increased head size. Even in older children, clinical manifestations may be nonspecific. However, the most common symptoms of infratentorial brain tumors are headache, especially on awakening, and vomiting that is not related to feeding. Tumors in this area of the brain often obstruct the flow of cerebrospinal fluid, causing increased ICP and the symptoms mentioned earlier. In addition, patients may have symptoms related to the specific structure involved. Tumors of the cerebellum often cause nystagmus, ataxia, dysarthria, and dysmetria. Supratentorial symptoms more commonly include seizures, personality or behavioral changes, visual disturbances, and hemiparesis. Tumors involving the structures of the midbrain, including the hypothalamus and pituitary gland, may cause endocrinopathies such as diabetes insipidus, delayed or precocious puberty, and growth failure. Table 29.4 shows the common presenting symptoms of brain tumors.

Diagnostic Evaluation

Diagnosis of a brain tumor is based on presenting clinical signs and diagnostic imaging. Because the signs and symptoms may be vague and easily overlooked, early diagnosis requires a high index of suspicion during history taking. A number of tests may be employed in the neurologic evaluation (see Table 30.1), but the gold standard diagnostic procedure is MRI, which permits early diagnosis of brain tumors and assessment of tumor growth during or after treatment. Diffusion-weighted imaging, spectroscopy, and perfusion imaging are other MRI tools used to investigate and diagnose tumor types (Poussaint, Panigrahy, & Huisman, 2015). The CT scan permits direct visualization of the brain parenchyma, ventricles, and surrounding subarachnoid space, and it is commonly used in urgent cases of suspected tumors when MRI is not available. Other tests may include an MRI of the spine and electroencephalography. In the presence of increased ICP, LP is avoided due to the danger of possible brainstem herniation after sudden release of pressure.

Definitive diagnosis is based on tissue specimens obtained during surgery. Occasionally, special techniques are required for determining the cell type. Because of the location of some brain tumors, such as brainstem tumors, a biopsy is not possible and the diagnosis is made by imaging findings alone.

Therapeutic Management

Treatment may involve the use of surgery, radiation therapy, and chemotherapy. All three may or may not be used, depending on the type of tumor. The treatment of choice is total removal of the tumor without residual neurologic damage. Patients with the most complete tumor removal have the greatest chance of survival. Several surgical advances have allowed the biopsy and removal of tumors in areas previously considered too dangerous for traditional operative techniques. Stereotactic surgery involves the use of CT and MRI in conjunction with other special computer techniques to reconstruct the tumor in three dimensions. With computer-assisted instruments, total resection of the tumor is sometimes possible. Stereotactic biopsy is performed with CT or MRI computer guidance for inserting the biopsy needle. This procedure has the benefit of a shorter hospital stay and a lower morbidity and mortality rate in comparison with an open craniotomy (Parsons, Pollack, Hass-Kogan, et al., 2016). Other procedures include the use of lasers to vaporize tumor tissue and brain mapping to determine the precise location of critical brain areas to avoid during surgery.

Radiation therapy is used to treat most tumors and to shrink the size of the tumor before attempting surgical removal. The use of chemotherapy has had an increasingly important role, either in combination with surgery and/or radiation, or alone. All three modes of therapy are associated with serious late effects. Surgery can cause injury to important areas of the brain, especially when the surgeon is attempting to remove invasive tumors. The long-term consequences of radiation therapy include tissue necrosis, subsequent malignancies, endocrine dysfunction, and behavioral or intellectual deficits. For these reasons, the use of irradiation is deferred for as long as possible in young children. Chemotherapy may allow a delay or reduction in radiation therapy. Proton beam radiation therapy, available at some sites, is being studied to learn whether it offers greater efficacy and less long-term toxicity (Parsons, Pollack, Hass-Kogan, et al., 2016).

Nursing Care Management

Nursing care of the child with a brain tumor is similar regardless of the type of intracranial lesion. Because a brain tumor is potentially fatal, the reader is urged to incorporate the psychologic interventions discussed in Chapter 19 with those elaborated on in this section. However, it is important to remember that many brain tumors are curable. Medulloblastoma, for instance, has a survival rate of approximately 80% in those patients without metastatic disease. Despite the grave nature of some brain tumors, new and emerging therapies are bringing hope to the families of many pediatric brain tumor patients.

Assess for Signs and Symptoms

A child admitted to the hospital with neurologic dysfunction is often suspected of having a brain tumor, even though the actual diagnosis is not yet confirmed. Establishing a baseline of data for comparing preoperative and postoperative changes is an essential step toward planning physical care and preventing complications. It also allows the nurse to assess the degree of physical incapacity and the family's emotional reaction to the diagnosis. For example, children with cerebellar astrocytoma may have displayed vague cerebellar symptoms for several years before a tumor is suspected. For these parents the revelation of a neoplasm may be as shocking as for those who witnessed a rapid deterioration in their child's abilities. Table 29.4 summarizes common presenting signs and assessment procedures to document significant changes in the child's condition.

Prepare the Family for Diagnostic and Operative Procedures

The suspected diagnosis of a brain tumor is always a crisis. Although some tumors are removed with excellent results, the physician can rarely give definitive answers regarding prognosis until after surgery. Therefore parents, the child, and other family members require much emotional support to face the diagnostic procedures and a craniotomy.

TABLE 29.4 Clinical Manifestations and Assessment of Brain Tumors

Signs and Symptoms	Assessment
Headache	
Recurrent and progressive In frontal or occipital areas Usually dull and throbbing Worse on arising, less during day Intensified by lowering head and straining, such as during bowel movement, coughing, sneezing	Record description of pain, location, severity, and duration. Use pain rating scale to assess severity of pain. (See Chapter 5.) Note changes in relation to time of day and activity. Observe changes in behavior in infants (e.g., persistent irritability, crying, head rolling).
Vomiting	
With or without nausea or feeding Progressively more projectile More severe in morning on arising Relieved by moving about and changing position	Record time, amount, and relationship to feeding, nausea, and activity.
Neuromuscular Changes	
Incoordination or clumsiness Loss of balance (e.g., use of wide-based stance, falling, tripping, banging into objects) Poor fine motor control Weakness Hyporeflexia or hyperreflexia Positive Babinski sign Spasticity Paralysis	Test muscle strength, gait, coordination, and reflexes. (See Chapter 4.)
Behavioral Changes	
Irritability Decreased appetite Failure to thrive Fatigue (frequent naps) Lethargy Coma Bizarre behavior (e.g., staring, automatic movements)	Observe behavior regularly. Compare observations with parental reports of normal behavioral patterns. Monitor growth and food intake. Monitor activity and sleep.
Cranial Nerve Neuropathy	
Cranial nerve involvement varied according to tumor location Most common signs: • Head tilt • Visual defects (e.g., nystagmus, diplopia, strabismus, episodic "graying out" of vision, visual field defect)	Assess cranial nerves, especially VII (facial), IX (glossopharyngeal), X (vagus), V (trigeminal, sensory roots), and VI (abducens). (See Chapter 4.) Assess visual acuity, binocularity, and peripheral vision. (See Chapter 4.)
Vital Sign Disturbances	
Decreased pulse and respiration Increased blood pressure Decreased pulse pressure Hypothermia or hyperthermia	Measure vital signs frequently. Monitor pulse and respirations for 1 full minute. Record pulse pressure (difference between systolic and diastolic blood pressure).
Other Signs	
Seizures Cranial enlargement* Tense, bulging fontanel at rest* Nuchal rigidity Papilledema (edema of optic nerve)	Record seizure activity. (See Chapter 30.) Measure head circumference daily (infant and young child). Perform funduscopic examination if skilled in procedure.

*Present only in infants and young children.

How the child is prepared for the diagnostic tests depends on the child's age and experience. Chapter 22 discusses preparing children for an MRI or a CT scan. Once surgery is scheduled, the child needs an explanation of what to expect. By the time most children are late preschoolers, they know that the head and brain are important parts of their body. It may be helpful to have children draw their concept of the brain to clarify misconceptions and base the explanation on their level of understanding. Although it may be tempting to justify the surgery by stating that removing the tumor will take away various symptoms, the nurse should refrain from emphasizing this point too strenuously. Postsurgical headaches and cerebellar symptoms, such as ataxia, may be aggravated rather than improved. Surgery may not improve vision. With optic gliomas the child will be blind in one eye even if the tumor is fully resected. Finally, surgical removal of the mass may be impossible, and after surgery, functioning may temporarily deteriorate or result in permanent damage. Being honest before surgery most often makes honesty after the procedure easier because no false hopes were created.

It is best to deliver information in small amounts to let the child pursue additional answers. For example, some children ask about what happens when part of the tumor is left. An honest reply is that after surgery the physician will try to shrink the tumor with special x-rays and medicines. Delay a further explanation of irradiation or chemotherapy until a decision regarding these treatments is made.

The hair is usually shaved in the operating room just before surgery, or sometimes in the child's room, usually the night before surgery. When shaving is done with the child awake, the procedure is approached in a sensitive, positive way. If the child's hair is long, braid it so that the long swatch can be saved. Showing children how they look at different stages of the process helps them prepare for their changed appearance.

Once the hair is clipped short or shaved, give the child a cap or scarf to camouflage the baldness. Take every precaution to provide privacy during the procedure and to protect the child from teasing or ridicule by other children before surgery. Also emphasize that the hair will regrow shortly after surgery. Depending on the child's immediate adjustment to the hair loss, the nurse may introduce the idea of wearing a wig until the hair grows in, particularly if additional irradiation or chemotherapy is anticipated.

Also tell children about the size of the dressing. Usually the entire scalp is covered to maintain tight wound closure, even if a small incision is made. Infratentorial head dressings may be attached to the upper back and extend forward to the neck to maintain slight extension and alignment as a precaution against wound rupture. Applying a similar dressing or "special hat" to a doll is often a less traumatic way of demonstrating the physical appearance.

Children also need a brief explanation of how they will feel after surgery and where they will be. Ordinarily they will return to a special intensive care unit, which they may visit beforehand, depending on hospital policy. They should be aware that they may be sleepy for some time after surgery and that a headache is likely, which may last a few days.

Parents need similar explanations before surgery, especially in terms of special equipment used in the intensive care unit, dressings, and their child's behavior. For example, they should know that it is not unusual for the child to be lethargic for a few days after surgery. The nurse may wish to encourage less frequent visiting during this period so that parents can rest and be able to support their child when the child is awake.

The nurse should participate in preoperative conferences with the physician and parents. The nurse needs to know what information the parents have been given in order to provide further explanations or emotional support when necessary.

! NURSING ALERT

Report sluggish, dilated, or unequal pupils immediately because they may indicate increased ICP and potential brainstem herniation—a medical emergency.

Prevent Postoperative Complications

After surgery the surgeon prescribes specific orders for taking vital signs, positioning, regulating fluids, and administering medication. These vary somewhat, depending on the location of the craniotomy. The following are general principles of care for patients undergoing infratentorial or supratentorial surgery. Chapter 30 discusses additional aspects of care, such as care of the child with seizures and care of the unconscious child in terms of respiratory status and neurologic assessment.

Assessment

Vital signs are taken as often as every 15 to 30 minutes until the patient is stable. Temperature measurement is particularly important because of hyperthermia resulting from surgical intervention in the hypothalamus or brainstem and from some types of general anesthesia. To prepare for this reaction, a cooling blanket may be placed on the bed before the child returns to the unit, or it may be used when needed. Because the temperature control centers are affected and hypothermia can occur suddenly, the nurse monitors body temperature often when any cooling measures are employed.

! NURSING ALERT

To keep an accurate account of drainage, circle the soiled area with a pen and monitor for signs of continuous bleeding. The presence of colorless drainage is reported immediately because it most likely is cerebrospinal fluid leaking from the incisional area. A foul odor from the dressing may indicate an infection. Such a finding is reported, and a culture is taken.

The most likely types of infection are meningitis and respiratory tract infection. The probable cause of meningitis is wound contamination. The risk of respiratory tract infections is high because of the imposed immobility, danger of aspiration, and possible respiratory depression from the brainstem. The usual precautions of deep breathing and turning as allowed are instituted. Regular pulmonary assessments are performed to identify adventitious sounds or any areas of diminished or absent breath sounds. Blood pressure is also taken at frequent intervals. The deflated cuff is left on the arm between readings to allow for the least movement and disturbance of the child. Ocular signs are recorded at least every hour.

As soon as possible the nurse should begin testing reflexes, hand grip, and functioning of the cranial nerves. Muscle strength is usually reduced after surgery because of general weakness but should improve daily. Ataxia may be significantly worse with cerebellar intervention, but it slowly improves. Edema near the cranial nerves may depress important functions such as the gag, blink, or swallowing reflex.

Neurologic checks are an essential aspect of care and include pupillary reaction to light, level of consciousness, sleep patterns, and response to stimuli. Although children may be comatose for a few days, once they regain consciousness there should be a steady increase in alertness. Regression to a lethargic, irritable state indicates increasing pressure, possibly caused by meningitis, hemorrhage, or edema.

Dressings are observed for evidence of drainage. If soiled, the dressing is not removed but reinforced with dry sterile gauze. The approximate amount of drainage is estimated and recorded.

Once the younger child is alert, the arms may need to be restrained to preserve the dressing. Even a child who has been cooperative before surgery must be closely supervised during the initial stages of regaining consciousness, when disorientation and restlessness are common. Elbow restraints are satisfactory to prevent the hands from reaching the head, although additional restraint may be necessary to preserve an infusion line and maintain a specific position.

Positioning

Correct positioning after surgery is critical to prevent pressure against the operative site, reduce ICP, and avoid the danger of aspiration. If a large tumor was removed, the child is not placed on the operative side because the brain may suddenly shift to that cavity, causing trauma to the blood vessels, linings, and the brain itself. The nurse confers with the surgeon to be certain of the correct position, including the degree of neck flexion. The first 24 to 48 hours after brain surgery are critical. If positioning is restricted, notice of this is posted above the head of the bed. When the child is turned, every precaution is used to prevent jarring or misalignment to prevent undue strain on the sutures. Two nurses, one supporting the head and the other the body, are needed. The use of a turning sheet may facilitate turning a heavy child.

> **! NURSING ALERT**
>
> The Trendelenburg position is contraindicated in both infratentorial and supratentorial surgeries because it increases ICP and the risk of hemorrhage. If shock is impending, the practitioner is notified immediately, before the head is lowered.

The child with an infratentorial craniotomy is usually positioned flat and on either side. Pillows should be placed against the child's back, not head, to maintain the desired position. Ordinarily the head and neck are kept in midline with the body and slightly extended. After a supratentorial craniotomy the head is usually elevated above the heart to facilitate cerebrospinal fluid drainage and decrease excessive blood flow to the brain to prevent hemorrhage.

Fluid Regulation

With an infratentorial craniotomy the child is allowed nothing by mouth for at least 24 hours or longer if the gag and swallowing reflexes are depressed or the child is comatose. With a supratentorial procedure, feeding may be resumed soon after the child is alert, sometimes within 24 hours. Clear water is always started first because of the danger of aspiration. If the child vomits, stop oral liquids. Vomiting not only predisposes the child to aspiration but also increases ICP and the risk for incisional rupture.

IV fluids are continued until fluids are well tolerated by mouth. Because of cerebral edema postoperatively and the danger of increased ICP, fluids are carefully monitored and usually infused less than the maintenance rate. If drugs, such as prophylactic antibiotics, are given intravenously the medication amount is calculated as part of the IV fluid. For example, if the child is to receive 20 ml/hr and the diluted drug is 5 ml, the IV solution is reduced to 15 ml for that hour.

A hypertonic solution such as mannitol may be necessary to remove excess fluid. These drugs cause rapid diuresis. After surgery the child may have a Foley catheter in place. Urinary output is monitored after administration of these drugs to evaluate their effectiveness.

When able to take fluids, the child should be fed to conserve strength and minimize movement. If there is any sign of facial paralysis, the child is fed slowly to prevent choking or aspiration. Scrupulous mouth care is essential to prevent oral infection. Sometimes gavage feeding is necessary when body functions are too depressed to permit safe oral feedings or the child refuses to eat or drink. In the latter instance the nurse should employ every measure to encourage acceptance of fluids or solids. (See Chapter 22 for nursing interventions.)

Comfort Measures

Headache may be severe and is largely the result of cerebral edema. Measures to relieve some of the discomfort include providing a quiet, dimly lit environment; restricting visitors; preventing any sudden jarring movement, such as banging into the bed; and preventing an increase in ICP. The last is most effectively achieved by proper positioning and prevention of straining, such as during coughing, vomiting, or defecating. The use of opioids, such as morphine, to relieve pain has been controversial because it is thought that they may mask signs of altered consciousness or depress respirations. However, opioids are considered safe because naloxone can be used to reverse opioid effects, such as sedation or respiratory depression. Acetaminophen and codeine are also effective analgesics. Regardless of the drugs used, adequate dosage and regular administration are essential to provide optimum pain relief. (See Pain Assessment and Pain Management, Chapter 5.)

Monitor bowel movements to prevent constipation. Stool softeners may be given as soon as liquids are tolerated to facilitate easy passage of stool.

Brain edema may severely depress the gag reflex, necessitating suctioning of oral secretions. Facial edema may also be present, necessitating eye care if the lids remain partially open. Ice compresses applied to the eyes for short periods help relieve the edema. A depressed blink reflex also predisposes the corneas to ulceration. Irrigating the eyes with saline drops and covering them with eye dressings are important steps in preventing this complication.

Support the Family

The family's informational and support needs are great when the diagnosis is a brain tumor, and are influenced by the extent of surgery, any neurologic deficits, the prognosis, and additional therapy. Because few definitive answers can be given before surgery, the surgeon's report is a significant finding that can vary from a completely benign, resected neoplasm to a highly malignant, invasive, and only partially removed tumor. Although parents try to prepare themselves for a potentially fatal diagnosis, it is understandably a shock for them.

Ideally, a nurse who will be involved in the continuing care of this child should be with the family when the physician discusses the prognosis and plan of therapy. Although parents may hear only a fraction of what they are told, they can begin to put the future into perspective. Regardless of the future prospects, direct the parents' thinking toward helping the child recover and resume a normal life to his or her fullest potential. Providing the opportunity for the family to share their concerns and questions with other families who have a child with a brain tumor may help the family cope, and the nurse can direct them to resources.*

It is also a time to encourage parents to verbalize their feelings about the diagnosis. Often they express guilt for attributing the insidious onset of symptoms, such as ataxia, visual difficulty, or headache, to

*Information about support groups is available from the National Brain Tumor Society, 22 Battery St., Suite 612, San Francisco, CA 94111; 800-934-CURE; e-mail: info@braintumor.org; http://www.braintumor.org; and the Pediatric Brain Tumor Foundation, 302 Ridgefield Court, Asheville, NC 28806; 800-253-6530; email: info@curethekids.org; http://www.curethekids.org.

minor "complaints" by the child. Parents may have punished their child for clumsiness, mistaking it for carelessness, or for their declining performance in school. The nurse listens to such statements and emphasizes the normality of the parents' reactions. Sometimes it may be helpful to start a discussion with a statement such as "It is difficult to know when a child's complaints are significant because so often they are caused by minor ailments and you would never have imagined they were the result of a brain tumor." The nurse avoids any comments that insinuate the parents should have sought medical advice sooner because such remarks only add to the parents' guilt feelings.

During this period the nurse should also discuss with parents what they plan to tell the child. If the child was prepared honestly, as described previously, the diagnosis can be expressed in a similar manner, such as "The surgeon removed most of the tumor, and the rest will be treated with special drugs and x-ray treatments." During recovery the child needs additional explanation about the treatment and the reason for residual neurologic effects, such as ataxia or blindness. Hair loss is a normal concern for the child, and its regrowth will be delayed, depending on the length of therapy. This is an appropriate time to reintroduce the idea of a wig.

Promote Return to Optimum Functioning

The ultimate goal is a cured child who has optimum functioning. As soon as possible, the child should resume usual activities within tolerable limits, especially returning to school.* Until the skull is completely healed, the child may need to wear a helmet when engaging in any active sport. This decision is made by the child's neurosurgeon. The school nurse and teacher should confer with the parents on activity restrictions, such as physical education, as well as the reactions of schoolmates to the child's appearance.

After discharge the family needs continuing medical and emotional support from health personnel. Children who are long-term survivors after treatment for a brain tumor require ongoing follow-up due to residual disabilities, such as short stature, cranial nerve palsies, sensory defects, motor abnormalities (especially ataxia), intellectual deficits, dysphagia, dysgraphia, and behavioral problems (Parsons, Pollack, Hass-Kogan, et al., 2016).

The realm of all possible consequences after the diagnosis of a brain tumor is not discussed here. The reader is referred to other sections of the text that deal with possible outcomes, such as the paralyzed, visually impaired, or unconscious child or the child with a ventricular shunt, seizure disorder, or meningitis. Numerous physical problems can occur with progression of the tumor that may necessitate additional procedures. For example, frequent vomiting, anorexia, and nausea may require nonoral routes of feeding, such as gastrostomy or parenteral alimentation. Trials with chemotherapy may necessitate the use of central venous access devices. Whenever these procedures are instituted, the nurse may be responsible for teaching the family appropriate home care to allow the child the highest quality of life for the longest time. (See discussion of discharge planning and home care in Chapter 21.)

NEUROBLASTOMA

Neuroblastoma is the most common extracranial childhood solid tumor. Approximately 800 new cases of neuroblastoma are diagnosed every year in the United States (Brodeur, Hogarty, Bagatell, et al., 2016). It is a disease of infancy and early childhood, with the median age at diagnosis of about 19 months (Brodeur, Hogarty, Bagatell, et al., 2016). Neuroblastoma can occur in a hereditary form, and two genes that play a part in hereditary neuroblastoma have been identified, as have other genes that contribute to neuroblastoma predisposition (Brodeur, Hogarty, Bagatell, et al., 2016). Within the tumor cells, a hallmark is amplification of an oncogene, *MYCN*. Neuroblastomas originate from embryonic neural crest cells that normally give rise to the adrenal medulla and the sympathetic nervous system. Consequently, the majority of the tumors arise from the adrenal gland or from the retroperitoneal sympathetic chain.

Clinical Manifestations

The signs and symptoms of neuroblastoma depend on the location and extent of disease (National Institutes of Health, 2017f). The most common primary site is within the abdomen; other sites include the head and neck region, chest, and pelvis. With abdominal tumors, the most common presenting sign is a firm, nontender, irregular mass in the abdomen that crosses the midline (in contrast to Wilms tumor, which is usually confined to one side). Other signs related to abdominal location include pain or discomfort, vomiting, anorexia, and respiratory compromise; compression of the kidney, ureter, or bladder may cause urinary frequency or retention. Tumors in the thoracic or cervical region can involve dyspnea, Horner syndrome (ptosis, miosis, anhidrosis), neck mass, stridor, and dysphagia. Spinal cord and brain sites can present with neurologic deficits, difficulty breathing, bladder and bowel dysfunction, paraparesis, paraplegia, or seizures. Neuroblastoma that infiltrates the bone marrow can produce anemia, thrombocytopenia, and neutropenia. Tumors in the orbit/optic nerves can produce exophthalmos, periorbital ecchymosis, and impaired vision. Tumors in bone can result in pain/limping. Metastases to the skin can appear as subcutaneous skin nodules, described as "blueberry muffin lesions" due to their color; this is usually only seen in infants.

Diagnostic Evaluation

Diagnostic evaluation is aimed at determining the primary site and extent of disease. Tumor imaging by CT or MRI is used to locate the primary tumor in neck, chest, abdomen, and pelvis. Evaluation for metastases includes examination of the bone marrow with bilateral aspirates and biopsies and the bony skeleton with iodine-131 metaiodobenzylguanidine (I-MIBG) scanning.

Neuroblastomas, particularly those arising on the adrenal glands or from a sympathetic chain, excrete the catecholamines epinephrine and norepinephrine. Urinary excretion of catecholamine metabolites (vanillylmandelic acid [VMA] and homovanillic acid [HVA]) is measured before therapy; these markers can be used to monitor response to therapy and detection of relapse after therapy (National Institutes of Health, 2017f). Diagnosis is based on the presence of tumor cells in a biopsy of tumor tissue (biopsy also provides tissue for determining *MYCN* copy number [amplification] and other chromosomal/genetic tests) or the presence of tumor cells in bone marrow plus increased urinary catecholamine metabolites (National Institutes of Health, 2017f).

Staging and Prognosis

Neuroblastoma is a "silent" tumor. In more than 70% of cases, diagnosis is made after metastasis occurs, with the first signs caused by involvement in a nonprimary site, usually the lymph nodes, bone marrow, skeletal system, or liver. The staging system in widespread use is the International Neuroblastoma Staging System, which is based on histology and extent of disease (Box 29.4). Newer staging systems that incorporate multiple other parameters are being used in clinical trials.

---

*The American Brain Tumor Association has information on returning to school, 8550 W. Bryn Mawr Ave. Suite 550, Chicago, IL 60631; 1-800-886-2282; e-mail: info@abta.org; http://www.abta.org.

BOX 29.4 Staging of Neuroblastoma by International Neuroblastoma Staging System

Stage 1: Localized tumor that is confined to the area of origin and complete gross excision; representative ipsilateral lymph nodes negative for tumor microscopically (nodes that are attached to and removed with the primary tumor may be positive)

Stage 2A: Unilateral tumor with incomplete gross resection; representative ipsilateral nonadherent lymph nodes and contralateral lymph nodes negative for tumor microscopically

Stage 2B: Unilateral tumor with or without complete gross excision, with ipsilateral nonadherent lymph nodes positive for tumor; enlarged contralateral lymph nodes must be negative microscopically

Stage 3: Tumor infiltrating across the midline, with or without regional lymph node involvement; or localized unilateral tumor with contralateral regional lymph node involvement; or midline tumor with bilateral lymph node involvement

Stage 4: Dissemination of tumor to distant lymph nodes, bone, bone marrow, liver, skin, and/or other organs

Stage 4S: Localized primary tumor (as defined for stage 1, 2A, or 2B) with dissemination limited to liver, skin, or bone marrow but not to bone

Factors that influence prognosis include age, site of primary tumor, tumor histology, regional lymph node involvement, response to treatment, and biologic features such as *MYCN* amplification (National Institutes of Health, 2017f). At 5 years after diagnosis, the survival rate for children younger than 1 year is 90%; older children with advanced-stage disease have a much lower chance for cure (National Institutes of Health, 2017f). Adrenal primary tumors are more often associated with unfavorable prognostic features, in contrast to thoracic tumors, which have fewer deaths and recurrences. Certain characteristics of neuroblastoma tumor histology are prognostically favorable (e.g., cellular differentiation/maturation). Children who have metastatic disease in lymph nodes that cross the midline and are on the opposite side of the body from the primary tumor have a poorer prognosis. Poor response to treatment (e.g., persistence of neuroblastoma cells in bone marrow) predicts a poor prognosis. Neuroblastoma is one of the few tumors that demonstrate spontaneous regression (especially stage 4S), possibly as a result of maturation of the embryonic cell or development of an active immune system.

Therapeutic Management

Accurate clinical staging is important for establishing initial treatment. Therefore the purpose of surgery is both to remove as much of the tumor as possible and to obtain biopsies. In stages 1 and 2, complete surgical removal of the tumor is the treatment of choice. If the tumors are large, partial resection is attempted, with a course of radiation therapy postoperatively to shrink the tumor in the hope of complete removal at a later date. Surgery is usually limited to biopsy in stages 3 and 4 because of extensive metastasis.

The precise role of radiation therapy is unclear. It does not appear to be of any benefit in children with stage 1 and 2 disease. It can be used with stage 3 disease, although it may not improve survival expectancy. Radiotherapy for paraspinal neuroblastoma is no longer recommended because the radiation therapy has long-term morbidity and chemotherapy is a safe and effective initial treatment modality (Brodeur, Hogarty, Bagatell, et al., 2016).

Chemotherapy is the mainstay of therapy for extensive local or disseminated disease. The drugs are administered in a variety of combinations according to specific protocols. In addition, the use of consolidative myeloablative therapy using autologous marrow or peripheral stem cells followed by 13-*cis*-retinoic acid has improved the outcome of patients with high-risk disease.

Nursing Care Management

Nursing care management is similar to that discussed under Nursing Care of the Child with Cancer, including psychologic and physical preparation for diagnostic and operative procedures; prevention of postoperative complications for abdominal, thoracic, or cranial surgery; and explanation of chemotherapy and radiation therapy and their side effects.

Because this tumor carries a poor prognosis for many children, the nurse evaluates and addresses the needs of the family in terms of coping with a life-threatening illness. (See Chapter 19.) Because of the high frequency of metastasis at the time of diagnosis, many parents suffer guilt for not having recognized signs earlier. Parents need skilled support in dealing with these feelings and expressing them to the appropriate members of the health care team.

BONE TUMORS

GENERAL CONSIDERATIONS

Osteosarcoma and Ewing sarcoma are the primary bone tumors that occur most often in young people. Although both are bone tumors, they are different in many ways. Osteosarcoma is the most common bone tumor in adolescents and young adults, with approximately 400 new cases annually in the United States (National Institutes of Health, 2017g). Ewing sarcoma is less common, with about 200 cases diagnosed annually among children under the age of 20 years in the United States (Hawkins, Brennan, Bolling, et al., 2016). Ewing sarcoma occurs predominantly in Caucasians and more than half are adolescents (National Institutes of Health, 2017h).

Clinical Manifestations

Most malignant bone tumors produce localized pain in the affected site, which may be severe or dull and may be attributed to trauma or the vague complaint of "growing pains." The pain is often relieved by a flexed position, which relaxes the muscles overlying the stretched periosteum. Frequently a bone tumor draws attention when the child limps, curtails physical activity, or is unable to hold heavy objects. A palpable mass is also a common manifestation of bone tumors. Systemic symptoms (such as fever) and other clinical symptoms (such as spinal cord compression and respiratory distress) are more frequent in patients with Ewing sarcoma.

Diagnostic Evaluation

Diagnosis begins with a thorough history and physical examination. A primary objective is to rule out causes such as trauma or infection. Careful questioning regarding pain is essential in attempting to determine the duration and rate of tumor growth. Physical assessment focuses on functional status of the affected area; signs of inflammation; size of the mass; and any systemic indication of generalized malignancy, such as anemia, weight loss, and frequent infection.

Definitive diagnosis is based on imaging studies, such as plain films and CT or MRI scan of the primary site, CT scan of the chest, and radioisotope bone scans to evaluate metastasis and bone marrow examination in patients with Ewing sarcoma. A needle or surgical biopsy is necessary to establish the diagnosis. Ewing sarcoma most commonly involves the pelvis, long bones of the lower extremities, and chest wall; imaging reveals involvement of the diaphysis with detachment of the periosteum from the bone (Codman triangle). In osteosarcoma, lesions are most commonly located in the metaphyseal region of the bone, often involving the long bones. Radial ossification in the soft tissue gives the tumor a "sunburst" appearance on plain radiograph.

Prognosis

A better understanding of the biology of neoplastic growth has resulted in more aggressive treatment and improved prognosis. The natural history of osteosarcoma and Ewing sarcoma suggests that multiple submicroscopic foci of metastatic disease are present at the time of diagnosis despite clinical evidence indicating only localized involvement. The lungs, distant bones, and bone marrow are the most common sites for metastatic bone tumor disease. With current therapies that include surgery and chemotherapy for osteosarcoma and surgery, radiation therapy, and chemotherapy for Ewing sarcoma, the majority of patients with localized disease can be cured.

OSTEOSARCOMA

Osteosarcoma occurs most often in adolescents and young adults, coinciding with the period of rapid bone growth (Gorlick, Janeway, & Marina, 2016; National Institutes of Health, 2017g). It presumably arises from bone-forming mesenchyme, which gives rise to malignant osteoid tissue. Most primary tumor sites are in the diametaphyseal region (wider part of the shaft, adjacent to the epiphyseal growth plate) of long bones, especially in the lower extremities. More than half occur in the femur, particularly the distal portion, with the rest involving the humerus, tibia, pelvis, jaw, and phalanges. Risk factors include ionizing radiation exposure, genetic predisposition syndromes, and a history of retinoblastoma, particularly the hereditary form (Gorlick, Janeway, & Marina, 2016).

Therapeutic Management

Optimum treatment of osteosarcoma includes surgery and chemotherapy. The surgical approach consists of surgical biopsy followed by either limb salvage or amputation. To ensure local control, all gross and microscopic tumors must be resected. A limb salvage procedure has become the standard approach to surgical intervention and involves resection of the primary tumor with prosthetic replacement of the involved bone (Gorlick, Janeway, & Marina, 2016). For example, with osteosarcoma of the distal femur, a total femur and joint replacement is performed. Frequently children undergoing a limb salvage procedure receive preoperative chemotherapy in an attempt to decrease the tumor size and make surgery more manageable (Gorlick, Janeway, & Marina, 2016).

Chemotherapy plays a vital role in treatment of osteosarcoma. Cytotoxic drugs, such as high-dose methotrexate with citrovorum factor rescue, doxorubicin, cisplatin, ifosfamide, and etoposide, may be administered singly or in combination and may be employed both before and after surgical resection of the tumor. When pulmonary metastases are found, thoracotomy and chemotherapy have resulted in prolonged survival and potential cure. These combined-modality approaches have significantly improved the prognosis in osteosarcoma to approximately 70% for patients with nonmetastatic disease (Gorlick, Janeway, & Marina, 2016).

Nursing Care Management

Nursing care depends on the type of surgical approach. The family may or may not have more difficulty adjusting to an amputation than a limb salvage procedure. In either instance, preparation of the child and family is critical. Straightforward honesty is essential in gaining the child's cooperation and trust. The responsibility of telling the child is generally left to the physician, depending on the family's preference. If at all possible, the nurse should be present at the discussion or be aware of exactly what is said in order to follow up with the child and family afterward. The child should be told a few days before surgery to allow time to think about the diagnosis and consequent treatment and to ask questions.

Sometimes children have many questions about the prosthesis, limitations on physical ability, and prognosis in terms of cure. At other times they react with silence or with a calm manner that belies their concern and fear. Either response must be accepted because it is part of grieving the loss of an aspect of their physical appearance and function. For those who desire information, it may be helpful to introduce them to another amputee or survivor with a limb salvage procedure before surgery or to show them pictures of the prosthesis.* However, the nurse must be careful not to overwhelm children with information. A sound approach is to answer questions without offering additional information. For those who do not pursue additional information, the nurse expresses a willingness to talk.

The child is also informed of the need for chemotherapy and its side effects before surgery. Exercise caution about offering too much information at one time. When discussing hair loss, emphasize coping strategies, such as wearing a wig. Because bone tumors occur most often in adolescents and young adults, when appearance and peer acceptance are key developmental issues, it is not unusual for them to become angry over all the radical body alterations.

If an amputation is performed, the child is usually fitted with a temporary prosthesis immediately after surgery, which permits early functioning and fosters psychologic adjustment. If this is not done, the child requires stump care, which is the same as for any amputee. A permanent prosthesis is typically fitted within 6 to 8 weeks. During hospitalization the child begins physical therapy to become proficient in the use and care of the device.

Phantom limb pain may develop in 60% to 80% of patients after amputation. The exact pathophysiology is still unclear, but may include a combination of physical and psychologic factors that need to be further clarified by research (Luo & Anderson, 2016). This symptom is characterized by sensations such as tingling, itching, and, more frequently, pain felt in the amputated limb. The child and family need to know that the sensations are real, not imagined. Although various pharmacologic and nonpharmacologic techniques have been used for phantom limb pain, none provide complete relief or are curative for phantom limb pain (Luo & Anderson, 2016). A study of pediatric patients with cancer-related amputation found that 76% had phantom limb pain during the first year after amputation, but only 10% still had phantom limb pain more than 1 year after amputation (Burgoyne, Billups, Jirón, et al., 2012). The nurse works with the institution's pain team to address the problem of phantom limb pain.

Discharge planning begins early in the postoperative period. Once the child has begun physical therapy, the nurse consults with the therapist and oncology team to evaluate the child's physical and emotional readiness to reenter school. It is an opportune time to involve a community nurse in the child's home care. Every effort is made to promote normality and gradual resumption of realistic preamputation activities. Role playing in anticipation of such experiences is beneficial in preparing the child for the inevitable confrontation by others. Environmental barriers, such as stairs, are assessed in terms of accessibility in the school and home, especially because the child may need to use crutches or a wheelchair before complete healing and prosthetic competency are

*Information about prostheses can be obtained from the National Amputation Foundation, 40 Church St., Malverne, NY 11565; 516-887-3600; http://www.nationalamputation.org.

achieved. Information about special programs for children with amputations is available from the American Childhood Cancer Organization (see footnote earlier in this chapter).

The nurse encourages the child to select clothing that best camouflages the prosthesis, such as pants or long-sleeved shirts. Well-fitted prostheses are so natural looking that girls can usually wear sheer stockings without revealing the device. Emphasizing feminine or masculine apparel helps the child regain a feeling of self-identity. Even during the postoperative period, encouraging the child to wear jeans and a T-shirt may distract attention from the deformity and focus it on familiar aspects of appearance.

The family and child need much support in adjusting not only to a life-threatening diagnosis but also to alteration in body form and function. Because loss of a limb entails a grieving process, those caring for the child need to recognize that the reactions of anger and depression are normal and necessary. Often parents view the anger as a direct affront to them for allowing the amputation to occur, or they see the depression as rejection. These are not personal attacks but the child's attempts to cope with a loss. Psychosocial support programs (or members of the health care team such as psychologists, social workers, and child life specialists) at the institution may be particularly helpful in supporting the patient and family's strengths in coping.

EWING SARCOMA (PRIMITIVE NEUROECTODERMAL TUMOR OF THE BONE)

Ewing sarcomas, or the Ewing sarcoma family of tumors, which includes primitive neuroectodermal tumor of the bone, are the second most common malignant bone tumor (after osteosarcoma) in childhood (Hawkins, Brennan, Bolling, et al., 2016). Ewing sarcoma arises in the marrow spaces of the bone rather than from osseous tissue. The tumor originates in the shaft of long and trunk bones, most often affecting the pelvis, femur, tibia, fibula, humerus, ulna, vertebra, scapula, ribs, and skull (Hawkins, Brennan, Bolling, et al., 2016).

Therapeutic Management

Limb salvage procedures may be feasible in extremity lesions, although amputation may be considered if the results of radiation therapy would render the extremity useless or deformed (e.g., from growth retardation in young children). The treatment of choice for the majority of localized lesions is involved field radiation therapy and chemotherapy. The standard chemotherapy protocol includes vincristine, doxorubicin, and cyclophosphamide alternating with ifosfamide, and etoposide. Approximately two-thirds of patients with localized Ewing sarcoma can expect to be cured (Hawkins, Brennan, Bolling, et al., 2016). Improving survival, especially for patients with metastatic or recurrent disease, is a focus of ongoing research.

Nursing Care Management

Ewing sarcoma differs from osteosarcoma because preservation of the affected limb is more likely. Families may accept the diagnosis with some relief in knowing that this type of bone cancer does not necessitate amputation. They need preparation for the various diagnostic tests, including bone marrow aspiration and surgical biopsy, and adequate explanation of the treatment regimen.

High-dose radiation therapy often causes a skin reaction of dry or moist desquamation followed by hyperpigmentation. The child should wear loose-fitting clothes over the irradiated area to minimize additional skin irritation. Because of increased sensitivity, the area should be protected from sunlight and sudden changes in temperature, such as from heating pads or ice packs. Encourage the child to use the extremity as tolerated. Occasionally the physical therapist may plan an active exercise program to preserve maximum function.

The child needs the same considerations for adjusting to the effects of chemotherapy as any other patient with cancer. The drug regimen usually results in hair loss, severe nausea and vomiting, peripheral neuropathy, and possible cardiotoxicity. Make every effort to outline a treatment plan that allows the child maximum resumption of a normal lifestyle and activities.

OTHER SOLID TUMORS

In addition to the cancers already discussed, several other types of solid tumors may occur in children. Wilms tumor, rhabdomyosarcoma, and retinoblastoma are unique in that they tend to be diagnosed early, typically before 5 years of age. Wilms tumor and retinoblastoma are also unusual in that they are among the few types of cancer that may occur in both hereditary and nonhereditary forms.

WILMS TUMOR

Wilms tumor (nephroblastoma) is the most common kidney tumor of childhood with approximately 600 to 650 new cases per year in the United States (Fernandez, Geller, Ehrlich, et al., 2016; National Institutes of Health, 2017i). The average age at diagnosis is 44 months in children with single kidney disease, but younger (31 months) in those with bilateral disease. Approximately 10% of children with Wilms tumor have congenital anomalies, some of which are associated with syndromes such as WAGR (Wilms tumor, aniridia, genitourinary anomalies, and cognitive impairment [mental retardation]) and Beckwith-Wiedemann syndrome (hemihypertrophy, macroglossia, omphalocele, and visceromegaly) (National Institutes of Health, 2017i). A number of genes and chromosomal alterations have been implicated in the biology of Wilms tumor (National Institutes of Health, 2017i). The incidence of bilateral involvement is higher in children with genetic predisposition syndromes.

Clinical Manifestations

The most common presenting sign is swelling or mass within the abdomen; pain is present in about 40% of patients (Fernandez, Geller, Ehrlich, et al., 2016). The mass is characteristically firm, nontender, confined to one side, and deep within the flank. If it is on the right side, it may be difficult to distinguish from the liver, although, unlike that organ, it does not move with respiration. The mass usually is discovered during routine bathing or dressing of the child.

Other clinical manifestations may result from compression by the tumor mass, metabolic alterations secondary to the tumor, or metastases. Hematuria occurs in less than one-fourth of children with Wilms tumor. Anemia, usually secondary to hemorrhage within the tumor, results in pallor, anorexia, and lethargy. Hypertension, probably caused by secretion of excess amounts of renin by the tumor, occurs occasionally. Other effects of malignancy include weight loss and fever. If pulmonary metastasis has occurred, symptoms of lung involvement, such as dyspnea, cough, shortness of breath, and pain in the chest, may be evident.

Diagnostic Evaluation

In a child suspected of having Wilms tumor, special emphasis is placed on the history and physical examination for the presence of congenital anomalies (e.g., aniridia, developmental delay, hypospadias, cryptorchidism); a family history of cancer; and signs of malignancy, such as weight loss, enlarged liver and spleen, indications of anemia, and lymphadenopathy. The diagnostic workup includes abdominal imaging studies (abdominal x-ray, ultrasound, CT or MRI of the abdomen);

BOX 29.5 Children's Oncology Group Staging of Wilms Tumor

Stage I: Tumor is limited to one kidney and completely resected without rupture or previous biopsy. All sampled lymph nodes negative for tumor.
Stage II: Tumor extends beyond kidney but is completely resected; lymph nodes do not contain tumor cells.
Stage III: There is postoperative residual tumor confined to abdomen. Lymph nodes in abdomen or pelvis contain tumor cells.
Stage IV: Hematogenous metastases with disease spread to the lung, liver, bone, brain, or distant lymph nodes.
Stage V: Bilateral renal involvement is present at diagnosis.

CT of the chest to look for lung metastases; and Doppler ultrasound of the inferior vena cava. Laboratory studies should include a CBC (polycythemia is sometimes present if the tumor secretes excess erythropoietin), biochemical studies, and urinalysis. Studies to assess intravascular extension of the tumor and tumor rupture also are essential.

Staging and Prognosis

There are two main staging systems for Wilms tumor, one used by the Children's Oncology Group and the other by the European group SIOP. In the Children's Oncology Group system, disease staging (ranging from stage I to V) is determined by results of imaging studies and pathologic findings at nephrectomy (Box 29.5), with stage I being localized to one kidney and stage V indicating bilateral involvement by tumor (National Institutes of Health, 2017i). The histology of the tumor cells is also classified into two groups: favorable histology (FH) and anaplastic (unfavorable) histology; the anaplastic group is subdivided into diffuse and focal (Fernandez, Geller, Ehrlich, et al., 2016). The best outcomes are associated with FH; diffuse anaplastic tumors have the worst outcomes.

Five-year survival rates for Wilms tumor with favorable histology are above 90% (National Institutes of Health, 2017i). In addition to histology, prognosis depends on stage of disease at diagnosis, molecular features of the tumor, and age, with older age conferring a worse prognosis (National Institutes of Health, 2017i).

Therapeutic Management

The standard of care is combined treatment with surgery and chemotherapy; radiation therapy may be used, based on clinical stage and tumor histology. In unilateral disease nephrectomy and lymph node sampling are performed; a transabdominal or thoracoabdominal incision is used for greatest visibility of the kidney. Great care is taken to keep the encapsulated tumor intact because intraoperative spill can seed cancer cells throughout the abdomen, lymph channel, and bloodstream. If imaging studies do not indicate bilateral kidney involvement, exploration of the contralateral kidney is not necessary during the operative procedure (National Institutes of Health, 2017i).

The child may be treated with chemotherapy preoperatively under some circumstances (e.g., tumor is bilateral or child has a single kidney) after biopsy confirmation of the diagnosis. Preoperative chemotherapy reduces the size and vascular supply of the tumor, thereby making tumor removal easier (National Institutes of Health, 2017i). Standard chemotherapy regimens for Wilms tumor include some or all of the following: vincristine, dactinomycin, doxorubicin, cyclophosphamide, and etoposide. Postoperative radiation therapy is indicated for children with tumors classified as stage II focal or diffuse anaplastic histology, stage III and IV (National Institutes of Health, 2017i). Options for stage V tumors may include preoperative chemotherapy and surgery, and/or renal transplantation.

Nursing Care Management

The nursing care of the child with Wilms tumor is similar to that of other cancers treated with surgery and chemotherapy, and possibly radiation therapy. However, some significant differences are discussed for each phase of nursing intervention.

Preoperative Care

As with many other cancers, the diagnosis of Wilms tumor is a shock. Frequently the child has no physical indication of the seriousness of the disorder other than a palpable abdominal mass. Because the parents usually discover the mass, the nurse needs to take into account their feelings regarding the diagnosis. Whereas some parents are grateful for detecting the tumor so it can be treated, others feel guilty for not finding it sooner or feel angry toward the health care professional, believing it was missed on earlier examinations.

The preoperative period is one of swift diagnostic workup. Typically, surgery is scheduled within 24 to 48 hours of admission. The nurse is faced with the challenge of preparing the child and parents for all laboratory and operative procedures. Explanations should be simple and repeated, with attention to what the child will experience. In addition to usual preoperative observations, monitor blood pressure because hypertension from excess renin production is a possibility.

There are several special preoperative concerns, the most important of which is not to palpate the tumor unless absolutely necessary because manipulation of the mass may cause dissemination of cancer cells to adjacent and distant sites.

! NURSING ALERT

To reinforce the need for caution, it may be necessary to post a sign on the bed that reads "Do not palpate abdomen." Careful bathing and handling are also important in preventing trauma to the tumor site.

Because chemotherapy and radiation therapy (if used) are usually begun immediately after surgery, parents need an explanation of what to expect, such as major benefits and side effects, although the timing of the information should be considered to avoid overwhelming the family. Ideally the nurse should be present during physician-parent conferences to answer questions as they arise afterward.

Postoperative Care

Despite the extensive surgical intervention necessary in many children with Wilms tumor, the recovery period is usually rapid. The major nursing responsibilities are those after any abdominal surgery. Because of the risk for intestinal obstruction from vincristine-induced adynamic ileus, radiation-induced edema, and postsurgical adhesion formation, the nurse monitors gastrointestinal activity, such as bowel movements, bowel sounds, distention, and vomiting. Other considerations are frequent evaluation of blood pressure and observation for signs of infection, especially during chemotherapy.

Support the Family

The postoperative period is frequently difficult for parents. The shock of seeing their child immediately after surgery may be the first realization of the seriousness of the diagnosis. From surgery, the stage and pathology of the tumor are determined. The physician discusses this information with the parents. The nurse's presence during this conversation is important to provide additional support and assess the parents' understanding of this information.

BOX 29.6 Subtypes of Rhabdomyosarcoma

Embryonal—Most common type; most frequently found in the head, neck, abdomen, and genitourinary tract

Alveolar—Second most common type; most often seen in deep tissues of the extremities and trunk

Pleomorphic—Rare in children (adult form); most often occurs in soft parts of extremities and trunk

Older children need an opportunity to deal with their feelings concerning the many procedures to which they have been subjected in rapid succession. Therapeutic play can be beneficial in helping children of any age understand what they have undergone and express their feelings.

RHABDOMYOSARCOMA

Sarcomas, including rhabdomyosarcoma (*rhabdo* means striated), are tumors arising from mesenchymal cells, which normally develop into muscle and other tissues (Wexler, Skapek, & Helman, 2016). Approximately 400 new cases are diagnosed in the United States each year, with almost two-thirds occurring in children less than 10 years of age; a smaller peak in incidence occurs in early to middle adolescence (Wexler, Skapek, & Helman, 2016).

Rhabdomyosarcomas originate from undifferentiated mesenchymal cells in muscles, tendons, bursae, and fascia, or in fibrous, connective, lymphatic, or vascular tissue. The most common primary sites are the head and neck (especially the orbit), the genitourinary tract, and the extremities, but these tumors can occur in other sites as well. Rhabdomyosarcoma is classified into histologic subtypes (Box 29.6): embryonal, alveolar, and pleomorphic. More than half are embryonal. The embryonal and alveolar subtypes are most common in children and have distinct genetic alterations in the tumor cells. At the molecular level, these genetic alterations appear to involve both muscle differentiation pathways and cell proliferation pathways (Wexler, Skapek, & Helman, 2016). Rhabdomyosarcoma is associated with several genetic conditions (e.g., Li-Fraumeni cancer susceptibility syndrome, neurofibromatosis type 1) (National Institutes of Health, 2017j).

Clinical Manifestations

The initial signs and symptoms are related to the site of the tumor and compression of adjacent organs (Table 29.5). Some tumor locations, such as the orbit, manifest early in the course of the illness. Other tumors, such as those of the retroperitoneal area, only produce symptoms when they are relatively big and cause organ compression. Unfortunately, many of the signs and symptoms attributable to rhabdomyosarcoma are vague and frequently suggest a common childhood illness, such as "earache" or "runny nose." Often it is not possible to identify the site of the primary tumor.

Diagnostic Evaluation

Diagnosis begins with a careful history and physical examination, imaging studies, and baseline laboratory studies. An extensive evaluation is then performed to determine the extent of disease. Metastatic evaluation includes chest x-ray and CT scan, CT/MRI for abdominal/pelvic tumors, MRI of the skull and brain for parameningeal tumors, imaging of regional lymph nodes, bilateral bone marrow aspirates and biopsies, and bone scan for selected patients. An excisional biopsy or surgical resection of the tumor, when possible, is done to confirm the diagnosis.

TABLE 29.5 Clinical Manifestations of Rhabdomyosarcoma According to Tumor Site

Location	Signs and Symptoms
Orbit	Rapidly developing unilateral proptosis Ecchymosis of conjunctiva Loss of extraocular movements (strabismus)
Nasopharynx	Stuffy nose (earliest sign) Nasal obstruction—dysphagia, nasal voice (obstruction of posterior nasal conches), serous otitis media (obstruction of eustachian tube) Pain (sore throat and ear) Epistaxis Palpable neck nodes Visible mass in oropharynx (late sign)
Paranasal sinuses	Nasal obstruction Local pain Discharge Sinusitis Swelling
Middle ear	Signs of chronic serous otitis media Pain Sanguinopurulent drainage Facial nerve palsy
Retroperitoneal area (usually a "silent" tumor)	Abdominal mass Pain Signs of intestinal or genitourinary obstruction
Perineum	Visible superficial mass Bowel or bladder dysfunction (from tumor compression)

BOX 29.7 Surgical-Pathologic Staging of Rhabdomyosarcoma

Group I: Localized disease; tumor completely resected and regional nodes not involved

Group II: Localized disease; tumor completely removed; microscopic residual that may have spread into nearby lymph nodes

Group III: Incomplete resection with gross residual disease

Group IV: Metastatic disease present at diagnosis

Staging and Prognosis

Careful staging is extremely important for planning treatment and determining the prognosis. Two staging systems are used in combination: a surgicopathologic staging system (Box 29.7) and a modified tumor, node, metastasis (TNM) pretreatment staging system. A stage is assigned, based on primary site, tumor size, and whether or not there is regional lymph node involvement or distant metastasis. A group is assigned based on the status of the surgical resection/biopsy, pathologic assessment of the tumor margin, and lymph node involvement before therapy. Then a risk group is assigned, based on stage, group, and histology (National Institutes of Health, 2017j). Risk refers to the risk of disease recurrence.

Prognosis is related to age, with children ages 1 to 9 years having the best prognosis; primary tumor site, size, and resectability; whether or not there is lymph node involvement or metastasis at diagnosis; and histologic subtype. The alveolar histologic subtype is associated with a worse outcome. Most rhabdomyosarcomas are curable with the use of contemporary multimodal therapy. More than 70% of patients with localized disease are expected to survive (Wexler, Skapek, & Helman, 2016). If relapse occurs, the prognosis for long-term survival is poor.

Therapeutic Management

Rhabdomyosarcoma is treated with multimodality therapy that includes chemotherapy plus surgery or radiation therapy, or both modalities. The intensity and duration of chemotherapy are based on risk group. Some or all of the following chemotherapeutic drugs are used: vincristine, dactinomycin, cyclophosphamide, and ifosfamide. Complete resection of the primary tumor before chemotherapy is advocated whenever possible, if it will not result in disfigurement, functional compromise, or organ dysfunction (National Institutes of Health, 2017j). Otherwise, only an initial biopsy is performed. Radiation therapy is also based on risk group and tailored to the primary site and sites of metastatic disease.

Nursing Care Management

The nursing responsibilities in caring for a child with rhabdomyosarcoma are similar to those for other types of cancer, especially the other solid tumors for which surgery is employed. Specific objectives include careful assessment for signs of tumor, especially during well-child examinations; preparation of the child and family for the multiple diagnostic tests; and supportive care during each stage of multimodal therapy. The reader is urged to review the Nursing Care Management section for cancer and Chapter 19 for emotional support of the family in the event of a poor prognosis.

RETINOBLASTOMA

Retinoblastoma, so named because it arises from the retina, is the most common intraocular malignancy of childhood, with approximately 300 new cases diagnosed annually in the United States (Hurwitz, Shields, Shields, et al., 2016). Retinoblastoma can be present at birth, can have single or multiple foci in one or both eyes, and occurs in a heritable form. Of all cases of retinoblastoma, 60% are unilateral and nonhereditary (also called sporadic), 25% are bilateral and hereditary, and 15% are unilateral and hereditary (Hurwitz, Shields, Shields, et al., 2016). Retinoblastoma occurs predominantly in very young children; most cases are diagnosed before 3 to 4 years of age (National Institutes of Health, 2017k). Children with hereditary retinoblastoma tend to be diagnosed at a younger age. In the hereditary form of retinoblastoma, germline mutation of the *RB1* gene is present. The mutation may have been inherited, occurred in a germ cell before conception, or occurred in utero during embryogenesis (Hurwitz, Shields, Shields, et al., 2016). The two-hit model (discussed earlier in this chapter) was developed to explain hereditary and sporadic retinoblastoma. According to the model, as few as two events can lead to tumor formation; in the hereditary form, the "first hit" occurs in the germline whereas both hits occur somatically in the sporadic form.

Clinical Manifestations

Retinoblastoma has few grossly obvious signs. Typically parents or relatives are the ones who first observe a whitish "glow" in the pupil, known as the cat's eye reflex, or leukocoria (Fig. 29.6), which prompts ophthalmoscopic examination. The reflex represents visualization of the tumor as light momentarily falls on the mass. When a tumor arises in the macular region (area directly at the back of the retina when the eye is focused straight ahead), a white reflex may be visible when the tumor is small. It is best observed when a bright light is shining toward the child as the child looks forward, which is why it may be discovered when a flash photograph is taken.

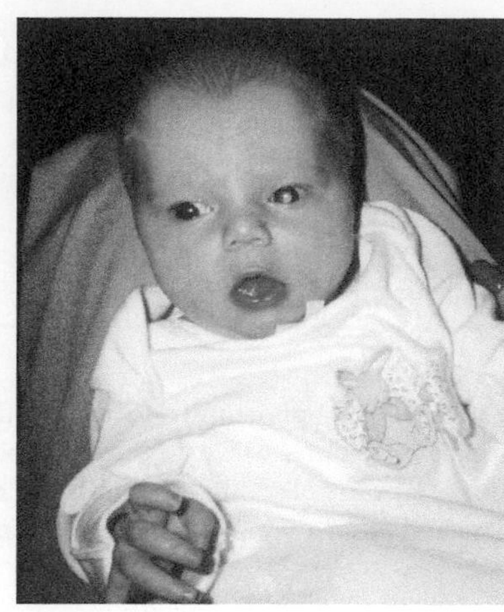

FIG. 29.6 Cat's eye reflex. Whitish appearance of lens is produced as light falls on tumor mass in left eye.

When the tumor arises in the periphery of the retina, it must grow to a considerable size before light can strike it sufficiently to produce the cat's eye reflex. In this situation it is visible only when the child looks sideways or if the observer stands at an oblique angle to the child's face as the child looks straight ahead. The fleeting nature of the reflex often results in a delayed diagnosis because health care professionals fail to appreciate the ominous significance of the parents' observation.

The next most common sign is strabismus resulting from poor fixation of the visually impaired eye, particularly if the tumor develops in the macula, the area of sharpest visual acuity. Blindness is usually a late sign, but it may not be obvious unless the parent consciously observes for behaviors indicating loss of sight, such as bumping into objects, slowed motor development, or turning of the head to see objects lateral to the affected eye. Other late signs and symptoms include pain, orbital cellulitis, and glaucoma.

Diagnostic Evaluation

A detailed family history and recording of eye signs and symptoms are essential. Children suspected of having retinoblastoma are referred to an ophthalmologist; the diagnosis usually is based on indirect ophthalmoscopy (under anesthesia), ultrasound, CT, and MRI scans. Blood and tumor samples can be tested for *RB1* gene mutations.

Metastatic disease at the time of retinoblastoma diagnosis is rare. For patients with suspected metastatic disease, bone marrow aspirates and biopsies, bone scan, and LP may be performed.

Staging and Prognosis

Staging of retinoblastomas is done under indirect ophthalmoscopy before surgery to accurately determine the tumor size (measured in disc diameters [DD]) and location (according to an imaginary line called the equator drawn on the midplane of the eye) (Hurwitz, Shields, Shields, et al., 2016).

Various classification systems have been used to stage or group retinoblastomas. The Reese-Ellsworth system classifies tumors according to five groups and is used to compare therapeutic results in patients treated with methods other than enucleation (i.e., radiation therapy). A revised classification system, the International Classification of Retinoblastoma, is based on the extent and location of the intraocular tumor; it better predicts globe salvage using contemporary treatments (Box 29.8). The overall 10-year survival rate is nearly 90% for unilateral and bilateral tumors (Hurwitz, Shields, Shields, et al., 2016). Retinoblastoma, like neuroblastoma, may spontaneously regress.

BOX 29.8 International Classification for Intraocular Retinoblastoma

Group A: Small (3 mm or less) intraretinal tumors away from the optic disc and foveola
Group B: All remaining tumors that are larger than 3 mm and/or close to the optic disc or foveola but remain confined to the retina
Group C: Discrete local disease with minimal disease under the retina (subretinal seeding) or in the gelatinous material of the eye (vitreous seeding)
Group D: Large or poorly defined tumors with significant vitreous or subretinal seeding; retina may have become detached from the back of the eye
Group E: Tumor is very large, extending near the front of the eye, is bleeding or causing glaucoma, or has other features that indicate it is not possible to save the eye

A major concern for long-term survivors is the development of SMNs. Children with bilateral disease (hereditary form) are more likely to develop subsequent cancers than are children with unilateral disease, and radiation therapy increases their risk.

Therapeutic Management

Treatment of retinoblastoma is complex. Enucleation may be used to treat advanced disease with optic nerve invasion in which vision cannot be salvaged. Radiation therapy can be used when there is vitreous seeding. Chemotherapy has been used to decrease the tumor size to allow treatment with local therapies such as plaque brachytherapy (surgical implantation of an iodine-125 applicator on the sclera until the maximum radiation dose has been delivered to the tumor), photocoagulation (use of a laser beam to destroy retinal blood vessels that supply nutrition to the tumor), and cryotherapy (freezing of the tumor, which destroys the microcirculation to the tumor and the cells themselves through microcrystal formation). Chemotherapy, along with radiation or high-dose chemotherapy with autologous stem cell rescue, is used to treat metastatic disease (Hurwitz, Shields, Shields, et al., 2016).

Nursing Care Management

Prepare the Family for Diagnostic and Therapeutic Procedures and Home Care

Because the tumor is usually diagnosed in infants or very young children, most of the preparation for diagnostic tests and treatment involves parents. Once the disease is staged, the physician confers with the parents regarding treatment. In most cases, enucleation can be avoided. In the event that enucleation is performed, the procedure and the benefits of a prosthesis are explained. Showing parents pictures of another child with an artificial eye may help with adjustment to the procedure (Fig. 29.7). Although the loss of vision is distressing, most parents realize that there is no alternative. Emphasizing that the unaffected eye retains normal vision and that the affected eye is probably already blind may be helpful in promoting acceptance of the imposed impairment.

After surgery the parents need to be prepared for the child's facial appearance. An eye patch is in place, and the child's face may be edematous and ecchymotic. Parents often fear seeing the surgical site because they imagine a cavity in the skull. On the contrary, the lids are usually closed, and the area does not appear sunken because a surgically implanted sphere maintains the shape of the eyeball. The implant is covered with conjunctiva, and when the lids are open, the exposed area resembles the mucosal lining of the mouth. Once the child is fitted for a prosthesis, usually within 3 weeks, the facial appearance returns to normal.

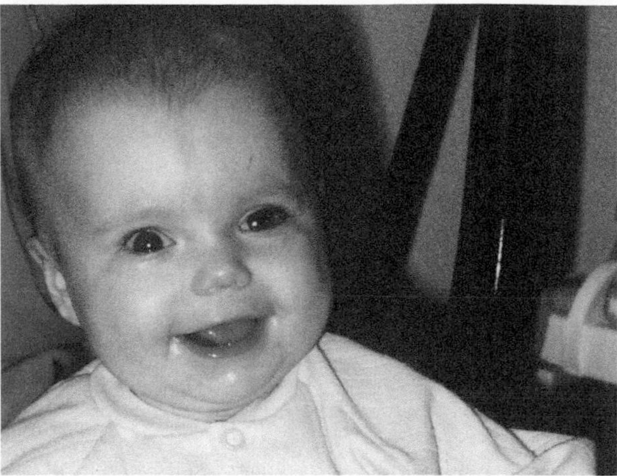

FIG. 29.7 Infant with left prosthetic eye.

After an uneventful recovery from enucleation, plans can be made for discharge from the hospital, usually within 3 to 4 days postoperatively. Parents need instruction regarding care of the surgical site and preparation for any additional therapy. They should be given the opportunity to see the socket as soon after surgery as possible. A good time to do this without unduly pressuring them is during dressing changes. They should then be encouraged to participate in the dressing changes.

Care of the socket is minimal and easily accomplished. The wound itself is clean and has little or no drainage. If an antibiotic ointment is prescribed, it is applied in a thin line on the surface of the tissues of the socket. The dressing consists of an eye pad changed daily. Once the socket has healed completely, a dressing is no longer necessary, although there are several reasons for having the child continue to wear an eye patch. Infants and toddlers explore their environment with their hands, and without an eye patch in place, the socket is available to exploring fingers. Although there is little danger of the child injuring the socket, parents may feel more secure with the socket covered. This also helps prevent infection.

The ocularist, who fits and manufactures the prosthesis, gives initial instructions for care of the device. Once in place, the prosthesis need not be removed unless cleaning is necessary, in which case it is taken out by gently pulling down on the lower lid, which frees the lower edge of the prosthesis, and applying pressure to the upper lid. The prosthesis is cleaned by placing it in hot water and soaking it for several minutes. Reinsertion is easier if the prosthesis remains wet. To reinsert the prosthesis, the lids are separated; and with the prosthesis held in the correct position (it should be marked to indicate the nasal side), it is pushed up under the upper lid, allowing the lower lid to cover its lower edge.

Safety is a major concern to prevent damage to the unaffected eye. Safety measures should be practiced at all times, and children should avoid rough contact sports or wear protective eyewear.

Support the Family

The diagnosis of retinoblastoma presents some special concerns in addition to those raised by any type of cancer. Families with a history of retinoblastoma may feel guilt for transmitting the mutation to their offspring, especially if they knowingly "played the odds" in conceiving an affected child. Conversely, when parents are aware of the probability and have an affected child, early treatment results in such favorable outcomes that parental adjustment may be rapid. In families with no history of retinoblastoma, the diagnosis is a shock, frequently complicated by guilt for not having discovered it sooner. Because parents frequently are the first to observe the cat's eye reflex, they may be angry at themselves or others, especially health care professionals, if a more thorough examination was delayed. The nurse should consider each of these variables while offering supportive care to the family.

Other concerns also relate to the hereditary aspects of the disease. Of great importance to parents is the risk of retinoblastoma in their subsequent offspring and in the offspring of the surviving affected child. With improving prognoses for these children, genetic counseling to is assuming greater importance. (See Chapter 3 for a discussion of the nurse's role in genetic counseling.)

Encourage these families to seek regular follow-up care for the affected child for early identification of possible SMNs. Offspring of unaffected parents and survivors should undergo regular ophthalmoscopy to detect retinoblastoma at its earliest stage.

GERM CELL TUMORS

Germ cell tumors (GCTs) account for approximately 3% of cancers in children younger than 15 years and 14% of cancers in adolescents 15 to 19 years (National Institutes of Health, 2017l). They can arise in gonadal and extragonadal sites and are broadly classified as teratomas (mature and immature) or malignant germ cell tumors (National Institutes of Health, 2017l). GCTs can appear in various body sites, including the testicles (e.g., yolk sac tumor, teratoma), ovaries (e.g., teratoma, germinoma, yolk sac tumor), sacrococcyx, mediastinum, and retroperitoneum (Frazier, Olson, Schneider et al., 2016; National Institutes of Health, 2017l). In general, most children with teratomas and localized gonadal tumors that are surgically resected can be observed without the need for further therapy. For patients with more advanced disease, the use of chemotherapy has produced excellent results.

LIVER TUMORS

Primary liver tumors are rare in childhood; they are divided into two main histologic subtypes, hepatoblastoma and hepatocellular carcinoma, with hepatoblastoma being most common (National Institutes of Health, 2017m). Surgical resection is the treatment of choice for liver tumors, usually performed after the administration of chemotherapy to increase the likelihood of complete resection (Meyers, Trobaugh-Lotrario, Malogolowkin, et al., 2016). Liver transplantation may be used in unresectable tumors. Survival rates for patients with hepatoblastoma can be as high as 90% with current therapies (Aronson & Meyers, 2016).

THE CHILDHOOD CANCER SURVIVOR

Survival rates for children with cancer have greatly improved over the past decades, so that long-term survival is expected for more than 80% of children with access to contemporary therapy for cancer (National Institutes of Health, 2017n). Curative therapy can also produce adverse health outcomes, referred to as late effects, which may become apparent months to years after cancer treatment is completed. Survivorship research has demonstrated that 60% to 90% of adult survivors of childhood cancer develop chronic health conditions; of these, 20% to 80% experience severe or life-threatening complications (Landier, Armenian, Meadows, et al., 2016). Late effects are related to therapeutic exposures (chemotherapy, surgery, radiation therapy, SCT) and are also influenced by host factors such as genetic predisposition, age at diagnosis/treatment, comorbid health conditions, and health habits (National Institutes of Health, 2017n).

Table 29.6 describes systemic late effects caused by cancer treatment that require careful nursing assessment. All survivors should have risk-based medical follow-up that includes a survivorship care plan for lifelong screening, surveillance, and health promotion. Because nurses in pediatric and adult primary care settings may encounter childhood cancer survivors, they should be aware of the risk-based, exposure-based guidelines developed by the Children's Oncology Group (2013) and endorsed by the American Academy of Pediatrics (2009). The guidelines include patient education materials ("Health Links") on guideline-specific topics that can be downloaded for use (Landier, Armenian, Meadows, et al., 2016).

Childhood cancer survivors have an elevated risk for disease and treatment-related morbidity and mortality that persists long after disease cure (Landier, Armenian, Meadows, et al., 2016). Survivorship research has contributed to better characterization of late effects, as well as to modification of treatment regimens to minimize the risk of late effects. As therapeutic options evolve, nurses will need to stay current with ongoing research to determine best practices for continued improvement in both the duration and quality of survival after childhood cancer.

TABLE 29.6 Late Effects of Cancer Treatment

Systemic Effects and Clinical Manifestations	Associated Mode of Treatment
Central Nervous System	
Leukoencephalopathy (syndrome ranging from lethargy, dementia, and seizures to quadriplegia and death)	Methotrexate, intrathecal chemotherapy, or CNS irradiation
Mineralizing microangiopathy (headaches, focal seizures, incoordination, gait abnormalities)	Methotrexate or CNS irradiation
Peripheral neuropathy (footdrop, tingling sensation in hands and/or feet, incoordination)	Vincristine
Cognitive deficits (decline with intelligence, memory, attention, nonlanguage skills)	Intrathecal chemotherapy or cranial irradiation (especially before 3 years old)
Cardiovascular	
Cardiomyopathy (tachycardia, tachypnea, dyspnea, shortness of breath, edema, palpitations)	Anthracyclines (doxorubicin and daunorubicin) or irradiation to heart High-dose cyclophosphamide
Pericardial damage (pleural effusion, cardiomegaly)	Mediastinal irradiation
Respiratory	
Pneumonitis (dyspnea, nonproductive cough, fever) Pulmonary fibrosis (dyspnea, restrictive ventilation, decreased exercise tolerance)	Lung irradiation, alkylating agents, possibly bleomycin, vinblastine, cisplatin

TABLE 29.6 Late Effects of Cancer Treatment—cont'd

Systemic Effects and Clinical Manifestations	Associated Mode of Treatment
Gastrointestinal	
Chronic enteritis (colic, abdominal pain, vomiting, diarrhea, obstipation, bleeding)	Abdominal irradiation, methotrexate, cytosine arabinoside
Hepatic fibrosis (jaundice, hepatomegaly)	Methotrexate, 6-mercaptopurine
Urinary	
Hemorrhagic cystitis (microscopic hematuria to gross hemorrhage)	Cyclophosphamide; ifosfamide; irradiation
Bladder fibrosis (decreased bladder capacity, ureteral reflux)	Cisplatin
Tubular necrosis (decreased creatinine clearance)	
Endocrine	
Thyroid dysfunction (see Chapter 31)	Irradiation to thyroid, pituitary gland, testes, ovaries
Reproductive	
Possible gonadal damage, both sexes (delayed puberty, amenorrhea, decreased sperm counts, increased follicle-stimulating and luteinizing hormones, decreased testosterone or estrogen)	Alkylating agents Irradiation to pituitary gland, testes, ovaries
Skeletal	
Growth retardation (short stature)	Irradiation, long-term steroids
Spinal deformities, scoliosis, kyphosis, asymmetric growth, pathologic fractures	Irradiation
Immune	
Asplenia (overwhelming infection, fever)	Splenectomy
Sensory Organs	
Cataracts (opacity over pupil)	Cranial irradiation, high-dose steroids
Hearing (decreased hearing, especially with high-frequency loss)	Cisplatin
Neurocognitive Effects	
Reduced intelligence quotient (IQ) scores	Cranial irradiation, antimetabolite chemotherapy; high-dose steroids
Slow processing speed; inattention; memory impairment; and deficits in visual spatial skills and psychomotor speed	Cranial irradiation although chemotherapy alone may be linked to subtle deficits
Additional Effects	
Dental Problems	
Increased caries, periodontal disease, hypoplastic teeth, hypodontia (delayed or absent tooth development)	Irradiation to maxilla and mandible
Second Malignancies	
Bone and soft tissue tumors	Irradiation, alkylating agents
Leukemia (ALL or AML)	

ALL, Acute lymphoblastic leukemia; *AML,* acute myeloid leukemia; *CNS,* central nervous system.

NCLEX REVIEW QUESTIONS

1. At a visit to the pediatric clinic, a mother is concerned by her 4-year-old's symptoms over the last few weeks. Which of the following symptoms described by the mother would lead the nurse to be concerned about an oncologic disorder? Select all that apply.
   A. Bruising in various stages, mainly on the legs
   B. Frequent complaints of respiratory infections, while siblings remain healthy
   C. Enlarged, firm lymph nodes
   D. Asthma symptoms with increase in wheezing
   E. Fever for more than 1 week
2. The nurse taking care of a 5-year-old cancer patient with ulcerative stomatitis is getting ready to perform mouth care. Which of the following principles should be followed? Select all that apply.
   A. Due to pain of the stomatitis, viscous lidocaine should be used to swish the mouth three times per day.
   B. A soft, bland diet, although not the favorite of the child, will help with the pain.
   C. Lemon glycerine swabs are helpful because they remind children of lemon drops.
   D. Using a soft sponge-type toothbrush will decrease the tendency for gums to bleed.
   E. A solution of 1 tsp of baking soda and ½ tsp of table salt in 1 quart of water is helpful for mouth rinse.
3. You are working with a new graduate and explaining prevention of infection for a child with acute lymphoblastic leukemia. Which statement by this new nurse indicates understanding?

A. "Prophylaxis against *Pneumocystis* pneumonia is routinely given to most children during treatment for cancer."
B. "If blood is drawn, firm pressure should be applied to the area for a minimum of 10 minutes."
C. "Having a roommate with a routine surgery would be acceptable for this child."
D. "The child should be vaccinated completely to avoid childhood diseases."

4. The parents of a child with Hodgkin disease ask how the physician will know what type of cancer their child has. Which of the following definitive signs and symptoms should the nurse describe? Select all that apply.
   A. The most common finding is enlarged, firm, nontender, movable nodes in the supraclavicular or cervical area.
   B. Tests include complete blood count, prothrombin time and G6PD, erythropoietin, and sedimentation rate.
   C. Generally a bone marrow biopsy is done to look for the presence of blast cells.
   D. The presence of Reed-Sternberg cells is considered diagnostic of Hodgkin disease.
   E. The presence of a white reflection as opposed to the normal red pupillary reflex in the pupil of a child's eye is a classic sign.
5. You are caring for a child on the pediatric unit with a suspected abdominal tumor. Which criterion would lead you to determine that this tumor is a neuroblastoma rather than a Wilms tumor?
   A. Most children present with neuroblastoma around age 4.
   B. Neuroblastoma is a firm, nontender, irregular mass confined to one side, generally deep in the flank.
   C. Hypertension is often noted due to secretion of excess amounts of rennin by the tumor.
   D. Most tumors develop in the adrenal gland or the retroperitoneal sympathetic chain.

Correct Answers

1. B, C, E; 2. B, D, E; 3. A; 4. A, D; 5. D

REFERENCES

Allen, C. E., Kamdar, K. Y., Bollard, C. M., et al. (2016). Malignant non-Hodgkin lymphomas in children. In P. A. Pizzo & D. G. Poplack (Eds.), *Principles and practices of pediatric oncology* (7th ed.). Philadelphia: Lippincott.

American Academy of Pediatrics (AAP). (2009). Long-term follow-up care for pediatric cancer survivors. *Pediatrics, 123*, 906–915.

American Academy of Pediatrics, Committee on Infectious Diseases. (2015). L. Pickering (Ed.), *2015 Red book: Report of the Committee on Infectious Diseases* (30th ed.). Elk Grove Village, IL: AAP.

Andrews, J., Galel, S. A., Wong, W., et al. (2016). Hematologic supportive care for children with cancer. In P. A. Pizzo & D. G. Poplack (Eds.), *Principles and practice of pediatric oncology* (7th ed.). Philadelphia: Lippincott.

Arceci, R. J., & Meshinchi, S. (2016). Acute myeloid leukemia and myelodysplastic syndromes. In P. A. Pizzo & D. G. Poplack (Eds.), *Principles and practice of pediatric oncology* (7th ed.). Philadelphia: Lippincott.

Ardura, M. I., & Koh, A. Y. (2016). Infectious complications in pediatric cancer patients. In P. A. Pizzo & D. G. Poplack (Eds.), *Principles and practice of pediatric oncology* (7th ed.). Philadelphia: Lippincott.

Aronson, D. C., & Meyers, R. L. (2016). Malignant tumors of the liver in children. *Seminars in Pediatric Surgery, 25*(5), 265–275.

Becze, E. (2017). *Nursing considerations for adverse events from CAR T-cell therapy*. ONS Voice, May 9. Retrieved from https://voice.ons.org/news-and-views/nursing-considerations-for-adverse-events-from-car-t-cell-therapy.

Bhatia, S., Landier, W., Shangguan, M., et al. (2012). Nonadherence to oral mercaptopurine and risk of relapse in Hispanic and non-Hispanic white children with acute lymphoblastic leukemia: A report from the Children's Oncology Group. *Journal of Clinical Oncology: Official Journal of the American Society of Clinical Oncology, 30*(17), 2094–2101.

Brodeur, G. M., Hogarty, M. D., Bagatell, R., et al. (2016). Neuroblastoma. In P. A. Pizzo & D. G. Poplack (Eds.), *Principles and practice of pediatric oncology* (7th ed.). Philadelphia: Lippincott.

Burgoyne, L. L., Billups, C. A., Jirón, J. L., Jr., et al. (2012). Phantom limb pain in young cancer related amputees: Recent experience at St Jude Children's Research Hospital. *Clinical Journal of Pain, 28*, 222–225.

Centers for Disease Control and Prevention (CDC), U.S. Department of Health & Human Services. (2016). *HPV vaccine recommendations*. December 15. 2016. Retrieved from. https://www.cdc.gov/vaccines/vpd/hpv/hcp/recommendations.html.

Centers for Disease Control and Prevention (CDC), U.S. Department of Health & Human Services. (2017). *What are the risk factors for skin cancer*, April 25. Retrieved from https://www.cdc.gov/cancer/skin/basic_info/risk_factors.htm.

Ceppi, F., Beck-Popovic, M., Bourquin, J. P., et al. (2017). Opportunities and challenges in the immunological therapy of pediatric malignancy: a concise snapshot. *European Journal of Pediatrics*.

Chaveli-Lopez, B., & Bagan-Sebastian, J. V. (2016). Treatment of oral mucositis due to chemotherapy. *J Clin Exp Denta, 8*(2), e201–e209.

Children's Oncology Group. (2013). *Long-term follow-up guidelines for survivors of childhood, adolescent and young adult cancers*. Retreived from http://www.survivorshipguidelines.org.

Crawford, J. (2013). Childhood brain tumors. *Pediatrics in Review, 34*(2), 63–78.

Effinger, K. E., Migliorati, C. A., Hudson, M. M., et al. (2014). Oral and dental late effects in survivors of childhood cancer: A Children's Oncology Group report. *Supportive Care in Cancer, 22*(7), 2009–2019.

Fernandez, C. V., Geller, J. I., Ehrlich, P. F., et al. (2016). Renal tumors. In P. A. Pizzo & D. G. Poplack (Eds.), *Principles and practice of pediatric oncology* (7th ed.). Philadelphia: Lippincott.

Feyer, P., & Jordan, K. (2011). Update and new trends in antiemetic therapy: The continuing need for novel therapies. *Annals of Oncology, 22*, 30–38.

Fielding, F., Sanford, T. M., & Davis, M. P. (2013). Achieving effective control in cancer pain: A review of current guidelines. *International Journal of Palliative Nursing, 19*, 584–591.

Foggo, V., & Cavenagh, J. (2015). Malignant causes of fever of unknown origin. *Clin Med (Lond), 15*, 292–294.

Freedman, J. L., Rheingold, S. R., & Fisher, M. J. (2016). Oncologic emergencies. In P. A. Pizzo & D. G. Poplack (Eds.), *Principles and practice of pediatric oncology* (7th ed.). Philadelphia: Lippincott.

Frazier, A. L., Olson, T. A., Schneider, D. R., et al. (2016). Germ cell tumors. In P. A. Pizzo & D. G. Poplack (Eds.), *Principles and practice of pediatric oncology* (7th ed.). Philadelphia: Lippincott.

Frew, J. A., Lewis, J., & Lucraft, H. H. (2013). The management of children with lymphomas. *Clinical Oncology, 25*, 11–18.

Gore, L., DeGregori, J., & Porter, C. C. (2013). Targeting developmental pathways in children with cancer: What price success? *The Lancet Oncology, 14*(2), e70–e78.

Gorlick, R., Janeway, K., & Marina, N. (2016). Osteosarcoma. In P. A. Pizzo & D. G. Poplack (Eds.), *Principles and practice of pediatric oncology* (7th ed.). Philadelphia: Lippincott.

Gottschalk, S., Naik, S., Hegde, M., et al. (2016). Hematopoietic stem cell transplantation in pediatric oncology. In P. A. Pizzo & D. G. Poplack (Eds.), *Principles and practice of pediatric oncology* (7th ed.). Philadelphia: Lippincott.

Gupta, S., & Bhatia, S. (2017). Optimizing medication adherence in children with cancer. *Current Opinion in Pediatrics, 29*, 41–45.

Hawkins, D. S., Bolling, T., Brennan, B. M. D., et al. (2016). Ewing sarcoma. In P. A. Pizzo & D. G. Poplack (Eds.), *Principles and practice of pediatric oncology* (7th ed.). Philadelphia: Lippincott.

Hill-Kayser, C., Tochner, Z., Both, S., et al. (2013). Proton versus photon radiation therapy for patients with high-risk neuroblastoma: The need for a customized approach. *Pediatric Blood and Cancer, 60*(10), 1606–1611.

Hockenberry, M. J., Kline, N. E., & Rodgers, C. (2016). Nursing support of the child with cancer. In P. A. Pizzo & D. G. Poplack (Eds.), *Principles and practice of pediatric oncology* (7th ed.). Philadelphia: Lippincott.

Hurwitz, R. L., Shields, C. L., Shields, J. A., et al. (2016). Retinoblastoma. In P. A. Pizzo & D. G. Poplack (Eds.), *Principles and practice of pediatric oncology* (7th ed.). Philadelphia: Lippincott.

Image Gently®. (2014). *Mission statement update.* Retrieved from http://www.imagegently.org/.

Karakukcu, M., & Unal, E. (2015). Stem cell mobilization and collection from pediatric patients and healthy children. *Transfusion and Apheresis Science, 53*, 17–22.

Kemper, K. J., Vohra, S., & Walls, R. (2008). American Academy of Pediatrics. The use of complementary and alternative medicine in pediatrics. *Pediatrics, 122*(6), 1374–1386.

Knudson, A. G., Hethcote, H. W., & Brown, B. W. (1975). Mutation and childhood cancer: A probabilistic model for the incidence of retinoblastoma. *Proc Natl Acad Sci, 72*(12), 5116–5120.

Krane, E. J., Casillas, J., & Zeltzer, L. K. (2016). Pain and symptom management. In P. A. Pizzo & D. G. Poplack (Eds.), *Principles and practice of pediatric oncology* (7th ed.). Philadelphia: Lippincott.

Landier, W., Armenian, S. H., Meadows, A. T., et al. (2016). Late effects of childhood cancer and its treatment. In P. A. Pizzo & D. G. Poplack (Eds.), *Principles and practice of pediatric oncology* (7th ed.). Philadelphia: Lippincott.

Lawson, C. M., Daley, B. J., Sams, V. G., et al. (2013). Factors that impact patient outcome: Nutrition assessment. *J Parenter Enteral Nutr, 37*(5 Suppl.), 30S–38S.

Luo, Y., & Anderson, T. A. (2016). Phantom limb pain: A review. *International Anesthesiol Clinics, 54*, 121–139.

Lutwak, N., Howland, M. A., Gambetta, R., et al. (2013). Even "safe" medications need to be administered with care. *BMJ Case Reports.*

McLean, T. W., & Kemper, K. J. (2016). Complementary and alternative medical therapies in pediatric oncology. In P. A. Pizzo & D. G. Poplack (Eds.), *Principles and practices of pediatric oncology* (7th ed.). Philadelphia: Lippincott.

Metzger, M., Krasin, M. J., Choi, J. K., et al. (2016). Hodgkin lymphoma. In P. A. Pizzo & D. G. Poplack (Eds.), *Principles and practices of pediatric oncology* (7th ed.). Philadelphia: Lippincott.

Meyers, R. L., Trobough-Lotrario, A. D., Malogolowkin, M. H., et al. (2016). Pediatric Liver tumors. In P. A. Pizzo & D. G. Poplack (Eds.), *Principles and practice of pediatric oncology* (7th ed.). Philadelphia: Lippincott.

National Institutes of Health (NIH), National Cancer Institute. (2017a). *Targeted cancer therapies.* Retrieved from https://www.cancer.gov/about-cancer/treatment/types/targeted-therapies/targeted-therapies-fact-sheet.

National Institutes of Health (NIH), National Cancer Institute. (2017b). *Childhood acute lymphoblastic leukemia treatment.* Retrieved from https://www.cancer.gov/types/leukemia/hp/child-all-treatment-pdq.

National Institutes of Health (NIH), National Cancer Institute. (2017c). *Childhood acute myeloid malignancies treatment.* Retrieved from https://www.cancer.gov/types/leukemia/hp/child-aml-treatment-pdq.

National Institutes of Health (NIH), National Cancer Institute. (2017d). *Childhood Hodgkin lymphoma treatment.* Retrieved from https://www.cancer.gov/types/lymphoma/hp/child-hodgkin-treatment-pdq.

National Institutes of Health (NIH), National Cancer Institute. (2017e). *Childhood Non-Hodgkin lymphoma treatment.* Retrieved from https://www.cancer.gov/types/lymphoma/patient/child-nhl-treatment-pdq.

National Institutes of Health (NIH), National Cancer Institute. (2017f). *Neuroblastoma treatment.* Retrieved from https://www.cancer.gov/types/neuroblastoma/hp/neuroblastoma-treatment-pdq.

National Institutes of Health (NIH), National Cancer Institute. (2017g). *Osteosarcoma and malignant fibrous histiocytoma of bone treatment.* Retrieved from https://www.cancer.gov/types/bone/hp/osteosarcoma-treatment-pdq.

National Institutes of Health (NIH), National Cancer Institute. (2017h). *Ewing sarcoma treatment.* Retrieved from https://www.cancer.gov/types/bone/hp/ewing-treatment-pdq.

National Institutes of Health (NIH), National Cancer Institute. (2017i). *Wilms tumor treatment.* Retrieved from https://www.cancer.gov/types/kidney/hp/wilms-treatment-pdq.

National Institutes of Health (NIH), National Cancer Institute. (2017j). *Childhood rhabdomyosarcoma treatment.* Retrieved from https://www.ncbi.nlm.nih.gov/pubmedhealth/PMH0032852/.

National Institutes of Health (NIH), National Cancer Institute. (2017k). *Retinoblastoma treatment.* Retrieved from https://www.ncbi.nlm.nih.gov/pubmedhealth/PMH0032680/.

National Institutes of Health (NIH), National Cancer Institute. (2017l). *Childhood extracranial germ cell tumors treatment.* Retrieved from https://www.cancer.gov/types/extracranial-germ-cell/hp/germ-cell-treatment-pdq.

National Institutes of Health (NIH), National Cancer Institute. (2017m). *Childhood liver cancer treatment.* Retrieved from https://www.ncbi.nlm.nih.gov/pubmedhealth/PMH0032595/.

National Institutes of Health (NIH), National Cancer Institute. (2017n). *Late effects of treatment for childhood cancer.* Retrieved from https://www.cancer.gov/types/childhood-cancers/late-effects-hp-pdq.

Parsons, D. W., Pollack, I. F., Hass-Kogan, D. A., et al. (2016). Gliomas, ependymomas, and other nonembryonal tumors of the central nervous system. In P. A. Pizzo & D. G. Poplack (Eds.), *Principles and practice of pediatric oncology* (7th ed.). Philadelphia: Lippincott.

Patel, P., Robinson, P. D., Thackray, J., et al. (2017). Guideline for the prevention of acute chemotherapy-induced nausea and vomiting in pediatric cancer patients: A focused update. *Pediatric Blood and Cancer*, epub ahead of print.

Plon, S. E., & Malkin, D. (2016). Childhood cancer and heredity. In P. A. Pizzo & D. G. Poplack (Eds.), *Principles and practice of pediatric oncology* (7th ed.). Philadelphia: Lippincott.

Poussaint, T. Y., Panigrahy, A., & Huisman, T. A. (2015). Pediatric brain tumors. *Pediatric Radiology, 45*(Suppl3), S443–S453.

Rabin, K. R., Gramatges, M. M., Margolin, J. F., et al. (2016). Acute lymphoblastic leukemia. In P. A. Pizzo & D. G. Poplack (Eds.), *Principles and practice of pediatric oncology* (7th ed.). Philadelphia: Lippincott.

Rau, R., & Loh, M. L. (2016). Myeloproliferative neoplasms of childhood. In P. A. Pizzo & D. G. Poplack (Eds.), *Principles and practice of pediatric oncology* (7th ed.). Philadelphia: Lippincott.

Sarvaria, A., Jawdat, D., Madrigal, J. A., et al. (2017). Umbilical cord blood natural killer cells, their characteristics, and potential clinical applications. *Frontiers in Immunology, 23*(8), 329.

Scheurer, M. E., Lupo, P. J., & Bondy, M. L. (2016). Epidemiology of childhood cancer. In P. A. Pizzo & D. G. Poplack (Eds.), *Principles and practice of pediatric oncology* (7th ed.). Philadelphia: Lippincott.

Ullrich, C. K., Sourkes, B. M., & Wolfe, J. (2016). Palliative care for the child with cancer. In P. A. Pizzo & D. G. Poplack (Eds.), *Principles and practice of pediatric oncology* (7th ed.). Philadelphia: Lippincott.

U.S. Food and Drug Administration (FDA). (2016). *Information about chemotherapy, biological therapy and immunotherapy*, November 10. Retrieved from https://www.fda.gov/forpatients/illness/cancer/ucm412505.htm.

U.S. Preventive Services Task Force (USPSTF). (2016a). *Final Update Summary: Breast cancer: Screening*, January. Retrieved from http://www.uspreventiveservicestaskforce.org/Page/Document/UpdateSummaryFinal/breast-cancer-screening.

U.S. Preventive Services Task Force (USPSTF). (2016b). *Final Recommendation Statement: Testicular Cancer: Screening*, December. Retrieved from http://.uspreventiveservicestaskforce.org/Page/Document/RecommendationStatementFinal/testicular-cancer-screening.

Wexler, L. H., Skapek, S. X., & Helman, L. J. (2016). Rhabdomyosarcoma. In P. A. Pizzo & D. G. Poplack (Eds.), *Principles and practice of pediatric oncology* (7th ed.). Philadelphia: Lippincott.

30

The Child With Cerebral Dysfunction

Maureen Sheehan

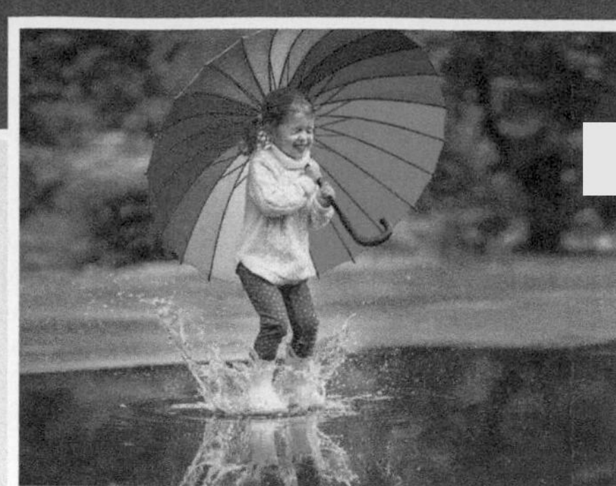

http://evolve.elsevier.com/wong/ncic

CONCEPTS

- Intracranial Regulation
- Sensory Perception
- Infection
- Safety

CEREBRAL STRUCTURE AND FUNCTION

The nervous system is made up of three intimately connected and functioning parts: the central nervous system (CNS), the peripheral nervous system, and the autonomic nervous system. The CNS is composed of two cerebral hemispheres, the brainstem, the cerebellum, and the spinal cord. The peripheral nervous system is composed of the cranial nerves (CNs) that arise from or travel to the brainstem and the spinal nerves that travel to or from the spinal cord. These nerves may be either motor (efferent) or sensory (afferent). The autonomic nervous system is composed of the sympathetic and parasympathetic systems, which provide automatic control of vital functions.

DEVELOPMENT OF THE NEUROLOGIC SYSTEM

In contrast to other body tissues, which grow rapidly after birth, the nervous system grows proportionately more rapidly before birth. Two periods of rapid brain cell growth occur during fetal life. From 15 to 20 weeks of gestation there is a dramatic increase in the number of neurons. Another increase in growth rate begins at 30 weeks of gestation and extends to 1 year of age. This rapid growth during infancy continues during early childhood and slows to a more gradual rate during later childhood and adolescence. Brain volume is readily reflected in head circumference, which increases six times as much during the first year as during the second year of life. During the first 3 months of life infants will gain 6 cm in head circumference, 3 cm during the next 3 months, and 1 cm per month from age 6 to 12 months. One-half of postnatal brain growth is achieved by age 1 year, 75% by age 3, and 90% by age 6. Cerebral blood flow (CBF) and oxygen consumption in childhood (up to age 6 years) is almost twice that of adults, which reflects an increased metabolic requirement consistent with growth and development.

The growth and final form of the brain depend on the development and multiplication of neurons. Creation of new cells occurs, in theory, only during the first 100 days of gestation. During the remainder of gestation, cells divide and multiply at the astonishing rate of 250,000 per minute. It is believed that no new nerve cells appear after the sixth month of fetal life. Postnatal growth consists of increasing the amount of cytoplasm around the nuclei of the 10 billion existing cells, increasing the number and intricacy of communications with other cells, and advancing their peripheral axons to keep pace with expanding body dimensions.

The brain constitutes 12% of the body weight at birth. It doubles its weight in the first year, and by age 5 or 6 years its weight at birth has tripled. Thereafter, growth slows until in adulthood the brain is only about 2% of the total body weight. The surface configuration of the brain also changes with development. The early embryonic brain surface is smooth, but the sulci deepen with advancing development. This process continues throughout childhood. At birth the cortex is only about one-half of its adult thickness, although all the major surface features are present. There is little cortical control over body movements at birth, with movements guided principally by primitive reflexes. (See Chapter 7.) With advancing development and maturation, the brain, through association pathways, exercises increasing control over much of the reflex activity. This allows the growing child to perform progressively complex tasks that require coordinated movements. Persistence of primitive reflexes may suggest defective cortical development.

Cortical control is closely associated with the acquisition of a myelin coating on the nerves. Although nerve fibers are able to conduct impulses without this myelin sheath, the impulses travel at a slower rate and with more likelihood of diffusion. Myelinization of the various nerve tracts in the CNS, which allows progressive neuromotor function, follows the cephalocaudal (head-to-toe) and proximodistal (near-to-far) sequence. It appears first with the fibers of the spinal cord and cranial nerves, then in the brainstem and corticospinal tracts.

Development of the nervous system proceeds on a continuum and generates the most complex structures within the embryo. The brain and spinal cord are among the first of the major organ systems to be recognized in the embryo and one of the last to finish significant development after birth. The rate of myelogenesis accelerates rapidly after birth. In general, the pathways concerned with sensation are myelinated early, before the motor pathways. The acquisition of motor skills depends on the maturation and myelination of the nervous system, and no amount of special training or practice will hasten the process. Most of an infant's advancing performance is a direct result of brain development indirectly influenced by environmental stimuli.

CENTRAL NERVOUS SYSTEM

The bony skull forms the strongest covering and provides the primary protection to the brain. It is an expansible structure in the infant and young child due to incomplete ossification of the bones of the skull, but becomes rigid in the older child and adolescent. Blood is supplied to the dura mater by the middle meningeal artery, a branch of the external carotid artery. It enters the skull at a point inferior to the temporal bone, then branches over the surface of the dura, usually encased in a groove in the temporal and parietal bones after 2 years of age. Damage to this artery or to its branches is a common cause of an epidural hematoma.

Brain Coverings

Within the skull, three membranes (the meninges) cover and protect the brain: the dura mater, arachnoid membrane, and pia mater (Fig. 30.1). The tough outer membrane, the **dura mater**, is a double layer that serves as the outer meningeal layer and the inner periosteum of the cranial bones. These two layers are separated by the epidural space. The dura is closely attached to the skull in infancy, causing slower spread of blood in epidural hemorrhage. Because of this adherence, epidural hemorrhages are uncommon in the first 2 years of life.

Between these layers of dura inside the skull lie large venous sinuses. Sheets of the dura mater also extend downward and inward to form partitions within the cranium. Projecting downward into the longitudinal fissure is a sheet of dura called the **falx cerebri**, which separates the cerebral hemispheres, and the **falx cerebelli**, which separates the cerebellar hemispheres. Another segment is a tentlike structure, the **tentorium**, which separates the cerebellum from the occipital lobe of the cerebrum. The large gap through which the brainstem passes is the tentorial hiatus.

The middle meningeal layer, the **arachnoid membrane**, is a delicate, avascular, weblike structure that loosely surrounds the brain. Between the arachnoid and the dura mater lies the subdural area, a potential space that normally contains only enough fluid to prevent adhesion between the two membranes. During cerebral trauma the fine blood vessels that bridge the subdural space are stretched and ruptured, causing venous blood to escape and spread freely, forming a subdural hemorrhage. The subdural space is small in children; therefore small amounts of blood can increase intracranial hemorrhage significantly.

The innermost covering layer, the **pia mater**, is a delicate, transparent membrane that, unlike the other coverings, adheres closely to the outer surface of the brain, conforming to the folds (gyri) and furrows (sulci). Within the pial layer lie the arteries and veins of the brain. Between the pia mater and the arachnoid membrane is the subarachnoid space. Cerebrospinal fluid (CSF) fills the entire subarachnoid space surrounding the brain and spinal cord and acts as a protective cushion for the brain tissue. Fibrous filaments known as arachnoid trabeculae provide further protection and help anchor the brain. When the head receives a blow, these attachments allow the arachnoid to slide on the dura, preventing excessive movement.

The Brain

Each section of the brain plays a vital role in regulation and control of body function. Each hemisphere is artificially divided into lobes. Pressure on or damage to these lobes produces observable signs or symptoms directly related to the area of pathology. These signs provide clues to the location of the damage.

The two large cerebral hemispheres that occupy the anterior and medial fossae of the skull are separated in the upper part by the longitudinal fissure. This separation is complete anteriorly and posteriorly,

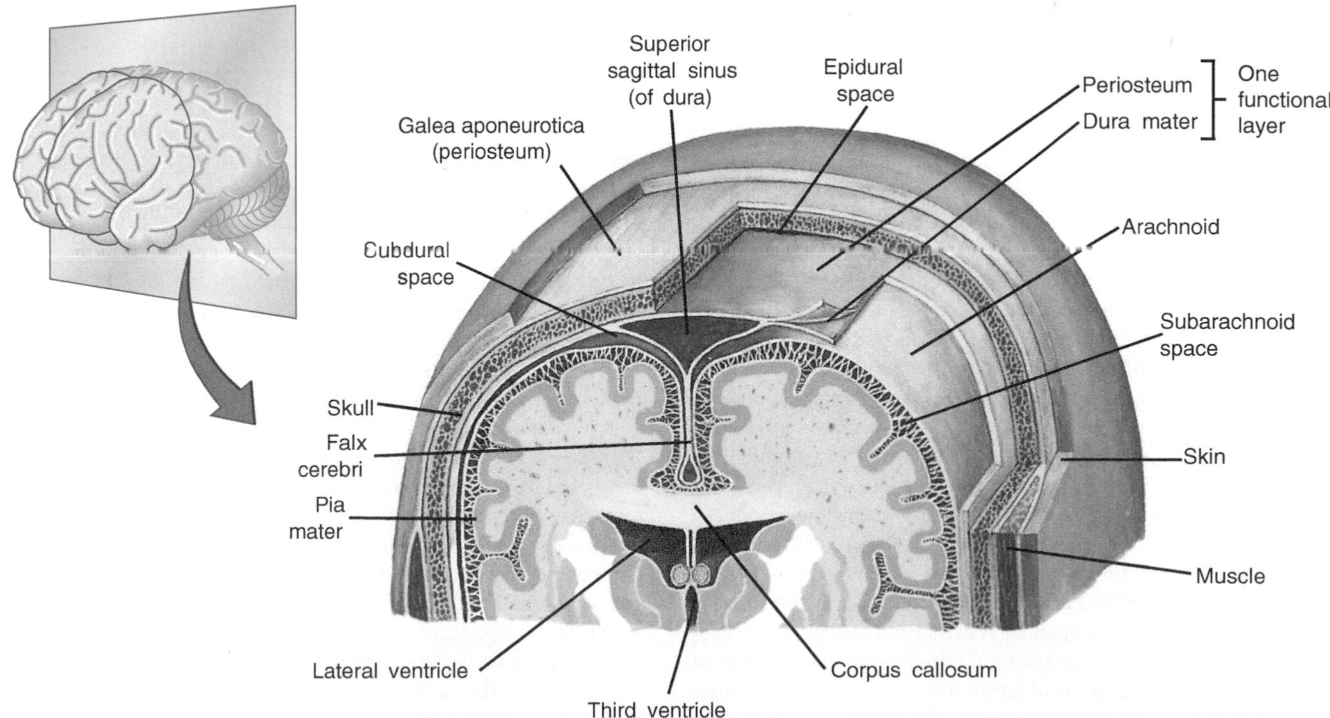

FIG. 30.1 Coronal section of top of head showing meningeal layers. (From Patton, K. T., & Thibodeau, G. A. [2010]. *Anatomy and physiology* [7th ed.]. St. Louis, MO: Mosby.)

but centrally the hemispheres are joined by the block of fibers known as the **corpus callosum**, the largest fiber bundle in the brain. These fibers interconnect cortical areas of the right and left hemispheres. Destruction of the corpus callosum causes hemispheric independence, or "split brain."

Situated deeply within each hemisphere and on each side of the midline are the basal ganglia (or cerebral nuclei), which serve as vital sorting areas for messages passing to and from the hemispheres. Connected to the hemispheres by thick bunches of nerve fibers is the brainstem, through which all nerve fibers traverse as they pass from the hemispheres to the cerebellum and spinal cord. The brainstem extends from the base of the hemispheres through the foramen magnum, where it is continuous with the spinal cord. Within the cranium and behind the brainstem is the cerebellum. Any pressure exerted on the intracranial structures can cause compression of the brainstem and prolapse of the cerebellum through the foramen magnum.

Cerebral Blood Flow

The blood supply to the brain tissue is carried by the internal carotid arteries, which branch to supply the various brain segments. The volume of blood to the brain, which constitutes only 17% of the cardiac output, supplies the brain with 25% of the body's oxygen supply. The brain, an "inactive" organ, uses 10 times the oxygen used by the body as a whole. Only the heart uses more oxygen per gram of tissue.

CBF is the result of two opposing forces: cerebral blood pressure (the difference between systemic arterial pressure and cerebral venous pressure) and cerebral vascular resistance. CBF remains constant at a cerebral blood pressure between 50 and 150 mm Hg. Because cerebral venous pressure is usually very low and relatively constant, cerebral blood pressure is determined mainly by systemic arterial pressure.

Autoregulation

One of the most important factors in the control of CBF is autoregulation, the unique ability of cerebral arterial vessels to change their diameter in response to fluctuating cerebral perfusion pressure (CPP). The CPP is the mean arterial pressure (MAP) minus the intracranial pressure (ICP):

$$CPP = MAP - ICP$$

As a result, cerebral vessels maintain a constant blood flow during alterations in blood pressure and perfusion caused by body posture, increased ICP, decreased cardiac output, or narrowing or occlusion in the major blood vessels of the neck. Autoregulation fails when the limits of cerebrovascular dilation are reached; at this point CBF decreases, causing clinical symptoms of ischemia (nausea, fainting, dizziness, dim vision). Conversely, increased MAP leads to "breakthrough of autoregulation," with increased CBF leading to microhemorrhages and cerebral edema. Autoregulation may be impaired locally or globally as a result of trauma or ischemia.

Changes in arterial oxygen pressure (Pao_2) or arterial carbon dioxide pressure ($Paco_2$) have a profound effect on autoregulation. Hypercapnia ($Paco_2$ >45 mm Hg) or increased levels of lactic acid have a pronounced dilating effect on cerebral arterioles, which increases CBF and thus cerebral volume. Hypocapnia ($Paco_2$ <35 mm Hg) constricts cerebral arterioles and decreases CBF. Pao_2 values between 70 and 100 mm Hg have little effect on the cerebrovascular system. Profound hypoxia (Pao_2 50 mm Hg) dramatically increases CBF. Consequently maintenance of the airway and effective hyperventilation are of primary importance in the initial management of the neurologically impaired patient. CPP is the most important physiologic determinant because the brain relies on the delivery of oxygen and nutrients to function.

Oxygen

Metabolic requirements for oxygen by the brain are not affected by rest or sleep, but they are reduced by narcosis and coma and are altered by changes in temperature. CBF is not altered when body temperature is between 35° and 40°C (95° and 104°F). Hyperthermia increases oxygen consumption by the brain. Hypothermia decreases oxygen consumption. The brain depends on a constant supply of oxygen-rich blood. Because the brain's need for oxygen is great in relation to the volume of blood supplied, the brain is capable of extracting more oxygen from each unit of circulating blood as needed.

Oxygen supply to the brain is compromised when the supply is inadequate as a result of impaired respiration, hypotension, increased ICP, or vascular damage, spasm, or compression. Neurons are highly susceptible to elevated $Paco_2$ (a potent vasodilator). The metabolic damage to brain tissue caused by an inadequate supply of well-oxygenated blood can often exceed the effects of trauma. Respiratory acidosis resulting from increased $Paco_2$ levels can produce symptoms indistinguishable from those of head injury.

Blood-Brain Barrier

The **blood-brain barrier (BBB)** is an anatomic-physiologic feature of the brain that separates the brain parenchyma from the blood. Unlike capillaries in other parts of the body, cerebral capillaries have no fenestrations or pores. The tight junctions of the vascular endothelium are responsible for the selective nature of the BBB. The mature BBB allows facilitated diffusion of glucose and passive diffusion of water and carbon dioxide but is impermeable to protein and does not permit passage of many active substances. However, the BBB of the fetus and newborn is normally indiscriminately permeable, allowing protein and other large and small molecules to pass freely between the cerebral vessels and the brain. Conditions that cause cerebrovascular dilation (hypertension, hypercapnia, hypoxia, acidosis) disrupt the BBB. Hyperosmotic fluids, which cause shrinkage of vascular endothelium and widen the vascular junctions, also disrupt the BBB.

INCREASED INTRACRANIAL PRESSURE

The brain, tightly enclosed in the solid bony cranium, is well protected but highly vulnerable to pressure that may accumulate within the enclosure. Its total volume—brain (80%), CSF (10%), and blood (10%)—must remain approximately the same at all times. A change in the proportional volume of one of these components (e.g., increase or decrease in intracranial blood) must be accompanied by a compensatory change in another (e.g., decrease or increase in CSF). In this way the volume and pressure normally remain constant. Examples of compensatory changes are reduction in blood volume, decrease in production of CSF, increase in CSF absorption, or shrinkage of brain mass by displacement of intracellular and extracellular fluid.

Children with open fontanels compensate for increased volume by skull expansion and widened sutures. However, at any age the capacity for spatial compensation is limited. An increase in ICP may be caused by tumors or other space-occupying lesions, accumulation of fluid within the ventricular system, bleeding, or edema of cerebral tissues. Once compensation is exhausted, any further increase in volume results in a rapid rise in ICP.

The early signs and symptoms of increased ICP are often subtle, such as headache, vomiting, personality changes, irritability, and fatigue (Box 30.1). In older children subjective symptoms are headache, especially when arising after lying flat (e.g., on awakening in the morning) or when coughing, sneezing, or bending over, and nausea and vomiting. The child may complain of double vision or blurred vision with

BOX 30.1 Clinical Manifestations of Increased Intracranial Pressure in Infants and Children

Infants

Tense, bulging fontanel
Separated cranial sutures
Macewen (cracked-pot) sign
Irritability and restlessness
Drowsiness
Increased sleeping
High-pitched cry
Increased frontooccipital circumference
Distended scalp veins
Poor feeding
Crying when disturbed
Setting-sun sign

Children

Headache
Nausea
Forceful vomiting
Diplopia, blurred vision
Seizures
Indifference, drowsiness
Decline in school performance
Diminished physical activity and motor performance
Increased sleeping
Inability to follow simple commands
Lethargy

Late Signs in Infants and Children

Bradycardia
Decreased motor response to command
Decreased sensory response to painful stimuli
Alterations in pupil size and reactivity
Extension or flexion posturing
Cheyne-Stokes respirations
Papilledema
Decreased consciousness
Coma

movement of the head. Seizures may occur. In children whose cranial sutures have not closed, there is an increase in head circumference and tense or bulging fontanels. Cranial sutures may widen. Head circumference can enlarge until the child is 5 years of age if the condition progresses slowly. As pressure increases, the pupils become progressively sluggish in reaction and eventually become fixed and dilated. The level of consciousness progressively deteriorates from drowsiness to eventual coma. Problems related to increased ICP are discussed later in this chapter in relation to head injury and hydrocephalus. (See also Brain Tumors, Chapter 29.)

Physiologic and biochemical changes within the cerebral vasculature serve to complicate the primary causes of increased ICP. Especially in cases of trauma, blood flow often initially increases as a result of venous congestion or vasomotor paralysis. If cerebral hypoxia is associated with the cerebral dysfunction, the compensatory vasodilation caused by oxygen deficiency will tend to increase the cerebral flow. However, blood flow is reduced as ICP progressively increases, with diminished blood supply to the brain tissues. The classic responses observed in adults (widening pulse pressure, increased blood pressure) rarely occur in children or are very late signs. Periodic or irregular breathing is an ominous sign of brainstem (especially medullary) dysfunction that often precedes apnea.

EVALUATION OF NEUROLOGIC STATUS

Earlier chapters discuss methods to evaluate neurologic function in relation to numerous aspects of child care. The neurologic examination is an integral part of the health assessment (see Chapter 4) and newborn assessment (see Chapter 7). Chapter 34 discusses some of the tests used to differentiate neuromuscular disorders. The assessment tools and examinations in this chapter are primarily those used to assess intracranial integrity.

ASSESSMENT: GENERAL ASPECTS

Children younger than 2 years of age require special evaluation because they are unable to respond to directions designed to elicit specific neurologic responses. Early neurologic responses in infants are primarily reflexive; these responses are gradually replaced by meaningful movement in the characteristic cephalocaudal direction of development. This evidence of progressive maturation reflects more extensive myelinization and changes in neurochemical and electrophysiological properties.

Most information about infants and small children comes from observation of spontaneous and elicited reflex responses. As they develop increasingly complex gross and fine motor skills and communication skills, more sophisticated techniques are used to assess acquisition of developmental milestones. Delay or deviation from expected milestones helps identify high-risk children. Persistence or reappearance of primitive reflexes indicates a pathologic condition. In evaluating the infant or young child, it is important to obtain the history of the pregnancy, delivery, respiratory status at birth, and neonatal health including any need for intensive care hospitalization to determine the possible impact of intrauterine and extrauterine environmental influences known to affect the orderly maturation of the CNS. These influences include maternal infections, chemical exposure, trauma, medication, illicit drug use, and metabolic insults.

History

A family history can sometimes offer clues regarding possible genetic disorders with neurologic manifestations. A review of family members often identifies conditions that might otherwise be overlooked, especially increased number of miscarriages or siblings or relatives who died at an early age. The nurse asks questions regarding specific neurologic problems, such as intellectual and developmental disabilities, deafness, epilepsy, blindness, unusual movements, weakness, ataxia, stroke, and progressive mental deterioration. History of consanguinity is also important.

A health history provides valuable clues regarding the cause of neurologic dysfunction. A history is assessed for injury with loss of consciousness, febrile illness, an encounter with an animal or insect, ingestion of neurotoxic substances, inhalation of chemicals, past illness, and known diabetes mellitus or sickle cell disease. Sudden or progressive alterations in movement or mental abilities may provide clues for investigation. It is also important to ascertain the chronologic course of the illness.

Physical Examination

Physical examination includes observation of the size and shape of the head (particularly in the infant and young child), spontaneous activity and postural reflex activity, and sensory responses. Note whether the

BOX 30.2 Abnormal Involuntary Muscular Movements

Ataxia—Gross incoordination that may become worse with the eyes closed
Spasm—Involuntary contraction of a muscle
Spasticity—Prolonged and steady contraction of a muscle characterized by clonus (alternating relaxation and contraction of the muscle) and exaggerated reflexes
Rigidity—Inability to flex or extend a joint
Tremors—Constant small involuntary movements
Twitching—Spasmodic movements of short duration
Tic—Involuntary, compulsive, stereotyped movement of an associated group of muscles
Choreiform movements—Quick, jerky, grossly uncoordinated, irregular movements that may disappear on relaxation
Athetosis—Slow, writhing, wormlike, constant, grossly uncoordinated movements that increase on voluntary activity and decrease on relaxation
Dystonia—Slow twisting movements of limbs or trunk
Associated movements—Voluntary movement of one muscle accompanied by involuntary movement of another muscle
Mirroring movements—Same as associated movements except with symmetric muscle group

BOX 30.3 Abnormalities of Gait That Indicate Cerebral Dysfunction

Ataxia—Impaired ability to coordinate movements; staggering gait and postural imbalance.
Spastic paraplegic gait—Narrow-based gait with a tendency to walk on toes, along with flexion at knees and hips, and shuffling. Hips are adducted, and knees may strike each other with each step; in younger children a "scissoring" position results when lower limbs cross because of increased adductor tone. Patients walk stiffly; take slow, deliberate steps; and have difficulty when attempting to walk on heels or run.
Spastic hemiplegic gait—Involved leg extended, circumducted, plantar flexion. The affected arm is flexed and adducted and does not swing.
Cerebellar gait—Staggering, unsteadiness, wide-based gait; tendency to veer in one lateral direction; often accompanied by swaying of the trunk.
Extrapyramidal gait—Rigidity, few automatic movements, and bradykinesia (slowness of all movements) with associated bending of trunk and head, arms adducted at shoulders and flexed at elbows and wrists, fingers extended; festination (upper body moving forward in advance of lower part), causing rapid steps and risk of falling.

patient is lethargic, drowsy, stuporous, alert, active, or irritable. The nurse also observes the overall tone, noting whether there is a normal flexed posture or one of extreme extension, opisthotonos, or hypotonia. Symmetry of movement is also assessed.

Facial features may suggest a specific syndrome. A high-pitched, piercing cry in an infant is often associated with CNS disorders. An abnormal respiratory cycle, such as prolonged apnea, ataxic breathing, paradoxic chest movement, and hyperventilation, may be the result of a neurologic problem.

Older children can be evaluated by the usual methods used in a neurologic examination. In addition, an estimation of the level of development provides essential information about neurologic function. This assessment is discussed throughout the book in relation to evaluation for specific disorders such as intellectual and developmental disabilities, failure to thrive, attention deficit hyperactivity disorder, cerebral palsy, cerebral tumors, and other physical or behavioral problems. Developmental screening tests can assess developmental progress in the young child.

Muscular activity and coordination, including ocular movements and gait, are valuable sources of information. Ocular movements, pupillary response, facial movements, and mouth functions provide clues regarding CNS involvement or impingement. (See Chapter 4 for CNS and reflex testing.) Testing reflexes, strength, and coordination and for the presence and location of tremors, twitching, tics, or other unusual movements is also an aspect of the neurologic assessment (Box 30.2). Box 30.3 describes abnormalities of gait that indicate cerebral dysfunction.

ALTERED STATES OF CONSCIOUSNESS

Consciousness implies awareness—the ability to respond to sensory stimuli and have subjective experiences. Consciousness has two aspects: alertness, an arousal-waking state that includes the ability to respond to stimuli, and cognition, which includes the ability to process stimuli and produce verbal and motor responses.

An altered state of consciousness usually refers to varying states of unconsciousness that may be momentary or may last for hours, days, or indefinitely. Unconsciousness is depressed cerebral function—the inability to respond to sensory stimuli and have subjective experiences. Coma is defined as a state of unconsciousness from which the patient cannot be aroused, even with powerful stimuli.

! NURSING ALERT

Lack of response to painful stimuli is abnormal and must be reported immediately.

The seat of consciousness, or "alerting area," of the brain is in the reticular formation—the central core of the brainstem. The reticular formation extends from the midbrain to the medulla. The reticular activating system receives collaterals from and is stimulated by every major somatic and special sensory pathway in the brain. Disturbances of consciousness may occur when any part of the reticular, thalamic, hypothalamic, and cortical circuits is sufficiently impaired. However, the effects may vary according to the areas involved. For example, small lesions of the reticular or hypothalamic regions produce a profound effect, whereas extensive impairment of the cortex is required to produce quantitatively similar results.

Etiology

An altered state of consciousness may be the outcome of several processes that affect the CNS. Impaired neurologic function can result from a direct or indirect cause. Some altered states, such as the diffuse changes observed in encephalitis, are directly related to cerebral insult. Others are the result of dysfunction in other organs or processes. For example, biochemical changes can impair neurologic function without morphologic findings, as in hypoglycemia.

Level of Consciousness

Assessment of level of consciousness (LOC) remains the earliest indicator of improvement or deterioration in neurologic status. LOC is determined by observations of the child's responses to the environment. Other diagnostic tests, such as motor activity, reflexes, and vital signs, are more variable and do not necessarily directly parallel the depth of the comatose state. The most consistently used terms are described in Box 30.4.

BOX 30.4 Levels of Consciousness

Full consciousness—Awake and alert, orientated to time, place, and person; behavior appropriate for age.

Confusion—Impaired decision making.

Disorientation—Confusion regarding time, place, and/or person; decreased level of consciousness.

Lethargy—Limited spontaneous movement, sluggish speech, drowsiness.

Obtundation—Arousable with stimulation.

Stupor—Remaining in a deep sleep, responsive only to vigorous and repeated stimulation.

Coma—No motor or verbal response to noxious (painful) stimuli.

Persistent vegetative state (PVS)—Permanently lost function of the cerebral cortex. Eyes follow objects only by reflex or when attracted to the direction of loud sounds; all four limbs are spastic but can withdraw from painful stimuli; hands show reflexive grasping and groping; the face can grimace, some food may be swallowed, and the child may groan or cry but utter no words.

Modified from Seidel, H. M., Ball, J. W., Dains, J. E., et al. (Eds.). (2006). *Mosby's guide to physical examination* (6th ed.). St. Louis, MO: Mosby.

Coma Assessment

Diminished alertness as a result of pathologic conditions occurs on a continuum and is designated as the comatose state, which extends from somnolence at one end to deep coma at the other. To produce coma, one of the following must occur: (1) extensive, diffuse, bilateral cerebral hemispheric destruction (the brainstem may be intact); (2) a lesion in the diencephalon; or (3) destruction of the brainstem down to the level of the lower pons.

Several scales have been devised in an attempt to standardize the description and interpretation of the degree of depressed consciousness. The most popular of these is the Glasgow Coma Scale (GCS), which consists of a three-part assessment: eye opening, verbal response, and motor response. The GCS was created to meet a clinical need to identify criteria for the consciousness level. For clinical purposes, the primary role of observation of the LOC is to detect a life-threatening complication such as cerebral edema. The GCS requires observational skills and is readily reproducible between observers.

A pediatric version of the GCS recognizes that expected verbal and motor responses must be related to the child's age (Fig. 30.2). The pediatric coma scale does not assess verbal responses as such but records smiling, crying, and interaction. It uses a 6-point motor scale that is inappropriate for children below the age of 6 months. In children under 5 years of age, speech is understood to be any sound at all, even crying. Young children demonstrate orientation by identifying their parents correctly or giving their own names. When assessing LOC in young children, the nurse may find it helpful to have a parent present to help elicit a desired response. An infant or child may not respond in an unfamiliar environment or to unfamiliar voices.

Numeric values are assigned to the levels of response in each category. The sum of these numeric values provides an objective measurement of the patient's LOC. The lower the score, the deeper the coma. A person with an unaltered LOC would score the highest, 15; a score of 8 or below is generally accepted as a definition of coma; the lowest score, 3, indicates deep coma or death.

The GCS in itself is not sufficient to determine depressed consciousness in all children. For example, because a child with quadriplegia cannot respond to commands physically, the child's GCS can be very low but the child may be cognitively intact. Nevertheless, the GCS provides a more objective method for evaluating the state of consciousness in most cases. Severely injured children (GCS ≤8) may have a consistent grading of motor response, verbal response, and eye opening.

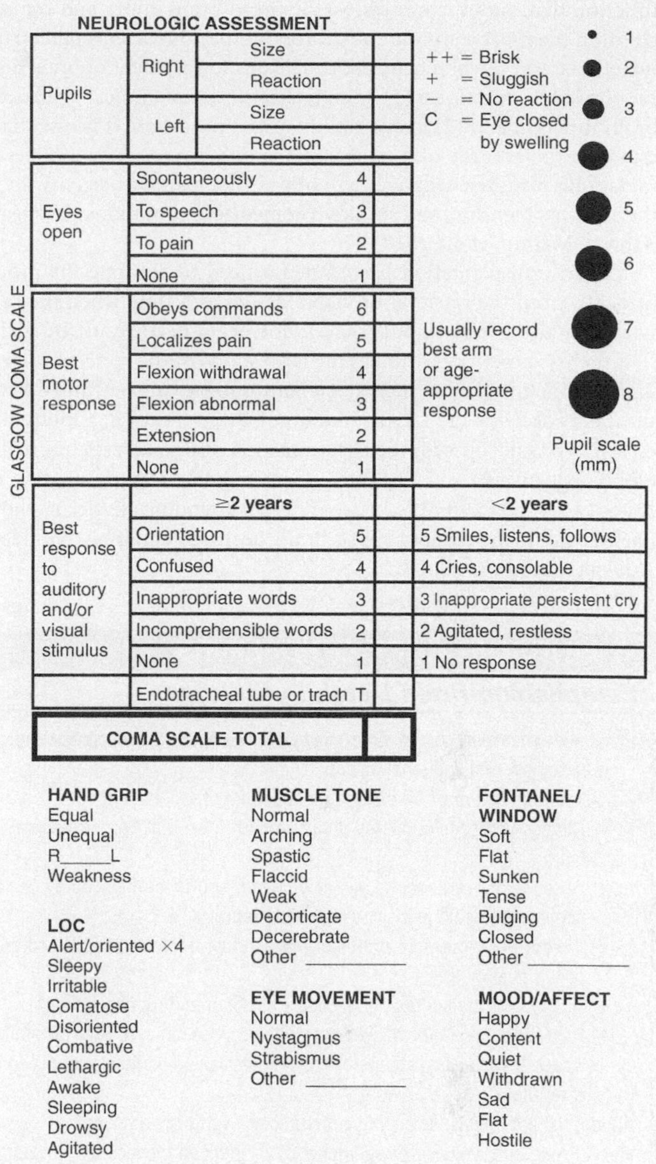

NEUROLOGIC ASSESSMENT

Pupils		
Right	Size	
	Reaction	
Left	Size	
	Reaction	

++ = Brisk
+ = Sluggish
− = No reaction
C = Eye closed by swelling

GLASGOW COMA SCALE

Category	Response	Score
Eyes open	Spontaneously	4
	To speech	3
	To pain	2
	None	1
Best motor response	Obeys commands	6
	Localizes pain	5
	Flexion withdrawal	4
	Flexion abnormal	3
	Extension	2
	None	1

Usually record best arm or age-appropriate response

Pupil scale (mm): 1, 2, 3, 4, 5, 6, 7, 8

Best response to auditory and/or visual stimulus	≥2 years		<2 years
	Orientation	5	5 Smiles, listens, follows
	Confused	4	4 Cries, consolable
	Inappropriate words	3	3 Inappropriate persistent cry
	Incomprehensible words	2	2 Agitated, restless
	None	1	1 No response
	Endotracheal tube or trach	T	

COMA SCALE TOTAL

HAND GRIP
Equal
Unequal
R____L
Weakness

LOC
Alert/oriented ×4
Sleepy
Irritable
Comatose
Disoriented
Combative
Lethargic
Awake
Sleeping
Drowsy
Agitated

MUSCLE TONE
Normal
Arching
Spastic
Flaccid
Weak
Decorticate
Decerebrate
Other ________

EYE MOVEMENT
Normal
Nystagmus
Strabismus
Other ________

FONTANEL/WINDOW
Soft
Flat
Sunken
Tense
Bulging
Closed
Other ________

MOOD/AFFECT
Happy
Content
Quiet
Withdrawn
Sad
Flat
Hostile

FIG. 30.2 Pediatric coma scale.

The GCS score performed during preadmission (i.e., assessment in the field), in the emergency department, and throughout the inpatient admission is universally accepted as one criterion to determine the patient's prognosis (Braine & Cook, 2017). GCS scores equal to or less than 5 are associated with poor outcome (Murphy, Thomas, Gertz, et al., 2017).

Irreversible Coma

There is no precise diagnosis for clinical death. Different tissues undergo permanent damage after varying periods of exposure to an ongoing insult; therefore the brain (especially the cerebrum) has become the tissue of most importance in determining the time of death. The current concept of dying is a process that takes place over a finite interval of time rather than an event that occurs spontaneously. Brain death is a clinical diagnosis based the total cessation of brainstem and cortical brain function that causes irreversible widespread brain injury and coma. In children the most common causes are trauma, anoxic encephalopathy, infections, and cerebral neoplasms. The pronouncement of brain death requires two conditions: (1) complete cessation of clinical evidence of brain function and (2) irreversibility of the condition. It is essential to establish the absence of a reversible condition, especially a toxic and metabolic disorder, sedative-hypnotic drugs, paralytic agents, hypothermia, hypotension, and surgically remediable conditions (Nakagawa, Ashwal, Mathur, et al., 2012).

Organ transplantation has created a need to separate the process of death from the retrieval of viable tissues at a time when the brain is already dead. The clinical criteria for brain death must be met so that there is no error. Although the legal status of the concept of death varies among individual states and communities in the United States, the Task Force for the Determination of Brain Death in Children has established Guidelines for the Determination of Brain Death in Children (see Nursing Care Guidelines box). (See Organ or Tissue Donation and Autopsy, Chapter 19.) At least two different attending physicians should participate in the diagnosing of brain death in children (Nakagawa, Ashwal, Mathur, et al., 2012).

NURSING CARE GUIDELINES

Establishing Brain Death in Children

Coma and apnea must coexist. Child must exhibit complete loss of consciousness, vocalization, and volitional activity.

Brainstem function must be absent, as defined by the following:

- Midposition or fully dilated pupils in both eyes that do not respond to light.
- Absence of spontaneous eye movements and those induced by oculocephalic and caloric (oculovestibular) testing.
- Absence of movement of bulbar musculature, including facial and oropharyngeal muscles.
- Absence of the corneal, gag, cough, sucking, and rooting reflexes.
- Absence of respiratory movements when child is removed from respirator. Apnea testing using standardized methods can be performed but is done after other criteria are met.

Child must not be significantly hypothermic or hypotensive for age.

Flaccid tone and absence of spontaneous or induced movements, including spinal cord events such as reflex withdrawal or spinal myoclonus, should exist.

Examination should remain consistent with brain death throughout the observation and testing period.

Observation periods according to age:

Term newborn 37 weeks of gestational age and up to 30 days of age—Two separate examinations separated by at least 24 hours

31 days to 18 years old—Two separate examinations separated by at least 12 hours

Ancillary testing with electroencephalogram or cerebral blood flow testing should be considered if there is concern about the validity of the examination.

Data from Nakagawa, T. A., Ashwal, S., Mathur, M., et al. (2012). Guidelines for the determination of brain death in infants and children: An update of the 1987 task force recommendations—executive summary. *Annals of Neurology, 71*(4), 573-585.

NEUROLOGIC EXAMINATION

The purpose of the neurologic examination is to establish an accurate, objective baseline of neurologic function. Therefore it is essential that the neurologic examination be documented in a descriptive and detailed fashion, thereby enhancing the ability to detect subtle changes in neurologic status over time. Descriptions of behaviors should be simple, objective, and easily interpreted—for example, "Drowsy but awake and conversationally rational/oriented" or "Sleepy but arousable with vigorous physical stimuli; pressure to nail base of right hand results in upper extremity flexion/lower extremity extension."

Vital signs, observation of posture and movement (both spontaneous and elicited), eye examination, CN testing, and reflex testing all provide valuable clues regarding the LOC, the site of involvement, and the probable cause, but they do not necessarily parallel the depth of a comatose state.

Vital Signs

Pulse, respiration, and blood pressure provide information regarding the adequacy of circulation and the possible underlying cause of altered consciousness. Autonomic activity is most intensively disturbed in deep coma and in brainstem lesions. Body temperature is often elevated; sometimes the elevation is extreme. High temperature is most often a sign of an acute infectious process or heatstroke, but it may be caused by ingestion of some drugs (especially salicylates, alcohol, and barbiturates) or by intracranial bleeding, especially subarachnoid hemorrhage. Hypothalamic involvement may cause elevated or decreased temperature. Serious infection may produce hypothermia.

The pulse is variable and may be rapid, slow and bounding, or feeble. Blood pressure may be normal, elevated, or very low. The Cushing reflex, or pressor response that causes a slowing of the pulse and an increase in blood pressure, is uncommon in children; when it does occur, it is a very late sign of increased ICP. Medications can also affect vital signs. For assessment purposes, actual changes in pulse and blood pressure are more important than the direction of the change.

Respirations are more often slow, deep, and irregular. Slow and deep breathing often occurs in the heavy sleep caused by sedatives, after seizures, or in cerebral infections. Slow, shallow breathing may result from sedatives or opioids. Hyperventilation (deep and rapid respirations) is usually the result of metabolic acidosis or abnormal stimulation of the respiratory center in the medulla caused by salicylate poisoning, hepatic coma, or Reye syndrome. A pattern of alternating hyperventilation and breath holding during wakefulness is common in Rett syndrome.

Breathing patterns have been described with a number of terms (e.g., *apneustic, cluster, ataxic, Cheyne-Stokes*). However, it is better to describe what is being observed rather than placing a label on it because the terms are often used and interpreted incorrectly. Periodic or irregular breathing is a sign of brainstem (especially medullary) dysfunction. This is an ominous sign that often precedes complete apnea. The odor of the breath may provide additional clues (e.g., the fruity and acetone odor of ketosis, the foul odor of uremia, the fetid odor of hepatic failure, or the odor of alcohol).

Skin

The skin may offer clues to the cause of unconsciousness. The body surface should be examined for injury, needle marks, petechiae, bites, and ticks. Evidence of toxic substances may be found on the hands, face, mouth, and clothing—especially in small children.

Eyes

Assess pupil size and reactivity (Fig. 30.3). Pupils either do or do not react to light. Pinpoint pupils are commonly observed in poisoning (e.g., opiate or barbiturate poisoning) or in brainstem dysfunction. Widely dilated and reactive pupils are often seen after seizures and may involve only one side. Widely dilated and fixed pupils suggest paralysis of CN III (oculomotor nerve) secondary to pressure from herniation of the brain through the tentorium. A unilateral fixed pupil usually suggests a

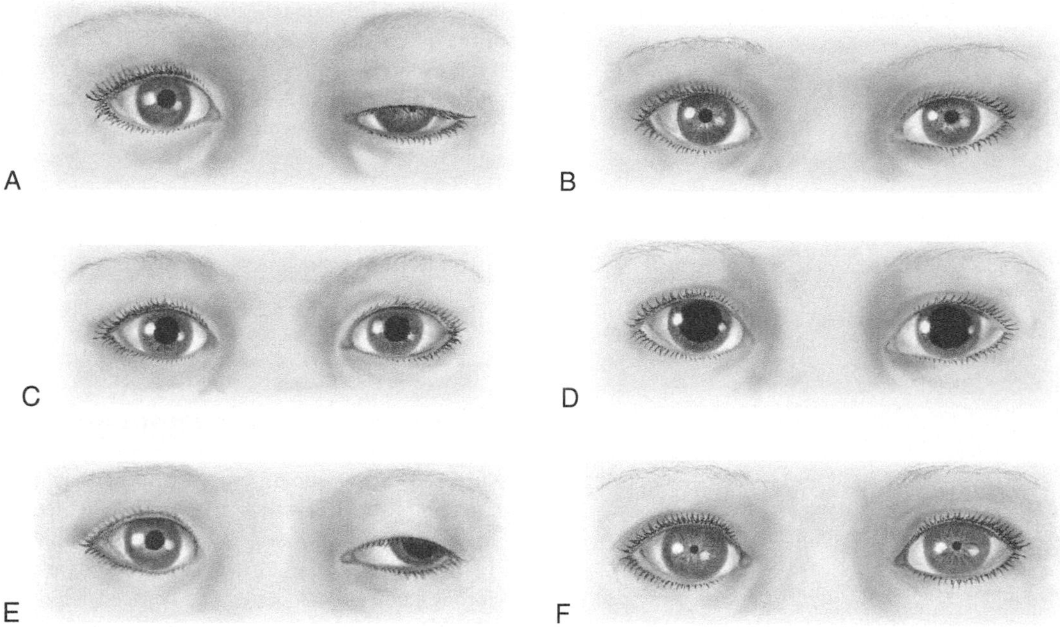

FIG. 30.3 Variations in pupil size with altered states of consciousness. **A,** Ipsilateral pupillary constriction with slight ptosis. **B,** Bilateral small pupils. **C,** Midposition, light fixed to all stimuli. **D,** Bilateral dilated and fixed pupils. **E,** Dilated pupils, left eye abducted with ptosis. **F,** Pinpoint pupils.

lesion on the same side. Bilateral fixed pupils if present for more than 5 minutes usually imply brainstem damage. Dilated and nonreactive pupils also occur in hypothermia, anoxia, ischemia, poisoning with atropine-like substances, or prior instillation of mydriatic drugs. Some of the therapies used (e.g., barbiturates) can alter pupil size and reaction.

The description of eye movements should indicate whether one or both eyes are involved and how the reaction was elicited. Ask the parents if the child has strabismus which may cause the eyes to appear misaligned.

> **! NURSING ALERT**
>
> The sudden appearance of a fixed and dilated pupil is a neurosurgical emergency.

Blinking observed at rest or in response to a sudden loud noise or bright light implies that the pontine reticular formation is intact. The corneal reflex, blinking of the eyelids when the cornea is touched with a wisp of cotton, can test the integrity of the ophthalmic division of CN V (trigeminal nerve). Posttraumatic strabismus indicates CN VI (abducens nerve) damage.

Eye movements are assessed by the doll's head maneuver, in which the child's head is rotated quickly to one side and then to the other. When the brainstem centers for eye movement are intact, there is conjugate (paired or working together) movement of the eyes in the direction opposite the head rotation. Absence of this response suggests dysfunction of the brainstem or CN III. Downward or lateral deviation is often observed in association with pupillary dilation in dysfunction of CN III.

> **! NURSING ALERT**
>
> Any tests that require head movement are not attempted until after cervical spine injury has been ruled out.

The caloric test, or oculovestibular response, is elicited by irrigating the external auditory canal with 10 ml of ice water over a period of approximately 20 seconds (with the head of bed elevated at a 30-degree angle). This test normally causes movement of the eyes toward the side of stimulation. This response is lost when the pontine centers are impaired and thus provides important information in assessment of the comatose patient.

> **! NURSING ALERT**
>
> The ice water caloric test is painful and is never performed if the child is awake or the tympanic membranes are ruptured.

Funduscopic examination reveals additional clues. Because it takes 24 to 48 hours to develop, papilledema (e.g., optic disc swelling, indistinct margins, hemorrhages, tortuosity of vessels, absence of venous pulsations), if it develops at all, will not be evident early in the course of unconsciousness. The presence of retinal hemorrhages in children is usually the result of accidental or inflicted trauma with intracranial bleeding (usually subarachnoid or subdural hemorrhage) but is sometimes caused by infection (Minns, Jones, Tandon, et al., 2017).

Motor Function

Observation of spontaneous activity, posture, and response to painful stimuli provides clues to the location and extent of cerebral dysfunction. Asymmetric movements of the limbs or the absence of movement suggests paralysis. In hemiplegia the affected limb lies in external rotation and falls uncontrollably when lifted and allowed to drop. Observations should be described rather than labeled.

In the deeper comatose states the child has little or no spontaneous movement, and the musculature tends to be flaccid. There is considerable variability in motor behavior in lesser degrees of coma. For example, the child may be relatively immobile or restless and hyperkinetic; muscle tone may be increased or decreased. Tremors, twitching, and spasms of muscles are common observations. The patient may display purposeless

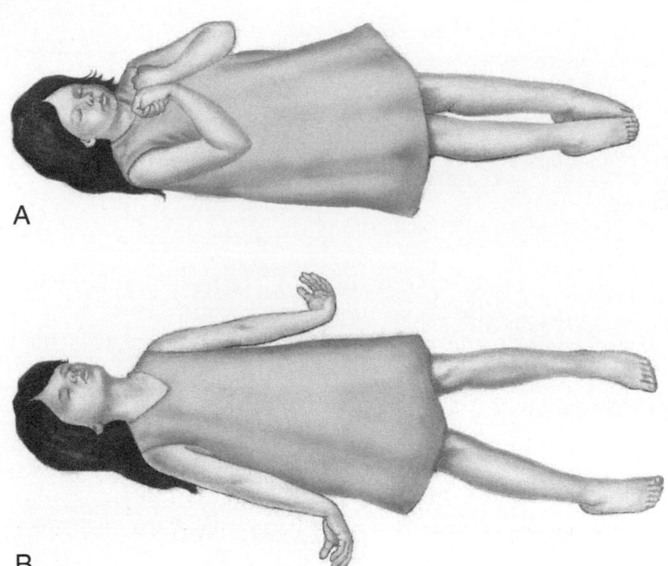

FIG. 30.4 **A,** Flexion posturing. **B,** Extension posturing.

plucking or tossing movements. Combative or negativistic behavior is not uncommon. Hyperactivity is more common in acute febrile and toxic states than in cases of increased ICP. Seizures are common in children and may be present in coma as a result of any cause. Any repetitive movements and movements during seizures are described.

Posturing

Primitive postural reflexes emerge as cortical control over motor function is lost in brain dysfunction. These reflexes are evident in posturing and motor movements directly related to the area of the brain involved. Posturing reflects a balance between the lower exciting and the higher inhibiting influences. Strong muscles overcome weaker ones. Flexion posturing (Fig. 30.4, *A*) occurs with severe dysfunction of the cerebral cortex or with lesions to corticospinal tracts above the brainstem. Typical flexion posturing includes rigid flexion, with arms held tightly to the body; flexed elbows, wrists, and fingers; plantar flexed feet; legs extended and internally rotated; and possibly fine tremors or intense stiffness. Extension posturing (Fig. 30.4, *B*) is a sign of dysfunction at the level of the midbrain or lesions to the brainstem. It is characterized by rigid extension and pronation of the arms and legs, flexed wrists and fingers, clenched jaw, extended neck, and possibly an arched back. Unilateral extension posturing is often caused by tentorial herniation.

Posturing may not be evident when the child is quiet but can usually be elicited by applying painful stimuli such as a blunt object pressed on the base of the nail. Nurses should avoid applying thumb pressure to the supraorbital region of the frontal bone (risk of orbital damage). Noxious stimuli (e.g., suctioning), turning, or touching will elicit a response. When the nurse is describing posturing, the stimulus needed to provoke the response is as important as the reaction.

Reflexes

Testing of certain reflexes, such as those present in an intact spinal cord, may be of limited value. (See Chapter 4.) In general, the corneal, pupillary, muscle-stretch, superficial, and plantar reflexes tend to be absent in deep coma. The state of reflexes is variable in lighter grades of unconsciousness and depends on the underlying pathologic process and the location of the lesion. The doll's eye reflex maneuver, described previously, reflects paralysis of CN III. The absence of corneal reflexes (CN V) and the presence of a tonic neck reflex are associated with severe brain damage. The Babinski reflex, in which the lateral portion of the bottom of the foot is stroked and causes the big toe to go up, may be of value if it is found to be present consistently in children older than 1 year. A positive Babinski reflex is significant in the assessment of pyramidal tract lesions when it is unilateral and associated with other pyramidal signs. A fluctuating Babinski reflex is often observed after seizures. (See Fig. 7.10, *B*.)

NURSING TIP

Three key reflexes that demonstrate neurologic health in young infants are the Moro, tonic neck, and withdrawal reflexes.

SPECIAL DIAGNOSTIC PROCEDURES

Numerous diagnostic procedures are used for assessment of cerebral function. Laboratory tests that may help determine the cause of unconsciousness include blood glucose, urea nitrogen, and electrolyte (pH, sodium, potassium, chloride, calcium, and bicarbonate) tests; clotting studies, hematocrit, and a complete blood count; liver function tests; blood cultures if there is fever; and sometimes studies to detect lead or other toxic substances, such as drugs.

An electroencephalogram (EEG) may provide important information. For example, generalized random, slow activity suggests suppressed cortical function, and localized slow activity suggests a space-occupying lesion. A flat tracing is one of the criteria used as evidence of brain death. Examination of spinal fluid is carried out when toxic encephalopathy or infection is suspected. Lumbar puncture is delayed if intracranial hemorrhage is suspected, and is contraindicated in the presence of increased ICP because of the potential for brainstem herniation.

Auditory and visual evoked potentials are sometimes used in neurologic evaluation of very young children. Brainstem auditory evoked potentials are useful for evaluating the continuity of brainstem auditory tracts and are particularly useful for detecting demyelinating disease and neoplasms of the brainstem and for distinguishing between brainstem and cortical lesions. For example, a normal evoked potential in a comatose patient suggests involvement of the cerebral hemispheres.

Highly sophisticated tests are carried out with specialized equipment. Two imaging techniques, computed tomography (CT) and magnetic resonance imaging (MRI) (Fig. 30.5), assist in diagnosis by scanning both soft tissues and solid matter. Most of these tests are listed in Table 30.1. Because these tests can be threatening to children, the nurse needs to prepare patients and their parents/guardians for the tests and provide support and reassurance during the tests. Consultation with a child life specialist can also be helpful. (See Preparation for Diagnostic and Therapeutic Procedures, Chapter 22.)

Children who are old enough to understand require careful explanation of the procedure, why it is being done, what they will experience, and how they can help. School-age children usually appreciate a more detailed description of why contrast material is injected. Because children are often frightened of needles, they and their families need to be informed of any medication or contrast medium that will be administered intravenously. Special anxiety reduction strategies may be necessary for children who have blood-injury-injection (needle) phobia (McMurtry, Taddio, Noel, et al., 2016). This phobia is the most inheritable of all phobias. The nurse should talk with parents to find out if they also have this phobia and will need help with anxiety management (Van Houtem, Laine, Boomsma, et al., 2013). When tests require venipuncture, the application of local anesthetics can prevent pain and increase the chance of venipuncture success (Baxter, Ewing, Young et al., 2013).

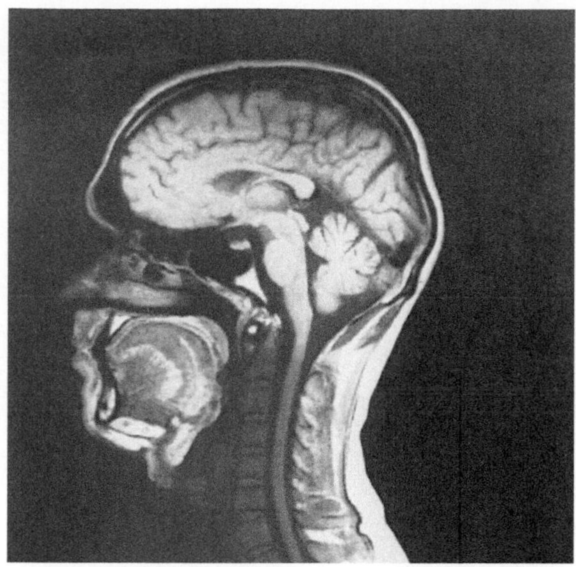

FIG. 30.5 Magnetic resonance imaging. Midsagittal image produces excellent anatomic detail. Note clear delineation of structures such as pituitary gland, brainstem, spinal cord, cerebellum, corpus callosum, and sylvian aqueduct. (Courtesy Philips Medical Systems. From Nolte, J. [1993]. *The human brain: An introduction to its functional anatomy* [3rd ed.]. St. Louis, MO: Mosby.)

The importance of lying still for tests needs to be stressed. Children unfamiliar with the machines can be shown a picture beforehand. Although radiographic examinations are not painful, the machinery often appears so frightening that the child protests because of anxiety. This is especially true of CT and MRI, both of which require that the child's head be placed within a special immobilizing device. Chin and cheek pads are sometimes used to prevent the slightest head movement, and straps are applied to the body to prevent a slight change in body position. The nurse can explain these events to a frightened child by comparing them to an astronaut's preparation for a space flight. It is important to emphasize to the child that at no time is the procedure painful.

It is helpful for nurses to become acquainted with the equipment and the general environment in which the test will take place so they can better explain the procedure to children and their families at their level of understanding. Written material describing the procedure should be available for parents and may be appropriate to share with children. Equipment is often strange and ominous to children. They need constant reassurance from a trusted companion.

The nurse should not expect cooperation from a young child. Sedation may be required. Many different agents are currently used for sedation of children undergoing neurologic diagnostic procedures. Chloral hydrate or benzodiazepines have been used for decades as short-term sedative agents and remain safe methods of pediatric sedation (Arlachov & Ganatra, 2012). Other sedative agents have been used safely, alone and

TABLE 30.1 Neurologic Diagnostic Procedures

Test	Description	Purpose	Comments
Lumbar puncture (LP)	Spinal needle is inserted between L3 and L4 or L4 and L5 vertebral spaces into subarachnoid space; cerebrospinal fluid (CSF) pressure is measured, and sample is collected for examination.	Measures spinal fluid pressure Obtains CSF for laboratory analysis Injection of medication	Contraindicated in patients with increased intracranial pressure (ICP) or infected skin over puncture site.
Subdural tap	Needle is inserted into anterior fontanel or coronal suture (midline to pupil).	Helps rule out subdural effusions Removes CSF to relieve pressure	Place infant in semierect position after subdural tap to minimize leakage from site; prevent child from crying if possible. Check site frequently for evidence of leakage.
Ventricular puncture	Needle is inserted into lateral ventricle via coronal suture (midline to pupil).	Removes CSF to relieve pressure	Risk of intracerebral or ventricular hemorrhage.
Electroencephalography (EEG)	EEG records changes in electrical potential of brain. Electrodes are placed at various points to assess electrical function in a particular area. Impulses are recorded by electromagnetic pen or digitally.	Detects spikes, or bursts of electrical activity that indicate the potential for seizures Used to determine brain death	Patient should remain quiet during procedure; may require sedation. Minimize external stimuli during procedure.
Nuclear brain scan	Radioisotope is injected intravenously, then counted and recorded after fixed time intervals. Radioisotope accumulates in areas where blood-brain barrier is defective.	Identifies focal brain lesions (e.g., tumors, abscesses) Positive uptake of material with encephalitis and subdural hematoma Visualizes CSF pathways	Requires intravenous (IV) access; patient may require sedation. In normal children or noncommunicating hydrocephalus, no retrograde filling of ventricles occurs. Areas of concentrated uptake of material are termed *hot spots.*
Endocephalography	Pulses of ultrasonic waves are beamed through head; echoes from reflecting surfaces are recorded graphically.	Identifies shifts in midline structures from their normal positions as a result of intracranial lesions May show ventricular dilation	Simple, safe, rapid procedure.

Continued

TABLE 30.1 **Neurologic Diagnostic Procedures—cont'd**

Test	Description	Purpose	Comments
Real-time ultrasonography (RTUS)	RTUS is similar to CT but uses ultrasound instead of ionizing radiation.	Allows high-resolution anatomic visualization in variety of imaging planes	Produces images similar to CT scan. Especially useful in neonatal central nervous system problems.
Radiography	Skull films are taken from different views—lateral, posterolateral, axial (submentoventricular), half-axial.	Shows fractures, dislocations, spreading suture lines, craniostenosis Shows degenerative changes, bone erosion, calcifications	Simple, noninvasive procedure.
Computed tomography (CT) scan	Pinpoint x-ray beam is directed on horizontal or vertical plane to provide series of images that are fed into computer and assembled in image displayed on video screen. CT uses ionizing radiation.	Visualizes horizontal and vertical cross section of brain in three planes (axial, coronal, sagittal) Distinguishes density of various intracranial tissues and structures—congenital abnormalities, hemorrhage, tumors, demyelinating and inflammatory processes, calcification	Requires IV access if contrast agent is used. Patient may require sedation.
Magnetic resonance imaging (MRI)	MRI produces radiofrequency emissions from elements (e.g., hydrogen, phosphorus), which are converted to visual images by computer.	Permits visualization of morphologic feature of target structures Permits tissue discrimination unavailable with many techniques	MRI is noninvasive procedure except when IV contrast agent is used. No exposure to radiation occurs. Patient may require sedation. Parent or attendant can remain in room with child. MRI does not visualize bone detail or calcifications. No metal can be present in scanner.
Positron emission tomography (PET)	PET involves IV injection of positron-emitting radionucleotide; local concentrations are detected and transformed into visual display by computer.	Detects and measures blood volume and flow in brain, metabolic activity, biochemical changes within tissue	Requires lengthy period of immobility. Minimum exposure to radiation occurs. Patient may require sedation.
Digital subtraction angiography (DSA)	Contrast dye is injected intravenously; computer "subtracts" all tissues without contrast medium, leaving clear image of contrast medium in vessels studied.	Visualizes vasculature of target tissue Visualizes finite vascular abnormalities	Safe alternative to angiography. Patient must remain still during procedure; may require sedation.
Single-photon emission computed tomography (SPECT)	SPECT involves IV injection of photon-emitting radionuclide; radionuclides are absorbed by healthy tissue at different rate than diseased or necrotic tissue; data are transferred to computer that converts image to film.	Provides information regarding blood flow to tissues; analyzing blood flow to organ may help determine how well it is functioning	Requires lengthy period of immobility. Minimum exposure to radiation occurs. Patient may require sedation.

in combination, for children and include intravenous (IV) sodium pentobarbital (Nembutal), IV fentanyl (Sublimaze), IV midazolam (Versed), and intranasal midazolam (Arlachov & Ganatra, 2012). Propofol is a good sedating agent for diagnostic procedures, but the medication can produce profound respiratory depression and should be administered only by trained personnel such as anesthesiologists (Arlachov & Ganatra, 2012). (See Pain Management, Chapter 5.)

Physical preparation for the diagnostic test may involve administration of a sedative. If so, children should be helped through the preparation and administration and assured that someone will remain with them (if this is possible). Children need continual support and reinforcement during procedures in which they remain conscious. Vital signs and physiologic responses to the procedure are monitored throughout. Many diagnostic procedures performed on an outpatient basis require sedation, and children need recovery time and observation. The nurse should review written instructions with parents if the child is discharged after a procedure. Children who have undergone a procedure with a general anesthetic require postanesthesia care, including positioning to prevent aspiration of secretions and frequent assessment of vital signs, oxygen saturation, and LOC. In addition, other neurologic functions such as pupillary responses, motor strength, and movement are tested at regular intervals. Any surgical wound resulting from the test is checked for bleeding, CSF leakage, and other complications. Children who undergo repeated subdural taps should have their hematocrit monitored to detect excessive blood loss from the procedure.

Consider children's emotional reactions to the procedure. They should be allowed and encouraged to express their feelings about the experience through verbal expression and therapeutic play. Parents also seek an explanation of the results of tests and procedures performed on their children. Nurses are in a unique position to provide support and education to parents regarding procedures.

THE CHILD WITH CEREBRAL COMPROMISE

NURSING CARE OF THE UNCONSCIOUS CHILD

The unconscious child requires nursing attendance with observation, recording, and evaluation of changes in objective signs. These observations provide valuable information regarding the patient's progress and often serve as a guide to diagnosis and treatment. Therefore careful and detailed observations are essential for the child's welfare. In addition, vital functions must be maintained and complications prevented through conscientious and meticulous nursing care. The outcome of unconsciousness is variable and ranges from early and complete recovery, to death within a few hours or days, or persistent and permanent unconsciousness, or recovery with varying degrees of residual mental or physical disability. The outcome and recovery of the unconscious child may depend on the level of nursing care and observational skills.

Direct emergency measures toward ensuring circulation, airway, and breathing (CAB); stabilizing the spine when indicated; treating shock; and reducing ICP (if present). Delayed treatment often leads to increased damage. Therapies for specific causes of unconsciousness begin as soon as emergency measures have been implemented; in many cases they occur concurrently. Because nursing care is closely related to the medical management, both are considered here.

Continual observation of the LOC, pupillary reaction, and vital signs is essential to management of CNS disorders. Regular assessment of neurologic status and vital signs is an integral part of the nursing care of unconscious children. The frequency depends on the cause of unconsciousness, the LOC, and the progression of cerebral involvement. Intervals between observations may be as short as every 15 minutes or as long as every 2 hours. Significant alterations are reported immediately.

The temperature is measured every 2 to 4 hours, depending on the child's condition. An elevated temperature may occur in children with CNS dysfunction; therefore a light covering may be sufficient. Vigorous efforts, such as tepid sponge baths or application of a hypothermia blanket, are needed to prevent brain damage if the rectal temperature exceeds 104°F (40°C).

The LOC is assessed periodically, including pupillary size, equality, and reaction to light. Signs of meningeal irritation, such as nuchal rigidity, need to be assessed. Assessment of LOC also includes response to vocal commands, spontaneous behavior, resistance to care, and response to painful stimuli. Note any abnormal movements, changes in muscle tone or strength, and body position. If a seizure occurs, describe the seizure, including the body areas involved from the beginning to the end of the seizure, and the duration of seizure (see Box 30.11 and Critical Thinking Case Study later in this chapter).

Pain management for the unconscious child requires astute nursing observation and management. Signs of pain include changes in behavior (e.g., increased agitation and rigidity) and alterations in vital signs and perfusion (usually, an increased heart rate, respiratory rate, and blood pressure, and decreased oxygen saturation). Because these findings are not specific for pain, the nurse should be alert for their appearance during times of induced or suspected pain and for their disappearance after the inciting procedure or the administration of analgesia. A pain assessment record is used to document indications of pain and the effectiveness of interventions. (See Pain Assessment, Chapter 5.) The use of opioids, such as morphine, to relieve pain is controversial because they can mask signs of altered consciousness or depress respirations. However, unrelieved pain activates the stress response, which can elevate ICP. To block the stress response, some authorities advocate the use of analgesics, sedatives, and, in some cases such as head injury, paralyzing agents via continuous IV infusion. A commonly used combination is fentanyl, midazolam, and vecuronium (Norcuron). If there are concerns about assessing the LOC or respiratory depression, naloxone can be used to reverse the opioid effects. Acetaminophen and ibuprofen may also be effective analgesics for mild to moderate pain (Whittaker, 2013). Codeine should not be used to treat pain in children under 12 years old (Lazaryan, Shasha-Zigelman, Dagan, et al., 2015). Regardless of the drugs used, adequate dosage and regular administration are essential to provide optimum pain relief.

> **! NURSING ALERT**
>
> When opioids are used, bowel elimination must be closely monitored because of the potential constipating effect. A stool softener should be given regularly with laxatives as needed to prevent constipation.

Other measures to relieve discomfort include providing a quiet, dimly lit environment; limiting visitors; preventing any sudden, jarring movement, such as banging into the bed; and preventing an increase in ICP. The latter is most effectively achieved by proper positioning and prevention of straining, such as during coughing, vomiting, or defecating. (See Pain Management, Chapter 5.) Antiepileptic drugs, such as fosphenytoin (Cerebyx) or phenobarbital, may be ordered for control of seizure activity.

Respiratory Management

Respiratory effectiveness is the primary concern in the care of the unconscious child, and establishment of an adequate airway is always the first priority. Carbon dioxide has a potent vasodilating effect and will increase CBF and ICP. Cerebral hypoxia at normal body temperature that lasts longer than 4 minutes often causes irreversible brain damage.

> **! NURSING ALERT**
>
> Respiratory obstruction and subsequent compromise lead to cardiac arrest. Always maintain an adequate, patent airway.

Children in lighter stages of coma may be able to cough and swallow, but those in deeper states of coma are unable to manage secretions, which tend to pool in the throat and pharynx. Dysfunction of CNs IX and X (glossopharyngeal and vagus nerves) places the child at risk of aspiration and cardiac arrest. Therefore position the child with the head and body to the side to prevent aspiration of secretions, and empty the stomach to reduce the likelihood of vomiting. In infants, the blockage of air passages from secretions can happen in seconds. In addition, upper airway obstruction from laryngospasm is a common complication in comatose children.

An oral airway can be used for the child who is suffering a temporary loss of consciousness, such as after a contusion, seizure, or anesthesia. For children who remain unconscious for a longer time, a nasotracheal or orotracheal tube is inserted to maintain the open airway and facilitate removal of secretions. A tracheostomy is performed in cases in which laryngoscopy for introduction of an endotracheal tube would be difficult or dangerous or for a child who needs long-term ventilatory support. Suctioning is used only as needed to clear the airway, exerting care to prevent increasing ICP. Respiratory status is observed and evaluated regularly. Signs of respiratory distress may indicate a need for ventilator assistance.

Mechanical ventilation is usually indicated when the respiratory center is involved. Blood gas analysis is performed regularly, and oxygen is administered when indicated. Moderately severe hypoxia and respiratory acidosis are often present, but they are not always evident from clinical manifestations. Hypoventilation often accompanies unconsciousness and may lead to respiratory alkalosis, or it may represent the body's attempt to compensate for metabolic acidosis. Therefore blood gas and pH determinations are essential guides for electrolyte therapy. Chest physiotherapy is carried out on a regular basis, and the child's position is changed at least every 2 hours to prevent pulmonary complications. Regular oral hygiene is recommended to reduce the risk of ventilator-associated pneumonia (VAP) (Hua, Xie, Worthington, et al., 2016).

Intracranial Pressure Monitoring

The selection of the type of ICP monitor should be guided by the clinical presentation and the therapeutic strategy chosen for each child. Indications for inserting an ICP monitor are (1) GCS evaluation ≤8, (2) GCS evaluation >8 with respiratory assistance, (3) deterioration of condition, and (4) subjective judgment regarding clinical appearance and response (Singhi & Tiwari, 2009).

Four major types of ICP monitors are intraventricular catheter with or without fibroscopic sensors attached to a monitoring system, subarachnoid bolt (Richmond screw), epidural sensor, and anterior fontanel pressure monitor. Transducers for both ventricular and subarachnoid monitoring should be set up without the use of a flush device. Direct ventricular pressure measurement remains the gold standard of ICP monitoring.

The catheter method involves introduction of a catheter into the lateral ventricle on the nondominant side, if known, or placement in the subdural space. The catheter has the advantage of providing a means of extraventricular (or continuous) drainage of CSF to reduce pressure. A drainage bag attached to the system is kept at the level of the ventricles and can be lowered to decrease ICP. This device requires full penetration of the brain, requires skill and experience with placement, and carries the risk of infection. Infection risks can be lowered by always using aseptic technique when handling the external ventricular drainage (EVD) system, manipulating the EVD as little as possible, and sterile dressing changes only weekly or when the dressing is compromised, whichever occurs first (Hepburn-Smith, Dynkevich, Spektor, et al., 2016).

> **! NURSING ALERT**
>
> If the external ventricular drain is unclamped for CSF drainage, carefully monitor the level of the collection container. If the container is positioned too low, improper CSF decompression could lower ICP too rapidly, causing bleeding and pain.

With the bolt method the end of the bolt is placed into the subarachnoid space. The bolt cannot be adequately secured in a small child's pliant skull, although special modifications have been developed for children under 6 years of age. The placement of the bolt is not adjusted by anyone except the neurosurgeon who placed the device. The neurosurgeon is notified if a satisfactory waveform is not observed.

> **! NURSING ALERT**
>
> With the bolt method, the bolt is stabilized with dressings, but these are not changed or disturbed—not even to check the site.

An epidural sensor can be placed between the dura and the skull through a burr hole and connected to a stopcock assembly and a transducer, which provides a readout of the pressure. Although less invasive, the epidural sensor may have inconsistent correlation of pressure readings. In infants a fontanel transducer can be used to detect impulses from a pressure sensor and convert them to electrical energy. The electrical energy is then converted to visible waves or numeric readings on an oscilloscope. ICP measurement from the anterior fontanel is noninvasive but may prove to be inaccurate if the equipment is poorly placed or inconsistently recalibrated. Intraparenchymal pressure monitoring devices (e.g., Camino) use fiberoptic technology and perform reliably.

ICP can be increased by direct instillation of solutions; therefore antibiotics are administered systemically if a positive CSF culture is obtained. However, ICP monitoring rarely causes infection. CSF is a body fluid; therefore implement Standard Precautions according to hospital policy. (See Infection Control, Chapter 22.)

Nurses caring for patients with intracranial monitoring devices must be acquainted with the system, assist with insertion, interpret the monitor readings, and be able to distinguish between danger signals and mechanical dysfunction. Because systemic blood pressure, ICP, and therefore CPP are normally lower in children, the child's age must be taken into account when deciding what constitutes abnormally high ICP or abnormally low CPP.

Several medical measures are available to treat increased ICP resulting from cerebral edema. These include sedation, CSF drainage, and osmotic diuretics. Osmotic diuretics may provide rapid relief of ICP in emergency situations. Although their effect is transient, lasting only about 6 hours, they can be lifesaving in emergencies. These substances are rapidly excreted by the kidneys and carry with them large quantities of sodium and water. Mannitol (or sometimes urea) administered intravenously is the drug most commonly used for rapid reduction of ICP. The infusion is generally given slowly but may be pushed rapidly if there is herniation or impending herniation. Because of the profound diuretic effect of the drug, an indwelling catheter is inserted to ensure bladder emptying. $Paco_2$ should be maintained at approximately 30 mm Hg to produce vasoconstriction, which reduces CBF, thereby decreasing ICP. Recording and analyzing the child's volume state, plasma sodium concentration, and serum osmolarity can avert potential fluid and electrolyte problems. Administration of adrenocorticosteroids is not recommended for cerebral edema secondary to head trauma.

Nursing Activities

In cases of high levels of increased ICP, nursing procedures tend to trigger reactive pressure waves in many children. For example, increased intrathoracic or abdominal pressure will be transmitted to the cranium. The goals of monitoring a child who is neurologically compromised include maintaining CPP; controlling ICP, cerebral edema, and factors that increase cerebral metabolism (e.g., fever, seizures); and maintaining hemodynamic stability. Take particular care in positioning these patients to avoid neck vein compression that may further increase ICP by interfering with venous return.

> **! NURSING ALERT**
>
> Elevate the head of the bed 15–30 degrees, and position the child so that the head is maintained in midline to facilitate venous drainage and avoid jugular compression. Turning side to side is contraindicated because of the risk of jugular compression.

Sandbags or other support devices can help maintain correct head position. The child can be propped to one side or the other, and the use of a pressure-relieving or pressure-decreasing mattress decreases the chance of prolonged pressure to vulnerable skin areas. Frequent clinical assessment of the child cannot be replaced by an ICP monitoring device.

It is important to avoid activities that may increase ICP by causing pain or emotional stress. Clustering nursing activities together and minimizing environmental stimuli by decreasing noxious procedures help control ICP. Range-of-motion exercises can be carried out gently but should not be performed vigorously. Any necessary disturbing procedures should be scheduled to take advantage of therapies that reduce ICP, such as osmotherapy and sedation. Make efforts to minimize or eliminate environmental noise, including managing the number of visitors. Assessment and intervention to relieve pain are important nursing functions to decrease ICP.

Suctioning and percussion are poorly tolerated; therefore these procedures are contraindicated unless the child has concurrent respiratory problems. Hypoxia and the Valsalva maneuver associated with cough acutely elevate ICP. Vibration, which does not increase ICP, accomplishes excellent results and should be tried first if treatment is needed. If suctioning is necessary, it should be used judiciously and preceded by hyperventilation with 100% oxygen, which can be monitored during suctioning with a pulse oxygen sensor reading to determine oxygen saturation.

Nutrition and Hydration

In the unconscious child, fluids and calories are supplied initially by the IV route. (See Chapter 25.) The type of fluid administered depends on the patient's general condition. Children on the ketogenic diet and with certain metabolic disorders, such as pyruvate dehydrogenase deficiency, should receive normal saline rather than fluids containing dextrose, which can cause seizures and worsen their condition. Fluid therapy requires careful monitoring and adjustment based on neurologic signs and electrolyte determinations. Often, unconscious children cannot tolerate the same amounts of fluid as when they are healthy. Over-hydration must be avoided to prevent fatal cerebral edema. When cerebral edema is a threat, fluids may be restricted to reduce the chance of fluid overload. Examine skin and mucous membranes for signs of dehydration. Adjustments to fluid administration are based on urinary output, serum electrolytes and osmolarity, blood pressure, and arterial filling pressure. Observation for signs of altered fluid balance related to abnormal pituitary secretions is a part of nursing care.

Provide long-term nutrition in a balanced formula given by nasogastric or gastrostomy tube. The nasogastric tube is usually taped in place, with care taken to prevent pressure on the nares. Most children have continuous feedings. When bolus feedings are used, the tube is rinsed with water after each feeding. Tubes are replaced according to institutional policy. Irritation of the nasal mucosa is prevented by alternating nares each time the nasogastric tube is replaced.

Avoid overfeeding to prevent vomiting and the associated risk of aspiration. Stomach contents are aspirated with a syringe and measured before feeding to ascertain the amount remaining in the stomach. The removed contents may be refed. If the residual volume is excessive (depending on the child's size), consult the dietitian and physician regarding the composition and amount to determine whether changes are required to provide calories and nutrients in a smaller volume.

Altered Pituitary Secretion

An altered ability to handle fluid loads is attributed in part to the syndrome of inappropriate antidiuretic hormone (SIADH) and diabetes insipidus (DI) resulting from hypothalamic dysfunction. (See Chapter 31.) SIADH often accompanies CNS conditions such as head injury, meningitis, encephalitis, brain abscess, brain tumor, and subarachnoid hemorrhage. In the child with SIADH, scant quantities of urine are excreted, electrolyte analysis reveals hyponatremia and hypoosmolality, and manifestations of over-hydration are evident. It is important to evaluate all parameters because the reduced urinary output might be erroneously interpreted as a sign of dehydration. The treatment of SIADH consists of fluid restriction until serum electrolytes and osmolality return to normal levels. If fluid restriction is not completely ineffective, medications such as sodium chloride and diuretics may be used.

TABLE 30.2 Effects of Altered Pituitary Secretion

Measurement	Diabetes Insipidus	Syndrome of Inappropriate Antidiuretic Hormone Secretion
Urinary output	Increased	Decreased
Specific gravity	Decreased	Increased
Serum sodium	Increased (hypernatremia)	Decreased (hyponatremia)

DI may occur after intracranial trauma. In DI there is increased urinary volume and the accompanying danger of dehydration. See Table 30.2 for comparison of fluid changes in SIADH and DI. Adequate replacement of fluids is essential, and observation of electrolyte balance is necessary to detect signs of hypernatremia and hyperosmolality. Exogenous vasopressin may be administered.

Medications

The cause of unconsciousness determines specific drug therapies. Children with infectious processes are given antibiotics appropriate to the disease and the infecting organism. Corticosteroids are prescribed for inflammatory conditions and edema. Cerebral edema is an indication for osmotic diuretics. Antiepileptic medications are prescribed for seizure activity. Sedation in the combative child provides amnesic and anxiolytic properties in conjunction with a paralytic agent. This combination decreases ICP and allows treatment of cerebral edema. Usual drugs include morphine and midazolam. Midazolam is attractive because of its short half-life.

Deep coma induced by the administration of barbiturates is controversial in the management of ICP. Barbiturates are currently reserved for the reduction of increased ICP when all else has failed. Barbiturates decrease the cerebral metabolic rate for oxygen and protect the brain during times of reduced CPP. Barbiturate coma requires extensive monitoring. EEG monitoring can assess depth of coma, record EEG background abnormalities that can help predict outcome, and evaluate any seizure activity. Cardiovascular and respiratory support and ICP monitoring are needed to assess response to therapy. Paralyzing agents such as vecronium may be needed to aid in performing diagnostic tests, improving effectiveness of therapy, and reducing the risks of secondary complications. Elevation of ICP or heart rate in patients who are being given paralyzing agents or are under sedation may indicate the need for another dose of either or both medications or need for pain medication.

Thermoregulation

Hyperthermia often accompanies cerebral dysfunction; if it is present, the nurse implements measures to reduce the temperature to prevent brain damage from hyperthermia and to reduce metabolic demands generated by the increased body temperature. Antipyretics are the method of choice for fever reduction; cooling devices are used for hyperthermia. (See Controlling Elevated Temperatures, Chapter 22.) Laboratory tests and other methods help determine the cause, if any, of the hyperthermia. Treatment with hypothermia and barbiturates increases the risk of iatrogenic complications.

Elimination

A urinary catheter is usually inserted in the acute phase, but diapers may be used and weighed to record urinary output. The child who previously had bowel and bladder control is generally incontinent. If the child remains comatose for a long period, the indwelling catheter may be removed and periodic bladder emptying accomplished by intermittent catheterization. Stool softeners are usually sufficient to maintain bowel function, but suppositories or enemas may be needed occasionally for adequate elimination and to prevent fecal impaction. The passage of liquid stool after a period of no bowel activity is usually a sign of impaction. To avoid this preventable problem, daily recording of bowel activity is essential.

Hygienic Care

Routine measures for cleansing and maintaining skin integrity are an integral part of nursing care of the unconscious child. Skinfolds require special attention to prevent excoriation. The child who is unable to move is prone to develop tissue breakdown and necrosis; therefore the child is placed on a resilient appliance (e.g., alternating-pressure or water-filled mattress) to prevent pressure on prominent areas of the body. The goal is prevention by regular change of position and inspection of vulnerable areas (e.g., the ankle, heels, trochanter, sacrum, and shoulder). Unconscious children undergo numerous invasive procedures, and the skin sites used for these procedures require special assessment and intervention to promote healing and prevent infection. Keep bed linen and any clothing dry and free of wrinkles. Rubbing the back and extremities with lotion stimulates circulation and helps prevent drying of the skin. However, to prevent further tissue damage, do not massage reddened and nonblanching skin. (See Maintaining Healthy Skin, Chapter 22.) If the child requires surgery or radiography, the nurse checks all dressings, bony sites, catheters, and IV access lines before and after the procedure.

Oral care is performed at least twice daily because the mouth tends to become dry or coated with mucus. The teeth are carefully brushed with a soft toothbrush or cleaned with gauze saturated with saline. Commercially prepared cleansing devices, such as Toothettes, are convenient for cleansing the mouth and teeth. Lips are coated with ointment to protect them from drying, cracking, or blistering.

The unconscious child is also prone to eye irritation. The corneal reflexes are absent; therefore the eyes are easily irritated or damaged by linen, dust, or other substances that may come in contact with them. Excessive dryness results from incomplete closure of the lids and/or decreased secretions, especially if the child is undergoing osmotherapy to reduce or prevent brain edema.

> **! NURSING ALERT**
>
> The eyes are examined regularly and carefully for early signs of irritation or inflammation. Artificial tears (methylcellulose) are placed in the eyes every 1–2 hours. Eye patches may be required to protect the eyes from possible damage.

Keep the child's hair combed and secure to prevent tangling. Keep the scalp clean with dry or wet shampoos as needed. The child's head may need to be shaved for tests or surgical procedures. The family may want the hair saved.

Positioning and Exercise

The unconscious child is positioned to minimize ICP and to prevent aspiration of saliva, nasogastric secretions, and vomitus. The head of the bed is elevated, and the child is placed in a side-lying or semiprone position. A small, firm pillow is placed under the head, and the uppermost limbs are flexed and supported with pillows. The weight of the body should not rest on the dependent arm. In the semiprone position the child lies with the dependent arm at the side behind the body; the opposite side is supported on pillows, and the uppermost arm and leg are flexed and resting on the pillows. This position prevents undue pressure on the dependent extremities. The dependent position of the face encourages drainage of secretions and prevents the flaccid tongue from obstructing the airway.

Normal range-of-motion exercises help maintain function and prevent contractures of joints. Perform exercises gently to minimize increasing ICP and with full range of motion. Place a small rolled pad in the palms to help maintain proper positioning of fingers. Splinting may be needed to prevent severe contractures of the wrists, knees, or ankles.

Stimulation

Sensory stimulation is as important in the care of the unconscious child as it is in the care of the alert child. For the temporarily unconscious or semiconscious child, sensory stimulation helps arouse the child to the conscious state and orient the child in terms of time and place. Auditory and tactile stimulation are especially valuable. Tactile stimulation is not appropriate for a child in whom it may elicit an undesirable response. However, for other children tactile contact often has a relaxing and calming effect. When the child's condition permits, holding or rocking the child is soothing and provides the body contact needed by young children.

Hearing is often intact in a state of coma. Hearing is the last sense to be lost and the first one to be regained; therefore speak to the child as any other child. Conversation around the child should not include thoughtless or derogatory remarks. Soft music is often used to provide auditory stimulation. Singing the child's favorite songs or reading a favorite story is a strategy used to maintain the child's contact with a familiar world. Playing songs or favorite stories recorded in the parents' voices can provide a continuous source of familiar stimulation.

Family Support

Helping the parents of an unconscious child cope with the situation is especially difficult. They may demonstrate all the guilt, fear, hostility, and anxiety of any parent of a seriously ill child. (See Chapter 19.) In addition, these parents face the uncertain outcome of the cerebral dysfunction. The fear of death, cognitive impairment, or permanent physical disability is present. Nursing intervention with parents depends on the nature of the pathologic condition, the parents' coping skills, and the parent-child relationship before injury or illness.

Recovering from coma is a complex process and may be confusing for parents and family members, who are already anxious and overwhelmed. Understanding the stages of recovery may assist parents in coping with the situation. It is important to remember that comatose children may not complete all stages of the recovery process and that they may manifest characteristics of more than one stage at a time.

Level 1: No response—Child does not respond to stimuli but may be able to hear what is said in the room.

Level 2: Generalized response—Child responds to painful or unpleasant stimuli; responses may not be consistent and may be delayed.

Level 3: Localized response—Child responds purposefully to painful or unpleasant stimuli by trying to pull away; turns toward sounds; responds inconsistently to simple commands.

Level 4: Confused, agitated—Child becomes restless, aggressive, frustrated; exhibits abnormal behavior; forgets answers to frequently asked questions.

Level 5: Confused, inappropriate—Child behaves more calmly; behavior starts to normalize, but child may become frustrated; voice and face lack expression; follows simple commands; performs simple tasks.

Level 6: Confused, appropriate—Child is less frustrated and is able to concentrate for longer periods (up to 30 minutes); short-term memory is improving; responses to questions are more appropriate but may not be correct.

Level 7: Automatic, appropriate—Child's memory continues to improve, although details may not be clear; continues to have difficulty concentrating; decreased safety awareness and judgment.

Level 8: Purposeful—Child's basic thinking skills will have recovered to the maximum extent; incidental changes in social skills, memory, and concentration may continue for months; child will fully understand what happened and may grieve over how things have changed. (Stages for recovery are based on the Rancho Levels of Cognitive Functioning, copyright Los Amigos Research and Educational Institute, 1990.)

Awakening from a coma is a gradual process; however, some children regain consciousness within a short time. If there is little or no residual effect, the child is discharged home fairly soon. The parents need the most intensive nursing intervention during the period of crisis and uncertainty. During the recovery phase the nurse gives them information, clarifies it as needed, and encourages them to become involved in the child's care. Often the child's hospitalization is brief; however, some children require extended hospitalization for intensive therapy and rehabilitation. The parents of children who die require support and guidance to cope with the reality of the death and to resolve their grief. (See Chapter 19.)

Probably the most difficult situations are those that involve children who never regain consciousness. Unlike losing a child through death, these children lack finality, which often leaves the parents in a state of suspended grief. Like parents of dying children, parents of comatose children search for any signs of hope. Well-meaning friends and relatives relate instances of miraculous recoveries. The parents seek confirmation and support for such possibilities and assign erroneous meanings to any sign in the child that might be interpreted as evidence of recovery (e.g., reflexive muscle contractions).

At these times nurses need to respond with compassion and honesty. They can acknowledge that miraculous recoveries do occur but are rare. The important message is to maintain open communication with the family.

Like parents who lose a child through death, the parents of a child who is unconscious attempt to construct a representation of the child. They bring items that belong to the child, such as favorite toys or music. This may be interpreted as an attempt to provide stimulation for the child in the hope of eliciting a response, to let the hospital staff know the child as the unique individual he or she was, and to reconstitute an image of the child "lost" to them and for whom they mourn. The nurses' recognition and understanding of these behaviors and coping mechanisms is important to support the parents in their grief process.

In addition to the process of grieving for the "lost" child, the parents may face difficult decisions. When the child's brain is so severely damaged that vital functions must be maintained by artificial means, the parents must make the final decision whether to remove the life-support systems and allow a natural death (Chen & Azueta, 2017). After parents are provided with information about what allowing a natural death and removal from life-support mean, the parents may turn to both the provider and the nurses with their questions and concerns. Nurses play a critical role in assisting families in participating in their child's care to the greatest extent possible and in planning the child's death when that is the inevitable outcome of their neurologic disorder (Bloomer, Endacott, Copnell, et al., 2016).

When the child has survived the cerebral insult but is physically and/or mentally limited, either minimally or severely, families must cope with and make decisions about the rehabilitation process and uncertain outcome. The family may need to make decisions whether to place their child in a chronic care facility or to care for their child at home. The drain on financial, emotional, and social resources can be enormous.

For parents who choose to care for their child at home, planning begins early in the recovery process. Family members should become involved with the child's care as soon as they indicate an interest and ability to do so. They need education and support in learning to care for the child, regular follow-up observation and planning for home equipment, nursing and respite care. Parents need to understand that it is important to plan for periodic relief from the continuous care of the child. (See Discharge Planning and Home Care, Chapter 21.)

HEAD INJURY

Head injury is a pathologic process involving the scalp, skull, meninges, or brain as a result of mechanical force. Unintentional injuries are the number one health risk for children and the leading cause of death in children older than 1 year of age (Chen, Shi, Stanley, et al., 2017). Children less than 1 year of age though had a significantly higher rate of severe head injury (Chen, Shi, Stanley, et al., 2017). In 2013 approximately 660,000 children 0 to 14 years old experienced a traumatic brain injury and 17,900 of those children were hospitalized; 1484 children died as a result of their brain injury (Taylor, Bell, Breiding, et al., 2017).

Etiology

The most common causes of head injury in children are falls, being struck by or striking an object with one's head, and motor vehicle accidents, in that order (Centers for Disease Control and Prevention, 2017a). Assaults are the leading cause of death from traumatic brain injury in children 4 years of age or younger (Taylor, Bell, Breiding, et al., 2017) (Fig. 30.6). Neurologic injury accounts for the highest mortality rate, with boys usually affected twice as often as girls. There are a number of head trauma strategies, including safety gates on stairs, restricting sleeping in the top bunk to children older than 6 years of age, seat belts and car seat use, and helmets during recreational activities such as biking and skiing. Furthermore, preventing child abuse is necessary and possible.

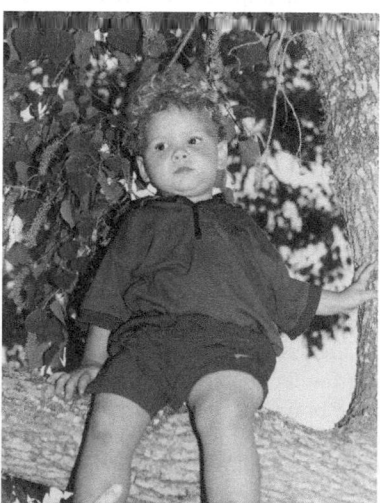

FIG. 30.6 Children possess a sense of adventure and wonder; however, falls remain the leading cause of head injury in children under 5 years of age.

Many of the physical characteristics of children predispose them to craniocerebral trauma. For example, infants are often left unattended on beds, in high chairs, and in other places from which they can fall. Because the head of an infant or toddler is proportionately large and heavy in relation to other body parts, it is the most likely to be injured. Incomplete motor development contributes to falls at young ages, and the natural curiosity and exuberance of children increase their risk for injury.

Pathophysiology

The pathology of brain injury is directly related to the force of impact. Intracranial contents (brain, blood, CSF) are damaged because the force is too great to be absorbed by the skull and musculoligamentous support of the head. Although nervous tissue is delicate, it usually requires a severe blow to cause significant damage.

A child's response to head injury is different from that of adults. The larger head size in proportion to body size and insufficient musculoskeletal support render the very young child particularly vulnerable to acceleration-deceleration injuries.

Primary head injuries are those that occur at the time of trauma and include skull fractures, contusions, intracranial hematomas, and diffuse injuries. Subsequent complications include hypoxic brain injury, increased ICP, and cerebral edema. The predominant feature of a child's brain injury is the diffuse amount of swelling that occurs. Hypoxia and hypercapnia threaten the energy requirements of the brain and increase CBF. The added volume across the BBB along with the loss of autoregulation exacerbates cerebral edema. Pressure inside the skull that is greater than arterial pressure results in inadequate perfusion. Because the cranium of very young children has the ability to expand and the thin skull is more compliant, they may tolerate increases in ICP better than older children and adults.

Physical forces act on the head through acceleration, deceleration, or deformation. Acceleration or deceleration is more descriptive of the circumstances responsible for most head injuries. When the stationary head receives a blow, the sudden acceleration causes deformation of the skull and mass movement of the brain. Continued movement of the intracranial contents allows the brain to strike parts of the skull (e.g., the sharp edges of the sphenoid or the irregular surface of the anterior fossa) or the edges of the tentorium.

Although the brain volume remains unchanged, significant distortion and cavitation occur as the brain changes shape in response to the force transmitted from the impact to the skull. This deformation can cause bruising at the point of impact (coup) or at a distance as the brain collides with the unyielding surfaces opposite or far removed from the point of impact (contrecoup) (Fig. 30.7). Thus a blow to the occipital region can cause severe injury to the frontal and temporal areas of the brain.

When a moving head strikes a stationary surface, such as during a fall, sudden deceleration occurs and causes the greatest cerebral injury at the point of impact. Deceleration is responsible for most severe brainstem injuries.

Children with an acceleration-deceleration injury demonstrate diffuse generalized cerebral swelling produced by increased blood volume or by a redistribution of cerebral blood volume (cerebral hyperemia) rather than by the increased water content (edema).

Another effect of brain movement is shearing forces, which are caused by unequal movement or different rates of acceleration at various levels of the brain. A shearing force may tear small arteries that travel from the cerebral surfaces through the meninges to the dural sinuses and cause subdural hemorrhages. Shearing or stretching effects can also be transmitted to nerve fibers. Maximum stress from the shearing force occurs at the interface between structures of different density so that the gray matter (cell body) rapidly accelerates, whereas the white matter (axons) tends to lag behind. Although maximum shearing forces are at the cerebral surface and extend toward the center of rotation within the brain, the most serious effects are often in the area of the brainstem. Severe compression of the skull can cause the brain to be forced through the tentorial opening and produce irreparable damage to the brainstem.

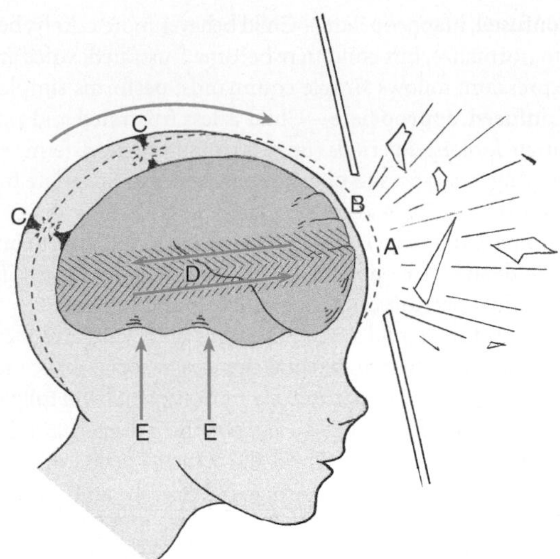

FIG. 30.7 Mechanical distortion of cranium during closed head injury. **A,** Preinjury contour of skull. **B,** Immediate postinjury contour of skull. **C,** Torn subdural vessels. **D,** Shearing forces. **E,** Trauma from contact with floor of cranium. (Redrawn from Grubb, R. L., & Coxe, W. S. [1974]. Central nervous system trauma: Cranial. In S. G. Eliasson, A. L. Presky, & W. B. Hardin [Eds.], *Neurological pathophysiology.* New York: Oxford University Press.)

A GCS value of 8 or less in pediatric patients indicates severe injury and requires aggressive therapeutic management (Hartman & Cheifetz, 2016). Three out of four children with a score of 3 or 4 will be severely disabled, be in a persistent vegetative state, or die within a year of their injury (Fulkerson, White, Rees, et al., 2015). There are a number of studies that indicate the Simplified Motor Scale (SMS) is equivalent to the GCS in predictive power but the GCS is better for prognosticating death (Singh, Murad, Prokop, et al., 2013).

Concussion

The most common and mildest traumatic brain injury is concussion, an alteration in mental status with or without loss of consciousness that occurs immediately after a head injury (McCrea, Nelson, & Guskiewicz, 2017). Direct head trauma and "whiplash" seen with rapid acceleration and deceleration of the head are the most frequent causes in children. Sports-related activities are responsible for the majority of concussions (Mullally, 2017).

The hallmarks of a concussion are confusion and amnesia. These are often not preceded by loss of consciousness and may occur immediately after the injury or several minutes later. The belief that loss of consciousness is the hallmark of concussion is a common misconception. A recent study among 182 adolescent athletes who sustained a concussion found that only 22% lost consciousness, whereas 34% experienced amnesia (Meehan, Mannix, Stracciolini, et al., 2013).

The pathogenesis of concussion is still unclear, but it may be a result of shearing forces that cause stretching, compression, and tearing of nerve fibers, particularly in the area of the central brainstem, the seat of the reticular activating system. It has also been suggested that the anatomic alterations of nerve fibers cause the release of large quantities of acetylcholine into the CSF and a reduction in oxygen consumption with increased lactate production.

Contusion and Laceration

The terms *contusion* and *laceration* are used to describe visible bruising and tearing of cerebral tissue. Contusions represent petechial hemorrhages or localized bruising along the superficial aspects of the brain at the site of impact (coup injury) or a lesion remote from the site of direct trauma (contrecoup injury). In serious accidents there may be multiple sites of injury.

The major areas of the brain susceptible to contusion or laceration are the occipital, frontal, and temporal lobes. In addition, the irregular surfaces of the anterior and middle fossae at the base of the skull are capable of producing bruises or lacerations on forceful impact. Contusions may cause focal disturbances in strength, sensation, or visual awareness. The degree of brain damage in the contused areas varies according to the extent of vascular injury. Signs vary from mild, transient weakness of a limb to prolonged unconsciousness and paralysis. However, the signs and symptoms may be clinically indistinguishable from those of concussion.

Infants who are roughly shaken, referred to as shaken baby syndrome or abusive head trauma, can sustain profound neurologic impairment, seizures, retinal hemorrhages (usually bilateral), and intracranial subarachnoid or subdural hemorrhages (Sieswerda-Hoogendoorn, Boos, Spivack, et al., 2012).

Cerebral lacerations are generally associated with penetrating or depressed skull fractures. However, they may occur without fracture in small children. When brain tissue is actually torn, with bleeding into and around the tear, more severe and prolonged unconsciousness and paralysis usually occur, leaving permanent scarring and some degree of disability.

Fractures

Skull fractures result from a direct blow or injury to the skull and are often associated with intracranial injury. Many of the falls that resulted in a skull fracture in children younger than 2 years of age involved short distances of less than 3 feet, such as falls from a caregiver's arms (Burrows, Trefan, Houston, et al., 2015).

The types of skull fractures that occur are linear, comminuted, depressed, open, basilar, and growing fractures. As a rule, the faster the blow, the greater the likelihood of a depressed fracture; a low-velocity impact tends to produce a linear fracture.

Linear skull fractures are a single fracture line that starts at the point of maximum impact and spreads; however, they do not cross suture lines. Linear skull fractures constitute the majority of childhood skull fractures and typically occur in the parietal bone. Most linear skull fractures are associated with an overlying scalp hematoma, particularly in infants younger than 2 years of age and in the parietal or temporal region (Burns, Grool, Klassen, et al., 2016). Scalp hematomas, in turn, are associated with the presence of intracranial injury whether there is a linear fracture or not (Burns, Grool, Klassen, et al., 2016).

Comminuted fractures consist of multiple associated linear fractures. They usually result from intense impact, often from repeated blows against an object or ejection from a car at a high rate of speed. They may suggest child abuse.

Depressed fractures are those in which the bone is locally broken, usually into several irregular fragments that are pushed inward. The greater the depression, the higher the risk of a tear in the dura or cortical laceration. Depressed skull fractures may be associated with direct underlying parenchymal damage and should be suspected when a child's head appears misshapen. Surgery may be needed to elevate the depressed bone fragment if there is an associated intracranial hematoma and if the depression is greater than 1 cm (0.4 inch).

Basilar fractures involve the bones at the base of the skull in either the posterior or the anterior region. The bones involved are the ethmoid, sphenoid, temporal, or occipital bones. These fractures usually result in a dural tear. Because of the proximity of the fracture line to structures surrounding the brainstem, a basal skull fracture is a serious head injury. Basilar fractures often involve frontal bone fractures. This can result in clinical features such as leakage of CSF from the nose (CSF rhinorrhea) or ear (CSF otorrhea), blood behind the tympanic membrane (hemotympanum), subcutaneous bleeding over the mastoid process that is located posterior to the ear, and subcutaneous bleeding around the orbit (Bonfield, Naran, Adetayo, et al., 2014). Meningitis, although rare, is always a potential risk with CSF leakage.

! NURSING ALERT

Suspect posttraumatic meningitis in children with increasing drowsiness and fever who also have basilar skull fractures.

Open fractures result in a communication between the skull and the scalp or the mucosa of the upper respiratory tract. The risk of CNS infection is increased with open fractures. Compound fractures consist of a skin laceration overlying the bone fracture. Open fractures that involve the paranasal sinuses or middle ear may lead to leakage of CSF (rhinorrhea or otorrhea). Prophylactic antibiotics are recommended to prevent osteomyelitis.

Growing skull fracture is an unusual complication of head trauma. The fracture is accompanied by an underlying tear in the dura or brain injury that fails to heal properly. A leptomeningeal cyst, dilated ventricles, or herniated brain may result and cause growth of the original fracture. The majority of growing skull fractures occur before 30 months of age and occur in the parietal bone (Vezina, Al-Halabi, Shash, et al., 2017). Physical examination usually shows a swelling scalp and skull defect. Clinical neurologic symptoms may be delayed for months to years after the initial skull fracture and include headache, seizures, hemiparesis, and learning and intellectual disabilities (Vezina, Al-Halabi, Shash, et al., 2017).

Complications

The major complications of trauma to the head are hemorrhage, infection, edema, and herniation through the brainstem. Infection is always a hazard in open injuries. Edema is related to tissue trauma. Vascular rupture may occur even in minor head injuries, causing hemorrhage between the skull and cerebral surfaces. Compression of the underlying brain produces effects that can be rapidly fatal or insidiously progressive.

Epidural Hematoma

Epidural (extradural) hematoma is a hemorrhage into the space between the dura and the skull. As the hematoma enlarges, the dura is stripped from the skull; this accumulation of blood results in a mass effect on the brain, forcing the underlying brain contents downward as it expands (Fig. 30.8, *A*). Because bleeding is generally arterial, brain compression occurs rapidly. The lower incidence of epidural hematoma in childhood is attributed to the fact that the middle meningeal artery is not embedded in the skull's bone surface until approximately 2 years old. Therefore a temporal bone fracture is less likely to lacerate the artery. However, occipital fractures are common with posterior fossa epidural hematomas (Sencer, Aras, Akcakaya, et al., 2012).

Epidural hematomas occur infrequently in infants and children, but they may occur after a low-velocity fall (Sencer, Aras, Akcakaya, et al.,

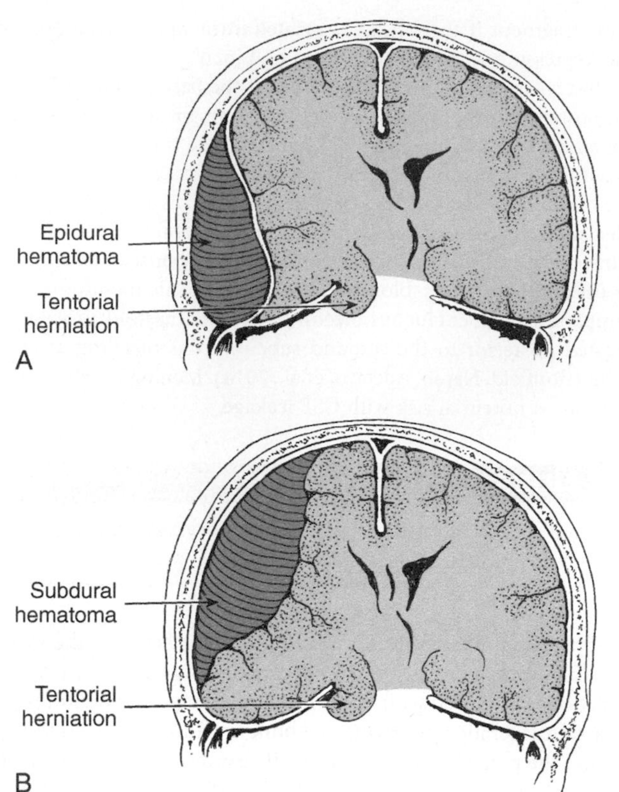

FIG. 30.8 A, Epidural (extradural) hematoma and compression of temporal lobe through tentorial herniation. **B,** Subdural hematoma.

2012). Child abuse accounts for a significant number of cases of epidural hematomas in infants and children, whereas motor vehicle accidents account for most epidural hematomas in adolescents.

Because bleeding is generally arterial, brain compression occurs rapidly. Most often the expanding hematoma is located in the parietal and temporal regions (Teichert, Rosales, Lopes, et al., 2012), which forces the medial portion of the temporal lobe under the edge of the tentorium, where it places pressure on nerves and blood vessels. Pressure on the arterial supply and venous return to the reticular formation causes loss of consciousness; pressure on CN III produces dilation and (later) fixation of the ipsilateral pupil. Pressure on the fibers of the pyramidal tract is evidenced by contralateral weakness or paralysis and increased deep tendon reflexes. Extreme pressure may cause brain herniation and death. Expanding epidural hemorrhages may be better tolerated in young children with open sutures that allow for expansion of the skull. In addition, young children have larger subarachnoid and extracellular spaces, which provide space for the expanding hematoma without compression on the brain parenchyma.

The classic clinical picture of an epidural hemorrhage is a lucid interval of minutes to hours followed by rapidly altered mental status, then loss of consciousness or coma due to blood accumulation in the epidural space and compression of the brain. The child may be seen with varying degrees of impaired consciousness, depending on the severity of the traumatic injury. Common symptoms in a child with no neurologic deficit are irritability, headache, and vomiting. In infants less than 24 months of age common symptoms are scalp swelling, irritability, and lethargy. They may also have seizures, reduced oral intake, and increasing head circumference (Sellin, Moreno, Ryan, et al., 2017).

An epidural hematoma can be detected by an initial CT scan. If the severity of the child's symptoms is not recognized, herniation and death will result. Cushing triad (systemic hypertension, bradycardia, and respiratory depression) is a late sign of impending brainstem herniation. See Table 30.3 for a comparison of epidural and subdural hematomas.

TABLE 30.3 Features of Acute Epidural and Subdural Hematomas

Feature	Epidural	Subdural
Supratentorial		
Frequency	Less frequent	More frequent than epidural
Skull fracture	70% of cases	30% of cases
Source of hemorrhage	Arterial or venous	Almost always venous
Age	Usually >2 years	Usually <1 year
Location	Usually temporoparietal	Usually frontoparietal
Laterality	Usually unilateral	75% bilateral
Seizures	<25%	75%
Preretinal or retinal hemorrhages	Uncommon	Very frequent
Increased ICP	Present	Present
CT configuration	Usually lenticular	Curvilinear or crescentic
Mortality	Relatively high	Usually lower
Morbidity	Low	High
Infratentorial		
Skull fracture	Almost always	Less common
Source of hemorrhage	Venous	Venous
Impaired consciousness	Frequent	Frequent
Acute hydrocephalus, medullary compression	Variable	Variable
Other posterior fossa signs	Variable	Variable

CT, Computed tomography; *ICP,* intracranial pressure.
From Swaiman, K. F. (1999). *Pediatric neurology: Principles and practice* (3rd ed.). St. Louis, MO: Mosby.

! NURSING ALERT

Children with a subdural hematoma and retinal hemorrhages should be evaluated for the possibility of child abuse, especially shaken baby syndrome.

Subdural Hematoma

A subdural hematoma is a hemorrhage between the dura and the arachnoid membrane that overlies the brain and the subarachnoid space. The hemorrhage may be from two sources: (1) tearing of the veins that bridge the subdural space and (2) hemorrhage from the cortex of the brain caused by direct brain trauma (see Fig. 30.8, *B*). Subdural hematomas are much more common than epidural hematomas in infants and children.

Unlike epidural hemorrhage, which develops inwardly against the less resistant brain tissue, subdural hemorrhage tends to develop more slowly and spreads thinly and widely, crossing cranial sutures, until it is limited by the dural barriers: the falx and the tentorium. The small subdural space and the dura, which is firmly attached to the skull in this area, are highly vulnerable to increased ICP.

Subdural hematoma is fairly common in infants. Most often it is the result of assaults or violent shaking. The caregiver's response to infant crying, often perceived as inconsolable, is an important risk factor (Barr, 2014). In neonates subdural hematoma can be a consequence of labor and delivery. Subdural hemorrhage can cause either acute or chronic subdural hematoma. Acute subdural hematoma may be associated with contusions or lacerations and develops within minutes or hours of injury. Chronic subdural hematoma is more common. The clinical course and manifestations vary depending on the damage sustained by the brain and the child's age.

Presenting signs of acute hematoma include irritability, vomiting, increased head circumference, bulging anterior fontanel (in the infant), lethargy, coma, or seizures. In infants with open fontanels, large amounts of intracranial blood may accumulate, causing hemorrhagic shock or fever before there are any changes in the neurologic examination (Squier & Mack, 2009). Retinal hemorrhages and skull and skeletal fractures are suggestive of physical abuse. An infant who has an altered LOC and in whom the CT scan shows subarachnoid hemorrhage or subdural hematoma may have been physically abused. A child with a GCS of 12 or less or a decrease in GCS score by 2 or more points requires emergency consultation with the neurosurgeon (Huang, Bi, Abd-El-Barr, et al., 2016).

Closely observe older children for signs of neurologic deterioration, including altered mental status, vomiting, lethargy, and signs of increased ICP. Hemiparesis, hemiplegia, and anisocoria (unequal pupils) are signs of brainstem compression and require emergency treatment targeted at decreasing ICP. The surgical management of subdural hematomas depends on the physical examination, size of the hematoma, and presence of other abnormalities on the CT scan. Not all children require surgery or are candidates for surgery. Various surgical options to treat subdural hematomas include transfontanel percutaneous aspiration, subdural drains, placement of burr hole, or craniotomy (Huang, Bi, Abd-El-Barr, et al., 2016).

Other Hemorrhagic Lesions

A subarachnoid hemorrhage is bleeding within the subarachnoid space, which is normally filled with CSF. Nontraumatic intracranial hemorrhages are rare in children. The most common causes of spontaneous intracranial hemorrhage in children are arteriovenous malformations and fistulas and brain tumors (Ding, Starke, Kano, et al., 2017). Sudden onset of a severe headache, headaches occurring out of sleep, first-time seizure, and abnormal neurologic examination are symptoms that require evaluation including neuroimaging (Blume, 2017).

Cerebral Edema

Some degree of brain edema is expected after craniocerebral trauma and often accompanies any of the previously mentioned disorders. Cerebral edema peaks at 24 to 72 hours after injury and may account for changes in a child's neurologic status. Cerebral edema associated with traumatic brain injury may be a result of two different mechanisms: cytotoxic edema or vasogenic edema. Cytotoxic edema is a result of direct cell injury and is caused by intracellular swelling. In many cases the brain cells are irreversibly damaged. Vasogenic edema is due to increased permeability of capillary endothelial cells, resulting in increased intracellular fluid. In vasogenic edema the nerve cells are not primarily injured. Either mechanism can result in increased ICP as a result of increased intracranial volume and changes in CBF as a result of loss of autoregulation and/or hypercapnia or hypoxia. Children at risk for deterioration can be identified by abnormalities seen on noncontrast CT scans.

Sequelae of Traumatic Brain Injury

Postconcussion syndrome is a sequela to brain injury with or without loss of consciousness. Concussions usually resolve in 1 to 3 weeks without complications. Up to a third of children may have ongoing somatic, behavioral, cognitive, and psychological symptoms including headaches, visual and balance problems, difficulty concentrating, irritability, and changes in their sleep patterns (Morgan, Zuckerman, Lee, et al., 2015). The pathophysiology of these symptoms is unclear. When these symptoms continue more than 4 weeks after the concussion the term *postconcussion syndrome* (PCS) is used (Zemek, Barrowman, Freedman, et al., 2016). Risk factors for PCS in youth athletes include a personal or family history of mood disorders and other psychiatric illnesses and migraines (Morgan, Zuckerman, Lee, et al., 2015). Previously concussion treatment guidelines recommended cognitive and physical rest as a path to recovery. Recent studies, though, have found that early participation in physical activity is significantly likely to prevent the development of PCS (Grool, Aglipay, Momoli, et al., 2016).

Posttraumatic headaches, one of the most common symptoms after mild traumatic brain injury (TBI), may occur within 1 week to 3 months after a mild TBI. They occur in 25% to 75% of individuals and are most commonly classified as migraines (Kuczynski, Crawford, Bodell, et al., 2013). Posttraumatic headaches are treated based on the primary headache type, migraine or tension/chronic headache (Kacperski & Arthur, 2016).

Posttraumatic seizures occur in a number of children who survive a head injury, often within 24 hours, but they can occur up to 1 week after the injury (Christensen, 2012). In comparison to children with no brain injury, seizures are two times more likely to occur in children with mild traumatic brain injury and seven times more likely to occur in children with severe head injury (Christensen, 2012).

Hydrocephalus may develop after subarachnoid hemorrhage or infection. Normal-pressure hydrocephalus can be a complication of traumatic brain injury. In infants, signs and symptoms include rapidly increasing head circumference irritability, refusal to feed, and sleepiness. The clinical signs and symptoms in children include changes in personality, developmental regression, ataxia, and incontinence. These signs are also seen during posttraumatic amnesia, making early recognition of this syndrome difficult. Focal deficits, including optic atrophy, CN palsies, motor deficits, DI, or aphasia, may be seen. The type of residual effect depends on the location and nature of the trauma.

Diagnostic Evaluation

A detailed health history, both past and present, is essential in evaluating the child with head trauma. Certain disorders such as drug allergies, hemophilia, diabetes mellitus, or epilepsy may produce similar symptoms. Even a minor traumatic injury can aggravate a preexisting disease process, thereby producing neurologic signs out of proportion to the injury.

After a minor injury, initial unconsciousness (if present) is brief. The child ordinarily exhibits a transient period of confusion, somnolence, and listlessness; this period is most often accompanied by irritability, pallor, and one episode of vomiting. A severe head injury requires immediate evaluation and treatment. Because head injuries are often accompanied by injuries in other areas (e.g., spine, viscera, extremities), the examination is performed with care to avoid further damage. Box 30.5 lists manifestations of head injury.

! NURSING ALERT

Stabilize the spine after head injury until spinal cord injury is ruled out.

Initial Assessment

Priorities in the initial phase in the care of a child with a head injury include assessment of the CAB (circulation, airway, breathing); neurologic examination focusing on mental status, papillary responses, and

BOX 30.5 Clinical Manifestations of Acute Head Injury

Minor Injury

May or may not lose consciousness
Transient period of confusion
Somnolence
Listlessness
Irritability
Pallor
Vomiting (one or more episodes)

Signs of Progression

Altered mental status (e.g., difficulty arousing child)
Mounting agitation
Development of focal lateral neurologic signs
Marked changes in vital signs

Severe Injury

Signs of increased intracranial pressure (see Box 30.1)
Bulging fontanel (infant)
Retinal hemorrhages
Extraocular palsies (especially cranial nerve III)
Hemiparesis
Quadriplegia
Elevated temperature
Unsteady gait (older child)
Papilledema (older child)
Retinal hemorrhages

Associated Signs

Scalp trauma
Other injuries (e.g., to extremities)

motor responses; and assessment for spinal cord injury. The assessment is carried out quickly in relation to vital signs (see Emergency Treatment box).

Ocular signs such as fixed, dilated, and unequal pupils; fixed and constricted pupils; and pupils that are poorly reactive or unreactive to light and accommodation indicate increased ICP or brainstem involvement. It is important to remain with the patient who demonstrates fixed and dilated pupils because these are ominous signs often associated with impending respiratory arrest. Dilated, nonpulsating blood vessels indicate increased ICP before the appearance of papilledema. Retinal hemorrhages often occur with acute head injuries, specifically with shaken baby syndrome.

Funduscopic examination should be performed routinely to detect retinal hemorrhages in a child with CNS trauma. Vestibulo-ocular symptoms such as diplopia, dizziness, motion sensitivity, eye-tracking and eye-focusing problems, photosensitivity, and visual inattention may develop (Ellis, Cordingley, Vis, et al., 2015). Transient vision loss may occur after mild head trauma but may not be obvious in children unless this diagnosis is evaluated. Theories of possible causes are vasospasm or localized cerebral edema.

Less urgent but important assessments include examination of the scalp for lacerations, widely separated sutures, and the size and tension of fontanels, which indicate intracranial hemorrhage or rapidly developing cerebral edema. Scalp lacerations may require surgical intervention. A significant amount of blood loss can occur from scalp lacerations. CT scan may be necessary to evaluate possible skull fractures and acute intracranial hemorrhage (Ryan, Jaju, Ciolino, et al., 2016).

EMERGENCY TREATMENT

Head Injury

1. Assess child:
   - C—Circulation
   - A—Airway
   - B—Breathing
   - Neurologic and thermoregulatory status
2. Stabilize neck and spine immediately. Use jaw thrust to open airway, not chin lift.
3. Clean any abrasions with soap and water.
   - Apply clean dressing.
   - If child is bleeding, apply ice to relieve pain and swelling.
4. Keep child NPO (nothing by mouth) until instructed otherwise.
5. Assess pain but give no analgesics or sedatives.
6. Check level of consciousness and pupillary reaction every 4 hours (including twice during night) for 48 hours.
7. Seek medical attention for any of the following:
   - Injury sustained at high speed (e.g., automobile)
   - Fall from a significant distance (height greater than that of the child)
   - Injury sustained from great force (e.g., baseball bat)
   - Injury sustained under suspicious circumstances
   - Loss of consciousness
   - Amnesia
   - Discomfort (crying) more than 10 minutes after injury
   - Headache that is severe, worsens, interferes with sleep, or lasts more than 24 hours
   - Vomiting three or more times or that begins or continues 4 to 6 hours after injury
   - Swelling in front of or above earlobe or swelling that increases in size
   - Fluid leak from ears or nose; blackened eyes
   - Confusion or abnormal behavior
   - Difficulty arousing child from sleep
   - Difficulty speaking
   - Blurring of vision or diplopia
   - Unsteady gait
   - Difficulty using extremities; weakness or incoordination
   - Neck pain or stiffness
   - Pupils dilated, fixed, or unequal
   - Infant with bulging fontanel
   - Seizures

! NURSING ALERT

Deep, rapid, periodic, or intermittent and gasping respirations; wide fluctuations or noticeable slowing of the pulse; and widening pulse pressure or extreme fluctuations in blood pressure are signs of brainstem involvement. Marked hypotension may represent internal injuries.

! NURSING ALERT

Observation of asymmetric pupils or one dilated, unreactive pupil in a comatose child is a neurologic emergency.

! NURSING ALERT

Bleeding from the nose or ears needs further evaluation, and a watery discharge from the nose (rhinorrhea) that is positive for glucose (as tested with reagent strips [e.g., Dextrostix]) suggests leaking of CSF from a skull fracture.

A documented accurate assessment of clinical signs provides baseline information. Serial evaluations, preferably by a single observer, help detect changes in neurologic status. Alterations in mental status, evidenced by increased difficulty in rousing the child, mounting agitation, development of focal neurologic signs, or marked changes in vital signs, usually indicate extension or progression of the basic pathologic process.

Evaluation of reflexes provides information about cerebral and pyramidal involvement, although transient abnormalities of the primitive reflexes and Babinski sign may be present in children with mild head trauma. Conscious, cooperative children are examined for cerebellar signs such as ataxia and dysmetria. Children may display unsteadiness, clumsiness, or tremor with intentional movement after head injury. Temperature may be moderately elevated for 1 or 2 days after an initial mild hypothermia after injury. A persistent fever may indicate subarachnoid hemorrhage or infection.

Special Tests

After a thorough clinical examination, a variety of diagnostic tests are helpful in providing a more definitive diagnosis of the type and extent of the trauma. A hematocrit and urinalysis are typically done. Serum electrolytes and glucose may also be measured in children with severe head injuries; hyperglycemia and disseminated intravascular coagulation are associated with a poor prognosis. The severity of a head injury may not be apparent on clinical examination of the child but detectable on a CT scan. Whenever the child has a history consistent with a serious head injury (as with an unrestrained occupant in a severe motor vehicle accident or a fall from greater than their own height), it is important to perform a scan even if the child initially appears alert and oriented. All children with head injuries who have any alteration of consciousness, headache, vomiting, skull fracture, seizure, or predisposing medical condition should undergo a diagnostic evaluation that includes CT scanning.

MRI may be done to further assess cerebral edema or other structural brain abnormalities. A neurodevelopmental assessment after early head injury may be useful in documenting cognitive impairment. Skull radiographs are of little benefit in diagnosing skull fractures. Other radiographic tests may be indicated, depending on the severity or cause of the trauma. Electroencephalography is not helpful for diagnosis of a head injury but is useful for defining seizures and looking for subclinical seizures, which can impair consciousness (Gainza-Lein, Sanchez-Fernandez, & Loddenkemper, 2017). Lumbar puncture is rarely used for craniocerebral trauma and is contraindicated in the presence of increased ICP because of the possibility of herniation.

Therapeutic Management

The majority of children with mild TBI who have not lost consciousness can be cared for and observed at home after careful examination reveals no serious intracranial injury. The nurse should give parents both verbal and written instructions of signs and symptoms that warrant concern and the need for reevaluation. These include persistent or worsening headaches, vomiting, change in mental status or behavior, unsteady gait, or seizure. The child should have a physical examination in 1 or 2 days after the injury. The manifestations of epidural hematoma in children do not generally appear until 24 hours or more after injury.

Maintaining contact with parents for continued observation and reevaluation of the child, when indicated, facilitates early diagnosis and treatment of possible complications from head injury, such as hematoma, cerebral edema, and posttraumatic seizures. Children are generally hospitalized for 24 to 48 hours of observation if their family lives far from medical facilities or lacks transportation or a telephone, which would provide access to immediate help. Other circumstances, such as language or other communication barriers or even emotional trauma, may hinder learning and make it difficult for families to feel confident caring for their child at home.

> **! NURSING ALERT**
>
> If a child loses consciousness or develops a severe headache after a head injury, medical attention should be sought.

Children with severe injuries, those who have lost consciousness for more than a few minutes, and those with prolonged and continued seizures or other focal or diffuse neurologic signs must be hospitalized until their condition is stable and their neurologic signs have diminished. The child is maintained on nothing-by-mouth (NPO) status or restricted to clear liquids (if able to take fluids by mouth) until it is determined that vomiting will not occur. IV fluids are indicated in the child who is comatose, displays dulled sensorium, or is persistently vomiting.

The volume of IV fluid is carefully monitored to minimize the possibility of over hydration in case of SIADH and cerebral edema. However, damage to the hypothalamus or pituitary gland may produce DI with its accompanying hypertonicity and dehydration. Fluid balance is closely monitored by daily weight, strict intake and output measurement, and serum osmolality (to detect early signs of water retention).

Sedating drugs are usually withheld in the acute phase. Headache is usually controlled with acetaminophen, although opioids may be needed. Antiepileptics are used for seizure control. Antibiotics are administered if there are lacerations or penetrating injuries. Prophylactic tetanus toxoid is given as appropriate. (See Chapter 6.) Cerebral edema is managed as described for the unconscious child. Hyperthermia is controlled with tepid sponges or a hypothermia blanket.

Surgical Therapy

Approximately 10% to 30% of pediatric head traumas will result in skull fractures. Because of the greater capacity of a child's skull fracture to heal, conservative nonsurgical management is often adequate. Children hit in the head or who have TBI as a result of a motor vehicle accident are more likely to require surgical intervention, especially if the frontal bones have been fractured (Bonfield, Naran, Adetayo, et al., 2014).

Scalp lacerations are sutured after careful examination of underlying bone. The use of topical lidocaine, adrenaline, and tetracaine (LAT) or lidocaine, epinephrine, and tetracaine (LET) provides noninvasive, effective anesthesia for suturing, particularly when combined with consultation from and the bedside presence of a child life specialist (Martin, 2017).

Depressed fractures require surgical reduction and removal of bone fragments. Torn dura is also sutured. A skull fracture depressed more than the thickness of the skull or an intracranial hematoma that causes more than a 5-mm (0.2-inch) midline shift is an indication for surgery. Direct pressure should never be applied to a depressed skull fracture. Parents should be advised that painful hardware and wound infections may need further surgical intervention. Parents and other caregivers must be taught the importance of meticulous hand washing after surgical repair of a skull fracture.

Prognosis

The outcome of craniocerebral trauma depends on the extent of injury and complications. Neurologic, cognitive, emotional, and behavioral symptoms can result in significant impairment. They may not present until the child is older and preparing to reach certain developmental milestones (Babikian, Merkley, Savage, et al., 2015). These symptoms can become chronic and include epilepsy, attention-deficit/hyperactivity disorder, and learning or psychiatric disorders. Children with learning and behavior problems before their head trauma are more likely to suffer these consequences (Beauchamp & Anderson, 2013). More than 90% of children with concussions or simple linear fractures recover without symptoms after the initial period.

Children may be more vulnerable than adults to long-term cognitive and behavioral dysfunction after diffuse brain injury. Contrary to what was previously thought about "brain plasticity," evidence now indicates that children's brains may be especially vulnerable to early injury due to their ongoing maturation processes, which can be disrupted by head trauma (Babikian, Merkley, Savage, et al., 2015). Parents of children who have suffered TBI should be advised to seek evaluation and treatment sooner rather than later if any of these symptoms present. TBI is recognized as a disability that may qualify a child for special education services under the Individuals with Disabilities Education Act (IDEA) of 1990.

True coma (i.e., not obeying commands, eyes closed, and not speaking) usually does not last more than 2 weeks. A child's eventual outcome can range from brain death to a persistent vegetative state to complete recovery. However, even the best recovery may be associated with personality changes, including mood lability and loss of confidence, impaired short-term memory, headaches, and subtle cognitive impairments. In general, 90% of the long-term neurologic outcome has been achieved within 6 months to 1 year after the injury.

Nursing Care Management

The hospitalized child requires careful neurologic assessment and evaluation repeated as frequently as every 15 minutes to establish a correct diagnosis, identify signs and symptoms of increased ICP, determine clinical management, and prevent many complications. The goals of nursing management of the child with a head injury are to maintain adequate ventilation, oxygenation, and circulation; to monitor and treat increased ICP; to minimize cerebral oxygen requirements; and to support the child and family during recovery. (See Quality Patient Outcomes box.)

QUALITY PATIENT OUTCOMES

Acute Head Injury

- Early recognition of signs and symptoms of increased intracranial pressure
- Adequate ventilation, oxygenation, and circulation maintained
- Cerebral oxygen requirements minimized
- Sedation and analgesia provided while allowing for neurologic assessment

The child is placed on bed rest, usually with the head of the bed elevated slightly and the head in midline position. Appropriate safety measures, such as side rails kept up and seizure precautions, are implemented. If the child is extremely restless, hard surfaces may be padded and restraints used to prevent further injury. Individualize care according to the child's specific needs.

A key nursing role is to provide sedation and analgesia for the child. The conflict between the need to promote the child's comfort and relieve anxiety versus the need to assess for neurologic changes presents a dilemma. Both goals can be achieved with close observation of the child's LOC and response to analgesics (using a pain assessment record) and effective communication with the provider. Decreasing restlessness after administration of an analgesic most likely reflects pain control rather than a decreasing LOC. (See Pain Assessment and Pain Management, Chapter 5.)

Children may be restless and irritable, but more often their reaction is to fall asleep when left undisturbed. A quiet environment can help reduce restlessness and irritability. Bright lights are irritating. This often makes checking the ocular responses more difficult and aggravating to the child.

Frequent examinations of vital signs, neurologic signs, and LOC are extremely important nursing observations. When possible, they should be performed by a single observer to better detect subtle changes that may indicate worsening of neurologic status. Pupils are checked for size, symmetry, reaction to light, and accommodation. Unless there is brainstem involvement, vital signs generally return to normal after the initial changes seen after injury.

The most important nursing observation is assessment of the child's LOC. In the progression of an injury, alterations in consciousness appear earlier than alterations of vital signs or focal neurologic signs (see evaluation of responsiveness later in this chapter). Frequent examinations of alertness are fatiguing to the child; therefore the child often desires to fall asleep, which may be confused with depressed consciousness. It is not uncommon to observe ocular divergence through the partially closed eyelids.

Observations of position and movement provide additional information. Note any abnormal posturing and whether it occurs continuously or intermittently. Questions nurses might ask include the following:

- Are the child's hand grips strong and equal in strength?
- Are there any signs of extension or flexion posturing?
- What is the child's response to auditory and physical stimulation?
- Is movement purposeful, random, or absent?
- Are movement and sensation equal on both sides or restricted to one side only?

The child may report a headache or other discomfort. The child who is too young to describe a headache may be fussy and resist being handled. The child who suffers from vertigo often vigorously resists being moved from a position of comfort. Forcible movement causes the child to vomit and display spontaneous nystagmus. Seizures are relatively common in children at the time of head injury and may be of any type. Carefully observe any seizure activity and describe it in detail. Children in postictal states are more lethargic, with sluggish pupils.

Document drainage from any orifice. Bleeding from the ear suggests the possibility of a basal skull fracture. Clear nasal drainage is suggestive of an anterior basal skull fracture. Observe the amount and characteristics of the drainage.

! NURSING ALERT

Suctioning through the nares is contraindicated because there is a risk of the catheter entering the brain through a fracture in the skull.

Head trauma is often accompanied by other undetected injuries; therefore any bruises, lacerations, or evidence of internal injuries or fractures of the extremities are noted and reported. Associated injuries are evaluated and treated appropriately.

The child with a normal LOC is usually allowed clear liquids unless fluid is restricted. If the child has an IV infusion, it is maintained as prescribed. The diet is advanced to that appropriate for the child's age as soon as the condition permits. Intake and output are measured and recorded with attention to the development of constipation. Any incontinence of bowel or bladder is noted for the child who has been toilet trained.

Assessment for unusual behavior can only be made in relation to the child's typical behavior. For example, urinary incontinence during sleep would be of no consequence in a child who routinely wets the bed but would be highly significant for one who is always dry. Parents are invaluable resources in evaluating objective behaviors of their children.

Information obtained from parents at or shortly after admission is essential in evaluating the child's behavior (e.g., the ease with which the child is roused normally, the usual sleeping position, how much the child sleeps during the day, the child's motor activities [rolling over, sitting up, climbing], hearing and visual acuity, appetite, and manner of eating [spoon, bottle, cup]). Documentation of the child's baseline developmental and behavioral level is crucial. There is less concern about a child who falls asleep several times during the day if this is consistent with the child's usual behavior.

When the child is discharged, advise the parents of probable post-traumatic symptoms they may observe, such as behavioral changes, sleep disturbances, phobias, and seizures. Parents should be taught seizure first aid. They should understand observations they need to make and when and how to contact the provider or health facility in case the child develops any unusual signs or symptoms. Emphasize the importance of follow-up evaluation.

Family Support

The emotional and educational support of the family presents a challenge. Witnessing the parents' grief and helplessness on seeing their child in an intensive care unit connected to monitoring equipment and in an altered state evokes empathy. The nurse can encourage the family to be involved in the child's care, to bring in familiar belongings, or to make a recording of familiar voices and sounds. Parents may need a demonstration on how to touch or cuddle their child and may want to talk about their grief. The nurse listens attentively, reinforces what is being done to assist the child, and directs parents toward signs and symptoms of recovery to instill hope without promises. Honesty and kindness, along with consistent and competent care, help families through this difficult time.

Rehabilitation

Rehabilitation and management of the child with permanent brain injury are essential aspects of care. Rehabilitation begins as soon as possible and usually involves the family and a rehabilitation team. The nurse makes a careful assessment of the child's capabilities and limitations and implements appropriate interventions to maximize the residual capacities. The Brain Injury Association of America* provides information and listings of rehabilitation services and support groups throughout the country.

Pediatric trauma rehabilitation is a national concern. Coordinating care and services for early rehabilitation involves identifying the child's and family's response to the traumatic injury and disability, securing available resources, and recognizing the parents' role in the process.

The child with a disability resulting from head trauma requires functional assessment of his or her physical, cognitive, emotional, and social levels. The child has experienced separation, pain, sensory deprivation and overload, changes in circadian cycle, and fear of the unknown. Recovery and transition require new coping strategies at the same time that regressive and acting-out behaviors may start. Parents and children need honest communication for decision making.

Rehabilitation is recommended when the child is making progress and no longer requires acute care hospitalization but continues to require daily therapies to return to his or her premorbid functional level. Children are more likely to continue in outpatient rehabilitation if they have had an inpatient assessment of their rehabilitation needs (Jimenez, Symons, Wang, et al., 2016). The Rancho Los Amigos Scale provides a systematic assessment of the progress that a child with a severe head injury may achieve.

Pediatric rehabilitation focuses on the child's strengths and needs. The rehabilitation team should include physical medicine; rehabilitation nursing; nutritional counseling; physical, occupational, and speech therapy; special education; and psychologic, neuropsychologic, child life, and social services support. Before the child's transfer, the hospital team should provide a detailed care plan of the child's needs and abilities, especially communication skills, and a description of the child's usual schedule, nursing care interventions, and the family's concerns and needs. To augment the care plan, a video introducing the child and family and showing any unique aspects of their care can be sent to the rehabilitation center.

Prevention

Preventive strategies are underused in almost all cases of accidental childhood injury. Head injuries occur in the most serious accidents—especially motor vehicle accidents, sports, and falls.

Strides are being made in the prevention of secondary brain tissue damage after the initial head injury in children. This secondary injury is caused by altered cerebral blood flow that results in ischemia, hypoxia, and eventually the death of brain cells (Popernack, Gray, & Reuter-Rice, 2015). Studies are ongoing in both humans and animals using therapeutic hypothermia, glucagon, blood pressure medications, and antioxidants (Toth, Szarka, Farkas, et al., 2016). The roles of calcium, oxyradicals, and prostaglandins are being investigated.

However, the greatest benefit lies in prevention of head injuries. Nurses can exert a valuable influence on behalf of children through education. Accidents occur that are preventable because unnecessary risks go unchecked. Inadequate supervision combined with a child's natural sense of curiosity and exploration can lead to lethal results. Nurses are in the unique position of influencing caregivers in terms of growth and development. The use of car seats; seat belts in strollers and feeding chairs; and helmets for biking, skateboarding, and other sports has been shown to reduce both the number and severity of head injuries in children (Ganti, Bodhit, Daneshvar, et al., 2013; Gaw, Chounthirath, & Smith, 2017).

Studies of ways to prevent abusive head trauma are ongoing. Promising interventions include teaching parents about infant crying and ways to cope with it (Lopes & Williams, 2016). Infants who have been hospitalized after birth have an increased risk of being abused after discharge. Neonatal nurses have an important role to play in teaching parents of these children about child abuse prevention.

Public education coupled with legislative support can aid in the prevention of childhood injuries. Research has shown increased household income can prevent abusive head trauma (Klevens, Schmidt, Luo, et al., 2017). For extensive discussions of childhood injuries, see the information on injury prevention in Chapters 10, 12, 13, 15, and 17.

SUBMERSION INJURY

Drowning is one of the major causes of unintentional injury-related death in children ages 1 to 19 years. In children ages 1 to 4 years it is the leading cause of unintentional injury-related death (Gilchrist & Parker, 2014) (see Research Focus box). The term *near-drowning* is no longer used; instead, the term *submersion injury* should be used up until the time of drowning-related death (Weiss, 2010). In 2002 the World Congress on Drowning and the World Health Organization established a uniform definition: "the process of respiratory impairment from submersion/immersion in liquid" and uniform classifications of death, no morbidity, or morbidity (Weiss, 2010).

*1608 Spring Hill Road, Suite 110, Vienna, VA 22182; 703-761-0750; fax: 703-761-0755; http://www.biausa.org.

RESEARCH FOCUS

Rate of Hospitalization for Pediatric Submersion Injuries

From 2005 to 2014 there were an estimated 10 drowning deaths daily in the United States, and about 1 in 5 of these deaths was a child age 14 or under (Centers for Disease Control and Prevention, 2016). For every childhood fatality related to submersion, another 5 children are seen in an emergency department for treatment of submersion injuries (Centers for Disease Control and Prevention, 2016). Between 2013 and 2015 over 75% of emergency department visits for submersion injuries from swimming in pools were children younger than 15, and the majority of these were under 5 years old (Consumer Product Safety Commission, 2016).

Most cases of submersion injury are accidental, usually involving children who are helpless in water, such as inadequately attended children in or near swimming pools or infants in bathtubs; small children who fall into ponds, streams, and flooded excavations, usually near home; occupants of pleasure boats who fail to wear life preservers; children who have diving accidents; and children who are able to swim but overestimate their endurance. Accidental submersion injury occurs predominantly in males, toddlers, and African Americans (Gilchrist & Parker, 2014) (Fig. 30.9).

Submersion injury can take place in any body of water. Children less than 1 year of age are most likely to have a submersion injury in a bathtub, whereas top-heavy toddlers fall headfirst into a pail of water and are unable to free themselves (Xu, 2014). Preschoolers are at risk for injury in swimming pools, and school-age children and adolescents are most commonly at risk in natural bodies of water such as lakes, ponds, and rivers (Xu, 2014). The suction created at the outlet of pools, hot tubs, or whirlpool spas is strong enough to trap even larger children underwater. Submersion injury as a form of fatal child abuse also occurs. Homicidal submersion injuries are not witnessed, usually occurring in the home, and the victims are either infants or toddlers.

Pathophysiology

Physiologically most organ systems are affected, especially the pulmonary, cardiovascular, and neurologic systems. The major pulmonary changes that occur in submersion injury are directly related to the length of submersion (regardless of the type and amount of fluid aspirated), the victim's physiologic response, and the development and degree of immersion hypothermia. Cerebral hypoxia is a major component of morbidity and mortality in these individuals. Therefore early and aggressive resuscitation is imperative.

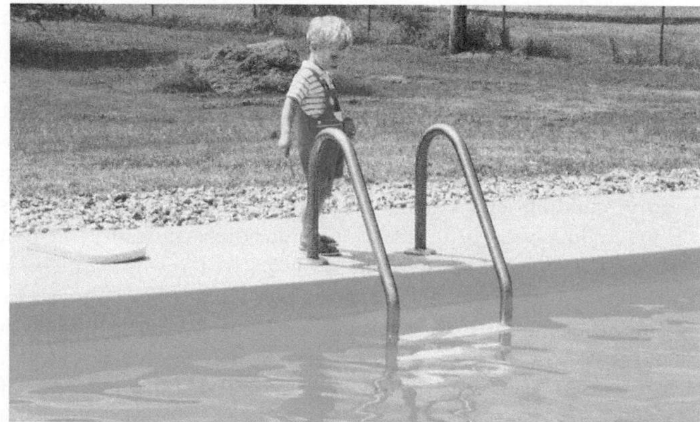

FIG. 30.9 Water is fascinating for children; however, drowning is the second leading cause of accidental death in unsupervised situations.

Physiologic factors in submersion injuries are hypothermia, aspiration, and hypoxia. The temperature of the liquid plays an important role. Cold water decreases metabolic demands and activates the diving reflex, which causes blood to be shunted away from the periphery to vital organs (i.e., the brain and heart). Hypothermia occurs rapidly in infants and children, partly because of their large surface area relative to size and partly as a result of the cold water itself. Profound hypothermia is usually evidence of lengthy submersion. Prolonged submersion in cold liquids can impair cognition, coordination, and muscle strength that ultimately results in loss of consciousness, decreased cardiac output, and cardiac arrest (Caglar & Quan, 2016). Submersion in cold water had previously been thought to be somewhat neuroprotective, but it is not (Quan, Mack, & Schiff, 2014).

Submerged children struggle initially to stay above water, and often breath-holding leads to air hunger. Reflex inspiration eventually occurs, which leads to aspiration (Caglar & Quan, 2016). Fluid is quickly absorbed in the pulmonary circulation, resulting in pulmonary edema, atelectasis, and airway spasm. Hypoxia is the primary problem because it results in global cell damage, with different cells tolerating variable lengths of anoxia. Neurons, especially cerebral cells, sustain irreversible damage after 4 to 6 minutes of submersion. The heart and lungs can survive up to 30 minutes. Regardless of the amount of water aspirated, the victim suffers arterial hypoxemia (resulting from atelectasis and shunting of blood through the nonventilated alveoli), combined respiratory acidosis (resulting from retained carbon dioxide), and metabolic acidosis (caused by buildup of acid metabolites because of anaerobic metabolism). Although electrolyte imbalances are contributing factors, they are not the major causes of morbidity and mortality. The pathologic events are directly related to the duration of submersion. Approximately 10% of submersion injury victims die without aspirating fluid but succumb from acute asphyxia as a result of prolonged reflex laryngospasm.

! NURSING ALERT

All children who have a submersion injury should be admitted to the hospital for observation. Although many patients do not appear to have suffered adverse effects from the event, complications (e.g., respiratory compromise, cerebral edema) may occur 24 hours after the incident.

Aspiration of fluid occurs in the majority of submersion injuries. The aspirated fluid results in pulmonary edema, atelectasis, airway spasm, and pneumonitis, which aggravates hypoxia. Submersion in salt water is associated with better outcomes than submersion in fresh water, although duration of the submersion is the main factor that predicts outcome (Quan, Bierens, Lis, et al., 2016).

Clinical Manifestations

Clinical manifestations are directly related to the duration of loss of consciousness and neurologic status after rescue and resuscitation.

Therapeutic Management

With rapid treatment some children can be saved. Resuscitative measures should begin at the scene, and the victim should be transported to the hospital with maximum ventilatory and circulatory support. In the hospital intensive pulmonary care is implemented and continued according to the patient's needs.

In general, management of the victim with a submersion injury is based on the degree of cerebral insult. The first priority is to restore oxygen delivery to the cells and prevent further hypoxic damage. A spontaneously breathing child does well in an oxygen-enriched atmosphere; the more severely affected child requires endotracheal intubation and mechanical ventilation. Blood gases and pH are monitored at frequent intervals as a guide to oxygen, fluid, and electrolyte therapies. Rewarming the hypothermic patient is initiated. Seizures may occur due to hypoxia and cerebral edema. Seizures result in increased cerebral oxygen consumption. Therefore it is imperative to aggressively control seizure activity. In addition, blood glucose should be monitored; both hypoglycemia and hyperglycemia are harmful to the brain.

All children who have a submersion injury should be hospitalized for observation. Although some children do not appear to have sustained adverse effects from the event, respiratory compromise or cerebral edema may occur within 24 hours after the incident. In the acute recovery period fever should be prevented although prophylactic antibiotics are not recommended. Aspiration pneumonia is a common complication that occurs approximately 48 to 72 hours after the episode. Bronchospasm, alveolar-capillary membrane damage, atelectasis, abscess formation, and acute respiratory distress syndrome are other complications that occur after aspiration of fluid.

Prognosis

Children who have submersion injuries usually have a good outcome with no or mild neurologic sequelae, no severe neurologic disabilities, and rarely morbidity (Caglar & Quan, 2016). The best predictors of a good outcome are length of submersion less than 5 minutes and the presence of sinus rhythm, reactive pupils, and neurologic responsiveness at the scene. The worst outcomes are for children submerged for more than 10 minutes and unresponsive to advanced life support within 25 minutes. All children without spontaneous purposeful movement and normal brainstem function 24 hours after sustaining a submersion injury suffered severe neurologic deficits or death (Caglar & Quan, 2016).

Nursing Care Management

Nursing care depends on the child's condition. A child who survives may need intensive respiratory nursing care with attention to vital signs, mechanical ventilation or tracheostomy, blood gas determination, chest physiotherapy, and IV infusion. Often the child has sustained a hypoxic insult and requires the same care as an unconscious child.

A difficult aspect in the care of the child who sustained a submersion injury is helping the parents cope with the grief, guilt, and anger reactions. Given the magnitude of the event, parents need repeated assurance that everything possible is being done to treat their child.

If the child dies, the sudden, unexpected nature of the death and the particular circumstances of the accident, especially in terms of guilt for not preventing it, compound the grief. (See Chapter 19.) The parents of the child who survives face the anxiety of not knowing the final outcome—to what extent will their child recover? This situation generates such intense feelings of loneliness and guilt that it is important for families to know they are not alone. They should be reminded frequently that there are people to assist them through this crisis. Additional sources of support that can be recommended include psychiatric and social work consultants, community services, and religious support. Self-help groups are excellent if available in the community.

Nurses often have difficulty relating to the parents if obvious neglect has precipitated the accident and subsequent problems; therefore it is important for those who care for these children and their families to assess their own feelings about the situation, in addition to assessing the family's coping abilities and resources. Caring for victims of a submersion injury and their families requires the nurse to be sensitive to the needs of the child and the family and to recognize his or her own reactions and emotions.

Prevention

Most submersion injuries are preventable. The most common cause of submersion injury in infants and young children is inadequate adult supervision, including a momentary lapse of supervision. Parents are often unaware that they must be within arm's reach and constantly supervising without being distracted (Caglar & Quan, 2016). Children with known risk factors such as epilepsy and autism require eyes-on surveillance. In general, children are not developmentally ready for formal swimming lessons until their fourth birthday, when the American Academy of Pediatrics recommends that lessons begin (Theurer & Bhavsar, 2013). All parents and swimming pool owners should be familiar with basic cardiopulmonary resuscitation (CPR) because rapid, basic CPR is one of the keys to improving outcomes (Tobin, Ramos, Pu, et al., 2017). Water safety and survival training should be required for all school-age children. Pool covers and fencing on all sides and the presence of lifeguards can prevent accidents.

Nurses can be active advocates in their communities. Nurses are also in a position to emphasize the importance of adequate adult supervision when children are around any body of water and should include the necessity of the adult not engaging in distracting activities.

INTRACRANIAL INFECTIONS

The nervous system is subject to infection by the same organisms that affect other organs of the body. However, the nervous system is limited in the ways in which it responds to injury. Laboratory studies are needed to identify the causative agent. The inflammatory process can affect the meninges (meningitis) or brain (encephalitis).

Meningitis can be caused by a variety of organisms, but the three main types are (1) bacterial, or pyogenic, caused by pus-forming bacteria, especially meningococci and pneumococci organisms; (2) viral, or aseptic, caused by a wide variety of viral agents; and (3) tuberculous, caused by the tuberculin bacillus. The majority of children with acute febrile encephalopathy have either bacterial meningitis or viral meningitis as the underlying cause.

BACTERIAL MENINGITIS

Bacterial meningitis is an acute inflammation of the meninges and CSF. The advent of antimicrobial therapy has had a marked effect on the course and prognosis. The introduction of conjugate vaccines against *Haemophilus influenzae* type b (Hib vaccine) in 1990 and *Streptococcus pneumoniae* (pneumococcus) in 2000 has led to dramatic changes in the epidemiology of bacterial meningitis (see Translating Evidence into Practice box). Today, *H. influenzae* type b infection has been virtually eradicated among young children in areas where the Hib vaccine is administered routinely. By 2013 there were fewer than 40 cases of Hib disease in children under 5 years old (Centers for Disease Control and Prevention, 2016). Before the vaccine, Hib was responsible for almost half of all cases of bacterial meningitis, but now it is the least likely pathogen to cause meningitis (Castelblanco, Lee, & Hasbun, 2014). Since the introduction of widespread vaccination for *S. pneumoniae*, the incidence of pneumococcal meningitis in children in the United States has decreased, but it remains the most common cause of meningitis in children ages 3 months to 11 years (Castelblanco, Lee, & Hasbun, 2014). It is also the most likely to result in death (Heckenberg, Brouwer, & Van de Beek, 2014).

Etiology

A variety of bacterial agents can cause bacterial meningitis. Since the introduction of vaccinations against most common causes of

TRANSLATING EVIDENCE INTO PRACTICE

Children With Bacterial Meningitis and Preventive Vaccines

Ask the Question

In children and adolescents with bacterial meningitis, has the administration of *Haemophilus influenzae* type b (Hib), pneumococcal, and meningococcal preventive vaccines reduced the incidence and mortality rates associated with bacterial meningitis?

Search for the Evidence

Search Strategies

Search selection criteria included English-language publications within past 10 years, research-based articles, children and adult populations.

Databases Used

PubMed and Cochrane Collaboration

Critically Analyze the Evidence

GRADE criteria: Evidence quality high; recommendation strong (Balshem, Hefland, Schunemann, et al., 2011)

A review of the literature revealed two literature reviews, one Cochrane review, and one population-based observational study.

- Watt, Wolfson, O'Brien, and colleagues (2009) performed a literature review with studies evaluating Hib disease incidence, fatality ratios, and the effect of Hib vaccine. In 2000 there were 173,000 cases of Hib meningitis and 78,300 deaths among children under the age of 5 years worldwide. Expanded use of Hib vaccine can reduce the incidence and mortality rates of Hib-related disease.
- A Cochrane review determined the effect, duration of protection, and age-specific effects of polysaccharide serogroup A vaccine (SgAV) to prevent meningococcal meningitis in children. The vaccine had a 95% protective effect during the first year in children over 5 years, but its efficacy after the first year could not be determined. Children ages 1 to 5 years in low-income countries also experienced protective effects from the SgAV, but the exact efficacy could not be determined (Patel & Lee, 2010).
- A literature review assessed the impact of the 7-valent pneumococcal conjugate vaccination on morbidity and mortality rates from invasive pneumococcal diseases. The six studies from North America consistently reported a decline in invasive pneumococcal disease mortality rate after the introduction of the pneumococcal vaccine, with reductions ranging from 57% to 62% among children and 37% to 76% among all age-groups (Myint, Madhava, Balmer, et al., 2013).
- A population-based observational study evaluated the incidence of bacterial meningitis from 1997 to 2010, after conjugate vaccination introduction. The incidence of *Streptococcus pneumoniae* decreased from 0.8 to 0.3 per 100,000 people; the incidence of *Neisseria* meningitis decreased from 0.721 to 0.123 per 100,000 people; and the mortality rate from pneumococcal meningitis decreased from 0.073 to 0.024 per 100,000 people (Castelblanco, Lee, & Hasbun, 2014).

Apply the Evidence: Nursing Implications

The evidence strongly suggests that all children should be immunized against the most common organisms responsible for bacterial meningitis (i.e., *H. influenzae* type b, *S. pneumoniae,* and *Neisseria meningitidis*) as prevention to decrease the incidence of bacterial meningitis. Nurses should stress to the parents, children, adolescents, and young adults the importance of adhering to the immunization schedule to protect against serious childhood diseases.

References

Balshem, H., Hefland, M., Schunemann, H. J., et al. (2011). GRADE guidelines: Rating the quality of evidence. *Journal of Clinical Epidemiology, 64,* 401–406.

Castelblanco, R. L., Lee, M., & Hasbun, R. (2014). Epidemiology of bacterial meningitis in the USA from 1997 to 2010: A population-based observational study. *The Lancet. Infectious Diseases, 14*(9), 813–819.

Myint, T., Madhava, H., Balmer, P., et al. (2013). The impact of 7-valent pneumococcal conjugate vaccine on invasive pneumococcal disease: A literature review. *Advances in Therapy, 30*(2), 127–151.

Patel, M., & Lee, C. K. (2010). Polysaccharide vaccines for preventing serogroup A meningococcal meningitis. *Cochrane Database of Systematic Reviews,* (1), art no. CD001093.

Watt, J. P., Wolfson, L. J., O'Brien, K. L., et al. (2009). Burden of disease caused by *Haemophilus influenzae* type b in children younger than 5 years. *Lancet, 374,* 903–911.

community-acquired pathogens, the incidence of bacterial meningitis has declined precipitously. It is now most common in children under 1 year of age (Marcdante & Kliegman, 2016). The leading causes of neonatal meningitis are group B streptococcus (GBS) and *Escherichia coli* (Ku, Boggess, & Cohen-Wolkowiez, 2015).

Meningococcal meningitis is the only type readily transmitted by droplet infection from nasopharyngeal secretions and so has the potential to occur in outbreaks (Vetter, Baxter, Denizer, et al., 2016). Before the development of a vaccine it occurred predominantly in school-age children and adolescents; now it is most common in children under 12 months old, with a secondary peak in incidence in 16- to 23-year-olds (Centers for Disease Control and Prevention, 2017b). Meningitis caused by pneumococcal and meningococcal infections can occur at any time but is more common in late winter and early spring.

Maternal factors, such as premature rupture of fetal membranes and maternal infection during the last week of pregnancy, are major causes of neonatal meningitis. It is a devastating disease with significant morbidity and mortality. Vaccination of pregnant women is being explored as a way to protect infants from meningitis (Jones, Munoz, Spiegel, et al., 2016). Children who survive neonatal meningitis are 10 times more likely to have moderate to severe disabilities than those who have not had meningitis (Ku, Boggess, & Cohen-Wolkowiez, 2015). The incidence of early-onset GBS meningitis has been reduced by more than 70% with the adoption of antenatal screening and administration of intrapartum prophylactic antibiotics (Ku, Boggess, & Cohen-Wolkowiez, 2015).

Risk factors for children developing meningitis include lack of immunization to the specific pathogen; recent exposure to someone with invasive *Neisseria meningitidis* or *H. influenzae* type b disease; penetrating head trauma; cochlear implant devices; and anatomic defects such as midline facial defects, inner ear fistulas, or recent placement of a ventricular shunt (Swanson, 2015).

Pathophysiology

The most common route of infection is vascular dissemination from a focus of infection elsewhere. For example, organisms from the nasopharynx invade the underlying blood vessels, cross the BBB, and multiply in the CSF. Invasion by direct extension from infections in the paranasal and mastoid sinuses is less common. Organisms also gain entry by direct implantation after penetrating wounds, skull fractures that provide an opening into the skin or sinuses, lumbar puncture or surgical procedures, anatomic abnormalities such as spina bifida, or foreign bodies such as an internal ventricular shunt or an external ventricular device. Once implanted, the organisms spread into the CSF, by which the infection spreads throughout the subarachnoid space.

The infective process is like that seen in any bacterial infection: inflammation, exudation, white blood cell accumulation, and varying degrees of tissue damage. The brain becomes hyperemic and edematous, and the entire surface of the brain is covered by a layer of purulent exudate that varies with the type of organism. For example, meningococcal exudate is most marked over the parietal, occipital, and cerebellar regions; the thick, fibrinous exudate of pneumococcal infection is confined chiefly to the surface of the brain, particularly the anterior lobes; and the exudate of streptococcal infections is similar to that of pneumococcal infections, but thinner. As infection extends to the ventricles, thick pus, fibrin, or adhesions may occlude the narrow passages and obstruct the flow of CSF.

Clinical Manifestations

The clinical manifestations of acute bacterial meningitis depend to a large extent on the child's age. The type of organism, the effectiveness of therapy for antecedent illness, and whether it occurs as an isolated entity or as a complication of another illness or injury also influence the clinical manifestation (Box 30.6).

Children and Adolescents

The onset of illness may be abrupt and rapid, or develop progressively over one or several days, and may be preceded by a febrile illness. Most children with meningitis are seen with fever, chills, headache, and vomiting that are associated with or quickly followed by alterations in sensorium; however, some may present only with lethargy and irritability (Weinberg & Thompson-Stone, 2018). The child is extremely irritable and agitated and may develop seizures, photophobia, confusion, hallucinations, aggressive behavior, drowsiness, stupor, or coma.

The child resists flexion of the neck (nuchal rigidity). Kernig and Brudzinski signs are positive. Reflex responses are variable, although they show hyperactivity. (See Reflexes, Chapter 4.) The skin may be cold and cyanotic with poor peripheral perfusion.

Other signs and symptoms may appear that are specific to individual organisms. Petechial or purpuric rashes occur in 50% of cases and indicate a meningococcal infection (meningococcemia), especially when the eruption is associated with a septic shock–like state. Joint involvement is seen in meningococcal and *H. influenzae* infection. A chronically draining ear commonly accompanies pneumococcal meningitis. *E. coli* infection may be associated with a congenital dermal sinus that communicates with the subarachnoid space.

Infants and Young Children

Between 3 months and 2 years of age the illness is characterized by fever or hypothermia, poor feeding, vomiting, marked irritability, restlessness, seizures, and a bulging or tense fontanel, which are often accompanied by a high-pitched cry.

Neonates

Meningitis in newborn and premature infants is extremely difficult to diagnose. The vague and nonspecific manifestations, which are characteristic of all neonatal sepsis, bear little resemblance to the findings in older children. These infants are usually well at birth but within a few days begin to appear ill. They refuse feedings, have poor sucking

BOX 30.6 Clinical Manifestations of Bacterial Meningitis

Children and Adolescents

Usually abrupt onset
Fever
Chills
Headache
Vomiting
Alterations in sensorium
Seizures (often the initial sign)
Irritability
Agitation
May develop the following:

- Photophobia
- Delirium
- Hallucinations
- Aggressive behavior
- Drowsiness
- Stupor
- Coma

Nuchal rigidity; may progress to opisthotonos
Positive Kernig and Brudzinski signs
Hyperactivity but variable reflex responses
Signs and symptoms peculiar to individual organisms:

- Petechial or purpuric rashes (meningococcal infection), especially when associated with a shock-like state
- Joint involvement (meningococcal or *Haemophilus influenzae* infection)
- Chronically draining ear (pneumococcal meningitis)

Infants and Young Children

Classic picture (above) rarely seen in children between 3 months and 2 years of age
Fever
Poor feeding
Vomiting
Marked irritability
Frequent seizures (often accompanied by a high-pitched cry)
Bulging fontanel
Nuchal rigidity possible
Brudzinski and Kernig signs not helpful in diagnosis
Difficult to elicit and evaluate in this age-group
Subdural empyema (*H. influenzae* infection)

Neonates

Specific Signs

Child well at birth but within a few days begins to look and behave poorly
Refuses feedings
Poor sucking ability
Vomiting or diarrhea
Poor tone
Lack of movement
Weak cry
Full, tense, and bulging fontanel may appear late in course of illness
Neck usually supple

Nonspecific Signs That May Be Present

Hypothermia or fever (depending on the infant's maturity)
Jaundice
Irritability
Drowsiness
Seizures
Respiratory irregularities or apnea
Cyanosis
Weight loss

ability, and may vomit or have diarrhea. They display poor muscle tone and lack of movement and have a poor cry. Other nonspecific signs that may be present include hypothermia or fever (depending on the infant's maturity), jaundice, irritability, drowsiness, seizures, respiratory irregularities or apnea, cyanosis, and weight loss. The full, tense, and bulging fontanel may or may not be present until late in the course of the illness, and the neck is usually supple. Untreated, the infant's condition will decline to cardiovascular collapse, seizures, and apnea. Even with improved antibiotics and more rapid diagnosis, the prognosis of neonatal meningitis has not improved in decades, likely due to the virulence of the infectious pathogen (Gordon, Srinivasan, & Harris, 2017).

Complications

The incidence of complications from acute bacterial meningitis has been significantly reduced with early diagnosis and vigorous antimicrobial therapy. If infection extends to the ventricles, thick pus, fibrin, or adhesions may occlude the narrow passages, thereby obstructing the flow of CSF and causing obstructive hydrocephalus. Subdural effusions often occur, and thrombosis may occur in meningeal veins or venous sinuses. Destructive changes may take place in the cerebral cortex, and brain abscesses may form by direct extension of the infection or by vascular dissemination. Extension of the infection to the areas of the cranial nerves or compression necrosis from increased pressure may cause deafness, blindness, or weakness or paralysis of facial or other muscles of the head and neck.

One of the most dramatic and serious complications usually associated with meningococcal infections is meningococcal sepsis, or meningococcemia. When the onset is severe, sudden, and rapid, it is known as the Waterhouse-Friderichsen syndrome. The syndrome is characterized by overwhelming septic shock, disseminated intravascular coagulation, massive bilateral adrenal hemorrhage, and purpura (Fig. 30.10). Meningococcemia requires immediate emergency treatment, hospitalization, and intensive care because of the serious sequelae that can quickly develop (Weinberg & Thompson-Stone, 2018).

! NURSING ALERT

Any child who is ill and develops a petechial or purpural rash may have meningococcemia and must receive immediate medical attention.

Other acute complications of meningitis include SIADH (see Chapter 31), subdural effusions, seizures, cerebral edema and herniation, and hydrocephalus. Obstruction to the flow of CSF occurs during the acute phase of illness by clumping of purulent material in the drainage channels and during the chronic phase by adhesive arachnoiditis or fibrotic obstruction through any of the ventricular foramina. Postmeningitic complications in neonates include ventriculitis, which results in cystic, walled-off areas of the brain with fluid accumulation and pressure.

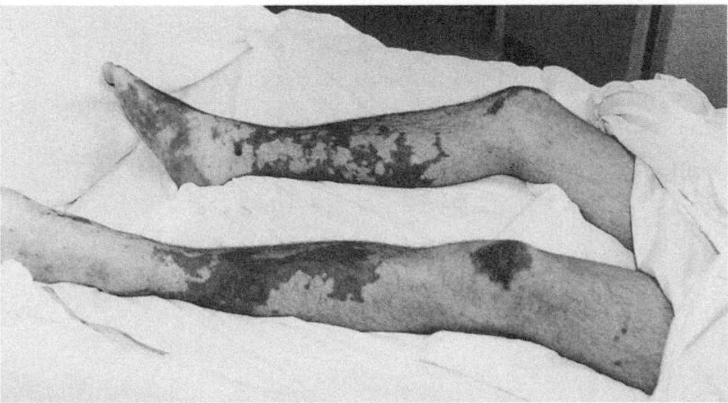

FIG. 30.10 Purpura of the lower extremities of child suffering from meningococcemia.

Extension of the inflammation to cranial nerves or compression and destruction of the nerves from ICP can produce permanent impairment of vision or hearing and other nerve palsies. CN VIII damage is usually followed by permanent deafness, the most common permanent neurologic sequela of bacterial meningitis (Weinberg & Thompson-Stone, 2018). Other long-term complications include cerebral palsy, cognitive impairments, learning disorders, attention-deficit/hyperactivity disorder, and seizures.

Hemiparesis and quadriparesis may result from damage caused by arteritis or thrombosis or other mechanisms. Behavioral changes occur in some children. Evidence indicates that psychometric and behavioral defects may be a significant concomitant sign of meningitis in childhood, although it is difficult to determine the degree to which meningitis affects the intelligence of young children. Meningitis in the neonatal period is more likely to cause lifelong impairments, including moderate to severe developmental delay, blindness, deafness, and epilepsy (Swanson, 2015).

Diagnostic Evaluation

A lumbar puncture is the definitive diagnostic test. The fluid pressure is measured, and samples are obtained for culture, Gram stain, blood cell count, and determination of glucose and protein levels. The findings are usually diagnostic. Culture and sensitivity are needed to identify the causative organism. Spinal fluid pressure is usually elevated, but interpretation is often difficult when the child is crying. Sedation with fentanyl and midazolam can alleviate the child's pain and fear associated with this procedure (see Atraumatic Care box). If there is evidence or suspicion of increased ICP, a CT scan of the head may be warranted before the procedure (Weinberg & Thompson-Stone, 2018).

ATRAUMATIC CARE

Lumbar Puncture

If time permits, LMX (4% lidocaine) or EMLA cream (a eutectic mixture of lidocaine and prilocaine), both topical anesthetics, should be applied to the skin overlying L3 to L5 to reduce pain before lumbar puncture. For maximum effect, apply EMLA cream at least 1 hour or LMX 30 minutes before the procedure.

The patient generally has an elevated white blood cell count, often predominantly polymorphonuclear leukocytes. The glucose level is reduced, generally in proportion to the duration and severity of the infection. The relationship between the CSF glucose and serum glucose levels is important in evaluating the glucose content of CSF; therefore a serum glucose sample is drawn approximately one-half hour before the lumbar puncture. Protein concentration is usually increased.

Blood culture is advisable for all children suspected of having meningitis if antibiotics are started before obtaining CSF. Blood culture will occasionally be positive when CSF culture is negative. Nose and throat cultures may provide helpful information in some cases.

Therapeutic Management

Acute bacterial meningitis is a medical emergency that requires early recognition and immediate therapy to prevent death and avoid residual disabilities. The initial therapeutic management includes the following:

- Isolation precautions
- Initiation of antimicrobial therapy
- Maintenance of hydration
- Maintenance of ventilation
- Reduction of increased ICP
- Management of systemic shock
- Control of seizures
- Control of temperature
- Treatment of complications

The child is usually moved to an intensive care unit for close observation. An IV infusion is started to facilitate administration of antimicrobial agents, fluids, antiepileptic drugs, and blood, if needed. The child is placed in respiratory isolation.

Drugs

Until the causative organism is identified, empirical therapy is administered. After identification of the organism, antimicrobial agents are adjusted accordingly.

DRUG ALERT

Dexamethasone Use in Meningitis

Dexamethasone may play a role in the initial management of increased ICP and cerebral herniation, but its ability to reduce long-term complications of bacterial meningitis remains controversial. There is evidence that dexamethasone given just before or with the first dose of antibiotics decreases the risk of hearing impairment in children with *H. influenzae* type b meningitis in the developed world (Marcdante & Klegman, 2016). Its use in meningococcal, neonatal, aseptic, or nonbacterial meningitis is not recommended (Weinberg & Thompson-Stone, 2018).

Signs of gastrointestinal hemorrhage or secondary infection may complicate steroid administration. Antibiotic treatment with cephalosporins demonstrates superiority for promptly sterilizing the CSF and reducing the incidence of severe hearing impairment. With increasing prevalence of antibiotic-resistant *S. pneumoniae,* vancomycin should be given until antibiotic susceptibility test results are available (Marcdante & Klegman, 2016).

Nonspecific Measures

Maintaining hydration is a prime concern. The patient's condition determines whether IV fluids are needed and the type and amount of fluid. The optimum hydration involves correction of any fluid deficits and electrolyte abnormalities, followed by fluid restriction until normal serum sodium levels and no signs of increased ICP are present. If needed, measures to decrease ICP are implemented (see earlier in the chapter); however, long-term fluid restriction is not the standard of care because a lack of fluid volume can reduce blood pressure and CPP, causing CNS ischemia (Prober, Srinivas, & Mathew, 2016a).

Complications, such as subdural effusion in infants and disseminated intravascular coagulation syndrome, are treated appropriately. Shock is managed by restoration of circulating blood volume and maintenance of electrolyte balance. Seizures can occur during the first few days of treatment. These are controlled with the appropriate antiepileptic drug.

Hearing loss is common. The patient should undergo auditory evaluation shortly after discharge so that audiology and speech and communication therapies can begin as soon as possible.

Lumbar puncture is carried out as needed to determine the effectiveness of therapy. The patient is evaluated neurologically during the convalescent period.

Prognosis

Less than 10% of cases of bacterial meningitis are fatal; the highest mortality rate is seen in pneumococcal meningitis and in infants under the age of 6 months (Prober, Srinivas, & Mathew, 2016a). Prognosis is dependent in large part on the length of time between onset of illness and initiation of antibiotic therapy, rapidity of diagnosis after onset, type of organism, prolonged or complicated seizures, low CSF glucose concentration, and adequacy of therapy. Up to half of those who recover from meningitis will have some neurodevelopmental sequelae ranging from mild behavioral and learning problems to profound hearing impairment, intractable epilepsy, and significant intellectual disability (Prober, Srinivas, & Mathew, 2016a).

DRUG ALERT

Antibiotic Use in Meningitis

A major priority of nursing care of a child suspected of having meningitis is to administer antibiotics as soon as they are ordered. The child is placed on respiratory isolation for at least 24 hours after initiation of antimicrobial therapy.

The sequelae of bacterial meningitis occur most often when the disease occurs in the first 2 months of life and least often in children with meningococcal meningitis. The residual deficits in infants are primarily a result of communicating hydrocephalus and the greater effects of cerebritis on the immature brain. In older children the residual effects are related to the inflammatory process itself or result from vasculitis associated with the disease. Bacterial meningitis continues to cause substantial morbidity in infants and children.

Prevention

Vaccination is the foundation of prevention of CNS infections. Vaccines are available for pneumococci, types A, C, Y, and W-135 meningococci, and *H. influenzae* type b. Routine meningococcal conjugate vaccination of children is recommended at age 11 to 12 years, with a booster at 16 years, but can be given to children 2 months to 10 years of age if they are considered high risk (e.g., asplenia, foreign travel to high-risk areas, or present during outbreaks). Routine vaccinations for *H. influenzae* type b and pneumococcal conjugate vaccines are recommended for all children beginning at 2 months of age. (See Immunizations, Chapter 6.)

Nursing Care Management

Nurses should take the necessary precautions to protect themselves and others from possible infection. Teach parents proper hand washing technique and remind them as needed.

Keep the room as quiet as possible and environmental stimuli at a minimum as most children with meningitis are sensitive to noise, bright lights, and other external stimuli. Help the family limit the number and frequency of visitors until the child is and feels better. Most children are more comfortable without a pillow under their head but with the head of the bed slightly elevated. Use pillows alongside a child in a side-lying position and between the child's knees for comfort in cases of nuchal rigidity. Avoid actions that cause pain or increase discomfort, such as lifting the child's head. Evaluating the child for pain and implementing appropriate relief measures are important ongoing interventions. Measures are used to ensure safety because the child is often restless, disoriented, and subject to seizures. Prevention of falls is essential.

The nursing care of the child with meningitis is determined by the child's symptoms and treatment (see Box 30.6). Observation of vital signs, neurologic signs, LOC, urinary output, and other pertinent data is carried out at frequent intervals. The child who is unconscious is managed as described previously, and all children are observed carefully for signs of the complications just described, especially increased ICP, shock, and respiratory distress. Frequent assessment of the open fontanels is needed in the infant because subdural effusions and obstructive hydrocephalus can develop as a complication of meningitis.

Administration of fluids and nourishment is determined by the child's status. The child who is not alert and oriented is given nothing by mouth. Other children are allowed clear liquids initially and, if tolerated, progress to a diet suitable for their age. Careful monitoring and recording of intake and output are needed to determine deviations that might indicate impending shock or increasing fluid accumulation, such as cerebral edema or subdural effusion.

One of the most challenging issues in the nursing care of children with meningitis is maintaining IV infusion for the length of time needed to provide adequate antimicrobial therapy (usually 10 days). Because continuous IV fluids are usually not necessary, an intermittent infusion device is used. In some cases children who are recovering uneventfully are sent home with the device, and the parents are taught IV drug administration. (See Quality Patient Outcomes box.)

QUALITY PATIENT OUTCOMES

Bacterial Meningitis

- Early recognition of signs and symptoms of meningitis
- Antibiotics administered as soon as diagnosis is established
- Cerebral edema prevented
- Exposure prevented by early isolation
- Side effects managed
- Neurologic sequelae prevented

Family Support

The sudden nature of the illness makes emotional support of the child and parents extremely important (see Family-Centered Care box). Parents are upset and concerned about their child's condition and often feel guilty for not having suspected the seriousness of the illness sooner. They need reassurance that the natural onset of meningitis is sudden and that they acted responsibly in seeking medical assistance when they did. The nurse encourages the parents to openly discuss their feelings to minimize blame and guilt. Some parents will benefit from referral to a hospital chaplain, social worker, psychologist, or psychiatrist. The nurse keeps parents informed of the child's progress and of all procedures, results, and treatments. In the event that the child's condition worsens, they need the same psychologic care as other parents facing the possible death of their child. (See Chapter 19.)

FAMILY-CENTERED CARE

Preventing Bacterial Meningitis

With immunization schedules calling for administration of *Haemophilus influenzae* type b vaccine and pneumococcal conjugate vaccine to infants at 2 months of age, encourage parents to bring their child to a health facility so that the full series of inoculations is completed. Given the 10% mortality rate associated with bacterial meningitis, early immunization can help families avoid the tragic death or permanent disability of a child. Nurses play a significant role in educating families regarding preventive measures, such as getting children immunized on schedule.

TABLE 30.4 Variation of Cerebrospinal Fluid Analysis in Bacterial and Viral Meningitis

Manifestations	Bacterial*	Viral
White blood cell count	Elevated; increased neutrophils	Slightly elevated; increased lymphocytes
Protein content	Elevated	Normal or slightly increased
Glucose content	Decreased	Normal
Gram stain; bacteria culture	Positive	Negative
Color	Turbid or cloudy	Clear or slightly cloudy
Opening pressure	Elevated	Normal

*Results may vary in the neonate.

NONBACTERIAL (ASEPTIC) MENINGITIS

The term *aseptic meningitis* refers to the onset of meningeal symptoms, fever, and pleocytosis without bacterial growth from CSF cultures. Aseptic meningitis is caused by many different viruses, including arbovirus, enterovirus, herpes simplex virus, cytomegalovirus, and human immunodeficiency virus. Enterovirus is the most common cause of aseptic meningitis (Prober, Srinivas & Mathew, 2016b). The onset may be abrupt or gradual, and many of the presenting signs and symptoms are the same as bacterial meningitis, including headache, fever, photophobia, and nuchal rigidity.

Diagnosis is based on clinical features and CSF findings. Table 30.4 lists variations in CSF values in bacterial and viral meningitis. It is important to differentiate this usually self-limiting disorder from the more serious forms of meningitis.

Treatment is primarily symptomatic, such as acetaminophen for headache and muscle pain, maintenance of hydration, and positioning for comfort. Until a definitive diagnosis is made, antimicrobial agents may be administered and isolation enforced as a precaution against the possibility that the disease might be of bacterial origin. Nursing care is similar to the care of the child with bacterial meningitis. The course of aseptic meningitis is usually much shorter and typically without significant complications.

TUBERCULOUS MENINGITIS

Tuberculous meningitis must be considered in children who have traveled or lived in, live with, or are immigrants from developing countries. In 2015 the incidence of tuberculous meningitis in the United States increased for the first time in over 2 decades (Smith, Pratt, Trieu, et al., 2017). Tuberculous is more likely to be disseminated (including CNS involvement) in very young or immunosuppressed children.

Ischemic infarction can occur with tuberculous meningitis. The most common clinical findings are meningeal signs, fever, altered consciousness, cranial nerve involvement, seizures, and focal neurologic deficit.

Early diagnosis of tuberculous meningitis in the child can significantly reduce the disability caused by hydrocephalus, a common complication of this type of meningitis. Nursing care is similar to the care of the child with bacterial meningitis and involves administration of medications, support of the child, control of pain, and neurologic monitoring.

BRAIN ABSCESS

Intracerebral abscesses form when pyogenic organisms gain access to neural tissue by way of the bloodstream from foci of infection or from direct inoculation of organisms from infections, penetrating trauma, or surgical procedures. Chronic ear infection, mastoiditis, sinusitis, and congenital heart disease are the most common predisposing factors for children with brain abscesses. The majority (70%) of brain abscesses are caused by aerobic and anaerobic streptococci (Prober & Mathew, 2016). In neonates *Citrobacter* is most common, and fungi are more common in immunocompromised children (Prober & Mathew, 2016).

The most common sites of intracerebral abscesses are the parietal, temporal, and frontal lobes. Early signs of the disease are vague; however, the most common symptom is a severe headache. As the inflammatory process proceeds, symptoms intensify and include vomiting, lethargy, fever, seizures, papilledema, focal neurologic signs (hemiparesis), and progression to coma (Prober & Mathew, 2016). Because mortality rates from brain abscesses may exceed 20%, prompt diagnosis and treatment are critical (Prober & Mathew, 2016). Successful management consists of surgical drainage and antibiotic therapy. Surgical drainage is necessary if the mass is greater than 2 cm in diameter or there are signs of increased ICP. Where possible, the source of the infection is eradicated. Children may experience epilepsy, hemiparesis, cranial nerve abnormalities, and behavior/learning problems as long-term complications (Prober & Mathew, 2016).

ENCEPHALITIS

Encephalitis is an inflammatory process of the CNS that is caused by a variety of organisms, including bacteria, spirochetes, fungi, protozoa, helminths, and viruses. Most infections are associated with viruses, and this discussion is limited to those agents.

Etiology

Encephalitis can occur as a result of direct invasion of the CNS by a virus or postinfectious involvement of the CNS after a viral disease. Enteroviruses are the most common etiology (Prober, Srinivas & Mathew, 2016b); however, the specific type of encephalitis may often not be identified. The cause of more than half the cases reported in the United States is unknown.

Autoimmune encephalitis syndromes are a recently recognized cause of new-onset neurologic deficits in children (Longoni, Levy, & Yeh, 2016). In some children antibodies are identified, and there is a small group (<20%) whose etiology is a tumor, particularly ovarian teratoma, but the majority of children will not have either of these conditions (Dubey, Sawhney, Greenberg, et al., 2015). Diagnosis is usually based on clinical symptoms, which can be neurologic, psychiatric, or both (Scheer & John, 2016). Neurologic symptoms include seizures, encephalopathy, and movement disorders (Dale, Gorman, & Lim, 2017). Behavioral changes, hallucinations, anxiety, and aggression are some of the more commonly seen psychiatric manifestations (Scheer & John, 2016).

Herpes simplex encephalitis is an uncommon disease, but 30% of cases involve children. The initial clinical findings are nonspecific (e.g., fever, altered mental status), but most cases evolve to demonstrate focal neurologic signs and symptoms. Children may experience focal seizures. The CSF is abnormal in most cases. Because of a rise in the number of children with herpes simplex encephalitis, suspected cases require prompt attention, especially because the diagnosis can be difficult. CSF polymerase chain reaction (PCR) testing can confirm the clinical diagnosis rapidly. The early use of IV acyclovir reduces mortality and morbidity rates. Empiric therapy with acyclovir is given before precise virologic diagnosis has been established.

The multiplicity of causes of viral encephalitis makes diagnosis difficult. Most are those involved with arthropod vectors (e.g., togaviruses and bunyaviruses) and those associated with hemorrhagic fevers (e.g., arenaviruses, filoviruses, and hantaviruses). In the United States the vector reservoir for most agents pathogenic for humans is the mosquito (St. Louis or West Nile encephalitis); therefore most cases of encephalitis appear during the hot summer months and subside during the autumn.

BOX 30.7 Clinical Manifestations of Encephalitis

Onset: Sudden or Gradual
Malaise
Fever
Headache
Dizziness
Apathy
Lethargy
Nuchal rigidity
Ataxia
Tremors
Hyperactivity
Speech difficulties: mutism
Altered mental status

Severe Cases
High fever
Stupor
Seizures
Disorientation
Spasticity
Coma (may proceed to death)
Ocular palsies
Paralysis

Clinical Manifestations

The clinical features of encephalitis are similar regardless of the agent involved. Manifestations can range from a mild benign form that resembles aseptic meningitis, lasts a few days, and is followed by rapid and complete recovery, to a rapidly progressing encephalitis with severe CNS involvement. The onset may be sudden or may be gradual with malaise, fever, headache, dizziness, apathy, nuchal rigidity, nausea and vomiting, ataxia, tremors, hyperactivity, and speech difficulties (Box 30.7). In severe cases the patient has high fever, stupor, seizures, disorientation, spasticity, and coma that may proceed to death. Ocular palsies and paralysis also may occur.

Diagnostic Evaluation

The diagnosis is made on the basis of clinical findings and, where possible, identification of the specific virus. Early in the course of encephalitis, CT scan results may be normal. Later, hemorrhagic areas in the frontotemporal region may be seen. Arboviruses are rarely detected in the blood or spinal fluid, but viruses of herpes, mumps, measles, and enteroviruses may be found in the CSF. Serologic testing may be required. The first blood sample should be drawn as soon as possible after onset, with the second sample drawn 2 or 3 weeks later.

Therapeutic Management

Patients suspected of having encephalitis are hospitalized promptly for observation, including ICP monitoring. In autoimmune encephalitis rapid initiation of immunotherapy, including corticosteroids, plasmapheresis, and IV immunoglobulin, improves outcomes. Herpes simplex virus encephalitis is the only viral encephalitis that has specific treatment available. In other cases, treatment is primarily supportive and includes conscientious nursing care, control of cerebral manifestations, and adequate nutrition and hydration, with observations and management as for other cerebral disorders.

Prognosis

Viral encephalitis can cause devastating neurologic injury. The prognosis for the child with encephalitis depends on the child's age, the type of encephalitis, and residual neurologic damage. Very young children (less than 2 years of age) with viral encephalitis have an increased risk of neurologic disability, including learning difficulties and epilepsy. About 80% of autoimmune encephalitis patients make a full or nearly full recovery (Longoni, Levy, & Yeh, 2016).

Follow-up care with periodic reevaluation and rehabilitation is important for patients who develop residual effects of encephalitis.

Nursing Care Management

Nursing care of the child with encephalitis is the same as for any unconscious child and for the child with meningitis. Additional nursing interventions include observation for deterioration in consciousness. Isolation of the child is not necessary; however, always use good hand washing technique. A main focus of nursing management is the control of rapidly rising ICP. Neurologic monitoring, administration of medications, and support of the child and parents are the major aspects of care. (See Quality Patient Outcomes box.)

QUALITY PATIENT OUTCOMES

Encephalitis

- Early recognition of signs and symptoms
- Cerebral edema prevented
- Side effects managed
- Neurologic sequelae prevented

RABIES

Rabies is an acute infection of the nervous system caused by a virus that is almost invariably fatal if left untreated. It is transmitted to humans by the saliva of an infected mammal introduced through a bite or skin abrasion. After entry into a new host, the virus multiplies in muscle cells and is spread through neural pathways without stimulating a protective host immune response.

Through dog vaccination, rabies from dog bites has been eliminated in the United States (World Health Organization, 2017). Carnivorous wild animals (e.g., raccoons, skunks, bats, and foxes) are the animals most often infected with rabies and the cause of most indigenous cases of human rabies in the United States (Singh, Singh, Cherian, et al., 2017).

The circumstances of a biting incident are important. An unprovoked attack is more likely than a provoked attack to indicate a rabid animal. Bites inflicted on a child attempting to feed or handle an apparently healthy animal can generally be regarded as provoked. Any child bitten by a wild animal is assumed to be exposed to rabies.

! NURSING ALERT

Unusual behavior in an animal is cause for suspicion; children should be warned to beware of wild animals that appear to be friendly.

Although rabies is common among wildlife species, human rabies is rarely acquired. The highest incidence of rabies occurs in children under age 15 years. The incubation period usually ranges from 1 to 3 months but may be as short as 5 days or longer than 6 months (Willoughby, 2016). Modern-day prophylaxis is nearly 100% successful. Only 10% to 15% of persons bitten develop the disease, but once symptoms are present, rabies progresses to a fatal outcome. In the United States human fatalities associated with rabies occur in people who fail to seek medical attention, usually because they are unaware of their exposure.

BOX 30.8 Clinical Manifestations of Rabies

Initial Signs
General malaise
Fever
Anorexia
Sore throat

Excitement Phase
Hypersensitivity
Increased reaction to external stimuli
Seizures
Fluctuating consciousness
Choking

Severe Spasm of Respiratory Muscles*
Apnea
Cyanosis
Anoxia

*From attempts at swallowing (characteristics from which the term *hydrophobia* was derived).

The disease is characterized by a period of nonspecific flulike symptoms, including general malaise, anorexia, fever, and sore throat, followed by a phase of excitement that features hypersensitivity and increased reaction to external stimuli, seizures, hallucinations, hypersalivation, and choking (Box 30.8). Attempts at swallowing may cause spasms of respiratory muscles so severe that they produce apnea, cyanosis, and anoxia—the characteristics from which the term *hydrophobia* was derived.

Diagnosis is made on the basis of history and clinical features. Hydrophobia is a cardinal sign of rabies. The diagnosis is confirmed by skin biopsy. Antibodies maybe detected 7 to 8 days after the onset of clinical symptoms (Crowcroft & Thampi, 2015).

Therapeutic Management

Treatment is of little avail once symptoms appear, but the long incubation period allows time for the induction of active and passive immunity before the onset of illness. Two types of immunizing products are available for use in humans: (1) the inactivated rabies vaccines, which induce an active immune response, and (2) the globulins, which contain preformed antibodies. The two types of products should be used concurrently for rabies postexposure treatment when prophylaxis is indicated.

The current therapy for a rabid animal bite consists of three steps: (1) thorough cleansing of the wound with soap and water (suturing should be avoided whenever possible); (2) administration of rabies vaccine; and (3) administration of rabies immunoglobulin. The rabies vaccine and immunoglobulin should be initiated as soon as possible after exposure. The rabies vaccine consists of four doses administered intramuscularly at days 0, 3, 7, and 14 but can be stopped if the animal remains healthy throughout the 10-day observation period or is proved to be negative for rabies by a reliable laboratory (Crowcroft & Thampi, 2015). Rabies immunoglobulin is administered locally at the wound and provides passive antibodies at the site of exposure. Rabies immunoglobulin is given once within 7 days after the first vaccine dose before the child develops an active immune response (Crowcroft & Thampi, 2015).

Nursing Care Management

Parents and children are frightened by the urgency and seriousness of the situation. They need anticipatory guidance for the therapy and support and reassurance regarding the efficacy of the preventive measures for this dreaded disease. The vaccine is well tolerated by children, although they need preparation for the series of injections. Mass immunization is unnecessary and unlikely to be implemented. In areas in which rabies is rare, the schedule given is sufficient. However, certain circumstances may warrant preexposure vaccination, such as when a child is being taken to an area of the world where rabies in stray dogs is still a problem.

REYE SYNDROME

Reye syndrome (RS) is a disorder defined as a metabolic encephalopathy associated with other characteristic organ involvement. It is characterized by fever, profoundly impaired consciousness, and disordered hepatic function.

The etiology of RS is not well understood, but most cases follow a common viral illness, typically influenza or varicella. RS is a condition characterized pathologically by cerebral edema and fatty changes of the liver. The onset of RS is notable for profuse effortless vomiting and lethargy that quickly progresses to neurologic impairment, including delirium, seizures, and coma, and can ultimately lead to increased ICP, herniation, and death (Ibrahim & Balistreri, 2016). The cause of RS is a mitochondrial insult induced by various viruses, drugs, exogenous toxins, and genetic factors. Elevated serum ammonia levels tend to correlate with the clinical manifestations and prognosis.

Definitive diagnosis is established by liver biopsy. The staging criteria for RS are based on liver dysfunction and on neurologic signs that range from lethargy to coma. As a result of improved diagnostic techniques, children who in the past would have been diagnosed with RS are now diagnosed with other illnesses such as viral or inborn metabolic errors affecting organic acid, ammonia, and carbohydrate metabolism. Cases of unrecognized, drug-induced encephalopathy by antiemetics given to children during viral illnesses have symptoms similar to those of RS.

The potential association between aspirin therapy for the treatment of fever in children with varicella or influenza and the development of RS precludes its use in these patients. However, by the time the Food and Drug Administration required aspirin product labeling in 1986, most of the decline in RS incidence had already occurred.

Nursing Care Management

The most important aspect of successful management of the child with RS is early diagnosis and aggressive therapy. Rapid progression to coma and high peak ammonia concentrations are associated with a more serious prognosis. Cerebral edema with increased ICP represents the most immediate threat to life.

Care and observations are implemented as for any child with an altered state of consciousness (see earlier in this chapter) and increasing ICP. Accurate and frequent monitoring of intake and output is essential for adjusting fluid volumes to prevent both dehydration and cerebral edema. Because of related liver dysfunction, monitor laboratory studies to determine impaired coagulation, such as prolonged bleeding time.

Keep the parents of children with RS informed of the child's progress and explain diagnostic procedures and therapeutic management. Recovery from RS is rapid and usually without sequelae if the diagnosis is determined early and therapy is initiated promptly. Patients who survive have full liver function recovery (Ibrahim & Balistreri, 2016).

DRUG ALERT

Salicylates

Families need to be aware that salicylates, the alleged offending ingredient in aspirin, are contained in other products (e.g., Pepto-Bismol). They should refrain from administering any product for influenza-like symptoms without first checking the label for "hidden" salicylates.

HUMAN IMMUNODEFICIENCY VIRUS ENCEPHALOPATHY

Documented routine human immunodeficiency virus (HIV) testing and counseling for all pregnant women in the United States is recommended. Consent is obtained before testing. The use of zidovudine (AZT) by HIV-infected pregnant women significantly reduces the chance that the mother will pass the virus on to her infant.

HIV infection is acquired through direct exposure to blood, semen, or vaginal fluid or via breast milk. The majority of pediatric HIV cases worldwide are acquired vertically from an infected mother. HIV deoxyribonucleic acid (DNA) PCR can identify HIV infection in more than 90% of infected newborns at 1 month of age, and HIV ribonucleic acid (RNA) assays can be a confirmatory test for infants who have an initial positive DNA PCR test. In the United States antiretroviral therapy is recommended for all HIV-infected infants less than 1 year of age.

Children with HIV infection can develop neurologic manifestations, including progressive multifocal encephalopathy, microcephaly, epilepsy, motor deficits such as spasticity and ataxia, and developmental delay or regression (Mann, Donald, Laughton, et al., 2017). Changes on CT examination, including generalized brain atrophy and bilateral calcifications of the basal ganglia, may be seen. Therapy consists of highly active antiretroviral therapy (HAART) (see Research Focus box).

RESEARCH FOCUS

Therapies Delay Onset of HIV Encephalopathy in Children

A cohort study conducted from 1993 to 2007 followed 2398 perinatally HIV-infected children in the United States to evaluate the impact of HAART on the incidence of HIV encephalopathy and CNS-penetrating antiretroviral regimens for the treatment of HIV encephalopathy (Patel, Ming, Williams, et al., 2009). HAART regimens were associated with a 50% decrease in the incidence of HIV encephalopathy compared with non-HAART regimens, and only 77 children in the study (3%) developed HIV encephalopathy. High-CNS-penetrating regimens were associated with a 74% reduction in the risk of death after being diagnosed with HIV encephalopathy compared with low-CNS-penetrating regimens.

CNS, Central nervous system; *HAART,* highly active antiretroviral therapy; *HIV,* human immunodeficiency virus.

SEIZURES AND EPILEPSY

A seizure is a "transient occurrence of signs and/or symptoms due to abnormal excessive and synchronous neuronal activity in the brain" (Fisher, Acevedo, Arzimanoglou, et al., 2014). Seizures are the most common pediatric neurologic disorder. About 4% to 10% of children will have at least one seizure in the first 16 years of life (Mikati & Hani, 2016). The manifestation of seizures depends on the region of the brain in which they originate and may include unconsciousness or altered consciousness, involuntary movements, and changes in perception, behaviors, sensations, and/or posture. Seizures are a symptom of an underlying disease process. They are individual events. Potential causes include infections, intracranial lesions or hemorrhage, metabolic disorders, trauma, brain malformations, genetic disorders, or toxic ingestion. (See Nursing Care Guidelines box.)

NURSING CARE GUIDELINES

Terminology for Seizures

Many words are used synonymously with the terms *seizure, epilepsy,* and *seizure disorder.* Epilepsy used to belong to the medical discipline of psychiatry, and therefore words such as *attacks* and *fits* are sometimes used to describe seizure events. These words, however, still create images of medieval superstitions, evil spirits, and the horrors of mental institutions. Parents are often hesitant to inform caregivers and the school that their child has a seizure disorder or epilepsy for fear of prejudice and misunderstandings. When working with families, health professionals should consider the words they use to discuss epilepsy and seizures. Correct terminology can help lessen the stigma and fear often associated with epilepsy and seizures.

The words *convulsion, convulsive disorder,* and *anticonvulsive drugs* are often used to cover all seizure types and antiepileptic drugs. However, the word *convulsion* conjures up images of a raving, wild person who is out of control and possibly dangerous. Therefore referring to all seizures as convulsions is questionable because most seizures are not convulsive in nature. In this chapter the word *event, episode,* or *experience* is used to describe a seizure; likewise, medications are referred to as *antiepileptic drugs.*

Epilepsy is defined as two or more unprovoked seizures more than 24 hours apart and can be caused by a variety of pathologic processes in the brain. A single seizure is not classified as epilepsy and is generally not treated with long-term antiepileptic drugs. Some seizures may result from an acute medical or neurologic illness and cease after the illness is treated. In other cases, children may have one or more seizures without the cause ever being found.

When a child has had a seizure, it is important to classify the seizure, according to the International Classification of Epileptic Seizures. Optimal treatment and prognosis require an accurate diagnosis and a determination of the cause whenever possible.

EPILEPSY

The clinical definition of epilepsy was recently updated by the International League Against Epilepsy (ILAE). "Epilepsy is a disease of the brain defined by the following conditions: (1) at least two unprovoked seizures occurring more than 24 hours apart OR (2) one unprovoked seizure and a probability of further seizures similar to the general recurrence risk (at least 60%) after two unprovoked seizures occurring over the next 10 years" (Fisher, Acevedo, Arzimanoglou, et al., 2014). Seizures are a symptom of an underlying disease process. A single seizure event should be classified as epilepsy only if it meets criteria in number 2. Single seizures in children are generally not treated with long-term antiepileptic drugs. Some seizures may result from an acute medical or neurologic illness and cease once the illness is treated. In other cases, children may have a single seizure without the cause ever being known.

Etiology

Seizures in children have many different causes (Box 30.9). Seizures had been classified according to type and etiology. The International League Against Epilepsy 2017 classification of seizures focuses on location of onset rather than etiology: focal (formerly known as partial), generalized, or unknown and unclassified (Fisher, Cross, French, et al., 2017). Focal seizures are divided into those with preserved awareness and those with impaired awareness and those with or without motor manifestations. Generalized from onset seizures are also divided by their motor symptoms: tonic for the stiffening movements and clonic for the rhythmic jerking that may accompany tonic stiffening, and absence for nonmotor seizures.

BOX 30.9 Etiology of Seizures in Children

Nonrecurrent (Acute)

Febrile episodes
Intracranial infection
Intracranial hemorrhage
Space-occupying lesions (cyst, tumor)
Acute cerebral edema
Anoxia
Toxins
Drugs
Tetanus
Lead encephalopathy
Shigella and Salmonella organisms
Metabolic alterations:

- Hypocalcemia
- Hypoglycemia
- Hyponatremia or hypernatremia
- Hypomagnesemia
- Alkalosis
- Disorders of amino acid metabolism
- Deficiency states
- Hyperbilirubinemia

Recurrent (Chronic)

Idiopathic epilepsy
Epilepsy secondary to the following:

- Trauma
- Hemorrhage
- Anoxia
- Infections
- Toxins
- Degenerative phenomena
- Congenital defects
- Parasitic brain disease
- Hypoglycemia injury

Epilepsy—sensory stimulus
Epilepsy-stimulating states

- Narcolepsy and catalepsy
- Psychogenic
- Tetany from hypocalcemia, alkalosis

Hypoglycemic states

- Hyperinsulinism
- Hypopituitarism
- Adrenocortical insufficiency
- Hepatic disorders

Uremia
Allergy
Cardiovascular dysfunction or syncopal episodes
Migraine

Unknown onset seizures are classified using the same motor criteria as generalized seizures.

The causes of seizures in children are many. Acute reactive seizures are caused by an acute condition such as electrolyte imbalance, acute stroke, head trauma, meningitis, or encephalitis. These seizures may continue and become epilepsy depending on the ability to treat the underlying condition. New-onset seizures may be the initial presentation of a child with a brain malformation. More than 100 genes have been found to cause epilepsy syndromes in children (Mikati & Hani, 2016). Many, but not all, of these genetic orders cause intellectual disability in addition to epilepsy. The proportion of seizures and epilepsy for which we have no identifiable cause becomes smaller each year as neuroimaging and genetic testing improve. Those children who do not have an identifiable cause for their seizures and epilepsy have a better prognosis for eventual resolution of their epilepsy.

Incidence

Epilepsy and seizures affect about 3 million Americans; it is the most common neurologic condition of children (Russ, Larson, & Halfon, 2012). Epilepsy affects people of all ages, but particularly the very young and the elderly. Approximately 1 in every 10 children experience one or more seizures in the first 17 years of life (Russ, Larson, & Halfon, 2012). The onset of epilepsy in children is highest during the first few months of life. The causative factors associated with childhood seizures are often linked to the child's age. In infants the most common causes are congenital brain malformations and genetic disorders, including metabolic disorders. Infections and epilepsy of unknown etiology are common causes of seizures in childhood. Children with intellectual disability, cerebral palsy, and/or autism spectrum disorder are more likely to have epilepsy than their typically developing peers.

Pathophysiology

Regardless of the etiologic factor or type of seizure, the basic mechanism is the same. Abnormal electrical discharges (1) may arise from the simultaneous activation of neurons in both hemispheres of the brain (generalized seizures); (2) may be restricted to one area of the cerebral cortex, producing manifestations characteristic of that particular anatomic focus; or (3) may begin in a localized area of the cortex as a focal seizure and spread to other portions of the brain and, if sufficiently extensive, produce generalized seizure activity.

A seizure occurs when there is sudden excessive excitation and loss of inhibition within neuronal circuits, allowing the circuits to amplify their discharges simultaneously. These discharges occur in response to the activity of sodium, potassium, calcium, and chloride ion channels. Normally these discharges are restrained by inhibitory mechanisms. In response to physiologic stimuli, such as brain injury or infection, genetic abnormalities, severe hypoglycemia, electrolyte imbalance, sleep deprivation, and toxic exposures, these abnormal neuronal discharges can spread to nearby cortex and subcortical structures. Primary generalized seizures begin with abnormal discharges in both hemispheres, which can involve connections between the thalamus and neocortex. On the basis of these characteristic neuronal discharges (manifested as stereotypical symptoms observed and reported during seizures and/or as recorded by the EEG), seizures are designated as focal, generalized, and unclassified epileptic seizures.

Seizure Classification and Clinical Manifestations

There are many different types of seizures, and each has unique clinical manifestations (Box 30.10). Seizures are classified into two major

BOX 30.10 Classification and Clinical Manifestations of Partial and Generalized Seizures

Partial Seizures

Simple Partial Seizures With Motor Signs

Characterized by the following:

- Localized motor symptoms
- Somatosensory, psychic, autonomic symptoms
- Abnormal discharges remaining unilateral

Manifestations

- Aversive seizure (most common motor seizure in children)—Eye or eyes and head turn away from the side of the focus; awareness of movement or loss of consciousness
- Rolandic (Sylvan) seizure—Tonic-clonic movements involving the face, salivation, arrested speech; most common during sleep
- Jacksonian march (rare in children)—Orderly, sequential progression of clonic movements beginning in a foot, hand, or face and moving, or "marching," to adjacent body parts

Simple Partial Seizures With Sensory Signs

Characterized by various sensations, including:

- Numbness, tingling, prickling, paresthesia, or pain originating in one area (e.g., face or extremities) and spreading to other parts of the body
- Visual sensations or formed images
- Motor phenomena such as posturing or hypertonia

Focal Seizures With Impaired Awareness

Observed more often in children from 3 years through adolescence

Characterized by the following:

- Period of altered behavior
- Amnesia for event (no recollection of behavior)
- Inability to respond to environment
- Impaired consciousness during event
- Drowsiness or sleep usually following seizure
- Confusion and amnesia possibly prolonged
- Complex sensory phenomena (aura)—Most frequent sensation is strange feeling in the pit of the stomach that rises toward the throat and is often accompanied by odd or unpleasant odors or tastes, complex auditory or visual hallucinations, ill-defined feelings of elation or strangeness (e.g., déjà vu, a feeling of familiarity in a strange environment), strong feelings of fear and anxiety, distorted sense of time and self, and in small children emission of a cry or attempt to run for help

Patterns of motor behavior:

- Stereotypic
- Similar with each subsequent seizure
- May suddenly cease activity, appear dazed, stare into space, become confused and apathetic, and become limp or stiff or display some form of posturing
- May be confused
- May perform purposeless, complicated activities in a repetitive manner (automatisms), such as walking, running, kicking, laughing, or speaking incoherently, most often followed by postictal confusion or sleep; may exhibit oropharyngeal activities, such as smacking, chewing, drooling, swallowing, and nausea or abdominal pain followed by stiffness, a fall,

Continued

BOX 30.10 Classification and Clinical Manifestations of Partial and Generalized Seizures—cont'd

and postictal sleep; rarely manifests actions such as rage or temper tantrums; aggressive acts uncommon during seizure

Generalized Seizures

Tonic-Clonic Seizures (Formerly Known as Grand Mal)

Most common and most dramatic of all seizure manifestations

Occur without warning

Tonic phase lasts approximately 10 to 20 seconds

Manifestations:

- Eyes roll upward
- Immediate loss of consciousness
- If standing, falls to floor or ground
- Stiffens in generalized, symmetric tonic contraction of entire body musculature
- Arms usually flexed
- Legs, head, and neck extended
- May utter a peculiar piercing cry
- Apneic, may become cyanotic
- Increased salivation and loss of swallowing reflex

Clonic phase: lasts about 30 seconds but can vary from only a few seconds to a half-hour or longer

Manifestations:

- Violent jerking movements as the trunk and extremities undergo rhythmic contraction and relaxation
- May foam at the mouth
- May be incontinent of urine and feces

As event ends, movements less intense, occurring at longer intervals, then ceasing entirely

Status epilepticus—Series of seizures at intervals too brief to allow the child to regain consciousness between the time one event ends and the next begins

- Requires emergency intervention
- Can lead to exhaustion, respiratory failure, and death

Postictal state:

- Appears to relax
- May remain semiconscious and difficult to arouse
- May awaken in a few minutes
- Remains confused for several hours
- Poor coordination
- Mild impairment of fine motor movements
- May have visual and speech difficulties
- May vomit or complain of severe headache
- When left alone, usually sleeps for several hours
- On awakening is fully conscious
- Usually feels tired and complains of sore muscles and headache
- No recollection of entire event

Absence Seizures (Formerly Called Petit Mal)

Characterized by the following:

- Onset usually between 4 and 12 years of age
- More common in girls than in boys
- Usually cease at puberty
- Brief loss of consciousness
- Minimum or no alteration in muscle tone
- May go unrecognized because of little change in child's behavior
- Abrupt onset; suddenly develops 20 or more attacks daily
- Event often mistaken for inattentiveness or daydreaming
- Events possibly precipitated by hyperventilation, hypoglycemia, stresses (emotional and physiologic), fatigue, or sleeplessness

Manifestations:

- Brief loss of consciousness
- Appear without warning or aura
- Usually last about 5 to 10 seconds
- Slight loss of muscle tone may cause child to drop objects
- Ability to maintain postural control; seldom falls
- Minor movements such as lip smacking, twitching of eyelids or face, or slight hand movements
- Not accompanied by incontinence
- Amnesia for episode
- May need to reorient self to previous activity

Atonic and Akinetic Seizures (Also Known as Drop Attacks)

Characterized by the following:

- Onset usually between 2 and 5 years of age
- Sudden, momentary loss of muscle tone and postural control
- Events recurring frequently during the day, particularly in the morning hours and shortly after awakening

Manifestations:

- Loss of tone causing child to fall to the floor violently; unable to break fall by putting out hand; may incur a serious injury to the face, head, or shoulder
- Loss of consciousness only momentary

Myoclonic Seizures

May be isolated as benign essential myoclonus

Characterized by the following:

- Sudden, brief contractures of a muscle or group of muscles
- Occur singly or repetitively
- No postictal state
- May or may not be symmetric
- May or may not include loss of consciousness

categories: (1) focal seizures (previously referred to as partial seizures), which have a local onset and involve a relatively small location in the brain, and (2) generalized seizures, which involve both hemispheres of the brain and are without local onset.

Focal Seizures (Formerly Known as Partial Seizures)

Focal seizures may arise from any area of the cerebral cortex, but the frontal, temporal, and parietal lobes are most often affected and are characterized by localized motor symptoms; somatosensory, psychic, or autonomic symptoms; or a combination of these. The abnormal EEG discharges begin unilaterally and are evident as focal spikes or sharp waves. Focal seizures are subdivided into three types:

Focal seizures without impaired awareness (formerly simple partial seizures)—Sensory symptoms that occur in one part of the brain and cause no alteration of consciousness, often referred to as aura. Sometimes accompanied by motor movements.

Focal seizures with impaired awareness (formerly complex partial seizures)—Sensory and/or motor symptoms that result in a change or loss of consciousness.

Focal to bilateral tonic-clonic seizures (formerly simple or complex seizures secondarily generalized)—Focal seizures with or without awareness that evolve into generalized seizures, usually a tonic-clonic event.

Focal seizures exhibit manifestations related to where they occur in the brain. A clear description of the seizure (ictal state) by an eyewitness is a valuable aid in localizing the brain area involved. Asking the child if he or she could hear, remember, and respond during the event is also helpful for localization. The initial event may provide the best clue for assessing the type of seizure and its localization. Correctly localizing the area of the brain involved with the seizure event is crucial for diagnostic and therapeutic reasons because many antiepileptic drugs are specific for each type of seizure.

In addition to the initial event, the circumstances that precipitated the episode are important. Identifying and eliminating triggering factors may be the only treatment needed. The postictal state (the period after a seizure) may be varied. The child may be drowsy, be uncoordinated, have transient aphasia or confusion, and display some sensory or motor impairment. Document neurologic changes. Weakness, hypotonia, or inactivity of a body part may indicate an epileptogenic focus in the corresponding contralateral cortical region.

Focal seizures without impaired awareness. Focal seizures with motor signs originate from the primary motor cortex, located in the temporal lobe, which is the area of the brain that controls muscle movement. They are the most frequent type of focal seizure. The simplest form of focal seizures with motor signs is clonus, the rhythmic alternating contraction and relaxation of muscle groups.

Eye movements provide clues to the focus or origin of the seizure. Discharge in the cortex of one hemisphere tends to cause the eyes to deviate to the opposite side. Bilateral discharges tend to cause the eyes to move upward or straight ahead. While deviated the eyes may rhythmically twitch.

Focal seizures with sensory symptoms are usually described as numbness, tingling, or pins and needles. This may be the only symptom of a seizure, or it may spread to involve an adjacent sensory cortex or motor cortex. Auditory seizures may manifest as sounds becoming painfully loud, humming, buzzing, or hissing. Visual seizures typically manifest as micropsia, macropsia, or flashes of light or colors. Focal seizures with autonomic symptoms may consist of feelings of nausea or epigastric rising. Flushing or pallor, sweating, or pupil dilation can be observed. Focal seizures with psychic symptoms may include speech arrest or vocalizations, the sensation that an experience has occurred before (déjà vu), fear, displeasure, anger, or irritability. The affective symptoms associated with focal seizures last only a few minutes and are unprovoked.

Focal seizures with impaired awareness. During the period of impaired consciousness the child may look vacant, dazed, or frightened and be unable to respond when spoken to or to follow instructions and will not react when touched. Focal seizures with impaired awareness are the most common type of seizures. Focal seizures are observed in children of all ages and are the most common type in infants. These seizures may begin with an aura—a sensation or sensory phenomenon that precedes the seizure activity. Common sensations include a strange feeling at the bottom of the stomach that rises toward the throat, odd or unpleasant odors or taste, complex auditory or visual hallucinations, or ill-defined feelings of strangeness (e.g., déjà vu). Small children may emit a cry as a manifestation of an aura. Strong feelings of fear and anxiety and a disturbed sense of time can be associated with an aura. The aura is part of the seizure event and is associated with EEG changes.

Another feature of a focal seizures may be automatisms (repetitive involuntary activities without purpose, carried out in a dreamy state). The predominant observations may be oropharyngeal activities such as lip smacking, chewing, drooling, swallowing, or picking at clothing or bed linens; ambulatory activities such as wandering or running; and verbal manifestations such as repeating words ("please, please," or "help, help"). These automatisms may appear to be antisocial behaviors, such as removing clothes in public or attempting to open the door of a moving car. The child may begin walking or running and unknowingly run out into traffic or into obstacles. It is important to realize that the child's consciousness is impaired and that these actions are not deliberate. It is sometimes difficult to determine whether such behavior is related to the seizure activity or to a behavioral deviation. If the behavior results from seizure activity, all attempts to control such behavior by physical restraint, with counseling, or with behavior plans will be ineffective. The child may suddenly cease activity, appear dazed, stare into space, become confused or apathetic, become limp or stiff, or display some form of posturing. Because the seizure starts in the same part of the brain each time, the child will do the same thing during every event. The term *psychomotor seizure* was formerly used because of the frequent association of psychic symptoms and motor automatisms with focal seizures.

If the seizure involves areas of the brain that control motor function, the child exhibits movements such as jerking of the hands and arms. Focal seizures generally last only a few minutes. After the seizure the postictal period occurs, with signs of confusion and lack of recollection of the ictal period. Depending on the area of the brain involved during the episode, the child may sleep for a time. (See Table 30.5 for a comparison of focal seizures without and with impaired awareness.)

Focal seizures that generalize. Focal seizures may spread and become generalized, usually into a tonic-clonic seizure. In such cases the focal seizure is considered the primary seizure event, and the generalized seizure is considered the secondary one. Thus it would be stated that the tonic-clonic seizure was not generalized at the onset but was a focal seizure that became a bilateral tonic-clonic or secondarily generalized seizure.

Generalized Seizures

Generalized seizures without a focal onset indicate that the initial involvement is from both hemispheres. Loss of consciousness and impairment of motor function occur from the outset. Unlike focal

TABLE 30.5 Comparison of Focal and Absence Seizures

Clinical Manifestations	Focal Seizures Without Impaired Awareness	Focal Seizures With Impaired Awareness	Absence
Frequency (per day)	Variable	Rarely over 1-2 times	Multiple
Duration	Usually <30 sec	Usually >60 sec, rarely <10 sec	Usually <10 sec, rarely >30 sec
Aura	May be sole manifestation of seizure	Frequent	Never
Impaired consciousness	Never	Always	Always, brief loss of consciousness
Automatisms	No	Frequent	Frequent
Clonic movements	Frequent	Occasional	Occasional
Postictal impairment	Rare	Frequent	Never
Mental disorientation	Rare	Common	Unusual

seizures that become generalized, there is no aura. Seizures can occur at any time, day or night. The interval between events may be minutes, hours, weeks, or even years.

Tonic-clonic seizures. The generalized tonic-clonic seizure, formerly known as *grand mal,* is the most dramatic of all seizure manifestations of childhood. The seizure usually occurs without warning and consists of two distinct phases: tonic and clonic. In the tonic phase the child stiffens, the eyes roll upward, and the child loses consciousness. If standing, the child falls to the ground. The musculature stiffens in a generalized and symmetric tonic contraction of the entire body. The arms usually flex, and the legs, head, and neck extend. The mouth snaps shut, and the tongue may be bitten. The thoracic and abdominal muscles contract and sometimes produce a "tonic cry" as air is forced over the vocal cords. Parents often misinterpret this as an expression of pain. The average tonic phase lasts 10 to 30 seconds, during which the child's respirations become slow and shallow and the child may become cyanotic. Autonomic phenomena that may be observed include increased blood pressure, increased heart rate, flushing, and increased salivation.

In the clonic phase the tonic rigidity is replaced by intense jerking movements as the trunk and extremities undergo rhythmic contraction and relaxation. During this time the child cannot control oral secretions and may be incontinent of urine and feces. As the seizure ends, the movements become less intense and occur at less frequent intervals until they cease entirely. The average clonic phase lasts 30 to 50 seconds.

In the postictal phase the child may remain semiconscious and difficult to arouse. The postictal phase can last 30 minutes to several hours (Mikati & Hani, 2016). The child may remain confused or sleep. He or she may have mild impairment of fine motor movements, have visual and speech difficulties, and may vomit or complain of headache. On awakening, he or she is fully conscious but usually feels tired and may complain of sore muscles and a headache. The child has no recollection of the event.

Absence seizures. Absence seizures, formerly called *petit mal,* are generalized seizures. They have a sudden onset and are characterized by a brief loss of awareness, a blank stare, and automatisms. Absence seizures are divided into typical and atypical. These seizures almost always first appear during childhood, usually between the ages of 5 to 8, and often stop spontaneously in the teenage years (Mikati & Hani, 2016).

The onset of typical absence seizures is abrupt, with the child suddenly experiencing 20 or more events daily. Characteristically the brief loss of consciousness appears without warning and usually lasts 5 to 10 seconds. The child has a motionless blank stare that may be confused with inattentiveness or daydreaming. Slight loss of muscle tone may cause the child to drop objects, but he or she seldom falls. There may be automatisms such as lip smacking, twitching of the eyelids or face, or fumbling with the clothes. The sudden arrest of activity and consciousness is not accompanied by incontinence. Although the child will not recall the episode, when the seizure ends, the child may be aware and able to report that he or she has missed things that happened. There is no postictal sleepiness. Most children can immediately resume previous activities but may be momentarily confused. Atypical absence seizures are accompanied by head nods and sudden myoclonic jerks. Atypical absence seizures, unlike typical absence seizures, can be difficult to treat (Mikati & Hani, 2016).

Hyperventilation and photic stimulation are potent precipitators of absence seizures (Mikati & Hani, 2016). If the child is involved in a group activity, such as classroom reading or discussion, he or she may need help to catch up with the group after the seizure. Frequent episodes can result in slowed intellectual processes and deterioration in schoolwork and behavior. This is often the first indication of the problem. Absence seizures can be distinguished from daydreaming and attention-deficit/hyperactivity disorder by attempting to physically interrupt the episode by touching the face and eyelashes. Children who are daydreaming will respond to touch, whereas those who are having an absence seizure cannot. The abnormal EEG pattern in absence epilepsy is diagnostic and distinguishes absence seizures from focal seizures.

Atonic seizures. Atonic seizures are a sudden, momentary, and total loss of muscle tone. The onset is usually between 2 and 5 years of age. During a mild seizure the child may simply experience several sudden brief head drops. During a more severe episode the child suddenly falls to the ground, loses consciousness briefly, and after a few seconds gets up as if nothing happened. Because of the sudden loss of tone, the child is unable to break the fall by putting out a hand, and can suffer injuries to the head, teeth, and face. Therefore if a child has frequent atonic seizures, wearing a helmet with a face guard when the child is up and walking around should be considered.

Myoclonic seizures. Myoclonic seizures are characterized by sudden, brief, shocklike movements of a muscle or group of muscles (Holmes, 2018). The seizures may involve only the face and trunk or one or more extremities. They may occur singly or repetitively. The seizures may or may not be symmetric. Myoclonic seizures often occur in combination with other seizure types. Myoclonic seizures should not be confused with myoclonic jerks that can occur normally in the course of falling asleep.

The myoclonic seizure can be confused with the exaggerated startle reflex often seen in children with severe developmental delays. The startle reflex occurs immediately after a stimulus such as a loud noise. The child will stiffly and rapidly extend all four extremities, sometimes with a cry, and then quickly return to his or her usual posture. An EEG with video recording can distinguish between the two events.

Tonic seizures. Tonic seizures are characterized by a sudden onset of increased tone. The child falls if standing. The child may involuntarily cry out because of contraction of the respiratory and abdominal muscles. Tonic seizures are longer than myoclonic seizures, with an average duration of 10 seconds. Postictal confusion, tiredness, and headache are common.

Clonic seizures. Clonic seizures are characterized by loss of consciousness and decreased tone followed by jerking movements of the extremities. These movements may be more predominant in one extremity. The duration is typically from 1 to several minutes and may be followed by a rapid recovery or may have a period of postictal confusion.

Unknown Onset Epileptic Seizures

Unknown-onset epileptic seizures are seizures that lack sufficient information to classify. For example, the location of the onset of epileptic spasms, a type of seizure found predominantly in children under 2 years old, is often unknown. In addition to the seizures listed in the International Classification of Epileptic Seizures, several types of epileptic syndromes display a group of signs and symptoms that collectively characterize or indicate a particular condition. Several syndromes associated with epilepsy occur in infants and children. Two of these are West syndrome and Lennox-Gastaut syndrome (LGS).

West syndrome. Infantile spasms are the most common epilepsy of infancy. It has a peak onset between 4 and 8 months of life and rarely occurs after 2 years of age (Singhal, Harini, & Sullivan, 2018). The etiology can be genetic, metabolic, or structural but is unknown in about one-third of affected children. The pathophysiology is poorly understood. An abnormal EEG with hypsarrhythmia is pathognomonic. Nearly all children with infantile spasms have some degree of cognitive impairment (Singhal, Harini, & Sullivan, 2018).

Flexor spasms consist of brief contractions of the neck, trunk, arms, and legs. The arms may either adduct or abduct, with the arms flexed at the elbow. Extensor spasms consist predominantly of extensor contractions resulting in abrupt extension of the neck and trunk with extensor adduction or abduction of the arms and legs. Eye deviation or nystagmus often occurs with infantile spasms. Infantile spasms may occur as a single event or in clusters, with as many as 150 seizures within a cluster. The infant often cries or is irritable during or after a cluster of spasms.

Adrenocorticotropic hormone (ACTH), an injectable hormonal treatment, is the first-line treatment recommended for infantile spasms. The use of high- versus low-dose therapy is controversial. Because of potential significant adverse side effects (e.g., immunosuppression, weight gain, hypertension, inconsolable crying, and irritability) short-term therapy followed by a taper is recommended (Shumiloff, Lam, & Manasco, 2013). ACTH is more likely to provide short-term resolution of infantile spasms, but longer-term resolution is no different when prednisolone (oral hormonal treatment) is used (Jones, Snead, Boyd, et al., 2015). Due to the cost and difficulty obtaining ACTH, prednisone is considered to be a reasonable option by many epileptologists.

Vigabatrin is usually the choice of treatment for infantile spasms in tuberous sclerosis (Hancock, Osborne, & Edwards, 2013). There is evidence that it works as well as hormonal treatment in the rare children with infantile spasms and normal development (Jones, Go, Boyd, et al., 2015). Long-term use can damage the retinas, causing clinically asymptomatic peripheral visual field cuts. The risk of this visual field cut must be balanced with the benefit of controlling infantile spasms. New evidence suggests that combining vigabatrin with hormonal treatment is more effective than either treatment alone (O'Callaghan, Edwards, Alber, et al., 2017).

The most recent Cochrane review of 18 randomized controlled studies found no single treatment proved to be more efficacious than any other in the treatment of infantile spasms; hormonal treatments resolve spasms more often than vigabatrin, but the hormonal treatments may cause more long-term side effects (Hancock, Osborne, & Edwards, 2013). Use of the ketogenic diet and other antiepileptic drugs as adjunctive therapy is increasing.

The diagnosis of infantile spasms is devastating for many families. Nurses play an important role in supporting these families while at the same time teaching them how to give injections, monitor blood pressure and blood glucose, avoid exposure to illness, and adhere to all recommended appointments and procedures after discharge.

Lennox-gastaut syndrome. Between 20% and 50% of infants who have infantile spasms eventually develop LGS (Germain & Maria, 2018). LGS is diagnosed on three criteria: (1) the presence of multiple seizure types (atonic, myoclonic, tonic, and atypical absence); (2) intellectual disability; and (3) slow spike wave discharges on EEG (Tenney & Glauser, 2018). Onset of LGS is between 1 and 8 years of age. Children with LGS typically have multiple seizures daily. Tonic seizures are the most common. There are many causes of LGS; about one-third of children with LGS have no known cause. Causes include brain malformations and injury, neurocutaneous disorders, brain infections, and genetic disorders. In addition to cognitive impairments, many of these children develop other problems, including hyperactivity, aggressive behavior, or autism spectrum disorder.

Treatment is challenging. Most children require more than one antiepileptic drug and even then many will continue to have some seizures. Drugs are chosen according to the types of seizures (Table 30.6). In addition, the ketogenic diet or implantation of a vagus nerve stimulator may be efficacious for some of these children. The prognosis

TABLE 30.6 Common Antiepileptic Medications

Drug	Indications	Adverse Effects
Carbamazepine	Complex partial, tonic-clonic	Nausea, diplopia, blurry vision, dizziness, drowsiness, hypersensitivity syndrome Black box warning for fatal dermatologic reactions, including toxic epidermal necrolysis and Stevens-Johnson syndrome Black box warning for blood dyscrasias, including anemia and agranulocytosis
Phenytoin	Partial, tonic-clonic; status epilepticus; neonatal seizures	Rashes, sedation, nystagmus, ataxia, hirsutism, gingival hyperplasia, coarse features, folate deficiency Black box warning: severe hypotension and cardiac arrhythmias with rapid infusion (greater than 3 mg/kg/min)
Valproic acid	Primary generalized, absence, myoclonic, febrile, complex partial, Lennox-Gastaut syndrome; not recommended for children less than 2 years of age	Nausea, tremor, weight gain, hair loss, thrombocytopenia, pancreatitis Black box warning: risk for hepatic failure resulting in death
Phenobarbital	Neonatal, febrile, partial, tonic-clonic	Sedation, inattention, hyperactivity, irritability, cognitive impairment, rash, rare hypersensitivity reactions
Clonazepam	Myoclonic	Sedation, irritability, tolerance, ataxia, diplopia Black box warning: concomitant use of opioids and benzodiazepines can cause profound sedation, respiratory depression, coma and death
Felbamate	Reserved for children with Lennox-Gastaut syndrome or adolescents with severe epilepsy	Anorexia, weight loss, nausea, insomnia, headache, fatigue Black box warning: aplastic anemia, hepatic toxicity
Gabapentin	Partial in patients greater than 3 years	Somnolence, dizziness, ataxia, fatigue, diplopia, weight gain
Lamotrigine	Partial, tonic-clonic, Lennox-Gastaut syndrome	Somnolence, dizziness, diplopia, tremor Black box warning: serious rashes including Stevens-Johnson syndrome
Topiramate	Partial, tonic-clonic, Lennox-Gastaut syndrome	Somnolence, anorexia, weight loss, fatigue, difficulty with concentration, kidney stones
Tiagabine	Partial	Dizziness, somnolence, headache, tremor, difficulty with concentration, depression
Oxcarbazepine	Partial, tonic-clonic	Somnolence, headache, dizziness, nausea, ataxia
Levetiracetam	Partial, myoclonic, tonic-clonic	Drowsiness, dizziness, behavioral problems

Modified from Browne, T. R., & Holmes, G. L. (2004). *Handbook of epilepsy.* Philadelphia, PA: Lippincott Williams & Wilkins; and Wilfong, A. (2017). Seizures and epilepsy in children: initial treatment and monitoring. *UpToDate,* T. W. Post (Ed.), Waltham, MA: UpToDate Inc. Retrieved from http://www.uptodate.com/contents/seizures-and-epilepsy-in-children-initial-treatment-and-monitoring?search=Handbook of epilepsy&source.

of LGS is typically poor. Additional family support is often required to maintain the child at home.

Diagnostic Evaluation

Establishing a diagnosis is critical for establishing a prognosis and planning appropriate treatment. The process of diagnosis in a child suspected of having epilepsy includes first determining whether the events thought to be seizures are epileptic seizures or nonepileptic events and then identifying the underlying cause, if possible. The assessment and diagnosis rely heavily on a thorough history, skilled observation, and several diagnostic tests.

It is especially important to differentiate seizures from other brief alterations in consciousness or behavior. Clinical entities that mimic seizures include staring, migraine headaches, toxic effects of drugs, syncope (fainting), breath-holding spells in infants and young children, movement disorders (tics, tremor, chorea), prolonged QT syndrome and other cardiac arrhythmias, sleep disturbances (sleepwalking, night terrors), psychogenic seizures, rage attacks, and transient ischemic attacks (rare in children). The toxic effects of maternal drug use and withdrawal from these drugs should be considered in the differential diagnosis of new-onset seizure activity in a newborn.

A detailed description of the seizure should be obtained from the caregiver(s) who witnessed it. Ask questions about the child's behavior during the event, especially at the onset, and the time at which the seizure occurred (e.g., early morning, while awake, or during sleep). Any factors that may have precipitated the seizure are important, including fever, infection, head trauma, anxiety, fatigue, sleep deprivation, menstrual cycle, alcohol, and activity (e.g., hyperventilation or exposure to strong stimuli such as bright flashing light or loud noises). Record any sensory phenomena that the child can describe and if the child was able to hear during the seizure. The duration and progression of the seizure (if any) and the postictal feelings and behavior (e.g., confusion, inability to speak, amnesia, headache, and sleep) should also be noted. For children who have epilepsy, document how often they have seizures: daily, weekly, or monthly. Knowing the age at which the child had his or her first seizure is important. It is important to determine whether more than one seizure type exists. It is often more informative to ask the parents to show you what the seizure looked like rather than relying on their verbal description. Demonstrating a seizure often reveals features, such as head turning, that would otherwise go unrecognized. Some seizures are overlooked by parents. For example, some parents may not identify brief head nods or brief single jerks as seizures unless specifically asked if their child has these symptoms.

A thorough medical history must be obtained, beginning with conception. Questions to consider include the following: Was the mother's pregnancy complicated by illness and drug use, either prescription or recreational? How old was the baby when discharged from the hospital after birth? Has the child had any overnight hospitalizations or surgeries? A complete history is designed to uncover possible risk factors for the development of seizures or epilepsy.

The family history should include whether other family members ever had a seizure of any kind, cognitive impairments, cerebral palsy, autism, or other neurologic disorders. Ask if there is a family history of sudden, unexpected deaths. A family history can offer clues to other paroxysmal disorders, such as migraine headaches, breath-holding spells, febrile seizures, or neurologic diseases.

A complete physical and neurologic examination, including developmental assessment of language, learning, behavior, and motor abilities, may provide clues to the cause of the seizures. A number of laboratory and neuroimaging tests may be ordered depending on the child's age, whether it is a new-onset seizure, characteristics of the seizure, and the history. Laboratory studies that may prove valuable include a white blood cell count (for signs of infection) and blood glucose measurements that may indicate hypoglycemic episodes. Serum electrolytes, blood urea nitrogen, calcium, serum amino acids, lactate, ammonia, and urine organic acids may indicate metabolic disturbances. Blood for chromosomal analysis may also be tested if a genetic etiology is suspected. A toxicology screen should be performed if alcohol or drug ingestion or withdrawal is suspected. Lumbar puncture can confirm a suspected diagnosis of meningitis. CT may be done to detect a cerebral hemorrhage, infarctions, brain tumors, and gross malformations. MRI provides greater anatomic detail and is used to detect developmental malformations, tumors, and cortical dysplasias.

Most children with seizures will have an EEG. The EEG is the most useful tool for evaluating the child's risk of recurrent seizures, helping determine the type of seizure the child had, and diagnosing the type of epilepsy. The EEG confirms the presence of abnormal electrical discharges and provides information on the seizure type and the location of onset. The EEG is carried out under varying conditions: with the child asleep, awake, awake with provocative stimulation (flashing lights, noise), and hyperventilation. Stimulation may elicit abnormal electrical activity that is recorded on the EEG. Various seizure types produce characteristic EEG patterns; for example, a three-per-second spike and wave pattern is observed in absence epilepsy and a slow spike and wave pattern in LGS.

A normal EEG does not rule out seizures. The EEG is only a surface recording, lasts approximately 1 hour, and therefore may show normal interictal activity. If there is concern about whether a child has seizures or the seizure type cannot be determined, a long-term video EEG may be done to record the child during wakefulness and sleep. The full-body image is recorded on video, with selected EEG channels displayed on the same screen for simultaneous recording and viewing. Amplitude-integrated electroencephalography (aEEG) monitoring is increasingly available in neonatal and pediatric intensive care units. This is a method of continuous monitoring of brain activity using recordings from a handful of leads compared with the 24 leads of standard EEGs. aEEG is useful for diagnosing seizures when standard EEG or a neurophysiologist to interpret it is unavailable. Although the EEG is valuable, it should not be used alone to determine the type of seizure. Rather, the EEG interpretation with a thorough clinical description of the child's behavior during the seizure will inform the correct classification of the seizure and the appropriate treatment choice.

Therapeutic Management

The goal of treatment of seizure disorders is to control the seizures or to reduce their frequency and severity, discover and correct the cause when possible, and help the child live as normal a life as possible. Discovering and, when possible, correcting the underlying cause of the seizures can lead to complete control of all seizures. If the seizure activity is a manifestation of an infectious, traumatic, or metabolic process, seizure therapy is instituted as part of the general therapeutic regimen. Management of epilepsy has four treatment options: drug therapy, the ketogenic diet, vagus nerve stimulation, and epilepsy surgery.

Drug Therapy

It is known that persons predisposed to epilepsy have seizures when their basal level of neuronal excitability exceeds a critical point; no event occurs if the excitability is maintained below this threshold. The administration of antiepileptic drugs serves to raise this threshold and prevent seizures. Consequently, the primary therapy for epilepsy is the administration of the appropriate antiepileptic drug or combination of drugs in a dosage that provides the desired effect without causing adverse side effects or toxicity (see Table 30.6). Antiepileptic drugs are believed to exert their effect primarily by reducing the responsiveness of neurons to the sudden, high-frequency nerve impulses that arise in the epileptogenic focus. Thus the seizure is effectively suppressed; however, the abnormal brain waves may or may not be altered. The chance of total control of seizures depends on the underlying cause of the seizures. Children with epilepsy without any underlying pathology such as brain malformations or genetic disorders and with normal development have the best prognosis.

The initiation of anticonvulsant therapy is based on several factors, including the child's age, type of seizure, risk of recurrence, and other comorbid or predisposing medical issues. For children who develop recurrent seizures or epilepsy, treatment is begun with a single drug known to be effective for the child's seizure type and have the lowest risk of adverse side effects. The dosage is gradually increased until the seizures are controlled. If a child develops intolerable side effects, the medication is stopped and another one tried. If the drug at maximum doses reduces but does not stop all seizures, a second drug is added in gradually increasing doses. When seizures are controlled, the first drug may be tapered to reduce the potential adverse effects and drug interactions of polytherapy. Monotherapy remains the treatment of choice for epilepsy, but a combination of medications may be a viable alternative for children who do not have total seizure control with only one medication (Mikati & Hani, 2016).

If complete seizure control is maintained on an antiepileptic drug for 2 years, it may be safe to slowly discontinue the drug for patients with no risk factors. Risk factors for recurrence of seizures include history of status epilepticus, older age at onset, duration of treatment before seizure control is achieved, presence of a neurologic dysfunction (e.g., motor or cognitive impairment), and abnormal EEG findings when the medication is stopped (Lee, Li, & Chen, 2017). Recurrence occurs most often within the first year of discontinuation (Braun & Schmidt, 2014). When seizure medications are discontinued, the dosage is decreased gradually over weeks or months. Sudden withdrawal of a drug is not recommended because it can cause seizures, which may be longer and more intense than previously, to recur.

Potential complications of drug therapy. The side effects of continued use of antiepileptic medications are often distressing to the child and family. Most side effects are transient and dose related, but drug reactions warrant immediate attention. A serious potential adverse side effect of antiepileptic medication is allergic drug rash. The rash can start with hives and is usually very pruritic. Allergic drug rashes from antiepileptic drugs can spread quickly and become severe, life-threatening events. The drug should be stopped with any signs of a rash. A physician or nurse practitioner should evaluate the child within 24 hours or sooner if the child develops edema or respiratory problems. Treatment includes antihistamines, epinephrine, glucocorticosteroids, anabolic steroids, and/or airway management, depending on the severity of the reaction (Blaszczyk, Lasoń, & Czuczwar, 2015).

Sleepiness, changes in mood or behavior, vision changes, and ataxia are some of the potential side effects of antiepileptic medications. These are very distressing to both children and families. They often disappear over time or when drug dosages are reduced. Blood cell counts, urinalysis, and liver function tests are obtained at regular intervals in children receiving some older antiepileptic medications that can affect organ function.

Knowledge of drug-to-drug interactions, including other medications such as antibiotics, is critical in caring for the child with epilepsy. Knowledge of potential adverse effects is also imperative. Severe, potentially life-threatening side effects can occur with specific antiepileptic medications. For example, carbamazepine, phenytoin, and lamotrigine may cause a severe, life-threatening rash. Valproic acid may cause liver toxicity, particularly in a child less than 2 years of age. To avoid possible complications of tissue damage and difficulties with administration of IV phenytoin, fosphenytoin should be used. Therefore critical thinking and careful monitoring are necessary in providing optimum care to the child with epilepsy.

DRUG ALERT

Fosphenytoin

Fosphenytoin is often used to treat seizures instead of IV phenytoin because of possible complications and drug interactions associated with IV phenytoin. If IV phenytoin is used, it should be administered via slow IV push and at a rate that does not exceed 50 mg/min. Because phenytoin precipitates when mixed with glucose, only normal saline is used to flush the tubing or catheter. Fosphenytoin may be given in saline or glucose solutions at a rate of up to 150 mg PE (phenytoin equivalent)/min, and it may be given intramuscularly if necessary.

Chronic treatment with phenytoin may cause gum hypertrophy. Surgical removal of the excess tissue may be needed in severe cases. Enlargement of the tonsillar and adenoidal tissue can cause partial airway obstruction, which produces snoring during sleep. Chronic treatment with antiepileptic medications, particularly enzyme-inducing medications, has been associated with decreased bone mineral density that worsened with prolonged use of antiepileptic medications (Ahmad, Petty, Gorelik, et al., 2017). Prophylactic administration of calcium and vitamin D supplements is recommended for all patients receiving antiepileptic medications, and bone mineral density testing is recommended for patients on long-term antiepileptic medications (Ahmad, Petty, Gorelik, et al., 2017).

Children whose mothers took antiepileptic medications in the first trimester of pregnancy have a twofold increased risk of being born with congenital malformations compared with children not exposed in utero to these drugs (Ban, Fleming, Doyle, et al., 2015). Folic acid can prevent birth defects but women taking antiepileptic medications tend to have low levels of serum folic acid. The Centers for Disease Control and Prevention and the American Academy of Neurology recommend all females capable of childbearing take 400 to 800 mcg of folic acid daily prior to conception.

Ketogenic Diet

The **ketogenic diet** is a high-fat, very-low-carbohydrate, and adequate-protein diet that has shown effectiveness for treatment of epilepsy (see Research Focus box) (Martin, Jackson, Levy, et al., 2016). It is also the first-line treatment for certain metabolic disorders, including pyruvate dehydrogenase deficiency, glucose transporter type I deficiency, and glutaric aciduria type I. Consumption of the ketogenic diet forces the body to shift from using glucose as the primary energy source to using fat, and the individual develops a state of ketosis. The diet is rigorous. All foods and liquids the child consumes must be carefully weighed and measured. There is a liquid formula available for children who cannot take solid food. The diet is deficient in vitamins and minerals; therefore vitamin and mineral supplementation is necessary. Potential adverse side effects of the diet include constipation, hypoglycemia during initiation of the diet, acidosis, and lethargy. Less common but more serious side effects include urinary tract infections, kidney stones, and insufficient weight gain (Luat, Coyle, & Kamat, 2016).

The ketogenic diet (and its variations) has been shown to be an effective and tolerable treatment for medically refractory epilepsy with seizure control comparable to or better than that obtained with antiepileptic medications in some children (Martin, Jackson, Levy, et al., 2016).

RESEARCH FOCUS

The Ketogenic Diet

The ketogenic diet may be effective in controlling seizures. A Cochrane review of the ketogenic diet, updated in 2016, reported on evidence from seven randomized controlled studies of children with epilepsy (Martin, Jackson, Levy, et al., 2016). The review found short-term benefits of seizure control from the ketogenic diet to be comparable with and, in some cases, better than antiepileptic medications. The most common adverse side effect was gastrointestinal problems, usually constipation. Some children found the diet difficult to tolerate and in others it did not work.

Vagus Nerve Stimulation

Vagus nerve stimulation (VNS) was developed as palliative treatment for patients with seizures not controlled by drugs and who are not candidates for diet or surgical therapy (Moshe, Perucca, Ryvlin, et al., 2015). The results in children have been mixed, with a usually modest reduction in seizures (Dhamne, Kaye, & Rotenberg, 2018). A programmable signal generator is implanted subcutaneously in the chest. Electrodes tunneled underneath the skin deliver electrical impulses to the left vagus nerve (CN X). The device is programmed noninvasively to deliver a precise pattern of stimulation to the left vagus nerve. The patient or caregiver can activate the device using a magnet at the onset of a seizure. No long-term adverse effects have been reported with VNS, but dysphonia, throat or neck pain, and cough can occur during stimulation.

Surgical Therapy

When seizures are caused by a hematoma, vascular malformation, tumor, or other cerebral lesion, surgical removal is usually recommended. Epilepsy surgery is the most effective treatment for children with medically refractory epilepsy due to focal cortical dysplasia and mesial temporal sclerosis. About 80% of these patients will be seizure free 4 years after surgery (Moosa & Gupta, 2014).

Epilepsy surgery does not always eliminate the need for antiepileptic drug therapy. The goal is to improve seizure control without worsening or producing serious deficits. Some children will see improvements in their cognition, behavior, and quality of life (Ryvlin, Cross, & Rheims, 2014). Types of surgeries include focal resection of the epileptogenic focus, functional hemispherectomy, and corpus callosotomy, which severs the connection between the hemispheres.

Status Epilepticus

Status epilepticus is a continuous seizure that lasts more than 30 minutes or a series of seizures from which the child does not regain a premorbid level of consciousness (Fernandez, Abend, & Loddenkemper, 2018). The term *impending status epilepticus* is used for a continuous seizure or series of seizures lasting between 5 and 30 minutes with the designation that treatment should begin within 5 minutes (Fernandez, Abend, & Loddenkemper, 2018).

The initial treatment is directed toward support of vital functions, that is, the CAB of life support, measuring blood glucose, administrating oxygen, and gaining IV access, immediately followed by IV administration of antiepileptic agents. Simultaneously with life support measures and emergency medications, the underlying cause of the status epilepticus is identified and corrected (Fernandez, Abend, & Loddenkemper, 2018).

Buccal or intranasal midazolam and rectal diazepam are simple, effective, and safe treatments for home or prehospital management of prolonged seizures and impending status epilepticus (Brigo, Nardone, Tezzon, et al., 2015). Time to cessation of the seizure with midazolam was 4 minutes shorter than with rectal diazepam (Brigo, Nardone, Tezzon, et al., 2015). Respiratory depression is a potential side effect of these medications when more than two doses are given (Abend & Loddenkemper, 2014); however, respiratory depression is not a side effect of rectal diazepam when it is administered as recommended (Shorvon, 2011). Intranasal midazolam is safe and effective for stopping seizures but also is easier to administer than rectal diazepam (Glauser, Shinnar, Gloss, et al., 2016).

For in-hospital management of status epilepticus, IV diazepam or lorazepam (Ativan) is the first-line drug of choice (Glauser, Shinnar, Gloss, et al., 2016). If IV access has not been established, rectal diazepam or intramuscular, intranasal, or buccal midazolam should be given. It appears that the exact medication chosen is less important than choosing the one that can be administered fastest (Fernandez, Abend, & Loddenkemper, 2018). The child must be closely monitored during administration to detect early alterations in vital signs that may indicate impending respiratory depression. When a benzodiazepine (diazepam or lorazepam) is ineffective, IV phenytoin or fosphenytoin followed by phenobarbital is given as the next line of treatment. Fosphenytoin is preferred over phenytoin because of better tolerability (Glauser, Shinnar, Gloss, et al., 2016). This combination of therapy places the child at high risk for apnea, and therefore respiratory support is generally necessary (see Translating Evidence into Practice box). Children may also receive other antiepileptic medications, including IV valproate or levetiracetam.

Children who continue to have seizures despite drug treatment may require general anesthesia with a continuous infusion of midazolam, propofol, or pentobarbital (Fernandez, Abend, & Loddenkemper, 2018). In this situation the patient may need to be intubated, and continuous EEG monitoring is typically done to monitor for and treat electrographic seizures (Fernandez, Abend, & Loddenkemper, 2018).

Nursing care of a child with status epilepticus includes, in addition to the CAB of life support, monitoring blood pressure and body temperature. During the first 30 to 45 minutes of the seizure the blood pressure may be elevated. Thereafter the blood pressure typically returns to normal but may be decreased depending on the medications being administered for seizure control. Hyperthermia requiring treatment may occur as a result of increased motor activity.

Status epilepticus is a medical emergency that requires immediate intervention to prevent possible brain injury or death. Diagnosis and correction of the underlying cause of the status epilepticus is essential.

Prognosis

Only about half of children who experience a first seizure will have additional seizures (El-Radhi, 2015). Children who have cognitive impairments and/or cerebral palsy are at highest risk for developing epilepsy. Prognosis for eventual remission of childhood epilepsy depends on the etiology and epilepsy syndrome diagnosis. Some syndromes almost always remit whereas others almost never do (Camfield & Camfield, 2015). **Intractable seizures** are failure to control seizures after two appropriately selected antiepileptic medications are trialed (Wassenaar, Leijten, Egberts, et al., 2013). **Refractory seizures** are usually defined as the persistence of seizures despite adequate trials of three antiepileptic medications, alone or in combination (Téllez-Zenteno, Hernández-Ronquillo, Buckley, et al., 2014).

Most deaths in children with epilepsy are due to factors associated with a child's coexisting neurologic conditions and poorly controlled seizures (Berg & Rychlik, 2015). Deaths from epilepsy in children who have no other neurologic conditions occur at the same rate as childhood deaths from other causes, with the exception of drowning (Franklin, Pearn, & Peden, 2017). The phenomenon of sudden unexpected death in epilepsy (SUDEP) is drawing increasing attention in child neurology and epilepsy clinics. It is an extremely rare condition in children with a

TRANSLATING EVIDENCE INTO PRACTICE

Use of Benzodiazepines and the Associated Risk for Respiratory Depression

Ask the Question

In children with status epilepticus (SE), what are the predictors for respiratory depression when treated with a benzodiazepine?

Search for the Evidence

Search Strategies

Search criteria included English-language publications within the past 10 years (2007 to 2017), research-based articles on children with SE.

Databases Used

PubMed, Cochrane, UpToDate, Canadian Medical Association, National Guideline Clearinghouse (AHRQ), Joanna Briggs Institute

Critically Analyze the Evidence

GRADE criteria: Evidence quality very low; recommendation strong (Balshem, Hefland, Schunemann, et al., 2011)

A review of the literature revealed one clinical guideline (Glauser, Shinnar, Gloss, et al., 2016) and three studies that examined the most effective, timely, and safe benzodiazepine to be used as first-line therapy (Appelton, MacLeod, & Martland, 2008; Chin, Neville, Peckham, et al., 2008; Spatola, Alvarez, & Rossetti, 2013). Two of the studies (Chin, Neville, Peckham, et al., 2008; Spatola, Alvarez, & Rossetti, 2013) specifically evaluated respiratory depression after first-line therapy.

- Chin, Neville, Peckham, and colleagues (2008) performed a prospective, population-based study of children treated for SE before being transported to the emergency department. Administration of two or more doses of benzodiazepines was associated with respiratory depression. Diazepam and lorazepam continued to be the most commonly used benzodiazepine as first-line therapy; however, intravenous (IV) lorazepam was found to be associated with a greater likelihood of seizure termination in comparison with rectal diazepam without an increased risk for respiratory depression.
- A retrospective study evaluated the morbidity and mortality effect of standard dosing of benzodiazepine versus excessive dosing (more than 30% above recommended dose) among 202 patients with SE (Spatola, Alvarez, & Rossetti, 2013). Among the excessive-dosed patients, 55% were intubated for respiratory depression, whereas only 8% from the standard-dosed group were intubated. In addition, the excessive-dosed group required significantly longer hospitalization (2 weeks) versus the standard-dosed group (1 week).
- An evidence-based clinical guideline developed by the American Epilepsy Society noted that IV lorazepam and IV diazepam are efficacious at stopping seizures in SE. Furthermore, among patients with SE treated with benzodiazepines, the rate of respiratory depression is lower than in patients with convulsive SE treated with placebo, indicating that respiratory problems are an important consequence of untreated convulsive SE (Glauser, Shinnar, Gloss, et al., 2016).

Apply the Evidence: Nursing Implications

Children receiving more than two doses of benzodiazepine are more likely to have respiratory depression requiring intubation than those receiving fewer doses; however, there is a significant risk of respiratory depression among children in SE who do not receive treatment.

References

Appleton, R., MacLeod, S., & Martland, T. (2008). Drug management for acute tonic-clonic convulsions including convulsive status epilepticus in children. *Cochrane Database of Systematic Reviews*, (3), CD001905.

Balshem, H., Hefland, M., Schunemann, H. J., et al. (2011). GRADE guidelines: Rating the quality of evidence. *Journal of Clinical Epidemiology, 64*, 401–406.

Chin, R. F. M., Neville, B. G. R., Peckham, C., et al. (2008). Treatment of community-onset, childhood convulsive status epilepticus: A prospective, population-based study. *Lancet Neurology, 7*(8), 696–703.

Glauser, T., Shinnar, S., Gloss, D., et al. (2016). Evidence-based guideline: Treatment of convulsive status epilepticus in children and adults: Report of the guideline committee of the American Epilepsy Society. *Epilepsy Currents, 16*(1), 48–61.

Spatola, M., Alvarez, V., & Rossetti, A. O. (2013). Benzodiazepine overtreatment in status epilepticus is related to higher need of intubation and longer hospitalization. *Epilepsia, 54*(8), e99–e102.

DRUG ALERT

Diazepam

Diazepam is incompatible with many drugs. To give intravenously, inject slowly and directly into the vein or through tubing as close as possible to the vein insertion site.

risk of between 1.1 and 3.4 per 10,000 patient-years (Morse & Kothare, 2016). The major risk factor for SUDEP is uncontrolled generalized tonic-clonic seizures, particularly in sleep (Harden, Tomson, Gloss, et al., 2017).

Nursing Care Management

An important nursing responsibility is to observe the seizure episode and accurately document the events. Record and note any alterations in behavior preceding the seizure and the characteristics of the episode, such as sensory-hallucinatory phenomena (e.g., an aura), motor effects (e.g., eye movements, muscular contractions), alterations in consciousness, and postictal state (Box 30.11). The nurse should describe only what is observed, rather than trying to label a seizure type. Note the time that the seizure began and the duration of the seizure.

Generalized seizures and other types with clear manifestations are easy to detect, but absence seizures may present more difficulties. They are easily misinterpreted as inattention. Any unusual behavior, even seemingly inconsequential, such as a momentary interruption of activity, staring, or mental blankness, should be described. The more detailed these descriptions, the more valuable they are for assessment (see Nursing Care Plan and Quality Patient Outcomes boxes).

The child must be protected from injury during the seizure. Nursing observations made during the event provide valuable information for diagnosis and management of the disorder (see Emergency Treatment box).

It is impossible to physically stop a seizure once it has begun, and no attempt should be made to do so. The nurse must remain calm, stay with the child, and prevent the child from injury during the seizure. If possible, isolate the child from the view of others by closing a door or curtain. A seizure can be upsetting to the child, other visitors, and their families. If other persons are present, reassure them that everything is being done for the child. After the seizure, they can be given a simple explanation about the event as needed.

If the nurse is able to reach the child in time, a child who is standing or seated in a chair is eased to the floor immediately. Do not remove a child from a wheelchair. During (and sometimes after) a tonic-clonic seizure, the swallowing reflex is lost, salivation increases, and the tongue

BOX 30.11 General Observations of the Child During a Seizure

Observations During Seizure

General Description

Order of events (before, during, and after)

Duration of seizure

- Tonic-clonic—from first signs of event until jerking stops
- Absence—from loss of consciousness until consciousness is regained
- Focal seizures with impaired awareness—from first sign of unresponsiveness, motor activity, automatisms until there are signs of responsiveness to environment

Onset

Time of onset

Significant precipitating events—missed medication dosage, illness, stress, sleep deprivation, menses

Behavior

Change in facial expression

Cry or other sound

Stereotypic or automatous movements

Random activity (wandering)

Position of eyes, head, body, extremities

Unilateral or bilateral posturing of one or more extremities

Movement

Change of position, if any

Site of commencement—hand, thumb, mouth, generalized

Tonic phase—length, parts of body involved

Clonic phase—twitching or jerking movements, parts of body involved, sequence of parts involved, generalized, change in character of movements

Lack of movement or muscle tone of body part or entire body

Face

Color change—pallor, cyanosis, flushing

Perspiration

Mouth—position, deviating to one side, teeth clenched, tongue bitten, frothing at mouth

Lack of expression

Asymmetric expression

Eyes

Position—straight ahead, deviation upward or outward, conjugate or divergent gaze

Pupils—change in size, equality, reaction to light

Respiratory Effort

Presence and length of apnea

Other

Incontinence

Postictal Observations

Duration of postictal period

State of consciousness

Orientation

Arousability

Motor ability

- Any change in motor function
- Ability to move all extremities
- Paresis or weakness

Speech

Sensations

- Complaint of discomfort or pain
- Any sensory impairment
- Recollection of preseizure sensations or aura

NURSING CARE PLAN

The Child With Seizures

Case Study

Jacob is a 7-year-old boy who was playing during physical education class at school when he suddenly stopped his activity, stared into space, repetitively moved his left arm up and down, and smacked his lips. After approximately 1 minute, he stopped the behavior and was drowsy but responsive to his environment. Jacob had no memory of the event. Jacob was accompanied to the school nurse by his teacher for further assessment.

Assessment

Based on these events, what are the most important subjective and objective data that should be assessed?

Seizure Defining Characteristics

From patient:

Aura

Sensory phenomena that the child can describe during the event (i.e., ability to hear)

Postictal feelings (i.e., confusion, inability to speak, amnesia, headache, sleepiness)

From person who observed the seizure:

Time of onset of seizure

Duration of seizure

Change in level of consciousness (LOC) before, during, and after the seizure

Movements (ask for demonstration of the seizure rather than relying on verbal description)

From parent or primary caregiver:

Previous seizures

Family history of seizures

Recent illness

Current medications

Nursing Interventions

What are the most appropriate nursing interventions for a child with seizures?

Nursing Interventions	Rationale
Monitor time (onset and duration), movements, and LOC during seizure.	To provide an accurate description of the seizure, including the order of events before, during, and after the seizure
If child is at risk of falling, ease child to floor. Prevent child from hitting head on objects. Do not attempt to restrain child or use force.	To prevent physical harm

NURSING CARE PLAN—CONT'D

The Child With Seizures

Nursing Interventions	Rationale
During seizure, place child in a side-lying position on a flat surface such as floor. Do not put anything in child's mouth.	To prevent possible aspiration
Stay with the child and reassure the child when awakening from seizure.	To decrease child's anxiety and fear
Evaluate postictal symptoms (e.g., confusion, return of speech).	To provide accurate description of the postictal state
Ensure antiepileptic drugs are being administered as directed.	To prevent further seizure activity
Involve child and parents in discussion of fears, anxieties, and resources and support options available to patient and family.	To promote coping by discussing fear and anxieties and encouraging participation in support resources

Expected Outcomes

Jacob will not experience physical injury as a result of seizure activity.
Jacob's airway will remain patent.
Jacob and his parents will cope with the condition and receive adequate support.

Case Study (Continued)

The following week, Jacob had another seizure while playing with his siblings in the backyard. His brother ran inside to get help and Jacob's mother ran outside to see Jacob staring into space with his head turned to the side and his left arm moving rhythmically up and down. This activity stopped for a few seconds and then started again. Jacob did not regain consciousness in between the episodes and was unable to speak. Jacob's mother called for emergency assistance (911), and Jacob was transported to a nearby hospital. Jacob had not regained consciousness during the transport.

Assessment

What are the most important signs and symptoms based in this child?

Status Epilepticus Defining Characteristics

Series of seizure activity
Lack of consciousness between seizures
Do the findings described in the case study concern you?

The fact that the child is not regaining a premorbid LOC between seizures is concerning and meets criteria for a diagnosis of status epilepticus. The child's circulation, airway, and breathing (CAB) should be monitored closely and supportive measures initiated (i.e., cardiopulmonary resuscitation) when indicated.

Nursing Interventions

What are the most appropriate nursing interventions for Jacob?

Nursing Interventions	Rationale
Monitor circulation, airway, and breathing (CAB) closely.	To provide supportive measures as needed to maintain airway, breathing, and circulation
Monitor and record characteristics, onset, and duration of each episode, including motor effects, alterations in consciousness, and postictal state.	To accurately describe the seizure activity and postictal state
Do not attempt to stop the seizure; ease the child to the floor if upright. A child in a wheelchair usually has adequate support and padding and does not need to be removed. If on a strethcher, the side rails should be padded.	To prevent injury during seizure
Place child in a side-lying position; suction the oral cavity and posterior oropharynx as needed.	During seizures, the swallowing reflex may be lost, salivation may increase, and the tongue is hypotonic, which causes the child to be at risk for aspiration and airway occlusion.
Administration of antiepileptic medications: • During transport: buccal or intranasal midazolam, buccal lorazepam, rectal diazepam • On arrival to the hospital: Intravenous (IV) lorazepam or diazepam	To decrease or stop the seizure activity
Closely monitor vital signs, including temperature, respirations, heart rate, and blood pressure.	Hyperthermia and hypertension are a common result of increased motor activity. In addition, side effects from the medications may cause respiratory depression.
If possible, isolate the child from view of others by closing door or curtain.	To maintain privacy for the child and family and to minimize distress to the family, and other visitors
Perform diagnostic testing as indicated.	To determine the underlying cause of status epilepticus

Expected Outcome

Jacob will have effective ventilation.
Jacob's airway will remain patent.
Jacob will not experience physical injury as a result of seizure activity.
Jacob's body temperature will remain in acceptable range.
Jacob's blood pressure will remain normal for age.

Case Study (Continued)

Jacob's parents are anxious and upset with the seizures. You are concerned that they do not understand what is happening to their son.

Assessment

What are the most important aspects of care to discuss with Jacob's parents at this time?

Family's Knowledge of Illness-Defining Characteristics

Understands definition of seizure and status epilepticus
Describes measures implemented to prevent harm during seizure
Describes treatment regimen including rationale for medications
Expresses fears and concerns
Shows appropriate reactions to child's condition

Continued

NURSING CARE PLAN—CONT'D

The Child With Seizures

Nursing Interventions

What are the most appropriate nursing interventions for this diagnosis?

Nursing Interventions	Rationale
Educate family about characteristics of seizures, including aura, seizure activity, and postictal state.	To promote understanding of seizures, including signs of impending seizure and characteristics to monitor during and after seizure
Educate family about safety precautions before and during a seizure, including side-lying positioning, padding area if needed, and not placing items in mouth or attempting to stop the seizure.	To promote understanding of measures needed to protect child from harm
Educate family about Jacob's medication administration including scheduled and as necessary (prn) medications and potential side effects of medications.	To promote understanding of medications including monitoring for side effects
Arrange for social worker to meet with family to assess emotional and financial needs. Consider consultation with child life specialist to assist with education of school personnel and classmates.	To identify and modify stressors associated with chronic illnesses and to assist with reentry into school
Education family about Jacob's daily care, including the following: • Have child wear medical identification. • Must have eyes-on supervision when swimming in pools and an adult within arm's reach in natural bodies of water. • Shower preferred. Bathe only with adult in the room. Do not lock the bathroom door when showering. • Use protective helmet and padding during bicycle riding, skateboarding, and in-line skating.	To promote understanding of safety measures for daily life

Expected Outcomes

Jacob's parents verbalize understanding of seizure and status epilepticus and necessary monitoring.

Jacob's parents verbalize safety measures for daily living and during seizure activity.

Jacob's parents verbalize understanding of medications, including schedule, route, and potential side effects.

Jacob's parents verbalize resources available for emotional, financial, and school support as indicated.

QUALITY PATIENT OUTCOMES

Seizures

- Etiology of seizure determined
- Seizures controlled or reduced in frequency and severity
- Family and child receive education to manage seizures
- Child adhering to treatment
- Side effects of treatment minimized

is hypotonic. Therefore the child is at risk for aspiration and airway occlusion. Placing the child on the side facilitates drainage and helps maintain a patent airway. Suctioning of the oral cavity and posterior oropharynx may be necessary. Take vital signs and allow the child to rest. When feasible, the child is integrated into the environment as soon as possible. Sending a child with a chronic seizure disorder home from school is not necessary unless requested by the parents.

Seizure precautions are required for children who are known to have seizures or who are under observation for seizures. The extent of these measures depends on the type and frequency of the seizure (Box 30.12).

Long-Term Care

Care of the child with epilepsy involves physical care and instruction regarding the importance of adherence to the treatment plan. Probably more significant is support and education regarding the potential for the development of psychosocial, educational, and emotional problems in children with epilepsy and their families. Few diseases generate as much anxiety among family, friends, and school personnel as epilepsy (Jones & Reilly, 2016). Fears and misconceptions about the disease and its treatment are common. Nursing care is directed toward educating the child and family about epilepsy and helping them develop strategies to cope with the psychologic and sociologic problems related to epilepsy.

Children with epilepsy are prescribed antiepileptic medications, which are administered at regular intervals to maintain adequate levels in the blood. The nurse can help the parents plan the administration of the medication at convenient times, usually breakfast and dinner

BOX 30.12 Seizure Precautions

The extent of precautions depends on type, severity, and frequency of seizures. Precautions may include the following:

- Side rails raised when child is sleeping or resting
- Side rails and other hard objects padded
- Waterproof mattress or pad on bed or crib

Appropriate precautions during potentially hazardous activities may include the following:

- Swimming with a companion
- Showers preferred; bathing only with close supervision
- Use of protective helmet and padding during bicycle riding, skateboarding, and skating
- Supervision during use of hazardous machinery or equipment

Have child carry or wear medical identification.

Alert other caregivers to need for any special precautions.

Child may not drive or operate hazardous machinery or equipment unless seizure free for designated period (varies by state).

EMERGENCY TREATMENT

Seizures

Tonic-Clonic Seizure

During the Seizure

Remain calm.
Time seizure episode.
If child is standing or seated, ease child down to the floor.
Place pillow or folded blanket under child's head.
Loosen restrictive clothing.
Remove eyeglasses.
Clear area of any hazards or hard objects.
Allow seizure to end without interference.
If vomiting occurs, turn child to one side.
Do *not*

- Attempt to restrain child or use force.
- Put anything in child's mouth.
- Give any food or liquids.

After the Seizure

Time postictal period.
Check for breathing. Check position of head and tongue.
Reposition if head is hyperextended.
If breathing is not present, give rescue breathing and call emergency medical services (EMS).
Keep child on side.
Remain with child.
Do not give food or liquids until child is fully alert and swallowing reflex has returned.
Look for medical identification, and determine what factors occurred before onset of seizure that may have been triggering factors.
Check head and body for possible injuries.
Check inside of mouth to see if tongue or lips have been bitten.

Focal Seizure With Impaired Consciousness

During the Seizure

Do not restrain the child's movements.
Remove harmful objects from area.
Redirect to safe area.
Do not agitate; instead, talk in calm, reassuring manner.
Do not expect child to follow instructions.
Watch to see if seizure generalizes.

After the Seizure

Stay with child and reassure until fully conscious.

Call EMS If

Child stops breathing.
There is evidence of injury or child is diabetic or pregnant.
Seizure lasts for more than 5 minutes (unless seizures typically last longer than 5 minutes) and written medical order is present.
Status epilepticus occurs.
Pupils are not equal after seizure.
Child vomits continuously 30 minutes after seizure has ended (sign of possible acute problem).
Child cannot be awakened and is unresponsive to pain after seizure has ended.
Seizure occurs in water.
This is child's first seizure.

Data from *Seizure First Aid,* Landover, MD, 2017, Epilepsy Foundation. Retrieved from http://www.epilepsyfoundation.org/aboutepilepsy/firstaid/index.cfm.

NURSING ALERT

Do not move or forcefully restrain the child during a tonic-clonic seizure, and do not place a solid object between the child's teeth.

or bedtime, to make taking the medication as easy as possible. It is important to talk with the family about the importance of giving the antiepileptic medication as scheduled to prevent recurrent seizures. Using a pill box can prevent accidentally missing doses. The seizure threshold may be lowered during any illness but particularly with fever. Therefore parents should be aware that if their child has an illness he or she may be at increased risk for seizures. Parents should contact their health professional if their child misses medications due to vomiting.

Rectal preparations of some antiepileptic medications are highly effective when a child is unable to take oral medications because of repeated vomiting, surgery, or status epilepticus. Parents can learn to administer rectal antiepileptic medication for home treatment. Buccal and intranasal midazolam and rectal diazepam are useful adjunctive home treatments for children at risk for prolonged seizures or clusters of seizures and can minimize the need for hospitalization while enhancing parental confidence.

Usually antiepileptic medications are continued until the child has been seizure free for 2 years (Lee, Li, & Chen, 2017). The medication is then slowly tapered over a period of weeks to decrease the chances of precipitating a seizure.

DRUG ALERT

Vitamin D and Folic Acid Deficiency

Children taking phenobarbital or phenytoin should receive adequate vitamin D and folic acid because deficiencies of both have been associated with these drugs. Phenytoin should not be taken with milk.

Nurses should educate the child and parents about the possible adverse reactions to the medications used to treat seizures. Parents must understand the rare but potentially serious side effect of allergic reaction to the medication. They must immediately report rashes to the child's health care provider. More common but less serious potential side effects include excessive sleepiness, changes in appetite, and worsening behavior and mood. Parents should be encouraged to share their observations with their child's health care provider. Parents should understand that the child needs periodic physical assessment. Depending on the medication prescribed, some children will need regular testing of their complete blood count and liver functions. Possible adverse effects on the hematopoietic system, liver, and kidneys may be reflected in symptoms such as fever, sore throat, enlarged lymph nodes, jaundice, and bleeding (e.g., abnormally easy bruising, petechiae, ecchymosis, and epistaxis). The most common cause of status epilepticus in children taking antiepileptic medications is missed medication.

Children with epilepsy are not at increased risk for injury with the exception of head injury (Baca, Vickrey, Vassar, et al., 2013). The degree to which activities are restricted is individualized for each child and depends on the type, frequency, and severity of the seizures; the child's response to therapy; and the length of time the seizures have been controlled. To prevent head injuries, children should always wear helmets and other safety devices when participating in sports, such as biking, skiing, skateboarding, horseback riding, and skating. Only children with frequent seizures must avoid these activities. Children with epilepsy should avoid activities involving heights, such as climbing on play structures taller than they are. Submersion injuries are a serious risk for children with a history of seizures. Children should never be left alone in the bathtub, even for a few seconds. Older children and adolescents should be encouraged to use a shower and reminded not to lock the bathroom door when showering. They must have eyes-on supervision at all times when swimming.

Because the child is encouraged to attend school, camp, and other normal activities, the school nurse and teachers should be made aware of the child's condition and therapy. They can help ensure regularity of medication administration and provision of any special care the child might need. Teachers, child care providers, camp counselors, youth organization leaders, coaches, and other adults who assume responsibility for children should be instructed regarding care of the child during a seizure so that they can react calmly, provide for the child's safety, and influence the attitude of the child's peers.

DRUG ALERT

Rectal Antiepileptic Medications

Rectal preparations of some antiepileptic medications are highly effective when a child is unable to take oral medications because of repeated vomiting, gastrointestinal surgery, or status epilepticus. Parents can learn to administer rectal antiepileptic medication for home treatment. Rectal diazepam is a useful adjunctive home treatment for children at risk for prolonged seizures or clusters of seizures. It also minimizes hospitalization and enhances parental confidence.

Triggering Factors

Careful and detailed documentation of seizures over time may indicate a pattern of seizures. About half of people 12 years old and older with epilepsy can recognize at least one trigger for their seizures (Wassenaar, Kasteleijn-Nolst Trenite, de Haan, et al., 2014). When this occurs, the child, nurse, or responsible adult can intervene to make changes in the lifestyle or environment that may prevent seizures or decrease their frequency. Often the necessary changes are simple but can make an enormous difference in the lives of the child and family.

The most precipitating factors for seizures in children include physical and psychologic stress, sleep deprivation, fever, and illness (Novakova, Harris, Ponnusamy, et al., 2013). Other precipitating factors include flickering lights, menstrual cycle, stimulant recreational drugs, and alcohol (Wassenaar, Kasteleijn-Nolst Trenite, de Haan, et al., 2014). Some individuals have pattern-sensitive or photosensitive epilepsy, that is, seizures precipitated by changes in dark/light patterns, such as those that occur with a flash on a camera, automobile headlights, reflections of light on snow or water, sunlight filtered through leafy trees, or rotating blades on a fan. Most of these individuals have absence, myoclonic, or generalized tonic-clonic seizures. A small minority of children have seizures while playing video games. Only these children need to be restricted from playing video games. (See Critical Thinking Case Study and Research Focus boxes.)

Family Support

Parental attitudes and management of a child with a seizure disorder vary. Whether the seizures result from illness, injury, or unknown cause, the parents may feel guilt, anxiety, and even humiliation. They want to know if the seizures will affect their child's ability to learn and develop. Many persons erroneously associate epilepsy with mental deficiency. Seizures commonly accompany other manifestations of severe brain damage from disease or injury, but children with seizures, like any population of healthy children, display a wide range of intelligence.

Parents also wonder how the illness will affect their child's future. The answer to this question depends on the cause of the seizures and other comorbid conditions. In many cases parents can be reassured

CRITICAL THINKING CASE STUDY

Seizures

Jane is a 14-year-old girl with focal epilepsy with focal seizures with impaired awareness. Her seizures have been well controlled for the past 6 years on monotherapy, with only an occasional breakthrough seizure every 3 or 4 months, often in association with a concurrent illness. Six months ago she entered high school. She is active with cheerleading and practices for 2 hours after school each day. In addition, she is taking honors English and math classes, both of which have daily homework. Jane typically does homework until midnight and gets up at 6 AM for school. For the past 3 months she has had an increasing number of seizures and is now having at least one seizure per week. She has not had any recent illnesses. Her physical and neurologic examination is normal.

1. What evidence should you consider regarding this condition?
2. What additional information is required at this time?
3. List the nursing intervention(s) that have the highest priority.
4. Identify important patient-centered outcomes with reference to your nursing interventions.

Answers are available at http://evolve.elsevier.com/wong/ncic.

RESEARCH FOCUS

Effect of Video Games on Seizures

Television and video games that produce either flashes or alternating patterns of lights have been known to be triggers for photosensitive seizures, especially among children ages 7 to 19 years who have an incidence of 5 per 100,000 (Harding & Harding, 2010). The majority of children (79%) have a tonic-clonic–type seizure, but 10% have an absence seizure, 6% have a myoclonic seizure, and 5% have a focal seizure (Harding & Harding, 2010). Prognosis is good for children who experience a photosensitive seizure but have no previous seizure activity.

that the illness will not shorten their child's life and that their child can attend school, marry, and have children. The child may need vocational guidance. Parents need to become familiar with the laws in their state regarding any limitations imposed on people with epilepsy. For children who are severely impaired, the family needs to become familiar with local early childhood programs. The nurse should emphasize that the seizures can be controlled or greatly reduced in the large majority of affected children.

Encourage a healthy attitude toward the child and the condition and help the parents feel competent in their ability to meet their responsibilities to their child. The child should be reared in the same manner as any normal child, with natural concern tempered by understanding of the need not to overprotect. Many parents refrain from correcting or punishing their child, especially if the child has had a seizure after being disciplined. The child must not be made to feel different in any way. Encourage parents to be honest and open about the disorder with their child and with others. Some parents try to conceal the nature of their child's illness because of their belief that the disorder is shameful or a disgrace to the family.

Educational materials and support groups may prove beneficial for families. The Epilepsy Foundation* is a national organization that works for the welfare of persons with epilepsy and their families; helps with

*8301 Professional Place, Landover, MD 20785; 800-332-1000; http://www.epilepsyfoundation.org/. In Canada: Epilepsy Canada, 2255B Queen St. E., Suite 336, Toronto, Ontario, Canada M4E 1G3; 877-734-0873; http://www.epilepsy.ca.

employment and legal problems; and provides education to patients, families, and communities.

The Child With Epilepsy

The child who is provided the security of a loving family, rewards and discipline no different from those of other children, and support in acquiring self-esteem is more likely to have a positive attitude toward the condition. Children derive their self-concept and self-esteem from observations of others' reactions to them and from their own perceptions of their capabilities. The suddenness and unpredictability of the seizures and the reactions of others further influence their feelings. When others consider children to be different, inferior, or objects of ridicule, the children come to view themselves in the same light.

Children with epilepsy need to learn about their condition and how medication contributes to their prolonged well-being. As they become more independent and spend more time away from home, children should begin to take responsibility for taking their own medication with supervision. Wearing or carrying medical identification with pertinent information about their condition is essential in case they have a seizure away from home and family. Planning activities with children and emphasizing those in which they can engage, rather than those from which they are restricted, will help them succeed and take pride in their achievements. They should be offered opportunities and encouraged to exercise judgment in their daily lives.

The adolescent period may prove to be a trying time for the child with epilepsy. Limits imposed on the young person's activities at a time when freedom and independence are desired may bring the disability into sharp focus. For example, all U.S. states have a defined seizure-free period before a driver's license can be obtained.

Epilepsy should not be a severe impairment to most youngsters. The nurse can help provide positive outcomes for the child and family by assuming the role of patient advocate, helping educate the public about the condition, working to make opportunities available to persons with the disorder, and lobbying for legislation that recognizes the needs of individuals with seizure disorders.

Febrile Seizures

A febrile seizure is a seizure associated with a febrile illness in the absence of a CNS infection. By definition, children who have a febrile seizure cannot have a history of afebrile seizures, must have a temperature of at least 38°C (100.4°F), and must be between the age of 6 and 60 months (Mikati & Hani, 2016). Febrile seizures are the most common type of seizure, affecting 2% to 4% of children (Weiss, Masur, Shinnar, et al., 2016).

There is evidence for both genetic and environmental causes of febrile seizures. Children with a family history of febrile seizures are at increased risk for both a single febrile seizure (10% to 46%) and for recurrent febrile seizures (Saghazadeh, Matrangelo, & Rezaei, 2014). In some families the predisposition to febrile seizures is inherited as an autosomal dominant trait. In most families, though, the predisposition involves multiple genes that have not yet been found (Mikati & Hani, 2016). Environmental factors include viral illness and age under 18 months old (Mewasingh, 2014).

> **! NURSING ALERT**
>
> If a febrile seizure lasts more than 5 minutes, parents should seek medical attention immediately. Instruct parents to call for emergency assistance (911) and not to place the child who is actively having a seizure in the car.

Most febrile seizures have stopped by the time the child is taken to a medical facility and require no treatment. There is no benefit of antiepileptic prophylaxis in these children; patients who were started on medication are exposed to several potential adverse side effects (Offringa, Newton, Cozijnsen, et al., 2017). Parents may be given a prescription to take home for a benzodiazepine for as-needed acute treatment of prolonged recurrent febrile seizures. If the child has recurrent febrile seizures that last more than 5 minutes, acute treatment with rectal diazepam, buccal lorazepam, or intranasal midazolam is recommended (Silverman, Sporer, Lemieux, et al., 2017). The child whose seizure does not stop within 10 minutes of administration of acute treatment will need treatment for febrile status epilepticus with IV administration of both short-acting and long-acting antiepileptic medications.

Antipyretic therapy during febrile illness offers symptomatic relief for fever-associated symptoms but appears to be ineffective in preventing seizures (Patel, Ram, Swiderska, et al., 2015). Parental education and emotional support are important interventions. Parents need reassurance regarding the benign nature of febrile seizures. Several large studies show no difference in intelligence, memory, behavior, or academic performance in children with febrile seizures compared with either population or sibling controls (Weiss, Masur, Shinnar, et al., 2016).

Parents need education on what to do during a seizure, that is, turn the child on his or her side, never put anything in the child's mouth, and time the seizure. Attempts to lower the temperature will not prevent a seizure. Tepid sponge baths are not recommended for several reasons: they are ineffective in significantly lowering the temperature, the shivering effect further increases metabolic output, and cooling causes discomfort to the child. Parental education and emotional support are important interventions, and information may need to be repeated, depending on the parents' anxiety and education level.

Long-term antiepileptic therapy is usually not required for children with simple febrile seizures. Children whose initial simple febrile seizure becomes febrile status epilepticus have an increased risk of subsequent febrile status epilepticus. Risk of recurrence of a simple febrile seizure is about 30% (Hesdorffer, Shinnar, Lax, et al., 2016). The risk of developing epilepsy after having simple febrile seizures is less than 3%, whereas the risk increases to 12% to 22% if the child has had prolonged febrile seizures and febrile status epilepticus. The risk of developing epilepsy for children with simple febrile seizures is increased if they have a family history of seizures (Seinfeld, Pellock, Kjeldsen, et al., 2016).

HEADACHE

Headaches are a common complaint of children. They can be either primary or secondary. Primary headaches are classified as migraine, tension-type headache, trigeminal autonomic cephalalgias, and other primary headache disorders by the International Headache Society (2018). A secondary headache is caused from another condition and should resolve once the underlying cause is treated. Headaches can be the result of a variety of conditions, including TBI, brain tumor, brain infections, cerebrovascular disorders, withdrawal from or exposure to substances, vision problems, hunger, psychiatric disorders, and medication overuse (Table 30.7).

ASSESSMENT

It is important to determine the pattern of the headache—acute, acute recurrent, chronic progressive, chronic nonprogressive (Langdon & DiSabella, 2017). Other assessment information includes the presence of seizures, ataxia, lethargy, weakness, nausea or vomiting, or any personality changes. Factors related to early development and past

TABLE 30.7 Characteristics of Headaches

Cause of Headache	Characteristics
Acute	
Acute sinusitis (may also be classified as inflammatory)	Usually accompanied by fever and tenderness over involved sinuses: *Ethmoid sinuses*—Referred pain to orbital and temporal areas *Frontal sinuses*—Periorbital pain
Ocular abnormalities	Headaches usually occurring late in day, precipitated by schoolwork, driving, or computer/television viewing
Dental disorders (may be classified as inflammatory)	Frontal or temporal headaches caused by malocclusion, caries, abscess, temporomandibular joint (TMJ) dysfunction TMJ headaches sometimes exacerbated by chewing or stress
Respiratory infections (pharyngitis, otitis media)	Pain localized to affected structures
Viral infections or febrile illnesses	Dull generalized pain
Inflammatory illness (meningitis, encephalitis)	Global headache usually accompanied by nuchal rigidity, fever, mental status changes
Trauma	Localized to area of trauma; related to nerve and tissue injury Postconcussion syndrome
Acute Recurrent	
Migraine (see migraine classification, Box 30.14)	Nausea, vomiting, fatigue, pallor Positive family history May be triggered by stress, fatigue, trauma, exercise, menses, medications, diet, sleep deprivation, environmental factors
Chronic Progressive	
Intracranial abnormalities	Symptoms of increased ICP
Tumors	Primarily early morning headaches
Hydrocephalus	Bulging fontanel, suture splitting in infants and young children, symptoms of increased ICP
Subdural hematoma	Usually results from trauma Seizures and focal neurologic deficits more common than headaches
Brain abscess	Rare but may be associated with chronic otitis media or sinusitis, cyanotic heart disease, and immunosuppression
Pseudotumor cerebri	Increased ICP without obstruction of CSF
Chronic Nonprogressive	
Tension type	Common in children Adjustment reaction, anxiety related
Psychiatric	Conversion reaction (anxiety converted to somatic symptoms)

CSF, Cerebrospinal fluid; *ICP,* intracranial pressure.
Modified from Browne, T. R., & Holmes, G. L. (2004). *Handbook of epilepsy.* Philadelphia, PA: Lippincott Williams & Wilkins.

BOX 30.13 Questions for Evaluating Headaches

1. Do you have more than one type of headache?
2. How did the headache begin? Trauma? Infection?
3. How long has it been present?
4. Are the symptoms getting worse or staying the same?
5. How often do they occur?
6. How long do they last?
7. Do they occur at any special time or when certain things happen?
8. Do you have warning signs?
9. Where does it hurt?
10. How does the pain feel? Pounding? Sharp?
11. Do you feel sick in other ways during the headache? Abdominal pain? Nausea, vomiting?
12. Do you stop what you are doing during the headache?
13. Do you have any other health problems?
14. Are you taking any medicines regularly?
15. Are there some things you do that make the headache worse or better?
16. Does anyone medicine make the headache better?
17. Does anyone else in your family have headaches?
18. What do you think is causing your headaches?

Modified from Rothner, A. D. (1993). Management of headaches in children and adolescents. *Journal of Pain and Symptom Management, 8*(2), 81-86.

illnesses and a family history of headaches may also be pertinent. A "headache diary," which includes time of onset and termination of headaches, intensity, associated events, and actions taken and their effects, can be helpful for the patient and provider.

Clues to etiology may be found in the family history, including information about the home or social situation (e.g., divorce, separation, alcoholism, school avoidance). Box 30.13 lists specific questions that often elicit needed information. Thorough physical and neurologic examinations are performed. An abnormal neurologic examination or unusual neurologic symptoms indicate the need for further diagnostic tests (e.g., CT, MRI, or EEG) (Hershey, Kabbouche, & O'Brien, 2016).

! NURSING ALERT

During the health history and neurologic assessment, the following abnormal signs require immediate follow-up for children:

- The headache progresses in frequency and severity over a brief period (2 to 3 weeks).
- It awakens the child from sleep (may also be migraine).
- It occurs in early morning.
- It is worse on arising.
- It is characterized by persistent, occipital, or frontal pain.
- It is accompanied by unexplained vomiting.
- It is associated with a change in gait, personality, or behavior.
- It is exacerbated by Valsalva maneuver (intensified by lowering head and straining, such as during a bowel movement, coughing, or sneezing).

Tension-type headaches are common in children. They are typically frontal, the pain is described as a pressing or tightness and nonthrobbing in character, and they are not typically accompanied by nausea or vomiting.

Management of tension-type headaches begins with headache hygiene or prevention (Gofshteyn & Stephenson, 2016). This includes adequate sleep, appropriate hydration, and regular meals and exercise. If headaches continue after the child is following a headache hygiene plan, ibuprofen is usually the most effective pharmacologic intervention. To prevent medication overuse headache, children with headaches should take no more than three doses of these medications per week (Kacperski, Kabbouche, O'Brien, et al., 2016). Biofeedback, cognitive-behavioral therapy, and relaxation techniques may be useful nonpharmacologic interventions in children with recurrent tension-type headaches (Langdon & DiSabella, 2017).

MIGRAINE HEADACHE

Migraine is in the top five common childhood diseases. Migraines can have their onset in very young children, including infants where they may manifest as colic. The onset tends to be earlier in boys than girls until puberty when girls have a twofold increase over boys in migraines. This is thought to be due to the effects of estrogen (Langdon & DiSabella, 2017).

The exact pathophysiology of migraines is not completely known. Genetics, neurotransmitters, and neurophysiologic mechanisms appear to be involved in varying degrees (Puledda, Messina, & Goadsby, 2017). Familial hemiplegic migraine has an identified autosomal dominant genetic cause. A number of other genes have been identified in diseases that that are often accompanied by migraine (Sutherland & Griffiths, 2017). Previously, it was thought that migraine headaches were caused by dilation of cerebral blood vessels; however, this is no longer thought to be correct. There is much attention on the specific vulnerability factors of the individual that leads to neuron dysfunction and the generation of the acute attack.

Revisions in the classification of migraine headaches introduced some new terms and eliminated, renamed, or reclassified others. Migraine headaches are now classified as migraine without aura and migraine with aura; the latter category includes the following subtypes: auras and prodrome, familial hemiplegic migraine, sporadic hemiplegic migraine, and basilar-type migraine (Box 30.14) (International Headache Society, 2018).

Migraines are paroxysmal. The symptoms vary depending on age. Typical symptoms include nausea, vomiting, and abdominal pain, which are relieved by sleep. Toddlers may be seen with episodic pallor, decreased activity, and vomiting. In children the onset may be bifrontal, temporal, and bilateral or unilateral. As children and adolescents advance in age, many will develop phonophobia and/or photophobia. Compared with adults, migraine headaches in children are generally shorter in duration. If the child falls asleep during the headache, the amount of time the child is asleep is counted as part of the duration (Hershey, Kabbouche, & O'Brien, 2016). A family history of migraine is elicited in up to 90% of children with migraine; 28% of all children who have migraines experience a headache before age 15 years (Hershey, Kabbouche, & O'Brien, 2016).

Like tension-type headaches, migraine management begins with headache hygiene. Keeping a headache diary can help with identifying triggers so they can be avoided. If these measures fail to prevent migraines, both abortive and prophylactic treatment may be needed. At the onset of the headache, the child should rest or sleep in a quiet, dark room when feasible. Migraine therapy, if administered early in the course of the headache, may provide rapid relief. Ibuprofen appears to be the safest and most effective treatment if given early (Patniyot & Gelfand, 2016). Prophylactic mediation can be considered if a child is having a migraine or more per week. Riboflavin and magnesium have helped some children (Merison & Jacobs, 2016). Topiramate, an antiepileptic drug, has been approved by the Food and Drug Administration for use in children to prevent migraine (Kacperski, Kabbouche, O'Brien, et al., 2016).

BOX 30.14 Migraine Patterns

Migraine With Aura

Aura may be visual (most common); hemiparetic (tingling and numbness of lips, lower face; second most common); hemiparetic; hemiplegic; or aphasic

Aura duration less than 1 hour and completely resolves. Followed by throbbing, unilateral or bilateral headache coupled with nausea, vomiting, photophobia, and phonophobia.

Migraine Without Aura

Prodrome that consists of pallor, alteration in personality, or change in appetite or thirst

Unilateral or bilateral headache coupled with nausea and/or vomiting, photophobia, and phonophobia

Pulsating quality

Moderate or severe pain intensity

Sporadic Hemiplegic Migraine

Migraine with aura

Motor weakness

No first- or second-degree relative who also has migraine with aura and motor weakness

Basilar-Type Migraine

Recurrent attacks

Headache typically occipital

Symptoms may include dysarthria, vertigo, diplopia, vomiting, and altered consciousness

DRUG ALERT

Triptans

Triptans are serotonin agonists and are effective in the abortive treatment of migraines. Almotriptan, zolmitriptan, and sumatriptan are Food and Drug Administration approved for use in children ages 12 to 17, and rizatriptan is approved for children ages 6 and older (Patniyot & Gelfand, 2016).

The outlook for a child with migraine is good, but the child and parents should be informed that predisposition to the headaches may be lifelong. Severe headaches can adversely affect the child's routine activities of daily living, including family relations and school. Many children and families will benefit from psychotherapy.

THE CHILD WITH CEREBRAL MALFORMATION

HYDROCEPHALUS

Hydrocephalus is a condition caused by an imbalance in the production and absorption of CSF in the ventricular system. The causes of hydrocephalus are varied and include either congenital (e.g., myelomeningocele, intrauterine viral infection [cytomegalovirus, toxoplasmosis], aqueduct stenosis) or acquired conditions such as intraventricular hemorrhage, tumor, CSF infection, or head injury. The result is either (1) impaired absorption of CSF fluid within the subarachnoid space, obliteration of the subarachnoid cisterns, or malfunction of the arachnoid villi (nonobstructive or communicating hydrocephalus) or (2) obstruction to the flow of CSF through the ventricular system (obstructive or noncommunicating hydrocephalus) (Kinsman & Johnston, 2016).

Any imbalance of secretion and absorption causes an increased accumulation of CSF in the ventricles, which become dilated (ventriculomegaly) and compress the brain tissue against the surrounding rigid

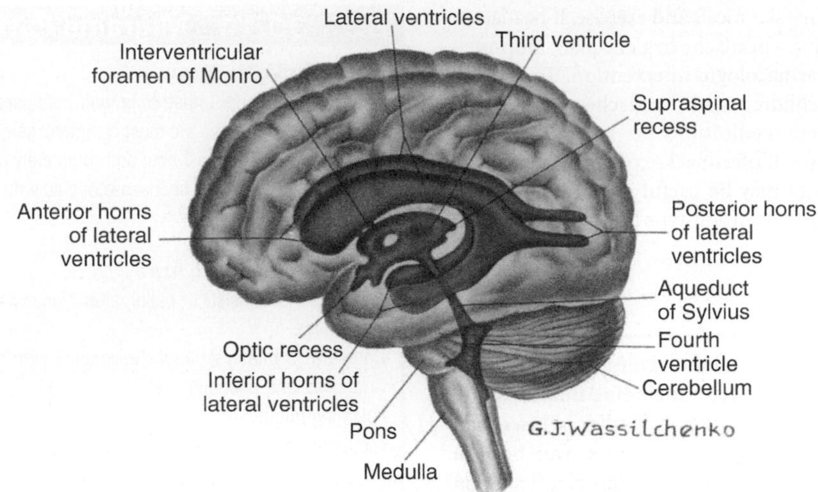

FIG. 30.11 Cerebral ventricular system. (From Thompson, J. M., McFarland, G., Hirsch, J. E., et al. [2002]. *Mosby's clinical nursing* [5th ed.]. St. Louis, MO: Mosby.)

bony cranium. When this occurs before fusion of the cranial sutures, it causes enlargement of the skull and dilation of the ventricles. In children younger than 12 years old, previously closed sutures, especially the sagittal suture, may become diastatic or opened. After 12 years old, the sutures are fused and will not open.

Pathophysiology

To appreciate the condition, an understanding of the dynamics of CSF and the relationship between the various structures that make up the ventricular and subarachnoid spaces is necessary (Fig. 30.11). The two mechanisms by which CSF is formed are secretion by the choroid plexuses and lymphatic-like drainage by the extracellular fluid of the brain. CSF circulates throughout the ventricular system and is then absorbed within the subarachnoid spaces by a mechanism that is not entirely clear.

Ventricular Circulation

The fluid flows from the lateral ventricles through the foramen of Monro to the third ventricle, where it combines with fluid secreted into the third ventricle. From there CSF flows through the aqueduct of Sylvius into the fourth ventricle, where more fluid is formed; it then leaves the fourth ventricle by way of the lateral foramen of Luschka and the midline foramen of Magendie and flows into the cisterna magna. From the cisterna magna, CSF flows to the cerebral and cerebellar subarachnoid spaces where it is absorbed. A large portion is absorbed through the arachnoid villi, but the sinuses, veins, brain substance, and dura also participate in absorption.

The terms *communicating* and *noncommunicating hydrocephalus* traditionally referred to obstructive and nonobstructive types of hydrocephalus. Because other diagnostic methods are now used, the terms may be used only as a reference point in the diagnosis. Hydrocephalus can also be classified according to the cause as either congenital or acquired hydrocephalus.

Etiology

Rarely, a tumor of the choroid plexus causes increased CSF secretion. Most cases of hydrocephalus are a result of developmental malformations. Although the defect usually is apparent in early infancy, it may become evident at any time from the prenatal period to late childhood or early adulthood. Other causes include neoplasms, CNS infections (e.g., meningitis, encephalitis), and trauma (e.g., shaken baby syndrome). An obstruction to the normal flow can occur at any point in the CSF pathway to produce increased pressure and dilation of the pathways proximal to the site of obstruction. Table 30.8 describes the most frequent sites of obstruction and the consequences.

Developmental defects (e.g., Chiari malformation [see following discussion], aqueductal stenosis, aqueductal gliosis, and atresia of the foramina of Luschka and Magendie [Dandy-Walker malformation]) account for most cases of hydrocephalus from birth to 2 years of age. Dandy-Walker malformation involves dilation of the fourth ventricle, partial or complete absence of the cerebellar vermis, and enlargement of the posterior fossa resulting in hydrocephalus in about 80% of children with Dandy-Walker (Shankar, Zamora, & Castillo, 2016).

Hydrocephalus is so often associated with myelomeningocele that all such infants should be observed for its development. In the remainder of cases there is a history of intrauterine infection (e.g., toxoplasmosis, cytomegalovirus), hemorrhage (e.g., posthemorrhagic hydrocephalus in preterm infants), and neonatal meningoencephalitis (bacterial or viral). In older children hydrocephalus is most often a result of intracranial masses (e.g., vascular anomalies, cysts, and tumors), preexisting developmental defects, intracranial infections, trauma, or hemorrhage.

Chiari I and II Malformations

Chiari malformations are structural defects in the base of the skull and cerebellum. They occur when the lower cerebellum extends below the foramen magnum and into the upper spinal canal (Chiari I) or when the lower cerebellum and brain stem protrude into the spinal canal through an enlarged foramen magnum (Chiari II). Chiari I malformation does not usually cause hydrocephalus. It is usually asymptomatic until adolescence when it can cause headaches, neck pain, frequent urination, and lower limb progressive spasticity (Kinsman & Johnston, 2016). Type II Chiari malformation is seen almost exclusively with myelomeningocele, and results in obstruction of CSF flow causing the hydrocephalus.

Clinical Manifestations

The three factors that influence the clinical picture in hydrocephalus are the acuity of onset, timing of onset, and associated structural malformations. In infancy, before closure of the cranial sutures, head enlargement (increasing occipitofrontal circumference [OFC]) is the predominant sign. The signs and symptoms in early to late childhood are caused by increased ICP. Specific manifestations are related to the location of the lesion.

TABLE 30.8 **Sites and Types of Hydrocephalus**

Site	Type	Causes and Comments
Aqueduct of Sylvius—Accounts for 33% of hydrocephalus	Stenosis or atresia	Congenital (X-linked recessive in small number) Insidious onset of symptoms from birth to adulthood
	Gliosis	Postinflammatory, usually secondary to perinatal infection or hemorrhage Prenatal maternal infection (toxoplasmosis)
	Obstructive	Tumors of third ventricle or midbrain Ependymitis from maternal toxoplasmosis Congenital aneurysm of Galen vein
	Posthemorrhagic	Blood from intraventricular hemorrhage in germinal matrix; most common type of hydrocephalus in preterm infants
Fourth ventricle or subarachnoid pathway—Intraventricular hemorrhage, postinflammatory conditions, or tumors	Posthemorrhagic	Blood from intraventricular hemorrhage in germinal matrix; most common type of hydrocephalus in preterm infants
Fourth ventricle and foramen magnum—Accounts for 50% of all hydrocephalus	Type I Chiari malformation	Neural tube defect with herniation of medulla through foramen magnum; may be asymptomatic in childhood; similar to type II but milder
	Type II Chiari malformation	More severe defect; downward displacement of brainstem, fourth ventricle, and lower parts of cerebellum through foramen magnum with fixed attachment of spinal cord at site of myelomeningocele
	Type III Chiari malformation (absence or occlusion of ventricles)	High cervical or occipitocervical myelomeningocele with cervical herniation through body defect Congenital (Dandy-Walker syndrome) caused by obstruction of foramina of Luschka and Magendie Tumors of posterior fossa (e.g., medulloblastoma) causing pressure on surrounding tissues to produce obstruction Less often—Subdural hematoma, bacterial or granulomatous meningitis
Arachnoid villi and cisterna magna—Obstruction by thick arachnoid membrane or meninges	Meningitis	Bacterial or granulomatous Acute phase—Clumping of purulent fluid in drainage channels Chronic phase—Organization of blood and exudate that results in fibrosis of subarachnoid spaces
	Prenatal maternal infections • Meningeal malignancy • Arachnoid cyst • Tuberculosis, fungal or parasitic infection	Toxoplasmosis, cytomegalic inclusion disease, mumps Secondary to leukemia or lymphoma Located in basal cistern or (uncommon) over cerebral cortex More common in children ages 2 to 10 years old

Infancy

In infants with hydrocephalus, the head grows at an abnormal rate, although the first signs may be bulging fontanels with or without head enlargement (Fig. 30.12). The anterior fontanel is tense, often bulging, and nonpulsatile. Scalp veins are dilated, especially when the infant cries. With the increase in intracranial volume, the bones of the skull become thin and the sutures become palpably separated to produce the cracked-pot sound (**Macewen sign**) on percussion of the skull. In severe cases there may be frontal protrusion, or **frontal bossing**, with depressed eyes, and the eyes may be rotated downward, producing a **setting-sun sign**, in which the sclera may be visible above the iris. Pupils are sluggish, with unequal response to light.

The infant is irritable and lethargic, feeds poorly, and may display changes in level of consciousness, opisthotonos (often extreme), and lower extremity spasticity. The infant cries when picked up or rocked and quiets when allowed to lie still. Early infantile reflexes may persist, and normally expected responses may not appear, indicating failure in the development of normal cortical inhibition.

Infants with Chiari malformations may exhibit behaviors that reflect cranial nerve dysfunction as a result of brainstem compression, including swallowing difficulties, stridor, apnea, aspiration, respiratory difficulties, and arm weakness.

The preterm infant with posthemorrhagic hydrocephalus may not exhibit any clinical signs and symptoms other than a gradual increase in head circumference. Alternatively, the nurse may note subtle seizure activity and alternating levels of consciousness. Ventricular size can be assessed by ultrasonography or CT scanning in preterm infants at high risk for intraventricular hemorrhage.

If hydrocephalus is allowed to progress, development of lower brainstem functions is disrupted, as manifested by difficulty in sucking and feeding and a shrill, brief, high-pitched cry. Eventually the skull becomes enlarged, and the cortex is destroyed. If the hydrocephalus is rapidly progressive, symptoms may include emesis, somnolence, seizures, and cardiopulmonary distress.

Childhood

The signs and symptoms in early to late childhood are caused by increased ICP, and specific manifestations are related to the location of the focal lesion. Most commonly resulting from posterior fossa neoplasms and aqueduct stenosis, the clinical manifestations are primarily those associated with space-occupying lesions (i.e., headache on awakening with improvement after emesis, papilledema, strabismus, and extrapyramidal tract signs such as ataxia. As with infants, the child is irritable, lethargic, apathetic, confused, and often incoherent. In one of the congenital

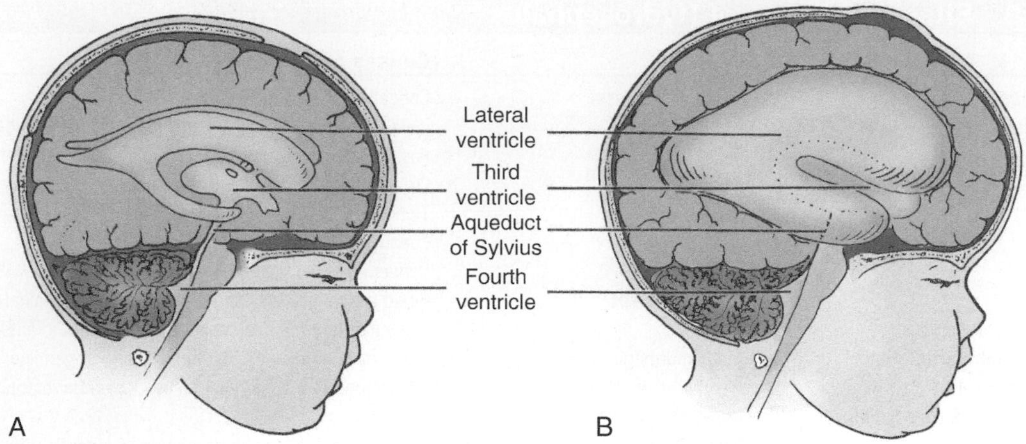

FIG. 30.12 Hydrocephalus: a block in flow of cerebrospinal fluid. **A,** Patent cerebrospinal fluid circulation. **B,** Enlarged lateral and third ventricles caused by obstruction of circulation—stenosis of aqueduct of Sylvius.

defects with later onset (by age 3 months), the Dandy-Walker syndrome, characteristic manifestations are a bulging occiput, nystagmus, ataxia, and cranial nerve palsies.

Manifestations of Chiari malformation in children over 3 years of age are related to spinal cord dysfunction rather than brainstem compression as observed in infants. Scoliosis proximal to the level of the myelomeningocele (usually associated with Chiari malformation) and development of upper extremity spasticity, which may progress to weakness and atrophy, are common. Cranial nerve deficits are rare.

Diagnostic Evaluation

Antenatal diagnosis of fetal ventriculomegaly, which is associated with postnatal hydrocephalus, is possible with fetal ultrasonography as early as 14 to 15 weeks of gestation, often followed by fetal MRI (Pisapia, Sinha, Zarnow, et al., 2017). There are ongoing trials in carefully selected pregnant women of fetal surgery for prevention of in utero brain damage from in utero hydrocephalus. Initial results were not promising, but recently outcomes have improved (Elbabaa, Gildehaus, Pierson, et al., 2017). Delivery is not currently recommended until fetal lung maturity has been achieved.

In infancy the diagnosis of hydrocephalus is based on head circumference that crosses one or more percentile lines on the head measurement chart within a period of 2 to 4 weeks and on associated neurologic signs that are progressive. However, other diagnostic studies are needed to localize the site of CSF obstruction. Routine daily head circumference measurements are carried out in infants with myelomeningocele, hemorrhage, or intrauterine viral or CNS infections. In evaluation of a preterm infant, specially adapted head circumference charts are consulted to distinguish abnormal head growth from rapid but normal head growth.

The primary diagnostic tools for detecting hydrocephalus in older infants and children are CT and MRI (Fig. 30.13). Mild sedation or general anesthesia is usually required for children under age 8 or with neurodevelopmental disabilities because the child must remain absolutely still for an accurate study. Diagnostic evaluation of children who have symptoms of hydrocephalus after infancy is similar to that employed in those with a suspected intracranial tumor. In the neonate, echoencephalography is useful in comparing the ratio of lateral ventricle to cortex.

Problems in differential diagnosis are related to the child whose head circumference is greater than the 95th percentile but whose head growth parallels the normal growth curve. It is sometimes valuable to measure the parental OFC to detect a possible normal familial characteristic (benign familial megalencephaly). (See Table 30.2 for diagnostic tests for neurologic evaluation.)

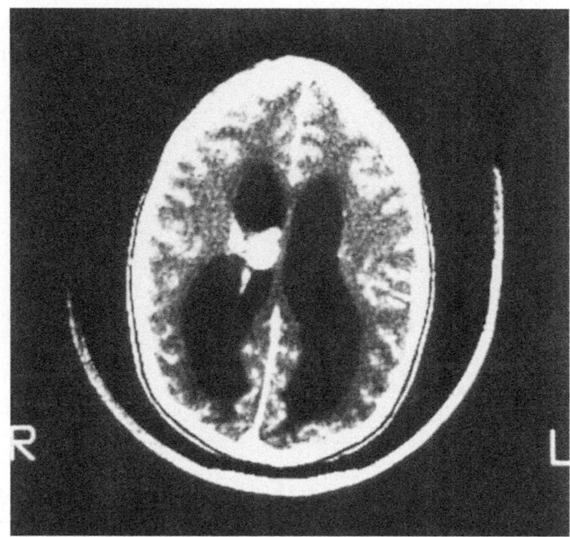

FIG. 30.13 Computed tomography scan reveals enlarged ventricles of child with hydrocephalus.

Therapeutic Management

The treatment of hydrocephalus is directed toward relief of ventricular pressure, treatment of the cause of the ventriculomegaly, treatment of associated complications, and management of problems related to the effect of the disorder on psychomotor development. The treatment is, with few exceptions, surgical.

Surgical Treatment

Improved neurosurgical techniques have established surgical treatment as the therapy of choice in almost all cases of hydrocephalus. This is accomplished by direct removal of an obstruction, such as resection of a neoplasm, cyst, or hematoma, or, in rare instances of fluid overproduction, by choroid plexus extirpation (plexectomy or electric coagulation). However, most children require a shunt procedure that provides primary drainage of the CSF from the ventricles to an extracranial compartment, usually the peritoneum.

Most shunt systems consist of a ventricular catheter, a flush pump, a unidirectional flow valve, and a distal catheter. All are radiopaque for easy visualization after placement, and all are tested for accuracy before insertion. A reservoir is frequently added to allow direct access to the ventricular system for administration of medications and removal of fluid. In all models the valves are designed to open at a predetermined intraventricular pressure and close when the pressure falls below that level, thus preventing backflow of fluid. Most shunts now in use have differential pressure and adjustable programmable valves with capability for changing the pressures with an external magnet, thus avoiding additional surgery.

! NURSING ALERT

Tablet computers, such as iPads, and magnetic toys may interfere with magnetically programmable shunt valve settings. They should be kept at least 2.5 cm from the shunt's valve (Strahle, Selzer, Muraszko, et al., 2012)

The standard procedure for many years has been the **ventriculoperitoneal (VP) shunt**, especially in neonates and young infants (Fig. 30.14). There is greater allowance for excess tubing, which minimizes the number of revisions needed as the child grows. Because it requires repeated lengthening, the ventriculoatrial (VA) shunt (ventricle to right atrium) is reserved for older children who have attained most of their somatic growth and children with abdominal pathologic conditions. The VA shunt is contraindicated in children with cardiopulmonary disease or elevated CSF protein.

The initial shunt is placed when indicated on the basis of individual assessment. The timing of revisions varies widely. In most instances revisions are performed when physical signs indicate shunt malfunction (i.e., signs of elevated ICP). Sometimes revisions are planned for specific times during development. The initial success rate is relatively high. However, shunts are associated with complications that interfere with continued shunt function or that threaten the child's life.

Endoscopic third ventriculostomy (ETV) is a procedure that has potential for allowing greater independence from VA or VP shunting in children with obstructive hydrocephalus. ETV involves creating a small opening in the floor of the third ventricle, allowing CSF to flow freely through the previously blocked ventricle. Studies to date have not demonstrated improved short-term outcomes with ETV compared with VP shunting (Kulkarni, Sgouros, Constantini, et al., 2016). Long-term outcomes need to be studied. VP shunts have a risk of infection and shunt failure whereas ETV does not; however, for the foreseeable future placement of a VP shunt for treatment of hydrocephalus remains a frequent neurosurgical procedure (Venable, Rossi, Morgan Jones, et al., 2016).

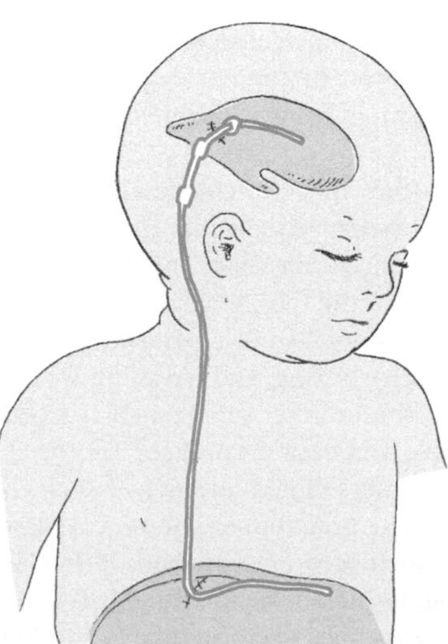

FIG. 30.14 Ventriculoperitoneal shunt. Catheter is threaded beneath skin.

Complications

The major complications of VP shunts are infection and malfunction. All shunts are subject to mechanical difficulties, such as kinking, plugging, or separation and migration of tubing. Malfunction is most often caused by mechanical obstruction either within the ventricles from particulate matter (tissue or exudate) or at the distal end from thrombosis or displacement as a result of growth. Functional obstruction of a shunt's antisiphon device remains a common complication. About 22% of shunt failures are reported within the first 90 days, the majority of these within the first month (Venable, Rossi, Morgan Jones, et al., 2016). The child with a shunt obstruction often is seen in an emergency visit with clinical manifestations of increased ICP, such as nausea, vomiting, irritability, and a bulging fontanel, that is frequently accompanied by worsening neurologic status.

One of the most common and serious complications, shunt infection, can occur at any time, but the period of greatest risk is within the first month after placement (Månsson, Johansson, Ziebell, et al., 2017). Within 2 years shunt infection rates are reported to be approximately 5% to 10% (Månsson, Johansson, Ziebell, et al., 2017). Infections include sepsis, bacterial endocarditis, wound infection, shunt nephritis, meningitis, and ventriculitis and may be a result of intercurrent infections at the time of shunt placement. Brain abscess associated with colonic perforation and infection with a gram-negative enteric organism suggests an ascending shunt infection in a child who has a VP shunt. Meningitis and ventriculitis are of greatest concern because any complicating CNS infection is a significant predictor of future intellectual disability. Infection is treated with antibiotics administered intravenously or intrathecally for a minimum of 7 to 10 days. The use of perioperative antibiotic prophylaxis or antibiotic-impregnated shunts has significantly decreased shunt infection rates, particularly acute infections, among all age ranges of patients and all types of shunts (Månsson, Johansson, Ziebell, et al., 2017). In addition measures to reduce the number of people in the operating room and strictly enforced hand washing can help. A persistent infection may require removal of the shunt until the infection is controlled, and an EVD, or external ventriculostomy, is used until CSF is sterile. EVD allows removal of CSF from a tube placed in the child's ventricle that flows by gravity into a collection device.

The primary reasons for inserting an EVD include unstable status, increased ICP that is difficult to stabilize, or infection from an existing VP shunt. The EVD may drain CSF intermittently or continuously according to need. The EVD is a closed system made up of transparent pliable tubing that should be labeled, a collection bag, and, at times, a drip chamber between the tubing and the collection bag. The EVD is placed at the level of the child's external auditory meatus with the head at a 20- to 30-degree elevation, depending on physician preference. Elevating the EVD above this level decreases the flow of CSF, and placing the device below the level of the external meatus increases the flow. Ambulation or sitting up in bed or a chair usually requires that the tubing be clamped to prevent imbalance in CSF drainage. In addition, the EVD is a closed sterile system. Aseptic technique should be used during any manipulation or maintenance of the EVD system, such as in relation to emptying the device or changing the scalp dressing (Hepburn-Smith, Dynkevich, Spektor, et al., 2016). Accurate and frequent documentation of the incision site; amount, color, and consistency of drainage into the device; and the child's vital and neurologic signs are an important part of the nursing care.

Another serious shunt-related complication is subdural hematoma caused by too-rapid reduction of ICP and, in some cases, tentorial herniation as a result of imbalance in CSF drainage. These complications can be averted by careful assessment of ICP before insertion of the shunt and use of correct valvular pressure. Other complications that may occur include peritonitis, abdominal abscesses, perforation of abdominal organs by catheter or trocar (at the time of insertion), fistulas, hernias, and ileus. Some children require shunt lengthening as body growth occurs. This procedure usually involves replacing the distal catheter below the valve.

Prognosis

The prognosis of children with treated hydrocephalus depends largely on the cause of the dilated ventricles before shunt placement and the amount of irreversible brain damage before shunting (Kinsman & Johnston, 2016). Those children with isolated aqueductal stenosis usually function cognitively like their typically developing peers (Kahle, Kulkarnia, Limbrick, et al., 2016). The neurologic disorders seen in children after shunting for hydrocephalus are most often due to the underlying cause of the hydrocephalus rather than the hydrocephalus itself (Paulsen, Lundar, & Lindegaard, 2015).

Survivors have a high incidence of intellectual disability and learning disorders, including challenges with memory, processing, and visual-spatial skills requiring special education services. Tumors, meningitis, and intraventricular hemorrhage are the conditions most closely associated with hydrocephalus accompanied by intellectual disability (Paulsen, Lundar, & Lindegaard, 2015). Children with myelomeningocele or intraventricular hemorrhage often have motor disabilities. As with all pediatric neurologic conditions, social and behavior problems are common, including attention-deficit/hyperactivity disorder. Up to a third of children with hydrocephalus will have epilepsy (Kahle, Kulkarnia, Limbrick, et al., 2016).

Surgically treated hydrocephalus in patients with little or no evidence of irreversible brain damage has a survival rate of about 80%, with most deaths occurring within the first year of treatment (Paulsen, Lundar, & Lindegaard, 2015). Those with poor outcomes included children shunted for posthemorrhagic hydrocephalus or meningitis. Most children who require shunting must depend on the shunt for the remainder of their life.

Nursing Care Management

The infant with suspected or confirmed hydrocephalus is observed carefully for signs of increasing ventricular size and increasing ICP. In infants the head is measured daily at the point of largest measurement—the OFC. (See Chapter 4 for technique.) To avoid the likelihood of wide discrepancies, the point at which the measurements are taken is indicated on the head with a marking pen. Fontanels and suture lines are palpated for size, signs of bulging, tenseness, and separation. Irritability, lethargy, seizure activity, and altered vital signs and feeding behavior may indicate an advancing pathologic condition.

In older children, who are usually admitted to the hospital for elective or emergency shunt revision, the most valuable indicators of increasing ICP are an alteration in the child's level of consciousness, complaint of headache, and changes in interaction with the environment. Changes are identified by observing and comparing present behavior with customary behavior, sleep patterns, developmental capabilities, and habits obtained through a detailed history and a baseline assessment. This baseline information serves as a guide for postoperative assessment and evaluation of shunt function.

The nurse is responsible for preparing the child for diagnostic tests such as MRI or a CT scan and for assisting with procedures such as a ventricular tap, which is often performed to relieve excessive pressure and to obtain CSF during the preoperative period. Sedation is required because the child must remain absolutely still during diagnostic testing. A variety of drugs are available for sedation. (See Chapter 22 for preparing children for procedures.) If surgery is anticipated, IV infusions should not be placed in a scalp vein.

Postoperative Care

In addition to routine postoperative care and observation, the infant or child is positioned carefully on the unoperated side to prevent pressure on the shunt valve. The child remains flat to help avert complications resulting from too-rapid reduction of intracranial fluid. The surgeon indicates the position to be maintained and the extent of activity allowed.

The nurse continues observation for signs of increased ICP that indicate obstruction of the shunt. Neurologic assessment includes pupil dilation (pressure causes compression or stretching of the oculomotor nerve, producing dilation on the same side as the pressure) and blood pressure (hypoxia to the brainstem causes variability in these vital signs). The nurse also observes for abdominal distention and constipation because CSF may cause peritonitis or a postoperative ileus as a complication of distal catheter placement.

Because infection is the greatest hazard of the postoperative period, nurses are continually on the alert for the usual manifestations of CSF infection, including elevated temperature, poor feeding, vomiting, decreased responsiveness, and seizure activity. There may be signs of local inflammation at the operative sites and along the shunt tract. Antibiotics are administered by the IV route as ordered, and the nurse may need to assist with intraventricular instillation. Inspect the incision site for leakage, and test any suspected drainage for glucose, an indication of CSF.

Family Support

Specific needs and concerns of parents during periods of hospitalization are related to the reason for the child's hospitalization (e.g., shunt revision, infection, diagnosis) and the diagnostic and surgical procedures to which the child must be subjected. Parents may have little understanding of anatomy; therefore they need further explanation and reinforcement of information that was given to them by the physician, neurosurgeon, and nurse practitioners, including information about what to expect. They are especially frightened of any procedure that involves the brain. The fear of disability or brain damage is real and pervasive. Nurses can calm their anxiety with explanations of the rationale underlying the various nursing and medical activities such as positioning or testing and by simply being available and willing to listen to their concerns.

To prepare for the child's discharge and home care, instruct the parents on how to recognize signs that indicate shunt malfunction or infection. Active children may have injuries, such as a fall, that can damage the shunt, and the tubing may pull out of the distal insertion site or become disconnected during normal growth. Contact sports such as football, rugby, boxing, and wrestling are usually prohibited if a person has a VP shunt; other sports such as swimming, soccer, and track are acceptable and even encouraged for the child's physical and emotional health. Families should consult with their child's neurosurgeon or neurosurgery nurse practitioner about activities after discharge as providers vary in their recommendations. Helmets must be worn for skating, skiing, biking, and skateboarding. It is also important for the nurse to encourage families to enroll infants and toddlers with hydrocephalus into an early childhood development program to monitor their development and quickly address any signs that they are not keeping up with their typically developing peers.

The management of hydrocephalus in a child is a demanding task for both the family and health professionals. Helping the family cope with the child's difficulties is an important nursing responsibility. Children with hydrocephalus have lifelong special health care needs. The nurse can provide optimum primary health care, including teaching families hand hygiene and hand washing, advice on immunizations, treatments for common infectious conditions, or child care and school precautions. The overall aim is to establish realistic goals and an appropriate educational program that will assist the child in achieving the maximum potential. Families can be referred to community agencies for support and guidance. The National Hydrocephalus Foundation* and the Hydrocephalus Association† in the United States and the Spina Bifida and Hydrocephalus Association of Canada‡ provide information on the condition for families; the National Hydrocephalus Foundation also assists interested groups in establishing local organizations.

Anticipatory guidance will prepare parents for possible problems and help them avoid being overprotective of the child. Few restrictions need be placed on the child's activities (mainly contact sports), and the child is encouraged to live as would any other youngster of the same age and abilities. Parents need support and encouragement in coping with the child and problems the child may encounter in relationships with peers and others. Reactions of other children when the child has a noticeably enlarged head or requires special restrictions are stressful for both the child and the parents. (See Chapter 19 for problems and coping with a child with a disability.)

*12413 Centralia Road, Lakewood, CA 90715-1653; 888-857-3434; http://www.nhfonline.org.

†4340 Eat West Highway, Suite 905, Bethesda, MD 20814; 888-598-3789; http://www.hydroassoc.org.

‡Suite 647-167 av. Lombard Avenue, Winnipeg MB, Canada R3B 0V3; 800-565-9488; http://www.sbhac.ca.

NCLEX REVIEW QUESTIONS

1. You are the nurse assigned to care for a child with a basilar skull fracture. Your most important nursing observation is change in level of consciousness. You will be highly alert for:
   A. Alterations in vital signs that often appear before alterations in consciousness or focal neurologic signs
   B. Bleeding from the ear, which is indicative of an anterior basal skull fracture
   C. Seizures that are relatively uncommon in children at the time of head injury
   D. Changes in posturing, such as any signs of extension or flexion posturing, unusual response to stimuli, and random versus purposeful movement
2. As the nurse assigned to a child diagnosed with bacterial meningitis, you know that:
   A. The child will not need to be placed in isolation because antibiotics have been started
   B. Enteric precautions will remain in place for up to 48 hours
   C. Respiratory isolation will remain in place for 24 hours after antibiotics are started
   D. Due to headache, the child will want the head of the bed elevated with two pillows
3. You are working with a pediatric nurse who has just transferred to the pediatric clinic. You are role-playing phone triage related to a child with a head injury. You ascertain that the nurse needs more teaching based on what response?
   A. "After initial physical examination, if there was no loss of consciousness with the head injury, the child can be observed at home."
   B. "If there is a language barrier, written instructions can be given, followed by discharge."
   C. "Another physical examination should take place in 1 or 2 days."
   D. "Parents should call the doctor if their child has any of these signs: blurred vision, walking unsteadily, or is hard to awaken."
4. You are caring for a child with hydrocephalus who is postoperative from a shunt revision. Which assessment finding is your priority for increased intercranial pressure?
   A. Nausea and refusal to eat postoperatively
   B. Complaint of a headache
   C. Irritability and wanting to sleep
   D. Decrease in heart rate over the last hour
5. You are working with a family that brought their child into the pediatric clinic. The mother describes what may be a type of seizure. What subjective data will help you determine the type? Select all that apply.
   A. The presence or absence of an aura
   B. If the child appeared disoriented after the seizure
   C. Presence of vomiting after the seizure
   D. The duration of the seizure
   E. If the seizure was related to certain foods or occurred after a certain activity

Correct Answers

1. D; 2. C; 3. B; 4. D; 5. A, B, D

REFERENCES

Abend, N. S., & Loddenkemper, T. (2014). Pediatric status epilepticus management. *Current Opinion in Pediatrics, 26*(6), 668–674.

Ahmad, B. S., Petty, S. J., Gorelik, A., et al. (2017). Bone loss with antiepileptic drug therapy: A twin and sibling study. *Osteoporosis International, 28*(9), 2591–2600.

Arlachov, Y., & Ganatra, R. H. (2012). Sedation/anaesthesia in paediatric radiology. *The British Journal of Radiology, 85*, e1018–e1031.

Babikian, T., Merkley, T., Savage, R. C., et al. (2015). Chronic aspects of pediatric traumatic brain injury: Review of the literature. *Journal of Neurotrauma, 32*(23), 1849–1860.

Baca, C. B., Vickrey, B. G., Vassar, S. D., et al. (2013). Injuries in adolescents with childhood-onset epilepsy compared with sibling controls. *The Journal of Pediatrics, 163*(6), 1684–1691.

Ban, L., Fleming, K. M., Doyle, P., et al. (2015). Congenital anomalies in children of mothers taking antiepileptic drugs with and without periconceptional high dose folic acid use: A population-based cohort study. *PLoS ONE, 10*(7), e0131130.

Barr, R. G. (2014). Crying as a trigger for abusive head trauma: A key to prevention. *Pediatric Radiology, 44*(Suppl4), S559–S564.

Baxter, A. L., Ewing, P. H., Young, G. B., et al. (2013). EMLA application exceeding two hours improves pediatric emergency department venipuncture success. *Advanced Emergency Nursing Journal, 35*(1), 67–75.

Beauchamp, M. H., & Anderson, V. (2013). Cognitive and psychopathological sequelae of pediatric traumatic brain injury. *Handbook of Clinical Neurology, 112*, 913–920.

Berg, A. T., & Rychlik, K. (2015). The course of childhood-onset epilepsy over the first two decades: A prospective, longitudinal study. *Epilepsia, 56*(1), 40–48.

Blaszczyk, B., Lasoń, W., & Czuczwar, S. J. (2015). Antiepileptic drugs and adverse skin reactions: An update. *Pharmacological Reports, 67*(3), 426–434.

Bloomer, M. J., Endacott, R., Copnell, B., et al. (2016). 'Something normal in a very, very abnormal environment' – Nursing work to honour the life of dying infants and children in neonatal and paediatric intensive care in Australia. *Intensive and Critical Care Nursing, 33*, 5–11.

Blume, H. K. (2017). Childhood headache: A brief review. *Pediatric Annals, 46*(4), e155–e165.

Bonfield, C. M., Naran, S., Adetayo, O. A., et al. (2014). Pediatric skull fractures: The need for surgical intervention, characteristics, complications, and outcomes. *Journal of Neurosurgery. Pediatrics, 14*(2), 205–211.

Braine, M. E., & Cook, N. (2017). The Glasgow Coma Scale and evidence-informed practice: A critical review of where we are and where we need to be. *Journal of Clinical Nursing, 26*(1–2), 280–293.

Braun, K. P., & Schmidt, D. (2014). Stopping antiepileptic drugs in seizure-free patients. *Current Opinion in Neurology, 27*(2), 219–226.

Brigo, F., Nardone, R., Tezzon, F., et al. (2015). Nonintravenous midazolam versus intravenous or rectal diazepam for the treatment of early status epilepticus: A systematic review with meta-analysis. *Epilepsy and Behavior: E&B, 49*, 325–336.

Burns, E., Grool, A. M., Klassen, T. P., et al. (2016). Scalp hematoma characteristics associated with intracranial injury in pediatric minor head injury. *Academic Emergency Medicine: Official Journal of the Society for Academic Emergency Medicine, 23*(5), 576–583.

Burrows, P., Trefan, L., Houston, R., et al. (2015). Head injury from falls in children younger than 6 years of age. *Archives of Disease in Childhood, 100*(11), 1032–1037.

Caglar, D., & Quan, L. (2016). Drowning and submersion injury. In R. Kliegman, B. Stanton, J. St. Geme, et al. (Eds.), *Nelson textbook of pediatrics* (20th ed.). Philadelphia PA: Elsevier/Saunders.

Camfield, P., & Camfield, C. (2015). Incidence, prevalence and aetiology of seizures and epilepsy in children. *Epileptic Disorders: International Epilepsy Journal With Videotape, 17*(2), 117–123.

Castelblanco, R. L., Lee, M., & Hasbun, R. (2014). Epidemiology of bacterial meningitis in the USA from 1997 to 2010: A population-based observational study. *The Lancet. Infectious Diseases, 14*(9), 813–819.

Centers for Disease Control and Prevention. (2016). *Unintentional drowning: get the facts*. Available at https://www.cdc.gov/homeandrecreationalsafety/water-safety/waterinjuries-factsheet.html. Retrieved July 22, 2017.

Centers for Disease Control and Prevention. (2017a). *TBI: Get the facts*. Retrieved from https://www.cdc.gov/traumaticbraininjury/get_the_facts.html.

Centers for Disease Control and Prevention. (2017b). *Meningococcal disease surveillance*. Retrieved from https://www.cdc.gov/meningococcal/surveillance/index.html.

Chen, C., Shi, J., Stanley, R. M., et al. (2017). US trends of ED visits for pediatric traumatic brain injuries: Implications for clinical trials. *International Journal of Environmental Research and Public Health, 14*(4), 414.

Christensen, J. (2012). Traumatic brain injury: Risks of epilepsy and implications for medicolegal assessment. *Epilepsia, 53*(Suppl. 4), 43–47.

Consumer Product Safety Commission. (2016). *Pool or spa submersion: estimated non-fatal drowning injuries and reported drownings, 2016 report*. Available at: https://www.poolsafely.gov/wp.../2016/05/2016-Pool-and-Spa-Submersion-Report.pdf. (Retrieved 22 July 2017).

Crowcroft, N. S., & Thampi, N. (2015). The prevention and management of rabies. *BMJ (Clinical Research Ed.), 350*, g7827.

Dale, R. C., Gorman, M. P., & Lim, M. (2017). Autoimmune encephalitis in children: Clinical phenomenology, therapeutics, and emerging challenges. *Currend Opinion in Neurology, 30*(3), 334–344.

Dhamne, S. C., Kaye, H. L., & Rotenberg, A. (2018). Neuromodulation in epilepsy. In K. F. Swaiman, S. Ashwal, D. M. Ferriero, et al. (Eds.), *Swaiman's pediatric neurology: Principles and practice* (6th ed.). Philadelphia, PA: Elsevier.

Ding, D., Starke, R. M., Kano, H., et al. (2017). International multicenter cohort study of pediatric brain arteriovenous malformations. Part 1: Predictors of hemorrhagic presentation. *Journal of Neurosurgery. Pediatrics, 19*(2), 127–135.

Dubey, D., Sawhney, A., Greenberg, B., et al. (2015). The spectrum of autoimmune encephalopathies. *Journal of Neuroimmunology, 287*, 93–97.

Elbabaa, S. K., Gildehaus, A. M., & Pierson, M. J. (2017). First 60 fetal in-utero myelomeningocele repairs at Saint Louis Fetal Care Institute in the post-MOMS trial era: Hydrocephalus treatment outcomes (endoscopic third ventriculostomy versus ventriculo-peritoneal shunt). *Child's Nervous System, 33*(7), 1157–1168.

Ellis, M. J., Cordingley, D., Vis, S., et al. (2015). Vestibulo-ocular dysfunction in pediatric sports-related concussion. *Journal of Neurosurgery. Pediatrics, 16*(3), 248–255.

El-Radhi, A. S. (2015). Management of seizures in children. *The British Journal of Nursing, 24*(3), 152–155.

Fernandez, I. S., Abend, N. S., & Loddenkemper, T. (2018). Status epilepticus. In K. F. Swaiman, S. Ashwal, D. M. Ferriero, et al. (Eds.), *Swaiman's pediatric neurology: Principles and practice* (6th ed.). Philadelphia, PA: Elsevier.

Fisher, R. S., Acevedo, C., Arzimanoglou, A., et al. (2014). ILAE official report: A practical clinical definition of epilepsy. *Epilepsia, 55*(4), 475–482.

Fisher, R. S., Cross, J. H., French, J. A., et al. (2017). Operational classification of seizure types by the International League Against Epilepsy: Position paper of the ILAE commission for classification and terminology. *Epilepsia, 58*(4), 522–530.

Franklin, R. C., Pearn, J. H., & Peden, A. E. (2017). Drowning fatalities in childhood: The role of pre-existing medical conditions. *Archives of Disease in Childhood, 102*(10), 888–893.

Fulkerson, D. H., White, I. K., Rees, J. M., et al. (2015). Analysis of long-term (median 10.5 years) outcomes in children presenting with traumatic brain injury and an initial Glasgow Coma Scale score of 3 or 4. *Journal of Neurosurgery. Pediatrics, 16*(4), 410–419.

Gainza-Lein, M., Sanchez-Fernández, I., & Loddenkemper, T. (2017). Use of EEG in critically ill children and neonates in the United States of America. *Journal of Neurology, 264*(6), 1165–1173.

Ganti, L., Bodhit, A. N., Daneshvar, Y., et al. (2013). Impact of helmet use in traumatic brain injuries associated with recreational vehicles. *Advances in Preventive Medicine, 2013*, 450195.

Gaw, C. E., Chounthirath, T., & Smith, G. A. (2017). Nursery product-related injuries treated in United States emergency departments. *Pediatrics, 139*(4), e20162503.

Germain, B., & Maria, B. L. (2018). Epileptic encephalopathies: Clinical aspects, molecular features and pathogenesis, therapeutic targets and translational opportunities, and future research directions. *Journal of Child Neurology, 33*(1), 7–40.

Gilchrist, J., & Parker, E. M. (2014). Racial/ethnic disparities in fatal unintentional drowning among persons aged≤ 29 years – United States, 1999–2010. *MMWR. Morbidity and Mortality Weekly Report, 63*(19), 421–426.

Glauser, T., Shinnar, S., Gloss, D., et al. (2016). Evidence-based guideline: Treatment of convulsive status epilepticus in children and adults: Report of the guideline committee of the American Epilepsy Society. *Epilepsy Currents, 16*(1), 48–61.

Gofshteyn, J. S., & Stephenson, D. J. (2016). Diagnosis and management of childhood headache. *Current Problems in Pediatric and Adolescent Health Care, 46*(2), 36–51.

Gordon, S. M., Srinivasan, L., & Harris, M. C. (2017). Neonatal meningitis: Overcoming challenges in diagnosis, prognosis, and treatment with omics. *Frontiers in Pediatrics, 5*, 139.

Grool, A. M., Aglipay, M., Momoli, F., et al. (2016). Association between early participation in physical activity following acute concussion and persistent postconcussive symptoms in children and adolescents. *JAMA: The Journal of the American Medical Association, 316*(23), 2504–2514.

Hancock, E. C., Osborne, J. P., & Edwards, S. W. (2013). Treatment of infantile spasms. *Cochrane Database of Systematic Review*, (6), CD001770.

Harden, C., Tomson, T., & Gloss, D. (2017). Practice guideline summary: Sudden unexpected death in epilepsy incidence rates and risk factors report of the guideline development, dissemination, and implementation subcommittee of the American Academy of Neurology and the American Epilepsy Society. *Neurology, 88*(17), 1674–1680.

Harding, G. F., & Harding, P. F. (2010). Photosensitive epilepsy and image safety. *Applied Ergonomics, 41*(4), 504–508.

Hartman, M. E., & Cheifetz, I. M. (2016). Pediatric emergencies and resuscitation. In R. M. Kliegman, B. F. Stanton, J. W. St Geme, et al. (Eds.), *Nelson textbook of pediatrics* (20th ed.). Philadelphia, PA: Elsevier/Saunders.

Heckenberg, S. G., Brouwer, M. C., & van de Beek, D. (2014). Bacterial meningitis. *Handbook of Clinical Neurology, 121*, 1361–1375.

Hepburn-Smith, M., Dynkevich, I., Spektor, M., et al. (2016). Establishment of an external ventricular drain best practice guideline: The quest for a comprehensive, universal standard for external ventricular drain care. *The Journal of Neuroscience Nursing: Journal of the American Association of Neuroscience Nurses, 48*(1), 54–65.

Hershey, A. D., Kabbouche, M. A., & O'Brien, H. L. (2016). Headaches. In R. M. Kliegman, B. F. Stanton, J. W. St Geme, et al. (Eds.), *Nelson textbook of pediatrics* (20th ed.). Philadelphia, PA: Elsevier/Saunders.

Hesdorffer, D. C., Shinnar, S., Lax, D. N., et al. (2016). Risk factors for subsequent febrile seizures in the FEBSTAT study. *Epilepsia, 57*(7), 1042–1047.

Holmes, G. L. (2018). Generalized seizures. In K. F. Swaiman, S. Ashwal, D. M. Ferriero, et al. (Eds.), *Swaiman's pediatric neurology: Principles and practice* (6th ed.). Philadelphia, PA: Elsevier.

Hua, F., Xie, H., Worthington, H. V., et al. (2016). Oral hygiene care for critically ill patients to prevent ventilator-associated pneumonia. *Cochrane Database of Systematic Review*, (10), CD008367.

Huang, K. T., Bi, W. L., Abd-El-Barr, M., et al. (2016). The neurocritical and neurosurgical care of subdural hematomas. *Neurocritical Care, 24*(2), 294–307.

Ibrahim, S. H., & Balestreri, W. F. (2016). Mitonchondrial hepatopathies. In R. M. Kliegman, B. F. Stanton, J. W. St Geme, et al. (Eds.), *Nelson textbook of pediatrics* (20th ed.). Philadelphia, PA: Elsevier/Saunders.

International Headache Society. (2018). *The international classification of headache disorders 3rd edition*. Available at: https://www.ichd-3.org/. (Accessed 18 May 2018).

Jimenez, N., Symons, R. G., Wang, J., et al. (2016). Outpatient rehabilitation for Medicaid-insured children hospitalized with traumatic brain injury. *Pediatrics, 137*(6), e20153500.

Jones, K., Go, C., & Boyd, J. (2015). Vigabatrin as first-line treatment for infantile spasms not related to tuberous sclerosis complex. *Pediatric Neurology, 53*(2), 141–145.

Jones, C. E., Munoz, F. M., & Spiegel, H. M. (2016). Guideline for collection, analysis and presentation of safety data in clinical trials of vaccines in pregnant women. *Vaccine, 34*(49), 5998–6006.

Jones, C., & Reilly, C. (2016). Parental anxiety in childhood epilepsy: A systematic review. *Epilepsia, 57*(4), 529–537.

Jones, K., Snead, O. C., III, & Boyd, J. (2015). Adrenocorticotropic hormone versus prednisolone in the treatment of infantile spasms post vigabatrin failure. *Journal of Child Neurology, 30*(5), 595–600.

Kacperski, J., & Arthur, T. (2016). Management of post-traumatic headaches in children and adolescents. *Headache, 56*(1), 36–48.

Kacperski, J., Kabbouche, M. A., O'Brien, H. L., et al. (2016). The optimal management of headaches in children and adolescents. *Therapeutic Advances in Neurological Disorders, 9*(1), 53–68.

Kahle, K. T., Kulkarni, A. V., Limbrick, D. D., et al. (2016). Hydrocephalus in children. *Lancet, 387*(10020), 788–799.

Kinsman, S. L., & Johnston, M. V. (2016). Hydrocephalus. In R. M. Kliegman, B. F. Stanton, J. W. St Geme, et al. (Eds.), *Nelson textbook of pediatrics* (20th ed.). Philadelphia, PA: Elsevier/Saundes.

Klevens, J., Schmidt, B., Luo, F., et al. (2017). Effect of the earned income tax credit on hospital admissions for pediatric abusive head trauma, 1995-2013. *Public Health Reports, 132*(4), 505–511.

Ku, L. C., Boggess, K. A., & Cohen-Wolkowiez, M. (2015). Bacterial meningitis in infants. *Clinics in Perinatology, 42*(1), 29–45.

Kuczynski, A., Crawford, S., Bodell, L., et al. (2013). Characteristics of post-traumatic headaches in children following mild traumatic brain injury and their response to treatment: A prospective cohort. *Developmental Medicine and Child Neurology, 55*(7), 636–641.

Kulkarni, A. V., Sgouros, S., Constantini, S., et al. (2016). International infant hydrocephalus study: Initial results of a prospective, multicenter comparison of endoscopic third ventriculostomy (ETV) and shunt for infant hydrocephalus. *Child's Nervous System, 32*(6), 1039–1048.

Langdon, R., & DiSabella, M. T. (2017). Pediatric headache: An overview. *Current Problems in Pediatric and Adolescent Health Care, 47*(3), 44–56.

Lazaryan, M., Shasha-Zigelman, C., Dagan, Z., et al. (2015). Codeine should not be prescribed for breastfeeding mothers or children under the age of 12. *Acta Paediatrica, 104*(6), 550–556.

Lee, I. C., Li, S. Y., & Chen, Y. J. (2017). Seizure recurrence in children after stopping antiepileptic medication: 5-year follow-up. *Pediatrics and Neonatology, 58*(4), 338–343.

Longoni, G., Levy, D. M., & Yeh, E. A. (2016). The changing landscape of childhood inflammatory central nervous system disorders. *The Journal of Pediatrics, 179*, 24–32.

Lopes, N. R., & Williams, L. C. (epub ahead of print, 2016). Pediatric abusive head trauma prevention initiatives: A literature review. *Trauma, Violence and Abuse.*

Luat, A. F., Coyle, L., & Kamat, D. (2016). The ketogenic diet: A practical guide for pediatricians. *Pediatric Annals, 45*(12), e446–e450.

Mann, T. N., Donald, K. A., Laughton, B., et al. (2017). HIV encephalopathy with bilateral lower limb spasticity: Upper limb motor function and level of activity and participation. *Developmental Medicine and Child Neurology, 59*(4), 412–419.

Månsson, P. K., Johansson, S., Ziebell, M., et al. (2017). Forty years of shunt surgery at Rigshospitalet, Denmark: A retrospective study comparing past and present rates and causes of revision and infection. *BMJ Open, 7*(1), e013389.

Marcdante, K., & Kliegman, R. M. (2016). Meningitis. In R. Kliegman, B. Stanton, J. St. Geme, et al. (Eds.), *Nelson textbook of pediatrics* (20th ed.). Philadelphia, PA: Elsevier/Saunders.

Martin, H. A. (2017). The power of lidocaine, epinephrine, and tetracaine (LET) and a child life specialist when suturing lacerations in children. *Journal of Emergency Nursing, 43*(2), 169–170.

Martin, K., Jackson, C. F., Levy, R. G., et al. (2016). Ketogenic diet and other dietary treatments for epilepsy. *Cochrane Database of Systematic Review*, (2), CD001903.

McCrea, M. A., Nelson, L. D., & Guskiewicz, K. (2017). Diagnosis and management of acute concussion. *Physical Medicine and Rehabilitation Clinics of North America*, *28*(2), 271–286.

McMurtry, C. M., Taddio, A., Noel, M., et al. (2016). Exposure-based interventions for the management of individuals with high levels of needle fear across the lifespan: A clinical practice guideline and call for further research. *Cognitive Behaviour Therapy*, *45*(3), 217–235.

Meehan, W. P., Mannix, R. C., Stracciolini, A., et al. (2013). Symptom severity predicts prolonged recovery after sport-related concussion, but age and amnesia do not. *The Journal of Pediatrics*, *163*(3), 721–725.

Merison, K., & Jacobs, H. (2016). Diagnosis and treatment of childhood migraine. *Current Treatment Options in Neurology*, *18*(11), 48.

Mewasingh, L. D. (2014). Febrile seizures. *BMJ Clinical Evidence*, *2014*, 0324.

Mikati, M. A., & Hani, A. J. (2016). Seizures in childhood. In R. M. Kliegman, B. F. Stanton, J. W. St Geme, et al. (Eds.), *Nelson textbook of pediatrics* (20th ed.). Philadelphia, PA: Elsevier/Saunders.

Minns, R. A., Jones, P. A., Tandon, A., et al. (2017). Raised intracranial pressure and retinal haemorrhages in childhood encephalopathies. *Developmental Medicine and Child Neurology*, *59*(6), 597–604.

Moosa, A. N., & Gupta, A. (2014). Outcome after epilepsy surgery for cortical dysplasia in children. *Child's Nervous System*, *20*(11), 1905–1911.

Morgan, C. D., Zuckerman, S. L., Lee, Y. M., et al. (2015). Predictors of postconcussion syndrome after sports-related concussion in young athletes: A matched case-control study. *Journal of Neurosurgery. Pediatrics*, *15*(6), 589–598.

Morse, A. M., & Kothare, S. V. (2016). Pediatric sudden unexpected death in epilepsy. *Pediatric Neurology*, *57*, 7–16.

Moshe, S. L., Perucca, E., Ryvlin, P., et al. (2015). Epilepsy: New advances. *Lancet*, *385*(9971), 884–898.

Mullally, W. J. (2017). Concussion. *The American Journal of Medicine*.

Murphy, S., Thomas, N. J., Gertz, S. J., et al. (epub ahead of print, 2017). Tripartite stratification of the Glasgow Coma Scale in children with severe traumatic brain injury and mortality: An analysis from a multi-center comparative effectiveness study. *Journal of Neurotrauma*.

Novakova, B., Harris, P. R., Ponnusamy, A., et al. (2013). The role of stress as a trigger for epileptic seizures: A narrative review of evidence from human and animal studies. *Epilepsia*, *54*(11), 1866–1876.

Nakagawa, T. A., Ashwal, S., Mathur, M., et al. (2012). Guidelines for the determination of brain death in infants and children: An update of the 1987 task force recommendations. *Annals of Neurology*, *71*(4), 573–585.

O'Callaghan, F. J., Edwards, S. W., Alber, F. D., et al. (2017). Safety and effectiveness of hormonal treatment versus hormonal treatment with vigabatrin for infantile spasms (ICISS): A randomised, multicentre, open-label trial. *The Lancet. Neurology*, *16*(1), 33–42.

Offringa, M., Newton, R., Cozijnsen, M. A., et al. (2017). Prophylactic drug management for febrile seizures in children. *Cochrane Database of Systematic Review*, (2), CD003031.

Paulsen, A. H., Lundar, T., & Lindegaard, K. F. (2015). Pediatric hydrocephalus: 40-year outcomes in 128 hydrocephalic patients treated with shunts during childhood. Assessment of surgical outcome, work participation, and health-related quality of life. *Journal of Neurosurgery. Pediatrics*, *16*(6), 633–641.

Patel, K., Ming, X., Williams, P. L., et al. (2009). Impact of HAART and CNS-penetrating antiretroviral regimens on HIV encephalopathy among perinatally infected children and adolescents. *AIDS (London, England)*, *23*(14), 1893–1901.

Patel, N., Ram, D., Swiderska, N., et al. (2015). Febrile seizures. *BMJ (Clinical Research Ed.)*, *351*, 1–7.

Patniyot, I. R., & Gelfand, A. A. (2016). Acute treatment therapies for pediatric migraine: A qualitative systematic review. *Headache*, *56*(1), 49–70.

Pisapia, J. M., Sinha, S., Zarnow, D. M., et al. (2017). Fetal ventriculomegaly: Diagnosis, treatment, and future directions. *Child's Nervous System*, *33*(7), 1113–1123.

Popernack, M. L., Gray, N., & Reuter-Rice, K. (2015). Moderate-to-severe traumatic brain injury in children: Complications and rehabilitation strategies. *Journal of Pediatric Health Care*, *29*(3), e1–e7.

Prober, C. G., & Mathew, R. (2016). Brain abscess. In R. M. Kliegman, B. F. Stanton, J. W. St Geme, et al. (Eds.), *Nelson textbook of pediatrics* (20th ed.). Philadelphia, PA: Elsevier/Saundes.

Prober, C. G., Srinivas, N. S., & Mathew, R. (2016b). Central nervous system infections. In R. M. Kliegman, B. F. Stanton, J. W. St Geme, et al. (Eds.), *Nelson textbook of pediatrics* (20th ed.). Philadelphia, PA: Elsevier/Saundes.

Prober, C. G., Srinivas, N. S., & Mathew, R. (2016a). Acute bacterial meningitis. In R. Kliegman, B. Stanton, J. St. Geme, et al. (Eds.), *Nelson textbook of pediatrics* (20th ed.). Philadelphia, PA: Elsevier/Saunders.

Puledda, F., Messina, R., & Goadsby, P. J. (2017). An update on migraine: Current understanding and future directions. *Journal of Neurology*, *264*(9), 2031–2039.

Quan, L., Bierens, J. J., Lis, R., et al. (2016). Predicting outcome of drowning at the scene: A systematic review and meta- analyses. *Resuscitation*, *104*, 63–75.

Quan, L., Mack, C. D., & Schiff, M. A. (2014). Association of water temperature and submersion duration and drowning outcome. *Resuscitation*, *85*(6), 790–794.

Russ, S. A., Larson, K., & Halfon, N. (2012). A national profile of childhood epilepsy and seizure disorder. *Pediatrics*, *129*(2), 256–264.

Ryan, M. E., Jaju, A., Ciolino, J. D., et al. (2016). Rapid MRI evaluation of acute intracranial hemorrhage in pediatric head trauma. *Neuroradiology*, *58*(8), 793–799.

Ryvlin, P., Cross, J. H., & Rheims, S. (2014). Epilepsy surgery in children and adults. *The Lancet. Neurology*, *13*(11), 1114–1126.

Saghazadeh, A., Mastrangelo, M., & Rezaei, N. (2014). Genetic background of febrile seizures. *Reviews in the Neurosciences*, *25*(1), 129–161.

Scheer, S., & John, R. M. (2016). Anti–N-Methyl-D-Aspartate receptor encephalitis in children and adolescents. *Journal of Pediatric Health Care*, *30*(4), 347–358.

Seinfeld, S. A., Pellock, J. M., Kjeldsen, M. J., et al. (2016). Epilepsy after febrile seizures: Twins suggest genetic influence. *Pediatric Neurology*, *55*, 14–16.

Sellin, J. N., Moreno, A., Ryan, S. L., et al. (2017). Children presenting in delayed fashion after minor head trauma with scalp swelling: Do they require further workup? *Child's Nervous System*, *33*(4), 647–652.

Sencer, A., Aras, Y., Akcakaya, M. O., et al. (2012). Posterior fossa epidural hematomas in children: Clinical experience with 40 cases. *Journal of Neurosurgery. Pediatrics*, *9*(2), 139–143.

Shankar, P., Zamora, C., & Castillo, M. (2016). Congenital malformations of the brain and spine. *Handbook of Clinical Neurology*, *136*, 1121–1137.

Shumiloff, N. A., Lam, W. M., & Manasco, K. B. (2013). Adrenocorticotropic hormone for the treatment of West Syndrome in children. *The Annals of Pharmacotherapy*, *47*(5), 744–754.

Shorvon, S. D. (2011). The etiologic classification of epilepsy. *Epilepsia*, *52*(6), 1052–1057.

Sieswerda-Hoogendoorn, T., Boos, S., Spivak, B., et al. (2012). Abusive head trauma part I: Clinical aspects. *European Journal of Pediatrics*, *171*, 415–423.

Silverman, E. C., Sporer, K. A., Lemieux, J. M., et al. (2017). Prehospital care for the adult and pediatric seizure patient: Current evidence-based recommendations. *The West Journal of Emergency Medicine*, *18*(3), 419–436.

Singh, B., Murad, M. H., Prokop, L. J., et al. (2013). Meta-analysis of Glasgow coma scale and simplified motor score in predicting traumatic brain injury outcomes. *Brain Injury: [BI]*, *27*(3), 293–300.

Singh, R., Singh, K. P., Cherian, S., et al. (2017). Rabies–epidemiology, pathogenesis, public health concerns and advances in diagnosis and control: A comprehensive review. *Veterinary Quarterly*, *37*(1), 212–251.

Singhal, N. S., Harini, C., & Sullivan, J. (2018). Epileptic spasms and myoclonic seizures. In K. F. Swaiman, S. Ashwal, D. M. Ferriero, et al. (Eds.), *Swaiman's pediatric neurology: Principles and practice* (6th ed.). Philadelphia, PA: Elsevier.

Singhi, S. C., & Tiwari, L. (2009). Management of intracranial hypertension. *Indian Journal of Pediatrics*, *76*(5), 519–529.

Smith, S. E., Pratt, R., Trieu, L., et al. (2017). Epidemiology of pediatric multidrug-resistant tuberculosis in the United States, 1993-2014. *Clinical Infectious Diseases*, *65*(9), 1437–1443.

Squier, W., & Mack, J. (2009). The neuropathology of infant subdural haemorrhage. *Forensic Science International, 187*(1–3), 6–13.

Strahle, J., Selzer, B. J., Muraszko, K. M., et al. (2012). Programmable shunt valve affected by exposure to a tablet computer. *Journal of Neurosurgery. Pediatrics, 10*(2), 118–120.

Swanson, D. (2015). Meningitis. *Pediatrics in Review, 36*(12), 514–524.

Sutherland, H. G., & Griffiths, L. R. (2017). Genetics of migraine: Insights into the molecular basis of migraine disorders. *Headache, 57*(4), 537–569.

Taylor, C. A., Bell, J. M., Breiding, M., et al. (2017). Traumatic brain injury–related emergency department visits, hospitalizations, and deaths—United States, 2007 and 2013. *MMWR. Surveillance Summaries: Morbidity and Mortality Weekly Report. Surveillance Summaries, 66*(9), 1–16.

Teichert, J. H., Rosales, P. R., Jr., Lopes, P. B., et al. (2012). Extradural hematoma in children: Case series of 33 patients. *Pediatric Neurosurgery, 48*(4), 216–220.

Téllez-Zenteno, J. F., Hernández-Ronquillo, L., Buckley, S., et al. (2014). A validation of the new definition of drug-resistant epilepsy by the International League Against Epilepsy. *Epilepsia, 55*(6), 829–834.

Tenney, J. R., & Glauser, T. (2018). Electroclinical syndromes: Childhood onset. In K. F. Swaiman, S. Ashwal, D. M. Ferriero, et al. (Eds.), *Swaiman's pediatric neurology: Principles and practice* (6th ed.). Philadelphia, PA: Elsevier.

Theurer, W. M., & Bhavsar, A. K. (2013). Prevention of unintentional childhood injury. *American Family Physician, 87*(7), 502–509.

Tobin, J. M., Ramos, W. D., Pu, Y., et al. (2017). Bystander CPR is associated with improved neurologically favourable survival in cardiac arrest following drowning. *Resuscitation, 115*, 39–43.

Toth, P., Szarka, N., Farkas, E., et al. (2016). Traumatic brain injury-induced autoregulatory dysfunction and spreading depression-related neurovascular uncoupling: Pathomechanisms, perspectives, and therapeutic implications. *American Journal of Physiology, Heart and Circulatory Physiology, 311*(5), H1118–H1131.

Van Houtem, C. M., Laine, M. L., Boomsma, D. I., et al. (2013). A review and meta-analysis of the heritability of specific phobia subtypes and corresponding fears. *Journal of Anxiety Disorders, 27*(4), 379–388.

Venable, G. T., Rossi, N. B., & Morgan Jones, G. (2016). The preventable shunt revision pate: A potential quality metric for pediatric shunt surgery. *Journal of Neurosurgery. Pediatrics, 18*(1), 7–15.

Vetter, V., Baxter, R., Denizer, G., et al. (2016). Routinely vaccinating adolescents against meningococcus: Targeting transmission & disease. *Expert Review of Vaccines, 15*(5), 641–658.

Vezina, N., Al-Halabi, B., Shash, H., et al. (2017). A review of techniques used in the management of growing skull fractures. *The Journal of Craniofacial Surgery, 28*(3), 604–609.

Wassenaar, M., Kasteleijn-Nolst Trenite, D. G., de Haan, G. J., et al. (2014). Seizure precipitants in a community-based epilepsy cohort. *Journal of Neurology, 261*(4), 717–724.

Wassenaar, M., Leijten, F. S., Egberts, T. C., et al. (2013). Prognostic factors for medically intractable epilepsy: A systematic review. *Epilepsy Research, 106*(3), 301–310.

Weinberg, G. A., & Thompson-Stone, R. (2018). Bacterial infections of the nervous system. In K. F. Swaiman, S. Ashwal, D. M. Ferriero, et al. (Eds.), *Swaiman's pediatric neurology: Principles and practice* (6th ed.). Philadelphia, PA: Elsevier.

Weiss, J. (2010). Prevention of drowning. *Pediatrics, 126*, e253–e262.

Weiss, E. F., Masur, D., & Shinnar, S. (2016). Cognitive functioning one month and one year following febrile status epilepticus. *Epilepsy & Behavior, 64*, 283–288.

Whittaker, M. R. (2013). Opioid use and the risk of respiratory depression and death in the pediatric population. *The Journal of Pediatric Pharmacology and Therapeutics, 18*(4), 269–276.

Willoughby, R. E., Jr. (2016). Rabies. In R. M. Kliegman, B. F. Stanton, J. W. St Geme, et al. (Eds.), *Nelson essentials of pediatrics* (20th ed.). Philadelphia, PA: Saunders/Elsevier.

World Health Organization. (2017). Human rabies: 2016 updates and call for data. *Weekly Epidemiological Record, 92*(7), 77–86.

Xu, J. (2014). Unintentional drowning deaths in the United States 1999–2010. *NCHS Data Brief, 149*, 1–8.

Zemek, R., Barrowman, N., Freedman, S. B., et al. (2016). Clinical risk score for persistent postconcussion symptoms among children with acute concussion in the ED. *JAMA: The Journal of the American Medical Association, 315*(10), 1014–1025.

31

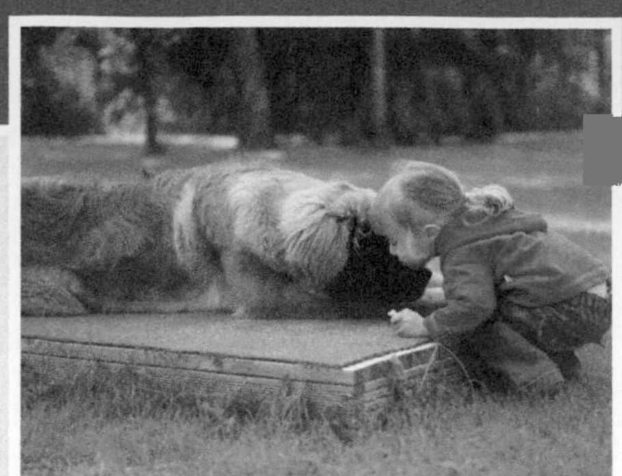

The Child With Endocrine Dysfunction

Amy Barry and Erin Connelly

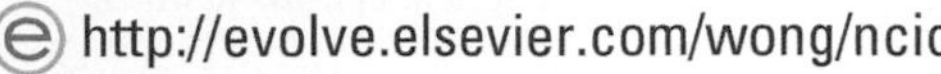

http://evolve.elsevier.com/wong/ncic

CONCEPTS

- Cellular Regulation
- Glucose Regulation
- Patient Education
- Health Promotion

THE ENDOCRINE SYSTEM

The endocrine system controls and regulates metabolism; this includes energy production, growth, fluid and electrolyte balance, response to stress, and sexual reproduction (Gardner, Anderson, & Nissenson, 2011). This system has three components: (1) the cell, which sends a chemical message using a hormone; (2) the target cells, or organs, which receive the chemical message; and (3) the environment through which the chemical is transported (e.g., blood, lymph, extracellular fluids) from the site of synthesis to the sites of cellular action.

The endocrine glands, which are distributed throughout the body, are listed in Box 31.1; also listed are several additional structures sometimes considered endocrine glands, although they are not usually included.

HORMONES

A **hormone** is a complex chemical substance produced and secreted into body fluids by a cell or group of cells that exerts a physiologic controlling effect on other cells (Garibaldi & Chemaitilly, 2016). Local hormones create their effect near the point of secretion. For example, secretin, a digestive hormone made by cells lining the duodenum, stimulates the pancreas. General hormones are released by endocrine glands into the bloodstream, where they are carried to responsive tissues (Fig. 31.1). Some of these hormones (such as thyroid hormone [TH] and growth hormone [GH]) affect most cells of the body, whereas others (such as the tropic hormones) produce their effects on specific tissues, called **target tissues**. These responsive, or target, tissues may be another endocrine gland, an organ, or tissue (Gardner, Anderson, & Nissenson, 2011). For example, pituitary hormones stimulate the adrenal glands and the thyroid gland to secrete adrenocorticotropic hormone (ACTH) and thyroid-stimulating hormone (TSH), respectively.

Control of Hormone Secretion

Regulation of hormonal secretion is often based on negative feedback. As a rule, endocrine glands have a tendency to oversecrete particular hormones. However, once the hormone's physiologic effect has been achieved, this information is transmitted to the producing gland, either directly or indirectly, to inhibit further secretion. If the gland undersecretes, the inhibition is stopped, and the gland increases production of the hormone again. As a result, the hormone is secreted according to the amount needed. This is the primary function of the tropic hormones.

The anterior pituitary gland, located below the hypothalamus, is often referred to as the master gland. It is primarily responsible for stimulation and inhibition of tropic hormones. Tropic (which literally means "turning") hormones secreted by the anterior pituitary regulate the secretion of hormones from various target organs (Fig. 31.2). As blood concentrations of the target hormones reach normal levels, a negative message is sent to the anterior pituitary to inhibit release of the tropic hormone. For example, TSH responds to low levels of circulating TH. As blood levels of TH reach normal concentrations, a negative feedback message is sent to the anterior pituitary, resulting in diminished release of TSH.

The pituitary gland is controlled by either hormonal or neuronal signals from the hypothalamus. Two types of substances are secreted from the hypothalamus: (1) releasing hormones and (2) inhibitory hormones. Both are secreted within the hypothalamus and transported by way of the pituitary portal system to the anterior pituitary, where they stimulate the secretion of tropic hormones. An example of this is the secretion of corticotropin-releasing factor (CRF) by the hypothalamus. CRF stimulates the pituitary to secrete ACTH. In this instance the anterior pituitary is the target of the hypothalamus. ACTH then stimulates the adrenals to secrete glucocorticoids, which have multiple target sites throughout the body. Pituitary hormones that lack feedback control from the product of a target tissue (e.g., GH, prolactin, and melanocyte-stimulating hormone) require hypothalamic inhibitors and stimulators for their control.

Not all hormones depend on other hormones for their release. For example, insulin is secreted in response to blood glucose concentrations. Other glandular hormones that are not under the control of the pituitary gland are glucagon, parathyroid hormone (parathormone, PTH), antidiuretic hormone (ADH), and aldosterone.

BOX 31.1 Endocrine Glands

Pituitary gland (hypophysis cerebri)—A pea-sized gland that lies within a deep bony depression at the base of the cranium (the sella turcica) and is attached to the hypothalamus on the undersurface of the brain by a slender infundibulum, or pituitary stalk

Thyroid gland—Two large lateral lobes and a connecting portion, the isthmus, situated on the anterior aspect of the neck just below the larynx

Parathyroid glands—Four or five (more or less) small round bodies attached to the posterior surfaces of the lateral lobes of the thyroid gland

Adrenal glands—Pyramid-shaped glands situated atop the kidneys, fitting like caps over these organs

Ovaries—Glands located in the female pelvis on each side of the uterus at the fimbriated end of the fallopian tubes

Testes—Oval-shaped glands situated within the male scrotum

Islets of Langerhans—Small clusters of endocrine cells within the pancreas situated between the acinar or exocrine-secreting portions of the gland

Structures Sometimes Considered Endocrine Glands

Pineal body (epiphysis cerebri)—A gland located in the cranial cavity behind the midbrain and third ventricle, the functions of which are largely speculative

Thymus—A gland situated behind the sternum and below the thyroid gland; plays an important role in immunity but only during fetal life and early childhood

Gastrointestinal glands—Mucosal lining of the gastrointestinal tract containing cells that produce hormones that play important roles in controlling and coordinating secretory and motor activities of digestion

Placenta—A body that secretes ovarian hormones and chorionic gonadotropin during gestation; only a temporary endocrine gland

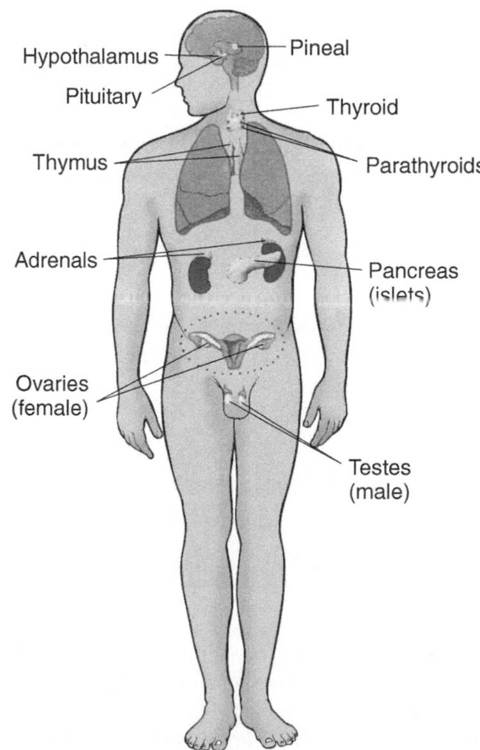

FIG. 31.1 Location of the endocrine glands and structures sometimes considered endocrine glands. (From Thibodeau, G. A., & Patton, K. T. [2008]. *Structure and function of the body* [13th ed.]. St. Louis, MO: Mosby.)

NEUROENDOCRINE INTERRELATIONSHIPS

Two regulatory systems maintain hemostasis: the endocrine and the autonomic nervous systems (collectively known as the neuroendocrine system) (Gardner, Anderson, & Nissenson, 2011). The autonomic nervous system consists of the sympathetic and parasympathetic systems that control nonvoluntary functions—specifically that of smooth muscle, myocardium, and glands. The parasympathetic system primarily regulates the digestive processes, whereas the sympathetic system functions to maintain homeostasis during times of stress.

The higher autonomic centers, located in the hypothalamus and limbic system, help control the functioning of both autonomic systems. Both sympathetic and parasympathetic nerve fibers secrete neurotransmitting substances: acetylcholine, released by cholinergic fibers, and norepinephrine, released by adrenergic fibers. Release of norepinephrine into the plasma produces the same effects as secretion of this substance by the adrenal medulla. Thus the interrelatedness between the two systems is demonstrated.

The neuroendocrine system acts by synthesizing and releasing various chemical substances that regulate body functions. Information is carried by means of neural impulses in the autonomic system and by the blood in the endocrine system. In general, neural responses are more rapid and localized, whereas endocrine responses are more lasting and widespread. The two systems function synergistically because neural impulses transmitted to the central nervous system (CNS) stimulate the hypothalamus to manufacture and release several releasing or inhibiting factors.

Because of the interdependent relationship of these glands, a malfunction in one gland produces effects elsewhere. Endocrine dysfunction may result from an intrinsic defect in the target gland or from a diminished or elevated level of tropic hormones. Endocrine problems occur when there is hypofunction or hyperfunction of the glands. Primary hypofunction is usually associated with a more profound deficiency of the target gland hormone because little or no hormone is secreted. In secondary dysfunction the target glands secrete some of their hormones but in smaller amounts and less rapidly.

DISORDERS OF PITUITARY FUNCTION

The pituitary gland is divided into two lobes: the anterior pituitary (adenohypophysis) and the posterior pituitary (neurohypophysis). It is regulated by hormones secreted from the hypothalamus. The anterior pituitary is responsible for secreting GH, TSH, ACTH, follicle-stimulating hormone (FSH), luteinizing hormone (LH), and prolactin. The posterior pituitary secretes ADH and oxytocin (Sathyapalan & Dixit, 2012).

Deficiencies of the anterior pituitary hormones may be due to organic defects or have an idiopathic etiology. Clinical manifestations depend on the hormones involved and the age of the patient. If the tropic hormones are involved, the resulting disorder reflects the altered stimulus of the target gland. For example, if TSH is deficient, the thyroid gland does not secrete TH and the child displays clinical signs of hypothyroidism.

An overproduction of the anterior pituitary hormones can result in gigantism (caused by excess GH production during childhood), hyperthyroidism, hypercortisolism (Cushing syndrome), and precocious puberty from excessive gonadotropins (LH and FSH). Overproduction may be caused by hyperplasia of the pituitary cells—which may eventually progress to a tumor (adenoma)—or a primary hypothalamic defect that results in an excess of the hormone's releasing factor. Although the initial clinical manifestations are a result of pituitary oversecretion, eventually pituitary insufficiency occurs, and the signs of panhypopituitarism become evident. Panhypopituitarism is defined clinically as

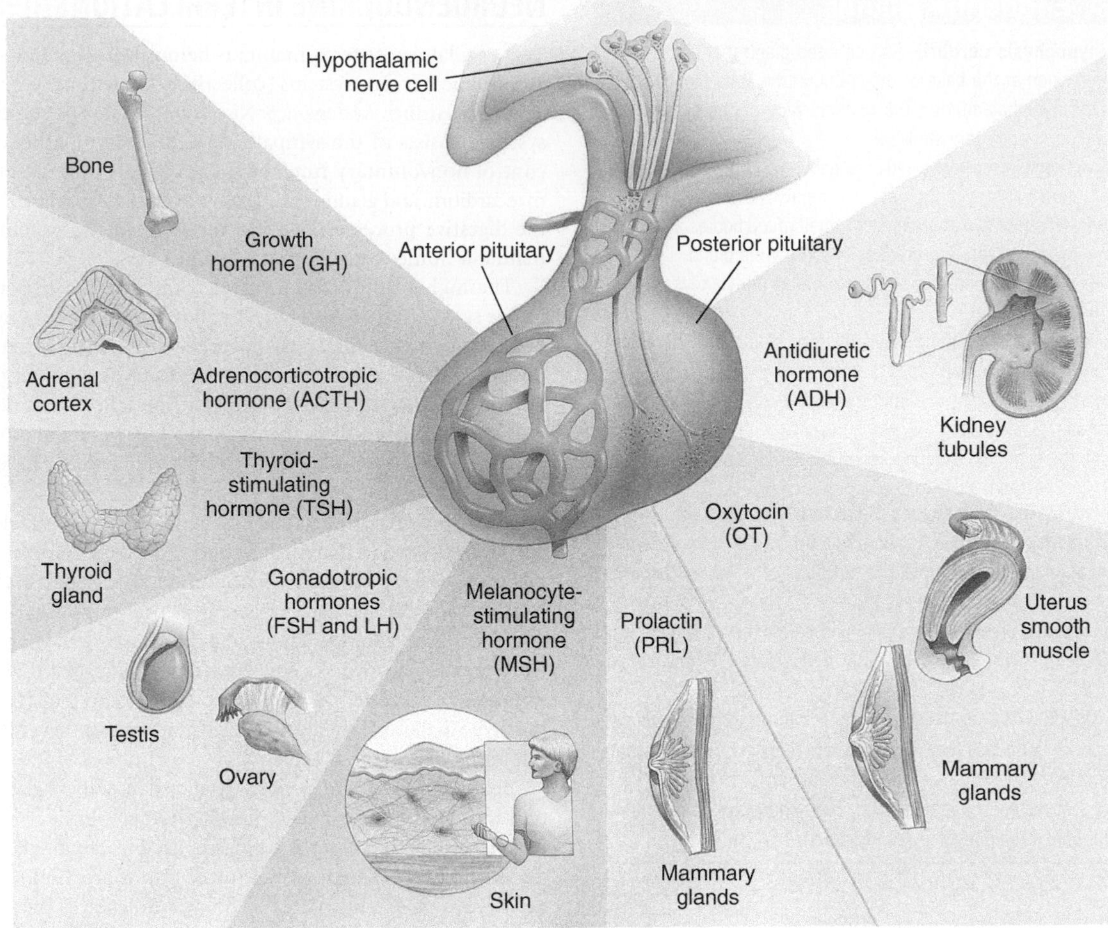

FIG. 31.2 Principal anterior and posterior pituitary hormones and their target organs. (From Thibodeau, G. A., & Patton, K. T. [2008]. *Structure and function of the body* [13th ed.]. St. Louis, MO: Mosby.)

the loss of all anterior pituitary hormones, leaving only posterior pituitary function intact (Toogood & Stewart, 2008).

> **! NURSING ALERT**
>
> Children with panhypopituitarism should wear medical identification, such as a bracelet.

HYPOPITUITARISM

Hypopituitarism is the diminished secretion of one or more pituitary hormones. The consequences of the condition depend on the degree of dysfunction. It often leads to the following:

- Gonadotropin deficiency (decrease in LH or FSH), where children show absence or regression of secondary sexual characteristics
- GH deficiency, which children display stunted somatic growth
- TSH deficiency, which produces hypothyroidism
- Corticotropin deficiency, which results in manifestations of adrenal hypofunction

Hypopituitarism can result from any of the conditions listed in Box 31.2. The most common organic cause of pituitary undersecretion is a tumor in the pituitary or hypothalamic region. Craniopharyngiomas are tumors known to invade these regions of the brain and cause panhypopituitarism (Box 31.3). A child may experience decreased growth velocity for some time before developing any symptoms or signs of increased intracranial pressure, local compression, or the destructive effects of a tumor. Other causes of panhypopituitarism include encephalitis, radiation to the head or neck, traumatic brain injury, and congenital hypoplasia of the hypothalamic area (Rose & Auble, 2012; Sathyapalan & Dixit, 2012).

> **BOX 31.2 Causes of Hypopituitarism**
>
> - Aplasia or hypoplasia
> - Developmental defects
> - Idiopathic—Sporadic; genetic
> - Destructive lesions
> - Trauma—Perinatal; child abuse; basal skull fracture
> - Irradiation—Central nervous system, eye, middle ear
> - Autoimmune hypophysitis
> - Surgery—Removal of pharyngeal pituitary, ablation of craniopharyngioma or other tumor
> - Vascular—Aneurysm, infarct
> - Functional deficiency
> - Psychosocial dwarfism
> - Anorexia nervosa

Congenital hypopituitarism can be seen in newborn infants and run in families, suggesting a genetic cause; however, the majority of cases have no genetic association (Schoenmakers, Alatzoglou, Chatterjee,

BOX 31.3 Clinical Manifestations of Panhypopituitarism

Growth Hormone
Short stature but proportional height and weight
Delayed epiphyseal closure
Retarded bone age proportional to height
Premature aging common in later life
Increased insulin sensitivity

Thyroid-Stimulating Hormone
Short stature with infantile proportions
Dry, coarse skin; yellow discoloration, pallor
Cold intolerance
Constipation
Somnolence
Bradycardia
Dyspnea on exertion
Delayed dentition, loss of teeth

Gonadotropins
Absence of sexual maturation or loss of secondary sexual characteristics
Atrophy of genitalia, prostate gland, breasts
Amenorrhea without menopausal symptoms
Decreased spermatogenesis

Adrenocorticotropic Hormone
Severe anorexia, weight loss
Hypoglycemia
Hypotension
Hyponatremia, hyperkalemia
Adrenal apoplexy, especially in response to stress
Circulatory collapse

Antidiuretic Hormone
Polyuria
Polydipsia
Dehydration

Melanocyte-Stimulating Hormone
Decreased pigmentation

et al., 2015). Neonates may have symptoms of hypoglycemia and seizure activity (Schoenmakers, Alatzoglou, Chatterjee, et al., 2015). A child with combined GH deficiency and hypothyroidism should be screened for congenital pituitary defects and genetic mutations (Pine-Twaddell, Romero, & Radovick, 2013).

Idiopathic hypopituitarism, or idiopathic pituitary growth failure, is usually related to GH deficiency, which inhibits somatic growth in all cells of the body (Amin, Mushtaq, & Alvi, 2015). Although most children with hypopituitarism are normal at birth, many show growth patterns that progressively deviate from the normal growth rate, often beginning in infancy. The chief complaint is often short stature. Of those who seek help, boys outnumber girls three to one. Idiopathic hypopituitarism can be associated with deficiencies of other pituitary hormones, such as TSH and ACTH; thus it is theorized that the disorder is probably secondary to hypothalamic deficiency.

Isolated GH deficiency without other associated pituitary hormone deficiencies or a known organic cause is also seen in children (Stanley, 2012). Growth failure is defined as an absolute height of less than −2 standard deviations (SD) for age, or a linear growth velocity consistently less than −1 SD for age. When this occurs without the presence of hypothyroidism, systemic disease, or malnutrition, an abnormality of the GH–insulin-like growth factor (IGF) axis should be considered (Grimberg, Divall, Polychonakos, et al., 2016).

Not all children with short stature have GH deficiency. In most instances the cause of short stature is considered idiopathic. Idiopathic short stature (ISS) is defined as a condition in which the height of an individual is more than 2 SD below the mean height for his or her age, sex, and population group, without evidence of systemic, endocrine, nutritional, or chromosomal abnormalities (Argente, 2016). Children with ISS fall into one of three groups: those with familial short stature, those with constitutional delay of growth and puberty, and those with a yet unidentified cause of short stature. Familial short stature refers to healthy children who have ancestors with adult height in the lower percentiles and whose height during childhood is appropriate for genetic background (Fig. 31.3). Constitutional delay of growth and puberty refers to individuals with delayed linear growth and delayed skeletal and sexual maturation for age (Amin, Mushtaq, & Alvi, 2015). GH therapy in children with ISS continues to be debated frequently by pediatric endocrinologists (Murray, Dattani, & Clayton, 2016). New guidelines are available that recommend the clinical management of children with growth failure related to growth hormone deficiency and idiopathic short stature. They now include recombinant IGF-1 therapy for primary IGF-1 deficiency (Grimberg, Divall, Polychronakos, et al., 2016).

Clinical Manifestations

Children with GH deficiency often grow normally during the first year and then follow a slowed growth curve that is below the 3rd percentile. In children with a partial GH deficiency, the growth retardation is less marked than in children with complete GH deficiency. Height may be stunted more than weight because, with good nutrition, these children can become overweight or even obese. Their well-nourished appearance is an important diagnostic clue to differentiation from other disorders such as failure to thrive. Skeletal proportions are normal for the age, but these children appear younger than their chronologic age. Later in life, premature aging is common. Bone age is delayed but is closely related to height age; the degree of growth delay depends on the duration and extent of the hormonal deficiency. Because of the underdeveloped jaw, teeth may be overcrowded and malpositioned.

Children with isolated GH deficiency have normal intelligence. However, emotional problems are common, especially as they near puberty, when their smallness becomes increasingly apparent in comparison with their peers. Height discrepancy has been correlated with emotional adjustment problems and may be a predictor of the extent to which GH-delayed children or children with short stature will experience emotional distress, relationship dysfunction (friendship and later dating/marriage), educational attainment, and type of employment (Sandberg & Gardner, 2015).

Diagnostic Evaluation

Only a small number of children with delayed growth or short stature have hypopituitary dysfunction. Diagnostic evaluation is aimed at isolating organic causes, which, in addition to GH deficiency, may include brain tumor, hypothyroidism, oversecretion of cortisol, gonadal aplasia, chronic illness, nutritional inadequacy, Russell-Silver dwarfism, or hypochondroplasia.

A complete diagnostic evaluation should include a family history, a history of the child's growth patterns and previous health status, a physical examination, and a psychosocial evaluation. Specific radiographic imaging, including magnetic resonance imaging (MRI), endocrine studies, and genetic testing, may also be warranted (Stanley, 2012).

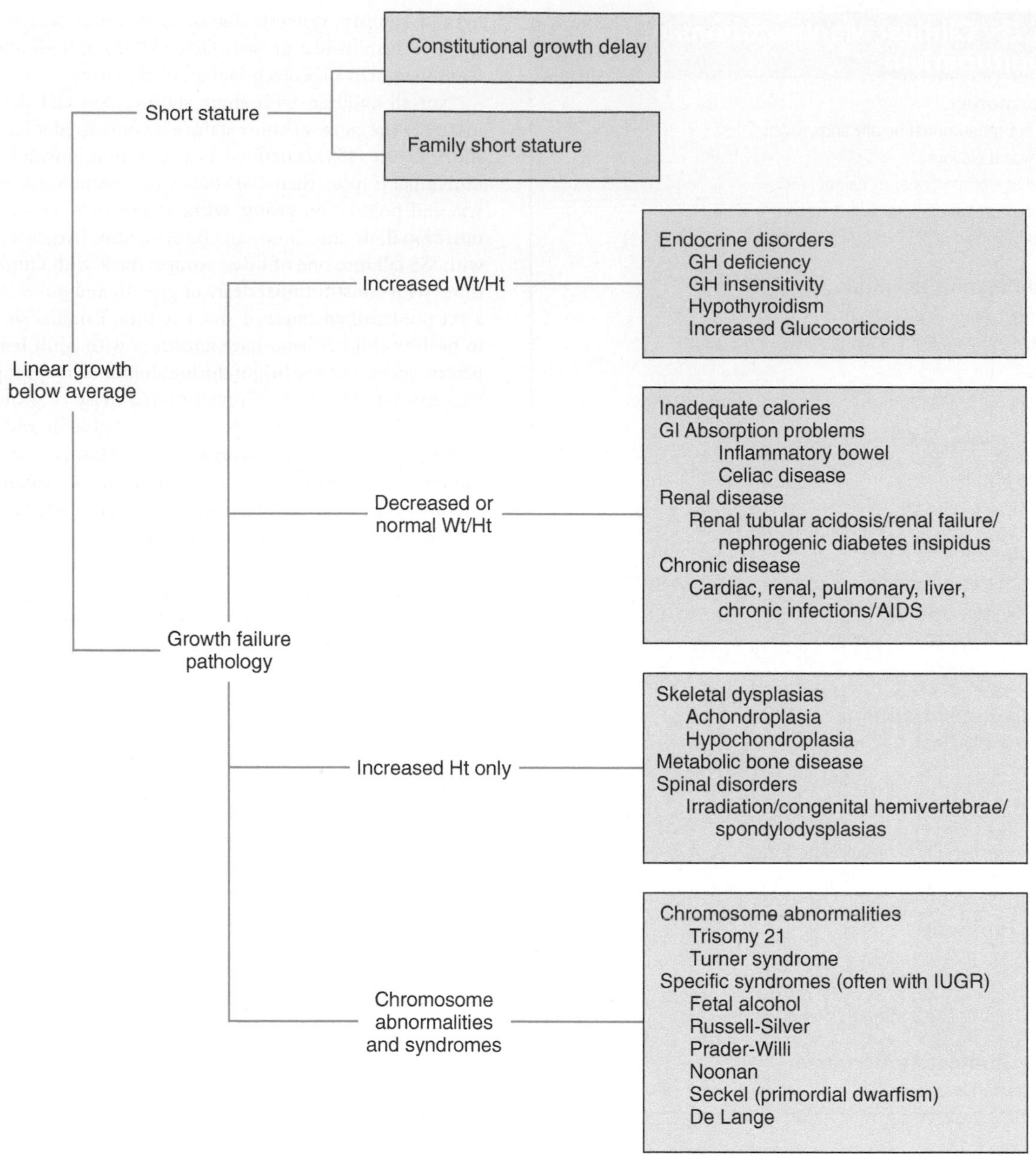

FIG. 31.3 Causes of short stature. *AIDS,* Acquired immunodeficiency syndrome; *GI,* gastrointestinal; *GH,* growth hormone; *IUGR,* intrauterine growth restriction; *Wt/Ht,* weight-to-height ratio. (From Vogiatzi, M. G., & Copeland, K. C. [1998]. The short child. *Pediatrics in Review, 19*[3], 92-99.)

Family History

A family history is of utmost importance in relating short stature to genetic background. The midparental height is an important prognosticator of the child's ultimate adult height. Normal adult height should fall within 5 cm (2 inches) of midparental height (Ferguson, 2011). Children with constitutional delays frequently are the products of parents who experienced similar slow growth patterns and delayed sexual maturation. A small percentage of those with GH deficiency demonstrate an autosomal recessive inheritance pattern. Height and weight of siblings should be compared with the child's growth patterns at comparable age periods.

Child's History

The child's history should include a thorough prenatal history to rule out maternal disorders that may have influenced growth, such as malnutrition. Compare birth height and weight with gestational age. Children with hypopituitarism are usually of normal size and normal gestational age at birth.

Investigate the child's health history for evidence of chronic illness that may have influenced growth patterns, although a chronic illness, such as congenital heart disease, malabsorptive disorders, severe anemia, or neurologic impairments, usually is identified long before the growth problem becomes a concern. Signs and symptoms suggesting a tumor, such as visual disturbances, headache, and signs of increasing intracranial pressure, are important. With lesions involving the hypothalamus, the history may also reveal somnolence, thermodysregulation, epilepsy, and polyphagia, resulting in obesity. Because a craniopharyngioma can affect the secretion of any of the pituitary hormones, assessment for hypothyroidism, hypoadrenalism, and hypoaldosteronism should also be included.

Whenever possible, evaluate the child's growth patterns since birth, especially growth velocity, and compare them with standard

BOX 31.4 Evaluating the Growth Curve

Ensure reliability of measurements: Accurately obtain and plot height and weight measurements.
Determine absolute height: The child's absolute height bears some relationship to the likelihood of a pathologic condition. However, the majority of children who have a height below the lowest percentile (either the third or fifth percentile on the height curve) do not have a pathologic growth problem.
Assess height velocity: The most important aspect of a growth evaluation is the observation of a child's height over time, or height velocity. Accurate determination of height velocity requires at least 4 and preferably 6 months of observation. A substantial deceleration in height velocity (crossing several percentiles) between 3 and 12 or 13 years of age indicates a pathologic condition until proven otherwise.
Determine weight-to-height relationship: Evaluation of the weight-to-height ratio has some diagnostic value in ascertaining the cause of growth retardation in a short child.
Project target height: The height of a child can be judged inappropriately short only in the context of his or her genetic potential. Determine the target height of the child with the formula:
[Father's height (cm) + Mother's height (cm) + 13]/2 for boys
or
[Father's height (cm) + Mother's height (cm) – 13]/2 for girls
Most children achieve an adult stature within approximately 10 cm (4 inches) of the target height.

Modified from Vogiatzi, M. G., & Copeland, K. C. (1998). The short child. *Pediatrics in Review, 19*(3), 92-99.

measurements. The age of onset of short stature provides a significant diagnostic clue. When the clinician evaluates the results of plotting height and weight, upward or downward changes in height velocity in children older than 3 years may indicate a growth abnormality (Cheetham & Davies, 2014).

Physical Examination

Accurate measurement of height (using a calibrated stadiometer) and weight and comparison with standard growth charts are essential (Box 31.4). Multiple height measures reflect a more accurate assessment of abnormal growth patterns (Cheetham & Davies, 2014). Other measurements may include crown-to-pubis and pubis-to-heel length to compare body proportions. Sexual development should be assessed and compared with age-appropriate development. Observation of general appearance yields valuable clues, especially signs of premature aging and infantile facial features. Funduscopic examination and testing for visual acuity are important to detect evidence of ocular damage from a tumor.

Radiographic Surveys

A skeletal survey in children less than 3 years of age and radiographic examination of the hand-wrist for centers of ossification (bone age) (Box 31.5) in older children are important in evaluating growth. Epiphyseal maturation is delayed in GH deficiency but consistent with height. This is in contrast with gonadal dysplasia, such as Turner syndrome, in which bone age is near normal. A skull series may help identify abnormalities such as an abnormally small sella turcica where the pituitary is located. MRI, computed tomography (CT), radionuclear scans, or carotid angiograms may be needed to establish diagnosis and localization of brain lesions (Stanley, 2012).

Endocrine Studies

Definitive diagnosis of GH deficiency is based on absent or subnormal reserves of pituitary GH. Measuring serum IGF-1 and IGF binding

BOX 31.5 Evaluating Bone Age for Growth Disorders

Bone age refers to a method of assessing skeletal maturity by comparing the appearance of representative epiphyseal centers obtained on x-ray examination with age-appropriate published standards. Most conditions that cause poor linear growth also cause a delay in skeletal maturation and a retarded bone age. Observation of even a profoundly delayed bone age is never diagnostic or even indicative of a specific diagnosis. A delayed bone age merely indicates that the associated short stature is to some extent "partially reversible," because linear growth will continue until epiphyseal fusion is complete. In comparison, a bone age that is not delayed in a short child is of much greater concern and may, in fact, be of some diagnostic value under certain circumstances.

Modified from Vogiatzi, M. G., & Copeland, K. C. (1998). The short child. *Pediatrics in Review, 19*(3), 92-99.

protein 3 (IGFBP3) levels may assist in the decision to pursue further testing for GH deficiency. It is recommended that GH stimulation tests be reserved for children with low serum IGF-1 and IGFBP3 levels and poor growth who do not have other endocrine or nonendocrine causes for short stature (Hokken-Koelega, 2011). However, although the IGF-1 test is useful in detecting severe GH insensitivity, it may not be accurate in detecting less severe cases of idiopathic short stature (Hokken-Koelega, 2011).

GH stimulation testing involves the use of pharmacologic agents such as levodopa, clonidine, arginine, insulin, propranolol, or glucagon followed by the measurement of GH in the blood (Parks & Felner, 2016). Studies have shown that traditional GH stimulation test results can be less reliable than previously accepted, and recommendations have been made to standardize assays (Stanley, 2012). Currently, findings in a child of poor linear growth, delayed bone age, and peak levels of GH at less than 10 ng/ml in two stimulation tests are consistent with GH deficiency (Parks & Felner, 2016). New reference standards that decrease the lower limit of normal GH levels have been proposed and continue to be debated (Murray, Dattani, & Clayton, 2016).

Therapeutic Management

Treatment of GH deficiency caused by organic lesions is directed toward correction of the underlying disease process (e.g., surgical removal or irradiation of a tumor). GH therapy in children with ISS continues to be debated frequently by pediatric endocrinologists (Murray, Dattani, & Clayton, 2016). New guidelines are available that recommend the clinical management of children with growth failure related to growth hormone deficiency and idiopathic short stature. They now include recombinant IGF-1 therapy for primary IGF-1 deficiency (Grimberg, Divall, Polychronakos, et al., 2016).

For more than 20 years cadaver-derived human growth hormone (HGH) was used successfully to enhance linear growth in short children. In 1985 the U.S. Food and Drug Administration stopped use of the hormone in response to reported deaths resulting from Creutzfeldt-Jakob disease (CJD) in three former HGH recipients. Patients have been identified who received HGH and became infected with CJD, a rare and fatal neurodegenerative condition iatrogenically transmitted through human tissue (Cali, Miller, Parisi, et al., 2015). Biosynthetic GH prepared by recombinant deoxyribonucleic acid (DNA) technology (and without the risk of CJD) is now used exclusively (Grimberg, Divall, Polychronakos, et al., 2016).

In the United States the recommended dosage range of recombinant GH is 0.037 to 0.18 to 0.3 mg/kg per week, divided into six or seven daily subcutaneous doses (Parks & Felner, 2016). Maximum growth velocity occurs in the first year of treatment; with each consecutive year of treatment, growth rates decline (Parks & Felner, 2016). A meta-analysis of the GH literature concluded that, although GH may improve growth velocity in children, individuals who receive treatment remain shorter than their peers (Bryant, Baxter, Cave, et al., 2007). For children to achieve their genetic growth potential, early diagnosis of and intervention for growth disorders are essential (Argente, 2016).

The child, family, and health care team make the decision jointly to stop GH therapy. Growth rates of less than 1 inch per year and a bone age of more than 14 years in girls and more than 16 years in boys are often used as criteria to stop GH therapy (Parks & Felner, 2016). Children with other hormone deficiencies require replacement therapy to correct the specific disorders. This may involve administration of thyroid extract, cortisone, testosterone, or estrogens and progesterone. The sex hormones are usually begun during adolescence to promote normal sexual maturation.

Nursing Care Management

The principal nursing consideration is identifying children with growth problems. Although the majority of growth problems are not a result of organic causes, any delay in normal growth and sexual development poses special emotional adjustments for these children.

The nurse is a key person in helping establish a diagnosis. For example, if serial height and weight records are not available, the nurse can question parents about the child's growth compared with that of siblings, peers, or relatives. Investigating clothing sizes is often helpful in determining growth at different ages. (See Quality Patient Outcomes box.)

QUALITY PATIENT OUTCOMES

Growth Hormone Deficiency

- Early recognition of growth problems
- Accurate diagnosis of growth hormone (GH) deficiency
- GH effective in stimulating growth
- Child and family demonstrate effective coping with diagnosis and treatment

Because the behavioral or physical changes that suggest a tumor are insidious, they are frequently overlooked. It is important to correlate the onset of any positive findings with the initial evidence of growth retardation. For example, visual problems and headaches are not uncommon in school-age children and can coincidentally occur after a growth problem is recognized. In fact, headache may represent the emotional trauma caused by short stature rather than be a symptom of a tumor. Pursue this line of questioning cautiously to avoid alarming parents unduly about the possibility of a brain tumor.

Part of a nurse's role in helping establish a diagnosis is assisting with diagnostic tests. Preparation of the child and family is especially important if a number of tests are being performed and the child requires particular attention during GH stimulation testing. Blood samples are usually taken every 30 minutes for a 3-hour period. Children also have difficulty overcoming hypoglycemia generated by tests with insulin, so they should be carefully observed for signs of hypoglycemia. Those receiving glucagon are at risk of nausea and vomiting. Patients receiving clonidine require close blood pressure monitoring. Nursing administration of intravenous (IV) fluids may be required if hypotension is detected. The use of arginine is often well tolerated by children, but it may cause hypoglycemia in some infants and toddlers. Therefore close monitoring for hypoglycemia is necessary.

Child and Family Support

If an organic cause of the problem has been confirmed, the parents and child need an opportunity to express their thoughts and feelings. Frequently a growth problem that was present since birth is missed until adolescence, at which time the child's difference in body development becomes dramatically evident in comparison with peers. Family members may feel anger and resentment toward members of the health staff for not detecting the problem sooner. Parents may experience guilt for not seeking medical attention earlier, especially if the child has been miserable from the ridicule and criticism of peers. Appropriate emotional support from the nurse can include an affirmation of each person's justified feelings, such as anger or guilt, and emphasis on the treatment plan and prospects for improvement in the future.

DRUG ALERT

Growth Hormone

GH is most effective when it is administered at bedtime. Physiologic release is more normally stimulated as a result of pituitary release of GH during the first 45 to 90 minutes after the onset of sleep.

Even when hormone replacement is successful, these children attain their eventual adult height at a slower rate than their peers; therefore they need assistance in setting realistic expectations regarding improvement. Psychologic counseling may be considered for children diagnosed with idiopathic short stature whether done in conjunction with GH therapy or treatment instead (Sandberg & Gardner, 2015). Both sexes need guidance toward appropriate vocational goals. Because these children appear younger than their chronologic age, others frequently relate to them in infantile or childish ways. Children having school problems need special counseling. Parents and teachers benefit from guidance directed toward setting realistic expectations for the child based on age and abilities. For example, in the home such children should have the same age-appropriate responsibilities as their siblings. As they approach adolescence, encourage them to participate in group activities with peers. If abilities and strengths are emphasized rather than physical size, such children are more likely to develop a positive self-image.

Professionals and families may find research, education, support, and advocacy from the Human Growth Foundation.* Treatment is expensive—up to $52,000 per year depending on the dosage or approximately $35,000 per inch (Ferguson, 2011). Usually the cost is partially covered by insurance if the child has a documented deficiency, and some pharmaceutical companies offer copay assistance.

PITUITARY HYPERFUNCTION

Excess GH before closure of the epiphyseal shafts results in proportional overgrowth of the long bones until the individual reaches a height of 2.4 m (8 feet) or more. Vertical growth is accompanied by rapid and increased development of muscles and viscera. Weight is increased but is usually in proportion to height. Proportional enlargement of head circumference also occurs and may result in delayed closure of the fontanels in young children. Children with a pituitary-secreting tumor may also demonstrate signs of increasing intracranial pressure, especially headache.

If oversecretion of GH occurs after epiphyseal closure, growth is in the transverse direction, producing a condition known as acromegaly. Typical facial features include the following:

- Overgrowth of the head, lips, nose, tongue, jaw, and paranasal and mastoid sinuses

*997 Glen Cove Ave., Suite 5, Glen Head, NY 11545; 800-451-6434; e-mail: hgf1@hgfound.org; http://www.hgfound.org.

- Separation and malocclusion of the teeth in the enlarged jaw
- Disproportion of the face to the cerebral division of the skull
- Increased facial hair; thickened, deeply creased skin
- Increased tendency toward hyperglycemia and diabetes mellitus (DM)

Excessive secretion of GH by a pituitary adenoma causes most cases of acromegaly. Acromegaly can develop slowly, with patients being diagnosed as much as 10 years after their symptoms first appear. Left untreated, these patients have a higher mortality rate due to potential cardiovascular, metabolic, and pulmonary complications (Pivonello, Auriemma, Grasso et al., 2017).

Diagnostic Evaluation

Diagnosis is based on a history of excessive growth during childhood and evidence of increased levels of IGF-1 concentration. If this is elevated, a specialized GH test will be done to assess for excess secretion (Ribeiro-Oliveira & Barkan, 2012). MRI may reveal a tumor in an enlarged sella turcica, normal bone age, enlargement of bones (such as the paranasal sinuses), and evidence of joint changes. Endocrine studies to confirm excess of other hormones, specifically thyroid, cortisol, and sex hormones, should also be included in the differential diagnosis.

Therapeutic Management

If a lesion is present, surgical treatment by cryosurgery or hypophysectomy is performed to remove the tumor when possible. Transsphenoid surgery (TSS) is the most common surgical treatment for pituitary adenoma. External radiation (XRT) or radioactive implants may be used to destroy GH-secreting tissue. Medical therapy using drugs that can suppress GH may be used in conjunction with TSS and/or XRT to treat this disease (Maffezzoni, Frara, Doga, et al., 2016). Depending on the extent of surgical excision and degree of pituitary insufficiency, hormone replacement with thyroid extract, cortisone, and sex hormones may be necessary.

Nursing Care Management

The primary nursing consideration is early identification of children with excessive growth rates. Although medical treatment of acromegaly will not reduce a patient's height, it will prevent further excess growth. Nurses in ambulatory settings who are frequently involved in growth screening should refer children who demonstrate excessive linear growth for a medical evaluation. They should also observe for signs of a tumor, especially headache, and evidence of concurrent hormonal excesses, particularly the gonadotropins, which cause sexual precocity.

Children with excessive growth rates require as much emotional support as those with short stature. However, girls may suffer from the effects of excessive height much more than boys. Like boys, some girls may find their height to be an asset when pursuing sports such as basketball. Children and their parents need an opportunity to express their thoughts. A compassionate nurse can be supportive to these children, especially before adolescence when they are larger than their peers. The nurse can emphasize to a tall girl that as boys grow older, they become taller and she will not always be looking down at them.

PRECOCIOUS PUBERTY

Manifestations of sexual development before age 9 years in boys or age 8 years in girls have traditionally been considered precocious development, and these children were recommended for further evaluation (Brito, Spinola-Castro, Kochi, et al., 2016), but guidelines on this have been debated (see Research Focus box).

Normally the hypothalamic-releasing factors stimulate secretion of the gonadotropic hormone from the anterior pituitary at the time of puberty. In the male, interstitial cell–stimulating hormone stimulates Leydig cells of the testes to secrete testosterone. In the female follicle-stimulating hormone and luteinizing hormone stimulate the ovarian follicles to secrete estrogens. This sequence of events is known as the **hypothalamic-pituitary-gonadal axis**. If for some reason the cycle undergoes premature activation, the child displays evidence of advanced or precocious puberty. Sex hormones affect bone growth, and premature exposure may cause short stature. Box 31.6 lists the causes of precocious puberty.

Isosexual precocious puberty is more common among girls than boys. Approximately 50% of children with precocious puberty have central precocious puberty (CPP), in which pubertal development is activated by the hypothalamic gonadotropin-releasing hormone (GnRH). This produces early maturation and development of the gonads, with secretion of sex hormones, development of secondary sexual characteristics, and sometimes production of mature sperm and ova (Garibaldi &

RESEARCH FOCUS

Precocious Puberty

Concern that the onset of puberty may be occurring earlier has been raised over the past two decades (Brito, Spinola-Castro, Kochi, et al., 2016). Earlier puberty in girls is now thought to be directly related to obesity, and newer data suggest that the timing of puberty has not changed for children who are not overweight (Walvood, 2010). Some data suggested that boys may be beginning maturation earlier as well (Herman-Giddens, Steffes, Harris, et al., 2012). However, no change in the guidelines for evaluation of precocious puberty in boys has been recommended (Herman-Giddens, Steffes, Harris, et al., 2012; Walvood, 2010).

BOX 31.6 Precocious Puberty

Central Precocious Puberty

Idiopathic, with or without hypothalamic hamartoma

Secondary

- Congenital anomalies
- Postinflammatory: Encephalitis, meningitis, abscess, granulomatous disease
- Radiotherapy
- Trauma
- Neoplasms

After effective treatment of long-standing pseudosexual precocity

Peripheral Precocious Puberty

Familial male-limited precocious puberty

Albright syndrome

Gonadal or extragonadal tumors

Adrenal

- Congenital adrenal hyperplasia
- Adenoma, carcinoma
- Glucocorticoid resistance

Exogenous sex hormones

Primary hypothyroidism

Incomplete Precocious Puberty

Premature thelarche

Premature menarche

Premature pubarche or adrenarche

Modified from Root, A. W. (2000). Precocious puberty. *Pediatrics in Review, 21*(1), 10-19.

Chemaitilly, 2016). CPP occurs more frequently in girls and is usually idiopathic, with 95% demonstrating no causative factor (Brito, Spinola-Castro, Kochi, et al., 2016). A CNS insult or structural abnormality occurs in more than 75% of boys with CPP (Garibaldi & Chemaitilly, 2016).

Peripheral precocious puberty (PPP) refers to early puberty resulting from hormone stimulation other than the hypothalamic GnRH–stimulated pituitary gonadotropin release. Clinical findings normally associated with puberty may be seen as variations in normal sexual development (Brito, Spinola-Castro, Kochi, et al., 2016). They appear without other signs of puberty and are probably caused by unusual end-organ sensitivity to prepubertal levels of estrogen or androgen. Included are premature thelarche (development of breasts in prepubertal girls), premature pubarche (premature adrenarche, early development of sexual hair), and premature menarche (isolated menses without other evidence of sexual development).

Therapeutic Management

Children with evidence of precocious puberty should be evaluated by a pediatric endocrinologist. In every case, an MRI of the brain should be performed to assess for hypothalamic brain tumor (Brito, Spinola-Castro, Kochi, et al., 2016). When there is no organic cause for CPP, patients will be monitored closely for growth. In 50% of cases, precocious pubertal development regresses or stops advancing without any treatment. CPP can be managed with monthly injections of a synthetic analog of luteinizing hormone–releasing hormone, which decreases the pituitary secretion of LH and FSH (Garibaldi & Chemaitilly, 2016). A slow-release formulation of leuprolide acetate (Lupron Depot) is given in a dosage of 0.2 to 0.3 mg/kg intramuscularly every 4 weeks. A longer-lasting preparation may be given intramuscularly every 3 months and has also been successful in the treatment of CPP in a majority of patients. Although expensive, the GnRH analog (GnRHa) histrelin has been formulated as a subdermal implant with effects lasting 12 months and may be beneficial for some patients who would like to avoid injections (Garibaldi & Chemaitilly, 2016).

After initiation of treatment, breast development regresses or does not advance, and growth returns to normal rates, enhancing predicted height. Treatment is discontinued at a chronologically appropriate time, allowing pubertal changes to resume. Despite the early sexual development, maturation of the gonads and the appearance of secondary sexual characteristics proceed in the usual order. The most difficult time for the child is usually the school years before adolescence. After puberty, physical differences from peers are no longer present. Some patients, however, do not attain adult targeted height during therapy. The use of GH to improved adult height is being investigated with children with precocious puberty and advanced bone age (Garibaldi & Chemaitilly, 2016).

Nursing Care Management

Psychologic support and guidance of the child and family are the most important aspects of management. Parents and children need anticipatory guidance, support and information resources, and reassurance. GnRH agonists are associated with side effects such as headache, emotional lability, and vasodilation causing hot flashes (Harrington & Palmert, 2016). Nurses are essential in providing medical education to the patient and family. Dress and activities for the physically precocious child should be appropriate to the chronologic age. Sexual interest is not usually advanced beyond the child's chronologic age, and parents need to understand that the child's mental age is congruent with the chronologic age.

Although the child's sexual behavior may be appropriate for the chronologic age, the nurse should emphasize to parents that the child may be fertile. Usually no form of contraception is necessary unless the child is sexually active. In this situation proper counseling is important because hormonal forms of birth control, such as estrogen pills, prematurely initiate epiphyseal closure, resulting in stunted linear growth.

DIABETES INSIPIDUS

The principal disorder of posterior pituitary hypofunction is diabetes insipidus (DI). Also known as neurogenic DI, central diabetes insipidus results from the undersecretion of antidiuretic hormone (ADH), also known as vasopressin. This disease results in the production of large volumes of urine (polyuria), which leads to a state of uncontrolled diuresis (Di Iorgi, Napoli, Allegri, et al., 2012). Central DI is not to be confused with nephrogenic DI, a rare hereditary disorder affecting primarily males and caused by unresponsiveness of the renal tubules to the hormone. (See Chapter 24.)

Neurogenic DI may result from a number of different causes. Primary causes are familial or idiopathic; approximately 20% to 50% of the total cases are idiopathic (Di Iorgi, Allegri, Napoli, et al., 2014). More than 55 genetic mutations have been identified, which result in a deficiency of vasopressin and cause familial central DI (Di Iogri, Napoli, Allegri, et al., 2012). Secondary causes include trauma (accidental or surgical), tumors, granulomatous disease, Langerhans cell histiocytosis (LCH), autoimmune disease, infections (meningitis or encephalitis), cranial malformations, and vascular anomalies (aneurysm). Certain drugs, such as alcohol or phenytoin (diphenylhydantoin), can cause a transient polyuria. DI may be an early sign of an evolving cerebral process (Di Iogri, Napoli, Allegri, et al., 2012).

Clinical Manifestations

The cardinal signs of DI are polyuria and polydipsia. In the older child, signs can include excessive urination accompanied by insatiable thirst so intense that the child does little more than go to the toilet and drink fluids. Frequently the first sign is enuresis. In the infant the initial symptom is irritability that is relieved with feedings of water but not milk. The infant is also prone to severe dehydration, electrolyte imbalance, hyperthermia, azotemia, and potential circulatory collapse. Other symptoms such as vomiting, constipation, fever, irritability, sleep issues, failure to thrive, and growth problems may be seen.

Dehydration is usually not a serious problem in older children, who are able to drink larger quantities of water. However, any period of unconsciousness, such as after trauma or anesthesia, may be life threatening because the voluntary demand for fluid is absent. During such instances careful monitoring of urine volumes, blood concentration, and IV fluid replacement is essential to prevent dehydration.

! NURSING ALERT

The child with DI complicated by congenital absence of the thirst center must be encouraged to drink sufficient quantities of liquid to prevent electrolyte imbalance.

Diagnostic Evaluation

The simplest test used to diagnose this condition is the water deprivation test, which restricts oral fluids and observes changes in urine volume and concentration. Normally, reducing fluids results in concentrated urine and diminished volume. In DI, fluid restriction has little or no effect on urine formation but causes weight loss from dehydration. Accurate results from this procedure require strict monitoring of fluid intake and urinary output, measurement of urine concentration (specific gravity or osmolality), and frequent weight checks. A weight loss between 3% and 5% indicates significant dehydration and requires termination of the fluid restriction.

! NURSING ALERT

Small children require close observation during fluid deprivation to prevent them from drinking, even from toilet bowls, flower vases, or other unlikely sources of fluid.

If this test is positive, the child should be given a test dose of injected aqueous vasopressin (Pitressin), which should alleviate the polyuria and polydipsia. Unresponsiveness to exogenous vasopressin usually indicates nephrogenic DI but a rise in urine osmolality after vasopressin administration indicates central DI (Arima, Azuma, Morishita, et al., 2016).

An important diagnostic consideration is differentiating DI from other causes of polyuria and polydipsia, especially diabetes mellitus. MRI to look for secondary causes of central DI such as a tumor or central brain anomaly is essential (Di Iorgi, Napoli, Allegri, et al., 2012). Often kidney function tests, urine osmolality tests, blood electrolyte levels, and specific endocrine studies are sent to isolate associated problems (Breault & Majzoub, 2016). In rare instances a psychologic consultation may be warranted to confirm the possibility of compulsive water drinking related to psychogenic causes.

Therapeutic Management

The usual treatment is hormone replacement using DDAVP, which is a synthetic analog of the endogenous hormone arginine vasopressin (AVP). DDAVP can be given orally, intranasally, or parenterally. The intranasal and oral forms of DDAVP are most commonly used in children. Oral DDAVP has few complications and is easier to give, which likely increases compliance (Di Iorgi, Napoli, Allegri, et al., 2012).

! NURSING ALERT

To be effective, vasopressin must be thoroughly mixed in the oil by being held under warm running water for 10 to 15 minutes and shaken vigorously before being drawn into the syringe. If this is not done, the oil may be injected minus the ADH. Small brown particles, which indicate drug dispersion, must be seen in the suspension.

The medication is usually administered twice daily—at bedtime to allow the child to sleep through the night and in the morning to allow fewer interruptions in the school day. Some "breakthrough" urination is allowed during the evening hours as a precaution against overmedication. The signs of overmedication are similar to manifestations associated with the syndrome of inappropriate ADH (SIADH). (See the next section.)

Nursing Care Management

The initial objective is identification of the disorder. Because an early sign may be sudden enuresis in a child who is toilet trained, excessive thirst with bed-wetting is an indication for further investigation. Another clue is persistent irritability and crying in an infant that is relieved only by bottle-feedings of water. After head trauma or certain neurosurgical procedures, the development of DI can be anticipated; therefore closely monitor these patients. (See Quality Patient Outcomes box.)

Assessment includes measurement of body weight, serum electrolytes, blood urea nitrogen (BUN), hematocrit, and urine specific gravity taken before surgery and every other day after the procedure. Fluid intake and output should be carefully measured and recorded. Alert patients are able to adjust intake to urine losses, but unconscious or very young patients require closer fluid observation. In children who are not toilet trained, collection of urine specimens may require application of a urine-collecting device.

QUALITY PATIENT OUTCOMES

Diabetes Insipidus

- Early recognition of signs and symptoms of diabetes insipidus (DI)
- Differentiation of DI from other causes of polyuria and polydipsia (e.g., diabetes mellitus)
- Effective hormone replacement

After confirmation of the diagnosis, parents need a thorough explanation regarding the condition, with specific clarification that DI is a different condition from DM. They must realize that treatment is lifelong. If children are to receive DDAVP, ideally two caregivers should learn the correct procedure for preparation and administration of the drug. Once children are old enough, encourage them to assume full responsibility for their care.

For emergency purposes, these children should wear medical alert identification. School personnel need to be aware of the problem so they can grant children unrestricted use of the lavatory. Failure to permit this may result in embarrassing accidents that often result in a child's unwillingness to attend school. Medication may need to be kept at school depending on dosing schedules.

SYNDROME OF INAPPROPRIATE ANTIDIURETIC HORMONE

Oversecretion of the posterior pituitary antidiuretic hormone (ADH) causes the disorder known as syndrome of inappropriate antidiuretic hormone (SIADH). This disorder occurs with increased frequency in a variety of conditions that disrupt CNS function such as infection, tumor, or surgery. It can also be the side effect of a variety of medications. SIADH is the most common cause of hyponatremia in hospitalized patients (Cuesta, Garrahy, & Thompson, 2016).

Excess ADH causes free water to be reabsorbed from the kidneys. As increased free water circulates, serum osmolality goes down, and urine osmolality inappropriately increases. Clinical signs of SIADH are directly related to fluid retention and hyponatremia. When hyponatremia occurs acutely, swelling of the brain occurs (Giuliani & Peri, 2014). When serum sodium levels are diminished to 120 mEq/L, affected children may display anorexia, nausea, vomiting, stomach cramps, irritability, and personality changes. With progressive hyponatremia, more serious neurologic signs, such as stupor and seizures, may occur.

Fluid restriction is the immediate management of choice. Subsequent management depends on the cause and severity. Fluids may be restricted in anticipation of SIADH development postoperatively. Some children may be treated with oral sodium replacement. Severe SIADH may require hypertonic saline infusion that is only given in the hospital setting under close supervision (Cuesta, Garrahy, & Thompson, 2016).

Nursing Care Management

The recognition of SIADH symptoms is the primary nursing goal. Close attention to measurements of intake and output, weight, and monitoring for the development of neurologic symptoms is essential, especially in patients at risk in the intensive care setting. (See Quality Patient Outcomes box.)

QUALITY PATIENT OUTCOMES

Syndrome of Inappropriate Antidiuretic Hormone

- Early recognition of signs and symptoms of syndrome of inappropriate antidiuretic hormone
- Fluid overload prevented
- Seizures prevented

! NURSING ALERT

Nausea, vomiting, and malaise may precede the onset of more severe stages such as disorientation, confusion, coma, and seizures (Robinson, 2011).

Seizure precautions are implemented in children at high risk for SIADH. The child and family need education and support regarding the rationale for fluid restrictions. The rare child with chronic SIADH is placed on long-term ADH-antagonizing medication. The patient and family will need instruction regarding medication administration.

DISORDERS OF THYROID FUNCTION

The thyroid gland secretes two types of hormones: thyroid hormone (TH) and calcitonin. TH is made up of the hormones thyroxine (T_4) and triiodothyronine (T_3). The anterior pituitary hormone TSH controls the secretion of TH. TSH is regulated by the hypothalamic hormone thyrotropin-releasing factor (TRF) as a negative feedback response. Hypothyroidism or hyperthyroidism may result from a defect in the thyroid or from a disturbance in the secretion of TSH or TRF. Because the functions of T_3 and T_4 are qualitatively the same, the term *thyroid hormone* (TH) is used throughout the discussion (Box 31.7).

BOX 31.7 Physiologic Effects of Thyroid Hormone

- Regulates metabolic rate of all cells; protein, fat, and carbohydrate catabolism; and nitrogen excretion
- Regulates body heat production and heat-dissipating mechanisms
- Regulates protein synthesis and catabolism, amino acid incorporation into protein, and transcription of messenger ribonucleic acid
- Increases gluconeogenesis and peripheral utilization of glucose
- Maintains appetite and secretion of gastrointestinal substances
- Maintains calcium mobilization
- Stimulates cholesterol synthesis and hepatic mechanisms that remove cholesterol from the circulation; stimulates lipid turnover and free fatty acid release
- Regulates hepatic conversion of carotene to vitamin A
- Maintains growth hormone secretion, skeletal maturation, and tissue differentiation
- Is necessary for muscle tone and vigor and normal skin constituents
- Maintains cardiac rate, force, and output
- Affects respiratory rate, depth of oxygen utilization, and carbon dioxide formation
- Affects central nervous system development and cerebration during first 2 to 3 years
- Affects milk production during lactation and menstrual cycle fertility
- Maintains sensitivity to insulin and insulin degradation
- Affects red cell production
- Affects cortisol secretion, probably by directly affecting the adrenal glands and by increasing adrenocorticotropic hormone secretion

The synthesis of TH depends on available sources of dietary iodine and tyrosine. The thyroid is the only endocrine gland capable of storing excess amounts of hormones for release. During circulation T_4 and T_3 are bound to carrier proteins (thyroxine-binding globulin). They must be unbound before they are able to exert their metabolic effect.

The main physiologic action of TH is to regulate metabolism and control the processes of growth and tissue differentiation, as outlined in Box 31.7. Unlike GH, TH is involved in many more diverse activities that influence the growth and development of body tissues. Therefore a deficiency of TH exerts a more profound effect on growth than that seen in GH deficiency.

Calcitonin helps maintain blood calcium levels by decreasing the calcium concentration. It inhibits skeletal demineralization and promotes calcium deposition in the bone. This effect is the opposite of parathyroid hormone (PTH).

JUVENILE HYPOTHYROIDISM

Hypothyroidism is one of the most common endocrine problems of childhood. It may be either congenital (see Chapter 8) or acquired and represents a deficiency in secretion of TH (Parks & Felner, 2016). Hypothyroidism from dietary insufficiency of iodine is now rare in the United States because iodized salt is a readily available source of the nutrient.

Beyond infancy, a number of defects may cause primary hypothyroidism. For example, a congenital hypoplastic thyroid gland may provide sufficient amounts of TH during the first year or two but be inadequate when rapid body growth increases demands on the gland. A partial or complete thyroidectomy for cancer or thyrotoxicosis can leave insufficient thyroid tissue to furnish hormones for body requirements. Radiotherapy for Hodgkin disease or other malignancies may lead to hypothyroidism (Metzger, Krasin, Choi, et al., 2016). Infectious processes may cause hypothyroidism. It can also occur when dietary iodine is deficient.

Low levels of circulating thyroid hormones and raised levels of TSH at birth characterize congenital hypothyroidism. If left untreated, congenital hypothyroidism causes mental retardation. Improvements in newborn screening have led to earlier detection and prevention of cognitive dysfunction (Hanley, Lord, & Bauer, 2016).

Thyromegaly (enlarged thyroid gland) and growth deceleration are seen in children with hypothyroidism. Growth and development are less impaired when hypothyroidism is acquired at a later age. Because brain growth is nearly complete by 2 to 3 years of age, intellectual disability and neurologic sequelae are not associated with juvenile hypothyroidism. Clinical manifestations may include dry skin, puffiness around the eyes, sparse hair, constipation, sleepiness, lethargy, and mental decline. Growth failure, delayed puberty, and excessive weight gain can also be seen.

Therapy is TH replacement, the same as for hypothyroidism in the infant. In children with severe symptoms, the restoration thyroid function is achieved more gradually with administration of increasing amounts of L-thyroxine over a period of 4 to 8 weeks. This is done to avoid symptoms of hyperthyroidism. Researchers have found that children treated early continue to have mild delays in reading, comprehension, and arithmetic but should catch up over time (Pardo Campos, Musso, Keselman, et al., 2017). Adolescents may demonstrate problems with memory, attention, and visuospatial processing.

Nursing Care Management

The importance of early recognition of congenital hypothyroidism in the infant is discussed in Chapter 8. Growth deceleration in a child whose growth has previously been normal should alert the observer to the possibility of hypothyroidism. Treatment is daily oral TH replacement.

The importance of daily compliance and the need for periodic monitoring of serum thyroid levels should be stressed to patients and their families.

GOITER

A goiter is an enlargement or hypertrophy of the thyroid gland. It may occur with deficient (hypothyroid), excessive (hyperthyroid), or normal (euthyroid) TH secretion. It can be congenital or acquired. Congenital disease usually occurs as a result of maternal administration of antithyroid drugs or iodides during pregnancy. Acquired disease can result from increased secretion of pituitary TSH in response to decreased circulating levels of TH or from infiltrative neoplastic or inflammatory processes. In areas where dietary iodine (essential for TH production) is deficient, goiter can be endemic.

Enlargement of the thyroid gland may be mild and noticeable only when there is an increased demand for TH (e.g., during periods of rapid growth). Where iodine deficiency is severe, a large percentage of the population display goiters. Enlargement of the thyroid at birth can be sufficient to cause severe respiratory distress. Sporadic goiter is usually caused by lymphocytic thyroiditis, and intrinsic biochemical defects in synthesis of the hormones are associated with goiters. TH replacement is necessary to treat the hypothyroidism and reverse the TSH effect on the gland.

Nursing Care Management

Large goiters are identified by their obvious appearance. Smaller nodules may be evident only on palpation. Nurses in ambulatory settings need to be aware of the possibility of goiters and report such findings. Benign enlargement of the thyroid gland may occur during adolescence and should not be confused with pathologic states. Nodules are rarely caused by a cancerous tumor but always require evaluation. Include questions regarding exposure to radiation in the assessment.

> **! NURSING ALERT**
>
> If an infant is born with a goiter, immediately begin precautions for emergency ventilation, such as having supplemental oxygen and a tracheostomy set nearby. Hyperextension of the neck often facilitates breathing.

Immediate surgery to remove part of the gland may be lifesaving in infants born with a goiter. When thyroid replacement is necessary, parents have the same needs regarding its administration as discussed for the parents of children who have hypothyroidism. (See Chapter 8.)

CHRONIC LYMPHOCYTIC THYROIDITIS

Chronic lymphocytic thyroiditis (also known as Hashimoto disease) is the most common cause of thyroid disease in children and adolescents and accounts for the largest percentage of juvenile hypothyroidism (Hanley, Lord, & Bauer, 2016). It accounts for many of the enlarged thyroid glands formerly designated as thyroid hyperplasia of adolescence or adolescent goiter. Although lymphocytic thyroiditis can occur during the first 3 years of life, it occurs more frequently after age 6, with peak incidence occurring during adolescence. Some children may have subclinical hypothyroidism, but the presence of a goiter and elevated thyroglobulin antibody with progressive increase in both thyroid peroxidase antibody and TSH are predictive factors for development of overt hypothyroidism (Hanley, Lord, & Bauer, 2016).

Pathophysiology

There is a strong genetic predisposition to the development of lymphocytic thyroiditis. In families this disease is closely related to other thyroid disorders (e.g., Graves disease, idiopathic hypothyroidism, idiopathic myxedema) and autoimmune disorders (e.g., pernicious anemia, Addison disease, type 1 DM, and hypoparathyroidism).

Thyroid cell damage and death are autoimmune mediated by T cells and cytokines. Lymphocytes infiltrate the thyroid gland and cause inflammation. Eventually, thyroid cells are replaced with fibrous tissue. Several antithyroid antibodies have been recognized in patients with thyroiditis and these antibodies are the best marker to determine a diagnosis (Caturegli, De Remiqis, & Rose, 2014). The identification of genes involved in this disease has led to improved diagnostic testing and may lead to new treatments in the future (Tomer, 2014).

Clinical Manifestations

Enlargement of the thyroid gland is often noted during routine examination. Parents may notice it when the youngster swallows. In most children the entire gland is enlarged symmetrically (but may be asymmetric) and is firm, freely movable, and nontender. There may signs of moderate tracheal compression (sense of fullness, hoarseness, and dysphagia). However, it is extremely rare for a nontoxic diffuse goiter to enlarge enough to cause tracheal compression. Most children are euthyroid, but some display symptoms of hypothyroidism. Others have signs suggestive of hyperthyroidism, such as nervousness, irritability, tachycardia, increased sweating, or hyperactivity.

Diagnostic Evaluation

Thyroid function tests are usually normal, although TSH levels may be slightly or moderately elevated. With progressive disease the T_4 decreases, followed by a decrease in T_3 levels and an increase in TSH. A variety of abnormalities in radioactive iodine uptake may be noted. The majority of children have serum antibody titers to thyroid antigens, but fewer children have a positive red blood cell hemagglutination test result. When both tests are used, almost all children with thyroid autoimmunity are detected. However, levels in children are lower than in adults; therefore repeated measurements may be needed in questionable cases because titers may increase later in the disease.

Therapeutic Management

In many cases the goiter is transient and asymptomatic and regresses spontaneously within a year or two. Therapy of a nontoxic diffuse goiter is usually simple, uncomplicated, and effective. Oral administration of TH decreases the size of the gland significantly and provides the feedback needed to suppress TSH stimulation, and the hyperplastic thyroid gland gradually regresses in size. Surgery is contraindicated in this disorder. Evaluate untreated patients periodically.

Nursing Care Management

Nursing care consists of identifying the youngster with thyroid enlargement, reassuring the child that the condition is probably only temporary, and reinforcing instructions for thyroid therapy.

HYPERTHYROIDISM

Graves disease (GD) is the most common cause of hyperthyroidism in children. This disease runs in families and is autoimmune. Most cases of GD in children occur in adolescence, with a peak incidence at 12 to 14 years of age. Transient GD may be present at birth in children of thyrotoxic mothers. The incidence is higher in girls than in boys (Leger & Carel, 2013).

The hyperthyroidism of GD is caused by the generation of autoantibodies to the TSH receptor. This leads to excess secretion of TH. Currently, there is no cure for GD. Choice of treatment continues to be debated among pediatric endocrinologists due to the risk of side effects associated with each option (Leger & Carel, 2013).

Clinical Manifestations

Signs and symptoms of hyperthyroidism develop gradually, with an interval between onset and diagnosis of approximately 6 to 12 months. Clinical features include irritability, hyperactivity, short attention span, tremors, insomnia, and emotional lability. Gradual weight loss despite a voracious appetite occurs in half the cases. Linear growth and bone age are usually accelerated. Muscle weakness often occurs. Hyperactivity of the gastrointestinal tract may cause vomiting and frequent stooling. Cardiac manifestations can include rapid pulse at rest, widened pulse pressure, systolic murmur, and cardiomegaly. Dyspnea may occur during slight exertion, such as climbing stairs. The skin is warm, flushed, and moist. Heat intolerance may be severe and is accompanied by diaphoresis. The hair is unusually fine and unable to hold a wave.

Exophthalmos (protruding eyeballs), observed in many children, is accompanied by a wide-eyed staring expression, increased blinking, lid lag, lack of convergence, and absence of wrinkling of the forehead when looking upward. If exophthalmos progresses, the eyelid may not completely cover the cornea. Visual disturbances may include blurred vision and loss of visual acuity. Eye disease associated with hyperthyroidism can develop before or after the clinical diagnosis.

Diagnostic Evaluation

The diagnosis of GD is established on the basis of increased levels of T_4 and T_3. TSH is suppressed to unmeasurable levels. Other tests are rarely indicated.

Therapeutic Management

Therapy for hyperthyroidism is controversial, but the end goal is the same: to decrease circulating TH. The three available treatments for children are antithyroid drugs, subtotal thyroidectomy, and ablation with radioiodine (^{131}I iodide, RAI) (Hanley, Lord, & Bauer, 2016). Each therapy has advantages and disadvantages.

When affected children exhibit signs and symptoms of hyperthyroidism (e.g., increased weight loss, pulse pressure, and blood pressure), their activity should be limited to schoolwork only. Vigorous exercise is restricted until thyroid levels are decreased to normal or near-normal values. The American Thyroid Association* has an extensive website with information relation to prevention, treatment, and cure of thyroid disease.

Drug Therapy

Antithyroid drug (ATD) therapy with carbimazole, methimazole, or propylthiouracil interferes with the biosynthesis of TH. Most centers use this as first-line treatment for hyperthyroidism. Generally, some improvement is noted within the first 2 weeks, with evidence of decreased nervousness, less fatigue, increased strength, a lowered pulse, and weight gain. In many children an initial treatment course of 1 to 2 years is followed by a complete remission of the disorder. Others require 2 to 4 years before remission is achieved (Leger & Carel, 2013).

ATD disadvantages include drug reactions (e.g., rash, hives, joint pain, nausea, vomiting) and chronic dependency on the drug. Remission is not achieved in many patients, and alternative treatments are required. The most serious side effect of ATDs is agranulocytosis (severe leukopenia), which generally occurs within the initial weeks or months of therapy. It is usually accompanied by a sore throat and fever. Treatment involves immediate discontinuation of the drug and the administration of antibiotics and glucocorticoids until symptoms resolve.

Thyroidectomy

Surgical treatment involves surgical ablation of the thyroid (thyroidectomy). Although this approach has the advantage of being a long-lasting form of therapy, it has a number of serious disadvantages. Hypothyroidism occurs along with the need for thyroxine therapy. Infrequently, recurrent laryngeal nerve palsy, permanent hypoparathyroidism, keloid formation, and surgical morbidity and mortality do occur. Surgery in most centers is reserved for children who fail ATD therapy or who are prone to recurrence.

Radioiodine Therapy

Radioiodine may be a therapy of choice in young patients with GD who relapse after medical treatment (Hanley, Lord, & Bauer, 2016). Low-dose RAI is administered to children to treat hyperthyroidism without resulting in hypothyroidism. The relapse rate is high in this case and may require multiple doses throughout life. RAI should be avoided in very young children due to the increased risk of cancer. More research on RAI in children is needed due to concerns over its potential long-term side effects, including thyroid cancer, hyperparathyroidism, and high mortality rates (Leger & Carel, 2013).

Thyrotoxicosis

Thyrotoxicosis (thyroid "crisis" or thyroid "storm") may occur from sudden release of TH. Although thyrotoxicosis is unusual in children, it can be life threatening. Clinical signs of thyroid storm are acute onset of severe irritability and restlessness, vomiting, diarrhea, hyperthermia, hypertension, severe tachycardia, and prostration. There may be rapid progression to delirium, coma, and death. A crisis may be precipitated by acute infection, surgical emergency, or discontinuation of antithyroid therapy. In addition to ATD therapy, the administration of beta blockers is used to control symptoms until normal thyroid function is achieved (Leger & Carel, 2013). Therapy is usually required for 2 to 3 weeks.

Nursing Care Management

Because the clinical manifestations of GD often appear gradually, the goiter and ophthalmic changes may not be noticed. Excessive activity may be attributed to behavioral problems. Nurses in ambulatory settings, particularly schools, need to be alert to signs that suggest this disorder. Weight loss despite an excellent appetite, inattention, hyperactivity, unexplained fatigue, sleepiness, and difficulty with fine motor skills may be seen. Exophthalmos, infrequent blinking, and impairment of convergence are common presenting signs (Huang & LaFranchi, 2016).

Nursing care focuses on treating physical symptoms before a response to drug therapy is achieved. These children need a quiet, unstimulating environment that is conducive to rest. (See Quality Patient Outcomes box.)

QUALITY PATIENT OUTCOMES

Hyperthyroidism

- Early recognition of signs and symptoms of hyperthyroidism
- Physical symptoms managed
- Regular routine established for child during recovery period
- Adherence to antithyroid drugs as prescribed

*6066 Leesburg Pike, Suite 550, Falls Church, VA 22041; 800-THYROID, 703-998-8890; e-mail: thyroid@thyroid.org; http://www.thyroid.org.

Until hyperthyroidism is controlled, symptoms often interfere with daily life. Emotional lability is often manifested by sudden episodes of crying or elation. Such behavior, coupled with irritability, disrupts interpersonal relationships, creating difficulties within and outside the home. The nurse can help parents understand the medical reason for behavior changes and offer ways to minimize them. A consultation with the child's teachers is important to provide education and suggest ways of helping the child adjust at school.

Heat intolerance may cause a child to dress differently. The use of light cotton clothing in the home, good ventilation, air conditioning or fans, frequent baths, and adequate hydration is helpful in providing comfort. Although the need for calories is increased, these should be provided in wholesome foods rather than "junk" foods.

Nurses should know the side effects of ATD therapy, including urticarial rash, fever, arthritis, or arthralgia. There may be enlargement of the salivary and cervical lymph glands, a diminished sense of taste, hepatitis, and edema of the lower extremities. Parents should also be aware of the signs of hypothyroidism, which can occur from overdose of the drugs. The most common indications are lethargy and somnolence.

DRUG ALERT

Propylthiouracil and Methimazole

Children being treated with propylthiouricil or methimazole must be carefully monitored for side effects. Because sore throat and fever accompany the grave complication of leukopenia, these children should be examined if such symptoms occur. Parents and children should learn to recognize and report symptoms immediately.

Surgical Care

If surgery is anticipated, iodine is administered for a few weeks before the procedure. Because oral iodine preparations are unpalatable, they should be mixed with a strong-tasting fruit juice, such as grape or punch flavors, and be given through a straw. Compliance with iodine therapy is essential to avoid the danger of thyroid crisis after sudden discontinuation.

Psychologic preparation of children for thyroidectomy is similar to that for any other surgical procedure. (See Chapter 22.) However, the fear of having one's throat cut is unique to thyroidectomy. The nurse should explain that the throat is not cut, only the skin, to remove the gland. Showing children a picture of the anatomic location of the thyroid around the trachea is often helpful. Children should be prepared for the dressing around the neck and the possibility of an endotracheal or "breathing" tube after surgery.

Postoperative care involves positioning with the neck slightly flexed to avoid strain on the sutures and observation for bleeding and complications. The children learn to support the neck in this position when they sit up. Damage to the laryngeal nerve is evidenced by severe stridor or hoarseness, although some hoarseness is expected. **Laryngospasm**, a spasmodic contraction of the larynx, can be a life-threatening complication of thyroidectomy. Signs of laryngospasm are stridor, hoarseness, and a feeling of tightness in the throat. Place a tracheostomy set near the bed for emergency use. The nurse should observe for signs of hypoparathyroidism, which causes hypocalcemia, in the immediate postoperative period.

DISORDERS OF PARATHYROID FUNCTION

The parathyroid glands secrete parathyroid hormone (PTH). Along with vitamin D and calcitonin, PTH regulates the homeostasis of serum calcium concentrations (Lal & Clark, 2011). The effect of PTH on calcium is opposite that of calcitonin. Box 31.8 lists the principal effects of PTH on its target sites.

BOX 31.8 Physiologic Effects of Parathyroid Hormone

Bones—Increases osteoclastic activity, causing phosphate-producing bone demineralization

Kidneys—Increases absorption of calcium and excretion of phosphate

Gastrointestinal tract—Promotes calcium absorption

NURSING ALERT

The earliest indication of hypoparathyroidism may be anxiety and mental depression, followed by paresthesia and evidence of heightened neuromuscular excitability, such as the following:

Chvostek sign—Facial muscle spasm elicited by tapping the facial nerve in the region of the parotid gland

Trousseau sign—Carpal spasm elicited by pressure applied to nerves of the upper arm

Tetany—Carpopedal spasm (sharp flexion of wrist and ankle joints), muscle twitching, cramps, seizures, and stridor

PTH and vitamin D work together to maintain serum calcium levels within a narrow normal range and mineralization of bone. Secretion of PTH is controlled by a negative feedback system involving the serum calcium ion concentration. Low ionized calcium levels stimulate PTH secretion, causing absorption of calcium by the target tissues; high ionized calcium concentrations suppress PTH.

HYPOPARATHYROIDISM

Hypoparathyroidism is a spectrum of disorders that result in deficient PTH. Congenital hypoparathyroidism may be caused by a specific defect in the synthesis or cellular processing of PTH or by aplasia or hypoplasia of the gland (Lal & Clark, 2011).

Hypoparathyroidism can occur secondary to other causes. Postoperative hypoparathyroidism may follow thyroidectomy with acute or gradual onset. It may be transient or permanent. Two forms of transient hypoparathyroidism may be present in the newborn, both of which are the result of a relative PTH deficiency. One type is caused by maternal hyperparathyroidism. A more common form appears almost exclusively in infants fed a milk formula with a high phosphate-to-calcium ratio.

Clinical Manifestations

Symptoms vary from none to significant morbidity if treatment is not initiated. Mild deficiency may be identified through laboratory studies. Muscle cramps are an early symptom, progressing to numbness, stiffness, and tingling in the hands and feet. A positive Chvostek or Trousseau sign or laryngeal spasms may be present. Convulsions with loss of consciousness may occur. These episodes may be preceded by abdominal discomfort, tonic rigidity, head retraction, and cyanosis. Headaches and vomiting with increased intracranial pressure and papilledema may occur and may suggest a brain tumor (Doyle, 2016a).

Children with long-standing hypoparathyroidism often have dry, scaly, coarse skin and horizontal lines in the nails. Mucocutaneous eruptions caused by *Candida* organisms are common (Doyle, 2016a). Dental and enamel hypoplasia often occurs. Cataracts develop in patients with untreated disease. Because hypoparathyroidism results in decreased bone resorption and inactive osteoclastic activity, skeletal remodeling and bone turnover are diminished. This may be the pathophysiology of poor growth that is associated with hypoparathyroidism in children (Waller, 2011).

Diagnostic Evaluation

The diagnosis of hypoparathyroidism is made on the basis of clinical manifestations associated with decreased serum calcium and increased serum phosphorus. Levels of plasma PTH are low in idiopathic hypoparathyroidism but high in pseudohypoparathyroidism. End-organ responsiveness is tested by the administration of PTH with measurement of urinary cyclic adenosine monophosphate. Kidney function tests are included in the differential diagnosis to rule out kidney disease. Although bone radiographs are usually normal, they may demonstrate increased bone density and suppressed growth.

Therapeutic Management

The objective of treatment is to maintain normal serum calcium and phosphate levels with minimum complications. Acute or severe tetany is corrected immediately by IV and oral administration of calcium gluconate and follow-up doses as necessary to achieve normal calcium levels. When diagnosis is confirmed, vitamin D therapy is begun. Vitamin D therapy is somewhat difficult to regulate because the drug has a prolonged onset and a long half-life. Some authorities advocate beginning with a lower dose with stepwise increases and careful monitoring of serum calcium until stable levels are achieved. Others prefer rapid induction with higher doses and rapid reduction to lower maintenance levels.

Long-term management administration of massive doses of vitamin D and oral calcium may be useful in maintaining adequate serum calcium levels. Blood calcium and phosphorus are monitored frequently until the levels have stabilized; they are then monitored monthly and less often until the child is seen at 6-month intervals. Renal function, blood pressure, and serum vitamin D levels are measured every 6 months. Serum magnesium levels are measured every 3 to 6 months to permit detection of hypomagnesemia, which may raise the requirement for vitamin D.

Nursing Care Management

The initial objective is recognition of hypocalcemia. Unexplained convulsions, irritability (especially to external stimuli), gastrointestinal symptoms (e.g., diarrhea, vomiting, cramping), and positive signs of tetany should lead the nurse to suspect this disorder. Initial nursing care includes institution of seizure and safety precautions and observation for signs of laryngospasm such as stridor, hoarseness, and a feeling of tightness in the throat. A tracheostomy set and injectable calcium gluconate should be located near the bedside for emergency use. The administration of calcium gluconate requires precautions against extravasation of the drug.

After initiation of treatment, the nurse discusses with the parents the need for continuous daily administration of calcium salts and vitamin D. Because vitamin D toxicity can be a serious consequence of therapy, parents should watch for signs that include weakness, fatigue, lassitude, headache, nausea, vomiting, and diarrhea. Polyuria, polydipsia, and nocturia are signs of early renal impairment.

HYPERPARATHYROIDISM

Hyperparathyroidism is rare in childhood but can be primary or secondary. The most common cause of primary hyperparathyroidism is adenoma of the gland (Doyle, 2016b). Primary hyperparathyroidism is rarely seen in children, but when it occurs, it is often due to a single parathyroid adenoma (Pashtan, Grogan, Kaplan, et al., 2013). The most common causes of secondary hyperparathyroidism are chronic renal disease, renal osteodystrophy, and congenital anomalies of the urinary tract. The common symptom of hyperparathyroidism is hypercalcemia. Box 31.9 lists the manifestations of hyperparathyroidism.

BOX 31.9 Clinical Manifestations of Hyperparathyroidism

Gastrointestinal—Nausea, vomiting, abdominal discomfort, and constipation

Central nervous system—Delusions, confusion, hallucinations, impaired memory, lack of interest and initiative, depression, and varying levels of consciousness

Neuromuscular—Weakness, easy fatigability, muscle atrophy (especially proximal muscles of the lower limbs), twitching of the tongue, and paresthesias in extremities

Skeletal—Vague bone pain, subperiosteal resorption of phalanges, spontaneous fractures, and absence of lamina dura around the teeth

Renal—Polyuria and polydipsia, renal colic, and hypertension

Diagnostic Evaluation

Blood studies to identify elevated calcium and decreased phosphorus levels are routinely performed. Measurement of PTH, as well as several tests to isolate the cause of the hypercalcemia, such as renal function studies, should be included. If parathyroid adenoma is suspected, imaging using ultrasound and a sestamibi nuclear substraction study are recommended (Pashtan, Grogan, Kaplan, et al., 2013). Other procedures used to substantiate the physiologic consequences of the disorder include electrocardiography and radiographic bone surveys.

Therapeutic Management

Treatment depends on the cause of hyperparathyroidism. The treatment of primary hyperparathyroidism is initially medication, but if this has no effect, surgical removal of the tumor or radioactive iodine is used (Huang & LaFranci, 2016). Parathyroidectomy may cause recurrent laryngeal nerve damage, voice impairment, and hypoparathyroidism, but the incidence of these complications is low if the surgeon has extensive experience (Huang & LaFranci, 2016). Treatment of secondary hyperparathyroidism is directed at the underlying contributing cause, which subsequently restores the serum calcium balance. However, in some instances, such as in chronic renal failure, the underlying disorder is irreversible. In this case treatment is aimed at raising serum calcium levels to inhibit the stimulatory effect of low levels on the parathyroid. This includes oral administration of calcium salts, high doses of vitamin D to enhance calcium absorption, a low-phosphorus diet, and administration of a phosphorus-mobilizing aluminum hydroxide to reduce phosphate absorption.

Nursing Care Management

The initial nursing objective is recognition of hyperparathyroidism. Because secondary hyperparathyroidism is a consequence of chronic renal failure, the nurse is always alert to signs that suggest this complication, especially bone pain and fractures. Because urinary symptoms are the earliest indication, assessment of other body systems for evidence of high calcium levels is indicated when polyuria and polydipsia coexist. Clues to the possibility of hyperparathyroidism include change in behavior, especially inactivity; unexplained gastrointestinal symptoms; and cardiac irregularities.

Much of the initial nursing care is related to the physical symptoms and prevention of complications. To minimize renal calculi formation, hydration is essential. Encourage the child to drink fruit juices that maintain a low urinary pH, such as cranberry or apple juice, because acidity of body fluids promotes calcium absorption. All urine should be strained for evidence of renal casts. Children with renal rickets (osteodystrophy) may wear braces to minimize skeletal deformities. These should be worn as prescribed. If the child is confined to bed, the nurse consults with the physical therapist regarding proper use of orthopedic appliances.

Vital signs are taken frequently, and the pulse should be counted for 1 full minute to detect irregularities. Report a decrease in pulse rate because it may signal severe bradycardia and cardiac arrest. The diet needs supervision to ensure compliance with low-phosphate foods, particularly dairy products.

If parathyroidectomy is anticipated, care is similar to that discussed for the child with hyperthyroidism. Because hypocalcemia is a potential complication, observing for signs of tetany, instituting seizure precautions, and having calcium gluconate available for emergency use are part of the nursing care.

DISORDERS OF ADRENAL FUNCTION

ADRENAL HORMONES

The adrenal glands consist of two distinct portions: the cortex, or outer section, and the medulla, or inner core. The adrenal cortex secretes hormones, called steroids, that are essential to life. The adrenal medulla, the inner core, produces the catecholamines epinephrine and norepinephrine. These three chemicals are also produced by the sympathetic nervous system, so if the adrenal supply fails, the body will continue to function.

Adrenal Cortex

The cortex secretes three groups of hormones that are classified according to their biologic activity: (1) glucocorticoids (cortisol, corticosterone), (2) mineralocorticoids (aldosterone), and (3) sex steroids (androgens, estrogens, and progestins). The glucocorticoids and mineralocorticoids affect metabolism and stress. The sex steroids influence sexual development but are not essential because the gonads secrete the major supply of these hormones.

Glucocorticoids

The most important glucocorticoids in humans are cortisol and corticosterone, the principal effects of which are listed in Box 31.10. Normally the hypothalamus secretes CRF, which causes the pituitary gland to produce ACTH, which stimulates the adrenal glands to produce glucocorticoids (primarily cortisol). Cortisol is the switch that controls this feedback. When blood levels of cortisol are low, the system turns on. When blood levels of cortisol rise, the system turns off.

In times of stress the anterior pituitary is stimulated by CRF from the hypothalamus, which causes the release of increased amounts of ACTH. Stressful stimuli capable of provoking this response include trauma; anesthesia; surgical intervention; sepsis; acute anoxia; hypothermia; hypoglycemia; and emotional states, especially panic, anxiety, or anger.

Body rhythms also regulate secretion of the glucocorticoids. Blood levels of cortisol demonstrate a typical diurnal or circadian pattern. In individuals who follow a regular routine of nighttime sleeping, cortisol levels are highest in the early morning hours before waking up and lowest in the evening hours before bedtime.

BOX 31.10 Physiologic Effects of Glucocorticoids

- Stimulation of gluconeogenesis by the liver (a hyperglycemic effect)
- Increased protein catabolism with resulting reduction in protein stores (except in the liver)
- Increased mobilization and utilization of fatty acids for energy
- Increased storage of adipose tissue in certain sites
- Decreased inflammatory and allergic reactions
- Regulation of fluid and electrolytes by promoting sodium retention and potassium excretion by the kidneys and by water diuresis through direct antagonistic action against antidiuretic hormone
- Increased gastric acid and pepsin production
- Suppression of lymphocytes, eosinophils, and basophils, but elevation of neutrophils, erythrocytes, and thrombocytes

Mineralocorticoids

The most important mineralocorticoid is aldosterone. Like cortisol, it promotes sodium retention and potassium excretion in the renal tubules. Aldosterone is significantly more potent than that of the glucocorticoids in maintaining extracellular fluid volume, acid-base balance, and normal potassium levels.

Aldosterone synthesis is regulated primarily by the renin-angiotensin system of the kidney. The juxtaglomerular cells of the kidney respond to decreased arterial pressure or blood volume and to decreased sodium concentrations by secreting the enzyme renin into the blood. Renin in turn converts angiotensinogen to angiotensin I and then to angiotensin II. Increased levels of angiotensin stimulate the adrenal cortex to secrete aldosterone, which preserves sodium, thereby retaining water. The renin-angiotensin mechanism also results in increased blood pressure.

Sex Steroids

Except for the first few days of life, the sex hormones are normally secreted in only minimum amounts until adolescence, at which time they play a role in pubertal changes. Their actions are the same as those of the gonadal hormones on internal and external sexual structures and skeletal growth.

Adrenal Medulla

The adrenal medulla secretes the catecholamines epinephrine and norepinephrine. Both hormones have essentially the same effects on different organs as those caused by direct sympathetic stimulation, except the hormonal effects last several times longer. Their major actions are listed in Box 31.11.

Although the catecholamines evoke similar responses from target sites, there are some important differences. Epinephrine has a greater effect on cardiac activity than norepinephrine, but it causes only weak

BOX 31.11 Physiologic Effects of Catecholamine Secretion

- Increased cardiac activity
- Vasoconstriction of blood vessels (elevation of blood pressure)
- Increased rate and depth of respirations
- Bronchial dilation
- Inhibition of gastrointestinal activity
- Increased muscular contraction
- Pupillary dilation
- Increased metabolic rate
- Heightened sensory awareness
- Diaphoresis

constriction of the blood vessels of muscles in comparison with the effect of norepinephrine. As a result, norepinephrine elevates blood pressure, whereas epinephrine increases cardiac output. Another important difference is their effect on metabolism. Epinephrine increases the metabolic rate to a much greater extent than norepinephrine. These differences in action have been attributed to the catecholamines' effects on α- or β-adrenergic receptors. Norepinephrine can only affect those effector cells that contain α-receptors, which are mostly excitatory (constriction and contraction). Epinephrine, however, can affect both α- and β-receptors, and β-receptors are mostly inhibitory (dilation and relaxation). Control of secretion of catecholamines, primarily in response to physiologic or emotional stress, is through the hypothalamus. Also, stimulation of the sympathetic nervous system results in the release of epinephrine and norepinephrine from the sympathetic nerves and adrenal medulla. Both systems support each other, and one can be substituted for the other. For this reason no condition is attributable to hypofunction of the adrenal medulla. Even in bilateral adrenalectomy, catecholamine replacement is not necessary because the sympathetic release of these chemicals is sufficient to meet all the physiologic functions required to cope with stressful events.

Pheochromocytoma is a rare tumor characterized by secretion of catecholamines. The tumor most commonly arises from the chromaffin cells of the adrenal medulla but may occur wherever these cells are found, such as along the paraganglia of the aorta or thoracolumbar sympathetic chain. In children, they are frequently bilateral or multiple and are generally benign. Often there is a familial transmission of the condition as an autosomal dominant trait (White, 2016a).

The clinical manifestations of pheochromocytoma are caused by an increased production of catecholamines, producing hypertension, tachycardia, headache, decreased gastrointestinal activity and resulting constipation, increased metabolism with anorexia, weight loss, hyperglycemia, polyuria, polydipsia, hyperventilation, nervousness, heat intolerance, and diaphoresis. In severe cases, signs of congestive heart failure are evident.

ACUTE ADRENOCORTICAL INSUFFICIENCY

The acute form of adrenocortical insufficiency (adrenal crisis) may have a number of causes during childhood. Although a rare disorder, some of the more common etiologic factors include hemorrhage into the gland from trauma, which may be caused by a prolonged, difficult labor and rapidly progressing infections, such as meningococcemia, which result in hemorrhage and necrosis (Waterhouse-Friderichsen syndrome). Abrupt withdrawal of exogenous sources of cortisone or failure to increase endogenous supplies during stressor congenital adrenogenital hyperplasia of the salt-losing type can also cause adrenal crisis.

Clinical Manifestations

Early symptoms of adrenocortical insufficiency include increased irritability, headache, diffuse abdominal pain, weakness, nausea and vomiting, and diarrhea. Generalized hemorrhagic manifestations are present in Waterhouse-Friderichsen syndrome. Abnormal serum electrolyte levels include hyponatremia and hyperkalemia. Fever increases as the condition worsens and is accompanied by signs of CNS involvement, such as nuchal rigidity, convulsions, stupor, and coma. The child is in a shocklike state with a weak, rapid pulse; decreased blood pressure; shallow respirations; cold, clammy skin; and cyanosis. Circulatory collapse is the terminal event.

In the newborn, adrenal crisis is accompanied by extreme hyperpyrexia (high temperature), tachypnea, cyanosis, and seizures. Usually there is no evidence of infection or purpura. However, hemorrhage into the adrenal gland may be evident as a palpable retroperitoneal mass.

Diagnostic Evaluation

There is no rapid, definitive test for confirmation of acute adrenocortical insufficiency. Samples for measurement of plasma cortisol and ACTH levels should be sent for analysis, but this is too time consuming to be practical for initial diagnosis. Therefore diagnosis is usually made based on clinical presentation, especially when hemorrhagic manifestations and signs of circulatory collapse despite adequate antibiotic therapy accompany a fulminating sepsis. Serum electrolytes can be helpful in narrowing the diagnosis as well. Because there is no real danger in administering a cortisol preparation for a short period, it is important to institute treatment immediately. Improvement with cortisol therapy confirms the diagnosis.

Therapeutic Management

Treatment involves replacement of cortisol, replacement of body fluids to combat dehydration and hypovolemia, administration of glucose solutions to correct hypoglycemia, and specific antibiotic therapy in the presence of infection. Initially, IV hydrocortisone (Solu-Cortef) is administered. Normal saline containing 5% glucose is given parenterally to replace lost fluid, electrolytes, and glucose. If hemorrhage has been severe, whole blood may be replaced. In the event that these measures do not reverse the circulatory collapse, vasopressors are used for immediate vasoconstriction and elevation of blood pressure.

After the child's condition has been stabilized, oral doses of cortisone, fluids, and salt are given, similar to the regimen used for chronic adrenal insufficiency. To maintain sodium retention, aldosterone is replaced by synthetic salt-retaining steroids.

Nursing Care Management

Because of the abrupt onset and potentially fatal outcome of this condition, prompt recognition is essential. Vital signs and blood pressure are taken every 15 minutes. Seizure precautions are instituted. The nurse should monitor the child's response to fluid and cortisol replacement. Rapid administration of fluids can precipitate cardiac failure and overdosage with cortisol may cause hypotension and a sudden fall in temperature.

When the acute phase is over and the hypovolemia has been corrected, the child is given oral fluids in small quantities. Rapid ingestion of oral fluids may induce vomiting, which increases dehydration. Therefore the nurse should plan a gradual schedule for reintroducing liquids. (See Quality Patient Outcomes box.)

QUALITY PATIENT OUTCOMES

Acute Adrenocortical Insufficiency

- Early recognition of signs and symptoms of acute adrenal crisis
- Hypokalemia or hyperkalemia prevented
- Fluid balance maintained
- Sufficient cortisol replacement

! NURSING ALERT

Monitor serum electrolyte levels and observe for signs of hypokalemia or hyperkalemia (e.g., weakness, poor muscle control, paralysis, cardiac dysrhythmias, and apnea). The condition is rapidly corrected with IV or oral potassium replacement.

! NURSING ALERT

When an oral potassium preparation is given, mix it with a small amount of strongly flavored fruit juice to disguise its bitter taste.

The sudden, severe nature of this disorder necessitates a great deal of emotional support for the child and family. The child may be placed in an intensive care unit where the surroundings are strange and frightening. Despite the need for emergency intervention, the nurse must be sensitive to the family's psychologic needs and prepare them for each procedure, even if this is as brief as a statement such as "The IV infusion is necessary to replace fluid that the child is losing." Because recovery within 24 hours is often dramatic, the nurse should keep the parents apprised of the child's condition, emphasizing signs of improvement, such as a lowered temperature and normal blood pressure.

If treatment needs to be continued past the acute stage, parents require the same preparation as in the case of children with chronic adrenal insufficiency. Preparation for discharge should begin as soon as possible after the child's condition has stabilized.

CHRONIC ADRENOCORTICAL INSUFFICIENCY (ADDISON DISEASE)

Chronic adrenocortical insufficiency is rare in children. Causes include infection, a destructive lesion of the adrenal gland, and autoimmune processes, but the cause may also be idiopathic. Because 90% of adrenal tissue must be nonfunctional before signs of insufficiency are manifested, onset of symptoms is often gradual. However, during periods of stress, when demands for additional cortisol are increased, symptoms of acute insufficiency may appear in a previously well child (Box 31.12).

Definitive diagnosis is based on measurements of functional cortisol reserve. The fasting serum cortisol and urinary 17-hydroxycorticosteroid levels are low and fail to rise, and plasma ACTH levels are elevated with corticotropin (ACTH) stimulation, the definitive test for the disease.

Therapeutic Management

Treatment involves replacement of glucocorticoids (cortisol) and mineralocorticoids (aldosterone). Some children are able to be maintained solely on oral supplements of cortisol (cortisone or hydrocortisone preparations) with a liberal intake of salt. During stressful situations (e.g., fever, infection, emotional upset, or surgery), the dosage must be tripled to accommodate the body's increased need for glucocorticoids. Failure to meet this requirement will precipitate an acute crisis. Overdosage produces appearance of cushingoid signs.

Children with more severe states of chronic adrenal insufficiency require mineralocorticoid replacement to maintain fluid and electrolyte balance. Other forms of therapy include monthly injections of desoxycorticosterone acetate or implantation of desoxycorticosterone acetate pellets subcutaneously every 9 to 12 months.

Nursing Care Management

After the disorder is diagnosed, parents need guidance concerning drug therapy. They must be aware of the continuous need for cortisol replacement. Sudden termination of the drug because of inadequate supplies or inability to ingest the oral form because of vomiting places

BOX 31.12 Clinical Manifestations of Acute and Chronic Adrenocortical Insufficiency

Clinical Manifestations of Acute Adrenocortical Insufficiency

Early Symptoms

Increased irritability
Headache
Diffuse abdominal pain
Weakness
Nausea and vomiting
Diarrhea
Generalized hemorrhagic manifestations (Waterhouse-Friderichsen syndrome)
Fever (increases as condition worsens)
Central nervous system signs:

- Nuchal rigidity
- Seizures
- Stupor
- Coma

Shocklike state
Weak, rapid pulse
Decreased blood pressure
Shallow respirations
Cold, clammy skin
Cyanosis
Circulatory collapse (terminal event)

Newborn

Hyperpyrexia
Tachypnea
Cyanosis
Seizures
Gland evident as palpable retroperitoneal mass (hemorrhagic)

Clinical Manifestations of Chronic Adrenocortical Insufficiency

Neurologic symptoms
Muscular weakness
Mental fatigue
Irritability, apathy, and negativism
Increased sleeping, listlessness
Pigmentary changes
Previous scars
Palmar creases
Mucous membranes
Hair
Hyperpigmentation over pressure points (elbows, knees, or waist)
Less frequently, vitiligo (loss of pigmentation)
Gastrointestinal symptoms
Dehydration
Anorexia
Weight loss
Circulatory symptoms
Hypotension
Small heart size
Dizziness
Syncopal (fainting) attacks
Hypoglycemia
Headache
Hunger
Weakness
Trembling
Sweating

Other Signs (Seen in Some Children)

Recurrent, unexplained seizures
Intense craving for salt
Acute abdominal pain
Electrolyte imbalances

the child in danger of an acute adrenal crisis. Parents should always have a spare supply of medication. Ideally, families will have a prefilled syringe of hydrocortisone and have training to administer this drug during a crisis. Unnecessary administration of cortisone will not harm the child, but if it is needed, it may be lifesaving. Any evidence of acute insufficiency is reported to the practitioner immediately.

Parents also need to be aware of side effects of the drugs. Undesirable side effects of cortisone include gastric irritation, which is minimized by ingestion with food or the use of an antacid; increased excitability and sleeplessness; weight gain, which may require dietary management to prevent obesity; and occasionally behavioral changes, including depression or euphoria. Parents should be aware of signs of overdose and report these to the practitioner. In addition, the drug has a bitter taste, which creates a challenge in its administration.

Because the body cannot supply endogenous sources of cortical hormones during times of stress, the home environment should be stable and relatively unstressful. Parents need to be aware that during periods of emotional or physical crisis, the child requires additional hormone replacement. The child should wear a medical identification bracelet, to notify medical personnel during emergency care.

CUSHING SYNDROME

Cushing syndrome is a characteristic group of manifestations caused by excessive circulating free cortisol. It can result from a variety of causes, which generally fall into one of five categories (Table 31.1).

Cushing syndrome is uncommon in children. When seen, it is often caused by excessive or prolonged steroid therapy that produces a cushingoid appearance (Fig. 31.4). This condition is reversible after the steroids are gradually discontinued. Abrupt withdrawal will precipitate acute adrenal insufficiency. Gradual withdrawal of exogenous supplies is necessary to allow the anterior pituitary an opportunity to secrete increasing amounts of ACTH to stimulate the adrenals to produce cortisol.

Clinical Manifestations

Because the actions of cortisol are widespread, clinical manifestations are equally profound and diverse. The symptoms that produce changes in physical appearance occur early in the disorder and are of considerable concern to school-age and older children (Fig. 31.5). The physiologic disturbances, such as hyperglycemia, susceptibility to infection, hypertension, and hypokalemia, may have life-threatening consequences unless recognized early and treated successfully. Children with short stature may be responding to increased cortisol levels, resulting in Cushing syndrome. Cortisol inhibits the action of GH.

Diagnostic Evaluation

Several tests are helpful in confirming Cushing syndrome. Serum cortisol levels should be measured at midnight and in the morning along with corticotropin hormone, urinary free cortisol, fasting blood glucose levels for hyperglycemia, serum electrolyte levels for hypokalemia and alkalosis, and 24-hour urinary levels of elevated 17-hydroxycorticoids and 17-ketosteroids (Lowitz & Keil, 2015). Imaging of the pituitary and adrenal glands to assess for tumors, bone density studies for evidence of osteoporosis, and skull radiographs to determine enlargement of the sella turcica may also aid in the diagnosis. Another procedure used to establish a more definitive diagnosis is the dexamethasone (cortisone) suppression test (Ceccato & Boscaro, 2016). Administration of an exogenous supply of cortisone normally suppresses ACTH production. However, in individuals with Cushing syndrome, cortisol levels remain elevated. This test is helpful in differentiating between children who are obese and those who appear to have cushingoid features.

TABLE 31.1 Clinical Manifestations of Cushing Syndrome

Signs and Symptoms	Physiologic Cause
Centripetal fat distribution Truncal obesity Supraclavicular fat pads Fat pads on neck and back (buffalo hump) Rounded or "moon" face	Increased appetite and deposition of fat
Muscular wasting Thin extremities Pendulous abdomen Muscle weakness Thin skin and subcutaneous tissue Poor wound healing	Increased protein catabolism resulting in negative nitrogen balance
Increased frequency of infection Decreased inflammatory response	Decreased production and circulating levels of antibodies by lysis of fixed plasma cells and lymphocytes
Excessive bruising Petechial hemorrhages	Capillary weakness resulting from loss of protein
Facial plethora ("red cheeks") Reddish purple abdominal striae	Thin skin allowing capillary blood to be visible; increased color from polycythemia
Hypertension—arteriosclerosis	Increased salt and water retention (hypervolemia)
Hypokalemia Alkalosis	Increased excretion of potassium and hydrogen ions
Osteoporosis Compression fractures of vertebrae Kyphosis Backache	Increased glomerular filtration rate and excretion of calcium and decreased absorption of calcium from intestinal tract
Stunted linear growth (short stature) Delayed bone age	Increased levels of cortisol interfering with action of growth hormone
Hypercalciuria—renal calculi	Excessive amount of calcium in urine
Psychoses Irritability Insomnia Euphoria Depression Frank psychoses	Cause unknown
Peptic ulcer	Increased production of hydrochloric acid and pepsin and decreased gastric mucus production
Glycosuria	Increased gluconeogenesis by liver and decreased rate of glucose utilization by cells
Latent or overt diabetes	Overstimulation of islets of Langerhans
Virilization Hirsutism (excessive body hair) Acne Deepening of voice Clitoral enlargement Tendency toward male physique in female Amenorrhea Impotence	Excess production of androgens

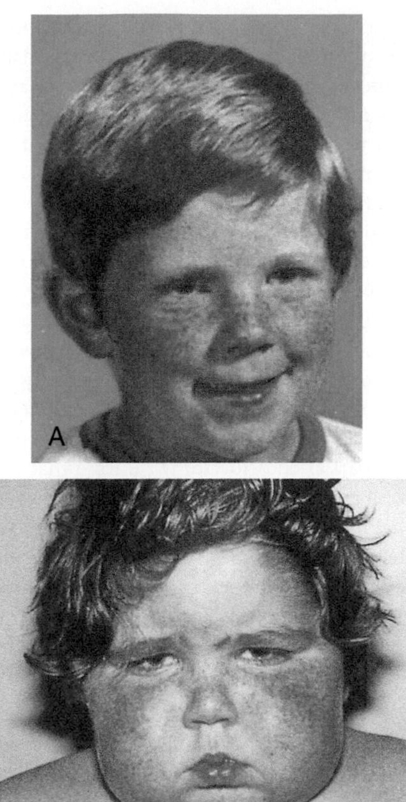

FIG. 31.4 A, Boy before development of Cushing syndrome. **B,** Same boy 4 months after onset of Cushing syndrome. (From Zitelli, B. J., & Davis, H. W. [2007]. *Atlas of pediatric physical diagnosis* [5th ed.]. St. Louis, MO: Mosby.)

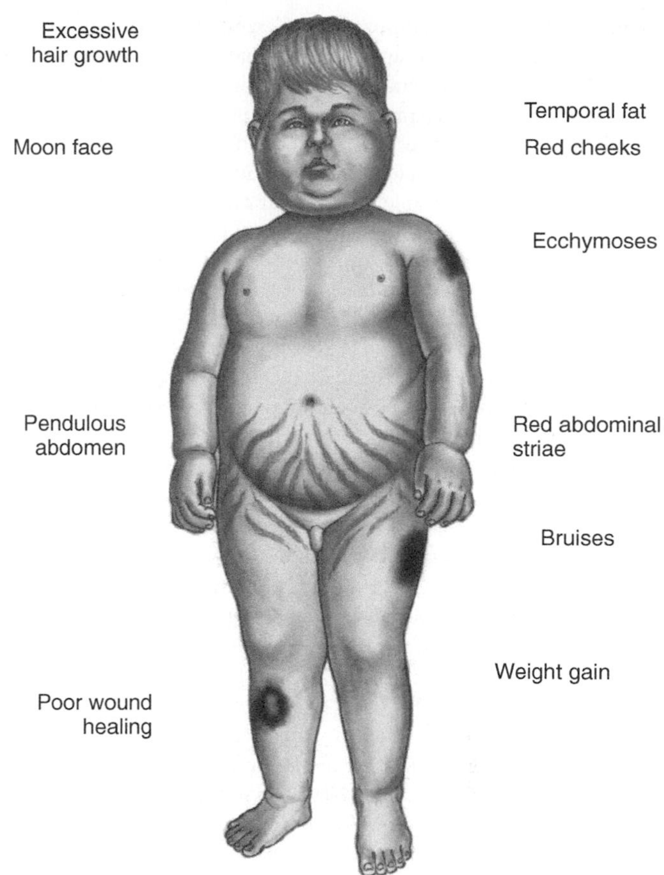

FIG. 31.5 Characteristics of Cushing syndrome.

Therapeutic Management

Treatment depends on the cause. In most cases, surgical intervention involves bilateral adrenalectomy and postoperative replacement of the cortical hormones (the therapy for this is the same as that outlined for chronic adrenocortical insufficiency). If a pituitary tumor is found, surgical extirpation or irradiation may be chosen. In either of these instances, treatment of panhypopituitarism with replacement of GH, TH, ADH, gonadotropins, and steroids may be necessary for an indefinite period (Lau, Rutledge, & Aghi, 2015).

Nursing Care Management

Nursing care also depends on the cause. When cushingoid features are caused by steroid therapy, the effects may be lessened with administration of the drug early in the morning and on an alternate-day basis. Giving the drug early in the day maintains the normal diurnal pattern of cortisol secretion. If given during the evening, it is more likely to produce symptoms because endogenous cortisol levels are already low, and the additional supply exerts more pronounced effects. An alternate-day schedule allows the anterior pituitary an opportunity to maintain more normal hypothalamic–pituitary–adrenal control mechanisms.

If an organic cause is found, nursing care is related to the treatment regimen. Although a bilateral adrenalectomy permanently solves one condition, it reciprocally produces another syndrome. Before surgery, parents need to be adequately informed of the operative benefits and disadvantages. Postoperative teaching regarding drug replacement is the same as discussed in the previous section.

> **! NURSING ALERT**
>
> Postoperative complications of adrenalectomy are related to the sudden withdrawal of cortisol. Observe for shocklike symptoms (e.g., hypotension, hyperpyrexia).

Anorexia and nausea and vomiting are common and may be improved with the use of nasogastric decompression. Muscle and joint pain may be severe, requiring use of analgesics. The psychologic depression can be profound and may not improve for months. Parents should be aware of the physiologic reasons behind these symptoms in order to be supportive of the child.

CONGENITAL ADRENAL HYPERPLASIA

Congenital adrenal hyperplasia (CAH) is a family of disorders caused by decreased enzyme activity required for cortisol production in the adrenal cortex. The adrenal gland produces excessive amounts of cortisol precursors and androgens to compensate. There are seven types of biochemical defects with the most common defect being 21-hydroxylase deficiency, which constitutes more than 90% of all cases of CAH (El-Maouche, Arlt, & Merke, 2017). This deficiency is an autosomal recessive disorder that results in improper steroid hormone synthesis (Mendes, Vaz Matos, Ribeiro, et al., 2015).

Clinical Manifestations

Excessive androgens cause masculinization of the urogenital system at approximately the tenth week of fetal development. The most pronounced abnormalities occur in girls, who are born with varying degrees of ambiguous genitalia. Masculinization of external genitalia causes the clitoris to enlarge so that it appears as a small phallus. Fusion of the labia produces a saclike structure resembling the scrotum without testes. However, no abnormal changes occur in the internal sexual organs, although the vaginal orifice is usually closed by the fused labia. The label *ambiguous genitalia* should be applied to any infant with hypospadias or micropenis and no palpable gonads, and a diagnostic evaluation for CAH should be contemplated (Carroll, Aron, Findling, et al., 2011).

Increased pigmentation of skin creases and genitalia caused by increased ACTH may be a subtle sign of adrenal insufficiency. A salt-wasting crisis frequently occurs, usually within the first few weeks of life (White, 2016b). Infants fail to gain weight, and hyponatremia and hyperkalemia may be significant. Cardiac arrest can occur.

Untreated CAH results in early sexual maturation, with enlargement of the external sexual organs; development of axillary, pubic, and facial hair; deepening of the voice; acne; and a marked increase in musculature with changes toward an adult male physique. However, in contrast to precocious puberty, breasts do not develop in girls, and they remain amenorrheic and infertile. In boys, the testes remain small, and spermatogenesis does not occur. In both sexes, linear growth is accelerated, and epiphyseal closure is premature, resulting in short stature by the end of puberty.

Diagnostic Evaluation

Clinical diagnosis is initially based on congenital abnormalities that lead to difficulty in assigning sex to the newborn and on signs and symptoms of adrenal insufficiency. Newborn screening is currently done in all 50 states by measurement of the cortisol precursor 17-hydroxyprogesterone. Definitive diagnosis is confirmed by evidence of increased 17-ketosteroid levels in most types of CAH (El-Maouche, Arlt, & Merke, 2017). In complete 21-hydroxylase deficiency, blood electrolytes demonstrate loss of sodium and chloride and elevation of potassium. In older children, bone age is advanced and linear growth is increased. DNA analysis for positive sex determination and to rule out any other genetic abnormality (e.g., Turner syndrome) is always done in any case of ambiguous genitalia.

Another test that can be used to visualize the presence of pelvic structures is ultrasonography, a noninvasive, painless imaging technique that does not require anesthesia or sedation. It is especially useful in CAH because it readily identifies the absence or presence of female reproductive organs or male testes in a newborn or child with ambiguous genitalia. Because ultrasonography yields immediate results, it has the advantage of determining the child's gender long before the more complex laboratory results for chromosome analysis or steroid levels are available.

Therapeutic Management

After diagnosis is confirmed, medical management includes administration of glucocorticoids to suppress the abnormally high secretions of ACTH and adrenal androgens. If cortisone is begun early enough, it is very effective. Cortisone depresses the secretion of ACTH by the anterior pituitary, which in turn inhibits the secretion of adrenocorticosteroids, which stems the progressive virilization. The signs and symptoms of masculinization in girls gradually disappear, and excessive early linear growth is slowed. Puberty occurs normally at the appropriate age.

The recommended oral dosage is divided to simulate the normal diurnal pattern of ACTH secretion. Because these children are unable to produce cortisol in response to stress, it is necessary to increase the dosage during episodes of infection, fever, surgery, or other stresses. Acute emergencies require immediate IV or intramuscular administration. Emergency situations include bacterial and viral infections, vomiting, surgery, fractures, major injuries, and sometimes insect stings.

Children with the salt-losing type of CAH require aldosterone replacement, as outlined under chronic adrenal insufficiency, and supplementary dietary salt. Frequent laboratory tests are conducted to assess the effects on electrolytes, hormonal profiles, and renin levels. The frequency of testing is individualized to the child.

Gender assignment and surgical intervention in the newborn with ambiguous genitalia is complex and controversial. It is a significant stress for families, who need support and education from a multidisciplinary team of experienced specialists. Factors that influence gender assignment include genetic diagnosis, genital appearance, surgical options, fertility, and family and cultural preferences. Generally, genetically female (46XX) infants should be raised as girls. Early reconstructive surgery should be considered only in the case of severe virilization (El-Maouche, Arlt, & Merke, 2017). Emphasis is on functional rather than cosmetic outcomes, and surgery can often be delayed. Reports concerning sexual satisfaction after partial clitoridectomy indicate that the capacity for orgasm and sexual gratification is not necessarily impaired. Male infants may require phallic reconstruction by an experienced surgeon.

Unfortunately, not all children with CAH are diagnosed at birth and raised in accordance with their genetic sex. Particularly in the case of affected females, masculinization of the external genitalia may have led to sex assignment as a male. In males, diagnosis is usually delayed until early childhood, when signs of virilism appear. In these situations, it is advisable to continue rearing the child as a male in accordance with assigned sex and phenotype. Hormone replacement may be required to permit linear growth and to initiate male pubertal changes. Surgery is usually indicated to remove the female organs and reconstruct the phallus for satisfactory sexual relations. These individuals are not fertile.

Nursing Care Management

Of major importance is recognition of ambiguous genitalia and diagnostic confirmation in newborns. Parents need assistance in understanding and accepting the condition and time to grieve for the loss of perfection in their newborn child. As soon as the sex is determined, parents should be informed of the findings and encouraged to choose an appropriate name, and the child should be identified as a male or female with no reference to ambiguous sex.

In general, rearing a genetically female child as a girl is preferred because of the success of surgical intervention and the satisfactory results with hormones in reversing virilism and providing a prospect of normal puberty and the ability to conceive. This is in contrast to the choice of rearing the child as a boy, in which case the child is sterile and may never be able to function satisfactorily in heterosexual relationships. If the parents persist in their decision to assign a male sex to a genetically female child, a psychologic consultation should be requested to explore their motivations and ensure their understanding of the future consequences for the child.

Nursing care management regarding cortisol and aldosterone replacement is the same as that discussed for chronic adrenocortical insufficiency. Because infants are especially prone to dehydration and salt-losing crises, parents need to be aware of signs of dehydration and the urgency of immediate medical intervention to stabilize the child's condition. Parents should have injectable hydrocortisone available and know how to prepare and administer the intramuscular injection (see Chapter 19). Parents, and later the child, need to understand that the medical regimen must be a lifelong commitment; therefore provide them with the education and counseling that is most likely to ensure informed and willing compliance.

In the unfortunate situation in which the sex is erroneously assigned and the correct sex determined later, parents need a great deal of help in understanding the reason for the incorrect sex identification and the options for sex reassignment or medical-surgical intervention.

Parents should be referred for genetic counseling before they conceive another child because CAH is an autosomal recessive disorder. Prenatal diagnosis and treatment are available.

! NURSING ALERT

Advise parents that there is no physical harm in treating for suspected adrenal insufficiency that is not present, but the consequence of not treating acute adrenal insufficiency can be fatal.

HYPERALDOSTERONISM

Excessive secretion of aldosterone may be caused by an adrenal tumor or, in some types of adrenogenital syndromes, result from enzymatic deficiency. The signs and symptoms are caused by increased sodium levels, water retention, and potassium loss. Hypervolemia causes hypertension and resultant headaches. Hypokalemia results in muscular weakness, paresthesia, episodes of paralysis, and tetany and may be responsible for polyuria and consequent polydipsia.

The clinical diagnosis is suspected when there are findings of hypertension, hypokalemia, and polyuria that fail to respond to ADH administration. Renin and angiotensin titers are abnormally low. Urinary levels of 17-hydroxycorticosteroids and 17-ketosteroids are normal in primary hyperaldosteronism caused by an aldosterone-secreting tumor but are usually abnormal in adrenogenital syndrome.

Therapeutic Management

Temporary treatment of the disorder involves replacement of potassium and administration of spironolactone (Aldactone), a diuretic that blocks the effects of aldosterone, thereby promoting excretion of sodium and water, while preserving potassium. Definitive treatment is similar to that for chronic adrenocortical insufficiency.

Nursing Care Management

An important nursing consideration is recognition of the syndrome, particularly in children with high blood pressure. Other clues include bed-wetting, excessive thirst, and unexplained weakness. After the diagnosis, nursing care is related to the treatment regimen. If diuretics are used, they should be administered in the morning to avoid accidents during the night. Children need unrestricted restroom privileges at school. Potassium supplements should be mixed with fruit juice such as grape juice to increase their acceptability, and potassium-rich foods should be encouraged. Parents need to be aware of the signs of hypokalemia and hyperkalemia. After an adrenalectomy, nursing care is similar to that for chronic adrenocortical insufficiency.

PHEOCHROMOCYTOMA

Pheochromocytoma is a rare tumor characterized by secretion of catecholamines. The tumor most commonly arises from the chromaffin cells of the adrenal medulla but may occur wherever these cells are found, such as along the paraganglia of the aorta or thoracolumbar sympathetic chain. In children, they are frequently bilateral or multiple and are generally benign. Often there is a familial transmission of the condition as an autosomal dominant trait (White, 2016a).

Clinical Manifestations

The clinical manifestations of pheochromocytoma are caused by an increased production of catecholamines, producing hypertension, tachycardia, headache, decreased gastrointestinal activity with resulting constipation, increased metabolism with anorexia, weight loss, hyperglycemia, polyuria, polydipsia, hyperventilation, nervousness, heat intolerance, and diaphoresis. In severe cases, signs of congestive heart failure are evident.

Diagnostic Evaluation

The clinical manifestations mimic those of other disorders, such as hyperthyroidism or DM. Tests specific to these conditions may be performed as part of the differential diagnosis. In a small number of instances a palpable tumor suggests the diagnosis. Usually the tumor is identified by CT scan or MRI. Definitive tests include 24-hour measurement of urinary levels of the catecholamine metabolites (Young, 2016).

Therapeutic Management

Definitive treatment consists of surgical removal of the tumor. In children, the tumors may be bilateral, requiring a bilateral adrenalectomy and lifelong glucocorticoid and mineralocorticoid therapy. The major complications that can occur during surgery are severe hypertension, tachyarrhythmias, and hypotension. The first two are caused by excessive release of catecholamines during manipulation of the tumor, and the latter results from catecholamine withdrawal and hypovolemic shock.

Preoperative medication to inhibit the effects of catecholamines is begun 1 to 3 weeks before surgery to prevent these complications. The major group of drugs used is the α-adrenergic blocking agents with or without β-adrenergic blocking agents. The most commonly used α-adrenergic blocker is phenoxybenzamine (Dibenzyline). To control catecholamine release after α-adrenergic blockage has been achieved, the child is given β-adrenergic blocking agents.

Success of therapy is judged by lowering of blood pressure to normal, absence of hypertensive attacks (e.g., flushing or blanching, fainting, headache, palpitations, tachycardia, nausea and vomiting, profuse sweating), heat tolerance, decrease in perspiration, and disappearance of hyperglycemia.

Nursing Care Management

An initial nursing objective is identification of children with this disorder. Children with hypertension and hypertensive attacks should be assessed for pheochromocytoma. Because of behavioral changes (nervousness, excitability, overactivity, and even psychosis), increased cardiac and respiratory activity may appear to be related to an acute anxiety attack. Therefore a careful history of the onset of symptoms and association with stressful events is helpful in distinguishing between an organic and a psychologic cause for the symptoms.

Preoperative nursing care involves frequent monitoring of vital signs and observation for evidence of hypertensive attacks and congestive heart failure. Therapeutic effects are evidenced by normal vital signs and absence of glycosuria. Note daily blood glucose levels, urine acetone, and any signs of hyperglycemia and report immediately.

! NURSING ALERT

Do not palpate the mass. Preoperative palpation of the mass releases catecholamines, which can stimulate severe hypertension and tachyarrhythmias.

The environment is made conducive to rest and free of emotional stress. This requires adequate preparation during hospital admission and before surgery. Parents are encouraged to room-in with their child and to participate in care. Play activities need to be tailored to the child's energy level without being overly strenuous or challenging because these can increase metabolic rate and promote frustration and anxiety.

After surgery, the child is observed for signs of shock from removal of excess catecholamines. If a bilateral adrenalectomy was performed, the nursing interventions are those discussed for chronic adrenocortical insufficiency.

DISORDERS OF PANCREATIC HORMONE SECRETION

DIABETES MELLITUS

DM is a chronic disorder of metabolism characterized by hyperglycemia and insulin resistance. It is the most common metabolic disease, resulting in metabolic adjustment or physiologic change in almost all areas of the body. In the United States during 2014, approximately 208,000 children younger than 20 years old had either type 1 or type 2 diabetes (Centers for Disease Control and Prevention, 2015). The odds are higher for African American and Hispanic children (Centers for Disease Control and Prevention, 2015). DM in children can occur at any age, but 40% of children diagnosed are between 10 and 14 years old and 60% are between 15 and 19 years old. Girls are 1.3 to 1.7 times more likely to develop type 2 diabetes than boys (Laffel & Svoren, 2015).

Traditionally, DM had been classified according to the type of treatment needed. The old categories were insulin-dependent diabetes mellitus (IDDM), or type I, and non–insulin-dependent diabetes mellitus (NIDDM), or type II. In 1997 these terms were eliminated because treatment can vary (some people with NIDDM require insulin) and because the terms do not indicate the underlying problem. The new terms are *type 1* and *type 2,* using Arabic symbols to avoid confusion (e.g., type II could be read as type eleven) (American Diabetes Association, 2007). The characteristics of type 1 DM and type 2 DM are outlined in Table 31.2.

In children younger than 10 years old, most diabetes cases are type 1 and occur frequently in non-Hispanic whites. In the age-group 10 to 19 years old, type 1 diabetes is more prominent in non-Hispanic whites followed by African Americans and then Hispanics; the lowest prevalence is among American Indians.

Type 1 diabetes is characterized by destruction of the pancreatic β cells, which produce insulin; this usually leads to absolute insulin deficiency (Fig. 31.6). Type 1 diabetes has two forms. Immune-mediated DM results from an autoimmune destruction of the β cells; it typically starts in children or young adults who are slim, but it can arise in adults of any age. Idiopathic type 1 refers to rare forms of the disease that have no known cause.

Type 2 diabetes usually arises because of insulin resistance in which the body fails to use insulin properly combined with relative (rather than absolute) insulin deficiency. People with type 2 can range from predominantly insulin resistant with relative insulin deficiency to predominantly deficient in insulin secretion with some insulin resistance. It typically occurs in those who are older than 45 years of age, are overweight and sedentary, and have a family history of diabetes.

The symptomatology of diabetes is more readily recognizable in children than in adults, so it is surprising that the diagnosis may sometimes be missed or delayed. Diabetes is a great imitator; influenza, gastroenteritis, and appendicitis are the conditions most often diagnosed when it turns out that the disease is really diabetes (Box 31.13).

Pathophysiology

Insulin is needed to support the metabolism of carbohydrates, fats, and proteins, primarily by facilitating the entry of these substances into the cells. Insulin is needed for the entry of glucose into the muscle and fat cells, prevention of mobilization of fats from fat cells, and storage of glucose as glycogen in the cells of liver and muscle. Insulin is not needed for the entry of glucose into nerve cells or vascular tissue. The chemical composition and molecular structure of insulin are such that it fits into receptor sites on the cell membrane. Here it initiates a sequence of poorly defined chemical reactions that alter the cell membrane to facilitate the entry of glucose into the cell and stimulate enzymatic systems outside the cell that metabolize the glucose for energy production.

TABLE 31.2 Characteristics of Types 1 and 2 Diabetes Mellitus

Characteristic	Type 1	Type 2
Age at onset	<20 years	Increasingly occurring in younger children
Type of onset	Abrupt	Gradual
Sex ratio	Affects males slightly more than females	Females outnumber males
Percentage of diabetic population	5%-8%	85%-90%
Heredity:		
Family history	Sometimes	Frequently
Human leukocyte antigen	Associations	No association
Twin concordance	25%-50%	90%-100%
Ethnic distribution	Primarily whites	Increased incidence in American Indians, Hispanics, African Americans
Presenting symptoms	Three Ps common—polyuria, polydipsia, polyphagia	May be related to long-term complications
Nutritional status	Underweight	Overweight
Insulin (natural):		
Pancreatic content	Usually none	>50% normal
Serum insulin	Low to absent	High or low
Primary resistance	Minimum	Marked
Islet cell antibodies	80%-85%	<5%
Therapy:		
Insulin	Always	20%-30% of patients
Oral agents	Ineffective	Often effective
Diet only	Ineffective	Often effective
Chronic complications	>80%	Variable
Ketoacidosis	Common	Infrequent

With a deficiency of insulin, glucose is unable to enter the cells, and its concentration in the bloodstream increases. The increased concentration of glucose (hyperglycemia) produces an osmotic gradient that causes the movement of body fluid from the intracellular space to the interstitial space and then to the extracellular space and into the glomerular filtrate to "dilute" the hyperosmolar filtrate. Normally, the renal tubular capacity to transport glucose is adequate to reabsorb all the glucose in the glomerular filtrate. When the glucose concentration in the glomerular filtrate exceeds the renal threshold (180 mg/dl), glucose spills into the urine (glycosuria) along with an osmotic diversion of water (polyuria), a cardinal sign of diabetes. The urinary fluid losses cause the excessive thirst (polydipsia) observed in diabetes. This water "washout" results in a depletion of other essential chemicals, especially potassium.

Protein is also wasted during insulin deficiency. Because glucose is unable to enter the cells, protein is broken down and converted to glucose by the liver (glucogenesis); this glucose then contributes to the hyperglycemia. These mechanisms are similar to those seen in starvation when substrate (glucose) is absent. The body is actually in a state of starvation during insulin deficiency. Without the use of carbohydrates

PATHOPHYSIOLOGY REVIEW

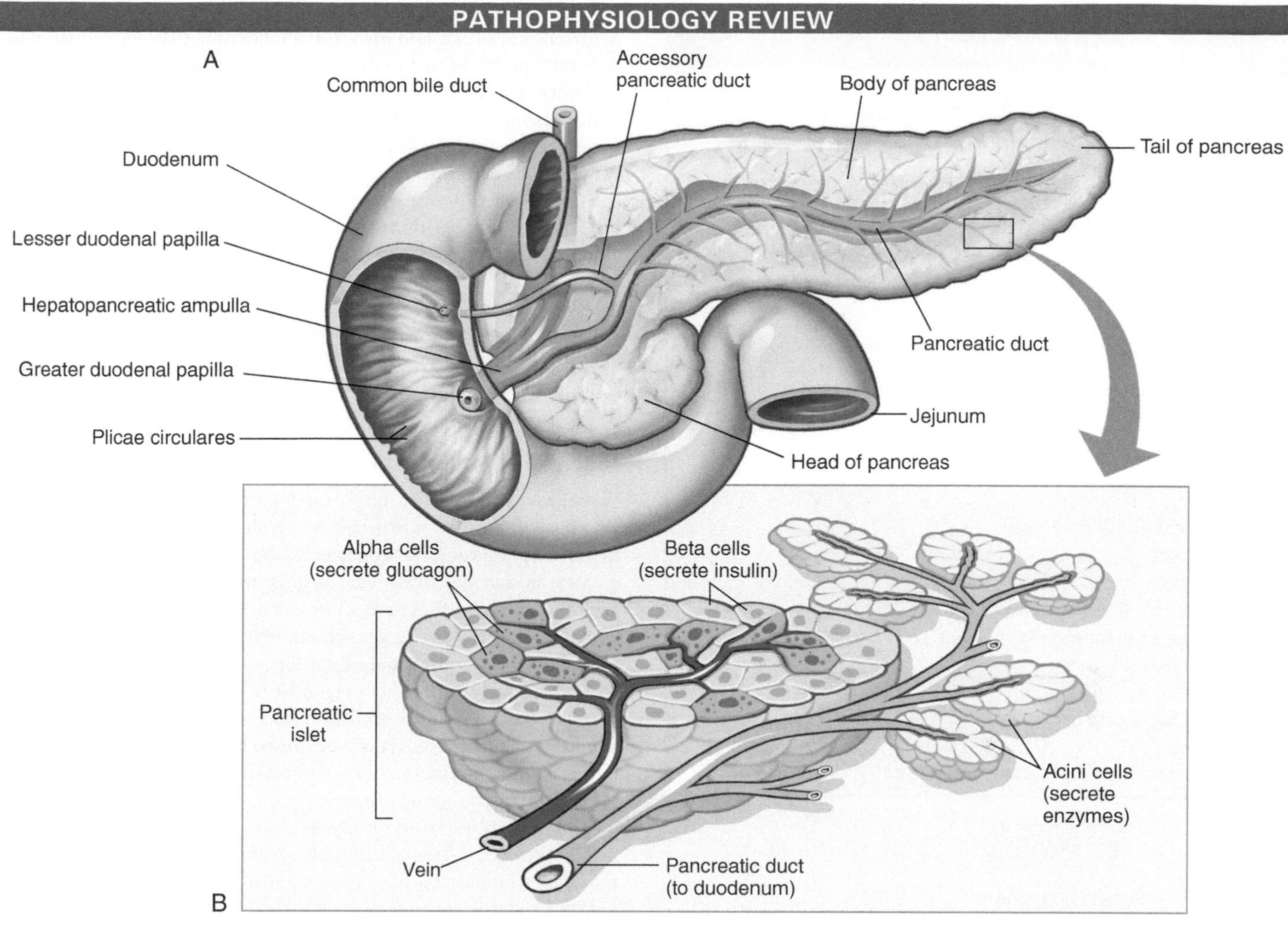

FIG. 31.6 The pancreas. **A,** The main and accessory ducts. **B,** Glandular cells of the pancreatic islets. (From Patton, K. T., & Thibodeau, G. A. [2010]. *Anatomy and physiology* [7th ed.]. St. Louis, MO: Mosby.)

for energy, fat and protein stores are depleted as the body attempts to meet its energy needs. The hunger mechanism is triggered, but increased food intake (polyphagia) enhances the problem by further elevating blood glucose (Fig. 31.7).

Ketoacidosis

When insulin is absent or insulin sensitivity is altered, glucose is unavailable for cellular metabolism, and the body chooses alternate sources of energy, principally fat. Consequently, fats break down into fatty acids, and glycerol in the fat cells is converted by the liver to ketone bodies (e.g., β-hydroxybutyric acid, acetoacetic acid, acetone). Any excess is eliminated in the urine (ketonuria) or the lungs (acetone breath). The ketone bodies in the blood (ketonemia) are strong acids that lower serum pH, producing ketoacidosis.

Ketones are organic acids that readily produce excessive quantities of free hydrogen ions, causing a fall in plasma pH. Then chemical buffers in the plasma, principally bicarbonate, combine with the hydrogen ions to form carbonic acid, which readily dissociates into water and carbon dioxide. The respiratory system attempts to eliminate the excess carbon dioxide by increased depth and rate—Kussmaul respirations, or the hyperventilation characteristic of metabolic acidosis. The ketones are buffered by sodium and potassium in the plasma. The kidneys attempt to compensate for the increased pH by increasing tubular secretion of hydrogen and ammonium ions in exchange for fixed base, thus depleting the base buffer concentration.

With cellular death, potassium is released from the cells (intracellular fluid) into the bloodstream (extracellular fluid) and excreted by the kidneys, where the loss is accelerated by osmotic diuresis. The total body potassium is then decreased even though the serum potassium level may be elevated as a result of the decreased fluid volume in which it circulates. Alteration in serum and tissue potassium can lead to cardiac arrest.

If these conditions are not reversed by insulin therapy in combination with correction of the fluid deficiency and electrolyte imbalance, progressive deterioration occurs, with dehydration, electrolyte imbalance, acidosis, coma, and death. Diabetic ketoacidosis (DKA) should be diagnosed promptly in a seriously ill patient and therapy instituted in an intensive care unit.

Long-Term Complications

Long-term complications of diabetes involve both the microvasculature and the macrovasculature. The principal microvascular complications are nephropathy, retinopathy, and neuropathy. Microvascular disease develops during the first 30 years of diabetes, beginning in the first 10 to 15 years after puberty, with renal involvement evidenced by proteinuria and clinically apparent retinopathy.

BOX 31.13 Clinical Manifestations of Type 1 Diabetes Mellitus

Polyphagia
Polyuria
Polydipsia
Weight loss
Enuresis or nocturia
Irritability; "not himself" or "not herself"
Shortened attention span
Lowered frustration tolerance
Dry skin
Blurred vision
Poor wound healing
Fatigue
Flushed skin
Headache
Frequent infections
Hyperglycemia
- Elevated blood glucose levels
- Glucosuria

Diabetic ketosis
- Ketones and glucose in urine
- Dehydration in some cases

Diabetic ketoacidosis
- Dehydration
- Electrolyte imbalance
- Acidosis
- Deep, rapid breathing (Kussmaul respirations)

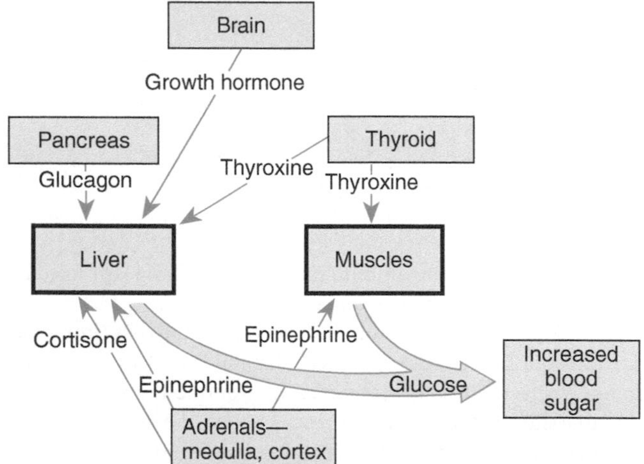

FIG. 31.7 Body systems respond to hypoglycemia in various ways to increase blood glucose level.

Macrovascular disease develops after 25 years of diabetes and creates the predominant problems in patients with type 2 DM. The process appears to be one of glycosylation, wherein proteins from the blood become deposited in the walls of small vessels (e.g., glomeruli), where they become trapped by "sticky" glucose compounds (glycosyl radicals). The buildup of these substances over time causes narrowing of the vessels, with subsequent interference with microcirculation to the affected areas (Svoren & Jospe, 2016).

With poor diabetic control, vascular changes can appear as early as 2½ to 3 years after diagnosis; however, with good to excellent control, changes can be postponed for 20 or more years. Intensive insulin therapy appears to delay the onset and slow the progression of retinopathy, nephropathy, and neuropathy. However, children who have type 2 DM have a higher risk of long-term cardiovascular disease, including hypertension, stroke, and myocardial infarction, than individuals who develop type 2 DM in adulthood (Reinehr, 2013).

Other complications have been observed in children with type 1 DM. Hyperglycemia appears to influence thyroid function, and altered function is frequently observed at the time of diagnosis and in poorly controlled diabetes. Limited mobility of small joints of the hand occurs in 30% of 7- to 18-year-old children with type 1 DM and appears to be related to changes in the skin and soft tissues surrounding the joint as a result of glycosylation.

! NURSING ALERT

Recurrent vaginal and urinary tract infections, especially with *Candida albicans*, are often an early sign of type 2 DM, especially in adolescents.

Diagnostic Evaluation

Three groups of children who are candidates for diabetes are (1) children who have glycosuria, polyuria, and a history of weight loss or failure to gain despite a voracious appetite; (2) those with transient or persistent glycosuria; and (3) those who display manifestations of metabolic acidosis, with or without stupor or coma. In every case, diabetes must be considered if there is glycosuria, with or without ketonuria, and unexplained hyperglycemia.

Glycosuria by itself is not diagnostic of diabetes. Other sugars, such as galactose, can produce a positive result with certain test strips, and a mild degree of glycosuria can be caused by other conditions, such as infection, trauma, emotional or physical stress, hyperalimentation, and some renal or endocrine diseases.

DM is diagnosed based on any of the following four abnormal glucose metabolites: (1) 8-hour fasting blood glucose level of 126 mg/dl or more, (2) a random blood glucose value of 200 mg/dl or more accompanied by classic signs of diabetes, (3) an oral glucose tolerance test (OGTT) finding of 200 mg/dl or more in the 2-hour sample, or (4) hemoglobin A1C of 6.5% or more (Laffel & Svoren, 2015). Postprandial blood glucose determinations and the traditional OGTTs have yielded low detection rates in children and are not usually necessary for establishing a diagnosis. Serum insulin levels may be normal or moderately elevated at the onset of diabetes; delayed insulin response to glucose indicates impaired glucose tolerance.

Ketoacidosis must be differentiated from other causes of acidosis or coma, including hypoglycemia, uremia, gastroenteritis with metabolic acidosis, salicylate intoxication encephalitis, and other intracranial lesions. DKA is a state of relative insulin insufficiency and may include the presence of hyperglycemia (blood glucose level ≥200 mg/dl), acidosis (pH <7.30 and bicarbonate <15 mmol/L), glycosuria, and ketonuria (Svoren & Jospe, 2016). Tests used to determine glycosuria and ketonuria are the glucose oxidase tapes (Keto-Diastix).

Therapeutic Management

The management of the child with type 1 DM consists of a multidisciplinary approach involving the family; the child (when appropriate); and professionals, including a pediatric endocrinologist, diabetes nurse educator, nutritionist, and exercise physiologist. Often psychologic support from a mental health professional is also needed. Communication among the team members is essential and extends to other individuals in the child's life, such as teachers, school nurse, school guidance counselor, and coach.

The definitive treatment is replacement of insulin that the child is unable to produce. However, insulin needs are also affected by emotions, nutritional intake, activity, and other life events, such as illnesses and puberty. The complexity of the disease and its management requires that the child and family incorporate diabetes needs into their lifestyle. Medical and nutritional guidance are primary, but management also includes continuing diabetes education, family guidance, and emotional support.

Insulin Therapy

Insulin replacement is the cornerstone of management of type 1 DM. Insulin dosage is tailored to each child based on home blood glucose monitoring. The goal of insulin therapy is maintaining near-normal blood glucose values while avoiding too frequent episodes of hypoglycemia. Insulin is administered as two or more injections per day or as continuous subcutaneous infusion using a portable insulin pump.

Healthy pancreatic cells secrete insulin at a low but steady basal rate with superimposed bursts of increased secretion that coincide with intake of nutrients. Consequently, insulin levels in the blood increase and decrease coincidentally, with the rise and fall in blood glucose levels. In addition, insulin is secreted directly into the portal circulation; therefore the liver, which is the major site of glucose disposal, receives the largest concentration of insulin. No matter which method of insulin replacement is used, this normal pattern cannot be duplicated. Subcutaneous injection results in absorption of the drug into the general circulation, thus reducing the concentrations of insulin to which the liver is exposed.

Insulin Preparations

Insulin is available in highly purified pork preparations and in human insulin biosynthesized by and extracted from bacterial or yeast cultures. Most clinicians suggest human insulin as the treatment of choice. Insulin is available in rapid-, intermediate-, and long-acting preparations; all are packaged in the strength of 100 U/ml. Some insulin is available as premixed insulins, such as 70/30 and 50/50 ratios, the first number indicating the percentage of intermediate-acting insulin and the second number the percentage of rapid-acting insulin. The different types of insulin are found in Box 31.14.

BOX 31.14 Types of Insulin

There are four types of insulin, based on the following criteria:

- How soon the insulin starts working (onset)
- When the insulin works the hardest (peak time)
- How long the insulin lasts in the body (duration)

However, each person responds to insulin in his or her own way. That is why onset, peak time, and duration are given as ranges.

Rapid-acting insulin (e.g., NovoLog) reaches the blood within 15 minutes after injection. The insulin peaks 30 to 90 minutes later and may last as long as 5 hours.

Short-acting (regular) insulin (e.g., Novolin R) usually reaches the blood within 30 minutes after injection. The insulin peaks 2 to 4 hours later and stays in the blood for about 4 to 8 hours.

Intermediate-acting insulins (e.g., Novolin N) reach the blood 2 to 6 hours after injection. The insulins peak 4 to 14 hours later and stay in the blood for about 14 to 20 hours.

Long-acting insulin (e.g., Lantus) takes 6 to 14 hours to start working. It has no peak or a very small peak 10 to 16 hours after injection. The insulin stays in the blood between 20 and 24 hours.

Some insulins come mixed together (e.g., Novolin 70/30). For example, you can buy regular insulin and NPH insulins already mixed in one bottle, which makes it easier to inject two kinds of insulin at the same time. However, you cannot adjust the amount of one insulin without also changing how much you get of the other insulin.

NPH, Neutral protamine Hagedorn.

! NURSING ALERT

The human insulins from various manufacturers may be interchangeable, but human insulin and pork insulin or pure pork insulin should never be substituted for one another.

Dosage. Conventional management is a twice-daily insulin regimen of a combination of rapid-acting and intermediate-acting insulin drawn up into the same syringe and injected before breakfast and before the evening meal. The amount of morning regular insulin is determined by patterns in the late morning and lunchtime blood glucose values. The morning intermediate-acting dosage is determined by patterns in the late afternoon and supper blood glucose values. Fasting blood glucose patterns at breakfast help determine the evening dose of intermediate insulin, and the blood glucose patterns at bedtime help determine the evening dose of rapid-acting (regular) insulin. For some children, better morning glucose control is achieved by a later (bedtime) injection of intermediate-acting insulin.

Regular insulin is best administered at least 30 minutes before meals. This allows sufficient time for absorption and results in a significantly greater reduction in the postprandial rise in blood glucose than if the meal were eaten immediately after the insulin injection. Intensive therapy consists of multiple injections throughout the day with a once- or twice-daily dose of long-acting (Ultralente) insulin to simulate the basal insulin secretion and injections of rapid-acting insulin before each meal. A multiple daily injection program reduces microvascular complications of diabetes in young, healthy patients who have type 1 DM.

The precise dose of insulin needed cannot be predicted. Therefore the total dosage and percentage of regular- to intermediate-acting insulin should be determined empirically for each child. Usually 60% to 75% of the total daily dose is given before breakfast, and the remainder is given before the evening meal. Furthermore, insulin requirements do not remain constant but change continuously during growth and development; the need varies according to the child's activity level and pubertal status. For example, less insulin is required during spring and summer months when children are more active. Illness also alters insulin requirements. Some children require more frequent insulin administration. This includes children with difficult-to-control diabetes and children during the adolescent growth spurt.

Methods of administration. Daily insulin is administered subcutaneously by twice-daily injections, by multiple-dose injections, or by means of an insulin infusion pump. The insulin pump is an electromechanical device designed to deliver fixed amounts of regular or lispro insulin continuously (basal rate), thereby more closely imitating the release of the hormone by the islet cells (Svoren & Jospe, 2016). Although the pump delivers a programmed amount of basal insulin, the child or parent must program a dose for the pump to deliver before each meal.

The system consists of a syringe to hold the insulin, a plunger, and a computerized mechanism to drive the plunger. The insulin flows from the syringe through a catheter to a needle inserted into subcutaneous tissue (the abdomen or thigh), and the lightweight device is worn on a belt or a shoulder holster. Using aseptic technique, the child or parent changes the needle and catheter every 48 to 72 hours and then tapes them in place.

Although the pump provides more consistent insulin delivery, it has certain disadvantages. Pump therapy is expensive and requires commitment from the parent and child. A certain level of math skills is required to calculate infusion rates. It should also not be removed for more than 1 hour at a time, which may limit some activities. Skin infections are common, and as with any other mechanical device, it is subject to malfunction. However, the pumps are equipped with alarms

TABLE 31.3 Plasma Blood Glucose and Hemoglobin A1C Goals for Type 1 Diabetes Mellitus by Age-Group

Age	Value* Before Meals (mg/dl)	Value* at Bedtime/ Overnight (mg/dl)	Hemoglobin A1C (%)	Implications
Toddlers and preschoolers (<6 years)	100-180	110-200	≤8.5% (but ≥7.5%)	High risk and vulnerability to hypoglycemia
School age (6-12 years)	90-180	100-180	<8%	Risks of hypoglycemia and relatively low risk of complications before puberty
Adolescents (>12 years) and young adults	90-130	90-150	<7.5%	Risk of hypoglycemia Developmental and psychologic issues

*Plasma blood glucose goal range.

Modified from American Diabetes Association. (2005). Standards of medical care in diabetes. *Diabetes Care, 28*(Suppl), S4-S36.

TABLE 31.4 Comparison of Hemoglobin Blood Glucose Levels to Hemoglobin A1C

Hemoglobin A1C Levels	Hemoglobin A1C (%)	Mean Blood Glucose (mg/dl)	Mean Blood Glucose (mmol/L)
Severely elevated	14	360	20
	13	330	18.3
	12	300	16.7
	11	270	15
Elevated	10	240	13.3
	9	210	11.7
Slightly elevated	8	180	10
	7	150	8.3
Normal	6	120	6.7
	5	90	5
	4	60	3.3

Modified from American Diabetes Association. (2005). Standards of medical care in diabetes: Clinical practice recommendations. *Diabetes Care, 28*(Suppl), S4-S36.

that signal problems, such as a depleted battery, an occluded needle or tubing, or a microprocessor malfunction.

Monitoring

Daily monitoring of blood glucose levels is an essential aspect of appropriate DM management. Plasma blood glucose and hemoglobin A1C vary according to age (Table 31.3). Plasma blood glucose and hemoglobin A1C goal ranges are found in Table 31.4.

Blood glucose. Self-monitoring of blood glucose (SMBG) has improved diabetes management and is used successfully by children from the onset of their diabetes. By testing their own blood, children are able to change their insulin regimen to maintain their glucose level in the euglycemic (normal) range of 80 to 120 mg/dl. Diabetes management depends to a great extent on SMBG. In general, children tolerate the testing well.

Glycosylated hemoglobin. The measurement of glycosylated hemoglobin (hemoglobin A1C) levels is a satisfactory method for assessing control of the diabetes. As red blood cells circulate in the bloodstream, glucose molecules gradually attach to the hemoglobin A molecules and remain there for the lifetime of the red blood cell, approximately 120 days. The attachment is not reversible; therefore this glycosylated hemoglobin reflects the average blood glucose levels over the previous 2 to 3 months. The test is a satisfactory method for assessing control, detecting incorrect testing, monitoring the effectiveness of changes in treatment, defining patients' goals, and detecting nonadherence. Nondiabetic hemoglobin A1C values are generally between 4% and 6% but can vary by laboratory. Diabetes control for children depends on age, with hemoglobin A1C levels of 6.0% to 7.5% as good control, levels of 7.6% to 9.9% as fair control, and levels of 10% or higher as poor control (Svoren & Jospe, 2016).

Urine. Urine testing for glucose is no longer used for diabetes management. There is poor correlation between simultaneous glycosuria and blood glucose concentrations. However, urine testing can be carried out to detect evidence of ketonuria.

! NURSING ALERT

It is recommended that urine be tested for ketones every 3 hours during an illness or whenever the blood glucose level is over 240 mg/dl when illness is not present.

Nutrition

Essentially, the nutritional needs of children with diabetes are no different from those of healthy children. Children with diabetes need no special foods or supplements. They need sufficient calories to balance daily expenditure for energy and to satisfy the requirement for growth and development. Unlike children without diabetes, whose insulin is secreted in response to food intake, insulin injected subcutaneously has a relatively predictable time of onset, peak effect, duration of action, and absorption rate depending on the type of insulin used. Consequently, the timing of food consumption must be regulated to correspond to the timing and action of the insulin prescribed.

Meals and snacks must be eaten according to peak insulin action, and the total number of calories and proportions of basic nutrients must be consistent from day to day. The constant release of insulin into the circulation makes the child prone to hypoglycemia between the three daily meals unless a snack is provided between meals and at bedtime. The distribution of calories should be calculated to fit the activity pattern of each child. For example, a child who is more active in the afternoon will need a larger snack at that time. This larger snack might also be split to allow some food at school and some food after school. Food intake should be altered to balance food, insulin, and exercise. Extra food is needed for increased activity.

Concentrated sweets are discouraged, and because of the increased risk of atherosclerosis in persons with DM, fat is reduced to 30% or less of the total caloric requirement. Dietary fiber has become increasingly important in dietary planning because of its influence on digestion, absorption, and metabolism of many nutrients. It has been found to diminish the rise in blood glucose after meals.

BOX 31.15 Nutritional Management in Type 1 Diabetes Mellitus

Goal
Attain metabolic control of glucose and lipid levels

Objectives
Appropriate meal and snack planning:
- Achieve a dietary balance of carbohydrates, fats, and proteins.
- Provide extra food during periods of exercise.
- Time meals consistently to prevent hypoglycemia.
- Avoid high-sugar, high-carbohydrate foods to prevent hyperglycemia.

Develop an appropriate insulin regimen and physical activity program:
- Administer insulin as directed before eating.
- Increase insulin dose or activity level when extra food is eaten.
- Decrease insulin dose during periods of strenuous activity.

For growing children, food restriction should never be used for diabetes control, although caloric restrictions may be imposed for weight control if the child is overweight. In general, the child's appetite should be the guide for the amount of calories needed, with the total caloric intake adjusted to appetite and activity. Box 31.15 outlines basic principles of diet management.

Exercise

Exercise is encouraged and never restricted unless indicated by other health conditions. Exercise lowers blood glucose levels, depending on the intensity and duration of the activity. Consequently, exercise should be included as part of diabetes management, and the type and amount of exercise should be planned around the child's interests and capabilities. However, in most instances, children's activities are unplanned, and the resulting decrease in blood glucose can be compensated for by providing extra snacks before (and if the exercise is prolonged, during) the activity. In addition to a feeling of well-being, regular exercise aids in utilization of food and often results in a reduction of insulin requirements.

Hypoglycemia

Occasional episodes of hypoglycemia are an integral part of insulin therapy, and an objective of diabetes management is to achieve the best possible glycemic control while minimizing the frequency and severity of hypoglycemia. Even with good control, a child may frequently experience mild symptoms of hypoglycemia. If the signs and symptoms are recognized early and promptly relieved by appropriate therapy, the child's activity should be interrupted for no more than a few minutes.

! NURSING ALERT

Hypoglycemic episodes most commonly occur before meals or when the insulin effect is peaking.

The signs and symptoms of hypoglycemia are caused by both increased adrenergic activity and impaired brain function. The increased adrenergic nervous system activity plus increased secretion of catecholamines produces tachycardia, tremors, sweating, irritability, aggression, and hunger (Svoren & Jospe, 2016). Drowsiness, personality changes, mental confusion, loss of coordination, seizures, and coma are more severe responses and reflect CNS glucose deprivation and the body's attempts to elevate the serum glucose levels.

It is often difficult to distinguish between hyperglycemia and a hypoglycemic reaction (Table 31.5). Because the symptoms are similar and usually begin with changes in behavior, the simplest way to differentiate between the two is to test the blood glucose level. The blood glucose level is low in hypoglycemia, but in hyperglycemia, the glucose level is significantly elevated. Urinary ketones may be present after hypoglycemia as a result of starvation ketone production. In doubtful situations, it is safer to give the child some simple carbohydrate. This will help alleviate the symptoms in the case of hypoglycemia but will do little harm if the child is hyperglycemic.

TABLE 31.5 Comparison of Manifestations of Hypoglycemia and Hyperglycemia

Variable	Hypoglycemia	Hyperglycemia
Onset	Rapid (minutes)	Gradual (days)
Mood	Labile, irritable, nervous, weepy	Lethargic
Mental status	Difficulty concentrating, speaking, focusing, coordinating Nightmares	Dulled sensorium Confusion
Inward feeling	Shaky feeling Hunger Headache Dizziness	Thirst Weakness Nausea and vomiting Abdominal pain
Skin	Pallor Sweating	Flushed Signs of dehydration
Mucous membranes	Normal	Dry, crusty
Respirations	Shallow, normal	Deep, rapid (Kussmaul)
Pulse	Tachycardia, palpitations	Less rapid, weak
Breath odor	Normal	Fruity, acetone
Neurologic	Tremors	Diminished reflexes Paresthesia
Ominous signs	Late: Hyperreflexia, dilated pupils, seizure Shock, coma	Acidosis, coma
Blood:		
• Glucose	Low: <60 mg/dl	High: ≥250 mg/dl
• Ketones	Negative	High, large
• Osmolarity	Normal	High
• pH	Normal	Low (≤7.25)
• Hematocrit	Normal	High
• Bicarbonate	Normal	<20 mEq/L
Urine:		
• Output	Normal	Polyuria (early) to oliguria (late)
• Glucose	Negative	Enuresis, nocturia
• Ketones	Negative or trace	High
Visual	Diplopia	Blurred vision

Children are usually able to detect the onset of hypoglycemia, but some are too young to implement treatment. Parents should become adept at recognizing the onset of symptoms—for example, a change in a child's behavior, such as tearfulness or euphoria. In the majority of cases, 10 to 15 g of simple carbohydrate, such as 1 Tbsp of table sugar, will elevate the blood glucose level and alleviate the symptoms. The simpler the carbohydrate, the more rapidly it will be absorbed (8 oz of milk equals 15 g of carbohydrate). The rapidly releasing sugar is followed by a complex carbohydrate, such as a slice of bread or a cracker, and by a protein, such as peanut butter or milk.

For a mild reaction, milk or fruit juice is a good food to use in children. Milk supplies them with lactose or milk sugar, as well as a more prolonged action from the protein and fat (aids in decreased absorption). Other glucose sources include Insta-Glucose (cherry-flavored glucose), carbonated drinks (not sugarless), sherbet, gelatin, or cake icing. All children with diabetes should carry with them glucose tabs, Insta-Glucose, sugar cubes, or sugar-containing candy, such as LifeSavers or Charms. A difficulty with candies or icing is that the child may learn to fake a reaction to get the sweets; therefore commercial treatment products such as Insta-Glucose or glucose tabs may be preferred.

Glucagon is sometimes prescribed for home treatment of hypoglycemia. It is available as an emergency kit that must be mixed at the time of use and is administered intramuscularly or subcutaneously. Glucagon functions by releasing stored glycogen from the liver and requires about 15 to 20 minutes to elevate the blood glucose level.

When in doubt, it is best to assume hypoglycemia and treat, but overtreatment could result in hyperglycemia. The treatment may be repeated in 10 to 15 minutes if the initial response is not satisfactory. Rest and the addition of food should be part of the plan.

! NURSING ALERT

Vomiting may occur after administration of glucagon; therefore precautions against aspiration must be taken (e.g., placing the child on the side) because the child often becomes unconscious.

Morning hyperglycemia. The management of elevated morning blood glucose levels depends on whether the increase is a true dawn phenomenon, insulin waning, or a rebound hyperglycemia (the Somogyi effect). Insulin waning is a progressive rise in blood glucose levels from bedtime to morning. It is treated by increasing the nocturnal insulin dose. The true dawn phenomenon shows relatively normal blood glucose level until about 3 AM, when the level begins to rise. The Somogyi effect may occur at any time but often entails an elevated blood glucose level at bedtime and a drop at 2 AM, with a rebound rise following. The treatment for this phenomenon is decreasing the nocturnal insulin dose to prevent the 2 AM hypoglycemia. The rebound rise in the blood glucose level is a result of counterregulatory hormones (epinephrine, GH, and corticosteroids), which are stimulated by hypoglycemia. More frequent blood monitoring (especially at times of anticipated peak insulin action) usually identifies these conditions. Trace amounts of urinary ketones aid in identifying undetected hypoglycemia.

Illness Management

Illness alters diabetes management, and maintaining control is usually related to the seriousness of the illness. In a well-controlled child, an illness will run its course as it does in an unaffected child.

The goals during an illness are to restore euglycemia, treat urinary ketones, and maintain hydration. Monitor blood glucose levels and urinary ketones every 3 hours. Some hyperglycemia and ketonuria are expected in most illnesses, even with diminished food intake, and are an indication for increased insulin. Insulin should never be omitted during an illness, although dosage requirements may increase, decrease, or remain unchanged, depending on the severity of the illness and the child's appetite. Often the child needs supplemental insulin between usual dose times. If the child vomits more than once, if blood glucose levels remain above 240 mg/dl, or if urinary ketones remain high, notify the health care practitioner. Simple carbohydrates may be substituted for carbohydrate-containing exchanges in the meal plan. Although insulin and diet are important tools in sick-day care, fluids are the most important intervention. Fluids must be encouraged to prevent dehydration and to flush out ketones.

Therapeutic Management of Diabetic Ketoacidosis

DKA, the most complete state of insulin deficiency, is a life-threatening situation. Management consists of rapid assessment, adequate insulin to reduce the elevated blood glucose level, fluids to overcome dehydration, and electrolyte replacement (especially potassium).

DKA constitutes an emergency situation, thus a child is admitted to an intensive care facility for management. The priority is to obtain a venous access for administration of fluids, electrolytes, and insulin. The child should be weighed, measured, and placed on a cardiac monitor. Blood glucose and ketone levels are determined at the bedside, and samples are obtained for laboratory measurement of glucose, electrolytes, BUN, arterial pH, Po_2, Pco_2, hemoglobin, hematocrit, white blood cell count and differential, calcium, and phosphorus.

Oxygen may be administered to patients who are cyanotic and in whom arterial oxygen is less than 80%. Gastric suction is applied to unconscious children to avoid the possibility of pulmonary aspiration. Antibiotics may be administered to febrile children after appropriate specimens are obtained for culture. A Foley catheter may or may not be inserted for urine samples and measurement. Unless the child is unconscious, a collection bag is usually sufficient for accurate assessments.

Fluid and Electrolyte Therapy

All patients with DKA experience dehydration (10% of total body weight in severe ketoacidosis) because of the osmotic diuresis, accompanied by depletion of electrolytes, sodium, potassium, chloride, phosphate, and magnesium. Serum pH and bicarbonate reflect the degree of acidosis. Prompt and adequate fluid therapy restores tissue perfusion and suppresses the elevated levels of stress hormones.

The initial hydrating solution is 0.9% saline solution. Traditionally, deficits have been replaced at a rate of 50% over the first 8 to 12 hours and the remaining 50% over the next 16 to 24 hours. Current trends suggest more cautious fluid management to reduce the risk of cerebral edema. Therefore the fluid deficit should be replaced evenly over a period of 36 to 48 hours (Hamilton, Knudsen, Vaina, et al., 2017).

! NURSING ALERT

Potassium must never be given until the serum potassium level is known to be normal or low and urinary voiding is observed. All maintenance IV fluids should include 30 to 40 mEq/L of potassium unless the potassium concentration is elevated or urinary output is absent. Never give potassium as a rapid IV bolus, or cardiac arrest may result.

Serum potassium levels may be normal on admission, but after fluid and insulin administration, the rapid return of potassium to the cells can seriously deplete serum levels, with the attendant risk of cardiac arrhythmias. As soon as the child has established renal function (is voiding at least 25 ml/hr) and insulin has been given, vigorous potassium replacement is implemented. The cardiac monitor is used as a guide to therapy, and configuration of T waves should be observed every 30 to 60 minutes to determine changes that might indicate alterations in potassium concentration (widening of the Q-T interval and the appearance of a U wave after a flattened T wave indicate hypokalemia; an elevated and spreading T wave and shortening of the Q-T interval indicate hyperkalemia).

Insulin should not be given until obtaining urinary ketones and a blood glucose level. Continuous IV regular insulin is given at a dosage of 0.1 U/kg/hr. Insulin therapy should be started after the initial rehydration bolus because serum glucose levels fall rapidly after volume expansion. Blood glucose levels should decrease by 50 to 100 mg/dl/hr. When blood glucose levels fall to 250 to 300 mg/dl, dextrose is added to the IV solution. The goal is to maintain blood glucose levels between 120 and 240 mg/dl by adding 5% to 10% dextrose. Sodium bicarbonate is used conservatively; it is used for pH less than 7.0, severe hyperkalemia, or cardiac instability. Because sodium bicarbonate has been associated with an increased risk for cerebral edema, children receiving this substance must be carefully monitored for changes in level of consciousness.

When the critical period is over, the task of regulating the insulin dosage in relation to diet and activity is started. Children should be actively involved in their own care and are given responsibility according to their ability and the guidance of the nurse.

! NURSING ALERT

Because insulin can chemically bind to plastic tubing and in-line filters, thereby reducing the amount of medication reaching the systemic circulation, an insulin mixture is run through the tubing to saturate the insulin-binding sites before the infusion is started.

Nursing Care Management

Children with DM may be admitted to the hospital at the time of their initial diagnosis; during illness or surgery; or for episodes of ketoacidosis, which may be precipitated by any of a variety of factors. Many children are able to keep the disease under control with periodic assessment and adjustment of insulin, diet, and activity as needed under the supervision of a practitioner. Under most circumstances, these children can be managed well at home and require hospitalization only for serious illnesses or upsets.

However, a small number of children with diabetes exhibit a degree of metabolic lability and have repeated episodes of DKA that require hospitalization, which interferes with their education and social development. These children appear to display a characteristic personality structure. They tend to be unusually passive and nonassertive and come from families that are inclined to smooth over conflicts without resolution. Children in this type of setting experience emotional arousal with little, if any, opportunity or ability to resolve it. Other children from psychosocially dysfunctional families display behavioral and personality problems. This emotional stress causes an increased production of endogenous catecholamines, which stimulate fat breakdown, leading to ketonemia and ketonuria.

Hospital Management

Children with DKA require intensive nursing care. Observe and record vital signs frequently. Hypotension caused by the contracted blood volume of the dehydrated state may cause decreased peripheral blood flow, which can be particularly hazardous to the heart, lungs, and kidneys. An elevated temperature may indicate infection and should be reported so that treatment can be implemented immediately.

Maintain careful and accurate records, including vital signs (pulse, respiration, temperature, and blood pressure), weight, IV fluids, electrolytes, insulin, blood glucose level, and intake and output. Use a urine collection device or retention catheter to obtain the urine measurements, which include volume, specific gravity, and glucose and ketone values. The volume relative to the glucose content is important because 5% glucose in a 300-ml sample is a significantly greater amount than a similar reading from a 75-ml sample. A diabetic flow sheet maintained at the bedside provides an ongoing record of the vital signs, urine and blood tests, amount of insulin given, and intake and output. Assess and record the level of consciousness at frequent intervals. The comatose child generally regains consciousness fairly soon after initiation of therapy but is managed like any unconscious child until then.

When the critical period is over, the task of regulating insulin dosage to diet and activity is begun. The same meticulous records of intake and output, urine glucose and acetone levels, and insulin administration are maintained. Capable children should be actively involved in their own care and are given responsibility for keeping the intake and output record; testing the blood and urine; and, when appropriate, administering their own insulin—all under the supervision and guidance of the nurse (see Nursing Care Plan box).

NURSING CARE PLAN

The Child With Diabetes Mellitus

Case Study

Tommy is an 8-year-old who has been healthy all his life. Recently his mother has noticed that he has lost weight and that he is getting up several times during the night to go to the bathroom. He was drinking a great deal more the past week, and she thought that was the reason for being awakened at night to use the bathroom. However, today Tommy says he is too tired to go to school and when she goes into his bedroom she notices that he has wet the bed during the night. She becomes alarmed and calls the pediatrician for an appointment the next day. Tommy's mom has a brother with diabetes and thinks that Tommy's symptoms are similar to brother's problems when he was first diagnosed as a child.

Assessment

What are the most important signs of type 1 diabetes mellitus (DM) that you need to look for in a child?

Type 1 Diabetes Mellitus Defining Characteristics

Polyphagia
Polyuria
Polydipsia
Weight loss
Enuresis or nocturia
Irritability; "not himself" or "not herself"
Shortened attention span
Lowered frustration tolerance
Fatigue
Dry skin
Blurred vision
Poor wound healing
Flushed skin
Headache
Frequent infections

Case Study (Continued)

At the pediatrician's office several tests are completed to evaluate Tommy. His blood glucose level is 220 mg/dl, and his hemoglobin (Hgb) A1C level is 10.5%. Tommy provides a urine specimen. And the urine dip test is positive for glucose and ketones in his urine. Tommy is admitted to the hospital for further evaluation to establish a diagnosis.

Continued

NURSING CARE PLAN—CONT'D

The Child With Diabetes Mellitus

Tommy has met the criteria for new-onset diabetes that will require insulin injections to help manage. Initially Tommy will start with a twice-daily insulin regimen combining a rapid-acting (regular) insulin with an intermediate-acting (neutral protamine Hagedorn [NPH]/Lente) insulin drawn up in the same syringe. One injection will be given at least 30 minutes before breakfast. The second one will be given 30 minutes before dinner. Tommy will learn how to self-monitor his blood glucoses. Even though he will start off only administering insulin twice daily, he will still need to check his blood glucose before meals and at bedtime. Based on Tommy's age, his glucose goal range before meals should be 90 to 180 mg/dl and 100 to 180 mg/dl at bedtime.

Nursing Interventions and Rationales

What are the most appropriate nursing interventions for administering insulin in a child newly diagnosed with type 1 DM?

Nursing Interventions	Rationales
Obtain blood glucose level before meals and at bedtime.	To determine most appropriate dose of insulin
Administer insulin as prescribed.	To maintain normal blood glucose level
Understand the action of insulin: differences in composition, time of onset, and duration of action for the various preparations.	To ensure accurate insulin administration
Employ aseptic techniques when preparing and administering insulin.	To prevent infection
Rotate insulin injection sites.	To enhance absorption of insulin

Expected Outcomes

Tommy's glucose levels will be maintained within the targeted range.
Diabetic ketoacidosis will be prevented.
Hgb A1C levels will range from 6.5% to 8%.

Case Study (Continued)

Tommy's parents are in shock and are asking lots of questions related to diabetes and the care Tommy will require. Tommy is quiet and listens as his mom and dad talk with you and express their fear and concern.

Nursing Interventions and Rationales

What are the most important interventions to focus on with Tommy and his family regarding his diagnosis? Where would you start to teach him and his family regarding diabetes management?

Treatment consists of glucose monitoring, insulin therapy, observing for common problems, encouraging healthy eating, and physical activity. Focus on these major categories when beginning your education with Tommy and his family.

Nursing Interventions	Rationales
Discuss glucose monitoring.	To determine most appropriate dose of insulin
Teach how to administer insulin.	To maintain normal blood glucose level
Discuss signs and symptoms of hypoglycemia and hyperglycemia.	To prevent complications
Promote healthy eating patterns.	To ensure accurate insulin administration
Encourage physical activity.	To enhance absorption of insulin

Expected Outcomes

Parents and Tommy demonstrate an understanding of the following:

- What diabetes is
- The need to administer insulin
- How to administer insulin
- How to monitor glucose
- Signs and symptoms to observe when glucose is low or high
- How to promote healthy eating
- How to remain physically active

Case Study (Continued)

Tommy is expecting to be discharged today. After the morning dose of insulin when the nurse is preparing the family for discharge, Tommy tells her that he feels funny and his head hurts. He is dizzy when he stands and his hands are shaking. In questioning Tommy's mother about the morning, you are told that he did not eat breakfast because he wanted to eat on the way home.

Assessment

What are the most important signs and symptoms of hypoglycemia?

Hypoglycemia

Shaky feeling
Hunger
Headache
Dizziness
Difficulty concentrating, speaking, and focusing
Tremors
Tachycardia
Shallow respirations
Can lead to convulsion, shock, and coma

Nursing Interventions and Rationales

What are the most appropriate nursing interventions for a child newly diagnosed with diabetes who is experiencing hypoglycemia?

Nursing Interventions	Rationales
Immediately administer ½ cup of fruit juice or a glass of nonfat or 1% milk.	To increase blood sugar
Check blood glucose after 15 minutes.	To check blood sugar
Give a starch-protein snack.	To stabilize blood sugar
Give parents instructions regarding signs and symptoms of hypoglycemia versus hyperglycemia.	To promote maintaining blood sugar within an acceptable range
Teach parents how to administer intramuscular glucagon if unresponsive, unconscious, or seizing.	To increase blood sugar

Expected Outcome

Tommy's blood sugar will return to the targeted range.

Case Study (Continued)

After 15 minutes, Tommy is feeling better and his blood sugar is within an acceptable range. Tommy's mother is concerned and is worried that she will not be able to identify whether his blood sugar level is too high or too low. She is quite worried about being discharge today.

Assessment

What are some key points that you can review with Tommy's mom about the signs and symptoms of low and high blood sugar?

NURSING CARE PLAN—CONT'D

The Child With Diabetes Mellitus

Family's Knowledge of Illness, Defining Characteristics

Hypoglycemia (see earlier)
Hyperglycemia
- Thirst
- Weakness
- Fatigue
- Nausea and vomiting
- Abdominal pain
- Frequent urination
- Confusion
- Flushed
- Rapid respirations
- Breath odor (fruity)

Nursing Interventions and Rationales

What should you focus on regarding the family's education needs at this time to assure Tommy's blood glucose is kept within the targeted range?

Nursing Interventions	Rationales
Review how to recognize high and low blood sugar levels to prevent glucose levels that lead to medical emergencies.	To ensure prompt and appropriate treatment
Reinforce the importance of keeping the blood sugar within a target range.	To keep blood glucose levels stable
Discuss when to contact the doctor, including fever for 2 days, vomiting and diarrhea, unable to keep fluids down, and glucose levels above target range.	To ensure prompt and appropriate treatment
Discuss that exercise and increased activity will affect blood glucose levels, so increased monitoring will be necessary.	To keep blood glucose levels stable

Expected Outcome

Tommy and his parents will understand the signs and symptoms of high or low blood sugar levels and will understand the actions needed when this occurs. His parents will be prepared to manage help Tommy manage his disease at home.

Child and Family Education

Children and their families vary in educational background and the capacity to learn and understand the various aspects of the therapeutic program. Some families respond best to simple explanations and directions, whereas others expect thorough, in-depth information about the physiologic processes and responses associated with the disease and its therapy. All the principles of teaching and learning are applied in the educational process; therefore before beginning, the nurse must determine the optimum time, place, method, and content to be taught. Self-management, the ultimate goal for children with diabetes, is more likely to occur when children understand the disease and the care it requires. Properly educated and motivated, most families should be able to follow a program of regulated control satisfactorily.

When to teach a family and child is best judged by their psychologic state and emotional readiness. When a child is newly diagnosed, the psychologic adjustment to the disease can block the learning process completely. For example, in a follow-up visit family members may state that they are hearing a certain bit of information for the first time even though the material had been covered several times in the course of teaching. The first 3 or 4 days after diagnosis are not usually an optimum time for complex learning. One successful program teaches only essential, or survival, information first and intense information 1 month later.

The setting for the educational process can facilitate learning. At times during the educational process individual instruction is needed, but contact with other children or parents can assist in adjustment to the reality of the disease and the implications of having a chronic condition.

A variety of teaching methods and teaching aids can be used. Varying the education with a variety of audiovisual materials, including verbal discussions, films, books, and websites stimulate the senses and helps the individual learn. Participation is an effective method for learning. For example, to teach blood glucose testing, the nurse explains the technique, demonstrates the procedure, and allows the learner to perform the procedure; this is followed by a review of the material using visual aids and validation of the learning by some testing method that includes feedback.

Several organizations are prepared to assist with education and dissemination of knowledge about diabetes. The American Diabetes Association,* Canadian Diabetes Association,† Juvenile Diabetes Research Foundation International,‡ and American Association of Diabetes Educators§ are valuable resources for a wide variety of educational materials. The National Institute of Diabetes and Digestive and Kidney Diseases¶ publishes a number of comprehensive annotated bibliographies, including "Educational Materials for and about Young People with Diabetes," a compilation of resource materials for children, siblings, parents, teachers, and health professionals, and "Sports and Exercise for People with Diabetes."

Medical Identification

One of the first things the nurse should call to the parents' attention is the need for the child to wear some means of medical identification. Usually recommended is the Medic-Alert identification, a stainless steel or silver- or gold-plated identification bracelet that is visible and immediately recognizable. It contains a collect telephone number that medical personnel can call around the clock for medical records and personal information.

Nature of Diabetes

The better the parents understand the pathophysiology of diabetes and the function and action of insulin and glucagon in relation to caloric intake

---

*1701 N. Beauregard St., Alexandria, VA 22311; 800-342-2383; http://www.diabetes.org.

†1400–522 University Ave., Toronto, ON M5G 2R5; 800-226-8464; http://www.diabetes.ca.

‡26 Broadway, 14th Floor, New York, NY 10004; 800-533-CURE; http://www.jdrf.org.

§200 W. Madison St., Suite 800, Chicago, IL 60606; 800-338-3633; email: education@aadenet.org; http://www.diabeteseducator.org.

¶Office of Communications and Public Liaison, NIDDK, NIH, Building 31, Room 9A06, 31 Center Drive, MSC 2560, Bethesda, MD 20892-2560; 301-496-3583; http://www.niddk.nih.gov.

and exercise, the better they will understand the disease and its effects on the child. Parents need answers to a number of questions (voiced or unvoiced) to increase their confidence in coping with the disease. For example, they may want to know about the various procedures performed on their child and treatment rationale, such as what is being put in the IV bottle and the expected effect.

Meal Planning

Normal nutrition is a major aspect of the family education program. The nutritionist conducts diet instruction, with reinforcement and guidance from the nurse. The emphasis is on adequate intake for age, consistent menus, complex carbohydrates, and consistent eating times. The family is taught how the meal plan relates to the requirements of growth and development, the disease process, and the insulin regimen. Meals and snacks are modified based on the child's preferences and current menu, preserving cultural patterns and preferences as much as possible. Extensive exchange lists are available that include foods compatible with most lifestyles.

Learning about foods within specific food groups helps in making choices. Weights and measures of foods are used as eye-training devices for defining serving sizes and should be practiced for about 3 months, with gradual progression to estimation of food portions. Even when the child and family become competent in estimating portion sizes, reassessment should take place weekly or monthly and when there is any change of brands.

Family members should also be guided in reading labels for the nutritional value of foods and food content. They need to become familiar with the carbohydrate content of food groups. Substitution with foods of equal carbohydrate content is the skill needed for successful carbohydrate counting. Substitution might be necessary if a food is not available in sufficient quantity or for the teenager who wishes to eat fast food with peers. The use of a multiple daily injection program lends flexibility to the timing of meals.

Lists of popular fast-food items and items served at the major fast-food chains can be obtained from the restaurants to help guide food selections. It is important that the child know the nutritional value of these items (the major chains are remarkably uniform), but the child should be cautioned to avoid high-fat and high-sugar/high-carbohydrate items. For example, the child could choose a plain hamburger instead of a double cheeseburger.

Children should use sugar substitutes in moderation in items, such as soft drinks. Artificial sweeteners have been shown to be safe, but if there is any question about amounts, the physician, dietitian, or nurse specialist can provide guidelines based on body weight. Sugar-free chewing gum and candies made with sorbitol may be used in moderation by children with DM. Although sorbitol is less cariogenic than other varieties of sugar substitutes, it is an alcohol sugar that is metabolized to fructose and then to glucose. Furthermore, large amounts can cause osmotic diarrhea. Most dietetic foods contain sorbitol. They are more expensive than regular foods. Also, although a product may be sugar free, it is not necessarily carbohydrate free.

Traveling

Traveling requires planning, especially when a trip involves crossing time zones. A number of tips are included in pamphlets available free of charge. Suggestions for traveling encompass what will be needed from the practitioner before leaving, what and how much to take along, needs in transit, what to consider at the destination, and planning for when the child returns home. Planning is needed no matter what type of travel is considered—automobile, plane, bus, or train.

Insulin

Families need to understand the treatment method and the insulin prescribed, including the effective duration, onset, and peak action. They also need to know the characteristics of the various types of insulins, the proper mixing and dilution of insulins, and how to substitute another type when their usual brand is not available (insulin is a nonprescription drug). Insulin need not be refrigerated but should be maintained at a temperature between 15° and 29.4°C (59° and 85°F). Freezing renders insulin inactive.

Insulin bottles that have been "opened" (i.e., the stopper has been punctured) should be stored at room temperature or refrigerated for up to 28 to 30 days. After 1 month, these vials should be discarded. Unopened vials should be refrigerated and are good until the expiration date on the label. Diabetic supplies should not be left in a hot environment.

Injection Procedure

Learning to give insulin injections is a source of anxiety for both parents and children. It is helpful for the learner to know that this important aspect of care will become as routine as brushing the teeth. First, the basic injection technique is taught using an orange or similar item and sterile normal saline for practice. To gain children's confidence, the nurse can demonstrate the technique by giving a skillful injection to the parent and then having the parent return the demonstration by giving the nurse an injection. With practice and confidence, the parents will soon be able to give the insulin injection to their children, and their children will trust them. Another effective strategy is to instruct the children and then have them teach the technique to the parents while the nurse observes. Both parents should participate, and as little time as possible should elapse between instruction and the actual injection, especially with parents and teenage learners.

Insulin can be injected into any area in which there is adipose (fat) tissue over muscle; the drug is injected at a 90-degree angle. Newly diagnosed children may have lost adipose tissue, and care should be exerted not to inject intramuscularly. The pinch technique is the most effective method for tenting the skin to allow easy entrance of the needle to subcutaneous tissues in children. The site selected will sometimes depend on whether children or parents administer the insulin. The arms, thighs, hips, and abdomen are usual injection sites for insulin. The children can reach the thighs, abdomen, and part of the hip and arm easily but may require help to inject other sites. For example, a parent can pinch a loose fold of skin of the arm while the child injects the insulin.

The parents and child are helped to work out a rotation pattern to various areas of the body to enhance absorption because insulin absorption is slowed by fat pads that develop in overused injection areas (Table 31.6). The most efficient rotation plan involves giving about four to

TABLE 31.6 Onset and Duration of Action Related to Injection Site

	SITE OF INJECTION			
	Abdomen	Arm	Leg	Buttock
Rate	Very fast	Fast	Slow	Very slow
Duration	Very short	Short	Long	Very long

From Albisser, A. M., & Sperlich, M. (1992). Adjusting insulins. *Diabetes Educator, 18*(3), 211-218.

six injections in one area (each injection about 2.5 cm [1 inch] apart, or the diameter of the insulin vial from the previous injection) and then moving to another area.

Remember that the absorption rate varies in different parts of the body (see Table 31.6). The methodical use of one anatomic area and then movement to another (as described in the previous paragraph) minimizes variations in absorption rates. However, absorption is also altered by vigorous exercise, which enhances absorption from exercised muscles. Therefore it is recommended that a site be chosen other than the exercising extremity (e.g., avoiding legs and arms when playing in a tennis tournament).

Injection sites for an entire month can be determined in advance on a simple chart. For example, a "paper doll" (body outline) can be constructed and insulin sites marked by the child. After injection, the child places the date on the appropriate site. To keep in practice, it is a good idea for the parent to give two or three injections a week in areas that are difficult for the child to reach.

The same basic methodology is used when teaching children to give their own insulin injections (Fig. 31.8). They should practice first on an orange or a doll, building courage gradually. Other devices are available for insulin injection and may offer advantages to some children. Children who do not wish to give themselves injections can be taught to use a syringe-loaded injector (Inject-Ease). With the device, puncture is always automatic. Adolescents respond well to a self-contained and compact device resembling a fountain pen (NovoPen), which eliminates conventional vials and syringes.

When the child's dosage requires the injection of both short- and intermediate-acting insulin at the same time, most families mix the two medications and use a single injection. Insulin can be premixed and stored in the refrigerator for later use. To obtain maximum benefit from mixing insulins, the recommended practice is to (1) inject the measured amount of air (equivalent to the dosage) into the long-acting insulin; (2) inject the measured amount of air into the rapid-acting (clear) insulin without removing the needle; (3) withdraw the clear insulin; and (4) insert the needle (already containing the clear insulin) into the long-acting (cloudy) insulin and then withdraw the desired amount.

Continuous subcutaneous insulin infusion. Some children are considered candidates for use of a portable insulin pump, and even some young children with unsatisfactory metabolic control can benefit from its use. The child and the parents learn to operate the device, including the mechanics of the pump, battery changes, and alarm systems. A number of devices are on the market that vary in the basal rates they are able to deliver and in the cost of the equipment. Families can investigate the various devices and select the model that best suits their needs. Product information is available from pump manufacturers and distributors.*

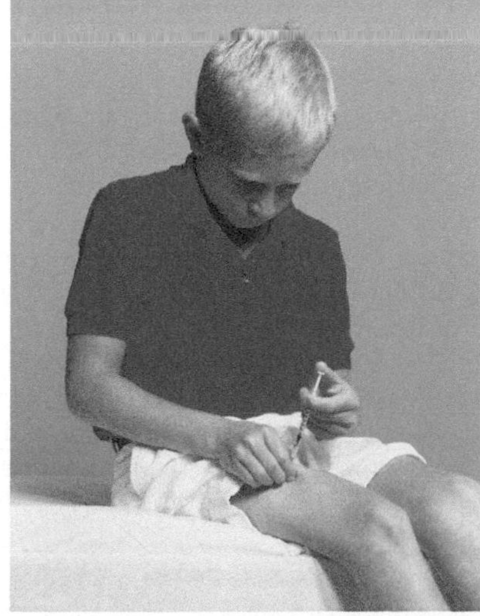

FIG. 31.8 School-age children are able to administer their own insulin.

! NURSING ALERT

When mixing types of insulin, always withdraw the clear, rapid-acting insulin into the syringe first, then the long-acting insulin. This avoids contaminating the short-acting insulin with the longer-acting insulin.

Parents and children learn (1) the technical aspects of the pump and SMBG; (2) prevention and treatment for hyperglycemia, sick-day management, and meal planning; (3) the effects of exercise, stress, and diet on blood glucose levels; and (4) decision-making strategies to evaluate blood glucose patterns and make adjustments in all aspects of the regimen.

Numerous blood glucose measurements (at least four times per day) are an essential part of infusion pump use. Intensive education and supervision are critical to obtaining maximum efficiency and control. This is particularly important if the family has been accustomed to a conventional insulin regimen. They must realize that simply wearing the pump will not normalize blood glucose. The pump is merely an insulin delivery device, and frequent, routine blood glucose determinations are necessary to adjust the insulin delivery rate.

The major problems with use of the insulin pump are inflammation from irritation and infection at the insertion site. The site should be cleaned thoroughly before the needle is inserted and then covered with a transparent dressing. The site is changed and rotated every 48 to 72 hours (this may vary) or at the first sign of inflammation. Nurses working where pumps are part of the therapeutic regimen should become familiar with the operation of the specific device being used and the protocol of disease management. Others should be aware of this management technique and be prepared to assist patients using the pump.

Monitoring

Nurses should also be prepared to teach and supervise blood glucose monitoring. SMBG is associated with few complications, and although it does not necessarily lead to improved metabolic control, it provides a more accurate assessment of blood glucose levels than can be obtained with the historical urine testing. Blood glucose monitoring has the added advantage that it can be performed anywhere (see Atraumatic Care box).

Blood for testing can be obtained by two different methods: manually or with a mechanical bloodletting device. A mechanical device is recommended for children, although the child and family should learn to use both methods in the event of mechanical failure. Several lancet devices are available, and each provides a means for obtaining a large drop of blood for testing (Fig. 31.9).

The blood sample may be obtained from fingertips or alternate sites, such as the forearm. Alternate site testing requires a meter that can test a small volume of blood. Not all meters are capable of this.

*Medtronic MiniMed, http://www.medtronicdiabetes.com/home; Disetronic, https://www.accu-chekinsulinpumps.com/ipus/; Animas, http://www.animas.com.

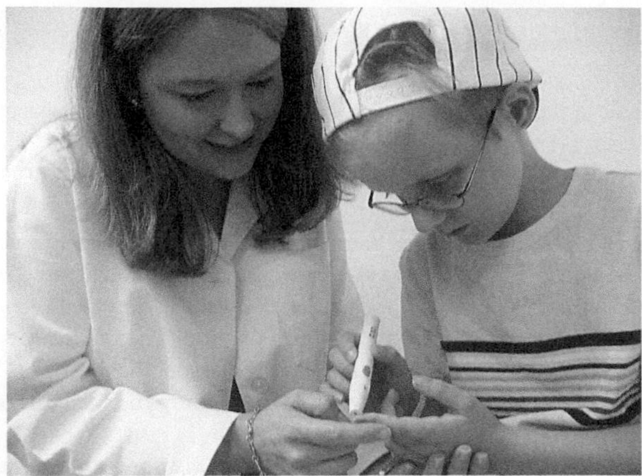

FIG. 31.9 Child using finger-stick device to obtain blood sample.

ATRAUMATIC CARE

Minimizing Pain of Blood Glucose Monitoring

- To enhance blood flow to the finger, hold it under warm water for a few seconds before the puncture.
- When obtaining blood samples, use the ring finger or thumb (blood flows more easily to these areas) and puncture the finger just to the side of the finger pad (more blood vessels and fewer nerve endings).
- To prevent a deep puncture, press the platform of the lancet device lightly against the skin and avoid steadying the finger against a hard surface.
- Use lancet devices with adjustable-depth tips. Begin with the shallowest setting.
- Use glucose monitors that require small blood samples (e.g., Ascensia Elite) to avoid repeated punctures.

! NURSING ALERT

Caution children not to allow anyone else to use their lancet because of the risk of contracting hepatitis B virus and/or human immunodeficiency virus infection.

The practitioner examines for signs of redness and soreness at the site of finger puncture. It may be evidence of poor technique, poor hygiene, or poor skin healing relative to poor control. Many types of blood-testing meters are available for home use. Newer technology has brought about improvements in meter size and ease of use. The family should be shown features of several meters, including advantages and disadvantages, and allowed to choose equipment that best meets their needs.

The least expensive testing method uses a reagent strip to which blood is applied (Fig. 31.10). After blotting, the color change is compared against a color scale for an estimation of the blood glucose level. The strips can be cut in half (although not all professionals recommend this) to obtain two readings per strip. This method is not accepted practice but may be necessary for some families or situations.

Urine testing. Testing for urinary ketones is recommended during times of illness and when blood glucose values are elevated. Information on a specific ketone-testing product should include correct procedure, storage, and product expiration. Families need a clear understanding of home management of ketones (fluids and additional insulin as directed by the health care team).

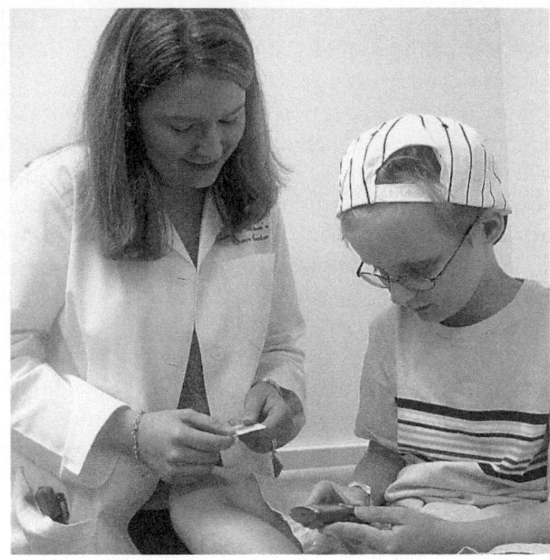

FIG. 31.10 Child using blood glucose monitor and reagent strips to test blood for glucose.

Hyperglycemia

Severe hyperglycemia is most often caused by illness, growth, emotional upset, or missed insulin doses. Emotional stress from school examinations or physical response to immunizations are examples of causes of hyperglycemia. With careful glucose monitoring, any elevation can be managed by adjustment of insulin or food intake. Parents should understand how to adjust food, activity, and insulin at the time of illness or when the child is treated for an illness with a medication known to raise the blood glucose level (e.g., steroids). The hyperglycemia is managed by increasing insulin soon after the increased glucose level is noted. Health care professionals should be aware that adolescent girls often become hyperglycemic around the time of their menses and should be advised to increase insulin dosages if necessary.

Signs of Hypoglycemia

Hypoglycemia is caused by imbalances of food intake, insulin, and activity. Ideally, hypoglycemia should be prevented, and parents need to be prepared to prevent, recognize, and treat the problem. They should be familiar with the signs of hypoglycemia and instructed in treatment, including care of the child with seizures. (See Chapter 30.) Early signs are adrenergic, including sweating and trembling, which help raise the blood glucose level, similar to the reaction when an individual is startled or anxious. The second set of symptoms that follow an untreated adrenergic reaction is neuroglycopenic (also called *brain hypoglycemia*). These symptoms typically include difficulty with balance, memory, attention, or concentration and slurred speech. Although rare in children, severe and prolonged hypoglycemia leads to seizures and coma (Svoren & Jospe, 2016). Hypoglycemia can be managed effectively as outlined in the Emergency Treatment box.

It is advisable for parents to plan for anticipated excitement or exercise. In addition, gastroenteritis may decrease insulin needs slightly as a result of poor appetite, vomiting, or diarrhea. If the blood glucose level is low but urinary ketones are present, the family should be aware of the increased need for simple carbohydrates and liquids.

Hygiene

All aspects of personal hygiene should be emphasized for children with diabetes. Children should be cautioned against wearing shoes without

EMERGENCY TREATMENT

Hypoglycemia

Mild Reaction: Adrenergic Symptoms

Give child 10 to 15 g of a simple, high-carbohydrate substance (preferably liquid; e.g., 3 to 6 oz of orange juice).

Follow with starch-protein snack.

Moderate Reaction: Neuroglycopenic Symptoms

Give child 10 to 15 g of a simple high-carbohydrate substance as above.

Repeat in 10 to 15 minutes if symptoms persist.

Follow with larger snack.

Watch child closely.

Severe Reaction: Unresponsive, Unconscious, or Seizures

Administer glucagon as prescribed.

Follow with planned meal or snack when child is able to eat or add a snack of 10% of daily calories.

Nocturnal Reaction

Give child 10 to 15 g of a simple carbohydrate.

Follow with snack of 10% of daily calories.

socks, wearing sandals, and walking barefoot. Correct nail and extremity care tailored to the individual child (with the guidance of a podiatrist) can begin health practices that last a lifetime. Eyes should be checked once a year unless the child wears glasses and then as directed by the ophthalmologist. Regular dental care is emphasized, and cuts and scratches should be treated with plain soap and water unless otherwise indicated. Diaper rash in infants and candidal infections in teens may indicate poor diabetes control.

Exercise

Exercise is an important component of the treatment plan. If the child is more active at one time of the day than at another time, food or insulin can be altered to meet that activity pattern. Food should be increased in the summer, when children tend to be more active. Decreased activity on return to school may require a decrease in food intake or increase in insulin dosage. Children who are active in team sports need a snack about a half hour before the anticipated activity. Races or other competition may call for a slightly higher food intake than at practice times.

Food intake will usually need to be repeated for prolonged activity periods, often as frequently as every 45 minutes to 1 hour. Families should be informed that if increased food is not tolerated, decreased insulin is the next course of action. If the timing of the exercise is changed so that the supper meal is delayed, the insulin in the second or third dose of the day may be moved back to precede the mealtime. Sugar may sometimes be needed during exercise periods for quick response. Elevated blood glucose levels after extreme activity may represent the body's adrenergic response to exercise. If the blood glucose level is elevated (>240 mg/dl) before planned exercise, urinary ketones should be checked, and the activity may need to be postponed until the blood glucose is controlled.

NURSING ALERT

Ketonuria in the presence of hyperglycemia is an early sign of ketoacidosis and a contraindication to exercise.

Record Keeping

Home records are an invaluable aid to diabetes self-management. The nurse and family devise a method to chart insulin administered, blood glucose values, urine ketone results, and other factors and events that affect diabetes control. The child and family are encouraged to observe for patterns of blood glucose responses to events such as exercise. If lapses in management occur (e.g., eating a candy bar), the child should be encouraged to note this and not be criticized for the transgression.

Self-Management

Self-management is the key to close control. Being able to make changes when they are needed rather than waiting until the next contact with health care professionals is important for self-management and gives the individual and family the feeling that they have control over the disease. Psychologically, this helps family members believe they are useful and participating members of the team. Allowing the child to learn to look at records objectively promotes independence in self-management support. As children grow and assume more responsibility for self-management, they develop confidence in their ability to manage their disease and confidence in themselves as persons. They learn to respond to the disease and to make more accurate interpretations and changes in treatment when they become adults.

Puberty is associated with decreased sensitivity to insulin that normally would be compensated for by an increased insulin secretion. Health care professionals should anticipate that pubertal patients may have more difficulty maintaining glycemic control and insulin doses may need to be adjusted. Patients should be taught to give themselves additional doses of rapid-acting insulin (5% to 10% of their daily dose) when their blood glucose levels are increased. The use of supplemental rapid-acting insulin is preferred to withholding food in adolescents.

Child or Adolescent and Family Support

Just as the physiologic responses affect the child, the parents and other family members of the child with newly diagnosed DM experience various emotional responses to the crisis. Care in the acute setting is short but may create fears and frustrations. The prospect of a chronic illness in their child engenders all the feelings and concerns that are faced by parents of children with other chronic illnesses (see Chapter 19). The threat of complications and death is always present, as well as the continuing drain on emotional and financial resources.

Certain fears may develop as a result of past experiences with the disease. A severe insulin reaction with seizures can contribute to fear of repetition. If parents observe a seizure or the adolescent has one in a public place, the desire to maintain better control is reinforced. They must understand how to prevent problems and how to handle problems calmly if they occur, and they must understand the complexities of the body, the disease, and its complications. Young children usually adjust well to problems related to the disease. With toddlers and preschoolers, insulin injections and glucose testing may be difficult at first. However, they usually accept the procedures when the parents use a matter-of-fact approach, without calling attention to a "hurt," and treat the procedure like any other routine part of the child's life. After the injection, time with some special and positive attention, such as reading or talking, or another pleasant activity, is one way to convert children who initially refuse injections to those who accept them.

In the years before adolescence, children probably accept their condition most easily. They are able to understand the basic concepts related to their disease and its treatment. They are able to test blood glucose and urine, recognize food groups, give injections, keep records, and distinguish fear or excitement from hypoglycemia. They understand how to recognize, prevent, and treat hypoglycemia. However, they still need considerable parental involvement.

! NURSING ALERT

Ongoing motivation to adhere to a regimen is difficult. An older child and parent (or another caregiver) may enjoy negotiating a day off when the responsibility for testing and recording blood glucose is delegated from the child to the caregiver (or vice versa).

Adolescents appear to have the most difficulty adjusting. Adolescence is a time of stress in trying to be perfect and similar to one's peers, and no matter what others say, having diabetes is being different. Some adolescents are more upset about not being able to have a candy bar than about injections, diet, and other aspects of management. If children can accept the difference as a part of life—in other words, that each person is different in some way—then, with adequate parental support, they should be able to adjust well (see Critical Thinking Case Study box).

Camping and other special group activities are useful. At diabetes camp, children learn that they are not alone. As a result, they become more independent and resourceful in other settings. Useful information about such camps and organizations can be obtained from the American Diabetes Association. A list of accredited camps specifically for children and teenagers with diabetes is also available from the American Camping Association.*

*5000 State Road 67 N., Martinsville, IN 46151; 800-428-2267; http://www.acacamps.org.

? CRITICAL THINKING CASE STUDY

Type 1 Diabetes

Shelly, a 14-year-old adolescent with a 3-year history of type 1 DM, has been admitted to the pediatric intensive care unit for treatment of DKA. This is her fifth hospital admission for DKA in the past year. Shelly's parents are divorced, and she has four younger siblings, none of whom has diabetes. Shelly's mother has maintained two jobs for the past 5 years and frequently leaves Shelly in charge of the household. In anticipation of her discharge, you are planning a patient education program for Shelly and her mother. What important issues regarding Shelly's unstable diabetes management must you consider to plan the education program?

Questions

1. Evidence: Is there sufficient evidence to draw conclusions about Shelly's recurrent episodes of DKA?
2. Assumptions: Describe an underlying assumption about each of the following:
   a. Type 1 DM in adolescence
   b. Type 1 DM and menses
   c. Emotional stress and elevated blood glucose levels
   d. Blood glucose monitoring for insulin management
3. What priorities for nursing care should be established for Shelly?
4. Does the evidence support your nursing intervention?

Answers are available at http://evolve.elsevier.com/wong/ncic.
DKA, Diabetic ketoacidosis; *DM,* diabetes mellitus.

NCLEX REVIEW QUESTIONS

1. Discharge teaching for parents of a school-age patient with diabetes insipidus (DI) should include which of the following? Select all that apply.
   A. Education and support regarding the rationale for fluid restrictions
   B. Information for school personnel regarding the diagnosis so they can grant children unrestricted use of the lavatory
   C. A thorough explanation regarding the condition with specific clarification that DI is a different condition from diabetes mellitus
   D. Understanding that treatment will only be needed until the child reaches puberty
   E. Knowing that school-age children may assume full responsibility for their care
2. You are working with a nurse who is new to your endocrine unit and has never worked with an infant born with congenital adrenal hyperplasia (CAH). You want to make sure he has a full understanding of this diagnosis. Which statement by the nurse indicates a need for further teaching?
   A. "Definitive diagnosis is confirmed by evidence of increased 17-ketosteroid levels in most types of CAH."
   B. "Blood studies to identify elevated calcium and decreased phosphorus levels are routinely performed."
   C. "Another test that can be used to visualize the presence of pelvic structures such as female reproductive organs is ultrasonography."
   D. "This deficiency is an autosomal recessive disorder that results in improper steroid hormone synthesis."
3. A father calls the pediatrician's office concerned about his 5-year-old type 1 diabetic child who has been ill. He reports that on checking the child's urine, it was positive for ketones. What is the nurse's best response to this father?
   A. "Come to the office immediately."
   B. "Encourage the child to drink calorie-free liquids."
   C. "Hold the next dose of insulin."
   D. "Administer an extra dose of insulin now."
4. A nurse working on a pediatric unit is assigned to an infant with hypothyroidism. She knows that the assessment may include:
   A. Thyroid function tests that are usually normal, although thyroid-stimulating hormone (TSH) levels may be slightly or moderately elevated
   B. Increased secretion of pituitary TSH in response to decreased circulating levels of TH or from infiltrative neoplastic or inflammatory processes
   C. Dry skin, puffiness around the eyes, sparse hair, constipation, sleepiness, lethargy, and mental decline
   D. Clinical features, including irritability, hyperactivity, short attention span, tremors, insomnia, and emotional lability
5. You are working in the emergency department, and a 10-year-old child with type 1 diabetes mellitus has just been admitted. He has been diagnosed with diabetic ketoacidosis. Which assessment data will you expect to note in this child?
   A. Shallow or normal respirations, hypertension, and tachycardia
   B. Fruity breath odor and decreasing level of consciousness
   C. Headache, hunger, and excessive irritability
   D. Normal urine output with specific gravity less than 1.020 and a trace of ketones

Correct Answers

1. B, C, E; 2. B; 3. B; 4. C; 5. B

REFERENCES

American Diabetes Association. (2007). Standards of medical care in diabetes—2007. *Diabetes Care, 30*(Suppl.), S4–S41.

Amin, N., Mushtaq, T., & Alvi, S. (2015). Fifteen-minute consultation: the child with short stature. *Arch Dis Child Educ Pract Ed, 100*(4), 180–184.

Argente, J. (2016). Challenges in the management of short stature. *Horm Res Paediatr, 85*(1), 2–10.

Arima, H., Azuma, Y., Morishita, Y., et al. (2016). Central diabetes insipidus. *Nagoya Journal of Medical Science, 78*(4), 349–358.

Breault, D. T., & Majzoub, J. A. (2016). Diabetes insipidus. In R. M. Kliegman, B. Stanton, J. W. St Geme, et al. (Eds.), *Nelson textbook of pediatrics* (ed. 20). Philadelphia: Saunders.

Brito, V. N., Spinola-Castro, A. M., Kochi, C., et al. (2016). Central precocious puberty: revisiting the diagnosis and therapeutic management. *Arch Endocrinol Metab, 60*(2), 163–172.

Bryant, J., Baxter, L., Cave, C. B., et al. (2007). Recombinant growth hormone for idiopathic short stature in children and adolescents. *Cochrane Database of Systematic Review*, (3), CD004440.

Cali, I., Miller, C. J., Parisi, J. E., et al. (2015). Distinct pathological phenotypes of Creutzfeldt-Jakob disease in recipients of prion-contaminated growth hormone. *Acta Neuropathologica Communications, 3*, 37.

Carroll, T. B., Aron, D. C., Findling, J. W., et al. (2011). Glucocorticoids & adrenal androgens. In D. G. Gardner & D. Shoback (Eds.), *Basic and clinical endocrinology* (9th ed.). New York: Lange Medical Books/McGraw-Hill.

Caturegli, P., De Remiqis, A., & Rose, N. R. (2014). Hashimoto thyroiditis: clinical and diagnostic criteria. *Autoimmunity Reviews, 13*(4–5), 391–397.

Ceccato, F., & Boscaro, M. (2016). Cushing's syndrome: screening and diagnosis. *High Blood Press Cardiovasc Prev, 23*(3), 209–215.

Centers for Disease Control and Prevention: *2014 national diabetes statistics report*, 2015, https://www.cdc.gov/diabetes/data/statistics/2014StatisticsReport.html.

Cheetham, T., & Davies, J. H. (2014). Investigation and management of short stature. *Archives of Disease in Childhood, 99*(8), 767–771.

Cuesta, M., Garrahy, A., & Thompson, C. J. (2016). SIAD: practical recommendations for diagnosis and management. *Journal of Endocrinological Investigation, 39*(9), 991–1001.

Di Iorgi, N., Napoli, F., Allegri, A. E., et al. (2012). Diabetes insipidus-diagnosis and management. *Horm Res Paediatr, 77*, 69–84.

Di Iorgi, N., Allegri, A. E., Napoli, F., et al. (2014). Central diabetes insipidus in children and young adults: etiological diagnosis and long-term outcome of idiopathic cases. *J Clin Ednocrinol Metab, 99*(4), 1264–1272.

Doyle, D. A. (2016a). Hypoparathyroidism. In R. M. Kliegman, B. Stanton, J. W. St Geme, et al. (Eds.), *Nelson textbook of pediatrics* (20th ed.). Philadelphia: Saunders.

Doyle, D. A. (2016b). Hyperparathyroidism. In R. M. Kliegman, B. Stanton, J. W. St Geme, et al. (Eds.), *Nelson textbook of pediatrics* (20th ed.). Philadelphia: Saunders.

El-Maouche, D., Arlt, W., & Merke, D. P. (2017). Congenital adrenal hyperplasia. *Lancet, 390*(10108), 2194–2210.

Ferguson, L. A. (2011). Growth hormone use in children: necessary or designer therapy? *Journal of Pediatric Health Care, 25*(11), 24–30.

Gardner, D. G., Anderson, M., & Nissenson, R. A. (2011). Hormones and hormone action. In D. G. Gardner & D. Shoback (Eds.), *Basic and clinical endocrinology* (9th ed.). New York: Lange Medical Books/McGraw-Hill.

Garibaldi, L. R., & Chemaitilly, W. (2016). Disorders of pubertal development. In R. M. Kliegman, B. Stanton, J. W. St Geme, et al. (Eds.), *Nelson textbook of pediatrics* (20th ed.). Philadelphia: Saunders.

Giuliani, C., & Peri, A. (2014). Effects of hyponatremia on the brain. *J Clin Med, 3*(4), 1163–1677.

Grimberg, A., Divall, S. A., Polychronakos, C., et al. (2016). Guidelines for growth hormone deficiency and insulin-like growth factor-1 treatment in children and adolescents: growth hormone deficiency, idiopathic short stature, and primary insulin-like growth factor-1 deficiency. *Horm Res Paediatr, 86*(6), 361.

Hamilton, H., Knudsen, G., Vaina, C. L., et al. (2017). Children and young people with diabetes: recognition and management. *British Journal of Nursing, 26*(6), 340–347.

Hanley, P., Lord, K., & Bauer, A. J. (2016). Thyroid disorders in children and adolescents: a review. *JAMA Pediatr, 170*(10), 1008–1019.

Harrington, J., & Palmert, M. R. (2016). Treatment of precocious puberty. In T. W. Post (Ed.), *UpToDate*. Waltham, MA.

Herman-Giddens, M. E., Steffes, J., Harris, D., et al. (2012). Secondary sexual characteristics in boys: data from the pediatric research in office settings network. *Pediatrics, 130*(5), e1058–e1068.

Hokken-Koelega, A. C. (2011). Diagnostic workup of the short child. *Horm Res Paediatr, 76*(Suppl. 3), 6–9.

Huang, S. A., & LaFranci, S. H. (2016). Hyperthyroidism. In R. M. Kliegman, B. Stanton, J. W. St Geme, et al. (Eds.), *Nelson textbook of pediatrics* (20th ed.). Philadelphia: Saunders.

Laffel, L., & Svoren, B.: *Epidemiology, presentation, and diagnosis of type 2 diabetes mellitus in children and adolescents*, 2015, http://www.uptodate.com/contents/epidemiology-presentation-and-diagnosis-of-type-2-diabetes-mellitus-in-children-and-adolescents.

Lal, G., & Clark, O. H. (2011). Endocrine surgery. In D. G. Gardner & D. Shoback (Eds.), *Basic and clinical endocrinology* (9th ed.). New York: Lange Medical Books/McGraw-Hill.

Lau, D., Rutledge, C., & Aghi, M. K. (2015). Cushing's disease: current medical therapies and molecular insights guiding future therapies. *Neurosurgical Focus, 38*(2), E11.

Leger, J., & Carel, J. C. (2013). Hyperthyroidism in childhood: causes, when and how to treat. *J Clin Res Pediatr Endocrinol, 5*(Suppl. 1), 50–56.

Lowitz, J., & Keil, M. F. (2015). Cushing syndrome: establishing a timely diagnosis. *Journal of Pediatric Nursing, 30*(3), 528–530.

Maffezzoni, F., Frara, S., Doga, M., et al. (2016). New medical therapies of acromegaly. *Growth Hormone and IGF Research, 30-31*, 58–63.

Mendes, C., Vaz Matos, I., Ribeiro, L., et al. (2015). Congenital adrenal hyperplasia due to 21-hydroxylase deficiency: genotype-phenotype correlation. *Acta Medica Portuguesa, 28*(1), 56–62.

Metzger, M. L., Krasin, M. J., Choi, J. K., et al. (2016). Hodgkin lymphoma. In P. A. Pizzo & D. G. Poplack (Eds.), *Principles and theories of pediatric oncology* (7th ed.). Philadelphia: Lippincott Williams & Wilkins.

Murray, P. G., Dattani, M. T., & Clayton, P. E. (2016). Controversies in the diagnosis and management of growth hormone deficiency in childhood and adolescence. *Archives of Disease in Childhood, 101*(1), 96–100.

Pardo Campos, M. L., Musso, M., Keselman, A., et al. (2017). Cognitive profiles of patients with early detected and treated congenital hypothyroidism. *Archivos Argentinos de Pediatria, 11591*, 12–17.

Parks, J. S., & Felner, E. I. (2016). Hypopituitarism. In R. M. Kliegman, B. Stanton, J. W. St Geme, et al. (Eds.), *Nelson textbook of pediatrics* (20th ed.). Philadelphia: Saunders.

Pashtan, I., Grogan, R. H., Kaplan, S. P., et al. (2013). Primary hyperparathyroidism in adolescents: the same but different. *Pediatric Surgery International, 29*(3), 275–279.

Pine Twaddell, E., Romero, C., & Radovick, S. (2013). Vertical transmission of hypopituitarism: critical importance of appropriate interpretation of thyroid function tests and levothyroxine therapy during pregnancy. *Thyroid, 23*(7), 892–897.

Pivonello, R., Auriemma, R. S., Grasso, L. F., et al. (2017). Complications of acromegaly: cardiovascular, respiratory, and metabolic comorbidities. *Pituitary, 20*(1), 42–62.

Reinehr, T. (2013). Type 2 diabetes mellitus in children and adolescents. *World J Diabetes, 4*(6), 270–281.

Ribeiro-Oliveira, A., Jr., & Barkan, A. (2012). The changing face of acromegaly-advances in diagnosis and treatment. *Nat Rev Endocrinology, 8*, 605.

Robinson, A. G. (2011). The posterior pituitary (neurohypophysis). In D. G. Gardner & D. Shoback (Eds.), *Basic and clinical endocrinology* (9th ed.). New York: Lange Medical Books/McGraw-Hill.

Rose, S. R., & Auble, B. A. (2012). Endocrine changes after pediatric traumatic brain injury. *Pituitary, 15*, 267–275.

Sandberg, D. E., & Gardner, M. (2015). Short stature: is it a psychological problem and does changing height matter? *Pediatric Clinics of North America, 62*(4), 963–982.

Sathyapalan, T., & Dixit, S. (2012). Radiotherapy-induced hypopituitarism: a review. *Expert Review of Anticancer Therapy, 12*(5), 669–683.

Schoenmakers, N., Alatzoglou, K. S., Chatterjee, V. K., et al. (2015). Recent advances in central congenital hypothyroidism. *The Journal of Endocrinology*, *227*(3), R51–R71.

Stanley, T. (2012). Diagnosis of growth hormone deficiency in childhood. *Curr Opin Endocrinol Diabetes Obes*, *19*, 47–52.

Svoren, B., & Jospe, N. (2016). Diabetes mellitus in children. In R. M. Kliegman, B. Stanton, J. W. St Geme, et al. (Eds.), *Nelson textbook of pediatrics* (20th ed.). Philadelphia: Saunders.

Tomer, Y. (2014). Mechanisms of autoimmune thyroid diseases: from genetics to epigenetics. *Ann Rev Pathol*, *9*, 147–156.

Toogood, A. A., & Stewart, P. M. (2008). Hypopituitarism: clinical features, diagnosis, and management. *Endocrinology and Metabolism Clinics of North America*, *37*, 235–261.

Waller, S. (2011). Parathyroid hormone and growth in chronic kidney disease. *Pediatric Nephrology (Berlin, Germany)*, *26*, 195–204.

Walvood, E. C. (2010). The timing of puberty: is it changing? Does it matter? *J Adoles Health*, *47*, 433–439.

White, P. C. (2016a). Pheochromocytoma. In R. M. Kliegman, B. Stanton, J. W. St Geme, et al. (Eds.), *Nelson textbook of pediatrics* (20th ed.). Philadelphia: Saunders.

White, P. C. (2016b). Congenital adrenal hyperplasia and related disorders. In R. M. Kliegman, B. Stanton, J. W. St Geme, et al. (Eds.), *Nelson textbook of pediatrics* (20th ed.). Philadelphia: Saunders.

Young, W. F. (2016). Pheochromocytoma in children. In T. W. Post (Ed.), *UpToDate*. Waltham, MA.

32

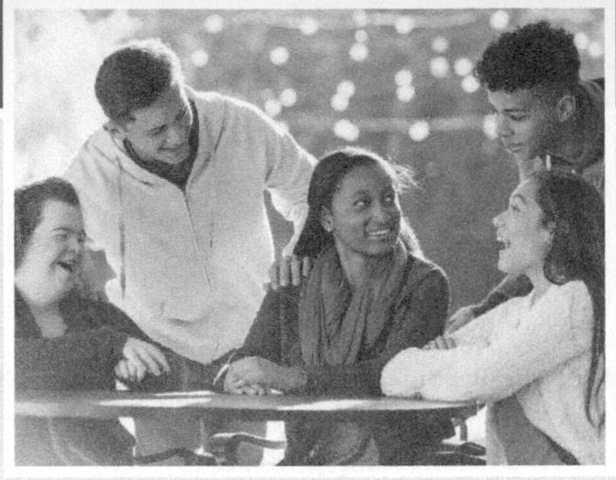

The Child With Integumentary Dysfunction

Cheryl C. Rodgers

http://evolve.elsevier.com/wong/essentials

CONCEPTS

- Tissue Integrity
- Inflammation
- Infection

INTEGUMENTARY DYSFUNCTION

SKIN LESIONS

Lesions of the skin result from a variety of etiologic factors. Skin lesions originate from (1) contact with injurious agents, such as infective organisms, toxic chemicals, and physical trauma; (2) hereditary factors; (3) external factors, such as allergens; or (4) systemic diseases, such as varicella, lupus erythematosus, and nutritional deficiency diseases. Responses are highly individualized in children. An agent that is harmless to one individual may be damaging to another, and a single agent may produce varying degrees of responses in different individuals.

Another factor in the etiology of skin manifestations is the child's age. For example, infants and young children are subject to "birthmark" malformations and atopic dermatitis that appear early in life. The school-age child is susceptible to tinea (ringworm) of the scalp, and acne is a characteristic skin disorder of puberty. Children's typical social environments also make them susceptible to skin disorders; the most recent national survey notes that up to 20% of American children experience atopy. Exposure to smoke and children with food allergies, particularly peanut allergy, have also been associated with higher rates of atopic dermatitis and eczema. Contact dermatitis, such as poison ivy, is seen only when the noxious agent is found in the environment. Similarly, insect bites are associated with seasonal activities during the summer and fall months.

Skin of Younger Children

The major skin layers arise from different embryologic origins. Early in the embryonic period, a single layer of epithelium forms from the ectoderm while simultaneously the corium develops from the mesenchyme. In infants and small children, the epidermis is loosely bound to the dermis. This poor adherence causes the layers to separate easily during an inflammatory process to form blisters. This is especially true in preterm infants, who have a propensity to blister formation and separation of the skin with minor trauma such as the removal of adhesive tape. In contrast, the skin of older children is thinner, and the cells of all the strata are more compressed.

Pathophysiology of Dermatitis

More than half of the dermatologic problems in children are various forms of dermatitis. This implies a sequence of inflammatory changes in the skin that are grossly and microscopically similar but diverse in course and causation. Acute responses produce intercellular and intracellular edema, the formation of intradermal vesicles, and an initial infiltration of inflammatory cells into the epidermis. In the dermis, there is edema, vascular dilation, and early perivascular cellular infiltration. The location and manner of these reactions produce the lesions characteristic of each disorder. The changes are usually reversible, and the skin ordinarily recovers without blemish unless complicating factors such as ulceration from the primary irritant, scratching, and infection are introduced or underlying vascular disease develops. In chronic conditions, permanent effects are seen that vary according to the disorder, the general condition of the affected individual, and the available therapy.

Diagnostic Evaluation

Although the history and subjective symptoms of skin lesions are explored first, the obvious objective characteristics of the lesions are often noted simultaneously. Many skin lesions are diagnosed after careful inspection.

History and Symptoms

Many cutaneous lesions are associated with local symptoms. The most common local symptom is itching (**pruritus**), which varies in frequency and intensity. Pain or tenderness often accompanies some skin lesions. Other skin sensations such as burning, prickling, stinging, or crawling are also described. Alterations in local feeling include absence of sensation (anesthesia); excessive sensitivity (hyperesthesia); diminished sensation (hypesthesia or hypoesthesia); or abnormal sensation, such as burning or prickling (paresthesia). These symptoms may remain localized or migrate. They may also be constant or intermittent and may be aggravated by a specific activity, such as exposure to sunlight.

It is important to determine whether the child has an allergic condition such as asthma or history of a previous skin disease. Atopic dermatitis, often associated with allergies, frequently begins in infancy. Important questions for the parent include when the lesion or symptom first appeared; whether it occurred with ingestion of a food or other substance, including any medication; and whether the condition was related to activity such as contact with plants, insects, or chemicals. Finally, inquire if other children in the home or classroom have similar symptoms and if the child's parents or siblings have a history of atopy or allergic skin conditions.

Objective Findings

The skin lesions' distribution, size, location, and morphology provide significant information. Skin lesions assume distinct characteristics that are related to the pathologic process. Nurses should become familiar with the common terms that are applied to skin lesions because these terms are used in the processes of record keeping and communication. These terms include the following:

Erythema—A reddened area caused by increased amounts of oxygenated blood in the dermal vasculature

Ecchymoses (bruises)—Localized red or purple discolorations caused by extravasation of blood into dermis and subcutaneous tissues

Petechiae—Pinpoint, tiny, and sharp circumscribed spots in the superficial layers of the epidermis

Primary lesions—Skin changes produced by a causative factor; common primary lesions in pediatric skin disorders are macules, papules, and vesicles

Secondary lesions—Changes that result from alteration in the primary lesions, such as those caused by rubbing, scratching, medication, or involution and healing

Distribution pattern—The pattern in which lesions are distributed over the body, whether local or generalized, and the specific areas associated with the lesions

Configuration and arrangement—The size, shape, and arrangement of a lesion or groups of lesions (e.g., discrete, clustered, diffuse, or confluent)

Extrinsic causes usually result from physical, chemical, or allergic irritants or from an infectious agent such as bacteria, fungi, viruses, or animal parasites. Intrinsic causes such as a specific infection (e.g., measles or chickenpox), drug sensitization, or other allergic phenomena can produce skin manifestations.

Laboratory Studies

When it is suspected that a skin problem might be related to a systemic disease, such as one of the collagen diseases or an immunodeficiency disease, studies are needed to rule out these possibilities. Diagnostic techniques include microscopic examination, cultures, skin scrapings or biopsy, cytodiagnosis, patch testing, and Wood light examination. Allergic skin testing and other laboratory tests such as blood count and sedimentation rate are used when indicated.

WOUNDS

Wounds are structural or physiologic disruptions of the skin that activate normal or abnormal tissue repair responses. Wounds are classified as acute or chronic. Acute wounds are those that heal uneventfully within 2 to 3 weeks. Chronic wounds are those that do not heal in the expected time frame or are associated with complications. Cofactors that disrupt or delay wound healing include compromised perfusion, malnutrition, and infection. In children, most wounds are acute and can be prevented from becoming chronic wounds through appropriate nursing care. Wounds are classified in the same manner as burns: superficial, partial thickness, full thickness, and complex wounds that include muscle and/or bone. Some types of acute wounds are the following:

Abrasion—Removal of the superficial layers of skin by rubbing or scraping

Avulsion—Forcible pulling out or extraction of tissue

Laceration—Torn or jagged wound; accidental cut wound

Incision—Division of the skin made with a sharp object; cut

Penetrating wound—Disruption of the skin surface that extends into underlying tissue or into a body cavity

Puncture—Wound with a relatively small opening compared with the depth

Epidermal Injuries

Abrasions are the most common epidermal wounds in children, usually in the form of a skinned knee or elbow. In most injuries, the margins of the abraded area are superficial, involving only the outer layers of epidermis, although the central portion may extend into the dermis. Initially the defect is filled by a blood clot and necrotic debris, which subsequently dehydrate to form a scab. Epithelial tissue is composed of labile cells, which are constantly destroyed and replaced throughout the life span. Injury to these tissues results in regeneration (i.e., rapid replacement by similar cells).

Injury to Deeper Tissues

Tissues composed of permanent cells such as muscle and nerve cells are unable to regenerate. These tissues repair themselves by substituting fibrous connective tissue for the injured tissue. This fibrous tissue, or scar, serves as a patch to preserve or restore the continuity of the tissue. Wounds involving permanent cells include surgical incisions, lacerations, ulcers, evulsions, and full-thickness burns. Injured cells of glandular organs and bones, composed of stable cells, multiply less vigorously and heal more slowly. With some wounds an overgrowth of nerve endings may occur, resulting in allodynia, or the sensation of pain from normally nonpainful stimuli, such as light touch.

Process of Wound Healing

The nonspecific repair mechanism of wound healing with scar formation involves the processes of inflammation, fibroplasia, scar contraction, and scar maturation. The initial response at the site of injury is inflammation, a vascular and cellular response that prepares the tissues for the subsequent repair process. There is a transient constriction of transected blood vessels, lasting 5 to 10 minutes, followed by active vasodilation of all local small vessels and increased blood flow to the area. This is accompanied by increased permeability of small venules, which allows plasma to leak into surrounding tissues (edema). A blood clot is formed along wound edges, providing a framework for future growth of capillaries (angiogenesis) and epithelial cells.

At the same time, vessel walls become lined with leukocytes, primarily neutrophils, which pass through the walls and concentrate at the injured site, where they ingest bacteria and debris (phagocytosis). Neutrophils are superseded by macrophages, which continue phagocytosis, and also by growth factors needed for skin repair and angiogenesis. Fibroblasts attracted to the area from blood vessels deposit fibrin throughout the clot. Adjacent capillaries begin to form buds that stretch across the supporting fibrin threads, and epithelial cells secrete a fibrolytic enzyme that allows their advancement across the wound. This initial phase of wound healing takes place during the first 3 to 5 days after injury. The wound is weakest at this time.

Fibroplasia (granulation or proliferation), the second phase of healing, continues 5 days to 4 weeks. Fibroblasts, immature connective tissue cells, migrate to the healing site and begin to secrete collagen into the meshwork spaces. Granulation tissue is highly vascular, "beefy" red, shiny connective tissue that organizes and restructures, forming thicker, stronger fibers arranged in orderly layers. A thin layer of epithelial tissue is regenerated over the surface of the wound, and leukocytes gradually disappear from the area. The wound is fragile at this time, and granulation tissue bleeds profusely if disturbed.

During contraction and maturation, the third and fourth phases of wound healing, collagen continues to be deposited and organized into layers, compressing the new blood vessels and gradually stopping blood flow across the wound. Fibroblasts disappear as the wound becomes stronger. Fibroblast movement causes contraction of the healing area, which helps bring wound edges closer together. A mature scar is then formed. Initially the scar is pink or hypopigmented and elevated. With maturation, the scar becomes pale, does not tan when exposed to sunlight, will not sweat or produce hair, and may itch. The maturation process continues for years, the extent to which the scar remodels varies among individuals.

Types of Wound Healing

Children have a highly elastic skin quality. This quality, combined with the rapid healing process during the latency and puberty developmental growth periods, results in abundant scar tissue that pulls on wounds during the healing process. Healing of wounds takes place in one of three ways: by primary, secondary, or tertiary intention (Fig. 32.1).

First intention (clean incision)

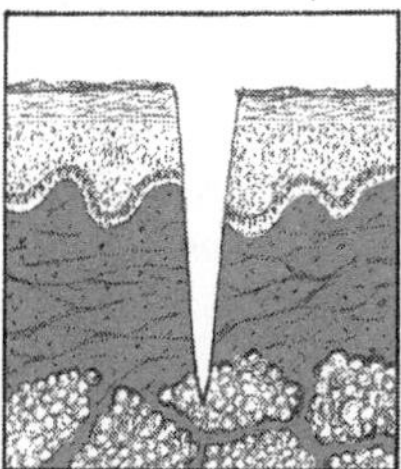

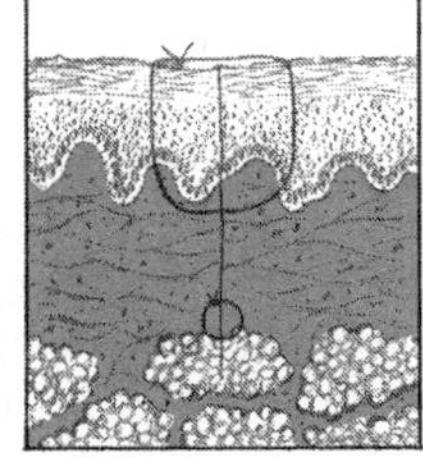

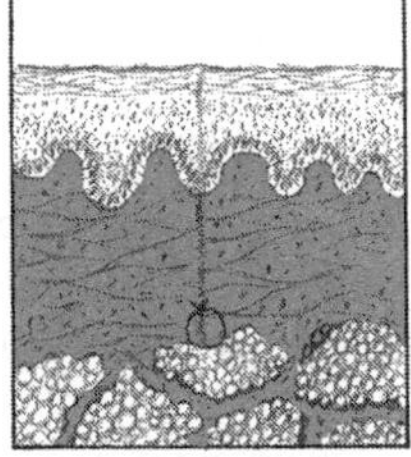

Second intention (wide, irregular wound)

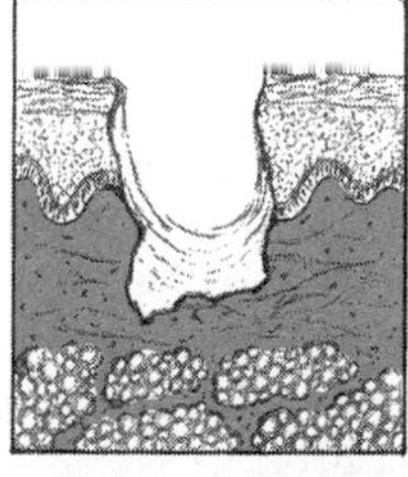

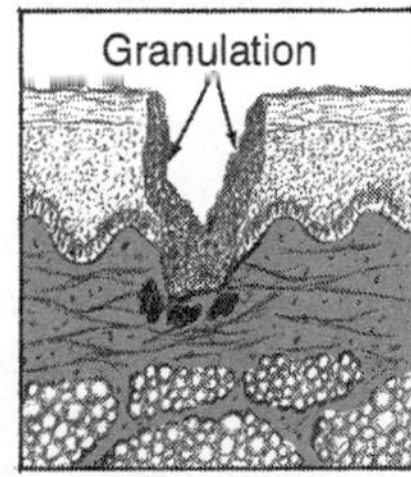

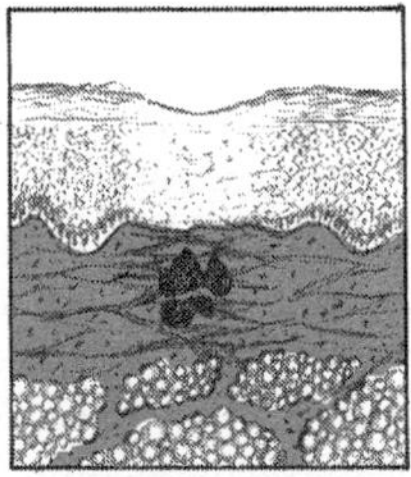

Third intention (puncture wound)

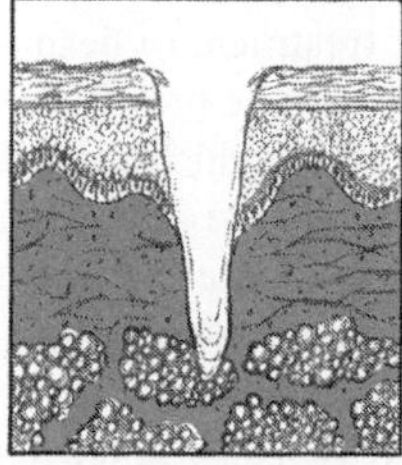

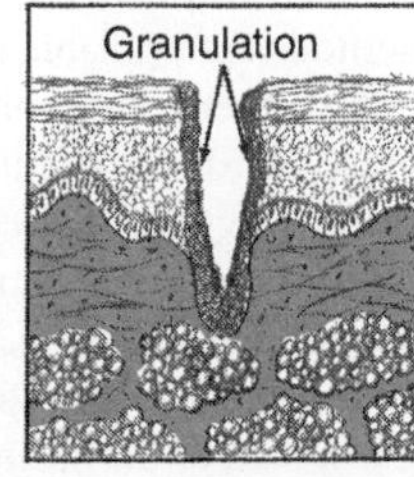

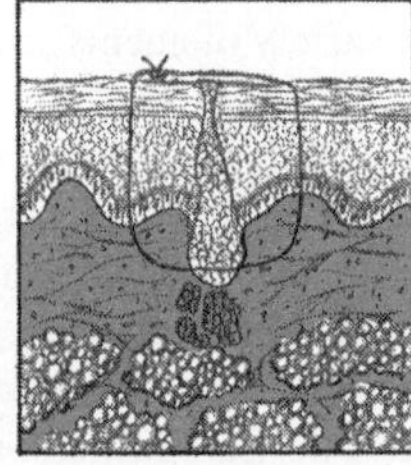

FIG. 32.1 Types of wound healing.

Primary intention healing takes place when all layers of the wound margins (skin, subcutaneous tissue, and muscle) are neatly approximated, as with a surgical incision. Unless infection interferes or the wound edges separate, these wounds heal with a minimum of scarring.

Repair by **secondary intention** takes place in wounds that occur from ulceration and lacerations in which the edges cannot be approximated, such as an avulsion or a third-degree burn. The inflammatory reaction may be greater, and the chance of infection is increased. Often debris, cells, and exudate must be cleaned away (debrided) before healing can take place. Healing takes place from the edges inward and from the bottom of the wound upward until the defect is filled. More granulation tissue and a larger scar are formed than in healing by primary intention.

Repair by **tertiary intention** takes place when suturing is delayed after injury or the wound later breaks down and is sutured or resutured when granulation is present. More granulation tissue is formed than in healing by primary intention, and there is a greater chance that microorganisms will invade the wound, resulting in a larger and deeper scar than healing by primary intention. Frequently, suturing of a contaminated wound is deliberately delayed to afford better removal of infection before closing.

Factors That Influence Healing

During the past decade, understanding of wound healing has revolutionized the interventions used to promote healing. Emphasis has shifted from interventions directed at maintaining a dry environment that promotes eschar formation to those that promote a moist, crust-free environment that enhances the migration of epithelial cells across the wound and facilitates resurfacing. An acute full-thickness wound kept in a moist environment usually reepithelializes in 12 to 15 days, whereas the same wound kept open to the air heals in approximately 25 to 30 days.

Eschar (thick, fibrin-containing necrotic tissue) also interferes with healing by preventing wound contraction. In most situations it is best to remove eschar and other dead tissue from the wound. Repeated application of occlusive dressings mobilizes the body's own enzymes to lyse the eschar, a process known as autolysis.

Adequate nutrition is essential for wound healing. In particular, sufficient protein, calories, vitamins C and D, and zinc are needed for healing of extensive wounds, such as burns. Supplemental nutrition is an integral aspect of treatment of severe wounds.

Numerous factors delay healing of the skin (Table 32.1). Some traditional practices are ineffective or even harmful; for example, antiseptics that were once used to help prevent infections (hydrogen peroxide and povidone-iodine [Betadine] solutions) are now known to have cytotoxic effects on healthy cells and minimal effect on controlling infections. Povidone-iodine may be absorbed through the skin in neonates and young children and must be used with caution in patients with thyroid or renal disease. Factors that delay wound healing, particularly in the home environment, include exposure to smoke or other allergens, dry or arid air, noncompliance or inconsistent adherence to the treatment regimen, and stress.

General Therapeutic Management

The human body intrinsically attempts to heal itself; therefore treatment is directed toward eliminating or ameliorating factors that interfere with normal healing processes. Some disorders may demand aggressive therapy, but by and large the major aim of any treatment is to prevent further damage, eliminate the cause, prevent complications, and provide relief from discomfort while tissues undergo healing. When possible, eliminate factors that contribute to the dermatitis and prolong the course of the disease. The most common offenders in pediatrics are

TABLE 32.1 Factors That Delay Wound Healing

Factor	Effect on Healing
Dry wound environment	Allows epithelial cells to dry out and die; impairs migration of epithelial cells across wound surface
Nutritional deficiencies	
• Vitamin A	Results in inadequate inflammatory response
• Vitamin B1	Results in decreased collagen formation
• Vitamin C	Inhibits formation of collagen fibers and capillary development
• Vitamin D	Regulates growth and differentiation of cell types, inhibits hyperproliferation of cells
• Protein	Reduces supply of amino acids for tissue repair
• Zinc	Impairs epithelialization
Immunocompromised	Results in inadequate or delayed inflammatory response
Impaired circulation	Inhibits inflammatory response and removal of debris from wound area Reduces supply of nutrients to wound area
Stress (pain, poor sleep)	Releases catecholamines that cause vasoconstriction
Antiseptics	
• Hydrogen peroxide	Toxic to fibroblasts; can cause subcutaneous gas formation (mimics gas-forming infection)
• Povidone-iodine	Toxic to white and red blood cells and fibroblasts
• Chlorhexidine	Toxic to white blood cells
Medications	
• Corticosteroids	Impair phagocytosis Inhibit fibroblast proliferation Depress formation of granulation tissue Inhibit wound contraction
• Chemotherapy	Interrupts the cell cycle; damages DNA or prevents DNA repair
• Antiinflammatory drugs	Decrease the inflammatory phase
Foreign bodies	Increase inflammatory response Inhibit wound closure
Infection	Increases inflammatory response Increases tissue destruction
Mechanical friction	Damages or destroys granulation tissue
Fluid accumulation in area	Inhibits tissues from approximating
Radiation	Inhibits fibroblastic activity and capillary formation May cause tissue necrosis
Diseases	
• Diabetes mellitus	Inhibits collagen synthesis Impairs circulation and capillary growth Hyperglycemia impairs phagocytosis
• Anemia	Reduces oxygen supply to tissues
• Peripheral vascular disease	Reduces oxygen supply to wounds
• Uremia	Decreases collagen and granulation tissue

DNA, Deoxyribonucleic acid.

environmental factors, including soaps (bubble baths and shampoos) and lotions; garments that are made of synthetic materials, have a rough texture (wool), or are tight-fitting; prolonged exposure to damp undergarments or swimsuits; and natural elements (plants and insects, dirt, sand, heat, cold, moisture, and wind). Dermatitis can also be aggravated by home remedies, poor nutrition, exposure to smoke, scratching or physical irritation of the site, and medications.

Dressings

No one dressing meets the needs of all wounds. The traditional dry gauze dressing should not be used on open wounds because it allows the wound surface to dry, does little to prevent bacterial invasion, and adheres to the dried scab so that removal disturbs the newly regenerating epithelial cells. In most instances, traditional gauze dressings have been replaced by dressings that promote moist wound healing. Moist wound healing increases the rate of collagen synthesis and reepithelialization and decreases pain and inflammation. It also creates an environment for autolytic debridement of necrotic tissue, which creates a clean wound bed and enhances granulation. However, a balance must be achieved between creating a moist wound bed and maintaining a dry periwound area that protects the skin and wound from maceration. The dressing type and frequency of dressing changes help achieve this balance. The frequency of dressing changes is based on the presence of infection, the type of dressing, the location of the wound, and the amount of drainage. Dressings should always be changed when they are loose or soiled. They should be changed more frequently in areas where contamination is likely (e.g., the sacral area, the buttocks, the tracheal area) or when wound infection is suspected or present.

Dressings serve the following functions: (1) provide a moist healing environment, (2) protect the wound from infection and trauma, (3) provide compression in the event of anticipated bleeding or swelling, (4) apply medication, (5) absorb drainage, (6) debride necrotic tissue, (7) reduce pain, and (8) control odor. To ensure a moist environment, cover wounds with an occlusive ointment or dressing (Table 32.2).

Occlusive dressings can be classified according to their degree of permeability. The term *occlusive* is synonymous with impermeable, *semiocclusive* is synonymous with semipermeable, and *nonocclusive* is synonymous with permeable. No one dressing meets the needs of all types of wounds. The traditional gauze dressing is a permeable dressing that reduces the moisture content in a wound by absorbing exudate and allowing it to evaporate. Dry gauze dressings have been replaced by new "active occlusive" dressings, which allow for moist wound healing rather than the traditional dry wound environment that created an increased risk for wound sepsis and trauma during removal. The use of silver-impregnated dressings for the treatment of wound care has reemerged. Although several studies suggest that silver decreases the bacteria and bioburden in the wound and improves short-term healing of wounds and ulcers, the long-term effects remain unclear. Due to the possibility of silver toxicity in children with silver-containing dressings, caution is strongly recommended when applying these dressings in the pediatric population (King, Stellar, Blevins, et al., 2014).

Topical Therapy

A variety of agents and methods are available for treatment of dermatologic problems. In selecting a therapeutic program, the practitioner considers (1) the active ingredient of the agent, (2) the vehicle or base, (3) the cosmetic effect, (4) the cost, (5) instructions for the agent's use, and (6) the family preference. Practitioners aim to avoid overtreatment, particularly in young children. For example, when the dermatitis is acute, short-term topical medications such as steroids are used to reduce irritation, inflammation, and spread of the disorder, then quickly tapered to mild or less frequent dosages to prevent side effects or long-term

TABLE 32.2 Dressing Category Definitions and Examples of Products

Category	Description	Examples
Gauze or sponge for external use	Nonresorbable Sterile or nonsterile Strip, piece, or pad Woven or nonwoven mesh cotton cellulose Simple chemical derivatives of cellulose Intended for medical purposes	Pads Island dressings
Hydrophilic wound dressing	Sterile or nonsterile Nonresorbable Material with hydrophilic properties No added drugs or biologics Intended to cover wound and absorb exudate	Alginate dressings Foam dressings Hydropolymer dressings Sheet gel dressings Hydrocolloid dressings Composite dressings
Occlusive wound dressing	Sterile or nonsterile Nonresorbable Synthetic polymeric material with or without adhesive backing Intended to cover wound, provide or support moist wound environment, and allow exchange of gases	Transparent adhesive dressings Thin film dressings Foam dressings Hydrocolloid dressings Composite dressings Hydropolymer dressings
Hydrogel wound dressing	Sterile or nonsterile Nonresorbable Matrix of hydrophilic polymers or other material combined with at least 50% water Intended to cover wound; absorb wound exudates; control bleeding or fluid loss; and protect against abrasion, friction, desiccation, and contamination	Alginate dressings Hydropolymer dressings Hydrogel dressings Gauze dressing impregnated with hydrogel (without active ingredients)
Porcine wound dressing	Made from pigskin Temporary burn dressing	

consequences. Chemicals that are nonirritating to intact skin (soaps and lotions) should be avoided because they can be quite irritating to inflamed or wounded skin, especially in children, whose skin is more absorbent.

Tepid or cool baths or the topical application of tepid or cool moist compresses may be used to treat the disorder, reduce the itching associated with many diseases, or decrease external stimuli. Baths are especially useful in the treatment of widespread dermatitis because they evenly distribute the soothing antipruritic and antiinflammatory solution, usually an oatmeal or mineral oil preparation. The temperature of the bathwater should be tepid, and the treatment usually lasts 15 to 30 minutes. Therapeutic baths are always more interesting for the child when toys are available in the tub for water play.

! NURSING ALERT

Application of heat tends to aggravate most conditions, and its use is generally reserved for reducing specific inflammatory processes, such as folliculitis and cellulitis.

Topical agents are applied to skin lesions to ease discomfort, prevent further injury, and facilitate healing. The emollient action of ointments and allergen-free lotions provides a soothing film over the skin surface that reduces external stimuli. Most preparations are placed directly on the skin and left uncovered; some may be applied under an occlusive dressing. The occlusive dressing promotes moisture retention and decreases evaporation of the therapeutic preparation. A thin application of the ointment or cream is covered with plastic film and anchored with adhesive or covered with a commercial transparent dressing. Apply any topical applications in a systematic manner following the contour of the body surface (not simply up and down). Children love to be "painted," so lotion applications can be fun when an ordinary soft-bristle paintbrush is employed. Regardless of the type of preparation used, parents need detailed information on the medication being applied, how to apply it, and how long the preparation should remain on the skin or under an occlusive dressing.

Topical corticosteroid therapy. Glucocorticoids are the therapeutic agents used most frequently for skin disorders. Their local antiinflammatory effects are merely palliative, so the medication is applied until the condition undergoes a remission or the causative agent is eliminated. Corticosteroids are applied directly to the affected area, are essentially nonsensitizing, and have only minor side effects. As with the use of any steroids, their use in large amounts may mask signs of infection, and symptoms may be exacerbated after termination of the drug. Families are cautioned that the medication cannot be used for all skin disorders. The concentrations available without prescription are not adequate for stubborn skin conditions (e.g., psoriasis, eczema) and may further aggravate inflammation caused by fungus or bacteria. When appropriate, it is important to counsel parents to apply only a thin film and to massage it into the skin because most parents and children apply more topical hydrocortisone than necessary for effective treatment. Parents and children should also be advised to use the application for no more than 5 to 7 days because these agents may cause depigmentation and other changes in the skin with extended use.

Other topical therapies. Other topical treatments include chemical cautery (especially useful for warts), cryosurgery, electrodesiccation (chiefly used for warts, granulomas, and nevi), ultraviolet (UV) light therapy (primarily used in psoriasis and acne), laser therapy (especially for birthmarks), and special acne therapies such as dermabrasion and chemical peels. Topical immunomodulators are effective in reducing the itching of atopic dermatitis (eczema) and preventing flare-ups in children resistant to first-line treatment options. However, the U.S. Food and Drug Administration issued a black box warning cautioning against the use of these topicals as first-line treatments in children younger than 2 years of age after chronic use of these medications was linked to possible skin cancer and lymphoma (Margolis, Abuabara, Hoffstad, et al., 2015). To date, no evidence has been published linking malignancy to the use of pimecrolimus cream (Elidel) in infants and children, but safety and efficacy are considered before using these medications in children (Margolis, Abuabara, Hoffstad, et al., 2015). Nonprescription and prescription topical antibiotics (lotions, gels, ointments, or creams) may also be used to treat minor wounds and acne. Again, families should be instructed to apply only a thin layer of medication at determined daily intervals for a limited number of days to the wound or affected area(s); each application of medication should be followed by careful hand washing.

! NURSING ALERT

Provide written instructions and demonstrate to parents the correct amount of topical medication to apply (e.g., size of a pea; thin film to cover). If more than one preparation is to be applied, mark the containers 1 and 2 to help parents remember the correct order for application to the skin. While educating children and their caregivers about medications, the nurse should emphasize that *more* medication or increased frequency of applications is *not better* when using topical medications and may carry the risk of being harmful, especially in the case of topical steroids.

Systemic Therapy

Systemic drugs may be used as an adjunct to topical therapy in some dermatologic disorders. The drugs most frequently used are corticosteroids, antibiotics, and antifungal agents. Corticosteroids are valuable in the treatment of severe skin disorders because of their capacity to inhibit inflammatory and allergic reactions. The dosage is carefully adjusted and gradually tapered to the minimum dosage that is effective and tolerated. Prolonged use of systematic corticosteroids may temporarily suppress the child's growth.

Antibiotics are used in cases of severe, chronic, or widespread skin infections. However, because these drugs tend to produce hypersensitivity in some patients, they are used with caution. Oral antifungal agents are the only effective means for treating systemic fungal infections and tinea capitus.

Nursing Care Management

To help establish a diagnosis, it is important for nurses to accurately describe any deviation in the character of the skin, using both inspection and palpation. Note the color, shape, size, character, and distribution of the lesions or wounds. Describe the individual lesions using the accepted terminology, understanding that there may be more than one type of wound, lesion, or rash. Assess wounds for depth of tissue damage, evidence of healing, and signs of infection (e.g., drainage, warmth, and odor).

To confirm or amplify the assessment findings made by inspection, gently palpate the skin to detect characteristics such as temperature, moisture, texture, elasticity, and the presence of edema. Indicate whether the findings are restricted to the area of the lesion(s) or are generalized.

A detailed history of the child's presenting illness, condition, or wound and their description (or appearance) of symptoms provide additional information. Older children may be able to tell you precipitating factors they may have been exposed to, timing of the disorder, and treatments

! NURSING ALERT

Signs of wound infection include the following:

- Increased erythema, especially beyond wound margin
- Edema
- Purulent exudate
- Odor
- Pain at the site or extending beyond the wound margin
- Increased temperature

they have already tried. They are also usually able to describe the condition as painful, itching, or tingling or use other descriptive terms and associated symptoms related to the condition. In younger children, the nurse can determine much by noting behavior during the intake interview and the caregivers' account of the symptoms or illness and the reaction to any home treatments. Besides asking about past medical history and noting the allergy and medication list of the patient, a careful nursing history may provide clues that will assist in determining an uncertain diagnosis. During the interview process, the nurse should ask the following questions:

- How long has this been occurring?
- Is the child scratching the area?
- Is the child restless or irritable?
- Does the child favor or avoid using a certain body part?
- Has the child had a fever or other illnesses recently?
- Has the child been around chemicals, woodlands, gardens, or woodpiles?
- Has the child traveled recently or visited someone's home for the first time?
- Has the child recently eaten a new food?
- Do any classmates, playmates, or siblings have similar lesions or illnesses?
- What has been done to treat the symptoms so far? Have any medications or home remedies been used?

Therapeutic treatments of skin disorders are typically aimed at providing comfort measures: rest, protection from infection or spread of the condition, and relief of discomfort. Specific treatments, such as a definitive medication or physical treatment or technique, may be prescribed for chronic conditions or wounds. Only a few skin disorders are contagious, so it is usually not necessary to isolate the affected child unless there is a danger that the child may acquire a secondary infection (e.g., the child who is receiving large doses of corticosteroids or other immunosuppressant drugs or the child with an immunologic deficiency disorder). However, when the skin manifestation is a viral exanthem such as chickenpox or an easily spread vector such as lice, the recommendation is to prevent exposing other susceptible children until the disorder is almost healed or the treatment is complete.

Wound Care

Parents can generally manage small skin wounds at home. Instruct parents to wash their hands and then wash the wound gently with mild soap and water. Topical antibiotics and nonadherent dressings are usually applied to the wound while it is in the primary healing stage. Caution parents to avoid povidone-iodine, alcohol, and hydrogen peroxide because these products are toxic to wounds. Wounds covering a very large area (>15% of the body) need medical attention with the child undergoing conscious sedation and analgesia.

! NURSING ALERT

Do not put anything in a wound that you would not put in the eye. The safest solution is normal saline.

Open wounds are typically covered with a nonadherent dressing, such as a commercial adhesive bandage, although larger wounds may benefit from the use of occlusive dressings. If occlusive dressings are applied, instruct parents on their correct application and removal. For example, hydrocolloid dressings adhere best if a wide margin is left around the wound and the dressing is pressed against intact skin until it adheres. The edges of the dressing can be secured to the healthy skin margins with waterproof tape. The dressings are removed if leakage occurs or after specific time intervals, usually for a period of 7 days.

! NURSING ALERT

Advise parents that the yellow gel forming under hydrocolloid dressings may look like pus and has a distinct odor (somewhat fruity) but is normal leakage.

Dressings are removed carefully to protect intact skin and the epithelial surface of the wound. If the affected skin has significant hair growth, the nurse may consider removing a small patch or strip of hair surrounding the wound to improve dressing adherence and decrease discomfort for the child during dressing changes. When removing transparent or hydrocolloid dressings, the nurse or parent raises one edge of the dressing and pulls *parallel* to the skin to loosen the adhesive. The child may assist the nurse or caregiver in the dressing change procedure by firmly holding their skin taut as the adhesive dressing is removed. If a dressing sticks to the wound base when it is being removed, saturate the dressing with normal saline or clean water to loosen it and then proceed with care. Another useful technique for applying dressings to wounds is "picture-framing." The wound is "framed" on all sides with the application of a skin barrier dressing that stays in place around the wound (e.g., DuoDERM, Coloplast). This technique protects the healthy skin from injury during repeated dressing changes because the adhesive can be secured to the skin barrier surrounding the wound rather than directly to the skin. Lacerations present a special challenge with cleaning and dressing. The injured child and family are usually distressed by the bleeding associated with the wound and may be in variable degrees of anxiety, fear, and shock. Because scalp and facial lacerations tend to bleed profusely, they are especially frightening. The initial nursing intervention is to calmly apply direct pressure to the area and to attempt to calm the child before further examination. Unless there is bleeding from a severed artery, the wound is cleansed with a forced stream of sterile tepid water or normal saline (via syringe). The wound is then examined for extent and depth of injury and presence of foreign material such as dirt, glass, or fabric fragments. Before suturing lacerations or wounds, a topical anesthetic or intradermal buffered lidocaine should be used to reduce discomfort and promote cooperation of the child during the procedure.

The location of the wound dictates careful physical assessment. For example, wounds over bony areas may contain bone chips, and clear fluid seeping from severe head wounds may indicate cerebrospinal fluid. For severe wounds that cannot be completely evaluated immediately and lacerations that require suturing, apply a clean pressure dressing over the affected area and transfer the child for emergency medical care. Puncture wounds should initially be irrigated with sterile saline and then soaked in a basin of warm soapy water for several minutes before applying a clean dressing. Causing the puncture wound to rebleed may be indicated to ensure no foreign body is embedded in the wound. Puncture wounds of the head, chest, or abdomen or those that could still contain a portion of the puncturing object must be evaluated further by a practitioner and may require an x-ray to confirm that all foreign material has been removed from the wound. Caution parents against opening ("popping") wounds, blisters, or vesicles, or kissing a wound "to make it better." The skin can easily become contaminated from germs in the human mouth. If scabs form, they are allowed to slough off without assistance; picking or early removal may cause scarring and secondary infection. Advise parents to seek medical help if there is evidence of infection.

Relief of Symptoms

Most of the therapeutic regimens are intended to promote wound healing, prevent infection, and provide relief of pruritus, the most common subjective complaint. Preventing scratching is of primary importance. Itching is believed to often result from stimulation of C fibers at the dermoepidermal junction and the release of histamine and endopeptidases. These fibers are similar to but distinct from pain fibers and may be stimulated with a single scratch. Cooling the affected area and increasing the skin pH with an alkaline-containing compress, such as a baking soda or Burow solution, or tepid bath reduce the child's external stimuli and the urge to scratch. Older children usually can avoid self-contaminating the wound, though they may occasionally need to be reminded to stop scratching or rubbing. In younger and uncooperative children, techniques and devices such as mittens (especially during sleep) or special hand coverings are required. Keeping fingernails short and clean helps reduce scratching and the chance of secondary infection of the wound. Clothing and bed linens should be soft, smooth, lightweight, and made of natural fibers to decrease the irritation from friction and stimulation. Antipruritic medications such as diphenhydramine (Benadryl) or hydroxyzine (Atarax) may be prescribed for severe itching, especially if it disrupts the child's sleep.

Wet compresses or dressings cool the skin by evaporation, relieve itching and inflammation, and cleanse the area by loosening and removing crusts and debris. A variety of ingredients, such as plain water or Burow solution (available without a prescription), can be applied on Kerlix gauze; plain gauze; or (preferably) soft cotton cloths such as freshly laundered towels, bed sheets, or pillowcases.

Pain and discomfort are usually managed with nonpharmacologic measures such as positioning and rest, distraction techniques, and individual preferences of comfort. Occlusive dressings applied over wounds reduce pain similar to cool or tepid compresses. Doses of mild analgesics such as acetaminophen or ibuprofen, prescribed based on the patient's weight, may be recommended. Severe pain requires prescribed analgesic medication and careful nursing assessment for infection or an underlying cause of discomfort. For severe wounds and burns, prescribed analgesic medications should be administered before each dressing change, debridement procedure, or cleansing, allowing adequate time for the medicine to take therapeutic effect. (See Pain Management, Chapter 5.)

Wound healing may be facilitated by recombinant growth factor or a vacuum-assisted closure device. These therapies may be employed when wounds are large and in a location that creates challenges for therapy (e.g., sacral or groin wound) or when the child has associated conditions such as malnutrition or a comprised immune system, putting "normal" wound healing at risk. Recombinant growth factors are human platelet–derived growth factors that are engineered outside the body. They foster the formation of new granulation tissue by stimulating the migration of fibroblasts, macrophages, smooth muscle cells, and capillary endothelial cells to the wound site.

The vacuum-assisted closure (VAC) device uses a technique that involves placing a foam dressing into the wound, covering it with an occlusive dressing, and applying gentle, continuous suction. The negative pressure of the suction is applied from the foam dressing to the wound surfaces. The mechanical force removes excess fluids from the wound, stimulates formation of granulation tissue, restores capillary flow, and fosters closure of the wound. VAC has been used to prepare wounds for a skin graft and to treat surgical wounds, burns, and pressure ulcers (Han & Ceilley, 2017). The safety and efficacy of the VAC technique for infants and children has been documented in recent studies (Satteson, Crantford, Wood, et al., 2015; Takahara, Sai, Kagatani, et al., 2014; Koehler, Jinbo, Johnson, et al., 2014).

Home Care and Family Support

Care of a child with a dermatologic condition always involves the family, but few situations require hospitalization, and most care is delivered at home. Because the family members must carry out the treatment plan, their cooperation is essential. Regimens that are routine for health care professionals to accomplish in the clinic, hospital, or primary care provider's office may be frustrating and baffling for caregivers in the home. The family may also need assistance in adapting equipment available for home therapy.

It is important that the child and family be given as detailed explanations as possible about both the expected and the unexpected results of treatment, including any side effects that might occur. If unexplained reactions develop, direct the family to discontinue treatment and report the reactions to the appropriate person. Discourage the use of over-the-counter medicines and homeopathic treatments unless the preparations have been discussed with the health care provider and have received approval.

Because the skin is the most visible portion of the body, defects in its surface alter its appearance and cause distress for the child. Skin problems may also result in rejection by others. Parents of other children may fear that their children will "catch" the disorder. Occasionally, the affected child's own family members reduce their interaction or physical contact with the child especially close physical contact, or demonstrate distaste for the condition, which the child may interpret as rejection or punishment. This is seldom a concern for children with dermatitis of short duration, but chronic conditions can frequently create problems and affect the child's self-esteem (see Family-Centered Care box).

FAMILY-CENTERED CARE

Skin Lesions and Self-Esteem in the School-Age Child

When I was 8 years old, a lot of small, oval, tannish-brown spots developed, especially around my neck and waist. The dermatologist said it was a rare condition and that it should disappear by the time I was 11 or 12. They actually disappeared when I was 10. Because the spots were kind of unusual, the dermatologist invited me to attend a dermatology meeting where people with strange skin problems were placed in private clinic rooms and doctors came in and looked at each person's skin. They were all nice, but I felt a little like an animal in the zoo. The thing I mostly remember about the spots was that I always tried to keep them covered. People stared, and kids made fun of me. The spots didn't hurt or itch, but I always knew they were there. I would not wear a two-piece swimsuit, even though my friends wore them. My mom and I tried to think of anything that might have caused the spots, but I never knew why they developed on me. I remember thinking it wasn't fair that it happened to me. I learned that many times, people cannot prevent the bad things that happen to them.

Marissa, age 16
Tulsa, Oklahoma

INFECTIONS OF THE SKIN

BACTERIAL INFECTIONS

Normally, the skin harbors a variety of bacterial flora, including the major pathogenic varieties of staphylococci and streptococci. The degree of pathogenicity of the organism depends on its invasiveness and toxicity, the integrity of the skin (the host's barrier), and the host's immune and cellular defenses. Children with congenital or acquired immunodeficiency disorders (e.g., acquired immunodeficiency syndrome [AIDS]), children receiving immunosuppressant therapy, and those with a malignancy such as leukemia or lymphoma are at risk for developing bacterial infections.

Because of the characteristic "walling-off" process of the inflammatory reaction (abscess formation), staphylococci are more difficult to treat, and the local infected area is associated with an increase in bacteria all over the skin surface that serves as a source of continuing infection. Since the early 2000s, the number of methicillin-resistant *Staphylococcus aureus* (MRSA) community-acquired infections rose dramatically until reaching a peak in 2007 and then steadily declining (Kaplan, 2016). These factors underline the importance of careful hand washing and cleanliness when caring for infected children and their lesions to prevent the spread of infection and as an essential prophylactic measure when caring for infants and small children. Common bacterial skin disorders are outlined in Table 32.3 (Figs. 32.2 and 32.3).

Nursing Care Management

The major nursing functions related to bacterial skin infections are to prevent the spread of infection and to prevent complications. Impetigo contagiosa and MRSA infection can easily spread by self-inoculation; therefore caution the child against touching the involved area. Hand washing is mandatory before and after contact with an affected child. Also emphasize hand washing to both the child and the family. Many children with atopic dermatitis are colonized with MRSA (Chaptini, Quinn, & Marshman, 2016). For many bacterial infections and MRSA infection in particular, the child should be provided with washcloths and towels separate from those of other family members. The child's clothes should be changed daily and washed in hot water. Razors used for shaving should be discarded after each use and not shared. To prevent recurrence, some infectious disease specialists recommend bathing in a chlorine bath daily for 5 to 14 days, although evidence of the effectiveness is inconclusive (Gupta, Lyons, & Rosen, 2015; Kaplan, Forbes, Hammerman, et al., 2014). For the chlorine bathing, 1 teaspoon of bleach is diluted in 13 gallons of water or $\frac{1}{4}$ cup of bleach is diluted in a standard 50-gallon tub one-fourth filled with water (Gupta, Lyons, & Rosen, 2015). In addition, mupirocin can be applied to the nares of patients and families twice daily for 5 to 10 days to prevent reinfection (Gupta, Lyons, & Rosen, 2015).

Children and parents are often tempted to squeeze follicular lesions. They must be warned that squeezing will not hasten the resolution of the infection and that there is a risk of making the lesion worse or spreading the infection. No attempt should be made to puncture the surface of the pustule with a needle or sharp instrument. A child with a sty may waken with the eyelids of the affected eye sealed shut with exudate. The child or the parents are instructed to gently wipe the eyelid from the inner to the outer edge with warm water and a clean washcloth until the exudate is removed.

The child with limited cellulitis of an extremity is usually managed at home on a regimen of oral antibiotics and warm compresses. The parents are taught the procedures and instructed in administration of the medication. Children with more extensive cellulitis, especially around a joint with lymphadenitis or on the face, are usually admitted

TABLE 32.3 Bacterial Infections

Disorder and Organism	Manifestations	Management	Comments
Impetigo contagiosa—*Staphylococcus* (see Fig. 32.2)	Begins as a reddish macule Becomes vesicular Ruptures easily, leaving superficial, moist erosion Tends to spread peripherally in sharply marginated irregular outlines Exudate dries to form heavy, honey-colored crusts Pruritus common Systemic effects—Minimal or asymptomatic	Topical bactericidal ointment mupirocin or triple antibiotic ointment Oral or parenteral antibiotics (penicillin) in severe or extensive lesions Vancomycin for methicillin-resistant *Staphylococcus aureus* (MRSA)	Tends to heal without scarring unless secondary infection Autoinoculable and contagious Common in toddlers and preschoolers May be superimposed on eczema
Pyoderma—*Staphylococcus, Streptococcus*	Deeper extension of infection into dermis Tissue reaction more severe Systemic effects—Fever, lymphangitis, sepsis, liver disease, heart disease	Soap and water cleansing Topical antiseptic, such as chlorhexidine Mupirocin Antibiotics depending on causative organism: Cephalexin, nafcillin, intramuscular benzathine penicillin Bathing with antibacterial soap as prescribed Do not share washcloths or towels	Autoinoculable and contagious May heal with or without scarring
Folliculitis (pimple), furuncle (boil), carbuncle (multiple boils)—*Staphylococcus aureus*, methicillin-resistant *S. aureus* (MRSA)	Folliculitis—Infection of hair follicle Furuncle—Larger lesion with more redness and swelling at a single follicle Carbuncle—More extensive lesion with widespread inflammation and "pointing" at several follicular orifices Systemic effects—Malaise if severe	Skin cleanliness Local warm, moist compresses Topical application of antibiotic agents Systemic antibiotics in severe cases Incision and drainage of severe lesions, followed by wound irrigations with antibiotics or suitable drain implantation MRSA infections: • 5-inch soak of ½ cup bleach diluted in a standard 50-gallon tub one-fourth filled with water once or twice weekly • No sharing of towels or washcloths, changing of clothes and underwear daily, and laundering in hot water • Disposal of razors after one use • Application of mupirocin to nares bid for 2-4 weeks	Autoinoculable and contagious Furuncle and carbuncle tend to heal with scar formation Lesions should never be squeezed
Cellulitis—*Streptococcus, Staphylococcus, Haemophilus influenzae* (see Fig. 32.3)	Inflammation of skin and subcutaneous tissues with intense redness, swelling, and firm infiltration Lymphangitis "streaking" frequently seen Involvement of regional lymph nodes common May progress to abscess formation Systemic effects—Fever, malaise	Oral or parenteral antibiotics Rest and immobilization of both affected area and child	Hospitalization may be necessary for child with systemic symptoms Otitis media may be associated with facial cellulites
Staphylococcal scalded skin syndrome—*S. aureus*	Macular erythema with "sandpaper" texture of involved skin Epidermis becomes wrinkled (in days or less), and large bullae appear Localized bullous impetigo in older child	Systemic antibiotics Gentle cleansing with saline, Burow solution, or 0.25% silver nitrate compresses	Infants subject to fluid loss; impaired body temperature regulation; and secondary infection, such as pneumonia, cellulitis, and septicemia Heals without scarring

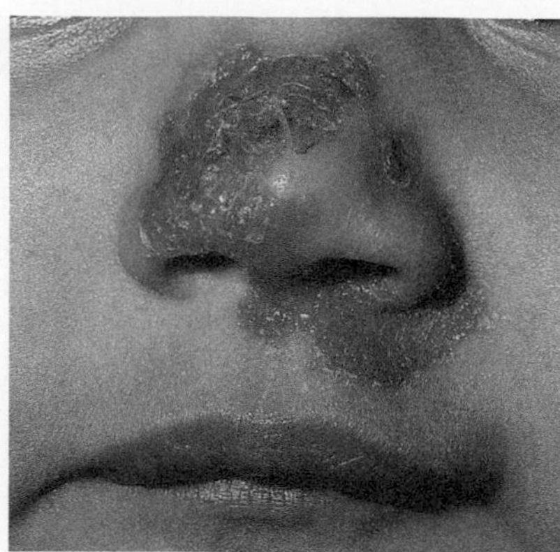

FIG. 32.2 Impetigo contagiosa. (From Weston, W. L., & Lane, A. T. [2007]. *Color textbook of pediatric dermatology* [4th ed.]. St. Louis, MO: Mosby.)

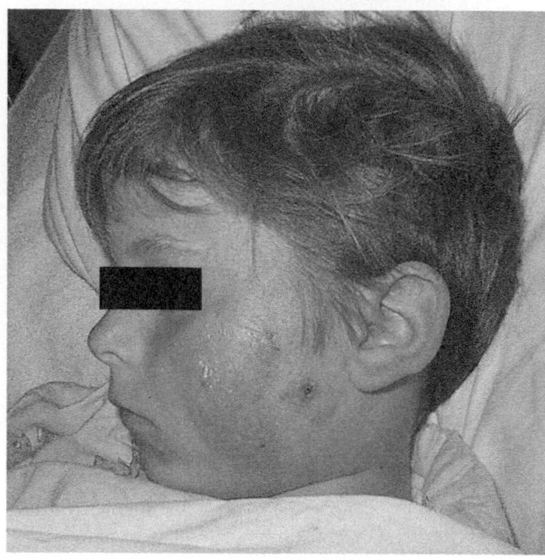

FIG. 32.3 Cellulitis of cheek from a puncture wound. (From Weston, W. L., & Lane, A. T. [2007]. *Color textbook of pediatric dermatology* [4th ed.]. St. Louis, MO: Mosby.)

to the hospital for parenteral antibiotics with continued treatment at home. Nurses are responsible for teaching the family to administer the medication and apply compresses.

VIRAL INFECTIONS

Viruses are intracellular parasites that produce their effect by using the intracellular substances of the host cells. Composed of only a deoxyribonucleic acid (DNA) or ribonucleic acid (RNA) core enclosed in an antigenic protein shell, viruses are unable to provide for their own metabolic needs or to reproduce themselves. After a virus penetrates a cell of the host organism, it sheds the outer shell and disappears within the cell, where the nucleic acid core stimulates the host cell to form more virus material from its intracellular substance. In a viral infection, the epidermal cells react with inflammation and vesiculation (as in herpes simplex) or by proliferating to form growths (warts).

Many of the communicable viral diseases of childhood are associated with rashes, and each rash is characteristic. The type of lesion and the configuration of rubeola, rubella, and chickenpox are described in Table 6.2. Other common viral disorders of the skin are outlined in Table 32.4.

DERMATOPHYTOSES (FUNGAL INFECTIONS)

The dermatophytoses (ringworm) are infections caused by a group of closely related filamentous fungi that invade primarily the stratum corneum, hair, and nails. These are superficial infections by organisms that live on, not in, the skin. Dermatophytoses are designated by the Latin word *tinea*, with further designation relating to the area of the body where they are found (e.g., tinea capitis [ringworm of the scalp]). Table 32.5 outlines common dermatophytoses (Fig. 32.4).

Dermatophyte infections are most often transmitted from one person to another or from infected animals to humans. Because the keratin is desquamated constantly, the fungus must multiply at a rate that equals the rate of keratin production to maintain itself; otherwise the infection would be shed with the discarded skin cells. Diagnosis is made from microscopic examination of scrapings taken from the advancing periphery of the lesion, which almost always produces a scale.

Nursing Care Management

When teaching families how to care for ringworm, the nurse should emphasize good health and hygiene. Because of the infectious nature of the disease, affected children should not exchange grooming items, headgear, scarves, or other articles of apparel that have been in proximity to the infected area with other children. Affected children are provided with their own towels and directed to wear a protective cap at night to avoid transmitting the fungus to bedding, especially if they sleep with another person. Because the infection can be acquired by animal-to-human transmission, all household pets should be examined for the disorder. Other sources of infection are seats in locker rooms, tanning beds, seats in public transportation vehicles, helmets, and gymnasium mats.

Both 2% ketoconazole and 1% selenium sulfide shampoos may reduce colony counts of dermatophytes. These shampoos can be used in combination with oral therapy to reduce the transmission of disease to others. The shampoo should be applied to the scalp for 5 to 10 minutes at least three times per week. The child may return to school after the therapy is initiated.

Alternatively, if the child is treated with the drug griseofulvin, the therapy frequently continues for weeks or months, and because subjective symptoms subside, children or parents may be tempted to decrease or discontinue the drug. The nurse should emphasize to family members the importance of maintaining the prescribed dosage schedule and of taking the medication with high-fat foods for best absorption. They are also instructed regarding possible drug side effects, such as headache, gastrointestinal upset, fatigue, insomnia, and photosensitivity. For children who take the drug over many months, periodic testing is required to monitor leukopenia and assess liver and renal function. Other antifungal medications such as terbinafine, itraconazole, and fluconazole can be used.

SYSTEMIC MYCOTIC (FUNGAL) INFECTIONS

Mycotic (systemic or deep fungal) infections have the capacity to invade the viscera, as well as the skin. The most common infections are the lung diseases, which are usually acquired by inhalation of fungal spores. These fungi produce a variable spectrum of disease, and some are common in certain geographic areas. They are not transmitted from person to person but appear to reside in the soil, from which their spores are airborne. The cutaneous lesions caused by deep fungal infections are granulomatous and appear as ulcers, plaques, nodules, fungating masses, and abscesses. The course of deep fungal diseases is chronic with slow progression that favors sensitization (Table 32.6).

TABLE 32.4 Viral Infections

Infection	Manifestations	Management	Comments
Verruca (warts) Cause—Human papillomavirus (various types)	Usually well-circumscribed, gray or brown, elevated, firm papules with a roughened, finely papillomatous texture Occur anywhere but usually appear on exposed areas such as fingers, hands, face, and soles May be single or multiple Asymptomatic	Not uniformly successful Local destructive therapy, individualized according to location, type, and number—surgical removal, electrocautery, curettage, cryotherapy (liquid nitrogen), caustic solutions (lactic acid and salicylic acid in flexible collodion, retinoic acid, salicylic acid plasters), laser ablation	Common in children Tend to disappear spontaneously Course unpredictable Most destructive techniques tend to leave scars Autoinoculable Repeated irritation will cause to enlarge
Verruca plantaris (plantar wart)	Located on plantar surface of feet and, because of pressure, are practically flat; may be surrounded by a collar of hyperkeratosis	Caustic chemical solution applied to wart and wear foam insole with hole cut to relieve pressure on wart; soak 20 minutes after 2-3 days; repeat until wart comes out	Destructive techniques tend to leave scars, which may cause problems with walking
Herpes simplex virus Type I (cold sore, fever blister) Type II (genital)	Grouped, burning, and itching vesicles on inflammatory base, usually on or near mucocutaneous junctions (lips, nose, genitalia, buttocks) Vesicles dry, forming a crust followed by exfoliation and spontaneous healing in 8-10 days May be accompanied by regional lymphadenopathy	Avoidance of secondary infection Burow solution compresses during weeping stages Oral antiviral (acyclovir [Zovirax]) for initial infection or to reduce severity in recurrence; may also be given prophylactically for recurrent Valacyclovir (Valtrex), an oral antiviral, used for episodic treatment of recurrent genital herpes; reduces pain, stops viral shedding, and has a more convenient administration schedule than acyclovir; primarily recommended for immunocompromised patients	Heal without scarring unless secondary infection Type I cold sores prevented by using sunscreens protecting against ultraviolet A and ultraviolet B light to prevent lip blisters Aggravated by corticosteroids Positive psychologic effect from treatment May be fatal in children with depressed immunity
Varicella-zoster virus (herpes zoster; shingles)	Caused by same virus that causes varicella (chickenpox) Virus has affinity for posterior root ganglia, posterior horn of spinal cord, and skin; crops of vesicles usually confined to dermatome following along course of affected nerve Usually preceded by neuralgic pain (rare in children), hyperesthesias, or itching May be accompanied by constitutional symptoms	Symptomatic Analgesics for pain Drying lotions sometimes helpful Ophthalmic variety: systemic corticotropin (adrenocorticotropic hormone) or corticosteroids Acyclovir or valacyclovir Preventive vaccine is available for persons >50 years old	Pain in children usually minimal Postherpetic pain does not occur in children Chickenpox may follow exposure; isolate affected child from other children in a hospital or school May occur in children with depressed immunity; can be fatal
Molluscum contagiosum Cause—Pox virus	Flesh-colored papules (1-20) with a central caseous plug (umbilicated) that occur on trunk, face and extremities; may be transmitted by sexual contact Usually asymptomatic	Cases in well children resolve spontaneously in about 18 months Treatment reserved for cosmetic purposes; alleviate discomfort; reduce autoinoculation; prevent secondary infection Numerous chemical removing agents including tretinoin gel 0.01% or cantharidin (Cantharone) liquid; podophyllin; imiquimod cream These are painful treatments: Use local anesthesia Curettage, electrodessication, or cryotherapy	Common in school-age children Spread by skin-to-skin contact, including autoinoculation and fomite-to-skin contact Outbreaks in child care centers have been reported

SKIN DISORDERS RELATED TO CHEMICAL OR PHYSICAL CONTACTS

CONTACT DERMATITIS

Contact dermatitis is an inflammatory reaction of the skin to chemical substances, natural or synthetic, that evoke a hypersensitivity response or direct irritation. The initial reaction occurs in an exposed region, most commonly the face and neck, backs of the hands, forearms, male genitalia, and lower legs. There is characteristically a sharp demarcation between inflamed and normal skin that ranges from a faint, transient erythema to massive bullae on an erythematous swollen base. Itching is a constant symptom.

The cause may be a primary irritant or a sensitizing agent. A **primary irritant** is one that irritates any skin. A **sensitizing agent** produces an irritation on those individuals who have encountered the irritant or something chemically related to it, have undergone an immunologic change, and have become sensitized. Prior exposure is not necessarily a factor in the reaction. A sensitizer irritates in relatively low concentrations only persons who are allergic to it.

The major goal in treatment is to prevent further exposure of the skin to the offending substance. Provided there is no further irritation,

TABLE 32.5 Dermatophytoses (Fungal Infections)

Disease and Organism	Manifestations	Management	Comments
Tinea capitis—*Trichophyton tonsurans, Microsporum audouinii, Microsporum canis* (see Fig. 32.4, *A*)	Lesions in scalp but may extend to hairline or neck Characteristic configuration of scaly, circumscribed patches or patchy, scaling areas of alopecia Generally asymptomatic but severe, deep inflammatory reaction may occur that manifests as boggy, encrusted lesions (kerions) Pruritic Diagnosis: Microscopic examination of scales	Oral griseofulvin or terbinafine Oral ketoconazole for difficult cases Selenium sulfide shampoos, used twice a week, may decrease infection and fungal shedding (American Academy of Pediatrics, 2015) Kerion: Griseofulvin and possibly oral corticosteroids for 2 weeks to achieve therapeutic effect (American Academy of Pediatrics, 2015)	Person-to-person transmission Animal-to-person transmission Rarely, permanent loss of hair *M. audouinii* transmitted from one human being to another directly or from personal items; *M. canis* usually contracted from household pets, especially cats Atopic individuals more susceptible
Tinea corporis—*Trichophyton rubrum, Trichophyton mentagrophytes, M. canis,* Epidermophyton (see Fig. 32.4, *B*)	Generally round or oval, erythematous scaling patch that spreads peripherally and clears centrally; may involve nails (tinea unguium) Diagnosis—Direct microscopic examination of scales Usually unilateral	Oral griseofulvin Local application of antifungal preparation such as tolnaftate, naftifine, miconazole, terbinafine, clotrimazole; applied 2.5 cm (1 inch) beyond periphery of lesion; application continued 1-2 weeks after no sign of lesion Topical antifungals with high-potency steroids are not recommended as they may lead to further infection and have local and systemic side effects (American Academy of Pediatrics, 2015)	Usually of animal origin from infected pets but may occur from human transmission, soil or fomites Majority of infections in children caused by *M. canis* and *M. audouinii* Tinea gladiatorum is commonly seen in wrestlers
Tinea cruris ("jock itch")—*Epidermophyton floccosum, T. rubrum, T. mentagrophytes*	Skin response similar to tinea corporis Localized to medial proximal aspect of thigh and crural fold; may involve scrotum in males Pruritic Diagnosis—Same as for tinea corporis	Local application of tolnaftate liquid, terbinafine, clotrimazole, ciclopirox twice daily for 2-4 weeks	Rare in preadolescent children Health education regarding transmission via person-to-person (direct or indirect) Occurs in close association with tinea pedis and tinea unguium
Tinea pedis ("athlete's foot")—*T. rubrum, Trichophyton interdigitale, E. floccosum* Tinea unguium: Nail infection	On intertriginous areas between toes or on plantar surface of feet Lesions vary: Maceration and fissuring between toes Patches with pinhead-sized vesicles on plantar surface Pruritic Diagnosis—Direct microscopic examination of scrapings	Local applications of terbinafine, ciclopirox or clotrimazole, or miconazole, or ketoconazole Oral itraconazole, terbinafine or griseofulvin for severe infections or those which do not respond to topical acute infections—Compresses or soaks with Burow solution (1 : 80) (American Academy of Pediatrics, 2015) Elimination of conditions of heat and perspiration by use of clean, light socks and well-ventilated shoes; avoidance of occlusive shoes	Most frequent in adolescents and adults; rare in children, but occurrence increases with wearing of plastic shoes Common in locations such as showers, locker rooms and swimming pools where fungi proliferate
Candidiasis (moniliasis)—*Candida albicans*	Grows in chronically moist areas Inflamed areas with white exudate, peeling, and easy bleeding Pruritic Diagnosis—Characteristic appearance; microscopic identification of scrapings; candidemia diagnosed from cultures (blood, cerebrospinal fluid, bone marrow); tissue biopsy Chronic or recurrent often seen with HIV infection and immunocompromised child	Neonates-thrush-oral nystatin Older children, clotrimazole troches applied to lesions (American Academy of Pediatrics, 2015) Fluconazole or itraconazole for immunocompromised Esophagitis: Treat with oral or IV fluconazole or itraconazole; IV amphotericin, voriconazole, micafungin Treat skin lesions with topical nystatin, miconazole, clotrimazole, ketoconazole, econazole, or ciclopirox (American Academy of Pediatrics, 2015) Vulvovaginal: Clotrimazole, miconazole, butoconazole, terconazole, and tioconazole used topically (American Academy of Pediatrics, 2015)	Common form of diaper dermatitis (see Fig. 32.10) Oral form common in infants (see Chapter 8) Vaginal form in females Disseminated disease in very-low-birth-weight infants and immunosuppressed children

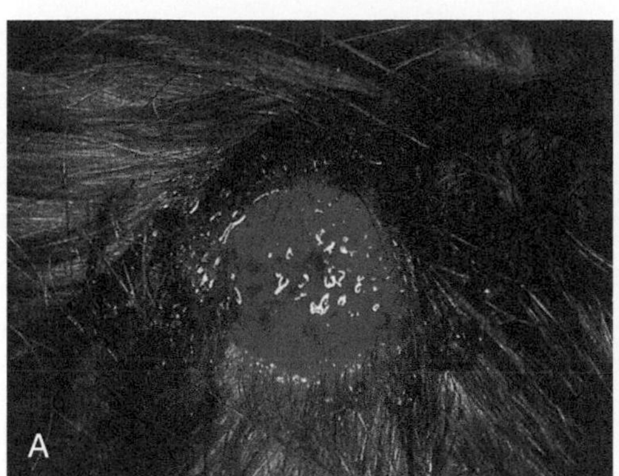

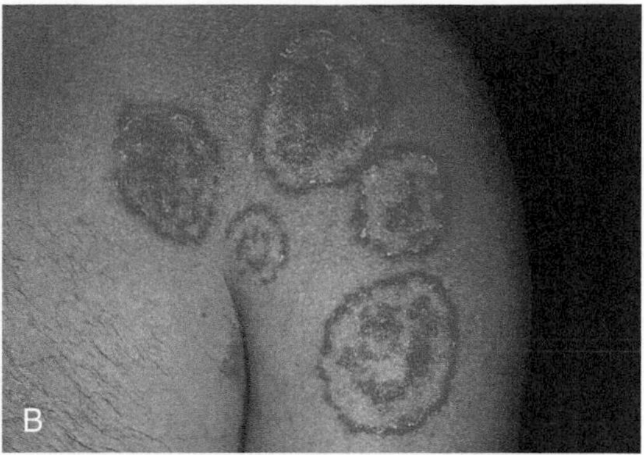

FIG. 32.4 A, Tinea capitis. **B,** Tinea corporis. Both infections are caused by *Microsporum canis,* the "kitten" or "puppy" fungus. (From Habif, T. P. [2004]. *Clinical dermatology: A color guide to diagnosis and therapy* [4th ed.]. St. Louis, MO: Mosby.)

TABLE 32.6 **Systemic Mycoses**

Disorder and Organism	Skin Manifestations	Systemic Manifestations	Management	Comments
North American blastomycosis—*Blastomyces dermatitidis*	Chronic granulomatous lesions and microabscesses in any part of body Initial lesion is a papule; undergoes ulceration and peripheral spread	Pulmonary symptoms, such as cough, fever, chest pain, weakness, and weight loss; rarely develop ARDS Possible skeletal involvement, with bone destruction and formation of cutaneous abscesses	IV amphotericin B Oral fluconazole or itraconazole for mild or moderate cases after amphotericin B (American Academy of Pediatrics, 2015)	Usual portal of entry is lungs Source of infection unknown Pulmonary infections may be mild and self-limiting and require no treatment Progressive disease often fatal
Cryptococcosis—*Cryptococcus neoformans* (*Torula histolytica*)	Usually on face; acneiform, firm, nodular, painless eruption	CNS manifestations—Headache, dizziness, stiff neck, and signs of increased intracranial pressure Low-grade fever, mild cough, lung infiltration	IV amphotericin B; may be administered intrathecal for CNS involvement Oral flucytosine then fluconazole for meningitis Excision and drainage of local lesions	Acquired by inhalation of contaminate soil (bird feces) Endemic in Mississippi and Ohio River valleys Increased incidence in persons with defects in T-lymphocyte–mediated immunity (HIV, leukemia, systemic lupus, AIDS, or organ transplant) No person-to-person transmission
Histoplasmosis—*Histoplasma capsulatum*	Not distinctive or uniform but most appear as punched-out or granulomatous ulcers Erythema nodosum in adolescents	General systemic symptoms may include pallor, diarrhea, vomiting, irregular spiking temperature, hepatosplenomegaly, and pulmonary symptoms Any tissue of body may be involved with related symptoms	IV amphotericin B for severe cases Itraconazole for mild to moderate infections	Organism cultured from soil, especially where contaminated with fowl droppings Fungus enters through skin or mucous membranes of mouth and respiratory tract Endemic in Mississippi and Ohio River valleys Disseminated diseases most common in infants and children younger than 2 years
Coccidioidomycosis (valley fever)—*Coccidioides immitis* and *C. posadasii*	Erythema nodosum Erythema multiforme Erythematous maculopapular rash	Primary lung disease usually asymptomatic: 60% of children Symptoms: Cough, fever, malaise, myalgia, headache, chest pain May be sign of acute febrile illness Disseminated disease is very serious; occurs in infants (meningitis)	Fluconazole or itraconazole for 3-6 months IV amphotericin B if no response to above Surgical resection of persistent pulmonary cavities	Inhalation of aerospores from soil Endemic in southwestern United States (*C. immitis* almost occurs exclusively in California) Usually resolves spontaneously Increased incidence in dark-skinned races (Filipino, African American, Hispanic), pregnant women, diabetics, persons with cardiopulmonary disease, and infants <1 year old

AIDS, Acquired immunodeficiency syndrome; *ARDS,* acute respiratory distress syndrome; *CNS,* central nervous system; *HIV,* human immunodeficiency virus; *IV,* intravenous.

the skin's normal recuperative powers will often produce healing without treatment. The most frequent offenders are plant (poison ivy, oak, or sumac), animal (wool, feathers, and furs), and metal irritants (nickel found in jewelry and the snaps on sleepers and denim). In infants, contact dermatitis occurs on the convex surfaces of the diaper area. Other agents that produce contact dermatitis include vegetable irritants (oleoresins, oils, and turpentine), synthetic fabrics (e.g., shoe components), dyes, cosmetics, perfumes, and soaps (including bubble baths).

Nursing Care Management

Nurses frequently detect evidence of contact dermatitis during routine physical assessments. Skin manifestations in specific areas suggest limited contact, such as around the eyes (mascara), areas of the body covered by clothing but not protected by undergarments (wool), or areas of the body not covered by clothing (ultraviolet [UV] injury). Generalized involvement is more likely to be caused by bubble bath, laundry soap, body soap, or lotion. Often nurses can determine the offending agent and counsel families regarding management. If the lesions persist, are extensive, or show evidence of infection, medical evaluation is indicated.

POISON IVY, OAK, AND SUMAC

Contact with the dry or succulent portions of any of three poisonous plants (ivy, oak, and sumac) produces localized, streaked or spotty, oozing, and painful impetiginous lesions that are often highly urticarial. The offending substance in these plants is an oil, **urushiol**, which is extremely potent. Sensitivity to urushiol is not inborn but is developed after one or two exposures and may change over a lifetime. All parts of the plants contain the oil, including dried leaves and stems (Fig. 32.5, *A*). Even smoke from burning brush piles can produce a reaction.

Animals do not seem to be affected by the oil; however, dogs or other animals that have run or played in the plants may carry the sap on their fur, and animals that eat the plants can transfer the oil in their saliva. Shoes, tools, and toys can transfer the oil. Golf balls that have been in the rough are another source of contact.

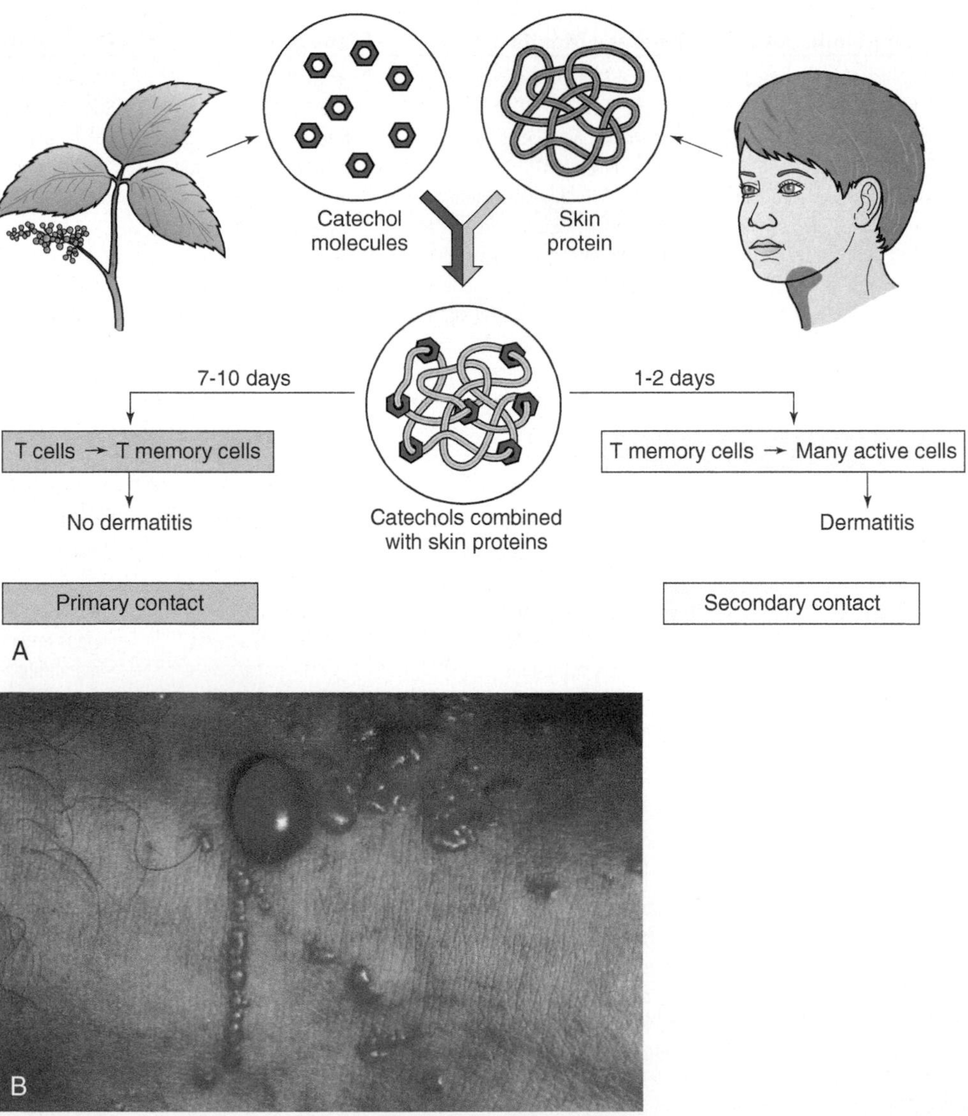

FIG. 32.5 A, Development of allergic contact dermatitis. **B,** Poison ivy lesions; note the "streaked" blisters surrounding one large blister. (*A,* From McCance, K., & Huether, S. [2010]. *Pathophysiology: The biological basis for disease in adults and children* [6th ed.]. St. Louis, MO: Mosby. *B,* From Habif, T. P. [2010]. *Clinical dermatology: A color guide to diagnosis and therapy* [5th ed.]. St. Louis, MO: Mosby.)

Urushiol takes effect as soon as it touches the skin. It penetrates through the epidermis as a mixture of compound molecules called *catechols*. These catechols bond skin proteins and initiate an immune response. The full-blown reaction is evident after about 2 days, with redness, swelling, and itching at the site of contact. Several days later, streaked or spotty blisters oozing serum from damaged cells produce the characteristic impetiginous lesions (see Fig. 32.5, *B*). The lesions dry and heal spontaneously, and itching stops by 10 to 14 days.

Therapeutic Management

Treatment of the lesions includes application of calamine lotion, soothing Burow solution compresses, and/or Aveeno baths to relieve discomfort. Topical corticosteroid gel is effective for prevention or relief of inflammation, especially when applied before blisters form. Oral corticosteroids may be needed for severe reactions, and those affecting the face, throat, or genital region. A sedative such as diphenhydramine may be ordered.

Nursing Care Management

The earlier the skin is cleansed, the greater the chance of removing the urushiol before it attaches to the skin. When it is known that the child has made contact with the plant, the area is immediately flushed (preferably within 15 minutes) with *cold* running water to neutralize the urushiol not yet bonded to the skin. Once the oil has been removed from the skin, the allergen has been neutralized. The rash that results from poison ivy cannot be spread to another child; only direct contact with the oil can cause the response. Harsh soap and scrubbing the exposed skin is contraindicated because it removes protective skin oils and dilutes the urushiol, allowing it to spread. All clothing that has come in contact with the plant is removed with care and thoroughly laundered in hot water and detergent. Every effort is made to prevent the child from scratching the lesions. Although the lesions do not spread by contact with the blister serum or from scratching, they can become secondarily infected.

Prevention

Prevention is best accomplished by avoiding contact and removing the plant from the environment. Teach all children, especially those known to be sensitive, to recognize the plant. Information regarding means for destroying plants can be obtained from the U.S. Department of Agriculture or U.S. Forestry Service. Home garden sprays that kill broad-leaf plants or all vegetation (e.g., Roundup or Spectracide) are ineffective. If poisonous plants are growing in public community area, the local authorities should be contacted to remove the plants.

DRUG REACTIONS

Although drugs can adversely affect any organ of the body, reactions to medications are seen more often in the skin than in any other organ. The reaction may be a result of toxicity related to drug concentration, individual intolerance to the therapeutic dosage of the drug, or an allergic or idiosyncratic response. The manifestations may be associated with side effects or secondary effects of a drug, either of which are unrelated to its primary pharmacologic actions.

Although any drug is capable of producing a reaction in the susceptible individual, some drugs have a tendency to produce a particular reaction consistently (e.g., hives after a dose of antibiotics in an individual with sensitivity), and others are more likely to produce an untoward effect (e.g., nausea, vomiting, or diarrhea). Many are allergenic responses that occur after a previous administration of the drug, even a topical application. Other factors influence a drug response in a particular individual. For example, the incidence of adverse reaction increases with the dosage amount and number of drugs given simultaneously.

> **! NURSING ALERT**
>
> Intravenous drugs are more likely to cause a reaction than oral drugs. If a reaction occurs, stop the drug but maintain the infusion with normal saline.

Manifestations of drug reactions may be delayed or immediate. A period of 7 days is usually required for a child to develop sensitivity to a drug that has never been administered previously. With prior sensitivity, the manifestations appear almost immediately. Rashes that are exanthematous, urticarial, or eczematoid are the most common manifestation of adverse drug reactions in children. However, individual drug reactions may vary from a single lesion to extensive, generalized epidermal necrosis such as that seen in Stevens-Johnson syndrome. Cutaneous manifestations can resemble almost any skin disease and can be seen in almost any degree of severity. With few exceptions, the distribution of a drug eruption is widespread because it results from a circulating agent; appears as an inflammatory response with itching; is sudden in onset; and may be associated with constitutional symptoms such as fever, malaise, gastrointestinal upset, anemia, or liver and kidney damage.

Another common adverse medication response in children is a fixed eruption (i.e., a recurrent eruption at the same site with each administration of the offending drug). The lesion, a purplish red round or oval plaque with a sharp border seen most frequently on the extremities, disappears slowly, and the pigmentation deepens with each episode.

In most cases, treatment for simple cutaneous reactions consists of discontinuing the drug. Sometimes a decision is made to continue the drug (e.g., an antibiotic in a small child) until the cause of the rash is clearly indicated and the negative or mild effects of the rash outweigh the benefits of the antibiotic (or other medication) treatment. Once the medication reaction is identified, it is well documented in the patient's medical record and avoided in the future. The provider will either substitute the offending medication with treatment in a comparative class or simply discontinue treatment, depending on the patient scenario. Often antihistamines may be ordered to relieve urticaric rashes. A tapering course of corticosteroids may be used for widespread and severe rashes. Severe anaphylactic reactions are a medical emergency (see Anaphylaxis, Chapter 23).

Nursing Care Management

The most effective means of management is prevention, documentation, and assessment. Frequent offenders in drug reactions are penicillin and sulfonamides, and nurses must be alert to this possibility. However, even commonplace drugs such as aspirin and barbiturates, chemical agents in some foods, flavoring agents, and preservatives are capable of producing an undesired response. Parents always remember details of their child's severe reaction. As the nurse takes a careful medical history, details of a previous drug reaction should include the name and dose of the drug, nature of the reaction, and how soon after administration the reaction occurred. This information should be carefully noted in the medical record. (See History Taking, Chapter 4.) A careful nursing assessment (observation, inspection, and palpation) of the skin is paramount for any child receiving medication, especially intravenously. Noting the child's behavior and frequency of scratching is also critical. Nurses who identify a new rash after medication is administered or suspect a medication sensitivity in a patient whose rash is enlarging, increasingly itchy, or widespread on the child's body should withhold any further dose and report the eruption to the practitioner. Persons who have severe reactions should wear a medical identification bracelet or necklace in case of emergency or inadvertent administration of the offending agent.

FOREIGN BODIES

Small wooden, glass, or metal splinters and thorns from plants can usually be safely removed with a pointed needle and tweezers that have been sterilized with either alcohol or a flame. The area around the sliver is washed thoroughly with soap and water before removal is attempted, and the child should be cooperative and calm before removal is attempted. The sliver is exposed with the needle and then grasped firmly by the tweezers and pulled out. Some foreign bodies, such as a fishhook, pieces of glass, a difficult-to-see object, or a deeply embedded object (e.g., a needle in a foot or near a joint), require medical evaluation.

Small cactus prickles or spines are troublesome to remove, and attempts may be distressing to the child and family. Large spines or clumps can be removed with tweezers. Small prickles or spines may be removed by the following methods:

- Apply a thin layer of water-soluble household glue and cover it with gauze; when the glue dries, peel off the gauze.
- Apply hair removal wax or body sugar, let it dry, and remove.
- Place cellophane tape, sticky side down, over the spines and lift it off.

SKIN DISORDERS RELATED TO ANIMAL CONTACTS

ARTHROPOD BITES AND STINGS

Arthropods include insects and arachnids, such as mites, ticks, spiders, and scorpions. Most arthropods in the United States, including tarantulas, are relatively harmless. Although all spiders produce venom that is injected via fangs, some are unable to pierce the skin, and others produce venom that is insufficiently toxic to be harmful. Only scorpions and two spiders—the brown recluse and the black widow—inject venom deadly enough to require immediate attention. Children bitten by these arachnids must receive medical attention as soon as possible. Major offending creatures, their manifestations, and management are outlined in Table 32.7. A brown recluse spider bite is shown in Fig. 32.6.

When a hymenopteran (bees in particular) stings, its barbed stinger penetrates the skin. As long as the stinger remains in the skin, the muscles push the stinger deeper, and the venom is pumped into the wound. The best approach is to remove the stinger as quickly as possible and to get away from the vicinity of other insects to prevent further

TABLE 32.7 Skin Lesions Caused by Arthropods

Mechanism and Characteristic	Manifestations	Management
Insect Bites—Flies, Gnats, Mosquitoes, Fleas		
Mechanism—Foreign protein in insects' saliva introduced when skin is penetrated for a blood meal Distribution: Almost everywhere—Fleas, mosquitoes, ants Suburbs and rural areas—Bees Urban areas—Hornets, wasps, yellow jackets	Hypersensitivity reaction Papular urticaria Firm papules; may be capped by vesicles or excoriated Little or no reaction in nonsensitized person	Treatment: Use antipruritic agents and baths Administer antihistamines Prevent secondary infection Prevention: Avoid contact Remove focus, such as untreated furniture, mattresses, carpets, and pets, where insects may live Apply insect repellent when exposure is anticipated
Chiggers—Harvest Mites		
Mechanism—Attach with claws and secrete a digestive substance that liquefies the host's epidermis	Erythematous papules Intense itching Favor warm areas of body, especially intertriginous areas and areas covered with clothing	Treatment: May require systemic steroids for extensive bites Prevention: Avoid contact, especially in areas of tall grass and underbrush Apply insect repellant when exposure is anticipated Spray insecticides such as diazinon in yards
Hymenopterans—Bees, Wasps, Hornets, Yellow Jackets, Fire Ants		
Mechanism: Injection of venom through stinging apparatus Venom contains histamine; allergenic proteins; and often a spreading factor, hyaluronidase Severe reactions caused by hypersensitivity or multiple stings	Local reaction—Small red area, wheal, itching, and heat Systemic reactions—May be mild to severe, including generalized edema, pain, nausea and vomiting, confusion, respiratory impairment, and shock	Treatment: Carefully scrape off stinger or pull out stinger as quickly as possible Cleanse with soap and water Apply cool compresses Apply common household product (e.g., lemon juice, paste made with aspirin or baking soda) Administer antihistamines Severe reactions—Administer epinephrine, corticosteroids; treat for shock Prevention: Teach child to wear shoes; to avoid wearing bright clothing, flowery prints, shiny jewelry, or perfumed grooming products (cologne, scented hairspray), which might attract the insect; and to avoid places where the insect may be contacted Hypersensitive children should wear medical identification to indicate allergy and therapy needed; family should keep emergency medication and be taught its administration

TABLE 32.7 **Skin Lesions Caused by Arthropods—cont'd**

Mechanism and Characteristic	Manifestations	Management
Black Widow Spider		
Mechanism—Venom injected through a clawlike appendage; has neurotoxic action Characteristics: Shiny black spider, with a body about 1.25 cm (0.5 inch) long and a red or orange hourglass-shaped marking on underside Avoids light and bites in self-defense	Mild sting at time of bite Area becomes swollen, painful, and erythematous Dizziness, weakness, and abdominal pain May produce delirium, paralysis, seizures, and (if large amount of venom absorbed) death	Treatment: Cleanse wound with antiseptic Apply cool compresses Administer antivenin Administer muscle relaxant, such as calcium gluconate; analgesics or sedatives; hydrocortisone or diazepam intravenously Prevention—Teach children to avoid places that harbor the spider (e.g., woodpiles)
Brown Recluse Spider		
Mechanism: Venom injected via fangs Venom contains powerful necrotoxin Characteristics: Slender spider, with long legs and body length of 1-2 cm; color is fawn to dark brown; recognized by fiddle-shaped mark on head Shy; bites only when annoyed or surprised Prefers dark areas where seldom disturbed	Mild sting at time of bite Transient erythema followed by bleb or blister; mild to severe pain in 2-8 hours; purple, star-shaped area in 3-4 days; necrotic ulceration in 7-14 days (see Fig. 32.6) Systemic reactions may include fever, malaise, restlessness, nausea, vomiting, and joint pain Generalized petechial eruption Wounds heal with scar formation	Treatment: Apply cool compresses locally Administer antibiotics, corticosteroids Relieve pain Wound may require skin graft Prevention—Teach children to avoid possible nesting sites
Scorpions		
Mechanism: Sting by means of a hooked caudal stinger that discharges venom Venom of more venomous species contains hemolysins, endotheliolysins, and neurotoxins Characteristics—Usual habitat southwestern United States	Intense local pain, erythema, numbness, burning, restlessness, vomiting Ascending motor paralysis with seizures, weakness, rapid pulse, excessive salivation, thirst, dysuria, pulmonary edema, coma, and death Some species produce only local tissue reaction with swelling at puncture site (distinctive) Symptoms subside in a few hours Deaths occur among children younger than 4 years of age, usually in first 24 hours	Treatment: Delay absorption of venom by keeping child quiet; place involved area in dependent position Administer antivenin Relieve pain Admit to pediatric intensive care unit for surveillance Prevention—Teach children to avoid possible nesting sites
Ticks		
Mechanism—In process of sucking blood, head and mouth parts are buried in skin Characteristics: Feed on blood of mammals Significant in humans because of pathologic organism carried May be vectors of various infectious diseases, such as Rocky Mountain spotted fever, Q fever, tularemia, relapsing fever, Lyme disease, tick paralysis Must attach and feed for 1-2 hours to transmit disease Usual habitat is wooded area	Tick usually attached to skin with head embedded Firm, discrete, intensely pruritic nodules at site of attachment May cause urticaria or persistent localized edema	Treatment: Grasp tick with tweezers (forceps) as close as possible to point of attachment Pull straight up with steady, even pressure; if using bare hands, use a tissue to touch tick during removal; wash hands thoroughly with soap and water Remove any remaining part (e.g., head) with sterile needle Cleanse wounds with soap and disinfectant Prevention—Teach children to avoid areas where prevalent Inspect skin (especially scalp) after being in wooded areas

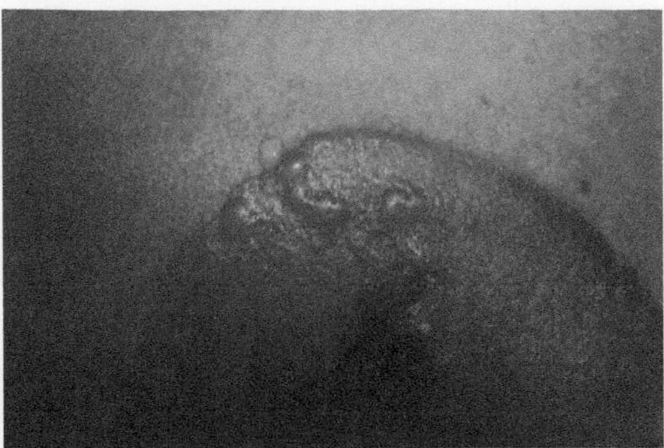

FIG. 32.6 Brown recluse spider bite. Note central necrosis surrounded by purplish area and blisters. (From Weston, W. L., & Lane, A. T. [2007]. *Color textbook of pediatric dermatology* [4th ed.]. St. Louis, MO: Mosby.)

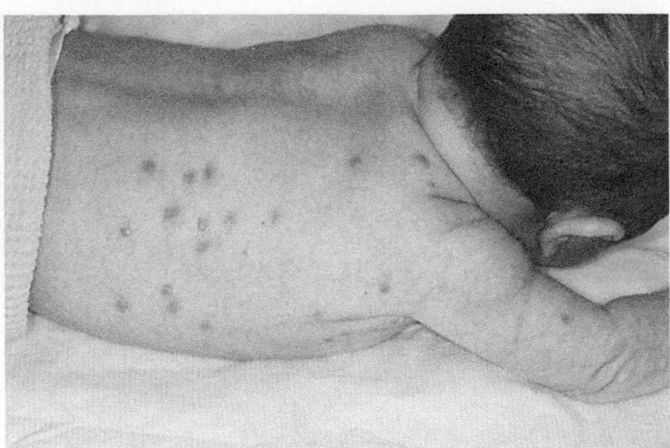

FIG. 32.7 Scabies. (From McCance, K., & Huether, S. [2010]. *Pathophysiology: The biological basis for disease in adults and children* [6th ed.]. St. Louis, MO: Mosby/Elsevier.)

BOX 32.1 Clinical Manifestations of Scabies

Lesion

Children—Minute grayish brown, threadlike (mite burrows), pruritic
- Black dot at end of burrow (mite)

Infants—Eczematous eruption, pruritic

Distribution

Generally in intertriginous areas—Interdigital, axillary-cubital, popliteal, inguinal

Children older than 2 years of age—Primarily hands and wrists

Children younger than 2 years—Primarily feet and ankles

injury. Children who have become sensitized to hymenopteran bites may demonstrate a severe systemic response that can be life threatening. One sting can produce generalized urticaria, respiratory difficulty (from laryngeal edema), hypotension, and death. Intramuscular administration of epinephrine provides immediate relief and must be available for emergency use.

Hypersensitive children should wear a medical identification bracelet. They should also have a kit that contains epinephrine and a hypodermic syringe. Families are reminded to check the expiration date on the kit and to replace an outdated one. They should determine whether a nurse is available at the school and find out what the school policy is regarding administration of drugs. If a school nurse is not present, someone at the school should be designated to inject the epinephrine in case of an emergency.

SCABIES

Scabies is an endemic infestation caused by the scabies mite, *Sarcoptes scabiei.* Lesions are created as the impregnated female burrows into the stratum corneum of the epidermis (never into living tissue) to deposit her eggs and feces. The inflammatory response causes intense pruritus that leads to punctate discrete excoriations secondary to the itching (Box 32.1). Maculopapular lesions are characteristically distributed in intertriginous areas: interdigital surfaces, the axillary-cubital area, popliteal folds, and the inguinal region. The observer must look for discrete papules, burrows, or vesicles (Fig. 32.7). Scabies is transmitted primarily through prolonged close personal contact, and it affects persons regardless of age, sex, personal hygiene, and socioeconomic status.

Nursing Care Management

The treatment of scabies is the application of a scabicide. The drug of choice in children and infants older than 2 months of age is permethrin 5% cream (Elimite). Alternative drugs are 10% crotamiton (cream or lotion), or oral ivermectin. Lindane can be neurotoxic and is contraindicated by the American Academy of Pediatrics.

Ivermectin, an oral medication, may be used to treat scabies in patients with secondary excoriations for whom topical scabicides are irritating and not well tolerated or whose infestation is refractory. However, the safety and efficacy of ivermectin for children weighing less than 15 kg (33 lb) has not been established.

Because of the length of time between infestation and physical symptoms (30 to 60 days), all persons who were in close contact with the affected child need treatment. This may include boyfriends or girlfriends, babysitters, grandparents, and immediate family members. The objective is to treat as thoroughly as possible the first time. Enough medication for the entire family should be prescribed, with 2 oz allowed for each adult and 1 oz for each child.

PEDICULOSIS CAPITIS

Pediculosis capitis (head lice) is an infestation of the scalp by *Pediculus humanus capitis,* a common parasite in school-age children. These lice infestations create embarrassment and concern in the family and community. They can also cause a child to be ridiculed by other children. An important nursing role is education about pediculosis. Nurses should emphasize that anyone can get pediculosis; it has no respect for age, socioeconomic level, or cleanliness.

The adult louse lives only about 48 hours when away from a human host, and the life span of the average female is 1 month. The female lays her eggs at night at the junction of a hair shaft and close to the skin because the eggs need a warm environment. The **nits**, or eggs, hatch in approximately 7 to 10 days. Itching, caused by the crawling insect and saliva on the skin, is usually the only symptom. The louse is a blood-sucking organism that requires approximately five meals a day. Common areas involved are the occipital area, behind the ears, and the nape of the neck (Box 32.2).

Diagnostic Evaluation

Diagnosis is made by observation of the white eggs (nits) firmly attached to the hair shafts (Fig. 32.8). Lice are small and grayish-tan, have no wings, and are visible to the naked eye. Observation of the white eggs (nits) firmly attached to the hair shafts confirms the diagnosis. The nits, or eggs, appear as tiny whitish oval specks adhering to the hair shaft about 6 mm (0.25 inch) from the scalp. The adherent nature of the nits distinguishes them from dandruff, which falls off readily. Empty nit cases, indicating hatched lice, are translucent rather than white and are located more than 6 mm from the scalp. Because of their brief life

BOX 32.2 Clinical Manifestations of Pediculosis

Pruritus (caused by crawling insects and insect saliva on skin)
Nits observable on hair shaft (see Fig. 32.8)

Distribution
Occipital area
Behind ears
Nape of neck
Eyebrows and eyelashes (occasionally) (caused by pubic lice)

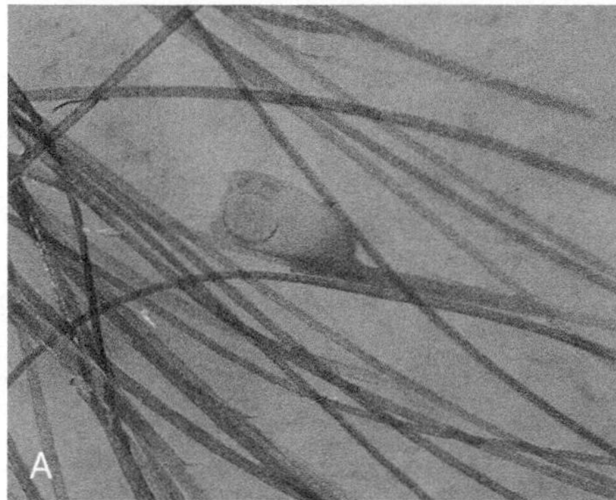

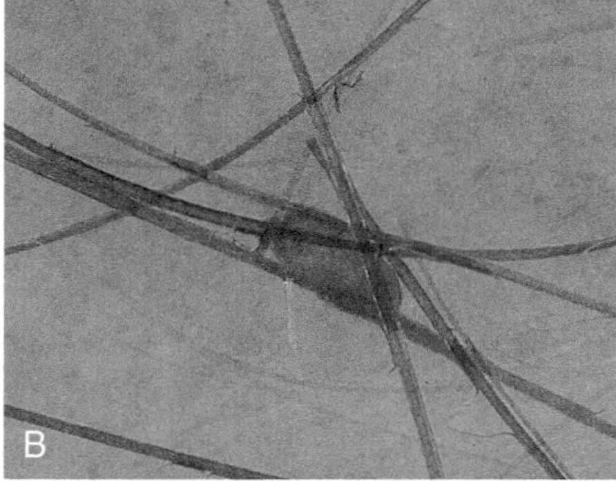

FIG. 32.8 A, Empty nit case. **B,** Viable nits. (From Stefani, A. D., Hofmann-Wellenhof, R., & Zalaudek, I. [2006]. Dermoscopy for diagnosis and treatment monitoring of pediculosis capitis. *Journal of the American Acadademy of Dermatology, 54*(5), 909-911.)

span and mobility, adult lice are more difficult to locate. Nits must be differentiated from dandruff, lint, hair spray, and other items of similar size and shape. Scratch marks or inflammatory papules, caused by secondary infection, are also be found on the scalp in the vulnerable areas.

Therapeutic Management

Treatment consists of the application of pediculicides and manual removal of nit cases. The drug of choice for infants and children is permethrin 1% cream rinse (Nix), which kills adult lice and nits. This product and preparations of pyrethrin with piperonyl butoxide (RID or A-200 Pyrinate) can be obtained without a prescription and are effective and safe. Most experts advise a second treatment at 7 to 10 days to ensure a cure (American Academy of Pediatrics, 2015). If neither permethrin nor pyrethrin products are effective, the prescription drug 0.5% malathion, which has been approved for treatment of head lice, can be used. However, malathion is not recommended for children younger than 2 years of age.

Because of concerns that head lice may be developing resistance to chemical shampoos and that repeated exposure of children to strong chemicals on the scalp may be unwise, effective nonchemical control measures are essential. Removal of nits from the child's hair with a metal nit comb daily is a control measure following treatment with a pediculicide.

Nursing Care Management

An important nursing role is educating the parents about pediculosis. Nurses should emphasize that *anyone* can get pediculosis; it has no respect for age, gender, socioeconomic level, or cleanliness. Lice do not jump or fly, but they can be transmitted from one person to another on personal items. Children are cautioned against sharing combs, hair ornaments, hats, caps, scarves, coats, and other items used on or near the hair. Lice are not carried or transmitted by pets (Devore, Schutze, & American Academy of Pediatrics, 2015).

Nurses or parents should carefully inspect children who scratch their heads more than usual for bite marks, redness, and nits. The hair is systematically spread with two flat-sided sticks or tongue depressors, and the scalp is observed for any movement that indicates a louse. Nurses should wear gloves when examining the hair. Lice are small and grayish tan, have no wings, and are visible to the naked eye. The nits, or eggs, appear as tiny whitish oval specks adhering to the hair shaft about 6 mm (0.25 inch) from the scalp. The adherent nature of the nits distinguishes them from dandruff, which falls off readily. Empty nit cases, indicating hatched lice, are translucent rather than white and are located more than 6 mm from the scalp (see Fig. 32.8).

If evidence of infestation is found, it is important to treat the child according to the directions on the label of the pediculicide. Parents are advised to read the directions carefully before beginning treatment. The child is made as comfortable as possible during the application process because the pediculicide must remain on the scalp and hair for several minutes. A useful strategy is playing "beauty parlor" while shampooing. The child lies supine with the head over a sink or basin and covers the eyes with a dry towel or washcloth. This prevents medication, which can cause chemical conjunctivitis, from splashing into the eyes. If eye irritation occurs, the eyes must be flushed well with tepid water. It is not necessary to remove the nits after treatment because only live lice cause infestation. However, because none of the pediculicides is 100% effective in killing all the eggs, the makers of some pediculicides recommend manual removal of the nits after treatment. An extra-fine-tooth comb that is included in many commercial pediculicides or is available at community pharmacies facilitates manual removal. Live lice survive for up to 48 hours away from the host, but nits are shed into the environment and are capable of hatching in 7 to 10 days; retreatment is required. Therefore measures must be taken to prevent further infestation (see Community and Home Health Considerations box). Spraying with insecticide is not recommended because of the danger to children and animals. Families should also be advised that the pediculicide is relatively expensive, especially when several members of the household require treatment. Families may be inclined to try home remedies such as petroleum jelly, oils, vinegar, butter, alcohol, and mayonnaise to treat the lice; however, there is no evidence demonstrating the effectiveness of these remedies (Devore, Schutze, & American Academy of Pediatrics, 2015).

RICKETTSIAL DISEASES

The organisms responsible for a number of disorders are transmitted to human beings via arthropods (Table 32.8). Mammals become infected only through the bites of infected lice, fleas, ticks, and mites, all of which serve as both infectors and reservoirs. Rickettsiae are intracellular

TABLE 32.8 **Eruptions Caused by Rickettsiae**

Disorder, Organism, and Host	Manifestations	Management	Comments
Rocky Mountain spotted fever—*Rickettsia rickettsii* Arthropod—Tick Transmission—Tick Mammal source—Wild rodents, dogs	Gradual onset—Fever, malaise, anorexia, myalgia Abrupt onset—Rapid temperature elevation, chills, vomiting, myalgia, severe headache Maculopapular or petechial rash primarily on extremities (ankles and wrists) but may spread to other areas, characteristically on palms and soles	Control—Protection from tick bite by wearing proper apparel, tick repellent Tetracycline or chloramphenicol Vigorous supportive therapy	Usually self-limiting in children Onset in children may resemble any infectious disease Severe disease rare in children Inspect children and dogs regularly if they play in wooded areas See Table 32.6 for management of ticks
Epidemic typhus— *Rickettsia prowazekii* Arthropod—Body louse Transmission—Infected feces into broken skin Mammal source—Humans	Abrupt onset of chills, fever, diffuse myalgia, headache, malaise Maculopapular rash becoming petechial 4-7 days later, spreading from trunk outward	Control—Immediate destruction of vectors Tetracycline or chloramphenicol Supportive treatment	Isolate patient until deloused See discussion in this chapter for management of pediculosis Excreta from infected lice also in dust; patient's clothing, bedding, and possessions are disinfected and washed in hot water
Endemic typhus—*Rickettsia typhi* Arthropod—Rat fleas or lice Transmission—Flea bite; inhaling or ingesting flea excreta Mammal source—Rats	Headache, arthralgia, backache followed by fever; may last 9-14 days Maculopapular rash after 1-8 days of fever; begins in trunk and spreads to periphery; rarely involves face, palms, soles	Control—Eliminate rat reservoir, insect vectors, or both Tetracycline or chloramphenicol Supportive treatment	Fairly common in United States Shorter duration than epidemic typhus Mild, seldom fatal illness Difficult to distinguish from epidemic typhus
Rickettsialpox—*Rickettsia akari* Arthropod—Mouse mite Transmission—Mite Mammal source—House mouse	Maculopapular rash following primary lesion; eschar at site of bite; fever, chills, headache	Control—Eradication of rodent reservoir and mite vector Tetracycline or chloramphenicol Supportive treatment	Self-limiting nonfatal disease Initial endemic in New York City but now found in many cities in United States

COMMUNITY AND HOME HEALTH CONSIDERATIONS

Focus Preventing the Spread and Recurrence of Pediculosis

- Machine wash all washable clothing, towels, and bed linens in water greater than 130°F and dry them in a hot dryer for at least 20 minutes. Dry clean nonwashable items.
- Thoroughly vacuum carpets, car seats, pillows, stuffed animals, rugs, mattresses, and upholstered furniture.
- Seal nonwashable items in plastic bags for 14 days if unable to dry clean or vacuum.
- Soak combs, brushes, and hair accessories in lice-killing products for 1 hour or in boiling water for 10 minutes.
- In daycare centers, store children's clothing items such as hats and scarves and other headgear in separate cubicles.
- Discourage the sharing of items such as hats, scarves, hair accessories, combs, and brushes among children in group settings such as daycare centers and schools.
- Avoid physical contact with infected individuals and their belongings, especially clothing and bedding.
- Inspect children in a group setting regularly for head lice.
- Provide educational programs on the transmission of pediculosis, its detection, and treatment.

Modified from Chin, J. (Ed.). (2000). *Control of communicable diseases manual.* Washington, DC: American Public Health Association; and Devore, C. D., Schutze, G. E., & American Academy of Pediatrics. (2015). Council on School Health and Committee on Infectious Diseases: Head lice. *Pediatrics, 135*(5), e1355-e1365.

parasites, similar in size to bacteria that inhabit the alimentary tract of a wide range of natural hosts. Rickettsial diseases are more common in temperate and tropical climates where humans live in association with arthropods. Infection in humans is incidental (except epidemic typhus) and not necessary for the survival of the rickettsial species. However, after the organism invades a human, it causes a disease that varies in intensity from a benign, self-limiting illness to a disease that is fulminating and fatal.

LYME DISEASE

Lyme disease is the most common tickborne disorder in the United States. It is caused by the spirochete *Borrelia burgdorferi,* which enters the skin and bloodstream through the saliva and feces of ticks, especially the deer tick (Steere, Strle Wormser, et al., 2016). Most cases of Lyme disease are reported in the Northeast from southern Maine to northern Virginia in the months of May through October and more commonly occur in children 5 to 15 years of age and adults 45 to 55 years of age (Steere, Strle, Wormser, et al., 2016).

Clinical Manifestations

The disease may be initially seen in any of three stages. The first stage, early localized disease, consists of the tick bite at the time of inoculation, followed in 3 to 30 days by the development of erythema migrans at the site of the bite. The lesion begins as a small erythematous papule that enlarges radially up to 30 cm (12 inches) over a period of days to weeks. It results in a large circumferential ring with a raised, edematous doughnut-like border resulting in a bull's-eye appearance (Fig. 32.9). The thigh, groin, and axilla are common sites. The lesion is described

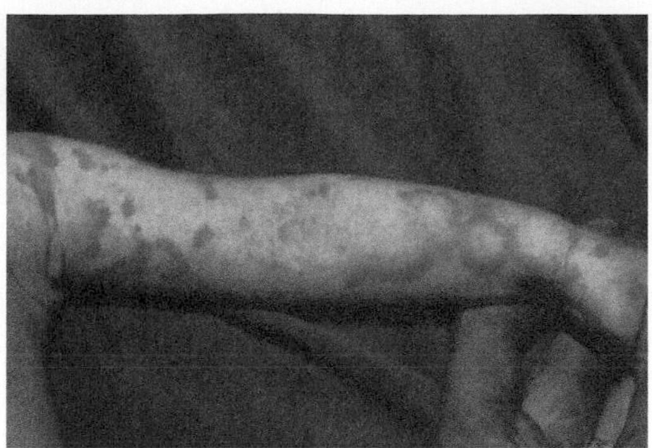

FIG. 32.9 Lyme disease. Note annular red rings in erythema chronicum migrans. (From Weston, W. L., & Lane, A. T. [2007]. *Color textbook of pediatric dermatology* [4th ed.]. St. Louis, MO: Mosby.)

as "burning," feels warm to the touch, and occasionally is pruritic. The single annular rash may be associated with fever, myalgia, headache, or malaise.

The second stage, early disseminated disease, occurs 3 to 10 weeks after inoculation. Many patients develop multiple smaller, secondary annular lesions without the indurated center. They may occur anywhere except on the palms and soles, and in untreated patients they disappear in 3 to 4 weeks. Constitutional symptoms, including fever, headache, malaise, fatigue, anorexia, stiff neck, generalized lymphadenopathy, splenomegaly, conjunctivitis, sore throat, abdominal pain, and cough, are often observed. A focal neurologic finding of cranial nerve palsy (seventh nerve palsy) occurs in 3% to 5% of cases. Additional manifestations include ophthalmic conditions such as optic neuritis, uveitis, conjunctivitis, and keratitis.

Finally, the third stage and the most serious stage of the disease, is characterized by systemic involvement of neurologic, cardiac, and musculoskeletal systems that appears 2 to 12 months after inoculation. Lyme arthritis is the most common manifestation with pain, swelling, and effusion. In children the arthritis is characterized by intermittently painful swollen joints (primarily the knees), with spontaneous remissions and exacerbations. Rare neurologic features of pediatric Lyme disease may include meningitis, encephalitis, and polyneuritis (Koedel, Fingerle, & Pfister, 2015). Cardiac complications, which may appear in a small percentage of persons during the early phase of the infection, are commonly acute atrioventricular conduction abnormalities and less commonly pericarditis or mild left ventricular dysfunction (Steere, Strle, Wormser, et al., 2016).

Diagnostic Evaluation

Diagnosis is based primarily on the history, observation of the lesion, and clinical manifestations. Serologic testing for Lyme disease at the time of a recognized tick bite is not recommended because antibodies are not detectable in most persons (American Academy of Pediatrics, 2015). Laboratory diagnosis can be established in later stages with a two-step approach that includes the screening test enzyme immunoassay or immunofluorescent immunoassay and, if the results are equivocal or positive, with Western immunoblot testing, as outlined by the Centers for Disease Control and Prevention (2017) and adopted by the American Academy of Pediatrics (2015).

Therapeutic Management

Early and appropriate treatment is essential to prevent complications. Children older than 8 years of age are treated with oral doxycycline; amoxicillin is recommended for children younger than 8 years of age (American Academy of Pediatrics, 2015). For patients who are allergic to penicillin, alternative drugs include cefuroxime or erythromycin.

The length of treatment depends on the clinical response and other disease manifestations, but it usually lasts from 14 to 21 days (American Academy of Pediatrics, 2015). The treatment is effective in preventing second-stage manifestations in most cases. Persons who have removed ticks from themselves should be monitored closely for signs and symptoms of tickborne diseases for 30 days; in particular, they should be monitored for erythema migrans, a red expanding skin lesion at the site of the tick bite that may suggest Lyme disease. People who develop a skin lesion or viral infection–like illness within 1 month of an attached tick should seek prompt medical attention. Treatment of erythema migrans most often prevents development of later stages of Lyme disease.

Neurologic, cardiac, and arthritic manifestations are managed with oral or intravenous antibiotics, such as ceftriaxone, cefotaxime, or penicillin G. Follow-up care is important in ensuring that treatment is initiated or terminated as needed.

Nursing Care Management

The major emphasis of nursing care should be educating parents to protect their children from exposure to ticks. Children should avoid tick-infested areas or wear light-colored clothing so that ticks can be spotted easily, tuck pant legs into socks, and wear a long-sleeved shirt tucked into pants when in wooded areas. Parents and children need to perform regular tick checks when they are in infested areas (with special attention to the scalp, neck, armpits, and groin areas). Parents should also be alert for signs of the skin lesion, especially if their children have been in tick-infested areas. The American Academy of Pediatrics (2015) points out that the risk of infection after a deer tick bite, even in endemic regions of the United States, is 1% to 4%; children bitten by a deer tick in nonendemic regions should not receive antibiotic prophylaxis.

Parents should also be educated regarding tick removal in the event of a tick bite. The tick should be grasped firmly with tweezers and pulled straight out. The application of nail polish or petroleum jelly is not recommended and does not appear to have an effect on tick withdrawal as has been hypothesized. Concerns about tick engorgement or tick remains left in the person's body (such as the tick head) appear to be unfounded; there is no need for medical examination of the tick itself. After the tick is removed, wash the bite area with an iodine scrub, rubbing alcohol, or plain soap and water.

Insect repellents containing diethyltoluamide (DEET) and permethrin can protect against ticks, but parents should use these chemicals cautiously. Although there have been reports of serious neurologic complications in children resulting from frequent and excessive application of DEET repellants, the risk is low when they are used properly. Products with DEET should be applied sparingly according to label instructions and not applied to a child's face, hands, or any areas of irritated skin. Plant essential oils, such as juniper and Chinese weeping cedar essential oil, have been reported as being safe and effective as an insect repellent without the effects of chemicals (Eisen & Dolan, 2016). Permethrin-treated clothing has also been shown to be effective in repelling ticks (Eisen & Dolan, 2016). After the child returns indoors, treated skin should be washed with soap and water. Information about Lyme disease can be obtained from the American Lyme Disease Foundation, Inc.,* or from the Centers for Disease Control and Prevention (https://www.cdc.gov/lyme/).

*PO Box 466, Lyme, CT 06371; http://www.aldf.com.

PET BITES

Animal bites are common in childhood. Wild animal bites are discussed in relation to rabies in Chapter 30. The present discussion is directed primarily toward dog bites because most animal bites to children are caused by dogs. Cat bites are less frequent, although cat scratches are extremely common (see Cat Scratch Disease, later in this chapter).

Most injuries caused by dogs or cats are to the upper extremities. Small children are likely to be bitten or scratched on the head, face, and neck because they tend to put their heads near the animal's head and flail their arms rather than protecting their heads. Most dogs involved are owned by the family of the victim or by a neighbor. Injuries vary in intensity from small puncture wounds to complete evulsion of tissue that is associated with significant crush injury. Animal bites are potentially serious because of the likelihood of significant infection.

Therapeutic Management

General wound care consists of rinsing the wound with copious amounts of saline or lactated Ringer solution under pressure via a large syringe and of washing the surrounding skin with mild soap. A clean pressure dressing is applied, and the extremity is elevated if the wound is bleeding. Medical evaluation is advised because of the danger of tetanus and rabies, although dogs in most urban areas are required to be immunized against rabies. Bites from wild animals, such as squirrels, bats, raccoons, foxes, and skunks, are potentially dangerous.

Prophylactic antibiotics are indicated for puncture wounds and wounds in areas that may prove to be cosmetically or functionally impaired if infected. Extensive lacerations are debrided and loosely sutured to allow drainage in the event of infection. Tetanus toxoid is administered according to standard guidelines (see Immunizations, Chapter 6), and rabies protocol is followed (see Rabies, Chapter 30). Injuries to poorly vascularized areas, such as the hands, are more likely to become infected than those in more vascularized areas, such as the face; puncture wounds are more likely to become infected than lacerations.

Nursing Care Management

The most important aspect related to animal bites is prevention. Children should understand animal behavior and develop respect for animals (see Community and Home Health Considerations box). Parents should monitor their children's behavior with dogs and instruct them not to tease or surprise dogs, invade their territory, interfere with their feeding or sleeping, take their toys, or interact with sick or injured dogs or dogs with pups. Parents who are considering getting a pet, especially a dog, for themselves or their children should select a dog that has a high level of sociability with, and is unlikely to be a danger to, children.

HUMAN BITES

Children often acquire lacerations from the teeth of other humans in rough play, during fights, or as victims of child abuse. Some young children bite others out of frustration or anger. Because human dental plaque and gingiva harbor pathogenic organisms, all human bites should receive attention. Delayed treatment increases the risk of infection.

The wound is washed vigorously with soap and water, and a pressure dressing is applied to stop bleeding. Ice applications minimize discomfort and swelling. Increased pain or redness at the wound site is an indication that the child should receive medical attention for antibiotic therapy. Tetanus toxoid is needed if the child is insufficiently immunized. Wounds larger than 6 mm should receive medical attention.

COMMUNITY AND HOME HEALTH CONSIDERATIONS

Animal Safety

- Teach children to avoid all strange animals, especially wild, sick, or injured ones, that may be carriers of rabies (use the same techniques used in teaching children not to talk to strangers).
- Teach children to avoid dangerous and nervous animals in the neighborhood.
- Vaccinate your own dog against rabies.
- Never permit children to break up an animal fight even when their own pet is involved. Use a rake, broom, or garden hose to separate animals.
- Teach children the danger of mistreating or teasing pets (animals will bite if mauled, annoyed, or frightened).
- Spay or neuter your pets (spaying or neutering reduces aggression).
- Avoid direct eye contact with a threatening dog and remain motionless until a threatening dog leaves the area.
- Never hold your face close to an animal.
- Teach children not to disturb an animal that is eating; sleeping; or caring for young puppies or kittens.
- Never tease; pull the tail; or take away food, a bone, or a toy with which an animal is playing.
- Never approach a strange dog that is confined or restrained; do not keep animals confined with short ropes or chains (this can make them aggressive or vicious).
- Do not run, ride a bicycle, or skate in front of a dog (it may startle the dog); teach children the importance of avoiding bike routes where dogs are known to chase vehicles.
- Do not allow an inexperienced child or adult to feed a dog (if the person pulls back when the animal moves to take the food, this can frighten and startle the animal).
- If a dog is asleep or unaware of your presence or has not seen you approach, speak to the animal to make it aware of your presence to avoid startling the animal.
- Allow a dog to see and sniff a child before the child attempts to pet the animal.
- Do not permit a child to lead a large dog.
- Train or socialize a dog for appropriate behavior; avoid aggressive play with pets.
- Do not adopt pets for children until children demonstrate their maturity and ability to handle and care for pets.

From Humane Society of the United States. (2015). *Preventing your dog from biting.* Washington, DC: Author.

CAT SCRATCH DISEASE

Cat scratch disease is the most common cause of regional lymphadenitis in children and adolescents. It usually follows the scratch or bite of an animal (a cat or kitten in 99% of cases) and is caused by *Bartonella henselae,* a gram-negative bacterium. The disease is usually a benign, self-limiting illness that resolves spontaneously in about 4 to 6 weeks (American Academy of Pediatrics, 2015).

The usual manifestations are a painless, nonpruritic erythematous papule at the site of inoculation, followed by regional lymphadenitis. The lymph nodes most commonly involved are axillary epitrochlear, cervical, submandibular, inguinal, and preauricular. The disease may persist for several months before gradual resolution. In some children, especially those who are immunocompromised, the adenitis may progress to suppuration. Some children may develop serious complications that include encephalitis, hepatitis, and Parinaud oculoglandular syndrome. This syndrome is characterized by granulomatous lesions on the palpebral conjunctiva associated with swelling of the ipsilateral preauricular nodes.

Diagnosis is made on the basis of (1) history of contact with a cat or kitten, (2) the presence of regional lymphadenopathy for several days, and (3) serologic identification of the causative organism by indirect fluorescent antibody assay or polymerase chain reaction test (American Academy of Pediatrics, 2015).

Treatment is primarily supportive. Some experts recommend a 5-day course of oral azithromycin to hasten recovery (American Academy of Pediatrics, 2015). Antibiotics do not shorten the duration or prevent progression to suppuration but may be helpful in severe forms of the disease. Trimethoprim-sulfamethoxazole, ciprofloxacin, gentamicin, and rifampin have shown some benefit in uncontrolled clinical studies. Enlarged painful nodes may be treated by needle aspiration.

Children should be cautioned about playing with aggressive kittens that bite or scratch. Wounds should be washed with soap and water. Analgesics may be given for discomfort. Most children can continue normal activities during the disease. The animals are not ill during the time they transmit the disease, and most authorities do not recommend disposal of a cherished pet.

MISCELLANEOUS SKIN DISORDERS

A number of miscellaneous skin lesions occur in children. Some occur as a result of congenital disorders and are inherited as an autosomal dominant trait (Table 32.9). Ichthyoses are a heterogeneous group of disorders characterized by scaling that create challenging problems in treatment. These disorders are not discussed in detail here because of their wide variability.

SKIN DISORDERS ASSOCIATED WITH SPECIFIC AGE-GROUPS

Several common dermatologic conditions are confined to children in specific age-groups. These conditions include diaper, atopic, and

TABLE 32.9 Miscellaneous Skin Disorders

Disease and Causative Agent	Local Manifestations	Management	Comments
Urticaria—Usually allergic response to drugs or infection	Development of wheals Vary in size and configuration and tend to appear quickly, spread irregularly, and fade within a few hours May be constant or intermittent, sparse or profuse, small or large, discrete or confluent May be acute, chronic, or recurrent in acute attacks	Topical soothing and antipruritic applications Antihistamines Cortisone in severe cases Severe involvement may require epinephrine	Known etiologic agents should be avoided May be accompanied by malaise, fever, lymphadenopathy Severe cases may involve mucous membranes, internal organs, and joints Obstruction to air passages constitutes medical emergency
Intertrigo—Mechanical trauma and aggravating factors of excessive heat, moisture, and sweat retention	Red, inflamed, moist, partially denuded, marginated areas, the shape of which is determined by location Appears where opposing skin surfaces rub together, such as intergluteal folds, groin, neck, and axilla Excessive moisture and obesity are often factors	Maintenance of cleanliness and dryness of affected areas Skinfolds kept separated with a generous supply of nonmedicated powder Expose to air and light Remove excess clothing	A form of diaper irritation Prevent recurrence by keeping susceptible areas clean and dry Frequently associated with overheating from too much clothing Common in tracheostomy patients with short necks and copious secretions
Psoriasis—Cause unknown; hereditary predisposition; may be triggered by stress	Round, thick, dry, reddish patches covered with coarse, silvery scales over trunk and extremities; first lesions commonly appear in scalp; facial lesions more common in children than in adults Affected cells proliferate at a much more rapid rate than normal cells	Tar preparations in combination with ultraviolet B light or natural sunlight Topical corticosteroids Topical vitamin D analog calcipotriene Phenol and saline solutions followed by a tar shampoo to remove scales Keratolytic agents (salicylic acid) Acitretin Emollients may provide relief	Uncommon in children younger than 6 years Affected patients are otherwise healthy Coal tar acts synergistically with ultraviolet light Keratolytic agents enhance absorption of corticosteroids Humidifiers may help in winter
Alopecia*			
Alopecia areata	Sudden onset of asymptomatic, noninflammatory, round, bald patches in hairy parts of body	Psychologic support Minoxidil (peripheral vasodilator)	Family history in 10%-26% of cases Some concern regarding drug therapy safety Refer to support groups*
Traumatic alopecia	Traction alopecia around scalp margins from tight hair styles (e.g., braids, pony tails, corn rows)	Counseling regarding hair styling, use of hair cosmetics, hot combs, rollers	More prevalent in African American children and adolescents Prolonged traction can produce fibrosis of hair root and permanent loss
Trichotillomania	Compulsive hair pulling	Determine and treat cause	Chronic hair pulling may require psychologic therapy
Tinea capitis	See Table 32.4	See Table 32.4	See Table 32.4

Continued

TABLE 32.9 Miscellaneous Skin Disorders—cont'd

Disease and Causative Agent	Local Manifestations	Management	Comments
Erythema multiforme (Stevens-Johnson syndrome)—Cause unknown; associated with ingestion of some drugs; often follows upper respiratory tract infection	Erythematous papular rash Lesions enlarge by peripheral expansion, develop central vesicle Involves most skin surfaces except scalp May extend to mucous membranes, especially oral, ocular, and urethral	Symptomatic and supportive Maintenance of adequate intake of fluids (oral or intravenous), calories, and protein Moist wound care, hydrogels such as CarraGauze, Vaseline, or Aquaphor Appropriate treatment of complications Diligent monitoring of urine volume and specific gravity, hemoglobin and hematocrit, serum electrolyte levels, total body weight	Rash often preceded by fever and malaise Complications include renal failure and severe eye disease Respiratory involvement in a number of cases Self-limiting, but recovery may extend for weeks; skin lesions may subside without scarring; mucous membrane lesions may persist for months Recurrence rate, 20%; mortality rate as high as 10%
Neurofibromatosis—Inherited disorder; autosomal dominant inheritance pattern	Café-au-lait spots, pigmented nevi, axillary freckling Slow-growing cutaneous and subcutaneous neurofibromas	Symptomatic treatment of associated manifestations (e.g., speech defects, seizures, skeletal defects [scoliosis, kyphosis], learning disabilities) Surgical removal of troublesome tumors	High mutation rate Refer to support groups† Family needs to know about genetic implications

*National Alopecia Areata Foundation, 65 Mitchell Blvd. Suite 200-B, San Rafael, CA 94903; 415-472-3780; e-mail: info@naaf.org; http://www.naaf.org.

†Children's Tumor Foundation, 120 Wall St., 16th Floor, New York, NY 10005-3904; 800-323-7938; e-mail: info@ctf.org; http://www.ctf.org.

seborrheic dermatitis, which occurs predominantly in infants, and acne, which is most common in adolescence.

DIAPER DERMATITIS

Diaper dermatitis is common in infants and one of several acute inflammatory skin disorders caused either directly or indirectly by wearing diapers. The peak age of occurrence is 9 to 12 months of age, and the incidence is greater in bottle-fed infants than in breastfed infants.

Pathophysiology and Clinical Manifestations

Diaper dermatitis is caused by prolonged and repetitive contact with an irritant (e.g., urine, feces, soaps, detergents, ointments, friction). Although the irritant in the majority of cases is urine and feces, a combination of factors contributes to irritation.

Prolonged contact of the skin with diaper wetness produces higher friction, greater abrasion damage, increased transepidermal permeability, and increased microbial counts. Healthy skin is less resistant to potential irritants.

Although ammonia was once thought to cause diaper rash because of the association between the strong odor on diapers and dermatitis, ammonia alone is not sufficient. The irritant quality of urine is related to an increase in pH from the breakdown of urea in the presence of fecal urease. The increased pH promotes the activity of fecal enzymes, principally the proteases and lipases, which act as irritants. Fecal enzymes also increase the permeability of skin to bile salts, another potential irritant in feces.

The eruption of diaper dermatitis is manifested primarily on convex surfaces or in folds. The lesions represent a variety of types and configurations. Eruptions involving the skin in most intimate contact with the diaper (e.g., the convex surfaces of buttocks, inner thighs, mons pubis, and scrotum) but sparing the folds are likely to be caused by chemical irritants, especially from urine and feces (Fig. 32.10). Other causes are detergents or soaps from inadequately rinsed cloth diapers or the chemicals in disposable wipes. Perianal involvement is usually the result of chemical irritation from feces, especially diarrheal stools. *Candida albicans* infection produces perianal inflammation and a maculopapular rash with satellite lesions that may cross the inguinal fold (Fig. 32.11). It is seen in up to 90% of infants with chronic diaper dermatitis and should be considered in diaper rashes that are recalcitrant to treatment.

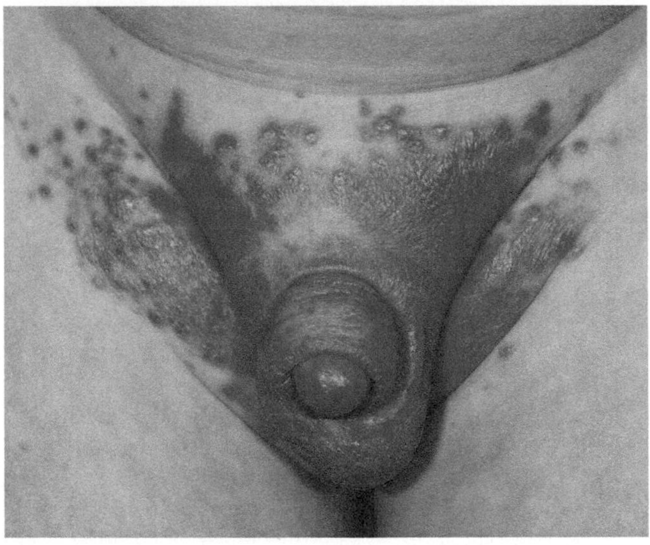

FIG. 32.10 Irritant diaper dermatitis. Note the sharply demarcated edges. (From Habif, T. P. [2010]. *Clinical dermatology: A color guide to diagnosis and therapy* [5th ed.]. St. Louis, MO: Mosby.)

Nursing Care Management

Nursing interventions are aimed at altering the three factors that produce dermatitis: wetness, pH, and fecal irritants. The most significant factor amenable to intervention is the moist environment created in the diaper area. Changing the diaper as soon as it becomes wet eliminates a large part of the problem, and removing the diaper to expose healthy skin to air facilitates drying. The use of a hair dryer or heat lamp is not recommended because these devices can cause burns.

Diaper construction has a significant impact on the incidence and severity of diaper dermatitis. Superabsorbent disposable paper diapers

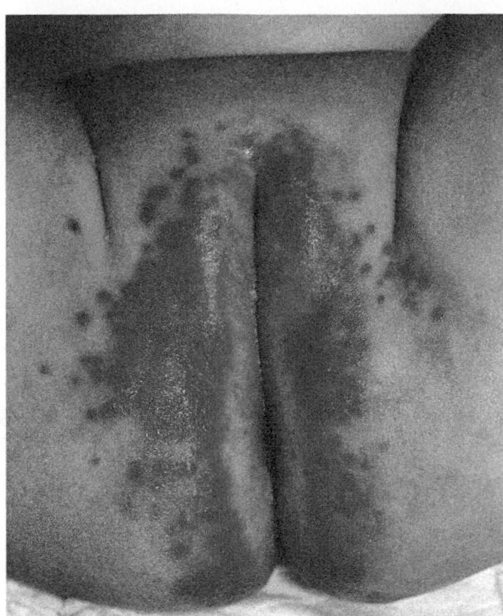

FIG. 32.11 Candidiasis of diaper area. Note the beefy red central erythema with satellite pustules. (From Paller, A. S., & Mancini, A. J. [2011]. *Hurwitz clinical pediatric dermatology* [4th ed.]. St. Louis, MO: Saunders Elsevier.)

reduce diaper dermatitis. They contain an absorbent gelling material that binds water tightly to decrease skin wetness, maintains pH control by providing a buffering capacity, and decreases skin irritation by preventing mixing of urine and feces in the diaper. Guidelines for controlling diaper rash are presented in the Family-Centered Care box. A common misconception about using cornstarch on skin is that it promotes the growth of *C. albicans.* Neither cornstarch nor talcum powder promotes the growth of fungi under conditions normally found in the diaper area. On the basis of safety in terms of inhalation injury, cornstarch is the preferred product. Talcum powder should not be used.

FAMILY-CENTERED CARE

Controlling Diaper Rash

Keep skin dry.*

- Use superabsorbent disposable diapers to reduce skin wetness.
- Change diapers as soon as soiled—especially with stool—whenever possible, preferably once during the night.
- Expose healthy or only slightly irritated skin to air, not heat, to dry completely.

Apply ointment, such as zinc oxide or petrolatum, to protect skin, especially if skin is very red or has moist, open areas.

- Avoid removing skin barrier cream with each diaper change; remove waste material and reapply skin barrier cream.
- To completely remove ointment, especially zinc oxide, use mineral oil; do not wash vigorously.

Avoid overwashing the skin, especially with perfumed soaps or commercial wipes, which may be irritating.

- May use a moisturizer or nonsoap cleanser, such as cold cream or Cetaphil, to wipe urine from skin.
- Gently wipe stool from skin using a soft cloth and warm water.
- Use disposable diaper wipes that are detergent and alcohol-free.

*Powder helps keep the skin dry, but talcum powder is dangerous if breathed into the lungs. Plain cornstarch or cornstarch-based powder is safer. When using any powder product, first shake it into your hand and then apply it to the diaper area. Store the container away from the infant's reach; keep the container closed when not in use.

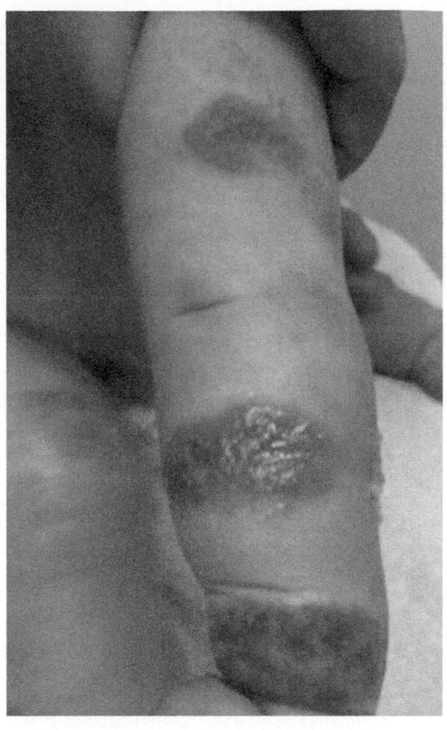

FIG. 32.12 Atopic dermatitis. (From Gupta, D. [2015]. Atopic dermatitis. *Medical Clinics of North America, 99*(6), 1269-1285.)

ATOPIC DERMATITIS (ECZEMA)

Atopic dermatitis (AD), also referred to as eczema, refers to a descriptive category of dermatologic diseases and not to a specific etiology. AD is a chronic relapsing inflammatory skin disorder that results in itching and lesions (Fig. 32.12; Grey & Maquiness, 2016). It occurs in 20% of children (Page, Weston, & Loh, 2016). AD manifests in three forms based on the child's age and the distribution of lesions:

1. **Infantile (infantile eczema)**—Usually begins at 2 to 6 months of age; generally undergoes spontaneous remission by 3 years of age
2. **Childhood**—May follow the infantile form; occurs at 2 to 3 years of age; 90% of children have manifestations by age 5 years
3. **Preadolescent and adolescent**—Begins at about 12 years of age; may continue into the early adult years or indefinitely

The diagnosis of AD is based on a combination of history and morphologic findings (Box 32.3). Although symptoms can vary among individuals, one symptom that is common is pruritus. Itching can be mild, moderate, or severe, and can intensify the inflammation and erythema associated with the lesions; itching can become so severe that the lesions bleed. Lesions gradually disappear when the scratching is stopped.

Although the cause is not fully understood, AD is believed to have genetic and environmental factors (Nguyen, Leonard, & Eichenfield, 2015). The majority of children with infantile AD have a family history of eczema, asthma, food allergies, or allergic rhinitis, which strongly supports a genetic predisposition. The cause is unknown but appears to be related to abnormal function of the skin, including alterations in perspiration, peripheral vascular function, and heat tolerance. Manifestations of the chronic disease improve in humid climates and get worse in the fall and winter, when homes are heated and environmental humidity is lower. The disorder can be controlled but not cured. A recent study of 250 patients with AD showed that the severity of AD significantly affected their quality of life, with more severe disease resulting in a lower quality of life (Holm, Agner, Causen, et al., 2016).

BOX 32.3 Clinical Manifestations of Atopic Dermatitis

Distribution of Lesions

Infantile form—Generalized, especially face, scalp, neck, and extensor surfaces of extremities

Childhood form—Flexural areas (antecubital and popliteal fossae, neck), wrists, ankles, and feet

Preadolescent and adolescent form—Face, sides of neck, hands, feet, face, and antecubital and popliteal fossae (to a lesser extent)

Appearance of Lesions

Infantile Form

Erythema
Vesicles
Papules
Weeping
Oozing
Crusting
Scaling
Often symmetric

Childhood Form

Symmetric involvement
Clusters of small erythematous or flesh-colored papules or minimally scaling patches
Dry and may be hyperpigmented
Lichenification (thickened skin with accentuation of creases)
Keratosis pilaris (follicular hyperkeratosis) common

Adolescent or Adult Form

Same as childhood manifestations
Dry, thick lesions (lichenified plaques) common
Confluent papules

Other Physical Manifestations

Intense itching
Unaffected skin dry and rough
African American children likely to exhibit more papular or follicular lesions than white children
May exhibit one or more of the following:

- Lymphadenopathy, especially near affected sites
- Increased palmar creases (many cases)
- Atopic pleats (extra line or groove of lower eyelid)
- Prone to cold hands
- Pityriasis alba (small, poorly defined areas of hypopigmentation)
- Facial pallor (especially around nose, mouth, and ears)
- Bluish discoloration beneath eyes ("allergic shiners")
- Increased susceptibility to unusual cutaneous infections (especially viral)

Furthermore, the study reported a lower quality of life among females and among patients with eczema on their face (Holm, Agner, Causen, et al., 2016).

Therapeutic Management

The major goals of management are to (1) hydrate the skin, (2) relieve pruritus, (3) reduce flare-ups or inflammation, and (4) prevent and control secondary infection. The general measures for managing AD focus on reducing pruritus and other aspects of the disease. Management strategies include avoiding exposure to skin irritants or allergens; avoiding overheating; and administrating medications such as antihistamines, topical immunomodulators, topical steroids, and (sometimes) mild sedatives as indicated.

Enhancing skin hydration and preventing dry, flaky skin are accomplished in a number of ways, depending on the child's skin characteristics and individual needs. A tepid bath with a mild soap (Dove or Neutrogena), no soap, or an emulsifying oil followed immediately by application of an emollient (within 3 minutes) assists in trapping moisture and preventing its loss. Bubble baths and harsh soaps should be avoided. The bath may need to be repeated once or twice daily, depending on the child's status; excessive bathing without emollient application only dries out the skin. Some lotions are not effective, and emollients should be chosen carefully to prevent excessive skin drying. Aquaphor, Cetaphil, and Eucerin are acceptable lotions for skin hydration. A nighttime bath followed by emollient application and dressing in soft cotton pajamas may help alleviate most nighttime pruritus.

Sometimes colloid baths, such as the addition of 2 cups of cornstarch to a tub of warm water, provide temporary relief of itching and may help the child sleep if given before bedtime. Cool wet compresses are soothing to the skin and provide antiseptic protection.

Oral antihistamine drugs (such as hydroxyzine or diphenhydramine) usually relieve moderate or severe pruritus. Nonsedating antihistamines such as loratadine (Claritin) or fexofenadine (Allegra) may be preferred for daytime pruritus relief. Because pruritus increases at night, a mildly sedating antihistamine may be needed.

Occasional flare-ups require the use of topical steroids to diminish inflammation. Low-, moderate-, or high-potency topical corticosteroids are prescribed, depending on the degree of involvement, the area of the body to be treated, the child's age, the potential for local side effects (striae, skin atrophy, and pigment changes), and the type of vehicle to be used (e.g., cream, lotion, ointment). Patients receiving topical corticosteroid therapy for chronic conditions should be evaluated for risk factors for suboptimal linear growth and reduced bone density. Topical immunomodulators, a nonsteroidal treatment for AD, are best used at the beginning of a "flare-up" just as the skin becomes red and itches. Second-line management for children with AD includes immunomodulator medications such as tacrolimus and pimecrolimus (Grey & Maquiness, 2016). These medications are approved for use in children 2 years of age and older (Grey & Maquiness, 2016). Both drugs can be used freely on the face without worrying about steroid side effects.

If secondary skin infections occur in children with AD, these infections are managed with appropriate systemic antibiotics. Obtaining cultures from affected areas and the child's nares is helpful to ensure appropriate therapy (Page, Weston, & Loh, 2016).

Nursing Care Management

Assessment of the child with AD includes a family history for evidence of atopy, a history of previous involvement, and any environmental or dietary factors associated with the present and previous exacerbations. The skin lesions are examined for type, distribution, and evidence of secondary infection. Parents are interviewed regarding the child's behavior, especially in relation to scratching, irritability, and sleeping patterns. Exploration of the family's feelings and methods of coping is also important.

The nursing care of the child with AD is challenging. Controlling the intense pruritus is imperative if the disorder is to be successfully managed because scratching leads to new lesions and may cause secondary infection. In addition to the medical regimen, other measures can be taken to prevent or minimize the scratching. Fingernails and toenails are cut short, kept clean, and filed frequently to prevent sharp edges. Gloves or cotton stockings can be placed over the hands and pinned to shirtsleeves. One-piece outfits with long sleeves and long pants also decrease direct contact with the skin. If gloves or socks are used, the child needs time to be free from such restrictions. An excellent time to remove gloves, socks, or other protective devices is during the bath or after receiving sedative or antipruritic medication.

Conditions that increase itching are eliminated when possible. Woolen clothes or blankets, rough fabrics, and furry stuffed animals are removed from the child's environment. Because heat and humidity cause perspiration (which intensifies itching), proper dress for climatic conditions is essential. Pruritus is often precipitated by exposure to the irritant effects of certain components of common products such as soaps, detergents, fabric softeners, perfumes, and powders. During cold months, synthetic fabrics (not wool) should be used for overcoats, hats, gloves, and snowsuits. Exposure to latex products, such as gloves and balloons, should also be avoided.

Clothes and sheets are laundered in a mild detergent and rinsed thoroughly in clear water (without fabric softeners or antistatic chemicals). Putting the clothes through a second complete wash cycle without using detergent reduces the amount of residue remaining in the fabric.

Preventing infection is usually accomplished by preventing scratching. Baths are given as prescribed; the water is kept tepid; and soaps (except as indicated), bubble baths, oils, and powders are avoided. Skinfolds and diaper areas need frequent cleansing with plain water. A room humidifier or vaporizer may benefit children with extremely dry skin. Skin lesions are examined for signs of infection—usually honey-colored crusts or pustules with surrounding erythema. Any signs of infection are reported to the practitioner.

! NURSING ALERT

If the child is being treated with baths, it is imperative that an emollient preparation be applied immediately after bathing (while the skin is still slightly moist) to prevent drying.

Wet soaks and compresses are applied and medications for pruritus or infection are administered as directed. The family is given explicit instructions on the preparation and use of soaks, special baths, and topical medications, including the order of application if more than one is prescribed. It is important to emphasize that one thick application of topical medication is *not* equivalent to several thin applications and that excessive use of an agent (particularly steroids) can be hazardous. If children have difficulty remaining still for a 10- or 15-minute soak, bath, or dressing application, these can be carried out at naptime or when the child is engrossed in watching television, listening to a story, or playing with tub toys.

Diet modification may prevent skin exacerbations. When a hypoallergenic diet is prescribed, parents need help to understand the reason for the diet and the guidelines for avoiding hyperallergenic foods. Because hypoallergenic diets take time before visible effects are apparent, parents need reassurance that results may not be seen immediately. If airborne allergens make eczema worse, the family is counseled about "allergy proofing" the home (see Asthma, Chapter 26).

Family Support

Parents are assured that the lesions will not produce scarring (unless secondarily infected) and that the disease is not contagious. However, the child may have repeated exacerbations and remissions. Spontaneous and permanent remission takes place at approximately 2 to 3 years of age in most children with the infantile disorder.

During acute phases, emotional stress can become intense for the family. They need time to discuss negative feelings and to be reassured that these feelings are normal. Stress tends to aggravate the severity of the condition. Therefore efforts to relieve as much anxiety as possible in both the parents and the child have a beneficial emotional and physical effect.

SEBORRHEIC DERMATITIS

Seborrheic dermatitis is a chronic, recurrent, inflammatory reaction of the skin. It occurs most commonly on the scalp (cradle cap) but may involve the eyelids (blepharitis), external ear canal (otitis externa), nasolabial folds, and inguinal region. The cause is unknown, although it is more common in early infancy, when sebum production is increased. The lesions are characteristically thick, adherent, yellowish, scaly, oily patches that may or may not be mildly pruritic. Unlike AD, seborrheic dermatitis is not associated with a positive family history for allergy and is common in infants shortly after birth and in adolescents after puberty. Diagnosis is made primarily on the basis of the appearance and the location of the crusts or scales.

Nursing Care Management

Cradle cap may be prevented with adequate scalp hygiene. Frequently, parents omit shampooing the infant's hair for fear of damaging the "soft spots," or fontanels. The nurse should discuss how to shampoo the infant's hair and emphasize that the fontanel is similar to skin anywhere else on the body—it does not puncture or tear with mild pressure.

When seborrheic lesions are present, direct the treatment at removing the scales or crusts. Parents are taught the appropriate procedure to clean the scalp. Education may need to include a demonstration. Shampooing should be done daily with a mild soap or commercial baby shampoo; medicated shampoos are not necessary, but an antiseborrheic shampoo containing sulfur and salicylic acid may be used. Shampoo is applied to the scalp and allowed to remain on the scalp until the crusts soften. Then the scalp is thoroughly rinsed. A fine-tooth comb or a soft facial brush helps remove the loosened crusts from the strands of hair after shampooing.

ACNE

Acne vulgaris is the most common skin problem treated by physicians during adolescence. Acne is caused by testosterone, a hormone present in boys and girls that increases during puberty. It stimulates the sebaceous glands of the skin to enlarge, or produce oil, and plug the pores. Comedogenesis (formation of comedones) results in a noninflammatory lesion that may be either an open comedone ("blackhead") or a closed comedone ("whitehead").

More than half of the adolescent population experiences acne by the end of the teenage years. Although the disorder can appear before the age of 10 years, the peak incidence occurs in middle to late adolescence (age 16 to 17 years in girls and 17 to 18 years in boys). It is more common in boys than in girls. After this age period, the disease usually decreases in severity, but it may persist into adulthood. The degree to which an individual is affected may range from nothing more than a few isolated comedones to a severe inflammatory reaction. Although the disease is self-limiting and not life threatening, it has great significance to adolescents. Health professionals should not underestimate the impact that acne has on teens.

Numerous factors affect the development and course of acne. Its distribution in families and a high degree of concordance in identical twins suggest hereditary factors. Premenstrual flare-ups of acne occur in nearly 70% of adolescent girls, suggesting a hormonal cause. Studies do not indicate a clear association between stress and acne, but adolescents commonly cite stress as a cause for acne outbreaks. Cosmetics containing lanolin, petrolatum, vegetable oils, lauryl alcohol, butyl stearate,

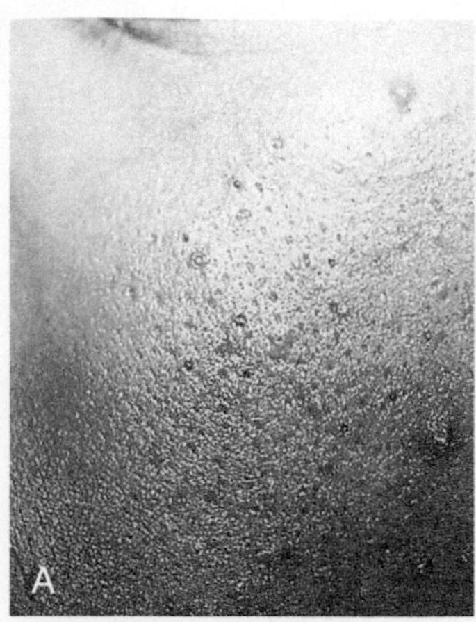

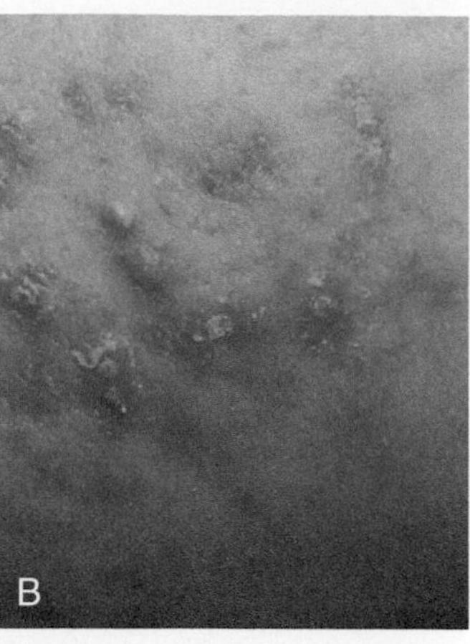

FIG. 32.13 Acne vulgaris. **A,** Acne vulgaris. **B,** Comedones with a few inflammatory pustules. (From Zitelli, B. J., McIntire, S. C., & Nowalk, A. J. [2012]. *Zitelli and Davis' atlas of pediatric physical diagnosis* [6th ed.]. St. Louis, MO: Saunders.)

and oleic acid can increase comedone production. Exposure to oils in cooking grease can be a precursor in adolescents who work over fast-food restaurant hot oils. There may be an association with the intake of dairy products and high glycemic index foods that may potentiate hormonal and inflammatory factors that contribute to acne severity (Fiedler, Stangl, Fiedler, et al., 2017).

Pathophysiology

Four pathophysiologic factors have the greatest influence on acne development: (1) excessive sebum production; (2) alterations in follicular growth; (3) differentiation with colonization of *Propionibacterium acnes;* and (4) an accompanying immune response and inflammation (Bhat, Latief, & Hassan, 2017). Acne severity is proportional to the sebum secretion rate, which is genetically determined and increases at the time of adrenocortical maturation. Inflammation occurs with the proliferation of *P. acnes,* which draws in neutrophils, causing inflammatory papules, pustules, nodules, and cysts (Fig. 32.13). Acne can be categorized as comedonal, inflammatory, or both and can be classified as mild, moderate, or severe based on the number and type of comedones and the extent of affected skin (Eichenfield, Krakowski, Piggott, et al., 2013).

Therapeutic Management

Successful management of acne depends on a cooperative effort among the health care provider, adolescent, and parents. Unlike many other dermatologic conditions, acne lesions resolve slowly, and improvement may not be apparent for at least 6 weeks. Individual comedones can take several weeks to months to resolve, and papules and pustules usually resolve in about 1 week. The multifactorial causes of acne necessitate a combined approach for successful treatment. Treatment consists of general measures of care and specific treatments determined by the type of lesions involved.

General Measures

The practitioner provides the adolescent with an overall explanation of the disease process, emphasizing the patient's involvement. Improvement of the adolescent's overall health status is part of the general management. Adequate rest, moderate exercise, a well-balanced diet, reduction of emotional stress, and elimination of any foci of infection are all part of general health promotion.

Cleansing

Dirt or oil on the surface of the skin does not cause acne. Gentle cleansing with a mild cleanser once or twice daily is usually sufficient. Antibacterial soaps are ineffective and may be drying when used in combination with topical acne medications. For some adolescents, hygiene of the hair and scalp appears to be related to the clinical activity of the acne. Acne on the forehead may improve with brushing the hair away from the forehead and more frequent shampooing.

Medications

Treatment success depends on commitment from the adolescent. Before prescribing treatment, the practitioner should determine the adolescent's level of comfort and readiness to begin treatment. The adolescent should be reminded that clinical improvement may take weeks to months. Early intervention, most often with topical medications, may prevent the development of more severe acne.

Tretinoin (Retin-A) is the only drug that effectively interrupts the abnormal follicular keratinization that produces microcomedones, the invisible precursors of the visible comedones. Tretinoin alone is usually sufficient for management of mild comedonal acne (Que, Whitaker-Worth, & Chang, 2016). Tretinoin is available as a cream, gel, or liquid. This drug can be extremely irritating to the skin and requires careful patient education for optimal usage. The patient should be instructed to begin with a pea-sized dot of medication, which is divided into the three main areas of the face and then gently rubbed into each area. The medication should not be applied for at least 20 to 30 minutes after washing to decrease the burning sensation. The avoidance of the sun and the daily use of sunscreen must be emphasized because sun exposure can result in severe sunburn. Adolescents should be advised to apply the medication at night and to use a sunscreen with a sun protection factor (SPF) of at least 15 in the daytime.

Topical benzoyl peroxide is an antibacterial agent that inhibits the growth of *P. acnes* organisms. It is effective against both inflammatory and noninflammatory acne and is an effective first-line agent. This medication is available as a cream, lotion, gel, or wash. Benzoyl peroxide and salicylic acid are the most effective acne treatment kits available over the counter. The patient should be informed that the medication may have a bleaching effect on sheets, bedclothes, and towels. The adolescent can be reassured that skin bleaching will not occur. Accommodation to the medication can be gained with a gradual increase in the strength and frequency of application.

When inflammatory lesions accompany the comedones, a topical antibacterial agent may be prescribed. These agents are used to prevent new lesions and to treat preexisting acne. Clindamycin, erythromycin, metronidazole, and azelaic acid are currently available topical antibacterial therapy. A 5% dapsone gel has recently been approved for the treatment of inflammatory acne lesions and is reported to be effective when used in combination with a topical retinoid (Que, Whitaker-Worth, & Chang, 2016). Retinoid in combination with antimicrobials also improves the penetration of these topical agents and is the only means to address three of the pathogenic causes of acne: keratinization, *P. acnes,* and inflammation. Side effects of the topical medications include erythema, dryness, and burning; using the medications every other day will decrease the adverse effects. Topical antimicrobials combined with benzoyl peroxide are more effective than either product alone; however, a yellowish discoloration of the skin occurs when topical dapsone is used in combination with benzoyl peroxide (Que, Whitaker-Worth, & Chang, 2016).

Systemic antibiotic therapy is initiated when moderate to severe acne does not respond to topical treatments. The foundation for using systemic antibiotics in acne treatment has been the elimination of the inflammatory effects of *P. acnes* by suppressing the bacteria. Tetracycline, minocycline, and doxycycline are systematic antibiotics used to treat acne (Que, Whitaker-Worth, & Chang, 2016). They are relatively free of side effects, with the exception of occasional gastrointestinal upset, photosensitivity, or vaginal candidiasis. Adolescent girls with mild to moderate acne may respond well to topical treatment and the addition of an oral contraceptive pill (OCP). OCPs reduce the endogenous androgen production and decrease the bioavailability of the woman's circulating androgens. Both of these actions result in decreased acne.

Isotretinoin, 13-*cis*-retinoic acid (Accutane), is a potent and effective oral agent that is reserved for severe cystic acne that has not responded to other treatments. Isotretinoin is the only agent available that affects factors involved in the development of acne. However, treatment with isotretinoin should be managed *only* by a dermatologist. Adolescents with multiple, active, deep dermal or subcutaneous cystic and nodular acne lesions are treated for 20 weeks. Multiple side effects can occur, including dry skin and mucous membranes, nasal irritation, dry eyes, decreased night vision, photosensitivity, arthralgia, headaches, mood changes, aggressive or violent behaviors, depression, and suicidal ideation. Adolescents taking this drug should be monitored for depression, depressive symptoms, and suicidal ideation (Oliveira, Sobreira, Velosa, et al., 2017). The drug should be given only at the recommended doses for no longer than the recommended duration. The most significant side effects of this drug are the teratogenic effects. Isotretinoin is absolutely contraindicated in pregnant women. Sexually active young women must use an effective contraceptive method during treatment and for 1 month after treatment. Patients receiving isotretinoin should also be monitored for elevated cholesterol and triglyceride levels. Significant elevation may require discontinuation of the medication.

Nursing Care Management

Because acne is so common and its appearance may seem so mild, the health care provider may underestimate the relative importance of the disease to the adolescent. The nurse should assess the individual adolescent's level of distress, current management, and perceived success of any regimen before initiating a referral. If adolescents do not perceive the acne to be a problem, they may lack motivation to follow the treatment plan.

The nurse can provide ongoing support for the adolescent when a treatment plan is initiated. Discuss the use of medications and basic skin care information in detail with the adolescent. Written instructions should accompany the verbal discussion. Information to dispel myths regarding the use of abrasive cleansing products can prevent unnecessary costs and trauma to the skin. Adolescents need education about the factors that aggravate and damage the skin, such as too vigorous scrubbing. In addition, picking, squeezing, and manual expression with fingernails break down the ductal walls of lesions and cause the acne to worsen. Mechanical irritation, such as vinyl helmet straps that rub areas predisposed to acne, can also cause the development of lesions.

COLD INJURY

In cold injuries the nature of the heat-regulating mechanisms of the body are such that the inner portion of the body, or core, produces heat, and the periphery, or outer area, conserves or dissipates heat. When the body attempts to conserve heat, the outer tissues are subjected to low temperatures, and local trauma may result.

Chilblain, redness and swelling of the skin, occurs when extremities, usually the hands, are exposed intermittently to temperatures of 1.1° to 15.5°C (30° to 60°F). The response may vary but is characterized by intense vasodilation that increases the temperature of involved tissues above that of unaffected tissue and produces edematous, reddish blue patches that itch and burn. As warming takes place, the sensations become more intense, but ordinarily they subside in a few days.

Frostbite is the term used to describe tissue damage caused when excessive heat loss to local tissues allows ice crystals to form in tissues. The frostbitten part appears white or blanched, feels solid, and is without sensation. Rapid rewarming is associated with less tissue necrosis than slow thawing. It restores blood flow and shortens the period of cellular damage. Rewarming produces a flush (sometimes deep purple) and a return of sensation, which is extremely painful. Large blisters may appear in 24 to 48 hours after rewarming and begin to reabsorb within 5 to 10 days followed by the formation of a hard black eschar. Superficial injury often heals without incident. Rewarming is accomplished by immersing the part in well-agitated water at 37.8° to 42.2°C (100° to 108°F). Discomfort is managed with analgesics and sedatives. Care of blistered skin is similar to that described for burns. It is seldom possible to estimate the extent of tissue loss until new skin layers are revealed after the eschar layer separates.

NCLEX REVIEW QUESTIONS

1. Identify the interventions that can be safely used to manage diaper dermatitis. Select all that apply.
   - **a.** Blow dry heat on skin with hair dryer.
   - **b.** Apply a skin barrier paste such as zinc oxide.
   - **c.** Keep skin surface irritants such as urine and stool off skin.
   - **d.** Expose skin to air.
   - **e.** Use only cloth diapers.
2. A new nurse is caring for a child with a wound and asks you to remind her about the phases of wound healing. You describe the order as:
   - **a.** Contraction: Fibroblast movement causes contraction of the healing area, which helps bring wound edges closer together.
   - **b.** Maturation: The scar becomes pale, does not tan when exposed to sunlight, will not sweat or produce hair, and may itch.
   - **c.** Inflammatory phase: Erythema, heat, edema, pain, and functional disturbance occur.
   - **d.** Proliferation: Fibroblasts, immature connective tissue cells, migrate to the healing site and begin to secrete collagen into the meshwork spaces.
3. Care of the child with a wound includes which of the following? Select all that apply.
   - **a.** Applying occlusive dressings, such as hydrocolloid dressings. Dressings adhere best if a wide margin is left around the wound and the dressing is gently pressed against intact skin until it adheres.
   - **b.** The safest solution for cleansing and loosening sticky dressings is normal saline.
   - **c.** To remove a transparent or hydrocolloid dressing, use one hand to hold the skin to which the dressing is secured firmly, then gently raise both edges of the dressing and pull the dressing away from the skin in a parallel direction.
   - **d.** Wounds covering a very large area (>25% of the body) need medical attention, with the child undergoing conscious sedation and analgesia.
   - **e.** Puncture wounds should initially be irrigated with sterile saline, then soaked in a basin of warm soapy water for several minutes before applying a clean dressing.

4. A 9-year-old child in the emergency department is diagnosed with Lyme disease. The nurse anticipates that the health care provider's orders will include the administration of:
   a. Cefotaxime
   b. Aqueous penicillin
   c. Doxycycline
   d. Trimethoprim-sulfamethoxazole

Correct Answers

1. B, C, D; 2. C, D, A, B; 3. A, B, E; 4. C

REFERENCES

American Academy of Pediatrics, Committee on Infectious Diseases (2015). L. Pickering (Ed.), *2015 Red book: report of the Committee on Infectious Diseases* (30th ed.). Elk Grove Village, IL: The Academy.

Bhat, Y. J., Latief, I., & Hassan, I. (2017). Update on etiopathogenesis and treatment of acne. *Indian Journal of Dermatology, Venereology and Leprology, 83*(3), 298–306.

Centers for Disease Control and Prevention. (2017). *Lyme disease (Borrelia burgdorferi)*. Retrieved from https://www.cdc.gov/nndss/conditions/lyme-disease/case-definition/2017/.

Chaptini, C., Quinn, S., & Marshman, G. (2016). Methicillin-resistant staphylococcus aureus in children with atopic dermatitis from 1999 to 2014: A longitudinal study. *The Australasian Journal of Dermatology, 57*(2), 122–127.

Devore, C. D., Schutze, G. E., & American Academy of Pediatrics, Council on School Health and Committee on Infectious Diseases. (2015). Head lice. *Pediatrics, 135*(5), e1355–e1365.

Eichenfield, L. F., Krakowski, A. C., Piggott, C., et al. (2013). Evidence-based recommendations for the diagnosis and treatment of pediatric acne. *Pediatrics, 131*(Suppl. 3), S163–S183.

Eisen, L., & Dolan, M. C. (2016). Evidence for personal protective measures to reduce human contact with blacklegged ticks and for environmentally based control methods to suppress host-seeking blacklegged ticks and reduce infection with lyme disease spirochetes in tick vectors and rodent reservoirs. *Journal of Medical Entomology, 53*, 1063–1092.

Fiedler, F., Stangl, G. I., Fiedler, E., et al. (2017). Acne and nutrition: A systematic review. *Acta Dermato-Venereologica, 97*(1), 7–9.

Grey, K., & Maquiness, S. (2016). Atopic dermatitis: Update for pediatricians. *Pediatric Annals, 45*(8), e280–e286.

Gupta, A. K., Lyons, D. C., & Rosen, T. (2015). New and emerging concepts in managing and preventing community-associated methicillin-resistant staphylococcus aureus infections. *International Journal of Dermatology, 54*(11), 1226–1232.

Han, G., & Ceilley, R. (2017). Chronic wound healing: A review of current management and treatments. *Advances in Therapy, 34*, 599–610.

Holm, J. G., Agner, T., Clausen, M. L., et al. (2016). Quality of life and disease severity in patients with atopic dermatitis. *Journal of the European Academy of Dermatology and Venereology, 30*(1), 1760–1767.

Kaplan, S. L. (2016). Staphylococcus aureus infections in children: The implications of changing trends. *Pediatrics, 137*(4), e20160101.

Kaplan, S. L., Forbes, A., Hammerman, W. A., et al. (2014). Randomized trial of "bleach baths" plus routine hygienic measures vs routine hygienic measures alone for prevention of recurrent infections. *Clinical Infectious Diseases, 58*(5), 679–682.

King, A., Stellar, J. J., Blevins, A., et al. (2014). Dressing and products in pediatric wound care. *Adv Wound Care, 3*(4), 324–334.

Koedel, U., Fingerle, V., & Pfister, H. (2015). Lyme neuroborreliosis – epidemiology, diagnosis and management. *Nature Reviews. Neurology, 11*, 446–456.

Koehler, S., Jinbo, A., Johnson, S., et al. (2014). Negative pressure dressing assisted healing in pediatric burn patients. *Journal of Pediatric Surgery, 49*(7), 1142–1145.

Margolis, D. J., Abuabara, K., Hoffstad, O. J., et al. (2015). Association between malignancy and topical use of pimecrolimus. *JAMA Dermatolog, 151*(6), 594–599.

Nguyen, T. A., Leonard, S. A., & Eichenfield, L. F. (2015). An update on pediatric atopic dermatitis and food allergies. *The Journal of Pediatrics, 167*(3), 752–756.

Oliveira, J. M., Sobreira, G., Velosa, J., et al. (2017). Association of isotretinoin with depression and suicide: A review of current literature. *Journal of Cutaneous Medicine and Surgery*, epub ahead of print.

Page, S. S., Weston, S., & Loh, R. (2016). Atopic dermatitis in children. *Australian Family Physician, 45*(5), 293–296.

Que, S. K. T., Whitaker-Worth, D. L., & Change, M. W. (2016). Acne: Kids are not just little people. *Clinics in Dermatology, 34*, 710–716.

Satteson, E. S., Crantford, J. C., Wood, J., et al. (2015). Outcomes of vacuum-assisted therapy in the treatment of head and neck wounds. *The Journal of Craniofacial Surgery, 26*(7), e599–e602.

Steere, A. C., Strle, F., Wormser, G. P., et al. (2016). Lyme borreliosis. *Nature Reviews, 2*, 1–18.

Takahara, S., Sai, S., Kagatani, T., et al. (2014). Efficacy and haemodynamic effects of vacuum-assisted closure for post-sternotomy mediastinitis in children. *Interactive Cardiovascular and Thoracic Surgery, 19*(4), 627–631.

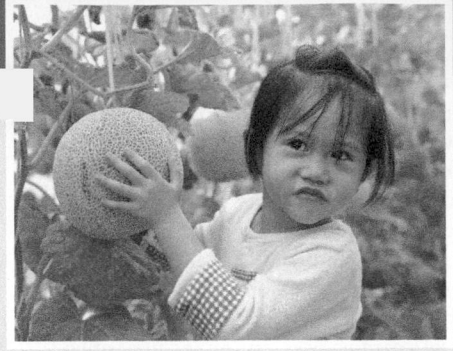

33

The Child With Musculoskeletal or Articular Dysfunction

Angela Drummond

http://evolve.elsevier.com/wong/ncic

CONCEPTS

- Infection
- Immunity
- Integrity
- Mobility

THE CHILD AND TRAUMA

TRAUMA MANAGEMENT

Epidemiology of Trauma

Trauma is a leading cause of death in children older than age 1 year (see Chapter 1) and an important cause of disability during childhood and adolescence. In many ways, childhood trauma differs little from trauma in adults. However, the child's developmental stage affects many aspects of injury, including the type of injury incurred and the physiologic response to injury.

Unintentional injuries are the leading cause of death in children 1 year to 19 years of age in the United States. Forty-two percent of all deaths in this age-group in 2015 were from unintentional injuries, with motor vehicle crashes accounting for the largest percentage of deaths (Centers for Disease Control and Prevention, 2015).

Childhood Characteristics

Certain developmental characteristics of children at various ages render them more susceptible to injury. For example, the large head of infants and toddlers predisposes them to head injury, especially in falls or motor vehicle injuries. Also, the relatively large spleen and liver and the broad costal arch make these structures prone to direct trauma. Because of their light weight and small size, infants and small children are easily thrown around in a moving vehicle. Their natural curiosity and their propensity for using large muscles lure them to attempt potentially hazardous activities.

Later, in school-age children and adolescents, whose bone growth outstrips muscle growth, difficulty controlling movement can contribute to physical injury. This is also a time when many children attempt to engage in activities beyond their physical capabilities to keep up with more agile companions and to meet the expectations of adults and older siblings. They are also vulnerable to a "dare." Risk taking compounded by a feeling of invulnerability is also characteristic of adolescence. Children of school age and early adolescence may also be encouraged to continue engaging in sports activities after suffering a contusion or injury and are therefore subject to repetitive injuries.

Unintentional or Accidental Injury

Among the leading causes of morbidity in children are medical problems resulting from traumatic injury that occurs at home or school, in an automobile, or in association with recreational activities. Children's everyday activities include vigorous play that may involve such things as climbing, falling, running into immovable objects, and receiving blows to any part of the body. All of these activities make them prone to injury. School-age children and adolescents are vulnerable to multiple and severe trauma because they are mobile on bikes, motorcycles, and all-terrain vehicles (ATVs) and in automobiles; they are also active in sports. Speed and congested surroundings often increase the chance of injury.

Young children and adolescents usually do not calculate risks as they learn to manipulate their environment and achieve developmental goals. Therefore accidents are a part of many childhood experiences. Fortunately, when children fall or are hit, their body's resilience protects them from serious damage to soft tissue, the musculoskeletal system, or other body organs. Their bones are more flexible with less density than those of adults and therefore do not offer the rigid resistance to external forces making it more likely for a child to sustain a fracture.

Child Abuse or Nonaccidental Trauma

Unfortunately, careless handling of an infant or child (in some instances intentional physical abuse) is not uncommon. A multitude of different types of bone and soft tissue injury are inflicted on children by adults, and smaller children who are unable to protect themselves are most vulnerable.

A traumatic incident that produces physical injury to an infant or child may be the outcome of an accident that was no one's fault, or it may be associated with child abuse. A well-documented history and a careful examination are essential to determine the cause of the injury. Emergency department and pediatric office personnel should be alert to situations in which the child's injuries are not congruent with the parent's description of the incident; the child's behaviors, such as fearful mannerisms or lack of crying, are not the expected ones; or radiographs

COMMUNITY AND HOME HEALTH CONSIDERATIONS

Distinguishing Unintentional From Intentional Fractures

Distinguishing abusive (nonaccidental) from unintentional fractures can be challenging. The history, location of the injury, radiographs, and associated injuries must be carefully considered. Details of the history to consider include delay in seeking medical care and an inappropriate clinical history or the report of a change in the child's health, behavior, or activity level but no report of injury.

Studies have shown that children less than 2 years of age and those that were born prematurely or have comorbid medical conditions are more likely to suffer a nonaccidental trauma. In addition, risk of abuse is increased if parents feel isolated, perceive an absence of support, or lack a connection to the community. No clear relationship with socioeconomic status has been found and all populations are at risk (Paul & Adamo, 2014). In one study, the child's age was determined to be a factor. The demographics in children most likely to suffer abuse requiring orthopedic treatment were less than 1 year of age, 1 to 2 years of age, and Medicaid as primary payer; winter and weekday presentation was also a strong predictor of child abuse presentation in this study (Bullock, Koval, Moen, et al., 2009). Loder and Feinberg (2007) found that the most common fractures in nonaccidental trauma involved the femur and humerus, and most of these fractures occurred in infants less than 2 years of age. One study found a high incidence of fractures and traumatic brain injury in children under 12 months of age; infants between 2 and 7 months of age were more likely to have injuries attributed to nonaccidental trauma than those younger than 2 months of age (Leventhal, Martin, & Asnes, 2010).

Although not diagnostic of an intentional injury, the location of a fracture can raise suspicions about the actual cause. In an infant, midshaft or metaphyseal humerus fractures and radius-ulna, tibia-fibula, and femur fractures are not common and raise suspicion about the likelihood of abuse. Rib fractures, scapular fractures, bilateral fractures, complex skull fractures, and vertebral fractures or subluxations are also suspicious. In contrast, in children older than 1 year of age, supracondylar humerus fractures and fractures of the clavicle, distal extremity, and femur are most frequently related to an unintentional or accidental injury.

In children of all ages, radiographic evidence of previous fractures at different stages of healing may indicate repeated trauma and raise concern about intentional injuries. The presence of bruises, burns, and additional soft tissue injuries in children may also prompt further evaluation to determine whether the child has been subjected to intentional harm. One mnemonic used to prompt consideration of the possibility of intentional physical abuse is the five *B*s:

- *Bumps*
- *Bruises*
- *Breaks*
- *Burns*
- Anything that happens in the *bathroom*

show multiple healed fractures. Accounts of injury inconsistent with developmental abilities can alert the provider to possible abuse as well. For example, a 6-month-old infant cannot "climb out of the crib and break her leg." Reporting these incidents will aid in securing help for the child and family. (See Community and Home Health Considerations box; also see Physical Abuse, Chapter 16.)

Prevention of Injury

Increasingly, health care providers are recognizing the importance of injury prevention efforts in preserving the health and well-being of children. Nurses have an important role to play in these efforts.

Leading causes of nonfatal injury to children include falls, being struck by or against an object, motor vehicle or transportation-related accidents, overexertion, bites or stings, and being cut or pierced. Falls are the leading cause of nonfatal injury among children ages 0 to 14 years. Being struck by or against a person or object is the leading cause of nonfatal injury in older children 15 to 19 years of age. Foreign body causes occur in young children, especially those between 0 and 4 years of age, whereas sports injuries or overexertion occur in school-age children and adolescents (Centers for Disease Control and Prevention, 2015).

Unintentional, preventable injury is the primary cause of pediatric mortality and a significant contributor to morbidity, including permanent disability. Both morbidity and mortality rates could be reduced dramatically by improved efforts at injury prevention. Studies have indicated a general lack of public awareness regarding risks, causes, and prevention of injury to children. Studies also show that injury prevention counseling is effective both in reducing hazards in the home and in increasing car seat use. Nurses can be active in legislative efforts, public awareness campaigns, group classes on injury prevention, and individual prevention counseling with children and families.

Many injury prevention strategies have been suggested for nurses. Nursing history or hospital admission forms can include screening questions about safety issues. Discharge planning or primary care visits might be a time to provide a family with information on safety practices. Well-child visits to the provider for physicals and immunizations are an excellent time to visit with children and parents about injury prevention in the home and the community. Home health care nurses can easily assist a family in conducting a home safety assessment. School nurses can develop safety education programs for different age-groups and discuss injury prevention with children that is applicable to their specific age-group. Nurses in emergency department and outpatient clinic settings can provide instructions related to injury prevention on an individual basis as developmentally appropriate. Additional resources for discussing injury prevention with adolescents include automobile insurance companies and the police and first-responder personnel.*

Accident prevention among adolescents presents a unique challenge to all health care workers. For accident prevention to be effective, adolescents must perceive the specific interventions as having an impact on their lives. Adolescents are concerned with body image and often feel indestructible unless their own life or the life of a close friend is touched by a catastrophic debilitating injury or death. With increased emphasis in society on having fun and enjoying life to its fullest (today) regardless of the consequences (tomorrow), it is difficult for adolescents to understand the need to follow the rules laid down by authority figures.

Concern is also increasing about injuries to older school-age children and adolescents from the use of all-terrain motor vehicles (for which many states have no laws on minimum age for riders), snowmobiles, personal water craft vehicles, in-line skates, trampolines, scooters, and motor vehicles. Activities involving such vehicles and equipment, although safe in and of themselves when conducted according to safety guidelines (of the manufacturer), may be dangerous for children and adolescents who are unable to appreciate the risks involved, not only to self, but to others as well. Adolescents are known for taking risks, and the approval of their peers often compounds risk-taking behaviors in games such as car surfing and the choking game. Parents may not be aware that their teens are partaking in such games and a frank discussion between parents and adolescents may be required. Nurses who work with adolescents and their families need to be aware of such games and be ready to discuss the effects of risk taking with teens.

*SafeKids Worldwide is an excellent resource for those interested in child safety; http://www.safekids.org.

EMERGENCY TREATMENT

Trauma

Before entering trauma area, observe for potential threats or dangers to rescuers and bystanders. Be aware of potential for further injuries to child.

Observe scene for signs and mechanism of injury (e.g., head-on motor vehicle injury), which helps determine proper course of action for treating child's injuries.

Do not move child before arrival of emergency medical services (EMS) personnel unless child is in danger of further injury. If it is necessary to move child, follow appropriate steps to prevent further injury (e.g., stabilize cervical spine to avoid exacerbation of spinal injury during movement).

Primary Assessment and Intervention

Assess level of consciousness. Use the AVPU method:

A—Child is **a**lert.
V—Child responds to **v**erbal stimulus.
P—Child responds to **p**ainful stimulus.
U—Child is **u**nresponsive to any stimulus.

Open airway, using appropriate method:

- In child with head, trunk, or multisystem trauma, modified jaw thrust is preferred method.
- At this point, cervical spine should be manually immobilized and held in alignment with rest of spinal column and should not be released until EMS personnel have immobilized child with appropriate equipment.

Activate the EMS system if child appears to be pubertal or older or if witnessed sudden collapse. If child has not reached puberty, perform 2 minutes of cardiopulmonary resuscitation (CPR) (as per assessment); then activate EMS and call for an automatic external defibrillator (AED).

If no response to stimulation and no pulse is detected, begin chest compressions. Compress at a rate of at least 100 compressions per minute.*

After 30 compressions administer 2 breaths—each breath is administered over 1 second. Avoid overventilating.*

Continue chest compressions and ventilations until person shows signs of responsiveness, breathing, or EMS arrives.

If an AED is available turn on the AED and follow the AED directions. Avoid interrupting chest compressions for more than 10 seconds.*

A pulse check may be made if 5 cycles of 30 compressions and 2 breaths have been administered.*

- Palpate carotid artery in children 1 year or older.
- Palpate brachial artery in infants younger than 1 year.

If pulse present, assess for breathing. If necessary, begin rescue breathing.*

Observe for hemorrhage. Control bleeding with a gloved or protected hand:

1. Apply direct pressure to wound site.
2. Elevate wound site.
3. Apply pressure to appropriate arterial pressure point.
4. Apply tourniquet only as a last resort. Once a tourniquet is applied, it should not be loosened.

Assess for further injury.

Do not remove objects protruding from child's body.

Check for evidence of decreased motor or sensory function in extremities:

- Infant and young child—Observe spontaneous movement in extremities.
- Older child—Ask if able to wiggle extremities.

Evaluate pain—Present, absent; severe, mild.

- Attempt to alleviate with nonpharmacologic techniques.
- Encourage use of analgesics when EMS personnel arrive.

Assess pulses in extremity distal to injury.

- Check color and temperature of extremities.

Manage any injuries appropriately (e.g., splint fractures) (see Emergency Treatment box, p. 1264).

Maintain body heat.

Identify child.

Obtain information regarding the injury from witnesses, if any.

*For detailed instructions for performing CPR, see Atkins, Berger, Duff, et al. (2015).

ASSESSMENT OF TRAUMA

The site of the injury usually influences the order of priority of interventions when emergency care is being instituted. Consider the safety of both the victim and the "Good Samaritan" rescuers to prevent further injury.

NURSING ALERT

Always consider personal safety a top priority because the victim cannot be helped if the rescuer is injured.

For example, removing a child from a burning building or the bottom of a swimming pool is an obvious, logical action, but anxious rescuers may not consider their own safety to be of prime importance. The major reason for thinking through the steps to be taken in an emergency before an incident actually occurs is to have preplanned actions available at a stimulus response level.

Emergency Management

The Emergency Treatment box outlines guidelines for care of the child at the scene of an injury. After level of consciousness is assessed, the concerns are for airway, breathing, and circulation (ABC), after which other injuries are managed as indicated by the assessment. When spinal trauma is a possibility, open the airway using the modified jaw thrust maneuver, which is accomplished by grasping the angles of the victim's lower jaw and lifting with both hands, one on each side, and displacing the mandible upward and outward (without head tilt or chin lift). Otherwise a head tilt–chin lift maneuver is effective in opening the victim's airway.

Spinal cord injury is always suspected in a patient with head, trunk, or multisystem trauma. Only in a fully equipped trauma center with radiography and other diagnostic testing such as computed tomography (CT) or magnetic resonance imaging (MRI) can spinal cord injury be ruled out or diagnosed. Therefore the patient is treated as if injury were present. Immobilize the cervical spine by maintaining the head in a neutral position and not allowing movement of the head or body in any direction.

Assess the child for signs of responsiveness, and if there are none detected, check for a pulse. If unresponsive, call for help and emergency medical services (EMS) activation. Begin chest compressions within 10

NURSING ALERT

In any situation in which spinal cord injury is suspected or is a possibility, the child should be calmed, reassured, and told not to move. *No one should be allowed to move the child unless the entire spine is stabilized.* A rigid cervical collar is used to immobilize the cervical spine, and the child is placed supine on a rigid immobilization board. Infants and small children are removed from a vehicle in their car seats; no attempt should be made to take them out of their seats unless medically necessary.

seconds and compress at a rate of 100 times per minute. If the child is not breathing, give two breaths over 2 seconds, then resume chest compressions. Oxygen should be provided when possible. If an automatic external defibrillator (AED) is available, follow the directions for its use after first turning on the apparatus. (Follow the complete detailed guidelines for cardiopulmonary resuscitation [CPR] available from the American Heart Association [Atkins, Berger, Duff, et al., 2015].)

Control of bleeding is first attempted by application of direct pressure with a gloved hand. If this does not work, a pressure dressing is applied. The next step is to elevate the body part and then attempt to control hemorrhage by pressing on arterial pressure points. A tourniquet is used only when the bleeding cannot be controlled with a pressure dressing. If used, the tourniquet should be applied only to control bleeding. Once applied, it should not be removed or loosened. Below the tourniquet site, skin and tissue necrosis begins. If the tourniquet is loosened or removed, the toxins can be released into the circulation in high concentrations and may induce a systemic, deadly tourniquet shock. With the tourniquet in place, the patient has a better chance of survival, even though it may mean the loss of a limb. Tourniquet use in prehospital settings has been shown to be safe (Fitzgibbons, Digiovanni, Hares, et al., 2012; Lee, Porter, & Hodgetts, 2007).

Assessment of the child involves observation from head to toe because infants and young children are unable to communicate except by crying and other behaviors. Therefore pinpointing areas of pain is difficult. To check for any motor or sensory dysfunction in the extremities, the nurse should note any spontaneous movement, which provides the best clue in infants and young children. Older children are able to follow directions to wiggle toes or fingers, demonstrate a grasp, "push down on the gas pedal," or lift legs off the floor or stretcher. The child is identified as soon as feasible by anyone who knows the child. It is important to determine whether the child has any existing health problems that might have implications for the circumstances of the injury and for therapeutic management. Ask any witnesses for details about the incident to aid in assessment of the child's emotional responses.

In the prehospital setting, the nurse's role consists of contacting EMS and providing basic life support until EMS personnel arrive on the scene. The nurse's role is limited to basic life support because the nurse has no standing orders or protocols under which to work in the prehospital setting (see Emergency Treatment box). Call EMS as soon as possible so that the patient can receive advanced life support before and during transport. A pediatric trauma triage system with personnel designated to care for an injured child is essential to provide excellent trauma patient care.

A paramedic-level ambulance provides at least one paramedic with skills in advanced cardiac life support, pediatric advanced life support, and neonatal resuscitation. A paramedic's skills include electrocardiogram interpretation and defibrillation, advanced airway management (including endotracheal intubation, as well as intravenous [IV] and pharmacologic therapy), placement of a pneumatic antishock garment, pleural decompression (with a chest tube), and placement of a nasogastric tube and Foley catheter. Other advanced life support skills include expertise in spinal immobilization, extrication, management of fractures and bleeding, and emergency scene management. The paramedic remains in constant contact with the emergency department physician by means of a radio or cellular telephone for situations requiring medical control. Attempting to transport a child by automobile wastes valuable time in obtaining help. Transportation by EMS is recommended. Services in most large communities can institute advanced life support immediately or en route to a medical facility.

! NURSING ALERT

It is imperative that EMS be called to respond as soon as possible. Family, friends, or strangers should *not* transport the trauma victim.

Systematic Assessment

Several factors can affect a child's response to trauma. An undetected congenital anomaly can contribute to a complicated injury. Acute gastric distention occurs frequently in children because of the crying and screaming that accompany an injury. The temperature of young children is unstable because of their large surface area in relation to body mass, and temperature maintenance is critical in trauma management. Children also experience rapid metabolic changes. When they are ill, children are really ill, but as they recover, they change very rapidly. In addition, children have a small volume of blood in absolute terms. Whereas blood volume is 60% of total body weight in the adult, it is 70% to 85% in the child.

The first priority on admission to an emergency facility is rapid assessment of ABC status. Because the overwhelming majority of childhood injuries are the result of blunt-impact trauma, multiple organ involvement is a common finding. Therefore it is essential to perform a systematic assessment of the trauma victim.

The secondary survey is a systematic head-to-toe search for any additional injuries not originally addressed in the primary survey. However, children are often an exception to the head-to-toe approach. It may be preferable to complete the secondary survey on the injured child in a toe-to-head direction. This approach may allow the rescuer to gain the child's trust as the survey progresses and the rescuer moves gradually into the child's personal space. Throughout the assessment, the nurse observes for areas of deformity, edema, ecchymosis, bleeding, hematoma, paralysis, or pain.

THE IMMOBILIZED CHILD

IMMOBILIZATION

One of the most difficult aspects of illness is the immobility it often imposes on a child. Children's natural tendency to be mobile influences all elements of growth and development—physical, social, psychologic, and emotional. Impaired physical mobility related to disability or imposed activity restrictions presents a definite challenge to children, their families, and their caregivers.

Causes of Immobilization

For some children immobilization may be due to a disability. For those children without disabilities, illness or injury is the usual reason for immobilization or restriction of activities. When children are ill, they are content to remain quiet, and most of them instinctively reduce their activity. It is children who are forced to remain inactive because of physical limitations or therapy who display the multiple effects of restricted movement.

The most frequent reasons for immobility are congenital defects (e.g., spina bifida); neuromuscular conditions (e.g., cerebral palsy, muscular dystrophy, spinal muscular atrophy); the need for prolonged mechanical ventilation and sedation; and infections or injuries that impair the integumentary system (e.g., severe burns), the musculoskeletal system (e.g., complex fractures or osteomyelitis), or the neurologic system (e.g., spinal cord injury, Guillain-Barré syndrome, or traumatic brain injury and coma). Sometimes therapies such as traction or surgery are responsible for prolonged immobilization, although the trend is toward early mobilization, early discharge, and outpatient care.

Physiologic Effects of Immobilization

Many clinical studies, including space program research, have documented predictable consequences that occur after immobilization and the absence of gravitational force. Functional and metabolic responses to restricted movement occur in most of the body systems. Each has a direct influence on the child's growth and development because homeostatic mechanisms thrive on normal use and need feedback to maintain dynamic equilibrium.

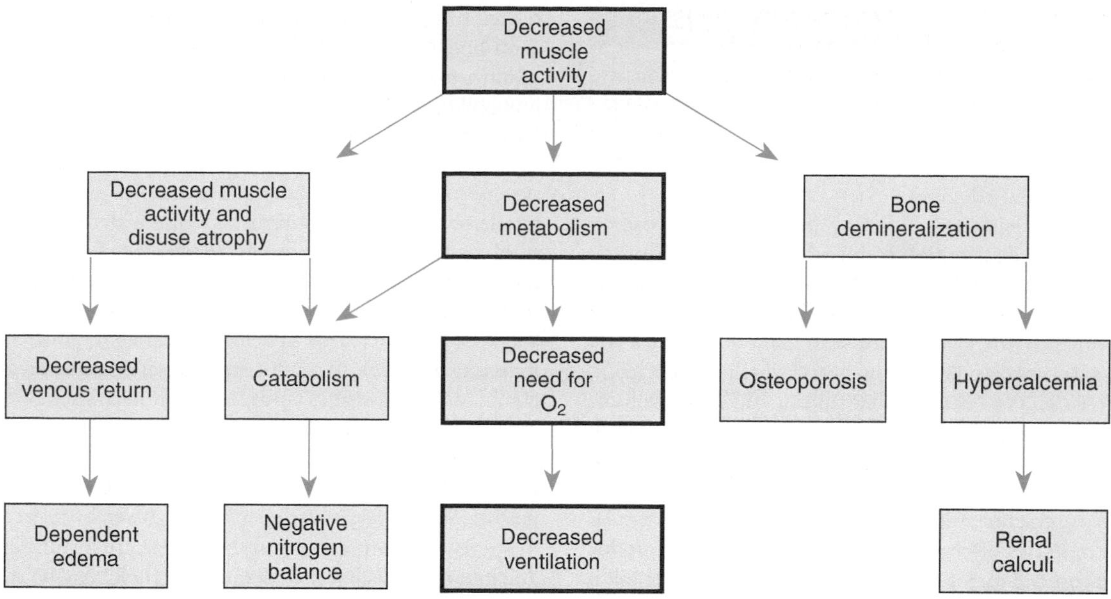

FIG. 33.1 Physiologic effects of immobilization.

Inactivity leads to a decrease in the functional capabilities of the whole body as dramatically as the lack of physical exercise leads to muscle weakness.

Immobilization from illness, injury, or a sedentary lifestyle can limit function and potentially delay a child from meeting age-appropriate milestones. Most of the pathologic changes that take place during immobilization arise from decreased muscle strength and mass, decreased metabolism, and bone demineralization. The three are closely interrelated, with one change leading to or affecting another. Some results of immobilization are primary and produce a direct effect; other pathophysiologic consequences occur frequently but seem to be more indirect and are therefore secondary effects. Many pathophysiologic changes affect more than one body system, with the primary or secondary effect being demonstrated in multiple systems.

The major effects of immobilization (Fig. 33.1) are related directly or indirectly to decreased muscle activity, which produces numerous primary changes in both muscular and bone structures, along with secondary alterations in the cardiovascular, respiratory, metabolic, and renal systems. The major consequences are as follows:

- Significant loss of muscle strength, endurance, and muscle mass (atrophy)
- Bone demineralization leading to osteoporosis
- Loss of joint mobility and contracture

The larger the portion of the body immobilized and the longer the immobilization, the greater the hazards of immobility.

Muscular System. Inactive muscle loses strength at the rate of 3% per day, and several weeks or months are sometimes required for function to be regained when there is no primary neuromuscular deficit. Stretching can occur as muscle loses its tone or as excessive strain is put on weakened muscle (e.g., stretching by tight bed covers or poor body position that produces footdrop as experienced by some children with disability). The disuse leads to tissue breakdown and muscle atrophy. The chief intracellular muscle enzyme, creatine, is released into the serum as the muscle atrophies; therefore serum levels provide an indication of the amount of muscle mass undergoing degeneration. Muscle inactivity also affects the cardiovascular system by decreasing venous return and cardiac output. In general, muscle atrophy causes decreased strength and endurance.

In children who have limited mobility, such as children who are unconscious or partially or fully paralyzed, joint mobility becomes restricted. In the absence of normal structural stretching, collagen fibers generated within the joint become fibrotic and further limit movement. This tissue fibrosis creates shortening of the muscles and contracture of the joint. Any decrease in circulation to the joint caused by edema, inflammation, or restrictive positioning contributes to further fibrotic changes. The problem rapidly becomes cyclic as the contracture leads to muscle fatigue and pain, which causes the child to protect the site, thus leading to more fibrosis. This process is further exaggerated because body flexor muscles are stronger than extensor muscles, and unless range of motion is reestablished within 3 to 7 days, contractures will develop. Passive or active range-of-motion exercises and proper positioning can help prevent joint stiffness and contractures. Frequent disabling contractures are hip flexion, knee flexion, plantar flexion of the feet, and shoulder stiffness.

Skeletal System. The daily stresses on bone created by motion and weight bearing maintain the balance between bone formation (osteoblastic activity) and bone resorption (osteoclastic activity). When these stresses are diminished, bone formation ceases while bone destruction continues leading to a disruption in the state of equilibrium. Bone calcium becomes severely depleted, and secretion of phosphorus and nitrogen is increased. This demineralization of the bone (osteopenia) makes the skeletal structures prone to pathologic fractures and increases calcium ion concentration in the blood (hypercalcemia).

Cardiovascular System. Immobility has three major cardiovascular consequences: orthostatic intolerance, increased workload of the heart, and thrombus formation. During movement, muscle contraction causes pressure on peripheral veins, which in turn causes the venous valves to close and thus assists in return of the blood to the heart when the individual is in an upright position. In the absence of this assistance, blood tends to pool in the dependent areas, reducing the blood supply to the trunk and brain. In addition, direct reflex stimulation to the splanchnic and peripheral vessels causes them to constrict when a person is upright. Impairment of this neurovascular orthostatic reflex activity from lack of motion causes further interference with venous return. The individual displays signs of excessive autonomic activity (e.g., pallor, sweating, and restlessness, which are frequently followed by fainting). The child with a spinal cord injury has unique problems with orthostatic intolerance, which is discussed in Chapter 34

> **! NURSING ALERT**
>
> Carefully evaluate sudden chest pain and dyspnea; sudden onset of shortness of breath; air hunger; or pain and swelling in the lower extremities, which sometimes indicates deep vein thrombosis.

Changes in vascular resistance caused by the horizontal position and immobility alter the distribution of blood within the body. The reduction in gravity pressure to the extremities causes much of the total blood volume to be redistributed from lower extremities to other parts of the body. Consequently, there is an increase in the venous return and the volume of blood to be handled by the heart, which is reflected in elevated blood pressure. As a result, cardiac output and stroke volume are increased, and a progressive increase in heart rate occurs. When immobilization extends over time, there is a compensatory decrease in blood volume and a decrease in heart rate and blood pressure.

Without muscle contraction, venous stasis and increased intravascular pressure in the extremities often lead to dependent edema. If undue pressure is exerted on the major veins by positioning or mechanical devices, the likelihood of interstitial edema is increased. Edematous tissue, especially tissue located over an area that receives much of the body's weight, is prone to skin breakdown.

Circulatory stasis combined with hypercoagulability of the blood, which results from factors such as damage to the endothelium of blood vessels (Virchow triad), can lead to thrombus and embolus formation. **Deep vein thrombosis** (DVT) involves the formation of a thrombus in a deep vein such as the iliac and femoral veins and can cause significant morbidity if it remains undetected and untreated. DVT may develop with prolonged venous stasis in conditions such as obesity, chronic heart failure, prolonged surgical procedure, long trips without exercise, or prolonged immobilization.

The state of deconditioned cardiac function, caused by skeletal muscle inactivity, can produce a variety of secondary problems in other systems. However, the major clinical manifestation is increased pulse and heart rate in response to an active exercise program. After prolonged immobility, the child should build up activity tolerance slowly to allow the heart to regain optimum capabilities.

Respiratory System. Initially the effects of immobilization are compensatory or adaptive. The basal metabolic rate is decreased because with reduced expenditure of energy the cells require less oxygen and produce less carbon dioxide. Lessened demand for oxygen–carbon dioxide exchange causes the respirations to become slower and more shallow. In children, chest expansion may be limited by the child's position (e.g., supine), abdominal distention caused by accumulation of feces, gas, or fluid, and by mechanical restriction such as from a brace or constricting binder. Pain (e.g., chest tube in place) may also limit deep breathing and adequate chest expansion. More effort is required to expand the lungs in the supine position. Reduced muscle power and coordination secondary to altered innervation can also hinder respiratory movement.

Prolonged immobility also reduces the normal movement of secretions from the tracheobronchial tree, particularly in the presence of impaired muscle function and without positional changes that normally facilitate removal of secretions. A weak and ineffectual cough reflex contributes to stasis of secretions and the possibility of airway obstruction in the smaller airways of children. Shallow respirations and obstruction of the airway with thick mucus are factors in the development of secondary complications such as atelectasis and pneumonia.

Gastrointestinal System. Prolonged immobility produces a state of negative nitrogen balance resulting from the increased catabolic activity related to muscle atrophy. This and the reduced energy requirements contribute to a diminished appetite and a resulting decrease in ingestion of nutrients (anorexia). Eating and feeding become more difficult with immobility, and the risk of aspiration is increased. Associated psychologic factors further influence intake.

The process of elimination depends on the integration of smooth and skeletal muscle activity and on visceral reflex patterns. Immobility may interfere with these mechanisms, as well as with the gravitational effect on stool passing through the intestines. Slowing of stool in the colon causes the feces to become hard (**fecal impaction**), and the bowel wall is not stimulated to further its peristaltic movement down the tract to the rectum. Weakened muscles used in defecation (diaphragmatic and abdominal muscles) are unable to produce the intraabdominal pressure needed for elimination. Sometimes embarrassment in using a bedpan or bedside commode may be the cause of not responding to the urge to defecate.

Renal System. The urinary system is designed to function in an upright posture. When the gravitational force is altered by the reclining position, the peristaltic contractions of the ureters are insufficient to overcome gravitational resistance. Consequently, there may be stasis of urine in the renal pelves, and any particulate matter that settles in the calyces may serve as nuclei for calculi formation or as foci for infection.

In the horizontal position the individual has difficulty relaxing the perineal musculature and external sphincter sufficiently to initiate the integrated reflex micturition mechanism, which involves the external sphincter, the internal sphincter, and the detrusor muscle of the bladder wall. If adequate intraabdominal pressure is exerted, voiding can occur, but if the individual does not respond to the sensation to void, bladder distention leads to stasis, and its complications add to embarrassing overflow incontinence. In time, reflux and back pressure may impair renal function, and urinary tract infection is always a hazard with urine retention.

Normally the kidney is able to handle the increased metabolites from protein breakdown and bone demineralization. However, the increased level of calcium excreted may predispose the person to calculus formation. Formation of **renal calculi** (kidney stones) is further favored by urinary stasis, infection, and alkaline urine caused by the decreased production of the acid by-products of metabolism. Hematuria may be the only clue to the condition.

Metabolism. Immobility or severe restriction of activity is often accompanied by decreased or inappropriate nutritional intake, which frequently leads to a decreased basal metabolic rate, a negative nitrogen balance associated with catabolism, and a high serum calcium level.

All body systems are influenced by a decrease in metabolism. The altered energy level leads to further fatigue and lack of motivation for moving. Immobilized persons often feel sluggish and have a poor appetite, particularly for protein foods. The protein breakdown in the body related to a loss of muscle and other tissues is more apt to be severe after injury or surgery. Protein breakdown produces nitrogenous wastes, and on the fifth or sixth day of catabolic protein metabolism, an increase in urinary nitrogen level develops that contributes to anemia and delayed healing.

Another metabolic problem is **hypercalcemia** associated with bone catabolism. Completely immobilized children or adolescents are especially prone to hypercalcemia. Symptoms, which include nausea and vomiting, polydipsia, polyuria, and lethargy, usually appear 4 to 8 weeks after immobilization. In quadriplegia, symptoms may occur within 10 days and last for as long as 6 months. The accelerated rate of bone metabolism in children makes the bone demineralization a greater hazard. Larger amounts of calcium are released into the blood than the kidney can excrete, and calcium continues to accumulate in serum. High levels of serum calcium decrease neuronal permeability, which can lead to a depression of the central and peripheral nervous systems. Symptoms, including smooth and skeletal muscle fatigue, diminished reflexes, and

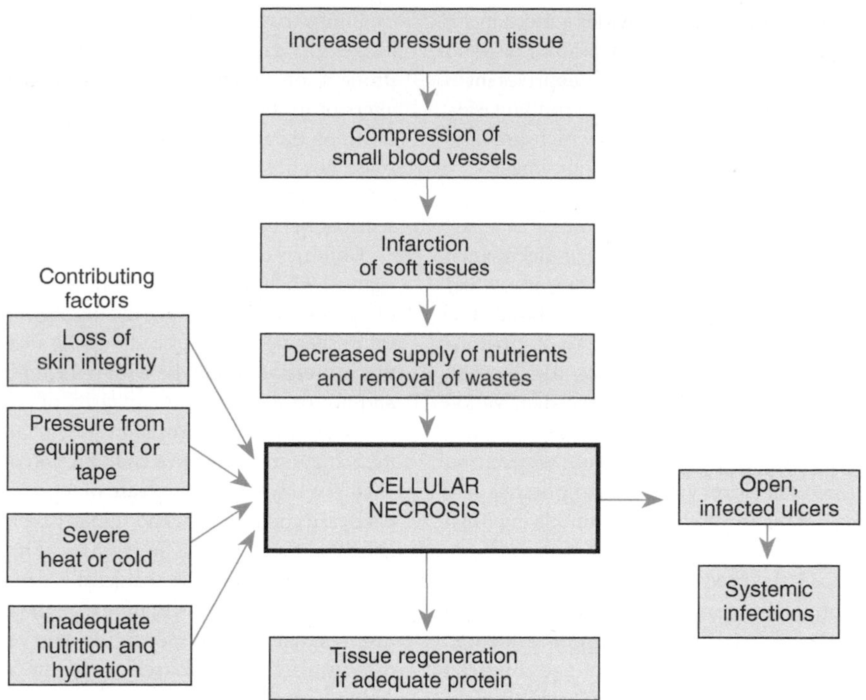

FIG. 33.2 Sequence of events in tissue breakdown.

atony of the gastrointestinal tract, are a result of the depressed nervous system.

A child with bone demineralization may not develop hypercalcemia, but the excess amount of calcium that the kidneys are required to excrete may produce a negative calcium balance, with more calcium than citric acid lost in the urine. This imbalance causes the urine to become alkaline, with the potential danger of renal calculi, especially if there is an accompanying retention of urine.

Integumentary System. The following factors play a major role in skin breakdown: moisture, friction, shear, and pressure (see also Chapter 22, Maintaining Healthy Skin). Circulation to the skin is reduced during inactivity and may be further impeded by dependent edema. Circulation is especially compromised in places where the bone surface is near the skin, such as areas over the sacrum, occiput, trochanter, and heel, and continued impairment causes rapid necrosis with ulcer formation. Friction and mechanical irritation from appliances, such as straps, rods, and tubing, and the friction of bedclothes during turning or other movement can produce skin breakdown. Healing capacity is also impaired by poor circulation, negative nitrogen balance, and anemia. Immobilization often makes it difficult to carry out adequate cleansing and hygienic measures, which may also contribute to tissue breakdown in areas that are difficult to reach.

Cellular breakdown caused by prolonged pressure has several characteristics. Normally when pressure is applied to the skin, the skin appears pale but becomes very red, or hyperemic, after the pressure is removed. This reactive hyperemia should disappear within 5 to 15 minutes. Prolonged redness (>30 minutes) indicates that a pressure area is developing and treatment should begin. Other manifestations of tissue ischemia include an increase in temperature in the area, blistering, swelling, and dark purple or black areas. The pressure area may be limited to the skin and subcutaneous layers or may be deeper and more extensive. The skin changes observed may represent the top of a cone-shaped area with widespread tissue destruction, beneath which tissue rapidly ulcerates and creates a large pressure ulcer that sometimes extends to the bone. Fig. 33.2 illustrates the sequence of events in tissue breakdown.

Neurosensory System. Studies indicate that immobilization does not produce neurosensory consequences directly; however, two occurrences—loss of innervation and sensory and perceptual deprivation—are common.

Peripheral nerves, in contrast to skeletal muscles, do not degenerate with disuse, but loss of innervation takes place if nerves are damaged by pressure or if their blood supply is disrupted. Improper body positioning, improperly applied casts or restraints, or fluid buildup within a compartment (compartment syndrome) can place excessive pressure on nerves and blood vessels that can lead to ischemia and nerve degeneration. Frequent sites of nerve compression phenomenon are the peroneal nerve, where pressure results in footdrop, and the radial nerve, where pressure leads to wristdrop. These complications significantly interfere with attempts to regain functional use of the extremities, but they can be prevented by conscientious nursing assessment and intervention. Preventing pressure on vulnerable areas and avoiding extreme positions of flexion and extension that apply inappropriate pressure on nerves and blood vessels reduce the likelihood of compression injury. Periodic plantarflexion and dorsiflexion of the feet and hands by passive or active range of motion will stimulate circulation and keep nerves from becoming pinched. Numbness, tingling, change in sensation, and loss of motion are symptoms of neurologic impairment and should be evaluated immediately.

Psychologic Effects of Immobilization

For children, one of the most difficult aspects of illness is immobilization. Throughout childhood, physical activity is an integral part of daily life and is essential for physical growth and development. It also serves children as an instrument for communication and expression and as a means for learning about and understanding their world. Activity helps them deal with a variety of feelings and impulses and provides a mechanism by which they can exert control over inner tensions. Children respond to anxiety with increased activity. Removal of this power deprives them of necessary input and a natural outlet for their feelings and fantasies. Through movement children also gain sensory input, which provides an essential element for developing and maintaining body image.

Active children have many opportunities for input from a wide variety of settings. When they are immobilized by disease or as a part of a treatment regimen, they experience diminished environmental stimuli with a loss of tactile, vestibular, and proprioceptive input and an altered perception of themselves and their environment. Sudden or gradual immobilization narrows the amount and variety of environmental stimuli they receive by means of all their senses: touch, sight, hearing, taste, smell, and proprioception. This sensory deprivation frequently leads to feelings of isolation, boredom, and being forgotten, especially by peers. Nursing interventions involving the use of diversion activities, schoolwork, structured television viewing, computer games, or interactive video programs can assist the child in maintaining usual activities.

The struggle for independence is thwarted by imposed immobility. For toddlers, exploration and imitative behaviors are essential to developing a sense of autonomy; preschooler's expression of initiative is evidenced by their penchant for vigorous physical activity; school-age children's development is strongly influenced by physical achievement and competition; and adolescents rely on mobility to achieve independence. The quest for mastery at every stage of development is related to mobility. To children, the inability to move is threatening to self-preservation and reactivates the struggle between activity and passivity, and between dependence and independence.

Behavioral changes occur when children experience prolonged sensory deprivation. Some of these behaviors are indications of a higher-than-normal level of anxiety (Box 33.1). Children are likely to become depressed over their loss of ability to function or the marked changes in body image. Significant others often notice regressive behavior and a greater reliance on them for tasks the children are able to perform. Children seek attention by reverting to earlier developmental behaviors, such as wanting to be fed, bed-wetting, and baby talk. In many ways, immobilized children are realistically dependent on others; therefore intelligent and sensitive care is required to prevent major developmental regressions during the period of immobility.

BOX 33.1 Behavioral Changes in Immobilized Children

Higher-than-normal level of anxiety leads to the following:
- Restlessness
- Difficulty with problem solving
- Inability to concentrate on activities
- Depression
- Regression
- Egocentrism

Monotony leads to the following:
- Sluggish intellectual responses
- Sluggish psychomotor responses
- Decreased communication skills
- Increased fantasizing
- Hallucinations
- Disorientation
- Dependence
- Acting-out behavior
- Depression

Limbs that are immobilized by casts, traction, or paralysis transmit less sensory data than typical. Sensory impairment may be a concomitant problem of the involved part. Numbness or loss of feeling markedly alters proprioception. Children who have limited ability to feel others touching them not only experience less tactile stimulation in a physical sense but are also deprived of warm, loving feelings that arise from being touched. The loss of feeling from touch can further add to their sense of being isolated and unwanted.

Children often react to immobility with active protest, anger, and aggressive behavior, or they may become quiet, passive, and submissive. Often children believe that the immobilization is a justified punishment for misbehavior. Children should be allowed to express their anger, but this expression should be within the limits of safety to their self-esteem and not damaging to the integrity of others.

Adults may be confused by, resent, and find it difficult to deal with the acting-out behavior of children. Too often this behavior is considered "bad" even when it is a release of tension. In some cases, such as with a paralyzed child, parents and nurses may feel inadequate to cope with the child's profound distress and feelings of hopelessness, and the professional help of a mental health specialist is necessary.

The most difficult situations are those involving major injuries and diseases that produce a disfigurement or a severe loss of function that directly affects a child's self-image, such as burns, amputation, or the sudden, catastrophic effects of an accident that leave a healthy, active child disabled. Children have difficulty expressing feelings of anger and hostility when they are at the mercy of the environment. They dare not speak out against or defy authority figures on which they depend so completely. Consequently, their aggression may be masked by cheerfulness or rigidity. When they are unable to express their anger, the aggression is often displayed inappropriately through regressive behavior and outbursts of crying or temper tantrums over insignificant irritations. Adolescents and older school-age children should vary their daily routine to fit their needs for independence; allowing this age-group to stay up late at night and sleep in during the daytime (within reasonable limits to accommodate treatment needs) may help decrease struggles over other inconsequential matters and at the same time allow a daily pattern of life. Encourage parents to continue setting limits and not abandon disciplinary measures with children who are confined to bed due to trauma or illness.

Effects of Immobilization on Families

Even brief periods of child immobilization may disrupt the functioning of a family, and a child's catastrophic illness or disability may severely tax their resources and coping abilities. The need for instruction concerning medical and nursing care, community resources to contact, and emotional support are paramount. Many families have unmet needs, operate from crisis to crisis, and are unable to use outside help appropriately. For these families, the new situation can be disruptive; therefore a multidisciplinary team must help the family members identify unmet needs and solve problems. The following are commonly occurring problems:

- Financial strains may decrease or totally eliminate the family's resources.
- Attention is focused, at least temporarily, on the affected member; therefore other members of the family, especially siblings, may feel that they are being neglected or that their needs may not be met.
- The family may have difficulty accepting the child's altered body condition.
- Individual family members may be unable to express their feelings and may have difficulty coping with the crisis.
- Parents often experience guilt over their child's condition and need for immobilization. Their perception of failing to protect the child forms the basis for their difficulty coping.

The family's needs often must be met through the services of a multidisciplinary team, and nurses play a key role in anticipating the services the family will need and coordinating appropriate care. In preparation for the child's discharge from the hospital, home management is frequently planned weeks in advance of the actual discharge, including special provisions for meeting cultural, economic, physical, and psychologic needs. A child with a severe disability is dependent, and caregivers need rest periods to revitalize themselves. Individual and group counseling is beneficial for problem-solving situations and provides an emotional support system. Parent groups are also helpful and often allow nonthreatening social contact. The families of children with permanent disabilities need long-term resources because some of the most difficult problems arise as they try to sustain high-quality care for many years (see Chapter 19).

Nursing Care Management

Physical assessment of the child who is immobilized for any number of reasons (e.g., injury or illness) includes a focus not only on the injured part (e.g., fracture) but also on the functioning of other systems that may be affected secondarily: the circulatory, renal, respiratory, muscular, and gastrointestinal systems. With long-term immobilization, there may also be neurologic impairment and changes in metabolism. In addition, the psychologic impact of immobilization should be assessed.

Encourage children to be as active as their condition and restrictive devices allow. This usually poses few problems for children, whose innate ingenuity and natural inclination toward mobility provide them with the impetus for physical activity. They need the opportunity, the materials or objects to stimulate activity, and the encouragement and participation of others. Those who are unable to move will need passive exercise and movement, often in consultation with a physical therapist. An occupational therapist and child life specialist may also assist in planning activities to decrease boredom and to help regain lost skills such as self-feeding. A child psychologist may be consulted to discuss with the child and family issues such as depression, anger management, and the effects of the illness on family function.

Children who require prolonged total immobility and are unable to move themselves in bed should be placed on a pressure reduction mattress to prevent skin breakdown. Frequent position changes also help prevent dependent edema and stimulate circulation, respiratory function, gastrointestinal motility, and neurologic sensation. Children at higher risk for skin breakdown include those with prolonged immobilization, mechanical ventilation, orthotic and prosthetic devices, including wheelchairs and casts, and children requiring intensive care. Additional risk factors include poor nutrition, friction (from bed linen with traction), and moist skin (from urine or perspiration) (Fig. 33.3).

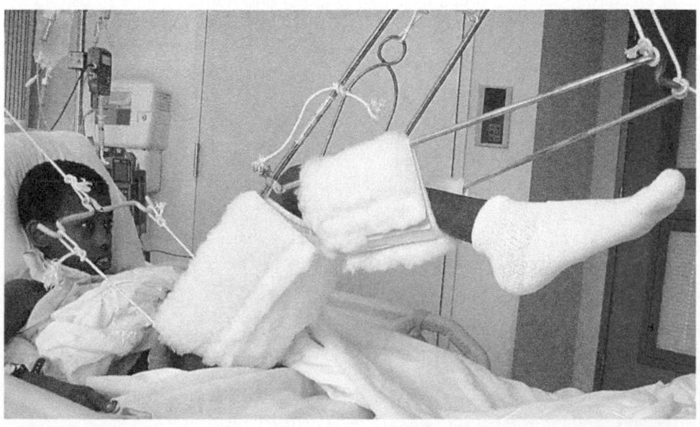

FIG. 33.3 Immobilized child.

Nursing care of children at risk includes proactive strategies for preventing skin breakdown when such conditions are present. The Braden Q Scale is a reliable, objective tool the nurse can use in assessing for pressure ulcer development in children who are acutely ill or who are at risk for skin breakdown from neurologic conditions and immobilization (Noonan, Quigley, & Curley, 2011).

Circulatory stasis and DVT development are prevented by instructing patients to change positions frequently, dorsiflex their feet and rotate the ankles, sit in a bedside chair periodically, or ambulate several times daily. The use of antiembolism stockings or intermittent compression devices also prevents circulatory stasis and dependent edema in the lower extremities and the development of DVT. Children who are unable to move should have passive range-of-motion exercises of the upper and lower extremities to increase circulation and minimize stasis. Anticoagulant therapy may also be implemented with low-molecular-weight heparin, vitamin K antagonists, or unfractionated heparin.

Transporting the child by stretcher, wheelchair, stroller, or wagon outside the confines of the room whenever possible increases environmental stimuli and provides social contact with others. While hospitalized, the child benefits from frequent visitors, accessibility of clocks and calendars, and a program of diversional therapy to help the child function more normally. A child life specialist should be consulted for recreational planning. An activity center or slanting tray can be helpful for the child with limited mobility to use for drawing, coloring, writing, and playing with small toys such as trucks and cars. A child is able to express frustration, displeasure, and anger through play, which is helpful in the child's recovery. As soon as possible, the child should wear street clothes and resume school and preinjury hobbies. Play is the most useful tool of nursing (see Chapter 22), and activities should be selected on the basis of interest, ability, and limitations. Activities should include some form of physical activity that encourages the use of uninvolved muscles and joints. Any activity that is tolerated (e.g., turning in bed or changing the position of the bed in the room) helps alter the monotony of immobilization and dissipates tension and frustration. Allow a parent and/or sibling to stay overnight and room-in with the hospitalized child to prevent the effects of family disruption from hospitalization. Make every effort to minimize family disruption resulting from the hospitalization. Although most of the suggestions discussed relate to hospital care, the same consultations (e.g., physical therapist, occupational therapist, child life specialist, speech/language pathologist, child psychologist) and environment may be considered in the home as well to help the child gain independence and the family to achieve normalization.

One of the most useful interventions to help children cope with immobility is participation in their own care. Self-care to the maximum extent possible is usually well received by children. They can help plan their daily routine, select their diet (when possible), and choose the clothes they are to wear, including innovative adornment, such as a baseball cap, brightly colored stockings, or other items that express their autonomy and individuality. Encourage them to do as much for themselves as they are able to keep muscles active and their interest alive. If feasible, they should be placed where they can benefit from the company of other children, which assures them that they are not being singled out for this medical treatment.

It is important for children to understand behavioral limitations or rules. Their questions should be answered. For example, children need to know the reasons for medical, nursing, occupational, and physical therapy and to know that some schedules are necessary. In some areas they have a choice; in others, they do not. Most of children's activities of daily living are play; therefore therapies that incorporate play are more apt to gain their cooperation.

Visits from significant persons, such as family members and friends from school or the neighborhood, offer occasions for emotional support and also provide opportunities for learning how to care for the child. If a traumatic incident caused the child's disability, guilt feelings may be displayed overtly or masked behind regressive or aggressive behavior. The feeling that "I must have been bad to receive this fate" is common, and honest feedback, such as "It just happened—it was an accident," needs repeating many times. Additional aspects of grieving are involved if there was a loss of another person or if permanent disability occurred as a result of the accident. All these feelings need to be brought out and dealt with by the child and family. Nurses working with the child or adolescent must not overprotect them but must help them cope with an altered body image and reestablish self-esteem.

For a child with greatly restricted movement (e.g., a child with quadriplegia or a child with a bilateral hip spica cast), creativity in nursing care is often required to keep the child stimulated and prevent the effects of immobilization. These situations may require long-term care in the hospital, in the rehabilitation center, or, increasingly, at home. Wherever the care occurs, consistent planning and coordination of activities with professionals and significant others is vital.

Nursing assessment includes gathering psychosocial data, in addition to assessing physical manifestations, because long-term immobilization has a profound effect on the child and the family. Nursing approaches are evaluated frequently and continued, discontinued, or modified to meet the changing problems and goals. Table 33.1 summarizes the physical effects of immobilization and appropriate nursing care management. With the increased trend toward early mobilization, early discharge, and home health care, many children are discharged home after a few days of hospitalization. Follow-up treatment may take place in the home or at an outpatient ambulatory facility.

THE CHILD IN A CAST

Children may be placed into a cast for different reasons, including treatment of a fracture or after a surgery to maintain alignment. In many situations, the joints above and below the site of injury are immobilized to eliminate the possibility of movement that might cause displacement at the site. Three major types of casts are used for immobilization: upper extremity to immobilize the wrist or elbow, lower extremity to immobilize the ankle or knee, and spica to immobilize the hip and knee (Fig. 33.4). Fig. 33.5 shows a full spica cast with a hip abduction, and Fig. 33.6 shows a single leg spica cast.

The Cast

Casts are constructed from gauze bandages impregnated with plaster of Paris or, more commonly, synthetic lighter-weight and water-resistant materials (e.g., waterproof liners, fiberglass and polyurethane resin). Both types of casting material produce heat from a chemical reaction activated

TABLE 33.1 Summary of Physical Effects of Immobilization With Nursing Interventions*

Primary Effects	Secondary Effects	Nursing Considerations
Muscular System		
Decreased muscle strength, tone, and endurance	Decreased venous return and decreased cardiac output	Use antiembolism stockings or intermittent compression devices to promote venous return (monitor circulatory and neurovascular status of extremities when such devices are used).
	Decreased metabolism and need for oxygen	Plan play activities to use uninvolved extremities.
	Decreased exercise tolerance	Place in upright posture when possible.
	Bone demineralization	Perform passive range-of-motion exercises.
Disuse atrophy and loss of muscle mass	Catabolism	Have patient perform range-of-motion, active, passive, and stretching exercises.
	Loss of strength	
Loss of joint mobility	Contractures, ankylosis of joints	Maintain correct body alignment.
		Use joint splints as indicated to prevent further deformity.
		Maintain range of motion.
Weak back muscles	Secondary spinal deformities	Maintain body alignment.
Weak abdominal muscles	Impaired respiration	See nursing considerations for respiratory system.
Skeletal System		
Bone demineralization—osteoporosis, hypercalcemia	Negative bone calcium uptake	With paralysis use upright posture on tilt table.
	Pathologic fractures	Handle extremities carefully when turning and positioning.
	Calcium deposits	Administer calcium-mobilizing drugs (diphosphonates) and normal saline infusions as ordered.
	Extraosseous bone formation, especially at hip, knee, elbow, and shoulder	Ensure adequate intake of fluid; monitor output.
	Renal calculi	Acidify urine.
		Promptly treat urinary tract infections.
Negative bone calcium uptake	Life-threatening electrolyte imbalance	Monitor serum calcium levels.
		Provide electrolyte replacement as indicated.
Metabolism		
Decreased metabolic rate	Slowing of all systems	Mobilize as soon as possible.
	Decreased food intake	Have patient perform active and passive resistance and deep-breathing exercises.
		Ensure adequate food intake.
		Provide a high-protein diet.
Negative nitrogen balance	Decline in nutritional state	Encourage small, frequent feedings with protein and preferred foods.
	Impaired healing	Monitor for and prevent pressure areas.

TABLE 33.1 Summary of Physical Effects of Immobilization With Nursing Interventions*—cont'd

Primary Effects	Secondary Effects	Nursing Considerations
Hypercalcemia	Electrolyte imbalance	See nursing consideration for skeletal system.
Decreased production of stress hormones	Decreased physical and emotional coping capacity	Identify causes of stress. Implement appropriate interventions to lower physical and psychosocial stresses.
Cardiovascular System		
Decreased efficiency of orthostatic neurovascular reflexes	Inability to adapt readily to upright position (orthostatic intolerance) Pooling of blood in extremities in upright posture	Monitor peripheral pulses and skin temperature changes. Use antiembolism stockings or intermittent compression devices to decrease pooling when upright.
Diminished vasopressor mechanism	Orthostatic intolerance with syncope, hypertension, decreased cerebral blood flow, tachycardia	Provide abdominal support. In severe cases use antigravitational pants. Position horizontally.
Altered distribution of blood volume	Increased cardiac workload Decreased exercise tolerance	Monitor hydration, blood pressure, and urinary output.
Venous stasis	Pulmonary emboli or thrombi	Encourage and assist with frequent position changes. Elevate extremities without knee flexion. Ensure adequate fluid intake. Have patient perform active or passive exercises or movement as needed. Prescribe routine wearing of antiembolism stockings or intermittent compression devices. Monitor for signs of pulmonary embolism—sudden dyspnea, chest pain, respiratory arrest. Promptly intervene to maintain adequate oxygenation if signs and symptoms of pulmonary emboli are noted. Measure circumference of extremities periodically. Give anticoagulant drugs as prescribed.
Dependent edema	Tissue breakdown and susceptibility to infection	Administer skin care. Turn every 2-4 hr. Monitor skin color, temperature, and integrity. Use pressure-reduction surface as necessary to prevent skin breakdown. (See Chapter 20.)
Respiratory System		
Decreased need for oxygen	Altered oxygen–carbon dioxide exchange and metabolism	Promote exercise as tolerated. Encourage deep-breathing exercises.
Decreased chest expansion and diminished vital capacity	Diminished oxygen intake Dyspnea and inadequate arterial oxygen saturation; acidosis	Position for optimum chest expansion. Semi-Fowler position may assist in lung expansion if patient can tolerate. Use prone positioning without pressure on abdomen to allow gravity to aid in diaphragmatic excursion. Ensure that patient maintains proper alignment when sitting to prevent pressure on respiratory mechanism.
Poor abdominal tone and distention	Interference with diaphragmatic excursion	Avoid restriction of chest and abdominal musculature. Supply torso support to promote chest expansion.
Mechanical or biochemical secretion retention	Hypostatic pneumonia Bacterial and viral pneumonia Atelectasis	Change position frequently. Use incentive spirometer. Monitor breath sounds. Encourage deep breathing exercises. Implement airway clearance techniques as necessary.
Loss of respiratory muscle strength	Poor cough	Encourage coughing and deep breathing. Support chest wall by splinting with pillow when patient coughs. Use incentive spirometer. Observe for signs of respiratory distress with pulse oximetry or blood gas measurement as necessary.
	Upper respiratory tract infection	Prevent contact with infected persons. Provide adequate hydration. Administer immunizations as necessary (pneumococcal, meningococcal).

Continued

TABLE 33.1 Summary of Physical Effects of Immobilization With Nursing Interventions*—cont'd

Primary Effects	Secondary Effects	Nursing Considerations
Gastrointestinal System		
Distention caused by poor abdominal muscle tone	Interference with respiratory movements	Monitor bowel sounds. Encourage small, frequent feedings.
	Difficulty in feeding in prone position	Have patient sit in upright position in bedside chair if possible.
No specific primary effect	Possible constipation caused by gravitational effect on feces through ascending colon or weakened smooth muscle tone	Carry out bowel training program with hydration, stool softeners, increased fiber intake, and mild laxatives if necessary.
	Anorexia	Stimulate appetite with favored foods.
Urinary System		
Alteration of gravitational force	Difficulty in voiding in prone position	Position as upright as possible to void.
Impaired ureteral peristalsis	Urinary retention in calyces and bladder infection Renal calculi	Hydrate to ensure adequate urinary output for age. Stimulate bladder emptying with warm running water as necessary. Catheterize only for severe urinary retention. Administer antibiotics as indicated.
Integumentary System		
Altered tissue integrity	Decreased circulation and pressure leading to tissue injury	Turn and reposition at least every 2-4 hours. Frequently inspect total skin surface. Eliminate mechanical factors causing pressure, friction, moisture, or irritation. Place on pressure-relief mattress.
	Difficulty with personal hygiene	Assess ability to perform self-care and assist with bathing, grooming, and toileting as needed. Encourage self-care to potential ability. Ensure adequate intake of protein, vitamins, and minerals.

*Individualize care according to child's needs; interventions may vary in different institutions.

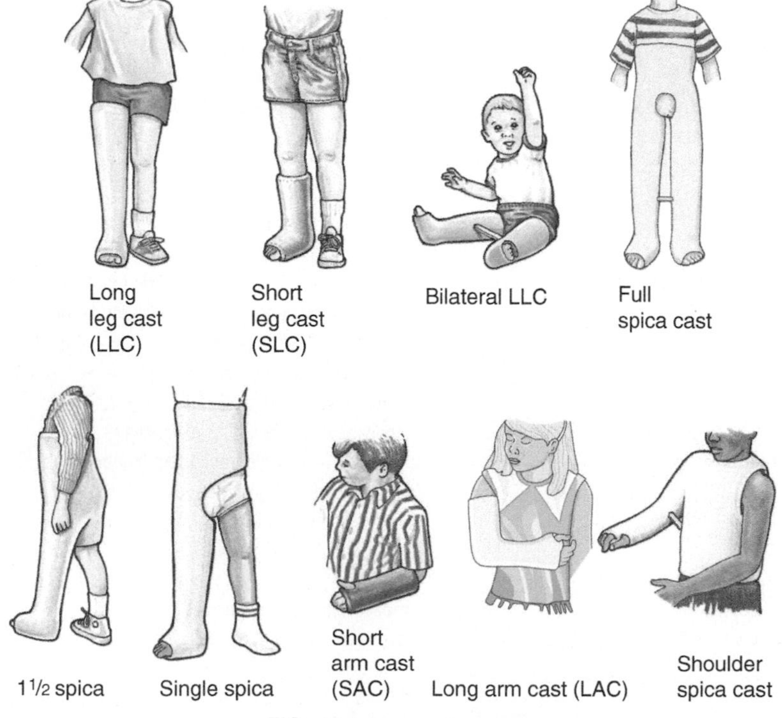

FIG. 33.4 Types of casts.

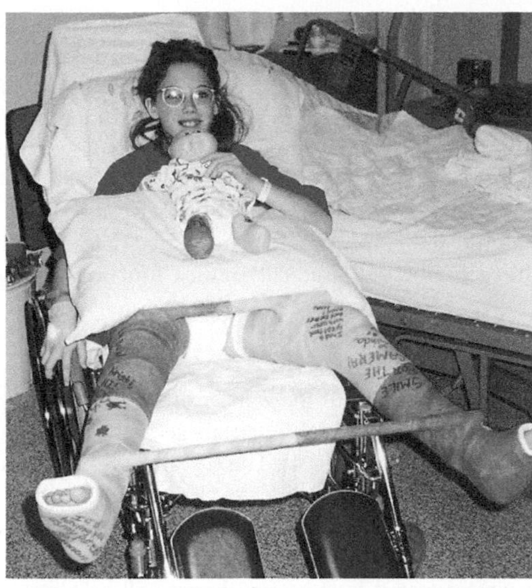

FIG. 33.5 Spica cast with hip abductor. Note casts on doll as well.

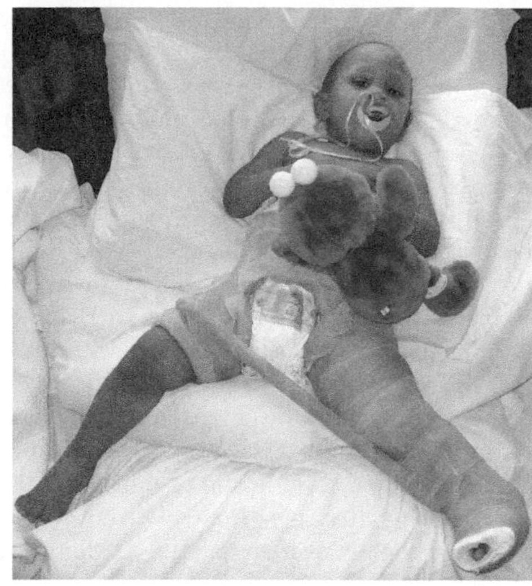

FIG. 33.6 Single spica cast. Note diaper to maintain dryness. (Courtesy Texas Children's Hospital, Houston.)

TABLE 33.2 Comparison of Plaster of Paris and Synthetic Casts

	Plaster of Paris	Synthetic
Composition and preparation	Cotton tape permeated with calcium sulfate crystals that interlock as tape dries (tepid water activated)	Polyester-cotton tape permeated with polyurethane resin (cool water activated) Knitted fiberglass tape with polyurethane resin (tepid water activated or photoactivated) Knitted thermoplastic polyester fabric (hot water activated)
Setting time	3-8 minutes	3-15 minutes
Drying time	10-72 hours (varies with cast size)	5-20 minutes (varies with type of cast) NOTE: The more rapid the drying time, the greater the likelihood of burning; therefore it is recommended to use tepid or cool water to slow drying time and decrease chemical heat produced; the warmer the water, the faster the material dries or hardens.
Indentations	Slow drying time increases possibility of indentations or alteration of intended fit	Rapid drying time reduces likelihood of indentations; allows rapid use (see previous statement under Drying time: synthetic)
Weight	Relatively heavy; bulky; makes it difficult to wear regular clothing	Lightweight; less bulky; permits regular clothing to be worn; allows for greater range of activity
Conformity	Molds readily to body part	Does not mold easily to some body parts such as fingers and toes; may be unsuitable for some fractures
Surface	Smooth exterior; does not snag clothing or scratch furniture	Smooth exterior
Cost	Relatively inexpensive; an advantage if cast changes anticipated	Inexpensive unless Gore-Tex added
Stability	Relatively stable; cast must be kept dry	Some cast material may tolerate being wet or immersed in water with permission from provider *(only those with use of nonabsorbent synthetic lining)*; can be cleaned with small amount of mild soap and water, dried with towel followed by blow dryer on cool or warm setting; takes considerable time to dry if immersed
Miscellaneous	Child may feel uncomfortable warming or burning sensation under cast while it dries (chemical reaction) Skin under cast may become irritated Cast must be protected when around water (bathing)	Child may feel uncomfortable warming or burning sensation under cast while it dries (chemical reaction) but this lasts only a few minutes (see Drying time) Skin under cast may become macerated from inadequate drying after water immersion

by water immediately after application. The lightweight casts are used more often for casting in children and are available in a variety of colors. Plaster casts are usually reserved for situations that require molding closely to the body part. Table 33.2 compares plaster and synthetic casts.

Cast Application. The child's developmental age should be considered before the cast is applied. For preschoolers who fear bodily harm and fantasize the loss of an extremity, use a plastic doll or stuffed animal to explain the procedure beforehand. Toddlers and preschoolers do not have easily defined body boundaries; if an extremity is wrapped in a bandage, splint, or cast, to the young child the extremity ceases to function or exist. During the application of the cast, use various distraction methods, including discussing favorite pets or activities at school and blowing bubbles. In this age-group, explanations such as "This will help your arm get better" are futile because the child has no concept of causality.

Before the cast is applied, check the extremities for any abrasions, cuts, or other alterations in the skin surface, and for the presence of rings or other items that might cause constriction with swelling; such objects are removed. A tube of cloth stockinette or waterproof liner is stretched over the area to be casted, and bony prominences are padded with soft cotton padding. Dry rolls of casting material are immersed in a pail of tepid water; the wet rolls are applied in bandage fashion and molded to the extremity. It is helpful to explain that some synthetic cast materials will become warm during application but will not burn the child. During application of the cast, the underlying stockinette is pulled over the raw edges of the cast and secured with a layer of casting material to form a smooth, padded edge to protect the skin. If the operator does not form such a protective edge with the stockinette, the raw edges of the cast can be protected by creating a "petaled" edge. Using a scissors, small pieces of moleskin or adhesive tape are cut with rounded edges; the individual "petals" are placed over the edge of the cast, with each petal slightly overlapping the previous one to form a smooth, neat edge.

! NURSING ALERT

Heated fans or dryers are not used because they cause the cast to dry on the outside and remain wet beneath. They may also cause burns from heat conduction by the cast to the underlying tissue.

Cast Removal. Cutting the cast to remove it or to relieve tightness is frequently a frightening experience for children. They fear the sound of the cast saw and are terrified that their flesh, as well as the cast, will be cut. Because it works by vibration, a cast saw cuts only the hard surface of the cast. The oscillating blade vibrates back and forth very rapidly and will not cut when placed lightly on the skin. Children have described it as producing a "tickly" sensation. The vibration also generates heat that the child may feel. Explain both of these sensations to the child.

Preparation for the procedure helps reduce anxiety, especially if the nurse has established a trusting relationship with the child. Many young children come to regard the cast as part of themselves, which intensifies their fear of removal (Fig. 33.7). They need continual reassurance that all is going well and that their behavior is accepted.

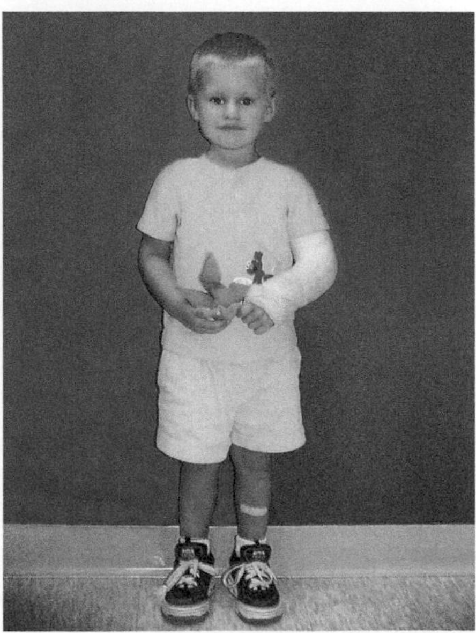

FIG. 33.7 Young children come to regard a cast as part of their body.

After the cast is removed, the skin surface is covered with desquamated skin and sebaceous secretions. Simple soaking in a bathtub is usually sufficient for their removal, but it may take several days to completely eliminate the accumulation. The parents and child should be instructed to not pull or forcibly remove this material with vigorous scrubbing because this may cause excoriation and bleeding. If the cast has been in place for a lengthy period of time, decreased muscle mass may be noted. The child and family should be reassured that resuming exercise and routine activities will gradually return function and appearance (provided there was no significant trauma beforehand).

Nursing Care Management

The complete evaporation of the water from a hip spica cast can take 24 to 48 hours when plaster materials are used. Drying occurs within minutes with fiberglass materials. The cast must remain uncovered to allow it to dry from the inside out. A wet plaster cast should be supported by a pillow covered with plastic and handled by the palms of the hands to avoid indenting the cast and creating pressure areas. Turning the child in a plaster cast at least every 2 hours will help dry a body cast evenly and prevent complications related to immobility. Use of a regular fan or a hair dryer on the cool setting to circulate air may be helpful when the humidity is high. A dry plaster of Paris cast produces a hollow sound when tapped with the finger.

! NURSING ALERT

Immediately report any observations that include the five *P*s of ischemia: pain, especially with passive range of motion; pallor; pulselessness (an ominous and late sign); paresthesia; and paralysis.

During the first few hours after a cast is applied, the chief concern is that the extremity may continue to swell to the extent that the cast becomes a tourniquet, shutting off circulation and producing neurovascular complications (compartment syndrome). One measure to reduce the likelihood of this problem is to elevate the body part and thereby increase venous return. If edema is excessive, casts are bivalved (i.e., cut to make anterior and posterior halves that are held together with an elastic bandage). The cast and the involved extremity are observed frequently to assess neurovascular integrity and detect any signs of compromise. Permanent muscle and tissue damage can occur within a few hours.

Appropriate cast care guidelines for the child's parents and caregivers are necessary before discharge. Instructions are also given for checking for signs and symptoms that indicate the cast is too tight (see Family-Centered Care box). Parents should also be told to take the child to their health care professional if the cast becomes too loose because a loose cast no longer serves its purpose.

Nurses can help families adapt the child's home environment to meet the temporary inconvenience of a large cast or one that restricts the child's mobility (e.g., a hip spica cast or long leg cast). Common situations (e.g., transporting a child safely and comfortably in a car) can become problematic. Standard seat belts and car seats may not be readily adapted for use by children in some casts. Specially designed car seats and restraints are available that meet safety requirements. Baths are possible only if the cast is kept out of the water and covered to prevent it from becoming wet from splashes. Some synthetic casts are waterproof, but proper care is necessary to avoid skin irritation beneath the cast.

Sitting can be impossible in a spica cast, and lower extremity casts require extra space in a small room, under a table, and in a bathroom. Children in spica casts may experience difficulty with feeding, and the

FAMILY-CENTERED CARE

Cast Care

- Keep the casted part of the body elevated on pillows or similar support for the first day or as directed by the health care professional.
- Expose the plaster cast to air until dry.
- A wet plaster cast should be lifted and supported with the palms of the hands only in order to avoid indenting with the fingers and creating pressure points.
- Observe the fingers or toes for any evidence of swelling or discoloration (darker or lighter than a comparable extremity) and contact the health care professional immediately if noted.
- Check movement and sensation of the visible fingers or toes frequently and contact the health care professional regarding any changes noted.
- Encourage frequent rest for a few days, and elevate the injured arm or leg while resting.
- Do not allow the affected limb to hang in a dependent position for more than 30 minutes (to prevent swelling and circulatory stasis).
- Keep an injured arm or hand elevated (e.g., in a sling) most of the time; supporting it on pillows at chest level is helpful.
- Elevate an injured leg when the child is sitting and avoid standing for too long.
- Do not allow the child to put anything inside the cast.
- Keep small items that might be placed inside the cast away from young children.
- Examine the skin at the cast edges to detect irritation or breakdown. Pad the cast accordingly.
- Instruct the child and parents to avoid placing the cast in water (e.g., tub, shower, swimming pool).
- If the patient is incontinent, protect the cast with waterproof tape and plastic. Use diapers, pull-ups, or other guards.

prone position may be easier for self-feeding from a small table; alternatively, they may manage a semisitting position in bed or in a wheelchair (see Figs. 33.5 and 33.6). Use of a conventional toilet is almost impossible for a child in a spica cast. Small bedpans or other containers offer alternatives for elimination. The nurse may suggest waterproofing methods by using plastic wraps, a protective skin barrier, and absorbent pads as means of reducing urine burns and heat rash and improving hygiene with a hip spica cast.

THE CHILD IN TRACTION

With the increased emphasis on outpatient care of acute and chronic illnesses to cut health care costs, developmental and social considerations, immobilization problems, and advanced surgical techniques, traction is used with decreasing frequency. Most skeletal traction is applied in children after a severe or complex injury to allow physiologic stability, align bone fragments, and permit closer evaluation of the injured site. New technology has developed orthopedic fixation devices that allow for partial or full mobility, thus preventing long-term immobilization and its consequences. In many cases, surgical intervention may be carried out within a matter of hours to days; therefore skeletal traction devices described herein may be used infrequently in pediatrics.

Purposes of Traction

The primary purposes of traction are as follows:

1. To realign bone fragments
2. To provide rest for an extremity
3. To help prevent or improve contracture deformity
4. To correct a joint deformity
5. To treat a dislocation
6. To allow preoperative or postoperative positioning and alignment
7. To provide immobilization of specific areas of the body
8. To reduce muscle spasms

The three primary purposes of traction for reduction of fractures are as follows:

1. To fatigue the involved muscle and reduce muscle spasm so that bones can be realigned
2. To position the distal and proximal bone ends in the desired realignment to promote satisfactory bone healing
3. To immobilize the fracture site until realignment has been achieved and sufficient healing has taken place to permit casting or splinting

When two forces of given direction and magnitude act on an object at the same point simultaneously from opposite directions, the object either changes its state of rest or motion or remains in equilibrium. The use of traction in the management of fractures is the direct application of such forces to reduce or realign the bone at the fracture site. The three essential components of traction management are traction, countertraction, and friction. **Traction** (forward force) is produced by attaching weight to the distal bone fragment. Body weight provides **countertraction** (backward force), and the patient's contact with the bed constitutes the frictional force (Fig. 33.8). These forces are used to align the distal and proximal bone fragments by adjusting the line of pull upward or downward and by adducting or abducting the extremity.

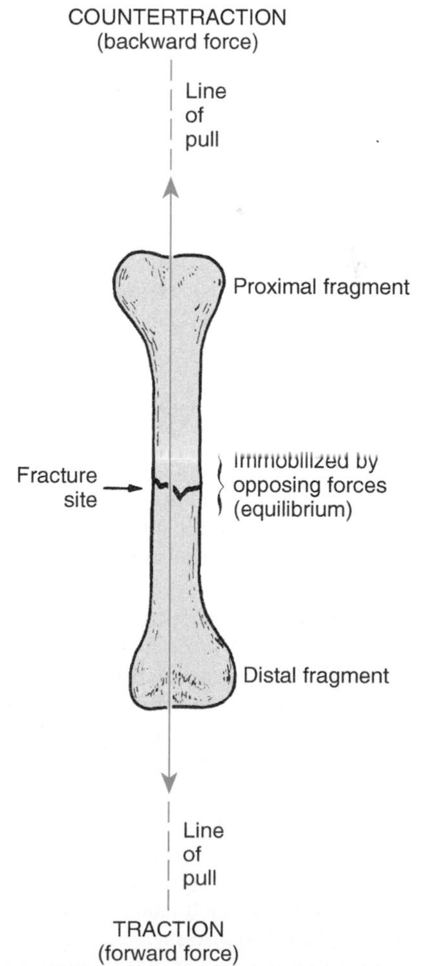

FIG. 33.8 Application of traction for maintaining equilibrium.

BOX 33.2 Types of Traction

Manual traction—Applied to the body part by the hands placed distal to the fracture site. Manual traction may be provided during application of a cast but more commonly when a closed reduction is performed.

Skin traction—Applied directly to the skin surface and indirectly to the skeletal structures. The pulling mechanism is attached to the skin with adhesive material or an elastic bandage. Both types are applied over soft, foam-backed traction straps to distribute the traction pull.

Skeletal traction—Applied directly to the skeletal structure by a pin, wire, or tongs inserted into or through the diameter of the bone distal to the fracture.

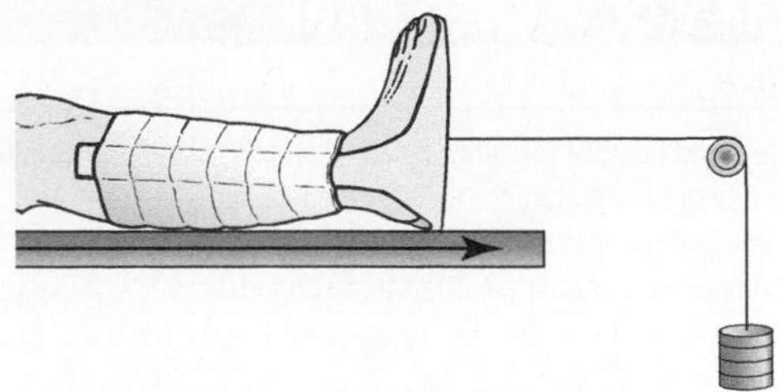

FIG. 33.9 Buck extension traction.

To attain equilibrium, the amount of forward force is adjusted by adding weight to or subtracting weight from the traction. Countertraction can be increased by elevating the foot of the bed to create a greater gravitational pull to the backward force.

The all-or-none law, characteristic of muscle contractility, applies to muscle relaxation as well. The muscle is fatigued by applying constant stress to the muscle so that the buildup of lactic acid will produce muscle relaxation. When muscles are stretched, muscle spasm ceases, which permits the realignment of the bone ends. The continuous maintenance of traction is important during this phase because releasing the traction allows the muscle to contract normally and again cause malpositioning of the bone ends.

The realignment of bone fragments is a gradual process that is achieved more rapidly in infants, who have limited muscle tone compared with muscular teenagers. The desired vector force, bone alignment, and callus formation are checked periodically by radiographic examination. The traction pull to some degree immobilizes the fracture site; however, adjunct immobilizing devices such as splints or casts are sometimes used with skeletal traction. Immobilization with traction is maintained until the bone ends are in satisfactory realignment, after which a less confining type of immobilization—a cast, pins, or external stabilization device—is applied. In injuries in which there is severe soft tissue swelling or vascular and nerve damage, it is customary to use traction until these complications have been resolved and it is safe to apply a cast.

Types of Traction

The pull needed for traction can be applied to the distal bone fragment in several ways. The main types of traction include manual, skin, and skeletal traction (Box 33.2). The type of traction applied is determined primarily by the child's age, the condition of the soft tissues, and the type and degree of displacement of the fracture. Fractures most commonly treated by application of traction are those involving the femur and vertebrae.

The use of upper extremity traction in children is uncommon. Current surgical techniques allow for early mobilization and acceptable results without the use of traction. Nursing care of children with upper extremity traction is similar to that for lower extremity traction, discussed later.

A common site for a femoral fracture is the middle third of the shaft (see Fig. 33.27, *A*, later in this chapter). With such a fracture there may be significant overriding but minimal displacement. In a fracture of the lower third of the femoral shaft, the pull of the gastrocnemius muscle causes the distal fragment to become downwardly displaced. Femur fractures in young children can often be reduced followed by application of a hip spica cast. When traction is necessary, several types may be used based on the initial assessment.

Buck extension traction is a type of skin traction applied with the legs in an extended position (Fig. 33.9). Buck extension traction is used primarily for short-term immobilization, such as preoperative management of a child with a dislocated hip, or for correction of contractures or bone deformities, such as in Legg-Calvé-Perthes disease. Except for fracture cases, a side-lying position may be permissible if the leg is held in an acceptable alignment. Buck extension traction can be utilized with either skin straps or a special boot designed for traction.

Russell traction uses skin traction on the lower leg and a padded sling under the knee. Two lines of pull, one along the longitudinal axis of the lower leg and one perpendicular to the leg, are produced. This combination of pulls allows realignment of the lower extremity and immobilizes the hip and knee in a flexed position. Hip flexion must remain at the prescribed angle to prevent fracture malalignment because there is no direct support under the fracture and the skin traction may slip. Nursing measures include carefully monitoring the position of the traction so that the appropriate amount of hip flexion is maintained and damage to the peroneal nerve under the knee does not cause footdrop.

A common skeletal traction is 90-degree–90-degree traction (90-90 traction). The lower leg is supported by a boot cast or a calf sling, and a skeletal Steinmann pin or Kirschner wire is placed in the distal fragment of the femur. This type of traction results in a 90-degree angle at both the hip and knee. It achieves the desired line of pull for reducing the fracture and provides adequate immobilization of the fracture site. The use of 90-90 traction also supports the lower extremity in a desired position with good venous return. From a nursing standpoint, this type of traction facilitates position changes, toileting, and prevention of complications related to traction.

Balanced suspension traction may be used with or without skin or skeletal traction. Unless it is combined with another type of traction, balanced suspension merely holds the leg in a desired flexed position to relax the hip and hamstring muscles and does not exert any traction directly on a body part. A Thomas splint extends from the groin to midair above the foot, and a Pearson attachment supports the lower leg. Towels or pieces of felt covered with stockinette are clipped or pinned to the splints for leg support. Ropes are attached to create a balanced traction. When the child is lifted from the bed, the traction lifts as well, without loss of alignment (see Fig. 33.3). This type of traction requires careful checking of splints and ropes to make certain no slippage or fraying has occurred. This mode of traction is of great value in an older and heavier child when it is essential to lift the patient for care.

The cervical area is a vulnerable site for flexion or extension injuries to muscles, vertebrae, or the spinal cord. Cervical muscle trauma without other complications is treated with a cervical soft or hard collar to relieve the weight of the head on the fracture site. When a child's cervical vertebra is displaced or fractured, it may be necessary to reduce and immobilize the site with cervical skeletal traction. The spinal cord runs through the intravertebral canal, and dislocation or fracture of the vertebrae can also cause spinal cord injury. Nursing assessment of

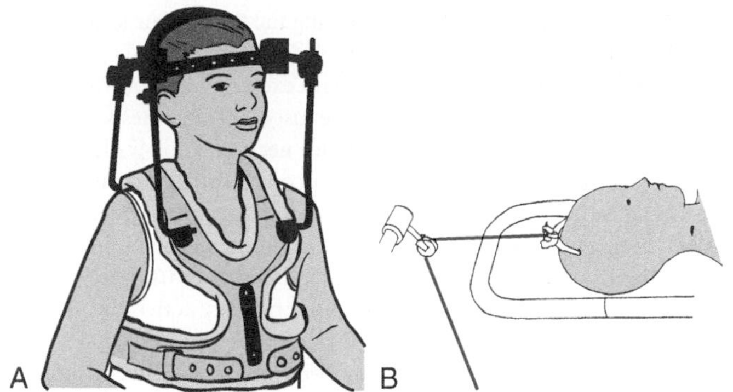

FIG. 33.10 **A,** Halo vest. **B,** Cervical traction with Gardner-Wells tong.

neurologic function is essential to prevent further injury during the application and use of cervical skeletal traction.

Most cervical traction is accomplished with the use of a halo brace or halo vest (Fig. 33.10, *A*). This device consists of a steel halo attached to the outer skull by four screws; several rigid bars connect the halo to a vest that is worn around the chest. This provides greater mobility of the rest of the body, while limiting cervical spinal motion completely. Gardner-Wells tongs may also be used to immobilize the cervical spine (Fig. 33.10, *B*). Gardner-Wells tongs are spring-loaded, so making burr holes and shaving hair are not required; a local anesthetic may be used during application. With cervical traction, the neck muscles fatigue with constant traction pull, the vertebral bodies gradually separate so the spinal cord is no longer pinched between the vertebrae. Immobilization until fracture healing or surgical fixation can occur is an essential goal of cervical traction. If immobilization is needed in a young child, a special cervical spine cast (Minerva cast) may be applied.

! NURSING ALERT

Skeletal traction is never released by the nurse (except under direct supervision by the provider). This precaution includes not lifting the weights that are applying traction (e.g., for moving the child in bed or repositioning).

Nursing Care Management

To assess the child in traction, it is essential to know the purpose or reason for application of traction and understand the basic principles of its use. Routine assessment of both the child and the traction apparatus is required. Many of the nursing problems associated with traction in a child are related to immobility. However, a number of physical needs related to traction require attention and vigilance.

In addition to routine skin observation and care, the child in skeletal traction will need special skin care at the pin site according to hospital policy or provider preference. Pin sites should be frequently assessed and cleaned to prevent infection; after the first 48 to 72 hours, pin site care may be performed once daily or weekly for mechanically stable pins. Several different methods and solutions can be used for cleaning pin sites; studies have shown no clear evidence that one pin care technique is better than another at reducing the chance of infection or complications (Lethaby, Temple, & Santy-Tomlinson, 2013). Before the child's discharge, parents and caregivers are taught pin site care, including how to observe for infection or pin instability, using a return demonstration method. A pressure-reduction device, such as a foam overlay or an alternating-pressure mattress, reduces the chance of skin breakdown.

When the child is first placed in traction, increased discomfort is common as a result of the traction pull fatiguing the muscle. Orthopedic

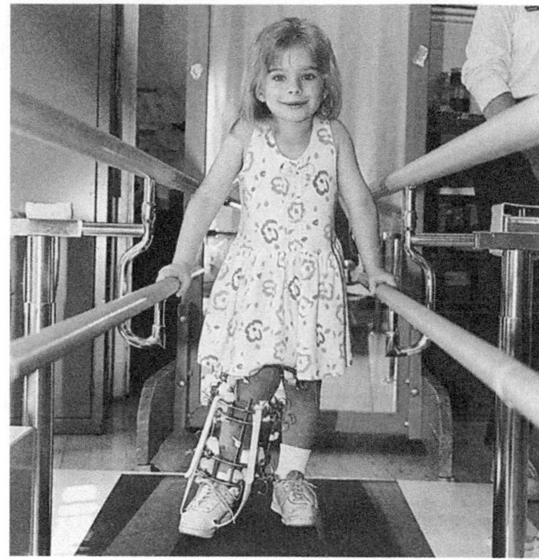

FIG. 33.11 Child with Ilizarov external fixator (on right leg) during physical therapy on parallel bars.

conditions are associated with a higher-than-average number of painful events and a higher percentage of bodily symptoms than other common conditions. Analgesics, including opioids, and muscle relaxants help during this phase of care and should be administered liberally with close attention paid to possible adverse effects.

DISTRACTION

Unlike traction, which helps bones realign and fuse properly, distraction is the process of separating opposing bone to encourage generation of new bone in the created space. An osteotomy is performed to allow for distraction and either an external or internal device is utilized. Distraction can be used when limbs are of unequal lengths or if there is an angular deformity of a limb.

Monolateral, Taylor spatial frame, and Ilizarov external fixators are common external fixation devices. The Ilizarov external fixator uses a system of wires, rings, and telescoping rods that permits limb lengthening to occur by manual distraction (Fig. 33.11). In addition to lengthening bones, the device can be used to correct angular or rotational deformities or to immobilize fractures. The device is attached surgically by securing a series of external full or half rings to the bone with wires. External telescoping rods connect the rings to each other. Manual distraction is accomplished by manipulating the rods to increase the distance between the rings. A special osteotomy or corticotomy involves cutting only the cortex of the bone, while preserving its blood supply, bone marrow, endosteum, and periosteum. Capillary blood flow to the transected area is essential for proper bone growth. The bone may be lengthened approximately 1 mm per day or about 1 inch per month.

The use of motorized internal fixation devices is a relatively new treatment for correcting limb length discrepancies. Intramedullary nails are placed within the bone and an electrical or magnetic remote is utilized to control the distraction of the bone. This technique is typically performed in adolescents or skeletally mature individuals.

Nursing Care Management

Successful use of external fixation depends on the child's and family's cooperation; therefore before surgery, they must be fully informed about the appearance of the device, the way it accomplishes bone growth, required alterations in activities, and home and follow-up care. Children are involved in learning to adjust the device to accomplish distraction.

Children and parents should be instructed in pin care, including observation for infection and loosening of pins. Close monitoring of neurovascular status and changes of the involved extremity are also important.

Children who participate actively in their care report less discomfort. Because the device may be external, the child and family need to be prepared for the reactions of others. Partial weight bearing is allowed, and the child needs to learn to walk with crutches. Alterations in activity include modifications at school and in physical education. Full weight bearing is not allowed until the distraction is completed and bone consolidation has occurred. Follow-up care is essential to maintain appropriate distraction until the desired limb length is achieved. The device is removed surgically after the bone has consolidated; the child may need to use crutches or have a cast for 4 to 6 weeks after removal of the device to reduce the risk of fracture.

AMPUTATION

A child may be born with the congenital absence of a body part, experience a traumatic loss of an extremity, or require a surgical amputation for a pathologic condition such as osteosarcoma. With today's surgical technology and the quick thinking of bystanders who save a traumatically amputated body part, some children have had fingers and arms sewn back on with variable degrees of functional use regained.

Surgical amputation or the surgical repair of a permanently severed limb focuses on constructing an adequately nourished residual limb. For lower extremities the presence of a smooth, healthy, padded stump, free of nerve endings, is important for prosthesis fitting and subsequent ambulation. In some situations in which there is no vascular or neurologic deficit, a cast is applied to the stump immediately after the procedure, and a pylon, metal extension, and artificial foot are attached so that the patient can walk on the temporary prosthesis within a few hours.

! NURSING ALERT

For a traumatically amputated limb or body part, do the following:

1. Rinse limb gently with normal saline.
2. Loosely wrap limb in sterile gauze.
3. Place wrapped limb in a watertight bag.
4. Chill bag, without freezing, in ice water. Do not pack in ice because this may harm tissue.
5. Label with child's name, date, and time, and transport with the child to the hospital.

Nursing Care Management

Extremity stump shaping is done postoperatively with special elastic bandaging using a figure eight compression bandage, which applies pressure in a conical fashion. This technique decreases stump edema, controls hemorrhage, and aids in developing desired contours so that the child will bear weight on the posterior aspect of the skin flap rather than on the end of the stump. Postoperative complications for which the nurse should be vigilant include hemorrhage and infection of the operative site.

Postoperatively, the stump may be elevated for the first 24 hours, but after this time the extremity should not be left in this position because contractures in the proximal joint will develop and seriously hamper ambulation. Monitoring proper body alignment further decreases the risk of flexion contractures. Children who undergo amputation of a lower extremity should be turned not only from side to side but also from front to back. As the child progresses, encourage him or her to lie prone at least three times a day, increasing the time prone to tolerance of an hour at a time.

For older children and adolescents, arm exercises, bed pushups, and exercises with parallel bars (which are used in prosthesis training programs) help build up the arm muscles necessary for walking with crutches. An overhead trapeze bar enhances mobilization and upper body strength building in the early postoperative period when a lower limb has been amputated. Full range-of-motion exercises of joints above the amputation must be performed several times daily, using active and isotonic exercises. Young children are spontaneously active and require little encouragement.

Depending on the child's age, the child or parents need to learn stump care, including careful washing with soap and water every day and checking for skin irritation, breakdown, or infection. A careful skin check must be performed every time the prosthesis is removed, and prosthesis tolerance time must be adjusted to prevent skin breakdown.

For children who have had an amputation, phantom limb pain is an expected experience because the nerve-brain connections are still present. Phantom pain is real pain and should be treated appropriately with analgesics and other pain-relieving measures. Gradually these sensations fade, although in many amputees they persist for years. Preoperative discussion of this phenomenon helps a child understand these feelings and not hide the experience from others. Limb pain, especially pain that increases with ambulation, should be evaluated for the possibility of a neuroma at the free nerve endings in the stump or a poorly fitting prosthesis. Chronic pain may also be related to weakness or joint instability, injury to the nerve, or fibrosis of soft tissues. Pain in the contralateral extremity may result from asymmetric weight bearing.

MOBILIZATION DEVICES

Orthotics and Prosthetics

Developments in the fields of **orthotics** (fabrication and fitting of braces) and **prosthetics** (fabrication and fitting of artificial limbs) have resulted in lighter and better-fitting devices and thus greater patient compliance in using them. Orthoses are often used to prevent deformity, increase the energy efficiency of gait, and control alignment. Braces that facilitate walking can sometimes stabilize paralyzed or markedly weakened extremities. Special joint hinges permit the hip, knee, and ankle to flex while sitting, whereas the leg is held rigid during ambulation. Well-fitted orthoses promote ambulation, whereas ill-fitting braces throw off the child's balance and frequently cause muscle stress and tissue breakdown. An orthosis must fit each body curvature to avoid undue pressure on tissues and imbalance between muscle groups. Bony prominences where a brace has contact, such as along the spine, chin, iliac crests, ankles, and feet, are observed closely for pressure or irritation and are padded as necessary. In the growing child, braces need frequent adjustment and replacement if long-term use is necessary.

Types of orthoses are described based on the joints controlled by the orthosis. The ankle-foot orthosis (AFO) is used to prevent footdrop due to bed rest, trauma to the foot, or paralysis of the muscles in the foot; to prevent heelcord tightening; or to support the foot in proper position for standing and walking (Fig. 33.12). Shorter styles of bracing for the foot include a supramalleolar orthosis (SMO) and foot orthosis.

The knee-ankle-foot orthosis (KAFO) is used to prevent buckling of the knee, to support the extremity when there is paralysis or marked weakness of the quadriceps muscle, or to protect the limb when the bone structure is weak (Fig. 33.13). The hip-knee-ankle-foot orthosis (HKAFO) is used to provide various types of control for the knee and ankle joints as described earlier, as well as the hip (e.g., flail lower limb

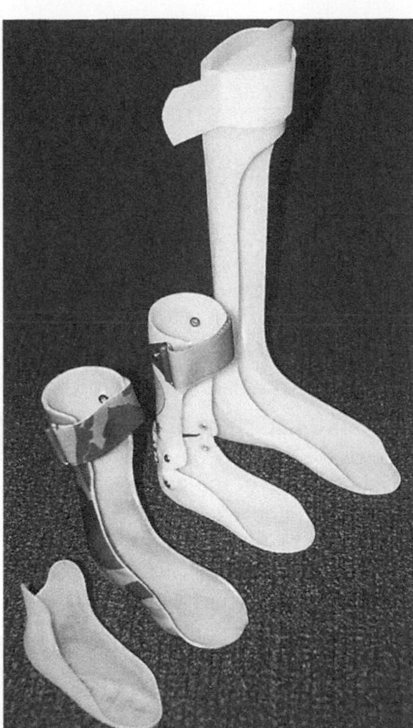

FIG. 33.12 *Left to right:* Supramalleolar orthosis (SMO), solid ankle-foot orthosis (AFO), articulating AFO, floor reaction AFO.

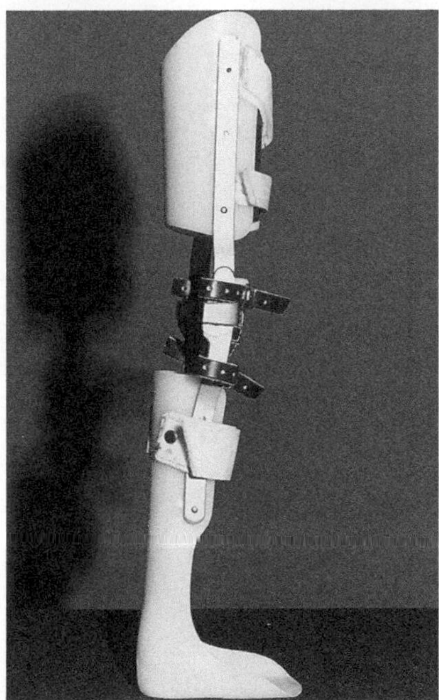

FIG. 33.13 Knee-ankle-foot orthosis (KAFO).

and paralysis). The reciprocal gait orthosis (RGO) is a type of HKAFO that has a mechanism allowing children with significant paraplegia to walk in a reciprocal fashion on a flat surface. RGOs are used in children with spinal cord injury, sacral agenesis, and spina bifida.

The thoracolumbosacral orthosis (TLSO) and cervical thoracolumbosacral orthosis (CTLSO) are custom molded and fit snugly around the trunk of the body to exert pressure on the ribs and back to support the spine in a straight position (Fig. 33.14). The Boston brace is an underarm orthosis customized from prefabricated plastic shells, with corrective forces for each patient supplied by lateral pads. These braces may prevent the progression of curves in the spine, such as scoliosis, or provide needed trunk support in a child with paraplegia. The Jewett-Taylor brace is sometimes used to support the spine and trunk during ambulation to prevent compression after fracture of the spinal column.

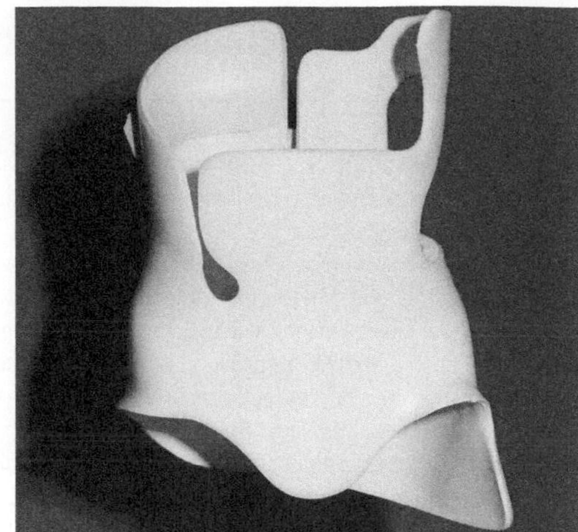

FIG. 33.14 Thoracolumbosacral orthosis (TLSO).

When prostheses are prescribed, the provider considers many factors: level of amputation, age, weight, activity, agility, and skin condition. Each prosthesis is custom made or fabricated of various plastic and foam materials. The style of the prosthesis depends on the most distal joint involved in the amputation or prosthetic fitting. Advances are constantly occurring in both the fabrication and fitting of prosthetics. Development of myoelectric devices, use of new cosmetic materials in terminal gloves and feet, and socket construction using computer-aided design and computer-aided manufacturing are but a few of the recent changes with positive effects for patients who require prostheses.

Nursing Care Management

Meticulous skin care under a brace is necessary. Protective clothing should be worn under braces to protect the skin from friction and pressure. Assessment of all areas that make contact with the brace every 1 to 2 hours for the first few days after application is recommended. If any area is reddened, the brace should be removed for at least 30 minutes. If the redness does not disappear, the nurse should notify the provider or orthotist (see Family-Centered Care box).

Before a prosthesis is applied, the condition of the skin must be assessed, with special note taken of areas of redness or breaks in the integrity of the skin. Prevention of skin breakdown is best accomplished through good hygiene of the residual limb, proper fitting of the artificial limb, and prosthetic training (see Family-Centered Care box).

Safety is another important consideration. Parallel bars provide secure handrails on both sides as the child learns to walk again with or without braces or a prosthesis. As the child becomes more proficient, a walker with or without wheels is substituted for the bars, and the child is no longer confined to a limited territory. The child then progresses to crutches if age and condition permit it.

Crutches, Canes, and Walkers

Crutches, canes, and walkers are used when children need support for balance while walking, are not allowed to bear weight, or can place only part of their body weight on an extremity, such as with a lower leg injury. There are many types of crutches, and the selection depends on the child's individual needs. Axillary swing-through crutches are used most frequently as temporary assistance. Forearm crutches (Fig. 33.15) are the usual selection for children who anticipate permanent use, such

FAMILY-CENTERED CARE

Orthoses

Care of Skin

AFO, KAFO, HKAFO

If the child has decreased sensation in the legs, check the skin condition more frequently than every 4 hours.

If the child complains of a burning sensation under the brace, remove the brace promptly and observe the skin for any reddened areas. If the child complains of burning several times, contact the provider or orthotist.

If a small blister or open area develops, cover it with a sterile bandage and check the skin more often. Do not put alcohol on open areas. The child should avoid wearing the device until the skin heals.

Sometimes open areas are slow to heal. If no sign of healing occurs after 3 days, contact the provider or orthotist.

Lotions and creams will soften the skin and should be used only if the skin is dry.

TLSO

Because the device works by pressing against the body and is kept very snug by straps and buckles, some skin pinkness is to be expected. The skin at the brace edges and under the pads should be inspected carefully and frequently, especially in the initial period when the child or adolescent is getting accustomed to the device. Any red mark that does not fade within 20 minutes, or any area that appears raw and sore, should be reported to the orthotist.

Have the child wear a cotton undershirt under the brace to protect the skin; keeping it clean, dry, and free of wrinkles will help prevent skin problems.

Care of Orthoses

AFO, KAFO, HKAFO

Clean the plastic sections of the brace with soap and water and dry them thoroughly.

Check all screws or fasteners periodically to make certain they are tight.

If the brace is broken, out of alignment, or causing skin problems, notify the orthotist.

TLSO

Clean the brace with soap and water, followed by a good rinsing with water, on a weekly basis. Thoroughly dry the brace before it is put on.

It is important to avoid leaving it in hot places, such as in direct, strong sunlight or by a warm heater.

AFO, Ankle-foot orthosis; *HKAFO,* hip-knee-ankle-foot orthosis; *KAFO,* knee-ankle-foot orthosis; *TLSO,* thoracolumbosacral orthosis.

as paraplegic children. In children with limited hand and arm strength or function, the use of trough crutches allows the weight to be assumed by the elbow. For small children who have not yet learned to walk or those who are unsteady, front or reverse walkers are typically used (Fig. 33.16).

Children must be properly fitted with a crutch, cane, or walker to prevent both poor posture and crutch pressure on the axilla during ambulation. A physical therapist usually measures the child and teaches crutch, cane, or walker use; however, nurses in some areas such as the emergency department do teach children crutch walking. Nurses also supervise the use of crutches and walkers in pediatric units and in the home. The type of crutch gait taught to a child depends on how stable the child is on crutches, whether or not the knees can be flexed, how much weight bearing is allowed, and what specific goal is established for the child.

FAMILY-CENTERED CARE

Prostheses

Care of Residual Limb

Wash with mild, nonperfumed soap, rinse, and dry thoroughly daily.

Check skin for redness, blisters, sensitive areas, or signs of infection.

Care of Prosthesis

Routinely wash the socket with water and mild soap, rinse, and dry thoroughly.

Check straps and rubber bands with each application.

Check joints to ensure that they operate smoothly.

Replace worn or broken parts (heels, soles, straps) as needed.

Use 100% cotton stump socks to absorb perspiration, prevent skin friction, and provide comfort.

Change socks daily, and wash and dry following instructions provided by prosthetist.

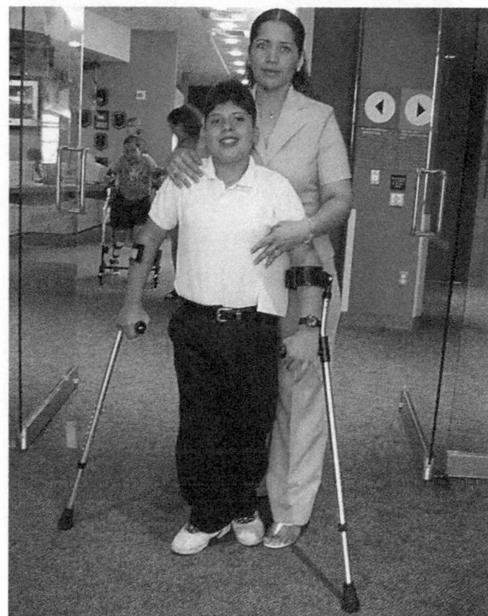

FIG. 33.15 Adolescent using forearm crutches for ambulation. (Courtesy Texas Children's Hospital, Houston.)

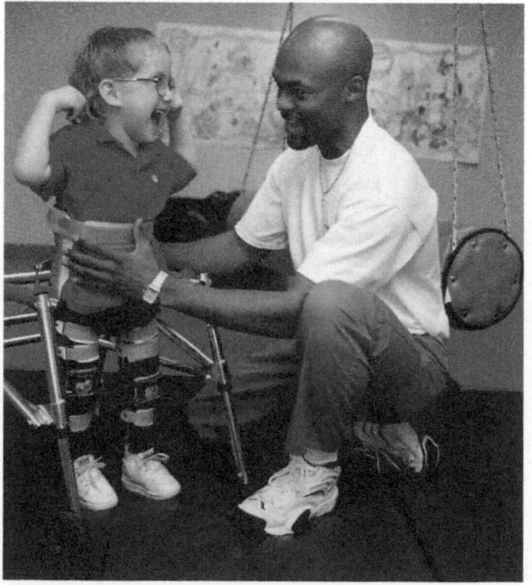

FIG. 33.16 Young child with rear-rolling walker. (Courtesy Texas Children's Hospital, Houston.)

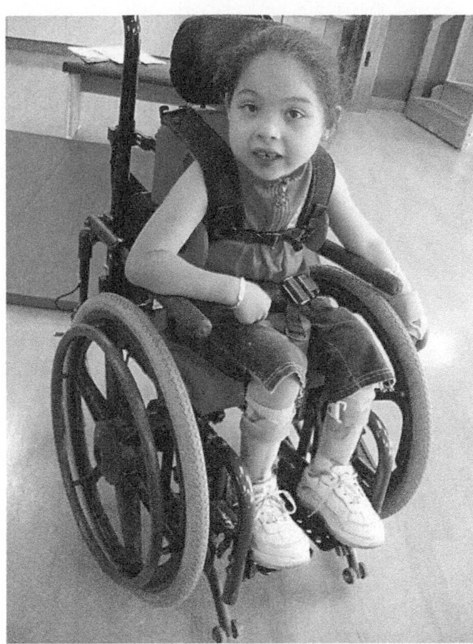

FIG. 33.17 Child in wheelchair, which should be scaled appropriately to child's size. Note AFOs and left wrist splint to prevent contractures. (Courtesy Texas Children's Hospital, Houston.)

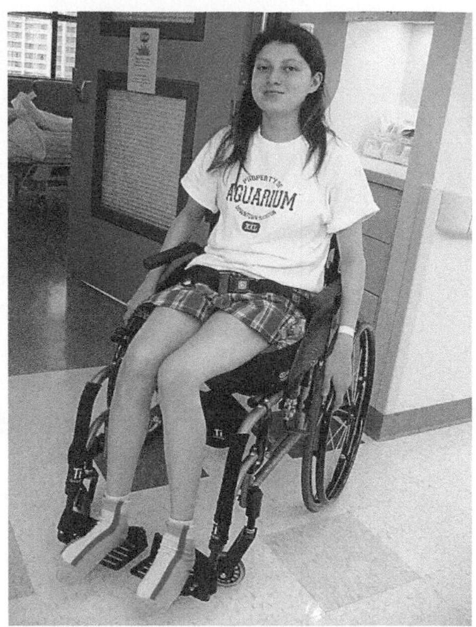

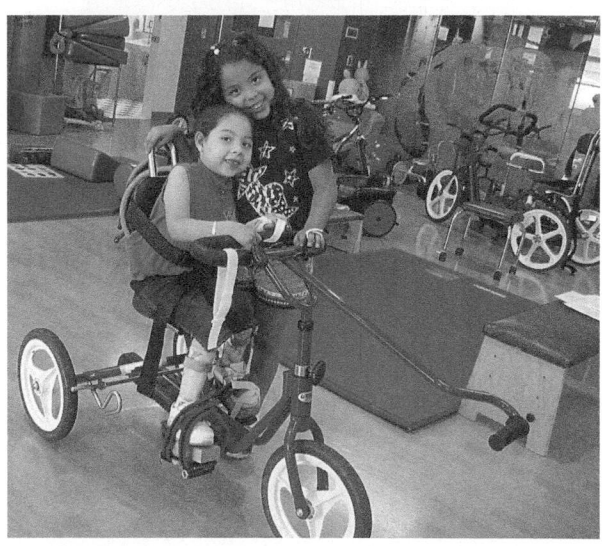

FIG. 33.18 Wheelchair allows adolescent mobility and independence. (Courtesy Texas Children's Hospital, Houston.)

Performing upper body strengthening exercises to condition and strengthen arms and shoulders before crutch use is important if immobilization has been prolonged. The child gains confidence in ambulating by wearing a safety belt held by the therapist. Instructions are conveyed in language children understand and with a demonstration. Most children adapt to the techniques readily.

Wheelchairs

Wheelchairs are used temporarily or permanently as a means of transportation. A wheelchair for temporary use should fit the child and contain any adaptations needed, such as an elevating leg rests or reclining back. The child learns how to transfer in and out of the chair and how to move it safely. Prescribing a wheelchair for permanent use is the joint responsibility of the provider and therapist after an assessment of home and surroundings. A wheelchair should be neither too small nor too large and preferably should be adaptable as the child grows (Fig. 33.17).

Detachable or rotating armrests, which permit easy transfer in and out, are needed for children with spinal cord injuries, cerebral palsy, and spina bifida. Other desirable features are detachable and swing-away footrests and detachable desk arms. Elevating leg rests are required for children who are prone to contractures, and a reclining backrest is needed for those who may have poor trunk balance. A pressure-relief cushion should be provided for a child who has decreased sensation. Hand-rim and brake-lever projections are helpful for children with upper extremity weakness. For children who have the use of only one arm, a special "one-arm drive" wheelchair is available. Children with lower extremity paraplegia require upper arm strengthening exercises and instruction on transfer techniques before wheelchair mobilization (Fig. 33.18). Often a tilt table is used to overcome the problem of orthostatic intolerance before the child is able to tolerate wheelchair sitting.

Various motorized chairs are available for children with marked upper extremity weakness, and mouth- or cheek-operated models are available for children who do not have the use of upper extremities so they can operate the wheelchairs independently. Very small children who have permanent paralysis of the lower extremities are provided with specially designed units that allow independent mobility. A detachable handle on these units permits their conversion to strollers.

FIG. 33.19 Tricycle used to provide mobility and to strengthen leg muscles. (Courtesy Texas Children's Hospital, Houston.)

Bicycles and tricycles (Figs. 33.19 and 33.20) can be modified for children with limited ambulatory mobility; these also promote muscle strengthening and prevent disuse contractures. Gait training may be accomplished with a number of special devices (Fig. 33.21).

THE CHILD WITH A FRACTURE

The process of ossification, the gradual conversion of precursor substances (i.e., cartilage) to bony structures, begins in the embryo and continues until the child is 18 to 21 years of age. In long bones this process progresses outward from the diaphysis, the hard, shaftlike portion that constitutes the major part of the bone. Within this hard, compact shaft is the hollow medullary canal composed of the bone marrow. The epiphyses, located at the ends of long bones, consist of layers of cartilage, subchondral bone, and spongelike cancellous bone.

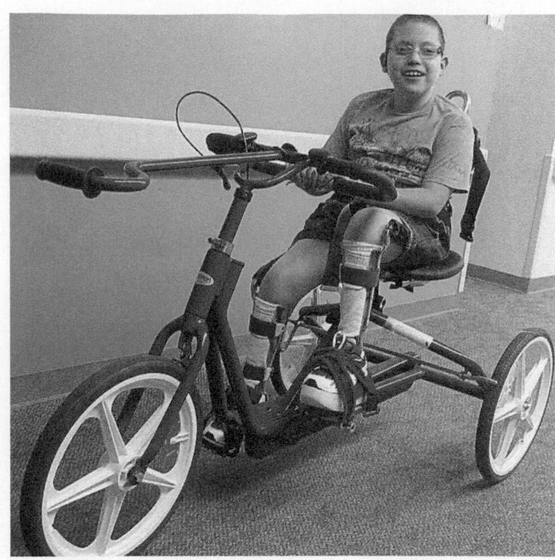

FIG. 33.20 Bike walker to provide mobility and to enhance leg muscle strength. (Courtesy Texas Children's Hospital, Houston.)

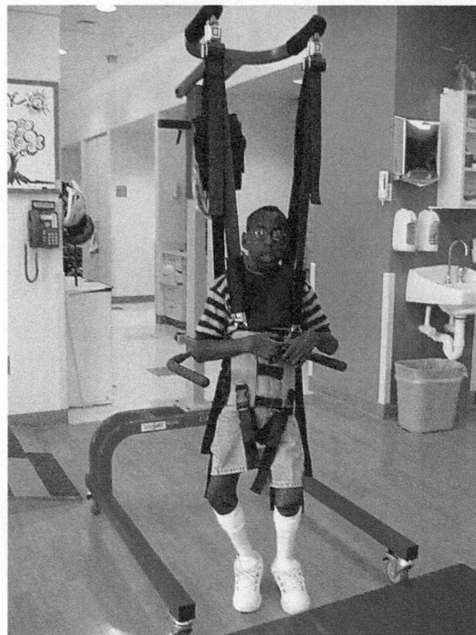

FIG. 33.21 Gait walker with suspension belts for balance and gait training. (Courtesy Texas Children's Hospital, Houston.)

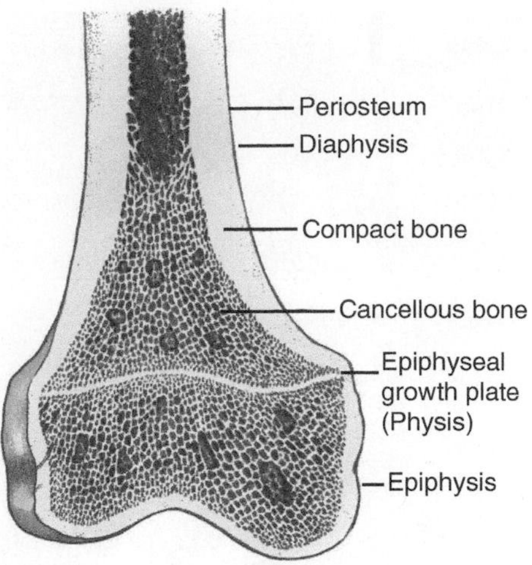

FIG. 33.22 Diagram of bone showing relationships of compact and cancellous bone, epiphysis, physis, and diaphysis.

BOX 33.3 Features of Fractures in Children

- The growth plate, a thick, elastic portion of bone where growth takes place, serves to absorb shock and protect joint surfaces from injury and is the means by which the limb is able to grow and to straighten itself. Growth is stimulated by a fracture in the diaphysis, whereas damage to the growth plate can cause shortening and often a progressive angular deformity.
- The periosteum of a child's bone is thicker and stronger and has more active osteogenic potential than that of an adult's bone.
- The pliable bones of the growing child are more porous than those of the adult, which allows them to bend, buckle, and break in a "greenstick" manner. The greater porosity increases the flexibility of the bone and dissipates and absorbs a significant amount of the force on impact.
- Healing is more rapid in children, and the rapidity is inversely related to the child's age. The younger the child, the more rapid the healing process. Nonunion of bone fragments is uncommon except in severe injuries in children.
- Stiffness is unusual and, unlike in adults, an uninjured joint in a child can be immobilized for a long period without producing stiffness that lasts longer than a few minutes. Injured joints do become stiff, however, and the current trend is toward early mobilization and active range-of-motion exercises as preventive measures.
- Children only complain when something is wrong. Unreasonable crying, restlessness, and calling for the parents are usually indications that something is amiss and requires investigation.

Situated between the diaphysis and the epiphysis is the **physis (growth plate)**, which plays a major role in the longitudinal growth of the developing child (Fig. 33.22). The **periosteum**, or thin, tough membrane covering all bones, contains blood vessels that nourish the living bone. Damage to this thin membrane can be a major problem in bone growth and healing.

Bones fracture when the resistance of the bone against the stress being exerted yields to the stress force. Fractures are a common injury at any age but are more likely to occur in children and the elderly. Because childhood is a time of rapid bone growth, the patterns of fractures, problems of diagnosis, and methods of treatment are different in children compared with adults. An adult's bones are strong and require a violent traumatic force to fracture, which is accompanied by massive injury to surrounding soft tissues. In children the bones are more easily injured, and fractures may result from minor falls or twists and are less likely to be accompanied by soft tissue damage. Features of children's fractures not observed in adults are listed in Box 33.3.

Aside from motor vehicle accidents or falls from heights, true injuries causing fracture are uncommon in infancy; therefore bony injuries in children of this age-group warrant further investigation. In any small child, radiographic evidence of fractures at various stages of healing, with few exceptions, indicates a nonaccidental trauma or child abuse (see Community and Home Health Considerations box, p. 1240). Any investigation of fractures in infants and young children, particularly multiple fractures, should include the suspicion of osteogenesis imperfecta (OI) after nonaccidental trauma has been ruled out.

A distal forearm (radius, ulna, or both) fracture is the most common fracture in children. The clavicle is also a common fracture in childhood, with approximately half of clavicle fractures occurring in children younger than 10 years of age. A common mechanism of injury is a fall with an outstretched hand or direct trauma to the bone (Fig. 33.23). In neonates, fractures of the clavicle may occur with a large newborn and a small maternal pelvis. Hip fractures are uncommon in children and require a

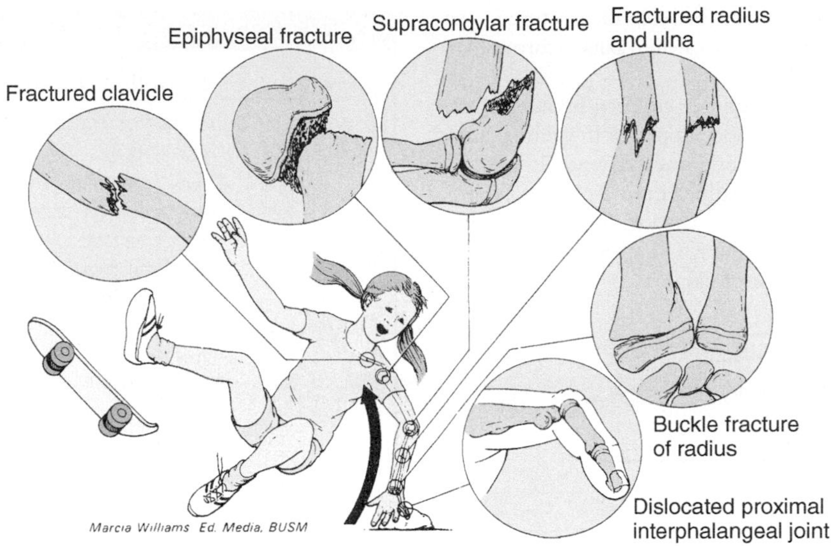

FIG. 33.23 Trauma resulting from progression of force in fall on outstretched hand.

great deal of force to produce. A femoral neck fracture may be sustained in children 6 or 7 years of age as a result of pedestrian-automobile accidents because in these children the hip is at the same level as an automobile bumper. In older children, the femur is the most likely target; in adolescents knee injuries are common with this type of accident.

Types of Fractures. A fractured bone consists of fragments: the fragment closest to the midline or trunk, called the proximal fragment, and the fragment farthest from the midline, or the distal fragment. When fracture fragments are separated, the fracture is complete; when fragments remain attached, the fracture is said to be incomplete. The fracture line can be any of the following:

Transverse—Crosswise, at right angles to the long axis of the bone

Oblique—Slanting but straight, between a horizontal and a perpendicular direction

Spiral—Slanting and circular, twisting around the bone shaft

The twisting of an extremity while the bone is breaking results in a spiral fracture. If the fracture injury does not produce a break in the skin, it is a simple, or closed, fracture. Open, or compound, fractures are those with an open wound through which the bone protrudes. If the bone fragments cause damage to other organs or tissues (e.g., the lung or bladder), the injury is said to be complicated. When small fragments of bone are broken from the fractured shaft and lie in the surrounding tissue, the fracture is called comminuted. This type of fracture is rare in children. The types of fracture that occur most often in children are shown in Box 33.4 and Fig. 33.24.

BOX 33.4 Types of Fracture in Children

Plastic deformation—Occurs when the bone is bent but not broken. A child's flexible bone can be bent 45 degrees or more before breaking. However, if bent, the bone will straighten slowly but not completely to produce some deformity but without the angulation seen when the bone breaks. Bends occur most commonly in the ulna and fibula, often in association with fractures of the radius and tibia.

Buckle, or torus, fracture—Produced by compression of the porous bone; appears as a raised or bulging projection at the fracture site. These fractures occur in the most porous portion of the bone near the metaphysis (the portion of the bone shaft adjacent to the epiphysis) and are more common in young children.

Greenstick fracture—Occurs when a bone is angulated beyond the limits of bending. The compressed side bends, and the tension side fails, causing an incomplete fracture similar to the break observed when a green stick is broken.

Complete fracture—Divides the bone fragments. These fragments often remain attached by a periosteal hinge, which can aid or hinder reduction.

Growth Plate or Physeal Injuries. The weakest point of long bones is the cartilage growth plate or the physis. Consequently, this is a frequent site of injury during childhood trauma. The Salter-Harris classification is typically used to describe growth plate injuries, as indicated in Fig. 33.25. Detection of physeal injuries is sometimes difficult but critical in determining whether bone growth will be affected. Close monitoring and early treatment, if indicated, are essential to prevent longitudinal or angular growth deformities (or both).

Bone Healing and Remodeling

Immediately after a fracture occurs, the muscles contract and physiologically splint the injured area. This phenomenon accounts for the muscle tightness observed over a fracture site and the deformity that is produced as the muscles pull the bone ends out of alignment. This muscle response must be overcome by traction or complete muscle relaxation (i.e., anesthesia) in order for the distal bone fragment to be realigned to the proximal bone fragment.

Bone healing follows a patterned sequence. Fig. 33.26 shows three broad overlapping phases: inflammatory, restorative, and remodeling. Bone healing can be described more definitively in terms of five stages (Table 33.3). When the bone breaks, the envelope of subcutaneous tissue, muscle, and periosteal tissue surrounding the site is torn; blood vessels rupture; and a hematoma forms. The ends of the fractured bone segments, deprived of circulation, die as far back as the nearest collateral circulation. Necrotic tissue accumulates, and an inflammatory response takes place at the site, with its characteristic vasodilation, plasma exudation, and edema. The organization and reabsorption of the hematoma proceeds, and the restorative phase begins with the reestablishment of local circulation. Repair requires an adequate blood supply and immobilization of the fracture fragments.

When there is a break in the continuity of bone, the periosteal and intraosseous osteoblasts are stimulated to maximum activity. New osteoblasts are formed in immense numbers almost immediately after the injury and begin building a bridge, as evidenced by a bulging growth of osteoblastic tissue and new bone matrix between the fractured bone fragments. This is followed by deposition of calcium salts to form callus, which provides stability (Fig. 33.27, *B*).

Bone healing is characteristically rapid in children because of the thickened periosteum and generous blood supply. In the young child, for example, there is frequently a solid union of the femoral shaft in 3 to 4 weeks, whereas in the adult, callus sufficient to avoid deformities from the constant muscle contraction associated with movement may not form for 10 to 16 weeks after the injury. The approximate healing times for a femoral shaft fracture are as follows:

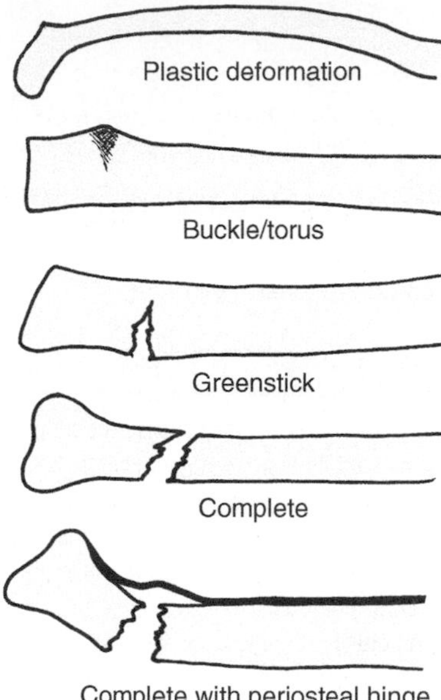

FIG. 33.24 Common types of fracture in children. Note that there are subclassifications of complete fractures based on characteristics of the fracture line.

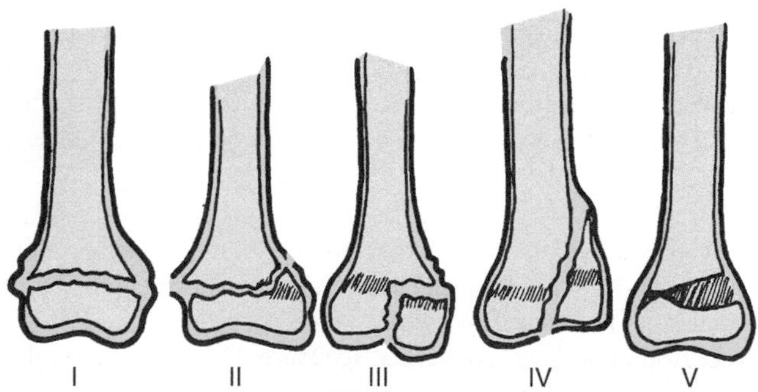

FIG. 33.25 Types of physeal injuries developed by orthopedists R. B. Salter and W. R. Harris: type I, separation or slip of growth plate without fracture of the bone; type II, separation of growth plate and breaking off of section of metaphysis; type III, fracture of physis extending through the epiphysis into the joint surface; type IV, fracture of growth plate, epiphysis, and metaphysis; type V, crushing, comminuted fracture of the physis.

TABLE 33.3 Stages of Bone Healing

Time*	Physiologic Events
Stage 1: Hematoma Formation	
Impact	Fracture occurs.
	Injury to soft tissue envelops site.
	Periosteal tissue tears.
	Vessels rupture.
3-5 minutes	Bleeding occurs from bone and tissues into area between and around bone fragments.
First 24 hours	Hematoma forms and clots; fibrin assists in clotting periosteal membrane to aid in repair.
	Clot provides fibrin network for cellular invasion.
	Granulation tissue forms by fibroblasts and new capillaries.
	Osteoblastic activity stimulated.
Stage 2: Cellular Proliferation	
After 24 hours	Blood supply increases, bringing available calcium, phosphate, and fibroblasts.
	Cells proliferate at ends of bone fragments and differentiate into cartilage and connective tissue.
Next few days	Hematoma becomes granulation tissue, which develops into a framework for bone-forming substances.
	Fibroblasts convert to osteoblasts (bone marrow–forming cells).
2-3 days	*Halisteresis* (softening of bone ends) occurs for ⅛ to ¼ inch; bone cells are resorbed.
Stage 3: Callus Formation	
6-10 days	Fibroblasts form in granulation tissue; form bone in areas adjacent to surface of bone shaft; form cartilage at surfaces more distal to blood supply.
	Provisional callus develops, bridging fracture ends; holds bone together but will not support body weight.
14-21 days	*True callus* develops, seen on radiographs; more than needed is formed, but with remodeling, excess callus is resorbed.
	Cartilage differentiates to bone tissue.
Stage 4: Ossification	
3-10 weeks	Callus forms into bone, which grows beneath periosteum of fragments; fuses (knits together) fracture defect.
	Also called *union stage.*
Stage 5: Consolidation and Remodeling	
After 9 months	Bone marrow cavity is restored.
	Compact bone forms according to stress patterns.
	Remodeling occurs according to Wolff's law.
	Fracture line is always visible on radiographs.

*Healing time is more rapid in infants and in cancellous (spongy) bone; may be delayed if complications occur.

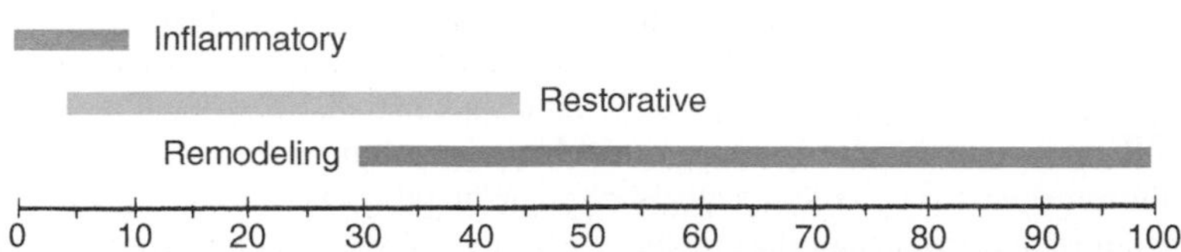

FIG. 33.26 Approximate time spent in inflammatory, restorative, and remodeling phases of bone healing. Scale indicates percentage of healing time.

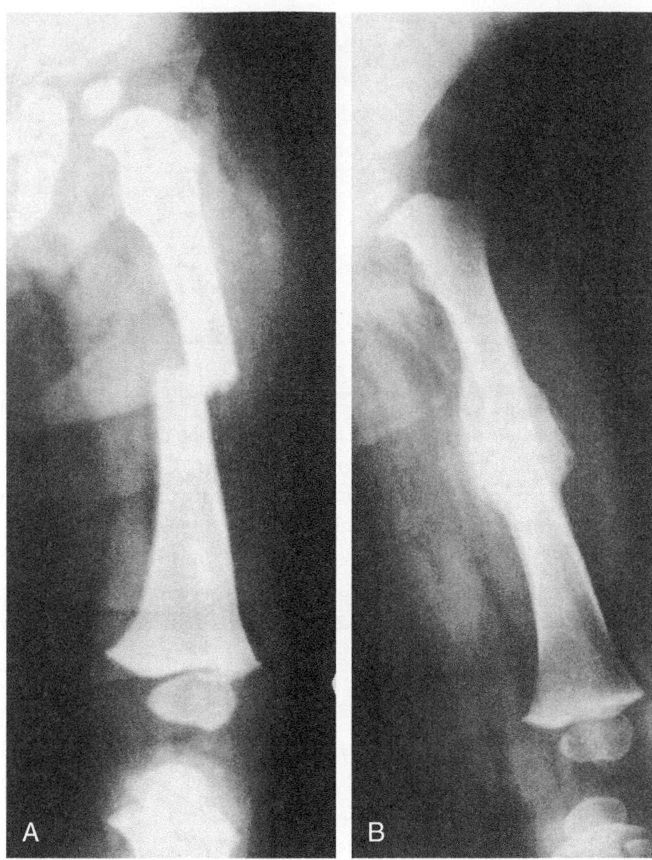

FIG. 33.27 Fractured femur. Most femur fractures in childhood are of the spiral type shown here. Note comparison of **A,** original x-ray film, and **B,** 6-month postfracture film showing callus formation.

- Neonatal period—2 to 3 weeks
- Early childhood—4 weeks
- Later childhood—6 to 8 weeks
- Adolescence—8 to 12 weeks

Remodeling is a unique process that occurs in the healing of long bone fractures in growing children. When a bone remodels, the irregularities produced by the fracture become distinct because hollows are filled in and angles are rounded off in the healing process, which gives the bone a straighter, more typical appearance. The buildup of new bone or callus restores a portion of the normal bone structure in most cases despite observable malalignment. The younger the child and the closer the proximity of the fracture to the growth plate, the greater the degree of remodeling that is able to take place. Various factors such as the type and location of the fracture, the child's age, and the amount of fragment angulation or rotation influence the degree of correction in alignment that can be obtained by remodeling.

The position of the bone fragments in relation to one another influences the rapidity of healing and the residual deformity. For example, a gap between fragments delays (or prevents) healing (Fig. 33.28, *A*). Healing is prompt and complete with end-to-end apposition (Fig. 33.28, *B*), but the fracture can stimulate accelerated growth of the neighboring physis, causing bony overgrowth and increased length of the extremity. Angulation deformity caused by an incomplete fracture (Fig. 33.28, *C*) may remodel in the young child, but the degree of residual deformity depends on the relationship of the angulation of the bone fragments to the angle of the joint. This requires careful evaluation and reduction to prevent permanent deformity.

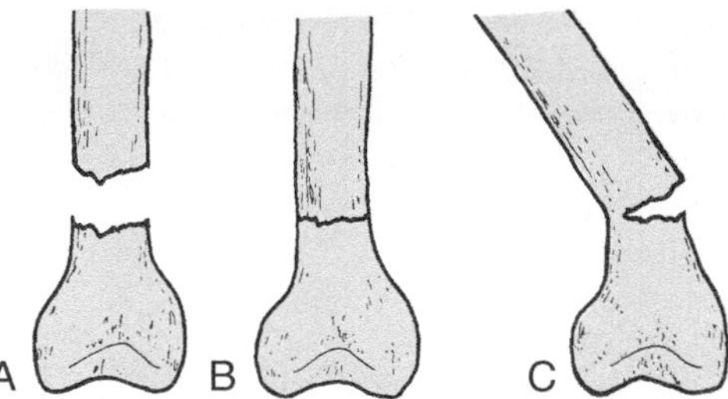

FIG. 33.28 Relationships of fracture fragments. **A,** Gap between fragments. **B,** End-to-end apposition. **C,** Angulation of incomplete fracture.

Wolff's law is applied in treating children with orthopedic problems. Paraphrased, it states that bone will grow in the direction in which stress is placed on it. Examples of the use of this law are the hip spica cast with an abduction bar for treating developmental dysplasia of the hip and application of casts or traction at a selected angle to influence the direction of bone healing.

Bone healing in any age-group is greatly influenced by the traumatized person's general health. The child with a fracture requires adequate nutrition for optimum bone healing. When nutritional intake is insufficient, vitamin and mineral supplementation may be necessary. Consumption of soda should be limited or completely eliminated as the phosphoric acid in these drinks may interfere with calcium absorption.

Diagnostic Evaluation

A history of the injury or events leading up to the injury is helpful but often may be lacking for childhood injuries. Infants and toddlers are unable to clearly communicate the details of what occurred. Older children may not be reliable informants or volunteer information (even under direct questioning) if the injury occurred during questionable activities. In cases of child abuse, parents or caregivers may deliberately give false information to protect themselves or family members. Whenever possible, it is helpful to get information from someone who witnessed the injury.

Children demonstrate the usual signs of injury: generalized swelling, pain or tenderness, and diminished functional use of the affected part. There may be bruising or severe muscular rigidity which are also frequent signs in adults. More often, the fracture is remarkably stable because of the usually intact periosteum. The child may even be able to use an affected arm or walk on a fractured leg.

Although neurologic and vascular damage is much less frequent in children than in adult patients, the integrity of these structures must be thoroughly assessed. This is often difficult in infants and young children, who are unable to cooperate. Vascular injury is most likely to occur with supracondylar fractures of the humerus and femur. Femoral and popliteal vessels and the sciatic nerve are prone to trauma in femoral fractures. Humeral fractures may cause damage to the medial, ulnar, or radial nerves and to the brachial artery.

Radiographic examination is the most useful diagnostic tool for assessing skeletal trauma. The calcium deposits in bone make the entire structure radiopaque. However, during normal growth and development, much of the skeleton of infants and young children is composed of radiolucent growth cartilage that does not appear on radiographs. Radiographs are sometimes less reliable than gross deformity and point tenderness in predicting extremity fractures. Health care providers may also obtain a film of the uninjured limb for a direct comparison to help identify minor alterations in alignment. Radiographic films are also taken after fracture reduction and during the healing process to confirm satisfactory progress.

BOX 33.5 Factors in Determining the Reduction Method for Fractures

- Age of child
- Degree of displacement
- Amount of overriding (bone)
- Degree of edema
- Condition of skin and soft tissue
- Sensation and circulation distal to fracture

! NURSING ALERT

A fracture should be strongly suspected in a small child who refuses to walk or crawl. However, the fact that a child walks on a suspected fractured extremity does not rule out a fracture.

Therapeutic Management

The goals of fracture management are as follows:

- To reestablish alignment and length of the bony fragments (reduction)
- To retain alignment and length (immobilization)
- To restore function to the injured parts
- To prevent further injury and deformity

The majority of children's fractures heal well, and nonunion is rare. Fractures are splinted (see Research Focus box) or casted to immobilize and protect the injured extremity. Children with displaced fractures may have a surgical reduction and fixation (internal or external) rather than being immobilized by traction. Box 33.5 describes factors that determine the type of reduction method for fractures. Some injuries may require immediate medical attention. These include open fractures, compartment syndrome with and without fracture, fractures associated with vascular or nerve injuries, and joint dislocations that cannot be reduced.

RESEARCH FOCUS

Removable Splints

Boutis, Willan, Babyn, and colleagues (2010) randomized treatment of minimally displaced distal radius fractures in children with either a short arm cast or wrist splint for 4 weeks. There was no difference between the two groups in fracture displacement or functional outcomes. The children and families were more satisfied and preferred splinting over cast immobilization.

In children, immobilization is used until adequate callus is formed. Weight bearing and active movement for the purpose of regaining function can begin after the fracture site is stable. The child's natural tendency to be active is usually sufficient to restore normal mobility, and physical or occupational therapy is rarely indicated.

Children are most frequently hospitalized for fracture of the femur. If simple reduction cannot be achieved or a neurovascular problem is detected after injury, observation in a hospital setting may be indicated. The trend is to avoid hospitalization. See Box 33.6 for medical interventions for the child with a fracture injury.

Nursing Care Management

Nurses often conduct the initial assessment of a child with a suspected fracture (see Emergency Treatment box). The child and parents may be frightened and upset, and the child is often in pain. Therefore if the child is alert and there is no sign of hemorrhage, the initial nursing interventions are directed at calming and reassuring the child and parents so that a more thorough assessment can be easily accomplished.

BOX 33.6 Medical Interventions for Fracture Injury

- Control of pain, hemorrhage, and edema
- Relief of muscle spasms
- Realignment of fracture fragments
- Promotion of bone healing
- Immobilization of fracture until adequate healing has begun
- Prevention of secondary complications
- Limitation of disuse syndrome
- Restoration of function

EMERGENCY TREATMENT

Fracture

Assess the extent of injury—five *P*s:

- Pain and point of tenderness
- Pulselessness—distal to the fracture site (late and ominous sign)
- Pallor
- Paresthesia—sensation distal to the fracture site
- Paralysis—movement distal to the fracture site

Determine the mechanism of injury.

Move the injured part as little as possible.

Cover open wounds with sterile or clean dressing.

Immobilize the limb, including the joints above and below the fracture site; do not attempt to reduce the fracture or push protruding bone under the skin.

- Soft splint (with pillow or folded towel)
- Rigid splint (rolled newspaper or magazine)
- Uninjured leg can serve as splint for leg fracture if no splint is available

Reassess neurovascular status.

Apply manual traction if circulatory compromise is present.

Elevate the injured limb if possible.

Apply cold to the injured area (no longer than 20 minutes with each application).

Call emergency medical services or transport to medical facility.

While maintaining a calm manner, the nurse can ask the parents and older child to describe what happened. The child may arrive with the limb supported in some manner; if not, carefully immobilize the affected site. If the limb is immobilized, it may be best not to touch the child initially but to ask him or her to point to the painful area and wiggle the fingers or toes distal to the injury. At this point, the child may feel relatively safe and allow someone to gently touch the area just enough to feel the pulses and test for sensation. A child's anxiety is greatly influenced by previous experiences with injury and health care personnel. However, the child needs to be told what will happen and what he or she can do to help. The affected limb need not be palpated and should not be moved unless properly splinted. A temporary splint should be applied carefully if the child must be transported to a medical facility or radiology department. Parental anxiety may heighten the child's reaction and fear. It is important to reassure the parents that their child will receive the necessary care, including pain management.

FRACTURE COMPLICATIONS

Circulatory Impairment

If the trauma or immobilizing device restricts blood flow in veins or arteries of the affected extremity, bone healing will be seriously impaired. Careful assessment of the pulses, capillary refill, skin color, and temperature is an important nursing responsibility. In the upper extremity, brachial, radial, ulnar, and digital pulses are felt. In the leg, femoral, popliteal, posterior tibial, and dorsalis pedis pulses are checked. After injury, swelling of tissues occurs more rapidly in the child than in the adult.

Closely associated with an inadequate blood supply is a low hematocrit value, which can result from the initial blood loss or surgically induced anemia. Although the blood flow may be adequate, a lowered amount of hemoglobin will not provide a sufficient supply of oxygen for tissue repair.

Nerve Compression Syndromes

Nerve damage can occur at the time of injury, develop in the process of realignment, or arise as a complication of use of an immobilizing apparatus. The syndromes are classified according to the anatomic area affected and can involve the median nerve (carpal tunnel syndrome), ulnar nerve (at wrist or elbow), radial nerve, posterior tibial nerve (tarsal tunnel syndrome), common peroneal nerve, or sciatic nerve. Peroneal nerve damage can result in footdrop, and radial nerve impairment produces wristdrop. Both these disabilities can significantly interfere with activities of daily living.

Sensory testing with touch and pinprick and evaluation of motor strength by asking the child to move the unaffected joint distal to the injury are common means of determining neurologic involvement. Subjective symptoms are pain or discomfort, muscular weakness, a burning sensation, limitation of motion, and altered sensation. Because the fear of pain limits the child's cooperation, play can be the nurse's most valuable tool.

Treatment is alleviation of pressure on the nerve. The health care provider determines whether correcting the alignment will alleviate pressure on the nerve or whether surgical intervention is necessary. At times, sensory or motor changes indicate ischemia, and the treatment is correction of the vascular disturbance.

Compartment Syndromes

A compartment is a group of muscles surrounded by tough, inelastic fascial tissue. **Compartment syndrome** occurs when pressure within this closed space increases and compromises circulation to the muscles and nerves within the space. Muscles and nerves of both upper and lower extremities are enclosed within such compartments. The most frequent causes of compartment syndrome are tight dressings or casts, skin traction, hemorrhage, trauma, burns, and surgery. Other causes include an increase in compartment contents (e.g., hemorrhage, venous obstruction, infiltrated IV infusion, exudate) and externally applied pressure, such as lying on the affected limb.

> **! NURSING ALERT**
>
> Assessing for compartment syndrome includes monitoring for the five *P*s of ischemia (pain, pallor, pulselessness, paresthesia, and paralysis).

Signs and symptoms of compartment syndrome reflect a deficit in or deterioration of neuromuscular status in the anatomic area surrounding the involved structures. Clinical manifestations of compartment syndrome may occur as early as 30 minutes after the ischemia develops and can be difficult to recognize in small children or in those who have a head injury. A palpable peripheral pulse and brisk capillary refill may be present despite increasing compartmental pressure. Tenseness may be noted on palpation of the area. The neuromuscular symptoms of compartment syndrome are severe pain that is out of proportion to the injury (although pain is not always a manifestation), pallor or cyanosis, edema, absence of pulses in the extremity, loss of sensation, and motor weakness. Sensory deficit in the affected limb is reported to be the most reliable physical finding of compartment syndrome (Mencio, Swiontkowski, & Green, 2015).

Unrelieved, the occlusive hypoxic process can cause some contracture if ischemia lasts as little as 6 hours. A great deal of muscle damage occurs after 12 to 24 hours; 48 hours of ischemia produces severe deformity, with muscle fibrosis and contractures in 5 to 10 days. If not treated, the contracture leads to severe deformity and paralysis.

The immediate treatment is to remove any mechanically obstructive materials, such as tight bandages, and extend the joint to free blood vessels. If the symptoms do not improve within a few hours, arteriography is done in anticipation of a possible need for surgical intervention (**fasciotomy**) to decrease arterial spasms and to improve the blood supply by separation of the fascial sheaths of the involved muscles. Elevation of the affected extremity is not recommended and may further decrease blood flow to the area. Because early detection is important in preventing permanent damage to tissues, in certain high-risk situations specialists may recommend continuous monitoring of compartment pressures by way of a small, slit-tip catheter; Wick catheter; or needle inserted into the compartment.

Volkmann contracture (ischemic muscular atrophy) is a serious, persistent flexion contraction of the forearm and hand caused by massive infarction of muscle. Pressure caused by a cast or tight bandage or by swelling from the injury in the area of the elbow begins with arterial occlusion and then progresses to muscle anoxia and reflex vasospasms. Finally, the lack of blood supply leads to muscle necrosis and replacement with fibrous tissue, which produces paralysis and a clawlike hand contracture. Any fracture that requires excessive traction can be complicated by Volkmann contracture; however, it occurs most often in the elbow.

Physeal Damage

Growth of bone originates from the physis or growth plate, and damage to this structure can result in unequal lengths of the extremities or angular deformity. This is most concerning in the lower extremities. Surgical intervention may be required if the limb length inequality becomes large enough. This may involve slowing the growth on the longer leg with a procedure called an epiphyseodesis or lengthening the bones in the shorter or affected extremity. Angular deformities may develop if a physeal bar or bony bridge forms across the growth plate. If less than 50% of the physis is involved a surgical procedure to resect the bar may be performed.

Nonunion

Bone healing and callus formation can span and repair only a limited space between bone fragments. When bone fragments cannot be maintained in correct alignment for repair due to inadequate reduction or poor immobilization, bone healing is impaired. The factors most likely to interfere with bone healing and to cause delayed union or nonunion, based on the physiologic needs for bone healing, are listed in Box 33.7.

The hematoma, which becomes the matrix for bone deposition in the break, must be free of infection or bits of adipose or connective tissue. Nutrients and bone-forming cells brought to the area by way of the bloodstream provide the vital ingredients for repair.

BOX 33.7 Factors That Interfere With Bone Healing

- Separation of bone fragments at fracture site
- Interposition of tissue between bone fragments
- Loss of bone tissue, especially from necrosis
- Infection
- Poor nutrition
- Interruption of blood supply
- Diseases that influence calcium metabolism (e.g., vitamin D deficiency)
- Bone cancer
- Administration of corticosteroids

Sometimes artificial means are employed to facilitate bone healing. Bone grafting becomes necessary when bone nonunion occurs. The donor site is usually the tibia or the iliac crest. Bleeding of bone ends may need to be artificially stimulated, and at times holes are drilled near the bone ends in an attempt to increase circulation. Postsurgical immobilization of the recipient area is crucial to the success of the graft. The Ilizarov external fixator may also be used to assist bone healing in patients with nonunion (see p. 1255).

Malunion

Malunion is fracture union with increased angulation or deformity at the fracture site. It can be detected at any stage in the healing process or after complete healing. Unsatisfactory reduction is the usual reason for malunion. A cast or splint that allows fracture movement will also likely result in malunion. Periodic radiographic examinations help detect this complication and prevent it from becoming a major long-term problem.

Excessive deformity can be corrected during the healing process through realignment and reimmobilization. However, attempts at correction may cause delayed union or nonunion; therefore the degree of deformity is carefully evaluated in light of these complications. The probability that sufficient spontaneous alignment will occur with growth and continuation of the healing process also is considered. Correction of the malunion when healing is near completion or completed requires surgical intervention.

Infection

Osteomyelitis, infection of the bone, is often secondary to a bloodstream infection but is a potential risk with open fractures, pressure ulcers, or when bone surgery has been performed. Any bacterial organism can cause this infectious process; however, *Staphylococcus aureus* is the pathogen most frequently identified (Pediatric Orthopaedic Society of North America, 2011) (see p. 1284 for a discussion of osteomyelitis).

Kidney Stones

Although uncommon in children, development of renal calculi is a potential risk whenever the child has a limb that is non–weight bearing for a long time, especially if the circumstances also produce urinary stasis. Measures to prevent the formation of renal calculi include maintaining optimal hydration, mobilizing the child as much as possible, and checking closely the amount and characteristics of urinary output. Any urinary tract infection should be treated promptly with appropriate antimicrobials and urine acidification because the nucleus of a calculus is often composed of bacterial debris or calcium and the buildup of stone is precipitated by alkaline urine. An associated problem, hypercalcemia, was reviewed in the section on problems of the immobilized child.

Pulmonary Emboli

Blood, air, or fat emboli can be a hazard to the child with a fracture. As postinjury bleeding and clotting occur, a small piece of the clot has the potential to travel to vital organs, such as the lung, heart, or brain, and produce a life-threatening vascular obstruction and ischemia. Generally the pulmonary system is the most frequent site of emboli deposition, but it may not occur until 6 to 8 weeks after the injury.

Fat emboli are the greatest threat in an individual with multiple fractures, particularly fractures of the long bones such as the femur. Fat droplets from the marrow are transferred to the general circulation by the venous-arterial route, where they can be transported to the lung or brain. This type of embolism occurs within the first 24 hours, generally in the second 12 hours after the injury occurs. Adolescents are those usually affected in the pediatric age-groups.

Intermittent compression devices are used to prevent venous pooling in the lower extremities when prolonged immobilization is required. These devices are inflatable sleeves that allow cyclic emptying and filling of leg veins; the devices are used in children with spinal cord injury once mobilization is initiated to decrease the effects of orthostatic intolerance. Anticoagulant drug therapy, passive and active range of motion, and early mobilization are also used to decrease venous stasis and prevent thrombus development.

! NURSING ALERT

Pulmonary embolism should be suspected in a child with a history of recent surgery, major trauma, or prolonged immobilization who suddenly develops chest pain and dyspnea. The severe dyspnea must be treated immediately by elevating the head when possible and administering oxygen by mask or nasal cannula; an IV line should be established. This is a medical emergency.

INJURIES AND HEALTH PROBLEMS RELATED TO SPORTS PARTICIPATION

Adolescents probably spend more time and energy practicing and participating in sports activities than members of any other age-group. Sports and game participation contributes significantly to growth and development, the education process, and good health. It provides exercise for growing muscles, interaction with peers, and a socially acceptable means of enjoying stimulation and conflict. In addition, competitive activities help the child and adolescent engage in self-appraisal and develop self-respect and concern for others.

Every sport has some potential for injury to the participant—whether the young person participates in serious competition or purely for enjoyment. Serious injury is not limited to the athlete who competes in rough contact sports; a large number of severe or fatal injuries occur to those who engage in milder physical activity but are not physically prepared for it. For example, a person's body build may not be suited to the sport, muscles and support systems (respiratory and cardiovascular) may not have been sufficiently conditioned to withstand the rigors of the physical stress, or the child or adolescent may not possess the insight and judgment to recognize when an activity is beyond his or her capabilities. Rapidly growing bones, muscles, joints, and tendons are especially vulnerable to unusual strain.

Awkward and inexperienced children or adolescents may suffer more injury than those who are more experienced. Strong muscles are less easily damaged than weak ones and provide better protection to the joints they cross. Fatigue significantly impairs muscle function and judgment. Although team sports give rise to frequent injuries, serious injuries resulting from recreational and individual sports are generally

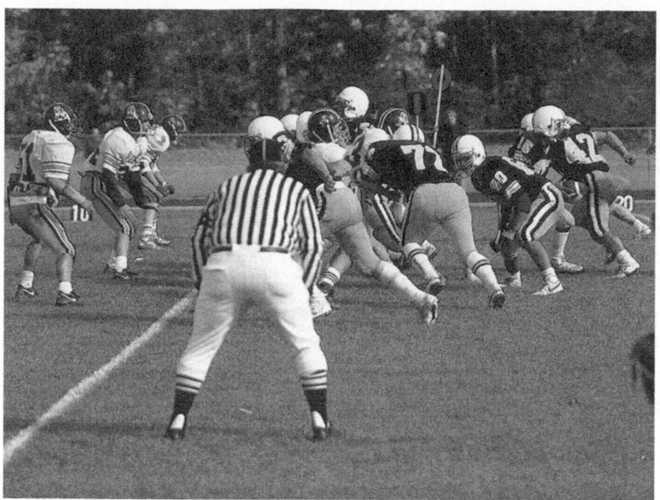

FIG. 33.29 Football is an example of a strenuous collision sport with a high risk of serious injury.

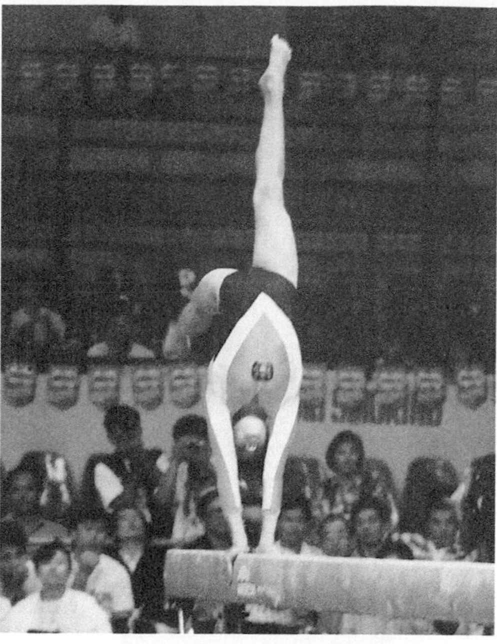

FIG. 33.30 Gymnastics is an example of a strenuous limited-contact, limited-collision sport with a high risk of serious injury.

more common. The increase in strength and vigor in adolescence may tempt children to overextend themselves.

Not only does the activity itself pose a hazard of greater or lesser degree, but the environment and the sports or recreational equipment present additional risks. Adolescents participate in physical activities in a variety of environments, both indoors and outdoors, on floors, the ground, snow or ice, on or beneath water surfaces, and sometimes in free air space. These activities frequently involve equipment that increases risk.

PREPARATION FOR SPORTS

Among adolescents of the same age, the degree of physical maturation varies greatly, and many of the physical characteristics important in sports are related to hormone production. Consequently, physical strength, coordination, endurance, and size vary considerably among children and adolescents who wish to compete against one another. Sports competition between young people who differ markedly in strength and agility is unfair and hazardous. Matching of candidates for sports should be based on physical maturity, height, weight, and physical fitness and skills, particularly in sports involving rigorous body contact.

Categorizing sports and activities according to the probability of collision and strenuousness can help estimate the risk of one sustaining an injury. Collision or contact sports such as tackle football, basketball, hockey, and soccer tend to have the highest injury rates, followed by other contact sports (Figs. 33.29 and 33.30). In addition, the American Academy of Pediatrics has published guidelines that provide criteria for determining inclusion or exclusion of the young athlete based on common medical and surgical conditions and relative risks in various sports categories. This serves as a useful guideline for the health professional in counseling youth regarding sports activities (Rice & Council on Sports Medicine and Fitness, 2008).

The American Academy of Pediatrics, Council on Sports Medicine and Fitness (2011) encourages sports participation by young persons and encourages adults close to sports activities to be aware of the early warning signs of fatigue, dehydration, and injury. Athletes should seek assistance when an injury is suspected and not "work through" injuries caused by overuse—for example, shin splints, stress fractures, tendinitis, and apophysitis.

The role of health care professionals, specifically nurses, in relation to sports injuries focuses on prevention, treatment, and rehabilitation. Of these areas, prevention is perhaps the most important. It is difficult to "sell" prevention, however, especially to children. Anticipatory guidance is an important aspect of preventive counseling for sports injuries because many injuries occur when children are tired and not concentrating on their activities. Injuries are also more common when participants are distracted by events off the field of play.

Youth who are actively involved in athletic programs need to undergo medical evaluation as a prerequisite to participation and to receive education in sports skills using correct training and conditioning methods. Children should use appropriate protective equipment that is properly maintained and fitted. The sports environment should make maximum provision for safety and availability of first aid and medical services.

The same protective principles apply to enthusiasts in noncompetitive sports. They need the same education in basic safety precautions, encouragement to acquire proper instruction in the skills required for performing the activity (such as water safety, skiing techniques), and proper maintenance of equipment.

TYPES OF INJURY

The injuries sustained in sports or recreational activities can involve any part of the body and range from relatively minor cuts, bruises, and abrasions to severe closed head injuries such as concussion or totally incapacitating central nervous system injuries or death. Some of these injuries are discussed in chapters devoted to the major topic (e.g., spinal cord injuries [Chapter 33] and head injuries [Chapter 30]).

Some sports are particularly dangerous for children and adolescents. Snowmobiling, snowboarding, use of ATVs, in-line skating, skateboarding, motorcycle riding, full-contact hockey, bicycle riding, wave running, and using trampolines are examples of sports and recreational activities that can lead to significant injuries in connection with inappropriate use, failure to wear protective equipment, or participation by children who are underage. One study reported a high incidence of injuries in

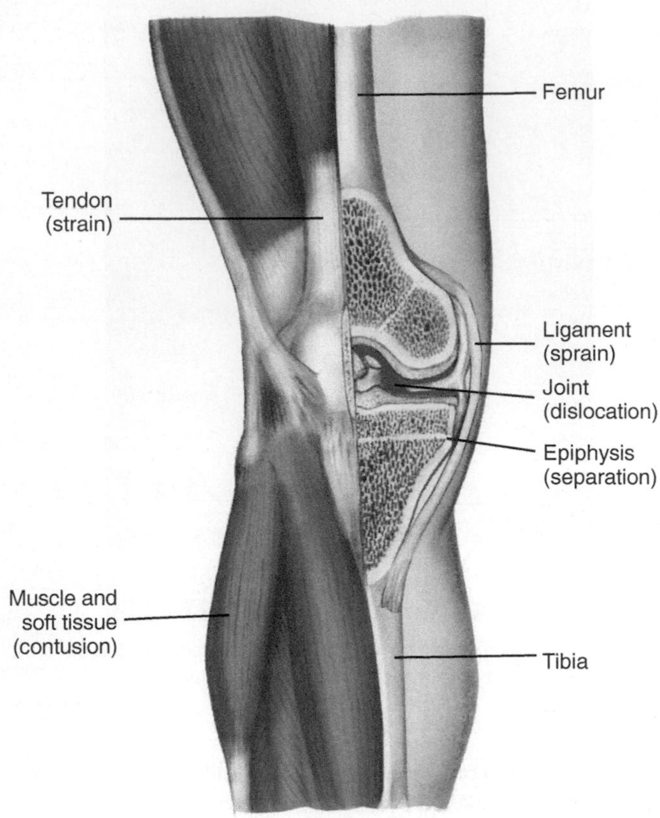

FIG. 33.31 Sites of injury to bones, joints, and soft tissues.

high school football athletic competition; boys' soccer had a high rate of head, neck, and face injuries; and high rates of concussion injuries occurred in boys' soccer (Rechel, Yard, & Comstock, 2008). Ankle injuries are the most common competitive sports–related injuries, with significant numbers occurring in boys' and girls' basketball (Nelson, Collins, Yard, et al., 2007). Recent attention has focused on the management and prevention of concussion injuries among adolescent as well as adult athletes. The majority of concussions occurred in boys' football and ice hockey, with girls' soccer being a major cause for collision injury and concussion (Marar, McIlvain, Fields, et al., 2012).

A variety of injuries can result when an external force is applied that causes severe stress on tissue, muscle, and skeletal structures (Fig. 33.31). The body structures attempt to absorb the force, but when they are unable to do so, injuries occur. Two general types of injury are recognized. The first is acute trauma, which is defined as a sudden, acute injury from a major force. Among such injuries are fractures of long bones and the axial skeleton; sprains of joint ligaments; strains of muscle tendon units; and contusions, including those of muscle tendon units and overlying soft tissue. The second type is repetitive overuse injuries, or microtrauma, which result from repetitive injury to tissue over a long period. Overuse injuries include stress fractures, bursitis, tendonitis, apophysitis, and at times injuries of the joint surface.

CONTUSIONS

Contusions are a common sports injury and are often considered to be "part of the game." A contusion is damage to the soft tissue, subcutaneous structures, and muscle. The tearing of these tissues and small blood vessels and the ensuing inflammatory response lead to hemorrhage, edema, and associated pain when the child or adolescent attempts to move the injured part. The escape of blood into the tissues is observed as ecchymosis, a black-and-blue discoloration.

The most serious contusions are those involving the quadriceps; they are common in strenuous, collision-type sports and usually result from being kicked or kneed in the thigh. Large contusions cause gross swelling, pain, and disability and usually receive immediate attention from health care personnel. The less spectacular, smaller injuries may go unnoticed, so continued participation is allowed. They can become disabling after rest, however, because of pain and muscle spasm. The young athlete is frequently instructed to "work it out" or disregard the pain. *Myositis ossificans* may occur from deep contusions to the biceps or quadriceps muscles; this condition may result in a restriction of flexibility of the affected limb.

Immediate treatment of a contusion consists of application of cold as in the treatment of sprains described later. Return to participation is allowed when the strength and range of motion of the affected extremity are equal to those of the opposite extremity.

DISLOCATIONS

Long bones are held in approximation to one another at the joint by ligaments. Joints can be tight or loose, and loose joints are more likely to be dislocated. A dislocation occurs when the force of stress on the ligament is great enough to disrupt the normal position of the opposing bone ends or the bone end and its socket. The predominant symptom is pain that increases with attempted passive or active movement of the extremity. In dislocations there may be an obvious deformity and inability to move the joint. Simple dislocations should be reduced as soon as possible with the child under mild sedation and often local anesthesia. Increased swelling, which makes reduction difficult and increases the risk of neurovascular problems, can complicate an unreduced dislocation. Treatment depends on the location and severity of the injury.

Dislocations are less common in children than in those who are skeletally mature, but some types are specific to the younger age-groups. Before final closure of the physis (growth plate), injuries to the joints are more likely to cause separation of the epiphysis from the metaphysis (growth plate injury) than dislocation.

One of the most vulnerable joints is the shoulder, which is structurally insecure, having only a rotator cuff to maintain the shoulder in place. The joint is shallow with relatively little muscle protection; therefore the capsule becomes stretched and the joint is vulnerable to dislocation. There is a high incidence of shoulder injuries in male gymnasts and a greater incidence of shoulder injuries in players of contact sports, such as football. Temporary restriction of the joint with a sling or bandage that secures the arm to the chest in a shoulder dislocation provides sufficient comfort and immobilization until the child or adolescent can receive medical help.

In children younger than 5 years of age, the hip can be dislocated by a fall. The greatest risk after this injury is the potential loss of blood supply to the head of the femur. Children with naturally lax joints, such as those with Down syndrome, are more prone to recurrent dislocation of the hip. In hip dislocation the best chance for prevention of damage to the head of the femur is to relocate the hip within 60 minutes after the injury occurs. As the length of time between injury and hip relocation increases, the risk of irreparable damage increases.

Dislocation of the patella occurs spontaneously in some children; in others it is a result of injury. The patella is typically dislocated laterally. Most dislocations are reduced either spontaneously or by a companion before a provider sees the child. Therapy is immobilization for 3 to 4 weeks. Surgery may be indicated to treat recurrent dislocations.

Radial head subluxation, also called *pulled elbow* or *nursemaid's elbow,* is a common injury in children ages 1 to 4 years. Typically, it occurs when a child receives a sudden longitudinal pull or traction at the wrist while the arm is fully extended and the forearm is pronated, causing the radial head to partially dislocate due to a weak or loose annular ligament. Often an adult is holding the child by the hand or wrist and gives a sudden jerk to prevent a fall or attempts to lift the child by pulling the wrist, or the child suddenly pulls away by dropping to the floor (or ground). The child has an anxious expression, whines, complains of pain in the elbow and wrist, refuses to move the arm, and holds it with the opposite hand and in a slightly flexed and pronated position against his or her body. The medical provider achieves reduction by applying firm finger pressure to the head of the radius and then supinating and flexing the forearm to return the bone structures to normal alignment. A click or clunk may be heard or felt, and functional use of the arm returns within minutes. Immobilization of the arm is not necessary. The longer the subluxation is present, however, the longer it takes for the child to recover mobility after treatment. A radiograph may be needed if attempts to reduce the dislocation are not successful.

SPRAINS AND STRAINS

Sprains and strains are the most common high school sports-related injury. A sprain occurs when trauma to a joint is so severe that a ligament is either stretched or partially or completely torn by the force created as a joint is twisted or wrenched. This is often accompanied by damage to associated blood vessels, muscles, tendons, and nerves. As a guideline for management and prognosis, sprains are classified according to the degree of injury (Box 33.8). Because of the number of ligaments required to maintain knee stability, the knee is one of the joints most commonly injured in sports. It is also the largest joint and consequently is more prone to injury. Ankle sprains in children account for approximately 75% of all ankle injuries (Guinta & Rocker, 2013). These injuries are common in individuals who participate in sports, especially in the pediatric age-group.

The presence of joint laxity is the most valid indicator of the severity of a sprain. With a severe injury the athlete complains that the joint "feels loose" or as if "something is coming apart" and may describe hearing a "snap," "pop," or "tearing." Pain is seldom the principal subjective symptom. There is a rapid onset with swelling, often diffuse, accompanied by immediate disability and appreciable reluctance to use the injured joint.

A strain is a microscopic tear to the musculotendinous unit and has features in common with sprains. The area is painful to the touch and is swollen. The severity is evaluated as grade I, II, or III, as for sprains, except that the degree of laxity does not apply. Even with severe grade III injuries, complaints of laxity are rare. Most strains happen over time rather than suddenly, and the rapidity of the appearance provides clues regarding severity. In general the more rapidly the strain occurs, the more severe the injury. When the strain involves the muscular portion, there is more bleeding, often palpable soon after injury and before edema obscures the hematoma.

BOX 33.8 Classification of Sprains

Grade I—Mild injury; involves overstretching or microscopic tearing but without hemorrhage or increased instability of the involved joint. Swelling may develop later.

Grade II—Moderate injury; involves partial, overt tearing of the ligament with at least some ligamentous continuity remaining; usually immediate pain and swelling with decreased function.

Grade III—Severe injury; total loss of ligamentous continuity (i.e., disruption of one or more ligaments or the musculotendinous unit). Pain is immediate but subsides because none of the pain fibers is being stretched. Swelling may be minimal because hemorrhage extravasates outside of the area into soft tissues.

Therapeutic Management

The first 6 to 12 hours is the most critical period for virtually all soft tissue injuries. Basic principles for managing sprains and other soft tissue injuries are summarized in the acronyms RICE and ICES:

R—Rest
I—Ice
C—Compression
E—Elevation
I—Ice
C—Compression
E—Elevation
S—Support

Soft tissue injuries should be iced immediately. This is best accomplished using crushed ice or a bag of frozen vegetables. An elastic wrap may be applied to provide compression and to keep the ice pack in place. A single layer of the wrap or cloth is placed over the injured area to protect the skin under the ice pack, and the remainder of the bandage secures the pack in place.

There is still controversy over whether heat or ice should be used during the rehabilitative phase of management. Regardless of the method used, it should be accompanied by appropriate exercise, depending on the severity of the injury, and carried out under the direction of a competent professional experienced in the care of sports injuries.

Ice has a rapid cooling effect on tissues that reduces pain and the magnitude of the stretch reflex by decreasing muscle spindle response, afferent nerve discharge, and the afferent loop response (monosynaptic reflex). Secondary effects are achieved by vasoconstriction, decrease in muscle nerve velocity, and increase in muscle viscosity. Also, the decreased temperature slows metabolism, which reduces tissue oxygen requirements. Edema formation is reduced when fewer histamine-like substances are released. Nine to 15 minutes of ice exposure produces deep-tissue vasodilation without increased metabolism. However, the effects last up to 7 hours. Ice therapy should be intermittent, and ice should never be applied for more than 30 minutes at a time to prevent tissue damage.

Elevating the extremity uses gravity to facilitate venous return and reduce edema formation in the damaged area. The point of injury must be kept several inches above the level of the heart for therapy to be effective (Fig. 33.32). Several pillows can be used effectively for elevation. Allowing the extremity to be dependent causes excessive fluid accumulation in the area of injury, which delays healing and causes painful swelling.

Major sprains or tears to the ligamentous tissue rarely occur in growing children. Ligaments are stronger than bone, and the physis (growth plate) is the weakest part of the bone. The more typical site of injury is at the growth plate (see Growth Plate or Physeal Injuries, p. 1261). The trend with ankle sprains is to encourage early mobilization and strengthening rather than prolonged immobilization and rest. Torn ligaments in the knee are usually treated by immobilization with a knee immobilizer or range-of-motion brace until the child is able to walk without a limp. Crutches are used for mobility to rest the affected extremity. Passive leg exercises, gradually increased to active ones, begin as soon as sufficient healing has taken place. Caution parents and children against using any form of liniment or other heat-producing preparation before examination. If the injury requires casting or splinting, the heat

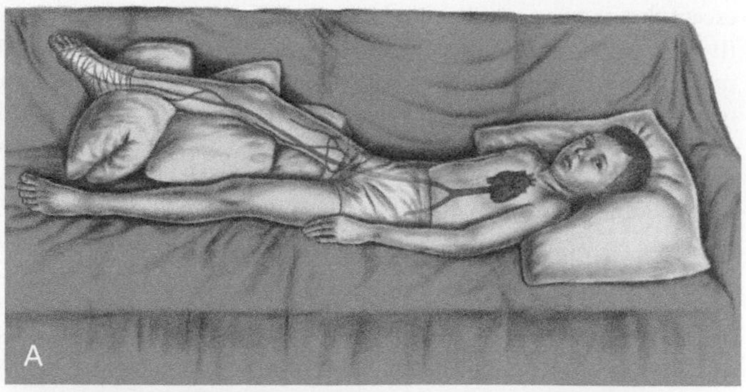

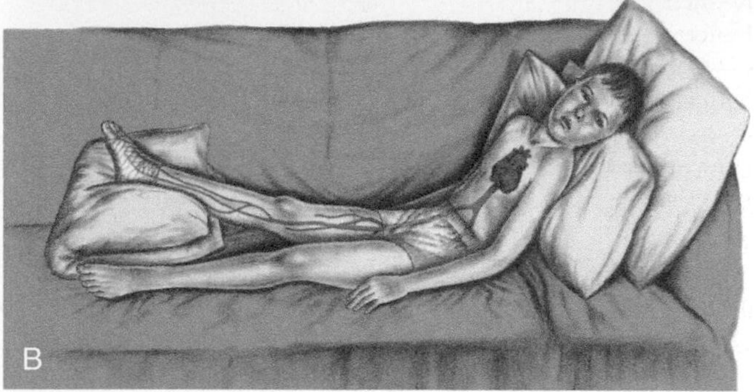

FIG. 33.32 Correct and incorrect methods for elevating a lower extremity. **A,** Correct method: lower leg elevated on pillows; ankle above heart level. **B,** Incorrect positioning: ankle below level of heart.

generated in the enclosed space can produce extreme discomfort and may even cause tissue damage.

In some cases torn knee ligaments are managed with arthroscopy and ligament repair or reconstruction as necessary, depending on the extent of the tear, the ligaments involved, and the person's age. Sometimes postoperative mobilization of the affected joint is implemented immediately using a continuous passive motion device. This device provides passive range-of-motion exercise to the injured extremity and decreases postoperative complications related to restricted mobility. The patient often is ambulatory within hours on crutches and is discharged late on the day of surgery or the following day.

OVERUSE INJURY

To excel in sports, the young athlete is forced to train longer, harder, and earlier in life than previously. The rewards are an increased level of fitness, better performance, faster times, and the satisfaction of attaining a personal goal. With the increase in the number of children participating in a wide variety of sports year-round, more overuse injuries are being seen in the pediatric age-group. More pediatric athletes are also specializing in one sport and participating year-round. Youth who participate in a variety of sports with adequate rest between seasons tend to have fewer injuries (Brenner & Council on Sports Medicine and Fitness, 2007; Hoang & Mortazavi, 2012).

The risk of overuse injury is always present and can be related to several factors: training errors, muscle-tendon imbalance, anatomic malalignment (e.g., femoral anteversion, excessive lumbar lordosis, tibial torsion), incorrect footwear or playing surface, an associated disease state, and growth (growth cartilage is less resistant to microtrauma). Chronic pain in athletes is often associated with overuse injury, which can occur at any level of athletic participation. The common feature in overuse injuries is the repetitive microtrauma that occurs to a particular anatomic structure. Performing the same movements time and time again can cause several types of injury: (1) frictional, or rubbing of one structure against another; (2) tractional, or repeated pull on a ligament or tendon; and (3) cyclic, or repetitive loading of impact forces (stress fractures). The end result is inflammation of the involved structure with complaints of pain, tenderness, swelling, and disability.

Bursae, tendons, muscles, ligaments, joints, and bones are all subject to overuse. Some of the more common overuse syndromes include plantar fasciitis, tennis elbow, Little League elbow, Osgood-Schlatter disease, swimmer's shoulder, and shin splints. Osgood-Schlatter disease (at the tibial tubercle in growing children) often occurs in children who are actively moving—for example, running and jumping. Athletes who run extensively frequently experience shin splints. The ligaments tear away from the tibial shaft, and this creates the pain. Ice, rest, and nonsteroidal antiinflammatory drugs (NSAIDs), such as ibuprofen or naproxen, are the usual treatment. The occurrence of overuse-type injuries, such as sore shoulders and strained elbows, may indicate that too much is being asked of the child in too short a period.

Stress Fractures

Given the intensity and duration of sports training, many young athletes suffer stress fractures, especially after a recent increase in training regimens. These fractures occur as a result of repeated muscle contraction and occur most often in sports involving repetitive weight bearing such as running, gymnastics, and basketball. They occur less often in swimming (in the upper extremities). Tibial stress fractures are most common.

The most common symptom of stress fracture is a sharp, persistent, progressive pain or a deep, persistent dull ache located over the bone. Sometimes there is pain on impact (heel strike), but the most important clinical sign is pain over the involved bony surface. Diagnosis is based on clinical observation. Plain radiographs are rarely diagnostic of stress fractures during the initial few weeks because callus formation is not yet evident. An MRI may more closely delineate a soft tissue injury/inflammation.

Therapeutic Management

Inflammation is common to all overuse syndromes; therefore management involves rest or alteration of activities, physical therapies, and medication. Rest is the primary therapy, usually interpreted as reduced activity and the use of alternative exercise—not bed rest or immobilization with casting. The main purpose is to alleviate the repetitive stress that initiated the symptoms. It is important to keep the child or adolescent mobile, and training can be continued. Alternative exercise is selected that maintains conditioning without aggravating the injury. For example, pool running (treading water in the deep end of a pool) uses the same movements as running but without the weight bearing. Bicycling, swimming, and rowing are viable alternatives.

Other modalities include cryotherapy and cold whirlpool baths, and sometimes taping, bracing, splinting, and other orthoses are employed, depending on the injury. Medications such as NSAIDs are sometimes prescribed to reduce inflammation and pain. Topical medications are of questionable value.

EXERCISE-INDUCED HEAT STRESS

Infants, children, and adolescents are at greater risk for heat-related illness than adults (American Academy of Pediatrics, Council on Sports Medicine and Fitness, 2011). Several characteristics of infants and children render them more vulnerable to heat stress. The greater ratio of surface area to body mass in infants and young children leads to increased transfer of heat between the body and the environment. Although infants do not exercise they may become overheated through environmental exposure (e.g., being left in a closed car). Children produce more metabolic heat for body mass during exercise and have a reduced capacity to convey heat from the body core to the skin. Also, children do not have the sweating capacity of adults and take longer to become acclimated to hot conditions. Young children may not feel the need to drink a sufficient amount of fluid during extended exercise.

Heat cramps are caused by sodium depletion, which in turn potentiates the effects of calcium on skeletal muscle. They most often occur as a result of strenuous exercise in a hot environment. Cramps most frequently involve the leg muscles. Vital signs are usually normal, but the core temperature may be elevated. The child sweats profusely, but mentation is normal. Treatment consists of rest and replacement of fluid and electrolytes. Ingestion of dilute sports drinks or electrolyte replacement liquids is helpful. Electrolyte replacement solutions are now available as popsicles and gelatin (like Jell-O), which are well tolerated with less vomiting. Replacement electrolyte strips that easily dissolve in the mouth are also available; small sips of a clear fluid such as water can be taken as tolerated.

Heat exhaustion, or heat stress, is a condition that usually occurs during vigorous exercise in a hot environment. It results from excessive loss of fluids, especially in poorly acclimated and dehydrated children. The onset may be gradual, with initial complaints that include thirst, headache, fatigue, dizziness, anxiety, or nausea and vomiting. The child usually has a clear sensorium but may be somewhat disoriented. The temperature can be normal or mildly elevated; sweating is profuse. Tachycardia, hypotension (usually postural), and syncope may be observed secondary to intravascular volume depletion. Treatment is to move the child to a cool environment, provide rest, and replace fluid volume. The child with a clear sensorium can receive oral replacement fluids, but often IV fluids are required due to vomiting. External cooling methods are not necessary.

Heatstroke represents a failure of normal thermoregulatory mechanisms. Heatstroke usually occurs during or immediately after physical activity, especially in the unacclimated adolescent who is exercising vigorously. The onset is rapid, with initial symptoms of headache, weakness, and disorientation. Central nervous system manifestations may be agitation, confusion, and lethargy. Loss of consciousness may occur without warning and may be accompanied by nuchal rigidity, posturing, and convulsions. Sweating may not be present. The temperature is typically higher than 104°F (40°C), and there is severe volume depletion. Immediate care is relocation to a cool environment, removal of clothing, application of cool water (wet towels or immersion), and use of fans. The child should be emergently transported to the nearest hospital.

Acute care includes rapid cooling until core temperature reaches 102°F (38.9°C) to prevent overcooling. Antipyretics are not used because they are metabolized by the liver, which is already not functioning properly. Renal and liver failure are common sequelae to heatstroke. Treatment includes careful monitoring of temperature and other vital signs, supportive care such as supplemental oxygen administration, and cautious fluid and electrolyte replacement. Prevention remains the best treatment for hyperthermia. If the temperature is elevated, time in the sun should be decreased. Activity should be stopped if the humidity is elevated as well. The athlete should drink plenty of fluids, preferably with low sugar content.

Nonexertional, or classic, heatstroke has a slow onset with insidious development of anorexia, nausea, vomiting, headache, mental manifestations, and loss of intravascular volume. Classic heatstroke occurs primarily in children with abnormal thermoregulation (e.g., children with cystic fibrosis) and infants subjected to prolonged neglect in a hot environment.

HEALTH CONCERNS ASSOCIATED WITH SPORTS

Nutrition

Some athletes are motivated to enhance their performance by any and all means available. They are eager to learn about nutrition, and many are influenced by misconceptions, fads, and superstitions regarding certain foods. Physical performance is affected by energy and body composition. The young athlete must maintain a diet that provides sufficient nutrients and energy to meet metabolic needs for optimum functioning. Physical training increases the need for energy and for more nutrients that convert food energy into chemical energy for physical performance.

There is no evidence to indicate that food supplements, extra vitamins, sports bars, or high-protein diets are needed to meet the demands of heavy physical exercise or improve physical performance in children or adolescents. In addition, there are no scientific data, other than anecdotal reports, supporting the benefits of such supplements in increasing physical performance (Academy of Nutrition and Dietetics, Dietitians of Canada, & American College of Sports Medicine, 2016). Athletes should be given accurate information regarding the lack of proven safety for such supplements. Young athletes need considerably more calories than the recommended dietary allowance (RDA). When the basic requirements for growth and activity are met by a balanced diet of protein, grains and cereals, fruits and vegetables, and dairy products, the additional calories needed for the extra exertion can be selected as desired. The athlete can obtain these extra calories by eating additional helpings from any of the basic four food groups, but many of the additional calories are provided by complex carbohydrates found in foods such as vegetables, pastas, and bread.

The recommended dietary energy intake for adolescents involved in sports is at least 50% of caloric intake from carbohydrates (6 to 10 g/kg/day), protein intake of 1.2 to 1.7 g/kg/day (average intake for athletes is 1.4 g/kg/day), and 25% to 30% from fat (Kleinman & Greer, 2014). It should be noted, however, that energy requirements vary depending on the sport and the child's or adolescent's age and body build. Adolescent athletes need additional iron and calcium intake from appropriate food sources to meet growth and developmental needs and to replace amounts lost in competition.

Water and Electrolytes. Considerable water is lost from the body through perspiration, urination, and evaporation from the respiratory tract. Water losses, especially from the skin, increase as the duration and intensity of exercise increase and as environmental temperature rises. Although thirst is experienced early in dehydration, it is unreliable as an indicator of fluid deficit. Water is recommended as *the best drink* for most athletes, and current recommendations are to take 5 to 8 oz of water every 15 to 20 minutes (150 ml for 40 kg [88 lb] athletes and 250 ml for athletes who weigh more than 40 kg) (American Academy of Pediatrics, Committee on Nutrition, & Council on Sports Medicine and Fitness, 2011). Very little water is exchanged in the stomach, and it must reach the intestines for absorption. The best fluids for rapid gastric emptying are cold, have low osmolality, and have a large volume. Fluids should never be restricted during activity. Drinking carbonated beverages is discouraged. Fluids containing 6% to 8% carbohydrates appear to have a faster gastric emptying time than water and may be tolerated by adolescent athletes (Kleinman & Greer, 2014).

Small amounts of electrolytes, especially sodium and chloride, are lost during exercise. Because sweat is quite dilute relative to plasma, excessive perspiration can result in excessive loss of water and an increase in plasma concentrations of sodium chloride. Therefore it is more important to replace water than sodium and chloride. Children should be well hydrated before beginning strenuous exercise or sports, especially in warm climates or environments. Athletes should hydrate with water regardless of thirst during strenuous exercise or activity. Periodic drinking breaks are encouraged, and adults or other team members should be alert to the child who has complaints such as headache, cramping, nausea, or vertigo. The use of salt tablets or table salt is unnecessary and may actually be harmful. Athletes usually derive sufficient salt replacement from the diet. Energy drinks are not recommended in children and adolescents participating in sports activities, and there is no evidence of an increase in performance with the use of such drinks in this population (American Academy of Pediatrics, Committee on Nutrition, & Council on Sports Medicine and Fitness, 2011; Kleinman & Greer, 2014).

Minerals. The basic diet does not satisfy the iron requirement of 10% to 15% of female athletes, most of whom are teenage girls who tend to become iron depleted after menarche. Young boys who are experiencing rapid adolescent growth and who have irregular and inadequate diets also are at risk of iron depletion. These children may need iron supplements; however, the American Academy of Pediatrics (Kleinman & Greer, 2014) does not recommend iron supplementation in athletes whose iron stores are adequate. Athletes who are participating in weight-restrictive sports or who are otherwise restricting dietary intake may need supplemental iron. There is currently no evidence that iron supplementation in healthy individuals enhances sports performance (Kleinman & Greer, 2014).

Adequate calcium intake during puberty is essential to promote mineralization of the growing skeleton. The recommended dietary reference intake (DRI) for calcium in adolescents ages 14 to 18 years is 1300 mg/day and vitamin D 400 to 1000 IU/day, yet few adolescents meet this goal. Calcium plays a vital role in nerve transmission, muscle contraction, and blood coagulation. Female athletes who engage in intensive training may develop amenorrhea, with subsequent decreased bone mineral density, osteopenia, and osteoporosis. Although the last two conditions may not occur immediately, stress fractures and impaired muscle contractions may be seen with low calcium intake. The best sources of additional calcium for athletes are nonfat dairy products. In addition, foods such as regular or low-fat yogurt and cheese, calcium-fortified orange juice, low-fat chocolate milk, and pudding may help meet daily calcium requirements. Consider the amount of calcium in the following: 1 glass of calcium-fortified orange juice contains 200 to 250 mg of calcium; 1 cup of skim milk has 300 mg of calcium; and 8 oz of yogurt contain approximately 410 mg of calcium. A well-balanced diet can provide the necessary calcium intake if adolescent athletes are made aware of the requirements and of the long-term consequences of poor nutrition.

Weight. Control of body weight by restricting water or food intake or increasing sweat loss is dangerous. Weight loss should not exceed 1.5% of total body weight per week (or 1 to 2 lb/week) (Kleinman & Greer, 2014). Young athletes need appropriate information about nutrition to dispel the allure of fads and fallacies about diet and performance. A sports nutritionist should be consulted for determining an optimal diet based on amount of energy expenditure and energy requirements. The optimum diet for an athlete is one that contains the essential food groups* and that is adjusted to the energy requirements of the sport in which the child or adolescent is engaged. Such a dietary plan should provide adequate nutrition for top physical efficiency and performance, maintenance of physical fitness and desirable body weight, and optimum function of all organ systems.

*See ChooseMyPlate.gov for recommended food groups and tips for serving sizes based on child or adolescent's level of physical activity.

Considerations for the Female Athlete

The syndrome known as female athlete triad was initially defined in 1997 as amenorrhea, osteoporosis, and low caloric intake or disordered eating. The definition has evolved to become more inclusive and represent the spectrum of this disorder ranging from health to disease. The three components of female athlete triad have been renamed to menstrual function, bone mineral density, and energy availability; female athletes may present with any or all of these components (Nattiv, Loucks, Manore, et al., 2007). There is some evidence that endothelial dysfunction and subsequent cardiovascular disease may be a fourth component of this condition (Zach, Smith Machin, & Hoch, 2011). The triad was originally described in athletes in sports for which thinness was desired (e.g., gymnasts, ballet dancers, figure skaters, and long-distance runners) but is now recognized in virtually all sports. The phenomenon has been attributed to a complex interplay of physical, genetic, hormonal, nutritional, psychologic, and environmental factors that include the stress of competition, decreased protein consumption, and altered lean-to-fat body ratio.

Menstrual irregularities can be common in adolescent girls but have been found to be more common in athletes. The incidence of menstrual dysfunction in sedentary adolescents was 21% whereas in adolescent athletes it was 54% (Hoch, Pajewski, Moraski, et al., 2009). Adolescent athletes with amenorrhea have a lower bone mineral density and are more likely to sustain a musculoskeletal injury than their peers. In addition, amenorrhea or oligomenorrhea has been associated with cardiovascular risk factors such as endothelial dysfunction.

Low estrogen levels and nutritional intake lead to a deficit in bone mineral density. The majority or nearly 90% of bone mass is reached by late adolescence. Girls with diminished estrogen secretion in delayed menarche will reach late adolescence with low bone density and will be subject to stress fractures and osteoporosis.

Energy availability is defined as the amount of energy left in the body after exercise training; a spectrum of eating disorders is commonly seen, ranging from poor eating habits to eating disorders (Deimel & Dunlap, 2012). Disordered eating is less severe and more subtle than eating disorders such as anorexia and bulimia. Disordered eating includes food restrictions, rigid food patterns, fasting, vomiting, and the use of diet pills and laxatives. The goal is to achieve a specific body image that is seen as desirable for the sport and is influenced by others such as coaches, teammates, or peers. Disordered eating results in poor protein intake, low fat intake, and inadequate caloric intake. Adolescent females should increase calcium intake to four to six servings per day of low-fat dairy products (recommendation for 1300 mg of calcium and at least 600 international units of vitamin D daily) (Weiss Kelly, Hecht, & AAP Council on Sports Medicine and Fitness, 2016). In such individuals, a 25-hydroxyvitamin D level greater than 30 ng/ml is considered adequate to promote bone health and prevent fractures (Ackerman & Misra, 2011). In addition, they should consume adequate protein and calories to meet the energy and metabolic needs of exercise (see Nutrition, p. 1271). Trainers and coaches also need to be aware of the potentially long-term results of intensive, prolonged exercise in pubertal girls.

Treatment may be long term and often involves development of an appropriate nutritional plan with a multidisciplinary team approach. However, education alone may not provide adequate incentive to change behavior, and psychologic health interventions may be required.

Substance Misuse by Athletes

Young athletes may use various performance-enhancing substances in an attecmpt to augment their athletic performance. Athletes believe that these substances, also known as *ergogenic aids,* increase strength and endurance, delay the onset of fatigue, increase the ability to concentrate, and decrease sensitivity to pain. Examples of substances athletes use include psychomotor stimulants (e.g., amphetamines), anabolic-androgenic steroids (AAS), ephedra, androstenedione (andro), dehydroepiandrosterone (DHEA), creatine, guarana, ginseng, amino acid and protein supplements, and excess amounts of vitamins (e.g., niacin, vitamin A, vitamin B_6).

Because many of these substances are considered natural, people willingly use them without further investigating potential hazards. The belief is that anything "natural," even if consumed in excess of the DRI, must be perfectly fine for the body because it will be rapidly metabolized and excreted without causing harm. This is not necessarily true for all substances, however, and parents, coaches, trainers, athletes, and health care workers should be knowledgeable about the effects of such substances. Rather than prohibiting their use, a better approach, especially for adolescents, is to provide open, informed discussion on the availability of appropriate substitutes that exist in foods that are indeed healthy to consume yet provide beneficial effects for athletic performance. Schools may include such discussions in existing curricula for their athletes and encourage participation in these educational programs.

Amphetamines and related drugs, such as methylphenidate (Ritalin), as well as caffeine, ephedra, or other stimulants, may be taken to provide a sense of increased alertness and relief of fatigue; however, obscuring fatigue may permit participants to exceed their limits and precipitate a sudden collapse. Some stimulants such as ephedra are used to burn fat when used in combination with caffeine. These substances can also make the users more aggressive, which can contribute to injuries to themselves and others.

Creatine is reported to be the most commonly used performance enhancing substance among athletes; it is a naturally occurring compound that supplies energy to muscles, builds muscle mass, increases recovery after strenuous exercise, and improves strength. A survey of high school students found a lifetime use of creatine of less than 5% in girls and nearly 18% of twelfth-grade boys (Johnston, O'Malley, Bachman, et al., 2014). Other misused drugs include stimulants intended for bronchodilation, decongestants, agents for weight gain or loss, physiologic agents used to enhance oxygen-carrying capacity, and nutritional supplements taken in doses greater than required.

Anabolic steroids are a source of concern to health professionals. Black market supplies of anabolic steroids are of poor quality and potency. The user develops larger-appearing muscles and increased body weight and body water, but reports on the side effects of these drugs outweigh any benefits for performance during athletic competition. Although the psychologic effect may be beneficial, many valid studies have failed to demonstrate any improvement in performance (Gregory & Fitch, 2007). The precise incidence of anabolic steroid use by adolescent athletes is unknown, but recent studies report a lifetime use of anabolic androgenic steroids ranging from less than 1% to 2.2% in high school girls and up to 4% in high school boys (Johnston, O'Malley, Bachman, et al., 2014; Kann, Kinchen, Shanklin, et al., 2014).

Adolescents and young adults rely on poor sources of information about the potential hazards of steroid use (e.g., friends, television, muscle magazines) and are generally poorly informed about their potential negative side effects. Health care professionals need to be aware of the clinical manifestations of steroid use. Clinical signs such as severe acne, a sudden increase in strength and muscle mass, a sudden decrease in body fat, a male pattern of baldness, and water retention are common. In females a male pattern of hair growth and a deepening voice are significant observations. The dangers of continued use are well known and include virilization in females; oligospermia, prostatic hypertrophy, myocardial infarction, stroke, testicular atrophy, infertility, and gynecomastia in males; and premature closure of the epiphyses, acne, increased blood cholesterol levels, hypertension, and hepatocellular carcinoma in both genders. Mood changes have been observed, including aggressiveness, changes in libido, depression, anxiety, and psychosis (Gregory & Fitch, 2007). Health hazards outweigh any potential gain that the drug might provide.

The American Academy of Pediatrics recommends that parents, coaches, and health care professionals be involved in educating athletes about the adverse effects of performance-enhancing substances. Prevention efforts that are focused on the lack of true benefit in performance with the use of performance enhancing substances may be most persuasive in curbing use. In addition, it is recommended that interventions for encouraging substance-free competition that are positive, rather than punitive, are promoted and encourage sound nutrition and training practices to achieve peak performance (LaBotz, Griesemer, & AAP Council on Sports Medicine and Fitness, 2016).

Sudden Death

A death associated with sports produces renewed anxiety in both parents and health care professionals. The term *sudden* or *instantaneous death* is applied to death that occurs within minutes of the onset of the cause of death or within 24 hours of the episode. *Sudden cardiac arrest* is also a term used to describe the athlete who experiences a sudden death. The incidence of sudden death among adolescent athletes has been estimated to be 2 to 7 per 100,000 per year (Angelini, Vidovich, Lawless, et al., 2013). Between 1980 and 2006 most causes of sudden death in athletes occurred as a result of cardiovascular disease (56%), followed by blunt trauma (22%), commotio cordis (3%), and heatstroke (2%) (Maron, Doerer, Haas, et al., 2009). One study of sudden cardiac deaths in young athletes reported an average of 69 cases per year during the years 2000 to 2006 (Drezner, Chun, Harmon, et al., 2008). Most studies show that causes of sudden cardiac death are due to hypertrophic cardiomyopathy (36%) and coronary anomalies (33%) (Angelini, Vidovich, Lawless, et al., 2013; Maron, Doerer, Haas, et al., 2009). Overall survival rates for young athletes experiencing sudden cardiac arrest during an athletic event between 2000 and 2006 were 11%, with a trend toward improved survival in the latter years of the study. More males (83%) than females (17%) experienced sudden cardiac arrest, and females were more likely to survive the arrest than were males (Drezner, Chun, Harmon, et al., 2008).

Causes of sudden death are related to three main risk factors: (1) sports with a high inherent risk for sports-related sudden death, (2) recognized or unknown underlying medical problems in child participants, and (3) the sports environment (e.g., the rules, equipment, practice fields or areas of sport participation, and ambient temperature of the geographic area). Some experts advocate screening all youth athletes with a 12-lead electrocardiogram to detect disorders such as Brugada syndrome, long QT syndrome, hypertrophic cardiomyopathy, and dilated cardiomyopathy, but this remains somewhat controversial. A comprehensive health history and physical examination may be helpful in identifying children and adolescents with risk factors for further diagnostic investigation, yet this has been reported to be inadequate for identifying risk factors (Morse & Funk, 2012). Chapter 19 discusses the impact of sudden death on the family and relevant nursing interventions.

Sports. Sports associated with the greatest risk of sudden death are those involving collision and frequent body contact. Examples of collision sports are football, ice hockey, rugby, and boxing. There is a high potential for serious injury or fatality in sports such as mountain or rock climbing and hang gliding. Sports that involve high-velocity objects, such as baseball and ice hockey, may result in death from serious head or chest injuries. Riding vehicles such as snowmobiles, mopeds, water jet skis, all-terrain vehicles, snowboards, minibikes, and motorcycles can also be considered high-risk sports.

Medical Conditions. The most frequent medical causes of sudden death during sports activity are cardiac abnormalities, especially idiopathic hypertrophic subaortic stenosis (hypertrophic cardiomyopathy). Manifestations suggestive of hypertrophic cardiomyopathy include a typical triad of severe chest pain, dizziness, and dyspnea. Unfortunately some affected individuals never display signs of disease until they collapse during a sports event. A history of sudden death of a relative or relatives in the second or third decade of life often offers a clue to recognition. Well-trained athletes often display evidence of hypertrophic cardiomyopathy, the so-called athlete's heart, but the condition is not pathologic.

Congenital coronary artery malformation is the second most common cause of sudden death in athletes. Additional causes include valvular heart disease, atherosclerotic coronary artery disease, dilated cardiomyopathy, Marfan syndrome, and myocarditis. Children with systemic hypertension, some types of cardiac arrhythmias such as prolonged QT syndrome, and some forms of heart block will face restrictions in the type and amount of exercise they can tolerate safely. Commotio cordis is a common cause of sudden death in athletes without previous history of heart disease. This occurs after a blunt, nonpenetrating blow to the chest, which produces ventricular fibrillation. Commotio cordis is more common in children and adolescents, with a mean age at occurrence of 13 years, and the blow may not be perceived as being that unusual or significant enough to produce such drastic results.

Appropriate use of an automatic external defibrillator (AED) by civilian bystanders or health care workers may save the life of an athlete who experiences a life-threatening cardiac emergency. A school-based AED program provides a high survival rate for student athletes and nonathletes who experience sudden cardiac arrest on school grounds (Drezner, Rao, Heistand, et al., 2009).

Environmental Causes. Environmental factors that are potential causes of sudden death include playing conditions, clothing, equipment, rules used by officials governing a sport, and outdoor temperature. Heatstroke and hypothermia (see Chapter 16) are the most serious environment-related causes of death in athletes.

The American Academy of Pediatrics has introduced an emergency response plan for schools that includes training teachers and school workers in cardiopulmonary resuscitation and first aid, collecting data to evaluate the risk for injuries in the school environment, and acting to reduce such risks (Council on School Health, 2008). Encourage nurses in school programs and in the community to become involved in the establishment of such programs and to assist in training, planning and implementation of effective risk prevention strategies designed to minimize child deaths in schools and local communities.

The American Academy of Pediatrics also recommends implementing a lay rescuer AED program in schools and that communication regarding the location of such equipment be properly managed (Council on School Health, 2008). The National Athletic Trainers' Association developed a consensus statement in conjunction with 15 national health care organizations for emergency preparedness and response in the event of sudden cardiac arrest in young athletes. This statement includes recommendations for those involved in high school and collegiate athletics for the prompt recognition and treatment of sudden cardiac arrest, including the use of an AED (Drezner, Courson, Roberts, et al., 2007).

NURSE'S ROLE IN CHILDREN'S SPORTS

Nurses may become involved in children's sports activities in preparation and evaluation of children for activities, provision of anticipatory guidance and counseling about athletic competition and nutrition, prevention of injuries, treatment of injuries, and rehabilitation after injuries. Selecting an appropriate sport for both recreation and competition is a joint effort of the child or adolescent, parents, and health professionals. Children are introduced to sports as part of family activities, neighborhood games, and school physical education programs, and both parents and children are influenced by media exposure to a variety of sports. Children are highly influenced by the popularity of and exposure afforded athletics in the school setting, especially in high school.

The best approach to counseling children and parents regarding sports participation is to encourage activities that are most likely to provide pleasure and physical benefits throughout childhood and into adulthood. Exposure to a variety of sports activities is probably better for young children than limitation to only one sport. Caution parents against overprogramming children to allow ample time for other activities and associations. Burnout among children and adolescents who continuously participate in sports is increasing in the United States. Children and adolescent are encouraged to take periodic breaks from such activities to allow physical healing, refresh the mind, and work on strength and conditioning (Brenner & Council on Sports Medicine and Fitness, 2007).

When children sustain athletic injuries, nurses are often responsible for instructing the children and their parents regarding care and rehabilitation. Instructions regarding, for example, the need and schedule for follow-up appointments, application of ice, and any restrictions in activity should be delivered clearly and preferably accompanied by written directions. Emphasize the importance of taking medications as prescribed because they may be needed for an extended period, and compliance may be difficult. For children continuing with activities, nonnarcotic pain medication administration an hour before practice or competition is advantageous.

Prevention of sports injuries is the most important aspect of any athletic program. Nurses collaborate with coaches and athletic trainers to ensure that safety measures are carried out. Stretching exercises, warming-up and cooling-down activities, and an appropriate training program are only some of the requisites for safe participation. Protective measures, such as padding, taping, wrapping, or use of other devices, are employed for areas at risk. Nurses are also on the alert for environmental safety risks.

For some athletes, their whole life revolves around sports participation. When a serious injury occurs, the athlete's self-esteem and self-image may suffer a devastating blow. Nursing assessment may reveal an athlete who appears to have difficulty dealing with this event and actually rejects any positive reinforcement. The nurse may help the child and family in establishing a support system. The athlete may need to learn new coping skills and explore other avenues to foster feelings of increased self-worth and a sense of accomplishment.

Lack of participation, exercise aversion, and declining interest in sports are sometimes the aftermath of participation during the school years and adolescence. Motivation can be altered or permanently destroyed by failure to appreciate the child's or adolescent's needs related to sports activities. Ridicule or derogation during acquisition of motor skills can shatter a child's or adolescent's self-esteem, producing anxiety and self-doubt that may result in a lifelong aversion to sports.

MUSCULOSKELETAL DYSFUNCTION

TORTICOLLIS

Torticollis, or wry neck, which can be either congenital or acquired, is a condition of limited neck motion. The condition is characterized by the neck being in a flexed position and the head drawn or tilted laterally to the affected side, while the chin is pointed toward the opposite side. Congenital muscular torticollis often occurs as a result of abnormal positioning in utero, causing a contracture of the sternocleidomastoid muscle. Torticollis is a manifestation rather than a disease entity and may be associated with a number of conditions, including congenital abnormality of the cervical spine or a traumatic lesion of the sternocleidomastoid muscle.

In early infancy a firm, nontender mass may be felt in the midportion of the sternocleidomastoid muscle. The mass regresses and is replaced by fibrous tissue. If the condition remains untreated, permanent limitation of neck movement results. Plagiocephaly and facial asymmetry often occur as a result of the contractured sternocleidomastoid muscle. Children may have other associated musculoskeletal conditions, including foot deformities or developmental dysplasia of the hips; a thorough physical examination should be performed for all infants.

Treatment of simple torticollis consists of gentle stretching exercises. The face is turned toward the affected muscle, while the head is tilted in the opposite direction, with the neck extended. A physical therapist typically establishes the treatment regimen to be followed by the family with the goal of achieving full, symmetric cervical range of motion. If stretching exercises are unsuccessful, surgical release of the sternocleidomastoid muscle may be needed. Increasingly, surgical correction by age 12 to 18 months is recommended to prevent muscle contracture and further progression of plagiocephaly. Other causes of torticollis occur in infancy or may develop at a later age but are not discussed in the text.

Nursing Care Management

Nurses should be alert to the possibility of torticollis in infants with limited head movement. After diagnosis, the nurse should supervise the family in performing stretching exercises and ensure proper technique. The nurse should also suggest that the child be positioned in a way that encourages turning the head and neck in the direction of limited range of motion; for example, placing interesting toys or activities toward one side. Parents can encourage the child to turn the head in the direction desired for correction through feeding and playing with the child.

KYPHOSIS AND LORDOSIS

The spine, which consists of numerous segments, can acquire deformation curves of three types: kyphosis, lordosis, and scoliosis (Fig. 33.33). Kyphosis is the lateral convex angulation in the curvature of the thoracic spine (see Fig. 33.33, *B*). If it is increased (greater than 45 degrees), it may occur secondary to disease processes such as tuberculosis, chronic arthritis, osteodystrophy, or compression fractures of the thoracic spine. Postural kyphosis is a common type of kyphosis in which the deformity is flexible and there are no radiographic vertebral body abnormalities or changes. Children, especially during the time when skeletal growth outpaces growth of muscle, are prone to postural roundback deformity. This is particularly common in self-conscious adolescent girls who assume a round-shouldered slouching posture in an attempt to hide their developing breasts and increasing height. No intervention is necessary other than education.

Scheuermann kyphosis is a thoracic curve of greater than 45 degrees, with wedging of more than 5 degrees of at least three adjacent vertebral bodies and vertebral irregularity. Onset occurs typically during the prepubertal growth spurt at approximately 10 to 12 years of age and is seen more frequently in males than females. Young adolescents often present with pain along with the visible kyphosis. The deformity has a degree of rigidity and lack of spine extension flexibility. Treatment for Scheuermann disease includes physical therapy working on increasing spine flexibility and strength as well as addressing potential lumbar hyperlordosis and hamstring or hip flexor tightness. Use of a spine brace may be indicated in children who are still growing. Surgical correction may be considered for severe, painful, or progressive deforming curves.

Lordosis is the lateral inward curve of the cervical and lumbar spine (see Fig. 33.33, *C*). Hyperlordosis may be a secondary complication of a disease process, the result of trauma, or idiopathic. Hyperlordosis is a normal observation in toddlers, and in older children it is often seen in association with flexion contractures of the hip, obesity, congenital dislocated hip, and SCFE.

Spondylolysis is a fracture sustained at the pars interarticularis. Spondylolisthesis is the forward slipping of one vertebral body on another. It most often involves L5 moving forward over S1. The condition may be asymptomatic, or it may cause lower back pain or neurologic compromise more typically seen with spondylolisthesis than spondylolysis. Treatment is usually nonsurgical; however, spinal fusion may be indicated in cases of severe, progressive slip.

IDIOPATHIC SCOLIOSIS

Scoliosis is a complex spinal deformity in three planes, usually involving lateral curvature, spinal rotation causing rib asymmetry, and when in

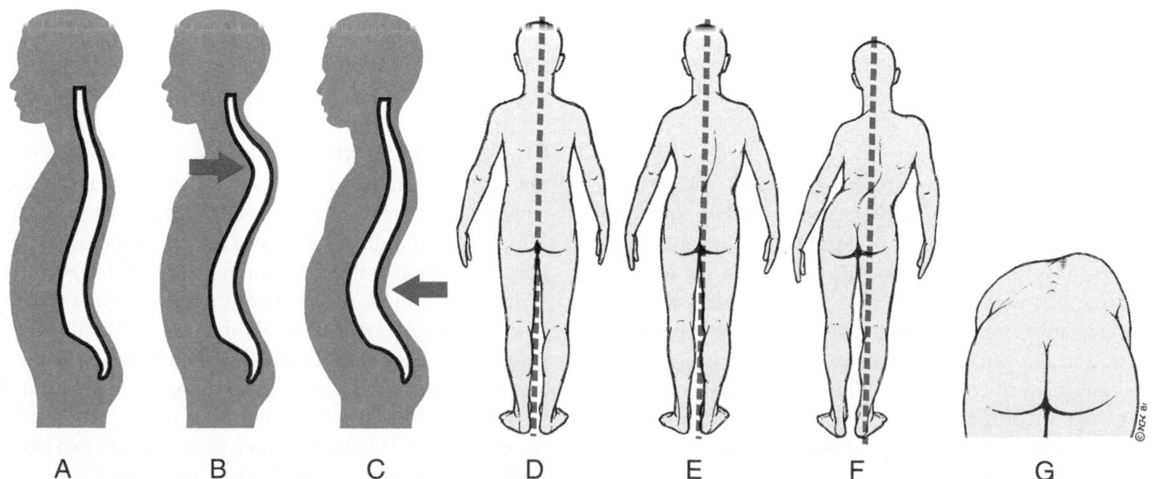

FIG. 33.33 Defects of spinal column. **A,** Normal spine. **B,** Kyphosis. **C,** Lordosis. **D,** Normal spine in balance. **E,** Mild scoliosis in balance. **F,** Severe scoliosis not in balance. **G,** Rib hump and flank asymmetry seen in flexion caused by rotary component.

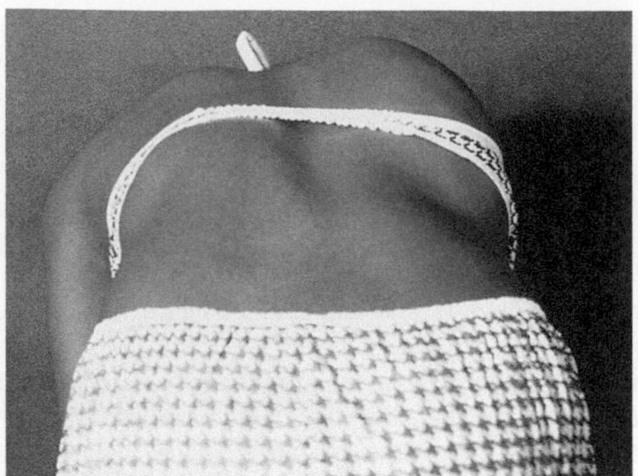

FIG. 33.34 Moderate thoracic idiopathic adolescent scoliosis. Forward flexion reveals a mild rib hump deformity.

the thoracic spine, often thoracic hypokyphosis (see Fig. 33.33, *E-G*, and Fig. 33.34). Scoliosis is the most common spinal deformity and is classified according to age of onset: *congenital* occurs in fetal development; *infantile* occurs at birth up to 3 years of age; *juvenile* occurs in children 3 to 10 years of age; and *adolescent* occurs at 10 years of age or older. Scoliosis may be caused by a number of conditions and may occur alone or in association with other diseases, particularly neuromuscular conditions (neuromuscular scoliosis). In most cases, however, there is no apparent cause, hence the name *idiopathic scoliosis.* The following discussion involves the adolescent type, which is often called adolescent idiopathic scoliosis. There appears to be a genetic component to the etiology of idiopathic scoliosis; however, the exact relationship has yet to be established.

Clinical Manifestations

Idiopathic scoliosis is most commonly identified during the preadolescent growth spurt. Parents frequently bring a child for follow-up on an abnormal school scoliosis screening or because of ill-fitting clothes, such as poorly fitting jeans. School screening is controversial because there are no controlled studies to demonstrate improved outcomes and a reported number of false positives lead to referrals. The American Academy of Orthopaedic Surgeons and the American Academy of Pediatrics published a joint position statement favoring scoliosis screening for preadolescents and adolescents in the school, physician's office, or nurses' clinic. Girls should be screened at ages 10 and 12 years, whereas boys should be screened once either at age 13 or 14 years. The benefits of early detection, referral, and medical treatment are considered to be significant, but the persons performing the screenings must be educated in the detection of spinal deformity (Richards & Vitale, 2008).

Diagnostic Evaluation

The standing child, wearing only shorts/briefs and viewed from behind, may exhibit asymmetry of shoulder height, scapular or flank shape, or hip height, or may demonstrate pelvic obliquity. Cutaneous changes may also be observed. When the child bends forward at the waist so that the trunk is parallel with the floor and the arms hang free (the Adams position), asymmetry of ribs and flanks may also be appreciated (see Fig. 33.33, *G*, and Fig. 33.34). A scoliometer is used in the initial screening to measure truncal rotation (as does the Adams test). Often a primary curve and a compensatory curve will place the head in alignment with the gluteal cleft. With an uncompensated curve, however, the head and hips are not aligned.

Definitive diagnosis is made by radiographs of the child in the standing position and use of the Cobb technique (standard measurement of angle curvature), which establishes the degree of curvature. The

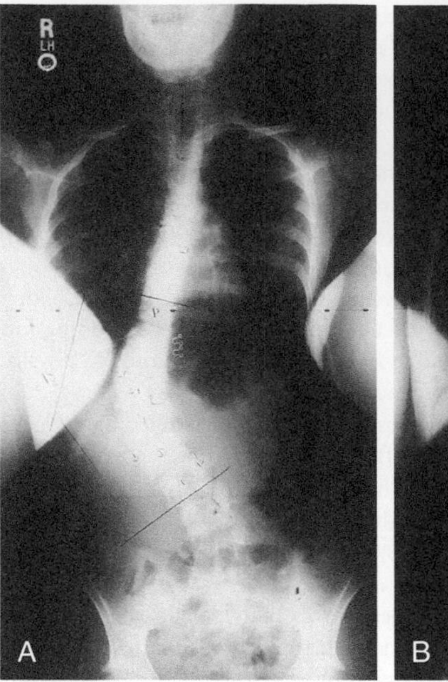

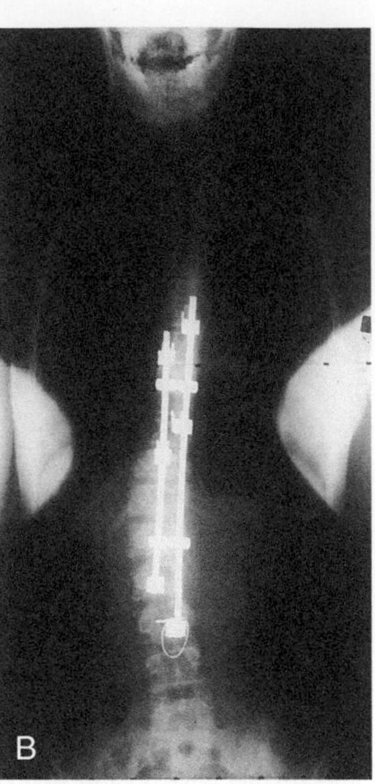

FIG. 33.35 Radiographs showing severe scoliosis before surgical correction **(A)** and after surgical correction of scoliosis, including internal fixation **(B)**.

Risser scale is used to evaluate skeletal maturity on the radiographs. This scale assists in making a determination of the likely progression of the spinal curvature as the child's bones mature. The sexual maturity rating is also used to evaluate the risk of curve progression in adolescents. Not all spinal curvatures are scoliosis. A curve of less than 10 degrees is considered a postural variation. Curves from 10 to 25 degrees are mild and, if nonprogressive, do not require treatment (Hresko, 2013).

Intraspinal conditions or other disease processes that may cause scoliosis must be ruled out. The presence of pain, sacral dimpling or hairy patches, cutaneous vascular changes, absent or abnormal reflexes, bowel or bladder incontinence, or left thoracic curve may indicate an intraspinal abnormality such as syringomyelia, diastematomyelia, or tethered cord syndrome. An MRI scan is usually obtained for evaluation.

Therapeutic Management

Current management options include observation with regular clinical and radiographic evaluation, orthotic intervention (bracing), and surgical spinal fusion (Fig. 33.35). Treatment decisions are based on the magnitude, location, and type of curve; the age and skeletal maturity of the child or adolescent; and any underlying or contributing disease process.

Bracing and Exercise. For moderate curves (25 to 45 degrees) in the growing child and adolescent, bracing may be the treatment of choice. Historically bracing has not been shown to be curative; the goal is to slow the progression of the curvature to allow skeletal growth and maturity. The two most common types of TLSOs are the Boston and Wilmington braces, which are customized underarm orthoses made of plastic with corrective external forces using lateral pads to help prevent progression (Fig. 33.36). The Milwaukee brace, which is an individually adapted brace that includes a neck ring, is rarely used in scoliosis but is sometimes used in the treatment of kyphosis. The Charleston nighttime bending brace is worn only when the child is in bed because it prevents walking due to the severity of the trunk bend.

Bracing, although used as the gold standard treatment for moderate curves in a growing child, has not proved to be entirely effective in the treatment of idiopathic scoliosis. Wearing the brace is challenging due

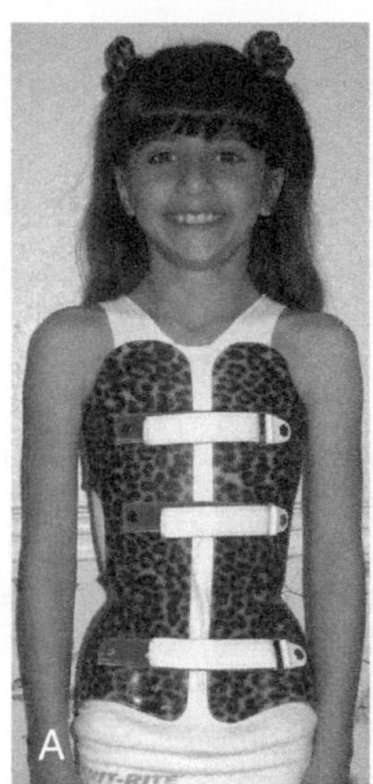
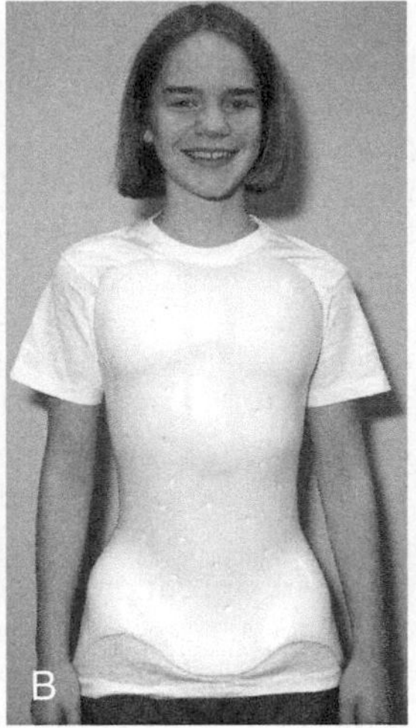
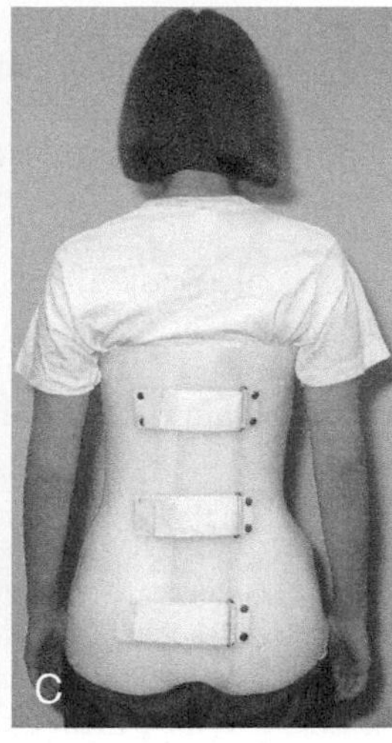

FIG. 33.36 A, Standard thoracolumbosacral orthosis (TLSO) brace for idiopathic scoliosis. Note the color and design incorporated into the brace to make it more acceptable to children and adolescents. **B** and **C,** Variation of a standard TLSO brace that fastens in the back to provide needed support for the spinal curvature.

to the child's age and preoccupation with body image and appearance. Experts recognize that brace treatment in some children with significant scoliosis may help avoid surgical intervention by slowing curve progression, but further studies are needed to clarify the effectiveness of bracing (Richards & Vitale, 2008). Some recent evidence suggests that bracing is effective in slowing a progressive spinal curvature in moderate scoliosis (Weinstein, Dolan, Wright, et al., 2013); however, the majority of studies involving bracing as the primary treatment of adolescent scoliosis are reportedly weak (Kotwicki, Chowanska, Kinel, et al., 2013).

There is very limited evidence regarding the effect of exercises and chiropractic treatment in the prevention of curve progression in scoliosis. Transcutaneous electrical nerve stimulation has proved to be an ineffective treatment. Exercises are of benefit when used in conjunction with bracing to maintain and increase the strength and range of motion of the spine.

Operative Management. Surgical intervention may be required for correction of severe curves or those measuring 45 degrees or more (see Fig. 33.35, *A*). The child's age, the location of the curvature, and curve magnitude influence the decision for surgery. In addition, thoracic curves with a magnitude greater than 50 degrees and lumbar curves greater than 30 degrees are more likely to progress after skeletal maturity (Newton, Wenger, & Yaszay, 2014). Any progressive or severe curve that does not respond to more conservative bracing measures requires surgical correction. Neuromuscular, dysplastic and congenital curves, which eventually progress, are best treated with early surgical stabilization. Difficulties with balance or seating, respiratory excursion, or pain are also considered.

There are a number of surgical techniques for severe scoliosis. One surgical intervention consists of realignment and straightening of the spine with internal fixation and instrumentation combined with bony fusion (**arthrodesis**). Posterior and/or anterior surgical approaches may be implemented. The goals of spinal fusion surgery are to improve the curvatures on the sagittal and coronal planes to provide a solid, pain-free fusion in a well-balanced torso (balanced shoulders and pelvis), with maximum mobility of the remaining spinal segments.

Spinal fusion can lead to decreased spinal mobility long-term. Other methods of surgical treatment are therefore being explored, including vertebral body stapling and anterior tethering. These types of surgical techniques do not require a fusion and may alter spinal growth by inhibiting growth of the anterior vertebral growth plate while still allowing for continued posterior growth thereby improving the spinal curvature or deformity (Newton, Wenger, & Yaszay, 2014).

Nursing Care Management

Treatment for scoliosis extends over a significant portion of the affected child's period of growth. In adolescents this period is the one in which their identity, both physical and psychologic, is formed. The identification of scoliosis as a "deformity," in combination with unattractive appliances and a significant surgical procedure, can have a negative effect on the already fragile adolescent body image. The adolescent and family require excellent nursing care to meet not only physical needs but also psychologic needs associated with the diagnosis, surgery, postoperative recovery, and eventual rehabilitation.

Although adolescents are encouraged to participate in most peer activities, necessary therapeutic modifications are likely to make them feel different and isolated. Nursing care of the adolescent who is facing scoliosis surgery, potential social isolation, pain, and uncertainty, not to mention misunderstood emotions and body image issues, must be evaluated from the adolescent's perspective to be successful in meeting the individual's needs.

When a child or adolescent first faces the prospect of a prolonged period in a brace or other device, the therapy program and the nature of the device must be explained thoroughly to both the child and the parents so that they will understand the anticipated results, how the appliance affects the curvature, the freedoms and constraints imposed by the device, and what they can do to help achieve the desired goal. The management involves the skills and services of a team of specialists, including the orthopedist, nurse, orthotist, social worker, and sometimes a physical therapist.

It is difficult for a child to be restricted at any phase of development, but the adolescent needs continual positive reinforcement, encouragement, and as much independence as can be safely assumed during this time. Guidance and assistance regarding anticipated problems, such as selection of clothing and participation in social activities, are appreciated by adolescents. Socialization with peers is strongly encouraged, and every effort is expended to help the adolescent feel worthwhile.

Preoperative Care. The preoperative workup usually involves a radiographic series, including bending or traction spine films, possible pulmonary function studies, and serologic laboratory studies (including prothrombin, partial thromboplastin, and bleeding times; blood count; electrolyte levels; urinalysis and urine culture; and blood levels of any medications). Spinal surgery typically results in considerable blood loss, so several options are considered preoperatively to maintain or replace blood volume. These options include autologous blood donations obtained from the patient before the surgery; intraoperative blood salvage; intraoperative hemodilution; erythropoietin administration; and controlled induced hypotension, which must be carefully monitored at all times to prevent physiologic instability.

Surgery for spinal fusion is complex, and often adolescents who require the procedure due to idiopathic scoliosis are not familiar with medical terms or procedures. Preoperative teaching is critical for the adolescent to be able to cooperate and participate in his or her treatment and recovery. Because the surgery is extensive, the patient is taught how to manage his or her own patient-controlled analgesia (PCA) pump; how to log-roll; and the use and function of other equipment, such as a chest tube (for anterior spinal fusion) and Foley urinary catheter. It is recommended that the child or adolescent bring personal items such as a favorite stuffed animal or toy, laptop computer, cell phone, or movie or music player for postoperative use. Meeting with a peer and his or her family members who have undergone a similar surgery may also be of value.

Postoperative Care. After surgery, patients are monitored in an acute care setting and log-rolled when changing position to prevent damage to the fusion and instrumentation. In some cases an immobilization brace or cast is used postoperatively depending on the type of surgical intervention. Skin care is important, and pressure-relieving mattresses or beds may be needed to prevent pressure wounds. (See Maintaining Healthy Skin, Chapter 22.)

In addition to the usual postoperative assessments of wound, circulation, and vital signs, the neurologic status of the patient's extremities requires special attention. Prompt recognition of any neurologic impairment is imperative because delayed paralysis may develop that requires surgical intervention. Common postoperative problems after spinal fusion include neurologic injury or spinal cord injury, hypotension from acute blood loss, wound infection, syndrome of inappropriate antidiuretic hormone, atelectasis, pneumothorax, ileus, delayed neurologic injury, and implanted hardware complications (Freeman, 2013). Superior mesenteric artery syndrome may occur several days after spinal surgery; this involves duodenal compression by the aorta and superior mesenteric artery and may result in acute partial or complete duodenal obstruction. Clinical manifestations include epigastric pain, belching, nausea, and copious vomiting; symptoms are aggravated in the supine position and often relieved with the patient in a left lateral decubitus or prone position.

The adolescent usually has considerable pain for the first few days after surgery and requires frequent administration of pain medication, preferably opioids administered intravenously on a regular schedule. For children able to understand the concept, PCA is recommended. (See Pain Assessment; Pain Management, Chapter 5.) In most cases the patient begins walking as soon as possible. Depending on the instrumentation used and the surgical approach, most patients are walking by the second or third postoperative day and are discharged by 5 to 7 days. In addition to pain management, the patient is evaluated for skin integrity, adequate urinary output, fluid and electrolyte balance, and ileus. Discharge planning should include a timetable for follow-up with the provider and resumption of regular activities.

Encourage the family to become involved in the patient's care to facilitate the transition from hospital to home management. An organization that provides education and services to both families and professionals is the National Scoliosis Foundation.*

SKELETAL LIMB DEFICIENCY

Congenital limb deficiencies are characterized by underdevelopment of skeletal elements of the extremities. The range of malformation or deficiency can extend from minor defects of the digit to serious abnormalities such as amelia (absence of an entire extremity) or hemimelia (partial absence of an extremity), which includes phocomelia, an interposed deficiency of long bones with relatively good development of hands and feet attached at or near the shoulder or the hip. Most reduction deficiencies involve anomalies in the development of the limb, but prenatal destruction of the limb can occur, such as full or partial amputation of a limb in utero from constriction by an amniotic band (amniotic band syndrome). Neonates with congenital limb deficiencies often have associated malformations and should be thoroughly assessed for cardiovascular, central nervous system, renal, and digestive abnormalities (Stoll, Alembik, Dott, et al., 2010).

Pathophysiology

Limb deficiencies can be attributed to both genetic and environmental causes and originate at any stage of limb development. Formation of limbs may be suppressed at the time of limb bud formation, or there may be interference in later stages of differentiation and growth. A family history of a deficiency increases the risk of a similar deficiency in a child demonstrating the inheritable or genetic nature of limb deficiencies. Prenatal environmental insults have been implicated in a number of cases, such as the well-publicized thalidomide tragedy in the late 1950s and early 1960s, which demonstrated a clear relationship between the time of exposure of the pregnant woman to the antiemetic drug and the presence and type of limb deformity in the newborn. There are still drugs that may have similar teratogenic effects in the first trimester of pregnancy; medication administration during this time period should be carefully evaluated by the provider (Bowen & Otsuka, 2014).

Therapeutic Management

The child with a limb deficiency should be fitted with prosthetic devices, and the devices should be applied at the earliest possible stage of development in an attempt to match the infant's motor readiness. This favors natural progression of prosthetic use. For example, an infant with an upper extremity deficiency is fitted with a simple passive device between 3 to 6 months of age, when limb exploration is active, sitting is beginning (with the extremities needed for support), and bilateral hand activities are encouraged. Lower limb prostheses are applied when the infant is ready to pull to a standing position.

In preparation for prosthetic devices, surgical modification may be necessary to ensure the most favorable use of the device because severe deformity can interfere with its effective use. Phocomelic digits are preserved for controlling switches of externally powered appliances in the upper extremities. Digits (in both the upper and lower extremities) provide the child with surfaces for tactile exploration and stimulation. Prostheses are replaced to accommodate the child's growth and increasing capabilities.

Nursing Care Management

Prosthetic application, training, and habilitation are most successfully carried out in a center that specializes in meeting the special needs of

*Five Cabot Place, Stoughton, MA 02072; 800-673-6922; http://www.scoliosis.org.

these children, especially very young children and those with multiple amputations. Management involves a prosthetist, who specializes in the development, fitting, and maintenance of prosthetic limbs, and other health care providers such as physical and occupational therapists. Parents need support and are encouraged to assist the child in making age-appropriate adjustments to the environment. Although these children need assistance, overprotection may produce overdependence, with later maladjustment to school and other situations.

DEVELOPMENTAL DYSPLASIA OF THE HIP

The broad term developmental dysplasia of the hip (DDH) describes a spectrum of disorders related to abnormal development of the hip that may occur at any time during fetal life, infancy, and childhood. A change in terminology from *congenital hip dysplasia* and *congenital dislocation of the hip* to DDH more properly reflects the varying onset and types of hip abnormalities in which there is a shallow acetabulum, femoral head subluxation or dislocation.

The incidence of hip instability is approximately 1 to 1.5 per 1000 live births, and approximately 17% to 23% of infants with DDH are born with a breech intrauterine position. Girls are more commonly affected than boys, and there is a positive family history in approximately 12% to 33% of affected individuals. Additional risk factors for DDH include firstborn child, oligohydramnios, hip asymmetry, and other musculoskeletal conditions including torticollis and metatarsus adductus or foot deformities (Weinstein, 2014a).

Pathophysiology

The cause of DDH is unknown, but certain factors such as female gender, first pregnancy, family history, breech intrauterine position, high birth weight, joint laxity, and postnatal positioning are believed to affect the risk of DDH. Predisposing factors associated with DDH may be divided into three broad categories: physiologic factors, including maternal hormone secretion and intrauterine positioning; mechanical factors, which involve breech presentation, multiple fetuses, oligohydramnios, and large infant size, as well as continued maintenance of the hips in adduction and extension that with time can cause dislocation (see Cultural Competence box); and genetic factors, which include a higher incidence of DDH in siblings of affected infants and even greater incidence of recurrence if a sibling and one parent were affected. One study found a twelvefold increase in risk of DDH for individuals with a first-degree relative affected (Stevenson, Mineau, Kerber, et al., 2009).

> **CULTURAL COMPETENCE**
>
> ***Developmental Dysplasia of the Hip and Infant Care Practices***
>
> A striking relationship exists between the development of dislocation and methods of handling infants. Among cultures with the highest incidence of dislocation (Navajo Indians and Canadian Natives [formerly referred to as Eskimos]), newly born infants are tightly wrapped in blankets or other swaddling material or are strapped to cradle boards. In cultures where mothers carry infants on their backs or hip in a widely abduction straddle position, such as the Far East and Africa, the disorder is virtually unknown.

Recently it has been recommended that infants' hips be placed in slight flexion and abduction during swaddling. Further, it was recommended that infants' knees be maintained in slight flexion and that forced or prolonged passive hip extension in the first months of life be avoided. These recommendations were made based on evidence that demonstrated a significant relationship between tight swaddling and hip dysplasia and are aimed at decreasing the incidence of DDH in infants (Price & Schwend, 2011).

DDH can be categorized into two major groups: idiopathic, in which the infant is neurologically intact, and teratologic, which involves a neuromuscular defect such as arthrogryposis or myelomeningocele. The teratologic forms usually occur in utero and are much less common.

Three degrees of DDH are illustrated in Fig. 33.37 and are outlined here:

1. Acetabular dysplasia: This is the mildest form of DDH, in which there is a delay in acetabular development evidenced by osseous hypoplasia of the acetabular roof that is oblique and shallow. The femoral head remains in the acetabulum with no subluxation or dislocation.
2. Subluxation: The largest percentage of DDH, subluxation implies incomplete dislocation. The femoral head remains in contact with the acetabulum, but a stretched capsule and ligamentum teres cause the head of the femur to be partially displaced. Pressure on the cartilaginous acetabulum inhibits ossification and produces a flattening of the socket.
3. Dislocation: This is the most severe form of DDH. The femoral head loses contact with the acetabulum and is displaced posteriorly and superiorly.

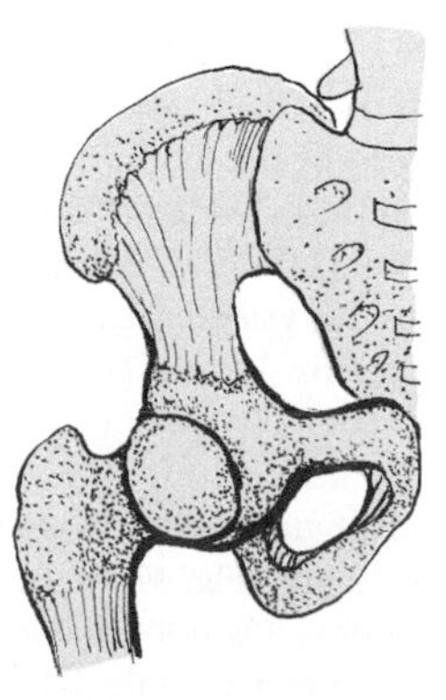

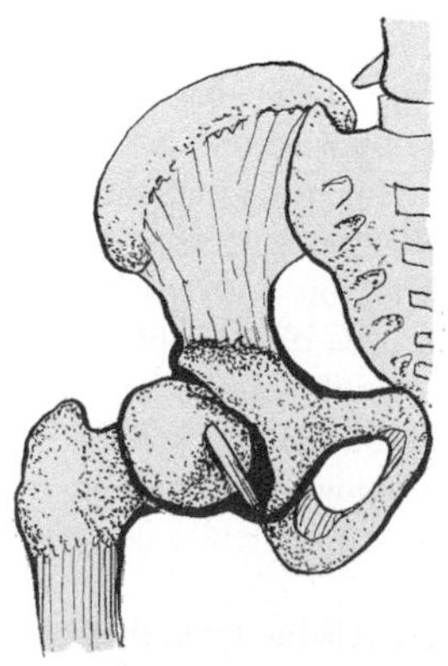

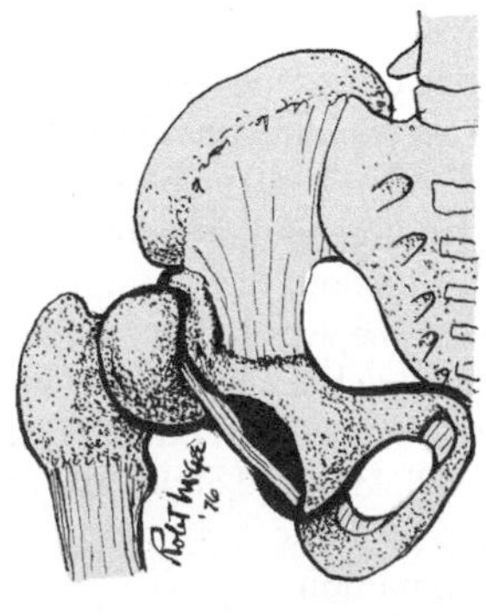

FIG. 33.37 Configuration and relationship of structures in developmental dysplasia of the hip.

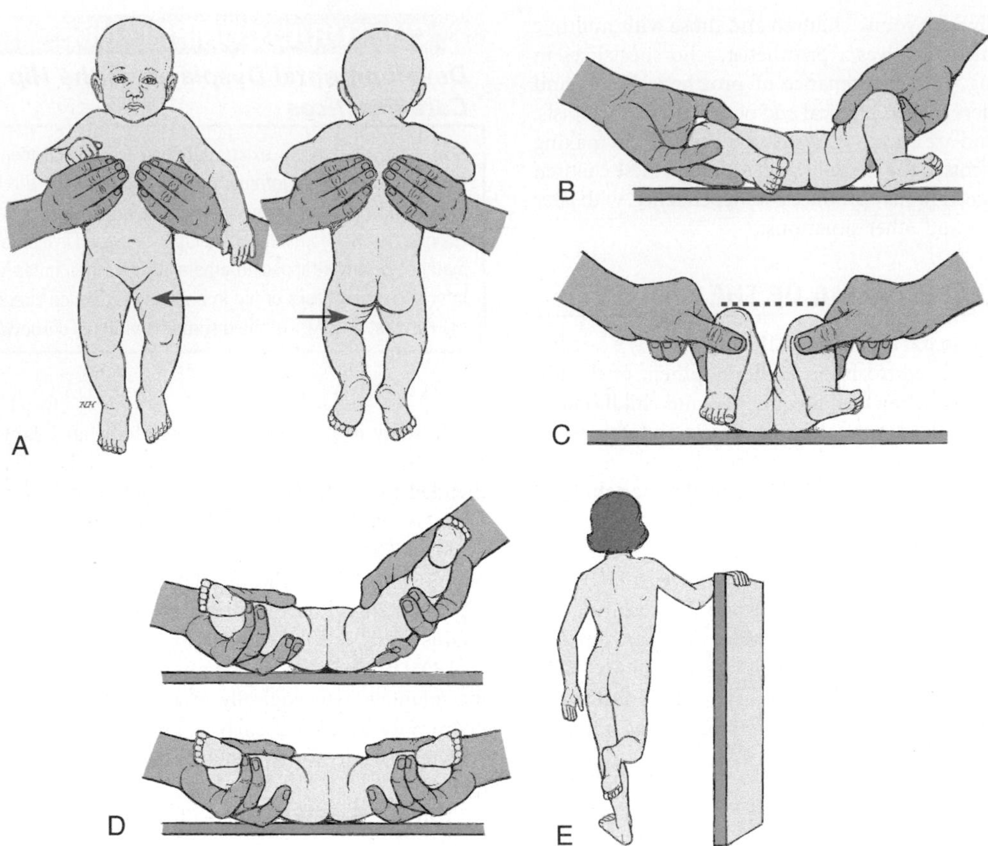

FIG. 33.38 Signs of developmental dysplasia of hip. **A,** Asymmetry of gluteal and thigh folds. **B,** Limited hip abduction, as seen in flexion. **C,** Apparent shortening of femur, as indicated by level of knees in flexion. **D,** Ortolani test. **E,** Positive Trendelenburg sign (if child is weight bearing).

Diagnostic Evaluation

The diagnosis of DDH should be made in the newborn period if possible because treatment initiated before 2 months of age achieves the highest rate of success. In the newborn period, hip dysplasia usually appears as hip joint laxity rather. Subluxation and the tendency to dislocate can be demonstrated by the Ortolani and Barlow tests (Fig. 33.38, *D*). With the infant quiet and relaxed in the supine position on a firm surface with the legs facing the examiner, the hips and knees are flexed (not forced) at right angles. The examiner places the middle finger of each hand over the greater trochanter and the thumbs on the inner side of the thigh at a point opposite the lesser trochanter. The knees are carried to midabduction, and each hip joint is submitted, one at a time, first to forward pressure exerted behind the trochanter and then to backward pressure exerted from the thumbs in front as the opposite joint is held steady. If the femoral head can be felt to slip forward into the acetabulum on pressure from behind, it is dislocated (Ortolani test). If with hip flexion and adduction, the femoral head is felt to slip out over the posterior lip of the acetabulum, the hip is said to be dislocatable or "unstable" (Barlow test). Sometimes an audible "clunk" can be heard on exit or entry of the femur out of or into the acetabulum. The audible clunk is not pathologic and occurs as a result of breaking surface tension across the hip joint, knee rotation, snapping of gluteal tendons, or patellofemoral motion.

The Ortolani and Barlow maneuvers are most reliable from birth to 4 weeks of age. Adduction contractures develop at about 6 to 10 weeks of age, and the Ortolani sign disappears. After this time, the most sensitive test is limited hip abduction (Fig. 33.38, *B*). Other signs are shortening of the thigh on the affected side (Galeazzi sign) (Fig. 33.38, *C*), asymmetric thigh and gluteal folds (Fig. 33.38, *A*), and broadening of the perineum (in bilateral hip dislocations).

> **! NURSING ALERT**
>
> The Barlow and Ortolani maneuvers should be performed only by an experienced clinician to prevent an injury to the infant's hips.

In the older infant and child, the affected leg appears shorter than the other. In both unilateral and bilateral dislocations the greater trochanter is prominent and appears above a line from the anterosuperior iliac spine to the tuberosity of the ischium. There may be telescoping or piston mobility, meaning that the head of the femur can be felt to move up and down in the buttock when the extended thigh is pushed first toward the child's head and then pulled distally. Instability of the hip on weight bearing produces a characteristic waddling gait and marked lumbar lordosis in bilateral hip dislocations. When the child stands first on one foot and then on the other (holding onto a chair, rail, or someone's hand), bearing weight on the affected hip, the pelvis tilts downward on the normal side instead of upward as it would with normal stability (positive Trendelenburg sign) (Fig. 33.38, *E*).

Radiographic examination in early infancy is not reliable because ossification of the femoral head does not normally take place until 4 to 6 months of life. However, the cartilaginous femoral head can be visualized directly by ultrasonography. Universal newborn screening with ultrasonography has been proposed; however, numerous studies reveal that this approach has a high rate of false-positive results and subsequent overtreatment. Therefore ultrasonography is considered an adjunct to the physical examination and recommended for young infants with known risk factors. In infants older than 6 months of age and in children, pelvis radiographs are obtained to confirm the diagnosis. The American Academy of Pediatrics has published extensive clinical guidelines for screening and early detection of DDH (Shaw, Segal, & AAP Section on Orthopaedics, 2016).

Therapeutic Management

Treatment is begun as soon as the condition is recognized because early intervention is more favorable to the restoration of normal bony architecture and function. The longer treatment is delayed, the more severe the deformity, the more difficult the treatment, and the less favorable the prognosis. The treatment varies with the child's age and the extent of the dysplasia. The goal of treatment is to obtain and maintain a safe, congruent position of the hip joint to promote normal hip joint development.

Newborn to 6 Months. The hip joint is maintained, by dynamic splinting, in a safe position with the proximal femur centered in the acetabulum in a degree of flexion. A variety of abduction devices are available; of these, the Pavlik harness is the most widely used, and with time, motion, and gravity, the hip works into a more abducted, reduced position (Fig. 33.39). The harness does not rigidly immobilize the hip but acts to prevent hip extension and adduction. The Pavlik harness is worn continuously until the hip is stable on both clinical and ultrasound examination, usually within 6 to 12 weeks. It is highly effective when the device is well constructed, follow-up care is adequate, and the parents follow instructions in its use. If young infants hips fail to locate with the Pavlik harness, then surgical closed reduction and spica casting may be warranted.

Ages 6 to 24 Months. In this age-group, the Pavlik harness has a low success rate. Therefore surgical treatment with a closed reduction is recommended, and the child is placed in a spica cast for approximately 12 weeks. If the hip is not reducible, a surgical open reduction may be necessary. A hip abduction orthosis may be used after spica casting in order to maintain the hip in an appropriate, stable position and further promote hip development.

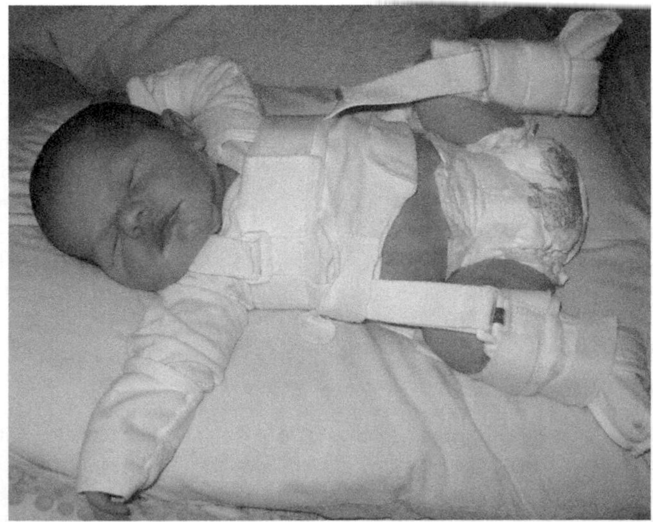

FIG. 33.39 Child in Pavlik harness. (Courtesy Amanda Polittle, St. Louis, MO.)

Older Child. Correction of the hip deformity in the older child is inherently more difficult than in the preceding age-groups because secondary adaptive changes and other etiologic factors (such as juvenile arthritis or cerebral palsy) complicate the condition. Operative reduction, which may involve preoperative traction, tenotomy of contracted muscles, and pelvic osteotomy procedures designed to construct an acetabular roof, often combined with proximal femoral osteotomy, is usually required. After cast removal, range-of-motion exercises help restore movement. Other rehabilitation measures may include muscle strengthening, a period of crutch or walker use, and gait training.

Nursing Care Management

Nurses are in a unique position to detect DDH in the newborn. During the infant assessment process and routine nurturing activities, the nurse inspects the hips and extremities for any deviations from normal. These observations are reported to the attending provider for further examination. The ambulatory child who displays a limp or waddling gait is also referred for evaluation. Nonambulatory children with cerebral palsy or spina bifida should be assessed for evidence of hip problems as well.

The major nursing challenges in the care of an infant or child in a cast or other device are related to maintenance of the device and adaptation of nurturing activities to meet the child's needs. Generally, treatment and follow-up care of these children are carried out in an outpatient setting.

The primary nursing goal is teaching parents to apply and maintain the reduction device or brace. The Pavlik harness allows for easy handling of the infant and usually produces less apprehension in the parent than heavy braces and casts. It is important that parents understand the correct use of the device, which may or may not allow for its removal during bathing. Removing the harness is determined individually on the basis of the provider's recommendations, the degree of hip instability, and the family's level of understanding. Parents should be instructed not to adjust the harness.

Skin care is an important aspect of the care of an infant in a Pavlik harness. The following instructions for preventing skin breakdown are stressed:

- Check frequently (at least two to three times per day) for red areas under the straps and at skin folds.
- Gently massage healthy skin under the straps once a day to stimulate circulation.
- In general, avoid lotions and powders because they can cake and irritate the skin.
- Always place the diaper under the straps.

Parents are encouraged to hold the infant who has a Pavlik harness and continue cares and activities. The nurse can assist by answering the parents' questions about necessary adaptations to daily care, thereby helping decrease the parents' anxiety and fears. Problems reported by parents include difficulty reapplying the harness, carrying the child, skin-crease dermatitis, feet slipping out of the harness, and difficulty in clothing the child (Hassan, 2009). These findings highlight the importance of close follow-up and written take-home instructions for the parents to follow in managing the Pavlik harness.

Casts offer more challenging nursing and caregiver problems because they cannot be removed for routine care and bathing. Care of an infant or small child with a cast requires nursing innovation to reduce irritation and to maintain cleanliness of both the child and the cast, particularly in the diaper area. The importance of spica cast care should be emphasized when providing instructions to parents and caregivers. The life of the cast should be prolonged to help prevent an unnecessary cast change.

It is important for nurses, parents, and other caregivers to understand that children in corrective devices need to be involved in all the activities of any child in the same age-group. Confinement in a cast or orthotic device should not exclude children from family activities. They can be held astride the lap for comfort and transported to areas of activity. An adapted wheelchair or stroller can offer mobility to an older infant or child.

LEGG-CALVÉ-PERTHES DISEASE

Legg-Calvé-Perthes disease is a self-limiting disorder in which there is avascular necrosis of the femoral head. The disease affects children ages 2 to 12 years, but most cases occur as an isolated event in boys between 4 and 8 years of age. The male-to-female ratio is 4 or 5 to 1. In approximately 10% of cases, the involvement is bilateral; most of the affected children have a skeletal age significantly below their chronologic age. Caucasian children are affected more frequently than African American children (Weinstein, 2014b).

Pathophysiology

The cause of the disease is unknown, but a temporary disturbance of circulation to the femoral capital epiphysis produces an ischemic aseptic necrosis of the femoral head. During middle childhood, circulation to the femoral epiphysis is more tenuous than at other ages, being supplied almost entirely by the lateral retinacular vessels. Activity causes microfractures of the soft ischemic epiphysis, which tends to induce synovitis, stiffness, and hip adductor contracture.

The pathologic events seem to take place in four stages (Box 33.9). The entire disease process may encompass as few as 18 months or continue for several years. The reformed femoral head may be severely altered or minimally affected.

Clinical Manifestations and Diagnostic Evaluation

The onset of Legg-Calvé-Perthes disease is usually insidious, and the history may reveal only intermittent appearance of a limp on the affected side or a symptom complex, including hip soreness, ache, or stiffness, which can be constant or intermittent. The parents may report seeing the child limping, and the limp may become more pronounced with increased activity. The pain may be experienced in the hip, along the entire thigh, or in the vicinity of the knee joint. The pain and limp are often more evident on arising and at the end of a long day of activities. The pain is usually accompanied by joint dysfunction and limited range of motion at the hip. There may be a vague history of trauma but not necessarily. The diagnosis is established by characteristic radiographic findings and, occasionally, by MRI.

BOX 33.9 Radiographic Stages of Legg-Calvé-Perthes Disease

Stage I—Aseptic necrosis or infarction of the femoral capital epiphysis with degenerative changes producing flattening of the upper surface of the femoral head (the avascular stage)

Stage II—Capital bone resorption and revascularization with fragmentation (vascular resorption of the epiphysis) that gives a mottled appearance on radiographs (the fragmentation, or revascularization stage)

Stage III—New bone formation, which is represented on radiographs as calcification and ossification or increased density in the areas of radiolucency; this filling-in process appears to take place from the periphery of the head centrally (the reparative stage)

Stage IV—Gradual reformation of the head of the femur without radiolucency and, it is hoped, to a spherical form (the regenerative stage)

Therapeutic Management

Because deformity occurs early in the disease process, the aims of treatment are to eliminate hip irritability; restore and maintain adequate hip range of motion; prevent capital femoral epiphyseal collapse, extrusion, or subluxation; and preserve as well-rounded femoral head as possible at time of healing. Treatment varies according to the child's age at the time of diagnosis and the appearance of the femoral head and position within the acetabulum.

The initial therapy is rest or activity restrictions and limited weight bearing, which helps reduce inflammation and irritability of the hip. The use of NSAIDs can provide relief of pain or discomfort; physical therapy or range-of-motion exercises help restore hip motion. In some cases, traction is applied to stretch tight adductor muscles and improve containment of the femoral head. Abduction braces or casting may also be used for containment. If nonsurgical or conservative management is unsuccessful, surgical reconstruction or containment procedures such as a pelvic or proximal femoral osteotomy may be necessary.

The disease is self-limiting, but the ultimate outcome of therapy depends on early and efficient treatment and the child's age at the onset of the disorder. Children 5 years and younger, whose epiphyses are more cartilaginous, tend to have the best prognosis or outcome. Children over 9 years old have a significant risk for degenerative arthritis, especially if they have femoral head deformity at the time of diagnosis. The later the diagnosis is made, the more femoral head damage will have occurred before treatment is implemented.

Nursing Care Management

Because these children are largely cared for on an outpatient basis, the major emphasis of nursing care is on teaching the family the required care and management. The family needs to comprehend the diagnosis and the importance of compliance with the prescribed regimen to achieve the desired outcome. The child and the family may rely on the nurse to help them understand and adjust to therapeutic measures.

One of the most difficult aspects associated with the disorder is the need to cope with a normally active child who feels well but must remain relatively inactive. It is important to emphasize that children should continue to attend school and engage in activities that can be adapted to the prescribed regimen. Suitable activities must be devised to meet the needs of the child in the process of developing a sense of initiative or industry. Activities that fulfill creative urges are well received.

SLIPPED CAPITAL FEMORAL EPIPHYSIS

Slipped capital femoral epiphysis (SCFE) refers to the spontaneous displacement of the proximal femoral epiphysis in relationship to the femoral neck and shaft. In most cases, the femoral head stays within the acetabulum while the femoral neck and shaft moves anteriorly and rotates externally relative to the femoral epiphysis. It develops most frequently shortly before or during accelerated growth and the onset of puberty (children between the ages of 10 and 16 years; median age 13 years for boys and 12 years for girls) and is commonly observed in boys and obese children. SCFE has a reported prevalence of 2 to 13 per 100,000 in the United States, with bilateral involvement occurring in up to 60% of cases (Kay & Kim, 2014).

Pathophysiology

Most cases of SCFE are idiopathic, although it can be associated with endocrine disorders such as hypothyroidism, growth hormone therapy, renal osteodystrophy due to secondary hyperparathyroidism, and previous radiation therapy to the femoral head. The cause of idiopathic SCFE is multifactorial, with a variety of mechanical factors playing a part, including obesity, physeal architecture and orientation, and pubertal hormone changes that affect physeal strength. Although obesity stresses the physeal plate, SCFE can also occur in children who are not obese.

Clinical Manifestations and Diagnostic Evaluation

SCFE is suspected when an adolescent or preadolescent displays clinical signs of a limp or complains of intermittent or continuous pain in the hip, groin, thigh, or knee. Onset may be acute, chronic, or acute-on-chronic. The child or adolescent often lies stiff with the lower extremity flexed, abducted, and externally rotated because of the pain; any attempts to move the limb are met with significant resistance. The limp of a child with SCFE often reveals a Trendelenburg gait with an external foot progression angle on the affected side. In an unstable SCFE, the child is unable to bear weight because of severe pain.

Physical examination reveals range of motion restrictions of both hip flexion and extension as well as limited internal rotation. The affected hip falls into obligate external rotation as it is flexed. The diagnosis is confirmed by anteroposterior and frog-leg or crosstable lateral radiographs that reveal a change in the position of the femoral neck relative to the proximal femoral epiphysis. With a more severe or progressive slip, displacement may lead to an uncovered upper portion of the femoral neck adjacent to the physis. The growth plate appears widened and irregularities may be seen at the metaphysis. Lateral view radiographs are more sensitive at detecting a mild SCFE.

Therapeutic Management

The treatment goals of SCFE are to prevent further slipping at the proximal femur until physeal closure, avoid further complications such as avascular necrosis, and maintain adequate hip function. Once the diagnosis is established, the child should be non–weight bearing to prevent further slippage. SCFE is an emergency and requires early diagnosis and treatment to increase the likelihood of an acceptable outcome.

Surgical treatment is necessary and varies with the degree of displacement or slippage. Current recommended treatment is with in situ fixation or pinning, which involves the placement of a single pin or alternatively multiple pins or screws through the femoral neck into the proximal femoral epiphysis to prevent further slippage. Most surgeons prefer to take the child to surgery within 24 hours of the onset of acute symptoms and avoid further risk of avascular necrosis. Postsurgical care includes non–weight bearing or limited weight bearing with crutches until acceptable, painless range of motion is achieved. Activities may be limited for a length of time. Fixation or pins remain in place at least until the physis is closed and often are not removed.

Nursing Care Management

Nursing care involves preparing the child and family for the surgical procedure and recovery. Postoperative care involves hemodynamic stabilization, pain management, and assessment for complications. The adolescent is taught the proper use of crutches and the importance of avoiding any weight bearing on the affected hip. Self-care and performance of activities of daily living to capability are encouraged to promote confidence and decrease a sense of helplessness.

METATARSUS ADDUCTUS

Metatarsus adductus is the most common congenital foot deformity. The deformity is characterized by medial adduction of the toes and forefoot, frequently in association with inversion and convexity of the lateral border of the foot (kidney shaped). In most instances, it is a result of abnormal intrauterine positioning, particularly in a firstborn child, and is usually detected at birth. Metatarsus adductus can be divided into three categories: type I, in which the forefoot is flexible and corrects easily into abduction with manipulation; type II, in which the forefoot is only partially flexible and corrects only to neutral position with active manipulation; and type III, in which the forefoot is rigid and will not stretch to a neutral position with manipulation. Unlike a clubfoot, with which it is often confused, the angulation occurs at the tarsometatarsal joint, while the heel and ankle remain in a neutral position. Ankle range of motion is normal. The deformity often causes a pigeon-toed or intoeing gait in the child. A thorough hip examination should be performed for all infants with metatarsus adductus, as an increased risk of hip dysplasia is associated with foot deformities.

Management depends on the flexibility of the deformity. The majority of cases spontaneously correct with no treatment over the first 4 years of life. Interventions such as stretching and bracing or corrective shoes have not been shown to be effective. However, the parents can perform gentle forefoot abduction stretching. For partly flexible or rigid deformities, serial manipulation and casting can be considered to correct the defect, after which a corrective shoe or orthosis may be used to help prevent a recurrence; risk of recurrence is reported to be as high as 37%. Surgical correction is rarely required for the condition, as even those with residual deformity tend to not have long-term functional disability. Surgery may be considered in children over 4 to 6 years of age who have considerable pain on ambulation or difficulties with shoe wear as a result of the deformity (Mosca, 2014).

Nursing Care Management

The nursing role primarily involves identifying the defect so that early education and instruction to the parents can be initiated. The nurse teaches the parents how to hold the heel firmly and to stretch only the forefoot; otherwise, undue force on the heel may produce a valgus deformity. If casting or an orthosis is needed, the nurse instructs the parents in cast care and care of the brace.

CLUBFOOT

Clubfoot, also referred to as congenital talipes equinovarus, is a complex deformity of the ankle and foot that includes forefoot adduction, cavus, hindfoot varus, and ankle equinus (Fig. 33.40). Clubfoot involves bone deformity and malposition with soft tissue contracture. It may occur as an isolated deformity or in association with other conditions or syndromes, such as spina bifida, arthrogryposis, constriction band or chromosomal abnormalities.

The incidence of clubfoot in the general population is approximately 1 per 1000 live births, with boys affected twice as often as girls. Bilateral clubfeet occur in 50% of the cases. The precise etiology of clubfoot is unclear but likely a result of multiple mechanisms. However, there is

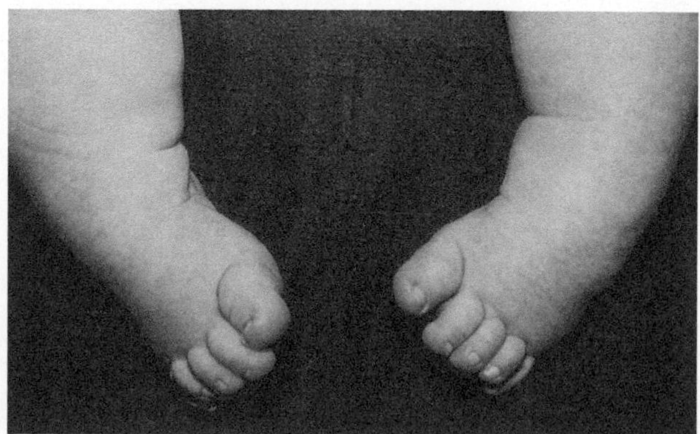

FIG. 33.40 Bilateral congenital talipes equinovarus (congenital clubfoot).

a strong genetic or familial tendency. Other possible theories as to the cause of clubfoot include arrested or abnormal fetal development or abnormal positioning and restricted movement in utero, although the evidence is inconclusive (Mosca, 2014).

Diagnostic Evaluation

A clubfoot deformity is readily apparent at birth if it has not been detected prenatally through ultrasonography. Once it is detected, a careful yet comprehensive physical assessment of the affected foot (or feet) should be completed to allow for appropriate decision making regarding treatment plans and prognosis. The affected foot (or feet) is usually smaller and shorter, with an empty heel pad and a midfoot plantar crease. When the deformity is unilateral, the affected limb may be shorter, and calf atrophy is present. Generally, imaging such as radiographs or ultrasonography is not necessary for diagnosis. A thorough hip examination should be performed for all infants with a clubfoot; an increased risk of hip dysplasia is associated with clubfoot deformities.

Therapeutic Management

The goal of treatment for clubfoot is to achieve a painless, plantigrade, and stable foot. Once the diagnosis is established, treatment is ideally initiated in the newborn period and involves three stages: (1) correction of the deformity, (2) maintenance of the correction until normal muscle balance is regained, and (3) follow-up observation to avert possible recurrence of the deformity. Some feet respond to treatment readily; some respond only to prolonged, vigorous, and sustained efforts; and the improvement in others remains disappointing even with maximum effort. Parents should realize that outcomes are not always predictable and depend on the severity of the deformity, age of the child at initial intervention, compliance with treatment protocols, and development of bones, muscles, and nerves.

The common approach to clubfoot management and treatment is the Ponseti method (Ponseti, 1996). Serial casting is begun within the first month of life. Weekly gentle manipulation and stretching of the foot along with placement of serial long-leg casts allow for gradual repositioning of the foot (Fig. 33.41). The extremity or extremities are casted until maximum correction is achieved, usually within 5 to 8 weeks. The majority of the time, a percutaneous heelcord tenotomy is performed at the end of casting to correct the equinus deformity. After the tenotomy, a long-leg cast is applied and left in place for 3 weeks. After the completion of casting, a Denis Browne bar with Ponseti sandals placed in abduction are fitted to maintain the correction and prevent recurrence. The foot abduction brace is used at nighttime for 3 to 5 years. Inability to achieve an acceptable foot alignment and ankle range of motion after casting and tenotomy indicates the need for additional surgical intervention.

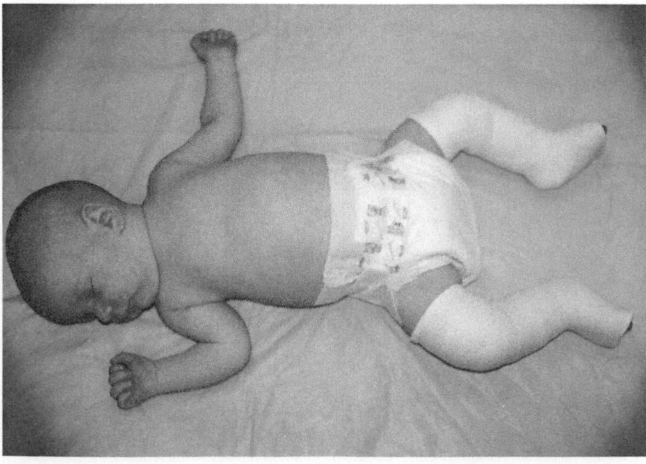

FIG. 33.41 Feet casted for correction of bilateral clubfeet.

NURSING CARE MANAGEMENT

Nursing care of the child with clubfoot is the same as for any child who has a cast. Because the child will spend considerable time in a corrective device, nursing care plans include both long- and short-term goals. Careful observation of the skin and circulation is particularly important in young infants because of their rapid growth rate.

Because treatment and follow-up care are handled in the orthopedic clinic or outpatient department, parent education and support are important in the nursing care of these children. Parents need to understand the diagnosis, the overall treatment program, the importance of regular cast changes, and the role they play in the long-term effectiveness of the therapy. Nursing responsibilities include reinforcing and clarifying the orthopedic provider's explanations and instructions, teaching parents about care of the cast or bracing (including vigilant observation for potential problems), and encouraging parents to facilitate normal development within the limitations imposed by the deformity or therapy.

ORTHOPEDIC INFECTIONS

OSTEOMYELITIS

Osteomyelitis, an infectious process involving the bone, may occur at any age but most frequently is seen in children 10 years of age or younger. *Staphylococcus aureus* is the most common causative organism. Neonates are also likely to have osteomyelitis caused by group B streptococci. Since the advent of *Haemophilus influenzae* type b immunization in the late 1980s, *H. influenzae* has become a less common causative pathogen. *Kingella kingae* and methicillin-resistant *S. aureus* (MRSA), however, are emerging as potential causative organisms in musculoskeletal infections (Stans, 2014).

Acute hematogenous osteomyelitis results when a blood-borne bacterium causes an infection in the bone. Common foci include infected lesions, upper respiratory tract infections, otitis media, tonsillitis, abscessed teeth, pyelonephritis, and infected burns. Exogenous osteomyelitis is acquired from direct inoculation of the bone from a puncture wound, open fracture, surgical contamination, or adjacent tissue infection. Subacute osteomyelitis has a longer course and may be caused by less virulent microbes with a walled-off abscess or Brodie abscess, typically in the proximal or distal tibia. Chronic osteomyelitis is a progression of acute osteomyelitis and is characterized by the presence of dead bone, bone loss, and drainage and sinus tracts. Generally healthy bone is not likely to become infected. Factors that contribute to infection include inoculation with a large number of organisms, presence of a foreign body, bone injury, high virulence of an organism, immunosuppression, and malnutrition. Certain types and locations of bone are also more vulnerable to infection. The limbs most commonly affected include the foot, femur, tibia, and pelvis.

Pathophysiology

In acute osteomyelitis, bacteria adhere to bone, causing a suppurative infection with inflammatory cells, edema, vascular congestion, and small-vessel thrombosis; the result is bone destruction, abscess formation, and dead bone (sequestra). Infection within the bone can rupture through the cortex into the subperiosteal space, stripping loose periosteum and forming an abscess. As dead bone is resorbed, new bone is formed along

PATHOPHYSIOLOGY REVIEW

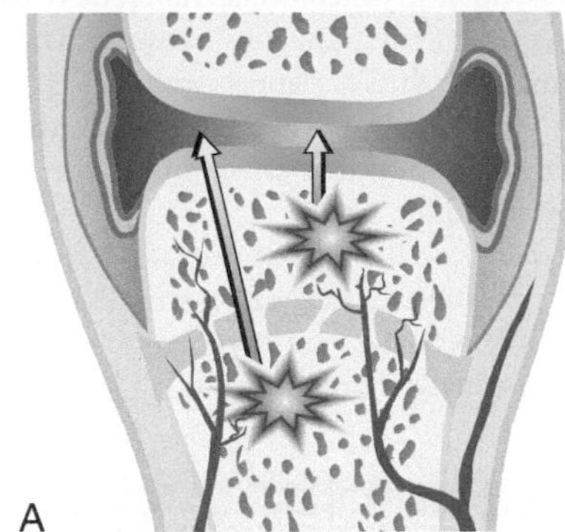

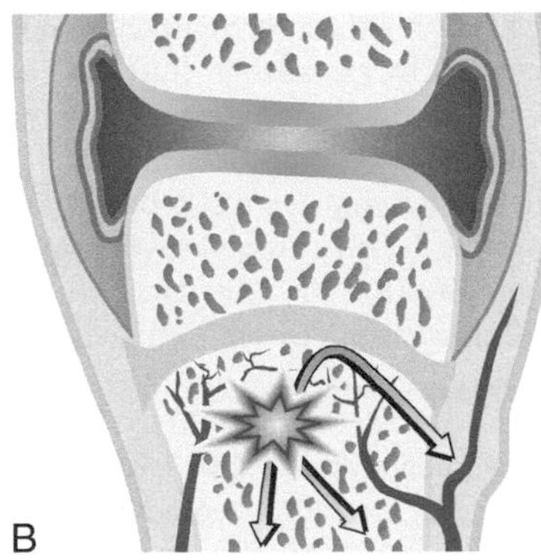

FIG. 33.42 Pathogenesis of acute osteomyelitis differs with age. **A,** In infants younger than 1 year, the epiphysis is nourished by penetrating arteries through the physis, allowing development of the condition within the epiphysis. **B,** In children up to 15 years of age, the infection is restricted to below the physis because of interruption of the vessels.

the live bone and infection borders. This surrounding sheath of live bone is called an involucrum. Sinus tracts from perforations in the involucrum may drain pus through soft tissue to the skin.

The pathology of osteomyelitis is different in infants, children older than 1 year of age, and adults. In infants blood vessels cross the growth plate into the epiphysis and joint space, which allows infection to spread into the joint. In children the infection is contained by the growth plate, and joint infection is less likely (unless the infection is intracapsular) (Fig. 33.42).

Clinical Manifestations

In children severe pain, fever, irritability, and tenderness with or without local signs of inflammation suggest osteomyelitis. The extremity is tender, and the child may hold it in a flexed position and resist movement. In infants these symptoms may be minimal or absent, and pain may be difficult to localize. The infant may demonstrate pain with movement of the extremity or hold it immobile. Fever is uncommon in infants, and they often do not appear to be ill. Infants may have an adjacent joint effusion. Typically the metaphysis of long bones—the tibia, femur, and/or humerus—are involved. In a small portion of children more than one bone may be affected.

Diagnostic Evaluation

Organism identification and antibiotic susceptibility testing are essential for effective therapy. Obtain cultures of aspirated subperiosteal pus along with cultures of blood, joint fluid, and infected skin samples. Bone biopsy may be indicated if blood culture results and radiographic findings are not consistent with osteomyelitis. Supporting evidence for osteomyelitis includes leukocytosis, elevated erythrocyte sedimentation rate, and elevated C-reactive protein. Radiographic signs, except for soft tissue swelling, are evident only after 2 to 3 weeks. A three-phase technetium bone scan can show areas of increased blood flow, such as occurs in early stages in infected bone, and is useful in locating multiple sites; however, it is not a diagnostic test. CT can detect bone destruction, and MRI provides anatomic details useful in delineating the area of involvement, especially if surgical intervention is planned. The differential diagnosis includes trauma, malignant lesions, leukemia, juvenile rheumatoid arthritis, and acute rheumatic fever. Sometimes osteomyelitis may be unrecognized if it occurs as a complication of a severe toxic and debilitating disease.

Therapeutic Management

Surgical management with aspiration and drainage of the bone or joint affected should be performed as soon as possible. Specimen cultures are obtained during the procedure to help identify the specific organism responsible for the infection. Aspiration also assists in determining whether there is an abscess or septic joint that requires surgical drainage.

After culture specimens are obtained, empiric therapy is started with IV antibiotics covering the most likely organisms. When the infective agent is identified, administration of the appropriate antibiotic is initiated and continued for at least 4 weeks, but the length of therapy is determined by the duration of the symptoms, the response to treatment, and the sensitivity of the organism. In selected cases oral antibiotic therapy may follow a shorter IV course. Due to the prolonged duration of high-dose antibiotic therapy, it is important to monitor for hematologic, renal, hepatic, ototoxic, and other potential side effects.

Nursing Care Management

During the acute phase of illness, any movement of the affected limb causes discomfort to the child, so the child is positioned comfortably with the affected limb supported. Moving and turning are carried out carefully and gently to minimize discomfort. The child may require pain medication (see Chapter 5) or sedation. Take vital signs and record them frequently, and implement measures to reduce a significant temperature elevation.

Antibiotic therapy requires careful observation and monitoring of the IV equipment and site. Because more than one antibiotic is usually administered, the compatibility of the drugs must be determined and care taken to avoid mixing incompatible drugs. The stability of the drugs and their toxic nature are also considered when determining the rate of administration. The infusion device must be well situated in the vein to ensure that the drug does not infiltrate into surrounding tissues, where it may produce tissue damage. For long-term antibiotic therapy, a venous access device, such as a peripherally inserted central catheter, is the preferred method of IV administration. (See Chapter 22)

The wound is managed according to the provider's directions. Administration of antibiotic solution directly into the wound is most efficiently accomplished using a regular infusion setup that is prepared and regulated in the same manner as for any IV infusion. Intake and output are measured and recorded, and the character of both the wound and drainage is noted. The amount and character of drainage on the wound dressing are also noted.

As the infection subsides, physical therapy is instituted to ensure restoration of optimum function. The child is usually discharged on a regimen of antibiotics (either IV or oral), and progress is monitored closely.

SEPTIC ARTHRITIS

Septic (suppurative) arthritis is a bacterial infection in the joint. It usually results from hematogenous spread or from direct extension of an adjacent cellulitis or osteomyelitis. Direct inoculation from trauma accounts for 15% to 20% of septic arthritis cases. The most common causative organism is *S. aureus.* Community-acquired MRSA is commonly a cause of septic arthritis. In addition to *S. aureus,* pathogens seen in neonates include group B and A *Streptococcus, Escherichia coli,* and *Streptococcus pneumoniae.* In children 2 months to 5 years of age, *S. aureus, Streptococcus pyogenes, S. pneumoniae,* and *K. kingae* are the primary organisms causing infection, whereas children older than 5 years are more likely to be infected by *S. aureus* and *S. pyogenes;* sexually active adolescents may be infected by *N. gonorrhoeae* (Montgomery & Epps, 2017).

Knees, hips, ankles, and elbows are the most commonly affected joints. Clinical manifestations include severe joint pain, swelling, warmth of overlying tissue, and occasionally erythema. The child is resistant to any joint movement. Features of systemic illness such as fever, malaise, headache, nausea, vomiting, and irritability may also be present.

Therapeutic and Nursing Care Management

The affected joint is aspirated and the specimen evaluated by Gram stain, culture, and determination of leukocyte count. In addition, blood cultures and complete blood counts with differential, erythrocyte sedimentation rate, and C-reactive protein levels should be monitored. Surgical decompression of the joint along with irrigation and debridement is recommended. Early radiographic findings are limited to soft tissue swelling but may reveal a foreign body, and such films always provide a baseline for comparison. MRI and CT scans provide more detailed images of inflammation, cartilage loss, joint narrowing, erosions, and marrow involvement.

IV antibiotic therapy is based on Gram stain results and clinical presentation. The benefits of serial aspiration to demonstrate sterility of synovial fluid and reduce pressure or pain are controversial. Pain management is an important aspect of nursing care, particularly with involvement of a large joint such as the hip. Surgical intervention may also be required if there was a penetrating wound or a foreign object was possibly involved. Physical therapy may be initiated to maintain range of motion and prevent contractures, similar to the nursing care for osteomyelitis.

SKELETAL TUBERCULOSIS

In children, tuberculous infection of the bones and joints is acquired by lymphohematogenous spread at the time of primary infection. Occasionally it is from chronic pulmonary tuberculosis. Skeletal tuberculous infection is not common in the United States but should be considered in communities with high tuberculosis case rates. The infection is most likely to involve the vertebrae, causing a paravertebral abscess formation. If the spine infection is progressive, it results in destruction of the vertebral bodies and results in hyperkyphosis deformity. Symptoms are insidious. The child may report persistent or intermittent pain. Other findings include joint swelling and stiffness; fever and weight loss are not common. Tuberculous arthritis can also affect single joints such as a knee or hip and tends to cause severe destruction of adjacent bone. Infection in the fingers causes spina ventosa, a tuberculous dactylitis.

As with pulmonary tuberculosis, the index case should be located. A family and environmental history needs to be obtained and skin tests performed. (See also Tuberculosis, Chapter 26.) Results of tuberculin skin tests are positive for the majority of children with tuberculous arthritis; however, the results are not diagnostic, and the clinical and laboratory features do not differentiate tubercular arthritis from a nontuberculous septic arthritis. Diagnosis requires isolation of *Mycobacterium tuberculosis* from the site. Patients with the susceptible organism start treatment with combined antituberculosis chemotherapy (isoniazid, rifampin, and pyrazinamide); directly observed therapy is preferred and should be continued for 1 year.

Nursing care depends on the site and extent of infection. Tuberculous spondylitis and hip infection may require immobilization and additional surgical management. Nursing care is the same as for osteomyelitis, with the addition of isolation requirements.

SKELETAL AND ARTICULAR DYSFUNCTION

OSTEOGENESIS IMPERFECTA

Osteogenesis imperfecta (OI) is the most common osteoporosis syndrome in children, characterized by excessive fractures and bone deformity; most affected children have moderate to severe growth restriction. There are at least 11 types of OI, accounting for significant disease variability. Clinical features include varying degrees of bone fragility, deformity, and fracture; blue sclerae; hearing loss; and dentinogenesis imperfecta (hypoplastic discolored teeth). The inheritance pattern is autosomal dominant in the majority of cases, although forms demonstrate autosomal recessive inheritance.

Most types of OI have defects in the *COL1A1* or *COL1A2* genes, which code for polypeptide chains in type 1 procollagen, a precursor of type 1 collagen, a major structural component of bone. The error results in faulty bone mineralization, abnormal bone architecture, and increased susceptibility to fracture. Recently genetic studies have found OI types caused by genetic mutations not associated with defective collagen production (Marini & Blissett, 2013). Additional autosomal recessive genetic types of OI have been described and include *CRTAP, PPIB, SERPINH1, LEPRE1, PLOD2, FKBP10, LRP5,* and *SP7* (Laron & Pandya, 2013).

Classifications for OI are based on clinical features and patterns of inheritance (Box 33.10). Clinically, type I is the most common, with wide variability of bone fragility; some affected family members have significant deformity and disability, whereas others lead agile, active lives. Type II variants are the most severe and are considered lethal in infancy. Type III OI is characterized by multiple fractures, bone deformity, and severe disability; affected individuals rarely live to 30 years of age. Type IV is similar to type I with blue or white sclerae. Another variant, or type V, has been described in which those affected have a hyperplastic callus, a radiodense metaphyseal band, and calcification of the interosseous membrane of the forearm; no collagen mutations are noted in this group (Marini, 2016). A type VI has been described with a characteristic mineralization defect, which does not respond to pamidronate therapy as types I to V do (Land, Rauch, Travers, et al., 2007). However, a small group of children with OI VI responded favorably to denosumab, a RANK ligand inhibitor (Semler, Netzer, Hoyer-Kuhn, et al., 2012). Children affected with this type have no dental involvement and normal sclerae; a bone biopsy is the only way to establish a diagnosis because of the similarities to other types. Types VII and VIII overlap types II and III in relation to clinical features, but those who survive these types have white sclerae, a normal-to-small head circumference, short stature, and rhizomelia (Marini, 2016).

Therapeutic Management

The treatment for OI has historically been primarily supportive, although patients and families are optimistic about new research advances. Bone marrow transplant for severe OI was first reported in 1999 with positive

BOX 33.10 Classification of Osteogenesis Imperfecta*

Type I†
- **A**—Mild bone fragility; blue sclerae; normal teeth; hearing loss (occurs between ages 20 and 30 years); autosomal dominant inheritance
- **B**—Same as A except dentinogenesis imperfecta instead of normal teeth
- **C**—Same as B but no bone fragility

Type II—Lethal; stillborn or die in early infancy; severe bone fragility, multiple fractures at birth; 10% of cases of OI; autosomal recessive inheritance

Type III—Severe bone fragility leading to severe progressive deformities; normal sclerae; marked growth failure; most autosomal recessive inheritance; few autosomal dominant inheritance

Type IV
- **A**—Mild to moderate bone fragility; normal sclerae; normal teeth; short stature; variable deformity; autosomal dominant inheritance
- **B**—Same as A except dentinogenesis imperfecta instead of normal teeth; approximately 6% of cases of OI

Type V—Clinically similar to type IV; hyperplastic callus; ossification of interosseous membranes between tibia/fibula and radius/ulna; collagen mutation negative

Type VI—Clinically similar to type IV; rare; sclerae and dentition normal; moderate to severe bone fragility; diagnosis by bone biopsy because of similarities to other types

Types VII and VIII (recessive form)—Clinically overlap types II and III but have white sclerae, rhizomelia, and small to normal head circumference; severe osteochondroplasia and short stature in survivors. Type VII is associated with *CRTAP* gene and Type VIII is associated with the LEPRE1 genetic mutation (Marini, 2016).

*Two-thirds of cases are type I.
†This classification is based on that proposed by Sillence, Senn, and Danks (1979), which originally included OI types I through IV. Additional types have been described but are not included herein.
OI, Osteogenesis imperfecta.

results; however, this is still considered an experimental treatment, and long-term follow-up of such children has not been published. The long-term effectiveness of bone marrow transplant for OI in comparison to the complications of the treatment have yet to be fully explored (Madonia, 2012).

Therapeutic management should focus on decreasing the number of fractures, decreasing pain, increasing growth, improving bone metabolism, and optimizing function. Bisphosphonate therapy with pamidronate, risedronate, olpadronate, neridronate, or alendronate to promote increased bone density and prevent fractures has become standard therapy for many children with OI. Bisphosphonate therapy reportedly is more beneficial for increasing vertebral bone density but is considered less effective for long bones (Marini, 2016). Others report effectiveness of pamidronate in children with moderate to severe OI (Alharbi, Pinto, Finidori, et al., 2009). Bachrach and Ward (2009) suggest that data are inadequate to recommend the use of bisphosphonate therapy in children with OI for sole treatment of bone mineral density reduction. Oral risedronate has been reported to be mildly effective in treating children with type I OI, but it is not superior to pamidronate therapy (Rauch, Munns, Land, et al., 2009).

The rehabilitative approach to management is directed to preventing positional contractures and deformities, muscle weakness and osteoporosis, and malalignment of lower extremity joints, prohibiting weight bearing. Lightweight braces and splints help support limbs, prevent fractures, and aid in ambulation. Physical therapy helps prevent disuse osteoporosis and strengthens muscles, which in turn improves bone density. Surgery is sometimes used to help treat the manifestations of the disease. Surgical techniques are used to correct deformities that interfere with bracing, standing, or walking. For the child with recurrent fractures, inserting an intramedullary rod provides stability to bones. Telescoping intramedullary rods may be used to accommodate normal growth; early reports show an improvement in ambulation, mobility, and gross motor function in OI patients with femoral deformities (Laron & Pandya, 2013). Because there is a 50% risk of an affected individual passing the gene to an offspring, genetic counseling is recommended.

Nursing Care Management

Infants and children with this disorder require careful handling to prevent fractures. They must be supported when they are being turned, positioned, moved, and held. Even changing a diaper may cause a fracture in severely affected infants. These children should never be held by the ankles when being diapered but should be gently lifted by the buttocks or supported with pillows; however, nurses should not be afraid to touch or handle the infant or child with OI. Such children need compassionate handling and care as much as any other patient. Parents who care for such children on a regular basis can often share tips for handling the child without causing fractures.

It is recommended that blood pressure be obtained with a manual cuff to prevent fractures. In addition nurses should be aware that such children, although smaller in stature than same-age children, have normal intelligence and should receive adequate information and instructions regarding their care. Involving parents in the daily care of the child is essential (Madonia, 2012). Children receiving bisphosphonate therapy should be closely monitored for respiratory infections and should receive appropriate immunizations for the prevention of childhood communicable diseases. Live virus vaccines may not be recommended in children on bisphosphonate therapy, and an infectious disease specialist should be consulted. Skin care for children with OI is essential; infants with OI may need frequent repositioning of the head to prevent posterior occipital flattening or other cranial molding. Oral and dental care should be performed on a regular basis and with extreme care due to bone and tooth fragility (Madonia, 2012). Parents of the child undergoing bone marrow transplant need adequate written information and instructions regarding special care in regard to the various chemotherapeutic drugs required (Madonia, 2012). (See also Bone Marrow Transplantation, Chapter 29.)

Children with current fractures or healing fractures should be screened for OI; the assumption that abuse or neglect is the cause of fractures in children must be carefully evaluated by a multidisciplinary team. A detailed history, no evidence of associated soft-tissue injury, and the presence of other symptoms related to OI help determine the diagnosis.

Both parents and the affected child need education regarding the child's limitations and guidelines in planning suitable activities that promote optimum development and protect the child from harm. Realistic occupational planning and genetic counseling are part of the long-term goals of care. The parents can obtain educational materials and information from the Osteogenesis Imperfecta Foundation, Inc.,* which also has a network to put families in contact with other families that have a similar problem.

JUVENILE IDIOPATHIC ARTHRITIS

Juvenile idiopathic arthritis (JIA) refers to chronic childhood arthritis. A group of heterogeneous chronic autoimmune diseases, JIA causes

*804 W. Diamond Ave., Suite 210, Gaithersburg, MD 20878; 800-981-2663; http://www.oif.org.

inflammation in the synovium, joints, and surrounding tissue. The cause of JIA is unknown. Some theories speculate that the disorder arises when an infectious agent activates an autoimmune inflammatory process in a genetically predisposed child. Although a genetic susceptibility to JIA is known, such as human leukocyte antigen (HLA) polymorphisms, the *PTPN22* gene, and the *IL2RA/CD 25* gene, the genetic contribution is complicated and still not well understood (Prahalad & Glass, 2008). The reported incidence of chronic childhood arthritis varies from 1 to 20 cases per 100,000 children, with a prevalence of 10 to 400 per 100,000 (Cassidy & Petty, 2011). JIA starts before age 16 years with two peak onsets: between 1 and 3 and between 8 and 10 years of age. There is a female predominance of 2:1.

Pathophysiology

The disease process is characterized by chronic synovial inflammation causing joint effusion and eventual erosion, destruction, and fibrosis of the articular cartilage. Adhesions between joint surfaces and ankylosis of joints occur if the process persists.

Clinical Manifestations

Whether single or multiple joints are involved, stiffness, swelling, and loss of motion develop in the affected joints. The swelling results from soft tissue edema, joint effusion, and synovial thickening. The affected joints may be warm and tender to the touch, but it is not uncommon for pain not to be reported. Erythema is not typical, and a warm, painful red joint is always suspect for infection. The limited motion early in the disease is a result of muscle spasm and joint inflammation; later it is caused by ankylosis or soft tissue contracture. Morning stiffness of the joint(s) is characteristic and present on arising in the morning or after inactivity. Functional change may be an obvious limp or subtle modifications of joint motion that protect the involved joint, such as fisting to avoid wrist extension with pressure. In severe, long-standing cases growth is significantly restricted. Corticosteroid therapy can be a contributing factor. There may be growth disturbances, either overgrowth or undergrowth, adjacent to the inflamed joints (e.g., altered leg length after knee involvement) and micrognathia (receding chin) from temporomandibular arthritis.

Classification. The International League of Associations for Rheumatology classification of JIA, developed in 1997, revised and published in 1998, and revised again in 2001, lists seven disease categories, each with its own set of criteria and exclusions: systemic arthritis, oligoarthritis, rheumatoid factor (RF)–negative polyarthritis, RF-positive polyarthritis, psoriatic arthritis, enthesitis-related arthritis, and undifferentiated arthritis (Petty, Southwood, Manners, et al., 2004) (Box 33.11).

Course and Prognosis

The outcome of JIA is variable and unpredictable. Even in severe forms, JIA is rarely life threatening and is significantly different from adult rheumatoid arthritis. Features that distinguish JIA from adult disease include onset before 16 years of age; a negative rheumatoid factor (in 90% of cases); classic symptoms of systemic arthritis, including quotidian fever, rash, and pericarditis; development of uveitis (inflammation of

BOX 33.11 International League of Associations for Rheumatology Classification of Juvenile Idiopathic Arthritis

Systemic Arthritis

Definition—Arthritis in one or more joints with or preceded by fever for at least 2 weeks' duration that is documented to be daily for at least 3 days, and accompanied by one or more of the following: evanescent (nonfixed) erythematous rash, generalized lymph node enlargement, hepatomegaly and/or splenomegaly, serositis.

Exclusions—a, b, c, d*

Oligoarthritis

Definition—Arthritis affecting one to four joints during the first 6 months of disease. Two subcategories are recognized: (1) persistent oligoarthritis, which never extends over four affected joints during disease course; and (2) extended oligoarthritis, which affects more than four joints after 6 months of disease.

Exclusions—a, b, c, d, e*

Polyarthritis (Rheumatoid Factor Negative)

Definition—Arthritis affecting five or more joints during the first 6 months of the disease and a negative rheumatoid factor.

Exclusions—a, b, c, e*

Polyarthritis (Rheumatoid Factor Positive)

Definition—Arthritis affecting five or more joints during the first 6 months of disease and two or more positive rheumatoid factor tests at least 3 months apart during the first 6 months of disease.

Exclusions—a, b, c, e*

Psoriatic Arthritis

Definition—Arthritis and psoriasis, or arthritis and at least two of the following: (1) dactylitis, (2) nail pitting or onycholysis, and (3) psoriasis in a first-degree relative.

Exclusions—b, c, d, e*

Enthesitis-Related Arthritis

Definition—Arthritis and enthesitis (inflammation at a tendon insertion site), or arthritis or enthesitis with at least two of the following: (1) presence or history of sacroiliac joint tenderness and/or inflammatory lumbosacral pain; (2) presence of HLA-B27 antigen; (3) onset of arthritis in a male over 6 years of age; (4) symptomatic anterior uveitis; and (5) a history of ankylosing spondylitis, enthesitis-related arthritis, sacroiliitis with inflammatory bowel disease, Reiter syndrome, or acute anterior uveitis in a first-degree relative.

Exclusions—a, d, e*

Undifferentiated Arthritis

Definition—Arthritis that fulfills criteria in no category or in two or more of the above categories.

*Exclusions: (a) Psoriasis or a history of psoriasis in the patient or first-degree relative; (b) arthritis in an HLA-B27–positive male beginning after the sixth birthday; (c) ankylosing spondylitis, enthesitis-related arthritis, sacroiliitis with inflammatory bowel disease, Reiter syndrome, or symptomatic anterior uveitis, or a history of one of these disorders in a first-degree relative; (d) the presence of immunoglobulin M rheumatoid factor on at least two occasions at least 3 months apart; (e) the presence of systemic juvenile idiopathic arthritis in the patient (Petty, Southwood, Manners, et al., 2004).

HLA, Human leukocyte antigen.

the iris and ciliary body) as a complication (in 8% to 20% of cases); and a tendency for the arthritis to become inactive.

Mortality is rare, occurring in less than 0.3% in North America. Deaths in the United States are typically associated with systemic JIA and infection. The arthritis tends to wax and wane and only becomes inactive in approximately 30% of the cases. These children may have severe or minimal joint damage remaining when active arthritis abates. Approximately 70% of the children have progressive arthritis into adulthood. Their arthritis can cause significant joint deformity and functional disability requiring medication, physical therapy, and perhaps future joint replacement. Chronic and acute uveitis is an extraarticular complication of JIA that may cause permanent vision loss if undiagnosed and not aggressively treated. Although many children have minimal arthritis, it can produce severe physical, functional, and emotional impairment.

Diagnostic Evaluation

JIA is diagnosis of exclusion; there are no definitive tests. Criteria include onset before 16 years, arthritis in one or more joints for 6 weeks or longer, and exclusion of other causes (Petty, Southwood, Manners, et al., 2004). Laboratory test results may provide supporting evidence of disease. An elevated sedimentation rate or C-reactive protein may or may not be present. Leukocytosis is frequently present during flares of systemic disease. Tests for RF give positive results in only 10% of the children with JIA. The presence of antinuclear antibodies is common in JIA, but they are not specific for arthritis; however, their presence helps identify children with pauciarticular disease, who are at greater risk for uveitis.

Therapeutic Management

There is no cure for JIA. The major goals of therapy are to control pain, preserve joint range of motion and function, minimize the effects of inflammation such as joint deformity, and promote normal growth and development. Achievement of these goals requires a family-centered approach with collaboration among the child, family, and health care team. The team includes the primary care physician; pediatric rheumatologist; rheumatology nurse educator; social worker; physical and occupational therapists; subspecialists (e.g., pediatric ophthalmologist); and a community of friends, relatives, and teachers. The treatment plan is individualized, but it can be complicated and intrusive, including medications, physical and occupational therapy, slit-lamp eye examinations, splints, comfort measures, dietary management, modification of school activities, and psychosocial support. Outpatient care is the mainstay of therapy; lengthy hospital admissions for rehabilitation are seldom financially feasible.

Chronic uveitis can cause permanent vision loss, glaucoma, and cataracts. Slit-lamp ophthalmologic examinations at regular intervals are required to diagnose chronic anterior uveitis (iridocyclitis), inflammation of the anterior segments of the eye, iris, and ciliary body. The majority of affected children have a relatively good visual prognosis if the inflammation is detected and treated early; however, most cases are asymptomatic. Consequently, routine slit-lamp examinations are critical. The children at greatest risk for development of uveitis have pauciarticular disease and a positive antinuclear antibody (Reininga, Los, Wulffraat, et al., 2008). Infections, injuries, and surgical procedures often precipitate a flare-up of the arthritis; therefore prompt recognition and treatment of infections are necessary.

Medications. In 2011 the American College of Rheumatology published recommendations for the treatment of JIA intended to lend guidance to the provider. The guidelines are divided into four groups: children with four or fewer affected joints, five or more affected joints, systemic arthritis with active systemic features, and systemic arthritis with active arthritis. Each path provides recommendations for stepwise escalation of medication therapy (Beukelman, Patkar, Saag, et al., 2011). The American College of Rheumatology further updated treatment recommendations for systemic arthritis in 2013 (Ringhold, Weiss, Beukelman, et al., 2013). All tracks consider poor prognostic indicators, such as erosions on radiographs; arthritis of the hip, cervical spine, ankle, or wrist; and a positive rheumatoid factor. Additionally, each track takes into account disease activity levels that include elevated acute phase reactants and global assessments of both the provider and the patient/parent.

A variety of antirheumatic drugs are available. NSAIDs are used alone or in combination with other drugs, depending on the amount of disease activity and poor prognostic features. Common NSAIDs include ibuprofen, naproxen, tolmetin, diclofenac, indomethacin, and meloxicam. (See Table 5.8) NSAIDs offer an immediate analgesic effect, but the antiinflammatory effect requires larger doses and more time to achieve. Patient and family education regarding potential gastrointestinal, renal, and hepatic side effects and reduced clotting is essential. Parents should monitor the child for abdominal pain and blood in the stool. Naproxen has the potential side effect of skin fragility; patients need to use sunscreen and report unusual skin lesions.

Additional medication is required in most children with arthritis. The agents used are disease-modifying antirheumatic drugs (DMARDs) and include the nonbiologic drugs methotrexate and sulfasalazine. The decision to use DMARDs at initiation of therapy or later in the escalation of therapy is guided by the amount of disease activity and poor prognostic features. Weekly low-dose methotrexate therapy is usually the first DMARD used. Families may be overwhelmed by the potential adverse effects, including liver disease, bone marrow suppression, gastrointestinal disturbance, teratogenic effects, and the alarming but unconfirmed risk of carcinogenesis. Methotrexate is effective, however, and the potential benefits outweigh the potential risks. Methotrexate therapy has also improved uveitis in children with uveitis resistant to steroid treatment. Laboratory monitoring of liver enzyme levels and blood counts is crucial. A daily folic acid supplement can help reduce the occurrence of oral ulcers. Taking methotrexate at bedtime may help reduce nausea.

Frank discussion about sexual activity and birth defects is critical. Sexually active teenagers need effective birth control and documented menstrual periods, as well as pregnancy tests if periods are not regular. As a precaution, pregnant caregivers and those trying to conceive need to avoid contact with methotrexate.

Alcohol consumption is another sensitive topic that needs to be discussed honestly because it increases the risk of hepatotoxicity. Patients should avoid additional over-the-counter NSAIDs and to take acetaminophen for episodes of fever. Parents should always discuss methotrexate drug interactions with providers prescribing medications for interval illness. During some illnesses, especially varicella, methotrexate should be discontinued because it can suppress the immune response. Sulfasazaline may be selected in children with axial arthritis, a positive test result for HLA-B27, or symptoms of inflammatory bowel disease, given this drug's success in these select groups of patients.

Biologic DMARDs. Biologic DMARDs are initiated when there is significant disease activity and/or poor prognostic indicators after unsuccessful treatment with methotrexate. Tumor necrosis factor alpha (TNF-α) inhibitors are the most frequently used biologic DMARDs and include etanercept, infliximab, and adalimumab. Etanercept blocks the binding of TNF-α with cell surface receptors, and adalimumab and infliximab are monoclonal antibody TNF-α blocking agents. All three reduce the proinflammatory response that promotes arthritis. Studies have shown TNF-α inhibitors to be effective and well tolerated (Lovell, Ruperto, Goodman, et al., 2008; Stoll & Gotte, 2008).

Although TNF-α inhibitors have been found safe and effective, parents need to inform providers of any unusual symptoms in the child given the relatively limited experience with these drugs and the potential for long-term side effects (Burmester, Mease, Dijkmans, et al., 2009; Lovell, Reiff, Ilowite, et al., 2008). The potential for malignancy, particularly lymphoma, is continuing to be monitored in children on TNF blockers. Increased infection risk is the most common adverse effect. Parents should withhold TNF-α inhibitors during a concurrent infection and promptly report symptoms of infection to their provider for assessment and treatment. A negative tuberculin skin test should be obtained before starting a biologic DMARD; yearly follow-up skin testing has been suggested. Interleukin-1 receptor antagonist, anakinra, is another biologic antirheumatic drug. In active systemic disease with poor prognostic features, anakinra may be initiated with systemic glucocorticoid steroids as initial therapy. Anakinra is approved by the U.S. Food and Drug Administration for the adult rheumatoid arthritis population and is available off-label for children with systemic JIA.

Glucocorticoids. Glucocorticoids are potent antiinflammatory agents; however, systemic steroids will not cure arthritis, and the significant adverse effects of long-term steroid use are undesirable. Steroids are administered when there is high disease activity or poor prognostic features. Prednisone is given orally in a burst and taper or at the lowest effective dosage. Use of an alternate-day schedule may help reduce side effects. High-dose IV steroids may provide sustained improvement for children with severe arthritis and pericarditis associated with systemic disease. Intraarticular injections of long-acting steroids have proven effective in treating limited arthritis with minimal adverse effects and frequently provided sustained control and, in some, a remission. Children may require procedural sedation or general anesthesia, which affects risk-benefit considerations, but it is critical to have a cooperative patient for good procedure outcome.

Physical Management. Programs of physical therapy are individualized for each child and are designed to reach the ultimate goal of preserving function and preventing deformity. Physical therapy is directed toward specific joints and focuses on strengthening muscles, mobilizing restricted joints, and preventing or correcting deformities. Occupational therapists assume responsibility of evaluating and improving performance of activities of daily living.

General treatment and maintenance programs vary. Physical therapists may be involved several times per week, or their visits may be limited to monthly evaluations to review the home program for compliance, effectiveness, and need. Muscle strength is frequently lost around the involved joints, and inactivity leads to generalized weakness. However, performance of the normal activities of daily living and the child's natural tendency to be active are usually sufficient to maintain muscle strength and joint mobility. Unless there is a specific risk of injury related to arthritis, the child should not be restricted from regular play, dance, exercise programs, and even individual and team sports. Activity modifications may be needed to accommodate joint limitations, but exercise should be encouraged; a sedentary lifestyle contributes to a deconditioned state, which further limits physical activity and ultimately influences the child's quality of life.

Exercising in a pool is excellent because it allows freedom of movement with support. When joints are inflamed, heavy resistance aggravates the pain. At such times, simple isometric or tensing exercises that do not involve joint movement are generally tolerated. Range-of-motion exercises are an important aspect of therapy and are continued after evidence of disease has disappeared in order to detect any signs of recurrence.

Providers may recommend nighttime splinting to help minimize pain and prevent or reduce flexion deformity. Vigilance is required to detect loss of motion, and vigorous attention must be given to specialized passive stretching, positioning, and resting splints to prevent deformity.

Surgery. The benefits of synovectomy, an established therapeutic procedure in adults, are questionable in children with arthritis. Synovectomy is used primarily in pauciarticular disease when all other therapy has been unsuccessful. In cases of synovitis, intraarticular steroid injection is an alternative to synovectomy and may be tried once or twice before surgery is performed. Joint replacement is proving to be successful in older children who are fully grown.

Nursing Care Management

Nursing care of children with JIA involves assessment of their general health, the status of involved joints, and their emotional responses to all of the ramifications of the disease: pain, physical restrictions, therapies, and self-concept, especially in preadolescents and adolescents.

The effects of the disease are manifested in every aspect of the child's life, including physical activities, social experiences, and personality development. Children's adjustment to the stresses and demands of the disease and the level of functioning they achieve are related largely to the reaction and support they receive from their family and the health care professionals involved in their care and management.

Relieve Pain. Multiple factors influence the pain of arthritis: disease severity, functional status, individual pain threshold, family variables, and psychologic adjustment. Although complete pain relief is desirable, it is probably unrealistic. The aim is to provide as much relief as possible with antiinflammatory medication and other therapies to help children tolerate the pain and complete the activities of daily living. At present, opioid administration is not a routine therapy for the chronic pain of arthritis. Nonpharmacologic modalities such as relaxation may be helpful. (See Pain Management, Chapter 5.)

Promote General Strength

Diet and exercise. The general health of children with arthritis and their siblings must be considered but may be overlooked as parents and health personnel concentrate on the disease. Maintenance of a well-balanced diet and assessment of nutritional status are integral parts of health supervision. A daily children's complete multivitamin with iron is a reasonable dietary supplement, but there is no "arthritis diet" or foods to avoid that are specifically associated with arthritis. Unfortunately children with arthritis have not been spared the nationwide obesity epidemic. After assessing the child growth chart, make a referral to a dietitian for children who are underweight or overweight due to malnutrition. Excessive weight causes additional strain on inflamed joints. Joint pain during or after exercise impedes active play, which perpetuates the vicious cycle of inactivity and weight gain. Encourage daily physical exercise, starting with a gradual program of walking and slowly advancing to more active play as tolerated. During the school year this can be accomplished with participation in physical education classes as tolerated. When school is out, parents and children should devise a family plan for exercise that includes a variety of options such as games, sports, dance, yoga, swimming, bike riding, and walking. This builds good habits for an active lifestyle for the entire family.

Sleep and rest. Children with JIA report frequent disrupted nighttime sleep, daytime sleepiness, fatigue, and sleep anxiety (Bloom, Owens, McGuinn, et al., 2002). Restorative sleep is essential. Children should get 8 to 10 hours of nighttime sleep. Daytime naps are discouraged, especially because inactivity provokes stiffness and prolonged naps can interfere with sleepiness at bedtime. Fatigue should be handled with rest rather than sleep. Thirty to 60 minutes of relaxation—viewing television, reading, playing video games, using the computer, or listening to music—is refueling and less likely to disrupt nighttime sleep than a nap.

Encourage School Attendance. School-aged children should attend school, even on days when there is joint pain. Staying home will not improve arthritis. If joint pain and stiffness prevent school attendance, the rheumatologist should be notified and the child assessed. The rheumatology team can make recommendations to the school to maximize attendance and participation. Enlisting the school nurse to administer scheduled medications and as-needed analgesics such as acetaminophen for pain rescue will help keep the child at school. Requesting one set of books for use at home and one for the classroom eliminates heavy backpacks and subsequent strain on arthritic joints. The child's participation in the physical education program as tolerated is another way to maximize attendance and performance. If more extensive modifications to the school routine are indicated, the development of an individualized education plan for the school setting may ensure that the child's needs are met. Examples of provisions included in such plans are half-day programs, special transportation, and in-school physical therapy. Although home teaching is rarely indicated, in some circumstances it is necessary; it is initiated with the goal of returning the child to the classroom as soon as possible.

Facilitate Compliance. For any medical or physical plan of therapy to be effective, the family must agree to it and understand the benefits of treatment and the problems associated with noncompliance. Review a simple written list of exercise benefits and complications of joint immobility. At the outset, elicit barriers to a plan from the child and parents. If a child cannot swallow pills or refuses injections, the given modality is not acceptable. If parents know they cannot monitor or enforce a complicated medication and physical therapy schedule, the plan needs to be simplified to honestly reflect the actual care that is being provided. If joint range-of-motion exercises are too painful and emotionally difficult for parents to implement despite use of pretherapy analgesics and comfort measures, then physical therapy home visits or outpatient physical therapy sessions need to be considered.

In addition to developing a plan that is attainable, recognizing a child's adherence by providing inexpensive weekly or monthly rewards fosters goal setting and ultimately boosts self-esteem. It is not just the child who needs therapy rewards; the nonprimary child care provider needs to step in and offer relief to the primary caregiver to prevent burnout, as well as to verbally acknowledge the extra parenting responsibilities being performed.

Everyone needs reminders; a simple written schedule of medications and physical therapy exercises should be provided and reviewed with the family at each visit.

Encourage Comfort Measures and Activities of Daily Living. Application of heat has been beneficial to children with arthritis. Moist heat is best for relieving pain and stiffness, and the most efficient and practical method is via the bathtub. Sometimes a daily whirlpool bath, paraffin bath, or hot packs may be used as needed for temporary relief of acute swelling and pain. Hot packs are easily applied at home using a towel that is wrung out after being immersed in hot water or heated in a microwave oven. Painful hands or feet can be immersed in a pan of warm water for 10 minutes two or three times daily as an adjunct to tub baths. A paraffin bath also provides relief to painful hands.

Pool therapy is the easiest method for exercising a large number of joints. Swimming activities strengthen muscles and maintain mobility in larger joints. Very small children who are frightened of the water can perform their exercises in the bathtub. Small children love to splash, kick, and throw things in the water.

Activities of daily living provide satisfactory exercise for older children to maintain maximum mobility with minimum pain. These children should be encouraged in their efforts and patiently allowed to dress and groom themselves, to assume daily tasks, and to care for their belongings. It is often difficult for stiff fingers to manipulate buttons, comb or brush hair, and turn faucets, but parents and other caregivers should not readily offer assistance. In addition, children should be helped to understand why others do not assist them. Many helpful devices, such as self-adhering fasteners, tongs for manipulating difficult items, and grab bars installed in bathrooms for safety, can be used to facilitate tasks. An elevated toilet seat often makes the difference between dependent and independent toileting because weak quadriceps muscles and sore knees inhibit the ability to raise the body from a low sitting position.

A child's natural affinity for play offers many opportunities for incorporating therapeutic exercises. Throwing or kicking a ball, hanging from monkey bars, and riding a tricycle (with the seat raised to achieve maximum leg extension) are excellent moving and stretching exercises for a young child whose daily living activities are physically limited.

The Arthritis Foundation and the American Juvenile Arthritis Organization* (an organization within the Arthritis Foundation) provide information and services for both parents and professionals, and nurses can refer families to these agencies as an added resource.

The child. For some, arthritis affects every aspect of the child's daily life. The physical pain and limitations interfere with performance of normal tasks and provision of self-care. Even simple tasks, such as dressing, combing the hair, using the bathroom, cutting food, climbing stairs, manipulating doors and faucets, and using public transportation, are difficult or impossible. The child may have school difficulties related to transportation to and from school, stair climbing, and loss of time as a result of exacerbations and hospitalization. Physical limitations interfere with participation in many activities, both curricular and extracurricular, which limits peer contacts and interaction and increases social isolation. These problems are especially critical for adolescents, for whom peer acceptance and relationships are vital to personality development. Many children with arthritis increasingly turn to solitary activities and to the family at a time when they are expected to move into greater independence and relationships with peers.

Changes in personality may accompany JIA, as with any chronic illness. These changes may be temporary, such as demanding, irritable behavior, or they may be persistent, such as passive hostility, uncommunicativeness, and manipulativeness. Families need confirmation that adjusting to a chronic illness is difficult. Consider and encourage support referrals to social workers, counselors, and psychologists. (See Chapter 19.)

The family. The diagnosis of chronic arthritis is often frightening for the family, and its variable course with cycles of remission and exacerbation is discouraging. Many parents become susceptible to experimenting with unorthodox cures advanced by advertisers and well-meaning friends. Access to the Internet and more than 200 sites

*PO Box 7669, Atlanta, GA 30357; 800-283-7800; http://www.arthritis.org. In Canada: The Arthritis Society, 393 University Ave., Suite 1700, Toronto, Ontario, Canada M5G 1E6; 416-979-7228; fax: 416-979-8366; http://www.arthritis.ca.

dedicated to arthritis provides families a welcome relief to the isolation of living with arthritis, but the Internet is also a bottomless source of unsubstantiated information that necessitates frank discussion and review with the family to help them sort out what is opinion versus fact and safe versus dangerous. Sometimes health care providers do not know the benefits or risks of a nutritional, herbal, or other complementary therapy. It is hoped that the new surge of legitimate scientific investigations of complementary alternative therapy will provide future answers.

Parents and patients need to hear that nurses promote independence. The child's participation in extracurricular activities, including play with friends, scouting, youth groups, dancing, and sports, is recommended. Nurses also support assigning children family chores and allowing older children to hold a part-time job, which foster self-reliance. Attendance at one of the several juvenile arthritis camps available to children with JIA is a confidence-boosting experience they will never forget.

Most of the reactions, problems, and concerns of families of a child with JIA are those of any parents of a child with a chronic illness or disability. The impact of the diagnosis is felt most acutely by the parents, who demonstrate anxiety, guilt, and all the manifestations of the grief process. The concerns and needs of these families are discussed extensively in Chapter 19, and the reader is directed to this chapter for additional guidance in planning care.

SYSTEMIC LUPUS ERYTHEMATOSUS

Systemic lupus erythematosus (SLE) is a chronic multisystem autoimmune disease of the blood vessels and connective tissue. The Lupus Foundation of America (2017) estimates that 1.5 million individuals have lupus, and 10% to 15% of these adults were diagnosed with SLE as children or adolescents. The prevalence of childhood SLE is reportedly 3.3 to 8.8 per 100,000 children (Levy & Kamphuis, 2012). It typically manifests between the ages of 10 and 19 years, and onset before age 5 years is unusual. There is a 4:3 female/male predominance in the first 10 years of life, which increases to 4:1 in the second decade.

Its course and symptoms are variable and unpredictable, with mild to life-threatening complications. SLE in children tends to be more severe at onset and has a more aggressive clinical course than adult-onset disease (Mina & Brunner, 2013). Other types of lupus erythematosus include chronic cutaneous lupus erythematosus (discoid lupus erythematosus), drug-induced lupus erythematosus, subacute cutaneous lupus erythematosus, and neonatal lupus erythematosus. Neonatal lupus erythematosus occurs when maternal autoantibodies cross the placenta and cause transient lupus-like symptoms in the newborn, with the potential lethal complication of heart block. The remaining discussion focuses on SLE.

Etiology

The cause of SLE is not known. It appears to result from a complex interaction of genetics with an unidentified trigger that causes the disease to activate. Suspected triggers include exposure to ultraviolet light, estrogen, pregnancy, infections, and drugs. Complement deficiencies C1q, C4, and C1s are associated with an increased risk of developing SLE. The major histocompatibility complex (MHC) Class II and III alleles are associated with an increased risk for developing SLE. There is a racial difference, with non-Caucasian children at increased risk of developing SLE.

Pathophysiology

SLE is the result of an abnormal immune response causing production of abnormal antibodies and formation of immune complexes. These immune complexes are deposited in tissues, causing inflammation and inciting other proinflammatory mediators that result in tissue injury and damage. Immune complex deposition in the glomerulus of the kidney causes lupus nephritis, a life-threatening complication of SLE. Almost any tissue in the body can be damaged by this abnormal inflammatory response, including the brain, heart, lungs, liver, gastrointestinal tract, spleen, joint tissues, muscles, and skin.

BOX 33.12 Manifestations of Systemic Lupus Erythematosus

Constitutional—Fever, fatigue, weight loss, anorexia
Cutaneous—Erythematosus butterfly rash over bridge of nose and across cheeks, discoid rash, photosensitivity, mucocutaneous ulceration, alopecia, periungual telangiectasias
Musculoskeletal—Arthritis, arthralgia, myositis, myalgia, tenosynovitis
Neurologic—Headache, seizure, forgetfulness, behavior change, change in school performance, psychosis, chorea, stroke, cranial and peripheral neuropathy, pseudotumor cerebri
Pulmonary and cardiac—Pleuritis, basilar pneumonitis, atelectasis, pericarditis, myocarditis, and endocarditis
Renal—Glomerulonephritis, nephrotic syndrome, hypertension
Gastrointestinal—Abdominal pain, nausea, vomiting, blood in stool, abdominal crisis, esophageal dysfunction, colitis
Hepatic, splenic, and nodal—Hepatomegaly, splenomegaly, lymphadenopathy
Hematologic—Anemia, cytopenia
Ophthalmologic—Cotton wool spots, papilledema, retinopathy
Vascular—Raynaud phenomenon, thrombophlebitis, livedo reticularis

Clinical Manifestations

The onset of SLE can be insidious, with intermittent constitutional symptoms such as fever, fatigue, weight loss, and arthralgia. However, rapid involvement of vital organs, primarily the kidneys, can herald an accelerated course with potentially fatal outcome. Reports suggest that survival rates in children with SLE have significantly improved; 5-year survival rates are over 90%, and 10-year survival rates are close to 90% (Levy & Kamphuis, 2012). Box 33.12 lists the manifestations related to the various tissues involved.

Rash is a common feature in SLE. The erythematous malar "butterfly" rash that spares the nasolabial fold is a suggestive feature but not pathognomonic. Maculopapular rashes are frequent and can occur anywhere but typically are found on sun-exposed skin. Nails and hair can be involved, with red, cracked cuticles; periungual telangiectasia; and patchy or diffuse alopecia. Raynaud phenomenon, or spasm of the blood vessels, causes cool hands and feet with pain and a characteristic tricolor (purple- or blue-white-red) change. Raynaud phenomenon usually appears as a response to cold exposure and can cause significant tissue damage. In addition to color changes in the extremities, vascular necrosis and digital ulceration can occur. Arthritis and tenosynovitis are common in SLE. The arthritis is usually painful and typically of short duration; joint deformity is unusual.

Renal involvement is a serious complication caused primarily by deposition of circulating immune complexes in the glomerular basement membrane with cellular infiltrates. Lupus nephritis is usually asymptomatic; consequently, monitoring of urine and renal function is required to detect disease. Kidney biopsy is required for lupus nephritis classification. There are six classes, depending on the type and extent of the renal lesion. Specific treatment is based on the class of nephritis. Although outcomes have improved for children with renal disease, the course is difficult to predict. Most children improve, although some remain the same or progress to renal failure, requiring dialysis and transplantation.

Neuropsychiatric lupus is another serious complication found in approximately 25% of pediatric SLE patients. The majority of these children manifest central nervous system involvement within the first or second year of diagnosis (Levy & Kamphuis, 2012). Symptoms can vary from manifestations as subtle as inability to concentrate to frank psychosis and seizure. Headaches are common with variable severity. Assess school performance and emotional stability at each visit as possible indicators of central nervous system involvement.

Cardiovascular disease results in significant mortality and morbidity in lupus. The immune dysregulation of SLE directly contributes to premature atherosclerosis. Children with SLE have an increased rate of dyslipidemia complicated by the secondary effects of corticosteroids (Sandborg, Ardoin, & Schanberg, 2008). Treatment includes exercise and dietary changes to promote a healthy weight, cardiovascular fitness, and management of hypertension. Studies are currently underway to assess the usefulness of statins in pediatric lupus for future evidence-based treatment of premature atherosclerosis in SLE.

Diagnostic Evaluation

SLE is a clinical diagnosis supported by specific abnormal results on laboratory tests. The American College of Rheumatology criteria for the classification of SLE in adults has a sensitivity of 96% and a specificity of 96% if 4 of the 11 criteria are present (Box 33.13). The SLE workup includes an extensive history taking and physical examination with inquiry about school performance and behavior change. Initial laboratory tests include complete blood count with differential; comprehensive metabolic chemistry panel; microscopic urinalysis; rapid plasma reagin test; quantitative determination of immunoglobulin levels; and tests for antinuclear antibodies, anti–deoxyribonucleic acid antibodies, complement 3 (C3), complement 4 (C4), lupus anticoagulant, and antiphospholipid antibodies.

A diagnosis of lupus should not be made without consideration of all medications being taken and their side effects. Some commonly used drugs such as minocycline, procainamide, hydralazine, and chlorpromazine can cause lupus-like symptoms. Minocycline, a common acne treatment, may not be considered important by the teenager and omitted from the history, so an accurate recent past and present medication history is essential for treatment. Drug-induced lupus resolves with time after the triggering medication has been discontinued.

BOX 33.13 Classification Criteria for Systemic Lupus Erythematosus*

Malar rash—Fixed malar erythema
Discoid rash—Patchy erythematous lesions
Photosensitivity—Rash with sunlight exposure
Oronasal ulcers—Painless ulcers in mouth and nose
Arthritis—Swelling, tenderness, or effusion in two or more peripheral joints (nonerosive)
Serositis—Pleuritis, pericarditis
Renal disorder—Proteinuria, casts in urine
Neurologic disorder—Psychosis, seizures
Hematologic disorder—Hemolytic anemia, thrombocytopenia, leukopenia, lymphopenia
Immunologic disorder—Anti–double-stranded deoxyribonucleic acid, anti-Sm, antiphospholipid antibodies; lupus anticoagulant; false-positive result on syphilis test (rapid plasma reagin)
Antinuclear antibodies—presence of antinuclear antibody by immunofluorescence or an equivalent assay

*The presence of four criteria is required for classification as systemic lupus erythematosus.

Therapeutic Management

There is no cure for SLE; the management goal is to reverse or minimize disease activity with appropriate medications while helping the child and family cope with the complications of the disease and treatment.

Medications. Since the 1950s, corticosteroids have been the mainstay of SLE therapy. They are effective antiinflammatory and immunosuppressive agents. Unfortunately, the use of steroids is hampered by side effects, which include growth delay, decreased resistance to infection, osteoporosis, weight gain, hypertension, development of cushingoid features and cataracts, and diabetes risks. Generally, a dosage sufficient to control symptoms is prescribed, and then the dosage is tapered to the lowest level possible to achieve an acceptable balance between disease activity and steroid side effects. For severe disease, IV pulse (high-dose) steroids are given on an intermittent schedule, which may allow reduction in the daily steroid dose with better compliance and fewer cushingoid features. Topical steroids are used for cutaneous lesions, but prolonged therapy thins the skin; consequently, facial application needs to be brief or with medication of lower concentration. Because of increased immunosuppression with steroid use, a tuberculin skin test should be performed before starting steroid therapy, especially in high-risk communities. A medical identification tag should be worn by children undergoing chronic steroid therapy so that administration of stress steroids can be considered in emergency situations.

Other medications used include NSAIDs such as naproxen and ibuprofen for pain associated with arthritis, arthralgia, and myalgia. Nurses need to instruct patients to take NSAIDs with food to help prevent gastrointestinal side effects. Hydroxychloroquine, an antimalarial drug, is an effective therapy for skin and joint manifestations. Possible untoward effects include skin, gastrointestinal, and retinal toxicity. A complete ophthalmologic examination is indicated before treatment begins and every 6 to 12 months thereafter. Methotrexate may be used in patients with stubborn arthritis that has not responded to NSAIDs and hydroxychloroquine and allows a lower dose of glucocorticoids to be used. Azathioprine, another steroid sparer, has been useful in treatment of SLE thrombocytopenia. Both methotrexate and azathioprine have significant potential adverse effects, including potential for increased infection, malignancy risks, liver and lung toxicity, and birth defects. Well documented discussions of these risks with patients and parents are required.

Cyclophosphamide, a potent immunosuppressive chemotherapy agent, used in combination with corticosteroids, is effective in treating proliferative lupus nephritis and neuropsychiatric lupus. A detailed cyclophosphamide education session should be held for patient and family to clearly describe potential benefits and risks, including infertility and future malignancy.

Mycophenolate mofetil, a purine inhibitor, has been used with success in adult lupus nephritis and is currently being used as a steroid-sparing agent in active pediatric lupus and as maintenance therapy after standard cyclophosphamide treatment for lupus nephritis. It is also being evaluated as an alternative to standard treatment of lupus nephritis with cyclophosphamide (Paredes, 2007). Mycophenolate mofetil is an attractive alternative, if successful, because it is less toxic and better tolerated than cyclophosphamide; however, it is not without potential side effects, including increased infection risk, liver toxicity, and birth defects. Sexually active females need to be on effective birth control.

New biologic treatments are being developed that focus on the immune dysregulation in SLE, cancer, and other autoimmune diseases. Belimumab is an IgG1-lambda monoclonal antibody that reduces the activity of B cell–mediated immunity and the autoimmune response by blocking receptors on B lymphocytes. It has been approved in adults with SLE and may be used off-label in select pediatric lupus, while pediatric studies are ongoing (Furie, Petri, Zamani, et al., 2011). Rituximab is a monoclonal antibody that eliminates CD20-positive B cells without affecting early B cells or plasma cells. This results in decreased antibody formation and has been used off-label in pediatric lupus patients who have not responded to standard therapy (Nwobi, Abitbol, Chandar, et al., 2008). Individuals with neuropsychiatric involvement may require antidepressants, psychotropics, and antiepileptic drugs (Levy & Kamphuis, 2012).

General Measures

In addition to medication, treatment includes general measures such as patient and family education, rest and exercise, proper diet, sun avoidance, and social support. SLE is complex and requires ongoing patient education. Families and patients need up-to-date, understandable information so they can become informed decision makers and participate in disease management. Nurses are duty bound to discuss with families any information they bring to appointments from the Internet, friends, and family. As health care providers critically evaluate disease information with families, families learn the skills needed to become self-advocates. Families also want to hear about the impact of SLE on growth and development, childbearing, schooling, and career choice. The message should be optimistic and clear, with few exceptions: "Prepare for the future; you will attend school, graduate, have children, and work."

Diet, exercise, and rest are the daily elements under direct patient control. The family needs to maximize the power of these normal functions to their benefit. There is no specific SLE diet, but a balanced diet that does not exceed calorie expenditure is essential for maintaining appropriate weight on corticosteroid therapy. A low-salt diet may be required if the patient becomes nephrotic or hypertensive. A low-fat diet is indicated in children with dyslipidemia. Maximizing peak bone mass in adolescent SLE is essential, especially because both SLE and its treatment with glucocorticoids increase the risk of osteoporosis. A diet rich in calcium and vitamin D is essential to prevent osteoporosis. If dietary calcium is not sufficient, calcium and vitamin D supplements need to be recommended. Consultation with a registered dietitian will help the family develop an individualized diet that meshes with their lifestyle.

The benefits of a regular exercise program include weight maintenance, cardiovascular fitness, and osteoporosis prevention, all of which help minimize SLE complications and corticosteroid side effects. Unfortunately many children stop participation in sports after diagnosis. Children with SLE report more fatigue and have lower aerobic fitness (Houghton, Tucker, Potts, et al., 2008). Encourage continuation of sports and recreational activities, if possible; if not, try to modify the activity or find alternatives to encourage the child and parents to view daily exercise as an essential part of the treatment plan and a continuation of the child's normal lifestyle. Additional rest is necessary during disease exacerbations but not to the extent that it interferes with regular sleep patterns.

A photosensitive rash is common, and the dangers of excessive ultraviolet A and B light exposure (including exposure to uncovered fluorescent lights) need to be stressed. This can be a sensitive topic for sun-loving teenagers and outdoor athletes. Discuss the use of sunscreen (with a sun protection factor [SPF] ≥30), hats, and protective clothing. Cosmetics and moisturizers that contain sunscreen are attractive options for adolescent girls. One useful rule to share with the adolescent who may be surrounded by peers who regularly seek out sun exposure is the "slip, slop, slap" rule: slip on a shirt, slop on sunscreen, and slap on a hat before going out in the sun. (See Chapter 18.) Scheduling outdoor activities in the morning and evening can reduce exposure without limiting participation in recreational activities. Make every effort to encourage children to participate in peer activities and to make sun-shielding modifications as inconspicuous as possible.

Social support from family, friends, teachers, counselors, and professional social workers and therapists can help the child and family through difficult times and promote adaptation to an illness that is not going to go away. Destructive coping mechanisms need to be identified and replaced with behaviors that enhance adaptation and healthy outcomes. Organizations that can help children and families learn about and adjust to the disease are the Lupus Foundation of America* and the Arthritis Foundation† (see p. 1291).

Nursing Care Management

Fostering adaptation and self-advocacy is the primary nursing goal. Patient and family acceptance and understanding of this life-threatening and therapeutically intrusive disease are big challenges for any nurse. Patient education is started at diagnosis and continued at every opportunity; repetition is good. Encourage family members to call with questions and concerns. Advise patients to write down their questions so they are prepared during the appointment. Consider adolescent development, with heightened concerns about body image and looking different. The nurse should be open about this. Skin care, cosmetics, and unobtrusive moisturizers with sunscreen and sunblock should be discussed.

Weight gain is an emotional issue, and it must be approached honestly with a workable plan for family dietary changes and a realistic exercise program. The nurse should work with a dietitian and a trainer or physical therapist to individualize a nutrition and fitness program for the child. A parent or sibling should be involved in the program, so the child does not feel that restrictions are punitive.

With older children, sexual activity and birth control must be discussed; birth defects are associated with mycophenolate and methotrexate. Additionally, pregnancy is a potential trigger for disease flare. Honest discussion about healthy, responsible reproductive choices with both the teenager and parents is important for establishing communication. The parents and teenager should know that the teenager can come to the nurse with reproductive concerns. Because estrogen can trigger disease flare, low-dose estrogen or progestin-only oral contraceptives are preferred. Some teenagers choose the compliance-friendly Depo-Provera (medroxyprogesterone) 3-month injections. Again, frank discussion about risks and benefits is essential.

Prevention of infection includes hand washing (especially at school) and preprocedure antibiotic coverage for routine events such as dental cleaning. Immunization vaccinations should be maintained in SLE, except live vaccines should be withheld in patients on immunosuppressive therapy.

To compensate for the side effects of some drugs, such as the corticosteroids, teenagers often go on fad or starvation diets. It is critical that nutritional counseling be available to ensure that the adolescent understands the role that a healthy diet plays in the management of SLE. School attendance may decrease because of loss of self-esteem, depression, feelings of inadequacy, or poor academic performance. Assessment of common adolescent risk-taking behaviors, including tobacco and recreational drug use, needs to be performed as it would

*2000 L St. NW, Suite 710, Washington, DC 20036; 202-349-1155; fax: 202-349-1156; http://www.lupus.org.

†A recommended booklet available from the Arthritis Foundation is *Meeting the Challenge: A Young Person's Guide to Living with Lupus.*

for any teenage patient. Treatment compliance is a significant issue in adolescence, especially given the medication side effects and restrictions on sun exposure. Adolescents need to understand what the function of each drug is, how each drug helps manage the disease, and what effect missing doses may have on their health. The nurse needs to keep track of prescription refills to evaluate compliance and medication efficacy. Barriers to medication compliance should be investigated, and patients should be helped to devise a workable plan. If friends are going to the beach, the patient should consider going late in the day with a beach umbrella, sunblock, and a wide-brim hat. Give instructions to reapply sunblock after swimming and to limit time in direct sun. (See Chapter 18.)

Teaching patients how to find ways to adapt positively to SLE with normal growth and development as the goal will give them self-advocacy skills. Nurses should apply the principles of adjusting to a chronic illness that are discussed in Chapter 19.

NCLEX REVIEW QUESTIONS

1. The potential physiologic and psychologic effects of prolonged immobilization on a 9-year-old child who has experienced significant trauma in a motor vehicle crash include which of the following? Select all that apply.
   A. Orthostatic intolerance
   B. Deep vein thrombosis
   C. Pressure ulcer formation
   D. Pneumonia
   E. Diarrhea
   F. Kidney stones
   G. Sense of euphoria and elation
   H. Constipation
2. A 12-year-old who was in an ATV accident has a long-leg fiberglass cast on his left leg for a tibia-fibula fracture. He requests pain medication at 2:00 AM for pain he rates at a 10/10 on the numeric scale. The nurse brings the pain medication and notes that he has removed the pillows that kept his leg elevated. He complains of pain in the left foot, and she notes that there is 3+ edema in the exposed leg and foot and she is unable to slip a finger under the cast. The nurse's priority interventions in this situation should include:
   A. Administer the pain medication and elevate the child's leg on the pillows
   B. Elevate the leg on the pillows and follow up within 2 to 3 hours to see if the edema has decreased
   C. Let the child know he cannot have any additional pain medication until 6:00 AM
   D. Notify the surgeon of the findings immediately
3. Disordered eating patterns, which may be observed in the female athlete triad, may include which of the following? Select all that apply.
   A. Use of diet pills and laxatives
   B. Fasting
   C. Binge eating
   D. Restriction of certain foods
   E. Inadequate caloric intake
   F. Excessive vitamin consumption
4. After the sudden death of a 14-year-old seemingly healthy basketball player, his parents ask the school administration to install an automatic external defibrillator (AED) in a central area of the athletic center. The school nurse is asked to participate in a meeting with the parents in which the administrators insist that such a device is not necessary. The school nurse advocates by providing which information about AEDs and children?
   A. An AED should be used only by health care persons trained in its use.
   B. An AED provides too much of an energy shock dose for children under 12 years of age.
   C. An AED can be effective in the resuscitation of a child or adolescent with a shockable rhythm.
   D. An AED is more commonly used in adults who have heart attacks than in children with undiagnosed heart conditions.
5. A 2-day-old infant in the newborn nursery is diagnosed with developmental dysplasia of the hip, and treatment is started by the orthopedist. The nurse assists the parents by providing home care instructions that include:
   A. Return to the orthopedist's office in 2 weeks to remove the hip spica cast
   B. The infant's bilateral foot casts should be elevated on pillows as much as possible
   C. Remove the Pavlik harness once a day for no more than an hour and inspect skin
   D. Remove the Pavlik harness while the infant is awake to allow "tummy time"

Correct Answers

1. A, B, C, D, F, H; 2. D; 3. A, B, D, E; 4. C; 5. C

REFERENCES

Academy of Nutrition and Dietetics, Dietitians of Canada, American College of Sports Medicine: Nutrition and Athletic Performance. (2016). *Medicine and Science in Sports and Exercise, 48*(3), 543–568.

Ackerman, K. E., & Misra, M. (2011). Bone health in adolescent athletes with a focus on female athlete triad. *The Physician and Sportsmedicine, 39*(1), 131–141.

Alharbi, M., Pinto, G., Finidori, G., et al. (2009). Pamidronate treatment of children with moderate-to severe osteogenesis imperfecta: A note of caution. *Hormone Research, 71*(1), 38–44.

American Academy of Pediatrics, Committee on Nutrition, Council on Sports Medicine and Fitness. (2011). Clinical report – Sports drinks and energy drinks for children and adolescents: Are they appropriate? *Pediatrics, 127*(6), 1182–1189.

American Academy of Pediatrics, Council on Sports Medicine and Fitness. (2011). Climatic heat stress and the exercising child and adolescent. *Pediatrics, 128*(3), 3741–3747.

Angelini, P., Vidovich, M. I., Lawless, C. E., et al. (2013). Preventing sudden cardiac death in athletes: In search of evidence-based, cost-effective screening. *Texas Heart Institute Journal, 40*(2), 148–155.

Atkins, D. L., Berger, S., Duff, J. P., et al. (2015). 2015 American Heart Association guidelines update for cardiopulmonary resuscitation and emergency cardiovascular care – part II: Pediatric basic life support and cardiopulmonary resuscitation quality. *Circulation, 132*, S519–S525.

Bachrach, L. K., & Ward, L. M. (2009). Clinical review 1: Bisphosphonate use in childhood osteoporosis. *The Journal of Clinical Endocrinology and Metabolism, 94*(2), 400–409.

Beukelman, T., Patkar, N. M., Saag, K. G., et al. (2011). 2011 American College of Rheumatology recommendations for the treatment of juvenile idiopathic arthritis: Initiation and safety monitoring of therapeutic agents for the treatment of arthritis and systemic features. *Arthritis Care & Research, 63*(4), 465–482.

Bloom, B. J., Owens, J. A., McGuinn, M., et al. (2002). Sleep and its relationship to pain, dysfunction and disease activity in juvenile rheumatoid arthritis. *The Journal of Rheumatology, 29*(1), 169–173.

Boutis, K., Willan, A., Babyn, P., et al. (2010). Cast versus splint in children with minimally angulated fractures of the distal radius: A randomized controlled trial. *Canadian Medical Association Journal, 182*(14), 1507–1512.

Bowen, R. E., & Otsuka, N. Y. (2014). The child with a limb deficiency. In S. L. Weinstein & J. M. Flynn (Eds.), *Lovell and Winter's Pediatric Orthopaedics*. Philadelphia, PA: Lippincott Williams & Wilkins.

Brenner, J. S., & Council on Sports Medicine and Fitness. (2007). Overuse injuries, overtraining, and burnout in child and adolescent athletes. *Pediatrics, 119*(6), 1242–1245.

Bullock, D. P., Koval, K. J., Moen, K. Y., et al. (2009). Hospitalized cases of child abuse in America: Who, what, when, and where. *Journal of Pediatric Orthopedics, 29*(3), 231–237.

Burmester, G. R., Mease, P. J., Dijkmans, B. A., et al. (2009). Adalimumab safety and mortality rates from global clinical trials of six immune-mediated inflammatory diseases. *Annals of the Rheumatic Diseases, 68*(12), 1863–1869.

Cassidy, J. T., & Petty, R. E. (2011). *The textbook of pediatric rheumatology* (6th ed.). Philadelphia, PA: Saunders Elsevier.

Centers for Disease Control and Prevention. (2015). *Web-based injury statistics query and reporting system (WISQARS)*. Centers for Disease Control and Prevention National Center for Injury Prevention and Control. http://www.cdc.gov/injury/wisqars/index.html.

Council on School Health. (2008). Medical emergencies occurring at school. *Pediatrics, 122*(4), 887–894.

Deimel, J. F., & Dunlap, B. J. (2012). The female athlete triad. *Clinic Sports Medicine, 31*(2), 247–254.

Drezner, J. A., Chun, J. S., Harmon, K. G., et al. (2008). Survival trends in the United States following exercise-related cardiac arrest in the youth, 2000-2006. *Heart Rhythm, 5*(6), 794–799.

Drezner, J. A., Courson, R. W., Roberts, W. O., et al. (2007). Inter Association Task Force recommendations on emergency preparedness and management of sudden cardiac arrest in high school and college athletic programs: A consensus statement. *Prehospital Emergency Care, 11*(3), 253–271.

Drezner, J. A., Rao, A. L., Heistand, J., et al. (2009). Effectiveness of emergency response planning for sudden cardiac arrest in United States high schools with automated external defibrillators. *Circulation, 120*(6), 518–525.

Fitzgibbons, P. G., Digiovanni, C., Hares, S., et al. (2012). Safe tourniquet use: A review of the evidence. *The Journal of the American Academy of Orthopaedic Surgeons, 20*(5), 310–319.

Freeman, B. L., III (2013). Scoliosis and kyphosis. In S. T. Canale & J. H. Beaty (Eds.), *Campbell's operative orthopaedics* (12th ed.). Philadelphia, PA: Mosby.

Furie, R., Petri, M., Zamani, O., et al. (2011). A phase III, randomized, placebo-controlled study of belimumab, a monicalonal antibody that inhibits B lymphocyte stimulator in patients with systemic lupus erythematosus. *Arthritis & Rheumatology, 63*(12), 3918–3930.

Gregory, A. J. M., & Fitch, R. W. (2007). Sports medicine: Performance-enhancing drugs. *Pediatric Clinics of North America, 54*(4), 797–806.

Guinta, Y. P., & Rocker, J. A. (2013). Sprains. *Pediatrics in Review, 34*(1), 47–49.

Hassan, F. A. (2009). Compliance of parents with regard to Pavlik harness treatment in developmental dyplasia of the hip. *Journal of Pediatric Orthopedics. Part B, 18*(3), 111–115.

Hoang, Q. B., & Mortazavi, M. (2012). Pediatric overuse injuries in sports. *Advances in Pediatrics, 59*(1), 359–383.

Hoch, A. Z., Pajewski, N. M., Moraski, L., et al. (2009). Prevalence of the female athlete triad in high school athletes and sedentary students. *Clinical Journal of Sport Medicine, 19*(5), 421–428.

Houghton, K. M., Tucker, L. B., Potts, J. E., et al. (2008). Fitness, fatigue, disease activity, and quality of life in pediatric lupus. *Arthritis & Rheumatology, 59*(4), 537–545.

Hresko, M. T. (2013). Idiopathic scoliosis in adolescents. *New England Journal of Medicine, 368*(9), 834–841.

Johnston, L. D., O'Malley, P. M., Bachman, J. G., et al. (2014). *Monitoring the future: national survey results on drug use, 1975-2013, vol I: Secondary school students*. Ann Arbor, MI: Institute for Social Research, The University of Michigan.

Kann, L., Kinchen, S., Shanklin, S. L., et al. (2014). Centers for Disease Control and Prevention: Youth risk behavior surveillance – United States, 2013. *MMWR Supplements, 63*(4), 1–168.

Kay, R. M., & Kim, Y. J. (2014). Slipped capital femoral epiphysis. In S. L. Weinstein & J. M. Flynn (Eds.), *Lovell and Winter's Pediatric Orthopaedics*. Philadelphia, PA: Lippincott Williams & Wilkins.

Kleinman, R. E., & Greer, F. R. (2014). *Pediatric nutrition*. Elk Grove Village, IL: American Academy of Pediatrics.

Kotwicki, T., Chowanska, J., Kinel, E., et al. (2013). Optimal management of idiopathic scoliosis in adolescents. *Adolescent Health, Medicine and Therapeutics, 4*, 59–73.

LaBotz, M., Griesemer, B. A., & AAP Council on Sports Medicine and Fitness. (2016). Use of performance-enhancing substances. *Pediatrics, 138*(1), e20161300.

Land, C., Rauch, F., Travers, R., et al. (2007). Osteogenesis imperfecta type VI in childhood and adolescence: Effects of cyclical intravenous pamidronate treatment. *Bone, 40*(3), 638–644.

Laron, D., & Pandya, N. K. (2013). Advances in the orthopedic management of osteogenesis imperfect. *Orthopaedic Clinics of North America, 44*(4), 565–573.

Lee, C., Porter, K. M., & Hodgetts, T. J. (2007). Tourniquet use in the civilian prehospital setting. *Emergency Medicine Journal, 24*(8), 584–587.

Lethaby, A., Temple, J., & Santy-Tomlinson, J. (2013). Pin site care for preventing infections associated with external bone fixators and pins. *Cochrane Database of Systematic Reviews*, (12), Art. No. CD004551.

Leventhal, J. M., Martin, K. D., & Asnes, A. G. (2010). Fractures and traumatic brain injuries: Abuse versus accidents in a US database of hospitalized children. *Pediatrics, 125*(1), e104–e115.

Levy, D. M., & Kamphuis, S. (2012). Systemic lupus erythematosus in children and adolescents. *Orthopaedic Clinics of North America, 59*(2), 345–364.

Loder, R. T., & Feinberg, J. R. (2007). Orthopaedic injuries in children with nonaccidental trauma: Demographics and incidence from the 2000 kids' inpatient database. *Journal of Pediatric Orthopedics, 27*(4), 421–426.

Lovell, D. J., Reiff, A., Ilowite, N. T., et al. (2008). Safety and efficacy of up to 8 years of continuous etanercept therapy in patients with juvenile rheumatoid arthritis. *Arthritis & Rheumatology, 58*(5), 1496–1503.

Lovell, D. J., Ruperto, N., Goodman, S., et al. (2008). Adalimumab with or without methotrexate in juvenile rheumatoid arthritis. *New England Journal of Medicine, 359*(8), 810–820.

Lupus Foundation of America. (2017). *Understanding lupus*. National Resource Center on Lupus. http://www.resources.lupus.org/collections/understanding-lupus.

Madonia, L. (2012). Osteogenesis imperfecta and bone narrow transplant. *Journal of Pediatric Oncology Nursing, 29*(1), 37–44.

Marar, M., McIlvain, N. M., Fields, S. K., et al. (2012). Epidemiology of concussions among United States high school athletes in 20 sports. *The American Journal of Sports Medicine, 40*(4), 747–755.

Marini, J. C. (2016). Osteogenesis imperfecta. In R. M. Kliegman, B. F. Stanton, J. W. St. Geme, et al. (Eds.), *Nelson textbook of pediatrics* (20th ed.). Philadelphia, PA: Saunders.

Marini, J. C., & Blissett, A. R. (2013). New genes in bone development: What's new in osteogenesis imperfecta. *Journal of Clinical Endocrinology and Metabolism, 98*(8), 3095–3103.

Maron, B. J., Doerer, J. J., Haas, T. S., et al. (2009). Sudden deaths in young competitive athletes: Analysis of 1866 deaths in the United States, 1980-2006. *Circulation, 119*(8), 1085–1092.

Mencio, G. A., Swiontkowski, M. F., & Green, N. E. (2015). *Green's skeletal trauma in children*. Philadelphia, PA: Elsevier/Saunders.

Mina, R., & Brunner, H. I. (2013). Update on differences between childhood-onset and adult-onset systemic lupus erythematosus. *Arthritis Research & Therapy, 15*(4), 218.

Montgomery, N. I., & Epps, H. R. (2017). Pediatric septic arthritis. *Orthopaedic Clinics of North America, 48*(2), 209–216.

Morse, E., & Funk, M. (2012). Preparticipation screening and prevention of sudden cardiac death in athletes: Implications for primary care. *Journal of the American Academy of Nurse Practitioners, 24*, 63–69.

Mosca, V. S. (2014). The foot. In S. L. Weinstein & J. M. Flynn (Eds.), *Lovell and Winter's Pediatric Orthopaedics*. Philadelphia, PA: Lippincott Williams & Wilkins.

Nattiv, A., Loucks, A. N., Manore, M. M., et al. (2007). American College of Sports Medicine position stand: The female athlete triad. *Medicine and Science in Sports and Exercise, 39*(10), 1867–1882.

Nelson, A. J., Collins, C. L., Yard, E. E., et al. (2007). Ankle injuries among United States high school sports athletes, 2005-2006. *Journal of Athletic Training, 42*(3), 381–387.

Newton, P. O., Wenger, D. R., & Yaszay, B. (2014). Idiopathic scoliosis. In S. L. Weinstein & J. M. Flynn (Eds.), *Lovell and Winter's Pediatric Orthopaedics*. Philadelphia, PA: Lippincott Williams & Wilkins.

Noonan, C., Quigley, S., & Curley, M. A. (2011). Using the Braden Q Scale to predict pressure ulcer risk in pediatric patients. *Journal of Pediatric Nursing, 26*(6), 566–575.

Nwobi, O., Abitbol, C. L., Chandar, J., et al. (2008). Rituximab therapy for juvenile-onset systemic lupus erythematosus. *Pediatric Nephrology, 23*(3), 413–419.

Paredes, A. (2007). Can mycophenolate mofetil substitute cyclophosphamide treatment of pediatric lupus? *Pediatric Nephrology, 22*(8), 1077–1082.

Paul, A. R., & Adamo, M. A. (2014). Non-accidental trauma in pediatrics: A review of epidemiology, pathophysiology, diagnosis and treatment. *Translational Pediatrics, 3*(3), 195–207.

Pediatric Orthopaedic Society of North America. (2011). *Bone, joint, and muscle infections in children*. American Academy of Orthopaedic Surgeons. http://orthoinfo.aaos.org/topic.cfm?topic=A00593.

Petty, R. E., Southwood, T. R., Manners, P., et al. (2004). International League of Associations for Rheumatology classification of juvenile idiopathic arthritis: Second revision, Edmonton, 2001. *The Journal of Rheumatology, 31*(2), 390–392.

Ponseti, I. V. (1996). *Congenital clubfoot: Fundamentals of treatment*. Oxford: Oxford University Press.

Prahalad, S., & Glass, D. N. (2008). A comprehensive review of the genetics of juvenile idiopathic arthritis. *Pediatric Rheumatology, 11*(6).

Price, C. T., & Schwend, R. M. (2011). Improper swaddling a risk factor for developmental dysplasia of hip. *AAP News, 32*(9), 11–12.

Rauch, F., Munns, C. F., Land, C., et al. (2009). Risedronate in the treatment of mild pediatric osteogenesis imperfecta: A randomized placebo-controlled study. *Journal of Bone and Mineral Research: The Official Journal of the American Society for Bone and Mineral Research, 24*(7), 1282–1289.

Rechel, J. A., Yard, E. E., & Comstock, R. D. (2008). An epidemiologic comparison of high school sports injuries sustained in practice and competition. *Journal of Athletic Training, 43*(2), 197–204.

Reininga, J. K., Los, L. I., Wulffraat, N. M., et al. (2008). The evaluation of uveitis in juvenile idiopathic arthritis (JIA) patients: Are current ophthalmologic screening guidelines adequate? *Clinical and Experimental Rheumatology, 27*(2), 367–372.

Rice, S. G., & Council on Sports Medicine and Fitness. (2008). Medical conditions affecting sports participation. *Pediatrics, 121*(4), 841–848.

Richards, B. S., & Vitale, M. G. (2008). Screening for idiopathic scoliosis in adolescents: An information statement. *The Journal of Bone and Joint Surgery. American Volume, 90*(1), 195–198.

Ringhold, S., Weiss, P. F., Beukelman, T., et al. (2013). 2013 update of the 2011 American College of Rheumatology recommendations for the treatment of juvenile idiopathic arthritis: Recommendations for the medical therapy of children with systemic juvenile idiopathic arthritis and tuberculosis screening among children receiving biologic medications. *Arthritis & Rheumatology, 65*(10), 2499–2512.

Sandborg, C., Ardoin, S. P., & Schanberg, L. (2008). Therapy insight: Cardiovascular disease in pediatric systemic lupus erythematosus. *Nature Clinical Practice. Rheumatology, 4*(5), 258–265.

Semler, O., Netzer, C., Hoyer-Kuhn, H., et al. (2012). First use of the RANKL antibody denosumab in osteogenesis imperfect type VI. *Journal of Musculoskeletal and Neuronal Interactions, 12*(3), 183–188.

Shaw, B. A., Segal, L. S., & AAP Section on Orthopaedics. (2016). Evaluation and referral for developmental dysplasia of the hip in infants. *Pediatrics, 138*(6), e20163107.

Sillence, D. O., Senn, A., & Danks, D. M. (1979). Genetic heterogeneity in osteogenesis imperfecta. *Journal of Medical Genetics, 16*(2), 101–116.

Stans, A. A. (2014). Musculoskeletal infection. In S. L. Weinstein & J. M. Flynn (Eds.), *Lovell and Winter's Pediatric Orthopaedics*. Philadelphia, PA: Lippincott Williams & Wilkins.

Stevenson, D. A., Mineau, G., Kerber, R. A., et al. (2009). Familial predisposition to developmental dysplasia of the hip. *Journal of Pediatric Orthopedics, 29*(5), 463–466.

Stoll, C., Alembik, Y., Dott, B., et al. (2010). Associated malformations in patients with limb reduction deficiencies. *European Journal of Medical Genetics, 53*(5), 286–290.

Stoll, M. L., & Gotte, A. C. (2008). Biological therapies for the treatment of juvenile idiopathic arthritis: Lessons from the adult and pediatric experiences. *Biologics: Targets & Therapy, 2*(2), 229–252.

Weinstein, S. L. (2014a). Developmental hip dysplasia and dislocation. In S. L. Weinstein & J. M. Flynn (Eds.), *Lovell and Winter's Pediatric Orthopaedics*. Philadelphia, PA: Lippincott Williams & Wilkins.

Weinstein, S. L. (2014b). Legg-Calve-Perthes syndrome. In S. L. Weinstein & J. M. Flynn (Eds.), *Lovell and Winter's Pediatric Orthopaedics*. Philadelphia, PA: Lippincott Williams & Wilkins.

Weinstein, S. L., Dolan, L. A., Wright, J. G., et al. (2013). Effects of bracing in adolescents with idiopathic scoliosis. *New England Journal of Medicine, 369*(16), 1512–1521.

Weiss Kelly, A. K., Hecht, S., & AAP Council on Sports Medicine and Fitness. (2016). The female athlete triad. *Pediatrics, 137*(6), e20160922.

Zach, K. N., Smith Machin, A. L., & Hoch, A. Z. (2011). Advances in management of female athlete triad and eating disorders. *Clinics in Sports Medicine, 30*(3), 551–573.

34

The Child With Neuromuscular or Muscular Dysfunction

Anne Feierabend Stanton and Teri A. Huddleston Lavenbarg

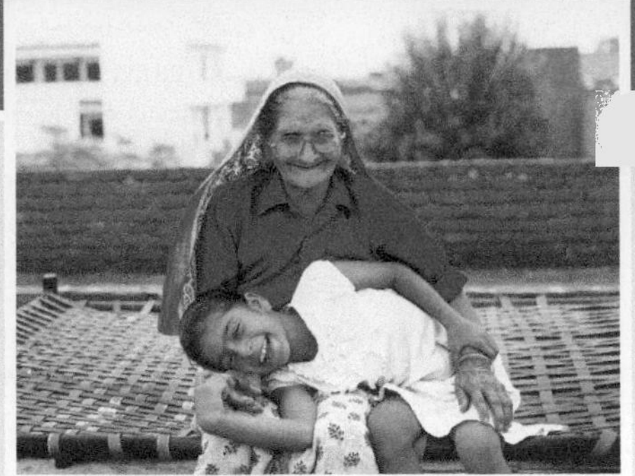

http://evolve.elsevier.com/wong/ncic

CONCEPTS

- Mobility
- Sensory Perception

NEUROMUSCULAR DYSFUNCTION

Weakness or abnormal skeletal muscle function may represent a defect in the muscle itself or reflect a pathologic disorder at some point along the neural pathway from the cortex of the brain to the neuromuscular junction. Identifying the source of muscular dysfunction includes not only the testing of muscle function but also the systematic elimination of possible disorders of neural structures on which muscle function depends for its stimulus. In a few disorders muscle disease may be accompanied by a neurologic disorder.

Some clinical features are shared by muscle disease (myopathy), which differs in many ways from muscular dysfunction resulting from disorders of neuronal structures—brain, cranial nerve nuclei, long nerve tracts, anterior horn cells of the spinal cord, and peripheral nerves. Motor function is accomplished by means of the simple reflex arcs or by way of impulses transmitted from the cerebral cortex and other centers in the brain through the various nerve pathways of the central nervous system (CNS). The upper motor neurons consist of cells that lie in the cerebral cortex and fibers that traverse the brainstem and spinal cord to terminate at their synapses with the anterior horn cells. The lower motor neurons consist of the anterior horn cells, axons, and peripheral nerve branches. The motor unit consists of the lower motor neuron, the neuromuscular (or myoneural) junction, and the muscle fibers it supplies (Fig. 34.1). The upper motor neuronal pathways from the cerebrum to the lower motor neuron are described as (1) pyramidal—those whose fibers extend from the cortex, come together in the medulla, cross from one side to the other, then extend down the cord to synapse with anterior horn motor neurons; and (2) extrapyramidal—a complex network of motor neurons that comprise relays between motor areas of the cortex, basal ganglia, thalamus, cerebellum, and brainstem.

CLASSIFICATION AND DIAGNOSIS

The site of pathologic disturbance determines the type of muscular dysfunction. In general, upper motor neuron lesions produce weakness associated with spasticity, increased deep tendon reflexes, and abnormal superficial reflexes. The primary disorder of upper motor neuron dysfunction is cerebral palsy (CP). Lower motor neuron lesions interrupt the reflex arc, causing weakness and atrophy of the skeletal muscles involved with associated hypotonia or flaccidity, which eventually progress to atrophy with varying degrees of contracture deformity. A disorder of the extrapyramidal pathway and the cerebellum rarely produces muscle weakness.

Lower motor neuron involvement is usually symmetric (except that of poliomyelitis and single peripheral nerve disease), whereas disorders of the pyramidal tract are more often asymmetric. Muscle wasting is characteristic of lower motor neuron lesions and more marked than in diseases of muscles. Deep tendon reflexes are briskly active in upper motor neuron disease, are diminished or absent in lower motor neuron disease, and depend on the progress of muscle degeneration in the myopathies.

These disorders can also be categorized according to onset: those in which there is acute onset of flaccid paralysis and those with more gradual onset and progressive degeneration. In most instances the sudden appearance of flaccid paralysis in a previously healthy child is due to an infectious process. Neurotoxins (e.g., botulism, tick paralysis, or heavy metal poisoning), pressure on the spinal cord from tumors or abscesses, and spinal cord injury (SCI) are less likely causes. Hereditary factors and metabolic disease are more often responsible for muscular weakness and atrophy of gradual onset.

Classification

The most useful classification of neuromuscular disorders is one that defines the site of origin of the pathologic lesion: the anterior horn cells of the spinal cord, the peripheral nerves, the neuromuscular junction, and the muscles.

Diseases of Anterior Horn Cells

Diseases and disorders that affect the anterior horn cells are the result of destruction or atrophy of the anterior horn of the spinal column along with the inability to transfer impulses from sensory neurons to motor neurons. Enteroviruses, which have a worldwide distribution, are prominent etiologic agents that selectively affect anterior horn cells.

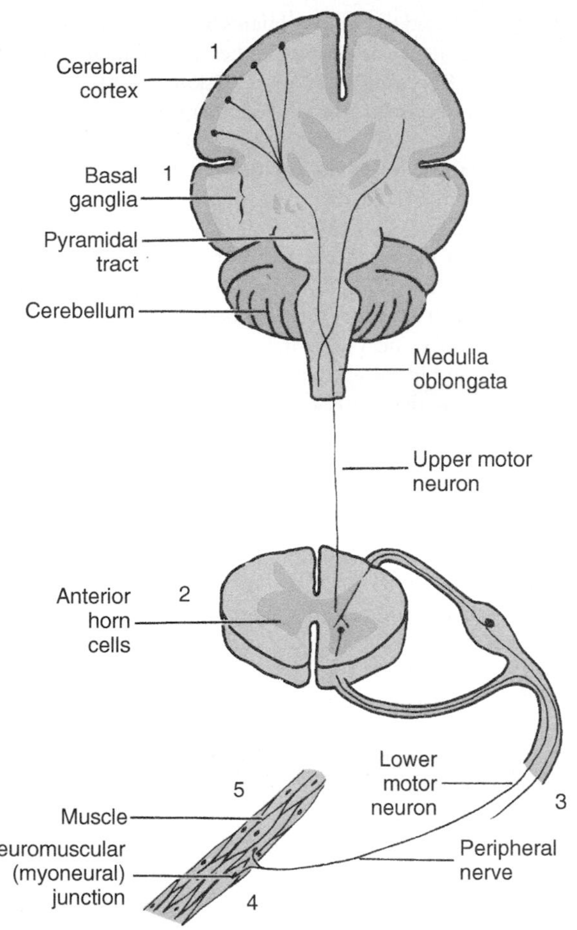

FIG. 34.1 Site of origin for neuromuscular disorders. *1,* Cerebral palsy; *2,* poliomyelitis, spinal muscular atrophy; *3,* mononeuropathies, polyneuropathies; *4,* myasthenia gravis, neurotoxic disorders; *5,* muscular dystrophies.

These include the nonpolioviruses, of which there are several types: human enterovirus A, B, C, and D, and the human parechoviruses 1 and 2 (Centers for Disease Control and Prevention, 2010). Inherited disorders, primarily the spinal muscular atrophies, cause degeneration of the anterior horn cells.

Neuropathies

Disorders affecting peripheral nerves may be mononeuropathies, which involve a single nerve and the muscles it innervates, or polyneuropathies, which involve multiple nerves and the muscles they supply. Neuropathies are caused by a number of hereditary diseases, traumatic injuries, infections, poisons, and (secondarily) some metabolic diseases. Polyneuropathy can be restricted to specific areas (as in diabetes mellitus). Some hereditary diseases involve skeletal muscles extensively. The distal limbs (feet and hands) are usually affected first, with gait disturbance and footdrop being early manifestations. The involvement gradually progresses proximally as the disorder becomes more severe.

In some polyneuropathies there is segmented or patchy loss of the myelin sheath of nerve fibers; in others the primary process appears to be progressive degeneration of nerve fibers. Examples of acute and chronic polyneuropathies are Guillain-Barré syndrome (infectious polyneuritis) and Charcot-Marie Tooth disease (peroneal muscular atrophy), respectively.

Neuromuscular Junction Disease

Disorders involving a neurohumoral deficiency interfere with transmission of nerve impulses to muscles at the neuromuscular junction. Normally nerve impulses are transmitted to skeletal muscles across the neuromuscular junction by acetylcholine. This is accomplished in three steps: (1) acetylcholine is released from vesicles in the terminal nerve endings; (2) it then diffuses across the junction and contacts receptor sites in the muscle membrane, stimulating the muscle to contract; and (3) it is removed by the action of cholinesterase. Interference at any of these three steps will block transmission of nerve impulses and prevent muscular contraction.

Several toxic substances act at the neuromuscular junction to inhibit nerve impulses to the skeletal muscles. Examples of toxins that prevent the release of acetylcholine are those that produce the paralysis of botulism and tick paralysis. Action at receptor sites is also blocked by the drug curare. Paralysis resulting from inhibition of cholinesterase release is caused by poisoning with organic phosphate insecticides.

Diseases of Muscles

Diseases of skeletal muscles can be inflammatory (such as polymyositis), the result of endocrine dysfunction (such as hypothyroidism and hyperthyroidism), or the result of congenital defects (e.g., absence of muscle, periodic paralysis, and the various muscular dystrophies [MDs] and myotonias). Inflammation occurs in a number of infectious illnesses such as trichinosis, toxoplasmosis, and those caused by the enteroviruses (coxsackieviruses and echoviruses).

Diagnostic Tools

Several general diagnostic tools aid in differentiating diseases with similar manifestations. In addition, a number of more definitive tests are used to establish a specific diagnosis. The neurologic examination is a basic test that helps assess the extent of motor and sensory function.

The electromyogram (EMG) measures the electric potentials generated in individual muscles. A small metal disk is placed on the skin overlying the muscle to be tested, or a sterile needle electrode is inserted directly into the muscle. The electric activity generated in the skeletal muscles is measured at rest, with slight voluntary contraction, and with maximum contraction. The electric activity is amplified and displayed on a cathode ray oscilloscope. Needle electrodes are sensitive enough to pick up the activity of a single muscle fiber; thus this is usually the method of choice. However, the procedure is traumatic for children. It is often not useful because it requires cooperation. A topical anesthetic should be considered to decrease pain. Nerve conduction velocity, or the velocity of electric impulse conduction along motor or sensory nerves, is often measured in conjunction with the EMG. Certain diseases affect the peripheral nerves, prolonging the conduction time from the point of stimulation of the nerve to the muscle and increasing the duration of the evoked potential of the muscle.

Muscle biopsy may be used to confirm and classify muscle disorders. The vastus lateralis is the most commonly sampled muscle. Procedural sedation may be accomplished with a number of medications used singly or in combination: midazolam and morphine; ketamine and midazolam; pentobarbital; etomidate; inhaled nitrous oxide; or midazolam and fentanyl. (See Surgical Procedures, Chapter 22.) Serum enzyme measurements are helpful in diagnosing and monitoring the course of muscular disease, but these are used as adjuncts in the diagnosis of most neuromuscular diseases. The intracellular enzyme creatine (phosphokinase) kinase (CK) is present in muscle tissues, including cardiac muscle, and the brain. It is released in large amounts in some muscular diseases, such as MD. CK is not elevated in neurogenic disease. Genetic testing is becoming increasingly valuable in the diagnosis of many neuromuscular conditions and may make muscle biopsies less necessary. Because of the increasing complexities of choosing appropriate genetic tests, genetic counseling may be appropriate.

CEREBRAL PALSY

Cerebral palsy (CP) has been defined as a disorder of posture and movement from static brain injury perinatally or postnatally, which limits activity (Ferris, 2015; Nordqvist & Christian, 2017; Patterson, Bridgemohan, & Armsby, 2017; Rosenbaum, Paneth, Leviton, et al., 2007). In addition to motor disorders, the condition often involves disturbances of sensation, perception, communication, cognition, and behavior; secondary musculoskeletal problems; and epilepsy (Nordqvist & Christian, 2017; Rosenbaum, Paneth, Leviton, et al., 2007). The etiology, clinical features, and course vary and are characterized by abnormal muscle tone and coordination as the primary disturbances. CP is the most common permanent physical disability of childhood, and the incidence is reported to range from 1.5 to over 4 per 1000 live births in various studies in the United States, affecting about 367,000 Americans (Centers for Disease Control and Prevention, 2016; Hirtz, Thurman, Gwinn-Hardy, et al., 2007; Nordqvist & Christian, 2017; Yeargin-Allsopp, Van Naarden Braun, Doernberg, et al., 2008). One systematic review and meta-analysis indicated a prevalence of 2.11 per 1000 live births, with the highest prevalence among infants born weighing 1000 to 1499 g at birth; the prevalence of CP was higher among infants born before completion of 28 weeks of gestation (Oskoui, Coutinho, Dykeman, et al., 2013). Van Naarden Braun, Doernberg, Schieve, and colleagues (2016) studied spastic CP prevalence over 17 years, 1985 to 2002, in Atlanta, Georgia, and found no significant trends by gestational age or birth weight; ethnic/racial disparities remained and warrant further investigation. In the 1960s the prevalence of CP rose approximately 20%, which most likely reflected the improved survival of extremely low-birth-weight (ELBW) and very low-birth-weight (VLBW) infants. However, in the past 2 decades there has been a decrease in the incidence of CP among ELBW and VLBW infants (Hack & Costello, 2008). The incidence is higher in males than females and more likely to occur in African Americans than in Caucasian or Hispanic children (Centers for Disease Control and Prevention, 2016; Van Naarden Braun, Doernberg, Schieve, et al., 2016).

Etiology

A variety of prenatal, perinatal, and postnatal factors contribute to the development of CP, singly or multifactorially (Box 34.1). The human brain undergoes development during the prenatal period and up to 2 years of age. A brain insult or injury occurring during this period may result in CP.

BOX 34.1 Etiologic Risk Factors for Cerebral Palsy

Prenatal

Maternal

1. Diabetes mellitus or hyperthyroidism
2. Exposure to radiation or toxins
3. Malnutrition
4. Seizure disorder or cognitive impairment
5. Infections
6. Incompetent cervix
7. Bleeding
8. Polyhydramnios
9. Genetic abnormalities
10. Previous child with development disabilities
11. Previous premature birth
12. Previous fetal loss
13. Medication use (e.g., thyroid, estrogen, progesterone)
14. Inflammatory response
15. Severe proteinuria

Gestational

1. Chromosome abnormalities
2. Genetic syndromes
3. Teratogens
4. Rh incompatibility
5. Infections
6. Congenital malformations
7. Fetal development abnormalities
8. Problems in placental functioning
9. Inflammatory response

Labor and Delivery

1. Premature delivery
2. Prolonged rupture of membranes
3. Prolonged fetal heart rate depression
4. Abnormal presentation
5. Long labor
6. Preeclampsia
7. Asphyxia

Perinatal

1. Prematurity and associated problems
2. Sepsis and/or central nervous system infection
3. Seizures
4. Intraventricular hemorrhage
5. Periventricular leukomalacia
6. Meconium aspiration
7. Number of days on mechanical ventilation
8. Persistent pulmonary hypertension
9. Intrauterine growth restriction
10. Low birth weight
11. Perinatal stroke
12. Unknown

Childhood or Postnatal

1. Brain injury
2. Meningitis or encephalitis
3. Toxins
4. Traumatic brain injury
5. Infections
6. Stroke

Unknown

1. Unknown prenatal factors that contribute to the development of CP; possibly as many as 70% to 80% of CP (Krigger, 2006)

CP, Cerebral palsy.
From Jackson, P. L., Vessey, J. A., & Schapiro, N. A. (Eds.). (2010). *Primary care of the child with a chronic illness* (5th ed.). St. Louis, MO: Mosby.

Although the prevalent traditional hypothesis has been that CP results from perinatal problems, especially birth asphyxia, it is now believed that CP results more often from existing prenatal brain abnormalities. However, the exact cause of these abnormalities remains elusive. It has been estimated that as many as 70% to 80% of the cases of CP are caused by unknown prenatal factors (Krigger, 2006; MacLennan, Thompson, & Gecz, 2015). Intrauterine exposure to maternal chorioamnionitis is associated with an increased risk of CP in infants of normal birth weight and preterm infants (Hermansen & Hermansen, 2006; Shatrov, Birch, Lam, et al., 2010); however, not all term infants exposed to chorioamnionitis develop CP.

In general, infants exposed to maternal and perinatal infections are at increased risk for the development of CP as a result of the effects on the developing brain. Although CP occurs in term births, preterm birth of ELBW and VLBW infants continues to be the single most important risk factor for CP. Still, in some cases no identifiable cause is determined. Periventricular leukomalacia and intracerebral hemorrhage in low-birth-weight infants are significant risk factors in the development of CP. Perinatal ischemic stroke is also associated with a later diagnosis of CP (Golomb, Saha, Garg, et al., 2007). One study found a higher risk for CP occurring among infants born at 42 weeks of gestation or later than among those born at 37 or 38 weeks of gestation (Moster, Wilcox, Vollset, et al., 2010). Additional factors that may contribute to the development of CP postnatally include bacterial meningitis, multiple births, viral encephalitis, motor vehicle accidents, and child abuse (shaken baby syndrome [traumatic brain injury]). One study found that 10% to 15% of children with CP acquired the condition after birth from causes such as falls, motor vehicle crashes, and infections such as meningitis (Centers for Disease Control and Prevention, 2013). A significant percentage (15% to 60%) of children with CP also have epilepsy. In summary, as many as 80% of the total cases of CP may be linked to a perinatal or neonatal brain lesion or brain maldevelopment, regardless of the cause (Krageloh-Mann & Cans, 2009). A number of biochemical disorders may cause motor abnormalities often seen in CP and may be initially misdiagnosed as CP (Nehring, 2010).

Pathophysiology

It is difficult to establish a precise location of neurologic lesions on the basis of etiology or clinical signs because there is no characteristic pathologic picture. In some cases, there are gross malformations of the brain. In others, there may be evidence of vascular occlusion, atrophy, loss of neurons, and laminar degeneration that produce narrower gyri, wider sulci, and low brain weight. Anoxia appears to play the most significant role in the pathologic state of brain damage, which is often secondary to other causative mechanisms.

There are a few exceptions. In some cases, the manifestations or etiology is related to anatomic areas. For example, CP associated with preterm birth is usually spastic diplegia caused by hypoxic infarction or hemorrhage with periventricular leukomalacia in the area adjacent to the lateral ventricles. The athetoid (extrapyramidal) type of CP is most likely to be associated with birth asphyxia but can also be caused by kernicterus and metabolic genetic disorders such as mitochondrial disorders and glutaric aciduria (Johnston, 2016; Keys & Chaves-Carballo, 2013). Hemiplegic (hemiparetic) CP is often associated with a focal cerebral infarction (stroke) secondary to an intrauterine or perinatal thromboembolism, usually a result of maternal thrombosis or hereditary clotting disorder (Johnston, 2016). Cerebellar hypoplasia and sometimes severe neonatal hypoglycemia are related to ataxic CP. Generalized cortical and cerebral atrophy often cause severe quadriparesis with cognitive impairment and microcephaly.

Clinical Classification

A revision of the Winter classification was proposed in 2005 to reflect the child's actual clinical problems and their severity, an assessment of the child's physical and quality-of-life status across time, and long-term support needs (Nehring, 2010; Romeo, Ricci, Brogna, et al., 2016)

The proposed new definition has four major dimensions of classification (Bax, Goldstein, Rosenbaum, et al., 2005):

Motor abnormalities—Nature and typology of the motor disorder; functional motor abilities

Associated impairments—Seizures; hearing or vision impairment; attentional, behavioral, communicative, and/or cognitive deficits; oral motor and speech function

Anatomic and radiologic findings—Anatomic distribution or parts of the body affected by motor impairments or limitations; radiologic findings sometimes including white matter lesions or brain anomaly noted on computed tomography (CT) or magnetic resonance imaging (MRI)

Causation and timing—Identification of a clearly identified cause such as a postnatal event (e.g., meningitis, traumatic brain injury)

The Gross Motor Functional Classification System (GMFCS) (Sehrawat, Marwaha, Bansal et al., 2014); Functional Mobility Scale (FMS) (Sehrawat, Marwaha, Bansal et al., 2014; Eliasson, Krumlinde-Sundholm, & Rösblad, 2006) Manual Ability Classification Scale (MACS); and Communication Functional Classification Scale (CFCS) (Hidecker, Paneth, & Rosenbaum, 2011) have been used by several authors to guide care of children with CP. Several studies used the Hammersmith Infant Neurological Examination (HINE) as an examination tool in diagnosing CP.

CP has four primary types of movement disorders: spastic, dyskinetic, ataxic, and mixed (Box 34.2) (Nehring, 2010). The most common clinical type, spastic CP (77.4% reported by the Centers for Disease Control and Prevention, 2013, 2016), represents an upper motor neuron muscular weakness. The reflex arc is intact, and the characteristic physical signs are increased stretch reflexes, increased muscle tone, and (often) weakness. Early neurologic manifestations are usually generalized hypotonia or decreased tone that lasts for a few weeks or may extend for months or even as long as a year.

Clinical Manifestations

The alert observer may suspect CP when a child demonstrates some of the groups of manifestations in Box 34.3.

Delayed Gross Motor Development

Delayed gross motor development is a universal manifestation of CP. The child shows a delay in all motor accomplishments, and the discrepancy between motor ability and expected achievement tends to increase with successive developmental milestones as growth advances. It is especially significant if other developmental behaviors, such as language and personal-social achievement, are normal. Delayed development of the ability to balance may also slow the progression of milestones.

Abnormal Motor Performance

Neuromotor dysfunction is particularly evident in motor performance. An early sign is preferential unilateral hand use that may be apparent at approximately 6 months of age. Hand dominance does not normally develop until the preschool years. Abnormal crawling with propulsion by hand movements only and with lower extremities and hips hiked along, much like a "bunny hop," occurs in diplegia. Children with hemiplegia have an asymmetric crawl, using the unaffected arm and leg to propel

BOX 34.2 Clinical Classification of Cerebral Palsy

Spastic (Pyramidal)

- Characterized by persistent primitive reflexes, positive Babinski reflex, ankle clonus, exaggerated stretch reflexes, eventual development of contractures
- Seventy percent to 80% of all cases of cerebral palsy (CP)
- **Diplegia**—All extremities affected; lower more than upper (30% to 40% of spastic CP)
- **Tetraplegia**—All four extremities involved: legs and trunk, mouth, pharynx, and tongue (10% to 15% of spastic CP)
- **Triplegia**—Three limbs involved
- **Monoplegia**—Only one limb involved
- **Hemiplegia**—Motor dysfunction on one side of the body; upper extremity more affected than lower (20% to 30% of spastic CP)
- Hypertonicity with poor control of posture, balance, and coordinated motion
- Impairment of fine and gross motor skills

Dyskinetic (Nonspastic, Extrapyramidal)

- **Athetoid**—Chorea (involuntary, irregular, jerking movements); characterized by slow, wormlike, writhing movements that usually involve the extremities, trunk, neck, facial muscles, and tongue
- **Dystonic**—Slow, twisting movements of the trunk or extremities; abnormal posture
- Involvement of the pharyngeal, laryngeal, and oral muscles causing drooling and dysarthria (imperfect speech articulation)

Ataxic (Nonspastic, Extrapyramidal)

- Wide-based gait
- Rapid, repetitive movements performed poorly
- Disintegration of movements of the upper extremities when the child reaches for objects

Mixed Type

- Combination of spastic CP and dyskinetic CP
- May be labeled *mixed* when no specific motor pattern is dominant; however, this term losing favor to more precise descriptions of motor function and affected area of brain involved (Rosenbaum, Paneth, Leviton, et al., 2007)

Data from Nehring, W. (2010). Cerebral palsy. In P. J. Allen, J. A. Vessey, & N. A. Schapiro (Eds.), *Primary care of the child with a chronic condition* (5th ed.). St. Louis, MO: Mosby; Jones, M. W., Morgan, E., Shelton, J. E., et al. (2007). Cerebral palsy: Introduction and diagnosis, part 1. *Journal of Pediatric Health Care, 21*(3), 146-152; and National Institute of Neurologic Disorders and Stroke. (2006). Cerebral palsy: Hope through research. Retrieved from http://www.ninds.nih.gov/disorders/cerebral_palsy/detail_cerebral_palsy.htm

BOX 34.3 Clinical Manifestations of Cerebral Palsy (at Time of Diagnosis)

Delayed Gross Motor Development

- A universal manifestation
- Delay in all motor accomplishments
- Increases as growth advances
- Delays more obvious as growth advances

Abnormal Motor Performance

- Very early preferential unilateral hand preference
- Abnormal and asymmetric crawl
- Standing or walking on toes
- Uncoordinated or involuntary movements
- Poor sucking
- Feeding difficulties
- Persistent tongue thrust

Alterations of Muscle Tone

- Increased or decreased resistance to passive movements
- Opisthotonic posturing (arching of back)
- Feels stiff on handling or dressing
- Difficulty in diapering
- Rigid and unbending at the hip and knee joints when pulled to sitting position (early sign)

Abnormal Postures

- Maintains hips higher than trunk in prone position with legs and arms flexed or drawn under the body
- Scissoring and extension of legs with feet plantar flexed in supine position
- Persistent infantile resting and sleeping position
- Arms abducted at shoulders
- Elbows flexed
- Hands fisted

Reflex Abnormalities

- Persistence of primitive infantile reflexes
- Obligatory tonic neck reflex at any age
- Nonpersistence beyond 6 months of age
- Persistence or hyperactivity of the Moro, plantar, and palmar grasp reflexes
- Hyperreflexia, ankle clonus, and stretch reflexes elicited in many muscle groups on fast, passive movements

Associated Disabilities

- Altered learning and reasoning
- Seizures
- Impaired behavioral and interpersonal relationships
- Sensory impairment (vision, hearing)

From Nehring, W. M. (2010). Cerebral palsy. In P. J. Allen, J. A. Vessey, & N. A. Schapiro (Eds.), *Primary care of the child with a chronic condition* (5th ed.). St. Louis, MO: Mosby. Adapted from Jones, M. W., Morgan, E., & Shelton, J. E. (2007). Primary care of the child with cerebral palsy: A review of systems (part II). *Journal of Pediatric Health Care, 21*(4), 226-237.

themselves on either the buttocks or the abdomen. Spasticity may cause the child to stand or walk on the toes. Uncoordinated or involuntary movements are characteristic of dyskinetic CP, and facial grimacing and writhing movements of the tongue, fingers, and toes are signs of athetosis. Other significant signs of motor dysfunction are poor sucking and feeding difficulties, with persistent tongue thrust. Head staggering, tremor on reaching, and truncal ataxia are also common. Hand preference in the first 2 years of life is reported to be a sign of hemiplegic CP (Berker & Yalçin, 2008).

Alterations of Muscle Tone

Increased or decreased resistance to passive movements is a sign of abnormal muscle tone. The child may exhibit opisthotonic postures (exaggerated arching of the back) and may feel stiff on handling or dressing. Also, there is difficulty in diapering because of spasticity of the hip adductor muscles and lower extremities. When pulled to a sitting position, the child may extend the entire body and be rigid and unbending at the hip and knee joints. This is an early sign of spasticity.

Abnormal Posture

Children with spastic CP assume abnormal postures at rest or when their position is changed. From an early age, a child lying in a prone position will maintain the hips higher than the trunk with the legs and arms flexed or drawn under the body. In the supine position spasticity is evident by scissoring (legs in crossed position; knees, hips, and ankles stiff) and extension of the legs, with the feet plantar flexed. This posture is exaggerated when the child is suspended vertically or when others try to make the child bear weight. Depending on the degree of impairment, spasticity may be mild or severe. A persistent infantile resting and sleeping posture (i.e., arms abducted at shoulders, elbows flexed, and hands fisted) is a sign of spasticity when it remains constant after 4 to 5 months of age. The hemiparetic child may rest with the affected arm adducted and held against the torso, with the elbow pronated and slightly flexed and the hand closed.

Reflex Abnormalities

Persistence of primitive reflexes is one of the earliest clues to CP (e.g., obligatory tonic neck reflex at any age or nonobligatory persistence beyond 6 months of age, and the persistence or even hyperactivity of the Moro, plantar, and palmar grasp reflexes). Hyperreflexia, ankle clonus, and stretch reflexes can be elicited from many muscle groups on fast passive movements (e.g., resistance to passive abduction when the hips are suddenly separated [adductor catch]).

Associated Disabilities and Problems

Some of the disabilities associated with CP are visual impairment, hearing impairment, behavioral problems, communication and speech difficulties, seizures, and intellectual impairment. Additional sensory deficits such as hypersensitivity, hyposensitivity, and balance difficulties may occur in children with CP (Nehring, 2010). According to data from the Centers for Disease Control and Prevention (2013) almost 8% of children with CP are also diagnosed with autism spectrum disorder (Delobel-Ayoub, Klapouszczak, van Bakel, et al., 2017).

Intellectual impairment is a concern, although children with CP have a wide range of intelligence, and 50% to 60% are within normal limits. Speech difficulties are often interpreted as a sign of cognitive impairment. Assessing the intelligence of a child with CP is often difficult because of the motor and sensory deficits. Tests carried out periodically over time should determine the degree of intelligence. Many persons with CP who have severely limiting physical involvement actually have the least intellectual impairment. As a group, children with athetosis and ataxia are intellectually superior to those with other types of CP. The incidence of severe or profound impairment is highest in rigid and atonic CP. Improved communication devices (e.g., communication jacket, computerized communication) have revealed that some people with quadriplegic spastic CP have normal intelligence. Rick Hoyt, for example, who has quadriplegic spastic CP, communicates with his eyes and slight head movement and a computer to spell what he wants to communicate; he graduated from University of Boston and serves as consultant for technology devices.

The manifestations of attention-deficit/hyperactivity disorder may occur in children with CP. The primary presenting symptoms are poor attention span, marked distractibility, hyperactive behavior, and defects of integration. (See Chapter 16.) Seizures are more likely to accompany postnatally acquired hemiplegia. They are an unusual finding in ataxia and diplegia. The most common types of seizures are generalized tonic-clonic seizures and minor motor types (Nehring, 2010). Epilepsy is reported to occur in 41% of children with CP; epilepsy was especially common in nonambulatory children (Centers for Disease Control and Prevention, 2013).

Poor control of oral musculature may contribute to a number of problems. Abnormal posture and motor performance and alterations in muscle tone affect chewing, swallowing, and talking. Occupational and speech-language therapy interventions may be necessary to assist some children with feeding and speech. Coughing and choking, especially while eating, may predispose the child with CP to aspiration, which may not be readily apparent. Respiratory problems may result from and coexist with feeding difficulties in children with CP; respiratory symptoms observed during feedings include apnea, dyspnea, tachypnea, coughing and choking, and hypoxemia (Nehring, 2010). Many children with CP may also have gastroesophageal reflux.

Motor impairment associated with CP contributes to other problems. Children with CP who are nonambulatory have an increased risk of developing orthopedic complications such as unilateral or bilateral hip dislocations, scoliosis, and joint contractures resulting from unbalanced muscle tone. One study examined the Cobb angle for use in predicting the course of scoliosis in adolescents with CP (Oda, Takigawa, Sugimoto, et al., 2017).

A variety of factors, including decreased mobility, decreased fluid intake, a fear of toileting, poor positioning on the toilet, and lack of fiber intake, may be responsible for constipation (Nehring, 2010). Stool softeners, laxatives, and a bowel management program may be required to prevent chronic constipation.

Increased incidence of dental caries results from improper dental hygiene, congenital enamel defects (hypoplasia of primary teeth), high carbohydrate intake and retention, dietary imbalance with poor nutritional intake, inadequate fluoride, and difficulty in mouth closure and drooling. Spastic or clonic movements can cause gagging or biting down on the toothbrush, thus interfering with cleaning techniques. Oral hypersensitivity is also common, which causes the child to resist dental hygiene. Malocclusion can occur in as many as 90% of these children. Gingivitis is secondary to inadequate dental hygiene and may be further complicated by the use of antiepileptic drugs (AEDs) such as phenytoin (Nehring, 2010). Sehrawat, Marwaha, Bansal, and colleagues (2014) presented an eloquent coverage of the complexities and importance of dental care in children with CP. The CP multidisciplinary clinic with the University of Kansas Medical Center included a dental assistant at each clinic as part of the Kansas State initiative to improve oral health. The nurse may check with the state to see if they could provide this for special needs children. It was most helpful for families to receive teaching regarding oral health.

Skin breakdown may occur with prolonged positioning, especially with underweight children with bony prominences and those who are unable to reposition themselves or who may have insensate areas of skin.

Nystagmus and amblyopia are common and may require surgery, corrective lenses, or both. Hearing impairment is also common in children with CP. Some loss is caused by sensorineural involvement. Affected infants may spend increased amounts of time lying flat. This predisposes them to otitis media, which may result in conductive hearing loss.

Diagnostic Evaluation

Infants at risk according to known etiologic factors associated with CP warrant careful assessment during early infancy to identify the signs of muscular dysfunction as early as possible. The neurologic examination and history are the primary modalities for diagnosis. Neuroimaging of the child with suspected brain abnormality and CP is now recommended for diagnostic assessment, with MRI being a strong predictor of CP when performed at term (corrected age); general movements assessment also had a strong predictive value in children over 2 years of age and under 5 years of age (Bosanquet, Copeland, Ware, et al., 2013). MRI has the capability of early identification of infants at risk for CP (George, Fiori, Fripp, et al., 2017). MRI was useful in predicting language development in people with certain brain lesions (Choi, Choi, & Park, 2017). Metabolic and genetic testing is recommended if no structural abnormality is identified by neuroimaging; laboratory tests are no longer recommended in the diagnostic process for CP.

Early recognition is made more difficult by the lack of reliable neonatal neurologic signs. However, the nurse should monitor infants with known etiologic risk factors and evaluate them closely in the first 2 years of life. Because cortical control of movement does not occur until later in infancy, motor impairment associated with voluntary control is usually not apparent until after 2 to 4 months of age at the earliest. More often the diagnosis cannot be confirmed until the age of 1 or 2 years because motor tone abnormalities may be indicative of another neuromuscular condition. In addition, some children who show signs consistent with CP before 2 years do not demonstrate such signs after 2 years (Nehring, 2010). However, there is no consensus regarding an age cutoff for the onset of symptoms.

Establishing a diagnosis may be easier with the persistence of primitive reflexes: either the asymmetric tonic neck reflex or persistent Moro reflex (beyond 4 months of age), and the crossed extensor reflex. The tonic neck reflex normally disappears between 4 and 6 months of age. An obligatory response is considered abnormal. This is elicited by turning the infant's head to one side and holding it there for 20 seconds. When a crying infant is unable to move from the asymmetric posturing of the tonic neck reflex, it is considered obligatory and an abnormal response. The crossed extensor reflex, which normally disappears by 4 months, is elicited by applying a noxious stimulus to the sole of one foot with the knee extended. Normally the contralateral foot responds with extensor, abduction, and then adduction movements. The possibility of CP is suggested if these reflexes occur after 4 months.

A number of assessment instruments are now available to evaluate muscle spasticity (Modified Ashworth Scale); functional independence in self-care, mobility, and cognition (Functional Independence Measure and WeeFIM [specific to children]); self-initiated movements over time (Gross Motor Function Measure); and capability and performance of functional activities in self-care, mobility, and social function (Pediatric Evaluation of Disability Inventory) (Krigger, 2006).

A thorough knowledge of normal variations of motor development is required for detecting abnormal progress, and a careful history is necessary to detect possible etiologic factors. Observe the child's spontaneous movements and behavior, including posture; attitude; and muscle size, function, and tone. Because children with CP often have sensory deficits, it is appropriate to evaluate the child for hearing and vision deficits.

Therapeutic Management: General Concepts

The goals of therapy for children with CP are early recognition and promotion of an optimum developmental course to enable affected children to attain their potential within the limits of their dysfunction. The disorder is permanent, and therapy is chiefly symptomatic and preventive.

The beneficial influences of a habilitation program on both child and family are based on recognizing the disability as early as possible and implementing treatment. Parents are essential to a treatment program. Consider their goals and desires, their cooperation, and their confidence in all aspects of management. With early diagnosis parents can begin to provide the sensorimotor experiences essential to cognitive development because CNS structures depend on stimulation and use to attain and maintain their functional integrity.

The broad aims of therapy are to (1) establish locomotion, communication, and self-help skills; (2) gain optimum appearance and integration of motor functions; (3) correct associated defects as early and effectively as possible; (4) provide educational opportunities adapted to the individual child's needs and capabilities; and (5) promote socialization experiences with other affected and unaffected children. Each child is evaluated and managed on an individual basis. The plan of therapy may involve a variety of settings, facilities, and specially trained persons. The scope of the child's needs requires multidisciplinary planning and care coordination among professionals and the child's family (Box 34.4). The outcome for the child and family with CP is normalization and promotion of self-care activities that empower the child and family to achieve maximum potential.

Mobilizing Devices

Many children with CP wear ankle-foot orthoses (AFOs) (braces) and a variety of orthotics. Orthotics are molded to fit the feet and are worn inside the shoes. Devices are often used to help prevent or reduce deformity, increase the energy efficiency of gait, and control alignment. Some of the more commonly used mobility devices include wheeled scooter boards that allow children to propel themselves while the abdomen or total body is supported and the legs are positioned with wedges to prevent scissoring. Wheeled go-carts provide good sitting balance and serve as an early "wheelchair" experience for young children. Strollers can be equipped with custom seats for dependent mobilization. Special devices for independent mobilization that may or may not allow the upper extremities to remain free are particularly valuable for children with lower extremity involvement (Fig. 34.2). A number of wheelchairs can be customized to meet the needs and preferences of older children. (See Mobilization Devices, Chapter 33.)

Surgery

Surgical intervention is usually reserved for the child who does not respond to the more conservative measures such as orthotics, but it is also indicated for the child whose spasticity causes progressive deformities. Orthopedic surgery may be required to correct contracture or spastic deformities, to provide stability for an uncontrollable joint, to address bone malalignment (e.g., lever arm dysfunction), and to provide balanced muscle power. This includes tendon-lengthening procedures (especially heel-cord lengthening), release of spastic wrist flexor muscles, and correction of hip and adductor muscle spasticity or contracture to improve locomotion. Orthopedic specialists with special interest in CP will implement hip observation protocols for children considered at risk for hip abnormalities. Hip surveillance and surgical salvage choices are individual for each person with CP. There is not one procedure that fits all. Orthopedic surgery is generally not performed until after the child is 6 years of age (Nehring, 2010). Surgery is used primarily to improve function rather than for cosmetic purposes and is followed by physical therapy. Surgery may also be performed to improve caloric intake, correct gastroesophageal reflux disease, prevent aspiration, and correct associated dental problems (Nehring, 2010).

Neurosurgical procedures are used only in selected cases. Selective dorsal rhizotomy has provided marked improvement in some children with CP (Nordmark, Josenby, Lagergren, et al., 2008). After selective dorsal rhizotomy, gait was improved in children with CP (Rumberg, Bakir, Taylor, et al., 2016). However, achieving the benefits from the surgery requires intensive physical therapy and family commitment. Because the procedure results in flaccid muscles, the child must relearn to sit, stand, and walk.

Medication

Intense pain may occur with muscle spasms in patients with CP. Children with CP may also experience pain as a result of painful procedures such

BOX 34.4 Therapeutic Interventions for Cerebral Palsy

Interdisciplinary developmental and physical assessment with recommendations may include the following:

Physical Therapy
Orthotic Devices
- Braces
- Splints
- Casting
- Molded orthoses

Adaptive Equipment
- Scooters, bicycles, and tricycles
- Wheelchairs
- Boards
- Standing devices

Functional (Neuromuscular) Electrical Stimulation (in Combination With Dynamic Splinting)

Occupational Therapy
Adaptive Equipment
- Utensils for functional use (e.g., eating, writing)
- Switches
- Computers

Speech-Language Therapy
- Oral-motor skills
- Adaptive communication techniques

Special Education
- Early intervention programs
- Specialized learning programs and support services in school
- Socialization to promote self-concept development

Surgical Intervention
- Orthopedic (e.g., tendon transfers, muscle lengthening, spinal deformities)
- Neurologic (e.g., neurectomies)
- Selective dorsal rhizotomy
- Feeding (e.g., gastrostomy)
- Dental

Medication Therapy
- Medications to treat the following:
  - Spasticity
  - Pain
  - Secondary conditions (e.g., seizure disorder, chronic constipation, urinary tract infections, gastroesophageal reflux)
- Primary care for health supervision and acute childhood illnesses

Behavioral Therapy
Care Coordination
- Care coordination of specialized services and community resources in collaboration with the child's family

Modified from Nehring, W. M. (2010). Cerebral palsy. In P. J. Allen, J. A. Vessey, & N. A. Schapiro (Eds.), *Primary care of the child with a chronic condition* (5th ed.). St. Louis, MO: Mosby.

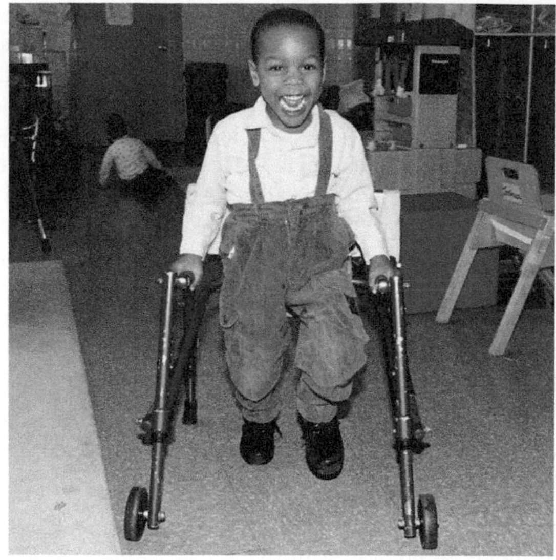

FIG. 34.2 Child ambulating with use of assistive device.

as injection with botulinum toxin type A (Botox), surgical procedures intended to reduce contracture deformities, abdominal pain related to position and gastroesophageal reflux, and pain associated with physical therapy. Therefore pain management is an important aspect of the care of the child with CP.

Pharmacologic agents given orally (dantrolene sodium [Dantrium], baclofen [Lioresal], and diazepam [Valium]) have had little effectiveness in improving muscle coordination in children with CP. However, they are effective in decreasing overall spasticity. The most common side effects of these agents include hepatotoxicity (dantrolene), drowsiness, fatigue, and muscle weakness. Less commonly, diaphoresis and constipation may occur with oral baclofen; other possible complications include hallucinations, mood changes, seizures, nausea, and urinary incontinence. Diazepam is used frequently but should be restricted to older children and adolescents.

Botulinum toxin A is also used to reduce spasticity in targeted muscles of the upper and lower extremities (Lukban, Rosales, & Dressler, 2009). Botulinum toxin A is injected into a selected muscle (commonly the quadriceps, gastrocnemius, or medial hamstrings), where it acts to inhibit the release of acetylcholine into a specific muscle group, thereby preventing muscle movement. When it is administered early in the course of the illness, this may prevent affected muscle contractures, particularly in lower extremities, thus avoiding surgical procedures with possible adverse effects. The goal is to allow stretching of the muscle; as it relaxes, it permits ambulation with an AFO. The major reported adverse effects of botulinum toxin A injection include pain at the injection site and a temporary weakness (Lukban, Rosales, & Dressler, 2009). Prime candidates for botulinum toxin A injections are children with spasticity confined to the lower extremities. The onset of action occurs within 24 to 72 hours, with a peak effect observed at 2 weeks and a duration of action of 3 to 6 months. Decreasing spasticity with botulinum toxin A may also result in less pain from spasms (Lundy, Doherty, & Fairhurst, 2009). One case study showed improvement with spinal balance after one botulinum toxin A injection (Chaléat-Valayer, Bernard, Deceuninck, et al., 2016). Using the Gross Motor Classification Scale, the history since 1993, and progression of botulism toxin A injections across the life span was explored as a safe, effective treatment to control spasticity in persons with CP, with expert decisions and precise muscle injections given for each developmental stage (Strobl, Theologis, Brunner, et al., 2015).

The neurosurgical and pharmacologic approach to managing the spasticity associated with CP involves the implantation of a pump to infuse baclofen directly into the intrathecal space surrounding the spinal cord to provide relief of spasticity. High doses of oral baclofen are associated with significant side effects, including drowsiness and confusion, yet are often unable to provide adequate relief of spasticity. Direct infusion of baclofen into the intrathecal space provides relief without as many side effects (Motta, Antonello, & Stignani, 2011). Intrathecal baclofen is especially helpful in improving comfort (Morton, Gray, & Vloeberghs, 2011).

One study combined baclofen and antibiotic in the pump to prevent infection and maintain lasting stability/benefit of the pump (Aristedis, Dimitrios, Nikolaos, et al., 2017). Patients may be screened before pump placement by the infusion of a "test dose" of intrathecal baclofen delivered via a lumbar puncture. Close monitoring for side effects (e.g., hypotonia, somnolence, seizures, nausea, vomiting, headache, and catheter- or pump-related problems) and relief of spasticity occurs for several hours after the infusion. If a positive effect occurs, the patient is considered a candidate for pump placement.

The pump is placed in the subcutaneous space of the midabdomen; it is about the size of a hockey puck. An intrathecal catheter is tunneled from the lumbar area to the abdomen and connected to the pump. The pump is filled with baclofen and programmed to provide a set dose using a telemetry wand and a computer. The patient remains hospitalized for several days to adjust the dosage and ensure proper healing. Outpatient visits to refill the pump and make dosage adjustments occur about every 4 to 6 weeks, depending on the patient's response to the treatment. Benefits of intrathecal baclofen include fewer systemic side effects, dosage titration for maximizing effects, and reversibility of therapy with removal of the pump if so desired. Abrupt withdrawal of intrathecal baclofen, especially at high doses, may result in adverse effects such as rebound spasticity, pruritus, hyperthermia, rhabdomyolysis, disseminated intravascular coagulation, multiorgan failure, and death; in some cases intrathecal baclofen withdrawal may mimic sepsis. Treatment of withdrawal centers on reestablishing the medication dosage, with improvements observed within 1 to 2 hours. Hospitalization and surgery may be required for withdrawal as a result of pump or catheter failure.

AEDs such as carbamazepine (Tegretol), divalproex (valproate sodium and valproic acid [Depakote]), oxcarbazepine (Trileptal), and lamotrigine (Lamictal) are prescribed routinely for children who have seizures. Gabapentin (Neurontin) has been used in adults with SCI to decrease spasticity with success. Yuan-Kim Liow, Gimeno, Lumsden, and colleagues (2016) found that gabapentin improved quality of life, pain, and dystonia in children with CP. The α_2-adrenergic agonists clonidine (Catapres) and tizanidine (Zanaflex) have been used to decrease spasticity in adults with SCI and multiple sclerosis; however, their use in children does not appear to have gained widespread acceptance in the United States. Oral tizanidine given in conjunction with botulinum type A has been reported to be more effective than oral baclofen and botulinum type A in one study of children with CP (Dai, Wasay, & Awan, 2008). Monitor all medications for maintenance of therapeutic levels and avoidance of subtherapeutic or toxic levels. (See Quality Patient Outcomes box.)

QUALITY PATIENT OUTCOMES

Seizures

- No physical injury as a result of seizure activity
- Prevention of seizure activity

Children with CP have been treated with a number of complementary and alternative medicine strategies, including Chinese herbs, acupuncture, growth hormone therapy, aquatic exercise, equine-assisted therapy, and hyperbaric oxygen (Nehring, 2010). Gasalberti (2006) reported some alternative therapies being used in children with disabilities that the practitioner may overlook during a health history but that may be beneficial to such children. These include pet therapy, massage, hippotherapy (horse riding), music, and color-light therapy. Other alternative therapies that may be used by families with children with disabilities include vitamins, prayer, meditation, hypnosis, and guided i magery.

Technical Aids

A wide variety of technical aids are available to improve the functioning of children with CP. These include electromechanical toys that employ the concept of biofeedback and operate from a head unit. The toy is manipulated only when the head and trunk are in correct alignment. Computerized toys and games can also enhance eye-hand coordination.

Microcomputers combined with voice synthesizers help children with speech difficulties to "speak." Smart phones and tablets with speech applications are appropriate for some children. These and other devices print messages onto screen monitors and paper. These devices have made it apparent that some children have been erroneously considered to be cognitively impaired. Microcomputers have also increased the possibilities for increased mobility via wheelchairs and specially designed mobilization devices.

Many other electronic devices allow independent functioning. Computerized games have been studied to help with fine motor skills in school-age children (Kanitkar, Szturm, Parmar, et al., 2017). Robots were studied to help improve movement in children with CP; there is a need for more cost-effective robots to further evaluate effectiveness (Michmizos & Krebs, 2017). Combined brain stimulation and robotics improved upper limb functioning in adults with CP; more study is needed with children (Friel, Lee, Soles, et al., 2017).

Sensors can be activated and deactivated using a head-stick, a voluntary muscle such as the tongue, or any other voluntary muscle movement over which the child has control. The application of this technology makes it possible for older persons with CP to eventually function in their own apartments and can be extended into the workplace.

Associated Problems

Children with CP often have sensory deficits, which require the attention of appropriate specialists. Speech-language therapy involves the services of a speech-language pathologist (SLP) who may also assist with feeding problems. (See Chapter 20) Dental care is especially important for children with CP and often is overlooked. Regular visits to the dentist and dental prophylaxis, including brushing, fluoride, and flossing (after several teeth are present), should begin as soon as the teeth erupt. This is especially important for children given phenytoin, who often develop gum hyperplasia. Additional problems common among children with CP include constipation caused by neurologic deficits and lack of exercise; poor bladder control and urinary retention; chronic respiratory tract infections and aspiration pneumonia, which occur as a result of gastroesophageal reflux, abnormal muscle tone, immobility, and altered positioning; and skin problems as a result of altered positioning, poor nutrition, and immobility. Hip dislocation occurs often in children with CP. Latex allergy has also been reported in children with CP (Nehring, 2010).

Therapeutic Management: Therapies, Education, Recreation

Physical Therapy

Physical therapy is one of the most commonly used treatment modalities in children with CP. In general, physical therapy is directed toward good skeletal alignment for the child with spasticity; training in purposeful acts, even in the face of involuntary motion, for the child with athetosis; and gait training and maximum development of proprioceptive sense for the child with ataxia.

An active therapy program involves the family, the physical therapist (PT), the occupational therapist (OT), and other members of the health care team. Developing a treatment program that can be carried out at home is of utmost importance. The major approach uses traditional types of therapeutic exercises that consist of stretching; passive, active, and resistive movements applied to specific muscle groups or joints to maintain or increase range of motion; strength; or endurance. Neuromuscular electrical stimulation combined with dynamic splinting may benefit some children (Wright, Durham, Ewins, et al., 2012). No therapeutic approach is able to achieve spectacular changes in the ultimate outcome of motor disability. Early efforts focus on alleviating abnormal postures by positioning and range-of-motion exercises. Passive range-of-motion exercises, stretching, and elongation exercises are valuable at any age, even when the child is too young to cooperate. Some active extension can be performed when the child is old enough to cooperate, with passive motion applied to complete joint extension. Prevention of contracture deformity is a prime function of physical therapy. Seating, mobility, strength, and endurance are other key goals.

Functional and Adaptive Training (Occupational Therapy)

Training in manual skills and activities of daily living (ADLs) proceeds along developmental lines and according to the child's functional level. Sitting, balancing, crawling, and walking are encouraged at appropriate ages and are accompanied by stimulation of protective extension and equilibrium reactions. Hand activities are began early to improve motor function and provide the child with sensory experiences and information about the environment. As the child progresses from simple feeding and self-care activities, training is extended to include other tasks (e.g., cooking or use of keyboard or computer mouse) that are within the child's developmental and functional capabilities.

Incorporating play into the therapeutic program often requires great ingenuity and inventiveness from those involved in the child's care. Objects and toys are chosen to provide needed sensory input using a variety of shapes, forms, and textures. Nurses can help parents integrate therapy into play activities in natural ways.

Children with CP may need considerable help (and patience) in learning to feed and dress themselves and care for personal hygiene needs. A feeding program may be developed by an OT in conjunction with an SLP. Children should be fed in the normal eating position. When they have difficulty sucking and swallowing, it is tempting to hold them in a semireclining posture to make use of gravity flow. However, this method does not promote active swallowing, and the neck hyperextension may even interfere with swallowing. A more flexed sitting position, with the arms brought forward to decrease the tendency toward back and neck extension, is more natural during bottle- or spoon-feeding and encourages active swallowing.

Because jaw control is compromised, more normal control can be achieved if the feeder provides stability for the oral mechanism from the side or front of the face. When directed from the front, the middle finger of the nonfeeding hand is placed posterior to the bony portion of the chin, the thumb is placed below the bottom lip, and the index finger is placed parallel to the child's mandible (Fig. 34.3). Manual jaw control from the side assists with head control, correction of neck and trunk hyperextension, and jaw stabilization. The middle finger of the nonfeeding hand is placed posterior to the bony portion of the chin, the index finger is placed on the chin below the lower lip, and the thumb is placed obliquely across the cheek to provide lateral jaw stability (Fig. 34.4).

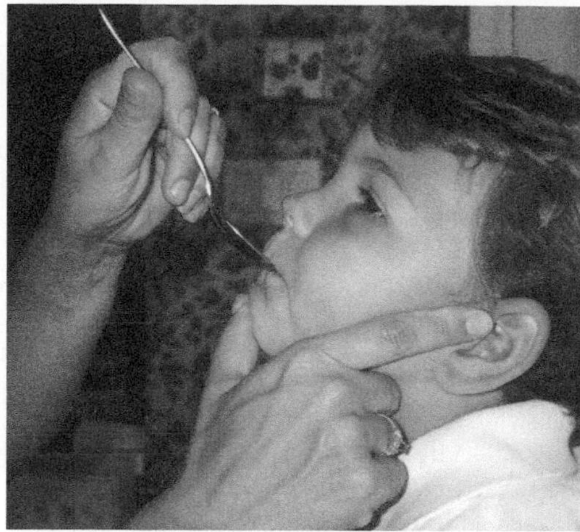

FIG. 34.3 Manual jaw control provided anteriorly.

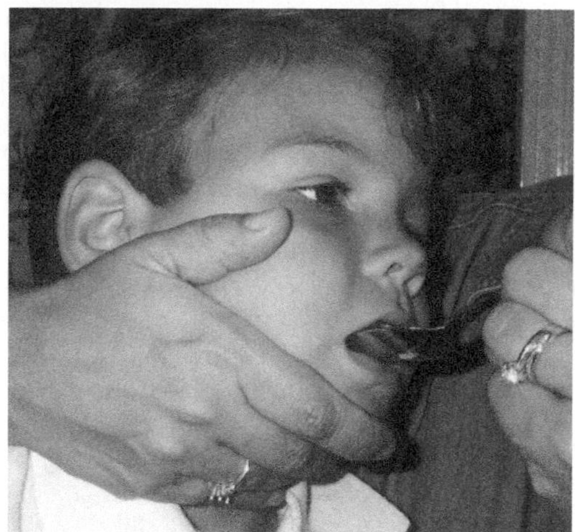

FIG. 34.4 Manual jaw control provided from the side.

In all ADLs it is important to capitalize on the child's assets and compensate for liabilities. The level of expected independence is related to both gross and fine motor manipulation. Even when complete independence in a specific activity is not realistic, the child should learn any part of the task that he or she can master. However, motor function is not the sole purpose of learning to be as independent as possible. Any accomplishment promotes self-reliance and self-esteem for healthier personality development.

Speech Therapy

Speech training under the supervision of an SLP begins early, before the child learns poor habits of communication. Parents and others can help by following the directions of the speech therapist and by talking to the child slowly while using pictures or handling objects about which the adult is speaking. Feeding techniques such as forcing the child to use the lips and tongue in eating facilitate speech. An example of this technique is placing food at the side of the tongue, first one side and then the other, and making the child use the lips to take food from a spoon rather than placing it directly on the tongue. If severe dysarthria prevents articulate speech and the child has reasonable intelligence, the child learns nonverbal communication (e.g., sign language). (See Chapter 20.)

Education

As in all aspects of care, educational requirements are determined by the child's needs and potential. This includes the severity of the child's disease and the presence and degree of associated conditions that affect learning and participation, such as learning impairment, abnormal actions or behaviors, impaired vision or hearing, and seizures. Children with mild to moderate cognitive involvement are generally able to participate, for varying amounts of time, in regular classes. Resource rooms are available in most schools to provide more individualized attention to a child's particular needs. Integration of these children into regular classrooms should be the initial goal. Teachers' assistants often work one-on-one with children in both settings. A training program may be appropriate for those children who are unable to benefit from formal education. Prevocational and vocational counseling and guidance are arranged at adolescence. Education is geared toward the child's assets at any phase or in any setting. Nurses should be aware of early intervention programs and provisions for special education and related services for children and should support parents in their efforts to obtain appropriate educational services for the child. Bourke-Taylor, Cotter, Lalor, and colleagues (2017) emphasized the importance of collaboration among team members of school-age children with CP in schools, in the community, in health care, and across the life span for best outcomes.

Recreation

Recreational activities are also a necessary part of growing up. Recreational outlets and after-school activities should be an option for the child who is unable to participate in regular athletic and other peer activities. Some can compete in athletic and artistic endeavors, and many games and pastimes are suited to their capabilities. Sports, physical fitness, and recreation programs are encouraged for children with CP, and young children should be exposed to all physical activities available to children without disabilities. Individual sports such as the martial arts (e.g., Tae Kwon Do) in which groups are small and the emphasis is on discipline and balance are also enjoyable to many children with CP. Many states mandate adaptive physical education classes.

Numerous developmental centers have facilities for indoor and outdoor activities designed to appeal to children of all ages. If these are not available, they should be developed. However, such programs require adequate supervision to avoid any harmful effects. Recreational activities serve to stimulate children's interest and curiosity, help them adjust to their disability, improve their functional abilities, and build self-esteem. Competitive sports are also becoming increasingly available to children with disabilities and offer an added dimension to physical activities. For more information access the United Cerebral Palsy website (http://www.ucp.org) and go to the Sports and Leisure link. Any accomplishment that helps children approach a normal way of life enhances their self-concept.

Prognosis

The prognosis for the child with CP depends largely on the type and severity of the condition. Children with mild to moderate involvement (85%) have the capability of achieving ambulation between the ages of 2 and 7 years (Berker & Yalçin, 2008). If the child does not achieve independent ambulation by this time, chances are poor for ambulation and independence. Approximately 30% to 50% of individuals with CP have significant cognitive impairments, and an even higher percentage have mild cognitive and learning deficits (Green, Greenberg, & Hurwitz, 2003; Liptak & Accardo, 2004). Children with profound cognitive impairment have a higher mortality rate, and less than one-half of those reach adulthood (O'Shea, 2008). However, many children with severe spastic tetraplegic CP have normal intelligence. Growth is affected in children with spastic tetraplegia, and many children remain below the 5th percentile for age and sex.

As children with CP become adults, about 30% remain in the home and are cared for by a parent or caregiver; 50% of individuals with spastic tetraplegia live in independent settings and function at appropriate social levels considering their disability (Green, Greenberg, & Hurwitz, 2003). Vocational rehabilitation and higher education are possible for adults with CP. Children with severe CP mobility impairment and feeding problems often succumb to respiratory tract infection in childhood. The few survival rate studies on children or adults with CP show that survival is influenced by existing comorbidities (Nehring, 2010). In general, the more medically fragile children are least likely to survive to adulthood (Westbom, Bergstrand, Wagner, et al., 2011). (See Quality Patient Outcomes box.)

QUALITY PATIENT OUTCOMES

Pain

- Acceptable pain threshold experienced as defined by patient or caregiver, or a pain score of 4 or less on Wong Baker Faces Pain Rating Scale.
- The occurrence of pain in people with cerebral palsy (CP) was measured and found to be similar to previous reports. More attention to the report and treatment of pain needs to be given (Westbom, Rimstedt, & Nordmark, 2017).
- Early detection, prevention, and treatment of pain in children with CP have been studied by several (Adolfsson, Johnson, & Nilsson, 2017).

Nursing Care Management

Assessment

Nursing assessment includes risk identification of infants with etiologic factors that are associated with CP. Ongoing assessment of infants for abnormal muscle tone, inability to achieve developmental milestones, and persistence of neonatal reflexes alert the nurse to investigate further.

Reinforce Therapeutic Plan and Assist in Normalization

Because children are being treated at an earlier age, parents are participating at an earlier stage in treatment programs for their disabled child. They learn the proper handling and home care of young children with CP and need carefully programmed steps so that their expanded parental role can be melded into the established relationship. Close work with other multidisciplinary team members is essential. Nurses reinforce the therapeutic plan and assist the family in devising and modifying equipment and activities to continue the therapy program in the home. (See also Chapter 20.)

Some children have difficulty keeping their head upright. Because of this, they can neither explore much of their environment nor process the information. Parents need to be complimented on their efforts to provide a stimulating environment for these children. These infants are at risk for delayed development in holding up their heads, righting their shoulders and trunks for stable posture, sitting, pulling, standing, and crawling. Most parents of children with impaired movements benefit from support and practical suggestions for feeding, moving, holding, and encouraging the infant to explore hands and feet and to play. Helping parents incorporate therapeutic suggestions into typical daily activities is an important normalizing strategy. (See Chapter 20 for a discussion of normalization.)

Although practical advice is important, the nurse, OT, or PT should offer suggestions at a pace that can be absorbed by the parents. Encourage the parents to define their concerns, acknowledge the concerns as genuine, and ask the parents what approaches they have tried and for how long. In this way the nurse is able to find out what works, what does not work, and what the parents would like to try next. Give the parents positive feedback for their observations of the infant, the progress they note, and how they differentiate the child's needs.

Address Health Maintenance Needs

Because children with CP expend so much energy in their efforts to accomplish ADLs, more frequent rest periods should be arranged to avoid the fatigue that may aggravate their limited capabilities. Meeting the child's nutritional needs may be a challenge because of gastroesophageal reflux, feeding and swallowing difficulties, chronic constipation and subsequent anorexia, and absence or diminished ability to independently feed himself or herself (Jones, Morgan, & Shelton, 2007). As a result of being ELBW or VLBW in combination with these feeding problems, children with CP are at risk for failure to thrive, and the nurse must ensure an adequate caloric intake. Children with spasticity expend more energy and often require more energy intake than same-age counterparts to maintain adequate growth. Nutritional supplements such as high-calorie milk products (e.g., Pediasure) may be necessary to provide adequate caloric intake after the child has reached 1 year of age. Additional nutritional concerns include providing adequate intake of fruits and fiber to enhance gastrointestinal (GI) motility, routinely monitoring child's growth on a standardized growth chart, and avoiding overfeeding and obesity (Jones, Morgan, & Shelton, 2007).

Routine assessment of skin status is imperative in children with CP who are limited in movement or who must remain in assistive devices such as a wheelchair for a prolonged period. The overall nutritional status may also be a risk factor for skin breakdown. Care must be taken to ensure that adequate objective skin assessments are routinely performed. If skin breakdown does occur, consult a skin and wound specialist for treatment and further prevention.

Gastrostomy feedings may be necessary to supplement regular feedings and ensure adequate weight gain, particularly in children at risk for growth failure and chronic malnutrition, those with severe CP and subsequent oral feeding difficulties, and children whose well-being is affected by illness and decreased fluid or medication intake (Rogers, 2004). Oral feedings may be continued to maintain oral motor skills. Weight gain is perceived as an important measure of adequate oral feeding efficiency (Rogers, 2004).

Parents may need assistance and advice with medication administration through a gastrostomy tube to prevent clogging. Pills may be crushed and mixed with small amounts of water but not other liquids, such as formula or elixir medications, because these may act together to form a sludge that can interfere with gastrostomy tube function. When crushed pills or tablets are administered, flush the feeding tube with more water after instilling the dissolved pill in water. The pharmacist can provide information regarding crushed pills and tablets and elixirs, which should not be mixed together when administered via gastrostomy or nasogastric tube. A skin-level gastrostomy is particularly suited for the child with CP. (See also Gastrostomy Feeding, Chapter 22.)

Safety precautions are implemented, such as having children wear protective helmets if they are subject to falls or capable of injuring their heads on hard objects. Because the child with CP is at risk for altered proprioception and subsequent falls, parents should adapt the home and play environment to the child's particular needs to prevent bodily harm. Transportation of the child with motor problems and restricted mobility may be especially challenging for the family and child. Attention must be given to the child's safety when riding in a motor vehicle; a federally approved safety restraint should be used at all times. Lovette (2008) recommends that children with CP ride in a rear-facing position as long as possible because of their poor head, neck, and trunk control. This author also provides a list of options for special car restraint systems for children with CP, including several restraints that are suitable for children with a hip spica cast.

Appropriate immunizations should be administered to prevent childhood illnesses and protect against respiratory tract infections such as influenza. Depending on the level of involvement, dental problems may be more common in children with CP, which creates a need for meticulous attention to all aspects of dental care.

Support the Family

The nursing interventions that are probably most valuable to the family are support and help in coping with the emotional aspects of the chronic disorder, many of which are discussed in Chapter 19. Initially the parents need information and support in understanding the implications of the diagnosis and all the feelings it engenders. Later they need clarification regarding what they can expect from the child and from health care professionals. Educating families in the principles of family-centered care and parent-professional collaboration is essential. The family also may require help modifying the home environment for care of the child. Transportation to the practitioner's office and other health care agencies often requires special considerations.

Care management for the child and family with CP is an important nursing role. In many cases the family assumes complete care of the child and becomes quite adept at caring for her or his individual needs. The home health nurse or case manager has an important role in the support and encouragement of families who assume the primary care of a child with CP. Having a child with CP implies numerous problems of daily management, with changes in family life, and the nurse needs to stress principles of normalization. (See Normalization, Chapter 19.)

The nurse can support the parents by acknowledging and addressing their concerns and frustrations and by noting and appreciating their problem-solving skills and their approaches to helping the child. Siblings of a child with a disability are also affected and may respond with overt or less evident behavioral problems. The family needs a relationship with nurses who can provide continued contact, support, and encouragement through the long process of habilitation.

Parents can also find help and support from parent groups, where they can share experiences, accomplishments, problems, and concerns while deriving comfort and practical information. For example, parents can understand from others what it is like to have a child with CP. United Cerebral Palsy has branches in most communities and provides a variety of services for children and families. A number of excellent books are available to guide parents and nurses who work with children with CP. Many of the books are written by people with CP who have triumphed (e.g., *My Left Foot,* a movie and book).

Care of the Hospitalized Child

CP is not a condition that requires hospitalization; therefore when children with CP are hospitalized, they are usually admitted for an associated illness or for corrective surgery. To facilitate the care and management of hospitalized children with CP, the therapy program should be continued (in so far as their condition allows) while they are hospitalized. This should be incorporated into the multidisciplinary care plan, with every effort expended to make certain the ground that has been so laboriously gained is not lost. Encouraging the parent to room-in and actively participate in the child's care facilitates a continuation of the home therapy program and helps the child adjust to an

BOX 34.5 Neural Tube Defects

Cranioschisis—A skull defect through which various tissues protrude
Exencephaly—Brain totally exposed or extruded through an associated skull defect; fetus usually aborted
Anencephaly—Congenital malformation in which both cerebral hemispheres are absent.
Encephalocele—Herniation of brain and meninges through a defect in the skull producing a fluid-filled sac
Rachischisis or spina bifida—Fissure in the spinal column that leaves the meninges and spinal cord exposed
Meningocele—Hernial protrusion of a saclike cyst of meninges filled with spinal fluid (see Fig. 34.5, *C*)
Myelomeningocele (meningomyelocele)—Hernial protrusion of a saclike cyst containing meninges, spinal fluid, and a portion of the spinal cord with its nerves (see Fig. 34.5, *D*)

unfamiliar environment. However, it is equally important to remember that a hospitalization may be the first time a parent can defer care to a nurse and not be the primary caregiver. This respite may be crucial to the parent's well-being. Respect the parent's preference in this regard.

DEFECTS OF NEURAL TUBE CLOSURE

Abnormalities that derive from the embryonic neural tube (neural tube defects [NTDs]) constitute the largest group of congenital anomalies with multifactorial inheritance. Normally the spinal cord and cauda equina are encased in a protective sheath of bone and meninges (Fig. 34.5, *A*). Failure of neural tube closure produces defects of varying degrees (Box 34.5). They may involve the entire length of the neural tube or may be restricted to a small area.

ETIOLOGY

Two of the defects, anencephaly and spina bifida (SB), occur in association with each other more often than would be expected by chance, suggesting a common origin. The CNS defects may alternate in siblings, which also tends to support the theory of a common origin. In the United States approximately 1500 infants with spina bifida are born each year (Parker, Mai, et al., 2010). The incidence of SB is higher in girls than in boys, and it is more likely to occur in Hispanic (3.8 per 10,000 births) women than in Caucasians (3.09 per 10,000) or African Americans (2.73 per 10,000) (National Center on Birth Defects and Developmental Disabilities, Centers for Disease Control and Prevention, 2016).

In the United States rates of NTDs declined by as much as 23% between 1995 and 1996 and 2000. NTD rates decreased an additional 6.9% between 2000 and 2005, primarily among African American mothers. One concern is that NTD rates have not decreased significantly among Hispanic and non-Hispanic Caucasian mothers since 1999 (Centers for Disease Control and Prevention, 2009). The decline in NTDs in the late 1990s has been attributed in large part to the addition of folic acid to cereal grain products (Centers for Disease Control and Prevention, 2016). In 2006 the rates for SB were estimated by the Centers for Disease Control and Prevention to be 3.05 per 10,000 live births, thus making this one of the most common birth defects in the United States (Matthews, 2009). Population-based studies have also witnessed a substantial decrease in NTDs since food fortification with folic acid and folic acid supplementation recommendations were made (Collins, Atkinson, Dean, et al., 2011). Increased use of prenatal diagnostic techniques and termination of pregnancies have also affected the overall incidence of NTDs.

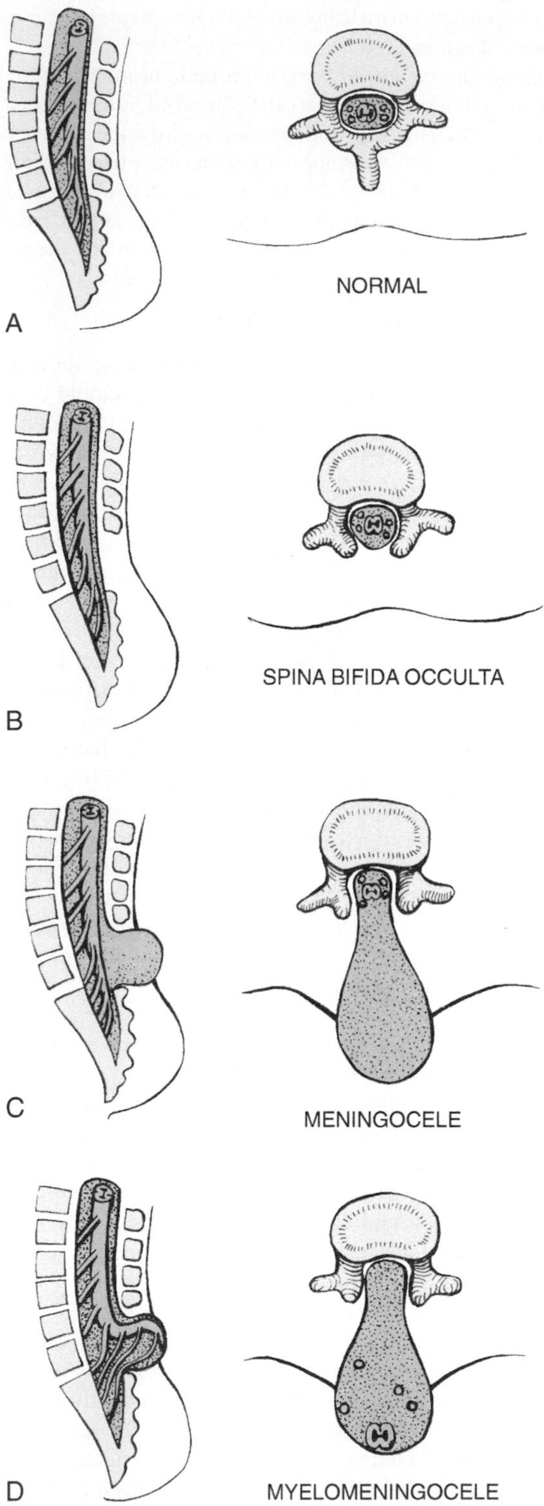

FIG. 34.5 A through **D,** Midline defects of osseous spine with varying degrees of neural herniations.

The National Spina Bifida Patient Registry is a data collection program funded by the Centers for Disease Control and Prevention. It was started in 2008 to provide a framework to standardize and improve treatment of children, adolescents, and adults over 21 years of age. Detailed questionnaires from the participating 10 specialized, multidisciplinary spina bifida clinics provide data, which are sent to a Centers for Disease

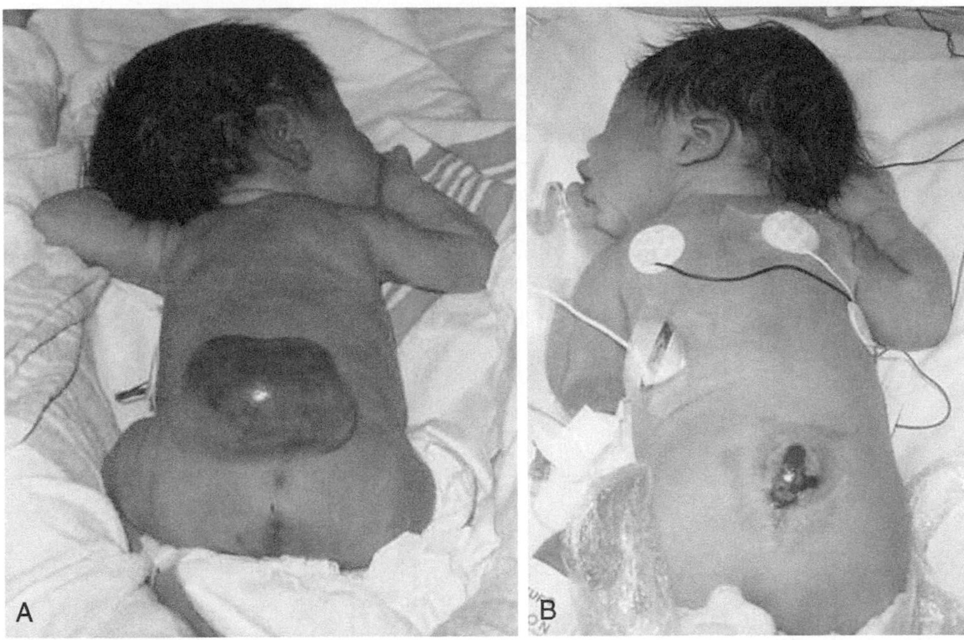

FIG. 34.6 A, Myelomeningocele with intact sac. **B,** Myelomeningocele with ruptured sac. (Courtesy Dr. Robert C. Dauser, Neurosurgery, Baylor College of Medicine, Houston, TX.)

Control and Prevention database for analysis. This process helps identify the most beneficial care for patients.

Most authorities believe that the primary defect in NTDs is a failure of neural tube closure during the embryo's early development (between the third and fourth week). However, evidence also implicates a multifactorial origin, including drugs, radiation, maternal malnutrition, chemicals, and possibly a genetic mutation in folate pathways in some cases, which may result in abnormal development (Kinsman & Johnston, 2015).

Additional factors predisposing the infant to NTDs include maternal obesity, previous NTD pregnancy, Hispanic ancestry, low folic acid intake, gestational diabetes, hot tub or sauna use, low maternal vitamin B_{12} status, and the use of antiepileptic drugs (e.g., valproic acid) in pregnancy (Agopian, Tinker, Lupo, et al., 2013). The degree of neurologic dysfunction depends on where the sac protrudes through the vertebrae, the anatomic level of the defect, and the amount of nerve tissue involved (Fig. 34.6). Most myelomeningoceles involve the lumbar or lumbosacral area.

The American Academy of Pediatrics (2007) recommends daily intake of folic acid for all women of childbearing age. The recommended 0.4-mg daily dose is supplied safely in many multivitamin preparations. Because the greatest risk factor is a previous pregnancy affected by NTDs, women in this category should increase their daily folic acid dose to 4 mg, under a practitioner's supervision, beginning at least 1 month before they plan a pregnancy and through the first trimester because the neural tube closes about 1 month after conception. In 2009 the U.S. Preventive Services Task Force published a statement indicating there is ample evidence to support the recommendations for folic acid supplementation to decrease the incidence of NTDs (Wolff, Witkop, Miller, et al., 2009). In 1998 the U.S. Food and Drug Administration authorized the fortification of cereal grains (including cornmeal, grits, and wheat flour) with folic acid. It remains important for all women of childbearing age to take a multivitamin with 0.4 mg folic acid daily (American Academy of Pediatrics, 2007). Sexually active females should be counseled regarding the risks of inadequate folate intake (Burke, Liptak, & Council on Children with Disabilities, 2011).

The following discussion of NTDs is limited to the two most common types: anencephaly, a defect incompatible with life, and SB, in particular myelomeningocele, an abnormality that causes significant disability.

ANENCEPHALY

Anencephaly, the most serious NTD, is a congenital malformation in which both cerebral hemispheres are absent. If the child with exencephaly (where brain protrudes from the skull), survives, degeneration of the brain to a spongiform mass occurs, with no bony covering. The condition is incompatible with life, and many affected infants are stillborn. For those who survive, no specific treatment is available. The infants have a portion of the brainstem and are able to maintain vital functions (such as temperature regulation and cardiac and respiratory function) for a few hours to several weeks but eventually die of respiratory failure.

Traditionally these infants have been provided comfort measures, but with no effort at resuscitation. Ethical and moral questions are encountered regarding treatment and withdrawal of support systems (e.g., feedings) if the newborn survives the first few days of life, as well as use of the organs for donor transplants. During this time the family requires emotional support and counseling to cope with the birth of an infant with a fatal defect. Referral to neonatal palliative care or hospice should be made as soon as possible.

SPINA BIFIDA AND MYELODYSPLASIA

Myelodysplasia refers broadly to any malformation of the spinal canal and cord. Midline defects involving failure of the osseous (bony) spine to close are called spina bifida, the most common defect of the CNS. SB is categorized into two types: SB occulta and SB cystica.

SB occulta refers to a defect that is not visible externally. It occurs most commonly in the lumbosacral area (L5 and S1) (Fig. 34.5, *B*). Routine radiographic examinations indicate that the disorder may occur in as many as 10% to 30% of the general population. However, it may not be apparent unless there are associated cutaneous manifestations or neuromuscular disturbances. Superficial cutaneous indications include a skin depression or dimple (which may also mark the outlet of a dermal sinus tract that extends to the subarachnoid space); port-wine angiomatous nevi; dark tufts of hair; and soft, subcutaneous lipomas. These signs may be absent, appear singly, or be present in combination.

If associated neurologic involvement is present, the defect is known as occult spinal dysraphism. Fibrous bands and adhesions, an intraspinal **lipoma** (fatty tumor) or subcutaneous lipoma (lipomyelomeningocele), a dermoid or epidermoid cyst, diastematomyelia (spinal cord split in two), or a tethered cord can distort the spinal cord or roots. The usual cause is abnormal adhesion, or tethering, to a bony or fixed structure, resulting in traction on the spinal cord and cauda equina. (See Figs. 34.7 and 34.8 for areas innervated by specific spinal nerves.)

Neuromuscular disturbances usually consist of progressive or static changes in gait with foot weakness, foot deformity, or bowel and bladder sphincter disturbances. Some manifestations may not be evident until the child walks or is toilet trained.

Plain radiography is employed to disclose the precise bony defect in the symptomatic lesion and to establish the diagnosis in the suspected, nonsymptomatic occult variety. Magnetic resonance imaging (MRI) is the most sensitive tool for evaluating the defect. Computed tomography (CT), ultrasonography, and myelography are also used to differentiate between SB occulta and other spinal disorders.

SB cystica refers to a visible defect with an external saclike protrusion. The two major forms of SB cystica are meningocele, which encases meninges and spinal fluid but no neural elements (Fig. 34.5, *C*), and myelomeningocele (or meningomyelocele), which contains meninges, spinal fluid, and nerves (Fig. 34.5, *D*). Neurologic deficit is not associated

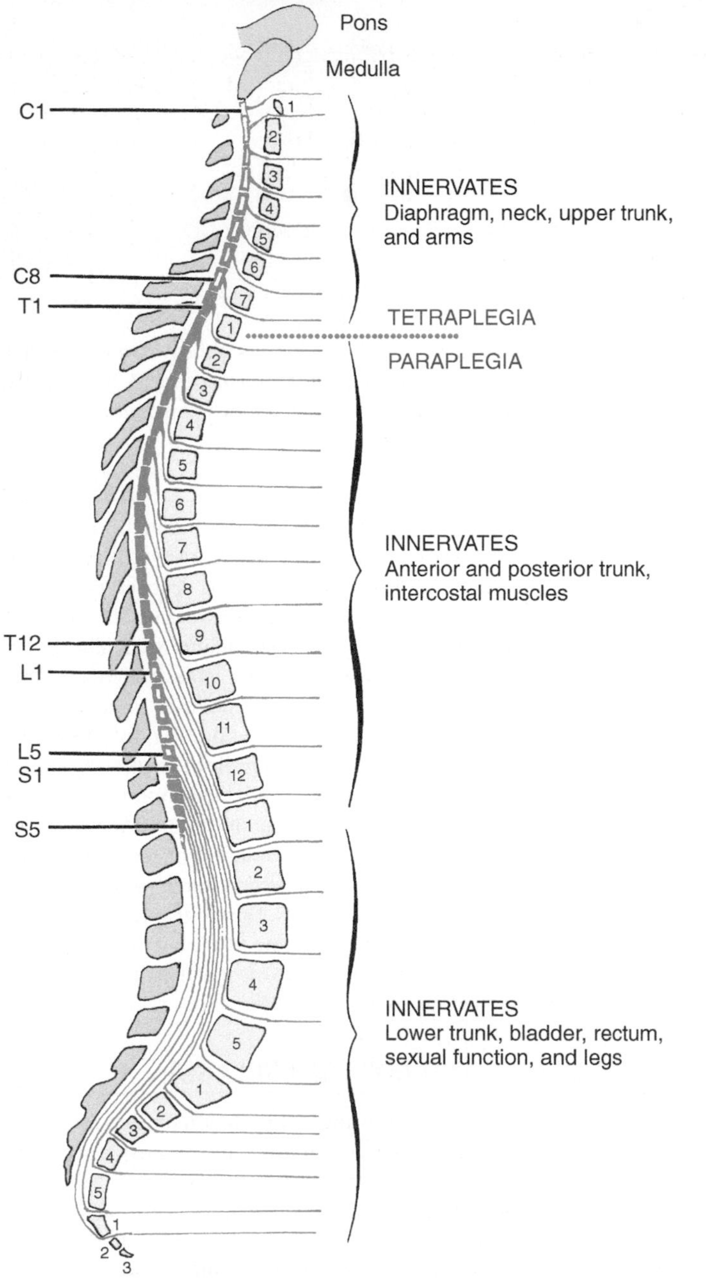

FIG. 34.7 Relationships of spinal cord segments and spinal nerves to vertebral bodies. Cervical nerves exit through intervertebral foramina above their respective vertebral bodies (seven cervical vertebrae and eight cervical nerves). Spinal cord ends at L1–L2 vertebral level.

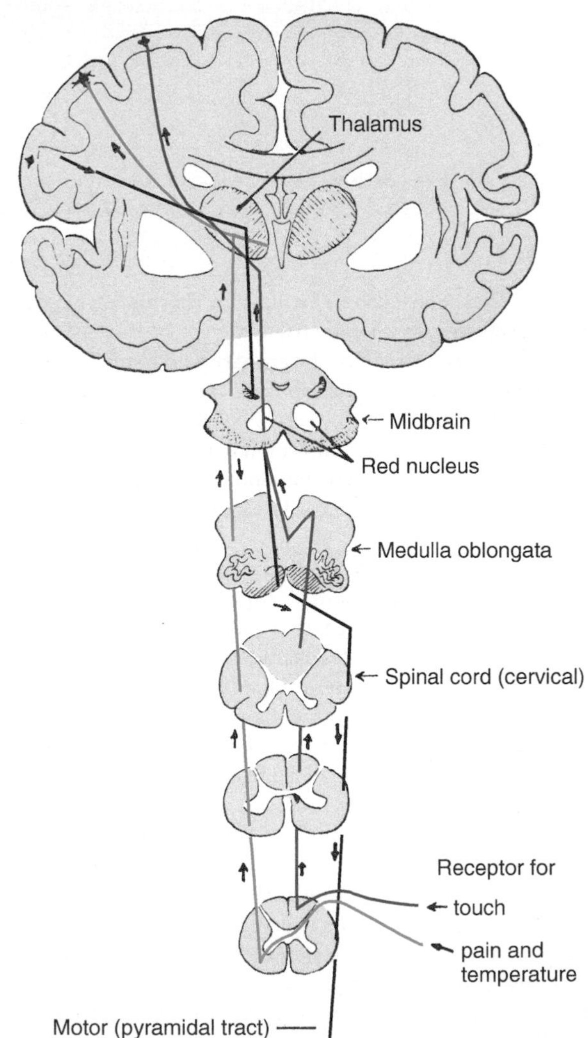

FIG. 34.8 Main motor and sensory pathways. Perception of touch, passive motion, position, and vibration is transmitted through posterior tract in spinal cord through medial lemniscus in brainstem to thalamus and through internal capsule to cortex (pathway is represented by *solid red line*). Pain and temperature sensations are transmitted through anterolateral tract and lateral lemniscus to thalamus, then through internal capsule to cortex *(blue line)*. Motor impulses are transmitted by pyramidal tract, descending from cerebral cortex, crossing in medulla to opposite side, and continuing to anterior horns of spinal cord *(black line)*. (From Conway, B. L. [1978]. *Carini and Owens' neurological and neurosurgical nursing* [7th ed.]. St. Louis, MO: Mosby.)

with meningocele but occurs in varying, often serious, degrees in myelomeningocele.

MYELOMENINGOCELE (MENINGOMYELOCELE)

Myelomeningocele (MMC) develops during the first 28 days of pregnancy when the neural tube fails to close and fuse at some point along its length. It may be detected prenatally or at birth, accounts for 90% of spinal cord lesions, and may be located at any point along the spinal column. Usually the sac is encased in a fine membrane that is prone to tears through which cerebrospinal fluid (CSF) leaks. In other instances the sac may be covered by dura, meninges, or skin, in which case there is rapid and spontaneous epithelialization. The largest number (75%) of myelomeningoceles occur in the lumbar or lumbosacral area (see Fig. 34.6). The location and magnitude of the defect determine the nature and extent of neurologic impairment. When the defect is below the second lumbar vertebra, the nerves of the cauda equina are involved, giving rise to symptoms such as flaccid, areflexic partial paralysis of the lower extremities and varying degrees of sensory deficit. Unlike a spinal cord injury, the degree of deficit is not necessarily uniform on both sides but may vary between extremities, depending on the compromise to specific nerves from malformation or tethering.

The anomaly most frequently associated with myelomeningocele is hydrocephalus; approximately 80% to 85% of children with SB develop hydrocephalus (Burke, Liptak, & Council on Children with Disabilities, 2011; Kinsman & Johnston, 2015). Although present at birth, hydrocephalus may not be apparent until shortly thereafter, or after the primary closure of the opening on the back. Careful monitoring of head circumference, fontanel tension, and ventricular size by head ultrasonography can indicate its presence. Hydrocephalus can occur because the NTD itself disrupts the flow of CSF (see p. 1159). In many cases Chiari malformation (type II) is responsible. Type II Chiari malformation (a downward herniation of the brain into the brainstem) is present, though asymptomatic, in many children with SB. It can, however, adversely affect respiratory function, causing episodic apnea. Other clinical symptoms of problematic Chiari malformation include stridor, hoarse cry from vocal cord paralysis, feeding difficulties, aspiration pneumonia, and, in older children, upper extremity spasticity. The appearance of such symptoms should not be taken for granted; immediate referral is required to prevent further neurologic deterioration.

Pathophysiology

The pathophysiology of SB is best understood when related to the normal formative stages of the nervous system. At approximately 20 days of gestation, a decided depression, the neural groove, appears in the dorsal ectoderm of the embryo. During the fourth week of gestation, the groove deepens rapidly, and its elevated margins develop laterally and fuse dorsally to form the neural tube. Neural tube formation begins in the cervical region near the center of the embryo and advances in both directions—caudally and cephalically—until by the end of the fourth week of gestation, the ends of the neural tube, the anterior and posterior neuropores, close.

Most experts believe the primary defect in neural tube malformations is a failure of neural tube closure. However, some evidence indicates that the defects are a result of splitting of the already closed neural tube as a result of an abnormal increase in CSF pressure during the first trimester.

There is evidence of a multifactorial etiology, including drugs, radiation, maternal malnutrition, chemicals, and possibly a genetic mutation in folate pathways in some cases, which may result in abnormal development. There is also evidence of a genetic component in the development of SB; myelomeningocele may occur in association with syndromes such as trisomy 18, PHAVER (limb **p**terygia, congenital **h**eart **a**nomalies, **v**ertebral defects, **e**ar anomalies, and **r**adial defects) syndrome, and Meckel-Gruber syndrome (Shaer, Chescheir, & Schulkin, 2007). The genetic predisposition is supported by evidence of the risk for recurrence after one affected child (3% to 4%) and a 10% risk for recurrence with two previously affected children (Kinsman & Johnston, 2015).

The degree of neurologic dysfunction depends on where the sac protrudes through the vertebrae, the anatomic level of the defect, and the amount of nerve tissue involved. One classification designates the level of functional mobility in relationship to the anatomic level of the defect. For example, children with a high lumbar-thoracic defect may be able to walk short distances using long-leg braces and by early adolescence must use a wheelchair for mobility; children with a low lumbar defect can walk with short leg braces and forearm crutches (Liptak & Dosa, 2010). This classification system, however, does not describe genitourinary and bowel function. About 80% of patients with myelomeningocele develop a type II Chiari malformation (Kinsman & Johnston, 2015). There is some evidence that prolonged exposure of the MMC sac to amniotic fluid predisposes to the development of hindbrain herniation and Chiari II malformation (Adzick, 2013).

Clinical Manifestations

The manifestations of SB vary widely according to the degree of the spinal defect. The defect is readily apparent on inspection. The degree of neurologic dysfunction is directly related to the anatomic level of the defect and thus the nerves involved. Sensory disturbances usually parallel motor dysfunction. The upper level of sensory and motor impairment can be determined by observation of the infant's response to a pinprick over the legs and trunk. The infant responds to the sensory stimulus with limb movement, arousal, and crying. When withdrawal activity is used to determine the lowest level of spinal cord function, the response to pinprick should begin above the lesion.

Defective nerve supply to the bladder affects both sphincter and detrusor tone, which often causes constant dribbling of urine or produces overflow incontinence. This can often be mistaken for normal voiding patterns in the newborn. Some infants with SB, however, are able to void in a stream and achieve complete bladder emptying with each void.

Frequently the infant has poor anal sphincter tone and poor anal skin reflex, which result in lack of bowel control and sometimes rectal prolapse. Avoid taking rectal temperatures in affected infants. Because bowel sphincter function is frequently affected, the thermometer can cause irritation and rectal prolapse. If the defect is below the third sacral vertebra, the infant has no motor impairment but may have saddle anesthesia with bladder and anal sphincter paralysis.

Sometimes the denervation to the muscles of the lower extremities produces joint deformities in utero. These are primarily flexion or extension contractures, talipes valgus or varus contractures, kyphosis, lumbosacral scoliosis, and hip dislocations. The extent and severity of these associated orthopedic deformities again depend on the degree of nerve involvement. Most flexion deformities result from the pull of stronger, fully innervated muscles acting without the counterpull of their nonfunctioning paralyzed antagonists. Box 34.6 provides a summary of clinical manifestations of SB cystica and occulta.

Diagnostic Evaluation

The diagnosis of SB is made on the basis of clinical manifestations (see Box 34.6) and examination of the meningeal sac (see Fig. 34.6, *A*). Diagnostic measures used to evaluate the brain and spinal cord include MRI, ultrasonography, and CT. A neurologic evaluation will determine the extent of involvement of bowel and bladder function, as

BOX 34.6 Clinical Manifestations of Spina Bifida

Spina Bifida Cystica
- Sensory disturbances usually parallel to motor dysfunction
- Below second lumbar vertebra:
  - Flaccid, partial paralysis of lower extremities
  - Varying degrees of sensory deficit
  - Overflow incontinence with constant dribbling of urine
  - Lack of bowel control
  - Rectal prolapse (sometimes)
- Below third sacral vertebra:
  - No motor impairment
  - Bladder and anal sphincter paralysis
- Joint deformities (sometimes produced in utero):
  - Talipes valgus or varus (foot) contractures
  - Kyphosis
  - Lumbosacral scoliosis
  - Hip dislocation

Spina Bifida Occulta
- Frequently no observable manifestations
- May be associated with one or more cutaneous manifestations:
  - Skin depression or dimple
  - Port-wine angiomatous nevi
  - Dark tufts of hair
  - Soft, subcutaneous lipomas
- May be neuromuscular disturbances:
  - Progressive disturbance of gait with foot weakness
  - Bowel and bladder sphincter disturbances

well as lower extremity neuromuscular involvement. Flaccid paralysis of the lower extremities is a common finding with absent deep tendon reflexes.

Prenatal Detection

It is possible to determine the presence of some major open NTDs prenatally. Ultrasonographic scanning of the uterus and elevated maternal concentrations of α-fetoprotein (AFP, or MS-AFP), a fetal-specific γ-1-globulin, in amniotic fluid may indicate anencephaly or myelomeningocele. The optimum time for performing these diagnostic tests is between 16 and 18 weeks of gestation before AFP concentrations normally diminish and in sufficient time to permit a therapeutic abortion. It is recommended that such diagnostic procedures and genetic counseling be considered for all mothers who have borne an affected child, and testing is offered to all pregnant women (American College of Obstetrics and Gynecology, 2007). Chorionic villus sampling is also a method for prenatal diagnosis of NTDs; however, it carries certain risks (skeletal limb depletion) and is not recommended before 10 weeks of gestation (Simpson, Richards, & Otaño, 2012).

Therapeutic Management

Management of the child who has a myelomeningocele requires a multidisciplinary team approach involving the specialties of neurology, neurosurgery, pediatrics, urology, orthopedics, rehabilitation, physical therapy, occupational therapy, and social services, as well as intensive nursing care in a variety of specialty areas. The collaborative efforts of these specialists focus on the following:

- The myelomeningocele and the problems associated with the defect—hydrocephalus, paralysis, orthopedic deformities (e.g., developmental dysplasia of the hip, clubfoot), and genitourinary abnormalities
- Possible acquired problems that may or may not be associated, such as Chiari II malformation, meningitis, seizures, hypoxia, tethered cord, and hemorrhage
- Other abnormalities, such as cardiac or GI malformations

Many hospitals have specialty clinics staffed by multidisciplinary teams to provide the complex follow-up care needed for children and families with myelodysplasia.

In 2008 the Centers for Disease Control and Prevention started a National Spina Bifida Patient Registry, based on results from a survey from spina bifida clinics across the United States. The Registry was initiated to provide a more organized approach to the care of all individuals with spina bifida. It seeks to improve and align the quality of care received at spina bifida clinics nationwide. The registry works to develop standards and best practices for patients with spina bifida. The data collected from the Registry clinics is sent to the Centers for Disease Control and Prevention to be analyzed so that it can be disseminated to other physicians and clinics. The Registry also hopes to gain insight into some of the secondary conditions of spina bifida, such as paralysis, neurogenic bladder and bowel, and hydrocephalus (Sawin, Liu, Ward, et al., 2015).

Many authorities believe that early closure, within the first 24 to 72 hours, offers the most favorable outcome. Surgical closure within the first 24 hours is recommended if the sac is leaking CSF (Kinsman & Johnston, 2015). Surgical closure within 24 hours also results in improved bladder capacities and lower detrusor leak point pressures. Increased incidence of febrile UTIs, vesicoureteral reflux, and hydronephrosis have been shown when closure is delayed past 72 hours (Tarcan, Onol, Ilker, et al., 2006).

A variety of neurosurgical and plastic surgical procedures are used for skin closure without disturbing the neural elements or removing any portion of the sac. The objective is satisfactory skin coverage of the lesion and meticulous closure. Wide excision of the large membranous covering may damage functioning neural tissue.

Prenatal surgical closure of the myelomeningocele sac through fetal surgery has been evaluated in relation to prevention of injury to the exposed spinal cord tissue and the improvement of neurologic and urologic outcomes in the affected child. The Management of Myelomeningocele Study (MOMS), a clinical trial supported by the National Institutes of Health, found that prenatal surgery for myelomeningocele reduced the need for shunting (for hydrocephalus), evaluated at 12 months, and decreased the incidence of hindbrain herniation. In addition there was an improvement in mental and motor function scores at 30 months in the children who had prenatal surgery (compared with children who had postnatal surgery) (Adzick, Thom, Spong, et al., 2011). However, the surgery is not without risks to the fetus and mother, and premature delivery is common. Outcome data for urologic and bowel function, motor function, cognition, and spina bifida–associated outcomes are being gathered in the MOMS2 study, which ended in 2013 (Clinical Trials, 2013).

Initial Care

Care of the newborn involves preventing infection; performing a neurologic assessment, including observation for associated anomalies; and dealing with the impact of the anomaly on the family. Although meningoceles are repaired early, especially if the sac is in danger of rupturing, the philosophy regarding skin closure of myelomeningocele varies. Most authorities believe that early closure, within the first 24 to 72 hours, offers the most favorable outcome. Surgical closure within the first 24 hours is recommended if the sac is leaking CSF (Kinsman & Johnston, 2015). Early closure, preferably in the first 12 to 18 hours, not only prevents local infection and trauma to the exposed tissues but also avoids stretching other nerve roots (which may occur as the meningeal sac expands during the first hours after birth), thus preventing further motor impairment. Broad-spectrum antibiotics are initiated, and neurotoxic substances such as povidone-iodine are avoided at the malformation.

Associated problems are assessed and managed by appropriate surgical and supportive measures. Shunt procedures provide relief from imminent or progressive hydrocephalus (see Chapter 30). When diagnosed, ventriculitis, meningitis, and urinary tract infection are treated with vigorous antibiotic therapy and supportive measures. Surgical intervention for Chiari II malformation is indicated only when the child is symptomatic (i.e., high-pitched crowing cry, stridor, respiratory difficulties, apnea, failure to thrive, gastroesophageal reflux, oral-motor difficulties, upper extremity spasticity).

Improved surgical techniques do not alter the major physical disability and deformity or chronic urinary tract infections that affect the quality of life for these children. Superimposed on these physical problems are the disorder's effects on family life and finances and on school and hospital services.

Musculoskeletal Considerations

According to most orthopedists, musculoskeletal problems that will affect later locomotion should be evaluated early and treatment, where indicated, instituted without delay. Neurologic assessment determines the neurosegmental level of the lesion, spasticity and progressive paralysis, potential for deformity, and functional expectations. Orthopedic and musculoskeletal management includes preventing joint contractures, correcting the existing deformity, preventing or minimizing effects of motor and sensory deficits, preventing skin breakdown, and obtaining the best possible function of affected lower extremities. Common musculoskeletal problems requiring attention in SB include deformities of the knees, hips, feet, and spine; fractures and insensate skin further complicate orthopedic care. Other problems that may occur later include kyphosis and scoliosis (Lazzaretti & Pearson, 2010; Liptak & Dosa, 2010). About 50% of infants born with myelomeningocele will have clubfoot (Sandler, 2010). Because children with MMC often have decreased sensitivity in lower extremities, preventive skin care is important. A high percentage (60%) of children seen in a wound clinic for skin breakdown had myelomeningocele at birth (Samaniego, 2003). The most common wound sites were the foot and ankle, with the buttocks being the second most common site. Pressure wounds are more common in patients who use wheelchairs for mobility (Ottolini, Harris, et al., 2013).

The status of the neurologic deficit remains the most important factor in determining the child's ultimate functional abilities; however, many children with lumbar and sacral myelomeningocele are able to achieve functional ambulation (Kinsman & Johnston, 2015). With technologic advances, a variety of lightweight orthoses, including braces, special "walking" devices, and custom-built wheelchairs, are available to provide mobility to children with spinal cord lesions (see also Chapter 30). Early in infancy, intervention with passive range-of-motion exercises, positioning, and stretching exercises may help decrease the incidence of muscle contractures. Corrective surgical procedures, when indicated, are best initiated at an early age so that the child will not lag significantly behind age-mates in developmental progress. The degree of lower extremity function guides decisions about whether orthopedic surgery will be needed.

Physical therapy and musculoskeletal management of children with myelomeningocele are continual processes to achieve optimum function and ambulation when possible. Problems such as type II Chiari malformation, hydrocephalus, and a tethered spinal cord can complicate expectations. A common complication is tethered cord syndrome in which there is a presumed traction injury to the distal spinal cord with subtle and progressive loss of neural function; this may occur any time but is more common during periods of rapid growth and can be precipitated by ventricular shunt failure (Burke, Liptak, & Council on Children with Disabilities, 2011).

Management of Genitourinary Function

Myelomeningocele is one of the most common causes of neuropathic (neurogenic) bladder dysfunction among children. Neurologic deficits can affect the innervation of the bladder, impairing the ability to store and empty urine. As many as 90% of children with SB will experience some form of voiding dysfunction. A child with a neuropathic bladder will require care across the life span. The goals of urologic treatment should be individualized to the child's developmental stage. In infants the goal of treatment is to preserve renal function. In older children the goal is to preserve renal function and achieve optimum urinary continence. Urinary incontinence is a chronic, often debilitating problem for the child. In addition, the neuropathic bladder may produce **urinary system distress**, characterized by symptomatic urinary tract infections, ureterohydronephrosis, vesicoureteral reflux, or renal insufficiency. The characteristics of bladder dysfunction in children vary according to the level of the neurologic lesion and the influence of bony growth and development of the spine. In addition, the presence of type II Chiari malformation and subsequent hydrocephalus has the potential to affect bladder function, although spinal influences predominate.

During infancy, urinary incontinence is normally physiologic, but urinary system distress may occur. Ongoing urologic monitoring is essential. Evidence is growing that early intervention, based on evaluation during the neonatal period and before complications occur, improves bladder function, reduces the subsequent risk of urinary system distress, and reduces the need for reconstructive surgery of the lower urinary tract. Ultrasonography of the bladder and ureters and routine urinalysis (and urine cultures when indicated) are used to detect urinary system distress before renal function is compromised. In addition, urodynamic testing is used to identify bladder dysfunction that predisposes the child to urinary system distress (Gray & Moore, 2009; Snodgrass & Gargollo, 2010). These conditions include high-pressure detrusor hyperreflexia (reflex contractions of the detrusor muscle) with vesicosphincter dyssynergia (incoordination of detrusor and sphincter muscles), low bladder wall compliance (poor distensibility of the bladder wall causing increased intravesical pressures during urine filling and storage), or detrusor areflexia (absence of detrusor contractions caused by the spinal defect).

Infants may have one of several predominant neuropathic bladder disorders. Detrusor contractions associated with vesicosphincter dyssynergia are particularly common. Some infants are able to empty the bladder efficiently despite incoordination between the sphincter mechanism and detrusor, but the majority experience chronic residual urine, urinary tract infections, or more serious types of urinary system distress. A minority of infants have poor detrusor contraction strength or detrusor areflexia. This condition is particularly damaging to the urinary system when it coexists with low bladder wall compliance and an elevated detrusor leak point pressure. Low bladder wall compliance occurs when collagen or fibrosis causes stiffening of the bladder wall. This stiffened bladder wall raises intravesical pressures, obstructing the bladder, ureters, and, ultimately, the nephron. The impact of low bladder wall compliance is directly related to the influence of the bladder outlet. Among children with myelodysplasia, the urethral muscles are typically weakened, and collagen replaces much of the muscle tissue. As a result, the sphincter is fixed, so it neither closes efficiently to prevent urinary leakage nor opens well to allow urinary flow with a detrusor contraction. When the magnitude of the pressure required to drive urine across the abnormal sphincter is greater than 40 cm H_2O (the detrusor leak point pressure) and the compliance of the bladder wall is low (<10 cm H_2O), the risk of urinary system distress is high.

In contrast, a small number of infants experience effective detrusor contractions without vesicosphincter dyssynergia. Effective bladder evacuation is likely among this group, and the incidence of urinary system distress during the first year of life is low.

As the child grows, detrusor hyperreflexia is often replaced by deficient detrusor contraction strength and stress urinary incontinence (SUI) (leakage produced by physical exertion). The bladder wall is often poorly compliant (producing chronically elevated intravesical pressures), and the bladder outlet, while incompetent, obstructs the outflow of urine. When the detrusor leak point pressure exceeds 40 cm H_2O, the child is predisposed to chronic urinary leakage and urinary distress symptoms, including recurrent urinary tract infections and reflux. When the detrusor leak point pressure is lower than 40 cm H_2O, urinary leakage is more severe, although the risk of urinary system distress is lessened. Thus the child with more severe urinary incontinence is less predisposed than the "drier" child to serious urinary tract infections.

Infants with myelomeningocele and a neurogenic bladder who are not at risk for urinary system distress are managed by diaper containment and watchful waiting. The infant empties the bladder into a diaper, the urine is routinely monitored for infection, and the upper urinary tracts are monitored for evidence of urinary system distress (dilation of the ureters, renal pelves, or collecting systems) via serial ultrasonography.

In contrast, children with evidence of urinary system distress, or those considered at risk based on early urodynamic testing, undergo clean intermittent catheterization (CIC), typically in combination with an antispasmodic medication such as oxybutynin or propantheline (De Jong, Chrzan, Klijn, et al., 2008; Gray & Moore, 2009). Anticholinergic medications are prescribed because they reduce detrusor muscle tone and reduce bladder pressures during both urine filling and storage and during micturition. CIC is not intended to prevent spontaneous voiding. Instead, it ensures routine, regular bladder evacuation, further preventing deleterious elevation of intravesical pressures. Usually, the parents learn to catheterize the infant every 4 hours during the day and once each night. Follow-up evaluation, consisting of serial ultrasonography and urinalysis, is completed every 3 to 6 months as indicated.

Infants with significant urinary system distress and neuropathic bladder dysfunction at birth sometimes require temporary urinary diversion to ensure adequate urine outflow and prevent further damage to the upper urinary tracts. A vesicostomy is a relatively simple procedure wherein the anterior bladder wall is brought to the abdominal wall, creating a small stoma for urinary drainage. Urine is contained via a diaper, but double diapering or use of a larger diaper that can be placed higher on the abdomen is necessary for adequate urine containment. Meticulous skin care is necessary because the perineal skin is exposed to continuous urinary leakage.

Among older children the quest for continence typically begins with a CIC program. The parents learn the procedure and teach the child to self-catheterize as soon as possible, usually by 6 years of age (Gray & Moore, 2009). The child with detrusor hyperreflexia and dyssynergia often responds well to antispasmodic medications and CIC. In contrast, the child with poor bladder wall compliance and SUI often requires a combination of antispasmodic medications to reduce intravesical filling pressures and a sympathetic agonist (such as imipramine, pseudoephedrine, or phenylpropanolamine) to enhance sphincter competence. Unfortunately, the combination of medications and CIC is typically only partially effective, and more aggressive interventions are often required to render the neuropathic bladder both continent and free from its predisposition toward producing urinary system distress. It is important that a careful history is taken by the provider to identify other problems that may be contributing to persistent incontinence. Factors that can affect bladder continence include caffeinated drinks, constipation, or lack of access to bathrooms (Metcalfe, 2017).

When the child cannot attain continence by conservative measures, surgery is considered. Augmentation enterocystoplasty (or gastrocystoplasty) is a surgical procedure that increases bladder capacity, reverses or halts the negative effects of the poorly compliant bladder wall, and reduces harmfully high bladder pressures caused by detrusor hyperreflexia with vesicosphincter dyssynergia. A detubularized segment of large or small bowel or a wedge of the fundus of the stomach has been used to successfully augment bladder capacity. The choice of segment varies according to the surgeon's preference and the status of the patient's urinary and GI systems. Large and small bowel segments produce significant volumes of mucus that may clog catheters used for CIC. Augmentation with the stomach produces less mucus, and its acidic secretions may reduce the urinary system's predisposition to infection. The bladder must be irrigated to decrease mucus within the bladder; this also decreases the possible complications of infection, stones, and bladder perforation.

Even though augmentation of the bladder may improve or resolve urinary leakage related to detrusor hyperreflexia or urinary system distress caused by low bladder wall compliance, the SUI produced by the abnormal sphincter mechanism typically persists. Several surgical procedures help correct this intrinsic sphincter deficiency. The Mitrofanoff procedure uses the appendix to provide an alternative route for intermittent catheterization. The appendix is removed from the colon and used to create a continent conduit between the abdominal wall and the bladder. The resulting stoma is relatively small and produces minimum mucus. The ureter may be used as an alternative to the appendix for some children. If the appendix is insufficient, a segment of tapered intestine, ileum, or colon may be used to create a conduit (Monti tube) (Gray & Moore, 2009). CIC through the easily accessible abdominal route fosters greater independence in children, especially in those unable to transfer from wheelchair to toilet to perform CIC.

When intrinsic sphincter deficiency produces only mild stress urinary leakage, the construction of a Mitrofanoff route alone may be sufficient to achieve continence between catheterization episodes. However, when SUI is more severe, a suburethral sling or suburethral collagen injection is used to alleviate intrinsic sphincter deficiency.

The suburethral sling is a slip of fascia or synthetic material that is placed below the proximal third of the urethra. The sling may be placed in a fashion that uses only slight tension to obstruct the urethra and prevent SUI. The sling may be used for both boys and girls, and the procedure can be completed at the same time the augmentation enterocystoplasty is constructed. After augmentation enterocystoplasty and placement of a suburethral sling, the patient can expect to evacuate the bladder by CIC of the appendiceal Mitrofanoff route (appendicovesicostomy) or the urethra if a Mitrofanoff route has not been constructed.

Suburethral injection of glutaraldehyde cross-linked (GAX) collagen also may be used to alleviate or prevent SUI caused by intrinsic sphincter deficiency. Collagen is used to bulk or expand the urethral tissue, promoting coaptation (approximation) of the mucosa. The collagen implant complements the urethra's ability to form a watertight seal, rather than obstructing the urethral lumen. Collagen may be injected using different approaches. Transurethral collagen is injected through the working channel of a cystoscope. Transperineal collagen is directed underneath the urethra using a needle inserted through the perineal skin. In this case the location of the urethra is confirmed by simultaneous cystoscopic visualization of the urethra. The antegrade approach requires creation of a suprapubic cystostomy tract. A flexible cystoscope is then inserted through the cystostomy tract, and collagen is injected into the proximal urethra. Multiple injections may be required to achieve optimum continence. Subsequent injections may be required when the collagen is dissipated or resorbed by the body over a period of years. Botulinum toxin (Botox) can also be injected into the detrusor muscle to increase bladder capacity and decrease intravesicular pressures, but this measure is only temporary (Frimberger, Cheng, & Kropp, 2012).

The artificial urinary sphincter provides another alternative for the management of intrinsic sphincter deficiency in the child with myelomeningocele. The device consists of a urethral cuff, abdominal reservoir, and control pump. In the activated position, the cuff is filled, and the pressure of this cuff closes the urethral lumen. During micturition, the control pump is used to baffle fluid from the urethral cuff to the abdominal reservoir, opening the urethra for micturition or catheterization. However, because of the significant risk for infection, need for revision with growth, and mechanical failure, the popularity of the artificial urinary sphincter has declined.

Because of advances in neurogenic bladder management, adolescents and young adults with myelomeningocele and neurogenic bladder have been followed for up to 30 years without evidence of deterioration in renal function. Nevertheless, urinary and fecal incontinence are common, and these conditions lead to significant, and sometimes devastating, problems with growth and developmental tasks, including establishing independence and social and intimate relationships. This observation underscores the need to aggressively manage both continence and the threat of urinary system distress from an early age and to establish an expectation of social continence critical to providing these patients with the skills they need to thrive as adolescents and adults. Newborns with SB and normal urodynamics require close follow-up care during the first several years of life to prevent deterioration in urodynamic status as a result of neurologic deterioration.

Bowel Control

Some degree of fecal continence can be achieved in most children with myelomeningocele with diet modification, regular toilet habits, and prevention of constipation and impaction. It is frequently a lengthy process. Dietary fiber supplements (recommended age of child in years + 5 g/day), laxatives, suppositories, or enemas aid in producing regular evacuation. Older children and adolescents seeking more independence may attain bowel continence and higher quality of life after undergoing an antegrade continence enema (ACE) procedure (Doolin, 2006). In a procedure similar to the Mitrofanoff, the appendix or ileum is used to create a catheterizable channel with attachment of the proximal end to the colon. The distal end of the channel exits through a small abdominal stoma. Every 1 or 2 days, a catheter is passed through the stoma, allowing enema solution to be instilled directly into the colon. After administration of the enema solution, the child sits on the toilet for 30 to 60 minutes as stool is flushed out through the rectum. The frequency of enemas and volume of solution used to completely evacuate the bowel vary among individuals.

Prognosis

The early prognosis for the child with myelomeningocele depends on the neurologic deficit present at birth, including motor ability, bladder innervation, and associated neurologic anomalies. Early surgical repair of the spinal defect, antibiotic therapy to reduce the incidence of meningitis and ventriculitis, prevention of urinary system dysfunction, and early detection and correction of hydrocephalus have significantly increased the survival rate and quality of life in such children. Mortality rates are reported to be 10% to 15%, with many deaths occurring before the age of 4 years (Kinsman & Johnston, 2015). Many young adults with SB achieve partial independent living and gainful employment. Reports of survival rates vary, and many include adults who were born before medical advances and surgical techniques seen in the past 25 years. Coordinated care for adults with SB is essential; however, multidisciplinary adult care is often inadequate (Lazzaretti & Pearson, 2010). One of the factors associated with early death among adults with MMC is hydrocephalus and shunt failure (Mourtzinos & Stoffel, 2010). This chronic condition has an array of associated complications, including hydrocephalus and shunt malfunctions, tethered cord syndrome, scoliosis, Chiari II development, bowel and bladder management issues, latex allergy, and epilepsy. However, based on current medical knowledge and ethical considerations, aggressive, early management is favored for the child with myelomeningocele.

Prevention

The Centers for Disease Control and Prevention (2009) continues to affirm that 50% to 70% of NTDs can be prevented by daily consumption of 0.4 mg of folic acid by women of childbearing age. The data indicate that serum folate concentrations among women of childbearing age decreased 16% from 2003 to 2004 in all ethnic groups studied. Lowest serum folate levels were seen in non-Hispanic Caucasians in 2003 to 2004; however, overall serum folate levels remained below recommended levels in non-Hispanic African Americans during all three periods studied (Centers for Disease Control and Prevention, 2007). These results indicate that nurses and other health care workers have an important task in disseminating information that may decrease the incidence of birth defects in children by promoting maternal consumption of folic acid.

To ensure adequate daily intake of the recommended amount of folic acid, women must take a folic acid supplement, eat a fortified breakfast cereal containing 100% of the recommended dietary allowance of folic acid (e.g., Kellogg's Product 19, General Mills Total, Multigrain Cheerios Plus), or increase their consumption of fortified foods (e.g., cereal, bread, rice, grits, pasta) and foods naturally rich in folate (e.g., green leafy vegetables and citrus fruits). For women who have had a previous pregnancy affected by NTDs, folic acid intake is increased to 4 mg/day under the supervision of a health care practitioner beginning 1 month before a planned pregnancy and continuing through the first trimester. Supplementation of 4 mg of folate should not be given solely in multivitamin preparations because of the risk for overdose of other vitamins. Drugs that affect folic acid metabolism and increase the risk for myelomeningocele should be avoided before pregnancy (if plans are to become pregnant in the near future) and during pregnancy; these include trimethoprim and the AEDs carbamazepine, phenytoin, phenobarbital, valproic acid, and primidone (Kinsman & Johnston, 2015).

Nursing Care Management

The basic needs of the infant with a myelomeningocele are essentially the same as for any newborn infant. (See Chapter 8) Special needs related to the defect and potential complications are discussed in the following section. As the child matures, the problems increase and involve all aspects of daily living; therefore care is directly related to the child's habilitation at each stage of development.

Assessment

At the time of delivery an examination is performed to assess the intactness of the membranous cyst. During transport to the nursery, make every effort to prevent trauma to this protective covering. In addition to the routine assessment of the newborn (see Chapter 7), assess the infant for the level of neurologic involvement. Note movement of extremities or skin response, especially an anal reflex that might provide clues to the degree of motor or sensory impairment.

Care of the Myelomeningocele Sac

The infant is usually placed in an incubator or radiant warmer so that temperature can be maintained without clothing or covers that might irritate the CNS lesion. When an overhead warmer is used, the dressings over the defect require more frequent moistening because of the dehydrating effect of the radiant heat. Before surgical closure, the myelomeningocele is kept from drying by the application of a sterile, moist, nonadherent dressing. The moistening solution is usually sterile normal saline. Dressings are changed frequently (every 2 to 4 hours), and the sac is closely inspected for leaks, abrasions, irritation, and signs of infection. The sac must be carefully cleansed if it becomes soiled or contaminated. Sometimes the sac ruptures during delivery or transport, and any opening in the sac greatly increases the risk of infection to the CNS (Fig. 34.6, *B*). When an overhead warmer is used, the dressings over the defect require more frequent moistening because of the drying effect of the radiant heat.

Positioning

One of the most important and challenging aspects of early care of the infant with myelomeningocele is positioning. Before surgery the infant remains in the prone position to minimize tension on the sac and the risk of trauma. The prone position allows for optimum positioning of the legs, especially in cases of associated hip dysplasia. A variety of aids, including diaper rolls, foam pads, or specially designed frames and appliances, are available to maintain the desired position.

The prone position affects other aspects of the infant's care. For example, in this position the infant is more difficult to keep clean, pressure areas are a constant threat, and feeding becomes a problem. The infant's head is turned to one side for feeding. Fortunately, most defects are repaired early, and the infant can be held for feeding and routine care soon after surgery. Physical therapy consultation may be necessary for difficult positioning problems. Speech-language pathologist consultation may be needed for difficulty with oral-motor skills that may indicate complications caused by a Chiari malformation.

General Care

Diapering the infant may be contraindicated until the defect has been repaired and healing is well advanced or epithelialization has taken place. The padding beneath the diaper area is changed as needed to keep the skin dry and free of irritation. When the nurse detects urinary retention (the bladder is still an abdominal organ in early infancy), CIC is employed. Because the bowel sphincter is frequently affected, there may be continual passage of stool, often misinterpreted as diarrhea, which is a constant irritant to the skin and a source of infection to the spinal lesion.

Areas of sensory and motor impairment are subject to skin breakdown and therefore require meticulous care. The infant may be placed on a pressure-reducing mattress or a mattress to prevent pressure on the knees and ankles. (See Skin Care, Chapter 7 and Maintaining Healthy Skin, Chapter 22)

Gentle range-of-motion exercises are carried out to prevent contractures, and stretching of contractures is performed when indicated. However, these exercises may be restricted to the foot, ankle, and knee joint. When the hip joints are unstable, stretching against tight hip flexors or adductor muscles, which act much like bowstrings, may aggravate a tendency toward subluxation. A physical therapy consultation is often necessary to develop a multidisciplinary plan to prevent long-term complications.

Some infants with unrepaired myelomeningocele are unable to be held in the arms and cuddled as unaffected infants are, so their need for tactile stimulation is met by caressing, stroking, and other comfort measures. To facilitate handling and reduce parental anxiety, the infant can recline on a pillow placed in the parent's lap.

Ophthalmic complications may occur in children with SB and hydrocephalus. The appearance of a squint, other ocular motility, or papilledema usually denotes hydrocephalus and is reported. Ophthalmologic follow-up care, particularly in children with shunts, is generally included in the multidisciplinary care plan.

Postoperative Care

Postoperative care for the infant with myelomeningocele involves the same basic care as for any postsurgical infant: monitoring vital signs, weight, and intake and output; maintaining body temperature; assessing and relieving pain; providing nourishment; and observing for signs of infection. The wound is managed according to the surgeon's directions, and general care is continued as preoperatively.

The prone position is maintained after operative closure, although many neurosurgeons allow a side-lying or partial side-lying position unless it aggravates a coexisting hip dysplasia or permits undesirable hip flexion. This offers an opportunity for position changes, which reduces the risk of pressure sores and facilitates feeding. Once the effects of anesthesia have subsided and the infant is alert, feedings may resume unless there are other anomalies or associated complications.

Nursing assessments are carried out for implementation of comfort measures in the postoperative period. The infant can be held upright against the body, taking care to avoid pressure on the operative site. In the case of an unusually large defect, skin grafting may be required for wound closure; the infant must then be kept prone postoperatively with as little movement as possible to prevent tension on the skin graft.

The nurse can assist in determining the extent of neuromuscular involvement. Note movement of the extremities or skin response, especially an anal reflex, that might provide clues to the degree of motor or sensory status. Measure head circumference daily (see Chapter 5), and examine the fontanels for signs of tension or bulging. The nurse is also alert to early signs of infection, such as elevated or decreased temperature (axillary), irritability, and lethargy, and to signs of increased intracranial pressure. Urinary catheterization may be needed for urine retention. Although it may not have been a problem preoperatively, swelling around the operative site may cause transient urine retention, which resolves in 2 to 5 days.

Family Support and Home Care

As soon as the parents are able to cope with the infant's condition, encourage them to become involved in care. They need to learn how to continue at home the care that has been initiated in the hospital: positioning, feeding, skin care, and range-of-motion exercises when appropriate. Parents also need to learn CIC technique when prescribed. The family needs to know the signs of complications and how to reach assistance when needed.

As the child grows and develops, parents need guidance to encourage and stimulate the infant to accomplish age-appropriate developmental tasks within the limits imposed by the disabilities. Upper limb movement can be stimulated early by placing the infant on the floor in a prone position with toys within reach. Activities that encourage body consciousness, such as rolling over and pulling to a sitting position, are encouraged at the appropriate times. Creeping and crawling help the child explore the environment. The parents may need help to modify appliances and activities normally expected of a growing child. A standing table, frame, or parapodium is helpful for a variety of activities, and it is best for the child to begin supported weight bearing and standing as close as possible to the expected time for standing to occur.

It is important for the family to understand the nature of sensory deficit in a child with a spinal defect. The child will be insensitive to pressure or other sources of tissue injury. Therefore the family must be alert to hot or cold items that could cause thermal injury to tissues and remember to inspect the skin regularly for signs of pressure, especially over bony prominences. Because of sensory impairment, the child is unaware of bladder discomfort. Therefore signs of urinary tract infections may go unnoticed. Urinary tract infection is often considered when the child becomes ill.

The long-range planning with and support of the parents and newborn begin in the hospital and extend throughout childhood and even into young adulthood. The life expectancy of children with SB extends well into adulthood; therefore planning should involve long-term goals and plans for optimum function as an adult. Long-range planning goals should include a discussion of achievement of functional mobility, urinary continence, and as much bowel continence as physically possible. Discussion about aspects of adulthood such as having a mate, sexual relationships, and bearing and rearing children is important and should not be overlooked (Rowe & Jadhav, 2008). The unique service needs of adolescents with SB as they attempt to gain independence from family and establish a life of their own have not been adequately addressed in the literature (Sawyer & Macnee, 2010). Betz, Linroth, Butler, and colleagues (2010) interviewed young people with SB making the transition to adulthood. Some common themes that emerged among these young people were challenges in preparation for self-management, limited social relationships, awareness of their cognitive challenges, and the cost of independence. Advances in neurology, orthopedics, and urology have enabled adolescents to progress into adulthood with fewer deficits than observed in previous decades; one key factor is the recognition of subtle signs of neurologic deterioration and rapid intervention (Rowe & Jadhav, 2008).

Nurses assume an important role as a central member of the health team. As a coordinator, the nurse reviews information with the family, takes responsibility for family teaching, and acts as a liaison between inpatient and outpatient services. The child may require numerous hospitalizations over the years, and each one will be a source of stress to which the younger child is especially vulnerable.

Changes in functional ability, particularly in the lower extremities, bowel, or bladder, may indicate the presence of a tethered cord, one that is bound low or restricted in an abnormal position by scar tissue. These symptoms usually occur after a growth spurt and can best be detected with MRI. Tethering can be repaired surgically but, unfortunately, may recur.

Habilitation involves solving not only problems of self-help and locomotion but also the most distressing problem of incontinence, which threatens the child's social acceptability. Assistance in preparing the child and the school regarding the special needs of children with disabilities helps the parents provide a better initial adjustment to broader social experiences. A Life Course Model has been developed for patients, families, caregivers, teachers, and clinicians to facilitate, through a developmental approach, the care of the child and young person with SB; this program has been made into a web-based tool that can be used to assist in the transition to adulthood (Dicianno, Fairman, Juengst, et al., 2010). Additional information regarding this program is available through the Spina Bifida Association's website at http://www.sbpreparations.org.

Numerous organizations and agencies offer assistance and support to children and families. The Spina Bifida Association provides services and support for families of children with spinal lesions.

The multiple aspects of care of the child with a disability are discussed in Chapter 19. Complex problems associated with partial or complete lower extremity paralysis are discussed in this chapter and Chapter 33 and include bowel and bladder control; orthopedic appliances; and the observation and management of complications, especially urinary tract infections (see Chapter 24) and pressure necrosis (see Wounds, Chapter 23).

LATEX ALLERGY

Latex allergy, or latex hypersensitivity, was identified as being a serious health hazard when a report linked intraoperative anaphylaxis with latex in children with SB. Latex, a natural product derived from the rubber tree, is used in combination with other chemicals to give elasticity, strength, and durability to many products. Children with SB are at high risk for developing latex allergy because of repeated exposure to latex products during surgery and procedures. Therefore such children should not be exposed to latex products from birth onward to minimize the occurrence of latex hypersensitivity. Allergic reactions range from urticaria, wheezing, watery eyes, and rashes to anaphylactic shock. More severe reactions tend to occur when latex comes in contact with mucous membranes, wet skin, the bloodstream, or an airway. There also can be cross-reactions to a number of foods (e.g., banana, avocado, kiwi, chestnut).

Allergic reactions to latex protein can also occur when the substance is transferred to food by food handlers wearing latex gloves, prompting several states to pass legislation that prohibits the use of latex gloves in food service. In addition to patients with SB, high-risk populations include patients with urogenital anomalies or multiple surgeries, as well as health care workers.

The most important goals are prevention of latex sensitivity and identification of children with a known hypersensitivity (see Nursing Care Guidelines box). High-risk and latex-allergic individuals must be managed in a latex-free environment. Take care that they do not come in direct or secondary contact with products or equipment containing latex at *any time* during medical treatment. Allergy testing can identify latex sensitivity with varying success. Skin prick testing and provocation testing carry the risk for allergic reaction or anaphylaxis. Several commercially available assays can be useful in confirming latex sensitivity. To date, none of these tests demonstrates complete diagnostic reliability, and they should not be the sole determinant of the presence or absence of an allergic response to latex.

NURSING CARE GUIDELINES

Identifying Latex Allergy

- Does your child have any symptoms, such as sneezing, coughing, rashes, or wheezing, when handling rubber products (e.g., balloons, tennis or Koosh balls, adhesive bandage strips) or when in contact with rubber hospital products, such as gloves or catheters?
- Has your child ever had an allergic reaction during surgery?
- Does your child have a history of rashes, asthma, or allergic reactions to medication or foods, especially milk, kiwi, bananas, or chestnuts?
- How would you identify or recognize an allergic reaction in your child?
- What would you do if an allergic reaction occurred?
- Has anyone ever discussed latex or rubber allergy or sensitivity with you?
- Has the child had any allergy testing?
- When did the child last come in contact with any type of rubber product? Were you present?

Because children who have SB are prone to develop sensitivity to latex, reducing exposure from birth on may decrease the chance of allergy development. Nonlatex products lists are available to parents and health care workers; these products may be substituted for those containing latex. In the health care arena, it is important to use products with the lowest potential risk for sensitizing patients and staff members.

The identification of those sensitive to latex is best accomplished through careful screening of all patients. During the health interview with the parent or child, ask *all* patients, not only those at risk, about sensitivity to latex. Be certain this is a routine part of all preoperative and preprocedural histories. Stress the importance of the allergy history to all personnel (e.g., phlebotomists, respiratory therapists). (See Nursing Care Guidelines box for questions related to latex allergy.) Children with latex hypersensitivity should carry some form of allergy identification, such as a MedicAlert bracelet. Education programs regarding latex hypersensitivity are aimed at those who care for high-risk groups, such as children with SB, and may include relatives, school nurses, teachers, child care workers, and babysitters. In addition to educating caregivers about the child's exposure to medical products that contain latex, nurses need to inform them of common nonmedical latex objects such as water toys, pacifiers, and plastic storage bags. Items brought to the hospital, such as floral bouquets, should also be screened for latex toys and balloons. Parents should also receive literature explaining signs and symptoms of latex hypersensitivity and appropriate emergency treatment. (See Anaphylaxis, Chapter 27)

HYPOTONIA

Decreased muscle tone may be observed in the neonatal period and is one of the most common presenting symptoms in neuromuscular disorders. Hypotonia in neonates born before 37 weeks may be due to neuromuscular immaturity or perinatal maternal medications. (See also Chapter 9.) Monitor such infants over time for neuromuscular tone and make further evaluation if physiologic immaturity is not determined to be a contributing factor. Hypotonia may also indicate a variety of systemic conditions. Common causes are cerebral trauma or perinatal hypoxia, but most neuromuscular disorders with hypotonia as the presenting symptom, especially Down syndrome and spinal muscular atrophy, are genetically determined. Additional conditions that may present in the neonatal period include inborn errors of metabolism such as glycogen storage disease; congenital and metabolic myopathies; cerebral dysgenesis such as lissencephaly; and congenital muscular dystrophies.

Clinical Manifestations

Hypotonia is marked by diminished muscle tone and weakness in both spontaneous and passive motion and reflex testing. The affected infant, when placed in a supine position, assumes a characteristic "frog-leg posture" or lies in some other unusual position at rest. Normally the neonate or infant who is held in horizontal suspension (i.e., with the examiner's hand supporting the infant under the chest) responds by slightly raising the head with the back relatively straight, the arms flexed and slightly abducted, and the knees partly flexed. The hypotonic infant droops over the supporting hand with head and extremities hanging loosely, resembling an inverted U. The muscles feel atrophied when palpated, and there is marked head lag when the infant is pulled to a sitting position. Poor sucking may be noted. *Floppy infant syndrome* was the term traditionally used to describe infants with hypotonia.

Diagnostic Evaluation

The infant with hypotonia presents a diagnostic challenge. The child's and family's history and the physical examination offer important clues to the general category of causes, such as central or motor neuron disorders. Laboratory diagnosis may include a CK level specific for skeletal muscle. Molecular deoxyribonucleic acid (DNA) analysis may eliminate the need for additional invasive tests when a definitive diagnosis is made for a hereditary myopathy or neuropathy (Sarnat, 2015a). Nerve conduction velocity, electromyography (EMG), and muscle biopsy may be used in diagnostic testing. Accurate diagnosis is essential for appropriate treatment, genetic implications, and family counseling.

Therapeutic and Nursing Care Management

The management of an infant with hypotonia is determined by the cause of the hypotonia. It is a nursing responsibility to record and report findings that suggest hypotonia in an infant so that further evaluation can be carried out and therapeutic measures implemented if indicated.

SPINAL MUSCULAR ATROPHY TYPE 1 (WERDNIG-HOFFMANN DISEASE)

Spinal muscular atrophy (SMA) type 1 (Werdnig-Hoffmann disease) is a disorder characterized by progressive weakness and wasting of skeletal muscles caused by degeneration of anterior horn cells. It is inherited as an autosomal recessive trait and is the most common paralytic form of the floppy infant syndrome (congenital hypotonia). The sites of the pathologic condition are the anterior horn cells of the spinal cord and the motor nuclei of the brainstem, but the primary effect is atrophy of skeletal muscles.

Clinical Manifestations

The age of onset is variable, but the earlier the onset, the more disseminated and severe the motor weakness. The disorder may be manifested early—often at birth—and almost always before 2 years of age; death may occur as a result of respiratory failure by age 2 years (Iannaccone & Burghes, 2002).

The manifestations (Box 34.7) and prognosis are categorized according to the age of onset, severity of weakness, and clinical course; some children may fluctuate between exhibiting symptoms of types 1 and 2 or types 2 and 3 in regard to clinical function (Sarnat, 2015a). Some experts also categorize SMA according to the highest level of motor function; type 1 includes "nonsitters," type 2 includes "sitters," and type 3 includes "walkers" (Iannaccone, 2007). A severe rare fetal form of SMA, classified as type 0, is reported to be quite lethal in the perinatal period; motor neuron degeneration may be noted as early as midgestation in type 0 (Sarnat, 2015a). Type 4 may present between 20 and 30 years of age and may be referred to as proximal adult-type SMA (Prior, 2010).

Diagnostic Evaluation

The diagnosis is based on the molecular genetic marker for the *SMN* (survival motor neuron) gene, which is located on chromosome *5q13.* Prenatal diagnosis may be made by genetic analysis of circulating fetal cells in maternal blood or circulating fetal cells in amniotic fluid. The risk for subsequent affected offspring in carriers of the mutant gene or in families with known cases of SMA may also be evaluated genetically. Further diagnostic studies include muscle electromyography (EMG), which demonstrates a denervation pattern, and muscle biopsy; however, the genetic analysis has become the gold standard for diagnosis of the condition (Sarnat, 2015a).

Therapeutic Management

There is no cure for the disease, and treatment is symptomatic and supportive, primarily preventing joint contractures and treating orthopedic problems, the most serious of which is scoliosis. Hip subluxation and dislocation may also occur. Many children benefit from powered wheelchairs, lifts, special pressure-adjustable mattresses, and accessible environmental controls. Muscle and joint contractures require careful attention and care to prevent further complications. Nutritional growth failure may occur in infants and toddlers as a result of poor feeding; supplemental gastrostomy feedings may be required to maintain adequate nutritional status and maintain weight gain. The use of lower

BOX 34.7 Clinical Manifestations of Spinal Muscular Atrophy

Type 1 (Werdnig-Hoffmann Disease)

- Clinical manifestations within first few weeks or months of life
- Onset within 6 months of life
- Inactivity the most prominent feature
- Infant lying in a frog-leg position with legs externally rotated, abducted, and flexed at knees
- Generalized weakness
- Absent deep tendon reflexes
- Limited movements of shoulder and arm muscles
- Active movement usually limited to fingers and toes
- Diaphragmatic breathing with sternal retractions (diaphragmatic paralysis may occur)
- Abnormal tongue movements (at rest)
- Weak cry and cough
- Poor suck reflex
- Fatigues quickly during feedings (if breastfed, may lose weight before noticeable)
- Failure to thrive (nutritional)
- Alert facies
- Normal sensation and intellect
- Affected infants not able to sit alone, roll over, or walk
- Early death possible from respiratory failure or infection

Type 2 (Intermediate Spinal Muscular Atrophy)

- Onset before age 18 months
  - **Early**—Weakness confined to arms and legs
  - **Later**—Becomes generalized
- Legs usually involved to greater extent than arms
- Prominent pectus excavatum
- Movements absent during complete relaxation or sleep
- Some infants able to sit if placed in position, but few can ambulate
- For most, life span varies from 7 months to 7 years, although many have normal life expectancy

Type 3 (Kugelberg-Welander Syndrome; Mild Spinal Muscular Atrophy)

- Onset of symptoms after 18 months of age
- Normal head control and ability to sit unassisted by 6–8 months of age
- Thigh and hip muscles weak
- Scoliosis common
- Failure to walk a common presentation
- In those who manage to walk:
  - Waddling gait
  - Genu recurvatum
  - Protuberant abdomen
  - Ambulation becoming increasingly difficult
  - Confined to a wheelchair by second decade
- Deep tendon reflexes may be present early but disappear

Type IV (Adult Spinal Muscular Atrophy)

- Rare, adult-onset spinal muscular atrophy usually in second or third decade of life; muscle weakness is first symptom

NOTE: These classifications are general, but some research suggests there may be variations in life span and other characteristics (Iannaccone & Burghes, 2002; Lunn & Wang, 2008; Russman, 1996; Russman, Iannaccone, Buncher, et al., 1992).

extremity orthoses may assist with ambulation, but eventually the child may be confined to a wheelchair as muscle atrophy progresses. Restrictive lung disease is the most serious complication of SMA (Iannaccone, 2007). Upper respiratory tract infections often occur and are treated with antibiotic therapy; they are the cause of death in many children. Rapid eye movement (REM)–related sleep-disordered breathing is common in children with SMA type 1; this progresses to sleep-disordered breathing during REM and non-REM sleep followed by respiratory failure, which often requires nocturnal noninvasive mechanical ventilation (Schroth, 2009). Noninvasive ventilation methods such as bilevel positive airway pressure (BiPAP) have decreased the morbidity and increased the survival rate of children with SMA types 1 and 2. Children with SMA type 1 who undergo tracheotomy and invasive ventilation often remain ventilator dependent for the rest of their lives; some families choose to withdraw support when invasive ventilation becomes necessary (Mercuri, Bertini, & Iannaccone, 2012). Palliative care is an important aspect of care for families of children with SMA type 1. A decreased ability to cough and clear secretions may be managed with airway clearance therapies such as the cough-assist machine and manual cough assistance. Guidelines for the standardization of respiratory care for patients with SMA have been published elsewhere (Schroth, 2009).

In addition to noninvasive respiratory support, some infants and children may benefit from tracheostomy and mechanical ventilation. If untreated, some infants may die of respiratory complications in infancy.

Associated medical conditions in survivors include gastroesophageal reflux, scoliosis, early-onset puberty, hip dysplasia, and recurrent oral candidiasis (Bach, 2007). A referral to pediatric palliative care may help the families of children with SMA make decisions about the benefits and burdens of treatment options.

A new therapy to treat SMA has recently been approved by the Food and Drug Administration. Spinraza (nusinersen) is an antisense oligonucleotide (ASO) that consists of small strings of synthetic nucleotides that selectively bind ribonucleic acid (RNA). It was designed to treat infants with SMA. In recent studies, treated infants experienced a statistically significant improvement in motor milestones compared with those not treated. The medication is given by intrathecal injection. This allows it to be delivered directly to the CSF around the spinal cord, where motor neurons degenerate in SMA patients due to insufficient levels of survival motor neuron (SMN) protein. Spinraza is designed to alter the splicing of SMN2 to increase the production of full-length SMN protein. Although not a cure, it is showing promise of improving motor skills in infants with SMA (Finkel, Chiriboga, Vajsar, et al., 2016).

Nursing Care Management

An infant or a small child with progressive muscle weakness requires nursing care similar to that of an immobilized patient (see Chapter 34). However, the underlying goal of treatment should be to assist the child and family in dealing with the illness while progressing toward a life of normalization within the child's capabilities. Special attention should be directed to preventing muscle and joint contractures, promoting independence in performance of ADLs, and becoming incorporated into the mainstream of school when possible. In addition, parents need support and resources to be able to provide for the child and remain an intact family. Because children with neuromuscular disease have abnormal breathing patterns that often contribute to early death, it is important to assess adequate oxygenation, especially during the sleep phase when shallow breathing occurs and hypoxemia may develop. Home pulse oximetry may be used to assess the child during sleep and provide noninvasive mechanical ventilation as necessary (Bush, Fraser, & Jardine, 2005; Young, Lowe, & Fitzgerald, 2007) (see Duchenne [Pseudohypertrophic] Muscular Dystrophy, p. 1338, for respiratory management). Supportive care also includes management of orthoses and other orthopedic equipment as required. Because children with SMA are intellectually normal, verbal, tactile, and auditory stimulation are important aspects of developmental care. Supporting them so they can see the activities around them and transporting them in appropriate equipment (e.g., wagon, power wheelchair) for a change of environment provide stimulation and a broader scope of contacts.

Children who are able to sit require proper support and attention to alignment to prevent deformities and other complications. Children who survive beyond infancy need attention to educational needs and opportunities for social interaction with other children. The parents of a child who is chronically ill require much support and encouragement (see Chapter 19). Parents who have not sought genetic counseling should be encouraged to do so to evaluate further risk potential.

JUVENILE SPINAL MUSCULAR ATROPHY (KUGELBERG-WELANDER DISEASE)

Spinal muscular atrophy type 3 (Kugelberg-Welander disease) is a result of anterior horn cell and motor nerve degeneration. The disease is characterized by a pattern of muscular weakness similar to that of infantile SMA (see Box 34.7). Several modes of inheritance have been reported for the disease: autosomal recessive, autosomal dominant, and X-linked recessive.

The onset occurs from younger than 1 year of age into adulthood, with symptoms resembling group 3 infantile SMA. Proximal muscle weakness (especially of the lower limbs) and muscular atrophy are the predominant features. The disease runs a slowly progressive course. Some children lose the ability to walk 8 to 9 years after the onset of symptoms, but many can still walk after 30 years or more. One source notes that approximately one-half of all children with SMA type 3 lose ambulation by age 14 years and may require a wheelchair when falls are more frequent (Mercuri, Bertini, & Iannaccone, 2012). Many affected persons have a normal life expectancy.

Therapeutic and Nursing Care Management

Promising results from ongoing clinical trials suggest treatments that increase SMN protein might provide clinical benefit to patients with spinal muscular atrophy (Chiriboga, Swoboda, Darras, et al., 2016). However, the management is primarily symptomatic and supportive and is related to maintaining mobility as long as possible, preventing complications such as skin breakdown, optimizing and maintaining respiratory function, and providing support to the child and family. The discussion of family support in the section for Duchenne muscular dystrophy is also applicable to families of children with SMA.

GUILLAIN-BARRÉ SYNDROME

Guillain-Barré syndrome (GBS), also known as *infectious polyneuritis,* is an uncommon acute demyelinating polyneuropathy with a progressive, usually ascending flaccid paralysis. The hallmark of GBS is acute peripheral motor weakness. The paralysis usually occurs approximately 10 days after a nonspecific viral infection; GBS has also been reported after administration of certain vaccines (e.g., rabies, influenza, polio, and meningococcal) (Sarnat, 2015b). Several subtypes of GBS include acute inflammatory demyelinating neuropathy, acute motor axonal neuropathy, acute motor sensory axonal neuropathy, and Miller Fisher syndrome. Children are less often affected than adults; among children, those between ages 4 and 10 years have higher susceptibility. The male-to-female ratio is reported to be 1.5 to 1. Two peak periods with an increased incidence of GBS have been identified: late adolescence and young adulthood.

Chronic inflammatory demyelinating polyradiculoneuropathies (CIDPs) are chronic types of GBS that recur intermittently or do not improve over a period of months to years (Sarnat, 2015b). The following discussion focuses on GBS.

Congenital GBS is rare, yet may occur in the neonatal period, and consists of hypotonia, weakness, and decreased or absent reflexes. Maternal neuromuscular disease may or may not be present. Diagnosis is established by the same criteria as in older children, but the symptoms gradually subside over the first few months of life and disappear by 12 months (Sarnat, 2015b).

Pathophysiology

Guillain-Barré syndrome is an immune-mediated disease often associated with a number of viral or bacterial infections or the administration of certain vaccines. It has been associated with infectious mononucleosis, measles, mumps, *Campylobacter jejuni* (gastroenteritis), cytomegalovirus, *Borrelia burgdorferi* (Lyme disease), Epstein-Barr virus, *Helicobacter pylori,* and *Mycoplasma* and *Pneumocystis* infections. Onset of GBS symptoms usually occurs within 10 days of the primary infection. Pathologic changes in spinal and cranial nerves consist of inflammation and edema with rapid, segmented demyelination and compression of nerve roots within the dural sheath. Nerve conduction is impaired, producing ascending partial or complete paralysis of muscles innervated by the involved nerves. GBS has three phases:

1. Acute—Phase starts when symptoms begin and continues until new symptoms stop appearing or deterioration ceases; it may last as long as 4 weeks.
2. Plateau—Symptoms remain constant without further deterioration; it may last from days to weeks.
3. Recovery—Patient begins to improve and progress to optimal recovery; it usually lasts a few weeks to months, depending on the deficits incurred by the illness.

Clinical Manifestations

A mild influenza-like illness or sore throat usually precedes the paralytic manifestations of GBS. The onset can be rapid, reaching peak activity within 24 hours, or there may be a gradual progression of symptoms over days or weeks. Neurologic symptoms initially involve muscle tenderness that sometimes is accompanied by paresthesia and cramps. Proximal muscle weakness progressing to paralysis usually occurs before distal weakness, and there is a tendency toward symmetric involvement. In most patients paralysis ascends from the lower extremities, often involving the muscles of the trunk and upper extremities and those supplied by cranial nerves. The seventh cranial (facial) nerve is often affected.

Tendon reflexes are depressed or absent, and paralysis is flaccid. Paralysis may involve facial, extraocular, labial, lingual, pharyngeal, and laryngeal muscles. Evidence of intercostal and phrenic nerve involvement includes breathlessness in vocalizations and shallow, irregular respirations. There may be variable degrees of sensory impairment. Most patients complain of muscle tenderness or sensitivity to slight pressure. Lower limb pain and back pain are common in children with GBS. Urinary incontinence or retention and constipation are often present. Abdominal pain and fatigue have also been reported in children with GBS (Lyons, 2008).

Autonomic nervous system disturbances may occur in children and adolescents with severe muscle involvement and respiratory muscle paralysis. These include orthostatic hypotension; hypertension; and vagal responses such as bradycardia, asystole, and heart block (Laskowski-Jones, 2007).

Diagnostic Evaluation

Diagnosis is based on the paralytic manifestations, CSF analysis, and EMG. Motor nerve conduction velocities are greatly reduced. Sensory nerve conduction time is often slowed. CSF analysis reveals an elevated protein concentration, and fewer than 10 WBCs/mm^3 and normal glucose level (Sarnat, 2015b). Other laboratory studies are usually noncontributory. The symmetric nature of the paralysis helps differentiate this disorder from spinal paralytic poliomyelitis, which usually affects sporadic muscles.

Therapeutic Management

Treatment of GBS is primarily supportive. In the acute phase, patients are hospitalized because respiratory and pharyngeal involvement may require assisted ventilation, sometimes with a temporary tracheostomy. Treatment modalities include aggressive ventilatory support in the event of respiratory compromise, intravenous (IV) administration of immunoglobulin (IVIG), and sometimes steroids; plasmapheresis and immunosuppressive drugs may also be used. Plasmapheresis has been shown to decrease the length of recovery in patients with severe GBS; however, it is expensive, and side effects include hypotension, fever, bleeding disorders, chills, urticaria, and bradycardia. Further evidence reports equal benefits to treatment of GBS with IVIG administration or plasmapheresis; both sped up recovery time in studies reviewed (Hughes & Cornblath, 2005). There is evidence, however, of significant improvement in children with high-dose IVIG therapy (vs. supportive treatment alone) (Hughes, Swan, & Van Doorn, 2012). IVIG is now recommended as the primary treatment of GBS when administered within 2 weeks of disease onset (Hughes, 2008). Corticosteroids alone do not decrease the symptoms or shorten the duration of the disease.

Additional medications that may be administered during the acute phase include a low-molecular-weight heparin to prevent deep vein thrombosis (DVT), a mild laxative or stool softener to prevent constipation, pain medication such as acetaminophen, and a histamine-antagonist to prevent stress ulcer formation. Chronic neuropathic pain after GBS may be treated with gabapentin, which is reported to be more effective than carbamazepine (Sarnat, 2015b).

Rehabilitation after the acute phase may involve physical therapy, occupational therapy, and speech therapy. Additional consideration should be given to problems of general weakness and retraining for toileting and feeding (Lyons, 2008).

Prognosis

Better outcomes are associated with younger age, no requirement for mechanical respiratory assistance, slower progression of disease, normal peripheral nerve function on EMG, and treatment with either IVIG or plasmapheresis. Recovery usually begins within 2 to 3 weeks, and most patients regain full muscle strength. The recovery of muscle strength progresses in the reverse order of onset of paralysis, with lower extremity strength being the last to recover. Poor prognosis with subsequent residual effects in children is reportedly associated with cranial nerve involvement, extensive disability at time of presentation, and intubation.

Most deaths associated with GBS are caused by respiratory failure; therefore early diagnosis and access to respiratory support are especially important. The rate of recovery is usually related to the degree of involvement and may extend from a few weeks to months. The greater the degree of paralysis, the longer the recovery phase.

Nursing Care Management

Nursing care is primarily supportive and is the same as that required for children with immobilization and respiratory compromise. The emphasis of care is on close observation to assess the extent of paralysis and on prevention of complications, including aspiration, ventilator-associated pneumonia (VAP), atelectasis, DVT, pressure ulcer, fear and anxiety, autonomic dysfunction, and pain.

During the acute phase of the disease, the nurse should carefully observe the child's condition for possible difficulty in swallowing and respiratory involvement. The child's respiratory function is closely monitored, and oxygen source, appropriate-size insufflation bag and mask, endotracheal intubation and suctioning equipment, tracheotomy tray, and vasopressor drugs are kept available. Vital signs are monitored frequently, as well as neurologic signs and level of consciousness. For children who develop respiratory impairment, the care is the same as that for any child with respiratory distress requiring mechanical ventilation.

Respiratory care, if intubation is required, requires close monitoring of oxygenation status (usually by pulse oximetry and sometimes arterial blood gases), maintenance of an open airway with suctioning, and postural changes to prevent pneumonia. Consideration should be given to preventing opportunistic infections such as VAP; meticulous oral care and hypopharynx suctioning, elevating the head of the bed 30 degrees, and strict asepsis with suctioning equipment (including catheters, a Yankauer device, or both) should be implemented to prevent VAP. Children with oral and pharyngeal involvement may be fed via a nasogastric or gastrostomy tube to ensure adequate feeding. It is also important to consider the possibility of stress ulcers in such patients and to administer a proton pump inhibitor. Immobilization, which occurs with GBS, decreases GI function; therefore problems such as decreased gastric emptying, constipation, and feeding residuals require nursing assessment and appropriate collaborative interventions. Temporary urinary catheterization may be required; urinary retention is common, and appropriate assessment of urinary output is vital. Sensory impairment and paralysis in the lower extremities make the child susceptible to skin breakdown; therefore attention should be given to meticulous skin care. Passive range-of-motion exercises and application of orthoses to prevent muscle contracture are important when paralysis is present. Prevention of DVT is accomplished with pneumatic compression (antiembolism) devices, administration of a low-molecular-weight heparin, and early mobilization and ambulation. Autonomic dysfunction may be life threatening; thus close monitoring of vital signs in the acute phase is essential.

A key to recovery in the child with GBS is the prevention of muscle and joint contractures, so passive range-of-motion exercises must be carried out routinely to maintain vital function. Although the child may have a generalized paralysis, cognitive function remains intact; therefore it is important for nursing care to involve communication with the child or adolescent regarding procedures and treatments that may be frightening, especially if mechanical ventilation is required. Encourage parents to talk to the child and make eye and physical contact and to reassure the child during this phase of the illness.

Pain management is crucial in the care of children with GBS. Although neuromuscular impairment may make pain perception more difficult to accurately evaluate, objective pain scales should be used. Gabapentin and carbamazepine may be used to manage neuropathic pain in patients with GBS.

Physical therapy may be limited to passive range-of-motion exercises during the evolving phase of the disease. Later, as the disease stabilizes and recovery begins, an active physical therapy program is implemented to prevent contracture deformities and facilitate muscle recovery. This may include active exercise, gait training, and bracing.

Throughout the course of the illness, child and parent support are paramount. The usual rapidity of the paralysis and the long recovery period greatly tax the emotional reserves of all family members. The parents and child benefit from repeated reassurance that recovery is occurring and from realistic information regarding the possibility of permanent disability. In the event of a residual disability, the family needs assistance in accepting and adjusting to the loss of function. (See Chapter 19.) The GBS/CIDP Foundation International is a nonprofit organization devoted to support, education, and research. It provides families with support from recovered persons, publishes informational literature and a newsletter, and maintains a list of health care practitioners experienced with the disease.

TETANUS

Tetanus, or lockjaw, is an acute, preventable, and sometimes fatal disease caused by an exotoxin produced by the anaerobic, spore-forming, gram-positive bacillus *Clostridium tetani.* It is characterized by painful muscular rigidity primarily involving the masseter and neck muscles. The development of tetanus has four requirements: (1) presence of tetanus spores or vegetative forms of the bacillus, (2) injury to the tissues, (3) wound conditions that encourage multiplication of the organism, and (4) a susceptible host.

Tetanus spores are found in soil, dust, and the intestinal tracts of humans and animals, especially herbivorous animals. The organisms are more prevalent in rural areas but are readily carried to urban areas by wind. They enter the body by way of wounds, particularly a puncture wound, burn, or crushed area. In the newborn, infection may occur through the umbilical cord, usually in situations in which infants are delivered in contaminated surroundings and the mother has not been properly immunized against tetanus. The disease has the greatest incidence during months in which persons are more involved in outdoor activities.

Prevention

Primary prevention is key and occurs through immunization and boosters and good wound care. Once an injury has occurred, further preventive measures are based on the child's immune status and the nature of the injury. Specific prophylactic therapy after trauma is administration of either tetanus toxoid or tetanus antitoxin. A dose of tetanus toxoid is not necessary for clean, minor wounds in children who have completed the immunization series (see Chapter 10) or who have received a booster within the previous 10 years. Protective levels of antibody are maintained for at least 10 years. Therefore antitoxin is not indicated for the fully immunized child. Children with more serious wounds (e.g., contaminated, puncture, crush, or burn wounds) are given a tetanus toxoid booster prophylactically as soon as possible after injury.

The unprotected or inadequately immunized child who sustains a "tetanus-prone" wound (including wounds contaminated with dirt, feces, soil, and saliva; puncture wounds; avulsions; and wounds resulting from missiles, crushing, burns, and frostbite) should receive tetanus immunoglobulin (TIG). Concurrent administration of both TIG and tetanus toxoid at separate sites is recommended both to provide protection and to initiate the active immune process (American Academy of Pediatrics, 2015). Completion of active immunization is carried out according to the usual pattern. Proper surgical cleansing and débridement of contaminated wounds reduce the chance of infection.

Pathophysiology

When prevention efforts are not effective and conditions are favorable, the organisms multiply and form two exotoxins: (1) tetanospasmin, a potent toxin that affects the CNS to produce the clinical manifestations of the disease, and (2) tetanolysin, which appears to have no significance. The ideal conditions for growth of the organisms are devitalized tissues without access to air (e.g., puncture wounds); wounds that have not been washed or kept clean; and those that have crusted over, trapping pus beneath. The exotoxin appears to reach the CNS by way of either the neuron axons or the vascular system. The toxin becomes fixed on nerve cells of the brainstem and the anterior horn of the spinal cord. The toxin acts at the neuromuscular junction to produce muscular stiffness and to lower the threshold for reflex excitability.

The incubation period is 3 days to 3 weeks and averages 8 days. Most cases occur within 14 days; in neonates it is usually 5 to 14 days. Shorter incubation periods have been associated with more heavily contaminated wounds, more severe disease, and a worse prognosis (American Academy of Pediatrics, 2015).

Clinical Manifestations

There are several forms of the disease. Local tetanus is a less common but severe form characterized by persistent rigidity of muscles near the inoculation site, which may persist for weeks or months. Some cases resolve without sequelae. Neonatal tetanus results from contamination of the umbilical cord, which is rare in the United States but is common and often fatal in developing countries. The first symptom is difficulty in sucking, progressing to total inability to suck, excessive crying, irritability, and nuchal rigidity.

Generalized tetanus is the most common and dangerous form of the disease. The manner of onset varies, but the initial symptoms are usually a progressive stiffness and tenderness of the muscles in the neck and jaw. The characteristic difficulty in opening the mouth (**trismus**), which is caused by sustained contraction of the jaw-closing muscles, is evident early and gives the disease its common name, lockjaw. Spasm of facial muscles produces the so-called sardonic smile (**risus sardonicus**). Progressive involvement of the trunk muscles causes **opisthotonos** and a boardlike rigidity of abdominal and limb muscles. The patient has difficulty swallowing and is highly sensitive to external stimuli. The slightest noise, a gentle touch, or bright light triggers convulsive muscular contractions that last seconds to minutes. The paroxysmal contractions recur with increased frequency until they become almost continuous.

Mentation is unaffected; the patient remains alert, and pain and distress are reflected in a rapid pulse, sweating, and an anxious expression. Laryngospasm and tetany of respiratory muscles and accumulated secretions predispose the child to respiratory arrest, atelectasis, and pneumonia. Fever is usually absent or mild and generally indicates a poor prognosis. As the child recovers from the disease, the paroxysms become less frequent and gradually subside. Survival beyond 4 days usually indicates recovery, but complete recovery may take weeks.

Therapeutic Management

The unprotected or inadequately immunized child who sustains a "tetanus-prone" wound (as described earlier) should receive TIG. Concurrent administration of both TIG and tetanus toxoid at separate sites is recommended both to provide protection and to initiate the active immune process (American Academy of Pediatrics, 2015). After the individual has received primary tetanus immunization, antitoxin is believed to provide protection for at least 10 years and for a longer period after booster immunization (American Academy of Pediatrics, 2015). (See also Immunizations, Chapter 6.)

Antibiotic treatment with penicillin G (or erythromycin or tetracycline in older children with allergy to penicillin) is important in the management of tetanus as an adjunct against clostridia; metronidazole is a viable alternative (Arnon, 2015a).

Aggressive supportive care is necessary to treat tetanus in the acute phase. The acutely ill child is best treated in an intensive care facility, where close and constant observation and equipment for monitoring and respiratory support are readily available.

General supportive care is indicated, including maintaining adequate airway and fluid and electrolyte balance, providing pain management, and ensuring adequate caloric intake. Indwelling oral or nasogastric feedings may be required to maintain adequate fluid and caloric intake; continued laryngospasm may necessitate total parenteral nutrition or gastrostomy feeding. Severe or recurrent laryngospasm or excessive secretions may require advanced airway management such as endotracheal intubation; in some cases a tracheotomy may be performed to provide an adequate airway.

TIG therapy to neutralize toxins is the most specific therapy for tetanus. In countries where TIG is not available, equine tetanus antitoxin (not available in the United States) should be administered. Antibiotics are administered to control the proliferation of the vegetative forms of the organism at the site of infection. When the child recovers, active immunization should take place because contraction of the disease does not confer a permanent immunity. Standard precautions for the child with tetanus are recommended; isolation is not recommended.

Local care of the wound by surgical débridement and cleansing with an antiseptic solution helps reduce the number of proliferating organisms at the site of injury. The cleansing should be repeated several times during the first 48 hours. Deep, infected lacerations are usually exposed and débrided. Infiltration of the wound with TIG is no longer considered necessary (American Academy of Pediatrics, 2015).

Diazepam is the drug of choice for seizure control and muscle relaxation (Arnon, 2015a), but lorazepam (Ativan) may be used in some cases. Other AEDs may be administered as well. Intrathecal baclofen, magnesium sulfate, dantrolene sodium, and midazolam may also be used in the management of tetanus; intrathecal baclofen may cause apnea and should only be used in the intensive care setting (Arnon, 2015a). Patients with severe tetanus and those who do not respond to other muscle relaxants may require the administration of a neuromuscular blocking agent, such as rocuronium or vecuronium. Because of their paralytic effect on respiratory muscles, use of these drugs requires mechanical ventilation with endotracheal intubation or tracheotomy and constant cardiopulmonary monitoring. Endotracheal tube insertion or tracheotomy is often indicated and should be performed before severe respiratory distress develops. Despite the absence of pain manifestation with these drugs, it is important to administer adequate analgesia. The administration of corticosteroids has met with success in some cases.

Nursing Care Management

The care of the child with tetanus requires supportive management with particular attention to airway and breathing. Respiratory status is carefully evaluated for any signs of distress, and appropriate emergency equipment is kept available at all times. The location, extent, and severity of muscle spasms are important nursing observations. Muscle relaxants, opioids, and sedatives that may be prescribed can also cause respiratory depression; therefore the child should be assessed for excessive CNS depression. Attention to hydration and nutrition involves monitoring an IV infusion, monitoring nasogastric or gastrostomy feedings, and suctioning oropharyngeal secretions when indicated.

In caring for a child with tetanus during the acute phase, every effort should be made to control or eliminate stimulation from sound, light, and touch. Although a darkened room is ideal, sufficient light is essential so that the child can be carefully observed; light appears to be less irritating than vibratory or auditory stimuli. The infant or child is handled as little as possible, and extra effort is expended to avoid any sudden or loud noise to prevent seizures.

If a potent muscle relaxant such as vecuronium is used, the total paralysis makes oral communication impossible. The drug is not a sedative, however, and anxiety should be considered in children who are intubated. Therefore all the child's needs must be anticipated and procedures carefully explained beforehand. Additional care is focused on preventing the complications associated with prolonged immobility, including decreased bowel and bladder tone and subsequent constipation, anorexia, DVT, pneumonia, and skin breakdown.

BOTULISM

Botulism is serious food poisoning that results from ingestion of the preformed toxin produced by the anaerobic bacillus *Clostridium botulinum.* Botulism toxin exerts its effect by inhibiting the release of acetylcholine at the neuromuscular junction, thereby impairing motor activity of the muscles innervated by the affected nerves. The disease has a wide variation in severity, from constipation to progressive sequential loss of neurologic function and respiratory failure. Human botulism is caused by neurotoxins A, B, E, and rarely F (American Academy of Pediatrics, 2015). Types A and B are the most common causes of infant botulism.

Several forms of botulism are recognized: food borne, infant, wound, human made (for bioterrorism), and botulism from undetermined causes. This chapter only covers the first three forms.

Food-Borne Botulism

This classic form of the disease usually occurs in adults but may occur in children and adolescents. The most common source of the toxin is improperly sterilized home-canned foods. CNS symptoms appear abruptly approximately 12 to 36 hours after ingestion of contaminated food and may or may not be preceded by acute digestive disturbance. Early symptoms include blurred vision, diplopia, weakness, dizziness, difficulty talking and speaking, vomiting, and dysphagia. These are followed by descending paralysis and dyspnea. Progressive respiratory paralysis is life threatening.

Infant Botulism

Infant botulism, unlike the disease in older persons, is caused by ingestion of spores or vegetative cells of *C. botulinum* and the subsequent release of the toxin from organisms colonizing the GI tract. *C. botulinum* types A and B are the most common causative strains of infant botulism. This form of botulism has become more prevalent than any other form. Many cases of infant botulism occur in breastfed infants who are being introduced to nonhuman milk substances (American Academy of Pediatrics, 2015). Cases of infant botulism are still being reported in Europe, where honey is commonly given to infants. There appears to be no common food or drug source of the organisms; however, the *C. botulinum* organisms have been found in honey. Botulism may occur in infants from 1 week to 12 months of age, with peak incidence between 2 and 4 months of age.

The severity of the disease varies widely, from mild constipation to progressive sequential loss of neurologic function and respiratory failure. The affected infant is usually well before the onset of symptoms. Constipation is a common presenting symptom, and almost all infants exhibit generalized weakness and a decrease in spontaneous movements. Deep tendon reflexes are usually diminished or absent. Cranial nerve deficits are common, as evidenced by loss of head control, difficulty in feeding, weak cry, and reduced gag reflex. SMA type 1 and metabolic disorders are often mistaken for infant botulism in the initial diagnostic phase because of the similarities in clinical manifestations of hypotonia, lethargy, and poor feeding (Arnon, 2015b). Presenting clinical signs also often mimic those of sepsis in young infants. Botulism toxin exerts its effect by inhibiting the release of acetylcholine at the myoneural junction, thereby impairing motor activity of muscles innervated by affected nerves.

Diagnosis and Therapeutic Management

The diagnosis is made on the basis of the clinical history, physical examination, and laboratory detection of the organism in the patient's stool and, less commonly, blood. However, isolation of the organism may take several days; therefore suspicion of botulism by clinical presentation should require emergency treatment (Arnon, 2015b). EMG may be helpful in establishing the diagnosis; however, results may be normal early in the course of the illness.

Treatment consists of immediate administration of botulism immune globulin intravenously (BIG-IV) (Arnon, 2015b) without delaying for laboratory diagnosis. Early administration of BIG-IV neutralizes the toxin and stops the progression of the disease. The human-derived botulism antitoxin (BIG-IV) has been evaluated and is now available nationwide for use only in infant botulism. Infants treated with BIG-IV usually have a shortened hospital stay from approximately 6 days to 2 weeks, reportedly as a result of decreased requirements for mechanical ventilation and intensive care (Arnon, 2015b). Approximately 50% of affected infants require intubation and mechanical ventilation; therefore respiratory support is crucial, as is nutritional support because these infants are unable to feed. Trivalent equine botulinum antitoxin and bivalent antitoxin, used in adults and older children, are not administered to infants. Antibiotic therapy is not part of the management because the botulinum toxin is an intracellular molecule and antibiotics would not be effective; aminoglycosides in particular should not be administered because they may potentiate the blocking effects of the neurotoxin (Arnon, 2015b).

The prognosis is generally good if the patient is adequately treated, although recovery may be slow, requiring a few weeks after severe illness. Untreated patients may require a longer hospitalization.

! NURSING ALERT

Although the precise source of *C. botulinum* spores has not been identified as originating from honey in many cases of infant botulism in the United States, it is still recommended that honey not be given to infants younger than 12 months because the spores have been found in honey.

Nursing Care Management

Nursing responsibilities include observing, recognizing, and reporting signs of poor feeding, constipation, and muscle impairment in the infant with botulism and providing intensive nursing care when an infant is hospitalized. (See Nursing Care Management for the infant with SMA, p. 1321, and Nursing Care of High-Risk Newborns, Chapter 9.) Parental support and reassurance are important. Most infants recover when the disorder is recognized and BIG-IV therapy is implemented. Nursing care of the infant on mechanical ventilation requires observation of oxygenation status and vigilance for any complications (see Chapter 26). Parents should be aware that, during recovery, infants fatigue easily when muscular action is sustained. This has important implications for timing the resumption of feedings because of the risk of aspiration. They should also be advised that normal bowel activity may not return for several weeks. Therefore a stool softener can be beneficial.

One cultural consideration that requires further parent education and anticipatory guidance is the use of honey pacifiers among mothers with small infants; there is evidence that honey pacifiers are still commonly used among many mothers to soothe their infants (Benjamins, Gourishankar, Yataco-Marquez, et al., 2013).

MYASTHENIA GRAVIS

Myasthenia gravis (MG) is relatively uncommon in childhood. The incidence in children under 18 years is 1 per 1 million in North America (Cirillo, 2008). Juvenile MG appears to be identical to that seen in adults and usually has its onset after age 10 years, but it may appear as early as age 2 years. Girls are affected three times more often than boys. Juvenile and adult forms of the disease are autoimmune disorders associated with the attack of circulating antibodies on the acetylcholine receptors on the muscle end plate, which blocks their function.

Clinical Manifestations

The most common symptoms associated with MG are general paralysis of the ocular muscles with ptosis and diplopia. Difficulty swallowing, chewing, and speaking are also prominent and are accompanied by varying degrees of weakness and paralysis of all skeletal muscles. The signs and symptoms are more pronounced in the late afternoon and evening. Rest can help relieve the symptoms, but exercise and stress worsen them. Some affected persons may have spontaneous remission of the symptoms with only mild residual ocular symptoms (Meriggioli & Sanders, 2012). Seizures are reported to occur in increasing frequency in children with MG (Meriggioli & Sanders, 2012).

Diagnostic Evaluation

The diagnosis is made on the basis of the characteristic distribution of muscle weakness and the progressive weakness on repeated or sustained muscular contraction. The definitive diagnosis is established on the basis of an EMG, which demonstrates a decrease in muscle potentials with repetitive nerve stimulation (Sarnat, 2015c). A clinical diagnosis may be established by observation of the response to the anticholinesterase drugs. IV administration of a small test dose of edrophonium (Tensilon) produces a beneficial effect in 1 minute, but the effect lasts less than 5 minutes. In infants and children under the age of 2 years, prostigmine methylsulfate (Neostigmine) should be administered intramuscularly instead of Tensilon because the latter may precipitate fatal cardiac arrhythmias in infants (Sarnat, 2015c). Electrophysiologic studies are helpful in diagnosis and help document transmission failure at the neuromuscular junction. Antibodies to human muscle acetylcholine are detected in the serum of almost one-third of affected individuals. Thyroid profiles should also be obtained.

Therapeutic Management

Patients with mild MG may not require specific treatment. For others treatment consists of the administration of cholinesterase-inhibiting drugs, such as neostigmine (Prostigmin), given intramuscularly or as oral neostigmine bromide. Pyridostigmine (Mestinon) may be administered because it is considered less toxic, but a higher dose is required to achieve the same results as neostigmine. The starting dosage of neostigmine is usually 0.04 mg/kg, administered intramuscularly every 4 to 6 hours; oral doses may be well tolerated (Sarnat, 2015c). The dosage is gradually increased until a satisfactory result is obtained. The child must be observed for signs of parasympathetic stimulation from overmedication. These signs include lacrimation, salivation, abdominal cramps, sweating, diarrhea, vomiting, bradycardia, and weakness of respiratory muscles. Long-term treatment with prednisone is effective in some patients. Thymectomy has been shown to be effective in achieving a cure in many children with MG (Castro, Derisavifard, Anderson, et al., 2013; Christison-Lagay, Dharia, Vajsar, et al., 2013). Other therapies directed at the immunologic mechanism include IVIG, long-term corticosteroid treatment, and plasmapheresis. Additional pharmacologic agents that may be used include azathioprine, methotrexate, cyclosporine A, tacrolimus, and rituximab (Gilhus, Owe, Hoff, et al., 2011).

Thymectomy is not effective for familial and congenital forms of MG. The prognosis for juvenile MG is relatively good. However, the course of the disease is marked by fluctuating remissions and exacerbations.

DRUG ALERT

Neuromuscular-Blocking Agents

Avoid neuromuscular-blocking agents such as pancuronium or succinylcholine in patients with MG because they may induce paralysis that can last for weeks. Avoid aminoglycoside antibiotics such as gentamicin because they potentiate MG symptoms (Sarnat, 2015c).

Nursing Care Management

Children with MG often require ongoing medical and nursing supervision, especially in the early stages of diagnosis and treatment considerations. Parents and children with MG are educated regarding the symptoms of a myasthenia crisis (respiratory failure) so that appropriate therapy may be instituted before deterioration is acute. Infections should be treated aggressively, and yearly influenza vaccination is recommended. Respiratory viral infections are a common precipitating cause of a myasthenia crisis (Meriggioli & Sanders, 2012).

Counsel parents to promote a lifestyle that minimizes stress and maximizes relaxation. They should receive instruction in providing respiratory assistance until help arrives or the child can be transported to medical aid.

Neonatal Myasthenia Gravis

A transient form of MG occurs in approximately 10% to 20% of infants born to mothers with MG, who may not know they have the disease. The muscular weakness results from transplacentally acquired maternal acetylcholine receptor antibodies. These infants display generalized muscular weakness and hypotonia at birth with a depressed Moro reflex, ptosis, ineffective sucking and swallowing reflexes, and weak cry. Some infants may require short-term mechanical ventilation (Sarnat, 2015c). Symptoms may be evident within a few hours of birth, following a period of normal appearance after delivery. There is no evidence of neurologic damage. Cholinesterase inhibitors may be given on a short-term basis to improve feeding ability. Symptoms usually disappear within 2 to 3 weeks. Infants with transient neonatal MG regain strength once maternal antibodies clear the system, and they are not at increased risk of MG later in life (Cirillo, 2008; Sarnat, 2015c).

Congenital Myasthenia Gravis

Congenital MG is a rare familial abnormality of neuromuscular transmission that is not immunologically mediated. It appears indistinguishable from the transient form, but the mother usually does not have the disease. The disease persists throughout life, and more than one sibling may be affected, which suggests a genetic etiology. Gender distribution is equal. The disorder is relatively resistant to drug therapy, and the eyelid and extraocular muscles seem to be the muscles most severely affected.

The prognosis in congenital MG is usually good. Despite gradual worsening of symptoms with age, the life span is not affected significantly.

SPINAL CORD INJURIES

SCIs with major neurologic involvement are not a common cause of physical disability in children. Pediatric spinal cord injury incidence is estimated at 24 per million, with the adolescent age group predominating (Piatt, 2015). However, many children with these injuries are admitted to major medical centers, and because of the increased survival rate as a result of improved management, nurses have an important role in the care of children with SCI.

The principles of management and nursing care of the child with a spinal cord lesion apply regardless of cause. In addition to care related to the immobilized child, as discussed in Chapter 33, children with damage to the spinal cord present additional problems—specifically, complications related to the neuropathology of the central and autonomic nervous systems. The extent of paralysis is determined by both neurologic and clinical assessment. Although the majority of children with SCI are paraplegic, some are tetraplegic (quadriplegic). Some children with tetraplegia are able to move only their face and neck muscles, whereas others are able to lift and bend their arms but are unable to perform fine hand movements. Almost every physiologic system is disrupted in a child with high-level tetraplegia. Not only are the central and peripheral nerves impaired, but there is also autonomic nervous system dysfunction. Vital structures such as blood vessels, lungs, bladder, and bowel are affected. Therefore an understanding of neuromuscular physiology is essential to effectively care for the child with damage or injury to the spinal cord.

Essential Neuromuscular Physiology

The spinal cord extends from the medulla oblongata to the lower border of the first lumbar vertebra and contains millions of nerve fibers. However, because of its protected location, a considerable amount of direct trauma is required to cause injury. Posteriorly the cord is protected by the spinous processes, which are stabilized by related ligaments and muscles. It is further protected by the spinal fluid, which surrounds it and absorbs some of the shock.

Spinal Nerves

The 31 nerves of the spinal cord are divided into five segments (Fig. 34.7). The cervical cord segments lie within the first seven vertebrae. The remaining cord segments—thoracic (12), lumbar (5), sacral (5), and coccygeal (1)—extend from the first thoracic vertebra to the lower level of the first lumbar vertebra. Therefore the cord constituents do not anatomically match by number the 33 associated vertebrae. However, nerves that arise from the spinal cord exit from the spinal column at the numerically corresponding vertebrae. In describing injuries to the spinal cord, the highest point at which there is normal function is referred to in relation to the vertebra; for example, an intact cord at the sixth cervical vertebra is designated a C6 injury.

Certain areas of the curved vertebral column are less stable and more prone to damage from severe flexion and twisting. These sites are the cervical area and the junction of the thoracic and lumbar regions. The cervical vertebrae are fractured most often, and this high level of injury causes extensive paralysis and many associated neurologic problems (Table 34.1). Also, traumatic tearing or embolic occlusion of the arteries supplying these areas can markedly jeopardize the cord tissue. Impaired blood supply often produces severe neurologic deficit, which can extend to complete loss of cord function at the level of injury.

Cell bodies of interneurons and motor neurons within the spinal cord are identified as H-shaped gray matter surrounded by columns of white myelinated nerve fibers. Each column serves as a route for a specific type of impulse, such as touch, vibration, pain, and temperature (Fig. 34.8). Nerve pathways in the spinal cord transmit sensory and motor impulses between peripheral receptors and the brain, conduct impulses through the reflex arc, and convey sympathetic and parasympathetic nerve impulses from the brain to peripheral structures.

Sensory transmission begins when peripheral receptors pick up a wide variety of stimuli and transfer the impulses, by means of peripheral nerves, to the spinal nerves, where they make ganglionic connections and enter the cord posteriorly. At this point the impulses travel in two

TABLE 34.1 **Functional Significance of Spinal Cord Lesions**

Highest Intact Cord Segment	Muscle Innervation	Functional Capacity	Functional Goals
Tetraplegia			
C1–C3	None below chin, including phrenic nerve to diaphragm	No voluntary control below chin Respiratory paralysis complete May cause bradycardia or tachycardia, vomiting	Mechanical ventilation; can be taught glossopharyngeal breathing to be used for short periods Electric wheelchair Adaptive equipment for special tasks in bed or wheelchair using mouth stick
C4	Intact sternocleidomastoid, trapezius, upper cervical paraspinal muscle	No voluntary function of upper extremities, trunk, or lower extremities All neck movements Mechanical ventilation dependent	Electric wheelchair Externally powered devices and adaptive equipment for special tasks in bed or wheelchair with mouth stick, such as turning pages, using computer Totally dependent for activities of daily living
C5	Partial deltoid, biceps, major muscles of rotator cuffs at shoulders Diaphragm	Abduction, flexion, and extension of arm Flexion and extension of forearm Unable to roll over or attain sitting position Abdominal respiration Poor respiratory reserve	Electric wheelchair Requires attendant to assist in moving and transfer to wheelchair Adaptive devices for self-feeding, grooming, using computer Vocational potential with adaptive devices
C6	Pectoralis major, serratus anterior, latissimus dorsi muscles Complete deltoid and brachioradialis muscles Partial triceps muscle	Significant increase in function over that with lesion at C5 level Adduction and medial rotation of arm Wrist extension Good elbow flexion	Cuff strapped to hand to permit use of implements for self-care and other activities Able to assist in dressing and transfer Hand rim extension to permit independence in wheelchair
C7	Triceps and finger flexion and extensor muscle Shoulder depressor muscles Still nerve disruption to intercostal muscles	With elbow stabilized in extension and intact shoulder depressor muscles, able to lift body weight Grasp and release still weak; dexterity lacking	Almost complete independence within limitations of wheelchair Requires some assistance in transfer and lower extremity dressing Hand splints helpful Can roll over in bed, sit up in bed, and eat independently Homebound employment possible; outside work usually not feasible
Paraplegia			
T1–T10	Full innervation of upper extremity muscles	Full use of upper extremities, including intrinsic muscles of hand Trunk balance poor—may have difficulty lifting trunk sufficiently to put on lower extremity clothing Considerable energy expenditure to put on long leg braces with extensive attachments	Completely wheelchair dependent Trunk balance benefits from training Able to drive automobile with hand controls May be braced for standing May hold job away from home Can manage adapted public transportation
T10–L2	Full abdominal and upper back muscle control	Good trunk balance Good respiratory reserve Can accomplish moderate hip hiking using external oblique and latissimus dorsi muscles	Ambulation with bilateral long braces using four-point or swing-through crutch gait Usually able to negotiate curbs Some able to use regular public transportation Few vocational limitations as long as does not require much walking or standing
L3–L4	Quadriceps muscle Partial gluteus and hamstring muscles	May have lumbar lordosis Floppy ankles	Ambulates well, often with short leg braces with or without cane Difficulty in getting out of wheelchair May never require wheelchair

directions: across the interneuron connection and then to the motor neurons (reflex arc), or up the spinal cord to predetermined areas of the brain. Motor impulses are transmitted from the cerebral cortex to the medulla (where nerve tracts cross) and proceed down descending motor pathways to the desired level within the spinal cord. Here they connect with the anterior horn cells and are transmitted to the muscle fibers by means of the lower motor neurons to complete a meaningful movement.

A network of nerves that serves the major muscle groups constitutes a plexus. Total involvement of any one of these plexuses seriously impairs

BOX 34.8 The Three Major Plexuses

1. **Cervical plexus (C1–C4)**—Innervates the neck and diaphragm
2. **Brachial plexus (C4–T1)**—Supplies the shoulders, chest, and arms
3. **Lumbosacral plexus (L1–S4)**—Transmits impulses to the lower trunk and legs

BOX 34.9 Differences in Clinical Manifestations Between Upper and Lower Motor Neuron Syndromes

Upper Motor Neuron Syndrome

- Spastic paralysis in muscle groups below lesion (intact reflex arcs below lesion)
- Hyperreflexia with tendon reflexes exaggerated, Babinski reflex present
- No wasting of muscle mass because of increased muscle tone
- Flexion contractures and spasms of muscle groups below lesion level common
- No skin or tissue changes

Lower Motor Neuron Syndrome

- Flaccid paralysis caused by muscle atonia (reflex arcs permanently damaged)
- Reflex with associated muscle response absent
- Marked atrophy of atonic muscle
- Fasciculations (local twitching of muscle groups) common
- No flexor spasms
- Loss of hair
- Skin and tissue changes
- Cornified nails

function to the areas it innervates. Box 34.8 describes the three major plexuses.

Upper Versus Lower Motor Neurons

Upper motor neurons extend from cerebral centers to cells in the spinal column; lower motor neurons consist of anterior horn cells and spinal and peripheral nerves. Motor fibers of the reflex arc are lower motor neurons. This is an important point because relative dominance of the CNS over reflex arcs suppresses some reflex responses. When the higher centers no longer exert an influence in SCI, spastic responses are observed in muscles innervated by the intact lower motor neurons. Most SCIs involve upper motor neurons; children born with spinal cord defects have primarily lower motor neuron deficits (see Fig. 34.7). Box 34.9 outlines manifestations of upper and lower motor neuron syndromes.

Effect on Sensory and Motor Tracts

Voluntary muscle control is lost after complete transection of the cord. In partial transection, function is altered to varying degrees depending on the areas innervated by involved nerves. The crossing of motor tracts at various levels makes it possible for an injured person to have motor paralysis in one leg but retain pain and temperature sensation in that leg, while the opposite leg retains its motor function but loses pain and temperature sensation.

Although a transected cord injury leads to sensory loss, it is not uncommon for the injured person to experience pain. For example, smooth or skeletal muscle spasms, destruction of the myelin sheath (impulses cross to adjacent nerves), and scar formation or irritation of nerve endings may cause pain. Pain suffered by a person with tetraplegia or paraplegia is often intensified because of loss of sensation in other parts. Severe and prolonged pain should be medically evaluated for a treatable pathologic condition.

BOX 34.10 Significant Effects of Autonomic Disruption

- Decreased muscle tone and impairment of vasoconstrictive effects of sympathetic innervation cause venous pooling; diminished venous return to the heart; decreased cardiac output; and hypotension, especially orthostatic hypotension (orthostatic intolerance).
- Thermoregulatory disruption in the hypothalamus and skin receptors causes blood vessels to remain dilated during the initial stage, an inability to sweat in response to increased environmental temperature, and a possible rapid elevation in body temperature.
- Voluntary bowel and bladder functions are lost because of damage to nerve fibers that innervate these organs.
- Altered sexual function (lack of erection, ejaculation, and orgasm) results from interference with numerous autonomic nerve fibers and plexuses.

Effect on Autonomic System

Sympathetic and parasympathetic systems receive both excitatory and inhibitory stimuli from autonomic centers in the cerebral cortex, limbic system, and hypothalamus. The stimuli are transmitted by means of a feedback mechanism within the ascending fibers of the cord that normally controls descending input. Axons of the many CNS neurons synapse with autonomic preganglionic fibers and thus are able to alter their patterned responses. Box 34.10 describes the most significant effects of autonomic disruption.

Etiology

The most common cause of serious spinal cord damage in children is trauma involving motor vehicle crashes (including automobile-bicycle, all-terrain vehicles, and snowmobiles), sports injuries (especially from diving, trampoline activities, gymnastics, and football), birth trauma, and nonaccidental trauma. MVCs accounted for 56% of SCIs in children and adolescents, and falls and firearm injury caused 14% and 9% of SCIs. The children injured (SCI) in MVCs were not properly restrained in 67.7% of the cases (Vitale, Goss, Matsumoto, et al., 2006). In the United States football injuries accounted for a high percentage of sport-related injuries in adolescents, whereas in Canada such injuries were associated with ice hockey (Mathison, Kadom, & Krug, 2008).

The increased use of recreational activities involving motorized vehicles such as jet water skis, all-terrain vehicles, and motorcycles has also increased the incidence of SCIs in children. Congenital defects of the spine such as myelomeningocele also may in some cases produce the effects of SCI (see p. 1313).

Transverse myelitis (inflammation of the spinal cord) may be caused by illness and has also been reported to develop from inadvertent intraarterial administration of long-acting penicillin injected into the buttocks. Damage can be extensive enough to result in paraplegia or even lower limb amputation.

In MVCs, most SCIs in children are a result of indirect trauma caused by sudden hyperflexion or hyperextension of the neck, often combined with a rotational force. Trauma to the spinal cord without evidence of vertebral fracture or dislocation (SCI without radiographic abnormality, or SCIWORA) is particularly likely to occur in an MVC when proper safety restraints are not used. An unrestrained child becomes a projectile during sudden deceleration and is subject to injury from contact with a variety of objects inside and outside the vehicle. Individuals who use only a lap seat belt restraint are at greater risk for SCI than those who use a combination lap and shoulder restraint. High cervical spine injuries have been reported in children younger than 2 years who are improperly restrained in forward-facing car seats. Infants who are improperly restrained in an infant car seat may experience cervical trauma in a car crash. Small children may also be severely injured by deploying front seat air bags.

Falling from heights occurs less often in children than in adults, but vertebral compression from blows to the head or buttocks can occur in water sports (diving and surfing), falls from horses, or other athletic activities. Birth injuries may occur in breech births from traction force on the spinal cord during birth of the head and shoulders. When shaken, infants commonly sustain cervical cord damage, as well as subdural hematoma and retinal hemorrhage; cognitive impairment and death may occur subsequent to the traumatic event. Infants have weak neck muscles, and during vigorous shaking, their large and heavy heads rapidly wobble back and forth. A significant number of adolescents receive SCIs secondary to gunshot wounds, stabbings, and other violent inflicted injury.

Because of the marked mobility of the neck, fracture or subluxation (partial dislocation) is the most common immediate cause of SCI, particularly in the lower cervical region. Although unusual in adults, SCI without fracture is common in children, whose spines are suppler, weaker, and more mobile than those of adults. Therefore the force is more easily dissipated over a larger number of segments. In infants and small children younger than 5 years, upper cervical spine fractures and spinal compression are more common, but adolescents tend to have lower cervical and thoracolumbar fracture dislocations (Rekate, 2015; Pruitt & McMahon, 2015). Children who suffer SCI before puberty are reported to experience a higher incidence of musculoskeletal complications such as scoliosis and hip dislocation (Vogel, Betz, & Mulcahey, 2012).

Pathophysiology

The severity of the force, the mechanisms of the injury, and the degree of the individual's muscular relaxation at the time of the injury greatly influence the extent of the trauma. SCIs are classified as either *complete* or *incomplete.* In a complete injury, there is no motor or sensory function more than three segments below the neurologic level of the injury (Mathison, Kadom, & Krug, 2008). Incomplete lesions have several typical characteristics (Mathison, Kadom, & Krug, 2008):

- Central cord syndrome—Central gray matter destruction and preservation of peripheral tracts; tetraplegia with sacral sparing common; some motor recovery gained
- Anterior cord syndrome—Complete motor and sensory loss with trunk and lower extremity proprioception and sensation of pressure
- Posterior cord syndrome—Loss of sensation, pain, and proprioception with normal cord function, including motor function; able to move extremities but have difficulty controlling such movements
- Brown-Séquard syndrome—Unilateral cord lesion with a motor deficit on the opposite side of the body from the primary insult; absence of pain and temperature sensation on the opposite side from the injury
- Spinal cord concussion—Transient loss of neural function below the level of the acute spinal cord lesion, resulting in flaccid paralysis and loss of tendon, autonomic, and cutaneous reflex activity; may last hours to weeks

The American Spinal Injury Association (ASIA) (Kirshblum, Waring, Biering-Sorensen, et al., 2011) International Standards for Neurological Classification of Spinal Cord Injury worksheet was recently revised and published in the cited reference. The ASIA Impairment Scale (Box 34.11) combines motor and sensory function and is used to determine the severity of impairment from the injury (complete or incomplete). It may also be used to measure neurologic changes and functional goals for rehabilitation (Mathison, Kadom, & Krug, 2008).

BOX 34.11 American Spinal Injury Association Impairment Scale

A—Complete: No motor or sensory function is preserved in the sacral segments S4–S5.

B—Sensory Incomplete: Sensory but not motor function is preserved below the neurologic level and includes the sacral segments S4–S5, or deep anal pressure, AND no motor function is preserved more than 3 levels below the motor level on either side of the body.

C—Motor Incomplete: Motor function is preserved below the neurologic level,* and more than half of key muscle functions below the single neurologic level of injury have a muscle grade less than 3.

D—Motor Incomplete: Motor function is preserved below the neurologic level,* and at least half (or more) of key muscles below the neurologic level have a muscle grade of 3 or more.

E—Normal: If sensation and motor function as tested with the International Standards for Neurological Classification of Spinal Cord Injury (ISNCSCI) are graded as normal in all segments, and the patient had prior deficits, then the AIS grade is E. Someone without an initial SCI does not receive an AIS grade.

*For further details and instructions see the online page at http://www.asia-spinalinjury.org/elearning/ISNCSCI_Exam_Sheet_r4.pdf. Used with permission, American Spinal Injury Association, 2011.

The injury sustained can affect any of the spinal nerves, and the higher the injury, the more extensive the damage. The child can be left with complete or partial paralysis of the lower extremities (paraplegia) or with damage at a higher level and without functional use of any of the four extremities (tetraplegia). A high cervical cord injury that affects the phrenic nerve paralyzes the diaphragm and leaves the child dependent on mechanical ventilation.

A mild but equally frightening form of cord trauma is spinal cord compression, a temporary neural dysfunction without visible damage to the cord. Complete tetraplegia can result but initially may not be differentiated from serious cord injury.

Clinical Manifestations

It is often difficult to determine the extent and severity of damage at first. Immediate loss of function is caused by both anatomic and impaired physiologic function, and improved function may not be evident for weeks or even months. Manifestation of the initial response to acute SCI is flaccid paralysis below the level of the damage. This stage is often referred to as spinal shock syndrome and is caused by the sudden disruption of central and autonomic pathways. Local effects of cord edema and ischemia produce a physiologic transection with or without an anatomic severance. Most children with an SCI experience some spinal shock. Manifestations include the absence of reflexes at or below the cord lesion, with flaccidity or limpness of the involved muscles, loss of sensation and motor function, and autonomic dysfunction (i.e., symptoms of hypotension, low or high body temperature, loss of bladder and bowel control, and autonomic dysreflexia). It is estimated that 25% to 50% of children with SCI will have a delay in the onset of neurologic abnormalities ranging from 30 minutes to 4 days (Vogel, Betz, & Mulcahey, 2012).

Autonomic paralysis also affects thermoregulatory functions. Afferent impulses from temperature receptors in the skin are not integrated; therefore the patient is subject to temperature increases or decreases in response to alterations in environmental temperature. Hyperthermia can result from excessive ambient temperature, such as too many covers.

Except in the situations previously mentioned, flaccid paralysis is replaced by spinal reflex activity and increasing spasticity or, in incomplete lesions, greater or lesser degree of neurologic recovery.

The paralytic nature of autonomic function is replaced by autonomic dysreflexia, especially when the lesions are above the midthoracic level. This autonomic phenomenon is caused by visceral distention or irritation, particularly of the bowel or bladder. Sensory impulses are triggered and travel to the cord lesion, where they are blocked, which causes activation of sympathetic reflex action with disturbed central inhibitory control. Excessive sympathetic activity is manifested by a flushing face, sweating forehead, pupillary constriction, marked hypertension, headache, and bradycardia. The precipitating stimulus may be merely a full bladder or rectum or other internal or external sensory input. It can be a catastrophic event unless the irritation is relieved.

Additional clinical findings of SCI may include numbness, tingling, or burning; priapism; weakness; and loss of bowel and bladder control (Hayes & Arriola, 2005).

Neurogenic shock occurs as a result of a disruption in the descending sympathetic pathways with loss of vasomotor tone and sympathetic innervations to the cardiovascular system (Hayes & Arriola, 2005). Hypotension, bradycardia, and peripheral vasodilation occur as a result of neurogenic shock.

Children with suspected SCI may have suffered multiple injuries (e.g., MVC); therefore multiple clinical manifestations may occur that may mask those of an SCI.

In the final stage neurologic signs are stabilized in terms of loss and recovery of function. The major emphasis is on rehabilitation. A problem unique to injury in childhood is progressive spinal deformity usually not seen in adults or in adolescents near the end of the growth period. Scoliosis develops in the majority of children with high thoracic and cervical lesions and is almost certain to occur in children with tetraplegia whose injury occurred in infancy or early childhood.

Diagnostic Evaluation

A history of the injury provides valuable clues regarding the possible type of damage incurred and directions for further assessment without the risk of additional damage. A complete neurologic examination determines whether damage was incurred and, if so, the level and extent of any nerve impairment. A neurologic unit of the CNS is considered normal if reflex arcs are functioning, sensory tracts are intact when each dermatome is examined separately, and voluntary motor response demonstrates an ability to move a body part against gravity on command.

Testing a reflex arc is accomplished by stimulating the peripheral receptors at a specific site, such as eliciting the patellar reflex. Symmetric testing is performed to determine unilateral or bilateral neurologic deficit. A sufficient number of reflexes are examined to test motor function thoroughly. The blunt end of a safety pin is used to assess pressure sensitivity, and the sharp point is used to elicit pain. Hot and cold water, a tuning fork, and cotton may also be used to determine specific sensory loss (e.g., temperature, vibration, and light touch).

The ASIA dermatome classification worksheet is used to determine the extent of neurologic damage (Fig. 34.9). Body surface zones, or dermatomes, accurately correspond to the spinal cord segment receiving the sensory input from the peripheral nerves in that zone. Systematically pinpricking the body surface in each zone determines intactness of sensory pathways. Fig. 34.9 illustrates the zones and the spinal cord segments they represent. The examiner tests for each specific sensory fiber in the dermatome areas in which neurologic deficit is suspected.

Matching cord level to vertebra is more difficult in infants and young children than it is in older children and adults because the sacral and several lower lumbar cord segments lie at a lower position, especially during the first 2 years of life. The spinal anatomy approaches adult configuration by the time the child reaches age 7 or 8 years; by late adolescence the conus medullaris has usually reached the level of L1.

Motor system evaluation includes observing gait if the child is able to walk; noting balance maintenance with the child's eyes open and closed; and noting the ability to lift, flex, and extend the arms and legs. Testing muscle strength with and without resistance and against gravity provides clues to the specific nature and degree of motor dysfunction. The number of muscles in any muscle group that remain completely intact in the upper extremities makes a marked difference in the individual's ability to provide self-care, especially at high injury levels. Hip movement is necessary for ambulation with braces and crutches.

The degree to which supportive aids are needed for ambulation is determined by the strength, stability, and movement of the pelvis, trunk, hip flexor muscles, and quadriceps muscles. A general guideline for determining the capacity for self-help is that a person with paraplegia who has function down to and including the quadriceps muscle or muscle function below the L3 level will have little difficulty in learning to walk with or without braces and crutches. It is especially vital that children with lumbar levels of injury be taught to walk functionally so that they are weight bearing at least part of the time; this minimizes the risk of osteoporosis and hypercalcemia. The functional significance of the spinal cord lesion level is given in Table 34.1.

If a CNS pathologic disorder is detected, a body system assessment is performed to determine the degree of autonomic impairment. Because the cord and CNS directly influence the function of the autonomic nerves, the specific sympathetically related organ systems are examined for skeletal muscle and vascular tone and body temperature regulation. For example, bladder and GI functions have sympathetic and parasympathetic innervation and local reflexes.

CT and MRI scans are important for localizing the lesion, but the nature of the spine in childhood often creates difficulty in interpretation. Guidelines for diagnostic imaging of children with suspected SCI have been published elsewhere (Rozelle, Arabi, Dhall, et al., 2013). Small children often have no radiographic evidence of vertebral or spinal injury despite significant injuries ranging from complete transection with major hemorrhage to minor hemorrhage, edema, or normal neural findings. This condition, SCIWORA, is reported to occur in approximately 64% of children 5 years of age or younger and in 19% to 32% of older children with SCIs (Launay, Leet, & Sponseller, 2005; Mathison, Kadom, & Krug, 2008; Vogel, Betz, & Mulcahey, 2012). The younger the child, the more likely for SCIWORA to occur—up to 72% of children 5 and under (Schottler, Vogel, & Sturm, 2012). SCIWORA is also a common finding in very young children who are victims of abuse (primarily shaken baby syndrome) because of the elasticity and incomplete ossification of the vertebrae. SCIWORA is more common in children under the age of 8 years, and injury to the cervical spine is common. Diagnostic scans must be taken carefully and with sufficient help to prevent further damage to the spine.

Therapeutic Management

Initial care begins at the scene of the accident with proper immobilization of the cervical, thoracic, and lumbar spine. Immobilization should take into account the age and size of the child; smaller children have a larger head size, which may make effective immobilization on a rigid board difficult (Rozelle, Arabi, Dhall, et al., 2013). Because of the complexity of these injuries, it is usually recommended that these persons be transported to a spinal injury center for care by specially trained health care personnel as soon as possible after the injury for appropriate diagnostic evaluation and intervention.

The initial management of the child with a suspected SCI should begin with an assessment of the ABCs: **a**irway, **b**reathing, and **c**irculation. The airway should be opened using the jaw-thrust technique to minimize

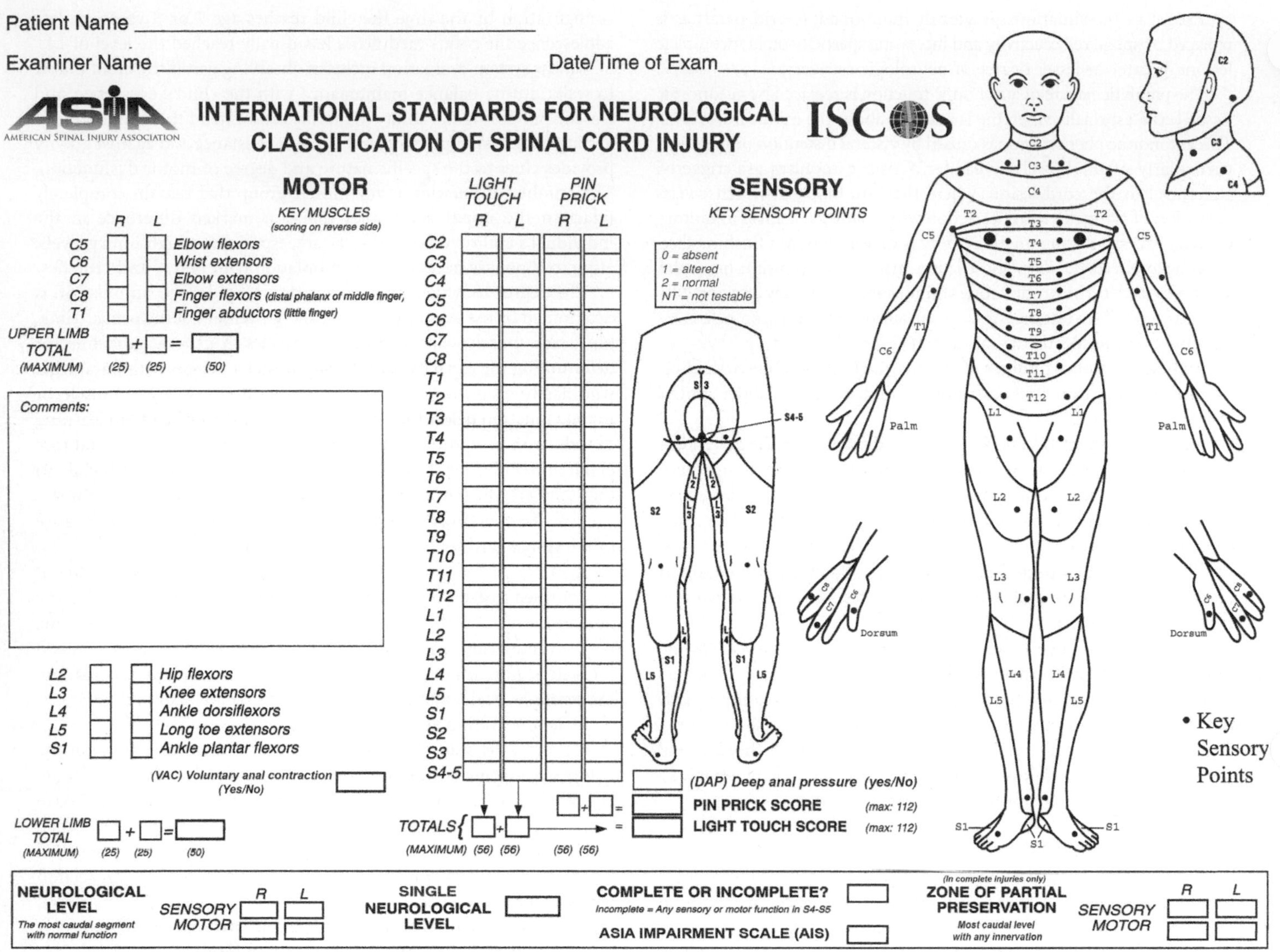

Patient Name ______________________

Examiner Name ______________________ Date/Time of Exam ______________________

ASIA AMERICAN SPINAL INJURY ASSOCIATION

INTERNATIONAL STANDARDS FOR NEUROLOGICAL CLASSIFICATION OF SPINAL CORD INJURY

ISCOS

MOTOR

KEY MUSCLES (scoring on reverse side)

	R	L	
C5			Elbow flexors
C6			Wrist extensors
C7			Elbow extensors
C8			Finger flexors (distal phalanx of middle finger)
T1			Finger abductors (little finger)

UPPER LIMB TOTAL (MAXIMUM) ☐ + ☐ = ☐ (25) (25) (50)

Comments:

	R	L	
L2			Hip flexors
L3			Knee extensors
L4			Ankle dorsiflexors
L5			Long toe extensors
S1			Ankle plantar flexors

(VAC) Voluntary anal contraction (Yes/No) ☐

LOWER LIMB TOTAL (MAXIMUM) ☐ + ☐ = ☐ (25) (25) (50)

	LIGHT TOUCH R	LIGHT TOUCH L	PIN PRICK R	PIN PRICK L
C2				
C3				
C4				
C5				
C6				
C7				
C8				
T1				
T2				
T3				
T4				
T5				
T6				
T7				
T8				
T9				
T10				
T11				
T12				
L1				
L2				
L3				
L4				
L5				
S1				
S2				
S3				
S4-5				

TOTALS ☐ + ☐ ☐ + ☐ (MAXIMUM) (56) (56) (56) (56)

SENSORY

KEY SENSORY POINTS

0 = absent
1 = altered
2 = normal
NT = not testable

(DAP) Deep anal pressure (yes/No) ☐

PIN PRICK SCORE (max: 112) ☐

LIGHT TOUCH SCORE (max: 112) ☐

NEUROLOGICAL LEVEL (The most caudal segment with normal function)	R	L
SENSORY		
MOTOR		

SINGLE NEUROLOGICAL LEVEL ☐

COMPLETE OR INCOMPLETE? ☐ Incomplete = Any sensory or motor function in S4-S5

ASIA IMPAIRMENT SCALE (AIS) ☐

(In complete injuries only) ZONE OF PARTIAL PRESERVATION (Most caudal level with any innervation)	R	L
SENSORY		
MOTOR		

This form may be copied freely but should not be altered without permission from the American Spinal Injury Association.

REV 04/11

FIG. 34.9 ASIA classification of spinal cord injury. (Used with permission, American Spinal Injury Association, 2011. Retrieved from http://asia-spinalinjury.org/?s=ASIA+spinal+cord+injury+classification)

damage to the cervical spine. The child is monitored for cardiovascular instability, and measures are taken to support systemic blood pressure and maintain optimal cardiac output. Because MVCs and other trauma in children may involve internal organ damage and potential bleeding, abdominal distention and other signs are acted on immediately to prevent further systemic shock. After the child is stabilized and transported to a regional trauma center, a thorough evaluation of neurologic status and any other associated trauma is carried out by the multidisciplinary team. In the emergency department, spinal immobilization should be maintained until a thorough neurologic assessment is completed and spinal cord injury is ruled out; in children, this typically involves a CT scan and possibly an MRI. Additional interventions are discussed in the Nursing Care Management section. Assessment of neurologic status using the Glasgow Coma Scale (see Chapter 30) is important; a helpful assessment is represented in the mnemonic AVPU: *a*lert; responds to *v*erbal stimuli; responds to *p*ainful stimuli; and *u*nresponsive. A secondary assessment tool in the emergency department follows the mnemonic AMPLE: *a*llergies, *m*edications, *p*ast medical history, *l*ast meal or fluids, and *e*nvironment and events leading to the incident (Avarello & Cantor, 2007).

The American Association of Neurological Surgeons and the Congress of Neurological Surgeons have published spinal cord injury management guidelines and standards of care for adult and pediatric patients with SCIs. Recently evidence-based guidelines for the management of SCI in children were published (Rozelle, Arabi, Dhall, et al., 2013).

IV methylprednisone may be started within the first 12 hours after the injury to decrease inflammation and minimize further injury; however, its use in small children is controversial. Studies of methylprednisone administration in adults with SCI have shown mixed results, with experts recommending against its use in acute SCI (Hurlbert, Hadley, Walters, et al., 2013).

In children with upper motor neuron involvement, the spasticity that develops may require administration of an antispasmodic medication such as diazepam. Baclofen is considered the drug of choice for reducing muscle spasticity (Vogel, Betz, & Mulcahey, 2012). Gabapentin may be used to treat neuropathic pain (Hayes & Arriola, 2005). Botulinum toxin type A and α_2-adrenergic agonists may be used in older children with SCI to decrease muscle spasticity.

A number of progressive rehabilitation modalities have been developed in recent years that have the potential for increasing the quality of life for children with SCI. One treatment is functional electrical stimulation (FES), also referred to as *functional neuromuscular stimulation* or *neuromuscular electrical stimulation.* With this treatment, an electrical stimulator is surgically implanted under the skin in the abdomen and electrode leads are tunneled to paralyzed leg muscles, enabling the child to sit, stand, and walk with the aid of crutches, a walker, or other orthoses. The stimulator can also be used to elicit a voluntary grasp and release with the hand. Before the latter can be accomplished, a number of surgical tendon transfers may be required for elbow extension, wrist extension, and finger and thumb flexion. In addition, FES has therapeutic benefits, which include increased muscle strength, improved gait function, and increased cardiovascular fitness (Thrasher & Popovic, 2008). Tendon transfers have been shown to be successful in enhancing hand and arm function, increasing pinch force, and facilitating independence in ADLs (Hosalkar, Pandya, Hsu, et al., 2009). Restoration of hand and arm function enables children with SCI to perform self-catheterization and achieve greater independence in personal hygiene.

Exercise is considered an integral part of SCI rehabilitation; exercise may enhance neuroplasticity and decrease further muscle atrophy. Examples of exercise modalities in SCI patients include upper body strength training and hand cycling (Hosalkar, Pandya, Hsu, et al., 2009).

Administration of pharmacologic agents such as clonidine hydrochloride may improve ambulation in patients with partial SCIs, and exercise therapy through interactive locomotor training has helped some individuals with SCI regain ambulatory function.

A number of orthoses or ambulation aids such as crutches may still be necessary to achieve upright mobility, yet as robotic technology advances, so do the chances for improved mobilization in children with SCI. Mechanical or robotic orthoses may be used in conjunction with FES to enable ambulation in persons with SCI (To, Kirsch, Kobetic, et al., 2005). Gait training may be achieved with a number of different modalities, including a stationary cycle; however, no specific method has proved superior to the others. FES has also been effective in reducing complications from bladder and bowel incontinence and in assisting males in achieving penile erection. Ambulation is an important part of rehabilitation in SCI; retrospective studies found that ambulation was dependent on age at injury and extent of neurologic injury (as measured by ASIA motor scales). Age (younger) and lesser neurologic impairment are key predictors for ambulation (Vogel, Betz, & Mulcahey, 2012). A knee ankle-foot orthosis and reciprocating-gait orthosis may also be used to assist with early rehabilitation and ambulation (Vogel, Betz, & Mulcahey, 2012). Additional detailed information regarding ambulation and orthotics for children have been published elsewhere (Calhoun, Schottler, & Vogel, 2013).

Surgical interventions for SCI include early cord decompression (decompression laminectomy) and cervical or thoracic fusion. Crutchfield, Vinke, or Gardner-Wells tongs and skeletal traction may be used for early cervical vertebral stabilization. A halo vest or Minerva jacket may be suited for ambulation after the acute phase. (See also Cervical Traction, Chapter 33) After cervical spinal fusion, a hard cervical collar or sterno-occipital-mandibular immobilizer brace may be worn until the fusion is solidified. When SCI occurs in young children and preteens, scoliosis develops over time and often requires surgical consideration (Parent, Mac-Thiong, Roy-Beaudry, et al., 2011).

Prognosis

The ultimate outlook for spinal cord function after injury depends on the completeness of the cord transection, site of injury, complicating damage to the neuronal tissue, and success of treatment regimens aimed at recovery of lost muscle movement and ability. Healing of the injury and the return of neurologic function are related to two factors:

1. Although individual nerve fibers do regenerate, they do not necessarily reconnect or make synaptic connections with the distal portion of the severed fibers; the chance of numerous fibers reconnecting is highly unlikely.
2. The damage resulting from cord ischemia produces necrosis in the gray and white matter of the cord tissue, which does not regenerate if the axon cylinder is not intact.

In children the prognosis for recovery is considered better than in adults because children have rapid healing of bone and ligaments and increased potential for nervous system regeneration. Paraplegia is more common in children under 12 years, whereas older children and adolescents tend to have incomplete injuries (Mathison, Kadom, & Krug, 2008). Shavelle, DeVivo, Paculdo, and colleagues (2007) reported an increased likelihood of mortality among children less than 16 years of age who suffered an SCI in comparison to adults with similar injuries. Children with incomplete injuries (and who are not ventilator dependent) had a projected 83% chance of normal life expectancy, whereas those with high-level cervical injuries who are not ventilator dependent had a 50% chance of having a normal life expectancy. One study found that adults who had an SCI as children (less than 18 years of age at time of incident) had comparable or greater degrees of education in comparison to the general population of the same age (Vogel, Chlan, Zebracki, et al., 2011). The same study found lower employment rates for adults with pediatric-onset SCI, lower rates of independent living and independent driving, and lower rates of marriage in this select population.

In general, recovery of motor function in children with thoracic lesions is variable. Cervical injuries are also variable in the extent of damage. Incomplete lesions produce hemiplegia, whereas complete transection implies some involvement of all extremities—from partial use of the upper extremities to complete paralysis, including the need for some type of assisted ventilation. Lumbar injury may involve partial or complete loss of function in the lower extremities and bladder. With rapidly advancing surgical technology, use of microcomputers in medicine, and newer treatment modalities such as FES, there are increasing hope and evidence that functional mobility and independence can be restored in children with SCI. (See Quality Patient Outcomes box.)

QUALITY PATIENT OUTCOMES

Neurologic Impairment

- Neurologic status maintained or improved
- No further injuries

Nursing Care Management

The nursing care of the child affected by SCI is complex and challenging. A multidisciplinary SCI team is equipped to manage the acute phase of the injury, and some members, including the nurse, may follow the patient to eventual recovery. Nursing management is concerned with ensuring adequate initial stabilization of the entire spinal column with a rigid cervical collar with supportive blocks on a rigid backboard. The traumatic event causing the injury may or may not be recalled if the child lost consciousness; such events are extremely frightening to the child. The young child may also be frightened by the immobilization process and the inability to move extremities; therefore it is important to reassure and comfort the child during this process.

During the acute phase of the injury it is imperative that airway patency be ensured, complications prevented, and function maintained.

Evaluate the extent of the neurologic damage early to establish a baseline for neurologic function. Continual assessment of sensory and motor function should occur to prevent further deterioration of neurologic status as a result of spinal cord edema. The ASIA Impairment Scale can be used to assess neurologic function on a routine basis during the patient's recovery. Once the patient is admitted, further evaluation of his or her ability to perform ADLs and need for assistance during recovery can be made with the Functional Independence Measure scale.

Nursing care during the acute phase should also focus on frequent monitoring of neurologic signs to determine any changes in neurologic function that require further intervention (e.g., level of consciousness using the Glasgow Coma Scale). In addition to airway maintenance, the nurse monitors for changes in hemodynamic status that may require immediate medical attention. Neurogenic shock consists of hypotension, bradycardia, and vasodilation. Inotropic medications may be required to maintain adequate perfusion. Renal function is closely monitored by measuring urinary output and fluids administered. The child with a head injury may experience elevated intracranial pressure; therefore changes in neurologic status are reported to the practitioner. Fluid restriction may be required if intracranial pressure is elevated, so fluid intake should be closely monitored.

The nursing care of the child with an SCI is, in most respects, the same as that of any immobilized child (see The Immobilized Child, Chapter 33). Additional aspects of care that should be addressed on an individual basis include hypercalcemia in adolescent boys, DVT, latex sensitization, pain, hypothermia and hyperthermia, spasticity, autonomic dysreflexia, and sleep-disordered breathing (Vogel, Betz, & Mulcahey 2012).

Respiratory Care

The child with a high-level cervical injury (C3 and above) requires continuous ventilatory assistance. In most instances a tracheostomy is the method of choice for greater ease in clearing secretions and for less trauma to tissues during long-term ventilatory dependence. Patient-triggered synchronous intermittent mandatory ventilation (SIMV–assist/control mode) may be required to maintain adequate oxygenation. In an acute care center, respiratory therapy personnel are often responsible for establishing and maintaining the equipment, but the nurse must understand how it works and recognize mechanical malfunction and deviations from the prescribed rate and volume. In case of malfunction the nurse must be prepared to maintain respirations manually with a self-inflating bag-valve-mask device. In many home care situations the family is responsible for the care of ventilatory assistance devices; therefore adequate family training and availability of the nurse (or durable medical equipment representative) for questions related to the equipment and evaluation of the child's breathing are essential. For some children, breathing pacemaker devices (phrenic nerve stimulators) are implanted to stimulate the phrenic nerve and produce diaphragmatic contractions and lung expansion without assisted ventilation.

Children with lesions below the C4 level are seldom ventilator dependent, but pulmonary vital capacity is significantly reduced. Position them for optimum chest expansion, and use a variety of breathing exercises and assistive devices to stimulate deep breathing. Chest physiotherapy is performed as needed to mobilize secretions, and flow-by oxygen may be needed occasionally. Regular monitoring of breath sounds to assess for adequate ventilation in all lung fields is part of routine care.

The cough reflex may be markedly diminished, which, combined with weak intercostal muscles, may mean the child has difficulty with secretions. Increasing the elastic qualities of the lung by breathing exercises, mechanical cough assist techniques, and incentive spirometry helps the child achieve a productive cough. (See discussion of airway management and airway clearance devices under Muscular Dystrophies: Therapeutic Management.)

Cardiovascular Care

Children with SCI may experience cardiovascular instability as a result of loss of vagal tone, vagal stimulation during procedures such as oral suctioning or insertion of a nasogastric tube, turning, and endotracheal suctioning. Close monitoring of heart rate and blood pressure is essential to detect any signs of decreased cardiac output. Pneumothorax may occur, resulting in a mediastinal shift and decreased cardiac output. Autonomic dysreflexia may occur and result in decreased cardiac output (see discussion later).

The child with loss of muscle tone and prolonged immobility may be at high risk for the development of DVT. In addition, major reparative surgery for associated injuries and spinal decompression place the child at risk for thrombus formation. DVT is prevented with the use of pneumatic compression devices and low-molecular-weight heparin during the acute phase of care. Fluid and electrolyte balance may be impaired as a result of trauma and associated injuries or decreased fluid intake during the recovery period. Fluid intake should be closely monitored, especially with regard to the development of pulmonary edema and intracranial pressure. The child may require nasogastric tube feedings due to anorexia and immobility.

Temperature Regulation

Temperature is often poorly regulated in children with SCI; therefore body temperature must be monitored closely for fluctuations. In small children hypothermia may occur relative to large body surface and inability to mount an appropriate metabolic response to the initial injury, so close attention should be given to preserving body temperature. Response to environmental temperature changes may be slow or absent, and the ability to dissipate heat through the process of shivering may be compromised.

During the spinal shock stage the dilated capillaries conducting body heat to the subcutaneous tissues cause heat loss. Without the capacity to sweat, the body retains heat in hot weather. An elevated temperature that cannot be corrected by environmental measures should be evaluated to rule out urinary or upper respiratory tract infection. However, excessive perspiration observed in sentient areas usually indicates an elevated ambient temperature.

Skin Care

Children with SCI have unique needs in relation to skin care. Because of decreased sensation and impaired mobility, they depend on others to assess and assist in the management of intact skin. Skin care practices are the same as those for any child who is immobilized. A skin score scale such as the Braden Q Scale can objectively evaluate risks for skin breakdown and skin conditions (Noonan, Quigley, &Curley, 2011). Keep an alternating-pressure mattress or other pressure relief/reduction device underneath the child, and inspect the skin thoroughly at least twice a day for signs of pressure, especially over bony prominences. Prevention of skin breakdown is much easier than treatment. A number of factors contribute to the risk of skin breakdown in these children: decreased sensation, inadequate nutrition, muscle spasticity, impaired peripheral circulation, diaphoresis, mechanical shearing from assistive devices, and improper positioning. (See Maintaining Healthy Skin, Chapter 22)

The areas most likely to be affected are the sacrum, scapulae, heels, and occiput when the child is supine; the trochanters and the lateral aspect of the ankles, heels, and knees when the child is in a side-lying position; and the ischial tuberosities when the child is sitting. The pressure wound may begin in deeper tissues and be visible on the surface only at a later stage. Therefore areas that feel firm, irregular, or warm or that appear to be only slightly reddened require careful evaluation. Keeping the skin clean and dry is particularly important in these children, especially those who are incontinent of urine or stool or those who have significant diaphoresis. When there is any evidence of skin breakdown, treatment to prevent further breakdown is implemented promptly. When orthotic devices such as AFOs and braces are used, skin care and vigilance for pressure areas are also important in the prevention of pressure ulcers. Prolonged use of wheelchairs without special sacral protection may also lead to skin ulceration.

The child who is heavily sedated or who is being given muscle paralytics should receive appropriate eye care to prevent corneal damage (e.g., artificial tears, ointment, and impermeable eye shield). Additional nursing care may involve the administration of histamine blockers and proton pump inhibitors to prevent stress ulcers by reducing the secretion of hydrochloric acid.

Physical Therapy

An important consideration for the child with SCI is achievement of mobility and ambulation. A developmental approach should be considered in the rehabilitation phase (Calhoun, Schottler, & Vogel, 2013). Range-of-motion, passive, and active exercises are carried out under the guidance of a physical therapist.

Unless there are contraindications, exercises during the period of immobilization are aimed at maintaining and increasing the strength of the child's intact musculature. Upper extremity strengthening is especially important to the paraplegic child, who must rely on these muscle groups for turning, transferring, dressing, parallel bar walking, gait training, and other activities. Children are usually eager to use their muscles and respond to interesting and innovative activities.

Neurogenic Bladder

When the bladder is denervated, as in the acute stage of spinal shock syndrome or after lower motor neuron damage, the bladder wall is flaccid. Lack of muscle tone inhibits the bladder's ability to respond to changes in passive pressure, causing overdistention. Therefore it is important to prevent distention by periodic emptying, even though there may be dribbling between emptying.

In contrast, an upper motor neuron lesion causes increased bladder tone and contractions that often include the urinary sphincter. Thus although the bladder empties periodically by reflex action, complete emptying is prevented, resulting in urinary retention and ureteral reflux. Administration of an anticholinergic drug such as dicyclomine (Bentyl) relaxes bladder musculature and promotes increased bladder capacity and more adequate emptying. Intervals of urination depend on many factors, including patterns of fluid intake and perspiration.

In school-age children and adolescents, achieving bladder and bowel continence is a significant developmental issue related to self-esteem and perception of self in relation to peers. Therefore it is imperative to consider options that best meet the child's physiologic and emotional needs.

Surgical options for children with neurogenic bladder include the creation of a urinary stoma, made possible by removing the appendix and creating a urinary diversion from the bladder to the exterior, usually the umbilicus, thus making self-catheterization more private, especially with the recovery of hand and elbow movement (with tendon transfers). Other options include surgical bladder augmentation to increase capacity and FES to restore micturition on command without a urinary catheter (Merenda & Hickey, 2005).

Emptying the bladder by clean intermittent catheterization (CIC) is also an option for children with SCI; older children who are functionally capable can learn to perform self-catheterization. Encourage the child to adhere to a schedule for CIC and to maintain a regular pattern of fluid intake throughout the day; they should avoid large intakes of fluid without considering the need for more frequent CIC. Caffeinated beverages and other caffeinated foods are used sparingly to avoid bladder overdistention with increased urine formation (Francis, 2007). Latex catheters should be avoided to prevent the development of latex allergy (if it is not already present). Bladder-training programs usually begin with intermittent bladder emptying at regular intervals that are gradually increased. (See Management of Genitourinary Function under Myelomeningocele [Meningomyelocele], p. 1313.) The Credé method (applying suprapubic pressure) for emptying the bladder may be used by some individuals with SCI, but this may result in high intravesical pressures, causing further bladder complications (Francis, 2007).

Urinary tract infections are common due to urinary stasis. A regular schedule of CIC may help prevent such infections. Encourage the child to increase fluid intake by approximately 240 ml/day and use CIC every 3 to 4 hours.

Maintenance of bladder dynamics and control of urinary tract infections are of utmost importance. Pyelonephritis and renal failure are the most significant causes of death in long-standing paraplegia.

Bowel Training

The loss of bowel function is considered to be one of the most stressful events when quality-of-life issues are considered in persons with SCI; however, successful bowel training is easier to institute than bladder management. The aim is to control defecation until an appropriate time and place are found. Merenda and Hickey (2005) propose four components in a successful bowel management program: desired stool consistency (i.e., a soft stool), a regular evacuation pattern, upright positioning for planned evacuation, and motivation and commitment from the child and family.

A diet with sufficient fiber (age in years plus 5 grams is recommended) for adequate stool bulk and insertion of a glycerin or bisacodyl (Dulcolax) suppository at a convenient time, either morning or evening, are often all that are necessary to induce a bowel movement within a short time. The probability of an accident between times diminishes once the bowel is completely evacuated. The key to adequate bowel training is to maintain consistency in the time of day for evacuation. Stool softeners, such as docusate sodium (Colace) and senna (Senokot), may be prescribed, and manual anal stimulation may help initiate evacuation, especially in spastic paraplegia. Sometimes an oral laxative such as bisacodyl may be necessary. Once an appropriate regimen is established, little modification is required.

One surgical option is the antegrade continence enema, which involves the creation of a stoma whereby colonic washouts may be performed with the child sitting on the toilet. FES has also been used successfully in some children with SCI to achieve bowel training.

Autonomic Dysreflexia

Children with high-level lesions are susceptible to the development of autonomic dysreflexia, which requires prompt action to prevent encephalopathy and shock. Clinical manifestations of autonomic dysreflexia include an increase in systemic blood pressure, headache, bradycardia, profuse diaphoresis, cardiac arrhythmias, flushing, piloerection, blurred vision, nasal congestion, anxiety, spots on the visual field, or absent or minimum symptoms. A quick assessment may rule out other causes, such as orthostatic intolerance. After that, vital signs, including blood pressure, are taken while the bladder is checked for distention (the usual precipitating cause). The bladder is drained slowly; if this does not relieve symptoms, any tight clothing is loosened, and the bowel is checked for the pressure of impacted feces.

Other potential causes of autonomic dysreflexia in SCI children include bowel impaction and abdominal distention, pressure ulcers, tight clothing, burns, DVT, menses, trauma, fractures, pregnancy, labor, surgery or invasive procedures, any painful stimulus, and hyperthermia (Vogel, Betz, & Mulcahey, 2012). If removal of the causative agent is unsuccessful in controlling the syndrome, IV administration of an antihypertensive drug is indicated, followed by oral maintenance doses. Antispasmodics may also be administered.

Remobilization

As soon as the condition warrants, the child is moved from a reclining to an upright position. Cardiovascular deconditioning and impaired autonomic responses below the level of injury will cause pooling of blood in the extremities (because of peripheral vasodilation); a drop in blood pressure; and a feeling of lightheadedness, dizziness, or fainting on sudden assumption of an upright posture, often referred to as orthostatic intolerance. Therefore an upright position must be accomplished gradually by first placing the child (who is secured by passive restraint) on a head-up tilt table. The table is slowly elevated from a horizontal to a 30-degree semireclining position. This is performed twice daily for 20 to 30 minutes, with the angle gradually increased until the vertical angle is reached.

During the procedure the vital signs are monitored, and the child's behavior is observed for subjective symptoms of syncope. The pooling of blood is reduced by using elastic antiembolism stockings and sequential pneumatic compression devices, which consist of inflatable sleeves that fit on the legs and compress the leg muscles for cyclic emptying and filling of leg veins. The process of achieving an upright posture may require several weeks. After tolerance is achieved, the child will be ready to begin using a wheelchair. Getting the child up should be accomplished slowly by gradually elevating the bed over 20 to 30 minutes before placing the child in the wheelchair and then gradually lowering the legs after the child has been in the chair a short time.

All adaptive devices help children increase their mobility, function, and endurance. The child with some lower extremity function progresses to parallel bars and then to a walker. The child with tetraplegia learns to use a wheelchair—among the most valuable aids available to the child with an SCI. The wheelchair should be selected carefully in relation to where it will be used, the architectural barriers, and the child's functional capacity. For lower extremity paralysis, the wheelchair described on p. 1259 is applicable. For children with severe upper extremity paralysis, a variety of motorized wheelchairs are used; however, the more complex they are, the greater their cost, weight, and tendency to break down. Wheelchair tolerance is gained over time and is accompanied by measures to prevent orthostatic hypotension and pressure sores.

A variety of orthoses and other appliances can be adapted for use by many children. The primary purpose of lower extremity bracing in the child with an SCI is for ambulation, although correction of deformities may be attempted. However, the efficacy is limited because of the tendency to develop pressure lesions over insensate areas. The higher the lesion, the more support required, with the accompanying difficulties of getting into the orthosis and the greater energy expended in using the appliance. The energy required in walking with crutches and braces is two to four times greater than that required for normal walking.

Children, with their natural and overwhelming desire for mobility, usually attain or even surpass the maximum expectation in ambulation. However, as they approach adulthood, the increasing weight and energy cost usually cause them to resort to predominant use of the wheelchair for mobility and the pursuit of more intellectual and vocational interests. Wheelchair mobility has the advantages of requiring no more energy than normal walking and allowing the person with paraplegia to maintain the speed of other pedestrians on level ground.

Physical Rehabilitation

The process of physical rehabilitation usually begins once the child is medically stable and associated problems have been managed. The major aims of physical rehabilitation are to prepare the child and family to achieve normalization and resume life at home and in the community. Additional goals of rehabilitation in children with SCI are to promote independence in mobility and self-care skills, academic achievement, independent living, and employment (Box 34.12).

Members of the multidisciplinary rehabilitation team cooperate with one another and the family to identify the child's needs and to plan realistic interventions. Integration of activities is coordinated by one team member, most often a specialist in physical medicine and rehabilitation. Members of the team attempt to achieve their collaborative goals through mutual trust, good communication, professional respect, and sincere interest in the child and family. Training in the rehabilitation center promotes maximum achievement commensurate with each child's physical capacities (Fig. 34.10). Instruction for home routine is stressed and includes all the precautions and management implemented in the acute care center (e.g., skin care, nutrition, bladder and bowel training, gait training) and an exercise program.

Inpatient physical rehabilitation of children with tetraplegia takes approximately 2 to 4 months; children with paraplegia can achieve these goals in 1 to 3 months but require constant vigilance to avoid complications. Emotional adjustments take longer, especially in older children and adolescents. In most children the outlook is favorable unless the life-threatening consequences of urinary pathologic condition are severe or the emotional adjustment is poor.

BOX 34.12 Goals of Rehabilitation for the Child With a Spinal Cord Injury

- Maximizing motor function and minimizing the disabling effects of the pathologic condition
- Assisting the child and family in setting realistic goals for the child, learning to be good problem solvers, and using the child's assets
- Helping the child cope with the stigma of being different and build a positive self-image

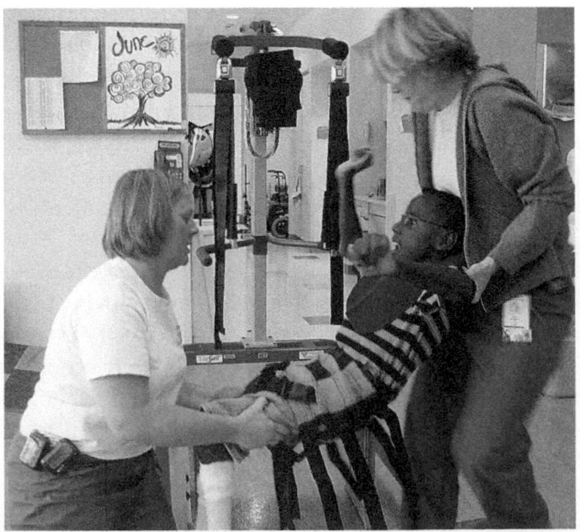

FIG. 34.10 Training in a rehabilitation facility can promote achievement and encourage the child to strive to reach his maximum physical abilities. (Courtesy E. Jacob, Texas Children's Hospital, Houston.)

Psychosocial Rehabilitation

Early-acquired or congenital disability is usually more readily accepted by children than paralysis that appears later in childhood. Rehabilitation efforts should include not only the child's emotional responses but also those of the persons closest to the child. Intensive education is important so that family members understand the nature of the disability, the therapeutic regimen, and complications and are able to provide the physical and emotional support the child needs.

As with any disability, treat children as normally as possible and encourage them in developmental tasks at the age at which they would typically be expected to acquire abilities and perform activities. However, the goals must be realistic, and children should not be forced beyond their capabilities. Vogel, Betz, & Mulcahey (2012) emphasize the need for children and adolescents with SCI to assume responsibility for their own care. When this is not physically possible, they should direct others in their care. Encouraging self-care is important in the emotional and physical rehabilitation of the child or adolescent with SCI.

Severe depression can be emotionally and intellectually immobilizing, but it indicates that the child is no longer hiding behind denial. In rehabilitation it is desirable for the child to begin to express negative feelings toward the situation because these feelings, redirected by efforts of the rehabilitation team, are the ones that will motivate the child toward learning a new way of life. Anxiety and depression in young children and adolescents with SCI are associated with a poorer quality of life (Anderson, Kelly, Klaas, et al., 2009).

The responses to loss are discussed in Chapter 19. The multiple problems related to altered self-image, especially in older children and adolescents, are discussed in relation to children with disabilities in Chapter 21. Children with severe disabilities need to alter certain concepts about self and social roles. If they perceive adults as persons with complete control over their bodies and the ability to do what they want when they want, they will need to develop a more realistic definition of interdependent adult living.

The needs of young children and adolescents who are permanently disabled must be reevaluated periodically by the total rehabilitation team, including the children and their families. Vocational rehabilitation is important for helping these adolescents find meaningful work activities and enroll in formal educational programs as desired.

The outlook for children and adolescents with SCI is increasingly favorable for integration into society. Increased awareness of the needs of persons with disabilities has removed many structural and occupational barriers. The success of a rehabilitation program is judged not by how well children and adolescents manage within the rehabilitation setting but by how well they function on the outside. In addition to agencies that offer assistance to children with disabilities in general, some agencies provide specific assistance to paralyzed persons, including children.

Sexuality

Issues related to loss of sexual function also apply to adolescents with debilitating neuromuscular diseases such as Duchenne muscular dystrophy (DMD) and SMA. The problems of self-image are particularly significant when children with SCI reach puberty, especially if the disability was acquired during early adolescence. Sexual development and awareness and changing perceptions of body image are prominent aspects of adolescence; a loss that affects these areas is often devastating. Development of secondary sexual characteristics does not seem to be altered by SCIs, and it is now believed that with comprehensive rehabilitation, motivated young people can look forward to successful participation in marital and family activities.

In females, if the injury occurs after the onset of menstruation, there is usually a temporary cessation and irregularity in menstrual flow, but menstruation resumes in the majority of cases. Ovulation and conception are possible, but only about 50% of females experience vaginal or clitoral orgasms, although they can learn to use other erogenous zones for a sexual experience. This is important to emphasize in sex education because many females have the misconception that they are unable to conceive because they lack sensation. FES may help some women with SCI achieve orgasm. Education is important because the pregnant paraplegic or tetraplegic patient may be unaware that she is in labor, and those with a high-level injury are subject to autonomic dysreflexia during labor.

More attention has been focused on rehabilitating male sexual function (erection and ejaculation) than female sexual function until the last two decades. A number of pharmacologic (prostaglandin E_1) and mechanical devices (e.g., penile implants, vacuum pump devices) now make it possible for males to participate in sexual intercourse and produce offspring, provided that fertility has not been affected by associated complications. Penile injections with vasoactive substances (prostaglandin E_1) are reported to be effective in 90% of men (DeForge, Blackmer, Garritty, et al., 2006). However, sildenafil (Viagra) is now considered the treatment of choice for the sexually active male. Adolescents with SCI should be counseled regarding condom use and the symptoms of latex allergy.

As soon as adolescent males become aware of their functional loss, they will be concerned about sexual capacities, regardless of the type of sexual activities experienced before the SCI. The health care professional should take the initiative in discussing sexuality with adolescents and their families. Parents of younger children may want to know about their children's sexual and reproductive potential. As their interest and understanding increase, adolescents need to know the specifics of physiology, the prognosis, and sexual techniques related to their particular problems. The practitioner should provide them with information about what can be expected regarding erection, ejaculation, and other sexual experiences.

A knowledgeable rehabilitation team is valuable to adolescents as they experience concerns regarding loss as a sexual being. This is especially true in paraplegia or tetraplegia. Most sexual counseling for adolescents with SCI focuses on developing the idea that sex means different things to different people. Most rehabilitation teams have an active counseling program to help adolescents learn intimacy and how to function sexually within their limitations. Through individual and group counseling they gain new attitudes concerning sexuality and experiences exclusive or inclusive of intercourse. Guidelines for sexual and reproductive health care of persons with SCI are published elsewhere (Consortium for Spinal Cord Medicine, 2010).

Transition to Adulthood

With the ultimate goal of making an effective transition to adulthood, adolescents with SCI often face challenges similar to others with chronic and debilitating conditions. Issues such as housing, education, personal assistance care, transportation, medical care, and specialized medical care must be addressed in a coordinated transition program (Vogel, Betz, & Mulcahey, 2012). The concepts of care coordination for children and adolescents requiring home care also apply to adolescents making the transition to adulthood because different health care services may be needed or requirements may change for benefits for those no longer dependent on parents.

MUSCULAR DYSFUNCTION

JUVENILE DERMATOMYOSITIS

Juvenile dermatomyositis (JDM) is a relatively rare systemic autoimmune vasculopathy that often occurs after a triggering event such as infection with group A β-hemolytic streptococci, enterovirus (coxsackievirus B), or parvovirus B19. An environmental trigger such as excessive sun exposure has also been proposed in some children. In children one of the human leukocyte antigens (DQA1*0501, B8, DRB*0301, or DQA1*0301) is present on chromosome 6 and may be associated with increased susceptibility to the disease (Feldman, Rider, Reed, et al., 2008; Robinson & Reed, 2015). Caucasian girls are twice as likely to be affected as boys. The peak age at onset is between 4 and 10 years of age. Children with onset before age 7 years may experience milder symptoms.

The diagnosis is often established through the following clinical presentations: bilateral symmetric proximal weakness; a characteristic heliotropic rash of the eyelids; Gottron papules on the knuckles, knees, and elbows; Gottron sign; elevated serum enzymes (aldolase, creatine kinase, aspartase aminotransferase, and lactate dehydrogenase); altered EMG; and abnormal muscle biopsy. An atraumatic alternative to muscle biopsy is an MRI. Nailfold capillaroscopy shows decreased capillary density and presence of disease activity and may be used to diagnose the condition (Feldman, Rider, Reed, et al., 2008).

For approximately half of affected children, the disease is acute and progresses rapidly. Children under 6 years of age often are seen initially with fever and signs of an upper respiratory tract illness. There is proximal limb and trunk muscle weakness and loss of reflexes. Consequently, the child may not be able to rise from the floor to a standing position without walking the hands up the legs (Gower sign). The disease often affects the neck muscles, and the child may have difficulty lifting the head or supporting it in an upright position. Muscles tend to be stiff and sore. A generalized vasculitis of small arteries and capillaries is one prominent feature of the disease. Masseter involvement with atrophy may occur, which makes it difficult to chew food during the active stage of the disease. Soft palate dysfunction may make speech difficult and interfere with breathing. Distal muscle strength and reflex responses remain unaffected. JDM is characterized by a red erythematous rash over the malar areas and nose and a violet discoloration of the eyelids. The skin over extensor muscle surfaces may be erythematous, scaly, and atopic. Calcium deposits (calcinosis) develop in muscle tissues as the disease progresses. Dystrophic calcifications may develop over areas exposed to pressure, including the elbows, knees, digits, and buttocks. These lesions may result in skin ulceration with subsequent infection, pain, and functional disability from joint contractures. The vasculitis may cause GI, renal, cardiac, and ophthalmologic symptoms as the disease progresses. A common problem in JDM is aspiration pneumonia, and measures should be taken to ensure the child has an adequate airway at all times. Additional pulmonary involvement includes interstitial lung disease, so pulmonary function testing should be part of the medical management. There is evidence that adults with pediatric-onset JDM may develop cardiac problems such as heart failure. If the child has difficulty feeding, a gastrostomy may be used to supplement caloric intake until the drug regimen controls the symptoms.

JDM responds to high-dose oral corticosteroid therapy and methotrexate; in some children high-dose intermittent intravenous methylprednisone may be required. All children with JDM should use a sunscreen to protect against ultraviolet A and B rays. Vitamin D and adequate dietary intake of calcium are also recommended to increase and maintain bone density and minimize osteopenia (Feldman, Rider, Reed, et al., 2008; Huber, 2012). IVIG has been effective in some children who were intolerant of high-dose corticosteroids. Other treatments that have been effective in adult myositis and in isolated cases of JDM include hydroxychloroquine, systemic tacrolimus, etanercept or infliximab, rituximab, and cyclosporin (Feldman, Rider, Reed, et al., 2008).

Physical therapy is essential to prevent contracture deformity and to rebuild muscle strength. Meticulous skin care is an important nursing consideration in the care of these patients.

Although the prognosis for survival has steadily improved, JDM remains a serious chronic illness. Death can occur in the acute phase as a result of myocarditis, progressive unresponsive myositis, perforation of the bowel, or, occasionally, lung involvement. The current mortality rate is approximately 1% (Robinson & Reed, 2015).

MUSCULAR DYSTROPHIES

The MDs constitute the largest and most important single group of muscle diseases of childhood (Table 34.2). They have a genetic origin in which there is gradual, progressive degeneration of muscle fibers, and they are characterized by progressive weakness and wasting of symmetric groups of skeletal muscles, with increasing disability and deformity. In all forms of MD there is insidious loss of strength, but each differs in regard to the muscle groups affected, age of onset, rate of progression, and inheritance patterns.

The basic defect in MD is still being clarified but appears to be caused by a metabolic disturbance unrelated to the nervous system. Initial sites of muscle involvement are illustrated in Fig. 34.11.

Treatment of the MDs consists mainly of providing supportive measures (including physical therapy; orthopedic procedures to minimize deformity; and ventilatory support, including airway clearance techniques) and assisting the affected child in meeting the demands of daily living.

Facioscapulohumeral (Landouzy-Dejerine) muscular dystrophy is inherited as an autosomal dominant disorder with onset in early adolescence. It is characterized by difficulty in raising the arms over the head, lack of facial mobility, and a forward slope of the shoulders. The progression is slow, and the life span is usually unaffected.

Limb-girdle muscular dystrophy (LGMD) is a heterogenous group of disorders with autosomal dominant and recessive inheritance whose clinical manifestations often appear in later childhood, adolescence, or early adulthood with variable but usually slow progression (Quan, 2011). All types of LGMD are characterized by weakness of proximal muscles of the pelvic and shoulder girdles. Other forms of MD include myotonic dystrophy, scapulohumeral MD (Emery-Dreifuss MD), facioscapulohumeral MD (Landouzy-Dejerine disease), and congenital MD; these forms consist of subtypes of MD and are discussed at length elsewhere (Sarnat, 2015c). Duchenne muscular dystrophy is discussed in the following section.

DUCHENNE MUSCULAR DYSTROPHY

DMD is the most severe and most common MD of childhood. It is inherited as an X-linked recessive trait, and the single-gene defect is located on the short arm of the X chromosome. DMD has a high mutation rate, with a negative family history in approximately 65% to 75% of all cases; therefore genetic counseling is an important aspect of the care of the family. Approximately 30% of DMD patients are new mutations and the mother is not the carrier (Sarnat, 2015d).

As in all X-linked disorders, males are affected almost exclusively. The female carrier may have an elevated serum CK, but muscle weakness is usually not a problem; however, about 10% of female carriers develop cardiomyopathy (Manzur, Kinali, & Muntoni, 2008). In rare instances a female may be identified with DMD disease yet with muscular weakness that is milder than in boys (Sarnat, 2015d). The incidence is approximately 1 in 3600 male births for the Duchenne form and approximately 1 in 30,000 live births for the Becker type, a milder variant (Sarnat, 2015d). Box 34.13 describes the characteristics of DMD.

TABLE 34.2 Characteristics of Major Muscular Dystrophies

Primary Myopathy and Inheritance Pattern	Age of Onset	Initial Manifestations	Progression	Therapy
Duchenne X-linked recessive, sporadic	Early childhood; ages 3-5 years	Lordosis Waddling gait Frequent falls Toe walking Difficulty in rising from floor and climbing stairs Fat deposits replace wasted gastrocnemius muscles	Rapid Ultimately involves all voluntary muscles Death usually occurs at ages 15-30 years	Supportive Physical therapy to prevent disuse atrophy of unaffected muscles
Becker X-linked recessive, sporadic	>7 years of age	Same as Duchenne	Much slower progression than Duchenne	Same as Duchenne
Myotonic Autosomal dominant Second most common muscular dystrophy in United States and Europe	Early infancy, except for severe congenital form	Facial wasting and hypotonia	Progressive muscle wasting into adolescence and adulthood; affects multiple organs	Treatment of cardiac, ocular, endocrine, and gastrointestinal complications
Limb-girdle Autosomal recessive (usually, but 16 genetic forms are recognized and some are autosomal dominant)	Late childhood or adolescence; >8 years of age	Weakness of proximal muscles of both pelvic and shoulder girdles	Variable but usually slow Most become incapacitated within 20 years of onset; in some, disability may remain slight	Supportive Physical therapy to prevent disuse atrophy of unaffected muscles
Facioscapulohumeral (Landouzy-Dejerine) Autosomal dominant	Early adolescence; >8 years of age	Lack of facial mobility Difficulty raising arms over head Forward slope of shoulders	Very slow May be intervals with no progression Considerable disability in time, but life span unaffected	Supportive

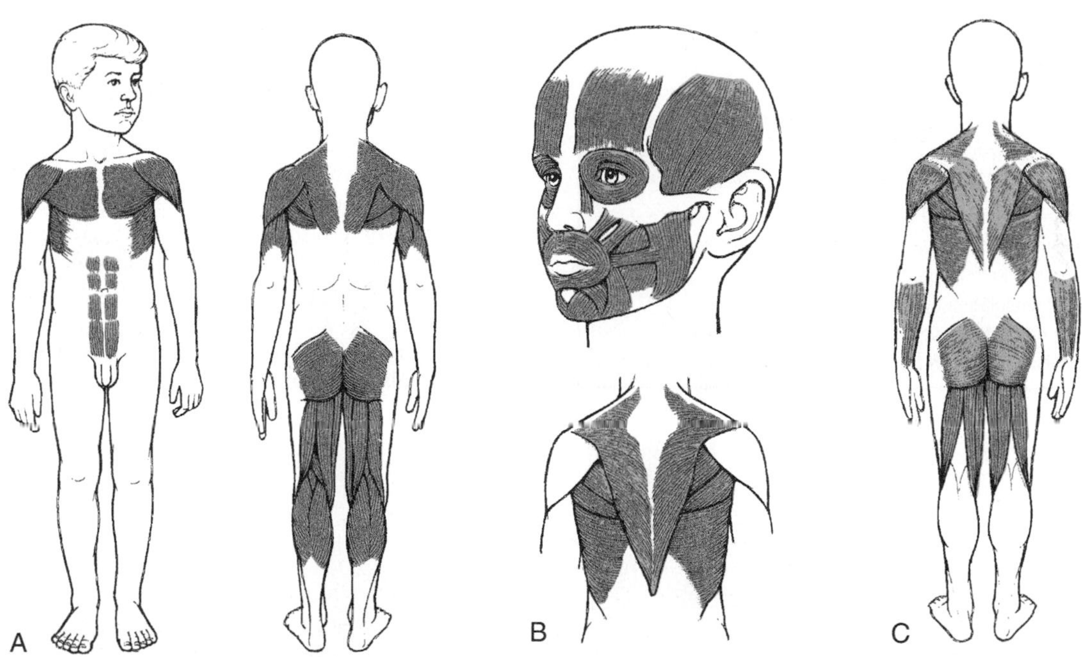

FIG. 34.11 Initial muscle groups involved in muscular dystrophies. **A,** Pseudohypertrophic (Duchenne). **B,** Facioscapulohumeral. **C,** Limb-girdle.

At the genetic level, both DMD and Becker MD result from mutations of the gene that encodes dystrophin, a protein product in skeletal muscle. Dystrophin is absent from the muscle of children with DMD and is reduced or abnormal in children with Becker MD. The absence of dystrophin leads to a number of problems in muscle, including muscle fiber degeneration. A deficiency of dystrophin isoforms in brain tissue causes cognitive and intellectual impairment (Manzur, Kinali, & Muntoni, 2008). Children with Becker MD have a later onset of symptoms, which are usually not as severe as those seen in DMD. There is a strong correlation between the clinical severity of these disorders and the type of genetic mutation and dystrophin protein alterations. Survival has increased with newer ventilation technologies, and median age is reported as high as 27 years in those being ventilated; types of ventilation used were not described in the report (Rall & Grimm, 2012).

Clinical Manifestations

Most children with DMD reach the appropriate developmental milestones early in life, although they may have mild, subtle delays. Evidence of muscle weakness usually appears during the third to seventh year, although there may have been a history of delay in motor development, particularly walking. Difficulties in running, riding a bicycle, and climbing stairs are usually the first symptoms noted. Later, abnormal gait on a level surface becomes apparent. In the early years, rapid developmental gains may mask the progression of the disease. Questioning the parents may reveal that the child has difficulty in rising from a sitting or supine position. Occasionally the parents notice enlarged calves.

Typically, affected boys have a waddling gait and lordosis, fall frequently, and develop a characteristic manner of rising from a squatting or sitting position on the floor (Gower sign) (Fig. 34.12). Lordosis occurs as a result of weakened pelvic muscles, and the waddling gait is a result of weakness in the gluteus medius and maximus muscles (Battista, 2010). Muscles, especially in the calves, thighs, and upper arms, become enlarged from fatty infiltration and feel unusually firm or woody on palpation. The term *pseudohypertrophy* is derived from this muscular enlargement. Profound muscular atrophy occurs in the later stages; contractures and deformities involving large and small joints are common complications as the disease progresses. Ambulation usually becomes impossible by 12 years of age. The loss of mobilization further increases the spectrum of complications, which may include osteoporosis, fractures, constipation, skin breakdown, and psychosocial and behavioral problems. Atrophy of facial, oropharyngeal, and respiratory muscles does not occur until the advanced stage of the disease. Ultimately the disease process involves the diaphragm and auxiliary muscles of respiration, and cardiomegaly is common.

BOX 34.13 Characteristics of Duchenne Muscular Dystrophy

- Early onset, usually between 3 and 5 years of age
- Progressive muscular weakness, wasting, and contractures
- Calf muscle hypertrophy in most patients
- Loss of independent ambulation by 9–12 years of age
- Slowly progressive, generalized weakness during adolescence
- Relentless progression until death from respiratory or cardiac failure

Mild to moderate mental impairment is commonly associated with MD. The mean intelligence quotient (IQ) is approximately 20 points below normal, and frank mental deficit is present in 20% to 30% of these children. Verbal IQ is markedly low in males with DMD, and emotional disturbance is more common than in other children with disabilities; however, children with DMD should be involved in early learning programs and eventually moved into regular classrooms as much as possible.

Complications

The major complications of MD include contractures, scoliosis, disuse atrophy, infections, obesity, and respiratory and cardiopulmonary problems. Contracture deformities of the hips, knees, and ankles occur from early selective muscle involvement and often exaggerate the weakness. Passive range-of-motion exercises, stretching, and active exercises under the supervision of a PT are effective in treating reducible contractures. Nonreducible contractures require wedge casting or surgical reduction. Scoliosis caused by muscle imbalance is common in children who lose ambulatory capability and tends to progress even when the child becomes dependent on a wheelchair. Bracing with an orthosis may be required, but in many cases spinal fusion surgery is performed to prevent complications associated with cardiac and pulmonary restriction.

Atrophy of disuse from prolonged inactivity occurs readily when children are immobilized or confined to bed with illness, injury, or surgery. To minimize this complication, physical therapy should begin if bed rest extends beyond a few days. To maintain muscle strength, a daily goal for well children with moderate disability should be at least 3 hours of ambulation.

Pulmonary infections become increasingly frequent as the dystrophic process produces a progressive decrease in pulmonary vital capacity as a result of weakness of the primary, secondary, and associated muscles of respiration. Consequently, even minor upper respiratory tract infections may become serious in these children. The eventual cause of death is usually respiratory tract infection or cardiac failure; however, much progress has been made in providing ventilatory methods to prolong and maintain quality of life. Prompt and vigorous antibiotic therapy, supplemented by postural drainage and aggressive airway clearance methods, is effective. Because of the respiratory musculature weakness, these children are unable to cough effectively and secretions collect easily.

Obesity is a common complication that contributes to premature loss of ambulation. Children who have restricted opportunities for

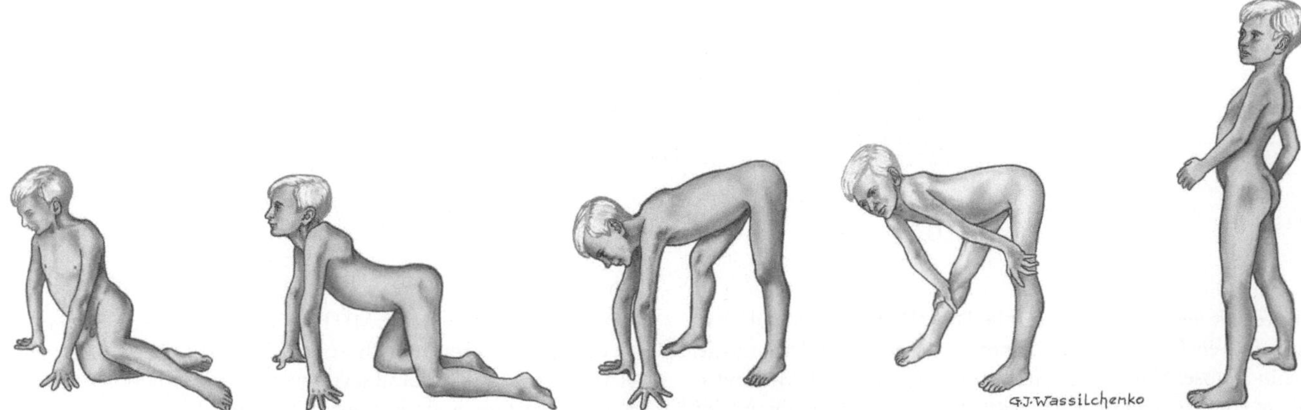

FIG. 34.12 Child with Duchenne muscular dystrophy attains standing posture by kneeling, then gradually pushing his torso upright (with knees straight) by "walking" his hands up his legs (Gower sign). Note marked lordosis in upright position.

physical activity and who suffer from boredom easily consume calories in excess of their needs. This may be compounded by overfeeding by well-meaning family and friends. Proper dietary intake and a diversified recreational program help reduce the likelihood of obesity and enable children to maintain ambulation and functional independence for a longer time.

Cardiac manifestations are usually late events but may occur in ambulatory children. The most significant of these, cardiac failure, is difficult to correct in advanced cases, but treatment with digoxin and diuretics is often beneficial in the early stages of the disease.

Diagnostic Evaluation

MD is suspected on the basis of clinical manifestations (see Box 34.13) and confirmed by molecular genetic detection of deficient dystrophin by DNA analysis from peripheral blood or in muscle tissue obtained by biopsy. The diagnosis of DMD is primarily established by blood polymerase chain reaction (PCR) for the dystrophin gene mutation (Sarnat, 2015d). Diagnostic techniques such as multiplex PCR have made it possible to diagnose 98% of the DMD mutations. Prenatal diagnosis is also possible as early as 12 weeks of gestation. However, ethical questions exist regarding diagnosing a condition in the fetus when no treatment exists.

Serum enzyme measurement, muscle biopsy, and EMG may also be used in establishing the diagnosis. Serum CK levels are extremely high in the first 2 years of life, before the onset of clinical weakness. If the child demonstrates the usual characteristics, has a positive family history for DMD, and the PCR is positive, the muscle biopsy may be deferred.

Muscle biopsy reveals degeneration of muscle fibers, with fibrosis and fatty tissue replacement. EMG readings show a decrease in amplitude and duration of motor unit potentials.

Therapeutic Management

Currently no curative treatment exists for childhood MD. Increased muscle bulk and muscle power have been reported after a course of corticosteroids. Several clinical trials demonstrated increased muscle strength and improved performance and pulmonary function, with significant decrease in the progression of weakness, when prednisone was administered for 6 months to 2 years (Manzur, Kuntzer, Pike, et al., 2008). Corticosteroid administration also prolonged ambulation, preserved respiratory function, and decreased the incidence of scoliosis and cardiomyopathy (Manzur, Kinali, & Muntoni, 2008). Major side effects in these studies included weight gain and a cushingoid facial appearance. The American Academy of Neurology has published a practice parameter for the administration of corticosteroids in the treatment of DMD (Moxley, Ashwal, Pandya, et al., 2005).

Maintaining optimum function in all muscles for as long as possible is the primary goal; secondary is the prevention of contractures. In general, children who remain as active as possible are able to avoid wheelchair confinement for a longer time. Maintenance of function often includes stretching exercises, strength and muscle training, breathing exercises and use of incentive spirometry to increase and maintain vital lung capacity, airway clearance, range-of-motion exercises, surgery to release contracture deformities, bracing, and performance of ADLs. Knee-ankle-foot orthoses have been shown to prolong ambulation for 18 to 24 months beyond the termination of independent ambulation. Serial casting of ankles has proven more effective than surgical release of Achilles tendons in many children with DMD to prevent contractures (Manzur, Kinali, & Muntoni, 2008).

Parents should always be involved in making decisions about the child's care, and teaching regarding home safety and prevention of falls is important as well. Also encourage parents to have the child keep follow-up appointments for medical care and physical and occupational therapy. Because respiratory tract infections are most troublesome in these children, encourage regular influenza and pneumococcal vaccines and avoidance of contact with persons with respiratory tract infections as much as possible. Baseline pulmonary function testing, electrocardiograms, and echocardiograms are also recommended.

Eventually, respiratory and cardiac problems become the central focus of the debilitating illness. Referral to Palliative Care may help the family evaluate the benefits and burdens of various treatments. The child and parents should be involved in discussion of long-term ventilation options. Cardiac and respiratory assessment during wake-sleep cycles is imperative. Children with neuromuscular disease eventually develop abnormal breathing patterns, particularly during REM sleep, and hypoxia occurs as a result of inadequate oxygenation. The sleep-disordered breathing of DMD results in symptoms such as frequent night awakenings, morning headache, and daytime sleepiness. Polysomnography should be performed once daytime symptoms of sleep-disordered breathing occur. Noninvasive positive pressure ventilation should be considered in such children to prevent further hypoventilation and cardiorespiratory deterioration (Culebras, 2008). Respiratory care for children with neuromuscular conditions such as SMA and DMD may involve the use of noninvasive ventilation with BiPAP on a temporary or full-time basis, mechanically assisted coughing (MAC), or tracheostomy and relief of airway obstruction with coughing and suctioning devices; the tracheostomy, however, is associated with more complications (Simonds, 2006; Young, Lowe, & Fitzgerald, 2007). Home pulse oximetry may be used to monitor oxygenation during sleep or to aid in decision making regarding the use of MAC to clear the airways. A polysomnogram may be used to evaluate the effectiveness of supplemental oxygen and noninvasive ventilation devices.

Several devices are available for children with neuromuscular disease to assist in clearing the airway when the cough reflex is ineffective or diminished. The *mechanical cough in-exsufflator* (MIE) (also referred to as cough assist) has been found to be safe and effective in the daily management of respiratory function (Kravitz, 2009; Miske, Hickey, Kolb, et al., 2004). The MIE delivers positive inspiratory pressures at a set rate, followed by negative pressure exsufflation coordinated with the patient's own breathing rhythm. The exsufflation is designed to mimic a cough reflex so mucus can be effectively cleared. Airway suctioning after exsufflation is accomplished as necessary to clear the airways. In children the MIE device may be connected directly to a tracheostomy or used with a mouthpiece or face mask. Boitano's (2009) article provides a variety of equipment options, including various masks that can be used to deliver noninvasive positive pressure.

Manual cough-assisting techniques include glossopharyngeal breathing or air stacking (frog breathing); the abdominal thrust, which is similar to the Heimlich maneuver (Kravitz, 2009); and manual hyperinflation with a self-inflating resuscitation bag (without oxygen) and a mouthpiece. Hyperinflation may be used in conjunction with abdominal thrusts to improve peak cough flows (Boitano, 2009).

The use of routine chest physiotherapy for DMD has not been adequately evaluated for its effectiveness in clearing the airway of mucus except when there is focal atelectasis and mucous plugging the airways (Kravitz, 2009).

Survival in individuals with DMD may be prolonged several years with the use of noninvasive ventilation and airway clearance devices such as cough assist as alternatives to tracheotomy and airway suctioning (Simonds, 2006). The American Thoracic Society (2004) has published extensive guidelines for respiratory monitoring and care of children and adults with DMD. See Finder's (2009) article for an elaboration on the 2004 American Thoracic Society statement.

The American Academy of Pediatrics (2005) recommends an extensive cardiac evaluation of the child diagnosed with either DMD or Becker MD. Patients with neuromuscular conditions may not have the typical signs and symptoms of cardiac dysfunction. Therefore symptoms such as weight loss, nausea and vomiting, cough, increased fatigue on performance of ADLs, and orthopnea should be carefully evaluated to detect early signs of cardiomyopathy.

Research evaluating a number of treatments for DMD is in progress. These include clinical trials with glutamine and creatine monohydrate to preserve muscle strength; utrophin, a protein that is similar to dystrophin and that in large quantities may counteract the effects of the dystrophin deficiency (Chakkalakal, Thompson, Parks, et al., 2005; Miura & Jardin, 2006); and the enzyme CT GalNAc transferase, which blocks muscle wasting in mice. Oral albuterol administered daily for 12 weeks increased lean body mass and decreased fat mass in a group of 14 ambulatory boys with Becker MD and DMD; however, overall muscle strength improvement was not observed (Skura, Fowler, Wetzel, et al., 2008).

Genetic counseling is recommended for parents, sisters, and maternal aunts and their daughters. (See Chapter 3.) Long-term care, end-of-life care, and palliative care options are issues that the health care team must discuss with the child and family affected by MD (Finder, 2009). Professional counseling is necessary in some cases to allow frank discussion of these issues, and referrals should be made as appropriate (Finder, Birnkrant, Carl, et al., 2004). (See Chapter 21.)

Guidelines for the standardization of diagnosis and therapeutic management of DMD have been published elsewhere (Bushby, Finkel, Birnkrant, et al., 2010).

Nursing Care Management

The care and management of a child with MD involve the combined efforts of a multidisciplinary health care team. Nurses can help clarify the roles of these health care professionals to family and others. The major emphasis of nursing care is to assist the child and family in coping with the progressive, incapacitating, and fatal nature of the disease; to help design a program that will afford a greater degree of independence and reduce the predictable and preventable disabilities associated with the disorder; and to help the child and family deal constructively with the limitations the disease imposes on their daily lives. Because of advances in technology, children with MD may live into early adulthood; therefore the goals of care should also involve decisions regarding quality of life, achievement of independence, and transition to adulthood.

Working closely with other team members, nurses assist the family in developing the child's self-help skills to give the child the satisfaction of being as independent as possible for as long as possible. It is tempting for parents to overprotect their affected children. Children derive pleasure and build self-esteem from performing actions that visibly please their parents. Therefore parents must be helped to develop a balance between limiting the child's activity because of muscular weakness and allowing the child to accomplish things alone. This requires continual evaluation of the child's capabilities, which are often difficult to assess. Most children with MD instinctively recognize the need to be as independent as possible and strive to do so.

Practical difficulties faced by families are the physical limitations of housing, transportation, and mobility. Housing accommodations must be made so the wheelchair-bound child can be mobile in the home setting. Transportation in a car restraint seat adapted for the child with weakened neck and back musculature will be necessary, and eventually a wheelchair-accessible vehicle will be required. Discuss diet, nutritional needs, and nutrition modification according to the needs of the individual child and family. Nutritional needs decrease once the child becomes wheelchair bound, and dietary modifications should be made in conjunction with a pediatric dietitian to ensure the child is receiving an adequate amount of the necessary nutrients to maintain bone health and prevent constipation.

Parents' social activities may be restricted, and the family's activities must be continually modified to meet the needs of the affected child. (See Chapter 21.) When the child becomes increasingly incapacitated, the family may consider home care to provide the care needed. The nurse as case manager can assist the family in making this difficult transition. Unless the child is severely incapacitated, he or she should also be involved in the decisions regarding such care. Nurses can assist with decision making by exploring all available options and resources and supporting the child and family in the decision.

Each child's therapy program is tailored to individual needs and capabilities, and family members should be active participants. Parents often need assistance with the physical therapy program and education regarding a home regimen of exercises and activity. Many parents erroneously believe that by exerting sufficient effort, the child can overcome the weakness and prevent progression of the disease process. They should also be advised to notify the nurse or other designated person when the child becomes even temporarily bedridden so that the exercise program can be modified and continued during this time.

Children with MD tend to become socially isolated as their physical condition deteriorates to the point that they can no longer keep up with friends and classmates. Their physical capabilities diminish, and their dependency increases at the age at which most children are expanding their range of interests and relationships. To gain peer associations, they often learn and employ behaviors that bring them the rewards of other children's company. These friends are often children who have been rejected by more able-bodied classmates.

Older boys with MD may also need psychiatric or psychologic counseling to deal with issues such as depression, anger, and quality of life. Parents need encouragement to become involved in support groups because there is evidence that adequate social support from family, community, and other parents is crucial to appropriate coping in families with children with chronic illness.

Regardless of the success of the program and how well the family adapts to the disorder, superimposed on the physical and emotional problems associated with the child's long-term disability is the constant specter of the disease's ultimate outcome. These families encounter all the manifestations of the child with a chronic and fatal illness. (See Chapter 19.)

Nurses are especially valuable health care professionals as they come to know the family and the family's challenges. Nurses can be alert to the problems and needs of the families and make necessary referrals when supplementary services are indicated. The Muscular Dystrophy Association has branches in most communities to provide assistance to families that have a member with MD.

NCLEX REVIEW QUESTIONS

1. The most common complication that should be anticipated and observed for in an infant with myelomeningocele after surgical repair of the defect is:
   A. Urinary stress
   B. Chiari malformation
   C. Hydrocephalus
   D. Latex allergy
2. A 14-year-old male with a spinal cord injury is placed on a standing table and suddenly begins to sweat profusely and complain of a headache. The nurse takes a set of vital signs and notes a significant increase in systolic blood pressure and a heart rate of 50 beats per minute. The most helpful intervention in this situation would be for the nurse to:
   A. **Place** the adolescent back in his wheelchair and take him to his room
   B. Palpate the bladder for distention
   C. Administer a routine analgesic for his headache and discontinue the therapy
   D. Place the standing table in a horizontal position and allow the adolescent to rest for a few minutes
3. The primary risk factor for the development of cerebral palsy is:
   A. Maternal chorioamnionitis
   B. Premature birth
   C. Birth asphyxia
   D. Intraventricular hemorrhage
4. Urinary system distress (neurogenic bladder) in children with spina bifida is managed by:
   A. DDAVP (1-deamino-8-D-arginine vasopressin)
   B. Clean intermittent catheterization
   C. Continuous urinary catheterization
   D. Mitrofanoff procedure
5. Which of these statements accurately describes Duchenne muscular dystrophy (DMD)? Select all that apply.
   A. The absence of dystrophin leads to muscle fiber degeneration.
   B. DMD is inherited as an X-linked recessive trait.
   C. Cognitive and intellectual impairment are rare in children with DMD.
   D. Affected children have a waddling gait and lordosis and fall frequently.
   E. Ambulation usually becomes impossible by 12 years of age, and affected children are confined to a wheelchair.
   F. Affected children must be hospitalized when ambulation becomes impossible.

Correct Answers

1. C; 2. B; 3. B; 4. B; 5. A, B, D, E

REFERENCES

Adolfsson, M., Johnson, E., & Nilsson, S. (2017). Pain management for children with cerebral palsy in school settings in two cultures: action and reaction approaches. *Disability and Rehabilitation*, 1–11.

Adzick, N. S. (2013). Fetal surgery for spina bifida: past, present, future. *Seminars in Pediatric Surgery*, *22*(1), 10–17.

Adzick, N. S., Thom, E. A., Spong, C. Y., et al. (2011). A randomized trial of prenatal versus postnatal repair of myelomeningocele. *The New England Journal of Medicine*, *364*(11), 993–1104.

Agopian, A. J., Tinker, S. C., Lupo, P. J., et al. (2013). Proportion of neural tube defects attributable to known risk factors. *Birth Defects Research. Part A, Clinical and Molecular Teratology*, *97*(1), 42–46.

American Academy of Pediatrics. (2005). Cardiovascular health supervision for individuals affected by Duchenne or Becker muscular dystrophy. *Pediatrics*, *116*(6), 1569–1573.

American Academy of Pediatrics, Committee on Genetics. (2007). Folic acid for the prevention of neural tube defects. *Pediatrics*, *119*(5), 1031.

American Academy of Pediatrics, Committee on Infectious Diseases (2015). D. W. Kimberlin (Ed.), *2015 Red book: report of the committee on infectious diseases* (30th ed.). Elk Grove Village, Ill: Author.

American College of Obstetrics and Gynecology. (2007). ACOG Practice Bulletin No. 77: screening for fetal chromosomal abnormalities. *Obstetrics and Gynecology*, *109*(1), 217–227.

American Thoracic Society. (2004). Respiratory care of the patient with Duchenne muscular dystrophy: ATS consensus statement. *American Journal of Respiratory and Critical Care Medicine*, *170*(4), 456–465.

Anderson, C. J., Kelly, E. M., Klaas, S. J., et al. (2009). Anxiety and depression in children and adolescents with spinal cord injuries. *Developmental Medicine and Child Neurology*, *51*(10), 826–832.

Aristedis, R., Dimitrios, P., Nikolaos, P., et al. (2017). Intrathecal baclofen pump infection treated by adjunct intrareservoir teicoplanin instillation. *Surgical Neurology International*, *8*, 38.

Arnon, S. S. (2015a). Tetanus (*Clostridium tetani*). In R. M. Kliegman, B. F. Stanton, J. W. St. Geme, et al. (Eds.), *Nelson textbook of pediatrics* (20th ed.). Philadelphia: Saunders.

Arnon, S. S. (2015b). Anaerobic bacterial infections: botulism (*Clostridium botulinum*). In R. M. Kliegman, B. F. Stanton, J. W. St. Geme, et al. (Eds.), *Nelson textbook of pediatrics* (20th ed.). Philadelphia: Saunders.

Avarello, J. T., & Cantor, R. M. (2007). Pediatric major trauma: an approach to evaluation and management. *Emergency Medicine Clinics of North America*, *25*(3), 803–836.

Bach, J. R. (2007). Medical considerations of long-term survival of Werdnig-Hoffmann disease. *American Journal of Physical Medicine and Rehabilitation*, *86*(5), 349–355.

Battista, V. (2010). Muscular dystrophy, Duchenne. In P. L. Jackson, J. A. Vessey, & N. A. Schapiro (Eds.), *Primary care of the child with a chronic illness* (5th ed.). St. Louis: Mosby.

Bax, M., Goldstein, M., Rosenbaum, P., et al. (2005). Proposed definition and classification of cerebral palsy. *Developmental Medicine and Child Neurology*, *47*(8), 571–576.

Benjamins, L. J., Gourishankar, A., Yataco-Marquez, V., et al. (2013). Honey pacifier use among an indigent pediatric population. *Pediatrics*, *131*(6), e1838–e1841.

Berker, A. N., & Yalçin, M. S. (2008). Cerebral palsy: orthopedic aspects and rehabilitation. *Pediatric Clinics of North America*, *55*(5), 1209–1225.

Betz, C., Linroth, R., Butler, C., et al. (2010). Spina bifida: what we learned from consumers. *Pediatric Clinics of North America*, *57*(4), 935–944.

Boitano, L. J. (2009). Equipment options for cough augmentation, ventilation, and noninvasive interfaces in neuromuscular respiratory management. *Pediatrics*, *123*(Suppl. 4), S226–S230.

Bosanquet, M., Copeland, L., Ware, R., et al. (2013). A systematic review of tests to predict cerebral palsy in young children. *Developmental Medicine and Child Neurology*, *55*(5), 418–426.

Bourke-Taylor, H. M., Cotter, C., Lalor, A., et al. (2017). School success and participation for students with cerebral palsy: a qualitative study exploring multiple perspectives. *Disability and Rehabilitation*, 1–9.

Burke, R., Liptak, G. S., & Council on Children with Disabilities. (2011). Providing a primary care medical home for children and youth with spina bifida. *Pediatrics*, *128*(6), e1645–e1658.

Bush, A., Fraser, J., & Jardine, E. (2005). Respiratory management of the infant with type 1 spinal muscular atrophy. *Archives of Disease in Childhood, 90*(7), 709–711.

Bushby, K., Finkel, R., Birnkrant, D. J., et al. (2010). Diagnosis and management of Duchenne muscular dystrophy, part 1: diagnosis, and pharmacologicical and psychosocial management. *The Lancet. Neurology, 9*(1), 77–93. Retrieved from http://www.treat-nmd.eu/downloads/file/standardsofcare/dmd/lancet/the_diagnosis_and_management_of_dmd_lancet_complete_with_erratum.pdf.

Calhoun, C. L., Schottler, J., & Vogel, L. C. (2013). Recommendations for mobility in children with spinal cord injury. *Topics in Spinal Cord Injury Rehabilitation, 19*(2), 142–151.

Castro, D., Derisavifard, S., Anderson, M., et al. (2013). Juvenile myasthenia gravis: a twenty-year experience. *Journal of Clinical Neuromuscular Disease, 14*(3), 95–102.

Centers for Disease Control and Prevention. (2007). Folate status in women of childbearing age, by race/ethnicity—United States, 1999-2000, 2001-2002, and 2003-2004. *MMWR. Morbidity and Mortality Weekly Report, 55*(51), 1377–1380.

Centers for Disease Control and Prevention. (2009). Racial/ethnic differences in the birth prevalence of spina bifida—United States, 1995-2005. *MMWR. Morbidity and Mortality Weekly Report, 57*(53), 1409–1413.

Centers for Disease Control and Prevention. (2010). Nonpolio enteroviruses and human parechovirus surveillance—United States, 2006-2008. *MMWR. Morbidity and Mortality Weekly Report, 59*(48), 1577–1580.

Centers for Disease Control and Prevention: *National Center on Birth Defects and Developmental Disabilities United States, page last updated*: October 12, 2016. Retrieved from http://www.cdc.gov/ncbddd/spinabifida/data.html.

Centers for Disease Control and Prevention: *Data and statistics for cerebral palsy: prevalence and characteristics*, 2013. Retrieved from http://www.cdc.gov/NCBDDD/cp/data.html.

Centers for Disease Control and Prevention, *Division of Birth Defects and Developmental Disabilities, National Center on Birth Defects and Developmental Disabilities*, May 2, 2016 https://www.cdc.gov/ncbddd/cp/data.html.

Chakkalakal, J. V., Thompson, J., Parks, R. J., et al. (2005). Molecular, cellular, and pharmacological therapies for Duchenne/Becker muscular dystrophies. *FASEB Journal : Official Publication of the Federation of American Societies for Experimental Biology, 19*(8), 880–891.

Chaléat-Valayer, E., Bernard, J. C., Deceuninck, J., et al. (2016). Pelvic-spinal analysis and the impact of Onabotulinum toxin A injections on spinal balance in one child with cerebral palsy. *Journal of Child Neurology Open* Jan-Dec; 3, 2016.

Chiriboga, C. A., Swoboda, K. J., Darras, B. T., et al. (2016). Results from a phase 1 study of nusinersen (ISIS-SMN Rx) in children with spinal muscular atrophy. *Neurology, 86*(10), 890–897.

Christison-Lagay, E., Dharia, B., Vajsar, J., et al. (2013). Efficacy and safety of thorcaoscopic thymectomy in the treatment of juvenile myasthenia gravis. *Pediatric Surgery International, 29*(6), 583–586.

Choi, J. Y., Choi, Y. S., & Park, E. S. (2017). Language development and brain magnetic resonance imaging characteristics in preschool children with cerebral palsy. *Journal of Speech, Language, and Hearing Research : JSLHR, 60*(5), 1330–1338. May 24.

Cirillo, M. L. (2008). Neuromuscular emergencies. *Clinical Pediatric Emergency Medicine, 9*(2), 88–95.

Clinical Trials: *Management of myelomeningocele study (MOMS)*, Washington, DC, 2013, US National Institute of Child Health and Human Development. Retrieved from http://clinicaltrials.gov/show/NCT00060606.

Collins, J. S., Atkinson, K. K., Dean, J. H., et al. (2011). Long-term maintenance of neural tube defects prevention in a high-prevalence state. *The Journal of Pediatrics, 159*(1), 143–149.

Consortium for Spinal Cord Medicine. (2010). Sexuality and reproductive health in adults with spinal cord injury: a clinical practice guideline for health-care professionals. *The Journal of Spinal Cord Medicine, 33*(3), 281–336.

Culebras, A. (2008). Sleep-disordered breathing in neuromuscular disease. *Sleep Medicine Clinics, 3*(3), 377–386.

Dai, A. I., Wasay, M., & Awan, S. (2008). Botulinum toxin type A with oral baclofen versus oral tizanidine: a randomized pilot comparison in patients with cerebral palsy and equines foot deformity. *Journal of Child Neurology, 23*(12), 1464–1466.

Delobel-Ayoub, M., Klapouszczak, D., van Bakel, M., et al. (2017). Prevalence and characteristics of autism spectrum disorders in children with cerebral palsy. *PLoS ONE, 59*(7), 738–742.

DeForge, D., Blackmer, J., Garritty, C., et al. (2006). Male erectile dysfunction following spinal cord injury: a systematic review. *Spinal Cord, 44*(8), 465–473.

De Jong, T. P., Chrzan, R., Klijn, A. J., et al. (2008). Treatment of the neurogenic bladder in spina bifida. *Pediatric Nephrology (Berlin, Germany), 23*(6), 889–896.

Dicianno, B. E., Fairman, A. D., Juengst, S. B., et al. (2010). Using the spina bifida Life Course Model in clinical practice: an interdisciplinary approach. *Pediatric Clinics of North America, 57*(4), 945–957.

Doolin, E. (2006). Bowel management for patients with myelodysplasia. *The Surgical Clinics of North America, 86*(2), 505–514.

Eliasson, A. C., Krumlinde-Sundholm, L., & Rösblad, B. (2006). The Manual Ability Classification System (MACS) for children with cerebral palsy: scale development and evidence of validity and reliability. *Developmental Medicine and Child Neurology, 48*(7), 549–554.

Feldman, B. M., Rider, L. G., Reed, A. M., et al. (2008). Juvenile dermatomyositis and other idiopathic inflammatory myopathies of childhood. *Lancet, 371*(9631), 2201–2212.

Ferris, F. (2015). Cerebral Palsy. In R. M. Kliegman, B. F. Stanton, J. W. St. Geme, et al. (Eds.), *Nelson textbook of pediatrics* (20th ed.). Philadelphia: Saunders.

Finder, J. D. (2009). A 2009 perspective on the 2004 American Thoracic Society statement, "Respiratory care of the patient with Duchenne muscular dystrophy,". *Pediatrics, 123*(Suppl. 4), S239–S241.

Finder, J. D., Birnkrant, D., Carl, J., et al. (2004). Respiratory care of the patient with Duchenne muscular dystrophy: ATS consensus statement. *American Journal of Respiratory and Critical Care Medicine, 170*(4), 456–465.

Finkel, R. S., Chiriboga, C. A., Vajsar, J., et al. (2016). Treatment of infantile-onset spinal muscular atrophy with nusinersen: a phase 2, open-label, dose escalation study. *Lancet, 388*, 3017–3026.

Francis, R. (2007). Physiology and management of bladder and bowel continence following spinal cord injury. *Ostomy/Wound Management, 53*(12), 18–27.

Friel, K. M., Lee, P., Soles, L. V., et al. (2017). Combined transcranial Direct Current Stimulation and robotic upper limb therapy improves upper limb function in an adult with cerebral palsy. *Neurorehabilitation.*

Frimberger, D., Cheng, E., & Kropp, B. K. (2012). The current management of the neurogenic bladder in children with spina bifida. *Pediatric Clinics of North America, 59*(4), 757–767.

Gasalberti, D. (2006). Alternative therapies for children and youth with special health care needs. *Journal of Pediatric Health Care, 20*(2), 133–136.

George, J. M., Fiori, S., Fripp, J., et al. (2017). Validation of an MRI brain injury and growth scoring system in very preterm infants scanned at 29- to 35-week postmenstrual age. *AJNR.*

Gilhus, N. E., Owe, J. F., Hoff, J. M., et al. (2011). Myasthenia gravis: a review of available treatment approaches. *Autoimmune Diseases, 2011*, 847393.

Golomb, M. R., Saha, C., Garg, B. P., et al. (2007). Association of cerebral palsy with other disabilities in children with perinatal arterial ischemic stroke. *Pediatric Neurology, 37*(4), 245–249.

Gray, M., & Moore, K. N. (2009). *Urologic disorders: adult and pediatric care.* St. Louis: Mosby.

Green, L., Greenberg, G. M., & Hurwitz, E. (2003). Primary care of children with cerebral palsy. *Clinic Family Practice, 5*(2), 1–21.

Hack, M., & Costello, D. W. (2008). Trends in the rates of cerebral palsy associated with neonatal intensive care of preterm children. *Clinical Obstetrics and Gynecology, 51*(4), 763–774.

Hayes, J. S., & Arriola, T. (2005). Pediatric spinal injuries. *Pediatric Nursing, 31*(6), 464–467.

Hermansen, M. C., & Hermansen, M. G. (2006). Perinatal infections and cerebral palsy. *Clinics in Perinatology, 33*(2), 315–333.

Hidecker, M. J., Paneth, N., Rosenbaum, P. L., et al. (2011). Developing and validating the Communication Function Classification System for individuals with cerebral palsy. *Developmental Medicine and Child Neurology, 53*(8), 704–710.

Hirtz, D., Thurman, D. J., Gwinn-Hardy, K., et al. (2007). How common are the "common" neurologic disorders? *Neurology, 68*(5), 326–337.

Hosalkar, H., Pandya, N. K., Hsu, J., et al. (2009). Specialty update: what's new in orthopaedic rehabilitation. *The Journal of Bone and Joint Surgery. American Volume, 91*(9), 2296–2310.

Huber, A. M. (2012). Idiopathic inflammatory myopathies in childhood: current concepts. *Pediatric Clinics of North America, 59*(2), 365–380.

Hughes, R. (2008). The role of IVIG in autoimmune neuropathies: the latest evidence. *Journal of Neurology, 255*(Suppl. 3), 7–11.

Hughes, R. A., & Cornblath, D. R. (2005). Guillain-Barré syndrome. *Lancet, 366*(9497), 1653–1666.

Hughes, R., Swan, A., & Van Doorn, P. (2012). Intravenous immunoglobulin for Guillain-Barre Syndrome. *Cochrane Database of Systematic Review*, (7), CD002063.

Hurlbert, R. J., Hadley, M. N., Walters, B. C., et al. (2013). Pharmacological therapy for acute spinal cord injury. *Neurosurgery, 72*(3 Suppl.), 93–105.

Iannaccone, S. T. (2007). Modern management of spinal muscular atrophy. *Journal of Child Neurology, 22*(8), 974–978.

Iannaccone, S. T., & Burghes, A. (2002). Spinal muscular atrophies. *Advances in Neurology, 88*, 83–98.

Jones, M. W., Morgan, E., & Shelton, J. E. (2007). Primary care of the child with cerebral palsy: a review of systems (part II). *Journal of Pediatric Health Care, 21*(4), 226–237.

Kanitkar, A., Szturm, T., Parmar, S., et al. (2017). The effectiveness of a computer game-based rehabilitation platform for children with cerebral palsy: protocol for a randomized clinical trial. *JMIR Research Protocols, 6*(5), e93.

Keys, D. E., & Chaves-Carballo, E. (2013). *Brain safari sick children sick brains and other maladies*. California: Bookstand Publishing.

Kinsman, S., & Johnston, M. (2015). Myelomeningocele. In R. M. Kliegman, B. F. Stanton, J. W. St. Geme, et al. (Eds.), *Nelson textbook of pediatrics* (20th ed.). Philadelphia: Saunders/Elsevier.

Kirshblum, S. C., Waring, W., Biering-Sorensen, F., et al. (2011). Reference for the 2011 revision of the international standards for neurological classification of spinal cord injury. *The Journal of Spinal Cord Medicine, 34*(6), 547–554.

Krageloh-Mann, I., & Cans, C. (2009). Cerebral palsy update. *Brain and Development, 31*(7), 537–544.

Kravitz, R. M. (2009). Airway clearance in Duchenne muscular dystrophy. *Pediatrics, 123*(Suppl. 4), S231–S235.

Krigger, K. W. (2006). Cerebral palsy: an overview. *American Family Physician, 73*(1), 91–100, 101–102.

Laskowski-Jones, L. (2007). Peripheral nerve and spinal cord problems. In S. L. Lewis, M. M. Heitkemper, S. R. Dirksen, et al. (Eds.), *Medical surgical nursing: assessment and management of clinical problems* (7th ed.). St. Louis: Mosby/Elsevier.

Launay, F., Leet, A. I., & Sponseller, P. D. (2005). Pediatric spinal cord injury without radiographic abnormality: a meta-analysis. *Clinical Orthopaedics and Related Research, 433*, 166–170.

Lazzaretti, C. C., & Pearson, C. (2010). Myelodysplasia. In P. J. Allen, J. A. Vessey, & N. A. Schapiro (Eds.), *Primary care of the child with a chronic condition* (5th ed.). St. Louis: Mosby.

Liptak, G. S., & Accardo, P. J. (2004). Health and social outcomes of children with cerebral palsy. *The Journal of Pediatrics, 145*(Suppl.), S36–S41.

Liptak, G. S., & Dosa, N. P. (2010). Myelomeningocele. *Pediatrics in Review, 31*(11), 443–450.

Lovette, B. (2008). Safe transportation for children with special needs. *Journal of Pediatric Health Care, 22*(5), 323–328.

Lukban, M. B., Rosales, R. L., & Dressler, D. (2009). Effectiveness of botulinum toxin A for upper and lower limb spasticity in children with cerebral palsy: a summary of evidence. *Journal of Neural Transmission, 116*(3), 319–331.

Lundy, C., Doherty, G., & Fairhurst, C. (2009). Botulinum toxin type A injections can be an effective treatment for pain in children with hip spasms and cerebral palsy. *Developmental Medicine and Child Neurology, 51*, 705–710.

Lyons, R. (2008). Elusive belly pain and Guillain-Barré syndrome. *Journal of Pediatric Health Care, 22*(5), 310–314.

MacLennan, A. H., Thompson, S. C., & Gecz, J. (2015). Cerebral palsy: causes, pathways, and the role of genetic variants. *American Journal of Obstetrics and Gynecology, 213*(6), 779–788. http://www.ajog.org/article/S0002-9378(15)00510-4/fulltext?cc=y=.

Manzur, A. Y., Kinali, M., & Muntoni, F. (2008). Update on the management of Duchenne muscular dystrophy. *Archives of Disease in Childhood, 93*(11), 986–990.

Manzur, A. Y., Kuntzer, T., Pike, M., et al. (2008). Glucocorticoid corticosteroids for Duchenne muscular dystrophy. *Cochrane Database of Systematic Review*, (1), CD003725.

Mathison, D. J., Kadom, N., & Krug, S. E. (2008). Spinal cord injury in the pediatric patient. *Clinical Pediatric Emergency Medicine, 9*(2), 106–123.

Matthews, T. J. (2009). *Trends in spina bifida and anencephalus in the United States, 1991-2006*. Hyatsville, Md: National Center on Health Statistics. Retrieved from https://www.cdc.gov/nchs/products/pubs/pubd/hestats/spine_anen.pdf.

Mercuri, E., Bertini, E., & Iannaconne, S. T. (2012). Childhood spinal muscular atrophy: controversies and challenges. *The Lancet. Neurology, 11*(5), 443–452.

Merenda, L. A., & Hickey, K. (2005). Key elements of a bladder and bowel management for children with spinal cord injuries. *SCI Nursing: A Publication of the American Association of Spinal Cord Injury Nurses, 22*(1), 8–14.

Meriggioli, M. N., & Sanders, D. B. (2012). Disorders of neuromuscular transmission. In R. B. Daroff, G. M. Fenichel, J. Jankovic, et al. (Eds.), *Bradley's neurology in clinical practice* (6th ed.). Philadelphia: Saunders.

Metcalfe, P. D. (2017). Neuropathic bladder: investigation and treatment through their lifetime. *Canadian Urological Association Journal, 11*(1–2Suppl1).

Michmizos, K. P., & Krebs, H. I. (2017). Pediatric robotic rehabilitation: current knowledge and future trends in treating children with sensorimotor impairments. *Neurorehabilitation, 41*(1), 69–76.

Miske, L. J., Hickey, E. M., Kolb, S. M., et al. (2004). Use of the mechanical in-exsufflator in pediatric patients with neuromuscular disease and impaired cough. *Chest, 125*(4), 1406–1412.

Miura, P., & Jardin, B. J. (2006). Utrophin upregulation for treating Duchenne or Becker muscular dystrophy: how close are we? *Trends in Molecular Medicine, 12*(3), 122–129.

Morton, R., Gray, N., & Vloeberghs, M. (2011). Controlled study of the effects of continuous intrathecal baclofen infusion in non-ambulant children with cerebral palsy. *Developmental Medicine and Child Neurology, 53*, 736–741.

Moster, D., Wilcox, A. J., Vollset, S. E., et al. (2010). Cerebral palsy among term and postterm births. *JAMA: The Journal of the American Medical Association, 304*(9), 976–982.

Motta, F., Antonello, C., & Stignani, C. (2011). Intrathecal baclofen and motor function in cerebral palsy. *Developmental Medicine and Child Neurology, 53*, 443–448.

Mourtzinos, A., & Stoffel, J. T. (2010). Management of goals for the spina bifida neurogenic bladder: a review from infancy to adulthood. *The Urologic Clinics of North America, 37*(4), 527–535.

Moxley, R. T., Ashwal, S., Pandya, S., et al. (2005). Practice parameter: corticosteroid treatment on Duchenne dystrophy. *Neurology, 64*(1), 13–20.

Nehring, W. M. (2010). Cerebral palsy. In P. L. Jackson, J. A. Vessey, & N. A. Schapiro (Eds.), *Primary care of the child with a chronic illness* (5th ed.). St. Louis: Mosby.

Noonan, C., Quigley, S., & Curley, M. (2011). Using the Braden Q scale to predict pressure ulcer risk in pediatric patients. *Journal of Pediatric Nursing, 26*(6), 566–575.

Nordmark, E., Josenby, A. L., Lagergren, J., et al. (2008). Long-term outcomes 5 years after selective dorsal rhizotomy. *BMC Pediatrics, 8*, 54.

Nordqvist, Christian (2017) *Cerebral palsy: Symptoms, causes, and treatments*. http://www.medicalnewstoday.com/articles/152712.php.

Oda, Y., Takigawa, T., Sugimoto, Y., et al. (2017). Scoliosis in patients with severe cerebral palsy: three different courses in adolescents. *Acta Medica Okayama, 71*(2), 119–126.

O'Shea, T. M. (2008). Diagnosis, treatment, and prevention of cerebral palsy. *Clinical Obstetrics and Gynecology, 51*(4), 816–828.

Oskoui, M., Coutinho, F., Dykeman, J., et al. (2013). An update on the prevalence of cerebral palsy: a systematic review and meta-analysis. *Developmental Medicine and Child Neurology, 55*(6), 509–519.

Ottolini, K., Harris, A. B., Amling, J. K., et al. (2013). Wound care challenges in children and adults with spina bifida: an open-cohort study. *Journal of Pediatric Rehabilitation Medicine, 6*(1), 1–10.

Parent, S., Mac-Thiong, J. M., Roy-Beaudry, M., et al. (2011). Spinal cord injury in the pediatric population: a systematic review of the literature. *Journal of Neurotrauma, 28*(8), 1515–1524.

Parker, S. E., Mai, C. T., Canfield, M. A., et al. (2010). Updated National Birth Prevalence estimates for selected birth defects in the United States, 2004-2006. *Birth Defects Research. Part A, Clinical and Molecular Teratology, 88,* 1008–1016. PubMed:20878909.

Patterson, M. C., Bridgemohan, C., & Armsby, C. (2017): *Clinical features and classification of cerebral palsy.* https://www.uptodate.com/contents/clinica l-features-and-classification-of-cerebral-palsy.

Piatt, J. H., Jr. (2015). Pediatric spinal injury in the US: epidemiology and disparities. *Journal of Neurosurgery. Pediatrics, 16*(4), 463–471.

Prior, T. (2010). Spinal muscular atrophy: newborn and carrier screening. *Obstetrics and Gynecology Clinics of North America, 37*(1), 23–26.

Pruitt, D. W., & McMahon, M. A. (2015). Spinal cord injury and autonomic crisis management. In R. M. Kliegman, B. F. Stanton, J. W. St Geme, et al. (Eds.), *Nelson textbook of pediatrics* (20th ed.). Philadelphia: Saunders/ Elsevier.

Quan, D. (2011). Muscular dystrophies and neurologic diseases that present as myopathy. *Rheumatic Diseases Clinics of North America, 37*(2), 233–244.

Rall, S., & Grimm, T. (2012). Survival in Duchenne muscular dystrophy. *Acta Myologica: Myopathies and Cardiomyopathies, 31*(2), 117–120.

Rekate, H. L. (2015). Spinal cord injuries in children. In R. M. Kliegman, B. F. Stanton, J. W. St. Geme, et al. (Eds.), *Nelson textbook of pediatrics* (20th ed.). Philadelphia: Saunders/Elsevier.

Robinson, A. B., & Reed, A. M. (2015). Juvenile dermatomyositis. In R. M. Kliegman, B. F. Stanton, J. St. Geme, et al. (Eds.), *Nelson textbook of pediatrics* (20th ed.). Philadelphia: Saunders/Elsevier.

Rogers, B. (2004). Feeding method and health outcomes of children with cerebral palsy. *The Journal of Pediatrics, 145*(2 Suppl.), S28–S32.

Romeo, D. M., Ricci, D., Brogna, C., et al. (2016). Use of the Hammersmith Infant Neurological Examination in infants with cerebral palsy: a critical review of the literature. *Developmental Medicine and Child Neurology, 58*(3), 240–245.

Rosenbaum, P., Paneth, N., Leviton, A., et al. (2007). A report: the definition and classification of cerebral palsy, April 2006. *Developmental Medicine and Child Neurology, 49*(S109), 1–44.

Rowe, D. E., & Jadhav, A. L. (2008). Care of the adolescent with spina bifida. *Pediatric Clinics of North America, 55*(6), 1359–1374.

Rozelle, C. J., Arabi, B., Dhall, S. S., et al. (2013). Management of pediatric cervical spine and spinal cord injuries. *Neurosurgery, 72*(3 Suppl.), 205–226.

Rumberg, F., Bakir, M. S., Taylor, W. R., et al. (2016). The effects of selective dorsal rhizotomy on balance and symmetry of gait in children with cerebral palsy. *PLoS ONE, 11*(4), e0152930.

Russman, B. S. (1996). Function changes in spinal muscular atrophy II and III: the DCN/SMA Group. *Neurology, 47*(4), 973–976.

Russman, B. S., Iannaccone, S. T., Buncher, C. R., et al. (1992). Spinal muscular atrophy: new thoughts on the pathogenesis and classification schema. *Journal of Child Neurology, 7*(4), 347–353.

Samaniego, I. A. (2003). A sore spot in pediatrics: risk factors for pressure ulcers. *Pediatric Nursing, 29*(4), 278–282.

Sandler, A. D. (2010). Children with spina bifida: key clinical issues. *Pediatric Clinics of North America, 57*(4), 879–892.

Sarnat, H. B. (2015a). Spinal muscular atrophies. In R. M. Kliegman, B. F. Stanton, J. St. Geme, et al. (Eds.), *Nelson textbook of pediatrics* (20th ed.). Philadelphia: Saunders.

Sarnat, H. B. (2015b). Guillain-Barre syndrome. In R. M. Kliegman, B. F. Stanton, J. St. Geme, et al. (Eds.), *Nelson textbook of pediatrics* (20th ed.). Philadelphia: Saunders.

Sarnat, H. B. (2015c). Myasthenia gravis. In R. M. Kliegman, B. F. Stanton, J. W. St. Geme, et al. (Eds.), *Nelson textbook of pediatrics* (20th ed.). Philadelphia: Saunders.

Sarnat, H. B. (2015d). Muscular dystrophies. In R. M. Kliegman, B. F. Stanton, J. W. St. Geme, et al. (Eds.), *Nelson textbook of pediatrics* (20th ed.). Philadelphia: Saunders.

Sawin, K. J., Liu, T., Ward, E., et al. (2015). The national spina bifida registry: profile of a large cohort of participants from the first 10 clinics. *The Journal of Pediatrics, 166*(2), 444–450.e1.

Sawyer, S., & Macnee, S. (2010). Transition to adult healthcare for adolescents with spina bifida: research issues. *Developmental Disabilities Research Reviews, 16*(1), 60–65.

Schottler, J., Vogel, L., & Sturm, P. (2012). Spinal cord injuries in young children: a review of children injured at 5 years of age and younger. *Developmental Medicine and Child Neurology, 54,* 1138–1143.

Schroth, M. K. (2009). Special considerations in the respiratory management of spinal muscular atrophy. *Pediatrics, 123*(Suppl. 4), S245–S249.

Sehrawat, N., Marwaha, M., Bansal, K., et al. (2014). Cerebral palsy: a dental update. *International Journal of Clinical Pediatric Dentistry, 7*(2), 109–118.

Shaer, C. M., Chescheir, N., & Schulkin, J. (2007). Myelomeningocele: a review of the epidemiology, genetics, risk factors for conception, prenatal diagnosis, and prognosis for affected individuals. *Obstetrical and Gynecological Survey, 62*(7), 471–479.

Shatrov, J. G., Birch, S. C., Lam, L. T., et al. (2010). Chorioamnionitis and cerebral palsy: a meta-analysis. *Obstetrics and Gynecology, 116*(2 Pt. 1), 387–392.

Shavelle, R. M., DeVivo, M. J., Paculdo, D. R., et al. (2007). Long-term survival after childhood spinal cord injury. *The Journal of Spinal Cord Medicine, 30*(Suppl. 1), S48–S54.

Simonds, A. K. (2006). Recent advances in respiratory care for neuromuscular disease. *Chest, 130*(6), 1879–1886.

Simpson, J. L., Richards, D. S., & Otaño, L. (2012). Prenatal genetic diagnosis. In S. G. Gabbe, J. R. Niebyl, J. L. Simpson, et al. (Eds.), *Obstetrics: normal and problem pregnancies* (6th ed.). Philadelphia: Saunders.

Skura, C. L., Fowler, E. G., Wetzel, G. T., et al. (2008). Albuterol increases lean body mass in ambulatory boys with Duchenne or Becker muscular dystrophy. *Neurology, 70*(2), 137–143.

Snodgrass, W., & Gargollo, P. (2010). Urologic care of the neurogenic bladder in children. *The Urologic Clinics of North America, 37*(2), 207–214.

Strobl, W., Theologis, T., Brunner, R., et al. (2015). Best clinical practice in botulinum toxin treatment for children with cerebral palsy. *Toxins, 7*(5), 1629–1648.

Tarcan, T., Onol, F. F., Ilker, Y., et al. (2006). The timing of primary neurosurgical repair significantly affects neurogenic bladder prognosis in children with myelomeningocele. *Journal of Urology, 176,* 1161.

Thrasher, T. A., & Popovic, M. R. (2008). Functional electrical stimulation of walking: function, exercise and rehabilitation. *Annales de Readaptation et de Medecine Physique: Revue Scientifique de la Societe Francaise de Reeducation Fonctionnelle de Readaptation et de Medecine Physique, 51*(6), 452–460.

To, C. S., Kirsch, R. F., Kobetic, R., et al. (2005). Simulation of a functional neuromuscular stimulation powered mechanical gait orthosis with coordinated joint locking. *IEEE Transactions on Neural Systems and Rehabilitation Engineering: A Publication of the IEEE Engineering in Medicine and Biology Society, 13*(2), 227–235.

Vitale, M. G., Goss, J. M., Matsumoto, H., et al. (2006). Epidemiology of pediatric spinal cord injury in the United States: years 1997 and 2000. *Journal of Pediatric Orthopedics, 26*(6), 745–749.

Van Naarden Braun, K., Doernberg, N., Schieve, L., et al. (2016). Birth prevalence of cerebral palsy: a population-based study. *Pediatrics, 137*(1), Jan.

Vogel, L. C., Betz, R. R., & Mulcahey, M. J. (2012). Spinal cord injuries in children and adolescents. In Verhaagen J, MacDonald JW, editors. *Handbook of Clinical Neurology, 109*(3), 131–148.

Vogel, L. C., Chlan, K. M., Zebracki, K., et al. (2011). Long-term outcomes of adults with pediatric-onset spinal cord injuries as a function of neurologic impairment. *The Journal of Spinal Cord Medicine, 34*(1), 60–66.

Westbom, L., Rimstedt, A., & Nordmark, E. (2017). Assessments of pain in children and adolescents with cerebral palsy: a retrospective population-based registry study. *Developmental Medicine and Child Neurology, 59*(8), 858–863.

Westbom, L., Bergstrand, L., Wagner, P., et al. (2011). Survival at 19 years of age in a total population of children and young people with cerebral palsy. *Developmental Medicine and Child Neurology, 53*, 806–814.

Wolff, T., Witkop, C. T., Miller, T., et al. (2009). Folic acid supplementation for the prevention of neural tube defects: an update of the evidence for the US Preventive Services Task Force. *Annals of Internal Medicine, 150*(9), 632–639, W112–W115.

Wright, P., Durham, S., Ewins, D., et al. (2012). Neuromuscular electrical stimulation for children with cerebral palsy: a review. *Archives of Disease in Childhood, 97*(4), 364–371.

Yeargin-Allsopp, M., Van Naarden Braun, K., Doernberg, N. S., et al. (2008). Prevalence of cerebral palsy in 8-year-old children in three areas of the United States in 2002: a multisite collaboration. *Pediatrics, 121*(3), 547–554.

Young, H. K., Lowe, A., & Fitzgerald, D. A. (2007). Outcome of noninvasive ventilation in children with neuromuscular disease. *Neurology, 68*(3), 198–201.

Yuan-Kim Liow, N., Gimeno, H., Lumsden, D. E., et al. (2016). Gabapentin can significantly improve dystonia severity and quality of life in children. *European Journal of Paediatric Neurology, 20*(1), 100–107.

INDEX

Page numbers followed by "*f*" indicate figures, "*t*" indicate tables, and "*b*" indicate boxes.

D

G

I

Blood Pressure (BP) Levels for Boys by Age and Height Percentile

AGE (yr)	BP PERCENTILE*	SYSTOLIC BP (mm Hg) PERCENTILE OF HEIGHT							DIASTOLIC BP (mm Hg) PERCENTILE OF HEIGHT						
		5th	10th	25th	50th	75th	90th	95th	5th	10th	25th	50th	75th	90th	95th
1	50th	80	81	83	85	87	88	89	34	35	36	37	38	39	39
	90th	94	95	97	99	100	102	103	49	50	51	52	53	53	54
	95th	98	99	101	103	104	106	106	54	54	55	56	57	58	58
	99th	105	106	108	110	112	113	114	61	62	63	64	65	66	66
2	50th	84	85	87	88	90	92	92	39	40	41	42	43	44	44
	90th	97	99	100	102	104	105	106	54	55	56	57	58	58	59
	95th	101	102	104	106	108	109	110	59	59	60	61	62	63	63
	99th	109	110	111	113	115	117	117	66	67	68	69	70	71	71
3	50th	86	87	89	91	93	94	95	44	44	45	46	47	48	48
	90th	100	101	103	105	107	108	109	59	59	60	61	62	63	63
	95th	104	105	107	109	110	112	113	63	63	64	65	66	67	67
	99th	111	112	114	116	118	119	120	71	71	72	73	74	75	75
4	50th	88	89	91	93	95	96	97	47	48	49	50	51	51	52
	90th	102	103	105	107	109	110	111	62	63	64	65	66	66	67
	95th	106	107	109	111	112	114	115	66	67	68	69	70	71	71
	99th	113	114	116	118	120	121	122	74	75	76	77	78	78	79
5	50th	90	91	93	95	96	98	98	50	51	52	53	54	55	55
	90th	104	105	106	108	110	111	112	65	66	67	68	69	69	70
	95th	108	109	110	112	114	115	116	69	70	71	72	73	74	74
	99th	115	116	118	120	121	123	123	77	78	79	80	81	81	82
6	50th	91	92	94	96	98	99	100	53	53	54	55	56	57	57
	90th	105	106	108	110	111	113	113	68	68	69	70	71	72	72
	95th	109	110	112	114	115	117	117	72	72	73	74	75	76	76
	99th	116	117	119	121	123	124	125	80	80	81	82	83	84	84
7	50th	92	94	95	97	99	100	101	55	55	56	57	58	59	59
	90th	106	107	109	111	113	114	115	70	70	71	72	73	74	74
	95th	110	111	113	115	117	118	119	74	74	75	76	77	78	78
	99th	117	118	120	122	124	125	126	82	82	83	84	85	86	86
8	50th	94	95	97	99	100	102	102	56	57	58	59	60	60	61
	90th	107	109	110	112	114	115	116	71	72	72	73	74	75	76
	95th	111	112	114	116	118	119	120	75	76	77	78	79	79	80
	99th	119	120	122	123	125	127	127	83	84	85	86	87	87	88
9	50th	95	96	98	100	102	103	104	57	58	59	60	61	61	62
	90th	109	110	112	114	115	117	118	72	73	74	75	76	76	77
	95th	113	114	116	118	119	121	121	76	77	78	79	80	81	81
	99th	120	121	123	125	127	128	129	84	85	86	87	88	88	89
10	50th	97	98	100	102	103	105	106	58	59	60	61	61	62	63
	90th	111	112	114	115	117	119	119	73	73	74	75	76	77	78
	95th	115	116	117	119	121	122	123	77	78	79	80	81	81	82
	99th	122	123	125	127	128	130	130	85	86	86	88	88	89	90
11	50th	99	100	102	104	105	107	107	59	59	60	61	62	63	63
	90th	113	114	115	117	119	120	121	74	74	75	76	77	78	78
	95th	117	118	119	121	123	124	125	78	78	79	80	81	82	82
	99th	124	125	127	129	130	132	132	86	86	87	88	89	90	90

Continued

Blood Pressure (BP) Levels for Boys by Age and Height Percentile—cont'd

AGE (yr)	BP PERCENTILE*	SYSTOLIC BP (mm Hg) PERCENTILE OF HEIGHT 5th	10th	25th	50th	75th	90th	95th	DIASTOLIC BP (mm Hg) PERCENTILE OF HEIGHT 5th	10th	25th	50th	75th	90th	95th
12	50th	101	102	104	106	108	109	110	59	60	61	62	63	63	64
	90th	115	116	118	120	121	123	123	74	75	75	76	77	78	79
	95th	119	120	122	123	125	127	127	78	79	80	81	82	82	83
	99th	126	127	129	131	133	134	135	86	87	88	89	90	90	91
13	50th	104	105	106	108	110	111	112	60	60	61	62	63	64	64
	90th	117	118	120	122	124	125	126	75	75	76	77	78	79	79
	95th	121	122	124	126	128	129	130	79	79	80	81	82	83	83
	99th	128	130	131	133	135	136	137	87	87	88	89	90	91	91
14	50th	106	107	109	111	113	114	115	60	61	62	63	64	65	65
	90th	120	121	123	125	126	128	128	75	76	77	78	79	79	80
	95th	124	125	127	128	130	132	132	80	80	81	82	83	84	84
	99th	131	132	134	136	138	139	140	87	88	89	90	91	92	92
15	50th	109	110	112	113	115	117	117	61	62	63	64	65	66	66
	90th	122	124	125	127	129	130	131	76	77	78	79	80	80	81
	95th	126	127	129	131	133	134	135	81	81	82	83	84	85	85
	99th	134	135	136	138	140	142	142	88	89	90	91	92	93	93
16	50th	111	112	114	116	118	119	120	63	63	64	65	66	67	67
	90th	125	126	128	130	131	133	134	78	78	79	80	81	82	82
	95th	129	130	132	134	135	137	137	82	83	83	84	85	86	87
	99th	136	137	139	141	143	144	145	90	90	91	92	93	94	94
17	50th	114	115	116	118	120	121	122	65	66	66	67	68	69	70
	90th	127	128	130	132	134	135	136	80	80	81	82	83	84	84
	95th	131	132	134	136	138	139	140	84	85	86	87	87	88	89
	99th	139	140	141	143	145	146	147	92	93	93	94	95	96	97

*The 90th percentile is 1.28 standard deviation (SD), the 95th percentile is 1.645 SD, and the 99th percentile is 2.326 SD over the mean. Retrieved from https://www.nhlbi.nih.gov/files/docs/guidelines/child_tbl.pdf.

Blood Pressure (BP) Levels for Girls by Age and Height Percentile

AGE (yr)	BP PERCENTILE*	SYSTOLIC BP (mm Hg) PERCENTILE OF HEIGHT 5th	10th	25th	50th	75th	90th	95th	DIASTOLIC BP (mm Hg) PERCENTILE OF HEIGHT 5th	10th	25th	50th	75th	90th	95th
1	50th	83	84	85	86	88	89	90	38	39	39	40	41	41	42
	90th	97	97	98	100	101	102	103	52	53	53	54	55	55	56
	95th	100	101	102	104	105	106	107	56	57	57	58	59	59	60
	99th	108	108	109	111	112	113	114	64	64	65	65	66	67	67
2	50th	85	85	87	88	89	91	91	43	44	44	45	46	46	47
	90th	98	99	100	101	103	104	105	57	58	58	59	60	61	61
	95th	102	103	104	105	107	108	109	61	62	62	63	64	65	65
	99th	109	110	111	112	114	115	116	69	69	70	70	71	72	72
3	50th	86	87	88	89	91	92	93	47	48	48	49	50	50	51
	90th	100	100	102	103	104	106	106	61	62	62	63	64	64	65
	95th	104	104	105	107	108	109	110	65	66	66	67	68	68	69
	99th	111	111	113	114	115	116	117	73	73	74	74	75	76	76
4	50th	88	88	90	91	92	94	94	50	50	51	52	52	53	54
	90th	101	102	103	104	106	107	108	64	64	65	66	67	67	68
	95th	105	106	107	108	110	111	112	68	68	69	70	71	71	72
	99th	112	113	114	115	117	118	119	76	76	76	77	78	79	79
5	50th	89	90	91	93	94	95	96	52	53	53	54	55	55	56
	90th	103	103	105	106	107	109	109	66	67	67	68	69	69	70
	95th	107	107	108	110	111	112	113	70	71	71	72	73	73	74
	99th	114	114	116	117	118	120	120	78	78	79	79	80	81	81